DISEASES OF THE
Kidney & Urinary Tract

DISEASES OF THE
Kidney &
Urinary Tract

Eighth Edition

Volume II

Edited by

Robert W. Schrier, MD
Professor of Medicine
Department of Medicine
University of Colorado School of Medicine
Denver, Colorado

Wolters Kluwer | Lippincott Williams & Wilkins
Health
Philadelphia · Baltimore · New York · London
Buenos Aires · Hong Kong · Sydney · Tokyo

Acquisitions Editor: Lisa McAllister
Developmental Editor: Louise Bierig
Managing Editor: Kerry Barrett
Production Editor: Fran Gunning
Marketing Manager: Kimberly Schonberger
Manufacturing Manager: Kathleen Brown
Design Coordinator: Risa Clow
Compositor: Techbooks
Printer: RR Donnelley-Willard

© 2007 by **LIPPINCOTT WILLIAMS & WILKINS**
530 Walnut Street
Philadelphia, PA 19106 USA
LWW.com

Printed in the USA

Library of Congress Cataloging-in-Publication Data

Diseases of the kidney & urinary tract.—8th ed. / edited by Robert W. Schrier.
    p. ; cm.
  Includes bibliographical references and index.
  ISBN 13: 978-0-7817-9307-0
  ISBN 10: 0-7817-9307-6 (alk. paper)
  1. Urinary organs—Diseases. 2. Kidneys—Diseases. I. Schrier, Robert W. II. Title:
Diseases of the kidney and urinary tract.
  [DNLM: 1. Kidney Diseases. 2. Urologic Diseases. WJ 300 D6115 2007]

RC900.D56 2007
616.6'1—dc22

2006028279

■ DEDICATION

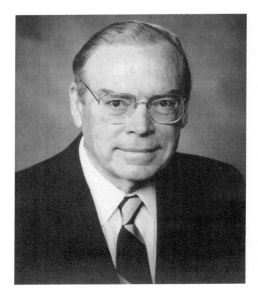

Carl William Gottschalk, MD was a man for all seasons—brilliant scholar, committed mentor of students, dedicated citizen of the University of North Carolina and the broader academic community, and a gentleman in every sense of the word. Carl was a native Virginian whose southern manners and warm demeanor emanated a personal charm to his friends, colleagues, and students. He graduated Phi Beta Kappa from Roanoke College in 1942 and received an Honorary Doctor of Science from that institution in 1966. An Alpha Omega Alpha graduate from the University of Virginia School of Medicine, Carl received his training in internal medicine at the Massachusetts General Hospital and his fellowship in Cardiology at the University of North Carolina. For the next 40 years (1952–1992), his loyalty and many talents were an integral part of the University of North Carolina, which accounted for the respect and affection that he received from his many colleagues and friends. He was the Kenan Professor of Medicine and Physiology from 1969 until his untimely death on October 15, 1997, in Chapel Hill, North Carolina.

Carl's scientific contributions were recognized by his election to the National Academy of Science. He was president of the American Society of Nephrology from 1976 until 1977 and was a Councilor of the International Society of Nephrology (ISN). Carl founded the History of Medicine Commission of the ISN and the ISN Archives in Amsterdam, *The Netherlands*, which are appropriately named the Carl W. Gottschalk Archives of the ISN. Among many honors, awards, and distinguished named lectureships, Carl received the Homer W. Smith Award from the New York Heart Association and the David H. Hume Award from the National Kidney Foundation. The American Physiological Society has established the Carl W. Gottschalk Distinguished Lectureship in Renal Physiology, and the University of North Carolina has inaugurated the Carl W. Gottschalk Lectureship in the Basic Sciences.

The written persona of Carl W. Gottschalk—scientist, medical historian, lepidopterist who has a butterfly (*Strymon cecrops Gottshalki*) named after him, recipient of many honors and awards—can only project a very modest picture of this Renaissance man. His kindness and consideration for others was unparalleled. It was my honor to have worked with him on three editions of *Diseases of the Kidney* and to dedicate this current edition to his memory.

Robert W. Schrier, MD

v

■ CONTENTS

SECTION VIII ■ HYPERTENSION

SECTION IX ■ GLOMERULAR, INTERSTITIAL, AND VASCULAR RENAL DISEASES

Volume III

SECTION X ■ SYSTEMIC DISEASES OF THE KIDNEY

SECTION XI ■ DISORDERS OF ELECTROLYTE, WATER, AND ACID-BASE

SECTION XII ■ UREMIC SYNDROME

SECTION XIII ■ MANAGEMENT OF END-STAGE RENAL DISEASE

■ PREFACE

The recent advances in all aspects of our knowledge of the kidney and its diseases mandate a new edition of *Diseases of the Kidney & Urinary Tract*. As in previous editions, a group of international experts was assembled to present this information in a comprehensive, authoritative, concise, and readily accessible fashion. The chapters have been extensively revised and updated.

Nephrology is a discipline that combines the basic and clinical sciences. Successful integration of this knowledge is the goal of this eighth edition. The 14 sections of the three volume book are actually individual texts which can stand on their own. Moreover, a unique feature of the book is a comprehensive inclusion of diseases of the urinary tract as well as the kidney.

The first section presents an overall view of the structural, physiologic, and biochemical aspects of the kidney. This section incorporates the latest developments in cellular and molecular biology, emphasizing the most current information and concepts on cell signaling, receptors, and ion channels. The subsequent 13 sections are disease-oriented, with each section beginning with a pathophysiology chapter. The goal of *Diseases of the Kidney & Urinary Tract* is to publish the most comprehensive material for practicing and academic physicians caring for patients with renal, hypertension, and urological diseases. The 14 sections of the book cover 104 chapters and are summarized as follows:

I. **Biochemical, Structural, and Functional Correlations in the Kidney** includes structural, hemodynamic, hormonal, ion transport and metabolic functions in nine chapters.

II. **Clinical Evaluation** is covered in six chapters on urinalysis, laboratory evaluation, urography, tomography, and angiography, with indications and interpretations for renal biopsy.

III. **Hereditary Diseases,** in five chapters, covers genetic mechanisms, medullary cystic and sponge disorders, polycystic kidney disease, Alport syndrome, Fabry disease, and nail-patella syndrome, as well as isolated renal tubular disorders.

IV. **Urological Diseases of the Genitourinary Tract** are described in six chapters, including congenital abnormalities, urinary tract obstruction, renal calculi, reflux nephropathy, and prostatic and micturition disorders.

V. **Neoplasms of the Genitourinary Tract** are addressed in five chapters covering molecular mechanisms in malignancy, testicular carcinoma, prostate and bladder cancer, and primary neoplasms of the kidney and renal pelvis.

VI. **Infections of the Urinary Tract and the Kidney** are contained in seven chapters, including host defense mechanisms; urinary bacterial infections, including tuberculosis and fungal infections; renal abscesses; and cystitis.

VII. **Acute Renal Failure** is described in 11 chapters, including the pathophysiology of renal cell ischemia and nephrotoxic injury, acute tubular necrosis, acute interstitial nephritis, and acute nephrotoxic renal disease.

VIII. **Hypertension** and its renal manifestations are covered in seven chapters, which include pathophysiology, renal vascular and endocrine-related hypertension, as well as hypertension in pregnancy and in diabetes.

IX. **Glomerular, Interstitial, and Vascular Renal Diseases** are discussed in 16 chapters, including collagen vascular diseases, chronic interstitial nephritis, primary glomerulonephritides, and vasculitides.

X. **Systemic Diseases of the Kidney** are covered in eight chapters, including diabetes, hepatorenal syndrome, sickle cell disease, gout, myeloma/amyloidosis, and tropical diseases.

XI. **Disorders of Electrolyte, Water, and Acid–Base** are covered in ten chapters, including SIADH, central and nephrogenic diabetes insipidus, cardiac failure, cirrhosis, and the nephrotic syndrome.

XII. **Uremic Syndrome** covers pathophysiology, anemia, osteodystrophy, the nervous system, cardiovascular complications and metabolic and endocrine dysfunctions in six chapters.

XIII. **Management of End-Stage Renal Disease** by transplantation, peritoneal dialysis and hemodialysis, including complications outcomes, and is discussed in four chapters.

XIV. **Nutrition, Drugs, and the Kidney** are covered in four chapters, including protein and caloric dietary issues, as well as drug dosing recommendations in renal failure.

I would like to thank our authoritative and remarkably talented contributing authors whose dedication to nephrology is unmatched.

Robert W. Schrier, MD

CONTRIBUTING AUTHORS

William T. Abraham, MD, FACP, FACC, FAHA
Professor of Internal Medicine
Director, Division of Cardiovascular Medicine
The Ohio State University
Columbus, Ohio

Gregory A. Achenbach, MD
Assistant Clinical Professor
Department of Pathology
University of Colorado School of Medicine
Chairman
Department of Pathology
Rose Medical Center
Denver, Colorado

Marcin Adamczak, MD
Department of Nephrology
Endocrinology and Metabolic Diseases
Medical University of Silesia
Katowice, Poland

Horacio J. Adrogué, MD
Professor
Department of Medicine
Baylor College of Medicine
Chief, Renal Service
Department of Medicine
The Methodist Hospital
Houston, Texas

Robert J. Alpern, MD
Dean, School of Medicine
Departments of Internal Medicine
   and Nephrology
Yale University School of Medicine
New Haven, Connecticut

Jamshid Amanzadeh, MD
Assistant Professor
Department of Medicine
University of Texas Southwestern
   Medical School
Staff Physician
Department of Medicine
VA North Texas Health Care System
Dallas, Texas

Robert J. Anderson, MD
Meiklejohn Professor
Chair, Department of Medicine
University of Colorado Health Sciences Center
Chief, Department of Medicine
University of Colorado Hospital
Denver, Colorado

Sharon Anderson, MD
Professor and Vice Chair
Department of Medicine, Division of Nephrology
Oregon Health and Science University
Portland, Oregon

Thomas E. Andreoli, MD, MACP
Distinguished Professor
Department of Internal Medicine
Department of Physiology and Biophysics
University of Arkansas College of Medicine
Little Rock, Arkansas

Dennis L. Andress, MD
Professor of Medicine
Department of Medicine
University of Washington
Seattle, Washington

Vincent T. Andriole, MD
Professor of Medicine
Department of Internal Medicine
Yale School of Medicine
Attending Physician
Department of Internal Medicine
Yale–New Haven Hospital
New Haven, Connecticut

William P. Arend, MD
Professor
Department of Medicine
University of Colorado Health Sciences Center
Denver, Colorado

William J. Arendshorst, PhD
Professor
Department of Cell and Molecular Physiology
University of North Carolina at Chapel Hill
Chapel Hill, North Carolina

Allen I. Arieff, MD
Professor Emeritus
Department of Medicine
University of California
San Francisco, California
Attending Physician
Department of Medicine
Cedars-Sinai Medical Center
Los Angeles, California

Anthony Atala, MD
Professor and Chair
Department of Urology
Wake Forest University School of Medicine
Chief, Department of Urology
North Carolina Baptist Hospital
Winston-Salem, North Carolina

Robert C. Atkins, MB, BS, DSc, FRACP
Professor of Medicine
Department of Epidemiology and
  Preventive Medicine
Monash University
Melbourne, Australia
Director Emeritus
Department of Nephrology
Monash Medical Centre
Victoria, Australia

Pierre Aucouturier, PhD
Professor
Department of Immunology
Université Pierre et Marie Curie
PU-PH
Department of Immunology
Hôpital Tenon
Paris, France

Faten Ayyoub, MD
Staff Nephrologist
Department of Medicine
Harper University Hospital
Detroit, Michigan

Kamal F. Badr, MD
Professor and Chair
Department of Internal Medicine
American University of Beirut
American University of Beirut Medical Center
Beirut, Lebanon

Ross R. Bailey, MD, FRACP, FRCP (deceased)
Clinical Lecturer, Department of Medicine,
Christchurch School of Medicine
Head, Department of Nephrology
Christchurch Hospital
Christchurch, New Zealand

Dean F. Bajorin, MD, FACP
Professor
Department of Medicine
Weill Medical College of Cornell University
Attending Physician
Department of Medicine
Memorial Sloan-Kettering Cancer Center
New York, New York

David S. Baldwin, MD
Professor Emeritus
Department of Medicine
New York University School of Medicine
Honorary Attending
Department of Medicine
New York University Medical Center
New York, New York

Rashad S. Barsoum, MD, FRCP, FRCPE
Professor of Medicine
Department of Internal Medicine
Cairo University
Chairman
Cairo Kidney Center
Cairo, Egypt

Anne M. Beck, MD
Associate Professor
Department of Pediatrics
Washington University School of Medicine
Medical Director of Pediatric Dialysis
Department of Pediatrics
Division of Nephrology
St. Louis Children's Hospital
St. Louis, Missouri

Darren T. Beiko, MD, FRCSC
Assistant Professor
Department of Urology
Queen's University
Urologist
Department of Urology
Kingston General Hospital
Kingston, Ontario, Canada

Mir Reza Bekheirnia, MD
Department of Medicine
Division of Renal Diseases and Hypertension
University of Colorado School of Medicine
Denver, Colorado

William M. Bennett, MD
Northwest Renal Clinic
Medical Director
Transplant Services
Legacy Good Samaritan Hospital
Portland, Oregon

Anatole Besarab, MD
Adjunct Professor
Department of Medicine
Wayne State University
Senior Staff
Department of Medicine
Henry Ford Health System
Detroit, Michigan

Daniel G. Bichet, MD, MSc
Professor
Departments of Medicine and Physiology
Canada Research Chair, Genetics of Renal Disease
University of Montreal
Nephrologist
Hôpital du Sacré-Coeur de Montréal
Montréal, Québec, Canada

Warren Kline Bolton, MD
Professor of Internal Medicine
Division of Nephrology
University of Virginia
Chief
Division of Nephrology
University of Virginia Health Systems
Charlottesville, Virginia

George J. Bosl, MD
Professor of Medicine
Department of Medicine
Joan and Sanford I. Weill Medial College
Chairman
Department of Medicine
Memorial Sloan-Kettering Cancer Center
New York, New York

Jean-Louis Bosmans, MD, PhD
Associate Professor
Department of Medicine
University of Antwerp
Section Director
Department of Nephrology
University Hospital of Antwerp
Antwerp, Belgium

Mayer Brezis, MD, MPH
Professor of Medicine
Braun School of Public Health
Hebrew University of Jerusalem
Director, Center for Quality and Safety
Hadassah Medical Center
Jerusalem, Israel

Verena A. Briner, MD
Professor
Department of Medicine
University of Basel
Basel, Switzerland
Head, Department of Medicine
Kantonsspital Luzern
Luzern, Switzerland

Keith E. Britton, MD, MSc, FRCR, FRCP
Emeritus Professor
University of London
Chairman of the Board
Cromwell Hospital
London, United Kingdom

Ruth Ellen Bulger, PhD
Professor
Department of Anatomy, Physiology, and Genetics
F. Edward Hebert School of Medicine
Uniformed Services University of the Health Sciences
Bethesda, Maryland

John M. Burkart, MD
Professor
Corporate Director, Dialysis Program
Department of Nephrology
Wake Forest University Medical Center
Winston-Salem, North Carolina

Melissa A. Cadnapaphornchai, MD
Associate Professor
Departments of Pediatrics and Medicine
University of Colorado Health Sciences Center
Attending Nephrologist
Department of Pediatrics
The Children's Hospital
Denver, Colorado

Andrés Cárdenas, MD
Associate Investigator
Faculty of Medicine
University of Barcelona
Associate Investigator
Liver Unit 7-3
Hospital Clinic
Barcelona, Spain

Michele Ceruti, MD
Mario Negri Institute for Pharmacological Research
Division of Nephrology and Dialysis
Azienda Ospedal, Ospedali Riuniti
Bergamo, Italy

Joumana Chaiban, MD
Endocrinology Fellow
Department of Internal Medicine
American University of Beirut
American University of Beirut Medical Center
Beirut, Lebanon

Laurence Chan, MD, PhD, FRCP, FACP
Professor of Medicine
Department of Medicine
Division of Renal Diseases and Hypertension
University of Colorado School of Medicine
Denver, Colorado

Silvia D. Chang, MD
Assistant Professor
Department of Radiology
University of British Columbia
Head of Abdominal MRI
Department of Radiology
Vancouver General Hospital
Vancouver, British Columbia, Canada

Cyril Chantler, MD, FRCP
GKT Department of Pediatric Nephrology
Guy's Tower
Guy's Hospital
Vice Principal
King's College
London, United Kingdom

Devasmita Choudhury, MD
Associate Professor of Medicine
University of Texas Southwestern Medical Center at Dallas
Director of Dialysis
Department of Medicine
Dallas Veterans Affairs Medical Center
Dallas, Texas

Godfrey Clark, MD
GKT Department of Pediatric Nephrology
Guy's Tower
Guy's Hospital
London, United Kingdom

Anthony R. Clarkson, MD, MBBS, FRACP
Associate Professor
Department of Medicine
University of Adelaide
Emeritus Consultant Nephrologist
Department of Renal Medicine
Royal Adelaide Hospital
Adelaide, South Australia

Kirk P. Conrad, MD
Professor
Department of Physiology and Functional Genomics
University of Florida College of Medicine
Gainesville, Florida

Howard L. Corwin, MD
Professor
Department of Medicine and Anesthesiology
Dartmouth Medical School
Hanover, New Hampshire
Medical Director, Intensive Care Unit
Dartmouth-Hitchcock Medical Center
Lebanon, New Hampshire

Luciano J. Costa, MD, ScD
Clinical Fellow, Division of Medical Oncology
Department of Medicine
University of Colorado
Aurora, Colorado

E. David Crawford, MD
Professor of Medicine
University of Colorado Hospital Cancer Center
Urologic Oncology
University of Colorado Health Sciences Center
Denver, Colorado

Byron P. Croker, MD, PhD
Professor
Department of Pathology, Immunology, and
    Laboratory Medicine
University of Florida
Chief
Department of Pathology and Laboratory Medicine Service
North Florida/South Georgia Veterans Health System
Gainesville, Florida

Robert E. Cronin, MD
Professor
Department of Internal Medicine
University of Texas Southwestern Medical Center
Staff Nephrologist
Medical Service
VA North Texas Health Care System
Dallas, Texas

Brian S. Cummings, PhD
Assistant Professor
Department of Pharmaceutical and Biomedical Sciences
University of Georgia
Athens, Georgia

Giuseppe D'Amico, MD, FRCP
Emeritus Director
Department of Nephrology
San Carlo Borromeo Hospital
Milan, Italy

Eugene Daphnis, MD
Assistant Professor
Department of Nephrology
Crete University
Chief
Department of Nephrology
University Hospital of Heraklion
Heraklion, Greece

Scott F. Davies, MD
Professor and Vice Chairman
Department of Medicine
University of Minnesota Medical School
Chief
Department of Medicine
Hennepin County Medical Center
Minneapolis, Minnesota

Marc E. De Broe, MD, PhD
Professor Emeritus
Faculty of Medicine
University of Antwerp
Wilrijk, Antwerp, Belgium

Paul E. de Jong, MD, PhD
Department of Internal Medicine
University Hospital Groningen
Groningen, The Netherlands

Angelo M. De Mattos, MD, MPH
University of Alabama (UAB) Birmingham
Division of Nephrology and Transplantation
Birmingham, Alabama

Louise-Marie Dembry, MD, MS
Associate Professor of Medicine and Epidemiology
Department of Internal Medicine
Yale University School of Medicine
Hospital Epidemiologist
Department of Quality Improvement and
    Support Services
Yale-New Haven Hospital
New Haven, Connecticut

Gary V. Desir, MD
Professor
Department of Medicine, Section of Nephrology
Yale University School of Medicine
New Haven, Connecticut
Chief
Department of Medicine
VA Connecticut Health Care System
West Haven, Connecticut

Hugh E. de Wardener, MD, FRCP
Emeritus Professor of Medicine
Imperial College School of Medicine
Department of Clinical Chemistry
Division of Investigative Sciences
London, United Kingdom

Giovanni Barbiano di Belgiojoso, MD
Associate Professor
Department of Medicine and Nephrology
University of Milan
Chief
Nephrology Unit
Luigi Sacco Hospital
Milan, Italy

Jacques Diezi, MD
Professor
Department of Pharmacology and Toxicology
University of Lausanne
Lausanne, Switzerland

Susan R. DiGiovanni, MD
Associate Professor of Medicine
Department of Medicine
Virginia Commonwealth University
Richmond, Virginia

Burl R. Don, MD
Professor of Medicine
Division of Nephrology
University of California, Davis
Director, Clinical Nephrology
Division of Nephrology
University of California, Davis Medical Center
Sacramento, California

Michael S. Donnenberg, MD
Department of Microbiology and Immunology
Division of Infectious Diseases
Department of Medicine
University of Maryland Medical System
Baltimore, Maryland

Harry A. Drabkin, MD
Professor of Medicine
Division of Medical Oncology
University of Colorado School of Medicine
Aurora, Colorado

Tevfik Ecder, MD
Professor of Medicine
Department of Internal Medicine
Istanbul School of Medicine
Istanbul, Turkey

Charles L. Edelstein, MD, PhD
Professor
Department of Medicine/Renal
University of Colorado Health Sciences Center
University Hospital
Denver, Colorado

Garabed Eknoyan, MD
Professor
Department of Medicine
Baylor College of Medicine
Houston, Texas

David H. Ellison, MD
Professor of Medicine and Physiology and Pharmacology
Head, Division of Nephrology and Hypertension
Department of Medicine
Oregon Health and Science University
Portland, Oregon

Raymond O. Estacio, MD
Associate Professor of Medicine
Department of Medicine
University of Colorado Health Sciences Center
Internal Medicine
Department of Community Health
Denver Health
Denver, Colorado

Ronald J. Falk, MD
Doc J. Thurston Professor of Medicine
Division of Nephrology and Hypertension
The University of North Carolina at Chapel Hill
    School of Medicine
Chief of Nephrology and Hypertension
Director, UNC Kidney Center
Department of Medicine
UNC Hospitals
Chapel Hill, North Carolina

Randall James Faull, MBBS, PhD
Associate Professor
Department of Medicine
University of Adelaide
Senior Consultant Nephrologist
Renal Unit
Royal Adelaide Hospital
Adelaide, South Australia

Franco Ferrario, MD
Chief
Renal Immunopathology Center
San Carlo Borromeo Hospital
Milan, Italy

Godela M. Fick-Brosnahan, MD
Western Nephrology and
    Metabolic Bone Disease
Lakewood, Colorado

Eli A. Friedman, MD
Distinguished Teaching Professor
Chief
Division of Renal Disease
Department of Medicine
SUNY, Health Science Center at Brooklyn
University Hospital of Brooklyn
Brooklyn, New York

Jørgen Frøkiaer, MD, DMSc
Professor of Cell Biology and Pathophysiology
The Water and Salt Research Centre
Institute of Experimental Clinical Research
Aarhus University Hospital, Skejby Sygehus
Aarhus C, Denmark

Gloria R. Gallo, MD
Adjunct Professor of Pathology
Department of Pathology
New York University School of Medicine
Attending Pathologist, Renal Pathology
Department of Pathology
New York University Medical Center
New York, New York

Matthew D. Galsky, MD
Assistant Member
Department of Medicine
Memorial Sloan-Kettering Cancer Center
New York, New York

Robert M. Gemmill, PhD
Associate Professor of Medicine
Department of Medicine
University of Colorado Health Sciences Center
Aurora, Colorado

Gregory G. Germino, MD
Professor
Department of Medicine–Renal
Johns Hopkins University
Active Staff Full Time
Department of Renal Medicine
Johns Hopkins Hospital
Baltimore, Maryland

L. Michael Glode, MD
Professor of Medicine and Robert Rifkin Chair
Department of Medicine
University of Colorado Cancer Center
Medical Oncology
Aurora, Colorado

Eric Gibney, MD
Assistant Professor
Virginia Commonwealth University
Richmond, Virginia

Pere Ginès, MD
Associate Professor
Faculty of Medicine
University of Barcelona
Chairman
Liver Unit 7-3
Hospital Clinic
Barcelona, Spain

Thomas A. Golper, MD
Professor
Department of Medicine–Nephrology
Medical Director
Department of Nephrology
Medicine Specialties Patient Care Center
Vanderbilt University Medical Center
Nashville, Tennessee

Martin C. Gregory, MD
Professor
Department of Medicine
The University of Utah
Nephrologist
Department of Medicine
University of Utah Health Sciences Center
Salt Lake City, Utah

Jean-Pierre Grünfeld, MD
Professor
Department of Nephrology
Université Paris-Descartes
Consultant
Department of Nephrology
AP-HP, Hôpital Necker
Paris, France

David Harris, MD
Professor and Head, Discipline of Medicine
Department of Medicine
University of Sydney
Western Clinical School Westmead Hospital
Consultant Nephrologist and
    Director of Nephrology
Western Sydney Renal Service
Department of Renal Medicine
Westmead Hospital
Westmead, NSW Australia

Choli Hartono, MD
Assistant Professor
Department of Medicine
Harvard Medical School
Assistant in Medicine
Department of Medicine
Massachusetts General Hospital
Boston, Massachusetts

Kathryn L. Hassell, MD
Associate Professor of Medicine
Division of Hematology
Director
Colorado Sickle Cell Treatment and
    Research Center
University of Colorado at Denver
    Health Sciences Center
Denver, Colorado

William L. Henrich, MD, MACP
Dean of the School of Medicine
VP for Medical Affairs Professor of Medicine
Department of Medicine
University of Texas Health Science Center
    at San Antonio
Physician Staff
University Health System
San Antonio, Texas

Samuel N. Heyman, MD
Associate Professor
Department of Medicine
Hebrew University Faculty of Medicine
Medical School, Hadassah Medical Campus,
    Ein Kerem
Senior Physician
Department of Medicine
Hadassah Hospital, Mount Scopus
Jerusalem, Israel

Friedhelm Hildebrandt, MD
Professor
Department of Pediatrics and Human Genetics
University of Michigan
Department of Diseases, Pediatric Nephrology
University of Michigan Health Systems
Ann Arbor, Michigan

Hedvig Hricak, MD, PhD
Professor
Department of Radiology
Weill Medical College of Cornell University
Chairman
Department of Radiology
Memorial Sloan-Kettering Cancer Center
New York, New York

Keith A. Hruska, MD
Professor
Department of Pediatrics, Medicine, Cell Biology
Washington University
Director
Department of Pediatric Nephrology
St. Louis Children's Hospital
St. Louis, Missouri

Michael H. Humphreys, MD
Professor of Medicine
University of California San Francisco
Division of Nephrology
San Francisco General Hospital
San Francisco, California

Alkesh Jani, MD
Assistant Professor of Medicine
Department of Medicine
Division of Renal Diseases and Hypertension
University of Colorado School of Medicine
Denver, Colorado

Robert W. Janson, MD
Associate Professor of Medicine
Division of Rheumatology
University of Colorado Health Sciences Center
Chief, Rheumatology Section
Denver VA Medical Center
Denver, Colorado

J. Charles Jennette, MD
Brinkhous Distinguished Professor and Chair
Department of Pathology and
    Laboratory Medicine
University of North Carolina
Chief of Service
Department of Pathology and
    Laboratory Medicine
UNC Hospitals
Chapel Hill, North Carolina

Richard J. Johnson, MD
Chief, Division of Nephrology, Hypertension
    and Transplantation
Department of Medicine
University of Florida
Gainesville, Florida

Paul Jungers, MD
Emeritus Professor of Nephrology
Faculté de Médicine Necker
Université Paris V
Paris, France

Igal Kam, MD
Professor
Division Head
Transplant Surgery
University of Colorado
Denver, Colorado

Mohammad Kamgar, MD
University of California–Irvine
Irvine, California

Duk-Hee Kang, MD, PhD
Associate Professor
Division of Nephrology, Department of
    Internal Medicine
Ewha Woman's University College of Medicine
Chief
Division of Nephrology, Department of
    Internal Medicine
Ewha Woman's University Tongdaemun Hospital
Seoul, Korea

Peter G. Kerr, MB, BS, PhD, FRACP
Professor
Department of Nephrology
Monash University
Director
Department of Nephrology
Monash Medical Center
Clayton, Victoria, Australia

Walid Khairallah, MD
Endocrinology Fellow
Department of Internal Medicine
American University of Beirut
American University of Beirut Medical Center
Beirut, Lebanon

Uday Khosla, MD
Assistant Professor
Renal Section
Baylor College of Medicine
Houston, Texas

Melanie S. Kim, MD
Associate Professor
Department of Pediatrics
Boston Medical Center
Boston University School of Medicine
Boston, Massachusetts

Paul L. Kimmel, MD
Professor of Medicine
George Washington University Medical Center
Attending Physician
Department of Medicine
George Washington University Hospital
Washington, District of Columbia

Saulo Klahr, MD
John E. and Adaline Simon Professor of Medicine
Department of Internal Medicine
Washington University School of Medicine
Physician
Department of Internal Medicine
Barnes-Jewish Hospital
St. Louis, Missouri

Mark A. Knepper, MD, PhD
Chief
Renal Mechanisms Section
National Heart, Lung, Blood Institute
National Institutes of Health
Bethesda, Maryland

Sidney Kobrin, MD
Associate Professor of Medicine
Renal, Electrolyte and Hypertension Division
University of Pennsylvania School of Medicine
Department of Medicine
Hospital of the University of Pennsylvania
Philadelphia, Pennsylvania

Radko Komers, MD, PhD
Assistant Professor
Division of Nephrology
Oregon Health and Science University
Portland, Oregon
Deputy Head
Diabetes Center
Institute for Clinical and Experimental Medicine
Prague, Czech Republic

Varuni Kondagunta, MD
Instructor
Department of Medicine
Joan and Sanford Weill Medical College of
    Cornell University
Assistant Attending Physician
Solid Tumor; Department of Medicine
Memorial Sloan-Kettering Cancer Center
New York, New York

Jeffrey B. Kopp, MD
Staff Clinician
National Institute of Diabetes and Digestive and
    Kidney Diseases
National Institutes of Health
Bethesda, Maryland

Joel D. Kopple, MD
Professor of Medicine and Public Health
The David Geffen School of Medicine at UCLA
 and UCLA School of Public Health
Los Angeles, California
Chief
Division of Nephrology and Hypertension
Harbor–UCLA Medical Center
Torrance, California

Matthias Kretzler, MD
Associate Professor
Department of Internal Medicine
University of Michigan
Attending
Department of Internal Medicine
University of Michigan Medical Center
Ann Arbor, Michigan

Wilhelm Kriz, MD
Professor Emeritus
Department of Anatomy and Cell Biology
University Heidelberg
Heidelberg, Germany

Tae-Hwan Kwon, MD, PhD
University of Alabama (UAB) Birmingham
Division of Nephrology and Transplantation
Birmingham, Alabama

Richard A. Lafayette, MD
Associate Professor
Department of Medicine
Associate Chief
Department of Nephrology
Stanford University Hospital
Stanford, California

Andrew Lazar, MD
Northeast Ohio Nephrology Associates
Akron, Ohio

Vincent Weng Seng Lee, MBBS, FRACP
Renal Fellow
Department of Renal Medicine
Westmead Hospital
Westmead, NSW Australia

Andrew S. Levey, MD
Professor
Department of Medicine
Tufts University
Chief
Division of Nephrology
New England Medical Center
Boston, Massachusetts

Moshe Levi, MD
Professor and Vice Chair for Research
Departments of Medicine, Physiology, and Biophysics
University of Colorado
Denver, Colorado

Francisco Llach, MD
Newark Beth Israel Medical Center
Newark, New Jersey

Stuart L. Linas, MD
Professor of Medicine
Department of Medicine
Division of Renal Diseases and Hypertension
University of Colorado School of Medicine
Denver, Colorado

Marshall D. Lindheimer, MD
Professor Emeritus
Department of Medicine/Obstetrics and Gynecology
University of Chicago
Chicago, Illinois

**Graham A. MacGregor, MA, MB, BChir,
 FRCP, FMedSci**
Professor of Cardiovascular Medicine
Blood Pressure Unit
St. George's University of London
St. George's Hospital
London, United Kingdom

Michael P. Madaio, MD
Chief of Nephrology
Department of Medicine
Temple University School of Medicine
Philadelphia, Pennsylvania

Sreedhar Mandayam, MD
Post-Doctoral Fellow
Division of Nephrology
University of Texas Medical Branch
Galveston, Texas

Bruno C. Medeiros, MD
Assistant Professor
Department of Medicine
Stanford Cancer Center
Stanford Hospital and Clinics
Stanford, California

Rajnish Mehrotra, MD, FACP, FASN
Associate Professor of Medicine
Division of Nephrology and Hypertension
Los Angeles Biomedical Research Institute at Harbor–UCLA
 Medical Center and David Geffen School of Medicine
 at UCLA
Torrance, California

Marie Merheb, MD
Endocrinology Fellow
Department of Internal Medicine
American University of Beirut
American University of Beirut Medical Center
Beirut, Lebanon

Timothy W. Meyer, MD
Professor of Medicine
Chief, Division of Nephrology
Stanford University of Medicine
Stanford, California
Veterans Affairs Palo Alto Health Center
Palo Alto, California

Dennis J. Mikolich, MD
Clinical Associate Professor
Department of Medicine
Brown University
Chief, Division of Infectious Diseases
Department of Medicine
Veterans Affairs Medical Center
Providence, Rhode Island

Anne Marie Miles, MD, FACP
Voluntary Assistant Professor of Medicine
 and Community Preceptor
University of Miami School of Medicine
Attending Physician in Nephrology
North Shore Hospital Medical Center
Miami, Florida

William E. Mitch, MD
Gordon A. Cain Professor of Medicine
Nephrology Division, Department of Medicine
Baylor College of Medicine
Houston, Texas

Harry L. T. Mobley, PhD
Frederick G. Novy Collegiate Professor
 and Chair
Department of Microbiology and Immunology
University of Michigan Medical School
Ann Arbor, Michigan

Jack Moore, Jr., MD
Associate Professor
Department of Medicine
Uniformed Services University of the
 Health Sciences
Bethesda, Maryland
Director, Section of Nephrology
Department of Medicine
Washington Hospital Center
Washington, District of Columbia

Christopher S. Morris, MD
Associate Professor of Radiology
Department of Radiology
University of Vermont College of Medicine
Attending Radiologist
Radiology Health Care Service
Fletcher Allen Health Care
Burlington, Vermont

Robert J. Motzer, MD
Professor of Medicine
Weil Medical College of Cornell University
New York Presbyterian Hospital
Attending Physician
Department of Medicine
Memorial Sloan-Kettering Cancer Center
New York, New York

Béatrice Mougenot, MD
Senior Pathologist
INSERM and University Pierre et Marie Curie
Senior Pathologist
Department of Pathology
Tenon Hospital (AP-HP)
Paris, France

Sean W. Murphy, MD, BSc, FRCPC
Assistant Professor of Medicine
Department of Nephrology and Clinical Epidemiology
Memorial University of Newfoundland
Health Sciences Center
St. John's, Newfoundland, Canada

Patrick H. Nachman, MD
Assistant Professor
Division of Nephrology and Hypertension
University of North Carolina
Chapel Hill, North Carolina

L. Gabriel Navar, PhD
Professor and Chair
Department of Physiology
Tulane University
New Orleans, Louisiana

Joel Neugarten, MD
Professor of Medicine
Department of Medicine
Albert Einstein College of Medicine
Site Director, Renal Division
Montefiore Medical Center
Bronx, New York

J. Curtis Nickel, MD, FRCSC
Professor
Department of Urology
Queen's University
Urologist
Department of Urology
Kingston General Hospital
Kingston, Ontario, Canada

Lindsay E. Nicolle, MO, FRCPC
Professor
Department of Internal Medicine and
 Medical microbiology
University of Manitoba
Consultant, Infectious Diseases
Department of Medicine
Health Science Centre
Winnipeg, Manitoba, Canada

Søren Nielsen, MD
Professor and Director
Water and Salt Research Center
University of Aarhus
Aarhus, Denmark

David J. Nikolic-Paterson, BSc, Dphil
Senior Research Fellow
Department of Nephrology
Monash Medical Centre
Clayton, Victoria, Australia

Charles R. Nolan, MD
Professor of Medicine and Surgery
Department of Medicine
University of Texas Health Science Center
 at San Antonio
Medical Director, Kidney Transplantation
Department of Organ Transplant
University Hospital
San Antonio, Texas

Mark D. Okusa, MD
John C. Buchanan Distinguished Professor of
  Internal Medicine
Department of Internal Medicine
University of Virginia
Attending Physician
University of Virginia Health System
Charlottesville, Virginia

Ali J. Olyaei, PharmD, BCPS
Associate Professor of Medicine
Director of Clinical Research
Clinical Pharmacotherapist
Division of Nephrology and Hypertension
Oregon Health Sciences University
Portland, Oregon

Biff F. Palmer, MD
Professor of Internal Medicine
Nephrology Fellowship Program Director
Division of Nephrology, Department of
  Internal Medicine
University of Texas Southwestern
  Medical School
Dallas, Texas

Patrick S. Parfrey, MD
University Research Professor
Department of Medicine
Memorial University of Newfoundland
Staff Nephrologist
Department of Medicine, Patient Research Centre
Health Sciences Centre
St. John's, Newfoundland, Canada

Chirag R. Parikh, MD, PhD, FACP
Assistant Professor
Department of Medicine
Yale University School of Medicine
West Haven, Connecticut

Mark S. Pasternack, MD
Associate Professor
Department of Pediatrics
Harvard Medical School
Chief, Pediatric Infectious Disease Unit
Pediatrician and Physician
Infectious Disease Units
Departments of Medicine and Pediatrics
Massachusetts General Hospital
Boston, Massachusetts

Mark A. Perazella, MD, FACP
Associate Professor
Department of Medicine
Yale University
Director
Acute Dialysis Services
Yale-New Haven Hospital
New Haven, Connecticut

Ronald D. Perrone, MD
Professor
Tufts New England Medical Center
Boston, Massachusetts

Marc A. Pohl, MD
Ray W. Gifford Chair
Head, Section of Clinical Hypertension and Nephrology
Department of Nephrology and Hypertension
Cleveland Clinic
Cleveland, Ohio

Patricia A. Preisig, PhD
Professor
Departments of Internal Medicine and Cellular and
  Molecular Physiology
Yale University
New Haven, Connecticut

Mahboob Rahman, MD, MS
Associate Professor
Department of Medicine
Case Western Reserve University School of Medicine
Department of Medicine
University Hospital of Cleveland
Cleveland, Ohio

Asghar Rastegar, MD
Professor of Medicine and Associate Chair for
  Academic Affairs
Department of Internal Medicine
Yale University School of Medicine
Attending Physician
Department of Internal Medicine and Nephrology
Yale-New Haven Hospital
New Haven, Connecticut

W. Brian Reeves, MD
Professor of Medicine
Department of Medicine
Penn State University College of Medicine
Chief of Nephrology
Department of Medicine
Milton S. Hershey Medical Center
Hershey, Pennsylvania

Robert F. Reilly, Jr., MD
Professor of Medicine
Department of Medicine
University of Texas Southwestern at Dallas
Chief, Section of Nephrology
Department of Internal Medicine
Dallas VA
Dallas, Texas

Giuseppe Remuzzi, MD, FRCP
Research Coordinator
Negri Bergamo Laboratories
Mario Negri Institute for Pharmacological Research
Director, Division of Nephrology and Dialysis
Azienda Ospedal. Ospedali Riuniti
Bergamo, Italy

Jeffrey M. Rimmer, MD
Professor of Medicine
Department of Medicine
University of Vermont
Department of Nephrology
Fletcher Allen Health Care
Burlington, Vermont

Brian I. Rini, MD
Associate Professor
CCF/CWRU Lerner College of Medicine
Staff
Department of Solid Tumor Oncology and Urology
Cleveland Clinic Foundation
Cleveland, Ohio

Eberhard Ritz, MD
Professor Emeritus
Department of Internal Medicine (Nierenzentrum)
Ruperto Carola University Heidelberg
Heidelberg, Germany

Alan M. Robson, MD, FRCP, FRCP-CH, FAAP
Professor of Pediatrics
Department of Pediatrics
Louisiana State University School of Medicine,
Tulane University School of Medicine
Medical Director, Senior Vice President
Children's Hospital
New Orleans, Louisiana

Françoise Roch-Ramel, PhD (deceased)
Professor
Institute of Pharmacology and Toxicology
University of Lausanne
Lausanne, Switzerland

Rudolph A. Rodriguez, MD
Associate Professor of Clinical Medicine
Department of Medicine
University of California, San Francisco
Clinical Director of Nephrology
Department of Medicine, Division of Nephrology
San Francisco General Hospital
San Francisco, California

Allan R. Ronald, MD, FRCPC, FRSC, MACP
Professor Emeritus
Department of Internal Medicine
University of Manitoba
Consultant
Internal Medicine and Infectious Diseases
St. Boniface General Hospital
Winnipeg, Manitoba, Canada

Pierre M. Ronco, MD, PhD
Professor of Renal Medicine
Chief, INSERM Unit 702
Department of Nephrology
University Pierre et Marie Curie/INSERM
Chief, Division of Nephrology and Dialysis
Department of Nephrology
Hôpital Tenon/AP-HP
Paris, France

Mitchell Rosner, MD
Assistant Professor of Medicine
Division of Nephrology
University of Virginia
Charlottesville, Virginia

Robert H. Rubin, MD
Gordon and Marjorie Osborne Professor of
    Health Sciences and Technology
Professor of Medicine
Harvard Medical School
Associate Director
Division of Infectious Disease
Brigham and Women's Hospital
Boston, Massachusetts

Piero Ruggenenti, MD
Assistant Professor
Division of Nephrology and Dialysis
Azienda Ospedal. Ospedali Riuniti
Head, Department of Renal Medicine
Mario Negri Institute for Pharmacological Research
Bergamo, Italy

Sandra Sabatini, PhD, MD
Professor
Departments of Internal Medicine and Physiology
Texas Tech University Health Sciences Center
Lubbock, Texas

Robert L. Safirstein, MD
Professor
Department of Internal Medicine
University of Arkansas for Medical Sciences
Chief
Department of Medicine Service
Central Arkansas Veterans Healthcare System
Little Rock, Arkansas

George A. Sarosi, MD, MACP
Professor of Medicine
Indiana University
Chief, Medical Service
Roudebush VA Medical Center
Indianapolis, Indiana

John A. Sayer, MB, ChB, PhD
Clinical Lecturer
Institute of Human Genetics
University of Newcastle upon Tyne
International Centre for Life
Clinical Lecturer
Department of Nephrology
Freeman Hospital
Newcastle Upon Tyne, United Kingdom

Laurent Schild, MD
Professor
Department of Pharmacology and Toxicology
University of Lausanne
Lausanne, Switzerland

Detlef Schlöndorff, MD
Chief
Medizinische Poliklinik-Innenstadt
Klinikum der Universität-Munchen
Munich, Germany

H. William Schnaper, MD
Professor and Vice Chair
Department of Pediatrics
Feinberg School of Medicine of Northwestern University
Attending Physician
Division of Kidney Diseases
Children's Memorial Hospital
Chicago, Illinois

Rick G. Schnellmann, PhD
Professor and Chair
Department of Pharmaceutical Sciences
Medical University of South Carolina
Charleston, South Carolina

Anton C. Schoolwerth, MD, MSHA
Visiting Professor
Department of Medicine
Dartmouth Medical School
Senior Consultant on Chronic Kidney Disease
Center for Disease Control and Prevention
Lebanon, New Hampshire

Robert W. Schrier, MD
Professor of Medicine
Department of Medicine
University of Colorado School of Medicine
Denver, Colorado

Jörg Schübert, MD, PhD
Professor and Chief
Department of Urology
Friedrich-Schilller-University
Jena, Germany

Stephan Segerer, MD
Assistant Professor
Attending
Medizinische Poliklinik-Innenstadt
Klinikum der Universität-Munchen
Munich, Germany

Alireza A. Shamshirsaz, MD
University of Iowa School of Medicine
Iowa City, Iowa

Donald J. Sherrard, MD
Professor
Department of Medicine
University of Washington
VA Medical Center
Seattle, Washington

Maybin Simfukwe, MD
Associate Professor
Department of Internal Medicine, Nephrology Section
Texas Tech University Health Sciences Center
Nephrologist
Department of Internal Medicine/Nephrology
Covenant Medical Center
Lubbock, Texas

Visith Sitprija, MD, PhD, FACP, FRCP, FRCPE, FRACP
Professor of Medicine
King Chulalongkorn Memorial Hospital
Director
Queen Saovabha Memorial Institute
Bangkok, Thailand

Eduardo Slatopolsky, MD
Joseph Friedman Professor of Renal Diseases
   in Medicine
Renal Division
Washington University
Physician
Barnes-Jewish Hospital
St. Louis, Missouri

Michael C. Smith, MD
Professor of Medicine
University Hospitals of Cleveland
Cleveland, Ohio

Walter E. Stamm, MD
Professor
Department of Medicine
University of Washington
Head, Division of Allergy and Infectious Diseases
University of Washington Medical Center
Seattle, Washington

Lodewijk W. Statius van Eps, MD
Department of History of Medicine
Free University of Amsterdam
Department of Internal Medicine
Slotervaart Hospital
Amsterdam, The Netherlands

Lesley A. Stevens, MD, FRCP
Assistant Professor
Sackler School of Graduate Biomedical Sciences
Tufts University
Boston, Massachusetts

Terry B. Strom, MD
Professor of Medicine and Surgery
Departments of Medicine and Surgery
Harvard School of Medicine
Director, Transplant Research Center
Beth Israel Deaconess Medical Center Director
Boston, Massachusetts

Frank Strutz, MD
Professor
Department of Nephrology and Rheumatology
University of Göettingen
Vice Chief
Department of Nephrology and Rheumatology
Hospital of the University of Göettingen
Göettingen, Germany

Manikkam Suthanthiran, MD
Stanton Griffis Distinguished Professor of Medicine
Department of Medicine, Division of Nephrology
Weill Medical College of Cornell University
Chief, Department of Transplantation Medicine and
   Extracorporeal Therapy
New York Presbyterian Hospital
New York, New York

Charles P. Swainson, MD, FRCP
Senior Lecturer
Department of Medicine
University of Edinburgh Medical School
Consultant Renal Physician
Department of Renal Medicine
Royal Infirmary
Edinburgh, United Kingdom

Isaac Teitelbaum, MD
Professor
Department of Medicine
University of Colorado Health Sciences Center
Director
Acute and Home Dialysis Programs
Department of Medicine
University of Colorado Hospital
Denver, Colorado

Joshua M. Thurman, MD
Assistant Professor
Division of Renal Diseases and Hypertension
University of Colorado Health Sciences Center
Denver, Colorado

C. Craig Tisher, MD
Professor and Dean
Departments of Medicine, Pathology, and
   Anatomy and Cell Biology
University of Florida College of Medicine
Shands Hospitals and Clinics
Gainesville, Florida

Vicente E. Torres, MD
Professor and Chair
Division of Nephrology and Hypertension
Mayo Clinic College of Medicine
Rochester, Minnesota

Jason Gari Umans, MD, PhD
Associate Professor
Departments of Medicine and of Obstetrics
   and Gynecology
Georgetown University
Scientific Director
Penn Medical Laboratory
MedStar Research Institute
Washington, District of Columbia

Heino E. Velázquez, PhD
Department of Internal Medicine
Yale University School of Medicine
New Haven Connecticut
VA Connecticut Healthcare System
West Haven, Connecticut

Joseph G. Verbalis, MD
Professor
Department of Medicine
Georgetown University
Interim Chair
Department of Medicine
Georgetown University Hospital
Washington, District of Columbia

Nicholas J. Vogelzang, MD
Professor
Division of Oncology, Department of
   Internal Medicine
University of Nevada School of Medicine
Director
Nevada Cancer Institute
Las Vegas, Nevada

Wei Wang, MD
Assistant Professor of Medicine
Department of Medicine
Division of Renal Diseases and Hypertension
University of Colorado School of Medicine
Denver, Colorado

John F. Ward, MD FACS
Chief of Urologic Oncology
Nevada Cancer Institute
Las Vegas, Nevada

John W. Warren, MD
Professor
Division of Infectious Diseases
Department of Medicine
University of Maryland School of Medicine
Baltimore, Maryland

Terry Watnick, MD
Assistant Professor of Medicine
Johns Hopkins University School of Medicine
Department of Medicine
Baltimore, Maryland

Judith A.W. Webb, MD, FRCR, FRCP
Honorary Consultant Radiologist
Diagnostic Radiology Department
St. Bartholomews Hospital
West Smithfield, London, United Kingdom

Richard P. Wedeen, MD
Professor
Departments of Medicine; Preventative Medicine and
   Community Health
University of Medicine and Dentistry of New Jersey
New Jersey Medical School
Newark, New Jersey
Associate Chief of Staff for Research and Development
Department of Research
Department of Veterans Affairs New Jersey Health
   Care System
East Orange, New Jersey

Myron H. Weinberger, MD
Professor of Medicine
Department of Medicine
Indiana University Medical Center
Indianapolis, Indiana

Scott J. Weissman, MD
Acting Assistant Professor
Department of Pediatrics
University of Washington School of Medicine
Acting Assistant Professor
Division of Infectious Diseases
Children's Hospital and Regional Medical Center
Seattle, Washington

Sterling G. West, MD
Professor
Department of Medicine
University of Colorado Health Sciences Center
Director, Rheumatology Fellowship Program
Department of Medicine
University of Colorado Hospital
Denver, Colorado

Andrzej Wiecek, MD, PhD
Professor
Department of Nephrology
Endocrinology and Metabolic Diseases
Medical University of Silesia
Katowice, Poland

Christopher Stuart Wilcox, MD, PhD
George E. Schrier Chair of Nephrology
Director, Cardiovascular Kidney Institute
Department of Medicine
Georgetown University
Chief of Nephrology and Hypertension
Department of Medicine
Georgetown University Hospital
Washington, District of Columbia

Shandra Wilson, MD
Assistant Professor
Department of Surgery/Urology
University of Colorado
Denver, Colorado

Alex Wiseman, MD
Associate Professor
Department of Medicine
University of Colorado Health Sciences Center
Division of Renal Diseases and Hypertension
Denver, Colorado

Yalem Woredekal, MD
Assistant Professor
Department of Medicine
SUNY, Health Science Center at Brooklyn
University Hospital of Brooklyn
Brooklyn, New York

Fred S. Wright, MD
Professor
Departments of Internal Medicine and C and M Physiology
Yale University School of Medicine
New Haven, Connecticut
Associate Chief of Staff for Research
VA Connecticut Healthcare System
West Haven, Connecticut

Michael Yudd, MD
Associate Professor
Department of Medicine
University of Medicine and Dentistry of
    New Jersey
Newark, New Jersey
Medical Director, Dialysis Unit
Department of Medicine
Veterans Health Administration New Jersey
    Healthcare System
East Orange, New Jersey

Dirk-Henrik Zermann, MD, PhD
Privatdozent
Department of Urology
Friedrich-Schiller University
Jena, Germany
Chief
Department of Urology
Vogtland-Klinik Bad Elster
Bad Elster, Germany

Stephen H. Zinner, MD
Charles S. Davidson Professor of Medicine
Department of Medicine
Harvard Medical School
Boston, Massachusetts
Chair, Department of Medicine
Mount Auburn Hospital
Cambridge, Massachusetts

DISEASES OF THE

Kidney &
Urinary Tract

SECTION VII
ACUTE RENAL FAILURE

CHAPTER 39 ■ PATHOPHYSIOLOGY OF ISCHEMIC ACUTE RENAL INJURY

CHARLES L. EDELSTEIN AND ROBERT W. SCHRIER

Acute renal injury may lead to the clinical syndrome, which has been termed *acute tubular necrosis* (ATN). This term emerged from the early observation on renal biopsy that necrosis of some renal tubular epithelial cells may occur in humans with acute renal injury (1). Tubular epithelial casts (muddy brown casts) are excreted in the urine of these patients. It is now known, however, that the tubular necrosis is quite patchy and alone could not account for glomerular filtration rates (GFR) less than 10 mL/minute/1.73m^2, the functional hallmark of clinically significant ATN (1). Moreover, a percentage, ranging from 30% to 70%, of the urinary tubular epithelial cells has been shown to be viable by culture and exclusion of vital dyes (2,3). This observation is somewhat surprising since generally cells, which are separated from their extracellular matrix, undergo apoptosis (4–7). Emerging results, however, suggest that adhesion molecules (e.g., cadherins and integrins) may allow cell to cell or cell to matrix adhesion, which not only avoids apoptosis but may contribute to intratubular obstruction (8–11). Intraluminal tubular casts on renal biopsy are a hallmark of clinical ATN and earlier nephron dissection studies by Jean Oliver demonstrated a preferential location of these casts in the medullary collecting duct (12). This location is of particular relevance to the overall low GFR in ATN, since thousands of nephrons drain into a single medullary collecting duct.

In the past, a debate emerged about whether the pathophysiology of clinical ATN was primarily tubular or vascular. In fact, initial rat micropuncture studies were unable to consistently detect an elevation in tubular pressures in experimental acute renal failure (ARF) and thus suggested that the term *vasomotor nephropathy* replace the ATN term for the clinical syndrome (13–15). However, against a purely vascular pathogenesis was the observation that the intrarenal infusion of a vasodilator (e.g., dopamine), which restored renal blood flow to normal, failed to reverse the ARF failure clinical syndrome in either human or experimental animals (16,17). Experimental results have emerged that both vascular and tubular factors are involved in the pathogenesis of clinical ATN. Most recently, the role of endothelial injury and dysfunction (18) in promoting an inflammatory response in ARF (19) has received prominence. Thus, this chapter will discuss the potential tubular and vascular factors, as well as inflammatory processes, involved in the pathogenesis of ischemic ARF (Fig. 39-1). Toxic ARF will be discussed in another chapter. However, it must be emphasized that ATN in humans is frequently multifactorial. Both ischemic and toxic insults combine to cause clinical ATN. In the present chapter, ATN and ischemic ARF will be used interchangeably with the assumption that causes of prerenal and postrenal (i.e., urinary tract obstruction) azotemia have been excluded (see Chapter 25).

Regarding the definition of ARF, criteria based on the serum creatinine and urine output, have been recently proposed for classifying ARF (19a). These RIFLE criteria (Risk, Injury, Failure, Loss of function, and End stage kidney disease) may facilitate early diagnosis and interpretation of future clinical trials.

The understanding of the pathogenesis of ischemic ARF is of considerable importance for several reasons. First of all, this clinical syndrome is quite frequent, occurring in 5% to 10% of hospitalized patients and 30% to 40% of intensive care unit patients (20–22). The incidence is likely to increase in the future because of the use of newer nephrotoxic drugs and the performance of more complex procedures in older patients (23). Secondly, ischemic ARF has a very high mortality particularly when requiring dialysis to treat the resultant uremic syndrome. Overall mortality averages 40% to 50%; however, patients in an intensive care unit with ischemic ARF may have mortality in excess of 80%, particularly if they have multiorgan failure (24–29). It is widely quoted that the mortality of ARF has only improved slightly in the last 40 years (30). However, a study suggests that there has been improvement in ARF mortality between the late 1970s and the early 1990s (31). Thirdly, there is considerable evidence that a functional component of the renal failure exists. Specifically, histologic examination of the kidney from patients with clinical ATN exhibits normal glomeruli, occasional tubular necrosis, some intraluminal casts, and modest interstitial edema (1). There is virtually no evidence for irreversible tissue damage and the morphological changes alone fail to support the presence of a GFR less than 10 mL/minute/1.73m^2. Lastly, the vast majority of patients who recover from ischemic ARF demonstrate grossly normal renal function (27). Thus, on recovery, patients with this clinical syndrome, which have a dramatically high mortality, are not left with residual dead tissue, which occurs after a myocardial infarction or stroke.

EXPERIMENTAL MODELS OF ACUTE RENAL FAILURE

Available models to study the pathophysiology of renal cell ischemia are listed in Table 39-1 (32). An understanding of these models will allow better interpretation of the multiple studies discussed in this chapter.

Proximal and distal tubular cells in culture have been widely used to study tubular injury. These cells change from their normal dependence on oxidative, mitochondrial metabolism to glycolysis under culture conditions (33). As a result, these cultured tubules become less susceptible to oxygen deprivation. Thus, exposure to drugs like antimycin-A, ionomycin, or a combination to induce "chemical" ATP depletion and subsequent necrosis or apoptosis is used. Cultured cells also undergo considerable structural change that includes simplification of both their apical and basolateral compartments (34). The presence of necrosis rather than apoptosis in these cells may be related to the level of ATP depletion. In cultured mouse proximal tubules subjected to ATP depletion below 15% of control values, the cells died of necrosis, whereas in ATP depletion from 25% to 70% of control values all the cells died of apoptosis

Pathogenesis of ischemic acute renal failure (ARF)

Tubular factors:
Back-leak of glomerular filtrate
Decreased proximal tubular sodium reabsorption
Increased tubuloglomerular feedback
Tubular cast formation and obstruction

Vascular factors:
Renal vasoconstriction

Inflammatory response:
Endothelial injury
Leukocyte adhesion/infiltration
Inflammatory mediators

FIGURE 39-1. Vascular and tubular factors and inflammatory processes are involved in the pathophysiology of ischemic acute renal failure.

(35). While cultured tubules are the least complex model and allow understanding of mechanisms involved, the therapeutic implications for *in vivo* ARF is limited.

Freshly isolated rat or rabbit proximal tubules in suspension are also widely used to study proximal tubular injury (36–44). The method of isolation of tubules is by collagenase digestion and Percoll centrifugation. The isolation of proximal tubules from mice has recently been described (41,45). Hypoxia is achieved by gassing the suspension with $95\%N_2/5\%CO_2$ for up to 15 minutes thereby reducing the pO_2 to approximately 30 mm Hg. Percent lactic dehydrogenase (LDH) release into the suspension medium is measured as an index of lethal membrane injury (46,47). The tubules are preincubated with cytoprotective agents and enzyme inhibitors before induction of hypoxia and the effect of these agents on cell membrane injury can be determined. The presence of necrosis rather than apoptosis during short periods of hypoxia (15 to 30 minutes) in this model was demonstrated using DNA-specific dyes, such as Hoechst 33342 and propidium iodide (48). Another study has also demonstrated that during hypoxia there is endonuclease activation without morphologic features of apoptosis

TABLE 39-1

AVAILABLE MODELS TO STUDY THE PATHOPHYSIOLOGY OF RENAL CELL ISCHEMIA (INCREASING ORDER OF COMPLEXITY)

Model	Origin
Cultured tubular cells	Primary culture of human, rat and mouse; Madin-Darby canine kidney (MDCK) cells (distal); porcine renal epithelial (LLC-PK1) cells (proximal); opossum kidney (OK) cells; human kidney (HK) cells.
Freshly isolated proximal tubules in suspension	Rabbits, rats, mice
Isolated perfused kidney	Rat
Whole animals	Rabbits, rats, mice, dogs (not much used anymore)
Human patients	Renal biopsy studies. Urine and serum biomarkers of ARF.

(Adapted from: Lieberthal W, Nigam SK. Acute renal failure: II. Experimental models of acute renal failure; imperfect but indispensable. *Am J Physiol* 2000;278:F1.)

in the same model of rat proximal tubules (49). Freshly isolated tubules are valuable for both structural and metabolic investigations as they retain the biochemical properties of the *in vivo* state, a high degree of structural integrity, and are highly polarized and fully differentiated (32). However, the tubules are highly sensitive to ATP depletion and severe hypoxia or anoxia results in necrosis of more than 50% of the cells after 30 minutes.

In whole animal studies, usually rats, rabbits, or mice, a clamp model of ischemic ARF is used (50–52). Ischemic ARF is generally induced by (i) clamping of both the right and left renal pedicles or renal arteries or (ii) unilateral renal pedicle or artery clamp preceded by contralateral nephrectomy. The renal vessels are clamped for varying periods of time, generally from 45 to 60 min, followed by varying periods of reperfusion. This results in a reversible model of ARF in which the BUN and serum creatinine reach a peak at 24 to 48 hours reperfusion and then gradually normalize over the next 7 days (50–53). However, renal vessel clamping in rats results in extensive necrosis of proximal tubules. This necrosis is much more extensive than is seen in humans with ischemic ARF. Nevertheless, while animal models of ischemic ARF are complex with many experimental limitations, they provide important leads for future therapeutic clinical interventions.

In the isolated perfused kidney model, the kidney is removed from the animal. The perfusate usually consists of Krebs-Henseleit buffer with albumin. Urine is collected by cannulation of the ureter. This model allows study of factors independent of changes in systemic hemodynamics and neural activity. The further advantages of this model are that it allows the study of specific circulatory factors or pharmacological agents that are added to the perfusate. These agents are thus delivered directly to the kidney. The disadvantages of the model are (i) the absence of red blood cells in the perfusate impairs oxygen delivery to the medullary thick ascending limb (MTAL) and (ii) perfusate flow greatly exceeds normal *in vivo* values. The isolated perfused kidney is regarded as a model of selective hypoxia to the medullary thick ascending limb (54).

Study of human patients with ARF, while having important experimental limitations, of course, has the most direct therapeutic value. Analysis of urine cytology represents a non-invasive method for potentially defining the cause of ARF (1). Myers and coworkers have examined patients with ischemic ARF postrenal transplantation by obtaining biopsies of these allografts at the time of transplantation (55–57). Biomarkers of kidney injury would greatly facilitate the early detection and precise diagnosis of ATN.

BIOMARKERS OF ARF

Acute renal failure is usually diagnosed by recording increases in serum creatinine and decreased urine output over several days. However, serum creatinine is not a good marker of renal function in ARF because its concentration can be affected by factors not related to renal function such as volume of distribution, muscle mass, and creatinine secretion (27). When the kidney is injured and the true GFR suddenly drops, there is a slow increase in serum creatinine over days. A new steady state, that may take up to 7 days, is reached when creatinine generation equals creatinine excretion. In contrast to serum troponin in myocardial infarction, an increase in serum creatinine is not directly related to tubular injury in ARF. Recent studies have examined urine and serum biomarkers of kidney injury that would facilitate the diagnosis of ATN.

Although the initial studies on some molecules like tubular enzymes (e.g., L-alanine aminopeptidase, N-acetyl-[beta]-D- glucosaminadase, and adenosine deaminase binding protein) were promising, the larger and more detailed studies have shown inadequate sensitivity or specificity to advocate clinical use (58–60). Recently described molecules such as the cytokine IL-18 (61), kidney injury molecule-1 (KIM-1) (62), cystein-rich protein 61 (Cry61) (63), neutrophil gelatinase-associated lipocalin (NGAL) (64), and sodium/hydrogen exchanger isoform 3 (NHE3) (65) have demonstrated compelling results as markers of ARF at the preclinical level. Studies are being initiated to explore these molecules in human ARF.

Urinary IL-18 is an excellent test for diagnosis of ATN and delayed graft function in humans (66). The mature form of IL-18, as detected by ELISA assay, is massively increased in the urine of patients with ischemic ATN compared to normal controls and other acute and chronic renal diseases. Urinary IL-18 increases in the first 24 hours after kidney transplantation in patients with delayed graft function (DGF). Lower levels of urinary IL-18 in the first 24 hours after kidney transplantation are associated with a better functioning kidney. On receiver operating characteristic (ROC) curve analysis, the discriminatory power of the urine IL-18 test to detect ATN is 97%. The accuracy of this test compares favorably with the recently described markers of ARF, actin, IL-6, and IL-8 (67).

Because of the crucial importance of earlier therapies and management of ARF, markers are being explored for early diagnosis of ARF. NGAL were investigated as an early biomarker for ARF following cardiopulmonary bypass in 45 patients (68). Urine and serum was collected at baseline and at frequent intervals for 5 days following cardiopulmonary bypass. All patients who developed ARF (defined as a 50% increase in serum creatinine) displayed a significant increase in serum and urine NGAL very early after cardiopulmonary bypass compared to patients without ARF. These results show that NGAL may be a sensitive, early urinary, and serum biomarker for ARF.

In a nested case-control study within the Adult Respiratory Distress Syndrome (ARDS) network trial, urinary IL-18 was investigated as an early marker of ARF (69). Median urine IL-18 levels were significantly higher in ARF cases (defined as a 50% increase in serum creatinine) as compared to controls. On multivariable analysis, urine IL-18 values predicted development of ARF 24 and 48 hours later after adjusting for demographics, sepsis, APACHE III score, serum creatinine, and urine output. After controlling for other parameters, a rise in urine IL-18 by 25 pg/mL is associated with increased odds of ARF by 19% in the next 24 hours. Urine IL-18 performs well as a diagnostic test with an area under the receiver operator characteristic curve of 73%. The conclusion of this study is that urinary IL-18 levels can be used for the early diagnosis of ARF.

A recent study demonstrated that serum cystatin C appears to increase 24 to 48 hours before creatinine in patients with ARF (70). However, cystatin C is a marker of clearance and not a marker of renal tubular injury.

An early biomarker of ischemic ATN may lead to earlier treatments (e.g., appropriate fluid balance, avoidance of nephrotoxic drugs, appropriate drug dosage, earlier nephrology consultation, and earlier initiation of dialysis) (71). Also, an early marker with a high sensitivity and specificity will help in designing interventional trials for the treatment of ARF by allowing for the timely initiation of the investigational drug. Future clinical trials and prospective studies in ARF should incorporate biomarker measurements to hasten the clinical development of these tests.

BACKLEAK OF GLOMERULAR FILTRATE POSTRENAL ISCHEMIA

It has been proposed that GFR in ischemic ARF is really not as low as measured since glomerular filtrate is leaking across damaged epithelium or tubular basement membranes. In some toxic experimental models of ischemic ARF, diffuse tubular necrosis and basement membrane damage have been associated with evidence for backleak of glomerular filtrate. The term *backleak* of glomerular filtrate refers to the unregulated passage of salt and water from the tubular lumen into the interstitium and later back into the renal venous capillaries and renal veins (72). However, the level of epithelial and basement membrane damage with these experimental toxic models (e.g., cisplatin and mercuric chloride) is virtually never observed in human ATN. Myers et al. have performed studies using solute sieving curves in search of tubular backleak of glomerular filtrate (73). They found that dextran sieving curves could sometimes exceed inulin sieving curves, thus providing evidence in support of backleak of solutes (i.e., inulin) which are normally unable to cross intact tubular epithelial basement membranes. Even when accepting the validity of this method for documenting tubular backleak of filtrate, however, the calculated amount would only account for a decrease in renal function of 8% to 10%. Thus, while tubular backleak of glomerular filtrate might occasionally occur in patients with severe ischemic ARF, it is unlikely to be a dominant pathogenic factor.

The tight junction of polarized tubular epithelial cells is the most apical component of the junctional complex and serves as an important permeability barrier (74). Tight junctions also control cell polarity (75). However, the tight junction in the proximal tubule is relatively "leaky" with as much as one-third of proximal sodium reabsorption occurring via the paracellular route. The tight junctional complex is a dynamic and regulated structure. Some of its protein components have been identified and include the transmembrane protein occludin. Nontransmembrane proteins on the cytosolic leaflet include zona occludens (ZO)-1, ZO-2, cingulin, 7H6, and several unidentified phosphoproteins. Interactions of some of these proteins with the actin cytoskeleton are major determinants of tight junction structure and may also play a role in the regulation of tight junction assembly (74). The integrity of the tight junction is disrupted during ischemic injury and must be reestablished for recovery (76). There is *in vitro* experimental evidence in cell culture studies for an impaired tight junction between tubular epithelial cells undergoing chemical anoxia (77). Ruthenium red, which normally is impermeable to tight junctions, has been shown to enter the zona occludans after chemical hypoxia and renal ischemia (77,78). Energy depletion abolishes the gate function of the tight junction, as determined by the dramatic decrease in transepithelial resistance, but it leaves the fence function intact, as determined by the maintenance of lipid polarity (79). In an ATP depletion-repletion model in Madin-Darby canine kidney cells, tight junction proteins, such as ZO-1, reversibly form large complexes and associate with cytoskeletal proteins (80). A model has been proposed in which a key, potentially regulated, step in the generation of the ischemic epithelial cell phenotype is the interaction between tight junction proteins and fodrin and/or other cytoskeletal proteins (80). Intracellullar calcium plays a role in tight junction reassembly after ATP depletion (76). In this study, the role of intracellular calcium in tight junction reassembly after ATP depletion-repletion was studied using the cell-permeable calcium chelator 1, 2-bis(2-aminophenoxy)ethane-N,N,N′,N′-tetraacetic acid-AM (BAPTA-AM). Lowering intracellular calcium during ATP depletion was associated with significant inhibition of the reestablishment of the permeability barrier following ATP repletion as measured by transepithelial electrical resistance and mannitol flux, marked alterations in the subcellular localization of occludin by immunofluorescent analysis and decreased solubility of ZO-1 and other tight junction proteins by Triton X-100 extraction assay. This suggested that lowering intracellular calcium potentiates the interaction of tight junction proteins with the cytoskeleton.

Recent studies have also shown the importance of small GTPases (Rho, Rac, and dc-42) in the integrity of the zona occludans (81). ATP depletion with chemical hypoxia has been demonstrated to inactivate these GTPases and thereby contribute to increased paracellular backleak of filtrate (75,82). Expression of constitutively active RhoA GTPase in ATP-depleted MDCK cells prevents tight junction disassembly (75). Cyanide-induced chemical hypoxia increases the kinase activity of c-Src and causes its translocation to cell-cell junctions where it binds to and phosphorylates beta-catenin and p120, suggesting that this may contribute to the loss of epithelial barrier function (83). It is likely that the effects on tight junction integrity seen in ATP depletion are due, at least in part, to the inhibition of Na-K-ATPase (84).The relevance of these cell culture observations to clinical ischemic ARF in patients remains to be proven.

DECREASED TUBULAR SODIUM REABSORPTION POSTRENAL ISCHEMIA

Proximal tubular injury, whether it be sublethal reversible dysfunction, necrosis, or apoptosis has been extensively studied. Mechanisms of proximal tubular injury that will be discussed in this section are outlined in Table 39-2. The study of proximal tubular injury is of special relevance in order to explain the decreased tubular sodium reabsorption that occurs in postrenal ischemia.

In the normal kidney, Na^+ is vectorially transported from the proximal tubule lumen across the apical membrane microvilli into the tubular epithelial cells and then across the basolateral membrane into the interstitium and the peritubular circulation (85). Na^+-influx into the polarized proximal tubular epithelial cells across the apical membrane is passive down the Na^+-gradient via the H^+/Na^+ exchanger and various Na^+-cotransporters. The Na^+- gradient is maintained by an active transport via the Na^+/K^+-ATPase at the basolateral membrane of the proximal tubular cells (Fig. 39-2).

The earliest signs of clinical ATN are urinary muddy brown casts and an increased fractional excretion of sodium (FE_{Na}) (86,87). The proximal tubule is the most frequent morphological site of injury in ischemic ARF in both humans and animals (88). The S_3 segment of the proximal tubule is particularly prone to ischemic injury, perhaps because of its location in the outer medulla, which is relatively hypoxic compared to the renal cortex (88). The proximal tubule nephron site is also associated with impaired vectorial sodium transport. The earliest morphological changes with ischemic injury are invagination and sloughing of the brush border membrane into the lumen, an abnormality compatible with impairment of apical sodium antiporters and cotransporters responsible for sodium entry into proximal tubular epithelium (89–91). The tubules lose their polarity (87). *In vitro* studies have shown that ATP depletion leads to dephosphorylation and inactivation of the actin binding protein, ezrin, and activation of actin depolarizing protein in the proximal tubule membrane (92,93). This leads to disruption of the microvillar actin and loss of the brush border membrane (94). Loss of polarity of proximal tubule cells during chemical anoxia and ischemia has also been shown with the translocation of the Na-K-ATPase to the apical membrane (95–97) (Fig. 39-3). The translocated Na-K-ATPase remains functional (98). In MDCK cells exposed to ATP depletion, there is loss of polarity of Na-K-ATPase and dissociation of the membrane-cytoskeleton complex at the spectrin-ankyrin interface (99). Thus, sodium transport into the proximal lumen and decreased proximal tubular sodium reabsorption have been proposed in response to hypoxia and ischemia.

TABLE 39-2

MECHANISMS OF HYPOXIC/ISCHEMIC PROXIMAL TUBULAR INJURY

SUBLETHAL REVERSIBLE INJURY
Cytoskeletal disruption and loss of polarity
Loss of tight junction function
Loss of cell-matrix adhesion
Abnormal gene expression

NECROSIS
Severe ATP depletion (15% of normal)
Calcium influx
Calcium-dependent phospholipase A_2(cPLA$_2$)
Calcium-dependent cysteine proteases e.g., calpain
Calcium-independent PLA$_2$
Caspase-1
Interleukin-18 (IL-18)
Metalloproteases
Oxygen radicals
Lipid peroxidation
Deficiency of glycine
Nitric oxide (generated by iNOS)
Endonuclease activation
Deficient heat stress response
Potassium efflux

APOPTOSIS
Mild ATP depletion (25% to 50% of normal)
Caspase-3
Caspase-1
Caspase-6
Endonuclease activation
Serine proteases
Insulin-like growth factor I receptor deficiency
Deficient heat stress response
Erythropoietin
Bcl-2 proteins
Mitochondrial injury

Studies in cadaveric transplanted kidneys with prompt and delayed graft function have been compared relative to the cellular location of the actin binding proteins, ankyrin and spectrin, and Na-K-ATPase using selective antibodies. In those kidneys with delayed graft function approximately 50% of the ankyrin, spectrin, and Na-K-ATPase was translocated from the basolateral membrane to the cytoplasm, whereas those kidneys with prompt graft function had only minimal translocation of these

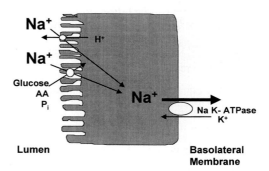

FIGURE 39-2. Normal reabsorption of sodium in the proximal tubule. The NaK-ATPase pump is located on the basolateral surface of the proximal tubule.

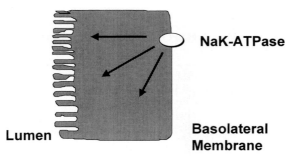

FIGURE 39-3. Tranlocation of the Na-K-ATPase pump away from the basolateral proximal tubule membrane during hypoxia/ischemia. Loss of polarity of proximal tubule cells during chemical anoxia and ischemia results in a translocation of the Na-K-ATPase. During ATP depletion in cultured cells the Na-K-ATPase translocates to the apical membrane. In human kidney allografts with delayed function, the Na-K-ATPase translocates to the cytoplasm. The translocated Na-K-ATPase remains functional.

proteins from the basolateral membrane (55) (Fig. 39-4). These observations, therefore, have contributed to our understanding of reversible and sublethal tubular dysfunction in ischemic kidneys *in vivo.*

Since proximal tubular cells in culture convert from primarily oxidative to glycolytic metabolism and alter their phenotype (33,34), confirmation of experimental results in other systems is advisable. The use of freshly isolated proximal tubules to study the response to hypoxia has also been enlightening. These tubules in general maintain their phenotype and oxidative metabolism but are more sensitive to hypoxia, as assessed by LDH release, than *in vivo* tubules (100–103). Hypoxia for 15 to 30 minutes causes a reproducible release of LDH and the cells die by necrosis (48,49). The central role of intracellular calcium and various protective maneuvers against hypoxic injury have been demonstrated in these isolated proximal tubules. However, before discussing the role of intracellular calcium in proximal tubular injury, we shall briefly consider adenine nucleotides. It is unquestioned that the first effect of ischemia, hypoxia, or mitochondrial inhibition in most *in vitro* and *in vivo* models is to compromise adenine nucleotide metabolism.

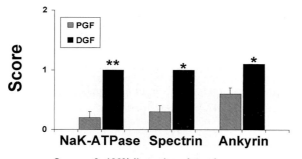

Score: 0=100% linear basolateral
        1=50% punctate basolateral and 50% cytosolic
        2=100% cytosolic

FIGURE 39-4. The cellular location on immunohistochemistry of the actin binding proteins, ankyrin and spectrin, and Na-K-ATPase in cadaveric transplanted kidneys with prompt graft function (PGF) and delayed graft function (DGF) was compared. In those kidneys with delayed graft function approximately 50% of the ankyrin, spectrin, and Na-K-ATPase was translocated from the basolateral membrane to the cytoplasm. Whereas those kidneys with prompt graft function had only minimal translocation of these proteins from the basolateral membrane. **p <0.01 vs PGF, **p <0.05 vs PGF. (Adapted from: Alejandro VS, Nelson WJ, Huie P, et al. Postischemic injury, delayed function and NaK-ATPase distribution in the transplanted kidney. *Kidney Int* 1995;48:1308.)

Decreased production of ATP precedes the increase in intracellular calcium.

Adenine Nucleotides

Removal of oxygen from renal cells or whole kidneys results in prompt decreases in the cellular ATP pool. Initially, adenosine diphosphate (ADP) and adenosine monophosphate (AMP) concentrations increase (52), and further catabolism of AMP to adenosine and then to hypoxanthine and, in some species, to xanthine occurs as the ischemic period is prolonged (104,105). Provision of exogenous ATP-MgCl$_2$ to ischemic rat kidneys protects against ischemic injury (106). Mechanisms whereby loss of ATP results in cellular injury include the loss of purine nucleosides themselves, in some species the generation of oxygen free radicals during reperfusion, and the loss of many metabolic functions (e.g., phosphorylation) of important enzymes and ion channels and the functions of ion transporters that are dependent on adequate ATP levels.

Ischemic preconditioning protects the heart and in some studies, the kidneys, from subsequent ischemia/reperfusion injury. Ischemic preconditioning appears to be mediated via activation of adenosine receptors, specifically A$_1$ adenosine receptors. In support of this are studies that the exogenous administration of adenosine, or A$_1$ adenosine agonists mimic ischemic preconditioning in cardiac muscle (107). It was recently demonstrated that rat kidneys can be preconditioned to attenuate ischemic-reperfusion injury. In this study, adenosine infusion before the ischemic insult protects renal function via A$_1$ adenosine receptor activation and adenosine A$_1$ antagonism blocks adenosine-induced protection. In addition, adenosine A$_3$ receptor activation before ischemia worsens renal ischemia-reperfusion injury and adenosine A$_3$ receptor antagonism protects renal function (107). A$_{2A}$ adenosine receptors mediate inhibition of ischemic ARF in rats due to an inhibitory effect on neutrophil adhesion (108,109). Combined infusion of an A$_{2A}$ adenosine receptor agonist and a type IV phosphodiesterase (PDE 4) inhibitor leads to enhanced protection against ischemia-reperfusion injury in mice (110). Protection against renal ischemia-reperfusion injury by adenosine A$_2$A receptor agonists or endogenous adenosine requires activation of receptors expressed on bone marrow–derived cells (111). The adenosine A$_2$ receptor may be a novel therapeutic target in renal ischemia-reperfusion injury (112).

Intracellular Calcium

The normal regulation of epithelial cell calcium is demonstrated in Figure 39-5. Calcium exists in the cell as cytosolic free calcium, which is the smallest amount, but the most critical for regulation of intracellular events. Calcium is also bound to proteins and anions in the cytosol and to membrane phospholipids and glycoproteins. The largest pool of intracellular calcium is in the mitochondria and the endoplasmic reticulum (113,114). The concentration of calcium in the cytosol is about 100 nM, which is 1/10,000 of the extracellular calcium that is in a mM concentration (113). The large electrochemical gradient between intracellular and extracellular calcium is maintained by binding of calcium to intracellular components and by apical and basolateral transport systems. Transport systems may be voltage dependent or ATP dependent. Calcium efflux is mediated in basolateral membranes by both calcium ATPase, which is ATP dependent, and by a Na$^+$/Ca^{2+} exchanger on the basolateral membrane, which is ATP independent (115). Normally, the cell membrane is impermeable to calcium and maintains the steep calcium gradient between cytosolic free calcium and the extracellular space (114). However, when cytosolic calcium increases in response to either increased cellular

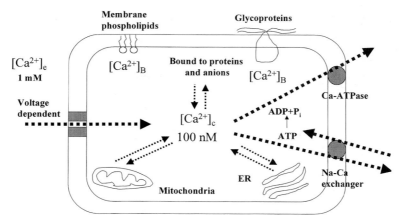

FIGURE 39-5. The normal regulation of epithelial cell calcium. The cytosolic free calcium $[Ca^{2+}]_c$ is the smallest amount, but the most critical for regulation of intracellular events. The concentration of calcium in the cytosol is about 100 nM, which is 1/10000 of the extracellular calcium, which is in a mM concentration $[Ca^{2+}]_e$ Calcium is also bound to proteins and anions in the cytosol and to membrane phospholipids and glycoproteins $[Ca^{2+}]_b$. The largest pool of intracellular calcium is in the mitochondria and the endoplasmic reticulum. The large electrochemical gradient is maintained by binding of calcium to intracellular components and by apical and basolateral transport systems. Transport systems, which maintain the large electrochemical gradient between intracellular and extracellular Ca^{2+} may be voltage dependent or ATP dependent like the Ca^{2+} ATPase pump and the Na^+/Ca^{2+} exchanger. During cell injury active mitochondrial sequestration appears to be quantitatively the most important process for buffering elevations in cytosolic calcium.

membrane permeability or decreased calcium efflux or both, the mitochondria and endoplasmic reticulum actively increase their calcium uptake. Mitochondrial uptake and retention of calcium becomes substantial only when cytosolic levels exceed 400 to 500 nM as occurs with cell injury (113). Mitochondrial uptake is regulated by a calcium uniporter in the mitochondrial inner membrane. Thus, during cell injury active mitochondrial sequestration appears to be quantitatively the most important process for buffering elevations in cytosolic calcium.

During epithelial cell injury, several factors favor increases in cytosolic free calcium (Fig. 39-6). There is (i) decreased mitochondrial electron transport leading to decreased ATP levels; (ii) increased membrane permeability; and (iii) depolarization or opening of voltage dependent channels. The decreased ATP leads to decreased calcium uptake by mitochondria and endoplasmic reticula and decreased ability to pump calcium out of the cell.

With this background on the normal regulation of cell calcium, we shall now consider the role of intracellular calcium in tubular injury. In 1981, it was proposed that calcium ions were important participants in the functional, biochemical and morphologic disturbances that characterize ARF (116,117).

Numerous studies over the past 15 years in different injury models and cell types have demonstrated an increase in cytosolic calcium in renal epithelial cell injury. These studies are summarized in Table 39-3.

Initial interest in this area began with the demonstration that chemically dissimilar Ca2+ channel blockers (CCB) are effective in preventing or attenuating the courses of experimental ARF (50,115). On the background of these experimental results, the efficacy of CCB has been shown in preventing ARF associated with cadaveric transplantation (118,119) and radiocontrast media (120). These results led to a series of experiments examining the role of cellular Ca^{2+} in the pathogenesis of ischemic ARF. Early studies demonstrated that renal mitochondrial Ca^{2+} accumulation characterizes ischemic ARF and that this Ca^{2+} uptake impairs renal mitochondrial oxidative phosphorylation and ATP synthesis (51,52,121,122). Moreover, protection against ischemic ARF with CCB was associated with an attenuation of this mitochondrial Ca^{2+} accumulation and improved mitochondrial respiratory function (50).

In vitro experiments using cultured renal tubules suggested a pathogenic role for cellular Ca^{2+} independent of any vascular effect (123,124). In other experiments, either removal of

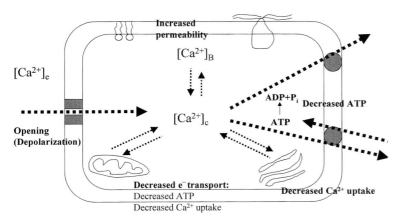

FIGURE 39-6. During epithelial cell injury, several factors favor increases in cytosolic free calcium. There is (1) depolarization or opening of voltage dependent channels; (2) increased membrane permeability and (3) decreased mitochondrial electron transport leading to decreased ATP levels. The decreased ATP leads to decreased calcium uptake by mitochondria and ER and decreased ability to pump calcium out of the cell.

TABLE 39-3

INCREASES IN CYTOSOLIC CALCIUM IN RENAL EPITHELIAL CELL INJURY

Injury model	Cell type	Reference
Calcium ionophore	Rabbit proximal tubules	(454)
Anoxia	LLCMK2 cells	(455)
Chemical ATP depletion	MDCK cells	(456)
Calcium ionophore	Cultured rabbit proximal tubules	(457)
Chemical ATP depletion		
Chemical anoxia	Rabbit proximal tubules	(178)
Hypoxia	Rabbit proximal tubules	(458)
Hydrogen peroxide	LLCPK1 cells	(459)
Anoxia and hypoxia	Rat proximal tubules	(127)
Chemical anoxia	Opossum kidney cells	(460)
Hypoxia-reoxygenation	Primary culture rat proximal tubules	(461)
Hypoxia	Rat proximal tubules	(103)
Anoxia	Rabbit proximal tubules	(462)

(Reproduced from: Edelstein CL. Editorial Comment: calcium-mediated proximal tubular injury—what is the role of cysteine proteases? *Nephrol Dial Transplant* 2000;15:141, with permission.)

Ca^{2+} from the medium during early reoxygenation (125) or the administration of CCB (126) was found to improve cell viability after anoxia. Further experiments were designed to examine the role of cellular Ca^{2+} and the direct effects of CCB on renal tubular epithelium without vascular influences; these experiments utilized isolated proximal tubules, a consistent tubular site of ischemic injury. The use of this preparation allowed the study of direct tubular effects of protective agents, which could not have been demonstrated to be independent of vascular effects in whole animal studies. Models of injury were developed in the isolated tubule preparation in response to hypoxia, anoxia, and phosphate depletion (127–129). Studies demonstrated that ^{45}Ca uptake is increased with hypoxia and that CCB prevent this increase (127). Moreover, the protective effect of a decreased pH was also shown to be associated with a decrease in hypoxia related enhanced ^{45}Ca influx (130). In addition, Wetzels et al. showed that hypoxia-induced proximal tubule membrane damage can be significantly reduced by lowering the extracellular Ca^{2+} concentration or by the addition of verapamil (46). In this latter study, the protective effect of verapamil was associated with improved cellular ATP and K^+ levels, an effect that is not observed with other protective agents, such as glycine or alanine. This finding suggested that verapamil could act directly on the mitochondria and affect the plasma membrane. Subsequent studies using isolated renal cortical mitochondria did, in fact, demonstrate that verapamil exerts a protective effect against Ca^{2+}-induced mitochondrial damage and that this effect may be mediated by the inhibition of mitochondrial Ca^{2+} uptake and mitochondrial phospholipase activity (131). Furthermore, studies in isolated tubules confirmed hypoxia-induced free fatty acid and lysophospholipid accumulation (132) and suggested a relationship between these events and the rate of cellular Ca^{2+} uptake (133).

One question is to what level the free cytosolic calcium rises during ATP depletion. Previously it was difficult to determine peak cytosolic calcium levels using the high affinity calcium fluorophore Fura-2. Weinberg's group showed that the cytosolic free calcium increases to greater than 100 μM in ATP depleted proximal tubules using the low-affinity calcium fluorophore Mag-Fura-2 (101). Experiments were done in the presence of 2mM glycine which approximates the physiological concentration *in vivo*. In the tubules studied, 91% had a free cytosolic calcium that exceeded 10 μM. Thirty-five percent had levels greater than 500 μM with no cell membrane damage. In this study, proximal tubules seemed to have a remarkable resistance to the deleterious effects of increased calcium during ATP de-

pletion in the presence of glycine. In the isolated perfused rat kidney, intracellular calcium increases have also been measured using 19^F NMR and 5^F BAPTA and demonstrated a partially reversible increase from 256 nM to 660 nM (134,135).

Another question is what level of oxygen deprivation is required to increase cytosolic calcium. Peters et al. demonstrated the rise in cytosolic calcium in anoxic but not hypoxic tubules (136). In hypoxic perfusion oxygen tension measured with a very sensitive electrode was 5 to 6 mm Hg. Complete anoxia was achieved with oxyrase in a nonperfused system. Calcium did not increase during hypoxia, but there was an increase in calcium during anoxia. This increase paralleled the collapse in mitochondrial membrane potential as measured by rhodamine fluorescence. Because cell membrane damage occurred during both anoxia and hypoxia, it was concluded that an increase in cell calcium is not always necessary for cell injury.

The crucial questions to implicate calcium as a primary factor in cell injury are (i) whether the increase in cytosolic calcium precedes the injury and (ii) whether preventing the rise in cytosolic calcium attenuates the injury (137,138). To investigate whether hypoxia is associated with an increase in free cytosolic calcium in proximal tubular cells, which precedes any evidence of membrane damage, a video imaging technique was developed in which free intracellular calcium could be measured simultaneously with the staining of nuclei with the membrane impermeable indicator, propidium iodide, as an index of hypoxia-induced membrane damage (139). Propidium iodide enters the cell through the damaged plasma membrane and stains the cell nucleus. The percent of nuclei that stain with propidium iodide is quantitated and is an index of plasma membrane damage. Hypoxia in rat proximal tubules is associated with a significant rise in cytosolic calcium that antecedes evidence of membrane damage as assessed by propidium iodide staining (103). Cytosolic calcium increased from 170 to 390 nM during 5 minutes of hypoxia. The increase in cytosolic calcium preceded propidium iodide detectable cell injury (Fig. 39-7). The increase in cytosolic calcium that preceded the hypoxic membrane damage was promptly reversible with reoxygenation after 8 minutes hypoxia. This is important because if cytosolic calcium is increased only after lethal cell membrane damage, reoxygenation should not have normalized cytosolic calcium. The 10-minute cytosolic calcium rise correlated significantly with subsequent cell damage observed at 20 minutes. The pivotal role of the rise in cytosolic calcium during hypoxia was further demonstrated by using the intracellular

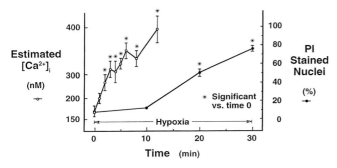

FIGURE 39-7. In isolated proximal tubules, the increase in free cytosolic calcium as measured by Fura-2 precedes the cell membrane damage as assessed by Propidium Iodide staining. (Adapted from: Kribben A, Wieder ED, Wetzels JF, et al. Evidence for role of cytosolic free calcium in hypoxia-induced proximal tubule injury. *J Clin Invest* 1994;93:1922.)

Ca^{2+} chelator 1,22-Bis (2-aminophenoxy) ethane-N,N,N',N'-tetraacetic acid (BAPTA) to prevent the rise in cytosolic calcium; this approach resulted in marked cytoprotection against hypoxic tubular injury.

Thus, low extracellular calcium also prevented the hypoxia induced increase in free intracellular calcium, indicating that hypoxic injury may be primarily due to net calcium entry (i.e., calcium influx > efflux) from the extracellular compartment into the cells (103). While this result suggests an increase in calcium influx during hypoxia, it does not exclude a decrease in calcium efflux. Direct measurement of the calcium efflux is not possible with the current technology. The estimation of the calcium influx with different techniques during hypoxia has provided contradictory results. Using $^{45}Ca^{2+}$ an increase in calcium influx was observed, while with manganese-quenching of fura-2, a decrease of the calcium influx was proposed (127,140). The latter study hypothesized that reducing calcium influx during hypoxia provides the cell with a means to prevent cellular calcium overload during ATP depletion when calcium extrusion is limited. In this regard, it was demonstrated that endoplasmic reticulum calcium stores play a role in determining the cytosolic calcium during hypoxia (141).

In summary, there are various factors that may explain the differences between the cytosolic calcium found in proximal tubules during hypoxic injury. These factors include (i) species differences between rat and rabbit tubules, (ii) differences in injury models caused by oxygen deprivation as compared to metabolic inhibitors (chemical hypoxia), (iii) the severity of the oxygen deprivation and the energy state of the mitochondria, and (iv) different methods in measuring cytosolic calcium.

What are the mechanisms whereby increases in cytosolic free calcium could lead to cell membrane injury? Potential calcium-dependent mechanisms include changes in the actin cytoskeleton of proximal tubule microvilli (142), activation of calcium-dependent PLA2(39), and activation of the cysteine protease, calpain (137,138,143,144).

Calcium-Dependent Changes in the Actin Cytoskeleton

The role of calcium in pathophysiological alterations of the proximal tubule microvillus actin cytoskeleton was studied in freshly isolated tubules (142). Precisely defined medium calcium levels were defined using a combination of the metabolic inhibitor, antimycin, and the ionophore, ionomycin, in the presence of glycine, to prevent lethal membrane damage. Increases of intracellular calcium to 10 μM were sufficient to initiate concurrent actin depolymerization, fragmentation of F-actin

into forms requiring high-speed centrifugation for recovery, redistribution of villin to sedimentable fractions, and structural microvillar damage consisting of severe swelling and fragmentation of actin cores. However, during ATP depletion induced by antimycin alone or hypoxia alone, initial microvillar damage was calcium-independent. This study suggests that both ATP depletion-dependent but Ca^{2+}-independent, as well as Ca^{2+}-mediated processes can disrupt the actin cytoskeleton during acute proximal tubule cell injury. It also suggests that both types of change occur, despite protection afforded by glycine and reduced pH against lethal membrane damage; and that Ca^{2+}-independent processes primarily account for prelethal actin cytoskeletal alterations during simple ATP depletion of proximal tubule cells.

In normal proximal tubule cells, actin is concentrated in apical brush border microvilli, along with the actin-binding protein villin. Villin plays an important role in actin bundling and in microvillar assembly, but can also act as an actin-fragmenting protein at higher calcium concentrations. The effects of ischemic injury and reperfusion on the distribution of villin and actin in proximal tubule cells of rat kidney were examined (145). This study demonstrated that villin may be involved in the initial disruption of the actin cytoskeleton during reperfusion injury and that its migration back to the apical domain of these cells accompanies the reestablishment of a normal actin distribution in the brush border.

ATP depletion results in the conversion of monomeric G-actin to polymeric F-actin during tissue ischemia (146). This conversion results from altering the ratio of ATP-G-actin and ADP-G actin, causing a net decrease in the concentration of thymosinactin complexes as a cosequence of the differential affinity of thymosin beta 4 for ATP and ADP-G actin (147). Recent studies suggest that the actin binding protein tropomysin binds to and stabilizes the apical actin microvilli under physiological conditions in proximal tubules (148).

Activation of Phospholipase A$_2$ (PLA$_2$)

PLA$_2$ enzymes are important regulators of prostaglandin and leukotriene synthesis and can directly modify the composition of cellular membranes (149). PLA$_2$enzymes are also potent regulators of inflammation. The cytosolic form, cPLA$_2$, preferentially releases arachidonic acid from phospholipids and is regulated by changes in intracellular calcium concentration (150).

PLA$_2$ enzymatic activity was measured in cell-free extracts prepared from rat renal proximal tubules (39). Both soluble and membrane-associated PLA$_2$ activity were detected. All PLA$_2$ activity detected during normoxia was calcium dependent. Fractionation of cytosolic extracts by gel filtration revealed three peaks of PLA$_2$ activity. Exposure of tubules to hypoxia resulted in stable activation of soluble PLA$_2$ activity, which correlated with disappearance of the highest molecular mass form (>100 kDa) and appearance of a low-molecular-mass form (approximately 15 kDa) of PLA$_2$. Hypoxia also resulted in release of a low-molecular-mass form of PLA$_2$ into the extracellular medium. Pretreatment of tubules with glycine before hypoxia blocked this release of PLA$_2$ but not activation of soluble PLA$_2$ activity. This study provides direct evidence for calcium-dependent PLA$_2$ activation during hypoxia. However, calcium-independent forms of PLA$_2$have also been found to play a role in hypoxic proximal tubular injury (151).

The mechanism of PLA$_2$-induced cell membrane damage is interesting. Membrane phospholipid breakdown has been observed to occur in a number of tissues during ischemia (152). In proximal tubules hypoxia has been shown to cause an increase in free fatty acids, which was initially believed to contribute to cell injury (153). However, a study from our laboratory has shown that unsaturated free fatty acids protect against hypoxic injury in proximal tubules and that this protection may be mediated by negative feedback inhibition of PLA_2 activity (40). This protective effect of unsaturated free fatty acids has been confirmed by Zager et al. (154). The injurious effect of PLA_2 could be related to a direct disruption of cell membrane integrity by attacking the phospholipid component of cell membranes or through accumulation of lysophospholipids, which have been shown to disrupt cell membranes and cause cytotoxicity (155).

cPLA$_2$ knockout mice have been developed (156). After transient middle cerebral artery ischemia, the cPLA2 knockout mice have smaller infarcts and developed less brain edema and fewer neurological deficits (156). The effect of ischemic ARF in cPLA2 knockout mice has not been reported.

Activation of Calpain

The cysteine proteases are a group of intracellular proteases that have a cysteine residue at their active site. The cysteine proteases consist of three major groups: cathepsins, calpains, and the newly discovered caspases. The major groups of cysteine proteases are shown in Table 39-4. The cathepsins are noncalcium-dependent lysosomal proteases that do not appear to play a role in lethal cell injury (157–159). Calpain is a calcium activated neutral protease (CANP) (160). It has absolute dependence on calcium. It is a heterodimer and has 2 subunits, an 80-kDa catalytic subunit and a 30-kDa regulatory subunit. There are two major ubiquitous or conventional isoforms of calpain, the low calcium sensitive μ-calpain and the high calcium sensitive m-calpain (161,162). The isoenzymes have the same substrate specificity, but differ in affinity for Ca^{2+}. μ-calpain is activated by micromolar concentrations of Ca^{2+} and m-calpain is activated by millimolar concentrations of Ca^{2+}. The millimolar concentrations of intracellular calcium needed for activation of m-calpain are not seen in normal cells and phosphophatidylinositol is thought to lower the calcium concentration required for half maximal autolysis of m-calpain (163).

Suzuki's membrane activation theory is thought to explain the regulation of calpain activity (164,165). Specifically, procalpain exists in the cytoplasm as an inactive proenzyme and becomes active proteolytically only after it has become autolysed at the cell membrane. Activity of the autolyzed calpain is subject to a final regulation by calpastatin (164,165). Calpastatin is a specific endogenous inhibitor of calpain. It is as widely distributed in nature as the enzyme itself. Calcium is required for calpastatin to bind to calpain and thus for the inhibitory effect of calpastatin on calpain.

Calpain substrates include cytoskeletal proteins (e.g., spectrin), receptor proteins (e.g., glutamate), and enzyme proteins (e.g., kinases and phosphatases). Postulated functions of calpain include platelet activation and aggregation, cytoskeleton and cell-membrane organization (166), and regulation of cell growth (167–170).

The calcium-dependent calpains have been shown to be mediators of hypoxic/ischemic injury to the brain, liver, and heart (171–174). The role of the calcium dependent cytosolic protease, calpain, in hypoxia-induced renal proximal tubular injury has also been investigated (42). Tubular calpain activity increased significantly by 7.5 minutes of hypoxia, before there was significant LDH release, and further increased during 20 minutes of hypoxia. Chemically dissimilar cysteine protease inhibitors markedly decreased LDH release after 20 minutes of hypoxia and completely prevented the rise in calpain activity during hypoxia. This role of calpain in proximal tubule injury has subsequently been confirmed by other groups (175,176). This increased calpain activity has subsequently been shown to be associated with breakdown of the cytoskeletal protein, spectrin, both *in vitro* (44) and *in vivo* (177) as well as increasing Na-K-ATPase into the cytoplasmic fraction of the cell.

Acidosis has been shown to protect the isolated proximal tubule from membrane damage (178). The effects of low intracellular pH (pH$_i$) or low free cytosolic calcium $[Ca^{2+}]_i$ on this hypoxia-induced calpain activity were also determined. Both low pH$_i$ and low $[Ca^{2+}]_i$ attenuated the hypoxia-induced increase in calpain activity. This attenuation of calpain activity was observed early before hypoxia-induced membrane damage and was associated with marked reduction in the typical pattern of hypoxia-induced cell membrane damage observed in this model (43).

Recent studies have demonstrated that calpain mediates progressive plasma membrane permeability and proteolysis of cytoskeleton-associated paxillin, talin, and vinculin during antimycin A or hypoxia-induced proximal tubular cell death (179). Novel nonpeptide calpain inhibitors are protective against antimycin A-induced calcium influx and hypoxia/reoxygenation-induced proximal tubular cell death (180).

Caspases

Caspases participate in two distinct signaling pathways: (i) activation of proinflammatory cytokines and (ii) promotion of apoptotic cell death (6,181–186). The term *caspase* embodies two properties of these cysteine proteases in which "c" refers to "cysteine" and "aspase" refers to their specific ability to cleave substrates after an aspartate residue. There are now

TABLE 39-4

THE MAJOR GROUPS OF CYSTEINE PROTEASES

	Cathepsins	Calpains	Caspases
Family	B,H,L,S (lysosomal)	μ and m-calpain Tissue specific isoforms	1 to 14
Location	Lysosome	Cytoplasm	Cytoplasm
Activation	Calcium-independent	Calcium-dependent	Caspase activated
Optimal pH	5 to 6	7.4	7.4
Functions	Intracellular protein degradation	Intracellular signaling Cytoskeletal stability Necrosis and apoptosis	Apoptosis/necrosis Cytokine activation

(Adapted from: Edelstein CL. Editorial Comment: Calcium-mediated proximal tubular injury—what is the role of cysteine proteases? *Nephrol Dial Transplant* 2000;15:141, with permission.)

14 members of the caspase family, caspases 1–14. Caspase-14 has recently been characterized and found to be present in embryonic tissues but absent from adult tissues (187). Caspases share a predilection for cleavage of their substrates after an aspartate residue at P1 (183,188). The members of the caspase family can be divided into three subfamilies based on substrate specificity and function (189). The peptide preferences and function within each group are remarkably similar (189). Members of Group 1 (of which caspase-1 is the most important) prefer the tetrapeptide sequences WEHD and YVAD. This specificity is similar to its activation sequence suggesting that caspase-1 may employ an autocatalytic mechanism of activation. Caspase-1 (previously known as interleukin-1 converting enzyme or ICE) plays a major role in the activation of proinflammatory cytokines. Caspase-1 is remarkably specific for the precursors of interleukin-1 (IL-1) and IL-18 (interferon-gamma-inducing factor), making a single initial cut in each procytokine that activates them and allows exit from the cytosol (190,191). Group III "initiator" caspases-8 and 9 prefer the sequence (L/V)EXD. This recognition motif resembles activation sites within the "executioner" caspase proenzymes, implicating this group as upstream components in the proteolytic cascade that serve to amplify the death signal. These "initiator" caspases pronounce the death sentence. They are activated in response to signals indicating that the cell has been stressed or damaged or has received an order to die. They clip and activate another family of caspases, the "executioners." The optimal peptide sequence motif for Group II or "executioner caspases" (of which caspase-3 is the most important) is DEXD (182,189,192). This optimal recognition motif is identical to proteins that are cleaved during cell death.

Activation of caspases-1, 8, 9, and 3 have been described in hypoxic renal epithelial cells (193–195) and cerebral ischemia (196). Caspase-1 may also cause cell injury by activation of the proinflammatory cytokines IL-1 and IL-18 (183,191). However, IL-1 was not found to play a role in ischemic ARF in mice (29). Caspase-3 knockout mice have decreased apoptosis in the brain and most have premature lethality dying at 1 to 3 weeks of age (197). However, caspase-3 deficient mice that have been backcrossed into C57BL/6 and reaching 6 to 12 weeks of age are protected against Fas-mediated fulminant hepatitis (198). These mice provide an ideal opportunity to evaluate the role of the "executioner" and the most abundant caspase, caspase-3, in ischemic and hypoxic cell injury. While cells contain many caspases, targeted disruption of specific caspase genes in mice has provided much insight into the functions of individual caspases during cell death (199).

While caspases play a crucial and extensively studied role in apoptosis, there is now considerable evidence that the caspase pathway may also be involved in necrotic cell death (200). Caspase inhibition has been demonstrated to reduce ischemic and excitotoxic neuronal damage (201–203). Moreover, mice deficient in caspase-1 demonstrate reduced ischemic brain injury produced by occlusion of the middle cerebral artery (203,204). Inhibition of caspases also protects against necrotic cell death induced by the mitochondrial inhibitor, antimycin A, in PC12 cells, Hep G2 cells, and renal tubules in culture (205,206). Caspases are also involved in hypoxic and reperfusion injury in cultured endothelial cells (207). Rat kidneys subjected to ischemia demonstrate an increase in both caspase-1 and caspase-3 mRNA and protein expression (208). Caspases play a role in hypoxia-induced injury of isolated rat renal proximal tubules (48). In this study, caspase activity was increased in association with cell membrane damage as assessed by lactate dehydrogenase (LDH) release. A specific caspase inhibitor attenuated the increase in caspase activity and markedly protected against cell membrane damage.

Like caspase-3, caspase-6 is also an "executioner" caspase (209). Caspase-6 was cloned and characterized in rat kidneys (210). In rat kidney ischemia-reperfusion injury, there is increased expression of caspase-6 and translocation from the cytoplasm to the nucleus (210).

A recent study investigated the role of caspase inhibition and apoptosis in ischemic ARF in mice *in vivo* (211). A relationship between apoptosis and subsequent inflammation was found. At the time of reperfusion, administration of the antiapoptotic agents IGF-1 and ZVAD-fmk (a caspase inactivator) prevented the early onset of not only renal apoptosis, but also inflammation and tissue injury. Conversely, when the antiapoptotic agents were administered after onset of apoptosis, these protective effects were completely abrogated.

There appears to be an interaction between caspases and calpain during hypoxia-induced injury in the proximal tubule, since caspase inhibition was shown to decrease calpain activity during hypoxia (48,144). Recent *in vivo* studies suggest that caspase mediated degradation of the endogenous inhibitor of calpain, calpastatin, is a mechanism whereby the calcium-mediated activity of calpain is increased (177).

Caspases in Cold Ischemia

Preservation injury, also known as cold ischemia, is an important clinical problem in kidney transplantation. Significant damage to the kidney may occur during harvest, cold storage and transport. An ongoing area of interest is identifying methods to reduce organ injury during this process. The primary consequence of cold ischemic injury is delayed graft function (DGF) in kidney transplants (212–214). These consequences have both short-term and long-term effects. In kidney transplant, for example, DGF increases patient morbidity in the short term as a hospital stay is longer and dialysis may be required. In the long term, DGF independently predicts reduced 1- and 5-year graft survival (215).

Both human and animal studies suggest that the adverse impact of cold ischemia may be associated with apoptosis. In human kidney transplant biopsies performed after 1 hour of reperfusion, apoptosis of tubular cells correlated significantly with cold ischemic time (216). Biopsies of human donor kidneys that subsequently developed postoperative ATN demonstrated increased renal tubular epithelial cell apoptosis (217). Prolonged cold ischemia has also been shown to increase apoptotic cell death in rat kidney allografts at 24 weeks posttransplant (218). Mitochondria undergo significant changes during ischemia and may contribute to preservation injury (219).

Caspases have been studied in cold ischemic kidneys (220). Kidneys of mice were perfused with cold University of Wisconsin (UW) solution containing a pancaspase inhibitor or vehicle via the left ventricle. The contralateral right kidney was used as a control. The left kidney was stored for 48 hours at 4°C to produce cold ischemia. Caspase-3 activity was massively (100-fold) increased in cold ischemic kidneys compared to controls. On immunoblot analysis, the processed form of caspase-3 was increased in cold ischemic kidneys compared to controls. The increase in caspase-3 was associated with significantly more renal tubular apoptosis and brush border injury. In addition, caspase-2, 8, and 9 activities were increased in cold ischemic kidneys. The pancaspase inhibitor prevented the formation of the processed form of caspase-3 and the increase in caspase activity, and reduced apoptosis and brush border injury. The results of this study suggest that caspase inhibition may prove useful in kidney preservation.

The relevance of these studies to organ preservation and the subsequent risk of graft dysfunction is substantial. In the models of liver organ harvest and storage, addition of a caspase inhibitor to the UW storage solution was effective at reducing caspase activation and cell death in both liver and kidney models (221,222). Phase I clinical trials regarding IDN-6556 developed by Idun Pharmaceuticals have been completed. IDN-6556 decreased the elevation of liver enzymes in patients with hepatic dysfunction (223). A placebo controlled phase II trial is being conduced to evaluate whether addition of IDN-6556 to the flush and cold storage solutions as well as administration to the recipient prior to transplant can improve markers of liver injury following liver transplantation. Caspase inhibitors are a particularly attractive approach to reducing the incidence of DGF in kidney transplantation.

Caspase-1 and IL-18

Caspase-1 is a proinflammatory caspase that cleaves precursor interleukin-1β (IL-1β) and precursor interleukin-18 (IL-18). Caspase-1 −/− mice develop less ischemic ARF as judged by renal function and renal histology (224) (Fig. 39-8A). IL-1β re-

ceptor knockout mice or mice treated with IL-1β receptor antagonist (IL-1Ra) are not protected against ischemic ARF (29). Since caspase-1 also activates IL-18, lack of the mature form of IL-18 in these caspase-1 −/− mice was investigated as a possible mechanism of this protection against ARF. Kidney IL-18 was more than 100% increased in wild-type ARF as compared to sham-operated controls. On immunoblot analysis, there was a conversion of the precursor to the mature form of IL-18 in ARF wild-type mice, but not in the caspase-1 −/− ARF mice and sham-operated controls. To further analyze the role of IL-18, wild-type mice were injected with rabbit anti-murine IL-18 neutralizing antiserum prior to the ischemic insult. These mice were protected against ARF to a similar degree as caspase-1 −/− mice (Fig. 39-8B).

Caspase deficient mice have provided extensive information on the role of individual caspases in disease processes. The study of caspase inhibitors is an important step toward the

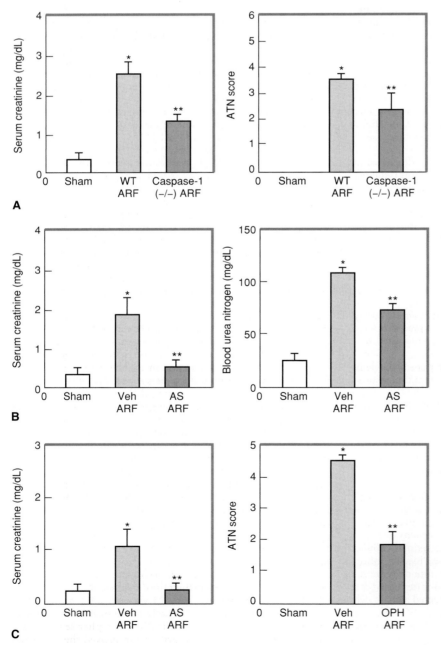

FIGURE 39-8. Caspases and IL-18 in ischemic ARF. A. Caspase-1 −/− mice are protected against ischemic ARF. Caspase-1 −/− mice developed less severe ARF, as determined by serum creatinine and ATN score compared with wild-type (WT) mice with ARF. *p <0.001 vs sham, **p <0.01 vs wild type ARF. B. Caspase-1 converts the pro to mature IL-18. Mice treated with IL-18 antiserum (AS) are functionally protected against ischemic ARF. In vehicle-treated mice with ischemic ARF (Veh ARF), serum creatinine and BUN was significantly increased at 24 hours compared with sham-operated controls. In mice treated with neutralizing IL-18 antiserum (AS), the serum creatinine and BUN were significantly reduced. *p <0.01 vs sham, **p <0.01 vs vehicle-treated mice with ARF (Veh ARF). C. Mice treated with the pancaspase inhibitor OPH-001 are protected against ischemic ARF. In vehicle-treated mice with ischemic ARF, serum creatinine and ATN score was significantly increased at 24 hours of post-ischemic reperfusion compared with sham-operated controls. In mice treated with OPH-001 (OPH) before induction of ischemic ARF, the serum creatinine and ATN score were significantly decreased compared with sham-operated controls. *p <0.001 vs sham, **p <0.01 vs vehicle-treated mice with ARF (Veh ARF), not significant vs sham. (Reproduced from: Melnikov VY, Faubel SG, Siegmund B, et al. Neutrophil-independent mechanisms of caspase-1- and IL-18-mediated ischemic acute tubular necrosis in mice. J Clin Invest 2002;110:1083, with permission.)

possible therapeutic effect of caspase inhibition in ischemic ARF. Mice with ischemic ARF treated with newly developed caspase inhibitor, Q-VD-(Ome)-OPH (OPH-001) had a marked (100%) reduction in blood urea nitrogen (BUN) and serum creatinine and a highly significant reduction in the morphological ATN score than did vehicle-treated mice (225) (Fig. 39-8C). OPH-001 significantly reduced the increase in caspase-1 activity and IL-18 and prevented neutrophil infiltration in the kidney during ischemic ARF. To further investigate whether this lack of neutrophil infiltration was contributing to the protection against ischemic ARF, a model of neutrophil depletion was developed. Neutrophil-depleted mice had a small (18%) reduction in serum creatinine during ischemic ARF but no reduction in the ATN score despite a lack of neutrophil infiltration in the kidney. Remarkably, caspase-1 activity and IL-18 were still significantly increased in the kidney in neutrophil-depleted mice with ARF. Thus, to investigate the role of IL-18 in ischemic ARF in the absence of neutrophils, neutrophil-depleted mice were treated with IL-18-neutralizing antiserum. IL-18-antiserum-treated neutrophil-depleted mice with ischemic ARF had a significant (75%) reduction in serum creatinine and a significant reduction in the ATN score compared to vehicle-treated neutrophil-depleted mice. These results suggest a novel neutrophil-independent mechanism of IL-18-mediated ischemic ARF.

The effects of different caspase inhibitors on ischemic ARF in the rat kidney has been studied (226). A caspase-1 inhibitor significantly reduced functional and histological evidence of ischemic ARF compared to a caspase-3 inhibitor.

Another group of investigators found that caspase-1-deficient mice were not protected against renal ischemia (227). In this study, the model of renal ischemia was 45 minutes of unilateral renal pedicle clamping with contralateral nephrectomy. This model produces a milder form of functional injury than bilateral clamping. At 24 hours, BUN and creatinine were lower in the caspase-1−/− mice than in wild type, but the decrease was not statistically significance. Studies of kidney tissue revealed that renal myelperoxidase (MPO) was reduced and DNA laddering was the same. On histological examination, immunohistochemistry for neutrophil infiltration and TUNEL positive cells were the same between both groups; necrosis, however, was not examined. In addition, in the same study (227), treatment with IL-1 receptor antagonist, anti-IL-1 receptor antibody, or anti-IL-18 antibody minimally reduced renal functional deterioration, inflammation, and apoptosis.

Caspase-1 also contributes to cisplatin-induced ARF and ATN (228). In this study, both caspase-1 and 3 activities were increased in the kidney. Caspase-1-deficient mice were protected against cisplatin-induced apoptosis and ARF. Surprisingly the caspase-1 deficient mice had less caspase-3 activation, less tubular apoptosis on day 2 after cisplatin injection and less ATN on day 3 after cisplatin injection.

Matrix Metalloproteinases

Matrix metalloproteinases are a large family of zinc-dependent matrix-degrading enzymes, which include interstitial collagenases, stromelysins, gelatinases, elastases, and secreted as well as membrane-type matrix metalloproteinases. They play a crucial role in remodeling of the extracellular matrix, which is an important physiological feature of normal growth and development. In the kidney, interstitial sclerosis and glomerulosclerosis have been associated with an imbalance of extracellular matrix synthesis and degradation (229). Alterations in renal tubular basement membrane matrix proteins, laminin and fibronectin, occur after renal ischemia-reperfusion injury (230). The role of matrix metalloproteinases in this process has been studied.

Meprin A is a zinc-dependent metallo-endopeptidase that is present in the brush border membrane of renal proximal tubular epithelial cells. The redistribution of this metalloendopeptidase to the basolateral membrane domain during ARF results in degradation of the extracellular matrix and damage to adjacent peritubular structures. The effect of meprin A, the major matrix degrading metalloproteinase in rat kidney, on the laminin-nidogen complex was examined. Nidogen-1 (entactin) acts as a bridge between the extracellular matrix molecules, laminin-1 and type IV collagen, and thus participates in the assembly of basement membranes. Following ischemic injury, meprin A undergoes redistribution and/or adherence to the tubular basement membrane. Nidogen breakdown products are produced as the result of partial degradation of tubular basement membrane by meprin A following renal tubular ischemia-reperfusion injury (231).

The susceptibility of inbred strains of mice to ischemic and nephrotoxic ARF was studied in mice with normal and low meprin A activity (232). The strains of mice with normal meprin A developed more severe renal functional and structural injury following renal ischemia or the injection of hypertonic glycerol compared to the two low meprin A strains. These findings suggest that meprin A plays a role in the pathophysiology of ARF following ischemic and nephrotoxic ARF insults to the kidney (232). A recent study demonstrated that meprin inhibition protects against ischemic ARF in vivo in rats (233). The characteristics of tubular metalloproteinases have been studied and indicate that it is distinct from classic matrix-degrading metalloproteinases (234).

Nitric Oxide (NO)

NO is a lipophylic, highly reactive free radical gas with diverse biomessenger functions (235). NO mediates diverse functions including vasodilatation, platelet aggregation inhibition, neurotransmission, inflammation, antimicrobial, antitumor, and apoptosis (235). Whether the net effects of NO are beneficial or deleterious is determined by the cell type, concentration of NO, duration of production, and the composition of surrounding microenvironment (235). There are three major nitric oxide synthase (NOS) isoforms in the kidney: neuronal NOS or nNOS (also known as NOS1), inducible NOS or iNOS (also known as NOS2), and endothelial NOS or eNOS (also known as NOS3) (236) (Table 39-5). The macula densa is the principal site of nNOS expression in the kidney (237,238). In situ hybridization studies in normal rat kidney demonstrate iNOS mRNA in the S3 segment of the proximal tubule, the cortical and medullary thick ascending limb, the distal convoluted tubule, and the cortical collecting duct and inner medullary collecting duct (239). eNOS mRNA has been detected in glomeruli and preglomerular vasculature, as well as proximal and distal tubules (240). eNOS protein is mainly present in the endothelium of intrarenal, afferent, efferent, glomerular arterioles, and medullary vas recta (237). Expression of eNOS protein in tubules has not yet been reported (236). nNOS and eNOS are continuously present, activated by calcium, and are also termed constitutive NOS (cNOS) (241,242). In contrast, iNOS is induced when the cells have been stimulated by certain cytokines, microbes, and microbial products, and thus is called inducible NOS (iNOS) (243,244). The time course of both calcium-dependent and independent NOS activity in rat renal cortex and medulla has been studied (245). Calcium-dependent NOS activity in cortex and medulla decreased in the early phase of ARF and then increased in the recovery phase in the cortex. iNOS activity increased in the early phase of ARF in both cortex and medulla and was maintained at higher levels in the medulla. In another study, L-arginine improved the deficiency

TABLE 39-5

NITRIC OXIDE SYNTHASE (NOS) ISOFORMS

| Isoform | Tissue distribution | | Phenotype of knockout mouse |
	Body	Renal	
nNOS (Type 1)	Neurons, skeletal muscle, penis	Macula densa	Protection against cerebral ischemia (463,464)
iNOS (Type 2)	Constitutive: ileum, uterus, skeletal muscle Induced: macrophage, VSMC	Constitutive: mTAL, proximal tubule	Less hypotensive response to LPS (465) Increased mortality in polymicrobial sepsis (466) No protection against LPS-induced ARF (398) Protection against ischemic ARF (247)
eNOS (Type 3)	Endothelium	Glomerular vessels, intrarenal arteries	Hypertension (467) Increased susceptibility to stroke (468) and myocardial ischemia (469)

of constitutive NOS activity and improved the recovery phase of ischemic ARF in rats (246).

Studies in freshly isolated proximal tubules from knockout mice have also been revealing about the role of nitric oxide in hypoxic/ischemic tubular injury. Hypoxia-induced proximal tubule damage, as assessed by LDH release, was no different between wild type and mice in which eNOS and nNOS has been "knocked out." However, proximal tubules from the inducible NOS (iNOS) knockout mice demonstrated resistance to the same degree of hypoxia (41). The iNOS knockout mice also had less renal failure and better survival than the wild type mice after renal artery clamping (247). An induction of heat shock protein was also observed in the iNOS knockout mice as a potential contributor to the protection. Star et al. produced further results in a renal artery clamp model in mice in which alpha melanocyte stimulating hormone (αMSH) was shown to block the induction of iNOS, decrease neutrophil infiltration and afford functional protection (248). A subsequent study examined the relative importance of αMSH on the neutrophil pathway by examining the effects of αMSH in ICAM-1 knockout mice and neutrophil poor isolated perfused kidneys where neutrophil effects are minimal or absent (249,250). In this study, it was found that αMSH decreases renal injury when neutrophil effects are minimal or absent indicating that αMSH inhibits neutrophil-independent pathways of renal injury.

Hypoxia was found to increase nitric oxide (NO) release from freshly isolated proximal tubules and this effect was blocked by L-NAME, a nonspecific NOS inhibitor, but not by the inactive D-NAME compound (38,251). The NO release during hypoxia was accompanied by LDH release and was reversed by L-NAME administration. Interestingly, however, L-NAME administration to the rat kidney clamp model actually worsened the renal failure (252). This result was interpreted as an overriding blocking effect of eNOS activity with the nonspecific effects of L-NAME (72). This would worsen the renal vasoconstriction and resultant injury, thus obscuring any salutary effect at the level of the proximal tubule (253). Thus, opposing abnormalities in NO production within the endothelial and tubular compartments of the kidney may contribute to renal injury (72). Reduced eNOS derived NO production causes vasoconstriction and worsens ischemia; increased iNOS derived NO production by tubular cells adds to the injurious effects of ischemia on these cells. Therapeutic interventions to modulate NO production in ischemic ARF may require selective modulation of different NOS isoforms in the tubular and vascular compartments of the kidney (254). On this background the group of Goligorsky performed studies using a specific antisense oligonucleotide to iNOS (252). The

ischemia-induced upregulation of iNOS and nitrite production were both blocked by the antisense oligonucleotide. Most importantly the BUN and serum creatinine did not rise after the renal ischemic insult in the animals treated with the antisense oligonucleotide against iNOS.

The Goligorsky group also studied the relationship between nitric oxide and osteopontin during ischemic ARF. Osteopontin is a negatively charged glycosylated phosphoprotein that is expressed in many tissues including renal epithelial cells. Osteopontin serves both a cell attachment function and a cell signaling function via the alpha v beta 3 integrin. Effects on gene expression include suppression of the induction of nitric oxide synthase by inflammatory mediators. Osteopontin may play an important role in the pathophysiology of ARF. Osteopontin knockout mice subjected to renal ischemia developed worse renal failure and more structural damage than wild type controls (255). This was associated with the augmented expression of inducible nitric oxide synthase and the prevalence of nitrotyrosine residues in kidneys from osteopontin knockout mice versus wild-type counterparts. This study provides strong evidence of renoprotective action of osteopontin in acute renal ischemia.

The microvillar actin and cellular integrins are potential substrates of NO action, which could contribute to the ischemia-mediated sloughing of the brush border membrane and detachment of proximal tubule epithelial cells from their extracellular matrix (8,256–258). Such an effect would not only result in impaired tubular sodium reabsorption, but also provide intraluminal cellular debris as a component of tubular cast formation.

Glycine

Glycine is a well-known cytoprotective agent against proximal tubular injury (259,260). The mechanism of this cytoprotective effect remains unknown. However, many of the pathophysiological events that occur in *in vitro* models of proximal tubule injury, for example, ATP depletion (261,262), cytoskeletal changes (92,102), prelethal influx of Ca^{2+} (103), activation of phospholipase A2 (PLA2)(132), activation of iNOS (38), calpain activation (43) are not affected by glycine. These events therefore are more likely to be potential mediators of *in vivo* proximal tubule injury where glycine is present at physiological concentrations (259,263). It is also well known that the availability of glycine in a cell is a major determinant of lethal cell membrane damage to anoxic, hypoxic, ischemic and toxin-induced insults in hepatocytes, proximal tubules, and endothelial cells (259,260,264–266). Since glycine is present at physiological concentrations *in vivo* (259,263), the mechanism of structural and functional changes during cell injury is better understood and needs to be assessed in the presence of glycine.

Heat Shock Proteins

The stress response is a highly conserved homeostatic mechanism that allows cells to survive a variety of different stresses (267). Stresses that trigger the heat shock response include hyperthermia, hypothermia, generation of oxygen radicals, hypoxia/ischemia, and toxins (268). On a molecular level, their function is to protect cells from environmental stress damage by binding to partially denatured proteins, dissociating protein aggregates, to regulate the correct folding, and to cooperate in transporting newly synthesized polypeptides to the target organelles.

The proteins induced by these stresses belong to a family of proteins called heat shock proteins (HSP). The proteins are identified by their molecular weight. The most important families include proteins of 90, 70, 60, and 27 kDa (268). HSP 90 is essential for cell viability. It is associated with the steroid hormone receptor and is a general chaperone with ATPase like activity. In stressed cells it associates with the cytoskeletal protein, actin. The HSP 70 family includes proteins that are both constitutively expressed and induced by stress. They are the most highly induced proteins by stress and function as chaperones binding to unfolded or misfolded proteins. The HSP 60 family is restricted to the mitochondrial matrix where it functions as an unfoldase. The HSP 27 family has functions similar to HSP 70. Ubiquitin is a stress protein that binds denatured proteins and targets them for proteolysis by the proteasome.

Renal ischemia results in both a profound fall in cellular ATP and a rapid induction of the 70 kD heat-shock protein family, HSP-70 (269,270). The relationship between cellular ATP and induction of the stress response in renal cortex during renal ischemia has been studied. Van Why et al. demonstrated that a 50% reduction in cellular ATP in the renal cortex must occur before the stress response is detectable, that reduction of ATP below 25% control levels produces a more vigorous response, and that reperfusion is not required for initiation of a heat-shock response in the kidney (271).

Ischemic ARF also induces differential expression of small HSPs. In sham-operated kidneys, HSP 25 localized to glomeruli, vessels, and collecting ducts, while another stress protein, alphaB-crystallin, localized primarily in medullary thin limbs of Henle's loop and collecting ducts. After ischemia, HSP 25 accumulated in proximal tubules in cortex and outer medulla, while alphaB-crystallin labeling became nonhomogeneous in outer medulla, and increased in Bowman's capsule. This study demonstrates that there is striking differential expression of HSP 25 and alphaB-crystallin in various renal compartments (272).

In vitro studies have demonstrated that HSP induction protects cultured renal epithelial cells from injury. It has been determined that prior heat stress protects opossum kidney (OK) cells, a cultured renal epithelial cell line, from injury mediated by ATP depletion (273). Also HSP 70 overexpression is sufficient to protect LLC- PK1 proximal tubular cells from hyperthermia but is not sufficient for protection from hypoxia (274).

During ischemic ARF, the question of whether prior HSP induction by hyperthermia is protective is controversial. One study found that prior heat shock protected kidneys against warm ischemia (275). Another study investigated the protective effect of heat-shock proteins on ischemic injury to renal cells in two different experimental models: ischemia-reflow in intact rats and medullary hypoxic injury as seen in the isolated perfused rat kidney. Prior induction of HSP by hyperthermia was not protective against the functional and morphological parameters of ischemic ARF in either of these models (276). These variable results may be explained by the complexity of the intact animal compared to cultured cells, the degree, duration, and timing of the hyperthermic stimulus and the differential response of mature and immature kidneys (23,277).

Pharmacological agents have been used to increase stress protein expression. Recently, inhibitors of the proteasome have been identified that can block the rapid degradation of abnormal cytosolic and ER-associated proteins. The hypothesis that proteasome inhibitors, by causing the accumulation of abnormal proteins, might stimulate the expression of cytosolic heat-shock proteins and/or ER molecular chaperones and thereby induce thermotolerance was tested in Madin-Darby canine kidney cell culture (278). Inhibition of proteasome function induced heat-shock proteins and ER chaperones and conferred thermotolerance in these cells. Thus, these agents may have applications in protecting against cell injury (278). Another study determined that proteasome inhibition protects against the morphological and functional abnormalities in ischemic ARF in rats (279). However, the effect of proteasome inhibition on HSP induction during ischemic ARF was not determined in this study.

The mechanism of HSP protection against ischemic ARF is interesting. It has been suggested that HSPs participate in the postischemic restructuring of the cytoskeleton of proximal tubules (280). It was found that HSP 72 complexes with aggregated cellular proteins in an ATP-dependent manner suggesting that enhancing HSP 72 function after ischemic renal injury assists refolding and stabilization of Na(+)-K(+)-ATPase or aggregated elements of the cytoskeleton, allowing reassembly into a more organized state (281). Another study examined the temporal and spatial patterns of HSP-25 induction in relation to the actin cytoskeleton (282). This study suggested that there are specific interactions between HSP 25 and actin during the early postischemic reorganization of the cytoskeleton. In another study, the Brown Norway rat was resistant to renal failure and ATN compared to the Sprague-Dawley rat (283). The Brown Norway rat had no distribution of Na-K-ATPase into detergent soluble cortical extracts and immunohistochemistry showed that baseline HSP-72 and 25 expression was increased in proximal tubules of the Brown Norway rats compared to the Sprague-Dawley rats.

Another potential mechanism of HSP protection against proximal tubular injury is the inhibition of apoptosis. Opossum kidney proximal tubule (OK) cells exposed to ATP depletion develop apoptosis by morphological and biochemical criteria. Prior heat stress reduced the number of apoptotic-appearing cells, significantly decreased DNA fragmentation, and improved cell survival compared with controls (284). This study demonstrated that novel interactions between HSP 72 and the antiapoptotic protein, Bcl2, may be responsible, at least in part, for the protection afforded by prior heat stress against ATP depletion injury.

Altered Gene Expression

During renal ischemia *in vivo*, the reaction of the renal epithelial cells is heterogeneous (285). Some cells, especially those of the proximal tubule, undergo necrosis. Other cells undergo apoptosis, and still others survive the ischemic injury intact. In addition, injured tubules are relined with new cells actively engaged in DNA synthesis. Thus, surviving tubular cells re-enter the cell cycle and replicate. These cells may undergo partial dedifferentiation that allows them to undergo mitosis (286). The complex events that mediate this heterogeneous response of tubular cells are being studied. This response of tubular cells may involve the early immediate gene response.

Immediate early genes and protooncogenes are induced during the early reperfusion period after renal ischemia (287). There is c-fos and c-jun activation as well as an increase in DNA synthesis (288). There is accumulation of early growth response factor-1 (Egr-1) and c-fos mRNAs in the mouse kidney after occlusion of the renal artery and reperfusion (289,290). Transient expression of the genes cfos and Egr-1 may code for DNA binding transcription factors and initiate the transcription of other genes necessary for cell division (291). JE and KC, growth-factor-responsive genes with cytokine-like properties that play a role in inflammation, are also expressed during early renal ischemia (292). These genes may code for proteins with chemotactic effects that can attract monocytes and neutrophils into areas of injury (290). Studies demonstrate that c-fos and c-jun are expressed following renal ischemia as a typical immediate early gene response, but they are expressed in cells that do not enter the cell cycle (286,293). The failure of the cells to enter the cell cycle may depend on the coexpression of other genes.

DNA synthesis occurs in the proximal tubule, whereas the induction of the early gene response is restricted to cells of the thick ascending limb and collecting duct (290). Thus, the immediate early gene response does not always occur in cells that undergo DNA synthesis, suggesting that the role of the early gene response is not necessarily proliferative in this setting. The role of the stress response during renal ischemia and the fate of the cells undergoing it are unknown. This immediate early gene response may play a role in the protection of tubular cells against injury. Alternatively, it may be important in mounting a response that will later help the regeneration of other tubular cells as the products of some of these genes are localized to cells that are not undergoing cell death from apoptosis or necrosis (294). The immediate early gene response may be the response to sublethal injury allowing the cell to dedifferentiate (291).

The pathways that lead to the early gene response are interesting. At least two quite different pathways lead to the activation of c-jun (295–297). Growth factors activate c-jun via the mitogen activated protein kinases (MAPKs), which include extracellular regulated kinases, (ERKs) –1 and 2. This pathway is proliferative in nature. In contrast, the stress-activated protein kinase (SAPK) pathway is separate from the MAPK pathway. These kinases include c-Jun N-terminal kinase (JNK)- 1 and 2. Activation and the effect on cell fate of the SAPK pathway is very different from the MAPK pathway. The SAPK pathway is essentially antiproliferative and can lead to either cell survival or cell death. During renal ischemia, SAPKs are activated and inhibition of SAPK after ischemia protects against renal failure (298,299). Thus, it is possible that manipulation of this pathway could lead to therapies that may ameliorate ARF.

Numerous recent studies have analyzed gene expression during ischemic ARF. Cell communication, apoptosis and inflammation genes distinguish primary allograft function in human kidney transplantation (300). In renal ischemia-reperfusion in the mouse, there was an increase in genes involved in cell structure, extracellular matrix, intracellular calcium binding, and cell division/differentiation (301). In another study in mice, there were consistent patterns of altered gene expression in the first 24 hours of postischemic reperfusion (302). These genes included transcription factors, growth factors, signal transduction molecules and apoptotic factors. In ischemia-reperfusion in the rat, alterations in the expression of 18 genes were identified by microarray analysis (303). Nine genes were up-regulated: ADAM2, HO-1, UCP-2, and thymosin beta4 in the early phase and clusterin, vanin1, fibronectin, heat-responsive protein 12, and FK506 binding protein in the established phase. Nine genes were down-regulated: glutamine synthetase, cytochrome p450 IId6, and cyp 2d9

in the early phase and cyp 4a14, Xist gene, PPARgamma, alpha-albumin, uromodulin, and ADH B2 in the established phase. Changes in gene expression of ADAM2, cyp2d6, fibronectin, HO-1, and PPARgamma were confirmed by quantitative real-time polymerase chain reaction (PCR). One of the problems with microarray analysis in the whole kidney during ischemic ARF in vivo is identifying which of the numerous cell types in the kidney is the source of the gene alteration. Laser capture microdissection of immunofluorescently defined cells (IF-LCM) can isolate pure populations of targeted cells from a sea of surrounding cells with excellent preservation of mRNA (304). This technique has been used to label and isolate thick ascending limb cells in the kidney for mRNA analysis (304).

Exploration of the early gene response in renal ischemia using DNA microarrays and other genome-scale technologies should narrow the gap in our knowledge of gene function and molecular biology (305). Gene expression in early ischemic ARF may provide clues toward pathogenesis, biomarker discovery and novel therapeutics (306).

Apoptosis

Apoptosis was first described by Kerr et al. (307). The term comes from the ancient Greek that means "the dropping off as of leaves from a tree." The term stresses the facts that apoptosis is a physiological form of cell death, occurs in the individual cell (or leaf) in a programmed pattern, and can be triggered according to a program regulated by external stimuli (autumn) (4). Thus, apoptosis is the name given to a process of physiologic or programmed cell death. Apoptotic cells undergo a series of morphologically identifiable changes in their pathway to cell death (308). The morphological, biochemical and molecular characteristics of apoptosis versus necrosis are very different (Table 39-6).

The triggers of apoptosis include (i) cell injury e.g. ischemia, hypoxia, oxidant injury, nitric oxide and cisplatinum; (ii) loss of survival factors e.g. deficiency of renal growth factors, impaired cell to cell or cell to matrix adhesion and (iii) receptor-mediated apoptosis (e.g., Fas [CD 295] and TGFβ) (309).

TABLE 39-6

MORPHOLOGICAL, BIOCHEMICAL, AND MOLECULAR DIFFERENCES BETWEEN APOPTOSIS AND NECROSIS

Apoptosis	Necrosis
Individual cells shrink and detach from other cells	Multiple cells swell but remain attached
Plasma membranes remain intact	Plasma membrane disruption
Cell excludes DNA specific dye, propidium iodide	Propidium iodide enters cell and stains nucleus
Nuclear condensation, fragmentation, and pyknosis	Nuclear swelling and autolysis
Apoptotic bodies	No apoptotic bodies
Nuclear DNA fragmentation	Nuclear DNA fragmentation
Programmed by gene activation	No gene activation
Phagocytosis of cellular fragments	Cellular lysis
No inflammation	Inflammation

The two major pathways of apoptosis involve Fas and p53 (6,7,310). In the TNF receptor superfamily, Fas antigen (CD 295) is the most important factor. Engagement of Fas by its ligand (FasL) results in apoptosis. The tumor suppressor gene, p53, mediates apoptosis in cells whose DNA has been damaged. The cascades involving Fas and p53, which are centrally important in cell death, are shown in Figure 39-9.

In the p53 pathway, cytochrome c release from mitochondria is an apoptosis trigger (311). Cytochrome c binds to a protein called apoptotic protease activating factor-1 (Apaf-1). This binding allows Apaf-1 to activate caspase-9, an "initia-

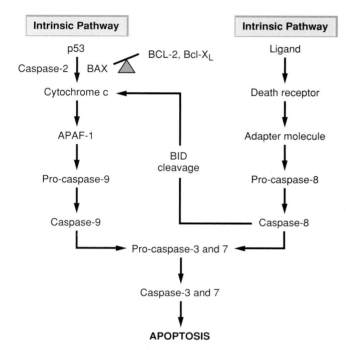

Intrinsic Pathway

p53

Caspase-2 ↓ BAX   BCL-2, Bcl-X$_L$

Cytochrome c

APAF-1

Pro-caspase-9

Caspase-9

Intrinsic Pathway

Ligand

Death receptor

Adapter molecule

BID cleavage

Pro-caspase-8

Caspase-8

Pro-caspase-3 and 7

Caspase-3 and 7

APOPTOSIS

FIGURE 39-9. Major pathways of apoptosis. There are two major pathways of caspase-mediated apoptosis [451]. In the mitochondrial or "intrinsic" pathway, stress-induced signals (for example p53) act via Bcl-2 proteins to cause cytochrome c release from mitochondria. In the "extrinsic" pathway, there is the binding of a ligand (for example, Fas ligand) to its death receptor (for example, Fas) that recruits an adaptor protein. In the "intrinsic" pathway cytochrome c release from mitochondria is an apoptosis trigger [311]. Cytochrome c binds to a protein called apoptotic protease activating factor-1 (Apaf-1). This binding allows Apaf-1 to activate caspase-9, an "initiator" caspase, which then activates caspase-3 and 7. The presence of an excess of the anti-apoptotic protein Bcl-2 on mitochondria inhibits cytochrome c release. Caspase-2 is a recently discovered caspase that is a critical initiator of the mitochondrial apoptosis pathway [452]. Activation and increased activity of caspase-2 is required for the permeabilization of mitochondria and release of cytochrome c [452]. In the "extrinsic" pathway, the death receptors (CD95/Fas/APO-1, TNFR1, DR3/WSL-1/TRAMP. DR4/TRAIL-R1, DR5/TRAIL-R2, DR6) are a subset of the TNF/NGF receptor family of cell surface molecules that possess a common motif within their cytoplasmic tails, called the death domain. The death domains of these receptors recruit adapter molecules that, in turn, recruit caspases to the receptor complex. For example, Fas antigen (CD 95) is engaged by its ligand (FasL) resulting in apoptosis. Activation of procaspase-8 requires association with its cofactor Fas-associated death domain (FADD). The pathways may be linked as caspase-8 may cleave a member of the Bcl-2 family, BID, which can release cytochrome c. Apoptosis mediated by both pathways has been described during renal ischemia/reperfusion in rats [312;313]. Both caspase-3 and 7 play a crucial and extensively studied role in the promotion of all forms of apoptotic cell death [184]. Caspase-7, like caspase-3, is an "executioner" caspase and is downstream of the "initiators" caspase-8 and 9.

tor" caspase which then activates caspase-3. During this form of apoptosis, the mitochondrial inner transmembrane potential collapses indicating the opening of a large conductance channel known as the mitochondrial permeability transition (PT) pore. The presence of an excess of the antiapoptotic protein Bcl-2 on mitochondria inhibits cytochrome c release. Bcl-2 can also prevent the mitochondrial PT pore opening. P53 levels are increased during renal ischemia reperfusion in rat kidneys (312). Mitochondrial dysfunction has been demonstrated during ischemic ARF (51). Thus, cytochrome c release from mitochondria and subsequent caspase-9 activation may be a common pathway in both apoptosis and necrosis in the kidney.

In the Fas pathway, Fas antigen (CD 295) is engaged by its ligand (FasL) resulting in apoptosis. Activation of procaspase-8 requires association with its cofactor Fas-associated death domain (FADD). The p53 and Fas pathways may be linked as caspase-8 may cleave a member of the Bcl-2 family, BID, which can release cytochrome c. Fas mediated apoptosis during renal ischemia/reperfusion has been described in rats (313).

Caspases are the major mediators of the cell death in apoptosis and also play a role in necrotic cell death. The central role of caspases in cell death is supported by caspase-8, 9, and 3 knockout mice that have strong phenotypes based on apoptotic cell death defects, developmental defects and usually fetal/perinatal mortality (186). Caspase-7, like caspase-3, is an "executioner" caspase and is downstream of the "initiators" caspase-8 and 9. Both the intrinsic and extrinsic pathways activate caspase-7. Caspase-3 and 7 exhibit very similar substrate specificities in peptide hydrolysis assays *in vitro* (314). However, the role of caspase-7 during the execution phase of apoptosis is obscure (315). Caspase-7 is unable to cleave the well-known caspase-3 substrates including fodrin, gelsolin, DNA fragmentation factor 45 (DFF45), inhibitor of apoptosis proteins (IAP) and signal transducer and activator of transcription-1 (STAT-1) (315). Also, caspase-7 is unable to activate caspases that would normally be activated by caspase-3 (316). It is known that caspase-3 and 7 can act independently as "executioners" of apoptosis (317). Both caspase-3 and caspase-7 deficient mice are perinatally lethal due to a lack of apoptosis (318). Caspase-7 may play a more specialized role in apoptosis than caspase-3 (315). Caspases have been described in detail earlier in this chapter.

Caspase-dependent or independent endogenous endonuclease activation, resulting in DNA fragmentation, is considered a characteristic biochemical marker for apoptosis (49). However, DNA fragmentation also occurs in cellular necrosis (49,319,320). The differentiation of apoptosis from necrosis in tubular cells therefore is still difficult (321) and requires both demonstration of DNA fragmentation, usually using a histochemical technique based on terminal deoxynucleotidyl transferase (TdT) reactivity with DNA breaks, as well as morphological evidence of apoptosis by light and electron microscopy. Pathways usually associated with apoptosis (e.g., endonuclease activation and increased mitochondrial permeability) may also be associated with necrosis, suggesting that apoptotic and necrotic cell death may share the same pathways (322). Both apoptosis and necrosis can occur in tissues exposed to ischemia/reperfusion or cultured cells exposed to hypoxia (323).

The number of *in vitro* and *in vivo* studies where apoptosis is described in renal tubules, is increasing. These studies are summarized in Tables 39-7 and 39-8. A feature of *in vitro* studies in tubules in culture (Table 39-7) is that severe or prolonged ATP depletion leads to necrosis while milder and shorter ATP depletion leads to apoptotic cell death. A similar pattern has emerged from the *in vivo* studies (Table 39-8) (i.e., the same insult in a mild form can lead to apoptosis and when severe can lead to necrosis).

TABLE 39-7

APOPTOSIS IN HYPOXIC/ANOXIC TUBULAR INJURY IN VITRO (CULTURED CELLS)

Cell type	Type of injury	Signals	Comment	Ref
MDCK and primary culture rat proximal tubules	Hypoxia		Necrosis also observed.	(470)
Primary culture mouse proximal tubules	Partial ATP depletion (Antimycin A)	Renal growth factors did not ameliorate apoptosis.	Severe ATP depletion caused necrosis.	(35)
LLC-PK1 (proximal) and MDCK cells	ATP depletion		Same pattern in LLC-PK1 and MDCK.	(471)
MDCK (distal)	Partial ATP depletion (Antimycin A)	Fas, FADD, Caspases, PARP	Severe ATP depletion caused necrosis.	(472)
Opossum kidney (proximal)	ATP depletion (cyanide, 2-deoxy-D-glucose)	Bcl-2/Bax	Prior heat shock attenuated apoptosis.	(284)
Rat proximal tubules	Hypoxia	Caspases Bcl-2	Serine protease inhibitors suppressed caspase-9 activation and apoptosis.	(473)
Rat proximal tubules	Antimycin A	Mitochondrial Ca^{2+} and permeability	L-type calcium channel blocker decreased apoptosis.	(474)
Human tubular cells	Fas transfection	Fas	High, but not basal Fas expression caused apoptosis.	(475)
MDCK	Overexpression of ankyrin death domain	Fas	Inhibition of ankyrin Fas interaction decreased apoptosis.	(476)
Rat proximal tubules	Hypoxia Cisplatin Staurosporine	Mitochondrial cytochrome c release	Minocycline upregulates Bcl-2 and decreases apoptosis.	(477)
Rat proximal tubules	ATP depletion	Bid cleavage	Bid cleavage and apoptosis blocked by anti apoptotic Bcl-2 overexpression and caspase-9 inhibition.	(478)

Numerous recent studies have demonstrated that erythropoietin (EPO) protects against ischemic ARF by affecting apoptotic cell death (324–326). A single dose of EPO either preischemia or just before reperfusion, improves renal function and tubular injury, prevents the activation of caspase-3, -8, and -9 and reduces apoptotic tubular cell death (324). EPO also protects against hypoxia-induced apoptosis in human proximal tubule cells (325). In the same study, EPO protected functionally against ischemic ARF in rats *in vivo* and reduced outer medullary thick ascending limb apoptosis while potentiating tubular mitosis and proliferation (325). In another study in rats with ischemic ARF, EPO decreased serum creatinine, decreased tubular apoptosis and necrosis, decreased tubular cell proliferation, increased antiapoptotic Bcl-2 protein expression, decreased caspase-3 activity and increased heat shock protein 70 (HSP70) expression (326). Thus, EPO may be a potential new therapy for ARF in humans.

Complement

The complement system is a mediator of ischemia-reperfusion injury in heart, lung, brain, intestine and muscle (327). A predominant role for C5b-9 in renal ischemia/reperfusion injury has been demonstrated (328). In this study, the primary damaging effect of complement was on parencymal cells rather than vascular endothelial cells. In another study, lack of a functional alternative complement pathway ameliorated is-

chemic ARF in mice (329). In this study, mice deficient in factor B, an essential protein in the alternative complement pathway, were functionally and histologically protected against ischemic ARF.

Relative Importance of Proximal Versus Distal Tubular Injury

There is an ongoing debate regarding which nephron segments are most severely injured in ischemic ARF (88). The target zone for hypoxic injury has also been extensively studied in the isolated rat perfused kidney (IPRK). This target zone predominantly involves the S3 segments of the proximal tubule and also distal tubules located within the outer stripe of the outer medulla and their cortical equivalent, the medullary rays, those straight sections of the proximal and distal tubules draining the superficial cortical glomeruli. While the sensitivity of the proximal tubules to injury is well recognized in all models of ARF, the debate over whether the proximal or distal nephron segments is the primary target for hypoxic/ischemic injury has been well reviewed recently (88). Of interest in the IPRK model of injury is the presence of a consistent artifact as a result of the absence of an oxygen carrier during erythrocyte-free perfusion. This artifact is the necrosis of medullary thick ascending limb (MTAL) cells first described by Alcorn (330). It had been observed by Leichtweiss et al. that tissue oxygen tension fell sharply in the region of the corticomedullary

TABLE 39-8

APOPTOSIS IN RENAL ISCHEMIA/REPERFUSION INJURY IN VIVO

Model	Type of injury	Location of apoptosis	Signals	Comment	Ref
Sprague Dawley rats	5 to 45 minutes I, 12 to 24 hours R	Distal	Sulfated glycoprotein 2	Longer periods of ischemia induced necrosis.	(479)
Wistar rats	60 minutes I, 7 to 14 days R	NT	NT	Necrosis at day 1 reperfusion.	(480)
Sprague Dawley rats	60 minutes I, 3 to 12 hours R	NT	Proliferating cell nuclear antigen (PCNA)	Uninephrectomy enhanced proliferation and decreased apoptosis.	(481)
Sprague Dawley rats	45 minutes I, 24 hours R	NT	P53 and c-myc	Verapamil attenuated apoptosis.	(312)
ICR mice	30 to 120 minutes I, 24 hours R	Distal	Fas	Proximal tubules developed necrosis. Less apoptosis in Lpr mice lacking Fas.	(313)
Human kidney allografts	Reperfusion after cold preservation	NT	NT	Less apoptosis in kidneys from living related donors.	(482)
Wistar rats	60 minutes I, 24 hours R	Proximal and distal	EGF, LGF1, and TGFβ	Osteogenic protein-1 reduced proximal but not distal apoptosis.	(483)
Sprague Dawley rats	60 minutes I, 1 and 5 days R	Proximal	Proapoptotic protein, SIVA	*Peaks of apoptosis at 1 and 7 days reperfusion.	(484)
Human kidney allografts	Cold ischemia	Distal	No change in Bcl-2	Apoptosis predicts early graft function.	(217)
Sprague Dawley rats	30 minutes I, 2 hours R	NT	NT	CCBs attenuated apoptosis.	(485)
Sprague Dawley rats	60 minutes I, 1 and 7 days R	Proximal		Fibroblast growth factor (FGF) attenuated proximal apoptosis and distal necrosis.	(486)
Swiss mice	45 minutes I, 2 hours R	Distal	Caspase-1 + 3.	Caspase inhibition attenuated renal failure and inflammation.	(211)
Sprague Dawley rats	60 minutes I, 7 days R			*Endothelin receptor antagonist attenuated apoptosis.	(487)
Sprague Dawley rats	30 minutes I, 4 to 14 days R	Proximal and distal	Bcl-2, Bcl-XL, and Bax	Distal tubules enhanced Bcl-2 expression.	(344)
NMRI mice	15 or 35 minutes I, 1 day R	NT	Fas	Small interfering RNA (siRNA) increased survival.	(488)
C57BL6 mice	22 minutes I, 1 day R	OSOM	Caspase-1 IL-18	Pancaspase inhibitor decreased tubular necrosis and apoptosis.	(225)
Sprague Dawley rats	45 minutes I, 6 hours R	NT	Nitrotyrosine, MDAde	Caspase-1 inhibitor decreased necrosis.	(226)
Death-associated protein kinase (DAPK) mutant mice	30 minutes I, 16 to 120 hours R	NT	DAPK	Mutant mice had less apoptosis and renal failure despite same degree of necrosis as wild type.	(489)

I, ischemia; R, reperfusion; NT, not tested; NMRI, Naval Medical Research Institute; OSOM, outer stripe of outer medulla; MDA, malondialdehyde; *, apoptosis not confirmed morphologically.

junction (331). Studies by Brezis et al. demonstrated that the MTAL lesion resulted from hypoxia and provided support for the hypothesis that countercurrent diffusion of oxygen from descending to ascending limbs of the vasa recta is responsible for the prevailing low oxygen tension of the renal medulla (332). Subsequently this group was able to induce a similar lesion in a number of models of renal injury. They have championed the notion that the MTAL segment lies on the brink of hypoxia as a result of the unique architecture of the kidney, which facili-

tates the countercurrent multiplier required for the formation of concentrated urine (333). Other groups have also suggested that arteriovenous diffusion of oxygen (between adjacent parallel arterial and veins) is responsible for lowering tissue PO_2 in the corticomedullary region and for maintaining the very low medullary PO_2 (334,335). However, Endre et al. demonstrated in the IPRK in the presence of low concentrations of erythrocytes that MTAL injury was prevented both under control conditions with high perfusate oxygen tension and in the presence of hypoxia (336). The proximal tubule continued to be injured by hypoxia in the presence of erythrocytes, confirming that MTAL necrosis is an artifact of cell-free perfusion in this model. Nevertheless, coupled with the evidence for preglomerular arteriovenous diffusion of oxygen, which reduces average cortical PO_2 to sub-venous levels (337), the IPRK studies suggest that an even greater amount of the kidney is under threat from hypoxia when renal perfusion is reduced. Such widespread borderline hypoxia may be adaptively useful in priming the oxygen sensor in renal erythropoietin producing cells. However, when there is reduced renal perfusion, critically low levels of oxygen can be reached in tubular regions, particularly where there is high energy demand from transepithelial transport. Clearly, both proximal straight tubules (S3) and MTAL exist in such a region under constant threat of hypoxia. Magnetic resonance (MR) microscopy studies of the IPRK have demonstrated swelling of the cells in these interbundle regions in the outer medulla and their cortical equivalent, the medullary rays, restricting flow through the vascular bundles (338). These MR observations complement the earlier observations by Mason et al. and others that there is erythrocyte aggregation and stasis in the outer stripe of the model after reperfusion following ischemia (339–341).

Of greater interest, however, is the observation that while frank necrosis of MTAL cells is rarely seen *in vivo*, several studies in the IPRK have observed DNA fragmentation in MTAL cells after brief hypoxia (54) and after 15 or 60 minutes reperfusion after ischemia (342). DNA fragmentation has been observed after 24 hours reperfusion following ischemia *in vivo* in rats (343,344) although little or no morphological evidence of apoptosis has been observed in any of these studies. Similar DNA fragmentation was observed in human autopsy specimens after renal hypoperfusion (345). Recent studies of the Bcl-2 multigene family and growth factors by Gobé et al. (343,345) in a 30-minute bilateral arterial clamp model of ischemia–reperfusion have suggested a way of reconciling the observations of proximal cell necrosis and DNA fragmentation without apoptosis in nearby MTAL. After 24 hours of reperfusion, distal tubules showed a marked increase in expression of antiapoptotic Bcl-2 and a moderate increase in antiapoptotic Bcl-X_L and proapoptotic Bax. Proximal tubules showed a marked increase in Bax expression and a moderate increase in Bcl-X_L. Twenty-four hours after expression of the Bcl-2 proteins was increased, IGF-1 and EGF protein levels were increased in the distal tubule, similar to the Bcl-2 antiapoptotic proteins, and were also detected in the adjacent proximal tubules suggestive of paracrine action in these tubules. TGF-beta expression was moderately increased in regenerating proximal tubules, but no relationship was seen with the pattern of expression of the Bcl-2 genes. An explanation of these results is that the distal tubule is adaptively resistant to ischemic injury via promotion of survival by antiapoptotic Bcl-2 genes, and its survival allows expression of growth factors critical not only to the maintenance and regeneration of its own cell population (autocrine action), but also to the adjacent ischemia-sensitive proximal tubular cells (paracrine action).

The hypothesis has therefore been proposed that both the S3 proximal tubule and MTAL cells reside in regions where oxygen availability is borderline. Hypoxia induces both necrosis and apoptosis in proximal tubular cells. Hypoxia triggers apoptosis in MTAL cells, but the presence of antiapoptotic Bcl-2 genes prevents completion of programmed cell death and the DNA fragmentation is repaired. The induction of the growth factors EGF and IGF in these MTAL and distal tubule cells then provides both autocrine and paracrine mechanisms respectively for the recovery of the MTAL and proximal tubules. Because proximal cells are necrotic or have sloughed due to loss of cell adhesion, proximal tubule recovery is delayed compared to the MTAL. This hypothesis also provides a mechanism for tubular obstruction by casts since viable MTAL cells are the source of Tamm-Horsfall protein.

TUBULOGLOMERULAR FEEDBACK

Tubuloglomerular feedback (TGF) ("tubular communication with the glomerulus") operates within the juxtaglomerular apparatus (JGA) of each nephron where changes are sensed in the salt content of fluid at the luminal macula densa and that information is transmitted to the afferent arteriole to cause compensatory changes in single nephron GFR (346). nNOS (NOS 1) is expressed in the macula densa and may influence TGF. However, micropuncture experiments using NOS antagonists have shown that nitric oxide (NO) may modulate TGF (346). Instead, local NOS blockade causes the curve that represents TGF to shift leftward and become more steep. Changes in macula densa NO production may underlie the resetting of TGF, which is required in order to keep the TGF curve aligned with ambient tubular flow as tubular flow changes to accommodate physiologic circumstances. Also, macula densa NO production may be substrate limited and dissociated from NOS protein content. The importance of NO to TGF resetting and the substrate dependence of NO production have both been found during changes in dietary salt (347,348). In addition, nNOS inhibition sensitizes the tubuloglomerular feedback mechanism after volume expansion (349). Macula densa cells detect changes in distal sodium chloride concentration, at least in part, through an apical Na:2Cl:K cotransporter (350). Macula densa NO directly inhibits Na:2Cl:K cotransport and NO and angiotensin II independently alter cotransporter activity (350). To determine the role of the local renin-angiotensin system on TGF, mice with absent renal tissue expression of ACE were studied (351). TGF was absent in mice without ACE in the kidney suggesting that renal tissue ACE is an important contributor to TGF (351). Mice deficient in adenosine A_1 receptors lack TGF (352). Mice deficient in ecto-5′nucleotidase/CD73, the enzyme responsible for adenosine formation from AMP have an impairment of TGF regulation of GFR (353).

Taken together, the proximal tubular injury and resultant dysfunction could contribute to the drastic fall in GFR, the hallmark of ischemic ARF. One potential mechanism is increased TGF. Specifically in ARF, the decreased proximal tubule reabsorption would increase solute delivery to the macular densa with the resultant constriction of the afferent arteriole and fall in GFR (354). In normal nephrons, the maximal fall in GFR with increased solute delivery to the macular densa is approximately 50%. Thus, increased TGF could be a major factor in mediating the pathway whereby proximal tubule damage could lower GFR. However, because clinical ATN or ischemic ARF is associated with a 90% fall in GFR, either additional factors or increased sensitivity of TGF postischemic injury to the kidney must occur. In that regard, dissected afferent arterioles from ischemic kidneys have been shown to have increased cytosolic calcium concentrations and enhanced vasoconstriction responses to angiotensin II and endothelin (355,356). It is thus theoretically tenable that the sensitivity of the TGF is indeed enhanced postischemia. However, the role of TGF in ischemic ARF remains controversial (357).

In support of a pathogenic role of TGF in ischemic ARF are studies by Brian Meyer's group that demonstrated the following (55,56): (i) Translocation of NaK-ATPase to the cytoplasm results in depolarization confined to the proximal tubule; (ii) Fractional excretion of lithium, a surrogate measure for the fraction of filtered sodium that is delivered to the macula densa, the site of tubuloglomerular feedback, is massively increased, and (iii) These abnormalities persist for the duration of the maintenance phase of postischemic ARF. This study provides evidence for decreased proximal reabsorption of sodium, resultant increased sodium delivery to macula densa, tubuloglomerular feedback and resultant filtration failure that accompanies ischemic ARF.

Another pathway whereby tubular injury can contribute to a fall in GFR is by causing intraluminal cast formation and tubule obstruction. This will be the next topic discussed.

TUBULAR CAST FORMATION AND OBSTRUCTION POSTRENAL ISCHEMIA

The classic radiological findings in early ARF, prior to the realization that contrast is nephrotoxic, was an early dense nephrogram not followed by a pyelogram. Because the nephrogram phase represents contrast entering the tubules by filtration, a persistent nephrogram suggests tubular obstruction with ongoing glomerular filtration.

Kidneys with ischemic ARF or ATN are swollen and, therefore, it was suggested that interstitial edema may lead to tubular collapse secondary to extraluminal-mediated compression. It is clear however that recovery from ATN can occur when the kidneys are still enlarged and swollen. Increased excretion of tubular epithelial casts are however a hallmark of recovery from ATN (23). The presence of tubular casts on renal biopsy as well as urinary casts has provided morphological support for a role of tubular obstruction due to intraluminal cast formation in the pathogenesis of ischemic ARF (358). As noted earlier, while earlier micropuncture studies failed to consistently demonstrate increased tubular pressures postischemia, several subsequent studies provided convincing evidence for the presence of tubular obstruction in experimental ischemic ARF. Finn and Gottschalk using micropuncture techniques during saline loading demonstrated clear evidence of increased tubular pressures in postischemic, as compared to normal kidneys (359). Renal vasodilation to restore renal blood flow also demonstrated increased tubular pressures in ischemic ARF in the rat. Perhaps the most compelling studies, however, were those micropuncture experiments performed by Tanner et al. (360). They found that perfusing the proximal tubule with artificial tubular fluid at a rate, which did not increase tubule pressure in normal animals, increased tubule pressures in animals after a renal ischemic insult. Moreover, venting those obstructed tubules led to improved nephron filtration rates. Burke et al. also demonstrated that prevention of ischemic ARF in dogs with mannitol led to a decrease in intratubular pressures, suggesting that the induced-solute diuresis led to relief of cast-mediated tubular obstruction (361).

While it is clear that brush border membranes, necrotic cells, viable cells and perhaps apoptotic tubular epithelial cells enter tubular fluid after an acute renal ischemic insult, the actual process and predominant location of the cast formation is however less clear. It is known, however, that the casts uniformly stain for Tamm Horsfall protein (THP) (358).

Integrins

Integrins are heterodimeric glycoproteins consisting of different combinations of alpha and beta subunits; they recognize the most common universal tripeptide sequence, arginine-glycine-aspartic acid (RGD), which is present in a variety of matrix proteins (9). These integrins can mediate cell-cell adhesion via an RGD inhibitable mechanism (8).

In normal kidneys, proximal tubular cells are stained by the RGD peptide, RhoG-RGD, basolaterally in a punctuate pattern

and with Bt-RGD only minimally. On the other hand, ischemic kidneys labeling with RhoG-RGD and Bt-RGD occurred at the basolateral and apical aspect of tubular cells as well as on desquamating or desquamated cells within the tubular lumen and also on the vasa rectae (362). In ischemic kidneys, antibodies to beta1 and αV subunits of integrins stained glomeruli and the apical aspect of the proximal and distal tubules. Desquamated cells and cellular conglomerates obstructing the tubular lumina were intensely stained with RGD peptides (363). Dual labeling experiments with Bt-RGD and antibodies against integrin receptors demonstrated αVβ3 binding sites for RGD peptides in the vasculature and some desquamated cells, whereas the majority of the desquamated cells bind Bt-RGD via β1 integrins (362).

Experimental results support a role for adhesion molecules in the formation of casts. It has been shown that a translocation of integrins to the apical membrane of tubular epithelial cells may occur with ischemia (8,257,258). Possible mechanisms for the loss of the polarized distribution of integrins include cytoskeletal disruption, state of phosphorylation, activation of proteases, and production of NO (364,365). These integrins are known to recognize arginine, glycine, aspartate (RGD) tripeptide sequences (10,363). Thus, viable intra-luminal cells could adhere to other luminal or paraluminal cells. The Goligorsky group provided experimental evidence for this cell-cell adhesion process as a contributor to tubule obstruction in ischemic ARF. Synthetic cyclical RGD peptides were infused prior to the renal ischemic insult in order to block cell to cell adhesion as a component of tubule obstruction (11,366–369). Using micropuncture techniques the cyclic RGD tripeptides blocked the rise in tubular pressure postischemic insult (10). In vivo study of RGD peptides (cyclic RGDDFLG and RGDDFV) in ischemic ARF in rats demonstrated attenuation of renal injury and accelerated recovery of renal function (11). Systemic administration of fluorescent derivatives of two different cyclic RGD peptides, a cyclic Bt-RGD peptide and a linear RhoG-RGD peptide, infused after the release of renal artery clamp ameliorated ischemic ARF in rats (11,368). The staining of these peptides suggests that cyclic RGD peptides inhibited tubular obstruction by predominantly preventing cell-to-cell adhesion, rather than cell-to-matrix adhesion (363).

In addition to cell-cell adhesion, it is worthy to note that Bonventre et al. have demonstrated increased fibronectin in the tubular lumen after an ischemic insult and fibronectin is known to possess RGD sequences, which are recognized by cellular integrins (370). Moreover, THP is known to possess an RGD sequence, which may or may not be in a position to be recognized by integrins. This possibility however led to in vitro cellular adhesion studies in which LLCPK$_1$ cell adhesion to several different matrices, (i.e., collagen I and collagen IV), was examined (364). Interestingly, THP diminished cell adhesion in artificial fluid mimicking distal tubular fluid but not tubular fluid similar to ATN or collecting duct fluid have significantly higher ionic concentrations (371). In this regard, it has been suggested that THP becomes a polymeric gel in the presence of high ionic strength fluid, but is a nongel monomeric substance in low ionic strength fluid. Recent studies documented that the gel formation by THP is an active process that can be abolished by boiling. A role of the oligosaccharide component of THP in the gel formation was demonstrated, since n-glycanase treatment to remove the oligosaccharide abolished the gel formation (371).

Thus, the intraluminal presence of brush border membranes, viable and nonviable cells in association with extracellular matrix, (e.g., fibronectin), THP and adhesion molecules support their involvement in cast formation in ischemic ARF. The actual tubular obstruction by the casts however may only occur in the presence of the impaired vascular responses to renal ischemia. More specifically, if net glomerular filtration pressure were normal, the majority of the tubular casts may be

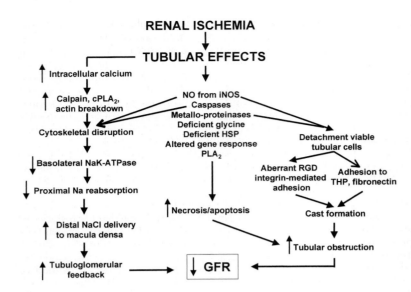

RENAL ISCHEMIA

TUBULAR EFFECTS

↑ Intracellular calcium

↑ Calpain, cPLA₂, actin breakdown

Cytoskeletal disruption

↓ Basolateral NaK-ATPase

↓ Proximal Na reabsorption

↑ Distal NaCl delivery to macula densa

↑ Tubuloglomerular feedback

NO from iNOS
Caspases
Metallo-proteinases
Deficient glycine
Deficient HSP
Altered gene response
PLA₂

Detachment viable tubular cells

Aberrant RGD integrin-mediated adhesion   Adhesion to THP, fibronectin

↑ Necrosis/apoptosis   Cast formation

↑ Tubular obstruction

↓ GFR

FIGURE 39-10. Tubular factors in the pathogenesis of ischemic ARF. *THP* = Tamm-Horsfall protein, *PLA₂* = phospholipase A₂. (Reproduced from: Kribben A, Edelstein CL, Schrier RW. Pathophysiology of acute renal failure. *J Nephrol* 1999;12[Suppl 2]:S142, with permission.)

excreted in the urine rather than lodging in the collecting duct and other nephron sites. Tubular factors in the pathogenesis of ischemic ARF are shown in Figure 39-10. The various perturbations in the renal vasculature, which occur in association with a renal ischemic insult, will now be discussed.

VASCULAR PERTURBATIONS POSTRENAL ISCHEMIA

Ischemic ARF is associated with renal vasoconstriction with a resultant decrease in glomerular hydrostatic pressure and renal plasma flow (16,17,372). Not only are circulatory vasoconstrictors, such as catecholamines, angiotensin II and endothelin, as well as renal sympathetic tone, frequently increased in the setting of ischemic ARF (72), but the renal vascular response has been shown to be enhanced. This increased response to vasoconstrictors is due in part to the earlier mentioned increase in cytosolic calcium concentration in the afferent arterioles of the glomerulus. The endothelial damage is also associated with a diminution of the renal vasodilators which oppose the action of vasoconstrictors. In experimental sepsis, the NO secondary to iNOS has been suggested to downregulate renal eNOS (373). Moreover, the renal clamp model of ARF in the rat has been shown to be associated with downregulation of endothelial-derived nitric oxide (eDNO) (355,374). Recent studies have also shown that endothelin receptor antagonists ameliorate the diminution in renal hemodynamics associated with renal ischemia in the isolated perfused rat kidney (375,376). Further support for endothelin as an important mediator of ischemia-reperfusion induced renal injury is the protective effect of an endothelin-A receptor antagonist in rats after clamping of the renal arteries (377). Impairment of prostaglandin synthesis by damaged endothelium can also profoundly enhance renal vascular resistance associated with renal ischemia. In this regard, infusion of prostaglandin E1 may protect against ischemic ARF (378). Also, inhibition of thromboxane A2 improves renal function in rats exposed to warm ischemia-reperfusion (379).

Oxygen Free Radicals

A large number of studies have been performed in the isolated perfused rat kidney (IPRK), which cast light on the role of

oxygen radicals in the biochemical and morphological changes which follow hypoxia and reperfusion. Studies with ^{31}P magnetic resonance spectroscopy (MRS) confirmed the rapid onset of ATP depletion with induction of hypoxia (380). These same studies also demonstrated that the extent of morphological injury during different degrees of hypoxic perfusion was proportional to the extent of ATP depletion. Further studies with [23]Na, ^{31}P and [87]Rb (a congener of potassium) MRS demonstrated that increases in intracellular sodium and decreases in potassium accompanied the decrease in ATP induced by hypoxia (381). Subsequent investigation revealed that the rate and extent of increase in sodium was reduced by pretreatment with dimethylthiourea (DMTU) and dimethylsulfoxide (DMSO), both scavengers of oxygen-derived free radicals (OFR) (382). These studies supported similar indirect evidence for injury induced by OFR during reperfusion (383,384). Whereas some studies have demonstrated that activated neutrophils produce OFR injury after ischemia (385,386), other studies in isolated proximal tubules (387) and the studies in the cell-free isolated perfused rat kidney, for example, (382) indicated that OFR were generated and contributed to the injury process even in the absence of neutrophils. The identification of the actual species of OFR involved in reperfusion injury required direct methods of detection rather than a reliance on scavengers.

Direct detection of hydoxyl radicals was initially achieved in isolated proximal tubules by using biochemical traps (387). Similar studies were subsequently performed in the intact kidney using 0.5 mM salicylate to react with hydroxyl radicals during reperfusion for 15 minutes after ischemia of 15 minutes (388). An increase in 2,5 dihydroxybenzoic acid was observed using high performance liquid chromotography (HPLC) with electrochemical detection. Subsequent studies by Endre et al. (389) utilized electron paramagnetic resonance (EPR) and 5,5-dimethyl-l-pyrroline N-oxide (DMPO) as a spin trap confirmed that hydroxyl radicals were generated during a briefer 3-minute reperfusion period following 20 minutes of ischemia. Interestingly, both studies demonstrated a significant generation of hydroxyl radicals in control kidneys, which was abolished by the addition of the scavenger, DMTU. An increase in an unidentified carbon-centered radical was also identified during reperfusion in the EPR study and could represent an early lipid peroxidation product (389).

With 60 minutes of reperfusion after 20 minutes of ischemia in the IPRK, tubular damage was prominent in both the cortical and medullary proximal tubule and in the MTAL (342). The morphological changes included cellular blebbing, brush border damage, tubular casts, and occasional apoptosis. The MTAL always demonstrates signs of injury during cell-free perfusion (see the subsequent text), so caution is required in interpreting damage in this region. DNA fragmentation was detected predominantly in the MTAL and distal tubule using the technique of in-situ end labeling (342). Pretreatment with either allopurinol, which acts both to inhibit xanthine oxidase and as an OFR scavenger, or DMTU, reduced both the morphological features of injury the extent of DNA fragmentation in the MTAL. Taken together, these results suggest that hydroxyl radicals formed during reperfusion after ischemia play a significant role in both necrotic and apoptotic cell injury.

On the background of these postischemic vascular perturbations is the observation that a decrease in renal perfusion pressure is not associated with autoregulation of either GFR or renal blood flow (17,355,372,390–392). In fact, rather than renal vasodilation, renal vasoconstriction occurs with a fall in renal perfusion pressure in the postischemic kidney. Thus, a degree of hypotension, which is of no clinical significance in the normal kidney, may cause renal damage in the kidney during the recovery phase of ATN. The same increased sensitivity in the postischemic kidney has also been shown to occur with nephrotoxic agents such as aminoglycosides.

The increased vulnerability to recurrent ischemic injury is a possible reason for the clinical finding of fresh tubular necrosis even 4 weeks after the initiation of ARF. Specifically, in patients with prolonged ARF after combat injury, a prominent finding in biopsy or autopsy specimens obtained 3 to 4 weeks after the initial insult was fresh tubular renal ischemic lesions that could not be related to the remote initial ischemic insult (393). A possible explanation for the fresh ischemic lesions was altered reactivity of the renal vasculature. Transient reduction of blood pressure within the normal autoregulatory range, which frequently occurs during intermittent hemodialysis treatment, can actually result in recurrent ischemic injury and prolongation of ARF due to the altered vascular reactivity of the injured kidneys (394). In humans, a deterioration of renal function parameters during hemodialysis are in accordance with this proposal of altered autoregulation (365).

Studies to examine the role of Ca^{2+} and CCB in the vascular perturbations in experimental ischemic ARF have been performed. These studies demonstrate that intrarenal CCB can reverse the increased sensitivity to renal nerve stimulation as well as the loss of renal autoregulation, both of which characterize experimental ARF (395). In addition, other studies in the rat showed that atrial natriuretic peptide (ANP), which attenuates vasoconstrictor-induced increases in $[Ca^{2+}]_i$ in cultured vascular smooth muscle cells (396), is also protective against ischemic ARF (397), despite the fact that its systemic administration causes a fall in arterial pressure.

Endotoxemia-Induced ARF

Recent experimental studies in septic mice have incriminated still another mediator of renal vasoconstriction. The intraperitoneal administration of lipopolysaccharide (LPS) as an endotoxin was associated with a profound decrease in GFR and renal blood flow both in wild type and iNOS knockout mice. A soluble receptor of tumor necrosis factor (TNF), however, was associated with profound improvement in renal hemodynamics in both wild type and iNOS knockout mice (398). Since septic patients with renal failure have a high mortality, this observation has potential therapeutic importance.

Sepsis in mice has also been shown to be associated with an impaired response of NO-mediated cyclic GMP in the renal cortex, the agent's secondary messenger for vasodilation (399). The renal nerves and activation of the renin-angiotensin system contribute to renal vasoconstriction during sepsis. In this study, renal denervation decreased the high plasma renin levels during endotoxemia and was protective against the decreased GFR and renal blood flow in a normotensive model of endotoxemia-induced sepsis (400).

Oxygen radicals may contribute to the vasoconstriction in endotoxemia-induced ARF (401). ARF during sepsis is associated with increased nitric oxide and oxygen radicals including superoxide. Renal extracellular superoxide dismutase (EC-SOD) is decreased in endoteoxemia (402). Antioxidant therapy with chemically dissimilar antioxidants, metalloporphyrin and tempol, preserved GFR and renal blood flow during endotoxemia (402). This protective effect was reversed by inhibition of iNOS suggesting the importance of the bioavailability of NO for preservation of renal function during endotoxemia (402).

The demonstration of global renal vasoconstriction in sepsis may depend on the model used. In a nonlethal hyperdynamic model of sepsis in sheep injected with *Escherichia coli*, renal failure developed despite markedly increased renal blood flow (403).

In another study in endotoxemia-induced ARF, the role of renal inflammation and apoptosis was determined (404). In this study, LPS acted on extrarenal Toll-like receptor 4 leading to systemic TNF release and subsequent ARF. Mice with a mutation in Toll-like receptor 4 were resistant to LPS-induced ARF and had less neutrophil infiltration and renal cell apoptosis (404).

INFLAMMATION IN POSTRENAL ISCHEMIA

Ischemic ARF has been described as an inflammatory disease (19). This is evidenced by numerous studies demonstrating endothelial injury, leukocyte infiltration in the kidney and the generation of inflammatory mediators by tubular cells (19).

Endothelial Cell injury

Silver nitrate staining of blood vessels was studied in rats at 4 hr after release of a renal artery clamp (405). Ischemic ARF resulted in disorganization of endothelial integrity with areas of denudation, partial disappearance of cell-cell borders and distortion of cell–cell contacts most prominent in the renal microvasculature. Intravital microscopy of blood flow in peritubular capillaries provided direct evidence for the existence of a "no flow" phenomenon caused by endothelial injury (405,406). Transplantation of endothelial cells or surrogate cells expressing endothelial NOS, either intravenously or intraarterially, resulted in functional protection against ischemic ARF (405). These studies suggested that endothelial cell injury is the primary cause of the "no-flow" phenomenon and that when ameliorated there is attenuation of renal function.

It has been demonstrated in mice that injury of renal microvascular endothelium alters barrier function after ischemia (407). In this study, circulating von Willebrand factor (vWF), a marker of endothelial injury, was increased in the circulation 24 hours after ischemia. In FVB-TIE2/GFP mice, in which the microvasculature can be visualized, there were alterations in the cytoskeleton and alterations in the integrity of adherens junctions that correlated with a permeability defect identified using fluorescent dextrans and two-photon intravital imaging (407).

The extension phase of ARF is marked by continued hypoxia and an inflammatory response, which are more marked in the corticomedullary junction (18). Severely reduced blood flow, stasis and accumulation of red blood cells has been documented in the corticomedullary region (18). Endothelial cell injury is thought to play an important role in the initiation and extension phase of ischemic ARF (18).

Neutrophil Activation

Renal ischemia-reperfusion injury is associated with an increase in infiltrating neutrophils (408). The adherence of neutrophils to the vascular endothelium is an essential step in the extravasation of these cells into ischemic tissue (28). Therefore, leukocyte adhesion molecules have been studied in renal injury (409). After adherence and chemotaxis, infiltrating leukocytes release reactive oxygen species and enzymes that damage the cells (28). Infusion of normal neutrophils accentuates severe ischemia/reperfusion injury and decreases GFR during ischemia. Activated neutrophils have been shown to enhance the decrease in GFR in response to renal ischemia at least in part due to release of oxygen radicals (386,410–412). In contrast, infusion of oxygen radical deficient neutrophils from patients with chronic granulomatous disease patients did not worsen the course of ischemic injury (411). The mechanism by which adherent leukocytes cause ischemic injury is unclear, but likely involves both the release of potent vasoconstrictors including the prostaglandins, leukotrienes, and thromboxanes (413), as well as direct endothelial injury via release of endothelin and a decrease in NO (72,414).

Intracellular adhesion molecule I (ICAM I) has been suggested to play an important role in the pathophysiology of ischemic ARF (408,415). Increased systemic levels of the cytokines, tumor necrosis factor (TNF-alpha) and interleukin-1 (IL-1) may upregulate ICAM-1 after ischemia and reperfusion in the kidney (415). ICAM-1 on endothelial cells promotes the adhesion of neutrophils to these cells and causes tissue damage. The administration of a monoclonal antibody against ICAM-1 protected against ischemic ARF in rats (408,411). Pretreatment with an ICAM-1 antisense oligodeoxyribonucleotide ameliorated the ischemia-induced infiltration of granulocytes and macrophages and resulted in less cortical renal damage as assessed by a quantitative pathologic grading scale (416). In parallel, ICAM-1 deficient mice are protected against renal ischemia (415). Thus, ICAM-1 is a mediator of ischemic ARF probably by potentiating neutrophil-endothelial interactions.

Red blood cell swelling has been suggested to cause the medullary blood flow congestion which occurs postrenal ischemia and worsens the relative hypoxia in that region of the kidney. The restoration of renal blood flow in experimental renal ischemia in the dog, however, occurs with either an isotonic or hypertonic mannitol induced-diuresis. There is now evidence that upregulation of adhesion molecules may contribute to this impaired medullary blood flow postischemic injury (409,417,418).

P-selectin, an important molecule involved in adherence of circulating leukocytes to tissue in inflammatory states, also seems to be involved in the infiltration of the leukocytes during ischemic injury. In fact, renal ischemia has also been shown to be associated with upregulation of endothelial P-selectin with enhanced adhesion of neutrophils (419). A soluble P-selectin glycoprotein ligand prevented infiltration of leukocytes and ameliorated ischemia induced renal dysfunction (365). In contrast to P-selectin, the L-selectin does not appear to mediate tubular damage in postischemic kidney (409). After adherence and chemotaxis, neutrophils release reactive oxygen species or oxygen free radicals.

There is evidence that neutrophils, mediate tubular injury in ARF (420). This evidence is derived from studies that show an accumulation of neutrophils in ischemic ARF and studies demonstrating a beneficial role of anti-ICAM-1 therapy in ARF (415). Also, mice depleted of peripheral neutrophils by antineutrophil serum were protected against ischemic ARF (415).

However, in another study, rats depleted of peripheral neutrophils by anti-neutrophil serum were not protected against ischemic ARF (421). In another study, mice were injected with 0.1 mg of the rat IgG2b monoclonal antibody RB6-8C5 (BD Pharmingen) intraperitoneally 24 hours before renal pedicle clamp (225). This results in depletion of neutrophils in the peripheral blood and in the kidney during ischemic ARF. In this study, there was the slight functional protection and no histological protection against ischemic ARF in neutrophil-depleted mice (225).

Lymphocytes

The role of lymphocytes in ischemic ARF is an ongoing area of study (422,423). Lymphocytes has been examined in genetically altered, immune deficient mice. In one study, mice with a combined deficiency of both CD4 and CD8 cells were protected against ischemic ARF at 48 hours, but not 24 hours, postischemic reperfusion (424). In a follow-up report by the same investigators, *nu/nu* mice that are athymic and deficient in both CD4 and CD8 T cells, were protected against ischemic ARF 24 and 48 hours postischemic reperfusion (425). To determine the pathogenic T cell type, mice with targeted genetic deficiencies of either CD4 or CD8 T cells were also studied. CD4 deficient mice, but not CD8 deficient, are protected against ischemic ARF (425). Therefore, it appears that the pathogenic T cell subtype in ischemic ARF is the CD4 T cell. However, RAG-1 −/− mice, which lack mature T and B lymphocytes, are not protected against ischemic ARF despite lacking both CD4 and CD8 T cells (426). In a recent study, mice deficient in B lymphocytes alone *were* protected against ischemic ARF (427). In summary, CD4 T cell deficient, *nu/nu* (lacking mature T cells), and B cell deficient mice are protected against ischemic ARF while CD8 T cell and RAG-1 −/− (lacking mature B and T cells) mice are not protected.

The effect of complete depletion of CD4 T cells with a monoclonal antibody in ischemic ARF is not known. In one report, the use of GK1.5 antibody alone to deplete CD4 T cells did not protect against ischemic ARF; however, complete depletion of CD4 T cells as judged by FACS analysis did not occur (428). Protection did occur when GK1.5 was used with two other antibodies, which resulted in the depletion of both CD4 and CD8 T cells (428). In another study, complete depletion of CD4 T cells using the GK1.5 antibody was not protective against ischemic ARF in mice (429). In summary, it is believed that CD4 T cells are important in the pathogenesis of ischemic ARF and that very few T cells in the kidney are enough to contribute to injury (425) (423,428).

Monocyte/macrophages

Another inflammatory cell that is a potential mediator of injury in ischemic ARF is the monocyte/macrophage (423). Macrophages infiltrate the postischemic rat kidney (430). Macrophage chemoattractants, for example, monocyte chemoattractant protein-1 (MCP-1) are increased in the postischemic rat kidney (423). In a model of macrophage depletion using liposomal clodronate, it was demonstrated that macrophages contribute to tissue damage during acute rejection (431). An anti-B7-1 antibody blocks mononuclear cell adherence in vasa recta in rats and attenuates ischemic ARF both functionally and histologically (432). Gene therapy in rats expressing an amino-terminal truncated MCP-1 reduced macrophage infiltration and ATN (433).Two recent studies have demonstrated that macrophage depletion using liposomal clodronate is protective against ischemic ARF in mice (434,435).

Inflammatory Mediators

In renal ischemia/reperfusion, tubular epithelial cells produce TNF-alpha, IL-1, IL-6, IL-8, IL-18 TGF-beta, MCP-1, RANTES and fractalkines (19,224,225). Leukocytes produce TNF-alpha, IL-1, IL-8, MCP-1, reactive oxygen species and eicosanoids (19). The antiinflammatory cytokine, IL-10, inhibits TNF-alpha, ICAM-1 and iNOS and protects against ischemic and cisplatin-induced renal failure and ATN (436).

Statins are potent antiinflammatory drugs (437). Both *in vitro* and *in vivo* studies suggest lipid lowering–independent antiinflammatory functions of statins (437). After adhesion to the vascular endothelium, inflammatory cells migrate to the site of inflammation (437). Statins act independently of lipid lowering to selectively inhibit leukocyte adhesion by direct interactions with the leukocyte-function antigen-1 (LFA-1) (437). Statins reduce macrophage influx and chemokine expression in rat kidneys (438). Statins are known to decrease the expression of pro-inflammatory cytokines by inflammatory cells (437). Simvastatin reduces expression of IL-6 and monocyte chemoattractant protein (MCP-1) in monocytes from hypercholesterolemic patients and in cultured endothelial cells (437). Pravastatin downregulates TNF-alpha and MCP-1 [439] in human monocytes *in vitro*. Some of the antiinflammatory effects of statins are mediated by nitric oxide.

Rats were treated with cerivastatin or vehicle for 3 days before induction of ischemic ARF (440). Statin treatment reduced the increase in serum creatinine by 40% and protected against tubular necrosis. In addition, monocyte and macrophage infiltration was almost completely prevented, ICAM-1 upregulation was decreased and iNOS expression was reduced (440). In another study, atorvastatin improved the course of ischemic ARF in aging rats by enhancing nitric oxide availability and improving renal hemodynamics (441).

RECOVERY FROM ISCHEMIC ARF

It has been demonstrated in rats that severe ischemic ARF results in permanent alteration in renal capillary density that contributes to a urinary concentrating defect and renal fibrosis (442,443). However, in contrast to other organs, the kidney can recover from tubular necrosis, at least in the short term. There are 2 potential mechanisms of recovery: (i) dedifferentiation and proliferation of the surviving non necrotic tubular

cells (444) and (ii) mobilization and delivery of bone marrow stem cells to the injured kidney (445).

After ischemic ARF there is proliferation of tubular cells that mimics events in the developing kidney (446). Epithelial cells are also dedifferentiated during the recovery period (444). In the postiscehmic kidney, there is also expression of genes that encode growth factors (301,303,306). Dedifferentiation and proliferation of tubular epithelial cells may result in the spreading of cells over the damaged basement membrane. Cell adhesion molecules like neural cell adhesion molecule (NCAM), cytokines and kidney injury molecule-1 (Kim-1) (62,447) may play a role in these processes. Targeted delivery of hepatocyte growth factor (HGF) to the proximal tubule in transgenic mice results in marked protection against ischemic ARF (448). Understanding the physiology of repair and recovery of surviving tubular cells may lead to therapies to hasten the recovery process in humans.

Bone marrow stem cells have the capacity to migrate to other organs (445). Bone marrow derived cells can populate and contribute to turnover of both the normal and injured renal tubular epithelium (449). Cells from the adult mouse bone marrow are mobilized into the circulation by transient renal ischemia and home specifically to the injured kidney where they differentiate into tubular epithelial cells (445). It was investigated whether an increase in circulating stem cells, using pharmacological mobilization from the bone marrow, would improve renal function in mice with ischemic ARF (450). The pharmacological increase in stem cells was associated with marked granulocytosis and worsening of renal failure. In the future, therapies aimed at stimulating the proliferation, mobilization and targeting of stem cells may enhance recovery from ischemic ARF (445).

SUMMARY

Tubular and vascular perturbations and inflammation combine to cause ischemic ARF. The tubular and vascular events in ischemic ARF are summarized in Figures 39-10 and 39-11. The inflammatory events are summarized in Figure 39-12. Recent laboratory studies using *in vivo*, cellular and molecular approaches have provided substantial insight into the pathogenesis of the syndrome. These studies have identified several potential therapeutic interventions, which need to be tested with prospective clinical trials. Interventions which have

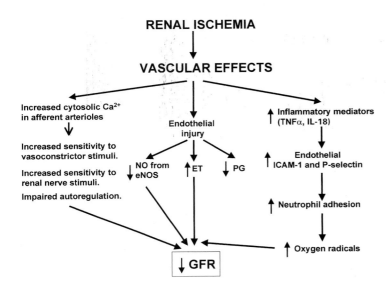

FIGURE 39-11. Vascular factors in the pathogenesis of ischemic ARF. *ET*, endothelin; *PG*, prostaglandins; *TNF α*, tumor necrosis factor. (Reproduced from: Kribben A, Edelstein CL, Schrier RW. Pathophysiology of acute renal failure. *J Nephrol* 1999;12[Suppl 2]:S142, with permission.)

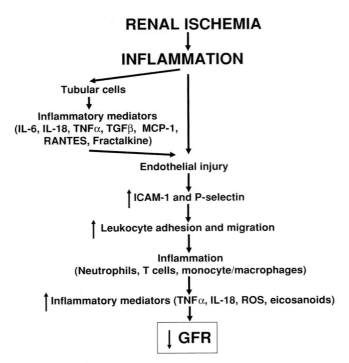

FIGURE 39-12. Inflammatory response in ischemic ARF. *IL-1,* interleukin-1; *IL-18,* interleukin-18; *TNFα,* tumor necrosis factor alpha; *TGFβ,* transforming growth factor beta; *RANTES,* regulated upon activation, normal T cell expressed and secreted, *ROS,* reactive oxygen species; *ICAM-1,* intracellular adhesion molecule-1; *MCP-1,* monocyte chemoattractant protein-1.

attenuated experimental ischemic/hypoxic proximal tubule damage include cysteine protease inhibitors, *α*MSH, specific iNOS inhibition, synthetic cyclical RGD sequences, mannitol, oxygen radical scavengers, TNF soluble receptors, inducers of HSP and anti-ICAM antibodies, endothelin antagonists, IL-18 antiserum, erythropoietin, CTLA4 immunoglobulin to mention a few (Table 39-9). The intrarenal administration of these compounds may be necessary to avoid systemic complications. In that regard, the hypotensive effect of atrial natriuretic pep-

tide in recent trials no doubt obscured any intrarenal beneficial effect of the compound.

TABLE 39-9

SOME EMERGING THERAPIES FOR ISCHEMIC ACUTE RENAL FAILURE

Cysteine protease inhibitors
Caspase inhibitors
IL-18 inhibition
*α*MSH
Specific iNOS inhibition
Synthetic cyclical RGD sequences
Oxygen radical scavengers
TNF soluble receptors
Inducers of HSP
Anti-ICAM antibodies
Endothelin antagonists
Endothelial cell infusion
Mannitol with natriuretic peptides or calcium channel blockers
Erythropoeitin
CTLA4 immunoglobulin

References

1. Racusen LC. Renal histopathology and urine cytology and cytopathology in acute renal failure. In: Goligorsky MS, Stein JH, eds. *Acute renal failure. New concepts and therapeutic strategies.* New York: Churchill Livingstone, 1995:194.
2. Racusen LC, Fivush BA, Li YL, et al. Dissociation of tubular cell detachment and tubular cell death in clinical and experimental "acute renal failure." *Lab Invest* 1991;64:546.
3. Graber M, Lane B, Lamia R, et al. Bubble cells: renal tubular cells in the urinary sediment with characteristic viability. *J Am Soc Nephrol* 1991;1:999.
4. Savill J. Apoptosis and the kidney (editorial). *J Am Soc Nephrol* 1994;5:12.
5. Hammerman MR. Renal programmed cell death and the treatment of renal disease (editorial). *Curr Opin Nephrol Hypertens* 1998;7:1.
6. Green DR, Reed JC. Mitochondria and apoptosis. *Science* 1998;281:1309.
7. Evan G, Littlewood T. A matter of life and cell death. *Science* 1998;281:1317.
8. Gailit J, Colflesh D, Rabiner I, et al. Redistribution and dysfunction of integrins in cultured renal epithelial cells exposed to oxidative stress. *Am J Physiol* 1993;33:F149.
9. Ruoslahti E. RGD and other recognition sequences for integrins. *Annu Rev Cell Dev Biol* 1996;12:697–715:697.
10. Goligorsky MS, DiBona GF. Pathogenic role of Arg-Gly-Asp recognizing integrins in acute renal failure. *Proc Natl Acad Sci USA* 1993;90:5700.
11. Noiri E, Gailit J, Sheth D, et al. Cyclic RGD peptides ameliorate ischemic acute renal failure in rats. *Kidney Int* 1994;46:1050.
12. Oliver J, Macdowell M, Tracy A. The pathogenesis of acute renal failure associated with traumatic and toxic injury: renal ischemia, nephrotoxic damage, and the ischemic episode. *J Clin Invest* 1951;30:1307.
13. Oken DE. Hemodynamic basis for human acute renal failure (vasomotor nephropathy). *Am J Med* 1984;76:702.
14. Oken DE. Theoretical analysis of pathogenetic mechanisms in experimental acute renal failure. *Kidney Int* 1983;24:16.
15. Oken DE. Acute renal failure (vasomotor nephropathy): micropuncture studies of the pathogenetic mechanisms. *AnnuRevMed* 1975;26:307.
16. Conger JD, Schrier RW. Renal hemodynamics in acute renal failure. *Annu Rev Physiol* 1980;42:603.
17. Conger JD. Prophylaxis and treatment of ARF by vasoactive agents. The facts and the myths. *Kidney Int* 1998;53:S23.
18. Molitoris BA, Sutton TA. Endothelial injury and dysfunction: role in the extension phase of acute renal failure. *Kidney Int* 2004;66:496.
19. Bonventre JV, Zuk A. Ischemic acute renal failure: an inflammatory disease? *Kidney Int* 2004;66:480.
19a. Ricci Z, Ronco C. Year in review: critical care 2004-nephrology. *Crit Care* 2005;9:523.
20. Binswanger U. ARF: changing causes? *Kidney Blood Press Res* 1997;20:163.
21. Corwin HL, Bonventre JV. ARF in the intensive care unit. Part 1. *Intens Care Med* 1988;14:10.
22. Groeneveld AB, Tran DD, van der Meulen J, et al. Acute renal failure in the medical intensive care unit: predisposing, complicating factors and outcome. *Nephron* 1991;59:602.
23. Kelly KJ, Molitoris BA. Acute renal failure in the new millennium: time to consider combination therapy. *Semin Nephrol* 2000;20:4.
24. Alkhunaizi AM, Schrier RW. Management of acute renal failure: new perspectives. *Am J Kidney Dis* 1996;28:315.
25. Elasy TA, Anderson RJ. Changing demography of ARF. *Sem Dial* 1996;9:438.
26. Levy EM, Viscoli CM, Horwitz RI. The effect of ARF on mortality. *JAMA* 1996;275:1489.
27. Star RA. Treatment of acute renal failure. *Kidney Int* 1998;54:1817.
28. Thadhani R, Pascual M, Bonventre JV. Medical progress–acute renal failure. *N Engl J Med* 1996;334:1448.
29. Haq M, Norman J, Saba SR, et al. Role of IL–1 in renal ischemic reperfusion injury. *J Am Soc Nephrol* 1998;9:614.
30. Schrier RW, Wang W, Poole B, et al. Acute renal failure: definitions, diagnosis, pathogenesis, and therapy. *J Clin Invest* 2004;114:5 (erratum appears in *J Clin Invest* 2004;114:598.)
31. McCarthy JT. Prognosis of patients with acute renal failure in the intensive-care unit: a tale of two eras. *Mayo Clinic Proc* 1996;71:117.
32. Lieberthal W, Nigam SK. Acute renal failure: II. Experimental models of acute renal failure; imperfect but indispensable. *Am J Physiol* 2000;278:F1.
33. Tang MJ, Suresh KR, Tannen RL. Carbohydrate metabolism by primary cultures of rabbit proximal tubules. *Am J Physiol* 1898;256:C535.
34. Kroshian VM, Sheridan AM, Lieberthal W. Functional and cytoskeletal changes induced by sublethal hypoxia in proximal tubules. *Am J Physiol* 1994;266:F21.
35. Lieberthal W, Menza SA, Levine JS. Graded ATP depletion can cause necrosis or apoptosis of cultured mouse proximal tubular cells. *Am J Physiol* 1998;274:F315.

36. Soares-da-Silva P. Actin cytoskeleton, tubular sodium and the renal synthesis of dopamine. *Biochem Pharmacol* 1992;44:1883.
37. Lehtonen E, Virtanen I, Saxen L. Reorganization of intermediate filament cytoskeleton in induced metanephric mesenchyme cells is independent of tubule morphogenesis. *Dev Biol* 1985;108:481.
38. Yaqoob MM, Edelstein CL, Wieder ED, et al. Nitric oxide kinetics during hypoxia in proximal tubules: effects of acidosis and glycine. *Kidney Int* 1996;49:1314.
39. Choi KH, Edelstein CL, Gengaro PE, et al. Hypoxia induces changes in phospholipase A_2 in rat proximal tubules: evidence for multiple forms. *Am J Physiol* 1995;269:F846.
40. Alkhunaizi AM, Yaqoob MM, Edelstein CL, et al. Arachidonic acid protects against hypoxic injury in rat proximal tubules. *Kidney Int* 1996;49: 620.
41. Ling H, Edelstein CL, Gengaro PE, et al. Effect of hypoxia on tubules isolated from nitric oxide synthase knockout mice. *Kidney Int* 1998;53: 1642.
42. Edelstein CL, Wieder ED, Yaqoob MM, et al. The role of cysteine proteases in hypoxia-induced renal proximal tubular injury. *Proc Natl Acad Sci USA* 1995;92:7662.
43. Edelstein CL, Yaqoob MM, Alkhunaizi A, et al. Modulation of hypoxia-induced calpain activity in rat renal proximal tubules. *Kidney Int* 1996; 50:1150.
44. Edelstein CL, Ling H, Gengaro PE, et al. Effect of glycine on prelethal and postlethal increases in calpain activity in rat renal proximal tubules. *Kidney Int* 1997;52:1271.
45. Stemmer PM, Klee CB. Dual calcium ion regulation of calcineurin by calmodulin and calcineurin B. *Biochemistry* 1994;33:6859.
46. Wetzels JF, Yu L, Wang X, et al. Calcium modulation and cell injury in isolated rat proximal tubules. *J Pharmacol Exp Ther* 1993;267:176.
47. Bergmeyer HU. *Methods in Enzymatic Analysis,* 2nd ed. New York: Academic, 1974.
48. Edelstein CL, Shi Y, Schrier RW. Role of caspases in hypoxia-induced necrosis of rat renal proximal tubules. *J Am Soc Nephrol* 1999;10:1940.
49. Ueda N, Walker PD, Hsu S, et al. Activation of a 15-kDa endonuclease in hypoxia/reoxygenation injury without morphologic features of apoptosis. *Proc Natl Acad Sci USA* 1995;92:7202.
50. Burke TJ, Arnold PE, Gordon JA, et al. Protective effect of intrarenal calcium membrane blockers before or after renal ischemia. Functional, morphological, and mitochondrial studies. *J Clin Invest* 1984;74:1830.
51. Arnold PE, Lumlertgul D, Burke TJ, et al. In vitro versus in vivo mitochondrial calcium loading in ischemic acute renal failure. *Am J Physiol* 1985; 248:F845.
52. Arnold PE, Van Putten VJ, Lumlertgul D, et al. Adenine nucleotide metabolism and mitochondrial Ca^{2+} transport following renal ischemia. *Am J Physiol* 1986;250:F357.
53. Wetzels JF, Yu L, Shanley PF, et al. Infusion of glycine does not attenuate in vivo ischemic acute renal failure in the rat. *J Lab Clin Med* 1993;121:263.
54. Beeri R, Symon Z, Brezis M, et al. Rapid DNA fragmentation from hypoxia along the thick ascending limb of rat kidneys. *Kidney Int* 1995;47:1806.
55. Alejandro VS, Nelson WJ, Huie P, et al. Postischemic injury, delayed function and NaK-ATPase distribution in the transplanted kidney. *Kidney Int* 1995;48:1308.
56. Kwon O, Corrigan G, Myers BD, et al. Sodium reabsoption and distribution of NaK-ATPase during postischemic injury to the renal allograft. *Kidney Int* 1999;55:963.
57. Alejandro V, Scandling JD, Sibley RK, et al. Mechanisms of filtration failure during postischemic injury of the human kidney. A study of the reperfused renal allograft. *J Clin Invest* 1995;95:820.
58. Westhuyzen J, Endre ZH, Reece G, et al. Measurement of tubular enzymuria facilitates early detection of acute renal impairment in the intensive care unit. *Nephrol Dial Transplant* 2003;18:543.
59. Rabb H. Evaluation of urinary markers in acute renal failure. *Curr Opin Nephrol Hypertens* 1998;7:681.
60. Rabb H. Novel urinary markers for early diagnosis of ARF. *Am J Kidney Dis* 2003;42:599.
61. Melnikov VY, Ecder T, Fantuzzi G, et al. Impaired IL-18 processing protects caspase-1-deficient mice from ischemic acute renal failure. *J Clin Invest* 2001;107:1145.
62. Han WK, Bailly V, Abichandani R, et al. Kidney injury molecule-1 (KIM-1): a novel biomarker for human renal proximal tubule injury. *Kidney Int* 2002;62:237.
63. Muramatsu Y, Tsujie M, Kohda Y, et al. Early detection of cysteine rich protein 61 (CYR61, CCN1) in urine following renal ischemic reperfusion injury. *Kidney Int* 2002;62:1601.
64. Mishra J, Ma Q, Prada A, et al. Identification of neutrophil gelatinase-associated lipocalin as a novel early urinary biomarker for ischemic renal injury. *J Am Soc Nephrol* 2003;14:2534.
65. du CD, Daubin C, Poggioli J, et al. Urinary measurement of Na+/H+ exchanger isoform 3 (NHE3) protein as new marker of tubule injury in critically ill patients with ARF. *Am J Kidney Dis* 2003;42:497.
66. Parikh CR, Jani A, Melnikov VY, et al. Urinary interleukin-18 is a marker of human acute tubular necrosis. *Am J Kidney Dis* 2004;43:405.
67. Kwon O, Molitoris BA, Pescovitz M, et al. Urinary actin, interleukin-6, and interleukin-8 may predict sustained arf after ischemic injury in renal allografts. *Am J Kidney Dis* 2003;41:1074.
68. Mishra J, Dent C, Tarabishi R, et al. Neutrophil gelatinase associated lipocalin (NGAL) as a biomarker for acute renal injury following cardiac surgery. *Lancet* 2005;365;1205.
69. Parikh C, Abraham E, Ancukiewicz M, et al. Urine IL-18 is an early diagnostic marker for acute kidney injury and predicts mortality in the intensive care unit *J Am Soc Nephrol* 2005;16:3046.
70. Herget-Rosenthal S, Marggraf G, Husing J, et al. Early detection of acute renal failure by serum cystatin C. *Kidney Int* 2004;66:1115.
71. Mehta RL, McDonald B, Gabbai F, et al. Nephrology consultation in acute renal failure: does timing matter? *Am J Med* 2002;113:456.
72. Lieberthal W. Biology of acute renal failure: therapeutic implications. *Kidney Int* 1997;52:1102.
73. Myers BD, Chui F, Hilberman M, et al. Transtubular leakage of glomerular filtrate in human acute renal failure. *Am J Physiol* 1979;237:F319.
74. Denker BM, Nigam SK. Molecular structure and assembly of the tight junction. *Am J Physiol* 1998;274:F1.
75. Gopalakrishnan S, Raman N, Atkinson SJ, et al. Rho GTPase signaling regulates tight junction assembly and protects tight junctions during ATP depletion. *Am J Physiol* 1998;275:C798.
76. Ye J, Tsukamoto T, Sun A, et al. A role for intracellular calcium in tight junction reassembly after ATP depletion-repletion. *Am J Physiol* 1999;277: F524.
77. Canfield PE, Geerdes AM, Molitoris BA. Effect of reversible ATP depletion on tight-junction integrity in LLC- PK1 cells. *Am J Physiol* 1991;261: F1038.
78. Molitoris BA. Ischemia-induced loss of epithelial polarity: potential role of the actin cytoskeleton (editorial). *Am J Physiol* 1991;260:F769.
79. Mandel LJ, Bacallao R, Zampighi G. Uncoupling of the molecular "fence" and paracellular "gate" functions in epithelial tight junctions. *Nature* 1993; 361:552.
80. Tsukamoto T, Nigam SK. Tight junction proteins form large complexes and associate with the cytoskeleton in an ATP depletion model for reversible junction assembly. *J Biol Chem* 1997;272:16133.
81. Molitoris BA. Putting the actin cytoskeleton into perspective: pathophysiology of ischemic alterations. *Am J Physiol* 1997;272:F430.
82. Raman N, Atkinson SJ. Rho controls actin cytoskeletal assembly in renal epithelial cells during ATP depletion and recovery. *Am J Physiol* 1999;276: C1312.
83. Sinha D, Wang Z, Price VR, et al. Chemical anoxia of tubular cells induces activation of c-Src and its translocation to the zonula adherens. *Am J Physiol Renal Fluid Electrolyte Physiol* 2003;284:F488.
84. Rajasekaran AK, Rajasekaran SA. Role of Na-K-ATPase in the assembly of tight junctions. *Am J Physiol Renal Fluid Electrolyte Physiol* 2003;285: F388.
85. Almers W, Stirling C. Distribution of transport proteins over animal cell membranes. *J Membr Biol* 1984;77:169.
86. Miller TR, Anderson RJ, Linas SL, et al. Urinary diagnostic indices in acute renal failure: a prospective study. *Ann Int Med* 1978;89:47.
87. Molitoris BA. Ischemia-induced loss of epithelial polarity: potential role of the cytoskeleton. *Am J Physiol* 1991;260:F769.
88. Lieberthal W, Nigam SK. Acute renal failure. Relative importance of proximal vs. distal tubular injury. *Am J Physiol* 1998;275:F623.
89. Kellerman P, Clark RA, Hoilen CA, et al. Role of microfilaments in maintenance of proximal tubule structure and functional integrity. *Am J Physiol* 1990;259:F279.
90. Molitoris BA, Leiser J, Wagner MC. Role of the actin cytoskeleton in ischemia-induced cell injury and repair. *Pediatr Nephrol* 1997;11:761.
91. Mills JW, Mandel LJ. Cytoskeletal regulation of membrane transport events. *FASEB J* 1994;8:1161.
92. Chen J, Doctor B, Mandel LJ. Cytoskeletal dissociation of ezrin during renal anoxia. Role in microvillar injury. *Am J Physiol* 1994;36:C784.
93. Chen J, Mandel LJ. Unopposed phosphatase action initiates ezrin dysfunction: a potential mechanism for anoxic injury. *Am J Physiol* 1997;273: C710.
94. Bacallao R, Garfinkel A, Monke S, et al. ATP depletion: a novel method to study junctional properties in epithelial tissues. I. Rearrangement of the actin cytoskeleton. *J Cell Sci* 1994;107:3301.
95. Molitoris BA, Geerdes A, McIntosh JR. Dissociation and redistribution of Na^+, K^+-ATPase from its surface membrane cytoskeletal complex during cellular ATP depletion. *J Clin Invest* 1991;88:462.
96. Molitoris BA, Dahl R, Geerdes AE. Cytoskeleton disruption and apical redistribution of proximal tubule Na^+ K^+ ATPase during ischemia. *Am J Physiol* 1992;263:F488.
97. Mandel LJ, Doctor RB, Bacallao R. ATP depletion: a novel method to study junctional properties in epithelial tissues. II. Internalization of Na+,K(+)-ATPase and E- cadherin. *J Cell Sci* 1994;107:3315.
98. Molitoris BA. Na(+)-K(+)-ATPase that redistributes to apical membrane during ATP depletion remains functional. *Am J Physiol* 1993;265:F693.
99. Woroniecki R, Ferdinand JR, Morrow JS, et al. Dissociation of spectrin-ankyrin complex as a basis for loss of Na-K-ATPase polarity after ischemia. *Am J Physiol Renal Fluid Electrolyte Physiol* 2003;284:F358.
100. Weinberg JM. Oxygen deprivation-induced injury to isolated rabbit kidney tubules. *J Clin Invest* 1985;76:1193.
101. Weinberg JM, Davis JA, Venkatachalam MA. Cytosolic-free calcium increases to greater than 100 micromolar in ATP-depleted proximal tubules. *J Clin Invest* 1997;100:713.

102. Nurko S, Sogabe K, Davis JA, et al. Contribution of actin cytoskeletal alterations to ATP depletion and calcium-induced proximal tubule cell injury. *Am J Physiol* 1996;270:F39.
103. Kribben A, Wieder ED, Wetzels JF, et al. Evidence for role of cytosolic free calcium in hypoxia-induced proximal tubule injury. *J Clin Invest* 1994;93:1922.
104. Linas SL, Whittenburg D, Repine JE. Role of xanthine oxidase in ischemia/reperfusion injury. *Am J Physiol* 1990;258:F711.
105. Doctor RB, Mandel LJ. Minimal role of xanthine oxidase and oxygen free radicals in rat renal tubular reoxygenation injury. *J Am Soc Nephrol* 1991;1:959.
106. Siegel NJ, Glazier WB, Chaudry IH, et al. Enhanced recovery from acute renal failure by the postischemic infusin of adenine nucleotides and magnesium chloride in rats. *Kidney Int* 1980;17:338.
107. Lee HT, Emala CW. Protective effects of renal ischemic preconditioning and adenosine pretreatment: role of A(1) and A(3) receptors. *Am J Physiol Renal Physiol* 2000;278:F380.
108. Okusa MD, Linden J, Huang L, et al. A(2A) adenosine receptor-mediated inhibition of renal injury and neutrophil adhesion. *Am J Physiol Renal Fluid Electrolyte Physiol* 2000;279:F809.
109. Okusa MD, Linden J, Macdonald T, et al. Selective A2A adenosine receptor activation reduces ischemia-reperfusion injury in rat kidney. *Am J Physiol* 1999;277:F404.
110. Okusa MD, Linden J, Huang L, et al. Enhanced protection from renal ischemia-reperfusion (correction of ischemia: reperfusion) injury with A(2A)-adenosine receptor activation and PDE 4 inhibition. (erratum appears in Kidney Int 2001 Aug;60[2]:820). *Kidney Int* 2001;59:2114.
111. Day YJ, Huang L, McDuffie MJ, et al. Renal protection from ischemia mediated by A2A adenosine receptors on bone marrow-derived cells. *J Clin Invest* 2003;112:883.
112. Okusa MD. A(2A) adenosine receptor: a novel therapeutic target in renal disease. *Am J Physiol Renal Fluid Electrolyte Physiol* 2002;282:F10.
113. Weinberg JM. The cell biology of ischemic renal injury. *Kidney Int* 1991;39:476.
114. Cheung JY, Bonventre JV, Malis CD, et al. Calcium and ischemic injury. *N Engl J Med* 1986;314:1670.
115. Schrier RW, Arnold PE, Van Putten VJ, et al. Cellular calcium in ischemic acute renal failure: role of calcium entry blockers. *Kidney Int* 1987;32:313.
116. Schrier RW, Gardenswartz MH, Burke TJ. Acute renal failure: pathogenesis, diagnosis and treatment. *Adv Nephrol Necker Hosp* 1981;10:213.
117. Schrier RW, Burke TJ, Conger JD, et al. New aspects of acute renal failure. In: Anonymous ed. *Proceedings of the 8th International Congress of Nephrology.* Athens: Basel, S. Karger, 1981:63.
118. Neumayer HH, Wagner K. Prevention of delayed graft function in cadaver kidney transplants by diltiazem: outcome of two prospective, randomized clinical trials. *J Cardio Pharm* 1987;10:S170.
119. Wagner K, Albrecht S, Neumayer HH. Prevention of posttransplant acute tubular necrosis by the calcium antagonist diltiazem: a prospective randomized study. *Am J Nephrol* 1987;7:287.
120. Bakris GL, Burnett JC. A role for calcium in radiocontrast-induced reduction in renal hemodynamics. *Kidney Int* 1985;27:465.
121. Burke TJ, Schrier RW. Pathophysiology of cell ischemia. In: RW Schrier, PE Arnold, CW Gottschalk, eds. *Diseases of the kidney.* Boston: Little, Brown & Co., 1992:1257.
122. Schrier RW, Arnold PE, Van Putten VJ, et al. Cellular calcium in ischemic acute renal failure: role of calcium entry blockers. *Kidney Int* 1987;32:313.
123. Cheung JY, Constantine JM, Bonventre JV. Regulation of cytosolic free calcium concentration in cultured renal epithelial cells. *Am J Physiol* 1986;251:F690.
124. Bonventre JV, Cheung JY. Cytosolic free calcium concentration in cultured renal epithelial cells. *Am J Physiol* 1986;250:F329.
125. Wilson PD, Schrier RW. Nephron segment and calcium as determinants of anoxic cell death in primary renal cell cultures. *Kidney Int* 1986;29:1172.
126. Schwertschlag U, Schrier RW, Wilson P. Beneficial effects of calcium channel blockers and calmodulin binding drugs on in vitro renal cell anoxia. *J Pharmacol Exp Ther* 1986;238:119.
127. Almeida AR, Bunnachak D, Burnier M, et al. Time-dependent protective effects of calcium channel blockers on anoxia and hypoxia-induced proximal tubule injury. *J Pharmacol Exp Ther* 1992;260:526.
128. Joseph JK, Bunnachak D, Burke TJ, et al. A novel method of inducing and assuring total anoxia during in vitro studies of O_2 deprivation injury. *J Am Soc Nephrol* 1990;1:837.
129. Almeida AR, Wetzels JF, Bunnachak D, et al. Acute phosphate depletion and in vitro rat proximal tubule injury: protection by glycine and acidosis. *Kidney Int* 1992;41:1494.
130. Burnier M, Van Putten VJ, Schieppati A, et al. Effect of extracellular acidosis on 45Ca uptake in isolated hypoxic proximal tubules. *Am J Physiol* 1988;254:C839.
131. Koo WS, Gengaro PE, Burke TJ, et al. Verapamil attenuates calcium-induced mitochondrial swelling and respiratory dysfunction. *J Pharmacol Exp Ther* 1995;273:206.
132. Wetzels JF, Wang X, Gengaro PE, et al. Glycine protection against hypoxic but not phospholipase A_2- induced injury in rat proximal tubules. *Am J Physiol* 1993;264:F94.
133. Bunnachak D, Almeida AR, Wetzels JF, et al. Ca^{2+} uptake, fatty acid, and LDH release during proximal tubule hypoxia: effects of mepacrine and dibucaine. *Am J Physiol* 1994;266:F196.
134. Dowd TL, Gupta RK. Multinuclear NMR studies of intracellular cations in perfused hypertensive rat kidney. *J Biol Chem* 1992;267:3637.
135. Gupta RK, Dowd TL, Spitzer A, et al. 23Na, 19F, 35Cl and 31P multinuclear nuclear magnetic resonance studies of perfused rat kidney. *Ren Physiol Biochem* 1989;12:144.
136. Peters SM, Tijsen MJ, Bindels RJ, et al. Rise in cytosolic calcium and collapse of mitochondrial potential in anoxic, but not hypoxic, rat proximal tubules. *J Am Soc Nephrol* 1998;7:2348.
137. Edelstein CL, Alkhunaizi AA, Schrier RW. The role of calcium in the pathogenesis of acute renal failure. *Ren Fail* 1997;19:199.
138. Edelstein CL, Yaqoob MM, Schrier RW. The role of the calcium-dependent enzymes nitric oxide synthase and calpain in hypoxia-induced proximal tubule injury. *Ren Fail* 1996;18:501.
139. Kribben A, Wetzels JF, Wieder ED, et al. New technique to assess hypoxia-induced cell injury in individual isolated renal tubules. *Kidney Int* 1993;43:464.
140. Peters SM, Tijsen MJ, Vas Os CH, et al. Hypoxia decreases calcium infux into proximal tubules. *Kidney Int* 1998;53:703.
141. Waters SL, Wong JK, Schnellmann RG. Depletion of endoplasmic reticulum calcium stores protects against hypoxia and mitochondrial inhibitor-induced cellular injury and death. *Biochem. Biophys. Res Comm* 1997;240:57.
142. Sogabe K, Roeser NF, Davis JA, et al. Calcium dependence of integrity of actin cytoskeleton of proximal tubule microvilli. *Am J Physiol* 1996;271:F292.
143. Edelstein CL, Ling H, Schrier RW. The nature of renal cell injury. *Kidney Int* 1997;51:1341.
144. Edelstein CL. Editorial Comment: Calcium-mediated proximal tubular injury-what is the role of cysteine proteases? *Nephrol Dial Transplant* 2000;15:141.
145. Brown D, Lee R, Bonventre JV. Redistribution of villin to proximal tubule basolateral membranes after ischemia and reperfusion. *Am J Physiol* 1997;273:F1003.
146. Molitoris BA: Actin cytoskeleton in ischemic acute renal failure. *Kidney Int* 2004;66:871.
147. Atkinson SJ, Hosford MA, Molitoris BA. Mechanism of actin polymerization in cellular ATP depletion. *J Biol Chem* 2004;279:5194.
148. Ashworth SL, Wean SE, Campos SB, et al. Renal ischemia induces tropomyosin dissociation-destabilizing microvilli microfilaments. *Am J Physio Renal Fluid Electrolyte Physio* 2004;286:F988.
149. Bonventre JV. Phospholipase A2 and signal transduction. *J Am Soc Nephrol* 1992;3:128.
150. Bonventre JV. Calcium in renal cells. Modulation of calcium-dependent activation of phospholipase A2. *Environ Health Perspect* 1990;84:155.
151. Portilla D, Shah SV, Lehman PA, et al. Role of cytosolic calcium-independent plasmalogen-selective phospholipase A2 in hypoxic injury to rabbit proximal tubules. *J Clin Invest* 1994;93:1609.
152. Matthys EY, Patel Y, Kreisberg J, et al. Lipid alterations induced by renal ischemia: pathogenic factor in membrane damage. *Kidney Int* 1984;26:153.
153. Humes HD, Nguyen VD, Cielinski DA. The role of free fatty acids in hypoxia-induced injury to proximal tubules. *Am J Physiol* 1989;256:F688.
154. Zager RA, Burkhart KM, Conrad DS, et al. Phospholipase A2-induced cytoprotection of proximal tubules: potential determinants and specificity for ATP depletion mediated injury. *J Am Soc Nephrol* 1996;7:64.
155. Chen Y, Morimoto S, Kitano S, et al. Lysophosphatidylcholine causes calcium influx, enhanced DNA synthesis and cytotoxicity in cultured vascular smooth muscle cells. *Atherosclerosis* 1995;112:69.
156. Bonventre JV, Huang Z, Taheri MR, et al. Reduced fertility and postischaemic brain injury in mice deficient in cytosolic phospholipase A2. *Nature* 1997;390:622.
157. Bronk SF, Gores GJ. pH dependent non-lysosomal proteolysis contributes to lethal ionic injury of rat hepatocytes. *Am J Physiol* 1993;264:G744.
158. Plomp PJ, Gordon PD, Meijen AJ, et al. Energy dependence of different steps in the autophagic-lysosomal pathway. *J Biol Chem* 1989;264:6699.
159. Hawkins HK, Ericsson JL, Biberfield P, et al. Lysosomal and phagosome stability in lethal cell injury. *Am J Path* 1972;68:255.
160. Suzuki K. Calcium activated neutral protease: domain structure and activity regulation. *Trends Biochem Sci* 1987;12.
161. Barrett MJ, Goll DE, Thompson VF. Effect of substrate on Ca2(+)-concentration required for activity of the Ca2(+)-dependent proteinases, mu- and m-calpain. *Life Sci* 1991;48:1659.
162. Yoshimura N, Hatanaka M, Kitahara A, et al. Intracellular localization of two distinct Ca2+ proteases (calpain I and II) as demonstrated using discriminative antibodies. *J Biol Chem* 1984;259:9847.
163. Sorimachi H, Saido TC, Suzuki K. New era of calpain research. Discovery of tissue-specific calpains. *FEBS Letters* 1994;343:1.
164. Suzuki K, Saido TC, Hirai S. Modulation of cellular signals by calpain. *Ann NY Acad Sci* 1992;674:218.
165. Mellgren RL. Calcium dependent proteases: an enzyme system active at cellular membranes? *FASEB* 1987;1:110.
166. Kumamoto T, Ueyama H, Watanabe S, et al. Immunohistochemical study of calpain and its endogenous inhibitor in the skeletal muscle of muscular dystrophy. *Acta Neuropathologica.* 1995;89:399.

167. Komatsu K, Inazuki K, Hosoya J, et al. Beneficial effect of new thiol protease inhibitors, epoxide derivatives, on dystrophic mice. *Exp Neurol* 1986; 91:23.
168. Nakamura M, Mori M, Nakazawa S, et al. Replacement of m-calpain byu-calpain during maturation of megakaryocytes and possible involvement in platelet formation. *Thromb Res* 1992;66:757.
169. Giancotti FG, Stepp MA, Suzuki S, et al. Proteolytic processing of endogenous and recombinant B4 integrin. *J Cell Biol* 1992;118:951.
170. Covault J, Liu QY, Eil Deeb S. Calcium activated proteolysis of intracellular domains of cell adhesion molecules NCAM and N-adherin. *Mol Brain Res* 1991;11:11.
171. Seubert P, Lee KS, Lynch G. Ischemia triggers NMDA receptor linked cytoskeletal proteolysis in hippocampus. *Brain Res* 1989;492:366.
172. Lee KS, Frank S, Vanderklish P, et al. Inhibition of proteolysis protects hippocampal neurons from ischemia. *Proc Natl Acad Sci USA* 1991;88:7233.
173. Lizuka K, Kawaguchi H, Yasuda H. Calpain is activated during hypoxic myocardial cell injury. *Biochem Med Metab Biol* 1991;46:427.
174. Tolnadi S, Korecky B. Calcium dependent proteolysis and its inhibition in ischemic rat myocardium. *Can J Cardiol* 1986;2:442.
175. Yang X, Schnellmann RG. Proteinases in renal cell death. *J Toxicol Environ Health* 1996;48:319.
176. Tijsen MJ, Peters SM, Bindels RJ, et al. Glycine protection against hypoxic injury in isolated rat proximal tubules: the role of proteases. *Nephrol Dial Transplant* 1997;12:2549.
177. Shi Y, Melnikov VY, Schrier RW, et al. Downregulation of the calpain inhibitor protein calpastatin by caspases during renal ischemia-reperfusion. *Am J Physio Renal Fluid Electrolyte Physio* 2000;279:F509.
178. Weinberg JM, Davis JA, Roeser NF, et al. Role of increased cytosolic free calcium in the pathogenesis of rabbit proximal tubule cell injury and protection by glycine or acidosis. *J Clin Invest* 1991;87:581.
179. Liu X, Schnellmann RG. Calpain mediates progressive plasma membrane permeability and proteolysis of cytoskeleton-associated paxillin, talin, and vinculin during renal cell death. *J Pharmacol Exp Ther* 2003;304:63.
180. Liu X, Harriman JF, Schnellmann RG. Cytoprotective properties of novel nonpeptide calpain inhibitors in renal cells. *J Pharmacol Exp Ther* 2002;302:88.
181. Barinaga M. Cell suicide: by ICE, not fire. *Science* 1994;263:754.
182. Salvesen GS, Dixit VM. Caspases: intracellular signaling by proteolysis. *Cell* 1997;91:443.
183. Fraser A, Evan G. A license to kill. *Cell* 1996;85:781.
184. Nicholson DW, Ali A, Thornberry NA, et al. Identification and inhibition of the ICE/CED-3 protease neccessary for mammalian apoptosis. *Nature* 1995;376:37.
185. Green DR. Apoptotic pathways: the roads to ruin. *Cell* 1998;94:695.
186. Kuida K, Haydar TF, Kuan CY, et al. Reduced apoptosis and cytochrome c-mediated caspase activation in mice lacking caspase 9. *Cell* 1998;94:325.
187. Hu S, Snipas SJ, Vincenz C, et al. Caspase-14 is a novel developmentally regulated protease. *J Biol Chem* 1998;273:29648.
188. Barinaga M. Death by dozens of cuts. *Science* 1998;280:32.
189. Thornberry NA, Rano TA, Peterson EP, et al. A combinatorial approach defines specificities of members of the caspase family and granzyme B. Functional relationships established for key mediators of apoptosis. *J Biol Chem* 1997;272:17907.
190. Dinarello CA. Biologic basis for interleukin-1 in disease. *Blood* 1996;87:2095.
191. Fantuzzi G, Puren AJ, Harding MW, et al. Interleukin-18 regulation of interferon gamma production and cell proliferation as shown in interleukin-1 beta-converting enzyme (caspase-1)-deficient mice. *Blood* 1998;91:2118.
192. Talanian RV, Quinlan C, Trautz S, et al. Substrate specifities of caspase family proteases. *J Biol Chem* 1998;272:9677.
193. Feldenberg LR, Thevananther S, del Rio M, et al. Partial ATP depletion induces Fas- and caspase-mediated apoptosis in MDCK cells. *Am J Physiol* 1999;276:F837.
194. Fukuoka K, Takeda M, Kobayashi M, et al. Distinct interleukin-1-beta-converting enzyme family proteases mediate cisplatin- and staurosporine-induced apoptosis of mouse proximal tubules. *Life Sci* 1998;62:1125.
195. Conaldi P, Bianconi L, Bottelli A, et al. HIV-1 kills renal tubular epithelial cells in vitro by triggering an apoptotic pathway involving caspase activation and Fas upregulation. *J Clin Invest* 1998;102:2041.
196. Krajewski S, Krajewska M, Ellerby LM, et al. Release of caspase-9 from mitochondria during neuronal apoptosis and cerebral ischemia. *Proc Natl Acad SciUSA* 1999;96:5752.
197. Kuida K, Zheng TS, Na S, et al. Decreased apoptosis in the brain and premature lethality in CPP32-deficient mice. *Nature* 1996;384:368.
198. Woo M, Hakem A, Elia AJ, et al. In vivo evidence that caspase-3 is required for Fas-mediated apoptosis of hepatocytes. *J Immunol* 1999;163:4909.
199. Colussi PA, Kumar S. Targeted disruption of caspase genes in mice: what they tell us about the functions of individual caspases in apoptosis. *Immunol Cell Biol* 1999;77:58.
200. Suzuki A. Amyloid B-protein induces necrotic cell death mediated by ICE cascade in PC12 cells. *Exp Cell Res* 1997;234:507.
201. Hara H, Friedlander RM, Gagliardini V, et al. Inhibition of interleukin 1beta converting enzyme family proteases reduces ischemic and excitotoxic neuronal damage. *Proc Natl Acad Sci USA* 1997;94:2007.
202. Loddick SA, MacKenzie A, Rothwell NJ. An ICE inhibitor, z-VAD-DCB attenuates ischaemic brain damage in the rat. *NeuroReport* 1996;7:1465.
203. Schielke GP, Yang GY, Shivers BD, et al. Reduced ischemic brain injury in interleukin-1 beta converting enzyme-deficient mice. *J Cereb Blood Flow Metab* 1998;18:180.
204. Kuida K, Lippke JA, Ku G, et al. Altered cytokine export and apoptosis in mice deficient in interleukin-1B converting enzyme. *Science* 1995;267:2000.
205. Kaushal GP, Ueda N, Shah SV. Role of caspases (ICE/CED 3 proteases) in DNA damage and cell death in response to a mitochondrial inhibitor, antimycin A. *Kidney Int* 1997;52:438.
206. Shimizu S, Eguchi Y, Kamiike W, et al. Retardation of chemical hypoxia-induced necrotic cell death by Bcl-2 and ICE inhibitors: possible involvement of common mediators in apoptotic and necrotic signal transductions. *Oncogene* 1996;12:2045.
207. Harrison-Shostak DC, Lemasters JJ, Edgell CJ, et al. Role of ICE-like proteases in endothelial cell hypoxic and reperfusion injury. *Biochem Biophys Res Comm* 1997;844.
208. Kaushal GP, Singh AB, Shah SV. Identification of gene family of caspases in rat kidney and altered expression in ischemia reperfusion injury. *Am J Physiol* 1998;274:F587.
209. Kaushal GP. Role of caspases in renal tubular epithelial cell injury. *Semin Nephrol* 2003;23:425.
210. Singh AB, Kaushal V, Megyesi JK, et al. Cloning and expression of rat caspase-6 and its localization in renal ischemia/reperfusion injury. *Kidney Int* 2002;62:106.
211. Daemen MA, Van t'Veer C, Denecker G, et al. Inhibition of apoptosis induced by ischemia-reperfusion prevents inflammation. *J Clin Invest* 1999;104:541.
212. Kyllonen LE, Salmela KT, Eklund BH, et al. Long-term results of 1047 cadaveric kidney transplantations with special emphasis on initial graft function and rejection. *Transplant Int* 2000;13:122.
213. Gjertson DW. Impact of delayed graft function and acute rejection on kidney graft survival. *Clin Transplants* 2000;467.
214. Hetzel GR, Klein B, Brause M, et al. Risk factors for delayed graft function after renal transplantation and their significance for long-term clinical outcome. *Transplant Int* 2002;15:10.
215. Ojo AO, Wolfe RA, Held PJ, et al. Delayed graft function: risk factors and implications for renal allograft survival. *Transplantation* 1997;63:968.
216. Castaneda MP, Swiatecka-Urban A, Mitsnefes MM, et al. Activation of mitochondrial apoptotic pathways in human renal allografts after ischemia-reperfusion injury. *Transplantation* 2003;76:50.
217. Oberbauer R, Rohrmoser M, Regele H, et al. Apoptosis of tubular epithelial cells in donor kidney biopsies predicts early renal allograft function. *J Am Soc Nephrol* 1999;10:2006.
218. Nakagawa K, Koo DD, Davies DR, et al. Lecithinized superoxide dismutase reduces cold ischemia-induced chronic allograft dysfunction. *Kidney Int* 2002;61:1160.
219. Jassem W, Heaton ND. The role of mitochondria in ischemia/reperfusion injury in organ transplantation. *Kidney Int* 2004;66:514.
220. Jani A, Ljubanovic D, Faubel SG, et al. Caspase inhibition prevents the increase in caspase-3,-2,-8 and 9 activity and apoptosis in the cold ischemic mouse kidney. *Am J Transplant* 2004;4:1246.
221. Natori S, Selzner M, Valentino KL, et al. Apoptosis of sinusoidal endothelial cells occurs during liver preservation injury by a caspase-dependent mechanism. *Transplantation* 1999;68:89.
222. Natori S, Higuchi H, Contreras P, et al. The caspase inhibitor IDN-6556 prevents caspase activation and apoptosis in sinusoidal endothelial cells during liver preservation injury. *Liver Transpl* 2003;9:278.
223. Valentino KL, Gutierrez M, Sanchez R, et al. First clinical trial of a novel caspase inhibitor: anti-apoptotic caspase inhibitor, IDN-6556, improves liver enzymes. *Int J Clin Pharmacol Ther* 2003;41:441.
224. Kwon MP, Bonventre JV. Castration protects male mice against ischemic acute renal failure. A critical role for testosterone and leukocyte trapping in the outer medulla. *J Am Soc Nephrol* 2000;11:594A.
225. Melnikov VY, Faubel SG, Siegmund B, et al. Neutrophil-independent mechanisms of caspase-1- and IL-18-mediated ischemic acute tubular necrosis in mice. *J Clin Invest* 2002;110:1083.
226. Chatterjee PK, Todorovic Z, Sivarajah A, et al. Differential effects of caspase inhibitors on the renal dysfunction and injury caused by ischemia-reperfusion in rat kidney. *Eur J Pharmacol* 2004;503:173.
227. Daemen MA, Denecker G, Van't Veer C, et al. Activated caspase-1 is not a central mediator of inflammation in the course of ischemia-reperfusion. *Transplantation* 2001;71:778.
228. Faubel SG, Ljubanovic D, Reznikov LL, et al. Caspase-1-deficient mice are protected against cisplatin-induced apoptosis and acute tubular necrosis. *Kidney Int* 2004;66:2202.
229. Lenz O, Elliot SJ, Stetler-Stevenson WG. Matrix metalloproteinases in renal development and disease. *J Am Soc Nephrol* 2000;11:574.
230. Walker PD. Alterations in renal tubular extracellular matrix components after ischemia-reperfusion injury to the kidney. *Lab Invest* 1994;70:339.
231. Walker PD, Kaushal GP, Shah SV. Meprin A, the major matrix degrading enzyme in renal tubules, produces a novel nidogen fragment in vitro and in vivo. *Kidney Int* 1998;53:1673.
232. Trachtman H, Valderrama E, Dietrich JM, et al. The role of meprin A in the pathogenesis of acute renal failure. *Biochem Biophys Res Commun* 1995;208:498.

233. Carmago S, Shah SV, Walker PD. Meprin, a brush-border enzyme, plays an important role in hypoxic/ischemic acute renal tubular injury in rats. *Kidney Int* 2002;61:959.

234. Walker PD, Kaushal GP, Shah SV. Presence of a distinct extracellular matrix-degrading metalloproteinase activity in renal tubules. *J Am Soc Nephrol* 1994;5:55.

235. Lane P, Gross SS. Cell signaling by nitric oxide. *Semin Nephrol* 1999;19: 215.

236. Kone BC. Localization and regulation of nitric oxide synthase isoforms in the kidney. *Semin Nephrol* 1999;19:230.

237. Bachman S, Bosse HM, Mundel P. Topography of nitric oxide synthesis by localizing constitutive NO synthases in mammalian kidney. *Am J Physiol* 1995;268:F885.

238. Wilcox CS, Welch WJ, Murad F, et al. Nitric oxide synthase in macula densa regulates glomerular capillary pressure. *Proc Natl Acad Sci USA* 1992;89:11993.

239. Ahn KY, Mohaupt MG, Madsen KM, et al. In situ hybridization localization of mRNA encoding inducible nitric oxide synthase in rat kidney. *Am J Physiol* 1994;267:F748.

240. Ujiie K, Yuen J, Hogarth L, et al. Localization and regulation of endothelial NO synthase mRNA expression in rat kidney. *Am J Physiol* 1994;267:F296.

241. Knowles RG, Moncada S. Nitric oxide synthases in mammals. *Biochem J* 1994;298:249.

242. Kone BC. Nitric oxide in renal health and disease. *Am J Kidney Dis* 1997; 30:311.

243. Moncada S, Palmer RM, Higgs EA. Nitric oxide: physiology, pathophysiology, and pharmacology. *Pharmacol Rev* 1991;43:109.

244. Morris SM, Billiar TR. New insights into the regulation of inducible nitric oxide synthase. *Am J Physiol* 1994;266:E829.

245. Komurai M, Ishii Y, Matsuoka F, et al. Role of nitric oxide synthase activity in experimental ischemic acute renal failure in rats. *Mol Cell Biochem* 2003;244:129.

246. Schneider R, Raff U, Vornberger N, et al. L-Arginine counteracts nitric oxide deficiency and improves the recovery phase of ischemic acute renal failure in rats. *Kidney Int* 2003;64:216.

247. Ling H, Edelstein CL, Gengaro P, et al. Attenuation of renal ischemia-reperfusion injury in inducible nitric oxide synthase knockout mice. *Am J Physiol* 1999;277:F383.

248. Chiao H, Kohda Y, McLeroy P, et al. Alpha-melanocyte-stimulating hormone protects against renal injury after ischemia in mice and rats. *J Clin Invest* 1997;99:1165.

249. Chiao H, Kohda Y, McLeroy P, et al. Alpha-melanocyte-stimulating hormone inhibits renal injury in the absence of neutrophils. *Kidney Int* 1998;54:765.

250. Kohda Y, Chiao H, Star RA. Alpha-Melanocyte-stimulating hormone and acute renal failure. *Curr Opin Nephrol Hypertens* 1998;7:413.

251. Yu L, Gengaro PE, Niederberger M, et al. Nitric oxide: a mediator in rat tubular hypoxia/reoxygenation injury. *Proc Natl Acad Sci USA* 1994;91: 1691.

252. Noiri E, Peresleni T, Miller F, et al. In vivo targeting of inducible NO synthase with oligodeoxynucleotides protects rat kidney against ischemia. *J Clin Invest* 1996;97:2377.

253. Gabbai FB, Blantz RC. Role of nitric oxide in renal hemodynamics. *Semin Nephrol* 1999;19:242.

254. Goligorsky MS, Noiri E. Duality of nitric oxide in acute renal injury. *Semin Nephrol* 1999;19:263.

255. Noiri E, Dickman K, Miller F, et al. Reduced tolerance to acute renal ischemia in mice with a targeted disruption of the osteopontin gene. *Kidney Int* 1999;56:74.

256. Noiri E, Peresleni T, Srivastava N, et al. Nitric oxide is necessary for the switch from stationary to locomoting phenotype in epithelial cells. *Am J Physiol* 1996;270:C794.

257. Goligorsky MS. Abnormalities of integrin receptors. In: MS Goligorsky, J Stein, eds. *Acute renal failure—new concepts and therapeutic strategies,* 1st ed. New York: Churchill Livingstone, 1995:255.

258. Goligorsky MS, Lieberthal W, Racusen LC, et al. Integrin receptors in renal tubular epithelium: new insights into pathophysiology of acute renal failure [editorial]. *Am J Physiol* 1993;264:F1.

259. Weinberg JM, Davis JA, Abarzua M, et al. Cytoprotective effects of glycine and glutathione against hypoxic injury to renal tubules. *J Clin Invest* 1987;80:1446.

260. Weinberg JM, Davis JA, Abarzua M, et al. Protection by glycine of proximal tubules from injury due to inhibitors of mitochondrial ATP production. *Am J Physiol* 1996;258:C1127.

261. Venkatachalam MA, Weinberg JM. Mechanisms of cell injury in ATP-depleted proximal tubules. Role of glycine, calcium, and polyphosphoinositides. *Nephrol Dial Transplant* 1994;9:15.

262. Garza-Quintero R, Weinberg JM, Ortega-Lopez J, et al. Conservation of structure in ATP-depleted proximal tubules: role of calcium, polyphosphoinositides, and glycine. *Am J Physiol* 1993;265:F605.

263. Weinberg JM, Roeser NF, Davis JA, et al. Relationships between intracellular aminoacid levels and protection against injury to isolated proximal tubules. *Am J Physiol* 1991;260:410.

264. Nichols JC, Bronk SF, Mellgren RL, et al. Inhibition of nonlysosomal calcium-dependent proteolysis by glycine during anoxic injury of rat hepatocytes. *Gastroenterology* 1994;106:168.

265. Miller GW, Lock EA, Schnellmann RG. Strychnine and glycine protect renal proximal tubules from various nephrotoxicants and act in the late phase necrotic cell injury. *Toxic Appl Physiol* 1996;125:192.

266. Weinberg JM, Varani J, Johnson KJ, et al. Protection of human umbilical vein endothelial cells by glycine and structurally similar amino acids against calcium and hydrogen peroxide-induced lethal cell injury. *Am J Pathol* 1992;140:457.

267. Craig EA, Weissman JS, Horwich AL. Heat shock proteins and molecular chaperones: mediators of protein conformation and turnover in the cell. *Cell* 1994;78:365.

268. Kashgarian M. Stress proteins induced by injury to epithelial cells. In: MS Goligorsky, J Stein, eds. *Acute renal failure-new concepts and therapeutic strategies,* 1st ed. New York: Churchill Livingstone, 1995:75.

269. Van Why SK, Hildebrandt F, Ardiro T, et al. Induction and intracellular localization of HSP-72 after renal ischemia. *Am J Physiol* 1992;263:F769.

270. Emami A, Schwartz JH, Borkan SC. Transient ischemia or heat stress induces a cytoprotectant protein in rat kidney. *Am J Physiol* 1991;260:F479.

271. Van Why SK, Mann AS, Thulin G, et al. Activation of heat-shock transcription factor by graded reductions in renal ATP, in vivo, in the rat. *J Clin Invest* 1994;94:1518.

272. Smoyer WE, Ransom R, Harris RC, et al. Ischemic acute renal failure induces differential expression of small heat shock proteins. *J Am Soc Nephrol* 2000;11:211.

273. Wang YH, Borkan SC. Prior heat stress enhances survival of renal epithelial cells after ATP depletion. *Am J Physiol* 1996;270:F1057.

274. Turman MA, Rosenfeld SL. Heat shock protein 70 overexpression protects LLC-PK1 tubular cells from heat shock but not hypoxia. *Kidney Int* 1999;55:189.

275. Chatson G, Perdrizet G, Anderson C, et al. Heat shock protects kidneys against warm ischemic injury. *Curr Surg* 1990;47:420.

276. Joannidis M, Cantley LG, Spokes K, et al. Induction of heat-shock proteins does not prevent renal tubular injury following ischemia. *Kidney Int* 1995;47:1752.

277. Gaudio KM, Thulin G, Mann A, et al. Role of heat stress response in the tolerance of immature renal tubules to anoxia. *Am J Physiol* 1998;274:F1029.

278. Bush KT, Goldberg AL, Nigam SK. Proteasome inhibition leads to a heat-shock response, induction of endoplasmic reticulum chaperones, and thermotolerance. *J Biol Chem* 1997;272:9086.

279. Takaoka M, Itoh M, Hayashi S, et al. Proteasome participates in the pathogenesis of ischemic acute renal failure in rats. *Eur J Pharmacol* 1999;384:43.

280. Schober A, Burger-Kentischer A, Muller E, et al. Effect of ischemia on localization of heat shock protein 25 in kidney. *Kidney Int* 1998;67(Suppl):S174.

281. Aufricht C, Lu E, Thulin G, et al. ATP releases HSP-72 from protein aggregates after renal ischemia. *Am J Physiol* 1998;274:F268.

282. Aufricht C, Ardito T, Thulin G, et al. Heat-shock protein 25 induction and redistribution during actin reorganization after renal ischemia. *Am J Physiol* 1998;274:F215.

283. Basile DP, Donohoe D, Cao X, et al. Resistance to ischemic acute renal failure in the Brown Norway rat: a new model to study cytoprotection. *Kidney Int* 2004;65:2201.

284. Wang Y, Knowlton AA, Christensen TG, et al. Prior heat stress inhibits apoptosis in adenosine triphosphate-depleted renal tubular cells. *Kidney Int* 1999;55:2224.

285. Safirstein R, Dimari J, Megyesi J, et al. Mechanisms of renal repair and survival following acute injury. *Semin Nephrol* 1998;18:519.

286. Safirstein R. Gene expression in nephrotoxic and ischemic acute renal failure (editorial). *J Am Soc Nephrol* 1994;4:1387.

287. Bonventre JV. Pathogenetic and regenerative mechanisms in acute tubular necrosis. *Kidney Blood Press Res* 1998;21:226.

288. Megyesi J, Di Mari J, Udvarhelyi N, et al. DNA synthesis is dissociated from the immediate-early gene response in the post-ischemic kidney. *Kidney Int* 1995;48:1451.

289. Ouellette AJ, Malt RA, Sukhatme VP, et al. Expression of two "immediate early" genes, Egr-1 and c-fos, in response to renal ischemia and during compensatory renal hypertrophy in mice. *J Clin Invest* 1990;85:766.

290. Safirstein R. Renal stress response and acute renal failure. *Adv Ren Replace Ther* 1997;4:38.

291. Witzgall R, Brown D, Schwarz C, et al. Localization of proliferating cell nuclear antigen, vimentin, c-Fos, and clusterin in the postischemic kidney. Evidence for a heterogenous genetic response among nephron segments, and a large pool of mitotically active and dedifferentiated cells. *J Clin Invest* 1994;93:2175.

292. Safirstein R, Megyesi J, Saggi SJ, et al. Expression of cytokine-like genes JE and KC is increased during renal ischemia. *Am J Physiol* 1991;261:F1095.

293. Safirstein R, Price PM, Saggi SJ, et al. Changes in gene expression after temporary renal ischemia. *Kidney Int* 1990;37:1515.

294. Bonventre JV, Sukhatme VP, Bamberger M, et al. Localization of the protein product of the immediate early growth response gene, Egr-1, in the kidney after ischemia and reperfusion. *Cell Regul* 1991;2:251.

295. Ip YT, Davis RJ. Signal transduction by the c-Jun N-terminal kinase (JNK)—from inflammation to development. *Curr Opin Cell Biol* 1998;10:205.

296. Kyriakis JM, Banerjee P, Nikolakaki E, et al. The stress-activated protein kinase subfamily of c-Jun kinases. *Nature* 1994;369:156.

297. Force T, Bonventre JV. Growth factors and mitogen-activated protein kinases. *Hypertension* 1998;31:152.

298. Bonventre JV, Force T. Mitogen-activated protein kinases and transcriptional responses in renal injury and repair. *Curr Opin Nephrol Hypertens* 1998;7:425.

299. Pombo CM, Bonventre JV, Avruch J, et al. The stress-activated protein kinases are major c-Jun amino-terminal kinases activated by ischemia and reperfusion. *J Biol Chem* 1994;269:26546.

300. Hauser P, Schwarz C, Mitterbauer C, et al. Genome-wide gene-expression patterns of donor kidney biopsies distinguish primary allograft function. *Lab Invest* 2004;84:353.

301. Yoshida T, Tang SS, Hsiao LL, et al. Global analysis of gene expression in renal ischemia-reperfusion in the mouse. *Biochem Biophys Res Commun* 2002;291:787.

302. Supavekin S, Zhang W, Kucherlapati R, et al. Differential gene expression following early renal ischemia/reperfusion. *Kidney Int* 2003;63:1714.

303. Yoshida T, Kurella M, Beato F, et al. Monitoring changes in gene expression in renal ischemia-reperfusion in the rat. *Kidney Int* 2002;61:1646.

304. Murakami H, Liotta L, Star RA. IF-LCM: laser capture microdissection of immunofluorescently defined cells for mRNA analysis rapid communication. *Kidney Int* 2000;58:1346.

305. Brown PO, Botstein D. Exploring the new world of the genome with DNA microarrays. *Nat Genet* 1999;21:33.

306. Devarajan P, Mishra J, Supavekin S, et al. Gene expression in early ischemic renal injury: clues towards pathogenesis, biomarker discovery, and novel therapeutics (Review). *Mol Genet Metab* 2003;80:365.

307. Kerr JF, Wyllie AH, Currie AR. Apoptosis: a basic biological phenomenon with wide-ranging implications in tissue kinetics. *Br J Cancer* 1972;26:239.

308. Fesus L, Davies PJ, Piacentini M. Apoptosis: molecular mechanisms in programmed cell death. *Eur J Cell Biol* 1991;56:170.

309. Lieberthal W, Koh JS, Levine JS. Necrosis and apoptosis in acute renal failure. *Semin Nephrol* 1998;18:505.

310. Thornberry NA, Lazebnik Y. Caspases: enemies within. *Science* 1998;281:1312.

311. Li P, Nijhawan D, Budihardjo I, et al. Cytochrome c and dATP-dependent formation of Apaf-1/caspase-9 complex initiates an apoptotic protease cascade. *Cell* 1997;91:479.

312. Raafat AM, Murray MT, McGuire T, et al. Calcium blockade reduces renal apoptosis during ischemia reperfusion. *Shock* 1997;8:186.

313. Nogae S, Miyazaki M, Kobayashi N, et al. Induction of apoptosis in ischemia-reperfusion model of mouse kidney: possible involvement of Fas. *J Am Soc Nephrol* 1998;9:620.

314. Lamkanfi M, Declercq W, Depuydt B, et al. The Caspase family. In: M Los, H Walczak, eds. *Caspases–their role in cell death and cell survival,* 1st ed. New York: Kuwer Academic, 2002:1.

315. Slee EA, Adrain C, Martin SJ. Executioner caspase-3, -6, and -7 perform distinct, non-redundant roles during the demolition phase of apoptosis. *J Bio Chem* 2001;276:7320.

316. Slee EA, Harte MT, Kluck RM. Ordering the cytochrome c-initiated caspase cascade: hierarchical activation of caspases-2,-3,-6,-7,-8 and -10 in a caspase-9-dependent manner. *J Cell Biol* 1999;144:281.

317. Adrian C, Creagh EM, Martin SJ. Caspase cascades in apoptosis. In: M Los, H Walczak, eds. *Caspases–their role in cell death and cell survival,* 1st ed. New York: Kuwer Academic, 2002:41.

318. Zheng TH, Hunot S, Kuida K, et al. Caspase knockouts: matters of life and death. *Cell Death Differ* 1999;6:1043.

319. Edelstein CL, Ling H, Gengaro P, et al. Calpain mediated changes in actin and spectrin in hypoxic and ionomycin-induced rat renal proximal tubular injury (abstract). *J Am Soc Nephrol* 1996;7:1824.

320. Ueda N, Kaushal GP, Shah SV. Apoptotic mechanisms in acute renal failure. *Am J Med.* 2000;108:403.

321. Gold R, Schmied M, Giegerich G, et al. Differentiation between cellular apoptosis and necrosis by the combined use of in situ tailing and nick translation techniques. *Lab Invest* 1994;71:219.

322. Kaushal GP, Basnakian AG, Shah SV. Apoptotic pathways in ischemic acute renal failure. *Kidney Int* 2004;66:500.

323. Saikumar P, Venkatachalam MA. Role of apoptosis in hypoxic/ischemic damage in the kidney. *Semin Nephrol* 2003;23:511.

324. Sharples EJ, Patel N, Brown P, et al. Erythropoietin protects the kidney against the injury and dysfunction caused by ischemia-reperfusion. *J Am Soc Nephro* 2004;15:2115.

325. Vesey DA, Cheung C, Pat B, et al. Erythropoietin protects against ischaemic acute renal injury. *Nephrol Dial Transplantation* 2004;19:348.

326. Yang CW, Li C, Jung JY, et al. Preconditioning with erythropoietin protects against subsequent ischemia-reperfusion injury in rat kidney. *FASEB Journal* 2003;17:1754.

327. Arumugam TV, Shiels IA, Woodruff TM, et al. The role of the complement system in ischemia-reperfusion injury (Review). *Shock* 2004;21:401.

328. Zhou W, Farrar CA, Abe K, et al. Predominant role for C5b-9 in renal ischemia/reperfusion injury. *J Clin Invest* 2000;105:1363.

329. Thurman JM, Ljubanovic D, Edelstein CL, et al. Lack of a functional alternative complement pathway ameliorates ischemic acute renal failure in mice. *J Immunol* 2003;170:1517.

330. Alcorn D, Emslie KR, Ross BD, et al. Selective distal nephron damage during isolated kidney perfusion. *Kidney Int* 1981;19:638.

331. Leichtweiss HP, Lubbers DW, Weiss C, et al. The oxygen supply of the rat kidney: measurements of int4arenal pO2. *Pflugers Arch* 1969;309:328.

332. Brezis M, Rosen S, Silva P, et al. Selective vulnerability of the medullary thick ascending limb to anoxia in the isolated perfused rat kidney. *J Clin Invest* 1984;73:182.

333. Brezis M, Rosen S. Hypoxia of the renal medulla-its implications for disease. *N Engl J Med* 1995;332:647.

334. Baumgartl H, Leichtweiss HP, Lubbers DW, et al. The oxygen supply of the dog kidney: measurements of intrarenal pO 2. *Microvasc Res* 1972;4:247.

335. Schurek HJ, Kriz W. Morphologic and functional evidence for oxygen deficiency in the isolated perfused rat kidney. *Lab Invest* 1985;53:145.

336. Endre ZH, Ratcliffe PJ, Tange JD, et al. Erythrocytes alter the pattern of renal hypoxic injury: predominance of proximal tubular injury with moderate hypoxia. *Clin Sci* 1989;76:19.

337. Schurek HJ, Jost U, Baumgartl H, et al. Evidence for a preglomerular oxygen diffusion shunt in rat renal cortex. *Am J Physiol* 1990;259:F910.

338. Endre RB, Solez K. Anatomical and functional imaging of transplant acute renal failure. *Transplantation Rev* 1995;9:147.

339. Thiel G, de Rougemont D, Kriz W, et al. The role of reduced medullary perfusion in the genesis of acute ischemic renal failure. Summary of a round-table discussion. *Nephron* 1982;31:321.

340. Mason J, Welsch J, Torhorst J. The contribution of vascular obstruction to the functional defect that follows renal ischemia. *Kidney Int* 1987;31:65.

341. Mason J, Torhorst J, Welsch J. Role of the medullary perfusion defect in the pathogenesis of ischemic renal failure. *Kidney Int* 1984;26:283.

342. Kadkhodaee M, Gobe G, Wilgoss DA, et al. DNA fragmentation reduced by anti-oxidants following ischemia-reperfusion in the isolated perfused rat kidney. *Nephrol* 1998;4:163.

343. Gobe G, Zhang XJ, Cuttle L, et al. Bcl-2 genes and growth factors in the pathology of ischaemic acute renal failure. *Immunol Cell Biol* 1999;77:279.

344. Gobe G, Zhang XJ, Willgoss DA, et al. Relationship between expression of Bcl–2 genes and growth factors in ischemic acute renal failure in the rat. *J Am Soc Nephrol* 2000;11:454.

345. Gobe G, Willgoss D, Hogg N, et al. Cell survival or death in renal tubular epithelium after ischemia- reperfusion injury. *Kidney Int* 1999;56:1299.

346. Welch WJ, Wilcox CS, Thomson SC. Nitric oxide and tubuloglomerular feedback. *Semin Nephrol* 1999;19:251.

347. Welch WJ, Tojo A, Lee JU, et al. Nitric oxide synthase in the JGA of the SHR: expression and role in tubuloglomerular feedback. *Am J Physiol* 1999;277:F130.

348. Wilcox CS, Welch WJ. Macula densa nitric oxide synthase: expression, regulation, and function. *Kidney Int* 1998;67(Suppl):S53.

349. Brown R, Ollerstam A, Persson AE. Neuronal nitric oxide synthase inhibition sensitizes the tubuloglomerular feedback mechanism after volume expansion. *Kidney Int* 2004;65:1349.

350. Kovacs G, Komlosi P, Fuson A, et al. Neuronal nitric oxide synthase: its role and regulation in macula densa cells. (see comment). *J Am Soc Nephrol* 2003;14:2475.

351. Hashimoto S, Adams JW, Bernstein KE, et al. Micropuncture determination of nephron function in mice without tissue angiotensin converting enzyme. *Am J Physiol Renal Physiol* 2004.

352. Vallon V, Richter K, Huang DY, et al. Functional consequences at the single nephron level of the lack of adenosine A1 receptors and tubuloglomerular feedback in mice. *Pflugers Arch* 2004;448:214.

353. Castrop H, Huang Y, Hashimoto S, et al. Impairment of tubuloglomerular feedback regulation of GFR in ecto-5′-nucleotidase/CD73-deficient mice. *J Clin Invest* 2004;114:634.

354. Greger R. How does the macula densa sense tubule function? *Nephrol Dial Transplant* 1997;12:2215.

355. Conger JD, Robinette JB, Schrier RW. Smooth muscle calcium and endothelium-derived relaxing factor in the abnormal vascular responses of acute renal failure. *J Clin Invest* 1988;82:532.

356. Yaqoob M, Alkhunaizi AM, Edelstein CL, et al. ARF: pathogenesis, diagnosis and management. In: RW Schrier, ed. *Renal and electrolyte disorders.* New York: Lippincott–Raven, 1997:449.

357. Vallon V, Osswald H, Blantz RC, et al. Luminal signal in tubuloglomerular feedback: what about potassium? *Kidney Int* 1998;67(Suppl):S177.

358. Kumar S. Tubular cast formation and Tamm-Horsfall glycoprotein. In: MS Goligorsky, ed. Acute renal failure. New concepts and therapeutic strategies. New York: Churchill Livingstone, 1995:274.

359. Arendhorst WJ, Finn WF, Gottschalk C, et al. Micropuncture study of acute renal failure following temporary renal ischemia in the rat. *Kidney Int* 1976;10:S100.

360. Tanner GA, Steinhausen M. Kidney pressure after temporary artery occlusion in the rat. *Am J Physiol* 1976;230:1173.

361. Burke TJ, Cronin RE, Duchin KL, et al. Ischemia and tubule obstruction during acute renal failure in dogs: mannitol in protection. *Am J Physiol* 1980;238:F305.

362. Romanov V, Noiri E, Czerwinski G, et al. Two novel probes reveal tubular and vascular Arg-Gly-Asp (RGD) binding sites in the ischemic rat kidney. *Kidney Int* 1997;52:93.

363. Goligorsky MS, Kessler H, Romanov VI. Molecular mimicry of integrin ligation: therapeutic potential of arginine-glycine-aspartic acid (RGD) peptides. *Nephrol Dial Transplant* 1998;13:254.

364. Wangsiripaisan A, Gengaro P, Nemenoff R, et al. Effect of nitric oxide donors on renal tubular epithelial cell-matrix adhesion. *Kidney Int* 1999;55:2281.

365. Manns M, Sigler MH, Teehan BP. Intradialytic renal haemodynamics–potential consequences for the management of the patient with acute renal failure (editorial). *Nephrol Dial Transplant* 1997;12:870.

366. Noiri E, Forest T, Miller F, et al. Effects of RGD peptides on the course of acute renal failure. In: J Stein, MS Goligorsky, eds. Acute renal failure. New concepts and therapeutic strategies. New York: Churchill Livingstone, 1995:379.

367. Noiri E, Romanov V, Forest T, et al. Pathophysiology of renal tubular obstruction. Therapeutic role of synthetic RGD peptides in ARF. *Kidney Int* 1995;48:1375.

368. Goligorsky MS, Noiri E, Kessler H, et al. Therapeutic effect of arginine-glycine-aspartic acid peptides in ARF. *Clin Exp Pharmacol Physiol* 1998;25:276.

369. Goligorsky MS, Noiri E, Kessler H, et al. Therapeutic potential of RGD peptides in acute renal injury. *Kidney Int* 1997;51:1487.

370. Zuk A, Bonventre JV, Brown D, et al. Polarity, integrin, and extracellular matrix dynamics in the postischemic rat kidney. *Am J Physiol* 1998;275:C711.

371. Wangsiripaisan A, Gengaro P, Edelstein CL, et al. The role of Tamm-Horsfall mucoprotein (THP) in LLC-PK1 cell adhesion (abstract). *J Am Soc Neph* 1999;10:642A.

372. Conger JD, Weil JU. Abnormal vascular function following ischemia-reperfusion injury. *J Invest Med* 1995;43:431.

373. Schwartz D, Mendoca M, Schwartz Y, et al. Inhibition of constitutive nitric oxide synthase (NOS) by nitric oxide generated by inducible NOS after lipopolysaccharide administration provokes renal dysfunction in rats. *J Clin Invest* 1997;100:439.

374. Lieberthal W, Wolf EF, Rennke HG, et al. Renal ischemia and reperfusion impair endothelium-dependent vascular relaxation. *Am J Physiol* 1989;256:F894.

375. Chan L, Chittinandana A, Shapiro JI, et al. Effect of endothelin-receptor antagonist on ischemic acute renal failure. *Am J Physiol* 1994;266:F135.

376. Gellai M, Jugus M, Fletcher T, et al. Reversal of postischemic acute renal failure with a selective endothelinA receptor antagonist in the rat. *J Clin Invest* 1994;93:900.

377. Birck R, Knoll T, Braun C, et al. Improvement of postischemic acute renal failure with the novel orally active endothelin-A receptor antagonist LU 135252 in the rat. *J Cardiovasc Pharmacol* 1998;32:80.

378. Vargas AV, Krishnamurthi V, Masih R, et al. Prostaglandin E1 attenuation of ischemic renal reperfusion injury in the rat. *J Am Coll Surg* 1995;180:713.

379. Garvin PJ, Niehoff ML, Robinson SM, et al. Evaluation of the thromboxane A2 synthetase inhibitor OKY-046 in a warm ischemia-reperfusion rat model. *Transplantation* 1996;61:1429.

380. Ratcliffe PJ, Endre ZH, Scheinman SJ, et al. 31P nuclear magnetic resonance study of steady-state adenosine 5′- triphosphate levels during graded hypoxia in the isolated perfused rat kidney. *Clin Sci* 1988;74:437.

381. Allis JL, Endre ZH, Radda GK. 87Rb, 23Na and 31P nuclear magnetic resonance spectroscopy of the perfused rat kidney. *Ren Physiol Biochem* 1989;12:171.

382. Cross M, Endre ZH, Stewart-Richardson P, et al. 23Na-NMR detects hypoxic injury in intact kidney: increases in sodium inhibited by DMSO and DMTU. *Magn Reson Med* 1993;30:465.

383. Paller MS, Hoidal JR, Ferris TF. Oxygen free radicals in ischemic acute renal failure in the rat. *J Clin Invest* 1984;74:1156.

384. Paller MS, Hedlund BE. Role of iron in postischemic renal injury in the rat. *Kidney Int* 1988;34:474.

385. Linas SL, Whittenburg D, Repine JE. Role of neutrophil derived oxidants and elastase in lipopolysaccharide- mediated renal injury. *Kidney Int* 1991;39:618.

386. Linas SL, Shanley PF, Whittenburg D, et al. Neutrophils accentuate ischemia/reperfusion injury in isolated perfused rat kidneys. *Am J Physiol* 1988;255:F725.

387. Paller MS, Neumann TV. Reactive oxygen species and rat renal epithelial cells during hypoxia and reoxygenation. *Kidney Int* 1991;40:1041.

388. Kadkhodaee M, Endre ZH, Towner RA, et al. Hydroxyl radical generation following ischaemia-reperfusion in cell- free perfused rat kidney. *Biochem Biophys Acta* 1995;1243:169.

389. Kadkhodaee M, Hanson GR, Towner RA, et al. Detection of hydroxyl and carbon-centred radicals by EPR spectroscopy after ischaemia and reperfusion of the rat kidney. *Free Radic Res* 1996;25:31.

390. Conger JD, Robinette J, Villar A, et al. Increased nitric oxide synthase activity despite lack of response to endothelium-dependent vasodilators in postischemic acute renal failure in rats. *J Clin Invest* 1995;96:631.

391. Adams PL, Adams FF, Bell PD, et al. Impaired renal blood flow autoregulation in ischemic acute renal failure. *Kidney Int* 1980;18:68.

392. Kelleher SP, Robinette JB, Conger JD. Sympathetic nervous system in the loss of autoregulation in acute renal failure. *Am J Physiol* 1984;15:F379.

393. Solez K, Marel-Maroger L, Sraer J. The morphology of acute tubular necrosis in man. Analysis of 57 renal biopsies and comparison with glycerol model. *Medicine (Baltimore)* 1979;58:362.

394. Conger JD. Does hemodialysis delay recovery from acute renal failure? *Semin Dial* 1990;3:146.

395. Schrier RW, Burke TJ. Role of calcium-channel blockers in preventing acute and chronic renal injury. *J Cardiovasc Pharmacol* 1991;18:S38.

396. Meyer-Lehnert H, Caramelo C, Tsai P, et al. Interaction of atriopeptin III and vasopressin on calcium kinetics and contraction of aortic smooth muscle cells. *J Clin Invest* 1988;82:1407.

397. Nakamoto M, Shapiro JI, Shanley PF, et al. In vitro and in vivo protective effect of atriopeptin III on ischemic acute renal failure. *J Clin Invest* 1987;80:698.

398. Knotek M, Rogachev B, Gengaro P, et al. Endotoxemic renal failure in mice: role of tumor necrosis factor indepenent of inducible nitric oxide synthase. *Kidney Int* 2001;59:2243.

399. Knotek M, Esson M, Gengaro P, et al. Desensitization of soluble guanylate cyclase in renal cortex during endotoxemia in mice. *J Am Soc Nephol* 2000;11,2133.

400. Wang W, Falk S, Jittikanont S, et al. Protective effect of renal denervation on normotensive endotoxemia-induced acute renal failure (ARF) in mice. *Am J Physiol Renal Physiol* 2002;283:F583.

401. Schrier RW, Wang W. Acute renal failure and sepsis (Review). *N Engl J Med* 2004;351:159.

402. Wang W, Jittikanont S, Falk SA, et al. Interaction among nitric oxide, reactive oxygen species, and antioxidants during endotoxemia-related acute renal failure. *Am J Physiol Renal Physiol* 2003;284:F532.

403. Di Giantomasso D, May CN, Bellomo R. Vital organ blood flow during hyperdynamic sepsis. *Chest* 2003;124:1053.

404. Cunningham PN, Wang Y, Guo R, et al. Role of Toll-like receptor 4 in endotoxin-induced acute renal failure. *J Immunol* 2004;172:2629.

405. Brodsky SV, Yamamoto T, Tada T, et al. Endothelial dysfunction in ischemic acute renal failure: rescue by transplanted endothelial cells. *Am J Physiol Renal Fluid Electrolyte Physiol* 2002;282:F1140.

406. Yamamoto T, Tada T, Brodsky SV, et al. Intravital videomicroscopy of peritubular capillaries in renal ischemia. *Am J Physiol Renal Fluid Electrolyte Physiol* 2002;282:F1150.

407. Sutton TA, Mang HE, Campos SB, et al. Injury of the renal microvascular endothelium alters barrier function after ischemia. *Am J Physiol Renal Fluid Electrolyte Physiol* 2003;285:F191.

408. Kelly KJ, Williams WW Jr, Colvin RB, et al. Antibody to intracellular adhesion molecule-1 protects the kidney against ischemic injury. *Proc Natl Acad Sci USA* 1994;91:812.

409. Rabb H, Postler G. Leucocyte adhesion molecules in ischaemic renal injury: kidney specific paradigms? *Clin Exp Pharmacol Physiol* 1998;25:286.

410. Linas SL, Whittenburg D, Parsons PE, et al. Mild ischemia activates primed neutrophils to cause acute renal failure. *Kidney Int* 1992;42:610.

411. Linas SL, Whittenburg D, Parsons PE, et al. Ischemia increases neutrophil retention and worsens acute renal failure: role of oxygen metabolites and ICAM 1. *Kidnet Int* 1995;48:1584.

412. Linas SL, Whittenburg D, Repine JE. Nitric oxide prevents neutrophil-mediated acute renal failure. *Am J Physiol* 1996;272:F48.

413. Klausner JM, Paterson IS, Goldman G, et al. Postischemic renal injury is mediated by neutrophils and leukotrienes. *Am J Physiol* 1989;256:F794.

414. Caramelo C, Espinosa G, Manzarbeitia F, et al. Role of endothelium-related mechanisms in the pathophysiology of renal ischemia/reperfusion in normal rabbits. *Circ Res* 1996;79:1031.

415. Kelly KJ, Williams WW Jr, Colvin RB, et al. Intracellular adhesion molecule-1 deficient mice are protected against ischemic renal injury. *J Clin Invest* 1996;97:1056.

416. Haller H, Dragun D, Miethke A, et al. Antisense oligonucleotides for ICAM-1 attenuate reperfusion injury and renal failure in the rat. *Kidney Int* 1996;50:473.

417. Rabb H, Martin JG. An emerging paradigm shift on the role of leukocyte adhesion molecules [editorial]. *J Clin Invest* 1997;100:2937.

418. Rabb H, O'Meara YM, Maderna P, et al. Leukocytes, cell adhesion molecules and ischemic acute renal failure. *Kidney Int* 1997;51:1463.

419. Takada M, Nadeau KC, Shaw GD, et al. The cytokine-adhesion molecule cascade in ischemia/reperfusion injury of the rat kidney. Inhibition by a soluble P-selectin ligand. *J Clin Invest* 1997;99:2682.

420. Heinzelmann M, Mercer-Jones MA, Passmore JC. Neutrophils and renal failure. *Am J Kidney Dis* 1999;34:384.

421. Paller MS. Effect of neutrophil depletion on ischemic renal injury in the rat. *J Lab Clin Med* 1989;113:379.

422. Ysebaert DK, De Greef KE, De Beuf A, et al. T cells as mediators in renal ischemia/reperfusion injury. *Kidney Int* 2004;66:491.

423. Friedwald JJ, Rabb H. Inflammatory cells in ischemic acute renal failure. *Kidney Int* 2004;66:486.

424. Rabb H, Daniels F, O'Donnell M, et al. Pathophysiological role of T lymphocytes in renal ischemia-reperfusion injury in mice. *Am J Physiol Renal Physiol* 2000;279:F525.

425. Burne MJ, Daniels F, El Ghandour A, et al. Identification of the CD4(+) T cell as a major pathogenic factor in ischemic acute renal failure. *J Clin Invest* 2001;108:1283.

426. Park P, Haas M, Cunningham PN, et al. Injury in renal ischemia-reperfusion is independent from immunoglobulins and T lymphocytes. *Am J Physiol Renal Physiol* 2002;282:F352.

427. Burne-Taney MJ, Ascon DB, Daniels F, et al. B cell deficiency confers protection from renal ischemia reperfusion injury. *J Immunol* 2003;171:3210.

428. Yokota N, Daniels F, Crosson J, et al. Protective effect of T cell depletion in murine renal ischemia-reperfusion injury. *Transplantation* 2002;74:759.

429. Faubel SG, Ljubanovic D, Poole B, et al. Peripheral CD4 T-cell depletion is not sufficient to prevent ischemic acute renal failure. *Transplantation* 2005;80:643.

430. Ysebaert DK, De Greef KE, Vercauteren SR, et al. Identification and kinetics of leukocytes after severe ischaemia/reperfusion renal injury. *Nephrol Dial Transplant* 2000;15:1562.
431. Jose MD, Ikezumi Y, Van Rooijen N, et al. Macrophages act as effectors of tissue damage in acute renal allograft rejection. *Transplantation* 2003;76:1015.
432. De Greef KE, Ysebaert DK, Dauwe S, et al. Anti-B7-1 blocks mononuclear cell adherence in vasa recta after ischemia. *Kidney Int* 2001;60:1415.
433. Furuichi K, Wada T, Iwata Y, et al. Gene therapy expressing amino-terminal truncated monocyte chemoattractant protein-1 prevents renal ischemia-reperfusion injury. *J Am Soc Nephrol* 2003;14:1066.
434. Dursun B, He Z, Ljubanovic D, et al. Macrophage depletion is protective against ischemic ARF in the mouse (abstract). *J Am Soc Nephrol* 2004;15:713A.
435. Day YJ, Huang L, Ye H, et al. Renal ischemia-reperfusion injury and adenosine 2A receptor-mediated tissue protection:role of macrophages. *Am J Physiol* 2005;288:F722.
436. Deng J, Kohda Y, Chiao H, et al. Interleukin-10 inhibits ischemic and cisplatin-induced acute renal injury. *Kidney Int* 2001;60:2118.
437. Schonbeck U, Libby P. Inflammation, immunity, and HMG-CoA reductase inhibitors: statins as antiinflammatory agents? (Review). *Circ* 2004;109: II18.
438. Park YS, Guijarro C, Kim Y, et al. Lovastatin reduces glomerular macrophage influx and expression of monocyte chemoattractant protein-1 mRNA in nephrotic rats. *Am J Kidney Dis* 1998;31:190.
439. Romano M, Diomede L, Sironi M, et al. Inhibition of monocyte chemotactic protein-1 synthesis by statins. *Lab Invest* 2000;80:1095.
440. Gueler F, Rong S, Park JK, et al. Postischemic acute renal failure is reduced by short-term statin treatment in a rat model. *J Am Soc Nephrol* 2002;13:2288.
441. Sabbatini M, Pisani A, Uccello F, et al. Atorvastatin improves the course of ischemic acute renal failure in aging rats. *J Am Soc Nephrol* 2004;15:901.
442. Basile DP, Donohoe D, Roethe K, et al. Renal ischemic injury results in permanent damage to peritubular capillaries and influences long-term function. *Am J Physiol Renal Physiol* 2001;281:F887.
443. Basile DP, Donohoe DL, Roethe K, et al. Chronic renal hypoxia after acute ischemic injury: effects of L-arginine on hypoxia and secondary damage. *Am J Physiol Renal Fluid Electrolyte Physiol* 2003;284:F338.
444. Bonventre JV. Dedifferentiation and proliferation of surviving epithelial cells in acute renal failure (Review). *J Am Soc Nephrol* 2003;14:S55.
445. Kale S, Karihaloo A, Clark PR, et al. Bone marrow stem cells contribute to repair of the ischemically injured renal tubule. *J Clin Invest* 2003;112:42.
446. Abbate M, Brown D, Bonventre JV. Expression of NCAM recapitulates tubulogenic development in kidneys recovering from acute ischemia. *Am J Physiol* 1999;277:F454.
447. Ichimura T, Bonventre JV, Bailly V, et al. Kidney injury molecule-1 (KIM-1), a putative epithelial cell adhesion molecule containing a novel immunoglobulin domain, is up-regulated in renal cells after injury. *J Biol Chem* 1998;273:4135.
448. Fiaschi-Taesch NM, Santos S, Reddy V, et al. Prevention of acute ischemic renal failure by targeted delivery of growth factors to the proximal tubule in transgenic mice: the efficacy of parathyroid hormone-related protein and hepatocyte growth factor. *J Am Soc Nephrol* 2004;15:112.
449. Poulsom R, Forbes SJ, Hodivala-Dilke K, et al. Bone marrow contributes to renal parenchymal turnover and regeneration. *J Pathol* 2001;195:229.
450. Togel F, Isaac J, Westenfelder C. Hematopoietic stem cell mobilization-associated granulocytosis severely worsens acute renal failure. *J Am Soc Nephrol* 2004;15:1261.
451. Green DR. Apoptotic pathways: paper wraps stone blunts scissors. *Cell* 2000;102:1.
452. Lassus P, Opitz-Araya X, Lazebnik Y. Requirement for caspase-2 in stress-induced apoptosis before mitochondrial permeabilization. *Science* 2002;297:1352.
453. Kribben A, Edelstein CL, Schrier RW. Pathophysiology of acute renal failure. *J Nephrol* 1999;12:S142.
454. Mandel LJ, Murphy E. Regulation of cytosolic free calcium in rabbit proximal tubules. *J Biol Chem* 1984;259:11188.
455. Snowdowne KW, Freudenrich CC, Borle AB. The effects of anoxia on cytosolic free calcium, calcium fluxes and cellular ATP levels in cultured kidney cells. *J Biol Chem* 1985;260:11619.
456. McCoy CE, Selvaggio AM, Alexander EA, et al. Adenosine triphosphate depletion induces a rise in cytosolic free calcium in canine renal epithelial cells. *J Clin Invest* 1988;82:1326.
457. Phelps PC, Smith MW, Trump BF. Cytosolic ionized calcium and bleb formation after acute cell injury of cultured rabbit renal tubule cells. *Lab Invest* 1989;60:630.
458. Jacobs WR, Sgambati M, Gomez G, et al. Role of cytosolic Ca in renal tubule damage induced by hypoxia. *Am J Physiol* 1991;260:C545.
459. Ueda N, Shah SV. Role of intracellular calcium in hydrogen peroxide-induced renal tubular cell injury. *Am J Physiol* 1992;263:F214.
460. Li H, Long D, Quamme GA. Effect of chemical hypoxia on intracellular ATP and cytosolic Mg levels. *J Lab Clin Med* 1993;122:260.
461. Greene EL, Paller MS. Calcium and free radicals in hypoxia/reoxygenation injury of renal epithelial cells. *Am J Physiol* 1994;266:F13.
462. Rose UM, Bindels RJ, Jansen JW, et al. Effects of Ca^{2+} channel blockers, low Ca^{2+} medium and glycine on cell Ca^{2+} and injury in anoxic rabbit proximal tubules. *Kidney Int*. 1994;46:223.
463. Huang PL, Dawson TM, Bredt DS, et al. Targeted disruption of neuronal nitric oxide synthase gene. *Cell* 1993;75:1273.
464. Huang Z, Huang PL, Panahian N, et al. Effects of cerebral ischemia in mice deficient in neuronal nitric oxide synthase. *Science* 1994;265:1883.
465. Wei XQ, Charles IG, Smith A, et al. Altered immune responses in mice lacking inducible nitric oxide synthase. *Nature* 1995;375:408.
466. Cobb JP, Hotchkiss RS, Swanson PE, et al. Inducible nitric oxide synthase (iNOS) gene deficiency increases the mortality of sepsis in mice. *Surgery* 1999;126:438.
467. Huang PL, Huang Z, Mashimo H, et al. Hypertension in mice lacking the gene for endothelial nitric oxide synthase. *Nature* 1995;377:239.
468. Samdani AF, Dawson TM, Dawson VL. Nitric oxide synthase in models of focal ischemia. *Stroke* 1997;28:1283.
469. Jones SP, Girod WG, Palazzo AJ, et al. Myocardial ischemia-reperfusion injury is exacerbated in absence of endothelial cell nitric oxide synthase. *Am J Physiol* 1999;276:H1567.
470. Allen J, Winterford C, Axelsen RA, et al. Effects of hypoxia on morphological and biochemical characteristics of renal epithelial cell and tubule cultures. *Ren Fail* 1992;14:453.
471. Wiegele G, Brandis M, Zimmerhackl LB. Apoptosis and necrosis during ischaemia in renal tubular cells (LLC-PK1 and MDCK). *Nephrol Dial Transplant* 1998;13:1158.
472. Feldenberg LR, Thevananther S, del Rio M, et al. Partial ATP depletion induced Fas- and caspase-mediated apoptosis in MDCK cells. *Am J Physiol* 1999;276:F837.
473. Dong Z, Saikumar P, Patel Y, et al. Serine protease inhibitors suppress cytochrome c-mediatedcaspase-9 activation and apoptosis during hypoxia-reoxygenation. *Biochem J* 2000;347:669.
474. Tanaka T, Nangaku M, Miyata T, et al. Blockade of calcium influx through L-type calcium channels attenuates mitochondrial injury and apoptosis in hypoxic renal tubular cells. *J Am Soc Nephrol* 2004;15:2320.
475. Khan S, Koepke A, Jarad G, et al. Apoptosis and JNK activation are differentially regulated by Fas expression level in renal tubular epithelial cells. *Kidney Int* 2001;60:65.
476. del Rio M, Imam A, DeLeon M, et al. The death domain of kidney ankyrin interacts with Fas and promotes Fas-mediated cell death in renal epithelia. *J Am Soc Nephrol* 2004;15:41.
477. Wang J, Wei Q, Wang CY, et al. Minocycline up-regulates Bcl-2 and protects against cell death in mitochondria. *J Biol Chem* 2004;279:19948.
478. Wei Q, Alam MM, Wang MH, et al. Bid activation in kidney cells following ATP depletion in vitro and ischemia in vivo. *Am J Physiol Renal Fluid Electrolyte Physiol* 2004;286:F803.
479. Schumer M, Colombel MC, Sawczuk IS, et al. Morphologic, biochemical and molecular evidence of apoptosis during the reperfusion phase after brief periods of renal ischemia. *Am J Path* 1992;140:831.
480. Shimizu A, Yamanaka N. Apoptosis and cell desquamation in repair process of ischemic tubular necrosis. *Virchows Arch B Cell Pathol Incl Mol Pathol* 1993;64:171.
481. Nakajima T, Miyaji T, Kato A, et al. Uninephrectomy reduces apoptotic cell death and enhances renal tubular cell regeneration in ischemic ARF in rats. *Am J Physiol* 1996;271:F846.
482. Burns AT, Davies DR, McLaren AJ, et al. Apoptosis in ischemia/reperfusion injury of human renal allografts. *Transplantation* 1998;66:872.
483. Vukicevic S, Basic V, Rogic D, et al. Osteogenic protein-1 (bone morphogenetic protein-7) reduces severity of injury after ischemic acute renal failure in rat. *J Clin Invest* 1998;102:202.
484. Padanilam BJ, Lewington AJ, Hammerman MR. Expression of CD27 and ischemia/reperfusion-induced expression of its ligand Siva in rat kidneys. *Kidney Int* 1998;54:1967.
485. Toronyi E, Hamar J, Perner F, et al. Prevention of apoptosis reperfusion renal injury by calcium channel blockers. *Exp Toxicol Pathol* 1999;51:209.
486. Cuevas P, Martinez-Coso V, Fu X, et al. Fibroblast growth factor protects the kidney against ischemia-reperfusion injury. *Eur J Med Res* 1999;4: 403.
487. Forbes JM, Leaker B, Hewitson TD, et al. Macrophage and myofibroblast involvement in ischemic acute renal failure is attenuated by endothelin receptor antagonists. *Kidney Int* 1999;55:198.
488. Hamar P, Song E, Kokeny G, et al. Small interfering RNA targeting Fas protects mice against renal ischemia-reperfusion injury. *Proc Natl Acad Sci USA* 2004;101:14883.
489. Kishino M, Yukawa K, Hoshino K, et al. Deletion of the kinase domain in death-associated protein kinase attenuates tubular cell apoptosis in renal ischemia-reperfusion injury. *J Am Soc Nephrol* 2004;15:1826.

CHAPTER 40 ■ PATHOPHYSIOLOGY OF NEPHROTOXIC CELL INJURY

BRIAN S. CUMMINGS AND RICK G. SCHNELLMANN

INTRODUCTION

Nephrotoxic epithelial cell injury induced by chemicals can result in acute renal failure (ARF) and can be mediated via a variety of mechanisms. After direct or indirect chemical-induced injury, renal epithelial cells either repair and regenerate or die. If the degree of cell death is sufficient, then overall renal function declines and ARF results. Indirect chemical insults may decrease renal blood flow, thereby causing renal ischemia and reperfusion-induced cell injury and death. Furthermore, recent studies demonstrate that the T and B cells and, to a lesser extent, macrophages and neutrophils inhibit renal function in ARF (1–3). The role of inflammatory cells in ARF is likely secondary to the initial insult and occurs during the maintenance phase of ARF (4,5). These examples highlight the premise that multiple mechanisms are involved in the pathophysiology of nephrotoxic epithelial cell injury and ARF.

A secondary effect of nephrotoxicant-induced cell death in ARF can be the generation of "backleak." After an insult, injured and dead epithelial cells release from the basement membrane and adhere via integrins to other released and attached epithelial cells (4–11). The cellular aggregates can form tubular casts that block the flow of filtrate and increase intraluminal pressure, decreasing the single nephron glomerular filtration rate (4). In addition, the loss of epithelial cells can leave gaps in the basement membrane allowing tubular filtrate to "backleak" into the circulation, further decreasing the apparent single nephron glomerular filtration rate as currently measured. Thus, "backleak" and the loss of epithelial cells contribute to the decreased renal function.

As a consequence of either direct or indirect renal epithelial cell injury, cells die or repair and regenerate. Renal epithelial cells are known to repair and regenerate, and significant advances have been made to enhance our understanding of this process (12–16). Regeneration begins when cells adjacent to the injured area de-differentiate, proliferate, and migrate into the denuded areas. Ultimately, the cells differentiate and tubular structure and function are restored. Chemicals also may protract the maintenance phase of renal dysfunction through their ability to inhibit cellular repair and regeneration. If a nephrotoxicant inhibits this process, then recovery of normal renal function may be delayed or inhibited. For example, the recovery of renal function after treatment with the aminoglycoside antibiotic tobramycin and cisplatin were compared (10,11). A 4-day treatment with tobramycin resulted in renal dysfunction with proximal tubular necrosis that was followed by a proliferative response. Renal dysfunction was fully reversible and serum creatinine levels and proximal tubular morphology returned to the control values by day 14. Although a 4-day regimen of cisplatin also resulted in renal dysfunction with proximal tubular necrosis, the renal dysfunction persisted. These studies provide evidence that renal proximal tubules damaged by cisplatin may not undergo normal regeneration, which results in protracted ARF.

In vitro studies support the hypothesis that nephrotoxicants can inhibit the proliferative and/or migratory processes during regeneration. For example, Counts and colleagues (17) used an *in vitro* model of renal proximal tubular cell (RPTC) regeneration to determine whether nephrotoxicants can inhibit the proliferative and/or migratory processes during regeneration. Subsequent to mechanically induced injury to a confluent monolayer, $HgCl_2$, the mycotoxin fumonisin B_1, and the haloalkene cysteine conjugate, S-(1,2)-dichlorovinyl-L-cysteine, inhibited the normal proliferative and migratory response that resulted in the closure of the denuded areas in the absence overt cytotoxicity to the monolayer. Therefore, it is important to determine if the mechanisms involved in the pathophysiology of nephrotoxic-induced ARF are directly inducing cell death or inhibiting regeneration after cell death.

The goal of this chapter is to review some of the mechanisms by which chemicals produce renal epithelial cell injury and death. Other chapters in this volume, and several excellent reviews, discuss renal cell death and ARF produced by specific chemicals; the reader is referred to these for additional insights and perspectives (18–20).

SUSCEPTIBILITY OF THE KIDNEY TO INJURY

The susceptibility of the kidney to various agents can be attributed to several functional properties of this organ. These properties include: (a) receiving 20% to 25% of the cardiac output, ensuring high levels of toxicant delivery over a period of time; (b) extensive reabsorptive capacity with specialized transporters promoting cellular uptake of the toxicant; (c) urinary concentrating capacity that results in high concentrations of toxicants in the medullary lumen and interstitium; (d) biotransformation enzymes resulting in the formation of toxic metabolites and reactive intermediates; (e) high metabolic rates and workload of renal cells resulting in increased sensitivity to toxicants; and (f) sensitivity of the kidney to vasoactive agents.

Nephrotoxicants generally damage specific segments of the nephron, with the proximal tubule epithelial cell being the primary target. Furthermore, different segments of the proximal tubule (S_1, S_2, and S_3) are targets for different nephrotoxicants. For example, aminoglycoside antibiotics, chromate, cadmium chloride, and the mycotoxin citrinin primarily affect the S_1 and S_2 segments, whereas cyclosporine, $HgCl_2$, uranyl nitrate, cisplatin, bromobenzene, and cysteine conjugates of halogenated hydrocarbons affect the S_3 segment (21). In addition, interferon-α, gold, and penicillamine may target cells in the glomeruli, whereas nonsteroidal antiinflammatory drugs (NSAIDs) and angiotensin converting enzyme (ACE) inhibitors may target cells in renal vessels (22). The reasons for these segmental differences may include: (a) differences in toxicant delivery to a given segment, (b) differences in transport and uptake among segments, and (c) differences in biotransformation enzymes among segments.

XENOBIOTIC TRANSPORT

For most xenobiotics, transport into the epithelial cell is required for the expression of toxicity and xenobiotics, in general, enter cells by passive diffusion or by active or facilitated transport. With xenobiotic accumulation, injury is initiated with altered cellular functions. Likewise, inhibition of the transporter(s) responsible for xenobiotic import blocks injury. As stated earlier, differences in transporter expression among different tubular segments are one indicator of whether a given tubular segment is the target of xenobiotic toxicity.

Several transporters that participate in basal physiological functions of renal cells, such as reabsorption and secretion, participate in the transport of nephrotoxicants (23–25). These transporters include, but are not limited to, the organic cation transporters (OCT [26–28]), organic anion transporters (OATs [29–31]), amino acid transporters (32,33), and transporters involved in multi-drug resistance such as P-glycoprotein (34).

OATs and OCTs transport a variety of physiological compounds into renal cells (35). In addition, they transport drugs, natural products, and industrial chemical and pollutants (23,29,31,35–37). For example, the mycotoxin ochratoxin A is transported into renal tubular cells by OAT1, OAT 3, and OAT 5 (35,36,38) and induces renal cell death. Ochratoxin A transport into renal cells is inhibited by probenecid (39), an inhibitor of most OAT proteins, and probenecid blocks ochratoxin A-induced cell death (40). The uptake and cell death induced by the trichloroethylene metabolite S-(1,2)-dichlorovinyl-L-cysteine also is inhibited by probenecid (41) and para-aminohippurate (PAH, an OAT substrate, [37]) in isolated RPTC. The ability of Hg^{+2} and its cysteine-conjugates to induce cell death *in vivo* and in canine kidney cells is altered by inhibitors or substrates of OAT proteins, suggesting that the nephrotoxicity of this environmental contaminant is regulated by these transporters (29,31).

OCT proteins also play a significant role in xenobiotic transport and injury in renal cells. For example, OCT 1 and OCT 2 are required for the nephrotoxicity of platinum compounds including cisplatin, oxaliplatin, and carboplatin in Madin-Darby canine kidney cells (27). OCT 1 and OCT 2 also mediate the transport of 1-methyl-4-phenyl-pyridinium, disopyramide, and chlorpheniramine into renal cells (42).

The role of P-glycoprotein in chemical-induced renal cell death is still being investigated. However, the nephrotoxicity of chemotherapeutics, such as cisplatin, is altered by over expression of P-glcyoprotein (43). Further, P-glycoprotein may mediate the nephrotoxicity of diallyl disulfide and S-allyl-cysteine, two investigational chemotherapeutics (44).

CELL DEATH

In many cases, transport of toxicants into renal cells results in cell death. Cell death is generally thought to occur through one of two mechanisms: oncosis or apoptosis (45–47). Apoptosis is a tightly controlled, organized process that was initially defined morphologically, and morphologic changes remain the hallmark of apoptosis. *Necrosis* or *necrotic cell death* affects masses of contiguous cells and is characterized by the swelling of organelles and increases in cell volume, after which the cell membrane becomes more permeable and ruptures with the release of cellular contents, followed by inflammation (Fig. 40-1). Majno and Joris (45) pointed out that necrotic cell death is a poor term to describe cell death characterized by cellular volume increases and cell rupture. Historically, necrosis has been used to describe drastic tissue changes occurring after cell death. These changes include karyorrhexis, karyolysis, pyknosis, condensation of the cytoplasm, and intense eosinophilia, and alterations representing the cadaver of a cell. Temporally speaking, cells die long before necrotic changes are observed.

Manjo and Joris (45) suggested that the term *oncosis* (from *ónkos*, meaning "swelling"), a word coined by von Recklinghausen in 1910 to describe cell death with swelling, be used generically to describe cell death characterized by cellular swelling, organelle swelling, blebbing, and rupture (48). Levin and associates (49) have supported the use of the term oncosis and further suggested that the term necrosis be used to designate groups of dead cells, defined on histological sections, regardless of the type of cell death (apoptosis or oncosis).

Despite the fact that both apoptosis and oncosis induce necrosis, the morphologic and biochemical characteristics of oncosis and apoptosis are very different (45–47) (Fig. 40-1). The morphology associated with oncosis has been explained previously. Apoptosis usually affects scattered individual cells, and morphologically, the cell shrinks while organelle integrity is retained. The chromatin becomes pyknotic and marginates against the nuclear membrane. Ultimately, the cell shrinks to a dense round mass (apoptotic body) or forms pseudopodia (i.e., buds) containing nuclear fragments and/or organelles that break off into small fragments (apoptotic bodies). In either case, adjacent cells, or macrophages phagocytize the apoptotic bodies, and inflammation does not occur. Numerous authors incorrectly use the terms *programmed cell death* and *apoptosis* synonymously. The phrase "programmed cell death" refers to situations in which cells are programmed to die at a fixed time (e.g., during development) (46). Although the process and morphology of programmed cell death and apoptosis may be similar, the term apoptosis is more appropriate for chemical- and ischemia-induced cell death.

Apoptosis

One key difference between oncosis and apoptosis is the activation of caspases in the latter. Caspases belong to a 14-member family of cysteine proteases and are key mediators of apoptosis (50–52). Caspases can be divided into three groups based on structural differences and substrate preferences: initiator caspases (caspase -2, -8, -9, -10, and possibly -12), executioner or effector caspases (caspases -3, -6, and -7), and cytokine processors (caspases -1, -4, -5, and -13). Initiator caspases are activated by numerous processes including receptor-directed mechanisms and chemical exposures, and mediate chemical-induced apoptosis in numerous cell types, including proximal tubular cells (53–55), glomerular cells (56), medullary cells (57,58), and cells present in the collecting ducts (57–61). Activation of initiator caspases results in the activation of executioner caspases that leads to several of the biochemical characteristics of apoptosis. However, recent studies in nonrenal cells suggest that caspase-2 can induce apoptosis independent of its catalytic activity via a mechanism involving permeabilization of the mitochondrial membrane and subsequent release of pro-apoptotic proteins inducing cytochrome c, Smac/Diablo (62,63) (see the subsequent text).

Caspase-8, an initiator caspase, plays an integral role in receptor-mediated apoptosis (64–67). Caspase-8 is activated by membrane receptors such as Fas-ligand and TNFα receptors (66;68–70) and, in turn, cleaves the Bcl-2 family protein Bid to form tBid (64-67). tBid acts on mitochondria to cause the release of pro-apoptotic proteins and result in the

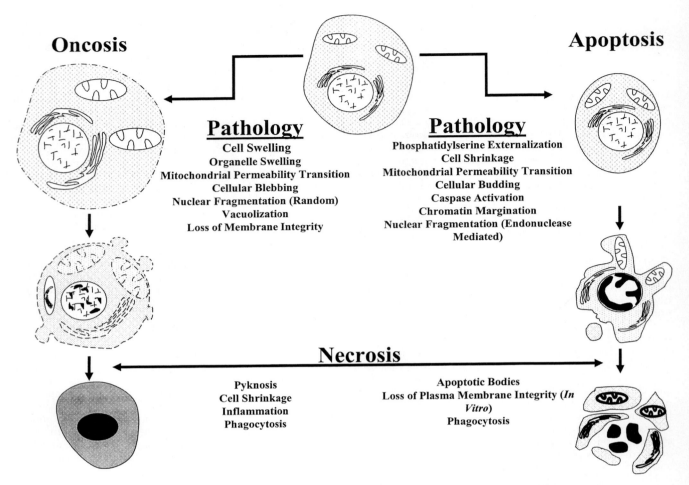

FIGURE 40-1. Comparison of the morphologic features of oncosis and apoptosis. At the top middle, a normal cell. **Left:** Cell and organelle swelling, followed by vacuolization, blebbing, and increased membrane permeability (lysis) and finally necrotic changes (i.e., coagulation, shrinkage, and karyolysis). **Right:** Cell shrinkage followed by budding and karyorrhexis and finally necrotic changes (i.e., breakup into cluster of apoptotic bodies). The pathology of each event is listed next to each pathway. (Adapted from: Cummings BS, Schnellmann RG. Measurement of cell death in mammalian cells. In: *Protocols in pharmacology*. New York: John Wiley & Sons, 2004;12:8, with permission.)

activation of caspase-9 and caspase-3. In contrast, caspase-8 may directly activate caspase-9 or caspase-3 independently of the mitochondrion (Figure 40-2). Chemicals may also activate caspase-8 independently of receptor-mediated mechanims. For example, cisplatin and etoposide activate caspase-8, caspase-9 and caspase-3 in LLC-PK1 cells (71) and U937 cells in the absence of receptor-stimulation (66). In contrast, cisplatin and cyclosporine activated caspase-3 in the absence of caspase-8 in mouse and rabbit RPTC (49–51). Thus, the role of caspase-8 in chemical-induced apoptosis is variable.

Executioner, or effector, caspases are responsible for the cleavage of a number of substrates that typically result in the morphologic features of apoptosis. For example, cleavage of the *Inhibitor of Caspase-Activated Deoxyribonuclease* (ICAD/DFF45) by caspases results in its deactivation and allows caspase-activated deoxyribonuclease to cleave DNA, resulting in the "ladder-like" pattern after agarose gel electrophoresis (72,73). Further, cleavage of poly(ADP-ribose) polymerase (PARP) by caspases-3 and -7 results in its activation and the addition of ADP-ribose monomers to a variety of proteins (74). Other substrates for caspases include DNA repair enzymes that prevent cells from making a futile attempt at repair, and scaffolding proteins that allow for the reorganization

of the cytoskeleton and the packaging of the cell constituents into apoptotic bodies (51).

Role of Mitochondria in Apoptosis

Mitochondria are integral in the apoptotic process through the production of ATP and the release of pro-apoptotic factors. For example, the release of cytochrome c from mitochondria results in the binding of cytochrome c to apoptotic protease activating factor 1 (APAF-1), which promotes the binding and proteolytic cleavage of pro-caspase-9 to caspase-9 (51; 75). Activated caspase-9 cleaves and activates executioner caspases (i.e., caspases-3, -6, and -7) (Fig. 40-2). A number of toxicants, including cisplatin and S-(1,2)-dichlorovinyl-L cysteine, cause cytochrome c release and apoptosis (51,66,76,77). Cytochrome c release from the mitochondria is associated with a decrease in the mitochondrial inner membrane potential and the accumulation of several pro-apoptotic proteins such as Bad, Bak, and Bax at the mitochondria (Fig. 40-2). Other pro-apoptotic proteins released from the mitochondria include apoptosis-inducing factor (AIF), Smac/Diablo, Omi and Endo G (64–66,78–85) (Fig. 40-2).

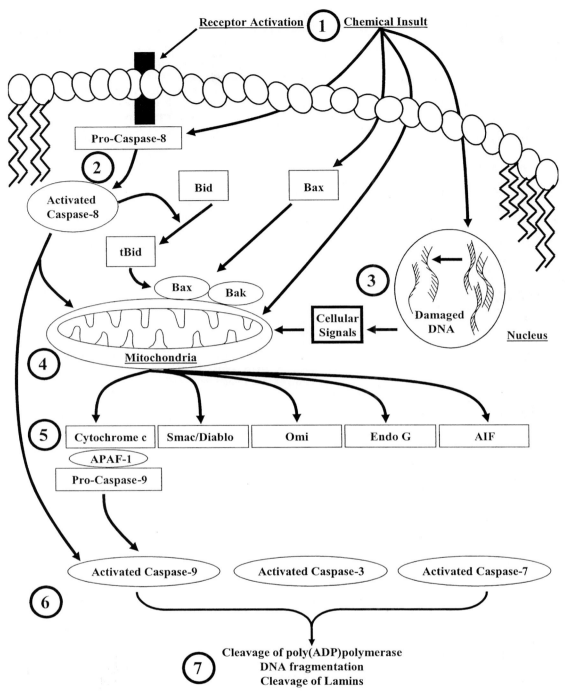

FIGURE 40-2. Cell signaling cascades involved in the activation of caspases and apoptosis. 1: Receptor-mediated death signals or chemicals can initiate apoptosis through multiple mechanisms. 2: Pro-caspase-8 is activated by receptor-mediated signals at the cellular membrane or directly by chemicals. Once activated, caspase-8 cleaves Bid to t-Bid, which interacts with Bax/Bak to induce mitochondrial-mediated apoptosis or directly activates caspase-9 and other caspases. 3: Some chemicals cause DNA damage that signals the release of pro-apoptotic proteins from the mitochondria. 4: Receptor-mediated signals, direct chemical injury, or signals resulting from DNA damage can all cause cytochrome c, Smac/Diablo, Endo G, and AIF release from the mitochondria. 5: Released cytochrome c forms a complex with APAF-1 and pro-caspase-9, resulting in caspase-9 activation. 6: Activated caspase-9 cleaves and activates pro-caspase-3 and -7, which can also be activated by caspase-8 independently of cytochrome c. 7: Activated caspases (e.g., 3 and 7), AIF, and Endo G cause the classical markers of apoptosis, such as cleavage and activation of poly(ADP)polymerase, inactivation of inhibitors of DNases leading to DNA fragmentation, cleaved lamins, and the activation of other caspases.

Bad, Bak, Bax, and Bid belong to the Bcl-2 family of pro-apoptotic proteins, which are characterized by specific regions of homology termed Bcl-2 homology domains (86). Under non-stressed conditions these proteins exist bound to proteins in the mitochondria and cytosol (64). After toxicant exposure Bax, Bid, or Bak can dissociate and translocate to the mitochondria. Translocation to the mitochondria typically initiates alterations in the mitochondrial membrane potential and release of cytochrome c, Endo G, Smac/Diablo, Omi, and AIF (61,64,87) (Fig. 40-2). The exact mechanisms involved in the regulation of these proteins, or whether caspases or cytochrome c can act independently of Bax, Bid, or Bak in renal cells is presently unclear. However, current studies suggest that these proteins are partially regulated by trans-activation factors such as p53 (88–91). Furthermore, studies show that Bid mediates apoptosis induced by hypoxia and ATP depletion in cultures of rat RPTC (92); Bax mediates proximal tubular apoptosis in mice treated with cisplatin *in vivo* (58); and Bak is elevated during apoptosis in primary bovine glomerular endothelial cells induced by TNFα or lipopolysaccharide (93) or during ischemia-reperfusion-induced renal cell apoptosis in mice (94).

In contrast to Bax, Bid, and Bak, Bcl-2 is an antiapoptotic protein (60). Increased levels of Bcl-2 prior to toxicant exposure protects numerous cells, including renal cells (94), from toxicant-induced apoptosis (78,86,94,95). The protective effect of Bcl-2 may be the result of its ability to bind Bax, Bid, and Bak, preventing them from altering mitochondrial membrane permeability, initiating the release of mitochondrial pro-apoptotic proteins, and activating caspases (95). In support of this hypothesis, over expression of Bcl-2 protects against ATP-depletion-induced apoptosis in cultures of rat RPTC (92), and up regulation of Bcl-2 protected kidney epithelial cells both *in vitro* and *in vivo* against apoptosis induced by hypoxia, azide, cisplatin, and staurosporine (67).

AIF is released from the mitochondria in response to decreases in the mitochondrial membrane potential induced by ATP depletion (78,96); ischemia-reperfusion; anti-Fas antibodies (97); or exposure to high concentrations of Ca^{2+} (98), *t*-butyl hydroperoxide (98), or atractyloside (98). Cellular pathologies associated with AIF release are similar to those seen with caspases (chromatin condensation and oligonucleosomal DNA fragmentation) (97). AIF is a distinct protease with properties similar to those of caspases. In opossum kidney cells AIF is released after ATP depletion-induced by sodium cyanide and 2-deoxy-D-glucose (79,96). However, the ability of AIF to participate in toxicant-induced renal cell death *in vivo* or in other renal cell models *in vitro* has not been fully explored.

Smac/Diablo is a pro-apoptotic protein released from the mitochondria to the cytosol during apoptosis where it blocks the antiapoptotic activity of inhibitors of apoptosis proteins (IAP) (81). However, the ability of Smac/Diablo to promote apoptosis may not exclusively be the result of its ability to bind IAP. This was demonstrated in human embryonic kidney cells (HEK293) in which a mutant Smac/Diablo was unable to bind IAP. In this model both receptor- and chemical-induced apoptosis was increased in the presence of mutant Smac/Diablo, supporting the hypothesis that this protein's ability to induce apoptosis is partially independent of its ability to bind IAP (82). Despite these data, released Smac/Diablo functions at the level of executioner caspases and downstream of the Bcl-2 family of proteins (83). Smac/Diablo is expressed in the mouse kidney and in several renal cell models (99) and mediates apoptosis *in vivo* in mice after treatment with high concentrations of folic acid or after exposure of cultures of renal epithelial cells to TNFα (81). Increased expression of Smac/Diablo potentiates TNFα- and etoposide-induced apoptosis in HEK293 cells (82). However, similar to several other pro-apoptotic proteins, ex-pression of Smac/Diablo is not essential for apoptosis in kidney cells. For example, acetaminophen-induced renal cell apoptosis proceeds in a caspase-dependent manner in the absence of Smac/Diablo activity (100).

Omi is a mammalian serine protease that has homology to bacterial HtrA endoprotease (101). Omi localizes to the endoplasmic reticulum and mitochondria and is expressed ubiquitously in a number of cell types including RPTC (84,85,101,102). After exposure to apoptotic stimuli Omi is released from the mitochondria and binds to, and cleaves, inhibitors of IAP (84). Omi-directed degradation of IAP facilitates caspase activation and the subsequent biochemical and morphological features of apoptosis. Inhibition of Omi using the synthetic inhibitor ucf-101, or siRNA against Omi, decreased cisplatin-induced apoptosis in primary cultures of mouse RPTC (84). Furthermore, treatment of mice with ucf-101 prior to cisplatin treatment decreased nephrotoxicity and renal cell death *in vivo* (84). These recent studies support the hypothesis that Omi may mediate other types of toxicant-induced renal cell apoptosis.

INITIATORS OF CELLULAR INJURY

Xenobiotics initiate cell injury by a variety of mechanisms. Some chemicals initiate toxicity directly because of their reactivity with selected cellular macromolecules. For example, the antifungal drug amphotericin B increases the permeability of the plasma membrane to cations (103), the mycotoxin fumonisin B_1 inhibits sphinganine (sphingosine) N-acyltransferase (104), and aminoglycosides bind initially to cellular anionic phospholipids (105,106). Other xenobiotics initiate toxicity following biotransformation to a reactive intermediate or a stable metabolite. Xenobiotics can also initiate toxicity indirectly through the production of reactive oxygen species.

Role of Biotransformation

Renal xenobiotic metabolism can contribute significantly to whole-body metabolism and/or renal toxicity of a chemical because a primary route of xenobiotic excretion is the kidney. Some chemicals need to be metabolized or biotransformed to a toxic reactive intermediate for cellular injury to occur (Fig. 40-3). The reactive intermediate binds covalently to critical cellular macromolecules, which are thought to interfere with the normal functioning of the macromolecules and thereby initiate cellular injury. In many cases, these reactive intermediates or "alkylating" agents are electrophiles that bind to cellular nucleophiles. The renal xenobiotic-metabolizing enzymes found in experimental animals and humans have been reviewed by Lock (107) and Lohr (108) and are summarized in Table 40-1.

Although the kidney contains many of the xenobiotic-metabolizing enzymes found in the liver, in general their concentration within the kidney is lower. For example, renal cytochrome P-450 levels are between 0.1 and 0.2 nmol/mg microsomal protein across a variety of species, which represents approximately 20% of cytochrome P-450 levels found in the liver (107,109). The distribution of cytochrome P-450 also varies in different renal cells. For example, cytochrome P-450 levels are highest in the S_2 segment, followed by the S_3 and S_1 segments, respectively with the other tubular segments having less than 10% of that of the S_1 segment (107).

The renal cytochrome P-450 system is very active against a variety of endogenous and exogenous compounds, and

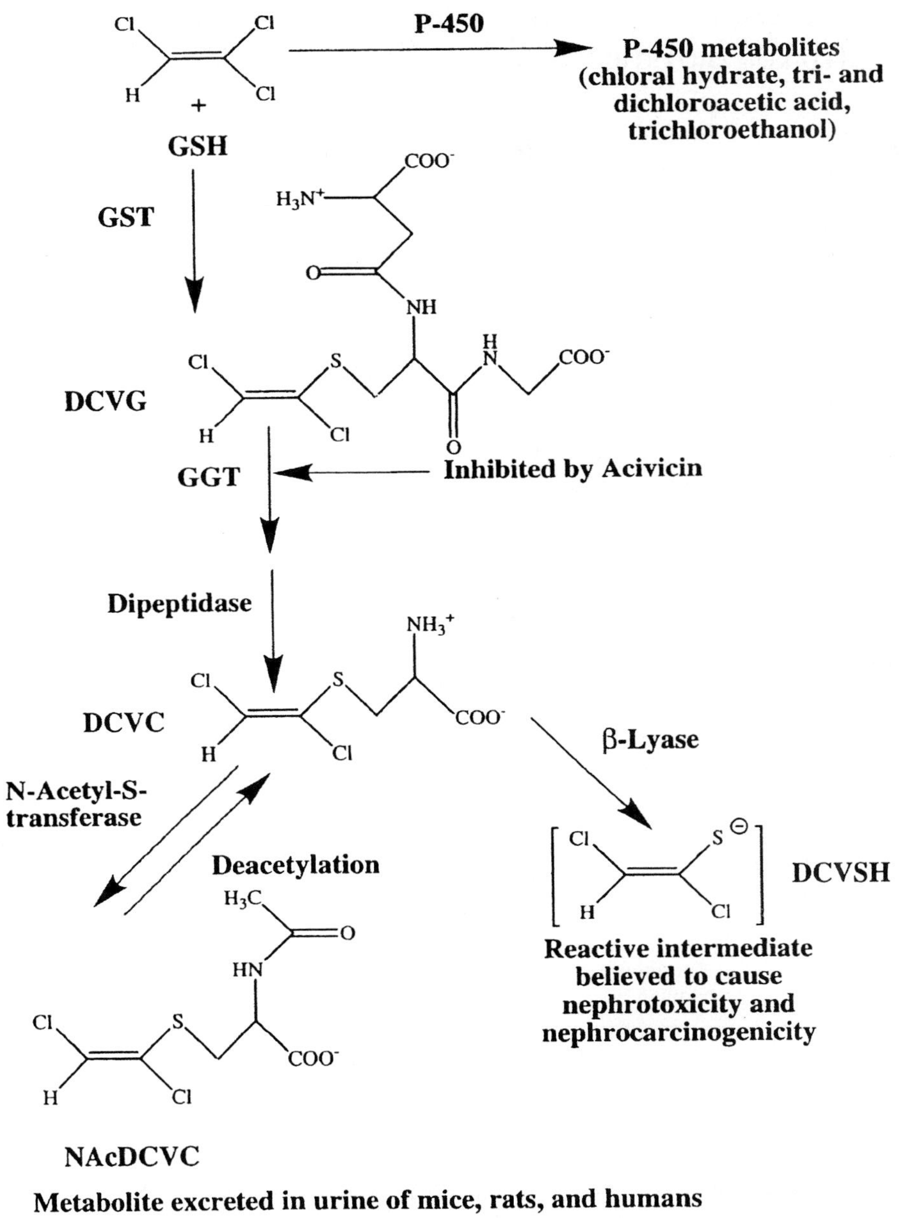

FIGURE 40-3. The bioactivation of trichloroethylene by the glutathione-(GSH-) conjugation pathway. Trichloroethylene (top left) can be metabolized by either cytochrome P-450 to the compound listed (top right) or be conjugated to GSH by the glutathione S-transferase (GST) to form S-(1,2)-dichlorovinyl-glutathione (DCVG). These reactions can occur either in the liver or in the kidney. DCVG formed in the liver is delivered to the kidney via the bile or the blood where the high concentrations of γ-glutamyltransferase (GGT) and dipeptidase in the kidney results in the cleavage of the GSH moiety and the formation of S-(1,2)-dichlorovinyl-L cysteine (DCVC). Metabolism of DCVC by N-acetyl-S-transferase produces N-acetyl-S-(1,2)-dichlorovinyl-L-cysteine (NAcDCVC), which is excreted in the urine of mice, rats, and humans exposed to trichloroethylene. NAcDCVC also can be deacetylated back to DCVC. Metabolism of DCVC by cysteine-conjugate ß-lyase results in the formation of a reactive thiol that can rearrange to form a protein acylating species. (From: Cummings BS, et al. Role of cytochrome P450 and glutathione S-transferase alpha in the metabolism and cytotoxicity of trichloroethylene in rat kidney. *Biochem Pharmacol* 2000;59:531, with permission.)

numerous cytochrome P-450 isoforms have been identified in renal tissue. For example, cytochromes P-450 IA1, IA2, IIB2, IIC2, IIC11, IID, IIE1, IIJ2, IIJ3, IIJ5, IIJ9, IIIA, IVA1, IVA2, IVA3, and IVF have been identified in RPT of the mouse, rat, and rabbit kidney (107,108,110–114). The distal tubular cells also express several cytochrome P-450 isoforms, including IIB1, IIC11, IIE1, IVA2, IVA3, and IVF (108,110,113,115). There are species- and sex-dependent differences in the expression of cytochrome P-450 isoforms. For example, cytochrome P-450 IIA, IIC, and IIE are present in male mouse kidneys but are absent, or present at very low levels, in female mouse kidneys (116). Several studies also report that there are differences in the expression of cytochrome P-450 isoforms between the human and rodent kidney. One important example is the expression of cytochrome P-450 IIE1, which has been detected in renal proximal and distal tubular cells of mice and rats but not human kidneys (107,108,110,111,117–119). In contrast, both human and rodent kidneys express high

amounts of cytochrome P-450 IVA isoforms. However, rat kidneys express IVA1, IVA2, and IVA3, whereas human kidneys appear to express IVA11 (110,119). Such differences in xenobiotic expression must be taken into account when the role of biotransformation in chemical-induced nephrotoxicity is assessed.

In contrast to the numerous compounds known to be biotransformed to reactive intermediates by P-450 isoforms in the liver, few compounds have been documented to produce nephrotoxicity through renal cytochrome P-450 bioactivation. Renal cytochrome P-450 plays a role in the nephrotoxicity of chloroform (120–127). Renal cytochrome P-450 metabolizes chloroform to trichloromethanol, which is unstable, and releases HCl to form phosgene. Phosgene can react with: (a) two molecules of glutathione to produce diglutathionyl dithiocarbonate, (b) water to produce two molecules of HCl and CO_2, (c) cysteine to produce oxothizolidine-4-carboxylic acid, or (d) cellular macromolecules to initiate toxicity (120,121,127).

TABLE 40-1

EXPRESSION OF SELECTED XENOBIOTIC BIOTRANSFORMATION ENZYMES IN THE KIDNEY

Enzyme	Cell type	Species	References
CYTOCHROME P450 MONOOXYGENASES			
IA	Proximal tubules	Rat, mouse, human	(107,108)
IA2	Proximal tubules		(112)
IIB	Proximal tubules	Rat and mouse	(110)
	Distal tubules	Rat and mouse	(110)
IIC2	Proximal tubules		
IIC9	Unknown[a]	Human but not rat	(107)
IIC11	Distal tubules	Male rat	(110)
IID	Proximal tubules		(114)
IIE1	Proximal tubules	Rat, mouse, not human	(110,119,375)
	Distal tubules		(110)
IIJ	Proximal tubules	Human, rat, mouse	(112,376–378)
IIIA1	Glomerulus	Rat, mouse, not human	(107,108,110)
IIIA4	Proximal tubules	Human, not rat or mouse	(107)
IVA2	Proximal tubules	Rat, mouse, not human	(107,110)
	Distal tubules		(107,110)
IVA3	Proximal tubules	Rat, mouse, not human	(107,110)
	Distal tubules		(107,110)
IVA11	Proximal tubules	Human, not rat or mouse	(117,119)
IVF	Proximal tubule	Human and mouse	(113,119)
	Distal tubules	Mouse	(113)
FLAVIN-CONTAINING MONOOXYGENASES			
FMO1	Unknown[a]	Rat, mouse, and human	(107,137)
FMO3	Unknown[a]	Rat, mouse, and human	(107,137)
FMO5	Unknown[a]	Human	(137)
GLUTATHIONE S-TRANSFERASES			
GSTα	Proximal tubules	Rat, mouse, and human	(115,117,136)
	Distal tubules		
GSTμ	Proximal tubules	Rat, mouse, not human[b]	(115,117,136,140)
GST π	Proximal tubules	Rat, mouse, and human	(115,117)
GST θ	Proximal tubules	Human	(117)

[a] Activity and expression have been measured in kidney microsomes only.
[b] GSTμ is expressed in some human kidney malignancies.

Chloroform bioactivation by renal cytochrome P-450 is dependent on the sex of the species. The marked sex difference in the nephrotoxicity of chloroform is reversed by castration of males or the treatment of females with testosterone, suggesting that the renal cytochrome P-450 responsible for chloroform bioactivation is under androgenic control (120,128). Because cytochrome P-450 isozymes IIB1 and IIE1 are present in male mice and are expressed in female mice treated with testosterone, these isozymes may be responsible for renal chloroform bioactivation (107,127).

Acetaminophen is metabolized in the mouse kidney by cytochrome P-450 IIE1 to the reactive intermediate N-acetyl-p-benzoquinonimine, which binds to cellular proteins (122,124,128). Numerous hepatic proteins to which N-acetyl-p-benzoquinonimine binds covalently have been identified. These include a cytosolic protein that has sequence homology to a selenium binding protein (58 kDa) (129–131), microsomal glutamine synthetase (44 kDa) (126), cytosolic N-10-formyl tetrahydrofolate dehydrogenase (100 kDa) (130,132), and mitochondrial glutamate dehydrogenase (50 kDa) (132). Recent studies suggest that acetaminophen can mediate renal cell death in mouse RPTC by inducing endoplasmic reticulum (ER) stress (100). In this model, acetaminophen treatment increased the expression of GADD153, an ER stress protein, and induced caspase-12 cleavage and apoptosis, independently of caspase-3, -9, or the release of the mitochondrial pro-apoptotic protein Smac/Diablo. It is not known if N-acetyl-p-benzoquinonimine mediates ER stress via cytochrome P-450 bioactivation or if novel mechanisms are involved.

Flavin-containing monooxygenases (FMOs) are a family of enzymes that oxidize the nucleophilic nitrogen, sulfur, and phosphorus moieties of a number of chemicals, including S-(1,2)-dichlorovinyl-L-cysteine, tamoxifen, and cimetidine (108,133–135). The role of FMOs in nephrotoxicity has received little attention, but FMO isozyme FMO3 activity has been detected in the kidneys of rats, dogs, mice, rabbits, and humans (136). Like cytochrome P-450, species differences do exist in FMO activity in the kidney with the rat exhibiting a two-fold to six-fold greater activity (as determined by methionine S-oxidase activity) than other species, including humans. Studies in human kidney microsomes demonstrate that FMO1, FMO3, and FMO5 are all expressed but at different levels (137). Further, samples from African American patients exhibited significantly higher levels of FMO1 activity compared to their Caucasian counterparts, suggesting that the expression of renal FMO isoforms may differ depending on ethnic background (137). However, the expression of FMO1, FMO3, or FMO5 does not appear to be sex-dependent as no difference in the activity or expression of these enzymes was detected between human male and female kidney microsomes (137).

In vitro, FMO1, FMO3, FMO4, and FM05 metabolize cysteine S-conjugated S-allyl cysteine, while FMO3 metabolizes S-(1,2)-dichlorovinyl-L-cysteine (137). However, little S-(1,2)-dichlorovinyl-L-cysteine was metabolized in human kidney microsomes, even though FMO3 was expressed in these tissues, suggesting that FMO may not contribute to the nephrotoxicity of this compound in human renal cells. In contrast, in studies using human proximal tubular cells, treatment with the FMO inhibitor methimazole decreased S-(1,2)-dichlorovinyl-L-cysteine-induced apoptosis (138). Recent studies also suggest that FMO catalyzed sulfoxidation of the sevoflurane (a commonly used anesthetic) degradation product fluoromethyl-2,2-difluoro-1-(trifluoromethyl)vinyl ether may be key to its renal toxicity (139). However the exact isoforms involved in the process, or the mechanisms involved, are not known.

The conjugation enzymes glucuronosyltransferase, sulfotransferase, and glutathione S-transferase are located in the kidney where they conjugate both endogenous and exogenous compounds. The action of these enzymes on nephrotoxicants increases their water solubility and promotes their excretion and elimination (108). Glutathione-S-transferases are a diverse family of enzymes with at least five different subfamilies. Glutathione-S-transferase α, μ, and π are expressed in RPTC of the rat, and α and μ are expressed in rat distal tubular cells (115,136). The expression of glutathione-S-transferases in human RPTC appear to be similar to that observed in rat RPTC (117). The μ class of glutathione-S-transferase is expressed in some patients exhibiting kidney neoplasias and/or tumor growth (140).

Although glutathione conjugation is normally recognized as a detoxification pathway in which electrophiles are neutralized, numerous extrarenally formed glutathione conjugates have proved to be nephrotoxic. In fact, glutathione conjugates and mercapturic acids may be considered targeting moieties for toxicant delivery to the kidney. For example, the extrarenal conjugation of glutathione is important for the nephrotoxicity of $HgCl_2$ (141), halogenated alkenes, and aromatics, and possibly acetaminophen (127,142–144). The nephrotoxicity of the halogenated alkene trichloroethylene in rats and humans is believed to be a direct result of its conjugation with glutathione to form S-(1,2)-dichlorovinyl-glutathione, and the subsequent processing of the glutathione-conjugate to S-(1,2)-dichlorovinyl-L-cysteine in RPTC (115,145) (Fig. 40-3). *In vivo*, trichloroethylene is conjugated with glutathione in the liver and delivered via the bile or blood to the kidney. The expression of enzymes, such as γ-glutamyl transferase and dipeptidase in the RPTC and biliary and intestinal tract results in the cleavage of the γ-glutamyl and glycyl moieties, respectively, and the formation of S-(1,2)-dichlorovinyl-L-cysteine. Metabolism of S-(1,2)-dichlorovinyl-L-cysteine by N-acetyl-S-transferase produces N-acetyl-S-(1,2)-dichlorovinyl-L-cysteine, which is excreted in the urine of mice, rats, and humans exposed to trichloroethylene (146,147). N-acetyl-S-(1,2)-dichlorovinyl-L-cysteine also can be deacetylated back to S-(1,2)-dichlorovinyl-L-cysteine. Metabolism of S-(1,2)-dichlorovinyl-L-cysteine by cysteine-conjugate ß-lyase results in the formation of a reactive thiol that can rearrange to form a protein acylating species. A strong correlation exists between increases in markers of renal injury (proteinuria, creatinine clearance, glucosuria) and the levels of glutathione metabolites of trichloroethylene in the blood and urine of humans exposed to high amounts of trichloroethylene (148). Key determinants in the nephrotoxicity of trichloroethylene and similar chemicals, such as sevoflurane, isoflurane, and desflurane, which utilize this common pathway of biotransformation (139,149),

appear to be the high levels of γ-glutamyl transferase, dipeptidase, and cysteine-conjugate ß-lyase activities found in the kidney.

Role of Reactive Oxygen Species

Reactive oxygen species (ROS) are mediators of cellular injury during inflammatory responses, ischemia-reperfusion, and after nephrotoxicant exposure. Cellular ROS are generated during the normal function of the mitochondrial and microsomal electron transport chains as a result of the incomplete reduction of O_2 to water (150–152) (Fig. 40-4). Superoxide anion free radical is produced by a one-electron reduction of O_2, and H_2O_2 is produced by a two-electron reduction of O_2. Superoxide anion can dismutate to form H_2O_2, or H_2O_2 can be formed directly. The hydroxyl radical is formed from H_2O_2, and the superoxide anion free radical via the metal-catalyzed Haber-Weiss reaction or the superoxide-driven Fenton reaction. Ferrous iron (Fe^{2+}) appears to be the major intracellular initiator of the reaction, but cuprous ions may participate as well. The precise source and form (e.g., ferritin) of the ferrous iron is still unclear.

One source of Fe^{2+} may be the heme-moiety that resides in the active site of cytochrome P-450 isoforms (153). Evidence for this source includes the observation that rats treated intraperitoneally with cisplatin for 4 days had significantly lower levels of renal cytochrome P-450 content compared to control rats, and the decrease in P-450 content correlated with increases in bleomycin-detectable iron content in the kidney. Piperonyl butoxide (a cytochrome P-450 inhibitor) decreased the cisplatin-induced release of iron in the kidney and the functional and morphologic markers of kidney toxicity (154). These same effects were observed in LLC-PK$_1$ cells, a porcine kidney cell culture line. Thus, P-450 may serve as one source of Fe^{2+} to initiate the formation of ROS.

Superoxide anion acts as a reductant for Fe^{3+}, and the Fe^{2+} generated reduces H_2O_2 to the hydroxyl radical. The hydroxyl radical is a highly reactive species and reacts rapidly with adjacent molecules. Superoxide anion and H_2O_2 are less reactive, and H_2O_2 may diffuse away from the initial site of formation to produce injury at a distant site within the cell. Although H_2O_2 readily crosses cell membranes, superoxide anion and hydroxyl radical do not. Because ROS production is a natural byproduct of metabolically active cells, such as the kidney, significant defenses against the normal production of ROS or those produced under pathologic conditions exist (Fig. 40-4).

The term oxidative stress is commonly used to describe those conditions in which there is an increase in ROS formation. Chemicals may initiate oxidative stress indirectly by augmenting the production of ROS. For example, Walker and Shah (155) showed that gentamicin enhances H_2O_2 generation in isolated rat renal cortical mitochondria, and Lund and associates (156) showed that mitochondria isolated from rats treated with $HgCl_2$ exhibit elevated levels of H_2O_2 production. Another mechanism by which chemicals may produce oxidative stress is through *redox cycling*. Certain compounds, especially quinones, can undergo a one-electron reduction to a semiquinone radical and a second one-electron reduction to the hydroquinone. The hydroquinone is oxidized to the quinone, and the cycle begins again, hence the term *redox cycling*. During the reduction process, superoxide anion is formed from O_2, and oxidative stress ensues. For example, Brown and colleagues (157) have provided evidence that menadione (2-methyl-1,4-naphthoquinone) produces toxicity in isolated rat renal epithelial cells through its ability to undergo redox cycling and cause oxidative stress. However, it should be recognized that the ability of quinones to undergo redox cycling varies with the

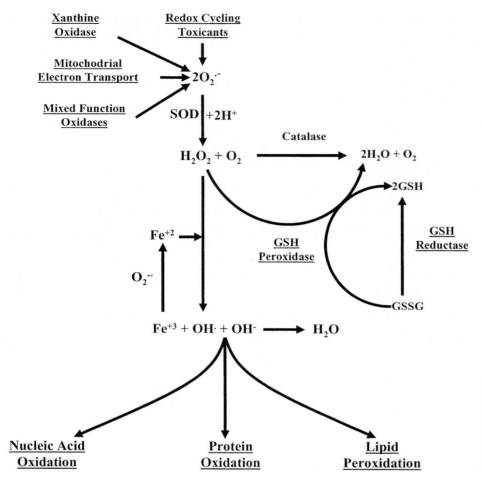

FIGURE 40-4. A schematic representation of the major pathways and possible intracellular targets and oxidants. Detoxification pathways and protective agents are also shown. See text for details. *GSH*, glutathione; *GSSG*, glutathione disulfide; *SOD*, superoxide dismutase.

quinone, and some quinones produce toxicity through their ability to arylate cellular macromolecules, particularly protein sulfhydryls (157–159).

ROS can induce lipid peroxidation, inactivate enzymes by directly oxidizing protein sulfhydryl or amino groups, depolymerize polysaccharides, and induce DNA strand breaks. Lipid peroxidation results from the interaction of free radicals with polyunsaturated fatty acid side chains of membrane phospholipids to form free radicals and relatively stable lipid hydroperoxides (160). Transition metals can catalyze the decomposition of lipid hydroperoxides, which results in the formation of alkoxyl and peroxyl free radicals that propagate the reaction. Lipid breakdown products such as hydroxylated fatty acids, 2-alkenyls, and 4-hydroxyalkenyls also are produced, are toxic, and may contribute to organelle and cellular dysfunction. Thus, ROS-induced degradation of membrane lipids can result in decreased cellular membrane integrity, altered enzymatic activity, and transport properties, and anisotropy (161,162). The oxidation of protein sulfhydryl and amino groups by ROS can produce dramatic alterations in enzymatic activity and membrane structure and function that also lead to cell death. Finally, ROS can produce DNA strand breaks that may lead to cell death. Although H_2O_2 does not directly damage DNA, because of its stability and ability to diffuse throughout the cell, it is generally thought that DNA damage results from the metal-catalyzed activation of H_2O_2 to the hydroxyl radical near the DNA.

A wide variety of structurally diverse nephrotoxicants appear to produce renal cell injury at least in part by oxidative stress, including $HgCl_2$ (141,156,160), haloalkene cysteine conjugates (163–166), cyclosporine A (166), and cisplatin (167–172). The diversity of these nephrotoxicants highlights the critical and common roles that ROS play in the mechanism of cell death. Further, the generation of ROS is typically an initiator signal for renal cell death.

MEDIATORS OF CELL INJURY

A number of common cellular pathways that mediate cell death have been identified. It is generally thought that after an initial cellular interaction, a sequence of events occurs that leads to cell injury and death. In the case of oncosis and apoptosis, there is a point along the sequence, yet to be identified, that is the point of no return; the point at which the cell will die irrespective of any intervention. Investigators have tried to identify the sequence of deleterious events, the point of no return, and the relative importance of each observed change in a variety of tissues for a number of years with some success. This has led to the identification of numerous intracellular mediators that are keys in the generation of renal cell injury and death.

p53 and p21

The tumor suppressor protein p53 and the cell cycle inhibitor protein p21 play important roles in renal cell death and acute renal failure (171,173–179). p53 and p21 appear to have opposite effects in that activation of p53 increases renal cell death (171) while activation of p21 appears to be protective (174,176). However, recent reports suggest that p53 can activate p21 during renal cell death induced by selected toxicants, such as cisplatin (175). Thus the exact mechanisms controlling p21 and p53 cross talk, and the effect of this cross talk on renal cell death and cellular proteins have yet to be determined.

p53 is activated in renal cells after exposure to agents that induce DNA damage, such as cisplatin (172,175). The mechanism of p53 activation involves its phosphorylation at numerous serine-residues and its subsequent release from a regulator protein and translocation to the nucleus. Once in the nucleus, p53 can induce the transcription of a number of genes, including p21 (175), and activate several apoptotic pathways such as those involving caspases. Inhibition of p53 activation with a pharmacological agent decreased cisplatin-induced apoptosis in rabbit RPTC through a mechanism that includes the inhibition of caspase-3 (171). Caspase-3 activity in this model preceded both phosphatidylserine externalization and chromatin condensation, but not p53 nuclear translocation. In support of this hypothesis others have demonstrated that inhibition of p53 translocation inhibits ARF and renal cell death induced by cisplatin in rat RPTC (180), and after renal ischemia in rats (181,182).

Induction of p21 occurs in response to DNA damage and p53-induced cell cycle arrest (174). Once activated, p21 inhibits one or more of the cyclin-dependent kinase activities (173,174) and it is hypothesized that inhibition of these processes prevents renal cell cycle activity and apoptosis, and protects against nephrotoxicity. In support of this hypothesis, knock-out mice lacking p21 exhibit increased renal cell cycle activity, apoptosis, and are more susceptible to cisplatin and ischemia-induced ARF compared to wild type controls (174). The downstream mediators of apoptosis include caspases, as treatment of RPTC from p21 knock-out mice with cisplatin resulted in significantly higher levels of caspase-3 activity and apoptosis compared to control cells expressing p21 (176). Al-though these studies illustrate that caspase activity is one mechanism by which p53 induces and p21 protects against renal cell death, the exact pathways needed to activate caspases have not fully determined.

Signaling Kinases

Signaling kinases refer to enzymes that alter the activity, expression, or localization of another protein by altering its phosphorylation, including other signaling kinases. Signaling kinases differ in terms of the amino acids targeted for phosphorylation (serine/threonine/tyrosine), the location within a cell (membrane-bound or cytosolic), and the protein targeted for phosphorylation. Table 40-2 lists several signaling kinases identified in the kidney, the site within the kidney or cell involved, the nephrotoxicant involved, and several references to studies that suggest critical roles for signaling kinases both in the development of renal cell death and in the recovery of renal cells after toxicant-induced injury (12,183–189).

Protein kinase C (PKC) refers to a family of serine/threonine kinases comprised of 11 different isoforms divided into conventional PKC (cPKC; α, $\beta_{1/2}$, and γ), novel PKC (nPKC; ε, δ, η, and θ), and atypical PKC (aPKC; τ, λ and ζ) groups (190). These isoforms differ in terms of preferred substrates and mechanisms of action (190–192). Activation of cPKC is Ca^{2+}- and diacylglycerol-dependent while activation of nPKC is Ca^{2+}-independent (190,193). In contrast, activation of aPKC is independent of both Ca^{2+} and diacylglycerol. RPTC have been reported to express α, β_1, β_2, ζ, δ, λ, and ϵ (194–197), and several other isoforms are expressed in the kidney of rats, mice, and humans (183,185,198,199).

TABLE 40-2

SELECTED SIGNALING KINASES INVOLVED IN RENAL CELL INJURY, SURVIVAL, OR REPAIR

Kinase	Location	Nephrotoxicant	Reference
PROTEIN KINASE C (PKC)			
CONVENTIONAL PKC			
PKCα	Proximal tubules	Cisplatin DCVC[a]	(185,379)
ATYPICAL PKC			
PKCζ	Proximal tubules	t-butylhydroperoxide	(184)
MITOGEN ACTIVATED PROTIEN KIANSE (MAPK)			
ERK1/2	Proximal tubules	Cisplatin H_2O_2 TGHQ[c]	(185,186,202, 205,380)
JNK/SAPK[a]	Proximal tubules	Cisplatin	(186)
P38	Proximal tubules	Cisplatin H_2O_2 TGHG[c]	(186,202,205)
OTHER KINASES			
Protein kinase B[b]	LLC-PK1 Proximal tubules	Cisplatin Mechanical Injury H_2O_2	(12,380)
Phosphoinositide-3-kinase	LLC-PK1 Proximal tubules	Cisplatin Mechanical Injury	(12)

[a]S-(1,2)-dichlorovinyl-L-cysteine
[b]Also known as AKT
[c]2,3,5-tris-(glutathion-S-yl)hydroquinone

The toxicity of both fumonison-B1 and TNF are mediated by PKC in human renal cells and LLC-PK1 cells (185,188,189). The exact role of PKC in renal cell death depends on the toxicant and the specific isoform(s) involved (183–185). For example, activation of PKCα in rabbit RPTC during cisplatin treatment results in mitochondrial dysfunction and cell death (185). In contrast, activation of PKC-ζ after exposure to t-butylhdyroperoxide mediates cellular repair (183,184).

One possible mechanism by which PKC mediates renal cell death following toxicant exposure is by activating a group of kinases called mitogen-activated protein kinases (MAPK). MAPK is the general name for a family of tyrosine/threonine kinases that are activated by oxidants, environmental chemicals, and anticancer agents (200–209). Family members of MAPK include ERK 1 and 2 (ERK1/2), the c-jun N-terminal kinase/stress activated protein kinases (JNK/SAPK), and p38 (206). Studies in RPTC support the hypothesis that activation of ERK1/2 is a participant in cisplatin-induced mitochondrial dysfunction (185). In particular cisplatin-induced PKCα activation was followed by ERK1/2 activation, which caused a decrease in mitochondrial membrane potential, caspase 3 activation, and apoptosis. Other studies supporting the hypothesis that MAPK mediates cisplatin-induced renal cell death include those performed *in vivo* in mouse kidneys (58,186,210). The targets of MAPK include mitochondrial-associated proteins (58,185), forkhead transcription protein (211), alpha-adducin (a prominent protein in the regulation of cytoskeleton filament, (210)), and proteins that are part of the mitochondrial electron transport chain (185).

Similar to PKC, the role of MAPK in toxicant-induced renal cell death is toxicant-specific. Arany et al. (186) demonstrated that ERK activation mediated cisplatin-induced renal cell death *in vivo* and *in vitro* in mouse models. However, the same investigators observed that ERK activation protected against oxidant-induced (H_2O_2) cell death (186). Interestingly, cisplatin-induced ERK activation and renal cell death was dependent on the epidermal growth factor-receptor (EGF-R) and c-Src. Although studies by Zhuang and colleagues (12) (personal communication) demonstrated that H_2O_2 exposure of RPTC results in Src, EGF-R, ERK1/2, protein kinase B (Akt) and phosphoinositide-3-kinase (PI3K) activation, ERK1/2 inhibition was associated with cell death and Src inhibition potentiated cell death. Finally, EGF-R-induced activation of ERK is believed to mediate 2,3,5-tris-(glutathion-S-yl)hydroquinone (TGHQ)-induced death in LLC-PK1 cells (202,205). The detailed mechanisms of Src, EGF-R, PI3K, ERK1/2 and p38 activation, the targets of these kinases and their role in cell death produced by different toxicants remain to be determined.

Altered Calcium Homeostasis

Intracellular Ca^{2+} homeostasis is important to cell viability because Ca^{2+} is a second messenger and plays a critical role in a variety of cellular functions (212–216). Cytosolic free Ca^{2+} concentration is approximately 100 nM and is tightly regulated in the face of a large extracellular-intracellular gradient (10,000:1) by a series of pumps and channels located on the plasma membrane and ER. Mitochondria are not thought to be involved significantly in the normal regulation of Ca^{2+}; however, they accumulate Ca^{2+} after toxicant exposure or hypoxia (212).

Considering the preceding, toxicants must increase cytosolic free Ca^{2+} levels supraphysiologically or produce sustained increases to initiate or mediate cell death. In turn, these increases in cytosolic free Ca^{2+} can activate a number of degradative Ca^{2+}-dependent enzymes, such as phospholipases, endonucleases, and proteinases, and alter the cy-

toskeleton. The precise role of Ca^{2+} influx remains unclear. However, decreasing the extracellular Ca^{2+} concentration or blocking extracellular Ca^{2+} influx decreases cell death (217–220). Increases in cytosolic free Ca^{2+} levels were observed in a hypoxia model using rat RPTC and in a mitochondrial inhibitor model using rabbit RPTC, and experimental manipulations that chelate intracellular Ca^{2+}, or decrease the influx of extracellular Ca^{2+}, decreased cell death (219–224). These results reveal that intracellular and extracellular Ca^{2+} mediate the late phase of cell injury. Studies demonstrating that inhibitors of Ca^{2+}-activated neutral proteases (calpains) decreased cell death produced by a variety of diverse toxicants, and anoxia, in rabbit RPTC, further supports the role of Ca^{2+} in cell death (219,220,224,225). Nephrotoxicants that have been shown to increase cytosolic free Ca^{2+} include $HgCl_2$ (226,227), pentachlorobutadienyl-glutathione (167), pentachlorobutadienyl-L-cysteine (228), tetrafluoroethyl-L-cysteine (229), S-(1,2)-dichlorovinyl-L-cysteine (230–233), oxidants (234,235), sevoflurane, miconazole (236,237), cyclosporine A (87,238), and gentamicin (155,239,240).

Proteinases

Nonphysiologic activation of proteinases in the cytosol or those associated with organelles or membranes could disrupt normal membrane, cytoskeleton, or organelle function and lead to cell death. Lysosomes are one source of proteinases because they normally degrade proteins with acid hydrolases. The lysosomal membrane could rupture under conditions of cell injury, releasing the proteinases into the cytosol to degrade susceptible critical proteins. Experimental studies have found little evidence of lysosomal rupture during injurious conditions (212). There was neither evidence of lysosomal rupture prior to cell death nor beneficial effects of lysosomal enzyme depletion in primary cultures of individually microdissected human and rabbit RPTC treated with cyclosporine A (241). The cysteine proteinase inhibitor t-trans-epoxysuccinyl-leucylamido(4-guandino)butane (E64), however, was cytoprotective.

A variety of cysteine and serine proteinase inhibitors were shown to be ineffective in protecting rabbit RPTC segments from antimycin A, tetrafluoroethyl-L-cysteine, bromohydroquinone, and t-butylhydroperoxide (242). However, E64 and the aspartic acid proteinase inhibitor pepstatin produced a small degree of cytoprotection in RPTC exposed to antimycin A or tetrafluoroethyl-L-cysteine. Although loss of lysosomal membrane potential was observed after antimycin A exposure, and extensive inhibition of lysosomal cathepsins B and L by E64 was correlated with cytoprotection, E64 cytoprotection was only observed after some cell death had occurred. These results reveal that lysosomal cysteine and aspartic acid proteinases do not play a significant role in RPTC death produced by nephrotoxicants.

Ca^{2+}-activated neutral cysteine proteinases (calpains) are a 14-member family of Ca^{2+}-activated proteinases that have cytoskeletal proteins, membrane proteins, and enzymes as substrates (243). The kidney expresses calpain-1 and -2, the two most-studied calpains and Schnellmann and colleagues (221,224,244,245) showed that calpain inhibitor II and the calpain inhibitor PD150606 decreased calpain activity and decreased cell death produced by a variety of toxicants including bromohydroquinone, antimycin A, tetrafluoroethyl-L-cysteine, and t-butylhydroperoxide. Inhibition of calpains may serve to protect the cell by preventing calpain-mediated extracellular Ca^{2+} influx and/or cytoskeletal alterations (221,244). Edelstein and associates (246) reported that calpain activity was increased early (within 10 minutes) in the genesis of hypoxic injury to rat RPTC and that inhibition of the initial calpain-mediated influx of extracellular Ca^{2+} protected these cells. Furthermore, Takaoka and associates (247) reported that treatment with calpeptin increased renal function in rats subjected to ischemia-reperfusion. These results suggest that calpains play a critical role in cell death produced by a wide range of nephrotoxicants and renal dysfunction produced by ischemia-reperfusion.

Recent evidence has revealed that mitochondrial Ca^{2+} accumulation results in the activation of a mitochondrial calpain, which causes mitochondrial dysfunction (248–250). This atypical mitochondrial calpain has been identified as calpain-10, and inhibition of it prevented mitochondrial dysfunction. Further, mitochondrial calpain-10 targets complex I of the electron transport chain. While cytosolic calpains-1 and -2 are mediators of cytoskeleton and membrane disruption in cell injury, it is now clear that mitochondrial calpain plays a role in cell injury.

In several reports, the activation of calpains resulted in the deactivation of caspases and increased oncosis (251,252). Likewise, in a neuronal apoptosis system, addition of calpain I inhibited the release of cytochrome c and the subsequent cleavage and activation of pro-caspase -3 and -9 (251). In contrast, inhibition of calpains in this same model increased apoptosis. Furthermore, calpains inactivate caspases -3, -7, -8, and -9 by cleaving them at sites distinct from their activation site (253). Thus, calpains may mediate key processes that determine whether a cell will die by either apoptosis or oncosis. The mechanisms and targets of calpains in renal cell injury are still to be determined. Caspases, a family of cysteine proteases, are discussed under the previous apoptosis section. Caspase activity, per se, is not always needed for apoptosis to occur. For example, caspase-2-directed permeabilization of the mitochondrial membrane results in the release of the pro-apoptotic proteins cytochrome c and Omi is independent of its catalytic activity (62,63,254). Furthermore, a recent study demonstrated that apoptosis induced by four diverse toxicants (cisplatin, vincristine, staurosporine, and A23187) proceeded in rabbit RPTC in the presence of caspase inhibitors and the absence of caspase-3, -8, and -9 activity (255). Further, cisplatin-induced apoptosis in RPTC was shown to be both dependent and independent of caspase-3 and p53 activity (171). Although these studies support the hypothesis that renal cell apoptosis can proceed in the absence of caspase activity, the exact mechanisms involved are not known. Recent data in renal cells show that cisplatin-induced apoptosis is mediated via endonuclease G as opposed to caspases (256,257).

Phospholipase A_2

Phospholipase A_2s (PLA_2) are a family of enzymes that hydrolyze the acyl bond at the sn-2 position of phospholipids, resulting in the release of arachidonic acid and a lysophospholipid (258). The enzymes in this group have different substrate preferences, Ca^{2+} dependencies, and biochemical characteristics. Several Ca^{2+}-dependent forms have been identified in the rat and rabbit kidney cytosolic fraction with molecular weights of 14, 85, and 100 kDa (258,259). The most thoroughly characterized renal cytosolic PLA_2 is the Ca^{2+}-dependent 85 kDa PLA_2 ($cPLA_2$). A Ca^{2+}-independent plasmalogen-selective PLA_2 has been described in the rabbit kidney (260), which is located in the cytosol and has a molecular weight of approximately 28 kDa. Recently an ER Ca^{2+}-independent 80 kDa PLA_2, distinct from the 85-kDa cytosolic $cPLA_2$, has been found in the rabbit kidney (261). Furthermore, Mancuso and associates (262) have reported that human kidneys express mRNA corresponding to an 85-kDa membrane bound Ca^{2+}-independent PLA_2. This PLA_2 was subsequently demonstrated to be localized to at least the ER of rabbit RPTC and in rat kidney (261,263). Thus, both Ca^{2+}-dependent and Ca^{2+}-

independent PLA_2 are present in the kidney. There are likely additional forms of PLA_2 found in the kidney, and additional characterization of all renal forms is needed.

It is generally thought that a toxicant-induced nonphysiological increase in PLA_2 activity could result in the loss of membrane phospholipids and consequently impair membrane function. Because many PLA_2 are Ca^{2+}-dependent, the increase in PLA_2 activity may be secondary to an increase in cytosolic free Ca^{2+} (258). For example, an increase in PLA_2 activity was observed in rabbit RPTC subjected to anoxia (264), and the phospholipase inhibitors mepacrine and dibucaine decreased hypoxia-induced rat RPTC death (265). The generated lysophospholipids and free fatty acids also may contribute to the injury by altering membrane permeability or uncoupling mitochondrial respiration (266–269). If ATP levels are limited during the injury process, reacylation of the lysophospholipids (270,271), de novo phospholipid synthesis (272), and esterification of free fatty acids (273,274) may all be inhibited.

The role of PLA_2 activation in various forms of renal cell injury and apoptosis is controversial (69,172,222,258–261,264,275–279). Nevertheless, the role PLA_2 in cell injury and death appears to be toxicant-specific. For example, inhibition of membrane-bound Ca^{2+}-independent PLA_2 with bromoenol lactone increased rabbit RPTC oncosis induced by the oxidants t-butylhydroperoxide, menadione, duraquinone, cumene hydroperoxide, and cisplatin (at high concentrations) but had no affect on oncosis induced by the nonoxidant antimycin A (261). The increase in cell death induced by these oxidants correlated to increased lipid peroxidation at early time points during injury, prior to decreases in membrane integrity. Thus, Ca^{2+}-independent PLA_2 in renal cells appears to protect against oxidant-induced renal cell oncosis. In contrast, inhibition of membrane-bound Ca^{2+}-independent PLA_2 in the same cell type decreased cisplatin-induced apoptosis and inhibited caspase-3 activation, phosphatidylserine externalization and chromatin condensation (172). Thus, membrane-bound $iPLA_2$ appears to induce apoptosis and protect against oxidant-induced oncosis in rabbit RPTC. The exact mechanisms controlling these opposing roles have yet to be fully determined. However, oxidants inactivate $iPLA_2$ activity in rabbit RPTC, whereas cisplatin, at an apoptotic inducing concentration, does not (275).

In contrast to the protective role of membrane-bound Ca^{2+}-independent PLA_2 following oxidative stress, increasing $cPLA_2$ activity increased the susceptibility of renal epithelial cells to oxidative stress (280). Increased H_2O_2 toxicity was not due to decreases in the activity of the antioxidant defense enzymes superoxide dismutase, catalase, or glutathione peroxidase. In contrast, chelation of cytosolic free Ca^{2+} decreased H_2O_2 toxicity, suggesting a key role for Ca^{2+} in the mediation of $cPLA_2$-mediated oncosis in renal cells. Kohjimoto and colleagues (281) demonstrated that preincubation of MDCK cells with an inhibitor of $cPLA_2$ (arachiondyl trifluoromethyl ketone) significantly reduced the toxicity of oxalate. Thus, $cPLA_2$ can mediate some forms of oncotic renal cell death.

Another possible role for PLA_2 in renal cell death is their ability to metabolize and release fatty acids from glycerophospholipids. Cell membranes are rich in polyunsaturated fatty acids and as such are susceptible to lipid peroxidation under normal and pathologic conditions. Peroxidized lipids are predisposed to degradation by PLA_2, resulting in increased PLA_2 activity and the formation of arachidonic acid metabolites and lysophospholipids. Ultimately, the lipids are reacylated and repaired. As discussed earlier, selective inhibition of an ER-Ca^{2+}-independent, plasmalogen-selective PLA_2-potentiated t-butylhydroperoxide induced rabbit RPTC death. Furthermore, t-butylhydroperoxide itself decreased $iPLA_2$ activity prior to the onset of cell death (275). These results reveal that the microsomal Ca^{2+}-independent, plasmalogen-selective PLA_2 may function to hydrolyze oxidized or damaged phospholipids and is therefore a *phospholipid repair enzyme*. The observation that *t*-butylhydroperoxide decreased the microsomal Ca^{2+}-independent, plasmalogen-selective PLA_2 activity suggests that one pathway by which *t*-butylhydroperoxide is toxic is through its ability to produce oxidized phospholipids and inhibit their removal. The importance of not only Ca^{2+}-independent PLA_2, but also all PLA_2 in renal cell death is still under investigation.

MITOCHONDRIA, ENDOPLASMIC RETICULUM, LYSOSOMES, AND THE CELL MEMBRANE

Mitochondria, ER, lysosomes, and the cell membrane all play a role in nephrotoxic cell injury that leads to oncosis and apoptosis. Apoptosis and oncosis do not proceed through mutually exclusive pathways consisting of single sequences of events. Cell death by apoptosis or oncosis is often determined by the organelles affected and the pathway(s) activated in these organelles. Typically, one pathway predominates over others, depending on the time of exposure, the concentration used, and the toxicant itself.

Because of the presence of multiple cell death pathways and multiple targets, inhibition of one pathway may not block nephrotoxicant-induced cell death. For example, if one blocks the oxidative stress associated with S-(1,2)-dichlorovinyl-L-cysteine, pentachlorobutadienyl-L-cysteine, or tetrafluoroethyl-L-cysteine exposure to RPTC, the rate of cell death is diminished, but the cells eventually die because of the mitochondrial dysfunction produced by these compounds (282) (Fig. 40-5). Thus, a given chemical can cause cell death by interacting at numerous organelles, and blocking one interaction at one organelle may not decrease cell death, rather it may alter the organelle targeted, and thus the mechanism of cell death.

Mitochondria

The renal tubular reabsorption of solutes and water requires a large expenditure of energy. Although ATP is generated by both oxidative phosphorylation and glycolysis, approximately 95% of renal ATP is formed by oxidative phosphorylation (283). The amount of oxidative phosphorylation that occurs within a given cell varies along the nephron. Thus, toxicants that interfere with mitochondrial function and anoxia will produce cell injury and death, particularly in tubular cells that have limited glycolytic capabilities, such as the S_1 and S_2 segments of the proximal tubules.

Mitochondria can act as primary or secondary mediators in apoptosis and oncosis (284,285). When mitochondria are the primary target of nephrotoxicants, release of cytochrome c and other apoptotic inducing proteins can occur early in the apoptotic process. If mitochondria are not a direct target of the nephrotoxicant, these proteins may be released but later in the apoptotic process. As stated, central to the role of the mitochondrion in apoptosis is its ability to release cytochrome c and other apoptotic inducing proteins, leading to the activation of caspases-9 and -3 and other downstream caspases (75) (Fig. 40-2). Other regulators of apoptosis that interact with the mitochondria have been discussed previously.

A key difference in mitochondrial function during apoptosis and oncosis is the maintenance of ATP during apoptosis. ATP production must be maintained long enough for apoptosis to ensue. Cellular ATP levels act with the mitochondrial membrane potential as one switch that dictates whether a cell dies by apoptosis or oncosis (286). If the mitochondrial membrane

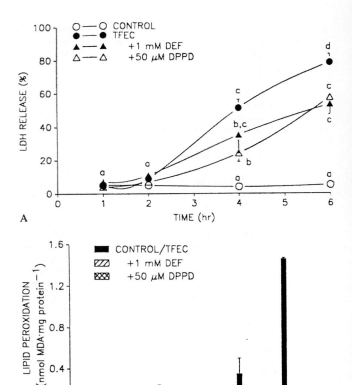

FIGURE 40-5. **A:** The time-dependent effects of deferoxamine (DEF) and N, N′-diphenyl-1,4-phenylenediamine (DPPD) on S-(1,1,2,2-tetrafluoroethyl)-L-cysteine (TFEC)-induced cell death (lactate dehydrogenase [LDH] release) from rabbit renal proximal tubules. DEF and DPPD were added at the same time as TFEC ($25\ \mu M$). Values are means ± SEM. Values at a given time point or within a given treatment with different superscripts are significantly different from one another ($P \leq 0.05$). **B:** The time-dependent effects of DEF and DPPD on TFEC-induced lipid peroxidation (malondialdehyde [MDA] formation) in rabbit renal proximal tubule suspensions. Values are means ± SEM. Only the TFEC alone is significantly different from controls ($P \leq 0.05$). (Adapted from: Groves CE, Lock EA, Schnellmann RG. Role of lipid peroxidation in renal proximal tubule cell death induced by haloalkene cysteine conjugates. *Toxicol Appl Pharmacol* 1991;107:54, with permission.)

potential is lost quickly and cellular ATP levels are drastically decreased (below 10% to 20% of normal), then oncosis occurs. Events that result in the rapid loss of mitochondrial membrane potential include the rapid influx of Ca^{2+} into the mitochondria and the rupture of the inner and/or outer mitochondrial membranes (286). In contrast, if the loss of membrane potential is slower and ATP levels are maintained through oxidative phosphorylation or glycolysis, then the cell dies through apoptosis. It should be noted that the majority of cells in culture derive their energy from glycolysis and can maintain ATP levels in the presence of mitochondrial dysfunction. Consequently, cultured cells are generally more susceptible to apoptosis than cells *in vivo*.

Many nephrotoxicants cause mitochondrial dysfunction (285). The mechanisms of cell death for many of these toxicants are still under investigation, whereas others are fairly well known. For example, $HgCl_2$ altered isolated renal cortical mitochondrial function and mitochondrial morphology prior to proximal tubule necrosis after an *in vivo* exposure

(287,288). When added to isolated rat renal cortical mitochondria, $HgCl_2$ produced similar changes in various respiratory parameters (287; 288). Rabbit RPTC exposed to $HgCl_2$ also exhibit decreased mitochondrial function prior to the onset of cell death (289). Pentachlorobutadienyl-L-cysteine initially uncouples oxidative phosphorylation in RPTC cells by dissipating the proton gradient (290–293). In contrast, tetrafluoroethyl-L-cysteine does not uncouple oxidative phosphorylation but rather inhibits state-3 respiration by inhibiting sites I and II of the electron transport chain (293). Other nephrotoxicants that have been shown to affect mitochondrial function include cisplatin (294–296), citrinin (297–301), ochratoxin A (302–304), cephaloridine (305,306), N-(3,5)-dichlorophenyl-succinimide (307), S-1,2-(dichlorovinyl)-L-cysteine (308,309), and 2-bromohydroquinone (159).

Because of the vast number of nephrotoxicants that induce mitochondrial dysfunction, studies are starting to focus on the exact protein targets within the mitochondria. For example, studies determining the effect of hypoxia on mitochondrial electron transport chain constituents in rabbit RPTC reveal that complex I may be particularly sensitive (310,311). Studies also illustrate that cisplatin-induced changes in oxidative phosphorylation, membrane potential, and ATP levels in rabbit RPTC are all preceded by inhibition of F(0)F(1)-ATPase (complex IV) (185).

Recent studies in renal cortical mitochondria suggest that an increase in Ca^{2+} influx activates a mitochondrial calpain that targets complex I of the electron transport chain and induces mitochondrial dysfunction (see the previous text) (248–250). These recent studies are of critical importance to the understanding of the pathology of mitochondrial-mediated renal cell death and to identifying novel therapeutic targets for inhibition of renal cell death and possibly ARF.

Endoplasmic Reticulum

The ER is the site of protein synthesis and processing, and bioactivation and detoxification pathways, including those involving cytochrome P-450 and FMO. The ER is also a key regulator of cellular Ca^{2+} homeostasis. Under physiologic conditions, ER Ca^{2+} is typically released following receptor activation through the binding of inositol triphosphate (IP_3) to IP_3 receptors on the ER. Cytosolic free Ca^{2+} increases as a consequence of the ER Ca^{2+} release and is subsequently decreased by ER uptake via the smooth ER Ca^{2+}-ATPases (SERCA) or extrusion via the plasma membrane Ca^{2+}-ATPase.

Schellmann and colleagues demonstrated that the release of ER Ca^{2+} is an important signaling pathway in oncosis (219,312). In this case, depletion of ER Ca^{2+} stores with the SERCA inhibitors thapsigargin or cyclopiazonic acid prior to antimycin A or hypoxia exposure resulted in the inhibition of oncosis (219,312). It was demonstrated that Ca^{2+} release from the ER activates calpains (Ca^{2+}-dependent cysteine proteases), which subsequently leads to further disruption of ion homeostasis, cleavage of cytoskeleton proteins, and cell swelling, which ultimately results in oncosis (221,224,244,312). Recent studies demonstrate that the cytoprotective effects of some stress proteins may be through their ability to regulate ER Ca^{2+}. For example, iodacetamide and S-(1,2)-dichlorovinyl-L-cysteine, both alkylating toxicants, can activate heat shock proteins (HSPs), calreticulin, and glucose related protein 78 (GRP78) in the renal epithelial cell line, LLC-PK1 (313,314). HSPs are typically ER localized proteins that are critical mediators of protein folding. Glucose related protein 78 and calreticulin are Ca^{2+} binding proteins that appear to aid in the sequestering of Ca^{2+} during toxic stress. Sequestering of Ca^{2+} by these proteins may also protect renal cells by preventing cellular oxidative stress that is induced by Ca^{2+}-mediated mitochondrial injury (315,316). The increased expression of Ca^{2+}-sequestering proteins and HSPs at the ER is a response to a previous injury and is meant to condition the cell to withstand further injury.

The ER is also a site within the kidney for genesis of apoptosis induced by a number of compounds. Caspase-12 is a murine caspase, is similar to caspase-1 and -11, and is localized to the ER. Further, caspases-12 is found in mice kidneys and is expressed in RPTC (317). Mice that do not express caspases-12 were resistant to renal cell apoptosis induced by the ER stress agents tunicaymcin, brefeldin A, and thapsigargin compared to wild type animals. In contrast, kidneys from mice null for caspases-12 underwent similar levels of apoptosis caused by the fas antibody, TNF-α plus cycloheximide, or staurosporine, agents that cause apoptosis by mechanisms other than ER stress. The key to the activation of caspases-12 as opposed to other caspases may be perturbations in the ER membrane and/or Ca^{2+} levels. Recently, acetaminophen has also been suggested to activate caspase-12 in mouse RPTC (100). Thus, ER can mediate both renal cell oncosis, via the release of Ca^{2+} and calpain activation, or renal cell apoptosis via the activation of caspases-12, and it appears that both mechanisms involve changes in the ability of the ER to regulate Ca^{2+}. The exact mechanistic differences between ER-mediated apoptosis and oncosis are under investigation.

Plasma and Organelle Membranes

Some compounds can interact with the plasma membrane directly, increase ion permeability, and disrupt ion homeostasis. For example, amphotericin B is an antifungal polyene that binds to cholesterol in the plasma membrane and forms a pore that increases potassium and proton permeabilities (103,318,319). Several heavy metals such as silver, gold, mercury, and copper also appear to react with the plasma membrane and increase potassium permeability (320,321). It remains to be determined how these changes in potassium and proton permeabilities ultimately lead to cell death; however, Reeves and Shah (322) reported that inhibition of potassium channels decreases hypoxic injury in rat RPTC.

Toxicants generally disrupt cell volume and ion homeostasis by inhibiting energy production either directly or indirectly. The loss of ATP results in the inhibition of membrane transporters that maintain the differential ion gradients across the plasma membrane. The Na^+-K^+-ATPase is responsible for maintaining the normal Na^+ and K^+ gradients and the secondary ion transport processes. As ATP levels decrease, Na^+-K^+-ATPase activity decreases, resulting in K^+ efflux and Na^+ influx and a decrease in the normally negative membrane potential (323,324). The decrease in the negative membrane potential allows Cl^-, as well as additional Na^+, to enter down a concentration gradient resulting in water influx and cellular swelling. For example, treatment of rabbit RPTC suspensions with the mitochondrial inhibitor antimycin A inhibits respiration within 1 minute, followed by ATP depletion, and the loss of the sodium and potassium gradients and transport over the next 5 to 10 minutes (224,325) (Fig. 40-6). Miller and Schnellmann (326) demonstrated that increased Cl^- influx does not occur during the initial 15 minutes but between 15 and 30 minutes, during the late stages of cellular injury, followed by cellular rupture. Decreasing extracellular NaCl concentrations by 50% with isoosmotic substitution of mannitol decreased Cl^- influx, cellular swelling, and cellular rupture (327). Furthermore, hyperosmotic incubation buffer decreased the cellular swelling and cellular lysis but not the increased Cl^- influx (327). Thus, the delayed increase in Cl^- influx may be the trigger for the water influx and additional Na^+ influx that provides the osmotic force for cellular swelling and rupture.

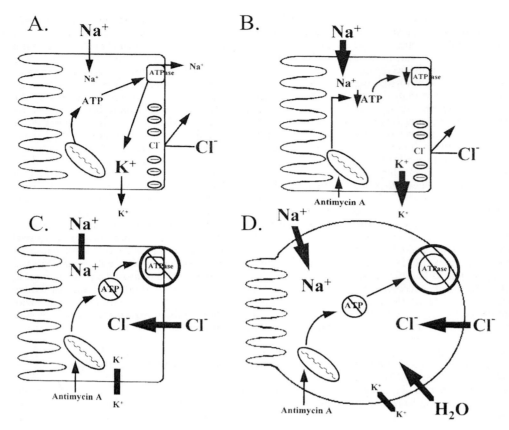

FIGURE 40-6. A: A schematic representation of a normally functioning renal cell. Note that the inside of the cell is negative with respect to the outside, which decreases the ability of Cl^- to enter the cell. **B:** The addition of a mitochondrial inhibitor such as antimycin A blocks cellular respiration, decreases ATP levels and Na^+-K^+-ATPase activity, increases Na^+ influx and K^+ efflux, and decreases the membrane potential. **C:** Subsequently, there is an increase in Cl^- influx (down the concentration gradient) by an unidentified pathway. **D:** The increase in Cl^- influx results in water influx, increased Na^+ influx, and cellular swelling. These processes provide the osmotic force that ultimately leads to cellular lysis.

Increased Cl^- influx occurs during the late stages of cell injury in RPTC and LLC-PK1 cells exposed to a variety of injury stimuli and toxicants, including $HgCl_2$, t-butylhydroperoxide, bromohydroquinone, tetrafluoroethyl-L-cysteine, and hypoxia (327,328). The mechanism by which Cl^- influx occurs under these conditions is not known, but it is inhibited by blockers of Ca^{2+}-activated Cl^- channels (e.g., niflumic acid, indanyloxyacetic acid (IAA-94), 5-nitro-2-(3)-phenylpropylamino-benzoate (NPPB), and diphenylamine-2-carboxylate (DPC)) (150–153). The Cl^- influx is insensitive to the Cl^- channel blockers 4-acetamide-4'-isothiocyanostilbene-2,2'-disulfonic acid (SITS) and diisothiocyanostilbene-2,2'-disulfonic acid (DIDS) or to the Cl^- transport inhibitors bumetanide and hydrochlorothiazide (327). Therefore, the Cl^- influx that occurs during the late phase of cell death may be through a Ca^{2+}-activated Cl^- channel.

Lysosomes

Lysosomes are membrane-bound vesicles that pinch off from the Golgi-apparatus and contain a variety of hydrolytic enzymes (329). Under normal conditions lysosomes contain hydrolytic enzymes that function as intracellular digestive enzymes. However, lysosomes can play an important role in the toxicity of several compounds including aminoglycoside antibiotics, and in α_{2u}-nephropathy. α_{2u}-nephropathy occurs in male rats when compounds such as unleaded gasoline, d-limonene, 1,4-dichlorobenzene, tetrachloroethylene, decalin, 2,2,4-trimethylpentane, and lindane bind to α_{2u}-globulin and prevent its normal renal proximal tubular lysosomal degradation (330–333). α_{2u}-Globulin is synthesized in the liver of male rats under androgen control. Serum α_{2u}-globulin (18.7 kDa) is freely filtered by the glomerulus with approx-

imately half being reabsorbed via endocytosis in the S_2 segment of the proximal tubule. The binding of these agents to α_{2u}-globulin inhibits its normal degradation and results in the accumulation of α_{2u}-globulin in the proximal tubule. Over time, the size and number of lysosomes increase, and characteristic protein-droplet morphology is observed. Ultimately, this leads to single-cell oncosis, the formation of granular casts at the junction of the proximal tubule and the thin loop of Henle, and cellular regeneration. Recent data show that an HS protein cognate of 73 kDa mediates the binding of α_{2u}-globulin to a 96-kDa membrane glycoprotein in male rat kidney lysosomes (334). This HSP also is involved in the degradation of other cellular proteins. Treatment of rats with 2,2,4-trimethylpentane increases the rate of transport of not only α_{2u}-globulin into the lysosome, but also increases the rate of lysosomal transport of many proteins. The increase in transport is a result of α_{2u}-globulin-mediated increases in the level of the receptor proteins in the lysosomal membrane. Thus, α_{2u}-globulin may induce lysosomal overload by increasing the rate of transport of cellular proteins to the lysosome. In this manner, chronic exposure to the preceding compounds may lead to a chronic nephropathy and in some cases results in an increased incidence of renal adenomas/carcinomas by nongenotoxic mechanisms.

α_{2u}-nephropathy is sex- and species-specific, occurring in particular strains of male rats but not female rats, male or female mice, rabbits, or guinea pigs. It does not occur in female rats, other species, or male Black Reiter rats because they do not produce α_{2u}-globulin. Because humans are exposed to these diverse compounds regularly, they may be at risk for α_{2u}-globulin-induced nephropathy and renal tumors. Current evidence suggests that humans are not at risk because: (a) humans do not synthesize α_{2u}-globulin; (b) humans secrete fewer proteins in general and, in particular, fewer low-molecular-weight proteins in the urine than the rat; (c) the low-molecular-weight proteins in human urine are either not related structurally to α_{2u}-globulin, do not bind to compounds that bind to α_{2u}-globulin, or are similar to proteins in female rats, male Black Reiter rats, rabbits, or guinea pigs that do not exhibit α_{2u}-globulin nephropathy; and (d) mice excrete a low-molecular-weight urinary protein that is 90% homologous to α_{2u}-globulin, but do not exhibit α_{2u}-globulin nephropathy and renal tumors after exposure to α_{2u}-globulin nephropathy-inducing agents (335).

The aminoglycoside antibiotics also induce lysosomal dysfunction and cause ARF failure (105,106,336) (Chapter 42, Antibiotic- and Immunosuppression-Related Renal Failure). In this case, the aminoglycosides are filtered, bound to anionic phospholipids in the brush border, reabsorbed by endocytosis in the S_1 and S_2 segments of the proximal tubule, and accumulated in the lysosomes. Over time, the size and number of lysosomes increase and electron-dense lamellar structures called myeloid bodies appear. The myeloid bodies contain undegraded phospholipids and are thought to occur through aminoglycoside-induced inhibition of lysosomal hydrolases such as sphingomyelinase and phospholipases. However, the steps between lysosomal phospholipid overload and tubule cell death are less clear.

CELLULAR DEFENSES

The RPT cell has numerous defenses against both reactive intermediates and ROS (Fig. 40-4). Glutathione, a primary cellular protectant and the most abundant cellular nonprotein thiol, is found at high concentrations in at least three subcellular compartments (cytosol, mitochondrion, nucleus) (337). Normally, glutathione detoxifies electrophiles by forming a glutathione conjugate either directly or with the aid of glutathione S-transferases. For example, RPT cells detoxify compounds containing a quinone nucleus, such as bromohydroquinone, by conjugating it to glutathione, forming mono- and di-substituted glutathione conjugates (159). Glutathione also acts in conjunction with glutathione peroxidase and glutathione reductase to neutralize ROS. In this case, an organic peroxide is reduced to water and an alcohol by glutathione peroxidase, forming glutathione disulfide (Fig. 40-4). Glutathione disulfide is reduced to glutathione by glutathione reductase in an NADPH-dependent reaction. Catalase and superoxide dismutase are two other enzymes that detoxify ROS. Superoxide dismutase converts the superoxide anion to H_2O_2, and catalase converts the hydrogen peroxide to water.

Several studies have investigated the differences in the activity of glutathione-dependent enzymes among different cells of the kidney. This area is of interest as differences in the activity of these enzymes may account for differences in the susceptibility of different kidney regions to oxidative stress. Cummings and associates (145) reported that the levels of glutathione peroxidase and γ-glutamylcysteinyl synthetase are higher in rat RPT cells than distal tubule cells. The activity of glutathione reductase and glutathione S-transferase appears to be equal between the two cell populations; however, the proximal tubular cells have a much higher concentration of glutathione than distal tubular cells (27 nmol/mg for proximal tubular cells versus 13 nmol/mg for distal tubular cells) (338). Lash and colleagues have demonstrated that overexpression of the dicarboxylate carrier, a protein responsible for the transport of glutathione into mitochondria, protected normal rat kidney-52E cell lines from both oxidant (t-butylhydroperoxide) and S-(1,2)-dichlorovinyl-L-cysteine-induced apoptosis (339). The mechanism of protection correlated to increased transport of glutathione into the mitochondria. The increased level of glutathione decreased oxidant-induced mitochondrial dysfunction and the subsequent release of cytochrome c and caspase activation.

Vitamin C (ascorbic acid) under normal circumstances is a very effective reducing agent and free radical scavenger and functions in the recycling of the Vitamin E radical back to Vitamin E (340,341). Like glutathione, Vitamin C can detoxify compounds containing a quinone nucleus such as bromohydroquinone, but in this case Vitamin C reduces the bromoquinone and the bromoquinone radical back to bromohydroquinone (159); however, Vitamin C can act as a prooxidant in the presence of iron under some circumstances.

Reports have suggested that Vitamin C may function in rabbit RPTC to promote repair and regeneration after exposure to t-butylhydroperoxide and S-(1,2)-dichlorovinyl-L-cysteine (14–16). Vitamin C added in pharmacological concentrations to primary cultures of rabbit RPTC prior to, during, and after exposure to toxicants improved recovery in these cultures as measured by increases in cell number and mitochondrial function (16). The effect of Vitamin C was not the result of its antioxidant function, because both t-butylhydroperoxide and S-(1,2)-dichlorovinyl-L-cysteine caused the same amount of damage in treated and untreated cultures. Rather, the increase in cellular function observed in cultures treated with Vitamin C was linked to its ability to aid cells in recovery after damage, potentially through its ability to promote collagen deposition in the extracellular matrix (16).

Vitamin E (α-tocopherol) is a lipid-soluble antioxidant found in cell membranes (342). Vitamin E is known as a chain-breaking antioxidant because it contributes an electron to a peroxyl radical formed during lipid peroxidation and thereby prevents further lipid peroxidation. The Vitamin E radical produced is unreactive and is recycled back to Vitamin E. Vitamin E can suppress cyclosporin A-mediated toxicity *in vivo* in rat renal kidneys by inhibiting lipid peroxidation (343). Vitamin E also can protect freshly isolated rat proximal tubule cells from the toxicity of cephaloridine, a beta-lactam antibiotic that causes cell specific acute tubular necrosis *in vivo* (344). The protective effect of Vitamin E on proximal tubule cells in this study also correlated with the decreases in the level of lipid peroxidation.

Glycine

During studies designed to examine the cytoprotective effects of glutathione, it was observed that glycine was cytoprotective in a number of models (345). In addition to glycine, a few other small amino acids of similar structure, including D- and L-alanine, ß-alanine, and 1-aminocylopropane-1-carboxylic acid, were protective, indicating a stringent structural requirement for cytoprotection. Studies have demonstrated that glycine is cytoprotective against a diverse group of chemical insults, such as anoxia, metabolic inhibitors, bromohydroquinone, halogenated alkene, and alkane cysteine conjugates, and to a lesser extent t-butylhydroperoxide and $HgCl_2$ (217,346). The mechanism of glycine cytoprotection has remained elusive, but recent studies demonstrate that glycine acts during the terminal phase of cell injury (346). Furthermore, Aleo and Schnellmann (347) and Miller and associates (326,327,348,349) observed that the neuronal glycine receptor antagonist strychnine was cytoprotective and acted in a similar manner to that of glycine under a variety of conditions. Thus, strychnine and glycine may be cytoprotective through a ligand–acceptor interaction. Strychnine binds to a low-affinity binding site on the basolateral membrane of the rabbit RPT cell in a saturable and reversible manner at concentrations equivalent to that necessary for cytoprotection (245). Proteins corresponding to two of the three subunits of the neuronal strychnine-sensitive glycine receptor have been identified on the basolateral membrane of the RPT and a recent report has provided evidence that one of these is the glycine receptor ß-subunit (348–350). The signal transduction pathway for the neuronal glycine receptor is Cl⁻. Because Cl⁻ influx plays a major role in providing the osmotic force for the swelling during cell injury and glycine and strychnine block Cl⁻ influx, glycine and strychnine are cytoprotective by directly or indirectly altering Cl⁻ influx.

Alternatively, Nichols and associates (351) proposed that glycine is cytoprotective in hepatocytes through its ability to inhibit calpains. However, Edelstein and coworkers (246) reported that glycine did not inhibit calpain activity in rat RPT exposed to hypoxia. Studies in rabbit RPT demonstrated that glycine and strychnine did not inhibit basal calpain activity but did inhibit the increase in calpain activity observed during the late phase of cellular injury (352). Later studies confirmed that glycine does not directly affect calpain activity, but rather inhibited toxicant-mediated extracellular Ca^{2+} influx, calpain translocation, and Cl⁻ influx (352). Further studies are needed to conclusively identify the mechanism of glycine cytoprotection.

Acidosis

Although acidosis is not a normal cellular defense mechanism per se, decreasing intracellular pH has been shown to be cytoprotective in a variety of in vitro models, and as such has contributed to our understanding of cell death (353,354). Using freshly isolated RPT, extracellular pH reduced to 6.8 to pH 7.0 results in cytoprotection (354–356). Interestingly, Weinberg (355) demonstrated that the protective effect of extracellular acidosis not only was limited to the addition of acids to the extracellular medium, but also was observed in high-density suspensions of RPT subjected to anoxia. Under these conditions, the RPT spontaneously lowered the pH of surrounding medium to pH 7.0, presumably due to the hydrolysis of ATP and the accumulation of protons. Thus, under conditions of ischemia in vivo, it is possible that localized acidosis may afford a degree of cytoprotection.

A number of findings have contributed to our understanding of the cytoprotective effect of extracellular acidosis. Rodeheaver and Schnellmann (353) demonstrated that extracellular acidosis (pH 6.4) ameliorated renal proximal tubular cell death produced by a series of mitochondrial inhibitors (antimycin A, rotenone, carbonyl cyanide-p-trifluoromethoxyphenylhydrazone, oligomycin) and ion exchangers (nigericin, monensin, valinomycin) but potentiated cell death produced by the oxidants t-butylhydroperoxide, hydrogen peroxide, and ochratoxin A. Associated with the extracellular acidosis-induced increases in cell death was an increase in glutathione disulfide formation, lipid peroxidation, and mitochondrial dysfunction and a decrease in glutathione peroxidase and reductase activities. Thus, the mechanism for this extracellular acidosis-induced potentiation of oxidant toxicity is most likely the result of a decrease in free radical detoxification.

Previous studies indicated that extracellular acidosis was not cytoprotective through its ability to preserve mitochondrial function or ATP levels (353–355). Studies have demonstrated that extracellular acidosis initiated at various times after toxicant exposure was still cytoprotective (212,354). For example, extracellular acidosis initiated 15 minutes after antimycin A or carbonyl cyanide-p-trifluoromethoxyphenylhydrazone addition, a time point after the cessation of respiration, depletion of ATP, and increases in intracellular sodium and decreases in intracellular potassium, was completely cytoprotective at 45 and 105 minutes later, respectively. However, the cytoprotection did not prevent the increase in Cl⁻ influx that occurs in the late stages of cell injury. Extracellular acidosis initiated 2 hours

after tetrafluoroethyl-L-cysteine or t-butylhydroperoxide addition also was cytoprotective 2 hours later. These results demonstrate that the cytoprotective effect of extracellular acidosis occurs very late in the cell injury process distal to Cl⁻ influx.

Peroxisomes and Peroxisomal Proliferating Activated Receptors (PPAR)

Peroxisomes are membrane-bound vesicles that contain degradative enzymes for fatty acids and amino acids (329). In addition peroxisomes contain catalase, which converts H_2O_2 to oxygen and water. Although the ability of peroxisomes to metabolize H_2O_2 is crucial in the protection of cells against oxidative stress, peroxisomal proliferation has been linked to the preservation of mitochondrial function (357) and the reduction in renal cell death following injury induced by gallic acid (358), cisplatin (256,359), and ischemia/reperfusion-induced injury.

Peroxisomes also may protect against renal cell death via mechanisms linked to the activation of peroxisomal proliferator receptors (PPAR). PPAR are members of a nuclear hormone-activated receptor and transactivation protein family (360). At this time, three different PPAR have been identified and cloned (PPAR-α, PPAR-β/δ, and PPAR-γ) (360). PPAR-β/δ appears to be expressed in almost all tissues including the kidney cortex (360–362). PPAR-γ is present in distal medullary collecting ducts, glomeruli, and the renal microvasculature (362,363). PPAR-α is expressed in the proximal tubule, medullary thick ascending limbs, and the glomerular mesangial cells. It is hypothesized that differences in the distribution PPAR isoforms may result in different mechanisms of protection between different cells.

Activators of PPAR are structurally diverse and include plasticizers (di[2-ethyhexl]phthalate) (364), herbicides (365), hypolipidemic drugs (fenofibrate, clofibrate, and clofibric acid) (360) and antidiabetic drugs (360,365,366) (e.g., troglitazone and rosiglitazone) (366–369). Activators of PPAR increase the number of peroxisomes within the cell and increase the expression of enzymes for fatty acid β-oxidation including fatty acyl-CoA oxidase, enoyl-CoA hydratase/3-hydroxyacyl-CoA dehydrogenase bifunctional enzyme, and 3-ketoacyl-CoA thiolase (364,365,370,371). Activators of PPAR isoforms also increase mitochondrial enzymes including carnitine palmitoyl transferase, medium chain acyl-CoA dehydrogenase, and pyruvate dehydrogenase complex (359,362). The increase in these proteins is believed to be key in the protection against nephrotoxicants (360,362,365,372).

The overall affect of the activation of PPAR, at least activation of PPAR-α, on renal cell death appears to be beneficial. The PPAR-α agonist clofibrate and WY14643 reduce renal cell dysfunction and injury induced by ischemia/reperfusion in male rat kidneys (362,373,374). In vivo studies demonstrate that induction of PPAR-α also correlated to increases in mitochondrial medium-chain acyl-CoA dehydrogenase and pyruvate dehydrogenase complex activity and decreases in cisplatin-induced proximal tubular necrosis (359). The exact mechanism involved in the PPAR-α mediated protection against nephrotoxicants has yet to be determined.

SPECIFIC TOXICANTS

It is critical to identify the ultimate toxic species and the cell type targeted in order to understand the mechanism by which a chemical produces nephrotoxicity. For example, is the glomerulus, proximal convoluted tubule, proximal straight tubule, the thick ascending limb of Henle, or the distal convoluted tubule the target of the parent compound, a primary or secondary metabolite? Thus, excellent biotransformation, toxicokinetic, and morphologic studies are paramount in determining the sites of biotransformation, which metabolites reach the kidney, the quantity of metabolites in the kidney, the target cell type in the kidney, and ultimately the mechanism of nephrotoxicity. Other chapters in this book focus on specific toxicants such as analgesics (Chapter 44, Nephrotoxicity of Nonsteroidal Antiinflammatory Agents, Analgesics, and Angiotensin-Converting Enzyme Inhibitors), antibiotics (Chapter 42, Antibiotic- and Immunosuppression-Related Renal Failure), antineoplastics (Chapter 43, Renal Diseases Induced by Antineoplastic Agents), heavy metals (Chapter 47, Nephrotoxicity Secondary to Environmental Agents and Heavy Metals), immunosuppressives (Chapter 42, Antibiotic- and Immunosuppression-Related Renal Failure), and radiocontrast media (Chapter 45, Radiocontrast Media-Induced Acute Renal Failure).

ACKNOWLEDGMENTS

The authors would like to thank Dr. Jennifer G. Schnellmann for critically reviewing this manuscript. Preparation of this chapter was supported by the National Institutes of Health grants ES-04410 (RGS), ES-12239 (RGS), DK-62028 (RGS), and a Georgia Cancer Coalition Distinguished Scientist Grant (BSC).

References

1. Friedewald JJ, Rabb H. Inflammatory cells in ischemic acute renal failure. *Kidney Int* 2004;66:486.
2. Kelly KJ, et al. Antibody to intercellular adhesion molecule 1 protects the kidney against ischemic injury. *Proc Natl Acad Sci USA* 1994;91:812.
3. Rabb H, et al. Role of CD11a and CD11b in ischemic acute renal failure in rats. *Am J Physiol* 1994;267:F1052.
4. Goligorsky MS, DiBona GF. Pathogenetic role of Arg-Gly-Asp-recognizing integrins in acute renal failure. *Proc Natl Acad Sci USA* 1993;90:5700.
5. Noiri E, et al. Cyclic RGD peptides ameliorate ischemic acute renal failure in rats. *Kidney Int* 1994;46:1050.
6. Romanov V, et al. Two novel probes reveal tubular and vascular Arg-Gly-Asp (RGD) binding sites in the ischemic rat kidney. *Kidney Int* 1997;52:93.
7. Yip KP, Marsh DJ. An Arg-Gly-Asp peptide stimulates constriction in rat afferent arteriole. *Am J Physiol* 1997;273:F768.
8. Kootstra CJ, et al. Effective treatment of experimental lupus nephritis by combined administration of anti-CD11a and anti-CD54 antibodies. *Clin Exp Immunol* 1997;108:324.
9. Rui-Mei L, Kara AU, Sinniah R. In situ analysis of adhesion molecule expression in kidneys infected with murine malaria. *J Pathol* 1998;185:219.
10. Kovacs CJ, et al. Proliferative defects in renal and intestinal epithelium after cis-dichlorodiammine platinum (II). *Br J Cancer* 1982;45:286.
11. Nonclercq D, et al. Renal tissue injury and proliferative response after successive treatments with anticancer platinum derivatives and tobramycin. *Virchows Arch B Cell Pathol Incl Mol Pathol* 1990;59:143.
12. Zhuang S, Dang Y, Schnellmann RG. Requirement of the epidermal growth factor receptor in renal epithelial cell proliferation and migration. *Am J Physiol Renal Physiol* 2004;287:F365.
13. Wang Z, et al. Importance of functional EGF receptors in recovery from acute nephrotoxic injury. *J Am Soc Nephrol* 2003;14:3147.
14. Nony PA, Schnellmann RG. Mechanisms of renal cell repair and regeneration after acute renal failure. *J Pharmacol Exp Ther* 2003;304:905.
15. Nony PA, Schnellmann RG. Interactions between collagen IV and collagen-binding integrins in renal cell repair after sublethal injury. *Mol Pharmacol* 2001;60:1226.
16. Nony PA, Nowak G, Schnellmann RG. Collagen IV promotes repair of renal cell physiological functions after toxicant injury. *Am J Physiol Renal Physiol* 2001;281:F443.
17. Counts RS, et al. Nephrotoxicant inhibition of renal proximal tubule cell regeneration. *Am J Physiol* 1995;269:F274.
18. Schrier RW, Berl T, Bonventre JV. *Atlas of diseases in the kidney*. Philadelphia: Current Medicine, 1999.
19. Sipes G, et al. *Comprehensive toxicology*. New York: Pergamon, 1997.
20. Tarloff JB, Lash LH. *Toxicology of the kidney*, 3rd ed. Boca Raton, FL: CRC Press, 2005.
21. Weinberg JM. Issues in the pathophysiology of nephrotoxic renal tubular cell injury pertinent to understanding cyclosporine nephrotoxicity. *Transplant Proc* 1985;17(4 Suppl 1):81.
22. Schnellmann RG, Kelly KJ. Phathophysiology of nephrotoxic acute renal failure. In: Schrier RW, ed. *Atlas of diseases of the kidney*. Washington, DC: Blackwell Sciences, 1999:5.
23. Wright SH, Dantzler WH. Molecular and cellular physiology of renal organic cation and anion transport. *Physiol Rev* 2004;84:987.
24. Burckhardt G, Wolff NA. Structure of renal organic anion and cation transporters. *Am J Physiol Renal Physiol* 2000;278:F853.
25. Sweet DH, Bush KT, Nigam SK. The organic anion transporter family: from physiology to ontogeny and the clinic. *Am J Physiol Renal Physiol* 2001; 281:F197.
26. Jonker JW, et al. Deficiency in the organic cation transporters 1 and 2 (Oct1/Oct2 [Slc22a1/Slc22a2]) in mice abolishes renal secretion of organic cations. *Mol Cell Biol* 2003;23:7902.
27. Ludwig T, et al. Nephrotoxicity of platinum complexes is related to basolateral organic cation transport. *Kidney Int* 2004;66:196.
28. Ludwig T, Oberleithner H. Platinum complex toxicity in cultured renal epithelia. *Cell Physiol Biochem* 2004;14:431.
29. Zalups RK, Ahmad S. Homocysteine and the renal epithelial transport and toxicity of inorganic mercury: role of basolateral transport organic anion transporter 1. *J Am Soc Nephrol* 2004;15:2023.
30. Aslamkhan AG, et al. Human renal organic anion transporter 1-dependent uptake and toxicity of mercuric-thiol conjugates in Madin-Darby canine kidney cells. *Mol Pharmacol* 2003;63:590.
31. Zalups RK, Barfuss DW. Renal organic anion transport system: a mechanism for the basolateral uptake of mercury-thiol conjugates along the pars recta of the proximal tubule. *Toxicol Appl Pharmacol* 2002;182:234.
32. Bridges CC, et al. Mercuric conjugates of cysteine are transported by the amino acid transporter system b(0,+): implications of molecular mimicry. *J Am Soc Nephrol* 2004;15:663.
33. Fleck C, Schwertfeger M, Taylor PM. Regulation of renal amino acid (AA) transport by hormones, drugs and xenobiotics—a review. *Amino Acids* 2003;24:347.
34. Ernest S, Bello-Reuss E. Xenobiotic transport differences in mouse mesangial cell clones expressing mdr1 and mdr3. *Am J Physiol* 1996;270: C910.
35. Lee W, Kim RB. Transporters and renal drug elimination. *Annu Rev Pharmacol Toxicol* 2004;44:137.
36. Youngblood GL, Sweet DH. Identification and functional assessment of the novel murine organic anion transporter Oat5 (Slc22a19) expressed in kidney. *Am J Physiol Renal Physiol* 2004;287:F236.
37. Dantzler WH, et al. Relation of cysteine conjugate nephrotoxicity to transport by the basolateral organic anion transport system in isolated S2 segments of rabbit proximal renal tubules. *J Pharmacol Exp Ther* 1998;286: 52.
38. Zhang X, et al. Relative contribution of OAT and OCT transporters to organic electrolyte transport in rabbit proximal tubule. *Am J Physiol Renal Physiol* 2004;287:F999.
39. Groves CE, Nowak G, Morales M. Ochratoxin A secretion in primary cultures of rabbit renal proximal tubule cells. *J Am Soc Nephrol* 1999;10: 13.
40. Jung KY, Endou H. Nephrotoxicity assessment by measuring cellular ATP content. II. Intranephron site of ochratoxin A nephrotoxicity. *Toxicol Appl Pharmacol* 1989;100:383.
41. Anders MW, Elfarra AA, Lash LH. Cellular effects of reactive intermediates: nephrotoxicity of S-conjugates of amino acids. *Arch Toxicol* 1987;60: 103.
42. Urakami Y. Molecular diversity of organic cation transporter (OCT) mediating renal excretion of drugs. *Yakugaku Zasshi* 2002;122:957.
43. Demeule M, Brossard M, Beliveau R. Cisplatin induced renal exspression of the P-glycoprotein and canalicular multispecific organic anion transporter. *Am J Physiol* 1999;277:F832.
44. Demeule M, et al. Diallyl disulfide, a chemopreventative agent in garlic, induces multidrug resistance-associated protein 2 expression. *Biochem Biophys Res Commun* 2004;324:937.
45. Majno G, Joris I. Apoptosis, oncosis, and necrosis. An overview of cell death. *Am J Pathol* 1995;146:3.
46. Corcoran GB, Ray SD. The role of the nucleus and other compartments in toxic cell death produced by alkylating hepatotoxicants. *Toxicol Appl Pharmacol* 1992;113:167.
47. Wyllie AH. Apoptosis (the 1992 Frank Rose Memorial Lecture). *Br J Cancer* 1993;67:205.
48. Recklinghausen FV. Untersuchungen uber Rachitis und Osteomalacie. *Jena: Gustav Fischer* 1910.
49. Levin S, et al. The nomenclature of cell death: recommendations of an ad hoc Committee of the Society of Toxicologic Pathologists. *Toxicol Pathol* 1999;27:484.
50. Kohler C, Orrenius S, Zhivotovsky B. Evaluation of caspase activity in apoptotic cells. *J Immunol Methods* 2002;265:97.
51. Salvesen GS, Dixit VM. Caspases: intracellular signaling by proteolysis. *Cell* 1997;91:443.
52. Wang J, Lenardo M. Roles of caspases in apoptosis, development, and cytokine maturation revealed by homozygous gene deficiencies. *J Cell Sci* 2000;113:753.
53. Yang B, et al. Inhibitors directed towards caspase-1 and -3 are less effective than pan caspase inhibition in preventing renal proximal tubular cell apoptosis. *Nephron Exp Nephrol* 2004;96:e39.

54. Lash LH, Hueni SE, Putt DA. Apoptosis, necrosis, and cell proliferation induced by S-(1,2-dichlorovinyl)-L-cysteine in primary cultures of human proximal tubular cells. *Toxicol Appl Pharmacol* 2001;177:1.

55. Tsuruya K, et al. Antioxidant ameliorates cisplatin-induced renal tubular cell death through inhibition of death receptor-mediated pathways. *Am J Physiol Renal Physiol* 2003;285:F208.

56. Bijian K, et al. Extracellular matrix regulates glomerular epithelial cell survival and proliferation. *Am J Physiol Renal Physiol* 2004;286:F255.

57. Horio M, et al. Apoptosis induced by hypertonicity in Madin Darley canine kidney cells: protective effect of betaine. *Nephrol Dial Transplant* 2001;16:483.

58. Sheikh-Hamad D, et al. Cellular and molecular studies on cisplatin-induced apoptotic cell death in rat kidney. *Arch Toxicol* 2004;78:147.

59. Park MY, et al. Apoptosis induced by inhibition of contact with extracellular matrix in mouse collecting duct cells. *Nephron* 1999;83:341.

60. Schwerdt G, et al. Inhibition of mitochondria and extracellular acidification enhance achratoxin A-induced apoptosis in renal collecting duct-derived MDCK-C7 cells. *Cell Physiol Biochem* 2004;14:47.

61. Michea L, et al. Mitochondrial dysfunction is an early event in high-NaCl-induced apoptosis of mIMCD3 cells. *Am J Physiol Renal Physiol* 2002;282:F981.

62. Robertson JD, et al. Processed caspase-2 can induce mitochondria-mediated apoptosis independently of its enzymatic activity. *EMBO Rep* 2004;5:643.

63. Enoksson M, et al. Caspase-2 permeabilizes the outer mitochondrial membrane and disrupts the binding of cytochrome c to anionic phospholipids. *J Biol Chem* 2004;279:49575.

64. Granville DJ, et al. Release of cytochrome c, bax migration, bid cleavage, and activation of caspases 2, 3, 6, 7, 8, and 9 during endothelial cell apoptosis. *Am J Pathol* 1999;155:1021.

65. Scarabelli TM, et al. Different signaling pathways induce apoptosis in endothelial cells and cardiac myocytes during ischemia/reperfusion injury. *Circ Res* 2002;90:745.

66. Sun XM, et al. Distinct caspase cascades are initiated in receptor-mediated and chemical-induced apoptosis. *J Biol Chem* 1999;274:5053.

67. Wang J, et al. Minocycline up-regulates Bcl-2 and protects against cell death in mitochondria. *J Biol Chem* 2004;279:19948.

68. Vanags DM, et al. Protease involvement in fodrin cleavage and phosphatidylserine exposure in apoptosis. *J Biol Chem* 1996;271:31075.

69. Atsumi G, et al. Fas-induced arachidonic acid release is mediated by Ca2+-independent phospholipase A2 but not cytosolic phospholipase A2, which undergoes proteolytic inactivation. *J Biol Chem* 1998;273:13870.

70. Ekert PG, Silke J, Vaux DL. Inhibition of apoptosis and clonogenic survival of cells expressing crmA variants: optimal caspase substrates are not necessarily optimal inhibitors. *Embo J* 1999;18:330.

71. Kaushal GP, et al. Role and regulation of activation of caspases in cisplatin-induced injury to renal tubular epithelial cells. *Kidney Int* 2001;60:1726.

72. Liu X, et al. DFF, a heterodimeric protein that functions downstream of caspase-3 to trigger DNA fragmentation during apoptosis. *Cell* 1997;89:175.

73. Enari M, et al. A caspase-activated DNase that degrades DNA during apoptosis, and its inhibitor ICAD. *Nature* 1998;391:43.

74. Walisser JA, Thies RL. Poly(ADP-ribose) polymerase inhibition in oxidant-stressed endothelial cells prevents oncosis and permits caspase activation and apoptosis. *Exp Cell Res* 1999;251:401.

75. Green DR, Reed JC. Mitochondria and apoptosis. *Science* 1998;281:1309.

76. Mantle D, Preedy VR. Free radicals as mediators of alcohol toxicity. *Adverse Drug React Toxicol Rev* 1999;18:235.

77. Zhan Y, et al. The roles of caspase-3 and bcl-2 in chemically-induced apoptosis but not necrosis of renal epithelial cells. *Oncogene* 1999;18:6505.

78. Susin SA, et al. Bcl-2 inhibits the mitochondrial release of an apoptogenic protease. *J Exp Med* 1996;184:1331.

79. Ruchalski K, et al. HSP72 inhibits apoptosis-inducing factor release in ATP-depleted renal epithelial cells. *Am J Physiol Cell Physiol* 2003;285:C1483.

80. Huang Q, et al. Assessment of cisplatin-induced nephrotoxicity by microarray technology. *Toxicol Sci* 2001;63:196.

81. Justo P, et al. Expression of Smac/Diablo in tubular epithelial cells and during acute renal failure. *Kidney Int Suppl* 2003:S52.

82. Roberts DL, et al. The inhibitor of apoptosis protein-binding domain of Smac is not essential for its proapoptotic activity. *J Cell Biol* 2001;153:221.

83. Srinivasula SM, et al. Molecular determinants of the caspase-promoting activity of Smac/DIABLO and its role in the death receptor pathway. *J Biol Chem* 2000;275:36152.

84. Cilenti L, et al. Omi/HtrA2 protease mediates cisplatin-induced cell death in renal cells. *Am J Physiol Renal Physiol* 2004.

85. Trencia A, et al. Omi/HtrA2 promotes cell death by binding and degrading the anti-apoptotic protein ped/pea-15. *J Biol Chem* 2004;279:46566.

86. Lutz RJ. Role of the BH3 (Bcl-2 homology 3) domain in the regulation of apoptosis and Bcl-2-related proteins. *Biochem Soc Trans* 2000;28:51.

87. Justo P, et al. Intracellular mechanisms of cyclosporin A-induced tubular cell apoptosis. *J Am Soc Nephrol* 2003;14:3072.

88. Vaghefi H, Hughes AL, Neet KE. Nerve growth factor withdrawal-mediated apoptosis in naive and differentiated PC12 cells through p53/caspase-3-dependent and -independent pathways. *J Biol Chem* 2004;279:15604.

89. Li CQ, et al. Apoptotic signaling pathways induced by nitric oxide in human lymphoblastoid cells expressing wild-type or mutant p53. *Cancer Res* 2004;64:3022.

90. Erster S, et al. In vivo mitochondrial p53 translocation triggers a rapid first wave of cell death in response to DNA damage that can precede p53 target gene activation. *Mol Cell Biol* 2004;24:6728.

91. Henry H, et al. Regulation of the mitochondrial checkpoint in p53-mediated apoptosis confers resistance to cell death. *Oncogene* 2002;21:748.

92. Wei Q, et al. Bid activation in kidney cells following ATP depletion in vitro and ischemia in vivo. *Am J Physiol Renal Physiol* 2004;286:F803.

93. Messmer UK, Briner VA, Pfeilschifter J. Tumor necrosis factor-alpha and lipopolysaccharide induce apoptotic cell death in bovine glomerular endothelial cells. *Kidney Int* 1999;55:2322.

94. Saikumar P, Venkatachalam MA. Role of apoptosis in hypoxic/ischemic damage in the kidney. *Semin Nephrol* 2003;23:511.

95. Korsmeyer SJ. BCL-2 gene family and the regulation of programmed cell death. *Cancer Res* 1999;59:1693s.

96. Li F, et al. Heat stress prevents mitochondrial injury in ATP-depleted renal epithelial cells. *Am J Physiol Cell Physiol* 2002;283:C917.

97. Susin SA, et al. The central executioner of apoptosis: multiple connections between protease activation and mitochondria in Fas/APO-1/CD95- and ceramide-induced apoptosis. *J Exp Med* 1997;186:25.

98. Petit PX, et al. Disruption of the outer mitochondrial membrane as a result of large amplitude swelling: the impact of irreversible permeability transition. *FEBS Lett* 1998;426:111.

99. Tikoo A, et al. Tissue distribution of Diablo/Smac revealed by monoclonal antibodies. *Cell Death Differ* 2002;9:710.

100. Lorz C, et al. Paracetamol-induced renal tubular injury: a role for ER stress. *J Am Soc Nephrol* 2004;15:380.

101. Faccio L, et al. Characterization of a novel human serine protease that has extensive homology to bacterial heat shock endoprotease HtrA and is regulated by kidney ischemia. *J Biol Chem* 2000;275:2581.

102. Faccio L, et al. Tissue-specific splicing of Omi stress-regulated endoprotease leads to an inactive protease with a modified PDZ motif. *Genomics* 2000;68:343.

103. Steinmetz PR, Husted RF. Amphotericin B toxicity for epithelial cells. In: Stein J, ed. *Nephrotoxic mechanisms of drugs and environmental toxins.* New York: Plenum, 1982.

104. Wang E, et al. Inhibition of sphingolipid biosynthesis by fumonisins. Implications for diseases associated with Fusarium moniliforme. *J Biol Chem* 1991;266:14486.

105. Laurent G, Kishore BK, Tulkens PM. Aminoglycoside-induced renal phospholipidosis and nephrotoxicity. *Biochem Pharmacol* 1990;40:2383.

106. Kosek JC, Mazze RI, Cousins MJ. Nephrotoxicity of gentamicin. *Lab Invest* 1974;30:48.

107. Lock EA. Renal drug-metabolizing enzymes in experimental animals and humans. In: Goldstein RS, ed. *Mechanisms of injury in renal diseases and toxicity.* Boca Raton, FL: CRC Press, 1994.

108. Lohr JW, Willsky GR, Acara MA. Renal drug metabolism. *Pharmacol Rev* 1998;50:107.

109. Muller P, et al. Injection of encapsulated cells producing an ifosfamide-activating cytochrome P450 for targeted chemotherapy to pancreatic tumors. *Ann N Y Acad Sci* 1999;880:337.

110. Cummings BS, et al. Cellular distribution of cytochromes P-450 in the rat kidney. *Drug Metab Dispos* 1999;27:542.

111. Endou H. Cytochrome P-450 monooxygenase system in the rabbit kidney: its intranephron localization and its induction. *Jpn J Pharmacol* 1983;33:423.

112. Moran JH, et al. Analysis of the cytotoxic properties of linoleic acid metabolites produced by renal and hepatic P450s. *Toxicol Appl Pharmacol* 2000;168:268.

113. Stec DE, et al. Distribution of cytochrome P-450 4A and 4F isoforms along the nephron in mice. *Am J Physiol Renal Physiol* 2003;284:F95.

114. Schaaf GJ, et al. Characterization of biotransformation enzyme activities in primary rat proximal tubular cells. *Chem Biol Interact* 2001;134:167.

115. Cummings BS, Parker JC, Lash LH. Role of cytochrome P450 and glutathione S-transferase alpha in the metabolism and cytotoxicity of trichloroethylene in rat kidney. *Biochem Pharmacol* 2000;59:531.

116. Henderson CJ, et al. Testosterone-mediated regulation of mouse renal cytochrome P-450 isoenzymes. *Biochem J* 1990;266:675.

117. Cummings BS, Lasker JM, Lash LH. Expression of glutathione-dependent enzymes and cytochrome P450s in freshly isolated and primary cultures of proximal tubular cells from human kidney. *J Pharmacol Exp Ther* 2000;293:677.

118. Amet Y, et al. Cytochrome P450 4A and 2E1 expression in human kidney microsomes. *Biochem Pharmacol* 1997;53:765.

119. Lasker JM, et al. Formation of 20-hydroxyeicosatetraenoic acid, a vasoactive and natriuretic eicosanoid, in human kidney. Role of Cyp4F2 and Cyp4A11. *J Biol Chem* 2000;275:4118.

120. Smith JH, et al. Effect of sex hormone status on chloroform nephrotoxicity and renal mixed function oxidases in mice. *Toxicology* 1984;30:305.

121. Smith JH. Role of renal metabolism in chloroform nephrotoxicity. *Comments Toxicol* 1986;1:125.

122. Hart SG, et al. Immunohistochemical localization of acetaminophen in target tissues of the CD-1 mouse: correspondence of covalent binding with toxicity. *Fundam Appl Toxicol* 1995;24:260.

123. Hu JJ, et al. Sex-related differences in mouse renal metabolism and toxicity of acetaminophen. *Toxicol Appl Pharmacol* 1993;122:16.

124. Hart SG, et al. Acetaminophen nephrotoxicity in CD-1 mice. I. Evidence of a role for in situ activation in selective covalent binding and toxicity. *Toxicol Appl Pharmacol* 1994;126:267.

125. Fahrig R, Madle S, Baumann H. Genetic toxicology of trichloroethylene (TCE). *Mutat Res* 1995;340:1.

126. Hoivik DJ, et al. Gender-related differences in susceptibility to acetaminophen-induced protein arylation and nephrotoxicity in the CD-1 mouse. *Toxicol Appl Pharmacol* 1995;130:257.

127. Lash LH. Role of metabolism in chemically induced nephrotoxicity. In: Goldstein RS, ed. *Mechanisms of injury in renal disease and toxicity*. Boca Raton, FL: CRC Press, 1994.

128. Hu JJ, Rhoten WB, Yang CS. Mouse renal cytochrome P450IIE1: immunocytochemical localization, sex-related difference and regulation by testosterone. *Biochem Pharmacol* 1990;40:2597.

129. Bartolone JB, et al. Purification, antibody production, and partial amino acid sequence of the 58-kDa acetaminophen-binding liver proteins. *Toxicol Appl Pharmacol* 1992;113:19.

130. Pumford NR, et al. Covalent binding of acetaminophen to N-10-formyltetrahydrofolate dehydrogenase in mice. *J Pharmacol Exp Ther* 1997;280:501.

131. Bulera SJ, et al. Identification of the mouse liver 44-kDa acetaminophen-binding protein as a subunit of glutamine synthetase. *Toxicol Appl Pharmacol* 1995;134:313.

132. Halmes NC, et al. Glutamate dehydrogenase covalently binds to a reactive metabolite of acetaminophen. *Chem Res Toxicol* 1996;9:541.

133. Ripp SL, et al. Oxidation of cysteine S-conjugates by rabbit liver microsomes and cDNA-expressed flavin-containing mono-oxygenases: studies with S-(1,2-dichlorovinyl)-L-cysteine, S-(1,2,2-trichlorovinyl)-L-cysteine, S-allyl-L-cysteine, and S-benzyl-L-cysteine. *Mol Pharmacol* 1997;51:507.

134. Mani C, Kupfer D. Cytochrome P-450-mediated activation and irreversible binding of the antiestrogen tamoxifen to proteins in rat and human liver: possible involvement of flavin-containing monooxygenases in tamoxifen activation. *Cancer Res* 1991;51:6052.

135. Ripp SL, et al. Methionine S-oxidation in human and rabbit liver microsomes: evidence for a high-affinity methionine S-oxidase activity that is distinct from flavin-containing monooxygenase 3. *Arch Biochem Biophys* 1999;367:322.

136. Rozell B, et al. Glutathione transferases of classes alpha, mu and pi show selective expression in different regions of rat kidney. *Xenobiotica* 1993;23:835.

137. Krause RJ, Lash LH, Elfarra AA. Human kidney flavin-containing monooxygenases and their potential roles in cysteine s-conjugate metabolism and nephrotoxicity. *J Pharmacol Exp Ther* 2003;304:185.

138. Lash LH, et al. Roles of necrosis, Apoptosis, and mitochondrial dysfunction in S-(1,2-dichlorovinyl)-L-cysteine sulfoxide-induced cytotoxicity in primary cultures of human renal proximal tubular cells. *J Pharmacol Exp Ther* 2003;305:1163.

139. Kharasch ED, Jubert C. Compound A uptake and metabolism to mercapturic acids and 3,3,3-trifluoro-2-fluoromethoxypropanoic acid during low-flow sevoflurane anesthesia: biomarkers for exposure, risk assessment, and interspecies comparison. *Anesthesiology* 1999;91:1267.

140. Rodilla V, et al. Glutathione S-transferases in human renal cortex and neoplastic tissue: enzymatic activity, isoenzyme profile and immunohistochemical localization. *Xenobiotica* 1998;28:443.

141. Zalups RK. Organic anion transport and action of gamma-glutamyl transpeptidase in kidney linked mechanistically to renal tubular uptake of inorganic mercury. *Toxicol Appl Pharmacol* 1995;132:289.

142. Koob M, Dekant W. Bioactivation of xenobiotics by formation of toxic glutathione conjugates. *Chem Biol Interact* 1991;77:107.

143. Monks TJ, Lo HH, Lau SS. Oxidation and acetylation as determinants of 2-bromocystein-S-ylhydroquinone-mediated nephrotoxicity. *Chem Res Toxicol* 1994;7:495.

144. Birge RB, et al. Acetaminophen hepatotoxicity: correspondence of selective protein arylation in human and mouse liver in vitro, in culture, and in vivo. *Toxicol Appl Pharmacol* 1990;105:472.

145. Cummings BS, Lash LH. Metabolism and toxicity of trichloroethylene and S-(1,2-dichlorovinyl)-L-cysteine in freshly isolated human proximal tubular cells. *Toxicol Sci* 2000;53:458.

146. Birner G, et al. Nephrotoxic and genotoxic N-acetyl-S-dichlorovinyl-L-cysteine is a urinary metabolite after occupational 1,1,2-trichloroethene exposure in humans: implications for the risk of trichloroethene exposure. *Environ Health Perspect* 1993;99:281.

147. Commandeur JN, Vermeulen NP. Identification of N-acetyl(2,2-dichlorovinyl)- and N-acetyl(1,2-dichlorovinyl)-L-cysteine as two regioisomeric mercapturic acids of trichloroethylene in the rat. *Chem Res Toxicol* 1990;3:212.

148. Bruning T, et al. Acute intoxication with trichloroethene: clinical symptoms, toxicokinetics, metabolism, and development of biochemical parameters for renal damage. *Toxicol Sci* 1998;41:157.

149. Lochhead KM, Kharasch ED, Zager RA. Spectrum and subcellular determinants of fluorinated anesthetic-mediated proximal tubular injury. *Am J Pathol* 1997;150:2209.

150. Halliwell B, Gutteridge JM. *Free radicals in biology and medicine*, 2nd ed. Oxford, UK: Clarendon, 1989.

151. Halliwell B, Gutteridge JM, Cross CE. Free radicals, antioxidants, and human disease: where are we now? *J Lab Clin Med* 1992;119:598.

152. Sies H. *Oxidative stress: oxidants and antioxidants*. New York: Academic Press, 1991.

153. Baliga R, et al. Role of cytochrome P-450 as a source of catalytic iron in cisplatin-induced nephrotoxicity. *Kidney Int* 1998;54:1562.

154. Baliga R, et al. In vitro and in vivo evidence suggesting a role for iron in cisplatin-induced nephrotoxicity. *Kidney Int* 1998;53:394.

155. Walker PD, Shah SV. Gentamicin enhanced production of hydrogen peroxide by renal cortical mitochondria. *Am J Physiol* 1987;253:C495.

156. Lund BO, Miller DM, Woods JS. Studies on Hg(II)-induced H2O2 formation and oxidative stress in vivo and in vitro in rat kidney mitochondria. *Biochem Pharmacol* 1993;45:2017.

157. Brown PC, Dulik DM, Jones TW. The toxicity of menadione (2-methyl-1,4-naphthoquinone) and two thioether conjugates studied with isolated renal epithelial cells. *Arch Biochem Biophys* 1991;285:187.

158. Schnellmann RG, et al. 2-Bromohydroquinone-induced toxicity to rabbit renal proximal tubules: the role of biotransformation, glutathione, and covalent binding. *Toxicol Appl Pharmacol* 1989;99:19.

159. Schnellmann RG. 2-Bromohydroquinone-induced toxicity to rabbit renal proximal tubules: evidence against oxidative stress. *Toxicol Appl Pharmacol* 1989;99:11.

160. Fukino H, et al. Effect of zinc pretreatment on mercuric chloride-induced lipid peroxidation in the rat kidney. *Toxicol Appl Pharmacol* 1984;73:395.

161. Sevanian A, et al. Lipid peroxidation and phospholipaes A2 activity in liposomes composes of unsaturated phospholipids: a structural basis for enzyme activation. In: Davies KJ, ed. *Biochem Biophys Acta* 1988;961:316.

162. Wratten ML, et al. DPH lifetime distributions in vesicles containing phospholipid hydroperoxides. *Biochem Biophys Res Commun* 1989;164:169.

163. Schmid A, Beuter W, Mayring L. [Mechanism of action of S-(dichlorovinyl)-L-cysteine]. *Zentralbl Veterinarmed A* 1983;30:511.

164. Beuter W, et al. Peroxidative damage and nephrotoxicity of dichlorovinyl-cysteine in mice. *J Appl Toxicol* 1989;9:181.

165. Chen Q, et al. The mechanism of cysteine conjugate cytotoxicity in renal epithelial cells. Covalent binding leads to thiol depletion and lipid peroxidation. *J Biol Chem* 1990;265:21603.

166. Wang C, Salahudeen AK. Cyclosporine nephrotoxicity: attenuation by an antioxidant-inhibitor of lipid peroxidation in vitro and in vivo. *Transplantation* 1994;58:940.

167. Lieberthal W, Triaca V, Levine J. Mechanisms of death induced by cisplatin in proximal tubular epithelial cells: apoptosis vs. necrosis. *Am J Physiol* 1996;270:F700.

168. Lau AH. Apoptosis induced by cisplatin nephrotoxic injury. *Kidney Int* 1999;56:1295.

169. Sugihara K, et al. Stimulatory effect of cisplatin on production of lipid peroxidation in renal tissues. *Jpn J Pharmacol* 1987;43:247.

170. Hannemann J, Baumann K. Cisplatin-induced lipid peroxidation and decrease of gluconeogenesis in rat kidney cortex: different effects of antioxidants and radical scavengers. *Toxicology* 1988;51:119.

171. Cummings BS, Schnellmann RG. Cisplatin-induced renal cell apoptosis: caspase 3-dependent and -independent pathways. *J Pharmacol Exp Ther* 2002;302:8.

172. Cummings BS, McHowat J, Schnellmann RG. Role of an endoplasmic reticulum Ca2+-independent phospholipase A2 in cisplatin-induced renal cell apoptosis. *J Pharmacol Exp Ther* 2004;308:921.

173. Price PM, Safirstein RL, Megyesi J. Protection of renal cells from cisplatin toxicity by cell cycle inhibitors. *Am J Physiol Renal Physiol* 2004;286:F378.

174. Megyesi J, et al. Positive effect of the induction of p21WAF1/CIP1 on the course of ischemic acute renal failure. *Kidney Int* 2001;60:2164.

175. Megyesi J, et al. The p53-independent activation of transcription of p21 WAF1/CIP1/SDI1 after acute renal failure. *Am J Physiol* 1996;271:F1211.

176. Nowak G, Price PM, Schnellmann RG. Lack of a functional p21WAF1/CIP1 gene accelerates caspase-independent apoptosis induced by cisplatin in renal cells. *Am J Physiol Renal Physiol* 2003;285:F440.

177. Nowak G, Price PM, Schnellmann RG. Lack of a functional p21WAF1/CIP1 gene accelerates caspase-independent apoptosis induced by cisplatin in renal cells. *Am J Physiol Renal Physiol* 2003;285:F440.

178. Megyesi J, et al. The lack of a functional p21(WAF1/CIP1) gene ameliorates progression to chronic renal failure. *Proc Natl Acad Sci USA* 1999;96:10830.

179. Megyesi J, Safirstein RL, Price PM. Induction of p21WAF1/CIP1/SDI1 in kidney tubule cells affects the course of cisplatin-induced acute renal failure. *J Clin Invest* 1998;101:777.

180. Jiang M, et al. Role of p53 in cisplatin-induced tubular cell apoptosis: dependence on p53 transcriptional activity. *Am J Physiol Renal Physiol* 2004;287:F1140.

181. Kelly KJ, et al. P53 mediates the apoptotic response to GTP depletion after renal ischemia-reperfusion: protective role of a p53 inhibitor. *J Am Soc Nephrol* 2003;14:128.

182. Dagher PC. Apoptosis in ischemic renal injury: roles of GTP depletion and p53. *Kidney Int* 2004;66:506.

183. Nowak G. Protein kinase C mediates repair of mitochondrial and transport functions after toxicant-induced injury in renal cells. *J Pharmacol Exp Ther* 2003;306:157.

184. Nowak G, Bakajsova D, Clifton GL. Protein kinase C-{epsilon} modulates mitochondrial function and active Na+ transport after oxidant injury in renal cells. *Am J Physiol Renal Physiol* 2004;286:F307.

185. Nowak G. Protein kinase C-alpha and ERK1/2 mediate mitochondrial dysfunction, decreases in active Na+ transport, and cisplatin-induced apoptosis in renal cells. *J Biol Chem* 2002;277:43377.

186. Arany I, et al. Cisplatin-induced cell death is EGFR/src/ERK signaling dependent in mouse proximal tubule cells. *Am J Physiol Renal Physiol* 2004;287:F543.

187. Arany I, Safirstein RL. Cisplatin nephrotoxicity. *Semin Nephrol* 2003;23:460.

188. Gopee NV, He Q, Sharma RP. Fumonisin B1-induced apoptosis is associated with delayed inhibition of protein kinase C, nuclear factor-kappaB and tumor necrosis factor alpha in LLC-PK1 cells. *Chem Biol Interact* 2003;146:131.

189. Woo KR, et al. Tumor necrosis factor mediates apoptosis via Ca++/Mg++ dependent endonuclease with protein kinase C as a possible mechanism for cytokine resistance in human renal carcinoma cells. *J Urol* 1996;155:1779.

190. Ferro T, et al. Protein kinase C-alpha mediates endothelial barrier dysfunction induced by TNF-alpha. *Am J Physiol Lung Cell Mol Physiol* 2000;278:L1107.

191. Coussens L, et al. Multiple, distinct forms of bovine and human protein kinase C suggest diversity in cellular signaling pathways. *Science* 1986;233:859.

192. Ullrich A, et al. Protein kinases in cellular signal transduction: tyrosine kinase growth factor receptors and protein kinase C. *Cold Spring Harb Symp Quant Biol* 1986;51:713.

193. Geiges D, et al. Activation of protein kinase C subtypes alpha, gamma, delta, epsilon, zeta, and eta by tumor-promoting and nontumor-promoting agents. *Biochem Pharmacol* 1997;53:865.

194. Pfaff IL, Wagner HJ, Vallon V. Immunolocalization of protein kinase C isoenzymes alpha, beta1 and betaII in rat kidney. *J Am Soc Nephrol* 1999;10:1861.

195. Padanilam BJ. Induction and subcellular localization of protein kinase C isozymes following renal ischemia. *Kidney Int* 2001;59:1789.

196. Serlachius E, et al. Protein kinase C in the developing kidney: isoform expression and effects of ceramide and PKC inhibitors. *Kidney Int* 1997;52:901.

197. Dong L, et al. Protein kinase C isozyme expression and down-modulation in growing, quiescent, and transformed renal proximal tubule epithelial cells. *Cell Growth Differ* 1994;5:881.

198. Efferth T, Volm M. Expression of protein kinase C in human renal cell carcinoma cells with inherent resistance to doxorubicin. *Anticancer Res* 1992;12:2209.

199. Goodnight J, et al. The cDNA sequence, expression pattern and protein characteristics of mouse protein kinase C-zeta. *Gene* 1992;122:305.

200. Zhuang S, et al. Involvement of protein kinase C in the activation of extracellular signal-regulated kinase 1/2 by UVC irradiation. *Biochem Biophys Res Commun* 1997;240:273.

201. Blumer KJ, Johnson GL. Diversity in function and regulation of MAP kinase pathways. *Trends Biochem Sci* 1994;19:236.

202. Ramachandiran S, et al. Mitogen-activated protein kinases contribute to reactive oxygen species-induced cell death in renal proximal tubule epithelial cells. *Chem Res Toxicol* 2002;15:1635.

203. Dong J, et al. Induction of ERK1/2 and histone H3 phosphorylation within the outer stripe of the outer medulla of the Eker rat by 2,3,5-tris-(glutathion-S-yl)hydroquinone. *Toxicol Sci* 2004;80:350.

204. Tikoo K, Lau SS, Monks TJ. Histone H3 phosphorylation is coupled to poly-(ADP-ribosylation) during reactive oxygen species-induced cell death in renal proximal tubular epithelial cells. *Mol Pharmacol* 2001;60:394.

205. Dong J, et al. EGFR-independent activation of p38 MAPK and EGFR-dependent activation of ERK1/2 are required for ROS-induced renal cell death. *Am J Physiol Renal Physiol* 2004;287:F1049.

206. English J, et al. New insights into the control of MAP kinase pathways. *Exp Cell Res* 1999;253:255.

207. Ludwig S, et al. 3pK, a novel mitogen-activated protein (MAP) kinase-activated protein kinase, is targeted by three MAP kinase pathways. *Mol Cell Biol* 1996;16:6687.

208. Park KM, Chen A, Bonventre JV. Prevention of kidney ischemia/reperfusion-induced functional injury and JNK, p38, and MAPK kinase activation by remote ischemic pretreatment. *J Biol Chem* 2001;276:11870.

209. Lee RH, et al. Cisplatin-induced apoptosis by translocation of endogenous Bax in mouse collecting duct cells. *Biochem Pharmacol* 2001;62:1013.

210. van de Water B, et al. Cleavage of the actin-capping protein alpha-adducin at Asp-Asp-Ser-Asp633-Ala by caspase-3 is preceded by its phosphorylation on serine 726 in cisplatin-induced apoptosis of renal epithelial cells. *J Biol Chem* 2000;275:25805.

211. Andreucci M, et al. Renal ischemia/reperfusion and ATP depletion/repletion in LLC-PK(1) cells result in phosphorylation of FKHR and FKHRL1. *Kidney Int* 2003;64:1189.

212. Weinberg JM, ed. *The cellular basis of nephrotoxicity*. Boston: Little Brown, 1993.

213. Orrenius S, Nicotera P. The calcium ion and cell death. *J Neural Transm Suppl* 1994;43:1.

214. Trump BF, Berezesky IK. Calcium-mediated cell injury and cell death. *Faseb J* 1995;9:219.

215. Herman B, et al. Calcium and pH in anoxic and toxic injury. *Crit Rev Toxicol* 1990;21:127.

216. Farber JL. The role of calcium in lethal cell injury. *Chem Res Toxicol* 1990;3:503.

217. Weinberg JM, et al. Role of increased cytosolic free calcium in the pathogenesis of rabbit proximal tubule cell injury and protection by glycine or acidosis. *J Clin Invest* 1991;87:581.

218. Takano T, et al. Intracellular respiratory dysfunction and cell injury in short-term anoxia of rabbit renal proximal tubules. *J Clin Invest* 1985;76:2377.

219. Harriman JF, et al. Endoplasmic reticulum Ca(2+) signaling and calpains mediate renal cell death. *Cell Death Differ* 2002;9:734.

220. Liu X, Harriman JF, Schnellmann RG. Cytoprotective properties of novel nonpeptide calpain inhibitors in renal cells. *J Pharmacol Exp Ther* 2002;302:88.

221. Waters SL, et al. Calpains mediate calcium and chloride influx during the late phase of cell injury. *J Pharmacol Exp Ther* 1997;283:1177.

222. Wetzels JF, et al. Calcium modulation and cell injury in isolated rat proximal tubules. *J Pharmacol Exp Ther* 1993;267:176.

223. Kribben A, et al. Evidence for role of cytosolic free calcium in hypoxia-induced proximal tubule injury. *J Clin Invest* 1994;93:1922.

224. Liu X, et al. Calpains mediate acute renal cell death: role of autolysis and translocation. *Am J Physiol Renal Physiol* 2001;281:F728.

225. Harriman JF, et al. Efficacy of novel calpain inhibitors in preventing renal cell death. *J Pharmacol Exp Ther* 2000;294:1083.

226. Smith MW, et al. HgCl2-induced changes in cytosolic Ca2+ of cultured rabbit renal tubular cells. *Biochim Biophys Acta* 1987;931:130.

227. Smith MW, Phelps PC, Trump BF. Cytosolic Ca2+ deregulation and blebbing after HgCl2 injury to cultured rabbit proximal tubule cells as determined by digital imaging microscopy. *Proc Natl Acad Sci USA* 1991;88:4926.

228. Jones TW, et al. The mechanism of pentachlorobutadienyl-glutathione nephrotoxicity studied with isolated rat renal epithelial cells. *Arch Biochem Biophys* 1986;251:504.

229. Groves CE, Lock EA, Schnellmann RG. The effects of haloalkene cysteine conjugates on cytosolic free calcium levels in suspensions of rat renal proximal tubules. *J Biochem Toxicol* 1990;5:187.

230. Lash LH, Anders MW. Cytotoxicity of S-(1,2-dichlorovinyl)glutathione and S-(1,2-dichlorovinyl)-L-cysteine in isolated rat kidney cells. *J Biol Chem* 1986;261:13076.

231. Vamvakas S, et al. Perturbations of intracellular calcium distribution in kidney cells by nephrotoxic haloalkenyl cysteine S-conjugates. *Mol Pharmacol* 1990;38:455.

232. van de Water B, et al. The relationship between intracellular Ca2+ and the mitochondrial membrane potential in isolated proximal tubular cells from rat kidney exposed to the nephrotoxin 1,2-dichlorovinyl-cysteine. *Biochem Pharmacol* 1993;45:2259.

233. Chen Q, Jones TW, Stevens JL. Early cellular events couple covalent binding of reactive metabolites to cell killing by nephrotoxic cysteine conjugates. *J Cell Physiol* 1994;161:293.

234. Ueda N, Shah SV. Role of intracellular calcium in hydrogen peroxide-induced renal tubular cell injury. *Am J Physiol* 1992;263:F214.

235. Greene EL, Paller MS. Calcium and free radicals in hypoxia/reoxygenation injury of renal epithelial cells. *Am J Physiol* 1994;266:F13.

236. Jan CR, Tseng CJ. Mechanisms of miconazole-induced rise in cytoplasmic calcium concentrations in Madin Darby canine kidney (MDCK) cells. *Life Sci* 1999;65:2513.

237. Jan CR, Wang KY, Tseng CJ. Effect of sevoflurane on Ca2+ mobilization in Madin-Darby canine kidney cells. *Biochem Pharmacol* 2000;59:393.

238. Carvalho da Costa M, et al. Cyclosporin A tubular effects contribute to nephrotoxicity: role for Ca2+ and Mg2+ ions. *Nephrol Dial Transplant* 2003;18:2262.

239. Cunha MA, Schor N. Effects of gentamicin, lipopolysaccharide, and contrast media on immortalized proximal tubular cells. *Ren Fail* 2002;24:687.

240. Ali BH, Al-Qarawi AA, Mousa HM. The effect of calcium load and the calcium channel blocker verapamil on gentamicin nephrotoxicity in rats. *Food Chem Toxicol* 2002;40:1843.

241. Wilson PD, Hartz PA. Mechanisms of cyclosporine A toxicity in defined cultures of renal tubule epithelia: a role for cysteine proteases. *Cell Biol Int Rep* 1991;15:1243.

242. Yang X, Schnellmann RG. Proteinases in renal cell death. *J Toxicol Environ Health* 1996;48:319.

243. Saido TC, Sorimachi H, Suzuki K. Calpain: new perspectives in molecular diversity and physiological-pathological involvement. *Faseb J* 1994;8:814.

244. Liu X, Schnellmann RG. Calpain mediates progressive plasma membrane permeability and proteolysis of cytoskeleton-associated paxillin, talin, and vinculin during renal cell death. *J Pharmacol Exp Ther* 2003;304:63.

245. Schnellmann RG, Williams SW. Proteases in renal cell death: calpains mediate cell death produced by diverse toxicants. *Ren Fail* 1998;20:679.

246. Edelstein CL, et al. Effect of glycine on prelethal and postlethal increases in calpain activity in rat renal proximal tubules. *Kidney Int* 1997;52:1271.

247. Takaoka M, et al. Proteasome participates in the pathogenesis of ischemic acute renal failure in rats. *Eur J Pharmacol* 1999;384:43.

248. Van Vleet T, Schnellmann RG. Identification of mitochondrial calpain-like activity during mitochondrial dysfunction. *Toxicol Sci* 2002;66:38.

249. Arrington DD, Van Vleet T, Schnellmann RG. Ca2+-induced mitochonrial-dysfunction is mediated by a calpain-like activity in renal cortical mitochondria. In: *Biology of the calpains in health and disease*. Tucson, AZ: 2004.

250. Arrington DD, Van Vleet T, Schnellmann RG. Localization and characterization of a novel mitochondrial calpain in renal cortical mitochondria. *J Am Soc Nephrol* 2003;14:351A.

251. Lankiewicz S, et al. Activation of calpain I converts excitotoxic neuron death into a caspase-independent cell death. *J Biol Chem* 2000;275:17064.

252. Chua BT, Guo K, Li P. Direct cleavage by the calcium-activated protease calpain can lead to inactivation of caspases. *J Biol Chem* 2000;275:5131.

253. Kaushal GP, Singh AB, Shah SV. Identification of gene family of caspases in rat kidney and altered expression in ischemia-reperfusion injury. *Am J Physiol* 1998;274:F587.

254. Orrenius S. Mitochondrial regulation of apoptotic cell death. *Toxicol Lett* 2004;149:19.

255. Cummings BS, et al. Identification of caspase-independent apoptosis in epithelial and cancer cells. *J Pharmacol Exp Ther* 2004;310:126.

256. Li S, et al. PPAR-alpha ligand ameliorates acute renal failure by reducing cisplatin-induced increased expression of renal endonuclease G. *Am J Physiol Renal Physiol* 2004;287:F990.

257. Basnakian AG, Kaushal GP, Shah SV. Apoptotic pathways of oxidative damage to renal tubular epithelial cells. *Antioxid Redox Signal* 2002;4:915.

258. Bonventre JV. Phospholipase A2 and signal transduction. *J Am Soc Nephrol* 1992;3:128.

259. Nakamura H, et al. Subcellular characteristics of phospholipase A2 activity in the rat kidney. Enhanced cytosolic, mitochondrial, and microsomal phospholipase A2 enzymatic activity after renal ischemia and reperfusion. *J Clin Invest* 1991;87:1810.

260. Portilla D, et al. Role of cytosolic calcium-independent plasmalogen-selective phospholipase A2 in hypoxic injury to rabbit proximal tubules. *J Clin Invest* 1994;93:1609.

261. Cummings BS, McHowat J, Schnellmann RG. Role of an endoplasmic reticulum Ca(2+)-independent phospholipase A(2) in oxidant-induced renal cell death. *Am J Physiol Renal Physiol* 2002;283:F492.

262. Mancuso DJ, Jenkins CM, Gross RW. The genomic organization, complete mRNA sequence, cloning, and expression of a novel human intracellular membrane-associated calcium-independent phospholipase A(2). *J Biol Chem* 2000;275:9937.

263. Kinsey GR, et al. Identification and distribution of endoplasmic reticulum iPLA2. *Biochem Biophys Acta* 2005;327:287.

264. Portilla D, et al. Anoxia induces phospholipase A2 activation in rabbit renal proximal tubules. *Am J Physiol* 1992;262:F354.

265. Bunnachak D, et al. Ca2+ uptake, fatty acid, and LDH release during proximal tubule hypoxia: effects of mepacrine and dibucaine. *Am J Physiol* 1994;266:F196.

266. Matthys E, et al. Lipid alterations induced by renal ischemia: pathogenic factor in membrane damage. *Kidney Int* 1984;26:153.

267. Katz AM, Messineo FC. Lipid-membrane interactions and the pathogenesis of ischemic damage in the myocardium. *Circ Res* 1981;48:1.

268. Corr PB, Gross RW, Sobel BE. Amphipathic metabolites and membrane dysfunction in ischemic myocardium. *Circ Res* 1984;55:135.

269. Chan SH, Higgins E Jr. Uncoupling activity of endogenous free fatty acids in rat liver mitochondria. *Can J Biochem* 1978;56:111.

270. Chien KR, et al. Accumulation of unesterified arachidonic acid in ischemic canine myocardium. Relationship to a phosphatidylcholine deacylation-reacylation cycle and the depletion of membrane phospholipids. *Circ Res* 1984;54:313.

271. Gunn MD, et al. Mechanisms of accumulation of arachidonic acid in cultured myocardial cells during ATP depletion. *Am J Physiol* 1985;249:H1188.

272. Otani H, et al. Mechanism of membrane phospholipid degradation in ischemic-reperfused rat hearts. *Am J Physiol* 1989;257:H252.

273. Idell-Wenger JA, Grotyohann LW, Neely JR. Coenzyme A and carnitine distribution in normal and ischemic hearts. *J Biol Chem* 1978;253:4310.

274. Bastin J, et al. Change in energy reserves in different segments of the nephron during brief ischemia. *Kidney Int* 1987;31:1239.

275. Cummings BS, et al. Inactivation of endoplasmic reticulum bound Ca(2+)-independent phospholipase A(2) in renal cells during oxidative Stress. *J Am Soc Nephrol* 2004;15:1441.

276. Enari M, et al. Different apoptotic pathways mediated by Fas and the tumor-necrosis-factor receptor. Cytosolic phospholipase A2 is not involved in Fas-mediated apoptosis. *Eur J Biochem* 1996;236:533.

277. Finkelstein SD, Gilfor D, Farber JL. Alterations in the metabolism of lipids in ischemia of the liver and kidney. *J Lipid Res* 1985;26:726.

278. Humes HD, et al. The role of free fatty acids in hypoxia-induced injury to renal proximal tubule cells. *Am J Physiol* 1989;256:F688.

279. Schnellmann RG, Yang X, Carrick JB. Arachidonic acid release in renal proximal tubule cell injuries and death. *J Biochem Toxicol* 1994;9:211.

280. Sapirstein A, et al. Cytosolic phospholipase A2 (PLA2), but not secretory PLA2, potentiates hydrogen peroxide cytotoxicity in kidney epithelial cells. *J Biol Chem* 1996;271:21505.

281. Kohjimoto Y, et al. Role of phospholipase A2 in the cytotoxic effects of oxalate in cultured renal epithelial cells. *Kidney Int* 1999;56:1432.

282. Groves CE, Lock EA, Schnellmann RG. Role of lipid peroxidation in renal proximal tubule cell death induced by haloalkene cysteine conjugates. *Toxicol Appl Pharmacol* 1991;107:54.

283. Mandel LJ. Metabolic substrates, cellular energy production, and the regulation of proximal tubular transport. *Annu Rev Physiol* 1985;47:85.

284. Schnellmann RG. Measurment of oxygen consumption. In: Tyson CA, Frazier JM, eds. *Methods in toxicology*. Boca Raton, FL: Academic Press, 1994.

285. Schnellmann RG, Griner RD. Mitochondrial mechanisms of tubular injury. In: Goldstein RS, ed. *Mechanisms of injury in renal diseases and toxicity*. Boca Raton, FL: CRC Press, 1994.

286. Lemasters JJ. Necrapoptosis and the mitochondrial permeability transition: shared pathways to necrosis and apoptosis. *Am J Physiol* 1999;276:G1.

287. Weinberg JM, Harding PG, Humes HD. Mitochondrial bioenergetics during the initiation of mercuric chloride-induced renal injury. I. Direct effects of in vitro mercuric chloride on renal mitochondrial function. *J Biol Chem* 1982;257:60.

288. Weinberg JM, Harding PG, Humes HD. Mitochondrial bioenergetics during the initiation of mercuric chloride-induced renal injury. II. Functional alterations of renal cortical mitochondria isolated after mercuric chloride treatment. *J Biol Chem* 1982;257:68.

289. Zalups RK, Knutson KL, Schnellmann RG. In vitro analysis of the accumulation and toxicity of inorganic mercury in segments of the proximal tubule isolated from the rabbit kidney. *Toxicol Appl Pharmacol* 1993;119:221.

290. Schnellmann RG, Lock EA, Mandel LJ. A mechanism of S-(1,2,3,4,4-pentachloro-1,3-butadienyl)-L-cysteine toxicity to rabbit renal proximal tubules. *Toxicol Appl Pharmacol* 1987;90:513.

291. Wallin A, et al. Toxicity of S-pentachlorobutadienyl-L-cysteine studied with isolated rat renal cortical mitochondria. *Arch Biochem Biophys* 1987;258:365.

292. Schnellmann RG, Cross TJ, Lock EA. Pentachlorobutadienyl-L-cysteine uncouples oxidative phosphorylation by dissipating the proton gradient. *Toxicol Appl Pharmacol* 1989;100:498.

293. Hayden PJ, Stevens JL. Cysteine conjugate toxicity, metabolism, and binding to macromolecules in isolated rat kidney mitochondria. *Mol Pharmacol* 1990;37:468.

294. Gordon JA, Gattone VH. Mitochondrial alterations in cisplatin-induced acute renal failure. *Am J Physiol* 1986;250:F991.

295. Safirstein R, et al. Cisplatin nephrotoxicity. *Am J Kidney Dis* 1986;8:356.

296. Brady HR, et al. Mitochondrial injury: an early event in cisplatin toxicity to renal proximal tubules. *Am J Physiol* 1990;258:F1181.

297. Lockard VG, et al. Citrinin nephrotoxicity in rats: a light and electron microscopic study. *Exp Mol Pathol* 1980;32:226.

298. Aleo MD, Wyatt RD, Schnellmann RG. The role of altered mitochondrial function in citrinin-induced toxicity to rat renal proximal tubule suspensions. *Toxicol Appl Pharmacol* 1991;109:455.

299. Chagas GM, et al. Mechanism of citrinin-induced dysfunction of mitochondria. IV–Effect on Ca2+ transport. *Cell Biochem Funct* 1995;13:53.

300. Chagas GM, et al. Citrinin affects the oxidative metabolism of BHK-21 cells. *Cell Biochem Funct* 1995;13:267.

301. Chagas GM, et al. Mechanism of citrinin-induced dysfunction of mitochondria. III. Effects on renal cortical and liver mitochondrial swelling. *J Appl Toxicol* 1995;15:91.

302. Moore JH, Truelove B. Ochratoxin A: inhibition of mitochondrial respiration. *Science* 1970;168:1102.

303. Aleo MD, Wyatt RD, Schnellmann RG. Mitochondrial dysfunction is an early event in ochratoxin A but not oosporein toxicity to rat renal proximal tubules. *Toxicol Appl Pharmacol* 1991;107:73.

304. Suzuki S, et al. Studies on the nephrotoxicity of ochratoxin A in rats. *Toxicol Appl Pharmacol* 1975;34:479.

305. Tune B. The nephrotoxicity of beta-lactam antibiotics. In: Hook J, Goldstein RS, eds. *Toxicology of the kidney*. New York: Raven Press, 1993.

306. Rush GF, Ponsler GD. Cephaloridine-induced biochemical changes and cytotoxicity in suspensions of rabbit isolated proximal tubules. *Toxicol Appl Pharmacol* 1991;109:314.

307. Aleo MD, et al. Toxicity of N-(3,5-dichlorophenyl)succinimide and metabolites to rat renal proximal tubules and mitochondria. *Chem Biol Interact* 1991;78:109.

308. Groves CE, et al. Differential cellular effects in the toxicity of haloalkene and haloalkane cysteine conjugates to rabbit renal proximal tubules. *J Biochem Toxicol* 1993;8:49.

309. Lock EA, Schnellmann RG. The effect of haloalkene cysteine conjugates on rat renal glutathione reductase and lipoyl dehydrogenase activities. *Toxicol Appl Pharmacol* 1990;104:180.

310. Weinberg JM, et al. Mitochondrial dysfunction during hypoxia/reoxygenation and its correction by anaerobic metabolism of citric acid cycle intermediates. *Proc Natl Acad Sci USA* 2000;97:2826.

311. Weinberg JM, et al. Anaerobic and aerobic pathways for salvage of proximal tubules from hypoxia-induced mitochondrial injury. *Am J Physiol Renal Physiol* 2000;279:F927.

312. Waters SL, Wong JK, Schnellmann RG. Depletion of endoplasmic reticulum calcium stores protects against hypoxia- and mitochondrial inhibitor-induced cellular injury and death. *Biochem Biophys Res Commun* 1997;240:57.

313. Liu H, et al. Endoplasmic reticulum chaperones GRP78 and calreticulin prevent oxidative stress, Ca2+ disturbances, and cell death in renal epithelial cells. *J Biol Chem* 1997;272:21751.

314. Chen Q, Yu K, Stevens JL. Regulation of the cellular stress response by reactive electrophiles. The role of covalent binding and cellular thiols in transcriptional activation of the 70-kilodalton heat shock protein gene by nephrotoxic cysteine conjugates. *J Biol Chem* 1992;267:24322.

315. Liu H, Lightfoot R, Stevens JL. Activation of heat shock factor by alkylating agents is triggered by glutathione depletion and oxidation of protein thiols. *J Biol Chem* 1996;271:4805.

316. Halleck MM, et al. Reduction of trans-4,5-dihydroxy-1,2-dithiane by cellular oxidoreductases activates gadd153/chop and grp78 transcription and induces cellular tolerance in kidney epithelial cells. *J Biol Chem* 1997;272:21760.

317. Nakagawa T, et al. Caspase-12 mediates endoplasmic-reticulum-specific apoptosis and cytotoxicity by amyloid-beta. *Nature* 2000;403:98.

318. Gil FZ, Malnic G. Effect of amphotericin B on renal tubular acidification in the rat. *Pflugers Arch* 1989;413:280.

319. Carlson MA, Condon RE. Nephrotoxicity of amphotericin B. *J Am Coll Surg* 1994;179:361.

320. Kone BC, Kaleta M, Gullans SR. Silver ion (Ag+)-induced increases in cell membrane K+ and Na+ permeability in the renal proximal tubule: reversal by thiol reagents. *J Membr Biol* 1988;102:11.

321. Kone BC, Brenner RM, Gullans SR. Sulfhydryl-reactive heavy metals increase cell membrane K+ and Ca2+ transport in renal proximal tubule. *J Membr Biol* 1990;113:1.

322. Reeves WB, Shah SV. Activation of potassium channels contributes to hypoxic injury in proximal tubules. *J Clin Invest* 1994;94:2289.

323. Leaf A. Maintenance of concentration gradients and regulation of cell volume. *Ann N Y Acad Sci* 1959;72:396.

324. Leaf A. On the mechanism of fluid exchange of tissues in vitro. *Biochem J* 1956;62:241.

325. Gullans SR, et al. Metabolic inhibitors: effects on metabolism and transport in the proximal tubule. *Am J Physiol* 1982;243:F133.

326. Miller GW, Schnellmann RG. Cytoprotection by inhibition of chloride channels: the mechanism of action of glycine and strychnine. *Life Sci* 1993;53:1211.

327. Miller GW, Schnellmann RG. Inhibitors of renal chloride transport do not block toxicant-induced chloride influx in the proximal tubule. *Toxicol Lett* 1995;76:179.

328. Reeves WB. Effects of chloride channel blockers on hypoxic injury in rat proximal tubules. *Kidney Int* 1997;51:1529.

329. Structure and function of the cell. In: Seeley RR, Stephens TD, Tate P, eds. *Anatomy and physiology*, 6 ed. Boston, MA: McGraw-Hill, 2003.

330. Borghoff SJ, Short BG, Swenberg JA. Biochemical mechanisms and pathobiology of alpha 2u-globulin nephropathy. *Annu Rev Pharmacol Toxicol* 1990;30:349.

331. Lehman-McKeeman L. Male rat-specific light hydrocarbon nephropathy. In: Hook J, Goldstein RS, eds. *Toxicology of the kidney*. New York: Raven Press, 1993.

332. Swenberg JA. Alpha 2u-globulin nephropathy: review of the cellular and molecular mechanisms involved and their implications for human risk assessment. *Environ Health Perspect* 1993;101:39.

333. Melnick RL. An alternative hypothesis on the role of chemically induced protein droplet (alpha 2u-globulin) nephropathy in renal carcinogenesis. *Regul Toxicol Pharmacol* 1992;16:111.

334. Cuervo AM, et al. Direct lysosomal uptake of alpha 2-microglobulin contributes to chemically induced nephropathy. *Kidney Int* 1999;55:529.

335. Goldstein SM, Schnellmann RG. Toxic responses of the kidney. In: Klaassen CD, ed. *Casarett and Doull's toxicology: the basic science of poisons*, 5th ed. New York: McGraw-Hill, 1996:471.

336. Kaloyanides GJ. Drug-phospholipid interactions: role in aminoglycoside nephrotoxicity. *Ren Fail* 1992;14:351.

337. Vina J. *Glutathione Metabolism and Physiological Functions*. Boca Raton, FL: CRC Press, 1990.

338. Lash LH, Tokarz JJ. Isolation of two distinct populations of cells from rat kidney cortex and their use in the study of chemical-induced toxicity. *Anal Biochem* 1989;182:271.

339. Lash LH, Putt DA, Matherly LH. Protection of NRK-52E cells, a rat renal proximal tubular cell line, from chemical-induced apoptosis by overexpression of a mitochondrial glutathione transporter. *J Pharmacol Exp Ther* 2002;303:476.

340. Rose RC, Bode AM. Biology of free radical scavengers: an evaluation of ascorbate. *Faseb J* 1993;7:1135.

341. Sauberlich HE. Pharmacology of vitamin C. *Annu Rev Nutr* 1994;14:371.

342. Liebler DC. The role of metabolism in the antioxidant function of vitamin E. *Crit Rev Toxicol* 1993;23:147.

343. Wang C, Salahudeen AK. Lipid peroxidation accompanies cyclosporine nephrotoxicity: effects of vitamin E. *Kidney Int* 1995;47:927.

344. Lash LH, Tokarz JJ, Woods EB. Renal cell type specificity of cephalosporin-induced cytotoxicity in suspensions of isolated proximal tubular and distal tubular cells. *Toxicology* 1994;94:97.

345. Weinberg JM. The cell biology of ischemic renal injury. *Kidney Int* 1991;39:476.

346. Miller GW, Lock EA, Schnellmann RG. Strychnine and glycine protect renal proximal tubules from various nephrotoxicants and act in the late phase of necrotic cell injury. *Toxicol Appl Pharmacol* 1994;125:192.

347. Aleo MD, Schnellmann RG. Regulation of glycolytic metabolism during long-term primary culture of renal proximal tubule cells. *Am J Physiol* 1992;262:F77.

348. Miller GW, Schnellmann RG. A novel low-affinity strychnine binding site on renal proximal tubules: role in toxic cell death. *Life Sci* 1993;53:1203.

349. Miller GW, Schnellmann RG. A putative cytoprotective receptor in the kidney: relation to the neuronal strychnine-sensitive glycine receptor. *Life Sci* 1994;55:27.

350. Sarang SS, et al. Expression and localization of the neuronal glycine receptor beta-subunit in human, rabbit and rat kidneys. *Nephron* 1999;82:254.

351. Nichols JC, et al. Inhibition of nonlysosomal calcium-dependent proteolysis by glycine during anoxic injury of rat hepatocytes. *Gastroenterology* 1994;106:168.

352. Waters SL, Schnellmann RG. Examination of the mechanisms of action of diverse cytoprotectants in renal cell death. *Toxicol Pathol* 1996;24:58.

353. Rodeheaver DP, Schnellmann RG. Extracellular acidosis ameliorates metabolic-inhibitor-induced and potentiates oxidant-induced cell death in renal proximal tubules. *J Pharmacol Exp Ther* 1993;265:1355.

354. Bonventre JV, Cheung JY. Effects of metabolic acidosis on viability of cells exposed to anoxia. *Am J Physiol* 1985;249:C149.

355. Weinberg JM. Oxygen deprivation-induced injury to isolated rabbit kidney tubules. *J Clin Invest* 1985;76:1193.

356. Burnier M, et al. Effect of extracellular acidosis on 45Ca uptake in isolated hypoxic proximal tubules. *Am J Physiol* 1988;254:C839.

357. Baumgart E, et al. Mitochondrial alterations caused by defective peroxisomal biogenesis in a mouse model for Zellweger syndrome (PEX5 knockout mouse). *Am J Pathol* 2001;159:1477.

358. Isuzugawa K, Inoue M, Ogihara Y. Catalase contents in cells determine sensitivity to the apoptosis inducer gallic acid. *Biol Pharm Bull* 2001;24:1022.

359. Li S, et al. PPAR alpha ligand protects during cisplatin-induced acute renal failure by preventing inhibition of renal FAO and PDC activity. *Am J Physiol Renal Physiol* 2004;286:F572.

360. Guan Y. Peroxisome proliferator-activated receptor family and its relationship to renal complications of the metabolic syndrome. *J Am Soc Nephrol* 2004;15:2801.

361. Sato K, et al. Expression of peroxisome proliferator-activated receptor isoform proteins in the rat kidney. *Hypertens Res* 2004;27:417.

362. Portilla D, et al. Alterations of PPARalpha and its coactivator PGC-1 in cisplatin-induced acute renal failure. *Kidney Int* 2002;62:1208.

363. Guan Y, et al. Expression of peroxisome proliferator-activated receptors in urinary tract of rabbits and humans. *Am J Physiol* 1997;273:F1013.

364. Reddy JK, et al. Transcription regulation of peroxisomal fatty acyl-CoA oxidase and enoyl-CoA hydratase/3-hydroxyacyl-CoA dehydrogenase in rat liver by peroxisome proliferators. *Proc Natl Acad Sci USA* 1986;83:1747.

365. Zhu Y, et al. Cloning of a new member of the peroxisome proliferator-activated receptor gene family from mouse liver. *J Biol Chem* 1993;268:26817.

366. Zhu C, et al. Involvement of apoptosis-inducing factor in neuronal death after hypoxia-ischemia in the neonatal rat brain. *J Neurochem* 2003;86:306.

367. Camp HS, et al. Differential activation of peroxisome proliferator-activated receptor-gamma by troglitazone and rosiglitazone. *Diabetes* 2000;49:539.

368. Chana RS, Lewington AJ, Brunskill NJ. Differential effects of peroxisome proliferator activated receptor-gamma (PPAR gamma) ligands in proximal tubular cells: thiazolidinediones are partial PPAR gamma agonists. *Kidney Int* 2004;65:2081.

369. Guan Y, et al. Peroxisome proliferator-activated receptor-gamma activity is associated with renal microvasculature. *Am J Physiol Renal Physiol* 2001;281:F1036.

370. Lazarow PB, De Duve C. A fatty acyl-CoA oxidizing system in rat liver peroxisomes; enhancement by clofibrate, a hypolipidemic drug. *Proc Natl Acad Sci USA* 1976;73:2043.

371. Hashimoto T. Individual peroxisomal beta-oxidation enzymes. *Ann N Y Acad Sci* 1982;386:5.

372. Portilla D. Energy metabolism and cytotoxicity. *Semin Nephrol* 2003;23(5):432.

373. Sivarajah A, et al. Agonists of peroxisome-proliferator activated receptor-alpha (clofibrate and WY14643) reduce renal ischemia/reperfusion injury in the rat. *Med Sci Monit* 2002;8:BR532.

374. Portilla D, et al. Etomoxir-induced PPARalpha-modulated enzymes protect during acute renal failure. *Am J Physiol Renal Physiol* 2000;278:F667.

375. Amet Y, et al. P-450-dependent metabolism of lauric acid in alcoholic liver disease: comparison between rat liver and kidney microsomes. *Alcohol Clin Exp Res* 1998;22:455.

376. Wu S, et al. Molecular cloning, expression, and functional significance of a cytochrome P450 highly expressed in rat heart myocytes. *J Biol Chem* 1997;272:12551.

377. Ma J, et al. Molecular cloning, enzymatic characterization, developmental expression, and cellular localization of a mouse cytochrome P450 highly expressed in kidney. *J Biol Chem* 1999;274:17777.

378. Wu S, et al. Molecular cloning and expression of CYP2J2, a human cytochrome P450 arachidonic acid epoxygenase highly expressed in heart. *J Biol Chem* 1996;271:3460.

379. Liu X, Godwin ML, Nowak G. Protein kinase C-alpha inhibits the repair of oxidative phosphorylation after S-(1,2-dichlorovinyl)-L-cysteine injury in renal cells. *Am J Physiol Renal Physiol* 2004;287:F64.

380. Zhuang S, Schnellmann RG, Zhougang S. H2O2-induced transactivation of EGF receptor requires Src and mediates ERK1/2, but not Akt, activation in renal cells. *Am J Physiol Renal Physiol* 2004;286:F858.

CHAPTER 41 ■ ACUTE RENAL FAILURE

VINCENT WENG SENG LEE, DAVID HARRIS, ROBERT J. ANDERSON, AND ROBERT W. SCHRIER

Acute renal failure (ARF) is defined as an abrupt decrease in renal function sufficient to result in retention of nitrogenous waste (e.g., blood urea nitrogen [BUN] and creatinine) in the body. Although there is unanimity of opinion regarding this general definition, there is no consensus regarding the magnitude of elevation of serum creatinine and BUN sufficient to ascribe a diagnosis of ARF (1–3). Moreover, there is a nonlinear relationship between decreasing glomerular filtration rate (GFR) and rising serum creatinine concentration in individuals with a normal basal serum creatinine. Thus, in individuals with a normal basal serum creatinine, significant decreases in GFR are often associated with either slight or modest increases in serum creatinine concentration (4). Also, not only renal elimination, but also rate of production and volume of distribution are significant determinants of serum creatinine concentration (5). Taken together, although practical and currently our most useful tool for diagnosis, increases in serum creatinine concentration can be a somewhat insensitive marker of ARF.

Not only differences in diagnostic criteria, but also differences in frequency of surveillance and populations studied render definitive conclusions about the incidence of ARF difficult. Nonetheless, the data depicted in Table 41-1 demonstrate that ARF occurs with relatively high frequency, especially in seriously ill hospitalized patients (6–34). Figure 41-1 depicts potential high incidence settings of ARF.

Acute renal failure not only occurs with high frequency, but is also associated with significant morbidity and mortality. A matched-pairs cohort study of mild-to-moderate radiocontrast-associated ARF found a mortality of 7% in controls that was increased about sixfold in patients with ARF (35). A prospective case control study of 17,126 intensive care unit (ICU) patients found that patients with ARF treated with dialysis had an over four times higher hospital mortality than control patients (62.8% vs. 15.6%, p <.001), which remained significantly higher even when dialysis patients were matched with control subjects for age, severity of illness, and treatment center (36). Contemporary mortality of patients with oliguric and nonoliguric ARF remains in the 40% to 80% and 15% to 20% ranges, respectively (Fig. 41-2) (37–44). It is noteworthy that a direct relationship exists between the magnitude of rise in serum creatinine concentration and mortality of ARF (Fig. 41-3) (37). This emphasizes the need for early assessment and intervention in all cases of ARF. Together, it is apparent that ARF is associated with substantial morbidity, mortality, and cost.

The financial costs of ARF are high. In a Canadian ICU, the cost of dialysis was $3,486 to $5,117 (Canadian) per week for continuous renal replacement therapy (CRRT), and $1,342 a week for ischemic heart disease (IHD). The total direct cost of care for the subsequent year for patients who remained on dialysis was substantially higher ($73,273) than for those patients with renal recovery ($11,192) (45). A prospective cohort study of 490 ARF patients requiring dialysis from five geographically distant teaching hospitals estimated costs per quality-adjusted life year saved to be from $62,000 to $274,000 (46). In a Finnish study carried out in 1992, the mean cost of the treatment for ARF was $36,000 per patient and $80,000 for ARF survivors (47). These latter data are now more than 12 years old, suggesting even greater contemporary cost.

Abrupt and progressive renal failure is the final common pathway for several disease processes (Tables 41-2 to 41-4; Fig. 41-4). Thus, multiple disease entities and diverse pathologic conditions can produce a similar clinical entity of ARF. The high frequency of occurrence, multiple causes, and potential for high morbidity and mortality demand a logical approach to the patient with ARF. In this chapter, we use the term ARF in its most generic sense to describe acute impairment of the kidney function independent of cause and mechanism. We discuss the causes, clinical settings, diagnostic approaches, consequences, and therapy of such clinically encountered ARF.

This chapter will discuss the general clinical aspects of acute renal failure. The pathophysiology of ARF (Chapters 39 and 40), antibiotic- and immunosuppression-related aspects of ARF (Chapter 42), renal diseases induced by antineoplastic agents (Chapter 43), nephrotoxicity of nonsteroidal anti-inflammatory agents, analgesics and angiotensin-converting enzyme inhibitors (Chapter 44), radiocontrast media–induced ARF (Chapter 45), nephrotoxicity secondary to drug abuse and lithium use (Chapter 46), nephrotoxicity secondary to environmental agents and heavy metals (Chapter 47), acute tubulointerstitial nephritis (Chapter 48), acute renal failure associated with pigmenturia or crystal deposits (Chapter 49) are discussed elsewhere.

DIAGNOSIS OF ACUTE RENAL FAILURE

Acute renal failure is most often diagnosed by finding increasing concentrations of serum creatinine and/or blood urea nitrogen (BUN). The usual BUN:serum creatinine ratio is about 15:1 and the BUN and serum creatinine increase by 10 to 15 and 1.0 to 1.5 mg/dL/day, respectively, in the absence of GFR. Several clinical situations can disproportionately affect either the BUN or serum creatinine thereby altering the BUN:serum creatinine ratio (48). Moreover, as is apparent from Figure 41-5, factors other than a reduction in GFR can be associated with increased concentrations of BUN (e.g., catabolic state with enhanced urea nitrogen formation) and occasionally serum creatinine (e.g., medication effects to impair renal tubular secretion of creatinine and chemically interfere with creatinine measurements).

The serum creatinine concentration is usually a better marker of glomerular filtration rate (GFR) than the BUN. In a steady state setting, a reasonable approximation is that each time the GFR halves the serum creatinine concentration doubles. Thus, steady state GFRs of 100, 50, 25, 12.5, and 6.25 mL/minute are associated with serum creatinine concentrations of about 1.0, 2.0, 4.0, 8.0, and 16.0 mg/dL, respectively. Acute renal failure often occurs in a non–steady state in which the three determinants of serum creatinine concentration (production, volume of distribution, and renal elimination) fluctuate (5). Computerized models derived from ARF patients

TABLE 41-1

INCIDENCE OF ACUTE RENAL FAILURE

Population with ARF	Any ARF (%)	Severe ARF (%)
General public (18,19)		
<50 yr of age	—	0.0017*
15–64 yr of age	—	0.0006*
>65 yr of age	—	0.0047*
>80 yr of age	—	0.095*
Pregnancy (20,21)		
Presumably healthy	—	0.00006
Underprivileged, inner city	—	0.0002
Heart disease (22–26)		
Admission to a coronary care unit	—	4
After coronary intervention	14	1
Cardiopulmonary resuscitation survivors	—	29
Infections (27–31)		
Hospitalized for pneumonia	8	—
Community-acquired bacteremia	24	4
Rocky Mountain spotted fever	20	—
Human immunodeficiency virus	20–40	10–30
Extensive trauma (32,33)	20–40	0.1–5.0
Significant burns (34,80)	15–30	1–5
Liver disease (96,224)		
Spontaneous bacterial peritonitis	30–40	0–1
End-stage liver disease	20–40	10–20
Hospital admission (37,54)		
General medical—surgical ward	1–4	0.1–1.0
Intensive care units	10–30	1–5
Nonrenal transplantation (96,185,192,195)		
Cardiac	25–50	1–15
Liver	30–50	20–40
Bone marrow autologous	5–15	2–7
Bone marrow allogeneic	30–60	15–30
Postoperative (24,25,161,167)		
Elective abdominal aortic aneurysm	10–30	2–10
Obstructive jaundice	5–10	2–3
General surgery	20–30	0.1–2.0

ARF, acute renal failure.
Severe ARF, ARF requiring dialysis except in those data marked by * where severe ARF is defined by a rise in serum creatinine to over 500 μmol/L with subsequent fall below 500 μmol/L.
— = not stated or assessed.

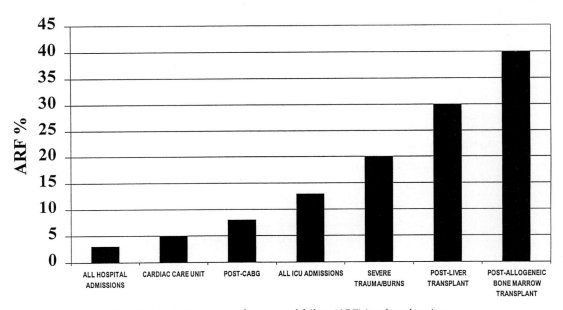

FIGURE 41-1. Frequency of acute renal failure (ARF) in selected settings.

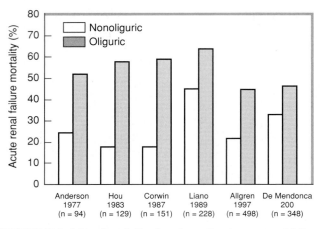

FIGURE 41-2. Mortality of oliguric and nonoliguric acute renal failure in six studies published in the past quarter of a century.

demonstrate that several patterns of change in GFR occur during development and recovery from ARF. These GFR changes are poorly reflected by daily changes in serum creatinine concentration (5). Moreover, the rise in serum creatinine that occurs in ARF is a *post facto* finding. Unfortunately, although real-time, noninvasive monitoring of GFR can be done in seriously ill patients, these techniques are currently expensive and not widely available (49).

In selected circumstances it is not clear if an elevated BUN:serum creatinine ratio is due to an acute or chronic process (Table 41-5). In this setting, review of previous records is helpful. In the absence of previous values, measurement of carbamylated hemoglobin can be helpful. Nonenzymatic carbamylation of the terminal valine of hemoglobin occurs in direct relationship to the magnitude and duration of increase in BUN (50,51). A carbamylated hemoglobin level greater than 80 to 100 μg carbamyl valine per gram hemoglobin suggests the diagnosis of acute rather than chronic renal failure (52,53). The presence of small kidney size on an imaging study strongly supports a diagnosis of chronic renal disease and the other factors noted in Table 41-5 may also help to differentiate acute from chronic renal failure. Because reversible factors often are operative in both acute and chronic renal failure, the clinician should assume the presence of potentially treatable conditions in all cases of renal failure.

Other biochemical markers of ARF that are more sensitive than serum creatinine have been sought (Table 41-6). Urinary

TABLE 41-2

CAUSES OF PRERENAL ACUTE RENAL FAILURE

Decreased intravascular fluid volume
Extracellular fluid loss—burns, diarrhea, vomiting, diuretics, salt-wasting renal disease, primary adrenal insufficiency, gastrointestinal hemorrhage
Extracellular fluid sequestration—pancreatitis, burns, crush injury, nephrotic syndrome, malnutrition, advanced liver disease

Decreased cardiac output
Myocardial dysfunction—myocardial infarction, arrhythmias, ischemic heart disease, cardiomyopathies, valvular disease, hypertensive disease, severe cor pulmonale

Peripheral vasodilation
Drugs—antihypertensive agents
Sepsis
Miscellaneous—adrenal cortical insufficiency, hypermagnesemia, hypercapnia, hypoxia

Severe renal vasoconstriction
Sepsis
Drugs—nonsteroidal antiinflammatory agents, β-adrenergic agonists
Hepatorenal syndrome

Mechanical occlusion of renal arteries
Thrombotic occlusion
Miscellaneous (emboli, trauma [e.g. angioplasty])

markers of early renal injury have been studied recently. Kidney injury molecule (KIM-1) is a transmembrane protein found in proximal tubule cells that was shown to be upregulated in a postischemic rat model (7). Han and colleagues found (8) that urinary KIM-1 protein concentration was significantly higher in urine samples from patients with ischemic acute tubular necrosis (ATN) compared to urine samples from patients with other forms of acute and chronic renal failure. Muramatsu and associates (9) found that the secreted, cysteine-rich, heparin binding protein Cyr61 was rapidly induced in proximal straight tubules following renal ischemia, and excreted in the urine where it might serve as an early biomarker of renal injury. No clinical studies have so far been undertaken. In a prospective study of critically ill patients, high values of urinary gamma glutamyl transpeptidase, alkaline phosphatase,

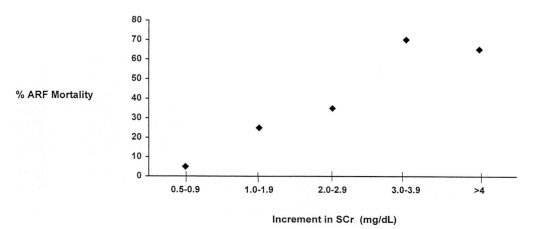

FIGURE 41-3. Relationship of acute renal failure mortality to magnitude of resultant rise in serum creatinine concentration. (From: Hou S, Bushinsky D, Wish JB, et al. Hospital-acquired renal insufficiency: a prospective study. *Am J Med* 1983;74:243, with permission.)

TABLE 41-3

CAUSES OF POSTRENAL ACUTE RENAL FAILURE

Intrarenal (intratubular)
Crystal deposition—uric acid, oxalic acid, methotrexate, acyclovir, triamterene, sulfonamides, indinavir, tenofovir
Protein deposition—light chains, myoglobin, hemoglobin

Extrarenal
Ureteral/pelvic
Intrinsic obstruction—tumor, stone, clot, pus, fungal ball, papilla
Extrinsic obstruction—retroperitoneal and pelvic malignancy, fibrosis, ligation, abdominal aortic aneurysm

Bladder
Prostate hypertrophy/malignancy
Stones
Clots
Tumor
Neurogenic
Medication

Urethral
Stricture
Phimosis

TABLE 41-4

RENAL CAUSES OF ACUTE RENAL FAILURE

Renal vascular disorders
Vasculitis
Malignant hypertension
Scleroderma
Thrombotic thrombocytopenic purpura
Hemolytic–uremic syndrome
Disseminated intravascular coagulation
Mechanical renal artery occlusion (surgery, emboli, thrombotic occlusion)
Renal vein thrombosis

Glomerulonephritis
Postinfectious
Membranoproliferative
Rapidly progressive glomerulonephritis (idiopathic, polyarteritis nodosa, systemic lupus erythematosus, Wegener's syndrome, microscopic polyarteritis, Goodpasture's syndrome, Henoch-Schonlein purpura)
Drugs

Interstitial nephritis
Drugs (penicillin, sulfonamide, rifampin, ciprofloxacin, phenindiones, cimetidine, proton pump inhibitors [omeprazole, lansoprazole], azathioprine, phenytoin, captopril, thiazides, furosemide, bumetanide, allopurinol, NSAIDs including selective cyclooxygenase-2 inhibitors, 5-aminosalicylates)
Hypercalcemia

Infections
Nonspecific due to frank septicemia or systemic antiinflammatory response syndrome
Specific organisms (Legionella, Leptospira, Rickettsia, Hantavirus, Candida, malaria)
Specific organ involvement (bacterial endocarditis, visceral abscess, pyelonephritis)

Infiltration
Sarcoid
Lymphoma
Leukemia

Connective tissue disease
Tubular necrosis
Renal ischemia (prolonged prerenal)
Nephrotoxins (aminoglycosides, radiocontrast agents, heavy metals, organic solvents, other antimicrobials)
Pigmenturia (myoglobinuria, hemoglobinuria)
Miscellaneous

N-acetyl-glucosaminidase, and alpha- and pi-glutathione S-transferase, indexed to urinary creatinine, were predictive of ARF. Urinary interleukin-18 was found to be elevated in patients with ATN and delayed graft function compared with other renal diseases (12). In patients with acute renal allograft dysfunction, selected chemokines that bind to the CXCR3 receptor appear to be useful (14). In patients with ARF, the apical sodium transporter Na^+/H^+ exchanger isoform 3 (NHE3) protein appears to be a marker of renal tubule damage, helping to differentiate prerenal azotemia, ATN, and intrinsic ARF other than ATN (13). Serum cystatin C appears to be more sensitive than serum creatinine for detecting early decrements in GFR (11), but is not validated in ARF. Further studies are required to assess the usefulness of these tests in clinical practice.

Kidney regulation of the normal volume and composition of body fluids and the process of urine formation begins with ultrafiltration of the blood delivered to the kidney, proceeds through intrarenal processing of the ultrafiltrate by tubular reabsorption and secretion, and ends by elimination of the formed urine through the ureters, bladder, and urethra. It follows that ARF can result from a decrease in renal blood flow (prerenal azotemia; Table 41-2), intrinsic renal parenchymal diseases (renal azotemia; Table 41-4), or obstruction to urine flow (postrenal azotemia; Table 41-3). Because appropriate therapy of ARF depends on delineating the underlying cause, the initial step in determining the cause of ARF is to attempt to classify the site of origin of ARF as prerenal, renal, or postrenal. From a practical perspective, patients with hospital-acquired ARF tend to have more than one cause, whereas those with community-acquired ARF often have a single cause of ARF (2,18,37,41,54–58). Individuals with community-acquired ARF have fewer numbers of comorbidities and greater prevalence of ARF of postrenal cause than those with hospital-acquired ARF (3,59). A number of clinical and laboratory clues may assist in determining the site of ARF.

Prerenal Acute Renal Failure

The process of urine formation begins with delivery of blood to the glomerulus. The highly selective permeability of the glomerular capillary combined with the glomerular capillary hydrostatic pressure (which exceeds glomerular capillary oncotic pressure and intratubular hydrostatic pressure) results in formation of glomerular filtrate. Under unusual circumstances such as mannitol intoxication, high-dose dextran infusion, or marked hyperproteinemia, a "hyperoncotic state" occurs in which glomerular capillary oncotic pressure exceeds hydrostatic pressure (60–62). This results in cessation of glomerular filtration and ARF, often accompanied by an anuric state. Rapid reversal of this form of ARF occurs with removal (plasmapheresis) of the osmotically active substance from plasma.

The central role of delivery of blood to the glomerulus as the starting point of formation of glomerular filtrate dictates that clinical disorders that can decrease renal perfusion are potential causes of ARF. In clinical practice, ARF owing to hypoperfusion with a resultant fall in glomerular capillary filtration pressure is one of the most common forms of ARF

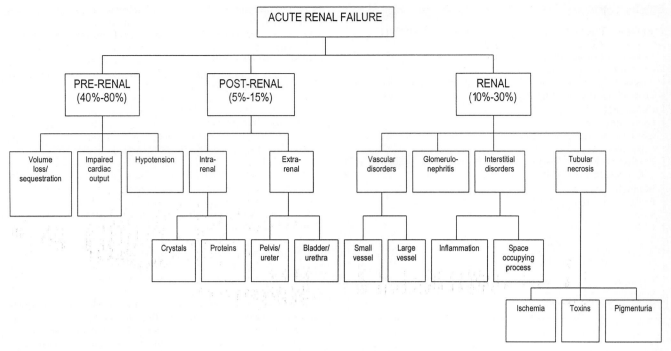

FIGURE 41-4. Causes of acute renal failure.

(1,2,18,35,38–40,44,55). The frequency of prerenal azotemia as a cause of ARF varies with the clinical setting. A prospective study by Hou et al. (37) found prerenal azotemia to be the single most common cause of ARF in a general medical-surgical hospital. Liano found that prerenal causes of ARF among the elderly accounted for 48% of community-acquired ARF and 58% of hospital-acquired ARF (63). In blacks, Obialo reported that 19% of community-acquired ARF and 35% of hospital-acquired ARF were prerenal in origin (3). Brivet observed that in critically ill patients, prerenal causes accounted for 17% of cases of ARF (44). Shusterman and associates found that the odds ratios for development of hospital-associated ARF were increased by 9.4- and 9.2-fold in the presence of the prerenal insults of volume depletion and congestive heart failure, respectively (55). Prerenal forms of ARF also appear to be common causes of community-acquired ARF and constituted 70%

of all such cases in the experience of Kaufman and associates (57). Not only is prerenal azotemia common but also it is often potentially reversible. Moreover, prolonged prerenal azotemia can lead to ischemic acute tubular necrosis (ATN) with significant morbidity. Thus, recognition and prompt therapy of prerenal causes of ARF are important.

Under normal circumstances, renal blood flow and glomerular filtration rate (GFR) are relatively constant over a wide range of renal perfusion pressures, a phenomenon termed *autoregulation* (64). Renal autoregulation not only allows constancy of GFR and filtered load of solutes but also maintains constancy of oxygen delivery in spite of variable renal perfusion pressures. This autoregulatory response normally renders an individual relatively resistant to prerenal forms of ARF; however, a marked decrease in renal perfusion pressure below the autoregulatory range can lead to an abrupt decrease

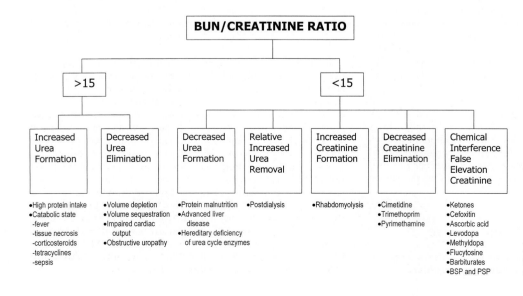

FIGURE 41-5. Causes of abnormalities in blood urea nitrogen (BUN) to serum creatinine ratio.

TABLE 41-5

DIFFERENTIATION OF ACUTE VERSUS CHRONIC RENAL FAILURE

	Favors chronic	Favors acute
History of kidney disease, hypertension, abnormal urinalysis	+	0
Small kidney size	+	0
Urinalysis with broad casts (i.e., more than two to three white blood cells in diameter)	+	0
Return of renal function to normal with time	0	+
Low carbamylated hemoglobin	0	+
Hyperkalemia, acidemia, hyperphosphatemia,[a] anemia[a]	+	+

[a] More common in chronic renal failure.

in GFR and ARF. Within the autoregulatory range, a reduction in renal perfusion, as occurs with either diminished cardiac output or depletion of extracellular fluid volume, normally results in dilation of the glomerular afferent arteriole and constriction of the glomerular efferent arteriole so that glomerular capillary-hydrostatic pressure and GFR usually remain constant (64). The afferent dilation is mediated in part by vasodilatory eicosanoids, whereas efferent constriction can be attributed in part to angiotensin II. It follows that in the setting of compromised cardiac output or intravascular volume depletion, prevention of afferent arteriolar dilation (as occurs

TABLE 41-6

EXPERIMENTAL URINARY MARKERS IN ARF (ADAPTED FROM [6])

Enzymes e.g., gamma glutamyl transpeptidase, alkaline phosphatase, N-acetyl-glucosaminidase, alpha- and pi-glutathione S-transferase
Tubular proteins, e.g., adenosine-deaminase binding protein, kidney injury molecule, cyr61 (cysteine-rich heparin binding protein),
Growth factors, e.g., human epidermal growth factor, hepatocyte growth factor
Low-molecular-weight proteins
Proteases, e.g., L-alanine aminopeptidase, N-acetyl-[beta]-D-glucosaminidase
Cytokines, e.g., IL-2, IL-6, IL-18
Chemokines, e.g., CXCR3 binding chemokines, monocyte chemotactic peptide-1
Adhesion molecules, e.g., intercellular adhesion molecule-1, CD8, CD25
Amino acids
Cytodiagnostics, e.g., proximal tubule cells
Coagulation factors
Ion and water transporters, e.g., NHE3

IL, interleukin.

following nonsteroidal antiinflammatory agent therapy, which impairs synthesis of selective eicosanoids) and attenuation of efferent arteriolar constriction (as occurs following angiotensin converting enzyme inhibition, angiotensin receptor inhibition, and perhaps calcium channel blocking agents) can potentially decrease glomerular capillary filtration pressure and potentially cause an abrupt decline in GFR.

From a clinical perspective, a potentially reversible "prerenal" form of ARF can be seen when nonsteroidal antiinflammatory drugs (NSAIDs) are given to patients with volume depletion, hypoalbuminemia, an edematous disorder, advancing age, underlying chronic renal failure, or recent diuretic (especially triamterene) use (65) (see Chapter 44). These clinical conditions are often associated with enhanced renal vasoconstriction owing to renal adrenergic neural tone, norepinephrine, and angiotensin II. If the nonsteroidal antiinflammatory drugs (NSAIDs) are stopped early, the renal failure readily reverses. With continued administration of the agent, a more severe form of ARF owing to ischemic ATN may occur. Selective cyclooxygenase-2 inhibitor therapy has also been associated with acute renal failure, hypertension, edema, hyponatremia, hyperkalemia, type 4 renal tubular acidosis, and acute tubulointerstitial nephritis (66).

A similar prerenal form of ARF can complicate angiotensin converting enzyme therapy (67,68). In the presence of a decrease in renal blood flow from severe bilateral renal artery stenosis, renal artery stenosis in a solitary kidney, and other high-renin, high-angiotensin II states (i.e., edematous states and volume depletion disorders), angiotensin II converting enzyme inhibition with a resultant decrease in both renal perfusion pressure and efferent arteriolar constriction can precipitously decrease GFR. For example, about one-third of patients with severe congestive heart failure experience an abrupt rise in serum creatinine concentration following angiotensin converting enzyme inhibitor therapy (68). In the setting of heart failure, this increase in serum creatinine following angiotensin converting enzyme inhibition tends to be mild and readily reversible on discontinuation of the drug.

Several clinical conditions can result in enhanced renal afferent arteriolar vasoconstriction, which potentially impairs renal autoregulation, thereby decreasing glomerular capillary hydrostatic pressure and inducing ARF. For example, in the setting of hemorrhagic hypotension or Gram-negative sepsis, the combined effect of intense renal adrenergic neural traffic, norepinephrine, angiotensin II, endothelin, a variety of lipid-derived mediators (thromboxanes, leukotrienes, and prostaglandin F_{2a}-like compounds), and endotoxin can all exert potent vasoconstrictor influences on the afferent arteriole of the kidney. Thus, the decrease in systemic and, therefore, renal perfusion pressure that accompanies septic or hemorrhagic shock, combined with intense afferent arteriolar constriction, can result in a precipitous fall in GFR and ARF.

It is noteworthy that experimental studies demonstrate that one effect of ischemic ATN may be to impair renal autoregulation (69). Some of this impaired autoregulation appears to be due to the effect of enhanced renal adrenergic neural tone and increased action of renal vasoconstrictors such as thromboxane to prevent afferent arteriolar dilation as renal perfusion pressure is reduced (69). Impaired generation of endothelial-derived relaxing factors such as nitric oxide may be important determinants of abnormal autoregulatory responses under normal and pathologic conditions. Sublethal endothelial injury and endothelial dysfunction, resulting in an impaired release of nitric oxide produced by endothelial-derived nitric oxide synthase, have been described in ischemic kidneys (70,71). From a clinical perspective in the setting of ATN, it is possible that modest decreases in renal perfusion pressure can serve to maintain a decrease in GFR in the maintenance phase of ARF, thus preventing or prolonging recovery from ATN.

It is also of interest that fixed renal artery stenosis is an important determinant of the renal autoregulatory response and thus predisposition to ARF. Studies by Textor and associates suggest a "critical renal perfusion pressure" in patients with fixed renal artery stenosis (72). In these studies, eight patients with unilateral renal artery stenosis tolerated sodium nitroprusside–induced arterial pressure reduction without a change in either GFR or estimated renal plasma flow. By contrast, a similar pressure reduction in eight patients with bilateral renal artery stenosis resulted in marked reductions in GFR and renal plasma flow. Sensitivity of GFR and renal plasma flow to blood pressure reduction was eliminated following revascularization in four patients with bilateral renal vascular stenosis (72). In addition to impairing renal autoregulation, fixed renal artery stenosis may also impair renal blood flow sufficient to cause a reversible form of prerenal azotemia (73). Correction of renal artery stenosis may not improve blood pressure or renal function if there is evidence of structural renal damage such as high resistance to renal blood flow (74). Although chronic renal hypoperfusion can lead to ischemic glomerulopathy, improvement in renal function often occurs in kidneys >9 cm in size once chronic vascular occlusion is relieved (73).

A number of disorders that result in extracellular fluid volume depletion can override normal autoregulatory responses and induce a prerenal form of ARF (64). For example, gastrointestinal losses of fluid can precipitate prerenal ARF. Prolonged nasogastric and biliary drainage (sodium concentration 150 mEq/L) of large amounts of fluid can cause ARF. Diarrhea of any cause can induce volume depletion and ARF. In this regard, aggressive restoration of extracellular fluid volume dramatically decreased the frequency of ARF owing to prerenal causes that complicate cholera (75). In a collected series of 22 patients with villous adenoma (stool sodium 70 to 150 mEq/L), all had azotemia with BUN as high as 200 mg/mL (76). Sequestration of extracellular fluid, as occurs with acute pancreatitis, can cause ARF. In some studies, 1% to 7% of cases of ARF have occurred in the setting of acute pancreatitis (77,78). In a case series of 363 individuals with severe acute pancreatitis, ARF occurred in 35.8% of patients and was an independent predictor of mortality (79). Extensive dermal losses of salt, albumin and water occur in the setting of burns (34,80,81). Early in the course of patients with burns, ARF is often due to volume depletion with prerenal azotemia and rarely ischemic ATN (34,80). Later, sepsis and aminoglycoside antimicrobial agents produce a nonoliguric form of ARF in the setting of burns. Burn size, inhalation injury, and albumin level at presentation are risk factors for ARF in burn patients (34,81). Delay in fluid resuscitation is associated with higher mortality (80). Excessive dermal losses with extracellular volume depletion and ARF also occur in heat stroke; however, rhabdomyolysis also is present in many cases of heat stroke (82–84).

Acute renal failure resulting from excessive renal loss of extracellular fluid also is common (55,62,85,86). Often this is due to overzealous use of diuretic agents. Mild degrees of azotemia often are seen in conditions of renal loss of fluid as occurs with diabetic ketoacidosis; fortunately, ischemic ATN is rare in this setting (86). Of note, ketoacidosis can interfere with automated serum creatinine assays, producing artifactually high values. Renal loss of salt and water also can lead to ARF in hyperosmolar, nonketotic states (87).

Interestingly, hemorrhagic shock, except in either occasional circumstances or in the obstetric setting, rarely leads to severe ARF. Of 590 patients with serious upper gastrointestinal hemorrhage, only 8 died with ARF (88). Of 175 episodes of gastrointestinal bleeding in 161 patients with cirrhosis, ARF occurred in 20 of these episodes, and 11 patients died (89). ARF occurring in the setting of acute myocardial infarction also is rare. Causes of ARF in the setting of myocardial infarc-

tion include prolonged hypotension with cardiogenic shock, contrast nephropathy, cholesterol embolism (from angiography or thrombolysis [90]), drugs, renal tract obstruction due to hemorrhage (91) and rarely, rhabdomyolysis from cardiopulmonary resuscitation or cardioversion (92). In two series of patients with acute myocardial infarction who underwent percutaneous coronary angioplasty, ARF occurred in 3% (93) in one series and 0.6% of patients required dialysis in another series (94). The risk of ARF increases with the degree of hemodynamic compromise. Of 118 patients with cardiogenic shock following acute myocardial infarction, 39 developed ARF and 35 died (95).

The hepatorenal syndrome (see Chapter 75) is a life-threatening complication of severe liver disease that shares many features with prerenal azotemia (96,97). In 234 patients with cirrhotic ascites, the probability of development of this syndrome was about 40% over a 5-year period (97). It is generally agreed that severe renal vasoconstriction occurs with the hepatorenal syndrome and is responsible in large part for the ARF. The renal vasoconstriction may be caused by a combination of enhanced renal vasoconstrictors (norepinephrine, angiotensin II, vasopressin, endotoxin, endothelin, selected thromboxanes, leukotrienes, and increased renal adrenergic traffic) as well as decreased renal vasodilators (eicosanoids, kinins, and nitric oxide). Other key hemodynamic features of hepatorenal syndrome are systemic arterial hypotension, portal hypertension, and splanchnic vasodilatation (98). Despite some understanding of the pathophysiology of this disorder, no therapeutic modality has been shown to be consistently beneficial. Liver transplantation has been lifesaving in selected cases. As a bridge to liver transplantation, intravenous albumin and vasoconstrictors of the splanchnic circulatory bed such as terlipressin are helpful short-term agents which may improve renal function in 50% to 75% of patients (98,99).

Postrenal Acute Renal Failure

Obstruction of urine flow is generally considered a less common cause of ARF. In several series, obstructive uropathy is encountered in 2% to 10% of all cases in ARF (18,22,37,38,44,54,56,57) (Table 41-3). However, obstructive uropathy is more common in selected patient populations such as the very young or older men with prostatic disease and patients with a single kidney or intraabdominal cancer, particularly pelvic cancer (18,100,101). Obstructive uropathy is most frequently encountered in community- and hospital ward-associated ARF and is less common in ICU-related ARF (56,63). For example, obstructive uropathy constitutes 20% to 40% of all community-acquired ARF. Finally, the cause of obstructive uropathy is often amenable to therapy. Thus, obstructive uropathy should be considered in each case of ARF.

The cause of obstruction of urine flow can be classified as intrarenal or extrarenal (Table 41-3; Fig. 41-4). Intratubular deposition of either crystalline or proteinaceous material can increase intratubular pressure, thereby decreasing effective glomerular filtration pressure. For example, intratubular precipitation of uric acid can cause tubule obstruction and ARF. Acute uric acid nephropathy is most often seen following chemotherapy for leukemias and lymphomas (102,103). In this setting, the liver converts the purine load generated by cytolysis into uric acid. The high filtered load of uric acid and tubular reabsorption combine to produce high tubular concentrations of soluble urate and uric acid. Acidification of tubular fluid converts urate to uric acid, which can occlude tubular lumens.

Abrupt exposure of the kidneys to high filtered loads of other insoluble crystalline substances can also cause an intrarenal form of obstructive uropathy (104). For example, ARF associated with calcium oxalate crystalluria can accompany ethylene glycol ingestion, administration of the anesthetic agent methoxyflurane, and small-bowel bypass operations (105,106). Administration of high doses of methotrexate can be associated with ARF, possibly owing to intratubular precipitation of the insoluble 7-hydroxy metabolite of methotrexate (104). Other crystalline substances that can potentially precipitate within renal tubules and lead to ARF include acyclovir, triamterene, sulfonamides, and protease inhibitors such as indinavir (104,107–109). Intratubular precipitation of myeloma proteins and perhaps other proteins also can lead to ARF (110). Dehydration with resultant high tubular water reabsorption and radiographic contrast material can facilitate intratubular myeloma protein deposition.

Recognition of intratubular obstruction as a potential cause of ARF has important therapeutic implications. For example, prophylactic therapy with the xanthine oxidase inhibitor allopurinol can prevent accumulation of uric acid in tumor lysis syndrome. Moreover, forced diuresis decreases tubular salt and water reabsorption, thereby diluting tubular fluid with decreases in crystal and protein concentrations. Finally, manipulations that increase urinary pH can increase solubility of crystalline substances such as methotrexate, uric acid, and sulfonamides (104).

Micropuncture and morphologic studies of an animal model of ARF owing to uric acid nephropathy illustrate these points (111,112). In this model, the underlying pathologic lesion is deposition of uric acid crystals within collecting ducts and deep cortical and medullary vessels. In these studies, high rates of urine flow, either induced by high-dose furosemide (which produced a solute diuresis) or in animals with central diabetes insipidus (which resulted in a water diuresis), protected against the development of uric acid–induced ARF. By contrast, either urinary alkalinization or induction of a mild diuresis with a furosemide provided only minimal protection. These observations suggest that maintenance of high urinary flow rates should be a major objective in cases of high uric acid loads. It is also noteworthy that clinical experience suggests that maintenance of high urine flow may protect against development of ARF in the setting of high doses of methotrexate infusion and myeloma cases. Finally, in patients with ARF owing to uric acid nephropathy, hemodialysis can remove large amounts of uric acid and restore renal function.

Extrarenal lesions are the most common cause of postrenal ARF and are listed in Table 41-3. Several factors determine renal response to extrarenal obstruction. The site, degree, and rapidity of onset of obstruction are all important. Without complicating infection, substantial improvement in renal function can follow decompression of the urinary tract after several days of complete obstruction. Prostatic obstruction is by far the most common cause of postrenal ARF encountered in men because of its critical location at the bladder outlet. Obstruction of the upper urinary tract is a less common cause of ARF because it requires simultaneous obstruction of both ureters or unilateral ureteric obstruction with either absence of or severe disease in the contralateral kidney. Intraureteric obstruction can be due to stone, necrotic papillae, tumor, pus, blood clots, and fungal balls. Papillary necrosis usually occurs in the setting of sickle cell disorders, diabetes mellitus, chronic urinary tract infections, analgesic abuse, obstructive uropathy, and possibly chronic alcoholism. Extraureteric lesions producing obstruction include retroperitoneal fibrosis, adenopathy, and tumors; pelvic tumors; and surgical ligation. Retroperitoneal fibrosis is often idiopathic but may be encountered in response to retroperitoneal neoplasia as well as in the setting of some pharmacologic agents (methysergide, methyldopa, ß-blockers) and connective tissue diseases. A high frequency of ARF due to prostatic carcinoma in males and pelvic carcinoma

(predominantly cancer of the cervix) in females causing ureteric occlusion has been reported (18,101). Less commonly encountered causes of extrinsic ureteric obstruction include inflammatory bowel disease (predominantly right-sided obstruction), an inflammatory reaction resulting from a leaking abdominal aortic aneurysm, and the late stages of pregnancy.

Norman and colleagues examined their experience with 50 cases of renal failure caused by ureteric obstruction experienced over a 5-year interval (113). The cause of obstruction was malignant disease (cervix, prostate, bladder, bowel, or ovary) in 76% of cases. Nonmalignant causes of obstructive uropathy included retroperitoneal fibrosis (16%), calculi (4%), and ligated ureters (4%). Substantial survival time was observed following relief of obstruction (often with percutaneous nephrostomy or ureteral stents) in many of the patients with extensive malignant disease.

Kaufman and associates (57) performed a prospective study looking at ARF that develops while living in the community. Of 100 patients with ARF, 20 cases were due to obstruction. Causes of obstruction included benign prostatic hypertrophy (12 patients); prostatic carcinoma (2 patients); and individual cases of lymphoma, ureteral stones, and bladder stones (57).

Recent reports emphasize that stone-induced obstruction may be a relatively frequent cause of ARF in selected populations (114,115). Grundy and collaborators described urosepsis as the setting of ARF in five quadriplegic patients. In three of these five patients, stone-induced obstructive uropathy played a role in the sepsis (114). Ansari et al. (115) have emphasized that uric acid obstruction of the ureters with anuric ARF can be seen in young male residents of the Near East. From 1978 to 1981, they encountered eight male patients with ARF, loin pain, and anuria owing to ureteral obstruction with uric acid calculi. Retrograde pyelography and either local or systemic alkalinization dissolved the stones, relieved the obstruction, and returned renal function to normal.

Pharmacologic agents with potential anticholinergic effects (e.g., tricyclic antidepressants, phenothiazines, antihistamines) and cold remedies containing α-adrenergic agents (e.g., phenylpropanolamine) often precipitate acute urinary retention by impairing detrusor function and enhancing bladder sphincter tone, respectively.

Acute Renal Failure

A variety of renal disorders can cause ARF (Table 41-4). These diagnoses should be considered when prerenal and postrenal disorders have been excluded. The frequency with which renal causes are encountered in patients with ARF varies between 25% and 80%. In a series of pediatric patients, as many as 50% of all cases of ARF can be attributed to such renal parenchymal disorders as acute glomerulonephritis and hemolytic-uremic syndrome. In hospitalized adults in whom prerenal and postrenal azotemia have been excluded, ARF is often caused by ATN. By contrast, in an outpatient setting in which prerenal and postrenal causes have been excluded, other renal parenchymal diseases more often cause ARF. The renal causes of ARF can be categorized most systematically by their anatomic site of origin. Thus, vascular, glomerular, interstitial, and tubular disorders occur. Acute renal failure due to renovascular (Chapters 52 and 70), glomerular (Chapters 58–69), and interstitial disorders (Chapter 48) are discussed in detail in other chapters.

The underlying disorders that usually predispose to ATN are listed in Table 41-4 and Figure 41-4. Basically, three major categories of insults predispose to ATN. These categories include renal ischemia (prolonged prerenal failure), nephrotoxins, and pigmenturia (myoglobinuria and hemoglobinuria). Studies of patients with ATN emphasize that multiple insults to renal function are usually present. For example, in more than 600 well-characterized patients with ATN, about half had more than a single insult to renal function (35,38–42,55). Several experimental studies in animal models of ARF demonstrate that multiple renal insults such as fever, bacteremia, endotoxemia, relative hypotension, and aminoglycoside agents individually produce relatively minor decrease in renal function. Collectively, however, these insults can produce marked decrements in renal function with resulting ARF (116,117).

The most common predisposing factor in the development of ATN appears to be renal ischemia resulting from prolonged prerenal azotemia (37,38,41–44,55). Sepsis, and particularly septic shock, has assumed an ever-increasing role as a major predisposing factor in the occurrence of ATN (37,38,42,55,56). Nephrotoxins (Chapters 42–47) account for about 25% of all cases of ATN (85,118). Contemporary nephrotoxins commonly encountered include the aminoglycoside antimicrobial agents, radiographic contrast materials, nonsteroidal antiinflammatory drugs (NSAIDs), organic solvents, and heavy metals such as cisplatin and carboplatin. A prospective case control study found that the relative risk for development of ARF was increased five- to sixfold by exposure to either aminoglycoside antimicrobials or radiocontrast agents (55). The increasing number of infections in patients with AIDS has served as a strong reminder of the significant nephrotoxicity and ARF that can accompany therapy with pentamidine, sulfamethoxazole-trimethoprim, amphotericin B, foscarnet, acyclovir, cidofovir, aminoglycosides, and β-lactam antibiotics (30,31,119). The use of recombinant cytokine therapy for advanced solid tumors has been associated with nephrotoxicity following gamma interferon and interleukin-2 treatment (120,121). Intravenous immunoglobulin therapy has been used to treat a variety of immunologic disorders. Such therapy can occasionally be associated with ARF, although the mechanism appears unclear (122). In addition to ischemia and nephrotoxins, a third common predisposing factor in ATN cases is pigmenturia caused by either hemoglobin or myoglobin. Finally, no specific identifiable cause is found in a few cases of ATN.

Rasmussen and Ibels examined risk factors for the development of ATN (123). In this study, the records of 143 patients who developed an acute increase in serum creatinine of more than 2.2 mg/dL and who did not have prerenal or postrenal azotemia, glomerulonephritis, and interstitial nephritis were examined by retrospective multivariate analyses. Approximately 60% of these patients were seen in a surgical setting. The following were considered possible acute insults: hypotension (74%), sepsis (31%), contrast media and aminoglycosides (25%), pigmenturia (hemoglobin, myoglobin, 22%), and dehydration (35%). Nearly two-thirds (64%) of the 143 patients had more than one acute insult before ATN. In three more recent series of ICU-associated ARF, 30% to 48% of patients experienced sepsis, 17% to 30% either impaired cardiac output or volume depletion, and 20% to 30% were exposed to one or more nephrotoxins (43,44,56).

CLINICAL SETTINGS OF ACUTE RENAL FAILURE

Multiple Organ Failure

Acute renal failure is increasingly recognized to occur commonly in the context of multiple organ failure. This is particularly true when ARF is encountered in critically ill patients. In the extensive experience of Liano and associates, only 11% of intensive care unit (ICU)–associated ARF occurred without failure of at least one additional organ system (56,124). By contrast, in Liano's series, 69% of hospital ward-associated

ARF occurred without failure of another organ system. Of more than 200 cases of intensive care unit-associated ARF, 11% had none, 24% had one, 40% had two, and 26% had concomitant failure of three or more concomitant organs (56). Allgren and colleagues reported that of ARF patients, 48% to 55% were on assisted ventilation, 26% to 35% had congestive cardiac failure, 27% to 42% were septic, and 13% to 33% had acute hepatic dysfunction at the time of presentation of ARF (42). Groeneveld and co-workers found that 90% of ICU patients who developed ARF had failure of other organ systems (125). In their experience, other organ systems failed 90% of the time before the ARF became apparent. Together these and other observations emphasize that intensive care unit-associated ARF usually occurs in the context of dysfunction of two or more additional organ systems. Moreover, this ARF usually appears after the onset of dysfunction of other organ systems.

A case-controlled study provides a unique perspective on the association of ARF and multiple organ dysfunction (35). This analysis of moderate radiocontrast-associated ARF found that preexisting sepsis (22%), respiratory failure (36%), mental status changes (41%), and clinically significant bleeding (15%) were commonly present before the onset of ARF (35). However, after the onset of ARF the percentage of patients that previously did not have the condition that experienced sepsis was 45%, respiratory failure 78%, mental status changes 68%, and bleeding 27%. These observations emphasize that although ARF often complicates the course of patients with multiple organ dysfunction, the occurrence of ARF often heralds either the onset or the further development of multiple organ failure.

The cause of ARF in the setting of multiple organ dysfunction can rarely be attributed to a single insult (37,38,41–44,55,125). Renal ischemia owing to hemodynamic instability and impaired cardiac output, intravascular volume depletion, sepsis, and exposure to potential nephrotoxins are nearly uniform accompaniments of ARF when it occurs in the setting of multiple organ dysfunction.

The basic principles of treatment for ARF occurring in the setting of multiple organ failure do not differ substantially from isolated ARF. However, with multiple organ failure, the associated hemodynamic instability and requirement for continuous adjustment of volume status often demands early continuous modalities of renal replacement therapy (125).

Older Age

The frequency of development of severe ARF is undoubtedly increased with advancing age. In a prospective, 2-year study of a 450,000 person population, Feest and co-workers found that individuals over 70 years of age comprised more than 70% of all cases of ARF (18). The frequency of severe ARF was 17 per million population in those under 50 years of age and was increased by 56-fold (949 per million population) in those aged 80 to 89 years (18). The mean age of several recent series of patients with severe ARF has ranged from 54 through 69 years. Pascual et al. (126) found that 14% of all ARF encountered in Madrid, Spain referral centers occurred in patients aged 80 years or older.

Elderly individuals have multiple other comorbidities that put them at higher risk of ARF. Fortescue et al. (127) found that in a prospective cohort of 8,797 patients undergoing coronary artery bypass grafting, 1.8 to 1.9% of patients over 70 years of age required dialysis versus 0.5 to 1.0% under the age of 70. However, in a stepwise logistic regression analysis, cardiogenic shock, history of renal disease, elevated left-ventricular end diastolic pressure in addition to age were also found to be independent predictors of development of ARF.

The causes and underlying predisposing factors of ARF in the elderly generally mirror those seen in a younger population. However, prerenal and postrenal causes of ARF may be especially common in the aging population. For example, Pascual et al. (126) found prerenal causes increased from 21% to 30% when individuals less than 65 years of age were compared with those over 80 years of age. Moreover, postrenal causes increased from 7% to 21% when those less than 65 were compared with those over 80 years of age. Together, prerenal and postrenal causes of ARF comprised 52% of all causes of ARF in the over 80 years of age population (128). Renal causes including those of vascular, glomerular, interstitial, and tubular origins are also encountered in the elderly population. Preston and collaborators found that 55 of 363 renal biopsies done on an over 65 years of age group were performed because of ARF (128). Of those 55, 42% revealed acute glomerulonephritis, 27% ATN, 16% renal vascular diseases, and 15% acute interstitial nephritis (128).

One specific concern with regard to ARF in an elderly population is use of NSAIDs and selective cyclooxygenase-2 inhibitors. About 10% to 15% of older adults in the United States consume these medications on a regular basis (19,129). Population-based case-control studies demonstrated that the incidence of ARF is rare (two per 100,000 person-years) but is increased fourfold by NSAID usage (19). In a population of individuals with an average age of 79 years, NSAID usage was associated with twofold-increased likelihood of having a blood urea nitrogen (BUN) >23 mg/dL and a serum creatinine >1.4 mg/dL (129). Selective cyclooxygenase-2 inhibitors appear to have a potential to reduce GFR similar to conventional NSAIDs in the elderly (66). There are several case reports in the elderly of ARF due to selective cyclooxygenase-2 inhibitors (130–132). A randomized trial of 8059 patients (39% aged over 65) compared a selective cyclooxygenase-2 inhibitor to a NSAID (133). Increased creatinine levels occurred in 0.7% of the selective cyclooxygenase-2 inhibitor versus 1.2% of the NSAID group (133).

The influence of increasing age on ARF outcome is debated. Some but not all studies demonstrate a direct relationship between advancing age and ARF mortality (126). There are, however, numerous outcome variables in the setting of ARF and a contribution of age, independent of comorbidity, on ARF outcome is difficult to ascertain. When stratified by severity of illness, recent studies do not suggest that age is an important ARF outcome determinant.

Sepsis or Infection

The occurrence of either frank septicemia or systemic inflammatory response syndrome is commonly noted in conjunction with development of ARF. Shusterman and collaborators found that septic shock was the clinical condition associated with the highest likelihood of development of hospital-acquired ARF with an adjusted odds ratio near infinity (55). Three studies of ICU-associated ARF found that sepsis was a predisposing factor in 30% to 48% of cases (40,43,44). In a multicenter study of 81 ICU's across Australia, septic shock accounted for 45% of cases of ARF requiring dialysis (134). In 234 patients with community-acquired bacteremia, 24% developed some degree of ARF (28). In about half of these patients, the ARF was mild to moderate in severity and readily reversible, whereas in the remainder it was severe and persisted (28). In a hospital-based study (135), ARF developed in 19% with sepsis, 23% with severe sepsis, and 51% with septic shock in culture-positive individuals.

Several types of infections with prominent systemic manifestations such as leptospirosis are occasionally complicated by ARF (see Table 41-4). A national pneumonia surveillance study found that 8% of patients hospitalized with pneumonia have some element of ARF (27). Some degree of ARF can be encountered in the context of specific causes of pneumonia such as that due to *Legionella* species and other organisms (136,137). Several systemic bacterial infections such as those due to bacterial endocarditis and visceral abscesses are associated with development of ARF (138). Severe bacterial pyelonephritis can be associated with bacteremia and ARF (139). Systemic infections of nonbacterial origin are also associated with ARF. Examples include Rocky Mountain spotted fever where ARF occurs in up to 20% of cases (29). Other examples of systemic, nonbacterial infections associated with ARF include Hantavirus and candidiasis (140,141). Malaria-associated ARF is common in many geographic areas (142).

The causes of ARF in patients with sepsis and infection are diverse (143–148)(see Table 41-7). Prospective studies have identified several risk factors for acute renal failure in patients with sepsis. Older age, elevated serum creatinine level despite elevated central venous pressure (CVP), and presence of hepatic failure were predictive for ARF in 2442 patients with sepsis admitted to an intensive care unit (149).

Therapeutic efforts for sepsis-related ARF, other than identification and treatment of the offending infectious agents, generally are supportive in nature. Some enthusiasm for continuous hemofiltration for treating sepsis-associated ARF has been generated (150,151). One rationale supporting such therapy is potential removal of proinflammatory cytokines; however, the brief half-life of many of these substances and direct measurements have demonstrated very limited removal of circulating mediators by continuous hemofiltration (151). In addition, large controlled trials of monoclonal antibodies and receptor antagonists directed against either tumor necrosis factor or interleukin-1 in patients with the sepsis syndrome have been disappointing (151).

TABLE 41-7

PATHOPHYSIOLOGIC FACTORS IN SEPTIC ARF

Prerenal
Hypoperfusion
Renal
Intrarenal vasoconstriction with redistribution of blood flow away from outer medulla (143)
Activation of coagulation and fibrinolysis (intraglomerular thrombosis and disseminated intravascular coagulation)
Norepinephrine
Angiotensin II
Endothelin
Interleukins (IL-6, Il-8, IL-10) (144)
Extrarenal toll-like receptor 4 (146)
Platelet activating factor
Eicosanoids
Tumor necrosis factor (145)
Apoptosis (144)
Acute tubular necrosis (312)
Interstitial nephritis (140,312)
Disseminated intrarenal microabscesses (147)
Rhabdomyolysis, hemoglobinuria, and myoglobinuria (142,148)
Glomerulonephritis (138)
Postrenal
Drug-induced intratubular crystallization (acyclovir, sulfonamides, protease inhibitors, foscarnet)
Fungus balls
Sloughed papilla
Renal calculi

Human Immunodeficiency Virus Infection

Acute renal failure is common in the setting of human immunodeficiency virus (HIV) infection (30,31,119,152–155) (see Table 41-8). The frequency of occurrence of ARF complicating the course of HIV infection is dependent on the stage of the disease, treatment regimen, comorbid complications, and sociodemographic features of the population studied. An early study that antedated current treatment protocols found 55% of 246 patients with advanced HIV infection experienced one or more episodes of a >0.3 mg/dL increase of serum creatinine over a 42-month interval (152). In this study, 20% of patients experienced a >2.0 mg/dL rise in serum creatinine and 7% had a peak serum creatinine that exceeded 6 mg/dL (152). Several other studies demonstrated a high frequency of occurrence of ARF in HIV populations in the context of the treatment regimens in use in the 1980s (30,31,154). Many clinicians experienced in the care of HIV-infected patients feel that advances in overall management have decreased the frequency and improved the prognosis of HIV-associated ARF (30). In a single center series of 92 HIV positive patients with ARF admitted between 1988 and 1997, most patients recovered with symptomatic treatment, but 18% of patients died within 2 months of their diagnosis of ARF (155).

Multiple potential causes are usually present in patients with HIV infection that develop ARF (30,31,152–155). The relative frequency of the cause depends on the characteristics of the HIV population being reported, the frequency with which renal biopsies are performed, and the academic interests of the reporting center. Often comorbid and/or associated conditions such as hypertension, diabetes mellitus, malignancy, intravenous drug abuse, and multiple infections are present that can contribute to renal dysfunction. Potential prerenal causes include gastrointestinal volume loss/sequestration, poor fluid intake, severe hypoalbuminemia, and early sepsis (30,31,152–155). Postrenal possibilities include intrarenal (tubular precipitation of sulfadiazine, acyclovir and protease inhibitors, and tubular precipitation of myeloma protein) (105), extrarenal (extraureteric blockage from fibrosis, tumor and nodes, and intraureteric obstruction from stones, pus, fungus balls, and papillae), and bladder/urethra (obstructing prostate) origin (30,31,152–155).

A renal source appears to be an especially common cause of ARF in the HIV population. Such renal causes include those of vascular (shiga–toxin independent hemolytic-uremic syndrome) and glomerular (HIV-associated glomerulosclerosis; cytomegalovirus [CMV], hepatitis B and C and other infection-associated glomerulopathies; tumor-associated glomerulopathy; and lupus-like glomerulopathies) origin (155). Although earlier studies suggested ATN as a common renal cause of ARF in HIV populations, more recent reports suggest a declining frequency of ATN (30). Potential causes of ATN include ischemia (prerenal disorders, sepsis), drugs (NSAIDs, radiocontrast, aminoglycoside, pentamidine, foscarnet, amphotericin), and pigmenturia from rhabdomyolysis. Other renal causes of ARF in HIV-infected individuals include allergic interstitial nephritis (trimethoprim–sulfamethoxazole, phenytoin, rifampin, and multiple other agents) and a rare but treatable disorder characterized by plasmacytic interstitial nephritis (154). The nucleotide analog tenofovir causes a reversible acute renal impairment and Fanconi syndrome (156,157). The use of highly active antiretroviral therapy (HAART) is associated with reconstitution of CD4 positive T cells. Reactivation of latent infection such as tuberculosis and cryptococcosis is a recognized consequence of HAART (158). Immune reconstitution may cause ARF due to reactivation of urinary tuberculosis (159).

A recent report of 92 HIV-infected individuals with ARF illustrates the spectrum of causes and potential utility of renal biopsy (155). The patients in this series were generally late in the course of HIV infection and had a mean CD4+ count of 76/mm^3. A renal biopsy was performed in 60 patients. The most common cause of ARF was hemolytic-uremic syndrome (36%). Other causes included ATN (27%), intrarenal or extrarenal obstruction (17%), HIV-associated glomerulosclerosis (16%), other glomerulopathies (4%), interstitial nephritis (2%), and myeloma kidney (1%).

The prognosis of ARF complicating HIV infection is dependent on the cause. A report of severe ARF (serum creatinine of 6 mg/dL or higher) found roughly comparable renal recovery in HIV-infected and noninfected ARF patients (56% and 47%, respectively) and comparable overall ARF mortality of 55% to 60% (30). A significantly higher percentage of the HIV ARF population than the non-HIV ARF group was considered to be terminal and was not dialyzed (36% vs. 18%, respectively). Many of the non-ATN causes of HIV-associated ARF appear to be responsive to therapeutic modalities (160).

TABLE 41-8

CAUSES OF ARF IN HIV-POSITIVE PATIENTS

Prerenal
Hypovolemia—gastrointestinal losses, poor fluid intake, severe hypoalbuminemia, renal salt wasting, diabetes insipidus
Hypotension and reduced renal perfusion—sepsis, cardiomyopathy, cirrhosis/hepatic insufficiency, pancreatitis, nephrotic syndrome

Intrarenal
Vascular—microangiopathy (hemolytic uremic syndrome and thrombotic thrombocytopenic purpura), drug-induced, infection, plasmacytic interstitial nephritis
Glomerular—HIV associated glomerulosclerosis, IgA nephropathy, immune complex glomerulonephritis
Tubulointerstitial—acute tubular necrosis (nephrotoxic, ischemic, pigment-related)

Postrenal
Intrarenal—tubular precipitation of uric acid, sulfadiazine, acyclovir, protease inhibitors, foscarnet
Extrarenal—extraureteric (fibrosis, tumor, lymph nodes), intraureteric (stones, pus, fungus balls, sloughed papilla), bladder (structural, e.g., stones and blood clots and functional, e.g., neuropathic), urethral obstruction (urethritis, stricture, blood clots)

IgA, immunoglobulin A.
(Adapted from: Perazella MA. Acute renal failure in HIV-infected patients: a brief review of common causes. Am J Med Sci 2000;319:385.)

Postoperative State

The postoperative period is currently one of the most prevalent settings of ARF. For example, 27% of the 748 cases of ARF reported by Liano and Pascual were encountered in the postoperative setting (40). Postoperative ARF accounted for 25% of all intensive care unit-associated ARF and 8% of all hospital ward-associated ARF in this study (40). Older studies by Charlson and associates indicated that 25% of elective, noncardiac surgical procedures were complicated by an acute rise in serum creatinine of 20% or greater (161). A 50% decline in endogenous creatinine clearance occurred in 11% of these patients (161). More recent studies indicate that mild ARF occurs in 7% to 8% of patients undergoing cardiac surgery and that about 1% of such patients will require renal replacement (24,25).

In studies by Chertow and associates (25), the development of postcardiac surgery ARF sufficient to require renal replacement therapy increased 30-day mortality by 15-fold (4% to 64%). Recursive partitioning could allocate patients into distinct risk groups for development of ARF (25). For example, use of intraaortic balloon pump, cardiomegaly plus New York Heart Association Class IV functional status or the presence of peripheral vascular disease plus a cardiac valve replacement operation were the three clinical settings associated with relatively high risk (>5%) of developing severe postoperative ARF (25). Leacche and colleagues (162) followed 13,847 consecutive patients undergoing cardiac surgery, 40 (0.3%) of whom developed postoperative ARF requiring dialysis. Of these 40 patients, 29 died and 7 of the remaining 11 survivors required permanent dialysis (162).

Several risk factors have been identified for ARF after cardiac surgery. The use of cardiopulmonary bypass was an independent predictor of ARF in a series of 2199 patients undergoing coronary artery bypass surgery (163). Mangano and colleagues (164) performed a multicenter prospective study of 2,222 patients undergoing cardiac surgery. Use of cardiopulmonary bypass for greater than 2 hours was associated with a 3.7 times relative risk of acute renal impairment (serum creatinine >2.0 mg/dL or increase of 0.7 mg/dL) or dialysis. Other risk factors identified included older age, congestive heart failure, previous coronary artery bypass surgery, preexisting renal impairment, diabetes, hyperglycemia, and poor ventricular function (164).

The use of hypothermia during cardiopulmonary bypass has been associated with worse post-operative renal function (165) (compare to effects of therapeutic hypothermia in section on cardiopulmonary resuscitation below). In a series of 1,442 patients undergoing coronary artery bypass surgery, the use of hypothermia was associated with worse renal function at 24 hours postoperatively, but similar renal function 1 week postoperatively (166). Duration on cardiopulmonary bypass was longer in the hypothermia group (because of the need for cooling down and rewarming), which may be the explanation for why the patients undergoing hypothermia had transiently worse postoperative renal function.

Another clinical situation in which a relationship between renal ischemia and ATN is well established involves surgical procedures on the aorta. In 25 series of more than 7,000 patients with an operation for an abdominal aortic aneurysm, 17% developed mild and 6% severe ARF. Mortality rate for ARF was 61% (167). Gornick and Kjellstrand reported their experience with 47 patients with ATN who required dialysis following repair of an abdominal aortic aneurysm (168). These 47 patients constituted approximately 15% of the patient population that required dialysis for ATN over an 11-year interval. Survival in patients with ATN after surgery for abdominal aortic aneurysms was low (21%).

Individuals undergoing aortic or thoracoabdominal aortic surgery commonly have renal arterial disease. A retrospective nonrandomized study (169) suggested that ARF requiring dialysis was less common in patients who had previously undergone renal artery endarterectomy for occlusive disease.

A third operative setting felt to be associated with a high frequency of ARF is that of the jaundiced patient. A review of 16 series made up of 2,300 jaundiced patients found an overall frequency of development of ARF of 8% (167). Recently, a very small (N = 23) prospective study of patients undergoing surgery for relief of obstructive jaundice studied the frequency of development of ARF (170). All patients were aggressively hydrated preoperatively and then assigned to receive either dopamine or no dopamine. No cases of ARF were seen in either group (170).

Abdominal operations may be associated with ARF postoperatively. Sugrue and colleagues (171) identified increased intraabdominal pressure as an independent risk factor contributing to postoperative ARF in patients undergoing abdominal surgery, a phenomenon known as the abdominal compartment syndrome. Operative exploration and decompression of 279 patients whose intraabdominal pressure exceeded 25 mm Hg resulted in diuresis and resolution of ARF in 7 patients (172). Proposed mechanisms include increased renal vascular resistance and increased levels of antidiuretic hormone, renin, aldosterone, and catecholamine concentrations (171,173–176). Pressure on the ureter is not thought to be an important factor (171).

What underlies the relatively high frequency of ARF that occurs in relation to elective surgical procedures? In many cases, underlying comorbidity (diabetes mellitus, chronic hypertension, vascular disease, congestive heart failure, myeloma, cirrhosis) leads to diminished baseline GFR and reduced renal reserve (161,177). With this background, the "surgical experience" may induce afferent arteriolar renal vasoconstriction and diminished GFR (178,179). Clinical ARF may then occur if an additional renal insult is encountered. These additional renal insults often are referred to as "second hits," and include reoperation, sepsis, nephrotoxin exposure, circulatory/volume deficits, and heart failure (161,177).

Trauma and Burns

The frequency with which ARF accompanies major trauma is dependent on the definition of ARF and the trauma population studied. A retrospective review of nearly 73,000 admissions to nine referral trauma centers over 5 years revealed only a 0.1% incidence of ARF sufficient to require renal replacement therapy (32). By contrast, 31% of prospectively studied trauma patients admitted to a single ICU developed either a rise in serum creatinine of >2 mg/dL or a 20% increase if baseline values were abnormal (32,33,180). The frequency of ARF complicating earthquake trauma is unknown but may be substantial in patients with significant degrees of rhabdomyolysis (181). In the earthquake in the city of Marmara, Turkey, 639 victims developed ARF, 477 required dialysis, and 97 died (182,183).

The causes of posttraumatic ARF depend on the timing of onset of ARF (32,33,180,181). When present early in the posttraumatic course, ischemia caused by hypotension and pigment-associated ARF, either alone or in combination, are the most common predisposing factors. When ARF occurs later in the course of the traumatized patient, it usually arises in the context of multiple organ failure and sepsis. Risk factors for development of posttraumatic ARF include high injury severity scores, hypotension at admission, high creatine phosphokinase (CPK) values (over 100,000 to 250,000), and requirement for mechanical ventilation.

About half of posttraumatic ARF is modest in degree with peak serum creatinine concentration less than 4 mg/dL (33). Generally speaking, any degree of posttraumatic ARF is associated with significant mortality. Thus, in the study of Vivino and associates, the mortality of mild ARF (peak serum creatinine <4.0 mg/dL) was 71%, whereas with greater degrees of severity of ARF it was 93% (33).

Acute renal failure complicating burn injury occurs in 5% to 15% of patients with third-degree burns exceeding 10% of body surface area (34,80). As with posttraumatic ARF, the occurrence of postburn ARF appears to be biphasic. Volume depletion, hypotension, and myoglobinuria usually are contributing factors when ARF occurs early postburn (34,80). Acute renal failure occurring later in the course of burn injury usually occurs in the context of sepsis, nephrotoxin exposure, and multiple organ failure (34,80). The degree of burn injury and the occurrence of infection are closely related to development of ARF (34,80). Mortality of burn injury complicated by ARF is exceptionally high and exceeds 85% in nearly all studies (34,80). Survivors tend to be younger, with less extensive burns and with clinical courses not complicated by sepsis (34,80).

Acute Renal Failure Complicating Nonrenal Solid Organ Transplantation

The widespread success and availability of transplantation of hearts, pancreases, lungs, bone marrow, and livers has been associated with substantial occurrence of renal failure that is both acute and chronic in nature. Much of the chronic renal failure seen after nonrenal solid organ transplantation appears attributable to cyclosporine and tacrolimus (184).

The frequency with which ARF complicates cardiac transplantation varies depending on the immunosuppressive regimen used and the underlying health of the recipient. Patients at highest risk are those with abnormal baseline renal function, recipients of high-dose cyclosporine, significant comorbidity, and associated posttransplant cardiac dysfunction (185). The frequency of occurrence of severe ARF after cardiac transplantation ranges from 5% to 15% in most series. In their series of 56 cardiac transplant patients, Stevens and colleagues (186) reported that 6 (11%) required renal replacement therapy. However, mild degrees of ARF are much more common and are seen in 25% to 50% of all cardiac transplant recipients (185,187,188). Typically, ARF after heart transplantation occurs within the first week posttransplantation and is characterized by an oliguric state, unremarkable urine sediment, and urinary diagnostic indices typical of prerenal azotemia (185). Often, a high BUN to creatinine ratio and disproportionate hyperkalemia are present. Late ARF can be seen in the setting of rhabdomyolysis in patients taking an HMG-COA (3-hydroxy-3-methyl-glutaryl-coenzyme A) reductase inhibitor and cyclosporine (189). General supportive treatment and reduction or elimination of cyclosporine are the mainstays of therapy (185–188). Even with severe ARF, survival may be good, perhaps because of the younger age of recipients and the presence of single organ failure (185). A small randomized trial did not demonstrate benefit of pretreatment with the renal vasodilator urodilatin (188).

Acute renal failure occurs commonly in patients awaiting and following liver transplantation. Over 18 months at a single large liver transplantation center, ARF occurred in 36% of end-stage liver disease patients who were not transplanted and in 30% of transplanted patients during their postoperative course (96). In this series, ARF was defined as either doubling of the serum creatinine within 24 hours or development of oliguria with need for dialysis. Patients with reversible prerenal azotemia were excluded. In another study, ARF occurred after liver transplantation in 51% of cases (190). Most (66%) of this ARF was modest in degree, although 34% of patients required dialysis (190). Patients at highest risk for the development of ARF in the setting of liver transplantation are those with higher comorbidity as reflected by higher Acute Physiology and Chronic Health Evaluation (APACHE) scores as well as those with abnormal basal renal function and impaired graft function.

The causes of ARF pretransplantation are usually attributed to either the hepatorenal syndrome or ischemic ATN (96,190). Acute renal failure after liver transplantation usually is due to ATN (about 60% of cases), which is most commonly ischemic and occasionally nephrotoxic in origin. Other common contributors to postliver transplantation ARF include cyclosporine (30% to 40%), hepatorenal syndrome (5% to 10%), sepsis (1% to 10%), and rhabdomyolysis (1% to 5%).

Liver transplant recipients who develop ARF exhibit postoperative mortality that exceeds that seen in those without ARF fourfold to sevenfold, an average of 30% to 50% (187,190). Interestingly, transplanted patients who develop ARF prior to liver transplant appear to have comparable mortality (29%) to those who develop ARF posttransplant (41%) (96).

Patients who develop ARF after liver transplantation not uncommonly progress to end-stage renal failure. Paramesh and colleagues studied 1,602 orthotopic liver transplant recipients, of whom 350 (22%) required dialysis postoperatively. Forty-three (2.7%) developed end-stage renal failure. Risk factors included cyclosporine and the presence of diabetes pretransplantation (191).

Acute renal failure is a common accompaniment of bone marrow transplantation, where it is estimated to complicate the course of 30% to 60% of allogeneic, 5% to 15% of autologous, and 5% of nonmyeloablative transplants (192–198) (see Table 41-9). About half of all patients with ARF have a sufficient degree of renal failure to require renal replacement

TABLE 41-9

HEMOPOIETIC CELL TRANSPLANTATION AND ARF

	Autologous	Allogeneic	Nonmyeloablative
Study	(198)	(194)	(193)
Number of patients	160	88	253
Population studied	Breast cancer (regional lymph node spread or metastases)	Lymphomas and leukemias ($N = 79$), breast cancer ($N = 7$), multiple myeloma ($N = 1$), myelodysplastic syndrome ($N = 1$)	Lymphomas and leukemias ($N = 183$), multiple myeloma ($N = 70$)
Grade 0 renal dysfunction	44%	8%	10%
Grade 1 renal dysfunction	35%	23%	50%
Grade 2 renal dysfunction	14%	36%	36%
Grade 3 renal dysfunction	7%	33%	4%
Mortality	7%	58%	34%

Grade 0 = decrement in GFR (as calculated by Cockcroft and Gault formula) of less than 25% from baseline.
Grade 1 = fall in GFR >25% from baseline but rise in serum creatinine less than twofold.
Grade 2 = fall in GFR >25% from baseline and rise in serum creatinine greater than twofold but without requiring dialysis.
Grade 3 = same as grade 2 but with dialysis.

therapy. Traditionally, the causes of ARF after bone marrow transplantation have been managed by time of onset (192,195–197). Very early ARF (within 1 week) is rare and usually attributable to either tumor lysis syndrome from cytoreductive therapy or bone marrow infusion toxicity. Bone marrow infusion toxicity often is caused by the presence of free hemoglobin from the red cell destructive action of freeze–thaw cycles and dimethylsulfoxide (DMSO) exposure. Acute renal failure is a relatively common occurrence 20 to 30 days after transplantation. This ARF is categorized as resulting from a form of hepatorenal syndrome owing to graft versus host disease or nephrotoxins or is multifactorial (prerenal factors, sepsis) in nature. Adenovirus associated nephritis is an unusual cause of ARF that occurs in allogeneic stem cell transplantation (199). These patients developed ARF in association with symptoms such as hematuria, flank pain, fever, and cystitis. Kidney biopsy revealed nuclear inclusions within renal tubular epithelial cells which were positive for adenovirus immunocytochemical stains (199). An even later form of ARF occurs usually in the context of thrombotic microangiopathy or cyclosporine nephrotoxicity. Mild forms of ARF (doubling of serum creatinine) after bone marrow transplant are associated with 20% to 45% mortality. Post–bone marrow transplant ARF sufficient to require hemodialysis is associated with greater than 80% mortality.

Cardiovascular Disease

Heart disease is the leading cause of mortality and hospitalization in patients over 65 years of age in the United States (200). Patients with cardiovascular disorders may be uniquely susceptible to the development of ARF. Thus, such patients often have substantial comorbidity (hypertension, atherosclerotic disease, and diabetes mellitus), which can decrease renal reserve. The presence of diminished cardiac output, therapy with multiple pharmacologic agents (angiotensin converting enzyme [ACE] inhibitors, receptor blockers, and diuretics), selected cardiac events (arrhythmias and arrest), exposure to nephrotoxins (radiocontrast media), and invasive procedures such as surgery and catheterizations all can result in development of ARF.

Several recent studies highlight many of these points. Behrend and Miller published a retrospective review of ARF as it occurred within a cardiac care unit (22). The frequency of ARF was 4%. More than 50% of these patients had hypertension and diabetes mellitus. Congestive heart failure accounted for 35% of ARF cases and contributed to an additional 25% of cases that had more than a single cause. Other etiologies included arrest or arrhythmia in 13%, radiocontrast in 11%, volume depletion in 6%, sepsis in 6%, and urinary tract obstruction in 3%. The overall mortality rate of these cardiac care unit patients with ARF was 50%.

McCullough and collaborators (23) reported on their experience with over 3,600 patients undergoing coronary intervention (angioplasty, atherectomy, or stenting). The incidence of ARF (defined as a 25% increase in serum creatinine concentration) was 14%, and 0.8% of patients required hemodialysis. Multivariable analysis found that decreased creatinine clearance, the presence of diabetes mellitus, and increasing dose of radiocontrast were independently associated with the development of ARF. In-hospital mortality was 1.1% for those without ARF, 7.1% for those with ARF who did not require dialysis, and 35.7% for those with ARF who needed dialysis (23).

Mattana and Singhal have reported on ARF accompanying cardiopulmonary arrest. These investigators found that 16 of 56 patients who survived cardiopulmonary arrest developed ARF (26). Those with ARF had longer duration of arrest (12 versus 7 minutes), received more epinephrine (1.8 vs. 0.9 mg),

and had more heart failure (44% vs. 13%) than those without ARF. Survival to discharge was observed in 6% of those with and 48% of those without ARF. In cardiopulmonary resuscitation, the use of mild therapeutic hypothermia (compared to normothermia) is associated with reversible acute renal dysfunction (201) (also see earlier section, "Postoperative State," for ARF associated with cardiopulmonary bypass surgery). The mechanism of this effect is unknown. In animal and human studies, hypothermia causes renal afferent arteriolar vasoconstriction, reducing renal plasma flow (201–203). In a rat model of hypothermia, mean blood pressure and heart rate fell, leading to reduced cardiac output and renal perfusion (204).

Other causes of ARF encountered in patients with cardiovascular diseases include prerenal forms of ARF caused by diuretics and ACE inhibitors, atheroembolic disease, and other vascular disorders (67,205–207).

Pregnancy

Acute renal failure occurring in the setting of pregnancy has dramatically declined in incidence in western societies but remains a major issue in selected less well-developed countries (20,21,208–212). Current estimates of the frequency with which ARF complicates pregnancy range from one in 5,000 pregnancies in an inner-city U.S. urban population to one in 18,000 pregnancies in an Italian population (20,21). The incidence in the Italian population decreased from one in 3,000 to one in 18,000 pregnancies when the 1956 to 1967 and 1988 to 1994 time periods, respectively, were examined (21). A strikingly high frequency of pregnancy-related ARF continues to be reported in some developing countries (208,209).

The causes and predisposing factors for pregnancy-associated ARF are multiple. Occasionally, prerenal factors from either associated illnesses or hyperemesis gravidarum are encountered. Rarely, the gravid uterus leads to obstructive uropathy, especially with twin pregnancies, polyhydramnios, or other intrapelvic processes (25). Pregnancy-associated ARF has occurred often in the context of septic abortion in the past and in some underdeveloped countries. Where septic abortions are rare, most contemporary pregnancy-related ARF occurs in the setting of the HELLP syndrome (hemolysis, elevated liver enzymes, and low platelets), eclampsia or preeclampsia, postpartum hemorrhage, or placental abruption. Cortical necrosis or idiopathic postpartum ARF occurs rarely. These disorders may lead to nonreversible renal failure (211,212). Pregnancy-associated pyelonephritis with sepsis can be associated with ARF infrequently.

Sibai and Ramadan provided information on ARF complicating the HELLP syndrome (211). Of 32 pregnant patients with HELLP, 6 had preexisting hypertension, and 26 were previously normotensive. Maternal and perinatal mortality rates were 13% and 35%, respectively, in these HELLP cases, whereas 72% of births were preterm. Acute dialysis was required in 10 of 32 patients with ARF complicating the HELLP syndrome. Eleven subsequent pregnancies occurred in eight normotensive women, and only one was complicated by preeclampsia. By contrast, preeclampsia occurred in three of six subsequent pregnancies in four hypertensive women. No residual renal dysfunction or hypertension was seen after 5 years of follow-up in 23 surviving normotensive women, whereas 2 of 5 surviving hypertensive women required chronic dialysis.

Overall, most contemporary series of ARF complicating pregnancy report relatively low mortality rates (approximately 25%). Nowadays, cortical necrosis with lack of recovery of renal function occurs much less commonly during pregnancy at present but continues to be seen when ARF accompanies pregnancies in developing countries (212).

See Chapter 74 for a detailed discussion of pregnancy-related ARF and Chapter 53 for discussion on syndromes of preeclampsia.

Malignant Disease

One setting in which ARF is encountered with high frequency is in patients with malignant disease (104,213–218) (see Chapters 43 and 49). For example, Lanore and collaborators found that 43% of 349 patients with hematologic malignancies encountered over 6 years developed some degree of ARF (213). Recent studies of patients with multiple myeloma find that about one-fourth develop ARF (214).

The causes of ARF in patients with neoplastic disease are diverse (213–217). Prerenal factors from lack of fluid intake, vomiting, and diarrhea are common. Less commonly encountered prerenal failures seen in patients with cancer include chemotherapeutic agent–induced heart failure owing to cardiomyopathy and cancer-related pericardial tamponade and interleukin-2–induced capillary leak syndrome (215,218). Postrenal factors potentially operative as causes of ARF in patients with neoplastic disorders include intrarenal obstruction from crystals (uric acid, methotrexate, myeloma protein) and extrarenal obstruction owing either to ureteric blockage (nodes, tumor mass, fibrosis) or bladder obstruction (prostatic or bladder cancer, neurogenic bladder caused by neoplastic spinal cord compression) (104,113,214–218). Acute tubular necrosis appears to be the most common renal cause of ARF in patients with neoplasm. This ATN is often attributable to sepsis or drugs (e.g., NSAIDs, radiocontrast, aminoglycosides, mithramycin, gallium, nitrosoureas, and amphotericin B). Other pharmacologic agents such as mitomycin, tacrolimus, and cyclosporine can induce renal vascular injury and ARF. Tumor-lysis syndrome, hyperuricemia, and hypercalcemia also are relatively common causes of neoplasia-associated ARF. Tumor-lysis syndrome may occur after cytotoxic therapy or may occur spontaneously (219–221). Other disorders (e.g., tumor infiltration, tumor-related glomerulopathy, and either tumor-related or chemotherapeutic agent-related thrombotic microangiopathy) are occasional causes of ARF in cancer patients (213–218,222,223). In patients with plasma cell dyscrasias, ARF can be attributable to light-chain tubular toxicity, amyloid renal involvement, and renal vein thrombosis (214).

Acute renal failure outcome occurring in the cancer setting is dependent on the cause and extent of the cancer, and is usually associated with a guarded prognosis; however, survival of up to 30% can be seen, even in patients requiring hemodialysis for the ARF (213). Recovery of renal function and at least 1-year survival can be seen in 40% to 50% of patients with multiple myeloma and ARF (214).

Liver Disease

Renal dysfunction is often encountered in patients with advanced liver disease (96,97,224–227). Acute renal failure occurred in 19% in 493 patients with end-stage liver disease who were being evaluated for possible liver transplantation (96). In this study, all cases of reversible prerenal forms of ARF were excluded. The likelihood of development of ARF owing to the hepatorenal syndrome was about 40% over a 5-year period in a prospective study of 234 patients with cirrhotic ascites (97,110).

There are several diagnostic considerations in patients with liver disease and ARF. With acute liver disease, prerenal factors (e.g., vomiting or diarrhea) always can play a role in ARF. Also toxins (e.g., acetaminophen, carbon tetrachloride and other hydrocarbons, and amanita phalloides), infections (e.g., sepsis; hepatitis A, B, and C; leptospirosis; and yellow fever), and circulatory disturbances (e.g., shock or hypotensive states and severe congestive heart failure) can result in concomitant acute renal and hepatic dysfunction. Prerenal and postrenal factors must be considered in the setting of chronic liver disease. Renal causes of ARF in patients with advanced liver disease usually fall into one of four categories: hepatorenal syndrome, ischemic ATN, nephrotoxin-induced ATN (especially NSAIDs and radiocontrast), and sepsis-associated ARF.

One common setting of ARF in patients with advanced liver disease is spontaneous bacterial peritonitis (224). With spontaneous bacterial peritonitis, about one-third of patients develop some degree of ARF. A recent prospective randomized trial found that intravenous albumin (1.5 g/kg initially and 1.0 g/kg on day 3) plus cefotaxime resulted in significantly less ARF (10% vs. 33%) and hospital death (10% vs. 29%) than cefotaxime alone in patients with cirrhosis and spontaneous bacterial peritonitis (36,224).

The prognosis of ARF complicating liver disease is dependent on the clinical setting and cause of the liver and renal dysfunction but generally is not good. Acute renal failure was associated with more than 80% mortality in patients with end-stage liver disease evaluated for transplantation (37,96).

Rhabdomyolysis

Dissolution of skeletal muscle with resultant extravasation of intracellular contents into the circulation constitutes the clinical syndrome of rhabdomyolysis. Rhabdomyolysis can be traumatic (muscle crush, and/or pressure injury, extreme physical exertion) or nontraumatic in nature (41,228–236). Nontraumatic causes of rhabdomyolysis are legion (Table 41-10 or see table in Chapter 49) and include ischemic, infectious, toxic, metabolic, and thermic insults (237–239). The frequency with which rhabdomyolysis is associated with ARF is variable, depending on associated medical conditions, the degree of muscle injury, the presence or absence of volume depletion and hemodynamic instability, and the duration of the rhabdomyolysis. In general, about 10% to 40% of patients undergoing significant rhabdomyolysis develop some degree of ARF (228–236). About half of the cases are mild in degree and responsive to volume repletion, whereas the remainder are more severe, with a clinical course typical of ATN. The logistic regression model for prediction of ARF in patients with rhabdomyolysis developed by Ward found that the magnitude of elevation of creatine kinase, potassium, and phosphorus; and the presence of volume depletion, hypoalbuminemia, and sepsis as causes of rhabdomyolysis were predictive of prolonged ARF (235).

Recent reviews highlight several key aspects of ARF that can be seen in the context of traumatic rhabdomyolysis (240). The immediate cause of morbidity is leak of the sarcolemmal membrane to potentially toxic factors (potassium and phosphorus) and metabolites (myoglobin and uric acid) as well as uptake by damaged muscles of extracellular fluid and calcium, which can lead to hypovolemic and hypocalcemic shock as well as neurovascular entrapment. Persons surviving the cardiotoxicity of hyperkalemia and the hypovolemic shock are susceptible to ATN, which is a consequence of ischemia (hypovolemia, hypotension), direct tubular toxicity of myoglobin, and myoglobin tubular cast formation. Management includes prehospital intravenous volume replacement and maintenance of high urine flow (>100 cc/hour) until myoglobinuria subsides. There is anecdotal evidence that a mannitol–alkaline diuresis can help prevent the associated ARF (229,232,236,240).

TABLE 41-10

CAUSES OF RHABDOMYOLYSIS

Physical causes	Nonphysical causes

Trauma and compression
   Traffic or working accidents
   Disasters
   Torture
   Abuse
   Long-term confinement to the same
   Position
 	
Occlusion or hypoperfusion of muscle
   Vessels thrombosis
   Embolism
   Vessel clamping
   Shock
 	
Excessive or prolonged contraction of
   muscles
   Exercise
   Epilepsy
   Psychiatric agitation
   Delirium tremens
   Tetanus
   Amphetamine overdose
   Ecstasy
   Status asthmaticus
 	
Electrical current
   High-voltage electrical injury
   Lightning
   Cardioversion
 	
Hyperthermia
   Exercise
   High ambient temperatures
   Sepsis
   Neuroleptic malignant syndrome
   Malignant hyperthermia
	Metabolic myopathies
	   McArdle's disease
	   Mitochondrial respiratory chain
	   Enzyme deficiencies
	   Carnitine palmitoyl transferase
	   Deficiency
	   Myoadenylate deaminase deficiency
	   Phosphofructokinase deficiency
	
	Drugs and toxins
	   Regular and illegal drugs (see Chapter 46)
	   Toxins
	   Snake and insect venoms
	   Buffalo fish (United States), burbot
	     (Northern Europe)—Haff disease
	
	Infections
	   Local infection with muscle invasion
	     (pyomyositis)
	   Metastatic infection (sepsis)
	   Systemic effects
	   Toxic shock syndrome
	   Legionella
	   Tularemia
	   Salmonella
	   Falciparum malaria
	   Influenza
	   HIV
	   Herpes viruses
	   Coxsackievirus
	   Dengue fever
	
	Electrolyte abnormalities
	   Hypokalemia
	   Hypocalcemia
	   Hypophosphatemia
	   Hyponatremia
	   Hypernatremia
	   Hyperosmotic conditions
	   Endocrine disorders
	   Hypothyroidism
	   Diabetic coma, related to electrolyte
	     disturbances
	   Polymyositis/dermatomyositis

(Adapted from: Vanholder R, Sever MS, Erek E, et al. Rhabdomyolysis *J Am Soc Nephrol* 2000;11:1553; Birewar S, Oppenheimer M, Zawada ET Jr. Hypothyroid acute renal failure *S D J Med* 2004;57:109; Davis JS, Bourke P. Rhabdomyolysis associated with dengue virus infection *Clin Infect Dis* 2004;38:e109.)

The International Society of Nephrology established the Renal Disaster Relief Task Force in 1995 and gave it responsibility for preparing stocks of goods (intravenous fluids, dialysis equipment) and lists of medical, nursing staff and volunteers who could intervene immediately in the event of a large-scale disaster (241). Victims of crush injury associated with earthquake damage were shown to benefit from early administration of mannitol and intravenous fluids (241,242).

Gabow and collaborators reported experience with 87 episodes of rhabdomyolysis in 77 patients seen over a 4-year interval (243). Rhabdomyolysis was defined as an at least sixfold increase in serum creatine kinase in the absence of myocardial infarction or cerebrovascular accident and an increase in MM isoenzymes of creatine kinase. Most patients (66 of 77) were men, with mean age of 48 years. Causes of rhabdomyolysis included alcoholism (67%), muscle compression (39%), seizures (24%), trauma (17%), drugs (5%), and metabolic (8%) factors. Muscle pain was noted in half the patients, but muscle swelling rarely was present. In the 87 episodes, 52 (60%) were not associated with ARF. Prerenal azotemia was seen in six (7%), whereas 29 (33%) developed ATN. Of the 29 patients who developed ATN, half had advanced ARF on hospital admission. Nearly one-half of the 29 patients with ARF were oliguric and 13 required dialysis. Rhabdomyolysis following major trauma appeared particularly to predispose to ARF. Six of the 29 ARF patients (21%) died. Only two patients required fasciotomy for neurovascular compression.

DIAGNOSTIC APPROACH

Presenting Features

There are numerous causes of ARF, as noted in the previous section, some of which are amenable to specific therapeutic interventions. For these interventions to be effective, they must usually be applied early in the course of the disease process. It follows that key considerations in the diagnosis of ARF are early detection and timely evaluation to determine the cause of the disorder.

With regard to early detection, hospital-acquired ARF usually comes to the attention of the clinician by finding a rising serum creatinine and/or BUN concentration. Less commonly, hospital-acquired ARF is detected by the development of oligoanuria. Rarely, hospital-associated ARF is detected when evaluation for one of the biochemical or clinical consequences of loss of renal function (i.e., hyperkalemia, metabolic acidosis, hyperphosphatemia, hypocalcemia, hyperuricemia, bleeding, or encephalopathy) is undertaken. Community-acquired ARF is usually detected by finding an elevated serum creatinine and/or BUN or abnormal urinalysis on multiphasic screening of patients with nonspecific complaints. Difficulties with the urinary stream also are a common presenting manifestation of ARF owing to postrenal causes in men in the outpatient setting.

It is important to acknowledge that early detection of the presence of ARF may be difficult. Currently, there is no reliable, practical "real time" method that provides accurate information on renal function. An abnormality in renal function certainly is present in the oliguric patient (244); however, most contemporary ARF is nonoliguric in nature. Also an increase in the serum creatinine concentration may not be a sensitive indicator of ARF, particularly in patients with normal baseline renal function and serum creatinine concentration. It follows that relatively large decreases in GFR in patients with a normal baseline GFR, as occurs early in the course of ARF, initially may be associated with only small increases in serum creatinine concentration; moreover, the serum creatinine concentration is also influenced by such variables as production rate and volume of distribution (5). Heightened awareness of the clinical settings of ARF and careful attention to small increases in serum cre-

atinine concentration and abnormalities of urinalysis in these settings are necessary for early detection of ARF.

Tests of tubular function have been developed to aid early diagnosis of ARF (see Table 41-6). Early reports are promising, but at present, these tests have no specific role in clinical practice. Similarly, radionuclide methods of real-time noninvasive monitoring of renal function are expensive and impractical for day-to-day use.

The importance of early detection and elucidation of the specific cause of ARF is illustrated by data in Figure 41-3. These data, from patients with hospital-acquired ARF, demonstrate that the mortality of ARF is directly proportional to the magnitude of subsequent rise in serum creatinine concentration (37). In addition to this observation, several disease entities that can produce ARF (e.g., acute glomerulonephritis, acute interstitial nephritis, and renal vascular disorders) may respond to specific therapeutic interventions. With regard to rapidly progressive glomerulonephritis, there is convincing evidence that therapy is beneficial primarily when given early in the course of the disorder. A recent study documents the relatively long delays that are often encountered before hospital or specialist referral for patients with potentially treatable disorders such as renal failure caused by Wegener's granulomatosis, Goodpasture's syndrome, and other forms of rapidly progressive glomerulonephritis (245) (see Chapters 60 and 68). Maximal effort should be directed to early detection in view of the high morbidity, mortality, and numerous causes of ARF. Once detected, timely determination of the cause of ARF depends on a systematic approach similar to that depicted in Figure 41-6. Other approaches that provide generalizations about the course of ARF include the "site" of onset (Table 41-11) and the associated clinical conditions.

Chart Review, History, and Physical Examination

Chart analysis for determination of the underlying disease states and recent clinical events is needed. A meticulous history with regard to prescription drugs, over-the-counter agents, and herbal preparations as well as possible environmental exposure is critical in view of the frequency with which nephrotoxins contribute to development of ARF (1,37,38,54,85,246,247)

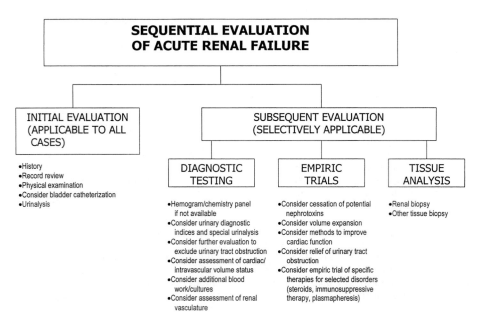

FIGURE 41-6. Suggested sequential diagnostic evaluation to determine the cause of acute renal failure.

TABLE 41-11

COMPARISONS OF ACUTE RENAL FAILURE BY SITE
OF ONSET

Factor	Community	Hospital ward	Intensive care unit
Age	Older	Older	Younger
Cause (%)			
Prerenal	30–50	30	20
Postrenal	20–40	10–20	1
Renal	15–30	30–50	70–80
Isolated (%)	80	70	10
Renal replacement therapy need (%)	10	20	70
Mortality (%)	20	30	70

(see Chapters 42–45, 47, 48). The relationship between medication exposure and ARF may not be readily apparent in some cases (248). Careful attention to a history of loss or sequestration of extracellular fluid volume, signs and symptoms of sepsis or heart failure, and symptoms related to the genitourinary tract (urine output, pyuria, dysuria, hematuria, and flank or abdominal pain) can provide helpful diagnostic information. Intense thirst, salt craving, orthostatic syncope, and muscle cramps often are symptoms of extracellular fluid volume depletion. Examination and careful recording, in flow sheet fashion, of available data on the clinical course of each patient with ARF are necessary. Examination of serial vital signs, hemodynamic data, intake and output, and daily weight can provide important data regarding the cause of ARF. A weight change of greater than 0.25 to 0.50 kg/day indicates gain or loss of salt and/or water. Recording of serial renal functional data and correlation of any deterioration in renal function with clinical events such as those altering systemic hemodynamics (Table 41-2) and use of potential nephrotoxins often are of great diagnostic value. As is discussed subsequently, analysis of the hemogram, routine biochemical data, and special serologic studies also can be of great diagnostic assistance.

Physical examination can be of value in determining the presence or absence of prerenal and postrenal causes of ARF as well as the presence of a systemic disorder that could result in a renal cause of ARF. The effect of either loss or sequestration of extracellular fluid volume on systemic hemodynamic responses depends on several variables, including the composition and rate of fluid loss and the underlying health state of the patient. For example, a 20% to 40% decrease in extracellular fluid volume by sodium depletion over 4 to 5 hours decreases mean arterial pressure by about 35% (249). This decrease in mean arterial pressure is associated with a decline in cardiac output and an increase in total peripheral resistance (249). By contrast, a 30% decrease in extracellular fluid volume by sodium depletion over 11 days causes no decrease in mean arterial pressure (249). The presence of a significant increase in pulse and a decrease in arterial pressure 2 to 3 minutes following change from a supine to either a sitting or standing position is compatible with the presence of extracellular fluid volume depletion. Dry mucous membranes, low jugular venous pressure, absence of axillary moisture, decreased turgor of skin over the forehead and sternum, and absence of skin sheet marks over the back are all findings compatible with either loss or sequestration of extracellular fluid volume.

A recent metaanalysis examined the sensitivity, specificity, and predictive value of physical examination in the setting of volume depletion (250). A large (>30 beats/minute) postural pulse rise and postural dizziness was highly associated with

blood loss hypovolemia, whereas dry mucous membranes and longitudinal tongue furrows were more than 80% sensitive for detecting non-blood loss hypovolemia (250). Physical examination also can provide evidence of cardiac dysfunction. Elevated jugular venous pressure, pulsus paradoxus, the presence of moist pulmonary rales, S_3 sounds, and murmurs are all compatible with prerenal azotemia owing to impaired cardiac function. The presence of significant edema is compatible with a number of disorders characterized by a decrease in effective arterial blood volume and prerenal azotemia. These include cardiac failure, hepatic cirrhosis, nephrotic syndrome, and severe hypoalbuminemia. Also, retroperitoneal fibrosis and intraabdominal lymphomas and other extensive cancers as well as acute inferior vena caval or renal vein thrombosis can present as ARF associated with pedal edema.

Physical examination must also include palpation for determining the state of peripheral circulation, renal size, and the possibility of abdominal aortic aneurysms. Palpation or percussion of the suprapubic area is necessary to detect bladder distention, and rectal and pelvic examinations are needed to detect prostatic and pelvic disorders. Examination of the skin may reveal palpable purpura suggestive of vasculitis; lower-extremity evaluation may reveal livedo reticularis and evidence of emboli, suggesting atheroembolic disease. It is beyond the scope of this chapter to detail all the physical findings that can be associated with causes of ARF other than ATN; however, the presence of neurologic or pulmonary disease, fever, skin lesions, joint abnormalities, or diffuse lymphadenopathy suggests the presence of a systemic disorder associated with ARF.

Urinalysis and Urinary Flow Rate

Chemical and microscopic examination of the urine is critical in assessment of the cause of ARF (6,37,251,252). Urinalyses in 103 patients with ATN yielded diagnostically useful information in approximately 75% of cases (37). Routine microscopic urinalysis may also provide prognostic information. Hou and associates found that about half of 97 patients with ARF had an abnormal microscopic urinalysis (37). An abnormal urinalysis (probable "renal" cause of ARF) was associated with 35% mortality, whereas a normal urinalysis (probable "prerenal" cause of ARF) was associated with 15% mortality (37). Such a relationship between routine urinalysis and prognosis was not found in another study of ARF (252). Marcussen et al. (251) recently used quantitative Papanicolaou smears of urine sediment in patients with ARF. Patients with ATN had higher numbers of collecting duct cells and casts than those without tubular necrosis; however, there was substantial overlap between the two groups. Moreover, significant numbers of patients with rapidly reversible ARF demonstrated tubular epithelial cells and casts on this type of urinary sediment examination (251). An entirely normal microscopic urinalysis in the setting of ARF suggests the presence of either prerenal azotemia or obstructive uropathy.

The "dipstick" can provide helpful information in ARF. A positive reaction for "blood" by an orthotoluidine test indicates the presence of red blood cells (>3/high-power field). If no red blood cells are present, this reaction will be positive in the presence of either myoglobin or hemoglobin. Because the myoglobin molecule is smaller (17,000 MW) and is not bound to plasma proteins, it is readily filtered and cleared from plasma. By contrast, the larger hemoglobin molecule (65,000 MW), which is bound to haptoglobin, is less readily cleared from the plasma and thus gives plasma a pink-red color. Definitive differentiation of hemoglobin from myoglobin in the urine is best done by electrophoretic or immunochemical techniques that are not widely available.

The dipstick protein reading reflects the presence of albumin. Urinary protein determination performed by the acid precipitation method (e.g., Exton's reagent) detects the presence of all types of protein in the urine. Thus, a quantitative estimate of proteinuria that is lower with the dipstick method than with Exton's reagent suggests the presence of light chains (globulins) in the urine. Immunoelectrophoretic techniques remain the definitive method for identifying urinary light chains. If heavy proteinuria (2 to 3 g/day) is present in ARF, the presence of vasculitis or glomerular or other renal parenchymal cause of ARF should be sought. It is important to correlate the dipstick proteinuria assessment with the urinary specific gravity. For example, a 1+ reading in a concentrated specimen may not indicate significant proteinuria. Conversely, a 1+ reading in a dilute specimen may indicate significant proteinuria. Recent studies indicate that the ratio of a urinary measurement of albumin-to-creatinine concentration in a spot urinary sample provides a reasonable estimate of the grams per day of urinary protein.

Examination of the urinary sediment is of great value in the differential diagnosis of acute impairment of renal function. Sediment containing few formed elements or only hyaline casts strongly suggests prerenal azotemia or obstructive uropathy. With ATN, brownish pigmented cellular casts and many renal tubular epithelial cells are observed in more than 75% of patients. Sufficient red blood cells to cause microscopic hematuria are traditionally thought to be incompatible with a diagnosis of ATN and usually result from glomerulonephritis or structural renal disorders (stones, tumor, infection, or trauma). However, a case report suggested that macroscopic hematuria might be a rare presenting manifestation of ATN (253). Red blood cell casts suggest the presence of glomerular or vascular inflammatory diseases of the kidney and rarely if ever occur with ATN. Red blood cell casts, however, can be seen rarely in acute interstitial nephritis. The presence of large numbers of polymorphonuclear leukocytes, singly or in clumps, suggests acute diffuse pyelonephritis or papillary necrosis. Eosinophilic casts on Hansel's stain of urine sediment may be diagnostically helpful (254). The stains that best detect the bilobed eosinophil include Hansel's stain and the May-Grunwald-Giemsa stain. These stains are less pH dependent than Wright's stain and often detect eosinophiluria in allergic interstitial nephritis. However, eosinophiluria also is seen in some forms of glomerulonephritis and in atheroembolic renal disease but is rarely encountered in ATN (205,254). The combination of brownish-pigmented granular casts and positive occult blood tests on urine in the absence of hematuria indicates either hemoglobinuria or myoglobinuria. In ARF, the finding in fresh, warm urine of large numbers of football-shaped uric acid crystals may suggest a diagnosis of acute uric acid nephropathy, whereas the finding of large numbers of "back-of-envelope–shaped" oxalic acid suggests ethylene glycol toxicity. Other agents (e.g., indinavir, sulfadiazine, acyclovir, and methotrexate) also can induce ARF with characteristic crystal appearance on urinalysis (104). The presence of broad casts (defined as more than three white blood cells in diameter) suggests chronic renal disease.

An older study used the technique of transmission electron microscopy to study urinary sediment in the setting of ARF (255,256). In this study, renal tubular epithelial cells were present in urine sediment only in the presence of ATN (255). There was a correlation between the severity of cellular damage to urinary renal tubular epithelial cells and clinical course. These observations suggest that transmission electron microscopy may be helpful in determining the cause and severity of ARF. Unfortunately, the test is not practical.

The urinary flow rate also may provide helpful information about the cause of ARF. Anuria should be defined as absence of urine by bladder catheterization. Sustained periods of anuria suggest urinary tract obstruction as the cause of ARF. Other rare causes of anuria include rapidly progressive glomerulonephritis, mechanical occlusion of renal blood flow, and diffuse renal cortical necrosis. Brief intervals of severe oliguria (<100 mL/day) may be encountered early in the course of some patients with ATN and may be especially common in the setting of ATN and heat stroke (82).

Oliguria (<400 mL/day) traditionally has been considered the cardinal feature of renal failure (257); however, the first clinical descriptions of progressive azotemia occurring with little or no oliguria were reported in the early 1940s (258). In the mid-1950s, additional reports suggested that nonoliguric varieties of ARF may be especially common following head injury, military combat casualties, and burns (259,260). Small series of selected patients in the 1960s and 1970s reemphasized the occurrence of nonoliguric ARF in burned and traumatized patients (261,262). Since then, it has become apparent that nonoliguric ARF is more common than generally appreciated. In a 1977 prospective study, we found that the majority (59%) of patients with ARF encountered in a general medical-surgical hospital were nonoliguric despite progressive azotemia (38). The nonoliguric state was seen with all types of ARF, including those following surgery, trauma, hypotension, nephrotoxins, and rhabdomyolysis. Additional studies report similar results and demonstrate a frequency of nonoliguric ARF ranging from 25% to 80% of all cases of ARF (Fig. 41-2). More recently in a nationwide study, Allgren et al. (42) enrolled ARF patients in a clinical trial of a renal vasodilator. Of enrolled patients, 24% were oliguric and 76% nonoliguric (42).

Why was the high frequency of nonoliguric ARF recognized only relatively recently? Daily biochemical monitoring of renal function in seriously ill patients, regardless of urine output, has contributed to greater recognition of nonoliguric ARF. Aminoglycoside nephrotoxicity, a frequent contemporary cause of hospital-acquired ARF, often is nonoliguric. Prophylactic use of volume expansion, high-dose potent diuretic agents, and renal vasodilators may also contribute to a high frequency of nonoliguric ARF, especially after aortic and open-heart surgery. It is possible also that aggressive resuscitation and improved supportive management of the seriously ill, traumatized patient have altered the natural history of ARF so that nonoliguric varieties are more common. For example, the Maryland Institute of Emergency Medical Services demonstrated an increasing incidence of nonoliguric and a decreasing incidence of oliguric ARF concomitant with more aggressive fluid resuscitation of traumatized patients (263). Another influence on the frequency of occurrence of nonoliguric ARF is the means of patient selection. When ARF patients are selected by need for dialytic therapy as the only criterion, few if any nonoliguric patients are encountered. When all patients with an increasing serum creatinine level are studied (2), the frequency of occurrence of nonoliguric ARF is very high (Fig. 41-2).

Oliguria with avid renal salt and water retention is the hallmark of reversible prerenal azotemia. Decreasing effective circulating arterial volume results in increased renal vascular resistance (occurring predominantly at the afferent arteriole) and diminished renal blood flow. A decrease in glomerular capillary hydrostatic pressures decreases glomerular filtration. The resultant decline in peritubular hydrostatic pressure and increase in filtration fraction (with an increased peritubular colloid oncotic pressure) may act to increase proximal tubular fluid reabsorption. Increases in plasma concentrations of aldosterone and antidiuretic hormone, decreases in glomerular capillary pressure and altered peritubular factors combine to result in avid tubular reabsorption of salt and water and decreased urine flow. Thus, urine flow in patients with prerenal azotemia usually is diminished, and the urine is concentrated with a low fractional excretion of sodium.

In 1980, Miller and associates reported nine patients with apparent polyuric prerenal failure (264). These patients ranged from 28 to 76 years of age. No evidence of diabetes insipidus, exposure to nephrotoxins or diuretic drugs, or glycosuria was present. Two patients had mild chronic interstitial renal disease, whereas the other seven had normal basal serum creatinine concentrations. Azotemia developed in each patient (mean serum creatinine, 2.5 mg/dL), and high urine outputs (ranging from 980 to 2140 mL/day at the time of peak serum creatinine) were present. A negative fluid balance, signs of intravascular volume depletion, low urinary sodium concentration (<22 mEq/L), and resolution of azotemia with intravenous fluid administration suggested prerenal azotemia. The authors postulated that a depletion of medullary interstitial solute prevented maximal urinary concentrating ability in these seriously ill patients, allowing the "polyuric" prerenal state to occur. However, because slow recovery of renal function following correction of prerenal factors was seen, some of these patients may have had nonoliguric ATN.

It is important to emphasize that all disease processes including prerenal, postrenal, and diseases of the kidney (vascular, glomerular, interstitial, and tubular) that can produce ARF are often nonoliguric (265). In nearly all of the reported cases, a nonoliguric clinical picture is associated with lower morbidity and mortality and better long-term outcome than an oliguric state (38,42,265).

Recent clinical studies and a review of experimental studies conducted in laboratory models of ARF have clarified several aspects of the pathophysiology underlying the variations of urine flow rate in ARF (266,267). In a study of 25 patients with predominantly renal ischemia-associated ARF, Rahman and Conger found that the urine flow rate strongly correlated with residual GFR (266). By contrast, urine flow rate did not correlate with selected aspects of renal tubular function such as urine:serum ratio of creatinine or fractional excretion of sodium. These clinical observations plus a large body of experimental data suggest that the residual level of GFR is the primary determinant of urine flow in patients with ARF (266,267). The higher level of residual GFR in nonoliguric patients is compatible with improved survival and lower morbidity in these patients.

Urinary Chemical Indices

Urinary concentrations of electrolytes and nitrogenous wastes were first measured in patients with ATN in the late 1940s (268,269). These studies found low urinary-plasma (U/P) creatinine and urea nitrogen ratios and high urinary concentrations of sodium (U_{Na}) and chloride (U_{Cl}) in the established phase of ATN. As renal function improved, U/P creatinine and urea–nitrogen ratios increased. These early observations were subsequently confirmed in nearly all studies (270–280). In the 1950s, Welt (281) and Waugh (282) first suggested that spot urinalysis, specific gravity, and U_{Na} would be helpful in distinguishing between reversible prerenal azotemia and ATN. In 1967 and 1976, Handa (273) and Espinel (276), respectively, suggested that the diagnostic accuracy of U_{Na} alone in determining the cause of ARF was limited. However, either the renal failure index ($U_{Na} \div$ U/P creatinine) or the fractional excretion of sodium (FE_{Na} or $U/P_{Na} \div$ U/P creatinine $\times$ 100) was found to have a high degree of accuracy in differentiating between reversible prerenal azotemia and ATN. Prospective studies have confirmed the utility of selected urinary indices as diagnostic aids in assessing the patient with ARF (270) (Table 41-12; Fig. 41-7). More recently, the fractional excretion of uric acid and trace lithium has been proposed to be even more sensitive and specific aids in determining the cause of ARF (278,279).

The primary use of spot urine chemistries in ARF is to assist in differentiation between potentially reversible prerenal states and ATN. For prerenal states, the combination of reduced renal

TABLE 41-12

FRACTIONAL EXCRETION OF SODIUM (FE_{Na}) IN ACUTE RENAL FAILURE

FE_{Na} <1%	FE_{Na} >1%
Prerenal azotemia	Diuretic use
ECF volume loss or sequestration	Nonreabsorbable solute
Impaired cardiac output	Bicarbonate
Severe renal vasoconstriction	Glucose
Hepatorenal syndrome	Mannitol
Nonsteroidal antiinflammatory agents	Mineralocorticoid deficiency
Disease of afferent arteriole (e.g., TTP, scleroderma)	Late obstructive uropathy
Sepsis	Chronic renal failure
Nephropathy	Acute tubular necrosis
Early phase of myoglobinuric renal failure	Severe ischemic
Acute glomerulonephritis	
Early obstructive uropathy	
10%–15% of nonoliguric acute tubular necrosis	

TTP, thrombotic thrombocytopenic purpura.

perfusion and intact tubular function results in enhanced renal tubular reabsorption of filtered salts and water in an effort to expand extracellular fluid volume, thereby restoring renal perfusion. This increase in tubular reabsorption of salts and other organic substances results in relatively low urine concentrations and fractional excretion of sodium, chloride, lithium,

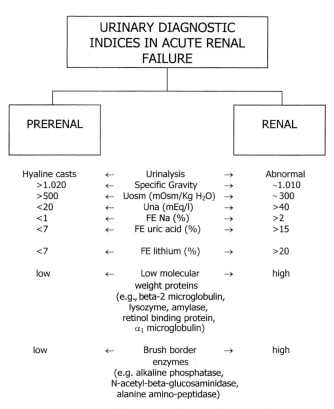

URINARY DIAGNOSTIC INDICES IN ACUTE RENAL FAILURE

PRERENAL			RENAL
Hyaline casts	← Urinalysis →		Abnormal
>1.020	← Specific Gravity →		~1.010
>500	← Uosm (mOsm/Kg H_2O) →		~ 300
<20	← Una (mEq/l) →		>40
<1	← FE Na (%) →		>2
<7	← FE uric acid (%) →		>15
<7	← FE lithium (%) →		>20
low	← Low molecular weight proteins (e.g., beta-2 microglobulin, lysozyme, amylase, retinol binding protein, α_1 microglobulin) →		high
low	← Brush border enzymes (e.g. alkaline phosphatase, N-acetyl-beta-glucosaminidase, alanine amino-peptidase) →		high

FIGURE 41-7. Urinary diagnostic indices to differentiate between prerenal and renal causes of acute renal failure.

and uric acid (Fig. 41-7). The enhanced tubular water reabsorption produces concentrated urine with relatively high U/P ratios of osmolality, urea nitrogen, and creatinine. By contrast, ATN is associated with impaired tubular reabsorption of salts and water with consequent higher urinary concentrations of sodium, chloride, lithium, and uric acid and lower U/P ratios of osmolality, urea nitrogen, and creatinine (Fig. 41-7). Some of the impaired tubular reabsorption of filtered salts in ATN can be attributed to loss of renal tubular epithelial cell polarity with translocation of the sodium pump (Na-K-ATPase) from a normal basolateral to an apical location (283). Also, a major Na exchanger in the proximal tubule (NHE-3), is transcriptionally downregulated with ischemic injury, as are other more distal transport systems that regulate tubular sodium reabsorption, such as the bumetanide sensitive Na-K-2Cl transporter and the thiazide sensitive Na-Cl-cotransporter (284,285).

Several caveats are in order in using spot urine chemistries as diagnostic aids in evaluating the cause of ARF. Despite widespread, routine use, no study has demonstrated that knowledge of these indices either changes management or improves outcome of ARF. There is currently no "gold standard" for the diagnosis of ATN and most data obtained on urine chemistries in ARF rely on variable and arbitrary criteria for determining the cause of the renal failure. Nearly all studies of spot chemistries have been performed at a single time point relatively late in the course of ARF. The lack of serial data is important because ARF state is often dynamic in nature (277). For example, early in the course of ARF, renal tubular function is intact. Later, ischemia may result in loss of tubular cell polarity. The resulting urine chemistries therefore are dependent on the phase of the course in which they were obtained. This may limit the sensitivity and specificity of urine chemical indices. For example, the early course of ARF occurring in the setting of sepsis, radiocontrast exposure, rhabdomyolysis, and NSAID use often is associated with renal vasoconstriction and low FE_{Na} (286–290). Later in the course, the FE_{Na} often increases, especially if tubular necrosis occurs.

Two other points deserve emphasis with regard to use of urine chemistries as ARF diagnostic aids. Early in the course of urinary tract obstruction, in some patients with nonoliguric ATN and in some vascular/glomerular disorders (acute glomerulonephritis, vasculitis, thrombotic thrombocytopenic purpura), urinary chemical indices can be indistinguishable from those seen with prerenal ARF (274,280,290). Conversely, several acute renal parenchymal disorders (e.g., interstitial nephritis, severe ischemic nephropathy, and exacerbations of chronic renal failure) can be associated with urine chemical parameters indistinguishable from ATN, suggesting a lack of specificity (291,292). Finally, it is important to acknowledge that potentially reversible prerenal ARF with a $FE_{Na} > 1\%$ occurs in selected settings such as recent diuretic use, bicarbonaturia, salt-wasting nephropathy, glycosuria, and mineralocorticoid deficiency (Table 41-12). In the setting of prerenal ARF associated with bicarbonaturia, the urinary chloride concentration is low, confirming a prerenal state (293). In the setting of prerenal ARF associated with diuretic use, the fractional excretion of trace lithium and uric acid continue to be low (279). Unfortunately, measurement of fractional excretion of trace lithium requires atomic absorption spectrophotometry and thus is not widely available for timely clinical use at present.

Although urine chemical indices are most often used as diagnostic adjuncts in patients with ARF, it is of interest that they may also provide prognostic information. For example, several studies suggest that, in oliguric patients with ARF, lower values for FE_{Na} and higher values for U/P osmolality predict a high likelihood of a diuretic response to loop diuretics, mannitol, and/or dopamine (38,294,295). Moreover, the more urine

chemistries resemble those seen in prerenal states, the higher the likelihood of survival from ARF (38,279).

One specific urine index deserves special comment. The ratio between urinary uric acid and urinary creatinine has been used as an aid to determine the nature of ARF (296). In an older study by Kelton et al. (296), ratios of higher than 1 in patients with renal failure were observed in patients with acute uric acid nephropathy compared with ratios below 1 in those who had ARF from other causes (296). For example, the ratio was found to be less than 1 in prerenal azotemia, chronic renal failure, and obstructive uropathy. It was concluded that a ratio of more than 1 in ARF signified a diagnosis of acute uric acid nephropathy. In a more recent study, the urinary uric acid–urinary creatinine ratio was studied in 23 patients with ARF (297). This ratio was >1 in 12 patients. These 12 patients had high fever, catabolism, hyperbilirubinemia, and nonoliguric ARF. The 11 patients with ratios of <1 tended to be less catabolic and oliguric. These results suggest limited diagnostic utility of the urinary uric acid–urinary creatinine ratio in determining the cause of ARF (297).

Consider Urinary Tract Obstruction

A postrenal cause is encountered in a significant percentage of all cases of ARF, especially in cases of community-acquired ARF (18,57) (see Chapter 25). The potential for therapeutic intervention suggests that the possibility of urinary tract obstruction should be considered in all cases of ARF. A cost-effectiveness analysis of a global strategy of excluding urinary tract obstruction in all cases of ARF has not been done. The presence of prostatic, pelvic, or intraabdominal cancer, a single kidney, anuria, widely fluctuating urinary volumes, recent surgery on the genitourinary tract or within the retroperitoneal space, or a normal urine sediment demand evaluation for potential obstruction.

The best means of excluding obstructive uropathy as a cause of ARF remains debatable. Physical examination (suprapubic palpation, and pelvic and rectal examinations) and postvoiding bladder catheterization continue to be the best methods for bladder neck obstruction. Ultrasonography in experienced hands is an excellent screening tool for the presence of extrarenal obstruction; however, it is recognized that significant obstructive uropathy may occur in the presence of minimal ureteral and renal pelvic dilation. For example, in studies by Curry and associates (298), 27 patients with obstructive uropathy were examined by ultrasound. Three of these 27 (11%) were found to have minimal dilation and high-grade obstruction that improved with percutaneous drainage. Other series of nearly 250 patients report a somewhat lower frequency (4%) of nondilated obstructive uropathy (299,300). Because the majority of patients with ARF and nondilated renal collecting systems do not have either retrograde pyelography or percutaneous nephrostomy, it is likely that the reported frequency of nondilated obstructive uropathy represents a minimal estimate. Abdominal and pelvic conventional and spiral computerized tomography scanning technologies appear to be exceptionally helpful in the diagnosis of acute obstructive uropathy (301). Occasionally, retrograde pyelography, stent replacement, or empiric percutaneous nephrostomy drainage may be necessary to exclude obstructive uropathy.

Miscellaneous Tests

In some circumstances, the cause of ARF is not apparent after chart review, history, physical examination, and urinalysis. Review of the hemogram may be helpful in this setting. A peripheral blood smear that reveals rouleaux formation may suggest the presence of a plasma cell dyscrasia. Serum and/or urinary protein electrophoresis are needed to substantiate this diagnosis. Eosinophilia is compatible with allergic interstitial nephritis, atheroembolic disease, and polyarteritis nodosa. A microangiopathic picture with thrombocytopenia suggests vasculitis, malignant hypertension, the HELLP syndrome, hemolytic-uremic syndrome, and thrombotic thrombocytopenic purpura. The presence of coagulopathy can suggest either disseminated intravascular coagulation or an antiphospholipid antibody syndrome as the cause of ARF. If glomerulonephritis is a diagnostic possibility, then the presence of antineutrophilic cytoplasmic antibodies may suggest a diagnosis of either Wegener's granulomatosis (primarily a cytoplasmic pattern) or pauci-immune glomerulonephritis (primarily a perinuclear pattern). Antibodies to glomerular basement membrane are strongly suggestive of Goodpasture's syndrome, whereas antinuclear antibodies and antibodies against DNA suggest the presence of systemic lupus erythematosus. The presence of cryoglobulins may point to the presence of circulating immune complexes, a plasma cell disorder, or primary cryoglobulinemia. A review of blood chemistries may be helpful. Hypercalcemia of diverse causes can be associated with the development of ARF, and very high uric acid concentrations may suggest the presence of diffuse tissue injury such as occasionally occurs in tumor lysis syndrome and rhabdomyolysis. If mechanical obstruction of the renal vasculature is suspected, then isotope studies, Doppler procedures, magnetic resonance angiography, or conventional angiography might be considered.

Therapeutic Trials

Response to specific interventions may provide diagnostically helpful information in the ARF setting. Restoration of renal function with either extracellular fluid volume replacement or improvement in cardiac output (dopamine/dobutamine) supports a diagnosis of prerenal azotemia. Improved renal function after relief of obstructive uropathy suggests postrenal azotemia. Improvement or amelioration of ARF after cessation of pharmacologic agents such as NSAIDs or ACE inhibitors suggests a pathogenetic role for those substances in ARF. Mechanical (angioplasty or surgical manipulations) or pharmacologic (thrombolytic) improvement in renal blood flow in the appropriate clinical setting supports an ischemic basis for worsening of renal function (72,73,302,303).

Renal Biopsy

Occasionally, despite a logical sequential approach, the cause of ARF remains unclear. Renal biopsy may be considered under such circumstances. A renal biopsy often is considered in the setting of ARF when some of the following are present: (a) no obvious cause of ARF, (b) either extrarenal clinical evidence or a history of systemic disease, (c) heavy proteinuria and persistent hematuria, (d) marked hypertension in the absence of volume expansion, (e) prolonged (>2 to 3 weeks) oliguria, and (f) anuria in the absence of obstructive uropathy. It is worth reemphasizing the necessity for aggressive, timely evaluation if glomerular disease is a diagnostic possibility as a cause of ARF (245). Once the serum creatinine exceeds 2 to 5 mg/dL in cases of rapidly progressive glomerulonephritis, and perhaps acute interstitial nephritis, the possibility of nonreversible scarring and lack of recovery of renal function increases significantly (245).

Several studies have examined the clinical utility of renal biopsy in the setting of ARF (304–309). Mustonen and associates (305) performed biopsies in 91 of 99 patients and compared biopsy results with the prebiopsy clinical diagnoses. A clinical impression of acute tubular and/or interstitial disease was confirmed by biopsy in 44 of 51 (86%) of cases. A clinical impression of acute glomerular disease was confirmed by biopsy in 16 of 23 (70%) of cases. In 30% of cases, either no clinical diagnosis was obvious or the clinical diagnosis differed from the biopsy diagnosis. Wilson et al. (307) performed a renal biopsy on 84 patients with ARF. All of these patients had undefined "atypical features" for ATN. On biopsy, 52% had glomerular disease, 30% had acute tubulointerstitial disease, and 18% had renal vascular disorders (307). In this study, a clinical diagnosis of an acute tubulointerstitial process was 77% sensitive and 86% specific. By contrast, a clinical diagnosis of acute glomerulonephritis was less sensitive (56%) and less specific (66%). In another prospective study, Cohen and associates (304) found that only one-third of the clinical diagnoses of the cause of ARF were substantiated by renal biopsy. Moreover, in this small series, the renal biopsy led to a significant change in therapy in more than half of the patients with ARF who were undergoing a biopsy (304).

Solez and colleagues (306) reported on their experience with 976 patients with ARF encountered over a 10-year interval. Twenty-two percent of these patients underwent biopsy because the cause of ARF was not apparent. Most of the patients had features atypical of ATN such as gradual onset of ARF, significant hypertension, marked proteinuria, significant hematuria, prolonged (>3 weeks) oliguria, and underlying systemic disease. Half of the patients, in whom the ARF diagnosis was not apparent, had glomerular disease on biopsy, whereas the remainder had tubulointerstitial disease.

In addition to indications for performing a renal biopsy in ARF, two other issues are of concern. The first is safety. Recent developments in treating the coagulopathy associated with renal failure plus improvements in biopsy techniques (e.g., biopsy guided by real time ultrasonography or CT imaging, use of smaller needles and biopsy guns) have improved safety. Indeed, reasonable safety has been demonstrated in the setting of uncooperative ICU patients requiring mechanical ventilation (310). In this small study, percutaneous renal biopsy performed on critically ill, ICU patients undergoing mechanical ventilation was compared with open biopsy. Sufficient renal tissue for diagnosis was obtained on all seven patients undergoing percutaneous biopsy and the rate of complications was roughly comparable to patients undergoing open biopsy (310). Renal biopsy utilizing a transjugular approach has been used in high-risk patients. Thompson and colleagues (311) reported on 25 patients who underwent transjugular renal biopsy—these procedures were performed by an interventional radiologist experienced in transjugular liver biopsies, and diagnostic tissue was obtained in 21 (84%) of cases. Seventeen out of 25 patients developed perforation of the renal capsule, 6 of whom required coil embolization. One patient developed renal vein thrombosis 6 days after a failed transjugular biopsy attempt (311).

The timing of biopsy in ARF remains a key issue (245). In the past, lack of recovery of renal function and persisting anuria after several days were considered as indicators for ARF biopsy. Presently, concerns about the irreversible nature of many forms of severe glomerulopathy and acute interstitial disorders, if left untreated, have led to a much more timely approach to biopsy when the cause of ARF is not clear.

COMPLICATIONS OF ACUTE RENAL FAILURE

Determination of the rate of occurrence of complications in patients with ARF sometimes is difficult. Patients with the highest rate of development of ARF often have significant co-morbidity and preexisting multiple organ dysfunction prior to development of ARF. For example, in a case cohort study of mild-to-moderate radiocontrast-induced ARF, preexisting sepsis (22%), respiratory failure (36%), mental status changes (41%), and bleeding (15%) were relatively common (35). However, the rate of new occurrence of these complications following development of ARF in patients that did not have the complication before ARF was strikingly high (sepsis 45%, respiratory failure 78%, mental status changes 68%, and bleeding 27%) (35).

Cardiovascular System Complication

Hemodynamic instability is often encountered before and after development of ARF. Liano found that 60% of ICU-associated and 19% of hospital ward-associated ARF cases experienced hypotension (56). Myocardial ischemia (13% to 19%) and cardiac arrhythmias that required treatment (22% to 29%) were observed commonly in a large multicenter study of patients with ARF (42). Volume overload and congestive cardiac failure are also common complications occurring in ARF patients (38,40,77,312,313). Of course, congestive heart failure and its treatment (angiotensin converting enzyme [ACE] inhibitors and diuretics) can be associated with ARF. Pericardial tamponade also can be associated with ARF. The causes of cardiac tamponade in ARF are pericardial effusion (usually of serosanguinous type), hemorrhage into the pericardial sac, and collagenization of pericardial exudate (314,315). The concomitant presence of significant cardiac dysfunction and ARF may be a manifestation of either systemic disease (i.e., systemic lupus erythematosus, scleroderma) or a complication of cardiac disease (i.e., subacute bacterial endocarditis, atrial fibrillation with emboli). Spontaneous and catheter-induced atheroemboli can cause abdominal and peripheral vascular manifestations as well as ARF. Indwelling arterial and venous catheters can lead to vascular occlusion, inflammation, and infection in the setting of ARF. Cardiac arrest in the setting of ARF always should arouse immediate suspicion of hyperkalemia, a potentially treatable cause of cardiac arrest.

Pulmonary System Complications

Pulmonary infiltrates caused by edema from volume overload and/or infection are encountered frequently in ARF. In eight series comprising 1,900 patients with severe ARF, more than 50% had concomitant respiratory failure sufficient to warrant mechanical ventilation (316).

Respiratory failure occurred commonly before (36%) and especially after (78%) the development of ARF in the experience of Levy and associates (35). Liano et al. (40) found that 82% of ICU-associated cases of ARF were on mechanical ventilation, whereas Allgren reported that 48% to 55% of all ARF patients were intubated for respiratory support (42). Pulmonary infiltrates appeared in 26 of 92 (28%) patients with ATN in our experience (38). Pulmonary complications including aspiration pneumonia, and adult respiratory distress syndrome occurred in 54% of 462 patients in another recent study (312). McMurray and associates found 81 episodes of pneumonia in 276 patients with ATN (77).

There are several disease processes that can cause simultaneous pulmonary involvement and impairment of renal function (316). These processes include Goodpasture's syndrome, systemic lupus erythematosus, Wegener's granulomatosis, allergic granulomatous angiitis (Churg-Strauss syndrome), polyarteritis nodosa, cryoglobulinemia, sarcoidosis, renal vein thrombosis with pulmonary emboli, and bronchogenic carcinoma with immune complex glomerulonephritis. The development of pulmonary complications is an adverse prognostic factor in ARF (312,313,316,317). In a study of prognostic risk factors in 462 patients with ATN, Bullock et al. (312) found the development of pulmonary complications to be the single most significant risk factor for death in ATN; and ARF occurring in the respiratory ICU was associated with an 80% mortality. In five series of patients with severe ARF, mortality increased from 49% in nonventilated patients to over 80% in patients who required mechanical ventilation (316).

Gastrointestinal System Complications

The primary gastrointestinal complications of ARF include symptoms of anorexia and nausea, vomiting, and upper gastrointestinal bleeding. Stress ulcers and gastritis are common. In a prospective study of 514 subjects with ARF (318), acute gastrointestinal bleeding occurred in 69 (13.4%) patients. Forty (7.8%) patients had bleeding that was severe, that is, resulted in hemodynamic compromise or required transfusion or surgery. The most common causes of bleeding were gastric erosions/ulcers, duodenal ulcers and esophageal varices. Independent risk factors for bleeding included thrombocytopenia, liver cirrhosis, de novo ARF, chronic liver disease, increased severity of ARF, and APACHE II score (318). Gastrointestinal bleeding complicated the course of 8% to 13% of patients with ARF recently reported by Allgren and associates (42).

Mild hyperamylasemia (two or three times normal) can be seen in ARF (319). Also noteworthy is the fact that several disease processes (e.g., atheroemboli, vasculitis, and common bile duct stones with bacteremia) can present with both acute pancreatitis and ARF. Acute and chronic renal failure can elevate the ratio of the renal clearances of amylase to creatinine (319). Thus, lipase determinations and clinical assessment often are necessary to assist in the diagnosis of pancreatitis in the setting of ARF. Acute pancreatitis can result in ARF. In two recent series of more than 1,000 patients with acute pancreatitis, 4% to 14% developed some degree of ARF (320,321). Allgren found that 2% to 10% of all ARF patients had a clinical diagnosis of acute pancreatitis (42).

Jaundice often occurs during the course of ARF. Jaundice occurred in 43% of 462 patients with ATN in the experience of Bullock et al. (312). Jaundice occurred in 28% of ICU-associated and 13% of hospital-ward associated ARF in the experience of Liano and associates (40). Jaundice is often multifactorial, with contributing factors including passive hepatic congestion, blood transfusions, hypotension, medications and toxins, and sepsis. A number of infections (Gram-negative sepsis, especially in patients with bile duct obstruction, leptospirosis, or hepatitis A, B, and C) and toxins (hydrocarbons, acetaminophen, Amanita phalloides toxin) can cause simultaneous hepatitis and ARF. The development of jaundice in the setting of ARF may be an ominous prognostic finding (312).

Neurologic System Complications

Central nervous system disorders have long been recognized as frequent accompaniments of ARF. Liano and associates emphasized that the presence of coma associated with ARF signals an exceptionally poor prognosis (40). Mental status changes were noted by Levy et al. (35) in 41% of patients before and 68% of patients after development of ARF. In another study, Liano found that about 25% of ARF patients were sedated, making assessment of mental status difficult, and that 5% were comatose (56). Levy et al. found that the course cases of 12% of ARF patients were complicated by an acute stroke, whereas a stroke occurred in only 2% of case controls (35).

There are a number of causes of neurologic dysfunction in the setting of ARF such as primary neurologic disease, other metabolic disturbances, and the presence of systemic disease involving both the kidneys and nervous system (vasculitis, systemic lupus erythematosus, subacute bacterial endocarditis, thrombotic thrombocytopenic purpura, hemolytic-uremic syndrome, malignant hypertension). Pharmacologic agent–induced (e.g., sedative-hypnotic drugs) encephalopathy is a common cause of central nervous system dysfunction in patients with renal failure (322). Neurologic symptoms appearing after dialytic therapy should arouse suspicion of a dialysis disequilibrium syndrome. Development of peripheral neuropathy in the setting of ARF should raise consideration of neurovascular entrapment (rhabdomyolysis), ischemic neuropathy (polyarteritis, emboli), and heavy metal intoxication.

Infectious Complications

Acute renal failure and infections are commonly associated. In the experience of Rasmussen and Ibels, septicemia appeared to be an important factor contributing to the development of ARF in 26% of 143 ARF patients (123). In a case-control study, Shusterman and colleagues (55) found that septic shock was the single clinical condition associated with the highest likelihood of development of hospital-acquired ARF.

Allgren found that sepsis occurred in 27% to 42% of patients with ARF and that the overall rate of associated infection ranged from 44% to 57% (42). In a recent prospective study of patients with septic shock, 21% of patients were oliguric at the time of study entry (323).

Not only is septicemia frequently associated with the onset of ARF, but also infections frequency complicates the course of patients with ARF. Levy and colleagues found a 22% frequency of preexisting infection before and an additional 45% frequency of infections after ARF (35). McMurray et al. (77) found infections in 74% of 276 patients with ATN. In their study, the most common sites of infection were pulmonary (29%), urinary tract (32%), and peritonitis (22%). A total of 56 patients had abscesses, and 97 had documented bacteremia. Infections from indwelling venous and arterial lines and indwelling bladder catheters also occur in ARF; however, urinary tract infections can occur even in patients without indwelling catheters. Patients with ARF on dialysis in ICU are especially susceptible to infection. Hoste (324) found that in 704 ICU patients treated for ARF with dialysis, 62 patients developed nosocomial bacteremia. The lungs were the most important source of bloodstream infection (26%), followed by the abdomen (23%), catheters for vascular access (16%), urogenital tract (10%), wounds (6%), and unknown (19%) (324). Pulmonary infections appear to occur later in the course of ARF. In a prospective analysis, we found that 11% of 92 patients with ARF developed septicemia. In the experience of Bullock et al. (312) with 462 ARF patients, 91% received an average of three antibiotics for 16 days. Keane et al. (325) recently published a small ($N = 35$) prospective, controlled study examining the efficacy of intravenous immunoglobulin G as adjunctive therapy in patients with ARF. A striking 71% of 35 ARF patients developed culture-proven infections (325). Interestingly, mortality was significantly lower in immunoglobulin-treated patients (12%) than controls (44%). Also of interest, there was no difference in the rate of infectious complications when the immunoglobulin-treated patients were compared with controls. Confirmation of these results as well as documentation of the mechanisms of improved survival is needed.

Infectious complications are a leading source of morbidity and mortality in ARF. McMurray et al. (77) found that infectious complications were the cause of death in 54% of 102 ATN deaths. In the extensive experience of Liano and associates in which progression of underlying disease was excluded, infection was the single leading case of death (40).

Endocrine System Complications

Acute tubular necrosis is often associated with disturbances in divalent ion metabolism (hypocalcemia, hyperphosphatemia, and hypermagnesemia) (326,327). Altered parathyroid hormone (PTH) action and vitamin D metabolism may play a pathogenetic role in the hypocalcemia and hyperphosphatemia. Several studies demonstrate a high plasma PTH in ATN (233,328–335). This probably occurs in response to hypocalcemia. The simultaneous presence of hypocalcemia with high PTH levels suggests impaired bone response to PTH, which has been demonstrated in humans with ATN (330). In some ARF patients, decreased 1,25-dihydroxy vitamin D is present and many ARF patients have hyperphosphatemia. These latter two factors may underlie the skeletal resistance to PTH that occurs with ATN (326–331,333–335). Monomeric calcitonin levels have been found to be increased with ARF (335). The role of calcitonin in the deranged calcium/phosphorus homeostasis of ARF remains to be determined.

Calcium homeostasis in ARF related to rhabdomyolysis has been investigated (233,329,335). In general, hypocalcemia, hyperphosphatemia and low levels of 1,25-dihydroxy vitamin D are present. Hypercalcemia can rarely occur early in the polyuric phase of ARF and is associated with increases in 1,25-dihydroxy vitamin D and PTH (both amino-terminal and carboxy-terminal) (233). Later in the polyuric phase, serum calcium vitamin D, and PTH levels returned to normal. A close correlation between serum calcium and vitamin D levels can be present (233). These observations suggest that the hypocalcemia seen during the early phase of ARF is due to hyperphosphatemia and decreased 1,25-dihydroxy vitamin D synthesis. In summary, high PTH, skeletal resistance to PTH, and low 1,25-dihydroxy vitamin D levels occur in ARF. Rarely, the recovery of rhabdomyolysis-associated ARF can be complicated by hypercalcemia. The cause of this late syndrome may be mobilization of calcium sequestered by necrotic muscle tissue rather than a disturbance of the PTH-vitamin D axis (336,337). Calciphylaxis has been reported as a rare complication of ARF (338).

Data on male gonadal function in ARF are available. Two groups of investigators found high blood prolactin levels and low testosterone in males with ARF (331,332). The abnormalities in prolactin and testosterone resolved as renal function normalized. In the study of Kokot and Kuska (331), increased blood concentrations of luteinizing hormone and estradiol also were present. These workers found a negative correlation between plasma prolactin and testosterone but no correlation between PTH and either testosterone or prolactin (331). By contrast, Levitan et al. (332) found a direct relationship between prolactin and PTH. Together, these observations demonstrate that male gonadal failure frequently occurs in the setting of ARF. Unfortunately, data on comparably ill control subjects are not available.

Thyroid function tests have been examined in the setting of ARF (339,340). Total thyroxine (T_4) and triiodothyronine (T_3) are decreased in ARF and return to normal with recovery of renal function. In one but not another study, free T_3 and free T_4 also were decreased in ARF (339,340); however, all patients appeared clinically to be euthyroid and thyroid-stimulating hormone was normal. Thus, patients with ARF resemble other critically ill patients, and thyroid function is normal.

Kokot and Kuska (331) studied glycogenic insulin release in patients with ARF. Insulin release from beta cells was studied by intravenous glucose infusions. Fasting insulin concentrations were normal. In response to glucose infusion, insulin concentrations were higher than in controls, and plasma disappearance was prolonged. These findings suggest the presence of insulin resistance such as is commonly seen in chronic renal failure. This conclusion was further documented by finding that insulin (0.1 μm/kg) decreased fasting plasma glucose from 96 to 58 mg/dL in patients with ARF and from 90 to 38 mg/dL in normal subjects. In acutely uremic rats, insulin resistance appears to be caused by skeletal muscle resistance to insulin-mediated glucose uptake (341). Also, there appears to be impaired hepatic glucose response to glucagon but not to cyclic adenosine monophosphate (cAMP). Together, these clinical and experimental studies suggest that ARF produces insulin resistance and the resistance occurs at the skeletal muscle level. Also, acute uremia appears to include a "pre-cAMP" defect in hepatic glucose response to glucagon (341). High plasma renin activity (PRA) and angiotensin II often occur in the setting of ARF. In a clinical study, Mitch and Walker (342) found elevated plasma levels of angiotensin II in 13 patients with shock and ARF. Of these 13 patients, 10 had increases in PRA; however, only slight increases in angiotensin II and PRA levels were frequently found. Furthermore, comparable increases in PRA and angiotensin II were observed in six patients undergoing elective drug-induced hypotension who did not develop ARF (342). The observations confirm that high levels of angiotensin II and PRA are often observed in the clinical setting of ARF. However, similar levels also occur in settings in which renal function is clinically well maintained. Whether the high angiotensin II levels contribute to hypertension that occasionally complicates ARF remains to be determined. Transient hyperreninemic hypoaldosteronism is common in patients with septic shock. These abnormal aldosterone levels are associated with greater sodium and fluid depletion and are followed by enhanced incidence of acute renal failure requiring renal replacement therapy and prolonged length of stay in the ICU (343).

Kokot and Kuska (331) examined growth hormone response in insulin in patients with ARF. Patients with ARF had a threefold greater increase in growth hormone compared with controls. Following hemodialysis, the exaggerated increase in growth hormone response was significantly less but still present.

BIOCHEMICAL ABNORMALITIES IN ACUTE RENAL FAILURE

Nitrogen Balance

Plasma urea nitrogen and serum creatinine increase because decreased urinary excretion of nitrogenous waste occurs in ARF. The magnitude of increase is dependent on the nitrogen intake, the degree of renal impairment, and the degree of protein catabolism (see Table 41-13). Urea nitrogen appearance rates ranging from 5 to 50 mg/day or greater can occur, depending on the catabolic state of the patient (344). In the noncatabolic patient with mild renal impairment, daily BUN usually increases <10 to 15 mg/dL per day and serum creatinine <1.5 mg/dL per day. Conversely, in the catabolic patient, daily increments of BUN can exceed 50 mg/dL. In 462 patients with ATN, Bullock et al. (312) found that 35 were "catabolic" as defined by an increase of BUN of >30 mg/dL on 2 consecutive days. Biesenbach et al. (317) found that 10% to 20% of 710 cases of ARF were hypercatabolic. The degree of renal impairment is also an important determinant of BUN and plasma creatinine in ARF. We found that the duration of BUN of >50 mg/dL in ARF was 18 ± 2.0 days in oliguric patients and 8 ± 0.8 days in nonoliguric patients who had a higher GFR (38).

TABLE 41-13

SELECTED BIOCHEMICAL COMPLICATIONS IN ACUTE RENAL FAILURE

	Change/day	
	Noncatabolic	Catabolic
Blood urea nitrogen (mg/dL)	10–20	>30
Creatinine (mg/dL)	<1.5	>1.5
K^+ (mEq/L)	<0.5	>0.5
HCO_3^- (mEq/L)	<2	>2
Phosphorus (mg/dL)	0.5	>1

The precise cause of the catabolic state in ARF cannot be stated with certainty. Many patients have necrotic tissue, muscle damage, fever, and sepsis and may be receiving corticosteroids. Several hormonal abnormalities are present in ARF (e.g., elevated levels of glucagon, catecholamines, growth hormone, cortisol, and insulin resistance) that could alter muscle protein metabolism (331,344). A major cause of protein catabolism in ARF is insulin resistance (345). Insulin resistance leads to reduced protein synthesis, enhanced degradation of muscle protein and excessive release of amino acids into the circulation (345). Gluconeogenesis and ureagenesis are increased due to hepatic uptake of these amino acids from the circulation (345). Circulating proteases released from leukocytes have been found in the blood of catabolic patients with ARF (346). ARF is associated with a reduction in protease inhibitors such as α-2-macroglobulin (347). The use of dialysis may remove amino acids and other nutritional elements (348). Finally, diminished nutritional intake can potentially contribute to the depressed level of muscle protein synthesis in ARF.

Enhanced muscle breakdown with release of creatine can lead to a disproportionate increase in serum creatinine relative to BUN in the setting of rhabdomyolysis-induced ARF. For example, Koffler and associates (349) found that about 25% of their patients with rhabdomyolysis-induced ARF had disproportionate increases in creatinine relative to BUN. Grossman and associates (234) found daily increments in plasma creatinine varying from 1.6 to 6.6 mg/dL. In 15 patients with rhabdomyolysis-related ARF, nine had daily increments of plasma creatinine of >3.0 mg/dL (234). However, Gabow et al. (243) did not find any difference in daily increment in plasma creatinine when ARF patients with (1.3 ± 0.7 mg/dL) and without (1.4 ± 0.8 mg/dL) rhabdomyolysis were compared. Clinicians usually follow daily serum creatinine concentrations to assess whether GFR is increasing, decreasing, or constant in patients with ARF. The serum creatinine concentration, however, is dependent on creatinine production, volume of distribution, and renal elimination, and all of these variables are subject to fluctuations in patients with ARF. Moran and Myers (5) developed a simple, computerized model of creatinine kinetics in patients with postischemic ARF. This model allows calculation of GFR based on serum creatinine concentration corrected for changes in creatinine volume of distribution and was validated by direct measurements of GFR. Using this model, two clinically noteworthy observations were made. First, in patients with ARF, changes in GFR often correlated poorly with changes in serum creatinine concentration. Second, several patterns (abrupt and large, slow and progressive, and stepwise) of change in glomerular filtration occurred during development of and recovery from postischemic ARF and were poorly reflected by daily changes in serum creatinine concentration (5). These observations suggest that definite conclusions regarding changes in GFR are difficult to make using serum creatinine concentration alone in the setting of ARF.

In this regard, isotopic methods (utilizing radioisotope or radiocontrast) can provide noninvasive, real-time monitoring of renal function in critically ill patients (49,350,351). Unfortunately, this methodology is not widely available at present.

Disorders of Electrolyte and Uric Acid Metabolism

Hyperkalemia, hyponatremia, metabolic acidosis, and hyperuricemia often occur in ARF. In our experience, a rise in plasma potassium concentrations to >5.5 mEq/L was seen in 50% of patients with ARF (38). Minuth and colleagues (252) found hyperkalemia in 75% of 94 patients. Wheeler and associates (352) found that 30% of patients with ATN develop an increase in plasma potassium concentration to >6.0 mEq/L; however, an increase in serum potassium may not occur in cases of mild ARF (326). The hyperkalemia is due to continued potassium release from cells in the face of impaired renal potassium elimination. For example, the potassium concentration of intracellular water is about 155 mEq/L in skeletal muscle. Thus, tumor lysis syndrome and rhabdomyolysis can induce dangerous levels of hyperkalemia quickly. A study of seven patients with rhabdomyolysis induced by extensive traumatic muscle crush injury revealed plasma potassium concentrations on admission of 4.5 to 8.3 mEq/L despite rapid evacuation from the site of injury (236). Three of the seven patients had potassium concentrations of >6.9 mEq/L. Gabow and colleagues (243) found significantly higher peak potassium concentrations in ARF associated with rhabdomyolysis than in other forms of ARF (5.6 ± 0.9 vs. 4.7 + 0.6 mEq/L, respectively; p <0.05). Other factors including a cellular shift of potassium owing to acidemia and hyperosmolality and potassium loads from exogenous sources such as blood, dietary intake, potassium salts (e.g., salt substitutes), or large doses of penicillin G can also contribute to hyperkalemia. Acute renal failure induced by NSAIDs can also be associated with marked hyperkalemia (353). An effect of these agents in suppressing renin and aldosterone secretion may be responsible in part.

Metabolic acidosis occurs often in ARF. In 92 patients with ARF, we found metabolic acidosis (plasma bicarbonate of <15 mEq/L, pH <7.40) in 19% (38). In a group of patients with mild ARF (rise in serum creatinine of 2 mg/dL), a 2 to 4 mEq/L decrease in serum bicarbonate occurred (339). Stable patients without kidney function on chronic hemodialysis usually have a decline of plasma bicarbonate of 2 mEq/L/day (344). The metabolic acidosis is often associated with an increased anion gap. Thus, Gabow and associates (243) found an anion gap of 17 ± 6 mEq/L in ARF; however, when rhabdomyolysis was present, the anion gap increased to 28 ± 14 mEq/L. By contrast, Dolson found an anion gap of 14 ± 0.6 mEq/L in series of patients with mild ARF (326). The metabolic acidosis results from continued production of nonvolatile acid and decreased renal ability to excrete acid. In severely catabolic states, the usual daily production of 1 mEq/L of nonvolatile acid can be increased markedly. It is noteworthy that other causes of anion gap metabolic acidosis such as ingestion of ethylene glycol and clinical settings associated with lactic acidosis are often associated with ARF.

Hyponatremia is a common complication of ARF and is caused by an absolute or relative increase in solute-free water intake. In a prospective analysis of hyponatremia, we found that 19% of all cases of hyponatremia occur in the setting of excess solute-free water intake in the presence of renal failure (354). Rare associations with hyponatremia and ARF include toxin ingestion (355,356), rhabdomyolysis, infection (357) and hypothyroidism (358). Hyperuricemia usually occurs in ARF. Peak uric acid was 9.2 ± 3.7 mg/dL in 38 patients with ATN

(243) and 8.6 mg/dL in 96 patients with mild ARF (326). Much higher blood uric acid concentrations occur in cell injury-associated ARF, and peak uric acid concentrations of 14.1 ± 4.4 mg/dL were found in patients with ARF and rhabdomyolysis (243). Uric acid concentrations of greater than 20.0 mg/dL were seen in five of 21 patients with rhabdomyolysis and ARF in other studies (234,349). Striking increases in uric acid concentrations also occur with ARF in the setting of heat stroke, tumor lysis, and catabolism. Despite high blood uric acid concentrations, there is little evidence of irreversible end-organ disease resulting from hyperuricemia (82,349).

Disorders of Divalent and Trivalent Ion Metabolism

Hyperphosphatemia in the range of 5 to 8 mg/dL often occurs in ARF (233,327,329,335). With mild ARF, the rise in serum phosphorus may be very modest, to the 4 to 5 mg/dL range (326). Decreased urinary excretion of phosphorus contributes to hyperphosphatemia. In addition, phosphorus is released from injured tissue, in which intracellular phosphate concentrations average 100 mmol/L. In the presence of tissue destruction, as in the tumor lysis syndrome and in rhabdomyolysis, extremely high serum phosphorus concentrations are seen. For example, 14 of 34 patients with ARF due to nontraumatic rhabdomyolysis had hyperphosphatemia (>9 mg/dL) in two studies (234,349). In another study, peak serum phosphorus in patients with ARF with and without rhabdomyolysis was 7.0 ± 2.7 and 4.5 ± 1.8 mg/dL, respectively (243). Acute acidosis can also contribute to hyperphosphatemia, by decreasing the glycolytic rate and increasing the rate of hydrolysis of sugar phosphates intracellularly.

Hypocalcemia is also an expected finding in ARF. In the absence of rhabdomyolysis, calcium concentrations usually exceed 6.5 mg/dL (327,329,335). In mild ARF, the serum calcium concentration usually is 8.5 mg/dL or higher (326). Profound hypocalcemia can be observed in rhabdomyolysis-associated ARF. Thus, eight of 35 patients with rhabdomyolysis and ARF had serum calcium concentrations of <6.5 mg/dL (233). The cause of the hypocalcemia of ARF is debated. Phosphate retention with calcium-phosphate deposition in soft tissues can cause some degree of hypocalcemia. However, in some studies, no relationship between hyperphosphatemia and hypocalcemia can be demonstrated, suggesting that additional mechanisms are operative (330). As noted previously, skeletal resistance to the calcemic effect of PTH is present in ARF.

Rarely, hypercalcemia complicates the course of ARF (243,359-361). Although this hypercalcemia usually occurs during the diuretic phase of rhabdomyolysis-induced ARF, it has been reported during the oliguric phase as well (359). The mechanism of this hypercalcemia is unclear. Both increased and decreased PTH levels are reported (243,359). Utilizing electron microscopy and technetium pyrophosphate scanning in four patients with rhabdomyolysis, Akmal et al. (359) demonstrated muscle tissue calcification that disappeared during recovery from ARF. Sperling (336) described one case of rhabdomyolysis in which plasma parathyroid hormone and 1,25-dihydroxyvitamin D levels were suppressed during the period of maximal hypercalcemia while in the recovery phase of ARF. A technetium pyrophosphate scan demonstrated extensive deposition of calcium throughout the pelvic and lower extremity muscles. Meroney et al. (362) administered radiolabeled calcium to dogs with experimental muscle trauma. They found that the isotope was deposited in injured skeletal muscle at a rate nine times that observed in control animals. As noted earlier, hypercalcemia occurring in the early polyuric phase of rhabdomyolysis-associated ARF is associated with increases in

1,25-dihydroxy vitamin D and PTH (233). Two studies demonstrated widespread tissue calcium deposition with calcium-related organ dysfunction in patients becoming hypercalcemic after rhabdomyolysis-associated ARF (243,349). These observations emphasize the importance of recognition and control of this complication of ARF.

Hypermagnesemia in the range of 2.5 to 4.0 mg/dL occurs frequently in ARF (326,327). This range of hypermagnesemia is almost always asymptomatic; however, striking hypermagnesemia can occur if magnesium-containing antacids are administered to patients with ARF.

High plasma aluminum concentrations are traditionally thought to occur exclusively in the setting of chronic renal failure. However, more recent reports demonstrate high plasma aluminum concentrations occurring in the setting of ATN (363,364). In the majority of these patients with ARF, the source of the aluminum appeared to be untreated water used for dialysis (363). Other potential sources include intravesicular alum therapy for hemorrhagic cystitis (364,365), oral feeding, and intravenous albumin (366).

Hematologic Status

Anemia is common with ARF. A recent study by Hales and associates (367) found anemia (hematocrit <35) in 91% of 56 patients with ARF. In this study, the degree of anemia correlated directly with the magnitude of elevation of BUN and was worse in oliguric than in nonoliguric patients (367). The causes of anemia in the ARF setting are multiple and include blood loss from surgical procedures/trauma, the gastrointestinal tract, and phlebotomy for laboratory testing. Contemporary reports establish that ARF may be associated with suppressed serum erythropoietin concentrations (334,368). For example, a report of 10 patients with ATN includes data on serial measurements (radioimmunoassay) of serum erythropoietin (368). Serum erythropoietin levels were very low in patients with ATN. Moreover, several weeks to months were required before serum erythropoietin levels returned to normal, and the normalization of serum erythropoietin lagged far behind the normalization of the GFR. In one patient with ATN, exogenous recombinant erythropoietin resulted in a brisk reticulocytosis and a progressive increase in hemoglobin, suggesting the lack of any endogenous inhibitor of erythropoiesis.

A number of disease states resulting in ARF are associated with significant abnormalities of the hemogram. Thus, ARF associated with a microangiopathic hemolytic process suggests a "vascular" form of ARF (Table 41-4). Eosinophilia suggests the possibility of allergic interstitial nephritis, polyarteritis nodosa, and atheroembolic disease (205,369–371). Anemia and rouleaux formation suggest a plasma cell dyscrasia. Leukopenia and thrombocytopenia often occur in systemic lupus erythematosus.

Coagulation disturbances occur frequently in ARF. Disseminated intravascular coagulation commonly accompanies ARF. Allgren found that of a large number of ARF patients (32% to 42%) were thrombocytopenic and 13% to 27% had coagulopathy (42). Acute renal failure associated with traumatic and atraumatic rhabdomyolysis is often accompanied by thrombocytopenia and disseminated intravascular coagulation (240). Cocaine-associated rhabdomyolysis appears to be associated with an especially high frequency of thrombocytopenia and coagulopathy (372). Preeclampsia and the HELLP syndrome may be associated in severe cases with ARF, thrombocytopenia and disseminated intravascular coagulation (373,374). The use of bioincompatible components in dialysis (intermittent or continuous therapies) may cause activation of platelets, plasmatic coagulation and fibrinolysis (375). Sepsis may cause activation of plasma coagulation, reduction of natural inhibitors of coag-

ulation, defective fibrinolysis, and thrombocytopenia. Consequently septic patients with ARF may develop a "consumptive thrombohemorrhagic disorder" where the initial presentation is hemorrhagic, whilst the initial pathologic event is thrombotic (376). In one study, 19 of 47 patients with intravascular coagulation developed ARF concurrently with or shortly after onset of the coagulopathy (377). However, the absence of either cortical necrosis or microthrombi in the 11 kidneys examined histologically argues against a role for coagulopathy in directly affecting renal function in these patients. Studies in three patients with ARF owing to cardiogenic shock also suggest that intravascular coagulation can contribute to ARF (378). A falling platelet count and a rise in fibrinogen degradation products occurred simultaneously with onset of ARF. Increasing urine output and improved renal function occurred after heparin therapy.

A bleeding diathesis complicating the course of ARF occurred in 16% of the patients reported by Liano and associates (40). A functional defect in platelets leading to a prolongation in the bleeding time is seen in ARF. Thus, hemorrhagic complications contributing to hemostatic abnormalities are seen in 5% to 20% of patients with ARF (77). Bleeding was encountered in 15% of patients before and in an additional 27% of patients after development of ARF in one study (35). Cardiac bypass surgery affects hemostasis by decreasing coagulation factors, due to hemodilution and consumption (provoked by endothelial activation from trauma and artificial surface exposure) (376). Massive transfusion may cause hemostatic failure due to dilution of clotting factors, while storage of blood leads to platelet dysfunction and reduced clotting factors (376). Associated liver disease is often present in patients with ARF.

TREATMENT OF ACUTE RENAL FAILURE

Prevention

In view of the high morbidity and mortality of ARF, it is imperative that maximal effort be directed to prevention of this disorder. General preventative strategies are outlined in Tables 41-14 and 41-15. With regard to nephrotoxins, about 20% to 30% of all cases of ARF can be attributed to one or more nephrotoxic agents (1,37,38,41,55,85) (see Chapters 42–45, 47, 48). The clinical characteristics that place a patient in a high-risk category for nephrotoxin-induced ARF are well known and include the presence of underlying renal ischemia (e.g., volume depletion, congestive heart failure, or an edematous disorder), concomitant exposure to more than a single nephrotoxin, and exposure to high doses of the nephrotoxin. Other characteristics such as advanced age and underlying renal insufficiency may also be important. When good indications for use of a potential nephrotoxin are present in high-risk patients, reasonable guidelines for usage include implementation of the smallest possible dose, clear end points for stopping the drug, measurement and maintenance of normal blood levels (if available), avoidance of concomitant nephrotoxins, maintenance of euvolemia, and serial monitoring of serum creatinine concentration. In some cases, such as with once daily dosage of aminoglycosides (379) or lipid encapsulated amphotericin B (380), dosing and formulation modification may modestly reduce nephrotoxicity (381).

A contemporary study has nicely illustrated the potential value of a computerized surveillance system with electronic notification of clinicians to attenuate nephrotoxin-induced ARF (382). In this study, e-mail messages were sent to clinicians to notify them whenever mild increases in serum creatinine occurred in their patients who were receiving a potential nephrotoxin (382). This notification led to earlier discontinuation of

TABLE 41-14

PREVENTION OF ACUTE RENAL FAILURE

Avoidance of nephrotoxicity
Recognition of agents with nephrotoxic potential
Recognition of high-risk populations
Avoidance of concomitant use of more than one nephrotoxin
Consideration of alternative therapies
Use of smallest dose and briefest duration
Formulation/dosing modification
Monitoring of blood levels if available
Frequent measurement of renal function
Surveillance systems to alert clinicians to changes in renal
    function
Hydration

Minimization of nosocomial infection
Meticulous handwashing
Conservative use and rapid removal of intravascular and
    intravesicular catheters
Cautious use of antibiotics based on culture data with
    automatic stop orders to ensure periodic reassessment
Aspiration pneumonia precautions (elevate head of bed,
    attention to gastric residual volume, conservative use of
    sedatives/hypnotics)

Selected application of pharmacologic intervention
Extracellular fluid expansion
Maintenance of high urine flow
Maintenance of cardiac index and mean arterial pressure
Renal vasodilators
Intravenous albumin
Growth factors
Calcium channel blockers
Miscellaneous agents

Selected application of nonpharmacologic interventions
Preoperative optimization
Maintenance of high oxygen delivery
Minimization of artificial ventilation
Supranormal optimization of cardiovascular hemodynamics
Prophylactic hemofiltration

the offending agent than when clinicians were not notified. Earlier notification and cessation of the offending agent decreased the frequency of development of severe ARF from 7.5% to 3.4%. It is likely that a more powerful intervention (e.g., automatic stop order, clinician telephone notification) could have even earlier, more meaningful impact.

Recommendations to prevent ARF are not uniformly followed. Weisbord and associates (383) reviewed the medical records of "at risk" patients who underwent radiologic investigations using radiocontrast. They found that of 144 patients eligible for intravenous volume expansion, 16% failed to receive any intravenous fluids. NSAIDs and COX-2 inhibitors were prescribed for 8% of patients (383).

Volume Expansion

A large body of experimental data and clinical studies suggest numerous clinical settings in which volume expansion and maintenance of high urine flow rates can protect the kidney from development of ARF (Tables 41-14 and 41-15). Based on a comparison with historic controls, Eisenberg and associates (384) suggested that volume expansion is 100% effective in preventing contrast agent-induced ARF. Currently, nearly all clinicians empirically utilize some form of volume expansion

before, during, and following contrast exposure if the patient's clinical condition permits such therapy (385,386) (see Chapter 45). However, there are no randomized, prospective trials that document effectiveness and compare the efficacy of any fluid administration regimens to "no therapy" (385). Similarly, early anecdotal clinical experience found that hydration decreased/prevented ARF that occurs occasionally in association with cisplatin (387,388). Currently, it is standard of care to hydrate all patients receiving cisplatin therapy if possible (387,388). As with contrast agents, there are no prospective randomized trials that either prove efficacy or hydration or compare various regimens. Amphotericin B often induces ARF (389–391). The nephrotoxicity associated with amphotericin B is directly related to cumulative dosage and worsened by concomitant diuretic administration (390). Although prospective, randomized trials are not available, case reports and anecdotal clinical experience strongly suggest that prophylactic volume expansion decreases the risk of amphotericin B-induced ARF (389–391). In patients with sepsis, the optimal form of volume replacement is unknown. Three meta-analyses have recently compared crystalloid versus colloid solutions: two showing no difference in mortality (392,393) and one showing that colloids increase mortality by 4% (394). A Cochrane review of albumin administration in systemically ill patients showed that albumin increased mortality in comparison to other intravenous solutions (395). In patients with severe sepsis, hydroxyethylstarch was associated with a higher risk of ARF than gelatin (396). Boldt and associates (397) found no difference between hydroxyethylstarch and albumin in a trial of volume replacement in critically ill patients. Finfer and colleagues (398) performed a multicenter randomized controlled trial of resuscitation fluids comparing albumin and saline in critically ill patients. There was no difference in 28-day mortality, organ failure, hospital stay, days on mechanical ventilation, or days on renal replacement therapy (398).

Another setting in which experimental (399–401) and retrospective clinical studies (229,232,236,240,243) suggest a role of volume expansion and maintenance of urine flow to potentially protect the kidneys from development of ARF is in pigmenturic states. In one study, seven individuals were given fluid resuscitation (1.5 to 3.0 L) during extrication and evacuation from crush injury (236). Subsequently, these patients were subjected to massive forced alkaline diuresis, and none developed ARF. The authors of this report have extensive experience dealing with crush injuries and felt that ARF would have been inevitable in these patients in the absence of forced alkaline diuresis. In another series of 21 patients admitted with nontraumatic rhabdomyolysis, 45% of patients responded to volume expansion with an increase in urine output (232). All patients who responded became nonoliguric, did not require dialysis, and survived. In patients who remained oliguric, 9% died, and all required dialysis. The timing of initiation of fluid resuscitation is also important. Gunal and colleagues (242) described a case series of 16 crush victims from the 2003 earthquake in Bingol, Turkey. Early and vigorous fluid resuscitation was performed as described by Better and Stein (402). Duration between rescue and initiation of fluids was significantly longer in the dialyzed victims as compared with nondialyzed ones (9.3 vs. 3.7 hours). To date, potential risks of forced alkaline diuresis in rhabdomyolysis, such as pulmonary edema, worsening muscle edema with neurovascular entrapment, and precipitation of calcium salts in damaged muscle, have not been observed. In view of controlled experimental data and the anecdotal human experience, it appears reasonable to attempt to maintain a carefully monitored diuresis in patients with myoglobinuria. Precise guidelines as to the magnitude of diuresis required to protect the kidneys are not available.

Deposition of relatively insoluble crystals within renal tubules with resulting tubular obstruction is another form of

TABLE 41-15

PHARMACOLOGIC AGENTS THAT HAVE BEEN ADVOCATED TO PREVENT/ATTENUATE CLINICAL ACUTE RENAL FAILURE IN SELECTED SETTINGS

	Prevention	Treatment	Reference
Renal vasodilators			
Dopamine[a]	Neutral	Neutral	(142,405,415,530, 533,534,536)
Fenoldopam	Beneficial (contrast nephropathy)	N/A	(425–428)
Atrial natriuretic peptides	Neutral	Neutral	(42,414,431,433, 434,542–547)
Sympathetic blocking agents			
Clonidine	Neutral	N/A	(178)
Calcium channel blockers	Neutral	N/A	(435–437,442,443)
Inotropic agents			
Dobutamine	Neutral	N/A	(444)
Dopexamine	Neutral	Neutral	(445–448,551)
Norepinephrine	N/A	Neutral	(536–538)
Vasopressin	N/A	Neutral	(539,540)
Diuretic agents			
Furosemide	Harmful	Neutral (beneficial as diuretic)	(406,459–461)
Mannitol	Neutral (beneficial in renal transplantation)	Neutral	(62,64,229,236,240, 242,295,411,413,414, 459,462–468,470, 472–476)
Growth factors			
Insulin-like growth factor	Neutral	Neutral	(479,480,548)
Growth hormone	N/A	Harmful	(549)
Thyroxine	N/A	Neutral	(550)
Theophylline	Beneficial (contrast nephropathy)	N/A	(412,481–484)
Albumin	Beneficial (hepatorenal syndrome)	N/A	(224)
Inflammation			
Endothelin antagonists	Harmful	N/A	(507)
Platelet activating factor	Neutral	N/A	(487–491)
Activated protein C	Beneficial (high APACHE score >25)	N/A	(485,486)
TNF blockade	Neutral	N/A	(493–495)
Nitric oxide synthase inhibitor	Harmful	N/A	(497)
Prostaglandin E1 antagonist	Neutral	N/A	(508)
Inhibitors of leukocyte adhesion	N/A	N/A	(498)
Tissue factor pathway inhibitor	N/A	N/A	(486)
Antithrombin	Neutral	N/A	(499)
Intensive insulin therapy	Beneficial	N/A	(518)
Steroid therapy	Neutral	N/A	(500,501)
N-acetylcysteine	Beneficial (contrast nephropathy)	N/A	(449–454)
Sodium bicarbonate	Beneficial (contrast nephropathy)	N/A	(477)

N/A, not applicable.
Beneficial = overall beneficial effect on renal function; harmful = overall harmful effect on renal function; neutral = no definite benefit or harm to renal function.
[a]See text for discussion of possible harmful effects.

ARF that may be preventable by maintenance of a high urine flow rate (103,104,111,296). Intratubular deposition of uric acid crystals has been clearly demonstrated to be prevented by maintaining a high rate of urine flow in the experimental setting (111,112). Although uric acid solubility is enhanced at an alkaline urinary pH, high urine flow appears to be significantly more protective against uric acid nephropathy than alkaline pH. Methotrexate, sulfadiazine, triamterene, indinavir, and other protease inhibitors, and acyclovir are therapeutic agents that, when administered in high doses, can occasionally be associated with ARF (104). Although the mechanisms of the ARF associated with these agents remain to be precisely defined, intratubular precipitation of insoluble parent drug or drug metabolite appears likely in many cases. Anecdotal experience suggests that maintenance of high urine flow can prevent the kidneys from the nephrotoxicity that occasionally follows high doses of these agents and is currently standard practice (104).

Several pharmacologic agents have been proposed to potentially protect the kidneys from ARF due to a variety of insults. Although much experimental data are available, few controlled clinical trials have evaluated the efficacy of the majority of these agents (Tables 41-14 and 41-15). Two renal vasodilators—low-dose intravenous dopamine and intravenous atrial natriuretic peptide—have been tried as renoprotective agents in several clinical settings.

Dopamine

Dopamine, at doses of 0.5 to 5.0 μg/kg/minute, acts on two populations of dopamine receptors. In the kidney, this action usually results in vasodilation, natriuresis, diuresis, and perhaps an increase in GRF (403). Recently, dopamine has been demonstrated to antagonize the renal vasoconstrictor effects of norepinephrine in healthy men (403). Dopamine has a potential beneficial effect on splanchnic blood flow and oxygen consumption in patients with septic shock, provided the fractional splanchnic flow is not already high before treatment (404). To date, the data on use of dopamine to prevent ARF have generally been disappointing. Although dopamine appears capable of inducing a diuretic effect after major vascular surgery (405), it does not exert a clear-cut renoprotective effect in the settings of cardiac surgery (406,407), elective major vascular surgery (408), or oliguric patients with septic shock (323,409).

It is in the area of prevention of radiocontrast-associated ARF in which most data on dopamine prophylaxis have been obtained. In one study of high-risk patients (those with chronic renal insufficiency, 40% of whom had diabetes), dopamine appeared to exert a renoprotective effect in patients with a serum creatinine $\leq$2.0 mg/dL (410). Similar findings were reported by Hall and associates in patients with chronic renal insufficiency (411). By contrast, dopamine did not protect high-risk patients (mean age 74 years, mean serum creatinine 1.9 mg/dL, 60% diabetic patients) undergoing coronary angioplasty (412). Stevens and associates found no benefit in prevention of ARF by forced diuresis with mannitol, dopamine, and intravenous saline in patients (average serum creatinine 2.5 mg/dL) undergoing angiography (413). Weisberg found that prophylactic dopamine increased the rate of ARF in diabetic patients but perhaps protected nondiabetic patients undergoing coronary angioplasty (414). In summary, although suggestive, the current data do not clearly establish a renoprotective effect of dopamine to prevent contrast-associated ARF.

In a meta-analysis of randomized controlled trials using dopamine in prevention of ARF, Kellum and Decker examined 58 studies ($N = 2,149$), of which 24 were randomized controlled trials ($N = 1,019$) and 5 involved radiocontrast dye ($N = 451$). There was no benefit in favor of dopamine in terms of mortality, incidence of ARF, or requirement for hemodialysis (415).

Dopamine is not without side effects. Dopamine administration requires venous cannulation and local extravasation of dopamine adjacent to an artery may provoke distal ischemia and gangrene (416). Dopamine can depress respiratory drive and may increase cardiac output and myocardial oxygen consumption (even at "renal-doses"), and trigger tachyarrhythmias and myocardial ischemia (417,418). Dopamine may potentially induce or exacerbate hypovolemia and prerenal ARF through its natriuretic effects and trigger hypokalemia and hypophosphatemia. In a porcine model of hemorrhagic shock (419) low-dose dopamine hastened the onset of gut ischemia. The latter complication appeared due to shunting of blood away from the bowel mucosa rather than an absolute reduction in mesenteric blood flow. Dopamine may worsen pituitary dysfunction in critical illness (420). The effect of dopamine wears off after 48 hours, suggesting tolerance of dopaminergic receptors (421,422). There is evidence that in normal subjects, dopamine has unpredictable pharmacokinetic properties and so administration based on body weight may not give a predictable response (423).

Fenoldopam

Fenoldopam mesylate is a dopamine agonist that holds promise for prevention of ARF, particularly in the setting of radiocontrast nephropathy. Fenoldopam blocks reduction in renal plasma flow after radiocontrast (424). One prospective trial and three retrospective trials of fenoldopam in radiocontrast nephropathy support its efficacy (425–428). In elderly patients with severe vascular disease undergoing aortic aneurysmal repair, the use of fenoldopam in an open label uncontrolled trial was associated with a relatively rapid return of renal function to baseline values, despite profound decreases during aortic cross-clamping (429). A study of patients undergoing elective repair of a thoracoabdominal aortic aneurysm found that the use of fenoldopam was associated with reductions in mortality, dialysis requirements, and lengths of stay in the hospital and intensive care unit (430).

Atrial Natriuretic Peptide

Another vasodilator, atrial natriuretic peptide (ANP), or anaritide, has also been studied as a renoprotective agent. Like dopamine, ANP improves renal blood flow and GFR (431) and has also been shown to improve patient hemodynamics during cardiopulmonary bypass (432). Early studies provided no convincing effects for a renoprotective effect of atrial natriuretic peptide and perhaps some worsening of renal function in selected settings (414,433,434). Also an atrial natriuretic peptide did not appear to exert a renoprotective effect after cardiac transplantation in a small study (188).

Clonidine

Several clinical settings are associated with enhanced activity of the sympathetic nervous system. One such setting is cardiac surgery (178,179). A randomized controlled study found that clonidine reduced sympathetic activity and better preserved creatinine clearance than placebo in the immediate postcardiac surgery period (178). No data on the effect of inhibitors of sympathetic activity on the occurrence of ARF are available, to our knowledge.

Calcium Channel Blockers

A wealth of experimental data suggests a renoprotective effect of calcium channel blockers. However, limited clinical data are available. Two prospective studies found that either 20 mg of oral nitrendipine or 10 mg of sublingual nifedipine prevented mild decreases in GFR and renal blood flow after radiocontrast exposure in normal subjects compared with untreated controls (435,436). In a large study, no significant change in serum creatinine was seen in either control or nifedipine treated (20 mg) patients exposed to nonionic contrast (437). The intravenous administration of diltiazem was shown to attenuate the temporary decrease in creatinine clearance that occurs immediately following cardiopulmonary bypass (179). In patients who have undergone cardiac surgery, use of diltiazem postoperatively increases urine output and preserves markers of renal tubular integrity such as urinary alpha-glutathion s-transferase, alpha-1-microglobulin, and N-acetyl-ß-glucosaminidase (438). The addition of intrarenal gallopamil (a potent calcium entry blocking agent) to intravenous furosemide treatment enhanced the recovery of renal function after acute renal failure (439). Fewer patients develop acute tubular necrosis after kidney transplantation when treated with oral (440,441) or intravenous (442) diltiazem, however, graft function, rate of rejection, and graft loss were unchanged (443). These modest human data are inadequate to suggest a potential protective role for calcium channel blockers in clinical settings.

Dobutamine

In many critically ill patients at risk for renal failure, impaired cardiac index is present (23,56,124). Some of these patients are treated with ß-adrenergic agonists such as dobutamine (444). In one comparative study of intensive care unit patients, dopamine induced a diuresis without any change in cardiac index or creatinine clearance, whereas in the same patients, dobutamine increased cardiac index and creatinine clearance without affecting urine output (444). To date there are no data on dobutamine relative to preventing ARF.

Dopexamine

Dopexamine is a dopamine-1 and less potent dopamine-2 agonist. It is also a $\beta 2$ agonist which acts on peripheral vessels and inhibits neuronal reuptake of norepinephrine. It reduces peripheral vascular resistance and increases cardiac output. Dopexamine does not protect against the development of ARF after abdominal surgery (445) or in the setting of cardiopulmonary bypass (446). A marginal benefit was seen in a small trial in patients undergoing aortic surgery (447). No benefit in renal vascular resistive index was seen in patients after coronary bypass surgery (448).

N-acetylcysteine

N-acetylcysteine has recently been advocated as a renoprotective agent, particularly in the setting of radiocontrast nephropathy (see Chapter 45). Tepel and associates (449) randomized 83 patients who underwent CT scanning with IV iopromide to receive N-acetylcysteine (600 mg twice daily) on the day prior to and day of the procedure, or placebo. He found a 90% reduction in radiocontrast nephropathy (defined as number of patients with 0.5 mg/dL rise in serum creatinine 48 hours postcontrast). Since then, several meta-analyses (450–454) have shown that N-acetylcysteine reduces the risk of radiocontrast nephropathy by about 50%. These meta-analyses were flawed by the heterogeneity of trials and variable definitions of what is "radiocontrast nephropathy." Those trials that showed lack of benefit of N-acetylcysteine in prevention of radiocontrast nephropathy may have done so for several reasons, including (a) negative results occurred in trials whose control group had less contrast nephropathy; (b) American studies which were negative used the liquid formulation which may be less efficacious; (c) in some negative studies acetylcysteine was not administered on the day prior to intervention—such a premedication may be required to induce sulfhydryl formation (451); (d) atheroemboli may be a more common cause than contrast nephropathy of ARF leading to dialysis following coronary angiography (455); (e) N-acetylcysteine is less effective in patients with moderate and severe renal impairment as shown in one study (456). The mechanism of action of N-acetylcysteine is unknown, but may include antioxidant effects and blockade of renal vasoconstriction (457). N-acetylcysteine may reduce serum creatinine (by increasing tubular secretion and/or enhancing metabolism) independent of its effect on prevention of radiocontrast nephropathy (458).

Furosemide

Diuretic agents such as furosemide and mannitol have long been used as possible renoprotective agents in high-risk settings for ARF. Recent controlled studies suggest that prophylactic furosemide exerts a deleterious effect on GFR in the setting of cardiac surgery (406). When administered in the setting of radiocontrast exposure, furosemide appears detrimental, even when care is taken to avoid concurrent extracellular fluid volume depletion (459–461). Furosemide is not effective in prevention of ATN due to cephalosporins and aminoglycosides (461).

Mannitol

Mannitol has long been utilized in clinical studies as a renoprotective agent (295,462–468). Early anecdotal experience suggested efficacy in several postoperative and other settings. For example, retrospective clinical experience suggests a beneficial effect of mannitol in some patients with rhabdomyolysis-associated ARF, although a randomized trial-documenting efficacy is not available (64,229,236,240,242,469). Mannitol has also been used in the setting of nephrotoxin exposure, including exposure to cisplatin, amphotericin B, and radiocontrast agents (414,464,466). With regard to amphotericin B, the only prospective randomized trial included 11 patients, and no benefit of mannitol was seen (468). With regard to radiocontrast exposure, mannitol appeared to increase the frequency of contrast nephropathy in one study and in diabetics with renal insufficiency in another study (411,459). In renal insufficiency in nondiabetics, mannitol may provide some renoprotective activity (414). Forced diuresis using a combination of mannitol, furosemide, and dopamine did not provide protection against radiocontrast nephropathy (413). In obstructive jaundice, mannitol does not protect against ARF (470,471). Mannitol does not reduce ARF but may reduce subclinical renal injury in individuals undergoing aortic aneurysm surgery (472). Mannitol in combination with moderate hydration administered prior to cross-clamp in cadaveric renal transplantation improved graft function postoperatively (473–476). In summary, clear-cut data supporting the widespread use of furosemide or mannitol as effective agents to prevent ARF are not available. Anecdotal observations suggest beneficial effects of mannitol in the setting of rhabdomyolysis. Mannitol is reported to cause ARF by inducing renal vasoconstriction and inducing vacuolar damage in renal tubular epithelial cells (62).

Sodium Bicarbonate

Intravenous sodium bicarbonate has been shown to be superior to sodium chloride in reducing the risk of radiocontrast nephropathy in a randomized controlled study of 119 patients with serum creatinine over 1.1 mg/dL (477). The postulated mechanism is alkalinization of urine within the renal medulla which inhibits contrast-induced free radical formation. Following the trial, a registry of 191 individuals receiving sodium bicarbonate for radiocontrast procedures demonstrated an incidence of radiocontrast nephropathy of 1.6% (477).

Growth Factors

Growth factors are among the most recent substances proposed to exert a protective influence to prevent ARF (478,479). Insulin-like growth factor was compared to placebo in 58 patients undergoing surgery of either the suprarenal aorta or the renal arteries (479). At 72 hours postoperatively, placebo-treated patients had decreased their creatinine clearance by 5 mL/minute, whereas growth factor-treated patients had increased their creatinine clearance by 8 mL/minute ($p <0.05$). However, there were no differences in discharge serum creatinine or length of stay when treated and untreated patients were compared. In another study, 43 recipients of cadaveric renal allografts were randomized to receive subcutaneous insulin-like growth factor or placebo (480). Inulin clearance on day 7, nadir serum creatinines after 6 weeks, and need for dialysis did not differ between the two groups. Clearly more study is needed to ascertain if growth factors can act as significant renoprotective agents.

Theophylline

Theophylline has been suggested to protect against development of radiocontrast-associated ARF (412,481–483). Some of these studies suggest that theophylline attenuates the nephrotoxic potential of radiocontrast agents; however, the effect appears to be modest in degree (1,88,481–483). Joachim Ix and colleagues (484) performed a meta-analysis of seven randomized controlled trials of theophylline and aminophylline in patients at risk of radiocontrast nephropathy (pooled sample size $N = 480$). The difference in mean change in serum creatinine was 11.5 μmol/L (95% confidence intervals 5.3–19.4 μmol/L, $p = 0.004$) lower in the theophylline- or aminophylline-treated groups than controls. One participant (0.6%) required dialysis.

Activated Protein C and Other Modulators of Sepsis

A large body of clinical and experimental data suggests that ARF in septic patients is driven by an intense inflammatory process, involving numerous regulatory mediators. Activated protein C (drotrecogin) has been shown in a large randomized controlled study of 1690 patients with sepsis and organ failure (485) to reduce 28-day mortality from 30.8% to 24.7%. Despite FDA approval, questions about study design have prevented universal acceptance of activated protein C as a therapy for patients with sepsis and organ failure (486). Inhibitors of platelet activating factor may decrease organ dysfunction in septic patients, decrease the need for dialysis (487) but do not significantly improve 28 day mortality (487–490). A large phase III trial was prematurely discontinued after interim data from >1250 patients failed to demonstrate improved 28-day all-cause mortality, the primary endpoint of the trial (491). In patients with septic shock, an elevated level of soluble tumor necrosis factor (TNF) receptors was shown to be an independent predictor for the development of ARF and death (492). However, TNF blockade had minimal benefit on mortality in septic patients (493) except in those whose serum interleukin-6 concentrations were elevated (494,495). The intricate relations between endothelial and epithelial cells, based in part on the relations between endothelial and inducible nitric oxide synthases, are perturbed in renal ischemia (496). An inhibitor of nitric oxide synthase was shown to increase mortality in a randomized controlled trial of 797 critically ill patients with septic shock (497). No clinical studies have yet been undertaken of inhibitors of leukocyte adhesion or endothelin (498). High-dose antithrombin III therapy had no effect on 28-day all-cause mortality in adult patients with severe sepsis and septic shock and did not reduce the risk of acute renal failure (499).

Steroid Therapy

Adrenal corticosteroid production is an important protective response during critical illness. Subnormal production of adrenal corticosteroids may result in hemodynamic instability and ongoing evidence of inflammation without an obvious source and lack of response to empirical therapy (498). The use of physiologic doses of steroids in critically ill patients, particularly those with adrenal hyporesponsiveness, has been shown to reduce 28-day mortality (500). However supranormal doses of corticosteroids may be harmful (501).

Minimizing Time of Mechanical Ventilation

Duration of time on mechanical ventilation is associated with increased mortality and renal failure in critically unwell patients (502). Daily interruption of sedation may reduce time on mechanical ventilation (503). Lower tidal volume on ventilation was shown to reduce mortality (504). Mechanical ventilation is associated with the disruption of pulmonary epithelium and endothelium, lung inflammation, atelectasis, hypoxemia, and the release of inflammatory mediators (504). These inflammatory mediators can cause injury to lung and other organs (504). In a rabbit model of acute respiratory distress syndrome, Imai (505) showed that low tidal volume ven-

tilation reduced injurious epithelial cell apoptosis in the kidney in vitro, possibly due to a inhibition of Fas ligand.

Endothelin Antagonists

Endothelin antagonists can prevent experimental ARF (506), and also can block intrarenal vasoconstriction (507). However, the endothelin antagonist SB209670 exacerbated contrast nephropathy in a clinical trial comparing it against placebo in patients receiving 0.45% saline before and after radiocontrast (507).

Prostaglandin E1

Prostaglandin E1 (PGE1) has been studied in a phase I trial of 130 patients with chronic renal impairment undergoing radiocontrast administration (508). The parenteral administration of PGE1 immediately before radiocontrast exposure and continued for a period of 5 to 5.5 hours significantly reduced the elevation of serum creatinine poststudy. The most effective of the three PGE1 dosing regimens tested was 20 ng/kg/minute (508).

Albumin

Impairment of renal function occurs commonly in patients with cirrhosis and spontaneous bacterial peritonitis. In a prospective controlled trial, intravenous albumin (1.5 g/kg at diagnosis followed by 1 g/kg on day 3) decreased the frequency of ARF (defined as a 50% greater increase in pretreatment BUN or serum creatinine to levels >30 and 1.5 mg/dL, respectively) from 33% to 10% ($p = 0.002$) (224).

Preoperative Optimization

With regard to prevention of ARF in a postoperative setting, older studies suggested that "preoperative optimization" could reduce the frequency of ARF in selected high-risk settings (169,509). For example, Berlauk and colleagues (509) have provided data that preoperative "optimization" of cardiovascular hemodynamics—guided by Swan-Ganz measurements—can be helpful in selected patients undergoing limb-salvage arterial surgery. In this randomized prospective study, patients who were "optimized" had less mortality (1.5% vs. 9.5%), graft loss (2.9% vs. 19.0%), and ARF (1.5% vs. 4.8%). Gattinoni and associates found that volume expansion to supranormal cardiac indices and normal mixed venous oxygen saturation had no effect on mortality or incidence/severity of ARF (510). Early institution of treatment to increase central venous oxygen saturation to greater than 70% resulted in lower mortality and less severe organ dysfunction in patients with severe sepsis or septic shock (patients had a mean serum Cr 260 μmol/L) (511). Other retrospective studies suggest similar results in the setting of abdominal aortic aneurysm surgery (169). Confirmation of these results, with delineation of patient populations and optimization regimens of benefit, is needed.

Perfusion with Ringer's Lactate

In a study of patients undergoing thoracoabdominal aorta repair, perfusion of the kidneys with cold Ringer's lactate solution was associated with less renal failure (512).

Improvement of Cardiac Index

With regard to critically ill patients, it has been proposed that the combination of inadequate oxygen delivery and increased tissue oxygen need potentially results in generalized organ ischemia and multiple organ failure. Consequently, in selected patients, fluid volume and pharmacologic therapy manipulated to increase cardiac index and the delivery and consumption of oxygen to "supranormal levels" (cardiac index

>4.5 L/minute/m^2 body surface area; oxygen delivery >600 mg/minute/m^2) is sometimes performed. These supranormal levels are viewed by some as whole-body overcompensation necessary to survive severe critical illness. Does this therapeutic strategy of achievement and maintenance of supranormal cardiac index and oxygen delivery improve outcome and protect the kidney? Five prospective randomized trials have been undertaken to test this hypothesis in heterogeneous groups of seriously ill patients (513–517). Improved survival is seen in some but not all studies. In one study, this therapeutic approach significantly decreased survival (517). Similar results are seen with regard to ARF. It should be noted that the sample sizes of most of these studies are relatively small. Moreover, these catastrophically ill patients often represent an extremely heterogeneous patient population, rendering precise matching of control and experimental subjects difficult. However, to date, compelling evidence that maintaining supranormal values of hemodynamic and oxygen delivery parameters in all cases of catastrophic illness will improve survival and protect the kidneys is not available.

Intensive Glycemic Control

Insulin therapy with aggressive glycemic control has been shown in intensive care patients to reduce mortality and decrease (by 41%) the incidence of ARF requiring dialysis (518). The mechanism of action is not just due to its hypoglycemic effect. Insulin is antiapoptotic and antiinflammatory (519), may reduce the oxidative stress due to hyperglycemia (520), is mitogenic (521) and normalizes lipids (522).

Prophylactic Dialysis

An area of controversy is the use of prophylactic dialysis to prevent ARF. Marenzi and colleagues (523) studied 114 patients with chronic renal failure and a serum creatinine greater than 2 mg/dL who were to undergo coronary angiography. These individuals were randomized to either hemofiltration plus saline hydration or saline hydration alone. Hemofiltration was carried out in an ICU, commenced 4 to 6 hours prior to, stopped during, and continued for 18 to 24 hours after the angiographic procedure. Temporary renal replacement therapy (hemodialysis or hemofiltration) was required in 25% of the control patients and in 3% of the patients in the hemofiltration group. The rate of in-hospital events was 9% in the hemofiltration group and 52% in the control group ($p<0.001$). In-hospital mortality was 2% in the hemofiltration group and 14% in the control group ($p = 0.02$), and the cumulative 1-year mortality was 10% and 30%, respectively ($p = 0.01$). The benefit of dialysis may be due to the ability of the physician to give adequate hydration without fear of volume overload as well as the ability of dialysis to remove radiocontrast after angiography. However, it is not possible based on this study to determine if the benefit of hemofiltration was due to the dialysis procedure, the intensity of medical and nursing care or the use of anticoagulation. Its invasiveness and cost prevents this strategy from being used more widely in the prevention of radiocontrast nephropathy, at least until further studies are done.

Conservative Management

An approach to the overall management of the patient with ARF is presented in Table 41-16. Of primary importance is the exclusion of potentially treatable prerenal, postrenal, and renal parenchymal causes of ARF that may be amenable to specific therapeutic interventions. Once specifically treatable conditions are excluded, it is important to achieve a euvolemic state and to correct any abnormalities in cardiac index that

TABLE 41-16

CONSERVATIVE TREATMENT OF ACUTE RENAL FAILURE

1. Exclude reversible/treatable causes of acute renal failure.
2. Obtain and maintain euvolemic state.
3. Attempt to establish a urine output if patient remains oliguric.
4. Provide adequate nutrition.
5. Minimize use of invasive lines and procedures.
6. Monitor drug usage carefully, and modify dosage or dosing interval appropriately.
7. Monitor and treat for clinical and biochemical complications.
8. Institute renal replacement therapy when appropriate.

are present. If the patient remains oliguric despite a euvolemic state, it has become common clinical practice to attempt to make the patient nonoliguric by administration of potent diuretic agents and/or renal vasodilators (524,525). The rationale for such therapy is the markedly lower morbidity associated with nonoliguric relative to oliguric ARF (38). Moreover, nonoliguric patients have higher GFRs and fewer biochemical and clinical complications than oliguric patients (38).

Diuretics and Renal Vasodilators

Substantial clinical experience allows several generalizations regarding diuretic/vasodilator therapy of patients who continue to be oliguric despite correction of prerenal and postrenal factors and exclusion of treatable renal parenchymal disorders. First, the greatest likelihood of success for converting an oliguric to a nonoliguric state occurs when the duration of oliguria is brief. Prospective randomized trials in oliguric patients in which furosemide was given late in the course of ARF demonstrate no benefit (525–527). In an analysis of 552 critically ill individuals, Mehta and colleagues found that those who were unresponsive to furosemide had a worse prognosis (528). Clinical observations clearly suggest that urinary chemical indices demonstrating more intact tubular function (i.e., lower spot urinary sodium concentration and FE_{Na}, and higher U/P osmolality) as well a briefer duration of oliguria predict a favorable response to furosemide (38,142,294,295). Second, the route of administration of the diuretic may be an important consideration because seriously ill patients with diminished renal function appear to respond more readily to a continuous infusion rather than a bolus of a loop diuretic (529). Third, a small controlled study and anecdotal experience suggest that dopamine may be synergistic with loop diuretics in converting an oliguric to a nonoliguric state (142,530). Although substantial controversy surrounds the issue as to whether dopamine exerts any beneficial effect in oliguric states (531,532), two recent studies clearly document that dopamine can increase urine flow in critically ill, oliguric patients (405,533). For example, Flancbaum and associates (533) used oliguric surgical intensive care unit patients as their own control and could clearly document a diuretic response to low-dose intravenous dopamine, which was reversible after cessation of dopamine. The combination of mannitol, furosemide, and dopamine has been shown to reduce the need for short term dialysis in patients with ARF after cardiac surgery (534). Finally, the complication rate of low-dose dopamine and continuous infusion of a loop diuretic appears to be low. Taken together, although no prospective, randomized controlled data document clinical outcome benefit, we continue to utilize a trial of a loop diuretic occasionally with low-dose dopamine in selected oliguric patients in whom obstructive uropathy has been excluded and prerenal factors corrected.

Inotropic Support

Many experimental and clinical data suggest a beneficial effect of norepinephrine on the urine output in sepsis. A beneficial effect on renal function (glomerular filtration) is a less consistent finding suggesting that blood pressure may be partially responsible for inducing a diuresis (535). It has yet to be demonstrated convincingly that therapeutic doses of norepinephrine compromise renal function in human shock (536) or that dopamine is renoprotective in norepinephrine-treated patients (421,536). Some studies suggest that in patients with septic shock, norepinephrine induces a diuresis more effectively than other vasoactive drugs such as dopamine (537,538). In critically ill septic individuals unresponsive to catecholamines, an infusion of vasopressin may increase urine output, creatinine clearance, blood pressure, and systemic vascular resistance (539,540).

Atrial Natriuretic Peptide

In addition to loop diuretics and dopamine, other renal vasoactive agents have also been used in oliguric patients in an attempt to attenuate ARF. In this regard, experimental and small clinical trials suggested the potential utility of atrial natriuretic peptide (541,542). Rahman and associates (542), in a prospective randomized trial of 53 ARF patients, found that intravenous atrial natriuretic peptide and diuretics, when compared with diuretics alone, decreased the need for dialysis (23% vs. 52%, $p <0.05$) and reduced mortality (17% vs. 35%, $p = 0.11$). Unfortunately, two large-scale multicenter studies failed to find benefit from intravenous infusion of atrial natriuretic peptides in established oliguric and nonoliguric ARF (42,543). Allgren and colleagues (42) examined 504 critically ill patients with ATN. They found that a 24 hour infusion of ANP (0.2 μg/kg/min) did not improve overall dialysis-free survival but did provide benefit in nonoliguric patients. Lewis (544) found that in 222 oliguric ARF patients there was a trend toward higher dialysis-free survival in patients on ANP. Sward (545) randomized 61 patients with nonoliguric ARF after cardiac surgery to ANP (lower dose 0.05 μg/kg/minute) or placebo. She found that ANP was associated with improved dialysis-free survival. Despite randomization, the placebo group had more diabetics ($N = 6$) than the ANP group ($N = 0$). Ularitide is a similar agent to ANP that showed no benefit in patients with ARF after abdominal surgery (546) but was beneficial in reducing the need for dialysis in a randomized study of 14 patients with ARF following cardiac surgery (547). One large-scale multicenter study failed to find benefit from intravenous infusion of ularitide in established oliguric and nonoliguric ARF (543). In summary, there is no consistent evidence for a beneficial role of atrial natriuretic peptides in the treatment of ARF.

Other Pharmacologic Agents

Insulin-like growth factor 1 has also been used in the setting of established ARF (548); however, a multicenter, randomized controlled trial found no benefit of this therapy (548). In patients with prolonged critical illness, high doses of growth hormone were associated with increased morbidity and mortality (549). Likewise, the thyroid hormone, thyroxine, has recently been demonstrated to be of no benefit in treating human ARF (550). Dopexamine (a dopamine agonist) did not improve creatinine clearance in critically ill patients (551).

Nutrition

Provision of adequate nutrition is another important therapeutic goal in the management of patients with ARF (552–556). The catabolic stress of infection and injury often seen in patients with ARF fosters the development of malnutrition with its potential consequences of immunosuppression, infection, poor wound healing, and skeletal muscle weakness (554). The goals of nutritional support in the setting of ARF include restoration of metabolic homeostasis with maintenance of fluid, electrolyte, and acid–base balance; preservation of lean body mass; maximization of protein synthesis; and prevention of vitamin, mineral, and trace element depletion. Obviously, accomplishment of these goals in critically ill, oliguric ARF patients represents a significant clinical challenge. Specific details on guidelines of nutritional assessment, calculation of protein and energy requirements, the products available, and means of administration of these products to meet the protein and energy requirements as well as the standards of care for monitoring nutritional therapy are beyond the scope of this chapter and can be found in readily available sources (552–556).

Monitoring Medication Use

Another aspect of the medical management of ARF that demands attention is careful monitoring of medication and drug usage. Nearly all pharmacologic agents are eliminated, at least in part, by the kidneys. Moreover, the presence of renal failure may impair hepatic metabolism and excretion of selected pharmacologic agents. Also, the consequences of the ARF state may potentiate end-organ responses to several pharmacologic agents, resulting in enhanced activity and possibly toxicity. Finally, the administration of some pharmacologic agents results in concomitant administration of "metabolic loads" (e.g., sodium and potassium) that are often poorly eliminated in patients with ARF. For these reasons, frequent, continuing scrutiny of the medication list is mandatory in all patients with ARF.

Complications of ARF

Clinical and laboratory monitoring are needed to detect the multiple potential complications of ARF. The frequency of this monitoring depends on several factors including the type and severity of underlying illness, whether the patient is oliguric, whether the patient is catabolic, and associated medical conditions.

Three of the most important complications of ARF are volume overload, hyperkalemia, and infection. All of these complications are associated with morbidity and are potentially fatal. All are preventable and/or treatable. With regard to volume overload, daily weight, intake and output, vital signs, oximetry, clinical assessments, and sometimes invasive monitoring are often necessary to evaluate extracellular fluid volume status and cardiac output. Occasional chest x-rays may also help. The most feared consequence of volume overload, pulmonary edema, is particularly difficult to manage in patients with ARF, especially if the patient is oliguric. Two studies emphasize the potential adverse consequences of volume overload in the postoperative setting (557,558). In 21 consecutive cases of postoperative ARF, Murkau and Latimer (557) found that 90% of these patients were grossly fluid overloaded at the time of institution of dialysis by an average of 10 to 11L. A study of Lowell and associates (558) suggested that volume overload per se is an important contributor to postoperative morbidity and mortality. In this study, 40% of 48 consecutive postoperative intensive care unit patients gained more than 10% body weight. Mortality in this group of patients was 32% versus 10% in those gaining <10% body weight. As noted previously, renal response to diuretic agents is markedly impaired in ARF, and the presence of volume overload and pulmonary edema often requires institution of either renal replacement or ultrafiltration therapy (557,558).

TABLE 41-17

TREATMENT OF HYPERKALEMIA IN ACUTE RENAL FAILURE

Modality	Onset	Duration	Mechanism
Calcium (10 mL of 10% calcium gluconate IV, 1–3 doses)	Immediate	30–60 min	Increases threshold potential
Sodium bicarbonate (1–2 ampoules; 45–90 mEq)	5–10 min	1–2 hr	Intracellular shift of potassium
Glucose–insulin (25–50 mL of 50% glucose with 5–10 U of insulin administered as intravenous push)	2–4 hr	30–60 min	Intracellular shift of potassium
Potassium exchange resin (25–50 g of kayexalate plus 70% sorbitol; 20–30 mL orally or 50–100 mL rectal enema)	1–4 hr	Few hours	Removal of potassium
Hemodialysis	2–3 hr	Several hours	Removal of potassium

Hyperkalemia is a frequent accompaniment of ARF and is due to continued potassium release from tissue with decreased renal potassium excretion. In some cases, such as in the presence of rhabdomyolysis, tumor chemotherapy, or extensive hemolysis, the endogenous potassium load results in profound hyperkalemia. Sometimes, exogenous potassium loads such as those occurring with inadvertent administration of potassium intravenously or blood transfusions contribute to hyperkalemia. Hyperkalemia exerts its deleterious effect by raising the resting electrical potential of excitable tissue toward the threshold potential. As the resting potential nears the threshold potential, there is danger of repolarization block with lack of electrical activity and cardiac arrest with asystole. The electrical effects of hyperkalemia are dependent on the rate and magnitude of rise in serum potassium concentration. Abrupt (only a few hours) increases to concentrations of 6.0 mEq/L or greater are often associated with electrocardiographic (ECG) and clinical manifestations, whereas slower (over several days) increases to this level may not be associated with either ECG or clinical findings. The ECG manifestations of hyperkalemia include a symmetrical increase in amplitude with peaking of the T waves (often seen only in leads V2 to V3), a decrease in P waves, widening of the QRS complex, prolongation of the PR interval, and development of left-axis deviation and left bundle branch block. Ultimately, a sine wave pattern and cardiac arrest occur. Rarely, paresthesias, muscular weakness, and flaccid paralysis can be seen with hyperkalemia.

Treatment of hyperkalemia (Table 41-17) is needed whenever ECG changes are present. The presence of neuromuscu-lar signs and symptoms also mandates therapy. Some form of therapy should also be considered when the serum potassium exceeds 5.5 to 6.0 mEq/L. Available therapies with their mode of action, speed of onset, and duration are presented in Table 41-17.

As noted previously, infectious complications commonly complicate the course of patients with ARF and are a frequent cause of death. Minimization of use and duration of invasive catheters is important in an attempt to decrease nosocomial infection. Not only are infections common complications, but also they may be especially difficult to detect in the ARF setting. For example, renal failure can dampen the febrile response to bacteremia (559). Moreover, the leukocytosis that often accompanies an acute bacterial infection may be absent in patients undergoing dialysis (560). A high index of suspicion, aggressive culturing, and early use of specific antimicrobial agents in appropriately modified doses should be the standard of care.

A bleeding tendency can complicate the course of some patients with ARF (40,42,561). This coagulopathy rarely results in spontaneous hemorrhage but can be of potential importance in the setting of operative and invasive procedures. Therapeutic options for the treatment of ARF-related bleeding are outlined in Table 41-18. Intravenous desmopressin rapidly shortens the bleeding time in renal failure. However, its duration of action is brief, and repeated doses lose effectiveness. Cryoprecipitate can shorten the bleeding time for 12 to 24 hours. Conjugated estrogens require 12 to 24 hours to exert their effect to reduce bleeding time in chronic renal failure. Estrogens have a long

TABLE 41-18

TREATMENT OPTIONS FOR HEMORRHAGIC DIATHESIS IN ACUTE RENAL FAILURE

Treatment	Onset	Duration	Comment
Desmopressin (0.3 U/kg body weight IV over 30 min)	1–4 hr	<8–12 hr	Tachyphylaxis with repeated doses
Cryoprecipitate (10 U IV over 10–30 min)	1–4 hr	12–24 hr	Possible risk for hepatitis
Conjugated estrogens (0.6 mg/kg body weight IV over 40 min)	12–24 hr	Several days with repetitive doses	Not well studied in acute renal failure
Elevation of hematocrit (packed RBC sufficient to elevate hematocrit to >30%–35%)	Few hours	Few days	Complications of transfusion

RBC, red blood cells.

duration of action but have not been studied in the setting of ARF. Elevation of the hematocrit to >35% can shorten the bleeding time in ARF.

The anemia of ARF is managed initially by excluding and treating reversible causes (for example hemolysis and blood loss). The anemia of ARF is usually modest and rarely symptomatic. Thus, therapy is reserved for either symptomatic patients (e.g., angina) or for large reductions in hematocrit/hemoglobin, which can usually be attributed to other conditions such as gastrointestinal blood loss. Blood transfusion is indicated in severe cases of anemia. Hebert and colleagues showed that a restrictive policy in transfusing patients if the hemoglobin was less than 7 g/dL rather than 10 g/dL was not associated with increased mortality and was probably superior (562). Recombinant human erythropoietin is effective at reducing transfusion requirements in critically ill patients not requiring dialysis (563). No studies specifically in ARF have been performed (564).

With regard to other biochemical complications of ARF, the development of hyponatremia usually implies administration of excess water, whereas hypobicarbonatemia that can be attributed to renal failure per se rarely requires therapy. In fact, rapid alkanization can, by decreasing ionized calcium, precipitate enhanced neuromuscular activity with carpopedal spasm, cramps, stridor, and seizures.

Usually the mild hypocalcemia that accompanies ARF remains asymptomatic and does not require therapy. The hypercalcemia that rarely occurs in the ARF setting can usually be best managed by dialysis using either a very low or calcium-free dialysate. The hyperphosphatemia of ARF is usually not specifically treated. Although oral aluminum hydroxide can reduce the serum phosphorus in ARF, this agent often leads to constipation. If the serum phosphorus exceeds 7 to 8 mg/dL, then short-term calcium citrate, calcium carbonate, or aluminum hydroxide therapy and/or some form of dialysis can be considered. The modest hypermagnesemia that is seen in ARF can best be managed by removal of all sources of magnesium intake.

The modest hyperuricemia of ARF rarely leads to clinical complications. Because of low GFR, little uric acid is filtered and available for precipitation within the renal tubules. Also, acute gouty arthritis rarely complicates the course of the secondary hyperuricemia of ARF. In cases of either exceptionally high uric acid (>20 to 30 mg/dL) or where it is not clear whether hyperuricemia-induced ARF is present, then dialytic therapy and reduced dosage allopurinol may be therapeutic considerations.

Renal Replacement Therapy

The issues regarding renal replacement therapy in ARF are currently the source of much debate and investigation. The areas of debate include when to start, what modality to use, and how much is enough (36,565–617).

When to Start

Generally agreed-on indications for institution of renal replacement therapy for ARF include persistent hyperkalemia, fluid overload unresponsive to conventional treatment, ongoing marked acidemia, symptoms of uremia, and occasionally, bleeding. Based on substantial retrospective data and historic data, most nephrologists also feel that "prophylactic" dialysis to keep the BUN and creatinine 90 to 100 and 9 to 10 mg/dL, respectively, can be readily justified (565,578,606). There are, however, no definitive data supporting these numbers. Moreover, a general trend to even earlier renal replacement therapy has occurred over the past decade based on recent studies. A prospective study of cardiac surgical patients randomized 61

patients to early (oliguria unresponsive to furosemide) or late dialysis (dialysis when serum creatinine greater than 5 mg/dl or potassium greater than 5.5 mmol/L) (577). The "early" group started dialysis earlier (0.9 vs. 2.5 days), stayed less in ICU (7.9 vs. 12 days) and had lower mortality (23 vs. 55%) (577). A retrospective analysis of 100 trauma patients with ARF found that, after controlling for injury severity score, a lower BUN at initiation of dialysis was associated with earlier commencement of dialysis and better survival (578). In a prospective trial of 425 patients comparing different rates of ultrafiltration on continuous hemofiltration, Ronco (579) found that a lower BUN before commencement of dialysis was associated with lower mortality. However, one study of 132 critically ill ARF patients found an inverse relationship between serum creatinine at initiation of hemodialysis and increased mortality (601). A high percentage of patients with ARF, particularly those with mild, nonoliguric ARF, do not require renal replacement therapy. By contrast, intensive and often continuous renal replacement therapy is frequently needed in catabolic intensive care unit patients with severe, oliguric ARF. Moreover, the fluid-volume requirement to maintain nutritional status often dictates early institution of some type of renal replacement therapy in many ICU patients with ARF.

What Modality to Use

There is debate about the optimal modes of renal replacement therapy for patients with ARF. Generally available modes of therapy include conventional intermittent hemodialysis (IHD), intermittent and continuous peritoneal dialysis (PD), continuous arteriovenous hemofiltration (CAVH), continuous arteriovenous hemodialysis (CAVHD), continuous venovenous hemofiltration (CVVH), and continuous venovenous hemodialysis (CVVHD). A survey conducted several years ago in the United States indicated that IHD followed by types of continuous renal replacement therapies and then, infrequently, PD were the modes most often used to treat ARF (576). There has been a widespread, increasing trend to use more continuous therapy, especially CVVHD in critically ill patients.

Several non–patient-related factors must be considered when selecting a mode of renal replacement therapy. Such factors include the availability of the necessary equipment, the expertise demanded by each modality, and the cost of each modality. Patient-related factors that must be considered include the patient's hemodynamic status, the indication for therapy and speed with which the indication must be corrected, the patient's catabolic state, the availability of vascular access, the requirement for patient mobility, the anticipated fluid-volume load that will be given to the patient, the associated clinical conditions of the patient, and the anticipated duration of therapy.

Peritoneal dialysis is rarely performed currently in adults as a treatment modality for ARF (576). However, this modality can be used in adults, especially those with a strong contraindication to anticoagulation, and peritoneal dialysis is more frequently used in children with ARF (602). Peritoneal catheter placement may be either temporary (percutaneous with maximal longevity generally limited to 48 to 72 hours because of infection) or indwelling (can be inserted under local anesthesia and maintained indefinitely). Peritoneal dialysis does not require anticoagulation, can be done on a continuous basis allowing for constant removal of volume and solute, and can be performed in patients with hemodynamic instability. However, the relative efficiency of peritoneal dialysis is such that removal of solute and fluid is only 10% to 20% that of hemodialysis. This inefficiency generally limits usage in patients with ARF who require significant volume and solute removal, although peritoneal dialysis has been used successfully to manage posttraumatic ARF (607). Additionally, the frequency of intraabdominal surgery and acute respiratory failure make PD impractical in critically unwell patients (580). Absorption of dextrose may lead to hepatic steatosis, increased carbon dioxide production causing worse respiratory failure, and hyperglycemia (581). Survival of PD patients was no different to hemodialysis patients in one small study (36).

The IHD modality has been in widespread use for the past four decades for the treatment of ARF (576). In recent years, the development of bicarbonate-based dialysate and volumetrically controlled machines for precise regulation of ultrafiltration has made IHD a safer procedure in the hemodynamically unstable ICU patient with multiorgan failure. In most centers in the United States, the standard approach to IHD for ARF uses moderate blood flow rates (200 to 250 mL/minute) and dialysate flow rates of 500 mL/minute. The most common reasons cited for preferential choice of IHD are efficacy, ease of use, familiarity with the modality, ready availability of nursing personnel familiar with the procedure, and ability to rapidly correct life-threatening fluid volume, electrolyte and acid–base disorders. Concerns about use of IHD include the fact that a reasonably good and stable level of mean arterial pressure is needed to safely and effectively use this modality. Moreover, any IHD-associated hemodynamic instability, combined with potentially impaired ability of the injured kidney to autoregulate blood flow, could either induce new ischemia or perpetuate previous ischemia (608).

Most recently, continuous modes of renal replacement therapy, especially CVVHD, have been increasingly utilized (565,572,574,575,602,603,605). Continuous modes of therapy such as CVVHD are especially useful for patients who have low mean arterial pressure, are hemodynamically unstable, are hypercatabolic, or have a requirement for large fluid volumes. Measurement of clearance and solute removal using CVVHD suggests treatment comparable to five quality IHD sessions per week (574,575).

The major disadvantage of CRRT is the need for well-trained ICU nursing personnel to perform the procedure. A lack of detailed understanding of the CRRT flow sheets and the computations necessary to determine replacement fluid volumes can lead to significant complications regarding significant volume depletion or excess. Occasionally, lactate-based replacement fluid may result in lactate accumulation and worsening acid–base status if the patient has liver disease and is unable to metabolize lactate as a source of base. On-site formulation of custom bicarbonate-containing replacement fluid is costly and time consuming. Ambulation and physical therapy is difficult while the patient is receiving CRRT.

CRRT is associated with activation of the inflammatory and coagulation pathways, and removal of antioxidants and cytokines (584,585). Removal of cytokines appears to be mediated by adsorption onto the dialysis membrane (586). Two recent studies suggest a hemodynamic and metabolic benefit of dialysis in patients with intractable circulatory shock without renal failure (587,588). It is uncertain if any such benefit is due to removal of cytokines or another mechanism (e.g. cooling, fluid removal) (589,590).

Because of difficulties precisely matching seriously ill patients with ARF, a clear-cut consensus as to whether IHD or CVVHD is a preferable mode of renal replacement therapy has not emerged. It is likely, however, that ARF patients are best served by considering these modalities as complementary rather than as competing therapeutic options. Martin and colleagues (582) have shown that continuous therapies are preferentially given to patients with marked hemodynamic compromise. The choice of modality may also be limited by availability of equipment and trained nursing staff (583). In this regard, the recent careful analysis of Swartz and associates is of interest (575). In this retrospective analysis of over 300 patients, the higher mortality seen with CVVH appeared clearly related to severity of

case mix and comorbidity rather than modality of treatment. When matched populations were analyzed retrospectively, no clear-cut outcome differences by modality of renal replacement therapy were apparent. A prospective randomized study of 166 patients compared continuous renal replacement therapy with intermittent hemodialysis after excluding individuals with severe hypotension (591). Despite randomization there were differences between groups that favored the intermittent hemodialysis group. After adjusting for confounders, there was no significant difference between modalities in terms of mortality or renal survival (591). Two systematic reviews (592,593) showed no difference between intermittent and continuous therapies, but after adjusting for study quality and severity of illness, Kellum found a decreased relative risk of death with continuous therapies. Different methodologies, small numbers of patients, study flaws, and lack of standardized approaches to timing and indications of dialytic intervention make accurate comparisons between modalities problematical (594,595).

New modalities of dialysis incorporating the advantages of hemodynamic stability of CRRT coupled with high rates of solute and fluid removal of intermittent hemodialysis have emerged. In slow low efficiency daily dialysis, or SLEDD, near conventional dialysis equipment is used at low blood and dialysate flow rates, for prolonged periods of time (6 to 12 hours/day). This modality offers more hemodynamic stability, better correction of hypervolemia, and more adequate solute removal, compared with IHD (596) and compares favorably with CRRT in terms of patient outcomes (597). SLEDD also uses less nursing resources and does not require intensive anticoagulation (600). The single-path batch dialysis system uses a closed-loop system comprising a 75-L dialysate tank which lasts for 18 hours of extended single-path high-flux hemodialysis. It was well tolerated by critically ill patients in two small series (598,599).

Another controversial issue with regard to RRT in ARF is selection of dialysis membrane (565,566,570,571,609–612). The polysaccharide structure of cellulosic (bioincompatible) membranes provides a trigger for complement activation via the alternative pathway, which leads to the liberation of anaphylotoxins and activation of leukocytes. The potential induction of a systemic inflammatory reaction during such dialysis treatment with bioincompatible dialysis membranes could conceivably cause further ischemia or inflammatory changes within the previously injured renal microcirculation.

In a recent study of 72 patients with ARF, patients were randomized to intermittent dialysis treatment with either bioincompatible Cuprophane dialysis membranes, which activate the complement system and leukocytes, or to dialysis with a biocompatible membrane composed of polymethyl methacrylate, which has a less marked effect on complement and leukocytes (610). The two dialysis membranes chosen for the study had similar clearance and ultrafiltration characteristics and the patient groups were similar. Fifty-seven percent of patients on dialysis with biocompatible membranes survived, compared with 37% of these dialyzed with Cuprophane membranes ($p = 0.11$). Recovery of renal function occurred in 62% of those dialyzed with a biocompatible membrane, compared with 37% of those who underwent dialysis with Cuprophane membranes ($p = 0.04$). The time to recovery of renal function after initiation of dialysis was also significantly shorter in the biocompatible membrane group compared with the Cuprophane group: five dialysis treatments over 11 days versus 17 dialysis treatments over 33 days, respectively. Subgroup analysis revealed that the benefits of biocompatible membrane dialysis were evident only in patients who were nonoliguric before the initiation of dialysis. These results suggest that use of the biocompatible dialysis membrane increases the likelihood of recovery of renal function and survival of patients with ARF. Other studies have confirmed and extended these observations to include other biocompatible dialysis membranes, including polysulfone, and polyacrylonitrile membranes (571); however, this issue may not be quite a clear-cut as those two studies suggest. For example, in recent prospective studies a clear-cut advantage of biocompatible membranes has not emerged (566,609,612). A meta-analysis by Jaber (567) demonstrated that the use of a biocompatible membrane did not significantly affect mortality among patients with ARF who require IHD. However, a meta-analysis by Subramanian (568) (which included an additional 169 patients from one trial) found a relative risk of mortality for cellulosic (bioincompatible) membranes of 1.37 (CI, 1.02–1.83). Given the known proinflammatory effects of these membranes in experimental models, the shift in clinical practice toward increased use of synthetic membranes in the setting of ARF, and the now reasonable cost of biocompatible membranes (in comparison to cellulose membranes), it is unlikely that this question will be resolved (569).

How Much Is Enough?

A final area of controversy with regard to RRT in ARF is how much is enough? Schiffl (613) randomized 160 patients with ARF to receive either daily hemodialysis or intermittent (second-daily) dialysis. Patients perceived to require CRRT because of hemodynamic instability were excluded. Daily hemodialysis resulted in better control of uremia, fewer hypotensive episodes during hemodialysis, and more rapid resolution of ARF (9 vs. 16 days) than did conventional hemodialysis. More patients in the conventional-hemodialysis group than in the daily-hemodialysis group had the systemic inflammatory response syndrome or sepsis, respiratory failure, changes in mental status, or gastrointestinal bleeding. The mortality rate, according to the intention-to-treat analysis, was 28% for daily dialysis and 46% for alternate-day dialysis. The mean time averaged urea concentration in the conventional hemodialysis group was 104 mg/dL, suggesting that this group was inadequately dialyzed and that the difference in outcomes was therefore more marked. Ronco (579) studied 425 patients with ARF commencing continuous venovenous hemofiltration, randomly assigning ultrafiltration at 20 mL/hour/kg, 35 mL/hour/kg, or 45 mL/hour/kg. Survival (calculated at 15 days after stopping dialysis) in the lowest ultrafiltration group was significantly lower (41%) than in the other groups respectively (57% and 58%). Renal survival was nonstatistically worse in the lowest ultrafiltration group. Increasing the dose of dialysis in these two studies improved both patient and renal survival. Measurement of dose in dialysis in ARF patients is not possible with the same techniques as in stable chronic hemodialysis patients due to lack of steady-state of urea generation and fluid compartments; however models have been developed (615–617).

Outcome and Prognosis of Acute Renal Failure

The outcome of ARF is highly dependent on the definition of the disorder and the patient population studied. In epidemiologic studies undertaken in general medical-surgical hospitals, ARF has often been defined as an increase of 0.25 to 1.0 mg/dL in serum creatinine. Although this appears to be a very mild increase in serum creatinine, it likely reflects at least a 30% to 60% decrement in GFR. In such ARF patients, mortality rates of 20% to 30% have been reported (37,55). These mortality rates exceed those for comparable hospitalized patients who do not develop ARF by a factor of 6 to 10 (55). Only 10% to 20% of these patients require dialytic therapy. When series of patients with ARF are identified by either reviewing consultations to a renal service or by retrospective reviews of discharge diagnoses, the selection bias generally results in a more seri-

TABLE 41-19

PROGNOSTIC FACTORS IN ACUTE RENAL FAILURE

Severity of renal dysfunction
Magnitude of rise in serum creatinine concentration
Urinalysis
Fractional excretion of sodium
Presence of oliguria or anuria
Requirement for renal replacement therapy
Duration of renal dysfunction
Underlying health of the patient
Age
Presence, severity, and reversibility of underlying disease
Clinical circumstances
Cause of the renal failure
Severity and reversibility of acute process(es)
Number and type of other organ systems failed
Development of sepsis and other complications

ously ill group of patients with more pronounced renal failure. In such patients, contemporary mortality rates of 30% to 60% are reported, with 30% to 50% of patients requiring dialytic therapy (35,39–44,312,618,619). Finally, many series report outcome and prognostic variables only in patients with ARF who have undergone dialytic therapy. In these patients, current mortality rates range from 50% to 90% (35,39–44,312,619).

A case-control study emphasizes some of the important outcome aspects of contemporary ARF (49). In this study, 183 patients with radiocontrast-associated ARF (defined as an increase in serum creatinine of at least 25% to at least 2 mg/dL) were matched to comparable patients exposed to radiocontrast that did not develop ARF. Mortality was 7% in control and 34% in ARF patients. After adjustment for comorbidity, the adjusted odds ratio for death with ARF was 5.5. The development of ARF was not only associated with death, but also with development of respiratory failure, sepsis, and bleeding (Fig. 41-9).

As alluded to previously, a major prognostic factor in patients with ARF is the severity and duration of the resultant renal dysfunction (Table 41-19, Figs. 41-8 and 41-9). Hou and collaborators (37), in a large prospective study, found that the presence of urinalysis abnormalities in patients with ARF had a marked influence on outcome. Death occurred in 31% of ARF patients with normal urine sediment and in 74% ($p < 0.025$) of patients with abnormal urine sediment (37). These observations have also been reported in other studies and probably

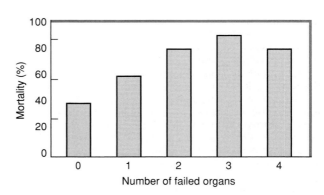

FIGURE 41-8. Acute renal failure mortality relative to number of organ systems failed. (From: Star RA. Treatment of acute renal failure. *Kidney Int* 1998;54:1817.)

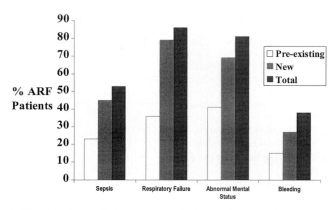

FIGURE 41-9. Morbidity occurring before and after radiocontrast-associated acute renal failure. (From: Levy EM, Viscoli CM, Horwitz RI. The effect of acute renal failure on mortality. *JAMA* 1996;275:1489, with permission.)

reflect outcome differences between prerenal azotemia (normal sediment) and renal azotemia (abnormal sediment). Hou and collaborators (37) also found a direct correlation between mortality and the magnitude of rise in serum creatinine in patients with ARF. The mortality rate was less than 20% to 30% until the increment in serum creatinine exceeded 3 mg/dL, at which time the mortality rate was 64%.

Other likely indicators of severity of renal insult in patients with ARF are the quantity and quality of urine output. Virtually all contemporary studies of patients with ARF find mortality rates of nonoliguric patients to be less than half of those of oliguric patients (Fig. 41-2).

It is unclear whether or not patients with acute renal failure due to sepsis appear to have a worse prognosis than those with non-septic acute renal failure. Confounding variables make an independent association among sepsis, ARF, and mortality difficult to tease out. In a prospective multicenter study of 345 patients with ARF, Levy (35) found that sepsis was an independent predictor of hospital mortality (OR, 2.51) and need for mechanical ventilation. Cytokine levels are also predictive of greater mortality in patients with septic ARF (620). Hoste (324) found that there was a high incidence of nosocomial bloodstream infection in a subgroup of severely ill patients with ARF who were treated with RRT in the ICU. However, nosocomial bloodstream infection did not lead to a statistically significant increased length of stay, costs, or mortality (324).

One advance in the study of ARF that has occurred over the past decade has been in the area of development of indices that predict ARF outcome (621–634). The issue of predicting outcome and estimating the probability of survival for individual patients with ARF is important with regard to cost-effective allocation of resources. Also, determination of severity of illness and likelihood of survival is important with regard to quality assurance assessment and comparability of patient populations for controlled prevention and treatment trials.

Most patients with ARF are seen in an ICU setting. Several multipurpose scoring systems for ICU patients have been designed to provide estimates of hospital mortality (621). These systems are all based on rigorous research involving several thousand patients from multiple sites for both development and validation studies (621). Some of three widely used systems (Acute Physiology and Chronic Health Evaluation or APACHE, Mortality Probability Models or MPM, and the Simplified Acute Physiology Score or SAPS) use logistic regression techniques and have evolved through three generations of development. These systems appear capable of assessing prog-

nosis, comparing different ICU performances, and stratifying patients for clinical studies. However, the number of patients with ARF included in the development of these ICU scoring systems was modest at best. Thus, it is perhaps not surprising that these general ICU scoring systems perform suboptimally with regard to ARF, inasmuch as they often underestimate the risks of death when applied to an exclusive ARF population (459). A study has validated the APACHE system for 153 patients with ARF (635). This has led to the development of "ARF specific" prognostic indices (622–634).

Perhaps the best of the ARF specific prediction tools is the one developed by Liano and colleagues (56,565,628,629). This tool was initially based on retrospectively obtained data and has been validated, prospectively. When applied to ARF mortality in both the ICU (actual 72%, predicted 65%) and the non-ICU (actual 32%, predicted 32%) setting, this instrument performed well (56). Renal failure accounts for 21% of this index, whereas comorbid conditions such as hypotension, jaundice, and assisted ventilation account for the remainder. Inclusion of comorbid conditions as a key aspect of ARF outcome is important. For example, in one large series, the cause of death could be directly attributed to underlying disease in 61% of the ARF deaths (56). The performance of the Liano scale and other scales in prediction of ARF mortality are discussed in Star (565). Recently, the observation that blacks may have especially high ARF morbidity and mortality has been emphasized (3).

One simple but powerful method to assess ARF mortality is in the context of the number of associated failed organs (565). An estimated association is depicted in Figure 41-8. In general, associated failure of more than two organ systems places ARF outcome in the vicinity of 10% to 20% likelihood of survival.

There has been recent discussion whether the prognosis of patients with ARF has improved. Improving general medical care and supportive therapy and changes in case-mix do not allow for a definitive answer to this issue. However, a Mayo Clinic study provides a qualified yes to the suggestion that modern therapy has been associated with improved ARF outcome (43). In this analysis of dialyzed patients with ARF, overall mortality declined from 68% to 48% when the years 1977 to 1979 were compared with 1991 to 1993. Stratification by APACHE II revealed markedly improved mortality in the two compared time frames in patients with either low (36% to 11%), or moderate (75% to 35%) but not high scores (100% to 85%). Modern medical management does not appear to be helping those with the greatest chance of dying.

In general, recovery from oliguric ARF due to acute tubular necrosis occurs relatively quickly (636). In our experience, the majority of patients with oliguric ATN require renal replacement therapy for roughly 5 to 15 days. Notable exceptions occur, particularly in elderly patients, patients with multiple organ failure or patients in whom ATN complicates the course of solid organ transplantation. In the experience of Kjellstrand and associates (636), the median time from initiation of dialysis to recovery of renal function in survivors was 12 days. Usually, renal function has reached maximal levels within 4 to 6 weeks after the last dialysis for ARF. However, there are notable published exceptions of protracted, slow, continuous recovery of renal function (637–639). There is also a small but significant group of patients with ARF that do not recover renal function. For example, Bhandry and Turney recently reported that 16% of 1095 patients with severe ARF failed to recover renal function and needed chronic RRT (639). Only six patients recovered sufficient renal function to become independent of dialysis after 3 to 18 months on regular dialysis therapy (6 to 21 months after onset of ARF) (639). The frequency of lack of renal recovery from ARF was highest for ARF attributed to renal parenchymal disease (35%) and less high for ARF occurring in either a medical (9%) or surgical (6%) setting. These latter settings likely reflected ATN as a cause of the ARF.

CONCLUSION

Acute renal failure is commonly encountered in contemporary medical practice. Acute renal failure is the end product of a variety of insults operating via several pathophysiologic mechanisms. At present, an incomplete understanding of the pathophysiology of human ARF hampers effective therapy to uniformly prevent, attenuate, and hasten recovery from ARF (640,641). However, effects directed toward prevention, early detection, timely diagnosis of the cause/predisposing factor(s), and specific intervention remain the keys to reducing the significant mortality and morbidity of ARF.

References

1. Thadani R, Pascual M, Bonventre JV. Acute renal failure. *N Engl J Med* 1996;334:1448.
2. Elasy TA, Anderson RJ. Changing demography of acute renal failure. *Semin Dial* 1996;9:438.
3. Obialo CI, Okonofua EC, Tayade AS, et al. Epidemiology of de novo acute renal failure in hospitalized African Americans: comparing community-acquired vs hospital-acquired disease. *Arch Intern Med* 2000;160:1309.
4. Couchoud C, Pozet N, Labeeuw M, et al. Screening early renal failure: cutoff values for serum creatinine as an indicator of renal impairment. *Kidney Int* 1999;55:1878.
5. Moran SM, Myers BD. Course of acute renal failure studied by a model of creatinine kinetics. *Kidney Int* 1985;27:928.
6. Rabb H. Evaluation of urinary markers in acute renal failure. *Curr Opin Nephrol Hypertens* 1998;7:681.
7. Ichimura T, Bonventre JV, Bailly V, et al. Kidney injury molecule-1 (KIM-1), a putative epithelial cell adhesion molecule containing a novel immunoglobulin domain, is up-regulated in renal cells after injury. *J Biol Chem* 1998;273:4135.
8. Han WK, Bailly V, Abichandani R, et al. Kidney Injury Molecule-1 (KIM-1): a novel biomarker for human renal proximal tubule injury. *Kidney Int* 2002;62:237.
9. Muramatsu Y, Tsujie M, Kohda Y, et al. Early detection of cysteine rich protein 61 (CYR61, CCN1) in urine following renal ischemic reperfusion injury. *Kidney Int* 2002;62:1601.
10. Westhuyzen J, Endre ZH, Reece G, et al. Measurement of tubular enzymuria facilitates early detection of acute renal impairment in the intensive care unit. *Nephrol Dial Transplant* 2003;18:543.
11. Coll E, Botey A, Alvarez L, et al. Serum cystatin C as a new marker for noninvasive estimation of glomerular filtration rate and as a marker for early renal impairment. *Am J Kidney Dis* 2000;36:29.
12. Parikh CR, Jani A, Melnikov VY, et al. Urinary interleukin-18 is a marker of human acute tubular necrosis. *Am J Kidney Dis* 2004;43:405.
13. du Cheyron D, Daubin C, Poggioli J, et al. Urinary measurement of Na$^+$/H$^+$ exchanger isoform 3 (NHE3) protein as new marker of tubule injury in critically ill patients with ARF. *Am J Kidney Dis* 2003;42:497.
14. Hu H, Aizenstein BD, Puchalski A, et al. Elevation of CXCR3-binding chemokines in urine indicates acute renal-allograft dysfunction. *Am J Transplant* 2004;4:432.
15. Tolkoff-Rubin NE, Cosimi AB, Delmonico FL, et al. Diagnosis of tubular injury in renal transplant patients by a urinary assay for a proximal tubular antigen, the adenosine-deaminase-binding protein. *Transplantation* 1986;41:593.
16. Di Paolo S, Gesualdo L, Stallone G, et al. Renal expression and urinary concentration of EGF and IL-6 in acutely dysfunctioning kidney transplanted patients. *Nephrol Dial Transplant* 1997;12:2687.
17. Taman M, Liu Y, Tolbert E, et al. Increase urinary hepatocyte growth factor excretion in human acute renal failure. *Clin Nephrol* 1997;48:241.
18. Feest TG, Round A, Hamad S. Incidence of severe acute renal failure in adults: results of a community based study. *BMJ* 1993;306:481.
19. Perez Gutthann S, Garcia Rodriguez LA, Raiford DS, et al. Nonsteroidal anti-inflammatory drugs and the risk of hospitalization for acute renal failure. *Arch Intern Med* 1996;156:2433.
20. Nzerue CM, Hewan-Lowe K, Nwawka C. Acute renal failure in pregnancy: a review of clinical outcomes at an inner-city hospital from 1986–1996. *J Natl Med Assoc* 1998;90:486.
21. Stratta P, Besso L, Canavese C, et al. Is pregnancy-related acute renal failure a disappearing clinical entity? *Ren Fail* 1996;18:575.
22. Behrend T, Miller SB. Acute renal failure in the cardiac care unit: etiologies, outcomes, and prognostic factors. *Kidney Int* 1999;56:238.
23. McCullough PA, Wolyn R, Rocher LL, et al. Acute renal failure after coronary intervention: incidence, risk factors, and relationship to mortality. *Am J Med* 1997;103:368.
24. Conlon PJ, Stafford-Smith M, White WD, et al. Acute renal failure following cardiac surgery. *Nephrol Dial Transplant* 1999;14:1158.
25. Chertow GM, Lazarus JM, Christiansen CL, et al. Preoperative renal risk stratification. *Circulation* 1997;95:878.
26. Mattana J, Singhal PC. Prevalence and determinants of acute renal failure following cardiopulmonary resuscitation. *Arch Intern Med* 1993;153:235.
27. Welage LS, Walawander CA, Timm EG, et al. Risk factors for acute renal insufficiency in patients with suspected or documented bacterial pneumonia. *Ann Pharmcother* 1994;28:515.
28. Rayner BL, Willcox PA, Pascoe MD. Acute renal failure in community-acquired bacteraemia. *Nephron* 1990;54:32.
29. Conlon PJ, Procop GW, Fowler V, et al. Predictors of prognosis and risk of acute renal failure in patients with Rocky Mountain spotted fever. *Am J Med* 1996;101:621.
30. Rao TK. Acute renal failure syndromes in human immunodeficiency virus infection. *Semin Nephrol* 1998;18:378.
31. D'Agati V, Appel GB. HIV infection and the kidney. *J Am Soc Nephrol* 1997;8:138.
32. Morris JA, Jr, Mucha P, Jr, Ross SE, et al. Acute posttraumatic renal failure: a multicenter perspective. *J Trauma* 1991;31:1584.
33. Vivino G, Antonelli M, Moro ML, et al. Risk factors for acute renal failure in trauma patients. *Intensive Care Med* 1998;24:808.
34. Holm C, Horbrand F, von Donnersmarck GH, et al. Acute renal failure in severely burned patients. *Burns* 1999;25:171.
35. Levy EM, Viscoli CM, Horwitz RI. The effect of acute renal failure on mortality. A cohort analysis. *JAMA* 1996;275:1489.
36. Rodgers H, Staniland JR, Lipkin GW, et al. Acute renal failure: a study of elderly patients. *Age Ageing* 1990;19:36.
37. Hou SH, Bushinsky DA, Wish JB, et al. Hospital-acquired renal insufficiency: a prospective study. *Am J Med* 1983;74:243.
38. Anderson RJ, Linas SL, Berns AS, et al. Nonoliguric acute renal failure. *N Engl J Med* 1977;296:1134.
39. Corwin HL, Teplick RS, Schreiber MJ, et al. Prediction of outcome in acute renal failure. *Am J Nephrol* 1987;7:8.
40. Liano F, Garcia-Martin F, Gallego A, et al. Easy and early prognosis in acute tubular necrosis: a forward analysis of 228 cases. *Nephron* 1989;51:307.
41. Sandhu JS, Sood A, Midha V, et al. Non-traumatic rhabdomyolysis with acute renal failure. *Ren Fail* 2000;22:81.
42. Allgren RL, Marbury TC, Rahman SN, et al. Anaritide in acute tubular necrosis. Auriculin Anaritide Acute Renal Failure Study Group. *N Engl J Med* 1997;336:828.
43. McCarthy JT. Prognosis of patients with acute renal failure in the intensive-care unit: a tale of two eras. *Mayo Clin Proc* 1996;71:117.
44. Brivet FG, Kleinknecht DJ, Loirat P, et al. Acute renal failure in intensive care units—causes, outcome, and prognostic factors of hospital mortality; a prospective, multicenter study. French Study Group on Acute Renal Failure. *Crit Care Med* 1996;24:192.
45. Manns B, Doig CJ, Lee H, et al. Cost of acute renal failure requiring dialysis in the intensive care unit: clinical and resource implications of renal recovery. *Crit Care Med* 2003;31:449.
46. Hamel MB, Phillips RS, Davis RB, et al. Outcomes and cost-effectiveness of initiating dialysis and continuing aggressive care in seriously ill hospitalized adults. SUPPORT Investigators. Study to Understand Prognoses and Preferences for Outcomes and Risks of Treatments. *Ann Intern Med* 1997;127:195.
47. Korkeila M, Ruokonen E, Takala J. Costs of care, long-term prognosis and quality of life in patients requiring renal replacement therapy during intensive care. *Intensive Care Med* 2000;26:1824.
48. Jurado R, Mattix H. The decreased serum urea nitrogen-creatinine ratio. *Arch Intern Med* 1998;158:2509.
49. Rabito CA, Panico F, Rubin R, et al. Noninvasive, real-time monitoring of renal function during critical care. *J Am Soc Nephrol* 1994;4:1421.
50. Han JS, Kim YS, Chin HJ, et al. Temporal changes and reversibility of carbamylated hemoglobin in renal failure. *Am J Kidney Dis* 1997;30:36.
51. Stim J, Shaykh M, Anwar F, et al. Factors determining hemoglobin carbamylation in renal failure. *Kidney Int* 1995;48:1605.
52. Tasanarong A, Seublinvong T, Eiam-Ong S. The role of carbamylated hemoglobin in identifying acute and chronic renal failure. *J Med Assoc Thai* 2002;85:462.
53. Wynckel A, Randoux C, Millart H, et al. Kinetics of carbamylated haemoglobin in acute renal failure. *Nephrol Dial Transplant* 2000;15:1183.
54. Anderson RJ, Schrier RW. Acute renal failure. In: Schrier RW, Gottschalk CW, eds. *Diseases of the kidney*. Boston: Little, Brown, 1996:1069.
55. Shusterman N, Strom BL, Murray TG, et al. Risk factors and outcome of hospital-acquired acute renal failure. Clinical epidemiologic study. *Am J Med* 1987;83:65.
56. Liano F, Junco E, Pascual J, et al. The spectrum of acute renal failure in the intensive care unit compared with that seen in other settings. The Madrid Acute Renal Failure Study Group. *Kidney Int Suppl* 1998;66:S16.
57. Kaufman J, Dhakal M, Patel B, et al. Community-acquired acute renal failure. *Am J Kidney Dis* 1991;17:191.

58. SelCuk NY, Odabas AR, Cetinkaya R, et al. Frequency and outcome of patients with acute renal failure have more causes than one in etiology. Ren Fail 2000;22:459.
59. Sesso R, Roque A, Vicioso B, et al. Prognosis of ARF in hospitalized elderly patients. Am J Kidney Dis 2004;44:410.
60. Horgan KJ, Ottaviano YL, Watson AJ. Acute renal failure due to mannitol intoxication. Am J Nephrol 1989;9:106.
61. Moran M, Kapsner C. Acute renal failure associated with elevated plasma oncotic pressure. N Engl J Med 1987;317:150.
62. Dorman HR, Sondheimer JH, Cadnapaphornchai P. Mannitol-induced acute renal failure. Medicine (Baltimore). 1990;69:153.
63. Liano F, Pascual J. Epidemiology of acute renal failure: a prospective, multi-center, community-based study. Madrid Acute Renal Failure Study Group. Kidney Int 1996;50:811.
64. Badr KF, Ichikawa I. Prerenal failure: a deleterious shift from renal compensation to decompensation. N Engl J Med 1988;319:623.
65. Murray MD, Brater DC. Effects of NSAIDs on the kidney. Prog Drug Res 1997;49:155.
66. Gambaro G, Perazella MA. Adverse renal effects of anti-inflammatory agents: evaluation of selective and nonselective cyclooxygenase inhibitors. J Intern Med 2003;253:643.
67. Toto RD. Renal insufficiency due to angiotensin-converting enzyme inhibitors. Miner Electrolyte Metab 1994;20:193.
68. Packer M, Lee WH, Medina N, et al. Functional renal insufficiency during long-term therapy with captopril and enalapril in severe chronic heart failure. Ann Intern Med 1987;106:346.
69. Kelleher SP, Robinette JB, Conger JD. Sympathetic nervous system in the loss of autoregulation in acute renal failure. Am J Physiol 1984;246:F379.
70. Conger J, Robinette J, Villar A, et al. Increased nitric oxide synthase activity despite lack of response to endothelium-dependent vasodilators in postischemic acute renal failure in rats. J Clin Invest 1995;96:631.
71. Noiri E, Peresleni T, Miller F, et al. In vivo targeting of inducible NO synthase with oligodeoxynucleotides protects rat kidney against ischemia. J Clin Invest 1996;97:2377.
72. Textor SC, Novick AC, Tarazi RC, et al. Critical perfusion pressure for renal function in patients with bilateral atherosclerotic renal vascular disease. Ann Intern Med 1985;102:308.
73. Roche Z, Rutecki G, Cox J, et al. Reversible acute renal failure as an atypical presentation of ischemic nephropathy. Am J Kidney Dis 1993;22:662.
74. Radermacher J, Chavan A, Bleck J, et al. Use of Doppler ultrasonography to predict the outcome of therapy for renal-artery stenosis. N Engl J Med 2001;344:410.
75. Carpenter CC. Clinical studies in Asiatic cholera II. Development of 2:1 saline:lactate regimen. Comparison of this regimen with traditional methods of treatment April and May, 1963. Bull Johns Hopkins Hosp 1966;118:174.
76. Babior BM. Villous adenoma of the colon. Study of a patient with severe fluid and electrolyte disturbances. Am J Med 1966;41:615.
77. McMurray SD, Luft FC, Maxwell DR, et al. Prevailing patterns and predictor variables in patients with acute tubular necrosis. Arch Intern Med 1978;138:950.
78. Akhtar M, Yashpal, Jetley V, et al. Renal failure in acute pancreatitis. J Assoc Physicians India 1995;43:176.
79. Company L, Saez J, Martinez J, et al. Factors predicting mortality in severe acute pancreatitis. Pancreatology 2003;3:144.
80. Chrysopoulo MT, Jeschke MG, Dziewulski P, et al. Acute renal dysfunction in severely burned adults. J Trauma 1999;46:141.
81. Kim GH, Oh KH, Yoon JW, et al. Impact of burn size and initial serum albumin level on acute renal failure occurring in major burn. Am J Nephrol 2003;23:55.
82. Schrier RW, Henderson HS, Tisher CC, et al. Nephropathy associated with heat stress and exercise. Ann Intern Med 1967;67:356.
83. Vertel RM, Knochel JP. Acute renal failure due to heat injury. An analysis of ten cases associated with a high incidence of myoglobinuria. Am J Med 1967;43:435.
84. Tan W, Herzlich BC, Funaro R, et al. Rhabdomyolysis and myoglobinuric acute renal failure associated with classic heat stroke. South Med J 1995;88:1065.
85. Davidman M, Olson P, Kohen J, et al. Iatrogenic renal disease. Arch Intern Med 1991;151:1809.
86. Woodrow G, Brownjohn AM, Turney JH. Acute renal failure in patients with type 1 diabetes mellitus. Postgrad Med J 1994;70:192.
87. Arieff AI, Carroll HJ. Nonketotic hyperosmolar coma with hyperglycemia: clinical features, pathophysiology, renal function, acid-base balance, plasma-cerebrospinal fluid equilibria and the effects of therapy in 37 cases. Medicine (Baltimore) 1972;51:73.
88. Kim U, Dreiling DA, Kark AE, et al. Factors influencing mortality in surgical treatment for massive gastroduodenal hemorrhage. Am J Gastroenterol 1974;62:24.
89. Cardenas A, Gines P, Uriz J, et al. Renal failure after upper gastrointestinal bleeding in cirrhosis: incidence, clinical course, predictive factors, and short-term prognosis. Hepatology 2001;34:671.
90. Gupta BK, Spinowitz BS, Charytan C, et al. Cholesterol crystal embolization-associated renal failure after therapy with recombinant tissue-type plasminogen activator. Am J Kidney Dis 1993;21:659.
91. Toupin LR, Blanchard DG. Acute anuric renal failure: a complication of combined thrombolytic and antithrombotic therapy. Int J Cardiol 1993;40:283.
92. Hojs R, Sinkovic A, Hojs-Fabjan T. Rhabdomyolysis and acute renal failure following cardioversion and cardiopulmonary resuscitation. Ren Fail 1995;17:765.
93. Lindsay J, Apple S, Pinnow EE, et al. Percutaneous coronary intervention-associated nephropathy foreshadows increased risk of late adverse events in patients with normal baseline serum creatinine. Catheter Cardiovasc Interv 2003;59:338.
94. Gruberg L, Mehran R, Dangas G, et al. Acute renal failure requiring dialysis after percutaneous coronary interventions. Catheter Cardiovasc Interv 2001;52:409.
95. Koreny M, Karth GD, Geppert A, et al. Prognosis of patients who develop acute renal failure during the first 24 hours of cardiogenic shock after myocardial infarction. Am J Med 2002;112:115.
96. Fraley DS, Burr R, Bernardini J, et al. Impact of acute renal failure on mortality in end-stage liver disease with or without transplantation. Kidney Int 1998;54:518.
97. Gines A, Escorsell A, Gines P, et al. Incidence, predictive factors, and prognosis of the hepatorenal syndrome in cirrhosis with ascites. Gastroenterology 1993;105:229.
98. Gines P, Guevara M, Arroyo V, et al. Hepatorenal syndrome. Lancet 2003;362:1819.
99. Halimi C, Bonnard P, Bernard B, et al. Effect of terlipressin (Glypressin) on hepatorenal syndrome in cirrhotic patients: results of a multicentre pilot study. Eur J Gastroenterol Hepatol 2002;14:153.
100. Bhandari S, Johnston P, Fowler RC, et al. Non-dilated bilateral ureteric obstruction. Nephrol Dial Transplant 1995;10:2337.
101. Chapman ME, Reid JH. Use of percutaneous nephrostomy in malignant ureteric obstruction. Br J Radiol 1991;64:318.
102. Kjellstrand CM, Cambell DC, 2nd, von Hartitzsch B, et al. Hyperuricemic acute renal failure. Arch Intern Med 1974;133:349.
103. Haas M, Ohler L, Watzke H, et al. The spectrum of acute renal failure in tumour lysis syndrome. Nephrol Dial Transplant 1999;14:776.
104. Perazella MA. Crystal-induced acute renal failure. Am J Med 1999;106:459.
105. Klahr S. Renal failure after jejunoileal bypass for obesity. Am J Med 1979;67:971.
106. Mandell I, Krauss E, Millan JC. Oxalate-induced acute renal failure in Crohn's disease. Am J Med 1980;69:628.
107. Famularo G, Di Toro S, Moretti S, et al. Symptomatic crystalluria associated with indinavir. Ann Pharmcother 2000;34:1414.
108. Hermieu J, Prevot M, Ravery V, et al. Urolithiasis and the protease inhibitor indinavir. Eur Urol 1999;35:239.
109. Reilly RF, Tray K, Perazella MA. Indinavir nephropathy revisited: a pattern of insidious renal failure with identifiable risk factors. Am J Kidney Dis 2001;38:E23.
110. Moist L, Nesrallah G, Kortas C, et al. Plasma exchange in rapidly progressive renal failure due to multiple myeloma. A retrospective case series. Am J Nephrol 1999;19:45.
111. Conger JD, Falk SA. Intrarenal dynamics in the pathogenesis and prevention of acute urate nephropathy. J Clin Invest 1977;59:786.
112. Conger JD, Falk SA, Guggenheim SJ, et al. A micropuncture study of the early phase of acute urate nephropathy. J Clin Invest 1976;58:681.
113. Norman RW, Mack FG, Awad SA, et al. Acute renal failure secondary to bilateral ureteric obstruction: review of 50 cases. Can Med Assoc J 1982;127:601.
114. Grundy DJ, Rainford DJ, Silver JR. The occurrence of acute renal failure in patients with neuropathic bladders. Paraplegia 1982;20:35.
115. Ansari ER, Kazim E, Husain I. Management of the choked ureter in obstructive renal failure due to uric acid lithiasis. J Urol 1982;128:257.
116. Zager RA. Endotoxemia, renal hypoperfusion, and fever: interactive risk factors for aminoglycoside and sepsis-associated acute renal failure. Am J Kidney Dis 1992;20:223.
117. Molitoris BA, Meyer C, Dahl R, et al. Mechanism of ischemia-enhanced aminoglycoside binding and uptake by proximal tubule cells. Am J Physiol 1993;264:F907.
118. Choudhury D, Ahmed Z. Drug-induced nephrotoxicity. Med Clin North Am 1997;81:705.
119. Perazella MA. Acute renal failure in HIV-infected patients: a brief review of common causes. Am J Med Sci 2000;319:385.
120. Ault BH, Stapleton FB, Gaber L, et al. Acute renal failure during therapy with recombinant human gamma interferon. N Engl J Med 1988;319:1397.
121. Textor SC, Margolin K, Blayney D, et al. Renal, volume, and hormonal changes during therapeutic administration of recombinant interleukin-2 in man. Am J Med 1987;83:1055.
122. Cayco AV, Perazella MA, Hayslett JP. Renal insufficiency after intravenous immune globulin therapy: a report of two cases and an analysis of the literature. J Am Soc Nephrol 1997;8:1788.
123. Rasmussen HH, Ibels LS. Acute renal failure. Multivariate analysis of causes and risk factors. Am J Med 1982;73:211.
124. Breen D, Bihari D. Acute renal failure as a part of multiple organ failure: the slippery slope of critical illness. Kidney Int Suppl 1998;66:S25.
125. Groeneveld AB, Tran DD, van der Meulen J, et al. Acute renal failure in the medical intensive care unit: predisposing, complicating factors and outcome. Nephron 1991;59:602.

126. Pascual J, Liano F. Causes and prognosis of acute renal failure in the very old. Madrid Acute Renal Failure Study Group. *J Am Geriatr Soc* 1998;46:721.
127. Fortescue EB, Bates DW, Chertow GM. Predicting acute renal failure after coronary bypass surgery: cross-validation of two risk-stratification algorithms. *Kidney Int* 2000;57:2594.
128. Preston RA, Stemmer CL, Materson BJ, et al. Renal biopsy in patients 65 years of age or older. An analysis of the results of 334 biopsies. *J Am Geriatr Soc* 1990;38:669.
129. Field TS, Gurwitz JH, Glynn RJ, et al. The renal effects of nonsteroidal anti-inflammatory drugs in older people: findings from the Established Populations for Epidemiologic Studies of the Elderly. *J Am Geriatr Soc* 1999;47:507.
130. Linares P, Vivas S, Jorquera F, et al. Severe cholestasis and acute renal failure related to rofecoxib. *Am J Gastroenterol* 2004;99:1622.
131. Morales E, Mucksavage JJ. Cyclooxygenase-2 inhibitor-associated acute renal failure: case report with rofecoxib and review of the literature. *Pharmacotherapy* 2002;22:1317.
132. Papaioannides D, Bouropoulos C, Sinapides D, et al. Acute renal dysfunction associated with selective COX-2 inhibitor therapy. *Int Urol Nephrol* 2001;33:609.
133. Silverstein FE, Faich G, Goldstein JL, et al. Gastrointestinal toxicity with celecoxib vs nonsteroidal anti-inflammatory drugs for osteoarthritis and rheumatoid arthritis: the CLASS study: a randomized controlled trial. Celecoxib Long-term Arthritis Safety Study. *JAMA* 2000;284:1247.
134. Silvester W, Bellomo R, Cole L. Epidemiology, management, and outcome of severe acute renal failure of critical illness in Australia. *Crit Care Med* 2001;29:1910.
135. Rangel-Frausto MS, Pittet D, Costigan M, et al. The natural history of the systemic inflammatory response syndrome (SIRS). A prospective study. *JAMA* 1995;273:117.
136. Fenves AZ. Legionnaires' disease associated with acute renal failure: a report of two cases and review of the literature. *Clin Nephrol* 1985;23:96.
137. Fung AS, Leikis MJ, McMahon LP. Acute renal failure associated with Legionella pneumonia and acute cholecystitis. *Nephrology (Carlton)* 2004;9:105.
138. Montseny JJ, Meyrier A, Kleinknecht D, et al. The current spectrum of infectious glomerulonephritis. Experience with 76 patients and review of the literature. *Medicine (Baltimore)* 1995;74:63.
139. Jones SR. Acute renal failure in adults with uncomplicated acute pyelonephritis: case reports and review. *Clin Infect Dis* 1992;14:243.
140. Bruno P, Hassell LH, Brown J, et al. The protean manifestations of hemorrhagic fever with renal syndrome. A retrospective review of 26 cases from Korea. *Ann Intern Med* 1990;113:385.
141. Ramsay AG, Olesnicky L, Pirani CL. Acute tubulo-interstitial nephritis from candida albicans with oliguric renal failure. *Clin Nephrol* 1985;24:310.
142. Lumlertgul D, Keoplung M, Sitprija V, et al. Furosemide and dopamine in malarial acute renal failure. *Nephron* 1989;52:40.
143. De Vriese AS. Prevention and treatment of acute renal failure in sepsis. *J Am Soc Nephrol* 2003;14:792.
144. Wan L, Bellomo R, Di Giantomasso D, et al. The pathogenesis of septic acute renal failure. *Curr Opin Crit Care* 2003;9:496.
145. Cunningham PN, Dyanov HM, Park P, et al. Acute renal failure in endotoxemia is caused by TNF acting directly on TNF receptor-1 in kidney. *J Immunol* 2002;168:5817.
146. Cunningham PN, Wang Y, Guo R, et al. Role of Toll-like receptor 4 in endotoxin-induced acute renal failure. *J Immunol* 2004;172:2629.
147. Feriozzi S, Muda AO, Massimetti C, et al. Sepsis-induced acute renal failure: unusual clinical presentation. *J Nephrol* 1998;11:261.
148. Betrosian A, Thireos E, Kofinas G, et al. Bacterial sepsis-induced rhabdomyolysis. *Intensive Care Med* 1999;25:469.
149. Yegenaga I, Hoste E, Van Biesen W, et al. Clinical characteristics of patients developing ARF due to sepsis/systemic inflammatory response syndrome: results of a prospective study. *Am J Kidney Dis* 2004;43:817.
150. Rogiers P. Hemofiltration treatment for sepsis: is it time for controlled trials? *Kidney Int Suppl* 1999;72:S99.
151. Sieberth HG, Kierdorf HP. Is cytokine removal by continuous hemofiltration feasible? *Kidney Int Suppl* 1999;72:S79.
152. Valeri A, Neusy AJ. Acute and chronic renal disease in hospitalized AIDS patients. *Clin Nephrol* 1991;35:110.
153. Connolly JO, Weston CE, Hendry BM. HIV-associated renal disease in London hospitals. *QJM* 1995;88:627.
154. Rao TK. Renal complications in HIV disease. *Med Clin North Am* 1996;80:1437.
155. Peraldi MN, Maslo C, Akposso K, et al. Acute renal failure in the course of HIV infection: a single-institution retrospective study of ninety-two patients and sixty renal biopsies. *Nephrol Dial Transplant* 1999;14:1578.
156. Barrios A, Garcia-Benayas T, Gonzalez-Lahoz J, et al. Tenofovir-related nephrotoxicity in HIV-infected patients. *Aids* 2004;18:960.
157. Gaspar G, Monereo A, Garcia-Reyne A, et al. Fanconi syndrome and acute renal failure in a patient treated with tenofovir: a call for caution. *Aids* 2004;18:351.
158. Shelburne SA, 3rd, Hamill RJ. The immune reconstitution inflammatory syndrome. *AIDS Rev* 2003;5:67.
159. Jehle AW, Khanna N, Sigle JP, et al. Acute renal failure on immune reconstitution in an HIV-positive patient with miliary tuberculosis. *Clin Infect Dis* 2004;38:e32.
160. Rao TK, Friedman EA. Outcome of severe acute renal failure in patients with acquired immunodeficiency syndrome. *Am J Kidney Dis* 1995;25:390.
161. Charlson ME, MacKenzie CR, Gold JP, et al. Postoperative changes in serum creatinine. When do they occur and how much is important? *Ann Surg* 1989;209:328.
162. Leacche M, Rawn JD, Mihaljevic T, et al. Outcomes in patients with normal serum creatinine and with artificial renal support for acute renal failure developing after coronary artery bypass grafting. *Am J Cardiol* 2004;93:353.
163. Stallwood MI, Grayson AD, Mills K, et al. Acute renal failure in coronary artery bypass surgery: independent effect of cardiopulmonary bypass. *Ann Thorac Surg* 2004;77:968.
164. Mangano CM, Diamondstone LS, Ramsay JG, et al. Renal dysfunction after myocardial revascularization: risk factors, adverse outcomes, and hospital resource utilization. The Multicenter Study of Perioperative Ischemia Research Group. *Ann Intern Med* 1998;128:194.
165. Bert AA. Systemic effects of normothermic cardiopulmonary bypass. *Artif Organs* 1998;22:77.
166. Christenson JT, Maurice J, Simonet F, et al. Normothermic versus hypothermic perfusion during primary coronary artery bypass grafting. *Cardiovasc Surg* 1995;3:519.
167. Kellerman PS. Perioperative care of the renal patient. *Arch Intern Med* 1994;154:1674.
168. Gornick CC, Jr, Kjellstrand CM. Acute renal failure complicating aortic aneurysm surgery. *Nephron* 1983;35:145.
169. Hesdorffer CS, Milne JF, Meyers AM, et al. The value of Swan-Ganz catheterization and volume loading in preventing renal failure in patients undergoing abdominal aortic aneurysmectomy. *Clin Nephrol* 1987;28:272.
170. Parks RW, Diamond T, McCrory DC, et al. Prospective study of postoperative renal function in obstructive jaundice and the effect of perioperative dopamine. *Br J Surg* 1994;81:437.
171. Sugrue M, Jones F, Deane SA, et al. Intra-abdominal hypertension is an independent cause of postoperative renal impairment. *Arch Surg* 1999;134:1082.
172. Kron IL, Harman PK, Nolan SP. The measurement of intra-abdominal pressure as a criterion for abdominal re-exploration. *Ann Surg* 1984;199:28.
173. Ulyatt D. Elevated intra-abdominal pressure. *Australas Anesth* 1992:108.
174. Bloomfield GL, Blocher CR, Fakhry IF, et al. Elevated intra-abdominal pressure increases plasma renin activity and aldosterone levels. *J Trauma* 1997;42:997.
175. Mikami O, Fujise K, Matsumoto S, et al. High intra-abdominal pressure increases plasma catecholamine concentrations during pneumoperitoneum for laparoscopic procedures. *Arch Surg* 1998;133:39.
176. Schein M, Ivatury R. Intra-abdominal hypertension and the abdominal compartment syndrome. *Br J Surg* 1998;85:1027.
177. Sadovnikoff N. Perioperative acute renal failure. *Int Anesthesiol Clin* 2001;39:95.
178. Kulka PJ, Tryba M, Zenz M. Preoperative alpha2-adrenergic receptor agonists prevent the deterioration of renal function after cardiac surgery: results of a randomized, controlled trial. *Crit Care Med* 1996;24:947.
179. Amano J, Suzuki A, Sunamori M, et al. Effect of calcium antagonist diltiazem on renal function in open heart surgery. *Chest* 1995;107:1260.
180. Regel G, Lobenhoffer P, Grotz M, et al. Treatment results of patients with multiple trauma: an analysis of 3406 cases treated between 1972 and 1991 at a German Level I Trauma Center. *J Trauma* 1995;38:70.
181. Tran DD, Cuesta MA, Oe PL. Acute renal failure in patients with severe civilian trauma. *Nephrol Dial Transplant* 1994;9(Suppl 4):121.
182. Sever MS, Erek E, Vanholder R, et al. Lessons learned from the catastrophic Marmara earthquake: factors influencing the final outcome of renal victims. *Clin Nephrol* 2004;61:413.
183. Sever MS, Erek E, Vanholder R, et al. Renal replacement therapies in the aftermath of the catastrophic Marmara earthquake. *Kidney Int* 2002;62:2264.
184. Wilkinson AH, Cohen DJ. Renal failure in the recipients of nonrenal solid organ transplants. *J Am Soc Nephrol* 1999;10:1136.
185. Cruz DN, Perazella MA. Acute renal failure after cardiac transplantation: a case report and review of the literature. *Yale J Biol Med* 1996;69:461.
186. Stevens LM, El-Hamamsy I, Leblanc M, et al. Continuous renal replacement therapy after heart transplantation. *Can J Cardiol* 2004;20:619.
187. Ouseph R, Brier ME, Jacobs AA, et al. Continuous venovenous hemofiltration and hemodialysis after orthotopic heart transplantation. *Am J Kidney Dis* 1998;32:290.
188. Brenner P, Meyer M, Reichenspurner H, et al. Significance of prophylactic urodilatin (INN: ularitide) infusion for the prevention of acute renal failure in patients after heart transplantation. *Eur J Med Res* 1995;1:137.
189. Alejandro DS, Petersen J. Myoglobinuric acute renal failure in a cardiac transplant patient taking lovastatin and cyclosporine. *J Am Soc Nephrol* 1994;5:153.
190. Bilbao I, Charco R, Balsells J, et al. Risk factors for acute renal failure requiring dialysis after liver transplantation. *Clin Transplant* 1998;12:123.
191. Paramesh AS, Roayaie S, Doan Y, et al. Post-liver transplant acute renal failure: factors predicting development of end-stage renal disease. *Clin Transplant* 2004;18:94.
192. Zager RA. Acute renal failure in the setting of bone marrow transplantation. *Kidney Int* 1994;46:1443.

193. Parikh CR, Sandmaier BM, Storb RF, et al. Acute renal failure after nonmyeloablative hematopoietic cell transplantation. *J Am Soc Nephrol* 2004;15:1868.
194. Parikh CR, McSweeney PA, Korular D, et al. Renal dysfunction in allogeneic hematopoietic cell transplantation. *Kidney Int* 2002;62:566.
195. Gruss E, Bernis C, Tomas JF, et al. Acute renal failure in patients following bone marrow transplantation: prevalence, risk factors and outcome. *Am J Nephrol* 1995;15:473.
196. Zager RA. Acute renal failure syndromes after bone marrow transplantation. *Adv Nephrol Necker Hosp* 1997;27:263.
197. Pulla B, Barri YM, Anaissie E. Acute renal failure following bone marrow transplantation. *Ren Fail* 1998;20:421.
198. Merouani A, Shpall EJ, Jones RB, et al. Renal function in high dose chemotherapy and autologous hematopoietic cell support treatment for breast cancer. *Kidney Int* 1996;50:1026.
199. Bruno B, Zager RA, Boeckh MJ, et al. Adenovirus nephritis in hematopoietic stem-cell transplantation. *Transplantation* 2004;77:1049.
200. Rich MW. Epidemiology, pathophysiology, and etiology of congestive heart failure in older adults. *J Am Geriatr Soc* 1997;45:968.
201. Zeiner A, Sunder-Plassmann G, Sterz F, et al. The effect of mild therapeutic hypothermia on renal function after cardiopulmonary resuscitation in men. *Resuscitation* 2004;60:253.
202. Broman M, Kallskog O. The effects of hypothermia on renal function and haemodynamics in the rat. *Acta Physiol Scand* 1995;153:179.
203. Broman M, Kallskog O, Kopp UC, et al. Influence of the sympathetic nervous system on renal function during hypothermia. *Acta Physiol Scand* 1998;163:241.
204. Sabharwal R, Johns EJ, Egginton S. The influence of acute hypothermia on renal function of anaesthetized euthermic and acclimatized rats. *Exp Physiol* 2004;89:455.
205. Wilson DM, Salazer TL, Farkouh ME. Eosinophiluria in atheroembolic renal disease. *Am J Med* 1991;91:186.
206. Bell SP, Frankel A, Brown EA. Cholesterol emboli syndrome—uncommon or unrecognized? *J R Soc Med* 1997;90:543.
207. Abuelo JG. Diagnosing vascular causes of renal failure. *Ann Intern Med* 1995;123:601.
208. Selcuk NY, Tonbul HZ, San A, et al. Changes in frequency and etiology of acute renal failure in pregnancy (1980–1997). *Ren Fail* 1998;20:513.
209. Turney JH, Marshall DH, Brownjohn AM, et al. The evolution of acute renal failure, 1956-1988. *Q J Med* 1990;74:83.
210. Jena M, Mitch WE. Rapidly reversible acute renal failure from ureteral obstruction in pregnancy. *Am J Kidney Dis* 1996;28:457.
211. Sibai BM, Ramadan MK. Acute renal failure in pregnancies complicated by hemolysis, elevated liver enzymes, and low platelets. *Am J Obstet Gynecol* 1993;168:1682.
212. Chugh KS, Jha V, Sakhuja V, et al. Acute renal cortical necrosis—a study of 113 patients. *Ren Fail* 1994;16:37.
213. Lanore JJ, Brunet F, Pochard F, et al. Hemodialysis for acute renal failure in patients with hematologic malignancies. *Crit Care Med* 1991;19:346.
214. Blade J, Fernandez-Llama P, Bosch F, et al. Renal failure in multiple myeloma: presenting features and predictors of outcome in 94 patients from a single institution. *Arch Intern Med* 1998;158:1889.
215. Weinman EJ, Patak RV. Acute renal failure in cancer patients. *Oncology (Huntingt)* 1992;6:47.
216. Harris KP, Hattersley JM, Feehally J, et al. Acute renal failure associated with haematological malignancies: a review of 10 years experience. *Eur J Haematol* 1991;47:119.
217. Obrador GT, Price B, O'Meara Y, et al. Acute renal failure due to lymphomatous infiltration of the kidneys. *J Am Soc Nephrol* 1997;8:1348.
218. Shalmi CL, Dutcher JP, Feinfeld DA, et al. Acute renal dysfunction during interleukin-2 treatment: suggestion of an intrinsic renal lesion. *J Clin Oncol* 1990;8:1839.
219. Hsu HH, Chan YL, Huang CC. Acute spontaneous tumor lysis presenting with hyperuricemic acute renal failure: clinical features and therapeutic approach. *J Nephrol* 2004;17:50.
220. Hsu HH, Huang CC. Acute spontaneous tumor lysis in anaplastic large T-cell lymphoma presenting with hyperuricemic acute renal failure. *Int J Hematol* 2004;79:48.
221. Davidson MB, Thakkar S, Hix JK, et al. Pathophysiology, clinical consequences, and treatment of tumor lysis syndrome. *Am J Med* 2004;116:546.
222. Sato A, Imaizumi M, Chikaoka S, et al. Acute renal failure due to leukemic cell infiltration followed by relapse at multiple extramedullary sites in a child with acute lymphoblastic leukemia. *Leuk Lymphoma* 2004;45:825.
223. Tokar M, Rogachev B, Levi I, et al. Rituximab in a patient with acute renal failure due to B-cell lymphomatous infiltration of the kidneys. *Leuk Lymphoma* 2004;45:819.
224. Sort P, Navasa M, Arroyo V, et al. Effect of intravenous albumin on renal impairment and mortality in patients with cirrhosis and spontaneous bacterial peritonitis. *N Engl J Med* 1999;341:403.
225. Gines P, Arroyo V. Hepatorenal syndrome. *J Am Soc Nephrol* 1999;10:1833.
226. Garzia P, Ferri GM, Ilardi M, et al. Pathophysiology, clinical features and management of hepatorenal syndrome. *Eur Rev Med Pharmacol Sci* 1998;2:181.
227. Gulberg V, Bilzer M, Gerbes AL. Long-term therapy and retreatment of hepatorenal syndrome type 1 with ornipressin and dopamine. *Hepatology* 1999;30:870.
228. Tozzo C, Mazzarella V, Splendiani G, et al. Acute renal failure caused by nontraumatic rhabdomyolysis. *Ren Fail* 1997;19:439.
229. Homsi E, Barreiro MF, Orlando JM, et al. Prophylaxis of acute renal failure in patients with rhabdomyolysis. *Ren Fail* 1997;19:283.
230. Zager RA. Rhabdomyolysis and myohemoglobinuric acute renal failure. *Kidney Int* 1996;49:314.
231. Owen CA, Mubarak SJ, Hargens AR, et al. Intramuscular pressures with limb compression clarification of the pathogenesis of the drug-induced muscle-compartment syndrome. *N Engl J Med* 1979;300:1169.
232. Eneas JF, Schoenfeld PY, Humphreys MH. The effect of infusion of mannitol-sodium bicarbonate on the clinical course of myoglobinuria. *Arch Intern Med* 1979;139:801.
233. Llach F, Felsenfeld AJ, Haussler MR. The pathophysiology of altered calcium metabolism in rhabdomyolysis-induced acute renal failure. Interactions of parathyroid hormone, 25-hydroxycholeciferol, and 1,25-dihydroxycholecalciferol. *N Engl J Med* 1981;305:117.
234. Grossman RA, Hamilton RW, Morse BM, et al. Nontraumatic rhabdomyolysis and acute renal failure. *N Engl J Med* 1974;291:807.
235. Ward MM. Factors predictive of acute renal failure in rhabdomyolysis. *Arch Intern Med* 1988;148:1553.
236. Ron D, Taitelman U, Michaelson M, et al. Prevention of acute renal failure in traumatic rhabdomyolysis. *Arch Intern Med* 1984;144:277.
237. Vanholder R, Sever MS, Erek E, et al. Rhabdomyolysis. *J Am Soc Nephrol* 2000;11:1553.
238. Birewar S, Oppenheimer M, Zawada ET, Jr. Hypothyroid acute renal failure. *S D J Med* 2004;57:109.
239. Davis JS, Bourke P. Rhabdomyolysis associated with dengue virus infection. *Clin Infect Dis* 2004;38:e109.
240. Abassi ZA, Hoffman A, Better OS. Acute renal failure complicating muscle crush injury. *Semin Nephrol* 1998;18:558.
241. Lameire N, Vanholder R, Clement J, et al. The organization of the European Renal Disaster Relief Task Force. *Ren Fail* 1997;19:665.
242. Gunal AI, Celiker H, Dogukan A, et al. Early and vigorous fluid resuscitation prevents acute renal failure in the crush victims of catastrophic earthquakes. *J Am Soc Nephrol* 2004;15:1862.
243. Gabow PA, Kaehny WD, Kelleher SP. The spectrum of rhabdomyolysis. *Medicine (Baltimore)* 1982;61:141.
244. Klahr S, Miller SB. Acute oliguria. *N Engl J Med* 1998;338:671.
245. Cassidy MJ, Gaskin G, Savill J, et al. Towards a more rapid diagnosis of rapidly progressive glomerulonephritis. *BMJ* 1990;301:329.
246. Landry JF, Langlois S. Acute exposure to aliphatic hydrocarbons: an unusual cause of acute tubular necrosis. *Arch Intern Med* 1998;158:1821.
247. Abuelo JG. Renal failure caused by chemicals, foods, plants, animal venoms, and misuse of drugs. An overview. *Arch Intern Med* 1990;150:505.
248. Woolf AD. The Haitian diethylene glycol poisoning tragedy: a dark wood revisited. *JAMA* 1998;279:1215.
249. Kelleher SP, Berl T. Acute renal failure associated with hypovolemia. In: Brenner BM, Lazarus JM, eds. *Acute renal failure*. Philadelphia: Saunders, 1983:223.
250. McGee S, Abernethy WB, 3rd, Simel DL. The rational clinical examination. Is this patient hypovolemic? *JAMA* 1999;281:1022.
251. Marcussen N, Schumann J, Campbell P, et al. Cytodiagnostic urinalysis is very useful in the differential diagnosis of acute renal failure and can predict the severity. *Ren Fail* 1995;17:721.
252. Minuth AN, Terrell JB, Jr, Suki WN. Acute renal failure: a study of the course and prognosis of 104 patients and of the role of furosemide. *Am J Med Sci* 1976;271:317.
253. Duflot J, Cohen AH, Adler S. Macroscopic hematuria as a presenting manifestation of oliguric acute tubular necrosis. *Am J Kidney Dis* 1993;22:607.
254. Nolan CR, 3rd, Anger MS, Kelleher SP. Eosinophiluria–a new method of detection and definition of the clinical spectrum. *N Engl J Med* 1986;315:1516.
255. Mandal AK, Sklar AH, Hudson JB. Transmission electron microscopy of urinary sediment in human acute renal failure. *Kidney Int* 1985;28:58.
256. Mandal AK. Transmission electron microscopy of urinary sediment in renal disease. *Semin Nephrol* 1986;6:346.
257. Swann RC, Merrill JP. The clinical course of acute renal failure. *Medicine (Baltimore)* 1953;32:215.
258. Goodpastor WE, Levenson SM, Tagnon HG. A clinical and pathologic study of the kidney in patients with thermal burns. *Surg Gynecol Obstet* 1946;82:652.
259. Sevitt S. Distal tubular necrosis with little or no oliguria. *J Clin Pathol* 1956;9:12.
260. Taylor WH. Management of acute renal failure following surgical operation and head injury. *Lancet* 1957;273:703.
261. Vertel RM, Knochel JP. Nonoliguric acute renal failure. *JAMA* 1967;200:598.
262. Gant NF Jr, Whalley PJ, Baxter CR. Nonoliguric renal failure. Report of a case. *Obstet Gynecol* 1974;34:675.
263. Shin B, Mackenzie CF, Cowley RA. Changing patterns of posttraumatic acute renal failure. *Am Surg* 1979;45:182.
264. Miller PD, Krebs RA, Neal BJ, et al. Polyuric prerenal failure. *Arch Intern Med* 1980;140:907.

265. Dixon BS, Anderson RJ. Nonoliguric acute renal failure. *Am J Kidney Dis* 1985;6:71.
266. Rahman SN, Conger JD. Glomerular and tubular factors in urine flow rates of acute renal failure patients. *Am J Kidney Dis* 1994;23:788.
267. Honda N, Hishida A. Pathophysiology of experimental nonoliguric acute renal failure. *Kidney Int* 1993;43:513.
268. Sirota JH. Carbon tetrachloride poisoning in man; the mechanisms of renal failure and recovery. *J Clin Invest* 1949;28:1412.
269. Bull GM, Joekes AM, Lowe KG. Renal function studies in acute tubular necrosis. *Clin Sci* 1950;8:379.
270. Miller TR, Anderson RJ, Linas SL, et al. Urinary diagnostic indices in acute renal failure: a prospective study. *Ann Intern Med* 1978;89:47.
271. Sporn IN, Lancestremere RG, Papper S. Differential diagnosis of oliguria in aged patients. *N Engl J Med* 1962;267:130.
272. Eliahou HE, Bata A. The diagnosis of acute renal failure. *Nephron* 1965;2:287.
273. Handa SP, Morrin PA. Diagnostic indices in acute renal failure. *Can Med Assoc J* 1967;96:78.
274. Hilton PJ, Jones NF, Barraclough MA, et al. Urinary osmolality in acute renal failure due to glomerulonephritis. *Lancet* 1969;2:655.
275. Jones LW, Weil MH. Water, creatinine and sodium excretion following circulatory shock with renal failure. *Am J Med* 1971;51:314.
276. Espinel CH. The FENa test. Use in the differential diagnosis of acute renal failure. *JAMA* 1976;236:579.
277. Lam M, Kaufman CE. Fractional excretion of sodium as a guide to volume depletion during recovery from acute renal failure. *Am J Kidney Dis* 1985;6:18.
278. Fushimi K, Shichiri M, Marumo F. Decreased fractional excretion of urate as an indicator of prerenal azotemia. *Am J Nephrol* 1990;10:489.
279. Steinhauslin F, Burnier M, Magnin JL, et al. Fractional excretion of trace lithium and uric acid in acute renal failure. *J Am Soc Nephrol* 1994;4:1429.
280. Hoffman LM, Suki WN. Obstructive uropathy mimicking volume depletion. *JAMA* 1976;236:2096.
281. Welt LG. *Clinical disorders of hydration and acid-base equilibrium*. Boston: Little, Brown, 1995.
282. Waugh WH. Functional types of acute renal failure and their early diagnosis. *AMA Arch Intern Med* 1959;103:686.
283. Spiegel DM, Wilson PD, Molitoris BA. Epithelial polarity following ischemia: a requirement for normal cell function. *Am J Physiol* 1989;256:F430.
284. Wang Z, Rabb H, Craig T, et al. Ischemic-reperfusion injury in the kidney: overexpression of colonic H^+-K^+-ATPase and suppression of NHE-3. *Kidney Int* 1997;51:1106.
285. Wang Z, Rabb H, Haq M, et al. A possible molecular basis of natriuresis during ischemic-reperfusion injury in the kidney. *J Am Soc Nephrol* 1998;9:605.
286. Fang LS, Sirota RA, Ebert TH, et al. Low fractional excretion of sodium with contrast media-induced acute renal failure. *Arch Intern Med* 1980;140:531.
287. Steiner RW. Interpreting the fractional excretion of sodium. *Am J Med* 1984;77:699.
288. Vaz AJ. Low fractional excretion of urine sodium in acute renal failure due to sepsis. *Arch Intern Med* 1983;143:738.
289. Corwin HL, Schreiber MJ, Fang LS. Low fractional excretion of sodium. Occurrence with hemoglobinuric- and myoglobinuric-induced acute renal failure. *Arch Intern Med* 1984;144:981.
290. Diamond JR, Yoburn DC. Nonoliguric acute renal failure associated with a low fractional excretion of sodium. *Ann Intern Med* 1982;96:597.
291. Lins RL, Verpooten GA, De Clerck DS, et al. Urinary indices in acute interstitial nephritis. *Clin Nephrol* 1986;26:131.
292. Liano F, Gamez C, Pascual J, et al. Use of urinary parameters in the diagnosis of total acute renal artery occlusion. *Nephron* 1994;66:170.
293. Anderson RJ, Gabow PA, Gross PA. Urinary chloride concentration in acute renal failure. *Miner Electrolyte Metab* 1984;10:92.
294. Graziani G, Cantaluppi A, Casati S, et al. Dopamine and furosemide in oliguric acute renal failure. *Nephron* 1984;37:39.
295. Luke RG, Briggs JD, Allison ME, et al. Factors determining response to mannitol in acute renal failure. *Am J Med Sci* 1970;259:168.
296. Kelton J, Kelley WN, Holmes EW. A rapid method for the diagnosis of acute uric acid nephropathy. *Arch Intern Med* 1978;138:612.
297. Tungsanga K, Boonwichit D, Lekhakula A, et al. Urine uric acid and urine creatine ratio in acute renal failure. *Arch Intern Med* 1984;144:934.
298. Curry NS, Gobien RP, Schabel SI. Minimal-dilatation obstructive nephropathy. *Radiology* 1982;143:531.
299. Rascoff JH, Golden RA, Spinowitz BS, et al. Nondilated obstructive nephropathy. *Arch Intern Med* 1983;143:696.
300. Maillet PJ, Pelle-Francoz D, Laville M, et al. Nondilated obstructive acute renal failure: diagnostic procedures and therapeutic management. *Radiology* 1986;160:659.
301. Koelliker SL, Cronan JJ. Acute urinary tract obstruction. Imaging update. *Urol Clin North Am* 1997;24:571.
302. Madias NE, Kwon OJ, Millan VG. Percutaneous transluminal renal angioplasty. A potentially effective treatment for preservation of renal function. *Arch Intern Med* 1982;142:693.
303. Schlanger LE, Haire HM, Zuckerman AM, et al. Reversible renal failure in an elderly woman with renal artery stenosis. *Am J Kidney Dis* 1994;23:123.
304. Cohen AH, Nast CC, Adler SG, et al. Clinical utility of kidney biopsies in the diagnosis and management of renal disease. *Am J Nephrol* 1989;9:309.
305. Mustonen J, Pasternack A, Helin H, et al. Renal biopsy in acute renal failure. *Am J Nephrol* 1984;4:27.
306. Solez K, Morel-Maroger L, Sraer JD. The morphology of "acute tubular necrosis" in man: analysis of 57 renal biopsies and a comparison with the glycerol model. *Medicine (Baltimore)* 1979;58:362.
307. Wilson DM, Turner DR, Cameron JS, et al. Value of renal biopsy in acute intrinsic renal failure. *Br Med J* 1976;2:459.
308. Richards NT, Darby S, Howie AJ, et al. Knowledge of renal histology alters patient management in over 40% of cases. *Nephrol Dial Transplant* 1994;9:1255.
309. Andreucci VE, Fuiano G, Stanziale P, et al. Role of renal biopsy in the diagnosis and prognosis of acute renal failure. *Kidney Int Suppl* 1998;66:S91.
310. Conlon PJ, Kovalik E, Schwab SJ. Percutaneous renal biopsy of ventilated intensive care unit patients. *Clin Nephrol* 1995;43:309.
311. Thompson BC, Kingdon E, Johnston M, et al. Transjugular kidney biopsy. *Am J Kidney Dis* 2004;43:651.
312. Bullock ML, Umen AJ, Finkelstein M, et al. The assessment of risk factors in 462 patients with acute renal failure. *Am J Kidney Dis* 1985;5:97.
313. Frankel MC, Weinstein AM, Stenzel KH. Prognostic patterns in acute renal failure: the New York Hospital, 1981-1982. *Clin Exp Dial Apheresis* 1983;7:145.
314. Baldwin DS, Edwards JE. Uremic pericarditis as a cause of cardiac tamponade. *Circulation* 1976;53:896.
315. Zakynthinos E, Theodorakopoulou M, Daniil Z, et al. Hemorrhagic cardiac tamponade in critically ill patients with acute renal failure. *Heart Lung* 2004;33:55.
316. Burkett E, Anderson RJ. Co-existing renal-respiratory failure: how to prevent and how to manage. *J Crit Illness* 1991;6:18.
317. Biesenbach G, Zazgornik J, Kaiser W, et al. Improvement in prognosis of patients with acute renal failure over a period of 15 years: an analysis of 710 cases in a dialysis center. *Am J Nephrol* 1992;12:319.
318. Fiaccadori E, Maggiore U, Clima B, et al. Incidence, risk factors, and prognosis of gastrointestinal hemorrhage complicating acute renal failure. *Kidney Int* 2001;59:1510.
319. Banks PA, Sidi S, Gelman ML, et al. Amylase-creatinine clearance ratios and serum amylase isoenzymes in moderate renal insufficiency. *J Clin Gastroenterol* 1979;1:331.
320. Ljutic D, Piplovic-Vukovic T, Raos V, et al. Acute renal failure as a complication of acute pancreatitis. *Ren Fail* 1996;18:629.
321. Kes P, Vucicevic Z, Ratkovic-Gusic I, et al. Acute renal failure complicating severe acute pancreatitis. *Ren Fail* 1996;18:621.
322. Richet G, Lopez de Novales E, Verroust P. Drug intoxication and neurological episodes in chronic renal failure. *Br Med J* 1970;2:394.
323. Marik PE, Iglesias J. Low-dose dopamine does not prevent acute renal failure in patients with septic shock and oliguria. NORASEPT II Study Investigators. *Am J Med* 1999;107:387.
324. Hoste EA, Blot SI, Lameire NH, et al. Effect of nosocomial bloodstream infection on the outcome of critically ill patients with acute renal failure treated with renal replacement therapy. *J Am Soc Nephrol* 2004;15:454.
325. Keane WF, Hirata-Dulas CA, Bullock ML, et al. Adjunctive therapy with intravenous human immunoglobulin G improves survival of patients with acute renal failure. *J Am Soc Nephrol* 1991;2:841.
326. Dolson GM. Electrolyte abnormalities before and after the onset of acute renal failure. *Miner Electrolyte Metab* 1991;17:133.
327. Massry SG, Arieff AI, Coburn JW, et al. Divalent ion metabolism in patients with acute renal failure: studies on the mechanism of hypocalcemia. *Kidney Int* 1974;5:437.
328. Pietrek J, Kokot F, Kuska J. Serum 25-hydroxyvitamin D and parathyroid hormone in patients with acute renal failure. *Kidney Int* 1978;13:178.
329. St John A, Davis TM, Binh TQ, et al. Mineral homoeostasis in acute renal failure complicating severe falciparum malaria. *J Clin Endocrinol Metab* 1995;80:2761.
330. Massry SG, Coburn JW, Lee DB, et al. Skeletal resistance to parathyroid hormone in renal failure. Studies in 105 human subjects. *Ann Intern Med* 1973;78:357.
331. Kokot F, Kuska J. The endocrine system in patients with acute renal insufficiency. *Kidney Int Suppl* 1976;6:S26.
332. Levitan D, Moser SA, Goldstein DA, et al. Disturbances in the hypothalamic-pituitary-gonadal axis in male patients with acute renal failure. *Am J Nephrol* 1984;4:99.
333. Fuss M, Bagon J, Dupont E, et al. Parathyroid hormone and calcium blood levels in acute renal failure. With special reference to one patient developing transient hypercalcemia. *Nephron* 1978;20:196.
334. Kokot F, Wiecek A, Grzeszczak W. Plasma parathyroid hormone and erythropoietin levels in patients with noninflammatory acute renal failure. *Int Urol Nephrol* 1993;25:89.
335. Shieh SD, Lin YF, Lin SH, et al. A prospective study of calcium metabolism in exertional heat stroke with rhabdomyolysis and acute renal failure. *Nephron* 1995;71:428.
336. Sperling LS, Tumlin JA. Case report: delayed hypercalcemia after rhabdomyolysis-induced acute renal failure. *Am J Med Sci* 1996;311:186.
337. Shrestha SM, Berry JL, Davies M, et al. Biphasic hypercalcemia in severe rhabdomyolysis: serial analysis of PTH and vitamin D metabolites. A case report and literature review. *Am J Kidney Dis* 2004;43:e31.

338. Chavel SM, Taraszka KS, Schaffer JV, et al. Calciphylaxis associated with acute, reversible renal failure in the setting of alcoholic cirrhosis. *J Am Acad Dermatol* 2004;50:S125.

339. Kaptein EM, Levitan D, Feinstein EI, et al. Alterations of thyroid hormone indices in acute renal failure and in acute critical illness with and without acute renal failure. *Am J Nephrol* 1981;1:138.

340. Makropoulos W, Heintz B, Stefanidis I. Selenium deficiency and thyroid function in acute renal failure. *Ren Fail* 1997;19:129.

341. Mondon CE, Dolkas CB, Reaven GM. The site of insulin resistance in acute uremia. *Diabetes* 1978;27:571.

342. Mitch WE, Walker WG. Plasma renin and angiotensin II in acute renal failure. *Lancet* 1977;2:328.

343. du Cheyron D, Lesage A, Daubin C, et al. Hyperreninemic hypoaldosteronism: a possible etiological factor of septic shock-induced acute renal failure. *Intensive Care Med* 2003;29:1703.

344. Knochel JP. Biochemical, electrolyte, and acid-base disturbances in acute renal failure. In: Brenner BM, Lazarus JM, eds. Acute renal failure. Philadelphia: Saunders, 1983.

345. Bozfakioglu S. Nutrition in patients with acute renal failure. *Nephrol Dial Transplant* 2001;16(Suppl 6):21.

346. Horl WH, Heidland A. Enhanced proteolytic activity–cause of protein catabolism in acute renal failure. *Am J Clin Nutr* 1980;33:1423.

347. Sponsel H, Conger JD. Is parenteral nutrition therapy of value in acute renal failure patients? *Am J Kidney Dis* 1995;25:96.

348. Druml W. Protein metabolism in acute renal failure. *Miner Electrolyte Metab* 1998;24:47.

349. Koffler A, Friedler RM, Massry SG. Acute renal failure due to nontraumatic rhabdomyolysis. *Ann Intern Med* 1976;85:23.

350. Agarwal R, Vasavada N, Chase SD. Evaluation of kidney function in patients with acute renal failure using high-performance liquid chromatography: a case report. *Pharmacotherapy* 2004;24:145.

351. Haug CE, Lopez IA, Moore RH, et al. Real-time monitoring of renal function during ischemic injury in the rhesus monkey. *Ren Fail* 1995;17:489.

352. Wheeler DC, Feehally J, Walls J. High risk acute renal failure. *Q J Med* 1986;61:977.

353. McCarthy JT, Torres VE, Romero JC, et al. Acute intrinsic renal failure induced by indomethacin: role of prostaglandin synthetase inhibition. *Mayo Clin Proc* 1982;57:289.

354. Anderson RJ, Chung HM, Kluge R, et al. Hyponatremia: a prospective analysis of its epidemiology and the pathogenetic role of vasopressin. *Ann Intern Med* 1985;102:164.

355. Kamijo Y, Soma K, Asari Y, et al. Severe rhabdomyolysis following massive ingestion of oolong tea: caffeine intoxication with coexisting hyponatremia. *Vet Hum Toxicol* 1999;41:381.

356. Elizalde-Sciavolino C, Racco A, Proscia-Lieto T, et al. Severe hyponatremia, neuroleptic malignant syndrome, rhabdomyolysis and acute renal failure: a case report. *Mt Sinai J Med* 1998;65:284.

357. Humphery TJ. Acute renal failure due to leptospirosis with hyponatraemia. *Med J Aust* 1975;1:621.

358. Woodrow G, Brownjohn AM, Turney JH. Acute-on-chronic renal failure and hyponatraemia associated with severe hypothyroidism. *Nephrol Dial Transplant* 1993;8:557.

359. Feinstein EI. Hypercalcemia and acute widespread calcifications during the oliguric phase of acute renal failure due to rhabdomyolysis. *Miner Electrolyte Metab* 1979;2:193.

360. Akmal M, Goldstein DA, Telfer N, et al. Resolution of muscle calcification in rhabdomyolysis and acute renal failure. *Ann Intern Med* 1978;89:928.

361. de Torrente A, Berl T, Cohn PD, et al. Hypercalcemia of acute renal failure. Clinical significance and pathogenesis. *Am J Med* 1976;61:119.

362. Meroney WH, Arney GK, Segar WE, et al. The acute calcification of traumatized muscle, with particular reference to acute post-traumatic renal insufficiency. *J Clin Invest* 1957;36:825.

363. Davenport A, Roberts NB. Accumulation of aluminium in patients with acute renal failure. *Nephron* 1989;52:253.

364. Perazella M, Brown E. Acute aluminum toxicity and alum bladder irrigation in patients with renal failure. *Am J Kidney Dis* 1993;21:44.

365. Moreno A, Dominguez P, Dominguez C, et al. High serum aluminium levels and acute reversible encephalopathy in a 4-year-old boy with acute renal failure. *Eur J Pediatr* 1991;150:513.

366. Erasmus RT, Kusnir J, Stevenson WC, et al. Hyperaluminemia associated with liver transplantation and acute renal failure. *Clin Transplant* 1995;9:307.

367. Hales M, Solez K, Kjellstrand C. The anemia of acute renal failure: association with oliguria and elevated blood urea. *Ren Fail* 1994;16:125.

368. Nielsen OJ, Thaysen JH. Erythropoietin deficiency in acute tubular necrosis. *J Intern Med* 1990;227:373.

369. Cosio FG, Zager RA, Sharma HM. Atheroembolic renal disease causes hypocomplementaemia. *Lancet* 1985;2:118.

370. Galpin JE, Shinaberger JH, Stanley TM, et al. Acute interstitial nephritis due to methicillin. *Am J Med* 1978;65:756.

371. Linton AL, Clark WF, Driedger AA, et al. Acute interstitial nephritis due to drugs: Review of the literature with a report of nine cases. *Ann Intern Med* 1980;93:735.

372. Roth D, Alarcon FJ, Fernandez JA, et al. Acute rhabdomyolysis associated with cocaine intoxication. *N Engl J Med* 1988;319:673.

373. Celik C, Gezginc K, Altintepe L, et al. Results of the pregnancies with HELLP syndrome. *Ren Fail* 2003;25:613.

374. Stratta P, Canavese C, Goia F, et al. Clinical and therapeutic correlations in consumption coagulopathy of obstetric acute renal failure. *Clin Exp Obstet Gynecol* 1986;13:43.

375. Ward DM. Anticoagulation in patients on hemodialysis. In: Nissenson AR, Fine RN, Gentile GE, eds. *Clinical dialysis,* 3rd ed. Norwalk, CT: Appleton & Lange, 1995:142.

376. Schetz MR. Coagulation disorders in acute renal failure. *Kidney Int Suppl* 1998;66:S96.

377. Mant MJ, King EG. Severe, acute disseminated intravascular coagulation. A reappraisal of its pathophysiology, clinical significance and therapy based on 47 patients. *Am J Med* 1979;67:557.

378. Krug H, Raszeja-Wanic B, Wochowiak A. Intravascular coagulation in acute renal failure after myocardial infarction. *Ann Intern Med* 1974;81:494.

379. Hatala R, Dinh T, Cook DJ. Once-daily aminoglycoside dosing in immunocompetent adults: a meta-analysis. *Ann Intern Med* 1996;124:717.

380. Sorkine P, Nagar H, Weinbroum A, et al. Administration of amphotericin B in lipid emulsion decreases nephrotoxicity: results of a prospective, randomized, controlled study in critically ill patients. *Crit Care Med* 1996;24:1311.

381. Barrett BJ, Carlisle EJ. Metaanalysis of the relative nephrotoxicity of high- and low-osmolality iodinated contrast media. *Radiology* 1993;188:171.

382. Rind DM, Safran C, Phillips RS, et al. Effect of computer-based alerts on the treatment and outcomes of hospitalized patients. *Arch Intern Med* 1994;154:1511.

383. Weisbord SD, Bruns FJ, Saul MI, et al. Provider use of preventive strategies for radiocontrast nephropathy in high-risk patients. *Nephron Clin Pract* 2004;96:c56.

384. Eisenberg RL, Bank WO, Hedgock MW. Renal failure after major angiography can be avoided with hydration. *AJR Am J Roentgenol* 1981;136:859.

385. Erley CM. Does hydration prevent radiocontrast-induced acute renal failure? *Nephrol Dial Transplant* 1999;14:1064.

386. Murphy SW, Barrett BJ, Parfrey PS. Contrast nephropathy. *J Am Soc Nephrol* 2000;11:177.

387. Madias NE, Harrington JT. Platinum nephrotoxicity. *Am J Med* 1978;65:307.

388. Blachley JD, Hill JB. Renal and electrolyte disturbances associated with cisplatin. *Ann Intern Med* 1981;95:628.

389. Branch RA. Prevention of amphotericin B-induced renal impairment. A review on the use of sodium supplementation. *Arch Intern Med* 1988;148:2389.

390. Fisher MA, Talbot GH, Maislin G, et al. Risk factors for amphotericin B-associated nephrotoxicity. *Am J Med* 1989;87:547.

391. Heidemann HT, Gerkens JF, Spickard WA, et al. Amphotericin B nephrotoxicity in humans decreased by salt repletion. *Am J Med* 1983;75:476.

392. Waikar SS, Chertow GM. Crystalloids versus colloids for resuscitation in shock. *Curr Opin Nephrol Hypertens* 2000;9:501.

393. Choi PT, Yip G, Quinonez LG, et al. Crystalloids vs. colloids in fluid resuscitation: a systematic review. *Crit Care Med* 1999;27:200.

394. Schierhout G, Roberts I. Fluid resuscitation with colloid or crystalloid solutions in critically ill patients: a systematic review of randomised trials. *BMJ* 1998;316:961.

395. Human albumin administration in critically ill patients: systematic review of randomised controlled trials. Cochrane Injuries Group Albumin Reviewers. *BMJ* 1998;317:235.

396. Schortgen F, Lacherade JC, Bruneel F, et al. Effects of hydroxyethylstarch and gelatin on renal function in severe sepsis: a multicentre randomised study. *Lancet* 2001;357:911.

397. Boldt J, Muller M, Mentges D, et al. Volume therapy in the critically ill: is there a difference? *Intensive Care Med* 1998;24:28.

398. Finfer S, Bellomo R, Boyce N, et al. A comparison of albumin and saline for fluid resuscitation in the intensive care unit. *N Engl J Med* 2004;350:2247.

399. Reineck HJ, O'Connor GJ, Lifschitz MD, et al. Sequential studies on the pathophysiology of glycerol-induced acute renal failure. *J Lab Clin Med* 1980;96:356.

400. Cushner HM, Barnes JL, Stein JH, et al. Role of volume depletion in the glycerol model of acute renal failure. *Am J Physiol* 1986;250:F315.

401. Zager RA. Studies of mechanisms and protective maneuvers in myoglobinuric acute renal injury. *Lab Invest* 1989;60:619.

402. Better OS, Stein JH. Early management of shock and prophylaxis of acute renal failure in traumatic rhabdomyolysis. *N Engl J Med* 1990;322:825.

403. Richer M, Robert S, Lebel M. Renal hemodynamics during norepinephrine and low-dose dopamine infusions in man. *Crit Care Med* 1996;24:1150.

404. Meier-Hellmann A, Bredle DL, Specht M, et al. The effects of low-dose dopamine on splanchnic blood flow and oxygen uptake in patients with septic shock. *Intensive Care Med* 1997;23:31.

405. Pavoni V, Verri M, Ferraro L, et al. Plasma dopamine concentration and effects of low dopamine doses on urinary output after major vascular surgery. *Kidney Int Suppl* 1998;66:S75.

406. Lassnigg A, Donner E, Grubhofer G, et al. Lack of renoprotective effects of dopamine and furosemide during cardiac surgery. *J Am Soc Nephrol* 2000;11:97.

407. Tang AT, El-Gamel A, Keevil B, et al. The effect of 'renal-dose' dopamine on renal tubular function following cardiac surgery: assessed by measuring retinol binding protein (RBP). *Eur J Cardiothorac Surg* 1999;15:717.

408. Baldwin L, Henderson A, Hickman P. Effect of postoperative low-dose dopamine on renal function after elective major vascular surgery. *Ann Intern Med* 1994;120:744.

409. Bellomo R, Chapman M, Finfer S, et al. Low-dose dopamine in patients with early renal dysfunction: a placebo-controlled randomised trial. Australian and New Zealand Intensive Care Society (ANZICS) Clinical Trials Group. *Lancet* 2000;356:2139.

410. Hans SS, Hans BA, Dhillon R, et al. Effect of dopamine on renal function after arteriography in patients with pre-existing renal insufficiency. *Am Surg* 1998;64:432.

411. Hall KA, Wong RW, Hunter GC, et al. Contrast-induced nephrotoxicity: the effects of vasodilator therapy. *J Surg Res* 1992;53:317.

412. Abizaid AS, Clark CE, Mintz GS, et al. Effects of dopamine and aminophylline on contrast-induced acute renal failure after coronary angioplasty in patients with preexisting renal insufficiency. *Am J Cardiol* 1999;83:260.

413. Stevens MA, McCullough PA, Tobin KJ, et al. A prospective randomized trial of prevention measures in patients at high risk for contrast nephropathy: results of the P.R.I.N.C.E. Study. Prevention of Radiocontrast Induced Nephropathy Clinical Evaluation. *J Am Coll Cardiol* 1999;33:403.

414. Weisberg LS, Kurnik PB, Kurnik BR. Risk of radiocontrast nephropathy in patients with and without diabetes mellitus. *Kidney Int* 1994;45:259.

415. Kellum JA, J MD. Use of dopamine in acute renal failure: a meta-analysis. *Crit Care Med* 2001;29:1526.

416. Greene SI, Smith JW. Letter: Dopamine gangrene. *N Engl J Med* 1976;294:114.

417. Lee MR. Dopamine and the kidney: ten years on. *Clin Sci (Lond)* 1993;84:357.

418. Rudis MI. Low-dose dopamine in the intensive care unit: DNR or DNRx? *Crit Care Med* 2001;29:1638.

419. Segal JM, Phang PT, Walley KR. Low-dose dopamine hastens onset of gut ischemia in a porcine model of hemorrhagic shock. *J Appl Physiol* 1992;73:1159.

420. Van den Berghe G, de Zegher F. Anterior pituitary function during critical illness and dopamine treatment. *Crit Care Med* 1996;24:1580.

421. Lherm T, Troche G, Rossignol M, et al. Renal effects of low-dose dopamine in patients with sepsis syndrome or septic shock treated with catecholamines. *Intensive Care Med* 1996;22:213.

422. Ichai C, Passeron C, Carles M, et al. Prolonged low-dose dopamine infusion induces a transient improvement in renal function in hemodynamically stable, critically ill patients: a single-blind, prospective, controlled study. *Crit Care Med* 2000;28:1329.

423. MacGregor DA, Smith TE, Prielipp RC, et al. Pharmacokinetics of dopamine in healthy male subjects. *Anesthesiology* 2000;92:338.

424. Tumlin JA, Wang A, Murray PT, et al. Fenoldopam mesylate blocks reductions in renal plasma flow after radiocontrast dye infusion: a pilot trial in the prevention of contrast nephropathy. *Am Heart J* 2002;143:894.

425. Walker PD, Brokering KL, Theobald JC. Fenoldopam and N-acetylcysteine for the prevention of radiographic contrast material-induced nephropathy: a review. *Pharmacotherapy* 2003;23:1617.

426. Madyoon H, Croushore L, Weaver D, et al. Use of fenoldopam to prevent radiocontrast nephropathy in high-risk patients. *Catheter Cardiovasc Interv* 2001;53:341.

427. Kini AS, Mitre CA, Kamran M, et al. Changing trends in incidence and predictors of radiographic contrast nephropathy after percutaneous coronary intervention with use of fenoldopam. *Am J Cardiol* 2002;89:999.

428. Chamsuddin AA, Kowalik KJ, Bjarnason H, et al. Using a dopamine type 1A receptor agonist in high-risk patients to ameliorate contrast-associated nephropathy. *AJR Am J Roentgenol* 2002;179:591.

429. Gilbert TB, Hasnain JU, Flinn WR, et al. Fenoldopam infusion associated with preserving renal function after aortic cross-clamping for aneurysm repair. *J Cardiovasc Pharmacol Ther* 2001;6:31.

430. Sheinbaum R, Ignacio C, Safi HJ, et al. Contemporary strategies to preserve renal function during cardiac and vascular surgery. *Rev Cardiovasc Med* 2003;4(Suppl 1):S21.

431. Sward K, Valson F, Ricksten SE. Long-term infusion of atrial natriuretic peptide (ANP) improves renal blood flow and glomerular filtration rate in clinical acute renal failure. *Acta Anaesthesiol Scand* 2001;45:536.

432. Sezai A, Shiono M, Orime Y, et al. Low-dose continuous infusion of human atrial natriuretic peptide during and after cardiac surgery. *Ann Thorac Surg* 2000;69:732.

433. Kurnik BR, Weisberg LS, Cuttler IM, et al. Effects of atrial natriuretic peptide versus mannitol on renal blood flow during radiocontrast infusion in chronic renal failure. *J Lab Clin Med* 1990;116:27.

434. Kurnik BR, Allgren RL, Genter FC, et al. Prospective study of atrial natriuretic peptide for the prevention of radiocontrast-induced nephropathy. *Am J Kidney Dis* 1998;31:674.

435. Russo D, Testa A, Della Volpe L, et al. Randomised prospective study on renal effects of two different contrast media in humans: protective role of a calcium channel blocker. *Nephron* 1990;55:254.

436. Neumayer HH, Junge W, Kufner A, et al. Prevention of radiocontrast-media-induced nephrotoxicity by the calcium channel blocker nitrendipine: a prospective randomised clinical trial. *Nephrol Dial Transplant* 1989;4:1030.

437. Khoury Z, Schlicht JR, Como J, et al. The effect of prophylactic nifedipine on renal function in patients administered contrast media. *Pharmacotherapy* 1995;15:59.

438. Piper SN, Kumle B, Maleck WH, et al. Diltiazem may preserve renal tubular integrity after cardiac surgery. *Can J Anaesth* 2003;50:285.

439. Lumlertgul D, Wongmekiat O, Sirivanichai C. Intrarenal infusion of gallopamil in acute renal failure. A preliminary report. *Drugs* 1991;42(Suppl 1):44.

440. Puig JM, Lloveras J, Oliveras A, et al. Usefulness of diltiazem in reducing the incidence of acute tubular necrosis in Euro-Collins-preserved cadaveric renal grafts. *Transplant Proc* 1991;23:2368.

441. Neumayer HH, Kuzendorf U. Renal protection with the calcium antagonists. *J Cardiol Pharmacol* 1991;18:11.

442. Duggan KA, Macdonald GJ, Charlesworth JA, et al. Verapamil prevents post-transplant oliguric renal failure. *Clin Nephrol* 1985;24:289.

443. Ladefoged SD, Andersen CB. Calcium channel blockers in kidney transplantation. *Clin Transplant* 1994;8:128.

444. Duke GJ, Briedis JH, Weaver RA. Renal support in critically ill patients: low-dose dopamine or low-dose dobutamine? *Crit Care Med* 1994;22:1919.

445. Takala J, Meier-Hellmann A, Eddleston J, et al. Effect of dopexamine on outcome after major abdominal surgery: a prospective, randomized, controlled multicenter study. European Multicenter Study Group on Dopexamine in Major Abdominal Surgery. *Crit Care Med* 2000;28:1417.

446. Dehne MG, Klein TF, Muhling J, et al. Impairment of renal function after cardiopulmonary bypass is not influenced by dopexamine. *Ren Fail* 2001;23:217.

447. Welch M, Newstead CG, Smyth JV, et al. Evaluation of dopexamine hydrochloride as a renoprotective agent during aortic surgery. *Ann Vasc Surg* 1995;9:488.

448. Sherry E, Tooley MA, Bolsin SN, et al. Effect of dopexamine hydrochloride on renal vascular resistance index and haemodynamic responses following coronary artery bypass graft surgery. *Eur J Anaesthesiol* 1997;14:184.

449. Tepel M, van der Giet M, Schwarzfeld C, et al. Prevention of radiographic-contrast-agent-induced reductions in renal function by acetylcysteine. *N Engl J Med* 2000;343:180.

450. Meine TJ, Washam JB. N-acetylcysteine to prevent contrast nephropathy. *Am Heart J* 2004;147:440.

451. Birck R, Krzossok S, Markowetz F, et al. Acetylcysteine for prevention of contrast nephropathy: meta-analysis. *Lancet* 2003;362:598.

452. Pannu N, Manns B, Lee H, et al. Systematic review of the impact of N-acetylcysteine on contrast nephropathy. *Kidney Int* 2004;65:1366.

453. Kshirsagar AV, Poole C, Mottl A, et al. N-acetylcysteine for the prevention of radiocontrast induced nephropathy: a meta-analysis of prospective controlled trials. *J Am Soc Nephrol* 2004;15:761.

454. Alonso A, Lau J, Jaber BL. Prevention of radiocontrast nephropathy with N-acetylcysteine in patients with chronic kidney disease: a meta-analysis of randomized, controlled trials. *Am J Kidney Dis* 2004;43:1.

455. Rudnick MR, Goldfarb S, Wexler L, et al. Nephrotoxicity of ionic and nonionic contrast media in 1196 patients: a randomized trial. The Iohexol Cooperative Study. *Kidney Int* 1995;47:254.

456. Fung JW, Szeto CC, Chan WW, et al. Effect of N-acetylcysteine for prevention of contrast nephropathy in patients with moderate to severe renal insufficiency: a randomized trial. *Am J Kidney Dis* 2004;43:801.

457. Efrati S, Dishy V, Averbukh M, et al. The effect of N-acetylcysteine on renal function, nitric oxide, and oxidative stress after angiography. *Kidney Int* 2003;64:2182.

458. Hoffmann U, Fischereder M, Kruger B, et al. The value of N-acetylcysteine in the prevention of radiocontrast agent-induced nephropathy seems questionable. *J Am Soc Nephrol* 2004;15:407.

459. Solomon R, Werner C, Mann D, et al. Effects of saline, mannitol, and furosemide to prevent acute decreases in renal function induced by radiocontrast agents. *N Engl J Med* 1994;331:1416.

460. Weinstein JM, Heyman S, Brezis M. Potential deleterious effect of furosemide in radiocontrast nephropathy. *Nephron* 1992;62:413.

461. Lieberthal W, Levinsky NG. Treatment of acute tubular necrosis. *Semin Nephrol* 1990;10:571.

462. Barry KG, Malloy JP. Oliguric renal failure. Evaluation and therapy by the intravenous infusion of mannitol. *JAMA* 1962;179:510.

463. Seitzman DM, Mazze RI, Schwartz FD, et al. Mannitol diuresis: a method of renal protection during surgery. *J Urol* 1963;90:139.

464. Hayes DM, Cvitkovic E, Golbey RB, et al. High dose cis-platinum diammine dichloride: amelioration of renal toxicity by mannitol diuresis. *Cancer* 1977;39:1372.

465. Baird RJ, Firor WB, Barr HW. Protection of renal function during surgery of the abdominal aorta. *Can Med Assoc J* 1963;89:705.

466. Powers SR, Jr, Boba A, Hostnik W, et al. Prevention of postoperative acute renal failure with mannitol in 100 cases. *Surgery* 1964;55:15.

467. Dawson JL. Post-Operative Renal Function in Obstructive Jaundice: Effect of a Mannitol Diuresis. *Br Med J* 1965;5427:82.

468. Bullock WE, Luke RG, Nuttall CE, et al. Can mannitol reduce amphotericin B nephrotoxicity? Double-blind study and description of a new vascular lesion in kidneys. *Antimicrob Agents Chemother* 1976;10:555.

469. Better OS, Rubinstein I, Winaver JM, et al. Mannitol therapy revisited (1940–1997). *Kidney Int* 1997;52:886.

470. Gubern JM, Sancho JJ, Simo J, et al. A randomized trial on the effect of mannitol on postoperative renal function in patients with obstructive jaundice. *Surgery* 1988;103:39.

471. Sitges-Serra A, Carulla X, Piera C, et al. Body water compartments in patients with obstructive jaundice. *Br J Surg* 1992;79:553.

472. Nicholson ML, Baker DM, Hopkinson BR, et al. Randomized controlled trial of the effect of mannitol on renal reperfusion injury during aortic aneurysm surgery. *Br J Surg* 1996;83:1230.

473. Salahi H, Malek Hosseini SA, Ahmad E, et al. Mannitol infusion and decreased incidence of allograft acute renal failure. *Transplant Proc* 1995;27:2569.

474. Weimar W, Geerlings W, Bijnen AB, et al. A controlled study on the effect of mannitol on immediate renal function after cadaver donor kidney transplantation. *Transplantation* 1983;35:99.

475. Tiggeler RG, Berden JH, Hoitsma AJ, et al. Prevention of acute tubular necrosis in cadaveric kidney transplantation by the combined use of mannitol and moderate hydration. *Ann Surg* 1985;201:246.

476. van Valenberg PL, Hoitsma AJ, Tiggeler RG, et al. Mannitol as an indispensable constituent of an intraoperative hydration protocol for the prevention of acute renal failure after renal cadaveric transplantation. *Transplantation* 1987;44:784.

477. Merten GJ, Burgess WP, Gray LV, et al. Prevention of contrast-induced nephropathy with sodium bicarbonate: a randomized controlled trial. *JAMA* 2004;291:2328.

478. Hammerman MR, Miller SB. The role of growth factors in preventing acute renal failure. *Semin Dial* 1996;9:464.

479. Franklin SC, Moulton M, Sicard GA, et al. Insulin-like growth factor I preserves renal function postoperatively. *Am J Physiol* 1997;272:F257.

480. Hladunewich MA, Corrigan G, Derby GC, et al. A randomized, placebo-controlled trial of IGF-1 for delayed graft function: a human model to study postischemic ARF. *Kidney Int* 2003;64:593.

481. Erley CM, Duda SH, Schlepckow S, et al. Adenosine antagonist theophylline prevents the reduction of glomerular filtration rate after contrast media application. *Kidney Int* 1994;45:1425.

482. Erley CM, Duda SH, Rehfuss D, et al. Prevention of radiocontrast-media-induced nephropathy in patients with pre-existing renal insufficiency by hydration in combination with the adenosine antagonist theophylline. *Nephrol Dial Transplant* 1999;14:1146.

483. Katholi RE, Taylor GJ, McCann WP, et al. Nephrotoxicity from contrast media: attenuation with theophylline. *Radiology* 1995;195:17.

484. Ix JH, McCulloch CE, Chertow GM. Theophylline for the prevention of radiocontrast nephropathy: a meta-analysis. *Nephrol Dial Transplant* 2004;19:2747.

485. Bernard GR, Vincent JL, Laterre PF, et al. Efficacy and safety of recombinant human activated protein C for severe sepsis. *N Engl J Med* 2001;344:699.

486. Warren HS, Suffredini AF, Eichacker PQ, et al. Risks and benefits of activated protein C treatment for severe sepsis. *N Engl J Med* 2002;347:1027.

487. Poeze M, Froon AH, Ramsay G, et al. Decreased organ failure in patients with severe SIRS and septic shock treated with the platelet-activating factor antagonist TCV-309: a prospective, multicenter, double-blind, randomized phase II trial. TCV-309 Septic Shock Study Group. *Shock* 2000;14:421.

488. Schuster DP, Metzler M, Opal S, et al. Recombinant platelet-activating factor acetylhydrolase to prevent acute respiratory distress syndrome and mortality in severe sepsis: Phase IIb, multicenter, randomized, placebo-controlled, clinical trial. *Crit Care Med* 2003;31:1612.

489. Vincent JL, Spapen H, Bakker J, et al. Phase II multicenter clinical study of the platelet-activating factor receptor antagonist BB-882 in the treatment of sepsis. *Crit Care Med* 2000;28:638.

490. Dhainaut JF, Tenaillon A, Hemmer M, et al. Confirmatory platelet-activating factor receptor antagonist trial in patients with severe gram-negative bacterial sepsis: a phase III, randomized, double-blind, placebo-controlled, multicenter trial. BN 52021 Sepsis Investigator Group. *Crit Care Med* 1998;26:1963.

491. Rabinovici R. Platelet activating factor inhibition in sepsis: the end? *Crit Care Med* 2003;31:1861.

492. Iglesias J, Marik PE, Levine JS. Elevated serum levels of the type I and type II receptors for tumor necrosis factor as predictive factors for ARF in patients with septic shock. *Am J Kidney Dis* 2003;41:62.

493. Reinhart K, Karzai W. Anti-tumor necrosis factor therapy in sepsis: update on clinical trials and lessons learned. *Crit Care Med* 2001;29:S121.

494. Panacek E, Marshall J, Fischkoff S. Neutralization of TNF by a monoclonal antibody improves survival and reduces organ dysfunction in human sepsis: results of the MONARCS trial. *Chest* 2000;118(Suppl 4):88S.

495. Reinhart K, Menges T, Gardlund B, et al. Randomized, placebo-controlled trial of the anti-tumor necrosis factor antibody fragment afelimomab in hyperinflammatory response during severe sepsis: The RAMSES Study. *Crit Care Med* 2001;29:765.

496. Goligorsky MS, Brodsky SV, Noiri E. Nitric oxide in acute renal failure: NOS versus NOS. *Kidney Int* 2002;61:855.

497. Lopez A, Lorente JA, Steingrub J, et al. Multiple-center, randomized, placebo-controlled, double-blind study of the nitric oxide synthase inhibitor 546C88: effect on survival in patients with septic shock. *Crit Care Med* 2004;32:21.

498. De Vriese AS, Bourgeois M. Pharmacologic treatment of acute renal failure in sepsis. *Curr Opin Crit Care* 2003;9:474.

499. Warren BL, Eid A, Singer P, et al. Caring for the critically ill patient. High-dose antithrombin III in severe sepsis: a randomized controlled trial. *JAMA* 2001;286:1869.

500. Annane D, Sebille V, Charpentier C, et al. Effect of treatment with low doses of hydrocortisone and fludrocortisone on mortality in patients with septic shock. *JAMA* 2002;288:862.

501. Lamberts SW, Bruining HA, de Jong FH. Corticosteroid therapy in severe illness. *N Engl J Med* 1997;337:1285.

502. Bernieh B, Al Hakim M, Boobes Y, et al. Outcome and predictive factors of acute renal failure in the intensive care unit. *Transplant Proc* 2004;36:1784.

503. Kress JP, Pohlman AS, O'Connor MF, et al. Daily interruption of sedative infusions in critically ill patients undergoing mechanical ventilation. *N Engl J Med* 2000;342:1471.

504. Ventilation with lower tidal volumes as compared with traditional tidal volumes for acute lung injury and the acute respiratory distress syndrome. The Acute Respiratory Distress Syndrome Network. *N Engl J Med* 2000;342:1301.

505. Imai Y, Parodo J, Kajikawa O, et al. Injurious mechanical ventilation and end-organ epithelial cell apoptosis and organ dysfunction in an experimental model of acute respiratory distress syndrome. *JAMA* 2003;289:2104.

506. Jerkic M, Miloradovic Z, Jovovic D, et al. Relative roles of endothelin-1 and angiotensin II in experimental post-ischaemic acute renal failure. *Nephrol Dial Transplant* 2004;19:83.

507. Wang A, Holcslaw T, Bashore TM, et al. Exacerbation of radiocontrast nephrotoxicity by endothelin receptor antagonism. *Kidney Int* 2000;57:1675.

508. Sketch MH, Jr, Whelton A, Schollmayer E, et al. Prevention of contrast media-induced renal dysfunction with prostaglandin E1: a randomized, double-blind, placebo-controlled study. *Am J Ther* 2001;8:155.

509. Berlauk JF, Abrams JH, Gilmour IJ, et al. Preoperative optimization of cardiovascular hemodynamics improves outcome in peripheral vascular surgery. A prospective, randomized clinical trial. *Ann Surg* 1991;214:289.

510. Gattinoni L, Brazzi L, Pelosi P, et al. A trial of goal-oriented hemodynamic therapy in critically ill patients. SvO2 Collaborative Group. *N Engl J Med* 1995;333:1025.

511. Rivers E, Nguyen B, Havstad S, et al. Early goal-directed therapy in the treatment of severe sepsis and septic shock. *N Engl J Med* 2001;345:1368.

512. Svensson LG, Crawford ES, Hess KR, et al. Thoracoabdominal aortic aneurysms associated with celiac, superior mesenteric, and renal artery occlusive disease: methods and analysis of results in 271 patients. *J Vasc Surg* 1992;16:378.

513. Tuchschmidt J, Fried J, Astiz M, et al. Elevation of cardiac output and oxygen delivery improves outcome in septic shock. *Chest* 1992;102:216.

514. Fleming A, Bishop M, Shoemaker W, et al. Prospective trial of supranormal values as goals of resuscitation in severe trauma. *Arch Surg* 1992;127:1175.

515. Yu M, Levy MM, Smith P, et al. Effect of maximizing oxygen delivery on morbidity and mortality rates in critically ill patients: a prospective, randomized, controlled study. *Crit Care Med* 1993;21:830.

516. Boyd O, Grounds RM, Bennett ED. A randomized clinical trial of the effect of deliberate perioperative increase of oxygen delivery on mortality in high-risk surgical patients. *JAMA* 1993;270:2699.

517. Hayes MA, Timmins AC, Yau EH, et al. Elevation of systemic oxygen delivery in the treatment of critically ill patients. *N Engl J Med* 1994;330:1717.

518. van den Berghe G, Wouters P, Weekers F, et al. Intensive insulin therapy in the critically ill patients. *N Engl J Med* 2001;345:1359.

519. Hansen TK, Thiel S, Wouters PJ, et al. Intensive insulin therapy exerts antiinflammatory effects in critically ill patients and counteracts the adverse effect of low mannose-binding lectin levels. *J Clin Endocrinol Metab* 2003;88:1082.

520. Allen DA, Harwood S, Varagunam M, et al. High glucose-induced oxidative stress causes apoptosis in proximal tubular epithelial cells and is mediated by multiple caspases. *FASEB J* 2003;17:908.

521. Augustin R, Pocar P, Wrenzycki C, et al. Mitogenic and anti-apoptotic activity of insulin on bovine embryos produced in vitro. *Reproduction* 2003;126:91.

522. Mesotten D, Swinnen JV, Vanderhoydonc F, et al. Contribution of circulating lipids to the improved outcome of critical illness by glycemic control with intensive insulin therapy. *J Clin Endocrinol Metab* 2004;89:219.

523. Marenzi G, Marana I, Lauri G, et al. The prevention of radiocontrast-agent-induced nephropathy by hemofiltration. *N Engl J Med* 2003;349:1333.

524. Solomon R. Managing acute renal failure: do vasodilators and diuretics have a role? *J Crit Illness* 1998;13:709.

525. Majumdar S, Kjellstrand C. Why do we use diuretics in acute renal failure? *Semin Dial* 1996;14:54.

526. Shilliday IR, Quinn KJ, Allison ME. Loop diuretics in the management of acute renal failure: a prospective, double-blind, placebo-controlled, randomized study. *Nephrol Dial Transplant* 1997;12:2592.

527. Kleinknecht D, Ganeval D, Gonzalez-Duque LA, et al. Furosemide in acute oliguric renal failure. A controlled trial. *Nephron* 1976;17:51.

528. Mehta RL, Pascual MT, Soroko S, et al. Diuretics, mortality, and nonrecovery of renal function in acute renal failure. *JAMA* 2002;288:2547.

529. Martin SJ, Danziger LH. Continuous infusion of loop diuretics in the critically ill: a review of the literature. *Crit Care Med* 1994;22:1323.

530. Lindner A. Synergism of dopamine and furosemide in diuretic-resistant, oliguric acute renal failure. *Nephron* 1983;33:121.

531. Chertow GM, Sayegh MH, Allgren RL, et al. Is the administration of dopamine associated with adverse or favorable outcomes in acute renal failure? Auriculin Anaritide Acute Renal Failure Study Group. *Am J Med* 1996;101:49.

532. Power DA, Duggan J, Brady HR. Renal-dose (low-dose) dopamine for the treatment of sepsis-related and other forms of acute renal failure: ineffective and probably dangerous. *Clin Exp Pharmacol Physiol Suppl* 1999;26:S23.

533. Flancbaum L, Choban PS, Dasta JF. Quantitative effects of low-dose dopamine on urine output in oliguric surgical intensive care unit patients. *Crit Care Med* 1994;22:61.

534. Sirivella S, Gielchinsky I, Parsonnet V. Mannitol, furosemide, and dopamine infusion in postoperative renal failure complicating cardiac surgery. *Ann Thorac Surg* 2000;69:501.

535. Schetz M. Vasopressors and the kidney. *Blood Purif* 2002;20:243.

536. Denton MD, Chertow GM, Brady HR. "Renal-dose" dopamine for the treatment of acute renal failure: scientific rationale, experimental studies and clinical trials. *Kidney Int* 1996;50:4.

537. Martin C, Papazian L, Perrin G, et al. Norepinephrine or dopamine for the treatment of hyperdynamic septic shock? *Chest* 1993;103:1826.

538. Albanese J, Leone M, Garnier F, et al. Renal effects of norepinephrine in septic and nonseptic patients. *Chest* 2004;126:534.

539. Patel BM, Chittock DR, Russell JA, et al. Beneficial effects of short-term vasopressin infusion during severe septic shock. *Anesthesiology* 2002;96: 576.

540. Tsuneyoshi I, Yamada H, Kakihana Y, et al. Hemodynamic and metabolic effects of low-dose vasopressin infusions in vasodilatory septic shock. *Crit Care Med* 2001;29:487.

541. Conger JD, Falk SA, Hammond WS. Atrial natriuretic peptide and dopamine in established acute renal failure in the rat. *Kidney Int* 1991;40: 21.

542. Rahman SN, Kim GE, Mathew AS, et al. Effects of atrial natriuretic peptide in clinical acute renal failure. *Kidney Int* 1994;45:1731.

543. Meyer M, Pfarr E, Schirmer G, et al. Therapeutic use of the natriuretic peptide ularitide in acute renal failure. *Ren Fail* 1999;21:85.

544. Lewis J, Salem MM, Chertow GM, et al. Atrial natriuretic factor in oliguric acute renal failure. Anaritide Acute Renal Failure Study Group. *Am J Kidney Dis* 2000;36:767.

545. Sward K, Valsson F, Odencrants P, et al. Recombinant human atrial natriuretic peptide in ischemic acute renal failure: a randomized placebo-controlled trial. *Crit Care Med* 2004;32:1310.

546. Herbert MK, Ginzel S, Muhlschlegel S, et al. Concomitant treatment with urodilatin (ularitide) does not improve renal function in patients with acute renal failure after major abdominal surgery—a randomized controlled trial. *Wien Klin Wochenschr* 1999;111:141.

547. Wiebe K, Meyer M, Wahlers T, et al. Acute renal failure following cardiac surgery is reverted by administration of Urodilatin (INN: Ularitide). *Eur J Med Res* 1996;1:259.

548. Hirschberg R, Kopple J, Lipsett P, et al. Multicenter clinical trial of recombinant human insulin-like growth factor I in patients with acute renal failure. *Kidney Int* 1999;55:2423.

549. Takala J, Ruokonen E, Webster NR, et al. Increased mortality associated with growth hormone treatment in critically ill adults. *N Engl J Med* 1999;341:785.

550. Acker CG, Singh AR, Flick RP, et al. A trial of thyroxine in acute renal failure. *Kidney Int* 2000;57:293.

551. Ralph CJ, Tanser SJ, Macnaughton PD, et al. A randomised controlled trial investigating the effects of dopexamine on gastrointestinal function and organ dysfunction in the critically ill. *Intensive Care Med* 2002;28:884.

552. Souba WW. Nutritional support. *N Engl J Med* 1997;336:41.

553. Heyland DK, MacDonald S, Keefe L, et al. Total parenteral nutrition in the critically ill patient: a meta-analysis. *JAMA* 1998;280:2013.

554. Seidner DL, Matarese LE, Steiger E. Nutritional care of the critically ill patient with renal failure. *Semin Nephrol* 1994;14:53.

555. Mitch WE, Klahr S. *Nutrition and the kidney.* 2nd ed. Boston: Little, Brown, 1995.

556. Druml W, Mitch WE. Metabolic abnormalities in acute renal failure. *Semin Dial* 1996;9:484.

557. Mukau L, Latimer RG. Acute hemodialysis in the surgical intensive care unit. *Am Surg* 1988;54:548.

558. Lowell JA, Schifferdecker C, Driscoll DF, et al. Postoperative fluid overload: not a benign problem. *Crit Care Med* 1990;18:728.

559. Wolk PJ, Apicella MA. The effect of renal function on the febrile response to bacteremia. *Arch Intern Med* 1978;138:1084.

560. Peresecenschi G, Blum M, Aviram A, et al. Impaired neutrophil response to acute bacterial infection in dialyzed patients. *Arch Intern Med* 1981;141: 1301.

561. Sagripanti A, Barsotti G. Bleeding and thrombosis in chronic uremia. *Nephron* 1997;75:125.

562. Hebert PC, Wells G, Blajchman MA, et al. A multicenter, randomized, controlled clinical trial of transfusion requirements in critical care. Transfusion Requirements in Critical Care Investigators, Canadian Critical Care Trials Group. *N Engl J Med* 1999;340:409.

563. Corwin HL, Gettinger A, Pearl RG, et al. Efficacy of recombinant human erythropoietin in critically ill patients: a randomized controlled trial. *JAMA* 2002;288:2827.

564. Liangos O, Pereira BJ, Jaber BL. Anemia in acute renal failure: role for erythropoiesis-stimulating proteins? *Artif Organs* 2003;27:786.

565. Star RA. Treatment of acute renal failure. *Kidney Int* 1998;54:1817.

566. Jorres A, Gahl GM, Dobis C, et al. Haemodialysis-membrane biocompatibility and mortality of patients with dialysis-dependent acute renal failure: a prospective randomised multicentre trial. International Multicentre Study Group. *Lancet* 1999;354:1337.

567. Jaber BL, Lau J, Schmid CH, et al. Effect of biocompatibility of hemodialysis membranes on mortality in acute renal failure: a meta-analysis. *Clin Nephrol* 2002;57:274.

568. Subramanian S, Venkataraman R, Kellum JA. Influence of dialysis membranes on outcomes in acute renal failure: a meta-analysis. *Kidney Int* 2002;62:1819.

569. Modi GK, Pereira BJ, Jaber BL. Hemodialysis in acute renal failure: does the membrane matter? *Semin Dial* 2001;14:318.

570. Kresse S, Schlee H, Deuber HJ, et al. Influence of renal replacement therapy on outcome of patients with acute renal failure. *Kidney Int Suppl* 1999; 72:S75.

571. Himmelfarb J, Tolkoff Rubin N, Chandran P, et al. A multicenter comparison of dialysis membranes in the treatment of acute renal failure requiring dialysis. *J Am Soc Nephrol* 1998;9:257.

572. Forni LG, Hilton PJ. Continuous hemofiltration in the treatment of acute renal failure. *N Engl J Med* 1997;336:1303.

573. Clark WR, Mueller BA, Kraus MA, et al. Extracorporeal therapy requirements for patients with acute renal failure. *J Am Soc Nephrol* 1997;8: 804.

574. Bellomo R, Farmer M, Bhonagiri S, et al. Changing acute renal failure treatment from intermittent hemodialysis to continuous hemofiltration: impact on azotemic control. *Int J Artif Organs* 1999;22:145.

575. Swartz RD, Messana JM, Orzol S, et al. Comparing continuous hemofiltration with hemodialysis in patients with severe acute renal failure. *Am J Kidney Dis* 1999;34:424.

576. Mehta RL, Letteri JM. Current status of renal replacement therapy for acute renal failure. A survey of US nephrologists. The National Kidney Foundation Council on Dialysis. *Am J Nephrol* 1999;19:377.

577. Demirkilic U, Kuralay E, Yenicesu M, et al. Timing of replacement therapy for acute renal failure after cardiac surgery. *J Card Surg* 2004;19:17.

578. Gettings LG, Reynolds HN, Scalea T. Outcome in post-traumatic acute renal failure when continuous renal replacement therapy is applied early vs. late. *Intensive Care Med* 1999;25:805.

579. Ronco C, Bellomo R, Homel P, et al. Effects of different doses in continuous veno-venous haemofiltration on outcomes of acute renal failure: a prospective randomised trial. *Lancet* 2000;356:26.

580. Van de Noortgate N, Verbeke F, Dhondt A, et al. The dialytic management of acute renal failure in the elderly. *Semin Dial* 2002;15:127.

581. Manji S, Shikora S, McMahon M, et al. Peritoneal dialysis for acute renal failure: overfeeding resulting from dextrose absorbed during dialysis. *Crit Care Med* 1990;18:29.

582. Martin C, Saran R, Leavey S, et al. Predicting the outcome of renal replacement therapy in severe acute renal failure. *ASAIO J* 2002;48:640.

583. Ronco C, Brendolan A, Bellomo R. Continuous renal replacement techniques. *Contrib Nephrol* 2001:236.

584. Druml W. Metabolic aspects of continuous renal replacement therapies. *Kidney Int Suppl* 1999;72:S56.

585. Metnitz GH, Fischer M, Bartens C, et al. Impact of acute renal failure on antioxidant status in multiple organ failure. *Acta Anaesthesiol Scand* 2000;44:236.

586. De Vriese AS, Colardyn FA, Philippe JJ, et al. Cytokine removal during continuous hemofiltration in septic patients. *J Am Soc Nephrol* 1999;10:846.

587. Honore PM, Jamez J, Wauthier M, et al. Prospective evaluation of short-term, high-volume isovolemic hemofiltration on the hemodynamic course and outcome in patients with intractable circulatory failure resulting from septic shock. *Crit Care Med* 2000;28:3581.

588. Cole L, Bellomo R, Journois D, et al. High-volume haemofiltration in human septic shock. *Intensive Care Med* 2001;27:978.

589. Schetz M. Non-renal indications for continuous renal replacement therapy. *Kidney Int Suppl* 1999;72:S88.

590. Ronco C, Bonello M, Bordoni V, et al. Extracorporeal therapies in non-renal disease: treatment of sepsis and the peak concentration hypothesis. *Blood Purif* 2004;22:164.

591. Mehta RL, McDonald B, Gabbai FB, et al. A randomized clinical trial of continuous versus intermittent dialysis for acute renal failure. *Kidney Int* 2001;60:1154.

592. Tonelli M, Manns B, Feller-Kopman D. Acute renal failure in the intensive care unit: a systematic review of the impact of dialytic modality on mortality and renal recovery. *Am J Kidney Dis* 2002;40:875.

593. Kellum JA, Angus DC, Johnson JP, et al. Continuous versus intermittent renal replacement therapy: a meta-analysis. *Intensive Care Med* 2002;28: 29.

594. Mehta RL. Outcomes research in acute renal failure. *Semin Nephrol* 2003; 23:283.

595. Teehan GS, Liangos O, Lau J, et al. Dialysis membrane and modality in acute renal failure: understanding discordant meta-analyses. *Semin Dial* 2003;16:356.

596. Vanholder R, Van Biesen W, Lameire N. What is the renal replacement method of first choice for intensive care patients? *J Am Soc Nephrol* 2001; 12(Suppl 17):S40.

597. Marshall MR, Ma T, Galler D, et al. Sustained low-efficiency daily diafiltration (SLEDD-f) for critically ill patients requiring renal replacement therapy: towards an adequate therapy. *Nephrol Dial Transplant* 2004;19: 877.

598. Lonnemann G, Floege J, Kliem V, et al. Extended daily veno-venous high-flux haemodialysis in patients with acute renal failure and multiple organ dysfunction syndrome using a single path batch dialysis system. *Nephrol Dial Transplant* 2000;15:1189.

599. Kielstein JT, Kretschmer U, Ernst T, et al. Efficacy and cardiovascular tolerability of extended dialysis in critically ill patients: a randomized controlled study. *Am J Kidney Dis* 2004;43:342.

600. Kumar VA, Craig M, Depner TA, et al. Extended daily dialysis: a new approach to renal replacement for acute renal failure in the intensive care unit. *Am J Kidney Dis* 2000;36:294.

601. Chertow GM, Lazarus JM. Intensity of dialysis in established acute renal failure. *Semin Dial* 1996;7:476.

602. Bhatla B, Nolph KD, Khanna R. Choosing the right dialysis option for your critically ill patient. What's right for a hyperkalemic patient may be wrong for one with shock. *J Crit Illn* 1996;11:21.

603. Kanagasundaram NS, Paganini EP. Critical care dialysis-a Gordian knot (but is untying the right approach?). *Nephrol Dial Transplant* 1999;14:2590.

604. Lameire N, Van Biesen W, Vanholder R. Dialysing the patient with acute renal failure in the ICU: the emperor's clothes? *Nephrol Dial Transplant* 1999;14:2570.

605. Abramson S, Singh AK. Continuous renal replacement therapy compared with intermittent hemodialysis in intensive care: which is better? *Curr Opin Nephrol Hypertens* 1999;8:537.

606. Kleinknecht D, Jungers P, Chanard J, et al. Uremic and non-uremic complications in acute renal failure: Evaluation of early and frequent dialysis on prognosis. *Kidney Int* 1972;1:190.

607. Howdieshell TR, Blalock WE, Bowen PA, et al. Management of post-traumatic acute renal failure with peritoneal dialysis. *Am Surg* 1992;58:378.

608. Conger J. Does hemodialysis delay recovery from acute renal failure? *Semin Dial* 1990;3:146.

609. Gastaldello K, Melot C, Kahn RJ, et al. Comparison of cellulose diacetate and polysulfone membranes in the outcome of acute renal failure. A prospective randomized study. *Nephrol Dial Transplant* 2000;15:224.

610. Hakim RM, Wingard RL, Parker RA. Effect of the dialysis membrane in the treatment of patients with acute renal failure. *N Engl J Med* 1994;331:1338.

611. Schiffl H, Lang SM, Konig A, et al. Biocompatible membranes in acute renal failure: prospective case-controlled study. *Lancet* 1994;344:570.

612. Jones CH, Newstead CG, Goutcher E. Continuous dialysis for ARF in the ICU: choice of membrane does not influence survival. *J Am Soc Nephrol* 1997;8:126A.

613. Schiffl H, Lang SM, Fischer R. Daily hemodialysis and the outcome of acute renal failure. *N Engl J Med* 2002;346:305.

614. Clark WR, Turk JE, Kraus MA, et al. Dose determinants in continuous renal replacement therapy. *Artif Organs* 2003;27:815.

615. Van Biesen W, Vanholder R, Lameire N. Dialysis strategies in critically ill acute renal failure patients. *Curr Opin Crit Care* 2003;9:491.

616. Clark WR, Ronco C. Renal replacement therapy in acute renal failure: solute removal mechanisms and dose quantification. *Kidney Int Suppl* 1998;66:S133.

617. Evanson JA, Ikizler TA, Wingard R, et al. Measurement of the delivery of dialysis in acute renal failure. *Kidney Int* 1999;55:1501.

618. Metnitz PG, Krenn CG, Steltzer H, et al. Effect of acute renal failure requiring renal replacement therapy on outcome in critically ill patients. *Crit Care Med* 2002;30:2051.

619. de Mendonca A, Vincent JL, Suter PM, et al. Acute renal failure in the ICU: risk factors and outcome evaluated by the SOFA score. *Intensive Care Med* 2000;26:915.

620. Simmons EM, Himmelfarb J, Sezer MT, et al. Plasma cytokine levels predict mortality in patients with acute renal failure. *Kidney Int* 2004;65:1357.

621. Lemeshow S, Le Gall JR. Modeling the severity of illness of ICU patients. A systems update. *JAMA* 1994;272:1049.

622. Halstenberg WK, Goormastic M, Paganini EP. Utility of risk models for renal failure and critically ill patients. *Semin Nephrol* 1994;14:23.

623. Douma CE. Prognostic methods for mortality of intensive care patients with acute renal failure. *J Am Soc Nephrol* 1994;5:402.

624. Parker RA. Survival of dialysis dependent acute renal failure patients predicted by APACHE II. *J Am Soc Nephrol* 1994;5:402.

625. Chertow GM, Christiansen CL, Cleary PD, et al. Prognostic stratification in critically ill patients with acute renal failure requiring dialysis. *Arch Intern Med* 1995;155:1505.

626. Cioffi WG, Ashikaga T, Gamelli RL. Probability of surviving postoperative acute renal failure. Development of a prognostic index. *Ann Surg* 1984;200:205.

627. Schaefer JH, Jochimsen F, Keller F, et al. Outcome prediction of acute renal failure in medical intensive care. *Intensive Care Med* 1991;17:19.

628. Liano F, Gallego A, Pascual J, et al. Prognosis of acute tubular necrosis: an extended prospectively contrasted study. *Nephron* 1993;63:21.

629. Douma CE, Redekop WK, van der Meulen JH, et al. Predicting mortality in intensive care patients with acute renal failure treated with dialysis. *J Am Soc Nephrol* 1997;8:111.

630. Halstenberg WK, Goormastic M, Paganini EP. Validity of four models for predicting outcome in critically ill acute renal failure patients. *Clin Nephrol* 1997;47:81.

631. Liano F. Severity of acute renal failure: the need of measurement. *Nephrol Dial Transplant* 1994;9(Suppl 4):229.

632. Lohr JW, McFarlane MJ, Grantham JJ. A clinical index to predict survival in acute renal failure patients requiring dialysis. *Am J Kidney Dis* 1988;11:254.

633. Chertow GM, Lazarus JM, Paganini EP, et al. Predictors of mortality and the provision of dialysis in patients with acute tubular necrosis. The Auriculin Anaritide Acute Renal Failure Study Group. *J Am Soc Nephrol* 1998;9:692.

634. Paganini EP, Halstenberg WK, Goormastic M. Risk modeling in acute renal failure requiring dialysis: the introduction of a new model. *Clin Nephrol* 1996;46:206.

635. Parker RA, Himmelfarb J, Tolkoff-Rubin N, et al. Prognosis of patients with acute renal failure requiring dialysis: results of a multicenter study. *Am J Kidney Dis* 1998;32:432.

636. Kjellstrand CM, Ebben J, Davin T. Time of death, recovery of renal function, development of chronic renal failure and need for chronic hemodialysis in patients with acute tubular necrosis. *Trans Am Soc Artif Intern Organs* 1981;27:45.

637. Hall JW, Johnson WJ, Maher FT, et al. Immediate and long-term prognosis in acute renal failure. *Ann Intern Med* 1970;73:515.

638. Levin ML, Simon NM, Herdson PB, et al. Acute renal failure followed by protracted, slowly resolving chronic uremia. *J Chronic Dis* 1972;25:645.

639. Bhandari S, Turney JH. Survivors of acute renal failure who do not recover renal function. *QJM* 1996;89:415.

640. Molitoris BA, Weinberg J. Acute renal failure. Experimental models of acute renal failure. *Am J Physiol* 2000;278:F1.

641. Kelly KJ, Molitoris BA. Acute renal failure in the new millennium: time to consider combination therapy. *Semin Nephrol* 2000;20:4.

CHAPTER 42 ■ ANTIBIOTIC- AND IMMUNOSUPPRESSION-RELATED RENAL FAILURE

JEAN-LOUIS BOSMANS AND MARC E. DE BROE

AMINOGLYCOSIDE ANTIBIOTICS

Nephrotoxic injury is a common complication of aminoglycoside antibiotic therapy. Studies that have used well-defined measures of nephrotoxicity indicate an incidence rate of 7% to 36% (1–9). This variability reflects differences with respect to the nephrotoxicity potentials of aminoglycoside antibiotics in clinical use as well as differences among patients receiving these drugs. A survey of clinical studies published between 1975 and 1982 reveals that the average incidence of nephrotoxicity caused by specific aminoglycoside antibiotics was gentamicin, 14%; tobramycin, 12.9%; amikacin, 9.4%; and netilmicin, 8.9% (10). In critically ill patients, the incidence of aminoglycoside nephrotoxicity may rise twofold (11).

Clinical Aspects

The clinical expression of aminoglycoside nephrotoxicity has been well described (12–16). The earliest and most common expression of aminoglycoside renal tubular cell alterations is increased urinary excretion of low-molecular-weight proteins (17,18) and of lysosomal and brush-border membrane enzymes (17–20). These changes may be detected within 24 hours of initiating drug therapy, and the frequency and magnitude of these changes increase as a function of dose and duration of therapy. Unfortunately, these changes do not predict which patients will progress to acute renal failure (ARF). This probably reflects the fact that several mechanisms underlie the expression of the enzymuria and proteinuria (13). With repeated dosing, the amount of enzymes and low-molecular-weight proteins excreted in the urine may increase quite sharply, which may signify the onset of proximal tubular cell necrosis (13).

Nonoliguric renal failure is a common expression of aminoglycoside nephrotoxicity (21) and may reflect a direct inhibitory effect on solute transport along the thick ascending limb of Henle's loop (22) or possibly tubulointerstitial cell injury (23), which results in impaired ability to maintain a hypertonic medullary interstitium. Inhibition of adenylate cyclase may also contribute to the polyuria (24). Neither mechanism, however, adequately explains the maintenance of normal to high urine output, even in the face of severe depression of whole-kidney glomerular filtration rate (GFR). The slow evolution of ARF, which has been attributed to a variable susceptibility of renal proximal tubular cells to aminoglycoside toxicity (12,25), may allow for the development of maximal compensatory adaptation by residual intact nephrons. In addition, micropuncture experiments (26) implicate a marked depression of solute and water transport along the proximal tubule such that the large increase in the fraction of filtrate escaping reabsorption along the proximal tubule may over-

whelm the reabsorptive capacity of the distal nephron and contribute to the pattern of nonoliguric renal failure. When oliguria occurs, it usually signifies the influence of one or more complicating factors, for example, ischemia or another nephrotoxin, especially if the oliguria appears early in the course of aminoglycoside administration. Studies in animals have shown that aminoglycoside therapy sensitizes the kidney to a subsequent ischemic or nephrotoxic insult (27–36), such that the severity of the ARF is substantially greater than that predicted by the sum of the individual insults. Deterioration of other proximal tubular transport processes may occur during aminoglycoside toxicity and in rare cases may mimic a Fanconi-like syndrome (37). Hypokalemia and hypomagnesemia secondary to renal potassium and magnesium wasting may also appear (38,39).

Depression of GFR is a relatively late manifestation of aminoglycoside nephrotoxicity. In humans, depression of GFR typically does not occur before 5 to 7 days of therapy have been completed (15) unless there has been a major complicating factor such as renal ischemia. Studies in animal models of aminoglycoside nephrotoxicity have implicated activation of the renin–angiotensin system (40), reduction in the size and density of glomerular endothelial fenestrae (41), tubular obstruction (42), tubular back leak (26), and release of platelet activating factor from mesangial cells (43) as pathogenic factors causing depression of GFR.

The majority of patients with aminoglycoside nephrotoxicity recover renal function clinically, although in some cases the time to recovery may be prolonged (16). Chronic renal failure is a distinctly uncommon complication of pure aminoglycoside nephrotoxicity in humans, so that when it occurs, it usually signifies the contribution of some additional factor. Animal studies indicate, however, that incomplete regeneration with interstitial fibrosis does occur (44), and the same may be true for humans (45).

Morphologic Alterations

Aminoglycosides cause tubular cell necrosis that in animal models is largely confined to the proximal convoluted tubule and pars recta (46–48). In humans, the renal tubular site of injury is less well established (23,49), due in part to the fact that little human biopsy material has been available for study. Moreover, in human subjects, the development of ARF in conjunction with aminoglycoside administration typically occurs in association with other insults such as sepsis and renal ischemia (23,50,51), and each of these insults has been shown to interact synergistically with aminoglycoside antibiotics to magnify the severity and sites of tubular cell injury (30–36).

The earliest lesion seen by electron microscopy is an increase in the number and size of secondary lysosomes, also

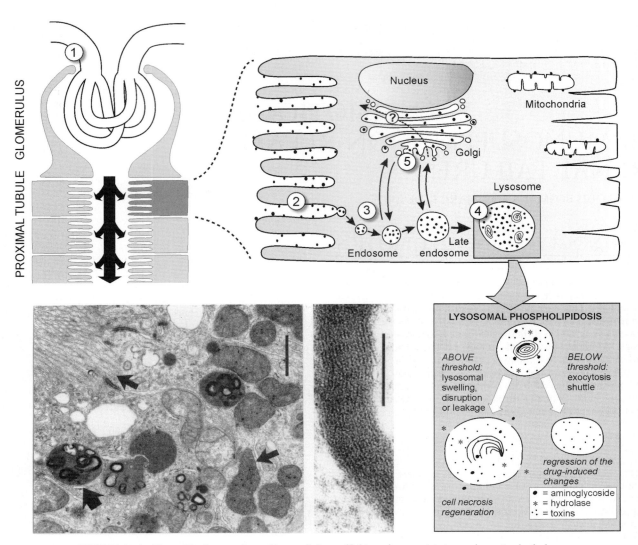

FIGURE 42-1. Above: Binding uptake and intracellular trafficking of gentamicin in renal proximal tubular cells. After glomerular filtration (1), gentamicin (•) is shown binding to the surface membrane (2) and being internalized by a receptor (megalin) mediated endocytic process (3). Gentamicin also enters the cell through fluid phase endocytosis. It moves through the endocytic system into late endosomes and from there into lysosomal structures (4). A small but quantifiable fraction (5%–10%) of gentamicin directly traffics from the surface membrane into the trans-Golgi network (5) and from there throughout the Golgi apparatus. **Below left:** Ultrastructural appearance of proximal tubular cells after 4 days of gentamicin treatment, showing lysosomes containing dense lamellar and concentric structures (*large arrow*), while brush border, mitochondria (*small arrow*) and peroxisomes are unaltered. Upon higher magnification, the structures in lysosomes show a periodic pattern. *Bar left* = 1 µm, *middle* = 0.1 µm. **Below right:** Internalization and lysosomal sequestration of gentamicin. (Adapted from: Verpooten GA, Tulkens PM, Molitoris BA. Aminoglycosides and vancomycin. In: DeBroe ME, Porter GA, Bennett VM, et al., eds. *Clinical nephrotoxins: renal injury from drugs and chemicals,* 2nd ed. Dordrecht, The Netherlands: Kluwer Acadmic Publishers, 2003:151.)

called cytosegrosomes or phagosomes (46–48). Examples of this lesion are shown in Figure 42-1. Secondary lysosomes are primary lysosomes that have coalesced with endocytic or autophagic vacuoles. Many of these lysosomes contain myeloid bodies, electron-dense lamellar structures of concentrically arranged and densely packed membranes. These lysosomal alterations probably represent autophagic vacuoles arising from sequestration of fragments of membranes and organelles damaged in the early phase of toxicity and are undergoing lysosomal processing. In experimental animals receiving single parenteral drug doses or continuous drug infusion, these changes have been observed as early as 6 to 12 hours posttreatment (52). Both the number and size of lysosomal myeloid bodies

increase as a function of dose and duration of drug therapy and are accompanied by progressive expansion of the volume of the cell occupied by engorged lysosomes (47,52,53). These morphologic alterations also have been convincingly demonstrated in human kidney material (54,55). Studies in experimental animals and in cultured cells have demonstrated that the myeloid bodies are composed of membranes rich in phospholipids (56,57) and form as a consequence of the lysosomal accumulation in high concentration of aminoglycosides. This lysosomal accumulation of aminoglycosides inhibits lysosomal phospholipases (58,59) and possibly other lysosomal enzymes and impairs the degradation of cell membranes (57,60). Similar alterations have been induced by a variety of compounds that accumulate within the lysosomal compartment and interfere with the activity of lysosomal enzymes (61–63).

Following lysosomal alterations, there occurs a decrease in the density and height of brush-border microvilli, dilation of the cisternae of rough endoplasmic reticulum, and the appearance of cytoplasmic vacuolization in tubular epithelial cells (48,52). As injury progresses, brush-border membrane fragments and extruded myeloid bodies, membrane vesicles, and cytoplasmic debris begin to be seen within tubular lumina (48,64). Later in the course of nephrotoxicity, mitochondrial swelling becomes evident, and patchy, but extensive tubular epithelial cell necrosis and desquamation occur. Many tubules, both proximal and distal, are filled with eosinophilic, granular material that, by electron microscopy, is composed of cytoplasmic debris, membrane fragments, and myeloid bodies. Transmission electron microscopy of the urine reveals the presence of myeloid bodies and fragments of brush-border membranes (64–66).

Proximal tubular cells manifest an apparent variable susceptibility to aminoglycoside toxicity evident by the appearance of cell regeneration simultaneously with ongoing cell necrosis (25,44,47,53,67). In several animal studies virtually complete recovery of renal structure and function has been observed during continued aminoglycoside administration (68,69). One explanation for these observations is that the renal tubular epithelium had acquired resistance to the nephrotoxic effects of the aminoglycoside antibiotic. Sundin and colleagues (70) report that the "acquired resistance" reflects selective inhibition of aminoglycoside uptake by renal proximal tubular cells, the mechanism of which does not involve a reduction in the membrane content of phosphatidylinositol or megalin. In animal models, cell regeneration can be detected by [^{3}H]thymidine incorporation into DNA after only 4 days of low-dose aminoglycoside administration and before cell necrosis is evident by light microscopy (53,70). The magnitude of DNA labeling correlates with the dose and duration of drug administration (71). Of particular interest is the observation that quantitatively similar labeling is observed in renal cortical interstitial cells as in tubular epithelial cells (53,71,72). This finding raises the question of the role of these interstitial cells in the pathogenesis of aminoglycoside toxicity. Eventually most areas of the affected kidney regain normal architecture and function, but residual scarring containing collections of collapsed, atrophic tubules may occur focally in the cortex (44,45,48). In animal models of aminoglycoside nephrotoxicity, the degree of tubular cell necrosis correlates reasonably well with the decline in renal excretory function. A similar correlation is lacking in human material (23,49,54).

Pathogenesis

The pathogenesis of aminoglycoside nephrotoxicity is intimately linked to the renal pharmacology of these drugs (73–76). Aminoglycoside antibiotics are organic polycations with a net cationic charge that, at pH 7.4, ranges from +4.47 in the case of neomycin to +2.39 for amikacin. Because these compounds are highly hydrophilic, they are poorly absorbed across the intestinal tract and therefore must be given parenterally. They are distributed in a volume slightly greater than extracellular volume and are eliminated from the body without metabolic transformation. The route of elimination is almost exclusively by the kidneys, and the principal mechanism of excretion is glomerular filtration. Of toxicologic significance is the fact that small amounts of aminoglycoside antibiotics are selectively transported into proximal tubular cells by adsorptive endocytosis (77–79), which has been shown to occur across the basolateral as well as the apical membrane (79). Several lines of evidence have implicated anionic phosphatidylinositol

as a membrane binding site for aminoglycosides (80,81). More-recent studies also suggest a role for megalin, an endocytic receptor for cationic ligands, in the uptake of aminoglycoside antibiotics across the brush-border membrane of renal proximal tubular cells (82). Indeed, by using the specific antagonist receptor-associated protein, blocking the activity of megalin in perfused rat proximal tubules, a reduction of 20% in gentamicin clearance ensued. Nagai demonstrated similar results in rats treated with maleate, impairing the receptor-mediated uptake of megalin ligands (83). Megalin knockout mice are protected against aminoglycoside nephrotoxicity (84).

Following endocytosis, the aminoglycosides are translocated into the lysosomal compartment, where they accumulate in millimolar concentrations and reside with a half-life measured in days (74). As noted, the lysosomal compartment is the site of myeloid body formation consequent to aminoglycoside-induced inhibition of lysosomal enzymes such as phospholipase, sphyngomyelase, etc. When the concentration of drug and/or the amount of lysosomal phospholipid reaches a critical threshold, an injury cascade is triggered that eventuates in irreversible cell injury with progression to necrosis (52). However, neither the sequence nor the specific mechanisms involved in the progression to cell death have been clearly established. Sandoval and colleagues report that within 15 minutes of endocytosis gentamicin traffics to the Golgi complex as well as to the lysosomal compartment of LLC-PK1 cells (85,86) and rat renal proximal tubular cells (87). These observations raise the possibility that the Golgi complex may provide a pathway for the redistribution of aminoglycoside antibiotics to other intracellular compartments and thereby broaden the potential for these drugs to disrupt a variety of organellar functions. For example, the depression of protein synthesis observed early in the course of gentamicin administration may signify retrograde transport of gentamicin to the endoplasmic reticulum (87). The reason gentamicin and presumably other aminoglycoside antibiotics are transported from the endosomal compartment to the Golgi complex is not known; but, it may reflect an effect of these agents to perturb endosomal fusion (88) possibly as a consequence of binding to megalin (88) or to membrane-acidic phospholipids (89,90).

A growing body of evidence supports the view that the pathogenesis of aminoglycoside toxicity is causally related to the capacity of these cationic drugs to bind to and perturb the function and structure of biologic membranes. Aminoglycosides have been shown to bind to anionic (58,80,91–98) but not to neutral phospholipids (58,80,92,94). Among the anionic phospholipids, aminoglycosides bind most avidly to phosphatidylinositol 4,5-bisphosphate (PIP$_2$) (80,93,99–101). Several approaches have been used to gain insight into the molecular interaction between aminoglycosides and anionic phospholipids (80,91,94,97,98,102–104). All models indicate an electrostatic interaction between a protonated amino group and the anionic phosphate group. Ramsammy and Kaloyanides (103) propose a model, that in addition to an electrostatic interaction between a protonated amino group and the phosphate group, also involves formation of hydrogen bonds between an amino group of gentamicin and the carbonyl groups of glycerol. This model explains aminoglycoside-induced changes in the biophysical properties of artificial membranes (i.e., an increase in the transition temperature and a decrease in glycerol permeability of phosphatidylinositol [PI]-containing liposomes) (96). Both changes signify that gentamicin induces a decrease in membrane fluidity, and this finding has been confirmed in brush-border membranes as assessed by changes in the fluorescence polarization of membrane probes (92) and by electron spin resonance spectroscopy (105). Aminoglycosides also have been shown to promote membrane aggregation (102,106), a process that requires neutralization of surface charge. In a comparative study of aminoglycoside-induced aggregation of

PI-containing liposomes (102), it was observed that the rank order with respect to efficacy in neutralizing membrane surface charge was neomycin > gentamicin = tobramycin = netilmicin = spermine. The rank order for inducing aggregation of liposomes was neomycin > gentamicin > tobramycin > netilmicin = spermine and was identical to the rank order of these agents with respect to depressing glycerol permeability (102). This rank order also coincides precisely with the established clinical nephrotoxicity potentials of these drugs. Since depression of glycerol permeability was shown to be dependent on hydrogen bonding between one or more amino groups of the drug and carbonyl groups of the glycerol backbone (103), these data suggest that the membrane toxicity of aminoglycosides is closely linked to their potentials to engage in hydrogen bonding. Importantly, the rank order in terms of nephrotoxicity potentials does not coincide with the net cationic charge of these agents (102). This observation emphasizes that spatial orientation of charge rather than net charge is a critical determinant of toxicity.

Schacht and colleagues (93,95,100,107) utilize a variety of methods to assess aminoglycoside-induced perturbations of PIP_2-containing membranes as a measure of the ototoxicity potentials of these antibiotics. Increased fluorescence of 1-anilino-8-naphthalenesulfonate (95), increased permeability to carboxy fluorescein (100), and increased surface tension of monomolecular film of phosphatidylcholine (PC)/PIP_2 (107) were shown to correlate precisely with the ototoxicity potentials of aminoglycoside antibiotics. These studies have led to the hypothesis that the ototoxicity of aminoglycosides is causally related to their binding to PIP_2 and disruption of this signaling mechanism (108).

The studies cited here provide the foundation for the hypothesis that the toxicity of aminoglycoside antibiotics is causally related to their capacity to interact electrostatically and by hydrogen bonding to membrane anionic phospholipids and, thereby, to perturb the biophysical properties and function of cell membranes. It is well established that these drugs interact with and perturb the function of plasma membranes (13,109–112), lysosomes (13,52,53–60,113–118), mitochondria (48,119–122), and microsomes (123–125). It remains unclear, however, whether toxicity results from disruption of a single critical membrane function or multiple membrane functions. It is possible that the injury cascade is triggered by the rupture of lysosomes engorged with aminoglycoside antibiotic and with myeloid bodies. The resultant release of potent acid hydrolases and high concentrations of drug into the cytoplasm might cause disruption of a number of critical intracellular processes including mitochondrial respiration (48,119–122), microsomal protein synthesis (123–125), intracellular signaling via the PI cascade (126–129) as well as generation of hydroxyl radicals (130–132), all of which have been observed in experimental models of aminoglycoside toxicity. However, the observation that gentamicin is transported to the Golgi complex shortly after endocytic uptake (85,86), provides an alternate mechanism by which these drugs gain access to other organelles. Recently, proteomic analysis following gentamicin administration indicated energy production impairment and a mitochondrial dysfunction occurring in parallel to the onset of nephrotoxicity (133).

Further insight into the pathogenesis of aminoglycoside nephrotoxicity has been gleaned from studies of interventions that modify the severity of this disorder in experimental animals. Williams and colleagues (134–136) first reported that polyasparagine and polyaspartic acid (PAA) inhibited binding of gentamicin to rat renal brush-border membrane *in vitro* and when injected *in vivo* conferred protection against the development of aminoglycoside nephrotoxicity without inhibiting the renal cortical accumulation of drug. These findings have been confirmed and extended by three groups of investigators

(137–145). The mechanism by which PAA protects against aminoglycoside nephrotoxicity was shown to be related to the ability of PAA, a polyanion, to form electrostatic complexes with the polycationic aminoglycoside antibiotics (142,146,147) presumably within the endocytic compartment (144), thereby preventing aminoglycosides from binding to anionic phospholipids, from inhibiting lysosomal phospholipase degradation of phospholipid, from forming lysosomal myeloid bodies, and from disrupting the PI cascade (146). Additional support for this theory is provided by the observation that PAA prevented gentamicin from depressing glycerol permeability or aggregating PI-containing liposomes (146), effects previously shown to be dependent on gentamicin binding electrostatically and by hydrogen bonding to PI (96,103). Subsequently, other compounds capable of forming electrostatic complexes with aminoglycosides have been reported to protect against nephrotoxicity (148–151).

Recently, an analog of pentoxifylline, HWA-448, was shown to protect against gentamicin toxicity in a cell culture model (152). Similar to PAA, HWA-448 did not depress the membrane binding or cellular uptake of gentamicin. It remains unknown whether HWA-448 forms a complex with gentamicin within the endosomal compartment.

Treatment and Prevention of Aminoglycoside Nephrotoxicity

The efficacy of PAA and other anionic compounds in preventing nephrotoxicity in humans has yet to be established. Therefore the primary focus of treatment is prevention, and this can be accomplished by understanding and modifying, when possible, the risk factors (Table 42-1) for this complication (153–155). Risk factors may be categorized into those that are determined by the individual patient and not easily influenced, if at all, and those that are determined by the clinician and potentially controllable (Table 42-1).

Prominent among the risk factors peculiar to the patient and not modifiable is advanced age (153). The mechanism is probably multifactorial and includes age-related decline of renal function that if not appreciated and corrected for results in excessive dosing (156). Animal studies suggest that aging is associated with altered renal pharmacokinetics accompanied by increased renal cortical accumulation of drug (157). Increased susceptibility of the aging kidney to aminoglycoside toxicity has also been suggested (158), possibly on the basis of an age-related impaired capacity for cellular repair and regeneration. Male gender has been shown to carry increased risk for aminoglycoside nephrotoxicity in the rat (159), whereas female gender has been identified as a risk factor in humans (153). The reason for this difference has not been established.

Obesity carries increased risk for aminoglycoside nephrotoxicity that is unexplained by differences in the volume of distribution or renal clearance of drug (160). The increased risk associated with chronic liver disease (153) may be related to the alterations in extracellular volume, hemodynamics, and electrolyte balance commonly observed in this disorder, all of which are known to promote renal cortical accumulation of drug (74). Preexisting chronic renal insufficiency is associated with increased risk primarily due to failure to adjust appropriately the dose of aminoglycoside for the level of impaired kidney function (161). Renal hypoperfusion from any cause carries an increased risk of aminoglycoside nephrotoxicity whether the renal ischemic insult occurs before (81), during (33), or after drug administration (31). The latter observation is particularly worthy of note because it implies that the increased risk of nephrotoxicity persists even after the drug has been discontinued. The prolonged half-life of aminoglycosides in renal cortex

TABLE 42-1

RISK FACTORS FOR AMINOGLYCOSIDE NEPHROTOXICITY

Patient factors
Older patients[a]
Preexisting renal disease
Magnesium, potassium, calcium deficiency[a]
Intravascular volume depletion,[a] hypotension[a]
Hepatic syndrome
Sepsis syndrome[a]

Aminoglycoside factors
Recent aminoglycoside therapy
Larger doses[a]
Treatment of 3 or more days[a]
Drug choice: e.g., gentamicin,[a] amikacin[a]
Frequent dosing interval[a]

Concomitant drugs
Amphotericin B
Cephalosporines
Cisplatin
Clindamycin
Cyclosporine
Foscarnet
Forosemide
IV radiocontrast agents
Piperacillin
Vancomycin

[a]Concurrent with experimental nephrotoxicity data.
(Adapted from: Verpooten GA, Tulkens PM, Molitoris BA. Aminoglycosides and vancomycin. In: De Broe ME, Porter GA, Bennett VM, et al., eds. *Clinical nephrotoxins—renal injury from drugs and chemicals*, 2nd ed. Dordrecht, The Netherlands. Kluwer Acadmic Publishers, 2003:151.)

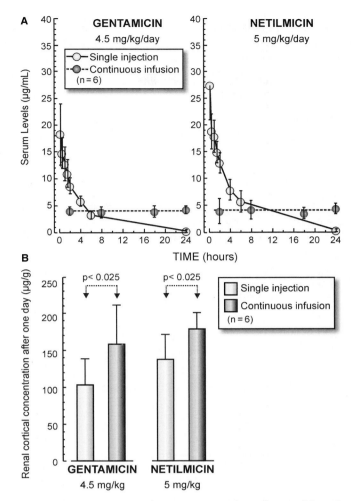

FIGURE 42-2. **A:** Course of serum concentrations of gentamicin and netilmicin after administration of the dose by a 30-minute intravenous injection or by continuous infusion of 24 hours. **B:** Cortical concentration of gentamicin and netilmicin after administration by the previously mentioned administration schedules. (Reprinted from: Verpooten GA, et al. Once-daily dosing decreases renal accumulation of gentamicin and netilmicin. *Clin Pharmacol Ther* 1989;45:22, with permission.)

(74) may contribute to this risk. Three components of the septic state—renal hypoperfusion, endotoxemia, and hyperthermia—have been identified as factors contributing to the heightened risk of nephrotoxicity during aminoglycoside therapy (34–36). Renal hypoperfusion (34,81) and endotoxemia (32,162) are associated with increased accumulation of drug in renal cortex; however, this factor alone does not explain the increased risk.

Of those risk factors that are potentially modifiable by the clinician, the most important are daily drug dose, interval of dosing, and the duration of therapy. A direct relationship between total dose (daily dose plus duration of therapy) and nephrotoxicity has been consistently found in experimental animals (25,44,48,52,67) and in humans (9,15,153,154,161). Animal studies have shown that the same dose of a drug administered in two or three divided doses leads to greater renal accumulation of the drug and greater nephrotoxicity than if it was given as a single dose (163,164). Two trials in humans found that the dosage schedule had a critical effect on the renal uptake of gentamicin, netilmicin (165), amikacin, and tobramycin (166). The study was carried out in patients with normal renal function (serum creatinine between 0.9 and 1.2 mg per dL, proteinuria lower than 300 mg per day) who had renal cancer and submitted to nephrectomy. Before surgery patients received gentamicin (4.5 mg per kg per day), netilmicin (5 mg per kg per day), amikacin (15 mg per kg per day), or tobramycin (4.5 mg per kg per day), as a single injection or as a continuous intravenous infusion over 24 hours. The single-injection schedule resulted in a 30% to 50% lower cortical drug con-

centration of netilmicin, gentamicin, and amikacin compared with administration by continuous infusion (Figs. 42-2 and 42-3). For tobramycin, in humans as well as in rats, no difference in renal accumulation could be found, indicating the linear cortical uptake of this particular aminoglycoside. Administration of drug by continuous IV infusion carries the highest risk of nephrotoxicity with respect to gentamicin, tobramycin, and netilmicin but not amikacin (76,164,167). These observations have stimulated studies in humans to assess the antimicrobial efficacy of once per day dosing with an aminoglycoside administered alone or in combination with a β-lactam antibiotic (168–171).

Several meta-analyses pooled the data of individual randomized control trials (RCT) (Table 42-2) (172–181), including a meta-analysis specifically of the studies in immunocompromised patients (181). It is apparent that only the meta-analyses that combine the results of the individual RCT by means of a fixed-effects model yielded significant results in favor of less nephrotoxicity in the single daily dose regimens. However, given the inhomogeneity of the study designs and the different aminoglycoside used, it seems prudent to use the random-effects model to combine the individual studies. The

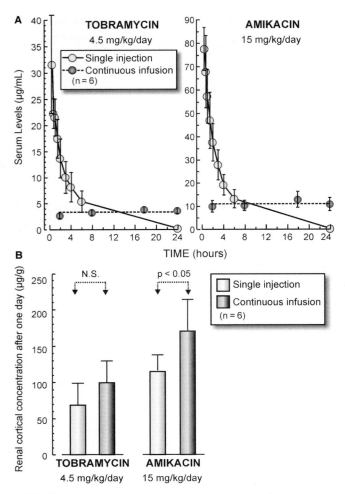

FIGURE 42-3. A: Course of serum concentrations of tobramycin and amikacin after administration of the dose by a 30-minute intravenous injection or by continuous infusion of 24 hours. **B:** Cortical concentration of tobramycin and amikacin after administration by the previously mentioned administration schedules. (Reprinted from: De Broe ME, Giuliano RA, Verpooten GA. Influence of dosage schedule on renal cortical accumulation of amikacin and tobramycin in man. *J Antimicrob Chemother* 1991;27[Suppl C]:41, with permission.)

(74). The mechanism underlying the increased risk associated with hypomagnesemia has not been definitively established but may relate to the competition between divalent cations and the cationic aminoglycoside antibiotics critical for membrane-binding sites (191). In the case of metabolic acidosis, the reduced pH promotes increased protonation of aminoglycoside antibiotics and augments the reactivity of these organic polycations with membrane anionic phospholipids (58,97,115).

Finally, the risk of nephrotoxicity has been shown to be augmented when aminoglycoside antibiotics are administered in conjunction with certain drugs and pharmaceutical agents, some of which have intrinsic nephrotoxicity potential. These include amphotericin B (171), cephalothin but not third-generation cephalosporins (192), vancomycin (195,194), cisplatin (195), furosemide (196), calcium channel blockers (197), radiocontrast agents (198), and nonsteroidal antiinflammatory drugs (199). Many of these synergistic interactions have been identified in animal studies so that the relevance of these observations to humans remains to be established. Nevertheless, prudence dictates that potentially nephrotoxic drugs should be avoided if possible in patients who are receiving or have recently completed therapy with aminoglycoside antibiotics.

The prevention of aminoglycoside nephrotoxicity requires that these drugs be used only for well-defined indications and that they be prescribed in the appropriate dose and for the appropriate duration to achieve the therapeutic goal. Dosing based on individualized drug pharmacokinetics derived from measurements of serum drug concentration would appear to be a rational approach. Unfortunately, prospective studies have failed to demonstrate that dosing based on drug pharmacokinetics reduces the incidence of nephrotoxicity (200). Indeed, eight prospective, randomized controlled trials specifically designed to investigate the effect of pharmacokinetic dosing (201) on aminoglycoside expression of nephrotoxicity could be identified from the literature (202–209). These individual studies have been unable to detect any change in the incidence of this adverse event. Nevertheless, close monitoring of serum drug concentration is still warranted, especially in high-risk patients to ensure that therapeutic concentrations are achieved. Even when those factors known to influence risk are absent, or have been minimized or eliminated, aminoglycoside nephrotoxicity will still occur in a certain percentage of appropriately dosed patients. These patients exhibit excessive renal accumulation of drug or increased sensitivity to a given level of drug accumulation (210). The clinician must be constantly alert to the possibility of aminoglycoside nephrotoxicity and monitor all patients on aminoglycoside therapy for this potential complication. The intensity of monitoring is dictated in part by the relative risk factors present. At a minimum, frequent measurements of serum creatinine concentration, generally every 2 to 3 days, should be performed. In high-risk patients, daily creatinine clearances and urinalysis may be required to detect early signs of toxicity before a rise in serum creatinine concentration or serum trough level of drug becomes evident. If renal injury occurs, then the drug should be stopped if possible or dosage should be reduced to prevent the accumulation of drug in serum and further toxic injury related thereto. Careful attention must be paid to maintaining fluid and electrolyte balance and avoiding potential insults to the kidney related to renal hypoperfusion or exposure to other potential nephrotoxins. Even when nephrotoxicity is recognized early and the drug is discontinued, renal failure may progress over the next 5 to 10 days, with the serum creatinine and blood urea nitrogen (BUN) rising to disturbingly high levels, where they may remain for a number of days before renal function slowly begins to improve. No specific therapy for hastening recovery has been identified to be effective in humans. In an animal model, epidermal growth factor was shown to accelerate recovery (211). The prognosis for recovery of renal function is generally good except in those

meta-analyses that used this technique did not show a significant difference in the two dosing regimens. Nevertheless, in all analyses the single daily dose regimen was associated with a decrease in nephrotoxicity. Even the most recent prospective study (182) evaluating the efficacy and nephrotoxicity of once-daily administration of gentamicin versus multiple-daily administration in 52 children could not show a difference in incidence of nephrotoxicity in both groups. Although a decrease in nephrotoxicity rates in once-daily dose regimens has not been established, extended interval dosing strategies have never been associated with an increased risk of nephrotoxicity. The main reason why the majority of acute care hospitals (183) have adopted this strategy is that once-daily dosing provides a cost-effective method for administration of aminoglycosides by reducing workload among service personnel and by reducing or even eliminating the need for therapeutic drug monitoring (184,185).

Volume depletion (187), hypokalemia (188), hypomagnesemia (189), and metabolic acidosis (190) all carry increased risk for aminoglycoside nephrotoxicity. In the case of volume depletion and hypokalemia, the increased risk appears to be related to increased accumulation of drug in renal cortex

TABLE 42-2

META-ANALYSIS OF THE INCIDENCE OF NEPHROTOXICITY IN SINGLE DAILY DOSING VERSUS MULTIPLE DOSING OF AMINOGLYCOSIDES

Author	N of RCT	Method	Results (95% CI)
Blaser and König, 1995 (172)	24	Summation	RR 0.82
Galloe et al., 1995 (173)	16	Not given	RR 1.00 (0.98–1.02)
Barza et al. 1996 (174)	21	Random-effects model	RR 0.78 (0.57–1.07)
Munckhof et al., 1996 (175)	15	Random-effects model	RD −1.3% (−5%–3.1%)
Ferriols-Lisart and Alos-Alminan, 1996 (176)	18	Fixed-effects model	OR 0.60 (0.40–0.86)
Freeman and Strayer, 1996 (177)	15	Fixed-effects Peto	OR 0.70 (0.51–0.94)
Hatala et al., 1996 (178)	13	Random-effects model	RR 0.87 (0.60–1.26)
Ali and Goetz, 1997 (179)	26	Random-effects model	RD −0.18% (−0.99%–3.75%)
Bailey et al., 1997 (180)	22	Random-effects model	RD −0.6% (−2.4%–1.1%)
Hatala et al., 1997 (181)	4	Random-effects model	RR 0.78 (0.31–1.94)

OR, odds ratio; *RD,* risk difference; *RR,* risk ratio.
(Adapted from: Verpooten GA, Tulkens PM, Molitoris BA. Aminoglycosides and vancomycin. In: De Broe ME, Porter GA, Bennett VM, eds. *Clinical nephrotoxins—renal injury from drugs and chemicals,* 2nd ed. Dordrecht, The Netherlands: Kluwer Acadmic Publishers, 2003:151.)

cases where the underlying disease exposes the kidney to persisting or recurrent insults related to sepsis, hypotension, and hypoperfusion.

β-LACTAM ANTIBIOTICS

The β-lactam antibiotics comprise the penicillins, cephalosporins, and carbapenems. ARF has been observed with this class of antibiotics as a result of acute proximal tubular cell necrosis or allergic interstitial nephritis. Studies in animals have established the relative nephrotoxicity potentials of β-lactam antibiotics as cephaloglycin > cephaloridine >> cefaclor > cefazolin > cephalothin >>> cephalexin, ceftazidime, and penicillins, which do not exhibit clinical nephrotoxicity (212). The selective toxic potential of β-lactam antibiotics toward renal proximal tubular cells appears to be causally linked to their concentrative uptake by the organic anion transport system and their intrinsic reactivity toward sensitive intracellular target proteins (212,213). The importance of the organic anion transport system to the nephrotoxic potential of these agents is supported by the observations that (a) toxicity is restricted to β-lactams that are secreted by this transport system, (b) toxicity can be prevented by inhibition of organic anion transport, and (c) maneuvers that increase the intracellular uptake of drug augment toxicity (212,213). The product of intracellular drug concentration and time, defined as the area under the curve (AUC), is an important determinant of toxicity. Among the cephalosporins, the greatest AUC is observed with cephaloridine (212,213). This agent is readily transported into proximal tubular cells across the basolateral membrane; however, its egress across the apical membrane is retarded due to the fact that cephaloridine is a zwitterion and the cationic moiety impedes its permeation across the luminal membrane (214). Therefore, at equivalent doses, the AUC for cephaloridine is significantly higher than that of other cephalosporins. Cephaloglycin, the most nephro-

toxic of the cephalosporins released for clinical use, has a renal cortical AUC only one-fifth that of cephaloridine (215). The greater nephrotoxicity of cephaloglycin reflects the fact that it is far more reactive than cephaloridine toward sensitive intracellular target proteins (212,216). Three molecular mechanisms have been implicated in the pathogenesis of cephaloridine nephrotoxicity: (a) lipid peroxidation (217), (b) competitive inhibition of mitochondrial carnitine transport and fatty acid oxidation (218,219), and (c) inhibition of mitochondrial respiration consequent to inactivation by acylation of mitochondrial anionic substrate transporters (220,221).

In the case of the other nephrotoxic β-lactam antibiotics, the pathogenesis of toxicity appears to be linked primarily to depression of mitochondrial respiration. This conclusion is supported by the following observations from *in vivo* animal studies (212,213,215,220,221):

1. The nephrotoxic potential of β-lactams correlates with the magnitude of inhibition of mitochondrial respiration.
2. Irreversible inhibition of mitochondrial respiration occurs within 1 hour after administration of a nephrotoxic dose.
3. Inhibition of respiration precedes the appearance of ultrastructural mitochondrial damage that resembles ischemic and cyanide injury.

Although only a limited number of β-lactam antibiotics cause toxic injury after *in vivo* exposure, many of these agents exhibit the capacity to inhibit *in vitro* mitochondrial respiration, especially that component supported by succinate (222). Inhibition of mitochondrial respiration is observed within 5 minutes of *in vitro* drug exposure. Increasing the concentration of succinate reverses the inhibition, presumably as a consequence of competitive displacement of drug from the mitochondrial membrane anionic carrier. However, as the exposure of mitochondria to drug is augmented by raising the product of drug concentration and time, inhibition of mitochondrial respiration becomes progressively irreversible, which has been attributed to drug-induced acylation and inactivation of the transporter (212,213). The rank order of cephalosporins with respect to their potential to acylate target proteins *in vitro* is ceftazidime > cefaclor > cephaloglycin > cephalothin > cephaloridine > cefazolin >> cephalexin and several penicillins (212,213). This order is at variance with their *in vivo* nephrotoxicity potential, which is cephaloglycin > cephaloridine >> cefaclor > cefazolin > cephalothin >>> cephalexin, ceftazidime, and the penicillins. The explanation for the differences between the *in vitro* and *in vivo* toxicity potentials of these drugs resides in the important role of concentrative uptake of these drugs into intact proximal tubular cells by the organic anion transport system. Although ceftazidime and cefaclor exhibit high acylation activity *in vitro*, the AUC of these agents is low (only 7% that of cephaloridine and only 37% that of cephaloglycin), and this severely restricts their interaction with the mitochondrial anion transporter (212,213). Mitochondrial injury also has been implicated as the major mechanism of nephrotoxicity caused by imipenem (223,224). This drug is marketed in combination with cilastin, which inhibits the enzymatic breakdown of imipenem by cytoplasmic and brush-border dihydropeptidase and also inhibits its nephrotoxicity.

The therapeutic–nephrotoxic ratio of these agents is much more favorable than that of aminoglycoside antibiotics. The incidence of serum creatinine elevations is difficult to say with certainty, but severe nephrotoxic ARF is uncommon (225,226). Similar to other antibiotics, high doses and prolonged therapy elevate the risk of nephrotoxicity. In animal studies, the incidence and severity of toxicity associated with β-lactam antibiotics were augmented by combined therapy with aminoglycoside antibiotics (227), by renal ischemia (228), and by endotoxemia (229). In three prospective studies in human subjects, the combination of an aminoglycoside antibiotic with cephalothin was associated with a significantly higher incidence of nephrotoxicity (230–232). Early reports suggested a possible interaction between several second-generation cephalosporins and aminoglycoside antibiotics (233). In contrast, a recent prospective study provides no evidence that combination therapy with third-generation cephalosporins and an aminoglycoside antibiotic potentiates the risk of nephrotoxicity (171).

The diagnosis of nephrotoxic ARF secondary to β-lactam antibiotics is suggested by the appropriate clinical setting in combination with a urine sediment and urinary indices typical of acute tubular cell necrosis. Establishing the precise diagnosis may be difficult in the presence of septicemia, hypotension, or other nephrotoxic drugs. It should be kept in mind that β-lactam antibiotics also cause ARF secondary to allergic interstitial nephritis (234). The pattern of the rise in the blood urea nitrogen (BUN) and serum creatinine may be indistinguishable from that seen with acute tubular cell necrosis. The presence of large numbers of red and white blood cells in the urinary sediment, especially if associated with eosinophiluria and systemic signs of hypersensitivity (rash, fever, and eosinophilia), strongly suggests the diagnosis of allergic interstitial nephritis. However, in many patients, these clues are equivocal so that it may be necessary to perform a kidney biopsy to establish the correct diagnosis.

VANCOMYCIN

Vancomycin use in clinical medicine has increased significantly in recent years as a consequence of the rise in the incidence of methicillin-resistant staphylococcal infections. Because this antibiotic is poorly absorbed from the gastrointestinal tract, it is usually administered intravenously for the treatment of systemic infections. Vancomycin is not appreciably metabolized, and it is excreted essentially entirely by the kidneys primarily by glomerular filtration, as there is no evidence that the drug un-

dergoes tubular absorption or secretion (235). Therefore, drug dosing must be modified in subjects with renal failure. Animal studies demonstrated that vancomycin had nephrotoxic and ototoxic potential (236). Early clinical experience in human subjects revealed a significant incidence of nephrotoxicity, which in retrospect may have been due to impurities generated during the initial manufacturing process (237). More recent reports indicate that the incidence of nephrotoxicity associated with vancomycin ranges between 0% and 7% when given as sole therapy (238). Animal studies initially suggested that vancomycin and aminoglycoside antibiotics interacted synergistically to cause ARF (239). Recent reports indicate that a similar interaction occurs in humans (194,195). Indeed, in a meta-analysis the incidence of nephrotoxicity associated with combination therapy was 13.3% greater than therapy with vancomycin alone. In a prospective study, comparing continuous versus intermittent infusion of vancomycin in severely ill patients, Wysocki et al. (240) found a significant rise in serum creatinine during treatment only in those patients who received vancomycin with other antibiotics including aminoglycosides. Monitoring vancomycin serum concentrations is not cost-effective in preventing vancomycin-induced nephrotoxicity in patients with normal renal function, since the correlation between serum levels and antibacterial efficacy or toxicity remains controversial (241). It should be noted that vancomycin has been reported to cause allergic interstitial nephritis (242); however, this appears to be an uncommon complication. Teicoplanin, a glycopeptide antibiotic similar to vancomycin, is devoid of nephrotoxicity.

SULFONAMIDE ANTIBIOTICS

The sulfonamide antibiotics and their metabolites are excreted primarily by the kidneys by a process involving glomerular filtration, tubular absorption, and tubular secretion (243). The high incidence of nephrotoxic ARF observed with the first-generation sulfonamides was due to their low solubility and the resultant precipitation of drug in the form of crystals that caused intratubular obstruction (244). Sulfadiazine, a poorly soluble sulfonamide, continues to be used today in combination with pyrimethamine for the treatment of *Toxoplasma encephalitis*; nephrotoxicity manifested as hematuria, crystalluria, renal colic, and ARF may complicate therapy in 5% of cases (245,246). These abnormalities usually subside with hydration and alkalinization of the urine.

Trimethoprim-sulfamethoxazole is administered intravenously in high concentrations as therapy for *Pneumocystis carinii* pneumonia. Although the solubility of sulfamethoxazole is high, ARF secondary to crystal deposition of the parent drug or a metabolite has been reported (247,248). More commonly, the elevation of serum creatinine observed in patients treated with this combination drug reflects inhibition of tubular secretion of creatinine by trimethoprim (249,250). This effect is more pronounced in subjects with baseline elevation of the serum creatinine secondary to underlying chronic renal insufficiency. Failure of the BUN to rise in proportion to the rise in serum creatinine should call attention to the correct diagnosis.

Sulfonamides including sulfamethoxazole also have been implicated in causing acute hypersensitivity reactions and ARF secondary to allergic interstitial nephritis (234).

ANTIFUNGAL AGENTS

Amphotericin B is widely used as the drug of choice for the therapy of systemic fungal infections, especially in immunocompromised patients (251,252). Unfortunately, the clinical application of this drug is accompanied by a number of dose-dependent toxic side effects, the most serious of which is ARF (253,254). Amphotericin B is a polyene that consists of a large lactone ring with seven conjugated double bonds, seven hydroxyl groups, and a sugar moiety. It exhibits the propensity to bind to membrane sterols and form membrane pores, which in mammalian cells are estimated to be composed of eight molecules of cholesterol alternating with eight molecules of drug (255). The resultant increase in membrane permeability to small electrolytes is thought to be a dominant factor in the toxicity of the drug. Amphotericin B binds preferentially to ergosterol, the major sterol of fungi, and this presumably explains the selective toxicity of this and similar drugs for fungi (256).

The reason amphotericin B causes nephrotoxicity in humans and experimental animals is not apparent from its pharmacokinetics (257,258). Because amphotericin B is poorly transported across the gastrointestinal tract, it must be administered intravenously. Its volume of distribution is about 4 L per kg. Up to 95% of drug in serum is bound, primarily to β-lipoproteins. The major depot site for amphotericin B is the liver, where up to 41% of administered drug can be recovered compared to 6% in the lung and 2% in the kidney. The elimination of amphotericin B from serum can be described by a triexponential curve, the half-lives of which are 24 hours, 48 hours, and 15 days, respectively. Less than 10% of administered drug is recovered in the urine, and there are no known metabolites.

Although the kidney is not a major route of amphotericin B elimination, it is the major site of toxicity, the incidence of which is influenced by daily drug dose, duration of therapy, and the presence of potentiating factors (259,260). The clinical expression of amphotericin B nephrotoxicity is dominated by the appearance of azotemia and creatininemia, which may occur early in the course of drug therapy (260–262) and reflects depression of renal blood flow and GFR secondary initially to a reversible rise in renal vascular resistance. With prolonged therapy, depression of renal function may persist as a consequence of injury to tubular epithelium (263) and possibly the renal vasculature (264). A variety of abnormalities of tubular function may be seen as well. These include incomplete distal renal tubular acidosis (265), hypokalemia and hypomagnesemia secondary to renal tubular wasting of these cations (266,267), and loss of urine concentrating capacity (268). The urinary sediment frequently contains evidence of microscopic hematuria, pyuria, and cylinduria. While most of these abnormalities are reversible after the drug is discontinued, full recovery may be delayed for a number of months. Chronic renal insufficiency may occur with prolonged or multiple courses of therapy.

Insight into the pathogenesis of amphotericin B nephrotoxicity has been gleaned from studies in experimental animals (269). It has been shown that intravenous administration of amphotericin B elicits an acute depression of renal blood flow and GFR in association with an increase in renal vascular resistance that is not mediated by the renal nerves, by angiotensin II, by endothelium-dependent factors, or by tubular glomerular feedback (270–273). These hemodynamic alterations have been shown to be modifiable by a variety of interventions including administration of calcium channel blockers (274), a selective dopamine-1 receptor agonist (275), saline loading (276,277), atrial natriuretic peptide (273,278), and theophylline suggesting its direct vasoconstrictive effect (273). Depolarization of vascular smooth muscle consequent to the formation of membrane pores was postulated as the basic mechanism by which amphotericin B augmented renal vascular resistance (269,273). Amphotericin B also induces tubular dysfunction in the rat that mimics alterations observed in humans (278). The dominant site of tubular injury in the rat is the inner stripe of the outer medulla (279), a zone that functions on the verge of hypoxia even under physiologic conditions. Investigators have postulated that hypoxic injury to this zone

TABLE 42-3

RISK FACTORS FOR AMPHOTERICIN B NEPHROTOXICITY

Daily drug dose
Duration of therapy
Chronic renal insufficiency
Sodium depletion
Renal hypoperfusion
Concomitant drug therapy/exposure
Diuretics
Aminoglycosides
Cisplatin
Radiocontrast agents
Cyclosporine

results from the demand for increased oxygen to support increased sodium transport stimulated by the heightened influx of sodium across the apical membrane made permeable by amphotericin B at a time when the supply of oxygen is reduced as a consequence of amphotericin B–induced reduction in renal blood flow (279,280).

A contributory factor to the toxicity of amphotericin B is deoxycholate, the vehicle in which the drug is suspended. Deoxycholate was shown to be cytotoxic to renal tubular cells *in vitro* (281). Various alternate vehicles and formulations for suspending amphotericin have been investigated in an attempt to reduce toxicity. Administration of amphotericin B in liposomes (257,282) or with other lipid preparations (283) has been reported to reduce the nephrotoxicity of this agent without compromising its therapeutic efficacy.

A number of factors have been identified as potentiating the risk of amphotericin B nephrotoxicity (Table 42-3), and the physician should strive to eliminate or minimize these risk factors whenever possible. Fisher et al. (259) observed a 1.8-fold increase in risk of nephrotoxicity for each 0.1 mg per kg increment in the daily dose of amphotericin B. The risk of nephrotoxicity was increased 15.4-fold in patients who had an elevated serum creatinine prior to the start of amphotericin B therapy and 12.5-fold in patients who received diuretics during the course of amphotericin B therapy. The latter observation may reflect the powerful influence of sodium depletion on this complication. Sodium loading has been shown to minimize amphotericin B nephrotoxicity (260) so that special attention should be paid to ensure that the patient is optimally volume-repleted prior to the initiation of therapy with this agent (Fig. 42-4).

ANTIVIRAL AGENTS

Acyclovir is a potent antiviral agent effective in the treatment of infections caused by herpes simplex viruses (285). Its major route of excretion is the kidney, which accounts for approximately 80% of total body clearance (286). Given the fact that the renal clearance of acyclovir exceeds the creatinine clearance by severalfold, it follows that a substantial fraction of drug must be eliminated by tubular secretion, which promotes the attainment of tubular fluid concentrations in excess of the drug's estimated solubility of 1.3 mg per L (286). Approximately 85% of the drug recovered in the urine is unchanged; the remainder is recovered as the principal metabolite, 9-carboxymethoxymethylguanine (286). In several large series, acyclovir has been reported to cause elevation of the BUN and serum creatinine in 10% to 15% of cases (287,288). In one series of 23 patients, an incidence of acute renal

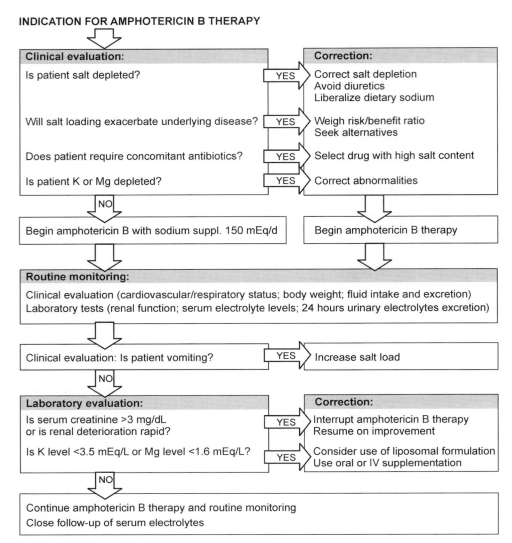

FIGURE 42-4. Proposed approach for management of amphotericin B therapy. (Reprinted from: Bernardo JF, Sabra R, Vyas SJ, et al. Amphotericin B. In: DeBroe ME, Porter GA, Bennett VM, eds. *Clinical nephrotoxins: renal injury from drugs and chemicals.* Dordrecht, The Netherlands: Kluwer Acadmic Publishers, 2003:199, with permission.)

insufficiency of 48% was reported (289). The clinical expression of nephrotoxicity may range from asymptomatic azotemia to renal colic with nausea and vomiting. Examination of the urinary sediment may reveal microscopic hematuria, pyuria, and birefringent crystals. The pathogenesis of acyclovir-induced ARF has been attributed to intratubular obstruction caused by precipitation of drug (288) as well as direct tubular cell toxicity (290,291). High drug dose, rapid drug infusion, and low urine volume predispose to the development of ARF. In about half the cases, the onset of azotemia occurs during the first few days of therapy; it is usually transient and frequently resolves in response to increased fluid intake even when drug therapy is continued. Severe renal failure has been reported, however, even in patients who were prehydrated (292). Fortunately, even in these cases, renal function usually recovers. In the rat infusion of acyclovir caused a decrease in whole kidney and single nephron GFR and renal plasma flow in association with an increase in renal vascular resistance (293).

Foscarnet is an antiviral agent that is being used with increasing frequency for the treatment of cytomegalovirus infections and acyclovir-resistant herpes virus infections, particularly in immunocompromised individuals (294,295). This agent is excreted unchanged in the urine by glomerular filtration and tubular secretion (296). Major complications of therapy include ARF, often severe and of uncertain pathogenesis (297,298), and electrolyte abnormalities that include hypercalcemia, hypocalcemia, hypophosphatemia, hypomagne-

semia, and hypokalemia (246,299). ARF secondary to crystal deposition has been described as well (300). Volume expansion by infusing saline has been reported to greatly reduce the incidence and severity of ARF (298,301).

Cidofovir is an antiviral nucleotide analog indicated for the treatment of cytomegalovirus retinitis in patients with acquired immunodeficiency syndrome (AIDS) (302). The drug is eliminated primarily by the kidneys by glomerular filtration and tubular secretion via the organic acid transport system (303). The major complication of therapy with this agent is nephrotoxic injury to proximal tubular cells; but, this complication can be significantly reduced by the coadministration of probenecid, which presumably blocks the renal tubular uptake of cidofovir and decreases the renal elimination of the agent (304).

PENTAMIDINE

Pentamidine has been used for the treatment of *P. carinii* pneumonia since the 1950s. In the preacquired immunodeficiency syndrome (AIDS) era, pentamidine therapy was complicated by ARF in about 25% of cases (305). The incidence of ARF in patients with AIDS treated with pentamidine appears to be substantially higher than this figure, and it is unexplained by greater drug dose, longer duration of therapy, or concomitant therapy with other potentially nephrotoxic agents

(306). The mechanism of pentamidine-induced ARF has not been established. Although pentamidine is concentrated in the kidney (307–309), pharmacokinetic studies utilizing a high-performance liquid chromatography assay indicate that <5% of the drug is excreted in the urine each day (308,310). The mechanism of renal elimination is not known.

Pentamidine nephrotoxicity presents as nonoliguric ARF beginning 7 to 10 days after the start of therapy. Urinalysis reveals mild proteinuria, microscopic hematuria, pyuria, and cylinduria. Most patients experience mild to moderate ARF, but occasionally severe renal failure necessitating dialysis therapy occurs. In one series, azotemia was accompanied by hyperkalemia in association with a picture of hyperchloremic metabolic acidosis (306). Renal magnesium wasting has been observed in several cases (311). Recovery of renal function usually begins within a week after stopping drug therapy and in most cases returns to baseline within several weeks.

Chronic renal insufficiency, volume depletion, cumulative dose, and concurrent use of other nephrotoxic drugs heighten the risk of pentamidine nephrotoxicity in humans (250,312). In the rat, pentamidine nephrotoxicity was potentiated by amphotericin B, tobramycin, and cyclosporine, whereas it was ameliorated by fosfomycin, D-glucaro-1,5-lactam, verapamil, and enalapril (313).

NEPHROTOXICITY OF CYCLOSPORINE

Since its clinical use as an immunosuppressant drug in the early 1980s, cyclosporine A (CsA) has tremendously improved the outcome of solid organ (kidney, heart, liver, lung, and pancreas) and bone marrow transplants (314,315). In more recent years, the immunosuppressive properties of CsA have also been used in the treatment of autoimmune diseases (psoriasis, uveitis, and severe rheumatoid arthritis) as well as steroid-resistant nephrotic syndrome.

The major side effect of CsA is its renal toxicity. Although in preclinical animal studies, renal side effects were not observed (316–318), early reports from clinical practice revealed the nephrotoxicity of CsA (319–321). Since that time, numerous observations have added to the overwhelming evidence of three different forms of cyclosporine nephrotoxicity (322–330). This toxicity is not restricted to only the field of kidney transplantation but has also unequivocally been documented in heart (331,332), bone marrow (332), liver (333,334), and pancreas transplantation (335), as well as in a variety of autoimmune diseases (336–339), in which *a priori* rejection of the kidney graft is absent.

Based on experimental data and clinical experience, this chapter intends to summarize our present knowledge about the three different forms of cyclosporine nephrotoxicity: ARF (with sometimes protracted course evolving to chronicity); the hemolytic–uremic-like syndrome; and chronic irreversible nephrotoxicity.

Clinical Pharmacology of Cyclosporine A

The selective immunosuppressive effects of CsA were described for the first time in 1976 (340). CsA is a lipophilic fungal peptide with a molecular weight of 1.203 daltons, consisting of 11 amino acids (Fig. 42-5). As a consequence of its high hydrophobicity, CsA interacts easily with phospholipid bilayer membranes, while some CsA amino acids form a hydrophilic active immunosuppressive site (341).

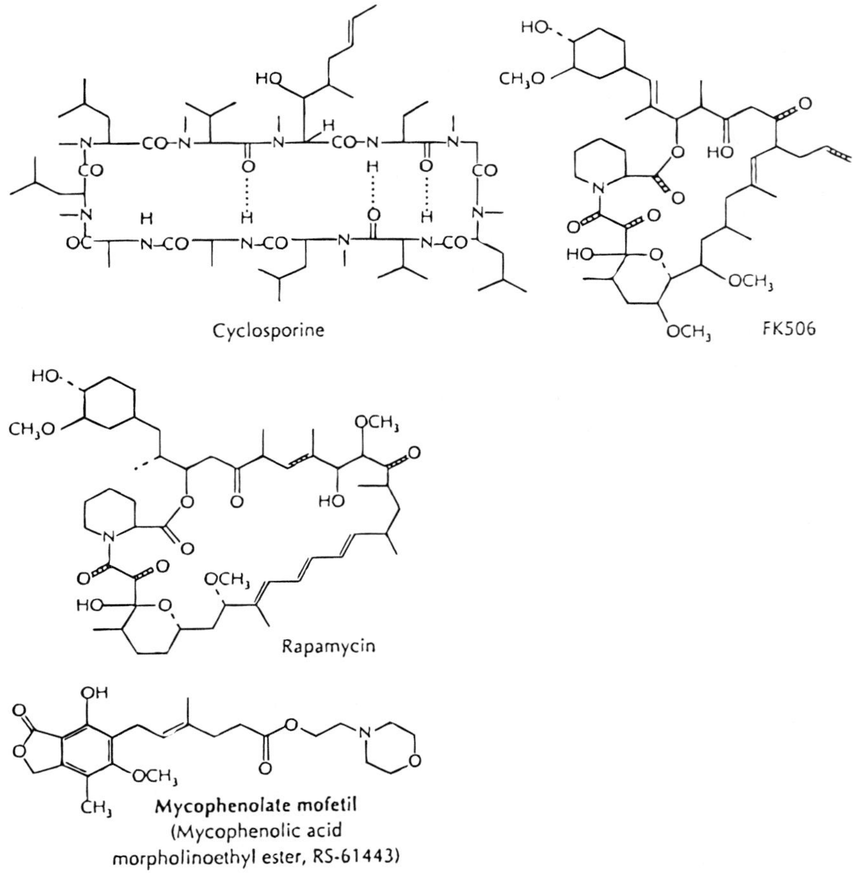

FIGURE 42-5. Structure of new immunosuppressive drugs.

CsA is available for clinical use in three formulations: one stabilized in castor oil (Cremophor) for intravenous injection, the second as a microemulsion formulation (Neoral), and a third formulation as soft gelatin capsules. The pharmacokinetic profile of the conventional CsA formulation (Sandimmune) exhibits a high degree of interpatient and intrapatient variability (342–344). Pharmacokinetic studies in healthy subjects and renal transplant recipients have shown that the more recent microemulsion formulation of CsA possesses superior pharmacokinetic characteristics, with more complete and predictable absorption of the drug from the gastrointestinal tract, resulting in less pharmacokinetic variability (345,346). In clinical trials, the microemulsion formulation of CsA increased drug exposure and reduced the incidence of acute rejections, without incremental toxicity (347–349).

In the circulation, CsA is mainly bound to high-, low-, or very low-density lipoproteins and to chylomicrons (350). Only a small fraction of CsA circulates unbound. The volume of distribution ranges from 4 to 8 L per kg of body weight (351). Due to its hydrophobicity, CsA dissolves extensively in cell membranes and tissue lipids (352). CsA accumulates in lymphocytes, liver, kidney, heart, lung, and neural and muscle cells (353).

CsA has a median half-life of 6.4 to 8.7 hours and is predominantly eliminated by hepatic metabolism through specific isoenzymes of the cytochrome P-450 superfamily (354). More than 90% of the parent compound and the metabolites are excreted in the bile, while only 6% is eliminated by the kidneys (352). Significant individual differences in CsA clearance rates (354,355), with a median value of 12 mL per minute per kg, can be explained by wide genetic differences among individuals in the content of cytochrome P-450 isoenzymes, as well as a variety of other factors such as patient age (356), the functional status of the liver (357), and interactions with other drugs (358). Independent of the intrinsic nephrotoxicity of CsA, its complex clinical pharmacokinetic profile entails the potential hazard of incorrect dosing, ultimately resulting in irreversible renal damage or acute rejection of the graft.

To optimize CsA therapy, monitoring of CsA trough levels in serum, plasma, or whole blood by means of radioimmunoassays or high-performance liquid chromatography is common clinical practice (359). Monitoring CsA trough levels has limited value, however, for the assessment of adequate immunosuppression or predicting protection from nephrotoxicity (360,361). The AUC is more informative and a better indicator of drug exposure (362) but is expensive and time consuming. Large-scale clinical trials using Neoral C_2 monitoring in renal and liver transplant recipients have demonstrated low acute rejection rates and good tolerability with a low adverse event profile to at least 1 year posttransplant (363–367). Neoral C_2 monitoring provided a more accurate assessment of delayed and/or low absorbers of CsA in these studies. Neoral C_2 monitoring in maintenance renal transplant recipients, showed that 26% to 49% of the patients, managed by monitoring of cyclosporine trough levels, were treated with excessive doses of CsA, adversely affecting graft function (368–370). Dose reduction to optimal C_2 levels, between 600 and 800 ng per mL, in these patients, resulted in improvement of graft function, without increased risk for rejection (368). These data provide evidence that monitoring of C_2 levels may result in more adequate dosing of cyclosporine.

Immunosuppressive Mechanism of Cyclosporine A

CsA blocks the activation of T cells, mainly through inhibition of transcription of lymphokines, most notably interleukin-2

(IL-2), the main growth factor for T cells (371). By inhibiting IL-2 expression in T cells, CsA prevents helper T cells from orchestrating a response to foreign antigens.

The immunosuppressive effect of FK506 (tacrolimus) is similar to that of CsA (372), as a logical consequence of a similar molecular mechanism of action of both drugs (373) (Fig. 42-6). CsA and FK506 bind with high affinity to intracellular target proteins, called immunophilins, which possess cis–trans isomerase activity. These immunophilins have been identified respectively as cyclophilins in the case of CsA (374) and FK-binding proteins in the case of FK506 and rapamycin (375). The binding of CsA or FK506 is a prerequisite of their immunosuppressive potential because it has been demonstrated that the CsA- or FK506-immunophilin complex competitively binds directly to the serine–threonine phosphatase calcineurin (376,377) in the presence of Ca^{2+}. The inhibition of calcineurin by the drug–immunophilin complex results in an altered modification pattern of the cytoplasmic components of transcription factors, thereby disturbing their nuclear translocation (373).

Potential substrates for calcineurin are the nuclear factor of activated T cells (NF-AT) and the nuclear factor of immunoglobulin (light chain in B cells (NF-κB), which were both reported as being affected in their IL-2 promoter binding activity by CsA and FK506, but not by rapamycin. This could explain the similarity of the immunosuppressive effect of CsA and FK506, in contrast to rapamycin, although rapamycin shares the same affinity as FK506 for the FK-binding protein (378,379).

Experimental Nephrotoxicity of Cyclosporine A

Much of our knowledge of cyclosporine nephrotoxicity derives from experimental studies in animal models. The understanding of the pathogenesis of chronic cyclosporine nephrotoxicity has long been hampered, however, by the lack of an experimental model until a number of investigators developed a suitable animal model of chronic cyclosporine nephrotoxicity (380–384).

Functional Alterations Induced by Cyclosporine A

It has been unequivocally established that CsA profoundly alters renal and glomerular hemodynamics. Acute and/or chronic CsA administration induces a decline in GFR, with a concomitant reduction in renal blood flow and an increase in renal vascular resistance as a consequence of vasoconstriction (385–388), preferentially at the level of afferent arterioles (324). These hemodynamic effects are mainly responsible for the acute cyclosporine nephrotoxicity and probably contribute also to the pathogenesis of chronic nephrotoxicity by inducing chronic renal ischemia. The possible underlying mechanisms of this vasoconstrictor effect of CsA are discussed under Pathophysiologic Studies of Cyclosporine Nephrotoxicity, below.

Although early pathologic studies suggested that CsA is a primary tubular toxin (389), the results of clearance experiments conflict with that premise (390). CsA reduces the end proximal tubular flow rate (391) and increases proximal fractional reabsorption (392). The latter is due to an inadequate adaptive reduction in the absolute rate of proximal reabsorption (393). CsA causes a resetting of the tubuloglomerular feedback with onset at lower tubular flow rates and greater maximum response (394).

CsA-treated rats show a reduction of sodium chloride reabsorption in the distal nephron, including Henle's loop (391,392), most likely as a secondary response to the decreased

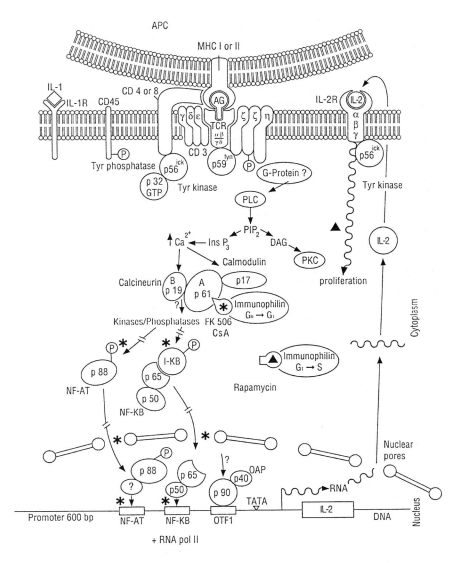

FIGURE 42-6. Cyclosporine (CsA) and FK506 both interfere, by binding to their respective immunophilins, with the function of intracellular molecules that transmit calcium-associated signals between the T-cell receptor (TCR) and the activation of lymphokine genes (interleukin-2) in the nucleus. Transcriptional regulation of interleukin-2 (IL-2) gene expression is modulated by the combination of transcription factors (e.g., NF-AT, NF-κ B, OTF-1) interacting with their corresponding recognition sites at the IL-2 promoter. These DNA/protein complexes, together with RNA polymerase II (RNA pol II), result in the antigen-inducible transcription of IL-2. Potential intervention sites for the pentameric complex (calcineurin A [p61], calcineurin B [p19], calmodulin [p17], immunophilin, drug), involving (e.g., modification and translocation) of antigen-inducible transcription factors (NF-AT [p88], NF-κ B [p50, p65]), are indicated by *asterisks*. CyA and FK506 interfere with the G_0 to G_1 transition of the cell cycle, whereas rapamycin interferes with the G_1 to S transition (indicated by a *triangle*). AG, antigen; APC, antigen presenting cell; DAG, diacylglycerol; Ins P_3, inositoltrisphosphate; MHC, major histocompatibility class; PiP_2, phosphatidylinositolbiphos-phate; PKC, protein kinase C; PLC, phospholipase C. (Reprinted from: Baumann G. Molecular mechanism of immunosuppressive agents. *Transplant Proc* 1992;24[Suppl 2]:4, with permission.)

proximal tubular fluid delivery. This reduced sodium delivery to and reabsorption from the distal nephron results in reduced distal acidification and potassium secretory capacity through a decreased generation of a negative transmembrane potential. This explains the observed hyperkalemic metabolic acidosis in CsA-treated rats (395) as well as in CsA-treated kidney transplant recipients (396).

In summary, CsA reduces renal blood flow and GFR predominantly through vasoconstriction of the afferent arterioles. Effects of CsA on tubular function consist of increased proximal tubular reabsorption and decreased distal sodium delivery, which induce hyperkalemic metabolic acidosis.

Morphologic Alterations Induced by Cyclosporine A

The renal pathology induced by CsA is largely dose-related and time-related. For clarity, we will focus on two distinct pathologic patterns, the acute (potentially reversible) toxic injury and the chronic (essentially irreversible) nephrotoxicity induced by CsA.

At supratherapeutic levels (100 mg per kg per day PO), CsA induces mainly tubular pathology consisting of isometric vacuolization of tubular cells, accumulation of eosinophilic bodies often representing giant mitochondria, and microcalcifications in proximal tubules by 21 days (389,397–399). The effects on the proximal tubule tend to be most prominent in the S3 seg-

ment (400) and become more widespread at very high doses. These pathologic alterations are reversible after dose reduction or withdrawal of CsA. In contrast to the acute toxic injury, chronic administration of CsA (12.5 mg per kg per day) for 3 to 10 weeks induces striking morphologic alterations in the medullary rays of the cortex of the rat (380). These changes progress in time and result in areas of focal or striped interstitial fibrosis with foci of atrophic proximal tubules, which are most prominent in the subcapsular cortex (401,402). The severity of the lesion progresses with treatment and is exacerbated by salt depletion (384). Withdrawal of CsA does not reverse the observed structural changes (401).

Besides the striped interstitial fibrosis, mild glomerular endothelial damage, glomerular hypercellularity, and mesangial matrix expansion (381) are observed after long-term CsA administration. Morphometric analysis with three-dimensional reconstruction of individual glomeruli (403) shows subsets of glomeruli with small volume with significant reduction in GFR (404), alternating with hypertrophic glomeruli.

At the vascular level, scanning electron microscopy shows focal narrowing of the afferent arteriolar diameter that progresses with time of CsA treatment and parallels the decrease in inulin clearance (326). CsA nephropathy is associated with degenerative hyaline changes in the walls of afferent arteriolar-sized blood vessels (405), which can disappear after discontinuation of CsA (406,407).

Pathophysiologic Studies of Cyclosporine Nephrotoxicity

Numerous studies have focused on different pathophysiologic mechanisms of cyclosporine nephrotoxicity. We will sequentially discuss mechanisms of renal vasoconstriction, cellular and molecular mechanisms, mechanisms of matrix protein accumulation, and studies on lipid peroxidation.

Mechanisms of Cyclosporine A–Mediated Renal Vasoconstriction. As mentioned previously, administration of CsA induces a marked afferent arteriolar vasoconstriction resulting in decreased renal blood flow and GFR. The renal sympathetic nervous system has been implicated in the renal functional effects of CsA because the α-adrenergic antagonists phenoxybenzamine (385) and prazosin (408) prevent a CsA-induced fall in renal blood flow and GFR. Moreover, a significant increase in renal afferent and efferent nerve activity has been demonstrated in CsA-treated rats (409). The relevance of the activated sympathetic nervous system to the pathophysiology of cyclosporine nephrotoxicity in kidney transplantation is questionable, however, because the renal allograft is denervated. Nevertheless, increased sensitivity of the denervated organ to circulating catecholamines (409) or significant reinnervation of renal allograft after transplantation (410) is a possible explanation.

Rodent models of cyclosporine nephrotoxicity consistently show activation of the renin–angiotensin–aldosterone axis, in contrast to results in humans. Besides increased plasma renin activity in CsA-treated rats (398,411), hyperplasia of the juxtaglomerular apparatus (383,412,413), as well as elevated renin synthesis and release in juxtaglomerular cells (414,415), has been documented in experimental animals during CsA therapy. However, angiotensin-converting enzyme inhibitors show conflicting effects on renal blood flow in CsA-treated rodents, with improvement in some studies (385,416) but not in others (386,417). More recent experimental studies suggest that CsA-related chronic interstitial injury is mediated by angiotensin II, since renin–angiotensin blockade prevents CsA-induced tubulointerstitial fibrosis (418,419). However, in human cardiac and renal allograft recipients treated with CsA, plasma renin is suppressed (331,420), suggesting that the renin–angiotensin system is not of primary importance in human cyclosporine nephrotoxicity.

Hypovolemia could contribute to renal vasoconstriction with CsA therapy because CsA-treated rats have reduced plasma volume and saline expansion reverses the deficits in renal blood flow and GFR (421). Studies with furosemide (422), mannitol (423), and chronic sodium depletion (380) have demonstrated that hypovolemia potentiates cyclosporine nephrotoxicity. Sodium depletion enhanced fibrosis and the expression of TGF-β1 and matrix proteins in experimental CsA nephropathy (424). However, there is evidence implicating hypovolemia and sodium-depletion as an exacerbating rather than as a causative factor of human cyclosporine nephrotoxicity.

Much attention has been paid to the potential role of an altered eicosanoid metabolism in cyclosporine nephrotoxicity. In animal models, CsA consistently increases the generation of thromboxane A$_2$ (TxA$_2$), a potent renal vasoconstrictor (425–427), while its effects on vasodilatory prostaglandins are controversial (421,428,429). Pharmacologic manipulation of thromboxane metabolism with a specific TxA$_2$ receptor antagonist (430,431) or a TxA$_2$ synthase inhibitor (432) partially prevented the CsA-induced acute decline in GFR and renal blood flow in normal rats. The TxA$_2$ receptor antagonist also attenuated chronic cyclosporine nephrotoxicity in rats with renal isograft (433). The relevance of these data to human cyclosporine nephrotoxicity, however, is controversial (434,435).

Another potential mediator of CsA-induced vasoconstriction is the platelet activating factor (PAF) because it has been demonstrated that rat mesangial cells release increased quantities of PAF when incubated with CsA, and CsA-stimulated cell contraction is abolished by the PAF antagonists, BN52021 and alprazolam (436). Chronic cyclosporine nephrotoxicity is also attenuated in rats treated with the PAF antagonist BN52063 (437).

More recently, the role of endothelin, the most potent vasoconstrictor yet identified, has been advocated in CsA-induced vasoconstriction. CsA treatment has been shown to stimulate endothelin production (438,439) and promote glomerular endothelin binding in vivo (440). Endothelin appears to mediate CsA-induced renal vasoconstriction in the rat (441). The resulting reduced single-nephron GFR and glomerular plasma flow rate, as well as the decreased glomerular capillary pressure, were attenuated by an antiendothelin antibody (442). Similarly, the endothelin receptor antagonist BQ123 has the potential to prevent hypoperfusion and hypofiltration induced by CsA (443). Recent work additionally demonstrated that CsA selectively modulates renal messenger RNA (mRNA) expression for endothelin peptide and one of its receptor subtypes in a site-specific way (442). In humans, the endothelin receptor antagonist bosentan markedly blunted the renal hypoperfusion effect of CsA (444).

Experimental data indicate that an enhanced 5-HT2 (serotonin)-mediated vasoconstriction plays an important role in the suppression of renal blood flow (RBF) autoregulation induced by CsA, since the administration of ritanserin, a pure 5-HT2 antagonist, restored the RBF autoregulation (445). In vivo studies in humans demonstrated reduced basal and stimulated nitric oxide (NO) production from the endothelium of forearm resistance vessels in cyclosporine-treated renal transplant recipients (446). This suggests endothelial dysfunction, and may provide a potential mechanism to explain cyclosporine-induced hypertension.

Elevated cytosolic calcium is yet another attractive candidate to explain the CsA-induced vasoconstriction. This has been demonstrated in cultured rat mesangial cells (447) as well as in vascular smooth muscle cells (448). The augmented transmembrane Ca^{2+} influx and intracellular Ca^{2+} mobilization could account for the protective effects of calcium channel antagonists in acute (449–451) as well as chronic (452,453) cyclosporine nephrotoxicity.

In summary, the acute or subacute effects of CsA on renal hemodynamics are likely mediated by a number of vasoactive substances such as endothelin, serotonin, impaired NO production, TxA$_2$, and PAF. At the cellular level, CsA induces increased intracellular Ca^{2+}, resulting in contraction of vascular smooth muscle cells as well as mesangial cells. Calcium channel blockers are able to protect against these effects.

Cellular and Molecular Mechanisms of Cyclosporine Nephrotoxicity. CsA modulates mitochondrial calcium fluxes, resulting in reduced mitochondrial swelling, respiration, and calcium discharge (454,455). Additionally, CsA modulates cytosolic calcium regulation in mesangial cells (447,456).

In T lymphocytes, CsA only affects calcium-dependent pathways on T-lymphocyte activation. As stated earlier under Immunosuppressive Mechanism of Cyclosporine A, the immunophilin-ligand complex inhibits the Ca^{2+}-dependent phosphatase calcineurin, which is an important step in signal transmission pathways. The analogy of immunosuppressive effect of FK506, as well as its nephrotoxicity, has led to an attractive hypothesis stating that cyclosporine nephrotoxicity could be inherent to its immunosuppressive effect (457); a similar hypothesis was formulated with regard to FK506 (458).

The mechanisms underlying the linkage of nephrotoxic effects to immunosuppressive effects of CsA or FK506 are still unknown. However, the blocking of T-cell activation by CsA or FK506 is an attractive explanation because it has been shown that a mononuclear cell infiltrate is part of cyclosporine nephrotoxicity (459). Alteration of the repair function of these cells could therefore be a possible mechanism inducing interstitial fibrosis.

Administration of CsA *in vivo* to rats causes a marked impairment of microsomal protein synthesis (460). Additional studies have shown a dose-dependent and time-dependent translational alteration of intracellular protein synthesis produced by cyclosporine (461).

The role of this decreased renal microsomal protein synthesis induced by CsA is speculative but could, if persistent with long-term cyclosporine treatment, alter renal cell matrix and interstitial cell interactions favoring fibrosis (461).

Recent *in vitro* studies showed that CsA induces apoptosis in tubular epithelial cells in a dose-dependent and time-dependent manner (462–465). This effect was mediated by the induction of inducible nitric oxide synthase (iNOS) (462), caspases (463), or TNF receptor super family member 6 (Fas) (464).

Mechanisms of Matrix Protein Accumulation. Interstitial fibrosis, the end point of chronic cyclosporine nephrotoxicity, results from an excessive extracellular matrix accumulation, which represents an imbalance between rates of extracellular matrix production and degradation. Cyclosporine has been shown to enhance the production of specific extracellular matrix components in mouse and rat kidney (466,467), as well as in renal cells in culture (468). In the presence of CsA, angiotensin II is known to induce interstitial collagen formation (469). Blockade of the renin–angiotensin system with angiotensin II receptor antagonists or angiotensin-converting enzyme inhibitors markedly abrogated the tubulointerstitial fibrosis without improving renal hemodynamics (418,419,470). The location of the angiotensin receptor type 1 mRNA in the outer medulla and medullary rays might explain the peculiar striped pattern of fibrosis noted in an experimental model of chronic cyclosporine nephrotoxicity (471). All together, these data strongly suggest that CsA-induced interstitial fibrosis could be mediated by angiotensin II, independent of its hemodynamic effects.

Several recent studies also implicated transforming growth factor-β1, a potent immunosuppressive and fibrogenic cytokine, as a potential mediator of CsA-induced interstitial fibrosis (472–478). Enhanced intragraft expression of TGF-β was associated with interstitial fibrosis in patients treated with CsA (472). In animals, CsA induced an increased expression of TGF-β1, both at the mRNA and the protein level, again associated with tubulointerstitial fibrosis (473–475,478). Similarly, CsA stimulated expression of TGF-β1 in renal cells (476,477). The fibrogenic effects, induced by CsA, were abrogated by a neutralizing anti-TGF-β1 antibody (477,478).

In contrast to the already mentioned enhanced collagen formation induced by CsA, recent work demonstrates an increased expression at both the transcriptional (mRNA) level and protein level of tissue inhibitor of metalloproteinases (TIMP-1) in a rat model of chronic cyclosporine nephrotoxicity (479,480). Moreover, Duymelinck and associates show that cholesterol feeding accentuates the cyclosporine-induced elevation of renal plasminogen activator inhibitor type 1 (PAI-1) (481). This increased expression and production of TIMP-1 and PAI-1, induced by CsA, could result in a decreased degradation of extracellular matrix, which would in turn lead to progressive extracellular matrix accumulation and interstitial fibrosis.

In summary, CsA-induced interstitial fibrosis results from a combination of increased synthesis of matrix components, as well as decreased degradation of extracellular matrix. Angiotensin II and transforming growth factor-β1 may play a role in the process of increased collagen formation induced by CsA,

while the TIMP-1 and the PAI-1 likely mediate the decreased degradation of extracellular matrix induced by CsA.

Studies on Lipid Peroxidation. It has been shown that *in vitro* incubation of rat renal microsomes or human liver microsomes with CsA induces dose-related lipid peroxidation (482,483). Lipid peroxidation seems to be the main mechanism of free-radical toxicity (484–486). Reactive oxygen species through a peroxidative process may increase the availability of arachidonate metabolites and enhance prostanoid production (487–489). Recent *in vivo* studies in the rat indicated that cyclosporine nephrotoxicity is accompanied by dose-related systemic and renal lipid peroxidation (490), preceding the fall in GFR (491). Concurrent treatment with antioxidants (i.e., Vitamin E [490], melatonin [492], or N-acetylcysteine [493]), suppressed CsA-induced lipid peroxidation and reduced functional and structural damage. The mechanism by which CsA-induced lipid peroxidation could contribute to cyclosporine nephrotoxicity is putative, including direct cellular toxicity (494), thromboxane-mediated ischemia (495), or peroxidation-linked excess extracellular matrix production (496). Several reports suggest that calcineurin inhibitors, CsA and tacrolimus, have prooxidant activity, and they increase the susceptibility of low-density lipoprotein to oxidation in humans (497–499).

Clinical Nephrotoxicity of Cyclosporine A

CsA can cause a wide spectrum of renal functional and morphologic impairments, including a marked and rapidly reversible decrease in GFR and renal plasma flow (323) and a chronic form of renal damage in patients treated for more than 6 months with a potential evolution to end-stage renal disease (328,331). Thrombotic microangiopathy is another, although relatively uncommon, nevertheless serious, adverse effect of cyclosporine (326,500).

Acute Renal Failure Induced by Cyclosporine A. Acute cyclosporine renal dysfunction is not infrequent in clinical practice and occurs not only in patients with kidney transplantation (319) but also in heart (501), liver (322), and bone marrow (320) transplant recipients. This acute form of nephrotoxicity may occur within weeks following initiation of CsA therapy and can also be observed after years of drug therapy (502). The incidence of this acute renal injury can be enhanced by extended graft preservation (325), preexistent renal histologic lesions (503), donor hypotension, and perioperative complications (504).

Acute cyclosporine nephrotoxicity has clinical features similar to those of acute renal allograft rejection, including an abrupt fall in GFR, impaired urinary concentrating capacity, and sodium retention (505). Hypertension is observed in up to 50% of patients, whereas metabolic acidosis, hyperkalemia, and hyperuricemia are less frequent (506). Characteristic of this syndrome of acute reversible renal dysfunction induced by CsA is the rapid recovery of renal function on reduction of the CsA dose (323,507).

Delayed kidney graft function is a less frequent severe form of protracted ARF with oliguria induced by CsA (504). Its incidence varies largely between centers (508,509), presumably reflecting different strategies of immunosuppressive treatment or variations in time of ischemia of the kidney before transplantation (510,511).

Although nephrotoxicity due to cyclosporine alone is rarely observed with CsA trough blood levels below 200 ng per mL per (344,512), blood level monitoring has proved unreliable in the differential diagnosis between acute cyclosporine nephrotoxicity and acute rejection of kidney allografts (344).

The difficulty in differentiating acute rejection from cyclosporine nephrotoxicity in the setting of kidney transplantation often compels performance of a kidney biopsy (513,514).

On the histologic basis, cyclosporine nephrotoxicity is often a diagnosis of exclusion with the absence of definite signs of acute rejection, such as intimal arteritis (515,516) or intratubular lymphocytes (517). Histologic features of cyclosporine nephrotoxicity are nonspecific and include arteriolar hyalinosis (518,519), as well as isometric vacuolization of proximal tubular cells (520).

Analogous to experimental data obtained in animal models, CsA causes a dose-related and time-related fall in GFR and renal plasma flow in humans induced by renal vasoconstriction (521,522). In two studies, the intrarenal blood flow was significantly reduced after oral cyclosporine intake, but hypoperfusion could not be elicited by tacrolimus (523,524). The beneficial effects of different calcium channel blockers on this CsA-induced renal hypoperfusion (525–530) suggest this vasoconstriction is mainly effected at the afferent arteriolar level because it has been demonstrated that calcium antagonists preferentially reduce glomerular afferent arteriolar tone (531).

In contrast, coadministration of indomethacin unmasks CsA-induced renal vasoconstriction and potentiates cyclosporine nephrotoxicity by reducing the intrarenal prostaglandins (532). This suggests a role for the eicosanoids in the CsA-induced vasoconstriction. Further arguments in favor of this possibility are the partial beneficial effects observed with a specific TxA_2 synthase inhibitor (435) and with dietary regimens with omega-3 polyunsaturated fatty acids (533).

Although a role for increased vascular renin activity in cyclosporine-induced renal and peripheral vasoconstriction has been suggested (534,535), investigators have never detected any significant preventive effect of angiotensin-converting enzyme inhibition on the decline in renal blood flow and the increase in renal vascular resistance induced by CsA.

Unlike in animal models, prazosin did not significantly affect GFR, renal plasma flow, or renal vascular resistance in patients who had undergone transplant and were treated with CsA (536), thus questioning the role of the sympathetic nervous system in cyclosporine nephrotoxicity.

Endothelin has been implicated as a causative agent in CsA-induced vasoconstriction (see Experimental Nephrotoxicity of Cyclosporine A, above). Although intrarenal injections of antiendothelin antibodies protected against the effects of cyclosporine (438), administration of specific endothelin receptor antagonists has shown conflicting results (443,537).

Chronic Cyclosporine Nephrotoxicity. The main clinical issue associated with CsA treatment is, however, the chronic nephrotoxicity (331) that is clinically defined by progressive renal dysfunction with hypertension. Histologic lesions can already appear after 6 months of CsA therapy (328,538), with progression over time, even after CsA dose reduction (335). As mentioned previously, chronic cyclosporine nephrotoxicity has been documented in other clinical settings besides kidney transplantation (331–339). Chronic cyclosporine nephrotoxicity is related to the cumulative CsA dose (335,539) and may be irreversible even after CsA discontinuation (540).

The clinical features of chronic cyclosporine nephrotoxicity are nonspecific, including a slowly progressive decline of renal function over months or years, severe arterial hypertension, mild proteinuria, and tubular dysfunction (505). In renal allografts, differential diagnosis with chronic rejection is often impossible on clinical grounds alone, thus necessitating the performance of a kidney biopsy (541).

The histopathologic lesions of chronic cyclosporine nephrotoxicity have been extensively studied and are now well known (329,330,542,543). Histopathologic findings in 2-year protocol biopsies from a randomized study showed comparable lesions in renal allografts under cyclosporine and tacrolimus treatment (544). They include renal arteriolar damage (the so-called CsA-associated arteriolopathy), tubular atrophy, and (striped) interstitial fibrosis, as well as glomerular sclerosis. These lesions are nonspecific, however, except for the CsA-associated arteriolopathy.

The vascular lesions are located almost exclusively in the arterioles and arteries, with up to two layers of smooth muscle cells, and usually consist of circular nodular protein deposits or mucoid thickening of the intima, which contributes to narrowing or occlusion of the lumen (329). CsA-associated arteriolopathy affects a limited number of arterioles in a dose-related manner (543).

Tubulointerstitial changes may be nearly diffuse, but usually there are narrow stripes of atrophy and fibrosis, apparently corresponding to areas of cortex with afferent arteriolar lesions (329). This interstitial fibrosis progresses over time (335). Tubular atrophy is nearly always found in areas with interstitial fibrosis (545) and likewise progresses with time (335). CsA-induced glomerulopathy consists of global or focal and segmental sclerosis (330,546). Again, the number of affected glomeruli increase with time (335).

Although the histologic features of chronic cyclosporine nephrotoxicity have been well characterized, the differential diagnosis with chronic rejection of the renal allograft in kidney transplantation still often remains difficult (547).

A great matter of debate is whether prolonged therapy with CsA can result in progressive, irreversible renal damage, ultimately leading to end-stage renal disease. This was advocated by some authors (548,549) but denied by others (536,550). Multicenter studies in renal transplant patients showed reduced but stable renal function after up to 3 to 5 years of CsA treatment (551,552). Conversion from CsA to azathioprine in kidney transplant recipients after 3 months significantly improved the creatinine clearance at 5 years' posttransplantation (553). In patients who have undergone pancreas transplant, a sequential functional and morphologic study has unequivocally shown the progressive character of the histologic lesions due to cyclosporine nephrotoxicity (335). This was strongly correlated with CsA blood levels, CsA dose, and magnitude of the decline in creatinine clearance during the first posttransplant year (335). Analysis of sequential protocol biopsies of renal allografts over a period of 10 years, in a prospective study of 120 kidney-pancreas transplant recipients, confirmed this progressive character of renal histologic lesions, induced by calcineurin-inhibitors (554). In this study, severe histologic damage was present in 58.4% of the renal allografts by 10 years.

Altogether, these data point out that chronic cyclosporine nephrotoxicity has a progressive and irreversible character once the histologic lesions have arisen. Assessment of the renal function, be it by means of serum creatinine or creatinine clearance, underestimates the magnitude of the problem due to the relatively low sensitivity of those methods and to the slow progression of the renal damage induced by cyclosporine.

The pathophysiology of chronic cyclosporine nephrotoxicity in humans is a matter of extensive investigation, mainly through experimental models (see Pathophysiologic Studies of Cyclosporine Nephrotoxicity, above).

Hemolytic–Uremic-like Syndrome Induced by Cyclosporine A. Thrombotic microangiopathy is a relatively uncommon but serious adverse effect of cyclosporine in renal (326) and nonrenal (500) transplant recipients, with an overall 43% graft survival rate (555,556). The most striking morphologic changes are an extensive thrombotic process in the renal microcirculation, with several glomerular capillaries occluded by thrombi extending from the afferent arterioles and containing platelet aggregates (329). Laboratory anomalies include thrombocytopenia, hemolytic anemia, and deterioration of the renal function (326). In the setting of kidney transplantation, the differential diagnosis of hemolytic–uremic syndrome and vascular rejection is not obvious (555). According to a retrospective study of 29 patients with calcineurin-inhibitor induced thrombotic microangiopathy, repeated plasma-exchange induced a recovery of the renal allograft function in 80% of the patients (557).

This hemolytic–uremic-like syndrome induced by CsA reinforces the concept that the vascular endothelium is the main target in this form of CsA toxicity. That CsA can damage vascular endothelium is confirmed by the high plasma concentration of factor VIII-related antigen, found in recipients of renal allograft given CsA and having clinical signs of nephrotoxicity (558). Recent work shows significantly higher plasminogen-activator inhibitor (PAI-1) levels in patients treated with CsA who underwent renal transplant, compared to patients who were not treated with CsA, suggesting a decreased fibrinolytic activity in the former patients (559). This could account for the increased risk of hemolytic–uremic syndrome induced by CsA.

Summary

CsA is a potent immunosuppressive drug with nephrotoxic side effects. Independent of the intrinsic nephrotoxic properties of CsA, its complex clinical pharmacokinetic profile could cause incorrect dosing, ultimately resulting in irreversible renal damage.

The clinical nephrotoxicity of CsA consists of three entities with different expressions of renal damage induced by CsA (i.e., ARF, hemolytic–uremic-like syndrome, and chronic cyclosporine nephrotoxicity). The ARF is essentially reversible and mainly hemodynamically mediated through afferent arteriolar vasoconstriction. Dosage reduction of CsA reverses the nephrotoxic effects. The hemolytic–uremic-like syndrome consists of an extensive thrombotic process at the level of the glomerular capillaries, causing loss of kidney function in more than half of the cases. Chronic cyclosporine nephrotoxicity is an irreversible renal damage characterized by a specific arteriolopathy and striped interstitial fibrosis, resulting in slow progressive decline of renal function. Although the pathophysiology of this process is extensively studied in experimental models, many questions still remain unanswered.

TACROLIMUS (FK506)

Tacrolimus (FK506) is a fungal product, a new macrolide immunosuppressant agent, which has shown important potential in transplantation and in the treatment of autoimmune diseases (560–562). Although it is many times more potent than cyclosporine, allowing the use of lower doses, both drugs have similar nephrotoxic properties (563,564). In 1991, the first international congress of FK506 was held in Pittsburgh, Pennsylvania (565).

Molecular Action

Cyclosporine and FK506 have dissimilar chemical structures (Fig. 42-5), nevertheless both agents bind to a similar class of ubiquitous intracellular receptors: immunophilins, molecules that are cis–trans prolyl isomerases. These intracellular binding proteins are well conserved through evolution and change the confirmation of cyclosporine and FK506. The cytosolic receptor for FK506 (FKBP) has been well characterized (566). This drug–immunophilin complex must bind to calcineurin, a calcium-dependent protein phosphatase, to allow the immunosuppressant actions of the drugs in lymphocytes (567,568) (Fig. 42-6). Similar calcineurin-mediated dephosphorylation of cyclosporine and FK506 may lead to inhibition of signal transduction in other cell types and organs, which mediates both the desirable immunosuppressant effects and the possibly toxic effects.

Cyclosporine and FK506 are powerful immunosuppressive drugs that inhibit the calcium–calmodulin-dependent phosphatase calcineurin in T cells, thereby preventing the activation of T cell-specific transcription factors such as NF-AT involved in lymphokine gene expression (Fig. 42-6). While this may, at least in part, explain the mechanism of cyclosporine and FK506 immunosuppression, additional mechanisms have to be invoked to explain the pharmacologic properties and toxic effect of these drugs such as nephrotoxicity and neurotoxicity. Schwaninger et al. (569) studied the effect of cyclosporine and FK506 on calcineurin phosphatase activity and gene transcription mediated by the cyclic adenosine monophosphate-responsive element (CRE), a binding site of the ubiquitous transcription factor CREB. An imported gene was placed under the transcriptional control of the CRE of the rat glucagon gene and transiently transfected into the glucagon expressing cell line αTC2. Cyclosporine and FK506 inhibited depolarization-induced gene transcription in a concentration-dependent manner. Both cyclosporine and FK506 inhibited calcineurin phosphatase activity at the drug concentrations that inhibited gene transcription. The FK506 analog rapamycin had no effect on calcineurin activity and gene transcription, but excess concentrations of rapamycin prevented the effect of FK506 on both calcineurin activity and gene transcription. These results further support the notion that the interaction of drug-immunophilin complexes with calcineurin may be the molecular basis of cyclosporine- and FK506-induced inhibition of CREB/CRE-mediated gene transcription. The ability to interfere with CREB/CRE-mediated gene transcription represents a new mechanism of cyclosporine and FK506 action that may underlie pharmacologic effects and toxic manifestations of these potent immunosuppressive drugs (569).

A recent report demonstrated that in vivo FK506 treatment eliminated antigen-stimulated T cells through DNA fragmentation (apoptosis), representing one of the mechanisms of immunologic tolerance (570).

Experimental Studies

Cell Culture

McCauley and colleagues (571) demonstrated a cyclosporine- and FK506-mediated, dose-dependent inhibition of renal cell proliferation using LLC-PK1 cells (an established cell line derived from the pig proximal tubule) in culture. Although FK506 inhibited renal cell proliferation to a greater degree than cyclosporine at the same concentration, when clinically relevant concentrations were compared, FK506 was significantly less inhibitory than cyclosporine. Moutabarrik and associates (572) observed similar effects in the same cell line but could not make a clear distinction between the FK506 and the cyclosporine effects on release of 3_H thymidine from prelabeled cells, N-acetyl-β-D-glucosaminidase release, and cell detachment. Ultrastructural changes such as vacuolization, swelling, and mitochondrial enlargement and inhibition of the growth of the cultured tubular cells were also observed at high concentrations of FK506 and cyclosporine. Low concentrations of FK506 and cyclosporine were not cytotoxic and induced only a minimal inhibitory effect on the growth of tubular cells in vitro. Cyclosporine and FK506 also induced a time-dependent stimulation of the secretion of endothelin by cultured tubular cells. The concentration of cyclosporine that induced these effects was 10 to 100 times higher than that required for FK506. The concentrations of FK506 and cyclosporine inducing endothelin secretion were not cytolytic for tubular cells in vitro. Yatscoff et al. (573) compare the effect of rapamycin and FK506 on the release of prostacyclin and endothelin *in vitro* using cultured rabbit mesangial and endothelial cells. The effects of both rapamycin and FK506 on the basal or stimulated release of prostacyclin or endothelin from mesangial cells and endothelial cells are similar with the following exceptions: Rapamycin results in a significant increase in the release of prostacyclin, while in contrast FK506 results in a significant decrease in the release of prostacyclin from the endothelial cells. Benigni and colleagues (574) review the vascular effects of FK506 as compared to cyclosporine in endothelial cell culture and intact organ. FK506, unlike cyclosporine, is without significant effect on thromboxane B_2, 6-ketoprostaglandin $F1_{1\alpha}$, or endothelin release in bovine aortic endothelial cells grown in culture and does not alter the renal vascular resistance *in vivo*. These findings suggest that FK506 causes much less pronounced endothelial cell injury, at least *in vitro*.

Atcherson and Trifillis (575) examine *in vitro* cytotoxicity of FK506 on normal human proximal tubule cells. They find that FK506 is reversibly and mildly toxic to monolayers of human renal proximal tubule cells.

Edkins and associates (576) compare the effect of FK506 (2.5 mg per kg for 7 days) and cyclosporine (50 mg per kg per day) on renal, hepatic, brain and cochlear-reduced glutathione content. Both cyclosporine and FK506 increase glutathione levels in kidney to approximately equivalent levels after 5 days of treatment. Only FK506 increases glutathione levels in liver, and neither drug changes levels in other tissues.

Ali Shah et al. (577) show that FK506 exhibits a broad, powerful inhibitory effect on human hepatic microsomal cytochrome P-450-dependent drug metabolism. However, the full potential for drug interactions can only be determined by investigating its effects on other P-450 families using both *in vivo* and *in vitro* studies. On the other hand, Yoshimura et al. (578) recently report that, in rats, both FK506 and rapamycin are without significant effects in contrast to cyclosporine on renal microsomal P-450–dependent drug metabolism.

Yoshimura et al. (579) review the effect of FK506 and rapamycin on renal P-450 systems in rat models. They find that although cyclosporine has a strong effect on renal P-450 systems and induces such a system in kidney cortex (microsomal P-450), FK506 and rapamycin have no substantial effect on the induction of renal P-450.

The role of intracellular calcium in the pathogenesis of cyclosporine nephrotoxicity has received great attention (580,581) and has resulted in therapeutic implications to prevent nephrotoxic effects of the drug. The effect of cyclosporine and FK506 on microsomes and mitochondria of rabbit renal cortex tissue has been studied by Prasad and associates (582). Both drugs decrease calcium uptake and A23187-induced calcium release from microsomes and mitochondria in a dose-dependent manner (0.5 to 10.0 μg per mL). The effect of FK506 is significantly less at equivalent concentrations, and microsomal calcium-stimulated ATPase is not changed by either drug.

The potential role of the FK506 binding protein (FKBP12) in cellular calcium homeostasis has been suggested. Indeed, Jayaraman and colleagues (583) find that a 12-kd protein tightly bound to the calcium release channel in skeletal muscles of rabbit is FKBP12. Obviously, if this observation can be confirmed in vascular smooth muscle, it may explain the mechanism of FK506-induced vasoconstriction in renal vasculature. This process also is probably calcineurin-drug complex mediated. A further role of calcineurin in α-adrenergic stimulation of Na^+-K^+-ATPase activity in renal tubular cells is illustrated by Aperia et al. (584). They demonstrate that FK506 inhibited Na^+-K^+-adenosine triphosphatase (ATPase) activity induced by oxymetazoline, an α-adrenergic agonist. This study may suggest a role for FK506-mediated renal nerve changes in sodium and potassium homeostasis. In this context, Palevsky and colleagues (585) report a resistance to the effect of aldosterone on renal cells in cultures exposed to FK506.

Animal Studies

Animal studies have shown both acute and chronic nephrotoxicity produced by FK506 (586). Somewhat different than cyclosporine, FK506 produces toxicity at blood levels that are clinically relevant; however, the doses necessary to achieve these blood levels on a weight basis are at least 10-fold larger than those used clinically. This contrasts with cyclosporine, with which acute and chronic nephrotoxicity can be produced with doses on a weight basis that are very close to those clinically used, particularly in the salt-depleted rat model; however, the blood levels achieved with these doses are at least three to four times those achieved clinically (587).

Preclinical animal studies gave few hints of nephrotoxicity (588). However, a troubling series of side effects soon appeared including vasculitis, myocardial necrosis, and severe weight loss. Fortunately, most of these side effects turned out to be species-specific. Nephrotoxicity of FK506 became apparent from the initial series of rescue patients treated with the drug (589).

Several studies have documented reduction in effective renal plasma flow and GFR in animal models. Ueda and colleagues (590) have measured renal cortical blood flow, using a hydrogen ion clearance method, serum creatinine, and juxtaglomerular cell cross-sectional area in mice treated with FK506, 3 mg per kg per day given subcutaneously as compared with saline-treated control animals. Cortical blood flow is significantly reduced in FK506-treated animals as compared with control animals, as is juxtaglomerular cell area. Kumano et al. (591) also note a reduction in GFR and effective renal plasma flow using inulin and p-aminohippuric acid in a heminephrectomized rat model in response to an acute infusion of FK506 and after 21 days of treatment. Proximal tubular vacuolization typical of cyclosporine nephrotoxicity is noted, and diltiazem improves both the functional and morphologic changes caused by FK506. Lieberman and associates (592) note a significant volume reduction in both cyclosporine-treated and FK506-treated glomeruli that are inhibited by verapamil. Mitamura and colleagues (593) review the FK506-induced nephrotoxicity in spontaneous hypertensive rats. These results indicate that the acute nephrotoxicity of FK506 is derived from impaired glomerular function associated with renal arteriolar constriction brought about by the drug. All of these renal disorders induced by FK506 recover completely or partially when the drug is withdrawn for 2 or 4 weeks. Thus, the acute nephrotoxicity of FK506 in spontaneous hypertensive rats is reversible.

Ryffel and colleagues (594) explore the nephrotoxicity of immunosuppressants in rats. Specifically, they compare the nephrotoxic effects of FK506 and rapamycin with that of cyclosporine in male Wistar rats. FK506 causes proximal tubular epithelial changes consisting of atrophy, vacuolization, inclusion bodies, microcalcification, and focal mononuclear interstitial infiltrate as described for cyclosporine. The most striking alteration is hypertrophy of the juxtaglomerular apparatus. The percentage of renin-containing juxtaglomerular apparatus and the extent of renin immunoreactivity along afferent vessels are significantly increased in FK506-treated and CsA-treated rats. By contrast, no renal morphologic lesions are found in rapamycin-treated animals. Renal cortical extracts contain abundant cyclophilin and FK506-binding protein, the main intracytoplasmic receptors for cyclosporine and FK506, respectively. The authors hypothesize that both the immunosuppressive and toxic effects of FK506 and cyclosporine, but not of rapamycin, are mediated through an immunophilin–drug–calcineurin complex. The renal substrate of calcineurin, which mediates renal vasoconstriction, is yet to be identified.

Andoh and associates (595) also compare the acute rapamycin nephrotoxicity with cyclosporine and tacrolimus. They find that cyclosporine and FK506 strikingly decrease urinary excretion of nitric oxide, renal blood flow, and GFR, whereas rapamycin does not. In contrast, all three of these drugs cause significant hypomagnesemia associated with inappropriately high fractional excretion of magnesium, suggesting renal magnesium wasting. In addition, with all three drugs there are lesions in the rat kidneys consisting of tubular collapse, vacuolization, and nephrocalcinosis. These researchers show that only the calcineurin inhibitors produce glomerular dysfunction in an acute experimental model of nephrotoxicity.

Of interest is the experiment of Hara and colleagues (596) that shows that FK506 is effective in the prevention of the development of rapid glomerular injury in rats with accelerated nephrotoxic serum glomerulonephritis.

Clinical Studies

Since the initial reports on the use of tacrolimus in clinical transplantation by Starzl and Shapiro (597,598), numerous large-scale trials compared the efficacy and safety of tacrolimus and cyclosporine mainly in liver (599,600), and kidney (601–603) transplantation. According to five out of six of these large trials, renal function and the incidence of renal impairment were comparable in both treatment arms at 1 year posttransplantation. Similar results were reported in a long-term comparison of nephrotoxicity between tacrolimus and cyclosporine in pediatric heart transplant recipients (604). In contrast, Ashan et al. reported a significantly better renal allograft function at 2 and 3 years, under tacrolimus compared to cyclosporine, both in combination with steroids and mycophenolate mofetil (603,605). However, graft survival at 2 and 3 years was comparable in both groups. In an intention-to-treat analysis, graft survival at 5 years was comparable between patients, initially randomized to tacrolimus or cyclosporine in the large U.S. multicenter trial (601,606).

In all these large trials, the incidence of acute rejection was significantly lower in the tacrolimus treated patients, compared to the cyclosporine treated patients. Similarly, there was a different profile of adverse effects with higher incidence of post-transplant diabetes mellitus and neurotoxicity under tacrolimus, compared to a higher incidence of hypertension, hyperlipidemia, hirsutism, and gum hyperplasia in cyclosporine treated patients.

According to three studies, the intrarenal hemodynamics are less affected by tacrolimus compared to cyclosporine, with better preservation of the renal plasma flow (523,524,607).

The histopathological changes, induced by tacrolimus, in the (transplanted) kidney, are entirely comparable to those induced by cyclosporine, that is, arteriolar hyalinosis and striped interstitial fibrosis (544,608-611). The intrarenal expression of TGF-beta, collagen, fibronectin, MMP-2, TIMP-1, and osteopontin was assessed by RT-PCR, and proved to be similar in kidneys treated with either tacrolimus or cyclosporine (612).

In conclusion, the nephrotoxicity of tacrolimus is functionally and morphologically comparable to the nephrotoxicity of cyclosporine as well in recipients of a renal allograft, as in recipients of a solid nonrenal organ. However, there is evidence that tacrolimus is a more powerful immunosuppressive agent, with a different toxicity profile.

OKT3

OKT3 is a murine monoclonal antibody directed against the epsilon-moiety of the CD3 receptor that comodulates with the antigen T-cell receptor (TCR) on the surface of T lymphocytes.

The immunosuppressive properties of OKT3 are related to its ability to deplete CD3+ cells from the circulation, to induce the internalization of CD3/TCR complexes, and to sterically inhibit residual CD3/TCR complexes (613). Since the CD3/TCR complex is a signal transducing system, binding of the OKT3 monoclonal antibody to this CD3 receptor activates the T lymphocytes before internalization or stripping of the CD3/TCR complex from the surface of the cell. In other words, before exerting immunosuppressive effects, OKT3 induces a transient activation of lymphocytes. In addition, monocyte activation is induced by the multivalent cross-linking of the CD3/TCR complex and the monocyte Fc receptor induced by OKT3 (614). This activation is accompanied by the release of several proinflammatory cytokines including tumor necrosis factor-α (TNF-α), interferon-γ (IFN-γ), IL-2, and interleukin-6 (IL-6) into the circulation within hours after the initial OKT3 injection (615–620). T cells are the main source of TNF-α in this clinical setting, although monocytes can also be activated, as shown by their production of IL-1 and IL-6 (621). That TNF-α and IFN-γ play a key role in this inflammatory reaction is suggested by the prevention of the hypothermia, hypomobility, diarrhea, and piloerection using monoclonal antibodies directed against TNF-α and IFN-γ (622–624).

Complement activation seems to play a minor role in the pathogenesis of OKT3-associated cytokine release syndrome. Indeed, Mackie and colleagues (625) describe a syndrome presenting all the clinical symptoms of a classic anti-CD3-induced toxicity in complement-deficient mice. Furthermore, Waid and associates (626) demonstrate the lack of toxicity of a complement-binding nonmitogenic anti–T-cell receptor immunoglobulin M (IgM) monoclonal antibody.

Clinical Observations

The clinical syndrome of this post-OKT3 inflammatory reaction is characterized by generalized capillary leak, fever, chills, rigors, diarrhea, headaches, aseptic meningitis, noncardiogenic pulmonary edema, cerebral edema/convulsions, and the so-called cytokine nephropathy.

OKT3 has been used to treat allograft rejection and has also been used prophylactically to delay the use of cyclosporine in the immediate postoperative period when the allograft is ischemic and most vulnerable to the use of vasculopathic and nephrotoxic effect of cyclosporine. However, Toussaint et al. (627) observe a higher rate of delayed graft function among OKT3 patients than those treated initially with cyclosporine immediately after transplantation. These investigators use low doses of steroid (1 mg per kg of methylprednisolone) before the first OKT3 injection in contrast with other centers where 4 to 8 mg per kg is used (628). The critical role of steroid pretreatment at sufficient dose in the partial protection of the late graft function among OKT3 patients is confirmed when 8 mg per kg of methylprednisolone is used (629). This increased dose of steroid is associated with a smaller increase of TNF and IFN-γ (629). Simpson et al. (630) report signs of tubular alterations as demonstrated by investigating the urinary sediment in renal allograft recipients and a striking increase in serum creatinine during the first 3 days of OKT3 therapy. Batiuk and associates (631) report a syndrome of reversible renal dysfunction associated with OKT3 induction therapy after renal transplantation and with OKT3 rejection after cardiac transplantation. Indeed, 7.5% of renal allograft recipients with immediate graft function developed a rising serum creatinine and decline in urine output not attributable to cyclosporine because cyclosporine therapy had not yet been initiated. The renal biopsies obtained in all of the patients showed no histologic abnormalities or mild interstitial edema. Four of sixteen cardiac transplant patients developed an increase in serum creatinine following the second dose of OKT3 given for rejection. However, two of the patients also received indomethacin. Renal dysfunction resolved spontaneously in all cases.

Goldman and colleagues (632) analyze the changes of serum creatinine levels in the first days of antirejection therapy with OKT3. Although initial serum creatinine levels were similar, the OKT3-treated group reached a mean peak increase in serum creatinine of 76% on day 4 as compared to the mean peak increase of 57% on day 3 in the pulse steroid treatment group. Chatenoud and others (616) examine the release of cytokines in the systemic circulation in 35 renal allograft recipients who received 5 mg per day of OKT3 starting at the time of transplantation. All but three patients were pretreated with a 1-g bolus of methylprednisolone from 1 to 3 hours before administration of OKT3 to ameliorate the clinical reactions. TNF reached a peak at 1 hour after OKT3 injection and remained elevated at 4 hours. Peak TNF was higher in the three patients who did not receive the steroid bolus and was higher in those who received the bolus concomitantly rather than 1 hour before OKT3. IFN-γ reached a maximum at 4 hours following the OKT3 injection and was highest in those not receiving the steroid bolus or who received it at the time of OKT3 injection. IL-2 increased in only five patients, three of whom did not receive the steroid bolus. IL-1β, IFN-α, and granulocyte–macrophage colony-stimulating factor levels did not increase with OKT3 injection. Fifteen to twenty hours after injection, TNF, IFN-γ, and IL-2 levels had returned to baseline.

The massive leukocyte activation resulting in cytokine release probably plays an important role in the acute renal dysfunction post-OKT3 administration. IL-1, IFN-γ, IL-2, IL-6, and TNF-α are involved in the capillary leak syndrome (633,634), which explains the clinical symptomatology of lung edema, reducing circulating volume, and hence compromising renal perfusion. Of note is the demonstrated release of endothelin after the first dose of OKT3 in renal transplant recipients (635). A direct cytotoxic effect of particular cytokines in kidney parenchyma has been put forward as a possible mechanism of allograft destruction (636). In addition, activation of leukocytes by cytokines induces an enhanced expression of adhesion molecules (637). The increased expression of adhesion molecules on endothelial and parenchymal cells may result in margination, diapedesis, migration, and appearance of those activated cells in the interstitium of the kidney. Indeed, activated neutrophils can play a mediator role by releasing oxygen radicals in the physiopathology of ischemic kidney injury. A recent report by Kelly et al. (638) shows that prohibiting neutrophils from infiltrating into the interstitium protects the kidney against ischemic injury, as is the case in other models (639).

Abramowicz and associates (640) demonstrate that OKT3 exerts procoagulant effects that can precipitate intragraft thromboses and result in transplant loss. The thrombotic events took place during the prophylactic administration of OKT3 occurring between day 1 and 11 postoperatively, always before the use of cyclosporine. The most striking finding in the renal biopsies was the formation of thrombi in some glomerular capillary loops and in afferent arterioles. Endothelial cells were swollen, causing diminished patency of capillary lumens. The interstitium was only slightly enlarged by edema without significant influx of inflammatory cells or tubular damage. Increased numbers of polymorphonuclear cells were present in the peritubular and glomerular capillaries. The authors look carefully for additional risk factors by comparing the clinical parameters of the 13 recipients with thrombosis to those of 218 patients free of this complication. The only relevant parameter appeared to be the methylprednisolone dose given as pretreatment before the first OKT3 injection. Six out of forty-two patients (14%) receiving 30 mg per kg of methylprednisolone ex-

perienced a thrombotic event, as compared to seven of the 189 patients (3.7%) who received the regular 8 mg per kg of methylprednisolone. The latter incidence compares to the 2% to 3% of vascular complications in renal transplantation reported in the absence of OKT3 prophylaxis (641,642), suggesting that the risk of thrombotic events related to OKT3 itself is rather low.

This clinically important side effect is related to the capacity of the first OKT3 dose to trigger the extrinsic pathway of the coagulation system and may precipitate early intragraft thrombosis, resulting in early transplant loss (641,643–645). Pradier and colleagues (643) find that all patients receiving OKT3 in the context of a kidney transplant have an increased plasma level of prothrombin fragments, peaking 4 hours after the first injection. There is no difference between the patients who receive 5 mg or 10 mg, neither when OKT3 is given as prophylaxis nor when given for treatment of rejection. Fibrin degradation products, indicative of a fibrinolytic process, are already above baseline values 4 hours after the first injection and continue to increase until 24 hours. The von Willebrand factor levels, an indicator of endothelial cell damage, are also significantly increased after OKT3 injection. The study of Raasveld and associates (644) confirms the previous findings, as they report an increased level of thrombin–antithrombin III complex, indicative of activation of the coagulation, as well as increased levels of tissue-type plasminogen activator and plasmin-α_2–antiplasmin complexes, indicative of fibrinolysis after the first injection of OKT3. According to the latter report, activation of the coagulation occurs via the extrinsic rather than the intrinsic pathway.

In vitro/Animal Studies

Pradier and associates (643) and Abramowicz and colleagues (645) studied this phenomenon *in vitro* and find that the activation of the coagulation by OKT3 is related to the induction of procoagulant activity of the tissue factor type on both endothelial cells and monocytes and that the high doses of methylprednisolone potentiate OKT3-induced tissue factor expression and activity on monocytes (646).

Indeed, using human umbilical vein endothelial cells, they could show that OKT3 and supernatants of unstimulated peripheral blood mononuclear cells are inactive. However, supernatants of OKT3-stimulated peripheral blood mononuclear cells induce a massive increase of tissue factor activity at the endothelial cell surface measured by thrombin generation. The inhibition of this procoagulant activity by anti-TNF monoclonal antibodies demonstrates that TNF is an important mediator of this effect of OKT3 at the endothelial cell membrane level. This is compatible with the well-known TNF effect on the expression of tissue factor on endothelium (647).

Itaka and colleagues observe (648) that monocytes also display increased procoagulant activity after culture in the presence of OKT3 antibody. This has been confirmed by other authors (645,646) as well. Again, this is due to an increased tissue factor expression by not clearly identified mechanisms. Indeed, TNF does not seem to play an important role (649). To what extent the monocyte procoagulant inducing factor (650), an as yet incompletely characterized cytokine (651), plays a role is still to be demonstrated. Furthermore, interactions between activated T cells and monocytes appear to be necessary to induce the monocyte procoagulant activity (651,652). The question of why only a small number of patients developed intragraft thrombosis after OKT3 was nicely addressed in a recent paper by Abramowicz and colleagues (645). They report that the procoagulant activity of unstimulated peripheral blood mononuclear cells reaches 3.0 ± 0.7 mU per mL after OKT3 stimulation and further increases to 7.4 ± 2.0 mU per mL when those cells are first preincubated overnight with methylprednisolone before OKT3 stimulation. They show that this process involves a tissue factor–factor VII pathway; specifically, they find increased membrane expression of tissue factor on monocytes and a marked reduction of the induced procoagulant activity when the clotting assay is performed with factor VII-deficient plasma (645). Furthermore, corticosteroids increase plasminogen activator inhibitor-1 (PAI-1) secretion by hepatocytes (653), while at the same time they decrease tissue-type plasminogen activator (654) as well as prostacyclin (655,656) and nitric oxide production (657,658). In addition, one has to remember that OKT3 induces the release of proinflammatory cytokines such as TNF, IL-1, and IFN-γ, which also contributes to the decrease of endothelial cell expression of thrombomodulin (622,647,659), markedly inhibiting the anticoagulant effects of protein C and S (659,660).

Administration of OKT3 induces increased group II secretory phospholipase A2 levels inducing the biosynthesis of vasoconstrictive prostaglandins, vasoactive lipid mediators that influence glomerular hemodynamics, and renal function (661).

Alegre et al. (662) investigate the possible direct renal damage of anti-CD3 monoclonal antibody in a murine model. In this study hamster anti-mouse CD3 monoclonal antibody 145-2C11 (663) is injected and induces an important transient release of several cytokines in the circulation (662,664). Tubular lesions are histologically identified mainly at the S3 segment of the nephron and are also evidenced by discrete renal function impairment. Pretreatment with steroids almost completely abolishes the cytokine release, and no changes in histology and renal function can be observed.

Finally, the kidney graft is by all means susceptible to the development of ARF. Warm and protracted cold ischemia associated with organ procurement and the immunosuppression administered may present additional risk factors to develop and maintain ARF after OKT3 administration.

Abramowicz and colleagues (665) performed a study in order to prevent as much as possible the nephrotoxic effects seen in the context of OKT3 administration. According to these authors, combined strategy of appropriate dosage of steroids before the first OKT3 injection, administration of a calcium-channel blocker, and optimization of volume status is safe and efficiently prevents OKT3 nephrotoxic effects.

OKT3 induces activation of both mononuclear cells and the common pathway of coagulation responsible for the first dose reactions and transient or severe nephrotoxic effects. Patient-related or donor-related risk factors and inappropriate doses of steroids contribute substantially to the severity of those side effects. New anti-CD3 agents such as humanized OKT3 and OKT3 F(ab')₂ are being developed and will contribute to a better clinical tolerance and comparable immunosuppression (666).

Daclizumab and basiliximab are new monoclonal antibodies approved for the prophylaxis of acute organ rejection in renal allograft recipients (667–671). The efficacy of these agents has been established in a number of well-controlled clinical trials. These multicenter studies assessed the efficacy of daclizumab and basiliximab versus placebo when used as part of a regimen of double therapy (cyclosporine and corticosteroids) or triple therapy (cyclosporine, corticosteroids, and azathioprine) to prevent acute allograft rejection. These studies demonstrate that daclizumab significantly decreases the incidence of acute rejection at 6 months. Daclizumab, when given in combination with other immunosuppressants, does not show an increase in the number of serious adverse events compared with placebo (670). With basiliximab, the incidence of acute rejection is 34% with double therapy in the basiliximab group and 52% in the placebo group. The incidence and types of adverse events are similar to those in placebo-treated patients. No drug interactions have been observed when daclizumab and basiliximab are administered with other immunosuppressive agents (667).

MYCOPHENOLATE MOFETIL

Mycophenolate mofetil (MMF), the morpholinoethyl ester of mycophenolic acid (Fig. 42-5), has been developed as an immunosuppressant for prevention of rejection in renal transplantation. *In vivo*, MMF is deesterified to mycophenolic acid (the active immunosuppressive component), which is a potent and specific inhibitor of the synthesis of guanosine nucleotides and thus a selective suppressor of proliferation of both T and B lymphocytes. MMF, given alone or with corticosteroids or cyclosporine, lowers the frequency of acute rejection after allogeneic organ transplantation in animals (672,673).

The immunosuppression of MMF appears to be additive with that of cyclosporine and tacrolimus, and MMF does not promote nephrotoxicity (674). Initial studies indicated that MMF, in combination with cyclosporine and steroids, reduces the incidence of acute rejection in renal transplantation (675–677).

In the meantime MMF has been used under several clinical conditions. In cardiac, liver, lung, and pancreas transplantation the use of MMF in association with reduced doses of cyclosporine has resulted in improved renal function and maintained immunosuppression (678–681). In renal transplantation, Halloran and others (682) summarize the three multicenter trials that confirm at 1-year posttransplant MMF is effective in preventing acute renal allograft rejection (675–677). Two studies address patients with chronic kidney graft dysfunction in whom MMF is introduced and cyclosporine exposure reduced (683,684). The rationale is that the increased, immunosuppressive potency of MMF would allow for a safe reduction of CsA doses. The conclusion from these two studies is that cyclosporine dose reduction in patients on MMF results in an improved graft function with no increased risk of rejection. It must be noted, however, that follow-up was short—less than 1 year—in both studies. In addition, whether MMF does better than azathioprine (AZA) in this setting remains an open question. Indeed, a similar improvement of chronic graft dysfunction is reported when AZA is introduced and cyclosporine doses reduced (685).

Is there a role for MMF in the attempt to withdraw calcineurin inhibitors in patients with stable renal transplantation? Several randomized (686–688), as well as nonrandomized (689), clinical trials in renal transplantation examined the efficacy and safety of calcineurin inhibitors in patients with stable graft function under triple immunosuppressive regimen, consisting of prednisolone, cyclosporine or tacrolimus, and MMF. All these studies reported a significant improvement of the graft function, as well as lower blood pressure, and an improved lipid profile after calcineurin inhibitor (CNI) withdrawal. In contrast, the incidence of acute rejection was higher in the CNI withdrawal group, without any impact on graft survival. Therefore, these studies provide evidence that CNI withdrawal is achievable in renal transplant recipients with stable graft function. CNI withdrawal appears to improve graft function, hypertension, and hyperlipidemia. However, caution should be paid to the increased incidence of acute rejection after CNI withdrawal, and the short term of follow-up, reported in these studies (6 to 32 months). Whether CNI withdrawal will result in improved graft survival, is not yet known.

Since MMF has multiple immunosuppressive and anti-inflammatory modes of actions including the inhibition of humoral and cellular immunity, antimutogenesis, reduction of mononuclear cell infiltration, and inhibition of vascular smooth muscle and mesangial cell proliferation, it is not surprising that the drug is now used in autoimmune-mediated renal disease (690). Briggs and colleagues (691,692) report their limited experience in eight patients with different types of nephrotic-type glomerulonephritis and unsatisfactory response to steroids as cyclosporine. Controlled prospective studies are underway to clarify the potential advantages of MMF compared with other immunosuppressive agents in these disease entities.

In conclusion, MMF is a potent, nonnephrotoxic immunosuppressive drug, which significantly reduced the incidence of acute rejection under triple immunosuppressive regimens with prednisolone and cyclosporine or tacrolimus. In addition, MMF appears to allow dose reduction or even withdrawal of CNI in renal transplant recipients with stable graft function, thereby avoiding the long-term nephrotoxicity induced by calcineurin inhibitors. Because immunosuppressant-induced nephrotoxicity has been associated with significant financial costs, cyclosporine-sparing and FK506-sparing regimens should result in substantial savings in health care costs (693) (Fig. 42-5). It is important to emphasize here that there are no long-term data for these experimental regimens, but they offer a new direction if these short-term results are confirmed over a more sufficient period of time.

RAPAMYCIN

Rapamycin (sirolimus, or SRL) is a macrocyclic fermentation product of *Streptomyces hygroscopicus*, and was first isolated in 1975 (694). SRL has a similar molecular structure to FK 506 and also binds to FKBP12 (695). However, the SRL-FKBP12 complex does not affect the calcineurin phosphatase, but instead binds to a protein, called the mammalian target of rapamycin (mTOR) (696). This binding of the SRL-FKBP12 complex to mTOR inhibits both DNA and protein synthesis, resulting in arrest of the cell cycle in late G1, as it progresses to the S phase (697).

SRL blocks T-cell proliferation, induced by cytokines, alloantigens, and mitogens in a dose-dependent manner (698). In addition, SRL acts on B-cells, causing an inhibition of antigen and cytokine driven B-cell proliferation (699). *In vitro* studies have demonstrated the synergistic immunosuppressive interaction of CsA and SRL (700), in contrast to the combination of FK506 and SRL, which produced an antagonistic effect at low doses (701). Animal studies have confirmed the immunosuppressive potential of SRL (702), as well as its synergistic interaction with CsA (703). In contrast to the *in vitro* studies, FK506 interacted synergistically with SRL in animal studies (704).

Clinical Efficacy of Sirolimus in Renal Transplantation

Based on the results from several multicenter, prospective, randomized trials, including a U.S. study, a global study, a combined European-U.S. study, and two European studies, SRL was approved in 1999 by the Food and Drug Administration (FDA) for the prevention of acute rejection in renal transplant recipients. SRL was used in combination with CsA and prednisolone in these studies and reduced the incidence of acute rejection at 1 year to 10% (705).

Three prospective, randomized trials in renal transplant recipients compared CsA to SRL in combination with prednisolone and azathioprine or mycophenolate mofetil (706–708). All these trials showed a comparable incidence of acute rejection in both treatment arms, and more importantly, a superior graft function at one year in the SRL-treated patients. In one study, graft function remained significantly bet-

ter at three years in the SRL-treated patients (709). In addition, the incidence of normal histology in protocol biopsies at 2 years was significantly higher in SRL-treated patients, compared to CsA-treated patients (66.6% vs. 20.8%) (709). These results from three trials provide evidence that avoidance of the long-term nephrotoxicity, induced by calcineurin inhibitors, is achievable in renal transplant recipients.

Several randomized trials in renal transplantation investigated the feasibility and the outcome of early calcineurin inhibitor withdrawal, in triple regimens with SRL and prednisolone (710–713). Overall, patient and graft survival, as well as the incidence of acute rejection at 1 year, were comparable in both treatment arms (CsA + SRL + P vs. SRL + P). In contrast, graft function was superior, and the incidence of hypertension was reduced in the patients weaned from CsA. Similarly, the incidence of chronic allograft nephropathy was significantly lower in protocol biopsies at 1 year from patients on SRL + P alone (713). Again, these data provide strong evidence that early withdrawal of calcineurin inhibitors can safely be achieved in renal transplant recipients under SRL, and may avoid long-term nephrotoxicity.

Nephrotoxicity of Sirolimus

Studies in pigs and rats have shown that sirolimus has no deleterious effects on glomerular filtration rate or renal blood flow, and caused minimal morphologic signs of toxicity (714,715). Sirolimus reduced medullary concentrating ability and increased tubular enzymuria in rat kidneys, suggesting that mild tubular injury may occur (716). In a salt-depleted rat model of CsA toxicity, the combination of CsA with SRL produced a functional and morphologic deterioration (717).

In clinical studies in renal transplant recipients, sirolimus proved to be an effective immunosuppressive drug, devoid of intrinsic nephrotoxicity (see Clinical Efficacy of Sirolimus in Renal Transplantation, above). However, sirolimus may prolong delayed graft function in renal transplant recipients (718). In addition, thrombotic microangiopathy has been described under the combination of sirolimus and tacrolimus, after intestinal transplantation (719). Of concern are the reports on de novo proteinuria, occurring after conversion from a calcineurin inhibitor to sirolimus in renal transplant recipients (720). Although the exact mechanism for the development of this proteinuria is currently putative, the increased intraglomerular pressure, resulting from the withdrawal of the intrarenal vasoconstriction, induced by CNIs, could be one reasonable explanation. However, proinflammatory effects of a rapamycin derivative, SDZ RAD, were described as well in experimental mesangial proliferative glomerulonephritis (721).

In conclusion, there is large evidence that sirolimus is a nonnephrotoxic immunosuppressive drug. Studies, performed in renal transplantation, have shown that sirolimus may allow the avoidance of the nephrotoxicity induced by calcineurin inhibitors. Of concern are the proteinuria, recently reported after conversion to sirolimus, and the side effects induced by this drug, such as myelosuppression and hyperlipidemia.

References

1. Lau WK, et al. Comparative efficacy and toxicity of amikacin/carbenicillin versus gentamicin/carbenicillin in leukopenic patients: a randomized prospective study. *Am J Med* 1977;62:959.
2. Smith CR, et al. Controlled comparison of amikacin and gentamicin. *N Engl J Med* 1977;296:349.
3. Kumin GD. Clinical nephrotoxicity of tobramycin and gentamicin: a prospective study. *JAMA* 1980;244:1808.
4. Smith CR, et al. Double-blind comparison of the nephrotoxicity and auditory toxicity of gentamicin and tobramycin. *N Engl J Med* 1980;302:1106.

5. Feig PU, et al. Aminoglycoside nephrotoxicity: a double blind prospective randomized study of gentamicin and tobramycin. *J Antimicrob Chemother* 1982;10:217.

6. Gatell JM, et al. Comparison of nephrotoxicity and auditory toxicity of tobramycin and amikacin. *Antimicrob Agents Chemother* 1983;23:897.

7. Lerner AM, et al. Randomized controlled trial of the comparative efficacy, auditory toxicity and nephrotoxicity of tobramycin and netilmicin. *Lancet* 1983;1:1123.

8. Tablan OC, et al. Renal and auditory toxicity of high-dose, prolonged therapy with gentamicin and tobramycin in Pseudomonas endocarditis. *J Infect Dis* 1984;149:257.

9. Eisenberg JM, et al. What is the cost of nephrotoxicity associated with aminoglycosides? *Ann Int Med* 1987;107:900.

10. Kahlmeter G, Dahlagers J. Aminoglycoside toxicity—a review of clinical studies published between 1975 and 1982. *J Antimicrob Chemother* 1984; 13(Suppl A):9.

11. Schentag JJ, Cerra FB, Plaut ME. Clinical and pharmacokinetic characteristics of aminoglycoside nephrotoxicity in 201 critically ill patients. *Antimicrob Agents Chemother* 1982;21:721.

12. Kaloyanides GJ, Pastoriza-Munoz E. Aminoglycoside nephrotoxicity. *Kidney Int* 1980;18:571.

13. Kaloyanides GJ. Aminoglycoside-induced functional and biochemical defects in the renal cortex. *Fund Appl Toxicol* 1984;4:930.

14. Humes HD. Aminoglycoside nephrotoxicity. *Kidney Int* 1988;22:900.

15. Lietman PS, Smith CR. Aminoglycoside nephrotoxicity in man. *Rev Infect Dis* 1983;5(Suppl 2):284.

16. Luft FC. Clinical significance of renal changes engendered by aminoglycosides in man. *J Antimicrob Chemother* 1984;13(Suppl A):23.

17. Gibey R, et al. Predictive value of urinary N-acetyl-beta-glucosaminidase (NAG), alanine-aminopeptidase (AAP) and beta-2-microglobulin (B₂M) in evaluating nephrotoxicity of gentamicin. *Clin Chem Acta* 1981;116:24.

18. Schentag JJ. Specificity of tubular damage criteria for aminoglycoside nephrotoxicity in critically ill patients. *J Clin Pharmacol* 1983;23:473.

19. Mondorf AW, et al. Effect of aminoglycosides on proximal tubular membranes of the human kidney. *Eur J Clin Pharmacol* 1978;13:133.

20. Nicot G, et al. Gentamicin and sisomicin induced renal tubular damage. *Eur J Pharmacol* 1982;23:161.

21. Anderson RJ, et al. Nonoliguric acute renal failure. *N Engl J Med* 1977; 296:1134.

22. Kidwell DT, et al. Acute effects of gentamicin on thick ascending limb function in the rat. *Eur J Pharmacol* 1994;270:97.

23. Rosen S, Brezis M, Stillman I. The pathology of nephrotoxic injury: a reappraisal. *Miner Electrolyte Metab* 1994;20:174.

24. Humes HD, Weinberg JM. The effect of gentamicin on antidiuretic hormone-stimulated osmotic water flow in the toad urinary bladder. *J Lab Clin Med* 1983;101:472.

25. Soberon L, et al. Comparative nephrotoxicities of gentamicin, netilmicin and tobramycin in the rat. *J Pharmacol Exp Ther* 1979;210:334.

26. Safirstein R, Miller P, Kahn T. Cortical and papillary absorptive defects in gentamicin nephrotoxicity. *Kidney Int* 1983;24:526.

27. Barr GA, et al. An animal model for combined methoxyflurane and gentamicin nephrotoxicity. *Br J Anaesth* 1973;45:306.

28. Hirsch GH. Enhancement of gentamicin nephrotoxicity by glycerol. *Toxicol Appl Pharmacol* 1974;29:270.

29. Luft FC, Yum MN, Kleit SA. The effect of concomitant mercuric chloride and gentamicin on kidney function and structure in the rat. *J Lab Clin Med* 1977;89:622.

30. Spiegel DM, Shanley PF, Molitoris BA. Mild ischemia predisposes the S3 segment to gentamicin toxicity. *Kidney Int* 1990;38:459.

31. Zager R, Sharma HM. Gentamicin increases renal susceptibility to an acute ischemic insult. *J Lab Clin Med* 1983;101:670.

32. Zager RA, Prior RB. Gentamicin and gram-negative bacteremia. A synergism for the development of experimental nephrotoxic acute renal failure. *J Clin Invest* 1986;78:196.

33. Zager RA. Gentamicin nephrotoxicity in the setting of acute renal hypoperfusion. *Am J Physiol* 1988;254:F574.

34. Zager RA. Gentamicin effects on renal ischemia/reperfusion injury. *Circ Res* 1992;70:20.

35. Zager RA. Endotoxemia, renal hypoperfusion, and fever: interactive risk factors for aminoglycoside and sepsis-associated acute renal failure. *Am J Kidney Dis* 1992;20:223.

36. Zager RA. Sepsis-associated acute renal failure: some potential pathogenic and therapeutic insights. *Nephrol Dial Transplant* 1994;9(Suppl 4):164.

37. Melnick JZ, Baum M, Thompson JR. Aminoglycoside-induced Fanconi's syndrome. *Am J Kidney Dis* 1994;23:118.

38. Bar RJ, Wilson HE, Mazzaferri EL. Hypomagnesemic hypocalcemia secondary to renal magnesium wasting: a possible consequence of high dose gentamicin therapy. *Ann Intern Med* 1975;82:646.

39. Patel R, Savage A. Symptomatic hypomagnesemia associated with gentamicin therapy. *Nephron* 1979;23:50.

40. Schor N, et al. Pathophysiology of altered glomerular function in aminoglycoside-treated rats. *Kidney Int* 1981;19:288.

41. Luft FC, et al. The renin-angiotensin system in aminoglycoside-induced acute renal failure. *J Pharmacol Exp Ther* 1982;20:443.

42. Neugarten J, Aynedjian HS, Bank N. Role of tubular obstruction in acute renal failure due to gentamicin. *Kidney Int* 1983;24:330.

43. Rodriguez-Barbero A, et al. Gentamicin activates rat mesangial cells—a role for platelet activating factor. *Kidney Int* 1995;47:1346.

44. Houghton DC, English J, Bennett WM. Chronic tubulointerstitial nephritis and renal insufficiency associated with long-term "subtherapeutic" gentamicin. *J Lab Clin Med* 1988;112:694.

45. Kourilsky O, et al. The pathology of acute renal failure due to interstitial nephritis in man, with comments on the role of interstitial inflammation and sex in gentamicin nephrotoxicity. *Medicine* 1982;61:258.

46. Kozek JC, Mazze RI, Cousins MJ. Nephrotoxicity of gentamicin. *Lab Invest* 1974;30:48.

47. Houghton DC, et al. A light and electron microscopic analysis of gentamicin nephrotoxicity in rats. *Am J Pathol* 1976;82:589.

48. Cuppage FE, et al. Gentamicin nephrotoxicity. II. Physiological, biochemical, and morphological effects of prolonged administration to rats. *Virchows Arch B Cell Pathol* 1977;234:121.

49. Olsen S, Solez K. Pathology of drug nephrotoxicity in humans. In: Whelton A, Neu HC, eds. *The aminoglycosides: microbiology, clinical use and toxicology.* New York: Marcel Dekker, 1982.

50. Solez K, Morel-Maroger L, Sraer JD. The morphology of "acute tubular necrosis" in man: analysis of 57 renal biopsies and a comparison with the glycerol model. *Medicine* 1979;58:362.

51. Racusen LC, Trpkov K, Solez K. Pathology of acute renal failure. In: Bellomo P, Ronco C, eds. *Acute renal failure in the critically ill. Update in intensive care and emergency medicine*, vol 20 Berlin: Springer, 1995.

52. Giuliano RA, et al. Recovery of cortical phospholipidosis and necrosis after acute gentamicin loading in rats. *Kidney Int* 1984;26:838.

53. Laurent G, et al. Kidney tissue repair after nephrotoxic injury: biochemical and morphological characterization. *CRC Crit Rev Toxicol* 1988;19:147.

54. Houghton DC, et al. Myeloid bodies in the renal tubules of humans: relationship to gentamicin therapy. *Clin Nephrol* 1978;10:140.

55. De Broe ME, et al. Early effects of gentamicin, tobramycin and amikacin on the human kidney. *Kidney Int* 1984;25:643.

56. Aubert-Tulkens G, Van Hoof F, Tulkens P. Gentamicin-induced lysosomal phospholipidosis in cultured rat fibroblasts: quantitative ultrastructural and biochemical study. *Lab Invest* 1979;40:481.

57. Josepovitz C, et al. Effect of netilmicin on the phospholipid composition of subcellular fractions of rat renal cortex. *J Pharmacol Exp Ther* 1985;235:810.

58. Laurent G, et al. Mechanism of aminoglycoside-induced lysosomal phospholipidosis: in vitro and in vivo studies with gentamicin and amikacin. *Biochem Pharmacol* 1982;31:3861.

59. Carlier MB, et al. Inhibition of lysosomal phospholipases by aminoglycoside antibiotics: in vitro comparative studies. *Antimicrob Agents Chemother* 1983;23:440.

60. Ramsammy LS, et al. Effect of gentamicin on phospholipid metabolism in cultured rabbit proximal tubular cells. *Am J Physiol* 1989;256:C204.

61. Hruban Z, Slessers A, Hopkins E. Drug induced and naturally occurring myeloid bodies. *Lab Invest* 1972;27:62.

62. Kacew S. Cationic amphiphilic drug-induced renal cortical lysosomal phospholipidosis: an in vivo comparison of gentamicin and chlorphentermine. *Toxicol Appl Pharmacol* 1987;91:469.

63. Hein L, Lullmann-Rauch R, Mohr K. Human accumulation of xenobiotics: potential of catamphiphilic drugs to promote their accumulation via inducing lipidosis of mucopolysaccharides. *Xenobiotica* 1990;20:1259.

64. Josepovitz C, et al. Contrasting effects of gentamicin and mercuric chloride on urinary excretion of enzymes and phospholipids in the rat. *Lab Invest* 1985;52:275.

65. Katz SM, Sufian S, Matsumoto T. Urinary myelin figures in gentamicin nephrotoxicity. *Am J Clin Pathol* 1979;72:621.

66. Mandel AK, Bennett WM. Transmission electron microscopy of urinary sediment in the assessment of aminoglycoside nephrotoxicity in the rat. *Nephron* 1988;49:67.

67. Houghton DC, et al. Chronic gentamicin nephrotoxicity: continued tubular injury with preserved glomerular filtrate function. *Am J Pathol* 1986; 123:183.

68. Gilbert DN, et al. Reversibility of gentamicin nephrotoxicity in rats: recovery during continuous drug administration. *Proc Soc Exp Biol Med* 1979;160:99.

69. Luft FC, et al. Recovery from aminoglycoside nephrotoxicity with continued drug administration. *Antimicrob Agents Chemother* 1975;14:284.

70. Sundin DP, et al. Cellular mechanism of aminoglycoside tolerance in long-term gentamicin treatment. *Am J Physiol* 1997;272 (Cell Physiol:41): C1809.

71. Laurent G, et al. Increased renal DNA synthesis in vivo after administration of low doses of gentamicin to rats. *Antimicrob Agents Chemother* 1983;24:586.

72. Porter GA, et al. Gentamicin-induced stimulation of DNA synthesis in rat kidney. Comparison between in vivo and in vitro models. *Toxicol Lett* 1984;23:205.

73. Neu HC. Pharmacology of aminoglycosides. In: Whelton A, Neu HC, eds. *The aminoglycosides.* New York: Marcel Dekker, 1982.

74. Kaloyanides GJ. Renal pharmacology of aminoglycoside antibiotics. *Contrib Nephrol* 1984;42:148.

75. Giuliano RA, Verpooten GA, De Broe ME. The effect of dosing strategy on kidney cortical accumulation of aminoglycosides in rats. *Am J Kidney Dis* 1986;8:297.

76. Giuliano RA, et al. In vivo uptake kinetics of amino-glycosides in the kidney cortex of rats. *J Pharmacol Exp Ther* 1986;236:470.

77. Just M, Erdmann G, Habermann E. The renal handling of polybasic drugs. 1. Gentamicin and aprotinin in intact animals. *Naunyn Schmiedebergs Arch Pharmacol* 1977;300:57.

78. Silverblatt FS, Kuehn C. Autoradiography of gentamicin uptake by the rat proximal tubule cell. *Kidney Int* 1979;15:335.

79. Ford DM, et al. Apically and basolaterally internalized aminoglycosides co-localize in LLC-PK1 lysosomes and alter cell function. *Am J Physiol* 1994;266:C52.

80. Sastrasinh M, et al. Identification of the aminoglycoside receptor of renal brush border membranes. *J Pharmacol Exp Ther* 1982;222:350.

81. Molitoris BA, et al. Mechanism of ischemia-enhanced amino-glycoside binding and uptake by proximal tubule cells. *Am J Physiol* 1993;264:F907.

82. Moestrup SK, et al. Evidence that epithelial glycoprotein 330/megalin mediates uptake of polybasic drugs. *J Clin Invest* 1995;96:1404.

83. Nagai J, et al. Role of megalin in renal handling of aminoglycosides. *Am J Physiol Renal Physiol* 2001;281:F337.

84. Schmitz C, et al. Megalin deficiency offers protection from renal aminoglycoside accumulation. *J Biol Chem* 2002;277:618.

85. Sandoval R, Leiser J, Molitoris BA. Aminoglycoside antibiotics traffic to the Golgi complex in LLC-PK1 cells. *J Am Soc Nephrol* 1998;9:167.

86. Sandoval RM, Dunn KW, Molitoris BA. Gentamicin traffics rapidly and directly to the Golgi complex in LLC-PK(1) cells. *Am J Physiol Renal Physiol* 2000;279(5):F884.

87. Sundin DP, Sandoval R, Molitoris BA. Gentamicin inhibits renal protein and phospholipid metabolism in rats: implications involving intracellular trafficking. *J Am Soc Nephrol* 2001;12(1):114

88. Hammond TG, et al. Gentamicin inhibits rat renal cortical homotypic endosomal fusion: role of megalin. *Am J Physiol* 1997;272(*Renal Physiol* 41):F117.

89. Jones AT, Wessling-Resnick M. Inhibition of in vitro endosomal fusion activity by aminoglycoside antibiotics. *J Biol Chem* 1998;273:25301.

90. van Bambeke F, et al. Aminoglycoside antibiotics prevent the formation of non-bilayer structures in negatively-charged membranes. Comparative studies using fusogenic (bis[β-diethylaminoethylether]hexestrol) and aggregating (spermine) agents. *Chem Physics Lipids* 1996;79:123.

91. Brasseur R, et al. Interactions of aminoglycoside antibiotics with negatively charged lipid layers. *Biochem Pharmacol* 1984;33:629.

92. Kirschbaum BB. Interactions between renal brush border membranes and polyamines. *J Pharmacol Exp Ther* 1984;229:409.

93. Wang BM, et al. Interaction of calcium and neomycin with anionic phospholipid-lecithin liposomes. *Biochem Pharmacol* 1984;33:3787.

94. Chung A, et al. Interaction of gentamicin and spermine with bilayer membranes containing negatively charged phospholipids. *Biochemistry* 1985;24:442.

95. Au S, Schacht J, Weiner N. Membrane effects of aminoglycoside antibiotics measured in liposomes containing the fluorescent probe, anilino-8-naphthalene sulfonate. *Biochim Biophys Acta* 1986;862:205.

96. Ramsammy LS, Kaloyanides G. Effect of gentamicin on the transition temperature and permeability to glycerol of phosphatidylinositol-containing liposomes. *Biochem Pharmacol* 1987;36:1179.

97. Mingeot-Leclercq MP, Brasseur R, Schank A. Molecular parameters involved in aminoglycoside nephrotoxicity. *J Toxicol Environ Health* 1995;44:263.

98. Mingeot-Leclercq MP, Tulkens P. Aminoglycosides: nephrotoxicity. *Antimicrob Agents Chemother* 1999;43:1003.

99. Schacht J. Isolation of an aminoglycoside receptor from guinea pig inner ear tissues and kidneys. *Arch Otorhinolaryngol* 1979;224:129.

100. Au S, Weiner ND, Schacht J. Aminoglycosides preferentially increase permeability in phosphoinositide-containing membranes: a study with carboxyfluorescein in liposomes. *Biochim Biophys Acta* 1987;902:80.

101. Gaver E, et al. Binding of neomycin to phosphatidylinositol 4, 5-bisphosphate (PIP2). *Biochim Biophys Acta* 1989;979:105.

102. Kaloyanides GJ, Ramsammy LS. Alterations of biophysical properties of liposomes predict aminoglycoside toxicity: inhibitory effect of polyaspartic acid. In: Bach PH, Delacrey L, Gregg NJ, et al., eds. *Proceedings of the Fourth International Symposium on Nephrotoxicity*. New York: Marcel Dekker, 1990.

103. Ramsammy LS, Kaloyanides GJ. The effect of gentamicin on the biophysical properties of phosphatidic acid liposomes is influenced by the 0-C'0 group of the lipid. *Biochemistry* 1988;27:8249.

104. Reid DG, Gajjar K. A proton and carbon 13 nuclear magnetic resonance study of neomycin B and its interactions with phosphatidylinositol 4,5-bisphosphate. *J Biol Chem* 1987;262:7967.

105. Moriyama T, et al. Decrease in the fluidity of brush-border membrane vesicles induced by gentamicin. A spin-labelling study. *Biochem Pharmacol* 1989;38:1169.

106. Mingeot-Leclercq MP, et al. Ultrastructural physico-chemical and conformational study of the interactions of gentamicin and bis(beta-diethylaminoethylether)hexestrol with negatively-charged phospholipid layers. *Biochem Pharmacol* 1989;38:729.

107. Wang BM, et al. Characterization of aminoglycoside-lipid interactions and development of a refined model for ototoxicity testing. *Biochem Pharmacol* 1984;33:3257.

108. Schacht J. Molecular mechanisms of drug-induced hearing loss. *Hearing Res* 1986;22:297.

109. Williams PD, Holohan PD, Ross CR. Gentamicin nephrotoxicity. I. Acute biochemical correlates in the rat. *Toxicol Appl Pharmacol* 1981;61:234.

110. Williams PD, Holohan PD, Ross CR. Gentamicin nephrotoxicity. II. Plasma membrane changes. *Toxicol Appl Pharmacol* 1981;61:243.

111. Williams PD, et al. Inhibition of renal Na$^+$, K$^+$-adenosine triphosphatase by gentamicin. *J Pharmacol Exp Ther* 1984;231:248.

112. Queener SF, Luft FC, Hamel FG. Effect of gentamicin treatment on adenylate cyclase and Na$^+$, K$^+$-ATPase activities in renal tissues of rats. *Antimicrob Agents Chemother* 1983;24:815.

113. Hostetler KY, Hall LB. Inhibition of kidney lysosomal phospholipases A and C by aminoglycoside antibiotics: possible mechanism of aminoglycoside toxicity. *Proc Natl Acad Sci USA* 1982;79:1663.

114. Mingeot-Leclercq MP, Laurent G, Tulkens PM. Biochemical mechanism of amino-glycoside-induced inhibition of phosphatidylcholine hydrolysis by lysosomal phospholipases. *Biochem Pharmacol* 1988;37:591.

115. Mingeot-Leclercq MP, et al. Effect of acidic phospholipids on the activity of lysosomal phospholipases and on their inhibition by aminoglycoside antibiotics—I. *Biochem Pharmacol* 1990;40:489.

116. Giurgea-Marion L, et al. Impairment of lysosome-pinocytic vesicle fusion in rat kidney proximal tubules after treatment with gentamicin at low doses. *Toxicol Appl Pharmacol* 1986;86:271.

117. Morin JP, et al. Gentamicin-induced nephrotoxicity: a cell biology approach. *Kidney Int* 1980;18:583.

118. Powell J, Reidenberg MN. In vitro response of rat and human kidney lysosomes to aminoglycoside. *Biochem Pharmacol* 1982;31:3447.

119. Bendirdjian JP, Fillastre JP, Foucher B. Mitochondria modifications with the aminoglycosides. In: Whelton A, Neu HC, eds. *The aminoglycosides: microbiology, clinical use and toxicology*. New York: Marcel Dekker, 1982.

120. Simmons CF, Bogusky RT, Humes HD. Inhibitory effects of gentamicin on renal mitochondrial oxidative phosphorylation. *J Pharmacol Exp Ther* 1980;214:709.

121. Weinberg JM, Humes HD. Mechanisms of gentamicin-induced dysfunction of renal cortical mitochondria. I. Effects on mitochondrial respiration. *Arch Biochem Biophys* 1980;205:221.

122. Mela-Riker LM, et al. Renal mitochondrial integrity during continuous gentamicin treatment. *Biochem Pharmacol* 1986;35:979.

123. Buss WC, Piatt MK, Kauten R. Inhibition of mammalian microsomal protein synthesis by aminoglycoside antibiotics. *J Antimicrob Chemother* 1984;14:231.

124. Buss UC, Piatt MK. Gentamicin administered in vivo reduces protein synthesis in microsomes subsequently isolated from rat kidneys but not from rat brains. *J Antimicrob Chemother* 1985;15:715.

125. Bennett WM, et al. Microsomal protein synthesis inhibition: an early manifestation of gentamicin nephrotoxicity. *Am J Physiol* 1988;255:F265.

126. Ramsammy LS, Josepovitz C, Kaloyanides GJ. Gentamicin inhibits agonist stimulation of the phosphatidylinositol cascade in primary cultures of rabbit proximal tubular cells and in rat renal cortex. *J Pharmacol Exp Ther* 1988;247:989.

127. Schwertz DW, et al. Effects of aminoglycosides on proximal tubule brush border membrane phosphatidylinositol-specific phospholipase C. *J Pharmacol Exp Ther* 1984;231:48.

128. Marche P, et al. Aminoglycoside-induced alteration of phosphoinositide metabolism. *Kidney Int* 1987;31:59.

129. Schibeci A, Schacht J. Action of neomycin on the metabolism of polyphosphoinositides in the guinea pig kidney. *Biochem Pharmacol* 1977;26:1769.

130. Ramsammy L, et al. Effect of gentamicin on lipid peroxidation in rat renal cortex. *Biochem Pharmacol* 1985;34:3895.

131. Walker PD, Shah SV. Gentamicin enhanced production of hydrogen peroxide by renal cortical mitochondria. *Am J Physiol* 1987;253:C495.

132. Walker PD, Shah SV. Evidence suggesting a role for hydroxyl radical in gentamicin-induced acute renal failure in rats. *J Clin Invest* 1988;81:334.

133. Charlwood J, et al. Proteomic analysis of rat kidney cortex following treatment with gentamicin. *J Proteome Res* 2002;1:73.

134. Williams PD, Hattendorf GH. Inhibition of renal membrane binding and nephrotoxicity of gentamicin by polyasparagine and polyaspartic acid in the rat. *Res Commun Chem Pathol Pharmacol* 1985;47:317.

135. Williams PD, Hattendorf GH, Bennett DB. Inhibition of renal membrane binding and nephrotoxicity of aminoglycosides. *J Pharmacol Exp Ther* 1986;237:919.

136. Williams PD, et al. Correlation between renal membrane binding and nephrotoxicity of aminoglycosides. *Antimicrob Agents Chemother* 1987;31:570.

137. Gilbert DN, et al. Polyaspartic acid prevents experimental aminoglycoside nephrotoxicity. *J Infect Dis* 1989;159:945.

138. Swan SK, et al. Long-term protection of polyaspartic acid in experimental gentamicin nephrotoxicity. *Antimicrob Agents Chemother* 1991;35:2591.

139. Swan SK, et al. Pharmacologic limits of the protective effect of polyaspartic acid on experimental gentamicin nephrotoxicity. *Antimicrob Agents Chemother* 1993;37:347.

140. Beauchamp D, et al. Protection against gentamicin-induced early renal alterations (phospholipidosis and increased DNA synthesis) by coadministration of poly-L-aspartic acid. *J Pharmacol Exp Ther* 1990;255:858.

141. Kally Z, Tulkens PM. Uptake and subcellular distribution of poly-L-aspartic acid. A protectant against aminoglycoside-induced nephrotoxicity in rat kidney cortex. In: Bach PH, Lock EA, eds. *Nephrotoxicity: in vitro to in vivo, animals to man.* New York: Plenum, 1989.

142. Kishore BK, et al. Mechanism of protection afforded by polyaspartic acid against gentamicin-induced phospholipidosis. I. Polyaspartic acid binds gentamicin and displaces it from negatively charged phospholipid layers in vitro. *J Pharmacol Exp Ther* 1990;255:867.

143. Kishore BK, et al. Mechanism of protection afforded by polyaspartic acid against gentamicin-induced phospholipidosis II. Comparative in vitro and in vivo studies with poly-L-aspartic acid, poly-L-glutamic acids and poly-D-glutamic acid. *J Pharmacol Exp Ther* 1990;255:875.

144. Kishore BK, et al. Comparative assessment of poly-L-aspartic and poly-L-glutamic acids against gentamicin-induced renal liposomal phospholipidosis, phospholipiduria and cell proliferation in rats. *J Pharmacol Exp Ther* 1992;262:242.

145. Ramsammy LS, et al. Polyaspartic acid protects against gentamicin nephrotoxicity in the rat. *J Pharmacol Exp Ther* 1989;250:149.

146. Ramsammy L, et al. Polyaspartic acid inhibits gentamicin-induced perturbations of phospholipid metabolism. *Am J Physiol* 1990;258:C1141.

147. Kaloyanides CJ, Ramsammy LS. Polyaspartic acid protects against gentamicin-induced toxicity: mechanism of action. *Contrib Nephrol* 1990;83:175.

148. Kacew S. Inhibition of gentamicin-induced nephrotoxicity by pyridoxal-5′-phosphate in the rat. *J Pharmacol Exp Ther* 1989;248:360.

149. Kojima R, Ito M, Suzuki Y. Studies on the nephrotoxicity of aminoglycoside antibiotics and protection from these effects (8): protective effect of pyridoxal-5′-phosphate against tobramycin nephrotoxicity. *Jpn J Pharmacol* 1990;52:11.

150. Kojima R, Ito M, Suzuki Y. Studies on the nephrotoxicity of aminoglycoside antibiotics and protection from these effects (9): protective effect of inositol hexasulfate against tobramycin-induced nephrotoxicity. *Jpn J Pharmacol* 1990;53:347.

151. Smetana S, et al. Effect of interaction between gentamicin and pyridoxal-5-phosphate on functional and metabolic parameters in kidneys of female Sprague-Dawley rats. *Ren Fail* 1992;14:147.

152. Ford DM, et al. HWA-448 reduces gentamicin toxicity in LLC-PK1 cells. *J Pharmacol Exp Ther* 1995;274:29.

153. Moore RD, et al. Risk factors for nephrotoxicity in patients treated with aminoglycosides. *Ann Intern Med* 1984;100:352.

154. Smith CR, Moore RD, Lietman PS. Studies of risk factors for aminoglycoside nephrotoxicity. *Am J Kidney Dis* 1986;8:308.

155. Bertino JS, et al. Incidence of and significant risk factors for aminoglycoside-associated nephrotoxicity in patients dosed using individualized pharmacokinetic modeling. *J Infect Dis* 1993;167:173.

156. Rowe JW. Clinical research on aging: strategies and directions. *N Engl J Med* 1977;297:1332.

157. Marra R, et al. Age-dependent nephrotoxicity and the pharmacokinetics of gentamicin in rats. *Eur J Pediatr* 1980;133:25.

158. McMartin DN, Engle SG. Effect of aging on gentamicin nephrotoxicity and pharmacokinetics in rats. *Res Commun Chem Pathol Pharmacol* 1982;38:193.

159. Bennett WM, et al. Sex-related differences in the susceptibility of rats to gentamicin nephrotoxicity. *J Infect Dis* 1982;145:370.

160. Corcoran GB, Salazar DE, Schentag JJ. Excessive aminoglycoside nephrotoxicity in obese patients. *Am J Med* 1988;85:279.

161. Moench TR, Smith CR. Risk factors for aminoglycoside nephrotoxicity. In: Whelton A, Neu HC, eds. *The aminoglycosides: microbiology, clinical use and toxicology.* New York: Marcel Dekker, 1982.

162. Tardif D, Beauchamp D, Bergeron MG. Influence of endotoxin on the intracortical accumulation kinetics of gentamicin in rats. *Antimicrob Agents Chemother* 1990;34:576.

163. Bennett WM, et al. The influence of dosage regimen on experimental gentamicin nephrotoxicity: dissociation of peak serum levels from renal failure. *J Infect Dis* 1979;140:576.

164. Gilbert DN. Once-daily aminoglycoside therapy. *Antimicrob Agents Chemother* 1991;35:399.

165. Verpooten GA, et al. Once-daily dosing decreases renal accumulation of gentamicin and netilmicin. *Clin Pharmacol Ther* 1989;45:22.

166. De Broe ME, Verbist L, Verpooten GA. Influence of dosage schedule on renal cortical accumulation of amikacin and tobramycin in man. *J Antimicrob Chemother* 1991;27(Suppl C):41.

167. De Broe ME, Giuliano RA, Verpooten GA. Choice of drug and dosage regimen. *Am J Med* 1986;80(Suppl 63):115.

168. Gilbert DN, et al. A randomized comparison of the safety and efficacy of once-daily gentamicin or thrice-daily gentamicin in combination with ticarcillin-clavulanate. *Am J Med* 1998;105:256.

169. Barclay ML, Kirkpatrick CM, Begg EL. Once daily aminoglycoside therapy. Is it less toxic than multiple doses and how should it be monitored? *Clin Pharmacokinet* 1999;36:89.

170. Murray KR, et al. Pharmacodynamic characterization of nephrotoxicity associated with once-daily aminoglycoside. *Pharmacotherapy* 1999;19:1252.

171. EORTC International Antimicrobial Therapy Project Group. Efficacy and toxicity of single daily doses of amikacin and ceftriaxone versus multiple daily doses of amikacin and ceftazidime for infections in patients with cancer and granulocytopenia. *Ann Int Med* 1993;119:584.

172. Blaser J, Konig C. Once-daily dosing of aminoglycosides. *Eur J Clin Microbiol Infect Dis* 1995;14:1029.

173. Galloe AM, et al. Aminoglycosides: single or multiple daily dosing? A meta-analysis on efficacy and safety. *Eur J Clin Pharmacol* 1995;48:39.

174. Barza M, et al. Single or multiple daily doses of aminoglycosides: a meta-analysis. *Brit Med J* 1996;312:338.

175. Munckhof WJ, Grayson ML, Turnidge JD. A meta-analysis of studies on the safety and efficacy of aminoglycosides given either once daily or as divided doses. *J Antimicrob Chemother* 1996;37:645.

176. Ferriols-Lisart R, Alos-Alminana M. Effectiveness and safety of once-daily aminoglycosides: a meta-analysis. *Am J Health Syst Pharm* 1996;53:1141.

177. Freeman CD, Strayer AH. Mega-analysis of meta-analysis: an examination of meta-analysis with an emphasis on once-daily aminoglycoside comparative trials. *Pharmacother* 1996;16:1093.

178. Hatala R, Dinh T, Cook DJ. Once-daily aminoglycoside dosing in immunocompetent adults: a meta-analysis. *Ann Intern Med* 1996;124:717.

179. Ali MZ, Goetz MB. A meta-analysis of the relative efficacy and toxicity of single daily dosing versus multiple daily dosing of aminoglycosides. *Clin Infect Dis* 1997;24:796.

180. Bailey TC, et al. A meta-analysis of extended-interval dosing versus multiple daily dosing of aminoglycosides. *Clin Infect Dis* 1997;25:786.

181. Hatala R, Dinh TT, Cook DJ. Single daily dosing of aminoglycosides in immunocompromised adults: a systematic review. *Clin Infect Dis* 1997;24:810.

182. Uijtendaal EV, et al. Once-daily versus multiple-daily gentamicin in infants and children. *Ther Drug Monit* 2001;23:506.

183. Chuck SK, et al. National survey of extended-interval aminoglycoside dosing. *Clin Infect Dis* 2000;30:433.

184. Nicolau DP, et al. Experience with a once-daily aminoglycoside program administered to 2184 adult patients. *Antimicrob Agents Chemother* 1995;39:650.

185. McCormack JP. An emotional-based medicine approach to monitoring once-daily aminoglycosides. *Pharmacother* 2000;20:1524.

186. Verpooten GA, Tulkens PM, Molitoris BA. Aminoglycosides and vancomycin. In: De Broe ME, et al., eds. *Clinical nephrotoxins—renal injury from drugs and chemicals,* 2nd ed. Dordrecht, The Netherlands: Kluwer Acadmic Publishers, 2003:151.

187. Bennett WM, et al. Effect of sodium intake on gentamicin nephrotoxicity in the rat. *Proc Soc Exp Biol Med* 1976;151:736.

188. Brinker KR, et al. Effect of potassium depletion on gentamicin nephrotoxicity. *J Lab Clin Med* 1981;98:292.

189. Rankin L, et al. Enhancement of gentamicin nephrotoxicity by magnesium depletion in the rat. *Miner Electrolyte Metab* 1984;10:199.

190. Elliott WC, et al. Effect of sodium bicarbonate and ammonium chloride ingestion in experimental gentamicin nephrotoxicity. *Res Commun Chem Pathol Pharmacol* 1980;28:483.

191. Humes HD, Sastrasinh M, Weinberg JM. Calcium is a competitive inhibitor of gentamicin-renal membrane binding interactions and dietary calcium supplementation protects against gentamicin nephrotoxicity. *J Clin Invest* 1984;73:134.

192. Rankin GO, Sutherland CH. Nephrotoxicity of aminoglycosides and cephalosporins in combination. *Adverse Drug React Acute Poisoning Rev* 1989;8:73.

193. Rybak MJ, et al. Nephrotoxicity of vancomycin, alone and with an aminoglycoside. *J Antimicrob Chemother* 1990;25:679.

194. Goetz MB, Sayers J. Nephrotoxicity of vancomycin and aminoglycoside therapy separately and in combination. *J Antimicrob Chemother* 1993;32:325.

195. Engineer MS, et al. A comparison of the effects of tetraplatin and cisplatin on renal function and gentamicin pharmacology in rats. *Toxicology* 1989;59:151.

196. Chiu PJ, Long JF. Effects of hydration on gentamicin excretion and renal accumulation in furosemide-treated rats. *Antimicrob Agents Chemother* 1978;14:214.

197. Farag MM, Kandil M, Fadali GA. Verapamil increases the nephrotoxic potential of gentamicin in rats. *Nephron* 1992;62:71.

198. Thomsen HS, et al. Gentamicin nephropathy and contrast media. *Acta Radiol* 1990;31:401.

199. Farag MM, et al. Assessment of gentamicin-induced nephrotoxicity in rats treated with low doses of ibuprofen and diclophenac sodium. *Clin Sci* 1996;91:187.

200. Leehey DL, et al. Can pharmacokinetic dosing decrease nephrotoxicity with aminoglycoside therapy? *J Am Soc Nephrol* 1993;4:81.

201. Burton ME, et al. A Bayesian feedback method of aminoglycoside dosing. *Clin Pharmacol Ther* 1985;37:349.

202. Dillon KR, et al. Individualized pharmacokinetic versus standard dosing of amikacin: a comparison of therapeutic outcomes. *J Antimicrob Chemother* 1989;24:581.

203. Burton ME, et al. A controlled trial of the cost benefit of computerized Bayesian aminoglycoside administration. *Clin Pharmacol Ther* 1991;49:685.

204. Whipple JK, et al. Effect of individualized pharmacokinetic dosing on patient outcome. *Crit Care Med* 1991;19:1480.

205. Leehey DJ, et al. Can pharmacokinetic dosing decrease nephrotoxicity associated with aminoglycoside therapy? *J Am Soc Nephrol* 1993;4:81.
206. Koo J, et al. Comparison of once-daily versus pharmacokinetic dosing of aminoglycosides in elderly patients. *Am J Med* 1996;101:177.
207. Hickling K, Begg E, Moore ML. A prospective randomised trial comparing individualized pharmacokinetic dosage prediction for aminoglycosides with prediction based on estimated creatinine clearance in critically ill patients. *Intensive Care Med* 1989;15:233.
208. Kemme DJ, Daniel CI. Aminoglycoside dosing: a randomized prospective study. *South Med J* 1993;86:46.
209. Destache CJ, et al. Impact of a clinical pharmacokinetic service on patients treated with aminoglycosides: a cost-benefit analysis. *Ther Drug Monit* 1990;12:419.
210. Schentag JJ, et al. Gentamicin tissue accumulation and nephrotoxic reactions. *JAMA* 1978;240:2067.
211. Morin PJ, et al. Epidermal growth factor accelerates renal tissue repair in a model of gentamicin nephrotoxicity in rats. *Am J Physiol* 1992;263: F806.
212. Tune BM. Nephrotoxicity of beta-lactam antibiotics: mechanisms and strategies for prevention. *Pediatr Nephrol* 1997;11:768.
213. Tune BM. The nephrotoxicity of beta-lactam antibiotics. In: Hook JB, Goldstein RS, eds. *Toxicology of the kidney*, 2nd ed. New York: Raven, 1993.
214. Tune BM, Fernholt M, Schwartz A. Mechanism of cephaloridine transport in the kidney. *J Pharmacol Exp Ther* 1974;191:311.
215. Tune BM, Fravert D. Cephalosporin nephrotoxicity. Transport, cytotoxicity and mitochondrial toxicity of cephaloglycin. *J Pharmacol Exp Ther* 1980;215:186.
216. Tune BM, Hsu CY. Effects of nephrotoxic beta-lactam antibiotics on mitochondrial metabolism of monocarboxylic substrates. *J Pharmacol Exp Ther* 1995;274:194.
217. Goldstein RS, et al. Biochemical mechanisms of cephaloridine nephrotoxicity: time and concentration dependence of peroxidative injury. *Toxicol Appl Pharmacol* 1986;87:297.
218. Tune BM, Hsu CY. Toxicity of cephaloridine to carnitine transport and fatty acid metabolism in rabbit renal cortical mitochondria: structure-activity relationships. *J Pharmacol Exp Ther* 1994;270:873.
219. Tune BM, Hsu CY. Toxicity of cephalosporins to fatty acid metabolism in renal cortical mitochondria. *Biochem Pharmacol* 1995;49:727.
220. Tune BM, Fravert D, Hsu CY. The oxidative and mitochondrial toxic effects of cephalosporin antibiotics in the kidney. A comparative study of cephaloridine and cephaloglycin. *Biochem Pharmacol* 1989;38:795.
221. Tune BM, Hsu CY. The renal mitochondrial toxicity of cephalosporins: specificity of the effect on anionic substrate uptake. *J Pharmacol Exp Ther* 1990;252:65.
222. Bendirdjian JP, et al. The mitochondrial respiratory toxicity of cephalosporins. Molecular properties and pathogenic significance. In: Fillastre JP, ed. *Nephrotoxicity, ototoxicity of drugs*. Rouen: INSERM, 1982.
223. Tune BM, Fravert D, Hsu CY. Thienamycin nephrotoxicity: mitochondrial injury and oxidative effects of imipenem in the rabbit kidney. *Biochem Pharmacol* 1989;38:3779.
224. Tune BM, Hsu CY. The renal mitochondrial toxicity of beta-lactam antibiotics: in vitro effects of cephaloglycin and imipenem. *J Am Soc Nephrol* 1990;1:815.
225. Norrby SR. Side effects of cephalosporins. *Drugs* 1987;34(Suppl 2):105.
226. Winston DJ, et al. Beta-lactam antibiotic therapy in febrile granulocytopenic patients: a randomized trial comparing cefoperazone plus piperacillin, cefazadime plus piperacillin and imipenem alone. *Ann Intern Med* 1991;115:849.
227. Bendirdjian JP, et al. Additive nephrotoxicity of cephalosporins and aminoglycosides in the rabbit. *J Pharmacol Exp Ther* 1981;218:631.
228. Browning MC, et al. Interaction of ischemic and antibiotic-induced injury in the rabbit kidney. *J Infect Dis* 1983;147:341.
229. Tune BM, Hsu CY. Augmentation of antibiotic nephrotoxicity by endoxemia in the rabbit. *J Pharmacol Exp Ther* 1985;234:425.
230. Klastersky J, Hensgens C, Debusscher L. Empiric therapy for cancer patients: comparative study of tircarcillin-tobramycin, tircarcillin-cephalothin, and cephalothin-tobramycin. *Antimicrob Agents Chemother* 1975;7:640.
231. Wade JC, et al. Cephalothin plus an aminoglycoside is more nephrotoxic than methicillin plus an aminoglycoside. *Lancet* 1978;2:604.
232. EROTC International Antimicrobial Therapy Group. Three antibiotic regimens in the treatment of infection in febrile granulocytopenic patients with cancer. *J Infect Dis* 1978;137:14.
233. Rankin GO, Sutherland CH. Nephrotoxicity of aminoglycosides and cephalosporins in combination. *Adverse Drug React Acute Poisoning Rev* 1989;8:73.
234. Grunfeld JP, Kleinknecht D, Droz D. Acute interstitial nephritis. In: Schrier RW, Gottschalk CW, eds. *Diseases of the kidney*, 5th ed. Boston: Little, Brown and Company, 1993.
235. Moellering RC, Krogstad DJ, Greenblatt DJ. Pharmacokinetics of vancomycin in normal subjects and in patients with reduced renal function. *Rev Infect Dis* 1981;3(Suppl):S230.
236. Wold JS, Turnipseed SA. Toxicology of vancomycin in laboratory animals. *Rev Infect Dis* 1981;3(Suppl):S224.
237. Cook FV, Farrar WE. Vancomycin revisited. *Ann Intern Med* 1978; 88:813.
238. Appel GB, et al. Vancomycin and the kidney. *Am J Kidney Dis* 1986;8:75.
239. Wood CA, et al. Vancomycin enhancement of experimental tobramycin nephrotoxicity. *Antimicrob Agents Chemother* 1986;30:20.
240. Wysocki M, et al. Continuous versus intermittent infusion of vancomycin in severe staphylococcal infections: prospective multicenter randomized study. *Antimicrob Agents Chemother* 2001;45:2460.
241. Elting LS, et al. Mississippi mud in the 1990s: risks and outcomes of vancomycin-associated toxicity in general oncology practice. *Cancer* 1998;83:2597.
242. Eisenberg RL, Robbins N, Lenci M. Vancomycin and interstitial nephritis. *Ann Intern Med* 1981;95:658.
243. Weinstein L, et al. The sulfonamides. *N Engl J Med* 1960;263:793.
244. Dowling HF, Lepper MH. Toxic reactions following therapy with sulfapyridine, sulfathiazole, and sulfadiazine. *JAMA* 1943;121:1190.
245. Molina JM, et al. Sulfadiazine-induced crystalluria in AIDS patients with Toxoplasma encephalitis. *AIDS* 1991;5:587.
246. Berns JS, et al. Renal aspects of therapy for human immunodeficiency virus and associated opportunistic infections. *J Am Soc Nephrol* 1991;1:1061.
247. Siegel WH. Unusual complication of therapy with sulfamethoxazole-trimethoprim. *J Urol* 1978;117:397.
248. Buchanan N. Sulfamethoxazole, hypoalbuminemia, crystalluria and renal failure. *Br Med J* 1978;2:172.
249. Bergland F, Killander J, Pompeius R. Effect of trimethoprim-sulfamethoxazole on the renal excretion of creatinine in man. *J Urol* 1975; 114:802.
250. Kainer G, Rosenberg AR. Effect of co-trimoxazole on the glomerular filtration of healthy adults. *Chemotherapy* 1981;27:229.
251. Como JA, Dismukes WE. Oral azole drugs as systemic antifungal therapy. *N Engl J Med* 1994;330:263.
252. Rowe JM, et al. Recommended guidelines for the management of autologous bone marrow transplantation: a report from the Eastern Cooperative Oncology Group. *Ann Intern Med* 1994;120:143.
253. Maddux MS, Barriere SL. A review of complications of amphotericin B therapy: recommendations for prevention and management. *Drug Intell Clin Pharmacol* 1980;14:177.
254. Medoff G, Kobayashi GS. Strategies in the treatment of systemic fungal infections. *N Engl J Med* 1980;302:145.
255. Bolard J. How do the polyene macrolide antibiotics affect the cellular membrane properties? *Biochim Biophys Acta* 1986;864:257.
256. Brajtburg J, et al. Amphotericin B: current understanding of mechanisms of action. *Antimicrob Agents Chemother* 1990;34:183.
257. Janknegt R, et al. Liposomal and lipid formulations of amphotericin B. *Clin Pharmacokinet* 1992;23:279.
258. Christiansen KJ, et al. Distribution and activity of amphotericin B in humans. *J Infect Dis* 1985;152:1037.
259. Fisher MA, et al. Risk factors for amphotericin B-associated nephrotoxicity. *Am J Med* 1989;87:547.
260. Branch RA. Prevention of amphotericin B-induced renal impairment: a review of the use of sodium supplementation. *Arch Int Med* 1988;148: 2389.
261. Butler WT, et al. Nephrotoxicity of amphotericin B: early and late effects in 81 patients. *Am J Med* 1964;61:175.
262. Medoff G, et al. Antifungal agents useful in the therapy of systemic fungal infections. *Annu Rev Pharmacol Toxicol* 1983;23:303.
263. Wertlake PT, et al. Nephrotoxic tubular damage and calcium deposition following amphotericin B therapy. *Am J Pathol* 1963;43:449.
264. Bhathena DB, et al. The effects of amphotericin B therapy on the intrarenal vasculature and tubules in man. A study of renal biopsies by light, electron and immunofluorescence microscopy. *Clin Nephrol* 1978;9:103.
265. Patterson RM, Ackerman GL. Renal tubular acidosis due to amphotericin B nephrotoxicity. *Arch Int Med* 1971;127:241.
266. Burgess JL, Birchall R. Nephrotoxicity of amphotericin B with emphasis on tubular function. *Am J Med* 1972;53:77.
267. Barton CH, et al. Renal magnesium wasting associated with amphotericin B therapy. *Am J Med* 1984;77:471.
268. Barbour GL, et al. Vasopressin-resistant nephrogenic diabetes insipidus—a result of amphotericin B therapy. *Arch Int Med* 1979;139:86.
269. Sawaya BP, Briggs JP, Schnermann J. Amphotericin B nephrotoxicity: the adverse consequences of altered membrane properties. *J Am Soc Nephrol* 1995;6:154.
270. Cheng JT, et al. Amphotericin B nephrotoxicity: increased resistance and tubule permeability. *Kidney Int* 1982;22:626.
271. Tolins JP, Raij L. Adverse effect of amphotericin B administration on renal hemodynamics in the rat. Neurohumoral mechanisms and influence of calcium channel blockade. *J Pharmacol Exp Ther* 1988;245:594.
272. Sabra R, et al. Mechanism of amphotericin B-induced reduction of the glomerular filtration rate: a micropuncture study. *J Pharmacol Exp Ther* 1990;253:34.
273. Sawaya BP, et al. Direct vasoconstriction as a possible cause for amphotericin B-induced nephrotoxicity in rats. *J Clin Invest* 1991;87:2097.
274. Tolins JP, Raij L. Chronic amphotericin B nephrotoxicity in the rat: protective effect of calcium channel blockade. *J Am Soc Nephrol* 1991;2:98.
275. Brooks DP, et al. Attenuation of amphotericin B nephrotoxicity in the dog by fenoldopam prodrug, SKF R-105058. *J Pharmacol Exp Ther* 1991;257:1243.
276. Ohnishi A, et al. Sodium status influences amphotericin B nephrotoxicity in the rat. *Antimicrob Agents Chemother* 1989;33:1222.

277. Llanos A, et al. Effect of salt supplementation on amphotericin B nephrotoxicity. *Kidney Int* 1991;40:302.

278. Gouge TH, Andriole VT. An experimental model of amphotericin B nephrotoxicity with renal tubular acidosis. *J Lab Clin Med* 1971;78:713.

279. Heyman SN, et al. Chronic amphotericin B nephropathy: morphometric, electron microscopic and fundamental studies. *J Am Soc Nephrol* 1993;4:69.

280. Brezis M, Rosen S, Silva P. Polyene toxicity in renal medulla: injury mediated by transport activity. *Science* 1984;224:66.

281. Zager RA, Bredl CR, Schimpf BA. Direct amphotericin B-mediated tubular toxicity: assessment of selected cytoprotective agents. *Kidney Int* 1992;41:337.

282. Walsh TJ, et al. Liposomal amphotericin B for empirical therapy in patients with persistent fever and neutropenia. National Institute of Allergy and Infectious Diseases Mycoses Study Group. *N Engl J Med* 1999;340: 764.

283. Moreau P, et al. Reduced renal toxicity and improved clinical tolerance of amphotericin B mixed with Intralipid compared with conventional amphotericin B in neutropenic patients. *J Antimicrob Chemother* 1992;30: 535.

284. Bernardo JF, et al. Amphotericin B. In: De Broe ME, et al., eds. *Clinical nephrotoxins—renal injury from drugs and chemicals,* 2nd ed. Dordrecht, The Netherlands: Kluwer Acadmic Publishers, 2003:199.

285. Dorski DI, Crumpacker CS. Drugs five years later: acyclovir. *Ann Intern Med* 1987;107:859.

286. De Miranda P, Blum MR. Pharmacokinetics of acyclovir after intravenous and oral administration. *J Antimicrob Chemother* 1983;12(Suppl B):29.

287. Keeney RE, Kirk LE, Brigden D. Acyclovir tolerance in humans. *Am J Med* 1982;73(Suppl 1A):176.

288. Brigden D, Rosling AE, Woods NC. Renal function after acyclovir intravenous injection. *Am J Med* 1982;73(Suppl 1A):182.

289. Bean B, Aeppli D. Adverse effects of high-dose intravenous acyclovir in ambulatory patients with acute herpes zoster. *J Infect Dis* 1985;151:362.

290. Campos SB, et al. Effects of acyclovir on renal function. *Nephron* 1992;62: 74.

291. Becker BN, et al. Rapidly progressive acute renal failure due to acyclovir: case report and review of the literature. *Am J Kidney Dis* 1993;22:611.

292. Sawyer MH, et al. Acyclovir-induced renal failure: clinical course and histology. *Am J Med* 1988;84:1067.

293. Dos Santos Mde F, et al. Nephrotoxicity of acyclovir and ganciclovirin rats: evaluation of glomerular hemodynamics. *J Am Soc Nephrol* 1997;8:361.

294. Wagstaff AJ, Bryson HM. Foscarnet—a reappraisal of its antiviral activity, pharmacokinetic properties and therapeutic use in immunocompromised patients with viral infections. *Drugs* 1994;48:199.

295. Safrin S, Crumpacker C, Chatis P. A controlled trial comparing foscarnet with vidarabine for acyclovir-resistant mucocutaneous herpes simplex in the acquired immunodeficiency syndrome. *N Engl J Med* 1991;325: 551.

296. Sjovall J, Bergdahl S, Gunille M. Pharmacokinetics of foscarnet and distribution to cerebrospinal fluid after intravenous infusion in patients with human immunodeficiency virus infection. *Antimicrob Agents Chemother* 1989;33:1023.

297. Jacobson MA, et al. A dose-ranging study of daily maintenance intravenous foscarnet therapy for cytomegalovirus retinitis in AIDS. *J Infect Dis* 1993;168:444.

298. Deray G, et al. Foscarnet nephrotoxicity: mechanism, incidence and prevention. *Am J Nephrol* 1989;5:316.

299. Gearhart MO, Sorg TB. Foscarnet-induced severe hypomagnesemia and other electrolyte disorders. *Ann Pharmacother* 1993;27:285.

300. Zanetta G, et al. Foscarnet-induced crystalline glomerulonephritis with nephrotic syndrome and acute renal failure after kidney transplantation. *Transplantation* 1999;67:1376.

301. Jayaweera DT. Minimising the dosage-limiting toxicities of foscarnet induction therapy. *Drug Safety* 1997;16:258.

302. Cundy KC. Clinical pharmacokinetics of the antiviral nucleotide analogues cidofovir and adefovir. *Clin Pharmacokinet* 1999;36:127.

303. Cihlar T, et al. The antiviral analogues cidofovir and adefovir are novel substrates for human and rat renal organic anion transporter 1. *Mol Pharmacol* 1999;56:570.

304. Lacy SA, et al. Effect of oral probenecid coadministration on the chronic toxicity and pharmacokinetics of intravenous cidofovir in cynomolgus monkeys. *Toxicolog Sci* 1998;44:97.

305. Walzer PD, et al. Pneumocystis carinii pneumonia in the United States. Epidemiologic, diagnostic and clinical features. *Ann Intern Med* 1974;80: 83.

306. Lachaal M, Venuto R. Nephrotoxicity and hyperkalemia in patients with AIDS treated with pentamidine. *Am J Med* 1989;87:60.

307. Farr SJ, et al. Dose-dependent distribution of (^{3}H)pentamidine following intratracheal administration to rats. *Xenobiotica* 1993;23:53.

308. Navin TR, et al. Effect of azotemia in dogs on the pharmacokinetics of pentamidine. *J Infect Dis* 1987;155:1021.

309. Waldman R, Pearce D, Martin R. Pentamidine isothionate levels in lungs, liver, and kidneys of rats after aerosol or intravenous administration. *Am Rev Respir Dis* 1973;108:1004.

310. Conte JE, Upton RP, Lin ET. Pentamidine pharmacokinetics in patients with AIDS with impaired renal function. *J Infect Dis* 1987;156:885.

311. Mani S. Pentamidine-induced renal magnesium wasting. *AIDS* 1992; 6:594.

312. O'Brien JG. A 5-year review of adverse drug reactions and their risk factors in human immunodeficiency virus-infected patients who were receiving intravenous pentamidine therapy for *Pneumocystis carinii* pneumonia. *Clin Infect Dis* 1997;24:854.

313. Feddersen A, Sack K. Experimental studies on the nephrotoxicity of pentamidine in rats. *J Antimicrob Chemother* 1991;28:437.

314. Merion RM, et al. Cyclosporine: five years experience in cadaveric renal transplantation. *N Engl J Med* 1984;310:148.

315. Kahan BD. Cyclosporine: the base for immunosuppressive therapy-present and future. *Transplant Proc* 1993;25:508.

316. Kostakis A, White D, Calne R. Toxic effects in the use of cyclosporine A in alcoholic solution as an immunosuppressant of rat heart allografts. *IRCS J Med Sci* 1977;5:243.

317. Calne R, et al. Prolonged survival of pig orthotopic heart grafts treated with cyclosporine A. *Lancet* 1978;1:1183.

318. Borel JF, Feurer C, Magnee C. Effects of the new anti-lymphocytic peptide cyclosporine A in animals. *Immunology* 1977;32:1010.

319. Calne R, Thiru S, McMaster P. Cyclosporine A in patients receiving renal allografts from cadaver donors. *Lancet* 1978;2:1323.

320. Powles R, et al. Cyclosporine A for the treatment of graft-versus-host disease in man. *Lancet* 1978;2:1327.

321. Calne R. Cyclosporine. *Nephron* 1980;26:67.

322. Powell-Jackson PR, et al. Nephrotoxicity of parenterally administered cyclosporine after orthotopic liver transplantation. *Transplantation* 1983;36:505.

323. Curtis JJ, et al. Cyclosporine in therapeutic doses increases renal allograft vascular resistance. *Lancet* 1986;2:477.

324. English J, et al. Cyclosporine-induced acute renal dysfunction in the rat: evidence for arterial vasoconstriction with preservation of tubular function. *Transplantation* 1987;44:135.

325. Novick CA, et al. Detrimental effect of cyclosporine on initial function of cadaveric renal allografts following extended preservation. *Transplantation* 1986;42:154.

326. Verpooten GA, et al. De novo occurrence of hemolytic uremic syndrome in a cyclosporine-treated renal allograft patient. *Transplant Proc* 1987;19:2943.

327. Klintmalm G, et al. Interstitial fibrosis in renal allografts after 12 to 46 months of cyclosporine treatment: beneficial effects of low doses in early post-transplantation period. *Lancet* 1986;2:950.

328. Ruiz P, et al. Associations between cyclosporine therapy and interstitial fibrosis in renal allograft biopsies. *Transplantation* 1988;45:91.

329. Mihatsch MJ, Thiel G, Ryffel B. Histopathology of cyclosporine nephrotoxicity. *Transplant Proc* 1988;20(Suppl 3):759.

330. Bertani T, et al. Nature and extent of glomerular injury induced by cyclosporine in heart transplant patients. *Kidney Int* 1991;40:243.

331. Myers BD, et al. Cyclosporine-associated chronic nephropathy. *N Engl J Med* 1984;311:699.

332. Nizze H, et al. Cyclosporine-associated nephropathy in patients with heart and bone-marrow transplants. *Clin Nephrol* 1988;30:248.

333. Platz KP, et al. Nephrotoxicity following orthotopic liver transplantation. A comparison between cyclosporine and FK 506. *Transplantation* 1994;58:170.

334. Gonwa TA, et al. End-stage renal disease (ESRD) after orthotopic liver transplantation (OLTX) using calcineurin-based immunotherapy. *Transplantation* 2001;72:1934.

335. Fioretto P, et al. Cyclosporine associated lesions in native kidneys of diabetic pancreas transplant recipients. *Kidney Int* 1995;48:489.

336. Mihatsch MJ, Thiel G, Ryffel B. Renal side-effects of cyclosporine A with special reference to auto-immune diseases. *Br J Dermatol* 1990;122:101.

337. Palestine AG, et al. Renal histopathologic alterations in patients treated with cyclosporine for uveitis. *N Engl J Med* 1986;314:1293.

338. Young EW, et al. A prospective study of renal structure and function in psoriasis patients treated with cyclosporine. *Kidney Int* 1994;46:1216.

339. Vercauteren SV, et al. A meta-analysis and morphological review of cyclosporine-induced nephrotoxicity in auto-immune diseases. *Kidney Int* 1998;54:536.

340. Borel JF, Feurer C, Goblet HV. Biological effects of cyclosporine A, a new antilymphocytic agent. *Agents Actions* 1976;6:468.

341. Wenger R. Cyclosporine: conformation and analogues as tools for studying its mechanisms of action. *Transplant Proc* 1988;20(Suppl 2):313.

342. Grevel J. Absorption of cyclosporine A after oral dosing. *Transplant Proc* 1986;18(Suppl 5):9.

343. Kahan B. Individualization of cyclosporine therapy using pharmacokinetic and pharmacodynamic parameters. *Transplantation* 1985;40:457.

344. Kahan BD, Reid M, Newburger J. Pharmacokinetics of cyclosporine in human renal transplantation. *Transplant Proc* 1983;15:446.

345. Kovarik JM, et al. Reduced inter- and intraindividual variability in cyclosporine pharmacokinetics from a microemulsion formulation. *J Pharm Sci* 1994;83:444.

346. Kovarik JM, et al. Cyclosporine pharmacokinetics and variability from a microemulsion formulation—a multicenter investigation in kidney transplant patients. *Transplantation* 1994;58:658.

347. Frei UA, et al. Randomized, double-blind, one-year study of the safety and tolerability of cyclosporine microemulsion compared with conventional cyclosporine in renal transplant patients. International Sandimmune Neoral Study Group. *Transplantation* 1998;65:1455.

348. Keown P, Niese D. Cyclosporine microemulsion increases drug exposure and reduces acute rejection without incremental nephrotoxicity in de novo renal transplantation. International Sandimmune Neoral Study Group. *Kidney Int* 1998;54:939.

349. Shah MB, et al. The evaluation of the safety and tolerability of two new formulations of cyclosporine: Neoral and Sandimmune. A meta-analysis. *Transplantation* 1999;67:1611.

350. Ryffel B, et al. Biological significance of cyclosporine metabolites. *Transplant Proc* 1988;20[]2):575.

351. Kahan B, Grevel J. Optimization of cyclosporine therapy in renal transplantation by a pharmacokinetic strategy. *Transplantation* 1988;46:631.

352. Kahan B. Cyclosporine. *N Engl J Med* 1989;321:1725.

353. Master G, et al. Disposition of cyclosporine in several animal species and man. Structural elucidation of its metabolites. *Drug Metab Dispos* 1984;12:120.

354. Kahan B, et al. Demographic factors affecting the pharmacokinetics of cyclosporine estimated by radioimmunoassay. *Transplantation* 1986;41:459.

355. Yee G, et al. Pharmacokinetics of intravenous cyclosporine in bone marrow transplant patients. *Transplantation* 1984;38:511.

356. Yee G, et al. Age-dependent cyclosporine pharmacokinetics in marrow transplant recipient. *Clin Pharmacol Ther* 1986;40:438.

357. Yee G, et al. Effect of hepatic dysfunction on oral cyclosporine pharmacokinetics in marrow transplant patients. *Blood* 1984;64:1277.

358. Sridhar N, et al. Influence of concomitant medication on cyclosporine dosage and blood concentration in renal allograft recipients. *Clin Transplant* 1992;6:134.

359. Oellerich M, et al. Lake Louise consensus conference on cyclosporine monitoring in organ transplantation: report of the consensus panel. *Ther Drug Monitor* 1995;17:642.

360. Keown D. Optimizing cyclosporine therapy: dose, levels, and monitoring. *Transplant Proc* 1988;20(Suppl 2):382.

361. Roesel T, et al. Thin-layer chromatographic detection of cyclosporine and its metabolites in whole blood using Rhodamine B and alpha-cyclodextrin. *Transplantation* 1987;43:274.

362. Grevel J, Welsh M, Kahan B. Cyclosporine monitoring in renal transplantation: area under the curve monitoring is superior to trough-level monitoring. *Ther Drug Monit* 1989;11:246.

363. Thervet E, et al. Clinical outcomes during the first three months posttransplant in renal allograft recipients managed by C2 monitoring of cyclosporine microemulsion. *Transplantation* 2003;76:903.

364. Mendez R, et al. Neoral therapy optimized by C2 monitoring and Simulect induction can result in a low acute rejection rate in renal transplant recipients. *Am J Transplant* 2004;4(Suppl 8):255.

365. Vitko S, et al. Everolimus with optimized cyclosporine dosing in renal transplant recipients: 6-month safety and efficacy results of two randomized studies. *Am J Transplant* 2004;4:626.

366. Levy GA, et al. Improved clinical outcomes for liver transplant recipients using cyclosporine monitoring based on two-hour post dose levels (C2). *Transplantation* 2002;73:953.

367. Levy G, et al. Results of LIS2T, a multicenter, randomized study comparing cyclosporine microemulsion with C$_2$ monitoring and tacrolimus with C$_0$ monitoring in de novo liver transplantation. *Transplantation* 2004; 778:1632.

368. Cole E, et al. Clinical benefits of Neoral C2 monitoring in the long-term management of renal transplant recipients. *Transplantation* 2003;75:2086.

369. Midtvedt K, et al. C2 monitoring in maintenance renal transplant recipients: is it worthwhile? *Transplantation* 2003;76:1236.

370. Einecke G, et al. The value of C2 monitoring in stable renal allograft recipients on maintenance immunosuppression. *Nephrol Dial Transplant* 2004;19:215.339.

371. Krónke M, Leonard WJ, Depper JM. Cyclosporine A inhibits T-cell growth factor gene-expression at the level of mRNA transcription. *Proc Natl Acad Sci USA* 1984;81:5214.

372. Goto T, et al. FK506: historical perspective. *Transplant Proc* 1991;23:2713.

373. Baumann G. Molecular mechanism of immunosuppressive agents. *Transplant Proc* 1992;24(Suppl 2):4.

374. Handschumacher R, et al. Cyclophilin: a specific cytosolic binding protein for cyclosporine A. *Science* 1984;226:544.

375. Siekirka J, et al. A cytosolic binding protein for the immunosuppressant FK506 has peptidyl-prolyl isomerase activity but is distinct from cyclophylin. *Nature* 1989;341:755.

376. Liu J, et al. Calcineurin is a common target of cyclophilin-cyclosporine A and FKBP-FK506 complexes. *Cell* 1991;6:903.

377. Friedman J, Weissman I. Two cytoplasmic candidates for immuno-philin action are revealed by affinity for a new cyclophilin: one in the presence and one in the absence of CsA. *Cell* 1991;66:799.

378. Mattila PS, Ullman KS, Fiering S. The actions of cyclosporine A and FK506 suggest a novel step in the activation of T-lymphocytes. *EMBO J* 1990;9:4425.

379. Baumann G, Geisse S, Sullivan M. Cyclosporine A and FK506 both affect DNA binding of regulatory nuclear proteins to the human interleukin-2 promotor. *New Biologist* 1991;3:270.

380. Rosen S, Greenfeld Z, Brezis M. Chronic cyclosporine-induced nephropathy in the rat. *Transplantation* 1990;49:445.

381. Bertani T, et al. Renal injury induced by long-term administration of cyclosporine A to rats. *Am J Pathol* 1987;127:569.

382. Simpson JG, et al. Chronic renal damage caused by cyclosporine. *Transplant Proc* 1988;20:792.

383. Gillum DM, et al. Chronic cyclosporine toxicity. A rodent model. *Transplantation* 1988;461:285.

384. Elzinga L, Rosen S, Bennett WM. Dissociation of glomerular filtration rate from tubulo-interstitial fibrosis in experimental chronic cyclosporine nephropathy: role of sodium intake. *J Am Soc Nephrol* 1993;4:214.

385. Murray BM, Paller MS, Ferris TF. Effect of cyclosporine administration on renal hemodynamics in conscious rats. *Kidney Int* 1985;28:767.

386. Barros EJ, et al. Glomerular hemodynamics and hormonal participation on cyclosporine nephrotoxicity. *Kidney Int* 1987;32:19.

387. Sabbatini M, Esposito C, Ucello F. Acute effects of cyclosporine on glomerular dynamics—micropuncture study in the rat. *Transplant Proc* 1988;20: 544.

388. Winston JA, Feingold R, Safirstein R. Glomerular hemodynamics in cyclosporine nephrotoxicity following nephrectomy. *Kidney Int* 1989; 35:1175, 357.

389. Blair JT, et al. Toxicity of the immune suppressant cyclosporine A in the rat. *J Pathol* 1982;138:163.

390. Dieperink H, et al. Effects of cyclosporine A, gentamicin and furosemide on rat renal function: a lithium clearance study. *Clin Exp Pharm Physiol* 1987;14:825.

391. Dieperink H, Starklint H, Leyssac PP. Nephrotoxicity of cyclosporine—an animal model: study of the nephrotoxic effect of cyclosporine on overall and renal tubular function in conscious rats. *Transplant Proc* 1983;15:736.

392. Dieperink H, et al. Nephrotoxicity of cyclosporine A. A lithium-clearance and micropuncture study in rats. *Eur J Clin Invest* 1986;16:69.

393. Thomson K, Holstein-Rathlou NH, Leyssac P. Comparison of three measures of proximal tubular reabsorption: lithium clearance, occlusion time and micro-puncture. *Am J Physiol* 1981;241:F348.

394. Kaskel F, et al. Inhibition of myogeneic autoregulation in cyclosporine nephrotoxicity in the rat. *Renal Physiol Biochem* 1989;12:250.

395. Battle DC, et al. Effect of short-term cyclosporine A administration on urinary acidification. *Clin Nephrol* 1986;25/1(Suppl 1):62.

396. Heering P, Grabensee B. Influence of cyclosporine A on renal tubular function after kidney transplantation. *Nephron* 1991;59:66.

397. Ryffel B, et al. Toxicological evaluation of cyclosporine A. *Arch Toxicol* 1983;53:107.

398. Siegl H, et al. Cyclosporine, the renin–angiotensin–aldosterone system and renal adverse reactions. *Transplant Proc* 1983;15:2719.

399. Thompson AW, Whiting PH, Simpson JG. Cyclosporine: immunology, toxicity and pharmacology in experimental animals. *Agents Actions* 1984;15: 306.

400. Duncan JL, et al. Cyclosporine-induced renal structural damage: influence of dosage, strain, age and sex with reference to the rat and guinea pig. *Clin Nephrol* 1986;25:S14.

401. Dieperink H, et al. Long-term Cyclosporine A nephrotoxicity in the rat: effects on renal function and morphology. *Nephrol Dial Transplant* 1988;3:317.

402. Mihatsch M, et al. Morphology of cyclosporine nephrotoxicity in the rat. *Clin Nephrol* 1986;25(Suppl):S2.

403. Remuzzi A, et al. Three dimensional morphometric analysis of segmental glomerulosclerosis in the rat. *Transplant Proc* 1990;23:3085.

404. Perico N, et al. Morphometrical analysis of glomerular changes induced by cyclosporine in the rat. *Am J Kidney Dis* 1991;27:537.

405. Mihatsch MJ, Ryffel B, Gudat F. The differential diagnosis between rejection and cyclosporine-nephrotoxicity. *Kidney Int* 1995;48(S52):S63.

406. Mourad G, et al. Chronic cyclosporine nephrotoxicity is reversible in renal transplant recipients. *Nephrol Dial Transplant* 1993;8:1045(abst).

407. Morozumi K, et al. Studies on morphologic outcome of cyclosporine-associated arteriolopathy after discontinuation of cyclosporine in renal allografts. *Clin Nephrol* 1992;38:1.

408. Murray BM, Paller MS. Beneficial effects of renal denervation and prazosin on GFR and renal blood flow after cyclosporine in rats. *Clin Nephrol* 1986;25:S37.

409. Moss NG, Powell SL, Falk RJ. Intravenous cyclosporine activates afferent and efferent renal nerves and causes sodium retention in innervated kidneys in rats. *Proc Natl Acad Sci USA* 1985;82:8222.

410. Gazdar AF, Dammin GJ. Neural degeneration and regeneration in human renal transplants. *N Engl J Med* 1970;283:222.

411. Perico N, et al. Acute cyclosporine A nephrotoxicity in rats: which role for renin-angiotensin system and glomerular prostaglandins? *Clin Nephrol* 1986;26:S83.

412. Verpooten GA, et al. Cyclosporine nephrotoxicity: comparative cytochemical study of rat kidney and human allograft biopsies. *Clin Nephrol* 1986;25:S18.

413. Nitta K, et al. Granular juxtaglomerular cell hyperplasia caused by cyclosporine. *Transplantation* 1987;44:417.

414. Duggin GG, et al. Influence of cyclosporine A on intrarenal control of GFR. *Clin Nephrol* 1986;25:S43.

415. Kurtz A, Bruna RD, Kuhn K. Cyclosporine A enhances renin secretion and production in isolated juxtaglomerular cells. *Kidney Int* 1988;33:947.

416. Kaskel FJ, et al. Cyclosporine nephrotoxicity: sodium excretion, autoregulation, and angiotensin II. *Am J Physiol* 1987;252:F733.

417. McAuley FT, et al. The influence of enalapril or spironolactone on experimental cyclosporine nephrotoxicity. *Biochem Pharmacol* 1987;36:699.

418. Burdmann EA, et al. Prevention of experimental cyclosporine-induced interstitial fibrosis by losartan and enalapril. *Am J Physiol* 1995;269:F491.

419. Pichler RH, et al. Pathogenesis of cyclosporine nephropathy: roles of angiotensin II and osteopontin. *J Am Soc Nephrol* 1995;6:1186.

420. Bantle JP, et al. Effects of cyclosporine on the renin–angiotensin–aldosterone system and potassium excretion in renal transplant recipients. *Arch Int Med* 1985;145:505.

421. Devarajan P, et al. Cyclosporine nephrotoxicity: blood volume, sodium conservation, and renal hemodynamics. *Am J Physiol* 1989;256:F71.

422. Whiting PH, et al. Enhancement of high dose cyclosporine A toxicity with furosemide. *Biochem Pharmacol* 1984;33:1075.

423. Brunner FP, et al. Mannitol potentiates cyclosporine nephrotoxicity. *Clin Nephrol* 1986;25(S1):S130.

424. Shihab FS, et al. Sodium depletion enhances fibrosis and the expression of TGF-β1 and matrix proteins in experimental chronic cyclosporine nephropathy. *Am J Kidney Dis* 1997;30:71.

425. Perico N, et al. Effect of short-term cyclosporine administration in rats on renin-angiotensin and thromboxane A: possible relevance to the reduction in glomerular filtration rate. *J Pharmacol Exp Ther* 1986;239:229.

426. Kawaguchi A, et al. Increase in urinary thromboxane B$_2$ in rats caused by cyclosporine. *Transplantation* 1985;40:214.

427. Metric R, et al. Effect of cyclosporine on urinary prostanoid excretion, renal blood flow, and glomerulotubular function. *Transplantation* 1988;45:883.

428. Lau DC, Wong KL, Hwang WS. Cyclosporine toxicity on cultured rat microvascular endothelial cells. *Kidney Int* 1989;35:604.

429. Zoja C, et al. Cyclosporine-induced endothelial cell injury. *Lab Invest* 1986;55:455.

430. Perico N, et al. Co-participation of thromboxane A$_2$ and leukotriene C4 and D4 in mediating cyclosporine-induced acute renal failure. *Transplantation* 1991;52:873.

431. Spurney RF, et al. Thromboxane receptor blockade improves cyclosporine nephrotoxicity in rats. *Prostaglandins* 1990;39:135.

432. Perico N, et al. Functional significance of exaggerated renal thromboxane A$_2$ synthesis induced by cyclosporine A. *Am J Physiol* 1986;20:F581.

433. Perico N, et al. Thromboxane receptor blockade attenuates chronic cyclosporine nephrotoxicity and improves survival in rats with renal isograft. *J Am Soc Nephrol* 1992;2:1398.

434. Heering P, et al. The role of thromboxane and prostacyclin in cyclosporine-induced nephrotoxicity. *Nephron* 1992;19:534.

435. Smith SR, et al. The effects of thromboxane synthase inhibition with CGS 13080 in human cyclosporine nephrotoxicity. *Kidney Int* 1992;41:199.

436. Rodriguez-Puyol D, et al. Actions of cyclosporine A on cultured rat mesangial cells. *Kidney Int* 1989;35:632.

437. Pirotzky E, et al. Cyclosporine-induced nephrotoxicity: preventive effect of a PAF-acether antagonist BN52063. *Transplant Proc* 1988;20(Suppl 3):665.

438. Kon V, et al. Role of endothelin in cyclosporine-induced glomerular dysfunction. *Kidney Int* 1990;37:1487.

439. Haug C, et al. Endothelin release by rabbit proximal tubule cells: modulatory effects of cyclosporine A, tacrolimus, HGF and EGF. *Kidney Int* 1998;54:1626.

440. Awazu M, et al. Cyclosporine promotes glomerular endothelin binding in vivo. *J Am Soc Nephrol* 1991;1:1253.

441. Perico N, Dadan J, Remuzzi G. Endothelin mediates the renal vasoconstriction induced by cyclosporine in the rat. *J Am Soc Nephrol* 1990;1:76.

442. Iwasaki S, Homma T, Kon V. Site specific regulation in the kidney of endothelin and its receptor subtypes by cyclosporine. *Kidney Int* 1994;45:592.

443. Kivlighn SD, Gabel AD, Siegl PK. Effects of BQ-123 on renal function and acute cyclosporine-induced renal dysfunction. *Kidney Int* 1994;45:131.

444. Binet I, et al. Renal hemodynamics and pharmacokinetics of bosentan with and without cyclosporine A. *Kidney Int* 2000;57:224.

445. Verbeke M, et al. Beneficial effect of serotonin 5-HT2-receptor antagonism on renal blood flow autoregulation in cyclosporine-treated rats. *J Am Soc Nephrol* 1999;10:28.

446. Morris ST, et al. Endothelial dysfunction in renal transplant recipients maintained on cyclosporine. *Kidney Int* 2000;57:1100.

447. Myer-Lehnert H, Schrier AW. Cyclosporine A enhances vasopressin-induced Ca^{2+} mobilization and contraction in mesangial cells. *Kidney Int* 1988;34:89.

448. Myer-Lehnert H, Schrier W. Potential mechanism of CsA induced vascular smooth muscle contraction. *Hypertension* 1989;13:352.

449. Dieperink H, et al. Antagonist capacity of Felodipine on cyclosporine A nephrotoxicity in the rat. *Nephrol Dial Transplant* 1992;7:124.

450. Petric R, et al. Amelioration of experimental cyclosporine nephrotoxicity by calcium channel inhibition. *Transplantation* 1992;54:1103.

451. Pedersen EB, et al. Interaction between cyclosporine and felodipine in renal transplant recipients. *Kidney Int* 1992;41(Suppl 36):S82.

452. Neumayer HH, Kunzendorf U, Schrieber M. Protective effects of Diltiazem and the prostacycline analogue Iloprost in human renal transplantation. *Renal Fail* 1992;14:289.

453. Shaik MG, et al. Chronic cyclosporine A (CsA) nephrotoxicity in the rat: the effect of calcium blockade with verapamil. *Int J Exp Pathol* 1993;74:389.

454. Fournier N, Ducet G, Crevat A. Action of cyclosporine on mitochondrial calcium fluxes. *J Bioenerg Biomembr* 1987;19:297.

455. Strzelecki S, Kumar S, Khauli R, et al. Impairment by cyclosporine of membrane-mediated functions in kidney mitochondria. *Kidney Int* 1988;34:234.

456. Kremer S, et al. Cyclosporine induced alterations in vasopressin signalling in the glomerular cell. *Clin Invest Med* 1989;12:201.

457. Schreier SJ, Baumann G, Zenke G. Inhibition of T-cell signalling pathways by immunophilin-drug complexes: are side-effects inherent to immunosuppressive properties? *Transplant Proc* 1993;25:502.

458. Dumont FJ, et al. The immunosuppressive and toxic effects of FK506 are mechanistically related: pharmacology of a novel antagonist of FK506 and Rapamycin. *J Exp Med* 1992;176:751.

459. Platt JL, et al. Renal interstitial cell populations in cyclosporine nephrotoxicity. *Transplantation* 1983;36:343.

460. Buss WC, Stepanek J, Bennett WM. A new proposal for the inhibition of cyclosporine A nephrotoxicity: inhibition of renal microsomal protein chain elongation following in vivo cyclosporine A. *Biochem Pharmacol* 1989;38:4085.

461. Bennett WM, Houghton DC, Buss WC. Cyclosporine-induced renal dysfunction: correlations between cellular events and whole kidney function. *J Am Soc Nephrol* 1991;1:1212.

462. Amore A, et al. Nitric oxide mediates cyclosporine-induced apoptosis in cultured renal cells. *Kidney Int* 2000;57:1549.

463. Ortiz A, et al. Cyclosporine A induces apoptosis in murine tubular epithelial cells: role of caspases. *Kidney Int* 1998;54(S68):S25.

464. Healy E, et al. Apoptosis and necrosis: mechanisms of cell death induced by cyclosporine A in a renal proximal tubular cell line. *Kidney Int* 1998;54:1955.

465. Lally C, Healy E, Ryan MP. Cyclosporine A-induced cell cycle arrest and cell death in renal epithelial cells. *Kidney Int* 1999;56:1254.

466. Wolf G, Neilson E. Increases in levels of collagen types I and IV messenger ribonucleic acid in murine kidneys after treatment with cyclosporine. *Nephron* 1992;60:87.

467. Nast C, et al. Cyclosporine induces elevated procollagen α1(I) mRNA levels in the rat renal cortex. *Kidney Int* 1991;39:631.

468. Ghiggeri GM, et al. Selective enhancement of collagen expression by cyclosporine with renal cells "in vitro." *J Am Soc Nephrol* 1993;4:753.

469. Wolf G, Killen PD, Neilson EG. Intracellular signalling of transcription and secretion of type IV collagen after angiotensin II-induced cellular hypertrophy in cultured proximal tubular cells. *Cell Regul* 1991;2:219.

470. Burdmann EA, et al. Dissociation between functional and structural changes in chronic cyclosporine nephrotoxicity. *J Am Soc Nephrol* 1993;4:751.

471. Meister B, et al. Cellular expression of angiotensin type-1 receptor mRNA in the kidney. *Kidney Int* 1993;44:331.

472. Cuhaci B, et al. Transforming growth factor-β levels in human allograft chronic fibrosis correlate with rate of decline in renal function. *Transplantation* 1999;68:785.

473. Vieira J, et al. Cyclosporine-induced interstitial fibrosis and arteriolar TGF-β expression with preserved renal blood flow. *Transplantation* 1999;68:1746.

474. Shihab FS, et al. Role of transforming growth factor-β1 in experimental chronic cyclosporine nephropathy. *Kidney Int* 1996;49:1141.

475. Khanna A, et al. In vivo hyperexpression of transforming growth factor-β1 in mice: stimulation by cyclosporine. *Transplantation* 1997;63:1037.

476. Johnson DW, et al. Cyclosporine exerts a direct fibrogenic effect on human tubulointerstitial cells: roles of insulin-like growth factor-1, transforming growth factor-β1, and platelet-derived growth factor. *J Pharmacol Exp Ther* 1998;289:535.

477. Wolf G, Thaiss F, Stahl RA. Cyclosporine stimulates expression of transforming growth factor-β in renal cells. Possible mechanism of cyclosporines antiproliferative effects. *Transplantation* 1995;60:237.

478. Khanna AK, et al. Transforming growth factor (TGF)-β mimics and anti-TGF-β antibody abrogates the in vivo effects of cyclosporine. Demonstration of a direct role of TGF-β in immunosuppression and nephrotoxicity of cyclosporine. *Transplantation* 1999;67:882.

479. Deng JT, et al. Expression of metalloproteinases and their inhibitor TIMP in the kidney of cyclosporine-treated rats. *J Am Soc Nephrol* 1994;5(3):804(abst).

480. Duymelinck C, et al. Inhibition of the matrix metalloproteinase system in a rat model of chronic cyclosporine nephropathy. *Kidney Int* 1998;54:804.

481. Duymelinck C, et al. Cholesterol feeding accentuates the cyclosporine-induced elevation of renal plasminogen activator inhibitor type 1. *Kidney Int* 1997;51:1818.

482. Inselman G, Hannemann J, Baumann K. Cyclosporine A induced lipid peroxidation and influence on glucose-6-phosphatase in rat hepatic and renal microsomes. *Res Commun Chem Pathol Pharmacol* 1990;68:189.

483. Ahmed SS, et al. Adenochrome reaction implicates oxygen radicals in metabolism of cyclosporine A and FK-506 in rat and human liver microsomes. *J Pharmacol Exp Ther* 1993;265:1047.

484. Weinberg JM. Issues in the pathophysiology of nephrotoxic renal tubular cell injury pertinent to understanding cyclosporine nephrotoxicity. *Transplant Proc* 1985;17(Suppl 1):S81.

485. Humes HD, Jackson NM, O'Connor RP. Pathogenetic mechanisms of nephrotoxicity: insights into cyclosporine nephrotoxicity. *Transplant Proc* 1985;17(Suppl 1):S51.

486. Halliwell B, Gutteridge JM, Cross CE. Free radicals, antioxidants, and human disease: where are we now? *J Lab Clin Med* 1992;119:598.

487. Baud L, et al. Stimulation by oxygen radicals of prostaglandin production by rat renal glomeruli. *Kidney Int* 1981;20:332.

488. Morrow JD, et al. Formation of novel non-cyclooxygenase-derived prostanoids (F2-Isoprostanes) in carbon tetrachloride hepatotoxicity. *J Clin Invest* 1992;90:2502.

489. Takahashi K, et al. Glomerular actions of a free radical-generated novel prostaglandin, 8-epi-prostaglandin F2a, in the rat: evidence for interaction with thromboxane A2 receptors. *J Clin Invest* 1992;90:136.

490. Süleymanlar G, et al. Possible role of lipid peroxidation in cyclosporine nephrotoxicity in rats. *Transplant Proc* 1994;26:2888.

491. Wang C, et al. Lipid peroxidation accompanies cyclosporine nephrotoxicity: effects of vitamin E. *Kidney Int* 1995;47:927.

492. Kumar KV, et al. Melatonin. An antioxidant protects against cyclosporine-induced nephrotoxicity. *Transplantation* 1999;67:1065.

493. Tariq M, et al. N-acetylcysteine attenuates cyclosporine-induced nephrotoxicity in rats. *Nephrol Dial Transplant* 1999;14:923.

494. Salahudeen AK. Role of lipid peroxidation in H2O2-induced renal epithelial (LLC-PK1) cell injury. *Am J Physiol* 1995;268:F30.

495. Petric R, et al. Effect of cyclosporine on urinary prostanoid excretion, renal blood flow, and glomerulo-tubular function. *Transplantation* 1988;45:883.

496. Houglum K, Brenner DA, Chojkier M. d-a-Tocopherol inhibits collagen a₁ (I) gene expression in cultured human fibroblasts. Modulation of constitutive collagen gene expression by lipid peroxidation. *J Clin Invest* 1991;87:2230.

497. Varghese Z, et al. Calcineurin inhibitors enhance low-density lipoprotein oxidation in transplant patients. *Kidney Int* 1999;56(S71):S137.

498. Apanay DC, et al. Cyclosporine increases the oxidisability of low-density lipoproteins in renal transplant recipients. *Transplantation* 1994;58:663.

499. Ghanem H, et al. Increased low-density lipoprotein oxidation in stable kidney transplant recipients. *Kidney Int* 1996;49:488.

500. Shulman H, et al. Nephrotoxicity of cyclosporine A after allogeneic marrow transplantation: glomerular thromboses and tubular injury. *N Engl J Med* 1981;305:1392.

501. Greenberg A, Egel JW, Thompson ME. Early and late forms of cyclosporine nephrotoxicity: studies in cardiac transplant recipients. *Am J Kidney Dis* 1987;9:12.

502. Flechner SM, et al. The nephrotoxicity of cyclosporine in renal transplant recipients. *Transplant Proc* 1983;15(Suppl 1):2689.

503. Leunissen KM, et al. Amplification of the nephrotoxic effect of cyclosporine by preexistent chronic histological lesions in the kidney. *Transplantation* 1989;48:590.

504. Canadian Multicenter Trial Group. A randomized clinical trial of cyclosporine in cadaveric renal transplantation. *N Engl J Med* 1983;309:809.

505. Myers BD. Cyclosporine nephrotoxicity. *Kidney Int* 1986;30:964.

506. Krupp P, Timonen P, Gulich A. Side-effects and safety of Sandimmune in long-term treatment of transplant patients. In: Schindler R, ed. *Ciclosporin in autoimmune disease.* Berlin: Springer, 1995:43.

507. Henny FC, Klehbloesem CH, Moolenaar AJ. Pharmacokinetics and nephrotoxicity of cyclosporine in renal transplant recipients. *Transplantation* 1985;40:261.

508. Bennett WM, Pulliam JP. Cyclosporine nephrotoxicity. *Ann Intern Med* 1983;99:851.

509. Gordon RD, Iwatsuki S, Shaw BJ. Cyclosporine-steroid combination therapy in 84 cadaveric renal transplants. *Am J Kidney Dis* 1985;5:307.

510. Belitsky P (for the Canadian Transplant Study Group). Initial nonfunction of cyclosporine-treated cadaver renal allografts preserved by simple cold storage. *Transplant Proc* 1985;17:1485.

511. Shiel AG, Hall BM, Tiller DJ. Australian Trial of Cyclosporine (CsA) in cadaveric donor renal transplantation. In: Kahan BD, ed. *Cyclosporine: biological activity and clinical applications.* Orlando: Grune & Stratton, 1984:307.

512. Keown PA, Stiller CR, Sinclair NR. The clinical relevance of cyclosporine blood levels as measured by radio-immunoassay. In: Kahan BD, ed. *Cyclosporine: biological activity and clinical applications.* Orlando: Grune & Stratton, 1984:599.

513. Taube D, et al. A comparison of the clinical, histopathologic, cytologic and biochemical features of renal transplant rejection, cyclosporine A nephrotoxicity, and stable renal function. *Transplant Proc* 1985;17:179.

514. Sibley RK, et al. Morphology of cyclosporine nephrotoxicity and acute rejection in patients immunosuppressed with cyclosporine and prednisone. *Surgery* 1983;94:225.

515. Burdick JF, et al. Characteristics of early routine renal allograft biopsies. *Transplantation* 1984;38:679.

516. Solez K, et al. Reflections on use of the renal biopsy as the "gold standard" in distinguishing transplant rejection from cyclosporine nephrotoxicity. *Transplant Proc* 1985;17:123.

517. Beschorner WE, et al. The presence of Leu 7 reactive lymphocytes in renal allografts undergoing acute rejection. *Transplant Proc* 1985;17:618.

518. Nield GH, Taube DH, Hartley RB. Morphological differentiation between rejection and cyclosporine nephrotoxicity in renal allografts. *J Clin Pathol* 1986;39:152.

519. Mihatsch MJ, Ryffel B. Evolution of cyclosporine nephrotoxicity. In: Hi-
tano M, ed. *Nephrology—Proceedings of the XI International Congress of Nephrology.* Tokyo: Springer 1991:576.

520. Nast CC, et al. Evaluation of cyclosporine nephrotoxicity by renal transplant fine needle aspiration. *Mod Pathol* 1989;2:577.

521. Perico N, et al. Daily renal hypoperfusion induced by cyclosporine in patients with renal transplantation. *Transplantation* 1992;54:56.

522. Conte G, et al. Acute cyclosporine renal dysfunction reversed by dopamine infusion in healthy subjects. *Kidney Int* 1989;36:1086.

523. Klein IH, et al. Different effects of tacrolimus and cyclosporine on renal hemodynamics and blood pressure in healthy subjects. *Transplantation* 2002;73:732.

524. Nankivell BJ, et al. Oral cyclosporine but not tacrolimus reduces renal transplant blood flow. *Transplantation* 2004;77:1457.

525. Ruggenenti P, et al. Calcium channel blockers protect transplant patients from cyclosporine-induced daily renal hypoperfusion. *Kidney Int* 1993;43:706.

526. McCulloch T, Furness PN, Feemally J. Volumetric analysis of renal interstitium in transplant kidney biopsies from cyclosporine treated patients with and without calcium channel blockade. *J Pathol* 1992;167:126A.

527. Chagnac A, et al. The effect of high-dose nifedipine on renal hemodynamics of cyclosporine-treated renal allograft recipients. *Transplantation* 1992;53:766.

528. Sørensen S, et al. Effect of felodipine on renal hemodynamics and tubular sodium handling in cyclosporine-treated renal recipients. *Nephrol Dial Transplant* 1992;7:69.

529. Berg K, et al. Effects of isradipine on renal function in cyclosporine-treated renal transplanted patients. *Nephrol Dial Transplant* 1991;6:725.

530. Wagner K, Albrecht S, Neumayer H. Prevention of delayed graft function in cadaveric kidney transplantation by calcium antagonist. Preliminary results of two prospective randomized trials. *Transplant Proc* 1986;18:510.

531. Carmines P, Navar L. Disparate effects of Ca channel blockade on afferent and efferent arteriolar response to Ang II. *Am J Physiol* 1989;253:F1015.

532. Sturrock ND, Lang CC, Struthers AD. Indomethacin and cyclosporine together produce marked renal vasoconstriction in humans. *J Hypertens* 1994;12:919.

533. Homan van der Heyde J, et al. The effect of dietary supplementation with fish oil on renal function and the course of early postoperative rejection episodes in cyclosporine-treated renal transplant recipients. *Transplantation* 1992;54:257.

534. Mason J, et al. Cyclosporine and the renin-angiotensin system. *Kidney Int* 1991;39(Suppl 32):S28.

535. Abrahams JS, Bentley FR, Garrison RN. In vivo assessment of videomicroscopy of acute renal microvascular responses to cyclosporine. *Br J Surg* 1992;79:1187.

536. Bantle JP, et al. Long-term effects of cyclosporine on renal function in organ transplant recipients. *J Lab Clin Med* 1990;115:233.

537. Davis LS, et al. Effects of selective endothelin antagonists on the hemodynamic response to cyclosporine A. *J Am Soc Nephrol* 1994;4:1448.

538. Zachariae H, et al. Morphologic renal changes during cyclosporine treatment of psoriasis. Studies on pretreatment and posttreatment kidney biopsy specimens. *J Am Acad Dermatol* 1992;26:415.

539. Kahan BD. Cyclosporine nephrotoxicity: pathogenesis, prophylaxis, therapy and prognosis. *Am J Kidney Dis* 1986;8:323.

540. Rao KV, Crasson JT, Kjellstrand JM. Chronic irreversible nephrotoxicity from cyclosporine A. *Nephron* 1985;41:75.

541. Mihatsch MJ, Ryffel B, Gudat F. Morphological criteria of chronic rejection: differential diagnosis, including cyclosporine nephropathy. *Transplant Proc* 1993;25:2031.

542. Mihatsch MJ, et al. Cyclosporine A nephropathy: standardization of the evaluation of kidney biopsies. *Clin Nephrol* 1994;41:23.

543. Strøm EH, Thiel G, Mihatsch MJ. Prevalence of cyclosporine-associated arteriolopathy in renal transplant biopsies from 1981 to 1992. *Transplant Proc* 1994;26:2585.

544. Solez K, et al. Histopathologic findings from 2-year protocol biopsies from a U.S. multicenter kidney transplant trial comparing tacrolimus versus cyclosporine: a report of the FK506 Kidney Transplant Study Group. *Transplantation* 1998;66:1736.

545. Klintmalm G, et al. Interstitial fibrosis in renal allografts after 12 to 46 months of cyclosporine treatment: beneficial effects of lower doses early after transplantation. In: Klintmalm G, ed. *Cyclosporine A nephrotoxicity in human transplant patients. Clinical, pharmacological and morphological findings.* Stockholm: Repro Print AB, 1984:215.

546. Myers BD, et al. Chronic injury of human renal microvessels with low-dose cyclosporine therapy. *Transplantation* 1988;46:694.

547. Keown PA, Stiller CR, Wallace AC. Nephrotoxicity of cyclosporine A. In: Williams GM, Burchick JF, Solez K, eds. *Kidney transplant rejection: diagnosis and treatment.* New York: Marcel Dekker, 1986:423.

548. Myers BD, Newton L. Cyclosporine-induced chronic renal nephropathy: an obliterative microvascular renal injury. *J Am Soc Nephrol* 1991;2:S45.

549. Greenberg A, et al. Cyclosporine nephrotoxicity in cardiac allograft patients. A seven-year follow-up. *Transplantation* 1990;50:589.

550. Solomon D. Cyclosporine nephrotoxicity and long-term renal transplantation. *Transplant Rev* 1992;6:10.

551. Calne R. Cyclosporine in cadaveric renal transplantation: 5-year follow-up of a multicentre trial. *Lancet* 1987;2:506.

552. The Canadian Multicentre Transplant Study Group. A randomized clinical trial of cyclosporine in cadaveric renal transplantation: analysis at three years. *N Engl J Med* 1986;314:1219.

553. Hollander AA, van Saase JL, Kootte AM. Beneficial effects of conversion from cyclosporine to azathioprin after kidney transplantation. *Lancet* 1995;345:610.

554. Nankivell BJ, et al. The natural history of chronic allograft nephropathy. *N Engl J Med* 2003;349:2326.

555. Katznelson S, et al. Cyclosporine-induced hemolytic uremic syndrome: factors that obscure its diagnosis. *Transplant Proc* 1994;26:2608.

556. Racusen LC, Solez K. Nephrotoxicity of cyclosporine and other immunosuppressive and immunotherapeutic agents. In: Hook IB, Goldstein RS, eds. *Toxicology of the kidney*, 2nd ed. New York: Raven, 1993:319.

557. Karthikeyan V, et al. Outcome of plasma exchange therapy in thrombotic microangiopathy after renal transplantation. *Am J Transplant* 2003;3:1289.

558. Brown Z, et al. Increased factor VIII as an index of vascular injury in cyclosporine nephrotoxicity. *Transplantation* 1986;42:150.

559. Verpooten GA, et al. Elevated plasminogen activator inhibitor levels in cyclosporine-treated renal allograft recipients. *Nephrol Dial Transplant* 1996;11:347.

560. Jegasothy BV, et al. Tacrolimus (FK506)—a new therapeutic agent for severe recalcitrant psoriasis. *Arch Dermatol* 1992;128:781.

561. Thomson AW, et al. FK506: a novel immunosuppressant for treatment of autoimmune disease: rationale and preliminary clinical exposure at the University of Pittsburgh. *Springer Semin Immunopathol* 1993;14:323.

562. Starzl TE. FK506 versus cyclosporine. *Transplant Proc* 1993;25:511.

563. McCauley J. The nephrotoxicity of FK506 as compared with cyclosporine. *Curr Opin Nephrol Hypertens* 1993;2:662.

564. Whiting PH. Acute and chronic nephrotoxicity associated with immunosuppressive drugs. *Curr Opin Nephrol Hypertens* 1994;3:174.

565. Starzl TE, Makowka L, Todo S, eds. First International Congress on FK506 (August 21–24, 1991, Pittsburgh, PA). *Transplant Proc* 1991;23:2709.

566. Siekierka J, Sigal N. FK506 and cyclosporine A: immunosuppressive mechanism of action and beyond. *Curr Opin Immunol* 1992;4:548.

567. Morris RE. Prime on new small molecule immunosuppressants. *Transplant Soc Bull* 1993;1:15.

568. Morris RE. New small molecule immunosuppressants for transplantation: review of essential concepts. *J Heart Lung Transplant* 1993;12:S275.

569. Schwaninger M, et al. The immunosuppressive drugs cyclosporine A and FK506 inhibit calcineurin phosphatase activity and gene transcription mediated through the cAMP-responsive element in a nonimmune cell line. *Naunyn Schmiedebergs Arch Pharmacol* 1993;348:541.

570. Migita K, et al. FK506 augments activation-induced programmed cell death of T lymphocytes in vivo. *J Clin Invest* 1995;96:727.

571. McCauley J, et al. Cyclosporine and FK506 induced inhibition of renal epithelial cell proliferation. *Transplant Proc* 1991;23:2829.

572. Moutabarrik A, et al. FK 506 induced kidney tubular cell injury. *Transplantation* 1992;54:1041.

573. Yatscoff RW, Fryer J, Thliveris JA. Comparison of the effect of rapamycin and FK-506 on release of prostacyclin and endothelin in vitro. *Clin Biochem* 1993;26:409.

574. Benigni A, et al. The acute effect of FK506 and cyclosporine on endothelial cell function and renal vascular resistance. *Transplantation* 1992;54:775.

575. Atcherson MM, Trifillis AL. Cytotoxic effects of FK506 on human renal proximal tubule cells in culture. *In Vitro Cell Dev Biol Anim* 1994;30A:562.

576. Edkins RD, Rybak LP, Hoffman DW. Comparison of cyclosporine and FK506 effects on glutathione levels in cochlea, brain, liver and kidney. *Biochem Pharmacol* 1992;43:911.

577. Ali Shah I, et al. Effects of FK506 on human hepatic microsomal cytochrome P-450 dependent drug metabolism in vitro. *Transplant Proc* 1991;23:2783.

578. Yoshimura R, et al. Effects of rapamycin on renal microsomal P-450 systems in the rat. *Transplant Proc* 1993;25:750.

579. Yoshimura R, et al. The effect of immunosuppressive agents (FK-506, rapamycin) on renal P450 systems in rat models. *J Pharm Pharmacol* 1999;51(8):941.

580. Epstein M. Calcium antagonist and renal protection. *Arch Intern Med* 1992;152:1573.

581. Weir MR. Therapeutic benefits of calcium channel blockers in cyclosporine-treated organ transplant recipients: blood pressure control and immunosuppression. *Am J Med* 1991;90:32S.

582. Prasad SJ, et al. In vitro effects of cyclosporine and FK506 on the renal cortex. *Transplant Proc* 1991;23:3128.

583. Jayaraman T, et al. FK506 binding protein associated with the calcium release channel (Ryanodine receptor). *J Biol Chem* 1992;267:9474.

584. Aperia A, et al. Calcineurin mediates alpha-adrenergic stimulation of Na^+, $K(+)$-ATPase activity in renal tubule cells. *Proc Natl Acad Sci USA* 1992;89:7394.

585. Palevsky P, et al. FK506 inhibits aldosterone-stimulated sodium transplant in A6 cells. *J Am Soc Nephrol* 1992;3:846(abst).

586. Andoh TF, et al. Enhancement of FK506 nephrotoxicity by sodium depletion. *Nephrol Dial Transplant* 1993;8:1034(abst).

587. Bennett WM, et al. Nephrotoxicity of immunosuppressive drugs. *Miner Electrolyte Metab* 1994;20:214.

588. Starzl TE, eds. First International Workshop on FK506: a potential breakthrough in immunosuppression. *Transplant Proc* 1987;29(Suppl):3.

589. McCauley J, et al. The effects of FK506 on renal function after liver transplantation. *Transplant Proc* 1990;22:17.

590. Ueda D, et al. Influence of FK506 on renal blood flow. *Transplant Proc* 1991;23:3121.

591. Kumano K, Endo T, Kashiba K. Functional and morphological changes in rat kidney induced by FK506 and its reversal by various vasodilators (in Japanese). *Nippon Hinyokika Gakkai Zasshi* 1992;83:650.

592. Lieberman KV, Lin WG, Reisman L. FK506 is a direct glomeruloconstrictor, as determined by electrical resistance pulse sizing. *Transplant Proc* 1991;23:3119.

593. Mitamura T, et al. Tacrolimus (FK506)-induced nephrotoxicity in spontaneous hypertensive rats. *J Toxicol Sci* 1994;19:219.

594. Ryffel B, Weber E, Mihatsch MJ. Nephrotoxicity of immunosuppressants in rats: comparison of macrolides with cyclosporine. *Exp Nephrol* 1994;2:324.

595. Andoh TF, et al. Comparison of acute rapamycin nephrotoxicity with cyclosporine and FK506. *Kidney Int* 1996;50:1110.

596. Hara S, et al. The effects of a new immunosuppressive agent, FK506, on the glomerular injury in rats with accelerated nephrotoxic serum glomerulonephritis. *Clin Immunol Immunopathol* 1990;57:351.

597. Starzl TE, et al. Kidney transplantation under FK506. *JAMA* 1990; 264:63.

598. Shapiro R, et al. FK506 in clinical kidney transplantation. *Transplant Proc* 1991;23:3065.

599. McDiarmid SV, et al. FK506 (tacrolimus) compared with cyclosporine for primary immunosuppression after pediatric liver transplantation. Results from the U.S. Multicenter Trial. *Transplantation* 1995;59:530.

600. Neuhaus P, et al. Comparison of FK-506- and cyclosporine-based immunosuppression in primary orthotopic liver transplantion: a single center experience. *Transplantation* 1995;59:31.

601. Pirsch JD, et al. A comparison of tacrolimus (FK-506) and cyclosporine for immunosuppression after cadaveric renal transplantation. FK 506 Kidney Transplant Study Group. *Transplantation* 1997;63:977.

602. Mayer AD, et al. Multicenter randomized trial comparing tacrolimus (FK 506) and cyclosporine in the prevention of renal allograft rejection: A report of the European Tacrolimus Multicenter Renal Study Group. *Transplantation* 1997;64:436.

603. Ahsan N, et al. Randomized trial of tacrolimus plus mycophenolate mofetil or azathioprine versus cyclosporine oral solution (modified) plus mycophenolate mofetil after cadaveric kidney transplantation: results at two years. *Transplantation* 2001;72:245.

604. English RF, et al. Long-term comparison of tacrolimus- and cyclosporine-induced nephrotoxicity in pediatric heart-transplant recipients. *Am J Transplant* 2002;2:769.

605. Gonwa T, et al. Randomized trial of tacrolimus + mycophenolate mofetil or azathioprine versus cyclosporine + mycophenolate mofetil after cadaveric kidney transplantation: results at three years. *Transplantation* 2003;75:2048.

606. Vincenti F, et al. A long-term comparison of tacrolimus (FK 506) and cyclosporine in kidney transplantation : evidence for improved graft survival at five years. *Transplantation* 2002;73:775.

607. Dello Strologo L, et al. Renal hemodynamic effect of tacrolimus in renal transplanted children. *Pediatr Nephrol* 2001;16:773.

608. Randhawa PS, et al. The histopathological changes associated with allograft rejection and drug toxicity in renal transplant recipients maintained on FK 506 Clinical significance and comparison with cyclosporine. *Am J Surg Pathol* 1993;17:60.

609. Kyo M, et al. Morphological findings in non-episode biopsies of kidney transplant allografts treated with FK-506 or cyclosporine. *Transpl Int* 1998;11:S100.

610. Hatori M, et al. Clinical and histopathological examination of renal allografts treated with tacrolimus (FK 506) for at least one year. *Int J Urol* 1998;5:526.

611. Toz H, et al. Comparison of tacrolimus and cyclosporine in renal transplantation by the protocol biopsies. *Transplant Proc* 2004;36:134.

612. Khanna A, et al. Expression of TGF-beta and fibrogenic genes in transplant recipients with tacrolimus and cyclosporine nephrotoxicity. *Kidney Int* 2002;62:2257.

613. Goldstein G. Overview of the development of Orthoclone OKT3: monoclonal antibody for therapeutic use in transplantation. *Transplant Proc* 1987;19(Suppl 1):1.

614. Van Wauwe J, De Mey J, Goossens J. OKT3: a monoclonal antibody with potent mitogenic properties. *J Immunol* 1980;124:2708.

615. Abramowicz D, et al. Release of tumor necrosis factor, interleukin-2, and gamma-interferon in serum after injection of OKT3 monoclonal antibody in kidney transplant recipients. *Transplantation* 1989;47:606.

616. Chatenoud L, et al. Systemic reaction to the anti-T-cell monoclonal antibody OKT3 in relation to serum levels of tumor necrosis factor and interferon-gamma. *N Engl J Med* 1989;320:1420.

617. Chatenoud L, et al. In vivo cell activation following OKT3 administration. *Transplantation* 1990;49:697.

618. Bloemena E, et al. Kinetics of interleukin 6 during OKT3 treatment in renal allograft recipients. *Transplantation* 1990;50:330.

619. Gaston RS, et al. OKT3 first-dose reaction: association with T cell subsets and cytokine release. *Kidney Int* 1991;39:141.

620. Goldman M, et al. Induction of interleukin-6 and interleukin-10 by the OKT3 monoclonal antibody: possible relevance to posttransplant lympho-proliferative disorders. *Clin Transplant* 1992;6:265.

621. Ferran C, et al. Anti-tumor necrosis factor modulates anti-CD3-triggered T cell cytokine gene expression in vivo. *J Clin Invest* 1994;93:2189.

622. Alegre M, et al. Hypothermia and hypoglycemia induced by anti-CD3 mon-oclonal antibody in mice: role of tumor necrosis factor. *Eur J Immunol* 1990;20:707.

623. Ferran C, et al. Cascade modulation by anti-tumor necrosis factor mono-clonal antibody of interferon-gamma, interleukin 3 and interleukin 6 re-lease after triggering of the CD3/T cell receptor activation pathway. *Eur J Immunol* 1991;21:2349.

624. Matthys P, et al. Modification of the anti-CD3-induced cytokine release syndrome by anti-interferon-gamma or anti-interleukin-6 antibody treat-ment: protective effects of biphasic changes in blood cytokine levels. *Eur J Immunol* 1993;23:2209.

625. Mackie JD, et al. Dose-related mechanisms of immunosuppression me-diated by murine anti-CD3 monoclonal antibody in pancreatic islet cell transplantation and delayed-type hypersensitivity. *Transplantation* 1990;49:1150.

626. Waid TH, et al. Treatment of acute cellular rejection with T10B9-1A-31 or OKT3 in renal allograft recipients. *Transplantation* 1992;53:80.

627. Toussaint C, et al. Possible nephrotoxicity of the prophylactic use of OKT3 monoclonal antibody after cadaveric renal transplantation. *Transplanta-tion* 1989;48:524.

628. Pesgovitz MD, et al. Corticosteroid inhibition of the OKT3-induced febrile and nephrotoxic responses during treatment of renal allograft rejection. *Clin Transplant* 1993;7:529.

629. Goldman M, et al. OKT3-induced cytokine release attenuation by high-dose methylprednisolone. *Lancet* 1989;2:802.

630. Simpson MA, et al. Sequential determinations of urinary cytology and plasma and urinary lymphokines in the management of renal allograft re-cipients. *Transplantation* 1989;47:218.

631. Batiuk T, Bennett W, Norman D. Cytokine nephropathy during anti-lymphocyte therapy. *Transplant Proc* 1993;25:27.

632. Goldman M, et al. Evolution of renal function during treatment of kid-ney graft rejection with OKT3 monoclonal antibody. *Transplantation* 1990;50:158.

633. Rosenstein M, Ettinghausen SE, Rosenberg SA. Extravasation of intravas-cular fluid mediated by the systemic administration of recombinant inter-leukin 2. *J Immunol* 1986;137:1735.

634. Rosenberg SA, et al. Use of tumor-infiltrating lymphocytes and interleukin-2 in the immunotherapy of patients with metastatic melanoma. A preliminary report. *N Engl J Med* 1988;319:1676.

635. Thervet E, et al. First dose OKT3-induced release of endothelin in renal transplant recipients. *Nephrol Dial Transplant* 1993;8:287.

636. Maessen JG, Buurman WA, Koostra G. Direct cytotoxic effect of cytokines in kidney parenchyma: a possible mechanism of allograft destruction. *Transplant Proc* 1989;21:309.

637. Heemann UW, et al. Early events in acute allograft rejection: leuko-cyte/endothelial cell interactions. *Clin Transplant* 1993;7:82.

638. Kelly KJ, et al. Antibody to intercellular adhesion molecule 1 protects against ischemic injury. *Proc Natl Acad Sci USA* 1994;91:812.

639. Ghielli M, et al. Inflammatory cells in renal regeneration. *Ren Fail* 1996; 18(3):355.

640. Abramowicz D, et al. Induction of thromboses within renal grafts by high-dose prophylactic OKT3. *Lancet* 1992;339:777.

641. Palleschi J, et al. Vascular complications of renal transplantation. *Urology* 1980;16:61.

642. Groggel GC. Acute thrombosis of the renal transplant artery: a case report and review of the literature. *Clin Nephrol* 1991;36:42.

643. Pradier O, et al. Procoagulant effect of the OKT3 monoclonal antibody: involvement of tumor necrosis factor. *Kidney Int* 1992;42:1124.

644. Raasveld MH, Hack CE, ten Berge I. Activation of coagulation and fibri-nolysis following OKT3 administration to renal transplant recipients: as-sociation with distinct mediators. *Thromb Haemost* 1992;68:264.

645. Abramowicz D, et al. High-dose glucocorticosteroids increase the proco-agulant effects of OKT3. *Kidney Int* 1994;46:1596.

646. Pradier O, et al. Procoagulant properties of OKT3 at the monocyte level: inhibition of pentoxifylline. *Transplant Proc* 1993;25:39.

647. Nawroth PP, Stern DM. Modulation of endothelial cell hemostatic proper-ties by tumor necrosis factor. *J Exp Med* 1986;163:740.

648. Itaka M, et al. Induction of monocyte procoagulant activity with OKT3 antibody. *J Immunol* 1987;139:1617.

649. Carlsen E, Flatmark A, Prydz H. Cytokine-induced procoagulant activity in monocytes and endothelial cells. Further enhancement by cyclosporine. *Transplantation* 1988;64:575.

650. Ryan J, Geczy CL. Characterization and purification of mouse macrophage procoagulant-inducing factor. *J Immunol* 1986;137:2864.

651. Gregory SA, et al. Monocyte procoagulant inducing factor: a lymphokine involved in the T cell-instructed monocyte procoagulant response to anti-gen. *J Immunol* 1986;137:3231.

652. Fan ST, Edgington TS. Clonal analysis of mechanisms of murine T helper cell collaboration with effector cells of macrophage lineage. *J Immunol* 1988;141:1819.

653. Konkle BA, et al. Plasminogen activator inhibitor-1 messenger RNA ex-pression is induced in rat hepatocytes in vivo by dexamethasone. *Blood* 1992;79:2636.

654. Vassalli JD, Hamilton J, Reich E. Macrophage plasminogen activator: mod-ulation of enzyme production by anti-inflammatory steroids, mitototic in-hibitors, and cyclic nucleotides. *Cell* 1976;8:271.

655. Blajchman MA, et al. Shortening of bleeding time in rabbits by hydrocor-tisone caused by inhibition of prostacyclin generation by the vessel wall. *J Clin Invest* 1979;63:1026.

656. Lewis GD, Campbell WB, Johnson AR. Inhibition of prostaglandin synthesis by glucocorticoids in human endothelial cells. *Endocrinology* 1986;119:62.

657. Knowles RG, et al. Anti-inflammatory glucocorticoids inhibit the induction by endotoxin of nitric oxide synthase in the lung, liver and aorta of the rat. *Biochem Biophys Res Commun* 1990;172:1042.

658. Geller DA, et al. Cytokines, endotoxin, and glucocorticoids regulate the expression of inducible nitric oxide synthase in hepatocytes. *Proc Natl Acad Sci USA* 1993;90:522.

659. Nawroth PP, et al. Interleukin 1 induces endothelial cell procoagulant while suppressing cell-surface anticoagulant activity. *Proc Natl Acad Sci USA* 1986;83:3460.

660. Wu KK. Endothelial cells in hemostasis, thrombosis, and inflammation. *Hosp Pract (Off Ed)* 1992;27:145.

661. Wever PC, et al. OKT3-induced nephrotoxicity is associated with release of group II secretory phospholipase A2. *Eur J Clin Invest* 1996;26(10):873.

662. Alegre M, et al. Cytokine release syndrome induced by the 145-2C11 anti-CD3 monoclonal antibody in mice: prevention by high doses of methyl-prednisolone. *J Immunol* 1991;146:1184.

663. Leo O, et al. Identification of a monoclonal antibody specific for a murine T3 polypeptide. *Proc Natl Acad Sci USA* 1987;84:1374.

664. Ferran C, et al. Cytokine-related syndrome following injection of anti-CD3 monoclonal antibody: further evidence for transient in vivo T cell activa-tion. *Eur J Immunol* 1990;20:509.

665. Abramowicz D, et al. Prevention of OKT3 nephrotoxicity after kidney transplantation. *Kidney Int* 1996;49(Suppl 53):S39.

666. Alegre M, et al. A non-activating "humanized" anti-CD3 monoclonal antibody retains immunosuppressive properties in vivo. *Transplantation* 1994;57:1537.

667. Nashan B, et al. Randomised trial of basiliximab versus placebo for control of acute cellular rejection in renal allograft recipients. CHIB 201 Interna-tional Study Group. *Lancet* 1997;350:1193.

668. Vincenti F, Nashan B, Light S. Daclizumab: outcome of phase III trials and mechanism of action. Double Therapy and the Triple Therapy Study Groups. *Transplant Proc* 1998;30(5):2155.

669. Vincenti F, et al. A phase I trial of humanized anti-interleukin 2 receptor antibody in renal transplantation. *Transplantation* 1997;63(1):33.

670. Vincenti F, et al. Interleukin-2-receptor blockade with daclizumab to pre-vent acute rejection in renal transplantation. Daclizumab Triple Therapy Study Group. *N Engl J Med* 1998;338(3):161.

671. Charpentier B, Thervet E. Placebo-controlled study of a humanized anti-TAC monoclonal antibody in dual therapy for prevention of acute rejection after renal transplantation. *Transplant Proc* 1998;30(4):1331.

672. Morris RE, et al. Mycophenolic acid morpholinoethylester (RS-6134) is a new immunosuppressant that prevents and halts heart allograft rejection by selective inhibition of T and B cell purine synthesis. *Transplant Proc* 1990;22:1659.

673. Platz DP, et al. RS-61443 reverses acute allograft rejection in dogs. *Surgery* 1991;110:736.

674. Gummert JF, Ikonen T, Morris RE. Newer immunosuppressive drugs: a review. *J Am Soc Nephrol* 1999;10:1366.

675. The Tricontinental Mycophenolate Mofetil Renal Transplantation Study Group. A blinded, randomized clinical trial of mycophenolate mofetil for the prevention of acute rejection in cadaveric renal transplantation. *Trans-plantation* 1996;61(7):1029.

676. European Mycophenolate Mofetil Cooperative Study Group. Placebo-controlled study of mycophenolate mofetil combined with cyclosporine and corticosteroids for prevention of acute rejection. *Lancet* 1995;345:1321.

677. Sollinger HW (for the U. S. Renal Transplant Mycophenolate Mofetil Study Group). Mycophenolate mofetil for the prevention of acute rejection in primary cadaveric renal allograft recipients. *Transplantation* 1995;60:225.

678. Aleksic I, et al. Improvement of impaired renal function in heart transplant recipients treated with mycophenolate mofetil and low-dose cyclosporine. *Transplantation* 2000;69(8):1586.

679. Torras J, et al. Mycophenolate mofetil overlap in liver transplant recipients with chronic cyclosporine nephrotoxicity. *Transplant. Proc* 1999;31(6):2430.

680. Soccal PM, et al. Improvement of drug-induced chronic renal failure in lung transplantation. *Transplantation* 1999;68(1):164.

681. Gruessner RW, et al. Mycophenolate mofetil in pancreas transplantation. *Transplantation* 1998;66(3):318.

682. Halloran P, et al. Mycophenolate mofetil in renal allograft recipients: a pooled efficacy analysis of three randomized, double-blind, clinical studies in prevention of rejection. The International Mycophenolate Renal Trans-plant Study Group. *Transplantation* 1997;63:39.

683. Weir MR, et al. A novel approach to the treatment of chronic allograft nephropathy. *Transplantation* 1997;64(12):1706.
684. Hueso M, et al. Low-dose cyclosporine and mycophenolate mofetil in renal allograft recipients with suboptimal renal function. *Transplantation* 1998;66(12):1727.
685. Mourad G, et al. Long-term improvement in renal function after cyclosporine reduction in renal transplant recipients with histologically proven chronic cyclosporine nephropathy. *Transplantation* 1998;65(5):661.
686. Schrama YC, et al. Conversion to mycophenolate mofetil in conjunction with stepwise withdrawal of cyclosporine in stable renal transplant recipients. *Transplantation* 2000;69:376.
687. Abramowicz D, et al. Cyclosporine withdrawal from a mycophenolate mofetil-containing immunosuppressive regimen in stable kidney transplant recipients: a randomized, controlled study. *Transplantation* 2002;74(12):1725
688. Schnuelle P, et al. Open randomized trial comparing early withdrawal of either cyclosporine or mycophenolate mofetil in stable renal transplant recipients initially treated with a triple drug regimen. *J Am Soc Nephrol* 2002;13:536.
689. Suwelack B, et al. Withdrawal of cyclosporine or tacrolimus after addition of mycophenolate mofetil in patients with chronic allograft nephropathy. *Am J Transplant* 2004;4:655.
690. Hauser IA, Sterzel RB. Mycophenolate mofetil: therapeutic applications in kidney transplantation and immune-mediated renal disease. *Curr Opin Nephrol Hypertens* 1999;8(1):1.
691. Briggs WA, Choi MJ, Scheel PJ. Successful mycophenolate mofetil treatment of glomerular disease. *Am J Kidney Dis* 1998;31:213.
692. Briggs WA, Choi MJ, Scheel PJ. Follow-up on mycophenolate treatment of glomerular disease (Letter). *Am J Kidney Dis* 1998;32:898.
693. de Mattos AM, Olyaei AJ, Bennett WM. Nephrotoxicity of immunosuppressive drugs: long-term consequences and challenges for the future. *Am J Kidney Dis* 2000;35:333.
694. Vezina C, et al. Rapamycin, a new antifungal antibiotic. Taxonomy of the producing Streptomycete and isolation of the active principle. *J Antibiot* (Tokyo) 1975;28:721.
695. Sehgal SN. Rapamune (sirolimus, rapamycin). An overview and mechanism of action. *Ther Drug Monit* 1995;17:660.
696. Chiu MI, et al. RAPT1, a mammalian homologue of yeast TOR interacts with the FKBP12-rapamycin complex. *Proc Natl Acad Sci USA* 1994;91:12574.
697. Terada N, et al. Rapamycin blocks cell cycle progression of activated T-cells prior to events characteristic of the middle to late G1 phase of the cell cycle. *J Cell Physiol* 1993;268:22825.
698. Sehgal SN. Rapamune: mechanism of action immunosuppressive effects results from blockade of signal transduction and inhibition of cell cycle progression. *Clin Biochem* 1998;31:335.
699. Aaguaard-Tillery KM, et al. Inhibition of human B lymphocyte cell cycle progression and differentiation by rapamycin. *Cell Immunol* 1994;152:493.
700. Kahan BD, et al. Synergistic interactions of cyclosporine and rapamycin to inhibit immune performances of normal human peripheral blood leukocytes in vitro. *Transplantation* 1991;51:87.
701. Dumont FJ, et al. The immunosuppressive macrolides FK506 and rapamycin act as reciprocal antagonists in murine T cells. *J Immunol* 1990; 144:1418.
702. Calne R, et al. Rapamycin for immunosuppression in organ allografting. *Lancet* 1989;2:227.
703. Stepkowski SM, Kahan BD. Rapamycin and cyclosporine synergistically prolong heart and kidney allograft survival. *Transplant Proc* 1991;23:3262.
704. Vu MD, et al. Tacrolimus and sirolimus in combination are not antagonistic but produce extended graft survival in cardiac transplantation in the rat. *Transplantation* 1997;64:1853.
705. Saunders RN, et al. Rapamycin in renal transplantation: a review of the evidence. *Kidney Int* 2001;59:3.
706. Groth CG, et al. Sirolimus (rapamycin)-based therapy in human renal transplantation: similar efficacy and different toxicity compared with cyclosporine. Sirolimus European Renal Transplant Study Group. *Transplantation* 1999;67:1036.
707. Kreis H, et al. Sirolimus in association with mycophenolate mofetil induction for the prevention of acute graft rejection in renal allograft recipients. *Transplantation* 2000;69:1252.
708. Flechner SM, et al. Kidney transplantation without calcineurin inhibitor drugs: prospective, randomized trial of sirolimus versus cyclosporine. *Transplantation* 2002;74:1070.
709. Flechner SM, et al. De novo kidney transplantation without use of calcineurin inhibitors preserves renal structure and function at two years. *Am J Transpl* 2004;4:1776.
710. Johnson RW, et al. Sirolimus allows early cyclosporine withdrawal in renal transplantation resulting in improved renal function and low blood pressure. *Transplantation* 2001;72:777.
711. Gonwa TA, et al. Improved renal function in sirolimus-treated renal transplant patients after early cyclosporine elimination. *Transplantation* 2002;74:1560.
712. Oberbauer R, et al. Long-term improvement in renal function with sirolimus after early cyclosporine withdrawal in renal transplant recipients: two year results of the Rapamune Maintenance Regimen Study. *Transplantation* 2003;76:364.
713. Ruiz JC, et al. Early Cyclosporine A withdrawal in kidney-transplant recipients receiving sirolimus prevents progression of chronic pathologic lesions. *Transplantation* 2004;78:1312.
714. Ryffel B, et al. Nephrotoxicity of immunosuppressants in rats: comparison of macrolides with cyclosporine. *Exp Nephrol* 1994;2:324.
715. Goldbaekdal K, et al. Effects of rapamycin on renal hemodynamics, water and sodium excretion and plasma levels of angiotensin II, aldosterone, atrial natriuretic peptide, and vasopressin in pigs. *Transplantation* 1994;58:1153.
716. Andoh TF, et al. Comparison of acute rapamycin nephrotoxicity with cyclosporine and FK506. *Kidney Int* 1996;50:1110.
717. Andoh TF, et al. Synergistic effects of cyclosporine and rapamycin in a chronic nephrotoxicity model. *Transplantation* 1996;62:311.
718. McTaggart RA, et al. Sirolimus prolongs recovery from delayed graft function after cadaveric renal transplantation. *Am J Transplant* 2003;3:416.
719. Paramesh AS, et al. Thrombotic microangiopathy associated with combined sirolimus and tacrolimus immunosuppression after intestinal transplantation. *Transplantation* 2004;77:129.
720. Butani L. Investigation of pediatric renal transplant recipients with heavy proteinuria after sirolimus rescue. *Transplantation* 2004;78:1362.
721. Daniel C, et al. Proinflammatory effects in experimental mesangial proliferative glomerulonephritis of the immunosuppressive agent SDZ RAD, a rapamycin derivative. *Exp Nephrol* 2000;8:52.

CHAPTER 43 ■ RENAL DISEASES INDUCED BY ANTINEOPLASTIC AGENTS

ROBERT L. SAFIRSTEIN

Treatment of previously resistant tumors with potent cytoreductive therapies for cure is now common clinical practice. Often this entails the use of nephrotoxic chemotherapeutic agents at high doses and in combinations that potentiate their ability to damage the kidney. In this setting, acute renal failure (ARF) has become an anticipated side effect of treatment along with the depressed hematopoiesis. Recent surveys of the incidence of ARF within hospitalized patients note that nearly 20% of such cases are due to antineoplastic therapy (1). This chapter reviews what is known about the nephrotoxicity of antineoplastic drugs, used alone or in combination with other nephrotoxic agents. The goal of this review is to rationalize therapy to prevent as much damage to the kidney as possible because, in almost all studies to date, acute renal failure, when it occurs, carries a grave prognosis for the patient with cancer.

FACTORS THAT POTENTIATE RENAL FAILURE IN PATIENTS WITH CANCER

Extracellular Volume Depletion and Diminished Effective Arterial Circulating Volume

The clinical context in which an anticancer drug is given contributes greatly to its nephrotoxic potential. Extracellular volume depletion as a consequence of nausea, vomiting, or diarrhea should always be suspected in patients with cancer. Fluid sequestered outside the vascular space, as might occur in peritonitis, bowel obstruction, and malignant effusion may also be present. Hepatobiliary disease and heart failure, both of which may be a consequence of the cancer or its treatment, also seem to potentiate nephrotoxicity. The ability of the renal circulation to respond normally to volume depletion may also be significantly impaired by the concurrent use of drugs that inhibit renal cyclooxygenase activity to achieve pain relief or diminish fever. To the extent that it is possible, steps should be taken to restore the circulation prior to the introduction of nephrotoxins and to stop these agents before antineoplastic treatment is instituted.

Patients with Cancer and Intrinsic Renal Disease

As will be seen, any preexisting decrease in renal function, even minor, contributes greatly to the incidence and severity of renal failure during antineoplastic therapy. In some cases, this may be a consequence of altered pharmacokinetics of drugs excreted primarily by the kidney, but in other circumstances, the reason for the potentiation is less clear. Recognition of underlying re-

nal disease, therefore, is important in cancer patients. Indeed renal failure may be provoked by characteristics unique to the specific nature of the cancer. For example, the invasion of the ureters by tumors of the ovary and cervix or the obstruction of the ureters caused by retroperitoneal fibrosis provoked by breast cancer is not uncommon.

Minor degrees of renal dysfunction, often recognized only on retrospective analysis of treatment-related nephrotoxicity, are a risk factor in the development of renal failure following chemotherapy (2). Prior chemotherapy and exposure to radiocontrast dyes, which provoke minor, and sometimes overlooked, renal injury are often the culprits. Prior radiation therapy is an important contributing factor because the dose of radiation necessary to damage kidneys is less when administered together with other cytoreductive drugs (3). Hypercalcemia, hyperphosphatemia, and hyperuricemia, as well as high blood concentrations of myoglobin, hemoglobin, and light chains, may all provoke renal failure. The clinical status of the patient also impacts on outcome. Infection and prolonged immobilization and their relationship to rhabdomyolysis, the use of hyperalimentation and subsequent hypophosphatemia, incompatible blood transfusions, and marrow infusion injury, all may occur during the course of therapy and impact negatively on renal function. Invasion of the kidney parenchyma with tumor is rarely a cause of renal failure, but renal failure has been reported with massive invasion of lymphomatous cells (4). The immunocompromised cancer patient is frequently infected and exposed to nephrotoxic antibiotics that can damage the kidney, and pyelonephritis-induced renal failure has been reported in such cases even in the absence of nephrotoxic drugs (5).

Urinary Tract Obstruction and Patients with Cancer

Ureteral and bladder outlet obstruction always need to be considered in the cancer patient, not only under the obvious circumstances of tumor invasion and obstruction in cancer of the urinary bladder, prostate, and cervix, but also ureteral obstruction due to stones and blood clot or to retroperitoneal fibrosis associated with malignancy locally and elsewhere (6). These complications often go unrecognized because of the asymmetric nature of the involvement.

Chronic Renal Failure and Patients with Cancer

Glomerular abnormalities are common in patients with cancer. Principal among them is membranous glomerulopathy, which may be associated with cancer in 10% of all patients with such nephropathy (7) and as high as 22% in older patients (8). As many as 50% of patients with multiple myeloma have renal

TABLE 43-1

NEPHROTIC ANTINEOPLASTIC AGENTS

Alkylating agents	Antimetabolites	Antitumor antibiotics	Biologic agents
Cisplatin	High-dose methotrexate	Mitomycin	Recombinant interferon-α and interferon-γ
Carboplatin	Cytosine arabinoside	Mithramycin	Interleukin-2
Cyclophosphamide	5-Fluorouracil		
Nitrosoureas	5-Azacytidine		
Carmustine (BCNU)			
Lomustine (CCNU)			
Semustine (methyl CCNU)			
Streptozocin			
Ifosfamide			

failure and nephrotic syndrome with κ or λ light chains in the urine, frequently with primary amyloidosis in the kidney (9). The paraproteinemic syndromes associated with cancers of the hematopoietic system, such as macroglobulinemia and cryoglobulinemia, may also be associated with glomerular abnormalities (10). These paraproteins may be produced in such large quantities that they exceed the ability of the tubules to reabsorb them sufficiently to prevent the formation of proteinaceous casts that obstruct the flow of urine and cause further decline in glomerular filtration. This so-called "cast nephropathy" is also associated with glomerular abnormalities.

Interstitial renal disease is also common in patients with cancer. Recurrent serious infections in the immunocompromised host requiring chronic exposure to potentially nephrotoxic antibiotics can cause damage to the kidney. Treatment with high-energy radiation may cause renal failure with hypertension, proteinuria, and profound anemia (11). The renal failure may not develop for years after exposure and occurs in patients exposed to greater than 20 Gy (2,000 rads) of high-energy radiation to both kidneys.

Fluid and Electrolyte Disorders Associated with Cancer

A variety of electrolyte disorders occur in the background of cancer. Hypophosphatemia with renal phosphate loss and osteomalacia can occur with mesenchymal tumors (12). The syndrome remits when the tumor is removed, which suggests the production of a phosphaturic substance by the tumor. Hyponatremia is associated with a number of tumors including small cell cancer of the lung (13) and various head and neck tumors (14). Hypokalemia and hypophosphatemia may occur together in cancer patients and, although rare, may be so severe that they induce rhabdomyolysis and acute renal failure. In a recent report, 16% of patients with small cell lung cancer had hyponatremia and had shorter survival than patients with the same stage of the disease who did not have hyponatremia (15). Although there is a relationship between hyponatremia and tumor cell production of arginine vasopressin (AVP) in some patients (15), there are some patients in whom hyponatremia is not associated with high levels of AVP (16). Interestingly, a patient with leiomyosarcoma was recently described who presented with hyponatremia and hypertension and very high levels of prorenin and renin who responded to both angiotensin-converting enzyme inhibitors and tumor removal (17). Central diabetes insipidus as a result of metastatic disease, especially breast cancer (18), may also occur.

Hypercalcemia is perhaps the most common electrolyte abnormality of cancer and can be divided into two forms (19). One is related to local osteolytic lesions, and the other is associated with a humoral factor, a parathyroid hormone-related protein, which is the cause of enhanced bone resorption. Hypercalcemia can reduce glomerular filtration itself, but it may cause renal failure by potentiating the nephrotoxic effects of other drugs or require treatment by drugs that are nephrotoxic themselves (see next section). Thus hypercalcemia is an important risk factor for the development of renal failure in cancer patients.

ANTINEOPLASTIC AGENTS THAT CAUSE ACUTE RENAL FAILURE

Several antineoplastic agents have predictable dose-related nephrotoxicity. Included in this group (Table 43-1) are the alkylating agents cisplatin and streptozotocin, the antimetabolite methotrexate, the antitumor antibiotic mithramycin, and the cytokine interleukin-2 (IL-2). These agents induce a fall in glomerular filtration that is usually dose-related and predictable. Others have nephrotoxic potential after chronic repeated exposure to the drug, especially in combination with other drugs, as single exposure rarely causes renal failure. Taxol (paclitaxel), a microtubule-binding agent recently introduced into multidrug cytoreductive regimens, has shown potentiation of the nephrotoxicity of cisplatin (20) and in the setting of bone marrow transplant (21). When recognized, the decline in renal function with some chemotherapeutic drugs is sometimes irreversible. Examples of these agents are the alkylating agents lomustine (CCNU) and semustine (methyl CCNU) and the anti-tumor antibiotic mitomycin. Chronic and irreversible decline in renal function has also been documented after cisplatin therapy and after bone marrow transplantation, perhaps as a result of repeated, but subclinical damage to the kidney.

ALKYLATING AGENTS

Cisplatin

Cisplatin, perhaps the most commonly used antineoplastic agent for the treatment of solid tumors, is the best-studied antineoplastic nephrotoxin. Long-term survivors have provided the opportunity to follow cisplatin nephrotoxicity over longer periods of time than has been possible with other agents.

Preclinical studies identified nephrotoxicity as cisplatin's major dose-limiting side effect early (22), and initial protocols not employing aggressive hydration prior to administration of cisplatin produced severe and frequently irreversible renal failure (23). Other significant side effects, such as ototoxicity and severe nausea and vomiting, may also limit its use.

Pathogenesis

The kidney accumulates and retains platinum to a greater degree than other organs and is the principal excretory organ for injected cisplatin (24). In the rat, the kidney excretes the drug rapidly within the first hour of its administration by a process consisting predominantly of glomerular filtration, with a minor component of secretion (25–27). There is no evidence of tubular reabsorption, suggesting that the kidney accumulates cisplatin by peritubular uptake (26). The uptake of cisplatin by the kidney is dependent on temperature and the normal consumption of oxygen and can be inhibited by drugs that participate in the organic base transport system, suggesting that at least some portion of renal cisplatin uptake is facilitated (26). Consistent with the view that cisplatin nephrotoxicity may be linked to how the kidney transports cisplatin is the high cisplatin content of proximal straight tubules after [^{195m}Pt] cisplatin injection (28), the principal site of necrosis following cisplatin (29). Changes in the distal nephron including apoptosis, if not frank necrosis, have also been described (23,30). The glomerulus is spared of obvious morphologic changes.

Excreted platinum is predominantly cisplatin, but inside the cell cisplatin is converted to another species (31). Once gaining access into the cell, cisplatin is thought to undergo aquation reactions in which the labile chloride ligands are replaced by water molecules, resulting in a positively charged and highly reactive electrophilic product (32). The primary lethal lesion produced by cisplatin in cancer cells is its intrastrand binding to adjacent purine bases (33), which alters the secondary structure of DNA, inhibiting its template function and inhibiting DNA replication (34,35). This lesion is not produced by the transplatin isomer, which is neither antineoplastic nor nephrotoxic. Whether the nephrotoxicity of cisplatin also depends on such damage to DNA is unknown. Cisplatin may also damage the kidney by depletion of critical sulfhydryl centers, including glutathione, and provoke damage to the cell in much the same manner as oxidant stress. Indeed the administration of manganese superoxide dismutase attenuates cisplatin-induced renal failure (36).

CELLULAR RESPONSES TO CISPLATIN TREATMENT

Role of the Protein Kinase Cascades in Cisplatin Nephrotoxicity

Cellular stress, including DNA-damaging chemotherapeutic drugs, activates several signaling pathways: the stress-activated protein kinase (SAPK), including the Jun N-terminal kinases (JNKs), p38 MAPK (mitogen-activated protein kinase), and the extracellular regulated kinases or (ERKs) (37). Cisplatin-mediated activation of JNK and concomitant cell death are related, since expression of a dominant negative expression vector of the JNK (Jun N-terminal kinase) MKK4 (mitogen-activated protein kinase kinase 4) blocked cell death (38). Similarly, cells derived from animals in which the gene for c-jun was deleted, a specific protooncogene target of JNK, were more resistant to cisplatin-induced cell death than normal cells (39).

A balance between the JNK and ERK pathways had been proposed to dictate the cellular decisions of death and survival: transient activation of JNK when also accompanied by activation of prosurvival ERK or AKT (v-akt kinase/protein kinase B) pathways may not be associated with cell death. Indeed, inhibition of JNK by dominant-negative mutants proved to be protective of cisplatin-induced injury (38). Pharmacologic inhibition of the cisplatin-induced ERK activity in ovarian carcinoma cells caused enhanced cisplatin cytotoxicity (40), and inhibition of the Akt/PKB pathway enhanced activation of caspase-3 and caspase-9 in proximal tubular cells (41).

However, inhibition of cisplatin-induced activation of ERK protected rabbit (42) and mouse proximal tubule (43) cells, suggesting that the interaction of cisplatin with such cells is fundamentally different from that seen in cancer cells. As these observations have important clinical implications, it will be necessary to explore these approaches *in vivo* to see whether the discrepancies are more a function of the limitations of *in vitro* models of tissue injury or signal important differences in cellular response.

Role of Casplase Activation in Cisplatin-induced Cell Death

Cisplatin induces apoptosis of renal proximal tubular cells (LL-CPK) *in vitro* via mitochondria-dependent and –independent pathways (41), and the activation of the caspases is crucial to this process. Studies in renal tubular epithelial cells demonstrate that cisplatin induces selective and differential activation of caspases including executioner caspase-3 and initiator caspase-8, -9, and -2 but not proinflammatory caspase-1 (41). The translocation of Bax to the mitochondria and release of cytochrome c from the mitochondria to the cytosol further support the activation of caspase-9 (42). Cisplatin–induced activation of caspase-8 and apoptosis has also been reported in freshly isolated proximal tubular epithelial cells, which involves the TNF- and Fas pathways (44). DEVD-CHO (acetyl-Asp-Glu-Val-Asp-aldehyde) or LEHD-CHO (acetyl-Leu-Asp-Glu-Asp-aldehyde), inhibitors of caspase-3 and caspase-9, respectively, provided only partial protection against cisplatin-induced cell death and DNA damage in LLC-PK1 cells (41) indicating mechanisms other than caspase activation are also involved in cisplatin-induced cell death. Thus, cisplatin-induced activation of caspase-8 and caspase-9 in renal proximal tubules indicate that both receptor and mitochondrial signaling pathways participate in the activation process. In a recent study p53 inhibition was shown to partially protect cisplatin-induced cell death (45) indicating that p53 may also be involved in cisplatin-induced activation of caspases in renal tubular epithelial cells. Working out the precise details of renal cisplatin-induced caspase activation is likely to reveal additional means to ameliorate its nephrotoxicity.

Cytokines and Cisplatin-induced Cell Death

Cisplatin administration significantly upregulates several cytokines and chemokines (tumor necrosis factor-α [TNF-α], transforming growth factor-β [TGF-β], regulated upon activation, normal T cell expressed and secreted [RANTES], macrophage inflammatory protein [MIP-2], monocyte chemotactic protein-1 [MCP-1]) in the kidney (46). Several antiinflammatory strategies have yielded positive protective results. Anti-ICAM I (intercellular adhesion molecule-1) antibodies reduce cisplatin toxicity (47), as does salicylate treatment (48) and interleukin-10 (IL-10) administration (49). These studies provide convincing evidence that cisplatin cytotoxicity is mediated in part by inflammatory mediators. Interestingly, TNFα itself provokes oxidant dependent damage to cells so that the possibility that the TNF-α–related toxicity is direct and unrelated to recruitment of inflammatory cells (50) cannot be ruled out.

Cell Cycle Events in Cisplatin Nephrotoxicity

Genotoxic damage either by intercalation of DNA or by oxidant-induced damage may be an important component of the stress imposed by cisplatin. Cisplatin provokes increased expression of the cyclin-dependent kinase inhibitor p21[WAF1/CIP1], which inhibits completion of the cell cycle, and promotes DNA repair. Interestingly, mice with deletion of the p21 gene are more susceptible to cisplatin nephrotoxicity (51), suggesting that it may be critical to the repair of cisplatin-induced damage to renal cells. Confronted with a hostile environment, the kidney mounts a response that is initiated by signaling molecules that engage multiple pathways including those that regulate the cell cycle. The cell undergoing these changes may decide to check the progression of the cycle and repair damage before proceeding or enter a pathway destined to cell death. This decision point is carefully regulated and cyclin-dependent kinase inhibitors, especially p21, are important in this decision. The interface between these pathways and the cell death pathways are first emerging but phosphorylation events critical to cell function reside in the cyclin dependent kinases and the kinases, phosphatases, inhibitors, and activators that regulate their activities. The identification of the precise pathways engaged in this process is an area of active research not only in acute renal failure but also in the field of cell biology in general.

Clinical Manifestations

Cisplatin predictably lowers glomerular filtration rate (GFR) in a dose-dependent manner (52) after even single drug exposure, and its nephrotoxicity is augmented by coadministration of drugs used in aggressive chemotherapy (53). The onset of the renal failure is gradual, usually occurring 3 to 5 days after its administration. Early proteinuria is mild (>500 mg/day), as is glycosuria. Enzymuria is common, even in the mildest forms of ARF. In a few patients, significant urinary electrolyte wasting may be provoked by cisplatin (54), including severe sodium, divalent cation excretion, and phosphate wasting, but this presentation is uncommon and seen primarily with high-dose therapy. Most common is the gradual onset of nonoliguric renal failure with water excretion in excess of solute (28). In micropuncture experiments, the site of altered water reabsorption is beyond the late distal tubule, probably in the apparently morphologically intact collecting duct (28). In rats, the cause of the fall in glomerular filtration is afferent vasoconstriction and possibly an altered ultrafiltration coefficient, before evidence of tubule obstruction (55). The mediators for these changes in segmental water transport and vascular resistance are unknown.

Cisplatin also produces hypomagnesemia (55) in a large percentage of patients receiving the drug. Although it may occur acutely, it is usually observed after repeated exposure over longer periods of time (56). It is often found when additional drugs with significant potential for magnesium wasting are used in conjunction with cisplatin, such as nephrotoxic antibiotics like gentamicin or amphotericin (57), or when cisplatin is used in combination with other chemotherapeutic agents (56). In the normomagnesemic animal ingesting a diet containing adequate magnesium, cisplatin does not induce hypomagnesemia. However, in the rat kept on a magnesium-deficient diet,

cisplatin induced a defect in maximal reclamation of an administered magnesium load, suggesting that hypomagnesemia is a consequence of diets deficient in magnesium in combination with a mild defect in magnesium reabsorption (58). This is consistent with the relative ease of treating the hypomagnesemia with oral magnesium supplementation. Hypomagnesemia may persist even when cisplatin is withdrawn (59) but usually remits when cisplatin administration is discontinued (53). Serum calcium is usually normal in such cases.

In almost all studies, repeated cisplatin administration has been shown to reduce GFR chronically in a dose-related manner (52,60–66). Patients receiving up to 850 mg in multiple courses had a 9% reduction in hippuran clearance, while patients receiving more than 850 mg of cisplatin had a 40% reduction in GFR over a 5-year period (52). This study also found significant potentiation of cisplatin nephrotoxicity in those patients receiving cisplatin combined with radiotherapy. In each of these studies, GFR remained stable after discontinuation of the therapy for up to 3 to 5 years of follow-up.

Protective Measures

The wide therapeutic application of cisplatin depends not only on its clinical efficacy but also on the development of strategies that diminish the severity of the ARF it produces. The most commonly used protective measure is to establish a solute diuresis (67). A commonly applied protocol is to establish a diuresis before (12 to 24 hours) administering cisplatin, which is then given in isotonic saline by a 3-hour infusion, followed by infusion of isotonic saline or mannitol for 24 hours after the drug is infused. Cisplatin is usually administered in daily divided doses for 5 days until the maximum dose is reached, usually not to exceed 120 mg per m² body surface area (BSA). Beyond this dose cisplatin provokes an unacceptable degree of renal failure, even in the presence of a diuresis.

The mechanism of the protection is not known. Although the concentration of cisplatin is lower in the urine, neither the tissue concentration of the drug nor the degree of cytotoxicity is altered by such maneuvers (67). Alternatively, the high chloride content of the urine might reduce its speciation into toxic metabolites, but mannitol is equally effective in diminishing the degree of renal failure where urine chloride concentration is reduced, so this explanation seems inadequate as well.

Additional maneuvers have been attempted to reduce cisplatin nephrotoxicity. Diethyldithiocarbamate (DDTC), which has been shown to compete for platinum binding to DNA (68), has shown promise experimentally (69) but has been much less successful in human trials due to its toxicity and failure to modify cisplatin ototoxicity (70). Inorganic thiophosphates like WR2721 (amifostine) has been shown to be effective in preventing renal failure even after repeated exposure (71). The mechanism of protection may involve promotion of better DNA repair and synthesis by amifostine (72) and/or by the release of free thiols after dephosphorylation with alkaline phosphatase, which then act as free radical scavengers and metal binding centers (73).

Erythropoietin improves renal function when co-administered with cisplatin and the improvement seems to be mediated by improved regeneration rather than an inherent reduction in toxicity (74).

Promising future strategies will be based on a better understanding of the pathophysiology of cisplatin-induced kidney injury. In Figure 43-1 are outlined likely therapeutic targets for intervention. Cisplatin by its pro-oxidant effects and direct interaction with proteins and DNA initiates a stress response characterized by activation of pro-death and pro-survival transduction and molecular pathways. In each instance the balance between these pathways can be manipulated to ameliorate

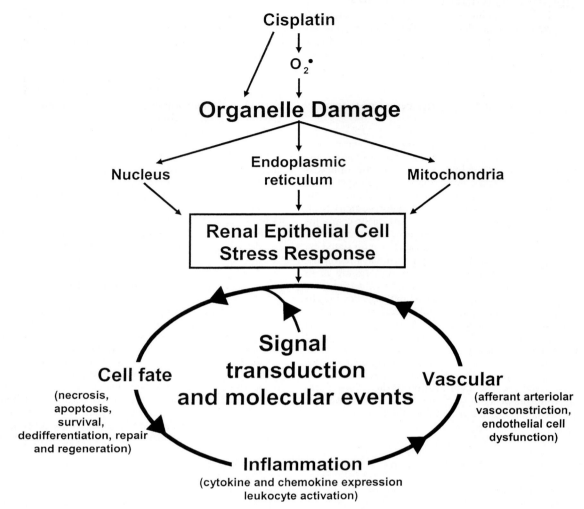

FIGURE 43-1. Cisplatin and the renal stress response. Sites of potential cisplatin-macromolecular interaction that initiates the renal stress response consisting of signal transduction and molecular pathways. These responses lead to the phenotypic changes characteristic of cisplatin-induced kidney injury including necrosis, apoptosis, survival, and repair, as well as inflammatory and vascular effects that may mediate and ameliorate these effects. The balance between the responses that promote repair and survival and those that cause cells to die can be manipulated by upregulating the former and downregulating the latter (see text).

the consequences of cisplatin exposure on kidney function and structure. Thus inhibitors of caspase activity, TNF-α inhibitors, inhibition of specific components of the MAPKs, upregulation of cell-cycle regulators, and antioxidants each show promise in ameliorating experimental cisplatin nephrotoxicity. Translating these observations to the bedside should be accomplished in the near future.

New platinum compounds with antineoplastic effects and less nephrotoxicity have been identified and are being increasingly applied. Prominent among them is carboplatin (*cis*-diaminecyclobutanedicarboxylplatinum II). While the kidney remains the primary excretory organ and dose modification must be applied in the presence of diminished renal function, the compound has much less nephrotoxicity than cisplatin (75). The dose-limiting side effect is myelosuppression, especially thrombocytopenia (76). Because of its overlapping toxicity with other antineoplastic agents and experience with such toxicity, carboplatin is increasingly included in protocols for lung, head and neck, and cervical cancer. Carboplatin and other similar compounds will almost certainly be increasingly used in patients with prior chemotherapy-induced renal dysfunction, especially in those patients with tumors expected to respond to anti-tumor platinum analogs. The full impact of the use of this drug on the occurrence of renal failure, however, is as yet unknown.

Cyclophosphamide

Cyclophosphamide is converted by hepatic mixed-function oxidases into an active alkylating agent with wide-ranging antitumor activities against many hematologic and solid tumors. Its primary toxicity is myelosuppression, but important toxicity involving the gastrointestinal tract and urinary bladder may also occur.

Cyclophosphamide diminishes the ability of the kidney to excrete water (77). Impaired water excretion occurs acutely and resolves after discontinuation of the drug. The water retention may involve a direct effect of cyclophosphamide on the collecting duct epithelium, as elevated serum AVP (arginine vasopressin) levels have not been detected (78). Recognition of this effect is important since hydration protocols with hypotonic solutions prior to the administration of cyclophosphamide are likely to provoke marked hyponatremia. Thus hydration with normal saline is preferable. It is important to remember, however, that any detectable AVP is inappropriate in the presence of hypo-osmolality. While the effect of cyclophosphamide is self-limited and rarely of clinical significance, the concentrated urine predisposes to hemorrhagic cystitis and uric acid nephropathy. Cyclophosphamide is increasingly included in high-dose treatment regimens combined with autologous bone marrow or stem cell transplants, and possible new potentiating patterns of renal failure may emerge (79).

Nitrosoureas

Semustine (methyl-CCNU), carmustine (BCNU), and lomustine (CCNU) have demonstrated efficacy against brain tumors, Hodgkin's disease and other lymphomas, and multiple myeloma (80). Their high lipid solubility and high permeability across the blood–brain barrier make them ideal for the treatment of such tumors. Carmustine, which is the most commonly used nitrosourea, is given intravenously at a dose of 150 to 200 mg per m^2 infused over 1 to 2 hours. Nephrotoxicity presents the main limitation to their greater efficacy at these doses, while hepatic failure and pulmonary fibrosis are common at higher doses. The nitrosoureas are rapidly metabolized (81), and their metabolites appear in the urine for up to 72 hours following administration (82). These metabolites are thought to be responsible for the nephrotoxicity, as the parent compound is not detected in the urine. The mechanism of the nephrotoxicity of the nitrosoureas is unknown.

Streptozotocin

Streptozotocin is a nitrosourea that is used for the treatment of metastatic islet cell carcinoma of the pancreas and carcinoid tumors. Nephrotoxicity is its chief limiting side effect and is present in 75% of patients who receive prolonged streptozotocin administration (83). Nephrogenic diabetes insipidus and obstructive uropathy from uric acid nephrolithiasis caused by its uricosuric effect have also been described.

The major excretory route of streptozotocin is the kidney, which accumulates the drug to high concentrations (84). Proximal tubules are the principal site of damage (85). Although there are no definitive data relating cumulative dose with nephrotoxicity, renal damage often occurs with a cumulative dose of 4 g per m^2 body surface area (BSA) (87). Clinical streptozotocin-induced nephrotoxicity includes tubular reabsorptive abnormalities similar to Fanconi's syndrome including hypophosphatemia as well as proteinuria (86); even after a single exposure to the drug (87), these tubular effects may precede the reduction in GFR. Extreme caution should be used before introducing it in patients with preexisting renal disease. A related analog, chlorozotocin, also causes renal failure in patients with metastatic islet cell carcinoma of the pancreas treated with total doses exceeding 1,500 mg (88).

Ifosfamide

Ifosfamide has been shown to be active against testicular carcinoma and pediatric soft tissue sarcomas, osteosarcoma, and Ewing's sarcoma (89). Used in conjunction with mesna, the dose-limiting side effect of hemorrhagic cystitis has been eliminated (90). The incidence of severe nephrotoxicity, which is dose related, has been significantly reduced by administering ifosfamide in divided daily doses rather than by bolus infusion (89). Reabsorptive defects have been reported even under these circumstances (91–93) and consist of aminoaciduria, bicarbonaturia, phosphaturia, and proteinuria. Small but consistent reductions in GFR and persistent proximal tubule defects have been documented in patients receiving multiple courses of nonplatinum-containing ifosfamide protocols (94–95). Previous renal disease, perhaps as a consequence of cisplatin exposure, has proved to be an important risk factor for the development of ifosfamide nephrotoxicity (2,96–98). A severe irreversible Fanconi-like syndrome with rickets may appear in the course of therapy with ifosfamide, especially when combined with cisplatin (97).

ANTIMETABOLITES

Methotrexate

Methotrexate (MTX), an analog of folic acid, is used in combination chemotherapy of embryonic hematologic and solid tumors, as well as in cytoreductive protocols in bone marrow transplant. It is given in two dose ranges, low and high, with clearly different degrees of nephrotoxic risk. At conventional doses, nephrotoxicity is rarely a problem (99), but at the doses given in leucovorin rescue therapy (1 to 7 g per m^2 BSA), high rates of nephrotoxicity and drug-related mortality can occur unless precautions are taken to minimize the nephrotoxicity.

Primarily the kidney excretes MTX by glomerular filtration and tubular secretion so that 90% of the drug appears unchanged in the urine after conventional intravenous doses (100). Thus reduced glomerular filtration raises the concentration of MTX in body fluids for a prolonged period of time. Under these conditions, marked bone marrow, gastrointestinal, and renal toxicity is observed (101). Removal by hemodialysis and peritoneal dialysis is poor, as is the efficacy of plasma exchange (102–104).

The mechanism of MTX nephrotoxicity is unclear. A commonly invoked mechanism is its limited solubility at acid urine pH, which provokes intratubular precipitation especially during high-dose infusion (104). According to this hypothesis, dehydrated patients who excrete acid urine are more at risk for this complication. Consistent with this notion is the decline in MTX nephrotoxicity observed since the institution of urinary alkalinization and hydration associated with high-dose MTX therapy (105). It should be pointed out that hydration alone ameliorates the nephrotoxicity of a wide variety of toxic and physical insults as discussed previously. MTX may be directly toxic to the tubule epithelium, as proximal tubule necrosis without intraluminal precipitation has been noted (106). Finally, infusion of high-dose MTX reduces glomerular filtration without changing blood pressure, suggesting a direct renal hemodynamic effect (107,108). Thus MTX nephrotoxicity is probably multifactorial.

Clinical Course

Typically symptoms of renal colic sometimes precede overt renal failure, which is nonoliguric. Since the onset of the renal failure is rapid, often only hours after administration, thus further limiting its excretion, it is often associated with severe organ toxicities including gastroenteritis, hepatitis, mucositis, and pancytopenia. Plasma levels exceeding 0.5 μM for 48 hours following MTX infusion are associated with a 40% incidence of severe systemic toxicity (103). Expansion of the extracellular fluid with 150 mM $NaHCO_3$ should precede use of drug. Removal of drug by dialysis is problematic because of its high volume of distribution and protein binding, but high-flux dialyzers show improved drug removal (109).

Treatment

When acute renal failure intervenes, the goal of therapy is to reduce MTX concentration as rapidly as possible. A newly introduced treatment of high-dose MTX nephrotoxicity with carboxypeptidase-G2 (CPDG-2), a recombinant bacterial enzyme that hydrolyzed MTX to an inactive metabolite shows early promise. In a recent study CPDG-2 reduced MTX blood levels by 98% following infusion. While early concern for delay in recovery due to the potential for the metabolite to crystallize in urine, this has not proven to be the case. Given the ease of administration and its greater efficacy in reducing MTX concentration, this treatment would appear to have definite advantages over dialytic approaches (110).

MTX is routinely used in chemoprevention of graft-versus-host disease (GVHD) following bone marrow transplant, and its participation in the renal failure induced on that background is discussed in the section Renal Failure Associated with Bone Marrow Transplant, below.

Cytosine Arabinoside

Cytosine arabinoside, also known as cytarabine and ara-C, is a pyrimidine nucleoside that inhibits DNA synthesis when activated by the enzyme deoxycytidine kinase (111). It is used in multidrug protocols in the treatment of acute leukemia, in the blast phase of chronic myelocytic leukemia, and non-Hodgkin lymphoma (112). Deamination of free cytosine arabinoside yields uracil arabinoside, which is the principal urinary metabolite of cytosine arabinoside (113).

Renal failure occurs in 50% of patients treated with multidrug regimens including cytosine arabinoside, even if used with drugs not known to produce renal failure (114). Potentiation of nephrotoxicity was especially common in a drug regimen using cytosine arabinoside in combination with cisplatin and hydroxyurea (115). High-dose cytosine arabinoside leads to even greater nephrotoxicity and neurotoxicity, especially in patients with prior renal injury (116). Rarely acute rhabdomyolysis may be a causative factor in cases exposed to cytosine arabinoside (117). Prominent apoptosis of muscle cells has been demonstrated in such cases secondary to cytochrome-c release. All other drugs that initiate muscle damage, such as cyclophosphamide, 5-azacytidine, interferon, and interleukin-2 should be discontinued.

5-Fluorouracil

The active metabolite of 5-fluorouracil (5-FU), fluorodeoxyuridine monophosphate, inhibits DNA synthesis by inhibiting thymidylate synthase. While not nephrotoxic when given as a single agent, renal insufficiency has been observed when it is combined with other agents of known nephrotoxic potential. When given with mitomycin-C, which provokes renal failure in a minority of patients (discussed later in this chapter in the section Mitomycin-C), fluorouracil provoked severe and fatal renal insufficiency in 10% of patients undergoing such treatment for carcinoma of the gastrointestinal tract and pancreas (118,119). In these reports, either an acute or chronic syndrome of microangiopathic hemolytic anemia with thrombocytopenia emerged. Histologic examination of the kidney revealed fibrin thrombi in arterioles, which also demonstrated intimal hyperplasia. Interstitial fibrosis, tubular atrophy, and glomerular necrosis were observed in the chronic forms. Renal failure was also noted when the drug was given in combination with cisplatin (120). This combination is increasingly applied

in otherwise resistant advanced solid tumors, especially of the head and neck (121) and invasive cervical cancers (122).

5-Azacytidine

A similar circumstance exists for azacytidine because there has been no nephrotoxicity described when this drug is used alone (123), but a high rate of tubular reabsorptive abnormalities has been noted when the drug is used in combination with others (124). Nephrotoxicity is manifested by glycosuria, acidemia, phosphaturia, and polyuria and with mild azotemia. The defects were compatible with an acquired renal tubular acidosis, which appears early in the course of treatment and resolves rapidly when the drug is discontinued.

ANTITUMOR ANTIBIOTICS

Mitomycin-C

Mitomycin-C is used in combination protocols, most often with 5-fluorouracil and doxorubicin, in the treatment of solid tumors of the genitourinary and gastrointestinal systems. In preclinical studies, acute tubular necrosis was induced by single intravenous injection (125). Although it is known that the drug is metabolized in the liver, the specifics of its renal handling have not been adequately addressed. The mechanism of the nephrotoxicity is also unknown.

The available data would seem to indicate that mitomycin-C occasionally induces a dose-related, mild form of ARF when administered alone (126). However, its nephrotoxicity is more frequent and severe when used in combination with other drugs. Clinically, the renal failure is accompanied by a microangiopathic hemolytic anemia, usually occurring late in the course of therapy (127). The incidence is reported to be between 2% and 10% of cases and patients receiving a cumulative dose of 30 to 50 mg per m^2 should be carefully monitored for fragmentation of red blood cells if unexplained anemia or thrombocytopenia appear. Histopathologically, the findings are consistent with a thrombotic microangiopathic process with fibrin deposition within glomeruli and interstitial blood vessels. Glomerular sclerosis and necrosis and interstitial scarring are prominent. While these changes are reminiscent of the hemolytic-uremic syndrome, plasma exchange does not improve renal function (127), nor is the experience with glucocorticoids and anti-platelet drugs good. Anecdotal evidence for improvement of renal function after immunoadsorbtion with staphylococcal protein-A columns suggest that immune complexes may play a role in the pathogenesis of the renal failure. A recent animal study of its nephrotoxicity, however, found a direct tubulotoxic effect only (128) and no good animal model exists that mimics the clinical situation.

Mithramycin

Mithramycin inhibits RNA synthesis and has some antineoplastic efficacy in testicular carcinomas and glioblastomas (129,130), but it is most frequently used to treat malignancy-associated hypercalcemia. The calcium-lowering effect of the drug seems to be due to its inhibition of osteoclast function (131) and is linked to its inhibition of messenger RNA (mRNA) synthesis (132). A single 25 μg per kg IV dose, which normalizes serum calcium in a large majority of cases, is usually not nephrotoxic. However, repeated daily injection of the drug has been reported to cause significant nephrotoxicity in up to

40% of patients in one study (129). Renal failure persists if it occurs on the background of preexistent renal disease and is the cause of death in 10% of the patients studied. Histologically, there is a picture typical of acute tubule necrosis with apparently normal glomeruli. The mechanism of the nephrotoxicity is unknown.

KIDNEY INJURY AND THE TREATMENT OF HYPERCALCEMIA OF MALIGNANCY

Zolendronnate

Zolendronnate, a highly effective bisphosphonate that is increasingly used to treat hypercalcemia in cancer patients, can also cause acute renal failure (133). The renal toxicity, which is characterized by proximal tubule necrosis and apoptosis but spares the glomerulus, is dose related and occurs in about 10% of cases receiving the usual 4 mg dose. Prolonging infusion time and reducing exposure dose have been found to reduce nephrotoxicity. Even under these circumstances, renal failure emerges slowly and requires cessation of drug. The renal failure, when recognized early, is partially reversible but is somewhat slow to resolve. The mechanism of its nephrotoxicity is unknown, but, like cisplatin, is almost certainly related to its active uptake and concentration in proximal tubule cells.

BIOLOGIC AGENTS

Interferons

The interferons are glycoproteins that have antiviral (134), as well as antitumor activity (135,136). Renal insufficiency has been produced by both interferon-α (IFN-α) and interferon-γ (IFN-γ), two of the three major classes of the interferons. IFN-α produces proteinuria, sometimes massive with nephrotic syndrome, and histopathologically a picture consistent with minimal-change nephropathy (137). The occurrence of ARF, however, is relatively rare (138). ARF with renal biopsy evidence of acute tubular necrosis has been described with IFN-γ treatment of acute lymphoblastic leukemia (139). Divided doses of up to 1×10^7 U per m^2 BSA total administered IFN-α and 1,000 μg per m^2 BSA IFN-γ are usually tolerated without significant nephrotoxicity (140).

Interleukin-2

IL-2 is a polypeptide cytokine that activates the natural killer function of lymphocytes. Infusion of IL-2 concurrently with such lymphokine-activated killer (LAK) cells is associated with regression of several solid tumors including malignant melanoma, renal cell cancer, and colorectal cancer (141). Profound reductions in blood pressure, GFR, and sodium excretion occur in patients during the period of drug infusion, which resolve fairly rapidly when the infusion is stopped (142).

A more comprehensive study of IL-2 nephrotoxicity documented falls in GFR in 90% of cases (143). Although the syndrome of hypotension, oliguria, salt retention, and azotemia suggests a prerenal component, massive infusion of fluid does not abrogate the fall in GFR (144). In Figure 43-2 is shown the time course of changes in salt excretion, GFR, and cardiac output in a patient receiving IL-2 infusion. It can be seen

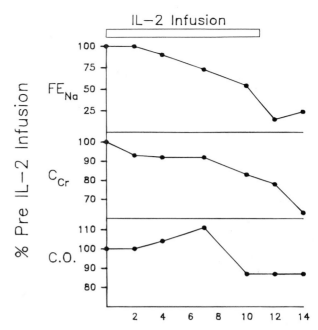

FIGURE 43-2. Hourly fractional sodium excretion (FE$_{Na}$), creatinine clearance (C$_{Cr}$), and cardiac output (CO) as a percent of preinfusion levels during the infusion of interleukin-2 (IL-2), 500,000 U in 12 hours, in a patient undergoing treatment for renal cell carcinoma. The patient also received mannitol and isotonic saline infusion prior to the infusion of IL-2.

that the fall in GFR and salt excretion precedes the period of reduced cardiac output, suggesting early effects of IL-2 on kidney function before effects on central hemodynamics are obvious. In a study of renal hemodynamics during high-dose IL-2 and IFN-α adoptive immunotherapy of renal cell carcinoma, GFR fell significantly following repeated infusion and was not accompanied by a fall in renal plasma flow, suggesting a fall in the net glomerular ultrafiltration pressure or permeability coefficient (145). The fall was accentuated by use of nonsteroidal anti-inflammatory drugs. Whether IL-2 mediates these effects directly or indirectly is not clear.

CHEMOTHERAPY-INDUCED TUMOR LYSIS AND RENAL FAILURE

The release of potential nephrotoxic products into the circulation from cancer cells lysed by chemotherapy is common. The blood concentration of uric acid, xanthine, phosphate, and potassium may increase to levels that impact on kidney function. This is especially true in the setting of prior renal insufficiency. This syndrome of metabolic derangements associated with renal failure during chemotherapy has been termed the "tumor lysis syndrome" and is not infrequently observed after the treatment of acute leukemia, malignant lymphoma, and bulky solid tumors (146,147).

Hyperuricemia and Acute Renal Failure

Renal insufficiency associated with acute hyperuricemia is most frequently associated with the therapy of leukemias and lymphomas (148), although it has been reported in disseminated carcinoma (149,150) and may even occur spontaneously (151).

The incidence in one series of patients treated for non-Hodgkin lymphoma was 6% of all patients but was highest in patients with high-grade tumors and renal insufficiency (152). Hyperuricemia-induced crystalluria and renal failure are discussed in Chapter 49, but pretreatment with allopurinol and establishing an alkaline diuresis have significantly reduced the incidence of this complication.

Xanthine Nephropathy

Although rare, xanthine nephropathy can occur during tumor lysis when allopurinol is used to prevent the production of uric acid. Xanthine concentration in the blood increases consequent to xanthine oxidase inhibition by allopurinol, and like uric acid, xanthine is poorly soluble in acid urines. Xanthine crystalluria can occur when its urinary excretion rises beyond its solubility (153). This is especially likely in patients who have minor degrees of hypoxanthine–guanine phosphoribosyltransferase deficiency (154).

Hyperphosphatemic Nephropathy

Hyperphosphatemia may occur as part of the tumor lysis syndrome and, when extreme, may result in ARF (155,156). This is especially true in patients with prior renal insufficiency (155). The cause of the reduced GFR seems directly related to the hyperphosphatemia itself because oral phosphate overdose also lowers GFR (157), and reduction in serum phosphate level reverses the renal failure (158,159). The mechanism of reduced GFR may be the intrarenal precipitation of calcium phosphate (155,160), which may be exacerbated by excessive alkalinization of the urine. Hemodialysis may be required to reduce plasma phosphate and to restore renal function under these circumstances.

Retinoic Acid Syndrome

Tretinoin (all-*trans*-retinoic acid) is a vitamin A derivative that is used in the treatment of acute promyelocytic leukemia. Tretinoin enhances the morphologic and functional maturation of leukemic promyelocytes and may provoke apoptosis in these cells. The appearance of a syndrome consisting of fever, respiratory distress, pulmonary infiltrates, and pleural and pericardial effusions occurs in as much as 25% of treated patients unless preventive measures are taken (161). Since the syndrome can be reproduced by the infusion of activated leukocytes, it is speculated that cytokine production by such stimulated white cells is responsible for its manifestations. The addition of intravenous dexamethasone and the reduction of the white cell count by prior chemotherapy usually before Tretinoin is added have decreased the occurrence of the syndrome markedly.

RENAL FAILURE ASSOCIATED WITH BONE MARROW TRANSPLANT

Bone marrow transplant is becoming an increasingly common modality for treatment of cancer and other disorders (162). Current indications include aplastic anemia, hematologic and nonhematologic malignancies, hereditary enzyme deficiencies, immunodeficiency states, and selected hemoglobinopathies. Renal failure occurs frequently in this group of patients, in most series as high as 40% (163,164) or higher (165).

It is useful to consider the frequency of ARF as it relates to the time of bone marrow transplant because it varies during the course of transplant (166). Also, the likelihood of the occurrence of ARF, especially its severity, appears to be related to whether the transplanted hematopoietic cells are derived from the patient (autologous) or not (allogeneic). In a recent study of autologous bone marrow transplants in high-dose patients with breast cancer (21), the incidence of ARF was significantly lower than that reported in an earlier report of predominantly allogeneic transplant patients (164). Thus the occurrence of graft-versus-host reactions and the use of immunosuppressive drugs with nephrotoxic potential may impact on the occurrence of ARF.

Up to 10 days following completion of conditioning with cytoreductive drugs and at the time of bone marrow infusion, a small percentage of patients (<5%) present with renal failure that is most often due to the tumor lysis syndrome or the infusion of the bone marrow. The latter would seem to be a result of toxic products that accumulate during cryopreservation of bone marrow cells or due to the cryopreservative that is used (167). Hemoglobin appears in the urine of 75% to 100% of such patients and may be due to disrupted red blood cells within the infusate or due to in vivo hemolysis induced by the dimethyl sulfoxide in the cryopreservation solution (168). This form of ARF is relatively uncommon, perhaps as a consequence of the induction of a solute and bicarbonate diuresis that is routinely induced prior to marrow infusion (167).

The most common time frame for ARF to develop after a bone marrow transplant is between 10 and 21 days after infusion (166), when as many as 20% of patients who survive the initial period of bone marrow transplant develop ARF. Whether the exposure of ordinarily nontoxic amounts of heme proteins might predispose the kidney to later injury has recently been the matter of some debate in the literature (169,170), since heme itself may be cytoprotective. During this time, almost all of the complications of prior cytoreductive therapy become most evident, including marrow aplasia, infection, and gastrointestinal and hepatic toxicity. This is also the period where dialysis will be most required (163,171). Mortality increases markedly if dialysis is required, approaching 90% in some studies (163,171). Despite the many possible causes of ARF, Zager and co-workers (163) find that the large majority of such patients develop renal failure in the background of liver failure reminiscent of the hepatorenal syndrome. The syndrome is characterized clinically by hyperbilirubinemia, hepatomegaly, usually with right upper quadrant pain, and sudden weight gain, often with peripheral edema and ascites. The urinary sodium remains low despite diuretic therapy, and in the presence of large requirements of fluid for administration of medications and blood products, there is the potential to develop significant degrees of circulatory congestion. Dialysis is most often required to relieve such congestion, rather than uremia.

The liver most often shows prominent changes of veno-occlusive disease characterized by venular thrombosis, variable degrees of hepatocellular necrosis, and portal hypertension (173,174). The cause of the syndrome is unknown, but it bears some resemblance to the veno-occlusive disease induced by radiochemical-induced endothelial cell damage. The severity of the liver disease, as assessed by serum bilirubin levels, correlates with the occurrence of renal failure. Also, preexisting liver disease, concurrent administration of estrogen–progestin, amphotericin, or MTX, and preexisting kidney disease all increase the risk of ARF (163,173,175). Zager et al. (163) point out the important role that sepsis plays in initiating the syndrome, either directly or by virtue of the exposure to additional toxins, especially amphotericin. Attempts to limit venous occlusion with heparin, prostaglandin E1 infusion, and tissue plasminogen activator have not been uniformly successful,

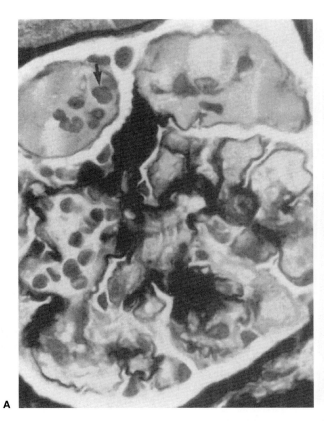
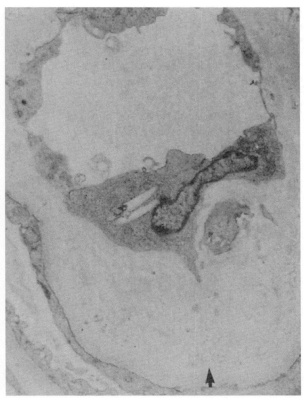

A   B

FIGURE 43-3. **A:** Light-microscopic appearance of a glomerulus from a patient who received a bone marrow transplant 6 months before and had a plasma creatinine of 2.1 mg/dL. Glomerular capillary loops are distended by the subendothelial deposition of proteinaceous material and formed elements of the blood including erythrocytes (*arrow*). There is loss of endothelial and mesangial cells. Focal sclerosis of the mesangium is present. (Jones silver methenamine, ×1,100.) **B:** Electron-microscopic appearance of a glomerular capillary from a patient 10 months after bone marrow transplant with a plasma creatinine of 4.3 mg/dL. Proteinaceous deposits, sometimes mineralized (*arrow*), lift the endothelium away from the glomerular basement membrane, tending to narrow the capillary lumen. (Magnification ×6,300.) (From: Cohen EP, et al. Clinical course of late-onset bone marrow transplant nephropathy. *Nephron* 1993;64:626, with permission.)

as is the attempt to reduce TNF-α by pentoxifylline (176). Recent studies have focused attention on the deficiency of the naturally occurring anticoagulants protein C and antithrombin III as causes of the syndrome (177), but preexisting liver and renal disease, the use of estrogens and progestin, amphotericin, MTX, mismatched grafts, and age greater than 25 years have each been shown to be risk factors. Once renal failure occurs, dialysis is the treatment of choice, as the administration of diuretics and dopamine infusion has not been successful in reversing it (166).

HEMOLYTIC-UREMIC SYNDROME ASSOCIATED WITH BONE MARROW TRANSPLANT

Renal failure may emerge as long as 2 years following bone marrow transplant in a manner that may be identical to the hemolytic-uremic syndrome (HUS). HUS was first reported by Shulman and colleagues (178) who described three patients who developed renal failure 6 weeks after bone marrow transplant with hypertension, congestive heart failure, and a severe microangiopathic hemolytic anemia. It is now a recognized complication in as many as 25% of transplant patients who survive 2 years following successful engraftment (179). The

syndrome is variable and may occur abruptly or take on a more chronic course (180). The microangiopathic hemolytic anemia may be clinically obscure, and the diagnosis may require careful and sequential analysis of the blood and urine and finally a renal biopsy. In both forms of presentation, it is common for patients to enter a more chronic phase with severe, but stable renal failure. Renal histopathology reveals enlarged, hypocellular glomeruli with deposition of spongy material along the inner aspect of the glomerular basement membrane extending into the glomerular capillary loops and producing a "double contour" appearance (Fig. 43-3). Arterioles also show thickening of the wall with expansion of the subendothelial space with mucoid deposits. These changes, consistent with severe mesangiolysis (181) and arterionecrosis, are similar to those seen in acute radiation nephritis (182). Deposition of fibrin, C3 (Complement 3), Clq (Complement 1q), and immunoglobulin M (IgM) can also be demonstrated. In the few patients who have been biopsied in the chronic phase of the disease, glomerular and interstitial fibrosis and arteriolar nephrosclerosis predominate (180).

The mechanism of the nephrotoxicity is unknown, but the role of cyclosporin A (CsA) is not thought to be primary, as the syndrome occurs in its absence (180,183,184). Total body radiation is thought to be a principal cause of the syndrome, as syngeneic transplants not receiving radiation do not have the disease and partial shielding of the kidney results in a lower incidence of HUS following bone marrow transplant (185). Interesting in this regard is that the radiation dose necessary to induce the damage is well below the known threshold of 20 Gy (11). Conditioning protocols used prior to transplantation that usually include cyclophosphamide and cytosine arabinoside, which may be radiomimetic, and the need to introduce CsA treatment to prevent GVHD, all probably potentiate the nephrotoxicity of ionizing radiation.

The similarity of post-transplant HUS and non–transplant-related HUS prompted attempts to treat patients with plasma exchange but without success (186). Another major treatment decision is whether to continue CsA. As already indicated, it does not seem that the role of CsA is primary, and the gravity of GVHD would dictate that patients should remain on the drug. Nonetheless, most centers attempt to reduce the CsA dose. Treatment includes aggressive management of the hypertension, as there is evidence that this slows the progression of the renal disease (179). Recently, there is some evidence to suggest that angiotensin-converting enzyme inhibition and angiotensin-receptor blockade can be used to prevent post-transplant HUS (187,188).

HEMOLYTIC-UREMIC SYNDROME SECONDARY TO CANCER AND CHEMOTHERAPY

HUS often occurs on the background of cancer and chemotherapy but may rarely occur in disseminated cancer even before the initiation of chemotherapy. In the latter circumstance, HUS may actually respond to chemotherapy (189). However, it is most often associated with mitomycin therapy as discussed above, but other agents have been implicated including bleomycin and cisplatin (190). As in autoimmune and familial forms of HUS, large molecular weight complexes of von Willebrand factor (vWF) trigger the characteristic microaggregation of platelets. But in contradistinction to these forms, the cause of the increase in the levels of circulating vWFs is not due to a deficiency of vWF-cleaving protease (ADAMTS13) but is due to release of these complexes from damaged endolethial cells (191,192). Standard plasma exchange therapy is less successful in cases of cancer chemotherapy-associated HUS and alternate therapy with plasma perfusion over staphylococcal protein-A is being advocated.

Cyclosporine Nephrotoxicity

GVHD is a serious complication of bone marrow transplant, carrying with it mortality rates of up to 50% (193). CsA, because of its lack of bone marrow toxicity and proven efficacy (193) over MTX alone in preventing GVHD, is the preferred drug to use in combination with MTX or prednisone. The use of CsA has been associated with a greater incidence of renal failure than the use of MTX alone (194) or MTX plus prednisone (195), and the risk of renal failure has correlated reasonably well with CsA levels in the blood (196), so that monitoring of CsA levels is recommended (166). However this is still a controversial point because the development of renal failure did not correlate with blood CsA levels in at least one large series (164). Currently the risk of CsA-induced renal failure is relatively low, perhaps as a consequence of close drug monitoring and the relatively brief period of full-dose therapy that is employed when no active GVHD is present (196). However, with the increasing use of unrelated donor grafts, it is likely that more chronic GVHD and prolonged CsA dosage will be accompanied by greater nephrotoxicity.

CONCLUSION

It is clear that several factors stand out as potentiating the nephrotoxicity of these agents. First is the presence of preexistent renal disease. Recognition of this and reduction of the administered dose of the nephrotoxin should lead to lower nephrotoxicity. Second is the fullness of the intravascular arterial circulation, and hydration of the patient prior to cytoreductive therapy is an important element in prevention of the most severe forms of renal disease. Data to support the notion that a full extracellular fluid space at the time of exposure ameliorate the subsequent course of the ARF are extensive and reviewed in Chapters 39 and 40. The mechanism of this protection is unknown, but several urinary indices have been identified to predict the outcome of exposure. Thus a high-solute excretion rate and increased renal blood flow are thought to be crucial elements in this regard (197). Interestingly, many different renal stresses respond to this regimen, including ischemic and nephrotoxic insults, and, experimentally at least, do not depend on altering the extent of the cytotoxic insult (34,197) or the pharmacodynamics of the drug (34), suggesting that the mechanism of protection depends on some interruption of the impact of cell injury on kidney function.

It is important to note that the coexistence of cardiovascular disease as well as pulmonary and liver disease will limit the kidney's ability to excrete salt so that monitoring the response of the kidney to salt infusion is crucial. Introduction of a diuretic may be necessary under conditions where there is no diuresis in response to the infusion of fluids alone. While there are advocates of one hydration protocol over another, there are very few randomized, prospective studies to demonstrate benefits of one protocol over another. One recent prospective trial found no benefit of the addition of either mannitol or furosemide to the infusion of 0.45% sodium chloride at a rate of 1 mL per kg body weight per hour for 12 hours before and 12 hours after exposure to radiocontrast dye (198). Adjustments to any standard protocol of fluid administration by careful monitoring of the urine output and assessment of solute excretion are crucial to achieve maximum benefit. If weight gain and peripheral or central edema are provoked, fluid administration may actually be deleterious to the outcome.

The full impact of the antineoplastic drugs on long-term renal function is more difficult to determine, but recent data with cisplatin and bone marrow transplant would indicate that significant degrees of renal dysfunction are to be expected. The challenge for the future is to uncover the mechanism of the permanent renal failure and prevent it.

References

1. Berns JS, Ford PA. Renal toxicities of antineoplastic drugs and bone marrow transplantation. *Semin Nephrol* 1997;17:54.
2. Goren MP, Pratt CB, Viar MJ. Tubular nephrotoxicity during long-term ifosfamide and mesna therapy. *Cancer Chemother Pharmacol* 1989;25:70.
3. Cohen EP, Fish BL, Moulder JE. Treatment of radiation nephropathy with captopril. *Radiat Res* 1992;132:346.
4. Randolph VL, Hall W, Bromson W. Renal failure due to lymphomatous infiltration of the kidneys. *Cancer* 1983;52:1120.
5. Baker LR, et al. Acute renal failure due to bacterial pyelonephritis. *Q J Med* 1979;48:603.
6. Thomas MH, Chisholm GC. Retroperitoneal fibrosis associated with malignant disease. *Br J Cancer* 1973;28:453.
7. Burstein DM, Korbet SM, Schwartz MM. Membranous glomerulonephritis and malignancy. *Am J Kidney Dis* 1993;22:5.
8. Keur I, Krediet R, Arisz L. Glomerulopathy as a paraneoplastic phenomenon. *Neth J Med* 1989;34:5.
9. Kyle RA, O'Fallon WM, Kurland LT. Incidence of multiple myeloma in Olmsted County, Minnesota: 1978 through 1990, with a review of the trends since 1945. *J Clin Oncol* 1994;12:1577.
10. Presti BC, Sciotto CC, Marsh SG. Lymphocytic lymphoma with associated gamma heavy chain and IgM-lambda paraproteins. An unusual biclonal gammopathy. *Am J Clin Pathol* 1990;93:137.

11. Krochak RJ, Baker DG. Radiation nephritis–clinical manifestations and pathophysiologic mechanisms. *Urology* 1986;27:389.

12. Cai Q, et al. Brief report: inhibition of renal phosphate transport by a tumor product in a patient with oncogenic osteomalacia. *N Engl J Med* 1994;330:1645.

13. Osterlind K. Factors confounding evaluation of treatment effect in lung cancer. *Lung Cancer* 1994;10:S97.

14. Talmi VP, Hoffman HT, McCabe BF. Syndrome of inappropriate secretion of arginine vasopressin in patients with cancer of the head and neck. *Ann Otol Rhinol Laryngol* 1992;101:946.

15. Gross AJ, et al. Atrial natriuretic factor and arginine vasopressin production in tumor cell lines from patients with lung cancer and their relationship to serum sodium. *Cancer Res* 1993;53:67.

16. Von Rohr A, et al. Syndrome of inappropriate ADH secretion (SIADH) in small-cell bronchus carcinoma. *Schweiz Med Wochenschr* 1991;121:1271.

17. Misiani R, et al. Hyponatremic hypertensive syndrome and massive proteinuria in a patient with renin-producing leiomyosarcoma. *Am J Kidney Dis* 1994;24:83.

18. Chaudhuri R, et al. MRI in diabetes insipidus due to metastatic breast carcinoma. *Clin Radiol* 1992;46:184.

19. Wysolmerski JJ, Broadus AE. Hypercalcemia of malignancy: the central role of parathyroid hormone-related protein. *Annu Rev Med* 1994;45:189.

20. Merouani A, et al. Increased nephrotoxicity of combination Taxol and cisplatin chemotherapy in gynecologic cancers as compared to cisplatin alone. *Am J Nephrol* 1997;17:53.

21. Merouani A, et al. Renal function in high dose chemotherapy and autologous hematopoietic cell support treatment for breast cancer. *Kidney Int* 1996;50:1026.

22. Schaeppi U, et al. Cis-dichlorodiamine platinum II (NSC 119875): preclinical toxicologic evaluation of intravenous injections in dogs, monkeys and mice. *Toxicol Appl Pharmacol* 1973;25:230.

23. Gonzales-Vitale JC, et al. The renal pathology in clinical trials of cis-platinum (II) diaminedichloride. *Cancer* 1977;39:1362.

24. Litterst CL, Torres IJ, Guarino AM. Plasma levels and organ distribution of platinum in the rat, dog, and dog fish following intravenous administration of cis-DDP(II). *J Clin Hemat Oncol* 1977;7:169.

25. Safirstein R, et al. Renal disposition and metabolism of liganded platinum: implications to toxicity. *Fed Proc* 1980;40:651A.

26. Safirstein R, Miller P, Guttenplan JB. Uptake and metabolism of cisplatin by rat kidney. *Kidney Int* 1984;25:753.

27. Jacobs C, et al. Renal handling of cis-diamine dichloroplatinum (II). *Cancer Treat Rep* 1980;64:1223.

28. Safirstein R, et al. Cisplatin nephrotoxicity insights into mechanism. *Int J Androl* 1987;10:325.

29. Safirstein R, et al. Cisplatin nephrotoxicity in rats: defect in papillary hypertonicity. *Am J Physiol* 1982;241:F175.

30. Megyesi J, Safirstein RL, Price PM. Induction of p21 WAF1/CIP1/SDI1 affects the course of cisplatin-induced acute renal failure. *Journal of Clinical Investigation* 1998;101:777.

31. Safirstein RL, Daye M, Guttenplan JB. Mutagenic activity and identification of excreted platinum in human and rat urine and rat plasma after administration of cisplatin. *Cancer Lett* 1983;18:329.

32. Rosenberg B. Cisplatin: its history and possible mechanism of action. In: Prestayko AW, et al., eds. *Cisplatin—current status and new developments*. New York: Academic Press, 1980.

33. Fichtinger-Shepman AM, et al. Immunochemical quantitation of adducts induced in DNA by cis-diaminedichloroplatinum (II) and analysis of adduct-related DNA unwinding. *Chem Biol Interact* 1985;55:275.

34. Harder HC, Smith RC, LeRoy A. Template-primer inactivation by cis- and trans-dichlorodiamine platinum for human DNA polymerase a, b, and Rausher murine leukemia virus reverse transcriptase as a mechanism of cytotoxicity. *Cancer Res* 1976;36:3821.

35. Harder HC, Rosenberg B. Inhibitory effects of anti-tumor platinum compounds on DNA, RNA, and protein synthesis in mammalian cells in vitro. *Cancer* 1970;6:207.

36. Davis CA, Nick HS, Agarwal A. Manganese superoxide dismutase attenuates cisplating-induced renal injury: importance of superoxide. *J Am Soc Nephrol* 2001;12:2683.

37. Tibbles LA, Woodgett JR. The stress-activated protein kinase pathways. *Cell Mol Life Sci* 1999;55(10):1230.

38. Zanke BW, et al. The stress-activated protein kinase pathway mediates cell death following injury induced by cis-platinum, UV irradiation or heat. *Curr Biol* 1996;6(5):606.

39. Sanchez-Perez I, Perona R. Lack of c-Jun activity increases survival to cisplatin. *FEBS Lett* 1999;453(1–2):151.

40. Persons DL, et al. Cisplatin-induced activation of mitogen-activated protein kinases in ovarian carcinoma cells: inhibition of extracellular signal-regulated kinase activity increases sensitivity to cisplatin. *Clin Cancer Res* 1999;5(5):1007.

41. Kaushal GP, et al. Role and regulation of activation of caspase in cisplatin-induced injury to renal tubular epithelial cells. *Kidney Int* 2001;60(5):1726.

42. Nowak G. Protein Kinase C-alpha and ERK1/2 mediate mitochondrial dysfunction, decreases in active NA$^+$ transport, and cisplatin-induced apoptosis in renal cells. *J Biol Chem* 2002;277(45):43377.

43. Arany I, et al. Cisplatin-induced cell death is EGF/src/ERK signaling dependent in mouse proximal tubule cells. *Am J Physiol* 2004;287:F543.

44. Tsuruya K, et al. Direct involvement of the receptor-mediated apoptotic pathways in cisplatin-induced renal tubular cell death. *Kidney Int* 2003;63(1):72.

45. Cummings B, Schnellmann R. Cisplatin-induced renal cell apoptosis: caspase 3-dependent and independent pathways. *J Pharmacol Exp Ther* 2002; 302:8.

46. Ramesh G, Reeves WB. TNF-α mediates chemokine and cytokine expression and renal injury in cisplatin nephrotoxicity. *J Clin Invest* 2002; 110(6):835.

47. Ulubas B, et al. The protective effects of acetylsalicylic acid on free radical production in cisplatin induced nephrotoxicity: an experimental rat model. *Drug Chem Toxicol* 2003;26(4):259.

48. Kelly KJ, et al. Antibody to intercellular adhesion molecule-1 protects the kidney against ischemic injury. *Proc Soc Nat Acad Sci* 1994;91:812.

49. Deng J, et al. Interleukin-10 inhibits ischemic and cisplatin-induced acute renal injury. *Kidney Int* 2001;60(6):2118.

50. Goossens V, et al. Direct evidence for tumor necrosis factor-induced mitochondrial reactive oxygen intermediates and their involvement in cytotoxicity. *Proc Soc Nat Acad Sci* 1995;92(18):8115.

51. Megyesi J, Safirstein RL, Price PM. Induction of p21WAF1/C3P1/SDI1 in kidney tubule cells affects the course of cisplatin-induced acute renal failure. *J Clin Invest* 1998;101:777.

52. Aass N, et al. Renal function related to different treatment modalities for malignant germ cell tumors. *Br I Cancer* 1990;62:842.

53. Merouani A, Davidson SA, Schrier RW. Increased nephrotoxity of combination taxol and cisplatin chemotherapy in gynecologic cancers is compared to cisplatin alone. *Am J Nephrol* 1997;17:53.

54. Winston JA, Safirstein R. Reduced renal blood flow in early cisplatin-induced acute renal failure in the rat. *Am J Physiol* 1985;249:F490.

55. Schilsky RL, Anderson T. Hypomagnesemia and renal magnesium wasting in patients receiving cisplatin. *Ann Intern Med* 1979;90:929.

56. Vogelzang NJ, Torkelson JL, Kennedy BJ. Hypomagnesemia, renal dysfunction, and Raynaud's phenomenon in patients treated with cisplatin, vinblastine, and bleomycin. *Cancer* 1985;56:2765.

57. Buckley JE, et al. Hypomagnesemia after cisplatin combination chemotherapy. *Arch Intern Med* 1984;144:2347.

58. Mavichak V, et al. Studies on the pathogenesis of cisplatin induced hypomagnesemia in rats. *Kidney Int* 1985;28:914.

59. Schilsky RL. Renal and metabolic toxicities of cancer chemotherapy. *Semin Oncol* 1982;9:75.

60. Meijer S, et al. Some effects of combination chemotherapy with cis-platinum on renal function in patients with nonseminomatous testicular carcinoma. *Cancer* 1983;51:2035.

61. Fjeldborg P, Sorensen J, Helkjaer PE. The long-term effect of cisplatin on renal function. *Cancer* 1986;58:2214.

62. Groth S, et al. Acute and long-term nephrotoxicity of cisplatinum in man. *Cancer Chemother Pharmacol* 1986;17:191.

63. Hansen SW, et al. Long-term effects on renal function and blood pressure of treatment with cisplatin, vinblastine, and bleomycin in patients with germ cell cancer. *J Clin Oncol* 1988;6:1728.

64. Macleod PM, Tyrell CJ, Kelling DH. The effect of cisplatin on renal function in patients with testicular tumors. *Clin Radiol* 1988;39:190.

65. Daugaard C, Rossing N, Rorth M. Effects of cisplatin on different measures of glomerular function in the human kidney with special emphasis on high-dose. *Cancer Chemother Pharmacol* 1988;21:163.

66. Hamilton CR, Bliss JM, Horwich A. The late effects of cis-platinum on renal function. *Eur J Cancer Clin Oncol* 1989;25:185.

67. Pera MF, Zook BC, Harder HC. Effects of mannitol or furosemide diuresis on the nephrotoxicity and physiological disposition of cis-dichloroplatinum(II) in rats. *Cancer Res* 1979;39:1269.

68. Bodenner DL, et al. Effect of diethyldithiocarbamate on cis-diaminedichloroplatinum(II)-induced cytotoxicity, DNA cross-linking and gamma-glutamyl transpeptidase inhibition. *Cancer Res* 1986;46:2745.

69. Bodenner DL, et al. Selective protection against cis-diaminedichloroplatinum(II)-induced toxicity in kidney, gut, and bone marrow by diethyldithiocarbamate. *Cancer Res* 1986;46:2751.

70. Berry JM, et al. Modification of cisplatin toxicity with diethyldithiocarbamate. *J Clin Oncol* 1990;8:1585.

71. Hartman JT, et al. The use of reduced doses of amifostine to ameliorate nephrotoxicity of cisplatin-ifosfamide-based chemotherapy in patients with solid tumors. *Anti-Cancer Drugs* 2000;11:1.

72. Weiss JF. Pharmacologic approaches to protection against radiation-induced lethality and other damage. *Environ Health Perspect* 1997; 105:6.

73. Santini V, Giles FJ. The potential of amifostine: from cytoprotectant to therapeutic agent. *Haematologica* 1999;84:1035.

74. Vaziri ND, Zhou XJ, Liao SY. Erythropoietin enhances recovery from cisplatin-induced acute renal failure. *Am J Physiol* 1994;266:F360.

75. Bunn PA Jr. Carboplatin: Current status and future directions. In: Bunn PA Jr, Canetta R, Ozols RF, et al., eds. *Carboplatin (JM-8). Current perspectives and future directions.* Philadelphia: Saunders, 1990:371.

76. Egorin MJ, et al. Pharmacokinetics and dosage reduction of cis-diamine (1,1-cyclobutanedicarboxylate) platinum in patients with impaired renal function. *Cancer Res* 1984;44:5432.

77. DeFronzo RA, et al. Proceedings: cyclophosphamide and the kidney. *Cancer* 1974;33:483.

78. Bode U, Seif SM, Levine AS. Studies on the antidiuretic effect of cyclophosphamide: vasopressin release and sodium excretion. *Med Pediatr Oncol* 1980;8:295.

79. Shea TC, et al. A dose-escalation study of carboplatin/cyclophos-phamide/etoposide along with autologous bone marrow or peripheral blood stem cell rescue. *Semin Oncol* 1992;19:139.

80. Carter SK, Wasserman TH. The nitrosoureas—thoughts for the future. *Cancer Treat Rep* 1973;4:13.

81. Oliverio VT. Toxicology and pharmacology of the nitrosoureas (part 3). *Cancer Chemother Rep* 1973;4:13.

82. Sponzo RW, DeVita VT, Oliverio VT. Physiologic disposition of 1-(2-chloroethyl)-3-cyclohexyl-1-nitrosourea (CCNU) and 1-(2-chloroethyl)-3-(4-methylcyclohexyl)-1-nitrosourea (Me CCNU) in man. *Cancer* 1973;31:1154.

83. Weiss RB. Streptozocin: a review of its pharmacology, efficacy and toxicity. *Cancer Treat Rep* 1982;66:427.

84. Bhuyan BK, et al. Tissue distribution of streptozotocin (NSC-85998). *Cancer Chemother Rep* 1974;58:157.

85. Loftus L, Cuppage FE, Hoogstraten B. Clinical and pathological effects of streptozotocin. *J Lab Clin Med* 1974;84:407.

86. Shein PS, et al. Clinical antitumor activity and toxicity of streptozotocin (NSC-85998). *Cancer* 1974;34:993.

87. Sadoff L. Nephrotoxicity of streptozotocin (NSC-85998). *Cancer Chemother Rep* 1970;54:457.

88. Bukowski RM, et al. Phase II trial of chlorozotocin and fluorouracil in islet cell carcinoma: a Southwest Oncology Group study. *J Clin Oncol* 1992;10:1914.

89. Zalupski M, Baker LH. Ifosfamide. *J Natl Cancer Int* 1988;556.

90. Brock N, Pohl J. The development of mesna for regional detoxification. *Cancer Treat Rep* 1983;10:33.

91. Antman KH, et al. Phase II trial of ifosfamide with mesna in previously treated metastatic sarcoma. *Cancer Treat Rep* 1985;69:499.

92. Goren MP, et al. Potentiation of ifosfamide neurotoxicity, hematotoxicity, and tubular nephrotoxicity by pro-cis-diaminedichloroplatinum (II) therapy. *Cancer Res* 1987;4:1457.

93. Patterson WP, Khojasteh A. Ifosfamide-induced renal tubular defects. *Cancer* 1989;63:649.

94. Arndt C, et al. Renal function in children and adolescents following 72 g/m2 of ifosfamide. *Cancer Chemother Pharmacol* 1994;34:431.

95. Rossi R, et al. Unilateral nephrectomy and cisplatin as risk factors for ifosfamide-induced nephrotoxicity: analysis of 120 patients. *J Clin Oncol* 1994;12:159.

96. Rossi RM, et al. Estimation of ifosfamide/cisplatinum-induced renal toxicity by urinary protein analysis. *Pediatr Nephrol* 1994;8:151.

97. Pratt CB, et al. Ifosfamide, Fanconi's syndrome and rickets. *Clin Oncol* 1991;9:1495.

98. Davies SM, Pearson AD, Craft AW. Toxicity of high-dose ifosfamide in children. *Cancer Chemother Pharmacol* 1989;24:58.

99. Condit PT, Chanes RE, Joel W. Renal toxicity of methotrexate. *Cancer* 1969;23:126.

100. Hande KR, Donehower RC, Chabner BA. Pharmacology and pharmacokinetics of high dose methotrexate in man. In: Pinedo HM, ed. *Clinical pharmacology of antineoplastic drugs*. Amsterdam: Elsevier, 1978.

101. Pitman SW, et al. Clinical trial of high dose methotrexate (NSC 740) with citrovorum factor (NSC 3590). Toxicologic and therapeutic observations. *Cancer Chemother Rep* 1975;6:43.

102. Hande KR, et al. Methotrexate and hemodialysis. *Ann Intern Med* 1977;87:495.

103. Stoller RG, et al. Use of plasma pharmacokinetics to predict and prevent methotrexate toxicity. *N Engl J Med* 1977;297:630.

104. Thierry IFX, et al. Acute renal failure after high-dose methotrexate therapy. Role of hemodialysis and plasma exchange in methotrexate removal. *Nephron* 1989;51:416.

105. Pitman SW, Frei E III. Weekly methotrexate–calcium leukovorin rescue: effect of alkalinization on nephrotoxicity; pharmacokinetics in the CNS and use in CNS non-Hodgkin's lymphoma. *Cancer Treat Rep* 1977;61:695.

106. Abelson HT, Garnick MB. Renal failure induced by cancer chemotherapy. In: Rieselbach RE, Garnick MB, eds. *Cancer and the kidney*. Philadelphia: Lea & Febiger, 1982.

107. Howell SB, Carmody J. Changes in glomerular filtration rate associated with high-dose methotrexate therapy in adults. *Cancer Treat Rep* 1977;61:1389.

108. Link MG, Fosburg MT, Ingelfinger JR. Renal toxicity of high dose methotrexate. *Pediatr Res* 1976;10:455.

109. Wall SM, et al. Effective clearance of methotrexate using high-flex Hemodialysis membranes. *Am J Kidney Dis* 1996;28:846.

110. Widemann BC, et al. High-dose Methotrexate-induced nephrotoxicity in patients with osteosarcoma. Incidence, treatment and outcome. *Cancer* 2004;100:2222.

111. Kizaki H et al. 1-beta-D-arabinosylcytosine and 5-azacyti-dine induce internucleosomal DNA fragmentation and cell death in thymocytes. *Immunopharmacology* 1993;25:19.

112. Hidemann W. Cytosine arabinoside in the treatment of acute myeloid leukemia: the role and place of high-dose regimens. *Ann Hematol* 1991;62:119.

113. Capizzi RL, et al. Effect of dose on the pharmacokinetic and pharmacodynamic effects of cytarabine. *Semin Hematol* 1991;28:54.

114. Slavin RE, Dias MA, Saral R. Cytosine arabinoside induced gastrointestinal toxic alterations in sequential chemotherapeutic protocols: a clinical-pathologic study of 33 patients. *Cancer* 1978;42:1747.

115. Albain KS, et al. Cisplatin preceded by concurrent cytarabine and hydroxyurea: a pilot study based on an in vitro model. *Cancer Chemother Pharmacol* 1990;27:33.

116. Damon LE, Mass R, Linker CA. The association between high dose cytarabine neurotoxicity and renal insufficiency. *J Clin Oncol* 1989;7:1563.

117. Morales-Pelanco M, et al. Rhabdomyolysis in patients with acute lymphoblastic leukemia. *Arch Med Res* 1997;28:377.

118. Hanna WT, et al. Renal disease after mitomycin C therapy. *Cancer* 1981;48:2583.

119. Jones BC, et al. Intravascular haemolysis and renal impairment after blood transfusion in two patients on long-term 5-fluorouracil and mitomycin-C. *Lancet* 1980;1:1275.

120. Brillet C, et al. Long-term renal effect of cisplatin in man. *Am J Nephrol* 1994;14:81.

121. Jassem J, et al. Combination of daily 4-h infusion of 5-fluorouracil and cisplatin in the treatment of advanced head and neck squamous-cell carcinoma: a South–East European Oncology Group study. *Cancer Chemother Pharmacol* 1993;31:489.

122. Park TK, et al. Role of induction chemotherapy in invasive cervical cancer. *Gynecol Oncol* 1991;41:107.

123. Von Hoff, DD, et al. Incidence of drug-related deaths secondary to high-dose methotrexate and citrovorum factor administration. *Cancer Treat Rep* 1977;61:745.

124. Peterson BA, et al. 5-azacytidine and renal tubular dysfunction. *Blood* 1981;57:182.

125. Philips FS, Schwartz HS, Steinberg SS. Pharmacology of mitomycin C: I. Toxicity and pathologic effects. *Cancer Res* 1960;20:1354.

126. Ratanatharathorn V. Clinical and pathological study of mitomycin C nephrotoxicity. In: Carter SK, Crooke ST, eds. *Mitomycin C: current status and new developments*. New York: Academic Press, 1979.

127. Price TM, et al. Renal failure and hemolytic anemia associated with mitomycin C. *Cancer* 1985;55:51.

128. Blanco C, et al. Kidney cortical necrosis induced by mitomycin-c: a morphologic experimental study. *Renal Fail* 1992;14:31.

129. Kennedy BJ. Metabolic and toxic effects of mithramycin during tumor therapy. *Am J Med* 1970;49:494.

130. Kennedy BJ, Brown JH, Yarbro JW. Mithramycin (NSC-24559) therapy for primary glioblastomas. *Cancer Chemother Rep* 1965;48:59.

131. Cortes EP, et al. Effects of mithramycin on bone resorption in vitro. *Cancer Res* 1972;32:74.

132. Hall TJ, Schaeublin M, Chambers TJ. The majority of osteoclasts require mRNA and protein synthesis for bone resorption in vitro. *Biochem Biophys Res Commun* 1993;195:1245.

133. Markowitz GS, et al. Toxic acute tubularnecrosis following treatment with zolendronate. *Kidney Int* 2003;64:281.

134. Bean B. Antiviral therapy: current concepts and practices. *Clin Microbiol Rev* 1992;5:146.

135. Krown SE. Interferons and interferon inducers in cancer treatment. *Semin Oncol* 1986;13:207.

136. Talpaz M, et al. Therapy of chronic myelogenous leukemia: chemotherapy and interferons. *Semin Hematol* 1988;25:62.

137. Selby P, et al. Nephrotic syndrome during treatment with interferon. *Br Med J* 1985;290:1180.

138. Sherwin SA, et al. A multiple-dose phase I trial of recombinant leukocyte A interferon in cancer patients. *JAMA* 1982;319:1397.

139. Ault BH, et al. Acute renal failure during therapy with recombinant human gamma interferon. *N Engl J Med* 1988;296:134.

140. Ernstoff MS, et al. A phase IA trial of sequential administration recombinant DNA-produced interferons: combination recombinant interferon gamma and recombinant interferon alpha in patients with metastatic renal cell carcinoma. *J Clin Oncol* 1990;8:1637.

141. Rosenberg SA. Immunotherapy of cancer by systemic administration of lymphoid cells plus interleukin-2. *J Biol Response Mod* 1984;3:501.

142. Textor SC, et al. Renal, volume, and hormonal changes during therapeutic administration of recombinant interleukin-2 in man. *Am J Med* 1987;83:1055.

143. Beildegrun A, et al. Effects of interleukin-2 on renal function in patients receiving immunotherapy for advanced cancer. *Ann Intern Med* 1987;106:817.

144. Ponce P, et al. Renal toxicity mediated by continuous infusion of recombinant interleukin-2. *Nephron* 1993;64:114.

145. Mercatello A, et al. Acute renal failure with preserved renal plasma flow induced by cancer immunotherapy. *Kidney Int* 1991;40:309.

146. Cohen L, et al. Acute tumor lysis syndrome. A review of 37 patients with Burkitt's lymphoma. *Am J Med* 1980;68:486.

147. Vogelzang NJ, Nelimark RA, Nath KA. Tumor lysis syndrome after induction chemotherapy of small-cell bronchogenic carcinoma. *JAMA* 1983;249:513.

148. O'Connor NT, Prentice HG, Hoffbrand AV. Prevention of urate nephropathy in the tumour lysis syndrome. *Clin Lab Haematol* 1989;11:97.

149. Hussein AM, Fern LG. Tumor lysis syndrome after induction chemotherapy in small-cell lung carcinoma. *Am J Clin Oncol* 1990;13:10.
150. Khan J, Broadbent VA. Tumor lysis syndrome complicating treatment of widespread metastatic abdominal rhabdomyosarcoma. *Pediatr Hematol Oncol* 1993;10:151.
151. Jasek AM, Day HI. Acute spontaneous tumor lysis syndrome. *Am J Hematol* 1994;47:129.
152. Hande KR, Yarrow CC. Acute tumor lysis syndrome in patients with high-grade non-Hodgkin's lymphoma. *Am J Med* 1993;94:133.
153. Hande KR, Hixson CV, Chabner BA. Postchemotherapy purine excretion in lymphoma patients receiving allopurinol. *Cancer Res* 1981;41:2273.
154. Gomez GA, Stutzman L, Chu TM. Xanthine nephropathy during chemotherapy in deficiency of hypoxanthine-guanine phosphoribosyltransferase. *Arch Intern Med* 1978;138:1017.
155. Cadman EC, Lundberg WB, Bertino JR. Hyperphosphatemia and hypocalcemia accompanying rapid cell lysis in a patient with Burkitt's lymphoma and Burkitt cell leukemia. *Am J Med* 1977;62:283.
156. Aubert JD, et al. Hyperphosphatemia and transient renal insufficiency following chemotherapy of acute lymphoblastic leukemia. *Schweiz Med Wochenschr* 1988;118:1953.
157. Ayala C, et al. Acute hyperphosphatemia and acute persistent renal insufficiency induced by oral phosphate therapy. *Ann Intern Med* 1975;83:520.
158. Ettinger DS, et al. Hyperphosphatemia, hypocalcemia, and transient renal failure: results of cytotoxic treatment of acute lymphoblastic leukemia. *JAMA* 1978;239:2472.
159. Kanfer A, et al. Extreme hyperphosphataemia causing acute anuric nephrocalcinosis in lymphosarcoma. *Br Med J* 1979;1:1320.
160. Boles JM, et al. Acute renal failure caused by extreme hyperphosphatemia after chemotherapy of an acute lymphoblastic leukemia. *Cancer* 1984;53:2425.
161. Fenaux P, Botton SD. Retinoic acid syndrome: recognition, prevention and management. *Drug Safety* 1998;18:273.
162. Bortin MM, et al. Increasing utilization of allogeneic bone marrow transplantation. *Ann Intern Med* 1992;116:505.
163. Zager RA, et al. Acute renal failure following bone marrow transplantation: a retrospective study of 272 patients. *Am J Kidney Dis* 1989;13:210.
164. Beelen DW, et al. Six weeks of continuous intravenous cyclosporine and short-course methotrexate as prophylaxis for acute graft-versus-host disease after allogeneic bone marrow transplantation. *Transplantation* 1990;50:421.
165. Tarbell NJ, et al. Renal insufficiency after total body irradiation for pediatric bone marrow transplantation. *Radiother Oncol* 1990;18:139.
166. Zager RA. Acute renal failure in the setting of bone marrow transplantation. *Kidney Int* 1994;46:1443(abst).
167. Davis JM, et al. Clinical toxicity of cryopreserved bone marrow graft infusion. *Blood* 1990;75:781.
168. Yellowlees P, Greenfield C, Mcintyre N. Dimethylsulphoxide-induced toxicity. *Lancet* 1980;2:1004.
169. Nath KA, et al. Induction of heme oxygenase is a rapid protective response in rhabdomyolysis in the rat. *J Clin Invest* 1992;90:267.
170. Zager RA. Intracellular myoglobin loading worsens H2O2-induced, but not hypoxia/reoxygenation-induced, in vitro proximal tubular injury. *Circ Res* 1993;73:926.
171. Kone BC, et al. Hypertension and renal dysfunction in bone marrow transplant recipients. *Q J Med* 1988;69:985.
172. Gruss E, et al. Acute renal failure and bone marrow transplantation. Proceedings of the Third Satellite Symposium Halkidiki, Greece, 1993.
173. McDonald CB, et al. Venocclusive disease of the liver after bone marrow transplantation: diagnosis, incidence, and predisposing factors. *Hepatology* 1984;4:116.
174. Jones RJ, et al. Venocclusive disease of the liver following bone marrow transplantation. *Transplantation* 1987;44:778.
175. McDonald CB, et al. Veno-occlusive disease of the liver and multiorgan failure after bone marrow transplantation: a cohort study of 355 patients. *Ann Intern Med* 1993;118:255.
176. Clift RA, et al. A randomized controlled trial of pentoxifylline for the prevention of regimen-related toxicities in patients undergoing allogeneic marrow transplantation. *Blood* 1993;82:2025.
177. Gordon B, et al. High frequency of antithrombin 3 and protein C deficiency following autologous bone marrow transplantation for lymphoma. *Bone Marrow Transplant* 1991;8:497.
178. Shulman H, et al. Nephrotoxicity of cyclosporin A after allogeneic marrow transplantation. Glomerular thrombosis and tubular injury. *N Engl J Med* 1981;305:1392.
179. Cohen EP, et al. Clinical course of late-onset bone marrow transplant nephropathy. *Nephron* 1993;64:626.
180. Antignac C, et al. Delayed renal failure with extensive mesangiolysis following bone marrow transplantation. *Kidney Int* 1989;35:1336.
181. Morita T, Churg J. Mesangiolysis. *Kidney Int* 1983;24:1.
182. Cogan MG, Arieff AI. Radiation nephritis and intravascular coagulation. *Clin Nephrol* 1978;10:74.
183. Chappell ME, et al. Haemolytic uraemic syndrome after bone marrow transplantation: an adverse effect of total body irradiation? *Bone Marrow Transplant* 1988;3:339.
184. Rabinowe SN, et al. Hemolytic–uremic syndrome following bone marrow transplantation in adults for hematologic malignancies. *Blood* 1991;77:1837.
185. Lawton CA, et al. Influence of renal shielding on the incidence of late renal dysfunction associated with T-lymphocyte depleted bone marrow transplantation in adult patients. *Int J Radiat Oncol Biol Phys* 1992;23:681.
186. Silva VA, et al. Plasma exchange and vincristine in the treatment of hemolytic uremic syndrome/thrombotic thrombocytopenic purpura associated with bone marrow transplantation. *J Clin Apheresis* 1991;6:16.
187. Moulder JE, et al. Prophylaxis of bone marrow transplant nephropathy with captopril, an inhibitor of angiotensin-converting enzyme. *Radiat Res* 1993;136:404.
188. Moulder JE, et al. Angiotensin II receptor antagonists in the prevention of radiation nephropathy. *Radiat Res* 1996;146:106.
189. Mungall S, Matheson H. Hemolytic uremic syndrome in metastatic adenocarcinoma of the prostate. *Am J Kidney Dis* 2002;40:1334.
190. Gordon LI, Kwaan HC. Cancer and drug-associated thrombotic thrombocytopenic purpura and hemolytic uremic syndrome. *Semin Hematol* 1997;34:140.
191. van der Plas RM, et al. Von Willebrand factor proteolysis is deficient in classic, but not in bone marrow transplant-associated thrombotic thrombocytopenic purpura. *Blood* 1999;93:3798.
192. Horninga JA, et al. Von Willebrand factor-clearing protease (ADAMTS-13) activity determination in the diagnosis of thrombotic microangiopathics: the Swiss experience. *Semin Hematol* 2004;41:75.
193. Sullivan KM. Graft-versus-host disease. In: Forman ST, Blume KG, Thomas ED, eds. *Bone marrow transplantation*. Oxford: Blackwell, 1994.
194. Deeg HJ, et al. Cyclosporine as prophylaxis for graft-versus-host disease: a randomized study in patients undergoing marrow transplantation for acute nonlymphoblastic leukemia. *Blood* 1985;65:1325.
195. Weisdorf D, et al. Combination graft-versus-host disease prophylaxis using immunotoxic (anti-CD5-RI[xomazyme-CD5I]) plus methotrexate and cyclosporine or prednisone after unrelated donor marrow transplantation. *Bone Marrow Transplant* 1993;12:531.
196. Dieterle A, et al. Chronic cyclosporine-associated nephrotoxicity in bone marrow transplant patients. *Transplantation* 1990;49:1093.
197. Patak R, et al. Study of factors which modify the development of norepinephrine-induced acute renal failure in the dog. *Kidney Int* 1979;15:227.
198. Solomon R, et al. Effects of saline, mannitol, and furosemide to prevent acute decreases in renal function induced by radiocontrast agents. *N Engl J Med* 1994;331:1416.

CHAPTER 44 ■ NEPHROTOXICITY OF NONSTEROIDAL ANTIINFLAMMATORY AGENTS, ANALGESICS, AND ANGIOTENSIN-CONVERTING ENZYME INHIBITORS

BIFF F. PALMER AND WILLIAM L. HENRICH

NEPHROTOXICITY OF NONSTEROIDAL ANTIINFLAMMATORY DRUGS

Nonsteroidal antiinflammatory drugs (NSAIDs) are some of the most widely utilized therapeutic agents in clinical practice today. While the gastrointestinal toxicity of these medications is well known, it has become increasingly apparent that the kidney is also an important target for untoward clinical events. The renal toxicity associated with the use of NSAIDs can be divided into one of several distinct clinical syndromes. These include a form of vasomotor acute renal failure, nephrotic syndrome associated with interstitial nephritis, chronic renal injury, and abnormalities in sodium, water, and potassium homeostasis. The common link in these syndromes is a disruption in prostaglandin metabolism, the class of compounds whose synthesis is inhibited by these agents.

Prostaglandin Biosynthesis and Compartmentalization

Prostaglandins are members of a class of compounds termed eicosanoids. Eicosanoids are biologically active fatty acids that are all derived from the oxygenation of arachidonic acid. The particular enzyme involved in the oxygenation process dictates which class of eicosanoid will be synthesized. Oxygenation of arachidonic acid by the enzyme cyclooxygenase is responsible for prostaglandin and thromboxane synthesis (Fig. 44-1). The enzyme lipoxygenase converts arachidonic acid to leukotrienes, lipoxins, and eventually to hydro fatty acid derivatives such as hydroxyeicosatetraenoic acid (HETE). Finally, oxygenation by the cytochrome P-450 system generates epoxyeicosatrienoic acids (EETs).

The availability of free arachidonic acid is the rate-limiting step in eicosanoid biosynthesis. Normally, arachidonic acid is found esterified to membrane phospholipids, where it undergoes deacylation primarily under the influence of phospholipase A_2. Phospholipase A_2-mediated arachidonic acid release is a calcium–calmodulin-dependent step that is stimulated by vasopressin, bradykinin, angiotensin, and norepinephrine (1). Corticosteroids inhibit this reaction by inducing the formation of an inhibitor of phospholipase A_2 called macrocortin or lipomodulin. Once released, free arachidonic acid is either reesterified back into membrane lipids or is converted into one of the biologically active eicosanoids.

The first step in the synthesis of prostaglandins and thromboxanes is a cyclooxygenase reaction in which arachidonic

acid is converted into the cyclic endoperoxide prostaglandin G_2 (PGG_2). PGG_2 then undergoes a peroxidase reaction to form a second endoperoxide called PGH_2, which is accompanied by the formation of a superoxide radical. Both of these reactions are catalyzed by the enzyme cyclooxygenase (COX), also known as prostaglandin endoperoxide H synthase (2,3). The cyclooxygenase and peroxidase reactions occur on distinct but neighboring sites on the COX enzyme. Once formed, PGH_2 has a short half-life and is rapidly acted on by a series of enzymes that produce biologically active prostaglandins or thromboxane. Prostacyclin synthase acts to form prostacyclin (PGI_2), thromboxane synthase forms thromboxane A_2, and isomerases are responsible for the formation of PGE_2, PGD_2, and PGF_{2a}. PGE_2 can be converted to $PGF_{2\alpha}$ by 9-ketoreductase, an enzyme that is stimulated by high-salt diet and inhibited by furosemide (4).

Prostaglandins are synthesized on demand and exert physiologic effects in discrete microenvironments along the nephron in close proximity to their points of synthesis (Table 44-1). Due to the virtual absence of distant effects, these compounds are best regarded as autacoids rather than hormones. Variations in the synthetic and degradative machinery along the length of the nephron account for the differing types and amounts of prostaglandins found in any given segment (5). PGI_2 is the most abundant prostaglandin produced in the cortex and is primarily synthesized in cortical arterioles and glomeruli (6). This location corresponds to the known effects of PGI_2 in regulating renal vascular tone, glomerular filtration rate (GFR), and renin release. PGE_2 and thromboxane A_2 are also produced in the glomerulus and therefore may exert effects at this site.

The most abundant prostaglandin found in the tubules is PGE_2 (5,6). The cortical and especially the medullary portion of the collecting duct is the dominant site of PGE_2 synthesis. Lesser amounts are found in the thin descending and thick ascending limb with the least amount of synthesis found in the proximal tubule. Medullary interstitial cells are also a rich source of PGE_2 production. This distribution provides the anatomic basis for PGE_2 to modulate sodium and chloride transport in the loop of Henle, regulate arginine vasopressin-mediated water transport, and control vasa recta blood flow. $PGF_{2\alpha}$ is synthesized primarily by medullary interstitial cells and less by the papillary collecting tubule and glomeruli. Prostaglandin-degradative enzymes are found in both the cortex and medulla but are most abundant in the cortex. Except for PGI_2, which undergoes spontaneous hydrolysis to 6-keto-$PGF_{2\alpha}$, prostaglandins are rapidly metabolized into inactive products by a 15-prostaglandin dehydrogenase (7). Increased concentration of this enzyme in the proximal nephron may facilitate degradation of prostaglandins delivered to the proximal tubule by glomerular filtration (8).

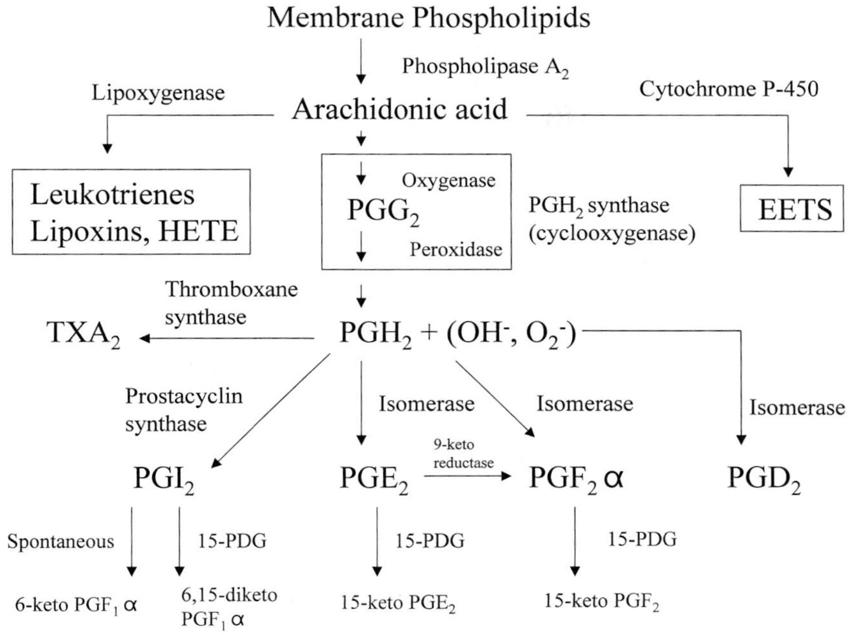

Membrane Phospholipids

Phospholipase A$_2$

Lipoxygenase   Arachidonic acid ——— Cytochrome P-450

Leukotrienes Lipoxins, HETE

Oxygenase
PGG$_2$ PGH$_2$ synthase (cyclooxygenase)
Peroxidase

EETS

Thromboxane synthase

TXA$_2$ ◄— PGH$_2$ + (OH$^-$, O$_2^-$) ———

Prostacyclin synthase   Isomerase   Isomerase   Isomerase

PGI$_2$ PGE$_2$ —9-keto reductase→ PGF$_2\alpha$ PGD$_2$

Spontaneous | 15-PDG   15-PDG   15-PDG

6-keto PGF$_1\alpha$ 6,15-diketo PGF$_1\alpha$ 15-keto PGE$_2$ 15-keto PGF$_2$

FIGURE 44-1. Synthetic and degradative pathways for the different types of eicosanoids. *15-PDG*, 15-prostaglandin dehydrogenase; *EETs*, epoxyeicosatrienoic acids; *HETE*, hydroxyeicosatetraenoic acid; *TXA$_2$*, thromboxane A$_2$.

Biologic Actions of Prostaglandins in the Kidney

Under baseline euvolemic conditions, prostaglandin synthesis is negligible, and as a result, these compounds play little to no role in the minute-to-minute maintenance of renal function. Where these compounds come to serve a major role is in the setting of a systemic or intrarenal circulatory disturbance. This interaction is best illustrated when examining renal function under conditions of volume depletion (Fig. 44-2). In this setting, renal blood flow is decreased while sodium reabsorption, renin release, and urinary concentrating ability are increased. To a large extent, these findings are mediated by the effects of increased circulating levels of angiotensin II (AII), arginine

vasopressin (AVP), and catechols. At the same time, these hormones stimulate the synthesis of renal prostaglandins, which in turn act to dilate the renal vasculature, inhibit salt and water reabsorption, and further stimulate renin release. Prostaglandin release under these conditions serves to dampen and counterbalance the physiologic effects of the hormones that elicit their production. As a result, renal function is maintained near normal despite the systemic circulation being clamped down. Predictably, inhibition of prostaglandin synthesis will lead to unopposed activity of these hormonal systems, resulting in exaggerated renal vasoconstriction and magnified antinatriuretic and antidiuretic effects. In fact, many of the renal syndromes that are associated with the use of NSAIDs can be explained by the predictions of this model.

TABLE 44-1

COMPARTMENTALIZATION AND FUNCTION OF RENAL PROSTAGLANDINS

Site	Eicosanoid	Action
Arterioles	PGI$_2$, PGE$_2$	Vasodilation
Glomeruli	PGI$_2$ > PGE$_2$ (human)	Maintain GFR Vasoconstriction
	PGE$_2$ > PGI$_2$ (rat) TXA$_2$	
Tubules	PGE$_2$, PGF$_{2\alpha}$	Enhance NaCl and water excretion
Interstitial cells	PGE$_2$	Enhance NaCl and water excretion, influence regional blood flow
Juxtaglomerular apparatus	PGI$_2$, PGE$_2$	Stimulate renin release

PGI, prostaglandin I; *PGE*, prostaglandin E; *PGF*, prostaglandin F; *TXA*, thromboxane A; *GFR*, glomerular filtration rate.

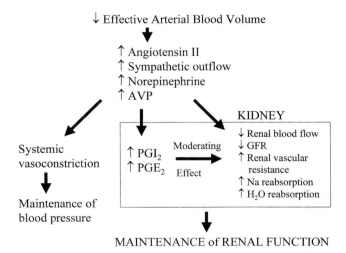

FIGURE 44-2. In the setting of absolute or effective volume depletion, a number of effectors are activated that serve to defend the circulation and at the same time stimulate the synthesis of renal prostaglandins. In turn, renal prostaglandins function to moderate the effects of these hormonal systems such that renal function is maintained in the setting of systemic vasoconstriction. *AVP*, arginine vasopressin; *GFR*, glomerular filtration rate.

Expression and Regulation of Cyclooxygenase (COX)-1 and COX-2 in the Kidney

Aspirin and other NSAIDs exert their prostaglandin-inhibitory effects by inhibiting the COX enzyme. The COX enzyme exists as two isoforms termed cyclooxygenase-1 (COX-1) and cyclooxygenase-2 (COX-2). These enzymes are encoded by two different genes and differ significantly in their regulation. The COX-1 enzyme is constitutively expressed in most tissues and is responsible for producing prostaglandins involved in maintaining normal tissue homeostasis. The COX-2 enzyme is principally an inducible enzyme rapidly upregulated in response to a variety of stimuli such as growth factors and cytokines typically found in the setting of inflammation (3). With the discovery of COX-2, a great deal of effort was put forth to develop compounds to selectively block the activity of this isoform without affecting the activity of COX-1. The availability of a COX-2–specific inhibitor would provide a therapeutic tool to inhibit the synthesis of arachidonic acid metabolites at sites of inflammation and yet leave unperturbed COX-1 derived prostanoids involved in normal homeostasis. In this manner the analgesic, antiinflammatory, and antipyretic effects of an NSAID could be obtained with minimal to no side effects. While initial experience with specific COX-2 inhibitors has been associated with a reduction in gastrointestinal complications, recent information suggests this paradigm is not applicable to the kidney.

COX-1 and COX-2 are both constitutively expressed in the kidney. COX-1 is localized to mesangial cells, arteriolar endothelial cells, parietal epithelial cells of Bowman's capsule and throughout the cortical and medullary collecting duct (9). COX-2 is primarily expressed in the macula densa and adjacent cells in the cortical thick ascending limb with lesser amounts in the podocytes and arteriolar smooth muscle cells (10–13). COX-2 is also abundantly expressed in interstitial cells in the inner medulla and papilla (Table 44-2).

The expression of COX-2 in different regions of the kidney varies in response to alterations in intravascular volume. This variation is particularly evident in the macula densa where studies show COX-2 plays an important stimulatory role in the release of renin via the tubuloglomerular feedback mechanism. Under conditions of low renal perfusion when the chloride concentration at the level of the macula densa is low, renin release is inhibited by a COX-2 selective inhibitor but unaffected by a COX-1 inhibitor (14). In genetically engineered mice lacking COX-2 there is a failure of renin release in response to a low salt diet whereas renin release is intact in animals lacking COX-1 (15,16).

Stimulation of renin with subsequent formation of angiotensin II is part of a feedback loop since angiotensin II exerts an inhibitory effect on COX-2 synthesis in the macula densa via the angiotensin type 1 (AT_1) receptor (17). In contrast to effects at the macula densa angiotensin II upregulates COX-2 and prostaglandin synthesis in vascular smooth muscle cells and mesangial cells (18,19). This latter effect provides a mechanism for COX-2 to both facilitate the tubuloglomerular feedback response to low salt delivery to the macula densa by increasing angiotensin II levels and preserve the glomerular filtration rate through generation of vasodilatory prostaglandins to antagonize the vasoconstrictive effect of angiotensin II (20).

The expression of COX-2 is also responsive to changes in volume in the medulla of the kidney. COX-2 expression decreases with salt depletion and increases with high salt diet and dehydration (13). COX-2–derived prostaglandins may play an important role in facilitating a natriuretic response to salt loading and help protect against volume overload. The increase in COX-2 in response to dehydration is thought to provide a cytoprotective effect in the setting of hypertonic stress (21,22). Treatment of water-deprived animals with a selective COX-2 inhibitor is associated with apoptotic patches of renal medullary interstitial cells. By contrast, no such changes are seen in animals treated with the inhibitor alone or in animals undergoing water deprivation without pharmacologic treatment.

In summary, COX-2 is constitutively expressed in the kidney and is highly regulated in response to physiologic perturbations in intravascular volume. As discussed in the remainder of this chapter the majority of experimental and clinical studies to date suggest that the specific COX-2 inhibitors may not offer any distinct advantage over traditional NSAIDs with regard to renal toxicity. In fact, most of the renal syndromes that have been linked to nonselective COX inhibitors have now been described with the selective COX-2 inhibitors (Table 44-3). The only exception is the development of chronic kidney disease and papillary necrosis. The failure to link COX-2 inhibitors use to these complications is not surprising since these agents have only been available for clinical use for a relatively short period

---

TABLE 44-2

INTRA-RENAL LOCALIZATION OF COX-1 AND COX-2

Localization of COX-1
Mesangial cells
Arteriolar endothelial cells
Parietal epithelial cells of Bowman's capsule
Cortical and medullary collecting duct cells

Localization of COX-2
Macula densa and adjacent cells of cortical thick ascending limb of Henle
Interstitial cells in inner medulla and papillae
Low-level expression in podocytes and arteriolar smooth muscle cells

---

TABLE 44-3

CLINICAL SYNDROMES ASSOCIATED WITH NONSELECTIVE COX INHIBITORS AND SELECTIVE COX-2 INHIBITORS

Syndrome	Nonselective COX inhibitor (traditional NSAID)	Selective COX-2 inhibitor
Vasomotor acute renal failure	Yes	Yes
Tubulointerstitial nephritis with nephrotic syndrome	Yes	Yes
Tubulointerstitial nephritis without nephrotic syndrome	Yes	Yes
NaCl retention and edema	Yes	Yes
Hypertension	Yes	Yes
Hyperkalemia	Yes	Yes
Decreased free water clearance and hyponatremia	Yes	Yes
Papillary necrosis	Yes	Not reported
Chronic kidney disease	Yes	Not reported

of time. As with traditional NSAIDs, the COX-2 inhibitors need to be used cautiously and require close monitoring of renal function in patients at high risk for adverse renal outcomes.

The overall clinical utility of selective COX-2 inhibitors has recently been called into question as a result of rofecoxib being removed from clinical use due to an increase risk of cardiovascular events. Whether such a risk applies to all COX-2 inhibitors is still a matter of debate.

Effects of Prostaglandins on the Renal Circulation

Prostaglandins primarily exert a vasodilatory effect on the renal vasculature (23). This vasodilatory effect alters the renal circulation in two major ways. First, these compounds influence the distribution of renal blood flow to different regions of the kidney. Prostaglandin stimulation results in a preferential increase in blood flow to the more juxtamedullary nephrons (24). By contrast, inhibition of prostaglandin synthesis results in a selective reduction of flow to inner cortical nephrons while flow remains well preserved in the outer cortex (25). Second, prostaglandins exert a vasoregulatory effect on the renal microcirculation to include the interlobular, afferent, and efferent arterioles as well as the glomerular mesangium. In isolated renal arterioles, both PGE_2 and PGI_2 attenuate AII-induced and norepinephrine-induced afferent arteriolar vasoconstriction. On the efferent side of the circulation, PGI_2 similarly antagonizes AII-induced and norepinephrine-induced vasoconstriction, but PGE_2 is without effect (26). In addition to local production, vascular reactivity of the efferent arteriole appears to be influenced by prostaglandins produced in the upstream glomerulus (27). In this regard, Arima and associates (27) find that orthograde infusion of AII (afferent arteriole-glomerulus-efferent arteriole) results in less vasoconstriction of the efferent arteriole as compared to when infused in a retrograde fashion (efferent arteriole-glomerulus-afferent arteriole). Pretreatment with indomethacin markedly increases the vasoconstrictive effect during orthograde infusion but is without effect during the retrograde infusion.

Prostaglandins have also been shown to attenuate mesangial cell contraction induced by AII, endothelin, AVP, and platelet-activating factor (28–31). Contraction of these cells will normally cause a decrease in the total glomerular capillary surface area and result in a fall in the GFR. Mesangial cell synthesis and release of PGI_2 in humans and PGE_2 in rats dampen the constrictor effects of these hormones such that the glomerular capillary surface area is maintained, thereby minimizing any fall in GFR. Thus, in the setting of enhanced hormonal constrictor activity, prostaglandins play a major role in maintaining glomerular hemodynamics by exerting a vasodilatory effect at the level of the afferent and efferent arteriole as well as within the glomerular mesangium.

Renal Syndromes Associated with Nonsteroidal Antiinflammatory Drugs

Vasomotor-Induced Acute Renal Failure

Prostaglandins appear to play a negligible role in maintenance of renal function under normal circumstances. This conclusion is based on studies in both experimental animals as well as humans. In conscious, sodium-replete dogs and rats, inhibition of renal prostaglandin synthesis with a variety of NSAIDs does not alter baseline renal blood flow or GFR (32–35). Similarly, renal hemodynamics are unaffected in healthy humans after both short-term (36,37) and long-term administration of as-

pirin (38). In related studies, administration of indomethacin to healthy volunteers was also found to produce no change in renal hemodynamics (39,40).

A sharply different effect of cyclooxygenase inhibition is observed when systemic hemodynamics are compromised. Under conditions of circulatory distress, renal blood flow represents a balance between vasoconstrictor influences on the one hand and vasodilatory prostaglandins on the other. Predictably, administration of NSAIDs in this setting will shift this balance toward unopposed vasoconstriction and potentially result in a precipitous decline in renal function.

This interplay between vasoconstrictive effectors and vasodilatory prostaglandins is particularly well illustrated in a series of studies utilizing a model of hemorrhage in dogs (41,42). In animals subjected to hemorrhage, prostaglandin synthesis inhibition was associated with a marked reduction in renal blood flow as compared to prostaglandin-intact dogs. This renal ischemic response was found to be partly reversed after infusion of an AII antagonist or after renal denervation. When renal denervation was combined with the AII antagonist, renal blood flow was restored to values comparable to that in the nonprostaglandin-inhibited animals. Clearly, these findings illustrate the pivotal role that prostaglandins play in opposing the renal ischemic effects of AII and renal nerves.

The modulating effect of vasodilatory prostaglandins on renal hemodynamics can be expected to roughly parallel the extent to which vasoconstrictor effectors are activated. In turn, the activity of these effectors will reflect the degree of circulatory distress. With only mild perturbations in the circulation, one can begin to detect a discernible effect of prostaglandins on renal blood flow. For example, unlike subjects ingesting an ad lib sodium diet, normal subjects placed on a salt-restricted diet will demonstrate a modest fall in creatinine clearance and renal blood flow following the administration of aspirin or indomethacin (43,44).

Diuretic therapy is a common clinical situation where NSAIDs may exert a deleterious effect on renal function in otherwise healthy subjects (45). Like sodium restriction, diuretics increase the dependence of renal blood flow and GFR on vasodilatory prostaglandins and potentiate the deleterious effects of prostaglandin inhibition with cyclooxygenase inhibitors (46). The degree to which renal function is disturbed, however, appears to vary depending on which diuretic–NSAID combination is used. In this regard, Favre and colleagues (45) find that the combination of triamterene and indomethacin given to healthy subjects results in a marked decline in creatinine clearance. By contrast, only a mild decrease in creatinine clearance is found when indomethacin is given in combination with furosemide, hydrochlorothiazide, or spironolactone. Interestingly, triamterene is the only diuretic associated with a marked increase in urinary prostaglandin secretion. Although there is little evidence to suggest that the renal failure patients in this study were volume-depleted, it appears that triamterene by some unknown mechanism renders the renal circulation critically dependent on vasodilatory prostaglandins. As a result, triamterene in combination with an NSAID should only be used with extreme caution.

As alterations in the circulation become more pronounced, rendering the renal circulation more dependent on vasodilatory prostaglandins, cyclooxygenase inhibition can be expected to result in more profound changes in renal hemodynamics. In congestive heart failure, a decrease in effective arterial circulatory volume is the proximate cause for activation of neurohumoral vasoconstrictor forces that participate in the maintenance of systemic arterial pressure and result in increased total peripheral vascular resistance. Important to note, the rise in renal vascular resistance is less than that seen in the periphery (47). Vasodilatory prostaglandins function in a counterregulatory role, attenuating the fall in renal blood flow and GFR that would otherwise occur if vasoconstrictor forces were left unopposed (48).

Cirrhosis is another clinical condition in which the integrity of the renal circulation can become critically dependent on vasodilatory renal prostaglandins. Cirrhotic patients with a low urinary sodium concentration tend to be the most susceptible to develop acute decrements in renal function following the administration of NSAIDs (49). These patients have a more marked decrease in effective arterial circulatory volume, primarily due to splanchnic vasodilation, which in turn leads to higher levels of circulating catechols, AII, and AVP (50,51). As a result, the renal circulation in this subset of patients is more critically dependent on the effect of vasodilatory prostaglandins. As seen in patients with congestive heart failure, these patients have high urinary concentrations of PGE_2, which decline in parallel with the fall in GFR (49).

Renal prostaglandins may play an important role in maintenance of renal hemodynamics in nephrotic syndrome. GFR and filtration fraction are moderately decreased in most patients with the nephrotic syndrome (52,53). Micropuncture studies in an experimental model of the nephrotic syndrome have indicated that relative preservation of renal plasma flow may serve an important role in attenuating the fall in GFR that would otherwise occur due to a reduction in the ultrafiltration coefficient (54). In this setting, locally produced vasodilatory prostaglandins may serve to reduce afferent arteriolar resistance, thereby increasing renal plasma flow and increasing filtration pressure (55,56). Administration of NSAIDs in this setting would lead to increased afferent arteriolar tone. The resulting fall in renal plasma flow and filtration pressure combined with the already decreased ultrafiltration coefficient would result in a dramatic fall in GFR (55). Indeed, administration of prostaglandin synthesis inhibitors to nephrotic subjects is commonly associated with a fall in GFR and may precipitate acute renal failure in some patients (57,58). Other settings in which there is increased vasoconstrictive input focused on the kidney rendering it particularly vulnerable to the deleterious effects of NSAIDs include endotoxic shock (59) and anesthesia (60).

Risk factors for the development of NSAID-induced ARF are not necessarily confined to conditions characterized by decreases in absolute or effective arterial circulatory volume (Table 44-4). One such example is the presence of underlying chronic kidney disease. In this setting, increased vasodilatory prostaglandins are thought to play an adaptive role in minimizing the decline in global renal function by increasing GFR in surviving nephrons through increased renal blood flow. The

TABLE 44-4

RISK FACTORS FOR NSAID-INDUCED ACUTE VASOMOTOR RENAL FAILURE

Decreased EABV	Normal or increased EABV
Congestive heart failure	Chronic renal failure
Cirrhosis	Glomerulonephritis
Nephrotic syndrome	Elderly
Sepsis	Contrast-induced nephropathy
Hemorrhage	Obstructive uropathy
Diuretic therapy	Cyclosporin A
Postoperative patients with "third space" fluid	
Volume depletion/ hypotension	

EABV, effective arterial blood volume.

TABLE 44-5

PREDISPOSING FACTORS FOR NSAID-INDUCED NEPHROTOXICITY IN THE ELDERLY

Age-related changes in renal function
↓ In glomerular filtration rate
↓ In renal blood flow
↑ In renal vascular resistance
Age-related changes in pharmacokinetics
↑ Free drug concentration
−Hypoalbuminemia
−Retained metabolites
↓ Total body water
↓ Hepatic metabolism with longer drug half-life

signal for increased prostaglandin production is generally not a disturbance in the systemic circulation leading to increased circulating levels of AII and catecholamines but rather intrarenal mechanisms leading to generation of vasoactive compounds within the glomerular microcirculation (61).

Increasing age is a risk factor for the development of nephrotoxicity when using NSAIDs (62,63). This susceptibility in part may be related to changes in renal function that normally accompany the aging process (64) (Table 44-5). Aging is associated with a progressive decline in the GFR and total renal blood flow. In addition, there is an increase in renal vascular resistance. Important to note, the renal vasculature becomes less responsive to vasodilators, while the response to vasoconstrictors remains intact. In an analysis of 1,908 patients treated with ibuprofen, renal impairment was found to occur in 343 (18%) patients (62). The two most important risk factors identified for the development of toxicity is age greater than 65 years and preexisting renal insufficiency. In a prospective study of 114 older patients (mean age 87 years) started on NSAID therapy, a greater than 50% increase in the serum urea nitrogen concentration was found in 15 (13%) patients (63). In this study, concurrent use of a loop diuretic and large doses of NSAIDs were found to be predictive of those who developed significant azotemia.

In addition to age-related changes in renal function, age-related changes in the pharmacokinetics of NSAIDs may also make this population more susceptible to renal toxicity (65,66). Older patients, particularly those with chronic illness, often have lower albumin levels, which reduce protein binding of the drugs and result in higher free-drug concentrations. This binding of the parent compound to circulating albumin is further impaired by retained metabolites, which accumulate as a result of the normal age-related impairment in renal function. Increased drug levels also occur as a result of the age-related decrease in total body water. Finally, decreased hepatic metabolism, which is often present in older adults, contributes to a longer half-life of the parent compound and can result in unexpectedly high drug levels.

Other conditions in which effective arterial circulatory volume is normal or increased and yet renal function is critically dependent on increased synthesis of prostaglandins include immune mediated glomerular injury, urinary obstruction (67), radiocontrast-induced injury (68), and administration of cyclosporin A (69). In these conditions, increased production of vasodilatory prostaglandins has been shown to counterbalance the effects of intrarenally generated vasoconstrictors such as thromboxane, leukotrienes, platelet-activating factor, and endothelin. Administration of NSAIDs in each of these settings can be expected to result in an exaggerated fall in renal function.

TABLE 44-6

CLINICAL FEATURES OF NSAID-INDUCED VASOMOTOR RENAL FAILURE

Oliguria
Usually occurs within a few days of beginning medicine
Hyperkalemia out of proportion to renal failure
Low fractional excretion of Na
Usually does not require dialysis
Usually reversible

NSAID-induced acute renal failure is most commonly an oliguric form of renal failure that begins within several days after initiation of the drug (Table 44-6). The urinalysis is unremarkable in the majority of cases. Unlike other causes of acute oliguric renal failure, the fractional excretion of sodium is often less than 1%. This low fractional excretion of sodium reflects the underlying hemodynamic nature of the renal failure. Hyperkalemia out of proportion to the decrement in renal function is also a typical feature of this lesion. If recognized early, the renal failure is reversible with discontinuation of the NSAID. As a result, dialysis is usually not required.

Are Certain Nonsteroidal Antiinflammatory Drugs Renal Sparing? An NSAID with effective antiinflammatory properties but associated with less nephrotoxicity would be highly desirable because there is a sizable population at risk for renal toxicity. This issue has been most commonly discussed with sulindac. It has been postulated that sulindac may have renal-sparing properties as a result of its unique metabolism. Sulindac is administered as a prodrug (sulindac sulfoxide), which must be first converted to sulindac sulfide to exert cyclooxygenase inhibitory effects. The sulfide metabolite can be converted back to the parent sulfoxide compound or be metabolized to an inactive sulfone metabolite (70). The liver and kidney are thought to be the major sites at which each of these biotransformations takes place. Based on the ability of the kidney to inactivate sulindac sulfide, renal prostaglandin synthesis should remain relatively intact (71). In fact, unlike other NSAIDs, the active metabolite of sulindac does not appear in the urine after oral administration of sulindac sulfoxide but rather is excreted as the parent compound or as the sulfone metabolite (72).

Despite the potential for less renal toxicity, studies examining this issue have produced conflicting results, some showing renal sparing effects (73,74) and others not (75–77). This discrepancy may in part be explained by changes in the pharmacokinetics of sulindac that occur as a function of duration of therapy and severity of underlying disease. Sulindac has a long half-life (16 to 18 hours) which is prolonged in the setting of renal or liver disease. In either circumstance, the active compound, sulindac sulfide, can progressively accumulate in the plasma over several days to weeks. In the setting of chronic renal failure, steady-state concentrations of ibuprofen are achieved within 24 to 48 hours, whereas concentrations of sulindac sulfide may not achieve a steady state even after 11 days of therapy (75,78,79). With regard to patients with baseline renal insufficiency, an adverse effect of sulindac on renal function has mostly been reported in studies of longer duration that included patients with more advanced degrees of renal insufficiency (75,78). In this setting, levels of sulindac sulfide up to 10 times normal have been reported (78). Such levels may exceed the capacity of remaining renal tissue to convert sulindac sulfide to inactive metabolites.

Similar observations have been noted in patients with cirrhosis and ascites (74). In patients who demonstrate a significant decline in both urinary prostaglandin excretion and GFR following the administration of sulindac, circulating levels of sulindac sulfide are much higher in comparison to patients with cirrhosis who fail to develop renal toxicity (74).

Thus, while there appears to be some reduced risk for vasoconstriction-induced renal insufficiency in patients who take sulindac versus other NSAIDs, this agent still needs to be given with caution. It is likely that the renal-sparing effect of sulindac may simply reflect that common clinical doses are at the low end of the dose-response curve in terms of inhibiting renal prostaglandins. By contrast, similar doses administered to high-risk patients, particularly those with renal insufficiency or liver disease, may result in much higher sulindac sulfide levels which may be capable of inhibiting renal prostaglandin synthesis. In addition to disease-induced changes in the pharmacokinetics of sulindac, there may be individual variability determined by genetic and/or environmental factors in the capacity of the kidney to convert sulindac sulfide to inactive metabolites (80). In this regard, a recent report found that 25 of 70 patients who were chronically ingesting sulindac for treatment of arthritis had detectable sulindac sulfide levels in the urine. It is interesting to speculate that this subgroup may be at risk for renal toxicity in the appropriate setting.

Nabumetone has also been postulated to have renal sparing properties due to modest selectivity of the drug toward the COX-2 enzyme. However, critical review of clinical studies examining this issue does not allow a definite answer to this question (81). As with sulindac, the use of nabumetone in patients at risk for adverse renal effects must be given cautiously with frequent monitoring of renal function.

COX-2 Inhibitors and Acute Renal Failure. Clinical studies comparing the specific COX-2 inhibitors with traditional NSAIDs have generally shown similar effects on renal function. One possible exception based on studies in healthy volume replete adults suggest prostaglandins derived from COX-2 may be more important in modulating urinary sodium excretion while COX-1 derived prostaglandins are more important in regulating renal blood flow and GFR. In one study 24 elderly subjects on a nonrestricted diet received either celecoxib or naproxen for a total of 10 days (82). A small but statistically significantly decrease in GFR developed only in the naproxen group. By contrast both drugs caused a similar decrease in urinary sodium excretion that was transient in nature. Urinary sodium levels returned to baseline after 72 hours and remained stable for the remainder of the study. Similar findings were found in 36 subjects maintained on a high-sodium diet and randomized to receive rofecoxib, indomethacin, or placebo (83). Both drugs caused a transient fall in urinary sodium excretion as compared to placebo while only the indomethacin-treated group demonstrated a decline in GFR.

Differing effects on GFR noted between selective and nonselective COX inhibitors in euvolemic patients are no longer apparent under conditions where renal function is more dependent upon prostaglandins. In elderly subjects placed on a low-sodium diet, rofecoxib lowers GFR to a similar extent as indomethacin (84). Similarly, treatment with celecoxib decreases GFR and renal plasma flow to the same extent as naproxen in young sodium-restricted healthy young men (85). Patients with stable chronic kidney disease treated for 7 days with either celecoxib or naproxen exhibit significant declines in GFR that are similar in magnitude (86).

There are now numerous reports of clinically relevant acute renal failure occurring in association with specific COX-2 inhibitor therapy (87). This complication has typically developed in patients with multiple risk factors for NSAID-induced nephrotoxicity to include decreases in absolute or effective circulatory volume. As with traditional NSAIDs, the renal failure is frequently accompanied by hyperkalemia and may be severe enough to require dialysis but is reversible following the discontinuation of the drug and restoration of extracellular fluid volume.

Glomerular and Interstitial Disease

The use of NSAIDs can be associated with the development of a distinct syndrome characterized by the development of interstitial nephritis and nephrotic range proteinuria. The incidence of this lesion is unknown but is thought to be rare. One estimate for fenoprofen-induced interstitial nephritis was one case per 5,300 patient-years of treatment (88). While virtually all NSAIDs have been reported to cause this syndrome, the vast majority of cases have been reported in association with use of the propionic acid derivatives (fenoprofen, ibuprofen, and naproxen) (133–142). Of these, fenoprofen has been implicated in greater than 60% of cases (89). Interstitial nephritis with and without nephrotic syndrome has also been reported with the COX-2 inhibitors, rofecoxib and celecoxib (90–94).

Unlike hemodynamically mediated ARF, there are no clear-cut risk factors that serve to identify those at risk for development of this syndrome. The mean age of patients is 65 years (89). The presence of an underlying renal disease prior to exposure of the NSAID has been notably absent. This syndrome has generally been referred to as an example of acute interstitial nephritis. There are, however, a number of features that distinguish this form of interstitial renal disease from that observed with other pharmacologic agents (89,95) (Table 44-7). First, the average duration of exposure prior to the onset of disease is typically measured in months and can be as long as a year. By contrast, allergic interstitial nephritis due to other drugs usually presents within several days to weeks after exposure to the drug. Second, nephrotic range proteinuria is found in >90% of cases of NSAID-induced interstitial disease, a degree of proteinuria that is distinctly uncommon in acute allergic interstitial nephritis due to other drugs. Third, symptoms of hypersensitivity that are commonly seen in acute allergic interstitial nephritis such as rash, fever, arthralgias, or peripheral eosinophilia are uncommon in NSAID-associated disease. Fourth, the vast majority of cases associated with NSAIDs have been reported in older patients. On the other hand, allergic interstitial nephritis is seen in all age groups.

Renal biopsy findings typically show a diffuse or focal lymphocytic infiltrate. The number of eosinophils in the infiltrate is variable but generally is not marked. The glomerular changes are most commonly those seen in minimal change disease.

TABLE 44-7

CLINICAL CHARACTERISTICS OF NSAID-INDUCED TUBULOINTERSTITIAL NEPHRITIS (TIN) VERSUS TYPICAL DRUG-INDUCED TIN

Characteristic	NSAID-induced TIN	Typical drug-induced TIN
Duration of exposure	5 days –>1 year	5–26 days
Hypersensitivity symptoms	7%–8%	80%
Eosinophilia	17%–18%	75%–80%
Proteinuria >3.5 g/24 hr	>90%	<10%
Eosinophiluria	0%–5%	80%–85%
Peak serum creatinine	1.5–>10 mg%	1.5–>10 mg%

In particular, the glomeruli are normal by light microscopy, while fusion of the podocytes is seen with electron microscopy. In some cases there is evidence of glomerulosclerosis. Since most patients who develop this syndrome are older, this latter finding may simply represent the normal age-related increase in glomerulosclerosis. Immunofluorescent studies are typically nonspecific. There has been an occasional report of weak and variable staining for immunoglobulin G and C_3 along the tubular basement membrane. Electron microscopy typically shows diffuse fusion of the podocytes in cases with heavy proteinuria. Mesangial, electron-dense deposits have been observed in only three patients, suggesting that this is not an immune-mediated disease (96–98).

While the combination of interstitial nephritis and nephrotic syndrome is the most common clinical manifestation, a second presentation is the development of nephrotic syndrome without evidence of interstitial renal disease (95,99). Once again, the glomerular histology is typical of minimal change disease, although a few patients have been described with changes typical of membranous glomerulopathy (90,95,100). It is likely that the pathophysiologic mechanism that underlies the development of glomerular disease in the absence of interstitial disease is similar, if not identical, to the more common finding of combined nephrotic proteinuria and interstitial nephritis.

A third presentation that has uncommonly been reported is the development of interstitial nephritis without nephrotic proteinuria (95,101–103). The onset of disease following the initiation of drug therapy tends to be much shorter and in this respect resembles the more common form of drug-induced allergic interstitial nephritis. In addition, these patients are more likely to exhibit a systemic hypersensitivity reaction. Given the closer temporal relationship between the administration of the offending NSAID and the development of renal insufficiency, one may confuse this latter presentation with that of NSAID-induced vasomotor ARF. Symptoms of hypersensitivity as well as histopathologic changes typical of interstitial renal disease should allow one to distinguish this lesion from hemodynamically mediated ARF.

Finally, NSAID toxicity may present as an exacerbation of an underlying disease. In a case report of a patient with systemic lupus erythematosus, the development of interstitial nephritis and nephrotic syndrome after administration of naproxen clinically appeared as a rapidly progressive lupus glomerulonephritis (104).

The clinical course of patients who present in any one of these manners is to develop a spontaneous remission after removal of the offending NSAID. The time until resolution is variable but can range from a few days to several weeks. In some patients, the degree of renal insufficiency can be severe enough that dialytic support is required. Steroid therapy has been used in many of the reported cases; however, the efficacy and necessity of this therapy are unknown. It should be noted that relapses have been reported after inadvertent exposure to the same NSAID or after exposure to a different NSAID (105–107).

Renal Sodium Retention

Sodium retention is a characteristic feature of virtually all NSAIDs, occurring in as many as 25% of patients who use them. The physiologic basis of this effect is directly related to the natriuretic properties of prostaglandins. Prostaglandins increase urinary sodium excretion by both indirect and direct mechanisms (Fig. 44-3). Through their activity as renal vasodilators, prostaglandins may cause an increase in the filtered load of sodium. In addition, these compounds preferentially shunt blood flow to the inner cortical and medullary regions of the kidney (24,25). As a result of increased medullary blood

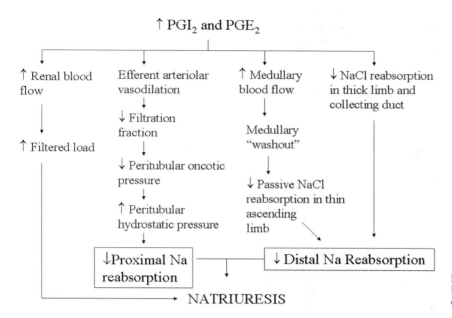

FIGURE 44-3. The direct and indirect mechanisms by which renal prostaglandins exert a natriuretic effect.

flow, there is a fall in the medullary interstitial solute concentration. Processes that reduce the degree of medullary hypertonicity lead to a concomitant reduction in the osmotic withdrawal of water from the normally sodium-impermeable thin descending limb of Henle. This in turn decreases the sodium concentration of fluid at the hairpin turn. The net effect is less passive reabsorption of sodium across the normally water-impermeable thin ascending limb of Henle. Consistent with this mechanism, infusion of PGE_1 lowers and prostaglandin synthesis inhibition raises sodium chloride and total solute concentration in the medulla (108–110).

Finally, prostaglandins can affect sodium reabsorption in the proximal tubule by virtue of their ability to influence the tone of the efferent arteriole. Changes in the tone of this vessel play a central role in determining the Starling forces that govern fluid reabsorption in this nephron segment. Increased resistance of this vessel, as that which occurs in the setting of high concentrations of AII, leads to a decrease in the downstream peritubular hydrostatic pressure. In addition, efferent constriction increases the filtration fraction by reducing glomerular plasma flow and increasing the upstream glomerular pressure. The increased filtration fraction leads to an increase in the peritubular oncotic pressure. A decrease in hydrostatic pressure and increase in oncotic pressure in the peritubular vessel favor fluid reabsorption in the proximal tubule. By modulating the degree to which the efferent arteriole is constricted and thus altering peritubular Starling forces acting on the proximal tubule, prostaglandins can decrease proximal tubular sodium reabsorption. Predictably, in a model of high circulating levels of AII induced by suprarenal aortic constriction, inhibition of prostaglandin synthesis was found to increase efferent arteriole oncotic pressure and decrease peritubular hydrostatic pressure, resulting in a significant increase in proximal fluid reabsorption (111).

In addition to these hemodynamically mediated changes in renal sodium handling, prostaglandins have direct effects on tubular sodium transport. In the isolated perfused tubule, PGE_2 has been shown to inhibit sodium transport in the cortical and outer medullary collecting duct (112,113). Using the same technique, PGE_2 has also been shown to decrease chloride transport in the thick ascending limb of Henle (114). *In vivo* studies also support a direct inhibitory effect of prostaglandins on sodium transport in the loop of Henle, distal nephron, and collecting duct (115,116). The mechanism of this direct inhibitory effect

is unclear but may involve decreased activity of the Na–K–ATPase pump (117). Prostaglandins have also been shown to mediate the natriuretic response to increased renal interstitial hydrostatic pressure that occurs during renal interstitial volume expansion (118,119). In addition, these compounds play a permissive role in the sodium excretion that follows volume expansion and an increase in renal perfusion pressure (120,121).

It would at first seem paradoxical that under conditions of volume depletion the kidney would elaborate a compound that would have further natriuretic properties. The role of prostaglandins in this setting, however, is to moderate the avid salt retention that would otherwise occur in the setting of unopposed activation of the renin–angiotensin–aldosterone and adrenergic systems. By virtue of their natriuretic properties, prostaglandins play a role in ensuring adequate delivery of filtrate to more distal nephron segments under conditions in which distal delivery is threatened (e.g., renal ischemia, hypovolemia). In addition, diminished NaCl reabsorption in the thick ascending limb of Henle reduces the energy requirements of this segment. This reduction in thick ascending limb workload in conjunction with a prostaglandin-mediated reallocation in renal blood flow helps to maintain an adequate oxygen tension in the medulla under conditions that would otherwise have resulted in substantial hypoxic injury (122,123).

NSAIDs are thought to cause salt retention primarily by inhibiting prostaglandin synthesis and therefore disrupting the foregoing mechanisms. The extent to which salt retention becomes clinically manifest depends on the degree of baseline prostaglandin production. In normal healthy humans, baseline prostaglandin production is minimal. As a result, NSAID-induced positive sodium balance is transient and usually of no clinical importance. By contrast, NSAID administration in clinical conditions such as congestive heart failure, cirrhosis, or nephrotic syndrome can result in marked sodium retention and potentially adverse clinical consequences.

In addition to causing sodium retention, NSAIDs have been shown to attenuate the natriuretic effect of diuretics (124–126). The mechanism of this resistance is multifactorial. The natriuretic effects of loop diuretics have, in part, been linked to the ability of these drugs to increase renal blood flow, an effect mediated by the stimulation of vasodilatory prostaglandins (127–129). By inhibiting prostaglandin synthesis, NSAIDs limit sodium excretion by preventing the increase in renal blood flow normally seen after the administration of the diuretic (128). In addition to this hemodynamic effect, micropuncture and microperfusion studies have shown that prostaglandin inhibition also blunts the effect of furosemide at the level of the thick ascending limb of Henle (130–132). This latter effect may be related to inhibition of furosemide-induced stimulation of natriuretic prostaglandins that act within this tubular segment. Finally, NSAIDs may limit the diuretic response to loop diuretics by competing for tubular secretion, thereby limiting the delivery of the drug to the luminal surface of the thick ascending limb (133).

Indomethacin has also been shown to attenuate the diuretic response to hydrochlorothiazide (134). The mechanism of this interaction may result from enhanced salt absorption in the loop of Henle, which would then limit the delivery of chloride to the site of the thiazide action in the distal nephron. A similar explanation may underlie the resistance that has been described with NSAIDs and spironolactone (135).

Sodium Balance and Hypertension. In considering the natriuretic and vasodilatory properties of prostaglandins, it is not surprising that administration of NSAIDs has been shown to interfere with blood pressure control. In pooled studies, administration of NSAIDs has been associated with an average increase in blood pressure of between 5 and 10 mm Hg (136–138). Of the various subgroups examined, this effect is most pronounced in patients who are already hypertensive and much less so in those who are normotensive. Of the hypertensive patients, those treated with β-blockers seem to be the most vulnerable to the hypertensive effect of NSAIDs (136,138). In this regard, it is particularly interesting to note that propranolol has been shown to increase prostacyclin formation (139). There is less of an interaction with diuretics and angiotensin-converting enzyme inhibitors, while no effect is seen with calcium channel blockers (136).

Subgroup analysis shows that patients with low renin hypertension (older adults and blacks) are at higher risk for worsening hypertension in association with NSAID use. Older hypertensive patients have reduced urinary PGE_2 excretion when compared to younger hypertensive patients (140). The pathogenesis of NSAID-induced hypertension is not known with certainty. In a recent metaanalysis, NSAIDs were found not to alter body weight or urinary sodium excretion significantly, implying that mechanisms other than salt retention were responsible for the increased blood pressure (138). In this regard, elimination of the vasodilator prostacyclin from the resistance blood vessels is believed to play some role in the development of hypertension in individuals at risk (141–143).

Sodium Balance, Edema, and Hypertension with COX-2 Inhibitors. The use of COX-2 inhibitors is complicated by the development of peripheral edema with a frequency similar to that seen with traditional NSAIDs. In approximately 6,000 patients with osteoarthritis lower extremity edema developed in 3.6% and 3.8% of patients treated with rofecoxib at 12.5 and 25 mg doses, respectively (87). These rates of edema were no different than the comparator NSAIDs ibupofren and diclofenac and greater than placebo. In over 5,000 patients with osteoarthritis treated with celecoxib the incidence of peripheral edema was 1.6% and 3.0% in patients receiving 100 or 200 mg celecoxib twice daily as compared to 2.2% for the NSAID comparator and 1.3% for placebo (144).

Increased blood pressure has also been reported to occur in a minority of patients in large trials designed to investigate the safety of rofecoxib and celecoxib. Conflicting results have been noted in smaller trials directly comparing these two drugs. In the Successive Celecoxib Efficacy and Safety Studies (SUCCESS) VI and VII only a minority of patients developed increased blood pressue but did so to a greater extent on rofecoxib as compared to celecoxib (145,146). These tri-

als have been criticized for using doses of the drugs that were not equivalent based on efficacy data, different baseline patient characteristics, and timing of blood pressure measurements favoring the shorter acting celecoxib. Subsequent studies using equipotent doses of the drugs and measuring blood pressure at intervals that would capture the peak effect of the drugs have shown no difference between these drugs with regards to increasing blood pressure (147,148). While more rigorously designed prospective trials would be useful, the majority of data suggest no difference between the various COX-2 inhibitors and the tendency to develop increased blood pressure. This complication is a class effect that is dose related and develops with the same frequency as traditional NSAIDs. As previously mentioned, rofecoxib is no longer available for clinical use.

Potassium Metabolism

The use of NSAIDs has been associated with the development of hyperkalemia in the setting of chronic renal insufficiency as well as normal renal function (149–154). The physiologic basis for this effect is inhibition of prostaglandin-mediated renin release with subsequent development of hypoaldosteronism. Both *in vivo* and *in vitro* studies have shown a direct stimulatory effect of prostaglandins (primarily PGI_2 and PGE_2) on renin release from the juxtaglomerular cells (155,156). Clinical studies in salt restricted subjects have shown the COX-2 selective inhibitors reduced urinary potassium excretion to a similar extent as traditional NSAIDs (84,85). Both celecoxib and rofecoxib have been reported to cause significant hyperkalemia in case reports. These finding are consistent with COX-2 in the macula densa playing an important role in stimulating renin release.

In addition to direct effects, these compounds play an essential intermediary role in those pathways that are of primary importance in the regulation of renin release. In particular, renin release stimulated by both decreased perfusion pressure and decreased delivery of filtrate to the macula densa is dependent on an intact cyclooxygenase system (157,158). By contrast, β-adrenergic stimulation of renin release can occur independently of prostaglandin synthesis (159,160).

NSAID-induced suppression of renin release with subsequent development of a hyporenin–hypoaldosterone state is thought to be the primary mechanism of hyperkalemia. Decreased renin release leads to decreased circulating levels of angiotensin I, which in turn results in low levels of AII. Since AII normally stimulates aldosterone release from the zona glomerulosa cells in the adrenal gland, serum aldosterone levels fall. In addition to low circulating levels, the effect of any given level of AII on aldosterone release is impaired because prostaglandins have been shown to play an intermediary role in this stimulatory effect (161). Low circulating levels of AII further contribute to the development of hypoaldosteronism because adequate levels of AII are required for the stimulatory effect of hyperkalemia on aldosterone release (162). In addition to interfering with the renin–angiotensin–aldosterone cascade, NSAIDs favor positive potassium balance in other ways. As discussed earlier, inhibition of prostaglandin synthesis is associated with increased sodium reabsorption in the loop of Henle and thus decreased distal delivery. A reduction in sodium delivery to the aldosterone-sensitive cortical collecting tubule is a known factor impairing potassium excretion. In addition, tubular flow rates are an important determinant of potassium excretion. Since NSAIDs increase the hydroosmotic effect of AVP, flow rates can fall, further impairing potassium excretion. Finally, decreased synthesis of prostaglandins may have effects of decreasing potassium secretion at the level of the potassium channel (163).

The development of hyperkalemia in patients receiving an NSAID is most likely to occur in the setting of renal

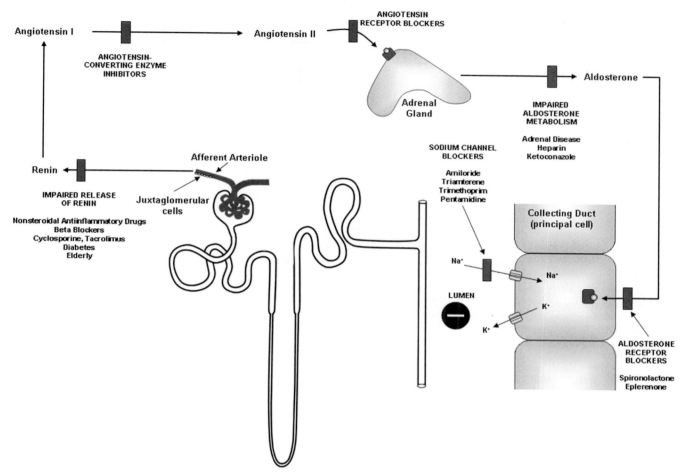

FIGURE 44-4. The renin-angiotensin-aldosterone system and regulation of renal potassium excretion. Aldosterone binds to a cytosolic receptor in the principal cell and stimulates sodium reabsorption across the luminal membrane through a well-defined sodium channel. As sodium is reabsorbed the electronegativity of the lumen increases thereby providing a more favorable driving force for potassium secretion through an apically located potassium channel. Disease states or drugs that interfere at any point along this system can impair renal potassium secretion and increase the risk of hyperkalemia when using angiotensin-converting enzyme (ACE)-inhibitors or angiotensin receptor blockers. In many patients, this risk is magnified due to disturbances at multiple sites along this system.

insufficiency or those with baseline abnormalities in the renin–angiotensin–aldosterone system (155). Diabetic patients are at risk due to the increased incidence of hyporeninemic hypoaldosteronism that occurs in this patient population (164,165). Similarly, older adults are at higher risk by virtue of the normal age-related decrease in circulating renin and aldosterone levels (166). Particular caution should be used when NSAIDs are combined with other pharmacologic agents known to interfere with the renin–angiotensin–aldosterone cascade (167) (Fig. 44-4). Examples would include β-blockers, cyclosporin A, angiotensin-converting enzyme inhibitors, angiotensin receptor blockers, heparin, ketoconazole, high-dose trimethoprim, and potassium-sparing diuretics.

Water Metabolism

Prostaglandins have important modulatory effects on renal water metabolism. Their primary effect is to impair the ability to maximally concentrate the urine. In doing so, two processes that are central in the elaboration of a concentrated urine are interfered with, namely, the generation of a hypertonic interstitium and maximal collecting duct water permeability. The decrease in interstitial hypertonicity is due to a washout effect

that results from the ability of prostaglandins to shunt blood flow to the inner cortical and medullary regions of the kidney. In addition, prostaglandins decrease sodium absorption in the thick ascending limb and decrease AVP-induced urea permeability in the medullary collecting duct. Decreased accumulation of sodium and urea in the interstitium further reduces the interstitial osmolality. The impairment in collecting duct water permeability is the result of prostaglandins opposing the hydroosmotic effect of AVP (168–170). Interesting to note, AVP is known to stimulate PGE_2 synthesis in collecting duct cells; by doing so, AVP induces its own antagonist. This interaction is another example in which prostaglandins exert a moderating effect on an effector mechanism that elicited their synthesis. In this case, prostaglandins play an important role in minimizing the water retention that would otherwise occur if the activity of AVP was unopposed (171). By opposing the vasoconstrictive action of AVP, prostaglandins also contribute to the maintenance of glomerular perfusion and filtration (172).

Based on the foregoing discussion, administration of NSAIDs would predictably impair solute-free water excretion by increasing the hydroosmotic effect of any given level of circulating AVP and increasing the degree of interstitial

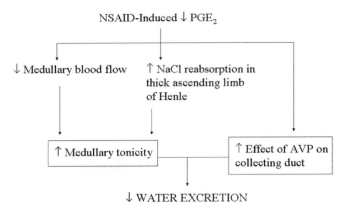

FIGURE 44-5. The mechanisms by which nonsteroidal antiinflammatory drugs lead to decreased renal water excretion. *AVP*, arginine vasopressin.

hypertonicity (Fig. 44-5). In most circumstances, however, hyponatremia is not associated with the use of NSAIDs. Under normal conditions, any decrease in serum osmolality would be sensed in the hypothalamus and result in inhibition of AVP release. As a consequence, excess solute-free water would be promptly excreted, restoring the serum osmolality back to normal. On the other hand, administration of NSAIDs in the setting of nonsuppressible AVP release may result in dramatic falls in the serum sodium concentration. Patients at risk for this complication would include those with high-circulating levels of AVP driven by a decreased effective arterial circulatory volume such as congestive heart failure or cirrhosis (173). Patients with syndrome of inappropriate antidiuretic hormone secretion (SIADH) or those taking medications capable of stimulating AVP secretion or impairing urinary dilution by other mechanisms are also at risk for the development of hyponatremia (60,174).

In this regard, a recent study examined the effects of ibuprofen and a thiazide diuretic on renal water handling in otherwise healthy young and older volunteers subjected to a water load (175). Three days of hydrochlorothiazide (100 mg per day) was found to impair both solute-free water clearance and the ability to elaborate a maximally dilute urine. A delay in the recovery of serum osmolality was noted in both the young and older subjects but to a significantly greater extent in the older subjects. When the young subjects were then given a water load after treatment with ibuprofen together with the thiazide, solute-free water clearance and serum osmolality were reduced further and to a degree similar to that seen in the older subjects on the thiazide regimen alone. It was postulated that the susceptibility to thiazide-induced hyponatremia known to occur in some elderly patients may, in part, be related to lower renal prostaglandin production. It can be expected that a greater number of older patients will be taking a combination of NSAIDs and hydrochlorothiazide given the efficacy of thiazide diuretics in the treatment of systolic hypertension.

NONSTEROIDAL ANTIINFLAMMATORY DRUG-INDUCED CHRONIC KIDNEY DISEASE AND ANALGESIC NEPHROPATHY

The most common form of drug-induced chronic kidney disease is analgesic nephropathy. This lesion has most commonly been linked to the chronic ingestion of compound analgesics containing aspirin, phenacetin, and caffeine (176). A still unresolved question is whether long-term use of NSAIDs alone can similarly result in a progressive and irreversible form of chronic kidney disease. In this regard, a number of observations have emerged that would appear to substantiate the belief that long-term use of NSAIDs can lead to a chronic form of renal injury. Furthermore, the clinical characteristics of NSAID-induced chronic kidney disease are sufficiently different from those in analgesic nephropathy to suggest that this is a distinct clinical entity. Before reviewing the data linking chronic NSAID use and renal insufficiency, a brief description of analgesic nephropathy will be provided.

Analgesic nephropathy is a chronic kidney disease characterized by renal papillary necrosis and chronic interstitial nephritis (176–178). The early reports linking analgesics and renal disease were generally found in patients who consumed combination products containing phenacetin. This fact focused attention on phenacetin as the primary cause of the syndrome and prompted many countries to officially remove the drug from nonprescription analgesics. Significantly, the removal of phenacetin has not been uniformly followed by the expected reduction in the incidence of the syndrome (179). Given that other agents such as acetaminophen or salicylamide have been substituted for phenacetin in many combination products, the lack of decline in incidence of analgesic nephropathy suggests that the use of combination products is as important as whether the compound contains phenacetin (179,180). This conclusion is further supported by the experience in Belgium where a strong geographic correlation exists between the prevalence of analgesic nephropathy and sales of analgesic mixtures containing a minimum of two analgesic components (181,182).

Numerous epidemiologic studies performed in the past demonstrated a wide variation in the geographic incidence of analgesic nephropathy (179,180,183–186). Much of this variability could be explained by differences in the annual per capita consumption of phenacetin (178,179). In those countries with the highest consumption such as Australia and Sweden, analgesic nephropathy was found responsible for up to 20% of cases of end-stage renal disease. In Canada, which had the lowest per capita consumption, analgesic nephropathy accounted for only 2% to 5% of end-stage renal disease patients. It has been estimated that between 2% and 4% of all end-stage renal disease cases in the United States can be attributable to habitual analgesic consumption. Within the United States, there are also regional differences in the reported incidence of analgesic nephropathy, which are thought to be reflective of differences in analgesic consumption (179,180,183,184). For example, the use of combination analgesics is more common in the southeastern United States, and the incidence of analgesic nephropathy is three to five times as common a cause of end-stage renal disease in North Carolina compared to Pennsylvania (179,180,183,184).

The development of analgesic nephropathy is associated with a number of well-defined clinical characteristics (187). The disease is more common in women by a factor of 2 to 6 and has a peak incidence at age 53 years. Patients typically consume compound analgesics on a daily basis, often for chronic complaints such as headache, dyspepsia, or to improve work productivity. It has been estimated that nephropathy occurs after the cumulative ingestion of 2 to 3 kg of the index drug. Often patients will exhibit a typical psychiatric profile characterized by addictive behavior. Gastrointestinal complications, such as peptic ulcer disease, are common. The patients are frequently anemic as a result of gastrointestinal blood loss as well as renal insufficiency. Ischemic heart disease and renal artery stenosis have both been reported to occur with higher frequency in these patients (178). In fact, regular use of analgesic drugs containing phenacetin is associated with an increased risk of hypertension and mortality and morbidity due to cardiovascular disease (186,188). Finally, long-term use of analgesics is known to be a risk factor for the subsequent generation of uroepithelial tumors (189).

Patients with analgesic nephropathy have predominantly tubulomedullary dysfunction characterized by impaired concentrating ability, acidification defects, and occasionally a salt-losing state. Proteinuria tends to be low to moderate in quantity. Interesting to note, the pattern of proteinuria is typically a mixture of glomerular and tubular origin. Pyuria is common and is often sterile. Occasionally hematuria is noted, but if persistent should raise the possibility of a uroepithelial tumor.

There are several features of analgesic nephropathy that make it difficult to diagnose. The disease is slowly progressive and the symptoms and signs are nonspecific. Patients are often reluctant to admit to heavy usage of analgesics and therefore are either misdiagnosed or not diagnosed at all until the renal failure is far advanced. In addition, the lack of a simple and noninvasive test that reliably implicates analgesics as the cause of the renal injury has been an important limiting factor. Noncontrast abdominal computed tomography (CT) may emerge as a useful diagnostic tool in this setting given its usefulness in the diagnosis of papillary necrosis (190). Characteristic findings by computerized tomography suggesting the diagnosis include small kidneys with an irregular contour and intrarenal calcifications particularly in the medulla.

As mentioned earlier, there are a number of reports that suggest that chronic use of NSAIDs alone may also lead to renal injury. In this regard, several NSAIDs have been associated with the development of papillary necrosis either when administered alone or in combination with aspirin (191). In addition to inhibiting prostaglandin synthesis, the ability of these agents to redistribute blood flow to the cortex, rendering the renal medulla ischemic, may underlie this association. While the reports linking papillary necrosis and NSAIDs are predominantly anecdotal in nature, more recent observations would suggest that chronic renal failure resulting from long-term use of NSAIDs may be more prevalent than once thought (192,193). In a multicenter case-control study, Sandler and associates (192) report a twofold increase in the risk for chronic kidney disease associated with the previous daily use of NSAIDs. Chronic kidney disease in these patients was newly diagnosed and was defined as a serum creatinine concentration of 1.5 mg/dL or greater. This increased risk was primarily limited to older men. An additional report linking chronic use of NSAIDs with development of chronic kidney disease described 56 patients from Australia (178). These patients had taken only NSAIDs over a period of 10 to 20 years for treatment of varying rheumatic diseases. In 19 patients (34%), radiographic evidence of papillary necrosis was found. In 37 patients, renal biopsy material was available that disclosed evidence of chronic interstitial nephritis. The clinical characteristics of these patients were quite different from those with analgesic nephropathy, suggesting that NSAID-induced chronic kidney disease is indeed a distinct entity. In particular, patients with NSAID-associated renal disease were older, had an equal female-to-male ratio, a lower incidence of papillary necrosis, less severe renal insufficiency, and a lower incidence of urinary tract infections (178). In addition, an increased risk of uroepithelial tumors has not been described in these patients.

Further evidence of chronic toxicity has been reported in a preliminary communication in which patients treated with NSAIDs for rheumatoid arthritis and osteoarthritis were compared to a matched control arthritis population (194). In this study, the NSAID-treated patients had a rise in the serum creatinine concentration from 1.28 to 2.58 mg/dL over a mean period of 47.5 months. The control group not taking NSAIDs had stable renal function. Finally, Segasothy and colleagues

(193) report on the risk of chronic renal disease in a prospective study of 259 heavy analgesic abusers. In this study, 69 patients developed radiographic evidence of papillary necrosis. Of these, 29 used NSAIDs either singularly (17 patients) or in combination with another NSAID (12 patients). Another nine patients used NSAIDs in combination with paracetamol, aspirin, caffeine, or a traditional herbal medicine. Renal insufficiency (serum creatinine concentration 1.4 to 8.8 mg/dL) was noted in 26 of the 38 patients who had used an NSAID chronically. Similar to the patients from Australia (178), this disorder was more common in males (1.9:1.0), distinguishing this disorder from classic analgesic nephropathy, which typically occurs in females. Similarly, these patients did not exhibit the usual psychological profile associated with analgesic abuse.

Thus, while further studies are needed to definitely assess the question of cumulative toxicity, it appears that some chronically treated patients may develop a change in renal function over a long-term period. Given the abuse potential of powerful NSAIDs and the fact that ibuprofen, naproxen, and ketoprofen are now available on an over-the-counter basis, it is possible that chronic NSAID abuse may become a more common cause of chronic kidney disease in the future.

In considering the definite association of compound analgesic abuse and the possible linkage of chronic NSAID use to the development of chronic kidney disease, it has become common clinical practice to recommend acetaminophen whenever possible for analgesia. In this regard, a recent case-control study examining the use of over-the-counter analgesics as a risk factor for end-stage renal disease found that acetaminophen may also cause chronic kidney disease when used on a continual basis (195). In this study, heavy average use of acetaminophen (>1 pill per day) and medium- to high-cumulative intake (1,000 or more pills in a lifetime) each doubled the odds of end-stage renal disease. These authors conclude that reduced consumption of acetaminophen could decrease the overall incidence of end-stage renal disease approximately 8% to 10%. The findings in this study confirmed an earlier report that also concluded that long-term daily use of acetaminophen is associated with an increased risk of chronic kidney disease (183). While these studies do not establish a cause-and-effect relationship between acetaminophen ingestion and chronic kidney disease, the data do suggest that ingestion of acetaminophen on a continual and chronic basis should be discouraged.

A recent organized review by a consensus panel of the National Kidney Foundation (NKF) surveyed over 600 articles and studied the implications of several different kinds of analgesic ingestion and renal failure risks (196,197). The highlights of the recommendations from the NKF consensus panel based on this review are that:

1. Ingestion of aspirin and nonsteroidal combinations are not encouraged because of an increased risk of renal failure when those combinations are ingested together.
2. Habitual consumption of analgesics is discouraged, and monitoring is recommended when such use is mandatory.
3. Combination analgesics are recommended to be available by prescription only with an explicit warning to physicians that the habitual consumption of these combination products could lead to the insidious development of chronic kidney disease.
4. There should be an explicit warning to consumers regarding NSAID ingestion.

The panel concluded that there is negligible clinical evidence that suggests habitual use of acetaminophen alone causes the clinical entity of analgesic nephropathy and that there is no evidence that occasional use of acetaminophen causes renal injury. Finally the panel points out that there is no risk from the

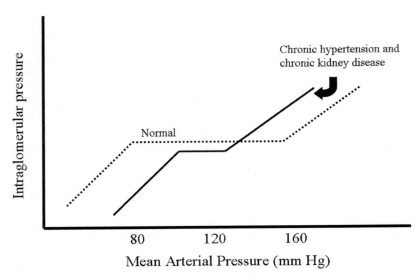

FIGURE 44-6. Renal autoregulation normally maintains intraglomerular pressure relatively constant despite variations in renal perfusion pressure. In patients with chronic hypertension or mild chronic kidney disease renal autoregulation changes in such a way that intraglomerular pressure begins to vary more directly with changes in mean arterial blood pressure. One can conceptualize this change as if the normal sigmoidal relationship between systemic blood pressure and intraglomerular pressure becomes progressively more linear. As a result, increases in mean pressure cause exaggerated rises in intraglomerular pressure while declines in mean pressure will cause exaggerated falls in intraglomerular pressure. The decline in intraglomerular pressure accompanying more stringent levels of blood pressure control will manifest itself by an increase in the serum creatinine concentration. Renal dysfunction that occurs in this setting is hemodynamic in origin and is reflective of a lower intraglomerular pressure.

regular use of aspirin in the relatively small doses recommended for prevention of cardiovascular events.

NEPHROTOXICITY OF ANGIOTENSIN-CONVERTING ENZYME INHIBITORS AND ANGIOTENSIN RECEPTOR BLOCKERS

The most common form of nephrotoxicity associated with angiotensin-converting enzyme (ACE) inhibitor therapy is an increase in the serum creatinine concentration occurring in the setting of antihypertensive therapy (198). This complication is becoming more common in clinical practice since guidelines governing adequate blood pressure control have been made more stringent. This decline in renal function is hemodynamic in origin and not secondary to structural injury to the kidney and can be traced to changes in renal autoregulation that accompany chronic kidney disease.

Normal renal autoregulation enables the kidney to maintain fairly constant renal blood flow and glomerular filtration rate in the setting of varying systemic blood pressure. One component of this process is an intrinsic property of the afferent arteriole called the myogenic reflex. The myogenic reflex causes this vessel to either constrict or dilate in response to changes in intraluminal pressure. An increase in arterial pressure elicits a vasoconstrictive response, whereas a decreased arterial pressure results in vasodilation. These changes in afferent tone provide an immediate response to maintain intraglomerular pressure and glomerular filtration rate relatively constant in the face of everyday fluctuations in systemic blood pressure (199).

In the setting of chronic hypertension, the small arteries of the kidney to include the afferent arteriole undergo a number of pathologic changes that give rise to alterations in the way the kidney autoregulates (200). As with vessels elsewhere, the afferent arteriole initially demonstrates evidence of endothelial dysfunction leading to impaired vasodilation. Over time this impairment is exaggerated by histologic changes of hyaline arteriosclerosis and myointimal hyperplasia. These changes lead to a blunted ability of the preglomerular circulation to either constrict or dilate in response to changes in renal perfusion pressure. In essence these vessels take on the characteristics of a pressure-passive vasculature where changes in mean arterial

pressure are matched by proportional change in GFR (201,202) (Fig. 44-6).

A blunted ability of the preglomerular circulation to dilate in response to a drop in the mean arterial pressure will cause an exaggerated decrease in the intraglomerular pressure and GFR. This impairment in autoregulation explains why patients with hypertension and chronic kidney disease are more likely to have an increase in the serum creatinine concentration when blood pressure is lowered. Any drug that lowers blood pressure can cause an increase in the serum creatinine concentration through this mechanism but ACE inhibitors are more commonly associated with this complication. ACE inhibitors will exaggerate the decline in intraglomerular pressure due to blood pressure reduction by concomitant vasodilation of the efferent side of the glomerular circulation.

As long as the increase in serum creatinine concentration is not excessive (>30% above the baseline value), or progressive, discontinuation of the ACE inhibitor is not necessarily warranted particularly considering the potential benefit, these agents have in slowing the progression of chronic renal failure. Long-term trials in both diabetic and nondiabetic patients have shown that the initial decline in renal function reaches a plateau within several weeks and is reversible with discontinuation of the ACE inhibitor even after several years of therapy (203,204). Thus a small, stable increase in the serum creatinine concentration after the start of an ACE inhibitor is hemodynamic in nature and reflects a fall in intraglomerular pressure.

If the rise in serum creatinine is >30% or the repeat value shows a progressive rise then the appropriate response is to discontinue the ACE inhibitor and initiate a search for other causes of renal dysfunction. There are several conditions in which use of ACE inhibitors may cause exaggerated or progressive declines in renal function (Table 44-8). The first

TABLE 44-8

RISK FACTORS FOR ACEI- OR ARB-INDUCED ACUTE RENAL FAILURE

Renal artery stenosis
Polycystic kidney disease
Decreased absolute or effective arterial blood volume
Nonsteroidal antiinflammatory drugs
Cyclosporin A, FK-506 (tacrolimus)
Sepsis

setting involves significant (usually >70%) bilateral renal artery obstruction or unilateral renal artery obstruction to a solitary functioning kidney. Under these conditions increased tone of the efferent arteriole acts to attenuate the decline in intraglomerular pressure that results from the arterial obstruction. The trade-off is that renal function and glomerular filtration rate become dependent upon sustained constriction of the efferent vessel by AII. A similar physiology can develop in patients with polycystic kidney disease where the renal arteries become extrinsically compressed by large cysts (205). Unless the underlying obstruction can be treated then other classes of antihypertensive agents will have to be utilized.

ACE inhibitors can also cause an azotemic response under conditions of an absolute (gastroenteritis, aggressive diuresis, poor oral intake) or effective reduction in arterial circulatory volume (moderate to severe congestive heart failure). In these settings angiotensin II-mediated constriction of the efferent arteriole serves to minimize the decline in glomerular filtration rate that would otherwise occur as a result of the fall in renal perfusion pressure. In the volume-contracted patient, the appropriate response to hold the ACE inhibitor and restart the drug once the extracellular fluid volume has been replenished. In a patient with congestive heart failure, ACE inhibitors will increase the serum creatinine when the decrease in intraglomerular pressure resulting from efferent vasodilation is not offset by an increase in renal perfusion. This can occur in patients with severely depressed cardiac function in which afterload reduction can no longer increase cardiac output or in the setting of aggressive diuresis.

A similar mechanism is responsible for renal dysfunction that occurs in patients given ACE inhibitors in the setting of NSAIDs, cyclosporin A, or early sepsis (206–208). In these settings, there is increased vasoconstriction of the renal vasculature. ACE inhibitor-induced efferent vasodilation in the face of decreased perfusion pressure accounts for the fall in GFR.

Angiotensin receptor blockers can cause renal dysfunction through the same mechanisms described with ACE inhibitors. Based on the biology of angiotensin II and its receptors there are reasons to suggest that such adverse effects on renal function may be slightly less common. These drugs block the AT_1 receptor, which is located primarily on the efferent vessel resulting in a vasodilatory response. AT_1 blockade is also associated with higher levels of angiotensin II that can then stimulate AT_2 receptors that are located to a greater extent on the afferent side of the glomerular circulation (209–211). Stimulation of the AT_2 receptor causes vasodilation (210). Efferent vasodilation (from AT_1 blockade) combined with afferent vasodilation (from AT_2 stimulation) might allow GFR to be better maintained in the setting of decreased blood pressure. In animal models of volume depletion, angiotensin receptor blockers have been shown to better preserve GFR as compared to ACE inhibitors (212,213). Whether such differences between angiotensin receptor blockers and ACE inhibitors are sufficient to be of clinical relevance in maintaining renal function has not been well studied (214).

A few cases of membranous nephropathy have been attributed to the use of ACE inhibitors (215,216), but the overall incidence of this complication and that of tubulointerstitial nephritis are believed to be low. To date there are no such reports linking angiotensin receptor blockers to the development of glomerular or interstitial renal disease.

References

1. Lote CJ, Haylor J. Eicosanoids in renal function. *Prost Leukot Essent Fatty Acids* 1989;36:203.
2. Smith WL. Prostanoid biosynthesis and mechanisms of action. *Am J Physiol* 1992;263:F181.
3. Kramer BK, Kammerl MC, Komhoff M. Renal cyclooxygenase-2 (COX-2). Physiological, pathophysiological and clinical implications. *Kidney Blood Press Res* 2004;27:43.
4. Weber PC, Larsson C, Scherer B. Prostaglandin E_2-9-ketoreductase as a mediator of salt intake-related prostaglandin-renin interaction. *Nature* 1977;266:65.
5. Schlondorff D. Renal prostaglandin synthesis: sites of production and specific actions of prostaglandins. *Am J Med* 1986;81(Suppl 2B):1.
6. Whorton AR, et al. Regional differences in prostacyclin formation by the kidney: prostacyclin is a major prostaglandin of renal cortex. *Biochim Biophys Acta* 1978;529:176.
7. Hansen HS. 15-hydroxyprostaglandin dehydrogenase. *Prostaglandins* 1976;12:647.
8. Uchida S, Nonoguchi H, Endou H. Localization and properties of NAD^+-dependent 15-hydroxyprostaglandin dehydrogenase activity in the rat kidney. *Pflugers Arch* 1985;404:278.
9. Komhoff M, et al. Localization of cyclooxygenase-1 and -2 in adult and fetal human kidney: implication for renal function. *Am J Physiol* 1997;272:F460.
10. Harris R, et al. Cyclooxygenase-2 is associated with the macula densa of rat kidney and increases with salt restriction. *J Clin Invest* 1994;94:2504.
11. Nantel F, et al. Immunolocalization of cyclooxygenase-2 in the macula densa of human elderly. *FEBS Lett* 1999;457:475.
12. Ferguson S, Hebert R, Laneuville O. NS-398 upregulates constitutive cyclooxygenase-2 expression in the M-1 cortical collecting duct cell line. *J Am Soc Nephrol* 1999;10:2261.
13. Yang T, et al. Regulation of cyclooxygenase expression in the kidney by dietary salt intake. *Am J Physiol* 1998;274:F481.
14. Traynor TR, et al. Inhibition of macula densa-stimulated renin secretion by pharmacological blockade of cyclooxygenase-2. *Am J Physiol* 1999;277:F706.
15. Cheng HF, et al. Prostaglandins that increase renin production in response to ACE inhibition are not derived from cyclooxygenase- 1. *Am J Physiol Regul Integr Comp Physiol* 2002;283:R638.
16. Cheng HF, et al. Genetic deletion of COX-2 prevents increased renin expression in response to ACE inhibition. *Am. J. Physiol Renal Physiol* 2001; 280:F449.
17. Harris RC, et al. Cyclooxygenase-2 is associated with the macula densa of rat kidneys and increases with salt restriction. *J Clin Invest* 1994;94:2504.
18. Kester M, et al. Endothelin stimulates prostaglandin endoperoxide synthase-2 mRNA expression and protein synthesis through a tyrosine kinase-signaling pathway in rat mesangial cells. *J Biol Chem* 1994;269:22574.
19. Ohnaka K, et al. Induction of cyclooxygenase-2 by angiotensin II in cultured rat vascular smooth muscle cells. *Hypertension* 2000;35:68.
20. Cheng HF, Harris RC. Cyclooxygenase, the kidney, and hypertension. *Hypertension* 2004;43:525.
21. Moeckel GW, et al. COX2 activity promotes organic osmolyte accumulation and adaptation of renal medullary interstitial cells to hypertonic stress. *J Biol Chem* 2003;278:19352.
22. Hao CM, et al. Dehydration activates an NF-kappaB-driven, COX2-dependent survival mechanism in renal medullary interstitial cells. *J Clin Invest* 2000;106:973.
23. Anderson RJ, et al. Prostaglandins: effects on blood pressure, renal blood flow, sodium and water excretion. *Kidney Int* 1976;10:205.
24. Oates JA, et al. Clinical implications of prostaglandin and thromboxane A_2 formation. *N Engl J Med* 1988;319:(Part I):689;(Part II):761.
25. Itskovitz HD, et al. Renal prostaglandins: determinants of intrarenal distribution of blood flow in the dog. *Clin Sci Mol Med* 1973;45:321S.
26. Edwards RM. Effects of prostaglandins on vasoconstrictor action in isolated renal arterioles. *Am J Physiol* 1985;248:F779.
27. Arima S, et al. Glomerular prostaglandins modulate vascular reactivity of the downstream efferent arterioles. *Kidney Int* 1994;45:650.
28. Scharschmidt L, Simonson M, Dunn MJ. Glomerular prostaglandins, angiotensin II, and nonsteroidal antiinflammatory drugs. *Am J Med* 1986; 81(Suppl 2B):30.
29. Uchida K, Ballermann BJ. Sustained activation of PGE2 synthesis in mesangial cells cocultured with glomerular endothelial cells. *Am J Physiol* 1992;263:C200.
30. Schlondorff D, et al. Prostaglandin synthesis by isolated rat glomeruli: effect of angiotensin II. *Am J Physiol* 1980;238:F486.
31. Schlondorff D, et al. In vivo demonstration of glomerular PGE2 responses to physiological manipulations and experimental agents. *Am J Physiol* 1987;252:F717.
32. Terragno NA, Tarragno DA, McGiff JC. Contribution of prostaglandins to the renal circulation in conscious, anesthetized, and laparotomized dogs. *Circ Res* 1977;40:590.
33. Swain JA, et al. Prostaglandin control of renal circulation in the unanesthetized dog and baboon. *Am J Physiol* 1975;299:826.
34. Berl T, et al. Prostaglandin synthesis inhibition and the action of vasopressin: studies in man and rat. *Am J Physiol* 1977;232:F529.
35. Haylor J, Lote CJ. Renal function in conscious rats after indomethacin: evidence for a tubular action of endogenous prostaglandins. *J Physiol* 1980;249:F1.
36. Berg KJ. Acute effects of acetylsalicylic acid on renal function in normal man. *Eur J Clin Pharmacol* 1977;11:117.

37. Haylor J. Prostaglandin synthesis and renal function in man. *J Physiol* 1980;298:383.
38. Muther RS, Bennett WM. Effects of aspirin on glomerular filtration rate in normal humans. *Ann Intern Med* 1980;92:386.
39. Donker AJ, et al. The effect of indomethacin on kidney function and plasma renin activity in man. *Nephron* 1976;17:288.
40. Epstein M, et al. Relationship between renal prostaglandin E and renal sodium handling during water immersion in normal man. *Circ Res* 1979;45:71.
41. Henrich WL, et al. The role of renal nerves and prostaglandins in control of renal hemodynamics and plasma renin activity during hypotensive hemorrhage in the dog. *J Clin Invest* 1978;61:744.
42. Henrich WL, et al. Angiotensin II, renal nerves, and prostaglandins in renal hemodynamics during hemorrhage. *Am J Physiol* 1978;235:F46.
43. Muther RS, Potter DM, Bennett WM. Aspirin-induced depression of glomerular filtration rate in normal humans: role of sodium balance. *Ann Intern Med* 1981;94:317.
44. Kramer HJ, et al. Interaction of renal prostaglandins with the renin–angiotensin and renal adrenergic nervous systems in healthy subjects during dietary changes in sodium intake. *Clin Sci* 1985;68:387.
45. Favre L, Glasson P, Vallotton MB. Reversible acute renal failure from combined triamterene and indomethacin. *Ann Intern Med* 1982;96:317.
46. Sedor JR, Davidson EW, Dunn MJ. Effects of nonsteroidal antiinflammatory drugs in healthy subjects. *Am J Med* 1986;81(Suppl 2B):58.
47. Berne RM, Levy MN. Effects of acute reduction of cardiac output on the renal circulation of the dog. *J Clin Invest* 1950;29:444.
48. Cannon PJ. Prostaglandins in congestive heart failure and the effects of nonsteroidal antiinflammatory drugs. *Am J Med* 1986;81(Suppl 2B):123.
49. Zipser RD. Role of renal prostaglandins and the effects of nonsteroidal antiinflammatory drugs in patients with liver disease. *Am J Med* 1986;81(Suppl 2B):95.
50. Arroyo V, et al. Renal function abnormalities, prostaglandins, and effects of nonsteroidal antiinflammatory drugs in cirrhosis with ascites. *Am J Med* 1986;81(Suppl 2B):104.
51. Gentilini P. Cirrhosis, renal function and NSAIDs. *J Hepatol* 1993;19:200.
52. Geers AB, et al. Functional relationships in the nephrotic syndrome. *Kidney Int* 1984;26:324.
53. Harris RC, Ismail N. Extrarenal complications of the nephrotic syndrome. *Am J Kidney Dis* 1994;23:477.
54. Bohrer MP, et al. Mechanisms of the puromycin-induced defects in the transglomerular passage of water and macromolecules. *J Clin Invest* 1977;l60:152.
55. Golbetz H, et al. Mechanism of the antiproteinuric effect of indomethacin in nephrotic humans. *Am J Physiol* 1989;256:F44.
56. de Jong PE, Anderson S, de Zeeuw D. Glomerular preload and afterload reduction as a tool to lower urinary protein leakage: will such treatments also help to improve renal function outcome? *J Am Soc Nephrol* 1993;3:1333.
57. Arisz L, et al. The effect of indomethacin on proteinuria and kidney function in the nephrotic syndrome. *Acta Med Scand* 1976;199:121.
58. Palmer BF. Nephrotic edema: pathogenesis and treatment. *Am J Med Sci* 1993;306:53.
59. Henrich WL, et al. Dissociation of systemic and renal effects in endotoxemia. *J Clin Invest* 1982;69:691.
60. Clive DM, Stoff JS. Renal syndromes associated with nonsteroidal antiinflammatory drugs. *N Engl J Med* 1984;310:563.
61. Patrono C, Pierucci A. Renal effects of nonsteroidal antiinflammatory drugs in chronic glomerular disease. *Am J Med* 1986; 81(Suppl 2B):71.
62. Murray MD, et al. Ibuprofen-associated renal impairment in a large general internal medicine practice. *Am J Med Sci* 1990;299:222.
63. Gurwitz JH, et al. Nonsteroidal antiinflammatory drug-associated azotemia in the very old. *JAMA* 1990;264:471.
64. Palmer BF, Levi M. Effect of aging on renal function and diseases. In: Brenner BM, Rector FC, eds. *The kidney*, 5th ed. Philadelphia: Saunders, 1996:2274.
65. Schlondorff T. Renal complications of nonsteroidal antiinflammatory drugs. *Kidney Int* 1993;44:643.
66. Bennett WM. Geriatric pharmacokinetics and the kidney. *Am J Kidney Dis* 1990;16:283.
67. Yanagisawa H, et al. Increases in glomerular eicosanoid production in rats with bilateral ureteral obstruction are mediated by enhanced enzyme activities of both the cyclooxygenase and 5-lipooxygenase pathways. *Proc Soc Exp Biol Med* 1993;203:291.
68. Cantley LG, et al. Role of endothelin and prostaglandins in radiocontrast-induced renal artery constriction. *Kidney Int* 1993;44:1217.
69. Altman RD, Perez GO, Sfakianakis GN. Interaction of cyclosporine A and nonsteroidal antiinflammatory drugs on renal function in patients with rheumatoid arthritis. *Am J Med* 1992;93:396.
70. Miller MJ, Bednar MM, McGiff JC. Renal metabolism of sulindac: functional implications. *J Pharmacol Exp Ther* 1984;231:449.
71. Eriksson LO, Bostrom H. Deactivation of sulindac-sulphide by human renal microsomes. *Pharmacol Toxicol* 1988;62:177.
72. Bunning RD, Barth WF. Sulindac: a potentially renal-sparing nonsteroidal antiinflammatory drug. *JAMA* 1982;248:2864.
73. Eriksson LO, et al. Effects of sulindac and naproxen on prostaglandin excretion in patients with impaired renal function and rheumatoid arthritis. *Am J Med* 1990;89:313.
74. Laffi G, et al. Effects of sulindac and ibuprofen in patients with cirrhosis and ascites. *Gastroenterology* 1986;90:182.
75. Klassen DK, et al. Sulindac kinetics and effects on renal function and prostaglandin excretion in renal insufficiency. *J Clin Pharmacol* 1989;29:1037.
76. Brater DC, et al. Effects of ibuprofen, naproxen, and sulindac on prostaglandins. *Kidney Int* 1985;27:66.
77. Henrich WL, Brater DC, Campbell WB. Sulindac accentuates renal ischemia during hemorrhage. *Kidney Int* 1985;27:295.
78. Whelton A, et al. Renal effects of ibuprofen, piroxicam, and sulindac in patients with asymptomatic renal failure. *Ann Intern Med* 1990;112:568.
79. Swainson CP, Griffiths P. Acute and chronic effects of sulindac on renal function in chronic renal disease. *Clin Pharmacol Ther* 1985;37:298.
80. Brandli DW, et al. Individual variability in concentrations of urinary sulindac sulfide. *Clin Pharmacol Ther* 1991;50:650.
81. Brater C. Effects of nonsteroidal antiinflammatory drugs on renal function: focus on cyclooxygenase-2-selective inhibition. *Am J Med* 1999;107[Suppl 6A]65S.
82. Whelton A, et al. Effects of celecoxib and naproxen on renal function in the elderly. *Arch Intern Med* 2000;160:1465.
83. Catella-Lawson F, et al. Effects of specific inhibition of cyclooxygenase-2 on sodium balance, hemodynamics, vasoactive eicosanoids. *J Pharmacol Exp Ther* 1999;289:735.
84. Swan SK, et al. Effect of cycloxygenase-2 inhibition on renal function in elderly persons receiving a low-salt diet. A randomized, controlled trial. *Ann Intern Med* 2000;133:1.
85. Rossat J, et al. Renal effects of selective cyclooxygenase-2 inhibition in normotensive salt-depleted subjects. *Clin Pharmacol Ther* 1999;66:76.
86. Harris RC, Zhang MZ, Cheng HF. Cyclooxygenase-2 and the renal renin-angiotensin system. *Acta Physiol Scand* 2004;181:543.
87. Perazella MA. COX-2 selective inhibitors: analysis of the renal effects. *Expert Opin Drug Safety* 2002;1:53.
88. Brezin JH, et al. Reversible renal failure and nephrotic syndrome associated with nonsteroidal antiinflammatory drugs. *N Engl J Med* 1979;301:1271.
89. Abraham PA, Keane WF. Glomerular and interstitial disease induced by nonsteroidal antiinflammatory drugs. *Am J Nephrol* 1984;4:1.
90. Markowitz GS, et al. Membranous glomerulopathy and acute interstitial nephritis following treatment in celecoxib. *Clin Nephrol* 2003;59:137.
91. Alper A Jr, Meleg-Smith S, Krane NK. Nephrotic syndrome and interstitial nephritis associated with celecoxib. *Am J Kidney Dis* 2002;40:1086–1090.
92. Henao J, et al. Celecoxib-induced acute interstitial nephritis. *Am J Kidney Dis* 2002;39:1313.
93. Alim N, et al. Rofecoxib-induced acute interstitial nephritis. *Am J Kidney Dis* 2003;41:720.
94. Rocha JL, Fernandez-Alonso J. Acute tubulointerstitial nephritis associated with the selective COX-2 enzyme inhibitor, rofecoxib. *Lancet* 2001;357:1946.
95. Levin ML. Patterns of tubulo-interstitial damage associated with nonsteroidal antiinflammatory drugs. *Semin Nephrol* 1988;8:55.
96. Katy S, et al. Tolmetin: association with reversible renal failure and acute interstitial nephritis. *JAMA* 1981;246:243.
97. Greenstone M, Hartley B, Gabriel R. Acute nephrotic syndrome with reversible renal failure after phenylbutazone. *Br Med J* 1981;282:950.
98. Finkelstein A, et al. Fenoprofen nephropathy: lipoid nephrosis and interstitial nephritis. *Am J Med* 1982;72:81.
99. Lomvardias S, et al. Nephrotic syndrome associated with sulindac. *N Engl J Med* 1979;304:1271.
100. Radford MG, et al. Membranous glomerulopathy associated with the use of nonsteroidal antiinflammatory drugs. *J Am Soc Nephrol* 1994;5:359.
101. Chan LK, et al. Acute interstitial nephritis and erythroderma associated with diflunisal. *Br Med J* 1980;1:84.
102. McCarthy JT, et al. Reversible nonoliguric acute renal failure associated with zomepirac therapy. *Mayo Clin Proc* 1982;57:351.
103. Fawaz-Estrup F, Ho G. Reversible acute renal failure induced by indomethacin. *Arch Intern Med* 1981;141:1670.
104. Ling BN, et al. Naproxen-induced nephropathy in systemic lupus erythematosus. *Nephron* 1990;54:249.
105. Raftery MJ, et al. Fenclofenac induced interstitial nephritis confirmed by inadvertent rechallenge. *Br Med J* 1985;2:81.
106. Reeves WB, Foley RJ, Weinman EJ. Nephrotoxicity from nonsteroidal antiinflammatory drugs. *South Med J* 1985;78:318.
107. Bender WL, et al. Interstitial nephritis, proteinuria, and renal failure caused by nonsteroidal antiinflammatory drugs. *Am J Med* 1984;76:1006.
108. Vander AJ. Direct effects of prostaglandin on renal function and renin release in anesthetized dog. *Am J Physiol* 1968;214:218.
109. Shimizu K, et al. Free water excretion and washout of renal medullary urea by prostaglandin E1. *Jpn Heart J* 1969;10:437.
110. Ganguli M, et al. Evidence that prostaglandin synthesis inhibitors increase the concentration of sodium and chloride in rat renal medulla. *Circ Res* 1977;40(Suppl 1):I35.
111. Ichikawa I, Brenner BM. Importance of efferent arteriolar vascular tone in regulation of proximal tubule fluid reabsorption and glomerulotubular balance in the rat. *J Clin Invest* 1980;65:1192.
112. Iino Y, Imai M. Effects of prostaglandins on Na transport in isolated collecting tubules. *Pflugers Arch* 1978;373:125.

113. Stokes JB, Kokko JP. Inhibition of sodium transport by prostaglandin E2 across the isolated, perfused rabbit collecting tubule. *J Clin Invest* 1977; 59:1099.
114. Stokes JB. Effect of prostaglandin E_2 on chloride transport across the rabbit thick ascending limb of Henle. *J Clin Invest* 1979;64:495.
115. Higashihara E, et al. Cortical and papillary micropuncture examination of chloride transport in segments of the rat kidney during inhibition of prostaglandin production. *J Clin Invest* 1979;64:1277.
116. Fulgraff G, Meiforth A. Effects of prostaglandin E2 on excretion and reabsorption of sodium and fluid in rat kidneys (micropuncture studies). *Pflugers Arch* 1971;330:243.
117. Cordova HR, Kokko JP, Marver D. Chronic indomethacin increases rabbit cortical collecting tubule Na^+-K^+-ATPase activity. *Am J Physiol* 1989; 256:F570.
118. Haas JA, et al. Mechanism of natriuresis during intrarenal infusion of prostaglandins. *Am J Physiol* 1984;247:475.
119. Pawlowska D, et al. Prostaglandin blockade blunts the natriuresis of elevated renal interstitial hydrostatic pressure. *Am J Physiol* 1988;254: F507.
120. Terashima R, Anderson FL, Jubiz W. Prostaglandin E release in the dog: effect of sodium. *Am J Physiol* 1976;231:1429.
121. Carmines PK, et al. Prostaglandins in the sodium excretory response to altered renal arterial pressure in dogs. *Am J Physiol* 1985;248:F8.
122. Silva P, et al. Influence of endogenous prostaglandins on mTAL injury. *J Am Soc Nephrol* 1990;1:808.
123. Stillman IE, et al. Effects of salt depletion on the kidney: changes in medullary oxygenation and thick ascending limb size. *J Am Soc Nephrol* 1994;4:1538.
124. Brown J, Dollery C, Valdes G. Interaction of nonsteroidal antiinflammatory drugs with antihypertensive and diuretic agents. *Am J Med* 1986;81(Suppl 2B):43.
125. Attallah AA. Interaction of prostaglandins with diuretics. *Prostaglandins* 1979;18:369.
126. Dixey JJ, et al. The effects of naproxen and sulindac on renal function and their interaction with hydrochlorothiazide and piretanide in man. *Br J Clin Pharmacol* 1987;23:55.
127. Patak RV, et al. Antagonism of the effects of furosemide by indomethacin in normal and hypertensive man. *Prostaglandins* 1975;10:649.
128. Nies AS, et al. Indomethacin-furosemide interaction: the importance of renal blood flow. *J Pharmacol Exp Ther* 1983;226:27.
129. Williamson HE, Bourland WA, Marchand GR. Inhibition of furosemide-induced increase in renal blood flow by indomethacin. *Proc Soc Exp Biol Med* 1975;148:164.
130. Greven J, Farjam A. Effect of inhibitors of prostaglandin synthesis on the furosemide action in the loop Henle of rat kidney. *Pflugers Arch* 1988; 411:579.
131. Kirchner KA, Martin CJ, Bower JD. Prostaglandin E_2 but not I_2 restores furosemide response in indomethacin-treated rats. *Am J Physiol* 1986; 250:F980.
132. Kirchner KA. Prostaglandin inhibitors alter loop segment chloride uptake during furosemide diuresis. *Am J Physiol* 1985;248:F698.
133. Levenson DJ, Simmons CE, Brenner BM. Arachidonic acid metabolism, prostaglandins and the kidney. *Am J Med* 1982;72:354.
134. Kirchner KA, et al. Mechanism of attenuated hydrochlorothiazide response during indomethacin administration. *Kidney Int* 1987;31:1097.
135. Favre L, et al. Interaction of diuretics and non-steroidal antiinflammatory drugs in man. *Clin Sci* 1983;64:407.
136. Houston MC. Nonsteroidal antiinflammatory drugs and antihypertensives. *Am J Med* 1991;90(Suppl 5A):42S.
137. Pope JE, Anderson JJ, Felson TD. A meta-analysis of the effects of nonsteroidal antiinflammatory drugs on blood pressure. *Arch Intern Med* 1993; 153:477.
138. Johnson AG, Nguyen TV, Day RO. Do nonsteroidal antiinflammatory drugs affect blood pressure? *Ann Intern Med* 1994;121:289.
139. Beckmann ML, et al. Propranolol increases prostacyclin synthesis in patients with essential hypertension. *Hypertension* 1988;12:582.
140. Mackenzie T, et al. The importance of age on prostaglandin E2 excretion in normal and hypertensive men. *Nephron* 1984;l38:178.
141. Minuz P, et al. Prostacyclin and thromboxane biosynthesis in mild essential hypertension. *Hypertension* 1990;15:469.
142. Kato T, et al. Prostaglandin H_2 may be the endothelium-derived contracting factor released by acetylcholine in the aorta of the rat. *Hypertension* 1990;15:475.
143. Diederich D, et al. Impaired endothelium-dependent relaxations in hypertensive resistance arteries involve cyclooxygenase pathway. *Am J Physiol* 1990;258:H445.
144. Whelton A, et al. Renal safety and tolerability of celecoxib, a novel cyclooxygenase-2 inhibitor. *Am J Ther* 2000;7:159.
145. Whelton A, et al. Cyclooxygenase-2—specific inhibitors and cardiorenal function; randomized, controlled trial of celecoxib and rofecoxib in order hypertenxive osteoarthritis patients. *Am J Ther* 2001;8:85.
146. Whelton A, et al. Effects of celecoxib and rofecoxib on blood pressure and edema patients > or = 65 years of age with systemic hypertension and osteoarthritis. *Am J Cardiol* 2002;90:959.
147. Geba GP, et al. Efficacy of rofecoxib, celecoxib, and acetaminophen in osteoarthritis of the knee; a randomized trial. *JAMA* 2002;287;64.
148. Schwartz JI, et al. Comparison of rofecoxib, celecoxib and naproxen on renal function in elderly subjects receiving a normal-salt diet. *Clin Pharmacol Ther* 2002;72:50.
149. Beroniade V, Corneille L, Haraoui B. Indomethacin-induced inhibition of prostaglandin with hyperkalemia. *Ann Intern Med* 1979;91:499.
150. Goldszer RC, et al. Hyperkalemia associated with indomethacin. *Arch Intern Med* 1981;141:802.
151. Kutyrina IM, Androsova SO, Tareyeva IE. Indomethacin-induced hyporeninaemic hypoaldosteronism. *Lancet* 1979;1:785.
152. Tan SY, et al. Indomethacin-induced prostaglandin inhibition with hyperkalemia. *Ann Intern Med* 1979;90:783.
153. Findling JW, et al. Indomethacin-induced hyperkalemia in three patients with gouty arthritis. *JAMA* 1980;244:1127.
154. Zimran A, et al. Incidence of hyperkalemia induced by indomethacin in a hospital population. *Br Med J* 1985;291:403.
155. Henrich WL. Role of prostaglandins in renin secretion. *Kidney Int* 1981; 19:822.
156. Yun J, et al. Role of prostaglandins in the control of renin secretion in the dog. *Circ Res* 1977;40:459.
157. Berl T, et al. Prostaglandins in the beta-adrenergic and baroreceptor-mediated secretion of renin. *Am J Physiol* 1979;236:F472.
158. Gerber JG, Nies AS, Olsen RD. Control of canine renin release: macula densa requires prostaglandin synthesis. *J Physiol* 1981;319:419.
159. Beierwaltes WH, et al. Interaction of the prostaglandin and renin-angiotensin systems in isolated rat glomeruli. *Am J Physiol* 1980;239: F602.
160. Henrich WL, Campbell WB. Relationship between PG and β-adrenergic pathways to renin release in rat renal cortical slices. *Am J Physiol* 1984; 247:E343.
161. Campbell WB, et al. Attenuation of angiotensin II- and III-induced aldosterone release by prostaglandin synthesis inhibitors. *J Clin Invest* 1979; 64:1552.
162. Pratt JH. Role of angiotensin II in potassium-mediated stimulation of aldosterone secretion in the dog. *J Clin Invest* 1982;70:667.
163. Ling BN, Webster CL, Eaton DC. Eicosanoids modulate apical Ca^{2+}-dependent K^+ channels in cultured rabbit principal cells. *Am J Physiol* 1992;263:F116.
164. DeFronzo RA. Hyperkalemia and hyporeninemic hypoaldosteronism. *Kidney Int* 1980;17:118.
165. Nadler JL, et al. Evidence of prostacyclin deficiency in the syndrome of hyporeninemic hypoaldosteronism. *N Engl J Med* 1986;314:1015.
166. Mimran A, Ribstein J, Jover B. Aging and sodium homeostasis. *Kidney Int* 1992;41(Suppl 37):107.
167. Palmer BF. Managing hyperkalemia caused by inhibitors of the renin-angiotensin-aldosterone system. *N Engl J Med* 2004;351:585.
168. Gross PA, Schrier RW, Anderson RJ. Prostaglandins and water metabolism: a review with emphasis on in vivo studies. *Kidney Int* 1981;19:839.
169. Kramer HJ, Glanzer K, Dusing R. Role of prostaglandins in the regulation of renal water excretion. *Kidney Int* 1981;19:851.
170. Breyer MD, Jacobson HR, Hebert RL. Cellular mechanisms of prostaglandin E2 and vasopressin interactions in the collecting duct. *Kidney Int* 1990;38:618.
171. Anderson RJ, et al. Evidence of an in vivo antagonism between vasopressin and prostaglandin in the mammalian kidney. *J Clin Invest* 1975;56:420.
172. Yared A, Kon V, Ichikawa I. Mechanism of preservation of glomerular perfusion and filtration during acute extracellular fluid volume depletion. *J Clin Invest* 1985;75:1477.
173. Perez-Ayuso RM, et al. Evidence that renal prostaglandins are involved in renal water metabolism in cirrhosis. *Kidney Int* 1984; 26:72.
174. Rault RM. Case report: hyponatremia associated with nonsteroidal antiinflammatory drugs. *Am J Med Sci* 1993;305:318.
175. Clark BA, et al. Increased susceptibility to thiazide-induced hyponatremia in the elderly. *J Am Soc Nephrol* 1994;5:1106.
176. Duggin GG. Mechanisms in the development of analgesic nephropathy. *Kidney Int* 1980;18:553.
177. Sabatini S. Analgesic-induced papillary necrosis. *Semin Nephrol* 1988;8:41.
178. Nanra RS. Analgesic nephropathy in the 1990's: an Australian perspective. *Kidney Int* 1993;44(Suppl 42):86.
179. Buckalew VM, Schey HM. Renal disease from habitual antipyretic analgesic consumption: an assessment of the epidemiologic evidence. *Medicine* 1986;11:291.
180. Pommer W, et al. Regular analgesic intake and the risk of end-stage renal disease. *Am J Nephrol* 1989;9:403.
181. Elseviers M, De Broe M. Analgesic nephropathy in Belgium is related to the sales of particular analgesic mixtures. *Nephrol Dial Transplant* 1994;9: 41.
182. De Broe M, et al. Analgesic nephropathy. *Nephrol Dial Transplant* 1996;11:2407.
183. Sandler DP, et al. Analgesic use and chronic renal disease. *N Engl J Med* 1989;320:1238.
184. Murray TG, et al. Epidemiologic study of regular analgesic use and end-stage renal disease. *Arch Intern Med* 1983;143:1687.
185. Morlans M, et al. End-stage renal disease and non-narcotic analgesics: a case control study. *Br J Clin Pharmacol* 1990;30:717.
186. Dubach UC, Rosner B, Pfister E. Epidemiologic study of analgesics containing phenacetin. *N Engl J Med* 1983;308:357.

187. Elseviers M, De Broe M. A long-term prospective controlled study of analgesic abuse in Belgium. *Kidney Int* 1995;48:1912.

188. Dubach UC, Rosner B, Stumer T. An epidemiologic study of abuse of analgesic drugs. *N Engl J Med* 1991;324:155.

189. Piper JM, Tonascia J, Matanoski GM. Heavy phenacetin use and bladder cancer in women aged 20 to 49 years. *N Engl J Med* 1985;313:292.

190. Elseviers M, et al. High diagnostic performance of CT scan for analgesic nephropathy in patients with incipient to severe renal failure. *Kidney Int* 1995;48:1316.

191. Carmichael J, Shankel SW. Effects of nonsteroidal antiinflammatory drugs on prostaglandins and renal function. *Am J Med* 1985;78:992.

192. Sandler DP, Burr R, Weinburg CR. Nonsteroidal antiinflammatory drugs and the risk for chronic renal disease. *Ann Intern Med* 1991;115:165.

193. Segasothy M, et al. Chronic renal disease and papillary necrosis associated with the long-term use of nonsteroidal antiinflammatory drugs as the sole or predominant analgesic. *Am J Kidney Dis* 1994;24:17.

194. Rice D, et al. Renal failure in patients with rheumatoid arthritis and osteoarthritis on nonsteroidal antiinflammatory drugs. *Fed Proc* 1984;43:1100.

195. Perneger TV, Whelton PK, Klag MJ. Risk of kidney failure associated with the use of acetaminophen, aspirin, and nonsteroidal antiinflammatory drugs. *N Engl J Med* 1994;331:1675.

196. Henrich W, et al. Analgesics and the kidney: summary and recommendations to the scientific advisory board of the NKF from an ad hoc committee of the NKF. *Am J Kidney Dis* 1996;162.

197. Henrich W. Analgesic nephropathy. *Trans Am Clin Climatol Assoc* 1998;109:147.

198. Palmer BF. Renal dysfunction complicating treatment of hypertension. *N Engl J Med.* 2002;347:1256.

199. Schnermann J. Juxtaglomerular cell complex in the regulation of renal salt excretion. *Am J Physiol* 1998;43:R263.

200. Fishberg G, Ditscherlein G. Renal histopathology in hypertensive diabetic patients. *Hypertension* 1985;7:II-29.

201. Christensen PK, Hansen HP, Parving H. Impaired autoregulation of GFR in hypertensive non-insulin dependent diabetic patients. *Kidney Int* 1997;52:1369.

202. Christensen PK, et al. Impaired autoregulation of the glomerular filtration rate in patients with nondiabetic nephropathies. *Kidney Int* 1999;56:1517.

203. Hansen H, et al. Increased glomerular filtration rate after withdrawal of long-term antihypertensive treatment in diabetic nephropathy. *Kidney Int* 1995;47:1726.

204. Apperloo A, De Zeeuw D, De Jong P. A short-term antihypertensive treatment-induced fall in glomerular filtration rate predicts long-term stability of renal function. *Kidney Int* 1997;51:793.

205. Chapman A, Gabow P, Schrier R. Reversible renal failure associated with angiotensin converting enzyme inhibitors in polycystic kidney disease. *Ann Intern Med* 1991;15:769.

206. Seelig CB, Maloley PA, Campbell JR. Nephrotoxicity associated with concomitant ACE inhibitor and NSAID therapy. *South Med J* 1990;83:114.

207. Curtis JJ, et al. Captopril-induced fall in glomerular filtration rate in cyclosporine-treated hypertensive patients. *J Am Soc Nephrol* 1993;3:1570.

208. Schor N. Acute renal failure and the sepsis syndrome. *Kidney Int* 2002;61:764.

209. Goldfarb DA, et al. Angiotensin II receptor subtypes in the human renal cortex and renal cell carcinoma. *J Urol* 1994;151:208.

210. Arima S, et al. Possible role of P-450 metabolites of arachidonic acid in vasodilator mechanism of angiotensin II type 2 receptor in the isolated microperfused rabbit afferent arteriole. *J Clin Invest* 1997;100:2816.

211. Zhuo J, et al. Presence of angiotensin II AT-II receptor binding sites in the adventitia of human kidney vasculature. *Clin Exp Pharmacol Physiol* 1996;3:S147.

212. Kon V, Fogo A, Ichikawa I. Bradykinin causes selective efferent arteriolar dilation during angiotensin I converting enzyme inhibition. *Kidney Int* 1993;44:545.

213. Demeilliers B, Jover B, Mimran A. Contrasting renal effects of chronic administration of enalapril and losartan on one-kidney, one clip hypertensive rats. *J Hypertens* 1998;16:1023.

214. Taal M, Brenner B. Renoprotective benefits of RAS inhibition: from ACEI to angiotensin II antagonists. *Kidney Int* 2000;57:1803.

215. Donker AJ. Nephrotoxicity of angiotensin converting enzyme inhibition. *Kidney Int* 1987;31:S132.

216. Cleland JGF, et al. Captopril in heart failure: a double-blind study of the effects on renal function. *J Cardiovasc Pharmacol* 1986;8:700.

CHAPTER 45 ■ RADIOCONTRAST MEDIA-INDUCED ACUTE RENAL FAILURE

SAMUEL N. HEYMAN, MAYER BREZIS, AND ROBERT E. CRONIN

Since the introduction of the first iodinated contrast medium in 1954, the use of iodinated radiocontrast media has markedly expanded, in parallel with the increasing use of imaging procedures, including computerized tomography and angiographic interventions. Some 80,000,000 imaging studies with iodinated contrast agents were performed worldwide during 2003, corresponding to about 8 millions liters of radiocontrast material (Idee JM, personal communications). This explains why contrast-induced nephropathy (CIN) remains an important iatrogenic cause of acute renal failure (1,2), despite its recognition, the implementation of preventive strategies and the use of safer agents. Hou reported in 1987 that of 129 cases of hospital-acquired renal insufficiency, 12% followed the use of radiocontrast (1), putting contrast media as the third leading cause of new-onset acute renal failure (ARF) in hospitalized patients. Fifteen years later, CIN remains an important cause of ARF acquired in a tertiary care hospital, together with reduced renal perfusion, medications, and surgery (3).

This chapter will first provide a brief review of the radiocontrast materials presently used. This will be followed by the important clinical features of CIN, and by an evaluation of laboratory investigations that provide insights into the pathogenesis of this disorder. The last section deals with methods currently used to prevent the development of CIN, and the search for additional preventive strategies.

TYPES OF CONTRAST AGENTS

The first widely used radiocontrast media were high-osmolar (≈1,600 mOsm) ionic derivatives of triiodobenzene, such as diatrizoate, meglumine, or metrizoate (Table 45-1, Fig. 45-1). Since the early 1990s their use has gradually been replaced by safer "low-osmolar" (600 to 800 mOsm) agents, such as the nonionic iohexol, ioversol, iopromide, or iopamidol, and the ionic dimer ioxaglate, particularly for high-risk patients. Third-generation isoosmolar (≈300 mOsm) nonionic agents, such as iodixanol and iotrolan have been introduced during the late nineties and their nephrotoxic potential as compared with the low-osmolar contrast media is currently being investigated.

The basic structure of high-osmolar agents, such as sodium-diatrizoate, is a single benzene ring that contains three iodine atoms and a short ionic residue that facilitates water solubility. The nonionic monomers, such as iohexol, do not have an ionic residue, and thus are only moderately hypertonic. Dimeric ionic compounds, for instance ioxaglate, are constructed of two linked benzene rings that together contain six iodine atoms and a cationic residue of either sodium or methylglucamine. Because the iodine content of these dimeric compounds is twice that of either the ionic or the nonionic agents, similar amounts of iodine can be given with only half the osmotic load. The recently developed nonionic dimers resemble the dimeric ionic compounds but are devoid of the ionic site. This structural modification further reduces the osmolar-

ity to a near-physiologic value, but at the price of a substantial increase in viscosity (Table 45-1). As outlined below, the new generation low- and isoosmolar agents are considered safer, as compared with the high-osmolar radiocontrast media. Indeed, the median lethal dose of intravenously administered iohexol, is three times greater than that of the ionic high osmolar agents (4). Nonionic contrast media seem to have a particular advantage in myelography, digital subtraction angiography, leg phlebography, arteriography and renal tomography. Systemic effects, such as a feeling of warmth (especially after intravenous use), that depend on iodine content, osmolality, and sodium ion concentration are less frequent with these agents (5). Unlike the ionic agents that are minimally reabsorbed by the nephron, the nonionic agents are to some extent reabsorbed by the proximal tubule, but there is species specificity to this property (6). Radiocontrast agents cause mild proteinuria when injected directly into the renal artery, but the magnitude of this effect with nonionic agents is smaller than with ionic radiocontrast (7). The nonionic agents also have significantly less cardiac effects, causing less depression of ventricular contractility and less reduction in coronary sinus calcium concentration (5). They also appear to have less effect on complement consumption, cause fewer hypersensitivity reactions, and have a less disruptive effect on the endothelial wall of blood vessels (8).

CLINICAL FEATURES OF CIN

Historical Perspective

In the early 1960s, radiocontrast material was suspected of causing acute renal failure (ARF), but controversy surrounded many of the early case reports. Ten years later, CIN was recognized as one of the leading causes of ARF in patients with renal insufficiency, diabetes mellitus, volume depletion, and low cardiac output. Soon after this recognition, however, the incidence of ARF in high-risk patients declined sharply, simply because physicians learned to volume expand these patients before administering radiocontrast (Fig. 45-2). This bell-shaped curve, which characterizes the history of clinical drug toxicities in general, disqualifies historical controls. For instance, the use of mannitol to prevent CIN was based on historical controls; more recent reports, using concurrent controls, suggest that mannitol may in fact be detrimental, especially in diabetic patients (9,10). Moreover, in prospectively studied, carefully prepared patients, the incidence of clinically significant ARF is very low; only about 1% of high-risk patients need dialysis following radiocontrast administration (9,10). Similar observations have led some investigators to suggest that following imaging studies, ARF may not occur much more often when radiocontrast medium is administered than when it is not (11). Prospective studies that focus on patient selection and optimal treatment often miss one of the most important factors

TABLE 45-1

TYPES OF RADIOCONTRAST AGENTS IN USE

Class of radiocontrast agent	Contrast agents	Osmolality (mosm)	Viscosity (mPa*s, 37°C)
High-osmolar Ionic monomer	Iothalamate Diatrizoate	1,400–2,000	~5–6
"Low-osmolar" Nonionic monomer	Iohexol, ioversol Iopamidol, iopromide Iomeprol	600–800	~4.5–6.5
Ionic dimer	Ioxaglate		
Isoosmolar Nonionic dimer	Iotrolan Iodixanol	~300	~9

involved in CIN—lack of awareness leading to the administration of large doses of radiocontrast to the sickest and least prepared patients (12).

Incidence of CIN

The incidence of CIN is highly dependent on the population studied and the criteria used to diagnose renal injury. CIN has been defined as a rise in serum creatinine of 0.3 mg/dL (13,14), 0.5 mg/dL (9,15–19), 0.6 mg/dL (20), 1.0 mg/dL (17,21–26), or 2.0 mg/dL (27,28), or a 10% (29), 25% (10,29–31) or a 50% increase in baseline serum creatinine 1 to 5 days following exposure to radiocontrast material (11,32). D'Elia and co-workers (22) report that 0.68% of nonazotemic patients and 17.4% of azotemic patients had a 1 mg/dL rise in serum creatinine following nonrenal angiography. A 12% incidence of ARF was reported in seriously ill, hospitalized patients, using a rise in serum creatinine of at least 1 mg/dL within 48 hours of the study as the criterion for nephrotoxicity (33). A prospective study of 537 consecutive patients undergoing major angiography, that used somewhat more stringent criteria for nephrotoxicity (i.e., 1 mg/dL serum creatinine rise within 24 hours), uncovered no episodes of ARF (23). Nevertheless, these patients received saline expansion during the angiographic procedure. The reported incidence of CIN seems to be declining (16, 34–36). In a group of patients with few risk factors other than an age >70 years, the incidence of ARF after angiography was as low as 1.2% (36). Mueller reported a comparable incidence of 0.7% to 2% of CIN in 1,620 patients undergoing coronary angiography, the majority without predisposing risk factors (18). Rudnick and colleagues (37) have emphasized that studies examining the incidence of CIN also report substantial ARF in the control patients not receiving radiocontrast. This suggests that earlier reports probably overestimated the true incidence of CIN in the general population. However, the reported incidence of CIN in high-risk patients remains much higher, at the range of 10% to 45% (21,26,36,38–43), despite the use of newer contrast media and the implementation of preventive measures, though only a small fraction of these patients require

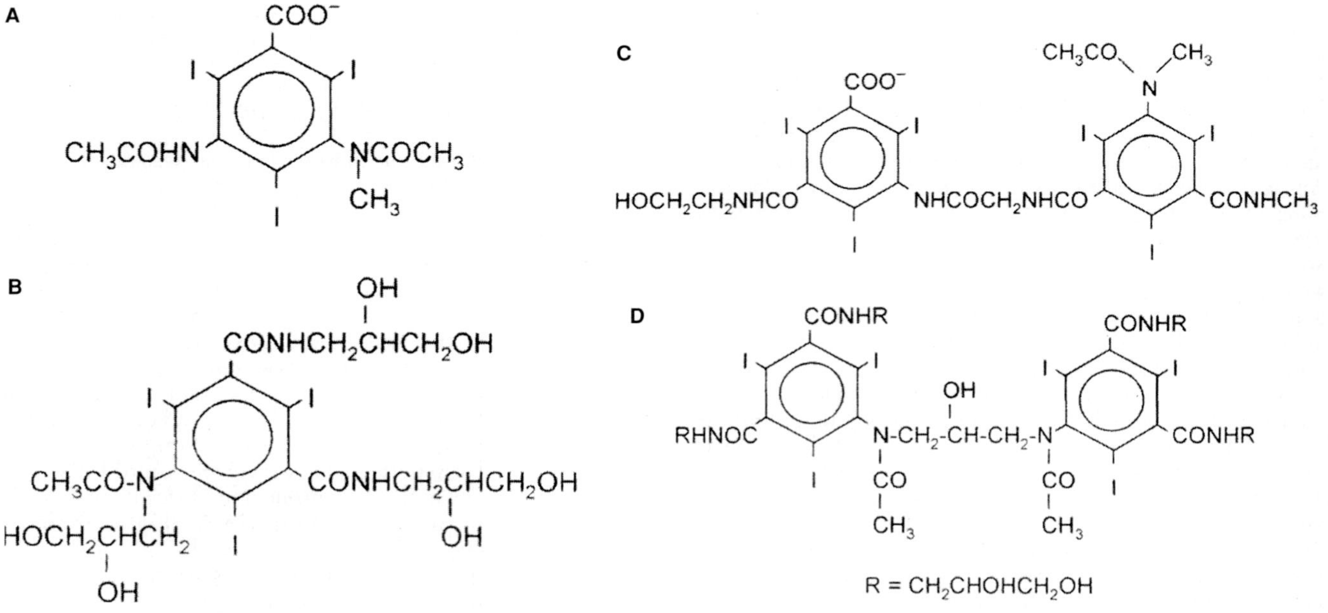

FIGURE 45-1. **A:** High-osmolar ionic radiocontrast agents are triiodinated benzoic acid anionic derivatives and a cation (metrizoate). **B:** Nonionic "low-osmolar" radiocontrast agents are also triiodinated benzoic acid derivatives (iohexol). **C:** Ionic "low-osmolar" dimeric radiocontrast agents contain two benzene rings, with a total of six iodine atoms and a cation (ioxaglate). **D:** Isoosmolar agents are nonionic dimmers also consisted of two iodinated benzene rings (iodixanol).

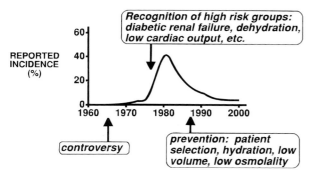

FIGURE 45-2. Schematized history of radiocontrast nephropathy. (From: reference 179, Heyman SN, Rosen S, Brezis M. Radiocontrast nephropathy: a paradigm for the synergism between toxic and hypoxic insults in the kidney. *Exp Nephrol* 1994;2:153, with permission.)

renal replacement therapy. Thus, the incidence of CIN and the assessment of the efficacy of preventive measures should be regarded in the perspective of predisposing risk factors, type and dosage of the radiocontrast agent, and the implementation of protective strategies. Indeed, diversity in the definition of CIN and the marked heterogeneity regarding patients' characteristics, the type and volume of administered radiocontrast, the type of imaging procedure and the applied protective measures, interfere with comparisons of clinical studies and in the assessment of efficacy of various interventions (44).

Risk Factors for CIN

Factors linked to the development of CIN can be divided into patient-related and procedure-related factors (Table 45-2). The former group include preexisting renal insufficiency (22,26,27,45–53), diabetes mellitus (21,24,26–28,33,46,47, 49,54–60), advanced age (13,27,28,33,45,46,54,55,61), multiple myeloma (62–65), volume depletion (45,49,53,66), presence of cardiovascular disease (13,14,28,46,49,53,56,59,67), hypertension (13,14,28,48,67,68), dehydration (54,57,59, 67,69), concomitant exposure to other nephrotoxins (56,57, 59,69), anemia (49,70), proteinuria (13,28,33,71), abnormal liver function (33,71), hyperuricemia (24,27,68), male sex (13,18), and renal transplantation (72,73). Hyperlipidemia also appears to be a risk factor in experimental CIN (74). Among procedure-related risk factors are the type of radiocontrast material used (i.e., high- vs. low- or isoosmolar agents) (26), volume of contrast media (19,21,45,49,56,57,66,75,76), repeated exposure to radiocontrast media over a few days (13,14,67,68,71), and injection site (i.e., intraarterial vs. intravenous) (27,49).

Many of these risk factors may be covariate rather than be independent variables. This probably accounts for reports that fail to confirm many of these as risk factors. The incidence of CIN is proportional to the number of coexisting clinical risk factors (36). As shown in Figure 45-3, among aged patients it was almost inevitable in the presence of three or more risk factors, while at their absence the chance to develop CIN became negligible.

Underlying renal insufficiency is the risk factor most commonly associated with CIN. Factors that may be involved in this predisposition include (a) a reduced glomerular filtration rate (GFR) that obligates each remaining nephron to excrete a proportionately greater load of contrast material, hence exposure to a greater amount of contrast, and (b) the lack of functional renal reserve in chronic stable renal insufficiency to buffer acute losses in glomerular filtration. Thus, any nephron

TABLE 45-2

RISK FACTORS FOR DEVELOPMENT OF RADIOCONTRAST AGENT-INDUCED ACUTE RENAL FAILURE

Patient-Related Factors	Procedure-Related Factors
Renal insufficiency	Type of radiocontrast medium (High-osmolar > low or isoosmolar)
Diabetes mellitus	Dose of radiocontrast medium
Age	Repeated exposures to radiocontrast material within 72 hr
Effective volume depletion Dehydration Congestive heart failure Chronic liver disease Nephrotic syndrome Concomitant hypotension	Mode of administration (Intraarterial > intravenous)
Concomitant exposure to nephrotoxins Medications Other exogenous nephrotoxins Sepsis	Primary coronary intervention for acute MI*
Myeloma	
Male gender	
Hypertension	
Transplanted kidney	
Hyperuricemia	
Proteinuria	
Anemia	

(*Marenzi, et al. N-acetylcysteine and contrast-induced nephropathy in primary angioplsty. *N Engl J Med* 2006;354:2773.)

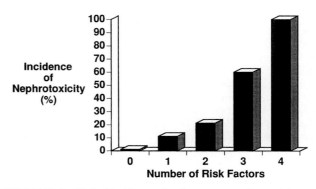

FIGURE 45-3. Clinical incidence of radiocontrast nephrotoxicity as a function of the number of preexisting risk factors present in the patient. (Redrawn from: Rich MW, Crecelius CA. Incidence, risk factors, and clinical course of acute renal insufficiency after cardiac catheterization in patients 70 years of age or older. *Arch Intern Med* 1990;150:1237, with permission.)

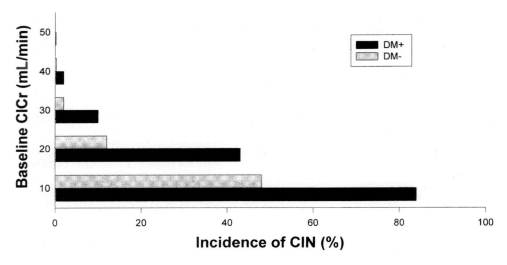

FIGURE 45-4. The impact of pre-existing renal dysfunction and diabetes on the incidence of CIN. (Modified with permission from: McCullough et al. Acute renal failure after coronary intervention: incidence, risk factors, and relationship to mortality. *Am J Med* 1997;103:368.)

damage or loss is translated immediately into a rise in serum creatinine. D'Elia and co-workers (22) have studied 378 hospitalized patients undergoing nonrenal angiography and identified the presence of preexisting azotemia as the only risk factor predisposing to nephrotoxicity (defined as a rise in serum creatinine of ≥1 mg/dL following the procedure). McCullough, evaluating the incidence and risk factors for CIN in 3,700 patients undergoing coronary intervention (75), reports that the lower the baseline creatinine clearance, the larger was the risk for the development of CIN (Fig. 45-4).

Taliercio and co-workers (77) show that class IV heart failure is an independent risk factor for CIN, particularly when the amount of contrast exceeds 125 mL. They report a 23% incidence of contrast nephropathy (>1 mg/dL rise in serum creatinine) in 139 patients with preexisting abnormal renal function (serum creatinine ≥2 mg/dL) who underwent cardiac angiography. The mean increment in serum creatinine was 2.6 mg/dL, the time to peak serum creatinine was 2.8 days, and 9% developed anuria or oliguria. Similarly, Gomes and colleagues (78) show an increased incidence of CIN in patients receiving digoxin for congestive heart failure or arrhythmias, and Rihal shows an increased risk for CIN in patients following acute myocardial infarction and hypotension (53).

Volume depletion and dehydration, often the result of purging enemas and restricted food and fluid intake prior to the radiographic study, appear to be less important risk factors nowadays, as current practice encourages volume expansion prior to most contrast requiring procedures. Nevertheless, effective volume depletion may still exist during contrast studies despite fluid administration in patients with poor cardiac output, cirrhosis or hypoalbuminuria, or in critically ill patients with sepsis syndrome or shock.

Whether diabetes mellitus per se predisposes to radiocontrast-induced ARF was for years a matter of debate. The incidence of CIN in diabetic patients rises sharply if the baseline serum creatinine is elevated. A serum creatinine >1.5 mg/dL increases by approximately 50% the likelihood of developing ARF (24,46). Harkonen and Kjellstrand (24) report that 22 of 29 (76%) of all diabetic patients with a serum creatinine >2 mg/dL developed ARF following intravenous pyelography. Diabetic patients with a baseline serum creatinine >5 mg/dL and those developing diabetes before the age of 40 years had an even greater risk of CIN. In 56% of these latter patients, renal failure was irreversible. The experience of 13 patients with type I diabetes with advanced nephropathy (mean serum creatinine of 6.8 mg/dL) undergoing coronary angiography was equally stark, with 12 of the 13 developing CIN (49). When renal insufficiency is advanced at the time CIN develops, it is often irreversible (49,58,79). The age

of onset of diabetes also seems to affect the severity and likelihood of developing CIN. It has been suggested that Type II diabetic patients are less likely to develop CIN than type I diabetic patients (24,80). Nonetheless, the risk of developing CIN in type II diabetes is not trivial. Shieh and others (80) report a 6% incidence of ARF after excretory urography in 49 type II diabetic patients who, as a group, had only minor renal impairment (mean baseline serum creatinine of 1.3 mg/dL and mean creatinine clearance of 79.6 ml/minute). Several reports suggest that diabetes in the absence of renal insufficiency does not predispose to CIN (11,22,26,32,35). By contrast, Rihal, reports that diabetes significantly predisposes to CIN after coronary intervention when baseline creatinine is below 2 mg/dL, but not above it (53). Other studies using sensitive measures to detect toxicity or using multivariate analysis of risk factors also suggest that diabetic patients with normal renal function are at increased risk for CIN (51,52). In summary, it seems most prudent to view the presence of diabetes as a synergistic factor in causing radiocontrast-induced ARF, although renal function may appear normal when insensitive measures such as the serum creatinine are used. This is well illustrated in McCullough's large cohort of patients undergoing coronary interventions (75): among patients with preexisting renal failure, the risk of CIN was doubled in diabetic patients at any given baseline renal function (Fig. 45-4).

Multiple myeloma historically has been singled out as a high-risk disease for the development of CIN (62–64). A central event in the pathogenesis of myeloma-induced renal failure is the co-precipitation of Bence-Jones proteins with Tamm-Horsfall protein in the renal tubule (81,82). However, an analysis of 476 patients with myeloma exposed to radiocontrast revealed an incidence of ARF of 0.6% to 1.25% (65). This low value is similar to the reported incidence of CIN found in patients who served as controls for radiocontrast-administered subjects (11) or in well hydrated low-risk population (18). The early reports of ARF following contrast exposure in myeloma patients may have underestimated the role of comorbid factors such as sepsis, hypercalcemia, and volume depletion. Nevertheless, it seems prudent in patients with unexplained renal disease undergoing contrast studies, particularly older patients, to screen the urine for Bence-Jones proteins with *p*-toluene sulfonic acid (TSA) or, if unavailable, the dipstick and sulfosalicylic acid (SSA) test (83). A positive TSA test, or a positive SSA test (which checks for all urinary proteins) with a negative dipstick (albumin), may be considered presumptive evidence of Bence Jones proteinuria, and radiocontrast studies should then be undertaken only with caution if no alternative imaging procedure is suitable.

As discussed below (under Prevention of CIN), the type of radiocontrast should be considered a renal risk factor, when the use of high-osmolar agents is to be considered. It is now clear that low-osmolar contrast media are significantly safer, as compared with the old generation high-osmolar agents, with an estimated 50% risk reduction for CIN (26,30). By contrast, the use of the more recently developed isoosmolar contrast materials is probably not advantageous over low-osmolar agents, regarding the risk of nephrotoxicity (42,43).

The importance of the volume of radiocontrast in the etiology of ARF was also debated for a while, with some studies showing a positive relationship (45,53,74,77,78) and others showing no relationship (22,24,84). Miller and colleagues (84) have studied prospectively 200 patients requiring intravenous or intraarterial contrast material and found no consistent change in renal function with increasing doses of contrast material. However, Cigarroa and associates (21) showed that careful limitation of the volume of contrast material used during cardiac catheterization could reduce the incidence of nephropathy (see Prevention of CIN, below). Recent studies, using much larger volumes of radiocontrast material for complicated angiographyic interventions, settled this debate, clearly defining contrast dose as an independent risk factor for CIN (19).

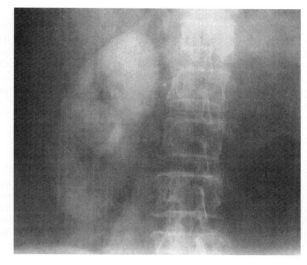

FIGURE 45-5. Persistent nephrogram in solitary kidney in a 73-year-old woman 8 hours following excretory urography performed to evaluate hematuria. The contralateral kidney had been removed previously because of nephrolithiasis. Baseline serum creatinine was 1.6 mg/dL. (Photograph courtesy of Dr. Thomas Curry.)

Clinical Presentation of CIN

CIN, manifested as an acute decline in renal function, has been reported following virtually every radiographic procedure using intravascular injection of iodinated radiocontrast. Renal toxicity appears to be favored in the presence of the risk factors outlined above. Nonoliguric CIN is far more common than the oliguric form, and is generally more common in patients initially having a lower serum creatinine prior to receiving the contrast. In oliguric ARF, the time course of the oliguria and the rise in serum creatinine depend on the baseline serum creatinine prior to receiving the contrast agent. Patients with normal or mild renal functional impairment prior to receiving radiocontrast agents usually have oliguria lasting 2 to 5 days, with recovery to baseline urine volumes and serum creatinine by day 7. When more serious impairment of underlying renal function is present, recovery is generally prolonged, and up to 30% of patients may end up with various degrees of residual renal impairment (85). Renal failure may even be irreversible, requiring long-term hemodialysis (22,23,41,45,49,51,77,78,86,87). As with ARF of other etiologies, protracted CIN is associated with a prolonged hospitalization course (88) and over fivefold increase in mortality (89).

Diagnosis of CIN

The most easily diagnosed case of CIN is that in which oliguria develops within 24 to 48 hours following a radiocontrast study. More often, a subtle, nonoliguric episode of ARF is diagnosed in retrospect by demonstrating a reversible 0.5 to 3.0 mg/dL rise in serum creatinine. In most situations, the serum creatinine remains the most practical test for detecting the presence of CIN. However, differential diagnoses are taken into account for this indication of declining glomerular filtration, including pre- and postrenal causes, comorbidities such as sepsis syndrome or advanced liver failure, exposure to other nephrotoxins, or cholesterol emboli in the case of angiographic studies performed through the aorta.

One feature that characterizes many patients with CIN is the paradoxical and, as yet, poorly explained propensity for the urinary sodium concentration and the fractional excretion of sodium to be low (28,46,47,90). Fang and colleagues (47) report 12 patients with radiocontrast-induced ARF who had

a low fractional excretion of sodium (mean 0.36%), which persisted for up to 5 days during the oliguric phase. Reduced renal perfusion and acute tubular obstruction have been offered as explanations for this phenomenon (47).

The urinalysis may occasionally show features of ATN (renal tubular cellular casts, muddy brown or coarsely granular casts), but these may often be absent (22,49). Conversely, in the absence of a rise in serum creatinine, radiocontrast agents may still alter the urinary sediment. Gelman and associates (91) demonstrate more formed elements (cells, casts, and debris) in the urine of 12 of 14 patients following angiography, although none of the patients experienced a reduction in GFR. All patients showed amorphous urate crystals, and two patients had a heavy shower of calcium oxalate crystals.

A persistent nephrogram 24 to 48 hours after the contrast study is a characteristic but not pathognomonic feature of CIN (20,22,92) (Fig. 45-5). In a healthy subject given a bolus of radiocontrast material, renal opacification is the densest immediately after the end of the injection and then fades rapidly, while it appears in the urinary collecting system. A very little nephrogram effect remains detectable at 6 hours (93). In most patients with radiocontrast-induced ARF as well as in patients with other forms of ARF, the nephrogram develops quickly but fails to disappear with time. A persistent nephrogram is a sensitive indicator of the presence of renal failure (83% of patients with renal failure had a positive nephrogram) with high specificity (93% of patients without renal failure lacked the persistent nephrogram) (22). The likelihood ratio of ARF being present, then, following a positive result is equal to 12 (sensitivity/[100 − specificity]). In other words, a positive nephrogram increases by 12 times the likelihood that ARF has occurred over baseline incidence (i.e., if it was 1.5%, it is now about 18%). The likelihood ratio following a negative test is equal to 0.18 ([100 − sensitivity]/specificity), or about one-fifth. Thus, the absence of a nephrogram decreases the likelihood of contrast nephropathy to one-fifth from baseline incidence (e.g., if it was 1.5%, it is now about 0.3%).

Detection of urinary biomarkers, released from tubular cells, such as gamma-glutamyltranspeptidase, alanine aminopeptidase, alkaline phosphatase, or N-acetyl-beta-glucosaminidase (NAG) has also been suggested in the diagnosis of CIN (94), but current technologies are considered to suffer from large basal variations and low specificity of increased urinary enzymes. For instance, increased urine volume per se may enhance enzymuria (95). However, protracted enzymuria five days after the exposure to the radiocontrast agent may be more indicative for tubular injury (96). Another limiting factor for the usefulness of urinary biomarkers is the selective or predominance of their expression by specific segments of the nephron, as with kidney injury molecule (KIM)-1, that serves as a sensitive marker of proximal tubular damage (97).

Human Pathology of CIN

The reportedly characteristic renal lesion with CIN is an intense vacuolization of proximal tubular cells, often called osmotic nephrosis (98,99). A review of 211 renal biopsies obtained within 10 days of urography or renal arteriography revealed osmotic nephrosis in 47; a diffuse form was found in patients with severe preexisting renal disease, while a milder focal form was seen in patients with less severe renal impairment or in patients with previously normal kidneys. However, the presence of the focal or even the diffuse form did not necessarily predict the presence of renal functional impairment. Conversely, virtually normal proximal tubular cells were found in patients who developed oligoanuric ARF after urography (99). Hyperosmolality or high ionic medium does not seem to be required for the development of these lesions because the newer low- and iso-osmotic contrast media are capable of inducing it as well (100–102). Notably, in 13 patients with histologically normal kidneys, vacuoles were not found in any of the tubular cells, implying that an underlying nephropathy was required to induce this histologic lesion. Iodine cannot be demonstrated in these vacuoles (103,104), which develop rapidly within 5 to 15 minutes under experimental settings (102,103). Heyman and co-workers (103) suggest that the origin of the vacuoles is not from endocytosis but from invagination of membranes of lateral cellular interdigitations. They suggest that the contrast media in the paracellular space may have damaged these membranes, leading to the vesicular outpouchings. Ultrastructural histochemistry, however, reveals that these vacuoles contain acid phosphatase activity (102), suggesting merging with lysosomes. Noteworthy, KIM-1, a marker of proximal tubular damage, was not found in the urine of patients with CIN (97), supporting the concept that proximal tubular vacuolization not necessarily reflects tubular cell injury. In summary, most human and animal studies indicate that proximal tubular vacuolization appears after radiocontrast exposure irrespective to changes in kidney function. In that perspective, and given the very limited (cortical) sampling of human material, that is often obtained at a very late phase of established ATN, we believe that proximal tubular vacuolization should serve as marker of radiocontrast exposure, rather than an indicator of CIN (105).

PATHOGENESIS OF CIN

Overview

Though recognized for some 40 years, the pathophysiology of CIN remains an issue of controversy. It is classified as "acute tubular necrosis" (ATN), or "toxic nephropathy," but, in fact, very little is known about its true nature and morphologic characteristics. Indeed, the low fractional excretion of sodium noted in many cases of CIN is not a typical finding in ATN. As detailed above, cortical tubular vacuolization, also present after radiocontrast administration under experimental settings, should better be regarded as a marker for contrast medium exposure, rather than an indicator of tubular damage. Unfortunately, human morphology of deeper kidney structures is lack-

ing, and urinary biomarkers of tubular injury are of limited value.

Typical toxic ATN, such as cis-platinum or gentamicin nephropathies are believed to be mediated primarily through well-characterized direct tubular-cell toxicity, as also documented with heavy metals in experimental and clinical settings. Renal handling of the toxin predominantly determines the distribution pattern of tubular damage. The injury is dose-dependent, and the contribution of perturbations is relatively marginal, with the exception of the hydration state (106). On the other hand, data regarding direct tubular toxicity of radiologic contrast agents is quite limited, and is predominantly based on in vitro prolonged incubation of tubular cells or tubular segments with iodinated dye. Contrast agents, once filtered through the glomerulus, are not reabsorbed or metabolized by tubular cells (perhaps with the exception of traces of nonionic agents) (6). Furthermore, although the dose of radiocontrast is considered proportional to the risk for renal dysfunction, CIN is rarely encountered in the absence of predisposing factors. These data suggest that factors other than direct tubular toxicity are predominantly responsible for CIN.

The current knowledge regarding the pathophysiology of CIN predominantly stems from animal studies that examined the effect of radiocontrast media upon renal function, hemodynamics and oxygenation. In complementary studies, the impact of contrast agents upon various mediators that could govern these changes was examined, and ultimately, adequate animal models of CIN were developed. Together with in vitro research and experiments in kidneys perfused ex vivo, these studies have led to the recognition that CIN represents the outcome of a unique combination of interactive pathogenic processes, including regional endothelial dysfunction, renal tissue hypoxia, and subsequent oxygen free radical-induced cytotoxicity (Table 45-3, Figure 45-6).

In this section we shall describe the intensification of the outer medullary hypoxemia that follows the administration of iodinated radiocontrast agents, review the various components believed to be involved in this process and their potential role in CIN, analyze related cytotoxic processes, and appraise the lessons learned from the development of animal models of CIN.

Physiologic Medullary Hypoxia

While oxygen is abundant in the renal cortex, the medulla is poorly oxygenated, working normally on the verge of anoxia. Medullary partial pressure of oxygen (PO_2) as low as 30 mm Hg has been detected with oxygen microelectrodes under normal physiologic conditions in rats, dogs, and humans, reflecting relatively low regional blood flow and countercurrent oxygen diffusion from decending to ascending vasa recta. The limited medullary oxygen delivery of some 8 mL/minute/100 g tissue is hardly sufficient for the metabolic needs for tubular transport, predominantly carried out in the outer medulla by medullary thick ascending limbs (mTALs) and S3 (straight) segments of the proximal tubule. Consequently, oxygen extraction by the renal medulla is near-maximal, reaching 79% of regional oxygen supply, leaving a very marginal oxygen reserve (107,108). This critical medullary oxygen balance is manifested by high levels of cytochrome AA3 in its redox state, and by the high levels of unsaturated hemoglobin, detected within the renal medulla by blood-oxygen-level dependent (BOLD) magnetic resonance imaging (MRI) (109,110). The kidney appears to have designed regulatory mechanisms to allow urinary concentration without medullary hypoxic injury. Optimal urinary concentration requires a perfect match between oxygen supply and demand, an effect achieved through a precise regulation of blood flow and tubular work in the outer medulla. Distal tubular reabsorption is affected by the control of GFR and

TABLE 45-3

CONTRAST-INDUCED PHYSIOLOGIC CHANGES

Extrarenal
 Decreased systemic oxygenation
  Altered pulmonary function
  Leftward shift of oxygen-hemoglobin dissociation curve
 Hemodynamic changes leading to transient renal
  hypoperfusion
 Rheologic alterations of the blood

Renal: physiologic changes
 Diuresis
 Altered GFR: biphasic response $\uparrow \rightarrow \downarrow$
 Intrarenal blood viscosity $\uparrow$
 Urine viscosity $\uparrow$
 Renal volume and interstitial pressure $\uparrow$
 Altered renal circulation
  Cortex: biphasic response $\uparrow \rightarrow \downarrow$
  Outer medulla: $\uparrow\uparrow\uparrow$
  Papilla: $\downarrow\downarrow\downarrow$
 Reduced renal oxygenation (cortex $\downarrow$; medulla $\downarrow\downarrow\downarrow$)
  Oxygen delivery $\downarrow$
  Oxygen consumption $\uparrow$
 Uric acid and oxalate excretion $\uparrow$
 Enzymuria

**Renal: altered mediators regulating renal hemodynamics and
 function**
 Adenosine $\uparrow$
 Nitric oxide: $\downarrow$ in cortex; $\uparrow$ in outer medulla
 Prostaglandins: PGE$_2$ $\uparrow$, PGI2 $\uparrow$ or $\downarrow$
 Atrial natriuretic peptide $\uparrow$
 Endothelin $\uparrow$
 Vasopressin $\uparrow$
 Histamine $\uparrow$
 Reactive oxygen species $\uparrow$

Renal: additional major changes at cellular level
 Free radical species $\uparrow$
 Hypoxia-inducible factors (HIF) and related stress-response
  genes $\uparrow$
 Poly-(ADP-ribose) polymerase (PARPP) $\uparrow$ (probably)

proximal tubular reabsorption (both governing solute delivery to the distal nephron) and by the regulation of distal tubular reabsorption. Locally produced prostaglandins and nitric oxide (NO), and the generation of adenosine from the breakdown of adenosine triphosphate (ATP) are major participants in the regulation of medullary oxygenation. All three induce medullary vasodilation and directly inhibit tubular reabsorptive activity. Adenosine can further improve medullary oxygenation by the induction of cortical vasoconstriction with the reduction of GFR, and subsequently diminished solute delivery for reabsorption by the distal nephron (107,108). The location were the mediator is released and the distribution and density of its receptors are important in maintaining medullary oxygenation. For instance, both the synthesis and the density of receptors for prostaglandine E$_2$ (PGE$_2$) are abundant in the outer medulla. The effect of various mediators upon cortical and medullary microcirculation may be diverse, depending on receptor types. Adenosine exerts cortical vasoconstriction through adenosine-A$_1$ receptors, while it induces medullary vasodilation through adenosine-A$_2$ receptors (111). Comparably, endothelin-1 exerts cortical vasoconstriction through ET$_A$ receptors, but enhances medullary blood flow activating ET$_B$ receptors (112). Angiotensin II also selectively induces cortical vasoconstriction, while medullary flow is maintained (113). Thus, in the normal intact kidney medullary blood flow is usually maintained, even during systemic and local vasoconstrictive stimuli, by the combined effects of locally produced vasodilators (NO, PGE$_2$) and a unique regional vasodilatory effect of renal vasoconstrictors. Corticomedullary redistribution of blood flow and the activation of the tubuloglomerular feedback mechanism may, therefore, be regarded as measures designed to maintain medullary oxygenation and prevent tubular hypoxic damage. Most risk factors for CIN are characterized by defective nitrovasodilation or prostaglandin synthesis (see below), major protectors of medullary oxygenation. Indeed, renal medullary PO$_2$ markedly declines during experimental inactivation of these mechanisms (114,115).

Ample experimental data indicate that enhancement of distal tubular reabsorptive workload, unmatched by adequate oxygen supply, or altered regional blood flow, may lead to ATN with a rather selective outer medullary hypoxic damage, predominantly affecting mTALs, and to a lesser extent S3 segments. Papillary injury may develop as well. The reader is referred to detailed reviews of the role medullary hypoxic injury plays in the evolution of ATN and in chronic renal parenchymal disease (107,108).

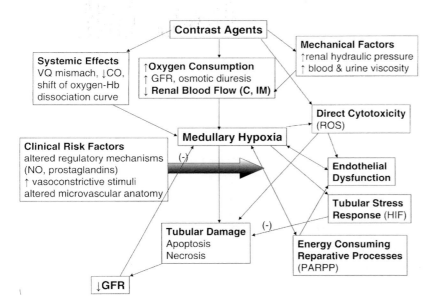

FIGURE 45-6. Schematic algorithm illustrating putative hypoxic and toxic mechanisms involved in the pathophysiology of CIN, and their interrelations.

Aggravation of Medullary Hypoxia by Radiocontrast Agents

Using Clark-type oxygen microelectrodes, Brezis found that injection of radiocontrast markedly affects renal parenchymal oxygenation (113). Following the administration of the high-osmolar ionic agent sodium iothalamate, cortical PO_2 declined from 40 to 25 mm Hg. More impressive was the change observed in outer medullary PO_2 which fell from 26 mm Hg at baseline to mean levels as low as 9 mm Hg (Figure 45-7). Comparable studies with oxygen microelectrodes were repeated by Liss and colleagues, showing a fall in medullary oxygenation from about 30 mm Hg to 15 mm Hg after the administration of ionic, as well as nonionic, low-osmolar and isoosmolar contrast agents (116). Radiocontrast-induced intensification of medullary hypoxemia has also been suggested by non-invasive BOLD MRI (110), which detects increased unsaturated hemoglobin concentration within the renal medulla, and by the detection of hypoxia inducible factors (HIF) shortly after contrast administration (117).

Systemic effects of the radiocontrast medium may contribute to the decline in renal tissue oxygenation, including the induction of pulmonary ventilation-perfusion mismatch (118), reduced cardiac output and renal perfusion pressure (119), rheologic alterations of the blood (120,121), and a leftward shift of the oxygen-hemoglobin dissociation curve (122). Systemic hypoxemia is less likely to occur with the use of nonionic agents (123), yet it may aggravate regional ischemic injury (124). However, the greater part of the decline in renal parenchymal oxygenation is attributed to altered intrarenal balance of oxygen supply and demand.

Radiocontrast-Induced Change in Oxygen Demand

Administration of radiocontrast media induces an abrupt transient increase in glomerular filtration, and urinary output (125). This response, comparable to the osmotic diuretic effect of mannitol, occurs despite a rise in vasopressin (126,127), and is mediated in part by an increase in plasma volume and the release of natriuretic peptides (128,129). Natriuresis and diuresis may also be related to an ET_B- mediated effect of endothelin (130), released in response to radiocontrast injection

(128,131). All these factors, perhaps in addition to the substantial osmotic load provided by many contrast media, lead to enhanced solute delivery to the distal nephron, with subsequent increased oxygen consumption for tubular reabsorption. The decline in outer medullary PO_2 despite enhanced regional blood flow (see below) only emphasizes the important role for increased reabsorptive activity in the ensuing regional hypoxia. Indeed, the inhibition of tubular transport with the loop diuretic furosemide abruptly reverses radiocontrast-induced medullary hypoxemia (114,132). The improvement of medullary hypoxemia with furosemide takes place even though it induces profound regional vasoconstriction (133), further emphasizing the central role of regulated tubular transport in the maintenance of medullary oxygen balance.

Radiocontrast-Induced Intrarenal Changes in Oxygen Supply

The decline in renal parenchymal oxygenation may also reflect radiocontrast-induced altered renal microcirculation. Indeed, it has been known for over 30 years that renal blood flow briefly and transiently increases following radiocontrast injection, with a prolonged subsequent decline to about 25% below baseline (134). This effect occurs whether the radiocontrast is administered intravenously or intra-arterially and is an intrinsic response of the kidney because it can be reproduced in isolated perfused kidneys (103). Weisberg and colleagues directly measured renal blood flow during cardiac catheterization in patients with chronic renal failure and found no association between reduced renal blood flow and the development of CIN (135). However, alterations in renal blood flow during contrast injection, predominantly reflecting changes in cortical flow, conceal very important changes in medullary flow, that constitute of only 10% of total renal perfusion. Thus, changes in renal blood flow cannot predict alterations in medullary oxygen supply (107,108). Moreover, medullary flow is usually preserved during a moderate decline in renal blood flow (within the "autoregulatory" range), despite a remarkable fall in cortical blood flow (136), a phenomenon called "corticomedullary redistribution of blood flow." Furthermore, a fall in cortical blood flow alone is expected to increase medullary oxygenation, the outcome of diminished glomerular filtration rate (GFR) and solute delivery for reabsorption by the distal nephron (136).

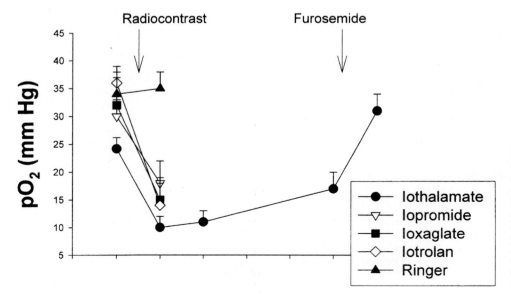

FIGURE 45-7. Changes in outer medullary partial pressure of oxygen (PO_2) following the administration of high-osmolar ionic agent (iothalamate), low-osmolar nonionic (iopromide), low-osmolar ionic (ioxaglate) and isoosmolar nonionic contrast medium (iotrolan), compared with Ringer's solution. Also illustrated is the reversal of iothalamate-induced decline in medullary oxygenation with furosemide. (Modified from: Heyman SN, et al. Early renal medullary hypoxic injury from radiocontrast and indomethacin. *Kidney Int* 1991;40:632, and from: Liss P, et al. Injection of low and isoosmolar contrast medium decreases oxygen tension in the renal medulla. *Kidney Int* 1998;53:698).

The possibility that radiocontrast-related medullary hypoxia reflects altered medullary microvasculature has therefore been explored by direct determination of the local microcirculation. Nygren (137) and subsequently Liss and colleagues (138) recorded papillary blood flow with laser-Doppler probes after the exposure of the papilla by the dissection of the renal pelvis. Indeed, they found that ionic high-osmolar, as well as nonionic and low-osmolar radiologic contrast media markedly reduced papillary blood flow. Using video microscopy of trans-illuminated papillary vasa recta and dual-window cross-correlation technique, they also documented near cessation of red blood cell movement in papillary blood vessels, associated with red cell aggregation (138).

At the outer medulla, however, microcirculatory response to radiocontrast was found to be quite different. Using needle laser-Doppler probes inserted through the cortex following partial renal decapsulation, Agmon found that outer medullary regional microcirculation markedly increases after the injection of the high-osmolar agent iothalamate, as long as NO- or prostaglandin-synthesis are intact (139). Increased outer medullary flow in response to radiocontrast was also reported by Heyman (140) and by Palm (141), using the nonionic low-osmolar iopromide, while Liss found a dose-related response, with a decline in regional flow at low and intermediate volumes of contrast, but enhancement at high volumes (142).

Altogether, these findings indicate that radiocontrast-induced accentuation of inner medullary hypoxia is mediated to large extent by a decline in regional blood flow and oxygen supply. By contrast, intensification of outer medullary hypoxia predominantly represents enhanced oxygen consumption, not fully compensated by increased regional oxygen delivery. The cause for the disparate papillary and outer medullary microcirculatory response to radiocontrast agents is unknown, but it may reflect structural and functional differences between regional pericytes (143), or diverse distribution of vasoactive mediators or their receptors. An additional artificial effect related to the technical procedures (i.e., papillary exposure and removal of the renal capsule, respectively), cannot be excluded with certainty.

Radiocontrast-Triggered Neurohumoral Responses and Their Potential Role in CIN

Numerous mediators are involved in the changes in renal microcirculation, associated with radiocontrast injection, some inducing renal vasoconstriction (vasopressin, histamine), others exerting renal vasodilation (nitric oxide [NO], natriuretic peptides, prostaglandins [PGE$_2$, PGI$_2$]), and others producing varying responses at different renal vascular beds (endothelin, adenosine).

The role of the renal sympathetic system is yet to be defined, though radiocontrast-induced constriction of innervated renal artery is not mediated through alpha receptors (144). Vasopressin levels rise after radiocontrast injection in response to the increase in plasma osmolality, and probably due to contrast-induced hypotension (126,127). Endothelin synthesis and release from endothelial cells is triggered by high- and low-osmolar ionic and nonionic agents, both *in vitro* and *in vivo* (128). This response is dose-related, and is not mediated through hypertonicity. Plasma and urinary endothelin increases in humans following radiocontrast studies (131). In a rat model of CIN, the low-osmolar agent ioversol stimulated endothelin remarkably less than iothalamate, and was less nephrotoxic, suggesting a role for endothelin in CIN (145). The renal microcirculatory response to endothelin-1 closely resembles radiocontrast-induced changes in renal hemodynamics (112). Total renal and cortical flows decline, an effect blocked by endothelin-ET$_A$ antagonist (146), and outer medullary flow increases, an effect triggered by ET$_B$-mediated release of NO (112).

Intrarenal adenosine also rises following the administration of radiocontrast media (125,147), reflecting ensuing renal hypoxia and/or increased tubular workload, with consequent breakdown of ATP. Like endothelin, and in resemblance to renal hemodynamic response to radiocontrast agents, released adenosine exerts dual effects on the renal vasculature, with A1-mediated cortical vasoconstriction and A2-dependent outer medullary vasodilation (111), with an overall decline in total renal blood flow and GFR (111,148). The administration of nonselective- or selective adenosine A1-receptor blockers did not attenuate the contrast-associated decline in renal blood flow and GFR in healthy rats (149), suggesting that under normal physiologic conditions renal hypoxia leads to adenosine release, rather than the other way around. By contrast, severe renal hypoxia induced by chronic inhibition of NO synthase increases renal vascular sensitivity to the radiocontrast-induced adenosine release, generating renal vasoconstriction and reduced GFR, both ameliorated with adenosine receptor antagonists (149). In the same fashion, theophylline blocks the decline in renal blood flow in volume-depleted anesthetized dogs (148). Adenosine breakdown generates oxygen free radicals that may lead to cytotoxic epithelial and endothelial injury (see below). Iodinated contrast agents also trigger the release of histamine that may also participate in the decline in renal blood flow (150).

Contrast media also alter renal vasodilatory mechanisms. Plasma levels of atrial natriuretic peptide (ANP) rapidly rise after the injection of the contrast material, in parallel with the abrupt transient rise in renal blood flow and diuresis (128). Intrarenal NO concentration is modified as well (140). Cortical NO declines, in parallel with the gradual fall in cortical blood flow. Cortical NO-synthase activity also tends to fall, and markedly declines in response to nonselective endothelin-receptor blockade, illustrating the cross-talk between these mediators. By contrast, medullary NO-synthase activity is unaffected by the contrast medium, though NO tracings with a selective electrode markedly increase, in parallel with the rise in regional flow (140). This might be explained by the evolving decline in regional PO$_2$ and extended local bioavailability of NO (151). Iodinated radiocontrast agents also affect vasoactive cyclooxygenase metabolites. Urinary PGE$_2$ increases sevenfold in the rat (146), indicating substantial upregulation of this important medullary vasodilator in response to ensuing hypoxia. The effect of radiocontrast agents on prostacyclin (PGI$_2$) production by endothelial cells is debated, with one report showing declining levels of 6-keto-PGF1-alpha in renal veins in dogs (134), and another study demonstrating rising plasma levels in humans with ionic as well as nonionic agents (152).

Intact nitrovasodilation and prostaglandin synthesis are essential for the maintenance of adequate medullary oxygenation during contrast administration. As shown in Figure 45-8, the outer medullary vasodilatory response to radiocontrast is blocked by the inhibition of each of these systems, and is replaced by intense vasoconstriction. This leads to a critical reduction in ambient PO$_2$ to levels as low as 8 mm Hg (115,139) and increases medullary hypoxia-induced factor (HIF) expression (117).

Mechanical Factors

Blood viscosity may be substantially influenced by contrast media (153,154) and may contribute to the reduction in papillary blood flow, noted by Liss (138). This may be related to the intrinsic physical properties of the dye (Table 45-1), or

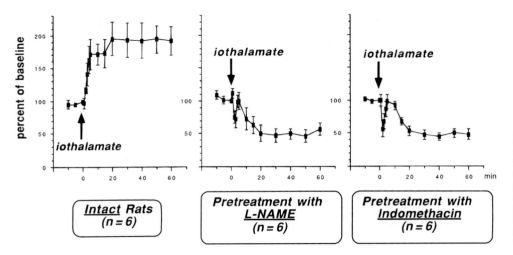

FIGURE 45-8. Reversal of outer medullary hyperemic response to radiocontrast administration after inhibition of nitric oxide or prostaglandin synthesis. (From: Agmon Y, et al. Nitric oxide and prostanoids protect the renal outer medulla from radiocontrast toxicity in the rat. *J Clin Invest* 1994;94: 1069, with permission.)

due to erythrocyte rigidity, endothelial injury or microthrombi (121,155,156). Additionally, the early radiocontrast-induced enhanced diuresis is associated with swelling of the renal parenchyma, presumably due to tubular luminal expansion and increased interstitial volume (157). It is conceivable that this could increase renal interstitial pressure with subsequent compression of the vasa recta and peritubular capillaries, compromising regional oxygenation. Tubular intraluminal urine viscosity also increases following radiocontrast administration, particularly at the distal nephron, as the result of water reabsorption with increasing concentration of the contrast medium (158). Rising urine viscosity, noted with high- and low-osmolar agents is markedly more pronounced with the new isoosmolar agents (154), reflecting their physical properties (Table 45-1). This could contribute to the increased intraluminal hydraulic pressure that might directly diminish GFR. Radiocontrast agents may also induce intratubular obstruction by precipitation of uric acid (76,91) or oxalate crystals, or co-precipitate with Tamm-Horsfall protein, synthesized and released by medullary thick ascending limbs following radiocontrast exposure (159). Radiocontrast agents may also bind with Bence-Jones protein in patients with multiple myeloma (160,161).

Toxic-Hypoxic Interactions and Endothelial Dysfunction

Increased urine viscosity and cast formation by cell debris and precipitation of contrast medium with urinary proteins could lead to prolonged exposure of tubular cells to the dye, as evidently happens during the persistent nephrogram phenomenon (20,62), increasing the risk for a direct cytotoxic effects on tubular cells. Indeed, *in vitro* studies show independent direct tubular damage caused by radiocontrast agents (162), with tubular membranal oxidative injury (163,164). *In vivo* studies also confirm the existence of oxygen free radical-mediated membranal damage (159,164–166), though this could indirectly result from reperfusion of critically hypoxic regions. Reactive oxygen species may cause DNA damage, activating high-energy consuming reparative processes such as the DNA mending poly-(ADP-ribose) polymerase (PARP). The induction of PARP may, in turn, initiate a vicious circle of additional intracellular energy store depletion and tubular damage (167,168).

Most importantly, endothelial cells may also be injured by the evolving hypoxic stress. Indeed, accumulation of HIF-2α

can be detected in medullary endothelial capillaries following exposure to contrast media (117). Subsequent endothelial damage, induced by reactive oxygen species (149,169) and energy consuming reparative mechanisms, such as PARP, may lead to endothelial dysfunction, which may further aggravate regional oxygen insufficiency (164,170). Finally, contrast studies are often carried out in critically ill patients, treated with other nephrotoxins or displaying co-morbid states such as sepsis or myohemoglobinuria that may exert additional tubulotoxic and hypoxic insults.

Thus, synergism exists between hypoxic, hemodynamic, toxic, and obstructive components of CIN. Renal dysfunction with minimal or absent tubular damage, noted in some of the animal models detailed below, implies that reversible cell injury has been restored, or that renal microvascular response predominates. Altered glomerular hemodynamics, mediated by tubuloglomerular feedback, helps in restoring medullary oxygenation by decreasing reabsorbtive workload (108). Yet, it is manifested as diminished GFR with a low fractional sodium excretion.

Risk Factors for CIN: Predisposition to Medullary Oxygen Insufficiency

As detailed above, CIN seldom develops among patients without risk factors. This highlights the value of protective mechanisms, designed to maintain medullary oxygen sufficiency, including vasodilating prostaglandins, NO, and adenosine. By adjustment of local transport activity to the limited available oxygen supply, these mechanisms enhance outer medullary blood flow and suppress tubular reabsorptive activity. Their inactivation in rats reverses the increase in outer medullary blood flow induced by radiocontrast, and aggravates regional hypoxia (115,139).

Dysregulation of medullary oxygen balance is also encountered in most clinical circumstances considered to predispose to CIN (105). As shown in Table 45-4, most risk factors for contrast nephropathy are characterized by structural or functional changes that can aggravate hypoxic stress during contrast administration. Diabetes, hypertension, aging, atherosclerosis, and hyperlipidemia are all characterized by defective nitrovasodilation, while defective prostaglandin synthesis is encountered in aging and in patients receiving nonsteroidal antiinflammatory agents. Indeed, intensified medullary hypoxia has been encountered is some of these conditions (114,171–173), associated with regional HIF expression (173,174),

TABLE 45-4

RISK FACTORS FOR CIN PREDISPOSE TO MEDULLARY OXYGEN INSUFFICIENCY

Defective protective mechanisms Altered nitrovasodilation 　　Diabetes, hypertension, aging, hyperlipidemia, 　　　atherosclerosis Altered renal prostaglandin synthesis 　　Aging, NSAIDs **Enhanced systemic vasoconstrictive stimuli** 　Volume depletion, heart failure, cirrhosis, nephrosis **Increased reabsorptive workload** 　Diabetes, chronic renal disease **Structural changes of the renal microvasculature** 　Chronic renal disease **Blood hyperviscosity** 　Myeloma

TABLE 45-5

ANIMAL MODELS OF CIN: INDUCTION OF PREDISPOSING FACTORS

Altered endothelial nitrovasodilation Congestive heart failure (182) Diabetes (256) Hypertension (184) Hypercholesterolemia (74) Transient global renal ischemia (189,191) Inhibition of nitric oxide synthase (115,139,149,186,227) **Altered prostaglandin synthesis** Aged animals (184) Inhibition of cyclooxygenase (103,115,139,181) **Increased single nephron GFR** Preexisting renal disease: prior reduction of renal mass 　(103,185) Acute-on-chronic renal failure (192) Amino-acid infusion (185) Diabetes (256) Aged animals (184) **Vasoconstrictive stimuli** Congestive heart failure (182) Salt depletion (103,148,181) AII infusion (183) Endothelin infusion (184) **Increased interstitial pressure** Urinary outflow obstruction (186)

and a defective medullary vasodilatory response (169,175). Consequently, the increase in outer medullary blood flow in response to radiocontrast is lost and even reversed, as shown by Palm in diabetic rats (141). Arginine depletion in these clinical conditions may also contribute to endothelial dysfunction (74). As reviewed elsewhere (107,108), enhanced systemic vasoconstrictive stimuli accompany effective arterial volume depletion, for instance in patients with heart failure, cirrhosis, hypovolemic shock, dehydration, or hypoalbuminemia. Preexisting renal parenchymal disease is characterized by deformed medullary microcirculation, the result of structural parenchymal changes, and local oxygen insufficiency may be intensified by increased reabsorbtive workload in hypertrophic remnant nephrons. Enhanced tubular reabsorption and oxygen consumption may accompany early or uncontrolled diabetes, associated with increased GFR, osmotic diuresis, or upregulation of tubular transport (171). Myeloma proteins may increase blood viscosity and alter the medullary microcirculation. Exposure to additional nephrotoxins may intensify medullary hypoxia by the induction of renal vasoconstriction (cyclosporine), by the increase in metabolic workload (mannitol) or by their combination (amphotericin, hypercalcemia). Finally, rhabdomyolysis, urine outflow obstruction, and sepsis are among other renal perturbations characterized by altered renal microcirculation and predisposition to medullary hypoxic damage (107,108).

Experimental Models of CIN: The Concept of Combined Insults

In isolated rat kidneys, contrast agents hasten the decline in kidney function and extend hypoxic tubular damage, which selectively involves mTALs and S3 segments in the outer medulla (103). *In vivo*, resembling humans, normal animals subjected to contrast media do not develop CIN (176), so much so that the intrinsic nephrotoxicity of radiocontrast agents has even been questioned (177). They either retain kidney function, or die when administered extremely large volumes of the dye. As in humans, proximal tubular vacuolization is a hallmark of radiocontrast exposure, rather than an indicator of CIN (103,178). In intact rats, the radiocontrast-associated decline in medullary PO_2 invokes adaptive cellular hypoxic stress response, initiated by post-transcriptional medullary accumulation of HIF, with preservation of renal integrity and function (117). By contrast, the induction of other insults that

mimic predisposing clinical conditions is a prerequisite for the development of CIN with tubular damage (106,179,180). As illustrated in Table 45-5, some perturbations were applied to generate vasoconstrictive stimuli, like volume depletion in rats and rabbits (163,181), heart failure in dogs (182), or the infusion of angiotensin II (183) or endothelin (184) in rats. Others were added to enhance oxygen requirements, by hypertrophy of single remnant kidney (103,185) or increased glomerular filtration (185). In additional models, renal medullary protective mechanisms were altered, such as the direct inhibition of prostaglandin- (103,115,139,181) or NO-synthesis (115,139,149,186). In others, endothelial dysfunction was reproduced by the induction of hypercholesterolemia (74) or with short- (187–190) or long-term ischemia (191). Ureteral obstruction served to enhance interstitial hydraulic pressure (186), while residual chronic damage produced by ischemia-reflow served to mimic preexisting tubulointerstitial disease (192). Unlike the consistently high reproducibility of other models of toxic nephropathies, most of these experimental models produce a rather heterogenous response with a wide spectrum of renal dysfunction and tubular injury, in reminiscence with the inconsistent occurence and pattern of CIN in humans.

We found the models of radiocontrast administration following the combined inactivation of prostaglandin- and NO-production (139) most convenient and clinically relevant, with respect to the characteristics of most risk factors, displaying altered renal microvascular regulation. In these rat models, renal sodium gradient, an indicator of an intact countercurrent exchange system and urinary concentrating capacity, is disrupted shortly after the administration of the radiocontrast medium (193), representing medullary functional failure, and subsequently diminished glomerular filtration (103,115,139). The severity of renal dysfunction is proportional to the number of the applied coperturbations (Figure 45-9A), resembling observations in humans (36). Renal dysfunction correlates with

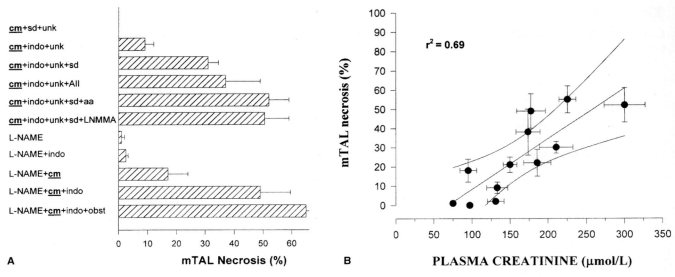

FIGURE 45-9. Rat models of CIN. **A:** the extent of medullary thick ascending limb (mTAL)-necrosis, induced by radiocontrast medium (CM), in animals preconditioned by prior uninephrectomy (UNK) salt depletion (SD), angiotensin II infusion (AII), amino acid infusion (AA), indomethacin (INDO), inhibition of NO synthase with NG-monomethyl-L arginine (L-NMMA) or NG-nitro-L-arginine methyl ester (L-NAME), and ureteral obstruction (Obst). **B:** Functional-morphologic correlations in these models. (Modified with permission from: Heyman SN, Reichman J, Brezis M. The pathophysiology of contrast nephropathy: a role for medullary hypoxia. *Invest Radiol* 1999;34:685.)

structural damage in the more severe protocols (Fig. 45-9B), but less so with the more moderate models of "partial" protocols, that cause limited tubular damage, underscoring a potential role for ensuing altered renal hemodynamics as the cause for the decline in kidney function (180).

Careful assessment of perfusion-fixed kidneys in our rat models reveals that morphologic tubular damage rapidly develops in the outer medulla as early as 15 minutes after the administration of the radiocontrast (114), predominantly affecting medullary thick ascending limbs and to a lesser extent S3 segments in the outer stripe of the outer medulla and in medullary rays. (103,114,115,139). These morphologic findings range from reversible injury (mitochondrial swelling with maintained cellular integrity) to a more severe damage pattern (nuclear pyknosis and disruption of cell membranes). A gradient of damage is noted, maximal among mTALs at the mid-interbundle zone, most remote from vasa recta. By 24 hours tubular necrosis is maximal, affecting about 50% of mTALs in the most severe models, occasionally associated with injured collecting ducts. Damaged inner medullary structures with necrosis of the papillary tip may develop as well (186). Apoptotic cell death is also noted with a pattern of distribution comparable to that of tubular necrosis (194). An additional morphologic hallmark of radiocontrast administration is outer medullary vascular congestion that appears as early as 15 minutes after the administration of contrast (114), representing altered microcirculation due to hypoxic endothelial dysfunction. Indeed, two-photon microscopy reveals renal endothelial injury with vascular leak, white blood cell adhesion, and rouleaux formation of red blood cells (195).

Conclusions

In summary, as schematically shown in Figure 45-6, the osmotic and volume loads of radiocontrast agents induce a host of systemic and renal physiologic responses that include diuresis and hemodynamic alterations, associated with profound medullary hypoxia (105,179,180). Numerous neurohumoral and physical mechanisms are involved in these reactions. In healthy subjects they are balanced by protective regulatory systems, structured to maintain renal parenchymal oxygenation, function, and integrity. These protective regulatory systems are characteristically altered in clinical risk factors that predispose to CIN. Consequently, renal parenchymal injury develops during contrast administration, the outcome of synergic hypoxic and toxic insults to tubular epithelial cells and to the renal microcirculation. In adequate models of CIN (106) animals are subjected to perturbations designed to mimic clinical risk factors. These models may improve our understanding of the pathophysiology of CIN, and enable the exploration of potential preventive strategies.

PREVENTION OF CIN

In generally healthy individuals, without risk factors, the threat of CIN is very low, probably less than 1%, and the possibility of severe and protracted renal dysfunction requiring renal replacement therapy is negligible (18,26,36,75). Among high-risk patients, a few strategies were found to be effective in reducing the incidence of CIN, including selection of patients, the choice of low- or isoosmolar radiocontrast materials rather than high osmolar agents, given at the lowest required dose, and proper hydration protocols (Table 45-6). Since the incidence of CIN remains substantial in high-risk individuals despite these precautions, a variety of additional measures, including vasodilators, antioxidants, and attenuators of tubular metabolism, are continually tested in animal models as well as in clinical trials, so far without unequivocal clinical success.

Selection of Patients

The first and most important step in the prevention of CIN is to identify those patients at risk and to consider the use

TABLE 45-6

CIN: PREVENTIVE STRATEGIES

Patients' selection
 Identification of patients at risk
 Consideration of alternative imaging procedures without
  radiocontrast
 Risk benefit assessment[a]

Avoidance of concomitant nephrotoxins
 NSAIDs in particular

Prophylactic hydration[a]
 Saline
 Bicarbonate

Type of Radiocontrast medium[a]
 The use of low- or nonionic agents rather than
  high-osmolar contrast material

Radiocontrast dosage/removal[a]
 The use of the smallest doses required
 Dose adjustment to renal function
 Prophylactic hemodialysis (failed)
 Prophylactic hemofiltration

Additional experimental approaches[a]
 Vasodilators
  Adenosine receptor antagonists
  Dopamine/fenoldopam
  Atrial natriuretic peptide
  Endothelin receptor antagonists (nonselective, selective
   ETA)
  Calcium-channel blockers
  Acetylcysteine
  L-Arginine
  Prostaglandins
  Angiotensin-converting enzyme inhibitors
 Attenuation of metabolic requirements
  Loop diuretics
  PARPP inhibition
  Hypothermia
  Prostaglandins
 Attenuation of free radical formation/attack
  Allopurinol
  Acetylcysteine
  Alkaluria: bicarbonate, acetazolamide
 Cellular adaptation to hypoxic/toxic stress
  Induction of heme-oxygenase
 Others
  Mannitol

[a]Strategies applied in high-risk patients/animal models of CIN.
All strategies classified as "additional experimental approaches" have
failed in human trials, exert debatable effects, or are under clinical or
laboratory investigation.

of alternative imaging technologies, such as sonography, nuclear imaging procedures, magnetic resonance imaging (MRI), or positron emission tomography (PET). The availability of these techniques, and their appropriateness in respect to convenience, costs, and their sensitivity and specificity should be taken into account and weighed against the risk of iodinated radiocontrast study. Obtaining medical history and physical examination is therefore a mandatory requirement before such procedures, in order to identify patients at risk, to correct reversible risk factors, to initiate effective protective measures and to consider alternative imaging approaches (196). Concurrent administration of drugs with potential nephrotoxicity

should be avoided, if possible. The concomitant use of overlooked over-the-counter nonsteroidal antiinflammatory agents is of particular concern, as are other medications that adversely affect renal parenchymal oxygenation, such as cyclosporine or amphothericin. For the above reasons, hospitalization prior to ambulatory imaging procedures is highly recommended for very high-risk patients. Monitoring of renal function over 48 to 72 hours following the imaging procedure should be scheduled as well.

Reports of lactic acidosis following contrast administration in diabetic patients taking metformin have raised concern about performing radiocontrast studies in patients on this drug (197,198). However, there is little evidence that this complication develops in patients taking metformin who have normal renal function before receiving contrast. It is more likely that the diabetic patient with prior renal insufficiency and superimposed radiocontrast nephropathy experiences delayed excretion of the drug that predisposes to the development of lactic acidosis. Rasuli (199) recommend that metformin be held for 48 hours after radiocontrast administration to determine whether renal function has been impaired. If renal function remains stable, the prior dose of metformin may be resumed. There is no pharmacologic reason to withhold metformin for 48 hours prior to the study in these patients, as is sometimes suggested.

Hydration Protocols

The administration of intravenous fluids has long been the standard treatment in the prevention of CIN in high-risk patients. This approach, based on retrospective and uncontrolled observations during the eighties (23,200) became widely accepted, though randomized controlled trials comparing hydration protocols with no fluids have never been performed. The rationale for fluid administration is to attenuate preexisting vasoconstrictive stimuli in patients with effective volume depletion and to compensate for fluid loss induced by the osmotic diuresis. In addition, fluid administration may decrease the tubular intraluminal concentration of the radiocontrast and hasten its clearance, reducing urine viscosity and minimizing the potential for direct tubular toxicity.

A routine protocol in hospitalized adult patients was for years the intravenous administration of 0.45% saline, applied at the rate of 1 mL/kg/hour for 24 hours and initiated 6 to 12 hours before the radiocontrast study (12). This simple routine is well tolerated even among patients with congestive heart failure (9), though minor adjustments may be needed to address the patient's clinical status.

For outpatient procedures this protocol was substituted with short oral hydration before the procedure, followed by intravenous 0.45% saline for 6 hours. This regimen was as successful as the inpatient intravenous hydration for the prevention of CIN following angiography in patients with mild-to-moderate renal failure (201). The choice of 0.45% saline has recently been challenged by a large study, in which 1,620 unselected patients, undergoing elective or emergency cardiac catheterization were randomized to hydration protocols using 0.45% versus 0.90% saline (18). The incidence of CIN was 2% and 0.7%, respectively, for the entire cohort ($p = 0.04$), indicating that normal saline may be better. However, most of the enrolled patients were at low risk for CIN. Subgroup analysis disclosed that in a subset of 286 patients with preexisting renal failure, the corresponding incidence of CIN was 4% and 2%, respectively (NS), but diabetic patients and those administered with large amounts of the contrast medium had a statistically significant favorable outcome with the 0.9% saline preparation (0% vs. 5.5%, and 0% vs. 3%, respectively). For obscure reason, women also had better results with the

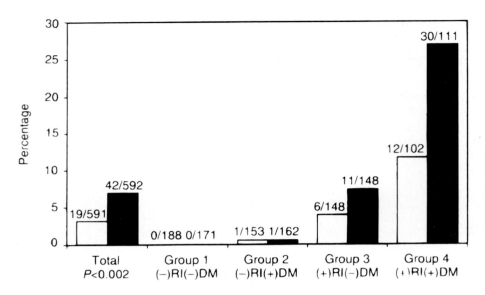

FIGURE 45-10. Percentage of patients able to be evaluated who developed nephrotoxicity for each treatment and stratification group following cardiac angiography. *DM,* diabetes mellitus; □, iohexol; ■, meglumine/sodium diatrizoate; RI, renal insufficiency. (From: Rudnick MR, et al. Nephrotoxicity of ionic and nonionic contrast media in 1,196 patients: a randomized trial. *Kidney Int* 1995;47:254, with permission.)

0.9% solution (0.6% vs. 5.1%). In another recent clinical trial, 119 patients with preexisting renal failure were randomized to a saline infusion protocol or equivalent load of bicarbonate solution (31). The rationale here was that alkaluria attenuates the generation of oxygen free radicals and may reduce subsequent tubular toxicity. CIN developed in 14% of patients on the saline hydration protocol, as compared with 2% only in the bicarbonate group. This finding was conceptually supported by a recent report that acetazolamide attenuates tubular damage and renal dysfunction in rats subjected to CIN (195). Bicarbonate infusion, however, may require a closer clinical monitoring to prevent clinically significant metabolic alkalosis. In conclusion, though additional large studies are required to confirm the above findings and to establish the superiority of isotonic saline over half-normal saline in patients with preexisting renal disease, it is reasonable to advocate the use of isotonic saline in high-risk patients, and to consider the alternative use of isoequivalent bicarbonate solution.

The Choice of Radiocontrast

The development of low-osmolar agents was aimed chiefly to reduce the incidence of adverse effects, including CIN. Indeed, as outlined above, these agents produce more moderate systemic hemodynamic effects, are given at smaller volumes (dimeric agents), produce smaller osmotic and sodium ionic loads, have a less disruptive effect on the vascular endothelium and, in the case of ioversol, do not stimulate endothelin release (145). Nevertheless, whether the use of low-osmolar contrast media causes a clinically important reduction in nephrotoxicity remained controversial for a long time, since their introduction in the late 1980s. Several well-designed studies were unable to demonstrate a lower incidence of nephrotoxicity when compared to high-osmolality contrast media (16,32,35,51,86). Others found a significant advantage of low-osmolality contrast medium over a conventional high-osmolality agent (30,202). Because the relatively small number of high-risk patients in the studies showing no benefit may have obscured a positive effect, a type II error, the Iohexol Cooperative Study enrolled 1,196 patients to compare the low-osmolar iohexol with the high osmolar agent meglumine/sodium diatrizoate in healthy and high-risk patients (26). This prospective, multicentered trial showed that individuals

with normal renal function, in the presence or absence of diabetes, had a very low risk of renal injury with either contrast agent (Fig. 45-10). However, patients with renal insufficiency who received diatrizoate were 3.3 times more likely to develop renal failure than those receiving iohexol. A metaanalysis of 45 controlled trials comparing high- and low-osmolality contrast media was consistent with this multicentered trial, showing that low-osmolality media is associated with reduced nephrotoxicity (203). Thus, for patients with normal renal function, there was no statistical benefit from the use of low-osmolality agents. By contrast, in patients with preexisting renal failure, the risk of developing ARF was reduced by 50%. Irrespective to these issues, the extensive use of cheap high-osmolar radiocontrast agents have been replaced to a large extent by the less toxic low-osmolar agents over the last decade, in parallel with the declining costs of the newer agents. Evidently, economic considerations in the long-lasting debate regarding the use of low-osmolar contrast media in all radiographic studies, or selectively for high-risk patients (26,204), are no longer valid.

A further reduction of the incidence of CIN in high-risk patients has been anticipated with the recent introduction of isoosmolar contrast media. Aspelin et al. (17) randomized 129 patients with chronic renal failure (mean plasma creatinine 1.5 mg/dL), undergoing cardiac catheterization, to the isoosmolar agent iodixanol or to the low-ionic material iohexol. The incidence of CIN (peak increase in serum creatinine >0.5 mg/dL) was significantly lower with the isoosmolar agent—2% versus 17%, respectively. Comparable results were also shown in a previous study by Chalmers and Jackson, who found that the incidence of CIN was 50% less in patients with chronic renal impairment given iodixanol, as compared to iohecol (29). However, in subsequent studies the incidence of CIN following iodixanol in comparable high-risk patients ranged from 12% to 33%. Indeed, in recent review and a meta-analysis, iso- and low-osmolar agents were found to be comparable regarding the risk for CIN (42,43). Possibly, the advantage of reducing radiocontrast volume and osmolar loads with the new isoosmolar agents is offset by the adverse effects of increased viscosity (154), as reflected by a comparable decline in medullary PO_2 (116). In conclusion, for high-risk patients, particularly those with renal dysfunction and diabetes, the use of low- or isoosmolar radiocontrast media is justified to minimize the risk of clinically significant CIN. By contrast, in patients with normal renal function the risk of CIN is extremely low and equal for low-osmolar and high-osmolar agents. The new isoosmolar contrast materials are not safer than low-osmolar agents, regarding nephrotoxicity.

Radiocontrast Dose

Since the dose of the iodinated radiocontrast agent is considered a risk factor for CIN, high-risk patients should be given the smallest loads of contrast material possible. There is a dose of radiocontrast below which severe radiocontrast nephropathy is very unlikely to occur. McCullough and colleagues (75), in a cohort of more than 3,600 patients undergoing coronary contrast intervention studies, reported that acute renal failure requiring dialysis does not occur in any patient who receives 100 mL of contrast or less. Cigarroa suggests adjusting the maximal permitted radiocontrast volume to the degree of renal dysfunction (21). Controlled dosing of the contrast medium using the following formula resulted in a 90% decline in the incidence of CIN.

$$\text{contrast medium dose (mL)} = \frac{5 \text{ mL} \times \text{body weight (kg)}}{\text{serum creatinine (mg/dL)}}$$

Radiocontrast Removal

The load of contrast material per functioning nephron inversely correlates with their numbers. Since iodinated contrast agents are effectively removed by hemodialysis (205), this procedure was expected to alleviate the risk of CIN when performed immediately after contrast studies in patients with advanced renal failure, given large volumes of the radiocontrast material. However, when hemodialysis was initiated in 30 patients with advanced renal failure one hour after the contrast study, the incidence of CIN was not reduced: 53% inpatients on hemodialysis vs. 40% in patients treated conservatively (206). In another larger cohort of 113 patients with advanced renal failure (creatinine above 3 mg/dL), prophylactic hemodialysis, started immediately after the contrast injection, also did not reduce the incidence of CIN. Moreover, subsequent dialysis was more than doubled among patients assigned to prophylactic hemodialysis, as compared with the control group (41). By contrast, Marenzi has recently reported favorable outcome with prophylactic venovenous hemofiltration among 114 patients with comparably advanced renal failure, undergoing coronary interventions with high volume (250 mL) of contrast (87). The need for subsequent renal replacement therapy was reduced eightfold (3% as compared with 25% in controls) and in-hospital mortality rate was 2% and 14%, respectively. Of the remaining patients, only one in the treatment group ended up on permanent hemodialysis, as compared with three patients in the control group. These study groups illustrates the results of angiographic interventions using large volumes of radiocontrast medium, often in hemodynamically unstable cardiac patients. The advantage of continuous venovenous hemofiltration over hemodialysis seems to be the hemodynamic stability, avoiding hypovolemia and hypotension. In addition, it enables vigorous hydration without causing pulmonary congestion. Thus, the study by Marenzi indicates that hemofiltration is probably the procedure of choice under such circumstances. As outlined by Asif (196), the associated increased costs must be viewed in the context of short- and long-term benefits obtained, that may justify its use in very high-risk patients with advanced renal failure.

Vasodilators—A Conceptual Debate

As shown in Table 45-6, numerous types of renal vasodilators were tried for the prevention of CIN. The late and protracted decline in renal blood flow and GFR after radiocontrast administration (132) provides the rationale for these trials. Increased GFR and subsequent urine generation may also reduce the intraluminal concentration of the radiocontrast medium, shorten its transit time, and remove sediments. However, increased renal blood flow predominantly reflects augmented cortical, rather than medullary blood flow, and endothelial dysfunction is not restored. Radiocontrast-induced reduction of cortical blood flow and GFR are mediated in part by renal defense mechanisms, designed to maintain medullary oxygen sufficiency (105). Their neutralization may enhance GFR and increase distal tubular reabsorption and oxygen consumption. Thus, a conceptual debate exists regarding the usefulness of induction of renal vasodilation in CIN. Should we, or should we not improve GFR at the price of intensification of medullary hypoxic injury? In the absence of unequivocal efficacy of vasodilators or available clinical tools for the noninvasive assessment of medullary hypoxic stress and injury, this debate remains open.

Theophylline

Since adenosine has been associated with the renal hemodynamic changes induced by the contrast material, the effect of the adenosine receptor antagonist, theophylline, was explored in few clinical trials, with small numbers of patients included, many at low risk for CIN (207,208). In these studies theophylline was not protective. Abizaid compared 20 high-risk patients (creatinine $\geq$1.5 mg/dL), half of them diabetics, treated with intravenous theophylline, with patients given fluids, only, ending with similar results (209). Early studied the effect of oral theophylline in a placebo-controlled study in 80 comparably high-risk patients, and found that theophylline provided no functional benefit over hydration, though it prevented enzymuria (210).

Most other studies, however, found that theophylline reduced the risk of CIN. Katholi studied its effect in 93 hydrated patients who were also treated with calcium channel blockers and randomized to low- and high-osmolar contrast agents (211). Theophylline totally prevented or attenuated by half the decline in creatinine clearance in patients receiving low- or high-osmolar agents, respectively. Kapoor studied 70 diabetic patients with a relatively preserved renal function, undergoing coronary angiography with high-osmolar agents. CIN developed in 3% of patients treated with theophylline, as compared with 31% in the control group (212). In intensive care unit (ICU) patients on aminophylline prophylaxis Huber reported CIN in 2% of 78 patients, as compared with 14% of 565 matched control patients (213). In a randomized, double-blind placebo-controlled study in 100 patients given low-osmolar contrast medium, the same group report corresponding incidence of 4% and 16% of CIN, respectively, with a significant protective impact of theophylline shown by multiple regression analysis (214).

As with most clinical studies of CIN, comparison of the different studies is difficult in the perspective of varied patients' characteristics, radiologic procedures, type and dose of the radiocontrast agent used, dosing and mode of theophylline administration, other interventions, and the definition of CIN. Nevertheless, it seems that the decline in GFR following CIN may be attenuated by adenosine-receptor antagonists. These findings underscore the role of adenosine in the contrast-related reduction of renal blood flow (149,208), but as discussed above, blocking its effect harbors a danger of enhancement of medullary hypoxia (111). Thus, the true impact of adenosine-receptor antagonists on the prevention of clinically significant CIN is yet to be proven.

Dopamine and Fenoldopam

Low-dose dopamine is a potent renal vasodilator and enhances GFR even in patients with renal impairment. In intact animals, dopamine increases outer medullary blood flow. However, physiologic medullary hypoxia is not improved, possibly as the result of enhanced distal tubular transport (215). Clinical trials with dopamine in the prevention of CIN provide mixed results. In a randomized study of 55 patients with chronic renal dysfunction, dopamine was not beneficial, though in a subgroup of patients with advanced renal failure (baseline creatinine ≥2 mg/dL) creatinine clearance was maintained, while in control patients it significantly declined (216). Weiseberg (10) randomized 50 patients with chronic renal failure, half of them with diabetes, to hydration alone, or together with dopamine, ANP, or mannitol. In nondiabetic individuals dopamine slightly reduced the plasma creatinine following the contrast study. By contrast, in diabetic patients, while renal blood flow was significantly improved, plasma creatinine paradoxically rose (10). Similar findings were noted with ANP and mannitol (see below), suggesting that in diabetic patients with endothelial dysfunction, improving cortical blood flow and GFR may adversely affect medullary oxygenation and intensify regional hypoxic damage (105).

Fenoldopam is a recently developed selective DA-1 agonist, devoid of DA-2 or adrenergic effects. It induces renal vasodilation and increases GFR, diuresis and natriuresis. In anesthetized dogs fenoldopam prevented the decline in renal blood flow, induced by radiocontrast (217). In a prospective study Kini compared 110 high-risk patients with baseline creatinine ≥1.5 mg/dL, undergoing coronary interventions, with historic controls. The incidence of CIN was 4.5% versus 19%, respectively (218). A small randomized multicenter study of 45 patients ended with comparable results (219). However, in a large, double-blind, placebo-controlled, randomized multicenter study, involving 315 high-risk patients (creatinine clearance ≤60 mL/min, half of them diabetics), the incidence of CIN among fenoldopam-treated patients was 34% as compared with 30% in the control group (40). Doses of fenoldopam higher than those studied so far seem impractical due to the risk of hypotension. Thus, currently both dopamine and fenoldopam are not recommended for the prevention of CIN in high-risk patients.

Natriuretic Peptides

Weisberg studied the effect of atrial natriuretic peptide (ANP) administered during contrast studies in patients with chronic renal failure, in addition to hydration (10). In nondiabetic patients ANP induces some decline in plasma creatinine. In diabetic individuals, however, as with dopamine and mannitol, ANP enhanced renal blood flow but paradoxically reduced kidney function, with plasma creatinine increasing twice as high as in the hydration-only group. Possibly, enhancing renal blood flow and GFR during contrast administration in patients with altered medullary microcirculation may intensify regional hypoxia and exacerbate medullary hypoxic damage. Comparable findings were noted in a more recent large-scale study, enrolling 247 patients with chronic renal failure undergoing contrast studies, half of them diabetics (220). Aneritide in addition to hydration did not prevent CIN in nondiabetic patients (8% vs.

9% in the saline-only group). Once again, in diabetic patients the incidence of CIN tended to be higher in the ANP group (39% vs. 26%, NS). Thus, ANP analogs are ineffective in the prevention of CIN in nondiabetic high-risk patients, and may be harmful in diabetic individuals.

Endothelin-Receptor Antagonists

Since radiocontrast media exert endothelin release that participates in contrast-related alterations in the renal microvasculature, the potential use of endothelin antagonists in the prevention of CIN was explored. In a recent placebo-controlled study, 158 hydrated patients with renal failure (mean serum creatinine 2.7 mg/dL) undergoing cardiac catheterization were randomized to receive the nonselective ET_A/ET_B receptor antagonist bosentan (39). The mean increase in serum creatinine 48 hours after the angiographic study was significantly higher in the treatment group (0.7 vs. 0.4 mg/dL in the placebo group) and the incidence of CIN was higher (56% vs. 29%, respectively). Endothelin ET-1 exerts cortical vasoconstriction by binding to endothelin ET_A receptors, while it induces medullary nitrovasodilation, mediated by ET_B receptors (112), with both actions conceivably leading to the amelioration of medullary hypoxemia. Nonselective inhibition of endothelin receptors is, therefore, likely to intensify medullary hypoxemia and to enhance CIN. Future research may therefore be directed to the evaluation of selective endothelin ET_A antagonists and their possible potential to prevent CIN.

Other Vasodilators

The prophylactic use of calcium channel blockers has been studied in few small studies (221–223), predominantly in patients without renal failure. Nifedipine acutely increased renal plasma flow when given before the radiocontrast, as compared with a decline or no change, noted in control patients given the high- and low-osmolar agents, respectively (222). Nevertheless, with the exception of one study (221) this treatment was found to be ineffective, and has not been explored further.

The protective potential of the vasodilating prostaglandin PGE_1 seems more promising. In a randomized, double-blind, placebo-controlled study, 130 patients with renal dysfunction (serum creatinine ≥1.5 mg/dL) were randomized to hydration alone or with the addition of PGE_1 infusion at 3 different doses. The mean increase in serum creatinine in the placebo group 48 hours following the radiographic study was 0.72 mg/dL, significantly higher than the 0.12 to 0.30 mg/dL increment in the three treatment groups (224). Comparable findings were achieved in a repeated experiment (225), establishing a potential protective effect of PGE_1 at a rate of 20 ng/kg/minute, administered 30 to 60 minutes prior the contrast study. This approach is compelling, in the perspective of the central role of prostaglandins in the maintenance of medullary oxygenation. This strategy may be particularly important in the aged population, characterized by reduced renal prostaglandin synthesis.

So far, a single randomized study was published in India, looking at the prophylactic use of angiotensin-converting enzyme inhibitors during contrast studies (226). Among 71 diabetic patients, the incidence of CIN was 29% in the control group, as compared with 6% in patients receiving captopril. The better outcome with captopril might reflect antioxidant properties of the sulfhydryl-containing compound, rather than, or in addition to, the class effect. Unfortunately, the wide use of these agents in the high-risk population precludes the conduction of comparable wide-scaled placebo-controlled studies. This report, however, possibly illustrates the safe use of angiotensin-converting enzyme inhibitors during contrast studies, and suggests a possible role for the renin-angiotensin system in the pathogenesis of CIN.

Finally, the NO precursor arginine may restore endothelial dysfunction and improve outer medullary vasodilatory response to contrast media. This is indirectly implicated from an experimental model of CIN in hypercholesterolemic rats, where L-arginine, but not D-arginine, prevented the contrast-mediated decline in renal blood flow and GFR (74). L-arginine also improved renal blood flow and GFR in salt-depleted rats given radiocontrast (227). However, it was ineffective in a small randomized clinical trial in patients undergoing coronary angiography, and may have caused a trend for larger deterioration in renal function. However, data presented is not stratified for patients with or without a propensity for renal endothelial dysfunction (228).

Loop Diuretics

While renal vasodilators may increase medullary tubular reabsorption and deepen medullary hypoxia, potentially intensifying CIN, inhibition of tubular transport seems a reasonable intervention in the attenuation of medullary hypoxemia and in the prevention of this disorder. Indeed, furosemide reverses the decline in medullary oxygenation caused by radiocontrast (114), even though it decreases regional blood flow (229). When given prior to the radiocontrast agent, furosemide does not prevent the decline in medullary PO_2, but since the starting point is higher, critical medullary hypoxia is prevented (230). In a rat model of CIN, furosemide averts the development of tubular necrosis in the outer medulla, though function is only partially restored, conceivably due to effective volume depletion (231). In young human subjects medullary hypoxia is improved with furosemide, as shown by BOLD MRI (109).

Solomon et al. (9) prospectively assigned 78 patients with chronic renal insufficiency undergoing cardiac catheterization, half of them with diabetes, to prior treatment with saline, saline plus mannitol, or saline plus furosemide. Eleven percent of patients treated with saline, 28% treated with mannitol, and 40% treated with furosemide developed ARF (i.e., 0.5 mg/dL rise in serum creatinine within 48 hours). Urine output and sodium excretion were unexpectedly similar in all three groups 24 hours postangiography, making volume depletion an unlikely explanation for the results. The worst outcome of patients receiving furosemide was consistent with an earlier report also showing that furosemide enhances radiocontrast-induced ARF (232). However, in the later study, substantial weight reduction in the furosemide group, as opposed to weight gain in the hydration-only group indicates that the decline in kidney function could result from volume depletion. Furosemide may also be deleterious in human CIN because of ensuing medullary vasoconstriction (151,229,233), and its failure to attenuate medullary hypoxemia in the aged (109).

Other Diuretics

Mannitol was one of the first agents used in an attempt to prevent radiocontrast-induced ARF. It reportedly decreased the incidence of ARF in a small group of patients when given within 1 hour of the radiocontrast (234,235). The precise interpretation and weight that should be given to these reports are unclear because in one report only five patients each were studied in the experimental and control groups (235). Mannitol-induced osmotic diuresis could have a beneficial effect in ARF by decreasing tubular obstruction. However, radiocontrast agents also promote a vigorous osmotic diuresis, making it unclear what additional benefit mannitol might afford in protecting

renal function. Mannitol, like dopamine and atrial natriuretic peptide, was superior to saline in preventing ARF in nondiabetics, but paradoxically, it worsened the severity of ARF in the diabetic patients when compared to saline alone (10). Other reports fail to demonstrate a protective effect from mannitol and suggest that saline expansion is the preferred agent to prevent contrast toxicity (9,25). Mannitol may be deleterious by increasing the osmotic load to the kidney and aggravating medullary hypoxia (229). In fact, mannitol itself, when given in large doses, can induce ARF (236).

The carbonic anhydrase-inhibitor acetazolamide was renoprotective in a rat model of CIN (195), perhaps by the attenuation of oxygen free radical formation through alkaluria.

Antioxidants: N-Acetylcysteine (NAC)

Evidence for renal parencymal injury by oxygen free radicals led to the evaluation of effectiveness of antioxidants in the prevention of CIN (164). In addition to a direct protection of tubular epithelial cells, this approach repairs vascular endothelial dysfunction, typical of clinical conditions that predispose to CIN (171,237), and may reduce the propensity to develop medullary hypoxic damage. NAC is a scavenger of reactive oxygen species, widely used in the prevention of acetaminophen liver toxicity. Being cheap and almost devoid of side effects, NAC became the subject of numerous clinical trials around the world since Tepel's report in 2000 (238), given orally or intravenously, before and after the radiocontrast study.

As underscored by Safirstein (239), NAC directly prevents cytotoxicity by neutralizing free radical species (162), and may replenish cellular glutathione levels. In addition, it might exert regional vasodilation through nitric oxide production, and may restore endothelial dysfunction and improve oxygen supply. Indeed, NAC was found to improve renal medullary microcirculation induced by reperfusion injury (240) and to attenuate renal vasoconstriction induced by radiocontrast media (241). Tepel randomized 83 hydrated patients with chronic renal failure, given a small intravenous dose (75 mL) of nonionic low-osmolar radiocontrast agent, to receive placebo or NAC orally, 600 mg every 12 hours, a day before, and a day after the procedure. The incidence of CIN after 48 hours was 2% in NAC-treated patients, significantly lower than 21% in the control group (238). Diaz Sandoval conducted a comparable study in 54 patients undergoing coronary angiography (38) with more than twice the volume of the contrast medium, showing a similarly striking difference in the incidence of CIN between the treatment and control groups (8% vs. 45%). In a study by Shyu (242) in patients with more advanced renal failure (serum creatinine ≥ 2.8 mg/dL) undergoing coronary intervention findings were similar (3% vs. 25%). Baker reported that high-dose intravenous NAC shortly before the contrast study was also highly effective in the prevention of CIN (5% vs. 21%) (243).

However, additional studies provide different results. Durham studied 79 patients with chronic renal failure (serum creatinine ≥ 1.7 mg/dL), undergoing cardiac studies with low mean volumes of contrast medium (85 mL). The incidence of CIN was 26% in the treatment group, as compared with 22% in the controls. Noteworthy, NAC oral administration was modified, given at two doses 1,200 mg each, 1 hour before and 3 hours after the procedure (244). However, NAC was non-protective also in other trials, such as Boccalandro's (245), that exactly followed Tepel's protocol. Briguori also conducted a randomized study in 183 consecutive patients with renal dysfunction, undergoing coronary or peripheral arterial procedures, adopting Tepel's dosing regimen of NAC (19). In this study the incidence of CIN was not statistically different (6.5% and 11% in the treatment- and control-groups, respectively). Subgroup analysis revealed that while in patients given contrast in excess of 140 mL NAC was not protective, at lower volumes of the contrast medium NAC treatment was significantly favorable (0% vs. 8%, respectively). However, logistic regression analysis showed that the amount of the radiocontrast agent and not the treatment strategy predicted the occurrence of CIN. The same Italian group conducted most recently two additional studies in large cohorts of patients with chronic renal failure, undergoing coronary or peripheral arterial procedures (246,247), and report that NAC administration at a double dose (1,200 mg twice a day) is more protective than Tepel's regimen in the prevention of CIN (3.5% vs. 11%), and more effective that fenoldopam infusion (4.3% vs. 14%, respectively). The double dose of NAC was this time protective, particularly when large volumes of the radiocontrast (>140 ml) were used (247).

In the perspective of additional studies with inconsistent results, Birck (248) and Alonso (249) performed meta-analysis of 7 and 12 well-conducted, randomized controlled reports, respectively, evaluating the outcome of over 800 patients. Both studies acknowledge the heterogeneity of patients' characteristics and of the variables related to the radiologic studies and NAC administration that were not controlled for in the meta-analysis. The potential bias of not reporting negative findings has also been addressed, as was the mixed outcome, with some reports showing clear benefit, while others concluded with no demonstrable efficacy. Birck and Alonso both reached the conclusion that NAC treatment was effective in the prevention of CIN, with an overall calculated risk reduction of 41% to 56%. A most recent meta-analysis by Kshirsagar (44), however, reaches a different conclusion, predominantly addressing the heterogeneity of the various study groups, regarding the definition of CIN, the patients' characteristics, the sort of radiologic procedure, the type and dose of radiocontrast studies, the hydration protocols used, and the dosing and timing of NAC administration. Comparing 16 well-designed studies, Kshirsagar concludes that research on NAC and the incidence of CIN is too inconsistent at present to warrant a conclusion on efficacy or a recommendation for its routine use (44). Hoffmann further questions the true value of NAC, showing that it may directly hasten creatinine excretion, irrespective to changes in GFR (250). Fishbane and colleagues (251) propose that currently the use of NAC should be recommended, in the perspective of the overall suggested benefit, the lack of effective alternatives, the safety and tolerability of the drug and its low costs. Thus, large-scale multicenter studies with strict definitions and control of variables are required, to confirm efficacy of NAC in the prevention of CIN (44). The use of intravenous NAC (243) or larger oral NAC doses, as suggested by Briguori, should be further explored (247).

Other Potential Strategies

Adenosine breakdown by xanthine oxidase elaborates free radical species, believed to exert tubular toxicity, as well as endothelial dysfunction. Bakris reported that the xanthine oxidase inhibitor allopurinol effectively prevented the fall in renal blood flow and GFR, and reduced urinary malondialdehyde, a marker of membranal injury, produced by oxygen free radicals (164). Katholi studied 39 patients with mild renal failure given ionic contrast agents (252). Allopurinol-treated patients with low plasma Mg^{2+} had somewhat milder decline in creatinine clearance as compared with control, low Mg^{2+} patients (33% vs. 79%, respectively). However, in nonhypomagnesemic patients allopurinol did not affect the decline in kidney function. PARP inhibition is another potential therapeutic approach. In a rat model of CIN, PARPP inhibition attenuated renal dysfunction, though the extent of tubular damage was unaffected (167). Activation of stress response genes is another alternative,

as shown in another rat model of CIN in rats, pretreated by the induction of heme-oxygenase (253). Other related potential options are erythropoietin or HIF stabilizers (254). Hypothermia was also found to prevent CIN in rabbits (255), supposedly through attenuation of renal oxygen consumption.

In summary, in high-risk patients attempts to reduce the incidence of CIN below 10% to 20% were futile, so far. A basic conceptual debate is whether deactivation of renal vasoconstrictive mechanisms is the appropriate mode of intervention, or is it the amelioration of medullary hypoxia. This debate calls for consideration of combined strategies that in addition to vigorous hydration will concomitantly enhance renal oxygen supply, reduce medullary oxygen consumption, and restore endothelial dysfunction.

CONCLUSIONS

Radiocontrast ARF may be a paradigm for the synergism between toxic and hypoxic insults to the kidney, illustrating the renal vulnerability to disruption of the delicate medullary oxygen balance and the pathogenic implications of endothelial dysfunction within the kidney. It develops almost exclusively in patients with risk factors, characterized by the propensity to develop medullary hypoxia. Prevention of CIN is initiated by an appropriate selection of patients and the identification of patients at risk, substitution of contrast studies with alternative imaging procedures, if possible, in high-risk individuals, and avoiding concomitant administration of other nephrotoxins. High-risk patients undergoing contrast studies should be given hydration regimen with normal saline, and receive low- or isoosmolar agents at the smallest dose possible. Hemofiltration may be used for very-high-risk patients that require large volumes of contrast medium for radiographic interventions. Regardless of all these measures, CIN develops in about 10% to 45% of high-risk patients, and remains a significant cause of iatrogenic acute renal failure. Measures to further reduce the incidence of CIN with additional preventive strategies are currently being explored.

References

1. Hou SH, et al. Hospital acquired renal insufficiency: a prospective study. *Am J Med* 1983;74:243.
2. Shusterman N, et al. Risk factors and outcome of hospital-acquired acute renal failure. Clinical epidemiologic study. *Am J Med* 1987;83:65.
3. Nash K, Hafeez A, Hou S. Hospital-acquired renal insufficiency. *Am J Kidney Dis* 2002;39:930.
4. Gomes AS, et al. Acute renal dysfunction in high-risk patients after angiography: comparison of ionic and nonionic contrast media. *Radiology* 1989;170:65.
5. Brogan WC, Hillis LD, Lange RA. Contrast agents for cardiac catheterization: conceptions and misconceptions. *Am Heart J* 1991;122:1129.
6. Golman G, Scient C. Metrizamide in experimental urography: V. Renal excretion mechanism of a nonionic contrast medium in rabbit and cat. *Invest Radiol* 1976;11:187.
7. Tornquist C, et al. Proteinuria following nephroangiography: VII. Comparison between ionic-monomeric, mono-acidic dimeric and nonionic contrast media in the dog. *Acta Radiol* 1980;362:S49.
8. Gabelmann A, Haberstroh J, Weyrich G. Ionic and non-ionic contrast agent-mediated endothelial injury. Quantitative analysis of cell proliferation during endothelial repair. *Acta Radiol* 2001;42:422.
9. Solomon R, et al. Effects of saline, mannitol, and furosemide on acute decreases in renal function induced by radiocontrast agents. *N Engl J Med* 1994;331:1416.
10. Weisberg LS, Kurnik PB, Kurnik BR. Risk of radiocontrast nephropathy in patients with and without diabetes mellitus. *Kidney Int* 1994;45:259.
11. Cramer BC, et al. Renal function following infusion of radiologic contrast material: a prospective controlled study. *Arch Intern Med* 1985;145:87.
12. Brezis M, Epstein FH. A closer look at radiocontrast nephropathy (Editorial). *N Engl J Med* 1989;320:179.
13. Cochran ST, Wong WS, Roe DJ. Predicting angiography-induced acute renal function impairment: clinical risk model. *Am J Roentgenol* 1983;14:1027.

14. Older RA, et al. Contrast-induced acute renal failure; persistent nephrogram as clue to early detection. *Am J Roentgenol* 1980;134:339.
15. Powe NR, et al. Contrast medium-induced adverse reactions: economic outcome. *Radiology* 1988;169:163.
16. Schwab SJ, et al. Contrast nephrotoxicity: a randomized controlled trial of a nonionic and an ionic radiographic contrast agent. *N Engl J Med* 1989;320:149.
17. Aspelin P, et al. Nephrotoxic effects in high-risk patients undergoing angiography. *N Engl J Med* 2003;348:491.
18. Mueller C, et al. Prevention of contrast media-associated nephropathy: randomized comparison of 2 hydration regimens in 1620 patients undergoing coronary angioplasty. *Arch Intern Med* 2002;162:329.
19. Briguori C, et al. Acetylcysteine and contrast agent-associated nephrotoxicity. *J Am Coll Cardiol* 2002;40:298.
20. Older RA, et al. Angiographically induced renal failure and its radiographic detection. *Am J Roentgenol* 1976;126:1039.
21. Cigarroa RG, et al. Dosing of contrast material to prevent contrast nephropathy in patients with renal disease. *Am J Med* 1989;86:649.
22. D'Elia JA, et al. Nephrotoxicity from angiographic contrast material. A prospective study. *Am J Med* 1982;72:719.
23. Eisenberg RL, Bank WO, Hedgcock MW. Renal failure after major angiography. *Am J Med* 1980;68:43.
24. Harkonen S, Kjellstrand CM. Exacerbation of diabetic renal failure following intravenous pyelography. *Am J Med* 1977;63:939.
25. Levitz CS, Friedman EA. Failure of protective measures to prevent contrast media-induced renal failure. *Arch Intern Med* 1982;142:642.
26. Rudnick MR, et al. Nephrotoxicity of ionic and nonionic contrast media in 1196 patients: a randomized trial. *Kidney Int* 1995;47:254.
27. Byrd L, Sherman RL. Radiocontrast-induced acute renal failure: a clinical and pathophysiologic review. *Medicine* 1979;58:279.
28. Carvallo A, et al. Acute renal failure following drip infusion pyelography. *Am J Med* 1978;65:38.
29. Chalmers N, Jackson RW. Comparison of iodixanol and iohexol in renal impairment. *Br J Radiol* 1999;72:701.
30. Harris KG, et al. Nephrotoxicity from contrast material in renal insufficiency: ionic versus nonionic agents. *Radiology* 1991;179:849.
31. Merten GJ, et al. Prevention of contrast-induced nephropathy with sodium bicarbonate. A randomized controlled trial. *JAMA* 2004;291:2328.
32. Parfrey PS, et al. Contrast material-induced renal failure in patients with diabetes mellitus, renal insufficiency, or both. *N Engl J Med* 1989;320:143.
33. Swartz RD, et al. Renal failure following major angiography. *Am J Med* 1978;65:31.
34. Moore RD, et al. Frequency and determinants of adverse reactions induced by high-osmolality contrast media. *Radiology* 1989;170:727.
35. Davidson CJ, et al. Cardiovascular and renal toxicity of a nonionic radiographic contrast agent after cardiac catheterization: a prospective trial. *Ann Intern Med* 1989;110:119.
36. Rich MW, Crecelius CA. Incidence, risk factors, and clinical course of acute renal insufficiency after cardiac catheterization in patients 70 years of age or older. *Arch Intern Med* 1990;150:1237.
37. Rudnick MR, et al. Nephrotoxic risks of renal angiography: contrast media-associated nephrotoxicity and atheroembolism—a critical review. *Am J Kidney Dis* 1994;24:713.
38. Diaz-Sandoval LJ, Kosowsky BD, Losordo DW. Acetylcysteine to prevent angiography-related renal tissue injury (the APART trial). *Am J Cardiol* 2002;89:356.
39. Wang A, et al. Exacerbation of radiocontrast nephrotoxicity by endothelin receptor antagonism. *Kidney Int* 2000;57:1675.
40. Stone CW, et al. Fenoldopam mesylate for the prevention of contrast-induced nephropathy. A randomized controlled trial. *JAMA* 2003;290:2284.
41. Vogt B, et al. Prophylactic hemodialysis after radiocontrast media in patients with renal insufficiency is potentially harmful. *Am J Med* 2001;111:692.
42. Bettmann MA. Contrast induced nephropathy: critical review of the existing clinical evidence. *Nephrol Dial Transplant* 2005;20(Suppl 1):i12.
43. Solomon RJ. Contrast-induced nephropathy (CIN): a metaanalysis of different contrast media. *J Am Soc Nephrol* 2004;15:579A.
44. Kshirsagar AV, et al. N-acetylcysteine for the prevention of radiocontrast induced nephropathy: a meta-analysis of prospective control trials. *J Am Soc Nephrol* 2004;15:761.
45. Martin-Paredero V, et al. Risk of renal failure after major angiography. *Arch Surg* 1983;118:1417.
46. VanZee BE, et al. Renal injury associated with intravenous pyelography in nondiabetic and diabetic patients. *Ann Intern Med* 1978;89:51.
47. Fang LS, et al. Low fractional excretion of sodium with contrast media-induced acute renal failure. *Arch Intern Med* 1980;140:531.
48. Teruel JL, et al. Renal function impairment caused by intravenous urography. *Arch Intern Med* 1981;141:1271.
49. Weinrauch LA, et al. Coronary angiography and acute renal failure in diabetic azotemic nephropathy. *Ann Intern Med* 1977;86:56.
50. Berns AS. Nephrotoxicity of contrast media. *Kidney Int* 1989;36:730.
51. Moore RD, et al. Nephrotoxicity of high-osmolality versus low-osmolality contrast media: randomized clinical trial. *Radiology* 1992;182:649.
52. Lautin EM, et al. Radiocontrast-associated renal dysfunction: incidence and risk factors. *Am J Roentgenol* 1991;157:49.
53. Rihal C, et al. Incidence and prognostic importance of acute renal failure after percutaneous coronary intervention. *Circulation* 2002;105:2259.
54. Ansari Z, Baldwin DS. Acute renal failure due to radiocontrast agents. *Nephron* 1976;17:28.
55. Kamdar A, et al. Acute renal failure following intravenous use of radiographic contrast dyes in patients with diabetes mellitus. *Diabetes* 1977;26:643.
56. Barshay ME, et al. Acute renal failure in diabetic patients after intravenous infusion pyelography. *Clin Nephrol* 1973;1:35.
57. Bergman LA, Ellison MR, Dunea G. Acute renal failure after drip-infusion pyelography. *N Engl J Med* 1968;279:1277.
58. Diaz-Buxo JA, et al. Acute renal failure after excretory urography in diabetic patients. *Ann Intern Med* 1975;83:155.
59. Pillay VK, et al. Acute renal failure following intravenous urography in patients with long-standing diabetes mellitus and azotemia. *Radiology* 1970;95:633.
60. Shafi T, et al. Infusion intravenous pyelography and renal function. Effects in patients with chronic renal insufficiency. *Arch Intern Med* 1978;138:1218.
61. Kini A, et al. Changing trends in the incidence and predictors of radiographic contrast nephropathy after percutaneous coronary intervention with the use of fenoldopam *Am J Cardiol* 2002;89:999.
62. Berdon WE, et al. Tamm-Horsfall proteinuria: its relationship to prolonged nephrogram in infants and children and to renal failure following intravenous urography in adults with multiple myeloma. *Radiology* 1969;92:714.
63. Gross M, McDonald H Jr, Waterhouse K. Anuria following urography with meglumine diatrizoate (Renografin) in multiple myeloma. *Radiology* 1968;90:780.
64. Myers GH Jr, Witten DM. Acute renal failure after excretory urography in multiple myeloma. *Am J Roentgenol* 1971;113:583.
65. McCarthy CS, Becker JA. Multiple myeloma and contrast media. *Radiology* 1992;183:519.
66. Lang EK, et al. The incidence of contrast medium-induced acute tubular necrosis following arteriography: a preliminary report. *Radiology* 1981;138:203.
67. Krumlovsky FA, et al. Acute renal failure: association with administration of radiographic contrast material. *JAMA* 1978;239:125.
68. Alexander RD, Berkes SL, Abuelo JG. Contrast media-induced oliguric renal failure. *Arch Intern Med* 1978;138:381.
69. Dudzinski PJ, et al. Acute renal failure following high dose excretory urography in dehydrated patients. *J Urol* 1971;106:619.
70. Nikolsky E, et al. Low hematocrit predicts contrast-induced nephropathy after percutaneous coronary interventions. *Kidney Int* 2005; 67:706.
71. Port FK, Wagoner RD, Fulton RE. Acute renal failure after angiography. *Am J Roentgenol* 1974;121:544.
72. Heidemann M, Claes G, Nilson AE. The risk of renal allograft rejection following angiography. *Transplantation* 1976;21:289.
73. Light JA, Hill GS. Acute tubular necrosis in a renal transplant recipient: complication from drip-infusion excretory urography. *JAMA* 1975;232:1267.
74. Andrade L, Campos SB, Seguro AC. Hypercholesterolemia aggravates radiocontrast nephrotoxicity: protective role of L-arginine. *Kidney Int* 1998;53:1736.
75. McCullough PA, et al. Acute renal failure after coronary intervention: incidence, risk factors, and relationship to mortality. *Am J Med* 1997;103:368.
76. Mudge GH. Uricosuric action of cholangiographic agents: a possible factor in nephrotoxicity. *N Engl J Med* 1971;284:929.
77. Taliercio CP, et al. Risks for renal dysfunction with cardiac angiography. *Ann Intern Med* 1986;104:501.
78. Gomes AS, et al. Acute renal dysfunction after major arteriography. *Am J Roentgenol* 1985;145:1249.
79. Manske CL, et al. Contrast nephropathy in azotemic diabetic patients undergoing coronary angiography. *Am J Med* 1990;89:615.
80. Shieh SD, et al. Low risk of contrast media-induced acute renal failure in nonazotemic type 2 diabetes mellitus. *Kidney Int* 1982;21:739.
81. Sanders PW, Booker BB. Pathobiology of cast nephropathy from human Bence Jones proteins. *J Clin Invest* 1992;89:630.
82. Huang ZO, et al. Bence Jones proteins bind to a common peptide segment of Tamm-Horsfall glycoprotein to promote heterotypic aggregation. *J Clin Invest* 1993;92:2975.
83. Cohen E, Raducha JJ. Detection of urinary Bence Jones protein by means of p-toluene sulfonic acid (TSA). *Am J Clin Pathol* 1963;37:660.
84. Miller DL, et al. Intravascular contrast media: effect of dose on renal function. *Radiology* 1988;167:607.
85. Porter GA. Contrast-associated nephropathy. *Am J Cardiol* 1989;64:22E.
86. Barrett BJ, et al. Contrast nephropathy in patients with impaired renal function: high versus low osmolar media. *Kidney Int* 1992;41:1274.
87. Marenzi G, et al. The prevention of radiocontrast-agent-induced nephropathy by hemofiltration. *New Engl J Med* 2003;349:1333.
88. Abizaid AS, et al. Effects of dopamine and aminophylline on contrast-induced acute renal failure after coronary angioplasty in patients with pre-existing renal insufficiency. *Am J Cardiol* 1999;83:260.
89. Levy EM, Viscoli CM, Horwitz RI. The effect of acute renal failure on mortality: a cohort analysis. *JAMA* 1996;275:1489.

90. D'Elia JA, et al. Inadequacy of fractional excretion of sodium test. *Arch Intern Med* 1981;141:818.
91. Gelman ML, et al. Effects of an angiographic contrast agent on renal function. *Cardiovasc Med* 1979;4:313.
92. Love L, Lind JA Jr, Olson MC. Persistent CT nephrogram: significance in the diagnosis of contrast nephropathy. *Radiology* 1989;172:125.
93. Cattell WR, et al. The functional basis for nephrographic patterns in acute tubular necrosis. *Invest Radiol* 1980;15:S79.
94. Hunter JV, Kind PR. Nonionic iodinated contrast media: potential renal damage assessed with enzymuria. *Radiology* 1992;183:101.
95. Jakobsen JA, et al. Renal tubular effects of diuretics and x-ray contrast media. A comparative study of equimolar doses in healthy volunteers. *Invest Radiol* 1993;28:319.
96. Severini G, Aliberti LM. Variation of urinary enzymes N-acetyl-beta-glucosaminidase, alanine-aminopeptidase, and lysozyme in patients receiving radio-contrast agents. *Clin Biochem* 1987;20:339.
97. Han WK, et al. Kidney injury molecule-1 (KIM-1): a novel biomarker for human renal proximal tubule injury. *Kidney Int* 2002;62:237.
98. Moreau JF, et al. Tubular nephrotoxicity of water-soluble iodinated contrast media. *Invest Radiol* 1980;15:S54.
99. Moreau JF, et al. Osmotic nephrosis induced by water-soluble tri-iodinated contrast media in man. *Radiology* 1975;115:329.
100. Moreau JF, Droz D, Noel LH. Nephrotoxicity of metrizamide in man. *Lancet* 1978;1:1201.
101. Moreau JF, et al. Nephrotoxicity of ioxaglic acid (AG 6227 or P286) in humans. *Invest Radiol* 1978;13:554.
102. Rees JA, Old SL, Rowlands PC. An ultrastructural histochemistry and light microscopy study of the early development of renal proximal tubular vacuolation after a single administration of the contrast enhancement medium Iotrolan. *Toxicol Pathol* 1997;25:2:158.
103. Heyman SN, et al. Acute renal failure with selective medullary injury in the rat. *J Clin Invest* 1988;82:401.
104. Moreau JR. Discussion: Symposium on radiocontrast agents and the kidney. *Invest Radiol* 1980;15:S84.
105. Heyman SN, Rosen S. Dye nephropathy. *Semin Nephrol* 2003;23:477.
106. Heyman SN, et al. Animal models of acute tubular necrosis. *Curr Op Crit Care* 2002;8:526.
107. Brezis M, Rosen S. Hypoxia of the renal medulla: implications for diseases. *N Engl J Med* 1995;332:647.
108. Heyman SN, Rosen S, Brezis M. The renal medulla: life at the edge of anoxia. *Blood Purif* 1997;5:232.
109. Epstein FH, Prasad P. Effects of furosemide on medullary oxygenation in younger and older subjects. *Kidney Int* 2000;57:2080.
110. Prasad PV, et al. Changes in intrarenal oxygenation as evaluated by BOLD MRI in a rat kidney model for radiocontrast nephropathy. *J Magn Reson Imaging* 2001;13:744.
111. Agmon Y, Dinour D, Brezis M. Disparate effects of adenosine A1 and A2-receptor agonists on intrarenal blood flow. *Am J Physiol* 1993;265:F802.
112. Gurbanov K, et al. Differential regulation of renal regional blood flow by endothelin-1. *Am J Physiol* 1996;271:F1166.
113. Duke LM, et al. Disparate roles of AT2 receptors in the renal cortical and medullary circulations of anesthetized rabbits. *Hypertension* 2003;42:200.
114. Heyman SN, et al. Early renal medullary hypoxic injury from radiocontrast and indomethacin. *Kidney Int* 1991;40:632.
115. Brezis M, et al. Role of nitric oxide in renal medullary oxygenation. *J Clin Invest* 1991;88:390.
116. Liss P, et al. Injection of low and isoosmolar contrast medium decreases oxygen tension in the renal medulla. *Kidney Int* 1998;53:698.
117. Rosenberger C, et al. Upregulation of HIF in acute renal failure—evidence for a protective transcriptional response to hypoxia. *Kidney Int* 2005;67:531.
118. Neagley SR, et al. Transient oxygen desaturation following radiographic contrast medium administration. *Arch Intern Med* 1986;146:1094.
119. Dawson P. Cardiovascular effects of contrast agents. *Am J Cardiol* 1989;64:2E.
120. Schiantarelli P, et al. Effects of iodinated contrast media on erythrocytes. *Invest Radiol* 1973;8:199.
121. Corot C, et al. Contrast media-related thromboembolic risks: effects of blood mixed with contrast media in contact with angiographic catheters. *Semin Hematol* 1991;28(Suppl 7):54.
122. Kim SJ, et al. Contrast media adversely affect oxyhemoglobin dissociation. *Anesth Analg* 1990;71:73.
123. Morettin LB, et al. Cardiorespiratory responses elicited by right atrial injections of iodinated contrast media. Comparative evaluation of four agents. *Invest Radiol* 1994;29:201.
124. Foitzik T, et al. Intravenous contrast medium impairs oxygenation of the pancreas in acute necrotizing pancreatitis in the rat. *Arch Surg* 1994;129:706.
125. Arakawa K, et al. Role of adenosine in the renal responses to contrast medium. *Kidney Int* 1996;49:1199.
126. Uretsky BF, et al. Plasma vasopressin response to osmotic and hemodynamic stimuli in heart failure. *Am J Physiol* 1985;248:H396.
127. Trewhella M, et al. Vasopressin release in response to intravenously injected contrast media. *Br J Radiol* 1990;63:97.
128. Heyman SN, et al. Radiocontrast agents induce endothelin release in vivo and in vitro. *J Am Soc Nephrol* 1992;3:58.
129. Kurnik BR, et al. Effects of atrial natriuretic peptide versus mannitol on renal blood flow during radiocontrast infusion in chronic renal failure. *J Lab Clin Med* 1990;116:27.
130. Hoffman A, et al. Mechanisms of big endothelin-1-induced diuresis and natriuresis: role of ET(B) receptors. *Hypertension* 2000;35:732.
131. Margulies KB, et al. Radiocontrast increases plasma and urinary endothelin. *J Am Soc Nephrol* 1991;2:1041.
132. Liss P. Effects of contrast media on renal microcirculation and oxygen tension. An experimental study in the rat. *Acta Radiol Suppl* 1997;409:1.
133. Brezis M, Agmon Y, Epstein FH. Determinants of intrarenal oxygenation I. Effects of diuretics. *Am J Physiol* 1994;267:F1054.
134. Workman RJ, et al. Relationship of renal hemodynamic and functional changes following intravascular contrast to the renin-angiotensin system and renal prostacyclin in the dog. *Invest Radiol* 1983;18:160.
135. Weisberg LS, Kurnik PB, Kurnik BR. Radiocontrast-induced nephropathy in humans: role of renal vasoconstriction. *Kidney Int* 1992;41:1408.
136. Brezis M, Heyman SN, Epstein F. Determinants of intrarenal oxygenation: 2 Hemodynamic effects. *Am J Physiol* 1994;267:F1063
137. Nygren A, et al. Effects of intravenous contrast media on cortical and medullary blood flow in the rat kidney. *Invest Radiol* 1988;23:753.
138. Liss P, et al. Effects of contrast media and mannitol on renal medullary blood flow and red cell aggregation in the rat kidney. *Kidney Int* 1996;49:1268.
139. Agmon Y, et al. Nitric oxide and prostanoids protect the renal outer medulla from radiocontrast toxicity in the rat. *J Clin Invest* 1994;94:1069.
140. Heyman SN, et al. The effect of radiocontrast on intra-renal nitric oxide (NO) and NO synthase activity. *Exp Nephrol* 1998;6:557.
141. Palm F, et al. Effects of the contrast medium iopromide on renal hemodynamics and oxygen tension in the diabetic rat kidney. *Adv Exp Med Biol* 2003;530:653.
142. Liss P, Nygren A, Hansell P. Hypoperfusion in the renal outer medulla after injection of contrast media in rats. *Acta Radiol* 1999;40:521.
143. Pallone TL, Silldroff EP. Pericyte regulation of renal medullary blood flow. *Exp Nephrol* 2001;9:165.
144. Drescher P, et al. Contrast medium induced renal vasoconstriction, role of alpha receptors. *Scand J Urol Nephrol Suppl* 1995;172:103.
145. Heyman SN, et al. Effects of ioversol versus iothalamate on endothelin release and radiocontrast nephropathy. *Invest Radiol* 1991;28:313.
146. Cantley LG, et al. Role of endothelin and prostaglandins in radio-contrast-induced renal artery constriction. *Kidney Int* 1993;44:1217.
147. Pflueger A, et al. Role of adenosine in contrast media-induced acute renal failure in diabetes mellitus. *Mayo Clin Proc* 2000;75:1275.
148. Arend LJ, et al. Role for intrarenal adenosine in the renal hemodynamic response to contrast media. *J Lab Clin Med* 1987;110:406.
149. Erley CM, et al. Prevention of radiocontrast-induced nephropathy by adenosine antagonists in rats with chronic nitric oxide deficiency. *J Am Soc Nephrol* 1997;8:1125.
150. Drescher P, Knes JM, Madsen PO. Histamine release and contrast media-induced renal vasoconstriction. *Acad Radiol* 1998;5:785.
151. Heyman SN, et al. Tissue oxygenation modifies nitric oxide bioavailability. *Microcirculation* 1999;6:199.
152. Parvez Z, et al. Effect of contrast media on prostaglandin synthesis in vivo. *Invest Radiol* 1988;23(Suppl 1):S178
153. Lancelot E, et al. Influence of the viscosity of iodixanol on medullary and cortical blood flow in the rat kidney: a potential cause of nephrotoxicity. *J Appl Toxicol* 1999;19:341.
154. Persson PB, Hansell P, Liss P. Pathophysiology of contrast medium-induced nephropathy. *Kidney Int* 2005;68:14
155. Riemann CD, et al. Ionic contrast agent-mediated endothelial injury causes increased platelet deposition to vascular surfaces. *Am Heart J* 1993;125:71.
156. Esplugas E, et al. Contrast media influence on thrombotic risk during coronary angioplasty. *Semin Thromb Hemost* 1993;1:192.
157. Ueda J, et al. Effect of intravenous contrast media on proximal and distal tubular hydrostatic pressure in the rat kidney. *Acta Radiol* 1993;34:83.
158. Ueda J, et al. Iodine concentrations in the rat kidney measured by x-ray microanalysis. Comparison of concentrations and viscosities in the proximal tubules and renal pelvis after intravenous injections of contrast media. *Acta Radiol* 1998;39:90.
159. Bakris GL, Gaber AO, Jones JD. Oxygen free radical involvement in urinary Tamm-Horsfall protein excretion after intrarenal injection of contrast medium. *Radiology* 1990;175:57.
160. Dawnay AB, et al. Tamm-Horsfall glycoprotein excretion and aggregation during intravenous urography. Relevance to acute renal failure. *Invest Radiol* 1985;20:53.
161. Holland MD, et al. Effect of urinary pH and diatrizoate on Bence Jones protein nephrotoxicity in the rat. *Kidney Int* 1985;27:46.
162. Haller C, Hizoh I. The cytotoxicity of iodinated radiocontrast agents on renal cells in vitro. *Invest Radiol* 2004;39:149.
163. Humes HD, Hunt DA, White MD. Direct toxic effect of the radiocontrast agent diatrizoate on renal proximal tubule cells. *Am J Physiol* 1987;252:F246.
164. Bakris GL, et al. Radiocontrast medium-induced declines in renal function: a role for oxygen free radicals. *Am J Physiol* 1990;258:F115.
165. Parvez Z, Rahman MA, Moncada R. Contrast media-induced lipid peroxidation in the rat kidney. *Invest Radiol* 1989;24:697.

166. Yoshioka T, Fogo A, Beckman JK. Reduced activity of antioxidant enzymes underlies contrast media-induced renal injury in volume depletion. *Kidney Int* 1992;41:1008.

167. Darmon D, et al. The effect of poly-(ADP-ribose) polymerase (PARP) inhibition on outer medullary hypoxic damage. *Nephron Physiol* 2003;93:1.

168. Filipovic DM, Meng X, Reeves WB. Inhibition of PARP prevents oxidant-induced necrosis but not apoptosis in LLC-PK1 cells. *Am J Physiol* 1999;277:F428.

169. Schnackenberg CG. Physiological and pathophysiological roles of oxygen radicals in the renal microvasculature. *Am J Physiol* 2002;282:R335.

170. Szabo G, et al. Poly(ADP-Ribose) polymerase inhibition reduces reperfusion injury after heart transplantation. *Circ Res* 2002;90:100.

171. Palm F, et al. Reactive oxygen species cause diabetes-induced decrease in renal oxygen tension. *Diabetologia* 2003;46:1153.

172. Welch WJ, et al. Renal oxygenation defects in the spontaneously hypertensive rat: role of AT1 receptors. *Kidney Int* 2003;63:202.

173. Heyman SN, et al. Diabetes predisposes to medullary hypoxia with activation of hypoxia inducible factors (HIF) and upregulation of endothelin-B receptors (ETB). *J Am Soc Nephrol* 4004;15:468A.

174. Miyazaki S, et al. Implication of hypoxia-inducible factor 1 alpha in tubulointerstitial injury in stroke-prone spontaneously hypertensive rats (SHR-SP). *J Am Soc Nephrol* 2004;15:236A.

175. Epstein FH, Veves A, Prasad PV. Effect of diabetes on renal medullary oxygenation during water diuresis. *Diabetes Care* 2002;25:575.

176. Vaamonde CA, et al. Acute and chronic renal effects of radiocontrast in diabetic rats. Role of anesthesia and risk factors. *Invest Radiol* 1989;24:206.

177. Katzberg RW. What do we really know about contrast medium-induced acute renal failure? *Invest Radiol* 1989;24:219.

178. Tervahartiala P, et al. Contrast media-induced renal tubular vacuolization. A light and electron microscopic study on rat kidneys. *Invest Radiol* 1991;26:882.

179. Heyman SN, Rosen S, Brezis M. Radiocontrast nephropathy: a paradigm for the synergism between toxic and hypoxic insults in the kidney. *Exp Nephrol* 1994;2:153.

180. Heyman SN, Reichman J, Brezis M. The pathophysiology of contrast nephropathy: a role for medullary hypoxia. *Invest Radiol* 1999;34:685.

181. Vari RC, et al. Induction, prevention and mechanisms of contrast media-induced acute renal failure. *Kidney Int* 1988;33:699.

182. Margulies KB, et al. Induction and prevention of radiocontrast-induced nephropathy in dogs with heart failure. *Kidney Int* 1990;38:1101.

183. Brezis M, et al. Angiotensin II augments medullary hypoxia and predisposes to acute renal failure. *Eur J Clin Invest* 1990;20:199.

184. Duarte CG, Zhang J, Ellis S. Effects of radiocontrast, mannitol, and endothelin on blood pressure and renal damage in the aging male spontaneously hypertensive rat. *Invest Radiol* 1999;34:455.

185. Heyman SN, et al. Effect of glycine and hypertrophy on renal outer medullary hypoxic injury in ischemia reflow and contrast nephropathy. *Am J Kidney Dis* 1992;19:578.

186. Heyman SN, et al. Renal microcirculation and tissue damage during acute ureteral obstruction: the effect of saline infusion, indomethacin and radiocontrast. *Kidney Int* 1997;51:653.

187. Lund G, et al. Role of ischemia in contrast-induced renal damage: an experimental study. *Circulation* 1984;69:783.

188. Cederholm C, et al. Acute renal failure in rats. Interaction between contrast media and temporary renal artery occlusion. *Acta Radiol* 1989;30:321.

189. Deray G, et al. Renal effects of radiocontrast agents in rats: a new model of acute renal failure. *Am J Nephrol* 1990;10:507.

190. Touati C, et al. Modulation of the renal effects of contrast media by endothelium-derived nitric oxide in the rat. *Invest Radiol* 1993;28:814.

191. Schultz SG, Lavelle KJ, Swain R. Nephrotoxicity of radiocontrast media in ischemic renal failure in rabbits. *Nephron* 1982;32:113.

192. Goldfarb M, et al. Acute-on-chronic renal failure in the rat: functional compensation and hypoxia tolerance. *Am J Nephrol* 2006;26:22.

193. Maril N, et al. Detection of evolving acute tubular necrosis with renal²³ sodium MRI: studies in rats. *Kidney Int* 2006;69:765.

194. Beeri R, et al. Rapid DNA fragmentation from hypoxia along the thick ascending limb of rat kidneys. *Kidney Int* 1995;47:1806.

195. Hellman RN, et al. Acetazolamide is renoprotective in a rat model of high dose contrast media induced renal failure. *J Am Soc Nephrol* 2004;15:717A.

196. Asif A, Epstein M. Prevention of radiocontrast-induced nephropathy. *Am J Kidney Dis* 2004;44:12.

197. Safadi R, et al. Metformin-induced lactic acidosis associated with acute renal failure. *Am J Nephrol* 1996;16:520.

198. McCartney MM, et al. Metformin and contrast media—a dangerous combination? *Clin Radiol* 1999;54:29.

199. Rasuli P, Hammond, DI. Metformin and contrast media: where is the conflict? *Can Assoc Radiol J* 1998;49:161.

200. Teruel JL, et al. An easy and effective procedure to prevent radiocontrast agent nephrotoxicity in high-risk patients. *Nephron* 1989;1:282.

201. Taylor AJ, et al. PREOARED: preparation for angiography in renal dysfunction. A randomized trial of inpatient vs outpatient hydration protocols for cardiac catheterization in mild-to-moderate renal dysfunction. *Chest* 1998;114:1570.

202. Lautin EM, et al. Radiocontrast-associated renal dysfunction: a comparison of lower-osmolality and conventional high-osmolality contrast media. *Am J Roentgenol* 1991;157:59.

203. Barrett BJ, Carlisle EJ. Metaanalysis of the relative nephrotoxicity of high- and low-osmolality iodinated contrast media. *Radiology* 1993;188:171.

204. Hunter TB, Dye J, Duval JF. Selective use of low-osmolality contrast agents for i.v. urography and CT: safety and effect on cost. *Am J Roentgenol* 1994;163:965.

205. Frank H, et al. Simultaneous hemodialysis during coronary angiography fails to prevent radiocontrast-induced nephropathy in chronic renal failure. *Clin Nephrol* 2003;60:176.

206. Lehnert T, et al. Effect of hemodialysis after contrast media administration in patients with renal insufficiency. *Nephrol Dial Transplant* 1998;13:358.

207. Shammas NW, et al. Aminophylline does not protect against radiocontrast nephropathy in patients undergoing percutaneous angiographic procedures. *J Invasive Cardiol* 2001;13:738.

208. Erley CM, et al. Adenosine antagonist theophylline prevents the reduction of glomerular filtration rate after contrast media application. *Kidney Int* 1994;45:1425.

209. Abizaid AS, et al. Effects of dopamine and aminophylline on contrast-induced acute renal failure after coronary angioplasty in patients with pre-existing renal insufficiency. *Am J Cardiol* 1999;83:260.

210. Erley CM, et al. Prevention of radiocontrast media induced nephropathy in patients with preexisting renal insufficiency by hydration in combination with the adenosine antagonist theophylline. *Nephrol Dial Transplant* 1999;14:1146.

211. Katholi RE, et al. Nephrotoxicity from contrast media: attenuation with theophylline. *Radiology* 1995;195:17.

212. Kapoor A, et al. The role of theophylline in contrast-induced nephropathy: a case-control study. *Nephrol Dial Transplant* 2002;17:1936.

213. Huber W, et al. Reduced incidence of radiocontrast-induced nephropathy in ICU patients under theophylline prophylaxis: a prospective comparison to series of patients at similar risk. *Intensive Care Med* 2001;27:1200.

214. Huber W, et al. Effect of theophylline on contrast material-induced nephropathy in patients with chronic renal insufficiency: controlled, randomized, double blind study. *Radiology* 2002;223:772.

215. Heyman SN, Kaminski N, Brezis M. Dopamine increases medullary blood flow without improving regional hypoxia. *Exp Nephrol* 1995;3:331.

216. Hans SS, et al. Effect of dopamine on renal function after arteriography in patients with preexisting renal insufficiency. *Am Surg* 1998;64:432.

217. Bakris GL, Lass NA, Glock D. Renal hemodynamics in radiocontrast medium-induced renal dysfunction: a role for dopamine-1 receptors. *Kidney Int* 1999;56:206.

218. Kini AA, Sharma SK. Managing the high-risk patient: experience with fenoldopam, a selective dopamine receptor agonist, in prevention of radiocontrast nephropathy during percutaneous coronary intervention. *Rev Cardiovasc Med* 2001;2:S19.

219. Tumlin JA, et al. Fenoldopam mesylate blocks reductions in renal plasma flow after radiocontrast dye infusion: a pilot trial in the prevention of contrast nephropathy. *Am Heart J* 2002;143:894.

220. Kurnik BR, et al. Prospective study of atrial natriuretic peptide for the prevention of radiocontrast-induced nephropathy. *Am J Kidney Dis* 1998;31:674.

221. Neumayer AA, et al. Prevention of radiocontrast-media-induced nephrotoxicity by the calcium channel blocker nitrendipine: a prospective randomized clinical trial. *Nephrol Dial Transplant* 1989;4:130.

222. Russo D, et al. Randomised prospective study on the renal effects of two different contrast media in humans: protective role of calcium channel blocker. *Nephron* 1990;55:254.

223. Khoury Z, et al. The effect of prophylactic nifedipine on renal function in patients administered contrast media. *Pharmacotherapy* 1995;15:59.

224. Koch JA, et al. Prostaglandin E₁: a new agent for the prevention of renal dysfunction in high-risk patients caused by radiocontrast media? *Nephrol Dial Transplant* 2000;15:43.

225. Sketch MH, et al. Prevention of contrast media-induced renal dysfunction with prostaglandin E₁: a randomized, double-blind, placebo-controlled study. *Am J Ther* 2001;8:155.

226. Gupta RK, et al. Captopril for the prevention of contrast-induced nephropathy in diabetic patients: a randomized study. *Indian Heart J* 1999;51:521.

227. Schwartz D, et al. Role of nitric oxide (EDRF) in radiocontrast acute renal failure in rats. *Am J Physiol* 1994;267:F374.

228. Miller HI, et al. Effects of an acute dose of L-arginine during coronary angiography in patients with chronic renal failure. A randomized, parallel, double-blind clinical trial. *Am J Nephrol* 2003;23:91.

229. Brezis M, Agmon Y, Epstein FH. Determinants of intrarenal oxygenation: 1 Effects of diuretics. *Am J Physiol* 1994;267:F1059.

230. Liss P, et al. Effect of furosemide ore mannitol before injection of a nonionic contrast medium on intrarenal oxygen tension. *Adv Exp Med Biol* 1999;471:353.

231. Heyman SN, et al. Protective role of furosemide and saline in radiocontrast-induced acute renal failure in the rat. *Am J Kidney Dis* 1989;14:377.

232. Weinstein JM, Heyman S, Brezis M. Potential deleterious effect of furosemide in radiocontrast nephropathy. *Nephron* 1992;62:413.

233. Brezis M, Agmon Y, Epstein FH. Determinants of intrarenal oxygenation: 2 Hemodynamic effects. *Am J Physiol* 1994;267:F1063.

234. Anto HR, et al. Infusion intravenous pyelography and renal function effects of hypertonic mannitol in patients with chronic renal insufficiency. *Arch Intern Med* 1981;141:1652.
235. Old CW, Lehrner LM. Prevention of radiocontrast induced acute renal failure with mannitol. *Lancet* 1980;1:885.
236. Dorman HR, Sondheimer JH, Cadnapaphornchai P. Mannitol-induced acute renal failure. *Medicine (Baltimore)* 1990;69:153.
237. Schnackenberg CG, Welch WJ, Wilcox CS. Normalization of blood pressure and renal vascular resistance in SHR with a membrane-permeable superoxide dismutase mimetic: role of nitric oxide. *Hypertension* 1998;32:59.
238. Tepel M, et al. Prevention of radiographic-contrast-agent-induced reductions in renal function by acetylcysteine. *N Engl J Med* 2000;343:180.
239. Safirstein R, Andrade L, Vieira JM. Acetylcysteine and nephrotoxic effects of radiographic contrast agents—a new use for an old drug. *N Engl J Med* 2000;343:210.
240. Conesa EL, et al. N-acetyl-L-cysteine improves renal medullary hypoperfusion in acute renal failure. *Am J Physiol* 2001;281:R730.
241. Heyman SN, et al. N-acetylcysteine (NAC) ameliorates renal microcirculation: studies in rats. *Kidney Int* 2003;63:634.
242. Shyu KG, Cheng JJ, Kuan P. Acetylcysteine protects against acute renal damage in patients with abnormal renal function undergoing a coronary procedure. *J Am Coll Cardiol* 2002;40:1383.
243. Baker CS, et al. A rapid protocol for the prevention of contrast-induced renal failure: the RAPPID study. *J Am Coll Cardiol* 2003;41:2118.
244. Durham JD, et al. A randomized controlled trial of n-acetylcysteine to prevent contrast nephropathy in cardiac angiography. *Kidney Int* 2002;62:2202.
245. Boccalandro F, et al. Oral acetylcysteine does not protect renal function from moderate to high doses of intravenous radiographic contrast. *Cathet Cardiovasc Interv* 2003;58:336.
246. Briguori C, et al. N-Acetylcysteine versus fenoldopam mesylate to prevent contrast agent-associated nephrotoxicity. *J Am Coll Cardiol* 2004;44:762.
247. Briguori C, et al. Standard vs double dose of N-acetylcysteine to prevent contrast agent associated nephrotoxicity. *Eur Heart J* 2004;25:206.
248. Birck R, et al. Acetylcysteine for prevention of contrast nephropathy: meta-analysis. *Lancet* 2003;362:598.
249. Alonso A, et al. Prevention of radiocontrast nephropathy with N-acetylcysteine in patients with chronic kidney disease: a meta-analysis of randomized,controlled trials. *Am J Kidney Dis* 2004;43:1.
250. Hoffmann U, et al. The value of N-acetylcysteine in the prevention of radiocontrast agent-induced nephropathy seems questionable. *J Am Soc Nephrol* 2004;15:407.
251. Fishbane S, et al. N-acetylecysteine in the prevention of radiocontrast-induced nephropathy. *J Am Soc Nephrol* 2004;15:251.
252. Katholi RE, et al. Oxygen free radicals and contrast nephropathy. *Am J Kidney Dis* 1998;32:64.
253. Goodman AI, et al. Acute renal failure is prevented by inducing heme oxygenase-1. *J Am Soc Nephrol* 2004;15:257A.
254. Goldfarb M, et al. A role for erythropoietin in the attenuation of contrast medium-induced acute renal failure in rats? *Renal Failure* 2006 (in press).
255. Dae MW, et al. Comparison of hypothermia, N-acetylcysteine, and fenoldopam for prevention of experimental radiocontrast nephropathy. *J Am Soc Nephrol* 2004;15:460A.
256. Shyh TP, Friedman EA. Uninephrectomy does not potentiate contrast media nephrotoxicity in the streptozotocin-induced diabetic rat. *Nephron* 1990;55:170.

CHAPTER 46 ■ NEPHROTOXICITY SECONDARY TO DRUG ABUSE AND LITHIUM USE

JOEL NEUGARTEN, GLORIA R. GALLO, AND DAVID S. BALDWIN

DRUG ABUSE

Abuse of narcotics, cocaine, and other illicit substances may be associated with a variety of renal disorders as listed in Table 46-1. In the 1970s and early 1980s, glomerulosclerosis associated with intravenous heroin abuse in young African American adults emerged as an important correlate of nephrotic syndrome and end-stage renal disease in urban areas and accounted for approximately 10% of patients aged 18 to 45 years undergoing dialysis (1,2). Also, in the early 1980s, secondary amyloidosis became an important cause of renal failure in heroin abusers who injected drugs via the subcutaneous route ("skin poppers") and developed chronic suppurative skin lesions (3–6). Later, glomerulosclerosis in intravenous drug abusers infected with the human immunodeficiency virus (HIV) was recognized as a clinicopathologic entity distinct from heroin-associated nephropathy in HIV-negative heroin addicts (7,8). HIV-associated nephropathy rapidly supplanted heroin-associated nephropathy as the major renal disorder affecting intravenous drug abusers. Concurrently, the incidence of heroin-associated nephropathy and of "skin poppers' amyloidosis" decreased dramatically (9–11). Friedman and Rao (9) reported on the sharp decline in the incidence of heroin-associated nephropathy since 1989 and the complete absence of new cases of end-stage renal disease due to this disease for the years 1991 to 1993. Friedman and Rao (9) suggested that heroin-associated nephropathy may be due to the adulterants contained in "street" heroin rather than the heroin itself, and attributed the virtual disappearance of heroin nephropathy to an increase in purity of "street" heroin leading to reduced exposure to nephrotoxic adulterants. However, the changing epidemiology of renal disease in drug abusers may instead reflect the high prevalence, ranging up to 50% to 60%, of HIV infection among drug abusers (12). The presence of HIV infection in such a large proportion of the addict population has greatly reduced the number at risk for heroin-associated nephropathy, which has been pre-empted by the occurrence of HIV infection and its nephropathy.

Focal Glomerulosclerosis in Intravenous Heroin Abusers

Nineteenth-century clinicians appreciated the occurrence of proteinuria among opium addicts. Early investigators found albuminuria in 7% to 17% of addicts (13,14). Later studies attempted to define the nature of renal disease in narcotics abusers (15,16–20). In cross-sectional studies, investigators determined the prevalence of glomerular abnormalities in postmortem specimens from heroin addicts and the prevalence of proteinuria and renal sediment abnormalities in populations of addicts attending drug rehabilitation centers (15–20). Markedly disparate data were reported. However, these studies probably have little relevance to renal disease in heroin addicts as we now understand it. The finding of nonspecific urinary abnormalities in surveys of the addict population cannot be accepted as representative of the incidence of heroin-associated nephropathy. The rarity with which cases could be detected in cross-sectional or prospective studies of heroin abusers is readily apparent when one considers that data available from the early 1980s, at the height of the epidemic of heroin-associated nephropathy, placed its prevalence at well below 1%, with an annual incidence of less than one new case per 1,000 heroin addicts (21,22).

In the early 1970s several investigators began to recognize a clinicopathologic entity in heroin addicts characterized by the nephrotic syndrome and glomerulosclerosis (16,19, 23,24). Rao and colleagues (25) identified focal and segmental glomerulosclerosis that progressed to global sclerosis as heroin-associated nephropathy. These authors described 14 African American intravenous heroin users in whom the nephrotic syndrome was present in all but one. Renal biopsy specimens showed focal and segmental or global glomerulosclerosis (FSGS) in 11 of 13 patients, associated with focal and segmental glomerular deposition of immunoglobulin M and complement. Numerous other investigators confirmed these characteristic morphologic features (3,4,26–33). A similar syndrome of glomerulosclerosis associated with the nephrotic syndrome and progressive renal insufficiency has been observed rarely in abusers of intravenous drugs other than heroin, among them cocaine and pentazocine with tripelennamine (1,23,29).

Clinical Features of Heroin-Associated FSGS

Detailed descriptions of the course of nephropathy in 298 intravenous drug abusers, most described prior to the advent of HIV, with biopsy-proven focal and segmental glomerulosclerosis are available in the literature (1–4,16,17,20,25–28,34–37); incomplete information is available in an additional 168 cases (Table 46-2). Over 90% were African American males. The mean age was 29 years. Intravenous heroin, often in conjunction with cocaine, was used in all but a few cases (1,23,29). The mean duration of drug abuse prior to presentation with renal disease was 6 years, ranging widely from 6 months to 24 years but generally exceeding 1 to 2 years.

Two-thirds of patients presented with edema due to the nephrotic syndrome, an additional one-fourth with an abnormal urinalysis, and most of the remainder with uremia. Hypertension was present in nearly two-thirds on initial presentation and developed in all those who progressed to uremia (1). Microscopic hematuria was described in one-third and pyuria in one-half of the cases, but nearly one-fourth had no documented sediment abnormalities. Renal function on presentation varied widely but was reduced in three-fourths of cases.

TABLE 46-1

RENAL DISEASE ASSOCIATED WITH DRUG ABUSE

1. Focal glomerulosclerosis in intravenous heroin users
2. Amyloidosis in subcutaneous heroin abusers
3. Endocarditis-associated glomerulonephritis in intravenous drug users
4. Acute renal failure due to nontraumatic rhabdomyolysis
5. Cocaine–associated nephropathy
6. Systemic necrotizing vasculitis
7. Nephropathy in glue and solvent "sniffers"
8. Hepatitis-related glomerulonephritis in drug abusers
9. Focal glomerulosclerosis in drug abusers infected with the human immunodeficiency virus

Ten percent presented with uremia. Urinary protein excretion averaged 9.3 g/24 hours and was less than 2 g/24 hours in only 6% of cases. Proteinuria exceeded 10 g in 43%. Serum complement levels were normal and rarely erythrocytosis was reported (28).

Follow-up observations demonstrated that heroin-associated nephropathy regularly progressed inexorably to uremia. Patients presenting with a serum creatinine level below 2.2 mg/dL or a creatinine clearance exceeding 50 mL/min advanced to end-stage renal failure (ESRD) over a mean period of 43 months (range 6 to 148 months). As would be expected, ESRD occurred over a commensurately shorter period in those who presented with more advanced renal insufficiency.

The effect of abstinence from drug use on the course of established nephropathy is not known. Several patients with heroin-associated nephropathy have been described who underwent sustained remission of proteinuria and/or stabilization or improvement in renal function following abstinence (4,35,37). Eleven other patients with heroin-associated FSGS progressed to ESRD despite discontinuation of drugs. It appears, however, that patients who abstained may have followed a more protracted course. Corticosteroid and immunosuppressive therapy have generally proved to be ineffective. Despite reported responses to such therapy (26), there is no convincing evidence that treatment induces remission of proteinuria or prevents progression to end-stage renal failure.

TABLE 46-2

FOCAL GLOMERULOSCLEROSIS IN INTRAVENOUS HEROIN ABUSERS

Clinical features	
African American	95%
Male sex	92%
Age	29 yr
Duration of drug abuse	6 yr
Hypertension on presentation	64%
Serum creatinine on presentation	3.6 mg/dL
Nephrotic syndrome	80%
Time to uremia:	
Initial creatinine clearance >50 mL/min	43 mo
Initial creatinine clearance 20–50 mL/min	23 mo
Initial creatinine clearance <20 mL/min	7 mo

Comparison with Other Forms of Focal Glomerulosclerosis

In studies performed prior to the recognition of HIV-associated nephropathy, we found that heroin-associated FSGS and idiopathic FSGS showed similar histology on presentation (39). Both frequently displayed segmental glomerulosclerosis with foam cells and hyalinosis as well as varying numbers of globally sclerotic glomeruli. In contrast, HIV-associated nephropathy is characterized by segmental and/or global collapse of tufts together with prominent visceral epithelial cell hypertrophy. In addition, patients with HIV-associated FSGS often present with severe renal failure even though they lack advanced stages of diffuse global glomerulosclerosis. In this respect, HIV-associated FSGS differed from idiopathic and heroin-associated FSGS. Furthermore, interstitial inflammation and distinctive cystic tubular dilatation was noted to be more prominent in HIV-associated FSGS than in idiopathic or heroin-associated FSGS.

D'Agati and co-workers (7,38) compared renal biopsy specimens from patients with idiopathic FSGS, heroin-associated FSGS, and HIV-associated FSGS. They found the specimens to be qualitatively similar but noted that the HIV group had more globally "collapsed" glomeruli, less hyalinosis, more severe visceral epithelial cell swelling, more prevalent and severe tubular microcytic dilation, and more severe tubular cell degenerative changes (7,38). The severity of tubular atrophy and interstitial fibrosis, edema, and inflammation did not differ among the three groups (7). Ultrastructural examination in the HIV group showed numerous tubuloreticular inclusions involving glomerular endothelium, interstitial capillary endothelium, and interstitial leukocytes (7). These inclusions were only rarely observed in biopsies from patients with idiopathic or heroin-associated FSGS and when present were seen only in glomerular capillaries (7,38). These authors concluded that, while no single morphologic feature distinguishes HIV-associated FSGS from idiopathic or heroin-associated FSGS, the constellation of clinical and pathologic features that characterize HIV-associated nephropathy is diagnostic (7,38).

Epidemiology

Epidemiologic studies performed during the 1970s and 1980s, prior to the HIV epidemic, suggested the existence of a form of FSGS that occurred in intravenous heroin abusers, predominantly young African American males. FSGS in nonaddicts is likewise more prevalent in African Americans than in Caucasians, but this race disparity is more marked in parenteral drug abusers (21). Intravenous drug abuse may unmask a genetic predisposition in blacks to develop glomerulosclerosis (1,21). The emergence of this latent tendency may be triggered by exposure to heroin itself or adulterants in "street" drugs, bacterial or viral contaminants, or other environmental factors related to heroin use. In this regard, Haskell and colleagues (40) have demonstrated an increased frequency of HLA-BW53 among African American intravenous drug abusers with heroin-associated nephropathy, and suggest a genetic predisposition to the development of FSGS in this population (40,41).

The epidemiology of nephropathy in intravenous heroin users has changed radically in the last two decades. HIV-associated collapsing FSGS and hepatitis C-related glomerulonephritis have supplanted heroin-associated FSGS as the major causes of glomerular disease among intravenous drug abusers. The virtual disappearance of heroin-associated FSGS may be due to an increase in purity of "street" heroin leading to reduced exposure to nephrotoxic adulterants, or the disease may have been pre-empted by the occurrence of HIV infection with its distinctive collapsing glomerulopathy.

Studies performed in the late 1980s and 1990s described renal histopathology in European intravenous heroin users who were selected for evaluation of proteinuria or examined postmortem (42,43,44,45). Glomerular lesions in some were classified as membranoproliferative glomerulonephritis and may have been due to infection with hepatitis C. However, serum antibody to the hepatitis C virus when sought postmortem could not be detected (42).

Perneger et al. (46) performed a case control study of 716 illicit drug users and 361 controls. Those who had ever used heroin or other opiates were at increased risk for end stage renal disease, with an adjusted odds ratio of 19.1. The association showed a dose-dependent effect. The use of cocaine, crack, or psychedelic drugs was also associated with ESRD but these associations could not be separated from the effects of heroin use. The authors estimated that heroin-associated renal disease accounts for 5.6% of all treated ESRD patients aged 20 to 64 and for 5% to 6% of new patients starting renal replacement therapy in this age group. However, these investigators failed to distinguish between HIV- or hepatitis C-related renal disease in heroin addicts and heroin-associated FSGS. In this regard, the United States Renal Data System (47) attributed 0.1% of new cases of ESRD from 1998–2002 to heroin/related abuse. The median age was 45 years, 75.5% were male, and 59.2% were black.

Pathogenesis

Early investigators suggested that FSGS in heroin abusers was immunologically mediated (22,25). The finding of immunoglobulin M (IgM) and C3 in segmental lesions suggested an immunologic mechanism of damage due to deposition of immune complexes; the putative antigen being a self-injected bacterial or viral contaminant, an adulterant used to dilute heroin, or the heroin itself (1). Although electron-dense material may be seen in areas of sclerosis, they are not found in uninvolved peripheral capillary walls in kidney biopsies of addicts with FSGS. The appearance and location in the lumens of sclerosing tufts suggest that these accumulations represent nonspecific trapping of immunoglobulins rather than immune deposits. Immunofluorescence findings are consistent with this interpretation.

Administration of morphine to rats by Marchand and co-workers (48) did not result in glomerular disease but instead caused tubulointerstitial lesions in the cortex, medulla, and papilla consisting of basement membrane thickening, loss of microvilli, and dense cytoplasmic inclusions in proximal, distal, and collecting duct tubules. However, other investigators have demonstrated increased glomerular podocyte microprojections in morphine-treated rats (49). Clearly, administration of morphine sulfate to rats is not analogous to the nonsterile self-injection of heroin and its adulterants by addicts.

Studies by Singhal and co-workers (50–58) suggest that morphine, the active metabolite of heroin, may directly mediate heroin nephrotoxicity. Exposure of mesangial cells to morphine stimulates cellular proliferation and synthesis of collagen and laminin and suppresses collagenase activity (50–56). Morphine enhances accumulation of macromolecules within the mesangium and stimulates production of pro-proliferative and fibrogenic cytokines (52–56). These alterations in mesangial cell function may contribute to the development of cell proliferation and matrix abnormalities observed in cultured mesangial cells after long-term exposure to morphine (50). In addition, morphine increases renal medullary interstitial cell and renal fibroblast proliferation and enhances the release of proinflammatory macrophage secretory products (57,58). However, the

relevance of these *in vitro* experimental observations to the development of heroin-associated nephropathy in humans remains to be established.

Deposition of talc granules has been observed in arterioles and glomeruli of intravenous drug abusers who inject drugs compounded for oral or rectal use (59–63). Granulomatous interstitial nephritis with particulate deposits in the renal interstitium has also been reported (60,62,64). In addition, a syndrome of microangiopathic hemolytic anemia, thrombocytopenia, and acute renal failure has also been observed with intravenous heroin use (65).

Amyloidosis in Subcutaneous Heroin Abusers ("Skin Poppers' Amyloidosis")

In the late 1970s and early 1980s, systemic amyloidosis emerged as a major cause of nephropathy in heroin abusers (3–6). The association was first reported in small numbers of addicts with proteinuria between 1975 and 1979 (66–72). By the early 1980s, approximately one-half of heroin abusers who underwent renal biopsy for proteinuria in New York City were found to have amyloidosis (3,4,6). However, with the advent of HIV infection among drug users, amyloidosis has become an infrequent cause of nephrotic syndrome and renal failure in drug abusers, paralleling the decline in heroin-associated FSGS.

Pathogenesis

We performed a prospective survey of 150 predominantly African American male intravenous drug addicts who were examined consecutively at postmortem in the early 1980s (5). We demonstrated that addicts with suppurative skin infections were at high risk for the development of amyloidosis (5). Twenty-six percent of the 23 addicts with chronic suppurative skin infections due to subcutaneous injections had renal amyloidosis. The skin infections, usually in the extremities, were generally extensive, involving 10% to 20% of the body surface area. The amyloid was amyloid A protein-related in all cases. All but one of those found to have renal amyloidosis had chronic skin infections. The near universal association of renal amyloidosis with chronic suppurative cutaneous lesions in subcutaneous drug abusers strongly implicates skin infection in the pathogenesis (3–6,70,73,74). Thus, to the extent examined, amyloidosis in addicts does not differ from amyloidosis secondary to chronic infections and inflammatory diseases in nonaddicts associated with chronic cutaneous dermatoses, secondarily infected burns, or decubitus ulcers (5).

The average duration of drug abuse in addicts with renal amyloidosis was 18 years, significantly longer than the average 6 years in addicts with FSGS. The mean age of addicts with amyloidosis was 41 years, while those with focal sclerosis averaged 29 years of age. In general, intravenous drug abuse antedated the subcutaneous route in those with amyloidosis. With advancing age and prolonged addiction, intravenous sites for injection of drugs become exhausted, necessitating a shift to the subcutaneous route. Cutaneous ulcerations that develop in response to local reactions to the injected heroin, bacterial contaminants, and/or diluents are followed by suppurative complications (72,75). Longer survival of addicts in the late 1970s and early 1980s due to improved management of bacterial endocarditis, hepatitis, and other narcotic abuse-related medical illnesses likely allowed the emergence of renal amyloidosis. However, there has been a dramatic decline in the incidence of "skin poppers' amyloidosis" in the HIV era.

Pathology

Deposits of amyloid are typically present in all renal compartments. Glomeruli typically exhibit prominent mesangial expansion or solidified lobules, which may be misinterpreted as sclerosis in hematoxylin–eosin-stained sections. However, routine stains readily differentiate the two processes because amyloid is silver-negative with periodic acid-silver methenamine stain, whereas the opposite is true of sclerosis. Peripheral capillary walls are often thickened and have a "spicular" deformity in silver-stained sections produced by the penetration of amyloid fibrils through the glomerular basement membrane. Tubular basement membranes, especially those of the distal segments, are thickened due to deposits of amyloid, and the degree of tubular atrophy appears to parallel the amount of amyloid deposited. While amyloid is seen focally in tubular basement membranes of some proximal tubules, the amount and distribution are far greater in distal segments.

All of the 17 kidneys with skin poppers' amyloidosis that we examined by immunofluorescence showed predominant staining for AA protein. Amyloid was isolated from the kidney and biochemically characterized in two instances. The amyloid protein was AA protein–related and did not differ from AA amyloid secondary to other chronic infections and inflammatory diseases (5,76).

Clinical Features

The following description of the clinical features of skin poppers' amyloidosis is based on data from 60 cases reported in the literature, (3,4,6,66–74,77–79) (Table 46-3). The mean age of these patients was 41 years (range, 5 to 57 years). When specified, nearly all patients were African American, and all but 10 were men. Heroin was abused in nearly all cases, often in association with cocaine; however, in two patients, crushed tablets of pentazocine and tripelennamine were the sole drugs abused. The vast majority injected drugs by the subcutaneous route and invariably had extensive skin ulcerations, usually with active chronic suppuration at the time of presentation. Chronic skin infections at intravenous injection sites or systemic illnesses known to be associated with systemic amyloidosis were seen in those who had not abused drugs by the subcutaneous route. The mean total duration of drug abuse was 18 years, and the average time from initiation of the subcutaneous route to presentation with amyloidosis was 3 years, with a range of 1 to 8 years.

Addicts with amyloidosis typically present with the nephrotic syndrome. Urinary protein excretion averaged 13 g/24 hours and was in the nephrotic range in over 80%. Microscopic hematuria and pyuria were uncommon. Hypertension on initial presentation was reported in 17%. Average serum creatinine levels did not differ between hypertensive and normotensive

patients. Dubrow and colleagues (3) comment on the infrequency of hypertension in heroin abusers with systemic amyloidosis in contrast to its presence at presentation in two-thirds of heroin abusers with FSGS. Our own experience differs insofar as we frequently observed hypertension at presentation among heroin addicts with systemic amyloidosis. Kidney size was normal in two-thirds of cases and was increased in the remainder. Serum creatinine on presentation varied widely and averaged 2.5 mg/dL. Only 4% were uremic at presentation.

Follow-up data are available in a limited number of patients who generally progressed to uremia over 2 to 3 years after presenting with serum creatinine levels ranging from 1.5 to 4.7 mg/dL. Abstinence from subcutaneous drug use and clearance of infection has been associated with remission of the nephrotic syndrome and improvement or stabilization of renal function in several patients (73–80). However, repeat renal biopsy showed persistent glomerular deposits of AA amyloid in one of these (74). In contrast, others have described persistent nephrotic syndrome, progressive loss of renal function and persistent renal amyloid deposits despite discontinuation of drug use and clearance of infection (72). Tan and colleagues (78) treated one patient with colchicine. Although renal function improved and the nephrotic syndrome remitted, repeat renal biopsy after 12 months failed to show any improvement in the amyloid burden (78).

Tubular Disorders

We assessed renal tubular function in 13 addicts with renal amyloidosis (6). Renal tubular acidosis was found in eight patients. Polyuria and polydipsia, glycosuria, and phosphaturia were additional clinical features. Nephrogenic diabetes insipidus insensitive to exogenous vasopressin administration was documented in one patient in whom amyloid deposits were demonstrated in renal tubular basement membranes, predominantly involving distal segments.

In summary, systemic amyloidosis emerged in the late 1970s and early 1980s as an important cause of nephropathy in drug abusers in urban areas related to use of the subcutaneous route of drug injection. However, with the advent of HIV infection, renal amyloidosis in the addict population has experienced a dramatic decline.

Endocarditis-Associated Glomerulonephritis in Heroin Abusers

In a review of the epidemiology and clinical features of glomerulonephritis during the course of bacterial endocarditis, we noted that patients were frequently parenteral drug abusers infected with *Staphylococcus aureus* (81,82). Others have reported a similarly high incidence of glomerulonephritis in parenteral drug abusers with bacterial endocarditis due to *S. aureus* (83–91). The predisposition of parenteral drug abusers to develop glomerulonephritis during the course of bacterial endocarditis may be related to preformed serum antibodies to bacterial antigens.

Pathology

Glomerulonephritis encountered in the course of endocarditis can be classified as diffuse or focal (81). Diffuse glomerulonephritis, as it occurs in addicts with acute bacterial endocarditis due to *S. aureus*, is generally indistinguishable from acute post streptococcal or other post infectious glomerulonephritis. Proliferation in glomeruli is global and regular, and electron-dense deposits are present in a subepithelial distribution. This contrasts with the morphologic features of diffuse glomerulonephritis seen with subacute bacterial endocarditis

TABLE 46-3

AMYLOIDOSIS IN SUBCUTANEOUS HEROIN ABUSERS

Clinical features	
African American	98%
Male sex	86%
Age	41 yr
Duration of intravenous route	18 yr
Duration of subcutaneous route	3 yr
Suppurative skin lesions	88%
Nephrotic syndrome on presentation	86%
Hypertension on presentation	17%
Serum creatinine on presentation	2.5 mg/dL

due to *Streptococcus viridans*. In this latter setting, deposits are predominantly subendothelial and mesangial, and proliferation in glomeruli is irregular with coexistence of segmental and global lesions (81). Focal glomerulonephritis in infective endocarditis is characterized by varying degrees of segmental glomerular hypercellularity, sclerosis, or capsular adhesions. Epithelial and fibroepithelial crescents, either small or circumferential, may be present.

Clinical Features

Clinical manifestations of focal glomerulonephritis are usually mild (82). Microscopic hematuria, pyuria, or modest proteinuria may be observed; heavy proteinuria and hypertension are rare. Renal functional impairment is uncommon, but when segmental glomerular involvement is severe and extensive, renal insufficiency may supervene (81). Occasionally, focal glomerulonephritis may be present in the absence of clinical abnormalities.

We reported our experience with the course of diffuse glomerulonephritis during bacterial endocarditis as seen predominantly in heroin abusers (81,82). Renal functional impairment on initial presentation ranged from mild to advanced renal failure. No correlation existed between the duration of symptoms prior to presentation and the initial and peak serum creatinine level. In the majority of patients, serum creatinine reached maximal levels prior to initiation of antibiotic therapy or during the early phase of treatment. Advanced renal insufficiency on initial presentation was associated with both failure of bacterial cure and failure to recover renal function. It is unclear whether the presence of severe renal insufficiency hindered the eradication of infection or whether more "severe" endocarditis gave rise to more severe glomerulonephritis. By contrast, effective antibiotic therapy led to recovery of renal function, normalization of the serum complement level, and remission of the clinical features of glomerulonephritis. Renal recovery occurred consistently in those patients in whom renal functional impairment was mild or moderate.

Microscopic hematuria and proteinuria are universal in endocarditis-associated diffuse glomerulonephritis (81). Gross hematuria may also be observed or may result from renal infarction or concurrent drug-induced interstitial nephritis. It is generally thought that the nephrotic syndrome is a rare feature; however, the nephrotic syndrome has been reported in 16% of histologically confirmed cases of glomerulonephritis in patients with bacterial endocarditis (81). Fifty-six percent of those with nephrotic syndrome were parenteral drug abusers with *S. aureus* bacterial endocarditis (81). Diffuse glomerulonephritis was present in most (81). These data, however, may overestimate the true incidence of nephrotic syndrome because patients with heavy proteinuria are more likely to be subjected to renal biopsy. Hypertension is rarely described despite its frequent occurrence in other forms of post infectious endocapillary glomerulonephritis (81). Because of the difficulty in differentiating cardiac, nephrotic, and "nephritic" edema in patients with endocarditis and renal disease, the contribution of primary renal sodium retention cannot be determined with certainty.

Outcome

With control of infection by antibiotic therapy, the urinary abnormalities normalize in most patients within several days to several weeks (81). Occasionally, microscopic hematuria or proteinuria may persist for months to years after bacteriologic cure (81). In the majority of cases, renal insufficiency of mild to moderate severity resolves promptly with successful antibiotic therapy. Infrequently, transient worsening of renal function may occur prior to recovery (81). Despite the worst prognosis in patients who present with uremia, even severe renal failure

may resolve with successful antibiotic therapy, sometimes with improvement continuing over weeks or months. Serial renal biopsies may reveal almost complete histological resolution of glomerulonephritis in association with clinical recovery (81).

Renal failure requiring dialysis may persist despite bacteriologic cure (81,82). This might occur more frequently were it not for the high mortality associated with uremia due to failure of antibiotic therapy. Among those cured of endocarditis, later deaths due to chronic renal failure secondary to glomerulonephritis acquired during the active phase of endocarditis have occasionally been reported (81). Persistent renal insufficiency, nephrotic syndrome, and sediment abnormalities have been described in parenteral drug abusers after bacteriologic cure of *S. aureus* endocarditis (92,93). Our own studies demonstrate that glomerulonephritis acquired during the course of endocarditis may occasionally prove to be irreversible despite bacteriologic cure and may result in persistent renal insufficiency or sediment abnormalities (82). A role for corticosteroids, cytotoxic agents, or plasmapheresis has been suggested in patients with bacterial endocarditis and diffuse proliferative glomerulonephritis with extracapillary proliferation in whom renal function fails to recover with antibiotic therapy alone (94). However, these recommendations are based solely on isolated case reports and require confirmation with controlled, randomized studies.

Acute Renal Failure Due to Nontraumatic Rhabdomyolysis in Drug Abusers

Nontraumatic rhabdomyolysis in drug users is a well-recognized clinical syndrome. Although cocaine (95–129) and heroin (122,130–161) are the agents most frequently responsible, the syndrome has also been described after intravenous or oral administration of amphetamine, methamphetamine, phencyclidine, methadone, and barbiturates and other sedatives singly or in combination (138,162–174). In particular, phencyclidine may cause rhabdomyolysis during periods of involuntary isometric activity against mechanical restraints (168,169). Intra-arterial injection of temazepan formulated as a gelatin capsule or hard gel may cause acute renal failure due to particulate embolization with rhabdomyolysis (173). However, temazapan is no longer available in these formulations. Tetanus or self-injection of water may rarely cause nontraumatic rhabdomyolysis in drug abusers (30,37).

Prolonged pressure on dependent muscles during extended periods of depressed consciousness and immobilization resulting in vascular compromise, is generally believed to be responsible for heroin-associated rhabdomyolysis (36,37,130–137). This sequence results in compression myonecrosis and ischemic injury. However, a number of cases of heroin-associated rhabdomyolysis have occurred in the absence of depressed consciousness or muscle compression (134,145–152). Rhabdomyolysis in these instances has been attributed to a direct toxic effect or an allergic reaction to heroin or a contaminant. Instead of the typical localized muscle involvement seen with pressure myonecrosis, generalized and symmetric muscle swelling may be observed in these cases (150–152). Lending further credence to a toxic or allergic pathogenesis is the occasional occurrence of swelling of an entire extremity after local injection of heroin (150). In several cases, myocarditis appeared to accompany nontraumatic rhabdomyolysis due to heroin (148,152,153); however, in only one case was myocardial involvement confirmed histologically (152).

Most heroin abusers with nontraumatic rhabdomyolysis are young men between the ages of 18 and 41 years (mean, 25 years). Prolonged muscle compression during extended periods of stupor and immobilization was present in the vast majority. The degree and duration of stupor usually determined the severity of rhabdomyolysis and the occurrence and severity of acute renal failure (37). Hypoxia, volume depletion, acidosis, hypotension, and disturbances in temperature regulation, which frequently accompany drug overdose, contributed to the occurrence of renal failure in this setting (134,154,155). Clinical evidence of muscle injury such as swelling and tenderness of involved muscles or localized pain and weakness was frequent; however, these findings may be absent or overlooked. Elevation of serum levels of muscle enzymes and myoglobinuria were characteristic features. Acute renal failure occurred in two-thirds of cases and was frequently oliguric. Prognosis was excellent, with full recovery in all but several patients who died during oliguric acute renal failure (150,152).

The first reports calling attention to the association between cocaine abuse and nontraumatic rhabdomyolysis appeared in 1987 (95–97). Well over 100 cases have been described to date (95–129,174–180). The vast majority were male, and their average age was 30 years. Ischemic myonecrosis due to cocaine-induced vasoconstriction may be primarily responsible for rhabdomyolysis; however, cocaine has also been shown to have direct toxic effects on muscle *in vitro* (181). Most patients experienced complications of cocaine use that may have contributed to the development of rhabdomyolysis or may have been primarily responsible for muscle injury. These complications included hypotension, seizures, hyperpyrexia, and muscle compression following prolonged immobilization. Others abused cocaine together with heroin or alcohol—drugs that are themselves associated with muscle injury. Cocaine may be contaminated with arsenic, strychnine, amphetamine, and phencyclidine, which may cause seizures and rhabdomyolysis (173). Myalgia or muscle tenderness accompanied cocaine-induced rhabdomyolysis in one-half of cases. Cocaine was most frequently administered by intravenous injection or by smoking of the cocaine alkaloid. It has been suggested that renal failure is unrelated to the route of administration (155); however, we found that intravenous cocaine was associated with more severe muscle injury and a greater incidence of renal failure (105,107).

Urinalysis typically showed a positive orthotolidine reaction for heme. Proteinuria was detected by dipstick in two-thirds of cases. Renal failure developed in nearly one-half of the patients. Of those who developed renal failure, one-half were oliguric and an equal number required dialysis. Roth and associates (104) found evidence of more severe muscle injury in patients with cocaine-induced rhabdomyolysis who developed acute renal failure. Mean serum creatine phosphokinase levels in those who developed renal failure were 150 times the upper limit of normal and twice as high as in the group as a whole (104). In our own series, mean peak serum creatine phosphokinase levels exceeded 90,000 IU/L in cocaine addicts with rhabdomyolysis who developed acute renal failure as compared to a mean peak value of approximately 1,000 IU/L among nonazotemic addicts (107). Hypotension, hyperpyrexia, volume contraction, diffuse intravascular coagulation, and severe hepatic dysfunction were associated with the development of acute renal failure in both series as well as in many individual case reports. Of the 13 patients with renal failure reported by Roth and associates (104), 6 died. In contrast, we observed an excellent renal prognosis (107). In view of the rapid proliferation of cocaine addiction among young adults, cocaine-induced rhabdomyolysis has become an increasingly frequent cause of acute renal failure in urban areas.

Cocaine-Associated Nephropathy

Although the most frequent renal manifestation of cocaine abuse is acute renal failure due to nontraumatic rhabdomy-

olysis, cocaine may induce nephropathy by other mechanisms (182–209). In several cases, cocaine use was associated with acute renal failure in the absence of rhabdomyolysis or accelerated hypertension (207–209). Renal failure was attributed to cocaine-induced vasoconstriction leading to acute tubular necrosis. Cocaine may also precipitate malignant hypertension with rapid progression to end-stage renal failure (175,182,183,210).

Cocaine may unmask, exacerbate, or induce scleroderma and has been responsible for precipitating scleroderma renal crises (184,186). Cocaine is a potent arterial vasoconstrictor and may contribute to thrombosis by its ability to increase platelet aggregability, enhance thromboxane production, and induce endothelial injury. Renal infarction has been attributed to cocaine-induced renal artery vasospasm or arterial thrombosis (200,204,211,213). Cocaine use has also been associated with the development of microangiopathic hemolytic anemia, thrombocytopenia, and acute renal failure due to thrombotic microangiopathy in the absence of hypertension (187,188). Isolated case reports have linked cocaine with a variety of glomerular and tubulointerstitial renal diseases, including anti-glomerular basement membrane disease, acute interstitial nephritis, and systemic necrotizing vasculitis; however, these associations have not been clearly established (189–191,205).

In the rat kidney, cocaine has been shown to enhance mesangial cell uptake of macromolecules, indirectly stimulate mesangial cell proliferation, and induce release of macrophage secretory products, including interleukin-6 and transforming growth factor β (192,193). In addition, chronic administration of cocaine to rats causes renal injury leading to glomerular sclerosis and chronic tubulointerstitial damage (194). However, these experimental observations may not translate to human disease. It has been suggested that cocaine use may be a risk factor for hypertensive end-stage renal disease in African Americans (10,183,214–216). However, convincing evidence of a cause and effect relationship remains to be established.

Vupputuri et al. (215) found that the relative risk for mild renal functional impairment among 637 men enrolled in a hypertension clinic was increased to 2.3 with the use of any illicit drug, to 3.0 with cocaine use and to 3.9 with psychedelic drug use. Use of marijuana, amphetamines, or heroin did not lead to a significant increase in risk. In a cross-sectional study of 193 ESRD patients, Norris et al. (216) found that a clinical diagnosis of hypertensive nephrosclerosis was strongly associated with a history of cocaine use. Cocaine users had an earlier onset of ESRD despite only a brief history of hypertension. In contrast, Breclin and colleagues (195) studied blood pressure measurements in 301 predominantly African American males hospitalized for cocaine addiction treatment and concluded that cocaine use is associated with acute but not chronic hypertension. There was no significant difference in age-adjusted blood pressure in the cocaine users compared to National Health and Nutrition Examination Survey groups. In addition, microalbuminuria was not detected in these patients who had used cocaine for a mean of 12 years.

Several reports have attributed accelerated arteriosclerosis of the renal vasculature to cocaine use even in the absence of hypertension (196–199). DiPaolo and associates (197) compared 40 renal autopsy specimens from cocaine-related deaths with 40 specimens obtained from road accident victims. Kidneys from cocaine addicts showed extensive arteriosclerosis with medial thickening, luminal narrowing, and vessel obstruction, which were absent in control cases. In association with these vessel changes, cocaine addicts showed significantly more glomerular hyalinosis, periglomerular fibrosis, and interstitial cellular infiltration. The pathogenesis of accelerated hyperplastic atherosclerotic damage in cocaine addicts is speculative but may relate to repeated episodes of cocaine-induced vasospasm, mast cell activation, activation of the renin-angiotensin system, or cocaine-stimulated thromboxane production, platelet aggregation, or collagen synthesis. In addition, cocaine may modulate mononuclear cell infiltration of atherosclerotic plaques and may adversely affect lipoprotein metabolism (196).

Teratogenicity

Exposure to cocaine *in utero* due to maternal use has been associated with a more than four-fold risk of developing congenital urinary tract abnormalities (217–226). Hydronephrosis, horseshoe kidney, prune belly syndrome, renal agenesis, prominent renal pelvis, nephromegaly, unilateral small kidney and genital organ abnormalities have been described in association with *in utero* cocaine exposure (218,221). Reduced urine output has been observed in fetuses exposed to cocaine (223,225). Stillborn fetuses exposed to cocaine show thickening of the renal interlobular artery walls with narrowing of the lumen (224). These vascular abnormalities are reflected in higher renal artery resistance indices (227). Severe hypertension due to renal artery stenosis and persistent postnatal hypertension have been described after prenatal cocaine exposure (226,228). Renal vascular disease and congenital urinary tract abnormalities are also observed in experimental models of in utero cocaine exposure (220). In addition, an increased incidence of urinary tract infections has been observed in infants after prenatal cocaine exposure (229). It has been postulated that cocaine-induced vasoconstriction of uterine and fetal blood vessels may lead to developmental abnormalities. Alterations in calcium metabolism may also contribute. Persistent postnatal hypertension in the absence of renal anomalies has been attributed to dysfunction of the sympathetic nervous system (228).

Ecstasy (3–4 methylenedioxymethamphetamine) (MDMA) has been associated with acute renal failure, accelerated hypertension and electrolyte disturbances (173,230–239). A syndrome of hyperthermia, coagulopathy, rhabdomyolysis with acute renal failure, and hepatic failure may complicate ingestion of this agent (230,231,234,235). Acute renal failure may also arise as a result of accelerated hypertension (237). MDMA may cause inappropriate release of antidiuretic hormone with resultant hyponatremia and has also been reported to cause urinary retention due to bladder neck closure (173).

Systemic Necrotizing Vasculitis in Parenteral Drug Abusers

Citron and co-workers (240) described systemic necrotizing vasculitis in parenteral drug abusers, which was clinically similar to classic polyarteritis nodosa, and attributed this syndrome to abuse of amphetamines. Although a variety of drugs were involved, methamphetamine had been abused by all but 2 of their 14 patients and was used exclusively by one of them. An experimental model of amphetamine-induced cerebral vasculitis was developed in the rhesus monkey (241). Cerebral angiography demonstrated vessel spasm, with occasional microaneurysm formation, while histology showed generalized cerebral edema, hemorrhage, and infarction. However, the validity of this model has been questioned because severe hypertension is produced, which itself may be responsible for the histological and angiographic features observed (242).

An association exists between classic polyarteritis nodosa and hepatitis B surface antigenemia (243). Hepatitis B surface antigen has been found in the serum of 4% to 13% of parenteral drug abusers (244–247). Accordingly, some investigators have proposed that systemic necrotizing vasculitis in parenteral drug abusers may be related to hepatitis B surface antigen, thus discounting a pathogenetic role for amphetamine

(248). When sought, hepatitis B surface antigen has been found in the serum of some, but not all, drug abusers with systemic necrotizing vasculitis (242,248–252). In one study, hepatitis B surface antigen was demonstrated in fewer than one-third of cases (250). However, Koff and colleagues (248) describe one abuser of heroin and amphetamine with systemic necrotizing angiitis in whom hepatitis B surface antigenemia was transient. More recently, systemic necrotizing vasculitis has been associated with hepatitis C infection and cryoglobulinemia. It is possible that hepatitis B surface antigen-negative drug users with systemic necrotizing vasculitis reported in earlier series may have been infected with hepatitis C. Thus, it is unclear what role methamphetamine use, hepatitis B infection, and hepatitis C infection play in the pathogenesis of systemic necrotizing angiitis in drug abusers.

The clinical course and angiographic features of systemic necrotizing vasculitis have been described in 39 parenteral drug abusers, and in addition, isolated cerebral angiitis has been described in 20 others (36,240,242,248–259). Patients with widespread vasculitis ranged in age from 18 to 47 years (mean, 24 years); one-half were male. The duration of parenteral drug abuse invariably exceeded 3 months. When specified, amphetamines were among the agents abused in all but two patients, usually in association with multiple other drugs. Hepatitis B surface antigen was demonstrated in the serum of fewer than one-third of the 30 patients evaluated by Citron and Peters (250). Hepatitis B surface antigen was sought in five additional patients and was present in all (242,248,249,251,252). In five asymptomatic patients, the diagnosis was made on the basis of typical angiographic findings consisting of arterial aneurysms and sacculations involving multiple organs (240). In symptomatic cases, the duration of illness prior to presentation ranged widely from several days to 1 year. The severity of hypertension observed in this syndrome and its refractoriness to therapy has been emphasized (249). Hypertension was present in 13 of 17 patients. Malignant hypertension associated with papilledema, encephalopathy, or rapidly progressive renal failure occurred in six patients.

Renal manifestations were present in 4 of the 14 patients reported by Citron and co-workers (240). Uremia developed in two cases and hematuria, proteinuria, or azotemia were present in the other two. Renal involvement was seen in a total of 11 patients; 7 of whom were uremic. Severe or accelerated hypertension was characteristic of all but one of those who developed renal failure. Small kidneys with segmental ischemic atrophy, reflecting old as well as more recent renal infarctions, were characteristic findings at postmortem examination. Necrotizing arteriolitis frequently involved the interlobular and arcuate arteries. Vascular changes of different ages often coexisted. Glomerulonephritis was not observed.

Of the 11 patients with renal involvement, 3 died in uremia and 4 others died due to visceral infarction, cardiovascular complications, or aneurysmal rupture. One patient underwent renal transplantation. Follow-up was not available in the remaining three uremic patients. The response to immunosuppressive therapy has been inconsistent. Four patients responded favorably to therapy with steroids or cytotoxic agents. In one of these, cytotoxic therapy induced a remission despite an equivocal response to steroids. However, relapse occurred after discontinuation of therapy. Two patients died and a third developed accelerated hypertension and renal failure during corticosteroid therapy.

Nephropathy in Glue and Solvent "Sniffers"

Inhalation of the fumes of toluene or toluene-containing compounds (spray paint, household and model glue, lacquer and paint thinners) may be associated with a variety of electrolyte and acid–base disturbances (260–281). Taher and co-workers (260) first recognized nonanion gap hyperchloremic metabolic acidosis in association with toluene "sniffing" in two patients, one of whom was studied in detail. Urine pH was inappropriately high, and studies of urinary bicarbonate excretion suggested a distal renal tubular acidosis. Azotemia was absent, and proximal tubular reabsorption of solutes was unimpaired. The acidifying defect was rapidly reversible but recurred with repeated episodes of toluene abuse. Renal potassium wasting was attributed to hyperaldosteronism, and generalized muscle weakness and flaccid quadriparesis resulted from severe hypokalemia. Numerous other cases of hyperchloremic metabolic acidosis due to toluene inhalation have subsequently been reported (261–280). In addition, transient congenital renal tubular dysfunction with hyperchloremic metabolic acidosis due to maternal toluene abuse has been described (267,268,270,281).

Moss and colleagues (263) reported proximal tubular dysfunction with toluene abuse. They describe a patient with hyperchloremic metabolic acidosis, hypokalemia, hypouricemia, hypophosphatemia, and hypocalcemia. Proximal reabsorption of uric acid, glucose, phosphate, calcium, and amino acids was impaired. The high fractional excretion of bicarbonate suggested a proximal defect, while submaximal urinary acidification during ammonium chloride loading suggested an additional distal defect. Microscopic hematuria and pyuria were present. Despite abstinence from toluene, hyperchloremic metabolic acidosis persisted, whereas the other tubular defects reversed, only to recur with repeated exposure. Two additional cases with hyperchloremic metabolic acidosis due to proximal bicarbonate wasting were described in this report (263).

Streicher and associates (265) reported 25 cases of toluene abuse associated with hypokalemia in 13 patients, hypophosphatemia in 10 patients, and hyperchloremic metabolic acidosis in 19 patients. Hypokalemia and hypophosphatemia contributed to muscle weakness, which was a frequent presenting complaint and which progressed in some to quadriparesis. Several patients developed nontraumatic rhabdomyolysis, perhaps related to the combined effects of hypokalemia and hypophosphatemia on skeletal muscle. In other cases, rhabdomyolysis occurred in the absence of these electrolyte disturbances, leading the authors to suggest that toluene may have direct toxic effects on skeletal and cardiac muscle. Hypokalemia was attributed to a redistribution of extracellular potassium. Despite normal values at presentation, serum calcium levels declined during fluid repletion, leading to symptomatic hypocalcemia in some patients.

Batlle and colleagues studied the mechanisms underlying toluene-induced distal renal tubular acidosis (274). Toluene abusers showed normal bicarbonate reabsorption but were unable to maximally acidify their urine. Inability to normally increase urinary partial pressure of carbon dioxide (PCO_2) in a highly alkaline urine excluded hydrogen ion back-diffusion as a cause of the acidification defect. Toluene decreased the rate of proton secretion in a turtle urinary bladder preparation, leading the authors to conclude that the defect in distal acidification observed in toluene abusers is due to impaired active hydrogen ion transport.

An elevated anion gap was found in approximately one-third of reported cases of toluene-induced metabolic acidosis (273). The elevated anion gap is due to the accumulation of products of toluene metabolism (benzoic acid and hippuric acid). These metabolites are more likely to accumulate and cause anion gap acidosis in those with impaired renal function. In contrast, in individuals with normal renal function, overproduction and urinary excretion of the anions of these organic acids may contribute to the development of nonanion gap hyperchloremic metabolic acidosis (261,273).

Heavy toluene exposure has been associated with pyuria in nearly one-third of reported cases, while microscopic hema-

turia and proteinuria were each observed in approximately one-fifth (264,282–284). In the series reported by Streicher and associates (265), abnormalities of the urinary sediment were particularly frequent, occurring in 18 of 21 patients, and included hematuria, pyuria, and proteinuria ranging up to 1 g/24 hours. Similarly, pyuria was universal, and hematuria and proteinuria each occurred in three-fourths of the 16 episodes of toluene intoxication reported by Voigts and Kaufman (264).

Acute renal failure has been observed in association with toluene inhalation (227,261,264,285–292). Transient renal insufficiency was observed in only one of the 25 cases reported by Streicher and associates (265). By contrast, Voigts and Kaufman (264) describe transient renal insufficiency in 38% of 16 episodes of toluene intoxication. Renal failure may be caused by nontraumatic rhabdomyolysis, hypotension-induced acute tubular necrosis, or in association with hepatic failure (261,285–286,289,290). Serial renal biopsies in one patient with irreversible acute renal failure demonstrated progressive tubulointerstitial injury (287). Of interest is a report of a long-term regular toluene abuser who developed recurrent nephrolithiasis due to toluene-induced distal renal tubular acidosis causing bone calcium mobilization and hypercalcuria (262). Renal calculi have also been observed in other chronic toluene abusers (269,292,293). Anti-glomerular basement membrane–mediated glomerulonephritis, focal glomerulosclerosis, and membranoproliferative glomerulonephritis have been associated with glue sniffing, however, a causal relationship has not been established (294–301).

Acute renal failure has been reported in inhalation abusers of trichloroethylene and other compounds contained in cleaning fluid and other solvents ("solvent sniffers") (302,303). Oliguria and renal insufficiency, with or without associated acute centrilobular necrosis of the liver, were reversible in all cases. Modest proteinuria was a universal feature, whereas microscopic hematuria was infrequent. Similarly, occupational inhalation exposure to trichloroethylene has been associated with reversible acute oliguric renal failure, abnormalities of the urinary sediment, and fatal combined hepatic and renal failure (304–308). Examination of renal tissue in one case showed acute tubular necrosis. Anti-glomerular basement membrane–mediated glomerulonephritis and hemolytic—uremic syndrome have also been associated with solvent abuse (309,310).

Hepatitis-Related Glomerulonephritis in Drug Abusers

Parenteral drug abusers are frequently infected with hepatitis B or hepatitis C (244–247). The association of these infections with glomerular disease is discussed in Chapter 59.

Human Immunodeficiency Virus-Associated Nephropathy in Drug Abusers

This subject is discussed in Chapter 59.

LITHIUM AND THE KIDNEY

Early histopathologic studies of the kidney in lithium-treated psychiatric patients raised great concern about the potential for serious nephrotoxicity (311,312). However, these disturbing estimates of the frequency and severity of lithium-induced renal injury were based on uncontrolled studies of patients who were selected because of prior acute lithium intoxication or severe polyuria (311,312). Clearly, lithium intoxication may be associated with acute deterioration of renal function, which can be followed by irreversible renal damage (313–316). However, the key question is whether maintenance therapy with doses in the therapeutic range may cause chronic renal injury and if so, how often this occurs. Based on the publication of more rigorous studies, a more accurate picture of lithium nephrotoxicity has emerged. However, even these studies have failed to fully define the spectrum of lithium nephrotoxicity.

Adequacy of Clinical Studies

Results of studies evaluating renal function in lithium-treated patients must be interpreted cautiously, with attention to differences in methodology and experimental design. Published reports differ with respect to sample size, criteria for patient selection, treatment duration, dose and type of lithium preparation, plasma lithium levels, concurrent therapy with other psychotropic agents, and the reference range used to determine normality. Exclusion of preexisting renal disease by pretreatment evaluation has not been a consistent feature.

Studies lacking a suitable control group are of limited informational value. An ideal control group would consist of patients suffering from affective disorders who have never received lithium and who are well matched for demographic factors including use or other psychotropic agents. In addition, behavioral factors such as psychogenic water drinking cannot be controlled. Prospective longitudinal studies, as opposed to the cross-sectional approach, provide the most reliable assessment of the effects of lithium on renal function. However, no longitudinal study has included a matched psychiatric group to control for the effects of aging and of other psychotropic agents on renal function.

Clinical Features of Lithium Nephrotoxicity

Acute Renal Failure

Acute lithium intoxication severe enough to require hospitalization is associated with renal insufficiency in up to 75% of cases (313,314,317–325). Circulatory collapse contributes to acute renal failure in some cases (319). Saline loading may improve renal function, suggesting that volume depletion due to lithium-induced natriuresis contributes to impaired renal function. However, a reduced glomerular filtration rate (GFR) frequently persists even after volume expansion (313,314,320). Examination of renal tissue in patients with acute renal failure associated with lithium intoxication has demonstrated proximal tubular necrosis, minimal histologic abnormalities, or nonspecific findings of distal tubular injury (319,321,325). In some, chronic tubulointerstitial nephritis has been found in the absence of acute tubular injury (313,314). Renal insufficiency may persist after recovery from an episode of lithium intoxication (313,314). In addition, rare cases of nontraumatic rhabdomyolysis have been described in association with lithium-induced hyperosmolar dehydration or neuroleptic malignant syndrome (326,327).

Chronic Renal Insufficiency

Whether or not lithium therapy may lead to progressive renal failure in the absence of clinical episodes of intoxication has been debated for decades. Identification of occasional patients with severely impaired renal function in cross-sectional or prospective studies of lithium-treated patients has limited informational value because renal disease unrelated to lithium cannot be excluded. The failure to identify patients with end-stage renal failure in longitudinal studies does not necessarily

exclude the possibility that a small subgroup may progress to uremia or that the duration of follow-up was insufficient. Until recently, remarkably few patients have been reported in whom advanced renal functional impairment or end-stage renal failure was attributed to lithium therapy (319,328–334).

Thirteen longitudinal studies measured serum creatinine or GFR prior to initiation of lithium therapy and again after periods of treatment ranging from 1 to 10 years (337–349). In addition, 13 longitudinal series measured serum creatinine or GFR on repeated occasions during the course of lithium therapy (315,334,335,338,346,350–357). No significant change in serum creatinine was observed in 16 of these reports after an average follow-up period of 4.5 years (315,335,340,343–348,351–356). A modest increase in serum creatinine, on the order of 10% to 20%, was reported in four studies over a follow-up period averaging 7 years (341,342,347,349). The rise in serum creatinine was not a general phenomenon but was restricted to a small number of patients. When filtration rate was measured by clearance techniques, GFR was unchanged in several series after an average follow-up period of 5 years (339–342,344,345). Other studies showed a 6% to 20% decline in GFR after a follow-up period that averaged 4 years (315,335,337,338,347,350,355–358). However, none of these studies was properly controlled for the effects of aging on renal function. Lokkegaard (347) evaluated 142 lithium-treated patients and found only a modest decline in GFR after 5 to 17 years, with none falling below the range of normal until after 7 years of therapy. It has been suggested that GFR only begins to decline after a decade or more of therapy (359,360). A prospective, longitudinal study of 14 lithium-treated patients performed by Presne et al. (334) found that creatinine clearance declined 1.93 mL/min/year over a mean follow-up period of 18.9 years (discussed in greater detail below).

Ten cross-sectional series compared GFR or serum creatinine levels in lithium-treated patients with a control group of patients suffering from affective disorders who had never received lithium (nine studies), with healthy controls (one study), or with both (one study) (316,351,355,361,370). In four of these studies, serum creatinine did not differ between lithium-treated patients and controls. In three others, a modest increase of serum creatinine, on the order of 10%, was observed in lithium-treated patients. Creatinine clearance was measured in six studies in which the average duration of lithium therapy was 6 years and was found not to differ between lithium-treated patients and controls (316,350,353,355,361,369). In another study, creatinine clearance was 42% lower in patients treated with lithium for 80 months than in lithium-naïve controls (370). In two studies, GFR was measured isotopically after an average duration of 7.5 years on lithium and was found to be modestly reduced (363,364).

Renal function has been assessed in lithium-treated patients in 24 cross-sectional reports that lacked any control group (329,330,359,366,371–391). Serum creatinine was found to be modestly elevated above the normal range in approximately 5% of patients. Five observers failed to demonstrate any reduction in GFR below the range of normal in lithium-treated patients (374,381,383,387,389). Other investigators found that GFR measured by creatinine clearance, isotopically, or by inulin clearance was modestly reduced below the range of normal in 3% to 36% of lithium-treated patients (359,366,367,371,372,376–380,382,384,385,388,390,391).

Data are inconsistent with respect to the relationship between various therapeutic variables and renal function. Several studies have found an inverse correlation between GFR and duration of lithium therapy (334,357,375,389,390,392). However, numerous other investigators have failed to confirm this observation (315,351,364,368–370,373,377,380,382,384,385,389,391). Most have failed to find any correlation between GFR and average serum lithium level or total cumulative dose (334,341,345,347,368–371,379,380,382,384); however, contrary data exist (334,347).

In summary, in most studies, adverse effects of lithium on GFR were modest and of little clinical significance. However, two recent studies suggest that chronic administration of lithium over decades may lead to end-stage renal failure (332,334).

Markowitz et al. (332) describe 24 lithium-treated patients who underwent renal biopsy due to renal insufficiency. The patients ranged in age from 26 to 57 and were predominantly white; 50% were men. The duration of lithium therapy ranged from 2 to 25 years (mean 13.6 years). Serum creatinine ranged from 1.3 to 8.0 mg/dL (mean, 2.8 mg/dL). Proteinuria exceeded 1 g/day in 10 patients, 6 of whom manifested the nephrotic syndrome. Only two patients had experienced prior episodes of acute lithium intoxication. Renal biopsy showed chronic tubulointerstitial nephropathy, associated in all but one case with cortical and medullary tubular cysts or dilation. Focal segmental glomerular sclerosis was seen in 50% and global glomerulosclerosis in 100% of biopsies. Despite discontinuation of lithium therapy in 19 of 20 patients, 8 progressed to end-stage renal failure over a mean of 30.6 months. A serum creatinine of 2.5 mg/dL or greater predicted progression to ESRD despite discontinuation of lithium. Renal function improved in only three patients, all of whom discontinued lithium before the serum creatinine exceeded 2.5 mg/dL. These authors conclude that renal dysfunction due to lithium is often irreversible, may be associated with proteinuria due to glomerular involvement, and may progress to end-stage renal failure.

Presne et al. (334) studied 54 patients with lithium-induced renal insufficiency and an additional 20 lithium-treated psychiatric patients, 14 of whom were studied prospectively. Eighteen percent had proteinuria, which exceeded 1 g/day approximately 10%. Microscopic hematuria was present in 24% and leucocyturia in 31%. After a mean of 10 years, calculated creatinine clearance fell from 62.6 to 41.4 mL/minute at a rate of 2.29 mL/min/year. Heavy proteinuria, which exceeded 750 mg/24 hours, was associated with a more rapid decline in renal function. Twelve patients reached end stage renal failure. They had higher serum creatinine levels at entry and two-third had proteinuria. Few had a history of lithium intoxication. Renal functional impairment generally required a duration of lithium therapy exceeding 20 years. Discontinuation of lithium when the calculated creatinine clearance exceeded 40 mL/min was usually associated with improvement in renal function, whereas discontinuation of therapy when renal function was more impaired was usually associated with continued deterioration. In the 14 patients studied prospectively, calculated creatinine clearance fell at a rate of 1.93 mL/min/year from 77.8 to 40.8 after a mean follow-up of 18.9 years. Presne et al. (334) performed renal biopsies in 29 patients (334). Interstitial fibrosis and tubular atrophy was present in 85%. Interstitial fibrosis was predictive of the final creatinine clearance and correlated with the duration of lithium administration and the cumulative dose. Tubular cysts were present in 28% and tubular dilation in 66% and correlated with the duration of lithium administration but not with renal function. The median percentage of sclerotic glomeruli was 10% (range 0% to 90%); only one patient had focal glomerulosclerosis.

These investigators surveyed dialysis centers in France and identified 24 patients in whom end-stage renal failure was attributed to lithium (0.22% of the dialysis population). The average duration of lithium administration prior to the development of end-stage renal failure was 20 years. By comparison, the incidence rate of end-stage renal disease attributed to lithium in Australia is 0.7% and in New Zealand, 0.2%.

In the series reported by Presne et al. (334), it is difficult to evaluate the relative contributions of concomitant neuroleptic therapy, hypercalcemia, and hypertension to progressive renal injury. Only 1 of the 12 patients who progressed to end-stage renal disease underwent renal biopsy. Segmental glomerulosclerosis was present in only 1 of the 29 renal biopsy specimens, including nine cases selected for lithium-induced renal insufficiency. It is difficult to reconcile the fact that focal and segmental glomerulosclerosis was common among the patients reported by Markowitz et al. (332), but rare in the series reported by Presne et al. (334). Nevertheless, prudence dictates an awareness of the potential for nephrotoxicity, as well as periodic monitoring of renal function and utilization of the lowest serum lithium levels capable of achieving a therapeutic response.

Urinary Concentrating Ability

Six longitudinal studies evaluated urinary concentrating ability before initiation of lithium therapy and again after treatment periods ranging up to 8 years (337,338,341,342,393,394). Most showed a 10% to 15% decline in maximum urinary osmolarity (Uosm) within weeks to months after initiation of therapy (338,393,394). Schou and Vestergaard (341) report a large cohort of patients before and up to 7 years after initiating lithium therapy. The investigators maintained a mean serum lithium level of 0.6 mmol/L, which was lower than previously recommended therapeutic serum levels (0.8 to 1.2 mmol/L). Maximum Uosm declined 7% from pretreatment levels and was abnormal in only 6% of patients (341). Similarly, two other reports in which serum lithium levels were maintained below 0.7 mmol/L found little decline in maximum Uosm after 3 and 8 years of treatment (337,342). In three studies, urine volume increased only modestly from prelithium levels after periods of treatment ranging up to 8 years, while in a fourth, urine volume increased by 23% (338,341,342,394). In patients maintained on a low therapeutic serum lithium level treatment regimen by Schou and Vestergaard (341), mean urine volume rose by only 10% to 20%, and the number of patients with severe polyuria did not increase.

Six longitudinal studies performed serial measurements of urinary concentrating ability in patients treated with lithium for 3 to 10 years and again after an additional treatment period ranging up to 10 years (315,335,338,355,356,357,363,395). Two failed to find any interval decline in urinary concentrating ability when first assessed 5 to 10 years after initiation of treatment and again after an additional treatment period of 2 to 10 years (315,335,363). By contrast, in three other studies, maximum Uosm declined by 7% to 20% between measurements first made 4 to 6 years after initiation of treatment and again after an additional treatment period of 2 to 8 years (355,356,357,395). Urine volume increased by 10% to 20% in two reports but showed no significant interval change in another (335,350,355,363).

Five longitudinal studies measured urinary concentrating ability in unselected patients during long-term lithium treatment and again after discontinuation of therapy (335,345,355,392,396,397). Maximum Uosm increased 10% to 30% within weeks to months after withdrawal of lithium but remained subnormal in all but one study. Bucht and Wahlin (392) examined a large cohort of lithium patients for periods up to 1 year after discontinuation of lithium. Maximum Uosm increased by nearly 30% in the first 8 weeks after lithium withdrawal, but no further improvement was observed thereafter (392). The percentage of patients with abnormal concentrating ability decreased from 96% while on lithium to 63% 1 year after discontinuation of lithium (392). Three studies reported urine volume measurements, which normalized after discontinuation of lithium in two studies and never increased in the third (335,355,396).

Sixteen cross-sectional studies compared concentrating ability in lithium-treated patients with control subjects suffering from affective disorders or with healthy controls (316,339, 351,355,360,361,363–367,369,392,395–400). In 10, urinary concentrating ability was reduced in lithium patients compared to psychiatric controls (316,339,355,360,363–365, 369,370,392,395–397). The average maximum Uosm was 589 mOsm/kg H$_2$O on lithium (range, 406 to 737 mOsm/kg H$_2$O) versus 818 mOsm/kg H2O in psychiatric controls (range, 683 to 850 mOsm/kg H2O). On average, 67% of patients treated with lithium for 5 to 10 years (range, 36% to 85%) showed abnormal urinary concentrating ability compared to 34% of psychiatric controls (range, 10% to 48%). By contrast, in three other studies, urinary concentrating ability did not differ between patients treated with lithium for 3 to 8 years and psychiatric controls (351,361,366,367,400). One of the latter reports maintained patients on low therapeutic serum lithium levels, while another utilized a single-dose schedule. Urine volume was increased in lithium-treated patients compared to psychiatric controls in nearly all studies (278,316, 339,360,361,363,364,366,367,369,392,396–398,400). Urine volume averaged 2.6 L/24 hours in lithium-treated patients compared to 1.8 L/24 hours in psychiatric controls. In the one study that failed to show any difference in urine volume between lithium-treated patients and psychiatric controls, patients were maintained on low therapeutic serum lithium levels (366,367).

Twenty-eight investigations evaluated concentrating ability in unselected lithium-treated patients (315,345,347–349,359, 366,367,371,372,374,375,377–379,381,383–391,393,401–405). When compared to the accepted range of normal, the prevalence of impaired urinary concentrating ability among patients treated with lithium for an average of 2 to 19 years ranged from 16% to 85% (mean, 53%), while the prevalence of increased urine volume ranged from 6% to 70% (mean, 24%). Only three groups failed to find any impairment in urinary concentrating ability in lithium-treated patients (366,367,374,381). Of note, two of these maintained patients on low therapeutic serum lithium levels.

Data are inconsistent with respect to the relationship between various therapeutic variables and concentrating ability. An inverse correlation between maximum Uosm and duration of lithium therapy or cumulative lithium dose has often been reported (316,345,347,349,355,357,371,378,379,385,390,392, 395–397,406). A positive correlation between urine flow rate and duration of lithium therapy has also been described (347, 348,374,375,385,389,396,407,408). However, many other studies have failed to confirm one or both of these observations (315,339,341,347,356,369,370,372,378,381,384,389, 391,406). Serum lithium levels correlated inversely with urinary concentrating ability or positively with urine flow rate in some reports (315,339,341,355,378,387,392,407), but not in others (341,347,357,369,370,372,381,384,393,406). Notwithstanding these inconsistent data, the preponderance of evidence suggests that maintenance of low serum lithium levels limits the adverse impact of lithium therapy on urinary concentrating ability and urine flow rate.

Polyuria and Polydipsia

Polyuria and impairment of urinary concentrating ability develop rapidly after initiating therapy and improve after lithium withdrawal (392,409,410). Hypernatremic dehydration may result if access to water is restricted (411–414). Inhibition of vasopressin-stimulated water flow in the collecting duct is primarily responsible for the concentrating defect (254,415–419). However, factors other than resistance to vasopressin may also contribute to lithium-induced polyuria. Typically the defect in concentrating ability is not severe enough to prevent elabora-

tion of a hypertonic urine, and in most patients polyuria cannot be explained solely by the degree of reduction in maximum Uosm. Those who show only a modest impairment in maximum Uosm may nevertheless produce large 24-hour urine volumes. Polyuria may be observed as well, even in patients with normal urinary concentrating ability. This constellation of observations can only be explained if excessive water drinking contributes to the polyuria in many lithium-treated patients. Although lithium clearly stimulates thirst in rat models, it is generally claimed that lithium-induced stimulation of thirst does not play a significant role in the development of polyuria in humans (319,420–424). The finding of normal or elevated plasma levels of vasopressin in lithium-treated polyuric patients is cited as evidence against a prominent role for primary polydipsia (313,366,398,415,425–427). However, since lithium induces resistance to vasopressin, it is reasonable to suggest that these patients operate at an elevated set point and that finding normal or mildly raised plasma vasopressin levels in this setting may still reflect some suppression by excessive water drinking. Increased fluid intake may be psychogenic in origin or due to dry mouth resulting from other psychotropic agents (424).

Thiazide diuretics may ameliorate lithium-induced polyuria through a reduction in solute-free water excretion (420,428–430). Thiazide diuretics induce a natriuresis, which results in a compensatory increase in sodium and lithium reabsorption in the proximal tubule (431). Thiazide diuretics may raise serum lithium levels and precipitate lithium intoxication by inducing extracellular volume depletion (420,429,430). Nonsteroidal antiinflammatory agents may also be used to treat lithium-induced polyuria, albeit, at the risk of precipitating lithium toxicity due to increased tubular reabsorption of lithium (432–443). Inhibition of prostaglandin synthesis increases cyclic adenosine monophosphate through increased production or inhibition of degradation (438). Nonsteriodal antiinflammatory agents also enhance sodium reabsorption leading to a secondary increase in passive water absorption (236). Both these factors contribute to antagonism of lithium-induced polyuria. Amiloride is the drug of choice to raise maximum urinary osmolarity and ameliorate lithium-induced polyuria (444–446). Amiloride antagonizes the inhibitory effect of lithium on vasopressin-induced water transport by blocking the cellular uptake of lithium through the amiloride-sensitive sodium channel (444).

Proteinuria

The effect of long-term lithium therapy on urinary protein excretion is controversial. However, it is clear that in the vast majority of patients any observed effects are modest and of little clinical significance. Administration of lithium to rats increases urinary protein excretion (447). In six longitudinal investigations of lithium-treated patients extending from 90 days to 7 years, no increase in the urinary excretion of protein, albumin, or β2-microglobulin was demonstrated (315,337,341,343,356,448). Similarly, in 11 cross-sectional reports of lithium-treated patients, albuminuria and low molecular-weight proteinuria were absent (361, 365–367,374,381–383,390,391,448). In contrast, one longitudinal and five cross-sectional studies showed modest proteinuria or albuminuria in lithium-treated patients (332,334,365,379,408,449). Markowitz et al. (332) reported proteinuria in 10 of 24 lithium-treated patients undergoing renal biopsy for renal insufficiency (six in the nephrotic range) (332). Similarly, Presne et al. (334) reported proteinuria in 11 of 62 lithium-treated patients; proteinuria exceeded 1 g in 10%. In six other studies, urinary excretion of low–molecular-weight proteins including β2-microglobulin and N-acetyl-β-glucosaminidase was increased (369,379,383,408,450,451).

At least 39 cases of the nephrotic syndrome have been described in association with lithium therapy (332,334,359,452–473). The duration of lithium therapy prior to the development of nephrotic syndrome ranged widely from weeks to 14 years. Serum lithium levels were in the therapeutic range in nearly all cases. Most renal biopsies showed minimal glomerular changes. Mesangial hypercellularity or focal or global glomerular sclerosis was observed in other cases. Resolution of the nephrotic syndrome after discontinuation of lithium and recurrence upon rechallenge in several cases strongly support an association between lithium and minimal change disease (452,454,462). In one case, the nephrotic syndrome due to focal glomerular sclerosis remitted after discontinuation of lithium (467), but failed to remit in other cases (332,453,463). Markowitz and colleagues (332) describe the nephrotic syndrome in six lithium-treated patients, all of whom showed focal or global glomerulosclerosis on renal biopsy. These investigators suggest that lithium may be responsible for a podocytopathy.

Pathophysiology

Concentrating Ability

Primary among the factors that contribute to impaired urinary concentrating ability is lithium-induced inhibition of vasopressin-stimulated water flow in the collecting duct (353,415–419). This effect has been attributed to inhibition of adenylate cyclase activity (353,415–419). As a result, lithium blunts vasopressin-stimulated synthesis of cyclic adenosine monophosphate (cAMP), which mediates the hydroosmotic actions of vasopressin in the collecting duct (415,419). Although the primary site of action of lithium on renal concentrating ability is at the luminal surface of the cortical collecting duct, lithium also influences vasopressin-stimulated cAMP synthesis in the medullary thick ascending limb and in medullary collecting tubules (416,484).

Vasopressin binds to the V2 receptor and induces a conformational change, which enables a stimulatory guanyl-nucleotide regulatory protein to be activated by intracellular guanosine triphosphate (438). Once activated, the stimulatory G protein in turn activates the catalytic subunit of adenyl cyclase to enhance cAMP generation (438). A study of the effects of lithium on medullary collecting tubules in a rat model of chronic oral lithium administration suggests that lithium-induced inhibition of vasopressin-sensitive adenylate cyclase activity is mediated via activation of an inhibitory G protein (475). In contrast, earlier studies suggested that lithium acts by inhibiting activation of the stimulatory G protein (353,476). Magnesium plays an essential role in transducing vasopressin-induced activation of the stimulatory G protein (476). Antagonism of magnesium's actions by lithium may explain the ability of magnesium loading to reverse the inhibitory effects of lithium on adenyl cylase activity.

Studies in a variety of vasopressin-responsive tissues demonstrate that lithium acts at points both proximal and distal to the generation of cAMP (353,393,416–418,477–482). In some vasopressin-responsive tissues, lithium fails to inhibit cAMP–analog-stimulated water flow, suggesting a site of action proximal to the generation of cAMP (481). However, in other tissues, including cortical collecting tubules from lithium-treated rabbits, lithium inhibits the hydroosmotic actions of cAMP analogs, suggesting a site of action beyond the generation of cAMP (393,417,480). Lithium does not appear to enhance degradation of cAMP via activation of phosphodiesterase; however, contrary data exist (418,483,484).

Aquaporin-2 is the apical water channel of the principal cell and the primary target for regulation of collecting duct water permeability by vasopressin (485). Cyclic AMP and protein kinase A are involved in the regulation of acquaporin-2 expression as well as vesicular trafficking of aquaporin-2 (486,487). Lithium-fed rats show decreased expression of aquaporin-2 protein and reduced mRNA levels in cortical and inner medullary collecting duct principal cells (485,488–493). Levels of acquaporin-3 levels are also decreased in the kidney of lithium-treated rats, whereas acquaporin-6 levels are increased and acquaporin-1 and acquaporin-4 levels are unchanged (485,488,492,494,495). In addition, the fraction of intercalated collecting duct cells is increased at the expense of a reduced fraction of aquaporin-2-expressing principal cells (488,496).

Lithium also inhibits delivery of aquaporin-2 to the plasma membrane (494). The presence of a cAMP response element in the 5' untranslated region of the aquaporin-2 gene suggests that the effects of lithium on aquaporin-2 expression and targeting may be due to inhibition of cAMP production (497). However, lithium's downregulation of aquaporin-2 expression is only partially reversed by 1-desamino-8d-arginine-vasopressin, whereas targeting to the apical plasma membrane is restored (494).

Lithium also decreases vasopressin V2 receptor density but has no effect on binding affinity (498). Some investigators suggest that enhanced synthesis of cyclooxygenase products may also play a role in mediating the effects of lithium on water transport; however, other studies fail to support this hypothesis (475,499–501). Carney and co-workers (502) have suggested that impaired urinary concentrating ability may result from lithium-induced upregulation of circulating parathyroid hormone, which competitively inhibits the hydroosmotic actions of vasopressin. Lithium-induced hyperparathyroidism may also impair concentrating ability via hypercalcemia-induced downregulation of aquarin-2 (485).

Factors other than resistance to vasopressin also contribute to the impairment of concentrating ability induced by lithium. In rare patients, central diabetes insipidus may coexist (319,362,393,399,444,503). Lithium-induced suppression of proximal tubular sodium and water reabsorption increases delivery of filtrate to the ascending limb, thereby increasing solute-free water generation (420,482). This increased delivery of tubular fluid to collecting tubule cells that are resistant to the hydroosmotic action of vasopressin may contribute to polyuria in those with excessive water intake (420,482). In patients with renal functional impairment and a reduced number of functioning nephrons, an osmotic solute diuresis in remaining nephrons may also contribute to impaired urinary concentrating ability. In addition, high urine flow rates and disturbances in sodium transport may impair medullary urea trapping and disrupt the medullary osmotic gradient (418). Whereas earlier direct measurements of the corticopapillary gradient have yielded conflicting results (418,420,504,505), Klein et al. (491) suggest that chronic administration of lithium reduces inner medullary interstitial osmolarity due to reduced interstitial urea and sodium chloride concentration. When administered to rats, lithium down-regulated expression of the urea transporters UT-A1 and UT-B in the renal inner medulla and inhibited vasopressin-stimulated UT-A1 phosphorylation in inner medullary collecting duct suspensions (491). Thus, reduced UTA-1 and UT-B protein and/or reduced sensitivity of UT-A1 to phosphorylation by vasopressin contribute to a decrease the in inner medullary interstitial urea concentration in lithium-treated rats (491).

Structural injury to tubules and interstitial tissue may contribute to reduced maximal Uosm after prolonged lithium administration. If this were the case, then the urinary concentrating defect might progress with increasing duration of therapy and persist in some patients after withdrawal of lithium. Although polyuria frequently corrects within several weeks after discontinuation of lithium, several longitudinal observations have shown a failure to normalize urinary concentrating ability up to 12 months after lithium withdrawal (311,345,392,396,397,506). Although controversial, several investigators have found a correlation between polyuria or impaired urinary concentrating ability and duration of lithium therapy, lithium dose, or histopathologic lesions (335,349,371,377,383,392,397,403,507). In addition, several patients have been reported in whom polyuria and impaired urinary concentrating ability persisted up to a decade after discontinuation of lithium (396,415,420,508–516). Persistence of impaired urinary concentrating ability was frequently associated with reduced GFR and correlated with chronic tubulointerstitial nephritis (510,511,513).

Normal or elevated plasma levels of vasopressin have been demonstrated in lithium-treated patients with impaired urinary concentrating ability (313,366,398,415,425–427). Hypothalamic responses to water loading and water deprivation are normal in most but not all cases (313–316,370). Lithium-induced central diabetes insipidus has been described in a small number of patients (370,393,399,481,503). Of note, diminished renal response to vasopressin and increased serum levels of vasopressin has been demonstrated in some lithium-treated patients with normal urinary concentrating ability (366). Thus, despite lithium-induced renal resistance to vasopressin, it appears that water balance may be maintained by compensatory increases in serum vasopressin levels in some patients (366).

Sodium Handling

Lithium inhibits reabsorption of sodium by the proximal tubule and by nephron segments beyond the loop of Henle (319,521,522). Although data are conflicting, lithium does not appear to impair sodium transport in the thick ascending limb of the loop of Henle (319,521–525). Lithium directly competes with sodium for tubular transport; however, the importance of this effect in humans is controversial (319,521,522). In addition, lithium antagonizes the tubular sodium-retaining properties of mineralocorticoids (319,526–530).

Lithium induces an immediate sodium and water diuresis, which lasts 1 to 2 days (531,532). Transient natriuresis is followed by a period of sodium and water retention lasting 4 to 5 days, associated with increased serum levels of aldosterone (531,533). This is followed by a return of serum aldosterone to pre-lithium levels and a return to sodium balance (319,533).

Downregulation of the amiloride-sensitive sodium channel (ENaC) contributes, at least in part, to the sodium wasting associated with lithium therapy (492,534). Nielson et al. (492) found a marked reduction in the β and γ subunits of ENaC in the principal cells of cortical and outer medullary collecting ducts of lithium-fed rats. These finding help explain the observation that lithium-treated animals show an impaired renal responsive to amiloride and mineralocorticoids (530). Downregulation of the Na-Cl cotransporter in the distal convoluted tubule may also contribute to lithium-induced sodium wasting, however this finding is controversial (485). In contrast, other major sodium transporters, including the type 3 Na/H exchanger, the α subunit of Na-K-ATPase and the bumetanide-sensitive Na-K-2Cl cotransporter do not contribute to the development of lithium-induced polyuria or increased sodium excretion (485,492). The expression of these transporters after administration of lithium to rats has generally (but not universally) been found to be unchanged or increased, presumably as a compensatory response to sodium wasting (490,493).

Acute administration of large doses of lithium raises plasma renin and aldosterone levels, secondary to lithium-induced natriuresis and perhaps to a direct effect of lithium on the juxtaglomerular apparatus (319,502,531,535,536). Most studies suggest that chronic administration of lithium is associated with normal plasma levels and appropriate responses of the renin–angiotensin axis to various stimuli (319,394,536–538). In contrast, other studies have demonstrated activation of the renin–angiotensin system in patients on long-term lithium therapy, possibly as a compensatory response to lithium-induced mineralocorticoid resistance (539–541).

Renal Lithium Handling

Lithium is not protein-bound and is freely filtered at the glomerulus (313,336,542,543). Approximately 80% of filtered lithium is reabsorbed by the nephron, primarily in the proximal tubule (313,336,542,543). Proximal reabsorption of lithium is enhanced by dietary sodium restriction or extracellular volume depletion leading to reduced urinary lithium excretion and elevated serum lithium levels (320,544). Thus, lithium intoxication may be precipitated by volume depletion induced by diuretic therapy (320,544). Nonsteroidal antiinflammatory agents may also raise serum lithium levels by increasing reabsorption of lithium by the proximal tubule (432–443). Toxic serum lithium levels may in turn exacerbate volume depletion by inducing a salt and water diuresis, which further elevates serum lithium levels (320,544). In addition, combined therapy with lithium and angiotensin-converting enzyme inhibitors has been associated with the development of renal insufficiency and lithium intoxication (545–556). Experimental studies have shown that angiotensin-converting enzyme inhibitors decrease renal lithium clearance by reducing the filtered load and increasing fractional reabsorption of lithium (557). It has been reported that losartan does not alter renal lithium handling or serum levels in the rat (558).

Calcium Metabolism

Lithium therapy is frequently associated with alterations in parathyroid hormone and calcium homeostasis (359,559–596). Therapeutic concentrations of lithium increase the concentration of calcium required for half-maximal inhibition of parathyroid hormone release by parathyroid cells in-vitro (561,562,570,571,585,591). The molecular mechanism responsible for this increase in the set-point for calcium is unclear. It has been suggested that lithium blunts the rise in intracellular calcium in response to an increase in extracellular calcium (570,585), however, other investigators discount any role for intracellular calcium, cAMP generation, or calcium receptor-mediated signal transduction (571,591).

Chronic treatment with lithium is associated with elevated serum calcium levels in 0% to 36% of patients, elevated ionized calcium levels in 25% to 42% of patients and elevated parathyroid hormone (PTH) level in 3% to 42% of patients (334,359,564,573,574,575,586,590,593,594). An even greater number of patients exhibit evidence of hyperparathyroidism as reflected by shift to the right in the relationship between PTH and ionized calcium (574). Serum magnesium levels are also frequently elevated (564–566).

The time course of lithium's effect on calcium and PTH are not entirely consistent (572,573,587,588). One longitudinal study found that ionized calcium rose after several weeks of lithium therapy, but PTH levels rose only after prolonged therapy (572). Other studies indicate that PTH levels rise shortly after initiation of lithium therapy (587,593). Another longitudinal study found that serum calcium and PTH levels rose in 80% of patients but remained within the normal range in the first few weeks after initiation of lithium therapy (573).

In thyro-parathyroidectomized rats, lithium inhibited PTH-stimulated renal resorption of calcium and magnesium and blunted PTH-stimulated phosphaturia (563). In lithium-treated patients, urinary calcium reabsorption is increased, whereas plasma phosphorus levels, urinary phosphorus excretion, and urinary cAMP levels are normal and renal stones are rare (569,572,583,593–595).

Lithium therapy has been associated with parathyroid adenomas and hyperplasia (336,559,584,592,595,597). Although parathyroid adenomas are more common than parathyroid hyperplasia in lithium-treated patients, the latter are overrepresented compared with the general population (596). Long-term administration of lithium leads to an increase in parathyroid gland volume (572). *In vitro* studies show that lithium stimulates cellular proliferation of hyperplastic and adenomatous parathyroid tissue but has no effect on the growth of normal parathyroid tissue (586).

In a cross-sectional study, Bendz et al. (596) examined calcium and parathyroid hormone homeostasis in 142 psychiatric patients on long-term lithium therapy compared to age and sex-matched psychiatric controls. Persistent hypercalcemia was found in 3.6% of lithium-treated patients. Serum calcium level was inversely correlated with glomerular filtration rate and urinary concentrating ability but not with serum lithium levels or the dose or duration of lithium therapy. The incidence of hyperparathyroidism over 19 years was 6.3%. Surgically-verified hyperparathyroidism was present in 2.7%. Despite withdrawal of lithium for 8.5 weeks, serum calcium levels remained higher than in controls. By contrast, other studies show that serum calcium levels normalize within several weeks after discontinuation of lithium therapy, however the duration of lithium therapy was shorter in those reports (559).

Mak et al. (594) prospectively studied 53 lithium-treated patients for 2 years. There was no change in serum calcium, serum phosphorus or tubular reabsorption of phosphorus. PTH levels rose by 1 month and were significantly elevated at 6 months. In the fasting state, renal calcium reabsorption was increased and calcium excretion decreased, suggesting that bone resorption was reduced. By contrast, bone mineral density was found to be reduced in lithium-treated patients by other investigators (559,564,565,569,583).

Urinary Acidification

Lithium induces a distal tubular acidification defect (316,337, 364,394,404,405,435,597–606). Although hyperchloremic metabolic acidosis develops in experimental animals treated with large doses of lithium, an incomplete form of distal renal tubular acidosis is usually observed in humans. Longitudinal studies have documented the development of a urinary acidification defect after initiation of lithium therapy in humans (316,364,396), which is reversible after lithium withdrawal (404). A correlation between reduced urinary acidification and duration of therapy has been suggested (316,364). The fractional excretion of bicarbonate is not markedly elevated in lithium-treated patients (304), and most are unable to achieve a normal urine-to-blood PCO_2 gradient in a maximally alkaline urine, suggesting a distal acidification defect (405,602). Some studies have found that lithium-treated patients are able to maximally acidify their urine and excrete normal amounts of ammonia and titratable acid after acid loading (405,602). However, these findings have not been universal (361,381,388,394,435,601). Studies carried out in isolated rabbit cortical collecting tubules and in the turtle bladder suggested that the impaired urinary acidification seen with lithium administration results from a voltage dependent defect (598,605,606). In this context, lithium-induced downregulation of the amiloride-sensitive sodium channel reduces sodium reabsorption in the collecting duct, which in turn decreases hydrogen ion secretion by decreasing lumen negative transepithelial potential (496). The expression of other renal acid transporters is unchanged or increased (496). Infusion of sodium sulfate corrected the acidification defect in several human studies (435,559,601). In addition, lithium may directly inhibit hydrogen ion secretion by inhibiting the activity of H-adenoisine triphosphatase (H-ATPase) despite increased protein expression (496,498).

Histopathology

Concern over irreversible renal damage following long-term lithium therapy led to the first systematic study of renal histopathology (312). This study was undertaken in selected patients with a history of lithium intoxication or with nephrogenic diabetes insipidus, many of whom showed marked reductions in GFR (312). This report described focal interstitial fibrosis, tubular atrophy and dilation, microcysts formation in distal and collecting tubules, and focally sclerotic glomeruli (312). The glomerular lesions appeared to be secondary to tubulointerstitial disease.

Although we now believe that lithium-induced inhibition of vasopressin-stimulated water flow is primarily responsible for impaired urinary concentrating ability, structural injury to tubules and interstitial tissue contribute to the reduced maximal Uosm. In this regard, early reports suggested that the degree of impaired concentrating ability correlated with the severity of tubular damage and the duration of lithium treatment (312,349).

The causal relationship between chronic tubulointerstitial abnormalities and lithium treatment has since been challenged because similar changes have been observed in psychiatric patients who have not received lithium (316,364,607,608). In a comparison of renal biopsies from 44 patients treated with lithium and 25 patients with affective disorders who had never received lithium, there was no difference in the degree of interstitial fibrosis (364). The only distinguishing feature was the presence of microcysts in lithium-treated patients (Fig. 46-1). In the same study, interstitial fibrosis did not differ between psychiatric patients who had never received lithium and 25 agematched transplant kidney donor controls, but was statistically greater in lithium-treated patients than in the transplant donor controls. These observations suggest that features shared by patients with affective disorders, such as the use of other psychotropic medications, may be partly responsible for the tubulointerstitial changes that have been attributed to lithium. Studies by other investigators have shown that renal abnormalities were more pronounced in patients treated with combinations of lithium and neuroleptics than with lithium alone, raising further questions concerning attribution of the nephropathy exclusively to lithium (507).

Chronic tubulointerstitial nephropathy is a nonspecific pattern of renal injury; however, specific renal lesions have been attributed to lithium (332,349,364). Lithium increases the mitotic rate of collecting duct cells both *in vitro* and *in vivo* (488) and causes marked principal cell hypertrophy (485). Tubular cysts have been observed in approximately 50% of lithium-treated patients with interstitial nephritis (332,349). These cysts show characteristics suggesting distal tubule and collecting duct origin (332). In addition, lesser degrees of tubular dilation are frequently observed (332). New Zealand white rabbits develop progressive chronic tubulointerstitial nephritis, identical tubular cysts, and progressive renal insufficiency with increasing duration of lithium exposure (609). The fact that tubular cysts are observed in lithium-treated psychiatric patients with chronic tubulointerstitial nephritis, but are not seen in psychiatric patients with chronic tubulointerstitial nephritis who were not treated with lithium, supports the specificity of these lesions (364). Farres et al. (610) utilized gadoliniumenhanced magnetic resonance imaging to evaluate patients with lithium-induced renal insufficiency. They identified abundant, uniformly and symmetrically distributed renal microcysts in both the cortex and medulla.

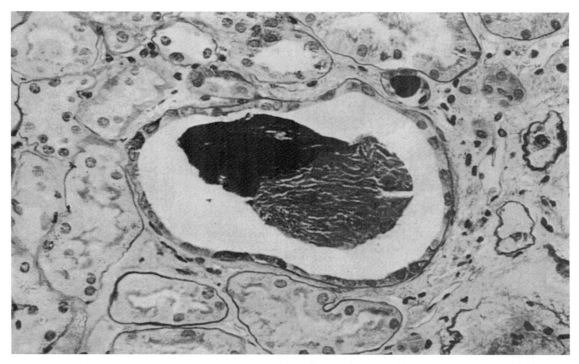

FIGURE 46-1. Cystic dilation of tubules, or "microcyst," formation, the only histologic feature suggesting chronic damage, which distinguished biopsies from patients receiving lithium from those of patients with manic-depressive psychosis who had not received lithium. (Periodic acid-Schiff, ×900.)

Reversible cytoplasmic lesions have been described in the distal tubules of lithium-treated patients, which are absent in non–lithium-treated psychiatric controls (316,449,611) (Fig. 46-2). These lesions, which consist of vacuolar swelling and glycogen accumulation, have been reproduced in the distal convoluted tubules and collecting ducts of lithium-treated rabbits (609). Glycogen accumulation has been attributed to lithium-induced decreases in intracellular cAMP (609). However, other investigators have only rarely observed these lesions (332).

Markowitz and colleagues (332) studied 24 renal biopsy specimens from lithium-treated patients referred for renal insufficiency. The predominant findings were tubular atrophy and interstitial fibrosis that tended to be patchy in early cases. A sparse, predominantly lymphocytic, interstitial infiltrate was often seen in association with interstitial fibrosis. Tubular cysts were seen in two-thirds of biopsies. The cysts were sparse and did not exceed 1 to 2 mm in diameter. All biopsies showed global glomerulosclerosis, whereas focal segmental glomerulosclerosis was present in half of the biopsies, involving 6% to 20% of glomeruli. Glomerulomegaly was frequent. Immunofluorescence showed focal nonspecific binding of IgM and C3. Electron microscopy showed variable podocyte effacement and no electron-dense deposits.

Dosing Regimen and Toxicity

It has been suggested that the type of lithium preparation and the dosing pattern may influence nephrotoxicity. However, results are conflicting. Slow-release lithium preparations have been said to be less nephrotoxic than rapidly dissolving preparations that deliver higher peak serum lithium levels (390,406,612,613). Although several cross-sectional studies show more severe impairment of urinary concentrating ability in patients treated with rapidly dissolving preparations, others find no difference between the preparations (341,347,372,389,390,406,613). It has been proposed that trough serum lithium concentrations are crucial in determin-

ing the severity of renal functional impairment and structural injury (612,614–616). This observation could be explained if tubular cell regeneration occurs only during periods of low serum lithium concentration (384,616). In several cross-sectional studies, multiple-dose regimens, which achieve relatively high trough but low peak serum lithium levels, were associated with greater histologic injury, lower GFR, or more pronounced impairment of urinary concentrating ability (335,363,384,403,615–621). Urine volume was correlated with trough serum lithium levels but not with peak levels or with lithium dose (614,616). In a prospective longitudinal study extending over 10 years, a multiple-dose regimen was associated with greater urine volumes and higher serum creatinine levels (335). In another report, urine volume decreased after lithium-treated patients were switched from a multiple-dose to a single-dose schedule in the absence of any difference in steady-state serum lithium concentration (363,615). However, treatment regimens were not randomly allocated, and in some of the studies cited, the lithium dose was greater in the multiple-dose group (614,618). Moreover, other investigators found no change in urine volume when lithium-treated patients were switched from a multiple- to a single-dose regimen or vice versa (622–625). In a randomized, cross-over study, Waldron et al. (626) failed to find any difference in urine volume with twice a day versus single daily dosing. In addition, several cross-sectional studies found no correlation between urine volume, renal concentrating ability, or GFR on the one hand and the number of lithium doses on the other (341,347,385,389,393). These discrepant data may be reconciled in part by the observation of Kusalic and Engelsmann (627) that conversion from a multiple- to single-dosing regimen was associated with an improvement in renal function only in those patients who had been treated with a multiple-dosing regimen for less than 5 years.

There is convincing evidence to suggest that maintenance of lower average serum lithium levels is associated with less nephrotoxicity. In prospective observations extending over

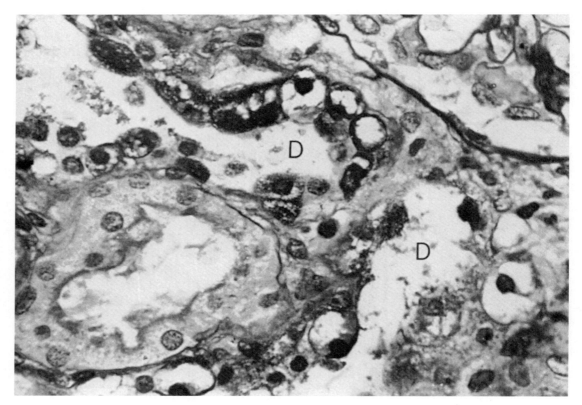

FIGURE 46-2. Ballooning, vacuolation, and accumulation of periodic acid-Schiff (PAS)–positive glycogen in epithelial cells in distal tubules (*D*) in a patient taking lithium. These changes appear within days of starting lithium and disappear soon after lithium is ceased. (PAS, ×900.)

7 years in which the average serum lithium concentration was maintained at a low level (0.68 mmol/L), GFR was unchanged, while urinary concentrating ability and urine flow rate showed only modest changes (341). In two cross-sectional series of patients maintained on low-dose regimens (0.4 to 0.6 mmol/L), renal function did not differ from controls suffering from affective disorders (302,303). Similar results have been obtained in uncontrolled cross-sectional studies (315,374), but contrary data do exist (357).

It has also been suggested that lithium nephrotoxicity may be enhanced by concurrent administration of neuroleptic agents. While several reports indicate that therapy with neuroleptic agents alone is associated with reduced urinary concentrating ability or increased urine volume, others have failed to confirm these observations (341,365,392,397). In several studies, concurrent neuroleptic therapy has been associated with more severe impairment of urinary concentrating ability, increased urine flow rate, worse renal histology, or lower GFR (341,344,348,351,362,365,371,379,392,395,397, 507,628). However, in some of these studies, the dose of lithium was greater in those who also received neuroleptic agents (351,392,507). Moreover, others investigators failed to find any differences in lithium nephrotoxicity between patients treated with lithium alone versus those also receiving other psychotropic agents (338,347,356,382,389,390,618).

Summary

In summary, in most patients the adverse effects of lithium on renal function are modest and of little clinical significance if maintenance serum levels are kept at the lowest effective level. However, it appears that advanced renal insufficiency may develop on maintenance lithium therapy after decades of treatment. Much more commonly, patients develop distressing polyuria. The relative contributions of lithium nephrotoxicity, behavioral factors (polydipsia), and the effects of other psychotropic agents in the development of renal symptoms vary among individual patients. Because nephrotoxicity may be associated with clinical episodes of lithium intoxication or high serum lithium levels, it is prudent to regularly monitor renal function and maintain the lowest effective serum lithium levels. Isolated polyuria due to impaired concentrating ability may respond to amiloride. In general, modest reduction of filtration rate in association with mildly impaired urinary concentrating ability may not be a harbinger of progressive renal failure. However, the risks of nephrotoxicity must be weighed in individual patients against the therapeutic benefit from continued lithium therapy.

References

1. Cunningham EE, et al. Heroin nephropathy—a clinicopathologic and epidemiologic study. *Am J Med* 1980;68:47.
2. Cunningham EE, Zielezny MA, Venuto RC. Heroin-associated nephropathy—a nationwide problem. *JAMA* 1983;250:2935.
3. Dubrow A, et al. The changing spectrum of heroin-associated nephropathy. *Am J Kidney Dis* 1985;5:36.
4. Kunis C, et al. Heroin nephropathy–clinical–pathologic correlations. Proceedings of the 9th International Congress of Nephrology, Los Angeles, CA, 1984:102A.
5. Menchel S, et al. AA protein-related renal amyloidosis in drug addicts. *Am J Pathol* 1983;112:195.
6. Neugarten J, et al. Amyloidosis in subcutaneous heroin abusers. *Am J Med* 1986;81:635.
7. D'Agati V, et al. The pathology of HIV-nephropathy: a detailed morphologic and comparative study. *Kidney Int* 1989;35:1358.
8. Rao TK, et al. Associated focal and segmental glomerulosclerosis in the acquired immunodeficiency syndrome. *N Engl J Med* 1984;310:669.
9. Friedman EA, Rao TK. Disappearance of uremia due to heroin-associated nephropathy. *Am J Kidney Dis* 1995;25:689.

10. Ward H, Pan D. Substance abuse is a risk factor for hypertensive renal disease. *J Am Soc Nephrol* 1998;9:162A(abst).
11. Qiu C, et al. Impact of the cocaine epidemic on end stage renal disease at San Francisco General Hospital. *J Am Soc Nephrol* 1990;1:373(abst).
12. Centers for Disease Control and Prevention. Drug abuse, AIDS and human immunodeficiency virus infection in the United States: 1988 update. *MMWR* 1989;38(S4):1.
13. Light AB, Torrance EG. Opium addiction. V. Miscellaneous observations on human addicts during the administration of morphine. *Arch Intern Med* 1929;43:878.
14. Stevens JW. Morphinism and kidney disease. *South Med J* 1916;9:300.
15. Arruda JA, Kurtzman NA, Pillay VK. Prevalence of renal disease in asymptomatic heroin addicts. *Arch Intern Med* 1975;135:535.
16. Avram MM, Iancu M, Weiss S. Heroin usage nephropathy—subclinical to end stage nephrotic syndrome. *Abstr Am Soc Nephrol* 1971:5.
17. Gardiner H, et al. Renal disease in heroin addicts. *Abstr Am Soc Nephrol* 1977:15A.
18. Sapira JD, Ball JC, Penn H. Causes of death among institutionalized narcotic addicts. *J Chronic Dis* 1970;22:733.
19. Thompson AM, et al. Focal membranoproliferative glomerulonephritis in heroin users. *Abstr Am Soc Nephrol* 1973:105.
20. Treser G, et al. Renal lesions in narcotic addicts. *Am J Med* 1974;57:687.
21. Zielezny MA, Cunningham EE, Venuto RC. The impact of heroin abuse on a regional end-stage renal disease program. *Am J Public Health* 1980;70:829.
22. Friedman EA, Rao TK, Nicastri AD. Heroin-associated nephropathy. *Nephron* 1974;13:421.
23. McGinn JT, et al. Nephrotic syndrome in drug addicts. *NY State J Med* 1974;74:92.
24. Kilcoyne MM, et al. Nephrotic syndrome in heroin addicts. *Lancet* 1972;1:17.
25. Rao TK, Nicastri AD, Friedman EA. Natural history of heroin-associated nephropathy. *N Engl J Med* 1974;290:19.
26. Grishman E, Churg J. Focal glomerular sclerosis in nephrotic patients: an electron microscopic study of glomerular podocytes. *Kidney Int* 1975;7:111.
27. Grishman E, Churg J, Porush JG. Glomerular morphology in nephrotic heroin addicts. *Lab Invest* 1976;35:415.
28. Matalon R, et al. Glomerular sclerosis in adults with nephrotic syndrome. *Ann Intern Med* 1974;80:488.
29. May DC, et al. Chronic sclerosing glomerulopathy (heroin-associated nephropathy) in intravenous T's and blues abusers. *Am J Kidney Dis* 1986;8:404.
30. Eknoyan G, et al. Renal involvement in drug abuse. *Arch Intern Med* 1973;132:801.
31. Heptinstall RH. *Pathology of the kidney*. Boston: Little, Brown and Company, 1983:676.
32. Grishman E, Churg J. Podocyte degeneration in focal glomerular sclerosis. *Abstr Am Soc Nephrol* 1973:44.
33. Bakir AA, et al. Focal segmental glomerulosclerosis: a common entity in nephrotic black adults. *Arch Intern Med* 1989;149:1802.
34. Davis JS, Lie JT. Extracellular glomerular microparticles in nephrotic syndrome of heroin users. *Arch Pathol* 1975;99:278.
35. Llach F, Descoeudres C, Massry SG. Heroin associated nephropathy: clinical and histological studies in 19 patients. *Clin Nephrol* 1979;11:7.
36. Olivero J, et al. Renal complications of drug addiction. *Urology* 1976;8:526.
37. Rao TK, Nicastri AD, Friedman EA. Renal consequences of narcotic abuse. In: Hamburger J, Crosnier J, Maxwell MH, eds. *Nephrology*. New York: Wiley, 1979:843.
38. Carbone L, et al. Course and progression of human immunodeficiency virus-associated nephropathy. *Am J Med* 1989;87:389.
39. Langs C, et al. Rapid renal failure in AIDS-associated focal glomerulosclerosis. *Arch Intern Med* 1990;150:287.
40. Haskell LP, Glicklich D, Senitzer D. HLA associations in heroin-associated nephropathy. *Am J Kidney Dis* 1988;12:45.
41. Glicklich D, et al. Possible genetic predisposition to idiopathic focal segmental glomerulosclerosis. *Am J Kidney Dis* 1988;12:26.
42. Dettmeyer R, Stojanovski G, Madea B. Pathogenesis of heroin-associated glomerulonephritis. Correlation between the inflammatory activity and renal deposits of immunoglobulin and complement? *Forensic Sci Int* 2000;113:227.
43. Dettmeyer R, Wessling B, Madea B. Heroin associated nephropathy-a postmortem study. *Forensic Sci Int* 1998;95:109.
44. Uzan M, et al. Renal disease associated with heroin abuse. *Nephrologie* 1988;9:217.
45. Faria MD, et al. Nephropathy associated with heroin abuse in Caucasian patients. *Nephrol Dial Transplant* 2003;18:2308.
46. Perneger TV, Klag MJ, Whelton PK. Recreational drug use: a neglected risk factor for end-stage renal disease. *Am J Kidney Dis* 2001;38:49.
47. United States Renal Data System. *USRDS 2004 Annual Data Report.* Bethesda, MD: National Institutes of Health, National Institute of Diabetes and Digestive and Kidney Diseases, 2004.
48. Marchand C, Cantin M, Cote M. Evidence for the nephrotoxicity of morphine sulfate in rats. *Can J Physiol Pharmacol* 1969;47:649.
49. Johnson JE, et al. Effects of morphine on rat kidney glomerular podocytes:

a scanning electron microscopic study. *Drug Alcohol Depend* 1987;19:249.
50. Singhal PC, Gibbons N, Abramovici M. Long term effects of morphine on mesangial cell proliferation and matrix synthesis. *Kidney Int* 1992;41:1560.
51. Sagar S, et al. Morphine modulates 72-kDa matrix metalloproteinase. *Am J Physiol* 1994;267:F654.
52. Pan CQ, Singhal PC. Coordinate and independent effects of cocaine, alcohol, and morphine on accumulation of IgG aggregates in the rat glomeruli. *Proc Soc Exp Biol Med* 1994;205:29.
53. Singhal PC, et al. Effect of morphine on mesangial immunoglobulin G aggregate kinetics. *Am J Physiol* 1993;265:C1211.
54. Singhal PC, Pan CQ, Gibbons N. Effect of morphine on uptake of immunoglobulin G complexes by mesangial cells and macrophages. *Am J Physiol* 1993;264:F859.
55. Singhal P, Shan Z, Garg P, et al. Morphine modulates migration of monocytes. *Nephron* 1996;73:526.
56. Singhal P, Mattana J, Garg P, et al. Morphine-induced macrophage activity modulates mesangial cell proliferation and matrix synthesis. *Kidney Int* 1996;49:94.
57. Singhal P, et al. Effect of morphine on renomedullary interstitial cell proliferation and matrix accumulation. *Nephron* 1997;77:225.
58. Singhal P, et al. Morphine modulates proliferation of kidney fibroblasts. *Kidney Int* 1998;53:350.
59. Hsu JY, et al. Pentazocine addict nephropathy: a case report. *Zhonghua Yi Xue Za Zhi (Taipei)* 1992;49:207.
60. Segal A, et al. Granulomatous glomerulonephritis in intravenous drug users: a report of three cases in oxycodone addicts. *Hum Pathol* 1998;29:1246.
61. Groth DH, et al. Intravenous injection of talc in a narcotics addict. *Arch Pathol Lab Med* 1972;94:171.
62. Steinmuller DR, et al. Chronic interstitial nephritis and mixed cryoglobulinemia associated with drug abuse. *Arch Pathol Lab Med* 1979;103:63.
63. Zientara M, Moore S. Fatal talc embolism in a drug addict. *Human Pathol* 1970;1:324.
64. McAllister CJ, et al. Granulomatous interstitial nephritis: a complication of heroin abuse. *South Med J* 1979;72:162.
65. Peces R, et al. Haemolytic-uraemic syndrome in a heroin addict. *Nephrol Dial Transplant* 1998;13:3197.
66. Brus I, et al. Amyloid fibrils in urinary sediment. Heroin addiction with renal amyloidosis. *NY State J Med* 1979;79:768.
67. Derosena R, Koss MN, Pirani CL. Demonstration of amyloid fibrils in urinary sediment. *N Engl J Med* 1975;293:1131.
68. Jacob H, et al. Amyloidosis secondary to drug abuse and chronic skin suppuration. *Arch Intern Med* 1978;138:1150.
69. Meador KH, Sharon Z, Lewis EJ. Renal amyloidosis and subcutaneous drug abuse. *Ann Intern Med* 1979;91:565.
70. Novick DM, Yancovitz SR, Weinberg PG. Amyloidosis in parenteral drug abusers. *Mt Sinai J Med* 1979;46:163.
71. Scholes JV, et al. Amyloidosis and the nephrotic syndrome in chronic heroin addicts. Proceedings of the 7th International Congress on Nephrology, Montreal, 1978:L9.
72. Scholes J, et al. Amyloidosis in chronic heroin addicts with the nephrotic syndrome. *Ann Intern Med* 1979;91:26.
73. Amigo JS, et al. Resolution of nephrotic syndrome secondary heroin-associated renal amyloidosis (Letter). *Nephrol Dial Transplant* 1990;5:158.
74. Crowley S, Feinfeld DA, Janis R. Resolution of nephrotic syndrome and lack of progression of heroin-associated renal amyloidosis. *Am J Kidney Dis* 1989;13:333.
75. Minkin W, Cohen HJ. Dermatologic complications of heroin addiction—report of a new complication. *N Engl J Med* 1967;277:473.
76. Yang GC, Gallo GR. Protein-A-gold immuno-electron microscopic study of amyloid fibrils, granular deposits, and fibrillar luminal aggregates in renal amyloidosis. *Am J Pathol* 1990;137:1223.
77. Formica R, Perazella M. Leg pain and swelling in an HIV-infected drug abuser. *Hosp Pract* 1998;33:195.
78. Tan AU, Cohen AH, Levine BS. Renal amyloidosis in a drug abuser. *J Am Soc Nephrol* 1995;5:1653.
79. Rakhit RD, et al. Complications of "skin popping" in a British heroin addict. *Nephrol Dial Transplant* 1993;8:572.
80. Dikman SH, et al. Resolution of renal amyloidosis. *Am J Med* 1977;63:430.
81. Neugarten J, Baldwin DS. Glomerulonephritis in bacterial endocarditis. *Am J Med* 1984;77:297.
82. Neugarten J, Gallo GR, Baldwin DS. Glomerulonephritis in bacterial endocarditis. *Am J Kidney Dis* 1984;5:371.
83. Heptinstall RH. Focal glomerulonephritis. In: *Pathology of the kidney*, 3rd ed. vol. 2 Boston: Little, Brown, 1982;557.
84. Freeman BG, et al. Poststaphylococcal glomerulonephritis in heroin addicts. *NY State J Med* 1974:74:2241.
85. Pelletier LL Jr, Petersdorf RG. Infective endocarditis: a review of 125 cases from the University of Washington Hospitals 1963–72. *Medicine (Baltimore)* 1977:56:287.
86. Cabane J, et al. Fate of circulating immune complexes in infective endocarditis. *Am J Med* 1979;66:227.

87. Tuazon CV, Cardella TA, Sheagren NJ. Staphylococcal endocarditis in drug users. *Arch Intern Med* 1975;66:277.

88. O'Connor DT, Weisman MH, Fierer J. Activation of the alternate complement pathway in Staph. aureus infective endocarditis and its relationship to thrombocytopenia, coagulation abnormalities, and acute glomerulonephritis. *Clin Exp Immunol* 1978;34:179.

89. Hurwitz D, Quismorio FP, Friou GJ. Cryoglobulinaemia in patients with infectious endocarditis. *Clin Exp Immunol* 1975;19:131.

90. Levine DP, et al. Community-acquired methicillin-resistant Staphylococcus aureus endocarditis in the Detroit Medical Center. *Ann Intern Med* 1982;97:330.

91. Eknoyan G, Olivero J. The kidney in infectious diseases. In: Suku WN, Eknoyan G, eds. *The kidney in systemic diseases*. New York: Wiley, 1976; 212.

92. Savin V. Glomerulonephritis in acute bacterial endocarditis in addicts. *Clin Res* 1974;22:208A(abst).

93. Savin V, Siegel L, Schreiner GE. Nephropathy in heroin addicts with staphylococcal septicemia. In: Kincaid-Smith P, Mathew TH, Becker EL, eds. *Glomerulonephritis, morphology, natural history and treatment*. New York: Wiley, 1973:397.

94. Le Moing VE, et al. Use of corticosteroids in glomerulonephritis related to infective endocarditis: three cases and review. *Clin Infect Dis* 1999;28:1057.

95. Merigian KS, Roberts JR. Cocaine intoxication: hyperpyrexia, rhabdomyolysis and acute renal failure. *Clin Toxicol* 1987;25:135.

96. Morrow JD. A case of rhabdomyolysis (CPC). *J Tenn Med Assoc* 1987;80:613.

97. Schwartz JG, McAfee RD. Cocaine and rhabdomyolysis. *J Fam Pract* 1987;24:209.

98. Barrido DT, et al. Renal disease associated acute and chronic "crack" abuse. *Kidney Int* 1988;33:181(abst).

99. Herzlich BC, et al. Rhabdomyolysis related to cocaine abuse. *Ann Intern Med* 1988;109:335.

100. Krohn KD, Slowman-Dovacs S, Leapman SB. Cocaine and rhabdomyolysis. *Ann Intern Med* 1988;108:639.

101. Parks JM, Reed G, Knochel JP. Cocaine-associated rhabdomyolysis. *Am J Med Sci* 1989;297:334.

102. Pogue VA, Nurse HM. Cocaine-associated acute myoglobinuric renal failure. *Am J Med* 1989;86:183.

103. Reinhart WH, Stricker H. Rhabdomyolysis after intravenous cocaine. *Am J Med* 1988;85:579.

104. Roth D, et al. Acute rhabdomyolysis associated with cocaine intoxication. *N Engl J Med* 1988;319:673.

105. Rubin RJ, Neugarten J. Cocaine-induced rhabdomyolysis masquerading as myocardial ischemia. *Am J Med* 1989;86:551.

106. Singhal P, et al. Acute renal failure following cocaine abuse. *Nephron* 1989;52:76.

107. Singhal P, et al. Cocaine-induced rhabdomyolysis and acute renal failure. *J Toxicol Clin Toxicol* 1990;28:321.

108. Zamora-Quezada JC, et al. Muscle and skin infarction after free-basing cocaine (crack). *Ann Intern Med* 1988;108:564.

109. Menashe PI, Gottlieb JE. Hyperthermia, rhabdomyolysis, and myoglobinuric renal failure after recreational use of cocaine. *South Med J* 1988;81:379.

110. Bauwens JE, Boggs JM, Hartwell PS. Fatal hyperthermia associated with cocaine use. *West J Med* 1989;150:210.

111. Lombard J, Wong B, Young JH. Acute renal failure due to rhabdomyolysis associated with cocaine toxicity. *West J Med* 1988;148:466.

112. Nolte KB. Rhabdomyolysis associated with cocaine abuse. *Hum Pathol* 1991;22:1141.

113. Campbell BG. Cocaine abuse with hyperthermia, seizures and fatal complications. *Med J Aust* 1988;149:387.

114. Horst E, Bennett RL, Barrett O Jr. Recurrent rhabdomyolysis in association with cocaine use. *South Med J* 1991;84:269.

115. Anand V, Siami G, Stone WJ. Cocaine-associated rhabdomyolysis and acute renal failure. *South Med J* 1989;82:67.

116. Janddreski MA, et al. Rhabdomyolysis in a case of free-base cocaine ("crack") overdose. *Clin Chem* 1989;35:1547.

117. Guerin JM, Lustman C, Barbotin-Larrieu F. Cocaine-associated acute myoglobinuric renal failure (Letter). *Am J Med* 1989;87:248.

118. Welch RD, Krause GS. Incidence of cocaine-associated rhabdomyolysis. *Ann Emerg Med* 1991;20:154.

119. Daras M, et al. Rhabdomyolysis and hyperthermia after cocaine abuse: a variant of the neuroleptic malignant syndrome? *Acta Neurol Scand* 1995;92:161.

120. Lampley EC, Williams S, Myers SA. Cocaine-associated rhabdomyolysis causing renal failure in pregnancy. *Obstet Gynecol* 1996;87:804.

121. McCrea MS, et al. Cocaine-induced rhabdomyolysis findings on bone scintigraphy. *Clin Nucl Med* 1992;17:292.

122. Ahijado F, Garcia de Vinuesa S, Luno J. Acute renal failure and rhabdomyolysis following cocaine abuse. *Nephron* 1990;54:268.

123. Brody S, et al. Predicting the severity of cocaine-associated rhabdomyolysis. *Ann Emerg Med* 1990;19:1137.

124. Censori B, et al. Acute rhabdomyolysis associated with acute cocaine intoxication. A case report. *Ital J Neurol Sci* 1993;14:325.

125. Enriquez R, et al. Skin vasculitis, hypokalemia and acute renal failure in rhabdomyolysis associated with cocaine. *Nephron* 1991;59:336.

126. Flague-Coma J. Cocaine and rhabdomyolysis: report of a case and review of the literature. *Bol Asoc Med P Rico* 1990;82:423.

127. Horowitz B, Panacek E, Jouriles N. Severe rhabdomyolysis with renal failure after intranasal cocaine use. *J Emerg Med* 1997;15:833.

128. Skluth HA, Clark JE, Ehringer GL. Rhabdomyolysis associated with cocaine intoxication. *Drug Intell Clin Pharmacol* 1988;22:778.

129. Ruttenber AJ, McAnally HB, Wetli CV. Cocaine-associated rhabdomyolysis and excited delirium: different stages of the same syndrome. *Am J Forensic Med Pathol* 1999;20:120.

130. Cadnapaphornchal P, Taher S, McDonald FD. Acute drug-associated rhabdomyolysis: an examination of its diverse renal manifestations and complications. *Am J Med Sci* 1980;280:66.

131. Dolich BH, Aiache AE. Drug-induced coma: a cause of crush syndrome and ischemic contracture. *J Trauma* 1973;13:223.

132. Grossman RA, et al. Nontraumatic rhabdomyolysis and acute renal failure. *N Engl J Med* 1974;291:807.

133. Klock JC, Sexton MJ. Rhabdomyolysis and acute myoglobinuric renal failure following heroin use. *Calif Med* 1973;119:5.

134. Koffler A, Friedler RM, Massry SG. Acute renal failure due to nontraumatic rhabdomyolysis. *Ann Intern Med* 1976;85:23.

135. Schreiber SN, Liebowitz MR, Bernstein LH. Limb compression and renal impairment (crush syndrome) following narcotic and sedative overdose. *J Bone Joint Surg* 1972;54A:1683.

136. Schreiber SN, et al. Limb compression and renal impairment (crush syndrome) complicating narcotic overdose. *N Engl J Med* 1971;284:368.

137. Weston CF, Chalker JC, Heaton KW. Multifactorial nature of renal impairment in heroin addicts. *J R Soc Med* 1986;79:185.

138. Deighan CJ, et al. Rhabdomyolysis and acute renal failure resulting from alcohol and drug abuse. *Q J Med* 2000;93:29.

139. Prynn WL, Kates DE, Pollack CV Jr. Gluteal compartment syndrome. *Ann Emerg Med* 1994;24:1180.

140. Valdovinos Mahave MC, et al. Non-traumatic rhabdomyolysis, compartment syndrome, and acute kidney failure caused by heroin. *Rev Clin Esp* 1997;197:533.

141. Klockgether T, et al. Gluteal compartment syndrome due to rhabdomyolysis after heroin abuse. *Neurology* 1997;48:275.

142. Kumar R, et al. Unusual consequences of heroin overdose: rhabdomyolysis, acute renal failure, paraplegia and hypercalcaemia. *Br J Anaesth* 1999;83:496.

143. Otero A, et al. Rhabdomyolysis and acute renal failure as a consequence of heroin inhalation. *Nephron* 1992;62:245.

144. Vucak MJ. Rhabdomyolysis requiring fasciotomy following heroin abuse. *Aust NZ J Surg* 1991;61:533.

145. D'Agostino RS, Arnett EN. Acute myoglobinuria and heroin snorting. *JAMA* 1979;241:277.

146. de Gans J, Stam J, van Wijngaarden GK. Rhabdomyolysis and concomitant neurological lesions after intravenous heroin abuse. *J Neurol Neurosurg Psychiatry* 1985;48:1057.

147. Gibb WR, Shaw IC. Myoglobinuria due to heroin abuse. *J R Soc Med* 1985;78:862.

148. Krige LP, et al. Rhabdomyolysis and renal failure—unusual complications of drug abuse. A case report. *S Afr Med J* 1983;64:253.

149. Nicholls K, Niall JF, Moran JE. Rhabdomyolysis and renal failure: complications of narcotic abuse. *Med J Aust* 1982;2:387.

150. Richter RW, et al. Acute myoglobinuria associated with heroin addiction. *JAMA* 1971;216:1172.

151. Rowland LP, Penn AS. Myoglobinuria. *Med Clin North Am* 1972;56:1233.

152. Schwartzfarb L, Singh G, Marcus D. Heroin-associated rhabdomyolysis with cardiac involvement. *Arch Intern Med* 1977;137:1255.

153. Tuller MA. Acute myoglobinuria with or without drug abuse. *JAMA* 1971;217:1868.

154. Greenwood RJ. Lumbar plexitis and rhabdomyolysis following abuse of heroin. *Postgrad Med J* 1974;50:772.

155. Penn AS, Rowland LP, Fraser DW. Drugs, coma and myoglobinuria. *Arch Neurol* 1972;26:336.

156. Chan P, et al. Acute heroin intoxication with complications of acute pulmonary edema, acute renal failure, rhabdomyolysis and lumbosacral plexitis: a case report. *Zhonghua Yi Xue Za Zhi (Taipei)* 1995;55:397.

157. Claros Gonzalez I, et al. Atraumatic rhabdomyolysis and acute renal failure secondary to a heroin overdose. *Rev Clin Esp* 1988;182:338.

158. Lie B, et al. Rhabdomyolysis in self-induced poisoning. A prospective study. *Tidsskr Nor Laegeforen* 1992;112:2359.

159. Rice EK, et al. Heroin overdose and myoglobinuric acute renal failure. *Clin Nephrol* 2000;54:449.

160. Shen CH, et al. Rhabdomyolysis-induced acute renal failure after morphine overdose—a case report. *Acta Anaesthesiol Sin* 1999;37:159.

161. Larbi EB. Drug induced rhabdomyolysis: case report. *East Afr Med J* 1997;74:829.

162. Richards JR, et al. Methamphetamine abuse and rhabdomyolysis in the ED: a 5-year study. *Am J Emerg Med* 1999;17:681.

163. Kendrick WC, Hull AR, Knochel JP. Rhabdomyolysis and shock after intravenous amphetamine administration. *Ann Intern Med* 1977;86:381.

164. Scandling J, Spital A. Amphetamine-associated myoglobinuric renal failure. *South Med J* 1982;75:237.
165. Patel R, Connor G. A review of thirty cases of rhabdomyolysis-associated acute renal failure among phencyclidine users. *J Toxicol Clin Toxicol* 1985–1986;23:547.
166. Akmal M, et al. Rhabdomyolysis with and without acute renal failure in patients with phencyclidine intoxication. *Am J Nephrol* 1981;1:91.
167. Lahmeyer H, Stock P. Phencyclidine intoxication, physical restraint and acute renal failure: case report. *J Clin Psychiatry* 1983;44:184.
168. Barton CH, Sterling ML, Vaziri ND. Rhabdomyolysis and acute renal failure associated with phencyclidine intoxication. *Arch Intern Med* 1980;140:568.
169. Cogen FC, et al. Phencyclidine-associated acute rhabdomyolysis. *Ann Intern Med* 1978;88:210.
170. Chaikin HL. Rhabdomyolysis secondary to drug overdose and prolonged coma. *South Med J* 1980;73:990.
171. Nanji AA, Filipenko JD. Rhabdomyolysis and acute myoglobinuric renal failure associated with methadone intoxication. *J Toxicol Clin Toxicol* 1983;20:353.
172. Rutgers PH, Van der Harst E, Koumans R. Surgical implications of drug-induced rhabdomyolysis. *Br J Surg* 1991;78:490.
173. Crowe AV, et al. Substance abuse and the kidney. *QJM* 2000;93:14.
174. Caramelo C, et al. Acute kidney failure due to rhabdomyolysis with normal blood calcium a possible diagnostic marker of the presence of cocaine abuse. *Rev Clin Esp* 1993;192:298.
175. de Mendoza Asensi D, et al. Acute renal insufficiency associated to cocaine consumption. *Rev Clin Esp* 2004;204:206211.
176. el-Hayek BM, et al. Rhabdomyolysis, compartment syndrome and acute kidney failure related to cocaine consume. *Nefrologia* 2003;23:469.
177. Gitlin M. Lithium and the kidney: an updated review. *Drug Saf* 1999;20:231.
178. McCann B, Hunter R, McCann J. Cocaine/heroin induced rhabdomyolysis and ventricular fibrillation. *Emerg Med J* 2002;19:264.
179. Turbat-Herrera EA. Myoglobinuric acute renal failure associated with cocaine use. *Ultrastruct Pathol* 1994;18:127.
180. Wholey MH, Ogasawara E, Ramadan MH. Acute rhabdomyolysis associated with cocaine intoxication: a case report. *Hawaii Med J* 1990;49:386.
181. Pagala M, et al. Effect on cocaine on leakage of creatine kinase from isolated fast and slow muscles of rat. *Life Sci* 1993;52:751.
182. Thakur V, et al. Case reports: cocaine-associated accelerated hypertension and renal failure. *Am J Med Sci* 1996;312:295.
183. Dunea G, Arruda JA, Bakir AA, et al. Role of cocaine in end-stage renal disease in some hypertensive African Americans. *Am J Nephrol* 1995;15:5.
184. Attoussi S, et al. Cocaine-induced scleroderma and scleroderma renal crisis. *South Med J* 1998;91:961.
185. Lam M, Ballou SP. Reversible scleroderma renal crisis after cocaine use (Letter). *N Engl J Med* 1992;326:1435.
186. Kilaru P, Kim W, Sequeira W. Cocaine and scleroderma: is there an association? *J Rheumatol* 1991;18(11):1753.
187. Tumlin J, Sands J, Someren A. Special feature: hemolytic-uremic syndrome following "crack" cocaine inhalation. *Am J Med Sci* 1990;299:366.
188. Volcy J, et al. Cocaine-induced acute renal failure, hemolysis and thrombocytopenia mimicking thrombotic thrombocytopenic purpura. *Am J Kidney Dis* 2000;35:E3.
189. Peces R, et al. Antiglomerular basement membrane antibody-mediated glomerulonephritis after intranasal cocaine use. *Nephron* 1999;81:434.
190. Alvarez D, et al. Acute interstitial nephritis induced by crack cocaine binge. *Nephrol Dial Transplant* 1999;14:1260.
191. Chevalier X, et al. Schönlein-Henoch purpura with necrotizing vasculitis after cocaine snorting [Letter]. *Clin Nephrol* 1995;43:348.
192. Mantana J, Gibbons N, Singhal PC. Cocaine interacts with macrophages to modulate mesangial cell proliferation. *J Pharmacol Exp Ther* 1994;271:311.
193. Pan C, Singhal P. Coordinate and independent effects of cocaine, alcohol, and morphine on accumulation of IgG aggregates in the rat glomeruli. *Proc Soc Exp Biol Med* 1994;205:29.
194. Barroso-Moguel R, Mendez-Armenta M, Villeda-Hernandez J. Experimental nephropathy by chronic administration of cocaine in rats. *Toxicology* 1995;98:41.
195. Brecklin CS, et al. Prevalence of hypertension in chronic cocaine users. *Am J Hypertens* 1998;11:1279.
196. Fogo A, Superdock KR, Atkinson JB. Severe arteriosclerosis in the kidney of a cocaine addict. *Am J Kidney Dis* 1992;20:513.
197. Di Paolo N, et al. Kidney vascular damage and cocaine. *Clin Nephrol* 1997;47:298.
198. van der Woude F. Cocaine use and kidney damage. *Nephrol Dial Transplant* 2000;15:299.
199. van der Woude F, Waldherr R. Severe renal arterio-arteriolosclerosis after cocaine use. *Nephrol Dial Transplant* 1999;14:434.
200. Kramer KR, Turner RC. Renal infarction associated with cocaine use and latent protein C deficiency. *South Med J* 1993;86:1436.
201. Goodman P, Rennie W. Renal infarction secondary to nasal insufflation of cocaine. *Am J Emerg Med* 1995;13:421.
202. Sharff J. Renal infarction associated with intravenous cocaine use. *Ann Emerg Med* 1984;13:1145.
203. Wohlman RA. Renal artery thrombosis and embolization associated with intravenous cocaine injection. *South Med J* 1987;80:928.
204. Nzerue CM, Hewan-Lowe K, Riley LJ. Cocaine and the kidney: a synthesis of pathophysiologic and clinical perspectives. *Am J Kidney Dis* 2000;35:783.
205. Garcia-Rostany Perez GM, Garcia Bragado F, Pras Gi AM. Pulmonary hemorrhage and antiglomerular basement membrane antibody-mediated glomerulonephritis after exposure to smoked cocaine (crack): a case report and review of the literature. *Pathol Int* 1997;47:692.
206. Leblanc M, Hebert MJ, Mongeau JG. Cocaine-induced acute renal failure without rhabdomyolysis (Letter). *Ann Intern Med* 1994;121:721.
207. Amoedo ML, et al. Cocaine-induced acute renal failure without rhabdomyolysis. *Nephrol Dial Transplant* 1999;14:2970.
208. Melandri R, et al. Cocaine poisoning in acute renal insufficiency. *Recenti Prog Med* 1993;84:188.
209. Dikow R, et al. Acute renal failure and hypertension crisis after a technoparty. *Dtsc Med Wochenschr* 2003;128:1221.
210. Rodriguez Jornet A, et al. Malignant arterial hypertension and acute renal failure caused by cocaine use. *Nefrologia* 2000;20:501.
211. Heng MC, Haberfeld G. Thrombotic phenomena associated with intravenous cocaine. *J Am Acad Dermatol* 1987;16:462.
212. Saleem TM, et al. Renal infarction: a rare complication of cocaine abuse. *Am J Emerg Med* 2001;19:528.
213. Mochizuki Y, et al. Acute aortic thrombosis and renal infarction in acute cocaine intoxication: a case report and review of literature. *Clin Nephrol* 2003;60:130.
214. Tylicki L, Rutkowski B, Horl WH. Multifactorial determination of hypertensive nephroangiosclerosis. *Kidney Blood Press Res* 2002;25:341.
215. Vupputuri S, et al. The risk for mild kidney function decline associated with illicit drug use among hypertensive men. *Am J Kidney Dis* 2004;43:629.
216. Norris KC, Thornhill-Joynes M, Tareen N. Cocaine use and chronic renal failure. *Semin Nephrol* 2001;21:362.
217. Brouhard BH. Cocaine ingestion and abnormalities of the urinary tract. *Clin Pediatr* 1994;33:157.
218. Battin M, Albersheim S, Newman D. Congenital genitourinary tract abnormalities following cocaine exposure in utero. *Am J Perinatol* 1995;12:425.
219. Chavez GF, Mulinare J, Cordero JF. Maternal cocaine use during early pregnancy as a risk factor for congenital urogenital anomalies. *JAMA* 1989;262:795.
220. Finnell RH, et al. Preliminary evidence for a cocaine-induced embryopathy in mice. *Toxicol Appl Pharmacol* 1990;103:228.
221. Greenfield SP, et al. Genitourinary tract malformations and maternal cocaine abuse. *Urology* 1991;37:455.
222. Jones KL. Developmental pathogenesis of defects associated with prenatal cocaine exposure: fetal vascular disruption. *Clin Perinatol* 1991;18:139.
223. Mitra SC. Effect of cocaine on fetal kidney and bladder function. *J Matern Fetal Med* 1999;8:262.
224. Mitra SC, et al. Maternal cocaine abuse and fetal renal arteries: a morphometric study. *Pediatr Nephrol* 2000;14:315.
225. Mitra SC, Ganesh V, Apuzzio JJ. Effect of maternal cocaine abuse on renal arterial flow and urine output of the fetus. *Am J Obstet Gynecol* 1994;171:1556.
226. Ho J, Afshani E, Stapleton FB. Renal vascular abnormalities associated with prenatal cocaine exposure. *Clin Pediatr* 1994;33:155.
227. Mizutani T, Oohashi N, Naito H. Myoglobinemia and renal failure in toluene poisoning: a case repot. *Vet Hum Toxicol* 1989;31:448.
228. Horn PT. Persistent hypertension after prenatal cocaine exposure. *J Pediatr* 1992;121:288.
229. Gottbrath-Flaherty E, et al. Urinary tract infections in cocaine-exposed infants. *J Perinatol* 1995;15:203.
230. Chadwick IS, et al. Ecstasy, 3–4 methylenedioxymethamphetamine (MDMA), a fatality associated with coagulopathy and hyperthermia. *J R Soc Med* 1991;84:371.
231. Dar KJ, McBrien ME. MDMA induced hyperthermia: report of a fatality and review of current therapy. *Intensive Care Med* 1996;22:995.
232. Fahal OH, et al. Acute renal failure after ecstasy. *BMJ* 1992;305:29.
233. Henry JA. Ecstasy and the dance of death. *BMJ* 1992;305:5.
234. Kunitz O, et al. Hyperpyrexia and rhabdomyolysis after ecstasy (MDMA) intoxication. *Anaesthesist* 2003;52:511.
235. Walubo A, Seger D. Fatal multi-organ failure after suicidal overdose with MDMA, "ecstasy": case report and review of the literature. *Hum Exp Toxicol* 1999;18:119.
236. Cunningham M. Ecstasy-induced rhabdomyolysis and its role in the development of acute renal failure. *Intensive Crit Care Nurs* 1997;13:216.
237. Woodrow G, Harnden P, Turney JH. Acute renal failure due to accelerated hypertension following ingestion of 3,4-methylenedioxymethamphetamine ("ecstasy"). *Nephrol Dial Transplant* 1995;10:399.
238. Maxwell DL, Polkey MI, Henry JA. Hyponatraemia and catatonic stupor after taking "ecstasy." *BMJ* 1993;307:1399.

239. Jones C, Little K. Hepatorenal problems presented in an urban high dependancy unit in a user of ecstasy and cocaine. *Accid Emerg Nurs* 2000;8:20.
240. Citron BP, et al. Necrotizing angiitis associated with drug abuse. *N Engl J Med* 1970;283:1003.
241. Rumbaugh CL, et al. Cerebral vascular changes secondary to amphetamine abuse in the experimental animal. *Radiology* 1971;101:345.
242. Pear BL. Radiologic recognition of extrahepatic manifestations of hepatitis B antigenemia. *Am J Roentgenol* 1981;137:135.
243. Inman RD. Rheumatic manifestations of hepatitis B virus infection. *Semin Arthr Rheum* 1982;11:406.
244. Husby G, Pierce PE, Williams RC Jr. Smooth muscle antibody in heroin addicts. *Ann Intern Med* 1975;83:801.
245. Millian SJ, Cherubin CE. Serologic investigations, in narcotic addicts: III. Latex fixation, C-reactive protein, "monotest," serum proteins and SH antigen. *Am J Clin Pathol* 1971;56:693.
246. Moser RH. Heroin addiction. *JAMA* 1974;230:728.
247. Wetli CV, Noto TA, Fernandez-Carol A. Immunologic abnormalities in heroin addiction. *South Med J* 1974;67:193.
248. Koff RS, Widrich WC, Robbins AH. Necrotizing angiitis in a methamphetamine user with hepatitis B-angiographic diagnosis, five-month follow-up results and localization of bleeding site. *N Engl J Med* 1973;288:946.
249. Bennett WM, Plamp C, Porter GA. Drug-related syndromes in clinical nephrology. *Ann Intern Med* 1977;87:582.
250. Citron BP, Peters RL. Angiitis in drug abusers. *N Engl J Med* 1971;284:112.
251. Duffy J, et al. Polyarthritis, polyarteritis and hepatitis B. *Medicine* 1976;55:19.
252. Fye KH, et al. Immune complexes in hepatitis B antigen-associated periarteritis nodosa. Detection by antibody-dependent cell-mediated cytotoxicity and the Raji cell assay. *Am J Med* 1977;62:783.
253. Halpern M. Angiitis in drug abusers. *N Engl J Med* 1971;284:113.
254. Halpern M, Citron BP. Necrotizing angiitis associated with drug abuse. *Am J Roentgenol* 1971;3:663.
255. Lignelli GJ, Buchheit WA. Angiitis in drug abusers. *N Engl J Med* 1971;284:112.
256. Margolis MT, Newton TH. Methamphetamine ("speed") arteritis. *Neuroradiology* 1971;2:179.
257. Rumbaugh CL, et al. Cerebral angiographic changes in the drug abuse patient. *Radiology* 1971;101:335.
258. Singleton EB, et al. Film interpretation session. Radiological Society of North America sixty-sixth scientific assembly and annual meeting. *Radiology* 1980;137:847.
259. Streiter ML, Bosniak MA. The radiology of drug addiction: urinary tract complications. *Semin Roentgenol* 1983;18:221.
260. Taher SM, et al. Renal tubular acidosis associated with toluene "sniffing." *N Engl J Med* 1974;290:765.
261. Fischman CM, Oster JR. Toxic effects of toluene—a new cause of high anion gap metabolic acidosis. *JAMA* 1979;241:1713.
262. Kroeger RM, et al. Recurrent urinary calculi associated with toluene sniffing. *J Urol* 1980;123:89.
263. Moss AH, et al. Fanconi's syndrome and distal renal tubular acidosis after glue sniffing. *Ann Intern Med* 1980;92:69.
264. Voigts A, Kaufman CE. Acidosis and other metabolic abnormalities associated with paint sniffing. *South Med J* 1983;76:443.
265. Streicher HZ, et al. Syndromes of toluene sniffing in adults. *Ann Intern Med* 1981;94:758.
266. Bennett RH, Forman HR. Hypokalemic periodic paralysis in chronic toluene exposure. *Arch Neurol* 1980;37:673.
267. Goodwin TM. Toluene abuse and renal tubular acidosis in pregnancy. *Obstet Gynecol* 1988;71:715.
268. Lindemann R. Congenital renal tubular dysfunction associated with maternal sniffing of organic solvents. *Acta Paediatr Scand* 1991;80:882.
269. Weinstein S, Scottolini AG, Bhagavan NV. Low neutrophil alkaline phosphatase in renal tubular acidosis with hypophosphatemia after toluene sniffing. *Clin Chem* 1985;31:330.
270. Wilkins-Haug L, Gabow PA. Toluene abuse during pregnancy: obstetric complications and perinatal outcomes. *Obstet Gynecol* 1991;77:504.
271. Lavoie FW, et al. Recurrent resuscitation and "no code" orders in a 27-year-old spray paint abuser. *Ann Emerg Med* 1987;16:1266.
272. Kirk LM, Anderson RJ, Martin K. Sudden death from toluene abuse. *Ann Emerg Med* 1984;13:119.
273. Carlisle EJ, et al. Glue-sniffing and distal tubular acidosis: sticking to the facts. *J Am Soc Nephrol* 1991;1:1019.
274. Batlle DC, Sabatini S, Kurtzman NA. On the mechanism of toluene-induced renal tubular acidosis. *Nephron* 1988;49:210.
275. Patel R, Benjamin J Jr. Renal disease associated with toluene inhalation. *J Toxicol Clin Toxicol* 1986;24:213.
276. Martinez J, et al. Renal tubular acidosis with an elevated anion gap in a 'glue sniffer.' *Hum Toxicol* 1989;8:139.
277. Kamijima M, et al. Metabolic acidosis and renal tubular injury due to pure toluene inhalation. *Arch Environ Health* 1994;49:410.
278. Meadows R, Verghese A. Medical complications of glue sniffing. *South Med J* 1996;89:455.
279. Suhara T, et al. A case of distal renal tubular acidosis associated with toluene sniffing. *Nippon Naika Gakka Zasshi* 1988;77:1452.
280. Kao KC, et al. Hypokalemic muscular paralysis causing acute respiratory failure due to rhabdomyolysis with renal tubular acidosis in a chronic glue sniffer. *J Toxicol Clin Toxicol* 2000;38:679.
281. Erramouspe J, Galvez R, Fischel DR. Newborn renal tubular acidosis associated with prenatal maternal toluene sniffing. *J Psychoactive Drugs* 1996;28:201.
282. Massengale ON, et al. Physical and psychologic factors in glue sniffing. *N Engl J Med* 1963;269:1340.
283. Press E, Done AK. Solvent sniffing. Physiologic effects and community control measures for intoxication from the intentional inhalation of organic solvents. II. *Pediatrics* 1967;39:611.
284. Hayden JW, Peterson RG, Bruckner JV. Toxicology of toluene (methylbenzene): review of current literature. *Clin Toxicol* 1977;11:549.
285. Knight AT, et al. Upholsterers' glue associated with myocarditis, hepatitis, acute renal failure and lymphoma. *Med J Aust* 1991;154:360.
286. O'Brien ET, Yeoman WB, Hobby JA. Hepatorenal damage from toluene in a "glue sniffer." *Br Med J* 1971;2:29.
287. Russ G, et al. Renal failure from "glue sniffing." *Med J Aust* 1981;2:121.
288. Will AM, McLaren EH. Reversible renal damage due to glue sniffing. *Br Med J* 1981;283:525.
289. Gupta RK, van der Meulen J, Johny KV. Oliguric acute renal failure due to glue-sniffing. *Scand J Urol Nephrol* 1991;25:247.
290. Reisin E, et al. Myoglobinuria and renal failure in toluene poisoning. *Br J Ind Med* 1975;32:163.
291. Taverner D, Harrison DJ, Bell GM. Acute renal failure due to interstitial nephritis induced by "glue sniffing" with subsequent recovery. *Scott Med J* 1988;33:246.
292. King MD. Reversible renal damage due to glue sniffing. *Br Med J* 1981;283:919.
293. Kaneko T, et al. Urinary calculi associated with solvent abuse. *J Urol* 1992;147:1365.
294. Beirne GJ. Goodpasture's syndrome and exposure to solvents. *JAMA* 1972;222:1555.
295. Beirne GJ. Glomerulonephritis associated with hydrocarbon solvents: mediated by antiglomerular basement membrane antibody. *Arch Environ Health* 1972;25:365.
296. Bonzel KE, et al. Anti-glomerular basement membrane antibody-mediated glomerulonephritis due to glue sniffing. *Eur J Pediatr* 1987;146:286.
297. Hamilton DV, Thiru S, Evans DB. Renal damage and glue sniffing. *Br Med J* 1982;284:117.
298. Venkataraman G. Renal damage and glue sniffing. *Br Med J* 1981;283:1467.
299. Rees AJ, Lockwood CM, Peters DK. Nephritis due to antibodies to GBM. In: Kincaid-Smith P, d'Apice AJ, Atkins RC, eds. *Progress in glomerulonephritis*. New York: Wiley, 1979:347.
300. Robert R, et al. Severe Goodpasture's syndrome after glue sniffing. *Nephrol Dial Transplant* 1988;3:483.
301. Bosch X, et al. Myelofibrosis and focal segmental glomerulosclerosis associated with toluene poisoning. *Hum Toxicol* 1988;7:357.
302. Baerg RD, Kimberg DV. Centrilobular hepatic necrosis and acute renal failure in "solvent sniffers." *Ann Intern Med* 1970;73:713.
303. Litt IF, Cohen MI. Danger vapor harmful: spot remover sniffing. *N Engl J Med* 1969;281:543.
304. Gutch CF, Tomhave WG, Stevens SC. Acute renal failure due to inhalation of trichlorethylene. *Ann Intern Med* 1965;63:128.
305. Ehrenreich T. Renal disease from exposure to solvents. *Ann Clin Lab Sci* 1977;7:6.
306. Cotter LH. Trichloroethylene poisoning. *Arch Ind Hygiene Occup Med* 1950;1:319.
307. Defalque RJ. Pharmacology and toxicology of trichloroethylene. A critical review of the world literature. *Clin Pharmacol Ther* 1961;2:665.
308. Hayden JW, Comstock EG, Comstock BS. The clinical toxicology of solvent abuse. *J Toxicol Clin Toxicol* 1976;9:169.
309. Locatelli F, Pozzi C. Relapsing haemolytic-uraemic syndrome after organic solvent sniffing. *Lancet* 1983;2:220.
310. Nathan AW, Toseland PA. Goodpasture's syndrome and trichloroethane intoxication. *Br J Clin Pharmacol* 1979;8:28408.
311. Hansen HE, et al. Renal function and renal pathology in patients with lithium-induced impairment of renal concentrating ability. *Proc Eur Dial Transplant Assoc* 1977;14:518.
312. Hestbech J, et al. Chronic renal lesions following long-term treatment with lithium. *Kidney Int* 1977;12:205.
313. Hansen HE. Renal toxicity of lithium. *Drugs* 1981;22:461.
314. Hansen HE, Amdisen A. Lithium intoxication. Report of 23 cases and review of 100 cases from the literature. *Q J Med* 1978;47:123.
315. Johnson GF, et al. Renal function and lithium treatment: initial and follow-up tests in manic-depressive patients. *J Affect Disord* 1984;6:249.
316. Walker RG, et al. A clinico-pathological study of lithium nephrotoxicity. *J Chron Dis* 1982;35:685.
317. Schou M, Amdisen A, Trap-Jensen J. Lithium poisoning. *Am J Psychiatry* 1968;125:520.
318. Gadallah MF, Feinstein EI, Massry SG. Lithium intoxication: clinical course and therapeutic considerations. *Miner Electrolyte Metab* 1988;14:146.
319. Singer I. Lithium and the kidney. *Kidney Int* 1981;19:374.
320. Thomsen K, Olesen OV. Precipitating factors and renal mechanisms in lithium intoxication. *Gen Pharmacol* 1978;9:85.

321. Amdisen A, et al. Grave lithium intoxication with fatal outcome. *Acta Psychiatr Scand* 1974;255:25.
322. Dias N, Hocken AG. Oliguric renal failure complicating lithium carbonate therapy. *Nephron* 1972;10:246.
323. Olsen S. Renal histopathology in various forms of acute anuria in man. *Kidney Int* 1976;10:S2.
324. Lavender S, Brown JN, Berrill WT. Acute renal failure and lithium intoxication. *Postgrad Med J* 1973;49:277.
325. Walker RG. Lithium nephrotoxicity. *Kidney Int* 1993;44(Suppl 42):S-93.
326. Bateman AM, et al. Rhabdomyolysis associated with lithium-induced hyperosmolal state. *Nephrol Dial Transplant* 1991;6:203.
327. Gill JS, Nugent K. Acute lithium intoxication and neuroleptic malignant syndrome. *Pharmacotherapy* 2003;23:811.
328. Aurell M, et al. Renal function and biopsy findings in patients on long-term lithium treatment. *Kidney Int* 1981;20:663.
329. Gitlin MJ. Lithium-induced renal insufficiency. *J Clin Psychopharmacol* 1993;13:276.
330. von Knorring L, et al. Uraemia induced by long-term lithium treatment. *Lithium* 1990;1:251.
331. Hestbech J, Aurell M. Lithium-induced uraemia. *Lancet* 1979;1:212.
332. Markowitz GS, et al. Lithium nephrotoxicity: a progressive combined glomerular and tubulointerstitial nephropathy. *J Am Soc Nephrol* 2000;11:1439.
333. Chugh S, Yager H. End-stage renal disease after treatment with lithium. *J Clin Psychopharmacol* 1997;17(6):495.
334. Presne C, et al. Lithium-induced nephropathy: rate of progression and prognostic factors. *Kidney Int* 2003;64:585.
335. Hetmar O, et al. Lithium: long-term effects on the kidney. A prospective follow-up study ten years after kidney biopsy. *Br J Psychiatry* 1991;158:53.
336. Neu C, Manschreck TC, Flocks JM. Renal damage associated with long term use of lithium carbonate. *J Clin Psychiatry* 1979;40:460.
337. Jorkasky DK, et al. Lithium-induced renal disease: a prospective study. *Clin Nephrol* 1988;30:293.
338. Smigan L, et al. Long-term lithium treatment and renal functions. A prospective study. *Neuropsychobiology* 1984;11:33.
339. Tyrer SP, et al. The effect of lithium on renal haemodynamic function. *Psychol Med* 1983;13:61.
340. Vaamonde CA, et al. Longitudinal evaluation of glomerular filtration rate during long-term lithium therapy. *Am J Kidney Dis* 1986;7:213.
341. Schou M, Vestergaard P. Prospective studies on a lithium cohort. 2 Renal function. Water and electrolyte metabolism. *Acta Psychiatr Scand* 1988;78:427.
342. Povlsen UJ, et al. Kidney functioning during lithium treatment: a prospective study of patients treated with lithium for up to ten years. *Acta Psychiatr Scand* 1992;85:56.
343. Khandelwal SK, Varma VK, Murthy RS. Renal function in children receiving long-term lithium prophylaxis. *Am J Psychiatry* 1984;141:278.
344. Jensen SB, Rickers H. Glomerular filtration rate during lithium therapy. A longitudinal study. *Acta Psychiatr Scand* 1984;70:235.
345. Grof P, et al. Long-term lithium treatment and the kidney. Interim report on fifty patients. *Can J Psychiatry* 1980;25:535.
346. Muller-Oerlinghausen B, Drescher K. Time course of clinical-chemical parameters under long-term lithium treatment. *Int J Clin Pharmacol Biopharm* 1979;17:228.
347. Lokkegaard H, et al. Renal function in 153 manic-depressive patients treated with lithium for more than five years. *Acta Psychiatr Scand* 1985;71:347.
348. Bakris GL, et al. Lithium prophylaxis and the kidney. *J Affect Disord* 1981;3:37.
349. Hansen HE, et al. Chronic interstitial nephropathy in patients on long-term lithium treatment. *Q J Med* 1979;48:577.
350. DePaulo JR, Correa EI, Sapir DG. Renal function and lithium: a longitudinal study. *Am J Psychiatry* 1986;143:892.
351. Gelenberg AJ, Coggins CH, LaBrie RA. Effects of lithium on the kidney. *Acta Psychiatr Scand* 1987;75:29.
352. Grounds AD. Deterioration in renal function in patients taking lithium and a diuretic. *Med J Aust* 1992;156:884.
353. Cogan E, Svoboda M, Abramow M. Mechanisms of lithium-vasopressin interaction in rabbit cortical collecting tubule. *Am J Physiol* 1987;252:F1080.
354. Hwu HG, Ardekani AB, Helzer JE. A longitudinal record study of renal function in patients treated with lithium. *J Affective Disord* 1981;3:101.
355. Vestergaard P, Amdisen A. Lithium treatment and kidney function. A follow-up study of 237 patients in long-term treatment. *Acta Psychiatr Scand* 1981;63:333.
356. Waller DG, Edwards JG, Papasthatis-Papayanni S. A longitudinal assessment of renal function during treatment with lithium. *Q J Med* 1988;68:553.
357. Bendz H, Aurell M, Lanke J. A historical cohort study of kidney damage in long-term lithium patients: continued surveillance needed. *Eur Psychiatry* 2001;16:199.
358. Braden G, et al. A prospective study of lithium-induced nephropathy: preliminary results. *Kidney Int* 1982;21:145(abst).
359. Kallner G, Petterson U. Renal, thyroid and parathyroid function during lithium treatment: laboratory tests in 207 people treated for 1–30 years. *Acta Psychiatr Scand* 1995;91:48.
360. Cattell WR, et al. Impairment of renal-concentrating capacity by lithium. *Lancet* 1978;2:44.
361. Coppen A, et al. Renal function in lithium and non-lithium treated patients with affective disorders. *Acta Med Scand* 1994;62:343.
362. Gellenberg AJ, et al. Renal function monitoring in patients receiving lithium carbonate. *J Clin Psychiatry* 1981;42:428.
363. Hetmar O, et al. Lithium: long-term effects on the kidney. III. Prospective study. *Acta Psychiatr Scand* 1987;75:251.
364. Walker RG, et al. Structural and functional effects of long-term lithium therapy. *Kidney Int* 1982;21(Suppl 11):S13.
365. Waller DG, Edwards JG, Polak A. Neuroleptics, lithium and renal function. *Br J Psychiatry* 1985;146:510.
366. Hullin RP, Birch NJ. Effects on renal and thyroid function and bone metabolism in long-term maintenance treatment with lithium salts. In: Cooper TB, et al., eds. *Lithium. Controversies and unresolved issues.* Amsterdam: Excerpta Medica, 1979:584.
367. Hullin RP, et al. Renal function after long-term treatment with lithium. *Br Med J* 1979;1:1457.
368. Decina P, et al. Effect of lithium therapy on glomerular filtration rate. *Am J Psychiatry* 1983;140:1065.
369. Coskunol H, et al. Renal side-effects of long-term lithium treatment. *J Affect Disord* 1997;43:5.
370. Turan T, et al. Effects of short-and long-term lithium treatment on kidney functioning in patients with bipolar mood disorder. *Prog Neuropsychopharmacol Biol Psychiatry* 2002;26:561.
371. Bendz H, et al. Kidney damage in long-term lithium patients: a cross-sectional study of patients with 15 years or more on lithium. *Nephrol Dial Transplant* 1994;9:1250.
372. Bendz H, Andersch S, Aurell M. Kidney function in an unselected lithium population. A cross-sectional study. *Acta Psychiatr Scand* 1983;68:325.
373. Colt EW, et al. Lithium-associated nephropathy. *Am J Psychiatry* 1979; 136:1098.
374. Conte G, Vazzola A, Sacchetti E. Renal function in chronic lithium-treated patients. *Acta Psychiatr Scand* 1989;79:503.
375. DePaulo JR Jr, Correa EI, Sapir DG. Renal toxicity of lithium and its implications. *Johns Hopkins Med J* 1981;149:15.
376. DePaulo JR Jr, Correa EI, Sapir DG. Renal glomerular function and long-term lithium therapy. *Am J Psychiatry* 1981;138:324.
377. Rafaelsen OJ, et al. Kidney function and morphology in long-term lithium treatment. In: Cooper TB, et al., eds. *Lithium. Controversies and unresolved issues.* Amsterdam: Excerpta Medica, 1979:578.
378. Albrecht J, Kampf D, Muller-Oerlinghausen B. Renal function and biopsy in patients on lithium-therapy. *Pharmacopsychiatry* 1980;13:228.
379. Waller DG. Renal function during lithium treatment. *Q J Med* 1994;53:369.
380. Thysell H, Brante G, Sjostedt L. Glomerular filtration rate and calcium metabolism in long-term lithium treatment. *Neuropsychobiology* 1981;7:105.
381. Donker AJ, et al. A renal function study in 30 patients on long-term lithium therapy. *Clin Nephrol* 1979;12:254.
382. Hallgren R, Alm PO, Hellsing K. Renal function in patients on lithium treatment. *Br J Psychiatry* 1979;135:22.
383. Hansen HE, et al. Albumin and beta 2-microglobulin excretion in patients on long-term lithium treatment. *Nephron* 1981;29:229.
384. Hetmar O, et al. Lithium: long-term effects on the kidney. I. Renal function in retrospect. *Acta Psychiatr Scand* 1986;73:574.
385. Jorgensen F, et al. Kidney function and quantitative histological changes in patients on long-term lithium therapy. *Acta Psychiatr Scand* 1984;70:455.
386. Kimbrell D, Colt EW, Fieve RR. Renal impairment and lithium. *Br Med J* 1979;2:1145.
387. Passavanti G, et al. Lithium induced polyuria and polydipsia. *Adv Exp Med Biol* 1989;252:215.
388. Uldall PR, et al. Renal function in patients receiving long-term lithium therapy. *Can Med Assoc J* 1981;124:1471.
389. Vestergaard P, et al. Lithium treatment and kidney function. A survey of 237 patients in long-term treatment. *Acta Psychiatr Scand* 1979;60:504.
390. Wallin L, Alling C, Aurell M. Impairment of renal function in patients on long-term lithium treatment. *Clin Nephrol* 1982;18:23.
391. Gerner RH, Psarras J, Kirschenbaum MA. Results of clinical renal function tests in lithium patients. *Am J Psychiatry* 1980;137:834.
392. Bucht G, Wahlin A. Renal concentrating capacity in long-term lithium treatment and after withdrawal of lithium. *Acta Med Scand* 1980;207:309.
393. Forrest JN Jr, et al. On the mechanism of lithium-induced diabetes insipidus in man and the rat. *J Clin Invest* 1974;53:115.
394. Miller PD, et al. Central, renal and adrenal effects of lithium in man. *Am J Med* 1979;66:797.
395. Wahlin A, et al. Kidney function in patients with affective disorders with and without lithium therapy. *Int Pharmacopsychiatry* 1980;15:253.
396. Bendz H. Kidney function in a selected lithium population. A prospective, controlled, lithium-withdrawal study. *Acta Psychiatr Scand* 1985;72:451.
397. Bucht G, Wahlin A. Impairment of renal concentrating capacity by lithium. *Lancet* 1978;1:778.
398. Morgan DB, et al. The responses to water deprivation in lithium-treated patients with and without polyuria. *Clin Sci* 1982;63:549.
399. Baylis PH, Heath DA. Water disturbances in patients treated with oral lithium carbonate. *Ann Intern Med* 1994;88:607.

400. Coppen A, Cattell WR. Lithium and the kidney (Letter). *Br Med J* 1980; 2:61.
401. Viol GW, Grof P, Daigle L. Renal tubular function in patients on long-term lithium therapy. *Am J Psychiatry* 1975;132:68.
402. Birch NJ, Hullin RP. Lithium and the kidney. *Br Med J* 1980;280:1148.
403. Hetmar O, et al. Long-term effects of lithium on the kidney: functional–morphological correlations. *J Psychiatr Res* 1989;23:285.
404. Carreras L, et al. Lithium-induced renal disease. *Clin Nephrol* 1989;32:149.
405. Batlle D, et al. Distal nephron function in patients receiving chronic lithium therapy. *Kidney Int* 1982;21:477.
406. Miller AL, Bowden CL, Plewes J. Lithium and impairment of renal concentrating ability. *J Affective Disord* 1985;9:115.
407. King JR, Aylard PR, Hullin RP. Side-effects of lithium at lower therapeutic levels: the significance of thirst. *Psychol Med* 1985;15:355.
408. Scherberich JE, et al. Effect of lithium on kidney function, serum proteinuria and excretion of tubular membrane proteins in psychiatric patients. *Kidney Int* 1986;29:1255(abst).
409. Price TR, Beisswenger PJ. Lithium and diabetes insipidus. *Ann Intern Med* 1978;88:576.
410. Ramsey TA, et al. Lithium carbonate and kidney function. *JAMA* 1972; 219:1446.
411. Kanfer A, Blondiaux I. Renal and metabolic complications of lithium. *Nephrologie* 2000;21:65.
412. Azam H, et al. Hyperosmolar nonketotic coma precipitated by lithium-induced nephrogenic diabetes insipidus. *Postgrad Med J* 1998;74:39.
413. Kamijo Y, et al. Dural sinus thrombosis with severe hypernatremia developing in a patient on long-term lithium therapy. *J Toxicol Clin Toxicol* 2003;41:359.
414. MacGregor DA, et al. Hyperosmolar coma due to lithium-induced diabetes insipidus. *Lancet* 1995;346:413.
415. Allen HM, et al. Indomethacin in the treatment of lithium-induced nephrogenic diabetes insipidus. *Arch Intern Med* 1989;149:1123.
416. Cogan E, Abramow M. Inhibition by lithium of the hydro-osmotic action of vasopressin in the isolated perfused cortical collecting tubule of the rabbit. *J Clin Invest* 1986;77:1507.
417. Cogan E, Nortier J, Abramow M. Impaired hydro-osmotic response to vasopressin of cortical collecting tubules from lithium-treated rabbits. *Pflugers Arch* 1990;416:694.
418. Christensen S, et al. Pathogenesis of nephrogenic diabetes insipidus due to chronic administration of lithium in rats. *J Clin Invest* 1985;75:1869.
419. Kincaid-Smith P, Nanra RS. Lithium-induced and analgesic-induced renal diseases. In: Schrier RW, Gottschalk CW, eds. *Diseases of the kidney,* 5th ed. Boston: Little, Brown, 1993:1099.
420. Forrest JN. Lithium-induced polyuria: cellular mechanisms and response to diuretics. In: Cooper TB, et al., eds. *Lithium. Controversies and unresolved issues.* Amsterdam: Excerpta Medica, 1979:632.
421. Cox M, Singer I. Lithium and water metabolism. *Am J Med* 1975;59:153.
422. Mishkind MH, et al. Studies of lithium (Li) induced polyuria. *Clin Res* 1977;25:596A(abst).
423. Smith DF, Balagura S. "Antidotal thirst:" a response to intoxication. *Science* 1970;167:297.
424. Waller DG, Edwards JG. Investigation of renal tubular function during treatment with lithium. *Neuropharmacology* 1984;23:277.
425. Hansen HE, et al. Plasma arginine-vasopressin, renal-concentrating ability and lithium excretion in a group of patients on long-term lithium treatment. *Nephron* 1982;32:125.
426. Padfield PL, et al. Lithium induced nephrogenic diabetes insipidus: changes in plasma vasopressin and angiotensin II. *Clin Nephrol* 1975;3:220.
427. Padfield PL, et al. Plasma levels of antidiuretic hormone in patients receiving prolonged lithium therapy. *Br J Psychiatry* 1977;130:144.
428. Constandis DD, Schriever HG. Severe lithium-induced diabetes insipidus in a surgical patient treated with hydrochlorothiazide. *Am J Surg* 1981;141:741.
429. Wahlin A, Rapp W, Jonsson EH. Failure of chlorothiazide to improve urinary concentrating capacity in lithium-treated patients. *Acta Med Scand* 1980;207:195.
430. Levy ST, Forrest JN Jr, Heninger GR. Lithium-induced diabetes insipidus: manic symptoms, brain and electrolyte correlates, and chlorothiazide treatment. *Am J Psychiatry* 1973;130:1014.
431. Timmer RT, Sands JM. Lithium intoxication. *J Am Soc Nephrol* 1999;10: 666.
432. Shelley RK. Lithium toxicity and mefenamic acid. A possible interaction and the role of prostaglandin inhibition. *Br J Psychiatry* 1987;151:847.
433. Ragheb M. Ibuprofen can increase serum lithium level in lithium-treated patients. *J Clin Psychiatry* 1987;48:161.
434. Reimann IW, Frolich JC. Effects of diclofenac on lithium kinetics. *Clin Pharmacol Ther* 1981;30:348.
435. Rapoport J, et al. Lithium-induced nephrogenic diabetes insipidus: studies of tubular function and pathogenesis. *Isr J Med Sci* 1979;15:765.
436. Frolich JC, et al. Indomethacin increases plasma lithium. *Br Med J* 1979;1:1115.
437. Boer WH, et al. Prostaglandin synthesis inhibition stimulates lithium reabsorption in Henle's loop in rats. *Kidney Int* 1993;43:301.
438. Burke D, Fulda GJ, Castellano J. Lithium-induced nephrogenic diabetes insipidus treated with intravenous ketorolac. *Crit Care Med* 1995;23:1924.

439. Slordal L, et al. A life-threatening interaction between lithium and celecoxib. A life-threatening interaction between lithium and celecoxib. *Br J Clin Pharmacol* 2003;413.
440. Lam SS, Kjellstrand C. Emergency treatment of lithium-induced diabetes insipidus with nonsteroidal anti-inflammatory drugs. *Ren Fail* 1997;19: 183.
441. Libber S, Harrison H, Spector D. Treatment of nephrogenic diabetes insipidus with prostaglandin synthesis inhibitors. *J Pediatr* 1986;108: 305.
442. Martinez EJ, et al. Lithium-induced nephrogenic diabetes insipidus treated with indomethacin. *South Med J* 1993;86:971.
443. Weinstock RS, Moses AM. Desmopressin and indomethacin therapy for nephrogenic diabetes insipidus in patients receiving lithium carbonate. *South Med J* 1990;83:1475.
444. Batlle D, et al. Amelioration of polyuria by amiloride in patients receiving long-term lithium therapy. *N Engl J Med* 1985;312:408.
445. Kosten TR, Forrest JN. Treatment of severe lithium-induced polyuria with amiloride. *Am J Psychiatry* 1986;143:1563.
446. Finch CK, Kelley KW, Williams RB. Treatment of lithium-induced diabetes insipidus with amiloride. *Pharmacotherapy* 2003;23:546.
447. Chmielnicka J, Nasiadek M. The trace elements in response to lithium intoxication in renal failure. *Ecotoxicol Environ Saf* 2003;55:178.
448. Pedersen EB, et al. Urinary excretion of albumin beta 2-microglobin and free light chains during lithium treatment. *Scand J Clin Lab Invest* 1978;38: 269.
449. Walker RG, et al. Renal pathology associated with lithium therapy. *Pathology* 1983;15:403.
450. Thysell H, Hultberg B, Regnell G. Urinary beta-hexosaminidase excretion in patients treated with lithium, thymoleptic and/or neuroleptic drugs. *Acta Psychiatr Scand* 1982;66:486.
451. Garvey MJ, et al. Use of renal enzymes to evaluate nephrotoxicity in lithium treated patients. *Br J Psychiatry* 1982;141:420.
452. Alexander F, Martin J. Nephrotic syndrome associated with lithium therapy. *Clin Nephrol* 1981;15:267.
453. Baer RA. Nephrotic syndrome and renal failure secondary to lithium carbonate therapy. *Can Med Assoc J* 1985;132:735.
454. Depner TA. Nephrotic syndrome secondary to lithium therapy. *Nephron* 1982;30:286.
455. Amsterdam JD. A prospective study of lithium-induced nephropathy. *Clin Sci* 1982;63:549.
456. Pawel BR, et al. Aggravation of diabetic nephropathy by lithium: a case report and review of the literature. *J Clin Psychiatry* 1989;50:101.
457. Hafner H, et al. Nierentoxizitat von lithium bei therapeutishen dosen. *Pharmakopsychiatr Neuropsychopharmakol* 1978;11:157.
458. Singer L, et al. Evolution favorable d'un syndrome nephrotique malgre la poursuite d'un traitement par le lithium. *Ann Med Psychol* 1979;137: 584.
459. Moscowitz R, Springer P, Urquhart M. Lithium induced nephrotic syndrome. *Am J Psychiatry* 1981;138:382.
460. Duflot JP, Dore C, Fellion G. L'utilisation due carbonate de lithium dans une institution psychiatrique. *Ann Med Psychol* 1973;131:311.
461. Jornet AR, Mate G, Olivares F. Sindrome nefrotico asociado a la terapeutica con litio. *Med Clin* 1985;85:125.
462. Richman AV, et al. Minimal-change disease and the nephrotic syndrome associated with lithium therapy. *Ann Intern Med* 1980;92:70.
463. Santella RN, Rimmer JM, MacPherson BR. Focal segmental glomerulosclerosis in patients receiving lithium carbonate. *Am J Med* 1988;84: 951.
464. Wood IK, Parmelee DX, Foreman JW. Lithium-induced nephrotic syndrome. *Am J Psychiatry* 1989;146:84.
465. Kalina KM, Burnett GB. Lithium and the nephrotic syndrome. *J Clin Psychopharmacol* 1984;4:148.
466. Tam VK, et al. Nephrotic syndrome and renal insufficiency associated with lithium therapy. *Am J Kidney Dis* 1996;27:715.
467. Schreiner A, et al. Focal segmental glomerulosclerosis and lithium treatment. *Am J Psychiatry* 2000;157:838.
468. Gill DS, Chhetri M, Milne JR. Nephrotic syndrome associated with lithium therapy. *Am J Psychiatry* 1997;154:1318.
469. Bosquet S, et al. Nephrotic syndrome during lithium therapy. *Nephrol Dial Transplant* 1997;12:2728.
470. Cledes J, Leyer C, Herve JP. Nephrotic syndrome during treatment with lithium. *Presse Med* 1990;19:86.
471. Herrero Mendoza MD, et al. Nephrotic syndrome and lithium therapy. *Med Clin* 2001;116:758.
472. Imbs JL, et al. Nephrotic syndrome under lithium therapy. *Presse Med* 1990;19:86.
473. Sakarean A, et al. Lithium-induced nephrotic syndrome in a young pediatric patient. *Pediatr Nephrol* 2002;17:290.
474. Godinich MJ, Batlle DC. Renal tubular effects of lithium. *Kidney Int* 1990;37:S-52.
475. Yamaki M, et al. Cellular mechanism of lithium-induced nephrogenic diabetes insipidus in rats. *Am J Physiol* 1991;261:F505.
476. Goldberg H, Clayman P, Skorecki K. Mechanism of Li inhibition of vasopressin-sensitive adenylate cyclase in cultured renal epithelial cells. *Am J Physiol* 1988;255:F995.

477. Bichet DG. Lithium, cyclic AMP signaling, A-Kinase anchoring proteins, and aquaporin-2. *J Am Soc Nephrol* 2006;17(4):920.
478. Bentley PJ, Wasserman A. The effects of lithium on the permeability of an epithelial membrane, the toad urinary bladder. *Biochim Biophys Acta* 1972;266:285.
479. Harris CA, Jenner FA. Some aspects of the inhibition of the action of antidiuretic hormone by lithium ions in the rat kidney and bladder of the toad Bufo marinus. *Br J Pharmacol* 1972;44:223.
480. Martinez-Maldonado M, et al. Renal effects of lithium administration in rats: alterations in water and electrolyte metabolism and the response to vasopressin and cyclic-adenosine monophosphate during prolonged administration. *J Lab Clin Med* 1975;86:445.
481. Singer I, Rotenberg D, Puschett JB. Lithium-induced nephrogenic diabetes insipidus: in vivo and in vitro studies. *J Clin Invest* 1972;51:1081.
482. Carney S, Rayson B, Morgan T. The effect of lithium on the permeability response induced in the collecting duct by antidiuretic hormone. *Pflugers Arch* 1976;366:19.
483. Dousa TP, Barnes LD. Lithium-induced antidiuretic effect of antidiuretic hormone in rats. *Am J Physiol* 1976;231:1754.
484. Beck N, Davis BB. Effects of lithium on vasopressin-dependent cyclic AMP in rat renal medulla. *Endocrinology* 1975;97:202.
485. Kwon TH, et al. Altered expression of renal AQPs and Na(+) transporters in rats with lithium-induced NDI. *Am J Physiol Renal Physiol* 2000;279:F552.
486. Nishimoto G, et al. Arginine vasopressin stimulates phosphorylation of aquaporin-2 in rat renal tissue. *Am J Physiol Renal Physiol* 1999;276:F254.
487. Yasui M, et al. Adenylate cyclase-coupled vasopressin receptor activates AQP2 promoter via a dual effect on CRE and AP1 elements. *Am J Physiol Renal Physiol* 1997;272:F443.
488. Christensen BM, et al. Changes in cellular composition of kidney collecting duct cells in rats with lithium-induced NDI. *Am J Physiol Cell Physiol* 2004;286:C952.
489. Gimenez M, et al. Endocarditis and acute renal failure due to Erysipelothrix rhusiopathiae. *Eur J Clin Microbiol Infect Dis* 1996;15:347.
490. Michimata M, et al. Reverse pharmacological effect of loop diuretics and altered rBSC1 expression in rats with lithium nephropathy. *Kidney Int* 2003;63:165.
491. Klein JD, et al. Down-regulation of urea transporters in the renal inner medulla of lithium-fed rats. *Kidney Int* 2002;61:995.
492. Nielsen J, et al. Segment-specific ENaC downregulation in kidney of rats with lithium-induced NDI. *Am J Physiol Renal Physiol* 2003;285:F1198.
493. Laursen UH, et al. Changes of rat kidney AQP2 and Na,K-ATPase mRNA expression in lithium-induced nephrogenic diabetes insipidus. *Nephron Exp Nephrol* 2004;97:e1.
494. Marples D, et al. Lithium-induced downregulation of aquaporin-2 water channel expression in rat kidney medulla. *J Clin Invest* 1995;95:1838.
495. Kwon TH, et al. Altered expression of renal aquaporins and Na+ transporters in rats with lithium-induced nephrogenic diabetes insipidus. *J Am Soc Nephrol* 1999;10:18A(abst).
496. Kim YH, et al. Altered expression of renal acid-base transporters in rats with lithium-induced NDI. *Am J Physiol Renal Physiol* 2003;285:F1244.
497. Frokiaer J, et al. Pathophysiology of aquaporin-2 in water balance disorders. *Am J Med Sci* 1998;316:291.
498. Hensen J, Haenelt M, Gross P. Lithium induced polyuria and renal vasopressin receptor density. *Nephrol Dial Transplant* 1996;11:622.
499. Anger MS, et al. Effects of lithium on cAMP generation in cultured rat inner medullary collecting tubule cells. *Kidney Int* 1990;37:1211.
500. Sugawara M, Hashimoto K, Ota Z. Involvement of prostaglandin E2, cAMP, and vasopressin in lithium-induced polyuria. *Am J Physiol* 1988;254:R863.
501. Nally JV, Rutecki GW, Ferris TF. The acute effect of lithium on renal renin and prostaglandin E synthesis in the dog. *Circ Res* 1980;46:739.
502. Carney SL, Ray C, Gillies AH. Mechanism of lithium-induced polyuria in the rat. *Kidney Int* 1996;50:377.
503. Posner L, Mokrzycki MH. Transient central diabetes insipidus in the setting of underlying chronic nephrogenic diabetes insipidus associated with lithium use. *Am J Nephrol* 1996;16:339.
504. Fenves AZ, Emmett M, White MG. Lithium intoxication associated with acute renal failure. *South Med J* 1984;77:1472.
505. Solomon S. Action of alkali metals on papillary-cortical sodium gradient of dog kidney. *Proc Soc Exp Biol Med* 1967;125:1183.
506. Bendz H, Sjodin I, Aurell M. Renal function on and off lithium in patients treated with lithium for 15 years or more. A controlled, prospective lithium-withdrawal study. *Nephrol Dial Transplant* 1996;11:457.
507. Bucht G, et al. Renal function and morphology in long-term lithium and combined lithium-neuroleptic treatment. *Acta Med Scand* 1980;208:381.
508. Cairns SR, Wolman R, Lewis JG. Persistent nephrogenic diabetes insipidus, hyperparathyroidism, and hypothyroidism after lithium treatment. *Br Med J* 1985;290:516.
509. Haghfelt T, et al. Lithiumforgiftning og nyrefunktion. *Nord Med* 1971;9:1465.
510. Neithercut WD, et al. Persistent nephrogenic diabetes insipidus, tubular proteinuria, aminoaciduria, and parathyroid hormone resistance following long term lithium administration. *Postgrad Med J* 1990;66:479.
511. Rabin EZ, et al. Persistent nephrogenic diabetes insipidus associated with long-term lithium carbonate treatment. *Can Med Assoc J* 1979;121:194.
512. Simon NM, Garber E, Arieff AJ. Persistent nephrogenic diabetes insipidus after lithium carbonate. *Ann Intern Med* 1977;86:446.
513. Neithercut WD, et al. Persistent nephrogenic diabetes insipidus, tubular proteinuria, aminoaciduria, and parathyroid hormone resistance following long term lithium administration. *Postgrad Med J* 1990;66:479.
514. Guirguis AF, Taylor HC. Nephrogenic diabetes insipidus persisting 57 months after cessation of lithium carbonate therapy: report of a case and review of the literature. *Endocr Pract* 2000;6:324.
515. Stone KA. Lithium-induced nephrogenic diabetes insipidus. *J Am Board Fam Pract* 1999;12:43.
516. Thompson CJ, France AJ, Baylis PH. Persistent nephrogenic diabetes insipidus following lithium therapy. *Scott Med J* 1997;42:16.
517. Abu R, et al. Brucella endocarditis causing acute renal failure. *Nephron* 1987;92:115.
518. Barthelmebs M, Grima M, Imbs JL. Ramipril-induced decrease in renal lithium excretion in the rat. *Br J Pharmacol* 1995;116:2161.
519. Censori B, et al. Acute rhabdomyolysis associated with acute cocaine intoxication. A case report. *Ital J Neurol Sci* 1993;14:325.
520. Choi HK, et al. Subacute bacterial endocarditis with positive cytoplasmic antineutrophil cytoplasmic antibodies and anti-proteinase 3 antibodies. *Arthritis Rheum* 2000;43:226.
521. Ramsey TA, Cox M. Lithium and the kidney. A review. *Am J Psychiatry* 1982;139:443.
522. Cox M, Singer I. Lithium-induced natriuresis. In: Cooper TB, Gershon S, Kline NS, et al., eds. *Lithium. Controversies and unresolved issues.* Amsterdam: Excerpta Medica, 1979:646.
523. Martinez-Maldonado M, Opava-Stitzer S. Distal nephron function of the rat during lithium chloride infusion. *Kidney Int* 1977;12:17.
524. Harris CA, Dirks JH. Effect of acute lithium infusion on proximal and distal tubular reabsorption in rats. *Fed Proc* 1973;32:381(abst).
525. Hecht B, et al. Effects of lithium on proximal and distal tubular function. *Clin Res* 1976;24:402A(abst).
526. Baer L, Glassman AH, Kassir S. Negative sodium balance in lithium carbonate toxicity. *Arch Gen Psychiatry* 1973;29:823.
527. Thomsen K, Jensen J, Olesen OV. Effect of prolonged lithium ingestion on the response to mineralocorticoids in rats. *J Pharmacol Exp Ther* 1976;196:463.
528. Steele TH, Stromberg BA, Underwood JL. Effects of lithium in the isolated perfused rat kidney. In: Cooper TB, Gershon S, Kline NS, et al., eds. *Lithium. Controversies and unresolved issues.* Amsterdam: Excerpta Medica, 1979:656.
529. Gutman Y, Tamir N, Benakein F. Effect of lithium on plasma renin activity. *Eur J Pharmacol* 1973;24:347.
530. Thomsen K, Jensen J, Olesen O. Effect of prolonged lithium ingestion on the response to mineralocorticoids in rats. *J Pharmacol Exp Ther* 1976;196:463.
531. Baer L, et al. Mechanisms of renal lithium handling and their relationship to mineralocorticoids: a dissociation between sodium and lithium ions. *J Psychiatr Res* 1971;8:91.
532. Lithium nephropathy (Editorial). *Lancet* 1979;2:619.
533. Murphy DL, Goodwin FK, Bunney WE Jr. Aldosterone and sodium response to lithium administration in man. *Lancet* 1969;2:458.
534. Thomsen K, Bak M, Shirley DG. Chronic lithium treatment inhibits amiloride-sensitive sodium transport in the rat distal nephron. *J Pharmacol Exp Ther* 1999;289:443.
535. Rutecki GW, et al. The acute effects of lithium (Li) on renal function. *Kidney Int* 1977;12:571(abst).
536. Jenner FA. Lithium and the kidney. In: Cooper TB, et al., eds. *Lithium. Controversies and unresolved issues.* Amsterdam: Excerpta Medica, 1979:567.
537. Myers JB, et al. Effects of lithium on the kidney. *Kidney Int* 1980;18:601.
538. Pedersen EB, et al. Plasma aldosterone during lithium treatment. *Neuropsychiatry* 1977;3:153.
539. Aronoff MS, Evans RG, Durell J. Effect of lithium salts on electrolyte metabolism. *J Psychiatr Res* 1971;8:139.
540. Stewart PM, et al. Lithium carbonate—a competitive aldosterone antagonist? *Br J Psychiatry* 1988;153:205.
541. Transbol I, et al. Endocrine effects of lithium. *Acta Endocrinol* 1978;88:619.
542. DePaulo JR Jr. Lithium. *Psychiatr Clin North Am* 1984;7:587.
543. Schou M, et al. Pharmacological and clinical problems of lithium prophylaxis. *Br J Psychiatry* 1970;16:615.
544. Boton R, Gaviria M, Batlle DC. Prevalence, pathogenesis, and treatment of renal dysfunction associated with chronic lithium therapy. *Am J Kidney Dis* 1987;10:329.
545. Correa FJ, Eiser AR. Angiotensin-converting enzyme inhibitors and lithium toxicity. *Am J Med* 1992;93:108.
546. Lehmann K, Ritz E. Angiotensin-converting enzyme inhibitors may cause renal dysfunction in patients on long-term lithium treatment. *Am J Kidney Dis* 1995;25:82.
547. Douste-Blazy P, et al. Angiotensin converting enzyme inhibitors and lithium treatment. *Lancet* 1986;1:1448.
548. Simon G. Combination angiotensin converting enzyme inhibitor/ lithium therapy contraindicated in renal disease. *Am J Med* 1988;85:893.

549. Pulik M, Lida H. Interaction lithium-inhibiteurs de l'enzyme de conversion. *Presse Med* 1988;17:755.

550. Conrad AJ. ACE-inhibitors and lithium toxicity. *Biol Ther Psychiatry* 1988;11:43.

551. Mahieu M, et al. Lithium-inhibiteurs de l'enzyme de conversion: une association a eviter? *Presse Med* 1988;17:281.

552. Navis GJ, deJong PE, deZeeuw D. Volume homeostasis, angiotensin converting enzyme inhibition, and lithium therapy. *Am J Med* 1989;86:621.

553. Baldwin CM, Safferman AZ. A case of lisinopril-induced lithium nephrotoxicity. *DICP Ann Pharmacother* 1990;24:946.

554. Drouet A, Bouvet O. Lithium et inhibiteurs de l'enzyme de conversion. *Encephale* 1990;16:51.

555. Griffin JH, Hahn SM. Lisinopril-induced lithium toxicity. *DICP Ann Pharmacother* 1991;25:101.

556. Finley PR, O'Brien JG, Coleman RW. Lithium and angiotensin-converting enzyme inhibitors: evaluation of a potential interaction. *J Clin Psychopharmacol* 1996;16:68.

557. Barthelmebs M, Grima M, Imbs JL. Ramipril-induced decrease in renal lithium excretion in the rat. *Br J Pharmacol* 1995;116:2161.

558. Barthelmebs M, et al. Absence of a losartan interaction with renal lithium excretion in the rat. *Br J Pharmacol* 1995;116:2166.

559. Ananth J, Dubin SE. Lithium and symptomatic hyperparathyroidism. *J R Soc Med* 1983;76:1026.

560. Baastrup PC, Christiansen C, Transbol I. Calcium metabolism in lithium-treated patients. Relation to uni-bipolar dichotomy. *Acta Psychiatr Scand* 1978;57:124.

561. Birnbaum J, et al. Lithium stimulates the release of human parathyroid hormone in vitro. *J Clin Endocrinol Metab* 1988;66:1187.

562. Brown EM. Lithium induces abnormal calcium-regulated PTH release in dispersed bovine parathyroid cells. *J Clin Endocrinol Metab* 1981;52:1046.

563. Carney S, Hackson P. Acute lithium administration impairs the action of parathyroid hormone on rat renal calcium, magnesium and phosphate transport. *Clin Exp Pharmacol Physiol* 1998;25:795.

564. Christiansen C, Baastrup PC, Transbol I. Osteopenia and dysregulation of divalent cations in lithium-treated patients. *Neuropsychobiology* 1975;143:344.

565. Christiansen C, Baastrup PC, Transbol I. Development of "primary" hyperparathyroidism during lithium therapy: longitudinal study. *Neuropsychobiology* 1980;6:280.

566. Christiansen C, Baastrup PC, Lindgreen P, et al. Endocrine effects of lithium: II. "Primary" hyperparathyroidism. *Acta Endocrinol* 1978;88:528.

567. Davis BM, et al. Lithium's effect of parathyroid hormone. *Am J Psychiatry* 1981;138:489.

568. Franks RD, et al. Long-term lithium carbonate therapy causes hyperparathyroidism. *Arch Gen Psychiatry* 1982;39:1074.

569. McHenry CR, et al. Lithiumogenic disorders of the thyroid and parathyroid glands as surgical disease. *Surgery* 1990;108:1001.

570. McHenry CR, et al. Lithium effects on dispersed bovine parathyroid cells grown in tissue culture. *Surgery* 1991;110:1061.

571. McHenry CR, Stenger DB, Racke F. Investigation of calcium-induced hydrolysis of phosphoinositides in normal and lithium-treated parathyroid cells. *Am J Surg* 1995;170:484.

572. Mallette LE, et al. Lithium treatment increases intact and midregion parathyroid hormone and parathyroid volume. *J Clin Endocrinol Metab* 1989;68:654.

573. Mallette LE, Eichhorn E. Effects of lithium carbonate on human calcium metabolism. *Arch Intern Med* 1986;146:770.

574. Nordenstrom J, et al. Biochemical hyperparathyroidism and bone mineral status in patients treated long-term with lithium. *Metabolism* 1994;43:1563.

575. Linder J, et al. Acute antidepressant effect of lithium is associated with fluctuation calcium and magnesium in plasma. A double-blind study on the antidepressant effect of lithium and clomipramine. *Acta Psychiatr Scand* 1989;80:27.

576. Christiansen C, Baastrup PC, Transbol I. Lithium, hypercalcemia, hypermagnesemia, and hyperparathyroidism. *Lancet* 1976;2:969.

577. Christensson TA. Letter: Lithium, hypercalcaemia, and hyperparathyroidism. *Lancet* 1976;2:144.

578. Christiansen C, Baastrup PC, Transbol I. Lithium-induced "primary" hyperparathyroidism. *Calcif Tissue Res* 1977;22:341.

579. Feldman ME, Pachman JS. Surgical management of lithium-induced hypercalcemia. *Conn Med* 1990;54:614.

580. Garfinkel PE, Ezrin C, Stancer HC. Hypothyroidism and hyperparathyroidism associated with lithium. *Lancet* 1973;2:331.

581. Prasad A. Chronic lithium intake and hyperparathyroidism. *Eur J Clin Pharmacol* 1984;27:499.

582. Shen FH, Sherrard DJ. Lithium-induced hyperparathyroidism: an alteration of the "set point." *Ann Intern Med* 1982;96:63.

583. Plenge P, Rafaelsen OJ. Lithium effects on calcium, magnesium and phosphate in man: effects on balance, bone mineral content, faecal and urinary excretion. *Acta Psychiatr Scand* 1982;66:361.

584. Nordenstrom J, et al. Hyperparathyroidism associated with treatment of manic-depressive disorders by lithium. *Eur J Surg* 1992;158:207.

585. Racke F, McHenry CR, Wentworth D. Lithium-induced alterations in parathyroid cell function: insight into the pathogenesis of lithium-associated hyperparathyroidism. *Am J Surg* 1994;168:462.

586. Saxe A, Gibson G, Silveira E. Effects of long-term lithium infusion on normal parathyroid tissue. *Surgery* 1995;117:577.

587. Seely EW, et al. A single dose of lithium carbonate acutely elevates intact parathyroid hormone levels in humans. *Acta Endocrinol* 1989;121:174.

588. Spiegel AM, et al. The effect of short term lithium administration on suppressibility of parathyroid hormone secretion by calcium in vivo. *J Clin Endocrinol Metab* 1984;59:354.

589. Hestbech J, et al. Chronic renal lesions following long-term treatment with lithium. *Kidney Int* 1977;12:205.

590. Johnson GF, et al. Renal function and lithium treatment: initial and follow-up tests manic-depressive patients. *J Affect Disord* 1984;6:249.

591. Wallace J, Scarpa A. Similarities of Li^+ and low Ca^{2+} in the modulation of secretion parathyroid cells in vitro. *J Biol Chem* 1983;258:6288.

592. Wolf ME, et al. Lithium therapy, hypercalcemia, and hyperparathyroidism. *Am J Ther* 1997;4:323.

593. Nielsen JL, et al. Parathyroid hormone in serum during lithium therapy. *Scand J Clin Lab Invest* 1977;37:369.

594. Mak TW, et al. Effects of lithium therapy on bone mineral metabolism: a two-year prospective longitudinal study. *J Clin Endocrinol Metab* 1998;83:3857.

595. Stancer HC, Forbath N. Hyperparathyroidism, hypothyroidism, and impaired renal function after 10 to 20 years of lithium treatment. *Arch Intern Med* 1989;149:1042.

596. Bendz H, et al. Hyperparathyroidism and long-term lithium therapy—a cross-sectional study and the effect of lithium withdrawal. *J Intern Med* 1996;240:357.

597. Chiu E, et al. Renal findings after 30 years on lithium. *Br J Psychiatry* 1983;143:424.

598. MacLaughlin M, de Mello Aires M. Impairment of renal tubular acidification by lithium: a microperfusion study in the rat. *Kidney Int* 1990;37:S-75.

599. Nascimento L, et al. On the mechanism of lithium-induced renal tubular acidosis. *J Lab Clin Med* 1977;89:455.

600. Orloff J, Kennedy TJ Jr. Effect of lithium on acidification of the urine. *Fed Proc* 1952;11:115.

601. Perez GO, Oster JR, Vaamonde CA. Incomplete syndrome of renal tubular acidosis induced by lithium carbonate. *J Lab Clin Med* 1975;86:386.

602. Perez GO, et al. Urinary carbon dioxide tension in lithium carbonate-treated patients. *J Pharmacol Exp Ther* 1977;201:456.

603. Roscoe J, et al. Studies on the mechanism of lithium-induced impairment of urinary acidification. *J Clin Invest* 1974;53:66A(abst).

604. Roscoe JM, et al. Lithium-induced impairment of urine acidification. *Kidney Int* 1976;9:344.

605. Bank N, et al. Studies on the urinary acidification defect induced by lithium. *Am J Physiol* 1982;242:F23.

606. Laski ME, Kurtzman NA. Characterization of acidification in the cortical and medullary collecting tubule of the rabbit. *J Clin Invest* 1983;72:2050.

607. Davies B, Kincaid-Smith P. Renal biopsy studies of lithium and prelithium patients and comparison with cadaver transplant kidneys. *Neuropharmacology* 1979;18:1001.

608. Kincaid-Smith P, et al. Renal-biopsy findings in lithium and prelithium patients. *Lancet* 1979;2:700.

609. Walker RG, et al. Chronic progressive renal lesions induced by lithium. *Kidney Int* 1986;29:875.

610. Farres MT, et al. Chronic lithium nephropathy: MR imaging for diagnosis. *Radiology* 2003;229:570.

611. Burrows GD, Davies B, Kincaid-Smith P. Unique tubular lesion after lithium. *Lancet* 1978;1:1310.

612. Perry PJ. Lithium nephrotoxicity. *Drug Intell Clin Pharmacol* 1982;16:740.

613. Wallin L, Alling C. Effects of sustained-release lithium tablets on renal function. *Br Med J* 1979;2:1332.

614. Plenge P, et al. Lithium treatment: does the kidney prefer one daily dose instead of two? *Acta Psychiatr Scand* 1982;66:121.

615. Perry PJ, et al. Lithium kinetics in single daily dosing. *Acta Psychiatr Scand* 1981;64:281.

616. Plenge P, Mellerup ET, Norgaard T. Functional and structural rat kidney changes caused by per oral or parenteral lithium treatment. *Acta Psychiatr Scand* 1981;63:303.

617. Plenge P, Mellerup ET. Lithium and the kidney. Is one daily dose better than two? *Compr Psychiatry* 1986;27:336.

618. Hetmar O, et al. Lithium: long-term effects on the kidney—II. Structural changes. *J Psychiatr Res* 1987;21:279.

619. Schou M, et al. Lithium treatment regimen and renal water handling: the significance of dosage pattern and tablet type examined through comparison of results from two clinics with different treatment regimens. *Psychopharmacology* 1982;77:387.

620. Hetmar O. The impact of long-term lithium treatment on renal function and structure. *Acta Psychiatr Scand* 1988;78:85.

621. Bowen RC, Grof P, Grof E. Less frequent lithium administration and lower urine volume. *Am J Psychiatry* 1991;148:189.

622. Griel W, et al. Single daily dose schedule in lithium long-term treatment: effects on pharmacokinetics and on renal and cardiac functions. *Pharmacopsychiatry* 1985;18:106.

623. Muir A, et al. Two regimens of lithium prophylaxis and renal function. *Acta Psychiatr Scand* 1989;80:579.
624. Abraham G, et al. Lithium treatment: a comparison of once and twice daily dosing. *Acta Psychiatr Scand* 1992;85:65.
625. O'Donovan C, Hawkes J, Bowen R. Effect of lithium dosing schedule on urinary output. *Acta Psychiatr Scand* 1993;87:92.
626. Abraham G, Waldron JJ, Lawson JS. Are the renal effects of lithium modified by frequency of administration? *Acta Psychiatr Scand* 1995;92:115.
627. Kusalic ME. Renal reactions to changes of lithium dosage. *Neuropsychobiology* 1996;34:113.
628. Lassen E, Vestergaard P, Thomsen K. Renal function of patients in long-term treatment with lithium citrate alone or in combination with neuroleptics and antidepressant drugs. *Arch Gen Psychiatry* 1986;43:481.

CHAPTER 47 ■ NEPHROTOXICITY SECONDARY TO ENVIRONMENTAL AGENTS AND HEAVY METALS

RICHARD P. WEDEEN

Environmental kidney diseases are usually recognized when they result from occupational exposure, a special case of environmental disease. Toxic effects detected in a few highly exposed workers suggest the diseases that can be anticipated from the lower exposures encountered by large populations from environmental pollution. Recognized chronic occupational renal diseases include those arising from exposure to heavy metals, organic solvents (aliphatic, aromatic, and halogenated hydrocarbons), and silica. Itai-itai disease from cadmium and Minimata disease from mercury are two environmental diseases arising from industrial pollutants first identified in Japan. To this group can be added Balkan nephritis, a disease of unknown etiology presumed to be of environmental origin and nephropathy caused by the ingestion of germanium compounds.

More than 45 naturally occurring elements are classified as heavy metals by virtue of their metallic qualities and specific gravities >5. Seven of these metals are generally recognized as nephrotoxic following environmental or occupational exposure: lead, cadmium, mercury, uranium, chromium, copper, and arsenic, although chronic renal failure has been described for only lead, mercury, cadmium, uranium, and arsenic. Therapeutic forms of platinum (Chapter 43, Renal Diseases Induced by Antineoplastic Agents), gold (Chapter 66, Renal Involvement in Systemic Sclerosis, Rheumatoid Arthritis, Sjögren's Syndrome, and Polymyositis-Dermatomyositis), lithium, and bismuth may also induce kidney damage. Although other heavy metals are potentially damaging to the kidneys, too little evidence of the clinical importance of these renal effects is available to warrant inclusion here. The potentially nephrotoxic heavy metals include barium, cobalt, manganese, nickel, silver, thallium, thorium, tin, and vanadium. The paucity of incriminating evidence against these elements may be more a testimony to our ignorance of the etiologic factors that lead to end-stage renal disease than to the benign nature of the metals.

Cause and effect are relatively easy to demonstrate when renal damage is acute. Establishing the contribution of an environmental toxin to kidney disease, however, is considerably more difficult if the toxicity is delayed. When renal disease is a consequence of long-term, low-dose, asymptomatic exposure modulated by complex interactions with other toxins, nutritional factors, other diseases, and genetic susceptibility, etiology remains difficult to prove. Kidney disease arising from exposure to environmental agents and heavy metals plays a special role in nephrology because of the potential for prevention.

URINARY BIOMARKERS

More than 25 urinary proteins and biochemical markers (eicosanoids) have been measured in urine using sensitive, specific assays to characterize early stages of toxic renal injury. We hope to detect specific causes of toxic nephropathy before the reduction in glomerular filtration rate (GFR) is sufficient to be manifest clinically by an increase in serum creatinine. The goal of establishing "fingerprints" for specific environmental nephrotoxins has been partially achieved. Urinary biomarkers are selected because they reflect specific sites of renal injury: (a) low-molecular-weight proteins and intracellular enzymes—proximal tubule damage, (b) Tamm-Horsfall glycoprotein and kallikrein—distal tubule injury, (c) high-molecular-weight proteins—increased glomerular permeability (if >200 mg/g creatinine), and (d) biochemical markers—eicosanoids suggesting vascular injury. Comprehensive urinary profiles have been evaluated in cooperative studies conducted in Europe (1–5) (Table 47-1). To achieve broad diagnostic value, the urinary markers are examined in subjects with known toxic exposures, over a wide range of dose rates and exposure times. Patients with known clinical renal failure, glomerular disease, multinephrotoxin or drug exposure, or systemic diseases that predispose to kidney damage (e.g., hypertension, diabetes mellitus, and gout) are excluded from these studies to reduce confounding variables. The specificity of tubular injury tends to disappear once renal damage is sufficient to cause an increase in the serum creatinine.

A sampling of 11 urinary markers (human intestinal alkaline phosphatase [HIAP], total nonspecific alkaline phosphatase [TNAP], N-acetyl-β-D-glucosaminidase [NAG], retinol binding protein [RBP], Tamm-Horsfall glycoprotein [THG], β_2-microglobulin, microalbumin, thromboxane B$_2$ [TBX$_2$], and three prostaglandins [prostaglandin E$_2$, PGE$_2$; prostaglandin F$_{2\alpha}$, PGF$_{2\alpha}$; 6-keto-prostaglandin F$_{1\alpha}$, 6-keto-PGF$_{1\alpha}$]) are presented to illustrate how differentiation of the toxic nephropathies can be accomplished (Table 47-1). The excretion patterns illustrated in Table 47-1 represent occupational exposure levels indicated by the mean blood or urine concentrations specified. The isoenzyme HIAP is a sensitive and specific indicator of injury to the S3 segment of the proximal tubule owing to occupational exposure to mercury and cadmium (3–5). Along with other markers of tubular and glomerular injury, HIAP is increased in the ischemic kidney and hypertension. Total nonspecific alkaline phosphatase is not increased in analgesic abuse or lead exposure, but it is increased after perchlorethylene exposure (6,7). N-acetyl-β-D-glucosaminidase is not elevated in the urine of workers exposed to perchlorethylene, or mercury (1,6); however, NAG and RBP are elevated after cadmium exposure (3,8). Tamm-Horsfall glycoprotein appears to be a marker of distal tubular injury in contrast to HIAP, TNAP, NAG, and RBP, which reflect proximal tubule injury. Although the pathophysiologic significance of the urinary eicosanoids is unclear, measurement of urinary PGE$_2$, PGF$_{2\alpha}$, and 6-keto-PGF$_{1\alpha}$ may provide insight into the mechanisms of hypertension and injury to the glomerulus or renal medulla.

TABLE 47-1

URINARY MARKERS IN TOXIC NEPHROPATHIES—EUROPEAN COOPERATIVE STUDY

	HIAP	TNAP	NAG	RBP	THG	β_2-M	mAlb	TXB$_2$	PG
Pb	−	−	+	−	−	−	−	++	6F−
Cd	+++	−	+++	+	−	+	++	−	6F++
Hg	+++	+	+	−	−	−	−	−	F−
					−			−	E−
PCE	−	+++	−	−	±	−	+	−	F−
									E−

HIAP, human intestinal alkaline phosphatase; *TNAP*, total nonspecific alkaline phosphatase; *NAG*, N-acetyl-β-D-glucosaminidase; *RBP*, retinol binding protein; *THG*, Tamm-Horsfall glycoprotein; β_2-*M*, β$_2$-microglobulin; mAlb, microalbumin; *TXB$_2$*, thromboxane B$_2$; *PG*, prostaglandin; *Pb*, lead; *Cd*, cadmium; *Hg*, mercury; *PCE*, perchloroethylene; *6F*, 6-keto-PGF$_{1\alpha}$; *F*, PGF$_{2\alpha}$; *E*, PGE$_2$.

The ability of these urinary markers to discriminate between various nephrotoxins increases with increasing exposure levels.

Low levels of urinary albumin may reflect either glomerular or tubular injury. Although generally considered to indicate early glomerular injury in diabetic patients, the appearance of small quantities of albumin in the urine may sometimes represent the failure of the tubule to reabsorb or metabolize albumin that passes through the glomerular filter in minute quantities but does not normally reach the bladder. Thus, low levels of urinary albumin may represent proximal tubular dysfunction rather than increased glomerular permeability.

A number of alternatives to the 11 urinary markers shown in Table 47-1 are available. For the present, they appear either to be redundant (e.g., alanine aminopeptidase, α_1-microglobulin, γ-glutamyltransferase) or to offer few advantages because their functional significance is unclear (e.g., fibronectin, glycosaminoglycans, kallikrein, or sialic acid). Reports by Mutti and associates (9) and the European Cooperative Study Group (1–3,6,8) suggest that the proximal tubule brush-border antigens designated BB50, BBA, and HF5 may be sensitive indicators of proximal tubular injury. However, standardization of these immunoassays has not been accomplished.

Urinary markers are determined in fresh-voided specimens (spot urines) and expressed relative to the creatinine concentration. Urine collections should be made at 8 AM when both GFR and protein excretion are highest. Circadian rhythm has been shown to occur for both GFR and low-molecular-weight proteinuria, with both being lowest during sleep (10).

LEAD NEPHROPATHY

Occupational exposure to lead began over 10,000 years ago in the region of the Aegean sea. The earliest description of lead poisoning is found in a poem dating from about 200 BC by the Greek philosopher Nikander of Colophon (11). Although possible recognition of renal effects of lead can be traced to the 17th century, Lancereaux provided the first description of lead nephrotoxicity in modern terms in 1862. Lancereaux's patient had saturnine (lead-induced) gout; his kidneys showed interstitial nephritis at postmortem examination. Controversy concerning the renal effects of lead stems from this 19th century description compounded by the recurrent failure to recognize the late sequelae of chronic absorption of relatively low levels of lead or to distinguish glomerular from extraglomerular renal disease. Additional confusion has been created by the failure to distinguish the transient Fanconi's syndrome of acute childhood lead poisoning from the chronic interstitial nephritis characteristic of lead nephropathy in adults. In addition to the difficulty in assigning cause when the effect is delayed in time,

identification of the renal effects of lead was further obscured because the late complications of excessive lead absorption, namely, gout and hypertension, can themselves produce renal damage unrelated to lead.

Diagnosis

In the past, lead nephropathy was identified in individuals who had repeated episodes of acute lead intoxication (11). The classic symptoms of inorganic lead poisoning (abdominal colic, extensor muscle weakness, and encephalopathy) in patients known to have excessive lead absorption made the diagnosis straightforward. In recent decades, the diagnosis was confirmed in the clinical laboratory by finding anemia in association with excessive urinary excretion of lead, coproporphyrins, or δ-aminolevulinic acid. Following the extensive studies of lead metabolism by Kehoe beginning in the 1930s (11), the mainstay of laboratory diagnosis was the blood lead concentration. Until 1978, a whole blood lead concentration of up to 80 μg/dL was considered "acceptable" in occupationally exposed adults. Blood lead levels below 80 μg/dL were considered incompatible with the diagnosis of lead poisoning in adults, although levels above 40 μg/dL were considered unacceptable in children. The battle over the determination of the "safe" blood lead level continues despite a growing consensus that blood levels over 10 μg/dL may be associated with lead-induced organ damage (12).

The blood lead concentration is relatively insensitive to cumulative body stores acquired over many years of moderate exposure (i.e., exposure insufficient to produce classic symptoms of acute poisoning). Blood lead concentrations tend to fall markedly within weeks of removal from exposure. Alternative approaches to the detection of excessive lead absorption have been examined because approximately 95% of the body stores of lead are retained in bone with a mean residence time approximating 20 years (13). At present, cumulative past lead absorption is best assessed by the calcium disodium edetate (CaNa$_2$EDTA) lead-mobilization test.

The ethylenediamine tetraacetic acid (EDTA) test is performed in adults by parenteral administration of 1 to 3 g of CaNa$_2$EDTA over 4 to 12 hours with subsequent collection of 24-hour urine samples over 1 to 4 days. A dosage of 20 to 30 mg of CaNa$_2$ EDTA per kg is generally used in children. Adults without undue prior lead absorption excrete up to 650 μg of lead-chelate in the urine. Neither the dose (1 to 3 g) nor the route of administration (intravenous or intramuscular) appears to critically modify the normal response to chelation testing (14), but in the presence of renal failure (serum creatinine >1.5 mg/dL) urine collections should be extended to

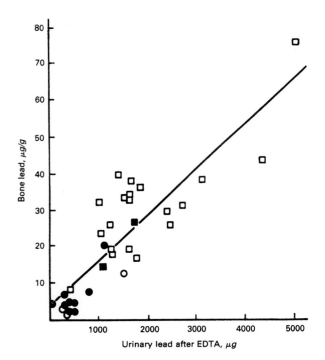

FIGURE 47-1. Relationship of bone lead to chelatable lead in 35 Belgians including 22 lead workers (*squares*). Lead was measured in transiliac bone biopsy specimens by atomic absorption spectroscopy and chelatable lead by the EDTA lead-mobilization test. The linear regression correlation coefficient (*r*) is 0.87. *Open symbols* represent subjects with normal glomerular filtration rates; *closed symbols*, those with reduced glomerular filtration rates. (From: Van de Vyver FL, et al. Bone lead in dialysis patients. *Kidney Int* 1988;33:601, with permission.)

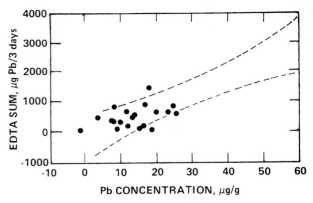

FIGURE 47-2. Bone lead determined by *in vivo* tibial K x-ray fluorescence compared to chelatable lead in American armed service veterans without known excessive exposure to lead. *Dotted lines* represent 95% confidence limits of data presented in Figure 47-1. Transiliac bone lead values in Figure 47-1 were multiplied by 1.75 to convert to tibial bone values. Pb, lead. (From: Wedeen RP. Bone lead, hypertension, and lead nephropathy. *Environ Health Perspect* 1988;78:57, with permission.)

at least 3 days. The intramuscular administration of 2 g of $CaNa_2EDTA$ (1 g of EDTA mixed with local anesthetic in each of two injections, 12 hours apart) may be the preferable method of performing the chelation test because it has been well standardized in both normal subjects and patients with renal failure (14–19). In the presence of reduced GFR, urinary excretion of lead chelate is measured for 3 consecutive days and the adequacy of collection checked by simultaneous measurement of urinary creatinine excretion (1.3 g of creatinine per day is an acceptable lower limit in normal adult males).

Because lead in bone has a biologic half-life measured in decades, compared to a biologic half-life of lead in blood of only 4 weeks (20), the bone more closely reflects cumulative body lead stores. Chelatable lead correlates well with bone lead (21,22) (Fig. 47-1). Diagnostic monitoring of the body lead burden can be accomplished by *in vivo* tibial K x-ray fluorescence, a new noninvasive technique that is both safe and accurate at bone lead concentrations associated with interstitial nephritis caused by lead (23–25) (Fig. 47-2). The characteristic K x-rays of lead are stimulated by the 88-keV gamma emissions from a ^{109}Cd radioactive source. The fluorescent x-rays are measured with a high-purity, liquid nitrogen-cooled, germanium detector and recorded in a computer equipped with a multichannel pulse height analyzer. The characteristic K x-rays differ from the characteristic L x-rays of lead in that the higher-energy K photons penetrate 2 cm of cortical bone (26). L x-rays only detect lead within the outermost 0.5 mm of subperiosteal bone. Calibration of the L x-rays is problematic because of major soft tissue absorption. K x-rays, on the other hand, can be accurately calibrated and normalized to the bone calcium content. The K x-ray fluorescence technique records the calcium-phosphorus content of the bone region under study (elastic scatter) and thus permits measurement of the lead-calcium atomic ratio. This ra-

tio is largely independent of target-source geometry and therefore permits calibration by either plaster-of-Paris phantoms or absolute physical properties (25). Whole-body radiation during the 30-minute K x-ray fluorescence test is 0.3 mrem, equivalent to background cosmic radiation absorbed over about 10 hours.

Although the blood lead reflects absorption of both organic and inorganic lead, the clinical symptoms of organic lead are primarily cerebral. Colic, peripheral neuropathy, and anemia are not seen in acute organic lead poisoning. Chelation therapy is ineffective in acute organic lead poisoning (27). DuPont's Chambers Works in Deepwater, New Jersey, became known as the "House of Butterflies" because of the frequency of hallucinations among workers producing tetraethyl lead shortly after discovery of the antiknock gasoline additive in 1923 (28). Renal disease has not been found following tetraethyl lead absorption (27).

Acute Lead Nephropathy

In children with lead encephalopathy, a proximal tubule reabsorptive defect characterized by aminoaciduria, phosphaturia, and glycosuria (Fanconi's syndrome) has been observed (29). Fanconi's syndrome is found in the presence of blood lead levels usually in excess of 150 μg/dL and appears to be rapidly reversed by chelation therapy designed to treat the far more dangerous encephalopathy. The proximal tubule reabsorptive defect has been induced experimentally in rats fed dietary lead (30). In both children and experimental animals, acute lead nephropathy is consistently associated with acid-fast intranuclear inclusions in proximal tubule epithelial cells (31). The intranuclear inclusion bodies consist of a lead–protein complex and may be seen in tubular epithelial cells in the urinary sediment during acute poisoning (32). Lead-containing intranuclear inclusions have been observed in liver, neural tissue, and osteoclasts as well as kidney. Acute poisoning is also associated with morphologic and functional defects in mitochondria.

Chronic Lead Nephropathy

The phrase *chronic lead nephropathy* refers to the slowly progressive interstitial nephritis occurring in adults following prolonged lead exposure. Occupational lead nephropathy has developed after as little as 3 years of intense exposure (18). Analysis of death certificates of 601 men employed at the Bunker Hill Lead Mine and Smelter in Kellogg, Idaho, up to 1977 indicated a twofold-increased risk of dying from chronic renal disease (33). The increased risk approached fourfold after 20 years of occupational exposure. Although most frequently recognized in lead workers after decades of occupational exposure, chronic lead nephropathy also has been recognized among young adults in Australia who sustained acute childhood lead poisoning (34) and among illicit whiskey ("moonshine") consumers in the southeastern United States. Chronic interstitial nephritis owing to lead has also been seen among American workmen whose exposure was never severe enough to produce acute symptoms of lead poisoning (18,19), and in U.S. armed service veterans suffering from renal failure attributed to gout or essential hypertension (16,17). In the veterans, exposure to lead had never produced acute symptoms of poisoning, and the source of exposure had never been recognized. The diagnosis was only established by performance of the $CaNa_2EDTA$ lead-mobilization test after renal failure was apparent. Medical histories were often misleading; patient recall frequently contradicted the objective evidence of chelation testing. Sporadic case reports of lead nephropathy arising from unusual accidental exposure such as geophagia (35) or Asian folk remedies and cosmetics continue to appear in the medical literature (11).

"Queensland nephritis" appears to represent the transition from the acute disease of childhood to the chronic nephropathy of adults (34). This evolution has been observed in experimental animals but has not been reported in American children. The difference between the American and Australian experience may well owe to the fact that the American children with pica who had long-term follow-up received chelation therapy in childhood. In an early follow-up study of untreated childhood lead poisoning, diagnostic criteria for both lead poisoning and renal disease were unacceptably vague (36). A 50-year follow-up of untreated lead-poisoned children in the United States found evidence of increased renal disease (37).

Chronic lead nephropathy from moonshine came to medical attention because of the dramatic symptoms of acute lead poisoning. As in severely exposed industrial workers, lead colic and anemia were associated with reduced GFR, which often improved following chelation therapy. Transient renal failure, apparently the result of renal vasoconstriction (38), was superimposed on more chronic renal damage that appeared to be less responsive to chelating agents. The chronic lead nephropathy of the moonshiners, more often than not, was accompanied by gout and hypertension, in accord with 19th century descriptions of plumbism and contemporary reports from Australia (11). A statistically significant odds ratio of 2.4 has been reported for moonshine consumption and end-stage renal disease, suggesting a causal association in the absence of acute lead poisoning (39).

Evaluation of renal function in workmen with excessive body lead stores has revealed previously unsuspected reductions in GFR (i.e., <90 mL/minute/1.73 m^2 body surface area) before renal dysfunction was clinically evident (19). In these occupationally exposed individuals, minimal (about 30%) reductions in GFR were restored to normal by long-term, low-dose chelation therapy (1 g of $CaNa_2EDTA$ with local anesthetic three times weekly until the chelation test returned to normal). This therapeutic response in preazotemic lead nephropathy may reflect reversal of functional impairment rather than reversal of established interstitial nephritis. Both the renin-angiotensin system and Na^+-K^+-ATPase are inhibited by lead (40), and these effects may have been modified by chelation therapy. Considerable epidemiologic evidence suggests that modest azotemia is significantly more prevalent among lead-exposed workers than among nonexposed counterparts, presumably owing to both morphologic and functional changes (11,41).

Renal biopsies in chronic lead nephropathy show nonspecific tubular atrophy and interstitial fibrosis with minimal inflammatory response as well as mitochondrial swelling, loss of cristae, and increased lysosomal dense bodies within proximal tubule cells (18,21) (Fig. 47-3). Arteriolar changes indistinguishable from nephrosclerosis are found, often in the absence of clinical hypertension. Intranuclear inclusion bodies are often absent when the renal disease is long-standing or following the administration of chelating agents. Clumped chromatin and nuclear invaginations of cytoplasmic contents may be found even in the absence of intranuclear inclusions. Morphologic alterations are minimal in glomeruli until the reduction in GFR is advanced.

The hypothesis derived from acute lead nephropathy—that proximal tubular injury accounts for the pathogenesis of chronic lead nephropathy—has gained little support. The appearance of arteriolar nephrosclerosis before hypertension develops and the relatively short duration of hypertension before renal failure supervenes suggest that the initial renal injury from lead may be in the microvascular endothelium (42,43). At the cellular level, lead metabolism mimics that of calcium (44). Proximal tubular transport defects in excess of that expected in comparable chronic renal failure have not been convincingly demonstrated in chronic lead nephropathy. The mechanism of microvascular injury remains speculative. Interference

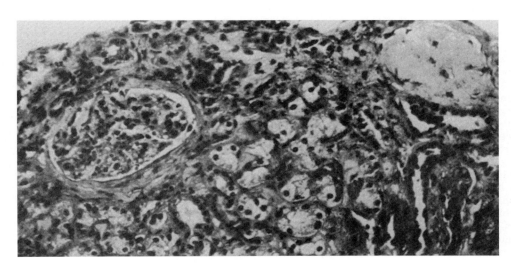

FIGURE 47-3. Renal biopsy obtained from a 28-year-old man who had prepared lead solder for 5 years. His ^{125}I-iothalamate clearance was 52 mL/minute/1.73 m^2; hemoglobin, 9.6 g/dL; uric acid, 13.2 mg/dL; and blood lead, 48 μg/dL when he was initially seen. Lead-chelate excretion following 2 g of $CaNa_2EDTA$ intramuscularly was 5.2 mg/24 hours. Light microscopy shows periglomerular fibrosis, a sclerotic glomerulus, and tubular atrophy. (Trichrome stain; magnification ×304.) (From: Wedeen RP, et al. Occupational lead nephropathy. *Am J Med* 1975;59: 630, with permission.)

with cation transport is a reasonable hypothesis because the metabolism of lead is similar to that of other cations. The paradox that increased dietary calcium reduces vascular smooth muscle tone, whereas increased free intracellular calcium increases it could, in part, be explained by lead–calcium interactions (15). Inhibition of red blood cell Na^+-K^+-ATPase in lead workers correlates with membrane-bound lead (45), and lead increases red blood cell Na^+-Li^+ countertransport *in vitro* (46). Similarly, lead interactions with vasoactive substances may modulate blood pressure and induce endothelial injury (47,48).

The functional changes in chronic lead nephropathy appear to be less specific than those observed in acute poisoning. As in other forms of interstitial nephritis, proteinuria and glycosuria are initially absent. In contrast to cadmium nephropathy, the excretion of urinary marker proteins such as HIAP, TNAP, THG, RBP, lysozyme, and β_2-microglobulin (2,8) is not increased in the absence of a reduced GFR (Table 47-1). The increase in urinary NAG with increasing blood lead reflects Fanconi's syndrome of acute lead poisoning rather than the chronic interstitial nephritis associated with occupational lead exposure (49,50). N-acetyl-β-D-glucosaminidase excretion correlates positively with the blood lead concentration but not with the bone lead concentration (50). Exhibiting a pattern of eicosanoid excretion noted in essential hypertension, lead-exposed workers showed an increase in TXB_2 and a decrease in PGE_2 and 6-keto-$PGF_{1\alpha}$ in the urine (2,50). In contrast to the reabsorptive defect of acute lead nephropathy, saturnine gout is characterized by renal retention of uric acid (34). The clearance (C_{PAH}) and maximal secretion rate (Tm_{PAH}) for p-aminohippurate (PAH) have been found to be variable in patients with occupational lead nephropathy.

The relationship of lead to gout nephropathy has provoked controversy for over a century (11,51). Hyperuricemia and gout are common among individuals with excessive exposure to lead, apparently the result of decreased excretion and increased production of uric acid. Similarly, although hyperuricemia invariably accompanies azotemia, gout is rare in patients with renal failure except in those with lead nephropathy. Half of uremic patients with lead nephropathy have clinical gout (34), but in the absence of renal failure, gout cannot usually be attributed to lead despite coexisting hypertension (52,53).

There is substantial evidence that renal failure in gout is sometimes secondary to overt or unsuspected lead poisoning. In Queensland, Australia, as many as 80% of gout patients with renal failure have elevated EDTA lead-mobilization tests (34). In New Jersey, chelatable lead was found to be significantly greater among gout patients with renal failure than among gout patients with normal renal function (16). Because patients with comparable renal failure owing to known causes other than lead show no increase in chelatable lead, the excessive mobilizable lead in these gout patients appears to be the cause rather than consequence of their renal failure. Measurement of lead levels in transiliac biopsy specimens from patients with end-stage renal disease confirms the fact that renal failure per se does not cause increased bone lead levels (22). Unrecognized lead poisoning, therefore, may explain the occurrence of renal failure in some gout patients who have neither urinary calculi nor intratubular uric acid deposition disease. Similarly, overt lead poisoning may explain the protean manifestations of gout in past centuries, the so-called irregular gout, as well as the long but almost forgotten association of gout with wine (11). Sporadic contamination of alcoholic drinks with lead throughout history may have been responsible for gout that terminated in cerebral disease (e.g., uremia, stroke, or encephalopathy).

The association between lead and hypertension has also been a subject of controversy since the first use of the sphygmomanometer. The early view that renal injury induced by lead causes hypertension has gained increasing support. The EDTA lead-mobilization test can sometimes indicate that lead is the most probable cause of hypertension with renal failure when lead exposure has not been previously suspected. Patients believed to have "essential hypertension with nephrosclerosis" may be identified as having lead nephropathy by the EDTA lead-mobilization test (17). The duration of hypertension in patients with lead nephropathy tends to be shorter than that in hypertensives without renal failure, suggesting that lead-induced renal injury precedes and therefore causes the hypertension. This view is consistent with the finding that creatinine clearance decreases with increasing blood lead in the general population, an effect that is independent of blood pressure (41,54).

Lead nephropathy does not account for renal failure in all hypertensives with kidney disease any more than it accounts for renal failure in all gout patients with kidney disease. The heavy metal may, however, contribute to the long and controversial association of gout with hypertension, as well as to the variable incidence of renal failure in each of these conditions. Mortality data show that death from hypertensive cardiovascular disease is more frequent among lead workers than the general population (33).

A role for lead in hypertension gains further credence from epidemiologic studies of low-level lead exposure (i.e., exposure too low in intensity to produce the classic symptoms of acute lead poisoning). The Second National Health and Nutrition Examination Survey (NHANES II) performed between 1976 and 1980 included blood lead and blood pressure measurements in almost 10,000 noninstitutionalized Americans aged 6 months to 74 years (55). The correlation between blood lead and blood pressure was robust even when both measurements were within the accepted "normal" range (56,57). Similar conclusions have been drawn from studies performed throughout the world, although statistically nonsignificant findings in small studies have also been reported. A longitudinal study of 590 men with a low mean blood lead concentration (6.3 μg/dL) found that bone lead was higher in those who developed hypertension than in those who did not, although the blood lead was not significantly different (58). Although some doubts have been raised about the magnitude of the dose-response relationship, there is a growing consensus that lead contributes to hypertension in the general population, particularly in the presence of renal dysfunction. Lead may also contribute to the disproportionate representation of black men with hypertensive nephrosclerosis and diabetic nephropathy in end-stage renal disease programs in the United States (15).

Treatment

Lead nephropathy is important because it is one of the few renal diseases that is preventable. Moreover, lead nephropathy can sometimes be reversed or its progression retarded by judicious use of chelation therapy (11,19,38,59). Lead nephropathy is unusual for a nonsystemic disease involving the kidneys in that an etiologic diagnosis can be established even after renal failure supervenes. The observation that chelation therapy improved renal function in renal failure patients with low body lead stores suggests that unrecognized low-level lead absorption contributes to renal failure owing to other causes (60).

Although chelation therapy effectively reverses acute lead nephropathy and the preclinical renal dysfunction of occupational lead nephropathy (19), there is no evidence that such therapy reverses established interstitial nephritis. The partial remissions achieved among moonshiners and symptomatic lead workers may represent reversal of acute poisoning superimposed on chronic lead nephropathy. No improvement in renal function can be expected once advanced interstitial nephritis is present and the steady-state serum creatinine concentration exceeds about 3 mg/dL (61). Chronic volume depletion and hyporeninemic hypoaldosteronism may contribute to the reversible component of renal dysfunction. The effect of lead on the renin–angiotensin system, however, remains controversial because increased renin responsiveness has also been observed in lead-exposed experimental animals and humans (40).

Before chelation therapy is undertaken, the diagnosis should be clearly established. It may be necessary to perform the EDTA lead-mobilization test, and other possible causes of renal disease must be rigorously excluded. For the present, attempts at chelation therapy probably should be avoided when the cause of the renal disease is unclear (e.g., in the presence of heavy proteinuria). Moreover, long-term, low-dose EDTA therapy should only be undertaken with a clear end point in mind, such as reversion of the EDTA test to normal and restoration of renal function. Although the EDTA test has been shown to be safe even in the presence of renal failure (62), the cumulative nephrotoxicity of prolonged EDTA therapy in patients with markedly reduced GFR is unknown. Reports that $CaNa_2EDTA$ therapy has been followed by deterioration of renal function warrant careful follow-up of treated patients (61,63). Despite these caveats, it may be appropriate to perform EDTA lead-mobilization tests in individuals with gout or hypertension and renal failure or interstitial nephritis of unknown etiology, because a positive test may provide the best available indication of etiology. Knowledge of etiology may permit identification and removal of the source of lead and prevention of lead nephropathy in others.

CADMIUM NEPHROPATHY

Industrial use of cadmium has increased steadily since its discovery by Stromyer in 1817. Cadmium-containing compounds are widely used in the manufacturing of pigments, plastics, glass, metal alloys, and electrical equipment. Acute absorption of as little as 10 mg as dust or fumes may induce severe gastrointestinal symptoms and, after a delay of 8 to 24 hours, fatal pulmonary edema (64,65). Chronic low-dose exposure, on the other hand, causes slowly progressive emphysema, anosmia, and proximal tubular reabsorptive defects characterized by low-molecular-weight proteinuria, enzymuria, aminoaciduria, and renal glycosuria (66). Hypercalciuria (with normocalcemia), phosphaturia, and distal renal tubular acidosis result in clinically important osteomalacia, pseudofractures, and urinary tract stones (67,68). Interstitial nephritis resulting from parenteral administration of cadmium to experimental animals was recognized in the 19th century (69), but only recently has the progression of early proximal tubular dysfunction to chronic renal failure been documented.

Metabolism

Nonoccupationally exposed individuals accumulate cadmium throughout their lives through food and cigarettes. The biologic half-life of cadmium in humans exceeds 15 years, and one-third of the total body stores (10 to 20 mg) is retained in the kidneys. Tubular proteinuria has resulted from low-level environmental exposure to cadmium as well as to the higher exposure levels encountered in industry (70).

Absorbed cadmium is initially sequestered in liver and kidney, where it is bound to a cysteine-rich apoprotein, metallothionein (64,66). Zinc, copper, mercury, and iron, as well as cadmium, induce metallothionein synthesis in these organs. With a molecular mass of 6,500 daltons, the cadmium–thionein complex is filtered at the glomerulus, taken up in the proximal tubule by endocytosis, and transferred to lysosomes, where it

is rapidly degraded. Cadmium–thionein is considerably more nephrotoxic than cadmium or metallothionein alone, but cytoplasmic cadmium ions released from lysosomes may be the mediator of tubular cell injury (71). Although uptake in liver initially exceeds that in kidney, most of the cadmium is eventually bound to protein in the proximal tubules, where it is accumulated until a "critical concentration," approximately 200 μg/g of renal cortex, is achieved. At this tissue level, renal effects become evident, including tubular proteinuria and increased cadmium excretion (66). Although urinary cadmium excretion is normally less than 2 μg/day, after the critical concentration has been exceeded, urinary cadmium in excess of 10 μg/day is usual. Significant abnormalities of proximal tubular function are associated with urinary cadmium excretion in excess of 30 μg/day (72). The blood cadmium concentration is less reliable as an indicator of health effects. Although the blood cadmium level rises promptly following occupational exposure, blood is a poor indicator of cumulative absorption. Nevertheless, blood levels greater than 1 μg/dL, as well as urine concentrations of over 10 μg/g of creatinine, are considered evidence of excessive exposure.

Increased urinary excretion of low-molecular-weight proteins such as β-2-microglobulin or RBP is an early renal effect of cadmium (64). β-2 Microglobulin has been the most extensively examined urinary protein in cadmium nephropathy, but because of its instability in acid urine, measurement of urinary RBP or NAG is probably more reliable (3,8,50,72). Low-level increases in the excretion of albumin and transferrin in cadmium workers with low-molecular-weight proteinuria and enzymuria (3) raise the possibility of glomerular injury but also could be explained by impaired tubular reabsorption or metabolism of these proteins that are normally filtered in small quantities. Proteinuria in cadmium workers rarely exceeds a few hundred milligrams per day and does not approach nephrotic levels (>3.5 g/day). The usual techniques for detecting albuminuria such as Albustix, heat and picric acid, or nitric acid are not sufficiently sensitive or specific to reliably detect tubular proteinuria. Although phosphotungstic, trichloroacetic, and sulfosalicylic acids are more sensitive, immunologic techniques are required for specific protein identification. The pathophysiologic implications for increased excretion of 6-keto-$PGF_{1\alpha}$ and sialic acid in cadmium workers remain to be determined (3).

Calcium Wasting

Clinical symptoms associated with cadmium nephropathy derive primarily from the increased calcium excretion that accompanies the renal tubular dysfunction. Hypouricemia, hypophosphatemia, intermittent renal glycosuria, or elevated serum alkaline phosphatase (in the absence of renal failure or hyperparathyroidism) may bring the acquired Fanconi's syndrome to the clinician's attention, but ureteral colic is more likely to be the cadmium worker's chief complaint (64,67). Although both osteomalacia and renal failure are distinctly uncommon in cadmium workers (62), urinary calculi have been reported in up to 40% of those subjected to industrial exposure (66,67,74). Osteomalacia is associated with diminished renal tubular reabsorption of calcium and phosphate, elevated circulating parathormone levels, and reduced hydroxylation of vitamin D metabolites (76).

Itai-Itai Disease

In Japan, a painful bone disease associated with pseudofractures caused by cadmium-induced renal calcium wasting was recognized in the 1950s. Attributed to local contamination of food staples by river water polluted with industrial effluents, particularly cadmium, the syndrome known as itai-itai or "ouch-ouch" disease afflicted postmenopausal, multiparous women. Sustained deficiencies in iron, zinc, calcium, and vitamin D rendered these women particularly vulnerable to cadmium toxicity. The women with itai-itai disease tended to have reduced GFR, anemia, lymphopenia, and hypotension as well as osteomalacia. They exhibited a waddling gait, short stature, anemia, glucosuria, and elevated serum alkaline phosphatase levels. Hypertension was absent. β_2-Microglobulin excretion exceeded the normal maximum (1 mg/g of creatinine) 100-fold, and GFR was substantially reduced in the most severely affected individuals. An increase in mean serum creatinine concentration from 1.19 to 1.68 mg/dL in 21 individuals averaging 65 years of age who were followed for 9 to 14 years after β_2 microglobulin was first detected demonstrated the progression of renal failure (76). The long-term follow-up demonstrated that β_2-microglobulin predicts the later development of renal failure in patients with itai-itai disease and that renal damage progresses even after exposure has ceased.

Chronic Interstitial Nephritis

Until recently, the role of cadmium in the induction of chronic interstitial nephritis has been controversial (Fig. 47-4). Epidemiologic studies do not show a consistent correlation between blood or urinary cadmium levels and blood pressure (77). Mortality studies designed to evaluate the long-term implications of industrial cadmium exposure have yielded conflicting results (78). Nevertheless, tubulointerstitial nephritis was found in 23 occupationally exposed and 26 environmentally exposed individuals in whom postmortem tissue or renal biopsy specimens were examined (79). These findings in conjunction with recent epidemiologic studies in the United States (74) and Belgium (80,81) and the long-term follow-up of itai-itai disease in Japan (76) leave little room for doubt that cadmium can induce chronic interstitial nephritis.

In the United States, Thun and coworkers (74) examined 45 current and retired nonferrous smelter workers exposed to cadmium for a mean of 19 years. Their blood cadmium levels averaged 7.9 μg/dL and urinary cadmium 9.3 μg/g of creatinine. Cumulative cadmium dose estimated from air measurements correlated with low-molecular-weight proteinuria and with decreased fractional calcium and phosphate reabsorption. The cadmium workers had significantly more kidney stones than did controls. Correlations between renal function and cadmium exposure were independent of other diseases in the workmen. A strong association between cumulative cadmium exposure and the later increase in serum creatinine supported the notion that cadmium-induced renal disease progresses slowly after a latent period of several decades. Roels and colleagues (80) provided further evidence that clinical renal disease results from cadmium. Workers who were exposed to cadmium in a nonferrous smelter in Belgium for up to 5 years and who had tubular proteinuria were examined annually for 5 years after exposure had ceased. Cadmium levels in liver ranged from 24 to 158 μg/g and from 133 to 355 μg/g in the kidney. Serum creatinine concentrations increased from a mean of 1.2 to 1.5 mg/dL over 5 years (Fig. 47-5). The reduction in GFR was accompanied by an increase in mean serum β_2-microglobulin from 0.189 to 0.300 mg/dL and an increase in mean urinary β_2-microglobulin excretion from 1.770 to 2.500 mg/L. The loss of glomerular filtration over the 5-year period was estimated to be 30 mL/minute, 30 times the predicted loss of kidney function for these elderly men. In contrast to the progression of renal disease in these cadmium workers, the same laboratory found that environmental exposure leading to urine cadmium concentrations of less than 1 μg/24 hours did not result in progressive renal failure over 5 years (81). Despite the low levels of cadmium absorption, the environmentally exposed group exhibited diminished bone density and increased risk of fractures (82).

Diagnosis

Most commonly, the diagnosis of cadmium nephropathy is established by the history of exposure in conjunction with laboratory tests indicative of proximal tubule dysfunction

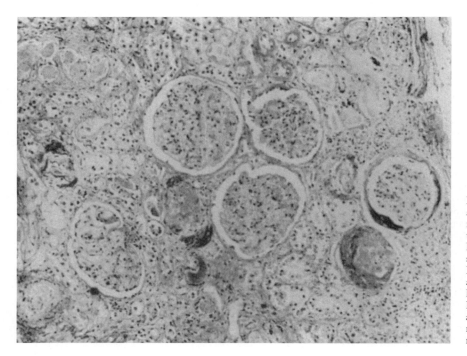

FIGURE 47-4. Autopsy section of kidney from a 46-year-old man who had manufactured cadmium pigments for 28 years. He was found to have renal glycosuria, proteinuria, mild hypertension, and severe pulmonary emphysema. Death was attributed to cor pulmonale. His kidneys contained 55 μg Cd/g wet wt and showed extensive interstitial fibrosis, tubular atrophy, and glomerular sclerosis. (From: Kazantzis G, et al. Renal tubular malfunction and pulmonary emphysema in cadmium pigment workers. *Q J Med* 1963;32:165, with permission.)

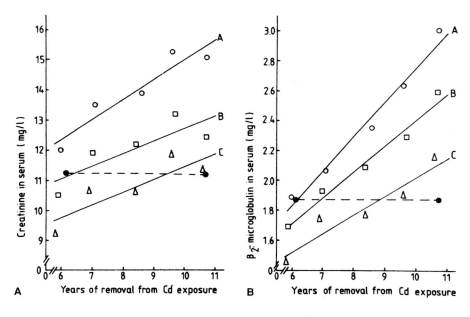

FIGURE 47-5. Progression of renal dysfunction in cadmium (Cd) workers over 5 years after removal from exposure. **A:** Total population of cadmium workers ($N = 23$). The mean serum creatinine increased from 1.2 to 1.5 mg/dL. **B:** Cadmium workers with serum creatinines <1.5 mg/dL ($N = 21$). **C:** Cadmium workers with tubular proteinuria and serum creatinine <1.3 mg/dL ($N = 11$). *Dashed line* represents two age-matched control groups of 23 subjects each.

(e.g., increased excretion of urinary biomarkers, hypercalciuria, or renal glycosuria). Suspicions are confirmed if the urinary cadmium concentration exceeds 10 μg/g of creatinine. Renal and hepatic accumulation of cadmium has been exploited for diagnostic purposes by *in vivo* neutron-activation analysis. This noninvasive technique for assessing organ cadmium content correlates well with tissue and urinary cadmium levels and β_2-microglobulin excretion. It should prove valuable for monitoring industrial exposure before toxic levels have been attained (80). In individuals without occupational exposure, renal cadmium content reaches a maximum of about 50 μg/g of cortex at about 45 years of age and thereafter declines as urinary elimination increases (66). Renal cadmium concentration tends to fall with the development of renal failure, so that the diagnostic value of neutron-activation analysis of kidney is diminished in azotemic or uremic patients. *In vivo* neutron-activation studies indicate that when the hepatic cadmium level exceeds about 60 ppm, and renal cortical content exceeds 200 ppm (20 mg/kidney), tubular proteinuria is likely to occur (80).

Treatment

Although CaNa$_2$EDTA given to experimental animals simultaneously with cadmium results in prompt excretion of the cadmium chelate and protection from nephrotoxicity, the chelating agent has little effect after cadmium has been complexed with metallothionein (83). Progression of renal disease has been described despite removal from exposure (76). Although osteomalacia may be arrested by calcium and vitamin D replacement (72), urinary tract stones represent a relative contraindication to such therapy.

MERCURY

The toxicity of mercury depends on both its chemical form and the route of absorption. Elemental mercury is virtually harmless when ingested (84), but inhalation of the metallic vapor can produce bronchial damage and later neurologic disease (85,86). After *in vivo* oxidation of metallic mercury to the ionic form, the inhaled vapor readily crosses the blood-brain barrier and is retained in the cerebrum and cerebellum. Although preferentially accumulated in the kidney, neurologic but not

nephrologic disease regularly follows exposure to elemental mercury; paresthesias, tremor, ataxia, visual impairment, erythrism, and ultimately stupor and death are the clinical course.

Once in the environment, elemental mercury undergoes biotransformation to both organic and inorganic salts that are absorbed by living organisms and thus enter the food chain. Methyl, ethyl, and phenoxyethyl mercury are important organomercurial contaminants arising from industrial and agricultural processes. Methyl and ethyl mercury compounds are widely used as fungicides but also enter the environment as industrial wastes and through biotransformation of less toxic mercurials. Although a diuretic effect of inorganic mercury was documented in the late 19th century, diuresis following therapeutic administration of organomercurials was first noted by a medical student in Vienna in 1920 as a side effect of Novasurol used in antisyphilitic therapy (86). Organomercurials subsequently became the mainstay of diuretic therapy until the advent of ethacrynic acid and furosemide in the 1960s. The inorganic mercurous salt, calomel (Hg$_2$Cl$_2$), is relatively nontoxic and was widely used as a medicinal agent until the twentieth century. The mercuric salt, corrosive sublimate (HgCl$_2$), on the other hand, is highly nephrotoxic and continues to be used to create animal models of acute tubular necrosis (ATN) (86). Phenyl and methoxy methyl mercuric salts produce similar nephrotoxicity.

Although all chemical forms of mercury are accumulated in the cells of proximal tubules, the cellular concentration by itself provides little insight into pharmacologic or toxic mechanisms. Inorganic mercury is retained in the kidney with a biologic half-life approximating 2 months (87). While HgCl$_2$, chlormerodrin, and *p*-chloromercuribenzoate (*p*-CMB) are each selectively concentrated in the proximal tubule, the inorganic HgCl$_2$ salt produces tubular necrosis, chlormerodrin is a diuretic, and *p*-CMB blocks the diuretic effect of chlormerodrin (87–89).

The inorganic and organic mercurials bind avidly to sulfhydryl groups in circulating proteins and amino acids as well as intracellular glutathione, cysteine, and metallothionein. Selective accumulation in the pars recta of proximal tubules is accomplished by transport primarily from the luminal side of mercury bound to amino acids or proteins. Mercury-ligand reaches lysosomes by endocytosis (88) with subsequent release into the cytosol by intralysosomal enzymatic degradation. It is less clear if mercury moves in the secretory direction, entering proximal tubular cells from the peritubular surface. Excretion is primarily through bile in the feces.

Diagnosis

Although blood mercury levels over 3 μg/dL or urine levels above 50 μg/g of creatinine are considered abnormal, the correlation of blood and urine concentrations with renal disease is poor (90). Workers exposed to mercury vapors frequently excrete more than 200 μg of mercury per liter of urine, but very few have renal disease. Consequently, the diagnosis of mercury-induced renal disease is usually dependent on known exposure in the presence of renal dysfunction. Case reports of ATN or the nephrotic syndrome attributed to occupational, accidental, or intentional exposure to mercury are necessarily limited to situations in which the toxic agent has been identified. Occupational exposure to elemental mercury for a decade with urinary concentrations exceeding 50 μg/dL is associated with increased HIAP excretion but little increase in urinary TNAP, NAG, RBP, THG, β_2 microglobulin, or microalbumin (1,5) (Table 47-1). There is no evidence that enzymuria from mercury exposure predicts the development of renal failure.

Acute Tubular Necrosis

Ingestion of as little as 0.5 g of $HgCl_2$ produces ATN in humans. Over the first few days, the clinical picture is dominated by gastrointestinal symptoms including erosive gastritis with hematemesis and melena. Before oliguria supervenes, chelation therapy with intravenous BAL (British antilewisite; dimercaprol) may limit renal damage. Initially, oliguria should be treated by volume expansion with close monitoring of central venous or pulmonary wedge pressure. Not only may diuresis induced by hydration, mannitol, and furosemide prevent the development of oliguric acute renal failure, but also persisting oliguria in the face of adequate therapy indicates renal parenchymal damage. An elevated urinary sodium concentration (>40 mEq/L) and diminished concentrating capacity (Uosm <450 mOsm/L) in association with failure to obtain diuresis in an acutely oliguric patient with adequate circulatory status confirm the diagnosis of ATN. Once oliguria has become established, rigid fluid restriction is mandatory (<500 mL/day). Acute oliguric renal failure may rapidly leads to death unless dialysis is provided.

Histologic examination of the kidneys reveals necrosis of the proximal tubules, particularly the pars recta. In the experimental model, the tubular basement membrane is spared compared with the damage incurred during ischemic tubular necrosis (87). However, backleak of inulin from the tubular lumen to peritubular capillaries has been observed in experimental animals, indicating loss of integrity of the proximal tubule. Such backleak contributes to the reduction in inulin or creatinine clearance induced by outer cortical ischemia. In the rat, $HgCl_2$-induced ATN is accompanied by sequestration of mercury sulfide within lysosomes of surviving proximal tubule cells (88). The extent of damage to individual nephrons is highly variable, although tubular necrosis extends to more proximal segments after larger doses (87).

During the recovery phase, oliguria is replaced by polyuria while the GFR is still low. Urine flow rates may double daily, reaching a maximum of about 5 L/day while the serum creatinine continues to rise, albeit more slowly than the initial rate of 1 to 2 mg/dL/day. During the diuretic phase, salt and water must be vigorously replaced, but potassium restriction and reduced doses of toxic drugs normally excreted by the kidneys should be maintained. If death from hypervolemia, hyperkalemia, hemorrhagic complications, uremia, and infection is avoided, spontaneous regeneration of tubular epithelium occurs with subsequent recovery. Dystrophic calcification of necrotic tubules may, however, limit restoration of function,

and the kidneys may show residual interstitial nephritis (88). The entire process from acute oliguria through polyuria and recovery may last from a few days to many months.

Nephrotic Syndrome

Sporadic case reports of nephrotic syndrome following exposure to elemental or organic mercury have appeared since the middle of the twentieth century. Proteinuria in children with acrodynia ("pink disease") following external use of mercurial ointments or powders has been attributed to allergic reactions. In the occupational setting, the causal relationship of mercury exposure to proteinuria and the nephrotic syndrome has been less compelling (84), largely because the dose-response is unpredictable and, in addition, the etiology of nephrotic syndrome unrelated to mercury is rarely known.

Renal biopsies have most often shown deposits within glomerular capillaries consistent with membranous nephropathy (92) (Fig. 47-6), but normal glomeruli (e.g., nil disease) and antiglomerular basement membrane (anti-GBM) antibody deposition also have been described. In most instances, proteinuria owing to mercury appears to be self-limited and disappears spontaneously when the source of exposure is removed.

Observations in rats may provide a framework for understanding mercury-induced glomerular disease in humans. In 1971, Bariety and associates (93) reported that multiple subcutaneous injections of $HgCl_2$ in rats, in doses too small to produce ATN, induced membranous nephropathy. Renal disease characterized by glomerular deposition of immune complexes and heavy proteinuria developed in about 2 months. Subsequent studies showed that the immune response is actually biphasic; immune complex deposition is preceded by anti-GBM antibody and complement deposition (94). The response to mercury in the rat is under precise genetic control and is dose

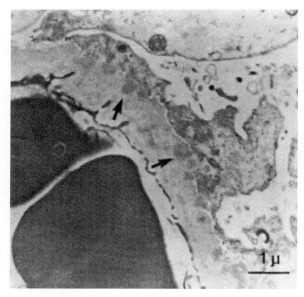

FIGURE 47-6. Electron micrograph of kidney from a 24-year-old man exposed to mercury vapor in an industrial electrolysis unit. The urinary mercury was 174 μg/24 hours; urinary protein, 3.11 μg/24 hours. Creatinine clearance was 116 mL/minute/1.73 m². Subepithelial electron-dense deposits (*arrows*), presumably immune complexes, overlie the glomerular basement membrane. (Lead citrate and uranyl acetate; magnification ×11,000.) (From: Tubbs RR, et al. Membranous glomerulonephritis associated with industrial mercury exposure. *Am J Clin Pathol* 1982;77:409, with permission.)

dependent (95,96). As little as 0.005 mg/100 g of body weight elicit immunologically mediated glomerular disease in selected strains. Metallic mercury vapor (1 mg/m^3) is as effective as HgCl$_2$ for inducing autoimmune disease in susceptible rats. Similar renal disease has been induced in other rodents and with alternate forms and routes of exposure, including organomercurials and inhalation. As in humans, mercury-induced glomerular disease in rats is self-limited. Immunoglobulin localization in the glomeruli is associated with heavy proteinuria, circulating immune complexes, and polyclonal B-cell activation owing to antiself Ia autoreactive T cells. The glomerular disease can be transferred to T cell-depleted rats by T cells and helper T cells taken from HgCl$_2$-treated rats of the same strain (97). Weening and co-workers found evidence that the autoimmune process is initiated by mercury inhibition of suppressor T-cell functions (97).

Minimata Disease

In 1956, endemic methyl mercury poisoning was recognized in Japan arising from the contamination of food by industrial effluents in the area of Minimata Bay (98). Severe neurologic defects including visual, speech, and gait disturbances afflicted several hundred adults whose diet consisted largely of contaminated fish. The mercury pollution had been going on for a decade before the health consequences were recognized. Fish from Minimata Bay contained up to 36 mg of mercury per kg. Cerebral palsy was common among the children of affected mothers. Similar clusters of cases were subsequently identified in Nigata, Japan, and in Iraq, where the disease was the result of bread prepared from grain that had been treated with methyl mercury fungicide.

Although methyl mercury is more avidly accumulated by renal than by neural tissue, the kidney manifestations of Minimata disease are minor. Tubular proteinuria occurs (99), but clinically important albuminuria and azotemia have not been reported. Postmortem examinations have shown minimal nonspecific renal abnormalities, although rats treated with methyl mercury show increased numbers of mercury-containing lysosomes in proximal tubule epithelial cells. In more heavily exposed rats, lysosomal and mitochondrial dysfunction has been observed and may account for the tubular proteinuria in patients with Minimata disease.

Treatment

British antilewisite is an effective chelator for acute inorganic mercury poisoning. Up to 5 mg/kg is given initially by the intramuscular route, followed by 2.5 mg/kg twice daily for 10 days. In the presence of acute renal failure, the mercury chelate can be removed by hemodialysis. BAL is of doubtful value in chronic poisoning, which is effectively treated by removing the patient from the source of exposure. Succimer (DMSA), an oral chelating agent, approved for the treatment of lead poisoning in children, is an effective chelator of mercury and may play an important role in the treatment of mercury toxicity in the future (89).

OTHER HEAVY METALS

As long as the etiology of most end-stage renal disease is unknown, the contribution of environmental and industrial toxicants to the induction of chronic renal disease will remain unclear. Uranium is used to induce experimental ATN and, like lead, is stored in bone. Uranium is selectively accumulated

in the proximal tubule with a biologic half-life approximating 1 week for 95% of the renal stores (100). After inhalation, the uranyl ion binds to circulating transferrin and to proteins and phospholipids in the second and third segments of the proximal tubule. Rats given uranyl nitrate subcutaneously develop intrarenal microcysts 8 weeks after injection (101). Acute tubular necrosis occurred in men working on the atomic bomb during the Manhattan Project in the 1940s (102), but chronic renal failure caused by uranium has not been reported. A workplace hazard evaluation performed by the National Institute of Occupational Safety and Health revealed significantly increased ß$_2$-microglobulin excretion compared to controls in workmen exposed to uranium dust (103). The clinical significance of this finding is doubtful, however, because the urinary ß$_2$-microglobulin levels were well within the normal range and there was no evidence of reduced renal function. Many of these men had urinary uranium levels in excess of the upper acceptable limit of 30 μg/L.

Acute tubular necrosis has been reported after voluntary ingestion of copper sulfate in young female science students attempting suicide in Delhi, India (104).

Minimal tubular proteinuria in the absence of reduced glomerular filtration has also been reported in chrome platers, but the implications of this finding for clinically important renal disease also remain speculative (105). Like other heavy metals, chromium is selectively accumulated in the proximal tubule. The hexavalent form induces ATN, but there is no convincing evidence of tubular injury from usual occupational exposure (9,106–109). Chromium has been recognized as an important cause of lung cancer for over 100 years, but chronic renal disease from occupational or environmental exposure has not been reported.

Bismuth compounds prepared as therapeutic agents have produced unequivocal ATN. Lower dosage induces Fanconi's syndrome with reduced glomerular filtration and bismuth-containing intranuclear inclusions in proximal tubule cells that are similar to, but distinguishable from, lead inclusions (110).

The acute cardiovascular collapse and hemolysis accompanying arsenic poisoning are associated with renal failure, but whether the mechanism of injury involves distinct cellular toxicity is unclear (111). Moonshine contaminated with arsenic produces painful polyneuropathy that is distinct from the isolated motor neuropathy of lead poisoning. Patchy cortical necrosis with persistent residual renal failure has been reported following consumption of arsenic-contaminated liquor (111,112). When arsenicals react with acid, the deadly, colorless, odorless gas arsine (AsH$_3$) evolves. Almost invariably the result of an industrial accident, arsine inhalation produces hemolysis, hematuria, and abdominal pain within a few hours, followed by acute oliguric renal failure and jaundice within 2 days (113). Reticulocytosis, basophilic stippling, bilirubinemia, and free hemoglobin in the plasma may assist diagnosis, which is established by detecting arsenic in the urine. Acute tubular necrosis followed by residual interstitial nephritis 2 years after exposure has been documented (Fig. 47-7). BAL is ineffective once renal failure is present. In addition to hemodialysis, exchange transfusion may be necessary to eliminate hemoglobin-bound arsenic from the body.

SOLVENTS

Halogenated hydrocarbons have often been implicated in the induction of ATN or Fanconi's syndrome in both humans and experimental animals. Low-level occupational absorption by inhalation of volatile hydrocarbons or absorption through the skin may also induce tubular proteinuria, which does not necessarily signify the presence of clinically important renal disease, glomerular damage, or immune system activation (114,115).

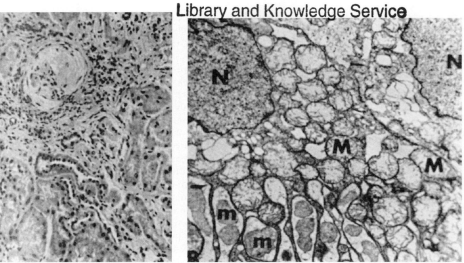

FIGURE 47-7. Renal biopsy obtained 2 years after acute renal failure from arsine poisoning in an industrial accident. The patient required peritoneal dialysis and hemodialysis for 6 weeks. The initial renal biopsy showed acute tubular necrosis. At the time of this biopsy the creatinine clearance was 24 mL/minute. **A:** Light microscopy shows local interstitial fibrosis, tubular atrophy, and sclerosis in 13 of 17 glomeruli. (Hematoxylin and eosin; magnification ×300.) **B:** Electron microscopy shows normal and damaged proximal tubule cells. In this illustration, normal and distorted mitochondria are present in a single cell adjacent to a normal nucleus. (Uranyl acetate and lead citrate; magnification ×9,000.) *m*, probably newly formed mitochondria; *M*, normal mitochondria; *N*, nuclei. (From: Muehrcke RO, Pirani CL. Arsine-induced anuria: a correlative clinicopathological study with electron microscopic observations. *Ann Intern Med* 1968;68:853, with permission.)

Light Hydrocarbon Nephropathy

Toxicologic studies of the effects of gasoline distillates performed over the past two decades under the auspices of the American petroleum industry have identified an effect of gasoline constituents on the renal tubule of male rats. Referred to as light hydrocarbon nephropathy, the tubular injury is induced by exposing Fischer 344 male rats to petroleum hydrocarbon vapors from a few hours up to a few years (116,117). Mice, guinea pigs, dogs, primates, and female rats do not develop the lesion. It is not known if similar morphologic tubular damage occurs in humans exposed to gasoline vapors. However, acute renal failure following intense exposure to diesel fumes has been reported in humans (118). The hydrocarbons studied in animal models include *n*-nonane, C_8, C_{10}–C_{11} isoparaffinic solvent, jet fuels, methylisobutyl ketone, varnish, unleaded gasoline, naphthas, and a variety of complex organic solvents and distillates. These volatile hydrocarbons are cytotoxic to proximal tubules, where they and their metabolic products are selectively accumulated. The most prominent lesion is hyaline droplet formation within epithelial cells of proximal tubules. Sustained renal failure with permanently reduced GFR has not been reported in light hydrocarbon nephropathy in humans or experimental animals.

A number of investigators have attempted to identify solvent-induced glomerulonephritis by assessing the urine of exposed workers for low-molecular-weight proteins and enzymes, markers for tubular, rather than glomerular disease. Light hydrocarbon nephropathy should not be confused with the relatively rare glomerular disease in humans referred to as solvent nephropathy (115). Increased excretion of TNAP has been reported in workers exposed to perchlorethylene in dry cleaning establishments (50). Although such tubular proteinuria is common, the massive albuminuria of solvent nephropathy is distinctly rare in association with perchlorethylene exposure.

Severe neurologic toxicity has been reported following glue sniffing among teenagers seeking intoxication. Permanent as well as transient neurologic and hepatic damage has resulted. Fanconi's syndrome caused by proximal tubular reabsorptive defects has been observed following recreational glue sniffing, apparently the result of toluene, mixed with acetone, isopropyl alcohol, ethyl acetate, and trichloroethylene. Immunologically mediated glomerulonephritis and the hemolytic–uremic syndrome have also been reported following glue sniffing (14). In addition, distal renal tubular acidosis and myoglobinuria have been reported with acute renal failure and residual chronic tubulointerstitial nephritis.

Toluene is metabolized to benzoic acid and then to hippuric acid, which are selectively accumulated in proximal tubules. These organic acids may contribute to "high anion gap metabolic acidosis" because they are "unmeasured anions" in the blood. Significant renal disease, however, has not been found in cross-sectional studies of industrial workers regularly exposed to styrene, toluene, or xylene or oil refinery workers (119). The failure to find increased tubular proteinuria in cohorts exposed to solvents, oils, or hydrocarbons, of course, has no bearing on the question of solvent-induced glomerulonephritis.

Solvent Nephropathy

At least 40 clinical epidemiologic studies have examined the relationship between glomerulonephritis and exposure to organic solvents (120–122). A number of these studies concluded that patients with chronic glomerulonephritis have been exposed to organic solvents (aliphatic and aromatic) more frequently than patients with other diseases. Initially, solvent nephropathy was associated with anti-GBM antibody-mediated glomerulonephritis and pulmonary hemorrhage (e.g., Goodpasture's syndrome) (114). As of 1992, at least 31 cases of Goodpasture's syndrome following solvent exposure had been reported (120). Organic solvents may expose the otherwise cryptic Goodpasture antigen (type IV collagen α3 chain) to the immune response system in susceptible individuals (123). On the other hand, inhaled hydrocarbons may alter alveolar immune reactivity, making lung a preferential target for antialveolar basement membrane antibody deposition (124).

Following the initial description of Goodpasture's syndrome resulting from solvent exposure, reports of solvent nephropathy have included many different types of glomerulonephritis. Although a graded dose-response to solvents has not been documented, this caveat may not be important for immunologically mediated disease. Progression of glomerulonephritis has been associated with continued solvent exposure (124,125). The huge number of chemically distinct compounds contained in petroleum may preclude identification of a specific toxic agent. Avoidance of exposure to volatile hydrocarbons and their derivatives remains an essential preventive approach.

The existence of solvent nephropathy has met with some skepticism. Indeed, caution is justified because of the absence of a good experimental model of immunologically mediated glomerulonephritis, combined with concern that the correlation between solvent exposure and chronic glomerulonephritis may be influenced by patient recall bias. The etiologic role of solvents remains controversial because the dose and composition of industrial solvents are usually unknown. Moreover, of the thousands of workers exposed, very few develop kidney disease. The genetic and environmental factors that make specific individuals susceptible to solvent nephropathy have not been delineated. The inability to obtain reliable measurements of solvent exposure makes it likely that the etiologic role of solvents in the induction of glomerular disease will remain controversial.

SILICON

Silicon is a semimetal found as the dioxide silica (SiO_2), in 28% of the earth's crust. Because it has a specific gravity of only 2.3 it is not a heavy metal. Silica is present in the serum at concentrations of 20 to $50 \mu g/dL$ in an unbound form as silicic acid and is cleared in the urine at the rate of glomerular filtration (126). Silica is believed to induce renal disease by direct deposition of crystalline material in the renal parenchyma (127) and by immunologic mechanisms acting as an adjuvant to stimulate the immune response. Tubular proteinuria is found in workers exposed to silica dust (128,129). The odds ratio to develop end-stage renal disease for a patient who worked as a sandblaster is 3.8 compared to matched controls (39). In the accelerated form of silicosis known as silicoproteinosis, rapidly progressive, immune complex-mediated focal glomerulosclerosis may appear (129). In addition to the severe nodular pulmonary fibrosis, these patients develop an overwhelming autoimmune response that simulates lupus erythematosus (Caplan's syndrome). Glomerular disease that is independent of silicosis also has been described as a result of exposure to silica (128–131). Antineutrophil cytoplasmic antibody (c-ANCA) positive Wegener's granulomatosis has been associated with exposure to silica dust as well as to silicon containing compounds such as grain dust (132).

GERMANIUM

Falling just below silica in the periodic table group IVA, which includes tin (Sn) and lead (Pb), germanium has a specific gravity of 5.23. Like silicon, it has semiconductor properties. It has been used in the treatment of cancer, a variety of medical ailments, and in unproved remedies for conditions such

as arthritis, acquired immunodeficiency syndrome (AIDS), and the chronic fatigue syndrome. Germanium-containing elixirs and health foods were reported to cause chronic tubulointerstitial nephritis first in Japan in the 1980s and more recently in Europe and the United States (133–137). Most cases have resulted from the ingestion of germanium oxide (GeO_2), but germanium-lactate-citrate and the organic germanium compound carboxyethyl germanium sesquioxide (Ge-132) have also been implicated. The renal disease differs from that induced by other heavy metals in that widening of the interstitium and tubular atrophy (apparently distal tubular) has been evident after prolonged (6 to 36 months), high-dose (16 g to hundreds of grams) consumption. The tubulointerstitial disease is slowly progressive even after exposure has been terminated. Fatal outcomes have been reported. The pathophysiologic mechanism of tubular damage is unclear because selective accumulation in the kidney does not occur and immunologic mechanisms have not been implicated. There is no evidence of primary proximal tubular injury. Proteinuria is absent. Electron-dense, periodic acid-Schiff (PAS) reagent-positive granules (containing germanium in the experimental rat) are found in distal tubular mitochondria (136). Vacuolization is present in proximal and distal tubular epithelia (133,134). Prolonged consumption of germanium compounds also induces severe hepatic steatosis, polymyositis, and peripheral neuropathy. Acute lactic acidosis has been reported from germanium-lactate-citrate (133,137).

BALKAN NEPHROPATHY

Balkan endemic nephropathy is a slowly progressive tubulointerstitial nephritis of unknown etiology described about 40 years ago among middle-aged men and women living in farming villages along the Danube River in Croatia, Serbia (the former Yugoslavia), Rumania, and Bulgaria (138). The disease occurs in families and is associated with urinary tract transitional cell carcinomas and tubular proteinuria (β_2-microglobulin). Heavy proteinuria, fluid retention and hypertension are absent. Unfortunately, control groups with renal disease of known etiology and comparable severity have not been studied in this region. A variety of environmental factors have been suspected including lead, cadmium, and mycotoxins, but no single etiologic agent has been incriminated. The possibility of low-level toxicity from suspect environmental nephrotoxins or a multifactorial etiology has not been excluded. The prevalence of generally recognized renal diseases has not been established in the Danube region, making differentiation of Balkan nephropathy from known renal diseases identified in other regions of the world problematic.

References

1. Cardenas A, et al. Markers of early renal changes induced by industrial pollutants. I. Application to workers exposed to mercury vapour. *Br J Ind Med* 1993;50:7.
2. Cardenas A, et al. Markers of early renal changes induced by industrial pollutants. II. Application to workers exposed to lead. *Br J Ind Med* 1993;50:28.
3. Roels H, et al. Markers of early renal changes induced by industrial pollutants. III. Application to workers exposed to cadmium. *Br J Ind Med* 1993;50:37.
4. Verpooten GF, Nouwen EJ, Hoylaerts MF. Segment-specific localization of intestinal-type alkaline phosphatase in human kidney. *Kidney Int* 1989;36:617.
5. Nuyts GD, et al. Intestinal-type alkaline phosphatase in urine as an indicator of mercury induced effects on the S3-segment of the proximal tubule. *Nephrol Dial Transplant* 1992;7:225.
6. Mutti A, et al. Nephropathies and exposure to perchloroethylene in dry cleaners. *Lancet* 1992;340:189.
7. Verpooten GE, et al. Immunoassay in urine of a specific marker for the human proximal tubular S3-segment. *Clin Chem* 1992;38:642.

8. Meuller PW, et al. Chronic effects in three studies of men and women occupationally exposed to cadmium. *Arch Environ Contam Toxicol* 1992;23: 125.

9. Mutti A, et al. Urinary excretion of brush-border antigen revealed by monoclonal antibody: early indicator of toxic nephropathy. *Lancet* 1985;26: 914.

10. Koopman MG, et al. Circadian rhythm of glomerular filtration rate in normal individuals. *Clin Sci* 1989;77:105.

11. Wedeen RP. *Poison in the pot: the legacy of lead.* Carbondale, IL: Southern Illinois University, 1984.

12. Agency for Toxic Substances and Disease Registry, Public Health Service, U.S. Department of Health and Human Services. *The nature and extent of lead poisoning in children in the United States: a report to Congress.* Atlanta: US Department of Health and Human Services, Public Health Service, 1988.

13. Rabinowitz MB. Kinetic analysis of lead metabolism in healthy humans. *J Clin Invest* 1976;58:260.

14. Wedeen RP. Occupational and environmental renal diseases. *Curr Nephrol* 1988;11:65.

15. Wedeen RP. Blood lead levels, dietary calcium, and hypertension. *Ann Intern Med* 1985;102:403.

16. Batuman V, et al. The role of lead in gout nephropathy. *N Engl J Med* 1981;304:520.

17. Batuman V, et al. Contribution of lead to hypertension with renal failure. *N Engl J Med* 1983;309:17.

18. Wedeen RP, et al. Occupational lead nephropathy. *Am J Med* 1975; 59:630.

19. Wedeen RP, Mallik DK, Batuman V. Detection and treatment of occupational lead nephropathy. *Arch Intern Med* 1979;139:53.

20. Chamberlain AC. Prediction of response of blood lead to airborne and dietary lead from volunteer experiments with lead isotopes. *Proc R Soc Biol (Lond)* 1985;244:149.

21. Inglis JA, Henderson DA, Emmerson BT. The pathology and pathogenesis of chronic lead nephropathy occurring in Queensland. *J Pathol* 1978; 124:65.

22. Van de Vyver FL, et al. Bone lead in dialysis patients. *Kidney Int* 1988;33: 601.

23. Skerfving S, et al. Biological monitoring, by in vivo XRF measurements, of occupational exposure to lead, cadmium, and mercury. *Biol Trace Element Res* 1987;13:241.

24. Somervaille LJ, et al. *In vivo* tibia lead measurements as an index of cumulative exposure in occupationally exposed subjects. *Br J Ind Med* 1988;45: 174.

25. Wedeen RP. *In vivo* tibial XRF measurement of bone lead. *Arch Environ Health* 1990;45:69.

26. Rosen JF, et al. L-line x-ray fluorescence of cortical bone lead compared with CaNa2, EDTA test in lead-toxic children: public health implications. *Proc Natl Acad Sci USA* 1989;86:685.

27. Grandjean P. *Biological effects of organolead compounds.* Boca Raton, FL: CRC Press, 1984.

28. Wedeen RP. The politics of lead. In: Sheehan HE, Wedeen RP, eds. *Toxic circles: environmental hazards from the workplace into community.* New Brunswick: Rutgers University, 1993:168.

29. Chisolm JJ, et al. Aminoaciduria, hypophosphatemia and rickets in lead poisoning. *Am J Dis Child* 1955;89:159.

30. Goyer RA, et al. Aminoaciduria in experimental lead poisoning. *Proc Soc Exp Biol Med* 1970;135:767.

31. Goyer RA, Wilson MH. Lead-induced inclusion bodies: results of ethylenediaminetetraacetic acid treatment. *Lab Invest* 1975;32:149.

32. Schumann GB, et al. Inclusion-bearing cells in industrial workers exposed to lead. *Am J Clin Pathol* 1980;74:192.

33. Selevan SG, et al. Mortality of lead smelter workers. *Am J Epidemiol* 1985; 122:673.

34. Emmerson BT. Chronic lead nephropathy. *Kidney Int* 1973;4:1.

35. Wedeen RP, et al. Geophagic lead nephropathy: a case report. *Environ Res* 1978;17:409.

36. Tepper L. Renal function subsequent to childhood plumbism. *Arch Environ Health* 1963;7:76.

37. Hu H. A 50-year follow-up of childhood plumbism: hypertension, renal function, and hemoglobin levels among survivors. *Am J Dis Child* 1991; 145:681.

38. Lilis R, et al. Nephropathy in chronic lead poisoning. *Br J Ind Med* 1968;25:196.

39. Steenland NK, et al. Occupational and other exposures associated with male end stage renal disease: a case/control study. *Am J Public Health* 1990; 80:153.

40. Wedeen RP. Lead, the kidney, and hypertension. In: Needleman H, ed. *Human lead exposure.* Boca Raton, FL: CRC Press, 1992:170.

41. Staessen J, et al. Renal function is inversely correlated with lead exposure in the general population. *N Engl J Med* 1994;327:151.

42. Chai S, Webb RC. Effects of lead on vascular reactivity. *Environ Health Perspect* 1988;78:85.

43. Kopp SJ, Barron JT, Tow JP. Cardiovascular actions of lead and relationship to hypertension: a review. *Scand J Work Environ Health* 1985;11:15.

44. Clarkson TW. Molecular and ionic mimicry of toxic metals. *Annu Rev Pharmacol Toxicol* 1993;32:545.

45. Weiler E, Khalil-Manesh F, Gonick H. Effects of lead and natriuretic hormone on kinetics of sodium/potassium-activated adenosine triphosphatase: possible relevance to hypertension. *Environ Health Perspect* 1988;78: 113.

46. Batuman V, et al. Lead increases the red cell sodium-lithium countertransport. *Am J Kidney Dis* 1989;14:200.

47. Khalil-Manesh F, et al. Lead-induced hypertension: possible role of endothelial factors. *Am J Hypertens* 1993; 6:723.

48. Vaziri ND, Liang K, Ding Y. Increased nitric oxide inactivation by reactive oxygen species in lead-induced hypertension. *Kidney Int* 1999;56:1492.

49. Endo G, Horiguchi S, Kiyota I. Urinary N-acetyl-β-D-glucosaminidase activity in lead-exposed workers. *J Appl Toxicol* 1990;10:235.

50. Wedeen RP, et al. Urinary biomarkers as indicators of renal disease. *Renal Fail* 1999;21:241.

51. Colleoni N, D'Amico G. Chronic lead accumulation as a possible cause of renal failure in gouty patients. *Nephron* 1986;44:32.

52. Peitzman SJ, Bodison W, Ellis I. Moonshine drinking among hypertensive veterans in Philadelphia. *Arch Intern Med* 1985;145:632.

53. Wright LF, Saylor RP, Cecere FA. Occult lead intoxication in patients with gout and kidney disease. *J Rheumatol* 1984;11:517.

54. Kim R, et al. A longitudinal study of low-level lead exposure and impairment of renal function. The normative aging study. *JAMA* 1996;275: 1177.

55. Mahaffey KR, et al. National estimates of blood lead levels: United States, 1976–1980. Association with selected demographic and socioeconomic factors. *N Engl J Med* 1982;307:573.

56. Harlan WR. The relationship of blood lead levels to blood pressure in the U.S. population. *Environ Health Perspect* 1988;78:9.

57. Pirkle JL, et al. The relationship between blood lead levels and blood pressure and its cardiovascular risk implications. *Am J Epidemiol* 1985;121: 246.

58. Hu H, et al. The relationship of bone and blood lead to hypertension. The normative aging study. *JAMA* 1996;275:1171.

59. Sehnert KW, Claque AF, Cheraskin E. The improvement in renal function following EDTA chelation and multi-vitamin-trace mineral therapy: a study in creatinine clearance. *Med Hypoth* 1984;15:301.

60. Lin JA, Ho HH, Yu CC. Chelation therapy for patients with elevated body lead burden and progressive renal insufficiency. A randomized controlled trial. *Ann Intern Med* 1999;130:7.

61. Germain MJ, Braden GL, Fitzgibbons JP. Failure of chelation therapy in lead nephropathy. *Arch Intern Med* 1984;144:2419.

62. Wedeen RP, Batuman V, Landy E. The safety of the EDTA lead-mobilization test. *Environ Res* 1983;30:58.

63. Yver L, et al. Insuffisance renale aigue au cours d'un saturnism professionel. *Nouvelle Presse Med* 1978;7:1541.

64. Friberg L. Introduction. In: Friberg L, et al., eds. *Cadmium and health: a toxicological and epidemiological appraisal.* Boca Raton, FL: CRC Press, 1986.

65. Nicaud P, et al. Les lesions osseuses de l'intoxication chronique par le cadmium: aspects radiologiques a type de syndrome de Milkman. *Bull Mem Soc Med Hop Paris* 1942;19:204.

66. Nordberg GF, Kjellstrom T, Nordberg M. Kinetics and metabolism: other toxic effects. In: Friberg L, et al., eds. *Cadmium and health: a toxicological and epidemiological appraisal.* Boca Raton, FL: CRC Press, 1986.

67. Jarup L, Elinder CG. Incidence of renal stones among cadmium exposed battery workers. *Br J Ind Med* 1993;50:598.

68. Kido T, et al. Long-term observation of serum creatinine and arterial blood pH in persons with cadmium-induced renal dysfunction. *Arch Environ Health* 1990;45:35.

69. Stephens GA. Cadmium poisoning. *J Ind Hyg* 1920;2:129.

70. Staessen JA, et al. Renal functional and historical environmental cadmium pollution from zinc smelters. *Lancet* 1994;343:1523.

71. Squibb KS, Pritchard JB, Fowler BA. Renal metabolism and toxicity of metallothionein. In: Foulkes EC, ed. *Biological roles of metallothionein.* New York: Elsevier/North Holland, 1982.

72. Blainey JD, et al. Cadmium-induced osteomalacia. *Br J Ind Med* 1980;37: 278.

73. Verschoor M, et al. Renal function of workers with low-level cadmium exposure. *Scand J Work Environ Health* 1987;13:232.

74. Thun MJ, et al. Nephropathy in cadmium workers: assessment of risk from airborne occupational cadmium exposure. *Br J Ind Med* 1989;46:689.

75. Nogawa K, et al. Serum vitamin D metabolites in cadmium-exposed persons with renal damage. *Arch Environ Health* 1990;62:189.

76. Kido T, et al. The association between renal dysfunction and osteopenia in environmentally cadmium-exposed subjects. *Environ Res* 1990;51:71.

77. Geiger H, et al. Cadmium and renal hypertension. *J Hum Hypertens* 1989;3: 23.

78. Anderson K, et al. Mortality among cadmium and nickel-exposed workers in a Swedish battery factory. *Toxicol Environ Chem* 1984;9:53.

79. Kjellstrom T. Renal effects. In: Friberg L, et al., eds. *Cadmium and health: a toxicological and epidemiological appraisal.* Boca Raton, FL: CRC Press, 1986.

80. Roels HA, et al. Health significance of cadmium-induced renal dysfunction: a five-year follow-up. *Br J Ind Med* 1989;46:755.

81. Hotz P, et al. Renal effect of low-level environmental cadmium exposure: 5-year follow-up of a subcohort from the Cadmibel study. *Lancet* 1999;354:150.

82. Staessen JA, et al. Environmental exposure to cadmium, forearm bone density, and risk of fractures: prospective population study. *Lancet* 1999;353:1140.
83. Cantilena LR Jr, Klaassen CD. The effect of repeated administration of several chelators on the distribution and excretion of cadmium. *Toxicol Appl Pharmacol* 1982;66:361.
84. Wright N, Yeoman WB, Carter GF. Massive oral ingestion of elemental mercury without poisoning. *Lancet* 1980;26:206.
85. Stonard MD, et al. An evaluation of renal function in workers occupationally exposed to mercury vapor. *Int Arch Occup Environ Health* 1983;52:177.
86. Goldwater LJ. *Mercury: a history of quicksilver*. Baltimore: York, 1972.
87. Biber TU, et al. A study by micropuncture and microdissection of acute renal damage in rats. *Am J Med* 1968;44:664.
88. Wedeen RP, Cheeks C. Intrarenal distribution of exchangeable calcium in HgCl2-induced acute tubular necrosis. *Histochem Cytochem* 1988;36:1103.
89. Zalups RK, Lash LH. Advances in understanding the renal transport and toxicity of mercury. *J Toxic Environ Health* 1994;42:1.
90. Wedeen RP, Goldstein MH. Renal tubular localization of chlormerodrin labelled with mercury-203 by autoradiography. *Science* 1963;141:438.
91. Roels HA, et al. Comparison of renal function and psychomotor performance in workers exposed to elemental mercury. *Int Arch Occup Environ Health* 1982;50:77.
92. Tubbs RR, et al. Membranous glomerulonephritis associated with industrial mercury exposure. *Am J Clin Pathol* 1982;77:409.
93. Bariety J, et al. Glomerulonephritis with α and β1C-globulin deposits induced in rats by mercuric chloride. *Am J Pathol* 1971;65:293.
94. Goldman M, Baran D, Druet P. Polyclonal activation and experimental nephropathies. *Kidney Int* 1988;34:141.
95. Hua H, et al. Autoimmune glomerulonephritis induced by mercury vapour exposure in the brown Norway rat. *Toxicology* 1993;79:119.
96. Bernaudin JF, et al. Inhalation or ingestion of organic or inorganic mercurials produces auto-immune disease in rats. *Clin Immunol Immunopathol* 1981;20:129.
97. Weening JJ, Fleuren GJ, Hoedemaeker PJ. Demonstration of antinuclear antibodies in mercuric chloride-induced glomerulopathy in the rat. *Lab Invest* 1978;39:405.
98. Nomiyama K. Recent progress and perspectives in cadmium health effects studies. *Sci Total Environ* 1980;14:199.
99. Iesato K, et al. Renal tubular dysfunction in Minimata disease: detection of renal tubular antigen and beta-2-microglobulin in the urine. *Ann Intern Med* 1977;86:731.
100. Leggett RW. The behavior and chemical toxicity of uranium in the kidney: a reassessment. *Health Phys* 1989;57:365.
101. Haley DP, Bulger RE, Dobyan DC. The long-term effects of uranyl nitrate on the structure and function of the rat kidney. *Virchows Arch (B Cell Pathol)* 1982;41:181.
102. Dounce AL. The mechanism of action of uranium compounds in the animal body. In: Voegtlin C, Hodge HC, eds. *Pharmacology and toxicology of uranium compounds*. New York: McGraw-Hill, 1949.
103. Thun MJ, et al. Renal toxicity in uranium mill workers. *Scand J Work Environ Health* 1985;11:83.
104. Dash SC. Copper sulfate poisoning and acute renal failure. *Int J Artif Organs* 1989;12:610.
105. Wedeen RP. Chromium-induced kidney disease. *Environ Health Perspect* 1991;92:71.
106. Petersen R, Mikkelsen S, Thomsen P. Chronic interstitial nephropathy after plasma cutting in stainless steel. *Occup Environ Med* 1994;51:259.
107. Vyskocil A, et al. Lack of renal changes in stainless steel welders exposed to chromium and nickel. *Scand J Environ Health* 1992;18:252.
108. Wang X, et al. Chromium-induced early changes in renal function among ferrochromium-producing workers. *Toxicology* 1994;90:93.
109. Verschoor MA, et al. Renal function of chrome-plating workers and welders. *Int Arch Occup Environ Health* 1988;60:67.
110. Randall RE, et al. Bismuth nephrotoxicity. *Ann Intern Med* 1972; 77:481.
111. Gerhardt RE, Crecelius EA, Hudson JB. Moonshine-related arsenic poisoning. *Arch Intern Med* 1980;140:211.
112. Muehrcke RC, Pirani CL. Arsine-induced anuria: a correlative clinico-pathological study with electron microscopic observations. *Ann Intern Med* 1968;68:853.
113. Fowler BA, Weissberg JB. Arsine poisoning. *N Engl J Med* 1974; 291:1171.
114. Daniell WE, Couser WG, Rosenstock L. Occupational solvent exposure and glomerulonephritis. *JAMA* 1988;259:2280.
115. Wedeen RP. Occupational renal diseases. *Am J Kidney Dis* 1984;3:241.
116. Gibson JE, Bus JS. Current perspectives on gasoline (light hydrocarbon)-induced male rat nephropathy. *Ann NY Acad Sci* 1988;534:481.
117. Short BG, Burnett VL, Swenberg JA. Elevated proliferation of proximal tubule cells and localization of accumulated α24-globulin in F344 rats during chronic exposure to unleaded gasoline or 2,2,4-trimethylpentane. *Toxicol Appl Pharmacol* 1989;101:414.
118. Hotz P, et al. Hydrocarbon exposure, hypertension and kidney function tests. *Int Arch Occup Environ Health* 1990;62:501.
119. Viau C, et al. A cross-sectional survey of kidney function in refinery employees. *Am J Ind Med* 1987;11:177.
120. Bombassei GJ, Kaplan AA. The association between hydrocarbon exposure and anti-glomerular basement membrane antibody-mediated disease (Goodpasture's syndrome). *Am J Ind Med* 1992;21:141.
121. Hotz P. Occupational hydrocarbon exposure and chronic nephropathy. *Toxicology* 1994;90:163.
122. Roy AT, Brautbar N, Lee DB. Hydrocarbons and renal failure. *Nephron* 1991;58:385.
123. Kalluri R, et al. The α3 chain of type IV collagen induces autoimmune Goodpasture's syndrome. *Proc Natl Acad Sci USA* 1994;91:6201.
124. Yamamoto T, Wilson C. Binding of anti-basement membrane antibody to alveolar basement membrane after intratracheal gasoline instillation in rabbits. *Am J Pathol* 1987;126:497.
125. Yaqoob M, et al. Hydrocarbon exposure and tubular damage: additional factors in the progression of renal failure in primary glomerulonephritis. *Q J Med* 1986;86:661.
126. DeBroe ME, et al. Occupational renal disease. *Current Opin Nephrol Hyertens* 1996;5:114.
127. Dobbie JW, Smith MJ. Silicate nephrotoxicity in the experimental animal: the missing factor in analgesic nephropathy. *Scottish Med J* 1982;27:10.
128. Hotz P, et al. Subclinical signs of kidney dysfunction following short exposure to silica in the absence of silicosis. *Nephron* 1995;70:438.
129. Ng TP, Lee HS, Phoon WH. Further evidence of human silica nephrotoxicity in occupationally exposed workers. *Br J Ind Med* 1993;50:907.
130. Osorio AM, et al. Silica and glomerulonephritis: a case report and review of the literature. *Am J Kidney Dis* 1987;9:224.
131. Calvert GM, Steenland K, Palu S. End stage renal disease among silica-exposed gold miners. A new method for assessing incidence among epidemiologic controls. *JAMA* 1995;277:1219.
132. Nuyts GD, et al. Wegener granulomatosis is associated to exposure to silicon compounds: a case-control study. *Nephrol Dial Transplant* 1995;10:162.
133. Hess B, et al. Tubulointerstitial nephropathy persisting 20 months after discontinuation of chronic intake of germanium lactate citrate. *Am J Kidney Dis* 1993;21:548.
134. Okada K, et al. Renal failure caused by long-term use of a germanium preparation as an elixir. *Clin Nephrol* 1989;31:219.
135. Takeuchi A, et al. Nephrotoxicity of germanium compounds: report of a case and review of the literature. *Nephron* 1992;60:436.
136. Sanai T, et al. Chronic tubulointerstitial changes induced by germanium dioxide in comparison with carboxyethyl sesquioxide. *Kidney Int* 1991;40:882.
137. Krapf R, Schaffner T, Iten PX. Abuse of germanium associated with fatal lactic acidosis. *Nephron* 1992;62:351.
138. Hall PW, Batuman V, eds. Balkan endemic nephropathy. *Kidney Int* 1991;34.

CHAPTER 48 ■ ACUTE TUBULOINTERSTITIAL NEPHRITIS

GARABED EKNOYAN AND UDAY KHOSLA

When first introduced, the pathologic diagnosis of "acute interstitial nephritis" was used to identify the morphologic features observed at postmortem in the kidney of patients with a disparate group of infectious diseases in which the kidney was sterile and free of the infectious organism causing the systemic illness (1). The earliest description of the lesion was reported in 1860 in a fatal case of scarlet fever that at postmortem examination revealed infiltration of the kidney by lymphocytic cells, in the absence of suppurative bacterial infection; the condition was termed *lymphomatous nephritis* (2). After the report of several similar cases, Councilman (1) in 1898 published his now classic paper in which he described the lesions of acute interstitial nephritis (AIN), based on a review of the literature and his observations made at postmortem examination of 42 cases. He found the lesion to occur with approximately equal incidence in patients with scarlet fever (25%) and diphtheria (23%), and less frequently in patients with other infectious diseases. Councilman summarized the pathologic process as "an acute inflammation of the kidney characterized by cellular and fluid exudation in the interstitial tissue, accompanied by, but not dependent on, degeneration of the epithelium; the exudation is not purulent in character, and the lesions may be both diffuse and focal," and identified the infiltrating cells as "plasma cells that had migrated from the blood vessels and multiplied locally by mitotic division." He localized the foci of cellular infiltrates to three sites: the boundary zone of the pyramids, the subcapsular region of the cortex, and around the glomeruli. These meticulous observations, lucid description, and insightful analysis are just as valid today as they were then and encapsulate the lesions of this disease of the kidneys more succinctly and thoroughly than anything that has been written over the century since they were first reported (1).

Subsequent reports confirmed Councilman's observation that nonsuppurative lesions of the kidney interstitium appeared after short but variable periods after the onset of acute infections that were primarily streptococcal in origin. These were most common in the cortex of the kidney and consisted mostly of focal infiltrates comprising for the most part lymphocytes and plasma cells, with only occasional polymorphonuclear leukocytes (3,4). The concept of acute tubulointerstitial injury after acute infection was so well accepted that several of the initial reports of acute tubular necrosis (ATN), which appeared immediately before the proper characterization of acute renal failure (ARF) due to tubular necrosis during the first part of World War II, called the lesion *acute hematogenous interstitial nephritis* and argued for the similarity of the lesions of ATN to those noted after streptococcal infections (5,6). In fact, there was a brief period during which the lesions of ATN and AIN were confused because they were considered variants of the same entity. This difficulty persists to this day if the kidney tissue is not examined carefully and is interpreted without benefit of the clinical history (7). The pathologic lesions of ATN and AIN now are classified as variants of tubulointerstitial disease in general (8).

The introduction of antibiotics during World War II and the eradication of serious and fatal streptococcal infections resulted in loss of interest in the entity described by Councilman, while attention focused on ischemic or nephrotoxic ATN as the predominant cause of ARF. It therefore is ironic that interest in AIN was revived in the 1960s when the very antibiotics used to treat streptococcal infections came to be recognized as a cause of AIN (9), after the lesions were described in a case of penicillin hypersensitivity in 1958 (10). In fact, the bulk of the current reports in the literature are on drug-induced AIN, and the number of drugs implicated as causing AIN continues to increase, as does that of the variations in their clinical and laboratory manifestation (11,12). AIN has since come to define the clinicopathologic syndrome that develops in diverse conditions, including infections, and is characterized by an acute deterioration of kidney function, the pathologic features of which remain those first described by Councilman in 1898 as "characterized by cellular and fluid exudation in the interstitial tissue, accompanied by, but not dependent on, degeneration of the epithelium; ... and the lesions may be both diffuse and focal" (1).

Although this clinicopathologic syndrome initially was referred to as *acute interstitial nephritis* (1,9,13), the more inclusive and precise descriptive terms *acute tubulointerstitial nephritis* (ATIN) and *acute tubulointerstitial nephropathy* are used now (12). The preferential use of the term *tubulointerstitial* stems from the fact that although the dominant morphologic features are those evident in the interstitium, the tubules also are affected, albeit to a degree that may be difficult to detect on light microscopy. However, the structural injury to the tubules can be severe; more important, and independent of the severity of their structural injury, it is disorders of tubular function that constitute a characteristic component of the disordered kidney function and that differentiate this entity from other forms of ARF due to glomerular or vascular disease (14–17). In fact, tubular dysfunction is an invariable accompanying feature of the reduction in glomerular filtration rate (GFR) and, as a rule, can be documented to precede a clinically evident decrease in GFR (15,18). In addition, although the interstitial cellular infiltrates contribute significantly to the pathogenesis of the disease, there is increasing evidence that the tubules play an important role in the processing and presentation of the antigenic stimulus and the immunopathogenesis of the disease process (19–22). Stimulated tubular epithelial cells also differentiate into infiltrating fibroblasts and are responsible for the release of cytokines that lead to recruitment of the infiltrating cells responsible for progression of the injury and its potential progression to irreversible damage (22–25).

Although ATIN may be suspected clinically, the diagnosis depends on the presence of characteristic morphologic changes of the kidney noted on biopsy specimens or at postmortem examination. The adjective *acute* refers to the sudden onset and rapid progression of the clinical features of this syndrome and not to its pathologic features, which are notable for mononuclear cell infiltration rather than the polymorphonuclear leukocytes characteristic of an acute inflammatory reaction (9).

PATHOLOGIC FEATURES

Independent of the causative agent or clinical condition responsible for ATIN, the principal morphologic features that characterize it are an increase in the interstitial volume, mainly because of edema; mononuclear cell infiltrates of varying degrees and distribution; and tubular injury and degeneration of differing severity, which in general are localized to the sites of the greatest cellular infiltrates. The glomeruli are spared, but many show some degree of periglomerular infiltrates and ischemic change, except in ATIN associated with nephrotic syndrome, where the lesions of minimal-change disease are seen on electron microscopy. Although the extent and severity of each of the tubulointerstitial lesions show some correlation with the level of reduction in GFR, the closest correlation is found with the infiltrative process (11,26). The interstitial infiltrative lesions may be diffuse but usually are patchy in distribution and most evident in the cortex and outer medulla of the kidney. When the infiltrating cells are meager, they show a focal peritubular distribution that is most evident in the corticomedullary region; when profuse, they literally obscure the normal appearance of the tubules, are even periglomerular, and may extend into the medulla, where they are always much less prominent. As first noted by Councilman (1), even in cases in which the infiltrates are diffuse they always are more prominent at certain foci. A diffuse infiltrative process has been shown to be associated with higher levels of serum creatinine and a poorer prognosis for recovery than patchy infiltrations. The infiltrating cells are composed mostly of mononuclear cells, lymphocytes, and plasma cells, and only rarely polymorphonuclear cells and macrophages. The prognosis appears to be less favorable when 1% to 6% of the interstitial infiltrating cells are composed of neutrophilic granulocytes (26). By the same token, an increase in the number of macrophages (usually <10%) and the presence of granulomatous reactions are associated with a prolonged course of ARF and varying degrees of residual impairment of kidney function (11,27–29). When present, eosinophils are sparse and constitute only a small component of the infiltrating cells, except in occasional cases of antibiotic-induced AIN, where they may be marked. The presence of infiltrating eosinophils shows no relation to the increased eosinophilia or the presence of urinary eosinophils that also occur in drug-induced ATIN. A role for a specific chemoattractant for eosinophil cells, eotaxin, which is expressed in the kidney, has been proposed as a mechanism for tissue eosinophilia (30). The production of eotaxin is upregulated in various forms of allergic and hypersensitivity inflammation such as asthma, conjunctivitis and drug-induced exanthems (31,32). Monoclonal antibodies to eotaxin have shown the presence of eotaxin mainly in the endothelial cells, infiltrating mononuclear cells, and in a small number of tubular epithelial cells in a case of renal interstitial eosinophilia with membranous glomerulopathy (33). Whether the same mechanism is operative in all cases of ATIN remains to be determined and deserves to be examined.

Immunologic characterization and analysis of the interstitial cellular infiltrates reveals that most (up to 80%) of the mononuclear cells are activated T lymphocytes. B lymphocytes also are present but constitute a much smaller portion of the interstitial cellular infiltrates, being highest in cases due to nonsteroidal antiinflammatory drugs (NSAIDs) (34). The infiltrating T cells are predominantly CD3+, with relatively smaller numbers of CD4+ cells of the helper/inducer subset and CD8+ cells of the cytotoxic/suppressor subset. In most cases, the CD4 variety predominates over the CD8 variety (34–38). Natural killer lymphocytes are rare and, when present, constitute only a small proportion of the infiltrating cells (35). A slight prevalence (just over 50%) of the CD8+ suppressor/cytotoxic subset has been noted in cases of ATIN associated with massive proteinuria after exposure to NSAIDs (34) or antibiotics (38). The relevance of this observation to massive proteinuria as a feature of ATIN is unknown (34–36). Convincing evidence has been advanced that the infiltrating cells are antigenically activated (39,40) and immunologically engaged in the pathogenesis of the lesions (41–43). However, no diagnostic pattern of markers or cell types has come to be identified with the lesions associated with any specific form of ATIN.

Variable degrees of tubular injury usually are present, but tubular atrophy is absent. The tubular lesions are most evident at the site of greatest concentration of infiltrating cells. They usually are focal and are more severe in the proximity of infiltrating cells (26,44). A distinguishing lesion that results from focal infiltrating lymphocytes is disruption of the tubular basement membrane (TBM) and its epithelial cell lining, so-called "tubulitis," which is characteristic of ATIN. Granulomatous reactions, multinucleated epithelioid cells, and polymorphonuclear leukocytes are detected in most cases with marked tubular injury. Rupture of the TBM and "tubulitis" may be seen in these severe cases. Even in the absence of evident epithelial cell injury on light microscopy, electron microscopy reveals structural cell changes, loss of the brush border, and fragmentation or lamination of the TBM (44,45). Occasional mitotic nuclei of the epithelial cells may be observed. As a rule, immunofluorescent studies are not revealing. Scant and nonspecific granular staining for immunoglobulins, usually without complement, may be detected along the TBM. In rare drug-induced cases, linear deposits of immunoglobulin G (IgG) and complement (C3) may be present, indicating antibodies directed against tubular membrane antigens. There is increasing evidence for a participatory role of the epithelial cells in the pathogenesis of ATIN (21,22). Enhanced expression of the human leukocyte antigen (HLA) class II antigens (HLA-DR) of injured tubular epithelial cells has been demonstrated (46,47), but shows no correlation with the intensity or phenotype of the infiltrating interstitial cells (37). The basilar vascular adhesion molecule (VCAM-1) and the luminal intercellular adhesion molecule (ICAM-1) have been shown to be induced (48). Both of these molecules are ligands to the integrin expressed on memory-activated T cells and their expression may serve to promote T-cell recruitment, adherence, and interaction with the tubule at sites of tissue injury.

The overall profile of immunocompetent cells identified in ATIN does not differ from that of chronic tubulointerstitial nephritis and suggests an important pathogenetic role for cell-mediated immunity in which both the epithelial and infiltrating cells are active and participating components. The role of mononuclear cells in lesions that pursue an acute time course is not unexpected. Activated lymphocytes are the dominant cell types observed, within the first 12 to 24 hours, in experimental models of delayed-type hypersensitivity (49). Their reversible presence over a limited time course in ATIN may reflect the balance of the mechanisms that regulate the immune response (50,51).

PATHOGENESIS

The immune response implicated in the pathogenesis of ATIN has been categorized into three phases: an antigen expression and recognition phase, an integrative or regulatory phase, and an effector or mediator phase (50). In the first phase, either the resident interstitial cells expressing major histocompatibility complex (MHC) class II or the tubular epithelial cells may function as antigen presenters. Tubular injury has been shown to stimulate MHC class II antigen expression by the tubular epithelial cells, providing a basis for a central role of the tubules in the initiation of the disease process (19,20,46).

The subsequent integrative or regulatory phase may suppress or intensify the reaction to the stimulus provided by the antigen-presenting cells. This is a rather complicated and still being deciphered as a phase of the immune response, in which T cells and antibodies directed at the presented antigen play a central role. Locally produced cytokines implicate a participatory role for the infiltrating, epithelial, and endothelial cells in this regulatory phase (21,22,52). The role of tubular epithelial cells (TECs) in this process has been examined. Exposure to selected insults or toxins result in activation of the TECs and their expression of various growth factors and chemokines, such as interleukins (IL), monocyte chemoattractant proteins (MCP), major histocompatibility complex (MHC), vascular endothelial growth factor (VEGF), transforming growth factor (TGF) and regulated on activation, normal T expressed and secreted (RANTES) (21,22). The subsequent bidirectional cross-talk between the TECs and recruited infiltrating inflammatory cells, either by soluble factors or direct contact, in this phase ultimately modulate the course of renal involvement and its potential for reversibility (32,50,51).

The final effector or mediator phase is mediated primarily by humoral factors released by the infiltrating cells, with the TECs playing a participatory role (Fig. 48-1). The cytotoxic cells may induce injury by the release of proteases, and the inducer cells by the release of lymphokines, which in addition to a direct detrimental action augment the role of the macrophages (50,53–55). In turn, the release of collagenases, elastases, and reactive oxygen species by the macrophages magnifies the injury initiated by the lymphocytes. Experimental studies indicate that the activated macrophages are responsible for the formation of a multinucleated epithelioid and granulomatous reaction (54,55). Lymphokines also promote fibroblast proliferation and alter the balance in favor of increased matrix synthesis rather than removal (21,22,25,50,56).

In the final analysis, it is the presence of a rather wide range of activated mononuclear cells and their interaction with each other and with parenchymal cells, during the integrative and regulatory phases, which is potentially damaging to the kidney (Table 48-1). Several of the cellular (epithelial, endothelial, lymphocytes, macrophages) signals have varying, often overlapping, functions that interact to modulate or amplify the in-

TABLE 48-1

IMMUNOMODULATORY SIGNALS INVOLVED IN THE PATHOGENESIS OF ACUTE TUBULOINTERSTITIAL NEPHRITIS

Antigenic cell surface markers
  MHC, major histocompatibility complex
  HLA Class II
  SPARC, secreted protein acidic and rich in protein

Adhesive cell surface makers
  ICAM-1, intracellular adhesion molecule 1
  VCAM-1, vacular adhesion molecule 1
  Integrins
  Selectins

Chemoattractants
  MCP-1, monocyte chemoattractant protein 1
  RANTES, normal T cell expressed and secreted
  MIP-1, macrophage inflammatory protein-1
  Eotaxin

Proinflammatory cytokines
  IL-6, interleukin-6
  IL-8, interleukin-8
  TGF-α, transforming growth factor α
  GM-CSF, granulocyte monocyte-colony stimulating factor
  PDGF-β, platelet derived growth factor β
  TNF-α, tumor necrosis factor α

Vasoactive substances
  Adenosine
  NO, nitric oxide
  ET-1, endothelin 1

Cytotoxic substances
  MP, metalloproteinases
  TIMP-1, tissue inhibitor metalloproteinases
  ROS, reactive oxygen species
  Ferric ion

Profibrotic cytokines
  TGF-β
  PDGF
  IL-1
  IL-6
  TNF
  PAI, plasminogen activator inhibitor

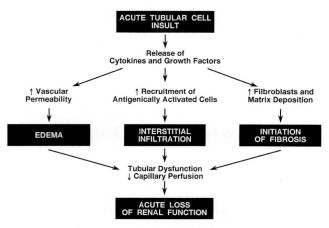

FIGURE 48-1. Pathogenetic pathways implicated in acute tubulointerstitial nephritis.

flammatory reaction of ATIN. Some of the ones that have been identified include cell surface markers that have either *antigenic* (MHC, HLA class II, secreted protein acidic and rich in protein [SPARC]) or *adhesive* (ICAM-1, VCAM-1, integrins; selectins) properties. Others are *chemoattractant* MCP-1; osteopontin; macrophage inflammatory protein-1 (MIP-1); eotaxin; RANTES, *proinflammatory* (interleukin [IL]-6 and IL-8; TGF-β; platelet-derived growth factor-β [PDGF-β]; granulocyte–monocyte colony-stimulating factor [GM-CSF]; tumor necrosis factor-α [TNF-α]), *vasoactive* (adenosine; nitrous oxide [NO]; endothelin-1 [ET-1]), *cytotoxic* (metalloproteinases [MP]; tissue inhibitor metalloproteinases [TIMP-1]; reactive oxygen radicals; ferric ion), or *fibrogenic* [TGF-β, PDGF, IL-1, IL-6, TNF, plasminogen activator inhibitor (PAI)]. Evidence also exists for possible protective cytokines that can favorably modify the proinflammatory sequence of events (57). The resultant integration, during the regulatory and effector phases, either suppresses the effector phase, as in mild forms of ATIN, or amplifies it, as in severe forms of ATIN. Ultimately, feedback mechanisms and removal of the inciting agent restore the response to injury to its baseline dormant state with consequent recovery of normal kidney function or residual permanent damage (31–33,52,58–62).

The bulk of the available information about the phases of the immune response and interstitial inflammatory reaction in ATIN derives from studies in experimental animals, particularly in models of recombinant rats and mice (43,51,56,63). Unfortunately, there are no animal models that correspond to the reaction that occurs in human ATIN. A principal limitation of human studies is that the data derived from kidney biopsies provide information only at fixed moments in the course of a lesion that is an evolving process. The same limitation applies to the serologic data provided in clinical studies that are obtained at a fixed period, usually when the lesion is well established and often at its worst, with limited or no data available on the onset or resolution phases of the lesion. These limitations notwithstanding, considerable evidence has accrued for a role of the principal immunologic mechanisms—cell-mediated injury, anti-TBM antibodies, immune complex deposition—in the pathogenesis of ATIN. Although there is evidence that all three mechanisms may be operative to varying degrees in different patients, the bulk of the available information favors a predominant role for cell-mediated injury.

Contrary to the extensive experimental data in support of anti-TBM disease from animal models of interstitial disease, anti-TBM antibodies have been detected only rarely in human ATIN (64,65). The evidence presented in favor of anti-TBM antibodies as a cause of ATIN derives from cases attributed to methicillin. The deposition of a metabolite of methicillin, dimethoxyphenylpenicilloyl, along the TBM was initially implicated as the antigenic stimulus but subsequently questioned to have a pathogenetic role when the deposits were found in the kidneys of totally asymptomatic patients exposed to the drug (66,67). By the same token, patients with a transplanted kidney who have anti-TBM antibodies that are shown to bind to the TBM of the allograft do not manifest the clinical features of ATIN (68). In two cases of ATIN attributed to phenytoin in which linear deposits of IgG were detected, the lesion could not be induced in rats by passive transfer, although binding of the antibodies to TBM could be demonstrated *in vitro* (69,70). Thus, the dearth of evidence for anti–TBM-mediated disease is far from convincing for an important role, if any, of this mechanism in human ATIN.

The same limitations apply for a role of immune complex–mediated ATIN. The cases in which granular deposits of IgG have been detected have been in patients with Sjögren's syndrome (71,72) and systemic lupus erythematosus (73–76), whose underlying disease mechanism accounts for the deposition of immune complexes in the kidneys as well as other body organs. Their presence in other, more common forms of ATIN is extremely rare and never a dominant feature.

By contrast, the evidence in favor of cell-mediated disease is overwhelming. The infiltrating cells are antigenically activated. T-cell reactivity has been demonstrated from *in vitro* studies of lymphocyte stimulation (52,63,77,78). Infiltrating cells have been analyzed by immunoperoxidase studies using monoclonal antibodies. Most are T lymphocytes that express the T-cell antigen–receptor complex (39,48,79). As a rule, the infiltrating lymphocytes are CD4+ and CD8+, with a slight preponderance of the former (46,80), except in cases due to NSAIDs (34,52) and on occasion in cases due to cimetidine (81) or antibiotics (79), in which CD8+ cells may show a slight preponderance. Comparative studies of ATIN due to NSAIDs or β-lactam antibiotics have failed to reveal significant differences in the CD4+/CD8+ ratio or in the overall percentage composition of T cells, B cells, and monocytes. The reported differences in infiltrating cell subtypes can be due to individual genetic background, nature of the insult, and the point in time during the course of the disease when biopsies were obtained. Nevertheless, it is clear that where sought, activated antigens have been demonstrated on the surface of the infiltrating cells (36,39), and plasma cells containing IgE (41,42,81), IgA (34), IgG, and IgM (42) have been detected. However, no diagnostic pattern of markers or infiltrating cells has emerged.

FUNCTIONAL MANIFESTATIONS

The principal manifestations of ATIN are those of tubular dysfunction, which is one reason that the term *tubulointerstitial nephritis* was introduced in preference to the initial appellation of *interstitial nephritis*. As a rule, tubular dysfunction precedes the onset of azotemia, which in turn precedes that of oliguria. As such, vigilance to clinically evident abnormalities of tubular function, including polyuria, are essential to the early detection of ATIN during its initial reversible stages.

Because of the focal nature of the lesions and the segmental nature of normal tubular function, the pattern of tubular dysfunction that results varies depending on the major site of injury, whereas the extent of damage determines the severity of tubular dysfunction. The principal hallmarks of glomerular disease, such as salt retention, edema, and hypertension, characteristically are absent (15,16,78,82). However, massive proteinuria does occur in ATIN due to NSAIDs and, occasionally, antibiotics (16,34,83). The magnitude of reduction in GFR that occurs seems to correlate with the extent of the interstitial cellular infiltrates (11,26). This is in contrast to chronic forms of tubulointerstitial nephritis, in which it is the magnitude of interstitial fibrosis that correlates with the severity of decreased GFR, whereas the enlargement of the interstitium by cellular infiltrate has less bearing on GFR (81,85). Under any circumstance, the structural changes of ATIN account for the functional changes observed in this clinicopathologic syndrome. In addition to the direct injury to epithelial cells that may account for tubular dysfunction, changes in the interstitial volume and composition contribute to the functional abnormalities that develop. A major part of the reabsorbed or secreted tubular fluid has to traverse a true interstitial space (86). The structure, composition, and permeability characteristics of the interstitial space must, of necessity, exert an effect on such an exchange. A change in any of these parameters of the interstitium or those of the epithelial cell tight junctions, by delaying equilibration or exchange processes, could well account for the functional alterations of the renal tubule that develop in ATIN. It also is possible that changes in the pressure of the supporting interstitium, which are transmitted to the periarterial space, could affect the blood flow to the adjacent tubule and thereby cause tubular dysfunction. In addition, the expansion of interstitial space would increase the distance between tubular epithelium and the peritubular capillary plexus, where the reabsorbed fluid is delivered.

Tubular alterations also may be reflected in reductions of the GFR through tubuloglomerular feedback as the function of the affected proximal tubular segments becomes compromised and both the rate and load of solute delivery to the macula densa are altered (87–89). Furthermore, the increase in hydrostatic pressure of the edematous interstitium, as has been demonstrated in allograft rejection (15), may adversely affect the intraarteriolar pressure and cause a reduction of the hydrostatic pressure transmitted to the glomerular capillaries (Fig. 48-1). In addition, a vasoactive effect of the cytokines, eicosanoids, and reactive oxygen species elaborated by the interstitial infiltrating cells and injured epithelial cells may affect renal hemodynamics through the increased production of vasoconstrictive substances, such as thromboxane A_2 and leukotrienes, and decreased production of vasodilators, such as NO, brought about by reduced production of its substrate L-arginine by the injured proximal tubule cells (90–92). Evidence for a role for

TABLE 48-2

CAUSES, PRINCIPAL SITES OF INJURY, AND PATTERNS OF TUBULAR DYSFUNCTION IN ACUTE
TUBULOINTERSTITIAL NEPHROPATHIES

Site of injury	Causes	Tubular dysfunction	Clinical manifestation
Cortex			
Proximal tubule	Antibiotics Multiple myeloma Immunologic diseases Neoplastic diseases Idiopathic	↓ Reabsorption: Na^+, glucose, HCO_3^-, urate, PO_4, amino acids	Glucosuria, hypouricemia, hypophosphatemia, aminoaciduria, alkaline urine, acidemia
Distal tubule	Antibiotics Immunologic diseases Nonsteroidal antiinflammatory drugs Idiopathic	↓ Secretion: H^+, K^+ ↓ Reabsorption Na^+	Alkaline urine, acidemia, hyperkalemia, inability to preserve sodium
Medulla and papilla	Infections Analgesics Nonsteroidal antiinflammatory drugs Disorders of uric acid, calcium, oxalate Immunologic diseases Idiopathic	↓ Reabsorption: Na^+ ↓ Concentrating ability	Polyuria, nocturia, inability to preserve sodium

cytokines released by the infiltrating cells in the reduction in renal blood flow and GFR has been advanced from studies of an experimental model of acute obstructive nephropathy that is characterized by acute mononuclear cell infiltrates (93). Certainly, the correlation between the severity and extent of cellular infiltrates and increments in serum creatinine attests to a role of the infiltrating cells in the reduction of GFR in ATIN (Fig. 48-1).

The tubulointerstitial lesions usually are localized either to the cortex or the medulla. Cortical lesions predominantly affect either the proximal tubule or the distal tubule. Medullary lesions affect the loop of Henle and the medullary collecting duct. The change in the normal function of each of the affected segments then determines the manifestations of tubular dysfunction (Table 48-2). Lesions principally affecting the proximal tubule result in bicarbonaturia (proximal renal tubular acidosis), glucosuria (renal glucosuria), aminoaciduria, β_2-microglobinuria, phosphaturia, and uricosuria (15,16). The latter two events can be valuable in suggesting the possibility of tubulointerstitial disease when the serum phosphate and urate levels are lower than expected in any patient with reduced kidney function. The presence of glucosuria when the blood sugar levels are normal should always lead to a consideration of ATIN. The distal nephron segment secretes hydrogen and potassium and regulates the final amount of sodium chloride excreted. Lesions primarily affecting the distal tubule result in the distal form of renal tubular acidosis, hyperkalemia, and salt wasting (15,16). Lesions that primarily involve the medulla and papilla disproportionately affect the loops of Henle, collecting ducts, and other medullary structures essential to achieving and maintaining medullary hypertonicity. Disruption of these structures therefore results in different degrees of nephrogenic diabetes insipidus, polyuria, and nocturia. A reduction in collecting duct aquaporins has been shown in an experimental model of acute renal injury (82). Actually, a polyuric phase almost always precedes the onset of oliguria in ATIN.

Although this general framework is useful in localizing the site of injury, considerable overlap is encountered clinically, with different degrees of proximal, distal, and medullary dysfunction present in any one patient, all of which usually pre-

cede any clinically detectable changes in GFR. In most cases, however, the reduction in GFR and consequent azotemia are the presenting clinical abnormalities calling attention to the acute kidney injury. Preexisting or coexistent evidence of tubular dysfunction, unless specifically sought, may go undetected and either delay the diagnosis or result in the wrong clinical diagnosis. One can only speculate on the number of cases of ATIN that go undetected clinically because of the presence of tubular dysfunction alone in the absence of frank azotemia or oliguria—hence the importance of monitoring for tubular dysfunction in patients exposed to agents known to be associated with ATIN, and the necessity of documenting tubular dysfunction in those with azotemia to marshal evidence for the diagnosis of ATIN.

CLINICAL FEATURES

The clinical presentation of individual cases of ATIN is diverse and varies to some degree depending on the causative factor. The manifestations best characterized in methicillin-induced ATIN can be considered the prototypically classic clinical manifestations, around which general variation occurs depending on the causative agent and individual variation depending on the particular case encountered clinically.

In most cases, symptoms develop several days or even weeks after exposure to the inciting agent, which in the case of drugs is not dose dependent. The classic triad of low-grade fever (70% to 100%), fleeting skin rash (30% to 50%), and mild eosinophilia (80%) described with methicillin-induced ATIN is not invariably present, and certainly it is less common for all three to occur together. Their documentation depends to some degree on the vigilance with which they are sought because they may be mild and transient. The full triad was noted to be present in approximately one-third of cases of methicillin-induced ATIN (94–97), but only in 5% of cases of ATIN induced by other drugs in which any one of them (fever, rash, or eosinophilia) is less likely to occur (11,12,83,98). The skin rash consists of erythematous maculopapular lesions, which often are pruritic, and affect preferentially the trunk and proximal portion of the extremities. Flank pain, reflecting edema-induced distention of the renal capsule, may be detected in over one-third of the cases when queried and may be the presenting symptom in some cases (99). Gross hematuria, another presenting feature, may be present in 10% to 15% of drug-induced ATIN cases when specifically sought. Gross hematuria was a distinct feature of the first reported case of methicillin-associated ATIN in a child with cystic fibrosis treated intermittently with methicillin, who experienced gross hematuria each time she was exposed to the drug (100), and occurs in more than half the cases of methicillin-induced ATIN (11). Although a transient eosinophilia often (40% to 60%) is present, it may go undetected unless specifically sought, which accounts for its inconsistency in reported cases.

Urinalysis can be helpful in the diagnosis. Proteinuria, hematuria, and pyuria are present in most cases. The proteinuria is mild, seldom exceeds 2 g/day, and only rarely is in the nephrotic range, except in those cases due to NSAIDs (95–97,101,102). Microscopic hematuria is detected in up to 90% of cases and gross hematuria in 15%; rarely, red blood cell casts may be detected (103). The pyuria is nonspecific except when eosinophils are detected in an appropriately prepared and carefully examined urinary sediment (104–106). Although eosinophils may be observed with Wright's stain of a well-spun urinary sediment, the use of Hansel's stain on the sediment of an alkalinized urine sample is superior in detecting eosinophils (104). The mere detection of eosinophiluria is not specific for ATIN (107,108). The sensitivity of eosinophiluria for the diagnosis of ATIN has been estimated to be 40% to 60%. Its specificity has not been well established, but its positive predictive value has been estimated to be only 38% (108). Eosinophiluria is present in approximately 15% of hospitalized patients, in whom it usually is caused by a variety of other inflammatory diseases of the urinary tract, and in only 14% of those with eosinophiluria is it due to ATIN (105). The presence of eosinophiluria is a better predictor of ATIN when more than 5% of the leukocytes are eosinophils, in which case 40% of the eosinophiluric patients have ATIN, as opposed to an incidence of 3.5% in those with less than 1% are eosinophils. Other conditions in which an eosinophiluria exceeding 5% may be present are urinary tract obstruction, cystitis, contrast-induced ARF, IgA nephropathy, and cholesterol emboli. Thus, the detection of selective eosinophiluria, although useful, is neither necessary nor sufficient for the diagnosis of ATIN. Equally useful urinary findings in the diagnosis of ATIN are the detection of renal glucosuria, increased fractional excretion of uric acid, and inability to concentrate the urine maximally and to conserve sodium, as reflections of tubular dysfunction detailed in the previous section.

The impairment in kidney function varies, ranging from discrete selective abnormalities of tubular function to frank kidney failure, with or without oliguria (109,110). As a rule, increments in blood urea nitrogen and serum creatinine develop after tubular dysfunction is detectable and while the patient is still nonoliguric or even polyuric. Oliguria develops if the presenting systemic symptoms, modest azotemia, and evidence of tubular dysfunction go undetected and if exposure to the causative agent or factor continues. Kidney failure is more likely to occur in older patients and is more severe in those who become oliguric. The duration of the oliguric period is variable, ranging from a few days to several weeks. Supportive renal replacement therapy may be required in approximately one-third of those patients. Reversal of kidney failure and return to baseline kidney function is the rule in the majority of cases (about 60% to 65%). Irreversible kidney failure can occur but is rare (about 5% to 10%), while partial recovery with persistent impairment of kidney function is relatively more common (10% to 20%) in cases where interstitial fibrosis and granulomas are present in biopsy specimens (11,12.83,111,112).

Increased kidney size on ultrasonography, reflecting interstitial edema, is common but nondiagnostic. Radioactive gallium uptake by the kidney, reflecting interstitial cellular infiltration, can be detected in one-third of cases, but lacks diagnostic specificity (78,113). However, when the gallium scan is negative it can be useful to rule out ATN (78,95,113). The lymphocyte stimulation test can be valuable in the diagnosis of drug-induced ATIN, especially in determining the responsible agent in cases of multiple-drug therapy (78,93). The serum level of IgE can be elevated and IgE-containing plasma cells have been demonstrated among the renal interstitial cellular infiltrates, providing further evidence for a hypersensitivity reaction (41,101,114).

There is suggestive evidence that a short course of treatment with steroids improves the kidney lesions and expedites recovery from drug-induced ATIN (115–117), although this is not a uniformly observed response (83,118,119). The use of steroids should be considered in patients with protracted kidney failure, especially when the failure persists after the inciting agent has been discontinued (26,94–96), and in those whose biopsy reveals granulomatous lesions that are associated with increased risk of permanent kidney injury (117,120,121). Reversal of apparently permanent kidney failure after steroid therapy in a patient on maintenance hemodialysis has been reported (122). However, in a retrospective evaluation of biopsy-proven cases of ATIN, the routine use of steroids was not associated with a statistical difference in kidney function or outcome (123). Unfortunately, no controlled clinical trials are available, and controversy over the use of steroids persists. If steroids are used, a response usually is evident relatively early after initiation of treatment. The course of treatment should be brief, and steroids should be discontinued if no response is observed after 3 to 4 weeks of therapy (124,125).

INCIDENCE AND DIAGNOSIS

The frequency with which ATIN accounts for cases of clinically encountered ARF is difficult to establish. The diagnosis of ATIN is based on the finding of characteristic morphologic features on kidney biopsy and on the identification of the causative factor. Both of these requirements for a correct diagnosis are fraught with difficulties and limitations.

Part of the difficulty associated with the diagnosis of ATIN stems from the relatively low index of suspicion with which its possibility is considered clinically and the general reluctance to perform a kidney biopsy in cases of ARF. Even if a biopsy is performed, there are difficulties in differentiating the lesions of ATIN from those of ATN, a distinct possibility in most cases of ARF in which the prevailing clinical condition could be conducive to either ATIN or ATN (7,126). An essential differential feature between the two entities is the magnitude of interstitial edema and cellular infiltrates, which are more prominent in ATIN, and the magnitude of tubular cell injury, which is more prominent in ATN (Fig. 48-2). However, given the variable degree to which each of these features may be present in each entity (7,126), there is sufficient overlap between the extent of edema and the severity of tubular injury in ATIN and ATN to make it difficult to differentiate among them on morphologic features alone, at least in some cases. This is best illustrated in the literature before World War II, when ATN came to be recognized as a distinct entity. In contemporary reports, classic ATN cases due to transfusion reactions were labeled *acute hematogenous interstitial nephritis*, emphasizing the similarity of the lesions to those reported by Councilman as being associated with systemic infections (5,6). Ironically, the subsequent focus on tubular cell injury in ATN has deviated attention from the interstitial infiltrates present in ATN and the

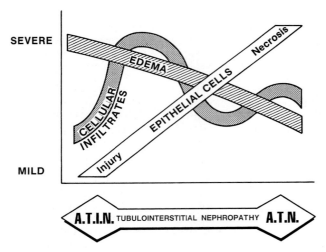

FIGURE 48-2. Schematic representation of the spectrum of structural changes associated with cases of acute renal failure due to acute tubulointerstitial nephritis (ATIN) and acute tubular necrosis (ATN). (Reproduced from: Eknoyan G. Acute renal failure associated with tubulointerstitial nephropathies. In: Brenner BM, Lazarus JM, eds. *Acute renal failure,* 2nd ed. New York: Churchill Livingstone, 1988:491, with permission.)

emerging evidence for their role in the pathogenesis of kidney injury in ATN (127). Broadly defined, the morphologic features of tubulointerstitial nephritis can be considered a spectrum of lesions characterized by interstitial edema, cellular infiltrates, and tubular injury (Figs. 48-2 and 48-3). Depending on the magnitude and severity of each of these structural features, at one end of the spectrum would be clear-cut cases of ATIN, and at the other end, ATN. Difficulty is encountered in cases that fit in the middle of this spectrum, and is further magnified in those with focal rather than diffuse lesions. In such cases, the history of exposure to an inciting agent and its identification become important in establishing a correct diagnosis.

There also are difficulties associated with identifying the causative factor. Clinically, removal of a suspected agent followed by reversal of the lesion strongly suggests the diagnosis. This can be particularly convincing in the presence of systemic

manifestations of a hypersensitivity reaction, such as fever, skin rash, and eosinophilia, in addition to ARF, all of which subside on removal of the inciting factor or agent. Difficulties arise when the only manifestation is ARF, which is potentially reversible, and when a number of corrective measures are instituted simultaneously. Moreover, most patients are on several drugs, and there is the expected tendency to incriminate the most common and better known agents that have been associated with ATIN. When the wrong drug is discontinued, the acute kidney injury continues unabated because the causative agent continues to be administered. The diagnostic limitations of removing agents wrongly surmised as a cause of ATIN have been shown by studies in which lymphocyte stimulation testing revealed causative agents that had not been suspected clinically (78). Proof depends on recurrence with reexposure to the same agent, as has occurred accidentally with some antibiotics (128).

Most of the figures quoted in the literature on the incidence of ATIN stem from retrospective studies based on kidney biopsies. Review of unselected kidney biopsy specimens reveals a low incidence of ATIN (26). Review of biopsy specimens from patients with unexplained ARF reveals a frequency that ranges from 8% to 22% (118,123,129–133), which generally is higher in the elderly population (134). The problem in deriving conclusions on incidence from kidney biopsies is illustrated by the following two studies. In a report of 976 patients with ARF, 218 of whom underwent kidney biopsy, a diagnosis of ATIN was made in 29 cases, an incidence of 14% of patients sampled for biopsy, but only 3% of all patients with ARF (135). The question remains whether such a report can be considered a cross-sectional study and whether the incidence of ATIN in the 758 patients who did not undergo biopsy was the same. In another study, 13% of the biopsies of patients with ARF revealed ATIN; the diagnosis was not suspected clinically in any of them (129). Thus, given the very small number of patients with ARF who are subjected to kidney biopsy, the necessity of kidney biopsy to diagnose ATIN, and the failure to suspect the diagnosis of ATIN clinically, all render conclusions derived from biopsy reports of limited value in estimating the true incidence of ATIN (135). Furthermore, because of the variable and often subjective reasons for which kidney biopsies are done in different centers, any attempt to compare or combine results from different reports would not be useful. Coupled with the fact that cases of ATIN with mild azotemia and only some

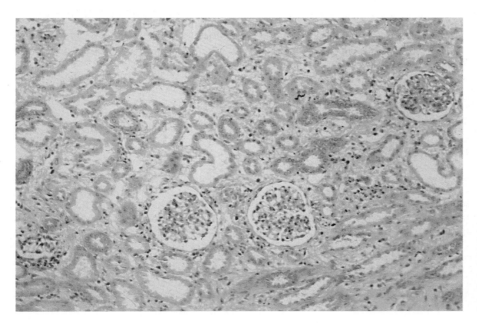

FIGURE 48-3. Kidney biopsy from a case of NSAID-induced acute tubulointerstitial nephritis. Note the increased interstitial space between the tubules showing edema and focal infiltration my mononuclear inflammatory cells. The glomerular structure is preserved, but there are periglomerular clusters of mononuclear cells.

TABLE 48-3

PRINCIPAL CONDITIONS ASSOCIATED WITH ACUTE TUBULOINTERSTITIAL NEPHROPATHY

Infections
    Invasive of renal parenchyma
    Reactive to systemic infections
Drugs
    Antibiotics
    Sulfonamides
    Nonsteroidal antiinflammatory drugs
    Other drugs
Systemic diseases
    Metabolic disorders
    Immune diseases
    Neoplastic disease
Idiopathic with uveitis

degree of tubular dysfunction may go entirely undetected, it is impossible to determine the true incidence of ATIN from biopsy reports. In cases of clinically evident ARF, ATIN probably accounts for approximately 15% to 20% of them. Among the causes of ATIN, infections and drugs are the most common (Table 48-3).

INFECTIONS

Infections as a possible cause of ATIN often are overlooked, and as a consequence their diagnosis is missed and their incidence as a cause of ATIN is underestimated. The eradication of serious streptococcal infections that were first associated with ATIN after the introduction of antibiotics and the recognition of antibiotics as a cause of ATIN have led to the preferential consideration of drugs used in the treatment of infections as a principal cause of ATIN. In addition, the hemodynamic changes associated with severe infections and the use of antibiotics with a direct nephrotoxic effect in their treatment usually are implicated as a cause of any deterioration of kidney function without adequate investigation of ATIN as a possible cause of ARF. Another reason that hinders the diagnosis of ATIN is the commonly held but questionable notion that postinfectious acute glomerulonephritis is the most common kidney lesion associated with infections. Finally, the modest reduction in kidney function and its return to baseline as the infection is treated limits the clinical consideration given to the observed changes in kidney function. Thus, unless the possibility of infection-induced ATIN is considered seriously, without undue bias toward coexistent and confounding conditions that may account for an acute deterioration of kidney function, and the diagnosis pursued actively, cases of infection-induced ATIN will go undetected, and its true incidence will remain underestimated. Nevertheless, several new causes of infection-induced ATIN have come to be identified since Councilman described their association.

Tubulointerstitial lesions of the kidney may develop in the kidney either because of direct invasion of the kidney parenchyma by the infective microorganisms or because of reactive changes to a nonrenal systemic infection.

Invasive Infections

The classic and by far the most common example of ATIN is due to direct bacterial invasion of the kidney, although fun-

gal, viral, and parasitic infections also may account for it. The usual forms of pyelonephritis are considered in Chapter 34, Infections of the Upper Urinary Tract, and are not detailed here, except to highlight their differential features from ATIN reactive to a systemic infection. Apart from the classic local and systemic symptoms of acute pyelonephritis that clinically differentiate direct infection of the kidney from reactive ATIN and culture of the invasive organism in the urine, there are distinct morphologic differences between the two entities that deserve emphasis. Acute bacterial pyelonephritis is a focal rather than diffuse lesion, which usually is limited to an individual pyramid and rarely affects all the pyramids of the kidney. The areas of infection are characteristically wedge shaped, with the apex directed to the medulla. The infected foci are focal and sharply demarcated from the adjoining uninfected parenchyma, and lack the tendency to spread laterally (9,136). Contrast-enhanced computed tomography reveals the typical wedge-shaped, nodular, hypodense areas corresponding to the distribution of the lesions and heavy cellular infiltrates in pyelonephritis (137). These are quite distinct from the generalized changes of ATIN (138). In the absence of obstruction, the infection tends to be confined to the originally affected lobule and to resolve gradually over a period of weeks. An acute reduction in kidney function is rare except in severe cases and those with obstruction, or when the infection is superimposed on preexisting chronic kidney disease (139). As recovery occurs, the initial polymorphonuclear leukocytic infiltrate is replaced by mononuclear cells and the development of streaks of fibrous tissue that account for the cortical scars encountered in such cases (140–144).

Occasional cases of acute ATIN have been reported in association with otherwise invasive infections such as mycoplasmal pneumonia (145), toxoplasmosis (146), cytomegalovirus infection (113,147,148), infectious mononucleosis (149–153), polyomavirus infection (154), hantavirus infection (155), Rocky Mountain spotted fever (156), leptospirosis (157,158), Legionnaires' disease (159,160), candidiasis (161,162), *Yersinia* pseudotuberculosis (163), *Ascaris lumbricoides* (164), and adenoviral infection (165,166). A greater number of such cases are now encountered clinically and recorded in the literature because of the increasing number of immunocompromised hosts [patients with acquired immunodeficiency syndrome (AIDS), transplant recipients, the elderly] in the general population. Of those, patients with AIDS constitute a special challenge in the diagnosis of ATIN, not only because of their propensity to contract unusual infections (167), but because of the number of drugs they consume, such as protease inhibitors, which not only are nephrotoxic but cause ATIN (168–172). Although the passage of the of implicated organisms through the renal parenchyma and their isolation from the urine have been demonstrated, their localization in the kidney is less well substantiated. The cellular infiltration is mononuclear rather than polymorphonuclear, and evidence has been advanced for an immunologic mechanism responsible for the renal reaction elicited by some of them (151). Antigenic material has been demonstrated in the renal parenchyma of humans with ATIN associated with some of these infectious agents, such as *Mycoplasma* (145), polyomavirus (154), the rickettsiae responsible for Rocky Mountain spotted fever (156), and leptospira (173–181). The complex nature of the lesions encountered in some of these infections can be better appreciated from a specific consideration of some of them.

Leptospirosis

Acute renal failure occurs in almost half the cases of leptospirosis, and the degree of kidney involvement often determines the gravity of the disease (173). In fact, in endemic areas of the disease, leptospirosis is one of the most common causes of ARF

(174). Although there might be evidence of renal involvement in the preicteric phase of the disease, it is in its icteric phase that ATIN develops in conjunction with a rapid deterioration of kidney function. Rodents are the principal reservoir of the organisms, which enter the host through the skin or mucosa and gain access to the kidney by the bloodstream. At first, they transiently invade the glomeruli, then pass to the peritubular capillaries, and ultimately penetrate the interstitium and tubules (175,176). The renal lesions of leptospirosis are limited exclusively to the tubules and interstitium. They are focal in distribution and are most pronounced at the corticomedullary junction, a structural feature characteristic of ATIN lesions that are reactive to infections. The tubular changes consist of degeneration, epithelial necrosis, and rupture of the basement membrane (174–177). The interstitial changes are restricted to the region of the affected tubules. Endothelial cell injury and capillary thrombosis are demonstrable in the affected foci. Initially, interstitial edema and cellular infiltration are minimal but ultimately become prominent, such that the whole kidney becomes enlarged, congested, and soft. The infiltrates consist of mononuclear cells, plasma cells, and eosinophils. The interstitial lesions may be present even in the absence of clinically detectable kidney failure (178). The tubular lesions occur during leptospiral migration through the renal parenchyma, and during this stage the spirochetes can be detected in the urine (176–179). Thus, direct tubular injury by *Leptospira* may account for the renal lesions. Leptospiral antigens have been demonstrated in the renal interstitium of a canine model of the disease, suggesting a role for immunologic mechanisms (180). Leptospiral outer membrane proteins and lipoproteins have been implicated in causing tubular dysfunction and initiating the immunologic injury (181–183). They have been shown to inhibit Na^+-K^+-Cl^- cotransporter activity and messenger RNA (mRNA) synthesis (182–183) in the thick ascending limb. This could account for the polyuria and hypokalemia frequently seen in these cases. Furthermore, the exposure of cultured proximal and thick ascending limb cells to the outer membrane proteins results in activation of a pro-inflammatory cascade, with increased induction gene expression of NF-?B, iNOS, MCP-1, and TNF-α (181,182) The superimposition of shock and volume depletion in severe cases of the disease may further contribute to the tubular lesions, and the structural changes observed may represent the cumulative effect of both direct invasion and ischemia, possibly coupled with an immune injury (178). Anti-glomerular basement membrane antibodies with linear, immunofluorescent deposits along the glomerular and TBM have been reported in one case (184) and diffuse nodular complement deposits in another (185).

Although the interstitial changes may persist for several months in an occasional patient, usually with persistent spirochetes in the urine, in most cases the renal changes subside within a few weeks after resolution of the disease with appropriate antibiotic therapy (140,152,157). In these usual cases, kidney function returns to normal, whereas in those who develop a chronic carrier state the leptospira localize in the kidney, fibrosis and tubular atrophy develop, and permanent impairment of kidney function ensues (157,177).

Hantavirus Infection

The once mysterious entities of "hemorrhagic fever with renal syndrome" in Asia and "nephropathia epidemica" in Europe are now recognized as due to infection with one of the related RNA viruses of the Hantavirus genus, which belong to the family of Bunyviridae (186–188). The availability of serologic tests for the specific antibodies, which appear early in the course of the infection and may persist indefinitely, now allows for the easy diagnosis of this once enigmatic disease that mimics several

of the features of leptospirosis—fever, petechiae, thrombocytopenia, and liver and kidney dysfunction (189–191).

The renal lesions consist of the classic changes of ATIN, with tubular injury, interstitial edema, and predominantly mononuclear cellular infiltrates with occasional polymorphonuclear leukocytes and eosinophils. They are most prominent in the medulla and corticomedullary junction, together with the hallmarks of Hantavirus nephropathy: vascular congestion and interstitial hemorrhage (155,188). This accounts for the microhematuria and, together with the enlarged kidneys, for the back pain present in most cases. The transient heavy proteinuria (>2 g/d) noted at the onset of the disease correlates with the urinary excretion of IL-6 (192). The severity of the lesions and frequency of renal failure are higher and the prognosis worse in the Asian than in the European and American varieties of the infection (193–197).

Polyoma Virus

Polyoma is a double-stranded DNA virus family, one strain of which, BK virus, commonly causes ATIN. Typically, the virus is acquired in childhood but remains latent as over 70% of adults are seropositive (198). However, when the immune system is compromised, as in AIDS and transplant recipients, the virus reemerges and causes ATIN (199,200). Its incidence in kidney transplant recipients is reported to be 3% to 5%, with an associated 50% graft loss among those affected (210,202). It is considered to result from over immunosuppression, and in transplant recipients its incidence has increased with the use of newer more potent immunosuppressants. Decreasing immunosuppression has been effective in the management of some cases but is associated with an increase in acute rejection episodes (201).

There are no specific clinical features the kidney disease except for increasing levels of serum creatinine. Diagnosis is based on findings on kidney biopsy that are distinct from those of acute rejection. The finding of cells in the urine that have viral inclusions, so-called decoy cells, are indicative of viral replication in the urinary tract but are not specific of ATIN. Detection and quantification of viral DNA load in plasma by PCR is potentially useful for the detection of significant viral reactivation, and can serve as a quantifiable surrogate marker of the course of the infection (201,202).

Brucellosis

Renal involvement is rare in brucellosis, although the organisms frequently are recovered from the urine of infected patients. By contrast, in those with renal involvement, it is unusual to recover the organisms from the urine (203). In the acute form of the disease, fever, proteinuria, hematuria, and pyuria are presenting features. The renal lesion consists of a focal glomerulitis coupled with a severe, sometimes diffuse, interstitial inflammatory reaction caused by infiltrating polymorphonuclear leukocytes (203). In the chronic form of the disease, extensive fibrosis develops that clinically and radiologically mimics the findings of tuberculosis (204).

Candidiasis

Disseminated candidiasis almost always affects the kidney (205,206). *Candida albicans* causes two types of lesions in the kidneys. The first type, which is relevant to this chapter, occurs during the candidemic phase with the initial seeding of the kidney, which rapidly elicits an inflammatory reaction with polymorphonuclear infiltration limited to the renal cortex. Depending on the severity and extent of the lesions, pyuria and candiduria may be the only findings, with varying degrees of renal insufficiency in approximately half the cases (207). When multiplication extends to the tubular lumen, they may invade the interstitial tissue and elicit a severe interstitial inflammatory reaction in the medulla. Based on experimental studies, it would seem that when smaller doses of *Candida* are injected, the mycelia pass down the tubules and enter the collecting system without eliciting the cortical lesions, which are seen only when larger doses of *Candida* are injected (208).

The second type of lesion develops in the more chronic form of the infection and results from the multiplication of the organisms in the urinary tract, where no limiting inflammatory reaction can be elicited. This can result in the proliferation of the organisms into mycelial filaments that form bezoars of *Candida* in the renal pelvis and calices (207,208). The large bezoars or fungus balls can completely fill and occlude the renal pelvis and calices and result in obstructive nephropathy and hydronephrosis (208,209).

Noninvasive Infections

Acute tubulointerstitial nephritis may complicate infections in the absence of bacteremia and parenchymal invasion of the kidneys. Before the widespread use of antibiotics, ATIN was a relatively common complication observed at autopsy of cases of scarlet fever, β-hemolytic streptococcal infections, and diphtheria (3,4,210). Although the lesions of ATIN were noted to be more common in cases of scarlet fever (3), the more severe destructive lesions occurred in cases of diphtheria (4). The availability of specific vaccines has eradicated diphtheria, whereas specific antibiotic therapy has ameliorated the severity of streptococcal infections such that, although renal lesions continue to occur, their clinical outcome is now more favorable (211–213). Unlike the relatively later renal changes of streptococcal infections, which occur in the second or third week after onset of the infection and cause typical postinfectious acute proliferative glomerulonephritis, the lesions of ATIN occur early in the course of infection, usually during the first few days of onset of the infection (3,4, 210–214), often between the 9th and 12th days of the disease (13,214), and in the absence of edema or hypertension.

The renal lesions may be focal or diffuse. Interstitial edema is more prominent than the cellular infiltrates, which are rather diffuse and localized to the corticomedullary junction. The cellular infiltrates are especially prominent in the perivascular areas and, on occasion, may be dense enough to mimic leukemic infiltration. The initial infiltrates consist of plasma cells, histiocytes, and lymphocytes, whereas in the later stages of the disease the number of plasma cells decreases and that of lymphocytes increases. The lesions can easily be differentiated from those of pyelonephritis by their distribution. In pyelonephritis, the inflammatory foci are arranged radially, whereas in noninvasive ATIN they form a circular band around the vessels at the corticomedullary region. Occasional eosinophils may be present (211–213). The proximal tubules may be dilated, with swelling and occasional necrosis of the lining cells (13). The interstitial ground substance may stain heavily with periodic acid-Schiff stain, suggesting depolymerization of the interstitial mucopolysaccharides (13).

In contrast to the detailed morphologic changes reported in the early literature describing this entity, the clinical information provided is sparse. Where noted, proteinuria and pyuria were said to be common (4). In a careful study of the urinary sediment of 14 children with scarlet fever, an abnormal sediment was reported to be present in all (215). In larger series, the urinary sediment is noted as being abnormal in only 50% to 60% of the cases (212).

The availability of antibiotics and supportive therapy has altered the picture of infection-associated ATIN, not only through the emergence of antibiotics as a more common cause of ATIN but by prolonging the course of the infective disease in severe cases that were once rapidly fatal and revealed ATIN at postmortem. The use of potentially nephrotoxic antibiotics allows time for tubular necrosis to develop and become the lesion most evident at autopsy. This is in contrast to the preantibiotic era, when patients died soon after the onset of severe infection, probably before epithelial cell necrosis had set in (216). Certainly, the lesions described by Councilman (1) are much less rarely noted in the current literature, and most of the available information on them dates back to the preantibiotic or early antibiotic periods. Nevertheless, they continue to be encountered, particularly in children (212,215,217), and must be considered in streptococcal infections with ARF in the absence of hypertension and edema, and with normal complement levels (218). In one series of 13 kidney biopsies of ATIN in children, 10 were attributed to systemic infections, of which 7 were considered to be streptococcal in origin (45).

Drugs

Drugs have emerged as the most common cause of ATIN, with most cases attributed to antimicrobials (219,220). First described in conjunction with the sulfonamides used in the 1940s (185,186), the lesion was next reported to occur during penicillin therapy in the 1950s (10) and was ultimately best characterized in patients treated with methicillin in the 1960s (100,109,223). Since then, the number of antimicrobials, as well as other drugs, implicated as a cause of ATIN continues to increase. Although the implicated mechanisms and general morphologic feature on kidney biopsy are the same as those described with methicillin, their clinical presentations differ with other drugs. Essentially, nonoliguric ARF is more common, while those of fever, eosinophilia and skin rash are less common. Other subtler differences are the less frequent occurrence of gross hematuria clinically, and of tubulitis on kidney biopsy (11,12,206).

The association of ATIN with most of the incriminated drugs is quite rare, often based on individual case reports, and the evidence for a causative role of the drug merely circumstantial, particularly in the absence of a kidney biopsy. Even in cases where a kidney biopsy is available, the possibility of ATIN due to the underlying infection or of ATN due to the hemodynamic instability of infected patients could make interpretation of the biopsy difficult and the attribution of ATIN to the implicated drug suspect, especially in instances where only a single case is reported in the literature. In cases where kidney biopsy is not available for documentation of interstitial lesions, the acute deterioration of kidney function and abnormal urinary sediment, even in the presence of the eosinophiluria used to implicate ATIN, may be due to any of the other possible causes, including preexisting kidney disease, ATN, postinfectious glomerulonephritis, or a direct nephrotoxic effect of the implicated agent or one of the coadministered drugs. The latter possibility is particularly confounding because any one of the multiple agents used in the treatment of most patients can be responsible for ATIN, even when least suspected (78,115). By contrast, the possibility that ATIN may be missed clinically because acute deteriorations of kidney function, particularly when only modest, are attributed to other possibilities and their diagnosis not pursued by kidney biopsy may occasionally prove detrimental to patient care, but it certainly limits any estimation of the true prevalence of drug-induced ATIN and its incidence in cases of clinical ARF (115).

Drug-induced ATIN is due to a hypersensitivity reaction, as evidenced by several facts: It occurs in only a small number of people exposed to the drugs; it is not dose related; it often is associated with other systemic manifestations of hypersensitivity such as fever, skin rash, eosinophilia, and arthralgia; the reaction recurs on reexposure to the same drug or one of its congeners; circulating antibodies to some of the incriminated drugs have been demonstrated in some instances; and laboratory evidence for a hypersensitivity reaction has been documented in some cases. In addition, the structural features of individual drugs (propionic acid derivatives) or those common to some groups of drugs (β-lactams) do seem to predispose to the development of ATIN. The most common causes of drug-induced ATIN are antibiotics and NSAIDs. The lesion is more commonly encountered with methicillin than penicillin (224) and with fenoprofen than other NSAIDs, including others that are propionic acid derivatives (225).

Antibiotics

Of the several antibiotics that have been incriminated as a cause of ATIN, most share the β-lactam structural ring—penicillin and its derivatives and the cephalosporins.

Methicillin

Methicillin is the agent with the highest incidence of drug-induced ATIN and the one in which the clinical features of this side effect of antibiotics are best characterized (11,12,226). The mean period of drug administration before the renal lesions occur is approximately 15 days, with a reported range of 10 to 45 days (227). The incidence of ATIN has been estimated to be approximately 2% of those exposed to the drug and increases to 15% in those who are exposed to it for over 2 weeks (53,224,228–230). In those who experience a reaction, subsequent exposure to methicillin results in recurrence after a much shorter period of exposure and at lower doses of the drug (229–233). With the reduced clinical use of methicillin, there has been a reduction in the number of cases encountered clinically and reported in the literature (28,98,233).

Systemic manifestations are a dominant feature of methicillin-induced ATIN. Characteristically, drug-induced fever appears after the initial fever caused by the infection has subsided. The recurrent episode of fever usually is accompanied by skin rash, eosinophilia, and arthralgias. The skin rash is fleeting and consists of erythematous, often pruritic, maculopapular lesions that are present in 30% to 50% of cases. Eosinophilia is common (80%) but transient, and, unless noted and specifically sought, goes undetected (11,94–97). Arthralgias are nonspecific and less common (10% to 20%) than the fever, skin rash, and eosinophilia. Eosinophiluria appears to be more common and more evident than in other forms of drug-induced ATIN (11,12,94).

As a rule, patients are polyuric as kidney function begins to deteriorate, and the ARF, when first detected, is nonoliguric in two-thirds of patients (95–97,101,234). Independent of the severity of the ARF, the outcome is favorable after withdrawal of methicillin in 90% of cases (95–97,227). The initial improvement, which is rapid over the first few weeks of discontinuing methicillin, is followed by a slower return of kidney function to normal in most (>2/3), but only to near normal in a some 20% of cases (12,26,235). The worst prognosis is in those with granulomatous lesions. Instances of persistent kidney failure are rare (<10%), and are more likely in those whose kidney biopsy reveals diffuse infiltrates, interstitial fibrosis, granulomatous reaction, and tubular injury (234,236,237). Recovery is faster and more likely in those whose dominant kidney lesions consist of interstitial edema rather than cellular infiltrates, and when the cellular infiltrates are focal rather than diffuse (26).

A metabolic derivative of methicillin, dimethoxyphenyl-penicilloyl, has been implicated as the inciting antigen on the basis of its demonstration by immunofluorescence techniques along the TBM (65,66) and the detection of circulating antibodies to dimethoxyphenylpenicilloyl in cases of ATIN (109).

However, neither of these findings appears to be specific to the incidence of ATIN because both have been shown to be present in methicillin-treated cases with no evidence of acute kidney injury (67,238).

Rifampin

Since the introduction of rifampin (rifampicin) as an antituberculous agent in 1976, over 100 cases of ARF have been ascribed to it in the literature. As a rule, ARF has occurred during intermittent administration of the drug (once or twice weekly), usually appearing several months after institution of therapy (239–242). A more abrupt onset occurs with rifampin readministration after a hiatus in its previous daily, uneventful use (243). ARF during continuous daily rifampin therapy also has been noted (18). However, most cases reported have occurred during intermittent therapy, and the number of cases noted has decreased since intermittent use of the drug has been abandoned (234,244).

Circulating antibodies to rifampin have been detected in most, but not all, affected patients, as well as in the serum of those without any adverse reaction to the drug (245–248). The suggestion has been made that the kidney lesions develop as a response to a critical level of antigen–antibody complexes that accumulate during intermittent rifampin therapy (245, 246,249). However, immunofluorescence staining of kidney biopsy specimens for deposits of antibodies to rifampin has been negative in most cases (18,239,243–246), although it has been positive in an occasional case (243–250). A role for cell-mediated immune injury appears more likely based on *in vitro* studies of lymphocyte activation on exposure to rifampin (234,251).

Accompanying and preceding symptoms of patients in whom renal involvement develops include fever, chills, nausea, vomiting, diarrhea, dizziness, lumbar or abdominal pain, and myalgias, which occasionally are accompanied by abnormalities of liver function, hemolysis, and thrombocytopenia (18,239–244). The symptoms are dramatic in their sudden appearance and severity in those patients exposed to the drug for a second time and sometimes are associated with hypotension and hemodynamic compromise. As a result, the initial reports of ARF attributed to rifampin were ascribed to ischemic tubular injury. A direct nephrotoxic effect that is slower in onset has been reported with rifampin. Kidney biopsy in such cases reveals marked proximal tubular injury but very little interstitial infiltration (249). Actually, the majority of lesions of rifampin-induced ARF are those of ATIN and consist of interstitial edema and focal infiltration with mononuclear cells and occasionally eosinophils, with focal segments of tubular epithelial cell injury and necrosis (18). In some cases, the necrotic tubular lesions may be severe and extensive (240–243,252). Whether this reflects the severity of ATIN or is due to ischemic injury secondary to vasomotor phenomena is difficult to establish. Certainly, the accompanying systemic manifestations—eosinophilia, recurrence on challenge, the reported humoral studies, as well as the morphologic features seen on kidney biopsy—are strongly supportive of ATIN due to an allergic hypersensitivity reaction to the drug. While ATIN is the most common lesion of rifampin-induced ARF, glomerular lesions have been reported also (242). As a drug that induces cytochrome P-450, the consequent reduced levels of tacrolimus and cyclosporine can result in ARF due to acute rejection in kidney transplant recipients (241,242)

The severity of ARF due to ATIN is variable. Dialysis may be required in some patients in whom prolonged oliguria develops (253). The course of renal failure usually is favorable, with return of kidney function to normal in most cases after withdrawal of rifampin, although residual impairment of renal function may occur in some (239,256,257). The role of steroids in accelerating recovery from rifampin-induced ATIN is undetermined. The lesion has occurred in a patient who was receiving steroids for other reasons (18).

Penicillin and Congeners

Acute tubulointerstitial nephritis clinically and pathologically undifferentiable from that described with methicillin also occurs with penicillin and its congeners, but is much less common than with methicillin. The dose of penicillin used has been fairly large, 12 to 60 million U/day, although ATIN has been reported at lower doses (16,109,113,146,234) and even after a single dose (258).

Other penicillin derivatives that have been associated with the lesions of ATIN are, in descending order of frequency, ampicillin (16,26,95,259–262), oxacillin (263), carbenicillin (264,265), nafcillin (102), and oxacillin and amoxicillin (102,234,237,265–268). The systemic manifestations of a hypersensitivity reaction in these cases have been less common than in ATIN due to methicillin and penicillin.

Cephalosporins

Acute tubulointerstitial nephritis also has been noted with the cephalosporins. It is more common with cephalothin (231,234,269–272), followed in descending order of frequency by cephalexin (95,273), cephradine (274), cefoxitin (275), cefazolin (276), cefaclor (102), cefotaxime (28,277), and cefotetan (278), cefoperazone (279), cephaloridine, cefamandole, and cephapirin (11).

Other Antibiotics

The incidence of ATIN with other antibiotics is much less than that encountered with methicillin, penicillin congeners, and rifampin, except for ciprofloxacin, with which an increasing number of cases continue to be reported (117,234,280–283). Isolated instances of ATIN have been reported with minocycline (284), doxycycline (26), gentamicin (26,230,285), polymyxin (286), vancomycin (287,288), lincomycin (287), mezlocillin (289), chloramphenicol (26), erythromycin (290–293), flurithromycin (294), netilmicin (291), norfloxacin (295,296), tetracycline (297), ethambutol (298), telithromycin (299), and levofloxacin (300).

Sulfonamides

The introduction of sulfonamides in the 1930s heralded a new and welcome era in the specific treatment of infectious diseases. Despite their utility and general safety, severe adverse reactions were quite common with these agents and often necessitated cessation of their use (301,302). The introduction of antibiotics during the following decade led to a consistent decline in the use of sulfonamides until the introduction of trimethoprim–sulfamethoxazole (TMP/SMX) (170), when a resurgence of adverse reactions attributed to sulfonamides was observed, necessitating modification of the warnings in the labeling of TMP/SMX (303). The advent of AIDS with the associated prophylactic use of TMP/SMX (170), as well as its use in transplant recipients (304), has led to the increased incidence of these side effects.

The renal effects observed with the initially available, less soluble sulfonamides (sulfathiazole, sulfapyridine, sulfadiazine) were due to the precipitation of sulfa crystals in the renal tubules, with consequent hematuria, obstructive uropathy, and kidney failure. The renal lesions consisted of focal tubular necrosis, sometimes with sulfa crystals noted in the lumen, and with peritubular interstitial infiltration and edema in the affected segments (305,306). The introduction of more soluble

sulfonamides (sulfisoxazole, sulfamethoxazole, sulfamerazine, sulfasalazine) made this complication much less common, but by no means eliminated it (301,305–309). An idiosyncratic hypersensitivity-type reaction as a cause of the acute renal injury, which was recognized from the outset, now is the principal cause of the renal adverse effects of sulfonamides (301,305–310). The symptoms develop at a mean of 14 days after initiating therapy. Fever followed by skin rashes of varying severity usually precede the onset of ARF. Eosinophilia has been noted as an accompanying finding in most cases. Unlike antibiotic-induced ATIN, there is evidence of multiple organ involvement (heart, liver, lungs) in patients who have sulfonamide-induced ATIN (301,310,311). The renal lesions noted in kidney biopsy specimens consist of interstitial edema and focal areas of mononuclear cell infiltration that are most pronounced around the segments of tubular injury and necrosis (306,310). The kidney failure is reversible after withdrawal of the drug and institution of steroid therapy (306), although residual fibrosis and tubular atrophy with persistent impairment of renal function may occur (310).

The predisposition of patients to idiosyncratic reactions has been attributed to individual differences in the metabolism of sulfonamides. Those who have idiosyncratic reactions are slow acetylators of sulfonamide, which leads to the accumulation of drug metabolites that can covalently bind to cell macromolecules and cause cell injury, or elicit a secondary immunologic phenomenon (311,312).

Acute renal failure due to a hypersensitivity reaction also occurs with TMP/SMX (26,232,234,313–317). The increase in serum creatinine that occurs with this agent does not necessarily indicate renal injury because trimethoprim interferes with the tubular secretion of creatinine, with a consequent increase in the serum creatinine level, without necessarily affecting true glomerular filtration rate (318). The clinical and morphologic features of ATIN induced by TMP/SMX are identical to those induced by other sulfonamides and are due to the sulfamethoxazole content. Multinucleated giant cells and granulomatous reactions, reflecting the severity of the reaction, have been described and are associated with only partial recovery of kidney function after withdrawal of the drug, despite steroid therapy (234).

Most of the reported cases of TMP/SMX-induced ATIN have been in patients with reduced kidney function, or transplant recipients (313,315,316). It has been suggested that the propensity of patients with reduced kidney function to ATIN may be due to the accumulation of a toxic metabolite, which predisposes them to the adverse effects of the drug (313,316), much like that noted in the genetically predisposed slow acetylators (311). Crystalluria occurs with the use of high doses of TMP/SMX. In patients with severe renal insufficiency, this could cause further deterioration of kidney function without necessarily eliciting an allergic reaction (319), as has been documented experimentally (320,321).

Nonsteroidal Antiinflammatory Drugs

The NSAIDs provide a relatively effective approach to the treatment of musculoskeletal pain and inflammation, which are among the most common complaints of an aging population. As a result, NSAIDs have become the most widely prescribed category of drugs. The impact of recent reports of increased relative risk for cardiac death associated with NSAID use remains to be determined, but is bound to have a significant dampening effect on their widespread level of utilization heretofore (322).

The most serious untoward effects of their use have been noted in the gastrointestinal tract and the kidney (323,324). The renal effects include reduction in GFR and renal blood flow, acute and chronic renal injury, and abnormalities of sodium and potassium homeostasis (323–326). By far the most common of these side effects is the hemodynamically mediated, reversible ARF related to the prostaglandin-inhibitory action of these agents, which occurs principally in patients with congestive heart failure, cirrhosis of the liver, nephrotic syndrome, septicemia, and volume depletion from any cause (326–328). Less common has been the development of another form of ARF due to tubulointerstitial nephritis, which, unlike other drug-induced ATINs, is frequently associated with massive proteinuria (215,326,329–331). A necrotizing vasculitis also has been reported in a few cases in association with fenoprofen, indomethacin, and diclofenac (331–335).

The duration of exposure to NSAIDs before the onset of ATIN is variable, ranging from 2 weeks to 18 months; as a rule, ATIN develops after prolonged exposure (mean, 5.4 months) to the incriminated agent (225,234,331). The propionic acid derivatives fenoprofen, ibuprofen, and naproxen account for approximately three-fourths of the cases reported (225, 331–336). Fenoprofen alone has been incriminated for over one-half of the reported cases. The lesions have been noted after the self-administration of over-the-counter ibuprofen (337,338) and of mefenamate in drug mixtures (339), and to recur after exposure to different NSAIDs of the same group (330,334) or on reexposure to the same agent (225). Other NSAIDs that have been incriminated include, in decreasing order of frequency, tolmetin (340–342), zomepirac (343–346), indomethacin (225,347,348), diclofenac (349–351), and diflunisal (3352,353). Isolated cases have been reported with the use of phenylbutazone (354,355), mefenamate (356), phenazone (357), sulindac (358), noramidopyrine (234), and piroxicam (259,260). Contrary to initial expectations they also occur with the selective cyclooxygenase-2–inhibitory agents such as celecoxib (361–363), rofecoxib (364,365) and nimesulide (366,367).

The proteinuria and clinical manifestations of the nephrotic syndrome usually are of insidious onset and precede the onset of kidney failure. Nephrotic syndrome, without renal insufficiency, may be the only manifestation in approximately 10% of cases. On the other hand, kidney failure without nephrotic syndrome occurs in approximately 15% of cases (11,12,83,225,331). The variation in clinical presentation has been attributed to the severity of the allergic hypersensitivity reaction, with a more rapid course presenting with reduced kidney function and nephrotic syndrome in hyperreactors (332). β_2-Microglobulinuria is a common and prominent feature. Flank pain has been a notable complaint in several cases. The clinical features of hypersensitivity reaction (fever, rash, eosinophilia) occur in only 20% of cases, compared with an incidence of over 85% in patients with methicillin-induced ATIN. The serum complement and IgE levels usually are normal, and anti-TBM antibodies are absent. Most of the patients reported have been older than 60 years of age, which is more a reflection of the greater use of NSAIDs in this age group than of age as a predisposing factor (333). The urine sediment reveals microscopic hematuria and pyuria and only rarely eosinophiluria (83). In the diagnosis of proteinuria due to NSAIDs, it should be kept in mind that tolmetin can produce pseudoproteinuria. This is due to the effect of its dicarboxylic metabolite on the detection of proteinuria by the acid precipitation (sulfosalicylic acid and trichloroacetic acid) methods. In such cases, no proteinuria is detected with dye-impregnated reagent strips, electrophoresis, or nephelometry (368,369).

Histologic examination of the kidney reveals diffuse edema, focal areas of interstitial infiltrates consisting predominantly of lymphocytes, and vacuolar degeneration of the tubules (Fig. 48-3). In some cases, the proportion of infiltrating B lymphocytes and CD8+ cells has been more than that noted in other forms of ATIN. Eosinophils have been observed in one-third of the cases reported and may constitute up to 20% of the infiltrating cells, even when eosinophiluria is absent. The glomeruli are minimally altered, if at all, except for the effacement of the epithelial foot processes consistent with minimal-change disease in nephrotic cases. Mesangial electron-dense deposits have been noted in rare instances in association with modest membranous and subendothelial deposits (370,371). Membranous glomerulonephritis, reversible after drug withdrawal, has been reported with sulindac and other NSAIDs (332,372). Immunofluorescent microscopy is negative, although a slight, nonspecific focal immunofluorescence of the glomeruli and TBM occasionally has been noted (334). Granulomatous reactions occur in severe cases (373).

The kidney failure, although insidious in onset, can be severe enough on clinical presentation to require supportive dialytic therapy in approximately a third of the patients. The severity of the kidney failure may stem from the additive effects of ATIN, reduced renal blood flow due to inhibition of prostaglandin, altered glomerular permeability, and absence of systemic effects, the latter of which leads to delayed diagnosis early in the course of the disease process until patients finally present with nephrotic syndrome and kidney failure. The response to discontinuation of the offending NSAIDs has been favorable in most cases, with improvement of kidney failure occurring within a few days, but with a slower subsidence of proteinuria over weeks or months. Cases of persistent kidney failure have been reported (225,374). Progression of the kidney lesion to focal glomerular sclerosis has been noted on repeat kidney biopsy in some patients (332,375,376). Steroids have been used in the treatment of severe cases. The response to steroid therapy, if any, appears to be slow, and the value of corticosteroids in this entity is questionable (83,377).

The pathogenesis of NSAID-associated ATIN remains undetermined. The rarity of the lesion despite the widespread use of these agents (estimated at 1 in 5,300 patient-years of treatment with fenoprofen) supports an idiosyncratic reaction (329). The clinical features of a hypersensitivity reaction, although present in only one-fifth of the cases, support an allergenic reaction. Their absence from most cases has been construed as an argument against a hypersensitivity reaction, but may actually reflect an amelioration of the hypersensitivity symptoms because of the antipyretic and antiphlogistic actions of NSAIDs. The presence of a diffuse interstitial eosinophilic infiltrate, in the absence of peripheral eosinophilia and eosinophiluria, also is compatible with the antiinflammatory effect of the NSAIDs. Evidence for a humoral antibody reaction is lacking. There is a slight preponderance of cytotoxic/suppressor (CD8+) T cells in the infiltrates, especially early in the course of the disease, which has been advanced as an argument for cell-mediated immunity (55,83,378,379). Potentially, the metabolism of these agents could yield metabolites that are injurious to the tubules and podocytes. Moreover, cyclo-oxygenase blockade can affect the arachidonic acid lipo-oxygenase pathways leading to the formation of proinflammatory and vasoactive compounds (313a). Whether the prostaglandin-inhibitory effect of these agents plays a role in the unique proteinuric features of this form of ATIN has not been ascertained but certainly is an attractive conceptual possibility that cannot be neglected (225,380).

Phenindione

An increasing number of severe sensitivity reactions were noted with the anticoagulant phenindione after its introduction in 1947. The more common reactions were skin rash, fever, diarrhea, blood dyscrasias, stomatitis, and hepatitis, in descending order of frequency. The reactions appeared after 3 to 5 weeks of therapy and continued to progress even after discontinuation of the drug, proving fatal in one-half of the cases. ARF due to ATIN, which was granulomatous in some cases, also was reported in approximately 30 cases, usually coincident with the development of jaundice and hepatotoxicity (381–388). ATIN was accompanied by the classic triad of skin rash, fever, and eosinophilia, usually with a prolonged period of oliguria and death in one-third of the cases reported (16,385), chronic kidney disease in some (358), and massive proteinuria in others (387).

Because of the high incidence (10%) of these adverse side effects and their severity, this agent was prescribed much less over the years, leading to the cessation of its manufacture in 1983 for economic reasons. It is, however, still available in some countries, or as an investigational drug in the United States. Phenindione is an indanedione derivative and since then other analogs (fluindione, anisoindione, diphenadione) have been introduced but ATIN has not been reported with any of them.

A metabolic product of phenindione that is excreted by the kidneys imparts a red-orange color to the urine. This is of no clinical importance except in the differential diagnosis of hematuria. Acidification of the urine eliminates the color and differentiates it from the true hematuria that develops in ATIN (389).

Allopurinol

Severe hypersensitivity reactions to allopurinol have been reported since its introduction in 1963 (337). They have the features of a diffuse vasculitis involving multiple organs (338). The symptoms appear approximately 4 weeks after initiation of therapy and consist of fever, rather severe generalized skin rashes that may be desquamative, eosinophilia, hepatic failure, and prolonged oliguric kidney failure (390–394).

The structural changes in the kidney are characteristic of ATIN, including those of a granulomatous reaction in severe cases (395). Although the renal lesions have been reported in patients with normal kidney function, most cases have occurred either in patients with preexisting kidney disease and reduced kidney function, or in those receiving other drugs that might themselves cause ATIN. The decreased excretion of a toxic metabolite of the drug, possibly oxypurinol, has been implicated as the inciting agent in those with reduced kidney function. A predisposing role of thiazides, furosemide, and ampicillin has been implicated in those who have experienced a reaction while receiving other drugs (390,396).

The finding of circulating anti-TBM antibodies, together with granular deposits of C3 along the TBM of a single case, has been advanced as evidence for the role of an immune-mediated mechanism (393). However, the absence of linear deposits of anti-TBM antibody in the kidney biopsy specimen and the fact that the patient had IgA nephropathy as the underlying primary kidney disease make the interpretation of the results from this individual case impossible, unless these findings are substantiated in other cases.

Proton Pump Inhibitors

Cases of classic ATIN have been reported with the antiulcer agent cimetidine (397–404). The renal lesions are patchy, with focal areas of tubule cell injury and interstitial inflammatory infiltrates consisting of lymphocytes and a few eosinophils.

In one carefully studied case, IgE-producing plasma cells were identified as part of the infiltrating cells, most of which were identified as being cytotoxic/suppressor T lymphocytes, and activated T cells were demonstrated in the circulation, strongly implicating a cell-mediated immune reaction as the pathogenetic mechanism of cimetidine-induced ATIN (81).

In addition to its inhibitory action on gastric acid secretion, there is evidence that cimetidine might have a role as an immunomodulator (81). It is possible that this action plays a role in cimetidine-induced ATIN; it seems unlikely, however, given that there are only a few case reports of ATIN related to this widely prescribed agent, now available over the counter. Hence, the more likely possibility is that the kidney injury is idiosyncratic. In addition, the clinical and morphologic features of the ATIN are characteristic of a hypersensitivity reaction: eosinophilia, eosinophiluria, fever, and IgE-containing plasma cells in the infiltrate, with recurrence of the symptoms on rechallenge (397–404). The lesions of ATIN have been reported also in association with other proton pump inhibitors such as ranitidine (98,405–407), lansoprazole (408), omeprazole (290,409–411), and pantoprazole (412,413).

Phenytoin

One of the adverse side effects associated with the anticonvulsant phenytoin, formerly known as diphenylhydantoin, is a delayed hypersensitivity reaction characterized by a systemic reaction and ARF. The systemic manifestations include fever, hepatitis, myositis, lymphadenopathy, skin rashes that may be exfoliative, eosinophilia, and anemia (69,70,414–416). The kidney injury is due to ATIN characterized by edema and focal inflammatory infiltrates consisting of mononuclear cells and occasional eosinophils. Nephrotic syndrome has been observed in some patients (69). The lesions are reversible on withdrawal of the drug, but steroid treatment has been successfully used in most reported cases (69,414–417).

In two cases, circulating antibodies to human TBM were detected and linear deposits of anti-TBM antibodies demonstrated along the renal TBM (69,70). In one case, deposits of phenytoin were demonstrated along the TBM, leading to the suggestions that the initial alteration of the host TBM is due to phenytoin deposition with secondary immune reaction directed at the phenytoin–TBM complex or to the phenytoin-altered TBM (69). Passive transfer of the anti-TBM from one patient failed to produce the disease in experimental animals (70), with increased DNA incorporation, on exposure to phenytoin could be induced only in the lymphocytes from patients demonstrating the hypersensitivity reaction (65,414).

Diuretics

Acute renal failure often is associated with the use of diuretics. The renal insufficiency that results usually is prerenal in origin and a result of the systemic and renal compensatory mechanisms mediated by extracellular fluid volume depletion induced by the diuretics (418). Less commonly, deterioration of kidney function is the result of other mechanisms, including direct renal toxicity, such as with mercurial diuretics (418,419); obstruction, such as with triamterene nephrolithiasis (420); necrotizing vasculitis, such as with thiazides (421); and occasionally ATIN that has been noted to occur with furosemide, thiazides, triamterene, chlorthalidone, ethacrynic acid, tienilic acid, and indapamide (422–428). Most of the reported cases have been associated with the use of thiazides and furosemide, both of which are structurally related to sulfonamides, another group of drugs associated with ATIN. A potentiating role of triamterene used in conjunction with thiazides or furosemide has been suggested (423).

Several of the patients with diuretic-induced ATIN had preexisting kidney disease (26,422), although the lesions also are noted in patients with normal kidney function (368,371). The deterioration of kidney function usually is insidious in onset but may be rapid and lead to oliguric ARF. Systemic symptoms of drug-related hypersensitivity reaction (fever, skin rash, and eosinophilia) were present in almost all the patients reported. The kidney biopsy findings were those of classic ATIN, including an eosinophilic infiltrate in one-half of the reported cases and a granulomatous reaction in an occasional case (422–430). Immunofluorescent studies have been negative. Abatement of symptoms and return of kidney function to baseline have occurred in all patients reported after removal of the incriminated diuretic and the administration of steroids to some patients.

Given the frequency with which diuretics are prescribed, the fact that less than 20 cases of ATIN have been reported with their use reflects the relative rarity of diuretic-induced ATIN.

Other Drugs

The list of other drugs associated with ATIN continues to expand. Most of these have been isolated, single case reports of patients who often were using more than one drug.

By far the most common among these to be associated with ATIN are glafenin (431,432) and its derivatives, antrafenin (433,434) and floctafenin (434). Although direct drug toxicity, with lesions of ATN, has been incriminated as the cause of ARF in some of these patients (434,435), clinical and laboratory evidence of an immunologically mediated hypersensitivity reaction causing ATIN has been sufficiently well documented to justify incriminating these agents as a cause of ATIN.

Other drugs that have been implicated are sulfinpyrazone (95,436,437), aminopyrine (11), azathioprine (438,439), quinine (440), clofibrate (441), propylthiouracil (442), carbamazepine (443,444), amidopyrine (445), amphetamine (446), phenobarbital (114,447), p-aminosalicylic acid (448), captopril (449–451), diltiazem (452), methyldopa (453), acyclovir (454,455), interferon (456), indinavir (457), griseofulvin (458), ifosfamide (459), intravenous immunoglobulin (446), phentermine and phendimetrazine (461), foscarnet (462), interleukin (463), and even aspirin (464,465).

SYSTEMIC DISEASES

Although most cases of ATIN are due to a hypersensitivity reaction to drugs or infections, whether renal or extrarenal, an acute deterioration of kidney function with the structural changes of ATIN also occurs in a variety of systemic diseases. In these, the renal involvement is due either to the metabolic disturbances associated with the underlying disease, the immunologic basis of the primary disease process, or the infiltrative nature of the disease (Table 48-3).

Metabolic Disorders

The metabolic disorders in which ATIN develops are those due to abnormalities in the metabolism of urate, oxalate, calcium, potassium, and heavy metals (466,467).

Uric Acid

The kidney, as the major organ responsible for uric acid excretion, becomes the principal target organ affected by disorders of urate metabolism. Renal involvement results from the precipitation of uric acid in the renal parenchyma and the urine outflow tract. Depending on the load of uric acid presented to the kidney and the duration of exposure, the parenchymal lesions that develop are those of either an acute or a chronic urate nephropathy. In the acute form of urate nephropathy, the renal changes are those of an ATIN (466–468). The most common condition in which this is encountered is in ARF associated

with the tumor lysis syndrome (469,470) and occasionally in massive tissue destruction such as rhabdomyolysis (471).

Oxalate

The increased metabolic production or intestinal absorption of oxalate and its consequent excretion by the kidney almost invariably results in the precipitation of calcium oxalate in the urine outflow tract (466). Microcrystallization first occurs in the proximal tubule, where oxalate is secreted. However, the lesions that develop are more prominent in the medulla, where the increased concentration of oxalate in the tubular fluid, as water is reabsorbed, and the acidification of the fluid, as hydrogen is secreted, favor the precipitation of calcium oxalate. This results in injury and atrophy of the affected tubules, with interstitial edema and inflammatory cell infiltration around the injured tubular segments (466,467,472,473). When the hyperoxaluria is sudden and massive, such as after ethylene glycol ingestion (474,475), methoxyflurane anesthesia (476) or the ingestion of star fruit (477), acute deterioration of kidney function occurs, the morphologic features of which are those of ATIN. Otherwise, when the hyperoxaluria is modest and chronic, such as in inflammatory bowel disease, the onset of kidney failure is insidious and the lesions are those of chronic tubulointerstitial nephritis (466,478), although ARF associated with enteric hyperoxaluria can occur (479,480).

The treatment of acute oxalate nephropathy consists of maintaining a high urine flow rate, hemodialysis, and supportive measures directed at elimination of the oxalate precursors.

Immune Diseases

Diseases due to an immune mechanism affect primarily the glomeruli, with secondary involvement of the tubules and interstitium. Primary tubulointerstitial nephritis mediated by an underlying altered immune mechanism is extremely rare in humans. The two conditions in which an immune mechanism may result in ARF primarily due to tubulointerstitial lesions, with only limited glomerular involvement, are the transplanted kidney (481,482) and systemic lupus erythematosus (73).

The diagnosis of ATIN in kidney transplant recipients can be challenging (483–490). Despite the numerous medications these patients receive, drug-induced ATIN is an uncommon cause of ARF in them. Drug-induced ATIN lesions can resemble acute cellular rejection morphologically, and both entities can show improvement after steroid therapy. While infiltrating eosinophils can be seen in acute cellular rejection, their presence and localization at the cortico-medullary junction and the presence of granulomatous lesions are suggestive of drug-induced ATIN (486–488), while that of tubulitis is a defining feature of allograft rejection (489). Clinically, the diagnosis is compounded by the fact that allograft recipients are prone to infection-induced ATIN, such as cytomegalic virus (483), adenovirus (484), and polyoma virus (485).

ARF with prominent tubulointerstitial lesions may occur in other diseases due to altered immune mechanisms, but very rarely in the absence of glomerular lesions. These diseases are Sjögren's syndrome (71), mixed cryoglobulinemia (71), Wegener's granulomatosis (491,492), crescentic glomerulonephritis (65), sarcoidosis (493), IgA nephropathy (494,495), and autoimmune pancreatitis (496).

Neoplastic Diseases

An acute deterioration of kidney function may occur in any neoplastic disease, either because of direct invasion of the kidney or the urinary tract by malignant cells or because of the metabolic disorders (hypercalcemia, hyperuricemia) that may be caused by the malignancy. The institution of antineoplastic therapy, which may itself be nephrotoxic or can magnify the existing tumor-related metabolic disorder (hyperuricemia), is another mechanism of the acute renal injury experienced by these patients (497). Lymphoproliferative disorders and plasma cell dyscrasias are the two neoplastic diseases in which ATIN due to neoplastic cellular infiltrates is a principal cause of the ARF (498–500).

Lymphoproliferative Disorders

The kidney is one of the most common extranodal sites of metastatic lymphomas (501–504), although primary lymphoma in the kidneys without evidence of extrarenal lesions also can occur (505–507). Infiltration of the kidney is more common in non-Hodgkin's lymphomas and acute lymphoblastic leukemia than in Hodgkin's disease (498,499). Leukemic infiltration of the kidney has been noted in two-thirds of patients with leukemia, usually in those with the acute form of the disease (495,508,509). Renal infiltrates usually are bilateral and symmetrical and may go undetected unless extensive parenchymal infiltration occurs, in which case flank pain, palpable, tender kidneys, gross hematuria, and ARF are the presenting findings (499,502–511). The infiltrates are localized to the interstitium, compressing the tubules but sparing the glomeruli, thereby mimicking the classic morphologic features of an ATIN. Irradiation of the kidneys or systemic chemotherapy can result in a dramatic reversal of the structural and functional abnormalities (504,512,513).

Plasma Cell Dyscrasias

The renal complications of plasma cell dyscrasias are a major cause of morbidity and mortality in patients with multiple myeloma (499,501,514). ARF occurs in approximately 10% of these patients, and chronic kidney disease is present in more than two-thirds of them (499,500,515–517).

The pathogenesis of ARF is multifactorial (517–523). The acute lesions directly related to multiple myeloma, the so-called myeloma cast nephropathy, are those that result from the excessive production of light chains and their precipitation as dimers in the distal tubules. As a result, varying degrees of injury, necrosis, and regeneration of the tubular epithelial cells occur, with interstitial edema and an inflammatory reaction, including polymorphonuclear, mononuclear, and multinucleate giant cells, around the affected tubules. Immunofluorescent study of the kidney tissue can provide the definitive diagnosis when fluorescence is positive for specific sera for either κ or λ light chains (499,518,519).

The propensity of light chains to lead to myeloma cast nephropathy depends on their concentration in the tubular fluid, the tubular fluid pH, and the intrinsic physiochemical properties of the light chains (521,522). These factors account for the fact that the patients who are dehydrated, those who are producing an acid urine, and those with λ light chains rather than κ chains are more prone to development of acute lesions of myeloma-induced kidney failure. They also provide a physiologic basis for treatment consisting of maintaining a high rate of urine flow and its alkalinization, which can prevent and reverse the lesions in their early stage of formation (514,522,523).

IDIOPATHIC ACUTE TUBULOINTERSTITIAL NEPHRITIS

Since the entity of idiopathic ATIN was first noted in the literature in 1972 (524), an increasing number of cases of ATIN in the absence of exposure to drugs, infections, or any of the other conditions usually associated with ATIN have been reported (26,36,101,234,524–530). In fact, in most reports of ATIN, where a series of cases from a single institution are presented, a varying number of cases included have been of unknown cause (26,45,101,528,529).

The only common feature of these cases has been the presence of reversible ARF and the finding of edema and a mononuclear inflammatory infiltration of the interstitium on kidney biopsy. Although certain of the laboratory features of a hypersensitivity reaction (elevated IgE levels, eosinophilic infiltrate, and eosinophiluria) are present in some of the cases (101,524,529), the systemic manifestations of a hypersensitivity reaction (fever, arthralgia, rash) have been characteristically absent. Linear deposits of IgG, C3, and anti-TBM antibodies have been detected on immunofluorescent study of the kidney biopsy in some cases (527,528), granular deposits of C3 and IgG were seen in others (524–526), but no deposits were present in the rest (36,524)

The clinical presentation of most has been nonspecific, except for the acute deterioration of kidney function. The renal failure has been severe enough in a third of the cases to necessitate supportive dialytic therapy. The outcome has been favorable in most cases, with recovery occurring spontaneously or after the institution of steroid therapy (45,122,525–532). There have been cases of irreversible kidney failure that have failed to respond to steroid therapy (525–527). Clinically, the nonspecific presentation of idiopathic ATIN coupled with its favorable prognosis and response to steroids, at least in some cases, mandates that its possibility be considered in the differential diagnosis of every patient with ARF in whom the cause of the kidney dysfunction is uncertain.

The number of cases reported is too low to formulate a common pattern for idiopathic ATIN. Idiopathic ATIN constitutes 15% to 25% of cases of ARF that are sampled for biopsy (132,133). Systemic diseases, such as chronic active hepatitis or ulcerative colitis, have been present in an occasional case (528). Uveitis, on the other hand, has been a feature of several patients with idiopathic ATIN. This group constitutes a variant that deserves separate consideration.

Idiopathic Acute Tubulointerstitial Nephritis with Uveitis

An acute eosinophilic interstitial nephritis that occurred in association with an anterior uveitis of unknown cause was first described in 1975 in two patients who also had bone marrow and lymph node granulomas (533). The syndrome of ATIN with uveitis has since been noted to occur rarely in other granulomatous conditions (534), and has been identified in patients with no bone marrow granulomas in most of the reported cases (535–545). Most of the patients have been adolescent girls of pubertal age, although the lesion occurs in adults (534,542,546). Familial occurrence and an association with certain HLA serotypes have been suggested (547,548), with a strong association with the HLA-DQ and HLA-DR alleles (549). Anorexia, asthenia, nocturnal fever, and weight loss may be present for several months before the onset of the ocular complaints. A moderate anemia is common and hyperglobulinemia usually is present (550,551). There also is evidence of tubular dysfunction, such as glucosuria, proteinuria, aminoaciduria, β_2-microglobulinuria, impaired urinary concentrating ability, and azotemia (530,546,548–551). Uveitis may occur as a manifestation of a variety of systemic diseases (552). It is unusual for any of these systemic disorders to be complicated by ATIN, and its occurrence with uveitis in those in whom ATIN develops has been termed *renal ocular syndrome* (535) or *tubulointerstitial nephritis and uveitis syndrome* (TINU syndrome) (536).

The cause of this syndrome complex remains undefined but has been presumed by some to be the result of an autoimmune process or reaction of an as yet undetermined viral infection. It has been described in individual cases of toxoplasmosis, giardiasis, chlamydiosis, and Epstein-Barr virus infection (553,554). No cause has been identified despite extensive investigation. The demonstration of circulating immune complexes in some cases has led to the suggestion of a role for an immune-mediated process (536). Mast cells may play a role in the development of interstitial injury in these cases (555). Both the ocular and renal changes respond to a brief course of steroid treatment (535,536) but can recur; spontaneous remission without steroid treatment also has been reported especially in children (536,551–556). The uveitis may be asymptomatic indicating the need for ophthalmologic examination in all cases of idiopathic ATIN (557). The uveitis can precede the onset of ATIN (558) or relapse without any renal manifestations, in which instances it responds to topical steroid treatment. In children and adolescents, the long-term prognosis is good, with recovery of kidney function and no documented visual loss. In adults, the prognosis is less favorable and kidney failure requiring dialysis may develop, particularly if steroid therapy is withheld (559,560).

References

1. Councilman WT. Acute interstitial nephritis. *J Exp Med* 1898;3:393.
2. Biermer A. Ein ungevohnlicher Fall von Scharlach. *Virchows Arch Pathol Anat* 1860;19:537.
3. Mallory GK, Keefer CS. Tissue reaction in fatal cases of *Streptococcus haemolyticus* infection. *Arch Pathol* 1941;32:334.
4. Kannerstein M. Histologic changes in the common acute infectious diseases. *Am J Med Sci* 1942;203:65.
5. Kimmelstiel P. Acute hematogenous interstitial nephritis. *Am J Pathol* 1938;14:737.
6. Mathews WR. Acute hematogenous interstitial nephritis. *South Med J* 1942;35:1055.
7. Olsen S. Renal histopathology in various forms of acute anuria in man. *Kidney Int* 1976;10:S2.
8. Churg J, et al. *Renal disease: classification and atlas of tubulointerstitial diseases.* New York: Igaku-Shoin, 1984:1.
9. Heptinstall RH. Interstitial nephritis: a brief review. *Am J Pathol* 1976;83:214.
10. Unger AM, Nemuth HI. Penicillinase treatment of acute renal insufficiency due to penicillin hypersensitivity. *JAMA* 1958;167:1237.
11. Rossert J. Drug-induced acute interstitial nephrits. *Kidney Int* 2001;60:804.
12. Baker RJ, Pusey CD. The changing profile of acute tubulointerstitial nephritis. *Nephrol Dial Transplant* 2004;19:8.
13. Zollinger HU. Interstitial nephritis. In: Mostofi FK, Smith DE, eds. *The kidney.* Baltimore: Williams & Wilkins, 1966:269.
14. Suki WN, Eknoyan G. Tubulo-interstitial disease. In: Brenner BM, Rector FC Jr, eds. *The kidney.* Philadelphia: Saunders, 1976:113.
15. Cogan MG. Tubulo-interstitial nephropathies: a pathophysiologic approach. *West J Med* 1980;132:134.
16. Appel GB, Kunis CL. Acute tubulointerstitial nephritis. *Contemp Issues Nephrol* 1983;10:151.
17. Cogan MG. Classification and patterns of renal dysfunction. *Contemp Issues Nephrol* 1983;10:35.
18. Quinibi WY, Godwin J, Eknoyan G. Toxic nephropathy during continuous rifampin therapy. *South Med J* 1980;73:791.
19. Neilson EG. Is immunologic tolerance self modulated through antigen presentation by parenchymal epithelium? *Kidney Int* 1993;44:927.
20. Wang S, Hirschberg R. Tubular epithelial cell activation and interstitial fibrosis: the role of glomerular ultrafiltration of growth factors in the nephrotic syndrome and diabetic nephropathy. *Nephrol Dial Transplant* 1999;14:2072.
21. Kuroiwa T, et al. Distinct T cell/renal tubular epithelial cell interactions define differential chemokine production: Implications for tubulointerstitial injury in chronic glomerulonephritides. *J Immunol* 2000;164:3323.
22. van Kooten C, Daha MR. Cytokine cross-talk between tubular epithelial cells and interstitial immunocompetent cell. *Curr Opin Nephrol Hypertens* 2001;10:55.
23. Toto RD. Acute tubulo-interstitial nephritis. *Am J Med Sci* 1990;299:392.
24. Tang WW, et al. Cytokine expression, upregulation of intracellular adhesion molecule-1, and leukocyte infiltration in experimental tubulointerstitial nephritis. *Lab Invest* 1994;70:631.
25. Muller GA, Markovic-Lipkowski J, Roderman HP. The progression of renal disease: on the pathogenesis of renal interstitial fibrosis. *Klin Wochenschr* 1991;69:576.
26. Laberke HG, Bohle A. Acute interstitial nephritis: correlation between clinical and morphological findings. *Clin Nephrol* 1980;14:263.
27. Colvin RB, Fang LS. Interstitial nephritis. In: Tisher CC, Brenner BM, eds. *Renal pathology with clinical and functional correlations,* vol. 1. Philadelphia: JB Lippincott, 1989:728.
28. Grünfeld JP, Kleinknecht D, Droz D. Acute interstitial nephritis. In: Schrier RW, Gottschalk CW, eds. *Diseases of the kidney,* 5th ed. vol. 2. Boston: Little, Brown, 1993.
29. Eddy AA, et al. A relationship between proteinuria and acute tubulointerstitial disease in rats with experimental nephrotic syndrome. *Am J Pathol* 1991;138:1111.
30. Garcia-Zepeda EA, et al. Human eotaxin is a specific chemoattractant for eosinophil cells and provides a new mechanism to explain tissue eosinophilia. *Nature Med.* 1997;2:449.
31. Lerch M, Pitcher WJ. The immunological and clinical spectrum of delayed drug–induced exanthems. *Curr Opin Allergy Immunol* 2004;4:411.
32. Lampiness M, et al. Cytokines-regulated accumulation of eosinophils in inflammatory disease. *Allergy* 2004;59:793.
33. Wada T, et al. Eotaxin contributes to renal interstitial eosinophilia. *Nephrol Dial Transplant* 1999;14:76.
34. Bender WL, et al. Interstitial nephritis, proteinuria and renal failure caused by nonsteroidal anti-inflammatory drugs: immunologic characterization of the inflammatory infiltrate. *Am J Med* 1984;76:1006.
35. Kobayashi Y, et al. Immunohistological study in sixteen children with acute tubulointerstitial nephritis. *Clin Nephrol* 1998;50:14.
36. Pamukcu R, et al. Idiopathic acute interstitial nephritis: characterization of the infiltrating cells in the renal interstitium as T helper lymphocytes. *Am J Kidney Dis* 1984;4:24.
37. Boucher A, et al. Characterization of mononuclear cell subsets in renal cellular interstitial infiltrates. *Kidney Int* 1986;29:1043.
38. Gimenez A, Mampaso F. Characterization of inflammatory cells in drug-induced tubulointerstitial nephritis. *Nephron* 1986;43:239.
39. Husby G, Tung KS, Williams RC. Characterization of renal tissue lymphocytes in patients with interstitial nephritis. *Am J Med* 1981;70:31.
40. D'Agati VD, et al. Interstitial nephritis related to nonsteroidal anti-inflammatory agents and beta-lactam antibiotics: a comparative study of the interstitial infiltrates using monoclonal antibodies. *Mod Pathol* 1989;2:390.
41. Faarup P, Christensin E. IgE-containing plasma cells in acute tubulointerstitial nephropathy. *Lancet* 1974;2:718.
42. Magil AB. Drug-induced acute interstitial nephritis with granulomas. *Hum Pathol* 1983;14:36.
43. Neilson EG, et al. Molecular characterization of a major nephritogenic domain in the autoantigen of anti-tubular basement membrane disease. *Proc Natl Acad Sci USA* 1991;88:2006.
44. Ivanyi B, et al. The distal nephron is preferentially infiltrated by inflammatory cells in acute interstitial nephritis. *Virchows Arch Pathol Anat Histopathol* 1992;420:37.
45. Ellis D, et al. Acute interstitial nephritis in children: a report of 13 cases and review of the literature. *Pediatrics* 1981;67:862.
46. Boucher A, et al. Characterization of mononuclear cell subsets in renal cellular interstitial infiltrates. *Kidney Int* 1986;29:1043.
47. Tokumoto M, et al. Acute interstitial nephritis with immune complex deposition and MHC class II antigen presentation along tubular basement membrane. *Nephrol Dial Transplant* 1999;14:2210.
48. Seron D, et al. Number of interstitial capillary cross sections assessed by monoclonal antibodies relation to interstitial damage. *Nephrol Dial Transplant* 1990;5:889.
49. Dvorak HF, et al. Morphology of delayed-type hypersensitivity reactions in man: quantitative description of the inflammatory response. *Lab Invest* 1974;31:111.
50. Neilson EG. Pathogenesis and therapy of interstitial nephritis. *Kidney Int* 1989;35:1257.
51. Kelly CJ. T cell regulation of autoimmune interstitial nephritis. *J Am Soc Nephrol* 1990;1:140.
52. Mene P. Molecular cell biology of renal diseases. *J Nephrol* 1999;12:140.
53. Appel GB, Kunis CL. Acute tubulo-interstitial nephritis. In: Cotran RS, Brenner BM, Stein JH, eds. *Tubulo-interstitial nephropathies.* New York: Churchill Livingstone, 1983:151.
54. Lang P, et al. Etude immunopathologique d'une nephropathie interstitielle aïgue induite par la clometacine. *Presse Med* 1986;15:915.
55. Cheng HF, et al. HLA-DR display by renal tubular epithelium and phenotype of infiltrate in interstitial nephritis. *Nephrol Dial Transplant* 1989;4:205.
56. Kuncio GS, Neilson EG, Haverty T. Mechanisms of tubulointerstitial fibrosis. *Kidney Int* 1991;19:550.
57. Shinozaki M, et al. IL-15, a survival factor for kidney epithelial cells, counteracts apoptosis and inflammation during nephritis. *J Clin Invest* 2002;109:951.
58. Michel DM, Kelly CJ. Acute interstitial nephritis. *J Am Soc Nephrol* 1998;9:506.

59. Palmer BF. The renal tubule in the progression of chronic renal failure. *J Invest Med* 1997;45:346.
60. Bruijn JA, et al. Matrix and adhesion molecules in kidney pathology: recent observations. *J Lab Clin Med* 1997;130:357.
61. Martin A, Escudero E, Mampaso F. Role of leucocyte adhesion molecules in amino nucleoside of puromycin (PAN)-associated interstitial nephritis. *Clin Exp Immunol* 1997;108:78.
62. Grandaliano G, et al. Monocyte chemotactic peptide-1 expression in acute and chronic human nephritides: a pathogenetic role in interstitial monocyte recruitment. *J Am Soc Nephrol* 1996;7:906.
63. Neilson EG. The nephritogenic T lymphocyte response in interstitial nephritis. *Semin Nephrol* 1993;13:496.
64. Zhou B, ey al. Identification of two alternatively spliced forms of human tubulointerstitial nephritis antigen (TIN-Ag). *J am Soc Nephrol* 2000;11:658.
65. Lehman DH, Wilson CB, Dixon FJ. Extraglomerular immunoglobulin deposits in human nephritis. *Am J Med* 1975;58:765.
66. Border WA, et al. Antitubular basement membrane antibodies in methicillin nephritis. *N Engl J Med* 1974;291:381.
67. Olsen S, Asklund M. Interstitial nephritis with acute renal failure following cardiac surgery and treatment with methicillin. *Acta Med Scand* 1976;199:305.
68. Rotellar C, et al. Role of antibodies directed against tubular basement membranes in human renal transplantation. *Am J Kidney Dis* 1986;7:157.
69. Hyman L, Ballow M, Kneiser MR. Diphenylhydantoin interstitial nephritis: roles of cellular and humoral immunologic injury. *J Pediatr* 1978;92:915.
70. Ooi BS, et al. Humoral mechanisms in drug-induced acute interstitial nephritis. *Clin Immunol Immunopathol* 1978;10:330.
71. Sawhney AS, et al. Sjögren's syndrome with immune complex tubulointerstitial renal disease. *Kidney Int* 1975;6:453.
72. Hu DC, Cathro HP, Okusa MD. Polymorphonuclear infiltration in acute interstitial nephritis of Sjögren syndrome. *Am J Med Sci* 2004;237:238.
73. Case records of the Massachusetts General Hospital. Case 2-1976. *N Engl J Med* 1976;294:100.
74. Kambham N, et al. Idiopathic hypocomplementemic interstitial nephritis with extensive tubulointerstitial deposits. *Am J Kidney Dis* 2001;37:388.
75. Wu CT, et al. Lupus vasculopathy combined with acute renal failure in lupus nephritis. *Pediatr Nephrol* 2003;18:1304.
76. Tolins JP, Hostetter MK, Hostetter TH. Hypokalemic nephropathy in the rat: role of ammonia in chronic tubular injury. *J Clin Invest* 79:1447, 1987.
77. Joh K, et al. Drug induced hypersensitivity nephritis lymphocyte stimulation testing and renal biopsy in 10 cases. *Am J Nephrol* 1990;10:222.
78. Shibasaki T, et al. Clinical characterization of drug induced allergic nephritis. *Am J Nephrol* 1991;11:174.
79. Stachura I, et al. Mononuclear cell subsets in human renal disease: enumeration in tissue sections with monoclonal antibodies. *Clin Immunol Immunopathol* 1984;30:362.
80. McCluskey RT, Bhan AK. Cell-mediated mechanisms in renal disease. *Kidney Int* 1982;21:S6.
81. Watson AJ, et al. Immunologic studies in cimetidine induced nephropathy and polymyositis. *N Engl J Med* 1983;308:142.
82. Fernandez-Llama P, et al. Decreased abundance of collecting duct aquaporins in post-ischemic renal failure in rats. *J Am Soc Nephrol* 1999;10:1658.
83. Porile JL, Bakris GL, Garella S. Acute interstitial nephritis with glomerulopathy due to nonsteroidal anti-inflammatory agents: a review of its clinical spectrum and effects of steroid therapy. *J Clin Pharmacol* 1990;30:468.
84. Mackensen S, et al. Influence of the renal cortical interstitium on the serum creatinine concentration and creatinine clearance of different chronic sclerosing interstitial nephritis. *Nephron* 1979;24:30.
85. Magil AB, Tyler M. Tubulo-interstitial disease in lupus nephritis: a morphometric study. *Histopathology* 1984;8:81.
86. Lemley KV, Kriz W. Anatomy of the renal interstitium. *Kidney Int* 1991;39:370.
87. Persson AE. Functional aspects of the renal interstitium. In: Maunsback AB, Olsen TS, Christensen AI, eds. *Functional ultrastructure of the kidney.* London: Academic Press, 1980:399.
88. Persson AE, Muller-Swur R, Selen G. Capillary oncotic pressure as a modifier for tubuloglomerular feedback. *Am J Physiol* 1979;236:F97.
89. Sahai T, et al. Extracellular fluid expansion and autoregulation in nephrotoxic nephritis in rats. *Kidney Int* 1984;25:619.
90. Blantz RC, Munger K. Role of nitric oxide in inflammatory conditions. *Nephron* 2002;90:373.
91. Gabbai FB, et al. Effect of acute iNOS inhibition on glomerular function in tubulointerstitial nephritis. *Kidney Int* 2002;61:851.
92. Meyers CM. New insights into the pathogenesis of interstitial nephritis. *Curr Opin Nephrol Hypertens* 1999;8:287.
93. Klahr S. New insights into the consequences and mechanisms of renal impairment in obstructive nephropathy. *Am J Kidney Dis* 1991;18:689.
94. Galpin JE, et al. Acute interstitial nephritis due to methicillin. *Am J Med* 1978;65:756.
95. Linton AL, et al. Acute interstitial nephritis due to drugs: review of the literature with a report of nine cases. *Ann Intern Med* 1980;93:735.
96. van Ypersele de Strihou C. Acute oliguric interstitial nephritis. *Kidney Int* 1979;16:751.
97. Ten RM, et al. Acute interstitial nephritis: Immunologic and clinical aspects. *Mayo Clin Proc* 1988;63:921.
98. Buysen JG, et al. Acute interstitial nephritis a clinical and morphological study in 27 patients. *Nephrol Dial Transplant* 1990;5:94.
99. Karras DJ. Severe low back pain secondary to acute interstitial nephritis following administration of ranitidine. *Am J Emerg Med* 1994;12:67.
100. Grattan WA. Hematuria and azotemia associated with administration of methicillin. *J Pediatr* 1964;64:285.
101. Ooi BS, et al. Acute interstitial nephritis: a clinical and pathological study based on renal biopsies. *Am J Med* 1975;59:614.
102. Baum M, Piel CF, Goodman JR. Antibiotic-associated interstitial nephritis and nephrotic syndrome. *Am J Nephrol* 1986;6:149.
103. Siegala JF, Biava CG, Hulter HN. Red blood cell casts in acute interstitial nephritis. *Arch Intern Med* 1988;138:1419.
104. Nolan CR, Anger MS, Kelleher SP. Eosinophiluria: a new method of detection and definition of the clinical spectrum. *N Engl J Med* 1986;315:1516.
105. Corwin HL, Korbet SM, Schwartz MM. Clinical correlates of eosinophiluria. *Arch Intern Med* 1985;145:1097.
106. Sutton JM. Urinary eosinophils. *Arch Intern Med* 1986;146:2243.
107. Loveless MO, Eidal CE, Peteet SA. Asymptomatic eosinophiluria during penicillin and cephalosporin therapy. *Curr Chemother Infect Dis* 1980;1:564.
108. Ruffing KA, et al. Eosinophils in urine revisited. *Clin Nephrol* 1994;41:163.
109. Baldwin DS, et al. Renal failure and interstitial nephritis due to penicillin and methicillin. *N Engl J Med* 1968;279:1245.
110. Cogan MC, Arieff AI. Sodium wasting, acidosis and hyperkalemia induced by methicillin interstitial nephritis: evidence for selective distal tubular dysfunction. *Am J Med* 1978;64:500.
111. Colvin RB, Fang LS. Interstitial nephritis. In: Tisher CC, Brenner BM, eds. *Renal pathology with clinical and functional correlations,* vol. 1. Philadelphia: Lippincott, 1989:728.
112. Kleinknecht D, Vanhille P, Druet P. Nephrites interstitielle aigues granulomateuses d'origine medicamenteuse. *Presse Med* 1988;17:201.
113. Platt JL, Sibley RK, Michael AF. Interstitial nephritis associated with cytomegalovirus infection. *Kidney Int* 1985;28:550.
114. Ooi BS, et al. IgE levels in interstitial nephritis. *Lancet* 1974;1:1254.
115. Pusey C, et al. Drug-associated acute interstitial nephritis: clinical and pathological features and the response to high-dose steroid therapy. *QJM* 1983;206:194.
116. Sarasin F, Schifferli JA. Nephrite interstitielle immunoallergique: steroide ou non? *Schweiz Med Wochenschr* 1990;120:1858.
117. Laberke HG. Treatment of acute interstitial nephritis. *Klin Wochenschr* 1980;58:531.
118. Cameron JS. Allergic interstitial nephritis: clinical features and pathogenesis. *QJM* 1988;250:97.
119. Handa S. Drug-induced acute interstitial nephritis: report of ten cases. *CMAJ* 1986;35:1278.
120. Mignon F, et al. Granulomatous interstitial nephritis. *Adv Nephrol* 1984;13:219.
121. Vanhille PH, et al. Nephrites interstitielles granulomateuses d'origine medicamenteuse. *Nephrologie* 1987;8:41.
122. Frommer P, et al. A case of acute interstitial nephritis successfully treated after delayed diagnosis. *CMAJ* 1979;121:585.
123. Clarkson MR, et al. Acute interstitial nephritis: Clinical features and response to corticosteroid therapy. *Nephrol Dial Transplant* 2004;19:2778.
124. Neilson EG. Pathogenesis and therapy of interstitial nephritis. *Kidney Int* 1989;35:1257.
125. Saharcan A, Marcelli, R, Stallworth S. Antibiotic-induced recurring interstitial nephritis. *Pediatr Nephrol* 2002;17:50.
126. Olsen TS, et al. Ultrastructure of the kidney in acute interstitial nephritis. *Ultrastruct Pathol* 1986;10:1.
127. Brezis M, Rosen S. Hypoxia of the renal medulla: its implications for disease. *N Engl J Med* 1995;332:647.
128. Assoud M, et al. Recurrent acute interstitial nephritis on rechallenge with omeprazole. *Lancet* 1994;344:549.
129. Wilson DB, et al. Value of renal biopsy in acute intrinsic renal failure. *BMJ* 1976;2:459.
130. Preston RA, et al. Renal biopsy in patients 65 years of age or older: an analysis of the results of 334 biopsies. *J Am Geriatr Soc* 1990;38:669.
131. Richet G, et al. La ponction biopsie rénales dans l'insuffisance rénale aigüe. *Ann Med Interne (Paris)* 1978;129:335.
132. Haas M, et al. Etiologies and outcomes of acute renal insufficiency in older adults: a renal biopsy study of 259 cases. *Am J Kidney Dis* 2000;35:433.
133. Farrington K, et al. Renal biopsy in patients with unexplained renal impairment and normal biopsy size. *QJM* 1989;70:221.
134. Davison AM, Jones CH. Acute interstitial nephritis in the elderly: a report from the UK MRC Glomerulonephritis Register and a review of the literature. *Nephrol Dial Transplant* 1999;13(Suppl 7):12.
135. Eapen SS, Hall PM. Acute tubulointerstitial nephritis. *Cleve Clin J Med* 1992;59:27.
136. Noshler NL, et al. Acute focal bacterial nephritis. *Am J Kidney Dis* 1988;11:36.
137. Huang J, et al. Acute bacterial nephritis: a clinicopathologic correlation based on computer tomography. *Am J Med* 1992;93:289.
138. Mallory GK, Crane AR, Edwards JE. Pathology of acute and of healed experimental pyelonephritis. *Arch Pathol* 1940;30:330.

139. Heyman SN, Brezis M. Asymptomatic group B streptococcal pyelonephritis: an unusual cause of acute renal failure. *Nephron* 1997;75:243.
140. Freedman LR, Beeson PB. Experimental pyelonephritis: IV. observations on infections resulting from direct inoculation of bacteria in different zones of the kidney. *Yale J Biol Med* 1958;30:406.
141. Heptinstal RH, Garrill RH. Experimental pyelonephritis and its effect on the blood pressure. *J Pathol Bacteriol* 1955;69:191.
142. Meyrier A, et al. Frequency of development of early cortical scarring in acute primary pyelonephritis. *Kidney Int* 1989;35:6967.
143. Kunin CM. *Detection, prevention and treatment of urinary tract infections,* 3rd ed. Philadelphia: Lea & Febiger, 1979.
144. Stamey TA. *Urinary infections.* Baltimore: Williams & Wilkins, 1972.
145. Pasternack A, et al. Acute tubulointerstitial nephritis in a patient with *Mycoplasma pneumoniae* infection. *Scand J Infect Dis* 1979;11:85.
146. Guignard JP, Torrado A. Interstitial nephritis and toxoplasmosis in a 10-year old child. *J Pediatr* 1974;85:381.
147. Cameron JS, et al. Severe tubulo-interstitial disease in a renal allograft due to cytomegalovirus infection. *Clin Nephrol* 1982;18:321.
148. Wong KM, et al. Cytomegalovirus-induced tubulointerstitial nephritis in a renal allograft treated with foscarnet therapy. *Am J Nephrol* 2000;20:222.
149. Woodroffe AJ, et al. Nephritis in infectious mononucleosis. *QJM* 1974;43:451.
150. Ramelli GP, Marone C, Truniger B. Acute kidney failure in infectious mononucleosis. *Schweiz Med Wochenschr* 1990;27:1590.
151. Mayer HB, et al. Epstein-Barr virus-induced infectious mononucleosis complicated by acute renal failure. *Clin Infect Dis* 1996;22:1009.
152. Norwood VF, Sturgill BC. Unexplained acute renal failure in a toddler: a rare complication of Epstein-Barr virus. *Pediatr Nephrol* 2002;17:628.
153. Okada H, et al. An atypical pattern of Epstein-Barr virus infection in a case with idiopathic tubulointerstitial nephritis. *Nephron* 2002;92:440.
154. Rosen S, et al. Tubulointerstitial nephritis associated with polyomavirus (Bk type) infection. *N Engl J Med* 1983;308:1192.
155. van Ypersele de Strihou C, et al. Diagnosis of epidemic and sporadic interstitial nephritis due to Hantaan-like virus in Belgium. *Lancet* 1983;2:1493.
156. Walker DH, Mattern WD. Acute renal failure in Rocky Mountain spotted fever. *Arch Intern Med* 1983;139:443.
157. Bain BJ, et al. Renal failure and transient paraproteinuria due to *Leptospira pomona. Arch Intern Med* 1973;131:740.
158. Vachvanichsanong P, Dissaneewate P, Mitarnun W. Tubulointerstitial renal failure in childhood leptospirosis. *Pediatr Emerg Care* 1999;15:332.
159. Poulker N, et al. Acute interstitial nephritis complicating Legionnaire's disease. *Clin Nephrol* 1981;15:216.
160. Nishitarumizu K, et al. Tubulointerstitial nephritis associated with Legionnaires' disease. *Intern Med* 2000;39:150.
161. Guziel LP, et al. Primary renal candidiasis with renal granulomata and salt-losing nephropathy. *Am J Med Sci* 1975;269:123.
162. Ramsay AG, Olesnicky L, Pirani CL. Acute tubulointerstitial nephritis from Candida albicans with oliguric renal failure. *Clin Nephrol* 1985;24:310.
163. Koo JW, et al. Acute renal failure associated with *Yersinia pseudotuberculosis* infection in children. *Pediatr Nephrol* 1996;10:582.
164. Jung O, et al. Acute interstitial nephritis in a case of Ascaris lumbricoides infection. *Nephrol Dial Transplant* 2004;19:1625.
165. Ito M, et al. Necrotizing tubulointerstitial nephritis associated with adenovirus infection. *Hum Pathol* 1991;22:1225.
166. Erdogan O, et al. Acute necrotizing tubulointerstitial nephritis due to systemic adenoviral infection. *Pediatr Nephrol* 2001;16:265.
167. Ahuja TS, et al. Acute renal failure in a patient with AIDS: histoplasmosis-induced granulomatous interstitial nephritis. *Am J Kidney Dis* 1998;32:E3.
168. Perazella MA. Acute renal failure in HIV-infected patients: a brief review of common causes. *Am J Med Sci* 2000;319:385.
169. Mouratoff JG, et al. Acute renal failure with interstitial nephritis in a patient with AIDS. *Am J Kidney Dis* 2000;35:557.
170. Nochy D, et al. Renal disease associated with HIV infection: a multicenter study of 60 patients from Paris hospitals. *Nephrol Dial Transplant* 1993;8:11.
171. Brewster UC, Pirazella MD. Acute interstitial nephritis with atazvir, a new protease inhibitor *Am J Kidney Dis* 2004;44:E81.
172. Laradat M, et al. Acute interstitial nephritis attributable to indinavir therapy *Am J Kidney Dis* 2000;35:E16.
173. Heatl CW, Jr, Alexander AD, Galton MM. Leptospirosis in the United States. *N Engl J Med* 1965;273:857.
174. Ooi BS, et al. Human renal leptospirosis. *Am J Trop Med Hyg* 1972;21:336.
175. Sitprija V, et al. Pathogenesis of renal disease in leptospirosis: clinical and experimental studies. *Kidney Int* 1980;17:827.
176. Areann VM. The pathologic anatomy and pathogenesis of fatal human leptospirosis (Weil's disease). *Am J Pathol* 1962;40:393.
177. Sheehan HL. Outbreak of Weil's disease in the British Army in Italy: II. post-mortem and histologic findings. *BMJ* 1946;1:83.
178. Sitprija V, Evans H. The kidney in human leptospirosis. *Am J Med* 1970;49:780.
179. Eknoyan G, Olivero J. The kidney in infectious diseases. In: Suki WN, Eknoyan G, eds. *The kidney in systemic disease,* 2nd edition. New York: Wiley, 1981:541.
180. Morrison WI, Wright NG. Canine leptospirosis: an immunopathological study of interstitial nephritis due to *Leptospira canicola. J Pathol* 1970;120:83.
181. Yang CW, Wu MS, Pan MJ. Leptospirosis renal disease. *Nephrol Dial Transplant* 2001;16(Suppl 5):73.
182. Yang CW, et al. The leptospira outer membrane protein LipL 32 induces tubulointerstitial nephritis mediated gene expression in mouse proximal tubule cells. *J Am Soc Nephrol* 2002;13:2037.
183. Wu M, et al. Reduced renal Na+-K+-Cl- co-transporter activity and inhibited NKCC2 mRNA expression by leptospira shermanii: from bedside to bench. *Nephrol Dial Transplant* 2004;19:2472.
184. Daoudal P, et al. Leptospirose avec immunisation anti-membrane basale glomérulaire. *Nouv Presse Med* 1978;7:3535.
185. Lai KN, et al. Renal lesions in leptospirosis. *Aust N Z J Med* 1982;12:276.
186. Oliver J, MacDowell M. The renal lesion in epidemic hemorrhagic fever. *J Clin Invest* 1957;36:99.
187. Tsai TF. Hemorrhagic fever with renal syndrome clinical aspects. *Lab Anim Sci* 1987;37:419.
188. Lahdevirta J. Nephropathia epidemica in Finland: a clinical histological and epidemiological study. *Ann Clin Res* 1971;3(Suppl 8):1.
189. Pasche FM, et al. Thrombocytopenia and acute renal failure in Puumal hantavirus infections. *Emerg Infect Dis* 2004;10:1420.
190. Olson GE et al. Human hantavirus infection, Sweden. *Emerg Infect Dis* 2003;9:1395.
191. Ledinchy JA. Hantavirus. A short review. *Arch Pathol Lab Med* 2003;127:30.
192. Makela S, et al. Urinary excretion of interleukin-6 correlates with proteinuria in acute Puumala hantavirus-induced nephritis *Am J Kidney Dis* 2004;43:809.
193. van Ypersele de Strihou C, Mery JP. Hantavirus related acute interstitial nephritis in western Europe: expansion of a world wide zoonosis. *QJM* 1989;73:941.
194. Bruno P, et al. The protean manifestation of hemorrhagic fever with renal syndrome: a retrospective review of 26 cases from Korea. *Ann Intern Med* 1990;113:385.
195. Lee HW. Hemorrhagic fever with renal syndrome (HFRS). *Scand J Infect Dis Suppl* 1982;36:82.
196. Bren AF, et al. Acute renal failure due to hemorrhagic fever with renal syndrome. *Ren Fail* 1996;18:635.
197. Patnaik M, Velsosa JA, Peter JB. Hantavirus-specific IgG, IgM and IgA in acute and chronic renal diseases versus congenital renal disease in the United States. *Am J Kidney Dis* 1999;33:734.
198. Elli A, et al. BK polyoma virus interstitial nephritis in renal transplant with previous acute rejection. *J Nephrol* 2002;15:313.
199. Mouratoff JG, et al. Acute renal failure in interstitial nephritis in a patient with AIDS. *Am J Kidney Dis* 2000;35,557.
200. Strache S, et al. Polyoma virus-associated interstitial nephritis in a patient with acute myeloid leukemia. *Nephrol Dial Transplant* 2003;18:2431.
201. Hirsch HH, et al. Prospective study of polyomavirus type BK replication and nephropathy in renal transplant recipients. *N Engl J Med* 2002;347:488.
202. Behring CK, et al. Influence of surveillance renal allograft biopsy on diagnosis and prognosis of polyoma virus-associated nephropathy. *Kidney Int* 2003;94:665.
203. Dunea G, et al. Brucella nephritis. *Ann Intern Med* 1969;70:783.
204. Abernathy RS, Price WE, Spink WW. Chronic brucellar pyelonephritis stimulating tuberculosis. *JAMA* 1955;159:1534.
205. Louria DB, Stiff DP, Bennett B. Disseminated moniliasis in the adult. *Medicine (Baltimore)* 1962;41:307.
206. Lehner T. Systemic candidiasis and renal involvement. *Lancet* 1964;1:1414.
207. Louria DB, Finkel G. Candida pyelonephritis. In: Kass EH, ed. *Progress in pyelonephritis.* Philadelphia: FA Davis, 1964:179.
208. Winblad B. Experimental renal candidiasis in mice and guinea pigs. *Acta Pathol Microbiol Scand* 1975;83:406.
209. Karlowicz MG. Candidal renal and urinary tract infection in neonates. *Semin Neonatol* 2003;7:393.
210. Brody H, Smith LW. The visceral pathology in scarlet fever and related *Streptococcus* infection. *Am J Pathol* 1936;12:373.
211. Knepshield JH, Carstens PH, Gentile DE. Recovery from renal failure due to acute diffuse interstitial nephritis. *Pediatrics* 1969;43:533.
212. Haddon JE, Robotham JL. Acute interstitial nephritis in children: a process produced by streptococcal infection and by chemotherapeutic agents. A review. *J Maine Med Assoc* 1978;69:1.
213. Haddon JE, Sher N, Gall DG. Streptococcal wound infection with evidence of widespread tissue involvement. *Pediatrics* 1971;48:458.
214. Ellis D, et al. Acute interstitial nephritis in children: a report of 13 cases and review of the literature. *Pediatrics* 1981;67:862.
215. Lytle JD. The Addis sediment count in scarlet fever. *J Clin Invest* 1938;12:95.
216. Markowitz GS, Perazella MA. Drug-induced renal failure: a focus on tubulointerstitial disease. *Clin Chim Acta* 2005;351:31.
217. Kabakus N, et al. Mumps interstitial nephritis: a case report. *Pediatr Nephrol* 1999;13:930.
218. Dharmarajan TS, et al. Acute post-streptococcal interstitial nephritis in an adult and review of the literature. *Int Urol Nephrol* 1999;31:145.
219. Kosey M, et al. Acute renal failure in patients with drug-induced acute interstitial nephritis. *Ren Fail* 1993;15:69.

220. Alexopoulos E. Drug-induced acute interstitial nephritis. *Ren Fail* 1998;20: 809.
221. Melnick PI. Acute interstitial nephritis with uremia. *Arch Pathol* 1943;36: 499.
222. More RH, McMillan GC, Duff GL. The pathology of sulfonamide allergy in man. *Am J Pathol* 1946;22:703.
223. Hewitt WL, Finegold SM, Monzon OT. Untoward side effects associated with methicillin therapy. *Antimicrob Agents Chemother* 1961;1:765.
224. Sanjad SA, Haddad GG, Nassar VH. Nephropathy, an underestimated complication of methicillin therapy. *J Pediatr* 1974;84:873.
225. Abraham PA, Keane WF. Glomerular and interstitial disease induced by non-steroidal anti-inflammatory drugs. *Am J Nephrol* 1984;4:1.
226. Appel GB. A decade of penicillin related acute interstitial nephritis: more questions than answers. *Clin Nephrol* 1980;13:151.
227. Ditlove J, et al. Methicillin nephritis. *Medicine (Baltimore)* 1977;56:483.
228. Nolan CM, Abernathy RD. Nephropathy associated with methicillin therapy. *Arch Intern Med* 1977;137:997.
229. Scholand JS, Tannenbaum JF, Grilli JG. Anaphylaxis to cephalothin in a patient allergic to penicillin. *JAMA* 1968;206:139.
230. Woodroffe AJ, et al. Interstitial nephritis due to methicillin, penicillin and ampicillin. *Ann Allergy* 1970;28:378.
231. Burton JR, et al. Acute renal failure during cephalothin therapy. *JAMA* 1974;229:679.
232. Saltissi D, Pusey CD, Rainford DJ. Recurrent acute renal failure due to antibiotic-induced interstitial nephritis. *BMJ* 1979;1:1182.
233. Vigeral PH, et al. Nephrogenic diabetes insipidus and distal tubular acidosis in methicillin-induced interstitial nephritis. In: Amerio A, Coratelli P, eds. *Acute renal failure, clinical and experimental.* New York: Plenum, 1987:129.
234. Kleinknecht D, et al. Acute interstitial nephritis due to hypersensitivity: an up-to-date review with a report of 19 cases. *Adv Nephrol* 1983;12:277.
235. Kida H, et al. Prediction of the long-term outcome in acute interstitial nephritis. *Clin Nephrol* 1984;22:55.
236. Nortier J, Depierreux M, Bourgeios V. Progression of naproxen and amoxicillin induced acute interstitial nephritis with nephrotic syndrome. *Clin Nephrol* 1991;5:187.
237. Lien YH, et al. Ciprofloxacin-induced granulomatous interstitial nephritis and localized elastolysis. *Am J Kidney Dis* 1993;22:598.
238. Colvin RB, et al. Penicillin-associated interstitial nephritis. *Ann Intern Med* 1974;81:404.
239. Campese VM, et al. Acute renal failure during intermittent rifampicin therapy. *Nephron* 1973;10:256.
240. Stradling P. Side effects observed during intermittent rifampicin therapy. *Scand J Respir Dis* 1973;84:129.
241. Covic A, et al. Rifampicin-induced acute renal failure: a series of 60 patients. *Nephrol Dial Transplant* 1998;13:924.
242. Muthukumar T, et al. Acute renal failure due to rifampicin: a study of 25 patients. *Am J Kidney Dis* 2004;40:690.
243. Nessi R, et al. Acute renal failure due to rifampicin: a case report and survey of the literature. *Nephron* 1976;16:148.
244. Kumar SK, et al. Rifampicin-induced acute tubulointerstitial nephritis. *J Indian Med Assoc* 1985;83:246.
245. Kanra T, Barris I, Kolacan B. Rifampicin-dependent antibodies in a patient with hepatorenal failure. *Br J Dis Chest* 1972;72:67.
246. Kleinknecht D, Homberg JC, Deeroix G. Acute renal failure after rifampicin. *Lancet* 1972;1:1238.
247. Gabriel M, Chew W. Relationship between rifampicin-dependent antibody scores, serum rifampicin concentrations and symptoms in patients with adverse reactions to intermitted rifampicin treatment. *Clin Allergy* 1973;3:353.
248. Worlledge S. Correlation between the presence of rifampicin-dependent antibodies and the clinical data. *Scand J Respir Dis* 1973;84:125.
249. Flynn CT, Rainford DJ, Hope E. Acute renal failure and rifampicin: danger of unsuspected intermittent dosage. *BMJ* 1974;2:482.
250. Gabow PA, Lacher JW, Neff TA. Tubulointerstitial and glomerular nephritis associated with rifampin: report of a case. *JAMA* 1976;235:2517.
251. Devulder B, et al. Insuffisance renal aige due a la rifampicine. *Nouv Presse Med* 1973;2:2691.
252. Minetti L, et al. Acute renal failure due to rifampicin. *Proc Eur Dial Transplant Assoc* 1975;12:210.
253. Sands M, Brown RB. Interactions of cyclosporine with antimicrobial agents. *Rev Infect Dis* 1989;11:691.
254. Chensu RY, et al. Renal allograft dysfunction associated with rifampicin-tacrolimus interaction. *Am Pharmacother* 2000;34:27.
255. Gallieni M, et al. Acute tubulointerstitial nephritis requiring dialysis associated with intermittent rifampicin use. *Int J Artif Organs* 1999;22:477.
256. Cochran M, Moorhead PJ, Platts M. Permanent renal damage with rifampicin. *Lancet* 1975;1:1428.
257. Bansal VK, Devasigamonie B, Molnar Z. Prolonged renal failure after rifampin. *Am Rev Respir Dis* 1977;116:137.
258. Brautbat N, et al. Renal failure and interstitial nephritis due to trichloroethylene anesthesia and high dose penicillin. *Isr J Med Sci* 1977;13: 604.
259. Mustonen J, et al. Renal biopsy in acute renal failure. *Am J Nephrol* 1984;4: 27.
260. Maxwell D, et al. Ampicillin nephropathy. *JAMA* 1974;230:586.

261. Ruley EJ, Lisi LM. Interstitial nephritis and renal failure due to ampicillin. *J Pediatr* 1974;84:878.
262. Woodroffe AJ, et al. Acute interstitial nephritis following ampicillin hypersensitivity. *Med J Aust* 1975;1:65.
263. Burton JR, et al. Acute interstitial nephritis from oxacillin. *Johns Hopkins Med J* 1974;134:58.
264. Appel GB, et al. Acute interstitial nephritis associated with carbenicillin therapy. *Arch Intern Med* 1978;138:1265.
265. Roselle GA, Clyne DH, Kauffman CA. Carbenicillin nephrotoxicity. *South Med J* 1978;71:84.
266. Appel GB, et al. Acute interstitial nephritis due to amoxicillin therapy. *Nephron* 1981;27:313.
267. Walker RJ, et al. Amoxicillin-induced acute interstitial nephritis. *N Z Med J* 1985;98:866.
268. Dharnidharka VR, Rosen S, Somers MJ. Acute interstitial nephritis presenting as presumed minimal change nephrotic syndrome. *Pediatr Nephrol* 1998;12:576.
269. Engle JE, et al. Reversible acute renal failure after cephalothin. *Ann Intern Med* 1975;83:232.
270. Milman N. Acute interstitial nephritis during treatment with penicillin and cephalothin. *Acta Scand Med* 1978:203:227.
271. Durham DS, Ibels LS. Cephalothin-induced acute allergic interstitial nephritis. *Aust N Z J Med* 1981;11:266.
272. Appel GB, Neu HC. The nephrotoxicity of antimicrobial agents. *N Engl J Med* 1977;296:663.
273. Verma S, Kieff E. Cephalexin-related nephropathy. *JAMA* 1975;234:618.
274. Wiles CM, et al. Cephradine-induced interstitial nephritis. *Clin Exp Immunol* 1979;36:342.
275. Haskell RJ, et al. Cefoxitin-induced interstitial nephritis. *Arch Intern Med* 1981;141:1557.
276. Rossi E, et al. Insufficienza renale acuta secondaria a somministrazione di cefazolina. *Min Nefrol* 1981;28:493.
277. Ferriozzi S, et al. Cephotaxime-associated allergic interstitial nephritis and MPO-ANCA positive vasculitis. *Ren Fail* 2000;22:245.
278. Nguyen VD, Nagelberg H, Agarwal BN. Acute interstitial nephritis associated with cefotetan therapy. *Am J Kidney Dis* 1990;16:259.
279. Torun D, et al. Acute interstitial nephritis due to cefoperazone *Ann Pharmacother* 2004;38:1446.
280. Allon M, Lopez EJ, Min KW. Acute renal failure due to ciprofloxacin. *Arch Intern Med* 1990;150:2187.
281. Lim S, Alam MG. Ciprofloxacin-induced acute interstitial nephritis and autoimmune hemolytic anemia. *Ren Fail* 2003;25:647.
282. Bailey JR, Tott SA, Philbrick JT. Ciprofloxacin-induced acute interstitial nephritis. *Am J Nephrol* 1992;12:271.
283. Andrews PA, Robinson GT. Intravascular haemolysis and interstitial nephritis in association with ciprofloxacin. *Nephron* 1999;83:359.
284. Walker RG, et al. Minocycline-induced acute interstitial nephritis. *BMJ* 1979;1:524.
285. Bell GM, Thomson D. Acute interstitial nephritis associated with gentamicin and lincomycin therapy. *Postgrad Med J* 1980;56:445.
286. Bierne GJ. Acute renal failure caused by hypersensitivity to polymyxin B sulfate. *JAMA* 1967;202:62.
287. Eisenberg ES, Robbins N, Lenci M. Vancomycin and interstitial nephritis. *Ann Intern Med* 1981;95:658.
288. Wai AO, et al. Vancomycin-induced acute interstitial nephritis. *Ann Pharmacother* 1998;32:1160.
289. Cushner HM, et al. Acute interstitial nephritis associated with mezlocillin, nafcillin and gentamicin treatment for pseudomonas infection. *Arch Intern Med* 1985;145:1204.
290. Kuiper JJ. Omeprazole-induced acute interstitial nephritis. *Am J Med* 1993;95:248.
291. Kleinknecht D, Landais P, Goldfarb B. Les insuffiances rénales aigües associées á des medicaments ou á des produits de contraste iodés: resultats d'une enquête cooperative multicenterique de la Societe de Nephrologie. *Nephrologie* 1986;7:41.
292. Rosenfeld J, et al. Interstitial nephritis with acute renal failure after erythromycin. *BMJ* 1983;286:938.
293. Singer DR. J, et al. Drug hypersensitivity causing granulomatous interstitial nephritis. *Am J Kidney Dis* 1988;11:357.
294. Fanos V, et al. Flurithromycin-induced acute interstitial nephritis. *Pediatr Infect Dis J* 2000;19:366.
295. Boelaert J, et al. Case report of renal failure during norfloxacin therapy. *Clin Nephrol* 1986;25:272.
296. Nakamura M, et al. Norfoxacin-induced acute interstitial nephritis. *Nephron* 2000;86:204.
297. Bihorac A, et al. Tetracycline-induced acute interstitial nephritis as a cause of acute renal failure. *Nephron* 1999;81:72.
298. Garcia-Martin F, et al. Acute interstitial nephritis induced by ethambutol. *Nephron* 1991;59:679.
299. Tintillier M, et al. Telithromycin-induced acute interstitial nephritis: a first case report. *Am J Kidney Dis* 2004;44:E25.
300. Ramalakshni S, Bastachy S, Johnson JP. Levofloxacin-induced granulomatous interstitial nephritis. *Am J Kidney Dis* 2003;41:E7.
301. Lehr D. Clinical toxicity of sulfonamides. *N Y Acad Sci* 1957;69:417.
302. Koch-Wesser J, et al. Adverse reactions to sulfisoxazole, sulfamethoxazole and nitrofurantoin. *Arch Intern Med* 1971;128:399.

303. Serious adverse reactions with sulfonamides. *FDA Drug Bull* 1984;14:5.

304. Josephson M, et al. Drug-induced acute interstitial nephritis in renal allografts: histopathologic features and clinical course in six patients. *Am J Kidney Dis* 1999;34:540.

305. French AJ. Hypersensitivity in the pathogenesis of the histopathologic changes associated with sulfonamide chemotherapy. *Am J Pathol* 1946;22:679.

306. Balsken K. The allergic reactions of the kidney to sulfonamide medications. *J Pathol Bacteriol* 1947;59:501.

307. Prien EL. The mechanism of renal complications in sulfonamide therapy. *N Engl J Med* 1945;63:236.

308. Crespo M, et al. Patterns of sulfadiazine acute nephrotoxicity. *Clin Nephrol* 2000;54:68.

309. Logan RF, Staa TP. Sulphsalazine and mesalazine: serious adverse reactions reevaluated on the basis of suspected adverse reaction reports. *Gut* 2003;52:1530 (263b).

310. Robson M, et al. Acute tubulo-interstitial nephritis following sulfadiazine therapy. *Isr J Med Sci* 1970;6:561.

311. Shear NH, et al. Differences in metabolism of sulfonamides predisposing to idiosyncratic toxicity. *Ann Intern Med* 1986;105:179.

312. Shear NH, Spielberg SP. In vitro evaluation of a toxic metabolite of sulfadiazine. *Can J Physiol Pharmacol* 1985;63:1370.

313. Kalowski S, et al. Deterioration of renal function in association with cotrimoxazole therapy. *Lancet* 1973;1:394.

314. Leynadier JD, Herman D, Pradalier A. L'association sulfamethoxazole-trimethoprime (cotrimoxazole): reaction immunoallergique inhabituelle. *Nouv Presse Med* 1975;4:36.

315. Richmond JM, et al. Co-trimoxazole nephrotoxicity. *Lancet* 1979;1:492.

316. Smith EJ, et al. Interstitial nephritis caused by trimethoprim–sulfamethoxazole in renal transplant recipients. *JAMA* 1980;244:360.

317. Chandra M. Rapid onset of co-trimoxazole induced interstitial nephritis. *Int J Pediatr Nephrol* 1985;6:289.

318. Berglund F, Killander J, Pompeius R. Effect of trimethoprim-sulfamethoxazole on the renal excretion of creatinine in man. *J Urol* 1974;114:802.

319. Cockerill FR, Edson RS. Trimethoprim-sulfamethoxazole. *Mayo Clin Proc* 1983;58:147.

320. Collomon FT. The pathologic changes produced by prolonged administration of sulfapyrazine and sulfamerazine in the kidneys of rabbits as compared to sulfathiazole and sulfadiazine. *J Lab Clin Med* 1944;29:574.

321. Endicott K, Kornberg A. A pathological study of renal damage produced by sulfadiazine in rats. *Am J Pathol* 1945;21:1091.

322. Fitzgerald GA. Coxibs and cardiovascular disease. *New Engl J Med* 2004;351:1709.

323. Nicklander R, McMahon FG, Ridolfo AS. Nonsteroidal anti-inflammatory agent. *Annu Rev Pharmacol Toxicol* 1979;19:469.

324. Whelton A, Hamilton CW. Nonsteroidal anti-inflammatory drug effects on kidney function. *J Clin Pharmacol* 1991;31:588.

325. Adams DH, et al. Non-steroidal anti-inflammatory drugs and renal failure. *Lancet* 1986;1:57.

326. Clive DM, Stoff JS. Renal syndromes associated with nonsteroidal anti-inflammatory drugs. *N Engl J Med* 1984;310:563.

327. Dunn MJ. Nonsteroidal anti-inflammatory drugs and renal function. *Annu Rev Med* 1984;35:411.

328. Carmichael J, Shankel SW. Effects of nonsteroidal anti-inflammatory drugs on prostaglandins and renal function. *Am J Med* 1985;78:992.

329. Brezin JH, et al. Reversible renal failure and nephrotic syndrome associated with nonsteroidal anti-inflammatory drugs. *N Engl J Med* 1979;301:1271.

330. Curt GA, et al. Reversible rapidly progressive renal failure with nephrotic syndrome due to fenoprofen calcium. *Ann Intern Med* 1980;92:72.

331. Eknoyan G. Acute and chronic tubulointerstitial disease and infections of the urinary tract. In: Glassock RI, ed. *Current practice of medicine-nephrology.* Philadelphia: Current Medicine, 1994:XV.15.1.

332. Ravnskov V. Glomerular, tubular and interstitial nephritis associated with nonsteroidal anti-inflammatory drugs: evidence of a common mechanism. *Br J Clin Pharmacol* 1999;47:203.

333. Ailabouni W, Eknoyan G. Non-steroidal anti-inflammatory drugs and acute renal failure in the elderly: a risk-benefit assessment. *Drugs Aging* 1996;9:341.

334. Lorch J, et al. Renal effects of fenoprofen. *Ann Intern Med* 1980;93:509.

335. Finkelstein A, et al. Fenoprofen nephropathy: lipid nephrosis and interstitial nephritis. A possible T-lymphocyte disorder. *Am J Med* 1982;72:81.

336. Wendland ML, Wagoner RD, Holley KE. Renal failure associated with fenoprofen. *Mayo Clin Proc* 1980;55:103.

337. Justiniani FR. Over-the-counter ibuprofen and nephrotic syndrome. *Ann Intern Med* 1986;304:303.

338. Griffiths ML. Endstage renal failure caused by regular use of anti-inflammatory analgesic medication for minor sports injuries. *S Afr Med J* 1992;81:377.

339. Diamond JR, Pallone TL. Acute interstitial nephritis following use of Tung Shueh pills. *Am J Kidney Dis* 1994;24:219.

340. Chatterjee GP. Nephrotic syndrome induced by tolmetin. *JAMA* 1981;246:1589.

341. Katz SM, et al. Tolmetin association with reversible renal failure and acute interstitial nephritis. *JAMA* 1982;246:243.

342. Feinfeld DA, et al. Nephrotic syndrome associated with the use of the nonsteroidal anti-inflammatory drugs. *Nephron* 1984;37:174.

343. McCarthy JT, et al. Reversible nonoliguric acute renal failure associated with zomepirac therapy. *Mayo Clin Proc* 1982;57:351.

344. Mease PF, et al. Zomepirac, interstitial nephritis and renal failure. *Ann Intern Med* 1982;97:454.

345. Warren SE, Mosley C. Renal failure and tubular dysfunction due to zomepirac therapy. *JAMA* 1983;249:396.

346. Miller FC, Schorr WJ, Lacher JW. Zomepirac-induced renal failure. *Arch Intern Med* 1983;143:1171.

347. Gary NE, Dodelson R, Eisinger RP. Indomethacin-associated renal failure. *Am J Med* 1980;69:135.

348. Baumelon A, Agrafiotis A, Jacobs C. Insuffisance renal aige au cours des traitements par l'indométhacine: six observations. *Nouv Presse Med* 1980;9:3611.

349. Rossi E, et al. Diclofenac-associated acute renal failure: report of 2 cases. *Nephron* 1985;40:491.

350. Wolters J, Van Breda Vriesman PJ. Minimal change nephropathy and interstitial nephritis associated with diclofenac. *Neth J Med* 1985;28:311.

351. Revai T, Harmos G. Nephrotic syndrome and acute interstitial nephritis associated with the use of diclofenac. *Wien Klin Wochenschr* 1999;111:523.

352. Chan LK, Winearls CG, Oliver DO. Acute interstitial nephritis and erythroderma associated with diflunisal. *BMJ* 1980;280:84.

353. Dixon AJ, Winearls CG, Dunnill MS. Interstitial nephritis. *J Clin Pathol* 1981;34:616.

354. Russel GI, et al. Interstitial nephritis in a case of phenylbutazone hypersensitivity. *BMJ* 1981;1:1322.

355. Neyer U, et al. Nephrotic syndrome and acute interstitial nephritis after phenylbutazone. *Schweiz Med Wochenschr* 1985;115:1551.

356. Venning V, Dixon AJ, Oliver DO. Mefenamic acid nephropathy. *Lancet* 1980;2:745.

357. Ortuno J, Botella J. Recurrent acute renal failure induced by phenazone hypersensitivity. *Lancet* 1973;2:1473.

358. Lomvardias S, et al. Nephrotic syndrome associated with sulindac. *N Engl J Med* 1981;304:424.

359. Fellner SK. Piroxicam-induced acute interstitial nephritis and minimal-change nephrotic syndrome. *Am J Nephrol* 1985;5:142.

360. Sarma PS. Fatal acute renal failure after piroxicam. *Clin Nephrol* 1989;31:54.

361. Alper AB, Meleg-Smith S, Krane NK. Nephrotic syndrome and intertitial nephritis associated with celecoxib *Am J Kidney Dis* 2002;40:1086.

362. Brewster UC, Perazella MA. Acute interstitial nephritis associated with celecoxib. *Nephrol Dial Transplant* 2004;19:1017.

363. Henao J, et al. Celecoxib induced acute interstitial nephritis *Am J Kidney Dis* 2002;39:1313.

364. Rocha JL, Fernandez-Alonso J. Acute tubulointerstitial nephritis associated with selective COX2 enzyme inhibitor rofecoxib. *Lancet* 2001;357:1946.

365. Alim N, et al. Rofecoxib-induced acute interstitial nephritis *Am J Kidney Dis* 2003;41:720.

366. Schattner A, Sokolovshaya N, Cohen J. Fatal hepatitis and renal failure during treatment with nimesulide. *J Intern Med* 2000;247:153.

367. Perazella MA, Eras J. Are selective COX-2 inhibitors nephrotoxic? *Am J Kidney Dis* 2000;35:937.

368. Ehrlich GE, Wortham GF. Pseudoproteinuria in tolmetin-treated patients. *Clin Pharmacol Ther* 1975;17:467.

369. Welbourne FR, Claypool RG, Copley JB. Nephrotic range pseudoproteinuria in a tolmetin-treated patient. *Clin Nephrol* 1983;19:211.

370. Jenkins DA, et al. Mefenamic acid nephropathy: an interstitial and mesangial lesion. *Nephrol Dial Transplant* 1988;2:217.

371. Marasco WA, et al. Ibuprofen-associated renal dysfunction: pathophysiologic mechanisms of acute renal failure, hyperkalemia, tubular necrosis, and proteinuria. *Arch Intern Med* 1987;147:2107.

372. Champion PJ, et al. Renal failure and nephrotic syndrome associated with sulindac. *Clin Nephrol* 1988;30:52.

373. Schwarz A, et al. Granulomatous interstitial nephritis after nonsteroidal anti-inflammatory drugs. *Am J Nephrol* 1988;8:410.

374. Wasser W, et al. Persistent renal failure following administration of naproxen. *Mt Sinai J Med* 1982;49:127.

375. Artinano M, et al. Progression of minimal change glomerulopathy to focal glomerulosclerosis in a patient with fenoprofen nephropathy. *Am J Nephrol* 1986;6:353.

376. Boletis J, et al. Irreversible renal failure following mefenamic acid. *Nephron* 1989;51:575.

377. Kleinknecht D, Landais P, Goldfarb B. Analgesic and nonsteroidal anti-inflammatory drug-associated acute renal failure: a prospective collaborative study. *Clin Nephrol* 1986;25:275.

378. Finkelstein A, et al. Fenoprofen nephropathy: a possible T-lymphocyte disorder. *Am J Med* 1983;75:9.

379. Strachura I, Subramonian J, Bourke E. T and B lymphocyte subsets in fenoprofen nephropathy. *Am J Med* 1983;75:9.

380. Tores VE. Present and future of the non-steroidal anti-inflammatory drugs in nephrology. *Mayo Clin Proc* 1982;57:389.

381. Kirkeby K. Agranulocytosis following treatment with phenylindanedione. *Lancet* 1954;2:580.

382. De C, Baker SB, Williams RT. Acute interstitial nephritis due to drug sensitivity. *BMJ* 1963;1:1655.

383. Hollman A, Wong HO. Phenindione sensitivity. *BMJ* 1964;2:730.
384. Smith K. Acute renal failure in phenindione sensitivity. *BMJ* 1965;2:24.
385. Galea EG, Young LN, Bell JR. Fatal nephropathy due to phenindione sensitivity. *Lancet* 1963;1:920.
386. Pearce JM. Nephropathy and phenindione sensitivity. *Lancet* 1963;1: 1158.
387. Mery JP, Morel-Maroger L. Les néphrites interstitielles aigües par hypersensibilité médicamenteuse. *Ann Med Interne* 1976;127:590.
388. Sraer JD, et al. Nephrite interstitielle chronique a la phenylindanedione faisant suite a une insuffisance renal aige. *Nouv Presse Med* 1972;1:193.
389. Levine WG. Anticoagulants: heparin and oral anticoagulants. In: Goodman LS, Gilman A, eds. *The pharmacological basis of therapeutics*, 4th ed. New York: Macmillan, 1970:1445.
390. Young JL, Boswell RB, Nies AS. Severe allopurinol hypersensitivity. *Arch Intern Med* 1974;134:553.
391. Mills RM. Severe hypersensitivity reactions associated with allopurinol. *JAMA* 1971;216:799.
392. Gelbart DR, Weinstein AB, Fajardo LF. Allopurinol-induced interstitial nephritis. *Ann Intern Med* 1977;86:196.
393. Grussendorf M, et al. Systemic hypersensitivity to allopurinol with acute interstitial nephritis. *Am J Nephrol* 1981;1:105.
394. Cameron JS, Simmonds HA. Use and abuse of allopurinol. *BMJ* 1987;294: 1504.
395. Magner P. Granulomatous interstitial nephritis associated with allopurinol therapy. *CMAJ* 1985;135:496.
396. Mousson C, et al. Néphrite interstitielle et hépatite aigüe granulomateuses d'origine médicamenteuse: role possible de l'association alluopurinol-furosémide. *Nephrologie* 1986;5:199.
397. McGowan WR, Vermillion SE. Acute interstitial nephritis related to cimetidine therapy. *Gastroenterology* 1980;79:746.
398. Richman AV, Narayan JI, Hirschfield JS. Acute interstitial nephritis and acute renal failure associated with cimetidine therapy. *Am J Med* 1981;70: 1272.
399. Hake DH. Interstitial nephritis and cimetidine. *Ann Intern Med* 1981;94: 416.
400. Seidelin R. Cimetidine and renal failure. *Postgrad Med J* 1980;56:440.
401. Teruel JL, et al. Renal failure and cimetidine. *Ann Intern Med* 1981;94:545.
402. Rudnick MR, et al. Cimetidine-induced acute renal failure. *Ann Intern Med* 1982;96:180.
403. Koarada S, et al. A case of acute interstitial nephritis and nonoliguric acute renal failure induced by cimetidine. *Nippon Jinzo Gakkai Shi* 1992; 34:1227.
404. Kitahara T, et al. A case of cimetidine-induced acute tubulointerstitial nephritis associated with antineutrophil cytoplasmic antibody. *Am J Kidney Dis* 1999;33:E7.
405. Freeman HJ. Ranidine-associated interstitial nephritis in a patient with celiac sprue. *Can J Gastroenterol* 1988;2:35.
406. Neelakantappa K, Gallo GR, Lowenstein JR. Ranitidine-associated interstitial nephritis and Fanconi syndrome. *Am J Kidney Dis* 1993;22: 333.
407. Gaughan WJ, et al. Ranitidine-induced acute interstitial nephritis with epithelial cell foot process fusion. *Am J Kidney Dis* 1993;22:337.
408. Torpey N, Parker T, Ross C. Drug-induced tubulointerstitial nephritis secondary to proton pump inhibitors: experience from a single UK unit. *Nephrol Dial Transplant* 2004;19:1441.
409. Assouad M, et al. Recurrent acute interstitial nephritis on rechallenge with omeprazole. *Lancet* 1994;344:549.
410. d'Adamo G, et al. Omeprazole-induced acute interstitial nephritis. *Ren Fail* 1997;19:171.
411. Montseny JJ, Meyrier A. Immunoallergic-granulomatous interstitial nephritis following treatment with omeprazole. *Am J Nephrol* 1998;18:243.
412. Moore I, et al. Pantoprozole-induced acute interstitial nephritis. *J Nephrol* 2004;17:580.
413. Ra A, Tobe SW. Acute interstitial nephitis due to pantoprazole. *Am Pharmacother* 2004;38:41.
414. Sheth KJ, Casper JT, Good RA. Interstitial nephritis due to phenytoin hypersensitivity. *J Pediatr* 1977;91:438.
415. Michael JR, Mitch WE. Reversible renal failure and myositis caused by phenytoin hypersensitivity. *JAMA* 1976;236:2773.
416. Agarwal BN, Cabebe FG, Hoffman BI. Diphenylhydantoin-induced acute renal failure. *Nephron* 1977;18:249.
417. Lehman DH, Wilson CB, Dixon FI. Interstitial nephritis in rats immunized with heterologous tubular basement membrane. *Kidney Int* 1974;5:187.
418. Frommer JP, Wesson DE, Eknoyan G. Side effects and complications of diuretic therapy. In: Eknoyan G, Martinez-Maldonado M, eds. *The physiological basis of diuretic therapy in clinical medicine*. Orlando, FL: Grune & Stratton, 1986:293.
419. Reubi FC. Pathogenesis and renal function in acute toxic nephropathies. *Contrib Nephrol* 1978;10:1.
420. Lucas CD, et al. Triamterene-induced nephrolithiasis. *J Urol (Paris)* 1982; 88:37.
421. Kjellbo H, Stakeberg H, Mellgren J. Possibly thiazide-induced renal necrotizing vasculitis. *Lancet* 1965;1:1034.
422. Lyons H, et al. Allergic interstitial nephritis causing reversible renal failure in four patients with idiopathic nephrotic syndrome. *N Engl J Med* 1973;288:124.
423. Magil A, et al. Acute interstitial nephritis associated with thiazide diuretics: clinical and pathological observations in three cases. *Am J Med* 1980;69:939.
424. Peskoe S, et al. Reversible acute renal failure associated with chlorthalidone therapy: possible drug-induced interstitial nephritis. *J Med Assoc Georgia* 1978;67:17.
425. Jennings M, Shortland JR, Maddocks JL. Interstitial nephritis associated with furosemide. *J R Soc Med* 1986;79:239.
426. Case records of the Massachusetts General Hospital. Case no. 42-1983. *N Engl J Med* 1983;309:970.
427. Newstead CG, Moore RH, Barnes AJ. Interstitial nephritis associated with indapamide *BMJ* 1990;300:1344.
428. Walker RG, Whitworth JA, Kincaid-Smith P. Acute interstitial nephritis in a patient taking tienilic acid. *Br Med J* 1980;280:1212.
429. Fialk MA, et al. Allergic interstitial nephritis with diuretics. *Ann Intern Med* 1974;81:403.
430. Fuller TJ, Barcenas CG, White MG. Diuretic-induced interstitial nephritis: occurrence in a patient with membranous glomerulonephritis. *JAMA* 1976;235:1998.
431. Renier JC, et al. Insuffisance rénale aigüe recidivante aprés ingestion de glafenine a dose therapeutique. *Nouv Presse Med* 1975;4:670.
432. Proesmans W, et al. Recurrent acute renal failure due to nonaccidental poisoning with glafenin in a child. *Clin Nephrol* 1981;16:207.
433. Lobel A, et al. Insuffisance rénal aigüe aprés ingestion d'antrafenine: possibilité d'un mécanisme immuno-allergique. *Nouv Presse Med* 1979;8:1098.
434. Leguy P, et al. Nephropathie aigüe tubulo-interstitielle aprés ingestion d'antrafenine de mécanisme apparement nomminnuno-allergique. *Nouv Presse Med* 1981;10:1336.
435. Ganeval D, et al. Glaphenine-induced acute renal failure in the fat: a new experimental model. *Am J Physiol* 1982;243:F416.
436. Howard R, et al. Acute renal dysfunction due to sulfinpyrazone therapy in post-myocardial infarction cardiomegaly: reversible hypersensitive interstitial nephritis. *Am Heart J* 1981;102:294.
437. Boelaert J, et al. Insuffiance rénal aigüe indiute par la sulfinpyrazone. *Nephrologie* 1981;2:92.
438. Sloth K, Thomsen AC. Acute renal insufficiency during treatment with azathioprine. *Acta Med Scand* 1971;189:145.
439. Meys E, et al. Fever, hepatitis and acute interstitial nephritis in a patient with rheumatoid arthritis: concurrent manifestations of azathioprine hypersensitivity. *J Rheumatol* 1992;19:807.
440. Pawar R, Jacobs GH, Smith MC. Quinine-associated acute interstitial nephritis. *Am J Kidney Dis* 1994;24:211.
441. Cumming A. Acute renal failure and interstitial nephritis after clofibrate treatment. *BMJ* 1980;281:1529.
442. Reinhart SC, et al. Acute interstitial nephritis with renal failure associated with propylthiouracil therapy. *Am J Kidney Dis* 1994;24:575.
443. Hogg RJ, et al. Carbamazepine-induced acute tubulointerstitial nephritis. *J Pediatr* 1981;98:830.
444. Ejgenraam JW, Buurke EJ, van der haan JS. Carbamazepine-associated acute tubulointerstitial nephritis. *Neth J Med* 1997;50:25.
445. Riou B, et al. Acute immunoallergic interstitial nephritis due to noramidopyrine. *Presse Med* 1984;13:1377.
446. Foley RJ, et al. Amphetamine-induced acute renal failure. *South Med J* 1984;77:258.
447. Sawaishi Y, et al. A case of tubulointerstitial nephritis with exfoliative dermatitis and hepatitis due to phenobarbital hypersensitivity. *Eur J Pediatr* 1992;151:69.
448. Owen D. Renal failure due to para-amino salicylic acid. *BMJ* 1958;2:483.
449. Luderer JR, et al. Acute renal failure, hemolytic anemia and skin rash, and eosinophilia associated with captopril therapy. *Am J Med* 1981;71:493.
450. Steinman TI, Silva P. Acute renal failure, skin rash, eosinophilia associated with captopril therapy. *Am J Med* 1983;75:154.
451. Islam S, Dubigeon MP, Gaenel J. Acute and reversible interstitial granulomatous nephropathy after treatment with captopril. *Rev Med Interne* 1990;11:231.
452. Abadin JA, Duran JA, Perez de Lelon JA. Probable diltiazem-induced acute interstitial nephritis. *Ann Pharmacother* 1998;32:656.
453. Wilson M, et al. Renal failure from alpha-methyldopa therapy. *Aust N Z J Med* 1974;4:415.
454. Sawyer MH, et al. Acyclovir-induced renal failure: clinical course and histology. *Am J Med* 1988;84:1067.
455. Rashed A, Azadeh B, Abu Romeh SH. Acyclovir-induced acute tubulointerstitial nephritis. *Nephron* 1990;56:436.
456. Averbuch SD, et al. Acute interstitial nephritis with the nephrotic syndrome following recombinant leukocyte A interferon therapy for mycosis fungoides. *N Engl J Med* 1984;310:32.
457. Jaradat J, et al. Acute tubulointerstitial nephritis attributable to indinavir therapy. *Am J Kidney Dis* 2000;35:E16.
458. Haskell LP, et al. Isolated erythroid hyperplasia and renal insufficiency induced by long-term treatment with griseofulvin. *South Med J* 1990;83: 1327.
459. Hill PA, Pinel HM, Power DA. Tubulointerstitial nephritis following high dose ifosamide in three breast cancer patients. *Pathology* 2000;32:166.
460. Tanaka H, et al. Acute tubulointerstitial nephritis following intravenous immunoglobulin therapy in a male infant with minimal-change nephrotic syndrome. *Tohoku J Exp Med* 1999;189:155.

461. Markowitz GS, Tartini A, D'Agati VD. Acute interstitial nephritis following treatment with anorectic agents phentermine and phendimetrazine. *Clin Nephrol* 1998;50:252.
462. Zarretta G, et al. Foscarnet-induced crystalline glomerulonephritis with nephrotic syndrome and acute renal failure after kidney transplantation. *Transplantation* 1999;27:1376.
463. Diekman MJ, et al. Acute interstitial nephritis during continuous intravenous administration of low dose interleukin. *Nephron* 1992;60:122.
464. McLeish KR, Senitzer D, Gohara AF. Acute interstitial nephritis in a patient with aspirin hypersensitivity. *Clin Immunol Immunopathol* 1979;14:64.
465. Mehta RP. Acute interstitial nephritis due to 5-amino salicylic acid. *CMAJ* 1990;15:1031.
466. Wedeen P, Bateman V. Tubulo-interstitial nephritis induced by heavy metals and metabolic disturbances. *Contemp Issues Nephrol* 1983;10:211.
467. Van Vleet TR, Schnellman RG. Toxic nephropathy: environmental chemicals. *Semin Nephrol* 2003;23:2003.
468. Foley RJ, Weinman EJ. Urate nephropathy. *Am J Med Sci* 1984;288:208.
469. Davidson MB, et al. Pathophysiology, clinical consequences, and treatment of tumor lysis syndrome. *Am J Med* 2004;116:546.
470. Locatelli F, Rossi F. Incidence and pathogenesis of tumor lysis syndrome. *Contrib Nephrol* 2005;147:61.
471. Moreau D. Pharmacological treatment of acute renal failure in intensive care unit patients. *Contrib Nephrol* 2005;147:161.
472. Khan SR, Finlayson B, Hackett RL. Scanning electron microscopy of calcium oxalate crystals formation in experimental nephrolithiasis. *Lab Invest* 1979;41:504.
473. Dykstra MJ, Hackett RL. Ultrastructural events in early calcium oxalate crystal formation in rats. *Kidney Int* 1979;15:640.
474. Wacker WE, Haynes H, Druyan R. Treatment of ethylene glycol poisoning with ethyl alcohol. *JAMA* 1965;194:1231.
475. Cox RD, Phillips WJ. Ethylene glycol toxicity *Milit Med* 2004;169:660.
476. Mazzer T, Shue GL, Jackson SH. Renal dysfunction associated with methoxyflurane anesthesia. *JAMA* 1971;216:278.
477. Chen CL, et al. Acute oxalate nephropathy after ingestion of star fruit. *Am J Kidney Dis* 2001;37:418.
478. Hodgkinson A. *Oxalic acid in biology and medicine.* New York: Academic Press, 1977.
479. Fogo A. Diabetic nephropathy and extensive, superimposed, intratubular, calcium oxalate crystals due to enteric hyperoxaluria. *Am J Kidney Dis* 2002;40:XI.
480. Cuvelier C, et al. Enteric hyperoxaluria: a hidden cause of early renal graft failure in two successive transplants: spontaneous late graft recovery. *Am J Kidney Dis* 2002;40:E3.
481. Farnsworth A, et al. Renal biopsy morphology in renal transplantation: a comparative study of light-microscopic appearance of biopsies from patients treated with cyclosporin A or azathioprine, prednisone and antilymphocyte globulin. *Am J Surg Pathol* 1984;8:243.
482. Wilson CB, et al. Antitubular basement membrane antibodies after renal transplantation. *Transplantation* 1974;18:447.
483. Trimarchi H, et al. Late onset cytomegalovirus-associated interstitial nephritis in a kidney transplant. *Nephron* 2002;92:490.
484. Asim M, Chong-Lopez A, Nickeleit V. Adenovirus infection in renal allograft. *Am J Kidney Dis* 2003;41:696.
485. Hill PA, et al. Delayed renal allograft failure due to polyoma virus-associated tubulointerstitial nephritis. *Pathology* 2003;35:172.
486. Mecham S, Josephson MA, Haas M. Granulomatous tubulointerstitial nephritis in a renal allograft. *Am J Kidney Dis* 2000;36:E27.
487. Chensuchon B, Staffelt-Loit C, Geiger X. Eosinophil-rich interstitial infiltrates in an allograft biopsy. *Am J Kidney Dis* 2003;41:1116.
488. Emovon OE, et al. Clinical significance of eosinophils in suspicious or borderline renal allograft biopsies. *Clin Nephrol* 2003;59:367.
489. Robertson H, Kirby JA. Post-transplant renal tubulitis: the recruitment, differentiation and persistence of intra-epithelial T cells. *Am J Transplant* 2003;3:3.
490. Sen S, et al. Drug-induced tubulointerstitial nephritis and vasculitis or vascular rejection in renal allografts. *Am J Kidney Dis* 2001;37:E4.
491. Andres G, et al. Histology of human tubulo-interstitial nephritis associated with antibodies to renal basement membranes. *Kidney Int* 1978;13:480.
492. Banergee A, et al. Wegener's granulomatosis presenting as acute suppurative interstitial nephritis. *J Clin Pathol* 2001;54:787.
493. Hannedouche T, et al. Renal granulomatous sarcoidosis: report of six cases. *Nephrol Dial Transplant* 1990;5:18.
494. Frasca GM, et al. Immunological tubulo-interstitial deposits in IgA nephropathy. *Kidney Int* 1982;22:184.
495. Druet P, et al. Les glomerulopathies primitives á depots mesangiaux d'IgA et d'IgG: etude clinique et morphologique de 52 cases. *Presse Med* 1970;78:583.
496. Takeda S, et al. IgG4-associated with idiopathic tubulinterstitial nephritis complicating autoimmune pancreatitis *Nephrol Dial Transplant* 2004;19:476.
497. Schrier RW. Cancer therapy and renal injury. *J Clin Invest* 2002;110:743.
498. Kapoor M, Chan GZ. Malignancy and renal disease. *Crit Care Clin* 2001; 17:571.
499. Pirani CL, Silva FG, Appel GB. Tubulo-interstitial disease in multiple myeloma and other non-renal neoplasias. *Contemp Issues Nephrol* 1983; 10:287.
500. Herrera GA, et al. Renal pathologic spectrum in an autopsy series of patients with plasma cell dyscrasia. *Arch Pathol Lab Med* 2004;128:875.
501. Martinez-Maldonado M, Ramirez-Arillano GA. Renal involvement in malignant lymphoma: a survey of 49 cases. *J Urol* 1966;95:485.
502. Richmond J, et al. Renal lesions associated with malignant lymphomas. *Am J Med* 1962;32:184.
503. Parish AE, et al. Relationship between glomerular function and histology in acute glomerulonephritis. *J Lab Clin Med* 1961;58:197.
504. Obrador GT. Acute renal failure due to lymphomatous infiltration of the kidneys. *J Am Soc Nephrol* 1997;8:1348.
505. Truong LD, et al. Primary lymphoma presenting as acute renal failure. *Am J Kidney Dis* 1987;9:502.
506. Mills NE, et al. B-cell lymphoma presenting as infiltrative renal disease. *Am J Kidney Dis* 1992;19:181.
507. Tomroth T, et al. Lymphomas diagnosed by percutaneous kidney biopsy. *Am J Kidney Dis* 2003;42:960.
508. Lundeberg WB, et al. Renal failure secondary to leukemic infiltration of the kidneys. *Am J Med* 1977;62:636.
509. Echman LN, Lynch ED. Acute renal failure in patients with acute leukemia. *South Med J* 1978;71:382.
510. Kanafer A, et al. Acute renal insufficiency due to lymphomatous infiltration of the kidneys. *Cancer* 1976;38:22588.
511. Tsokos GC, et al. Renal and metabolic complications of undifferentiated and lymphoblastic lymphomas. *Medicine (Baltimore)* 1981;60:218.
512. Pagniez DC, et al. Reversible renal failure due to specific infiltration in chronic lymphocytic leukemia. *Am J Med* 1988;85:579.
513. Tucker B, et al. Reversible renal failure due to renal infiltration and associated tubulointerstitial disease in chronic lymphocytic leukaemia. *Nephrol Dial Transplant* 1990;5:616.
514. Kyle RA. Multiple myeloma: review of 869 cases. *Mayo Clin Proc* 1975; 50:29.
515. Martinez-Maldonado M, et al. Renal complications in multiple myeloma: pathophysiology and some aspects of clinical management. *J Chronic Dis* 1971;24:221.
516. DeFronzo RA, et al. Acute renal failure in multiple myeloma. *Medicine (Baltimore)* 1975;54:209.
517. Winearls CG. Acute myeloma kidney. *Kidney Int* 1995;48:1347.
518. Markowitz GS. Dysproteinemia and the kidney. *Adv Anat Pathol* 2004; 11:49.
519. Pozzi C, et al. Light chain deposition disease with renal involvement: clinical characteristics and prognostic factors *Am J Kidney Dis* 2003;42:1154.
520. Clyne DH, Pesce AJ, Thompson RE. Nephrotoxicity of Bence-Jones protein in the rat. Importance of protein isoelectric point. *Kidney Int* 1979;16: 345.
521. Hill GS, et al. Renal lesions in multiple myeloma: their relationship to associated protein abnormalities. *Am J Kidney Dis* 1983;2:423.
522. Bernstein SP, Humes HD. Reversible renal insufficiency in multiple myeloma. *Arch Intern Med* 1982;142:2083.
523. Sakhiya V, et al. Renal involvement in multiple myeloma: a 10 year study. *Ren Fail* 2000;22:465.
524. Chazan JA, Geller AS, Esparza A. Acute interstitial nephritis: a distinct clinicopathological entity? *Nephron* 1972;9:10.
525. Graber ML, Cogan MG, Connor DG. Idiopathic acute interstitial nephritis. *West J Med* 1978;129:72.
526. Hyun J, Gallen MA. Acute interstitial nephritis: a case characterized by increase in serum IgG, IgM, IgE concentrations, eosinophilia and IgE deposition in renal tubules. *Arch Intern Med* 1978;141:679.
527. Bergstein J, Litman N. Interstitial nephritis with antitubular basement membrane antibody. *N Engl J Med* 1975;292:875.
528. Levy M, et al. Immunologically medicated tubulo-interstitial nephritis in children. *Contrib Nephrol* 1979;16:132.
529. Koskimies O, Holmberg C. Interstitial nephritis of acute onset. *Arch Dis Child* 1985;60:752.
530. Spital A, Panner BJ, Sterns RH. Acute idiopathic tubulointerstitial nephritis: report of two cases and review of the literature. *Am J Kidney Dis* 1987;9: 71.
531. Enriquez R, et al. Relapsing steroid-responsive idiopathic acute interstitial nephritis. *Nephron* 1993;63:4622.
532. Okada K, et al. Steroid-responsive renal insufficiency due to idiopathic granulomatous tubulointerstitial nephritis. *Am J Nephrol* 1993;13:164.
533. Dobrin RS, Vernier RL, Fish AL. Acute eosinophilic interstitial nephritis and renal failure with bone marrow-lymph node granulomas and anterior uveitis: a new syndrome. *Am J Med* 1975;59:325.
534. Segeu A, et al. Acute eosinophilic interstitial nephritis and uveitis (TINV syndrome) associated with granulomatous hepatitis. *Clin Nephrol* 1999;51:310.
535. Steinman TI, Silva P. Acute interstitial nephritis and iritis: renal-ocular syndrome. *Am J Med* 1984;77:189.
536. Vanhaesebrouck P, et al. Acute tubulointerstitial nephritis and uveitis syndrome (TINU syndrome). *Nephron* 1985;40:418.
537. Burnier M, et al. Idiopathic acute interstitial nephritis and uveitis in the adult. *Am J Nephrol* 1986;6:312.
538. Van Acker KJ, et al. Acute tubulointerstitial nephritis with uveitis. *Acta Paediatr Belg* 1980;33:171.
539. Kikkawa Y, et al. Interstitial nephritis with concomitant uveitis. *Contrib Nephrol* 1977;4:1.

540. Gafter U. Anterior uveitis, a presenting symptom in acute interstitial nephritis. *Nephron* 1986;42:249.
541. Catalano C, et al. Acute interstitial nephritis associated with uveitis and primary hypoparathyroidism. *Am J Kidney Dis* 1989;14:317.
542. Yoshioka K, et al. Acute interstitial nephritis and uveitis syndrome activated immune cell infiltration in the kidney. *Pediatr Nephrol* 1991;5:232.
543. Montagnon F, et al. Acute interstitial nephritis with uveitis. *Rev Med Interne* 1992;13:384.
544. Bunchman TE, Bloom JN. A syndrome of acute interstitial nephritis and anterior uveitis. *Pediatr Nephrol* 1993;75:520.
545. Sessa A, et al. Acute renal failure due to idiopathic tubulointerstitial nephritis and uveitis: case report and review of the literature. *J Nephrol* 2000;13:377.
546. Lessard M, Smith JD. Fanconi syndrome with uveitis in an adult woman. *Am J Kidney Dis* 1989;13:158.
547. Morino M, et al. Acute tubulointerstitial nephritis in two siblings and concomitant uveitis in one. *Acta Paediatr* 1991;33:93.
548. Itsuka T, et al. HLA tissue types in patients with acute tubulointerstitial nephritis accompanying uveitis. *Nippon Jinzo Gakkai Shi* 1993;35:723.
549. Levinson RD, et al. Strong association between specific HLA-DQ and HLA-DR alleles in tubulointerstitial nephritis and uveitis syndrome. *Invest Ophthalmol Vis Sci* 2003;44:653.
550. Vohra S, et al. Tubulointerstitial nephritis and uveitis in children and adolescents: four new cases and a review of the literature. *Pediatr Nephrol* 1999;13:426.
551. Takemura T, et al. Course and outcome of tubulointerstitial nephritis and uveitis syndrome. *Am J Kidney Dis* 1999;34:1016.
552. James DG. Uveitis is a systemic disorder. *Am J Med* 1978;65:567.
553. Stupp R, et al. Acute tubulo-interstitial nephritis with uveitis (TINU syndrome) in a patient with serologic evidence for Chlamydia infection. *Klin Wochenschr* 1990;68:971.
554. Grefer J. Tubulointerstitial nephritis and uveitis in association with Epstein-Barr virus infection. *Pediatr Nephrol* 1999;13:336.
555. Kondo JJ, et al. The role of mast cells in acute tubulointerstitial nephritis and uveitis. 2003:162:496.
556. Brughard R, et al. Acute interstitial nephritis in childhood. *Eur J Pediatr* 1984;142:103.
557. Gallego N, et al. Tubulointerstitial nephritis and asymptomatic uveitis. *J Nephrol* 2000;13:373.
558. Azar R, Verove C, Boldron A. Delayed onset of uveitis I TINU syndrome. *J Nephrol* 2000:13:381.
559. Cacoub P, et al. Idiopathic acute interstitial nephritis associated with anterior uveitis in adults. *Clin Nephrol* 1989;31:307.
560. Eknoyan G. Acute renal failure associated with tubulointerstitial nephritis. In: Brenner BM, Lazarus JM, eds. *Acute renal failure,* 2nd ed. New York: Churchill Livingstone, 1988:491.

CHAPTER 49 ■ ACUTE RENAL FAILURE ASSOCIATED WITH PIGMENTURIA OR CRYSTAL DEPOSITS

BURL R. DON, RUDOLPH A. RODRIGUEZ, AND MICHAEL H. HUMPHREYS

ACUTE RENAL FAILURE RESULTING FROM HEME PIGMENTS

Myoglobinuric Acute Renal Failure

The destruction of skeletal muscle and the release of muscle cell contents, notably myoglobin, into the circulation can cause an acute deterioration in renal function. The seminal description of the consequences of traumatic muscle injury on kidney function is attributed to Bywaters and Beall (1), who vividly documented the brown-black granular casts, the reduction in urinary output, hyperkalemia, and ultimately death in the victims of crush injuries at the time of the German blitz of London during World War II. In addition, Bywaters et al. (2,3) were the first to establish a definite pathophysiologic relationship between crush injury, myoglobinuria, and acute tubular necrosis. Since that time, it has become evident that muscle damage from nontraumatic, (4) as well as traumatic, causes can produce the syndrome of myoglobinuric acute renal failure, thus establishing rhabdomyolysis as a common cause of acute renal failure on medical and surgical services of large hospitals.

Causes of Rhabdomyolysis and Myoglobinuria

A variety of conditions and diseases can lead to rhabdomyolysis and acute renal failure, and the list of causes is constantly being expanded with new case reports (Table 49-1). Although the list is lengthy, it can be divided into eight basic categories: (a) direct muscle injury, (b) drugs and toxins, (c) genetic disorders (decreased energy production), (d) infections, (e) excessive muscular activity, (f) ischemia, (g) electrolyte and endocrine/metabolic disturbances, and (h) immunologic diseases. The common denominator for all the causes is a disruption of normal skeletal muscle cell structure or metabolism that leads to influx of Ca^{2+} across the sarcolemmal membrane and impairment of the normal sequestration of calcium in the sarcoplasmic reticulum. Adenosine triphosphate (ATP) depletion further interferes with Ca^{2+} sequestration, leading to lethal intracellular Ca^{2+} overload. The high intracellular Ca^{2+} concentration activates neutral proteases, phospholipases, and other degradative enzymes that cause myofibril and membrane damage (5). The subsequent death and lysis of the skeletal muscle cells results in the release of intracellular contents into the circulation. In the United States, the three most common causes of rhabdomyolysis are drug abuse (with a substantial percentage related to ethanol use), muscle compression, and seizures (6,7).

Crush injuries (8–12) and prolonged compression of the limbs (13) can lead to massive rhabdomyolysis and its sequelae, including acute renal failure. Related to such injuries are hy-

povolemia, hypocalcemia, and shock as sodium chloride, calcium, and water flow from the extracellular compartment into the damaged muscle cells. In addition, hyperkalemia and hyperphosphatemia commonly are seen as a result of the efflux of these solutes from injured cells. Prolonged compression of a limb has been shown to increase intramuscular pressures to a point sufficient to cause muscle and capillary ischemia and necrosis by local obstruction of the circulation (13).

Drugs and toxins that have been implicated in causing rhabdomyolysis are legion (14–16). Several mechanisms have been implicated for drug- and toxin-induced rhabdomyolysis, including (a) drug-induced coma leading to compression of a limb (13); (b) excessive muscular activity [e.g., phencyclidine (17), LSD, hemlock (18)]; (c) drug-induced hyperthermia (19); (d) drug-induced vasoconstriction with muscle ischemia [e.g., cocaine (20)]; (e) impaired ATP formation (e.g., cyanide, salicylates); (f) induction of potassium or phosphorus depletion (e.g., diuretics); (g) hypersensitivity reaction resulting in myositis; and (h) a direct toxic effect on skeletal muscle cell, as has been attributed to ethanol (21). Although certain drugs such as heroin (22) or ethanol may have a direct toxic effect on skeletal muscle cells, a more important factor in causing rhabdomyolysis is the occurrence of coma after their use, which leads to muscle compression and ischemia. In addition, drug use may be associated with other conditions that predispose to rhabdomyolysis. For example, in the alcoholic patient, concomitant hypokalemia (23), hypophosphatemia (24–26), starvation (27), and ethanol-induced enzyme defects (28) may contribute to rhabdomyolysis. The presence of multiple etiologic factors may be a common scenario, as noted in a large clinical series by Gabow et al. (29) in which more than one factor capable of injuring muscles was present in 51 of 87 episodes of rhabdomyolysis.

Various hereditary enzyme deficiencies and defects have been associated with rhabdomyolysis and myoglobinuria. In patients with hereditary deficiency of myophosphorylase (McArdle's syndrome) (30), phosphofructokinase (31), and carnitine palmityl transferase (32), physical exercise can induce rhabdomyolysis. The common denominator of these disorders is decreased energy production on the part of skeletal muscle cells due to impaired substrate utilization. In the setting of increased energy demands (exercise), the inability of muscle cells to generate sufficient ATP leads to cell damage and rhabdomyolysis.

The myositis occasionally associated with infectious diseases such as influenza (33) and leptospirosis can lead to disruption of skeletal muscle cells and thus rhabdomyolysis and myoglobinuria. In addition, infections like gas gangrene produce a clostridial toxin that is directly myotoxic (34).

Excessive muscular activity has been increasingly recognized as a common and preventable cause of rhabdomyolysis (35). Strenuous and exhaustive exercise, especially in

TABLE 49-1

CAUSES OF RHABDOMYOLYSIS

Traumatic muscle injury	Phosphohexoseisomerase deficiency
Crush injuries	Infections (partial list)
Compression/pressure necrosis	Influenza
Severe burns	Tetanus
Contact sports	Gas gangrene
Direct muscle trauma	Legionnaires' disease
Drugs and toxins (partial list)	Shigellosis and salmonellosis
Ethanol	Coxsackievirus
Heroin	Leptospirosis
Barbiturates	Streptococcus
Cocaine	HIV
Amphetamines	Excessive muscular activity
Benzodiazepines	Vigorous exercise
Phencyclidine	Seizures/status epilepticus
HMG-CoA reductase inhibitors (statins)	Delirium tremens
Fibric acid derivatives (clofibrate, gemfibrozil)	Status asthmaticus
Hemlock	Psychotic muscle contractions
Salicylates	Tetany
Carbon monoxide	Ischemia
Ethylene glycol	Arterial occlusion
Isopropyl alcohol	Compression
Snake and insect venoms	Electrolyte and endocrine/metabolic
Succinylcholine	disorders
Colchicine	Hypokalemia
Propofol	Hypophosphatemia
Para-phenylenediamine	Hypothyroidism
Colchicum autumnale (autumn crocus)	Diabetic ketoacidosis
Monensin	Diabetic hyperosmolar nonketotic
Genetic disorders	coma
Phosphorylase deficiency (McArdle's disease)	Hypothermia and hyperthermia
Phosphofructokinase deficiency	Immunologic disease
α-Glucosidase deficiency	Polymyositis
Carnitine palmityltransferase deficiency	Dermatomyositis
Amylo-1,6-glucosidase deficiency	

deconditioned men (so-called "white collar" rhabdomyolysis), can result in major morbidity from hyperkalemia, metabolic acidosis, disseminated intravascular coagulation (DIC), acute respiratory distress syndrome, and rhabdomyolysis (36). Contributing factors to this syndrome include exercising in a hot or humid environment, volume depletion, fasting, eccentric muscle contractions (running downhill), preexistent muscle injury (alcoholic myopathy), and male sex (36). Intense muscle contractions deplete energy reserves, thus disrupting normal cellular transport processes and permitting calcium to accumulate in the cell, resulting in activation of proteolytic enzymes and cell death. Based on a number of studies reviewed by Knochel (36), physical training raises the threshold and induces a degree of resistance to the development of exertional rhabdomyolysis. Training may induce this adaptation by increasing blood flow and oxygen delivery to muscles, increasing muscle glycogen content (improved fuel storage), and increasing the capacity for oxidative metabolism (improved fuel utilization). Other conditions associated with excessive muscle contractions and significant rhabdomyolysis include seizures, tetanus, and delirium tremens.

Severe potassium deficiency can lead to rhabdomyolysis, myoglobinuria, and acute renal failure. During exercise, there is an increase in blood flow to the contracting muscles that is mediated by potassium released from the contracting muscle fibers. In the setting of potassium depletion, the potassium release from contracting muscle fibers is suboptimal, leading to

blunted vasodilation and thus muscle ischemia (cramps) and necrosis (23). Hypophosphatemia, especially in the setting of severe alcoholism, has been associated with muscle cell injury and rhabdomyolysis (24–26). Other metabolic conditions that have been reported to cause rhabdomyolysis include hypothyroidism (37) and both hyperthermia (19) and hypothermia (38).

Myoglobin Metabolism

Myoglobin is composed of a folded polypeptide portion (globin) and a prosthetic group, heme, which contains an atom of iron. The molecular weight of myoglobin is 17,800 daltons, which is approximately one-fourth that of the other major heme pigment, hemoglobin (39). Based on tracer studies, the half-life of myoglobin in the circulation varies from 1 to 3 hours; after 6 hours, it has completely disappeared (40). Small quantities of myoglobin (milligram amounts) released during normal conditions are probably cleared by the reticuloendothelial system (41). Because of its relatively small molecular weight and size, larger quantities of myoglobin released from muscle in states of injury or disease are readily filtered at the glomerulus and thus can be cleared by renal mechanisms.

In the human circulation, myoglobin appears to be bound to an α_2-globulin that has a binding capacity of 23 mg/dL. Because myoglobin is loosely bound to α_2-globulin, at concentrations below 23 mg/dL, approximately 15% to 50% of the myoglobin is in an unbound state and is filtered (fractional clearance relative to inulin, 0.75) and excreted in the urine. This interesting kinetic relationship between myoglobin and its binding protein probably explains why myoglobin is detected in the urine when plasma levels are less than 23 mg/dL (39). According to Kagen (42), the effective renal threshold for myoglobin occurs when the plasma concentration exceeds 0.5 to 1.5 mg/dL. Based on a distribution volume of myoglobin of 28.5 L and a muscle myoglobin content of 4 mg/g, Knochel (43) has calculated that injury of approximately 102 g of muscle would be required to exceed a renal threshold of 1.5 mg/dL. Beyond this threshold, the factors that determine the urinary concentration and excretion rate of myoglobin include (a) the plasma concentration of myoglobin, (b) the extent of myoglobin binding in plasma, (c) glomerular filtration rate (GFR), and (d) urine flow rate.

Myoglobin is visible in plasma or urine to the unaided eye when the concentration exceeds 100 mg/dL. Because of relatively rapid renal clearance of myoglobin, visible plasma levels of myoglobin have never been reported. Knochel (43) has estimated that a visible plasma level of myoglobin would require the destruction of 7.1 kg of muscle in an anephric patient. In contrast, because myoglobin is cleared rapidly in patients with normal renal function, visible myoglobinuria is achieved with far less muscle necrosis. For example, necrosis of only 178 g of muscle, achieving a plasma myoglobin level of only 2.5 mg/dL, is sufficient to produce visible myoglobinuria in a patient with normal renal function excreting concentrated urine (43). However, reduced renal function or a high urine flow rate decreases the concentration of myoglobin in urine, diminishing the utility of a visual inspection of the urine to detect myoglobinuria for a given amount of muscle necrosis. In these situations, benzidine, guaiac, or orthotoluidine (dipstick) tests detect levels as low as 0.5 mg/100 mL. These tests, however, do not distinguish between myoglobin and hemoglobin. This can be accomplished either by immunodiffusion or spectrophotometry (39).

Although the presence of myoglobinemia or myoglobinuria is indicative of skeletal or cardiac muscle injury, it may not be the most sensitive method to detect rhabdomyolysis. Given that myoglobin has a relatively rapid renal clearance (1 to 6 hours), a patient with rhabdomyolysis may have a normal plasma level by the time he or she is hospitalized. In the series by Gabow et al. (29), 26% of the patients with documented rhabdomyolysis had a negative orthotoluidine reaction for myoglobin in the urine. In contrast, creatine kinase, an intracellular muscle enzyme, appears to be a more sensitive plasma marker for rhabdomyolysis because of its slower clearance (serum half-life, 1.5 days) (44). Thus, at initial clinical evaluation, patients with rhabdomyolysis have increased serum creatine kinase levels, whereas urine myoglobin levels may or may not be detected.

Pathophysiology of Myoglobinuric and Hemoglobinuric Acute Renal Failure

The exact pathophysiology of pigment-induced acute renal failure is unclear and probably is multifactorial. Given the biochemical similarity between myoglobin and hemoglobin, most investigators suspect that both myoglobinuric and hemoglobinuric acute renal failure share a common pathogenesis. In fact, the major animal model used to study pigment-induced oliguric acute renal failure is produced by subcutaneous or intramuscular injections of glycerol, and results in both intravascular hemolysis (hemoglobinuria) and rhabdomyolysis (myoglobinuria). Thus, the pathogeneses of myoglobinuric and hemoglobinuric acute renal failure are considered together in this discussion.

The proposed mechanisms by which myoglobinuria or hemoglobinuria causes acute renal failure include (a) hypovolemia and renal ischemia, (b) direct tubular toxicity of myo-

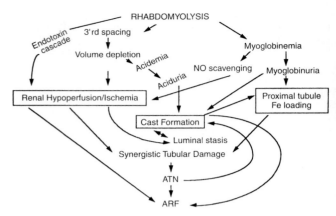

FIGURE 49-1. Pathophysiologic process of myoglobinuric and hemoglobinuric acute renal failure. (Reprinted from: Zager RA. Rhabdomyolysis and myohemoglobinuric acute renal failure. *Kidney Int* 1996;49:317, with permission.)

globin/hemoglobin, (c) tubular obstruction from heme pigment casts or uric acid crystals, and (d) glomerular fibrin deposition. As in many clinical syndromes, it is probably the interplay of these proposed mechanisms that results in acute renal failure, rather any one single factor; these interactions are schematized in Figure 49-1.

Hypovolemia and Renal Ischemia

During the initial phase of glycerol-induced acute renal failure, there is a marked reduction in cardiac output (36%) and renal blood flow (20%) and an increase in renal vascular resistance (45). Subcutaneous or intramuscular (but not intravenous) glycerol not only produces muscle injury but causes sequestration of fluid into the injection site (46). Thus, the hemodynamic changes are due, in part, to the migration of plasma water into the site of injury, with consequent severe intravascular volume contraction that occurs in this model of myohemoglobinuric acute renal failure. Comparable events occur in the clinical setting inasmuch as muscle injury that occurs in the crush syndrome causes a shift of fluid from the vascular space into the injured muscle, leading to intravascular volume depletion (12). Moreover, the conditions that predispose a person to rhabdomyolysis, such as drug-induced coma with accompanying poor oral intake or excessive insensible fluid losses from exhaustive exercise, contribute to intravascular volume depletion and compromise of renal function.

In the initial phases of glycerol-induced acute renal failure, the reduction in renal blood flow is associated with a redistribution of regional blood flow from the outer to the inner cortex (47) and vasoconstriction of the afferent and efferent arteriole. As reviewed by Honda (48), the proposed mediators of this initial renal vasoconstriction include (a) increased sympathetic nerve activity, (b) augmented activity of the renin–angiotensin system, (c) reduced nitric oxide production, (d) suppressed renal prostaglandin production, (e) increased plasma vasopressin concentration, and (f) glomerular microthrombi and reduced nitric oxide activity. The reduction in nitric oxide may be due to the fact that heme proteins can scavenge this important endogenous vasodilator. Marlee et al. (49) have shown that nitric oxide synthase inhibition worsens and nitric oxide supplementation protects against glycerol-induced acute renal failure, lending support to the importance of nitric oxide in the pathogenesis of myoglobin-induced acute renal failure. The exact mediators have not been established and the renal vasoconstriction may be due to the interplay among a number of vasoconstricting/vasodilating systems.

The critical role that intravascular volume depletion plays in the pathogenesis of myohemoglobinuric acute renal failure is demonstrated by studies in which volume status is manipulated in the glycerol-treated rat. In initial studies, Oken et al. (50,51) noted that renal damage was ameliorated if the rats ingested adequate quantities of water before the administration of glycerol. Similarly, Hsu et al. (45,52) found that the reduction in renal blood flow and function in response to the administration of glycerol was attenuated in rats chronically drinking saline compared with rats drinking water. The study by Reineck et al. (53) provided a better understanding of the important temporal relationship between volume expansion and improvement of renal function in the glycerol-treated rat. Like other investigators, they noted that there was a significant reduction in renal blood flow and GFR after the administration of glycerol. These variables could be restored to normal levels by volume expansion with Ringer's solution at 3 and 6 hours after administration of glycerol. They concluded that the initial decrease in GFR and low fractional excretion of sodium in this model of myohemoglobinuric acute renal failure was due to a decrease in renal blood flow (renal hypoperfusion). Volume expansion, however, was not successful in restoring GFR when given 18 hours after the administration of glycerol, suggesting that other events (e.g., tubular necrosis) had occurred that were not amenable to volume therapy. These studies in the rat support the clinical observation that, initially, patients with myoglobinuric acute renal failure have features of prerenal azotemia, including a low urinary fractional excretion of sodium (54). In addition, they provide the rationale for early use of volume expansion in patients with significant rhabdomyolysis and hemoglobinuria.

As noted above, renal ischemia as well as oxygen metabolites play an important role in the renal injury during myoglobinuric acute renal failure. Recent studies in experimental animal models of myoglobinuric-induced acute renal failure have shown that antioxidant bioflavonoids, such as polyphenols found in red wine, attenuate the severity of the renal damage (55–57). Rodrio et al. noted that red wine reduces both biochemical and morphologic renal damage caused by rhabdomyolysis in rats given Chilean red wine. This attenuation of renal damage is less impressive when the animals were treated with alcohol-free red wine suggesting a synergy between ethanol and nonalcoholic components of red wine in reducing renal damage (56).

Myoglobin and Hemoglobin Nephrotoxicity. Bywaters and co-workers expanded on their original description of the clinical syndrome of rhabdomyolysis-induced acute renal failure (1) to examine the role of myoglobin as a direct nephrotoxin. In a study published in 1942 (2), they noted that rabbits ingesting an acid diet with a urine pH below 6.0 had acute renal failure after infusion of human myoglobin, whereas rabbits ingesting a normal diet were spared from renal injury. Other investigators (58–61) have confirmed this observation that intravenous infusions of myoglobin are relatively benign, but can become highly nephrotoxic in the setting of acidemia/aciduria and volume depletion. Vetterlein et al. (62) demonstrated that infusions of myoglobin had no effect on renal blood flow in normal rats, but worsened renal blood flow in hypotensive animals. Thus, it appears that heme proteins can intensify the degree of vasoconstriction in the setting of hypovolemia. This may explain the clinical observation that the presence merely of myoglobinuria or a markedly elevated creatine kinase at the time of hospital admission had little predictive value in determining who experiences acute renal failure (29), suggesting that other conditions (i.e., volume depletion, acidemia) are required for renal injury to occur.

To address the question of why heme pigments are nephrotoxic only in certain metabolic conditions, Braun et al. (46) performed a detailed study investigating the effect of breakdown products of heme pigments on renal tubular transport. First, they noted that, 4 hours after subcutaneous glycerol administrations to rats, there was both swelling and pallor of the proximal tubule and depression of normal tubular uptake of hippurate and tetraethylammonium. Then, the investigators measured the uptake of hippurate in renal cortical slices incubated with various specific heme proteins or their derivatives. Incubation with hemoglobin did not depress uptake if the pH of the medium was kept at 7.4. However, uptake was depressed when the pH was lowered to 5.4 or during hypoxic conditions. In an acidic medium (pH <5.6), both myoglobin and hemoglobin dissociate into ferrihemate (hematin; molecular weight, 670 daltons) and their respective globin moieties (63). Incubation with ferrihemate, regardless of the pH of the medium, depressed the uptake of hippurate in the renal cortical slices, whereas incubation with either globin or albumin alone had no significant effect on transport. The inhibitory action of ferrihemate on hippurate transport could be mitigated if the incubation medium also contained albumin, which presumably bound the ferrihemate. Intravenous injection of ferrihemate has been shown to cause glomerular and tubular damage in the dog (64). Therefore, it has been proposed that after filtration by the glomerulus, myoglobin or hemoglobin is converted to ferrihemate in the presence of an acid tubular fluid, or after exposure to the acid pH of cellular lysosomes, and it is this metabolite that is directly nephrotoxic.

These early studies implicated the heme moiety as the nephrotoxic factor in myoglobinuric and hemoglobinuric acute renal failure. More recent studies have suggested that the iron component of heme may be the specific culprit in causing renal injury. Iron can promote hydroxyl free radical formation by the Fenton/Haber/Weiss reactions (65), leading to lipid peroxidation and cell necrosis. Both myoglobin (66) and hemoglobin (67) can act as Fenton reagents. Shah and Walker (68) and Paller (69) have proposed that the iron in these heme pigments could cause renal injury in vivo through the damaging effects of free radicals. Administration of hydroxyl free radical scavengers such as dimethylthiourea and sodium benzoate attenuated the renal injury in glycerol-treated rats (68). In addition, both laboratories demonstrated that the iron chelator, deferoxamine, ameliorated both myoglobinuric and hemoglobinuric acute renal failure and lipid peroxidation. Zager (70) has also shown that deferoxamine attenuates renal damage in the glycerol-induced model of acute renal failure, but concluded that iron toxicity is mediated by factors other than free radical generation. For example, it has been suggested that heme protein endocytosis in the proximal tubule sensitizes the tubular cell membranes to the damaging effects of phospholipase A_2 (71). In addition, heme proteins appear to deplete cellular ATP stores and thus have an adverse effect on cellular energetics (5). A more recent study suggest that the iron toxicity may be due to a redox cycling of the heme moiety from ferrous to ferric and to ferryl oxidation states (72).

The kidney may have its own system to contend with exposure to iron-containing heme pigments. Normally, iron is released from heme by the rate-limiting enzyme heme oxygenase, which acts by opening up the heme ring, generating iron and biliverdin. In turn, the liberated iron molecule can be taken up by ferritin, the major cellular repository for iron. Nath et al. (7) have demonstrated that the renal production of both heme oxidase and ferritin is increased in the glycerol-induced model of myohemoglobinuric acute renal failure. The increase in heme oxygenase and ferritin production is proposed to be an adaptive response on the part of the kidney on exposure to heme pigments and is a mechanism by which the kidney normally degrades heme and sequesters the potentially nephrotoxic iron. They noted that prior stimulation of the activity of heme oxygenase coupled with increased ferritin synthesis attenuated renal damage, whereas inhibition of the enzyme worsened renal function. This increased activity of heme oxygenase or possibly a broad-based proximal tubular cytoresistance (73) in the kidney may explain the experimental observation that, after induction of myohemoglobinuric acute renal failure, rechallenging the animals with a second dose of glycerol does not result in acute renal failure (74). One speculation is that in the setting of clinical myoglobin-induced acute renal failure, there may be factors contributing to inhibition of heme oxygenase and ferritin synthesis or a diminution in proximal tubular resistance, resulting in both accumulation of nephrotoxic iron and tubular necrosis.

Tubular Obstruction. Filling of the tubular lumen by pigmented casts that become inspissated and obstruct urinary flow with subsequent injury to tubular epithelium is one of the earliest mechanisms proposed to explain the nephrotoxicity of the heme pigments (75). In their original clinical description of rhabdomyolysis-induced acute renal failure, Bywaters and Beall (1) described the prominent histologic features, including the appearance of tubular obstruction by cellular debris and pigmented casts. It has been suggested that hypovolemia and acidemia and the concomitant acidic concentrated urine facilitate precipitation of filtered myoglobin or hemoglobin, leading to obstructive cast formation (76). The presence of Tamm-Horsfall protein in the tubular lumen is critical for heme protein cast formation in the distal nephron. Moreover, an obstructing cast induces urinary stasis, providing for an extended time for proximal tubular heme reabsorption and its attendant tubular toxicity, as noted previously (77). In addition, it has been speculated (43) that the increased urinary uric acid concentration observed in rhabdomyolysis (especially that caused by exertion) may result in uric acid precipitation in the tubules.

Tubular obstruction can decrease GFR either by increasing the tubular pressure and thus decreasing the glomerular transcapillary hydraulic pressure, or by inducing the release of factors (e.g., thromboxane) that cause renal vasoconstriction, thereby reducing glomerular blood flow. The importance of tubular obstruction as a possible mechanism of heme pigment–induced acute renal failure is suggested by the studies of Zager and colleagues (70,78) that explored the reasons why mannitol exerts a protective effect against this syndrome. They evaluated three hypotheses: (a) mannitol attenuates renal hypoperfusion, (b) mannitol scavenges hydroxyl free radicals, and (c) mannitol prevents intrarenal heme trapping and cast formation. The major beneficial effect of mannitol was attributed to its diuretic effect, which presumably decreased cast formation and proximal tubular uptake of heme proteins. Similarly, alkalinization of the urine may mitigate against myoglobinuric acute renal failure by increasing the solubility of myoglobin (reduced cast formation) and inducing a solute diuresis (76).

Although there is evidence that tubular obstruction may be a factor in the pathogenesis of the acute renal failure, it probably is not the primary cause of the initial decrease in GFR in myohemoglobinuric acute renal failure. Rather than high intratubular pressures from obstructing casts, intratubular pressures were found to be low in the glycerol-induced model of acute renal failure (50). This observation was interpreted to indicate that the presence of casts is the result, rather than the cause, of the decrease in GFR and urine flow. Instead of causing the initial decrease in renal function, cast formation may play a role in the maintenance of the renal failure once it develops (79).

Glomerular Fibrin Deposition. Because of the liberation of tissue factors, both rhabdomyolysis and intravascular hemolysis can initiate DIC (43). Fibrin strands have been demonstrated in glomeruli from patients (80) and experimental animals (81) with rhabdomyolysis-induced acute renal failure. Intravenous infusion of a muscle extract in rabbits resulted in DIC, renal dysfunction, and glomerular microthrombi, whereas an intravenous infusion of pure myoglobin had no untoward effect (82). This led to the conclusion that myoglobin, *per se*, is not the cause of the renal damage in the crush syndrome, but rather it is the release of other muscle constituents that induces DIC and the subsequent deposition of glomerular microthrombi that is responsible for rhabdomyolysis-induced acute renal failure.

Clinical and Laboratory Features of Rhabdomyolysis and Acute Renal Failure

The diagnosis of myoglobinuria can be suspected from history and physical examination but must be confirmed by laboratory testing. The diagnosis should be entertained in any patient with obvious muscle damage from trauma or ischemia in whom the involved region, usually an extremity, shows reddened overlying skin with local swelling and induration. In patients with rhabdomyolysis resulting from a drug overdose, these findings also are common. Less obvious is muscle involvement in cases of diffuse rhabdomyolysis, as from exertion, hypophosphatemia, or viral infections. In such patients, mild, diffuse muscle tenderness, or no tenderness at all, may mask the rhabdomyolysis and lead the examiner to dismiss the symptoms as resulting from viral myalgias (4). In one series (29), 50% of patients with rhabdomyolysis did not admit to the presence of muscle pain and only 5% had obvious muscle swelling on admission, thus emphasizing the importance of continued clinical inquiry, observation, and laboratory follow-up.

Risk Factors for Acute Renal Failure. The frequency of acute renal failure in the setting of rhabdomyolysis is unknown, and reports of frequency have ranged from 5% (4,83) to 33% (29). Gabow and colleagues (29) emphasized that no single laboratory value could predict which patients are at high risk for the development of acute renal failure. However, using discriminant analysis, patients could be separated into high- and low-risk groups, with the high-risk group (elevated serum potassium and creatinine and reduced serum albumin concentrations) having a 41% prevalence of acute renal failure.

Based on a large historical cohort (157 patients), Ward (84) identified clinical and laboratory differences between those patients in whom renal failure did or did not develop, and factors predictive of progression to renal failure. As shown in Table 49-2, patients with rhabdomyolysis and renal failure were older, had a higher incidence of hypertension, and were more hypotensive and dehydrated. A significantly greater proportion of them had a creatine kinase level greater than 16,000 IU/L, although as noted in the study, elevations to this degree were seen in 10.7% of patients in whom renal failure did not develop (Table 49-3). The renal failure group also had significantly higher serum potassium and phosphorus levels and lower serum calcium and albumin concentrations, and was more acidemic with a concomitant lower urinary pH. Sepsis, burns, and drug ingestion were the causes of rhabdomyolysis more closely associated with the development of renal failure. Using multiple logistic regression analysis, a scoring system was developed predicting the risk of renal failure in patients with rhabdomyolysis based on the variables of serum phosphorus, potassium, albumin, and creatine kinase concentrations, and the presence of dehydration and sepsis. A point score of 7 or greater predicted a greater than 50% likelihood for development of renal failure. In a more recent multivariate analysis of 72 consecutive patients with rhabdomyolysis due to illicit drug use, patients with a creatine kinase greater than 25,000 U/L, hypotension, and leukocytosis were at a greater risk of developing acute renal failure, whereas hyperthermia (temperature >38.5°C) was associated with a reduced risk (85).

TABLE 49-2

UNIVARIATE ANALYSIS OF CLINICAL VARIABLES IN PATIENTS WITH RHABDOMYOLYSIS DEVELOPING AND NOT DEVELOPING RENAL FAILURE

Variables	Group		
	Renal failure (N = 26)	Nonrenal failure (N = 131)	p^a
Age, yr (SD)	53.7 ± 20.6	41.4 ± 18.1	0.002
Male (%)	69.2	61.1	0.418
Hypertension (%)	46.2	22.9	0.026
Diabetes mellitus (%)	11.5	7.6	0.562
Previous renal disease (%)	19.2	3.8	0.051
Dehydration (%)	38.5	4.6	0.001
Hypotension (%)	34.6	14.5	0.040
Nephrotoxin exposure (%)	19.2	39.7	0.020
Diuretic use (%)	30.8	16.8	0.147
Nonsteroid drug use (%)	19.2	6.1	0.101
IV hydration (%)^b	80.7	54.2	0.289
Osmotic treatment (%)	26.9	22.9	0.674
Bicarbonate treatment (%)	50.0	12.2	0.001

^{a}p value for difference in means or proportions between renal failure and nonrenal failure groups.
^{b}>150 mL/hr averaged over the first 24 hr after admission. IV indicates intravenous.

Urinalysis. Examination of the urine provides the first laboratory clue to the presence of myoglobinuria. Classically, the initial urine is dark (Table 49-4) and usually with an acid pH; the benzidine or orthotoluidine reagent gives a positive reaction for blood, (3+ to 4+), but microscopic examination of the urinary sediment fails to reveal any red blood cells (RBCs) or, at best, only a few (less than five per high-power field), indicating the presence of a heme pigment not contained in RBCs. This could result from hemoglobin released from RBCs lysed in the urine, but more likely reflects myoglobin excreted by glomerular filtration. Specific tests for urine myoglobin determination are available in some clinical laboratories but, as noted earlier, urine myoglobin levels are not the most sensitive clinical markers for rhabdomyolysis. Although the strongest clinical clue for myoglobinuria is the presence of a strongly heme-positive urine and the absence of RBCs, in one major series (29), hematuria was present in 32%, and the dipstick was heme negative in 18% of the patients with rhabdomyolysis. In addition, proteinuria was detected by dipstick in 45% of

patients (29), which may be attributed to altered glomerular permeability or tubular transport of small proteins (86). The urinary sediment demonstrates brown "debris" and, with the evolution of renal injury, pigmented brown granular casts and renal tubular epithelial cells are seen with great frequency.

Serum Potassium Concentration. The most life-threatening consequence of rhabdomyolysis is the release of large amounts of intracellular potassium into the circulation. Because more than 98% of total body potassium resides in cells, and skeletal muscle represents 60% to 70% of the total cellular mass, breakdown of even a small area of skeletal muscle releases a considerable potassium load. The presence of acidosis may shift more potassium extracellularly and worsen the hyperkalemia. As noted in the section on Risk Factors for Acute Renal Failure, above, admission serum potassium levels tend to be higher in the patients who go on to experience acute renal failure (84). Approximately half of an acute potassium load is handled by renal excretion (87,88); therefore, in acute renal failure, serious

TABLE 49-3

UNIVARIATE ANALYSIS OF LABORATORY VARIABLES IN PATIENTS WITH RHABDOMYOLYSIS DEVELOPING AND NOT DEVELOPING RENAL FAILURE

Variables	Group		
	Renal failure (N = 20)	Nonrenal failure (N = 131)	p
Peak creatine kinase >16,000 U/L, %	57.7	10.7	<0.001
Serum bicarbonate (mmol/L)	21.4 ± 7.2	23.7 ± 4.0	0.1306
Serum potassium (mmol/L)	4.73 ± 1.2	3.92 ± 0.6	0.0018
Serum phosphorus (mmol/L)	1.85 ± 1.08	0.06 ± 0.35	0.0006
Serum calcium (mmol/L)	2.02 ± 0.4	2.14 ± 0.2	0.1452
Serum albumin (g/L)	30.8 ± 10.0	35.9 ± 8.0	0.0107
Arterial pH	7.33 ± 0.10	7.38 ± 0.11	0.0495
Urinary pH	5.19 ± 0.06	5.75 ± 1.0	0.0009

All values are mean SD except peak creatine kinase.

TABLE 49-4

DIFFERENTIAL DIAGNOSIS OF PIGMENTURIA

Factors	Myoglobinuria	Hemoglobinuria	Porphyria
Urine color	Brown	Reddish-brown	Dark red
Serum color	Clear	Pink	Clear
Orthotoluidine reaction	Positive	Positive	Negative
Watson-Schwartz porphobilinogen	Negative	Negative	Positive
Muscle pain/tenderness	Present	Absent	Absent
Serum creatine kinase level	Elevated	Normal	Normal
Serum haptoglobin	Normal	Decreased	Normal

(Reprinted from: Schultze VE. Rhabdomyolysis as a cause of acute renal failure. *Postgrad Med* 1982;72:145, with permission.)

hyperkalemia can result and is usually the major indication for dialysis.

Creatine Kinase. The relatively slower clearance of creatine kinase compared with myoglobin makes this enzyme level a more sensitive marker of muscle injury (44). Although no correlation has been established between the absolute level of the creatine kinase and the risk for development of acute renal failure, creatine kinase levels are significantly higher in the patients in whom renal failure develops (89). It has been stated anecdotally that it is unusual to see acute renal failure develop in patients with serum creatine kinase levels less than 3,000 IU/L (90,91). Following serial serum creatine kinase levels is crucial to monitoring patients with rhabdomyolysis, inasmuch as the concentration of creatine kinase may continue to increase after admission to the hospital, reflecting ongoing or worsening muscle necrosis. Increasing or decreasing creatine kinase concentrations provide some insight into whether the rhabdomyolysis is worsening or resolving, and following these levels is essential to observe for the "second wave" phenomenon (see later).

Acid–Base Balance. The conditions that cause rhabdomyolysis involve tissue trauma or ischemia and predispose the patient to an augmented acid load. In the study by Ward (84), the patients with rhabdomyolysis who progressed to renal failure tended to be significantly more acidemic. An elevated serum anion gap is usual in patients with rhabdomyolysis and is due to impaired renal excretion of intracellular organic acids released from damaged muscles (92), as well as retention of inorganic anions such as phosphate.

Uric Acid. Hyperuricemia is expected in patients with rhabdomyolysis, especially when the muscle injury is due to strenuous exercise or exertion. The increase in uric acid levels is due to the release of intracellular purines from damaged muscle cells, which are converted to uric acid in the liver (43).

Blood Urea Nitrogen: Creatinine Ratio. The rate of rise of serum creatinine relative to the rise in blood urea nitrogen (BUN) is often disproportionately greater in rhabdomyolysis-induced acute renal failure compared with other causes of acute renal failure. This phenomenon has been attributed to the release of large quantities of creatine from damaged muscles and the subsequent conversion of the creatine to creatinine, resulting in a more rapid increase in the serum creatinine concentration (4,48). Based on creatine:creatinine kinetics and their respective concentrations in skeletal muscle, Oh (93) has challenged this conventional view. He has pointed out that the pa-

tient population in which rhabdomyolysis develops tends to have a larger percentage of younger men with a greater muscle mass, whereas other forms of acute renal failure are more often associated with older and more cachectic patients who have less muscle mass and thus reduced creatinine production rates.

Calcium–Phosphorus Metabolism. The perturbations of calcium and phosphorus metabolism usually seen in most types of acute renal failure appear to be exaggerated in rhabdomyolysis-induced acute renal failure (94). Muscle damage leads to breakdown of intracellular phosphate compounds and release of large quantities of inorganic phosphorus into the circulation, resulting in hyperphosphatemia. This abnormality is accentuated when acute renal failure develops owing to impaired urinary excretion. Hypocalcemia also occurs early in the course of myoglobin-induced acute renal failure (29); its pathogenesis has been attributed to a number of mechanisms. Early observations by Meroney et al. (95) suggested that the hypocalcemia may be due to the deposition of calcium salts in the damaged muscles. Using electron radiography and technetium-99m diphosphonate scans, Akmal et al. (96) provided evidence of deposits of calcium in the damaged muscles of patients during the oliguric phase of myoglobinuric acute renal failure. When renal function improved, the calcium deposits disappeared. They concluded that, initially, the damaged muscles serve as a nidus for calcium deposition (dystrophic calcification), which is accentuated by the concomitant hyperphosphatemia and elevated calcium–phosphorus product. Subsequently, during the recovery phase of acute renal failure as GFR increases, the concentration of phosphorus and resultant calcium–phosphorus product decrease. This permits the release of the sequestered calcium deposits back into the circulation, leading to an increased serum calcium concentration, sometimes to the point of hypercalcemia.

More recently, it has been suggested that the hypocalcemia may be due to abnormalities of vitamin D and parathyroid hormone metabolism. Very low levels of 1,25-dihydroxycholecalciferol ($1,25[OH]_2D_3$) and high levels of parathyroid hormone have been noted during the oliguric phase of myoglobinuric acute renal failure (97,98). This may be due, in part, to the hyperphosphatemia associated with rhabdomyolysis, inasmuch as hyperphosphatemia has been demonstrated to reduce the renal synthesis of $1,25(OH)_2D_3$ and stimulate the production of parathyroid hormone (99). Thus, the hypocalcemia of myoglobin-induced acute renal failure may be due both to a deficiency of $1,25(OH)_2D_3$ and to concomitant skeletal resistance to parathyroid hormone (97). Regardless of the mechanism, in the absence of frank tetany, hypocalcemia usually does not require treatment. In fact, correction of the hypocalcemia with vigorous intravenous calcium replacement may increase both dystrophic (calcium deposition in the damaged muscle) and metastatic calcification.

Approximately 20% to 30% of patients with myoglobinuric acute renal failure experience transient hypercalcemia during the recovery (diuretic) phase of their acute tubular necrosis (4,83). Early studies (4,83,96) suggested that the hypercalcemia was due to an augmentation of the normal remobilization of the calcium deposits in the injured muscle that occurs during the recovery phase of acute renal failure. Alternatively, it has been proposed that as renal function improves, the combination of a decreasing serum phosphorus concentration and the ambient secondary hyperparathyroidism stimulates the synthesis of $1,25(OH)_2D_3$, resulting in an "overshoot" hypercalcemia (97,100,101). This augmented $1,25(OH)_2D_3$ production may be due, in part, to release of vitamin D from damaged muscle tissue (102).

Urinary Sodium Excretion. Impaired renal tubular reabsorption of sodium is typically seen in most types of oliguric acute renal failure as manifested by a high fractional excretion of sodium. However, in both myoglobinuric and hemoglobinuric acute renal failure, a low fractional excretion of sodium ($<1\%$) has been observed (54). As noted earlier in this chapter, hypovolemia and renal ischemia are important factors in the development of renal failure in heme pigment–induced acute renal failure, and thus the increased sodium avidity may be due to renal hypoperfusion. In addition to this mechanism, it is known that tubular obstruction and urinary tract obstruction are associated transiently with a low fractional excretion of sodium; therefore, this also may be a factor contributing to the augmented sodium reabsorption (103,104). A low fractional excretion of sodium is not seen in all cases of myoglobinuric and hemoglobinuric acute renal failure, however, and the presence of a low fractional excretion of sodium does not indicate less severe renal injury.

Disseminated Intravascular Coagulation. Disseminated intravascular coagulation is commonly present in patients with rhabdomyolysis and may be due to the release of intracellular thromboplastins that activate the clotting cascade (43). Moreover, DIC may be an important factor in the pathogenesis of the acute renal failure (see section on Glomerular Fibrin Deposition, above).

Differential Diagnosis

Myoglobin-induced acute renal failure should be suspected in patients subjected to trauma presenting with the classic triad of heme-positive urine, an elevated serum creatine kinase level, and dark (pigmented) urine containing dirty-brown granular casts. More subtle cases, usually associated with diffuse, nontraumatic rhabdomyolysis, may be more difficult to detect. The differential diagnosis of pigmenturia is limited (Table 49-4). Although certain drugs may impart an orange, red, or brown hue to the urine, they do not react with the benzidine or orthotoluidine reagent on the urine dipstick. Among such agents are rifampin, phenazopyridine (Pyridium), nitrofurantoin, and some sulfa compounds. Porphyrins also color the urine brown but do not react to give a positive test for occult blood. The most difficult challenge is to discriminate myoglobin from hemoglobin in the urine. Because these are heme compounds, they both react with the benzidine or orthotoluidine reagent and both are associated with the absence of RBCs in the urine sediment. One helpful clue may be the color of the serum in these two conditions. Because myoglobin is relatively rapidly cleared by the kidney, serum levels of myoglobin are not sufficiently elevated to alter the color of the serum in patients with rhabdomyolysis.

In contrast, because of its much larger size and its avid binding to haptoglobin, hemoglobin is not as rapidly cleared by the kidney, and serum levels may be high enough to result in a pink discoloration of the serum in patients with hemoglobinuria.

Clinical Course and Complications of Myoglobinuric Acute Renal Failure

Myoglobinuric acute renal failure can run a course ranging from mild renal dysfunction with only transient oliguria and quick recovery to a much more catastrophic disease requiring frequent dialysis for periods of 2 or 3 weeks. Typically, the duration of oliguria is 7 to 10 days; during this interval, patients may excrete virtually no urine for up to 3 days at a time. Resumption of more normal urine formation heralds the recovery of renal function as patients enter the diuretic phase, with subsequent clearing of azotemia and a cessation of the requirement for hemodialysis.

In addition to muscle injury and acute renal failure, patients with rhabdomyolysis may have peripheral neuropathies. These can result from compartment syndromes in which involved muscle becomes edematous in confined tissue spaces with compromise of blood supply to both muscle and nerves in the area (96). Measurement of tissue pressure has been advocated as a tool in identifying those areas of damaged muscle at risk; surgical fasciotomy may be required to avoid this complication (13). The swelling of the muscles can lead to an impairment in the blood supply of the muscles, resulting in a recurrence or "second wave" of muscle necrosis as reflected by a second rise in the serum creatine kinase concentration (43). Neuropathy also can result from traction if rhabdomyolysis is caused by prolonged coma, as from drug overdose (13).

Prevention and Treatment of Myoglobinuric Acute Renal Failure

In addition to their landmark description of the medical consequences of the "crush syndrome" and implication of myoglobin as a nephrotoxin, Bywaters and colleagues in 1941 (1) were one of earliest groups to recognize the benefits of brisk alkaline fluid resuscitation in victims of crush injuries to mitigate the development of acute renal failure. They demonstrated that prompt and early oral and intravenous administration of fluids containing sodium salts of bicarbonate, lactate, and citrate dramatically reduced mortality rates and the development of renal injury in victims of the blitz of London (6). The rationale for this therapy was based on their notion that both an augmentation of urinary flow and an increase in the urine pH would facilitate the clearance and minimize the nephrotoxicity of myoglobin. As is discussed later, the current recommended therapy to prevent acute renal failure in the setting of rhabdomyolysis has not changed appreciably since Bywaters and colleagues' original recommendations.

Understanding the possible mechanisms by which rhabdomyolysis causes acute renal failure can provide the basis for the various therapies that have been advocated for this disorder. Because hypovolemia and renal ischemia are important factors in the pathogenesis of myoglobinuric acute renal failure, it has long been recognized that early and vigorous intravenous fluid therapy is important in attenuating renal injury. Based on the notion that myoglobin is more nephrotoxic at an acid pH (increased formation of ferrihemate; see earlier), most groups advocate the addition of sodium bicarbonate to the intravenous fluids for alkalinization of the urine (8–11,91). By correcting cellular acidosis, bicarbonate therapy may reduce renal tubular epithelial swelling and attenuate renal tubular and vascular collapse (105). Further, this therapy may ameliorate the hyperkalemia commonly seen in rhabdomyolysis. There is a theoretical concern that inducing a metabolic alkalosis with such treatment may enhance metastatic calcification, but the salutary benefit of bicarbonate therapy probably outweighs any untoward effect (9).

Mannitol has long been recognized to be an effective agent in the prophylaxis against the development of experimental and clinical acute renal failure, and has been used in combination with fluid/alkaline therapy to prevent renal injury in patients with rhabdomyolysis. Potential beneficial effects of mannitol include (a) a decrease in blood viscosity and oncotic pressure across the glomerulus, causing an increase in GFR; (b) dilatation of glomerular capillaries and stimulation of prostaglandin release; (c) increase in urine flow and prevention of obstructing cast formation; (d) reduction in renal tubular epithelial swelling and injury; and (e) scavenging of oxygen free radicals (8). In addition, mannitol may have extrarenal benefits, including (a) extracellular volume expansion, (b) increased cardiac contractility, (c) increased release of atrial natriuretic factor, and (d) reduction in skeletal muscle cell edema and decompression of muscle tamponade (8,106).

Furosemide, a loop-acting diuretic, has the theoretic advantage of inhibiting sodium transport in the thick ascending limb of Henle's loop. Oxygen consumption is dictated primarily by the rate of sodium transport, and a precarious balance exists in this segment between the rate of oxygen delivery and its consumption (107). By inhibiting sodium transport, furosemide may reduce oxygen consumption in the face of limited delivery and thereby preserve cell viability. In addition, the augmented urinary flow induced by the diuretic may reduce the risk of tubular obstruction. Loop diuretics, however, have the theoretic disadvantage of increasing acidification of the urine, worsening intravascular volume depletion, and inducing ototoxicity, and thus the use of these agents has not been generally recommended (8,9,90).

Plasma exchange therapy (108) and continuous hemodiafiltration (109) have been performed in patients with rhabdomyolysis for the purpose of removing myoglobin to prevent renal failure. These studies are anecdotal and have not shown a demonstrable benefit.

Although there are no controlled trials to show a direct benefit of a forced alkaline–mannitol diuresis in the prevention of acute renal failure in rhabdomyolysis, there are many case reports suggesting such therapy was instrumental in averting renal injury (11,91,110). Adequate fluid hydration and bicarbonate therapy, however, did not ameliorate the development of renal failure in a large retrospective study (84). Moreover, in a recent retrospective evaluation of 382 ICU trauma admissions with a creatine kinase of >5,000 U/L, the use of bicarbonate and mannitol in 40% of this group had no effect on rates of renal failure, need for dialysis, and mortality, although there was a trend to lower mortality rate in patients with creatine kinase greater than 30,000 I/U treated with bicarbonate and mannitol (111). The Divisions of Nephrology at San Francisco General Hospital and at the University of California, Davis Medical Center recommend the infusion of both mannitol and sodium bicarbonate in most cases of myoglobinuria. Initially, optimization of intravascular fluid volume deficits should be carried out with dispatch using isotonic crystalloid solutions, usually normal saline. Variables useful in following this course of therapy include physical examination of the state of the circulation, hematocrit, and recording of external fluid balance. If the clinical assessment suggests that a euvolemic state has been achieved but no improvement in oliguria has occurred, the decision must be made about further intervention. Usually by this time, laboratory results offer further support for the diagnosis of myoglobinuria and acute renal insufficiency, and we recommend the prompt infusion of a mannitol–bicarbonate solution. This is made by adding two ampules, each containing 12.5 g mannitol in 50 mL, and two ampules of 50 mEq $NaHCO_3$ in 50 mL to 800 mL of 5% dextrose in water for

intravenous infusion. This reconstituted liter is roughly isosmotic with plasma once the glucose is metabolized and contains both mannitol and 100 mEq $NaHCO_3$. It should be infused at 250 mL/hour; urine flow rate should increase by the end of the 4-hour infusion if the treatment is successful. If this is the case, the solution should continue to be administered at a rate equal to urine output and sufficient to achieve a urine pH greater than 6.5 until such time as azotemia has started to clear and all evidence of myoglobinuria has disappeared. If urine flow does not increase after the 4-hour infusion, the patient has entered the established phase of oliguric acute renal failure and should be treated conservatively until dialysis can be arranged, based on conventional criteria. This approach corrected oliguria, hastened the clearing of azotemia, and avoided the need for dialysis in roughly half of patients with myoglobinuric acute renal failure (91). As a group, these patients had somewhat lower indices of muscle damage and somewhat better preservation of renal function than the half that did not respond. Whether this reflects earlier intervention or a less severe degree of muscle injury, or both, is not known, and it also is possible that vigorous volume expansion with normal saline alone might have caused the same result in some patients. Given that complications from the mannitol–bicarbonate infusion are few, even in those patients who do not respond, its use should be seriously entertained in patients with myoglobin-induced acute renal failure.

When acute renal failure has become established, dialysis must be used. Early and intensive hemodialysis may be associated with significantly lower morbidity and mortality rates (112). Experience with peritoneal dialysis indicated that solute clearance using this modality was inadequate to keep pace with the rapid rate of solute appearance in these highly catabolic patients (113) and, thus, hemodialysis should be the modality of treatment. Even so, daily hemodialysis often is required for the first several days until the consequences of extensive muscle injury have abated and rates of urea and potassium accumulation have fallen. Thereafter, a schedule of thrice-weekly dialysis usually is adequate unless other factors, such as continued catabolism from infection or surgical wound debridement, or volume overload from parenteral nutritional therapy demand more frequent treatments. The prognosis for the renal failure is good, and full recovery of function is the rule. However, the ultimate prognosis for the patient probably depends more on other coexisting conditions such as sepsis, bleeding, and respiratory failure.

Hemoglobinuric Acute Renal Failure

Compared with the frequency of myoglobinuric acute renal failure, hemoglobinuric acute renal failure is an uncommon event. This is because the most common cause of hemoglobinuric acute renal failure is intravascular hemolysis from mismatched blood transfusions, and with modern blood banking techniques, such untoward events are rare. An additional point to emphasize in this regard is that significant hemoglobinuria and renal failure are seen primarily in the setting of major intravascular hemolysis. During most types of extravascular hemolysis, the released hemoglobin is quickly taken up by the reticuloendothelial system and metabolized to bilirubin. Thus, extravascular hemolysis rarely results in acute renal failure.

Causes of Hemoglobinuria

Hemoglobinuria results from filtration of free hemoglobin in plasma, due almost exclusively to intravascular hemolysis, which occurs in a variety of conditions (Table 49-5). Although each of the listed causes may be associated with acute

TABLE 49-5

CAUSES OF HEMOGLOBINURIA AND ACUTE RENAL FAILURE

Genetic defects
Glucose-6-phosphate dehydrogenase deficiency
Paroxysmal cold hemoglobinuria
March hemoglobinuria
Infection
Malaria
Clostridia
Transfusion reactions
Chemical agents
Arsine
Glycerol
Quinine sulfate
Analine
Benzene
Hydralazine
Fava beans
Cresol
Sodium chlorate
Methyl chloride
Coal tar products
Venoms
Rattlesnake, copperhead, water moccasin, coral snake
Tarantula
Brown recluse spider
Traumatic/mechanical destruction
Prosthetic valves
Disseminated intravascular coagulation
Extracorporeal circulation
Miscellaneous
Heat stroke
White phosphorus
Hemoglobin infusions

(Reprinted from: Dubrow A, Flamenbaum W. Acute renal failure associated with myoglobinuria and hemoglobinuria. In: Brenner BM, Lazarus JM, eds. *Acute renal failure*, 2nd ed. New York: Churchill Livingstone, 1988:285, with permission.)

renal dysfunction, hemoglobinuria is more likely to occur in only a few settings. These are hemolytic transfusion reactions (114–116), DIC (117), march hemoglobinuria (118), and infections with clostridia (119,120) and *Plasmodium falciparum* malaria, the latter causing blackwater fever (121–124). In addition, infusion of hemoglobin solutions as a plasma volume expander has been noted to cause acute renal dysfunction owing to associated hemoglobinuria (125).

Hemoglobin Physiology and Metabolism

Hemoglobin has a molecular weight of 68,000 daltons and is a tetramer of two α and two β globin chains surrounding a ferrihemate core. As noted earlier, free hemoglobin in plasma is tightly bound to haptoglobin, and the hemoglobin–haptoglobin complex is too large to be filtered by the glomerulus. Thus, free hemoglobin appears in the urine only after the plasma concentration of hemoglobin exceeds the maximum binding capacity of haptoglobin, which is approximately 100 mg/dL (in contrast to 1.5 mg/dL for myoglobin). In the setting of intravascular hemolysis, the relatively low renal clearance of hemoglobin (fractional clearance relative to inulin, 0.03) results in an increase in plasma hemoglobin levels sufficient to be visible to the naked eye as pink-colored plasma, whereas with rhabdomyolysis, the rapid renal clear-

ance of myoglobin (fractional clearance, 0.75) prevents myoglobin retention in the plasma and the plasma color is not visibly altered. The color of the plasma is an important "bedside" clue that helps to distinguish between these two forms of pigmenturia.

Clinical and Laboratory Features of Hemoglobinuric Acute Renal Failure

As with myoglobin, the mechanisms by which hemoglobin causes acute renal failure are not clearly understood. Because both are heme-containing compounds and the heme moiety has been implicated as a major factor in inducing renal injury, it is generally accepted that the mechanisms by which they both cause nephrotoxicity are similar, if not the same. As with myoglobinuric acute renal failure, clinical experience indicates that coexistent compromise of renal function from volume depletion, acidosis, or hypotension must be present for hemoglobinuric acute renal failure to develop. Moreover, in the clinical settings most commonly associated with it, other pathogenetic mechanisms have been proposed to account for the acute renal failure. For example, with hemolytic transfusion reactions, the interaction of antigens on the red cell stroma with preformed antibodies may be responsible for adverse effects on kidney function (116). In DIC, afferent arteriole and glomerular capillary fibrin deposition are the events most directly related to acute renal failure (117). March hemoglobinuria occurs from traumatic hemolysis of RBCs, most likely in people with a genetic susceptibility (118); acute renal failure in this setting results from volume depletion as well as hemoglobinuria. In blackwater fever, hemolysis is caused by the abrupt release of *falciparum* trophozoites and perhaps also from the quinine used to treat it (121–124). These patients are dehydrated and volume depleted from sweating and high fevers. Clostridial sepsis also has multiple effects on renal function, including hypotension, acidosis, and DIC, as well as hemolysis (119,120).

Laboratory features of intravascular hemolysis and hemoglobinuria include (a) increased serum lactate dehydrogenase (LDH) levels, (b) low serum haptoglobin levels, (c) increased unconjugated (indirect) serum bilirubin, (d) increased reticulocyte count, and (e) hyperkalemia. As with myoglobinuria, hemoglobinuria and hemoglobinuric acute renal failure are associated with pigmented urinary casts. The differential diagnosis and clinical course of hemoglobin-induced acute renal failure are similar to those described for myoglobinuria.

Prevention and Treatment of Hemoglobinuric Acute Renal Failure

Prevention of hemoglobinuric acute renal failure involves many of the same preventative measures for myoglobinuric acute renal failure, such as correcting volume depletion and the administration of mannitol and bicarbonate. In fact, Bywaters' therapy to treat crush injuries using saline and bicarbonate in the 1940s was based on earlier reports demonstrating such therapy was beneficial in preventing renal failure in mismatched blood transfusion reactions (6). In an experimental animal model of hemoglobinuric acute renal failure, the simultaneous administration of the amino acid, lysine, prevented the development of acute renal failure. This was attributed to the ability of lysine to inhibit proximal tubular reabsorption of hemoglobin or its heme moiety (126). The clinical utility of such therapy remains to be determined.

Management of sustained acute renal failure usually requires hemodialysis. These patients in general are less catabolic than patients with rhabdomyolysis. The acute renal failure usually lasts 1 to 2 weeks, but full recovery of renal function can be expected.

CRYSTALLINE ACUTE RENAL FAILURE

Uric Acid Nephropathy

Acute uric acid nephropathy is the term given to the development of acute renal failure caused by renal tubular obstruction by urate and uric acid crystals. The main clinical setting in which uric acid nephropathy occurs is the treatment of malignancy, especially of leukemia and lymphoma. Treatment of these malignancies results in cell death and release of large amounts of uric acid precursors. Some patients with these malignancies also have renal insufficiency and high serum uric acid levels before chemotherapy, possibly because of early uric acid nephropathy on the one hand, and the rapidly dividing cell population on the other (127).

Properties of Uric Acid

The final breakdown product of purine degradation in humans is uric acid (Fig. 49-2). Most other mammals degrade purines to the soluble end product allantoin, but humans lack the enzyme uricase. Uric acid (2,6,8-trioxypurine) is a weak acid with a pK_a of 5.75. Urates are the ionized form of uric acid, and at a physiologic pH of 7.4, over 95% of uric acid dissociates into urates, with 98% existing as monosodium urate. However, uric acid predominates in an acid urine. Although initial *in vitro* and *in vivo* studies had shown urate binding to plasma proteins, urate binding to human serum proteins probably is not significant (128–130).

At a temperature of 37°C and a plasma pH of 7.40, the saturation point of urate is at a concentration of 8.8 mg/dL, which is only slightly above the normal physiologic range in humans (131). However, urate crystal precipitation in the bloodstream does not occur even with concentrations much higher than the saturation point. Urates form stable supersaturated solutions in plasma, possibly because of solubilizing substances (128,132). On the other hand, precipitation of urate occurs in extracellular fluid when the solubility concentration is exceeded. The most important factor affecting the solubility of uric acid is pH. For example, in a buffer medium at a pH of 5.0, saturation with uric acid occurs at a concentration below 10 mg/dL, whereas at a pH above 7.0, saturation occurs at a concentration above 150 mg/dL (131).

There are four components to the renal handling of urate. First, urate is filtered freely at the glomerulus. Virtually all of this filtered urate is then reabsorbed in the proximal tubule. An amount equal to 50% is then secreted, and after further absorption, 10% is finally excreted (133,134). Animal data have provided evidence for this bidirectional transport of urate, although net transport differs among species. In humans, there is net reabsorption of urate with the fractional excretion of urate being approximately 10%, whereas in rabbits there is net secretion with the fractional excretion of urate being over 100% (135). Animal micropuncture studies have localized the primary nephron site of urate absorption and secretion to the proximal tubule (135–137). An anion exchanger and a

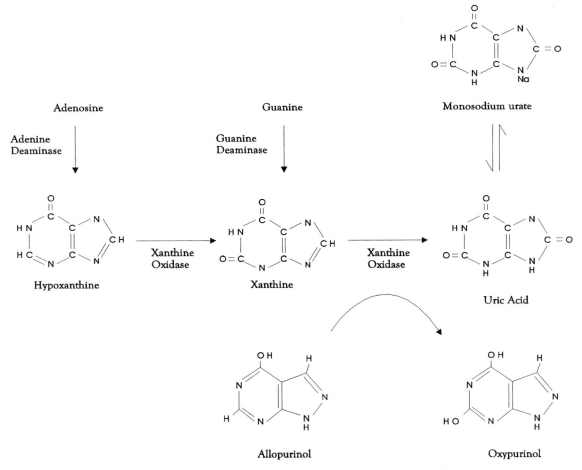

FIGURE 49-2. Pathway of purine degradation showing the competitive inhibition of urate formation by allopurinol and the site of action of rasburicase.

voltage-dependent pathway seem to be the mechanisms involved in urate transport (138,139).

Pathogenesis of Uric Acid Nephropathy

Experimental animal models of uric acid nephropathy are characterized by hyperuricemia, hyperuricosuria, and uric acid deposits in and dilation of the kidney tubules, as observed in the clinical entity (140). Along with the presence of extensive distal tubule deposits of uric acid and urate, micropuncture studies in the rat have shown increased proximal and distal tubular pressures. The vasa recti also show deposits, and efferent arteriolar and peritubular capillary pressures also are increased (141). In this model, uric acid nephropathy was prevented by maintaining a high tubular fluid flow, and only a modest benefit was shown by alkalinization of the urine (142).

Humans with malignancies and hyperuricemia have an increased urinary excretion rate and urinary concentration of uric acid both in the presence and absence of renal insufficiency (143). Autopsy studies have documented the presence of uric acid crystals in patients with leukemia. The uric acid crystals were found only within the lumens of renal tubules, in contrast to patients with gout, in whom no uric acid crystals were found in tubular lumens (144,145). In addition, internal hydronephrosis has been described in association with the intraluminal uric acid crystals, but the glomeruli and tubules usually are intact (146). Supporting the concept that mechanical intraluminal obstruction causes uric acid nephropathy are the observations that the renal failure reverses after a short time and that there is earlier and greater depression of inulin clearance compared with p-aminohippurate clearance (146). This evidence is consistent with the concept that uric acid nephropathy occurs because of uric acid crystals obstructing the renal tubular segments with maximum acidifying and concentrating abilities, namely, the distal tubule and collecting duct. The obstruction then leads to increased intraluminal pressure, decreased filtration pressure, and a reduction in GFR.

Clinical and Laboratory Manifestations

The initial reports of uric acid nephropathy focused on patients treated for acute lymphoblastic leukemia, 10% of whom had uric acid nephropathy (146). In these early patient series, risk factors for uric acid nephropathy included urine pH less than 5.0, dehydration, rapid response to chemotherapy, elevated serum uric acid, increased urinary excretion of uric acid, and preexisting renal insufficiency (145–147). Tumor lysis syndrome and acute uric acid nephropathy develop primarily during the treatment of leukemia and lymphoma, but can also occur in association with the treatment of other types of malignancies or in other situations associated with elevated plasma level and urinary excretion of uric acid. Metastatic breast carcinoma, bronchogenic carcinoma, disseminated adenocarcinoma, pancreatic carcinoma, and other nonhematopoietic neoplasms have been reported to cause acute uric acid nephropathy and tumor lysis syndrome (148–154). In addition to myoglobinuria, elevated serum uric acid concentration and increased renal excretion of uric acid are thought to play a role in the etiology of the renal failure caused by heat stress (155). Hyperuricemic acute renal failure also has been reported after epileptic seizures, during pregnancy, and in the setting of cyclosporine use and renal transplantation (156–158).

Uric acid nephropathy during tumor lysis syndrome is characterized by elevations in serum urea nitrogen, creatinine, potassium, uric acid, and phosphate concentrations, and by a decrease in the serum calcium concentration. Hyperuricemia before chemotherapy occurs in 30% to 50% of patients with leukemia and lymphoma, and renal insufficiency seems to be more common in patients with hyperuricemia before chemotherapy (127,147). Before the routine use of aggressive prophylactic measures, patients with uric acid nephropathy presented with serum uric acid levels of 20 to 80 mg/dL, but although most patients still present with uric acid levels greater than 8.0 mg/dL, uric acid concentrations in most patients can be normalized before chemotherapy with allopurinol, alkalinization, and diuresis (127,159). Patients receiving chemotherapy are at risk for other forms of renal failure in addition to acute uric acid nephropathy, and the urinary uric acid-to-creatinine ratio is a useful test to differentiate these various forms of renal failure. A ratio greater than 1 is consistent with acute uric acid nephropathy (160). This is supported by the observation that both the serum uric acid concentration and the urinary excretion of uric acid are elevated in acute uric acid nephropathy as opposed to other forms of renal failure, where serum uric acid concentrations may be high but urinary excretion is not elevated (161). The urinary uric acid-to-creatinine ratio is more helpful in the diagnosis of uric acid nephropathy than urinalysis, which usually is nondiagnostic. The urine sediment may be normal or occasionally reveal amorphous material containing uric acid crystals (150,160). Uric acid crystals appear as rhomboid crystals or as microcrystallites (Fig. 49-3).

Elevations in BUN and serum creatinine typically develop 2 days after the initiation of chemotherapy, with return to baseline after 7 to 10 days. Prior renal insufficiency seems to predispose to the development of uric acid nephropathy (162,163). The acute renal failure is usually of the oliguric variety, even when treated with diuretics (163). When indicated, dialysis usually is initiated within the first week from the start of chemotherapy, but only one to four dialysis treatments usually are required before the spontaneous return of renal function (159,163).

As noted previously, the electrolyte abnormalities associated with the tumor lysis syndrome and uric acid nephropathy are hyperkalemia, hyperphosphatemia, and hypocalcemia. These abnormalities result from the release of intracellular contents after tumor necrosis, and patients with large tumor burdens are at higher risk for tumor lysis syndrome (127). Hyperkalemia actually occurs in less than 5% of patients after chemotherapy, but if it develops, it can occur within 24 hours of initiation of chemotherapy and can be severe enough to necessitate emergent dialysis. In fact, sudden death has been reported as a consequence of tumor lysis–induced hyperkalemia, occurring within 48 hours of chemotherapy (164). Hyperkalemia also is more likely to occur in patients with preexisting renal insufficiency (127,162,163).

Hyperphosphatemia, on the other hand, is very common in the tumor lysis syndrome, and occurs in virtually all patients in whom acute renal failure develops and in 30% of patients with normal renal function (127). The development of hyperphosphatemia also is correlated with the tumor burden (127). In patients with renal failure, the phosphorus concentrations average 12 mg/dL, with a range of 7 to 22 mg/dL (127,162,163). Hypocalcemia also is common, and development of hypocalcemia correlates with hyperphosphatemia (127,159). In the presence of hyperphosphatemia, the etiology of hypocalcemia may be the precipitation of calcium phosphate salts, as discussed in the section on Myoglobinuric Acute Renal Failure, above; when this occurs in the kidney, it may contribute to the acute renal failure seen in tumor lysis syndrome (165,166). Hyperphosphatemia also may contribute to the development of hypocalcemia by depressing the production of $1,25(OH)_2D_3$, as was discussed earlier. Hyperphosphatemia has been shown to worsen experimental acute renal failure, but the mechanism is not clear because calcium phosphate deposition could not be demonstrated in the rat kidneys (167). Calcium deposits have been found at autopsy in the calices and tubules of a patient who had acute renal failure in association with tumor lysis syndrome, hyperphosphatemia (20 mg/dL), and hypocalcemia (168).

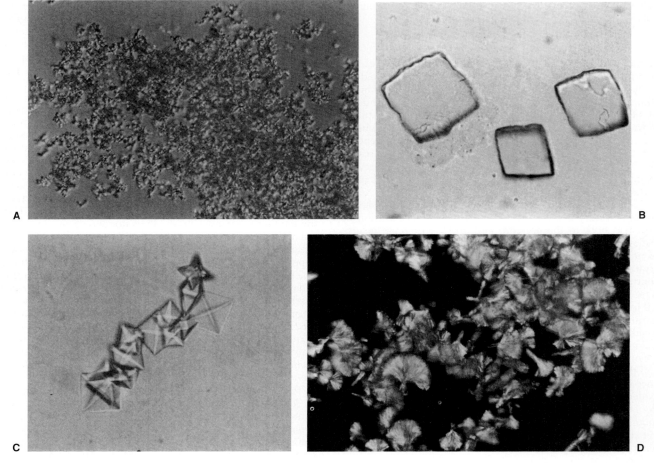

FIGURE 49-3. **A:** Amorphous urate crystals in urine. (Interference contrast microscopy, magnification ×200.) **B:** Uric acid crystals, cuboidal shape. (Magnification ×160.) **C:** Envelope-shaped calcium oxalate dihydrate form of crystal. (Note: needle-shaped monohydrate calcium crystals are not pictured.) **D:** Sulfadiazine crystals in urine. (Polarized microscopy, magnification ×40.) These birefringent crystals often assume a "fan" or "shock of wheat" shape. (Courtesy of Professor M. H. Haber, Department of Pathology, Rush Medical College, Chicago, IL.)

Despite these characteristic manifestations of the tumor lysis syndrome, it is difficult to predict in which patients acute uric acid nephropathy will develop. Even when appropriate prophylactic measures are taken with hydration, alkalinization, and allopurinol, the following still may develop: hyperuricemia in 9%, hyperphosphatemia in 25% to 50%, hypocalcemia in 10% to 60%, and hyperkalemia in 8%. However, the incidence of clinically significant tumor lysis syndrome after chemotherapy is only 5% (127,162). The likelihood for development of acute uric acid nephropathy is increased in the presence of renal insufficiency, in patients with oliguria before therapy, and in patients with lymphoma with high serum LDH levels (127,162,163).

Differential Diagnosis

The diagnosis of acute uric acid nephropathy should be suspected when acute renal failure in concert with tumor lysis syndrome develops within the first 1 to 3 days after initiation of chemotherapy for lymphoma or leukemia. The diagnosis sometimes is made difficult by the variety of drugs, radiographic studies, and associated clinical problems common during the early presentation of malignancies. Renal complications associated with malignancies include direct lymphomatous or leukemic renal infiltration, obstruction due to stones, and obstruction due to malignancy. However, despite the common occurrence of direct lymphomatous or leukemic renal infiltration, it rarely causes acute renal failure (146,163). Although early reports suggested an association of tumor lysis and ureteral obstruction due to calculi, this also occurs only rarely (159,166). Contrast nephropathy, dehydration, myeloma kidney, light-chain disease, ureteral obstruction due to tumor compression or invasion, sepsis-related renal failure, and acute tubular necrosis due to nephrotoxic drugs all should be considered in this high-risk population. The diagnosis also is made difficult by the common occurrence of hyperuricemia unrelated to tumor lysis syndrome, but caused by any of the following: preexisting renal failure, volume depletion, diuretics, salicylates, levodopa, cyclosporine, nicotinic acid, pyrazinamide, or ethambutol.

The diagnosis of uric acid nephropathy also should be considered when patients present with renal insufficiency before treatment of the malignancy. Spontaneous hyperuricemia occurs more commonly with lymphomas, and some patients present with renal insufficiency before treatment, possibly because of uric acid nephropathy (149,159,162). Ultimately, the diagnosis of acute uric acid nephropathy is made in the presence of tumor lysis syndrome, with the urinary uric acid-to-creatinine concentration ratio greater than 1, and exclusion of other causes acute renal failure.

Prophylactic Measures and Treatment

Before the dialysis era, the mortality rate from acute renal failure associated with uric acid nephropathy was 50%, but with modern treatment, including proper prophylaxis and dialysis, uric acid nephropathy is rare, and when it does occur, the prognosis for the acute renal failure is excellent (159). The treatment approach to uric acid nephropathy is divided into two stages. The first is to prevent or minimize the metabolic consequences of the tumor lysis syndrome, and the second is to treat these consequences when they do occur. The approach to both prophylaxis and treatment of tumor lysis syndrome includes inhibition of xanthine oxidase, forced diuresis, and urinary alkalinization. When these measures fail to prevent the consequences of tumor lysis, and acute renal failure from uric acid nephropathy develops, dialysis must be initiated to treat uremia and severe electrolyte problems, and control hyperuricemia (Table 49-6). However, in the future, rasburicase, a recombinant form of urate oxidase, may be an additional option for adult patients with acute renal failure from uric acid nephropathy (169) (see below). In July 2002, the U.S. Food and Drug Administration approved rasburicase for the initial management of plasma uric acid levels in pediatric patients with leukemia, lymphoma, and solid tumor malignancies who are receiving anti-cancer therapy expected to result in tumor lysis.

TABLE 49-6

THE APPROACH TO URIC ACID NEPHROPATHY AND TUMOR LYSIS SYNDROME

Approach to prophylaxis for tumor lysis syndrome and uric acid nephropathy

Patients presenting prior to chemotherapy with hyperuricemia and evidence of a large tumor burden: allopurinol, 300–600 mg

4–5 L/24 hr of normal saline. Add diuretics if the patient is well hydrated and not maintaining an adequate urine output. If there is no response to diuretics, match fluid input with urine output.

Urinary pH should be maintained above 7.0 by titrating intravenous bicarbonate therapy. Start with 100 mEq/L of sodium bicarbonate in D5W per hour. Bicarbonate therapy should be discontinued after serum uric acid is normalized.

If clinically feasible, postpone chemotherapy until uric acid is normalized along with any other electrolyte abnormalities.

Patients presenting prior to chemotherapy and with a normal uric acid level but still at risk for tumor lysis syndrome:

A llopurinol, 300–600 mg

4–5 L/24 hr of normal saline as described above.

If clinically feasible, postpone chemotherapy until 2 days after start of allopurinol.

Treatment of uric acid nephropathy and tumor lysis syndrome

Hemodialysis initiated per the routine indications including hyperkalemia, acidosis, hyperphosphatemia, volume overload, or uremia.

Hemodialysis for control of hyperuricemia unresponsive to the above measures. Adjust allopurinol doses for renal failure:

Creatinine clearance	Allopurinol dose
0	100 mg q3d
10	100 mg q2d
50	200 mg qd

After hemodialysis, supplement with 50% of allopurinol dose.

Inhibition of Xanthine Oxidase. Allopurinol is a substrate for and a competitive inhibitor of the enzyme xanthine oxidase (Fig. 49-2). It blocks the conversion of hypoxanthine and xanthine to uric acid, resulting in a reduction in both serum uric acid concentration and urinary excretion of urates. In the presence of allopurinol, hypoxanthine and xanthine accumulate instead of uric acid, and the urinary excretion of these precursors also increases (170). Hypoxanthine is highly soluble, and even with increased renal excretion, does not cause clinical problems. Xanthine, on the other hand, is less soluble than uric acid. Precipitated xanthine can be found in the urine of patients receiving allopurinol, but these precipitates do not correlate with the development of renal failure (170). However, well documented cases of xanthine nephropathy and xanthine calculi associated with allopurinol use have been reported (170–173).

The half-life of allopurinol is less than 2 hours owing to prompt renal elimination and rapid conversion to its chief metabolite, oxypurinol. Oxypurinol is an active metabolite, and reduces serum uric acid concentration and urinary uric acid excretion half as much as allopurinol (174). Unlike allopurinol, oxypurinol is eliminated solely by the kidney and its half-life is approximately 24 hours (174). Renal clearance of oxypurinol is approximately 30 mL/minute, and its clearance correlates directly with creatinine clearance such that with a creatinine clearance of less than 10 mL/minute, the half-life of oxypurinol is approximately 1 week.

In patients with normal renal function and hyperuricemia associated with malignancy, allopurinol decreases serum uric acid within 48 hours with a peak effect at 5 days (175). The clinical effects of allopurinol probably are mediated by oxypurinol because the half-life of allopurinol is short. Despite the use of allopurinol, hyperuricemia and acute uric acid nephropathy sometimes cannot be avoided, and reasons for this failure include a large tumor burden, aggressive chemotherapy, and the inability to delay chemotherapy until allopurinol has decreased the serum uric acid concentration (159,162,163).

For optimal prophylaxis, allopurinol should be administered at least 3 days before chemotherapy. The level of existing renal function also must be considered when dosing the drug. Allopurinol can lead to a life-threatening toxicity syndrome that is characterized by a diffuse, desquamative skin rash, fever, hepatic dysfunction, eosinophilia, and worsening renal function of unknown etiology, although consistent with a diffuse vasculitis. Eighty percent of patients reported with this toxicity had renal insufficiency (176–178). Improper dosing of allopurinol also can lead to xanthine nephropathy (171–173,176).

Optimal allopurinol dosing is reflected by a therapeutic serum oxypurinol concentration, which ranges from 30 to 100 μmol/L (178). Patients with end-stage renal disease achieve therapeutic levels of oxypurinol after one dose of allopurinol (300 to 600 mg) and maintain this level until the next dialysis, at which time the serum level is reduced by 40% (176,179). Therefore, the maintenance dose must be reduced in patients with renal insufficiency to avoid accumulation of oxypurinol. For example, plasma oxypurinol levels greater than 300 μmol/L can be achieved after the usual dose of allopurinol (300 mg) in the presence of mild renal insufficiency, and these potentially toxic levels persist for days after cessation of the drug (179). The oral route is equivalent to intravenous dosing of allopurinol; therefore, intravenous dosing should be considered only in patients unable to take anything by mouth. Rectal administration of allopurinol is not effective and should not be used (180,181). Allopurinol started at 300 to 600 mg is safe and achieves therapeutic levels of oxypurinol, but the peak clinical effect on uric acid production is not seen for 3 days. Optimally, allopurinol should be started 3 days before chemotherapy, and dose adjustments must be made in the presence of renal insufficiency (Table 49-6).

Rasburicase

As mentioned above, most mammals degrade purines to the soluble end product allantoin utilizing the enzyme uricase (Fig. 49-2) which humans lack. Rasburicase, the recombinant form of urate oxidase, has several advantages over allopurinol. Rasburicase has a rapid onset of action and has been shown to return uric acid to normal levels with hours (182). Unlike allopurinol which inhibits the production of uric acid, rasburicase quickly reduces the existing uric acid levels and does not rely on the renal clearance of existing uric acid or alkalization of the urine. In one compassionate use trial, rasburicase (0.20 mg/kg) was administered intravenously once a day for 1 to 7 days. The mean uric acid level in 29 hyperuricemic children decreased from 15.1 to 0.4 mg/dL, and in 27 hyperuricemic adults, the mean level decreased from 14.2 to 0.5 mg/dL (183). Rasburicase is a very expensive drug and although clinical trials have compared rasburicase to allopurinol, the outcomes have been a decrement in uric acid level rather than important metabolic outcomes or acute renal failure (184). Additional clinical trials are necessary before rasburicase will be approved for use in adults.

Forced Diuresis. Animal data have suggested that high renal tubular fluid flow induced by a solute or water diuresis is important in the prevention of acute urate nephropathy. In fact, rats treated with high-dose furosemide, and Brattleboro rats with central diabetes insipidus and water diuresis both had complete protection from uric acid nephropathy, whereas rats treated solely with urine alkalinization had only partial protection (142). Diuresis probably imparts protection by lowering the urate concentration in the collecting duct where uric acid precipitation occurs, or by effects on tubular urate handling. Whether these results can be applied to humans is not known because species differences in urate handling exist.

Despite efforts to maintain high urine flow with hydration and diuretics, a lower urine flow rate preceding chemotherapy is more common in patients who have renal failure than in those who do not (163). Although this observation probably reflects the existence of mild spontaneous uric acid nephropathy before chemotherapy, it is reasonable to assume that increased urine flow would add protection from uric acid nephropathy. Patients should be hydrated with 4 to 5 L of normal saline per 24 hours. If the patient is well hydrated and not maintaining the expected urine output, diuretics should then be initiated. If urine output remains low, fluid intake should be adjusted to match output in the effort to avoid fluid overload.

Urinary Alkalinization. Although evidence is lacking to confirm its theoretic role in preventing uric acid nephropathy, urinary alkalization remains a prominent component in prophylactic regimens. The theoretical benefit of urinary alkalization is to increase the solubility of uric acid. However, in animal studies, the most important intrarenal dynamic in prevention of acute uric acid nephropathy was high urine tubular flow (142). In this study, the use of acetazolamide achieved only partial protection, which was likely due to the drug's diuretic effect and not its effect on urine pH (142). Along with the inherent risk of causing a severe metabolic alkalosis when attempting to alkalinize the urine with sodium bicarbonate administration, other potential disadvantages include increasing the risk of symptomatic hypocalcemia and calcium phosphate precipitation, which can cause acute renal failure by itself in this setting (165,166,168,185). Urinary alkalinization also does not have an effect on xanthine precipitation because the pK_a of xanthine is 7.4, as opposed to 5.6 for uric acid.

Bicarbonate therapy should be included in the prophylactic regimen only when attempting to correct hyperuricemia. If hyperuricemia is present before chemotherapy, bicarbonate should be added to intravenous fluids with the aim of keeping the urine pH above 7.0. Once hyperuricemia has been corrected, bicarbonate therapy should be discontinued.

Hemodialysis. Dialysis assists in the management acute uric acid nephropathy in two ways. First, dialytic therapy is initiated for the typical indications common in acute renal failure such as hyperkalemia, severe hyperphosphatemia, azotemia, and fluid overload, although these indications may be more severe and occur more rapidly than in other forms of acute renal failure. Cases of fatal hyperkalemia have occurred within hours after initiation of chemotherapy (163,164). Second, dialysis is an effective way to reduce the serum uric acid level. This is an important role for dialysis because patients usually do not recover from acute uric acid nephropathy until the serum uric acid level is reduced (186). Once this occurs, usually after only one to four dialysis treatments, recovery of renal function is signaled by a brisk diuresis (159).

Depending on the dialyzer and blood flow used, hemodialysis has a uric acid clearance rate of 90 to 150 mL/minute, whereas the peritoneal dialysis clearance is only 10 to 20 mL/minute (159,186,187). The superior clearance of hemodialysis compared with peritoneal dialysis is evidenced by the typical total uric acid cleared on hemodialysis versus peritoneal dialysis: 7 to 8 g versus 4 g. When starting a patient on hemodialysis, caution should be taken not to use a high-calcium bath if severe hyperphosphatemia is present because of the risk of increasing the calcium–phosphorus product. Selected patients may benefit from continuous forms of dialytic therapy such as continuous arteriovenous hemodialysis. On continuous arteriovenous hemodialysis with a dialysate flow of 4 L/hour, the uric acid clearance is 40 mL/minute, and the possible advantage over the intermittent nature of dialysis is the continuous clearance and control of phosphorus and potassium (188).

Ethylene Glycol Toxicity

Acute ethylene glycol intoxication is a medical emergency that, if not treated aggressively, leads to serious neurologic, cardiopulmonary, and renal dysfunction and may result in death. In 1993, 501 ethylene glycol exposures, including 254 hospitalizations and 11 deaths, were reported to the American Poison Control Centers (189). Ethylene glycol, an odorless and clear liquid, is the major ingredient in antifreeze, and is most commonly consumed either intentionally by alcoholics seeking an ethanol substitute or accidentally by children. An ingestion of 100 mL is considered the minimal lethal dose of ethylene glycol (190). Diethylene glycol is a condensation product of ethylene glycol production, and ingestion causes the same toxicities as ethylene glycol. Diethylene glycol was used as the diluent in the first sulfa antibiotic, sulfanilamide, and consequently led to mass poisonings in 1937. One hundred five patients died from the therapeutic use of Elixir Sulfanilamide, and one important consequence of this tragedy was the 1938 Federal Food, Drug and Cosmetic Act, requiring proof of product safety before release of a drug (191,192). Unfortunately, this kind of governmental supervision of pharmaceutical companies does not exist in other countries such as Nigeria and Haiti, where 47 and 85 children, respectively, died when diethylene glycol was used as a solvent in a preparation of cough syrup (193,194).

Metabolism of Ethylene Glycol

The metabolism of ethylene glycol is complex and incompletely understood. As is the case with other alcohols such as ethyl and methyl alcohol, nicotinamide adenine dinucleotide (NAD)-dependent alcohol dehydrogenase is responsible for the first

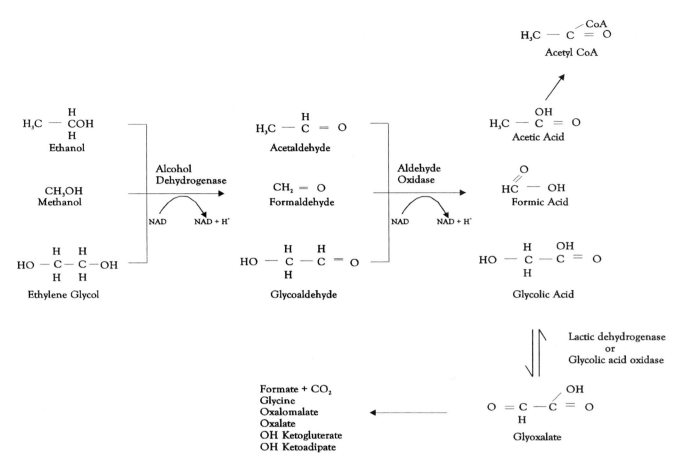

FIGURE 49-4. Pathway of ethylene glycol degradation.

oxidative step, converting ethylene glycol to glycoaldehyde (Fig. 49-4). After this first step, the pathways have not been well elucidated in humans, but are thought to include the following: glycoaldehyde oxidized to glycolic acid by aldehyde oxidase, glycolic acid to glyoxylate by glycolic acid oxidase or LDH, and then numerous subsequent pathways for glyoxylate metabolism, including one to oxalate by LDH and glycolic acid oxidase (190) (Fig. 49-4). Glycolate is converted to glyoxylate very slowly and is probably the rate-limiting step in the metabolism of ethylene glycol, whereas glycoaldehyde and glyoxylate have very short half-lives (195,196). Lactic acid production had been thought to be increased in ethylene glycol intoxication because of the altered NADH:NAD ratio resulting from increased NADH formation from alcohol dehydrogenase, but lactic acidosis is not a consistent finding and may be associated with alcoholism or hemodynamic instability (190,195,197).

Ethylene glycol metabolites are thought to mediate the toxicity seen with ethylene glycol ingestion, and ethylene glycol itself is not toxic. In fact, inhibition of ethylene glycol metabolism with ethyl alcohol or pyrazole prevents toxicity (198,199). The observation that the mortality rate in rats is reduced by performing a partial hepatectomy before administration of ethylene glycol and glycolate illustrates the importance of ethylene glycol metabolites on toxicity: The partially hepatectomized rats metabolized ethylene glycol more slowly to its toxic byproducts, which allowed more time for renal excretion of the nontoxic and unchanged ethylene glycol (200). Glycolate and oxalate are thought to be important mediators of ethylene glycol toxicity.

The pathophysiologic process of ethylene glycol toxicity is multifactorial and is thought to include accumulation of toxic ethylene glycol metabolites, calcium oxalate crystal deposition in tissues, and the effects of severe acidosis. After administration of a lethal dose of ethylene glycol in rats, profound renal oxalosis is produced, and the same occurs with administration of glycolic acid and glyoxylic acid. Renal pathology in these rats demonstrated calcium oxalate crystals in the proximal and distal convoluted tubules, with smaller amounts in the collecting tubule and none in glomeruli or renal interstitium (201). The degree of crystal formation correlated with diffuse convoluted tubular dilatation, but occasional epithelial necrosis seemed to bear a relation to the degree of crystal formation. Administration of glycoaldehyde did not produce significant crystal formation or the same degree of microscopic changes, but did lead to pronounced tubular epithelial swelling. In addition to the renal findings, oxalate crystals were found in brain tissue (201). In dogs given nonlethal doses of ethylene glycol, renal biopsy specimens revealed interstitial edema, tubular dilatation, hydropic degeneration, and tubular cell necrosis even in areas free of crystals. Electron microscopic findings were most prominent in proximal tubule cells and included vacuolization, cellular rupture, cytoplasmic buds, and increased density of mitochondria (202). This pattern of proximal tubule damage is similar to other models of ischemic and nephrotoxic forms of renal failure (202).

These findings are similar to human autopsy series that also have found calcium oxalate crystals in renal tubules. In these studies, renal epithelial cells appear either normal or extensively necrotic, depending on the interval between ingestion and death; minimal if any damage of the glomeruli has been reported (203–205). Despite severe clinical neurologic disturbances, the brain characteristically has only mild perivascular and meningeal deposition of calcium oxalate crystals, but edema, capillary engorgement, hemorrhage, and infarctions also have been described (205,206). Although crystal deposition usually is not reported, myocardial tissue findings are consistent with myocarditis (205).

Renal biopsies in survivors of ethylene glycol intoxication helped clarify the renal pathologic process because most reported autopsy subjects had died within 48 hours of ingestion of ethylene glycol. Survivors consistently show widespread renal epithelial cell necrosis with preservation of the basement membrane; calcium oxalate deposition is present but in a scattered distribution, with preservation of epithelial cells at the point of contact (207). Crystals are prominent in proximal tubules and sparse in the distal tubules, and tubular dilatation and obstruction are not consistently observed (208,209). Serial biopsies have shown a clear sequence from initial severe tubular damage to regeneration of tubular epithelium over a 60-day period (209). In aggregate, the autopsy and renal biopsy studies do not support the hypothesis that calcium oxalate crystallization is the primary cause of ethylene glycol toxicity; despite widespread renal tubule damage, calcium oxalate crystal deposition is patchy; and despite the presence of crystals, there is no tubule obstruction or dilation.

High–anion-gap metabolic acidosis is a major feature of ethylene glycol intoxication, and also is thought to contribute directly to the clinical toxicity. In rats poisoned with ethylene glycol, survival rates are five times greater after treatment with sodium bicarbonate alone or with ethanol alone compared with no treatment, and giving ethanol and sodium bicarbonate together improved the survival rate to six times that seen in rats with no treatment (210). Also possibly illustrating the relationship between acidosis and ethylene glycol toxicity is a report of a patient who ingested a large amount of ethylene glycol and lithium carbonate, a potential source of 320 mEq of bicarbonate. Despite an ethylene glycol level of 500 mg/dL on admission, the patient did not have an anion gap metabolic acidosis or renal failure (211). The major determinant of the metabolic acidosis is glycolic acid; in dogs and monkeys, administration of ethylene glycol produces severe metabolic acidosis, and the depressed bicarbonate is matched by the increase in glycolic acid production (212). Oxalic acid is very toxic to kidneys and is lethal in doses much lower than toxic doses of ethylene glycol, but in rats and monkeys, only 0% to 2.5% of the original dose of ethylene glycol is excreted as oxalic acid (190,196,213). In humans with ethylene glycol poisoning, plasma glycolate concentration correlated with the increased anion gap, and the serum concentrations of oxalate and glyoxylate were negligible in these patients (195,214). Although studies have suggested that organic acids such as lactic acid contribute to the severe metabolic acidosis of ethylene glycol intoxication, glycolic acid seems to be the main cause of the acidosis, with lactic and β-hydroxybutyric acids being elevated in special circumstances such as associated hypotension or alcoholic ketoacidosis (197,214).

It has been postulated that production of glycoaldehyde, glyoxal, glycolate, and glyoxylate from ethylene glycol metabolism is important in the pathophysiologic process of the toxicity. Aldehyde production is greatest 6 to 12 hours after ethylene glycol ingestion, and this is when cerebral symptoms are most severe (190). However, as mentioned, glycolate is the only metabolite that accumulates; its direct toxicity has not been well studied, but it is known to be toxic in animals (196). For example, glycolic acid given to rats is lethal and also causes renal tubular oxalosis (201). The role that glycolic acid plays in the human renal, cerebral, and cardiac toxicity remains to be proven, but it probably is one of the

multifactorial causes along with acidosis and calcium oxalate crystals.

Clinical and Laboratory Manifestations

The initial reports of ethylene glycol poisoning in the 1940s and 1950s noted that the clinical manifestations of acute ethylene glycol poisoning could be divided into three stages (207). During the first stage, occurring 30 minutes to 12 hours after ethylene glycol ingestion, the central nervous system manifestations predominate. During the second stage, occurring over the next 12 hours, cardiopulmonary dysfunction develops, and includes tachypnea, pulmonary edema, and cardiac failure. In patients who survive past the first 24 hours, the third stage is characterized by prolonged renal failure. Before the advent of aggressive treatment with hemodialysis and intravenous ethanol, these stages were very typical of the clinical course of most patients, but with modern treatment and depending on the amount of ethylene glycol ingested, the sequence and occurrence of these clinical features and stages vary considerably (206,215).

In addition to apparent inebriation but without an alcoholic odor, central nervous system manifestations include nystagmus, depressed reflexes, seizures, and coma (190,216,217). Delayed appearance of multiple cranial nerve deficits also has been reported, and the deficits have not always been reversible (218). Ocular effects are a main feature of methanol ingestion, but ophthalmoplegia, papilledema, loss of visual acuity, and eventual optic atrophy also have been reported with ethylene glycol ingestion (219). Abdominal signs and symptoms, including nausea, vomiting, and pain, are very common (215). For unexplained reasons, mild hypertension, tachycardia, and a low-grade fever sometimes are present, and one study noted a poor prognosis in patients with hypertension. Three of 6 patients with hypertension died in a series of 36 patients in which the total deaths were 6 (190,206).

High–anion-gap metabolic acidosis with a high osmolar gap is the most striking initial laboratory finding and is the main diagnostic feature. The severity of the clinical presentation depends on the quantity of ingested ethylene glycol and elapsed time since its ingestion, but typically patients present with a pH of less than 7.2, bicarbonate less than 10 mEq/L, anion gap greater than 20, mean osmolal gap of 35, measured osmolality greater than 300 mOsm, and hyperkalemia (206,220,221). Hypocalcemia is a frequent finding and can be severe and symptomatic, leading to tetany or cardiac arrhythmia (206,217). The onset of hypocalcemia is usually within the first 12 hours, and the serum calcium usually remains low despite treatment (222,223). The hypocalcemia probably is caused by a combination of chelation of calcium by oxalate and an abnormal parathyroid hormone response (222).

Lumbar puncture frequently is performed because of the mental status changes, and the cerebrospinal fluid sometimes reveals pleocytosis with a sterile culture (203,205,215). A normal hematocrit and platelet count but a moderate leukocytosis of 10,000 to 40,000/mm^3 with a predominance of polymorphonuclear cells is seen commonly in the initial complete blood count (190,205).

The urinalysis typically includes a low specific gravity, mild proteinuria, microscopic hematuria, and pyuria (215,217,224). Crystalluria is not invariably present, but usually is seen on presentation. The envelope-shaped calcium oxalate dihydrate form of crystals (octahedral dihydrate) traditionally has been thought of as the most commonly seen crystal in ethylene glycol intoxication, but in fact the needle-shaped monohydrate calcium oxalate crystals predominates in ethylene glycol intoxication (224–226) (Fig. 49-3). Monohydrate calcium oxalate crystals are thermodynamically stable, and with time the dihydrate form transforms to the monohydrate form (227). *In vitro*, the dihydrate form is seen only at high

TABLE 49-7

DOSING GUIDELINES FOR ETHANOL TREATMENT

Ethanol solution and route of administration	Specific gravity of ethanol (g/dL)	Loading dose (100 mg/dL of ethanol × 0.6 L/kg) (mL/kg)	Maintenance dose in nondrinkers 66 mg/kg/hr (mL/kg/hr)	Maintenance dose in drinkers 154 mg/kg/hr (mL/kg/hr)	During dialysis add the following to the maintenance dose (mL/hr)
5% IV	3.9	15.4	1.7	3.9	185
10% IV	7.8	7.7	0.84	2.0	90
20% PO	15.8	3.8	0.42	1.0	45
50% PO	39.5	1.5	0.17	0.4	18

IV, intravenous; *PO*, orally.
Oral ethanol dose should be increased by 50% after charcoal therapy.

concentrations of both calcium and oxalate (227). The pattern of oxalate crystals in individual patients transforms from the envelope-shaped crystals to the needle-shaped crystals in a matter of hours (214).

The cardiopulmonary consequences of ethylene glycol intoxication now are rarely seen with prompt, aggressive treatment. However, early reports described rapidly progressive tachypnea, cyanosis, pulmonary edema, hypotension, and cardiac failure in most cases (203,204,207). In a recent report from an ethylene glycol poisoning epidemic in Sweden, pulmonary edema occurred in only 1 of 36 patients and circulatory failure and hypotension in 2 of 36 patients (206). The etiology of the pulmonary dysfunction is not known, but is probably adult respiratory distress syndrome (228). However, this is not necessarily due to direct ethylene glycol toxicity because these patients are at risk for aspiration and pneumonia (206). Myocarditis, with focal muscle cell necrosis and diffuse infiltrates of mononuclear cells, has been reported as a consequence of ethylene glycol poisoning (206,229).

After ingestion of ethylene glycol sufficient to cause metabolic acidosis, oliguric renal failure develops in most patients (206,215). If aggressive treatment, including dialysis and ethanol, is provided soon after the ethylene glycol is ingested, renal failure can be avoided. However, most patients do not seek medical attention until symptoms develop, which usually is many hours after ingestion. Thus, renal failure is common, and may develop as soon as 24 hours after ingestion (203,214,215,230). The course of the renal failure is typical of oliguric acute tubular necrosis. The oliguria lasts 4 to 5 days and is followed by a diuretic phase. The BUN and serum creatinine usually peak at 7 to 10 days, and most patients require only 1 to 2 weeks of dialytic support (199,206,207,215). However some patients require dialysis for many months, and despite the return of sufficient renal function to stop dialysis, renal function does not always return to baseline values (214).

Diagnosis

In the absence of ketoacidosis and in the presence of the characteristic signs and symptoms, it should be assumed that all patients presenting with metabolic acidosis combined with increased anion and osmolal gaps have either methanol or ethylene glycol poisoning (221). The prognosis of both these poisonings is improved with early diagnosis and treatment, and therefore, if diagnosis cannot be confirmed with serum levels of methanol or ethylene glycol, treatment with bicarbonate and ethanol infusion and hemodialysis should be initiated. Screening tests for the identification of ethylene glycol are being developed, but are not commonly used (231). Determination of ethylene glycol in serum is best performed with gas

chromatography, but this method is not routinely available at most hospitals (232). Sodium fluorescein is a fluorescent dye that is added to some commercial antifreeze preparations, and a Wood's lamp can be used to detect fluorescence visually in urine, a finding that supports the diagnosis of ethylene glycol ingestion (233).

Once the diagnosis of ethylene glycol poisoning has been confirmed and the blood concentration of any concomitantly ingested ethanol determined, the serum ethylene glycol level can be estimated using the osmolal gap (234–236) (Table 49-7). Ethylene glycol levels above 20 mg/dL can be lethal if not treated aggressively (235).

Clinical Course and Treatment

Initial Emergency Department Treatment. If the patient is seen in the first few hours after ethylene glycol ingestion, gastric lavage and oral charcoal should be initiated to reduce further drug absorption. Ethylene glycol is metabolized quickly to acid intermediaries, and thus the high–anion-gap acidosis develops rapidly after ingestion of ethylene glycol. Hemodialysis to provide a source of bicarbonate and to clear ethylene glycol and its metabolites is the therapy of choice for treatment of the acidosis. However, hemodialysis usually is delayed, and during this waiting period patients usually require hundreds of milliequivalents of sodium bicarbonate. Despite intravenous administration of 300 to 500 mEq of sodium bicarbonate in the first 6 hours, severe metabolic acidosis usually persists and is not corrected until hemodialysis is initiated (214,237).

Correction of the acidosis may increase the likelihood of symptomatic hypocalcemia such as seizures, tetany, and cardiac dysfunction. Intravenous calcium supplementation should be given cautiously because of the potential risk of further calcium oxalate precipitation. Calcium should be given if clinical signs or symptoms of hypocalcemia develop, but not prophylactically (217). Thiamine and pyridoxine are cofactors required in the nontoxic metabolic pathways of ethylene glycol (away from oxalate), and early replacement of these cofactors is advocated to prevent potential depletion (190,216).

Administration of ethanol and hemodialysis have traditionally made up the definitive treatments for ethylene glycol intoxication. Compared with ethylene glycol, ethanol has a higher affinity for alcohol dehydrogenase and therefore inhibits the metabolism of ethylene glycol to the toxic metabolites, permitting the ethylene glycol to be renally excreted or dialyzed. With a blood ethanol level of 100 mg/dL, liver alcohol dehydrogenase is saturated, and the half-life of ethylene glycol increases from 3 to 17 hours (238). In rats, the median lethal dose of ethylene glycol is doubled when ethanol also is given, and in monkeys, a dose of 3.2 mL/kg of ethylene glycol was lethal except for those also receiving ethanol. The urinary excretion of ethylene glycol was 10 times greater in ethanol-protected monkeys than in those receiving ethylene glycol alone (239). Since the first report of ethyl alcohol treatment in humans, ethyl alcohol has been used in conjunction with dialysis in the treatment of ethylene glycol poisoning, and ethanol is not recommended as a sole treatment (199). Although there have been reports of successful treatment with ethyl alcohol without dialysis, these were isolated cases in which ingestion only of small amounts of ethylene glycol occurred (206,215).

For maximal inhibition of ethylene glycol metabolism, the plasma ethanol concentration should be maintained between 100 and 200 mg/dL. This is achieved with a loading dose of 0.6 g/kg, followed by a maintenance dose of 66 mg/kg in nondrinkers, and 154 mg/kg in regular alcohol consumers. During dialysis, 7.2 g/hour should be added to the maintenance dose (238,240). Oral ethanol also can be used, but the dose should be increased by 50% if given soon after the administration of charcoal (238). Intravenous ethanol comes in 5% and 10% solutions diluted in dextrose and water, whereas a 20% or 50% solution usually is used for oral or nasogastric administration. The specific gravity of ethanol is used in calculating the correct dose (234,238) (Table 49-7). Until the correct dose to achieve a level between 100 and 200 mg/dL has been ascertained, hourly ethanol concentrations should be checked.

4-Methylpyrazole. An alternative to ethanol therapy is fomepizole (4-methylpyrazole; Antizol) which is a potent inhibitor of alcohol dehydrogenase. It is now considered by many to be the first line therapy over ethanol for treatment of ethylene glycol toxicity (241,242). Animal studies have shown that fomepizole prevents ethylene glycol–related mortality and toxicities, and increases the urinary excretion of ethylene glycol by preventing its metabolism (198,212). In humans, fomepizole has been studied in a small number of patients, and has been shown to normalize acidosis within hours, prevent decreases in renal function if used early, and decrease serum levels of ethylene glycol toxic metabolites (243). In humans without renal failure, treatment results in an increase in the ethylene glycol half-life from 3 to 14 hours, an increase in urinary excretion of ethylene glycol, and prevention of clinical toxicity (244,245).

Fomepizole offers advantages over ethanol treatment, including predictable pharmacokinetics, avoiding the need to achieve and maintain the desired blood ethanol level, and avoiding the ethanol-induced central nervous system depression. Fomepizole is available as a parenteral solution. The loading dose is 15 mg/kg intravenously, followed by 4 more doses of 10 mg/kg every 12 hours, after which it is continued at a rate of 15 mg/kg every 12 hours until the ethylene glycol concentration is undetectable or the patient is asymptomatic with a resolution of the high–anion-gap metabolic acidosis. Like ethanol, the dose of fomepizole is adjusted during dialysis therapy. At the start of dialysis, the next scheduled dose is given if it has been longer than 6 hours since the last dose, but if it has been less than 6 hours, the next scheduled dose is held. Fomepizole is then given every 4 hours during dialysis. At the completion of dialysis, no additional dose is given if it has been less than 1 hour since the last dose, one-half of the next scheduled dose is given if it has been 1 to 3 hours since the last dose, and the next scheduled dose is given if it has been longer than 3 hours since the last dose. The maintenance dose off dialysis is continued 12 hours after the last dose (246).

Fomepizole has been used to treat ethylene glycol poisoning successfully without hemodialysis or ethanol, but these patients had normal renal function and fomepizole treatment was initiated soon after ethylene glycol ingestion (244,245). In mild cases of ethylene glycol poisoning as evidenced by normal renal function and no high–anion-gap acidosis, ethanol or fomepizole is used by some as sole therapy without dialysis, but in these cases forced diuresis with intravenous fluids and mannitol or furosemide should be used to avoid dehydration, minimize renal calcium oxalate crystal formation, and maintain renal clearance of ethylene glycol (223,230,245). However, recent data suggest that an abnormal presenting serum creatinine concentration ($\geq$1.5 mg/dL) predicts significantly prolonged ethylene glycol elimination during fomepizole therapy, and in the presence of metabolic acidosis, patients should undergo hemodialysis (247).

Hemodialysis is indicated in all cases of confirmed or strongly suspected ethylene glycol poisoning presenting with renal failure, metabolic acidosis, and/or deteriorating clinical status. Ethylene glycol and glycolate have low molecular weights, no protein binding, and a volume of distribution of 0.8 and 0.55 L/kg, respectively, which make them easily dialyzable (195,238,248). Large surface-area dialyzers (>2 m^2) can achieve clearance of ethylene glycol of greater than 200 mL/minute, and with smaller surface-area dialyzers (1.1 to 1.6 m^2) clearance of ethylene glycol and glycolate typically ranges from 150 to 190 mL/minute and from 140 to 170 mL/minute, respectively (195,214,238,248,249). The renal clearance of ethylene glycol can be as high as 30 mL/minute in patients with preserved renal function, but the importance of hemodialysis is illustrated by the fact that most patients present with renal insufficiency, and in these patients the renal clearance of ethylene glycol and glycolate is negligible (214,249). The length of the hemodialysis session should be determined by the quantity of ethylene glycol ingested, but this rarely is known. Although blood ethylene glycol levels are helpful, they do not necessarily reflect the total quantity ingested because the blood ethylene glycol level is influenced by time since ingestion and amount metabolized. Dialysis should be continued for 8 hours if ethylene glycol levels are not available, and when levels are available, the dialysis prescription should be calculated using the total body water, blood ethylene glycol level, and the manufacturer-specified dialyzer urea clearance (mL/minute) at the initial observed blood flow rate (250). Bicarbonate-based dialysate is probably optimal compared with acetate dialysate, which is associated with greater hemodynamic instability, more central nervous system symptoms, and more oscillations in plasma bicarbonate (216,251). Although peritoneal dialysis clears ethylene glycol and oxalate, it should not be used over hemodialysis because of the high efficacy of hemodialysis (211).

Sulfonamide Antibiotics, Indinavir, and Acyclovir

Crystalline acute renal failure also can be caused by drugs used for therapeutic purposes. If the solubility limit of a given drug is exceeded in the renal tubules, the drug can then crystallize and possibly cause obstructive nephropathy. Certain sulfonamide antibiotics and acyclovir are the most common drugs that can cause crystalline acute renal failure, but other drugs such as methotrexate, triamterene, and high-dose vitamin C potentially can crystallize and cause stones or obstructive nephropathy (252–255,256). Before the acquired immunodeficiency syndrome (AIDS) era, crystalline acute renal failure had become fairly rare, but with the frequent use of high-dose sulfadiazine, sulfamethoxazole, indinavir, and acyclovir in this population, it is again an important cause of acute renal failure (257).

The sulfonamides were introduced into medical practice in 1936, and early animal experiments recognized that sulfonamides of low solubility were able to crystallize in the urinary tract and renal parenchyma, causing obstructive nephropathy (258,259). Reports of patients with hematuria, crystalluria, renal colic, and renal failure were common until the 1950s, when sulfonamides with greater solubility became available (258,260). In patients with AIDS, high-dose sulfadiazine is again being used commonly in conjunction with pyrimethamine for the treatment of toxoplasmosis. After an oral dose, sulfadiazine is rapidly absorbed and then partially acetylated in the liver. The half-life of sulfadiazine is 8 to 17 hours in patients with normal renal function and 22 to 34 hours in patients with severe renal insufficiency (257). Renal crystal formation in the nephron is promoted as the filtrate is concentrated and acidified. The solubility of sulfadiazine is almost 10-fold higher at a pH of 7.5 than a pH of 6.5.

Patients with sulfonamide-induced renal failure classically present with renal colic, hematuria, acute renal failure, and oliguria or anuria (261,262). Although renal failure develops in most patients in the first week after the start of the sulfadiazine, patients also can present months after the start of the medication. Delayed presentation of acute renal failure usually occurs with the concurrent development of volume depletion, often due to diarrhea, and these patients can be managed with hydration without stopping the sulfadiazine (263,264). The urinalysis usually shows hematuria, mild pyuria, and "shock of wheat" crystals (Fig. 49-3). Renal ultrasonography may reveal multiple echogenic foci in the renal parenchyma, but occasionally shows frank hydronephrosis with ureteral stones (261,265,266).

The acute renal failure should be managed with intravenous fluids containing sodium bicarbonate with the aim of maintaining urine pH over 7.15 and urine output over 1 L/day. Urologic intervention sometimes is required in patients who remain anuric. Bilateral retrograde ureteral catheterization with warm 5% sodium bicarbonate solution, ureteral stents, and stone extraction with a stone basket all have been used in cases of ureteral obstruction with stones (267–270). Although temporary hemodialysis sometimes is necessary, recovery of renal function to baseline is the rule within 7 days (262,266).

Patients starting sulfadiazine therapy should receive prophylaxis against renal toxicity. To minimize crystal formation, patients should be encouraged to maintain fluid intake over 2 to 3 L/day and should be started on sodium bicarbonate (6 to 12 g/day) to maintain urine pH higher than 7.15 (262). Patients with renal insufficiency, diarrhea, or volume depletion should be monitored closely with urinalyses, looking for hematuria and crystalluria, and sulfadiazine levels should be considered in patients with renal insufficiency (262).

Indinavir is one of the most common protease inhibitors used in patients with AIDS as part of highly active antiretroviral therapy. Indinavir causes nephrolithiasis in 3% to 4%, and symptomatic urinary tract disease, including nephrolithiasis with renal colic, flank pain without evidence of stones, and dysuria or urgency, in 8% of patients taking the drug (271,272). Most patients presenting with symptomatic urinary tract disease have crystalluria, and many have radiographic evidence of either stones or renal parenchyma filling defects. However, only a minority have mild to moderate renal insufficiency. Hydration can prevent symptomatic urinary tract disease, but permanent discontinuation of indinavir is necessary in some because of recurrence of symptoms. Asymptomatic indinavir crystalluria is found in 20% of patients receiving the drug in the normal dosage of 800 mg orally, three times a day, and the drug should not be discontinued for asymptomatic crystalluria. In vitro, indinavir is more soluble at a pH of 4.5, but this is below the in vivo potential of the kidney (272). The presence of crystalluria and pyuria may signal the presence of interstitial nephritis, which may not reverse with conservative treatment with hydration alone (273).

High-dose acyclovir also is associated with acute renal failure and crystalluria. Early preclinical toxicology studies in animals clearly demonstrated that high-dose acyclovir given to rats resulted in precipitation of drug crystals in the distal nephron and also caused reversible obstructive nephropathy (274,275). Although it has been assumed that intratubular acyclovir crystallization also is responsible for the renal failure observed in humans, the pathophysiologic process is not entirely clear. Most reported kidney biopsy or autopsy specimens have not demonstrated intrarenal crystals, but typically show normal glomeruli, no obstruction, occasional ruptured tubules, and minimal focal areas of interstitial hemorrhage, congestion, and inflammatory infiltrates (276,277). In one case report of acyclovir nephrotoxicity, the renal biopsy was consistent with acute tubular necrosis without any evidence of intratubular crystals (278). Crystal dissolution during tissue fixation or the time interval between discontinuation of acyclovir and obtaining the renal biopsy could account for the inconsistent demonstration of crystals in renal tissue (278).

Renal impairment after intravenous acyclovir was commonly observed when bolus injections were used instead of slow infusions; one series reported that increased BUN or serum creatinine developed in 58 of 354 (16%) of patients 24 to 48 hours after administration of acyclovir (275,279). Unlike all other subsequent reports, one infant in this series with renal failure did show birefringent crystals in the renal tubules in the postmortem examination (275). In contrast to bolus injections, renal failure after slow intravenous infusions or oral acyclovir is less common, but does occur, especially in patients with renal insufficiency or volume depletion (276,280–282).

The acute renal failure caused by acyclovir typically develops 24 to 72 hours after the first dose of intravenous acyclovir. Unlike with the sulfonamide antibiotics, most patients do not have renal colic, stones, or ultrasonographic findings of obstruction. Many patients also have neurotoxicity, including headache, irritability, tremulousness, ataxia, nystagmus, lethargy, dysarthria, confusion, and coma (276,283,284). The urinalysis usually reveals both mild hematuria and pyuria, and examination of the urine with a polarizing microscope may show birefringent, needle-shaped crystals within leukocytes (276,283). Despite the development of massive acyclovir crystalluria in some patients, renal function may remain unaffected (277,285).

Risk factors for the development of acyclovir-induced acute renal failure include dehydration, bolus dosing, chronic renal failure, and an acyclovir serum level of greater than 25 μg/mL (275,282,286). Renal function in patients with acute renal failure usually normalizes within 4 to 9 days after drug discontinuation (276,286). Conservative management, with hydration and discontinuation of acyclovir, is sufficient in most patients, but in patients with combined severe neurotoxicity and nephrotoxicity, hemodialysis can be used to reduce serum acyclovir levels. This results in prompt reversal of acyclovir-associated neurologic symptoms (283). In cases of mild renal failure, acyclovir nephrotoxicity can be managed by hydration and dose reduction of acyclovir (282).

The half-life of acyclovir is 3 hours, and renal excretion is the major route of elimination. For example, over 90% of a given dose of acyclovir can be recovered unchanged in the urine of subjects with normal renal function 12 hours after dosing (287). There is a linear relationship between creatinine clearance and the renal clearance of acyclovir. The renal clearance of acyclovir is three times that of a given creatinine clearance, indicating significant tubular secretion (287). In subjects with preexisting renal insufficiency, the half-life of acyclovir can be as high as 20 hours, and dosing in renal insufficiency should be adjusted according to the level of renal function (287,288). Hemodialysis effectively removes acyclovir, reducing the

half-life to 5 hours, and can effectively remove 40% of acyclovir in body stores (283,287,289).

References

1. Bywaters EG, Beall D. Crush injuries with impairment of renal function. *BMJ* 1941;1:427.
2. Bywaters EG, Stead JK. The production of renal failure following injection of solutions containing myohemoglobin. *Q J Exp Physiol* 1944;33:53.
3. Bywaters EG, Popjak G. Experimental crushing injury: peripheral circulatory collapse and other effects of muscle necrosis in the rabbit. *Surg Gynecol Obstet* 1942;75:612.
4. Grossman RA, Hamilton RW, Morse BM, et al. Nontraumatic rhabdomyolysis and acute renal failure. *N Engl J Med* 1974;291:807.
5. Zager R. Rhabdomyolysis and myohemoglobinuric acute renal failure. *Kidney Int* 1996;49:314.
6. Bywaters EG. 50 years on: the crush syndrome. *BMJ* 1990;301:1412.
7. Nath KA, Balla G, Vercellotti GM, et al. Induction of heme oxygenase is a rapid, protective response in rhabdomyolysis in the rat. *J Clin Invest* 1992; 90:267.
8. Better OS, Rubinstein, I, Winaver J. Recent insights into the pathogenesis and early management of the crush syndrome. *Semin Nephrol* 1992;12:217.
9. Better OS, Stein JH. Early management of shock and prophylaxis of acute renal failure in traumatic rhabdomyolysis. *N Engl J Med* 1990;322:825.
10. Better OS. The crush syndrome revisited (1940–1990). *Nephron* 1990;55: 97.
11. Ron D, Taitelman U, Michaelson M, et al. Prevention of acute renal failure in traumatic rhabdomyolysis. *Arch Intern Med* 1984;144:277.
12. Odeh M. The role of reperfusion-induced injury in the pathogenesis of the crush syndrome. *N Engl J Med* 1991;324:1417.
13. Owen CA, Mubarak SJ, Hargens AR, et al. Intramuscular pressures with limb compression. *N Engl J Med* 1979;300:1169.
14. Curry SC, Chang, D, Connor D. Drug- and toxin-induced rhabdomyolysis. *Ann Emerg Med* 1989;18:1068.
15. Prendergast BD, George CF. Drug-induced rhabdomyolysis: mechanisms and management. *Postgrad Med J* 1993;69:333.
16. Graham, DJ, et al. Incidence of hospitalized rhabdomyolysis in patients treated with lipid-lowering drugs. *JAMA* 2004;292(21):2585.
17. Cogen FC, Rigg G, Simmons JL, et al. Phencyclidine-associated acute rhabdomyolysis. *Ann Intern Med* 1978;88:210.
18. Billis AG, Kastanakis S, Giamarellou H, et al. Acute renal failure after a meal of quail. *Lancet* 1971;2:702.
19. Mason J, Thomas E. Rhabdomyolysis from heat hyperpyrexia. *N Engl J Med* 1976;235:633.
20. Roth D, Alarcon FJ, Fernandez JA, et al. Acute rhabdomyolysis associated with cocaine intoxication. *N Engl J Med* 1988;319:673.
21. Song SK, Rubin E. Ethanol produces muscle damage in human volunteers. *Science* 1972;175:327.
22. D'Agostino RS, Arnett EN. Acute myoglobinuria and heroin snorting. *JAMA* 1979;241:277.
23. Knochel JP, Schlein EM. On the mechanism of rhabdomyolysis in potassium depletion. *J Clin Invest* 1972;51:1750.
24. Singhal PC, Kumar A, Desroches L, et al. Prevalence and predictors of rhabdomyolysis in patients with hypophosphatemia. *Am J Med* 1992;92: 458.
25. Knochel JP, Barcenas C, Cotton JR, et al. Hypophosphatemia and rhabdomyolysis. *J Clin Invest* 1978;62:1240.
26. Knochel JP. Hypophosphatemia and rhabdomyolysis. *Am J Med* 1992;92: 455.
27. Haller RG, Drachman DB. Alcoholic rhabdomyolysis: an experimental model in the rat. *Science* 1980;208:412.
28. Perkoff GT, Hardy P, Velez-Garcia E. Reversible acute muscular syndrome in chronic alcoholism. *N Engl J Med* 1966;274:1282.
29. Gabow PA, Kaehny WD, Kelleher SP. The spectrum of rhabdomyolysis. *Medicine (Baltimore)* 1982;61:141.
30. Grunfeld JP, Ganeval D, Chanard J, et al. Acute renal failure in McArdle's disease. *N Engl J Med* 1972;286:1237.
31. Layzer RB, Rowland LP, Ranney HM. Muscle phosphofructokinase deficiency. *Arch Neurol* 1967;17:512.
32. Bank WJ, DiMauro S, Bonilla E, et al. A disorder of muscle lipid metabolism and myoglobinuria. *N Engl J Med* 1975;292:443.
33. Cunningham E, Kohli R, Venuto MF. Influenza-associated myoglobinuric renal failure. *JAMA* 1979;242:2428.
34. Weinstein L, Michael MA. Gas gangrene. *N Engl J Med* 1973;289:1129.
35. Demos MA, Gitin EL, Kagen LJ. Exercise myoglobinemia and acute exertional rhabdomyolysis. *Arch Intern Med* 1974;134:669.
36. Knochel JP. Catastrophic medical events with exhaustive exercise: "white collar rhabdomyolysis." *Kidney Int* 1990;38:709.
37. Halverson PB, Kozin, F, Ryan LM, et al. Rhabdomyolysis and renal failure in hypothyroidism. *Ann Intern Med* 1979;91:57.
38. Ralfman MA, Berant M, Lenarsky C. Cold weather and rhabdomyolysis. *J Pediatr* 1978;93:970.
39. Kagen LJ. Clinical considerations. In: Kagen LJ, ed. *Myoglobin: biochem-*

ical, physiological, and clinical aspects. New York: Columbia University Press, 1973:79.
40. Koskelo P, Kekki M, Wager O. Kinetic behaviour of ^{131}I-labelled myoglobin in human beings. *Clin Chim Acta* 1967;17:339.
41. Daly JS, Little JM, Troxle RF, et al. Metabolism of ^{3}H-myoglobin. *Nature* 1967;216:1030.
42. Kagen LJ. Myoglobinemia and myoglobinuria in patients with myositis. *Arthritis Rheum* 1971;14:457.
43. Knochel JP. Rhabdomyolysis and myoglobinuria. In: Suki WN, Eknoyan G, eds. *The kidney in systemic disease.* New York: Wiley, 1976:263.
44. Hess JW, MacDonald RP, Frederick RJ, et al. Serum creatine phosphokinase activity in disorders of heart and skeletal muscle. *Ann Intern Med* 1964;61:1015.
45. Hsu CH, Kurtz TW, Waldinger TP. Cardiac output and renal blood flow in glycerol-induced acute renal failure in the rat. *Circ Res* 1977;40: 178.
46. Braun SR, Weiss FR, Keller AI, et al. Evaluation of the renal toxicity of heme proteins and their derivatives: a role in the genesis of acute tubule necrosis. *J Exp Med* 1970;131:443.
47. Ayer G, Grandchamp A, Wyler T, et al. Intrarenal hemodynamics in glycerol-induced myohemoglobinuric acute renal failure in the rat. *Circ Res* 1971;29:128.
48. Honda N. Acute renal failure and rhabdomyolysis. *Kidney Int* 1983;23: 888.
49. Marlee A, Peer G, Schwartz D, et al. Role of nitric oxide in glycerol-induced acute renal failure in rats. *Nephrol Dial Transplant* 1994;9:78.
50. Oken DE, Arce ML, Wilson DR. Glycerol-induced hemoglobinuric acute renal failure in the rat: I. micropuncture study of the development of oliguria. *J Clin Invest* 1966;45:724.
51. Thiel G, Wilson DR, Arce ML, et al. Glycerol induced hemoglobinuric acute renal failure in the rat: II. the experimental model, predisposing factors and pathophysiologic features. *Nephron* 1967;4:276.
52. Hsu CH, Kurtz TW, Goldstein JR, et al. Intrarenal hemodynamics in acute myohemoglobinuric renal failure. *Nephron* 1976;17:65.
53. Reineck HJ, O'Connor GJ, Lifschitz MD, et al. Sequential studies on the pathophysiology of glycerol-induced acute renal failure. *J Lab Clin Med* 1980;96:356.
54. Corwin HL, Schreiber MJ, Fang ST. Low fractional excretion of sodium: occurrence with hemoglobinuric and myoglobinuric induced acute renal failure. *Arch Intern Med* 1984;144:981.
55. Avramovic V, Vlahovic P, Mihailovic D, et al. Protective effect of bioflavonoid proanthocyanidin-BP1 in glycerol-induced acute renal failure in the rat: renal stereological study. *Ren Fail* 1999;21627.
56. Rodrigo R, Bosco C, Herrera P, et al. Amelioration of myoglobinuric renal damage in rats by chronic exposure to flavonol-rich red wine. *Nephrol Dial Transplant* 2004;19:2237.
57. Chander V, Singh D, Chopra K. Catechin, a natural antioxidant protects against rhabdomyolysis-induced myoglobinuric acute renal failure. *Pharm Res* 2003;48:503.
58. Perri GC, Gorini P. Uraemia in the rabbit after injection of crystalline myoglobin. *Br J Exp Pathol* 1952;33:440.
59. Lalich JJ. The role of oxyhemoglobin and its derivatives in the pathogenesis of experimental hemoglobinuric nephrosis. *Am J Pathol* 1955;31:153.
60. Corcoran AC, Page IH. Renal damage from ferroheme pigments myoglobin, hemoglobin, hematin. *Tex Rep Biol Med* 1945;3:528.
61. Lalich JJ. The influence of in vitro hemoglobin modification on hemoglobinuric nephrosis in rabbits. *J Lab Clin Med* 1952;40:102.
62. Vetterlein R, Hoffman F, Pedina J, et al. Disturbance in renal microcirculation induced by myoglobin and hemorrhagic hypotension in anesthetized rat. *Am J Clin Pathol* 1995;268:F839.
63. Bunn HF, Jandl JH. Exchange of heme among hemoglobin molecules. *Biochemistry* 1966;56:974.
64. Anderson WA, Morrison DB, Williams EF. Pathologic changes following injections of ferrihemate (hematin) in dogs. *Arch Pathol* 1942;33:589.
65. Aust SD, Morehouse LA, Thomas CE. Role of metals in oxygen radical reactions. *J Free Radic Biol Med* 1985;1:3.
66. Grisham MB. Myoglobin-catalyzed hydrogen peroxide dependent arachidonic acid peroxidation. *J Free Radic Biol Med* 1985;1:227.
67. Sadrzadeh SM, Graf G, Panter SS, et al. Hemoglobin: a biologic Fenton reagent. *J Biol Chem* 1984;259:14354.
68. Shah SV, Walker PD. Evidence suggesting a role for hydroxyl radical in glycerol-induced acute renal failure. *Am J Physiol* 1988;255:F438.
69. Paller MS. Hemoglobin- and myoglobin-induced acute renal failure in rats: role of iron in nephrotoxicity. *Am J Physiol* 1988;255:F539.
70. Zager RA. Combined mannitol and deferoxamine therapy for myohemoglobinuric renal injury and oxidant tubular stress. *J Clin Invest* 1992;90: 711.
71. Zager R, Burkhart K, Conrad D, et al. Phospholipase A2-induced cytoprotection of proximal tubules potential determinants and specificity for ATP depletion-mediated injury. *J Am Soc Nephrol* 1996;7:64.
72. Holt S, Moore K. Pathogenesis of renal failure in rhabdomyolysis: the role of myoglobin. *Exp Nephrol* 2000;8:72.
73. Zager RA. Heme protein-induced tubular cytoresistance: expression at the plasma membrane level. *Kidney Int* 1995;47:1336.
74. Hayes JM, Boonshaft, B, Maher JF, et al. Resistance to glycerol induced hemoglobinuric acute renal failure. *Nephron* 1970;7:155.

75. Venuto RC. Pigment-associated acute renal failure: is the water clearer 50 years later? *J Lab Clin Med* 1992;119:452.
76. Zager RA. Studies of mechanisms and protective maneuvers in myoglobinuric acute renal injury. *Lab Invest* 1989;60:619.
77. Zager R, Gameli L. Pathogenetic mechanisms in experimental hemoglobinuric acute renal failure. *Am J Physiol* 1989;256:F446.
78. Zager RA, Foerder C, Bredl C. The influence of mannitol on myoglobinuric acute renal failure: functional, biochemical, and morphological assessments. *J Am Soc Nephrol* 1991;2:848.
79. Stein JH, Lifschitz MD, Barnes LD. Current concepts on the pathophysiology of acute renal failure. *Am J Physiol* 1978;234:F171.
80. Clarkson AR. Glomerular coagulation in acute ischemic renal failure. *QJM* 1970;39:585.
81. Wardle EN, Wright NA. Intravascular coagulation and glycerin hemoglobinuric acute renal failure. *Arch Pathol* 1973;95:271.
82. Blachar Y, Fong JS, De Chadarevian JP, et al. Muscle extract infusion in rabbits: a new experimental model of the crush syndrome. *Circ Res* 1981;49:124.
83. Koffler A, Friedler RM, Massry SG. Acute renal failure due to nontraumatic rhabdomyolysis. *Ann Intern Med* 1976;85:23.
84. Ward MM. Factors predictive of acute renal failure in rhabdomyolysis. *Arch Intern Med* 1988;148:1553.
85. Fine DM, Gelber AC, Melamed ML, et al. Risk factors for renal failure among 72 consecutive patients with rhabdomyolysis related illicit drug use. *Am J Med* 2004;117:607.
86. Ravnskov U. Low molecular weight proteinuria in association with paroxysmal myoglobinuria. *Clin Nephrol* 1975;3:67.
87. DeFronzo RA, Taufield PA, Black H, et al. Impaired renal tubular potassium secretion in sickle cell disease. *Ann Intern Med* 1979;90:310.
88. DeFronzo RA, Sherwin RS, Dillingham M, et al. Influence of basal insulin and glucagon secretion on potassium and sodium metabolism. *J Clin Invest* 1978;61:472.
89. Schulze VE Jr. Rhabdomyolysis as a cause of acute renal failure. *Postgrad Med* 1982;72:145.
90. Humphreys MH. Pigment- and crystal-induced acute renal failure. In: Jacobson HR, Striker GE, Klahr S, eds. *The principles and practice of nephrology.* Philadelphia: BC Decker, 1991:650.
91. Eneas JF, Schoenfeld PY, Humphreys MH. The effect of infusion of mannitol-sodium bicarbonate on the clinical course of myoglobinuria. *Arch Intern Med* 1979;139:801.
92. McCarron DA, Elliott WC, Rose JS, et al. Severe mixed metabolic acidosis secondary to rhabdomyolysis. *Am J Med* 1979;67:905.
93. Oh MS. Does serum creatinine rise faster in rhabdomyolysis? *Nephron* 1993;63:255.
94. Knochel JP. Serum calcium derangements in rhabdomyolysis. *N Engl J Med* 1981;305:161.
95. Meroney WH, Arney GK, Segar WE, et al. The acute calcification of damaged muscle, with particular reference to acute post-traumatic renal insufficiency. *J Clin Invest* 1957;36:825.
96. Akmal M, Goldstein DA, Telfer N, et al. Resolution of muscle calcification in rhabdomyolysis and acute renal failure. *Ann Intern Med* 1978;89:928.
97. Lllach F, Felsenfeld AJ, Haussler MR. The pathophysiology of altered calcium metabolism in rhabdomyolysis-induced acute renal failure. *N Engl J Med* 1981;305:117.
98. Feinstein EI, Akmal M, Telfer N, et al. Delayed hypercalcemia with acute renal failure associated with nontraumatic rhabdomyolysis. *Arch Intern Med* 1981;141:753.
99. Gray RW, Wilz DR, Caldas AE, et al. The importance of phosphate in regulating plasma 1,25-(OH)$_2$-vitamin D levels in humans: studies in healthy subjects in calcium-stone formers and in patients with primary hyperparathyroidism. *J Clin Endocrinol Metab* 1977;45:299.
100. Hadjis T, Grieff M, Lockhat D, et al. Calcium metabolism in acute renal failure due to rhabdomyolysis. *Clin Nephrol* 1993;39:22.
101. Leonard CD, Eichner ER. Acute renal failure and transient hypercalcemia in idiopathic rhabdomyolysis. *JAMA* 1970;211:1539.
102. Akmal M, Bishop JE, Telfer N, et al. Hypocalcemia and hypercalcemia in patients with rhabdomyolysis with and without acute renal failure. *J Clin Endocrinol Metab* 1986;63:137.
103. Suki W, Eknoyan G, Rector RC Jr, et al. Patterns of nephron perfusion in acute and chronic hydronephrosis. *J Clin Invest* 1966;45:122.
104. Hoffman LM, Suki WN. Obstructive uropathy mimicking volume depletion. *JAMA* 1976;236:2096.
105. Sullivan LP, Wallace DP, Clancy RL, et al. Effect of cellular acidosis on cell volume in S2 segments of renal proximal tubules. *Am J Physiol* 1990;258:F831.
106. Better OS, Ziman C, Reis DN, et al. Hypertonic mannitol ameliorates intracompartmental tamponade in model compartment syndrome in the dog. *Nephron* 1991;58:344.
107. Brezis M, Rosen S. Hypoxia of the renal medulla: its implications for disease. *N Engl J Med* 1995;332:647.
108. Cornelissen JJ, Haanstra W, Haarman HJ, et al. Plasma exchange in rhabdomyolysis. *Intensive Care Med* 1989;15:528.
109. Bellomo R, Daskalakis M, Parkin G, et al. Myoglobin clearance during continuous hemodiafiltration. *Intensive Care Med* 1991;17:509.
110. Gunal AI, et al. Early and vigorous fluid resuscitation prevents acute renal failure in the crush victims of catastrophic earthquakes. *J Am Soc Nephrol* 2004;15:1862.
111. Brown CV, et al. Preventing renal failure in patients with rhabdomyolysis: do bicarbonate and mannitol make a difference? *J Trauma* 2004;56:1191.
112. Conger JD. A controlled evaluation of prophylactic dialysis in post-traumatic acute renal failure. *J Trauma* 1975;15:1056.
113. Nolph KD, Whitcomb ME, Schrier RW. Mechanisms for inefficient peritoneal dialysis in acute renal failure associated with heat and exercise. *Ann Intern Med* 1969;71:317.
114. Goldfinger D. Acute hemolytic transfusion reactions-a fresh look at pathogenesis and considerations regarding therapy. *Transfusion* 1977;17:85.
115. Honig CL, Bove JR. Transfusion-associated fatalities: review of bureau of biologic reports 1976–1978. *Transfusion* 1980;20:653.
116. Schmidt PJ, Holland PV. Pathogenesis of the acute renal failure associated with incompatible transfusions. *Lancet* 1967;2:1169.
117. McGehee WG, Rapaport SI, Hjort PF. Intravascular coagulation in fulminant meningococcemia. *Ann Intern Med* 1967;67:250.
118. Pollard TD, Weiss IW. Acute tubular necrosis in a patient with march hemoglobinuria. *N Engl J Med* 1970;283:803.
119. Pritchard JA, Whalley PJ. Abortion complicated by *Clostridium perfringens* infection. *Am J Obstet Gynecol* 1971;111:484.
120. Bennett JM, Healey PJ. Spherocytic hemolytic anemia and acute cholecystitis caused by Clostridium welchii. *N Engl J Med* 1963;268:1070.
121. Canfield CJ, Miller LH, Bartelloni PJ, et al. Acute renal failure in *Plasmodium falciparum* malaria. *Arch Intern Med* 1968;122:199.
122. Boonpucknavig V, Sitprija V. Renal disease in acute *Plasmodium falciparum* infection in man. *Kidney Int* 1979;16:44.
123. Dukes DC, Sealey BJ, Forbes JI. Oliguric renal failure in blackwater fever. *Am J Med* 1968;45:903.
124. Rosen S, Hano JE, Inman MM, et al. The kidney in blackwater fever. *Am J Clin Pathol* 1968;49:358.
125. Savitsky JP, Doczi J, Black J, et al. A clinical safety trial of stroma-free hemoglobin. *Clin Pharmacol Ther* 1978;23:73.
126. Cheng TS, Ko WH, Swaminathan R, et al. Effect of lysine on hemolysis-induced kidney damage. *J Lab Clin Med* 1992;19:502.
127. Cohen LF, Balow JE, Magrath IT, et al. Acute tumor lysis syndrome: a review of 37 patients with Burkitt's lymphoma. *Am J Med* 1980;68:486.
128. Alvsaker JO. Uric acid in human plasma: V. isolation and identification of plasma proteins interacting with urate. *Scand J Clin Lab Invest* 1966;18:227.
129. Postlethwaite AE, Gutman RA, Kelley WN. Salicylate-mediated increase in urate removal during hemodialysis: evidence for urate binding to protein in vivo. *Metabolism* 1974;23:771.
130. Kovarsky J, Holmes EW, Kelley WN. Absence of significant urate binding to human serum proteins. *J Lab Clin Med* 1979;93:85.
131. Klinenberg JR, Bluestone R, Schlosstein L, et al. Urate deposition disease. *Ann Intern Med* 1973;78:99.
132. Allen DJ, Miloxovich G, Mattocks AM. Inhibition of monosodium urate needle crystal growth. *Arthritis Rheum* 1965;8:1123.
133. Levinson DJ, Sorensen LB. Renal handling of uric acid in normal and gouty subjects: evidence for a 4-component system. *Ann Rheum Dis* 1980;39:173.
134. Rieselbach RE, Steele TH. Influence of the kidney upon urate homeostasis in health and disease. *Am J Med* 1974;56:665.
135. Weiner IM. Urate transport in the nephron. *Am J Physiol* 1979;237:F85.
136. Weinman EJ, Senekjian HO, Sansom SC, et al. Evidence for active and passive urate transport in the rat proximal tubule. *Am J Physiol* 1981;240:F90.
137. Senekjian HO, Knight TF, Weinman EJ. Urate transport by the isolated perfused S2 segment of the rabbit. *Am J Physiol* 1981;240:F530.
138. Roch-Ramel F, Werner D, Guisan B. Urate transport in brush-border membrane of human kidney. *Am J Physiol* 1994;266:F797.
139. Knorr BA, Beck JC, Abramson RG. Classical and channel-like urate transporters in rabbit renal brush border membranes. *Kidney Int* 1994;45:727.
140. Stavric B, Johnson WJ, Grice HC. Uric acid nephropathy: experimental model. *Proc Soc Exp Biol Med* 1969;130:512.
141. Conger JD, Falk SA, Guggenheim SJ, et al. A micropuncture study of the early phase of acute urate nephropathy. *J Clin Invest* 1976;58:681.
142. Conger JD, Falk SA. Intrarenal dynamics in the pathogenesis and prevention of acute urate nephropathy. *J Clin Invest* 1977;59:786.
143. Rieselbach RE, Bentzel CJ, Cotlove E, et al. Uric acid excretion and renal function in the acute hyperuricemia of leukemia. *Am J Med* 1964;37:872.
144. Seegmiller JE, Frazier PD. Biochemical considerations of the renal damage of gout. *Ann Rheum Dis* 1966;25:668.
145. Gold GL, Fritz RD. Hyperuricemia associated with the treatment of acute leukemia. *Ann Intern Med* 1957;47:428.
146. Frei E, Bentzel CJ, Rieselbach RE, et al. Renal complications of neoplastic disease. *J Chronic Dis* 1963;16:757.
147. Lynch EC. Uric acid metabolism in proliferative diseases of the marrow. *Arch Intern Med* 1962;109:43.
148. Hricik DE, Goldsmith GH. Uric acid nephrolithiasis and acute renal failure secondary to streptozotocin nephrotoxicity. *Am J Med* 1988;84:153.
149. Crittenden DR, Ackerman GI. Hyperuricemic acute renal failure in disseminated carcinoma. *Arch Intern Med* 1977;137:97.
150. Dirix LY, Prove A, Becquart D, et al. Tumor lysis syndrome in a patient with metastatic Merkel cell carcinoma. *Cancer* 1991;67:2207.
151. Barton JC. Tumor lysis syndrome in nonhematopoietic neoplasms. *Cancer* 1989;64:738.

152. Stark ME, Dyer MC, Coonley CJ. Fatal acute tumor lysis syndrome with metastatic breast carcinoma. *Cancer* 1987;60:762.
153. Tomlinson GC, Solberg LA. Acute tumor lysis syndrome with metastatic medulloblastoma. *Cancer* 1984;53:1783.
154. Vogelzang NJ, Nelimark RA, Nath KA. Tumor lysis syndrome after induction chemotherapy of small-cell bronchogenic carcinoma. *JAMA* 1983;249:513.
155. Knochel JP, Dotin LN, Hamburger RJ. Heat stress, exercise and muscle injury: effects on urate metabolism and renal function. *Ann Intern Med* 1974;81:321.
156. Alexopoulos E, Tampakoudis P, Bili H, et al. Acute uric acid nephropathy in pregnancy. *Obstet Gynecol* 1992;80:488.
157. Ventataseshan VS, Feingold R, Dikman S, et al. Acute hyperuricemic nephropathy and renal failure after transplantation. *Nephron* 1990;56:317.
158. Warren DJ, Leitch AG, Leggett RJ. Hyperuricemic acute renal failure after epileptic seizures. *Lancet* 1975;2:385.
159. Kjellstrand CM, Cambell DC, von Hartitzsch B, et al. Hyperuricemic acute renal failure. *Arch Intern Med* 1974;133:349.
160. Kelton J, Kelley WN, Holmes EW. A rapid method for the diagnosis of acute uric acid nephropathy. *Arch Intern Med* 1978;138:612.
161. Steele TH, Rieselbach RE. The contribution of residual nephrons within the chronically diseased kidney to urate homeostasis in man. *Am J Med* 1967;43:876.
162. Hande KR, Garrow GC. Acute tumor lysis syndrome in patients with high-grade non-Hodgkin's lymphoma. *Am J Med* 1993;94:133.
163. Stapleton FB, Strother DR, Roy S III, et al. Acute renal failure at onset of therapy for advanced stage Burkitt lymphoma and B cell acute lymphoblastic lymphoma. *Pediatrics* 1988;82:863.
164. Arseneau JC, Bagley JW, Anderson T, et al. Hyperkalemia: a sequel to chemotherapy of Burkitt's lymphoma. *Lancet* 1973;1:10.
165. Monballyu J, Zachee P, Verberckmoes R, et al. Transient acute renal failure due to tumor-lysis-induced severe phosphate load in a patient with Burkitt's lymphoma. *Clin Nephrol* 1984;22:47.
166. Ettinger DS, Harker WG, Gerry HW, et al. Hyperphosphatemia, hypocalcemia, and transient renal failure: results of cytotoxic treatment of acute lymphoblastic leukemia. *JAMA* 1978;239:2472.
167. Zager RA. Hyperphosphatemia: a factor that provokes severe experimental acute renal failure. *J Lab Clin Med* 1982;100:230.
168. Boles J, Dutel J, Briere J, et al. Acute renal failure caused by extreme hyperphosphatemia after chemotherapy of an acute lymphoblastic leukemia. *Cancer* 1984;53:2425.
169. de Bont JM, Pieters R. Management of hyperuricemia with rasburicase review. *Nucleosides Nucleotides Nucleic Acids* 2004;23(8–9):1431.
170. Andreoli SP, Clark JH, McGuire WA, et al. Purine excretion during tumor lysis in children with acute lymphocytic leukemia receiving allopurinol: relationship to acute renal failure. *J Pediatr* 1986;109:292.
171. Band PR, Silverberg DS, Henderson JF, et al. Xanthine nephropathy in a patient with lymphosarcoma treated with allopurinol. *N Engl J Med* 1970;283:354.
172. Greene ML, Fujimoto WY, Seegmiller JE. Urinary xanthine stones-a rare complication of allopurinol therapy. *N Engl J Med* 1969;280:426.
173. Potter JL, Silvidi AA. Xanthine lithiasis, nephrocalcinosis, and renal failure in a leukemia patient treated with allopurinol. *Clin Chem* 1987;33:2314.
174. Elion GB, Yu TF, Gutman AB, et al. Renal clearance of oxypurinol, the chief metabolite of allopurinol. *Am J Med* 1968;45:69.
175. DeConti RC, Calabresi P. Use of allopurinol for prevention and control of hyperuricemia in patients with neoplastic disease. *N Engl J Med* 1966;274:481.
176. Hande KR, Noone RM, Stone WJ. Severe allopurinol toxicity: description and guidelines for prevention in patients with renal insufficiency. *Am J Med* 1984;76:47.
177. Mills RM. Severe hypersensitivity reactions associated with allopurinol. *JAMA* 1971;216:799.
178. Hande KR, Reed E, Chabner B. Allopurinol kinetics. *Clin Pharmacol Ther* 1978;23:598.
179. Simmonds HA, Cameron JS, Morris GS, et al. Allopurinol in renal failure and the tumor lysis syndrome. *Clin Chim Acta* 1986;160:189.
180. Appelbaum SJ, Mayersohn M, Dorr RT, et al. Allopurinol kinetics and bioavailability: intravenous, oral and rectal administration. *Cancer Chemother Pharmacol* 1982;8:93.
181. Murrell GA, Rapeport WG. Clinical pharmacokinetics of allopurinol. *Clin Pharmacokinet* 1986;11:343.
182. Coiffier B, et al. Efficacy and safety of rasburicase (recombinant urate oxidase) for the prevention and treatment of hyperuricemia during induction chemotherapy of aggressive non-Hodgkin's lymphoma: results of the GRAAL1 (Groupe d'Etude des Lymphomes de l'Adulte Trial on Rasburicase Activity in Adult Lymphoma) study. *J Clin Oncol* 2003;21(23):4402.
183. Bosly A, et al. Rasburicase (recombinant urate oxidase) for the management of hyperuricemia in patients with cancer: report of an international compassionate use study. *Cancer* 2003;98(5):1048.
184. Goldman SC, et al. A randomized comparison between rasburicase and allopurinol in children with lymphoma or leukemia at high risk for tumor lysis. *Blood* 2001;97(10):2998.
185. Tsokos GC, Balow JE, Spiegel RJ, et al. Renal and metabolic complications of undifferentiated and lymphoblastic lymphomas. *Medicine (Baltimore)* 1981;60:218.
186. Steinberg SM, Galen MA, Lazarus JM, et al. Hemodialysis for acute anuric uric acid nephropathy. *Am J Dis Child* 1975;129:956.
187. Deger GE, Wagoner RD. Peritoneal dialysis in acute uric acid nephropathy. *Mayo Clin Proc* 1972;47:189.
188. Pichette V, Leblanc M, Bonnardeax A, et al. High dialysate flow rate continuous arteriovenous hemodialysis: a new approach for the treatment of acute renal failure and tumor lysis syndrome. *Am J Kidney Dis* 1994;23:591.
189. Litovitz TL, Clark LR, Soloway RA. 1993 Annual report of the American Association of Poison Control Centers toxic exposure surveillance system. *Am J Emerg Med* 1994;12:546.
190. Parry MF, Wallach R. Ethylene glycol poisoning. *Am J Med* 1974;57:143.
191. Wax PM. Elixirs, diluents, and the passage of the 1938 federal Food, Drug and Cosmetic Act. *Arch Intern Med* 1995;122:456.
192. Winek CL, Shingleton DP, Shanor SP. Ethylene and diethylene glycol toxicity. *Clin Toxicol* 1978;13:297.
193. Okuonghae HO, Ighogboja IS, Lawson JO, et al. Diethylene glycol poisoning in Nigerian children. *Ann Trop Paediatr* 1992;12:235.
194. O'Brien K, Selanikio J, Hecdivert C, et al. Epidemic of pediatric deaths from acute renal failure caused by diethylene glycol poisoning. *JAMA* 1998;279:1175.
195. Jacobsen D, Ovrebo S, Ostborg J, et al. Glycolate causes the acidosis in ethylene glycol poisoning and is effectively removed by hemodialysis. *Acta Med Scand* 1984;216:409.
196. McChesney EW, Golberg L, Parekh CK, et al. Reappraisal of the toxicology of ethylene glycol: II. metabolism studies in laboratory animals. *Food Cosmet Toxicol* 1971;9:21.
197. Gabrow PA, Clay K, Sullivan JB, et al. Organic acids in ethylene glycol intoxication. *Ann Intern Med* 1986;105:16.
198. Chou JY, Richardson KE. The effect of pyrazole on ethylene glycol toxicity and metabolism in the rat. *Toxicol Appl Pharmacol* 1978;43:33.
199. Wacker WE, Haynes H, Druyan R, et al. Treatment of ethylene glycol poisoning with ethyl alcohol. *JAMA* 1965;194:173.
200. Richardson KE. The effect of partial hepatectomy on the toxicity of ethylene glycol, glycolic acid, glyoxylic acid and glycine. *Toxicol Appl Pharmacol* 1973;24:530.
201. Bove KE. Ethylene glycol toxicity. *Am J Clin Pathol* 1966;45:46.
202. Smith BJ, Anderson BG, Smith SA, et al. Early effects of ethylene glycol on the ultrastructure of the renal cortex in dogs. *Am J Vet Res* 1990;51:89.
203. Hagemann PO, Chiffelle TR. Ethylene glycol poisoning. *J Lab Clin Med* 1948;33:573.
204. Pons CA, Custer RP. Acute ethylene glycol poisoning, a clinico-pathologic report of eighteen fatal cases. *Am J Med Sci* 1946;211:544.
205. Friedman EA, Greenberg JB, Merrill JP, et al. Consequences of ethylene glycol poisoning. *Am J Med* 1962;32:891.
206. Karlson-Stiber C, Persson H. Ethylene glycol poisoning: experiences from an epidemic in Sweden. *Clin Toxicol* 1992;30:565.
207. Berman LB, Schreiner GE, Feys J. The nephrotoxic lesion of ethylene glycol. *Ann Intern Med* 1957;46:611.
208. Flanagan P, Libcke JH. Renal biopsy observations following recovery from ethylene glycol nephrosis. *Am J Clin Pathol* 1964;41:171.
209. Collins JM, Hennes DM, Holzgang CR, et al. Recovery after prolonged oliguria due to ethylene glycol intoxication: the prognostic value of serial percutaneous renal biopsy. *Arch Intern Med* 1970;125:1059.
210. Borden TA, Bidwell CD. Treatment of acute ethylene glycol poisoning in rats. *Invest Urol* 1968;6:205.
211. Leon M, Graeber C. Absence of high anion gap metabolic acidosis in severe ethylene glycol poisoning: a potential effect of simultaneous lithium carbonate ingestion. *Am J Kidney Dis* 1994;23:313.
212. Clay KL, Murphy RC. On the metabolic acidosis of ethylene glycol intoxication. *Toxicol Appl Pharmacol* 1977;39:39.
213. McChesney EW, Golberg L. Reappraisal of the toxicology of ethylene glycol: IV. The metabolism of labelled glycolic and glyoxylic acids in the rhesus monkey. *Food Cosmet Toxicol* 1972;10:655.
214. Jacobsen D, Hewlett TP, Webb R, et al. Ethylene glycol intoxication: evaluation of kinetics and crystalluria. *Am J Med* 1988;84:145.
215. Moriarty RW, McDonald RH. The spectrum of ethylene glycol poisoning. *Clin Toxicol* 1974;7:583.
216. Frommer JP, Ayus JC. Acute ethylene glycol intoxication. *Am J Nephrol* 1982;2:1.
217. Jacobsen D, McMartin KE. Methanol and ethylene glycol poisonings: mechanism of toxicity, clinical course, diagnosis and treatment. *Med Toxicol* 1986;1:309.
218. Spillane L, Roberts JR, Meyer AE. Multiple cranial nerve deficits after ethylene glycol poisoning. *Ann Emerg Med* 1991;20:208.
219. Ahmed MM. Ocular effects of antifreeze poisoning. *Br J Ophthalmol* 1971;55:854.
220. Gennari FJ. Serum osmolality: uses and limitations. *N Engl J Med* 1984;310:102.
221. Jacobsen D, Bredesen JE, Eide I, et al. Anion and osmolal gaps in the diagnosis of methanol and ethylene glycol poisoning. *Acta Med Scand* 1982;212:17.
222. Simpson E. Some aspects of calcium metabolism in a fatal case of ethylene glycol poisoning. *Ann Clin Biochem* 1985;22:90.
223. Stokes JB III, Aueron F. Prevention of organ damage in massive ethylene glycol ingestion. *JAMA* 1980;243:2065.

224. Jacobsen D, Akesson I, Shefter E. Urinary calcium oxalate monohydrate crystals in ethylene glycol poisoning. *Scand J Clin Lab Invest* 1982;42:231.

225. Godolphin W, Meagher EP, Sanders HD, et al. Unusual calcium oxalate crystals in ethylene glycol poisoning. *Clin Toxicol* 1980;16:479.

226. Terlinsky AS, Grochowski J, Geoly KL, et al. Identification of atypical calcium oxalate crystalluria following ethylene glycol ingestion. *Am J Clin Pathol* 1981;76:223.

227. Burns JR, Finlayson B. Changes in calcium oxalate crystal morphology as a function of concentration. *Invest Urol* 1980;18:174.

228. Catchings TT, Beamer WC, Lundy L, et al. Adult respiratory distress syndrome secondary to ethylene glycol ingestion. *Ann Emerg Med* 1985;14:594.

229. Denning DW, Berendt A, Chia Y, et al. Myocarditis complicating ethylene glycol poisoning in the absence of neurological features. *Postgrad Med J* 1988;64:864.

230. Underwood F, Bennett WM. Ethylene glycol intoxication. *JAMA* 1973;226:1453.

231. Jarvie DR, Simpson D. Simple screening tests for the emergency identification of methanol and ethylene glycol in poisoned patients. *Clin Chem* 1990;36:1957.

232. Porter WH, Auansakul A. Gas-chromatographic determination of ethylene glycol in serum. *Clin Chem* 1982;28:75.

233. Winter ML, Ellis MD, Snodgrass WR. Urine fluorescence using a Wood's lamp to detect the antifreeze additive sodium fluorescein: a qualitative adjunctive test in suspected ethylene glycol ingestions. *Ann Emerg Med* 1990;19:663.

234. Brewer I. Toxicology of the alcohols. Part 1: methanol and ethylene glycol. *Clin Toxicol Update* 1985;7:1.

235. Glasser L, Sternglanz PD, Combie J, et al. Serum osmolality and its applicability to drug overdose. *Am J Clin Pathol* 1973;60:695.

236. Robinson AG, Loeb JN. Ethanol ingestion: commonest cause of elevated plasma osmolality? *N Engl J Med* 1971;284:1253.

237. Michelis MF, Mitchell B, Davis BB. "Bicarbonate resistant" metabolic acidosis in association with ethylene glycol intoxication. *Clin Toxicol* 1976;9:53.

238. Peterson CD, Collins AJ, Himes JM, et al. Ethylene glycol poisoning: pharmacokinetics during therapy with ethanol and hemodialysis. *N Engl J Med* 1981;304:21.

239. Peterson DI, Peterson JE, Hardinge MG, et al. Experimental treatment of ethylene glycol poisoning. *JAMA* 1963;186:169.

240. McCoy HG, Cipolle RJ, Ehlers SM, et al. Severe methanol poisoning: application of a pharmacokinetic model for ethanol therapy and hemodialysis. *Am J Med* 1979;67:804.

241. Watson WA. Ethylene glycol toxicity: closing in on rational, evidence-based treatment. *Ann Emerg Med* 2000;36(2):139.

242. Megarbane BS, Borron SW, Baud FJ. Current recommendations for treatment of severe toxic alcohol poisonings. *Intensive Care Med* 2004.

243. Brent J, McMartine K, Phillips S, et al. Fomepizole for the treatments of ethylene glycol poisoning. *N Engl J Med* 1999;340:832.

244. Baud FJ, Galliot M, Astier A, et al. Treatment of ethylene glycol poisoning with intravenous 4-methylpyrazole. *N Engl J Med* 1988;319:97.

245. Harry P, Turcant A, Bouachour G, et al. Efficacy of 4-methylpyrazole in ethylene glycol poisoning: clinical and toxicokinetic aspects. *Hum Exp Toxicol* 1994;13:61.

246. Barceloux D, Krenzelok E, Olson K, et al. American Academy of Clinical Toxicology practice guidelines on the treatment of ethylene glycol poisoning. *Clin Toxicol* 1999;37:537.

247. Sivilotti ML, Burns MJ, McMartin KE, et al. Toxicokinetics of ethylene glycol during fomepizole therapy: implications for management. For the Methylpyrazole for Toxic Alcohols Study Group. *Ann Emerg Med* 2000;36(2):114.

248. Jacobsen D, Ostby N, Bredesen JE. Studies on ethylene glycol poisoning. *Acta Med Scand* 1982;212:11.

249. Cheng JT, Beysolow TD, Kaul B, et al. Clearance of ethylene glycol by kidneys and hemodialysis. *Clin Toxicol* 1987;25:95.

250. Hirsch DJ, Jindal KK, Wong P, et al. A simple method to estimate the required dialysis time for cases of alcohol poisoning. *Kidney Int* 2001;60(5):2021.

251. Graefe U, Milutinovich J, Follette WC, et al. Less dialysis-induced morbidity and vascular instability with bicarbonate dialysate. *Ann Intern Med* 1978;88:332.

252. Ettinger B, Weil E, Mandel NS, et al. Triamterene-induced nephrolithiasis. *Ann Intern Med* 1979;91:745.

253. Abelson HT, Fosburg MT, Beardsley P, et al. Methotrexate-induced renal impairment: clinical studies and rescue from systemic toxicity with high-dose leucovorin and thymidine. *J Clin Oncol* 1983;1:208.

254. Pitman SW, Frei E III. Weekly methotrexate-calcium leucovorin rescue: effect of alkalinization on nephrotoxicity; pharmacokinetics in the CNS; and use in CNS non-Hodgkin's lymphoma. *Cancer Treat Rep* 1977;61:695.

255. Roy LF, Villeneuve J, Dumont A, et al. Irreversible renal failure associated with triamterene. *Am J Nephrol* 1991;11:486.

256. Nakamoto Y, Motohashi S, Kasahara H, et al. Irreversible tubulointerstitial nephropathy associated with prolonged, massive intake of vitamin C. *Nephron Dial Transplant* 1998;13(3):754.

257. Berns JS, Cohen RM, Stumacher RJ, et al. Renal aspects of therapy for human immunodeficiency virus and associated opportunistic infections. *J Am Soc Nephrol* 1991;1:1061.

258. Appel GB, Neu HC. The nephrotoxicity of antimicrobial agents. *N Engl J Med* 1977;296:784.

259. Weinstein L, Madoff MA, Samet CM. The sulfonamides. *N Engl J Med* 1960;263:793.

260. Dorfman LE, Smith JP. Sulfonamide crystalluria: a forgotten disease. *J Urol* 1970;104:482.

261. Carbone LG, Bendixen B, Appel GB. Sulfadiazine-associated obstructive nephropathy occurring in a patient with the acquired immunodeficiency syndrome. *Am J Kidney Dis* 1988;12:72.

262. Simon DI, Brosius FC, Rothstein DM. Sulfadiazine crystalluria revisited: the treatment of toxoplasma encephalitis in patients with acquired immunodeficiency syndrome. *Arch Intern Med* 1990;150:2379.

263. Oster S, Hutchison F, McCabe R. Resolution of acute renal failure in toxoplasmic encephalitis despite continuance of sulfadiazine. *Rev Infect Dis* 1990;12:618.

264. Molina J, Belenfant X, Doco-Lecompte T, et al. Sulfadiazine-induced crystalluria in AIDS patients with toxoplasma encephalitis. *AIDS* 1991;5:587.

265. Farinas MC, Echevarria S, Sampedro I, et al. Renal failure due to sulphadiazine in AIDS patients with cerebral toxoplasmosis. *J Intern Med* 1993;233:365.

266. Christin S, Baumelou A, Bahri S, et al. Acute renal failure due to sulfadiazine in patients with AIDS. *Nephron* 1990;55:233.

267. Siegel WH. Unusual complication of therapy with sulfamethoxazole-trimethoprim. *J Urol* 1977;117:397.

268. Sahai J, Heimberger T, Collins K, et al. Sulfadiazine-induced crystalluria in a patient with the acquired immunodeficiency syndrome: a reminder. *Am J Med* 1988;84:791.

269. Winterborn MH, Mann JR. Anuria due to sulfadiazine. *Arch Dis Child* 1973;48:915.

270. Hein R, Brunkhorst R, Thon WF, et al. Symptomatic sulfadiazine crystalluria in AIDS patients: a report of two cases. *Clin Nephrol* 1993;39:254.

271. Merck and Co. Crixivan (indinavir sulfate): U.S. package insert. West Point, PA: Merck and Co., 1996.

272. Kopp J, Miller K, Mican J, et al. Crystalluria and urinary tract abnormalities associated with indinavir. *Ann Intern Med* 1997;127:119.

273. Tashima K, Horowitz J, Rosen S. Indinavir nephropathy. *N Engl J Med* 1997;336:138.

274. Tucker WE, Macklin AW, Szot RJ, et al. Preclinical toxicology studies with acyclovir: acute and subchronic tests. *Fundam Appl Toxicol* 1983;3:573.

275. Brigden D, Rosling AE, Woods NC. Renal function after acyclovir intravenous injection. *Am J Med* 1982;73(Suppl 1A):182.

276. Sawyer MH, Webb DE, Balow JE, et al. Acyclovir-induced renal failure: clinical course and histology. *Am J Med* 1988;84:1067.

277. Potter JL, Krill CE. Acyclovir crystalluria. *Pediatr Infect Dis* 1986;5:710.

278. Becker BN, Fall P, Hall C, et al. Rapidly progressive acute renal failure due to acyclovir: case report and review of the literature. *Am J Kidney Dis* 1993;22:611.

279. Peterslund NA, Black FT, Tauris P. Impaired renal function after bolus injections of acyclovir. *Lancet* 1983;1:243.

280. Giustina A, Romanelli G, Cimino A, et al. Low-dose acyclovir and acute renal failure. *Ann Intern Med* 1988;108:312.

281. Hernandez E, Praga M, Moreno F, et al. Acute renal failure induced by oral acyclovir. *Clin Nephrol* 1991;36:155.

282. Bean B, Aeppli D. Adverse effects of high-dose intravenous acyclovir in ambulatory patients with acute herpes zoster. *J Infect Dis* 1985;151:362.

283. Krieble BF, Rudy DW, Glick MR, et al. Case report: acyclovir neurotoxicity and nephrotoxicity: the role for hemodialysis. *Am J Med Sci* 1993;305:36.

284. Eck P, Silver SM, Clark EC. Acute renal failure and coma after a high-dose of oral acyclovir. *N Engl J Med* 1991;325:1178.

285. Peterslund NA, Larsen ML, Mygind H. Acyclovir crystalluria. *Scand J Infect Dis* 1988;20:225.

286. Bianchetti MG, Roduit C, Oetliker OH. Acyclovir-induced renal failure: course and risk factors. *Pediatr Nephrol* 1991;5:238.

287. Blum MR, Liao SH, de Miranda P. Overview of acyclovir pharmacokinetic disposition in adults and children. *Am J Med* 1982;73(Suppl 1A):186.

288. Laskin OL, Longstreth JA, Whelton A, et al. Effect of renal failure on the pharmacokinetics of acyclovir. *Am J Med* 1982;73(Suppl. 1A):197.

289. Krasny HC, Liao SH, de Miranda P, et al. Influence of hemodialysis on acyclovir pharmacokinetics in patients with chronic renal failure. *Am J Med* 1982;73(Suppl 1A):202.

CHAPTER 50 ■ BLOOD PRESSURE AND THE KIDNEY

HUGH E. DE WARDENER AND GRAHAM A. MACGREGOR

Ten to fifteen percent of the world's population suffers from hypertension, but the cause can be identified in only 5%. Absurdly, hypertension is referred to as essential hypertension when the cause cannot be identified, as if other causes were nonessential. It now seems increasingly likely that the initiating fault underlying hypertension of unknown cause (essential hypertension) is a covert abnormality of the kidney. It appears therefore that nearly all patients with high blood pressure have a renal abnormality for the cause of hypertension, when known, usually is an overt abnormality of the kidney.

HISTORICAL BACKGROUND

Bright, Hypertension, and Advanced Renal Disease

Bright first proposed the notion in 1841 that hypertension is in some way connected with the kidney (1). He performed postmortem examinations on patients who had died from "dropsy and coagulable urine" in whom he stated there was always "some obvious derangement of the kidneys." He also noted that the left ventricle was enlarged and the wall hypertrophied. "What is most striking," he pointed out was that, " ... there were twenty two (patients) without any probable organic cause (e.g., a valvular lesion) for the marked hypertrophy." In trying to find an explanation for the association of disease of the kidney and left ventricular hypertrophy, Bright is credited with a proposal that, after many vicissitudes, appears to be increasingly relevant today.

Bright had noted that the radial pulse of these patients was hard. Although he could not measure the arterial pressure, fluctuating hydrostatic pressure within the artery was a well-accepted phenomenon; therefore, a hard pulse denoted raised arterial pressure. Harvey (2) had demonstrated the presence of arterial pressure by cutting an artery, and Hales had measured the arterial pressure of a horse (3) with a glass tube inserted into the femoral artery (Fig. 50-1). Bright (1), searching for a cause for cardiac hypertrophy and hypertension, concluded that,

> This leads us to look for some less local cause for the unusual effects to which the heart has been impelled; and the two most ready solutions appear to be; either that the altered quality of the blood affords irregular and unwanted stimulus to the organ (the heart) immediately; or that it so effects [sic] the minute and capillary circulation as to render greater action necessary to force the blood through the distant subdivisions of the vascular system.

The "altered quality of the blood" referred to those substances he rightly assumed severely diseased kidneys could no longer excrete. The idea that an "unwanted stimulus" to the heart (i.e., an increase in cardiac output) might raise blood pressure was not taken up until the 1960s (4), when it was put forward as a possible factor for the onset of a pressure rise in

some patients (see later discussion). The second proposal, that a greater action of the heart is necessary to force blood through the vascular system, indicates that Bright considered that raised arterial pressure might cause ventricular hypertrophy.

Bright did not specify which "distant sub-division of the vascular system" he had in mind. One reads the word "distant" and assumes that he was referring to all the vessels in the body. Bright's contemporaries, however, clearly thought he was referring " ... solely to the resistance of the small renal arteries" (5); in other words, the rise in blood pressure was necessary to force the blood through the kidneys. It is possible that this interpretation was derived from some anatomic dissections of kidneys made by Toynbee (6) working in collaboration with Bright. He found that in the final stages of Bright's disease when the kidneys were contracted, the renal arteries and vessels in the "malpighian tubules" (the glomeruli) were so contracted that they were very difficult or impossible to inject via the renal artery. Subsequently, Johnson in 1868 (5) drew attention to the fact that, in contrast to Bright's opinion, all the minute arteries of the body were involved in that the walls of the very small arteries of the brain and pia mater, as well as those in the kidneys, were hypertrophied. Like Bright, he thought this change directly resulted from an abnormality of the blood that was "contaminated by urinary excreta and otherwise deteriorated."

Traube (7) made a fascinating suggestion in 1871. He pointed out that "the shrinking of the renal parenchyma will ... act by decreasing the amount of liquid which is ... removed from the arterial system by urinary excretion. As a result ... the mean pressure of the arterial pressure must increase." This inspired teleologic hypothesis anticipated Fahr (8), Borst and Borst-de-Gues (9), and Guyton's (4) identical (although more detailed) proposals by about 100 years, even though it leaves unexplained the mechanisms that cause blood pressure to rise. Traube's assertion that hypertension is a compensatory phenomenon to increase an impaired urinary excretion toward normal is now considered to be relevant to most forms of hypertension, including those in which there is no overt renal disease such as essential hypertension. Borst and Borst-de-Gues's (9) summing up of this idea and its overall effect was that the arterial pressure rises to correct the kidney's "unwillingness to excrete sodium. Thus a seemingly normal sodium output is maintained at the expense of the hypertension."

Essential Hypertension and Nephrosclerosis

The next step forward was that of Mahomed in 1879 (10). He observed that, "it is very common to meet people, apparently in good health, who have no albumin in the urine or any other sign of organic disease, who constantly present a condition of high arterial tension." He found at postmortem examination that the kidneys of such patients, who had not had albuminuria, were "red" rather than "yellow," like those who had died with

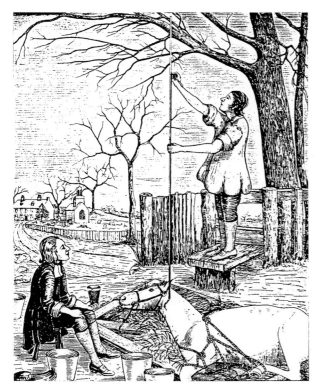

FIGURE 50-1. Stephen Hales and assistant measuring blood pressure of a horse. (From: Pickering GW. Systemic arterial hypertension. In: Fishman AP, Richards DW, eds. *Circulation of the blood, men and ideas.* New York: Oxford University Press, 1964:487, with permission.)

albuminuria and dropsy; that is, they did not look very abnormal, although they were somewhat contracted. Patients without proteinuria had come under treatment for "symptoms of cerebral haemorrhage, heart disease, lung disease and sundry medical and surgical disease." This is the first description of essential hypertension, a condition of sustained hypertension not due to overt renal disease. Mahomed concluded that

> high pressure is a constant condition in the circulation of some individuals and that this condition is a symptom of a certain constitution or diathesis. ... These persons appear to pass through life much as others do and generally do not suffer from their high blood pressure except in their petty ailments upon which it imprints itself. ... As age advances the enemy gains accession of strength. ... The individual has now passed 40 years of age, his lungs begin to deteriorate, he has a cough in the winter time, but by his pulse you will know him. Alternatively headache, vertigo, epistaxis, a passing paralysis, a more severe apoplectic seizure, and then the final blow. ... Of this I feel sure, that the clinical symptoms and the pathological changes resulting from high arterial pressure are frequently seen in cases in which slight, if any, disease is discoverable in the kidney.

Mahomed's proposals overlapped certain conclusions put forward a few years earlier by Huchard (11) in Paris, who had written that: "It has been wrongly assumed that chronic hypertension only appears following interstitial nephritis (glomerular nephritis). The opposite is true; arterial hypertension is the cause of arteriosclerosis; it precedes by a varying time interval the evolution of different diseases (heart disease, arterial nephritis, etc.) which are in turn secondary to vascular sclerosis."

In addition to the suggestion attributed to Bright that occlusive changes in the renal arteries are responsible for the associated rise in arterial pressure, Huchard put forward the concept

that hypertension itself could cause widespread occlusive arterial changes (including in the renal arterial tree) that he called "arterial nephritis," what we now call hypertensive vascular changes or nephrosclerosis, when present in the kidney.

Malignant Hypertension

These seminal observations were confirmed, elaborated, forgotten, and revived during the next 100 years. The next step forward was Volhard's (12) demonstration in 1931 that primary hypertension could have either a benign or malignant course. The benign form of hypertension, although accompanied by enlargement of the heart, might remain unchanged for years (as Mahomed had noted), the patient eventually dying of heart failure or a cerebrovascular accident while renal function remained relatively unimpaired throughout. Malignant hypertension was heralded by acute retinal changes and then increasing renal functional deterioration, the patient rapidly dying of renal failure. Volhard considered that benign essential hypertension was caused by a primary thickening of the systemic arteriolar walls that he called elastosis (i.e., full of elastic tissue), which he suggested was due to the effects of age on a "genetic constitution." He thought that malignant hypertension resulted from the action of a renal pressor substance released because of renal ischemia, which in turn resulted from severe "elastosis" of the renal arteries or glomerular nephritis that reduced renal blood flow by contracting the kidneys. He was also the first to suggest that vascular spasm of the renal vasculature produced by a pressor substance released by the kidney could lead to a vicious cycle effect that released more pressor substance. The concept of a circulating pressor substance resulted from the work of Tigerstedt and Bergman (13), who showed in 1898 that saline extracts of fresh rabbit kidney or an alcohol-dried powder produced a prolonged rise of pressure when injected into rabbits that were lightly anesthetized with urethane. They named this substance renin.

Volhard's hypothesis about the origin of malignant hypertension was supported first by the observation of Goldblatt et al. (14) in 1934 that renal ischemia in dogs, induced by partially constricting renal arteries, induced persistent hypertension that was caused by some substance released by the kidney. However, it took another 56 years before Tigerstedt and Bergman's observations led to the identification and structure of horse and ox angiotensin II by Skeggs et al. (15) and Peart (16), respectively. Volhard's vicious cycle hypothesis was supported by Wilson and Byrom's (17) experiments in rats, in which hypertension was induced by a partially occluding renal artery clip placed on one renal artery while the other kidney was left intact. In the first few weeks thereafter, removal of the "clipped" kidney was associated with a return of arterial pressure to normal, but removal of the clipped kidney did not lower arterial pressure if the clip was removed later (after the unclipped kidney had suffered irreversible vascular damage). Rettig et al. (18) confirmed, by transplanting the unclipped kidney into a normal rat that then develops hypertension, that the persistence of hypertension after the clip is removed is caused by the hypertensive vascular changes in the unclipped kidney.

Renal Origin of Hypertension

Mahomed's notion that the kidney in nonmalignant essential hypertension is normal before being damaged by the rise in pressure was continuously reaffirmed (19–21). Bell (19), a pathologist, concluded in 1946 that "hypertension may develop in persons whose renal vascular lesions are no greater than is found in non-hypertensive controls." It was not until the emergence of hereditary strains of hypertension in the rat that Borst and Borst-de-Gues (9) and Guyton's (4) claim began to be accepted that the kidney is abnormal in essential hypertension. This followed the finding that hereditary hypertension in the rat strongly resembles essential hypertension in humans, and that the kidneys in these strains, as in essential hypertension, are abnormal before the onset of hypertension, thus excluding the possibility that the high blood pressure itself is responsible for the renal abnormality.

Renal Origin of Hypertension in Hereditary Strains in Animals

The principal evidence that the initiating hypertensive trigger in hereditary rat strains of hypertension resides in the kidney has been obtained in renal cross transplantation experiments (22,23) (Fig. 50-2). This experiment was carried out from 1960 on by many different groups of research workers using four different strains of rat—the Dahl salt-sensitive rat, spontaneously hypertensive rat, stroke-prone spontaneously hypertensive rat, and Milan hypertensive rat (24–30). A unilateral nephrectomy is performed on both rats, and the remaining kidney from each is then cross-transplanted. Transplanting a kidney from a hypertensive to a normotensive strain rat raises blood pressure of the normotensive rat. To avoid the possibility that preexisting hypertensive vascular changes in the graft induce pressure rises in recipients, some of the kidneys from hypertensive strain rats were taken from prehypertensive 7-week-old or 20-week-old rats, blood pressure of which was kept within normal limits from the age of 4 weeks with a converting enzyme inhibitor. Nevertheless, blood pressure of the rat that received the kidney still rose to the same extent. In the reverse set of experiments, a kidney from a normotensive strain rat, when placed into a young hypertensive strain rat before the onset of hypertension, prevented the onset of hypertension. If placed into an older rat

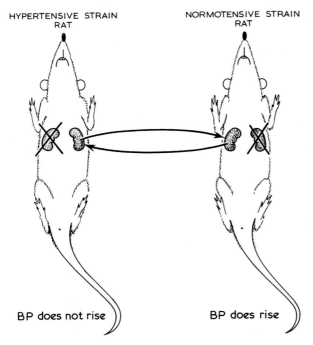

FIGURE 50-2. Cross-transplantation experiment between an inherited hypertensive strain rat and a control normotensive strain rat demonstrating that the kidney carries a genetic abnormality that causes blood pressure (BP) to rise. One kidney is removed from each rat, and the remaining kidney is then cross-transplanted into the other rat. The experiments are performed before the arterial pressure has risen in the hypertensive strain rat. (From: de Wardener HE. *The kidney,* 5th ed. Edinburgh: Churchill Livingstone, 1985:260, with permission.)

with established hypertension, it lowered the blood pressure. These experiments clearly demonstrate that an underlying genetic defect in the kidney is responsible for high blood pressure in these rats with hereditary hypertension.

Renal Origin of Essential Hypertension

In essential hypertension, the nearest equivalent to the cross transplantation experiments in animals is the relation of the recipient's blood pressure, after renal transplantation, to blood pressure of the donor's family. In one study of 50 recipients, those from normotensive families who received a kidney from a donor with a hypertensive parent needed significantly more hypertensive therapy than those who received a kidney from a normotensive family (31). In addition, there is a study of six black hypertensive patients with terminal renal failure owing to nephrosclerosis from severe essential hypertension (32). Their blood pressure fell to normal without the need for hypertensive treatment after they received a kidney from young normotensive donors. The average follow-up was 4.5 years.

Nature of the Renal Abnormality Responsible for Hypertension in Inherited Hypertension

The principal overall abnormality appears to be an impaired ability to excrete sodium. In cross transplantation experiments in the rat, sodium is retained as blood pressure rises by the recipients of hypertensive strain kidneys (33,34), which suggests that the rise in blood pressure is directly related to an impaired ability of the renal graft to excrete sodium. Recent observations in the spontaneously hypertensive rat (SHR) demonstrated that the impaired ability to excrete sodium is present at 3 to 7 weeks of age and that such kidneys have a blunted natriuretic response to arterial pressure associated with an increase in renal vascular resistance owing to a narrowing of the afferent arterioles. The most marked changes occur in the papillae, where there is a reduction in blood flow and interstitial hydrostatic pressure. Such vascular changes certainly could contribute to the impaired ability of the kidneys to excrete sodium (35–39). In addition, the kidney in essential hypertension and several strains of hypertensive rats is the site of several other, inherited abnormalities that could alter the ability of the kidney to excrete sodium (see the following).

In humans renal vascular resistance is raised in normotensive children of hypertensive parents (40) and there is considerable evidence that they also have an impaired ability to excrete sodium. In some patients with essential hypertension who have an exaggerated increase in blood pressure following an intravenous infusion of saline (41), there is a detectable impairment in their ability to excrete an acute sodium load (42).

Urinary sodium excretion is closely related to dietary intake. When the kidney has difficulty excreting sodium, the consequences that follow are more severe, that is, the greater the amount that has to be excreted. Thus, as the evidence accumulates, studies demonstrate that hypertension is closely related to the dietary intake of sodium.

Summary

Bright proposed (or at least is given credit for proposing) that hypertension associated with severe renal disease is caused by occlusive changes to the distant subdivisions of the vascular system of the kidney (1). Subsequently it was found that hypertension without severe renal disease (i.e., essential hypertension), can occur without microscopic vascular abnormalities in the kidneys; therefore, it was deemed that essential hypertension is unrelated to any abnormality of the kidney, in contrast to hypertension with severe renal disease.

In the past 40 years, however, evidence has accumulated that although the renal vessels in an animal model of hypertension that closely resembles essential hypertension appear to be normal on microscopy before the rise in pressure, they are functionally abnormal in that they have an increased tone. Such an increase, together with several other documented renal abnormalities in both essential hypertension and hypertensive strains of rats, could be responsible, in part, for the "unwillingness" of these kidneys to excrete salt. There is now evidence that even a single monogenetic lesion, intrinsic to the kidney, such as Liddle's syndrome, which impairs sodium excretion, is sufficient itself to cause blood pressure to rise (43). Thus, both hypertension associated with severe renal disease, first described by Bright, and essential hypertension are renal diseases, and the principal functional abnormality appears to be an impaired ability to excrete sodium.

SALT INTAKE AND BLOOD PRESSURE

If essential hypertension is caused by an impaired ability to excrete sodium, then there should be some relation between salt intake and hypertension.

History of Salt in Human Affairs

The human race is considered to have been on the earth for about 3 million years, and those living inland had to eat a low-salt diet (approximately 10 to 15 mmol/day) until about 5,000 years ago. In other words, the human race is genetically programmed to eat a low-salt diet. This was accomplished by increasing the tongue's exceptional ability to detect minute quantities of salt, and by a remarkable capacity to conserve sodium by reducing sodium lost in sweat and urine. (It is possible to reduce 24-hour urine loss to less than 1 mmol.) Salt intake rose when humans discovered that salt had the "magical" property of being able to preserve food. Initially, salt was obtained with great difficulty from the sea and was one of the precious cargoes carried inland by camel caravans across the Arabian and African deserts. The Roman army, which at first issued a monthly ration of salt to each man, eventually found it more convenient to pay each man a monthly lump sum (a salary) with which to purchase salt. Salt's ability to preserve food was of vital economic importance. It is probable, however, that the consumption of highly salted preserved food meant that fresh food tasted bland, and not surprisingly, those who could afford it started to add salt to unsalted food. The increasing use of salt made it an important object of commerce, especially for those countries that bordered on the sea or had salt mines. The salt trade was the underlying foundation of the Venetian empire that lasted nearly 800 years (44). The Chinese had a salt tax circa 2000 BC. Governments used the desire for salt as a source of revenue, much as they now use that for alcohol. The demand for salt was so powerful and pervasive that smugglers took enormous risks to bypass the tax. In the 17th century, about one-third of the galley slaves in France had been sentenced for violation of the salt tax. It was the most hated of all taxes, and in the next century was one of the major causes of the French Revolution (45).

By 1850, salt was no longer expensive, and it was estimated that salt consumption in England and France per capita was about 20 g/day (330 mmol), half added to the food at table, the other half present in food. The introduction of refrigeration reversed this trend, and during the 20th century salt consumption tended to fall. Nevertheless, in Western communities, it is still 100 to 400 mmol/day, with an average intake of 150 mmol in Europe and the United States, at least six times more than late Paleolithic man (46). Now, less is added at the table than in 1850, but processed foods are responsible for the 70% to 80% of the total intake.

THE INFLUENCE OF SALT INTAKE ON BLOOD PRESSURE

The relation of salt intake to blood pressure has been revealed by (a) epidemiologic studies, (b) measuring the effect of increasing and decreasing the intake of salt on the normal blood pressure, and (c) decreasing salt intake in patients with hypertension.

Epidemiologic Studies

There have been nearly 40 accounts of certain unacculturated populations in which blood pressure did not rise with age—in other words, such populations did not have essential hypertension (47). Their dietary intake of salt was below 3 g/day, in a few it was below 1 g/day, and in one it was about 0.05 g/day. At the other end of the scale, there have been studies among Japanese and Portuguese communities with a high prevalence of hypertension in one of which the salt intake averaged 26 g/day. The bulk of Westernized societies, which consume around 7 to 12 g of salt/day with an average of 9 g/day, are in between. The connection between salt intake and hypertension in these intermediate populations is evident but more difficult to discern mainly because of the relatively narrow range of salt intake (approximately 6 to 10 g/day) and the wide fluctuations of 24-hour urinary salt excretion (used to measure salt intake), which is owing to the variable day-to-day salt intake of individuals in most developed countries.

Unacculturated Populations

Low-salt-eating unacculturated populations used to inhabit the tropics of Africa, South America, and the Pacific and Arctic regions. The outstanding example is the Yanomamo Indians in South America. Their staple foods are cooked bananas and manioc; they have little access to salt. Their mean 24-hour urinary excretion of salt is around 0.05 g/day and their potassium intake is about 3 g/day. The Yanomamo culture encourages chronic warfare and violence (48), yet there is no rise in blood pressure with age.

Nigeria

In two related rural tribes in Nigeria only one had access to salt. There was a highly significant difference in blood pressure between the two tribes, the one with access to salt having the higher arterial pressure. The two tribes were identical in all other respects.

The Iranian Qash' qai

The relation of salt intake to blood pressure in this primitive nomadic tribe complements the others. Throughout the area that this tribe has inhabited for approximately 400 years are natural surface deposits of salt, which the tribe uses liberally in baking and cooking as well as at the table. The average urinary sodium excretion is 186 mmol/day in the men and 141 mmol/day in the women. The prevalence of hypertension in those over 30 years of age is 12% and 18%, respectively, with no tendency for increased weight with age.

Thus, whatever subsidiary factors may be suggested, other than the dietary intake of salt to account for the stability in blood pressure with age in unacculturated people on low-salt intakes, they did not prevent a rise in blood pressure in the unacculturated tribe, which consumes a high-salt diet.

Migratory Studies

There are examples of groups of individuals from low-salt-eating communities whose blood pressure rises when a change in their circumstances causes them to eat more salt. The best of these was a carefully controlled study from Kenya where subsistence farmers ate a low-salt/high-potassium diet. Some of the farmers migrated to an urban community where there was a marked increase in salt intake and a fall in potassium intake to levels similar to those in Western countries. Blood pressure in these migrants rose, whereas there was no change in blood pressure in a control group that did not migrate. It was concluded that a major part of blood pressure rise that occurred on migration resulted from the increase in salt intake (49).

High-Salt-Intake Societies

There are several societies that continue to have a high salt intake, comparable to that of most Western societies during the 19th century, before the introduction of refrigeration and canning. These include Portugal, northern China, and Japan. Japan has been studied the longest.

Japan

In the late 1950s, the Japanese became aware that certain northeastern parts of the country, which had a very high consumption of salt, had the highest incidence of death from stroke (owing, at that time, to brain hemorrhage from a ruptured cerebral artery), and that in these areas the prevalence of high blood pressure also was greater than in the rest of the country (Fig. 50-3). For instance, the number of hypertensive individuals aged between 50 and 60 years in one community in the northeast in which the salt intake was 26 g/day was 70%, whereas it was only 10% in the south where the salt intake was 14 g/day.

THE RELATIONSHIP OF BLOOD PRESSURE TO SALT INTAKE WITHIN AND BETWEEN POPULATIONS

Studies of rural Asian communities in which there is a wide range of salt intake but each individual's intake is relatively constant have repeatedly shown a direct within-center relationship between 24-hour urinary sodium excretion and blood pressure (50–54). In Western cultures, however, in which the within-individual daily salt intake varies considerably, it has been difficult until recently to detect a significant relationship within populations. In addition, early attempts to correlate data among several international centers were criticized in that the various centers from which the data were obtained had used different criteria and there had been a failure to take into account many confounding variables. Thus, interesting cross-center linear relationships between blood pressure and sodium intake, which were repeatedly demonstrated from data collected worldwide (55,56), consistently failed to be universally convincing.

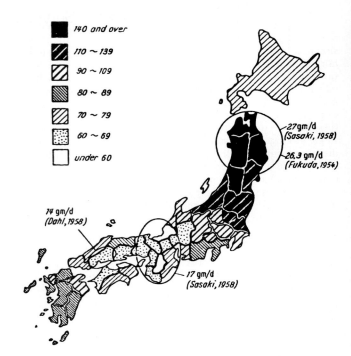

FIGURE 50-3. Regional distribution of cerebral hemorrhage in Japan in 1957–highest in the north and lowest in the south. The intake of sodium in four areas is also indicated, 14 g/day in the south and 27 g/day in the north. (Reprinted from: Takahashi E, et al. The geographic distribution of cerebral hemorrhage and hypertension in Japan. *Hum Biol* 1957;29[2]:139, with permission.)

An extensive and very well controlled international epidemiologic study (the Intersalt Study) that avoided the weaknesses of previous investigations was carried out in 10,079 men and women aged 20 to 59 years sampled from 52 centers around the world. They were studied using a standardized protocol, central training, and a central laboratory (57,58). After standardization for age, sex, body mass index, alcohol intake, and potassium excretion, within-center analyses showed that sodium excretion was significantly related to systolic pressure among individuals in a population, and cross-center analysis showed that sodium excretion is significantly related to the rise in systolic and diastolic pressure with age (Fig. 50-4). A conservative estimate of the size of this effect is that, on average, a reduction in sodium intake of 100 mmol/day between the ages of 25 and 55 years corresponds to a 9 mm Hg lower rise in systolic pressure. This is an underestimate because only one 24-hour urine sample was obtained from each person to measure the sodium excretion. Within-individual variations in daily sodium excretion, however, may be considerable (e.g., more than fivefold). When multiple regression analyses are calculated, factors that fluctuate to a large degree in this way tend to appear less important than those, such as weight, that fluctuate much less (an effect known as regression dilution bias). In order to obtain a correct regression coefficient in Western communities in which daily urinary sodium excretion fluctuates most widely, it would be necessary to sample five to 14 24-hour samples (59–62). This is impractical in a large survey. In the Intersalt Study, a partial adjustment was attempted by calculating a coefficient of reliability from the results of two 24-hour urine samples collected from 807 participants at random.

Once again, the Intersalt Study demonstrated that in geographically isolated centers where urinary sodium excretion rates were below approximately 60 mmol/day, of which there were four in the Intersalt Study, blood pressure does not rise with age, and hypertension is rare. In the past, the applicability

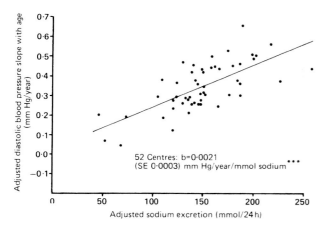

FIGURE 50-4. Cross-center plots of diastolic blood pressure slope with age, and median sodium excretion and fitted regression lines standardized for age, sex, body mass index, and alcohol consumption for 52 centers. (From: Intersalt Cooperative Research Group. Intersalt: an international study of electrolyte excretion and blood pressure. Results for 24-hour urinary sodium and potassium excretion. *Br Med J* 1988;297:319, with permission.)

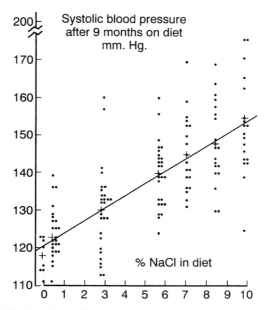

FIGURE 50-5. The effect of various intakes of salt for 9 months on the systolic blood pressure of normal rats. (From: Bell CD, Meneely GR. Observations on dietary sodium chloride. *J Am Diet Assoc* 1957;33:366, with permission.)

of such observations to other societies, particularly Western societies, tended to be dismissed on the assumption that the general health and daily life patterns of such isolated unacculturated societies was probably more relevant to their low blood pressure than their intake of sodium (63). It appears that this assumption is unwarranted, at least regarding their physical features. The local organizers at each of the four Intersalt centers with sodium intakes below 60 mmol/day reported that the participants were physically active, appeared healthy, and showed no sign of malnutrition or protein deficiency (64).

The Effect of Increased Salt Intake on Normal Blood Pressure

Normal Animals

The prolonged ingestion of increased quantities of salt causes hypertension in the normal dog (65,66), chicken (67), rabbit (68), baboon (69), rat (70–72), and chimpanzee (73). The rate of rise in blood pressure depends on the amount ingested. Hypertension usually comes on within a few weeks, is sustained thereafter, and is proportional to the intake. The effect is more marked in animals exposed just after birth (69,70,74) and in males (69,75).

Salt intake was first unequivocally demonstrated in animals as an initiator of hypertension by Meneely and associates (71), who fed groups of ordinary stock rats a range of dietary sodium intakes. At the end of 9 months, the mean blood pressure of each batch was directly related to the intake of sodium (Fig. 50-5). Dahl (76) confirmed these findings and made an additional observation of immense importance. He found that in each batch of rats' blood pressure rose in some rats but not others, and that this "sensitivity" and "resistance" of blood pressure to a high-salt diet was genetically determined. At about the same time, Smirk and Hall (77) bred a strain of rats that became hypertensive with age on a normal sodium intake (the first strain of "spontaneously hypertensive" rat) and another strain that did not develop hypertension with age.

A recent study in chimpanzees (73) phylogenetically our closest relation (98.4% genetic identity) is the most convincing testimony that excess sodium probably causes hypertension in humans. Normally chimpanzees, which live up to

50 years and weigh up to 50 kg, eat a diet of fruit and vegetables with sodium content around 10 mmol/day. A gradual increase in sodium intake in a colony of chimpanzees over 20 months to 200 mmol/day increased blood pressure by 33/10 mm Hg. Blood pressure returned to values present at the beginning of the study when the salt intake was lowered to 10 mmol/day (Fig. 50-6). This experiment shows that if the animal species most closely related to humans (which normally consumes a low-salt diet, as both they and humans are genetically programmed to do) increases its salt intake into the same range as present-day humans, then they will develop hypertension, just as humans do.

Normal Humans

There do not appear to be any studies comparable to those made in animals of the effect of an imposed, prolonged increase in salt intake on blood pressure of normotensive humans previously accustomed to a low salt intake; that is, a situation comparable to the chimpanzees. Salt intake has been increased for relatively short periods in the normal high-sodium diet of young adults (150 mmol/day), and this has induced only small changes in blood pressure. For instance, in four out of five studies (78–82), increases in sodium intake up to 420 mmol/day for up to 4 weeks in young or middle-aged (<47 years) normotensive subjects did not cause a rise in arterial pressure.

Normotensive Offspring of Hypertensive Parents

Observations in monozygotic and dizygotic twins have established that in normal subjects there are "strong heritable influences on the renal excretion of sodium which are most readily identified in the volume expanded state" (83); and that following a relatively slow infusion of saline (2 L in 4 hours), normotensive, first-degree relatives of patients with essential hypertension excrete less sodium than control subjects do (84). The relation of habitual salt intake to blood pressure, as measured by 24-hour urinary sodium excretion, has also been studied in normotensive offspring of two hypertensive parents (n = 41), normotensive offspring of one hypertensive parent (n = 52), and normotensive offspring of two normotensive

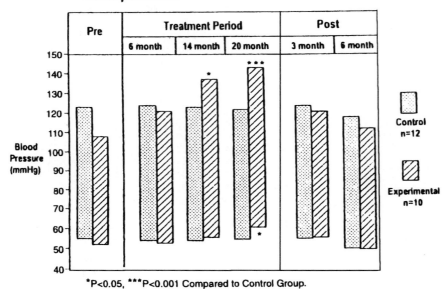

Chimpanzees

*P<0.05, ***P<0.001 Compared to Control Group.

FIGURE 50-6. Blood pressure in chimpanzees who either continued on their usual diet (sodium 10 mmol/day) or were given an increased salt intake (sodium 200 mmol/day). At the end of the 20-month study, the salt supplements were stopped, and blood pressure declined to that of the control group. (From: Denton D, et al. *Nat Med* 1995;I:1009, with permission. Figure reproduced from: MacGregor GA. Salt: blood pressure, the kidney, and other harmful effects. *Nephrol Dial Transplant* 1998;13:2471, with permission.)

parents (n = 61). The mean age of the three groups was 21, 22, and 23 years, respectively. The 24-hour urinary sodium excretion was similar in the three groups, but although there was a positive association between 24-hour urinary sodium excretion and systolic blood pressure in the offspring of two hypertensive parents, no such association was apparent in the offspring of two normotensive parents (85).

In contrast to a group of normotensive children of normotensive parents, a high dietary intake of sodium (270 mmol/day for 7 days) by normotensive children (mean age 25 ± 3 years) of hypertensive parents causes an increase in blood pressure (86). The effect of a relatively slow intravenous infusion of saline (2 L in 4 hours) has been studied frequently (87–89). Again in contrast to normotensive children of normotensive parents, an intravenous infusion to normotensive offspring of hypertensive parents causes a rise in blood pressure associated with a lesser rise in sodium excretion. The reduced excretion of sodium is consistent with the evidence that the kidneys in essential hypertension have an inherited abnormality of their ability to excrete sodium.

The Effect of Reducing Salt Intake on the Blood Pressure of Normal Humans

The effect of a reduction in salt intake on the arterial pressure of normal subjects has been studied in neonates, school-age children, and adults.

Neonates

The blood pressure in normal newborn babies has been found to be particularly sensitive to a prolonged small reduction in sodium intake. Hofman et al. (90) allocated 476 babies into two groups, one of which had a normal sodium intake and the other a lower intake for 6 months. The normal intake was three times greater than the lower. There was a progressive and increasing difference in systolic pressure between the two groups, so that the mean systolic pressure at 6 months was significantly higher in those on the higher sodium intake. Of the original 476 subjects, 167 were reinvestigated when they were 15 years old; blood pressure difference persisted in spite of the same salt intake in both groups in the interval (91) (Fig. 50-7).

This apparent prolonged effect on blood pressure of an increase in salt intake early in human life is consistent with many examples in animals that there is a period of high susceptibility to the effects of increased salt intake in youth (74).

Children

In four studies in children, the significance of the results was greatly influenced by the number of participants. In one study

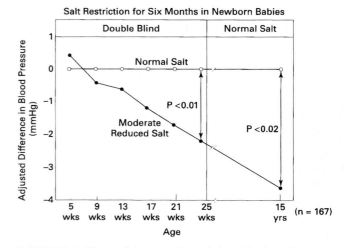

FIGURE 50-7. This study began with 476 babies. The figure illustrates the differences in blood pressure between two subgroups who were studied for the first 6 months of life and 15 years later. The heading "Double Blind" covers the first 6 months during which half the babies consumed a normal intake of salt and the other half a lower intake. At the end of 6 months blood pressure of the group that received the lower intake of salt was lower than that of the group that received a normal intake. For the next 14.5 years both groups ate a diet with a normal intake of salt. The blood pressure difference between the two groups, as measured in 167 of the original 476, in the 15th year is illustrated under the heading "Normal Salt." It can be seen that the difference in blood pressure that was present at 6 months is still present, although both groups have been eating the same amount of salt since that time. (Drawn from data in Hofman A, et al. *JAMA* 1983; 250:370, and Geleijnse et al. *Hypertension* 1996;29:913, with permission.)

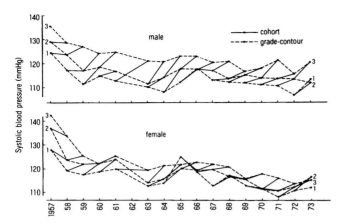

FIGURE 50-8. Mean systolic blood pressure levels in school children in grade 1 (12 to 13 years old), grade 2 (13 to 14 years old), and grade 3 (14 to 15 years old). The blood pressure of each new intake into these grades was measured at the beginning of the year. (From: Sasaki N. In: Yamori Y, et al., eds. *Prophylactic approach of hypertensive diseases.* New York: Raven Press, 1979:467. Reprinted by permission of Lippincott Williams & Wilkins.)

with a total of only 80 children, a reduction in sodium intake from 86 mmol/day to 56 mmol/day had no effect on blood pressure at the end of 1 year (92). In the second study with a total of 124 adolescents, a reduction in sodium intake of 65 mmol/day to an intake of 45 mmol/day for 24 days induced a nonsignificant fall in blood pressure (93). In a third group of 149 children, a reduction in sodium intake from 105 mmol/day to 50 mmol/day induced a significant fall in blood pressure after 12 weeks but only after adjustment for age and weight (94). With a total group of 750 children in the fourth study, however, a reduction in sodium intake from 166 mmol/day to 127 mmol/day induced a significant fall in blood pressure at 24 weeks (95). Records from one school in Japan between 1957 and 1972, during which there was a national reduction in dietary salt intake, show a steady decline in blood pressure in children between of 12 and 14 years of age (96) (Fig. 50-8).

Adults

There are over 100 trials in adults on the effect of a reduction in salt intake on blood pressure of a relatively small number of normal subjects. Four older meta-analyses limited to random controlled trials (97) agree that there is a significant fall in blood pressure of 2/1 mm Hg. It is difficult to know what to conclude from such trials because most of them lasted for less than 2 weeks and some involved very large acute reductions in salt intake that transiently stimulate the sympathetic nervous system. A more recent meta-analysis of studies of 1 month or more did show highly significant falls in blood pressure and a dose response—i.e. the greater the reduction in salt intake, the larger the fall in blood pressure. Indeed, a 6 gram reduction in salt intake would cause a fall in blood pressure of 7/4 mm Hg in hypertensives and 4/2 mm Hg in normotensives (98).

There is some evidence of the effect of prolonged reductions in salt intake, but it was obtained by studying whole communities, which precluded it being randomly controlled.

The Effect of Reducing Salt Intake on the Blood Pressure of Populations

The most vigorously controlled trial was carried out in Portugal, which is notorious for its high salt consumption (99). The trial was carried out in two communities within the same district, each with about 800 inhabitants, who had a very high salt intake of about 21 g/day, and in which 30% had high blood pressure. Each community was close-knit and rural, which was particularly favorable for health education. One village was used as the control for the other in which the intake of salt was reduced. Community awareness of stroke and hypertension probably enhanced cooperation and the acceptance of guidance. Active intervention lasted 2 years and involved the whole community, but the responses were assessed in random samples. About half the total salt intake was added in the kitchen, which was easy to influence; another 30% came from salted codfish; the rest was in bread. Those responsible for cooking were advised to add less salt and instead to use herbs and other alternative flavorings (often previously unknown in the village), which became popular. The community as a whole was advised to eat less cod and fewer sausages, which also contained much salt, and the bakers were asked to reduce the salt added to bread by about 50% during the 2 years of the trial (Fig. 50-9). The reduction in salt intake in the trial village was associated with a highly significant difference in blood pressure. At the end of the second year the difference in blood pressure between the two villages was 13 mm Hg in systolic and 6 mm Hg in diastolic pressure. The fall was maintained in the second year. There was an upward trend in blood pressure of the control village over the 2-year period. The fall in blood pressure involved the whole community, not just those with hypertension, and the response was similar between young and old or men and women. It was estimated that a downward shift of blood pressure by 5 mm Hg, as observed in this trial, could reduce the prevalence of hypertension by about one-fourth.

Japan

The most comprehensive and wide-ranging endeavor to reduce the salt intake of whole communities took place in Japan. As a result of much public health activity to reduce salt intake the natural average salt consumption was reduced from 13.5 to 12.1 g/day. The change was greatest where the salt intake was highest. For instance, between 1960 and 1989, the salt intake in the province of Akita was reduced from 18 to 14 g/day. This reduction was accompanied by a gradual fall in average blood pressure and hypertension, and a marked decline in stroke mortality (100).

The Effect of Reducing Salt Intake in Essential Hypertension

Historical Background

Ambard and Beaujard first demonstrated the connection between salt and hypertension in humans in 1904 (101). They varied the intake of salt in patients with hypertension by means of three diets: 2 L/day of milk only, milk plus meat and eggs without the addition of salt, or 2 L of salty broth (containing approximately 10.6 g of salt/L). The urinary output of chloride was measured. Six hypertensive patients were studied for a period of about 3 weeks. It was found that a negative chloride balance lowered the blood pressure, whereas a positive chloride balance increased the blood pressure. One patient's blood pressure was relatively unaffected. They concluded: "We have shown that there is a close relationship between chloride balance and the arterial pressure. Does this mean that chloride is the initiator of hypertension or is it no more than yet another index that certain putative poisons are being retained though they have never been demonstrated?"

In the next 20 years, salt deprivation was occasionally used to lower blood pressure, mainly in patients with renal disease,

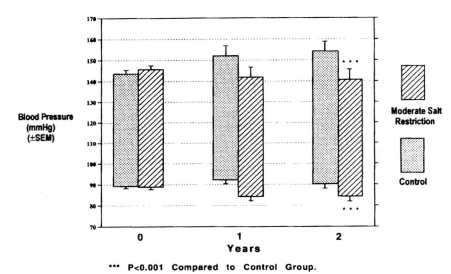

FIGURE 50-9. Blood pressure changes in two Portuguese villages, in one of which the dietary intake of salt was reduced. (Drawn from: Forte JG, et al. Salt and blood pressure: a community trial. *J Hum Hypertens* 1989;3:179.)

but the poor success reported, particularly by German workers (102), was sufficient to discourage its general use. The notion that there was a connection between salt intake and hypertension in humans was discredited. The "protein intoxication" theory of hypertension, referred to by Ambard and Beaujard (101), undoubtedly dominated the scene. This idea had originally been put forward by Bright (1) in relation to hypertension associated with severe renal disease when it had some justification. Its extension to essential hypertension, particularly at a time when it was considered that the kidneys were normal, is difficult to understand. Allen scathingly pointed out in 1920 (103) that treatment for hypertension at this time consisted "chiefly in low protein diets, the elimination of supposed toxins or the artificial reduction of pressure by drugs, bleeding, electricity and the like. Mental and bodily rest is advised to a degree which largely terminates usefulness of life." Houghton (104) and Allen and Sherrill (105) deplored this approach and published detailed accounts of their experience of reducing salt intake to patients with essential hypertension. Both groups agreed that the effective hypotensive level of sodium intake might vary from patient to patient; it might be necessary for some patients to lower the intake of sodium to less than 2 g/day. Allen and Sherrill (105) described the effect of a low-sodium diet in 180 severe cases of hypertension. All patients had essential hypertension and were given a normal protein intake. The blood pressure returned to normal in 19%. The relief of hypertension and other symptoms was sufficient to be regarded as a distinct therapeutic success in 42%. Complete failure occurred in 30%. Allen and Sherrill concluded that pure hypertension is "essentially a salt nephritis." Houghton (104), discussing all the effects of salt reduction in several forms of hypertension, concluded that arterial hypertension is a "tertiary condition of which the immediate cause is a larger sodium chloride intake than the damaged kidneys can excrete," a very modern view. The nature of the renal abnormality that might impair the kidney's ability to excrete salt in primary hypertension (i.e., essential hypertension) was not discussed. Fahr (8) in 1919 was the first to suggest that essential hypertension might result from a primary renal disturbance, but he did not elaborate on its nature.

The connection between salt and hypertension continued to be denied in spite of Ambard and Beaujard, Allen and Sherrill, Houghton, and others. Kempner (106) finally clarified the position in 1948, although somewhat against his own incli-

nations. He studied patients with and without renal "involvement" (nephrosclerosis) who were given a low-fat, low-protein (20 g/day), low-sodium (180 mg/day) rice diet for months and years. Kempner claimed that he had devised this diet because of his findings on "protein, fat and carbohydrate metabolism of isolated kidney cells under various pathologic conditions (cell injury and or changes in pH, sodium bicarbonate concentration, oxygen tension, and metabolizable substrate)," a non sequitur that many, including Pickering (107), found incomprehensible. Kempner was clearly more interested in the low protein content of the diet and was reluctant to admit that it might be the low sodium alone that lowered blood pressure. He attributed such an assertion to others who used his diet. He stressed that what he called the "active principle" of the rice diet was its rigid restriction of protein, fat, sodium, and chloride. His only acknowledgment that others before him had observed that a low-salt diet alone lowered blood pressure was to use derogatory quotes by some contemporary prominent hypertension experts: (a) Fishberg (108) in 1939, who had stated that "No dietary treatment is known which has a specifically favorable effect on essential hypertension;" (b) Goldring and Chasis (109) in 1944, who had concluded that in the absence of edema and paroxysmal dyspnea the restriction of salt was unwarranted; and Page and Corcoran (110) in 1945, who had written that the hypotensive results obtained were owing not to salt restriction but to "rest in bed and the psychotherapy of constant attention." It is ironic, therefore, that Kempner is now remembered as the person who brilliantly demonstrated that high blood pressure can often be lowered by a low-salt diet.

The sodium content of Kempner's rice diet was so low that the 24-hour urinary excretion of sodium at the end of 2 months usually fell to below 100 mg. The effect of the diet in 500 patients with hypertensive vascular disease as opposed to glomerular nephritis (i.e., intrinsic overt renal disease) with and without renal "involvement" was reported. The probable reason that Kempner's paper had such an impact was that it was visually so compelling and that it came 44 years after Ambard and Beaujard's initial seed had been sown (101). The paper contained (a) blood pressure charts showing the relentless fall of blood pressure (Fig. 50-10), (b) chest x-rays showing pronounced reductions in heart size, (c) electrocardiograms showing T-wave inversions reverting to normal, and (d) photographs of the retinae showing loss of papilledema,

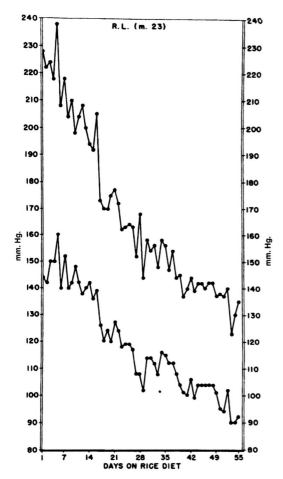

FIGURE 50-10. The fall in blood pressure in a patient with severe hypertension who was placed on Kempner's rice diet. (From: Kempner W. Treatment of hypertensive vascular disease with rice diet. *Am J Med* 1948;4:545, with permission.)

hemorrhages, and exudates. There is no doubt that in his hands the rice diet achieved remarkable and sustained results; however, Kempner made no mention of the overwhelming difficulty of trying to get patients to follow the rice diet or of the complications associated with such severe reductions in sodium intake, although he did admit that the rice diet was contraindicated unless frequent checks of the patient's blood and urine were possible. Nor did Kempner discuss the role of the kidney in the etiology of essential hypertension. Nevertheless, the paper irrevocably linked the intake of sodium to hypertension and therefore reinforced the suggestion that the connection between the two was the abnormal handling of sodium by the kidney.

The use of severe salt restriction as recommended by Kempner had a temporary vogue but ceased with the introduction of oral diuretics in the 1950s. In the 1970s and subsequently numerous studies have shown the effect of much more moderate restrictions in salt intake.

There has been a slow acceptance that lowering the salt intake of hypertensive patients lowers blood pressure and increases the effectiveness of hypotensive drugs. There is no doubt that part of the reluctance to reduce salt intake has stemmed from the difficulty in getting patients to change their dietary habits. Even when the patient is cooperative, it is difficult because of the high salt content of bread, and nearly all processed foods, as well as fast food, restaurant food, and so on. For instance, in 1997 Liebman and Jacobson ascertained

TABLE 50-1

SODIUM CONTENT OF VARIOUS FOODS SOLD AT RESTAURANTS IN UNITED STATES

Item	Sodium (mg)
Tuna salad sandwich	1,320
Lasagna	2,055
Ham sandwich	2,200
Spaghetti with sausage	2,435
House fried rice	2,680
General Tso's chicken	3,150
House lo mein	3,460
Beef burrito platter	3,920
Fried seafood platter	4,405

the sodium content of various foods sold in restaurants in the United States (Table 50-1) (111). Thus, in a single meal many customers at that time were exceeding the 2,400 mg of sodium (6 g of sodium chloride) recommended for an entire day.

In one double-blind randomized study in 20 patients with a mean age of 57 and a blood pressure of 164/101 mm Hg in which salt excretion was reduced to 3 g/day for 1 year, 1 patient was lost to follow-up, and 3 required the addition of drug therapy to control blood pressure, but blood pressure fell to 142/85 mm Hg in the remaining 16 patients (112). There are several other studies that agree that reducing the salt intake of elderly hypertensive patients induces a substantial fall in blood pressure. Cappuccio et al. reported the response of a group of elderly patients in whom a reduction in salt intake of 83 mmol/day for 1 month induced a fall in blood pressure of 7.2/3.2 mm Hg. In another study in 975 elderly patients aged 60 to 80 who were being successfully treated with antihypertensive drugs, treatment was stopped and they were randomly allocated to one of four regimens: (a) sodium restriction, (b) weight reduction, (c) both sodium restriction and weight reduction, and (d) the control group. They were monitored over the next 30 months to detect those whose blood pressure returned to hypertensive levels. There was a 50% decrease in patients whose blood pressure returned to hypertensive level in the group on 40 mmol sodium/day (113).

A meta-analysis of studies of sodium restriction of a month or more confirmed that for a reduction in salt intake of 6 grams/day in untreated patients with essential hypertension, blood pressure fell by 7/4 mm Hg (98).

There was also a successful mass campaign in Belgium against salt in 1969. A total of 3,328 elderly subjects between the age of 70 and 81 were studied. Between 1967 and 1986 the prevalence of hypertension in these subjects decreased substantially and severe hypertension disappeared. The reduction in salt intake was from 16 to 11 g/day in the men and from 12 to 9 g/day in the women (114).

CONSEQUENTIAL THERAPEUTIC AND PUBLIC HEALTH IMPLICATIONS OF SALT INTAKE AND HYPERTENSION

Both the epidemiologic evidence and the rise in blood pressure that accompanies a rise in salt intake in normal animals and humans demonstrate that salt intake is a major determinant of blood pressure. Reducing the salt intake of patients with essential hypertension induces a fall in blood pressure; therefore, all such patients should reduce their salt intake. Furthermore,

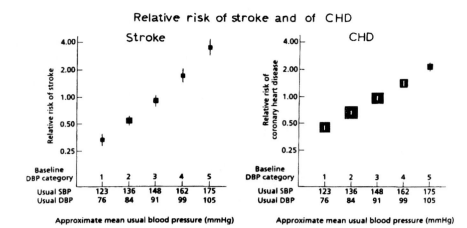

FIGURE 50-11. This figure summarizes studies that had been performed up to 1990, in which blood pressure had been measured and the subjects followed up subsequently to find out how many went on to develop a stroke or coronary heart disease (CHD). The *horizontal axis* shows that blood pressure has been arranged in five ascending groups: both the systolic (SBP) and diastolic (DBP) pressures are shown. The *vertical axis* on the *left* shows the relative risk of developing a stroke, and on the *vertical axis* on the *right* the risk of developing CHD. It is clear that the risk of developing a stroke (left) or CHD (right) is directly related to the level of blood pressure throughout the normal and hypertensive range. Note that the risk of developing a stroke is 16 times less with a low normal blood pressure than with a moderately raised blood pressure. The size of the *black boxes* denotes the number of persons who died during the period of observation: The boxes for CHD are much larger, indicating the larger number who died from CHD compared to stroke. (From: MacMahon S, et al. Blood pressure, stroke, and coronary heart disease. Part 1: Prolonged differences in blood pressure: prospective observational studies corrected for the regression dilution bias. *Lancet* 1990;335:765, with permission.)

the close connection between blood pressure and salt intake in normal subjects and animals and the blood pressure lowering effect of salt reduction all indicate that it should be possible to prevent a rise in arterial pressure by reducing the population's salt intake.

However, the slight fall in arterial pressure achieved after a few days of salt reduction in normotensive subjects has led some (115) to oppose the proposal that the nation's salt intake should be reduced (97). Although the effects of a few days of salt reduction are irrelevant to the proposal that the nation's salt intake should be permanently reduced, it is incorrect to suggest that the smallness of such a reduction is unimportant because it neglects the fact that the relation of salt intake to strokes and myocardial infarctions is continuous not only in the hypertensive but also in the average range starting at a systolic pressure of 115 mm Hg (Fig. 50-11). In other words, although patients with hypertension have a much greater risk of developing a stroke, the greater number of subjects in the upper range of normal blood pressure have a greater number of strokes (Fig. 50-12). A population-based reduction in salt intake of 6 grams/day would lower blood pressure in adults by an average of 5/3 mm Hg. This would result in an 24% in stroke deaths and an 18% reduction in coronary heart disease deaths (116).

The principal overt objections to the widespread agreement among scientific bodies that the population's salt intake should be lowered from 10 to 12 g/day to 5 to 6 g/day are that the long-term effects of such a maneuver are not known and that they might be dangerous. Taking the second point first there is the U.S. Food and Drug Administration's (117) conclusion that "no convincing evidence has been presented that a moderate but significant reduction in salt intake would have any adverse health effects." Nevertheless, a myth continues to be disseminated which is encapsulated in Muntzel and Drüeke's (118) assertion that "lowering salt intake may result in health risks that outweigh the benefit of blood pressure reduction." This remarkable assertion is founded in part on the results of

experiments carried out in animals subjected to intense sodium deprivation or massive intravenous injections of angiotensin. It is also based on interpretations of some observations in humans that have been repeatedly exposed as irrelevant or based on data that turn out not to support the assertion (119,120).

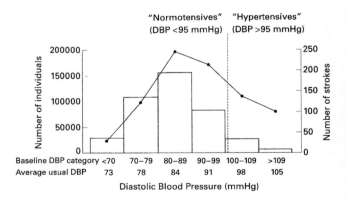

FIGURE 50-12. This figure shows how blood pressure of a large number of persons is distributed. The distribution of the population has been divided into six solid blocks. The tallest and largest block contains the greatest number of people and their diastolic pressure lies between 80 and 89 mm Hg. The line that connects the *small black circles* indicates the number of strokes that occurred in each block. What is clearly illustrated is that the greatest total number of strokes occurred in those subjects with a diastolic pressure of 80 to 89 mm Hg, the upper range of normal, and that a slightly lower number occurred in those with a diastolic pressure of 90 to 99 mm Hg, which is a mild elevation of blood pressure. Patients with severe hypertension, however, with a diastolic pressure above 100 mm Hg have far fewer strokes in total (although individually they have a much greater risk of developing a stroke) because there are far fewer patients with severe hypertension. (Redrawn from: MacMahon S, Rogers A. *J Hypertens* 1994;12:S5.)

The long-term effects of salt intake reduction are not known. In order to find out unequivocally it would be necessary to have a randomized trial in several thousand subjects, starting at birth and lasting about 50 years. There is no support for such a trial, which would be unethical, an administrative nightmare, prohibitively expensive, and that would have to rely on those control participants who were consuming a high (normal) sodium intake being willing to continue on such an intake when they grew up and understood the dangers. In the absence of such a trial decisions have to be made on what evidence there is, keeping Geoffrey Rose's words in mind (121): "The level of evidence approximate to a particular decision depends on the consequences of making the wrong decision. For example, there is substantial evidence, but still well short of proof, that a reduction in national salt consumption leads to a somewhat lower mean blood pressure, with important expected health benefits. The change is safe and its cost minimal (except to a small but noisy section of the business community). The evidence for this policy is important, but one may judge it to be sufficient."

Worldwide there is now a scientific consensus that the population's salt intake should be reduced. The World Health Organization (WHO) has recommended that all adults should eat less than 5 g of salt per day (122). In the United States similar recommendations have been put forward by the National Heart Lung and Blood Institute, the National Academy of Sciences, the National Research Council, the Department of Health and Human Services, the Department of Agriculture, the American Dietetic Investigation, the American Public Health Association, the American Society of Clinical Investigation, and the American Medical Association. Similar views have been expressed in the United Kingdom by government appointed nutritional committees of independent experts (123). The UK Food Standards Agency through its Specialist Advisory Committee (SACN) recommended in 2003 that all adults should eat less than 6 g of salt/day and set much lower targets for children depending on age. Currently in the United Kingdom salt concentrations of many processed, canteen, and fast foods are gradually being reduced so that salt intake will fall below 6 g/day by 2110 (124).

It has to be pointed out that the case for a general reduction in salt intake is much wider than simply preventing a rise in blood pressure (125). There is evidence in humans that a decrease in sodium intake provides the following additional benefits, which are largely independent of any fall in blood pressure: (a) regression of left ventricular hypertrophy (126,127), (b) reduction of proteinuria (128), (c) reduction of urinary calcium (129) with a decrease in osteoporosis (129), (d) reduction in the risk of renal stones (130), (e) protection against cancer of the stomach (131), (f) reduction in the incidence of stroke (114,132), (g) enhancement of the antihypertensive effect of antihypertensive agents (133), and (h) decrease in diuretic-induced potassium loss (134). In addition, reducing salt intake may influence the genesis of nephrosclerosis and renal failure because it has been shown in normotensive and hypertensive rats that a high dietary salt intake leads to widespread fibrosis and increase in transforming growth factor-beta (TGF-$_{\beta 1}$) (135) in the heart and kidney.

RENAL ABNORMALITIES THAT DIMINISH AND ACCOMPANY THE KIDNEY'S ABILITY TO EXCRETE SODIUM

The effect of a change in salt intake on the blood pressure of normal subjects and hypertensive patients, the epidemiologic studies on the prevalence of hypertension in relation to salt intake, the influence of cross-transplantation of kidneys between normal and hypertensive animals or humans, and the finding that the rise in blood pressure takes place during a period of salt retention in hereditary forms of hypertension in the rat suggest that the hypertensive effect of sodium on blood pressure is related to a renal impairment in sodium excretion.

There is considerable evidence for the presence of multiple inherited renal abnormalities, each of which could interfere with sodium excretion. In essential hypertension and the hypertensive strains of rats it is probable that to have an overall impairment in the ability to excrete sodium, it is necessary for the kidney to have several functional disturbances, each of which has this effect. But there is no doubt that, as was stated earlier, an isolated impairment in sodium transport limited to the kidney can cause hypertension. In the rare human monogenic condition known as Liddle syndrome, mutations of the gene-encoding subunits of the sodium channel cause an increase in sodium reabsorption and hypertension. The effect of these mutations in raising blood pressure appears to be limited to the kidney in that renal transplantation lowers blood pressure (136). It is important to distinguish an inherited functional abnormality from one that has been acquired as a result of the rise in arterial pressure. The arterial pressure in inherited hypertensive rats tends to rise steeply around the sixth week of life; therefore, the distinction between an inherited lesion and a lesion secondary to the rise in pressure has to be made in young rats. In essential hypertension, the studies have to be made in young normotensive relatives of patients with hypertension.

Renal Blood Flow, Glomerular Filtration Rate, and Patterns of Urinary Sodium Excretion

Changes in renal hemodynamics in the normotensive children of hypertensive parents have yielded inconsistent results. Bianchi and Barlassina (137) reported an increase in renal blood flow and glomerular filtration rate (GFR). In contrast, some investigators (40,138) have found that renal blood flow and GFR rate are normal but that there is an increase in vascular resistance, whereas others (139) have reported that the renal blood flow is reduced and renal vascular resistance is raised. This variability has been claimed to be artificial because of differences in the techniques used to measure the renal plasma flow and filtration rate (140); there is probably some increase in renal vascular resistance overall.

Approximately half of the patients with essential hypertension have a group of abnormalities that consist of: (a) a failure of renal blood flow to increase normally in response to a high salt intake, (b) a failure of renal blood flow to decrease normally in response to an infusion of angiotensin II, and (c) a lower than normal rise in plasma aldosterone in response to an infusion of angiotensin II when on a low sodium diet (141). Eighty-five percent of hypertensive patients who have some features of this characteristic set of abnormalities have a positive family history of hypertension (142), and such factors are more likely to be present in both of hypertensive sibling pairs than would be expected from the frequency of their presence in the general hypertensive population (143). These abnormalities also occur in normotensive offspring of parents with hypertension (144).

Renal blood flow and GFR in hypertensive strains of rats are reduced before the rise in pressure (145,146). The glomerulus of young SHR and Milan hypertensive rats has a reduction in glomerular ultrafiltration coefficient, GFR, and single-nephron filtration rate. The Dahl salt-sensitive hypertensive rat has an impaired ability to excrete a high intake of sodium and a

persistently low plasma renin value. On a normal sodium intake, however, blood pressure tends to be normal. In the Milan
(147) and Heidelberg (148) hypertensive strain rats, in which
blood pressure rises on a normal intake of sodium, there is a
transient period ending about the sixth to the seventh week
of life when the fractional excretion of sodium is lower, the
cumulative retention of sodium is greater, and plasma renin
activity is lower in the hypertensive strain than in the control
normotensive rat. At the end of this period, blood pressure of
the hypertensive strain rat has risen considerably.

The phenomenon of accelerated natriuresis in response to
an infusion of saline is prominent in inherited hypertensive
strains of rats and occurs, as in humans, both before and after
the rise in arterial pressure (149,150). As in humans, it has been
shown that the phenomenon of accelerated natriuresis in rats
is unrelated to changes in peritubular capillary hydrostatic or
colloid osmotic pressure (150).

Structural Glomerular Changes

There is a scanning and electron microscopic study in the 6-
week-old SHR in which the arterial pressure was 131 mm Hg,
as opposed to 121 mm Hg in control Wistar-Kyoto (WKY)
rats (151). The fenestrae of the glomerular capillary endothelium of the SHR were already significantly smaller with an increased number of cytoplasmic ridges and bulbous projections
lying across the endothelial surface. These changes should reduce the filtration surface per unit area of endothelium. At 12
weeks, when the arterial pressure of the SHR was 175 mm Hg
and that of the WKY rat was 138 mm Hg, these abnormalities
were more pronounced, whereas the endothelium of the WKY
rat was unchanged (in spite of the WKY rat having an arterial
pressure slightly higher at 12 weeks than that of the SHR at
6 weeks). Not only is the filtration surface per unit area reduced, some workers have also found that the SHR has a diminished number of nephrons (152).

Proteinuria

In a study of microalbuminuria, Fauvel et al. (153) found that
normotensive individuals with a genetic risk of hypertension
had a mean albuminuria of 36 ± 37 μ/min, whereas a control
group of normotensive individuals without a genetic risk of
hypertension had a mean proteinuria of 6 μ/min.

Tubular Sodium Reabsorption

Fractional lithium and uric acid clearance are considered to be
a measure of proximal tubule sodium reabsorption. A decrease
in renal fractional lithium clearance (i.e., an increase in reabsorption) has been observed in the normotensive offspring of
hypertensive parents by one group (154) but not by three others (155–157). On the other hand, the two groups who have
studied fractional uric acid excretion agree that it is reduced
in the offspring of two and one hypertensive parents (85,158).
There is increased sodium reabsorption in the proximal tubule
in both the SHR and Milan hypertensive rat (145,146). The
amount of sodium delivered to the distal tubule is reduced, but
to keep in balance this should normally be adjusted by a diminished reabsorption from the distal tubule and collecting duct.
The inability of the distal nephron to adjust sodium excretion
to the reduced filtration rate therefore must be owing to an
additional functional abnormality of the distal and collecting
tubule.

Vascular Changes

Altered Relation of Arterial Pressure to Urinary Sodium Excretion

The urinary sodium excretion of an isolated kidney is directly
related to the perfusion pressure (159–161). Changes in pressure alter sodium excretion by changing the hydrostatic pressure of the venous capillaries and the interstitial pressure surrounding the tubules, an effect that is independent of the GFR
or renal blood flow, both of which tend to remain unchanged
throughout the autoregulatory range of perfusion pressure. The
relation between urinary sodium excretion and renal perfusion
pressure is sometimes referred to as a "pressure natriuresis"
curve. Some isolated kidneys need greater pressure to promote
the same rate of sodium excretion, a change that can be referred to as a right shift of the pressure natriuresis curve. If,
therefore, the pressure natriuresis curve of an isolated kidney,
perfused with blood from a normal animal, has shifted to the
right, it is probable that there is a rise in resistance in a vascular
site between the arterial perfusion pressure and the peritubular venous capillaries. It is probable that such a site of raised
resistance is present in kidneys in situ in all forms of hypertension; otherwise, hypertension would be accompanied by severe
sodium depletion.

In essential and inherited hypertension in the rat, there is a
primary shift of the natriuresis curve to the right. Tobian and
colleagues (162) and Roman and Cowley (163) have shown
that isolated kidneys of young prehypertensive salt-sensitive
and spontaneously hypertensive Dahl rats have a shift to the
right of the pressure natriuresis curve (Fig. 50-13). In the SHR,
there is evidence that the increased vascular resistance is owing
to narrowing of the afferent arteriole; these vessels are already
smaller than control at 6 to 7 weeks of age (164,165) because
of an increase in tone rather than medial hypertrophy. The increase in resistance that results is particularly marked in the
papillary circulation and is evident between 4 and 10 weeks of
age, when the arterial pressure is rising (37). There is an accompanying reduction in papillary blood flow and interstitial
pressure (38), which tends to enhance sodium reabsorption.
In the Dahl salt-sensitive rat, in contrast to the SHR, the shift

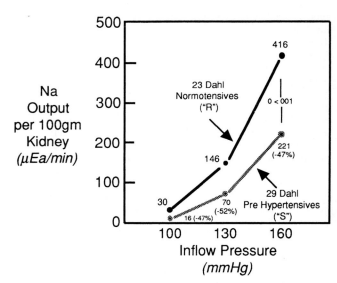

FIGURE 50-13. Sodium excretion of isolated kidneys from salt-
sensitive prehypertensive and salt-resistant normotensive Dahl rats.
(From: Tobian L. The relationship of salt to hypertension. *Am J Clin
Nutr* 1979;32:2739, with permission.)

to the right of the pressure natriuretic curve does not appear to be associated with a particular reduction of the papillary interstitial pressure (166), but to a reduced sensitivity of the renal tubules to the interstitial pressure (167). These observations are consistent with the finding of increased renal vascular resistance in the normotensive children of hypertensive parents.

Abnormalities of Arachidonic Acid Metabolism

The increased renal vasoconstriction of the young SHR may result from one or more abnormalities of arachidonic acid metabolism.

Cyclooxygenase Activity

At 6 weeks of age, bolus injections of arachidonic acid into the renal artery of isolated kidneys perfused at constant flow cause a greater rise in the perfusion pressure of the SHR kidney than in the WKY rat (168). This is accompanied by a greater release of the vasoconstrictor, thromboxane B_2. This difference is no longer evident at 18 weeks. These changes do not occur in kidneys from rats made hypertensive with deoxycorticosterone acetate (DOCA) or a clip on the renal artery of one kidney.

Cytochrome P-450-Dependent Monooxygenase Activity

There are two forms of these enzymes of particular interest, epoxygenases and hydroxylases (169). Epoxygenase activity leads to the production of 11,12-epoxyeicosatrienoic acid (EET), which can be hydrolyzed to 11,12-dihydroxyeicosatrienoic acid (DHT). Hydroxylase activity leads to the production of 20-hydroxyeicosatetraenoic acid (20-HETE) and 19-hydroxyeicosatetraenoic acid (19-HETE). These products of cytochrome P-450 metabolism of monooxygenase activity are present in greater amounts in SHR microsomes from rats aged 5 to 13 weeks (170). Tin ($SnCl_2$), which reduces the concentration of cytochrome P-450 monooxygenase when given for 4 days to 7-week-old SHR, prevents the customary rise in blood pressure, an effect that lasts for 7 weeks after the administration of tin. Tin has no effect on the blood pressure of 20-week-old rats (171).

It has been found that from birth until the ninth week, hydroxylase activity in cortical microsomal fractions is greater in the SHR than the WKY rat, whereas there is no difference in epoxygenase activity (172). The production of 20- and 19-HETE is greater in the SHR. In addition, the conversion of the hydroxylase metabolite 20-HETE by cyclooxygenase is much greater in the SHR from birth until the seventh week. The production of the resultant metabolite 20-OH prostaglandin (P5) and 20-OH (PGH_2) in the SHR rises substantially. Because these are potent vasoconstrictors, it is possible that in the SHR during the early weeks when the pressure is rising (173), these metabolites are responsible in part for the observed renal vascular constriction. In addition, although epoxygenase activity is the same in the SHR and WKY rat, the production of EET in the SHR is less than in the WKY because its conversion to DHT is greater in the SHR (174). Thus, in the SHR the increased presence of 19-HETE, which stimulates Na-K-ATPase, and the diminished presence of ETE, which inhibits Na-K-ATPase (175), may be responsible for the documented increase in renal Na-K-ATPase activity in the young SHR and in part for the sodium retention.

Urinary Kallikrein Excretion

Urinary kallikrein influences urinary sodium excretion. Its excretion is reduced in essential hypertension (176) in the SHR and the Dahl salt-sensitive rat (177). It is also reduced in normotensive children of hypertensive parents (178). The lower kallikrein excretion in essential hypertension extends through a range of 9 to 259 mmol/day of urinary sodium excretion (179). Urinary kallikrein is synthesized in the distal tubule and secreted into its lumen, where it acts on kininogen to release kinins (180). Kinins are natriuretic substances (181) closely linked to several other intrarenal substances that have an effect on sodium excretion, such as angiotensin II, prostaglandins, and antidiuretic hormone (182). Plasma aldosterone is the major regulator of urinary kallikrein excretion (183). A decrease in sodium intake raises and an increase lowers urinary kallikrein excretion (184,185). Kallikrein induces a loss of amiloride-sensitive sodium current and an increase in amiloride-insensitive "leak" current on the mucosa of the mammalian bladder (186). The net effect is to reduce sodium transport, from which it is concluded that kallikrein may hydrolyze amiloride-sensitive channels, thus diminishing the rate of entry of sodium into the cell. If this takes place in the apical membranes of the distal tubules there is diminished sodium reabsorption so that a reduction in urinary kallikrein may be an additional factor, together with the reduced presence of the natriuretic kinins, which could increase sodium reabsorption and thus impair the ability of the kidney to excrete sodium. There is some fragmentary information on the genetic origin for the reduced urinary kallikrein in essential hypertension (187) and hereditary hypertension (188).

Tubuloglomerular Feedback

An increase in GFR increases the rate of delivery of tubular fluid to the macula densa, the cells of which then signal the afferent arteriole to constrict. This reduces the filtration rate and the delivery of tubular fluid to the macula densa, which results in a reduction of urinary sodium excretion (189). In the normal animal, the sensitivity and reactivity of this adjustment increase when there is a need to conserve sodium (hemorrhage and dehydration) (190,191) and diminish when there is a prolonged need to increase sodium excretion (chronic salt loading and DOCA administration) (192–195). When dietary sodium is increased, the depression in tubuloglomerular feedback activity results from the presence of an inhibitory factor in the tubular fluid (192), whereas with prolonged DOCA administration (196) the fall in tubuloglomerular feedback activity is associated with a change in the characteristics of the juxtaglomerular apparatus.

In the young SHR (196,197) and Milan hypertensive rat (198) at a time when there is most evidence of sodium retention and blood pressure is beginning to rise, there is a paradoxical increase in tubular feedback activity that would tend to aggravate the sodium retention. This increase in tubuloglomerular activity instead of a compensatory fall, which would increase sodium excretion, appears to be owing to a relative lack of the humoral inhibiting factor in the tubule fluid (199). By the 12th week, however, when blood pressure has risen considerably, the tubuloglomerular feedback has almost returned to normal. The Milan hypertensive rat has been studied at 3.5 to 5 weeks and at 5 to 7 weeks, just before and after blood pressure begins to rise (198). At 3.5 to 5 weeks, tubuloglomerular feedback activity is absent, and 2 weeks later, when the blood pressure has started to rise, tubuloglomerular feedback increases inappropriately to supranormal levels as in the SHR, thus diminishing the kidney's ability to excrete sodium.

Dopamine Metabolism

Urinary dopamine is formed in the kidney. The renal actions of dopamine include a substantial increase of regional blood flow, a less marked rise in GFR, inhibition of proximal tubule sodium reabsorption, and inhibition of renin release by the juxtaglomerular apparatus. These are all natriuretic mechanisms, but the effect on the proximal tubule is by far the most prominent (200).

Basal dopamine excretion in essential hypertension may be normal or even increased (201). Nevertheless, although the sodium loading of normal Whites increases urinary dopamine excretion, in patients with essential hypertension it either induces a smaller increase or a reduction in dopamine excretion (202). In a group of Japanese patients with hypertension who were divided into sodium-resistant and -sensitive, depending on the response of their blood pressure to a sodium load, the salt-resistant patients (who showed a mean rise of blood pressure of only 0.5 mm Hg) had a prompt increase in dopamine excretion, whereas the sodium-sensitive patients (in whom there was a mean rise in blood pressure of 10.5 mm Hg) had no increase in dopamine excretion (203). Other Japanese workers (204) have found that dopamine excretion in hypertensive patients in response to salt loading is lower than in normal subjects, particularly in the low renin group (205,206). Normotensive relatives of patients with hypertension also have a lower urinary dopamine excretion and do not have a normal regression between urinary sodium and dopamine excretion. There is also some evidence that this renal dopamine abnormality is present in hypertensive black Americans, but there are important ethnic differences. The increasing dopamine abnormalities detected in the Japanese hypertensive patients and their normotensive offspring are also present in normotensive American blacks, Thais, and Zimbabweans but not Ghanaians and Iranians. Various studies suggest that in essential hypertension it is the intrarenal generation of dopamine that is defective (201,206). The carboxylation of exogenous L-dopa is reduced (207), and the intravenous administration of dopamine induces a greater increase in urinary sodium excretion and fractional excretion, which suggests an enhanced dopamine receptor activity. These renal abnormalities of dopamine metabolism are also present in normotensive relatives of hypertensive patients (202).

Abnormalities of dopamine metabolism also have been detected in the Dahl (208) and SHR (209) forms of hypertensive strain rats, but they are not the same as those in essential hypertension. Although the overall excretion of a salt load in the SHR is less than normal, the initial rise in urinary sodium excretion, in contrast to the response in essential hypertension, is *greater* than in the WKY; and, instead of an impairment of dopamine generation, there appears to be a defect of the dopamine A_1 receptor in both the SHR and the Dahl salt-sensitive rat. For instance, the natriuretic effect of a dopamine A_1 receptor agonist in the SHR is less than in the WKY rat. Furthermore, there is a dopamine A_1 receptor coupling defect to adenyl cyclase in the proximal tubules of the SHR kidney, even at 3 weeks of age, well before the onset of hypertension (210).

Atrial Natriuretic Peptide

There is diminished atrial natriuretic peptide (ANP) immunoreactivity at distal tubule segments in essential hypertension, which suggests a diminished binding capacity (211). A continuous low dose of ANP induces a similar natriuretic response in normotensive subjects as it does in hypertensive patients, whereas there is a greater rise in solute-free water excretion in

the SHR (212). As in a normal animal, the natriuretic effect of ANP is directly related to blood pressure (213), the absence of a greater natriuretic effect in the SHR and the increase in solute-free water suggest that the distal tubules in the SHR have an increased sodium reabsorption.

There is a lowered renal response to ANP in the mature hypertensive SHR (214). This is associated with a maximum binding capacity of SHR glomeruli for I^{131}-ANP that is reduced by about 50% (215) and similarly diminished immunoreactivity at distal tubule segments (216). Urinary cyclic guanosine monophosphate (cGMP) excretion response to intravenous synthetic ANF (synthetic 26 amino acid peptide contained with rat ANP), however, is increased and is associated with an increase in affinity (217,218).

The intravenous injection of atrial extracts to Dahl rats has also shown that the mature Dahl salt-sensitive hypertensive rat has a natriuretic response that is about 50% less than that of the Dahl salt-resistant strain (219). This is associated with a defect of intracellular cGMP synthesis. There is a similar hyporesponsiveness to sodium nitroprusside, but cyclic adenosine monophosphate response to arginine vasopressin (AVP) of the Dahl sensitive rat is the same as from the Dahl resistance rat (220). These changes are present in the 5- to 6-week prehypertensive rat and appeared to be specific to the medullary structure in that the response of mesangial cells is the same in the Dahl-sensitive and resistant rats.

The Effect of Age

Blood pressure rises with advancing age (Fig. 50-14). It is probable that this relationship owes in part to a gradual involutional diminution in renal function (221), which aggravates the overall effect of any inherited difficulty in excreting sodium. After the age of 30 years there is a gradual decline in renal blood

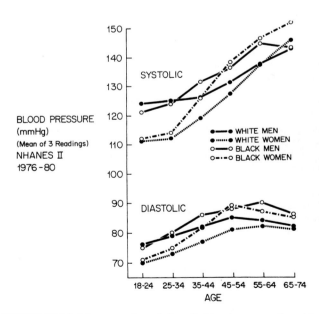

FIGURE 50-14. Mean systolic and diastolic blood pressures for white and black men and women in various age groups in the 1976 to 1980 National Health and Nutrition Examination Survey (NHANES II). (From: Rowland M, Roberts J. *Blood pressure levels and hypertension in persons aged from 6–74 years. United States 1976–80 NCHS, Advance Data No. 84, Vital and Health Statistics of the National Center for Health Statistics. Washington, DC: U.S. Department of Health and Human Services, Oct. 8, 1982.)*

flow, GFR, secretion tubular maximum (T_m), and the ability to concentrate the urine (222). By the age of 90 years, these functions have decreased to approximately half their value at the age of 30 years.

The Renal Contribution to the Fetal Origins of Essential Hypertension

At all ages beyond infancy, people who had lower birth weights have a higher blood pressure (223,224). This relationship becomes larger with increasing age. Measuring renal growth by counting the number of glomeruli has raised the possibility that the principal cause of this phenomenon is impaired intrauterine renal development. Sixty percent of nephron growth develops in the third trimester (225). Severe intrauterine growth retardation in human fetuses has been shown to exert a profound effect on renal development (226). This effect is magnified thereafter by the lack of any compensatory increase in either nephron numbers or size during the early phase of postnatal life. There is one report, however, that maternal blood pressure is inversely correlated, though weakly, with infant birth weight, which suggests that the link between birth weight and hypertension may in part result from an inherited tendency to hypertension (227).

A similar phenomenon can be produced experimentally in the pregnant guinea pig, which has a bicornuate uterus, by tying the uterine artery on one side of the uterus while allowing the fetuses on the other side to grow normally. The animals on the ischemic side have low birth weight and develop higher blood pressure in later life. In rats, maternal low-protein diets, which have been shown to impair renal function of the fetus (228) if maintained throughout pregnancy, also lead to an inverse relationship between blood pressure and the low protein intake at 9 weeks (229).

Conclusion

Many of the renal functional abnormalities in the various forms of hereditary hypertension are the same, for instance, there are defects of dopamine and renin–angiotensin metabolism that could impair urinary sodium excretion in essential hypertension, the spontaneously hypertensive rat, and the Dahl salt sensitive rat but the molecular disturbances and thus, presumably the genetic faults that gives rise to them are usually different. In other words, although patients with essential hypertension share several functional abnormalities with hypertensive strains of rats, the precise nature of the few genetic disturbances that have been detected in essential hypertension, and the many detected in the hypertensive strains of rats are different, with the exception of the adducin gene.

GENETIC ABNORMALITIES AND HYPERTENSION

Polygenic Changes and Hypertension

The following account demonstrates that, although many genetic abnormalities have been detected in hypertensive strains of rats thus far, only three have been identified in essential hypertension and they appear to play a minor part in raising blood pressure.

Essential Hypertension

Angiotensinogen

A variant of the angiotensinogen (AGT) gene locus, so-called AGT 235T, has been found to be more frequent in hypertensive patients than in controls in Europe, the United States, Japan (230), and the Afro-Caribbean (231). There is no evidence that this variant confers a similar risk in African Americans and Nigerians (232). The variant is associated with high AGT levels, which suggests that the mutation results in an increase in activity with a higher basal transcription rate. "The AGT gene has been the most scrutinized and the most promising finding of the primary hypertension genes thus far, however the AGT 235T variant explains a relatively small part of blood pressure variance" (233). An increase in angiotensinogen activity in the kidney could increase sodium reabsorption.

The Epithelial Sodium Channel

A variant (the T594m mutation) of the β subunit of the epithelial sodium channel has been found in about 8% of black London residents with a raised blood pressure as opposed to 2% of those with normal blood pressure (234). Plasma renin activity was also significantly lower in those with hypertension and the T594m variant. In addition, lymphocytes with the variant show increased sodium transport, suggesting that the variant may increase sodium reabsorption in the renal tubules, thus reducing renal sodium excretion.

Adducin

The membrane-skeleton protein adducin was originally chosen for genetic studies in the Milan hypertensive rat because it was the only membrane skeletal protein eliciting an immunologic response in cross-immunization experiments between Milan hypertensive strain rats and Milan normotensive controls. It is an $a\beta$ heterodimer that promotes the organization of a spectrin-actin lattice. In the Milan hypertensive rat there is a mutation in each of the two genes that codes for adducin. There is a high degree (94%) of amino acid homology between rat and human adducin, and many of the renal cell membrane ion transport alterations in the Milan hypertensive strain rat are shared by a subset of patients with essential hypertension. Linkage and association studies were performed in hypertensive patients and controls in Italy and a point mutation (G460W) was found in the human α-adducin gene. The 460W variant was shown to be more frequent in hypertensive patients than in controls (235). But no association between α-adducin allele variants was found in a group of patients with essential hypertension in Japan (236) or Scotland (237). Experiments in patients with essential hypertension with the α-adducin variant have shown them to flatten pressure natriuresis relationships (235). This is consistent with the findings in renal cell transfection experiments (238) that the α-adducin variant increases Na-K-ATPase activity, which increases tubular sodium reabsorption, and decreases fractional excretion of lithium and uric acid in hypertensive patients exhibiting the variant, which is consistent with an increase in proximal tubule sodium reabsorption (239).

Hypertensive Strains of Rats

An identified genetic locus influencing a quantitative trait such as blood pressure is known as a quantitative trait locus (QTL)

(240). Many QTLs that influence blood pressure have been identified in hypertensive strains of rats. On chromosome 1 there is the SA gene responsible for a protein of unknown function that is expressed 10 times more in the proximal tubules of SHR than in WKY, and the kallikrein gene that is also linked to hypertension in the SHR. On chromosome 2 there is the ANP receptor A gene, which is more expressed in the glomeruli of SHR. On chromosome 4 of the SHR there is a QTL associated with the neuropeptide Y gene and on chromosome 8 a significant QTL with the dopamine receptor and potassium channel genes, which explain about one-eighth of the genetic variance in blood pressure in the SHR. On chromosome 10 there are strong associations between blood pressure and some markers on a region near the ACE gene in the SHR and Dahl salt-sensitive strain. On chromosome 13 the renin locus influences blood pressure but appears to be expressed only in conjunction with as yet unknown alleles. The interaction of the missense mutations found in the coding regions of the α-adducin genes on chromosome 14 and α-adducin on chromosome 4 explain up to 50% of blood pressure difference between the Milan hypertensive and normotensive rats. And there are other genes on chromosome 17 and 20, the testis-specific histone locus and the heat-shock protein 70 and 27, respectively, that are significantly related to blood pressure but their relation to renal function is not apparent. There is also a linkage of hypertension to the Y chromosome in some strains of SHR but not in others.

Monogenic Changes and Hypertension

In contrast to the apparently diffuse, uncertain, and subsidiary position of the polygenic contribution in essential hypertension and hypertensive strains of rats, there are rare monogenic abnormalities in humans, which are entirely responsible for raising blood pressure, and others that lower it (241). In view of the extent of the evidence that links sodium and the kidney to hypertension it is not surprising that all the monogenic mutations identified so far, which induce changes in blood pressure, both up and down, do so by interfering with sodium reabsorption in the kidney.

The most relevant mutation regarding essential hypertension is Liddle's syndrome, in which the patient presents early with moderate to severe hypertension. It is caused by mutations of either the β or γ subunits of the amiloride-sensitive sodium channel on chromosome 16 that increase the passage of sodium into the cell and therefore increase sodium reabsorption in the kidney. Renal transplantation corrects the rise in blood pressure, which suggests that, as regards the origin of the hypertension, the defect is intrinsic to the kidney, and that therefore impairment in the kidney's ability to excrete sodium alone can cause hypertension.

There are two other monogenic causes of hypertension, glucocorticoid-remediable aldosteronism (GRE) and the syndrome of apparent mineralocorticoid excess (AME). In GRE, mutations of two genes on chromosome 8, the products of which are involved in adrenal biosynthesis cause aldosterone synthesis to be brought under the control of ACTH as well as angiotensin II. This leads to a rise in plasma aldosterone and therefore increases sodium reabsorption and the blood pressure. AME patients also have excess stimulation of mineralocorticoid receptors, although the plasma aldosterone is low. Normally the cells that contain mineralocorticoid receptors contain an enzyme, 11 β hydroxycorticoid dehydrogenase, that metabolizes cortisol to cortisone and prevents cortisol from binding onto the mineralocorticoid receptors. Patients with AME have a mutation of the gene responsible for 11ßhydroxycorticoid dehydrogenase so that cortisol can now bind onto aldosterone receptors (as well as aldosterone), but as cortisol circulates at concentrations that are orders of magnitude greater than aldosterone the net effect is one of mineralocorticoid excess. Glycyrrhetinic acid, which is a constituent of liquorice, inhibits 11β hydrocorticoid dehydrogenase and is the cause of the hypertension that is associated with the excessive consumption of licorice particularly in Holland.

In contrast to the monogenic lesions that increase sodium reabsorption and raise the blood pressure, there are monogenic lesions that diminish sodium reabsorption, and lead to sodium loss and hypotension (e.g., Gitelman's syndrome and pseudo-hypoaldosteronism). Patients with Gitelman's syndrome have a low blood pressure, neuromuscular abnormalities, and hypokalemia. There is an array of mutations of a gene on chromosome 16 that encodes the renal thiazide-sensitive Na-Cl co-transporter on the distal convoluted tubule. These result in loss of function and an increase in sodium excretion. Pseudo-hypoaldosteronism type I (PHA-1) is characterized by severe dehydration in the neonatal period, marked by hypotension, metabolic acidosis, and a high serum potassium concentration. These patients have mutations in chromosome 12 or 16, which each encodes different subunits of the same amiloride-sensitive sodium channel as that which is affected in Liddle's syndrome. In PHA-1, however, the mutations instead of activating the sodium channel impair its function and thus diminish sodium reabsorption and increase sodium excretion, this is accompanied by secondary defects in the secretion of hydrogen and potassium ions.

The Mechanisms Responsible for the Rise in Blood Pressure Resulting from Impaired Ability to Excrete Sodium

The renal cross-transplantation experiments described earlier and the demonstration that there is a connection between the kidney's ability to excrete sodium and the onset of hypertension are among the most significant advances made in the pathogenesis of essential hypertension in the past 80 years. However, they beg the question, how does an "unwillingness" to excrete sodium cause hypertension? It is not a question that is very often addressed. Two disconcerting but logical conclusions emerge from the cross-transplantation experiments in rats. The first is that in hereditary strains of hypertension the rise in arterial pressure stems from one or more genetic abnormalities of the kidney. It does not follow that the genetic faults that lead to the functional hypertensinogenic renal disturbance are only expressed in the kidney. There is much evidence that there are generalized membrane abnormalities in hereditary hypertension in both rats and humans (242–245). Nor does it follow that the same genetic abnormalities are responsible for all forms of hereditary hypertension. The second conclusion that emerges from cross-transplantation experiments is that if there are genetic abnormalities expressed in vascular smooth muscle, the brain, or sympathetic system in hereditary forms of hypertension, they do not, per se, cause hypertension, because blood pressure of a hypertensive strain rat does not rise in the presence of a normal kidney. Conversely, an imposed surgical procedure on a kidney can induce hypertension in an animal with no genetic abnormalities of its vascular smooth muscle or nervous system.

In other words, the mechanisms that cause blood pressure to rise as a consequence of a primary abnormality in the kidney are secondary. It is useful to divide these into afferent and efferent mechanisms. The evidence suggests that the kidney's impaired ability to excrete sodium stimulates cardiothoracic (or renal) afferents to the hypothalamus that induce a multiplicity of pressor changes; these increase sympathetic activity and thus arterial tone, which raises the blood pressure, a rise buttressed by rises in plasma noradrenaline (246) and ouabain

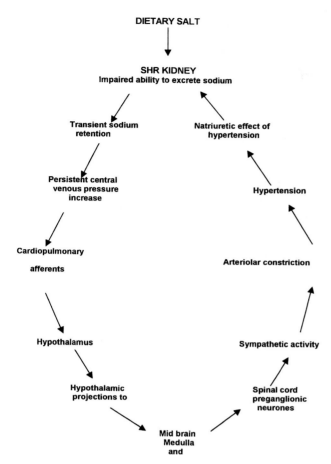

FIGURE 50-15. Flow diagram of a hypothesis that illustrates a chain of possible links between an impaired ability to excrete sodium and hypertension. (From: de Wardener HE. The hypothalamus and hypertension. *Physiol Rev* 2001;81:1599, with permission.)

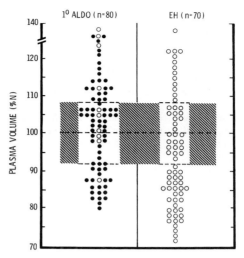

FIGURE 50-16. Plasma volume values during normal dietary sodium intake in patients with primary hyperaldosteronism (1° Aldo) and essential hypertension (EH). Values are expressed as percent of normal. The *crosshatched area* represents the variability of the method (± 8%). The *open circles* are primarily aldosteronism owing to hyperplasia; the *closed circles*, aldosteronism owing to adenomas. In primary aldosteronism, there were as many patients who were hypovolemic (25%) as there were those who were hypervolemic (30%). (From: Bravo EL, et al. The changing clinical spectrum of primary aldosteronism. *Am J Med* 1983;74:641, with permission.)

(247,248); the natriuretic effect of a rise in pressure then tends to correct the kidney's impaired ability to excrete sodium (Fig. 50-15), which is also countered by the well-documented decrease in plasma renin and rise in plasma atrial natriuretic peptide (249).

Afferent Mechanisms

Theoretically, the immediate effect of an impaired ability to excrete sodium should be to alter hydrostatic pressure or change sodium concentration. Cardiopulmonary hydrostatic pressure changes in hereditary strains of hypertensive rats and essential hypertension do occur, and it has been demonstrated in normal humans that it is the intrathoracic blood volume that controls urinary sodium excretion, not total blood volume (250). Blood volume in established essential hypertension and the inherited forms of hypertension is usually normal or low, although it is raised in a minority of patients (251). This appears inconsistent with the proposal that the kidneys have a persistent difficulty in excreting sodium in essential hypertension, because one would intuitively suppose that such a persistent tendency toward volume expansion would lead to volume expansion. In primary hyperaldosteronism, however, a parallel situation in which hypertension is certainly associated with a persistent tendency to retain sodium, the blood volume in the majority of patients is either normal or low, as in essential hypertension (252)

(Fig. 50-16). It is raised in only a minority of patients; nevertheless, patients with essential hypertension and those with primary hyperaldosteronism behave as if they were volume expanded. The phenomenon of accelerated natriuresis (253,254) occurs in both, and the plasma of both has an increased concentration of mammalian ouabain (255). The rise in plasma ANP in essential hypertension is also consistent with a central blood volume disturbance, because the stimulus for the release of ANP is distention of the atria (256).

Venous Tone and Central Venous Pressure

The discrepancy between having a normal or low total blood volume and yet responding to certain stimuli as if the blood volume were expanded is perhaps explained by the observation that in essential hypertension and in hypertensive strains of rats, there is an increase in tone of the venous vasculature with a diminished venous compliance that causes a shift of blood from the periphery to the thorax (257,258). These changes are accompanied by a rise in left atrial pressure both in humans (259) and the rat (260,261). It appears, therefore, that a normal or even low blood volume in hereditary forms of hypertension is associated with such a shift of blood to the chest that the intrathoracic venous pressure rises in spite of an overall fall in blood volume. That this rise in central venous pressure leads to a persistent increase in neural traffic from the chest to the hypothalamus is a supposition that appears reasonable. There is evidence that acute afferent neural stimulation from the chest can induce certain hypothalamic changes. The proposal that cardiothoracic afferents might be responsible for pressor hypothalamic changes in essential hypertension and hypertensive strains of rats mirrors the well-documented phenomenon that renal afferents appear to induce pressor hypothalamic changes in certain forms of experimental renal failure (262–264). Renal deafferentation by dorsal root section prevents the rise in arterial pressure after 5/6 removal of renal mass (264) and lowers the arterial pressure by about 50% in the one-kidney, one-clip hypertensive rat but it has no effect on the development of hypertension in the SHR—one form of hereditary hypertension (265). There also is some evidence that renal afferents are involved in the hypertension that accompanies chronic renal failure in humans (266).

Efferent Mechanisms

In most forms of hypertension, particularly early on, there is an increase in sympathetic activity that is owing to the extensive functional changes in the hypothalamus.

Sympathetic Activity

The increase in sympathetic nervous activity in essential hypertension has been recorded by measuring noradrenaline "spillover" (i.e., the amount that is released from the nerve endings that does not return into the sympathetic nerves and is not metabolized), and by measuring neuronal activity of the posterior tibial or peroneal nerve. Both methods reveal that in patients with essential hypertension below the age of 30 to 40 there is an increase in activity that diminishes thereafter (267–269). Direct evidence for an increase in sympathetic nervous activity in the spontaneously hypertensive rat, the Dahl salt-sensitive rat, renovascular hypertension, chronic renal failure from reduction of renal mass, and mineralocorticoid hypertension has been obtained by measurement of electrical activity in sympathetic nerves (270–272).

Hypothalamic Changes

Experiments in hypertensive strains of rats and certain experimental forms of hypertension have shown that the particular site in the hypothalamus where a functional change takes place, and the direction of the change, determine the direction of the alteration in arterial pressure. The same neurotransmitter is able to have either pressor or depressor activity depending on the neuronal system targeted (273). Hypothalamic abnormalities include increases in neuronal firing and the secretion and production of neurotransmitters and neuromodulators such as catecholamines, acetylcholines, angiotensin, natriuretic peptide, vasopressin, nitric oxide synthase, ouabain, serotonin, γ-aminobutyric acid, neuropeptide Y, tachykinin, opioids, thyrotropin-releasing hormone, bradykinin, vasoactive intestinal peptide, histamine, corticotrophin-releasing factor, and their receptors and associated enzymes (249). Increased gene expression in the hypothalamus of the SHR has been detected for angiotensinogen (274), angiotensin receptors (275), vasopressin (276), atrial natriuretic peptide (277), nitric oxide synthase (278), pre-proneuropeptide (279) pre-proenkephalin (280), vasoactive intestinal peptide (281), and thyrotrophin releasing hormone precursor (282). The type and direction of most of the changes found in hypertensive animals are pressor and they appear to be, both individually and collectively, responsible for the increase in sympathetic activity and rise in arterial pressure. A few are probably depressor, effectively compensatory adjustments (278).

Most of the changes in hypothalamic activity that occur in hypertension take place in the rostral hypothalamus and the forebrain. The effect of the anesthetic used is critical and the age of the rat at the time of observation is also of paramount importance. A few changes can be detected before the onset of the rise in pressure and others only appear as the pressure is rising or thereafter. Overall the evidence suggests that with age there is a progressive pattern of change. Early pressor increases in catecholamine (283) and serotonin (284) activity become less pronounced with time and, as a sustained pressor increase is seen in cholinergic activity (285) and diminution in gamma-aminobutyric acid (GABA) activity (286) take over. The earlier diminution in nitrate oxide synthase (NOS) activity changes

to a depressor increase. The lessening with age, of the early increase in sympathetic activity (see the preceding) makes it likely that overall there is an evolutionary decrease in the intensity of the initial pressor associated hypothalamic change. The functional changes in the various forms of hypertension are similar but there are differences. In DOCA + salt hypertension there is no increase in catecholamine activity and there is the pressor effect of the circulating DOCA on hypothalamic mineralocorticoid receptors (287). In the Dahl salt-sensitive rat there is greatly increased permeability of the blood-brain barrier and an associated increase in water content of the brain (288).

Summary

It is proposed that in patients with essential hypertension and inherited forms of hypertension in rats there is an initial retention of sodium that stimulates compensatory mechanisms. They not only cause an increase in arteriolar tone, but also an increase in venous tone that tends to shift blood centrally; they also are responsible for a wide variety of central nervous and humoral changes, including abnormalities in the hypothalamus, sympathetic nervous system, and the concentration of a variety of substances that circulate in the plasma. Collectively, these changes raise blood pressure, which overcomes the impaired ability of the kidneys to excrete sodium.

ACQUIRED HYPERTENSION AND THE KIDNEY

The diseases that afflict and destroy the kidney cause acquired hypertension in humans. Many of the same conditions can be imposed experimentally in animals. A variety of glomerular nephritides can be induced. Hyperaldosteronism is usually reproduced in animals by administration of DOCA; and increasing the salt intake speeds and accentuates the process. Coarctation of the aorta in humans can be surgically reproduced in dogs by an operation that narrows the aorta. The relatively uncommon human condition of renal artery stenosis can occur with a normal contralateral kidney. This condition can be reproduced in animals by placing a partially constricting clip on the renal artery of one kidney and either leaving the other kidney intact or removing it. Salt intake is often increased to accelerate the onset and increase the severity of the hypertension in such experimental maneuvers. The nearest experimental equivalent to a renin-producing tumor of the kidney is a slow chronic infusion of angiotensin II. Acromegaly is another form of hypertension with salt and water retention.

Mechanisms that Raise Blood Pressure

The mechanisms responsible for the rise in arterial pressure in the acquired forms of hypertension are much the same as those discussed for essential hypertension. Most forms of acquired hypertension involve some form of renal abnormality that gradually distorts and destroys the kidney and consequently impairs sodium excretion. This sets in motion similar mechanisms that raise blood pressure in essential hypertension and hereditary forms of hypertension in the rat. And these are reinforced by increased renal afferent stimulation to the hypothalamus (see the following). In addition, the reduction in renal mass appears to bring in to operation three other mechanisms: (a) the renal control of interstitial space compliance, (b) the secretion of certain hypotensive hormones from the renal medulla, and (c) the reciprocal relationship between fluid volumes and the concentration and effectiveness of angiotensin II.

Renal Control of Interstitial Space Compliance

The compliance of the interstitial space determines the proportion of the extracellular fluid volume that is apportioned between the plasma and the interstitial space. Interstitial space compliance, therefore, is one determinant of blood volume. Blood volume, more particularly its distribution, is an important factor in the control of arterial pressure.

An index of the compliance of the interstitial space can be obtained by measuring the ratio of the plasma volume (PV) to the portion of the extracellular fluid volume (ECFV) that lies in the interstitial space (i.e., the interstitial fluid volume [IFV]); thus IFV = ECFV − PV. Measuring changes in interstitial fluid pressure, particularly during an acute infusion of saline, can also assess interstitial space compliance. To maintain constant extracellular fluid osmolality, it is probable that changes in interstitial space compliance (i.e., its swelling to pressure characteristics) are accompanied by a change in the capacity of the space to bind sodium. Hyaluronic acid molecules can bind large amounts of sodium ions (289). Changes in the compliance of the interstitial tissues and their ability to bind sodium probably represent a physiologic way to store water and sodium. These mechanisms can be demonstrated in some animals adapted to withstand heat and dehydration. There are studies of changes in body water and electrolytes after water deprivation and heat stress in Somali donkeys and Zebu cattle, animals that live under desert conditions for several days without drinking (290). Donkeys lose up to 21% of body water and 29% of extracellular fluid but up to only 14% of plasma volume, whereas serum sodium concentration increases by only 7%. They can then drink large amounts of water and restore their total body water deficiency in a few minutes, whereas serum sodium falls by only 5% (291).

The following observations suggest that the kidney controls the compliance of the interstitial space. Plasma volume: extracellular fluid volume ratio increases significantly more after bilateral nephrectomy than after unilateral nephrectomy and placement of the remaining ureter in the inferior vena cava. The interstitial pressure rises more after bilateral nephrectomy, although there is greater expansion of the interstitial fluid volume after unilateral nephrectomy and placement of the remaining ureter in the vena cava (290,292,293). Interstitial space compliance has been measured by measuring changes in interstitial fluid volume and tissue pressure (TP) 10 minutes after a saline infusion (compliance = IFV/TP). After unilateral nephrectomy and placing the remaining ureter in the vena cava, there was little change in compliance from values obtained after unilateral nephrectomy alone; following bilateral nephrectomy, however, compliance falls severalfold. Similar observations have been made 60 days after partial constriction of one renal artery with a clip and removal of the opposite kidney. Tissue pressure and venous pressure are significantly higher in the rats that develop hypertension; in these animals, plasma volume also increases, but interstitial fluid volume remains unchanged (i.e., the plasma volume: interstitial fluid volume [PV/IFV] ratio is higher). After removal of the clip, tissue pressure falls despite a rise in interstitial fluid volume, and there is a fall in PV/IFV.

A study of patients with chronic renal failure has yielded similar results (294). Patients were divided into two groups, one with GFR >32 mL/minute and the other with GFR <20 mL/minute. The PV/IFV ratio of the group with the lower GFR was significantly higher than that in the group with the higher GFR. On increasing salt intake, the PV/IFV ratio of the group with the lower GFR rose still higher, whereas in the patients with the higher GFR the ratio did not change. It was also noted that the associated rise in blood pressure induced by the increase in salt intake was directly related to the change in the PV/IFV ratio. In other words, the lower the renal mass, the less the compliance of the interstitial fluid space, so that, with the increase in sodium intake and the tendency to retain sodium (and water) that are associated with reduced renal mass, a large proportion of the extracellular fluid volume is apportioned to the plasma volume. The greater the plasma volume, the higher the arterial pressure, possibly through the mechanisms discussed earlier.

The nature of the substance responsible for the change in interstitial space compliance is not known. The experiments demonstrating its presence make it likely that the concentration of the substance is dependent on the excretory function of the kidney or on the kidney's ability to secrete renin. It is probably a hormone, the rate of release of which is dependent on the amount of renal mass and its effective perfusion with blood.

Hypotensive Hormones from the Renal Papilla

If fragments of renal papilla (0.5 to 1.0 mm in size) from a healthy donor animal are transplanted subcutaneously or intraperitoneally into an animal suffering an experimentally induced form of hypertension, blood pressure falls toward normal (295–297). This observation has been made in renoprival hypertension in the dog and the rabbit and in one-clip, one-kidney hypertension in the rat (295,298). The hypotensive effect is reversed by removal or rejection of the papillary transplant. In time there is a change in the morphologic characteristics of the transplant. The tubules disappear, and the transplant consists mostly of renal interstitial cells embedded in a network of capillaries. Similar results have been obtained by injecting live monolayer cultures of renomedullary interstitial cells subcutaneously. In contrast, chemical ablation of the papillae in a rat on a normal diet leads to hypertension (299). It has been concluded that the renal medullary cells induce this hypotensive effect by releasing into the circulation a substance or substances that cause vasodilation (300).

Renal medullary cells lie alongside and between Henle's loop, the vasa recta, and the collecting ducts (295,301). They are surrounded by proteoglycans, which they secrete, and they extend cytoplasmic processes that touch adjoining structures. Renal interstitial cells have lipid-containing granules that are a source of substrate for conversion into membrane lipid, prostaglandins, and possibly antihypertensive lipids. The granules per se, either intact or disrupted, however, do not have a hypotensive effect on their own when injected intravenously. Many forms of experimental hypertension are associated with a significant decrease in the lipid granules, which also show several degenerative changes. Such changes also occur in a papillary renal transplant or in cultured renal medullary cells when they are no longer able to lower the blood pressure.

The renomedullary vasodepressor hormone secreted by the renomedullary interstitial cells in the renal papillae is a lipid named medullolipin I. It is conveyed to the liver, where it is converted into its active form, medullolipin II, a vascular dilator that suppresses sympathetic activity and causes natriuresis. Its action also opposes that of angiotensin II (302). The secretion and conversion of medullolipin in both the kidney and liver are related to cytochrome P450-dependent enzyme systems.

The main factor that controls the secretion of medullolipin is renal arterial perfusion pressure. Renal venous blood medullolipin I has been obtained in greatly increased amounts after suddenly raising renal arterial perfusion pressure by unclipping a one-kidney, one-clip hypertensive rat or rabbit preparation (303). The effect of this sudden release of medullolipin I has been demonstrated by an extracorporeal pump perfusion of an isolated clipped kidney in circuit with a conscious normotensive rat (303). On removing the renal artery clip, there is a significant fall in pressure of the normotensive rats from 125 to 70 mm Hg within 1 hour without an associated rise in heart rate. The sudden appearance of medullolipin in the renal venous blood as blood pressure is falling is associated with an acute degranulation of the renomedullary interstitial cells of the kidney that has just been unclipped. It is concluded that the medullolipin acutely released into the general circulation after unclipping the renal artery is an important factor in the fall of arterial pressure, which occurs for about 24 hours after the clip is removed. Maintenance of the low arterial pressure subsequently appears to be caused by other mechanisms. In contrast therefore with the effect of lowered perfusion pressure on renin secretion, elevation of the renal arterial perfusion pressure causes a compensatory increase in medullolipin I secretion, and lowering the perfusion pressure shuts off secretion.

A deficiency of medullolipin that contributes to an associated hypertension can be caused by: (a) the decrease in the number of and damage to renomedullary cells that occurs in accelerated experimental hypertension and malignant hypertension in humans, (b) inhibition of medullolipin secretion by angiotensin II, sympathetic stimulation, and nitric oxide synthase inhibition, and (c) removal of renomedullary cells by bilateral nephrectomy, surgical and chemical papillectomy, and papillary atrophy or necrosis (295,302,304,305).

Medullolipin I by mouth lowers blood pressure of the SHR without altering cardiac output or heart rate (306). One case of hypotension resulting from hypermedullolipinemia, which in turn is caused by a lipinomedullolipinoma of renal medullary interstitial cells, has been described in a 46-year-old woman (307).

Fluid Volumes and Angiotensin II

There is a relationship between the concentration of plasma angiotensin II and the state of fluid volumes that is particularly relevant in most forms of acquired hypertension. In normal humans and animals, there is a reciprocal relationship between plasma angiotensin II and the effectiveness of angiotensin II. Normally, the effects of changes in blood volume or sodium intake on the arterial pressure are nicely balanced. Although moderate blood volume expansion induces a fall in angiotensin II, it increases its effectiveness; although a contraction of the blood volume increases angiotensin II, it reduces its effect; thus, in both instances the resultant change in blood pressure is buffered.

These relationships may become distorted with renal disease; therefore, serious disturbances in blood pressure usually occur. Eighty percent of patients with diseased kidneys have a tendency to volume expansion, whereas the distortion and architectural compression of the renal vascular tree causes a simultaneous rise in plasma renin activity and angiotensin II. This is the worst of all worlds. There is an increased vascular response to the raised levels of angiotensin II because of the tendency toward volume expansion. This is presumably why blood pressure rises early, quickly, and often to heights that cause severe complications in most patients with chronic renal failure.

There is a persistent restraint on urinary sodium excretion in primary hyperaldosteronism. Similarly, it can be shown in experimental animals given DOCA or fludrocortisone, or following renal artery stenosis, that there is a brief initial period of positive sodium balance with a gain in weight; however, the weight gain usually levels out, then the weight is restored to near its control value (308–310). As in essential hypertension, systemic venous compliance diminishes, and there is a tendency

for the central blood volume to rise (297,310,311). Edema does not form. Blood volume, like that in essential hypertension, tends to be normal or low or is raised in only a minority of patients (308,310). Total exchangeable sodium tends to be raised (308,309). Plasma renin is reduced, and it is possible that the hypertension is due in part to the raised level of plasma ouabain (312) and vascular reactivity factor (313,314), but there is still insufficient information on this point.

In unilateral renal artery stenosis, with the other kidney *in situ*, plasma renin activity rises, and there is initial sodium retention. Then, as mentioned, blood pressure rises, and sodium balance is adjusted by increasing the excretion of sodium through the unclipped kidney, presumably because of the rise in arterial pressure and an increase in plasma natriuretic activity. Then there is a continued rise in plasma renin that can be demonstrated to be an important cause of the rise in arterial pressure. The eventual outcome with renal artery stenosis of a sole remaining kidney is a tendency toward salt and water retention and a fall in plasma renin, so that the main hypertensive mechanisms are related to volume retention.

Hypertension and Dialysis

Most patients on maintenance hemodialysis continue to fight a relentless battle against hypertension (315). The mechanisms responsible for the rise in pressure are the same as those that caused the rise in pressure before dialysis, but now they are magnified and tend to be glaringly obvious. This is the reason why nephrologists have no difficulty in accepting the role of salt and water in the control of blood pressure. On the one hand, a normal intake of fluids and the gross reduction in daily urine volume inevitably cause a rapid increase in extracellular fluid volume between each dialysis (easily monitored as a gain in weight), and on the other hand, severely diseased kidneys tend to secrete large amounts of renin. Furthermore, the need to lower the patient's weight at each dialysis by rapidly removing a considerable amount of fluid may cause a further brisk rise in plasma renin activity (316). If this recurring seesaw reciprocal movement of extracellular fluid volume and renin release is sufficiently violent, it eventually seems to resonate. Then the more one attempts to control blood pressure by fluid removal, the greater the rise in renin and angiotensin II so that at each dialysis the blood pressure, instead of falling, rises and becomes uncontrollable. In one patient, in an attempt to control the hypertension, the weight was lowered from 60 kg to 40 kg in about 2 months (316) (Fig. 50-17). This so reduced the extracellular fluid and blood volume that the patient fainted when he stood up, but his renin secretion was now so great that when he lay down he had severe hypertension with intolerable headaches and a tendency to develop acute pulmonary edema. The problem was resolved by bilateral nephrectomy, an operation that is now rarely performed to control hypertension in patients on maintenance hemodialysis. Weight reductions are performed now with more circumspection, and there are better hypotensive agents. By using measurements of blood volume, extracellular fluid volume, and plasma renin activity before and immediately after a dialysis and administering substances that nullify the pressor effect of angiotensin II, it is possible to show that hypertension in patients on maintenance hemodialysis are either dependent on an increased volume or a raised plasma angiotensin II, or sometimes a combination of both.

In Figure 50-18 are illustrated the findings in a patient whose blood pressure was volume dependent. Before dialysis when blood pressure was 200/100 mm Hg, the blood volume was obviously high, and there was a gross expansion of extracellular water, whereas plasma renin activity was abnormally low. And the lack of effect of an intravenous infusion of saralasin

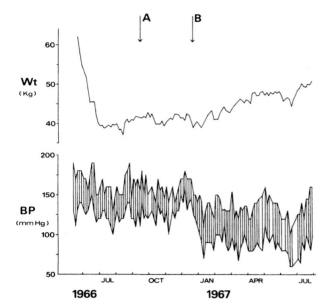

FIGURE 50-17. The effect of bilateral nephrectomy (*B*) on uncontrollable hypertension in a patient on maintenance hemodialysis with a very high plasma renin. There is an immediate fall in blood pressure, which is maintained although there is a rise in weight. At point *A* the patient had an attack of acute infectious hepatitis. (From: Brown JJ, et al. Plasma renin concentration and the control of blood pressure in patients on maintenance haemodialysis. *Nephron* 1969;6:329.)

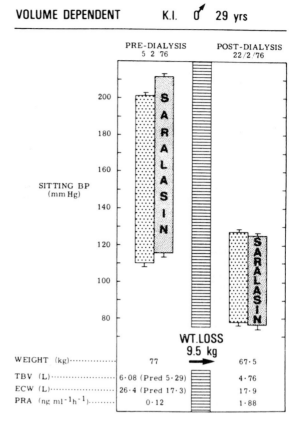

FIGURE 50-18. Patient on maintenance hemodialysis with hypertension caused by excess volume. Blood pressure (BP), weight, total blood volume (TBV), extracellular water (ECW), plasma renin activity (PRA), and the effect of an infusion of saralasin on the blood pressure, measured before and after the loss of 9.5 kg of weight in 17 days, are shown. Saralasin, a competitor of angiotensin II, was infused to gauge the dependency of blood pressure on angiotensin II. On the first occasion, when blood pressure was 200/100 mm Hg, the blood volume obviously was high, and there was a gross expansion of extracellular water, plasma renin activity was abnormally low, and the lack of effect of the infusion of saralasin on blood pressure indicated that blood pressure was not dependent on the plasma level of angiotensin II. On the second occasion, after the loss of weight, when blood pressure was 128/78 mm Hg, blood volume, extracellular water, and plasma renin activity were now normal, and the saralasin infusion again demonstrated that blood pressure was not dependent on angiotensin II.

(a competitor of angiotensin II) on blood pressure indicated that blood pressure was not dependent on the plasma level of angiotensin II. After several dialyses, the patient lost 9.5 kg when blood pressure was 128/78 mm Hg, and the blood volume, extracellular fluid volume, and plasma renin activity became normal; the saralasin infusion again demonstrated that blood pressure was not dependent on angiotensin II.

In Figure 50-19 are illustrated the findings in a patient in whom blood pressure was dependent on a raised level of angiotensin II. Before dialysis, when blood pressure was 180/100 mm Hg, the blood volume was normal, plasma renin activity was greatly raised, and the fall in pressure induced by saralasin indicated that blood pressure was under the influence of angiotensin II. After a dialysis, the patient lost 2.2 kg, blood pressure fell to 170/95 mm Hg, and the blood volume was still "normal," but the plasma renin activity was now extremely high and the greater fall in blood pressure induced by the saralasin infusion indicated that blood pressure was even more dependent on angiotensin II.

Renal Hypotension

Renal hypotension is an infrequent complication of some forms of renal disease and usually follows bilateral nephrectomy in a patient on maintenance hemodialysis. The renal diseases that are most prone to this unusual complication are those that affect predominantly the renal medulla (e.g., the reflux nephropathy, obstructive uropathy, and phenacetin nephropathy). Although the condition is sometimes referred to as salt-losing nephritis, it is rarely owing to glomerular nephritis. The fall in arterial pressure is due to a urinary leak of sodium. It occurs only with bilateral renal disease and after the onset of renal failure. It is associated with a gross generalized hypertrophy of the juxtaglomerular apparatus and the adrenals. Plasma renin activity and aldosterone are raised. Often there is hypokalemia

caused in part to the hyperaldosteronism and in part to the renal disease. The condition tends to fluctuate wildly. Exacerbations often are caused by an upper urinary tract infection when the combination of infection, hypotension, a fall in extracellular fluid volume, and hypokalemia may cause severe but usually entirely and easily reversible reductions in renal function. In spite of these alarming episodes, these patients survive longer than other patients with renal failure whose progress is calmer but who develop hypertension. Survival of patients with renal hypotension depends on the skill and speed of reaction of those who look after them. The continuous administration of oral supplements of sodium chloride such as Slow Sodium (Novartis), repeated monitoring of the urine for infection, and prompt treatment of a relapse may prevent any progressive deterioration in renal function.

Renal hypotension is such a serious and frequent complication of the anephric state that bilateral nephrectomy is no longer used for the treatment of intractable hypertension in

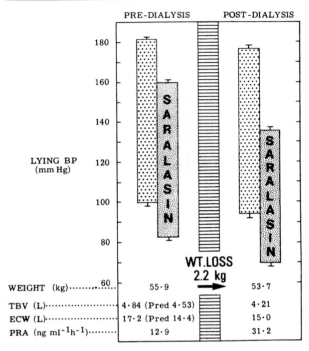

ANGIOTENSIN II DEPENDENT   G.F. ♂ 27 yrs

FIGURE 50-19. Patient on maintenance hemodialysis with hypertension caused by high plasma renin activity. Blood pressure (BP), weight, total blood volume (TBV), extracellular water (ECW), plasma renin activity (PRA), and the effect of an infusion of saralasin on blood pressure measured before and after a loss of 2.5 kg of weight during a single dialysis of 7 hours are shown. Saralasin, a competitor of angiotensin II, was infused to gauge the dependency of blood pressure on angiotensin II. Before dialysis, when blood pressure was 180/100 mm Hg, the blood volume was normal, although the extracellular water was 2.5 kg greater than predicted (a not unusual gain in weight between dialyses), plasma renin activity was greatly raised, and the fall in blood pressure induced by the infusion of saralasin indicated that blood pressure was under the influence of angiotensin II. After dialysis, having lost a "normal" amount of weight, blood pressure was 170/95 mm Hg, the blood volume and extracellular water were normal, but the plasma renin activity was now extremely high, and the greater fall in blood pressure induced by saralasin infusion indicated that blood pressure was even more dependent on angiotensin II.

patients on maintenance hemodialysis. After bilateral nephrectomy and the fall in plasma angiotensin II, the relation between the arterial pressure and the blood volume is such that the volume has to be greater than normal to maintain a normal blood pressure (317) (Fig. 50-20). Many anephric patients therefore live precarious lives of fluctuating hypotension in spite of an overexpanded extracellular fluid volume, sometimes to the point of demonstrable clinical edema and breathlessness. The low arterial pressure presumably is due primarily to the almost total absence of renin and angiotensin II, but there is evidence that it may also result in part from the associated reduction in plasma aldosterone.

These two forms of hypotension beautifully illustrate the interdependence of angiotensin and extracellular fluid volume in the control of blood pressure. On the one hand, in "salt-losing nephritis," the urinary leak of sodium and the decrease in extracellular fluid volume are so great that the arterial pressure falls in spite of enormous rises in plasma renin activity. On the other hand, after bilateral nephrectomy in the absence of angiotensin, gross overexpansion of the extracellular fluid volume does not

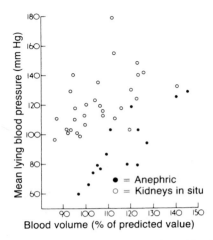

Dialysis patients
(Blood pressure vs. blood volume)

FIGURE 50-20. Blood volume versus mean lying blood pressure in patients on maintenance hemodialysis. At normal blood volumes blood pressure of anephric patients (●) was lower than in patients whose kidneys were still *in situ* (○).

prevent the arterial pressure from being intolerably low. Some workers have claimed that the relationship between fluid volume and arterial pressure after bilateral nephrectomy depends on whether the patient suffered from hypertension before the operation. Occasionally, amyloidosis of the sympathetic chains causes hypotension in a patient on dialysis. Until now this has been an intractable and irreversible condition that leads to endless difficulties and death.

References

1. Bright T. Tabular view of the morbid appearance in 100 cases connected with albuminous urine: with observations. *Guy's Hosp Rep* 1836;1:380.
2. Harvey W. *Exercitatio anatomica de motu cordis et sanguinis in animalibus.* Frankfurt: W. Fitzeri, 1628.
3. Hales S. Containing haemasticks; or an account of some hydraulick and hydrostatical experiments made on the blood and blood-vessels of animals. In: *Statistical essays,* vol. 2. London: Innis and Mauby, 1769.
4. Guyton AC. *Arterial pressure and hypertension. Circulatory physiology III.* Philadelphia: Saunders, 1980.
5. Johnson GI. On certain points in the anatomy and pathology of Bright's disease. II. On the influence of the minute blood-vessels upon the circulation. *Med-Chir Trans* 1868;51:57.
6. Toynbee J. On the intimate structure of the human kidney, and on the changes which its several component parts undergo in "Bright's Disease." *Med-Chir Trans* 1846;29:303.
7. Traube L. *Ueber den zusammenhang von herz-und-nierenkrankheiten, gesammelte beitrage zur pathologie und physiologie,* vol. 2 Berlin: Hirschwald, 1871.
8. Fahr Th. Uber Nephrosklerose. *Virchows Archiv* 1919;226:119.
9. Borst JG, Borst-de-Gues A. Hypertension explained by Starling's theory of circulatory homeostasis. *Lancet* 1963;1:677.
10. Mahomed FA. On chronic Bright's disease, and its essential symptoms. *Lancet* 1879;i:46.
11. Huchard H. *Maladies du coeur & des vaisseaux.* Paris: Doin, 1889.
12. Volhard P. Nieren und Ableitende Harnwege. In: von Bergmann G, Staehelin R, eds. *Hanbuch der inneren medizin.* Berlin: Springer, 1931.
13. Tigerstedt R, Bergman PG. Niere und kreislauf. *Arch Physiol (Scand)* 1898;8:223.
14. Goldblatt H, et al. Studies on experimental hypertension: the production of persistent elevation of systolic blood pressure by means of renal ischemia. *J Exp Med* 1934;59:347.
15. Skeggs LT, et al. The amino acid sequence of hypertension. II. *J Exp Med* 1956;104:193.
16. Peart WS. The isolation of a hypertensin. *Biochem J* 1956;62:520.
17. Wilson C, Byrom FB. The vicious circle in chronic Bright's disease: experimental evidence from the hypertensive rat. *Q J Med* 1941;10:65.

18. Rettig R, et al. Are renal mechanisms involved in primary hypertension? Evidence from kidney transplantation studies in rats. *Klin Wochenschr* 1991;69:597.
19. Bell ET. *Renal diseases.* London: Henry Kimpton, 1946.
20. Castleman B, Smithwick R. Relation of vascular disease to hypertension. *J Amer Med Assoc* 1943;121:1256.
21. Fishberg AM. *Hypertension and nephritis,* 5th ed. London: Bailliere, Tindell & Cox, 1954.
22. de Wardener HE. The primary role of the kidney and salt intake in the aetiology of essential hypertension. Part 1. *Clin Sci* 1990;79:193.
23. de Wardener HE. The primary role of the kidney and salt intake in the aetiology of essential hypertension. Part II. *Clin Sci* 1990;79:289.
24. Tobian L, et al. A comparison of the antihypertensive potency of kidneys from one strain of rats susceptible to salt hypertension and kidneys from another strain resistant to it. *J Clin Invest* 1966;45:1080A.
25. Dahl LK, Heine M, Thompson K. Genetic influence of renal homografts on blood pressure of rats from different strains (36566). *Proc Soc Exp Biol Med* 1972;140:852.
26. Bianchi G, et al. The hypertensive role of the kidney in spontaneously hypertensive rats. *Clin Sci* 1973;45:135s.
27. Dahl LK, Heine M, Thompson K. Genetic influence of the kidneys on blood pressure. *Circ Res* 1974;34:94.
28. Morgan DA, DiBona GF, Mark AL. Effects of inter-strain renal transplantation on NaCl-induced hypertension in Dahl rats. *Hypertension* 1990;15:436.
29. Greene AS, et al. Role of blood volume expansion in Dahl rat model of hypertension. *Am J Physiol* 1990;258:H508.
30. Rettig R, et al. Role of the kidney in primary hypertension: a renal transplantation study in rats. *Am J Physiol* 1990;258:F606.
31. Guidi E, et al. Hypertension in man with kidney transplant: role of familial versus other factors. *Nephron* 1985;41:14.
32. Curtis JJ, et al. Remission of essential hypertension after renal transplantation. *N Engl J Med* 1983;309:1009.
33. Bianchi G, et al. Changes in renin, water balance and sodium balance during development of high blood pressure in genetically hypertensive rat. *Circ Res* 1975;36(Suppl 1):153.
34. Graf C, et al. Sodium retention and hypertension after kidney transplantation in rats. *Hypertension* 1993;21:724.
35. Imig JD, et al. Elevated renovascular tone in young spontaneously hypertensive rats. *Hypertension* 1993;22:357.
36. Gebremedhin D, et al. Enhanced vascular tone in the renal vasculature of spontaneously hypertensive rats. *Hypertension* 1990;16:648.
37. Roman RJ, Kaldunski ML. Renal cortical and papillary blood flow in spontaneously hypertensive rats. *Hypertension* 1988;11:657.
38. Khiraibi AA, Knox FG. Renal interstitial hydrostatic pressure during pressure natriuresis in hypertension. *Am J Physiol* 1988;255:R756.
39. Nørrelund H, et al. Early narrowed afferent arteriole is a contributor to the development of hypertension. *Hypertension* 1994;24:301.
40. Hollengerg NK, Williams GH, Adams DF. Essential hypertension: abnormal renal vascular and endocrine responses to a mild psychological stimulus. *Hypertension* 1981;3:11.
41. Weinberger MH, et al. Definitions and characteristics of sodium sensitivity and blood pressure resistance. *Hypertension* 1986;9:127.
42. Fujija T, et al. Factors influencing blood pressure in salt sensitive patients with hypertension. *Am J Med* 1980;69:334.
43. Lifton RP. Molecular genetics of human blood pressure variation. *Science* 1996;272:676.
44. MacGregor GA, de Wardener HE. *Salt, diet & health.* Cambridge, England: Cambridge University Press, 1998.
45. Multhauf RP. *Neptune's gift: a history of common salt.* Baltimore: Johns Hopkins University, 1978.
46. Eaton SB, Kohner M, Shostak M. Stone ages in the fast lane: chronic degenerative diseases in evolutionary perspective. *Am J Med* 1988;84:739.
47. Denton D. *The hunger for salt.* Heidelberg: Springer Verlag, 1982.
48. Chagnon NA. *Yanomamö. The fierce people.* New York: Holt, Rinehart & Winston, 1968.
49. Poulter NK, et al. The Kenyan Luo migration study: observations on the initiation of a rise in blood pressure. *Br Med J* 1990;300:967.
50. Kesteloot H, et al. The relationship between cations and blood pressure in the People's Republic of China. *Hypertension* 1987;9:654.
51. Kesteloot H, et al. A comparative study of blood pressure and sodium intake in Belgium and in Korea. In: Kesteloot H, Joosens JV, eds. *Epidemiology and arterial blood pressure.* The Hague: Martinus Nijhoff, 1980:453.
52. Mir MA, Newcombe R. The relationship of dietary salt and blood pressure in three farming communities in Kashmir. *J Hum Hypertens* 1984;2:241.
53. Shibata H, Hatano SA. Salt restriction trial in Japan. In: Gross F, Strasser T, eds. *Mild hypertension: natural history and management.* Bath: Pitman Medical, 1979:147.
54. Yamori Y, et al. Hypertension and diet: multiple regression analysis in a Japanese farming community. *Lancet* 1981;i:1204.
55. Gleiberman L. Blood pressure and dietary salt in human populations. *Ecol Food Nutr* 1973;2:143.
56. Dahl LK. Possible role of salt intake in the development of essential hypertension. In: Brock KD, Cottier PT, eds. *Essential hypertension: proceedings of an international symposium.* London: Ciba, 1960:53.
57. The Intersalt Study. *J Hum Hypertens* 1989;3:279.
58. Elliott P, Stamler R. Manual of operations for "Intersalt," an international cooperative study on the relation of sodium and potassium to blood pressure. *Controlled Clin Trials* 1988;9:1.
59. Liu K, et al. Can overnight urines replace 24-hour urine collections to assess salt intake? *Hypertension* 1979;ii:529.
60. Luft FC, Fineberg NS, Sloan RS. Estimating dietary sodium intake in individuals receiving a randomly fluctuating intake. *Hypertension* 1982;4:805.
61. Siani A, et al. Comparison of variability in urinary sodium, potassium and calcium in free living man. *Hypertension* 1989;13:38.
62. Watson RL, Langford HG. Usefulness of overnight urines in population groups. *Am J Clin Nutr* 1970;23:290.
63. Swales JD. Salt saga continued. *Br Med J* 1988;297:307.
64. Carvalho JJ, et al. Blood pressure in four remote populations in the Intersalt study. *Hypertension* 1989;14:238.
65. Allen FM, Cope OM. Influence of diet on blood pressure and kidney size in dogs. *J Urol* 1942;47:751.
66. Wilhelmj CM, Waldmann EB, McGuire TF. Effect of prolonged high sodium chloride ingestion and withdrawal upon blood pressure of dogs (18784). *Proc Soc Exp Biol Med* 1951;77:379.
67. Lenel R, Katz LN, Rodbard S. Arterial hypertension in the chicken. *Am J Physiol* 1948;152:557.
68. Fukuda TR. L'hypertension par le sel chez les lapins et ses relations avec la glande surrenale. *Union Med Can* 1951;80:1278.
69. Cherchovich GM, et al. High salt intake and blood pressure in lower primates. *J Appl Physiol* 1976;40:601.
70. Dahl LK, et al. Effects of chronic excess salt ingestion: modification of experimental hypertension in the rat by variations in the diet. *Circ Res* 1968;22:11.
71. Meneely GR, et al. Chronic sodium chloride toxicity: hypertension, renal and vascular lesions. *Ann Intern Med* 1953;39:991.
72. Sapirstein LA, Brandt WL, Drury DR. Production of hypertension in the rat by substituting hypertonic sodium chloride solutions for drinking water. *Proc Soc Exp Biol Med* 1950;73:82.
73. Denton D, et al. The effect of increased salt intake on blood pressure of chimpanzees. *Nat Med* 1995;1:1009.
74. Zicha J, Kunes J. Ontogenic aspects of hypertension development: analysis in the rat. *Physiol Rev* 1999;79:1227.
75. Dahl LK, Shackow E. Effects of chronic excess salt ingestion: experimental hypertension in the rat. *Can Med Assoc J* 1964;90:155.
76. Dahl LK. Excessive salt intake and hypertension: a dietary and genetic interplay. *Brookhaven Lecture Ser* 1962;12:22.
77. Smirk FH, Hall WH. Inherited hypertension in rats. *Nature* 1958;182:727.
78. Burstyn P, Hornall D, Watchorn C. Sodium and potassium intake and blood pressure. *Br Med J* 1980;2:537.
79. Gros G, Weller JM, Hoobler SW. Relationship of sodium and potassium intake to blood pressure. *Am J Clin Nutr* 1971;24:605.
80. Kirkendall WM, et al. The effect of dietary sodium chloride on blood pressure, body fluids, electrolytes, renal function and serum lipids of normotensive man. *J Lab Clin Med* 1976;87:418.
81. Sagnella GA, et al. Plasma immunoreactive atrial natriuretic peptide and changes in dietary sodium intake in man. *Life Sci* 1987;40:139.
82. Sullivan JM, et al. Hemodynamic effects of dietary sodium in man. *Hypertension* 1980;2:506.
83. Murray RH, et al. Blood pressure responses to extremes of sodium intake in normal man (40364). *Proc Soc Exp Biol Med* 1978;159:432.
84. Grim CE. Genetic influences on renin aldosterone and the renal excretion of sodium and potassium following volume expansion and contraction in normal man. *Hypertension* 1979;1:583.
85. Renal sodium handling, intra-cellular sodium, sodium-potassium ATP-ase activity, and unsaturated fatty acids in offspring of hypertensive and normotensive parents. In: van Hooft IM, ed. *The Dutch hypertension and offspring study.* Rotterdam: University of Rotterdam, thesis.
86. Pusterela C, et al. Blood pressure regulation on low and high sodium diets in normotensive members of normotensive or hypertensive families. *J Hypertens* 1986;4:S310.
87. Widgren BR, et al. Blunted renal sodium excretion during acute saline loading in normotensive men with positive family histories of hypertension. *Am J Hypertens* 1991;4:570.
88. Grim CE, et al. An approach to the evaluation of genetic influences on factors that regulate arterial blood pressure in man. *Hypertension* 1980;2:1.
89. Grim CE, et al. Effects of sodium loading and depletion in normotensive first-degree relatives of essential hypertensives. *J Lab Clin Med* 1979;94:764.
90. Hofman A, Hazebroek A, Valkenburg HA. A randomized trial of sodium intake and blood pressure in newborn infants. *JAMA* 1983;250:370.
91. Geleijnse JN, et al. Long-term effects of neonatal sodium restriction on blood pressure. *Hypertension* 1997;29:913.
92. Gillum RF, Elmer PJ, Prineas RJ. Changing sodium intake in children. *Hypertension* 1981;3:698.
93. Cooper R, et al. Randomized trial on the effect of decreased dietary sodium intake on blood pressure in adolescence. *J Hypertens* 1984;2:361.
94. Miller JZ, et al. Blood pressure response to dietary sodium restriction in healthy normotensive children. *Am J Clin Nutr* 1988;47:113.

95. Ellison RC, et al. Effects on blood pressure of a decrease in sodium use in institutional food preparation. The Exeter and Andover project. *J Clin Epidemiol* 1989;42:201.

96. Sasaki N. The salt factor in apoplexy and hypertension: epidemiological studies in Japan. In: Yamori Y, ed. *Prophylactic approach to hypertensive diseases*. New York: Raven Press, 1979:467.

97. Swales J. Population advice on salt restriction: the social issues. *Am J Hypertens* 2000;13:2.

98. He FJ, MacGregor GA. Effect of modest salt reduction on blood pressure: a meta-analysis of randomized trials. Implications for public health. *J Human Hypertens* 2002;16:761.

99. Forte JG, et al. Salt and blood pressure: a community trial. *J Hum Hypertens* 1989;3:179.

100. Takahashi EJ, et al. The geographic distribution of cerebral hemorrhage and hypertension in Japan. *Hum Biol* 1957;29:139.

101. Ambard L, Beaujard E. Causes de l'hypertension arterielle. *Arch Gen Med* 1904;1:520.

102. Brodski J. Experimentelle untersuchungen uber das Verhalten des Blutdruckes und uber den Einfluss der Nahrung bei Verschiedenen Nephritsarten. Dtsch. *Arch Klin Med* 1908;93:310.

103. Allen FC. Arterial hypertension. *JAMA* 1920;74:652.

104. Houghton HA. The treatment of arterial hypertension with low sodium chloride diet. *Med Record* 1922;101:441.

105. Allen FC, Sherrill JW. The treatment of arterial hypertension. *J Metab Res* 1922;2:429.

106. Kempner W. Treatment of hypertensive vascular disease with rice diet. *Am J Med* 1948;4:545.

107. Pickering G. *High blood pressure*, 2nd ed. London: J&A Churchill, 1968.

108. Fishberg AM. *Hypertension and nephritis*, 4th ed. Philadelphia: Lea and Febiger, 1939.

109. Goldring W, Chasis H. *Hypertension and hypertensive disease*. New York: Commonwealth Fund, 1944.

110. Page IH, Corcoran AC. *Arterial hypertension*. Chicago: Year Book, 1945.

111. Liebman BF, Jacobson MF. Sodium contents of restaurant foods in United States are high. *Br Med J* 1997;7106:488.

112. MacGregor GA, et al. Double-blind study of three sodium intakes and long-term effects of sodium restriction in essential hypertension. *Lancet* 1989;25:1244.

113. Whelton PK, et al. Sodium reduction and weight loss in the treatment of hypertension in older persons. *JAMA* 1998;279:839.

114. Joosens JV, Kesteloot MD. Trends in systolic blood pressure, 24-hour sodium excretion, and stroke mentality in the elderly in Belgium. *Am J Med* 1991;90:5S.

115. Kotchen TR. Research and public health directions. In: Cutler A, Kotchen TA, Charzanek E, eds. The National Heart, Lung and Blood Institute Workshop on Salt and Blood Pressure. *Hypertension* 1991;17:216.

116. He FJ, MacGregor GA. How far should salt intake be reduced? *Hypertension* 2003;42:1093.

117. Food labelling: declaration of sodium content of food and label claims for foods on the basis of sodium content. Department of Health and Human Services. Food and Drug Administration 21 CFR, parts 101 and 105. *Fed. Reg.* 76:15510,1984.

118. Muntzel M, Drüeke TA. A comprehensive review of the salt and blood pressure relationship. *Am J Hypertens* 1992;5:15.

119. de Wardener HE. Salt reduction and cardiovascular risk: the anatomy of a myth. *J Hum Hypertens* 1999;13:1.

120. de Wardener HE, Kaplan NM. On the assertion that a moderate restriction of sodium intake may have adverse health effects. *Am J Hypertens* 1993;6:810.

121. Rose G. Preventive cardiology: what lies ahead? *Preventive Med* 1990;19:97.

122. Joint WHO/FAO expert consultation on diet, nutrition and the prevention of chronic diseases. 2003, Geneva. Available at http://www.who.int/hpr/NPH/docs/who_fao_experts_report.pdf.

123. Committee on Medical Aspects of Food Policy (COMA). *Nutritional aspects of cardiovascular disease*. Dept. of Health, Report on Health and Social Subjects. London: Her Majesty's Stationery Office, 1994:46.

124. Scientific Advisory Committee on Nutrition, Salt and Health. 2003. Her Majesty's Stationery Office. Available at http://www.sacn.gov.uk/pdf/saltfinal.pdf.

125. de Wardener HE, MacGregor GA. Harmful effects of dietary salt in addition to hypertension. *J Hum Hypertens* 2002;16:213.

126. Daniels SD, et al. Determinants of cardiac involvement in children and adolescents with essential hypertension. *Circulation* 1990;82:1243.

127. Schmieder E, et al. Sodium intake modulates left ventricular hypertrophy in essential hypertension. *J Hypertens* 1988;6:S148.

128. Weir MR, et al. Salt-induced increases in systolic blood pressure affect renal hemodynamics and proteinuria. *Hypertension* 1995;25:1339.

129. Devine A, et al. A longitudinal study. *Am J Clin Nutr* 1995;62:740.

130. Sakhaee K, et al. The potential role of salt abuse on the risk for kidney stone formation. *J Urol* 1993;150:310.

131. Joosens JB, et al. On behalf of European Cancer Prevention (ECP) and the Intersalt Co-operative Research Group's dietary salt, nitrate and stomach cancer mortality in 24 countries. *Int J Epidemiol* 996;25:494.

132. Perry IJ, Beevers DG. Salt intake and stroke: a possible direct effect. *J Hum Hypertens* 1992;6:123.

133. Weir MR, et al. Influence of race and dietary salt on the antihypertensive efficacy of an angiotensin-converting enzyme inhibitor or a calcium channel antagonist in salt-sensitive hypertensives. *Hypertension* 1998;31:1088.

134. Ram CV, Garrett BN, Kaplan NM. Moderate sodium restriction and various diuretics in the treatment of hypertension. *Arch Intern Med* 1981;141:1015.

135. Yu HC, et al. Salt induces myocardial and renal fibrosis in normotensive and hypertensive rats. *Circulation* 1998;98:2621.

136. Botero-Velez M, Curtis JJ, Warnock DG. Brief report: Liddle's syndrome revisited—a disorder of sodium reabsorption in the distal tubule. *N Engl J Med* 1994:330:178.

137. Bianchi G, Barlassina C. Renal function in essential hypertension. In: Genest J, et al., eds. *Hypertension*. New York: McGraw-Hill, 1983:54.

138. Uneda S, et al. Renal hemodynamics and renin-angiotensin system in adolescents genetically predisposed to essential hypertension. *J Hypertens* 1984;2:S437.

139. Van Hooft IMS, et al. Renal hemodynamics and the renin-angiotensin-aldosterone system in normotensive subjects with hypertensive and normotensive parents. *N Engl J Med* 1991;324:1305.

140. Berger EY, Farber SJ, Earle DP. Comparison of the constant infusion and urine collection techniques for the measurement of renal function. *J Clin Invest* 1948;27:710.

141. Williams GH, Hollenberg NK. "Sodium sensitive" essential hypertension: emerging insights into pathogenesis and therapeutic implications. *Contemp Nephrol* 1985;3:303.

142. Moore TJ, et al. Altered renin-angiotensin-aldosterone relationships in normal renin essential hypertension. *Circ Res* 1977;41:167.

143. Lifton RP, et al. Evidence for heritability of non-modulating essential hypertension. *Hypertension* 1989;13:884.

144. Beretta-Pocolla C, et al. Blunted aldosterone responsiveness to angiotensin II in normotensive subjects with predisposition to essential hypertension. *J Hypertens* 1988;6:57.

145. Baer PG, Bianchi G. Renal micropuncture study of normotensive and Milan hypertensive rats before and after development of hypertension. *Kidney Int* 1978;13:452.

146. Dilley JR, Stier CT, Arendshorst WI. Abnormalities in glomerular function in rats developing spontaneous hypertension. *Am J Physiol* 1984;246:F12.

147. Bianchi G, et al. The role of the kidney in the rat with genetic hypertension. *Postgrad Med J* 1977;53:123.

148. Dietz R, et al. Studies on the pathogenesis of spontaneous hypertension of rats. *Circ Res* 1978;43:98.

149. Ben-Ishay D, Knudsen KD, Dahl LK. Exaggerated response to isotonic saline loading in genetically hypertension prone rats. *J Lab Clin Med* 1973;82:597.

150. Willis LR, Bauer JH. Aldosterone in the exaggerated natriuresis of spontaneously hypertensive rats. *Am J Physiol* 1978;234:F29.

151. Evan AP, et al. The glomerular filtration barrier in the spontaneously hypertensive rat. *Hypertension* 1981;3:1.

152. Rosenberg W, et al. Quantitative structural aspects of the renal glomeruli of hypertensive mice. *Nephron* 1982;30:161.

153. Fauvel JP, et al. Microalbuminuria in normotensives with genetic risk of hypertension. *Nephron* 1991;57:375.

154. Weder AB. Red cell lithium-sodium countertransport and renal lithium clearance in hypertension. *N Engl J Med* 1986;314:198.

155. Niutta E, et al. Renal lithium clearance in the different stages of hypertension. *J Hypertens* 1991;9:1135.

156. Weinberger MH, et al. Red-cell sodium-lithium countertransport and fractional excretion of lithium in normal and hypertensive humans. *Hypertension* 1989;13:206.

157. Strazullo P, et al. Erythrocyte sodium-lithium countertransport and renal lithium clearance in a random sample of untreated middle-aged men. *Clin Sci* 1989;77:337.

158. Cusi D, et al. Erythrocyte Na^+, K^+, Cl cotransport and kidney function in essential hypertension. *J Hypertens* 1993;11:805.

159. Aperia AC, Broberger CG, Soderlund S. Relationship between renal artery perfusion pressure and tubular sodium reabsorption. *Am J Physiol* 1971;220:1205.

160. Blake WD, et al. Effect of renal arterial constriction on excretion of sodium and water. *Am J Physiol* 1950;163:422.

161. McDonald SJ, de Wardener HE. The relationship between the renal arterial perfusion pressure and the increase in sodium excretion which occurs during an infusion of saline. *Nephron* 1965;2:1.

162. Tobian L, et al. Reduction of natriuretic capacity and renin release in isolated blood perfused kidneys of Dahl hypertension prone rats. *Circ Res* 1978;43:192.

163. Roman RJ, Cowley AW Jr. Abnormal pressure-diuresis-natriuresis response in spontaneously hypertensive rats. *Am J Physiol* 1985;248:F189.

164. Gattone VH, et al. Renal afferent arteriole in the spontaneously hypertensive rat. *Hypertension* 1983;5:8.

165. Norrelund H, et al. Reduced renal afferent arteriole diameter at 7 weeks is a predictor of increased blood pressure at 23 weeks in F2 generation spontaneously hypertensive and Wistar-Kyoto rats. *J Hypertens* 1993;11:S462.

166. Roman JR, Kaldunski M. Pressure natriuresis and cortical and papillary blood flow in inbred Dahl rats. *Am J Physiol* 1991;261:R595.

167. Kato T, et al. Decreased sensitivity to renal interstitial hydrostatic pressure in Dahl salt-sensitive rats. *Hypertension* 1994;23:1082.

168. Shibouta Y, et al. Enhanced thromboxane A2 biosynthesis in the kidney of spontaneously hypertensive rats during development of hypertension. *Eur J Pharmacol* 1981;70:247.

169. Schwartzman ML, et al. Cytochrome P450 dependent arachidonic acid metabolism in human kidney. *Kidney Int* 1990;37:94.

170. Sacerdoti D, et al. Renal cytochrome P450 dependent metabolism of arachidonic acid by microsomes from renal vessels. *FASEBJ* 1990;4:A486.

171. Sacerdoti D, et al. Treatment with tin prevents the development of hypertension in spontaneously hypertensive rats. *Science* 1989;243:388.

172. Omata K, et al. Age-related changes in renal cytochrome P450 arachidonic acid metabolism in spontaneously hypertensive rats. *Am J Physiol* 1991;262:F8.

173. Beierwaltes WH, Arendshorst WJ, Klemmer PJ. Electrolyte and water balance in young spontaneously hypertensive rats. *Hypertension* 1982;4:908.

174. Rapp JP, Dahl LK. Mutant forms of cytochrome P-450 controlling both 18 and 11B-steroid hydroxylation in the rat. *Biochemistry* 1976;15:1235.

175. Garg LC, Harang N, McArdle S. Na-K-ATPase in nephron segments of rats developing spontaneous hypertension. *Am J Physiol* 1985;249:F863.

176. Elliot AH, Nuzum FR. Urinary excretion of a depressor substance (kallikrein of Frey and Kraut) in arterial hypertension. *Endocrinology* 1934;18:462.

177. Carretero OA, et al. Urinary kallikrein in rats bred for their susceptibility and resistance to the hypertensive effect of salt: a new radio-immuno assay for its direct determination. *Circ Res* 1978;42:727.

178. Zinner SH, et al. Stability of blood pressure rank and urinary kallikrein concentration in childhood: an eight year follow-up. *Circulation* 1978;58:908.

179. Margolius HS, et al. Urinary kallikrein in hypertensive man: relationship to sodium intake and sodium retaining steroids. *Circ Res* 1974;35:820.

180. Margolius HS. Kallikrein as a participant in renal and circulatory function. *Cardiovas Rev Rep* 1982;3:559.

181. Gill JR, et al. Bradykinin and renal function in normal man: effects of adrenergic blockade. *Am J Physiol* 1965;209:844.

182. Scicli AG, Carretero OA. Renal kallikrein-kinin system. *Kidney Int* 1986;29:120.

183. Margolius HS, Chao J, Kaizu T. The effects of aldosterone and spironolactone on renal kallikrein in the rat. *Clin Sci Mol Med* 1976;51:279S.

184. Adetuyibi A, Miles IH. Relation between urinary kallikrein and renal function hypertension and excretion of sodium and water in man. *Lancet* 1972;2:203.

185. Rabito SF, Scicli AG, Carretero OA. Immunoreactive glandular kallikrein in plasma during alterations in urinary kallikrein excretion. *Hypertension* 1983;5:V-153.

186. Lewis SA, Alles WP. Urinary kallikrein: a physiological regulator of epithelial Na absorption. *Proc Natl Acad Sci* 1986;14:5345.

187. Berry TD, et al. A gene for high urinary kallikrein may protect against hypertension in Utah kindreds. *Hypertension* 1989;13:3.

188. Pravenec M, et al. Cosegregation of blood pressure with a kallikrein family polymorphism. *Hypertension* 1991;17:242.

189. Haberle DA, von Baeyer H. Characteristics of glomerulotubular balance. *Am J Physiol* 1983;244:F355.

190. Kaufman JS, Hamburger RJ, Flamenbaum W. Tubuloglomerular feedback response after hypotensive haemorrhage. *Renal Physiol* 1982;5:173.

191. Persson AE, et al. Interstitial pressure as a modulator of tubuloglomerular feedback control. *Kidney Int* 1982;22:S122.

192. Haberle DA, Davis JM. Resetting of tubuloglomerular feedback: evidence for a humoral factor in tubular fluid. *Am J Physiol* 1984;246:F495.

193. Schnerman J, Schubert G, Briggs JP. Tubuloglomerular feedback response with native and artificial tubular fluid. *Am J Physiol* 1986;250:F16.

194. Schnerman J, et al. Impaired potency for feedback regulation of glomerular filtration rate in DOCA escaped rat. *Pflugers Arch* 1975;359:325.

195. Moore LC, Mason G. Tubuloglomerular feedback control of distal fluid delivery: effect of extracellular volume. *Am J Physiol* 1986;250:F1024.

196. Dilley JR, Arendshorst WJ. Enhanced tubuloglomerular feedback activity in rats developing spontaneous hypertension. *Am J Physiol* 1984;247:F672.

197. Ploth DW, et al. Tubuloglomerular feedback and autoregulation of glomerular filtration rate in Wistar-Kyoto spontaneously hypertensive rats. *Pflugers Arch* 1978;375:261.

198. Boberg U, Persson AE. Increased tubuloglomerular feedback activity in Milan hypertensive rats. *Am J Physiol* 1986;250:F967.

199. Ushiogi Y, Takabatake T, Haberle DA. Blood pressure and tubuloglomerular feedback mechanism in chronically salt-loaded spontaneously hypertensive rats. *Kidney Int* 1991;39:1184.

200. Soares-da-Silva P. Source and handling of renal dopamine: its physiological importance. *News Physiol Sci* 1994;9:128.

201. Gill JR, Grossman E, Goldstein DS. High urinary dopa and low urinary dopamine-to-dopa ratio in salt-sensitive hypertension. *Hypertension* 1991;18:614.

202. Harvey JN, et al. A paradoxical fall in urine dopamine output when patients with essential hypertension are given added dietary salt. *Clin Sci* 1984;67:83.

203. Saito I, et al. Urinary dopamine excretion in normotensive subjects with or without family history of hypertension. *J Hypertens* 1986;4:57.

204. Imura O, Shimamoto K. Suppressed dopaminergic activity and water-sodium handling in the kidneys at the prehypertensive stage of essential hypertension. *J Auton Pharmacol* 1990;10:S73.

205. Imura O, et al. The pathophysiological role of renal dopamine kallikrein/kinin and prostaglandin systems in essential hypertension. *Agents Actions* 1987;22:247.

206. Aoki K, et al. Attenuated renal production of dopamine in patients with low renin essential hypertension. *Clin Exp Hypertens* 1989;ii:403.

207. Kuchel O, Shigetomi S. Defective dopamine generation from dihydroxyphenylalanine in stable essential hypertensive patients. *Hypertension* 1992;19:634.

208. De Feo ML, Jadhav AL, Lokhandwala MF. Dietary sodium intake and urinary dopamine and sodium excretion during the course of blood pressure development in Dahl salt sensitive and salt resistant rats. *Clin Exp Hypertens* 1987;9:2049.

209. Yoshimura M, et al. Effect of decreased dopamine synthesis on the development of hypertension induced by salt loading in spontaneously hypertensive rats. *Clin Exp Hypertens* 1987;9:1141.

210. Kinoshita S, Sidhu A, Felder RA. Defective dopamine-1 receptor adenylate cyclase coupling in the proximal convoluted tubule of the hypertensive rat. *J Clin Invest* 1989;84:1849.

211. Fiueroa CD, et al. Cellular localisation of atrial natriuretic factor in the human kidney. *Nephrol Dial Transplant* 1990;5:25.

212. Janssen WM, et al. Renal tubular sensitivity to atrial natriuretic factor in essential hypertension. *J Hypertens* 1994;12:439.

213. Janssen WM, et al. Atrial natriuretic factor influences renal diurnal rhythm in essential hypertension. *Hypertension* 1992;20:80.

214. Lochance D, Garcia R. Atrial natriuretic factor and volume expansion-induced natriuresis in the spontaneously hypertensive rat. *Eur J Pharmacol* 1991;192:301.

215. Swithers SE, Stewart RE, McCarty R. Binding sites for atrial natriuretic factor (ANP) in kidneys and adrenal glands of spontaneously hypertensive (SHR) rats. *Life Sci* 1987;40:1673.

216. Agnati LF, et al. Receptor autoradiographical evidence of a preferential reduction of binding site for atrial natriuretic factor in renal papilla of the spontaneously hypertensive rat. *Acta Physiol Scand* 1988;134:61.

217. Marsh EA, et al. Renal and blood pressure responses to synthetic atrial natriuretic factor in spontaneously hypertensive rats. *Hypertension* 1985;7:386.

218. Brown J, Salas SP, Polak JM. Renal atrial natriuretic peptide receptor subtypes in spontaneously hypertensive rats. *Am J Physiol* 1990;259:F605.

219. Hirata Y, et al. Dahls rats have increased natriuretic factor in atria but are markedly hyporesponsive to it. *Hypertension* 1984;6:I-148.

220. Appel RG, Dunn MJ. Papillary collecting tubule responsiveness to atrial natriuretic factor in Dahl rats. *Hypertension* 1987;10:107.

221. Levi M, Rowe JW. Aging and the kidney. In: Schrier RW, Gottschalk CW, eds. *Diseases of the kidney*, 5th ed. Boston: Little, Brown, 1993:2405.

222. Luft FC, Weinberger MH, Fineberg NS. Effects of age on renal sodium homeostasis and its relevance to sodium sensitivity. *Am J Med* 1987;82:9.

223. Barker DJ. The fetal origins of adult hypertension. *J Hypertens* 1992;10:S39.

224. Law CM, et al. Initiation of hypertension in utero and its amplification throughout life. *Br Med J* 1993;306:24.

225. Hinchcliffe SA, et al. Human intra-uterine renal growth expressed in absolute number of glomeruli assessed by "Disector" method and Cavalieri principle. *Lab Invest* 1991;64:777.

226. Hinchcliffe SA, et al. The effects of intrauterine growth retardation on the development of renal nephrons. *Br J Obst Gynaecol* 1992;99:296.

227. Churchill D, Beevers DG. The relationship between maternal blood pressure and infants birth weight. *Clin Sci* 1995;88:2.

228. Hall SM, Zeiman FJ. Kidney function of the frequency of rats fed a low protein diet. *J Nutr* 1969;95:49.

229. Langley SC, Jackson AA. Increased systolic blood pressure in adult rats induced by fetal exposure to maternal low protein diets. *Clin Sci* 1994;86:217.

230. Hata A, et al. Angiotensinogen as a risk factor for essential hypertension in Japan. *J Clin Invest* 1994;93:1285.

231. Jeunemaitre X, et al. Molecular basis of human hypertension: role of angiotensinogen. *Cell* 1992;71:169.

232. Rotimi C, et al. Angiotensinogen gene in human hypertension: lack of an association of the 235T allele among African Americans. *Hypertension* 1994;24:591.

233. Luft FC, et al. Genetic influences on the response to dietary salt reduction, acute salt loading, or salt depletion in humans. *J Cardiovasc Pharmacol* 1988;12:S49.

234. Baker EH, et al. Association of hypertension with T594 mutation in β sub-unit of epithelial sodium channels in black people in London. *Lancet* 1998;351:1388.

235. Manunta P, et al. Alpha-adducin polymorphism and renal sodium handling in essential hypertensive patients. *Kidney Int* 1998;53:1471.

236. Kato N, et al. Lack of association between the α-adducin locus and essential hypertension in the Japanese population. *Hypertension* 1998;31:730.

237. Kamitani A, et al. Human α-adducin gene, blood pressure and sodium metabolism. *Hypertension* 1998;32:138.

238. Tripodi G, et al. Hypertension-associated point-mutations in the adducin α and β sub-units affects. *J Clin Invest* 1996;97:2815.

239. Manunta P, et al. Adducin polymorphism affects renal proximal tubule reabsorption in hypertension. *Hypertension* 1999;33:694.

240. Cusi D, Bianchi G. A primer on the genetics of hypertension. *Kidney Int* 1999;54:328.

241. Lipton RP. Molecular genetics of human blood pressure variation. *Science* 1996;272:676.
242. Kobayashi A, et al. Increased Na-H exchange activity in cultured vascular smooth muscle cells from stroke-prone spontaneously hypertensive rats. *J Hypertens* 1990;8:153.
243. Edmonson RP, et al. Abnormal leukocyte composition and sodium transport in essential hypertension. *Lancet* 1975;i:1003.
244. Canessa M, et al. Kinetic abnormalities of the red blood cell sodium-proton exchange in hypertensive patients. *Hypertension* 1991;17:340.
245. Devynck MA, et al. Diffuse structural alteration in cell membranes of spontaneously hypertensive rats. *Proc Natl Acad Sci USA* 1982;79:5057.
246. Isler M, Jennings G, Lambert G. Noradrenaline release and the pathophysiology of primary hypertension. *Am J Hypertens* 1989;2:140S.
247. Woolfson RG, et al. Ouabain and responses to endothelium-dependent vasodilators in the human forearm. *Br J Clin Pharmacol* 1991;32:758.
248. Woolfson RG, Hilton PJ, Poston L. Effect of ouabain and low sodium on contractility of human resistance arteries. *Hypertension* 1990;15:583.
249. de Wardener HE. The hypothalamus and hypertension. *Physiol Rev* 2001; 81:1599.
250. Behn C, et al. Effects of sustained intrathoracic vascular distension. *Pflugers Arch* 1969;313:123.
251. Folkow B. Physiological aspects of primary hypertension. *Physiol Rev* 1982;62:347.
252. Bravo EL, et al. The changing clinical spectrum of primary aldosteronism. *Am J Med* 1983;74:641.
253. Biglieri EG, McIllroy MB. Abnormalities of renal function and circulatory reflexes in primary aldosteronism. *Circulation* 1966;33:78.
254. Schalekamp MA, et al. Studies on the mechanism of hypernatriuresis in essential hypertension in relation to measurements of plasma renin concentration, body fluid compartments and renal function. *Clin Sci* 1971;41:219.
255. Rossi G, et al. Immunoreactive endogenous ouabain in primary aldosterones, and essential hypertension: relationship with plasma renin, aldosterone, and blood pressure levels. *J Hypertens* 1995;13:1181.
256. Dietz JR. Release of natriuretic factor from rat heart-lung preparation by atrial distension. *Am J Physiol* 1984;247:R1093.
257. Safar ME, et al. Rapid dextran infusion in essential hypertension. *Hypertension* 1979;i:615.
258. Tripoddo NC, Yamamoto J, Frolich ED. Whole body venous capacity and effective total tissue compliance in SHR. *Hypertension* 1981;3:104.
259. London GM, et al. Blood pressure in the "low pressure system" and cardiac performance in essential hypertension. *J Hypertens* 1985;3:337.
260. Rickstein SE, Yao T, Thoren P. Peripheral and central vascular compliances in conscious normotensive and spontaneously hypertensive rats. *Acta Physiol Scand* 1981;112:169.
261. Noresson E, Rickstein SE, Thoren P. Left atrial pressure in normotensive and spontaneously hypertensive rats (SHR). *Acta Physiol Scand* 1981;112:473.
262. Ciriello J, Calaresu FR. Hypothalamic projections of renal afferent nerves in the cat. *Can J Physiol Pharmacol* 1980;58:574.
263. Calaresu FR, Ciriello J. Renal afferent nerves affect discharge rate of medullary and hypothalamic single units in the cat. *J Auton Nerv Sys* 1981; 3:311.
264. Campese VM, Kogosov E. Renal afferent denervation prevents hypertension in rats with chronic renal failure. *Hypertension* 1995;25:878.
265. Janssen BJ, et al. Role of afferent renal nerves in spontaneous hypertension in rats. *Hypertension* 1989;13:327.
266. Campese VM, et al. Mechanisms of autonomic nervous system dysfunction in uremia. *Kidney Int* 1981;20:246.
267. Esler M, et al. Assessment of human sympathetic nervous system activity from measurements of norepinephrine turnover. *Hypertension* 1988; 11:3.
268. Anderson EA, et al. Elevated sympathetic nerve activity in borderline hypertensive humans. *Hypertension* 1989;14:177.
269. Matsukawa T, Ishii M. Age-related changes in muscle sympathetic nerve activity in essential hypertension. *Hypertension* 1989;13:870.
270. Judy WV, et al. Sympathetic nerve activity. Role in regulation of blood pressure in the spontaneously hypertensive rat. *Circ Res* 1976;38:21.
271. Judy WV, et al. Sympathetic nerve activity and blood pressure in normotensive backcross rats genetically related to the spontaneously hypertensive rat. *Hypertension* 1979;1:598.
272. Lundin S, Rickstein SE, Thoren P. Renal sympathetic activity in spontaneously hypertensive rats and normotensive controls, as studied by three different methods. *Acta Physiol Scand* 1984;120:265.
273. Okamoto K, et al. Participation of neural factor in the pathogenesis of hypertension in the spontaneously hypertensive rat. *Jpn Heart J* 1967;8:168.
274. Shibata K, et al. Developmental differences of angiotensinogen mRNA in the preoptic area between spontaneously hypertensive and age-matched Wistar-Kyoto rats. *Brain Res Mol Brain Res* 1993;19:115.
275. Raizada MK, Sumners C, Lu D. Angiotensin II type I receptor mRNA levels in the brains of normotensive and spontaneously hypertensive rats. *J Neurochem* 1993;60:1949.
276. van Tol HH, et al. Vasopressin and oxytocin gene expression in the supraoptic and paraventricular nucleus of the spontaneously hypertensive rat (SHR) during development of hypertension. *Brain Res* 1988;464:303.
277. Komatsu K, et al. Increased level of atrial natriuretic peptide messenger RNA in the hypothalamus and brainstem of spontaneously hypertensive rats *J Hypertens* 1992;10:17.
278. Plochocka-Zulinska D, Krukoff TL. Increased gene expression of neuronal nitric oxide synthase in brain of adult spontaneously hypertensive rats. *Brain Res Mol Brain Res*48:291,1997.
279. McLean KJ, Jarrott B, Lawrence AJ. Neuropeptide Y gene expression and receptor autoradiography in hypertensive and normotensive rat brain. *Brain Res Mol Brain Res* 1996;35:249.
280. Boone JB, McMillen D. Proenkephalin gene expression is altered in the brain of spontaneously hypertensive rats during the development of hypertension. *Brain Res Mol Brain Res* 1994;24:320.
281. Avidor R, et al. VIP-mRNA is increased in hypertensive rats. *Brain Res* 1989;503:304.
282. Garcia SI, et al. Thyrotropin-releasing hormone hyperactivity in the preoptic area of spontaneously hypertensive rats. *Hypertension* 1995;26:1105.
283. Qualy JM, Westfall TC. Release of norepinephrine from the paraventricular hypothalamic nucleus of hypertensive rats. *Am J Physiol* 1988;254:H993.
284. Koulu M, et al. Serotonin turnover in discrete hypothalamic nuclei and mesencephalic raphe nuclei of young and adult spontaneously hypertensive rats. *Brain Res* 1986;379:257.
285. Wei D, Milici A, Buccafusco JJ. Alterations in the expression of the genes encoding specific muscarinic receptor subtypes in the hypothalamus of spontaneously hypertensive rats. *Circ Res* 1995;76:142.
286. Czyzewska-Szafran H, et al. Down-regulation of the GABA-ergic system in selected brain areas of spontaneously hypertensive rats (SHR). *Pol J Pharmacol Pharm* 1989;41:619.
287. Qualy JM, Westfall TC. Overflow of endogenous norepinephrine from PVH nucleus of DOCA-salt hypertensive rats. *Am J Physiol* 1995;268:H1549.
288. Simchon S, et al. Handling 22NaCl by the blood-brain barrier and kidney. Its relevance to salt-induced hypertension in Dahl rats. *Hypertension* 1999;33:517.
289. Ogston AG, Wells JD. The osmotic properties of sulphoethyl-Sephadex: a model for cartilage. *Biochem J* 1972;128:685.
290. Lucas J, Floyer MA. Renal control of changes in the compliance of the interstitial space: a factor in the etiology of reno-prival hypertension. *Clin Sci* 1973;44:397.
291. Maloiy GM, Boarer CD. Response of the Somali donkey to dehydration: hematological changes. *Am J Physiol* 1971;221:37.
292. Floyer MA. The mechanism underlying the response of the hypertensive subject to a saline load. In: Miliez P, ed. *L'hypertension arterielle*. Paris: L'Expansion Scientifique Francaise, 1966:56.
293. Lucas J, Floyer MA. Changes in body fluid distribution and interstitial tissue compliance during the development and reversal of experimental renal hypertension in the rat. *Clin Sci Mol Med* 1974;47:1.
294. Koomans HA, et al. Salt sensitivity of blood pressure in chronic renal failure: evidence for renal control of body fluid distribution in man. *Hypertension* 1982;4:190.
295. Muirhead EE. The renomedullary antihypertensive system and its putative hormone(s). In: Genest J, et al. eds. *Hypertension*. New York: McGraw-Hill, 1983:394.
296. Muirhead EE, et al. Antihypertensive lipid from tissue culture of renomedullary interstitial cells of the rat. *Clin Sci Mol Med* 1976;51:287S.
297. Yamamoto J, et al. Decreased total venous capacity in Goldblatt hypertensive rats. *Am J Physiol* 1981;240:H487.
298. Russell GI, et al. Surgical reversal of two-kidney one-clip hypertension during inhibition of the renin-angiotensin system. *Hypertension* 1982;4:69.
299. Bing RF, et al. Chemical renal medullectomy: effect upon reversal of two-kidney one-clip hypertension in the rat. *Clin Sci* 1981;61:335S.
300. Muirhead EE, et al. Cardiovascular effects of antihypertensive polar and neutral renomedullary lipids. *Hypertension* 1983;5:112.
301. Pitcock JA, et al. Functional-morphological correlates of renomedullary interstitial cells. *Clin Sci Mol Med* 1976;51:291S.
302. Muirhead EE. Renal vasodepressor mechanism: the medullolipin system. *J Hypertens* 1993;11:S53.
303. Gothberg G, Lundun S, Folkow B. An acute vasodepressor effect in normotensive rats following extracorporal perfusion of the declipped kidney of two-kidney, one-clip hypertensive rats. *Hypertension* 1982;4:101.
304. Muirhead EE. Antihypertensive functions of the kidney. *Hypertension* 1980;2:444.
305. Muirhead EE, et al. Captopril in angiotensin-salt hypertension: a possible linkage between angiotensin, salt, vascular disease, and renomedullary interstitial cells. In: Laragh JH, Buhler FR, Seldin DW, eds. *Frontiers in hypertension*. New York: Springer, 1981:559.
306. Muirhead EE. Renomedullary vasodepressor lipid: medullipin. In: Swales JD, ed. *Textbook of hypertension*. Oxford: Blackwell Scientific, 1993:204.
307. Muirhead E, et al. Persistent hypotension associated with hypermedullipinaemia: a new syndrome. *Blood Pressure* 1992;1:138.
308. Bianchi G, Tilde-Tenconi L, Lucca R. Effect in the conscious dog of constriction of the renal artery to a sole remaining kidney on hemodynamics, sodium balance, body fluid volumes, plasma renin concentration and pressor responsiveness to angiotensin. *Clin Sci* 1970;38:741.

309. Ledingham JM, Cohen RD. Changes in extracellular fluid volume and cardiac output during development of experimental renal hypertension. *Can Med Assoc* 1964;90:292.

310. Simon G. Altered venous function in hypertensive rats. *Circ Res* 1976;38:412.

311. Overbeck HW. Hemodynamics of early experimental renal hypertension in dogs: normal limb blood flow, elevated limb vascular resistance and decreased venous compliance. *Circ Res* 1972;31:653.

312. Haddy FJ, Pamnani MB, Clough DL. Role of a humoral factor in low renin hypertension. In: Lichardus B, Schrier RW, Ponec J, eds. *Hormonal regulation of sodium excretion*. Amsterdam: Elsevier, 1980:379.

313. Hinke JA. In vitro demonstrations of vascular hyperresponsiveness in experimental hypertension. *Circ Res* 1965;17:359.

314. Michelakis AM, et al. Further studies on the existence of a sensitizing factor to pressor agents in hypertension. *J Clin Endocrinol Metab* 1975;41:90.

315. de Wardener HE. *The kidney*, 5th ed. Edinburgh: Churchill Livingstone, 1985:273.

316. Brown JJ, et al. Plasma renin concentration and the control of blood pressure in patients on maintenance hemodialysis. *Nephron* 1969;6:329.

317. Russell GI, et al. Indomethacin or aprotinin infusion: effect on reversal of chronic two-kidney, one-clip hypertension in the conscious rat. *Clin Sci* 1982;62:361.

CHAPTER 51 ■ HYPERTENSION ASSOCIATED WITH RENAL PARENCHYMAL DISEASE

MICHAEL C. SMITH, ANDREW LAZAR, AND MAHBOOB RAHMAN

In 1836, Richard Bright (1) reported that the presence of small granular kidneys at postmortem examination was associated with cardiac enlargement and theorized that the kidney was the "chief promoter" of left ventricular hypertrophy. Subsequently, the discovery of renin in 1898 (2) and the classic experiments by Goldblatt et al. in 1934 (3) established the central role of the kidney in the control of arterial blood pressure. Multiple neurohumoral factors increase blood pressure by limiting salt excretion and shifting the renal function curve to the right (4–9). In addition, not only can renal parenchymal disease initiate and sustain hypertension (8), but also the consequent elevation of blood pressure exposes the remaining renal tissue to further hydraulically mediated damage (10).

This chapter reviews the important pathophysiologic mechanisms, clinical features, and therapy of hypertension caused by both unilateral and bilateral renal parenchymal disease. Although relevant models of experimental renal parenchymal hypertension are discussed, the primary focus of this chapter is to emphasize key advances in the understanding of hypertension in human renal disease.

UNILATERAL KIDNEY DISEASE

Unilateral Kidney Disease

Unilateral renal parenchymal disease resulting from reflux nephropathy, congenital malformations, or bacterial pyelonephritis can cause hypertension. Butler first described the association between unilateral kidney disease and hypertension (11). He reported that unilateral nephrectomy could cure hypertension in patients with unilateral chronic pyelonephritis. However, the exact prevalence of this form of secondary hypertension is unclear (12). Extensive early experience with unilateral nephrectomy in hypertensive patients with presumed unilateral parenchymal disease produced a disappointing cure rate of only 26% (13). Additional investigation, however, has clearly shown that with proper selection and careful preoperative evaluation a subset of patients benefits substantially from surgical intervention. Although initial investigations utilized split renal function studies (14,15) or clinical characteristics (16) to predict response to unilateral nephrectomy, these criteria have been abandoned because of poor predictive value and have been replaced by renal vein renin ratios.

Vaughan et al. (17) and Delin et al. (18) evaluated hypertensive patients with unilateral renal parenchymal disease of diverse etiologies. Both groups of investigators found that cure or improvement of hypertension was limited to patients with preoperative lateralizing renal venous renins. Additional data have confirmed and extended the positive predictive value of renal venous renins by demonstrating amelioration of hypertension in 90% of patients with lateralizing renal venous renin ratios of 1.5 or greater (19,20). In an important study, Gordon et al. (21) evaluated 20 hypertensive patients with unilateral renal parenchymal disease. All patients had measurements of supine and stimulated renal venous renins and underwent unilateral nephrectomy without regard to the renin values. These investigators found that recumbent lateralizing renal venous renin ratios of 1.5 or more identified patients likely to benefit from nephrectomy with a sensitivity of 100%, a specificity of 84%, and a positive predictive value of 100%. Despite the fact that not all studies support the utility of renal venous renins in predicting response to surgery (22), we believe it is reasonable to restrict operative intervention or renal artery embolization to hypertensive patients, with uncontrolled blood pressure, who demonstrate evidence of functional ischemia. Hypertension in patients with unilateral kidney disease and nonlateralizing renins probably reflects occult bilateral disease or essential hypertension.

A note of caution is warranted, however, in the evaluation of hypertensive patients with apparent unilateral kidney disease. DeJong et al. (23) reported eight young women with hypertension and unilateral renal parenchymal disease. Renal venous renins were measured in four and did not lateralize to the side with the apparent unilateral parenchymal disease. Renal angiography revealed fibromuscular disease of the contralateral renal artery in all eight patients. Surgical revascularization of the stenotic kidney normalized blood pressure in all patients. The fact that unilateral renal parenchymal disease can coexist with contralateral fibromuscular dysplasia underscores the importance of this diagnostic consideration, especially in patients with nonlateralizing renal venous renins. In this latter group of patients, nephrectomy should not be considered until renal artery stenosis has been excluded by angiography.

Hypertension in Patients with Solitary Kidneys

Hypertension, proteinuria, focal glomerulosclerosis (FGS), and progressive loss of renal function occur in experimental renal ablation in rats (24–26) and frequently in humans with unilateral renal agenesis (26–32). Because of these observations, some authorities have raised the issue of whether patients undergoing unilateral nephrectomy for renal disease or transplant donation are at risk for the development of hypertension, loss of renal function, or both (30,33–35). Renal ablation by five-sixths nephrectomy in rats consistently results in hypertension, proteinuria, and FGS (24,36,37). Moreover, in the same model, supplementation of renal mass by isograft transplantation reduces blood pressure, attenuates proteinuria, and ameliorates glomerulosclerosis (38). Glomerulosclerosis and progressive renal insufficiency have been associated with characteristic intraglomerular hemodynamic alterations consisting

TABLE 51-1

HYPERTENSION IN PATIENTS WITH SOLITARY KIDNEYS

	No. of patients	No. with hypertension	Percent	References
Unilateral agenesis	193	96	50	27–29,31,32,49–54
Unilateral nephrectomy	156	22	14	34,56,57,59
Kidney donation	833	137	16	35,58,60–65

of an increased single-nephron glomerular filtration rate (GFR), an increment in glomerular capillary flow rate (Q_A), and elevated glomerular capillary pressure (P_{GC}) by most (37,39,40), but not all (41,42) investigators. On the other hand, some studies have suggested a link between glomerular hypertrophy (41,42), manifest as increments in glomerular volume (V_G) or glomerular capillary radius (R_{GC}), or both glomerular hypertrophy and altered intrarenal hemodynamics (26,43,44) and progressive kidney disease in this model. Therapeutic maneuvers that reduce P_{GC}, such as dietary protein restriction or angiotensin-converting enzyme (ACE) inhibition, decrease proteinuria and retard progressive renal injury (25,26,37). Nevertheless, the relation among altered intrarenal hemodynamics, glomerular hypertrophy, and progressive FGS in experimental renal ablation is unsettled and requires further investigation (45,46). It is important to note, however, that three-fourths reduction in renal mass in a canine model does not lead to inexorable loss of renal function (47). Thus, although these observations in experimental models of renal ablation are provocative, their relevance to human renal disease is not established.

Table 51-1 depicts the prevalence of hypertension in patients with unilateral renal agenesis and in those who underwent unilateral nephrectomy for renal disease or transplant donation. In 1960, Ashley and Mostofi (48) reported the first association between unilateral renal agenesis and progressive renal insufficiency. They noted that, of 232 patients with unilateral renal agenesis, 16% developed chronic renal failure and that one-third of these had "chronic glomerulonephritis;" however, the prevalence of hypertension was not reported. Since then, the association between unilateral renal agenesis and the development of proteinuria, hypertension, and chronic kidney disease (CKD) owing to FGS has been emphasized repeatedly (27–29,31,32,49–54). Hypertension is more prevalent in patients with unilateral renal agenesis compared with uninephrectomized individuals (Table 51-1). Kiprov et al. (27) found that four of eight patients with unilateral renal agenesis and histologically proven FGS were hypertensive. In addition, in a series of 586 cases of renal biopsy or nephrectomy specimens, they found 29 cases of FGS; there were 24 cases of FGS in the 581 patients with two kidneys (4.1%), whereas all 5 patients with unilateral agenesis demonstrated FGS ($p < 2 \times 10^{-7}$) (27). These findings have been confirmed by other investigators (28–32) and suggest a clear relation among an increased prevalence of hypertension, FGS, and unilateral renal agenesis. Argueso et al. confirmed this increased risk for proteinuria, hypertension, and CKD in a study of 159 patients with unilateral renal agenesis (54). It is possible that the number of remaining nephrons in the contralateral kidney is reduced in patients with unilateral renal agenesis. Alternatively, an *in utero* reduction in renal mass could subject the remaining nephrons to abnormal hemodynamic forces or neurohumoral factors with the consequent development of glomerulosclerosis (26,55). Occasionally, the hypertension is renin dependent and subsides with removal of the dysplastic kidney (53), whereas in other cases proteinuria and renal insufficiency antedate the increase in blood pressure

(27,28). In most instances of unilateral renal agenesis, however, the pathophysiologic mechanisms relating hypertension, proteinuria, and FGS are speculative but unproved (30,32).

The prevalence of hypertension is lower in patients subjected to unilateral nephrectomy for renal disease or transplant donation (Table 51-1). Despite periods of prolonged observation, multiple studies have shown that high blood pressure was not more common overall in patients undergoing nephrectomy for unilateral kidney disease compared with the general population (28,29,34,50–52,56,57). A more important issue, and the subject of considerable debate, is whether kidney donors are at increased risk for the development of hypertension or CKD. One group of investigators noted a 47% prevalence of hypertension in 38 renal transplant donors followed for more than 10 years (58); however, this prevalence was not different from that of an age- and gender-matched control group. Other authorities have made similar observations (59). Despite the fact that one report suggests that kidney donors demonstrate an accelerated rate of development of hypertension (60), the majority of studies show no increase in the risk for the development of proteinuria, hypertension, or CKD (61–65). With an average follow-up ranging from 8 to more than 15 years, the prevalence of hypertension does not exceed that of the general population (Table 51-1). In a meta-analysis of 48 studies with 3,124 patients who had undergone a nephrectomy and 1,703 controls, Kasiske et al. (66) demonstrated that there was a small rise in systolic blood pressure (2.4 mm Hg) that increased further (1.1 mm Hg/decade) with longer duration of follow-up in the nephrectomized group but there was no increase in the overall prevalence of hypertension. Thus, in normal individuals, unilateral nephrectomy does not cause progressive renal dysfunction, but may be associated with a small increase in blood pressure. However, patients with a family history of hypertension may be more likely to develop hypertension following uninephrectomy (67).

Taken together, the available data suggest that although the findings from experimental models of renal ablation might be applicable to patients with more than 50% reductions in renal mass (68,69), they cannot be extrapolated to all patients with solitary kidneys. Although unilateral renal agenesis is definitely associated with an increased risk for the development of proteinuria, hypertension, and FGS (70), unilateral nephrectomy for renal disease or transplant donation does not increase the risk for developing systemic hypertension or CKD in the remaining kidney. The reason for these apparently contrasting observations is unclear but might relate to unrecognized contralateral renal disease, the developmental stage at which the reduction in renal mass occurs, or other unrecognized factors (26).

Miscellaneous Lesions

Hypertension has been described in association with several lesions that could potentially stimulate renin secretion from the unilaterally involved kidney. Renin secreting tumors arising from the juxtaglomerular cells are rare. Patients present with hypertension, hypokalemia, and hyperreninemic hyperaldosteronism (71). Control of blood pressure usually requires ACE inhibition and definitive treatment is surgical resection. Most patients with Wilms' tumor also develop a renin dependent form of hypertension that resolves after excision of the tumor (72,73). Simple cysts (74,75), renal tuberculosis (76), renal infarction (77,78), and segmental hypoplasia (79,80) have been linked to the development of hypertension. In the majority of cases, unilateral hypersecretion of renin was demonstrated and blood pressure normalized after surgical intervention (74–76,78–80). Some reports, however, have not documented lateralizing renal venous renins in all patients (79). These findings are reminiscent of similar observations in renovascular hypertension and might reflect the effect of dietary salt intake or hypertension maintained by increased activity of the sympathetic nervous system.

Bilateral Kidney Disease

Hypertension is common in both acute and chronic renal disease. In acute renal parenchymal disease, hypertension is chiefly mediated by expansion of the extracellular fluid volume (ECFV). Volume depletion usually normalizes blood pressure, and hypertension resolves with improvement of renal function. Because hypertension is often transient in acute kidney disease, its pathogenesis has not been studied extensively. On the other hand, in CKD, not only is hypertension more frequent, but its pathogenesis is more complex and its long-term cardiovascular effects are of greater significance. Consequently, the following sections focus largely on the pathogenesis, sequelae, and management of hypertension in patients with CKD.

Acute Renal Disease

Hypertension occurs more frequently in acute glomerulonephritis than in acute tubular necrosis (81–83). In the largest analysis to date, Bonomini et al. (81) retrospectively reviewed 262 patients with acute renal failure and serum creatinine concentrations >5 mg/dL. Hypertension developed at some time during the course of acute renal failure in 103 patients (39%) and was more common in patients with acute renal failure due to glomerular or vascular disease (73%) compared with those whose renal insufficiency was the result of tubulointerstitial processes (15%). High blood pressure was consequent to expansion of the ECFV from salt and water retention and responded to salt subtraction during dialysis in hypertensive patients with acute renal failure, especially in the subset with acute tubular necrosis (81). These investigators found that overall 17% of patients who experienced an episode of acute renal failure were hypertensive at 3 months; however, the prevalence of hypertension was 30% after 3 years of follow-up. Hypertension was more common in patients who developed acute renal failure consequent to glomerular disease compared with those with acute tubulointerstitial disease after both 3 months (42% vs. 3%) and 3 years (53% versus 17%) of observation.

The pathogenesis of hypertension in acute renal failure due to clinically apparent acute poststreptococcal glomerulonephritis has been studied extensively (82–85). Hypertension occurs in 80% of patients with epidemic poststreptococcal glomerulonephritis and is thought to be primarily volume mediated because of consistent findings of suppressed plasma renin activity (PRA) and reduced aldosterone levels (82–84). Rodriguez-Iturbe et al. (85) studied 13 children with acute poststreptococcal glomerulonephritis during the acute illness and after resolution of the disease. Reduction in blood pressure from a mean of 121/80 mm Hg to 90/54 mm Hg was associ-

ated with an average weight loss of 1.4 kg and an increase in creatinine clearance from 47 to 123 mL/minute. Initially, PRA and aldosterone were suppressed but increased to normal values within 4 to 6 weeks. Because the elevation of blood pressure during the acute illness was significantly correlated with fluid retention, estimated by changes in weight ($R = 0.74, p <0.01$), these investigators concluded that hypertension in poststreptococcal glomerulonephritis was chiefly volume dependent. They postulated that an acute decline in glomerular filtration rate (GFR) causes salt and water retention, expands the ECFV, suppresses the renin-angiotensin-aldosterone system (RAAS) and results in hypertension. Further investigations by the same group (86) confirmed their initial observations and also demonstrated reduced urinary excretion of prostaglandin E_2 (PGE_2) and $PGF_{2\alpha}$ as well as kallikrein in 14 patients with acute poststreptococcal glomerulonephritis. They found no correlation, however, between decreased prostanoid or kallikrein excretion and activity of the RAAS, or changes in weight or blood pressure. Converting enzyme inhibition with captopril decreased blood pressure in hypertensive patients with poststreptococcal glomerulonephritis, reduced plasma aldosterone, and increased urinary PGE_2 and kallikrein (87). The unexpected antihypertensive efficacy of ACE inhibition in this setting of presumably volume-dependent hypertension could be the result of a further decrease in an inappropriately elevated angiotensin II level, interruption of the vascular RAAS, or increased synthesis of vasodilator and natriuretic prostaglandins and kinins.

Twenty percent to 30 percent of adults with minimal change disease are hypertensive at the time of initial presentation (88). Both vasoconstrictor (83,89) and volume-dependent (90) forms of hypertension have been described. Some investigators have shown hypertension and increased PRA in minimal change disease that are ameliorated by volume expansion or steroid-induced remission (83,89). These observations support the notion that hypertension in this setting is the result of angiotensin II–induced vasoconstriction consequent to underfilling of the systemic vasculature that results from hypoalbuminemia. On the other hand, some studies have clearly shown a volume-dependent component of hypertension in some patients with minimal change disease. Dorhout Mees et al. (90) measured plasma albumin, blood pressure, plasma volume, and blood volume in 10 patients, 5 of whom were hypertensive, with minimal change disease before and after treatment with corticosteroids (Fig. 51-1). Steroid therapy resulted in a substantial increase in plasma albumin and significant reductions in blood pressure (17/14 mm Hg), plasma volume, and blood volume. Blood pressure normalized in the 5 hypertensive patients, and GFR increased an average of 42 mL/minute in all 10 subjects. There were no consistent changes in the normal or decreased PRA levels with steroid administration.

Consequently, the evidence to date suggests that the majority of hypertensive patients with acute renal disease exhibit volume-dependent hypertension that improves with salt removal during dialysis or with spontaneous or steroid-induced natriuresis. However, vasoconstrictor-mediated hypertension is evident in some. It is also likely that, given the multiple etiologies of acute renal disease, both volume and vasoconstrictor mechanisms are responsible for hypertension in many patients in a fashion similar to the development of hypertension in chronic renal disease.

Chronic Kidney Disease

Hypertension associated with renal parenchymal disease is the most common form of secondary hypertension; 5% of all hypertensive patients have underlying kidney disease (91). Renal parenchymal hypertension is important for several reasons. First, renal parenchymal hypertension increases the risk of

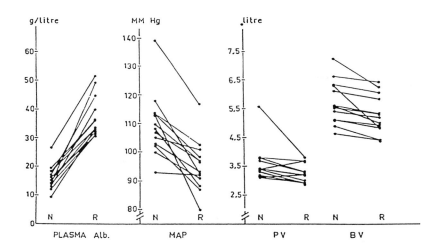

FIGURE 51-1. Plasma albumin (Alb), mean arterial pressure (MAP), plasma volume (PV), and blood volume (BV) in 10 patients with minimal change disease before *(N)* and after *(R)* steroid-induced remission. (Reprinted with permission from: Dorhout Mees EJ, et al. Observations on edema formation in the nephrotic syndrome in adults with minimal lesions. *Am J Med* 1979;67:378.)

cardiovascular morbidity and mortality to an equal or even greater extent compared with the risk attributable to essential hypertension (91,92). Second, hypertension secondary to kidney disease is associated with a greater prevalence of retinopathy, especially malignant retinopathy, compared with essential hypertension at all levels of blood pressure (93), suggesting that neurohumoral factors involved in its pathogenesis are particularly vasculotoxic. Finally, hypertension in kidney disease accelerates the loss of renal function in both diabetic and nondiabetic nephropathy (94,95). Renal parenchymal hypertension can occur even with a normal serum creatinine concentration and normal GFR (94,96) and increases in prevalence as renal function decreases (94,95,97–99). More than 80% of patients with CKD are hypertensive (98), and hypertension is present in up to 90% of patients by the time end stage renal disease (ESRD) supervenes (100,101).

Similar to hypertension in acute renal disease, the prevalence of hypertension in CKD varies depending on the underlying pathology. Table 51-2 summarizes the approximate prevalence of hypertension in different chronic renal diseases. The data are derived from series in the recent literature and include patients with various levels of renal function (83,97–99,102–108). It is apparent that hypertension is more frequent in pa-

tients with chronic glomerular disease compared with those with polycystic kidney disease or chronic interstitial nephritis (99,102,109). Moreover, among the glomerular diseases, hypertension is more common in FGS and membranoproliferative glomerulonephritis compared with mesangioproliferative glomerulonephritis or immunoglobulin A (IgA) nephropathy (108).

Pathophysiology

Discussion of hypertension in CKD requires a brief examination of the central role of the kidney in the regulation of arterial blood pressure (110). This critical function is primarily the result of the kidney's unique position in regulating salt balance. Blood pressure is expressed by the equation

$$BP = CO \times TPR$$

where *BP* is blood pressure, *CO* is cardiac output, and *TPR* is total peripheral resistance. Although cursory examination of this equation could lead to the conclusion that increments in cardiac output, TPR, or both can result in hypertension, its simplicity obscures two important observations. First, isolated elevation in TPR will not cause sustained hypertension without a simultaneous constraint on renal sodium excretion. Second, a primary defect in salt excretion can result ultimately in an increased blood pressure maintained by an elevated TPR with a normal cardiac output. Both of these critical concepts have been developed and refined by Guyton et al. in a series of elegant experiments over the last 20 years (9,111–114).

In an isolated perfused kidney, Guyton et al. (111) developed a renal function curve by plotting arterial pressure as a function of urinary sodium excretion (Fig. 51-2). The solid line in Figure 51-2 depicts sodium excretion over a wide range of perfusion pressures in the isolated perfused kidney free of any neurohumoral constraints on salt excretion. The curve intersects the line at a point (a) where sodium intake and excretion are in equilibrium. Utilizing a computer-generated model of arterial pressure regulation, Guyton et al. (111,113) found that alterations in TPR alone would not change long-term arterial pressure in the presence of a constant sodium intake and an unchanged renal function curve. For example, if an increase in TPR raised arterial pressure to 150 mm Hg (b), sodium excretion would increase substantially (c) until a sufficient decrease in ECFV returned arterial pressure to the original set point (a). On the other hand, a decrease in arterial pressure owing to a reduction in TPR (d) would lower sodium excretion below sodium intake, eventually increasing ECFV and returning arterial pressure to baseline (a). Therefore, according to this model, changes in salt intake or salt excretion (i.e., the position of the

TABLE 51-2

PREVALENCE OF HYPERTENSION IN CHRONIC RENAL PARENCHYMAL DISEASE

Disease	Percent with hypertension	References
Glomerular disease		83,97,98,
Focal glomerular sclerosis	75–80	99,102,103,
		104,105,106,
Membranoproliferative glomerulonephritis	70–75	107,108
Diabetic nephropathy	70–75	
Membranous nephropathy	50–60	
Mesangioproliferative glomerulonephritis	40–45	
IgA nephropathy	40	
Polycystic kidney disease	70	
Chronic interstitial nephritis	50–60	

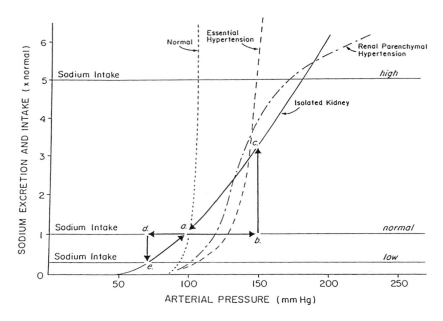

FIGURE 51-2. Renal function curves plotting sodium intake and excretion against mean arterial pressure. Curves for the isolated perfused kidney and normal individuals are shown along with hypothetical renal function curves for salt-sensitive essential hypertension and renal parenchymal hypertension. (Modified with permission from: Guyton AC. Dominant role of the kidneys and accessory role of whole-body autoregulation in the pathogenesis of hypertension. *Am J Hypertens* 1989;2:575.)

renal function curve) are required for the development of sustained hypertension.

Renal function curves can be developed in humans by determining arterial blood pressure, once salt balance is achieved, over a range of dietary salt intake. The series of dashed lines in Figure 51-2 are examples of renal function curves in normotensive subjects, patients with salt-sensitive essential hypertension, and patients with renal parenchymal hypertension. The curve from the normotensive subjects was derived at extremes of dietary salt intake (115) and underscores the fact that wide variation in sodium intake has little or no effect on blood pressure in normal individuals, presumably because of the integrated neurohumoral response to changes in salt intake. The curves for essential hypertension and renal parenchymal hypertension are theoretic and are shifted to the right of the normal renal function curve. In both conditions, salt balance occurs at higher than normal arterial pressure with either normal or high salt intake. Salt restriction, however, reduces arterial pressure to the normotensive range at the equilibrium point.

Despite the fact that hypertension is sustained by an elevated TPR in the majority of patients with renal parenchymal hypertension (see Hemodynamic Patterns, below) (116–120), initiation of hypertension is probably the result of a positive salt balance and expanded ECFV. Guyton et al. (111,113) examined the effect of salt loading on circulating hemodynamics in a canine model of renal ablation. Substantial hypertension developed in this model after 4 days of a high-salt diet at a time when TPR was normal. This early increase in arterial pressure was consequent to an increased ECFV and elevated cardiac output. Over the next 2 weeks, blood pressure remained increased, and ECFV and cardiac output decreased toward, but not quite to, baseline (113). These observations are consistent with longitudinal studies in patients with mild to moderate renal insufficiency (121,122), and suggest that whereas hypertension is initiated by volume expansion in this model, it is maintained primarily by vasoconstriction. It is not clear how the transition from a volume-mediated to vasoconstrictor form of hypertension occurs. Possible explanations include local autoregulation of tissue blood flow (111) or the production of an endogenous digitalislike substance (EDLS) (123–125) that simultaneously increases TPR and enhances renal sodium excretion.

Eventually, renal parenchymal hypertension results from the integrated action of elements that influence cardiac output,

TPR, or both. Table 51-3 lists some of the factors implicated in the pathogenesis of hypertension in CKD and their effect on cardiac output and TPR. It is important to note that each has a dual effect; both vascular resistance and salt balance are affected. Moreover, the effects are generally concordant with regard to the potential influence on blood pressure; vasoconstrictor compounds are antinatriuretic, whereas vasodilator substances are natriuretic; hence, it is difficult, if not impossible, to selectively alter TPR without simultaneously affecting renal salt excretion. The development of hypertension in a given patient with CKD results from the complex interplay of several or more of these elements in addition to the absolute level of GFR, underlying renal disease, genetic predisposition to hypertension, and dietary salt intake. Despite the fact that

TABLE 51-3

FACTORS THAT REGULATE ARTERIAL BLOOD PRESSURE

Affect cardiac output	Affect TPR
Extracellular volume (stroke volume)	Vasoconstrictor
	Angiotensin II
Antinatriuretic	Arginine vasopressin
Angiotensin II	Endogenous digitalis-like substance
Norepinephrine	Endothelin
	Norepinephrine
Antidiuretic	Thromboxane A2
Arginine vasopressin	
	Vasodilator
Natriuretic	Atrial and brain natriuretic peptides
Atrial and brain natriuretic peptides	Kinins
Endogenous digitalis-like substance	Nitric oxide
Kinins	PGE$_2$, PGI$_2$
Nitric oxide	
PGE$_2$, PGI$_2$	
Sympathetic nervous system (heart rate)	

TPR, total peripheral resistance.

multiple factors (Table 51-3) are conceivably involved in the pathogenesis of renal parenchymal hypertension, only those for which there is substantial support are discussed.

Salt Balance

Renal ablation in both rats (126) and dogs (113) clearly demonstrates the central role of salt balance in the development of hypertension under circumstances of reduced nephron mass. Ylitalo et al. (126) subjected rats to subtotal nephrectomy and found that a high-salt diet suppressed the RAAS and consistently produced severe hypertension in animals with a 70% reduction in GFR. In contrast, in the same experimental model, a normal salt intake caused only mild hypertension, and a low-salt diet resulted in no increase in blood pressure. Similarly, Guyton et al. (113) showed that dogs with renal ablation fed a high-salt diet develop hypertension initiated by expansion of the ECFV and an elevated cardiac output but maintained by an increased TPR.

Although hypertension produced by renal ablation in animals is clearly dependent on a positive salt balance, the situation with regard to human renal parenchymal hypertension is more complicated. Human renal disease often causes hypertension that not only is related to a positive salt balance consequent to a decreased GFR but also is the result of the production of hormones and autacoids that increase TPR, reduce sodium excretion, and shift the renal function curve to the right (Fig. 51-2). However, despite the complexity of the situation in an individual patient with a specific renal disease, there is persuasive evidence that suggests that overall a positive salt balance is critical to the development of hypertension in human renal disease. Many (127–129), but not all (130) studies have shown that hypertensive subjects with mild to moderate renal impairment have increased total exchangeable sodium compared with normotensive subjects, patients with essential hypertension, or normotensive patients with similar levels of renal function. These subtle alterations in total body sodium antedate frank hypertension or an increase in serum creatinine concentration. Harrap et al. (131) compared young adults with polycystic kidney disease to unaffected subjects from the same kindreds. They found that the affected subjects had a significant increase in total exchangeable sodium, PRA, and systolic blood pressure compared with unaffected offspring despite exhibiting similar, normal GFRs. Consequently, these investigators theorized that the increase in total exchangeable sodium, presumably owing to activation of the RAAS, could cause the increase in systolic pressure possibly mediated by elaboration of an EDLS (131).

Plasma volume, blood volume, or ECFV are often normal (130,132) or expanded (133,134) early in the course of CKD, but are consistently elevated by the time ESRD supervenes (135–138). In addition, salt loading in patients with ESRD results in a disproportionate increase in plasma volume and blood volume compared with interstitial fluid volume, further exacerbating hypertension (139). Last, blood pressure directly correlates with plasma volume (132) and exchangeable sodium (140) in patients with mild to moderate renal insufficiency and with ECFV (136,141) and exchangeable sodium (142) in those with ESRD; however, not all studies have confirmed these findings. Some have shown no correlation between blood volume or ECFV and blood pressure after the institution of maintenance dialysis (138,143) and only detected a relation between sodium and blood pressure in renoprival hypertension (143). Nevertheless, the bulk of the data support the concept that an increase in total exchangeable sodium occurs early in the course of renal disease when most measurements of plasma volume or ECFV are normal. As kidney function declines, an increase in ECFV is more readily detected and correlates significantly, although often weakly (140), with arterial pressure.

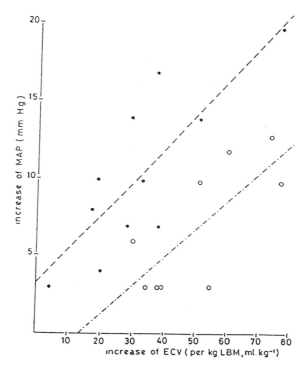

FIGURE 51-3. The relation between increments in mean arterial pressure (MAP) and extracellular fluid volume (ECV) per kilogram of lean body mass (LBM) in patients with chronic renal failure subjected to a high salt intake. For any given increase in ECV, there was a larger increment in MAP (p <0.005) in group 2 (● creatinine clearance <22 mL/minute) compared with group 1 (○ creatinine clearance >32 mL/minute). (Reprinted with permission from: Koomans HA, et al. Salt sensitivity of blood pressure in chronic renal failure: evidence for renal control of body fluid distribution in man. *Hypertension* 1982;2:190, with permission of the American Heart Association, Inc.)

Studies that have examined the effect of changes in salt balance on blood pressure in patients with chronic renal disease provide additional support for the importance of salt in the genesis of renal parenchymal hypertension. Koomans and et al. (141) measured arterial pressure, blood volume, and ECFV in patients with stage 3 (creatinine clearance >32 mL/minute) or stage 4 (creatinine clearance <22 mL/minute) CKD at two levels of salt intake. Institution of a high-salt diet increased ECFV and arterial pressure in both groups. The increment in arterial pressure, however, was larger for any given increase in ECFV in the group with stage 4 disease (Fig. 51-3) compared with those with stage 3 CKD. These data suggest that a positive salt balance consequent to an increase in dietary salt augments both ECFV and blood pressure; this hypertensive effect is inversely related to GFR and is most pronounced in severe renal insufficiency. In patients with ESRD, the prohypertensive effect of a positive salt balance is the result, not only of an increase in plasma volume and cardiac output (144), but also of an enhanced vasoconstrictor response to angiotensin II (100,145).

Just as a positive salt balance increases blood pressure in patients with renal disease, reduction of salt intake or administration of diuretics decreases exchangeable sodium, plasma volume, ECFV, and arterial pressure in hypertensive patients with CKD (134,146–148). Vasavada and Agarwal recently demonstrated that daily administration of loop diuretics to patients with stage 2 and 3 CKD significantly decreased ECFV and ambulatory systolic blood pressure over a 3-week period (134). Further support for the dependence of blood pressure on salt balance is the fact that salt subtraction with reduction of dry weight by hemodialysis (144,147,149–152) or peritoneal dialysis (153,154) normalizes blood pressure in the majority of ESRD patients without the need for pharmacologic therapy. Vertes et al. (149) initially showed that hypertension could be controlled in 35 of 40 patients undergoing maintenance hemodialysis with salt removal during ultrafiltration. Recently, Ozkahya et al. confirmed these findings by documenting substantial improvements in blood pressure in both hemodialysis and peritoneal dialysis patients with aggressive ultrafiltration and sodium restriction (154,155). Further, in a large cohort of patients undergoing chronic hemodialysis, interdialytic weight gain, reflecting salt and water intake, was an independent predictor of blood pressure (156). Finally, in the Hemodialysis Study, there was a strong, statistically significant correlation among intradialytic changes in blood pressure, body weight, and plasma volume (152). These important observations have been confirmed and extended by other investigators (150–154) and reinforce the concept that adequate fluid removal is the cornerstone of therapy in the hypertensive patient with ESRD.

The preceding data strongly support the central role that salt balance plays in renal parenchymal hypertension. However, salt balance is a major, but not exclusive, determinant of blood pressure in patients with CKD. Even in patients whose blood pressure is well controlled by salt removal during dialysis, binephrectomy reduces blood pressure without significant alterations in exchangeable sodium or ECFV (100,146). This latter observation might result from a decrease in the RAAS or a reduction in central sympathetic outflow and emphasizes the important relation between volume and vasoconstrictor factors in the control of arterial pressure even under circumstances where hypertension appears to be primarily sodium dependent (100,144,145).

Sympathetic Nervous System

Increasing evidence suggests that the sympathetic nervous system plays an important role in renal parenchymal hypertension. Activation of the sympathetic nervous system directly increases cardiac output and TPR and indirectly elevates vascular resistance by stimulation of the RAAS (157–159). Angiotensin II enhances both peripheral and central sympathetic activity reciprocally; the increment in central sympathetic outflow may be consequent to an angiotensin II-induced decrease in nitric oxide content in the posterior hypothalamus (160). Further, elevated renal sympathetic nerve traffic directly increases tubular reabsorption of sodium, reduces renal blood flow, and decreases GFR (160). Taken together, there are multiple mechanisms by which increased adrenergic activity contributes to hypertension through both vasoconstrictor and volume-dependent mechanisms.

The sympathetic nervous system plays an important role in several models of experimental renal hypertension. Vari et al. (161) studied the effect of renal denervation on the development of hypertension in uninephrectomized rats maintained on a low-salt diet. Simultaneous renal denervation and contralateral nephrectomy decreased renal norepinephrine stores and prevented the development of hypertension. When denervation was delayed until 6 weeks postnephrectomy, both renal norepinephrine content and arterial pressure declined (161). These investigators concluded that both the development and maintenance of hypertension in this experimental model were dependent on intact renal nerves. Theoretically, this beneficial effect of renal denervation might be consequent to elimination of the decrements in GFR and sodium excretion mediated by increased renal efferent sympathetic nerve activity. However, accumulating evidence suggests that renal afferent sympathetic neurons are important in renal hypertension. Campese et al. studied the role of the afferent renal nerves in the development

of hypertension in rats that had undergone 5/6 nephrectomy (162). Endogenous norepinephrine concentrations and norepinephrine turnover in the hypothalamus were significantly increased in rats with intact renal afferent nerves. However, in rats subjected to dorsal rhizotomy, which interrupts the renal afferent nerves, the increment in hypothalamic norepinephrine was blunted and norepinephrine turnover was similar to control rats. Importantly, the increase in blood pressure induced by 5/6 nephrectomy was substantially attenuated by renal afferent denervation. The same group of investigators (163) repeated a similar set of experiments after the induction of acute renal injury by intrarenal injection of phenol. There was a significant increase in blood pressure and secretion of norepinephrine from the hypothalamic nuclei in rats with intact renal afferent nerves. As in their previous model, in rats that underwent renal denervation, renal injury by phenol did not induce a rise in blood pressure or norepinephrine secretion. These data provide persuasive evidence that afferent signaling from diseased kidneys is important in mediating central sympathetic outflow and hypertension in experimental renal disease. Whether the proximate cause of the increased afferent traffic is local ischemia or cytokine production remains to be determined (164,165).

Most studies (130,166,167), but not all (171), have found increased plasma concentrations of norepinephrine in hypertensive patients with mild to moderate renal dysfunction. Ishii et al. (166) found significantly increased plasma norepinephrine in hypertensive patients with chronic glomerulonephritis compared with normotensive patients with similar renal function or normal subjects. Further, they noted a significant correlation between arterial pressure and plasma norepinephrine concentration. Ligtenberg et al. demonstrated that muscle sympathetic nerve activity (MSNA) and serum norepinephrine levels were higher in patients with hypertension and CKD compared to normal controls (167). Treatment with enalapril for 4 to 6 weeks resulted in reduction of blood pressure and improvement of MSNA (Fig. 51-4) and the baroreflex curve. In contrast, amlodipine lowered blood pressure but MSNA remained elevated. These important observations have been confirmed and extended by other investigators (168–170). Klein et al. showed that MSNA is increased in hypertensive patients with polycystic kidney disease irrespective of renal function (168). In patients with CKD, the enhanced MSNA is due to intrinsic renal disease and is not solely a function of reduced nephron mass. Moreover, the elevated MSNA in CKD that is ameliorated by interruption of the RAAS can be completely normalized by inhibition of central sympathetic outflow with monoxidine (170). Finally, hypertensive patients with renal disease demonstrate an increased pressor response to exogenous norepinephrine (171).

Accumulating data suggest that increased activity of the sympathetic nervous system contributes to hypertension in patients undergoing long-term dialysis. Plasma norepinephrine levels are usually increased in hypertensive patients with CKD before initiation of dialysis (166,167,172) and normal (173) or elevated (174–176) in hypertensive dialysis patients. Selective postganglionic sympathetic blockade reduces blood pressure in patients on maintenance hemodialysis. Schohn and et al. (174) gave debrisoquine, a postganglionic sympathetic blocker, to normal subjects and both normotensive and hypertensive patients undergoing long-term dialysis. Blood pressure declined by an average of 33/19 mm Hg in the hypertensive patients but did not change significantly in the two former groups. Further, Converse et al. (175) measured MSNA to skeletal muscle in 11 normal subjects and 23 patients receiving long-term hemodialysis. Five patients on dialysis had undergone bilateral nephrectomy, but 18 retained their native kidneys; 14 of the latter group were hypertensive. Sympathetic nerve discharge was significantly higher in the dialysis patients who retained their kidneys compared with their nephrectomized counterparts or

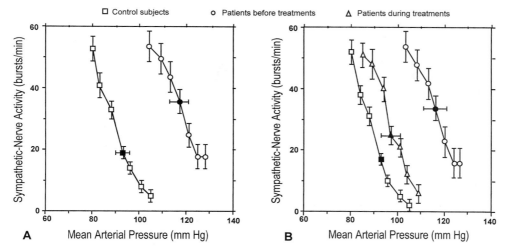

FIGURE 51-4. Baroreflex response to changes in mean arterial pressure (MAP) in patients with chronic renal insufficiency (average creatinine 3.9 ± 1.9 mg/dL) before and after treatment with enalapril and in control subjects. Sodium nitroprusside and phenylephrine were infused to provide gradations in MAP. Results are shown at baseline (**A**) in 14 patients with renal insufficiency and 14 control subjects and before and during treatment with enalapril (**B**) in 11 patients and 11 controls. Values are means ± SE. (Reproduced with permission from: Ligtenberg G, et al. Reduction of sympathetic hyperactivity by enalapril in patients with chronic renal failure. *N Engl J Med* 1999;340:1321, with permission of the Massachusetts Medical Society.)

normal subjects. Mean arterial pressure and vascular resistance in the calf were significantly lower in the nephrectomized dialysis patients compared with the patients who had not undergone nephrectomy. These and other data (177) suggest that retention of diseased kidneys, and not the uremic environment, is responsible for the increase in MSNA. Taken together, these observations provide persuasive support for the concept that afferent sympathetic nerve traffic from diseased kidneys signals the anterior hypothalamus with a consequent increase in peripheral sympathetic nerve activity (159,162,163,176).

Hence, there is abundant evidence that sympathetic overactivity contributes importantly to renal parenchymal hypertension. Early in the course of renal disease, circulating norepinephrine is often elevated, MSNA is increased, and the vascular response to exogenous norepinephrine is augmented. Increased sympathetic activity results in hypertension in patients with pre-ESRD not only by increasing TPR but also by directly stimulating renal sodium reabsorption and indirectly limiting salt excretion through activation of the RAAS. In ESRD, because urine volume is minimal, sympathetic overactivity raises blood pressure primarily, if not solely, by increasing TPR.

Pressor Compounds

Arginine Vasopressin. Despite extensive investigation, the exact role of arginine vasopressin (AVP) in renal parenchymal hypertension remains to be determined (178). Cowley et al. (179) infused AVP into normal dogs with an *ad libitum* intake of water; serum sodium decreased, weight increased, but blood pressure was unchanged. Any pressor effect of AVP, however, under these circumstances is difficult to interpret because any increase in TPR is offset by dose-dependent decrements in cardiac output with no net change in mean arterial pressure (180). On the other hand, in dogs with subtotal renal ablation, chronic infusion of subpressor doses of AVP resulted in hyponatremia, an increased blood volume, suppression of the RAAS, and hypertension (181). These data suggest that, in the face of substantial reductions in renal mass, AVP can contribute to hypertension by stimulation of V_2 receptors in the collect-

ing duct with consequent hypotonic expansion of the ECFV. In rats subjected to bilateral nephrectomy (182) or subtotal renal ablation (183) and later rendered hypernatremic, administration of an AVP antagonist significantly reduced mean arterial pressure. In one study (182), there was an inverse correlation between blood pressure and plasma volume indicating that, in rats with decreased renal mass, AVP increases arterial pressure by stimulating V_1 receptors, inducing vasoconstriction, and increasing TPR.

Studies in humans have confirmed and extended these observations in experimental models. Padfield et al. (184) studied normal volunteers, patients with malignant hypertension, and patients with the syndrome of inappropriate antidiuretic hormone secretion. They found no correlation between the plasma concentration of AVP and blood pressure in either group of patients. In addition, an infusion of AVP in normal subjects did not increase arterial pressure. In normally hydrated volunteers, AVP antagonism had no significant effect on blood pressure, heart rate, or cutaneous blood flow (185). In contrast, application of an orally active V_1 antagonist to patients with essential hypertension reduced the peak blood pressure response and increased heart rate after the administration of hypertonic saline (186). These data suggest that AVP has a limited role in blood pressure homeostasis in normal individuals or those with essential hypertension; however, in patients with chronic renal failure, AVP might play a greater part in control of blood pressure. Plasma concentrations of AVP are increased in hypertensive patients with severe chronic renal insufficiency compared with normal volunteers and exhibit an enhanced response to an infusion of hypertonic saline (187). In patients with ESRD undergoing long-term hemodialysis (188,189) or continuous ambulatory peritoneal dialysis (190), plasma AVP levels are also increased and correlate significantly with plasma osmolality in some studies (189), but not in others (188). These observations, although provocative, shed no light on the role of AVP in the control of arterial blood pressure in patients with chronic renal failure.

Investigations that utilized specific AVP antagonists (191,192) provide more direct evidence of a role for AVP in renal parenchymal hypertension. Gavras et al. (193) infused an AVP inhibitor in salt-loaded patients with ESRD receiving maintenance hemodialysis and demonstrated a modest decline (13/8 mm Hg) in blood pressure. Further, Miura et al. (194) administered an orally active V_1 receptor antagonist to a fluid-overloaded, hypertensive patient with diabetic nephropathy and a serum creatinine concentration of 5.5 mg/dL. Blood pressure decreased markedly without any change in heart rate, suggesting a substantial reduction in TPR owing to V_1 blockade. These preliminary but important observations suggest that, although in the presence of euvolemia and normal renal function AVP might not contribute significantly to control of arterial pressure, its vasoconstrictor effect is revealed in the setting of CKD. Additional investigation is required to determine whether AVP is consistently involved in the initiation or maintenance of renal parenchymal hypertension and to elucidate whether its effect is primarily mediated through expansion of the ECFV or an increment in TPR (178).

Renin-Angiotensin-Aldosterone System. Multiple lines of evidence suggest an important role for the RAAS in the initiation and maintenance of hypertension in patients with renal parenchymal disease. Plasma renin activity (131,166,195) and angiotensin II concentrations (130,196) are increased and correlate with arterial pressure in hypertensive patients with pre-ESRD. In addition, angiotensin II blockade with saralasin in hypertensive patients with early renal disease results in a decrease in blood pressure that is inversely proportional to baseline PRA (195). Some of the most persuasive evidence linking the RAAS system to renal parenchymal hypertension derives from studies in early polycystic kidney disease. Many (131,197,198), but not all (199) reports have found increased PRA in hypertensive patients with polycystic kidney disease and normal or only slightly impaired renal function. Filtration fraction is increased (131,199), reflecting the fact that angiotensin II preferentially constricts the efferent arteriole (200). Finally, administration of lisinopril decreases mean arterial pressure, renal vascular resistance, and filtration fraction (200). These data, along with the observation that renal volume is increased in hypertensive patients with polycystic disease compared with their normotensive counterparts, have led some authorities to speculate that enlarging cysts compress intrarenal arterioles, producing ischemia and ultimately activating the RAAS (197).

Not all studies, however, have supported a significant role for the RAAS in the hypertension of pre-ESRD. Vascular reactivity to exogenous angiotensin II is not increased (130,171), and PRA is often normal (199) or decreased (201). Recently, Wagner et al. (202), utilizing the quantitative polymerase chain reaction, demonstrated that renin gene expression in human renal biopsy specimens was decreased early in the course of glomerulonephritis. Consequently, hypertension in early stage kidney disease might be due to increased activity of the RAAS in some circumstances, but not others. Analysis of the relation is complicated by the fact that most studies have measured PRA and not assessed the role of the vascular renin-angiotensin system (203). Moreover, the involvement is complex because angiotensin II directly and indirectly stimulates renal sodium absorption, increases total exchangeable sodium, regulates GFR, and potentiates the activity of the renal sympathetic nerves (204). Finally, the role of aldosterone, per se, in the pathogenesis of renal parenchymal hypertension is incompletely understood. Aldosterone not only increases sodium reabsorption with consequent expansion of plasma volume but also enhances vasoconstriction in response to adrenergic stimulation (205). Administration of exogenous aldosterone to rats with remnant kidneys treated with losartan increased blood pressure, proteinuria, and glomerulosclerosis compared with rats that did not receive aldosterone (206). These data suggest a possible role for aldosterone in renal parenchymal hypertension, independent of angiotensin II. Hence, activation of the

RAAS can mediate hypertension in CKD through both vasoconstrictor and volume-dependent mechanisms.

The majority of patients with ESRD demonstrate normal PRA and angiotensin II levels (144), are salt sensitive, and remain normotensive with reduction to dry weight during dialysis (149,150,155). Ten to twenty percent of hypertensive patients with ESRD, however, clearly exhibit renin-dependent hypertension. Blood pressure in this latter group does not respond to salt removal, and most patients (147,149,207,208), but not all (209) have elevated PRA. Arterial blood pressure and PRA correlate significantly in this subset of patients (143). Weidmann and et al. (207) examined the relation between blood pressure and PRA in 51 patients undergoing long-term dialysis. Thirty-one of 33 patients with normal blood pressure or hypertension that was easily controlled by ultrafiltration demonstrated normal PRA. Moreover, 18 patients demonstrated hypertension that was resistant to salt removal and eventually required bilateral nephrectomy to control blood pressure; 17 had elevated PRA. Before the availability of minoxidil and ACE inhibitors, bilateral nephrectomy was often required to control blood pressure in patients with increased PRA and resistant hypertension (207,208). Lifschitz et al. (208) found that hypertensive patients whose blood pressure normalized after bilateral nephrectomy could be identified by their preoperative decrease in blood pressure in response to angiotensin II blockade and their increased PRA. Decrements in arterial pressure in response to binephrectomy have been associated with a reduction in TPR but no change in cardiac output (210,211). Taken together, the humoral and hemodynamic response to bilateral nephrectomy has been interpreted by some investigators to further implicate the RAAS in this form of hypertension. However, these observations are also consistent with the important role of the sympathetic nervous system in the hypertension of ESRD (175). Predictably, ACE inhibition normalizes arterial pressure in patients with increased PRA and dialysis-resistant hypertension (100,212,213). Whether this owes exclusively to interruption of the RAAS or is mediated in part by reduced sympathetic nervous system (SNS activity) (167) remains to be determined.

Hence, there is substantial support for the pathogenetic role of the RAAS in the hypertension of CKD. Early in the course of some forms of renal disease, activation of the RAAS causes hypertension not only by increasing TPR but also by limiting renal sodium excretion. Patients with chronic interstitial nephritis are often normotensive with normal or only slightly increased PRA (207,214). When hypertension develops, it is usually responsive to salt depletion. At the other end of the spectrum, hypertensive patients with chronic glomerular disease, especially those with severe hypertension, often demonstrate markedly elevated PRA, respond poorly to salt removal, and require interruption of the RAAS for control of blood pressure (207). In the 10% to 20% of hyperreninemic hypertensive patients with ESRD, the vasoconstrictor action of angiotensin II is dominant, and hormonally mediated changes in salt balance are insignificant. However, the lack of consistent relation between blood pressure and either ECFV or PRA in patients with ESRD clearly suggests that multiple other factors are involved in the pathogenesis of hypertension in this setting (211,215).

Endothelin. Yanagisawa and et al. (216) initially identified endothelin, a 21 amino acid, vasoactive, mitogenic peptide, in 1988. Endothelin exists in three distinct isoforms and, although originally thought to be produced solely by vascular endothelium, is secreted by various cells in multiple tissues (217,218) including glomerular endothelial, epithelial, and mesangial cells. Synthesis of endothelin is increased by shear stress and a variety of agonists such as thrombin, angiotensin II, AVP, and transforming growth factor-ß (219,220). Endothelin is the most potent vasoconstrictor yet described (218,221) and exerts a wide range of physiologic effects including increasing the secretion of atrial natriuretic peptide (ANP), nitric oxide (NO), renin, and prostaglandins as well as stimulating mitogenesis in diverse cell lines (218,222). Infusion of endothelin in dogs increases blood pressure, TPR, and PRA and simultaneously decreases renal blood flow, GFR, and urinary sodium excretion (223,224). Therefore, it is possible that endothelin could be pathogenetically related to renal parenchymal hypertension consequent to hormonal, paracrine, or autocrine actions. Actions of endothelin are mediated through two different receptors. The ET_A and ET_B receptors in vascular smooth muscle mediate vasoconstriction, whereas ET_B receptors on endothelial cells mediate vasodilatation. However, there are species differences in receptor actions since in rats, but not dogs, renal vasoconstriction is due to endothelin binding to the ET_B receptor (225). Therefore, endothelin provides a counterregulatory mechanism serving the maintenance of normal renal function (226) depending on the differential effects of endothelin on various receptor subtypes.

Administration of endothelin at pathophysiologic doses in dogs markedly decreases renal blood flow (RBF) and GFR and increases PRA and plasma aldosterone (224). Experiments that have examined the effect of inhibition of endothelin converting enzyme or blockade of endothelin receptors, however, provide greater insight into the potential pathophysiologic role of endothelin in hypertensive renal disease. Erythropoietin-induced hypertension is ameliorated by ET_A blockade but not ET_B blockade (226). Inhibition of endothelin converting enzyme reduces blood pressure in both spontaneously hypertensive rats (SHR) and rats with renovascular hypertension (227). On the other hand, administration of an endothelin receptor antagonist decreases arterial pressure in the SHR (228,229) and in some (228), but not all (229) models of renovascular hypertension. Benigni and et al. (230) treated rats with subtotal renal ablation with a specific ET_A receptor antagonist and found that endothelin receptor blockade not only decreased blood pressure and proteinuria but also ameliorated the biochemical and histologic progression of renal disease. However, more recent studies utilizing both ET_A and $ET_{A/B}$ antagonists have been unable to confirm these earlier observations (231,232). Nevertheless, these preliminary observations suggest possible application of endothelin receptor antagonists in human renal parenchymal hypertension.

Infusion of endothelin into normal subjects at low doses that double the normal plasma concentration significantly decreases urinary sodium excretion without affecting RBF, GFR, or blood pressure (233). Higher infusion rates that achieve the pathophysiologic plasma endothelin concentrations found in renal failure result in significant increments in renal vascular resistance and systemic blood pressure while preferentially reducing RBF compared with GFR (234). The resultant increase in filtration fraction is associated with a significant decrease in urinary sodium excretion. Two reports provide additional support for a contributory role of endothelin in some forms of human hypertension. In one patient with carcinoma of the lung, episodic hypertension during bouts of disseminated intravascular coagulation correlated with plasma endothelin levels (235). Yokokawa and et al. (236) described two patients with malignant hemangioendothelioma, increased plasma endothelin levels, and hypertension. Removal of the tumor, which contained increased concentration of endothelin and endothelin messenger RNA, normalized both blood pressure and plasma endothelin concentration. Recurrence of the tumor in one patient was again associated with hypertension and increased plasma levels of endothelin. Multiple studies have compared radioimmunoassayable plasma concentrations of endothelin in normotensive subjects, patients with essential hypertension, and hypertensive patients with renal disease. Endothelin levels have been increased in patients with essential hypertension compared with

normal control subjects in some studies (237,238), but not in others (239,240). Although no consistent correlation has been found between plasma concentrations of endothelin and arterial pressure in essential hypertension (237,238), administration of bosentan, a mixed $ET_{A/B}$ receptor antagonist, to essential hypertensives, decreased blood pressure to a level similar to that achieved with ACE inhibition (240). Plasma concentrations (239,241,242) and urinary excretion (243) of endothelin are more consistently elevated in hypertensive patients with renal disease compared with normal volunteers but still correlate poorly with blood pressure (241,243). These inconsistent findings are not surprising, however, considering that endothelin probably functions as an autocrine or paracrine substance and not as a circulating hormone (217,222). Vajo and coworkers demonstrated that endothelin levels were elevated in an anephric patient with severe hypertension, implying a role for endothelin in the development of hypertension in this patient (244). However, methods to exclude volume overload contributing to hypertension were not well described in this study (245). In contrast, Hand et al. administered a selective ET_A antagonist to patients with pre-ESRD and healthy control subjects (246). Forearm blood flow increased in both groups but the increment was significantly greater in the healthy subjects than in the patients with chronic renal failure, suggesting a reduced role of endothelin in the maintenance of resting vascular tone in patients with pre-ESRD. Hence, the role of endothelin in renal parenchymal hypertension remains to be elucidated.

Endogenous Digitalis-like Substance (EDLS). The concept that an inhibitor of Na^+-K^+-ATPase, an EDLS, might be involved in the pathogenesis of renal parenchymal hypertension was initially postulated by several groups of investigators (123,247,248) more than 20 years ago. Despite intensive study, the precise identification of this compound(s) remains elusive (125,249,250). The EDLS is clearly distinct from ANP, brain natriuretic peptide (BNP), and steroidal natriuretic compounds (249). Candidate factors share several common features; they inhibit Na^+-K^+-ATPase, are natriuretic, and cross-react with antibodies to digitalis (249). The theoretic mechanism by which an EDLS causes renal hypertension has been debated but has received increasing support. According to this hypothesis, an intrinsic or acquired defect in renal sodium excretion causes an increase in the ECFV that signals the release of an EDLS from the hypothalamus that inhibits Na^+-K^+-ATPase (250). Inhibition of Na^+-K^+-ATPase in renal tubular epithelia decreases sodium chloride reabsorption and increases urinary sodium excretion, thus attenuating the expansion of the ECFV. On the other hand, inhibition of Na^+-K^+-ATPase in vascular smooth muscle increases intracellular sodium concentration, reduces the transplasmalemmal sodium gradient, and raises the intracellular calcium content because of decreased sodium-dependent calcium efflux (123,125,250). The eventual increment in intracellular calcium results in an increase in vascular tone and TPR. Hence, salt balance is returned toward baseline at the expense of an elevated TPR and increase in arterial pressure.

Rats subjected to subtotal renal ablation and maintained on a high-salt diet develop an increase in ECFV and hypertension and demonstrate decreased Na^+-K^+-ATPase activity in cardiac microsomes and arteries (251). In addition, diabetic rats with a 25% reduction in renal mass demonstrate an increase in ECFV, suppressed PRA, and hypertension (124). Plasma levels of EDLS are increased, and cardiac and renal medullary microsomal Na^+-K^+-ATPase activity is decreased. Further, EDLS significantly correlates with mean arterial pressure (124). Gomez-Sanchez et al. (252) immunized salt-sensitive Dahl rats with an ouabain conjugate and ameliorated, but did not completely prevent, the development of hypertension when the animals were fed a high-salt diet. Finally, Digibind significantly reduced mean arterial pressure in rats with reduced renal mass (253).

Since the initial report by Graves et al. (254) of an EDLS in the plasma of patients with CKD, increased levels of EDLS have been found in most (131,255–259), but not all (260), studies of patients with essential hypertension and hypertensive patients with CKD. Young adults with polycystic kidney disease and normal GFR have significantly increased total exchangeable sodium, higher systolic blood pressure, decreased RBF, and reduced ouabain-sensitive sodium efflux that is inversely related to total exchangeable sodium compared with their unaffected siblings (131). These observations are consistent with the presence of a circulating EDLS. Similar results have been reported in hypertensive patients with mild to moderate renal insufficiency (256). Other investigators have demonstrated radioimmunoassayable evidence of digoxin-like activity in patients with renal insufficiency who were not receiving digitalis (257). Although digitalis-like activity correlated inversely with GFR, there was no relation to blood pressure. Kelly et al. (258) demonstrated both increased levels of digoxin-like immunoreactivity and greater Na^+-K^+-ATPase inhibitory activity in hypertensive patients with moderate renal dysfunction compared with hypertensive patients with normal renal function or with normal subjects. However, in patients receiving maintenance dialysis, digoxin-like immunoreactivity was normal. There was no correlation between digoxin-like immunoreactivity and blood pressure in any group. On the other hand, in patients undergoing continuous ambulatory peritoneal dialysis, Na^+-K^+-ATPase increased with sustained volume expansion and significantly correlated with both mean arterial pressure and change in body weight (259). Finally, Bisordi and Holt found elevated levels of an EDLS in 15 hemodialysis patients (261). Plasma concentrations of EDLS correlated with both pre- and post-dialysis ECFV and were paralled by similar changes in ANP levels. Taken together, increasing evidence suggests that an EDLS is elaborated in response to increments in salt balance in patients with normal or reduced renal function, but its role in the pathogenesis of renal parenchymal hypertension requires further clarification.

Erythropoietin. Recombinant human erythropoietin (r-HuEPO) was introduced two decades ago for the treatment of the anemia of chronic renal failure (262). It was soon apparent that the development or exacerbation of hypertension was a frequent adverse effect of therapy with r-HuEPO (263,264). This prohypertensive effect of r-HuEPO occurs in patients with mild to moderate renal dysfunction as well as in those with ESRD (265,266). Increments of blood pressure can occur in normotensive patients with ESRD, but elevations are more evident in hypertensive individuals. Although early reports (262,263) occasionally noted the development of severe hypertension with seizures or encephalopathy, this rarely occurs now, given the increased awareness of this potential complication. The incidence of reported hypertension in patients with renal disease treated with r-HuEPO ranges from 17% to 48% (265–268). However, some studies have shown no correlation between the dose of r-HuEPO and blood pressure (269). On the other hand, an analysis of placebo-controlled multicenter trials (268) found that 21% of patients on chronic hemodialysis treated with r-HuEPO developed clinically significant increases in blood pressure. This latter estimate is a more accurate reflection of the prohypertensive effect of r-HuEPO because some previous trials were uncontrolled.

Although endogenous erythropoietin concentrations correlate with blood pressure in patients with essential hypertension (270), the mechanism(s) by which r-HuEPO results in hypertension remains uncertain (271). Since blood transfusion to correct uremic anemia increases arterial pressure in patients on chronic dialysis (272), some investigators have examined the relation between either red cell mass or hematocrit and blood pressure in patients with chronic renal failure. Treatment with r-HuEPO increases red cell volume, but because of a concomitant decrease in plasma volume, blood volume remains unchanged (265,273). Moreover, despite a significant increase in hematocrit, increments in blood pressure do not correlate with the net change in hematocrit, the rate of increase in hematocrit, or the dose of r-HuEPO (265,267,269). Finally, Kaupke et al. (274) studied the effect of an increase in red cell mass owing to iron repletion in anemic iron-deficient patients with ESRD who were receiving a constant dose of r-HuEPO. In 15 patients, repletion of iron stores resulted in an increase of hematocrit from 25% to 32% (p <0.001) but did not significantly change either systolic or diastolic blood pressure. Hence, therapy with r-HuEPO causes hypertension by additional mechanisms other than an increase in red cell mass.

Although r-HuEPO is not a direct vasoconstrictor, incubation of r-HuEPO with rabbit aorta or carotid artery (275) increases endothelin production. Incubation with a selective ET_A antagonist blocks the vasoconstrictor response induced by r-HuEPO (275). These observations have led some investigators to speculate that endothelin might play a role in the hypertension associated with therapy with r-HuEPO (275,276). Carlini et al. (276) found increased plasma levels of endothelin in patients on chronic hemodialysis treated with intravenous r-HuEPO compared with their counterparts receiving subcutaneous r-HuEPO. There was a significant correlation between mean arterial pressure and plasma levels of endothelin only in the patients receiving intravenous erythropoietin. Other investigators have also been unable to demonstrate any change in plasma concentration of endothelin during the subcutaneous or intraperitoneal administration of r-HuEPO (268). Hence, if endothelin is causally related to r-HuEPO-induced hypertension, the route of administration might be important.

Correction of the anemia of ESRD with r-HuEPO is associated with an increase in blood pressure mediated by an increased TPR and a decrease in cardiac output (265,268,277). The decrement in cardiac output, however, is proportionately less than the increment in TPR, resulting in an increase in blood pressure. Several mechanisms potentially contribute to the increased TPR. Correction of anemia increases whole blood viscosity (264,277), which increases TPR (264,265). Further, an increase in red cell mass improves tissue oxygenation and could reverse hypoxic vasodilation, thereby increasing vascular tone (265). Hence, enhanced production of endothelin, increased blood viscosity, and reversal of hypoxic vasodilation together with a genetic predisposition to hypertension (278), an augmented vascular responsiveness to norepinephrine (275), and possibly other undefined factors (265,271) increase blood pressure during therapy with r-HuEPO. The observation that hypertension does not develop to a significant extent in normal volunteers, patients with multiple myeloma, or individuals with the acquired immune deficiency syndrome (279,280) treated with r-HuEPO underscores the concept that other factors associated with renal disease are required for therapy with r-HuEPO to increase blood pressure (281). Hypertension associated with the treatment of the anemia of chronic renal failure with r-HuEPO should be anticipated. Blood pressure must be carefully monitored, and if hypertension develops or worsens, it should be treated in the same fashion as in patients not receiving r-HuEPO (see Treatment of Hypertension, below).

Depressor Compounds

In addition to producing vasoconstrictor and antinatriuretic compounds, the kidney also synthesizes vasodilator and natriuretic factors (7,201,283,284). Therefore, it is theoretically possible that deficient production of vasodepressor medullary lipids, nitric oxide, kinins, or renal prostaglandins could contribute to the generation or maintenance of renal parenchymal hypertension. However, despite the important antihypertensive function of nonprostaglandin renal medullary lipids in some forms of experimental hypertension (6,284,285) and the prohypertensive effect of chemical renal medullectomy (286), there is no substantial evidence linking a deficiency of these compounds to the genesis of hypertension in human renal disease. On the other hand, considerable evidence suggests that alterations in the production of nitric oxide, kinins, ANP, and prostaglandins occur in renal parenchymal hypertension.

Nitric Oxide. Nitric oxide is produced by the vascular endothelium from L-arginine by the enzyme NO synthase (NOS) and functions as an endogenous nitrovasodilator (287–289). To date, three isoforms of NOS have been described: neuronal NOS (nNOS); inducible NOS (iNOS); and endothelial NOS (eNOS). Within the kidney, NO mediates the vasodilator action of kinins, participates in pressure-mediated natriuresis, exerts a tonic vasodilator effect on the afferent arteriole, decreases tubular sodium reabsorption, and opposes endothelin-induced vasoconstriction (283,288,289). Accumulating data suggest that impaired production of NO might be related to both experimental and human renal parenchymal hypertension. For example, in rats, stimulation of endogenous NO production increases RBF and salt excretion, whereas inhibition of NO synthesis produces the opposite effect (288,290,291). Increased dietary salt stimulates renal NO production, and inhibition of NOS under conditions of salt loading results in increased renal vascular resistance, decreased RBF and GFR, increased urinary protein excretion, systemic hypertension, and chronic progressive nephropathy (290–294). Angiotensin II receptor blockade or ACE inhibition ameliorate the deleterious renal effects of chronic inhibition of NOS (294), implying a particularly noxious effect of angiotensin II in the face of reduced NO production. In rats subjected to subtotal renal ablation, systemic NO production is augmented whereas renal synthesis is decreased (295,296) and chronic NOS inhibition aggravates both systemic and glomerular hypertension, resulting in both functional and histologic renal deterioration (297).

Decreased NOS activity and reduced NO production have recently been demonstrated in an experimental model of immunologically mediated glomerulonephritis (298). Data in humans provide some support for these experimental observations. Some (299) but not all (300) studies suggest that NO synthesis is reduced in essential hypertension. Further, NOS inhibition in normotensive volunteers resulted in a marked increase in blood pressure (301). Endogenous inhibitors of NOS that are normally excreted in the urine accumulate in the plasma of patients with CKD and ESRD (302,303). Infusion of one of these compounds, asymmetric dimethyl arginine (ADMA), results in systemic hypertension in guinea pigs and decreases forearm blood flow in normal volunteers (304). Schmidt and Baylis (305) found that 13 patients with stage 3–5 CKD demonstrated increased ADMA levels, reduced total NO production and higher blood pressure compared with normal control subjects. However, other investigators have found no difference in plasma ADMA concentrations between normotensive and hypertensive patients with CKD (302). There are conflicting data with regard to NO production in patients with ESRD. Both increased (306) and decreased (307,308) NO synthesis have been reported. Hence, at this juncture no firm conclusions can be drawn regarding the role of NO in the initiation or maintenance of human renal parenchymal hypertension.

Kinins. Kinins stimulate the release of NO and PGI$_2$ from vascular endothelium and thereby cause vasodilation (283,309). However, their role in the regulation of arterial pressure under physiologic or pathophysiologic circumstance is uncertain. Intrarenal infusion of bradykinin in conscious dogs for 7 days had no significant effect on urinary sodium excretion, GFR, or arterial blood pressure (310). These observations suggest that circulating kinins do not exert an important long-term effect on blood pressure but do not exclude a potentially significant vasodepressor role of local intrarenal kinin production. In this regard, rats subjected to chronic NOS inhibition or 5/6 renal ablation, both models of salt-sensitive hypertension, demonstrate decreased renal kallikrein expression and kinin excretion (311). Levy et al. (312) demonstrated a direct relation between RBF and urinary kallikrein excretion in patients with essential hypertension. Further, excretion of both active and inactive urinary kallikrein is decreased in salt sensitive subjects with essential hypertension (313,314) and in Japanese (314) and whites, but not blacks (315), with renal parenchymal hypertension. Almeida and et al. (316) demonstrated reduced plasma kininogen concentration in patients with malignant hypertension and an average serum creatinine concentration of 4 mg/dL compared with essential hypertensives or normal subjects. After 3 months of adequate control of blood pressure, plasma kininogen concentrations were still decreased, suggesting that the reduced levels were not the result of the severe hypertension but might have contributed to its pathogenesis.

Natriuretic Peptides. The natriuretic peptide system consists of ANP, brain natriuretic peptide (BNP), and C-type natriuretic peptide (CNP) (317). Of the three peptides, ANP and BNP have been best characterized. Multiple studies have shown that both ANP and BNP increase GFR and urinary sodium excretion, inhibit the release of renin, aldosterone, and AVP, and directly relax vascular smooth muscle (317–319). Hence, it is theoretically possible that a deficiency of ANP, or BNP, or both is related to the development of hypertension because all of the actions of these natriuretic peptides tend to reduce blood pressure and administration of synthetic ANP to patients with essential hypertension decreases arterial pressure and increases sodium excretion (320). Basal levels of ANP and BNP, however, are significantly higher in patients with essential hypertension compared with normotensive individuals and correlate with blood pressure and left ventricular mass index (130,318,321). Concentrations of both peptides are elevated in pre-ESRD CKD (322,323), and in patients with ESRD (323–325). Suda and et al. (322) measured plasma ANP concentrations in hypertensive patients with an average creatinine clearance of 39 mL/minute and in normal subjects. They found that ANP levels in the hypertensive patients with renal disease were significantly greater than in the normotensive controls and that plasma ANP correlated with blood pressure. Similarly, Takami et al. (323) demonstrated that plasma BNP concentrations were five-fold greater in hypertensive patients with pre-ESRD than in hypertensive controls. Brain natriuretic peptide levels correlated with echocardiographic estimates of left ventricular overload independent of the degree of renal dysfunction (323). In ESRD, the concentrations of both natriuretic peptides are elevated to an even greater extent, increase with volume expansion, decrease significantly with fluid removal during dialysis, and directly correlate with the degree of volume expansion (324,326). Changes in natriuretic peptide concentrations with salt removal during dialysis undoubtedly reflect decreases in secretion because they are not cleared significantly across conventional dialysis membranes (324,325). Taken together, these observations suggest that both ANP and BNP are increased in hypertensive patients with renal disease and respond appropriately to changes in cardiac filling pressure. Hence, there is no deficiency of these natriuretic peptides; rather, their levels are increased, and they modulate the salt-retaining and vasoconstrictor actions of other neurohumeral influences (Fig. 51-5).

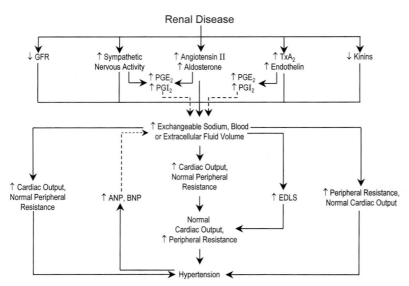

FIGURE 51-5. Pathophysiologic mechanisms responsible for the initiation of renal parenchymal hypertension and the hemodynamic patterns that sustain the elevated arterial pressure. Direct effect (−); decreases or attenuates (—). *ANP*, atrial natriuretic peptide; *BNP*, brain natriuretic peptide; *EDLS*, endogenous digitalislike substance; *GFR*, glomerular filtration rate; *PGE2*, prostaglandin E_2; *PGI2*, prostacyclin; *TxA2*, thromboxane A_2. (Modified from: Smith MC, Dunn MJ. Hypertension in renal parenchymal disease. In: Laragh JH, Brenner BM, eds. *Hypertension: pathophysiology, diagnosis, and management.* New York: Raven Press, 1995:2091.)

Prostaglandins. Renal and extrarenal prostaglandin synthesis exerts an important influence on vascular tone and salt excretion. Prostacyclin (PGI_2), PGE_2, and PGD_2 are vasodilator and natriuretic, whereas thromboxane A_2 and $PGF_{2\alpha}$ are vasoconstrictor and antinatriuretic (7,282,327). Not only do prostaglandins directly modulate vascular tone and sodium chloride excretion, they also indirectly affect vascular resistance by regulating renin secretion and sympathetic tone (282). However, because stimulation of endogenous prostaglandin production tends to decrease blood pressure (328) and administration of both nonselective and selective nonsteroidal antiinflammatory drugs (NSAIDs) increases blood pressure in treated hypertensives (329–332), a deficiency of systemic or renal prostaglandin synthesis could conceivably contribute to hypertension in patients with renal disease.

This notion is supported by the observation that urinary excretion of PGE_2 is reduced in about a third of patients with essential hypertension (333) and that plasma concentrations of 6-keto-$PGF_{1\alpha}$, a stable metabolite of PGI_2, are reportedly decreased in some populations with essential hypertension as well (334). In contrast, urinary excretion of PGE_2 is normal (335) or increased (336) in hypertensive patients with CKD and increases further with salt loading (337). These latter data imply that deficient prostaglandin synthesis is not etiologically related to human renal parenchymal hypertension but rather that normal or enhanced prostaglandin production modulates the vasoconstrictor and salt-retaining effects of angiotensin II, the sympathetic nervous system, and other pressor compounds (Fig. 51-6). The fact that virtually all NSAIDs, except aspirin and sulindac, increase blood pressure in treated patients with essential hypertension (282,327,329–332,338,339) and in hypertensive patients with renal disease (335,339) further supports this contention. Ruilope and et al. (335) treated hypertensive patients with stage 2–3 CKD with indomethacin at a dosage of 2 mg/kg for 3 days and demonstrated a simultaneous decrease in urinary excretion of PGE_2 and creatinine clearance together with a significant increment in weight and diastolic blood pressure. Thus, inhibition of renal prostaglandin production by NSAIDs in hypertensive patients with renal disease can further reduce GFR and salt excretion in addition to exacerbating hypertension (327,335,338–341). Sulindac and piroxicam are less nephrotoxic than ibuprofen (341) but should still be used cautiously in patients with renal parenchymal hypertension. On the other hand, selective cyclooxygenase-2 inhibitors can also exacerbate hypertension and cause acute on chronic renal failure (330,342) and do not offer distinct advantages over nonselective NSAIDs in this patient population (343).

Hemodynamic Patterns

In hypertensive patients with renal disease, the increased arterial pressure must be caused by an elevated cardiac output or TPR, or both, consequent to expansion of the ECFV owing to salt retention or as the result of vasoconstriction from increased sympathetic tone or increased synthesis of pressor compounds (Fig. 51-5). Both cross-sectional and longitudinal studies have examined this issue. Cross-sectional studies in stage 2–3 CKD (116–118) and ESRD (119,120,344) show that hypertension is maintained chiefly by an increase in TPR and bilateral nephrectomy or salt subtraction during hemodialysis reduces both blood pressure and TPR without changing cardiac output (119,120). Longitudinal observations in patients with early stage kidney disease (121,122) in addition to

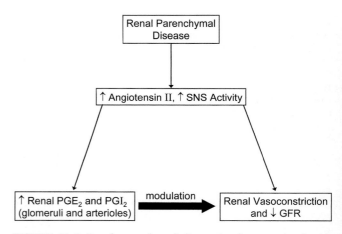

FIGURE 51-6. Renal parenchymal disease is often associated with augmented production of angiotensin II and increased activity of the sympathetic nervous system (SNS). The effect is twofold: first, a direct intrarenal vasoconstrictor effect that decreases renal blood flow (RBF) and GFR and second, an increased synthesis of vasodilator and natriuretic prostaglandins (PG). The latter modulates intrarenal vasoconstriction. Inhibition of intrarenal PG production by nonsteroidal antiinflammatory drugs results in unopposed intrarenal vasoconstriction with a further decline in RBF and GFR.

hemodynamic measurements in patients with ESRD subjected to salt loading (9,113,345), however, suggest that alternative hemodynamic patterns exist. For example, some data imply that an elevated cardiac output can precede an increase in TPR or, under certain circumstances, maintain hypertension. Brod and et al. (121,122) repetitively measured hemodynamic parameters over a period of 2 to 8 years in 97 patients with stage 1 CKD (GFR 90–117 mL/minute). Initially 12 of 32 normotensive patients demonstrated an increased cardiac output, expanded blood volume, and reduced TPR. During the follow-up period, 11 of these 12 patients eventually developed hypertension. Of the group of patients with initially mild to moderate hypertension, one-third had an increased cardiac output and normal vascular resistance. On the other hand, patients with severe hypertension uniformly had an increased TPR. Taken together, these data support the hypothesis that early in the development of renal parenchymal hypertension the elevated blood pressure is consequent to salt retention, an expanded ECFV, and an increased cardiac output. In the established phase, especially with moderate to severe hypertension, the increased blood pressure is the result of an augmented TPR.

The sequential hemodynamic changes subsequent to volume expansion observed in experimental models of renal ablation (9,113) also have been demonstrated in humans with renoprival hypertension and nonnephrectomized patients with ESRD (345,346). Coleman et al. (346) studied three nephrectomized patients before and after volume expansion. During expansion of the ECFV, blood pressure increased as a result of an elevated cardiac output, whereas TPR remained constant. Established hypertension, however, was associated with an elevated vascular resistance and normal cardiac output. Similar maneuvers in a larger group of nonnephrectomized patients with ESRD have confirmed and extended these findings and have indicated that an increase in cardiac output is not a necessary initial event in the development of hypertension. Kim et al. (345) found four hemodynamic patterns consequent to salt loading in 10 patients undergoing chronic hemodialysis: Two showed no increase in blood pressure; two developed an increment in blood pressure along with an increase in cardiac output; one patient developed hypertension that was initiated by an increase in cardiac output and sustained by an elevated TPR; and five had increases in blood pressure and vascular resistance without a measurable change in cardiac output. However, in the latter group, it is possible that transient increments in cardiac output occurred but were missed before the new steady state developed.

The relation between the factors that initiate hypertension in renal disease and the hemodynamic patterns that maintain the increased blood pressure is complex and multidirectional (Fig. 51-5). A decline in GFR together with increased activity of the sympathetic nervous system, the RAAS, or other vasoconstrictor or salt-retaining compounds causes an increase in exchangeable sodium and ECFV or an abnormal volume–renin relationship. These phenomena trigger a sequence of hemodynamic events culminating in hypertension. In anephric patients or those with a decreased PRA, hypertension is initiated or sustained by an elevated cardiac output. On the other hand, if the underlying renal disease increases the activity of the sympathetic nervous system or is associated with the elaboration of vasoconstrictors (e.g., angiotensin II, endothelin), hypertension is mediated chiefly by an increase in TPR. Under certain circumstances, however, an increment in cardiac output antedates the sustained elevation of TPR and is reminiscent of the autoregulation theory of blood pressure control espoused by Guyton et al. (113). The factors that mediate the transition from hypertension maintained by an increased cardiac output to elevated blood pressure sustained by an increment in TPR remain elusive. Increased sodium and calcium content of vascular smooth muscle consequent to a circulating EDLS that inhibits Na^+-K^+-ATPase could mediate the increase in vascular resistance (125,261).

Effect of Systemic Hypertension on Renal Function

The concept that systemic hypertension accelerates the decline in renal function has become well accepted since the initial reports by Wilson and Byrom (347) and Ellis (348) more than 50 years ago (349). Progressive renal dysfunction is uncommon in benign essential hypertension (350); however, GFR declines more rapidly in hypertensive patients with renal disease compared with their normotensive counterparts. Multiple epidemiologic studies and clinical trials have convincingly demonstrated by multivariate analysis that elevated systolic blood pressure (351,352) or mean arterial pressure (353) strongly predict progression of renal disease and rate of decline in GFR. Poorly controlled blood pressure contributes to progressive loss of kidney function in both diabetic nephropathy (354) and nondiabetic renal disease (10,349,353,355–358). The exact mechanism whereby elevated systemic blood pressure aggravates renal injury has not been firmly established. Initially, it was speculated that hypertension caused arteriolar nephrosclerosis with consequent ischemic glomerular sclerosis superimposed on primary renal disease (359). Investigators theorized that luminal obliteration owing to arteriolar nephrosclerosis further decreased renal blood flow (RBF) and GFR and contributed additionally to the decline in renal function. Few experimental data, however, support this notion. Rather, accumulating evidence over the past two decades suggests that multiple interrelated mechanisms, including impaired autoregulation of RBF and GFR with consequent glomerular capillary hypertension, glomerular hypertrophy, and the production of fibrogenic cytokines cause the accelerated loss of kidney function in hypertensive patients with renal disease.

Azar and et al. (360,361) first demonstrated that in some experimental models of hypertension, increments in systemic blood pressure were transmitted directly to the glomerulus. Utilizing micropuncture, they found that rats with one-kidney post-salt hypertension had significantly greater P_{GC} compared with normotensive controls. The higher P_{GC} was consequent to reduced afferent arteriolar resistance (R_A) and was associated with increased transcapillary hydraulic pressure differences (ΔP). Histologically, the animals developed glomerulosclerosis rather than arteriolar sclerosis (361). Olson et al. (362) confirmed and extended these observations. They demonstrated greater glomerular damage in experimental models of hypertension in rats that showed a reduced R_A (deoxycorticosterone-salt, renal ablation) compared with models that had a normal or increased R_A (aortic ligature, stroke-prone spontaneously hypertensive rats). These data imply that in experimental hypertension, unassociated with primary renal disease, impaired auto-regulation of RBF and GFR is decreased R_A causes hydraulically mediated renal damage and progressive glomerular injury.

Substantial evidence suggests that similar intrarenal hemodynamic abnormalities are linked to progressive renal dysfunction when hypertension develops in conjunction with renal disease or is superimposed on preexisting renal disease. Dogs with a marked reduction in renal mass exhibit significant loss of autoregulation of RBF and GFR in response to changes in renal perfusion pressure (363). In rats, nephrotoxic serum nephritis (364), aminonucleoside nephrosis (365), or subtotal renal ablation (366–368) disturbs renal autoregulation with a consequent increment in Q_A and GFR as systemic blood pressure increases. Bidani and et al. (366) showed that rats subjected to 5/6 nephrectomy and fed a normal protein diet demonstrated impaired autoregulation in response to graded changes in renal perfusion pressure and greater glomerular injury compared with their counterparts fed a low-protein diet. In contrast, they found no significant short-term loss of renal function in normotensive rats with subtotal renal ablation (368). However, recent studies from the same group (369) in a "normotensive" rat remnant kidney model showed that the percent glomerulosclerosis correlated significantly with average systolic blood pressure. These investigators speculated that impaired autoregulation of RBF and GFR antedates morphologic injury and explains the observation that progressive glomerular damage occurs in this model despite no significant increase in blood pressure. Their conclusions are further strengthened by the fact that superimposition of hypertension, by clipping a renal artery (370) or institution of a high-salt diet (371), in experimental immunologically mediated renal disease results in increasing proteinuria and accelerated glomerulosclerosis. Finally, in rats with streptozotocin-induced diabetes and two-kidney, one-clip hypertension, the clipped kidney exhibits fewer morphologic manifestations of diabetic nephropathy as compared with the unclipped kidney (372).

These indirect observations are bolstered by direct measurements of Q_A and P_{GC} by micropuncture in experimental models of hypertensive renal disease. In rats with subtotal renal ablation or in uninephrectomized spontaneously hypertensive rats, increases in systemic pressure are transmitted directly to glomerular capillaries as the result of a greater reduction in R_A compared with efferent arteriolar resistance (R_E) (37,43,373). The consequent increment in P_{GC} is associated with progressive proteinuria and glomerular injury. Similarly, in diabetic rats, glomerular hypertension with increments in ΔP and P_{GC} occurs in the absence of systemic hypertension because of relatively greater reductions in R_A compared with R_E (374). Moreover, in fawn-hooded rats that spontaneously develop proteinuria, hypertension, and progressive glomerulosclerosis, proteinuria and glomerular damage are linked to an increase in P_{GC} and aggravated by uninephrectomy with its attendant preferential reduction in R_A (39,375,376). Hence, in diverse models of renal parenchymal disease, renal morphologic and functional deterioration occurs together with impaired renal autoregulation owing to a greater decrease in R_A compared with R_E with a resultant increase in P_{GC} (46,377).

The relation between intraglomerular hemodynamic abnormalities and progressive glomerulosclerosis in experimental renal disease is not straightforward. For example, Yoshida et al. (41,43) demonstrated that glomerulosclerosis correlated with glomerular hypertrophy and not P_{GC} in a rat remnant kidney model. Similarly, other investigators have dissociated progression of experimental renal disease from increments in P_{GC} and have suggested that measures of nephronal hypertrophy such as V_G and R_{GC} or the production of growth factors are more tightly linked to ongoing glomerular injury (26,378–382). In this regard, mesangial cells in culture proliferate (383) and produce excess type I and IV collagen (384) in response to mechanical stretching. Further, both angiotensin II (385,386) and endothelin (387,388) stimulate mitogenesis of cultured mesangial cells. The degree of glomerular sclerosis correlates significantly with urinary excretion of endothelin in rats with subtotal renal ablation (388). Moreover, emerging data suggest that aldosterone has an important role, independent of angiotensin II, to mediate glomerulosclerosis and production of TGFβ (206). Finally, in a rat model of Heymann nephritis the combination of an ACE inhibitor and an ET_A receptor antagonist reduces glomerular sclerosis and interstitial damage to a greater extent than either drug alone (381). Consequently, the above data imply that in various experimental models renal disease progresses by different mechanisms; increments in P_{GC} or V_G or augmented production of angiotensin II, aldosterone or endothelin stimulate the production of growth factors that results in progressive glomerular obsolescence.

Both salt restriction (42,378) and pharmacologic therapy (26,37,38,374,376,389–391) limit proteinuria, preserve renal function, and retard glomerular injury in experimental renal parenchymal hypertension. Salt restriction exerts its beneficial effect by reducing renal hypertrophy without significantly decreasing P_{GC} (42,378). Pharmacologic treatment, on the other hand, has ameliorated progressive renal disease while decreasing P_{GC} (37,44,374,376,389,392), minimizing glomerular hypertrophy (43,44,380), and limiting (381,393,394) or reversing (395) glomerular and interstitial injury. Although the protective effect of drug treatment differs according to the experimental model (37,391), stage of the disease at which therapy is instituted (396), and probably other unidentified variables, some classes of antihypertensive agents might be more renoprotective than others. For example, ACE inhibitors and angiotensin II antagonists consistently ameliorate progressive renal injury (37,43,44,374,376,380,389–393,397,398), whereas calcium channel blockers or combinations of other drugs have prevented glomerular damage in some (30,43,44,380,391,392,399), but not all (37,389, 390,397,398) studies. Anderson and et al. (37) compared ACE inhibition by enalapril with a combination of reserpine, hydralazine, and hydrochlorothiazide with regard to development of proteinuria and glomerular sclerosis in rats subjected to subtotal renal ablation. They found that enalapril reduced P_{GC} by preferentially decreasing R_E relative to R_A, decreased systemic blood pressure, minimized proteinuria, and prevented progressive glomerular damage. In contrast, triple drug therapy did not decrease P_{GC} or R_E, despite similar effects on systemic blood pressure, and failed to ameliorate progressive renal injury. Based on these and similar data (374,376,389,393,395), many authorities have concluded that ACE inhibitors and angiotensin II receptor antagonists are especially renoprotective because of their unique ability to modulate hydraulically mediated glomerular damage, decrease glomerulosclerosis, and minimize interstitial damage. On the other hand, Dworkin et al. (391), in the uninephrectomized spontaneously hypertensive rat, demonstrated that higher doses of triple drug therapy decreased P_{GC} and ΔP to a similar extent compared with ACE inhibition and that both retarded the progression of renal disease. In addition, these same investigators (44) showed that nifedipine and enalapril were equally renoprotective in rats with subtotal renal ablation. However, all investigators have not substantiated the latter observation (37,389,390,397). The lack of calcium channel blockade to consistently ameliorate renal injury in experimental models of renal disease could be due to further impairment of renal autoregulation or inconsistent effects on systemic blood pressure. For example, Griffin and et al. (390,397) showed that dihydropyridine calcium channel blockers (DHPCCBs) caused a further loss of renal autoregulation in the rat remnant kidney model associated with increased proteinuria and glomerular sclerosis. In addition, radiotelemetric blood pressure monitoring in this model demonstrates marked lability of blood pressure that is incompletely ameliorated by calcium channel blockade compared with ACE inhibition (369,390,394,397). The finding that glomerular damage in the renal ablation model is tightly linked to achieved blood pressure reduction (369,389,394) could explain some of the inconsistent experimental data with regard to the renoprotective effects of calcium channel blockade. In addition, combination therapy with both an ACE inhibitor and an angiotensin II receptor blocker, despite similar control of blood pressure, is more renoprotective with regard to limiting proteinuria and renal injury than monotherapy with either drug alone (400). Taken together, the available data indicate that ACE inhibitors and angiotensin II antagonists consistently limit renal injury in experimental renal parenchymal disease through both hemodynamic (37,374,376,389,393) and nonhemodynamic (392) mechanisms. Other antihypertensive regimens are less effective. It is uncertain whether this is the result of inconsistent control of systemic blood pressure, adverse hemodynamic effects

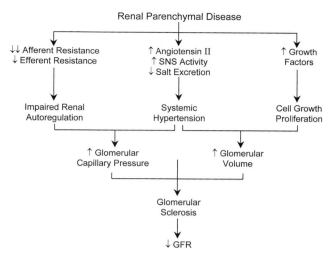

FIGURE 51-7. Mechanisms responsible for the progression of renal disease when systemic hypertension coexists with renal parenchymal disease. GFR, glomerular filtration rate; SNS, sympathetic nervous system. (Reprinted with permission from: Smith MC, Dunn MJ. Hypertension in renal parenchymal disease. In: Laragh JH, Brenner BM, eds. *Hypertension: pathophysiology, diagnosis, and management.* New York: Raven Press, 1995:2094.)

in the renal microcirculation, or incomplete suppression of fibrogenic cytokines (401).

Figure 51-7 summarizes our current understanding of the pathophysiologic mechanisms responsible for the accelerated loss of renal function in renal parenchymal hypertension. Hypertension results from decreased excretion of salt, increased production of vasoconstrictor compounds, or both. The preferential reduction in R_A relative to R_E owing to increased intrarenal prostaglandin (367) or nitric oxide (289) synthesis impairs autoregulation of renal blood flow. Consequently, even small increments in systemic blood pressure are transmitted to the glomerulus and increase P_{GC}. The mitogenic effects of angiotensin II, aldosterone, endothelin, tumor growth factor β (TGFβ), and other growth factors result in mesangial cell proliferation and glomerular hypertrophy (206,386,387,401,402). Increased P_{GC} and nephronal hypertrophy alone or together are associated with progressive glomerular injury and fibrosis. Sustained reduction of systemic blood pressure limits glomerular damage.

Beneficial Effects of Treatment of Hypertension in Chronic Kidney Disease. Both systolic and diastolic blood pressures are continuous, strong, independent risk factors for the development of cardiovascular morbidity and mortality in the general population (403). The Prospective Studies Collaboration Group (404) developed a meta-analysis of individual data for one million adults in 61 prospective studies to examine the relationship between blood pressure and mortality. They found that, at ages 40–69 years, each difference of 20 mm Hg usual systolic blood pressure or 10 mm Hg usual diastolic blood pressure, was associated with more than a twofold difference in the death rate from stroke and a twofold difference in the death rates from ischemic heart disease and other vascular causes. The relationship existed down to a blood pressure of 115/75 mm Hg. The Seventh Report of the Joint National Committee on Prevention, Detection, Evaluation, and Treatment of High Blood Pressure (JNC VII) embraced these data in their 2003 recommendations (405). Over the past 40 years, numerous studies have clearly demonstrated that effective pharmacologic therapy significantly decreases cardiovascular morbidity

and mortality in patients with essential hypertension. Despite the fact that upward of 80% of CKD patients will have hypertension as their GFR declines (98,406), similar data pertaining to patients with CKD are scant (92). Nevertheless, it is logical to assume that existing data for the general population support an aggressive approach to blood pressure control in the CKD population. Unfortunately, the Third National Health and Nutrition Examination Survey (NHANES III) data indicate that only 11% of individuals with hypertension and an elevated serum creatinine had a blood pressure <130/85 and only 27% had a blood pressure <140/90 mm Hg (407). Patients with ESRD are at a 500-fold risk of a cardiovascular event in some age ranges (408) and the cardiovascular risk increases at the earliest stages of CKD (409–412). In fact, a patient with early stage CKD is more likely to die from a cardiovascular event than progress to ESRD (413). Thus, the ultimate goals of the treatment of hypertension in CKD are reduction of cardiovascular events and slowing the progression of CKD to ESRD. The following sections will use evidence primarily from studies of nondiabetic kidney disease to discuss the concepts of: (a) the racial disparity in ESRD, especially hypertensive renal disease; (b) the importance of dietary sodium restriction and the use of diuretics to ameliorate hypertension; (c) the appropriate blood pressure goal; (d) proteinuria as a contributor to renal disease progression and a target for therapy; (e) the primary role of ACE inhibitors, angiotensin receptor blockers, and their combination; (f) add-on therapy with calcium channel blockers and sympatholytics; and (g) emerging agents such as aldosterone antagonists in the treatment of hypertension in CKD patients.

Racial Differences in ESRD. Blacks have a sixfold greater risk of developing hypertensive ESRD compared with whites, a 3.8-fold increase in risk for ESRD owing to diabetic nephropathy, and a 2.6-fold greater risk for renal failure from chronic glomerulonephritis (414). Blacks have the highest incidence rates for ESRD but the rate of rise may be slowing (410). There are multiple potential reasons for the marked difference in the occurrence of hypertensive renal disease in blacks compared with whites. Several investigators postulate that lower socioeconomic status and reduced access to preventive health care are important determinants of the higher prevalence of ESRD, particularly hypertensive ESRD, in the black population (415,416). However, one study (350) showed that neither accurately predicted the development of renal disease, and others (417,418) contend that controlling for these factors does not eliminate the influence of race on the development of ESRD. In addition, the availability of effective antihypertensive therapy over the past two decades has decreased the occurrence of stroke and congestive heart failure in blacks as well as whites but has not reduced the incidence of hypertensive ESRD (419). Although the prevalence of hypertensive in blacks is 1.3- to 2-fold greater than whites (420,421), this fact alone does not explain the greater than six-fold increase in the occurrence of hypertensive ESRD in blacks (416,420,421). Misclassification bias could contribute to the higher prevalence of hypertensive ESRD in blacks compared with whites (420). In this regard, Perneger et al. (422) have shown that, given the same written case histories, black patients were twice as likely to receive a diagnosis of hypertensive ESRD compared with their white counterparts. However, the African American Study of Kidney Disease (AASK) Trial showed that renal biopsies in nondiabetic hypertensive blacks with mild to moderate renal insufficiency and minimal proteinuria revealed changes consistent with hypertensive renal disease in over 90% of the specimens (423). Treated hypertensive blacks have significantly elevated nocturnal blood pressures compared with their white counterparts (424), an observation that may explain their higher prevalence of hypertensive ESRD. Finally, it is possible that an inherent genetic susceptibility of certain black kindreds to develop ESRD contributes to the observed racial disparity (425,426).

Blacks with essential hypertension demonstrate greater arteriographic (427) and histologic (428) evidence of arteriolar nephrosclerosis compared to whites with essential hypertension. There are several functional correlates of these anatomic differences. Both normotensive (429,430) and hypertensive (431,432) blacks excrete less of a sodium load compared with their white counterparts. This sluggish response to salt loading is associated with a higher prevalence of salt-sensitive hypertension and lower plasma renin activity compared with white hypertensives in blacks with essential hypertension (421,431,432). Hypertensive blacks exhibit an increase in filtration fraction under basal conditions (427) and in response to dietary salt loading (432,433). Campese et al. (432) examined the renal hemodynamic response to a high dietary salt intake in 26 subjects with essential hypertension. Fifteen patients (nine white, six black) were salt resistant; 11 patients, all of whom were black, were salt-sensitive. Renal blood flow increased and GFR was unchanged with a consequent decline in filtration fraction from 21% to 19% in the salt-resistant group. On the other hand, in the salt-sensitive patients, GFR remained stable whereas renal blood flow decreased, resulting in an increase in filtration fraction from 19% to 23%. Calculated P_{GC} decreased from 58 to 52 mm Hg in the salt-resistant subjects but increased from 48 to 58 mm Hg in the salt-sensitive group. These intrarenal hemodynamic abnormalities in the latter group were due to a disproportionate increase in R_E compared with R_A in response to salt loading. Interestingly, nifedipine reversed the abnormal renal adaptation to a high-salt diet in the salt-sensitive patients (432). Hence, the renal hemodynamic response of salt-sensitive blacks to an augmented salt intake (decreased R_A with respect to R_E and a consequent increment in P_{GC}) is reminiscent of the micropuncture data in experimental models of renal hypertension and offers a plausible explanation for the enhanced susceptibility of blacks to develop hypertensive ESRD as well as chronic renal failure from diabetes or other glomerular diseases.

Salt Restriction and Diuretic Use. The pathophysiology of hypertension in patients with CKD is largely consequent to a positive sodium balance and ECFV expands as GFR decreases (434). In addition, the magnitude of increase in blood pressure in response to ECFV expansion is greater as renal function declines (141,434,435) (Fig. 51-3), but the impairment in ECFV control antedates the development of hypertension and reduction in GFR (436,437). These observations underscore the important therapeutic implications of dietary salt restriction and diuretic administration in the treatment of renal parenchymal hypertension. Sodium retention not only causes hypertension in CKD, but it also reduces the antihypertensive response to nondiuretic antihypertensive agents such as ACE inhibitors, angiotensin receptor blockers, vasodilators, and centrally acting sympatholytics but not calcium channel blockers (438–441). Heeg et al. (442) found that the antiproteinuric effect of lisinopril was abolished by increasing sodium intake but that it was restored by dietary salt restriction. Other investigators (443) demonstrated that diuretic therapy could restore the beneficial effect of ACE inhibition or nondihydropyridine CCBs (444) on proteinuria and blood pressure control that had been blunted by a high-sodium diet.

Despite the data supporting the pathophysiologic role of a positive salt balance in renal parenchymal hypertension, large, controlled, prospective studies on the effects of a low-salt diet have not been conducted with CKD patients. Although Koomans et al. (435) found that lower sodium intake markedly diminished blood pressure in patients with advanced CKD, these data have not been rigorously validated. Further, Kumagai et al. (445) showed that restriction of daily salt intake

decreased mean blood pressure by 16 mm Hg in 10 hypertensive patients with chronic glomerulonephritis and an average creatinine clearance of 50 mL/minute, but did not change blood pressure in normotensive patients with glomerular disease or in normal volunteers. Nevertheless, it is reasonable to recommend that hypertensive patients with CKD limit their daily sodium consumption to 80–100 mmol/day. Early in the course of renal disease, modest salt restriction alone can normalize blood pressure in a minority of hypertensive patients. However, diuretic therapy is required in the majority of cases and is the cornerstone of antihypertensive therapy, especially as renal function deteriorates (405,406). In the AASK trial, the importance of diuretic use, and dose, was confirmed. Patients required higher doses of diuretics at lower estimated GFR to achieve the target blood pressure for the trial (on average, 50 mg/day for GFR of 50–65 mL/minute, 60 mg/day for GFR of 50–65 mL/minute, and 70 mg/day for GFR <35 mL/minute) (446). The requirement for a diuretic to achieve goal blood pressure and optimize the antiproteinuric and antihypertensive effect of ACE inhibitors, may explain the lack of superiority of the ACE inhibitor in the ALLHAT CKD subgroup since diuretics were prohibited in the ACE inhibitor group (413).

Thiazide diuretics are effective in patients with stage 1–3 CKD (447). Loop-blocking diuretics, often in a multiple daily dosing regimen, are required to achieve an adequate natriuresis with more severe renal impairment (447,448). It is important to emphasize that the diuretic regimen should be advanced until the patient is free of edema, because even small increments in ECFV can contribute to poor blood pressure control (449). In patients with stage 5 CKD (i.e., creatinine clearances <15 mL/minute), the combination of a loop diuretic with a thiazide minimizes diuretic resistance and has a synergistic effect on salt excretion (450,451). Effective diuretic therapy alone will normalize blood pressure in approximately one-third of hypertensive patients with chronic renal insufficiency (148); the remainder require additional pharmacologic treatment. Nevertheless, dietary or pharmacologically induced salt depletion is crucial both from a pathophysiologic perspective and to limit the development of pseudotolerance if short-acting vasodilators or centrally acting sympatholytics are utilized as antihypertensive agents (452,453).

Blood Pressure Goal. Recently, the JNC VII guidelines (405) and the Kidney Disease Outcomes Quality Initiative (K/DOQI) Clinical Practice Guidelines on Hypertension in Chronic Kidney Disease (406) recommended a blood pressure goal of less than 130/80 mm Hg for patients with CKD. The stated goals of aggressive blood pressure management in these guidelines are to slow deterioration of renal function and prevent cardiovascular events. These recommendations are based on data from several randomized prospective trials. Schrier et al. (454), in the normotensive Appropriate Blood Pressure Control in Diabetes (ABCD) trial, demonstrated that an achieved blood pressure of 128/75 mm Hg versus 137/81 mm Hg significantly reduced the progression of incipient to overt diabetic nephropathy. A secondary analysis of the Reduction of Endpoints in Non–Insulin-Dependent Diabetes Mellitus (NIDDM) with the Angiotensin II Antagonist Losartan (RENAAL) study of 1,513 type 2 diabetics with overt nephropathy found an increased risk of progression of kidney disease among those with a treated systolic blood pressure of greater than 140 mm Hg compared with values less than 130 mm Hg (455). Thus, there are reasonably good data to support a blood pressure goal of less than 130/80 mm Hg in the setting of diabetic nephropathy.

Emerging data also support lower goal blood pressures for patients with nondiabetic renal disease. Schrier et al. (456) randomized 72 patients with polycystic kidney disease to either rigorous blood pressure control (<120/80 mm Hg) or standard control (<135–140/85–90 mm Hg). Primary end points were change in creatinine clearance and change in LV mass index (LVMI) as a cardiovascular surrogate. At seven years, the rigorous control group achieved a blood pressure of 119/77 mm Hg compared with 130/82 mm Hg for the standard control group. Although there was no significant difference in change in creatinine clearance between the two groups, the patients with the lower goal blood pressure had a significantly greater decrease in LVMI. A lower blood pressure was achievable, safe, and theoretically could prevent cardiovascular events since LVH is a significant risk factor for cardiovascular morbidity and mortality (457).

In the Modification of Diet in Renal Disease (MDRD) (458,459) trial, 585 patients with nondiabetic renal disease and a mean GFR of 39 mL/minute were randomized to usual blood pressure control (MAP = 107 mm Hg) or aggressive control (MAP ≤92 mm Hg). Achieved blood pressures were approximately 130/80 mm Hg versus 125/75 mm Hg, respectively. When patients were stratified according to baseline proteinuria, those with >3 g/day showed significantly slower progression of renal disease in the lower blood pressure group compared with those randomized to the usual blood pressure goal. Patients excreting between 1 and 3 g of protein per day demonstrated a modest benefit from the lower blood pressure goal while those with <1 g/day of proteinuria had the slowest rate of progression and derived no benefit from the lower blood pressure goal (459).

The African American Study of Hypertension and Kidney Disease (AASK) trial enrolled nearly 1,100 African-Americans with hypertension, minimal proteinuria (mean of approximately 500 mg/day), mean serum creatinines of approximately 1.7–2.7 mg/dL, and a clinical diagnosis of hypertensive nephropathy (460). Patients were randomized to ramipril, metoprolol, or amlodipine and to one of two blood pressure goals, 125/75 (MAP <92 mm Hg) or 140/90 mm Hg (MAP 102–107 mm Hg). At four years the groups achieved blood pressures of 128/78 mm Hg and 141/85 mm Hg. Patients randomized to ramipril had a significantly decreased risk of reaching the composite end point of a 50% reduction in GFR, decrease in GFR of 25 mL/minute, the onset of renal failure, or death (461). However, there was no difference between the two goal blood pressure groups with respect to the primary outcome of rate of change in GFR.

A meta-analysis by Jafar et al. for the Ace Inhibition in Progressive Renal Disease (AIPRD) study group (462) analyzed 1,860 nondiabetic patients to assess the relationship between systolic and diastolic blood pressures, urinary protein excretion, and progression of kidney disease. A systolic blood pressure of 110 to 129 mm Hg and urine protein excretion of less than 2 g/day were associated with lowest risk for kidney disease progression. In patients with proteinuria >1 g, the risk for kidney disease progression decreased as systolic blood pressure declined from 160 to 110 mm Hg. In contrast, patients with <1 g of proteinuria showed no significant benefit with regard to loss of kidney function over the same range of blood pressure. Finally, a long-term follow-up (mean 10.6 years) of the MDRD study found that patients assigned to the low target blood pressure (MAP <92 mm Hg) had a significantly decreased risk of progression to ESRD or a composite end point of ESRD or all cause mortality compared with those assigned to the usual blood pressure goal (MAP <107 mm Hg) (463). Collectively, the MDRD, AASK, and AIPRD study group data support a more aggressive blood pressure goal of <125/75 mm Hg among patients with greater than 1 g of proteinuria per day.

Taken together, the available data suggest that a blood pressure of <130/80 mm Hg is appropriate for most CKD patients; however, for patients with greater than 1g/day of proteinuria, <125/75 should be the goal. If a blood pressure of <125/75 mm Hg can be achieved without unacceptable side effects, all CKD patients may derive cardiovascular and renal benefit.

Reduction of Proteinuria as a Treatment Goal. Both observational studies and prospective trials support the concept that the extent of urinary protein excretion is the best predictor of future progression to ESRD (464). A 20-year observational study in a large white population found that dipstick-positive proteinuria was a powerful predictor of both ESRD and overall mortality (465). A Japanese screening study of over 100,000 people found that the risk of ESRD over a 7-year follow-up was almost entirely restricted to subjects with dipstick-positive urine at enrollment, regardless of their initial renal function (466). Whether proteinuria is a reflection of the kidney disease, or plays a role in its progression is controversial. There are data to suggest, however, that proteinuria itself propagates renal injury.

Chronic nephropathies share common pathogenetic mechanisms that contribute to disease progression that are independent of the original etiology of the renal disease. A reduction in renal mass causes remaining nephrons to undergo hypertrophy with concomitant decrease in R_A, increase in glomerular plasma flow, and increase in P_{GC} (467). This adaptation initially maintains GFR but is ultimately detrimental, causing an increase in protein trafficking (468). Filtered proteins are reabsorbed by proximal tubules and degraded by lysosomes which causes gene activation encoding NK-kappa β, MCP-1, RANTES and other proinflammatory mediators (469,470). These pathways, along with increased TGF-β upregulation by angiotensin II (471), may cause fibrogenesis and subsequent scarring. Hence, reduction of proteinuria has become an important treatment goal in hypertensive patients with CKD.

Studies of ACE inhibition and angiotensin receptor blockade in patients with proteinuric renal disease support the concept that the reduction of proteinuria, itself, should be a primary goal of therapy for these patients. Table 51-4 summarizes the salient features of recent trials that examined the effect of pharmacologically induced reduction of blood pressure, or the addition of ACE inhibition, or both on the progression of nondiabetic renal disease. Zucchelli et al. (472) conducted a prospective, randomized trial assessing the effect of captopril compared with slow-release nifedipine on the progression of nondiabetic renal disease. After a 1-year prerandomization period with conventional antihypertensive therapy during which blood pressure averaged 165/100 mm Hg, 121 patients were randomly allocated to treatment with captopril or slow-release nifedipine. After 3 years of follow-up, both groups demonstrated significantly lower blood pressure and slower decline in renal function compared with the conventional antihypertensive treatment administered during the prerandomization period. There was no difference between the captopril and nifedipine groups with regard to progression of renal disease assessed by the reciprocal of the serum creatinine, creatinine clearance, or radionuclide clearance. Urinary protein excretion was unchanged over the duration of the study in both the ACE inhibitor group and the calcium channel blocker group. The authors concluded that improved control of arterial pressure slows the rate of decline of renal function in nondiabetic renal disease and that ACE inhibitors and calcium channel antagonists are equally renoprotective. The primary results of the MDRD study (458), based on an intention to treat analysis, showed no significant difference over a 3-year period with respect to change in GFR between subjects randomized to a usual (107 mm Hg) mean arterial pressure (MAP) goal compared with a low (92 mm Hg) MAP. However, the relatively short mean duration of follow up (2.2 years), small separation of MAP (4.7 mm Hg) between the two blood pressure goals, and the greater than anticipated initial decline in GFR in the low MAP group obscured important observations. In this

TABLE 51-4

LONG-TERM OUTCOME IN RANDOMIZED CONTROLLED TRIALS EXAMINING THE EFFECT OF PHARMACOLOGICALLY INDUCED REDUCTION IN BLOOD PRESSURE ON THE PROGRESSION OF NONDIABETIC RENAL DISEASE

Study (reference)	Mean follow-up (Y)	Patients (N)	Primary outcome measure(s)	Intervention group				Comparitor group				Conclusion
				Intervention	Change in BP and MAP (mm Hg)			Comparitor	Change in BP and MAP (mm Hg)			
					Baseline	Δ	Follow-up		Baseline	Δ	Follow-up	
Zucchelli (472)	3	121	Change in renal function[a]	Captopril	166/101 121	NA −21	NA 100	Nifedipine	164/99 121	NA −18	NA 103	Both slow progression; no difference between ACEI and CCB
Kamper (515)	2.2	70	Change in renal function	Enalapril	151/92 112	−18/10 −13	133/82 99	Conventional therapy[b]	140/90 107	−4/4 −4	136/86 103	Enalapril slows progression of renal disease
Klahr (458)	2.2	840	Change in renal function	MAP 92	133/81 98			MAP 107 ← Δ MAP −4.7→	133/80 98			MAP goal of 92 not more renoprotective
Hannedouche (516)	3	100	Progression to ESRD, change in renal function	Enalapril	167/103 124	−20/15 −16	147/88 108	Conventional therapy[c]	166/101 121	−13/11 −11	153/90 111	Enalapril slows progression of renal disease
Bannister (511)	1	34	Change in renal function	Enalapril	NA 116	NA −14	NA 102	Nifedipine	NA 114	NA −8	NA 106	No difference between ACEI and CCB
Ihle (517)	2	70	Change in renal function	Enalapril	147/87 107	−8.9/4.4 −6	NA 102	Placebo + conventional therapy[d]	154/88 110	−0.7/1.4 −1	NA NA	Enalapril slows progression of renal disease
Maschio (474)	3	583	Change in renal function, Progression to ESRD	Benazepril	142/87 105	−4.5−8.0/ −3.5−5.0 NA	NA NA	Placebo + conventional therapy	144/88 107	+0.2−1.5/ +1.0−3.7 NA	NA NA	Benazepril slows progression of renal disease

Study	N	Follow-up (yr)	Endpoint[a]		BP				BP			Result
Vanessen (518)	89	3.9	Change in renal function	Enalapril	151/89 110	−16/11 −13	135/78 97	Atenolol	153/91 112	−16/11 −13	137/80 99	No difference between ACEI and β-blocker
REIN Stratum 2 (476)	166	1	Change in renal function	Ramipril	150/92 111	−6/4 −4	144/88 107	Placebo + conventional therapy[d]	148/91 110	−3/2 −2	145/89 108	Ramipril reduced rate of decline in GFR
REIN Stratum 1 (477)	186	2.6	Change in renal function, Progression to ESRD	Ramipril	142/87 106	NA NA	NA NA	Placebo + conventional therapy[d]	145/90 108	NA NA	NA NA	No difference in ΔGFR; less ESRD with ramipril
SHEP-CKD (634)	4,336	5	Cardiovascular event	Chlorthalidone	172/77	−27/7	145/70	Placebo + conventional therapy[e]	172/77	−14/5	158/72	Fewer CV events in diuretic group; lower BP achieved
Cinotti (635)	131	1.9	Change in renal function	Lisinopril	141/84	−3/0	138/84	Conventional therapy	142/85	−1/1	141/84	Lisinopril slowed decline in GFR
ALLHAT (413) GFR <60 mL/min	5,662	4.9	ESRD and/or 50% decrease in GFR	Chlorthalidone	147/83	−11/9	136/74	Lisinopril + conventional therapy	147/83	−12/9	134/73	No difference in renal outcomes
ALLHAT (413) GFR <60 mL/min	5,662	4.9	ESRD and/or 50% decrease in GFR	Chlorthalidone	147/83	−11/9	136/74	Amlodipine + conventional therapy	146/82	−12/9	134/73	No difference in renal outcomes

NA, Not available; ESRD, end-stage renal disease.
[a] Change in renal function, assessed by change in creatinine clearance, 1/SCR, GFR, or plasma creatinine.
[b] Conventional, α-blockers, diuretics, vasodilators.
[c] Conventional, β-blocker, furosemide, calcium channel blocker, or α2-agonist.
[d] Conventional, α1-blocker, β-blocker, diuretics, calcium channel blockers, or α2 agonists.
[e] Conventional, atenolol, or reserpine.

regard, secondary analyses of the MDRD data demonstrated a faster decline in GFR in patients with a higher achieved blood pressure (p <0.001), particularly in blacks and subjects with proteinuria >1 g/24 hours (459,473).

The Angiotensin-Converting-Enzyme Inhibition in Progressive Renal Insufficiency (AIPRI) study, a trial of ACE inhibition in nondiabetic renal disease patients, included 563 patients followed for an average of 3.5 years (474). The primary end point was a doubling of baseline creatinine or the need for dialysis. Patients receiving benazepril had a 53% reduced risk of reaching the primary endpoint; however, the benefit was seen primarily in those patients with >3 g of proteinuria per day. Unfortunately, there was a significant difference in final blood pressures between the benazepril and placebo group making it difficult to assign a unique renoprotective effect to ACE inhibition independent of a reduction in blood pressure.

In 1997, Giatras et al. (475) published a meta-analysis for the AIPRD study group assessing the effect of ACE inhibitors on the development of ESRD in nondiabetic kidney disease. Among 1,594 patients from 10 studies, patients receiving ACE inhibitors had a 30% reduction in the risk of developing ESRD. Again, blood pressures were lower in the ACE inhibition group casting doubt on whether ACE inhibitors themselves, or better blood pressure control, were to be credited with lowering the risk of ESRD.

Results from the Ramipril Efficacy in Nephropathy (REIN) study (476) provide the most persuasive evidence for a uniquely renoprotective effect of ACE inhibition. Three hundred fifty-two patients with chronic nondiabetic renal disease were stratified according to baseline proteinuria (stratum 1: 1 to 3 g/24 hours; stratum 2: ≥3 g/24 hours) and randomly assigned to ramipril or placebo plus conventional antihypertensive therapy to achieve a goal diastolic blood pressure less than 90 mm Hg. By the time of the second interim analysis, there was already a significant difference in the rate of decline of GFR between the two groups despite similar blood pressure control. Glomerular filtration rate decreased by 0.53 mL/minute per month in the ramipril-treated group compared with 0.88 mL/minute per month in the placebo group (p = 0.03). Moreover, reduction of proteinuria predicted the decrease in risk of doubling the serum creatinine or progressing to ESRD. The renoprotective effect of ACE inhibition was attenuated, however, in patients with only 1 to 3 g of proteinuria (stratum 1). In REIN stratum 1 the decline in GFR was not significantly different between the ramipril group (0.26 mL/minute per month) and the placebo group (0.29 mL/minute/month); however, progression to ESRD was significantly decreased with ACE inhibition (477). In the most recent analysis of the REIN data, both proteinuria >2 g and hypertension were independent predictors of a more rapid decline in GFR (478). Not surprisingly, hypertensive patients with proteinuria >2 g benefited most from ramipril. On the other hand, ACE inhibition did not confer a significant benefit to patients with <2 g proteinuria, non–insulin-dependent diabetes, or polycystic kidney disease.

With inclusion of the REIN data and the AIPRD study, a meta-analysis of 11 trials confirmed the role of proteinuria in the progression of renal disease (479). Among 1,860 nondiabetic patients with proteinuric renal disease, relative risk in the ACE inhibitor group was .69 for ESRD and .70 for the composite outcome of doubling of baseline creatinine or ESRD (479,480). Patients with greater baseline proteinuria benefited most from ACE inhibitor therapy. There was a trend toward benefit of ACE inhibition at baseline proteinuria of approximately 500 mg but the data were inconclusive. Moreover, the relative risk reduction for ESRD was greater at increasing levels of baseline proteinuria. Finally, in the AIPRD study, change in proteinuria during treatment predicted renal outcome. The 1,710 patients whose proteinuria declined had an improved renal outcome while the 638 patients without a decrease in proteinuria saw no improvement in renal outcome (481). In fact, the percent change of proteinuria at 3 months predicted the change in GFR at 31 months (482). This analysis further strengthens the concept that proteinuria is a modifiable risk factor for progression of renal disease.

In the AASK trial, subjects with >300 mg/d of proteinuria at baseline had more rapid decline in renal function and ESRD events (461). Importantly, participants with a urine protein:creatinine rate > 0.66 g/g assigned to amlodipine had a rate of decline in GFR double that of those assigned to ramipril. After controlling for randomization, baseline GFR, and change in GFR over the first 6 months of follow-up, the change in urine protein excretion rate from baseline to 6 months was an independent predictor of subsequent development of ESRD (461). Thus, the results of the AASK trial are in agreement with other important trials of proteinuric renal disease, suggesting that a primary goal of treatment should be reduction of proteinuria. Taken together, the data support the recommendation that ACE inhibitors and angiotensin II receptor blockers (ARBs) are first-line therapy in patients with CKD.

Combination ACE Inhibition and Angiotensin Receptor Blockade. Long-term ACE inhibition results in the accumulation of angiotensin I that may "escape" ACE inhibition and be converted to angiotensin II at the tissue level via alternative pathways including cathepsin G and chymase (483). Theoretically, an angiotensin II receptor antagonist would block the alternate pathway effects. Huang et al. have shown that chymase is upregulated in patients with CKD, particularly those with diabetic nephropathy (484). In addition, ACE inhibition may regulate important metalloproteinase activities in CKD patients, where ARBs are not effective (485). Thus, combination ACE inhibitor and an angiotensin II receptor blocker therapy could have additive renoprotective effects.

Short-term studies in patients with both diabetic nephropathy (486) and nondiabetic nephropathies (487–489) have demonstrated additive beneficial effects of ACE inhibition and angiotensin II receptor blockade on microalbuminuria, proteinuria, and serum creatinine. In the largest trial to date, Nakao et al., in the COOPERATE study (490), randomized 301 nondiabetic patients with a mean GFR of 38 mL/minute to losartan, trandolapril, or a combination of these medications. At 36 months patients treated with combination therapy, despite similar blood pressure control, had a 76% reduction in proteinuria versus 42% and 44% decreases for losartan and trandolapril, respectively. More importantly, the combination therapy group had a significantly lower risk (11%) of ESRD or doubling of creatinine compared with both the losartan and trandolapril groups (23%) (p <0.02). Combination therapy was particularly efficacious among patients with greater than 1 g of proteinuria per day. These data provide strong support for the concept that combination therapy with an ACE inhibitor and an ARB more effectively retards the progression of nondiabetic kidney disease compared with monotherapy with either class of drugs.

Calcium Channel Blockers (CCB). In most instances, patients with CKD will require between two and four anti-hypertensives to achieve goal blood pressure (405). Thus, the role of CCBs as add-on therapy in the treatment of hypertensive patients with CKD is important. Recent studies have demonstrated the efficacy of both nondihydropyridine (491) and DHPCCBs (492,493) in reducing cardiovascular events in high-risk patients. However, data with regard to the effect of CCBs on the progression of CKD are conflicting. In the REIN study (494), patients with proteinuric nondiabetic nephropathies treated with DHPCCBs and placebo (no ACE inhibitor) had significantly greater proteinuria when compared with patients not administered DHPCCBs. In the AASK trial (460), patients with proteinuria greater than 300 mg/day randomized to ramipril had a significantly slower decline in GFR over 3 years compared with patients treated with amlodipine. On the other hand, non-DHPCCBs reduce proteinuria and slow the rate of renal disease progression in diabetic nephropathy (495,496). However, in patients with nondiabetic nephropathies, Boero et al. (497) found no difference in the reduction of proteinuria between those treated with trandolapril and verapamil compared with those who received trandolapril and amlodipine.

Herlitz et al. (498) showed that the addition of felodipine to ramipril resulted in a slower progression of nondiabetic renal disease compared with felodipine alone without any suggestion of adverse effect from the DHPCCB. In the RENAAL study (499), patients with type 2 diabetic nephropathy who received a DHPCCB without losartan had a higher risk of reaching the primary composite end point of ESRD, death, or a doubling of serum creatinine. In contrast, patients receiving a DHPCCB with losartan showed a slower progression to ESRD than did the entire losartan arm.

In summary, CCBs are important add-on medications to diuretics and ACE inhibitors or angiotensin II receptor blockers in order to achieve goal blood pressure. For patients with significant proteinuria, non-DHPCCBs may decrease proteinuria further and thus slow progression of renal disease, while DHPCCBs are effective antihypertensive agents and may slow progression of renal disease when added to a regimen already containing a drug that interrupts the RAAS. Among CKD patients without significant proteinuria, either class of CCB is likely safe when added to an ACE inhibitor or angiotensin II receptor blocker.

Emerging Agents. Emerging data supporting an important role for aldosterone in the pathogenesis of progressive renal disease (500,501) have stimulated interest in the study of aldos-

terone antagonism in patients with CKD. Shiigai et al. (502) found that between 24% and 43% of patients had a loss of the antiproteinuric effects of ACE inhibition within months of treatment initiation. Sato et al. (503) studied 45 patients with diabetic nephropathy treated with an ACE inhibitor. Forty percent of the subjects who demonstrated an initial decline in microalbuminuria subsequently showed an increase in albumin excretion within several months. The loss of the antiproteinuric effect of ACE inhibition corresponded to an increase in plasma aldosterone. The addition of spironolactone at a dose of 25 mg/day reduced urinary albumin excretion rate and ameliorated the effect of "aldosterone escape." Rachmani et al. (504) compared the effect of spironolactone, cilazapril, and the combination on albuminuria in patients with hypertension and diabetic nephropathy. Despite a similar reduction in blood pressure, spironolactone was superior to cilazapril alone with regard to decreasing urinary albumin excretion, and the combination was more effective than either drug alone. Eplerenone, a selective aldosterone receptor antagonist, has less anti-androgenic effects than spironolactone (505). As monotherapy in essential hypertensives, eplerenone was as effective as enalapril but decreased albuminuria more effectively than the ACE inhibitor (506). Less than 1% of patients had adverse events such as hyperkalemia. Taken together, the data suggest that complete suppression of the RAAS might be an important goal in retarding the progression of CKD. However, hyperkalemia could be a limiting factor in a population that already has multiple constraints on potassium homeostasis. Thus, while the concept of aldosterone antagonism in patients with CKD appealing, randomized controlled trials are necessary to confirm the utility and safety of this approach.

Approach to Treatment. Available classes of antihypertensive drugs are shown in Table 51-5 along with general comments regarding their utility or special attributes in patients with renal

TABLE 51-5

CLASSES OF ANTIHYPERTENSIVE AGENTS

Class	Comments (References)
Thiazide diuretics	Usually not effective with creatinine clearances <25–30 mL/min (447). Additive or synergistic effect on salt excretion in severe renal insufficiency when combined with a loop diuretic (448,450,451).
Loop-blocking diuretics	Short duration of action often requires multiple daily dosing (BID or TID) in patients with avid salt retention (447,448). Continuous infusions more effective than bolus therapy in severe renal dysfunction when parenteral treatment required (448).
β-Adrenoreceptor antagonists	No significant effect on renal hemodynamics or salt excretion (519,520).
α_1-Adrenoreceptor antagonists	Salt retention (pseudotolerance) with short-acting agents can limit long-term efficacy in chronic renal failure (521). Improve lipoprotein profile.
Central α_2-adrenergic agonists	Can cause pseudotolerance. Concomitant diuretic therapy usually necessary in patients with renal insufficiency (452,513). Have therapeutic advantage because of important role of sympathetic nervous system in renal parenchymal hypertension (167,169,170,175,177).
α- and β-Adrenoreceptor antagonists	Logical choice from pathophysiologic perspective. Side effects might limit utility.
Vasodilators	Not suitable as monotherapy. Diuretics and sympatholytics required to limit salt retention and reflex tachycardia.
ACE inhibitors	Renoprotective effect independent of reduction in blood pressure (461,462,476). Cardioprotective in high-risk patients (507). Suitable as monotherapy. Can cause hyperkalemia (522). Exaggerated hypotensive effect with salt removal (522,523).
Angiotensin II receptor antagonists	Antihypertensive effects and renoprotective effects probably similar to ACE inhibitors (455,483). May be beneficial in combination with ACE inhibitors (487–490).
Calcium channel blockers	Antihypertensive effect not blunted by high salt intake (509,510). Verapamil might accumulate in severe renal insufficiency and produce acute toxicity (524).
Aldosterone antagonists	Spironolactone and eplerenone might have specific renoprotective effects (503–505). Can cause hyperkalemia alone or if added to ACE inhibitor or angiotensin II receptor antagonist (506).

parenchymal hypertension. In patients with pre-ESRD, an ideal antihypertensive agent should be logical from a pathophysiologic perspective, produce few or no adverse clinical or metabolic effects, exert a favorable effect on cardiovascular morbidity and mortality, and beneficially influence the progression of renal disease. In this regard, ACE inhibitors, ARBs, centrally acting sympatholytics, and calcium channel antagonists are particularly useful for several reasons. Because both increased central sympathetic activity and activation of the RAAS are important pathophysiologically in the initiation and maintenance of hypertension in renal disease, pharmacologic interruption of these systems is logical from a therapeutic standpoint. Angiotensin-converting enzyme inhibitors and ARBs not only inhibit the RAAS but also modulate activity of the SNS (167,170). They are rational agents from a pathophysiologic perspective, exert a beneficial effect on the progression of renal disease independent of their antihypertensive effect, and decrease cardiovascular morbidity and mortality in this high-risk population (507,508). Consequently, ACE inhibitors or ARBs should be considered as first-line antihypertensive therapy in the majority of patients with CKD and hypertension (462,478). Calcium channel antagonists effectively decrease blood pressure despite extremes of dietary salt intake (509,510) and consequently have proved effective antihypertensive agents in patients with CKD (472,511). Centrally acting sympatholytics such as clonidine or monoxidine are logical from a pathophysiologic and practical perspective (169,170,512); however, they are not effective as long-term monotherapy (452,513) and exhibit significant side effects that often limit long-term utility. Nevertheless, they are quite effective as adjunctive therapy in selected patients.

Based on the previous discussion, we recommend the following approach to the treatment of renal parenchymal hypertension. Limitation of sodium intake to 100 mEq/day or less is essential to achieve the blood pressure goal, derive full benefit from ACE inhibition or angiotensin II receptor blockade, and limit the development of pseudotolerance. An ACE inhibitor or angiotensin receptor blocker is recommended as first line therapy for all patients, particularly those with more than 30 mg/day of albuminuria or overt proteinuria. A diuretic will likely be necessary to achieve the blood pressure goal. Thiazide diuretics are effective in patients with mild to moderate renal insufficiency and creatinine clearances >30 mL/minute (447). Loop-blocking diuretics, often in a multiple daily dosing regimen, are required to achieve an adequate natriuresis with more severe renal impairment (447,448). It is important to emphasize that the diuretic regimen should be advanced until the patient is free of edema, because even small increments in ECFV can contribute to poor blood pressure control (449,452). In patients with advanced renal insufficiency (i.e., creatinine clearances <15 mL/minute), the combination of a loop diuretic with a thiazide minimizes diuretic resistance and has a synergistic effect on salt excretion (450,451). Effective diuretic therapy alone may normalize blood pressure in approximately one-third of hypertensive patients with chronic renal insufficiency (148). Dietary and/or pharmacologically induced salt depletion is crucial both from a pathophysiologic perspective and to limit the development of pseudotolerance if short-acting vasodilators or centrally acting sympatholytics are utilized as antihypertensive agents (452,453).

As necessary, a CCB can be added to help achieve blood pressure goal. A non-DHPCCB may be preferred for those with overt proteinuria. The use of a beta-blocker should be considered 'earlier' if patients have heart failure or another indication for its use. The addition of a beta-blocker may offer little additional antihypertensive effect when added to an ACE inhibitor if the pulse is greater than 84 beats/minute (514). A vasodilator or central sympatholytic agent may be necessary add-on therapy for some patients, as studies have found that as many

as four or more drugs may be necessary to achieve goal. Klein et al. (169) and others (167,175) have shown that sympathetic nerve activity is inappropriately increased in chronic kidney disease. Agents such as clonidine, or the recently studied moxonidine (170), provide theoretical benefit to CKD patients with elevated sympathetic tone.

Hypertension is a common clinical problem in patients undergoing chronic hemodialysis (525–528); 60% to 90% of patients are hypertensive at the onset of ESRD. In a large, nationally representative sample from the U.S. Renal Data System, 63% of prevalent hemodialysis patients were hypertensive. Of these, 27% of patients had stage I, 25% had stage II, and 11% had stage III hypertension, respectively (525). Several studies show that blood pressure remains uncontrolled in the majority of hemodialysis patients in the Unite States (529–531). Hypertension is clearly established as a risk factor for cardiovascular disease morbidity and mortality in the general population; however, whether hypertension is an independent predictor of survival in patients undergoing chronic hemodialysis is uncertain. Several studies show the association between hypertension and adverse cardiovascular outcomes in hemodialysis patients. In a long-term follow up of 432 ESRD patients, after adjusting for age, diabetes, and ischemic heart disease, as well as hemoglobin and serum albumin levels measured serially, each 10 mm Hg rise in mean arterial blood pressure was independently associated with the presence of concentric LV hypertrophy, and the development of de novo cardiac failure and ischemic heart disease (532). Other studies have confirmed that hypertension is a risk factor for left ventricular hypertrophy (533,534), heart failure, coronary heart disease, and arrhythmias in hemodialysis patients (535). Conversely, reduction of arterial pressure is associated with regression of LV hypertrophy (536). In addition, hypertension has been associated with stroke and cerebral infarction (537,538) and progression of atherosclerosis (539) in patients on hemodialysis. Given this adverse impact on cardiovascular events, it is surprising that several epidemiologic studies show no association between hypertension and survival, and in fact have shown that low blood pressure is strongly associated with mortality (540–542). In a national random sample of 4,499 U.S. hemodialysis patients, no association with an elevated mortality risk could be observed for predialysis systolic hypertension (RR = 0.98 to 0.99, p value not significant) (540). Similarly, in a cohort of 5433 patients followed by a national dialysis provider (Dialysis Clinic, Inc.), predialysis hypertension was not associated with an increase in cardiovascular mortality (541). In a cohort of 932 patients, the lowest mortality was associated with predialysis systolic pressure of 160 to 189 mm Hg, whereas normal to low predialysis pressure values were associated with significantly increased mortality (543). Even in home hemodialysis patients, low and high blood pressure were associated with increased mortality and patients with mid-range blood pressure values survived the longest (544). Thus hypertension is associated with increased cardiovascular events, but not increased mortality in hemodialysis patients (545). The reasons underlying this apparently paradoxical relationship between low pressure and mortality in this population have not been clearly elucidated. It is possible that advanced cardiac disease may confound the interpretation of these data. Patients with ESRD who develop congestive heart failure have a very high mortality; they also have a decline in blood pressure after the onset of congestive heart failure that is well documented in the Canadian cohort study (546–548). In addition, advancing age is associated with lower blood pressure in ESRD patients (525). Therefore, the effects of age and congestive heart failure on mortality may mask the true relationship between blood pressure and mortality in these studies. Another limitation of previous studies may have been inadequate duration of follow up. When early mortality was analyzed in an Italian study, (in the first 2 years) only low BP (diastolic BP <74.5 mm Hg) was significantly associated with mortality, a finding that is consistent with the literature. However, when late mortality was analyzed, only high BP (systolic BP >160 mm Hg) was significantly associated with mortality (549). Therefore, well-designed prospective studies of appropriate duration, carefully controlling for comorbid conditions, are needed to resolve this critical issue (550). A high pulse pressure is an independent predictor of adverse cardiovascular outcomes in dialysis patients, perhaps reflecting decreased arterial compliance in this population (551,552).

Measurement of blood pressure presents some unique problems in hemodialysis patients (553). Inaccurate readings may result from lack of standardization of blood pressure measurement (554,555). In addition, blood pressure readings vary considerably before and after dialysis and in the interdialytic period. Predialysis blood pressures correlate better with LV hypertrophy than postdialysis blood pressure readings (556). However, postdialysis systolic pressure, not predialysis systolic pressure, may be associated with an elevated mortality risk (540,541). Using multiple blood pressure readings, such as a 2-week average predialysis BP of greater than 150/85 mm Hg or a postdialysis BP of greater than 130/75 mm Hg increases the sensitivity in diagnosing hypertension compared to single readings (557,558). Despite these conflicting data, pending further definitive information, some authors recommend a target predialysis blood pressure of less than 140/90 mm Hg, unless the patient has symptomatic hypotension during or after dialysis (559). The use of ambulatory blood pressure monitoring (ABPM) has been gaining popularity in hemodialysis patients to overcome the difficulties of conventional measurements described above (560,561). Blood pressure is often low at the end of the dialysis treatment and gradually rises during the interdialytic period (562). The "nondipping" profile with the lack of normal nocturnal decline in blood pressure is common and contributes to the accelerated target organ damage in these patients. For example, Covic et al. demonstrated that reduced blood pressure diurnal variability was an independent risk factor for progressive left ventricular dilatation in hemodialysis patients (563). In addition, Amar et al., albeit in a small sample, demonstrated that nocturnal blood pressure and 24-hour pulse pressure were predictive of mortality in ESRD patients (564). Finally, the nondipping phenomenon is closely related to a high incidence of cardiovascular diseases and a poor long-term survival (565). While the overall reproducibility of the nondipper profile is variable (566), most patients diagnosed as nondippers will continue to demonstrate that profile over time (567). However, until larger studies comparing the predictive value of ABPM with conventional blood pressure measurements in predicting outcomes of cardiovascular disease in ESRD patients are available, the expense and inconvenience of ambulatory blood pressure monitoring in all hemodialysis patients may not be justifiable. Home blood pressure monitoring may be a useful adjunct in the management of hypertension (568).

While pathogenesis of hypertension in hemodialysis patients is clearly multifactorial, expansion of intravascular volume status due to sodium and water retention is thought to be the major determinant of blood pressure in this population (569–571). This concept is supported by the fact that blood pressure is directly correlated with total body water content (572), and that higher interdialytic weight gains are associated with higher blood pressure (525,573). Differences in interdialytic weight gain often contribute to seasonal variations in blood pressure (574,575). However, hypertensive dialysis patients have a higher rise in blood pressure for a given interdialytic weight gain than normotensive dialysis patients, suggesting that altered arterial compliance may contribute to the pressor response to a large interdialytic weight gain (529). The

best clinical demonstration of the importance of the volume regulation in the pathogenesis of hypertension is by Charra et al. in Tassin, France. By performing long and slow dialysis, and meticulous ultrafiltration, this group has been able to achieve excellent volume control, blood pressure reduction with minimal antihypertensive medication use, and high survival rates in their patients (576,577). Similarly daily dialysis has been shown to have a beneficial impact on blood pressure control (555). Other factors that may contribute to hypertension in hemodialysis patients include increased or inappropriate response of the renin-angiotensin system (578), over activity of the sympathetic nervous system (579), and imbalance of factors such as endothelin (580), nitric oxide (581), and other vasoactive substances including asymmetric dimethylarginine (582–585). An elevation in blood pressure in association with erythropoeitin therapy, particularly given intravenously, has been well established; however, the precise mechanism of this action remains poorly defined (586). In addition, elevated levels of parathyroid hormone may cause an elevation in blood pressure (587,588). Unlike the general population, higher body mass index has not been associated with higher blood pressure in hemodialysis patients (589).

Management of Hypertension in Hemodialysis Patients

The primary focus of management of hypertension in hemodialysis patients should be to optimize intravascular volume status (590,591); this is accomplished by a strategy of restricting salt intake, limiting interdialytic weight gain, and adjusting utrafiltration and dialysate sodium concentration to consistently attain dry weight (592). Patients who do not become normotensive by this strategy will require antihypertensive drug therapy.

Dry Weight Estimation and Maintenance

The crucial role of achieving and maintaining patients at dry weight is illustrated by the Tassin experience discussed above. In addition, patients with "resistant hypertension" may still be volume expanded as demonstrated by Fishbane et al. who showed that atrial natriuretic peptide levels (ANP) were elevated in patients with refractory hypertension, suggesting that intravascular volume remained expanded (593). When these patients were subjected to more intensive ultrafiltration, blood pressure and ANP levels were reduced, suggesting that patients were now closer to their dry weight.

A practical problem in optimizing the intravascular status of a patient is the lack of a consistent definition of, and a reliable diagnostic tool for the determination of "dry weight." Dry weight is defined as "that body weight at the end of dialysis at which the patient can remain normotensive until the next dialysis despite the retention of salt and water" (594). Clinically, this is often estimated by the weight below which further fluid removal would produce hypotension, muscle cramps, nausea, and vomiting. Other diagnostic tools that have can be used include bioimpedance (595), estimation of inferior venacaval diameter (596), measurement of ANP (597), and on-line hematocrit (598) or blood volume monitoring (599); the utility of these techniques in usual clinical practice is not well established.

At the initiation of dialysis, ultrafiltration and restriction of dietary salt intake should be used to reduce excess extracellular fluid volume while antihypertensive drug therapy is being tapered. Reduction of blood pressure may be seen several weeks following optimization of intravascular volume status—this has been described as the "lag phenomenon" of blood pressure and may be due to gradual changes in peripheral resistance (600–603). An individualized sodium concentration of the dialysate based on predialysis plasma sodium levels can decrease thirst, interdialytic weight gain and blood pressure (602). Once dry weight has been established, it should be reassessed every few months since lean body mass may change due to changes in nutritional status. Patients who remain hypertensive despite apparently reaching dry weight should be restarted on antihypertensive drug therapy.

Minimizing Interdialytic Weight Gain

Excessive interdialytic weight gain is independently associated with higher blood pressure (525,529). In addition, excessive intradialytic weight gains may result in intradialytic hypotension when large-volume ultrafiltration is attempted. This may result in symptoms of nausea and cramping and limit the amount of fluid that can be removed. Therefore, patients should be instructed not to gain more than 2.5% to 3% of their body weight in between dialysis sessions.

Daily and Prolonged Dialysis

Increased frequency and duration of dialysis, such as nocturnal dialysis, has been associated with improvement in blood pressure (604). Gentle and persistent ultrafiltration may allow time for refilling of the intravascular compartment and permits normalization of extracellular volume (605). It is also possible that intensive dialysis enables removal of pressor molecules and improves endothelial function (606). Thus, prolonged and frequent dialysis permits better control of hypertension via volume and volume-independent mechanisms (606). In addition, nocturnal dialysis has been shown to improve endothelial function (555), and induce regression of left ventricular hypertrophy (607).

Antihypertensive Drug Therapy

Antihypertensive drugs are frequently used as an adjunct to dialysis to control hypertension (526,608,609). Interestingly, Salem et al. have shown that antihypertensive treatment has a favorable effect on survival in the hemodialysis population irrespective of the level of blood pressure (610). This provocative study hints at perhaps beneficial effects of antihypertensive drug therapy at the end organ level, in addition to lowering blood pressure.

Other than diuretics, all classes of antihypertensive agents appear to be effective in lowering blood pressure in hemodialysis patients. High doses of individual medications and combination therapy are often required (611). No single class of antihypertensives appears to offer particular advantage over another with regard to lowering blood pressure (569). Observational data indicate that the use of calcium channel blockers (612), ACE inhibitors (613), and beta-blockers (614) is associated with lower total and cardiovascular-specific mortality in hemodialysis patients. Most calcium channel blockers are not removed by dialysis (615), and the use of calcium channel blockers has been associated with better graft patency (616). However, there are no randomized prospective clinical trials comparing the effects of different classes of antihypertensive agents on clinical outcomes. Pending such studies, it is reasonable that the recommendations of JNC-7 (other than choice of thiazide diuretic as initial therapy) may be used as a guideline with regard to the choice of antihypertensive drug therapy in specific situations (617). Several antihypertensive medications may require dosage modification in hemodialysis patients. The *Physicians Desk Reference* (PDR) or other sources of pharmacologic information should be consulted prior to prescription of antihypertensive drug therapy (618).

Several issues regarding ACE inhibitor therapy are unique to the hemodialysis population. ACE inhibitors can trigger an anaphylactic reaction in patients dialyzed with a polyacrylonitrile membrane dialyzer (619). In addition, ACE inhibitors have been associated with worsening of anemia and erythropoietin resistance in hemodialysis patients (620), though other reports have not confirmed this (621). However, long-term therapy with ACE inhibitors has been show induce regression of LV hypertrophy in this population (622), and may reduce interdialytic weight gain by minimizing the effect of angiotensin II on the thirst mechanism (623).

Refractory Hypertension. Several factors may contribute to resistant hypertension; these include inadequate fluid removal, excessive interdialytic weight gains, poor compliance with dialysis and medication regimens, and underprescription of antihypertensive drugs (529). In patients who are poorly compliant, three times a week supervised administration of atenolol or lisinopril may be a safe and effective technique of lowering blood pressure (624–626). Patients who remain refractory or have suggestive signs or symptoms should be evaluated for secondary hypertension (627,628). In the occasional patient who remains refractory to all conventional measures, bilateral nephrectomy may be considered (629).

Patients on peritoneal dialysis tend to have better blood pressure control, perhaps due to better ultrafiltration (630–632). Recent development of new solutions have enhanced the ability to achieve adequate volume removal in peritoneal dialysis (633).

Conclusion

In conclusion, hypertension remains a common and difficult clinical problem in patients undergoing chronic hemodialysis. Meticulous attention to optimizing intravascular volume status often results in improvement in blood pressure. Prospective clinical studies are needed to define treatment goals, and develop rational therapeutic strategies based on understanding of pathophysiology. Development of reliable and clinically useful tools to define intravascular volume may be invaluable in obtaining better control of hypertension in this population.

References

1. Bright R. Cases and observations illustrative of renal disease accompanied with the secretion of albuminous urine. *Guy's Hosp Rep* 1836;1:338.
2. Tigerstedt R, Bergman PG. Niere und Krieslauf. *Skand Arch Physiol* 1898; 8:223.
3. Goldblatt H, et al. Studies on experimental hypertension. I. The production of persistent elevation of systolic blood pressure by means of renal ischemia. *J Exp Med* 1934;59:347.
4. Guyton AC, et al. Arterial pressure regulation. Overriding dominance of the kidneys in long-term regulation and in hypertension. *Am J Med* 1972;52:584.
5. Kaplan NM. The Goldblatt Memorial Lecture. Part II. The role of the kidney in hypertension. *Hypertension* 1979;1:456.
6. Muirhead EE. Antihypertensive functions of the kidney. *Hypertension* 1980;2:444.
7. Smith MC, Dunn MJ. Renal kallikrein, kinins and prostaglandins in hypertension. In: Brenner BM, Stein JH, eds. *Contemporary issues in nephrology: hypertension.* New York: Churchill Livingstone, 1981:168.
8. Ferris TF. The kidney and hypertension. *Arch Intern Med* 1982;142:1889.
9. Hall JE, Brande MW, Henegar JR. Angiotensin II and long-term arterial pressure regulation: the overriding dominance of the kidney. *J Am Soc Nephrol* 1999;10:S258.
10. Remuzzi G, Bertani T. Pathophysiology of progressive nephropathies. *N Engl J Med* 1998;339:1448.
11. Butler AM. Chronic pyelonephritis and arterial hypertension. *J Clin Invest* 1937;16:889.
12. Pfau A, Rosenmann E. Unilateral chronic pyelonephritis and hypertension: coincidental or causal relationship? *Am J Med* 1978;65:499.
13. Smith HW. Unilateral nephrectomy in hypertensive disease. *J Urol* 1956;76:685.

14. Connor TB, et al. Hypertension due to unilateral renal disease with a report on a functional test helpful in diagnosis. *Bull Johns Hopkins Hosp* 1957;100:241.

15. McDonald DF. Renal hypertension without main arterial stenosis. Function tests predict cure. *JAMA* 1968;203:932.

16. Luke RG, et al. Results of nephrectomy in hypertension associated with unilateral renal disease. *Br Med J* 1968;3:764.

17. Vaughan ED, et al. Hypertension and unilateral renal parenchymal disease. Evidence for abnormal vasoconstriction-volume interaction. *JAMA* 1975;233:1177.

18. Delin K, Aurell M, Granerus G. Renin-dependent hypertension in patients with unilateral kidney disease not caused by renal artery stenosis. *Acta Med Scand* 1977;201:345.

19. Siamopoulos K, et al. Experience in the management of hypertension with unilateral chronic pyelonephritis: results of nephrectomy in selected patients. *Q J Med* 1983;52:349.

20. Pujadas JO, et al. Small kidney and hypertension: selection of patients for surgery. *Urol Int* 1986;41:95.

21. Gordon RD, et al. Unstimulated renal venous renin ratio predicts improvement in hypertension following nephrectomy for unilateral renal disease. *Nephron* 1986;44:S25.

22. Bailey RR, et al. Renal vein renin concentration in the hypertension of unilateral reflux nephropathy. *J Urol* 1978;120:21.

23. deJong PE, van Bockel JH, deZeeuw D. Unilateral renal parenchymal disease with contralateral renal artery stenosis of the fibrodysplasia type. *Ann Intern Med* 1989;110:437.

24. Shimamura T, Morrison AB. A progressive glomerulosclerosis occurring in partial five-sixths nephrectomized rats. *Am J Pathol* 1975;79:95.

25. Hostetter TH, et al. Hyperfiltration in remnant nephrons: a potentially adverse response to renal ablation. *Am J Physiol* 1981;241:F85.

26. Fogo AB. Glomerular hypertension, abnormal glomerular growth, and progression of renal diseases. *Kidney Int* 2000;57:S-15.

27. Kiprov DD, Colvin RB, McCluskey RT. Focal and segmental glomerulosclerosis and proteinuria associated with unilateral renal agenesis. *Lab Invest* 1982;46:275.

28. Gutierrez-Millet V, et al. Focal glomerulosclerosis and proteinuria in patients with solitary kidneys. *Arch Intern Med* 1986;146:705.

29. Rugiu C, et al. Clinical features of patients with solitary kidneys. *Nephron* 1986;43:10.

30. Oldrizzi L, et al. The solitary kidney: a risky situation for progressive renal damage. *Am J Kidney Dis* 1991;17:57.

31. Arfeen S, et al. Familial unilateral renal agenesis and focal segmental glomerulosclerosis. *Am J Kidney Dis* 1993;21:663.

32. Rodby RA, Schwartz MM. Nephrotic syndrome in a patient with unilateral renal dysplasia. *Am J Kidney Dis* 1995;25:88.

33. Brenner BM, Meyer TW, Hostetter TH. Dietary protein intake and the progressive nature of renal disease. The role of hemodynamically mediated glomerular injury in the pathogenesis of progressive glomerular sclerosis in aging, renal ablation and intrinsic renal disease. *N Engl J Med* 1982;307: 652.

34. Zucchelli P, et al. Focal glomerulosclerosis in patients with unilateral nephrectomy. *Kidney Int* 1983;24:649.

35. Vincenti F, et al. Long-term function in kidney donors: sustained compensatory hyperfiltration with no adverse effects. *Transplantation* 1983;36: 626.

36. Purkerson ML, et al. Inhibition of thromboxane synthesis ameliorates the progressive kidney disease of rats with subtotal renal ablation. *Proc Natl Acad Sci USA* 1985;82:193.

37. Anderson S, Rennke HG, Brenner BM. Therapeutic advantage of converting enzyme inhibitors in arresting progressive renal disease associated with systemic hypertension in the rat. *J Clin Invest* 1986;77:1993.

38. Ots M, et al. Impact of supplementation of kidney mass on blood pressure and progression of kidney disease. *Nephrol Dial Transplant* 2004;19:337.

39. Pelayo JC, et al. Glomerular hemodynamic adaptations in remnant nephrons: effects of verapamil. *Am J Physiol* 1988;254:F425.

40. Simons JL, et al. Pathogenesis of glomerular injury in the fawn-hooded rat: early glomerular capillary hypertension predicts glomerular sclerosis. *J Am Soc Nephrol* 1993;3:1775.

41. Yoshida Y, et al. Serial micropuncture analysis of single nephron function in subtotal renal ablation. *Kidney Int* 1988;33:855.

42. Lax DS, et al. Effects of salt restriction on renal growth and glomerular injury in rats with remnant kidneys. *Kidney Int* 1992;41:1527.

43. Yoshida Y, et al. Effects of antihypertensive drugs on glomerular morphology. *Kidney Int* 1989;36:626.

44. Dworken LD, et al. Calcium antagonists and converting enzyme inhibitors reduce renal injury by different mechanisms. *Kidney Int* 1993;43:808.

45. Tapia E, et al. Determinants of renal damage in rats with systemic hypertension and partial renal ablation. *Kidney Int* 1990;38:642.

46. Brenner BM, Lawler EV, Mackenzie HS. The hyperfiltration theory: a paradigm shift in nephrology. *Kidney Int* 1996;49:1774.

47. Robertson JL, et al. Long-term renal responses to high dietary protein in dogs with 75% nephrectomy. *Kidney Int* 1986;29:511.

48. Ashley DJ, Mostofi FK. Renal agenesis and dysgenesis. *J Urol* 1960;83: 211.

49. Maschio G, et al. Proteinuria, hypertension and renal failure in a patient with unilateral renal agenesis. *Am J Nephrol* 1987;7:243.

50. Thorner PS, et al. Focal segmental glomerulosclerosis and progressive renal failure associated with a unilateral kidney. *Pediatrics* 1984;73:806.

51. Schmitz A, et al. No microalbuminuria or other adverse effects of long-standing hyperfiltration in humans with one kidney. *Am J Kidney Dis* 1989;13:131.

52. Oberle G, et al. Mild proteinuria in patients with unilateral kidney. *Klin Wochenschr* 1985;63:1048.

53. Fernbach SK, Holland EA, Benuck I. Hypertension induced by occult renal tissue. *J Urol* 1987;138:842.

54. Argueso L, et al. Prognosis of patients with unilateral renal agenesis. *Pediatr Nephrol* 1992;6:412.

55. Moritz KM, Wintour EM, Dodic M. Fetal uninephrectomy leads to postnatal hypertension and compromised renal function. *Hypertension* 2002;39:1071.

56. Smith S, Laprod P, Grantham J. Long-term effect of uninephrectomy on serum creatinine and blood pressure. *Am J Kidney Dis* 1985;6:143.

57. Robitaille P, et al. Long-term follow-up of patients who underwent unilateral nephrectomy in childhood. *Lancet* 1985;1:1297.

58. Williams SL, Oler J, Jorkasky DK. Long-term renal function in kidney donors: a comparison of donors and their siblings. *Ann Intern Med* 1986; 105:1.

59. Hakim RM, Goldzer RC, Brenner BM. Hypertension and proteinuria: long-term sequelae of uninephrectomy in humans. *Kidney Int* 1984;25:930.

60. Torres VE, et al. Blood pressure determinants in living-related renal allograft donors and their recipients. *Kidney Int* 1987;31:1383.

61. Weiland D, et al. Information on 628 living-related kidney donors at a single institution, with long-term followup in 472 cases. *Transplant Proc* 1984;16:5.

62. Talseth T, et al. Long-term blood pressure and renal function in kidney donors. *Kidney Int* 1986;29:1072.

63. Bonomini V, Gozzetti G. Is living donation still justifiable? *Nephrol Dial Transplant* 1990;5:407.

64. Anderson CF, et al. The risks of unilateral nephrectomy: status of kidney donors 10 to 20 years postoperatively. *Mayo Clinic Proc* 1985;60:367.

65. Watnick TJ, et al. Microalbuminuria and hypertension in long-term renal donors. *Transplantation* 1988;45:59.

66. Kasiske BL, et al. Long-term effects of reduced renal mass in humans. *Kidney Int* 1995;48:814.

67. Oshishi A, et al. Status of patients who underwent uninephrectomy in adulthood more than 20 years ago. *Am J Kidney Dis* 1995;26:889.

68. Novick AC, et al. Long-term follow-up after partial removal of a solitary kidney. *N Engl J Med* 1991;325:1058.

69. Foster MH, et al. Prolonged survival with a remnant kidney. *Am J Kidney Dis* 1991;17:261.

70. Fotino S. The solitary kidney: a model of chronic hyperfiltration in humans. *Am J Kidney Dis* 1989;13:88.

71. Corvol P, et al. Renin-secreting tumors. *Endocrinol Metab Clin North Am* 1994;23:255.

72. Sheth KJ, et al. Polydipsia, polyuria, and hypertension associated with a renin-secreting Wilm's tumour. *J Pediatr* 1978;92:921.

73. Spahr J, Demers LM, Shochat SJ. Renin-producing Wilms' tumor. *J Pediatr Surg* 1981;16:32.

74. Babka JC, Cohen MS, Sode J. Solitary intrarenal cyst causing hypertension. *N Engl J Med* 1974;291:343.

75. Rose HJ, Pruitt AW. Hypertension, hyperreninemia and a solitary renal cyst in an adolescent. *Am J Med* 1976;61:579.

76. Marka LS, Poutasse EF. Hypertension from renal tuberculosis. Operative cure predicted by renal vein renin. *J Urol* 1973;109:149.

77. Peterson NE. Fate of functionless post-traumatic renal segment. *Urology* 1986;27:237.

78. Stockigt JR, et al. Segmental renal sampling and partial nephrectomy in renal hypertension. *Arch Intern Med* 1976;136:1297.

79. Godard C, Vallotton MB, Broyer M. Plasma renin activity in segmental hypoplasia of the kidneys with hypertension. *Nephron* 1973;11: 308.

80. Zezulka AV, Arkell DG, Beevers DG. The association of hypertension, the Ask-Upmark kidney and other congenital abnormalities. *J Urol* 1986;135:1000.

81. Bonomini V, et al. Hypertension in acute renal failure. *Contr Nephrol* 1987;54:152.

82. Rodriguez-Iturbe B. Epidemic poststreptococcal glomerulonephritis. *Kidney Int* 1984;25:129.

83. Cameron JS. Hypertension in glomerulonephritis. *Contr Nephrol* 1987;54: 103.

84. Birkenhager WH, et al. Interrelations between arterial pressure, fluid volumes, and plasma-renin concentration in the course of acute glomerulonephritis. *Lancet* 1970;1:1086.

85. Rodriguez-Iturbe B, et al. Studies on the renin-aldosterone system in the acute nephritic syndrome. *Kidney Int* 1981;19:445.

86. Colina-Chourio JA, et al. Urinary excretion of prostaglandins (PGE_2 and $PGE_{2\alpha}$) and kallikrein in acute glomerulonephritis. *Clin Nephrol* 1983;20: 27.

87. Parra G, et al. Short-term treatment with captopril in hypertension due to acute glomerulonephritis. *Clin Nephrol* 1988;29:58.

88. Nolasco F, et al. Adult onset minimal change nephrotic syndrome: a long-term follow-up. *Kidney Int* 1986;29:1215.

89. Meltzer JI, et al. Nephrotic syndrome: vasoconstriction and hypervolemic types indicated by renin-sodium profiling. *Ann Intern Med* 1979;91:688.
90. Dorhout Mees EJ, et al. Observations on edema formation in the nephrotic syndrome in adults with minimal lesions. *Am J Med* 1979;67:378.
91. Sinclair AM, et al. Secondary hypertension in a blood pressure clinic. *Arch Intern Med* 1987;147:1289.
92. Levey AS. Controlling the epidemic of cardiovascular disease in chronic renal disease: where do we start? *Am J Kidney Dis* 1998;32:S5.
93. Heidland A, Heidbreder E. Retinopathy in hypertension: increased incidence in renoparenchymal disease. *Contr Nephrol* 1987;54:144.
94. Campese VM, Bigazzi R. The role of hypertension in the progression of renal diseases. *Am J Kidney Dis* 1991;17:43.
95. Smith MC, Dunn MJ. Hypertension in renal parenchymal disease. In: Laragh JH, Brenner BM, eds. *Hypertension.* New York: Raven Press, 1995:2081.
96. Kelleher CL, et al. Characteristics of hypertension in young adults with autosomal dominant polycystic kidney disease compared with the general U.S. population. *Am J Hypertens* 2004;17:1029.
97. Danielson H, et al. Arterial hypertension in chronic glomerulonephritis. An analysis of 310 cases. *Clin Nephrol* 1983;19:284.
98. Buckalew VM, et al. Prevalence of hypertension in 1,795 subjects with chronic renal disease: the Modification of Diet in Renal Disease study baseline cohort. *Am J Kidney Dis* 1996;28:811.
99. Orofino L, et al. Hypertension in primary chronic glomerulonephritis: analysis of 288 biopsied patients. *Nephron* 1987;45:22.
100. Acosta JH. Hypertension in chronic renal disease. *Kidney Int* 1982;22:702.
101. Agarwal R. Hypertension and survival in chronic hemodialysis patients—past lessons and future opportunities. *Kidney Int* 2005;67:1.
102. Arze RS, et al. The natural history of chronic pyelonephritis in the adult. *Q J Med* 1982;51:396.
103. D'Amico G, Vendemia F. Hypertension in IgA nephropathy. *Contr Nephrol* 1987;54:113.
104. Subias R, et al. Malignant accelerated hypertension in IgA nephropathy *Clin Nephrol* 1987;27:1.
105. Ecder T, Schrier RW. Hypertension in autosomal-dominant polycystic kidney disease: early occurrence and unique aspects. *J Am Soc Nephrol* 2001;12:194.
106. Korbet SM, Schwartz MM, Lewis EJ. Primary focal segmental glomerulosclerosis: clinical course and response to therapy. *Am J Kidney Dis* 1994;23:773.
107. Galla JH. IgA nephropathy. *Kidney Int* 1995;47:377.
108. Rambausek M, et al. Hypertension in chronic idiopathic glomerulonephritis: analysis of 311 biopsied patients. *Eur J Clin Invest* 1989;19:176.
109. Eto T, et al. Factors contributing to blood pressure levels in chronic glomerulonephritis: an analysis of 105 biopsied patients. *Nephron* 1990;55:129.
110. Smith MC, Dunn MJ. Role of the kidney in blood pressure regulation. In: Jacobson HR, Striker GE, Klahr S, eds. *The principles and practice of nephrology.* Philadelphia: Decker, 1995:362.
111. Guyton AC. Dominant role of the kidneys and accessory role of whole body autoregulation in the pathogenesis of hypertension. *Am J Hypertens* 1989;2:575.
112. Coleman TG, Samar RE, Murphy WR. Autoregulation versus other vasoconstrictors in hypertension. *Hypertension* 1979;1:324.
113. Guyton AC, et al. Salt balance and long-term blood pressure control. *Annu Rev Med* 1980;31:15.
114. Cowley AW Jr. The concept of autoregulation of total blood flow and its role in hypertension. *Am J Med* 1980;68:906.
115. Murray RH, et al. Blood pressure responses to extremes of sodium intake in normal men. *Proc Soc Exp Biol Med* 1978;159:432.
116. Frolich ED, Tarazi RC, Dustan HP. Hemodynamic and functional mechanisms in two renal hypertensions: arterial and pyelonephritis. *Am J Med Sci* 1971;261:189.
117. Valvo E, et al. Hypertension in primary immunoglobulin A nephropathy (Berger's disease): hemodynamic alterations and mechanisms. *Nephron* 1987;45:229.
118. Valvo E, et al. Hypertension in polycystic kidney disease. *Contrib Nephrol* 1987;54:95.
119. Kim KE, Onesti G, Schwartz AB. Hemodynamics of hypertension in chronic end-stage renal disease. *Circulation* 1972;46:456.
120. Cangiano JL, et al. Normal renin uremic hypertension: study of cardiac hemodynamics, plasma volume, extracellular fluid volume and the renin angiotensin system. *Arch Intern Med* 1976;136:17.
121. Brod J, et al. Mechanisms for the elevation of blood pressure in human renal disease. *Hypertension* 1982;4:839.
122. Brod J, et al. Development of hypertension in renal disease. *Clin Sci* 1983;64:141.
123. Kramer HJ, et al. Endogenous natriuretic and ouabain-like factors: their roles in body fluid volume and blood pressure regulation. *Am J Hypertens* 1991;4:81.
124. Chen S, et al. Role of digitalislike substance in the hypertension of streptozotocin-induced diabetes in reduced renal mass rats. *Am J Hypertens* 1993;6:397.
125. Blaustein M. Endogenous ouabain: role in the pathogenesis of hypertension. *Kidney Int* 1996;49:1748.
126. Ylitalo P, et al. Effects of varying sodium intake on blood pressure and

127. Friis T, Nielsen B, Willumsen J. Total exchangeable sodium in chronic nephropathy with and without hypertension. *Acta Med Scand* 1970;188:65.
128. Davies DL, et al. Abnormal relation between exchangeable sodium and the renin-angiotensin system in malignant hypertension and in hypertension with chronic renal failure. *Lancet* 1973;1:683.
129. Feldt-Rasmussen B, et al. Central role for sodium in the pathogenesis of blood pressure changes independent of angiotensin, aldosterone and catecholamines in type I (insulin-dependent) diabetes mellitus. *Diabetalogra* 1987;30:610.
130. Weidmann P, et al. Hypertensive dysregulation and its modification by calcium channel blockade in nonoliguric renal failure. *Am J Nephrol* 1989;9:269.
131. Harrap SB, et al. Renal, cardiovascular and hormonal characteristics of young adults with autosomal dominant polycystic kidney disease. *Kidney Int* 1991;40:501.
132. Tarazi RC, et al. Plasma volume and chronic hypertension: relationship to arterial pressure levels in different hypertensive diseases. *Arch Intern Med* 1970;125:835.
133. Wang D, Strandgaard S. The pathogenesis of hypertension in autosomal dominant polycystic kidney disease. *J Hypertens* 1997;15:925.
134. Vasavada N, Agarwal R. Role of excess volume on the pathophysiology of hypertension in chronic kidney disease. *Kidney Int* 2003;64:1772.
135. Lazarus JM, Hampers CL, Merrill JP. Hypertension in chronic renal failure. Treatment with hemodialysis and nephrectomy. *Arch Intern Med* 1974;133:1059.
136. dePlanque BA, Mulder E, Dorhout Mees EJ. The behavior of blood and extracellular volume in hypertensive patients with renal insufficiency. *Acta Med Scand* 1969;186:75.
137. Cannella G, et al. Blood pressure control in end stage renal disease in man: indirect evidence of a complex pathogenetic mechanism besides renin or blood volume. *Clin Sci Mol Med* 1977;52:19.
138. Schultze G, Piefke S, Molzahn M. Blood pressure in terminal renal failure: fluid spaces and the renin-angiotensin-system. *Nephron* 1980;25:15.
139. Koomans HA, et al. A study on the distribution of body fluids after rapid saline expansion in normal subjects and in patients with renal insufficiency: preferential intravascular deposition in renal failure. *Clin Sci* 1983;64:153.
140. Beretta-Piccoli C, et al. Hypertension associated with early stage kidney disease: complementary roles of circulating renin, the body sodium/volume state and duration of hypertension. *Am J Med* 1976;61:739.
141. Koomans HA, et al. Salt sensitivity of blood pressure in chronic renal failure. Evidence for renal control of body fluid distribution in man. *Hypertension* 1982;4:190.
142. Dathan JRE, Johnson DB, Goodwin FJ. The relationship between body fluid compartment volumes, renin activity and blood pressure in chronic renal failure. *Clin Sci Mol Med* 1973;45:77.
143. Wilkinson R, et al. Plasma renin and exchangeable sodium in the hypertension of chronic renal failure. *Q J Med* 1970;39:377.
144. Schalekamp MADH, et al. Hypertension in chronic renal failure. An abnormal relation between sodium and the renin-angiotensin system. *Am J Med* 1973;55:379.
145. Schalekamp MA, et al. Interrelationships between blood pressure, renin, renin substrate and blood volume in terminal renal failure. *Clin Sci Mol Med* 1973;45:417.
146. Bianchi G, et al. Role of the kidney in "salt and water dependent hypertension" of end-stage renal disease. *Clin Sci* 1972;42:47.
147. Chrysanthakopoulos SG, et al. Hypertension in patients on maintenance hemodialysis: evaluation of peripheral renin activity and bilateral nephrectomy. *Am J Med Sci* 1972;264:9.
148. Bank N, Lief PD, Piczon O. Use of diuretics in treatment of hypertension secondary to renal disease. *Arch Intern Med* 1978;138:1524.
149. Vertes V, Cangiano JL, Berman LB, et al. Hypertension in end-stage renal disease. *N Engl J Med* 1969;280:978.
150. Charra B, et al. Control of hypertension and prolonged survival on maintenance hemodialysis. *Nephron* 1983;33:96.
151. Charra B, et al. Survival as an index of adequacy of dialysis. *Kidney Int* 1992;41:1286.
152. Leypoldt JK, et al. Relationship between volume status and blood pressure during chronic hemodialysis. *Kidney Int* 2002;61:266.
153. DiPaolo B, et al. Pathophysiological features of hypertension in CAPD: hemodynamic pattern evaluated by impedance cardiography. *Contrib Nephrol* 1994;106:186.
154. Gnol AI, et al. Strict volume control normalizes hypertension in peritoneal dialysis patients. *Am J Kidney Dis* 2001;37:588.
155. Özkahya M, et al. Treatment of hypertension in dialysis patients by ultrafiltration: role of cardiac dilatation and time factor. *Am J Kidney Dis* 1999;34:218.
156. Rahman M, et al. Interdialytic weight gain, compliance with dialysis regimen, and age are independent predictors of blood pressure in hemodialysis patients. *Am J Kidney Dis* 2000;35:257.
157. Textor SC, et al. Norepinephrine and renin activity in chronic renal failure: evidence for interacting roles in hemodialysis hypertension. *Hypertension* 1981;3:294.
158. Oparil S, et al. Central mechanisms of hypertension. *Am J Hypertens* 1989;2:477.

159. Dibona GF. Nervous kidney. Interaction between renal sympathetic nerves and the renin-angiotensin system in the control of renal function. *Hypertension* 2000;36:1083.
160. Dibona GF. The sympathetic nervous system and hypertension. Recent developments. *Hypertension* 2004;43:147.
161. Vari RC, et al. Role of renal nerves in rats with low sodium, one-kidney hypertension. *Am J Physiol* 1986;250:H189.
162. Campese VM, Kogosov E. Renal afferent denervation prevents hypertension in rats with chronic renal failure. *Hypertension* 1995;25:878.
163. Ye S, et al. A limited renal injury may cause a permanent form of neurogenic hypertension. *Am J Hypertens* 1998;11:723.
164. Joles JA, Koomans HA. Causes and consequences of increased sympathetic activity in renal disease. *Hypertension* 2004;43:699.
165. Koomans HA, Blankestijn PJ, Joles JA. Sympathetic activity in chronic renal failure: A wake-up call. *J Am Soc Nephrol* 2004;15:524.
166. Ishii M, et al. Elevated plasma catecholamines in hypertensives with primary glomerular diseases. *Hypertension* 1983;5:545.
167. Ligtenberg G, et al. Reduction of sympathetic hyperactivity by enalapril in patients with chronic renal failure. *N Engl J Med* 1999;340:1321.
168. Klein IH, et al. Sympathetic activity is increased in polycystic kidney disease and is associated with hypertension. *J Am Soc Nephrol* 2001;12:2427.
169. Klein IH, Ligtenberg G, Neumann J, et al. Sympathetic nerve activity is inappropriately increased in chronic renal disease. *J Am Soc Nephrol* 2003;14:3239.
170. Neumann J, et al. Monoxidine normalizes sympathetic hyperactivity in patients with eprosartan-treated chronic renal failure. *J Am Soc Nephrol* 2004;15:2902.
171. Beretta-Piccoli C, et al. Enhanced cardiovascular pressor reactivity to norepinephrine in mild renal parenchymal disease. *Kidney Int* 1982;22:297.
172. Zucchelli P, et al. Pathophysiology and management of hypertension in hemodialysis patients. *Contrib Nephrol* 1987;54:209.
173. McGrath BP, Ledingham JG, Benedict CR. Catecholamines in peripheral venous plasma in patients on chronic hemodialysis. *Clin Sci Mol Med* 1978;55:89.
174. Schohn D, et al. Norepinephrine-related mechanism in hypertension accompanying renal failure. *Kidney Int* 1985;28:814.
175. Converse RL, et al. Sympathetic overactivity in patients with chronic renal failure. *N Engl J Med* 1992;327:1812.
176. Zoccali C, et al. Plasma norepinephrine predicts survival and incident cardiovascular events in patients with end-stage renal disease. *Circulation* 2002;105:1354.
177. Hausberg M, et al. Sympathetic nerve activity in end-stage renal disease. *Circulation* 2002;106:1974.
178. Thibonnier M. Vasopressin and blood pressure. *Kidney Int* 1988;34:S52.
179. Cowley AW, et al. Role of vasopressin in regulation of sodium excretion. *Am J Med Sci* 1988;31:308.
180. Cowley AW. Vasopressin and blood pressure regulation. *Clin Physiol Biochem* 1988;6:150.
181. Manning RD, et al. Hypertension in dogs during antidiuretic hormone and hypotonic saline infusion. *Am J Physiol* 1979;236:H314.
182. Hatzinikolaou P, et al. Role of vasopressin, catecholamines, and plasma volume in hypertonic saline induced hypertension. *Am J Physiol* 1981;240:H827.
183. DiPette DJ, et al. Vasopressin in salt-induced hypertension of experimental renal insufficiency. *Hypertension* 1982;4:125.
184. Padfield PL, et al. Blood pressure in acute and chronic vasopressin excess. *N Engl J Med* 1981;304:1067.
185. Bussien JP, et al. Does vasopressin sustain blood pressure of normally hydrated healthy volunteers? *Am J Physiol* 1984;246:H143.
186. Thibonnier M, et al. Effects of the nonpeptide V1 vasopressin receptor antagonist SR49059 in hypertensive patients. *Hypertension* 1999;34:1293.
187. Argent NB, et al. Osmoregulation of thirst and vasopressin release in severe chronic renal failure. *Kidney Int* 1991;39:295.
188. Shimamota K, Watarai I, Miyahara M. A study of plasma vasopressin in patients undergoing chronic dialysis. *J Clin Endocrinol Metab* 1977;45:714.
189. D'Amore TF, et al. Response of plasma vasopressin to changes in extracellular volume and/or plasma osmolality in patients on maintenance dialysis. *Clin Nephrol* 1985;23:299.
190. Zabetakis PM, et al. Increased levels of plasma renin, aldosterone, catecholamines and vasopressin in chronic ambulatory peritoneal dialysis (CAPD) patients. *Clin Nephrol* 1987;28:147.
191. Manning M, Sawyer WH. Discovery, development, and some uses of vasopressin and oxytocin antagonists. *J Lab Clin Med* 1989;114:617.
192. Yamamura Y, et al. OPC-21268, an orally effective, nonpeptide vasopressin V1 receptor antagonist. *Science* 1991;252:572.
193. Gavras H, et al. Effects of a specific inhibitor of the vascular action of vasopressin in humans. *Hypertension* 1984;6:I-156.
194. Miura Y, et al. The effect of OPC-21268, an oral nonpeptide arginine vasopressin V1 receptor antagonist, on a patient with congestive heart failure. *Clin Nephrol* 1993;40:60.
195. Wong SF, et al. Sodium and renin in the hypertension of early renal disease. *Clin Sci Mol Med* 1978;55:301s.
196. Catt KJ, et al. Metabolism and blood levels of angiotensin II in normal subjects, renal disease and essential hypertension. *Circ Res* 1970;26:177.
197. Chapman AB, et al. The renin-angiotensin-aldosterone system and autosomal dominant polycystic kidney disease. *N Engl J Med* 1990;323:1091.
198. Watson ML, et al. Effects of angiotensin converting enzyme inhibition in adult polycystic kidney disease. *Kidney Int* 1992;41:206.
199. Bell PE, et al. Hypertension in autosomal dominant polycystic kidney disease. *Kidney Int* 1988;34:683.
200. Navar LG, Rosivall L. Contribution of the renin-angiotensin system to the control of intrarenal hemodynamics. *Kidney Int* 1984;25:857.
201. Mitas JA, et al. Urinary kallikrein in the hypertension of renal parenchymal disease. *N Engl J Med* 1978;299:162.
202. Wagner J, et al. PCR analysis of human renal biopsies—renin gene regulation in glomerulonephritis. *Kidney Int* 1994;46:1542.
203. Campbell RC. The renin-angiotensin system: a 21st century perspective. *J Am Soc Nephrol* 2004;15:1963.
204. Johnston CI, Fabris B, Jandeleit K. Intrarenal renin-angiotensin system in renal physiology and pathophysiology. *Kidney Int* 1993;44:S59.
205. Freel EM, Connell JM. Mechanisms of hypertension: the expanding role of aldosterone. *J Am Soc Nephrol* 2004;15:1993.
206. Hollenberg NK. Aldosterone in the development and progression of renal injury. *Kidney Int* 2004;66:1.
207. Weidmann P, et al. Plasma renin activity and blood pressure in terminal renal failure. *N Engl J Med* 1971;285:757.
208. Lifschitz MD, et al. Effect of saralasin in hypertensive patients on chronic hemodialysis. *Ann Intern Med* 1978;88:23.
209. Boer P, Koomans HA, Dorhout Mees EJ. Renin and blood volume in chronic renal failure: a comparison with essential hypertension. *Nephron* 1987;45:7.
210. Kim KE, et al. Hemodynamics of hypertension in chronic end-stage renal disease. *Circulation* 1972;46:456.
211. Onesti G, et al. Blood pressure regulation in end stage renal disease and anephric man. *Circ Res* 1975;37:I-145.
212. Vaughan ED, et al. Hemodialysis-resistant hypertension: control with an orally active inhibitor of angiotensin-converting enzyme. *J Clin Endocrinol Metab* 1979;48:869.
213. Wauters JP, et al. Uncontrollable hypertension in patients on hemodialysis: long-term treatment with captopril and salt subtraction. *Clin Nephrol* 1981;16:86.
214. Siampoulos KC, Wilkinson R. Hypertension in chronic pyelonephritis. *Contrib Nephrol* 1987;54:119.
215. Zuccala A, et al. Pathogenesis of hypertension in dialysis patients. A pharmacological study. *Kidney Int* 1988;34:S-190.
216. Yanagisawa M, et al. A novel potent vasoconstrictor peptide produced by vascular endothelial cells. *Nature* 1988;332:411.
217. Simonson MS. Endothelins: multifunctional renal peptides. *Physiol Rev* 1993;73:375.
218. Kohan DE. Endothelins in the kidney: physiology and pathophysiology. *Am J Kidney Dis* 1993;22:493.
219. Abassi ZA, et al. Regulation of the urinary excretion of endothelin in the rat. *Am J Hypertens* 1993;6:453.
220. Kon V, Badr KF. Biological actions and pathophysiologic significance of endothelin in the kidney. *Kidney Int* 1991;40:1.
221. Nord EP. Renal actions of endothelin. *Kidney Int* 1993;44:451.
222. Remuzzi G. Endothelins in the control of cardiovascular and renal function. *Lancet* 1994;342:589.
223. Miller WL, Redfield MM, Burnett JC. Integrated cardiac, renal, and endocrine actions of endothelin. *J Clin Invest* 1989;83:317.
224. Miller WL, et al. Endothelin-mediated cardiorenal hemodynamic and neuroendocrine effects are attenuated with nitroglycerin in vivo. *Am J Hypertens* 1993;6:156.
225. Kaasjager KA, et al. Role of endothelin receptor subtypes in the systemic and renal responses to endothelin-1 in humans. *J Am Soc Nephrol* 1997;8:32.
226. Rabelink TJ, et al. Endothelin in renal pathophysiology: from experimental to therapeutic application. *Kidney Int* 1996;50:1827.
227. Benigni A. Endothelin antagonists in renal disease. *Kidney Int* 2000;57:1778.
228. McMahon EG, et al. Effect of phosphoramidon (endothelin converting enzyme inhibitor) and BQ-123 (endothelin receptor subtype A antagonist) on blood pressure in hypertensive rats. *Am J Hypertens* 1993;6:667.
229. Clozee M. Endothelin receptor antagonism: a new therapeutic approach in experimental hypertension. *Am J Hypertens* 1994;7:2A.
230. Benigni A, et al. A specific endothelin subtype A receptor antagonist protects against injury in renal disease progression. *Kidney Int* 1993;44:440.
231. Pollock DM, Polakowski JS. ET$_A$ receptor blockade prevents hypertension associated with exogenous endothelin-1 but not renal mass reduction in the rat. *J Am Soc Nephrol* 1997;8:1054.
232. Cao Z, et al. Blockade of the renin-angiotensin and endothelin systems in progressive renal injury. *Hypertension* 2000;36:561.
233. Rabelink TJ, et al. Effects of endothelin-1 on renal function in humans: implications for physiology and pathophysiology. *Kidney Int* 1994;46:376.
234. Bijlsma JA, Rabelink AJ, Kaasjager KA, et al. L-Arginine does not prevent the renal effects of endothelin in humans. *J Am Soc Nephrol* 1995;5:1508.
235. Ishibashi M, et al. Endothelin-1 and blood pressure. *Am J Hypertens* 1992;5:772.
236. Yokokawa K, et al. Hypertension associated with endothelin-secreting malignant hemangioendothelioma. *Ann Intern Med* 1991;114:213.

237. Kohna M, et al. Plasma immunoreactive endothelin in essential hypertension. *Am J Med* 1990;88:614.
238. Saito Y, et al. Increased plasma endothelin levels in patients with essential hypertension. *N Engl J Med* 1990;322:205.
239. Schiffrin EL, Thibault G. Plasma endothelin in human essential hypertension. *Am J Hypertens* 1991;4:303.
240. Krum H, et al. The effect of an endothelin-receptor antagonist, bosentan, on blood pressure in patients with essential hypertension. *N Engl J Med* 1998;338:784.
241. Koyama H, et al. Plasma endothelin levels in patients with uraemia. *Lancet* 1989;1:991.
242. Kohan DE. Endothelins in the normal and diseased kidney. *Am J Kidney Dis* 1997;28:2.
243. Ohta K, et al. Urinary excretion of endothelin-1 in normal subjects and patients with renal disease. *Kidney Int* 1991;39:307.
244. Vajo Z, et al. Elevated endothelin-1 levels and persistent stage IV hypertension in a nonvolume overloaded anephric patient. *Am J Hypertens* 1996;9:935.
245. Mees EJ. The role of endothelin-1 in hypertension. *Am J Hypertens* 1997;10:825.
246. Hand MF, Haynes WE, Webb DJ. Reduced endogenous endothelin-1-mediated vascular tone in chronic renal failure. *Kidney Int* 1999;55:613.
247. Haddy FJ, Pamnani MB, Clough DL. Volume overload hypertension: a defect in the sodium-potassium pump? *Cardiovasc Rev Rep* 1980;1:376.
248. DeWardener HE, MacGregor GA. Dahl's hypothesis that a saluretic substance may be responsible for a sustained rise in arterial pressure: its possible role in essential hypertension. *Kidney Int* 1980;18:1.
249. Graves SW, Williams GH. Endogenous digitalis-like natriuretic factors. *Annu Rev Med* 1987;38:433.
250. Woolfson RG, Poston L, de Wardener HE. Digoxinlike inhibitors of active sodium transport and blood pressure: the current status. *Kidney Int* 1994;46:297.
251. Huot SJ, et al. The role of sodium intake, the Na+-K+ pump and a ouabain-like humoral agent in the genesis of reduced renal mass hypertension. *Am J Nephrol* 1983;3:92.
252. Gomez-Sanchez EP, Gomez-Sanchez CE, Fort C. Immunization of Dahl SS/gn rats with an ouabain conjugate mitigates hypertension. *Am J Hypertens* 1994;7:591.
253. Kaide JI, et al. Effects of digoxin-specific antibody Fab fragment (Digibind) on blood pressure and renal water-sodium metabolism in 5/6 reduced renal mass hypertensive rats. *Am J Hypertens* 1999;12:611.
254. Graves SW, Brown B, Valdes R. An endogenous digitalis-like substance in patients with renal impairment. *Ann Intern Med* 1983;99:604.
255. Goto A, et al. Digitalis-like activity in human plasma: relation to blood pressure and sodium balance. *Am J Med* 1990;89:420.
256. Brod J, Schaeffer J, Hengstenberg JH, et al. Investigations on the Na+, K+-pump in erythrocytes of patients with renal hypertension. *Clin Sci* 1984;66:351.
257. Kramer HJ, et al. Digoxin-like immunoreactivity substance(s) in the serum of patients with chronic uremia. *Nephron* 1985;40:297.
258. Kelly RA, et al. Endogenous digitalis-like factors in hypertension and chronic renal insufficiency. *Kidney Int* 1986;30:723.
259. Glatter KA, et al. Sustained volume expansion and (Na,K) ATPase inhibition in chronic renal failure. *Am J Hypertens* 1994;7:1016.
260. Manunta P, et al. Plasma ouabain-like factor during acute and chronic changes in sodium balance in essential hypertension. *Hypertension* 2001;38:198.
261. Bisordi JE, Holt S. Digitalislike immunoreactive substance and extracellular fluid volume status in chronic hemodialysis patients. *Am J Kidney Dis* 1989;18:396.
262. Winearls DG, et al. Effect of human erythropoietin derived from recombinant human DNA on the anaemia of patients maintained by chronic dialysis. *Lancet* 1986;2:1175.
263. Eschbach JW, et al. Correction of the anaemia of end stage renal disease with recombinant human erythropoietin. Results of a combined phase I and II clinical trial. *N Engl J Med* 1987;316:73.
264. Schaefer RM, et al. Blood rheology and hypertension in hemodialysis patients treated with erythropoietin. *Am J Nephrol* 1988;8:449.
265. Raine AE, Roger SD. Effects of erythropoietin on blood pressure. *Am J Kidney Dis* 1991;18:76.
266. Roth D, et al. Effects of recombinant human erythropoietin on renal function in chronic renal failure predialysis patients. *Am J Kidney Dis* 1994;24:777.
267. Abraham PA, Macres MG. Blood pressure in hemodialysis patients during amelioration of anemia with erythropoietin. *J Am Soc Nephrol* 1991;2:927.
268. Lebel M, et al. Hemodynamic and hormonal changes during erythropoietin therapy in hemodialysis patients. *J Am Soc Nephrol* 1998;9:97.
269. Mittal SK, et al. Prevalence of hypertension in a hemodialysis population. *Clin Nephrol* 1999;51:77.
270. Schmieder RE, Langenfeld MR, Hilgers KF. Endogenous erythropoietin correlates with blood pressure in essential hypertension. *Am J Kidney Dis* 1997;29:376.
271. Varizi ND. Mechanism of erythropoietin-induced hypertension. *Am J Kidney Dis* 1999;33:821.
272. Neff MS, et al. Hemodynamics of uremic anemia. *Circulation* 1971;43:883.
273. Abraham PA, et al. Body fluid spaces and blood pressure in hemodialysis patients during amelioration of anemia with erythropoietin. *Am J Kidney Dis* 1990;16:438.
274. Kaupke CJ, Kim S, Varizi ND. Effect of erythrocyte mass on arterial blood pressure in dialysis patients receiving maintenance erythropoietin therapy. *J Am Soc Nephrol* 1994;4:1874.
275. Bode-Böger SM, et al. Recombinant human erythropoietin enhances vasoconstrictor tone via endothelin-1 and vasoconstrictor prostanoids. *Kidney Int* 1996;50:1255.
276. Carlini R, Obialo C, Rothstein M. Intravenous erythropoietin (rHuEPO) administration increases plasma endothelin and blood pressure in hemodialysis patients. *Am J Hypertens* 1993;6:103.
277. Fellner SK, et al. Cardiovascular consequences of correction of the anemia of renal failure with erythropoietin. *Kidney Int* 1993;44:1309.
278. Ishimitsu T, et al. Genetic predisposition to hypertension facilitates blood pressure elevation in hemodialysis patients treated with erythropoietin. *Am J Med* 1993;94:401.
279. Ludwig H, et al. Erythropoietin treatment of anemia associated with multiple myeloma. *N Engl J Med* 1990;322:1693.
280. Fischl M, et al. Recombinant human erythropoietin for patients with AIDS treated with zidovudine. *N Engl J Med* 1990;322:1488.
281. Erslev AJ. Erythropoietin. *N Engl J Med* 1991;324:1339.
282. Smith MC, Dunn MJ. The role of prostaglandins in human hypertension. *Am J Kidney Dis* 1985;5:A32.
283. Shepherd JT, Katusic ZS. Endothelium-derived vasoactive factors. I Endothelium-dependent relaxation. *Hypertension* 1991;18:III-78.
284. Muirhead EE. Renomedullary system of blood pressure control. *Hypertension* 1986;8:I-38.
285. Susic D. The role of the renal medulla in blood pressure control. *Am J Med Sci* 1988;295:234.
286. Bing RF, et al. Chemical renal medullectomy. Effect on urinary prostaglandin E2 and plasma renin in response to variations in sodium intake and in relation to blood pressure. *Hypertension* 1983;5:951.
287. Moncada S, Higgs A. The L-arginine-nitric oxide pathway. *N Engl J Med* 1993;329:2002.
288. Bachmann S, Mundel P. Nitric oxide in the kidney: synthesis, localization, and function. *Am J Kidney Dis* 1994;24:112.
289. Kone BC. Nitric oxide in health and disease. *Am J Kidney Dis* 1997;30:311.
290. Tolins JP, Shultz PJ. Endogenous nitric oxide synthesis determines sensitivity to the pressor effect of salt. *Kidney Int* 1994;46:230.
291. Baylis C, Harvey J, Engels K. Acute nitric oxide blockade amplifies the renal vasoconstrictor actions of angiotensin II. *J Am Soc Nephrol* 1994;5:211.
292. Ribeiro MO, et al. Chronic inhibition of nitric oxide synthesis—a new model of arterial hypertension. *Hypertension* 1992;20:298.
293. Fujihara CK, et al. Sodium excess aggravates hypertension and renal parenchymal injury in rats with chronic NO inhibition. *Am J Physiol* 1994;266:F697.
294. Graciano ML, et al. Intrarenal renin-angiotensin system is upregulated in experimental models of progressive renal disease induced by chronic inhibition of nitric oxide synthesis. *J Am Soc Nephrol* 2004;15:1805.
295. Aiello S, et al. Renal and systemic nitric oxide synthesis in rats with renal mass reduction. *Kidney Int* 1997;52:171.
296. Varizi ND. Effect of chronic renal failure on nitric oxide metabolism. *Am J Kidney Dis* 2001;38:S74.
297. Fujihara CK, DeNucci G, Zatz R. Chronic nitric oxide synthase inhibition aggravates glomerular injury in rats with subtotal nephrectomy. *J Am Soc Nephrol* 1995;5:1498.
298. Wagner L, et al. Reduced nitric oxide synthase activity in rats with chronic renal disease due to glomerulonephritis. *Kidney Int* 2002;62:532.
299. Panza JA, et al. Role of endothelium-derived nitric oxide in the abnormal endothelium-dependent vascular relaxation of patients with essential hypertension. *Circulation* 1993;87:1468.
300. Cockcroft JR, et al. Preserved endothelium-dependent vasodilation in patients with essential hypertension. *N Engl J Med* 1994;330:1036.
301. Sander M, Chavoshan B, Victor RG. A large blood pressure-raising effect of nitric oxide synthase inhibition in humans. *Hypertension* 1999;33:937.
302. Kielstein JT, et al. Marked increase of asymmetric dimethylarginine in patients with incipient primary chronic renal disease. *J Am Soc Nephrol* 2002;13:170.
303. Zoccali C, et al. Plasma concentration of asymmetrical dimethylarginine and mortality in patients with end-stage renal disease: a prospective study. *Lancet* 2001;358:2113.
304. Vallance P, et al. Accumulation of an endogenous inhibitor of nitric oxide synthesis in chronic renal failure. *Lancet* 1992;339:572.
305. Schmidt R, Baylis C. Total nitric oxide production is low in patients with chronic renal disease. *Kidney Int* 2000;58:1261.
306. Madore F, et al. Impact of nitric oxide on blood pressure in hemodialysis patients. *Am J Kidney Dis* 1997;30:665.
307. Schmidt RJ, et al. Nitric oxide production is low in end stage renal disease patients on peritoneal dialysis. *Am J Physiol* 1999;276:F794.
308. Sarkar SR, Kaitwatcharachai C, Levin N. Nitric oxide and hemodialysis. *Seminars in Dialysis* 2004;17:224.
309. Madeddu P, et al. A kallikrein-like enzyme in human vascular tissue. *Am J Hypertens* 1993;6:344.
310. Granger JP, Hall JE. Acute and chronic actions of bradykinin on renal function and arterial pressure. *Am J Physiol* 1985;248:F87.

311. Ardiles LG, Figueroa CD, Mezzano SA. Renal kallikrein-kinin system damage and salt sensitivity: Insights from experimental models. *Kidney Int* 2003;86:S2.

312. Levy SB, et al. Urinary kallikrein and plasma renin activity as determinants of renal blood flow. The influence of race and dietary sodium intake. *J Clin Invest* 1977;60:1291.

313. Bellini C, et al. Impaired inactive to active kallikrein conversion in human salt-sensitive hypertension. *J Am Soc Nephrol* 1996;7:2565.

314. Shimamoto K, et al. Mechanisms of suppression of renal kallikrein activity in low renin essential hypertension and renoparenchymal hypertension. *Hypertension* 1989;14:375.

315. Mitas JA, et al. Urinary kallikrein in the hypertension of renal parenchymal disease. *N Engl J Med* 1978;299:162.

316. Almeida FA, et al. Malignant hypertension: a syndrome associated with low plasma kininogen and kinin potentiating factor. *Hypertension* 1981;3:II46.

317. McFarlane SI, Winer N, Sowers JR. Role of the natriuretic peptide system in cardiorenal protection. *Arch Intern Med* 2003;163:2696.

318. Kohno M, et al. Brain natriuretic peptide as a cardiac hormone in essential hypertension. *Am J Med* 1992;92:29.

319. Levin ER, Gardner DG, Samson WK. Natriuretic peptides. *N Engl J Med* 1998;339:321.

320. Weder AB, et al. Antihypertensive and hypotensive effect of atrial natriuretic factor in men. *Hypertension* 1987;10:582.

321. van der Zander K, et al. Does brain natriuretic peptide have a direct renal effect in human hypertensives? *Hypertension* 2003;41:119.

322. Suda S, et al. Atrial natriuretic factor in mild to moderate chronic renal failure. *Hypertension* 1988;11:483.

323. Takami Y, et al. Diagnostic and prognostic value of plasma brain natriuretic peptide in non–dialysis-dependent CRF. *Am J Kidney Dis* 2004;44:420.

324. Franz M, Woloszczuk W, Hörl WH. N-terminal fragments of the proatrial natriuretic peptide in patients before and after hemodialysis treatment. *Kidney Int* 2000;58:374.

325. Ishizaka Y, et al. Plasma concentration of human brain natriuretic peptide in patients on hemodialysis. *Am J Kidney Dis* 1994;24:461.

326. Nishikimi T, Futoo Y, Tamano K, et al. Plasma brain natriuretic peptide levels in chronic hemodialysis patients: influence of coronary artery disease. *Am J Kidney Dis* 2001;37:1201.

327. Whelton A. Nephrotoxicity of nonsteroidal anti-inflammatory drugs: physiologic foundations and clinical implications. *Am J Med* 1999;106:13S.

328. Lorenz R, et al. Platelet function, thromboxane formation and blood pressure during supplementation of the western diet with cod liver oil. *Circulation* 1983;67:504.

329. Johnson AG, Nguyen TV, Day RO. Do nonsteroidal anti-inflammatory drugs affect blood pressure? A meta-analysis. *Ann Intern Med* 1994;121:289.

330. Komers R, Anderson S, Epstein M. Renal and cardiovascular effects of selective cyclooxygenase-2 inhibitors. *Am J Kidney Dis* 2001;38:1145.

331. Cheng HF, Harris RC. Cyclooxygenases, the kidney, and hypertension. *Hypertension* 2004;43:525.

332. Izhar M, et al. Effects of COX inhibition on blood pressure and kidney function in ACE-inhibitor treated blacks and Hispanics. *Hypertension* 2004;43:573.

333. Tan S, Bravo E, Mulrow P. Impaired renal prostaglandin E$_2$ biosynthesis in human hypertensive states. *Prostaglandins Med* 1978;1:76.

334. Uehara Y, et al. Plasma levels of 6-keto-prostaglandin F$_{1\alpha}$ in normotensive subjects and patients with essential hypertension. *Prostaglandins Leuko-Med* 1983;10:455.

335. Ruilope L, et al. Role of renal prostaglandin E$_2$ in chronic renal disease hypertension. *Nephron* 1982;32:202.

336. Niwa T, Maeda K, Shibata M. Urinary prostaglandins and thromboxane in patients with chronic glomerulonephritis. *Nephron* 1987;46:281.

337. Schneider M, et al. Urinary prostaglandins E$_2$ and F$_{2\alpha}$ in chronic renal failure. Influence of chronic and acute changes in Na balance. *Nephron* 1985;40:152.

338. Schlondorff D. Renal complications of nonsteroidal anti-inflammatory drugs. *Kidney Int* 1993;44:643.

339. Radack KL, Deck CC, Bloomfield SS. Ibuprofen interferes with the efficacy of antihypertensive drugs. *Ann Intern Med* 1987;107:628.

340. Blackshear JL, Davidman M, Stillman MT. Identification of risk for renal insufficiency from nonsteroidal anti-inflammatory drugs. *Arch Intern Med* 1983;143:1130.

341. Whelton A, et al. Renal effects of ibuprofen, piroxicam and sulindac in patients with asymptomatic renal failure. *Ann Intern Med* 1990;112:568.

342. Perazella MA, Eras J. Are selective COX-2 inhibitors nephrotoxic? *Am J Kidney Dis* 2000;35:937.

343. Dunn MJ. Are COX-2 selective inhibitors nephrotoxic? *Am J Kidney Dis* 2000;35:976.

344. Quarello F, et al. Cardiovascular disease in elderly dialysis patients. *Contrib Nephrol* 1994;106:84.

345. Kim KE, et al. Sequential hemodynamic changes in end stage renal disease and the anephric state during volume expansion. *Hypertension* 1980;2:102.

346. Coleman TG, Bower JD, Langford HG, et al. Regulation of arterial pressure in the anephric state. *Circulation* 1970;42:509.

347. Wilson C, Byrom FB. Renal changes in malignant hypertension. *Lancet* 1939;1:136.

348. Ellis A. Natural history of Bright's disease. *Lancet* 1942;1:1.

349. Marcantoni C, et al. The role of systemic hypertension in the progression of nondiabetic renal disease. *Kidney Int* 2000;57:S-44.

350. Rostand SG, et al. Renal insufficiency in essential hypertension. *N Engl J Med* 1989;320:684.

351. Ruggenenti P, et al. Pretreatment of blood pressure reliably predicts progression in chronic nephropathies. *Kidney Int* 2000;58:2093.

352. Young JH, et al. Blood pressure and decline in kidney function: findings from the Systolic Hypertension in the Elderly Program (SHEP). *J Am Soc Nephrol* 2002;13:2776.

353. Hunsicker, LG, et al. Predictors of the progression of renal disease in the Modification of Diet in Renal Disease Study. *Kidney Int* 1997;51:1908.

354. Parving HH, et al. Effective antihypertensive treatment postpones renal insufficiency in diabetic nephropathy. *Am J Kidney Dis* 1993;22:188.

355. Oldrizizi L, et al. The place of hypertension among risk factors for renal function in chronic renal failure. *Am J Kidney Dis* 1993;21:119.

356. Brazy PC, Stead WW, Fitzwilliam JF. Progression of renal insufficiency: role of blood pressure. *Kidney Int* 1989;35:670.

357. Tozawa M, et al. Blood pressure predicts risk of developing end-stage renal disease in men and women. *Hypertension* 2003;41:134.

358. D'Amico G. Influence of clinical and histological features on actuarial survival adult patients with idiopathic IgA nephropathy, membranous nephropathy, and membranoproliferative glomerulonephritis: survey of the recent literature. *Am J Kidney Dis* 1992;20:315.

359. McManus JF, Lupton CH Jr. Ischemic obsolescence of renal glomeruli. The natural history of the lesions and their relation to hypertension. *Lab Invest* 1960;9:413.

360. Azar S, Tobian L, Johnson MA. Glomerular, efferent arteriolar, peritubular and tubular pressures in hypertension. *Am J Physiol* 1974;227:1045.

361. Azar S, et al. Single-nephron pressures, flows and resistances in hypertensive kidneys with nephrosclerosis. *Kidney Int* 1977;12:28.

362. Olson JL, Wilson SK, Heptinstall RH. Relation of glomerular injury to preglomerular resistance in experimental hypertension. *Kidney Int* 1986;29:849.

363. Brown SA, Finco DR, Navar G. Impaired renal autoregulatory ability in dogs with reduced renal mass. *J Am Soc Nephrol* 1995;5:1768.

364. Baldwin DS, Neugarten J. Hypertension and renal diseases. *Am J Kidney Dis* 1987;10:186.

365. Amato D, et al. Mechanisms involved in the progression to glomerular sclerosis induced by systemic hypertension during mild puromycin aminonucleoside nephrosis. *Am J Hypertens* 1992;5:629.

366. Bidani AK, Schwartz MM, Lewis EJ. Renal autoregulation and vulnerability to hypertensive injury in remnant kidney. *Am J Physiol* 1987;252:F1003.

367. Noth KA, Chmielewski DH, Hostetter TH. Regulatory role of prostanoids in glomerular microcirculation of remnant nephrons. *Am J Physiol* 1987;252:F829.

368. Bidani AK, et al. Absence of glomerular injury or nephron loss in a normotensive kidney model. *Kidney Int* 1990;38:28.

369. Griffen KA, Picken MM, Bidani AK. Blood pressure lability and glomerulosclerosis after normotensive 5/6 renal mass reduction in the rat. *Kidney Int* 2004;65:209.

370. Neugarten J, et al. Aggravation of experimental glomerulonephritis by superimposed clip hypertension. *Kidney Int* 1982;22:257.

371. Raij L, Azar S, Keane W. Mesangial immune injury, hypertension, and progressive glomerular damage in Dahl rats. *Kidney Int* 1984;26:137.

372. Mauer SM, et al. The effects of Goldblatt hypertension on development of the glomerular lesions of diabetes mellitus in the rat. *Diabetes* 1978;27:738.

373. Dworken LD, Feiner HD. Glomerular injury in uninephrectomized spontaneously hypertensive rats. A consequence of glomerular capillary hypertension. *J Clin Invest* 1986;77:797.

374. Zatz R, et al. Prevention of diabetic glomerulopathy by pharmacological amelioration of glomerular capillary hypertension. *J Clin Invest* 1987;77:1925.

375. Simons JL, et al. Pathogenesis of glomerular injury in the fawn-hooded rat: effect of unilateral nephrectomy. *J Am Soc Nephrol* 1993;4:1362.

376. Simons JL, et al. Modulation of glomerular hypertension defines susceptibility to progressive glomerular injury. *Kidney Int* 1994;46:396.

377. Anderson S. Systemic and glomerular hypertension in progressive renal disease. *Kidney Int* 1988;34:S-119.

378. Benstein JA, et al. Superiority of salt restriction over diuretics in reducing renal hypertrophy and injury in uninephrectomized SHR. *Am J Physiol* 1990;258:F1675.

379. Dworken LD. Effects of calcium antagonists on glomerular hemodynamics and structure in experimental hypertension. *Am J Kidney Dis* 1991;17:89.

380. Brown SA, et al. Long-term effects of antihypertensive regimens on renal hemodynamics and proteinuria. *Kidney Int* 1993;43:1210.

381. Benigni A, et al. Renoprotective effect of contemporary blocking of angiotensin II and endothelin-1 in rats with membranous nephropathy. *Kidney Int* 1998;54:353.

382. Bidani AK, Griffin KA. Pathophysiology of hypertensive renal damage: implications for therapy. *Hypertension* 2004;44:595.

383. Harris RC, et al. The role of physical forces in alterations of mesangial cell function. *Kidney Int* 1994;45:S-17.

384. Cortes P, et al. Glomerular volume expansion and mesangial cell mechanical strain: mediators of glomerular pressure injury. *Kidney Int* 1994;45:S-11.

385. Kakinuma Y, et al. Blood pressure-independent effect of angiotensin inhibition on vascular lesions of chronic renal failure. *Kidney Int* 1992;42:46.
386. Wolf G, Neilson EG. Angiotensin II as a renal growth factor. *J Am Soc Nephrol* 1993;3:1531.
387. Simonson MS, et al. Endothelin stimulates phospholipase C, Na$^+$H$^+$ exchange, c-fos expression, and mitogenesis in rat mesangial cells. *J Clin Invest* 1989;83:708.
388. Orisio S, et al. Renal endothelin gene expression is increased in remnant kidney and correlates with disease progression. *Kidney Int* 1993;43:354.
389. Lafayette RA, et al. Angiotensin II receptor blockade limits glomerular injury in rats with reduced renal mass. *J Clin Invest* 1992;90:766.
390. Griffin KA, Picken PM, Bidani AK. Deleterious effects of calcium channel blockers on pressure transmission and glomerular injury in rat remnant kidneys. *J Clin Invest* 1995;96:793.
391. Dworkin LD, et al. Renal vascular effects of antihypertensive therapy in uninephrectomized SHR. *Kidney Int* 1989;35:790.
392. Dworkin LD, et al. Effects of nifedipine and enalapril on glomerular structure and function in uninephrectomized SHR. *Kidney Int* 1991;39:1112.
393. Nakamura T, et al. Blocking angiotensin II ameliorates proteinuria and glomerular lesions in progressive mesangioproliferative glomerulonephritis. *Kidney Int* 1999;55:877.
394. Bidani AK, et al. Lack of blood pressure independent protection by renin-angiotensin system blockade after renal ablation. *Kidney Int* 2000;57:1651.
395. Adamczak M, et al. Reversal of glomerulosclerosis after high-dose enalapril treatment in subtotally nephrectomized rats. *Kidney Int* 2003;14:2833.
396. Perico N, et al. Evidence that an angiotensin-converting enzyme inhibitor has a different effect on glomerular injury according to the different phase of the disease at which the treatment is started. *J Am Soc Nephrol* 1994;5:1139.
397. Griffin KA, et al. Class differences in the effects of calcium channel blockers in the rat remnant kidney model. *Kidney Int* 1999;55:1849.
398. Tolins JP, Raij L. Comparison of converting enzyme inhibitor and calcium channel blocker in hypertensive glomerular injury. *Hypertension* 1990;16:452.
399. Dworken LD, et al. Effects of nifedipine and enalapril on glomerular injury in rats with deoxycorticosterone-salt hypertension. *Am J Physiol* 1990;259:F598.
400. Tobilli JE, et al. ACE inhibitor and angiotensin type I receptor antagonist in combination reduce renal damage in obese Zucker rats. *Kidney Int* 2004;65:2343.
401. Junard A, Rosenberg ME, Hostetter TH. Interaction of angiotensin II (AII) and transforming growth factor Beta (TGFβ) in the remnant kidney. *J Am Soc Nephrol* 1993;4:772.
402. Mackie FE, Meyer TW, Campbell DJ. Effects of antihypertensive therapy on intrarenal angiotensin and bradykinin levels in experimental renal insufficiency. *Kidney Int* 2002;61:555.
403. Stamler J, Stamler R, Neaton JD. Blood pressure, systolic and diastolic, and cardiovascular risks. U.S. population data. *Arch Intern Med* 1993;153:598.
404. Lewington S, et al. Age specific relevance of usual blood pressure to vascular mortality: a meta-analysis of individual data for one million adults in 61 prospective studies. *Lancet* 2000;360:1903.
405. Chobanian AV, et al. The Seventh Report of the Joint National Committee on Prevention, Detection, Evaluation, and Treatment of High Blood Pressure: the JNC 7 report. *JAMA* 2003;289(19):2560.
406. Clinical Practice Guidelines on Hypertension and Antihypertensive Agents in Chronic Kidney Disease. *Am J Kidney Dis* 2004;5(Suppl 1):43.
407. Coresh J, et al. Prevalence of high blood pressure and elevated serum creatinine level in the United States: findings from the third National Health and Nutrition Examination Survey (1988–1994). *Arch Intern Med* 2001;161(9):1207.
408. Foley RN, Parfrey PS, Sarnak MJ. Clinical epidemiology of cardiovascular disease in chronic renal disease. *Am J Kidney Dis* 1998;32(5 Suppl 3):S112.
409. Ma KW, Greene EL, Raij L. Cardiovascular risk factors in chronic renal failure and hemodialysis populations. *Am J Kidney Dis* 1992;19:505.
410. USRDS 2004 Annual Data Report. *Am J Kidney Dis* 2005;45(1 Suppl 1).
411. Jungers P, et al. Incidence and risk factors of atherosclerotic cardiovascular accidents in predialysis chronic renal failure patients: a prospective study. *Nephrol Dial Transplant* 1997;12:2597.
412. Go AS, et al. Chronic Kidney Disease and the Risks of Death, Cardiovascular Events, and Hospitalization. *N Eng J Med* 2004;351:1296.
413. Rahman M, et al. Cardiovascular disease (CVD) outcomes in hypertensive patients with renal disease (ALLHAT substudy). *Am J Kidney Dis* 2003;41:A31.
414. U.S. Renal Data System, USRDS 1994 Annual Data Report IV. Incidence and causes of treated ESRD. *Am J Kidney Dis* 1994;24:S48.
415. Rostand SG. U.S. minority groups and end-stage renal disease: a disproportionate share. *Am J Kidney Dis* 1992;19:411.
416. Feldman HI, et al. End stage renal disease in U.S. minority groups. *Am J Kidney Dis* 1992;19:397.
417. Brancati FL, et al. The excess incidence of diabetic end stage renal disease among blacks. A population based study of potential explanatory factors. *JAMA* 1991;268:3079.
418. Whittle J, Whelton PK, Klag MJ. Does racial variation in risk factors explain black-white differences in hypertensive end-stage renal disease? *Arch Intern Med* 1991;151:1359.
419. Blythe WB, Maddux FW. Hypertension as a causative diagnosis of patients entering end stage renal disease programs in the United States from 1980 to 1986. *Am J Kidney Dis* 1991;18:33.
420. Smith SR, Svetkey LP, Dennis VW. Racial differences in the incidence and progression of renal disease. *Kidney Int* 1991;49:815.
421. Rahman M, Douglas JG, Wright JT. Pathophysiology and treatment implications of hypertension in the African-American population. *Endocrinol Metab Clin North Am* 1997;26:125.
422. Perneger TV, et al. Diagnosis of hypertensive renal disease in blacks and whites. *J Am Soc Nephrol* 1993;4:256.
423. Fogo A, et al. Accuracy of the diagnosis of hypertensive nephrosclerosis in African Americans: a report from the African American Study of Kidney Disease (AASK) Trial. *Kidney Int* 1997;51:244.
424. Hebert LA, et al. Nocturnal blood pressure in treated hypertensive African Americans compared to treated European Americans. *J Am Soc Nephrol* 1996;7:2130.
425. Freedman BI, et al. The familial risk of end stage renal disease in African Americans. *Am J Kidney Dis* 1993;21:387.
426. Bergman S, et al. Kidney disease in first-degree relatives of African Americans with hypertensive end-stage renal disease. *Am J Kidney Dis* 1996;27:341.
427. Levy SB, et al. Renal vasculature in essential hypertension: racial differences. *Ann Intern Med* 1978;88:12.
428. Tracy RE, et al. Nephrosclerosis in three cohorts of black and white men born in 1925–1944, 1934–1953, and 1943–1962. *Am J Hypertens* 1993;6:185.
429. Luft FC, et al. Differences in response to sodium administration in normotensive white and black subjects. *J Lab Clin Med* 1977;90:555.
430. Luft FC, et al. Salt sensitivity and resistance of blood pressure: age and race as factors in physiologic responses. *Hypertension* 1991;17:1102.
431. Weinberger MH, et al. Definitions and characteristics of sodium sensitivity and blood pressure resistance. *Hypertension* 1986;8:II-127.
432. Campese VM, et al. Abnormal renal hemodynamics in black salt-sensitive patients with hypertension. *Hypertension* 1991;18:805.
433. Weir MR. Salt intake and hypertensive renal injury in African Americans: a therapeutic perspective. *Am J Hypertens* 1995;8:635.
434. Vasavada N, Agarwal R. Role of excess volume in the pathophysiology of hypertension in chronic kidney disease. *Kidney Int* 2003;64(5):1772.
435. Koomans HA, et al. Sodium balance in renal failure. A comparison of patients with normal subjects under extremes of sodium intake. *Hypertension* 1985;7:714.
436. Cianciaruso B, et al. Renal adaptation to dietary sodium restriction in moderate renal failure resulting from chronic glomerular disease. *J Am Soc Nephrol* 1996;7:306.
437. Konishi Y, et al. Sodium sensitivity of blood pressure appearing before hypertension and related to histological damage in IgA nephropathy. *Hypertension* 2001;38:81.
438. Jerums G, et al. ACE inhibition and calcium channel blockade in incipient diabetic nephropathy. *Kidney Int* 1992;41:904.
439. Singer DR, et al. Reduction of salt intake during ACE inhibitor treatment compared with hydrochlorothiazide. *Hypertension* 1995;25:1042.
440. Navis G, et al. Moderate sodium restriction in hypertensive subjects: Renal effects of ACE-inhibition. *Kidney Int* 1985;31:815.
441. Weir MR. The influence of dietary salt on the antiproteinuric effect of calcium channel blockers. *Am J Kidney Dis* 1997;(5):800.
442. Heeg JE, et al. Efficacy and variability of the antiproteinuric effect of ACE inhibition by lisinopril. *Kidney Int* 1989;36:272.
443. Buter H, et al. The blunting of the antiproteinuric efficacy of ACE inhibition by high sodium intake can be restored by hydrochlorothiazide. *Nephrol Dial Transplant* 1998;13(7):1682.
444. Bakris GL, Smith A. Effects of sodium intake on albumin excretion in patients with diabetic nephropathy treated with long-acting calcium antagonists. *Arch Intern Med* 1996;125:201.
445. Kumagai H, et al. Effects of salt restriction on blood volume, hemodynamics, and humoral factors in hypertensive patients with chronic glomerulonephritis. *Am J Hypertens* 1989;2:699.
446. Wright JT, et al. Successful blood pressure control in the African American Study of Kidney Disease and Hypertension. *Arch Intern Med* 2002;162:1636.
447. Ellison DH. Diuretic drugs and the treatment of edema: from clinic to bench and back again. *Am J Kidney Dis* 1994;23:623.
448. Brater DC. Diuretic therapy. *N Engl J Med* 1998;339:387.
449. Ulvila JM, et al. Blood pressure in chronic renal failure: effect of sodium intake and furosemide. *JAMA* 1972;220:233.
450. Ellison DH. The physiologic basis of diuretic synergism: its role in treating diuretic resistance. *Ann Intern Med* 1991;114:886.
451. Fliser D, et al. Coadministration of thiazides increases the efficacy of loop diuretics even in patients with advanced renal failure. *Kidney Int* 1994;46:482.
452. Finnerty FA, et al. Influence of extracellular volume on response to antihypertensive drugs. *Circ Res* 1970;26:71.
453. Dustan HP, Tarazi RC, Bravo EL. Dependence of arterial pressure on intravascular volume in treated hypertensive patients. *N Engl J Med* 1972;286:861.

454. Schrier RW, et al. Effects of aggressive blood pressure control in normotensive type 2 diabetic patients on albuminuria, retinopathy, and stroke. *Kidney Int* 2002;61:1086

455. Bakris GL, et al. RENAAL Study Group. Effects of blood pressure level on progression of diabetic nephropathy: results from the RENAAL study. *Arch Intern Med* 2003;163:1555.

456. Schrier R, et al. Cardiac and renal effects of standard versus rigorous blood pressure control in autosomal-dominant polycystic kidney disease: results of a seven-year prospective randomized study. *J Am Soc Nephrol* 2002;13:1733.

457. Kannel WB. LVH as a risk factor: the Framingham experience. *J Hypertens* 1991;9(Suppl):S3.

458. Klahr S et al. The effects of dietary protein restriction and blood pressure control on the progression of renal disease. *N Engl J Med* 1994;330:877.

459. Peterson JC, et al. Blood pressure control, proteinuria, and the progression of renal disease. The Modification of Diet in Renal Disease Study. *Ann Intern Med* 1995;123:754.

460. Agodoa LY, et al. Effect of ramipril vs amlodipine on renal outcomes in hypertensive nephrosclerosis (AASK). *JAMA* 2001;285:2719.

461. Wright JT, et al. Effect of blood pressure lowering and antihypertensive drug class on progression of hypertensive kidney disease: results from the AASK trial. *JAMA* 2002;288:2421.

462. Jafar TH, et al. Progression of chronic kidney disease: the role of blood pressure control, proteinuria, and angiotensin-converting enzyme inhibition: a patient-level meta-analysis. *Ann Intern Med* 2003;139(4):244.

463. Sarnak MJ, et al. The effect of a lower target blood pressure on the progression of kidney disease: long-term follow-up of the Modification of Diet in Renal Disease study. *Ann Intern Med* 2005;142:342.

464. Ruggenenti P, et al. Urinary protein excretion rate is the best independent predictor to ESRF in non-diabetic chronic nephropathies. *Kidney Int* 1998;57:1209.

465. Tarver-Carr ME, et al. Proteinuria and the risk of chronic kidney disease (CKD) in the United States. *J Am Soc Nephrol* 2000;11:168A.

466. Iseki K, et al. Relationship between predicted GFR and proteinuria on the risk of developing ESRD in Okinawa, Japan. *Kidney Int* (in press).

467. Remuzzi G, Bertani T. Pathophysiology of progressive nephropathies. *N Engl J Med* 1998;339(20):1448.

468. Remuzzi G, Bertani T. Is glomerulosclerosis a consequence of altered glomerular permeability to macromolecules? *Kidney Int* 1990;38:384.

469. Wang Y, et al. Induction of MCP-1 in proximal tubular cells by proteinuria. *J Am Soc Nephrol* 1997;8:1537.

470. Zoja C, et al. Protein overload stimulates RANTES production by proximal tubular cells depending on NF-κB activation. *Kidney Int* 1998;53:1608.

471. Eddy A. Molecular insights into renal interstitial fibrosis. *J Am Soc Nephrol* 1996;7:2495.

472. Zucchelli P et al. Long-term comparison between captopril and nifedipine in the progression of renal insufficiency. *Kidney Int* 1992;42:452.

473. Hebert L, et al. Effects of blood pressure control on progressive renal disease in blacks and whites. *Hypertension* 1997;30:428.

474. Maschio G, et al. The effect of the angiotensin-converting enzyme inhibitor benazepril on the progression of chronic renal insufficiency. *N Engl J Med* 1996;334:939.

475. Giatras I, Lau J, Levy AS. Effect of angiotensin-converting enzyme inhibitors on progression of nondiabetic renal disease: a meta-analysis of randomized trials. *Ann Intern Med* 1997;127:337.

476. The GISEN Group. Randomized placebo controlled trial of effect of ramipril on decline in glomerular filtration rate and risk of terminal renal failure in proteinuric, nondiabetic nephropathy. *Lancet* 1997;349:1857.

477. Ruggenenti P et al. Renoprotective properties of ACE inhibitors in non-diabetic nephropathy with non-nephrotic proteinuria. *Lancet* 1999;354:359.

478. Ruggenenti P, et al. Chronic proteinuric nephropathies: Outcomes and response to treatment in a prospective cohort of 352 patients with different patterns of renal injury. *Am J Kidney Dis* 2000;35:1155.

479. Jafar TH, et al. Angiotensin-converting enzyme inhibition and progression of renal disease: Proteinuria as a modifiable risk factor for the progression of non-diabetic renal disease. AIPRD Study Group. *Kidney Int* 2001;60:1131.

480. Jafar TH, et al. Angiotensin-converting enzyme inhibitors and progression of nondiabetic renal disease. A meta-analysis of patient-level data. *Ann Intern Med* 2001;135:73.

481. Ruggenenti P. Progression, remission, regression of chronic renal diseases. *Lancet* 2001;357:1601.

482. Ruggenenti P, et al. Retarding progression of chronic renal disease: the neglected issue of residual proteinuria. *Kidney Int* 2003;63:2254.

483. Taal MW, Brenner BM. Renoprotective benefits of RAS inhibition: from ACEI to angiotensin II antagonists. *Kidney Int* 2000;57(5):1803.

484. Huang XR, et al. Chymase is upregulated in diabetic nephropathy. *J Am Soc Nephrol* 2003;14:1738.

485. Lods N, et al. ACE inhibition but not angiotensin II receptor blockade regulates matric metalloproteinase activity in patients with glomerulonephritis. *J Am Soc Nephrol* 2003;14:2861.

486. Mogensen CE, et al. Randomized control trial of dual blockade of renin angiotensin system in patients with hypertension, microalbuminuria, and non-insulin dependent diabetes: the CALM study. *BMJ* 2000;321:1440.

487. Russo D, et al. Additive antiproteinuric effect of converting enzyme inhibitor and losartan in normotensive patients with IgA nephritis. *Am J Kidney Dis* 1999;33:851.

488. Woo KT, et al. ACEI/ATRA therapy decreases proteinuria by improved glomerular permselectivity in IgA nephritis. *Kidney Int* 2000;58:2485.

489. Rutkowski P, et al. Low-dose dual blockade of the renin-angiotensin system in patients with primary glomerulonephritis. *Am J Kidney Dis* 2004;43:260.

490. Nakao N, et al. Combination treatment of angiotensin II receptor blocker and ACE inhibitor in non-diabetic renal disease (COOPERATE). *The Lancet* 2003;361:117.

491. Black HR, et al. Principal results of the controlled onset verapamil investigation of cardiovascular end points trial (CONVINCE). *JAMA* 2003;289:2073.

492. Julius S, et al. Outcomes in hypertensive patients at high cardiovascular risk treated with regimens based on valsartan or amlodipine: the VALUE randomized trial. *Lancet* 2004;363:2022.

493. Nissen SE, et al. Effect of antihypertensive agents on cardiovascular events in patients with coronary disease and normal blood pressure (CAMELOT). *JAMA* 2004;292:2217.

494. Ruggenenti P, et al. Effects of dihydropyridine calcium channel blockers, ACE inhibition, and blood pressure control on chronic nondiabetic nephropathies. *J Am Soc Nephrol* 1998;9:2096.

495. Bakris GL, et al. Effects of an ACE inhibitor/calcium antagonist combination on proteinuria in diabetic nephropathy. *Kidney Int* 1998;54:1289.

496. Bakris GL, et al. Calcium channel blockers versus other antihypertensive therapies on progression of NIDDM associated nephropathy. *Kidney Int* 1996;50:1641.

497. Boero R, et al. The verapamil versus amlodipine in nondiabetic nephropathies treated with trandolapril study (VVANNTT). *Am J Kidney Dis* 2003;42:67.

498. Herlitz H, et al. The effects of an ACE inhibitor and a calcium antagonist on the progression of renal disease: the Nephros study. *Nephrol Dial Transplant* 2001;16:2158.

499. Bakris GL, et al. Effects of blood pressure level on progression of diabetic nephropathy: results from the RENAAL study. *Ann Intern Med* 2003;163:1555.

500. Epstein M. Aldosterone and the hypertensive kidney: its emerging role as a mediator of progressive renal dysfunction: a paradigm shift. *J Hypertens* 2001;19:829.

501. Epstein M. Aldosterone as a mediator of progressive renal disease: pathogenetic and clinical implications. *Am J Kidney Dis* 2001;37:677.

502. Shiigai T, et al. Late escape effect from the antiproteinuric effect of ACE inhibitors in nondiabetic renal disease. *Am J Kidney Dis* 2001;37:477.

503. Sato A, et al. Effectiveness of aldosterone blockade in patients with diabetic nephropathy. *Hypertension* 2003;41:64.

504. Rachmani R, et al. The effect of spironolactone, cilazapril, and their combination on albuminuria in patients with hypertension and diabetic nephropathy is independent of blood pressure reduction. *Diab Med* 2004;21:471.

505. Krum H, et al. Efficacy of eplerenone added to renin-angiotensin blockade in hypertensive patients. *Hypertension* 2002;40:117.

506. Williams GH, et al. Efficacy of eplerenone versus enalapril as monotherapy in systemic hypertension. *Am J Cardiol.* 2004;93(8):990.

507. The Heart Outcomes Prevention Evaluation Study Investigators. Effects of an angiotensin-converting enzyme inhibitor, ramipril, on cardiovascular events in high risk patients. *N Engl J Med* 2000;342:145.

508. Estacio RO, et al. The effect of nisoldipine as compared with enalapril in cardiovascular outcomes in patients with non-insulin-dependent diabetes and hypertension. *N Engl J Med* 1998;338:645.

509. Nicholson JB, Resnick LM, Laragh JH. The antihypertensive effect of verapamil at extremes of dietary sodium intake. *Ann Intern Med* 1987;107:329.

510. MacGregor GA. Nifedipine, sodium intake, diuretics, and sodium balance. *Am J Nephrol* 1987;7:44.

511. Bannister KM, et al. Effect of angiotensin-converting enzyme and calcium channel inhibition on progression of IgA nephropathy. *Contrib Nephrol* 1995;111:184.

512. Rahman M, Smith MC. Chronic renal insufficiency: a diagnostic and therapeutic approach. *Arch Intern Med* 1998;158:1743.

513. Ikeda T, et al. Effects of guanfacine monotherapy on blood pressure, heart rate, plasma renin activity, aldosterone, and catecholamines in hypertensive patients with chronic glomerulonephritis. *Clin Pharmacol Ther* 1988;43:228.

514. Belz GG, et al. Influence of the ACE inhibitor cilazapril, the beta blocker propranolol, and their combination in haemodynamics in hypertension. *J Hypertens* 1989;7:817.

515. Kamper AL, Strangaard S, Leyssac PP. Effect of ramipril on the progression of chronic renal failure. A randomized controlled trial. *Am J Hypertens* 1992;5:423.

516. Hannedouche T, et al. Randomized controlled trial of enalapril and β blockers in nondiabetic chronic renal failure. *Br Med J* 1994;309:833.

517. Ihle BU, et al. Angiotensin-converting enzyme inhibition in nondiabetic progressive renal insufficiency: a controlled double-blind trial. *Am J Kidney Dis* 1996;27:489.

518. Van Essen GG, et al. Are angiotensin-converting enzyme inhibitors superior to beta blockers in retarding progressive renal function decline? *Kidney Int* 1997;63:S58.

519. Weber MA, Drayer JI. Renal effects of beta-adrenoreceptor blockade. *Kidney Int* 1980;18:686.
520. Bauer JH. Effects of propranolol on renal function and body fluid composition. *Arch Intern Med* 1983;143:927.
521. Bailey RR, Nairn PL, Walker RJ. Effect of doxazosin on blood pressure and renal hemodynamics of hypertensive patients with renal failure. *N Z Med J* 1986;99:942.
522. Williams GH. Converting-enzyme inhibitors in the treatment of hypertension. *N Engl J Med* 1988;319:1517.
523. Brunner HR. ACE inhibitors in renal disease. *Kidney Int* 1992;42:463.
524. Pritza DR, Bierman MH, Hammke MD. Acute toxic effects of sustained release verapamil in chronic renal failure. *Arch Intern Med* 1991;151:2081.
525. Rahman M, et al. Interdialytic weight gain, compliance with dialysis regimen, and age are independent predictors of blood pressure in hemodialysis patients. *Am J Kidney Dis* 2000;35:257.
526. Agarwal R, et al. Prevalence, treatment, and control of hypertension in chronic hemodialysis patients in the United States. *Am J Med* 2003;115:291.
527. Mittal SK, et al. Prevalence of hypertension in a hemodialysis population. *Clin Nephrol* 1999;51:77.
528. Tozawa M, Iseki K, Fukiyama K. Hypertension in dialysis patients: a cross-sectional analysis. *Nippon Jinzo Gakkai Shi* 1996;38:129.
529. Rahman M, et al. Factors associated with inadequate blood pressure control in hypertensive hemodialysis patients. *Am J Kidney Dis* 1999;33:498
530. Salem MM. Hypertension in the hemodialysis population: a survey of 649 patients. *Am J Kidney Dis* 1995;26:461.
531. Yassa H, et al. Prevalence and control adequacy of hypertension in a large renal unit. *Transplant Proc* 2004;36:1812.
532. Foley RN, et al. Impact of hypertension on cardiomyopathy, morbidity and mortality in end-stage renal disease. *Kidney Int* 1996;49:1379.
533. Kong CH, Farrington K. Determinants of LV hypertrophy and its progression in high-flux haemodialysis. *Blood Purif* 2003;21:163.
534. Cannella G, et al. Inadequate diagnosis and therapy of arterial hypertension as causes of LV hypertrophy in uremic dialysis patients. *Kidney Int* 2000;58:260.
535. Zoccali C, et al. Cardiac consequences of hypertension in hemodialysis patients. *Semin Dial* 2004;17:299.
536. Cannella G, et al. Regression of LV hypertrophy in hypertensive dialyzed uremic patients on long-term antihypertensive therapy. *Kidney Int* 1993;44:881.
537. van der Sande FM, et al. Noncardiac consequences of hypertension in hemodialysis patients. *Semin Dial* 2004;17:304.
538. Seliger SL, et al. Risk factors for incident stroke among patients with end-stage renal disease. *J Am Soc Nephrol* 2003;14:2623.
539. Malatino LS, et al. Smoking, blood pressure and serum albumin are major determinants of carotid atherosclerosis in dialysis patients. CREED Investigators. Cardiovascular Risk Extended Evaluation in Dialysis patients. *J Nephrol* 1999;12:256.
540. Port FK, et al. Predialysis blood pressure and mortality risk in a national sample of maintenance hemodialysis patients. *Am J Kidney Dis* 1999;33:507.
541. Zager PG, et al. "U" curve association of blood pressure and mortality in hemodialysis patients. Medical Directors of Dialysis Clinic, Inc. *Kidney Int* 1998;54:561.
542. Goodkin DA, et al. Association of comorbid conditions and mortality in hemodialysis patients in Europe, Japan, and the United States: the Dialysis Outcomes and Practice Patterns Study (DOPPS). *J Am Soc Nephrol* 2003;14:3270.
543. Kalantar-Zadeh K, et al. Reverse epidemiology of hypertension and cardiovascular death in the hemodialysis population: the 58th annual fall conference and scientific sessions. *Hypertension* 2005;45:811.
544. Lynn KL, et al. Hypertension as a determinant of survival for patients treated with home dialysis. *Kidney Int* 2002;62:2281.
545. Takeda A, et al. Discordance of influence of hypertension on mortality and cardiovascular risk in hemodialysis patients. *Am J Kidney Dis* 2005;45:112.
546. Foley RN, et al. Long-term evolution of cardiomyopathy in dialysis patients. *Kidney Int* 1998;54:1720.
547. Foley RN, Parfrey PS, Sarnak MJ. Epidemiology of cardiovascular disease in chronic renal disease. *J Am Soc Nephrol* 1998;9:S16.
548. Foley RN. Serial change in echocardiographic parameters and cardiac failure in end-stage renal disease. *J Am Soc Nephrol* 2000;11:912.
549. Mazzuchi N, Carbonell E, Fernandez-Cean J. Importance of blood pressure control in hemodialysis patient survival. *Kidney Int* 2000;58:2147.
550. Agarwal R. Hypertension and survival in chronic hemodialysis patients-Past lessons and future opportunities. *Kidney Int* 2005;67:1.
551. Klassen PS, et al. Association between pulse pressure and mortality in patients undergoing maintenance hemodialysis. *JAMA* 2002;287:1548.
552. Tozawa M, et al. Pulse pressure and risk of total mortality and cardiovascular events in patients on chronic hemodialysis. *Kidney Int* 2002;61:717.
553. Lazar AE, Smith MC, Rahman M. Blood pressure measurement in hemodialysis patients. *Semin Dial* 2004;17:250.
554. Rahman M, et al. A comparison of standardized versus "usual" blood pressure measurements in hemodialysis patients. *Am J Kidney Dis* 2002;39:1226.
555. Chan CT, et al. Short-term blood pressure, noradrenergic, and vascular effects of nocturnal home hemodialysis. *Hypertension* 2003;42:925.
556. Conion PJ, et al. Predialysis systolic blood pressure correlates strongly with mean 24-hour systolic blood pressure and LV mass in stable hemodialysis patients. *J Am Soc Nephrol* 1996;7:2658.
557. Agarwal R, Lewis RR. Prediction of hypertension in chronic hemodialysis patients. *Kidney Int* 2001;60:1982.
558. Agarwal R. Assessment of blood pressure in hemodialysis patients. *Semin Dial* 2002;15:299.
559. Mailloux LU, Levey AS. Hypertension in patients with chronic renal disease. *Am J Kidney Dis* 1998;32:S120.
560. Covic A, Goldsmith DJ. Ambulatory blood pressure measurement in the renal patient. *Curr Hypertens Rep* 2002;4:369.
561. Covic A, Haydar AA, Goldsmith D. Ambulatory blood pressure monitoring in hemodialysis patients: a critique and literature review. *Semin Dial* 2004;17:255.
562. Santos SF, et al. Profile of interdialytic blood pressure in hemodialysis patients. *Am J Nephrol* 2003;23:96.
563. Covic A, Goldsmith DJ, Covic M. Reduced blood pressure diurnal variability as a risk factor for progressive LV dilatation in hemodialysis patients. *Am J Kidney Dis* 2000;35:617.
564. Amar J, et al. Nocturnal blood pressure and 24-hour pulse pressure are potent indicators of mortality in hemodialysis patients. *Kidney Int* 2000;57:2485.
565. Liu M, et al. Non-dipping is a potent predictor of cardiovascular mortality and is associated with autonomic dysfunction in haemodialysis patients. *Nephrol Dial Transplant* 2003;18:563.
566. Peixoto AJ, et al. Reproducibility of ambulatory blood pressure monitoring in hemodialysis patients. *Am J Kidney Dis* 2000;36:983.
567. Rahman M, et al. Diurnal variation of blood pressure; reproducibility and association with LV hypertrophy in hemodialysis patients. *Blood Press Monit* 2005;10:25.
568. Agarwal R. Role of home blood pressure monitoring in hemodialysis patients. *Am J Kidney Dis* 1999;33:682.
569. Mailloux LU. Hypertension in chronic renal failure and ESRD: prevalence, pathophysiology, and outcomes. *Semin Nephrol* 2001;21:146.
570. Rahman M, Smith MC. Hypertension in hemodialysis patients. *Curr Hypertens Rep* 2001;3:496.
571. Wilson J, Shah T, Nissenson AR. Role of sodium and volume in the pathogenesis of hypertension in hemodialysis. *Semin Dial* 2004;17:260.
572. Dionisio P, et al. Influence of the hydration state on blood pressure values in a group of patients on regular maintenance hemodialysis. *Blood Purif* 1997;15:25.
573. Lopez-Gomez JM, et al. Interdialytic weight gain as a marker of blood pressure, nutrition, and survival in hemodialysis patients. *Kidney Int* 2005(Suppl):S63, 574.
574. Argiles A, Mourad G, Mion C. Seasonal changes in blood pressure in patients with end-stage renal disease treated with hemodialysis. *N Engl J Med* 1998;339:1364.
575. Argiles A, et al. Seasonal modifications in blood pressure are mainly related to interdialytic body weight gain in dialysis patients. *Kidney Int* 2004;65:1795.
576. Charra B, et al. Survival in dialysis and blood pressure control. *Contrib Nephrol* 1994;106:179.
577. Charra B. Control of blood pressure in long slow hemodialysis. *Blood Purif* 1994;12:252.
578. Vertes V, et al. Hypertension in end-stage renal disease. *N Engl J Med* 1969;280:978.
579. Converse RL Jr, et al. Sympathetic overactivity in patients with chronic renal failure. *N Engl J Med* 1992;327:1912.
580. Tsunoda K, Abe K, Yoshinaga K. Endothelin in hemodialysis-resistant hypertension. *Nephron* 1991;59:687.
581. Erkan E, Devarajan P, Kaskel F. Role of nitric oxide, endothelin-1, and inflammatory cytokines in blood pressure regulation in hemodialysis patients. *Am J Kidney Dis* 2002;40:76.
582. Bargman JM. The role of Na,K-ATPase inhibitors in hypertension and end-stage renal disease. *Perit Dial Int* 1997;17:536.
583. Shimosawa T, et al. Adrenomedullin amidation enzyme activities in hypertensive patients. *Hypertens Res* 2000;23:167.
584. Blankestijn PJ, Ligtenberg G. Volume-independent mechanisms of hypertension in hemodialysis patients: clinical implications. *Semin Dial* 2004;17:265.
585. Osanai T, et al. Relationship between salt intake, nitric oxide and asymmetric dimethylarginine and its relevance to patients with end-stage renal disease. *Blood Purif* 2002;20:466.
586. Smith KJ, et al. The cardiovascular effects of erythropoietin. *Cardiovasc Res* 2003;59:538.
587. Raine AE, Bedford L, Simpson AW, et al. Hyperparathyroidism, platelet intracellular free calcium and hypertension in chronic renal failure. *Kidney Int* 1993;43:700.
588. Coen G, et al. Parathyroidectomy in chronic renal failure: short- and long-term results on parathyroid function, blood pressure and anemia. *Nephron* 2001;88:149.
589. Salahudeen AK, et al. Underweight rather than overweight is associated with higher prevalence of hypertension: BP vs BMI in haemodialysis population. *Nephrol Dial Transplant* 2004;19:427.

590. Purcell W, et al. Accurate dry weight assessment: reducing the incidence of hypertension and cardiac disease in patients on hemodialysis. *Nephrol Nurs J* 2004;31:631.

591. Morse SA, et al. Hypertension in chronic dialysis patients: pathophysiology, monitoring, and treatment. *Am J Med Sci* 2003;325:194.

592. Ahmad S. Dietary sodium restriction for hypertension in dialysis patients. *Semin Dial* 2004;17:284.

593. Fishbane S, Natke E, Maesaka JK. Role of volume overload in dialysis-refractory hypertension. *Am J Kidney Dis* 1996;28:257.

594. Charra B, et al. Clinical assessment of dry weight. *Nephrol Dial Transplant* 1996;11(Suppl 2):16.

595. Zhu F, et al. Adjustment of dry weight in hemodialysis patients using intradialytic continuous multifrequency bioimpedance of the calf. *Int J Artif Organs* 2004;27:104.

596. Chang ST, et al. Enhancement of quality of life with adjustment of dry weight by echocardiographic measurement of inferior vena cava diameter in patients undergoing chronic hemodialysis. *Nephron Clin Pract* 2004;97:c90.

597. Wolfram G, et al. Assessment of dry weight in haemodialysis patients by the volume markers ANP and cGMP. *Nephrol Dial Transplant* 1996;11 (Suppl 2):28.

598. Leypoldt JK, et al. Determination of circulating blood volume by continuously monitoring hematocrit during hemodialysis. *J Am Soc Nephrol* 1995;6:214.

599. Zellweger M, Querin S, Madore F. Measurement of blood volume during hemodialysis is a useful tool to achieve safely adequate dry weight by enhanced ultrafiltration. *ASAIO J* 2004;50:242.

600. Khosla UM, Johnson RJ. Hypertension in the hemodialysis patient and the "lag phenomenon": insights into pathophysiology and clinical management. *Am J Kidney Dis* 2004;43:739.

601. Charra B, Bergstrom J, Scribner BH. Blood pressure control in dialysis patients: importance of the lag phenomenon. *Am J Kidney Dis* 1998;32:720.

602. de Paula FM, Peixoto AJ, Pinto LV, et al. Clinical consequences of an individualized dialysate sodium prescription in hemodialysis patients. *Kidney Int* 2004;66:1232.

603. Locatelli F, et al. Optimal composition of the dialysate, with emphasis on its influence on blood pressure. *Nephrol Dial Transplant* 2004;19:785.

604. Fagugli RM, et al. Short daily hemodialysis: blood pressure control and LV mass reduction in hypertensive hemodialysis patients. *Am J Kidney Dis* 2001;38:371.

605. Nesrallah G, et al. Volume control and blood pressure management in patients undergoing quotidian hemodialysis. *Am J Kidney Dis* 2003;42:13.

606. Saad E, Charra B, Raj DS. Hypertension control with daily dialysis. *Semin Dial* 2004;17:295.

607. Chan CT, et al. Regression of LV hypertrophy after conversion to nocturnal hemodialysis. *Kidney Int* 2002;61:2235.

608. Rahman M, Griffin V. Patterns of antihypertensive medication use in hemodialysis patients. *Am J Health Syst Pharm* 2004;61:1473.

609. Horl MP, Horl WH. Drug therapy for hypertension in hemodialysis patients. *Semin Dial* 2004;17:288.

610. Salem MM, Bower J. Hypertension in the hemodialysis population: any relation to one-year survival? *Am J Kidney Dis* 1996;28:737.

611. Ikeda Y, et al. Successful combined therapy of nifedipine and diltiazem for severe hypertension in a maintenance hemodialysis patient. *Clin Nephrol* 1999;51:127.

612. Griffith TF, et al. Characteristics of treated hypertension in incident hemodialysis and peritoneal dialysis patients. *Am J Kidney Dis* 2003;42:1260.

613. Efrati S, et al. ACE inhibitors and survival of hemodialysis patients. *Am J Kidney Dis* 2002;40:1023.

614. Foley RN, Herzog CA, Collins AJ. Blood pressure and long-term mortality in United States hemodialysis patients: USRDS Waves 3 and 4 Study. *Kidney Int* 2002;62:1784.

615. Sica DA, Gehr TW. Calcium-channel blockers and end-stage renal disease: pharmacokinetic and pharmacodynamic considerations. *Curr Opin Nephrol Hypertens* 2003;12:123.

616. Saran R, et al. Association between vascular access failure and the use of specific drugs: the Dialysis Outcomes and Practice Patterns Study (DOPPS). *Am J Kidney Dis* 2002;40:1255.

617. Chobanian AV, et al. Seventh report of the Joint National Committee on Prevention, Detection, Evaluation, and Treatment of High Blood Pressure. *Hypertension* 2003;42:1206.

618. Aronoff GR, Berns JS, Brier ME. *Drug prescribing in renal failure*. Philadelphia: American College of Physicians, 1999.

619. Brunet P, et al. Anaphylactoid reactions during hemodialysis and hemofiltration: role of associating AN69 membrane and angiotensin I-converting enzyme inhibitors. *Am J Kidney Dis* 1992;19:444.

620. Matsumura M, et al. Angiotensin-converting enzyme inhibitors are associated with the need for increased recombinant human erythropoietin maintenance doses in hemodialysis patients. Risks of Cardiac Disease in Dialysis Patients Study Group. *Nephron* 1997;77:164.

621. Cruz DN, et al. Angiotensin-converting enzyme inhibitor therapy in chronic hemodialysis patients: any evidence of erythropoietin resistance? *Am J Kidney Dis* 1996;28:535.

622. Cannella G, et al. Prolonged therapy with ACE inhibitors induces a regression of LV hypertrophy of dialyzed uremic patients independently from hypotensive effects. *Am J Kidney Dis* 1997;30:659.

623. Sica DA, Gehr TW, Fernandez A. Risk-benefit ratio of angiotensin antagonists versus ACE inhibitors in end-stage renal disease. *Drug Saf* 2000;22:350.

624. Agarwal R. Supervised atenolol therapy in the management of hemodialysis hypertension. *Kidney Int* 1999;55:1528.

625. Agarwal R, et al. Lisinopril therapy for hemodialysis hypertension: hemodynamic and endocrine responses. *Am J Kidney Dis* 2001;38:1245.

626. Ross EA, Pittman TB, Koo LC. Strategy for the treatment of noncompliant hypertensive hemodialysis patients. *Int J Artif Organs* 2002;25:1061.

627. Box JC, Braithwaite MD, Duncan T, et al. Pheochromocytoma, chronic renal insufficiency, and hemodialysis: a combination leading to a diagnostic and therapeutic dilemma. *Am Surg* 1997;63:314.

628. Bommer J. Unexplained hypertension in a previously normotensive dialysis patient. Diagnosis: pheochromocytoma. *Nephrol Dial Transplant* 2000;15:1705.

629. Zazgornik J, et al. Bilateral nephrectomy: the best, but often overlooked, treatment for refractory hypertension in hemodialysis patients. *Am J Hypertens* 1998;11:1364.

630. Page DE, Lavoie SL, Knoll GA. Team approach in a peritoneal dialysis unit provides better control of hypertension than in a hemodialysis unit. *Adv Perit Dial* 2004;20:117.

631. Lameire N, Van Biesen W. Importance of blood pressure and volume control in peritoneal dialysis patients. *Perit Dial Int* 2001;21:206.

632. Gunal AI, et al. Strict volume control normalizes hypertension in peritoneal dialysis patients. *Am J Kidney Dis* 2001;37:588.

633. Lameire N. Volume control in peritoneal dialysis patients: role of new dialysis solutions. *Blood Purif* 2004;22:44.

634. Pahor M, et al. Diuretic-based treatment and cardiovascular events in patients with mild renal dysfunction enrolled in the systolic hypertension in the elderly program. *Arch Int Med* 1998;158:1340.

635. Cinotti GA, Zucchelli PC. Collaborative Study Group: effect of lisinopril on the progression of renal insufficiency in mild proteinuric non-diabetic nephropathies. *Nephrol Dial Transplant* 2001;16:961.

CHAPTER 52 ■ RENAL ARTERY STENOSIS, RENAL VASCULAR HYPERTENSION, AND ISCHEMIC NEPHROPATHY

MARC A. POHL AND CHRISTOPHER STUART WILCOX

Since 1934, when Goldblatt and et al. first experimentally produced hypertension by clamping the renal artery, the relationship between renal artery stenosis and hypertension has intrigued countless investigators and clinicians (1). The physiology and pathophysiology of the renin-angiotensin system have been widely discussed, and much of our understanding of the role and regulation of the renin-angiotensin system has evolved from models of experimental hypertension produced by renal artery clamping. The development of pharmacologic agents that interfere with the activity of the renin-angiotensin system (e.g., beta-blockers, angiotensin-converting enzyme (ACE) inhibitors, and angiotensin II receptor antagonists), fascination with numerous diagnostic screening studies designed to predict a relationship between renal artery stenosis and hypertension, and controversies about renal revascularization versus medical management of renal artery stenosis may all be viewed, in one way or another, as emanating from the original Goldblatt experiment.

The detection of renal artery stenosis in a patient with hypertension typically raises the question as to whether the renal artery stenosis causes the hypertension. However, renal artery stenosis can be observed angiographically in normotensive individuals (2–4). In a postmortem study, Holley and associates found moderate or severe stenosis of the renal artery in nearly 50% of patients who had been normotensive (4). Dustan et al. reported that 39 (35%) of 111 normotensive patients had unsuspected renal artery stenosis in one or both renal arteries revealed by aortography that was performed to evaluate peripheral arterial occlusive disease (3). Thus, significant renal arterial stenosis in patients with normal arterial pressure or in patients with mild hypertension is well recognized. Conversely, many hypertensive patients with renal artery stenosis are not cured of their hypertension by renal revascularization (surgical or endovascular) procedures. Most patients with hypertension and atherosclerotic renal artery disease have essential or primary hypertension despite the anatomic presence of renal artery stenosis. Therefore, it is critical to distinguish between renal artery stenosis wherein a stenotic lesion is present, but not necessarily causing hypertension, and renovascular hypertension in which sufficient arterial stenosis is present to produce renal tissue ischemia and initiate the sequence of pathophysiologic events leading to elevated blood pressure.

The syndrome of renovascular hypertension may be broadly defined as the secondary elevation of the blood pressure (BP) produced by any of a variety of conditions interfering with arterial circulation to kidney tissue and causing renal tissue ischemia. Most of the time, the condition interfering with the arterial circulation is main renal artery stenosis. However, Page demonstrated persistent arterial hypertension in experimental animals in which one kidney was wrapped in cellophane; within 3 to 5 weeks of cellophane wrapping, severe hypertension occurred, and was later alleviated by removal of the wrapped kidney (5). Unilateral renal trauma, chronic subcapsular hematoma, perirenal hematoma, unilateral ureteral obstruction, unilateral chronic atrophic pyelonephritis, unilateral renal hypoplasia, and unilateral segmental hypoplasia (Ask-Upmark kidney) may be associated with hypertension and viewed as clinical counterparts of the experimental Page kidney, wherein one may observe the syndrome of renovascular hypertension without main renal artery stenosis. Thus, renovascular hypertension and renal artery stenosis are not synonymous.

Historically, clinical discussions of renal artery stenosis have focused on its role in the pathogenesis of hypertension, that is, renovascular hypertension. More recently, the notion that renal artery stenosis can produce renal insufficiency has generated considerable interest and enthusiasm. Surgical renal revascularization, percutaneous transluminal renal angioplasty (PTRA), and renal artery stent placement sometimes produce improvement in overall renal function in selected patients, and occasionally, patients can discontinue dialysis after renal revascularization. This syndrome of clinically significant reduction in renal function due to compromise of the renal circulation has been called ischemic renal disease or ischemic nephropathy. In comparison to the voluminous literature addressing the relationship between renal artery stenosis, renal ischemia, and hypertension (i.e., renovascular hypertension), the syndrome of ischemic nephropathy, and the notion that renal artery stenosis can produce renal failure have received relatively little attention.

This chapter reviews the types of renal artery disease producing renal artery stenosis; the pathophysiology of renovascular hypertension; clinical features and diagnostic approaches to renal artery stenosis, renovascular hypertension, and ischemic nephropathy; management of patients with renal artery stenosis; and therapeutic strategies for the clinical syndromes of renovascular hypertension and ischemic renal disease.

HISTORICAL ASPECTS OF RENOVASCULAR HYPERTENSION

The history of renal disease and hypertension can be traced to Richard Bright, who demonstrated in 1827 the association between hardness of the pulse, proteinuria, and dropsy with hardening of the kidneys (6). These observations suggested a link between renal disease and disturbances of the circulation. Bright also noted that the altered quality of blood so affects the minute and capillary circulation as to render greater action necessary to force the blood through the distal division of the vascular system (6). Mahomed reported in 1874 a high tension in the arterial system in patients with renal disease (7). Blood pressure measurements were not described in the observations of either Bright or Mahomed. In 1898, Tigerstedt and

Bergmann described a renal pressor substance in the rabbit that they called renin (8). The development of ideas on renovascular hypertension has been reviewed by Peart (9).

In 1934, Goldblatt et al. produced hypertension in dogs by constriction of the renal artery (1). They also noticed extensive renal vascular abnormalities at autopsy of patients with hypertension. About 40 years later, reflecting on his own work, Goldblatt stated, "Contrary, therefore, to what I had been taught, I began to suspect that vascular disease comes first, and when it involves the kidneys, the resultant impairment of the renal circulation probably, in some way, causes elevation of blood pressure" (10). Goldblatt's studies, investigating the relationship between hypertension and the kidney, largely preceded renal revascularization procedures. However, they strongly suggested that hypertension secondary to renal ischemia could be corrected by nephrectomy (11).

Although renin was first identified by Tigerstedt and Bergman in 1898, most of the information on it and the renin-angiotensin cascade have accumulated over the past 50 years. Tigerstedt's initial experiments proved difficult to reproduce by others, and renin lost credibility until Goldblatt's classic experiment. The biochemistry of the renin-angiotensin system was elucidated over the next 20 years, forming the basis for many physiologic and clinical studies that continue today (12,13). The complexity of the renin-angiotensin system in terms of its regulation, expression in different tissues, and sites of action has been widely studied over the past decade with application of modern molecular biology. Although much is currently known about the renin-angiotensin system and its role in the elevation of BP, fundamental questions about its mode of action in the pathogenesis of elevated BP and other diseases of the circulation remain unanswered.

PATHOLOGIC CLASSIFICATION OF RENAL ARTERY DISEASE

A variety of pathologic lesions (Table 52-1) cause renal artery stenosis, with or without associated renovascular hypertension. The two main types of renal arterial lesions forming the anatomic basis of renal artery stenosis are atherosclerotic renal artery disease and fibrous dysplasia or fibrous renal artery disease. Atherosclerotic renal artery disease is the most common cause of renal artery stenosis, accounting for about 80% of

TABLE 52-1

CAUSES OF RENAL ARTERY STENOSIS

Atherosclerotic renal artery disease
Fibrous renal artery disease (fibromuscular dysplasia, fibrous dysplasia)
    Medial fibroplasia
    Perimedial fibroplasia
    Intimal fibroplasia
    Medial hyperplasia
Acute arterial embolism
Arterial trauma
Aortic dissection
Neurofibromatosis
Arterial aneurysm
Arteriovenous malformation
Cholesterol emboli
Systemic necrotizing vasculitis
    Polyarteritis nodosa
    Takayasu's arteritis

renal arterial lesions. Fibrous renal artery diseases, as a group, account for about 20% of renal arterial lesions (14–19). Recent reports of "resistant hypertension" have indicated figures of 84% for atherosclerotic renal artery disease and 16% for fibrous renal artery disease of any kind (20). Fibrous renal artery disease has been reported in 2% to 6% of potential renal transplant donors (usually normotensive individuals) (19,21–26). The vast majority of "incidental" renal artery lesions in angiographic series are atherosclerotic.

In addition to atherosclerotic and fibrous renal artery disease, a number of less common clinical entities can produce renovascular hypertension. These include acute arterial thrombosis or embolism, cholesterol emboli, aortic dissection, renal arterial trauma, arterial aneurysm, arteriovenous malformation of the renal artery, neurofibromatosis, polyarteritis nodosa, and Takayasu's arteritis. Renal artery thrombosis occurring as a complication of umbilical artery catheterization has been recognized as causing renovascular hypertension in infants (27). Transplant renal artery atherosclerosis, intimal hyperplasia, or vascular kinking may contribute to renal transplant renovascular hypertension (see Chapter 98).

Table 52-2 presents a classification of atherosclerotic and fibrous renal artery diseases with a description of their morphology and histology. These types of renal artery occlusive diseases represent a heterogeneous group of diseases, occurring in different age groups and behaving differently with regard to their individual natural history. An appreciation of these differences may be important for therapeutic decision making in patients with renal artery occlusive disease.

ATHEROSCLEROTIC RENAL ARTERY DISEASE

Atherosclerotic renal artery disease is the most common form of renal artery stenosis and the most common cause of renovascular hypertension in the Western world. Although on average it accounts for 70% to 80% of renal artery lesions, it may account for as many as 90% of all renal artery stenoses in certain populations. Atherosclerosis of the renal artery, frequently observed in conjunction with generalized atherosclerosis obliterans, predominantly affects men after the fifth decade of life, but is not uncommon in women of similar ages or in younger adults.

Renal artery atherosclerosis is often observed in patients with peripheral vascular disease and in patients with coronary artery disease. A prospective study by Olin et al. reviewed 395 consecutive patients who underwent arteriography for routine evaluation of abdominal aortic aneurysms, aortoocclusive disease, lower extremity occlusive disease, or suspected renal artery stenosis (28). Unilateral renal artery stenosis of more than 50% was observed in 38% of the patients with abdominal aortic aneurysm, in 33% of patients with aortoocclusive disease, and in 39% with lower extremity atherosclerotic-occlusive disease. Bilateral renal artery stenosis of more than 75% was noted in 13% of the patients studied. Fifty percent of patients with diabetes and claudication had unilateral renal artery stenosis of more than 50%. Other observers note significant atherosclerotic renal artery disease in up to 30% of patients with carotid and lower extremity atherosclerosis (29) and in patients with coronary artery disease (30,31).

The precise epidemiologic correlations between hypercholesterolemia or cigarette smoking and atherosclerotic renal artery disease are not clear, but one might presume that they are risk factors for renal artery atherosclerosis just as they are for atherosclerosis in other vascular beds. In one series of patients with atherosclerotic renal artery disease, 88% were smokers, compared with only 42% of patients with essential

TABLE 52-2

CHARACTERISTICS OF THE TWO MAIN TYPES OF RENAL ARTERY DISEASE

Lesion type	Frequency (%)	Sex	Age (yr)	Anatomic location	Morphology	Histology	Natural course
Atherosclerosis	70–80	M > F	>50	Proximal 2 cm of renal artery, ostial and adjacent aorta; branch disease uncommon; 50%–75% bilateral	Eccentric or concentric focal stenosis	Complex fibrous plaque with mural calcification, hemorrhage, cholesterol crystals, and luminal thrombus	Progression in 40%–50%, often to total occlusion
Fibrous dysplasias	20–30						
Medial fibroplasia	25 (65–85[a])	F	25–50	Mid and distal main renal artery and branches; 60% bilateral	Serial stenoses with intervening mural aneurysm; "string-of-beads" appearance	Areas of disorganized proliferation, medial fibroblasts surrounded by dense fibrous connective tissue (stenosis), alternating with areas of marked medial thinning (aneurysm)	Progression in one-third; dissection, thrombosis and complete occlusion rare
Perimedial fibroplasia	5 (15[a])	F	15–30	Mid and distal main renal artery or branches; 30% bilateral	Serial stenoses without mural aneurysm	Excess elastic tissue in subadventitial region	Progression in most cases; dissection and/or thrombosis common
Intimal fibroplasia and medial hyperplasia	5 (5–10[a])	F > M	Children and young adults	Mid main renal artery, occasionally proximal main renal artery; rarely bilateral	Focal or tubular	Subendothelial accumulation of mesenchymal cells within loose connective tissue; intact internal elastic lamina	Progression in most cases; dissection and/or thrombosis common

[a]Percent of fibrous dysplasia lesions.

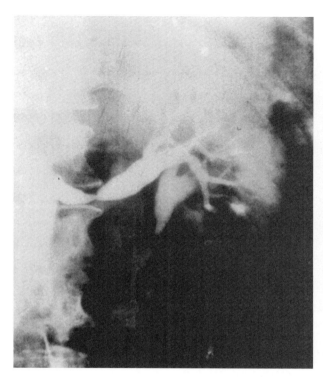

FIGURE 52-1. Aortogram demonstrating severe nonostial atherosclerotic renal artery disease of the left main renal artery.

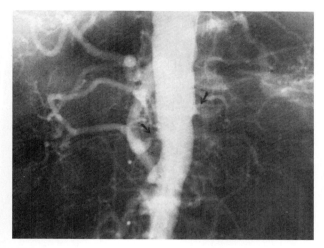

FIGURE 52-2. Abdominal aortogram demonstrating severe bilateral atherosclerotic renal artery disease with total occlusion of the left renal artery at the ostium and tight right orificial (ostial) stenosis.

hypertension (32). The investigators of this study also note a higher-than-expected prevalence of cigarette smoking in patients with fibrous renal artery disease. Atherosclerotic renal artery disease is infrequently observed in women younger than 50 years of age unless they have experienced premature menopause or are heavy cigarette smokers, or both. Men are affected twice as often as women, but this gender difference declines with advancing age. Recent series indicate a distinct shift toward women in series referred for revascularization (33–35). Several studies suggest that atherosclerotic renal vascular disease is associated with adverse coronary events (36) and increased mortality (37,38).

Renal artery atherosclerosis presents anatomically in two locations. The first appears as an eccentric or concentric lesion approximately 1 cm distal to the ostium of the renal artery ("nonostial" atherosclerotic renal artery disease) (Fig. 52-1). The second location for renal artery atherosclerosis is at the orifice (ostium) of the renal artery, occurring as an aortic plaque spillover lesion involving that orifice (ostial atherosclerotic renal artery disease) (Fig. 52-2). The histologic appearance at both locations of renal artery atherosclerosis is similar, with typical complex plaque features of mural hemorrhage and calcification, deposition of cholesterol crystals, and accumulations of luminal thrombus. Some 75% to 80% of patients with renal artery atherosclerosis and renovascular hypertension have ostial atherosclerotic lesions, and 25% to 30% of lesions are in the nonostial location (39–41). Differentiating between ostial and nonostial atherosclerotic renal artery disease is clinically important in planning interventive strategies for renal revascularization.

With recent interest in obstructive atherosclerotic renal artery disease as a threat to long-term renal function and the ability to improve kidney function with renal revascularization, an understanding of the natural history of atherosclerotic renal artery disease as a guide to the long-term management of such patients is important. Unfortunately, prospective angiographic studies on the natural history of atherosclerotic renal artery

disease are not available. Four reports, retrospectively describing the natural history of atherosclerotic renal artery disease with serial arteriographic studies, suggest that atherosclerotic renal artery disease is a progressive disorder. Progressive stenosis occurs in 40% to 50% of patients with progression to total arterial occlusion in approximately 15% of patients (42–45). A contemporary prospective study reported a 16% progression to total occlusion in medically managed (no vascular intervention) patients over one year (46). It is important to distinguish here between the "natural history" of renal vascular lesions and the natural history of kidney function in these patients.

In the largest of these retrospective studies, Schreiber et al. (44) observed that progressive atherosclerotic lesions developed in 37 (44%) of 85 patients over a mean follow-up period of 52 months; progression to complete occlusion of the involved renal artery occurred in 14 patients (16%). Examples of progressive atherosclerotic renal artery disease are indicated in Figures 52-3 and 52-4. In patients in whom progressive disease developed, it occurred primarily within the first 2 years of angiographic follow-up. A careful analysis of the diseased renal arteries suggested that the rate of progression of atherosclerotic renal artery disease bore a relationship to the degree of stenosis on the initial renal angiogram. Most renal arteries with less than 50% stenosis on the initial angiogram demonstrated less than 50% stenosis on the follow-up angiogram (i.e., the lesion remained essentially unchanged). In contrast, 7 (39%) of 18 renal arteries initially demonstrating 75% to 99% stenosis progressed to total occlusion. Thus, progression to complete occlusion occurred more often and more rapidly in renal arteries initially demonstrating higher degrees of stenosis. Renal arteries with more than 50% stenosis on the initial angiogram that eventuated in complete occlusion did so within 2 years of the initial angiogram. The serum creatinine concentration increased in 54% of patients with progressive disease, but in only 25% of patients without evidence of angiographic progression. The size of the involved kidney decreased in 70% of patients with progressive renal arterial disease, but in only 27% of patients without progressive disease. There was no significant difference in how well BP was controlled between patients with and those without progressive renal artery disease. In a more recent study by Tollefson and Ernst, 48 patients with a minimum of two renal arteriograms at least 1 year apart were followed for a mean of 7.3 years (45). Stenosis progression was found in 42 (53%) of the 79 renal artery lesions, with 7 progressing to total occlusion.

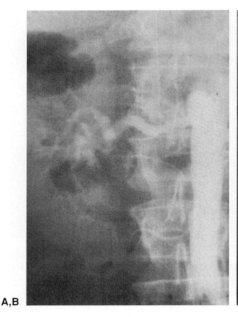
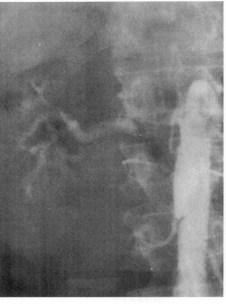

A,B

FIGURE 52-3. A: Mild stenosis (less than 50%) due to atherosclerotic disease of the right main renal artery (B) progressed to high-grade (75% to 99%) stenosis, as shown on a later arteriogram. (From: Schreiber MJ, Pohl MA, Novick AC. The natural history of atherosclerotic and fibrous renal artery disease. *Urol Clin North Am* 1984;11:383, with permission.)

Some centers use renal duplex ultrasonography and color-coded duplex ultrasonography to noninvasively diagnose, grade, and monitor the progress of atherosclerotic renal artery lesions (47–53) The overall sensitivity and specificity of renal artery duplex ultrasonography (compared with renal arteriography—the gold standard) was 98% in one study (51). Another recent study reported a 92% sensitivity in identifying renal artery stenosis of more than 75%, with none of the high-grade stenoses missing detection (52). Prospective studies of progressive renal artery stenosis that used duplex ultrasonography also suggested that atherosclerotic renal artery disease is a progressive disorder; one report suggested a cumulative incidence of progression to total occlusion of 5% ± 3% at 12 months and 11% ± 6% at 24 months (53). A more recent report from the same institution, which provided longer follow-up on two-and-a-half times as many kidneys, prospec-

tively monitored a total of 295 kidneys in 170 patients with atherosclerotic renal artery stenosis for a mean follow-up period of 33 months (54). Overall, the cumulative incidence of atherosclerotic renal artery stenosis progression was 35% at 3 years and 51% at 5 years. The 3-year cumulative incidence of renal artery disease progression stratified by baseline disease classification was 18%, 28%, and 49% for renal arteries initially classified as normal, less than 60% stenosis, and greater than or equal to 60% stenosis, respectively. The cumulative incidence of progression of lesions with less than 60% reduction in lumen diameter progressing to more than 60% reduction in lumen diameter was 30% at 1 year, 44% at 2 years, and 48% at 3 years. Progression to total occlusion occurred only in nine arteries all of which had a baseline reduction in lumen diameter of greater than 60%. The cumulative incidence of progression to total occlusion in patients with baseline stenosis

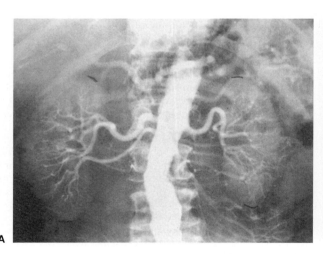
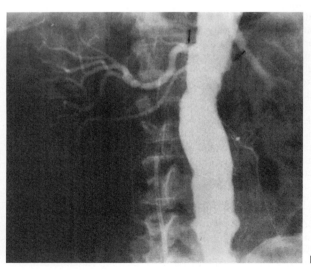

A   **B**

FIGURE 52-4. A: Aortogram taken in 1974 demonstrates two normal right renal arteries and minimal atherosclerotic irregularity of the left main renal artery. B: Repeat aortogram taken in 1978 shows progression to moderate stenosis of the upper right renal artery and progression to total occlusion of the left main renal artery. (From: Pohl MA, Novick AC. Natural history of atherosclerotic and fibrous renal artery disease: clinical implications. *Am J Kidney Dis* 1985;5:A120, with permission.)

of 60% or more was 4% at 1 year, 4% at 2 years, and 7% at 3 years. Factors significantly associated with the risk of renal artery disease progression during the time of monitoring included: systolic BP greater than or equal to 160 mm Hg, diabetes mellitus, and high-grade (more than 60%) stenosis in either the ipsilateral or contralateral renal artery. Blood pressure control and serum creatinine did not predict progression. Further observations by these authors demonstrated that kidneys distal to high-grade renal artery stenosis and subjected to severe ischemia and poorly controlled hypertension are at increased risk of renal atrophy, and that loss of renal mass correlates with elevations in the serum creatinine concentration (55).

Cholesterol emboli and atheroembolic renal disease frequently occurs in patients with diffuse atherosclerosis. Renal cholesterol embolization may occur spontaneously, after abdominal aortography or selective renal angiography, after aortic surgery or following trauma (56–60). Chapter 70 provides a detailed discussion of atheroembolism. Clinically, cholesterol emboli through the renal arterial circulation are associated with deteriorating renal function, sudden onset of hypertension, or an exacerbation of hypertension (58,61,62). Malignant hypertension resulting from atheromatous embolization has also been described (63). The pathogenesis of hypertension in patients with renal cholesterol embolism has not been investigated extensively, but might be the result of activation of the renin-angiotensin system, producing a vasoconstrictor-type of hypertension. Bilateral renal vein renin sampling in one patient with malignant hypertension and papilledema demonstrated evidence of unilateral hypersecretion of renin; at autopsy, the ipsilateral renal artery was occluded by atheromatous debris and evidence of cholesterol embolism was found in the high renin-producing kidney. The authors speculate that cholesterol embolism causes increased renin release from the involved kidney, in turn causing renin-dependent hypertension (63).

FIBROUS RENAL ARTERY DISEASE (FIBROMUSCULAR DYSPLASIA)

Fibrous diseases of the renal artery are the most common cause of renovascular hypertension in persons younger than 40 years (Table 52-2). These abnormalities of the renal artery are a heterogeneous group of nonatherosclerotic, noninflammatory vascular occlusive diseases. Fibrous dysplasias account for 20% to 30% of renal artery lesions producing renovascular hypertension, and are the most frequent cause of renovascular hypertension in children, accounting for 40% to 80% of cases. Fibrous renal artery disease producing renovascular hypertension is much more common in women than men and in white patients rather than African American or Asian patients with hypertension. It is only rarely observed in patients older than 60 years (64).

The etiology of the fibrous dysplasias is not completely understood. Genetic factors and cigarette smoking have been implicated as etiologic factors (19,65). The preponderance of fibrous renal artery disease in women suggests hormonal influences, but no proof is available and no animal models exist. An association between ptotic kidneys and fibrous dysplasia suggests that arterial stretching may be a factor in the development of fibrous renal artery disease (66,67). Mural ischemia resulting from functional defects in the vasa vasorum supplying the arterial wall has been implicated (68,69).

There are four different types of fibrous renal artery diseases: medial fibroplasia, perimedial fibroplasia, medial hyperplasia, and intimal fibroplasia (Table 52-2). Although the true incidence rates for these four types have not been clearly defined, medial fibroplasia is most common, accounting for ap-

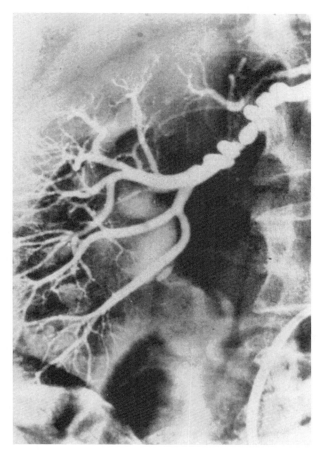

FIGURE 52-5. Right renal arteriogram demonstrating the weblike stenoses with interposed segments of dilation (large beads) typical of medial fibroplasia ("string-of-beads" lesion).

proximately 75% of fibrous renal artery lesions. Medial fibroplasia affects the distal half of the main renal artery, frequently extends into the major branches, is often bilateral, and angiographically gives the appearance of multiple aneurysms (a "string of beads") wherein the diameter of the aneurysms is wider than the apparently unaffected portion of the main renal artery (Fig. 52-5). Most cases of medial fibroplasia are diagnosed in women between the ages of 30 and 50 years. Although medial fibroplasia progresses to higher degrees of stenosis in about one-third of patients, complete arterial occlusion and ischemic atrophy of the kidney ipsilateral to the renal artery stenosis are rare. The stenotic lesions in medial fibroplasia are secondary to thickened fibromuscular ridges replacing the normal structure of the intima and media of the artery. These areas alternate with thinned areas that do not have an internal elastic membrane, thereby becoming aneurysmal.

Perimedial fibroplasia (subadventitial fibroplasia) accounts for approximately 15% of fibrous renal artery lesions. This lesion also occurs predominantly in women, typically between the ages of 15 and 30 years. Angiographically, it is often characterized by a small string-of-beads appearance, with the beads being of similar or smaller diameter compared to the diameter of the apparently unaffected portion of the renal artery (Fig. 52-6). This lesion typically affects the distal half of the main renal artery, is frequently bilateral and highly stenotic, and may progress to total arterial occlusion. Collateral blood vessels and renal atrophy on the involved side are commonly observed (19,42,70,71).

Medial hyperplasia and intimal fibroplasia account for only 5% to 10% of fibrous renal artery lesions. Intimal fibroplasia

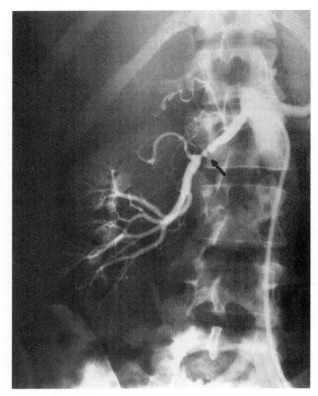

FIGURE 52-6. Selective right renal arteriogram shows tight stenosis in the midportion of the renal artery, with a small string-of-beads appearance typical of perimedial fibroplasia. Note that the beads are of a smaller diameter than the unaffected proximal portion of the renal artery. Note also the presence of collateral vessels often seen with perimedial fibroplasia. (From: Pohl MA, Novick AC. Natural history of atherosclerotic and fibrous renal artery disease: clinical implications. *Am J Kidney Dis* 1985;5:A120, with permission.)

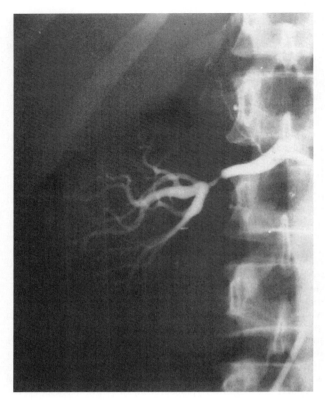

FIGURE 52-7. Selective right renal arteriogram shows smooth tight stenosis of the distal right renal artery from intimal fibroplasia.

occurs primarily in children and teenagers and angiographically appears as a localized, highly stenotic, smooth lesion with poststenotic dilation. It may occur in the proximal portion of the renal artery and when it does, it can resemble atheroma. Intimal fibroplasia is progressive, and is occasionally associated with dissection or renal infarction, and renal atrophy (Fig. 52-7). Medial hyperplasia, also rare, is found predominantly in teenagers, and angiographically also appears as a smooth, linear stenosis, sometimes appearing as though a ligature were tied around the renal artery. There is considerable difficulty in distinguishing between intimal fibroplasia and medial hyperplasia by angiography, and in the literature, these two types of fibrous artery disease may be grouped together (70,71).

As emphasized by Goncharenko and associates, who reviewed the progression of fibrous renal artery disease in 42 patients studied by serial angiography, perimedial fibroplasia, medial hyperplasia, and intimal fibroplasia produce high-grade renal artery stenosis that eventually leads to renal atrophy, renal infarction, and loss of renal parenchyma ipsilateral to the stenosis (70). Because these disorders are generally encountered in children, adolescents, and young adults with significant hypertension, who would, without intervention, require lifelong antihypertensive therapy, surgical renal revascularization is recommended for relief of hypertension and preservation of renal function.

On the other hand, the most common form of fibrous renal artery disease, medial fibroplasia, rarely progresses to total

arterial occlusion. Further, progressive arterial stenosis from medial fibroplasia does not adversely affect total renal function as measured by serum creatinine concentrations, nor is it associated with a significant reduction in kidney size (44). Despite the progressive nature of medial fibroplasia, the available data indicate that the risk of losing renal function over time due to progressive arterial occlusion is small. Accordingly, surgical renal revascularization or PTRA need not be considered for the goal of restoring or preserving renal function in patients with medial fibroplasia. In most centers, PTRA is the initial interventive maneuver for patients with medial fibroplasia and hypertension refractory to drug therapy or for hypertensive patients wishing to avoid antihypertensive drug therapy. Because medial fibroplasia and perimedial fibroplasia can produce a "beaded" appearance on angiography, differentiating between these two forms of fibrous renal artery disease may be difficult. Accordingly, prudence dictates careful monitoring of serum creatinine levels, kidney size, and BP control for patients thought to have medial fibroplasia.

Acute and chronic renal artery occlusion secondary to renal artery emboli, aortic or renal artery dissection, neurofibromatosis, arterial trauma, arteriovenous malformations, polyarteritis nodosa, and Takayasu's arteritis are discussed in conjunction with corresponding angiograms in Chapter 14. Rupture of a renal artery aneurysm is a rare but serious complication that requires urgent surgery. Novicki et al. reported 200 cases of perirenal hematoma, 20% due to renal artery aneurysm rupture (72). Stanley et al. reported a series in which the incidence of rupture of renal artery aneurysm was 5.6% (73). There is disagreement about the natural history and factors that predispose to rupture. Hageman and associates followed 25 patients with renal artery aneurysms less than 2 cm in diameter for periods of 1 to 17 years without demonstration of rupture or increase of aneurysm size (74). Rupture of a renal artery aneurysm tends to occur in noncalcified or incompletely calcified aneurysms larger than 1.5 to 2.0 cm in diameter (75–78). Pregnancy also predisposes to rupture of renal artery aneurysms (77).

Takayasu's arteritis, a nonspecific inflammatory disease affecting large arteries such as the aorta and its main branches, including the renal arteries, mainly affects young women. It can cause discrete stenosis of the aorta and its main branches, including the common carotid, subclavian, and renal arteries. Renal artery involvement is not uncommon in Asian and African patients and is a major cause of renovascular hypertension in these countries. Koide reports renovascular hypertension in 278 (18.8%) of 1,475 patients in a Japanese nationwide survey of Takayasu's arteritis (79). Takayasu's arteritis is the most common cause of renovascular hypertension in India and China, accounting for as many as 60% of all cases of renovascular hypertension (80–82).

THE ATROPHIC KIDNEY IN RENOVASCULAR HYPERTENSION

A variety of imaging techniques (see Chapters 12–14) are employed in clinical medicine to evaluate diseases of the kidney and urinary tract and pathologic processes in the abdominal and pelvic cavities. Not infrequently, an atrophic kidney or a substantial discrepancy in renal size is observed. Although the relationship between an atrophic kidney and its possible role in hypertension has long been appreciated, in the hypertensive patient with unilateral renal atrophy, the renal atrophy is not necessarily due to main renal artery stenosis.

In a postmortem study of 84 cases of unilateral atrophy reported by Baggenstoss and Barker, ischemic atrophy from occlusive disease of the renal artery was not mentioned as a cause of renal atrophy (83). In 1944, Sensenbach reviewed the literature and found that 48 of 75 (64%) diseased (but not necessarily atrophic) kidneys removed for relief of hypertension showed chronic pyelonephritis (84). These investigators noted only one instance each of renal infarction and occlusion of the renal artery. Subsequent reviews by Smith (1948) (85), Sabin (1948) (86), and Barker (1951) (87) attributed most cases of an atrophic kidney, wherein the atrophic kidney was presumably related to hypertension, as due to either unilateral pyelonephritis, post obstructive atrophy, or congenital hypoplasia.

With the advent of renal angiography in the late 1950s and early 1960s for the evaluation of patients with hypertension, renal artery occlusive disease became more evident as a cause of the atrophic kidney. In 1965, Gifford and associates found that in 53 (71%) of 75 patients with an atrophic kidney, the renal atrophy was due to stenosing atherosclerotic renal artery disease (88). In 22 (29%) of these 75 patients, the atrophic kidney was associated with a patent renal artery and the renal atrophy was thought to be secondary to pyelonephritis or congenital hypoplasia. Of special interest in that report was the observation that of the 53 patients with atherosclerosis of the renal artery supplying the atrophic kidney, 17 (32%) had unsuspected atherosclerotic disease involving the renal artery of the contralateral normal-sized kidney. Lawrie and associates reviewed 40 patients with renal atrophy due to total arterial occlusion and observed contralateral renal artery stenosis in 31 patients (78%) (89). An example (Case 1) is included in the section Ischemic Renal Disease (Ischemic Nephropathy) later in this chapter.

In children, the observation of hypertension in conjunction with an atrophic kidney raises the possibilities of congenital hypoplasia, segmental hypoplasia of the kidney (Ask-Upmark kidney) (90–93), postobstructive atrophy (88),

chronic pyelonephritis, and fibrous renal artery disease as the basis for the small kidney. With advancing age, and certainly for patients older than 45 to 50 years, particularly in the setting of generalized atherosclerosis, atherosclerotic renal artery stenosis is the leading cause of an atrophic kidney.

THE RENIN-ANGIOTENSIN SYSTEM IN RENOVASCULAR HYPERTENSION

Activation of the renin-angiotensin system by proteolysis of circulating angiotensinogen is summarized in Figure 52-8. Renin, an enzyme produced and released by the juxtaglomerular cells of the kidney, hydrolyzes the circulating peptide angiotensinogen or renin substrate to form angiotensin I. Angiotensin I, a decapeptide, reaches an active form after two additional amino acids are cleaved by a carboxypeptidase, angiotensin-converting enzyme (ACE), yielding angiotensin II. Many details concerning the renin-angiotensin cascade have been established by pharmacologic blockade of the action or formation of angiotensin II (94–97). These sites of intervention are illustrated on the right side of Figure 52-8. A non-ACE pathway is an alternative route for the generation of angiotensin II (98–100).

The renin-angiotensin-aldosterone system (RAAS) has a central role in renovascular hypertension(101). Angiotensin II is among the most potent, naturally occurring vasoconstrictors interacting with specific vascular receptors in nearly all vascular beds. At high levels, angiotensin II produces elevations in vascular resistance, thereby raising BP directly. Another major role of angiotensin II is the regulation of aldosterone production by the adrenal glomerulosa. Although not the only factor stimulating aldosterone production, angiotensin II is a potent stimulus for the secretion of aldosterone, thereby producing sodium and volume retention and "secondary aldosteronism," clinically manifested by hypokalemia. A more detailed discussion of the biochemical pathways that generate angiotensin II, actions of angiotensin at specific locations in the kidney, actions of angiotensin II on the central nervous system and on sympathetic nerve modulation, and interactions of angiotensin II with other hormones (e.g., bradykinin, prostaglandins, vasopressin) is beyond the scope of this chapter, but is explored more thoroughly in Chapters 2 and 9.

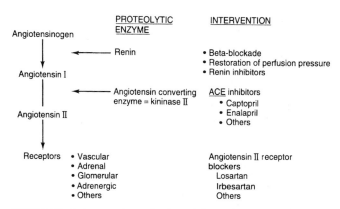

FIGURE 52-8. Progressive activation of the renin-angiotensin system initiated by proteolysis of circulating angiotensinogen. Sites of pharmacologic intervention are illustrated on the right side of the diagram. (Adapted from: Textor SC. Pathophysiology of renovascular hypertension. *Urol Clin North Am* 1984;11:373, with permission.)

PATHOPHYSIOLOGY OF RENOVASCULAR HYPERTENSION

Current understanding of the pathophysiology of renovascular hypertension has been derived largely from animal studies. The pioneering experiments of Goldblatt et al. in 1934 demonstrated that persistent hypertension could be produced in dogs by renal artery clamping (1). They proposed that a circulating substance might be responsible for the hypertension, and this concept was later confirmed by Page and Helmer (102), Pickering (103), and Braun-Menendez et al. (104). Subsequently, "Goldblatt hypertension" was extensively studied in animals, and it has been assumed that many of the experimental observations apply to human renovascular hypertension.

Critical Perfusion Pressure

The generation of elevated BP by constriction of a renal artery in experimental animals and in humans requires sufficient compromise of the renal arterial lumen to initiate the pathophysiologic sequence of events resulting in an increase in the BP. Studies of arterial lesions in several vascular beds indicated that compromise of the arterial lumen must reach an advanced level, exceeding 80% to 85% cross-sectional obstruction, before hemodynamic changes are evident (105,106). Renal blood flow and the pressure gradient across a graded stenosis of the artery supplying a dog's kidney are not changed until the degree of stenosis exceeds 70% to 80% (107). Renin secretion increases as renal perfusion pressure falls, and becomes maximal at the limit of autoregulation (101,108). These experimental studies demonstrated that a substantial reduction in both lumen diameter and cross-sectional area is necessary before any measurable decrease in arterial flow or pressure occurs (Fig. 52-9). In experimental animals, the Goldblatt clamp is manually tightened to produce a presumable reduction in lumen diameter of at least 80% to 85% and to induce hemodynamically significant renal artery constriction (109). In humans, the ability of

currently available imaging techniques to visualize hemodynamically critical renal artery stenosis (i.e., greater than 75% to 80%) may be more problematic; renal artery stenosis is often present, but not sufficiently tight to be hemodynamically significant. It is notoriously difficult to establish the true dimensions of a stenotic lesion from two-dimensional arteriograms, but poststenotic dilation suggests hemodynamically significant main renal artery stenosis (see Chapter 14). Simon has concluded that an 80% stenosis of a renal artery is required to stimulate renin secretion and lead to renovascular hypertension in humans (110).

The feature common to all experimental models of renovascular hypertension and to clinical examples of the syndrome of renovascular hypertension is a reduction in renal perfusion pressure. Whether or not this reduced renal perfusion pressure predictably causes intrarenal ischemia is unclear. Although the clinical conditions producing human renovascular hypertension vary widely, these conditions all share the common denominator of rendering renal perfusion sufficiently low to activate the renin-angiotensin system. In the case of a main renal artery stenosis, it is important to recognize that detection of hemodynamic effects related to renal artery stenosis implies far-advanced (greater than 75% to 80%) reduction in lumen diameter. High-grade renal artery occlusion may result in loss of poststenotic perfusion and possibly, eventual total arterial occlusion. The concomitant renal hypotension injures the kidney and causes progressive loss of renal parenchyma (111). These concepts are explored in greater detail in Chapters 2 and 39.

Experimental Models

Although there are differences among species (rat, dog, rabbit) in experimental renovascular hypertension, two basic models of Goldblatt hypertension are recognized: the two-kidney, one-clip (2K-1C) model (in which one renal artery is constricted and the contralateral renal artery and kidney are left intact) and the one-kidney, one-clip (1K-1C) model (in which one renal

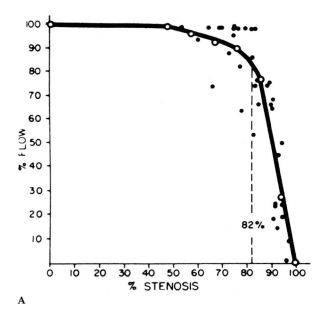

A

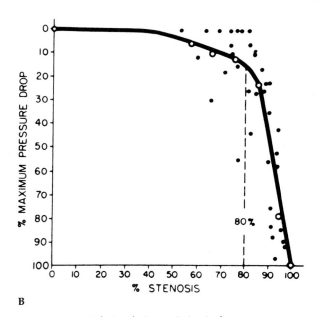

B

FIGURE 52-9. **A:** Changes in arterial flow and (**B**) pressure across a stenotic lesion during variation in the degree of stenosis in the dog. These studies demonstrate that blood flow and pressure gradients induced by vascular stenosis are negligible until the lumen narrows to more than 75% to 80% of total occlusion. Further stenosis produced abrupt loss in blood flow. (Adapted from: May AG, Van de Berg L, DeWeese JA, et al. Critical arterial stenosis. *Surgery* 1963;54:250, with permission.)

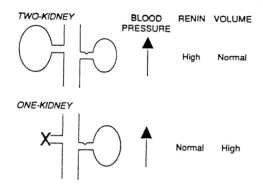

FIGURE 52-10. Two animal models of renovascular hypertension. In the two-kidney model the hypertension is mainly renin-dependent; in the one-kidney model, hypertension is mainly volume-dependent.

artery is constricted and the contralateral kidney is removed). These two experimental models of renovascular hypertension are diagrammed in Figure 52-10.

In 2K-1C ("two-kidney") Goldblatt hypertension, the renal artery on one side is partially occluded (clipped) and the renal artery to the contralateral kidney remains patent. Initially, elevated arterial pressure is associated with increased renal and plasma renin levels and normal plasma and extracellular fluid volumes. This form of experimental renovascular hypertension is mainly renin- or angiotensin II-dependent (112). In 1K-1C ("one-kidney") Goldblatt hypertension, the renal artery on one side is partially occluded and the contralateral kidney is removed. In this model, the elevated BP is associated with volume expansion and circulating renin levels which become normal over time. A renin-initiated vasoconstrictor state is implicated in the two-kidney model (112,113). The volume component is not a major initial mechanism because the intact contralateral kidney undergoes a pressure natriuresis (114,115). In the one-kidney model, pressure-induced natriuresis is absent owing to the removal of the contralateral kidney (96,116).

Human unilateral renovascular hypertension most closely resembles the 2K-1C model. Clinical counterparts of experimental two-kidney renovascular hypertension are listed in Table 52-3. The 1K-1C model may be comparable to human bilateral renal artery stenosis, renal artery stenosis in a solitary functioning kidney, hypertension in a transplanted kidney, and renovascular disease with coexisting bilateral renal parenchy-

TABLE 52-3

CLINICAL COUNTERPARTS OF EXPERIMENTAL 2K-1C ("TWO-KIDNEY") RENOVASCULAR HYPERTENSION (IMPLIES CONTRALATERAL [NONAFFECTED] KIDNEY IS PRESENT)

Unilateral atherosclerotic renal artery disease
Unilateral fibrous renal artery disease
Renal artery aneurysm, arterial embolus
Arteriovenous fistula (congenital or traumatic)
Segmental renal arterial occlusion
Pheochromocytoma compressing renal artery
Unilateral ureteral obstruction, atrophic pyelonephritis, or
    hypoplastic kidney
Unilateral metastatic tumor, perirenal hematoma, or
    subcapsular hematoma (compressing renal parenchyma)[a]

[a]Clinical analogs of experimental Page kidney.

TABLE 52-4

CLINICAL COUNTERPARTS OF EXPERIMENTAL 1K-1C ("ONE-KIDNEY") RENOVASCULAR HYPERTENSION (IMPLIES TOTAL RENAL MASS HYPOPERFUSED)

Stenosis to a solitary functioning kidney
Bilateral renal arterial stenosis
Aortic coarctation
Vasculitis (polyarteritis nodosa and Takayasu's arteritis)
Unilateral renal arterial disease (atherosclerotic or fibrous)
    with coexisting renal parenchymal disease
Atheroembolic renal disease

mal disease (Table 52-4). Nevertheless, most patients with apparently significant bilateral renal artery stenosis, or stenosis of a transplanted kidney have elevated levels of PRA (117,118).

Most discussions of renovascular hypertension focus on two-kidney hypertension. In Figure 52-11 are schematically represented the classic model of two-kidney Goldblatt hypertension. In the presence of hemodynamically sufficient unilateral renal artery stenosis, the kidney distal to the stenosis ("stenotic kidney") is rendered ischemic, consequent to impaired renal perfusion, activating the renin-angiotensin system, generating high levels of angiotensin II, and producing a "vasoconstrictor" type of hypertension. Numerous studies established the causal relationship between angiotensin II–mediated vasoconstriction and hypertension in the early phase of experimental renovascular hypertension (94,112,113,115,119). The high levels of angiotensin II stimulate the adrenal cortex to elaborate large amounts of aldosterone (secondary aldosteronism), promoting sodium retention by the stenotic kidney. Moreover, angiotensin directly enhances renal NaCl and fluid reabsorption (120). Both the direct pressor effects of angiotensin II and sodium retention lead to restoration of renal perfusion pressure at the expense of producing systemic hypertension (119). Mild or moderate degrees of renal artery stenosis (less than 75% to 80%) do not initiate this sequence of events. The human correlate of experimental two-kidney hypertension assumes a similar sequence of events, with renal artery stenosis producing a hemodynamically significant reduction in perfusion, and activating the renin-angiotensin system. Secondary aldosteronism ensues, and hypokalemia is frequently observed.

The model of 2K-1C Goldblatt hypertension implies that the "contralateral" (unaffected) kidney is present and that its renal artery is patent or only minimally narrowed. As indicated in Figure 52-11, the contralateral kidney exhibits suppressed renin secretion and a pressure natriuresis. The suppressed renin from the contralateral kidney is explained by the exposure of this kidney to systemic arterial pressures that are higher than normal and higher than the pressure reaching the stenotic kidney. Accordingly, there should be no stimulus for renin release by the contralateral kidney, and renin content should be suppressed on this side. Renal venous renin levels are typically the same as arterial levels, indicating no net renin secretion from the contralateral kidney (121,122). In experimental studies, the contralateral kidney is devoid of renin content and juxtaglomerular cell granulation (123,124). Further, the contralateral kidney, if truly functioning normally and devoid of renal parenchymal damage, should undergo a "pressure natriuresis," excreting salt and volume at levels higher than normal (125). Numerous studies confirmed that excretion of sodium predominates in the contralateral kidney, but it has been difficult to establish in humans whether this pressure natriuresis is caused purely by exaggerated natriuresis of the contralateral kidney or by extreme sodium avidity by the stenotic kidney, or by both (126,127).

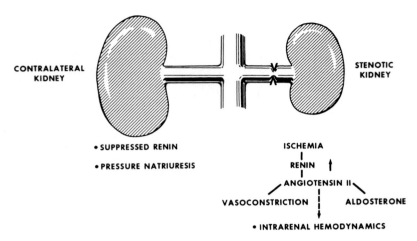

FIGURE 52-11. Schematic representation of two-kidney renovascular hypertension. The presence of a unilateral, hemodynamically significant renal arterial narrowing initiates a sequence of events within the affected kidney ("stenotic kidney") based on activation of the renin-angiotensin system. Initially vasoconstriction and sodium retention result, leading to the systemic elevation of blood pressure and suppression of renin and enhanced excretion of sodium by the "contralateral kidney."

Therefore, the hemodynamic, biochemical, and functional observations in two-kidney Goldblatt hypertension differ between the stenotic and contralateral kidneys. The kidneys effectively work against one another; the contralateral kidney excretes sodium and water continuously and thereby prevents the systemic arterial pressure from reaching levels sufficient to restore renal perfusion to the stenotic kidney adequate to suppress the release of renin (128). Based on this pathophysiology, two-kidney renovascular hypertension should be characterized by the following: (a) unilateral release of renin and contralateral suppression; (b) sodium avidity by the stenotic kidney and continuous excretion of sodium by the unaffected, contralateral kidney; (c) euvolemia or relative intravascular volume depletion, depending on the balance between sodium avidity in the stenotic kidney and the pressure natriuresis in the contralateral kidney; and (d) BP dependent on circulating angiotensin II (and marked decreases in BP with administration of angiotensin II antagonists or ACE inhibitors). These observations have been largely confirmed in humans, although not entirely (129–133).

A similar sequence of events probably produces elevated arterial pressure in one-kidney renovascular hypertension. The critical difference between one-kidney and two-kidney renovascular hypertension is that in one-kidney renovascular hypertension there is no contralateral kidney to offset the systemic BP elevation and sodium retention by the kidney distal to the renal artery stenosis. There is no contralateral kidney to undergo a pressure natriuresis. Renal perfusion pressures are thus able to reach levels sufficient to suppress renin to "normal" levels although these can be considered markedly elevated relative to the high BP. The elevated arterial pressure is sustained by sodium and volume excess and inappropriate, ongoing secretion of renin (113,134,135). BP elevation is less dependent on circulating angiotensin II (94,112,113). Under conditions of sodium depletion, however, the pressor role of angiotensin II may be demonstrated (136). The normal renin and angiotensin II levels in one-kidney renovascular hypertension might be viewed as being inappropriately normal for the level of BP elevation, arguing for a vasoconstrictor contribution of angiotensin II in one-kidney hypertension.

Evolution of Renovascular Hypertension

The notions that 2K-1C renovascular hypertension is renin-dependent and that 1K-1C renovascular hypertension is volume-dependent are oversimplifications. Considerable data in animals (mainly rats and dogs) indicate that the pathogenetic processes producing renovascular hypertension do not remain static. Operationally, the pathogenesis of both models of Goldblatt hypertension can be viewed as evolving through an acute phase (phase I), a transition phase (phase II), and a chronic phase (phase III) (114,116,137). In both the two-kidney and one-kidney models of experimental renovascular hypertension, induction of renal hypoperfusion produced by constriction of a renal artery produces prompt elevation of the BP in concert with activation of the renin-angiotensin system. Administration of ACE inhibitors or the angiotensin II receptor blocker saralasin prevents this rise in BP, indicating that this initial elevation of arterial pressure is renin- or angiotensin II-dependent (138,139). Cervenka demonstrated that mice with genetic knockout of the AT1 receptor failed to develop renovascular hypertension with the renal artery clipped (139). Removal of the renal artery clip or unilateral nephrectomy of the stenotic kidney promptly normalizes the BP in this acute phase of 2K-1C experimental renovascular hypertension (94,96,113,114,116,119).

Although one presumes that excess renin is released from the stenotic kidney, peripheral plasma concentrations of renin are not always increased (140,141). Removal of the stenotic kidney does not always reduce the BP (119,131,142,143). Further, widespread clinical experience supports the observation that surgical renal revascularization to the stenotic kidney or balloon dilation of the renal artery ipsilateral to the stenotic kidney often fails to lower the BP, particularly in patients with atherosclerotic renal artery stenosis (131,144–146).

These observations may be reconciled by separating two-kidney renovascular hypertension into sequential phases as depicted in Figure 52-12 (116). In phase I, renal ischemia and activation of the renin-angiotensin system are of fundamental importance, and the BP elevation is renin-dependent. Acute administration of angiotensin II antagonists or ACE inhibitors, removal of the renal artery stenosis (i.e., removal of the clip in the experimental animal), or removal of the stenotic kidney will promptly normalize the BP. In the absence of these maneuvers, a transition phase (phase II) subsequently develops, bridging the acute (phase I) and chronic (phase III) phases of experimental renovascular hypertension. This transition phase variably lasts from a few days to several weeks, depending on the experimental model and animal species. During this transition phase, plasma renin levels progressively fall, but the BP remains elevated. Salt and water retention are observed as a consequence of the effects of hypoperfusion of the stenotic kidney, augmented proximal renal tubular reabsorption of sodium and water, and secondary aldosteronism (137,147). In addition, the high levels of angiotensin II stimulate thirst, further contributing to an expansion of the extracellular fluid volume. The expanded extracellular fluid volume results in a progressive

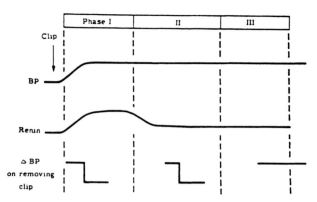

FIGURE 52-12. Sequential phases in two-kidney, one-clip (two-kidney) experimental renovascular hypertension and the effect on blood pressure and renin secretion. After the clip is put on one main renal artery with the contralateral kidney left untouched, blood pressure and renin secretion increase. In phase II, the blood pressure remains high, but renin secretion falls. In phase III, the blood pressure remains elevated, despite removal of the clip, presumably reflecting vascular damage in the contralateral kidney. (From: Brown JJ, Davies DL, Morton JJ, et al. Mechanism of renal hypertension. *Lancet* 1976;1:1219, with permission.)

suppression of peripheral plasma renin activity (PRA). During this transition phase, the hypertension is still responsive to removal of the unilateral renal artery stenosis, to angiotensin II blockade, or to unilateral nephrectomy, although these maneuvers do not normalize the BP as promptly and consistently as in the acute phase (137,148). These changes may depend on recruitment of additional mechanisms of angiotensin II action, including the generation of reactive oxygen species (149,150), quenching of nitric oxide (151), and generation of endothelium-derived substances such as endothelin (152,153) and thromboxanes (154,155). Some of these mechanisms depend upon slowly developing effects of angiotensin II at levels that do not reverse with direct angiotensin II blockade (156).

After several days or weeks, a chronic phase (phase III) evolves, wherein removal of the stenosis by unclipping the renal artery in the experimental animal or nephrectomy of the stenotic kidney fails to reduce the BP (116). The mechanism maintaining elevated arterial pressure, that is, the failure of "unclipping" to lower the BP in this chronic phase of 2K-1C hypertension, is almost certainly multifactorial but is in large part due to widespread arteriolar damage in the contralateral kidney consequent to elevated systemic pressure and the initial high levels of angiotensin II. In this chronic phase of 2K-1C renovascular hypertension, extracellular fluid volume expansion and systemic vasoconstriction are the main pathophysiologic abnormalities (112), The BP remains elevated even though the PRA has returned to a normal level. The pressure natriuresis of the contralateral kidney blunts the extracellular fluid volume expansion initially generated by the stenotic kidney (Fig. 52-11), but as the contralateral kidney suffers vascular damage from prolonged exposure to the increased BP, its excretory function diminishes and extracellular fluid volume expansion persists. In phase III of 2K-1C hypertension, acute blockade of the renin-angiotensin system fails to lower the BP. Sodium depletion may ameliorate the hypertension but does not normalize it (112,157).

Systemic vasoconstriction also contributes to the elevated BP in phase III of two-kidney hypertension, despite normalization of renin levels. Conceptually, the normal levels of renin and angiotensin II may be viewed as inappropriately high for the level of arterial pressure. In rat studies 9 to 12 months into 2K,1C hypertension, although there is no immediate response

to an angiotensin receptor blocker (ARB), the BP gradually falls to near normal values over 3 days of ARB infusion (155). This suggests that angiotensin II remains a critical determinant of the hypertension, but that this is no longer due to direct effects of circulating angiotensin II. Interestingly, blockade of thromboxane-prostanoid (TP) receptors over 3 days also reduces BP in this model, suggesting a role for vasoconstrictor prostaglandins. Whether the peripheral renin level is elevated or not, this phase of renovascular hypertension is associated with increased sensitivity to angiotensin II (157), increased levels of vasopressin (137,158,159), and increased peripheral and central sympathetic nervous system activity (127,160–164). Experimental studies demonstrated that angiotensin II acts on both the central and the peripheral nervous system to activate sympathetic outflow. Plasma norepinephrine concentration and norepinephrine content in the hypothalamus are increased in 1K-1C hypertensive rats, and in the same model, central sympatholytic interventions such as creation of lesions in the posterior hypothalamus prevent or attenuate the hypertension. Further, renal denervation lowers BP, plasma norepinephrine levels, and hypothalamic norepinephrine content in the absence of changes in sodium or water intake, sodium excretion, PRA, or creatinine clearance (164). A recent study demonstrated elevated sympathetic nerve activity by means of intraneural recordings of muscle sympathetic nerve activity in patients with renovascular hypertension (165). Administration of clonidine lowers BP, PRA, and urinary norepinephrine excretion, providing further support for a role of central nervous system pressor mechanisms in the chronic phase of experimental renovascular hypertension. Hypertension-induced structural changes in the vascular wall may also contribute to the maintenance of elevated pressure in this chronic phase of 2K-1C renovascular hypertension. These changes may develop via mechanical, neural, humoral, or pressure-related factors (137,147). This may explain why it takes some days for an angiotensin II receptor blocker to reduce BP in chronic renovascular hypertension in rats (155).

In human 2K-1C renovascular hypertension, the duration of hypertension is probably a surrogate for the chronic phase (phase III) of experimental 2K-1C renovascular hypertension. Hypertension, lasting more than 3 to 5 years in patients with unilateral renal artery stenosis, particularly if poorly controlled, has a mediocre cure rate after renal revascularization or nephrectomy (131,144–146). This is illustrated in studies of the outcome of two sets of selected patients having tests indicating functionally important renal artery stenosis. Among 63 patients with atherosclerotic RAS, hypertension was cured by intervention in 21% (166) while it was cured by intervention in 52% with fibromuscular RAS (167). In both series, the strongest factor predicting cure was a short history of hypertension. These observations are particularly true for patients with unilateral atherosclerotic renal artery disease, and may be accounted for by the development over time of unrecognized nephrosclerosis in the contralateral kidney (168–171). As emphasized by Vertes and associates (170), many patients with unilateral atherosclerotic renal artery stenosis have the unequal development of bilateral, obliterative, intrarenal vascular disease. Detection of such pathologic changes in renal biopsy specimens from the contralateral kidney in patients with atherosclerotic renal artery stenosis was consistently associated with failure to achieve BP reduction by either renal revascularization of the stenotic kidney or its removal (171,172). However, the concept that the late stage of renovascular hypertension in humans is strictly analogous to phase III renovascular hypertension in animals may be an oversimplification because nephrectomy of the kidney ipsilateral to the renal artery stenosis usually leads to a significant fall in BP.

Thus, although in the early phase of 2K-1C Goldblatt hypertension the generation of the hypertension appears to be

TABLE 52-5

PATHOGENETIC MECHANISMS IN SEQUENTIAL PHASES OF RENOVASCULAR HYPERTENSION

Acute phase
  Renin dependency
Transition phase
  Sodium and water retention
  Angiotensin II effects
    Aldosterone
    Intrarenal hemodynamics
    Tubular function
    Thirst
  Progressive suppression of plasma renin activity
  Changes in the contralateral kidney
    Blunted pressure natriuresis
    Impaired autoregulation
Chronic phase
  Volume expansion
    Suppressed plasma renin activity
    Reciprocation of sodium dependency with renin
      dependency
  Systemic vasoconstriction
  Renin-angiotensin system
    Increased angiotensin II sensitivity
    Local vascular renin-angiotensin system
    Vasopressin
    Peripheral and central sympathetic activity
    Quenching of nitric oxide
    Oxidative stress
    Thromboxanes
    Endothelin
    Impaired sodium transport
    Total body autoregulation
    Structural changes in vascular wall
  Development of nephrosclerosis

predominantly renin-dependent and the hypertension is ameliorated by interference with the renin-angiotensin system, revascularization, or nephrectomy, the maintenance of BP elevation in the chronic phase of experimental renovascular hypertension and in hypertensive patients with long-standing unilateral renal artery stenosis is multifactorial and less clearly defined. The complexities of the pathogenetic mechanisms in sequential phases of renovascular hypertension are summarized in Table 52-5.

Extrapolating these observations to patients, one might presume that the sooner an arterial lesion presumably causing renovascular hypertension is removed, the more likely the chance for relief of the hypertension. Admittedly, this clinical suggestion may be stretching the experimental observations too far. Nevertheless, clinical experience indicates that corrective surgery for unilateral renal artery stenosis as the presumptive cause for hypertension is far more successful in patients with a brief history of hypertension (e.g., less than 5 years) in contrast to patients with hypertension of a longer duration or with coexisting azotemia (131,144–146).

Thus far in this chapter, our discussion of the pathophysiology of renovascular hypertension has focused on the 2K-1C model of renovascular hypertension (Fig. 52-11). The most common clinical counterpart to this type of hypertension is unilateral renal artery stenosis due to atherosclerotic or fibrous renal artery disease. It should be appreciated, however, that several other clinical circumstances (Table 52-3) may be associated with this type of hypertension, including unilateral renal artery aneurysm (75,173,174), congenital and traumatic arteriove-

nous fistula (175,176), and segmental arterial occlusion. Unilateral renal trauma, with perirenal or subcapsular hematoma formation, and development of a calcified fibrous capsule surrounding the injured kidney causing compression of the renal parenchyma may produce the syndrome of two-kidney renovascular hypertension (177–182), a clinical situation analogous to the experimental Page kidney. Clinical counterparts of 1K-1C experimental renovascular hypertension (Table 52-4), wherein the total renal mass is implicitly underperfused and possibly ischemic, are common in clinical medicine. In polyarteritis nodosa, Takayasu's arteritis (81,183), and atheroembolic renal artery disease (61,63,184) the syndrome of renovascular hypertension is initiated by renal underperfusion, but without main renal artery stenosis. In patients with bilateral renal artery stenosis or renal artery stenosis of a solitary functioning kidney (native or transplanted kidney), multiple physiologic factors contribute to the hypertension; these include systemic vasoconstriction, volume expansion, and probable coexisting intrarenal ischemia due to nephrosclerosis or the vascular changes of chronic rejection.

In summary, the pathogenesis and pathophysiology of human renovascular hypertension are complex, and to a large degree incompletely defined. The relative contribution of various physiologic factors implicated in experimental models is uncertain. These uncertainties apply to human renovascular hypertension as well. Not surprisingly, predicting which patients might have renovascular hypertension is even more difficult. Nonetheless, compelling evidence exists for the important participation of the renin-angiotensin system as well as of volume-renin interrelationships in the pathogenesis of renovascular hypertension. The contribution of other factors and, in particular, a clearer understanding of intrarenal physiology and pathology distal to main renal artery stenosis are areas for future investigation.

Diagnosis of Renal Artery Stenosis and Renovascular Hypertension

There are two reasons to diagnose renal artery stenosis. First, renal artery stenosis in some hypertensive patients, if hemodynamically significant, might be the cause of the hypertension (i.e., renovascular hypertension). Second, renal artery stenosis has the potential to adversely affect renal function. Clinical concern over these two issues "hypertension and renal function" dictates the appropriate choice of diagnostic tests.

A number of epidemiologic observations, clinical features, laboratory tests, and diagnostic maneuvers are associated with the anatomic presence of renal artery stenosis or predict the likelihood that the renal artery stenosis is causing or contributing substantially to hypertension (Tables 52-6 to 52-8). Some clinical features and diagnostic tests (e.g., an atrophic kidney in a hypertensive patient with generalized atherosclerosis or an abnormal-appearing renal artery duplex ultrasound scan [34]) indicate main renal artery stenosis. Auscultation of a

TABLE 52-6

STEPS IN MAKING THE DIAGNOSIS OF RENOVASCULAR HYPERTENSION

1. Demonstration of renal arterial stenosis by angiography
2. Determination of pathophysiologic significance of the stenotic lesion
3. Cure of the hypertension by intervention (i.e., surgical revascularization, percutaneous transluminal angioplasty, or nephrectomy)

TABLE 52-7

DIAGNOSIS OF RENAL ARTERIAL STENOSIS

Clinical clues
  Age at onset of hypertension <30 or >55 yr
  Abrupt onset of hypertension
  Acceleration of previously well-controlled hypertension
  Hypertension refractory to an appropriate three-drug regimen
  Accelerated retinopathy
  Malignant hypertension
  Systolic-diastolic abdominal bruit
  Flash pulmonary edema
  Evidence of generalized atherosclerosis obliterans
  Acute renal failure with angiotensin-converting enzyme inhibitor treatment

Diagnostic tests
  Duplex ultrasonography
  Magnetic resonance angiography
  Computerized tomography angiography
  Radionuclide renography
  Captopril renography
  Captopril provocation test (captopril plasma renin activity)
  Rapid-sequence intravenous pyelography
  Intravenous digital subtraction angiography
  Carbon dioxide angiography
  Conventional arteriography

systolic/diastolic abdominal bruit in the abdomen of a young white woman not only suggests renal artery stenosis due to fibrous renal artery disease, but also predicts a cure for the hypertension with renal revascularization (185). Similarly, captopril renography is highly predictive of both renal artery stenosis and renovascular hypertension (28,186). Formal renal angiography detects renal artery stenosis but does not differentiate renal artery stenosis from renovascular hypertension. Confounding the interpretation of clinical clues and diagnostic tests suggesting renal artery stenosis and renovascular hypertension is the frequent occurrence of renal artery stenosis in patients with essential hypertension and the fact that the diagnosis of renovascular hypertension is only firmly established, retrospectively, by observing cure or marked amelioration of the hypertension following renal revascularization or nephrectomy. There is abundant literature devoted to clinical features and diagnostic maneuvers predicting that renal artery stenosis is causing the hypertension. On the other hand, clinical clues and diag-

TABLE 52-8

DETERMINATION OF PATHOPHYSIOLOGIC SIGNIFICANCE OF THE STENOTIC LESION (THE DECISION TO RECOMMEND INTERVENTION, i.e., OPERATION OR PERCUTANEOUS TRANSLUMINAL RENAL ANGIOPLASTY [PTRA], OR RENAL ARTERY STENT)

Duration of hypertension <3–5 yr
Positive findings on captopril renogram
Positive result on captopril test
Renal vein renin ratio >1.5
Hypokalemia
Systolic-diastolic bruit in abdomen
Abnormal rapid-sequence intravenous pyelogram
Appearance of lesion on angiogram (>75% stenosis)

nostic tests predicting that renal artery stenosis will eventuate in renal insufficiency are lacking.

Because the great majority of patients diagnosed as having renovascular hypertension have this syndrome consequent to main renal artery stenosis, the first step in making the diagnosis of renovascular hypertension is to demonstrate that renal artery stenosis is present. Until recently, the anatomic diagnosis of renal artery stenosis was confirmed only by conventional renal arteriography. Newer imaging modalities (see Chapters 12–14), including intravenous digital subtraction angiography, magnetic resonance angiography, computerized tomography angiography, and duplex ultrasound, have evolved in recent years, allowing for variable reductions in expense, risk, and invasiveness in diagnosing renal artery stenosis. The second step in making the diagnosis of renovascular hypertension is to determine the pathophysiologic significance of the renal artery stenosis. The third step in diagnosing renovascular hypertension is to cure or markedly ameliorate the hypertension with surgical or endovascular renal revascularization or removal of the involved kidney. Thus, hypertension presumed to be renovascular in origin is a retrospective diagnosis. Although renovascular hypertension is hypertension that is improved or cured by a technically successful intervention, at some point the hypertension may be analogous to phase III renovascular hypertension in animals when the hypertension becomes autonomous.

Issues of Prevalence, Epidemiology, Clinical Features, and Physical Examination

Epidemiology and Prevalence

The prevalence of renovascular hypertension is not known with precision, but available data suggest that it occurs in 0.5% to 5.0% of the general hypertensive population (187–196). Centers with special interest in hypertensive disorders have generated the available data on the prevalence of renovascular hypertension. Consequently, the incidence of renovascular hypertension in the community remains unknown. Many centers search for the presence of renovascular hypertension only when BP is poorly controlled. Screening procedures were less sensitive when these prevalence figures were obtained. It is difficult to determine whether prevalence figures in various reports are referring to renal artery stenosis, renovascular hypertension, or both. A negative result on a screening procedure at some point during a patient's clinical course does not exclude future development of renal artery stenosis, particularly from atherosclerotic renal artery disease.

Data from the Mayo Clinic revealed relative rarity of renovascular hypertension; only 0.18% of their hypertensive population underwent surgery for presumed renovascular hypertension. This low prevalence may be accounted for in part by the fact that not all the screened patients underwent arteriography (197). Although the small prevalence range for renovascular hypertension implies that this condition is rare, hypertension affects approximately 15% of the general population in Western countries, and it is estimated that more than 60 million people in the United States have hypertension (187,198). With the exception of hypertension due to oral contraceptive use, excessive alcohol ingestion, and the relief of hypertension by treatment of end-stage renal disease, renovascular hypertension is the most common correctable cause of secondary hypertension.

Although the prevalence of renovascular hypertension is probably less than 1% for patients with mild-to-moderate hypertension (187,193,195), the incidence of renovascular hypertension may be as high as 10% to 45% in white patients with acute onset of hypertension or severe or refractory hypertension, even if worsening BP is superimposed on preexisting mild-to-moderate hypertension (199–202). Most studies suggested that renal artery stenosis and renovascular hypertension are less common in African American patients, in whom severe hypertension is usually due to essential hypertension (203–205). Grim and co-workers (205) found functional renal artery stenosis in 11.7% of 377 hypertensive whites, but in none of 87 hypertensive blacks. However, because hypertension affects a greater proportion of the black population, the number of blacks with renovascular disease may be underestimated. One study indicated that the prevalence of renovascular hypertension in selected whites and blacks was similar, but that blacks had a much higher prevalence of both renal artery stenosis and renovascular hypertension compared to rates in previous reports (206). Another report indicated that 30% of blacks with significant coronary disease had concomitant renal artery stenosis (207). These data are supported by population surveys in the elderly in North Carolina (208).

Clinical Signs and Symptoms

When sustained diastolic hypertension (with diastolic pressure greater than 110 mm Hg) appears before age 30 or after age 55, renovascular disease should be suspected. Renovascular hypertension may appear between the ages of 30 and 55 years, but the onset of hypertension between these years typically indicates primary (essential) hypertension. In the Cooperative Study of Renovascular Hypertension, the average age of onset for fibrous renal artery disease as the cause of renovascular hypertension was 33 years, and 16% of these patients were younger than 20 years. For atherosclerotic renal artery disease as the cause of renovascular hypertension, the average age at onset was 46 years, and 39% of these patients were older than 50 years. For essential hypertension, the average age at onset was 35 years, and only 7% were older than 50 years; 12% were younger than 20 years (133,209). The decision for or against renal angiography should not be based on gender, because atherosclerotic renovascular disease occurs with enough frequency in either sex to justify renal angiography if other clinical clues are present.

Virtually all discussions and definitions of renovascular hypertension have focused on persistent elevation of the diastolic BP or on elevations of both diastolic and systolic BP. Therapies directed at curing or improving presumed renovascular hypertension have always defined "cure" or "improvement" in terms of reduction in the diastolic BP or improved levels of both diastolic and systolic pressure. The notion that isolated systolic hypertension or wide pulse pressure hypertension (e.g., 180/70 mm Hg) could be renovascular in origin has been largely ignored. In the Cooperative Study of Renovascular Hypertension (209), no mention was made that renovascular hypertension might be a reflection of isolated systolic hypertension or wide pulse pressure hypertension. With the widespread employment of renal artery stenting, particularly in elderly patients with generalized atherosclerosis obliterans, new thoughts and data regarding degrees of improvement in systolic BP in patients with normal diastolic BPs could emerge. Conceivably, new definitions of renovascular hypertension could include reductions in systolic pressure alone or reductions in pulse pressure in addition to the time-honored definitions of renovascular hypertension which have required improvement in diastolic BP levels or both diastolic and systolic BP levels.

A strong family history of hypertension suggests primary (essential) hypertension and argues against renovascular hypertension. However, a negative family history is not always useful as evidence for renovascular hypertension unless one can ascertain that close relatives are normotensive. The Cooperative Study of Renovascular Hypertension reported a statistically significant difference in the presence of family histories of hypertension between patients with renovascular hypertension (46%) and a group of patients with essential hypertension (71%) matched for race, age, and sex (133,209). However, family history by itself has limited usefulness in guiding subsequent diagnostic studies for a specific hypertensive patient because the overlap is large and many patients with essential hypertension develop superimposed atherosclerotic renal artery stenosis later in life. Several reports suggest the familial occurrence of fibrous renal artery disease, the exact mode of transmission being unclear (210,211). Cigarette smoking has been proposed as an etiologic factor in fibrous renal artery disease (19,32,65), and one presumes that cigarette smoking is a risk factor for atherosclerosis of the renal artery as it is for atherosclerosis in other vascular beds.

In general, the duration of hypertension is shorter for patients with renovascular hypertension than for patients with essential hypertension (131,133,211,212). When the clinical characteristics of essential and renovascular hypertension (cured by surgery) were compared, a duration of hypertension less than 1 year was observed in 10% of patients with essential hypertension and 25% of patients with renovascular hypertension (212). Duration of hypertension is an important prognostic factor regarding the response to surgery and it has been suggested that the success of surgical treatment in reducing blood pressure is inversely proportional to the duration of renovascular hypertension (131,133). The likely pathophysiologic explanation for this clinical observation was discussed earlier in this chapter. Patients whose hypertension suddenly becomes more severe or resistant to a previously effective drug regimen, or both, are candidates for renal artery stenosis and renovascular hypertension; the possibility that renovascular hypertension has been superimposed on underlying essential hypertension should also be considered. Although the Cooperative Study of Renovascular Hypertension did not find that acceleration of hypertension occurred more frequently in patients with renovascular hypertension than in patients with essential hypertension, 133 many patients with renovascular hypertension demonstrate resistance to drug therapy (64,213).

Accelerated or malignant hypertension and hypertensive crisis may be manifestations of renovascular hypertension (133,199,214). Rapid onset or progression of hypertension associated with severe funduscopic changes is a strong clue to the presence of renal artery stenosis. Davis et al. reported renovascular hypertension in 23% of 123 patients with severe hypertension and grade III or IV funduscopic retinal changes (199). This figure is considerably higher than the prevalence of renovascular hypertension among the general hypertensive population and argues for a thorough evaluation for renovascular hypertension in patients presenting with accelerated or malignant hypertension.

Pulmonary edema ("flash pulmonary edema") has been suggested as a pattern of clinical presentation for patients with advanced renal artery stenosis (215–217). In a series of 55 consecutive patients who were also azotemic, pulmonary edema was present in 13 (25%). Most of these patients had high-grade renal artery stenosis bilaterally or involving the artery to a solitary kidney. Successful renal revascularization prevented further occurrence of pulmonary edema. Although pulmonary edema is frequently observed in the setting of severe hypertension and hypertensive heart disease, in this series (217) the occurrence of pulmonary edema was not related to the severity of the hypertension or coexisting renal failure. However, in a study of 90 patients with renal artery stenosis, 23 had bilateral renal artery stenosis and recurrent pulmonary edema (218). Ninety percent of this latter group had renal insufficiency; only 20% had moderate or severe reduction in ejection fraction. Therefore, the findings of hypertension, recurrent pulmonary edema, azotemia, and a well-preserved ejection fraction should raise the possibility of bilateral renal artery stenosis.

Generalized vascular disease is closely associated with atherosclerotic renal artery stenosis (28,207,219). Of interest, atherosclerotic renovascular disease is not more common in diabetic patients despite the increased prevalence of vascular disease in this patient population (187,195).

There are no symptoms that are pathognomonic of renovascular hypertension. Flank pain does not occur more often in patients with renal vascular disease than in patients with essential hypertension (133,209). Flank pain or hematuria or both may indicate segmental renal infarction due to segmental renal artery occlusion (220), renal artery dissection associated with several of the fibrous dysplasias (221), or intimal dissection of the renal artery after selective angiography (222). Hypertension following traumatic injury is an indication to exclude traumatic renal artery occlusion. A delayed onset of hypertension following traumatic injury to the retroperitoneal area suggests subcapsular or perirenal hematoma (Page kidney). Takayasu's arteritis, frequently involving the renal artery and associated with renovascular hypertension, is characterized by nonspecific symptoms such as fever, myalgias, arthralgias, weight loss, general fatigue, vertigo, and cold extremities. Hypertension developing in a young woman, an abdominal bruit, increased erythrocyte sedimentation rate, and absent radial artery pulse are important clinical findings for establishing this diagnosis (223).

Rapid deterioration of renal function following BP reduction with conventional antihypertensive agents or particularly following BP reduction with ACE inhibitors strongly suggests the presence of bilateral renal artery stenosis, or stenosis in a solitary functioning kidney (162,224–229). In one series, more than one-half of patients demonstrating an acute elevation in the plasma creatinine concentration that was either unexplained or occurred shortly after institution of therapy with an ACE inhibitor had main renal artery disease, while the remainder presumably had disease of the intrarenal vessels due to nephrosclerosis (230). The mechanism of acute renal dysfunction after treatment with ACE inhibitors appears to be a combination of a fall in BP and a direct action of these compounds on intrarenal hemodynamics. It is presumed that the glomerular filtration rate (GFR) in the presence of renal artery stenosis is maintained, in part by the actions of angiotensin II on the efferent glomerular arterioles. Attenuation of this action of angiotensin II by converting enzyme inhibition may explain renal dysfunction occurring with ACE inhibitor therapy in the setting of bilateral renal artery stenosis, or stenosis of a solitary kidney.

In an instructive series of 104 patients at high risk for bilateral renal artery stenosis, all were given an ACE inhibitor for 2 weeks (although this was discontinued after 4 days if the serum creatinine concentration had increased >20%) (231). If after 2 weeks, the serum creatinine had not increased >20%, and the BP remained elevated, patients were given a diuretic to correct fluid retention. All patients subsequently had a renal arteriogram. Of the 52 patients with severe (>50%) bilateral renovascular disease or severe stenosis of the artery to a solitary functioning kidney, each had a rise in serum creatinine of >20% with ACE inhibitor therapy. The authors concluded that a controlled exposure to an ACE inhibitor is generally safe and that an ACE inhibitor-induced increase in serum creatinine is 100% sensitive and 70% specific for the detection of severe bilateral renovascular disease.

Physical Examination

The physical examination affords four clues to the presence of renovascular disease: the severity of the hypertension, an abdominal bruit, abnormalities of the optic fundi, and evidence of atherosclerotic disease of the aorta and peripheral arteries. As in essential hypertension, the hypertension in patients with renovascular disease can be of any degree. As alluded to earlier, however, severe hypertension and accelerated or malignant hypertension are not uncommon manifestations of renovascular hypertension (189,214,232,233). An acute rise in BP over previously controlled or stable baseline BP suggests renovascular disease.

Detection of an abdominal bruit, although not diagnostic, suggests renal artery disease and possible renovascular hypertension. A systolic/diastolic bruit in the epigastrium or one or both upper quadrants is virtually pathognomonic of renovascular disease and provides a strong indication for renal angiography even if other clinical clues to renovascular disease are lacking. Further, the abdominal systolic/diastolic bruit predicts a successful result from surgical renal revascularization (185), and hence is an index of renovascular hypertension as well as of renovascular disease. The absence of a systolic/diastolic bruit in the epigastrium does not exclude renovascular disease, but, particularly in the case of fibrous renal artery disease, makes it less likely that surgery or angioplasty will relieve the hypertension.

The diastolic component to an epigastric bruit is frequently difficult to appreciate; a soft, wide, pansystolic bruit also suggests renovascular disease. The helpfulness of an abdominal bruit in the diagnosis of renovascular hypertension has been stressed by several authors (133,209,234–236). Maxwell reported detecting an abdominal bruit in 41% of patients with renovascular hypertension due to atherosclerotic renal artery disease and in 57% of patients with renovascular hypertension due to fibrous dysplasia. Hunt et al. reported abdominal bruits with diastolic components in 25 (36%) of 69 patients with atherosclerotic renal artery disease and in 76 (74%) of 104 patients with fibrous renovascular disease (235). Eipper et al. found that 25 of 47 patients with fibrous renovascular lesions had systolic/diastolic bruits in the abdomen while such bruits were present in only 5 of 40 patients with atherosclerotic renovascular disease (185). Moser and Caldwell and the Renovascular Study Cooperative Group, although emphasizing the importance of abdominal bruits, were less impressed with the significance of the diastolic component (236).

Systolic bruits are frequently heard in the abdomen and it is often difficult to determine whether the systolic bruit is emanating from the renal artery, other intraabdominal arteries, or the aorta. In contrast to the importance of a systolic/diastolic bruit in patients with fibrous renal artery disease, systolic epigastric bruits, without a diastolic component, are of marginal clinical utility.

In the absence of an arteriovenous fistula, a diastolic component to an arterial bruit signifies stenosis of approximately 70% or more (237,238). A diastolic component to the arterial bruit, although highly suggestive of hemodynamic renal artery disease, may also reflect hemodynamically significant stenosis of other visceral arteries, particularly the celiac access or the superior mesenteric artery. Fibrous renal artery disease may affect these vessels, as well as the renal arteries, and occasionally the carotid arteries. The importance of a bruit in the back or flank is probably overstated and when present in these locations is almost certainly audible in the epigastrium or upper abdominal quadrants (214).

Severe hypertensive retinopathy (Keith-Wagener-Barker grades III and IV), detected on examination of the optic fundi, is a strong clue to renovascular hypertension (199,206). Davis et al. 199 reported that 41 (48%) of 85 hypertensive patients with retinal hemorrhages and exudates with or without papilledema had stenotic lesions on renal arteriograms and 26 (31%) had a strong likelihood of renovascular hypertension, which was defined by the presence of lateralizing differential renal function or renal venous renin activity. Nearly 25% of these patients with severe hypertensive retinopathy turned out to have proven renovascular hypertension. In the Cooperative Study of Renovascular Hypertension (209), the prevalence of Keith-Wagener-Barker retinopathy of grades III and IV was twice as high among those having renovascular hypertension compared to those with primary or essential hypertension. The presence of malignant hypertension (diastolic BP greater than 140 mm Hg and papilledema) suggests renovascular disease, particularly when accelerated hypertension and accelerated retinopathy occur in a white patient with well-documented hypertension of less than 2 years, and is a strong indication for renal angiography.

In the absence of hemorrhages, exudates, and papilledema (Keith-Wagener-Barker grades III and IV), severe retinal arteriolar constriction with minimal or no retinal arteriolar sclerosis suggests recent onset of severe hypertension, and is a clue to the presence of renovascular hypertension. This funduscopic observation has been called *arteriospastic angiopathy*. Hunt et al. observed these changes in 15 (20%) of 81 patients with atherosclerotic renovascular disease and in 60 (45%) of 133 patients with fibrous renal artery disease (235).

Moderate to severe hypertension in patients with evidence of atherosclerotic disease of the aorta and peripheral arteries, particularly in patients older than 50 years, implies atherosclerotic renovascular disease as a possible cause of the hypertension. This is especially true for patients with abdominal aortic aneurysms or occlusive disease in the distribution of the aorto-iliac-femoral popliteal system (2,3,34,239). In one prospective study of 100 patients presenting with signs of peripheral vascular disease, bilateral renal artery stenosis was present in 24, of whom 7 had complete occlusion on one side (34). Others reported as much as a 50% incidence of at least 50% stenosis in one renal artery in patients with peripheral vascular disease, with or without hypertension (28,239). Some of these patients were normotensive and many had essential hypertension. Thus, although these atherosclerotic renal artery lesions may not be instrumental in the pathogenesis of hypertension, the existence of these stenoses may threaten long-term renal function.

Laboratory Tests, Radiologic Examinations, and Diagnostic Maneuvers

Laboratory Tests

Urinalysis is of little benefit in evaluating renal artery stenosis and renovascular hypertension. Mild-to-moderate proteinuria is common and probably reflects the severity of the hypertension or associated nephrosclerosis (133). Nephrotic range or heavy proteinuria has been described in association with renal artery stenosis and renovascular hypertension, usually in the setting of accelerated or malignant hypertension (prior to availability of effective antihypertensive drugs) (240). Several authors reported nephrotic-range proteinuria due to renal artery stenosis wherein the urinary protein excretion normalized after renal revascularization or nephrectomy (241–244). In these uncommon situations, excessive production of angiotensin II may be responsible for promoting high levels of protein excretion (245,246). Focal segmental glomerulosclerosis (FSGS) with heavy proteinuria has been described in association with renal artery stenosis (247,248). In a series of 24 patients with biopsy-proven FSGS who were over 50 years old, 8 had renovascular disease (249). These eight patients had typical glomerular lesions with focal segmental tuft collapse and synechiae. All patients had heavy proteinuria and developed a further decline in renal function at follow-up. The au-

thors proposed that FSGS may be an unrecognized complication of renovascular disease in elderly patients and may contribute to irreversible changes in the kidneys. Nephrotic-range proteinuria can occur in adults with diabetic renal disease and atherosclerotic renal artery stenosis, wherein the proteinuria is likely due to the diabetic glomerular disease, rather than to main renal artery stenosis.

Unexplained azotemia in elderly patients with generalized atherosclerosis and minimal proteinuria suggests vascular occlusive disease of the kidneys, including bilateral renal artery stenosis, stenosis of an artery to a solitary kidney, or a combination of renal artery stenosis and nephrosclerosis. Uncontrolled BP itself may contribute to renal insufficiency, particularly if there is an underlying baseline impairment in GFR (233,239,250–252). In the Cooperative Study of Renovascular Hypertension, 15% of patients with atheromatous renal artery disease had an elevated serum creatinine concentration, compared with 11% of patients with essential hypertension; only 2% of patients with fibrous renal artery disease had an elevated serum creatinine concentration (209).

Hypokalemia (serum potassium level less than 3.4 mEq/L) is a marker of hemodynamically significant renal artery stenosis, reflecting stimulation of the renin-angiotensin system with secondary aldosteronism. Although the concomitant use of diuretics to treat the hypertension may confound the interpretation of hypokalemia in patients with renovascular disease, hypokalemia in a patient (not receiving a diuretic) with severe hypertension is highly suggestive of renovascular hypertension. In the Cooperative Study of Renovascular Hypertension, a serum potassium concentration of less than 3.4 mEq/L was observed in 16% of patients with renovascular hypertension cured by surgery, in contrast to 8% of patients with essential hypertension (133,209).

A significant discrepancy in kidney size in hypertensive adults, and particularly the observation of an atrophic kidney, strongly indicate renal artery stenosis as the basis for the smaller kidney. Not infrequently, the small kidney is the cause of the hypertension, which may be relieved by renal revascularization or nephrectomy (88). A number of currently available renal imaging techniques, including ultrasonography, scintigraphy, radiography of the kidneys, ureters, and bladder (KUB), intravenous pyelography, and computed tomography, all allow for easy detection of a unilateral small kidney. This observation, in conjunction with additional clinical clues suggesting renovascular hypertension, may be sufficient reason to proceed quickly to renal angiography to confirm that renal artery stenosis is the cause of the smaller kidney. Significant renal artery stenosis involving the artery to the contralateral kidney is observed frequently (30% to 50% of the time) in the setting of high-grade stenosis or total arterial occlusion of the artery supplying the atrophic kidney (88,89).

Plasma Renin Activity

Although unilateral hypersecretion of renin is an expected finding in hemodynamically significant renal artery stenosis when renovascular hypertension is eventually proved (247), baseline plasma renin activity (PRA) is elevated in only approximately 50% of patients with renovascular hypertension (213,229,253). Tabulation of the number of patients whose hypertension was cured or improved by surgical renal revascularization indicates that probably no more than 50% of patients with renovascular hypertension have elevated PRA (205,212,213,254-259).

There are several reasons for the relatively low specificity and sensitivity of peripheral PRA in the diagnosis of renovascular hypertension. Most high-renin hypertension is not renovascular in origin; increased renin substrate can be due to estrogen intake, pregnancy, cortisol excess, intrarenal ischemia

TABLE 52-9

SENSITIVITY AND SPECIFICITY OF THE CAPTOPRIL PLASMA RENIN ACTIVITY TEST

Investigators	No. of patients studied	No. of patients with renal artery stenosis	Sensitivity (%)	Specificity (%)
Muller, et al. (269)	152	49	100	95
Derkx, et al. (271)	179	89	93	84
Frederickson, et al. (117)	100	29	100	80
Gosse, et al. (272)	114	11	73	84
Hansen, et al. (273)	47	11	91	89
Postma, et al. (274)	149	44	38	93
Svetkey, et al. (275)	66	11	73	72
Thibonnier, et al. (276)	65	14	40	100
Elliott, et al. (277)	100	59	76	58

(From: Nally JV Jr, Olin JW, Lammert GK. Advances in noninvasive screening for renovascular disease. *Cleve Clin J Med* 1994;61:328, with permission.)

(parenchymal disease), or accelerated or malignant hypertension, and the 15% to 20% of patients with primary (essential) hypertension and high renin levels constitute the majority of high-renin hypertensives. Renin secretion fluctuates widely (260), and is also influenced by sodium intake and posture (261), a variety of antihypertensive drugs, age (262), sex, and race (263). The utility of peripheral PRA is reportedly enhanced when measured in the morning with the patient in the seated position and when indexed against urinary sodium excretion; when measured under these exacting circumstances, a high peripheral PRA is found in 75% to 80% of patients with proven renovascular hypertension (122,264). Other investigators, measuring peripheral PRA under similar circumstances, failed to demonstrate significantly increased sensitivity of the peripheral PRA in predicting renovascular hypertension, even under controlled circumstances (122,265,266). Complicating the interpretation of peripheral plasma renin values is the long list of coexisting medical conditions and drugs that either stimulate or inhibit renin release. A very low PRA (e.g., less than 0.3 ng/mL/hour) indexed against a normal urinary sodium excretion in the absence of drugs known to suppress renin argues strongly against renovascular hypertension (267–269).

Captopril Provocation Test, Captopril Plasma Renin Activity

The predictive value of the peripheral PRA can be increased by measuring the rise in PRA 1 hour after the oral administration of 50 mg of captopril (a rapidly acting ACE inhibitor) (118,229,253,269,270). Case and Laragh (270) first showed that the reactive rise of renin following the administration of captopril is greater in patients with renovascular hypertension than in those with essential hypertension. The criteria that this group recommended (269) for distinguishing patients with renovascular hypertension (i.e., criteria for a positive captopril test result) are: (a) a stimulated PRA of 12 ng/mL/hour; (b) an absolute increase in PRA of 10 ng/mL/hour; and (c) an increase in PRA of 150% or more if the baseline PRA is more than 3 ng/mL/hour, or a percent increase in PRA of 400% if the baseline PRA is less than 3 ng/mL/hour. These investigators emphasized that all three of these criteria should be satisfied and that blood samples should be drawn with the patient seated (not supine). It is important to realize that the renin assay to which these results relate was that used in Laragh and Sealey's laboratory. Other renin assays may provide very different values for cut off points as described in Frederickson et al. (117). A sim-

pler criterion of a post-captopril PRA (PRA >5.7 ng/mL/hour) yields a test without any loss of sensitivity (117,118). In a series of more than 200 patients, the sensitivity and specificity of this test were better than 95% (269). Other groups, however, reported lower levels of sensitivity, in part using different criteria; the sensitivity and specificity of the captopril PRA test from nine separate series are summarized in Table 52-9 (117,186,269,271–277). The general utility of this test is further limited by: (a) the need to discontinue antihypertensive medications that can affect the PRA (e.g., beta-blockers and diuretics), (b) the need to standardize the procedure, (c) the variable sensitivity, and (d) the somewhat decreased predictive value when compared to captopril renography (102,201). When applied prospectively, the accuracy of renin-based measurements for predicting the outcomes of renal revascularization is limited to between 35 to 60% sensitivity and specificity (278).

In interpreting the captopril test, the poststenotic kidney is likely to have excess stores of renin and thereby could be considered to be primed to demonstrate a reactive rise of renin following administration of captopril, particularly with a concomitant fall in arterial pressure (270). This possible mechanism, however, may not be the major cause for the enhanced response to ACE inhibition, since equivalent reductions of BP produced by other agents, such as clonidine, do not elevate PRA excessively in patients with functionally significant unilateral renal artery stenosis (279,280). More likely, a positive captopril provocation test signifies the same intrarenal hemodynamic changes as a positive ACE inhibitor renogram, that is, a fall in GFR in the poststenotic kidney. This GFR decline will reduce NaCl delivery to the macula densa and stimulate renin secretion preferentially in a functionally stenotic kidney. A decrease in BP 1 hour after captopril administration may be expected to be greater for patients with renovascular hypertension than for patients with essential hypertension, and this assumption is supported by the observation in one study that patients with renovascular disease demonstrated an average decrease in BP of 18 mm Hg, whereas patients with essential hypertension had a decrease in BP of 7 mm Hg (202,275,281). However, considerable overlap exists in the decrease in BP in patients with renovascular versus essential hypertension that limits the utility of this observation as a reliable screening test for renovascular hypertension. A dramatic decrease in BP after captopril administration, however, may predict a good BP response to renal revascularization or angioplasty (281). The captopril-stimulated PRA test becomes less reliable in patients with renal insufficiency, and it does not discriminate between patients with unilateral versus those with bilateral renal artery stenosis (269,271).

Three prospective studies showed that the BP of hypertensive subjects with renal artery stenosis during established monotherapy with ACE inhibitors correlates quite closely with the BP after reconstructive surgery (129,282), nephrectomy (129,282), or percutaneous transluminal angioplasty (PTRA) (283). The overall correlation coefficient in these three trials for BP during ACE inhibitor monotherapy and BP after intervention is 0.64 (229). Therefore, some insight into the effectiveness of a planned intervention to correct renal artery stenosis for reduction in BP can be obtained from the BP achieved during ACE inhibitor therapy.

Saralasin Infusion Test

Before captopril administration became popular to enhance the sensitivity of the peripheral PRA in the diagnosis of renovascular hypertension, the BP response to the angiotensin II antagonist saralasin was advocated both as a screening test for presumed renovascular hypertension and to identify patients who might be candidates for renal angiography (270,284,285). Saralasin, an angiotensin II analog, competitively binds to angiotensin II vascular receptors and inhibits the pressor effect of angiotensin II. In addition, saralasin has weak agonist (vasoconstrictor) properties. If renal artery stenosis is instrumental in causing the hypertension, angiotensin II levels are presumably high, and an infusion of saralasin should markedly lower the diastolic BP. When angiotensin II levels are low, saralasin either has a minimal response in reducing the BP or, via its agonist properties, could produce a pressor effect. This construct would then allow for differentiation between angiotensin II-dependent and angiotensin II-independent hypertension. Initial enthusiasm for this test waned because its performance requires careful adherence to an infusion protocol and discontinuation of antihypertensive medications other than diuretics 1 week before testing. Although mild volume depletion may augment the discriminatory potential of the test (285), several sizable series indicated a sensitivity of only 50% to 60% and a specificity of about 85% (205,286,287). For these reasons, the saralasin infusion test is not recommended as a screening procedure for renovascular hypertension (213,288).

Differential Renal Vein Renin Determinations

For almost 30 years, determination of the renal vein renin ratio (ipsilateral renal vein renin to contralateral renal vein renin) was used to assess the functional significance of renal vascular stenoses. The rationale of obtaining renal vein renin ratios is derived from the pathophysiology of classic two-kidney Goldblatt hypertension, wherein renal hypotension distal to the renal artery stenosis generates hypersecretion of renin by the affected kidney. Characteristics of renin-dependent unilateral renovascular hypertension are (a) increased renin secretion from the affected side and (b) suppression of contralateral renin release (122,259,268,289–293). Blood is sampled from each renal vein and from the inferior vena cava, and the plasma renin levels from the two renal veins are compared to each other and to the corresponding level in the inferior vena cava (below the level of the renal veins), which has been shown to be the same as the renin level in the main renal artery. Vaughan et al. (122,293) added a third criterion suggesting renin-dependent unilateral renovascular hypertension based on their analysis of renal vein and renal arterial renin relationships in patients with hypertension. These workers calculated that the mean renal venous renin is about 25% higher than the arterial renin, indicating that the hypoperfused kidney is truly overproducing renin (122,290,293). They derived a specific formula to estimate renin production from the two kidneys. Most centers

simply employ a renal vein renin ratio of at least 1.5 to 2.0 (ipsilateral to contralateral) with suppression of renin production (i.e., renin from contralateral kidney is equal to or below the plasma renin level from the inferior vena cava below the renal arteries) as the criterion for "lateralizing" renal renin secretion and as a predictor of a beneficial surgical outcome for relief of hypertension.

Since the report of Helmer and Judson in 1960 (294), wherein a renal vein renin ratio of 2.0 or higher was used as a predictor of surgical cure of renovascular hypertension, the renal vein renin ratio has been widely accepted as a criterion to diagnose hemodynamically significant unilateral renal artery stenosis. In 1976, Marks et al. reviewed 21 previously published series encompassing 468 patients with unilateral renovascular disease who had been subjected to a broad spectrum of renin-stimulating maneuvers (e.g., sodium depletion, upright posture) (132). They concluded that a lateralizing renal vein renin ratio predicted surgical cure or substantial improvement in the BP in 93% of patients. Fifty-seven percent of patients with a nonlateralizing renal vein renin ratio (less than 1.5 ipsilateral to contralateral) also benefited from surgery (132). In another review of 58 studies, a ratio of 1.5 or more (ischemic kidney to contralateral kidney) as the diagnostic criterion predicting renovascular hypertension had a sensitivity of 80% and a specificity of 62% (295). Remarkably low renin levels sampled from the renal veins (less than 1 ng/mL/hour), particularly if equally low bilaterally, militate against renovascular hypertension (267,269,296).

The high predictive value of a lateralizing renal vein renin ratio as well as the high false-negative rate (i.e., nonlateralizing renal vein renin ratio) have been observed in many subsequent studies. An analysis of 10 reports between 1976 and 1986 (147) including 282 patients with renovascular disease subjected to various renin-stimulating maneuvers indicated an average false-positive rate of only 14% but an impressively high false-negative rate of 67%. Some of the false-negative results may be attributed to technical errors; nevertheless, the high false-negative rate of renal vein renin determination is a consistent finding from many centers. Possible explanations for this high false-negative rate include technical difficulties in placing the catheters far enough distally in the renal vein or failure to use two catheters so samples can be drawn simultaneously from the renal veins (297); renal vein sampling while the patient is taking antihypertensive drugs (298); branch lesions of the renal arteries or bilateral renal artery stenoses, which are notorious for minimizing differences in renal venous PRA between the two kidneys (268,299); dilution errors, or substances interfering with the assays; and non–renin-mediated renovascular hypertension (e.g., hypoplastic kidney, atrophic pyelonephritis) (88).

Several stimulatory maneuvers have been designed to increase the sensitivity of differential renal vein renin determinations (209,300). These include sodium depletion (low-sodium diet and/or diuretic presampling) (131,209,259,300,301), upright posture (tilt) (290,302–304), and a variety of pharmacologic agents. Saralasin (270,285), acute administration of captopril (270,276,285,305–307), intravenous hydralazine (308), and bolus furosemide (298,309) have been utilized. Aurell (303) and Michelakis (304) and their respective colleagues demonstrated a reduced incidence of false-negative renal vein renin results with upright posture stimulation wherein the disparity in renal vein renin secretion from the two sides was exaggerated by tilting during the collection of renal venous blood. Captopril administration, which results in a reactive rise in renin in renovascular hypertension, potentiates the disparity in the renin secretion from the two kidneys, reducing the false-negative rate of renal vein renin determination. The mechanism of augmented renin secretion with bolus furosemide at the time of renal venous sampling is not clear, but may be due to inhibition of the macula densa NaCl reabsorption, intrarenal vasodilation, and prostaglandin secretion all of which can potentiate renin release. Assuming that the kidney ipsilateral to the stenosis is primed to release large amounts of renin, these stimulatory maneuvers should theoretically increase the renal vein renin value from the ipsilateral kidney more than from the contralateral kidney, thereby reducing false-negative renal vein renin results. In addition to augmenting the renal vein renin differential, captopril administration also obviates the need to discontinue previous antihypertensive drugs in preparation for renal vein renin sampling, except, possibly, diuretics (306,307). This maneuver is particularly pertinent, because stopping all antihypertensive medications in preparation for renal vein renin sampling may be hazardous in patients with presumed renovascular hypertension, who often have significant and dangerous elevations in the BP.

In patients with stenoses of both renal arteries, the pattern of renal vein renin levels often shows the same degree of asymmetry as in patients with unilateral stenosis, and the renin values usually lateralize to the kidney demonstrating the greater degree of stenosis on the arteriogram (268). The most marked asymmetry is seen in patients who have complete occlusion of one renal artery, wherein renal vein renin levels from the side of the occluded artery may represent low flow through the kidney rather than hypersecretion of renin. Contralateral suppression of renin secretion may occur even in the presence of severe stenosis of the contralateral kidney. This asymmetry is less pronounced in the presence of azotemia. Although less valuable in patients with bilateral renal artery stenosis, determination of renal vein renin levels may be useful for identifying which kidney is the "most ischemic," which can be useful in planning which kidney to subject to intervention (268).

Taken together, the data regarding renal vein renin determinations indicate that the renal vein renin ratio has a strong positive predictive value in forecasting a beneficial interventional outcome. On the other hand, many patients (at least 50%) demonstrating a nonlateralizing renal vein renin ratio have marked improvement or cure of their hypertension following intervention for the renal artery stenosis. This fact, and the ready availability of captopril scintigraphy, and the common practice of PTRA or renal artery stenting done at the time of diagnostic renal angiography, have led to a decline in the use of renal vein renin tests.

Intravenous Pyelography

The rapid-sequence (hypertensive) intravenous pyelogram (IVP) has historically been used as a test for renovascular hypertension. In 1964, Maxwell et al. described the radiographic features suggesting renal artery stenosis (310). In the 1960s and 1970s, the hypertensive IVP was the standard screening test for renal artery stenosis and renovascular hypertension, and its initial popularity was attributed to its simplicity and safety, as demonstrated in the renovascular cooperative study (209,310,311). Abnormalities in the IVP suggesting renovascular disease are (a) a difference in renal lengths of 1.5 cm or more (the left kidney is normally 0.5 cm longer than the right); (b) delayed appearance of contrast medium in the intrarenal collecting system on the early sequence films; and (c) prolonged concentration of contrast medium, that is, persistent nephrogram, on late sequence films. Of these features, the delayed appearance of contrast medium on early sequence films was the most discriminating between essential and renovascular hypertension in the Cooperative Study of Renovascular Hypertension (209,311). In this study, 78% of patients who had at least 50% stenosis of one renal artery had one or more abnormalities on the IVP, compared with 11.4% of patients with essential hypertension. The more severe the renal artery stenosis, the greater likelihood that the IVP was abnormal. In

patients with a totally occluded renal artery, 96% of pyelograms appeared abnormal, readily demonstrating a nonfunctioning kidney ipsilateral to the totally occluded renal artery. Although 78% of patients with significant renal artery stenosis had an abnormal IVP, there was a 17% false-negative and an 11% false-positive rate in surgically proved unilateral renovascular hypertension (311).

Reanalysis of the same data by Thornbury et al. derived a false-negative rate of 22% and a false-positive rate of 13% (312). Havey et al., in a review of 20 studies, reported a sensitivity of 74.5% and a specificity of 86.2% for IVP in detecting renovascular hypertension (313). The IVP is insensitive in detecting bilateral or branch stenosis (187,200,253,313). The suboptimal sensitivity and specificity, sizable dye load, and radiation dosage have all contributed to the current unpopularity of the hypertensive IVP as a routine screening procedure for renal artery stenosis and renovascular hypertension.

Renal Scans

Isotope renograms or renal scans have been available for many years and are helpful in selecting hypertensive patients for renal angiography (209,314,315). However, routine renal scanning never gained widespread acceptance because of the high incidence of false-negative results (315,316). The most widely used isotopes have been iodohippurate sodium (hippuran) and diethylenetriamine pentaacetic acid (DTPA). Iodohippurate sodium gives an approximation of the renal flow rate, while DTPA gives an approximation of the GFR. The value of radionuclide imaging of the kidneys is that it is a noninvasive and relatively simple method of assessing renal ischemia. In addition, computer-assisted qualitative and quantitative measurements of renal function (renal blood flow and GFR) can be performed (317). Radionuclide renal scanning has comparable sensitivity to the rapid-sequence IVP in diagnosing renovascular hypertension, but lower specificity; false-positive rates approximating 25% have been reported (209,212). In selecting patients for renal angiography, radionuclide renal scanning has a marginal advantage over the rapid-sequence IVP in that it obviates the need for contrast medium, and entails less radiation exposure. A renal scan can also be utilized to estimate the contribution of one kidney to overall renal function prior to a planned nephrectomy. The IVP on the other hand provides much more information about the anatomy of the kidneys and urinary tract, which in selected situations is useful in evaluating hypertensive patients.

Captopril Renography

The sensitivity and specificity of the routine renal radionuclide scan have been improved by combining scintigraphy with the administration of captopril (captopril renography, captopril scintigraphy). The rationale for this maneuver is that the GFR of the ischemic kidney ipsilateral to the renal artery stenosis is dependent on the effects of angiotensin II on the efferent glomerular arterioles; captopril reduces the angiotensin II-mediated constriction of the efferent arteriole, thus lowering glomerular pressure (229,318). The resulting decrease in glomerular filtration of the hypoperfused kidney is demonstrated by renal handling of radioactive tracers with the characteristic observation of a decreased uptake of DTPA (reflecting the GFR) with a delayed time to peak and slowed, or absent, washout (226,319–322). Simultaneously, inhibition of the pressor effects of excess circulating angiotensin II might improve the function of the contralateral (nonischemic) kidney, thereby exaggerating the asymmetry in renal function between the two kidneys (143,323–326). Studies of the effects of diuretic administration have shown that the characteristic captopril-induced changes are little affected by furosemide, but are abolished by mannitol (229). This indicates that the

TABLE 52-10

SENSITIVITY, SPECIFICITY, AND PREDICTIVE VALUE OF CAPTOPRIL RENOGRAPHY

Investigators	No. of patients	No. of patients with RAS	Radionuclide used	Sensitivity (%)	Specificity (%)	Predicted blood pressure response
Geyskes, et al. (328)	34	15	OIH	80	100	Yes: 12/15
Sfakianakis, et al. (319)	31	16	OIH	67	100	—
			Tc-DTPA	48	—	—
Erbslöh-Möller, et al. (329)	40	28	OIH	96	95	Yes: 10/11
Svetkey, et al. (275)	61	11	Tc-DTPA	74	44	—
			OIH	71	41	—
Setaro, et al. (330)	90	44	Tc-DTPA	91	94	Yes: 15/18
Mann, et al. (331)	55	35	Tc-DTPA	94	95	—
			OIH	83	85	—
Fommei, et al. (332)	472	259	Tc-DTPA	83	91	—
			Tc-MAC$_3$	83	100	—
Dondi (333)	102	54	Tc-MAC$_3$	90	92	Yes
Elliott, et al. (242)	100	59	Tc-pentetate	92	80	Yes: 51/53

RAS, renal artery stenosis; OIH, iodine-131-orthoiodohippurate; Tc-DTPA, technetium 99m-diethylenetriaminepentaacetic acid; Tc-Mag3, technetium 99m-mercaptoacetyltriglycine.
(From: Nally JV Jr, Olin JW, Lammert GK. Advances in noninvasive screening for renovascular disease. *Cleve Clin J Med* 1994;61:328, with permission.)

captopril-induced reduction in renal clearance of the tracer is due to accumulation in the proximal nephron because of a reduced GFR leading to a reduced tubular fluid flow that can be reversed by mannitol (118).

Although protocols for performing captopril renography are complex, and diagnostic criteria are not well standardized (327), the accuracy of captopril renography is clearly an improvement over routine renal scans. As indicated in Table 52-10, the accuracy of captopril renography is quite acceptable, with a sensitivity of approximately 90% to 93% (range 48% to 94%) and a specificity of approximately 93% to 98% (range 41% to 100%) (186,275,277,319,328–333). Unlike the captopril PRA test, captopril renography can be conveniently done without discontinuing antihypertensive medications (330,331), with the exception of ACE inhibitors. Administration of furosemide during the procedure may improve sensitivity without compromising specificity (118,329,334). In performing captopril renography, a baseline renal scan is obtained. Subsequently, a second renal scan is obtained, usually on another day and after oral administration of captopril (25 to 50 mg), and the two scans are compared. Typical renographic time-activity curves with technetium 99m-DTPA at baseline and after captopril stimulation are depicted in Figure 52-13. Alternatively, a renal scan after oral administration of captopril can be performed initially, and if the initial scan is abnormal, a repeat renal scan without captopril is performed subsequently to ascertain if there are discrepancies in renal function observed after captopril administration disappear or if they persist in the absence of captopril provocation. The former scenario suggests hemodynamically significant unilateral renal artery stenosis, whereas the latter does not (325,327,330,331,335).

The isotopic label most widely used in captopril renography is DTPA, although some authors claim that iodohippurate sodium can be as sensitive (329,336). More recently, technetium 99m-mercaptoacetyltriglycine (99 mTc-MAG3) has been utilized as the labeling isotope to provide images superior to those made with hippurate, with less radiation dosage and better resolution than provided by DTPA (333,337,338). Nearly always, captopril is the converting enzyme inhibitor employed because of its rapid onset of action, but enalapril or intravenous enalaprilat have also been used (336).

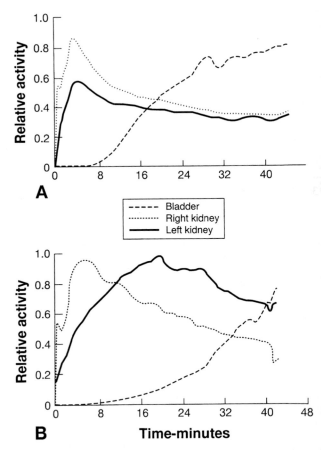

FIGURE 52-13. Renogram of a patient with unilateral left renal artery stenosis. **A:** Technetium 99m-diethylenetriamine pentaacetic acid (99mTc-DTPA)-timed activity curves during baseline. **B:** 99mTc-DTPA-timed activity curves following captopril administration. (From: Nally JV Jr, Olin JW, Lammert GK. Advances in noninvasive screening for renovascular disease. *Cleve Clin J Med* 1994;61:328, with permission.)

Diagnostic criteria in interpreting the captopril scintigram are based on a comparison of either (a) affected versus contralateral kidney (for asymmetry of uptake or excretion), or (b) pre– versus post–captopril administration scintigram (for captopril-induced changes) (253). Specific quantitative diagnostic criteria to distinguish essential from renovascular hypertension have not been firmly established; some investigators prefer the use of qualitative criteria (335).

Asymmetry of uptake or excretion or both may occur when uptake is measured between 1.5 and 2.5 minutes after injection. Asymmetric uptake has been defined as an uptake of less than 40% by the affected kidney and more than 60% of the total renal uptake by the contralateral kidney. A lesser degree of asymmetry occurs frequently and is not diagnostically helpful (330,331). The more severe the stenosis, the more reduced the uptake of the isotope (339). When stenosis is less severe, delayed excretion may be the only renographic abnormality. When stenosis approaches total occlusion, renal function is dramatically reduced, and renal function as assessed isotopically may cease (331).

Renal insufficiency reduces the sensitivity of captopril renography, and the dose of orthoiodohippurate that can be administered, as an index of effective renal plasma flow, is limited by the cumulative radiation exposure associated with renal insufficiency. MAG$_3$, because of its enhanced tubular secretion and lesser duration of radioactive exposure compared to orthoiodohippurate (338), probably has some advantages with better resolution than does DTPA. Patients with severe bilateral renal artery stenosis or renal artery stenosis of a solitary kidney are at risk of developing a transient but significant decline in renal function with captopril administration during this test (335), but this concern has not been a major clinical problem. Some studies indicate that captopril renography can discriminate between renovascular and renal parenchymal disease. In a study of 20 azotemic patients, all had abnormal baseline hippuran scans (329). However, a captopril-induced change in the scan predicted the presence of renal artery stenosis with a good BP response to intervention after renal artery angioplasty with a sensitivity and specificity >90%.

Taken together, experience with captopril renography to date is a major advance in diagnostic maneuvers designed to predict renal artery stenosis and renovascular hypertension (340). A positive finding by captopril renography strongly suggests the anatomic presence of renal artery stenosis and is an indication for renal angiography. A positive finding further indicates that renal artery stenosis is physiologically significant and instrumental in producing hypertension, thereby providing an indication for intervention (e.g., angioplasty, surgery) in an attempt to cure the hypertension. Whether captopril renography is a reliable probe for predicting progressive renal insufficiency due to renal artery stenosis is undetermined at this time.

Renal Arterial Pressure Gradient

One might assume that the more severe the renal artery stenosis, the greater the fall in arterial flow and pressure across the area of stenosis (105). The more severe the stenosis, the more likely that this lesion is generating the hypertension. Stewart et al. (341) confirmed this notion in humans by measuring the gradient across the stenotic lesion at surgery. Subsequent experience with this approach in the 1960s demonstrated that the preoperative measurement of a pressure gradient across a stenosis of the renal artery is associated with catheter-induced artifacts in the pressure distal to the lesion and the hazard of dissecting or perforating a highly stenotic artery. Even when measurements are made under direct vision on the operating table, the gradient varies considerably, depending on the state of the renal parenchymal vascular bed (342). If the intrarenal

vascular bed is dilated by drugs or anesthetic agents, the gradient will be high; if the renal vascular bed is constricted, the pressure gradient across the renal artery stenosis will be low. Therefore, renal arterial pressure gradient measurements were rarely used to influence decision making regarding intervention.

The pressure gradient across a stenosis is proportional to the resistance of the stenosis, but inversely proportional to the downstream resistance in the renal microvessels. A successful outcome following an intervention requires that the stenosis be high grade (i.e., high stenosis resistance) and that the renal microvessels be compliant, reactive and not irreversibly fibrosed and remodeled (i.e., low intrarenal resistance). Accordingly, the degree of pressure gradient across a stenosis should be a useful predictor of functional severity of the stenosis and the degree of preservation of normal microvascular function within the affected kidney and should predict a good outcome after intervention. These assumptions have been validated in a recent treatment trial (343), using a group of patients with positive clinical criteria of renovascular disease and positive color-coded Doppler velicometry studies. All patients were investigated by angiography, and patients with renal artery stenosis >70% and transluminal pressure gradient >30 mm Hg were selected for PTRA and stenting. This selection procedure yielded a population that had favorable results from the intervention, suggesting that a combination of careful measurements of the degree of stenosis and preintervention trans-stenotic pressure gradient may be useful in selecting patients likely to benefit from intervention to correct renal artery stenosis.

In comparison, in a series of 231 patients with advanced atherosclerotic renal artery disease, mean serum creatinine concentration of 2.6 mg/dL, and a pre-intervention average pressure gradient of 109 mm Hg, which fell to 12 mm Hg after endovascular intervention, no relationship was apparent between severity of BP, number of antihypertensive medications, renal function and the gradients measured (344). Although many interventional angiographers obtain renal artery pressure gradients before and after PTRA or PTRA/stenting to predict the response to these interventional maneuvers, the relationship of the pressure gradient before and after endovascular intervention to later effects on BP and renal function is unclear.

Renal Biopsy

Vertes et al. (168–171) once advocated bilateral renal biopsy to predict the curability of hypertension in patients with renal arterial stenosis, the rationale being that if either kidney had severe arteriolar sclerosis, hypertension would probably not be relieved by surgery to repair the stenotic renal artery. Although, as previously discussed (see Pathophysiology of Renovascular Hypertension), there is substantial rationale for this maneuver, there are less invasive and much safer surrogates (duration of hypertension, duration of severe hypertension, renal insufficiency) to suggest bilateral renal parenchymal disease (i.e., nephrosclerosis) or unilateral renal artery stenosis with small-vessel disease in the contralateral kidney. Bilateral percutaneous renal biopsy and biopsy of the kidney ipsilateral to the renal artery stenosis, searching for significant arteriolar nephrosclerosis, are relatively formidable procedures such that this approach is virtually never employed today. There are more than enough clinical clues, laboratory suggestions, and noninvasive diagnostic maneuvers suggesting cure of hypertension following renal revascularization that renal biopsy to predict outcome of surgery or angioplasty is not recommended. Further, the observation of vascular changes in the renal parenchyma does not necessarily confer a poor outcome from surgical treatment of unilateral renal vascular disease (345). The role of renal biopsy in guiding renal revascularization for improvement or preservation of renal function however is under continuing investigation (250).

Imaging of the Renal Vasculature

Several angiographic and nonangiographic imaging procedures are currently employed for the anatomic diagnosis of renal artery stenosis. The techniques, methodology, advantages, disadvantages, and complications of conventional renal arteriography, intravenous digital subtraction arteriography (IV-DSA), intraarterial digital subtraction angiography (IA-DSA), computed tomographic angiography, and magnetic resonance angiography (MRA) are detailed in Chapters 12–14.

Conventional Renal Arteriography

Although the need for conventional renal arteriograms for diagnosis of renal artery stenosis has decreased since the advent of IA-DSA, conventional arteriography gives the maximum information about vascular architecture, the intrarenal vasculature (e.g., segmental arterial branches), and collateral blood vessels (346). Selective renal arteriography is generally performed if there is no significant orificial stenosis and when the angiographer is searching for branch arterial lesions or better definition of main renal artery lesions viewed with abdominal aortography. If significant stenosis is present at the orifice of the renal artery, selective renal arteriography probably should be avoided because the catheter is advanced into the proximal renal artery and there is a risk of dissecting or occluding the artery or generating atheroemboli to the renal vascular bed. Renal angiography is generally performed when DSA is not available or when the DSA technique provides suboptimal images.

Digital Subtraction Angiography

DSA is a major advance in the radiologic evaluation of renal artery disease. IA-DSA has several advantages over conventional angiography: (a) there is significant time savings for the angiographer because the images can be recalled immediately on the monitor, and there is no need for the development of film before proceeding to the next injection of contrast medium; (b) only selected images are eventually recorded on film, resulting in significant cost savings; (c) digitalized images allow for computer processing such as enhancement of vessel edges, measurement of vessel diameters, and optimization of picture contrast and intensity; (d) IA-DSA requires less than half of the amount of contrast material needed for conventional angiography, and often no more than 50 mL (346).

There are two disadvantages to DSA: motion artifact and inferior spatial resolution on a digitally subtracted image compared to a conventional film. This latter disadvantage not infrequently results in suboptimal delineation of small distal arterial branches in the renal parenchyma and lessens the ability to detect the intrarenal changes of vasculitis and nephrosclerosis. The development of newer DSA equipment that uses smaller pixel sizes is quickly eliminating this disadvantage.

IV-DSA has been extensively used in the diagnosis of renovascular disease (347,348).

Renal IV-DSA is performed by injecting contrast material via a catheter placed in the antecubital vein or in the right atrium. During the imaging, the patient must remain motionless to avoid motion artifacts, a not insignificant disadvantage of IV-DSA. Although IV-DSA was quite popular in the early to mid-1980s because of its convenience as a simple outpatient procedure, its relatively low cost, and the fact that it made femoral artery cannulation with its attendant risks of atheroemboli unnecessary, recent experience suggests that its sensitivity is not be as high as originally proposed. In experienced hands, there is approximately 80% agreement between IV-DSA and either conventional arteriography or IA-DSA (347,349,350). Disadvantages of IV-DSA include opacification by the contrast bolus of all arteries within the field of view, resulting in considerable overlapping of mesenteric and renal arteries; a relatively long time gap between the injection of contrast material into the venous system and its arrival in the abdominal aorta; and artifact from patient motion, respiration, and bowel peristalsis. IV-DSA images are of poor quality in patients with impaired cardiac output, and the relatively large volume of contrast material required poses a relative contraindication in patients with renal insufficiency. Nevertheless, IV-DSA is a useful screening procedure for renovascular disease or as a follow-up procedure to surgical revascularization or balloon angioplasty. In addition, limited excretory urography can be performed concomitantly by obtaining a plain film of the abdomen with renal laminography after the injection of contrast material for IV-DSA.

Magnetic Resonance Angiography (MRA)

MRA (see Chapters 13 and 14) is entirely noninvasive and less operator-dependent than duplex ultrasound scanning. Several series examined the performance of MRA of the renal arteries with conventional angiographic confirmation, and demonstrated sensitivity and specificity rates for MRA of 80% to 90% (351–355). MRA exaggerates the severity of renal artery stenosis, particularly the distal half of the main renal artery, and its ability to detect branch stenosis is not clear. Technical improvements in MRA including gadolinium enhanced MRA (breath-hold MRA with perimagnetic contrast material [gadopentetate dimeglumine]), improve the ability to visualize some accessory renal arteries, but certainly not as clearly as conventional angiography or IA-DSA (356,357). The detection of hemodynamically significant renal artery lesions may be enhanced by using phase-contrast MRA (358). Although more expensive than duplex ultrasound scanning, MRA is increasingly reported to provide results as good as or better than duplex Doppler ultrasonography. Whereas most studies of the accuracy of MRA have been conducted retrospectively by radiologists, and have given very good results, a recent prospective trial evaluated MRA and CT angiography compared with IA-DSA in patients studied consecutively (359). This study yielded reduced values for both sensitivity and specificity (in. 70%) for both MRA and CT angiography in the detection of renal artery stenosis lesions that were deemed to be significant by angiography. MRA is contraindicated for patients with claustrophobia or metallic implants such as cardiac pacemakers, cranial aneurysm clips, cochlear implants, and older types of Starr-Edwards heart valves.

Carbon Dioxide Angiography

Carbon dioxide (CO_2) is currently being utilized not only for diagnostic imaging of the renal artery but also to guide percutaneous interventional vascular procedures. The use of CO_2 angiography was pioneered by Hawkins (360), and the potential for CO_2 to serve as a clinically useful arterial contrast agent has advanced over the past 15 years (310,361,362). In experienced centers, DSA using CO_2 as an intravascular contrast agent has proved to be both safe and clinically useful in the evaluation of patients with renovascular disease. In a dog study in which 5 to 10 times the maximum quantity of CO_2 normally used was injected directly into the renal artery, only minor reductions in blood flow, and no morphologic changes in the kidneys or vascular endothelium were detailed subsequently (363). In most centers, CO_2 angiography is not available, and research is continuing utilizing CO_2 for diagnostic arterial and venous imaging and as a guide to percutaneous vascular interventional procedures in selected centers.

Duplex Ultrasound Scanning

Duplex ultrasound scanning of the renal arteries is a noninvasive screening test for the detection of the anatomic presence of renal artery stenosis. It combines direct visualization of the renal arteries (B-mode imaging) with measurement of various hemodynamic factors in the main renal arteries and within the kidney (Doppler), thus providing both an anatomic and a functional assessment of renal arterial disease. Duplex scanning also allows measurement of kidney size at the same time. Unlike other noninvasive tests, duplex scanning is not affected by medications, the level of renal function, or whether the disease is unilateral, bilateral, or affecting a solitary functioning kidney (47,48,51,364–368). As indicated earlier in this chapter, increasing experience with duplex ultrasound scanning demonstrates an overall sensitivity and specificity when compared with renal arteriography of 98%, with a positive predictive value of 0.99 and a negative predictive value of 0.97 (51). Olin et al. (51) prospectively studied 102 consecutive patients by both duplex ultrasound scanning of the renal arteries and renal arteriography. All patients in the study had difficult-to-control hypertension, unexplained azotemia, or associated peripheral vascular disease, giving them a high pretest likelihood of renovascular disease. Sixty-two of 63 arteries showing stenosis of less than 60% by arteriography were correctly identified by duplex ultrasound scanning. Thirty-one of 32 arteries with 60% to 79% stenosis on arteriography were identified as having 60% to 99% stenosis on duplex ultrasound; 67 of 69 arteries with 80% to 99% stenosis on arteriography were identified as having 60% to 99% stenosis on ultrasound. Twenty-two of 23 arteries with total occlusion on arteriography were correctly identified by duplex ultrasound (Table 52-11) (51).

Of the arteries with an end-diastolic velocity of 150 cm/second or more, 81% (38/47) had 80% to 99% stenosis, while only 19% (9/47) had 60% to 79% stenosis by arteriography. At the present time, most centers experienced in the duplex ultrasound scanning technique are able to discriminate between renal arterial stenoses of less than 60% or of 60% or more by ultrasound. Gradations of stenosis by duplex ultrasound scanning are generally reported as 0% to 59% stenosis, 60% to 99% stenosis, and total occlusion. The ability to discriminate by duplex ultrasound renal arterial lesions causing 60% to 79% stenosis from those causing 80% or more stenosis (most likely the degree of stenosis that is hemodynamically significant) is approaching with advances in duplex ultrasound technology.

Radermacher et al. have validated the renal resistive index (RI) obtained by Doppler velicometry over the intrarenal vessels as a predictor of future renal outcomes in patients with renal transplant nephropathy (369), chronic renal insufficiency (370), and renal artery stenosis (371). The RI is calculated as: (1 – [end diastolic velocity] maximal systolic velocity) ×100. Of 138 patients with renal artery stenosis subject to angioplasty or surgery, the RI scanning procedure was technically successful in 131 patients. The results demonstrated that a RI of >80% reliably identifies patients with renal artery stenosis in whom intervention will not improve renal function, BP, or kidney survival. The index effectively quantitates the microvascular resistance within the kidneys, which is emerging as a critical factor in determining outcome in these patients.

The availability of high-quality duplex ultrasound scanning has dramatically altered the approach to renal artery stenosis in several centers. When the history and physical examination suggest renal artery stenosis, duplex ultrasound scanning may well be the procedure of choice for detecting the anatomic presence of renal artery disease. When duplex ultrasound scanning indicates 0% to 59% stenosis, hemodynamically significant renal artery stenosis is highly unlikely. However, the technique is technically demanding and has a steep learning curve. Each vascular laboratory needs to correlate the results obtained from duplex ultrasound of the renal arteries with arteriography to ensure a reasonable degree of internal correlation. It is important to examine the renal artery from the anterior, lateral decubitus, and at times, posterior approaches so that all segments of the renal artery can be visualized and adequate Doppler samples obtained. Accessory renal arteries are difficult to identify and remain a limitation of the test (51,368). After detecting renal artery stenosis by duplex ultrasound, an angiographic imaging procedure in concert with a maneuver designed to detect the physiologic significance of the renal artery stenosis (e.g., captopril renography, renal vein renin determination) is recommended.

Spiral Computed Tomography Scanning

Spiral (helical) CT scanning with intravenous contrast injection (CT angiography) combines the diagnostic accuracy of formal arteriography with the low-risk of intravenous digital subtraction angiography. In several reports, the spiral CT scan had a sensitivity and specificity for renal artery stenosis ranging from 87% to 98% (sensitivity) and 94% to 98% specificity, respectively (372–374).

In summary, the ideal approach to the choice of appropriate workup in this patient population is to select in advance the specific questions to be answered: (a) is significant renal artery stenosis present? (b) is it bilateral or unilateral? (c) is it associated with and suspected of causing hypertension? (d) is

TABLE 52-11

COMPARISON OF DUPLEX ULTRASONOGRAPHY WITH ARTERIOGRAPHY IN 102 CONSECUTIVE PATIENTS[a]

Percent stenosis by ultrasonography	Percent stenosis by arteriography				
	0–59	60–79	80–99	100	Total
0–59	62	0	1	1	64
60–99	1	31	67	0	99
100	0	1	1	22	24
Total	63	32	69	23	187

[a]Numbers refer to arteries visualized (N = 187). The sensitivity was 98%, specificity 98%, positive predictive value 99%, and negative predictive value 97%.
(From: Olin JW, Piedmonte MR, Young JR, et al. The utility of duplex ultrasound scanning of the renal arteries for diagnosing significant renal artery stenosis. *Ann Intern Med* 1995;122:833, with permission.)

it associated with and suspected of causing renal insufficiency? and (e) are we seeking information about the likely outcomes of revascularization? Answers to these questions help in selecting the most useful test in each individual circumstance. Generally, conventional renal angiography is reserved as a prelude to renal revascularization, for example, PTRA, PTRA/stenting or surgical renal revascularization.

ISCHEMIC RENAL DISEASE (ISCHEMIC NEPHROPATHY)

Ischemic renal disease and *ischemic nephropathy* are terms that imply gradual loss of renal function caused by vascular occlusion. Although interrelationships between main renal artery stenosis, arteriolar nephrosclerosis, hypertension, and renal insufficiency have, historically, been appreciated, the notion that main renal artery stenosis might threaten renal function, possibly independent of BP control, is relatively recent. The frequency of atherosclerotic renovascular disease, and in particular the appearance of atherosclerotic renal artery disease in patients with atherosclerosis in other vascular beds and the suggestion that atherosclerotic renal artery stenosis might be responsible for advanced renal failure, particularly in patients older than 50 years (34,239,251,375), and reports of patients coming off dialysis following renal revascularization (233,250,376–38) have contributed to current interest in ischemic nephropathy and enthusiasm for renal revascularization (surgical or endovascular) for preservation or restoration of renal function. Regardless of whether or not renovascular hypertension is likely, the anatomic presence of atherosclerotic renal artery disease as a threat to renal function has become a more pressing concern than that of atherosclerotic renovascular hypertension (28,30,34,381,382). Accordingly, in some centers, trends in surgical revascularization for renal artery disease have shifted from the issue of renovascular hypertension to the issue of preservation of renal function (383).

Ischemic renal disease or ischemic nephropathy may be defined as a clinically significant reduction in GFR due to hemodynamically significant obstruction to renal blood flow, or renal failure due to renal artery occlusive disease. The following case histories are examples of this clinical syndrome.

Case 1

A 62-year-old white woman presented in 1977 with the recent appearance of hypertension and a BP of 170/115 mm Hg. Three years previously, she had been found to have polycythemia vera, and an IVP at that time appeared normal. She had been followed closely until 1977 by her local internist and was always normotensive until the hypertension suddenly appeared. A rapid- sequence IVP demonstrated a reduction in the size of the left kidney from 14.0 to 11.5 cm. Further evaluation demonstrated a serum creatinine level of 2.6 mg/dL and an asymptomatic left carotid bruit. Renal arteriography disclosed a left kidney 11.5 cm in height and 100% stenosis of the left renal artery; the right kidney measured 14.5 cm in height and there was 95% stenosis of the right renal artery (Fig. 52-14). Renal vein renin determinations lateralized strongly to the smaller (left) kidney. The BP was well controlled with propranolol and a diuretic. Right aortorenal reimplantation was undertaken solely to preserve renal function. Postoperatively, the serum creatinine level fell to 1.5 mg/dL and remained at this level for the next 12 years. The BP remained controlled postoperatively with propranolol, 40 mg daily, and a small dose of chlorthalidone. The patient died in 1989 of

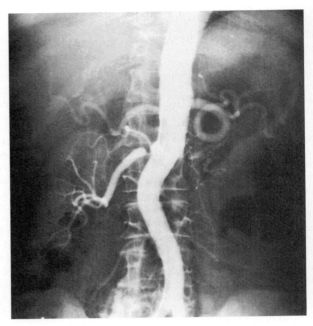

FIGURE 52-14. Case 1: Aortogram of a 62-year-old woman, demonstrating total occlusion of the left renal artery supplying an atrophic left kidney and high-grade ostial stenosis of the proximal right renal artery from atherosclerosis.

complications of polycythemia vera, with a serum creatinine of 1.5 mg/dL.

Case 2

A 67-year-old white woman, known to have a single (left) kidney and a serum creatinine level of 1.0 mg/dL, was in her usual state of good health until October 1988, when she observed a marked diminution in urine volume after 4 to 5 days of nausea, vomiting, diarrhea, and diminished food and fluid intake, all of which were attributed to viral gastroenteritis. The gastrointestinal symptoms subsided, but oliguria persisted. She sought medical attention and was observed to be severely azotemic. Over the next several days, oligoanuria developed, and acute hemodialysis was initiated. Over the next 6 weeks, there was no increase in urine volume, and regular hemodialysis was required. The patient's nephrologist presumed that she had sustained an episode of severe acute tubular necrosis, but when renal function failed to improve after 6 weeks of hemodialysis, open renal biopsy was performed. The biopsy specimen was surprisingly unremarkable, revealing only mild interstitial fibrosis, intact tubular basement membranes, absence of glomerular sclerosis, and retracted glomeruli consistent with ischemia (Fig. 52-15). There was no evidence of active glomerular proliferation or crescents, and no evidence of vasculitis. Six months later a renal arteriogram demonstrated tight left renal artery stenosis beginning just beyond the takeoff of the renal artery and extending to the first major bifurcation, with evidence of collateral circulation. The patient was referred for further evaluation in June 1989, at which time laminography indicated the left kidney to be 10.5 cm in height, with surprisingly good function demonstrated by DTPA isotope renal scanning. Left renal revascularization (bench repair and autotransplantation) was performed. During the first 4 postoperative weeks, the serum creatinine level gradually fell from the range of 12 to 16 mg/dL to 3 mg/dL, and the urine volumes increased to 1,500 to 2,000 mL/day. There have been no subsequent

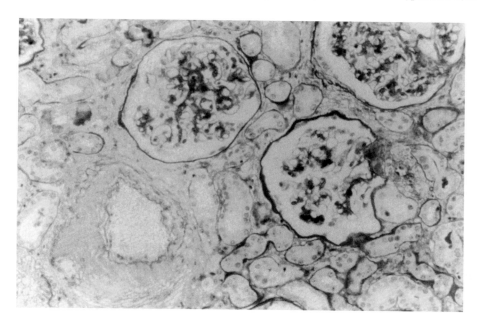

FIGURE 52-15. Case 2: Left renal biopsy specimen obtained after 6 weeks of hemodialysis from a 67-year-old woman who had been anuric. The biopsy specimen shows hypoperfused retracted glomeruli consistent with ischemia. There is no evidence of active glomerular proliferation or glomerular sclerosis. Note the intact tubular basement membranes, and negligible interstitial inflammation. Left renal revascularization resulted in recovery of renal function and discontinuance of dialysis.

dialysis treatments. The serum creatinine level 10 years postoperatively was 2.3 mg/dL.

Discussion

These two patients represent two ends of the spectrum of ischemic nephropathy. In the first patient, surgical revascularization of the right kidney was done solely to improve moderately severe renal insufficiency and preserve long-term renal function, ignoring the prediction that left renal revascularization would cure the hypertension. In the second patient, renal revascularization removed a patient from lifelong dialysis.

The observation of improved renal function after renal revascularization is not new. In 1962, Morris et al. (384) reported on eight azotemic patients with bilateral renal artery stenosis who experienced improvement in renal function following surgical renal revascularization. However, the major indication for operation in this report was the presence of severe associated hypertension—the concept of undertaking renal revascularization primarily to stabilize or improve renal function had not yet arisen. Additional reports in the 1960s and 1970s (133,385) described improvement in renal function in patients undergoing renal revascularization for presumed renovascular hypertension. Although the beneficial effect of surgery on renal function in these reports was in part due to improvement in BP control, the possibility that improved renal perfusion pressure promoted increased GFR was also entertained. Case 1 reflects an approach taken by Novick et al. (250), wherein 51 patients with significant renal artery stenosis and hypertension underwent surgery primarily to preserve or salvage renal function. In all patients, the BP was well controlled preoperatively with antihypertensive drug therapy, and hypertension was not considered an indication for surgery. In 24 of these 51 patients, progressive deterioration in kidney function, despite adequate BP control, was observed during the 6 months prior to surgery (250). Shortly thereafter, Ying et al. (233) described eight patients with bilateral atherosclerotic renal artery disease or unilateral arterial stenosis in a solitary functioning kidney, in whom antihypertensive drug therapy substantially worsened preexisting renal insufficiency despite enhanced BP control; surgical renal revascularization produced improvement or stabilization of renal function in these patients. These investigators concluded that refractory

hypertension with renal insufficiency is a common problem and suggested that renal revascularization is warranted, particularly if renal function deteriorates with medical management.

The reports of Novick (1983) (250) and Ying (1984) (233) et al. in conjunction with the advent of PTRA fueled enthusiasm for detecting and correcting main renal artery stenosis to preserve renal function. Reports of the role of PTRA in improving renal function in patients with atherosclerotic renal artery disease were encouraging, and a number of centers reported improvement or stabilization in renal function following surgical renal revascularization or balloon angioplasty in patients with ischemic renal disease. More recently, atherosclerotic renal artery disease has been claimed to contribute to the end-stage renal disease population (251,375–378,380,386,387). Case 2 is representative of this type of patient.

Despite these rewarding anecdotes, most patients who progress to end-stage renal failure in conjunction with main renal artery stenosis have irreversible ischemic parenchymal damage (Fig. 52-16) that precludes recovery of renal function even if main renal arterial blood flow is restored. Many of these patients have associated atheroembolic renal disease (388), severe small-vessel disease (nephrosclerosis), or both, and many patients have secondary focal segmental glomerulosclerosis or global glomerulosclerosis (Fig. 52-17). These pathologic alterations in the renal parenchyma limit the effectiveness of surgical renal revascularization, PTRA, or stenting of the main renal artery in improving renal function (389). The studies of Radermacher utilizing measurement of renal resistance index (RI) demonstrated that a RI >80% predicted an unfavorable effect of renal artery stenting on post stent creatinine clearance, whereas a pre-stent RI <80% was associated with an improved creatinine clearance post renal artery stenting (369). In contrast to the voluminous literature devoted to predicting which patients might gain improvement in BP control following renal revascularization, a clear understanding is lacking about the pathogenesis of ischemic nephropathy on the basis of large-vessel occlusive disease and of which diagnostic tests might predict improvement in renal function following renal revascularization. The relative contributions of main renal artery stenosis, arteriolar nephrosclerosis, glomerular collapse, and interstitial fibrosis—all associated with main renal artery stenosis—await further definition. The renal RI studies of Radermacher (369) and the study of Cheung (390) in patients with total renal artery occlusion of one renal artery and varying degrees of stenosis

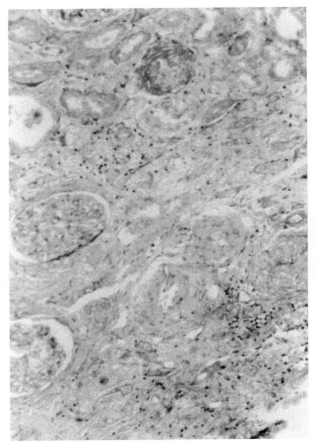

FIGURE 52-16. Pathologic specimen of a kidney from beyond a main renal artery occlusion demonstrating glomerular sclerosis, tubular atrophy, and interstitial fibrosis. The magnitude of glomerular and interstitial scarring is consistent with irreversible loss of kidney viability.

in the contralateral renal artery emphasize the importance of renal parenchymal damage as a major contributor to the overall impairment in GFR (i.e., renal function) in patients with main renal artery stenosis. Further, paradigms applied to acute renal ischemic injury may have limited applicability to chronic vascular injury.

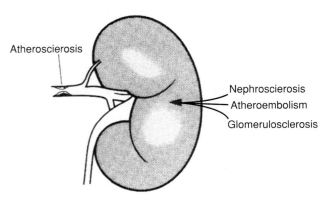

FIGURE 52-17. Schematic representation of ischemic nephropathy. Patients with atherosclerotic artery stenosis often have coexisting renal parenchymal disease with varying degrees of nephrosclerosis (small-vessel disease), atheroembolic disease, or glomerulosclerosis.

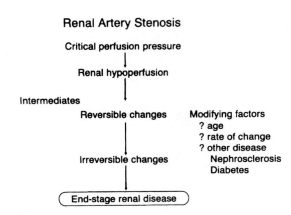

FIGURE 52-18. Theoretical scheme wherein renal artery stenosis leads to end-stage renal disease. Central to this model is the notion that vascular compromise produces intermediate events that injure the kidney. How these events promote "reversible" to "irreversible" tissue damage awaits further clarification. (Adapted from: Textor SC. Pathophysiology of renal failure in renovascular disease. *Am J Kidney Dis* 1994;24:642, with permission.)

The pathophysiology of ischemic nephropathy is incompletely understood. Presumably, a sufficiently severe vascular lesion reduces renal perfusion pressure below a "critical perfusion pressure" when the kidney is perfused at these reduced arterial pressures, a series of changes develop, some irreversible, eventuating in end-stage renal disease (Fig. 52-18). Textor proposes a sequence of events for chronic ischemic renal injury wherein repetitive episodes of renal hypoperfusion might produce irreversible renal parenchymal damage beyond a stenotic main renal arterial lesion (Fig. 52-19). Data to support the role of each of these steps have been obtained from models of acute ischemic renal failure (see Chapter 39), although their role in chronic renovascular disease is not yet established (109,111). Renal fibrosis induced by ischemia evolves with intrarenal ischemia increasing the generation of angiotensin II that is fibrogenic, owing to interaction with endothelin-1 and TGF-beta (391).

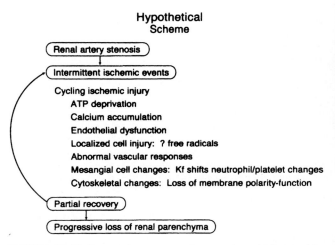

FIGURE 52-19. Proposed sequence of events by which repetitive episodes of renal hypoperfusion might produce irreversible renal parenchymal injury beyond a stenotic arterial lesion. Data to support the role of each step were obtained from models of acute ischemic renal failure, although their role in chronic renovascular disease is not yet established. (Adapted from: Textor SC. Pathophysiology of renal failure in renovascular disease. *Am J Kidney Dis* 1994;24:642, with permission.)

The pathologic changes in the kidney beyond an arterial occlusion include glomerular collapse with loss of tuft volume, tubular atrophy, and interstitial fibrosis. The fibrosis of Bowman's capsule can obstruct the origin of the proximal tubule, leading to atubular glomeruli and tubular atrophy, while fibrosis around tubules themselves likely impairs their function and viability. Loss of tubular structures, interstitial inflammation, and glomerulosclerosis are consistent with irreversible loss of kidney viability (109,392–395). Typical changes of arteriolar nephrosclerosis coexist (Fig. 52-16) (396,397). Experimental studies using progressive renal arterial occlusion in a swine model indicate a complex interaction between atherosclerosis and renal arterial disease in activating fibrogenic pathways of the kidney, potentiating the renal scarring (398,399).

Clinical Presentation

The clinical presentation of patients likely to develop progressive renal failure from atherosclerotic ischemic nephropathy is that of an older (more than 50 years) patient demonstrating progressive azotemia in conjunction with antihypertensive drug therapy, history of cigarette smoking, known renal artery disease, refractory hypertension, and generalized atherosclerosis obliterans (233,250,251). Men or women over the age of 50 who smoke and have unexplained azotemia with mild-to-moderate proteinuria, hypertension (usually), and a bland urinary sediment with few casts or cells are frequently found to have atherosclerotic renal artery disease. Clinically, ischemic renal disease is present in patients with high-grade (greater than 75%) arterial stenosis involving both kidneys or more than 75% arterial stenosis to a solitary kidney. The threat to overall kidney function in patients with high-grade (greater than 75%) unilateral renal artery stenosis in the setting of azotemia, wherein renal functional impairment is most likely due to a combination of nephrosclerosis and unilateral main renal artery stenosis, is less clear (250). Accordingly, an ag-

gressive interventive approach with either surgical or endovascular renal revascularization appears to be most appropriate for patients with high-grade bilateral renal artery stenosis or high-grade renal artery stenosis to a solitary functioning kidney. Clinical clues to bilateral renovascular disease include (a) generalized atherosclerosis obliterans, (b) presumed renovascular hypertension, (c) a unilateral small kidney, (d) unexplained azotemia, (e) deterioration in renal function with BP reduction, particularly with ACE inhibitor therapy (225,251,400), and (f) recurrent episodes of flash pulmonary edema (216–218).

Preserving Renal Function

In considering patients as candidates for revascularization (surgical or endovascular) to preserve renal function, some determination should be made of the potential for salvable renal function. Total occlusion of the renal artery usually eventuates in irreversible ischemic damage of the involved kidney; however, in some patients with gradual arterial occlusion, the viability of the kidney can be maintained through the development of collateral arterial supply (401–404). Clinical clues suggesting renal function preservation include (a) kidney height more than 9 cm (by IVP or renal laminography); (b) evidence of function of the involved kidney, on either intravenous urogram or isotope renography; (c) angiographic filling of the distal renal arterial tree by collateral circulation in patients with total renal arterial occlusion proximally (Fig. 52-20); and (d) a specimen obtained by intraoperative renal biopsy demonstrating well-preserved glomeruli with minimal arteriolar sclerosis (see Case 2) (Fig. 52-15) (89,250,403–407). When these criteria are present, restoration of normal renal arterial flow can result in recovery of renal function.

As has been emphasized, the coexistence of arteriolar nephrosclerosis, secondary glomerulosclerosis, and in many patients atheroembolic renal disease, in conjunction with main renal artery atherosclerotic renal artery stenosis, makes predictions difficult as to which patients will show improvement in

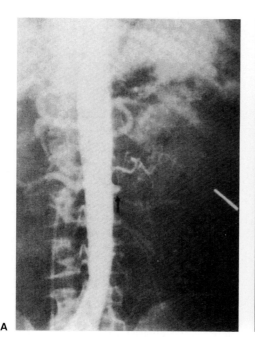
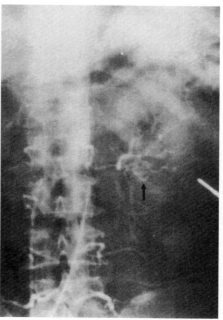

FIGURE 52-20. A: Abdominal aortograms reveal complete occlusion of the left main renal artery, **(B)** with filling of the distal renal artery branches from the collateral blood supply seen on a delayed film. The observation of collateral circulation when the main renal artery is totally occluded proximally suggests viable renal parenchyma.

renal function following surgical or endovascular renal revascularization. Data from the Mayo Clinic of 304 patients who underwent surgical renal revascularization (408) and 44 patients who underwent PTRA389 indicated that approximately 27% improved renal function (serum creatinine decreased more than or equal to 1 mg/dL), 53% had no change in renal function (change in serum creatinine less than 1 mg/dL), and 20% experienced worsened renal function (serum creatinine increased more than 1 mg/dL). Many of the patients who had worsening of renal function developed rapid deterioration in renal function within 1 year of the interventive procedure. Similar observations have been reported by Sandy et al. (409).

In general, surgical or endovascular renal revascularization to preserve renal function in patients with atherosclerotic renal artery stenosis is most likely to be useful in patients who have not yet demonstrated severe and permanent impairment of overall renal function. In a study from the Cleveland Clinic (410) baseline renal function predicted the outcome of surgical revascularization in older adult patients; a preoperative serum creatinine level of less than 3 mg/dL correlated with a stable or improved postoperative serum creatinine level. In contrast, patients with moderately severe azotemia (serum creatinine greater than 3.0 to 3.5 mg/dL) are likely to have severe renal parenchymal disease (Fig. 52-16), which renders improvement in renal function following surgical or endovascular revascularization unlikely (389,411,412). The study of Radermacher (369) using the renal RI measurement prior to endovascular renal revascularization is consistent with these observations. For patients over age 65, in whom serum creatinine concentrations are between 2 and 3 mg/dL indicating severe renal functional impairment, desired benefits on renal function from renal revascularization maneuvers are also frequently disappointing (413,414). Exceptions to these observations are patients with total main renal artery occlusion in whom renal viability is maintained via collateral circulation. In situations of uncertain renal viability, an intraoperative renal biopsy may be helpful. On occasion, we have used the findings by intraoperative kidney biopsy to help guide subsequent decision making regarding surgical revascularization for the goal of improving kidney function (250). Several groups reported their results in such patients, confirming that when criteria indicative of renal function preservation are present, successful revascularization can in fact lead to reversal of renal failure (89,250,404–406,415–422).

In addition to the absolute level of renal function as measured by serum creatinine as a criterion for renal function preservation, the rate of decline in overall renal function was recently suggested as an important determinant of outcome following renal revascularization in atherosclerotic ischemic renal disease. This was particularly true in dialysis-dependent patients for whom dialysis is presumed to be required for ischemic nephropathy (380,423). Dean et al. and Hansen et al. (380,423) suggested that predictors of recovery of renal function in dialysis-dependent patients with atherosclerotic renal artery stenosis are (a) bilateral (vs. unilateral) renal artery stenosis; (b) a rapid rate of deterioration in estimated GFR during the 6 months preceding surgical revascularization; and (c) less severe nephrosclerosis angiographically. Postoperative recovery of renal function was not associated with the severity of renal artery stenosis, preoperative length, or extent of extrarenal atherosclerosis. Other groups suggest that patients presumed to have end-stage renal disease from ischemic nephropathy may be removed from dialysis when there is chronic bilateral total renal arterial occlusion or total occlusion of the artery to a solitary kidney. In these patients, fortuitously, the viability of one or both kidneys has been maintained through collateral vascular supply (see Case 2) (376,421). Unfortunately this clinical presentation is rare, and a less favorable

outcome of total arterial occlusion on renal viability is far more common.

End-Stage Renal Disease

The frequency with which main renal artery stenosis causes end-stage renal disease (ESRD) is unclear. Mailloux et al. (378) and Appel et al. (386) suggested that ESRD may be a relatively common consequence of atherosclerotic renal artery stenosis. Appel et al. reported that renovascular disease accounts for 11% of all ESRD patients more than 50 years of age, and 20% of ESRD cases among whites older than 50 years. These figures were rough estimates, however, and there have been no prospective studies carefully addressing the relationship between renal artery disease and ESRD. More likely, the incidence of renovascular disease as a cause of ESRD is much lower as supported by the United States Renal Data System 1997 Annual Data Report (424). In this report, renal artery stenosis or occlusion was listed as the primary disease in only 1.7% of all ESRD incident patients ($N = 305,876$) for the years 1991 to 1995. Fatica et al. reported an annualized percentage growth of ESRD attributable to atherosclerotic renal artery disease (ASO/RAD-ESRD) to 12.4% (vs. 8.4% for diabetes mellitus and 5.4% for all-cause ESRD) from 1991 to 1997 (USRDS database), and that the percentage of incident patients with ASO/RAD-ESRD increased from 1.4% to 2.1% over this time period (425).

Documentation of atherosclerotic renovascular disease in patients on dialysis is often plagued with coexisting comorbid conditions that in conjunction with the requirement for dialysis, predict a poor long-term survival (378,386,426). In these patients, at the initiation of dialysis, the most frequently occurring associated comorbid conditions were documented preexisting cardiac disease, peripheral vascular disease, hypertension, cerebrovascular disease and transient ischemic attack, and congestive heart failure. Patients with atherosclerotic renovascular disease had these risk factors at a significantly increased frequency (378) compared to patients on dialysis with renal diagnoses other than ischemic renal disease. Novick et al. described the survival of 25 patients with end-stage renal failure and coexisting atherosclerotic renovascular disease in whom it was presumed that the renal failure was due to main renal artery occlusion (426). Eight of these 25 patients underwent surgical revascularization. At the time of analysis, 6 of the 8 patients were alive (mean survival time 58.2 months) and 2 patients had died (mean survival time 96 months); of the 17 "chronic dialysis" patients who did not undergo surgical revascularization, 3 were alive (mean survival time 29.5 months) and 13 were dead (mean survival time 8.7 months) at the time of analysis.

In view of the increasing median patient age and associated comorbid cardiovascular risk factors that impact poorly on dialysis survival (427–431), one might consider detection and correction of atherosclerotic renal artery stenosis in patients requiring dialysis for the goals of discontinuance of dialysis as well as improved long-term survival. This suggestion warrants close scrutiny, however, because the precise etiology of the ESRD in these reports was frequently unclear, the assumption that coexisting renal artery stenosis produced the renal insufficiency was not proved, and in most cases, irreversible parenchymal damage was present at the time of dialysis, precluding removal of these patients from dialysis following surgical or endovascular renal revascularization. Most patients with ESRD and atherosclerotic renal artery stenosis without total arterial occlusion are not appropriate candidates for revascularization to restore function. In such patients, main renal arterial blood flow is preserved at a reduced level, but the supplied renal parenchyma is without function. The renal parenchymal involvement is, in most situations, severely diseased with varying degrees of nephrosclerosis (170,171,395,432) or atheroembolic disease (388) in conjunction with severe interstitial fibrosis, tubular atrophy, and glomerular sclerosis. A more encouraging view has been reported by Hansen et al. who have performed surgical renal revascularization in 222 patients; 27 of these patients (12%) who had been dialysis-dependent were removed from dialysis (433).

Hemodynamic Probes

Hemodynamic probes may be helpful in confirming the functional significance of large-vessel occlusive disease. Clearly, such probes need to be designed and tested prospectively, to help identify patients at highest risk for loss of renal function prior to the development of moderate to severe azotemia (i.e., serum creatinine greater than 3 to 4 mg/dL) presumably consequent to main renal artery stenosis. In the 1980s, Textor and associates (224,434) described a test involving an intravenous infusion of sodium nitroprusside that was designed to define the hemodynamic limits posed by vascular disease on overall renal function in patients with main renal artery stenosis. Sixteen hypertensive patients underwent a graded reduction in BP with sodium nitroprusside. Eight patients with high-grade (greater than 70%) unilateral renal artery stenosis tolerated BP reduction (205/103 to 146/84 mm Hg) without a change in either renal plasma flow or GFR. Eight patients with high-grade bilateral renal arterial stenosis had similar BP reduction, but renal plasma flow fell (152 to 66 mL/minute) and GFR declined (38 to 16 mL/minute). Four patients with high-grade bilateral renal artery stenosis who initially experienced a decline in renal plasma flow and GFR were studied after unilateral renal revascularization; a reduction in BP with nitroprusside no longer reduced total renal blood flow or GFR (Fig. 52-21). Six of these 16 patients had been receiving captopril prior to referral, and 5 of these 6 patients developed severe acute renal failure while on captopril therapy. The data from these studies suggest that renal hemodynamic and functional evaluation during graded BP reduction with sodium nitroprusside provides a means of identifying a pathophysiologic limit on perfusion pressure required for renal function in patients with severe renal artery stenosis in whom the entire renal mass is threatened by renal artery occlusion. Despite these appealing observations, the invasive nature of this test and the time necessary to perform it have limited its clinical application in this patient population.

Another hemodynamic probe that might be predictive of loss of renal function is the simple observation of worsening renal function following BP reduction with any type of antihypertensive agent with or without the concomitant use of ACE inhibitor drugs (225,233,239,251,400). Deterioration in renal function with BP reduction, particularly with ACE inhibitor drugs or angiotensin receptor blocking agents, is not only an important clue to the presence of bilateral renovascular disease but also a marker for the hemodynamic significance of the lesion. Acute renal failure with converting enzyme inhibitor therapy may also be seen without main renal artery stenosis and may indicate intrarenal vascular disease (i.e., nephrosclerosis) or occasionally, other types of renal parenchymal damage (435). Whether or not captopril renography, widely employed as a means of detecting renal artery stenosis and predicting that renal artery stenosis is the cause of hypertension, can be utilized to predict which patients are at risk for losing renal function has not been tested. Serial captopril renography could theoretically become a sensitive, noninvasive means of following patients with high-grade renal artery stenosis over time, with recommendations regarding the timing of interventive therapy determined by changes in the captopril renogram in a given patient. This conjecture requires further study.

If a fixed increase in intrarenal microvascular resistance is critical for making ischemic nephropathy or renovascular hypertension irreversible, then how can this be assessed? Two strategies have been proposed, both depending on the demonstration of preserved diastolic blood flow into the kidneys as an index of microvascular function. The first strategy is the use of duplex Doppler velicometry estimates of the resistance index (RI) of the two kidneys. Resistance index can be quantitated by a skilled technician from the profile of blood flow velocities over time in the vessels within the kidneys. The index is calculated from the ratio of maximal systolic to diastolic blood flow velocity (see section on ultrasound testing for details). Using a cutoff RI of 80%, Radermacher et al. (371) investigated 130 patients with renal artery stenosis (RAS) prior to percutaneous transluminal angioplasty and stenting. The odds ratio for worsening of renal function or failure to reduce BP at follow up after 1 year was in excess of 100 for those with an RI >80%. The second strategy is the use of small, pediatric intraarterial catheters to measure the pressure gradient across a stenosis of the main renal artery >70%. The gradient is directly proportional to the resistance offered by the renal vasculature downstream. For example, the *reductio ad absurdum* would be that even a very tight stenosis of 95% would have no gradient

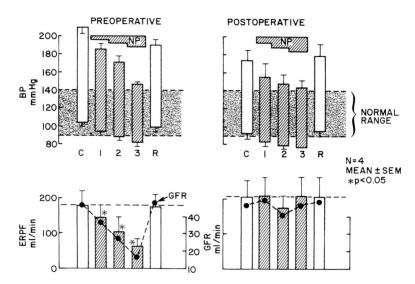

FIGURE 52-21. Blood pressure, renal plasma flow, and GFR in patients with bilateral renal artery stenosis undergoing nitroprusside (NP) infusion before and after renal revascularization. BP, blood pressure; ERPF, effective renal plasma flow. (From: Pohl MA, Novick AC. Natural history of atherosclerotic and fibrous renal artery disease: clinical implications. *Am J Kidney Dis* 1985;5:A120, with permission.)

if a ligature were placed downstream to provide infinite resistance, whereas even a modest stenosis would have a large gradient if the arterioles were widely patent and there was a brisk blood flow run off. The use of the gradient to select patients with preserved diastolic flow implies that the stenosis itself is hemodynamically sufficiently significant to reduce renal perfusion pressure and trigger autoregulatory vasodilatation of downstream renal resistance vessels. Ramos et al. (343) selected a group of patients with >70% stenosis of a main renal vessel due to atherosclerosis and >30 mm Hg maximum pressure gradient across the stenosis. One year after PTRA and stenting, this group experienced either a significant fall in BP if renal function was not impaired, or a significant improvement in renal function if it was initially impaired.

Both of these tests, that is, estimates of renal RI and measurement of pressure gradients, need to be validated by other investigators in prospective studies. The advantage of the RI is that it is entirely noninvasive, but it requires practice and skill. The advantage of the assessment of the stenosis and pressure gradient is that it can be done at the time of arteriography, but it also requires skill and practice and may increase the morbidity of the arteriography procedure.

Ischemic renal disease or ischemic nephropathy is an important clinical problem, particularly in older patients with generalized atherosclerosis obliterans. Noninvasive diagnostic maneuvers to screen for the anatomic presence of renal artery stenosis, particularly renal duplex ultrasonography, have made it possible to readily identify these patients. However, the importance of ischemic nephropathy as a major contributor to progressive renal insufficiency and ESRD remains to be rigorously determined. In some patients, severe renal artery stenosis poses a threat to renal function, and in others it does not. As detailed in this chapter, renal artery stenosis and renovascular hypertension are not synonymous. Similarly, renal artery stenosis and renal insufficiency are not synonymous.

Several factors must be considered in evaluating the renal functional benefit of intervention to relieve arterial obstruction. These include the severity and extent of renal artery obstruction, the level of renal function, the renal histopathologic information, the relative contribution of renal parenchymal damage and main renal artery stenosis to the renal insufficiency, the role of competing risks and high mortality from other cardiovascular diseases, and the merits of medical management of frequently associated hypertension versus renal revascularization in such patients (414,436–438). Although intervention to restore normal renal arterial blood flow may be indicated in selected patients to prevent deterioration of renal function that may culminate in the need for dialysis therapy, and although there is an occasional dialysis-dependent patient in whom renal revascularization might remove from dialysis, a large, prospective, randomized controlled study of patients assigned to receive medical (nonsurgical) therapy or to undergo renal revascularization (surgical or endovascular) is needed to test the hypothesis that atherosclerotic renal artery disease is a correctable cause of progressive renal failure. Several small, prospective, randomized studies of either endovascular or surgical renal revascularization showed no difference in either survival or renal functional outcomes as compared to medical management alone (439,440). A large multicenter study comparing optimal medical management plus stenting to optimal medical management alone is currently in progress (441).

A number of unresolved issues relative to ischemic nephropathy remain: Can we be certain that atherosclerotic renal artery disease is indeed a progressive disorder in a specific individual? For which patients does progression pose a hazard greater than the risks of vascular intervention? What is the optimal time to intervene to preserve renal function in patients with progressive azotemia? That is, is there a "window of opportunity in which one should intervene? And, at what point is it too early or too late to intervene? In patients with controlled hypertension and mild degrees of renal insufficiency, is an aggressive approach for preservation of renal function justified? How often does atherosclerotic renal artery disease cause end-stage renal failure? What is occurring in the renal parenchyma distal to the stenosis, metabolically and structurally? Although the information reviewed herein suggests that interventive therapy might favorably affect the natural course of atherosclerotic renal artery disease and prevent or stabilize ischemic nephropathy, much more information needs to be accumulated and analyzed about this subject.

TREATMENT OF RENOVASCULAR HYPERTENSION AND ISCHEMIC NEPHROPATHY

There are currently four therapeutic options available for patients with presumed renovascular hypertension or renal insufficiency, or both, resulting from renal artery disease. These are (a) medical management, (b) surgical revascularization, (c) PTRA, and (d) renal artery stents. Several factors must be weighed in determining whether medical or interventive management is more appropriate for a given patient. These include the causal relationship of renovascular disease to hypertension, that is, the likelihood that intervention will cure or markedly ameliorate the hypertension; the severity of the hypertension; the adequacy of BP control with medical antihypertensive therapy; the specific type of renal artery disease (fibrous or atherosclerotic); the natural history of untreated renovascular disease with regard for the risk of losing renal function; the general medical condition of the patient; and the known efficacy and risks of medical antihypertensive therapy, surgical revascularization, PTRA, and stents in various clinical subgroups.

The best method of treating patients with presumed renovascular hypertension remains an elusive goal. What constitutes appropriate management—medical, surgical revascularization, endovascular revascularization—is a matter of ongoing debate. Each therapeutic modality has its advocates, advantages, and disadvantages. In addition, factors influencing therapeutic decision making in patients with renal artery stenosis include the expertise and experience in performing surgical renal revascularization or endovascular revascularization (PTRA and stent placement) in an individual medical center. The goals of treatment are to cure or markedly improve the BP, to prevent target organ complications, to reverse or prevent impairment of renal function, and occasionally, to alleviate flash pulmonary edema. The anatomic presence of renal artery stenosis is not necessarily a mandate for intervention.

Surgical Treatment

Surgical treatment of presumed renovascular hypertension includes unilateral nephrectomy, partial nephrectomy (segmental hypoplasia, branch renal artery stenosis), endarterectomy, *in situ* aortorenal bypass procedures, alternative bypass procedures, atherectomy, and extracorporeal microvascular reconstruction and autotransplantation for branch renal artery disease. A detailed discussion of the surgical techniques involved, and results and complications of each of these procedures, is beyond the scope of this chapter.

The indications for primary nephrectomy are limited, and a procedure to preserve renal function as a secondary goal in patients with presumed renovascular hypertension is preferable. Nephrectomy is generally employed to relieve hypertension in the setting of a small (less than 8- to 9-cm pole-to-pole length by laminography) hyperreninemic kidney or because of a congenitally hypoplastic kidney, atrophic pyelonephritis, surgically uncorrectable renovascular disease, occlusion after attempted surgical or endovascular revascularization, or a nonfunctioning kidney consequent to renal trauma (88,179,180,182,442,443). Partial nephrectomy can be attempted to cure hypertension if there is stenosis of one of multiple distal renal arteries or branches, or to excise a hypoplastic segment (Ask-Upmark kidney). Partial nephrectomy has variable results in improving BP, in part because ischemic zones may remain in nonexcised renal tissue (92,444. Laparoscopic nephrectomy reduces postoperative complications compared to an open major surgical procedure and certainly reduces postoperative recuperation time.

Endarterectomy was the first revascularization procedure described as an alternative to nephrectomy (445). Several techniques of endarterectomy (aortorenal endarterectomy, transaortic endarterectomy, and aortic endarterectomy by transection of aorta) have variable popularity, depending on the experience and preference of the vascular surgeon (446–448). Currently, however, there are several revascularization procedures, most of which employ aortorenal bypass using a saphenous vein or hypogastric artery (446,449–451). The choice of revascularization procedure is influenced by the position and anatomic characteristics of the lesion as well as by the available surgical expertise. Lesions involving the proximal or middle third of the renal artery can generally be revascularized satisfactorily by conventional *in situ* procedures. Lesions involving the distal third of the renal artery or its branches are optimally treated by *ex vivo* reconstructive procedures using microsurgical techniques (452–455). Polytetrafluoroethylene aortorenal bypass grafts have been successfully employed by some surgeons, usually when an autogenous graft is not available (456–458).

In older patients, severe atherosclerosis of the abdominal aorta may render an aortorenal bypass or endarterectomy technically difficult and potentially hazardous to perform. In such cases, some surgeons prefer alternative surgical approaches that allow renal revascularization to be safely and effectively accomplished while avoiding surgery on a badly diseased aorta. Splenorenal bypass for left renal revascularization (459,460) and hepatorenal bypass for right renal revascularization (461) have been effective alternative bypass techniques. The absence of occlusive disease involving the origin of the celiac artery is an important prerequisite for either splenorenal or hepatorenal bypass surgery. A recent study indicates the presence of significant celiac artery stenosis in 50% of patients with atherosclerotic renal artery stenosis (462). This information mandates the importance of preoperative lateral aortography in evaluating the celiac artery origin in patients who are being considered for hepatorenal or splenorenal bypass (Fig. 52-22).

Iliorenal bypass is occasionally used for revascularization in patients with severe aortic atherosclerosis, providing there is acceptable blood flow through the diseased aorta and no significant iliac disease (463,464). Mesenterorenal bypass is occasionally used in patients with a severely diseased aorta in whom a bypass to the kidney from the celiac or iliac arteries is not possible. Ideally, when this procedure is considered, an enlarged superior mesenteric artery, if present, may be employed for arterial bypass to either kidney. When the superior mesenteric artery is sufficiently enlarged to allow for mesenterorenal bypass, there is generally no compromise of intestinal blood flow (464,465).

Use of the supraceliac or lower thoracic aorta for renal revascularization is a new surgical alternative in patients with significant atherosclerosis of the abdominal aorta and its major visceral branches (466–468). The supraceliac aorta is often relatively disease-free in these patients and can be used to achieve renal vascular reconstruction with an interposition saphenous vein graft. Simultaneous aortic replacement and renal revas-

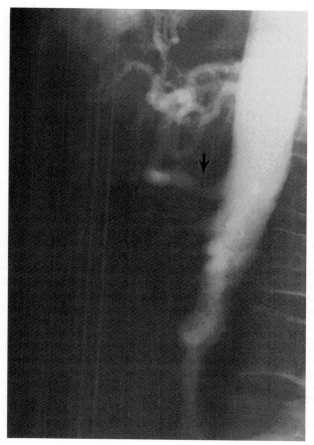

FIGURE 52-22. Lateral aortogram demonstrating a patent celiac artery, a prerequisite for employing hepatorenal or splenorenal bypass procedures.

cularization may be recommended for patients with a fixed indication for aortic replacement such as a significant abdominal aortic aneurysm or symptomatic aortoiliac occlusive disease in conjunction with renal artery occlusive disease (469). Several centers reported an increased operative mortality rate with simultaneous aortic replacement and renal revascularization (469–471).

Reports from several centers indicated that the techniques described above for surgical renal vascular reconstruction can be safely performed with a high technical success rate (383,469,472). The choice of surgical technique depends, to a large degree, on the experience and preference of the surgeon. Patients with fibrous dysplasia are generally healthy, without comorbid risk factors for major visceral vascular surgery; operative morbidity and mortality rates following revascularization in this patient group have been minimal (383,472). On the other hand, operative mortality rates of 2.1% (383), 3.1% (472), 3.4% (473), 5.5% (469), and 6.1% (474) have been reported following surgical revascularization in patients with atherosclerotic renal artery disease. An increased risk of operative mortality has been observed with bilateral simultaneous renal revascularization (475) or when renal revascularization is performed in conjunction with another major vascular surgery such as aortic replacement (469,471).

Most studies have indicated a high technical success rate for surgical vascular reconstruction, with postoperative thrombosis or stenosis rates of less than 10% (383,455,474). In analyzing the results of surgical revascularization for renovascular hypertension and in comparing these results to medical management, most studies considered patients as surgically cured

TABLE 52-12

RESULTS OF SURGICAL SERIES FOR TREATMENT OF RENOVASCULAR HYPERTENSION

Type of renal arterial disease (reference numbers)	No. of patients	Cured (%)	Improved (%)	Failed (%)
Fibromuscular dysplasia (40,431, 460–463,465,466,467,520)	663	59	30	11
Atheroma (focal) (460,463,465,468,575)	382	41	46	13
Atheroma (diffuse) (460,464,468,575)	435	24	45	36

(From: Pickering TG, Laragh JH, Sos TA. Renovascular hypertension. In: Schrier RW, Gottschalk CW, eds. *Diseases of the Kidney*. Boston: Little, Brown, 1993:1451, with permission.)

if the BP was 140/90 mm Hg or less postoperatively. Patients were considered improved if they showed either a reduction in diastolic pressure of 10 to 15 mm Hg or more or became normotensive with medication. Failures of surgical revascularization generally were viewed as those patients who did not qualify for either of the aforementioned criteria for "cured" or "improved."

The results of surgical treatment for presumed renovascular hypertension vary according to the underlying nature of the renal artery disease (Table 52-12) (64,209,228,383,451,472, 476–484,485–487). For patients with fibrous renal artery disease, 50% to 60% are cured, 30% to 40% are improved, and the failure rate is approximately 10%. For example, the Cooperative Study of Renovascular Hypertension, a study of 502 patients who underwent 577 surgical procedures in various centers in the United States published in 1975, reported a favorable BP response in 80% of patients with unilateral fibrous dysplasia, with an operative mortality of 3.4% (209,476). In patients undergoing revascularization for atherosclerotic renovascular disease, the failure rate is somewhat higher, fewer patients are cured, and fewer improve postoperatively. For example, in the Cooperative Study of Renovascular Hypertension, a favorable BP response was observed in 63% of patients with unilateral atherosclerotic stenosis and in 56% of patients with bilateral atherosclerotic stenosis (209,476). The operative mortality rate was 9.3% for atherosclerotic renovascular disease. In the patients with atherosclerotic renal artery disease, the presence of coronary disease or preoperative renal insufficiency (defined by a serum creatinine concentration greater than 1.4 mg/dL) raised the mortality rate to about 23%. Concurrent extrarenal surgery was associated with mortality in the range of 16% to 25% (209,476).

Clearly, fewer patients with atherosclerotic renal artery stenosis are cured of their hypertension in comparison to patients with fibrous dysplasia (Table 52-12). The presumed renovascular hypertension in patients with atherosclerotic renal artery disease either is superimposed on existing essential hypertension or is entirely due to primary (essential) hypertension with coexisting anatomic atherosclerotic renal artery stenosis. On the other hand, a recent study by van Bockel et al. demonstrates excellent long-term results following renal revascularization for atherosclerotic renal artery stenosis; with a mean follow-up of 8.9 years, postoperative hypertension was cured or improved in 83 (79%) of 105 patients (455).

The benefits of surgical treatment should also be assessed by long-term follow-up of BP control, renal function, and patient survival. In over 300 revascularization procedures performed during a 10-year period at the Cleveland Clinic, the operative mortality rate was 2.1% in patients with atherosclerotic disease and 0% in patients with fibrous dysplasia. Long-term cure or improvement in BP was observed in 72.4% of patients,

but cured in only 35.7% with atherosclerotic renal artery disease. Hypertension was cured in 93% of patients with fibrous dysplasia. Renal function was preserved or improved in 89% of patients who underwent surgery primarily for improving renal function (383,488). Starr et al. report that during a 20-year follow-up period, the actuarial patient survival rate was 93% at 5 years, 80% at 10 years, and 70% at 20 years (489). Seventy-four percent of these patients remained normotensive at 15 years. Even in elderly patients who are generally considered to be at increased operative risk, surgical revascularization can be successfully accomplished in those properly selected (383,488,490). These results are consistent with an earlier report from the Mayo Clinic (64) indicating the value of operative treatment in properly selected patients with presumed renovascular hypertension. The surgical benefits are inversely proportional to the duration of hypertension, and for patients with atherosclerotic renal artery disease in particular, long-term patient survival appears to be somewhat better for surgically treated patients than for medically treated patients (64).

Taken together, with proper patient selection, that is, high likelihood that the hypertension is renovascular in origin, and in experienced surgical centers, excellent long-term benefits relative to BP control can be achieved from surgical renal revascularization. Further, surgical morbidity has been considerably reduced over the past 30 years with negligible mortality (18,383,479,491–493).

The past 30 years have witnessed more centers performing surgical renal revascularization for the goal of preserving renal function (i.e., to correct or prevent ischemic nephropathy) in patients with high-grade atherosclerotic arterial occlusive disease affecting both kidneys or a solitary kidney. These are generally older patients with diffuse atherosclerosis, ostial renal artery lesions, and varying degrees of renal functional impairment. In 1983, Novick et al. (250) described improved renal function in 34 of 51 (67%) patients in whom BP was controlled medically preoperatively. The indication for surgery in this study was solely to improve or preserve renal function. Renal function improved most dramatically in patients with chronic bilateral total renal arterial occlusion.

In analyzing their data over a 10-year period, Novick et al. reported that indications for surgical renal revascularization fell substantially (41% to 26%) when the goal of surgery was for relief of hypertension alone, and increased substantially (14% to 36%) when the goal of surgery was only to preserve renal function, when this 10-year period was divided into two time segments (1975 to 1980 vs. 1981 to 1984) (378). Studies from several centers (Table 52-13) indicate improvement or stabilization of renal function postoperatively in 75% to 89% of patients (216,239,383,473,474,494–496). A more contemporary series of surgical renal revascularization in 96 patients operated on between 1990 and 2001 describes long-term

TABLE 52-13

RESULTS OF SURGICAL SERIES FOR TREATMENT OF ISCHEMIC NEPHROPATHY

Investigators, year	No. of patients	Surgical outcome, n (%)			
		Improved	Stable	Worse[a]	Death
Luft, et al., 1983 (494)	12	8 (67)	2 (17)	2 (17)	2 (17)
Jamieson, et al., 1984 (495)	23	15 (65)	0 (0)	8 (35)	4 (17)
Novick, et al., 1987 (383)	153	93 (61)	50 (33)	10 (6)	5 (3)
Hansen, et al., 1989 (496)	25	12 (48)	11 (44)	2 (8)	2 (8)
Messina, et al., 1992 (216)	17	12 (71)	2 (12)	3 (18)	1 (6)
Bredenberg, et al., 1992 (473)	25	9 (36)	12 (48)	4 (16)	NA
Libertino, et al., 1992 (474)	97	45 (46)	31 (32)	21 (22)	6 (6)
Total	352	194 (55)	108 (31)	50 (14)	20 (6)

NA, not available.
[a]Includes all deaths.
(Adapted from: Rimmer JM, Gennari FJ. Atherosclerotic renovascular disease and progressive renal failure. *Ann Intern Med* 1993;118:712, with permission.)

clinical success in the preservation of renal function in 70% of patients, with prediction of long-term success being the initial postoperative response in renal function and bilateral renal artery repair (497). Considering the potential risks of progressive occlusive disease and renal failure (ischemic nephropathy) that have been associated with medical management in similar patients, these results demonstrate a favorable influence of surgical revascularization on the natural history of untreated atherosclerotic renal artery disease.

Before recommending surgical revascularization for patients with atherosclerotic renal artery disease, one must appreciate that these patients are at high risk because of age and frequently associated coronary, cerebrovascular, or peripheral vascular disease (37,437,438,469). Their aortas are often laden with extensive atherosclerotic plaque, making angiographic investigation hazardous. Technical difficulties and complications of angiographic investigation in these patients include contrast medium-induced acute renal failure and atheroembolic renal disease. Spontaneous atheroembolic renal disease or atheroembolic renal disease associated with angiography or PTRA is not uncommon in this patient population (388,498). It is well known that coronary heart disease is often the determining factor affecting early and late mortality after elective surgical reconstruction of the abdominal aorta for an aneurysm or for occlusive peripheral artery disease (499–501). Surgical morbidity and mortality in patients with atherosclerotic renal artery disease can be minimized by selective screening and correcting significant coexisting coronary and cerebrovascular disease before undertaking elective surgical renal revascularization, either for the goal of improving BP or for ischemic nephropathy in patients with atherosclerotic renal artery disease (383,501,502).

Percutaneous Transluminal Renal Angioplasty (PTRA)

Since the introduction of percutaneous transluminal renal angioplasty (PTRA) by Dotter and Judkins in 1964 (503) and the subsequent development of a modified technique by Gruntzig et al. in 1978 (483), considerable interest has ensued in the application of this procedure to patients with renal artery stenosis. PTRA has the advantages of avoiding general anesthesia, the ability to be repeated, and a shorter duration of hospitalization. Many reports have reviewed the role of PTRA in patients with renal artery disease, and some have suggested that PTRA should be the initial treatment of choice for all patients with

renal artery stenosis, atherosclerotic or fibrous, whether the indication for intervention is for presumed renovascular hypertension or ischemic nephropathy or both. The technique of PTRA, efficacy in the treatment of renovascular hypertension due to fibrous dysplasia or atherosclerotic renal artery disease, experience in transplant renal artery stenosis, and complications of PTRA are reviewed in Chapter 14.

In many instances, it is difficult to interpret and compare information from various published series, owing to differences in methodology and reporting of data. Many studies employed different patient selection criteria in terms of the degree of stenosis necessary for treatment. They used different definitions of BP response to treatment and variable post-PTRA follow-up intervals to categorize BP response to PTRA. Many reports did not provide pre- and post-PTRA renal function data. The distinction between technical success rates (e.g., residual stenosis, reduction of pressure gradient before versus after PTRA) and clinical success (improvement in BP, improvement in serum creatinine) following PTRA is not always clear. Few studies provided follow-up angiographic results on all patients treated with PTRA, and long-term results regarding BP control and renal function are often lacking. Results in specific patient subgroups such as those with ostial versus those with nonostial atherosclerotic lesions have not always been reported. For these reasons, including the lack of prospective randomized comparative data, it is difficult to compare the efficacy of PTRA with that of surgical vascular reconstruction for renal artery disease.

In general, data on technically successful dilation in patients with atherosclerotic renal artery disease have been excellent (70% to 90%) for nonostial plaques located exclusively within the renal artery (Fig. 52-23) (39,40,485). On the other hand, ostial lesions have responded poorly to PTRA, with an average technical success rate of 30% to 50% (39,485,504). A higher incidence of recurrent renal artery stenosis after PTRA is observed in patients with ostial lesions than in those with nonostial lesions (74% vs. 55%) (504). An earlier study by Cicuto et al. emphasized that PTRA provides less effective treatment for ostial atherosclerotic lesions than for nonostial atherosclerotic lesions (505).

Canzanello et al. reported a large experience with PTRA in the management of 100 consecutive patients with presumed renovascular hypertension due to high-grade (greater than 75%) atherosclerotic renal artery stenosis (40). Technical success was determined from an immediate post-PTRA arteriogram, and clinical success was determined from the BP response at a mean follow-up of 35 months. In the overall group

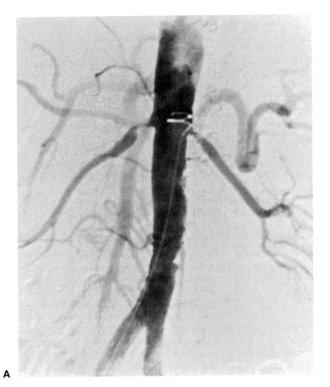

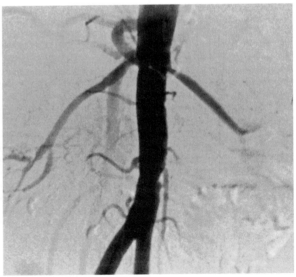

FIGURE 52-23. A: Intraarterial digital subtraction aortogram showing severe proximal right renal artery stenosis and moderately severe narrowing of the left renal artery due to atherosclerosis. **B:** Balloon angioplasty of the right renal artery was successfully performed, with reduction in the pressure gradient across the stenotic lesion from 150 mm Hg before to 10 mm Hg after the procedure. Repeat aortogram 2 years later demonstrated patency of the right renal artery.

of 100 patients, the technical success rate of PTRA was 73% (nonostial 72%, ostial 62%), and the clinical success rate (BP cured or improved) was 43% (nonostial 53%, ostial 25%). Post-PTRA angiographic studies indicated that restenosis was the main cause of failure in patients with ostial lesions.

Ramsay and Waller (506) summarized the results of PTRA as treatment for renovascular hypertension in 10 large studies published from 1981 to 1987 (Table 52-14) (39,485,507–514). PTRA was technically unsuccessful in 84 (12%) of 691 pa-

tients. Excluding technical failures and patients lost to follow-up, BP response data were available for 391 patients with atheromatous renal artery stenosis and 175 patients with fibrous renal artery disease. These aggregate data indicated post-PTRA cure, improvement, and failure rates of 50%, 42%, and 9%, respectively, in patients with fibrous disease; the aggregate post-PTRA cure, improvement, and failure rates in patients with atheromatous renal artery lesions were 19%, 52%, and 30%, respectively. The pooled analysis of these 10 studies supports the notion that the outcome of PTRA depends on the type of renal artery disease treated. In all studies, cure rates were higher for fibromuscular disease than for atherosclerotic disease. In patients in whom angioplasty was technically successful, the overall cure rate for fibrous renal artery disease was 50%. Accordingly, for fibrous renal artery disease, many centers view PTRA as the treatment of choice when intervention is pursued for presumed renovascular hypertension. For atheromatous disease, the cure rate after technically successful angioplasty was only 19%.

Brawn and Ramsay indicated that in completely unselected patients, atherosclerotic lesions were associated with a very high rate of technical failure, as high as 60% (515). The true cure rate might, therefore, be substantially lower than 19% for atheromatous renal artery disease. A more current review from the Mayo Clinic described the technical results and clinical outcome following renal artery angioplasty in 320 patients (389). The investigators observed significant reductions in mean arterial pressure and in antihypertensive medications after PTRA. The percentage of patients who benefited after renal artery angioplasty was 70% for patients with atherosclerotic renal artery disease (8.4% cured) and 63% for patients with fibrous renal artery disease (22% cured). No significant overall change in serum creatinine level was noted after the procedure in any group. The authors concluded that PTRA rarely leads to a "cure" of hypertension, but provides effective control of BP and decreases the medication requirements in selected patients.

Three prospective comparisons of PTRA versus medical therapy for hypertensive patients with atherosclerotic renal artery stenosis failed to demonstrate substantial benefits in BP control following PTRA (46,439,516). Webster randomized 55 patients to either PTRA or medical management; there was no benefit of PTRA in patients with unilateral renal artery stenosis in comparison to the medically treated patients. A modest benefit on BP was observed in patients with bilateral renal artery stenosis, particularly a reduction in systolic BP (439). In the DRASTIC study, van Jaarsveld randomly assigned 106 hypertensive patients with atherosclerotic renal artery disease to medical antihypertensive drug therapy versus PTRA. According to intention to treat analysis, at 12 months there were no significant differences between the PTRA and drug therapy groups in systolic and diastolic BPs, daily drug doses, or renal function (46). The results of this study were confounded by about 40% of patients initially allocated to medical treatment who eventually received PTRA. The Plouin study was particularly notable for randomizing patients who, by clinical criteria, had a high likelihood of substantial improvement in BP following renal artery intervention (516). Taken together, these studies indicate that renal angioplasty is no more effective for control of BP than antihypertensive drug therapy alone in patients with atherosclerotic renal artery stenosis.

The limited benefit of PTRA on BP in these studies was probably not attributable to restenosis. Restenosis did occur in about half of the patients who underwent PTRA, but there was no difference in BP control or renal function between patients who had restenosis and in those who did not (46,516). Currently available potent antihypertensive drugs, not available in the early days of PTRA, might have contributed to the negative results of these randomized trials. The tendency toward

TABLE 52-14

SUMMARY OF OUTCOMES AFTER ANGIOPLASTY IN 10 PUBLISHED SERIES OF HYPERTENSIVE PATIENTS ACCORDING TO TYPE OF RENAL ARTERY DISEASE (ATHEROMATOUS OR FIBROMUSCULAR RENAL ARTERY STENOSIS)[a]

Investigators	Atheromatous renal artery stenosis				Fibromuscular renal artery stenosis			
	Technically successful angioplasty	Blood pressure response			Technically successful angioplasty	Blood pressure response		
		Cured	Improved	Failure		Cured	Improved	Failure
Martin, et al. (513)	13	2 (15)	4 (31)	7 (54)	8	5 (63)	1 (13)	2 (25)
Colapinto, et al. (510)	44	8 (18)	29 (66)	7 (16)	9	4 (44)	5 (56)	0 (0)
Geyskes, et al. (511)	44	4 (9)	19 (43)	21 (48)	21	10 (48)	10 (48)	1 (5)
Sos, et al. (39)	34	7 (21)	10 (29)	17 (50)	27	16 (59)	9 (33)	2 (7)
Tegtmeyer, et al. (485)	61	15 (25)	46 (75)	0 (0)	27	10 (37)	17 (63)	0 (0)
Miller, et al. (512)	34	5 (15)	15 (44)	14 (41)	13	11 (85)	2 (15)	0 (0)
Martin, et al. (513)	60	9 (15)	30 (50)	21 (35)	20	5 (25)	12 (60)	3 (15)
Kaplan-Pavlohcic, et al. (514)	48	11 (23)	21 (44)	16 (33)	21	10 (48)	8 (38)	3 (14)
Kuhlmann, et al. (507)	31	9 (29)	15 (48)	7 (23)	22	11 (50)	7 (32)	4 (18)
Bell, et al. (508)	22	3 (14)	13 (59)	6 (27)	7	5 (71)	2 (29)	0 (0)
Totals	391	73 (19)	202 (52)	116 (30)	175	87 (50)	73 (42)	15 (9)
Range (%)		9–29	29–75	0–54		25–8	13–63	0–25

[a]Results are numbers (percentages) of patients.
(From: Martin EC, Mattern RF, Baer L, et al. Renal angioplasty for hypertension: predictive factors for long-term success. *AJR Am J Roentgenol* 1981;137:921, with permission.)

improvement in systolic BP compared to medical therapy alone in patients undergoing PTRA in the Webster study raises the question of which BP level (systolic or diastolic) should be treated, or treated preferentially, in hypertensive patients with atherosclerotic renal artery stenosis. Consistent with this thought are the observations of Burket et al. (35) who observed significant improvement in systolic BP among patients with highest baseline systolic BP treated with renal artery angioplasty and stent placement.

There are relatively few published reports on the results of PTRA undertaken primarily for preservation of renal function in patients with atherosclerotic renal artery disease. Donovan and coauthors reported stabilization or improvement of renal function in 11 of 17 patients, most of whom had nonostial lesions (517). Pickering et al. and Sos et al. reported improvement or stabilization of renal function in 45 (82%) of 55 patients who underwent PTRA for atherosclerotic renovascular hypertension and azotemia (518,519). The outcome of angioplasty in ischemic renal disease is summarized in

Table 52-15 (494,508,517,518). Paulsen et al. described their results with 227 PTRA procedures of 223 stenoses in 135 patients performed between 1982 and 1993 at a single center; improved renal function was achieved in 23% of patients, stabilization in 56%, and failure in 21%. Stabilized or improved renal function was higher when baseline serum creatinine was less than or equal to 250 μmol/L than when it was greater than 250 μmol/L (520).

The potential benefits of angioplasty must be assessed in comparison to the risks. *Complications* of transluminal angioplasty of the renal arteries are listed in Table 52-16. The most common complications have been hematoma (4% of patients) and transient worsening of renal function from contrast media (518). With angioplasty done in conjunction with IA-DSA, the dye load is reduced and contrast medium-induced acute renal failure is observed less frequently. Dissection of the intima of the renal artery occurs in 5% of patients, and usually resolves spontaneously, although it may require emergency surgery (508).

TABLE 52-15

ISCHEMIC RENAL DISEASE: OUTCOME OF ANGIOPLASTY

Investigators, year	No. of patients	Angioplasty outcome, N (%)			
		Improved	Stable	Worse[a]	Death
Luft, et al., 1983 (494)	12	3 (25)	5 (42)	4 (33)	0 (0)
Pickering, et al., 1986 (518)	55	26 (47)	19 (35)	10 (18)	NA
Bell, et al., 1987 (508)	20	7 (35)	10 (50)	3 (15)	0 (0)
O'Donovan, et al., 1992 (517)	17	9 (53)	2 (12)	6 (35)	5 (29)
Total	104	45 (43)	36 (35)	23 (22)	5 (5)

NA, not available.
[a]Includes all deaths.
(Modified from: Rimmer JM, Gennari FJ. Atherosclerotic renovascular disease and progressive renal failure. *Ann Intern Med* 1993;118:712, with permission.)

TABLE 52-16

COMPLICATIONS OF TRANSLUMINAL ANGIOPLASTY OF THE RENAL ARTERY OR RENAL ARTERY STENTING

Contrast medium-induced acute renal failure (mild or severe)
Atheroembolic renal failure
Rupture of the renal artery
Dissection of the renal artery
Thrombotic occlusion of the renal artery
Occlusion of a branch renal artery
Balloon malfunction (may lead to inability to remove balloon)
Balloon rupture
Puncture site hematoma, hemorrhage, or vessel tear
Median nerve compression (axillary approach)
Renal artery spasm
Mortality (<1%)

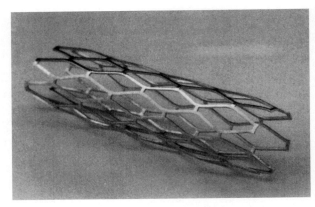

FIGURE 52-24. Palmaz stent, expanded.

The most worrisome complication of angioplasty of the renal arteries is that of cholesterol emboli. Cholesterol emboli are seen mainly in patients with diffuse atheroma and may be the cause of deterioration in renal function, with or without contrast medium-induced acute renal failure. The mortality rate related to angioplasty of the renal arteries is exceedingly low. In the series of Pickering et al., in 55 high-risk patients, the mortality rate was 0% (518); in the series of Canzanello et al., the mortality rate was 2% (40). In the Mayo Clinic report of 320 patients, the 30-day all-cause mortality rate was 2.2%; all deaths occurred in patients with atherosclerotic renal artery disease (389).

The published data on PTRA in patients with renal artery stenosis due to fibrous dysplasia are excellent and in general, equivalent to those obtained with surgical revascularization. Therefore, PTRA appears to be the treatment of choice, particularly for medial fibroplasia. However, as many as 30% of patients with medial fibroplasia or perimedial fibroplasia have disease in the distal main renal artery, often extending into renal artery branches, which increases the technical difficulty of PTRA and may render this procedure technically difficult or hazardous to perform. Some focal fibrodysplastic lesions that are confined to one or two accessible branches may be managed successfully with PTRA. However, surgical renal revascularization is probably the primary interventive treatment for most patients with branch renal artery disease.

In patients with nonostial atherosclerotic renal artery lesions, the technical and clinical success rates of PTRA have been excellent and comparable to those for surgical revascularization in patients with nonostial lesions. Unfortunately, nonostial lesions comprise only 15% to 25% of all atherosclerotic renal artery lesions. For the more commonly encountered ostial atherosclerotic lesions, the efficacy of PTRA is less favorable, and as indicated previously, restenosis rates are substantial. Whether patients with ostial atherosclerotic disease should undergo attempted PTRA versus surgical revascularization versus renal artery stenting has been a matter of local expertise and preference. Currently, most patients with ostial atherosclerotic lesions that undergo endovascular intervention will undergo primary renal artery stenting (PTRA plus stent) as opposed to PTRA alone.

Controlled trials comparing PTRA versus surgical revascularization are sparse. Weibull and co-workers reported the results of a recent single-center randomized prospective study comparing PTRA with surgical revascularization as treatment for unilateral ostial atherosclerotic renal artery stenosis in 58 patients with severe hypertension (521). Detailed clinical and angiographic follow-up data were available on all patients

in this study. PTRA was technically successful in 24 (83%) of 29 patients. Primary renal artery patency was achieved in 18 of these patients after 2 years, and 5 additional patients with recurrent stenosis underwent successful repeat PTRA. There was no difference in follow-up BP response between patients treated with PTRA and those treated with surgery. This report suggested a better outlook for PTRA in patients with ostial atherosclerotic renal artery lesions than has been the experience from other centers.

Renal Artery Stents

Much of the current work in the area of renal angioplasty is focused on catheter-delivered expandable metallic stents that mechanically hold open the vascular lumen. Metallic stents for intravascular use were first proposed by Dotter in 1969, employing simple stainless-steel coils (522). Subsequently, many other stent devices have been created, with variable success. Currently, there are three basic categories of stent designs: shape-memory alloy stents, balloon-expanded stents, and self-expanding stents. The Palmaz stent (Fig. 52-24) is a balloon-expandable stent developed in the 1980s by Julio Palmaz (523). This stent was initially approved for use in the United States by the Food and Drug Administration (FDA), specifically for the iliac and coronary arteries. Trials on use of the Palmaz stent in renal arteries have been in progress for the past decade (524).

The basic concept of stents (Palmaz stent, Strecker stent, Wallstent) is similar. They are composed of metallic wires or struts that can be collapsed and affixed to a catheter for the purpose of insertion. In most models, the unexpanded stent is mounted on the uninflated balloon of an angioplasty catheter. The stent mounted on the balloon is then positioned across the lesion, and the balloon is inflated. This maneuver expands and deploys the stent. The balloon is then deflated and removed, with the expanded stent left in place (Fig. 52-25). Over the next several weeks, endothelialization occurs, and the stent struts become covered with intima (525,526).

The rationale for renal artery stent placement relates to the generally poor technical results of balloon angioplasty (PTRA), particularly for ostial atherosclerotic lesions, with significant residual stenosis and high short-term restenosis rates characteristic of balloon angioplasty of orificial atherosclerotic renal artery lesions. Ostial renal artery stenoses consist of two entities: (a) aortic plaque encroaching on the renal artery orifice, and (b) disease of renal artery origin. Balloon angioplasty works by "controlled trauma." The atheroma is fractured longitudinally and circumferentially. Soon after deflation of the balloon, the atheroma recoils, and stenosis recurs. Stents are useful in preventing this recoil (527).

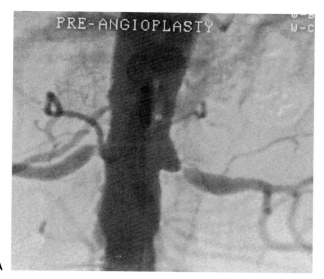

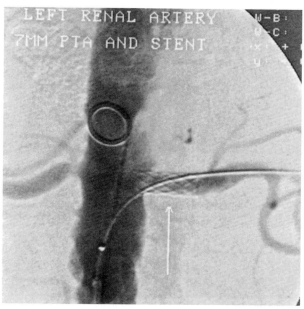

FIGURE 52-25. A: Intraarterial digital subtraction aortogram (before angioplasty) showing bilateral orificial renal artery stenosis, more severe on the left, due to atherosclerosis. **B:** Balloon angioplasty of the left renal artery was performed but significant stenosis remained. A Palmaz stent restored luminal caliber to normal.

Current clinical trials on the placement of stents in renal arteries are focused on lesions where the technical results of balloon angioplasty alone are unsatisfactory; that is, there is a significant residual stenosis commonly occurring in orificial lesions or significant postangioplasty dissection. Renal artery stents are therefore best suited when there are ostial stenoses, restenosis following PTRA, and complications of PTRA. Accumulating data suggest that use of stents for ostial stenoses has a higher initial technical success rate, a greatly improved immediate patency rate, and lower restenosis rate in comparison to balloon angioplasty alone (528–532). Most angiographers now consider the accumulating information sufficiently impressive to justify primary placement of stents for ostial or nonostial disease regardless of the results of angioplasty (38,533).

Several other factors affect the decision to utilize balloon angioplasty or primary renal artery stent placement as treatment

for ostial atherosclerotic disease. Balloon angioplasty does not usually affect subsequent surgical renal artery revascularization, but a stent in the ostial location prevents the performance of aortorenal endarterectomy, a procedure that is popular in some centers. A proximally placed renal artery stent will not usually interfere with most surgical bypass procedures, unless the stent extends near the branching of the main renal artery. Placement of stents in the distal main renal artery will severely limit the options for subsequent surgical reconstruction.

The complications of stent placement are the same as those of PTRA (Table 52-16), most importantly atheroembolic renal disease and contrast medium-induced acute renal failure. Additional problems with stent placement include malpositioning, migration, embolization of the stent, and difficulty removing the balloon from the stent (534).

Results of stent placement in the renal arteries are currently being generated and are encouraging. Data presented in 1994 by Rees et al. in the United States Multicenter Trial reported on 304 stents placed in 296 renal arteries in 263 patients (535). The technical success rate was 95%, with 80% of the lesions in the ostial location and 98% of the lesions atherosclerotic. At 6-month follow-up, 64% of patients had improvement or cure of hypertension. In 123 patients with renal insufficiency (serum creatinine greater than 1.5 mg/dL), renal function improved in 34%, remained stable in 39%, and deteriorated in 27%. Angiographic follow-up at 6 months was performed in 150 patients, unfortunately showing restenosis in 32.7%.

Olin et al. and Bacharach et al. deployed renal artery stents for ostial atherosclerotic renal artery stenosis in approximately 120 patients (490,536). The mean clinical follow-up period was 13.8 months, with a maximum follow-up of 36.5 months. The 6-month patency rate by angiography and duplex ultrasonography was 95%, with a 12-month patency rate of 82%. When restenosis was identified by routine duplex ultrasound surveillance studies, the patients underwent repeat arteriography and the stent was reexpanded if significant stenosis was present. The primary assisted patency rate was 100%. The BP was improved in approximately 85% of patients. Renal function improved in 35% of patients, remained stable in 35%, and worsened in 30% of patients. Complications included nine pseudoaneurysms, four episodes of acute tubular necrosis, and three episodes of clinically significant atheromatous embolization. Additional results reported by Dorros et al. in a multicenter Palmaz stent renal revascularization registry describe a 4-year follow up of more than 1000 stented patients (537).

A recent study selected 105 patients for intervention on the basis of clinical criteria, positive Doppler flow studies, a transstenotic pressure gradient of >30 mm Hg with >70% renal artery narrowing at arteriography (343). At a mean follow-up of 1 year, systolic and diastolic BP were reduced significantly ($p <0.0001$) in those with normal or mildly reduced renal function (GFR >50 mL/min). In patients with an initial reduction in GFR, the calculated GFR increased significantly ($p <0.007$) from 33 ± 10 to 54 ± 24 (mean ± SD) mL/minute. The authors concluded that in patients with atherosclerotic RAS fulfilling these strict criteria for severity, there may be a favorable BP response following angioplasty and stenting in those with normal renal function prior to stenting and a favorable renal function response in those with impaired renal function prior to stenting.

A review of renal artery stenting in 10 studies is presented in Table 52-17 (538). This report did not offer comparisons of stenting with angioplasty or with surgery. Overall, stents were placed in 416 renal arteries in 379 patients, mean age 64 years. Of the stenoses, 97% were atheromatous with 80% being ostial lesions. Technical success was reported in 96% to 100% of procedures. Restenosis (greater than or equal to 50% narrowing), evaluated in 312 of 416 (75%) arteries, generally between 6 and 12 months, was 16% overall. Hypertension was

TABLE 52-17A

RENAL ARTERY STENTING—BASELINE CLINICAL DATA IN 10 STENT STUDIES

Investigator, year	No. of patients/ no. of arteries	Age (range)	Male (%)	Atheromatous (%)	Ostial (%)	Bilateral (%)
Rees, et al., 1991 (524)	28/28	66 (48–80)	46	100	100	21
Hennequin, et al., 1994 (611)	21/21	55 (27–74)	52	71	33	24
Raynaud, et al., 1994 (612)	18/18	58 (31–77)	56	83	22	44
Dorros, et al., 1995 (613)	76/92	67 (37–84)	53	100	100	21
van de Ven, et al., 1995 (614)	24/28	66 (45–81)	54	100	100	87
Rundback, et al., 1996 (615)	20/24	70 (57–84)	45	100	92	20
Henry, et al., 1996 (616)	59/64	65 (27–84)	66	93	53	12
Blum, et al., 1997 (617)	68/74	60 (31–80)	65	100	100	18
Boisclair, et al., 1997 (618)	33/35	63 (37–77)	42	100	54	45
Harden, et al., 1997 (619)	32/32	67 (49–79)		100	75	78
Total (all 10 studies)	379/416	64 (27–84)	97	56	80	31

(Adapted from: Isles CG, Robertson S, Hill D. Management of renovascular disease: a review of renal artery stenting in 10 studies. *QJM* 1999;92:159, with permission.)

cured by stenting (diastolic BP less than or equal to 90 mm Hg without drugs) in 34 of 379 (9%) patients overall and in 34 of 207 (16%) patients whose renal function was normal initially. Renal function, as judged by serum creatinine concentration improved in 26%, stabilized in 48%, and deteriorated in 26% of patients whose renal function was impaired initially (serum creatinine greater than 133 μmol/L.)

Similar results were reported by Leertouwer and associates in a meta-analysis of 14 studies dealing with renal artery stent placement involving 678 patients (532). This report also compared, by meta-analysis, PTRA (10 articles, 644 patients) with the stent meta-analysis. Studies published well into 1998 were selected. Most articles reviewed described a decrease in systolic and diastolic pressure after stent placement. Because of large variation in definitions for "cure" and "improvement" of hypertension, PTRA and stents could not be critically compared regarding their effect on BP. The renal arterial stent meta-

analysis indicated an overall improvement in renal function in 30% of patients, stabilization in 38%, and worsening renal function in 32%. The restenosis rate at a follow-up of 6 to 29 months was 17% after renal artery stenting versus 26% following PTRA. The cure rate for hypertension was higher and the improvement rate for renal function was better after stent placement than after PTRA (20% vs. 10%, and 30% vs. 38%, respectively; p <0.001).

Taken together, current reports are encouraging with regard to immediate and intermediate results of renal artery stent placement. Longer follow-up is needed to test the patency of stents in comparison with surgical revascularization and to compare long-term effects on BP, renal function, and patient survival with surgical revascularization and/or medical management alone. Burket et al. have emphasized the improvement in systolic BP, but not diastolic BP, after renal artery stenting (35). Dorros et al., in a follow-up of Palmaz stent

TABLE 52-17B

TECHNICAL ASPECTS IN 10 STENT STUDIES[a]

Investigator, year	Inclusion stenosis (%)	Indications for stent				Stents evaluated (% total stents)	Restenosis (% stents evaluated)	Average[b] time to evaluation (months)
		Rec	Dis	Res	Pri			
Rees, et al., 1991 (524)	≥40	71	0	29	0	18 (64)	7 (39)	8
Hennequin, et al., 1994 (611)	≥70	38	0	62	0	20 (95)	4 (20)	29
Raynaud, et al., 1994 (612)	≥60	66	11	6	17	18 (100)	2 (11)	11
Dorros, et al., 1995 (613)	≥70	0	0	0	100	56 (61)	14 (25)	7
van de Ven, et al., 1995 (614)	≥50	58	0	0	42	23 (82)	3 (13)	6[c]
Rundback, et al., 1996 (615)	≥60	83	0	17	0	16 (67)	3 (19)	6
Henry, et al., 1996 (616)	≥70	66	3	31	0	54 (84)	5 (9)	14
Blum, et al., 1997 (617)	≥50	85	1	14	0	74 (100)	8 (11)	24
Boisclair, et al., 1997 (618)	≥60	83	0	17	0	9 (23)	0 (0)	8
Harden, et al., 1997 (619)	≥50	94	6	0	0	24 (75)	3 (13)	6[a]
Total (all 10 studies)	≥50 in 9 studies	58	2	15	25	312 (75)	49 (16)	6–12 in 7 studies

Rec, elastic recoil; *Dis*, dissection; *Res*, restenosis; *Pri*, primary procedure.
[a]Palmaz stent used in all studies except Hennequin and Raynaud (Wallstent).
[b]Follow-ups are means except[c] medians.
(Adapted from: Isles CG, Robertson S, Hill D. Management of renovascular disease: a review of renal artery stenting in ten studies. *QJM* 1999;92:159, with permission.)

revascularization as treatment for atherosclerotic renal artery stenosis, found that 38 patients indicated a 3-year cumulative probability of survival which worsens with increasing baseline serum creatinine concentrations and extent (bilateral vs. unilateral renal artery stenosis) of atherosclerotic disease. In this report, the survival probability at 3 years was only 46 ± 15% for patients with bilateral atherosclerotic renal artery disease and baseline serum creatinine concentrations equal to or greater than 2.0 mg/dL. Kennedy et al. reported similar results in a series of 230 patients (539).

Restenosis of stents tends to be secondary to intimal hyperplasia and located at or just beyond the end of the stent (525). Active research is ongoing to improve on current stent design and possibly the use of covered, biodegradable, and chemically impregnated stents. Based on current experience, renal artery stent placement is recommended for endovascular revascularization of atherosclerotic ostial lesions, either as an adjunct to PTRA or as a primary procedure.

Renal Artery Disease in Children

The most common cause of renal artery disease in children is fibrous dysplasia. Other lesions in this age group include arterial aneurysm, arteriovenous malformation, Takayasu's arteritis, neurofibromatosis, thromboembolic disease, and renal trauma (540). Bilateral or branch renal artery stenosis, particularly in fibrous dysplasia, is not infrequently present, nor is extrarenal vascular disease. As reviewed earlier, many renal artery lesions in children, such as intimal and perimedial fibroplasia, cause progressive vascular obstruction. Accordingly, treatment is directed not only at relief of hypertension but also at preserving renal function.

Although PTRA is effective in some children, angioplasty is often not technically feasible because of the small size of the diseased vessels, involvement of renal artery branches, or the presence of multiple lesions, aneurysmal disease, or perivascular scarring in cases of arteritis. Medical antihypertensive therapy is generally not recommended as the definitive treatment in young children with renovascular hypertension because it would be lifelong and there is a risk of losing renal function from progressive renal arterial disease. Accordingly, surgical revascularization is probably the best option.

The results of surgical revascularization in children have improved, owing to the development of microvascular techniques and a better appreciation of specific operative approaches most likely to be effective in this group (541). Aortorenal bypass grafting with an autogenous hypogastric artery is the usual revascularization technique. Saphenous vein grafts are generally avoided in the small child, in whom postoperative aneurysmal graft expansion may occur. When aortorenal bypass is not possible because of peripheral renal artery disease or aortic hypoplasia, renal autotransplantation is the treatment of choice. Extracorporeal microvascular arterial reconstruction with autotransplantation is recommended for children with branch renal artery disease (245,542).

MEDICAL MANAGEMENT

The issue of medical versus surgical treatment of presumed renovascular hypertension has generated intense interest and discussion for many years. The advent of balloon angioplasty and renal artery stents has amplified this discussion. To date, no truly randomized study has addressed the benefits and risks of medical versus surgical versus angioplasty therapy. Until recently, few reports assessed the natural history of renal artery stenosis without surgical intervention. The search for the presence of renal artery stenosis and assessing its likelihood in causing hypertension implies an intent to intervene by either surgical or endovascular renal revascularization. The major concerns with medical management (antihypertensive drug treatment) of these patients are the progression of renal artery stenosis, the hemodynamic effects of BP reduction on renal function, and the diminished likelihood of success of renal revascularization in curing the hypertension the longer one waits to intervene.

There is little question that the more severe the hypertension, the greater the likelihood that it is renovascular in origin. Further, in general, younger patients with fibrous renal artery disease respond well to intervention with either surgery or angioplasty. However, the results of renal revascularization in patients with atherosclerotic renal artery disease are less favorable, as many of them are older and almost certainly have coexisting primary or essential hypertension (46,131, 187,232,439,516,543,544).

Several scenarios should be considered in the care of patients with renal artery stenosis and hypertension: (a) true renovascular hypertension, in which atherosclerotic or fibrous renal artery disease is the sole cause of the hypertension; (b) pure essential hypertension, in which atherosclerotic or fibrous renal artery disease is present but does not contribute to the hypertension at all; (c) essential hypertension with superimposed renal artery stenosis producing a renovascular contribution to the underlying essential hypertension; and (d) the hypertension of renal parenchymal disease, that is, chronic renal insufficiency (see Chapter 51), with superimposed renal artery stenosis contributing to the hypertension. Accordingly, the medical management of patients with presumed renovascular hypertension and renovascular disease is really an effort to control the BP. Despite the uncertainty in knowing whether a patient with hypertension and coexisting renal artery stenosis has renovascular hypertension, the goals of medical therapy in such patients similar to those with hypertension in general. They are to control the BP, minimize target organ damage, prolong life, avoid adverse drug side effects, and maintain renal function.

In 1974, Hunt et al. reported results comparing medical versus surgical treatment in 214 patients followed prospectively for 7 to 14 years (235). This was not a randomized study because of 100 patients selected for surgical therapy, 82 had failed to respond to 3 months of medical treatment. During the subsequent 7 to 14 years, 16% of the surgically treated and 40% of the medically treated patients with atherosclerotic renal artery disease died. Fifty-one of the 84 surviving patients treated surgically were normotensive without medication at latest follow-up. Satisfactory BP control (diastolic BP less than 100 mm Hg) was maintained for 7 years or longer in 52 of 98 patients managed medically. Most late deaths were caused by cardiac or cerebral events or uremia. Survival rates for a younger group of patients with fibromuscular disease undergoing surgical or medical therapy were 92% and 83%, respectively.

Dean et al. reported on 41 patients with atherosclerotic renal arterial disease and presumed renovascular hypertension who were treated medically (545). Progression of the renal arterial stenosis to total occlusion was observed in 4 (12%) of 31 patients who underwent serial angiographic studies. Seventeen patients (41%) had deterioration of renal function or loss of renal size that led to surgery. Despite deterioration, most patients had acceptable BP control. Sheps et al. reviewed their experience with medical management in 54 patients for an average follow-up of 20 months (546). The effectiveness of medical therapy was emphasized by excellent control of BP in 32 (65%) of 49 surviving patients. Funduscopic changes improved in half the patients. Despite BP control, additional cardiovascular complications developed in 12 patients with atherosclerotic disease, and 5 patients died. Three patients had progressive deterioration in renal function despite good BP control.

Shapiro et al. reported on 72 medically treated patients (543). Compared with a surgical subgroup at the same institution, the medically treated patients were older and had more evidence of significant target organ involvement, indicating that they were at greater long-term risk. In a follow-up period of 1 to 6 years, 29 (40%) of the 72 nonsurgical patients had died. Similarly, Dustan et al. studied 32 medically managed patients (547). Coronary and cerebrovascular disease were common in these patients, and although 12 (37%) apparently achieved normal BPs over 5 years of follow-up, 10 (31%) had died at the end of the follow-up period.

Altogether, the aforementioned reports suggest that the most dependable treatment for presumed renovascular hypertension, particularly when the likelihood of renovascular hypertension is high, is to relieve the ischemia by means of surgery. In this context, conceptually, indications for intervention on the renal artery stenosis should be similar and applied equally to either surgical or endovascular renal revascularization. Assessment of operative risk for postoperative morbidity and mortality is standard medical practice for patients being considered for surgical renal revascularization. Similar comorbid risk factor assessment (advanced age, increased serum creatinine, i.e., >2 mg/dL, history of congestive heart failure or myocardial infarction) has been emphasized in predicting morbidity and subsequent cardiovascular mortality post–renal artery stenting (438,537,539).

Although hypertension in patients with true renovascular hypertension is more severe than in most patients with primary or essential hypertension (131,148,546,548,549), renovascular hypertension does, indeed, respond to standard antihypertensive drug therapy. The degree of hypertension and the response to drug therapy are highly variable in patients with presumed renovascular hypertension, and one should not assume that every patient with renal artery stenosis and coexisting hypertension will need surgical revascularization, angioplasty, or nephrectomy to control their BP. This is particularly true now with the availability of a number of potent antihypertensive agents with a variety of pharmacologic properties that, when used appropriately and in proper combinations, can successfully control the BP. In addition, medical antihypertensive therapy is necessary to optimize BP control before planned surgery or angioplasty and for patients whose BP is not normalized by surgery or angioplasty.

The main indications for antihypertensive drug therapy (medical management) of presumed renovascular hypertension include advanced age, poor surgical risk, atherosclerotic lesions, situations wherein renal revascularization or angioplasty is not feasible owing to technical difficulties of these treatment modalities, irreversible atrophy of the kidney distal to the stenosis, doubtful significance of the renal artery stenosis lesion by angiographic criteria, hypertension of long duration (suggesting concomitant essential hypertension or arteriolar nephrosclerosis or both), and patients who simply choose medical management (131,232,544,546,548,549). Before the early 1970s, pharmacologic therapy for presumed renovascular hypertension was empirical and quite similar to that of essential hypertension. The degree of hypertension and response to drug therapy are, not unexpectedly, highly variable for patients with renal artery stenosis, and one should not assume that every patient with renal artery stenosis will respond readily to antihypertensive treatment or to treatment with only one or two drugs. Neither can the physician assume that patients with hypertension and renal artery stenosis will necessarily need surgery, angioplasty, stenting, or nephrectomy to control the BP, even when clinical clues predicting that such intervention will cure or markedly improve the hypertension are present.

Patients undergoing medical treatment of presumed renovascular hypertension must be closely monitored for continuing or worsening hypertension, intolerable drug side effects, progressive atrophy of the kidney distal to the stenosis, and the development of azotemia or worsening azotemia. Surgical therapy, angioplasty, or renal artery stenting for presumed renovascular hypertension should, therefore, be strongly considered for patients whose hypertension is refractory to medical management, younger patients with fibrous renal artery disease, patients of any age who are good surgical risks, and when progressive arterial stenosis poses a threat to renal function.

Responses to Medical Treatment

There is considerable successful experience in the medical treatment of hypertension associated with renovascular disease (550). The first substantial series of patients with presumed renovascular hypertension, treated medically, was reported by Dustan et al. in 1963 (547). These investigators used a thiazide diuretic and either hydralazine or guanethidine or both in 32 patients followed for 1 to 6 years. Treatment successfully controlled the hypertension in 13 (41%) and failed in 9 (28%); 10 (31%) of the patients died during follow-up.

Results of antihypertensive drug therapy during the late 1960s and the 1970s yielded somewhat better results, that is, controlled or much improved BPs (543,551–555). Dramatic improvements in the medical treatment of presumed renovascular hypertension evolved with the development of beta-adrenergic blocking agents (beta-blockers) and subsequently with the use of ACE inhibitors and angiotensin receptor blockers (128,129,228,261,555–564 565,566). These classes of antihypertensive agents are particularly effective because they interfere with specific steps in the renin-angiotensin-aldosterone system, which plays a pivotal role in the pathogenesis of hypertension.

As depicted in Figures 52-8 and 52-11, the pathophysiology of classic two-kidney Goldblatt hypertension produces hypoperfusion of the stenotic kidney, activating the renin-angiotensin-aldosterone axis and producing a vasoconstrictor type of hypertension. Beta-adrenergic blockade, by suppressing renin release (261,561,562,564,567), blunts the generation of angiotensin I and subsequently, angiotensin II, the primary vasoconstrictor substance operative in the early stages of classic 2K-1C Goldblatt hypertension. In addition, beta-blockers also lower BP by reducing cardiac output, suppressing the central nervous system, reducing peripheral vascular resistance, resetting the baroreceptor levels, and preventing the pressor response to catecholamines with exercise and stress (548,563,564,568).

Angiotensin-Converting Enzyme Inhibitors and Beta-Adrenergic Blockers

As shown in Figure 52-8, ACE inhibitors interfere with the conversion of angiotensin I to angiotensin II, again reducing the concentration of this potent endogenous vasoconstrictor. Improved responses to medical management with beta-blockers and ACE inhibitors are not surprising, at least in the early stages of renovascular hypertension, because these two classes of antihypertensive agents directly affect the renin-angiotensin system. Although experience with the angiotensin II receptor blockers is limited in this patient population, one would anticipate them to be effective in controlling BP in the early stages of renovascular hypertension when the elevated arterial pressure is driven by angiotensin II. Interference with the generation of angiotensin is not, however, the entire explanation for the BP-lowering effect of ACE inhibitors; they also potentiate bradykinin, and some ACE inhibitors are associated with increased levels of vasodilatory prostaglandins (565).

TABLE 52-18

REPORTED RESPONSES TO MEDICAL THERAPY FOR RENOVASCULAR HYPERTENSION

Investigators, year	N	Follow-up	Agents[a]	Controlled or much improved	Intermediate	Failure	Deaths
Dustan, et al., 1963 (547)	32	1–6 yr	Hydralazine, guanethidine	41	31	28	31
Peart, 1967 (551)	42	0–8 yr	—	45	36	19	—
Shapiro, et al., 1969 (543)	72	34 mo	—	—	—	—	40
Kjellbo, et al., 1970 (552)	165	0.5–10 yr	—	46	30	24	30
Owen, 1973 (553)	83	5 yr	—	35	34	31	34
Buhler, et al., 1973 (556)	11	1–180 days	Propranolol	45	27	18	—
Hunt and Strong, 1976 (554)	114	1–8 yr	Methyldopa	81	19	3	—
	59	7–14 yr		46	—	39	—
Streeten and Anderson, 1979 (555)	4	6 mo	Propranolol	9	3	8	—
			No propranolol	9	8	3	—
Struder, et al., 1981 (557)	2	6 mo	Captopril	9	38	0	—
Atkinson, et al., 1982 (129)	15	6 wks	Captopril	62	23	15	—
Hollifield, et al., 1982 (558)	53	2–3 yr	Captopril	68	20	17	—
Case, et al., 1982 (559)	21	28 ± 3 mo	Captopril	90	10	0	—
Hollenberg, 1983 (570)	269	0.3–2 yr	Captopril	77	18	0.37	—

Results (%)

[a]In most patients, a thiazide diuretic was also used.
(Adapted from: Hollenberg NK. Treatment of renovascular hypertension: surgery, angioplasty, and medical therapy with converting enzyme inhibitors. *Am J Kidney Dis* 1987;10[Suppl 1]:52, with permission.)

Despite the physiologic rationale for the use of beta-blockers, ACE inhibitors, and angiotensin II receptor blockers in patients with presumed angiotensin II-dependent hypertension, widespread experience indicates that medical antihypertensive therapy even with these agents becomes more difficult if hypertension has lasted longer than 3 to 5 years (particularly for patients with atherosclerotic renal artery disease), if a patient has coexisting chronic renal insufficiency with concomitant extracellular fluid volume expansion, or if there is a major element of essential hypertension or arteriolar nephrosclerosis or both. Treatment with a beta-blocker or an ACE inhibitor alone (or in combination) is often ineffective in controlling the BP in these circumstances. The same observations are true for patients with bilateral atherosclerotic renal artery stenosis.

As reviewed earlier in this chapter, the pathophysiology of 2K-1C hypertension indicates that the high pressure initially generated by the stenotic kidney is transmitted to the contralateral kidney via the contralateral patent renal artery, producing substantial small-vessel disease or augmenting preexisting small-vessel disease (i.e., arteriolar nephrosclerosis). Therefore, over time, and especially in the presence of uncontrolled BPs, the 2K-1C hypertension escalates to an analog of one-kidney hypertension, wherein the pathophysiologic features are similar to those of chronic renal failure associated with extracellular fluid volume expansion (reviewed in Chapter 51) (128). Volume control is necessary for such patients, usually with dietary salt restriction and diuretics, and it has been well documented that the effectiveness of beta-blockers and ACE inhibitors is markedly augmented when they are used in conjunction with diuretics (556,557,559). Thus, in contrast to the choice of antihypertensive drugs in initiating therapy for patients with essential hypertension, wherein the pathogenesis and pathophysiology are multifactorial and poorly understood, the pathophysiology of renovascular hypertension allows for a more mechanism-oriented approach to drug selection and focused treatment interfering with elements of the renin-angiotensin system (569).

Reports of the effectiveness of captopril in patients with renovascular hypertension are especially encouraging, particularly because some of these patients were resistant to alternative medical regimens that included beta-blockers (550,559,570). In a series of 269 patients, the efficacy of captopril was unequivocal, even though 40% of the patients were azotemic and 51% (136/269) had either a solitary kidney or advanced bilateral renal arterial disease (570). Captopril was ineffective in only 5% of patients, and more than 80% of the patients achieved marked improvement or goal BP. Like captopril, enalapril has also been shown to be useful in the medical management of patients with renovascular hypertension (571). Reported responses to medical therapy in patients with presumed renovascular hypertension are summarized in Table 52-18 (129,543,547,551–559,570).

Although certain pharmacologic differences exist between captopril and enalapril, both drugs exert equal antihypertensive effects in patients with renovascular hypertension. Franklin and Smith compared the results of enalapril plus hydrochlorothiazide therapy with standard triple therapy in 75 patients with presumed renovascular hypertension (571). Blood pressure control was better in the enalapril group. Poor response to therapy occurred in patients with bilateral renal artery stenosis or impaired renal function. Renal function deteriorated (increase in serum creatinine level of 0.3 mg/dL or more from pretreatment value) in 10 (20%) of the 49 enalapril-treated patients compared to 1 (3%) of 39 patients receiving triple therapy (571). In the enalapril-treated patients demonstrating an increase in serum creatinine, this increase occurred during the first 2 to 3 weeks of therapy, after which point the level plateaued without any evidence of progressively worsening renal function. No occurrence of acute oliguric renal failure was observed in any of the patients receiving enalapril-plus-hydrochlorothiazide therapy, even among the 18 patients with bilateral renal artery stenosis.

The pharmacodynamic and pharmacokinetic properties of beta-blockers (564,565,567) and ACE inhibitors (183) are detailed in standard pharmacology reviews. Propranolol is the prototype of a number of beta-adrenergic blocking agents (556,572). Regardless of the etiology of the hypertension, the initial antihypertensive effects of propranolol and ACE inhibitors (573) relate to the preexisting level of the plasma renin activity considered in relation to the urinary sodium excretion. The antihypertensive action of propranolol and other beta-blockers affects both the vasoconstrictor and the volume components of hypertension because inhibition of renin secretion also retards aldosterone secretion, thus preventing sodium and water retention. The beta-blockers are particularly effective in combination with a diuretic and occasionally with a vasodilating agent such as hydralazine. The available beta-blockers have different effects on renal function (564,567,573). There is little evidence to suggest that administration of beta-blockers in patients with preexisting renal disease or renal artery stenosis results in a deterioration of renal function, or carries the risk of irreversible renal failure.

ACE inhibitors are excreted mainly by the kidneys. Because many of their side effects are dose-dependent, the dosage should be reduced in patients with impaired renal function. Important adverse effects with captopril include skin rash, dysgeusia, and neutropenia. Undesirable reactions to ACE inhibitors as a class are cough, the prevalence of which varies from 45% to 16% (183); functional renal insufficiency; and hyperkalemia. Angioedema is a rare, but potentially serious complication of ACE inhibitors. Cough and angioedema are most likely attributable to decreased degradation of bradykinin (565).

Angiotensin II Receptor Blockers

Because of the potential of interfering more specifically with the actions of angiotensin II at the receptor level (574), angiotensin II receptor blockers are now widely used in the treatment of hypertension. Of historical interest, the first angiotensin II receptor blocker, saralasin, was used in the early 1970s, mainly to explore the effects of inhibition of the renin-angiotensin-aldosterone system (575). Although widely used in clinical investigation, its complex peptide structure and quick hydrolysis after oral administration made it impractical as an antihypertensive drug (270). Several nonpeptide molecules that interfere with angiotensin II receptors and lower BP have now been synthesized (576). The first blocker of this type to become available for clinical use was losartan. Currently, many other angiotensin II receptor blockers are now available. There is hope that since these agents interfere farther down the renin-angiotensin system cascade than do the ACE inhibitors (Fig. 52-8), they may not cause some of the troublesome side effects associated with ACE inhibition (e.g., cough and angioedema). Whether these agents will be as effective as currently available ACE inhibitors in patients with presumed renovascular hypertension remains to be determined. At present, there is no unequivocal information as to whether the angiotensin receptor blockers differ significantly from the available ACE inhibitors in causing hyperkalemia, mild reduction in GFRs (577), or frank acute renal failure, but at least one report suggests they have less adverse effects on renal function (578).

Calcium Antagonists

Calcium antagonists have been found to be quite effective in patients with presumed renovascular hypertension (579,580). Their antihypertensive effect is primarily due to direct arteriolar vasodilatation. The calcium antagonists are a chemically, pharmacologically, and therapeutically heterogeneous group of agents. Their clinical effects are related to blocking the L class of voltage-gated calcium channels in a variety of tissues. In general, the calcium antagonists act by selective inhibition

of calcium influx through the cell membrane. This interference appears to interact with selective blockade of the slow channels for transmembrane calcium influx. Because calcium ions play an important role in the contractile process of smooth muscle, calcium antagonists, by preventing this influx, produce arteriolar relaxation (581,582).

The precise mechanisms of action of the calcium antagonists are under active investigation, but the effects of calcium antagonists on the elements of the renin-angiotensin system are complex. In general, an increase in intracellular calcium produces an increase in hormone release and synthesis, and blockage of calcium entry might be expected to blunt this response. However, calcium antagonists stimulate the synthesis and release of renin in juxtaglomerular cells (583,584). Therefore, the antihypertensive effect of calcium antagonists in renovascular hypertension is probably not due to decreasing renin release, but is more likely secondary to direct peripheral arteriolar vasodilation.

One potential benefit of calcium antagonists in the treatment of hypertensive patients with renovascular disease is their favorable effect on renal function in comparison to ACE inhibitors (585–587). Although there have been occasional reports of calcium antagonists adversely affecting renal function, particularly in patients with renal insufficiency (588), calcium antagonists are generally safe in patients with renal artery stenosis. In patients with bilateral renal artery stenosis, calcium antagonists lower BP effectively without causing as much deterioration of GFR as ACE inhibitors (585–587).

Calcium antagonists have had a major impact on the treatment of all types of hypertension and of ischemic heart disease. Their well-documented effectiveness in lowering BP has resulted in their widespread use (258,585–587). The pharmacodynamic, pharmacokinetic, cardiac, and hemodynamic effects of calcium antagonists are detailed in a number of reviews (258,579,581,582,589,590). Three categories of calcium antagonists are clinically available: dihydropyridines (e.g., nifedipine, felodipine, amlodipine), benzothiazepines (e.g., diltiazem), and phenylalkylamines (e.g., verapamil). All three categories are useful in hypertensive patients with or without renal artery stenosis and in the presence of a wide variety of concomitant conditions, including ischemic heart disease, peripheral vascular disease, diabetes mellitus, and chronic renal disease.

Nifedipine, a dihydropyridine calcium antagonist, has little suppressive effect on myocardial tissue, having its major effects in blocking vasoconstriction in large to medium-sized arteries. Verapamil is less directly vasodilatory than the dihydropyridines. Verapamil depresses sinoatrial and atrioventricular nodal activity and should be used with caution in patients with heart block. Diltiazem, with properties closely related to those of verapamil, has a more variable and evidently dose-dependent effect on heart rate (579,581,582,589,590). Whether the three classes of clinically available calcium antagonists have differing BP-lowering capabilities or different side-effect profiles in patients with renal artery stenosis has not been determined.

A detailed discussion of the many additional types of antihypertensive agents (e.g., diuretics, alpha1-agonists, alpha-blockers, peripheral neurogenic inhibitors, and the vasodilators hydralazine and minoxidil) is beyond the scope of this chapter. In general, the use of these agents in the medical management of patients with renovascular disease and presumed renovascular hypertension follows the usual guidelines for these agents when used for essential hypertension. However, when renovascular hypertension is suspected, the first step should be to use either a beta-blocker, ACE inhibitor, angiotensin II receptor blocker, or calcium antagonist. The combination of an ACE inhibitor and a calcium antagonist is extremely effective. The conjoint use of an ACE inhibitor and a beta-blocker is also effective.

Caution must be exercised in using a beta-blocker in combination with verapamil or diltiazem, especially in patients prone to bradycardia or with any electrocardiographic evidence of heart block, because the conjoint use of these two drug classes might dangerously slow the heart rate or precipitate congestive heart failure.

The next drug to be added would ideally be a diuretic agent, especially in conjunction with an ACE inhibitor, beta-blocker, or angiotensin II receptor blocker. Clonidine is also effective, often as a third drug in patients with severe hypertension in association with renovascular disease. Clonidine administration may produce an acute reduction in BP in patients with renovascular hypertension; the reduction in BP occurs without a significant change in plasma renin activity, but is associated with a decrease in plasma norepinephrine levels (591). Clonidine is especially effective in lowering the systolic BP in older adult hypertensive patients.

Complications and Liabilities of Medical Management of Renovascular Hypertension and Renovascular Disease

The side effects of the many antihypertensive drugs used in treating renovascular hypertension are well known and beyond the scope of this chapter. However, several untoward metabolic or physiologic effects of medical antihypertensive therapy are of particular interest in managing patients with renovascular disease including, but not limited to, hypokalemia, hyperkalemia, acute renal failure, reduced renal perfusion pressure, flash pulmonary edema, and ischemic shrinkage of the kidney distal to the stenosis.

In two-kidney Goldblatt hypertension, aldosterone levels increase as a consequence of activation of the renin-angiotensin system. Secondary aldosteronism ensues, and hypokalemia is a cardinal feature of true renovascular hypertension. Diuretics may further activate the renin-angiotensin-aldosterone cascade and increase sodium delivery to the site of aldosterone action in the nephron, and produce severe hypokalemia. The clinical syndrome of hyporeninemic hypoaldosteronism is not uncommon in older adult diabetic patients, many of whom have renovascular disease and underlying essential hypertension (not true renovascular hypertension); these patients may develop hyperkalemia, which can be aggravated to dangerous levels with the use of ACE inhibitors and beta-blockers, both of which increase the serum potassium concentration.

Acute renal failure in conjunction with ACE inhibition in patients with bilateral renal artery stenosis or high-grade stenosis of an artery to a solitary kidney is well described (225,228,230,434,435,592–596). This drawback is often the limiting factor in drug treatment of patients with presumed renovascular hypertension. Acute deterioration in renal function in patients undergoing medical treatment for presumed renovascular hypertension is frequently the clinical observation that prompts the physician to discontinue medical therapy and consider angioplasty or surgical revascularization in suitable candidates. This phenomenon has been observed in up to 23% of patients with high-grade renal artery stenosis who take ACE inhibitors (597). Fortunately, renal function usually recovers when the ACE inhibitor is discontinued (435,594–596). Although clear evidence of permanent structural damage in the kidney distal to the stenosis in such situations is lacking in humans, renal artery thrombosis has been described (597–600). Whether shrinkage of the kidney distal to the stenosis in patients treated with ACE inhibitors for a long time is due to ACE inhibition per se or to progressive arterial stenosis (or to both) is unclear, but progressive renal atrophy is an indication

to abandon medical management and proceed with angioplasty or surgery if technically feasible.

Calcium antagonists appear to induce less impairment of renal function in patients with renovascular hypertension than do ACE inhibitors (585,586). In two studies comparing the effects of captopril and nifedipine, both agents demonstrated excellent antihypertensive efficacy (585,586). Nifedipine, however, produced a smaller decrement in the GFR than did captopril in patients with unilateral, bilateral, or solitary kidney renal artery stenosis. Dihydropyridine calcium antagonists may better maintain renal blood flow and glomerular filtration because of their preferential afferent arteriolar vasodilatory effect (579).

Any type of antihypertensive therapy that effectively lowers the BP may decrease renal blood flow and glomerular filtration if the BP is lowered below a "critical" renal perfusion pressure (224,233). Diuretic-induced extracellular fluid volume contraction would potentiate this untoward effect of reduced perfusion pressure on renal function.

Flash pulmonary edema has been discussed as a clinical clue to unilateral or bilateral renal artery stenosis (216,217), or in association with uncontrolled BP. Episodes of acute pulmonary edema in the absence of obvious overt cardiac disease in patients with a reasonable left ventricular ejection fraction are being observed more frequently in the older adult population with disseminated vascular disease involving the renal arteries. These episodes occur more frequently in patients with bilateral renal artery stenosis or high-grade stenosis of an artery to a solitary kidney than in patients with unilateral renal artery stenosis (218). This clinical syndrome complicates the medical management of patients with renal artery stenosis and may be the critical factor prompting an intervention procedure on the renal artery (218,536).

Some authors have suggested that atherosclerotic RAS is associated with increased cardiovascular events and decreased survival in comparison to patients without RAS (36–38). Edwards et al. conducted a prospective, multicenter cohort study of cardiovascular disease risk factors, morbidity, and mortality among Americans older than 65 years (36). Renovascular disease was associated with an increase in the risk of adverse coronary events in this study population. The increment in risk was not dependent on the effects of associated atherosclerotic risk factors, other prevalent cardiovascular disease, or increased BP. Whether these authors' findings relate specifically to the anatomic presence of atherosclerotic RAS versus other comorbid cardiovascular risk factors associated with generalized atherosclerosis merits continued examination. Such reports could, however, fuel enthusiasm for renal revascularization to prevent adverse coronary outcomes.

An explosive increase in endovascular renal revascularization procedures over the past decade has been emphasized recently by Murphy et al. (601). Whether or not this explosion in endovascular intervention is due to a substantial increase in renovascular hypertension, increased concern that systolic hypertension in an increasingly aging population may be helped by renal artery stenting, that more patients are developing endstage renal disease (ESRD) as a consequence of atherosclerotic renal artery disease (ASO-RAD), concerns about chronic kidney disease (CKD) (elevated serum creatinine concentrations) as promoting cardiac disease and adversely affecting patient survival, or other considerations, is unclear. What is clear, however, is that despite the widespread occurrence of ASO-RAD, there is no consensus on the best treatment approach.

The discussion of medical management has focused on a pathophysiologic approach to the drug treatment of renal artery stenosis and presumed renovascular hypertension. Regardless of the pharmacologic regimen employed to control BP in such patients, long-term adherence to therapy remains a major problem, as it does for patients with essential hypertension.

Failure to control BP leaves such patients at risk for the cardiovascular complications of stroke, congestive heart failure, and progressive renal insufficiency.

Which drugs to use and the choice of medical or surgical treatment or angioplasty or stent placement must be considered carefully for each individual. In general, medical management is preferred for older patients, especially those with serious cardiovascular risk factors for surgery. Older patients with tight ostial renal artery atherosclerosis in conjunction with severe aortoiliac disease are at high risk during angiography, angioplasty, renal artery stent placement, and surgery, and probably should be managed medically if at all possible. Balloon angioplasty or surgical renal revascularization is preferred for patients with fibrous renal artery disease and for younger patients with atherosclerosis, particularly if they have acceptable surgical risk factors.

For all patients managed medically, meticulous follow-up is required to ensure that the systolic BP remains less than 140 mm Hg and the diastolic pressure less than 90 mm Hg. Optimal medical management of such patients, particularly those with atherosclerotic renal artery disease, demands modification of cardiovascular risk factors such as smoking and serum lipid levels. Whether current or future antihyperlipidemic drugs (e.g., hepatic hydroxymethylglutaryl coenzyme A reductase inhibitors) will have a meaningful impact on atherosclerotic renal artery stenosis (602,603) remains to be determined, but their benefits in promoting regression of atherosclerosis in other vascular beds are promising (604–609).

References

1. Goldblatt H, Lynch J, Hanzal RF, et al. Studies on experimental hypertension. I. The production of persistent elevation of systolic blood pressure by means of renal ischemia. *J Exp Med* 1934;59:347.
2. Eyler WR, Clark MD, Garman JE, et al. Angiography of the renal areas including a comparative study of renal artery stenosis in patients with and without hypertension. *Radiology* 1962;78:879.
3. Dustan HP, Humphries AW, DeWolfe VG. Normal arterial pressure in patients with renal arterial stenosis. *JAMA* 1964;187:1028.
4. Holley KE, Hunt JC, Brown AL Jr, et al. Renal artery stenosis: a clinical-pathological study in normotensive and hypertensive patients. *Am J Med* 1964;34:14.
5. Page IH. The production of persistent arterial hypertension by cellophane perinephritis. *JAMA* 1939;113:2046.
6. Bright R. *Reports of medical cases selected with a view of illustrating symptoms and the cure of diseases by a reference to morbid anatomy.* London: Longman, 1827.
7. Mahomed FA. Etiology of Bright's disease and the pre-albuminuric stage. *Med Chir Trans* 1874;57:197.
8. Tigerstedt R, Bergmann PG. Niere und kreislauf. *Skand Arch Physiol* 1898;8:223.
9. Peart S. Development of ideas on renovascular hypertension. *Semin Nephrol* 2000;20:388.
10. Goldblatt H. Symposium on the management of renovascular hypertension. Reflections. *Urol Clin North Am* 1975;2:219.
11. Butler AM. Chronic pyelonephritis and arterial hypertension. *J Clin Invest* 1937;16:889.
12. Swales JD. *Classic papers in hypertension: blood pressure and renin.* London: Science Press, 1985.
13. Basso N, Terragno NA. History about the discovery of the renin-angiotensin system. *Hypertension* 2001;38:1246.
14. Pohl MA, Novick AC. Natural history of atherosclerotic and fibrous renal artery disease: clinical implications. *Am J Kidney Dis* 1985;5:A120.
15. Harrison EG, Jr, McCormack LJ. Pathologic classification of renal arterial disease in renovascular hypertension. *Mayo Clin Proc* 1971;46:161.
16. Stanley JC, Gewertz BL, Bove EL, et al. Arterial fibrodysplasia. Histopathologic character and current etiologic concepts. *Arch Surg* 1975;110:561.
17. Novick AC, Stewart BH. Surgical treatment of renovascular hypertension. *Curr Prob Surg* 1979;16:1.
18. Novick AC. Atherosclerotic renovascular disease. *J Urol* 1981;126:567.
19. Slovut DP, Olin JW. Current concepts: fibromuscular dysplasia. *N Engl J Med* 2004;350:1862.
20. Krijnen P, Van Jaarsveld BC, Steyerberg EW, et al. A clinical prediction rule for renal artery stenosis. *Ann Intern Med* 1998;129:705.
21. Nahas WC, Lucon AM, Mazzucchi E, et al. Kidney transplantation: the use of living donors with renal artery lesions. *J Urol* 1998;160:1244.
22. Indudhara R, Kenney, Bueschen AJ, et al. Live donor nephrectomy in patients with fibromuscular dysplasia of the renal arteries. *J Urol* 1999;162:678.
23. Parasuraman R, Attallah N, Venkat KK, et al. Rapid progression of native renal artery fibromuscular dysplasia following kidney donation. *Am J Transplant* 2004;4:1910.
24. Neymark E, LaBerge JM, Hirose R, et al. Arteriographic detection of renovascular disease in potential renal donors: incidence and effect on donor surgery. *Radiology* 2000;214:755.
25. Andreoni KA, Weeks SM, Gerber DA, et al. Incidence of donor renal fibromuscular dysplasia: does it justify routine angiography? *Transplantation* 2002;73:1112.
26. Kolettis PN, Bugg CE, Lockhart ME, et al. Outcomes for live donor renal transplantation using kidneys with medial fibroplasia. *Urology* 2004;63:656.
27. Seibert JJ, Northington FJ, Miers JF, et al. Aortic thrombosis after umbilical artery catheterization in neonates: prevalence of complications on long-term follow-up. *AJR Am J Roentgenol* 1991;156:567.
28. Olin JW, Melia M, Young JR, et al. Prevalence of atherosclerotic renal artery stenosis in patients with atherosclerosis elsewhere. *Am J Med* 1990;88:46N.
29. Zierler RE, Bergelin RO, Polissar NL, et al. Carotid and lower extremity arterial disease in patients with renal artery atherosclerosis. *Arch Intern Med* 1998;158:761.
30. Harding MB, Smith LR, Himmelstein SI, et al. Renal artery stenosis: prevalence and associated risk factors in patients undergoing routine cardiac catheterization. *J Am Soc Nephrol* 1992;2:1608.
31. Vetrovec GW, Landwehr DM, Edwards VL. Incidence of renal artery stenosis in hypertensive patients undergoing coronary angiography. *J Intervent Cardiol* 1989;2:69.
32. Nicholson JP, Teichman SL, Alderman MH, et al. Cigarette smoking and renovascular hypertension. *Lancet* 1983;2:765.
33. Buller CE, Nogareda JG, Ramanathan K, et al. The profile of cardiac patients with renal artery stenosis. *J Am Coll Cardiol* 2004;43:1606.
34. Choudhri AH, Cleland JG, Rowlands PC, et al. Unsuspected renal artery stenosis in peripheral vascular disease. *BMJ* 1990;301:1197.
35. Burket MW, Cooper CJ, Kennedy DJ, et al. Renal artery angioplasty and stent placement: predictors of a favorable outcome. *Am Heart J* 2000;139:64.
36. Edwards MS, Craven TE, Burke GL, et al. Renovascular disease and the risk of adverse coronary events in the elderly: a prospective, population-based study. *Arch Intern Med* 2005;165:207.
37. Conlon PJ, Athirakul K, Kovalik E, et al. Survival in renal vascular disease. *J Am Soc Nephrol* 1998;9:252.
38. Dorros G, Jaff M, Mathiak L, et al. Four-year follow-up of Palmaz-Schatz stent revascularization as treatment for atherosclerotic renal artery stenosis. *Circulation* 1998;98:642.
39. Sos TA, Pickering TG, Sniderman K, et al. Percutaneous transluminal renal angioplasty in renovascular hypertension due to atheroma or fibromuscular dysplasia. *N Engl J Med* 1983;309:274.
40. Canzanello VJ, Millan VG, Spiegel JE, et al. Percutaneous transluminal renal angioplasty in management of atherosclerotic renovascular hypertension: results in 100 patients. *Hypertension* 1989;13:163.
41. Stanley JC. The evolution of surgery for renovascular occlusive disease. *Cardiovasc Surg* 1994;2:195.
42. Meaney TF, Dustan HP, McCormack LJ. Natural history of renal arterial disease. *Radiology* 1986;91:881.
43. Wollenweber J, Sheps SG, Davis GD. Clinical course of atherosclerotic renovascular disease. *Am J Cardiol* 1968;21:60.
44. Schreiber MJ, Pohl MA, Novick AC. The natural history of atherosclerotic and fibrous renal artery disease. *Urol Clin North Am* 1984;11:383.
45. Tollefson DF, Ernst CB. Natural history of atherosclerotic renal artery stenosis associated with aortic disease. *J Vasc Surg* 1991;14:327.
46. Van Jaarsveld BC, Krijnen P, Pieterman H, et al. The effect of balloon angioplasty on hypertension in atherosclerotic renal-artery stenosis. Dutch Renal Artery Stenosis Intervention Cooperative Study Group. *N Engl J Med* 2000;342:1007.
47. Kohler TR, Zierler RE, Martin RL, et al. Noninvasive diagnosis of renal artery stenosis by ultrasonic duplex scanning. *J Vasc Surg* 1986;4:450.
48. Taylor DC, Kettler MD, Moneta GL, et al. Duplex ultrasound scanning in the diagnosis of renal artery stenosis: a prospective evaluation. *J Vasc Surg* 1988;7:363.
49. Strandness DG, Jr. The renal arteries. In: Strandness DG Jr, ed. *Duplex scanning and vascular disorders.* New York: Raven Press, 1983:197.
50. Hoffmann U, Edwards JM, Carter S, et al. Role of duplex scanning for the detection of atherosclerotic renal artery disease. *Kidney Int* 1991;39:1232.
51. Olin JW, Piedmonte MR, Young JR, et al. The utility of duplex ultrasound scanning of the renal arteries for diagnosing significant renal artery stenosis. *Ann Intern Med* 1995;122:833.
52. Spies KP, Fobbe F, El-Bedewi M, et al. Color-coded duplex sonography for noninvasive diagnosis and grading of renal artery stenosis. *Am J Hypertens* 1995;8(12):1222.
53. Zierler RE, Bergelin RO, Isaacson JA, et al. Natural history of atherosclerotic renal artery stenosis: a prospective study with duplex ultrasonography. *J Vasc Surg* 1994;19:250, discussion 257.

54. Caps MT, Perissinotto C, Zierler RE, et al. Prospective study of atherosclerotic disease progression in the renal artery. *Circulation* 1998;98:2866.

55. Caps MT, Zierler RE, Polissar NL, et al. Risk of atrophy in kidneys with atherosclerotic renal artery stenosis. *Kidney Int* 1998;53:735.

56. Fine MJ, Kapoor W, Falanga V. Cholesterol crystal embolization: a review of 221 cases in the English literature. *Angiology* 1987;38:769.

57. Thurlbeck WM, Castleman B. Atheromatous emboli to the kidneys after aortic surgery. *N Engl J Med* 1957;257:442.

58. Kassirer JP. Atheroembolic renal disease. *N Engl J Med* 1969;280:812.

59. Harrington JT, Sommers SC, Kassirer JP. Atheromatous emboli with progressive renal failure. Renal arteriography as the probable inciting factor. *Ann Intern Med* 1968;68:152.

60. Anonymous. Case records of the Massachusetts General Hospital. Weekly clinicopathological exercises. Case 34-1991. A 51-year-old man with severe hypertension and rapidly progressive renal failure. *N Engl J Med* 1991; 325:563.

61. Handler FP. Clinical and pathologic significance of atheromatous embolization with emphasis on an etiology of renal hypertension. *Am J Med* 1956;20:366.

62. Smith MC, Ghose MK, Henry AR. The clinical spectrum of renal cholesterol embolization. *Am J Med* 1981;71:174.

63. Dalakos TG, Streeten DH, Jones D, et al. "Malignant" hypertension resulting from atheromatous embolization predominantly of one kidney. *Am J Med* 1974;57:135.

64. Hunt JC, Strong CG. Renovascular hypertension. Mechanisms, natural history and treatment. *Am J Cardiol* 1973;32:562.

65. Sang CN, Whelton PK, Hamper UM, et al. Etiologic factors in renovascular fibromuscular dysplasia. A casecontrol study. *Hypertension* 1989;14:472.

66. Tsukamoto Y, Komuro Y, Akutsu F, et al. Orthostatic hypertension due to coexistence of renal fibromuscular dysplasia and nephroptosis. *Jpn Circ J* 1988;52:1408.

67. de Zeeuw D, Donker AJ, Burema J, et al. Nephroptosis and hypertension. *Lancet* 1977;1:213.

68. Sottiurai V, Fry WJ, Stanley JC. Ultrastructural characteristics of experimental arterial medial fibroplasia induced by vasa vasorum occlusion. *J Surg Res* 1978;24:167.

69. Stanley JC, Fry WJ. Pediatric renal artery occlusive disease and renovascular hypertension. Etiology, diagnosis, and operative treatment. *Arch Surg* 1981;116:669.

70. Goncharenko V, Gerlock AJ Jr, Shaff MI, et al. Progression of renal artery fibromuscular dysplasia in 42 patients as seen on angiography. *Radiology* 1981;139:45.

71. Stewart BH, Dustan HP, Kiser WS, et al. Correlation of angiography and natural history in evaluation of patients with renovascular hypertension. *J Urol* 1970;104:231.

72. Novicki DE, Turlington JT, Ball TP Jr. The evaluation and management of spontaneous perirenal hemorrhage. *J Urol* 1980;123:764.

73. Stanley JC, Rhodes EL, Gewertz BL, et al. Renal artery aneurysms. Significance of macroaneurysms exclusive of dissections and fibrodysplastic mural dilations. *Arch Surg* 1975;110:1327.

74. Hageman JH, Smith RF, Szilagyi E, et al. Aneurysms of the renal artery: problems of prognosis and surgical management. *Surgery* 1978;84:563.

75. Poutasse EF. Renal artery aneurysms. *J Urol* 1975;113:443.

76. Hidai H, Kinoshita Y, Murayama T, et al. Rupture of renal artery aneurysm. *Eur Urol* 1985;11:249.

77. Love WK, Robinette MA, Vernon CP. Renal artery aneurysm rupture in pregnancy. *J Urol* 1981;126:809.

78. Cerny JC, Chang CY, Fry WJ. Renal artery aneurysms. *Arch Surg* 1968;96: 653.

79. Koide K. Takayasu arteritis in Japan. *Heart Vessels* 1992;7:48.

80. Chugh KS, Sakhuja V. Aortoarteritis, a common cause of renovascular hypertension in Asia. *Intern J Artif Organs* 1988;11:319.

81. Chugh KS, Jain S, Sakhuja V, et al. Renovascular hypertension due to Takayasu's arteritis among Indian patients. *Q J Med* 1992;85:833.

82. Chugh KS, Sakhuja V. Takayasu's arteritis as a cause of renovascular hypertension in Asian countries (editorial). *Am J Nephrol* 1992;12:1.

83. Baggenstoss AH, Barker NW. Unilateral atrophy associated with hypertension. *Arch Pathol* 1941;32:966.

84. Sesenbach W. Effects of unilateral nephrectomy in the treatment of hypertension: an evaluation. *Arch Intern Med* 1944;73:123.

85. Smith HW. Hypertension and urologic diseases. *Am J Med* 1948;4:721.

86. Sabin HS. Hypertension in unilateral kidney disease. *J Urol* 1948;59:8.

87. Barker NW. Symposium on diseases of the kidney; hypertension and unilateral renal disease. *Med Clin North Am* 1951;35:1041.

88. Gifford RW Jr, McCormack LJ, Poutasse EF. The atrophic kidney: its role in hypertension. *Mayo Clin Proc* 1965;40:834.

89. Lawrie GM, Morris GC Jr, DeBakey ME. Long-term results of treatment of the totally occluded renal artery in forty patients with renovascular hypertension. *Surgery* 1980;88:753.

90. Sobel JD, Hampel N, Kursbaum A, et al. Hypertension due to Ask-Upmark kidney. *Br J Urol* 1977;49:477.

91. Arant BS, Jr, Sotelo-Avila C, Bernstein J. Segmental "hypoplasia" of the kidney (Ask-Upmark). *J Pediatr* 1979;95:931.

92. Anonymous. Case records of the Massachusetts General Hospital. Weekly clinicopathological exercises. Case 40-1973. *N Engl J Med* 1973;289:736.

93. Zezulka AV, Arkell DG, Beevers DG. The association of hypertension, the Ask-Upmark kidney and other congenital abnormalities. *J Urol* 1986;135: 1000.

94. Brunner HR, Gavras H, Laragh JH. Specific inhibition of the renin-angiotensin system: a key to understanding blood pressure regulation. *Prog Cardiovasc Dis* 1974;17:87.

95. Hollenberg NK, Williams GH, Burger B, et al. Blockade and stimulation of renal, adrenal, and vascular angiotensin II receptors with 1-Sar, 8-Ala angiotensin II in normal man. *J Clin Invest* 1976;57:39.

96. Miller ED Jr, Samuels AI, Haber E, et al. Inhibition of angiotensin conversion and prevention of renal hypertension. *Am J Physiol* 1975;228:448.

97. Textor SC, Brunner H, Gavras H. Evidence for bradykinin potentiation by angiotensin congeners in conscious rats. *Am J Physiol* 1981;240:H255.

98. Husain A. The chymase-angiotensin system in humans [editorial]. *J Hypertens* 1993;11:1155.

99. Urata H, Boehm KD, Philip A, et al. Cellular localization and regional distribution of an angiotensin II-forming chymase in the heart. *J Clin Invest* 1993;91:1269.

100. Hoit BD, Shao Y, Kinoshita A, et al. Effects of angiotensin II generated by an angiotensin converting enzyme-independent pathway on left ventricular performance in the conscious baboon. *J Clin Invest* 1995;95:1519.

101. Welch WJ. The pathophysiology of renin release in renovascular hypertension. *Semin Nephrol* 2000;20:394.

102. Page IH, Helmer OM. A crystalline pressor substance, angiotensin, resulting from reaction of renin and renin activator. *Proc Soc Clin Invest* 1939;12:17.

103. Pickering GW. The role of the kidney in acute and chronic hypertension following renal artery constriction in the rabbit. *Clin Sci* 1945;5:229.

104. Braun-Menendez E, Fasciolo JC, Leloir LF, et al. *Renal hypertension*. Springfield, IL: Charles C Thomas, 1946.

105. May AG, DeWeese JA, Rob CG. Hemodynamic effects of arterial stenosis. *Surgery* 1963;53:513.

106. May AG, Van de Berg L, DeWeese JA, et al. Critical arterial stenosis. *Surgery* 1963;54:250.

107. Velazquez H, Naray-Fejes-Toth A, Silva T, et al. Rabbit distal convoluted tubule coexpresses NaCl cotransporter and 11 beta-hydroxysteroid dehydrogenase II mRNA. *Kidney Int* 1998;54:464.

108. Finke R, Gross R, Hackenthal E, et al. Threshold pressure for the pressure-dependent renin release in the autoregulating kidney of conscious dogs. *Pflugers Arch* 1983;399:102.

109. Textor SC, Smith-Powell L. Pathophysiology of renal failure in ischemic renal disease. In: Novick AC, Scoble J, Hamilton G, eds. *Renovascular Disease*. Philadelphia: Saunders, 1996:289.

110. Simon G. What is critical renal artery stenosis? Implications for treatment *Am J Hypertens* 2000;13:1189.

111. Textor SC. Pathophysiology of renal failure in renovascular disease. *Am J Kidney Dis* 1994;24:642.

112. Gavras H, Brunner HR, Thurston H, et al. Reciprocation of renin dependency with sodium volume dependency in renal hypertension. *Science* 1975;188:1316.

113. Brunner HR, Kirshman JD, Sealey JE, et al. Hypertension of renal origin: evidence for two different mechanisms. *Science* 1971;174:1344.

114. Swales JD, Thurston H, Queiroz FP, et al. Dual mechanism for experimental hypertension. *Lancet* 1971;2:1181.

115. Tobian L, Coffee K, McCrea P. Contrasting exchangeable sodium in rats with different types of Goldblatt hypertension. *Am J Physiol* 1969;217:458.

116. Brown JJ, Davies DL, Morton JJ, et al. Mechanism of renal hypertension. *Lancet* 1976;1:1219.

117. Frederickson ED, Wilcox CS, Bucci M, et al. A prospective evaluation of a simplified captopril test for the detection of renovascular hypertension. *Arch Intern Med* 1990;150:569.

118. Wilcox CS. Functional testing: renin studies. *Semin Nephrol* 2000;20:432.

119. Dzau VJ, Siwek LG, Rosen S, et al. Sequential renal hemodynamics in experimental benign and malignant hypertension. *Hypertension* 1981;3:I63.

120. Granger JP, Schnackenberg CG. Renal mechanisms of angiotensin II-induced hypertension. *Semin Nephrol* 2000;20:417.

121. Vaughan ED, Buhler FR, Laragh JH, et al. Hypertension and unilateral parenchymal renal disease. Evidence for abnormal vasoconstriction-volume interaction. *JAMA* 1975;233:1177.

122. Vaughan ED Jr, Buhler FR, Laragh JH, et al. Renovascular hypertension: renin measurements to indicate hypersecretion and contralateral suppression, estimate renal plasma flow, and score for surgical curability. *Am J Med* 1973;55:402.

123. Regolio D, Brunner HK, Peters G, et al. Changes in renin content in kidneys of renal hypertensive rats. *Proc Soc Exp Biol Med* 1962;109:142.

124. Heptinstall RH. The role of the juxtaglomerular apparatus in experimental hypertension in the rat. *Lab Invest* 1965;14:2150.

125. Thompson JM, Dickinson CJ. The relation between the excretion of sodium and water and the perfusion pressure in the isolated, blood-perfused, rabbit kidney, with special reference to changes occurring in clip-hypertension. *Clin Sci Mol Med* 1976;50:223.

126. Stamey TA, Nudelman JJ, Good PH, et al. Functional characteristics of renovascular hypertension. *Medicine* 1961;40:34794.

127. Textor SC, Novick A, Mujais SK, et al. Responses of the stenosed and contralateral kidneys to (Sar1, Thr8) AII in human renovascular hypertension. *Hypertension* 1983;5:796.

128. Textor SC. Pathophysiology of renovascular hypertension. *Urol Clin North Am* 1984;11:373.

129. Atkinson AB, Brown JJ, Cumming AM, et al. Captopril in the management of hypertension with renal artery stenosis: its long-term effect as a predictor of surgical outcome. *Am J Cardiol* 1982;49:1460.

130. Genest J, Cartier P, Roy P, et al. Renovascular hypertension. In: Genest J, Kuchel O, Hamet P, et al., eds. *Hypertension: pathophysiology and treatment.* New York: McGraw-Hill, 1983:1007.

131. Hughes JS, Dove HG, Gifford RW Jr, et al. Duration of blood pressure elevation in accurately predicting surgical cure of renovascular hypertension. *Am Heart J* 1981;101:408.

132. Marks LS, Maxwell MH, Varady PD, et al. Renovascular hypertension: does the renal vein renin ratio predict operative results? *J Urol* 1976;115:365.

133. Simon N, Franklin SS, Bleifer KH, et al. Clinical characteristics of renovascular hypertension. *JAMA* 1972;220:1209.

134. Brown JJ, Davies DL, Lever AF, et al. Plasma renin concentration in human hypertension. II. Renin in relation to aetiology. *Br Med J* 1965;2:144.

135. Akahoshi M, Carretero OA. Body fluid volume and angiotensin II in maintenance of one- kidney, one clip hypertension. *Hypertension* 1989;14:269.

136. Gavras H, Brunner HB, Vaughan ED, et al. Angiotensin-sodium interaction in blood pressure maintenance of renal hypertensive and normotensive rats. *Science* 1973;180:1369.

137. Nabel EG, Gibbons GH, Dzau VJ. Pathophysiology of experimental renovascular hypertension. *Am J Kidney Dis* 1985;5:A111.

138. DeForrest JM, Knappenberger RC, Antonaccio MJ, et al. Angiotensin II is a necessary component for the development of hypertension in the two kidney, one clip rat. *Am J Cardiol* 1982;49:1515.

139. Cervenka L, Horacek V, Vaneckova I, et al. Essential role of AT1A receptor in the development of 2K1C hypertension. *Hypertension* 2002;40:735.

140. Brown TC, Davis JO, Olichney MJ, et al. Relation of plasma renin to sodium balance and arterial pressure in experimental renal hypertension. *Circ Res* 1966;18:475.

141. Bianchi G, Tenconi LT, Lucca R. Effect in the conscious dog of constriction of the renal artery to a sole remaining kidney on haemodynamics, sodium balance, body fluid volumes, plasma renin concentration and pressor responsiveness to angiotensin. *Clin Sci* 1970;38:741.

142. Floyer MA. Effect of nephrectomy and adrenalectomy upon blood pressure in hypertensive and normotensive rats. *Clin Sci* 1951;10:405.

143. Sweitzer G, Gertz KH. Changes of hemodynamics and glomerular ultrafiltration in renal hypertension of rats. *Kidney Int* 1979;15:134.

144. Grim CE, Yune HY, Weinberger MH, et al. Balloon dilatation for renal artery stenosis causing hypertension: criteria, concerns, and cautions. *Ann Intern Med* 1980;92:117.

145. Grim CE, Luft FC, Yune HY, et al. Percutaneous transluminal dilatation in the treatment of renal vascular hypertension. *Ann Intern Med* 1981;95:439.

146. Grim CE, Yune HY, Donahue JP, et al. Treatment of renovascular hypertension: A comparison of patients treated by surgery or by percutaneous transluminal angioplasty. In: Schilfgaarde RV, et al., eds. *Clinical aspects of renovascular hypertension.* Boston: Martinus Nijhoff, 1983:238.

147. Madias NE. Renovascular hypertension. *American Kidney Foundation, Nephrology Letter* 1986;3(4):27.

148. Smith MC, Dunn MJ. Renovascular and renal parenchymal hypertension. In: Brenner BM, Rector FC, Jr., eds. *The Kidney.* Philadelphia: Saunders, 1986:1221.

149. Lerman LO, Nath KA, Rodriguez-Porcel M, et al. Increased oxidative stress in experimental renovascular hypertension. *Hypertension* 2001;37:541.

150. Welch WJ, Mendonca M, Aslam S, et al. Roles of oxidative stress and AT1 receptors in renal hemodynamics and oxygenation in the postclipped 2K,1C kidney. *Hypertension* 2003;41:692.

151. Sigmon DH, Beierwaltes WH. Renal nitric oxide and angiotensin II interaction in renovascular hypertension. *Hypertension* 1993;22:237.

152. Ortiz MC, Sanabria E, Manriquez MC, et al. Role of endothelin and isoprostanes in slow pressor responses to angiotensin II. *Hypertension* 2001;37:505.

153. Chade AR, Best PJ, Rodriguez-Porcel M, et al. Endothelin-1 receptor blockade prevents renal injury in experimental hypercholesterolemia. *Kidney Int* 2003;64:962.

154. Wilcox CS, Welch WJ. Angiotensin II and thromboxane in the regulation of blood pressure and renal function. *Kidney Int* 1990;30:S81.

155. Wilcox CS, Cardozo J, Welch WJ. AT1 and TxA2/PGH2 receptors maintain hypertension throughout 2K,1C Goldblatt hypertension in the rat. *Am J Physiol* 1996;271:R891.

156. Reckelhoff JF, Romero JC. Role of oxidative stress in angiotensin-induced hypertension. *Am J Physiol Regul Integr Comp Physiol* 2003;284:R893.

157. Okamura T, Miyazaki M, Inagami T, et al. Vascular renin-angiotensin system in two-kidney, one clip hypertension. *Hypertension* 1986;8:560.

158. Ichikawa I, Ferrone RA, Duchin KL, et al. Relative contribution of vasopressin and angiotensin II to the altered renal microcirculatory dynamics in two-kidney Goldblatt hypertension. *Circ Res* 1983;53:592.

159. Taquini CM, Gallo A, Basso N, et al. Influence of sodium on experimental renovascular hypertension in rats. *Clin Sci* 1980;59(Suppl 6):149s.

160. Dargie HJ, Franklin SS, Reid JL. Plasma noradrenaline concentrations in experimental renovascular hypertension in the rat. *Clin Sci Mol Med* 1977;52:477.

161. Dargie HJ, Franklin SS, Reid JL. Proceedings: the sympathetic nervous system and renovascular hypertension in the rat. *Br J Pharmacol* 1976;56:365P.

162. Katholi RE, Winternitz SR, Oparil S. Decrease in peripheral sympathetic nervous system activity following renal denervation or unclipping in the one-kidney one-clip Goldblatt hypertensive rat. *J Clin Invest* 1982;69:55.

163. Katholi RE, Whitlow PL, Winternitz SR, et al. Importance of the renal nerves in established two-kidney, one clip Goldblatt hypertension. *Hypertension* 1982;4:166.

164. Oparil S. The sympathetic nervous system in clinical and experimental hypertension. *Kidney Int* 1986;30:437.

165. Johansson M, Elam M, Rundqvist B, et al. Increased sympathetic nerve activity in renovascular hypertension. *Circulation* 1999;99:2537.

166. Barri YM, Davidson RA, Senler S, et al. Prediction of cure of hypertension in atherosclerotic renal artery stenosis. *South Med J* 1996;89:679.

167. Davidson RA, Barri Y, Wilcox CS. Predictors of cure of hypertension in fibromuscular renovascular disease. *Am J Kidney Dis* 1996;28:334.

168. Vertes V, Grauel JA, Galvin J. Observations on renal hypertension: a practical test for the diagnosis of functional unilateral renal ischemia. *J Urol* 1963;90:591.

169. Vertes V, Grauel JA, Goldblatt H. Renal arteriography, separate renal-function studies, and renal biopsy in human hypertension. *N Engl J Med* 1964;270:656.

170. Vertes V, Grauel JA, Goldblatt H. Studies of patients with renal hypertension undergoing vascular surgery. *N Engl J Med* 1965;272:186.

171. Vertes V, Grauel JA. Renal hypertension: role of renal biopsy. *Circulation* 1963;28:536.

172. Baker GP Jr, Page LP, Leadbetter GW Jr. Hypertension and renovascular disease: follow-up study of 23 patients with analysis of factors influencing results of surgery. *N Engl J Med* 1962;267:1325.

173. Bulbul MA, Farrow GA. Renal artery aneurysms. *Urology* 1992;40:124.

174. Cummings KB, Lecky JW, Kaufman JJ. Renal artery aneurysms and hypertension. *J Urol* 1973;109:144.

175. McAlhany JC Jr, Black HC Jr, Hanback LD Jr, et al. Renal arteriovenous fistula as a cause of hypertension. *Am J Surg* 1971;122:117.

176. Takaha M, Matsumoto A, Ochi K, et al. Intrarenal arteriovenous malformation. *J Urol* 1980;124:315.

177. Spark RF, Berg S. Renal trauma and hypertension: the role of renin. *Arch Intern Med* 1976;136:1097.

178. Massumi RA, Andrade A, Kramer N. Arterial hypertension in traumatic subcapsular perirenal hematoma (Page kidney). Evidence for renal ischemia. *Am J Med* 1969;46:635.

179. Grant RP Jr, Gifford RW Jr, Pudvan WR, et al. Renal trauma and hypertension. *Am J Cardiol* 1971;27:173.

180. Sufrin G. The Page kidney: a correctable form of arterial hypertension. *J Urol* 1975;113:450.

181. Freed TA, Tavel FR. Diagnosis and surgical treatment of page kidney: selected aspects. *Urol* 1976;7:330.

182. Engel WJ, Page IH. Hypertension due to renal compression resulting from subcapsular hematoma. *J Urol* 1955;73:735.

183. Gavras H. Angiotensin-converting enzyme inhibitors. In: Goodfriends TL, Sowers J, Messerly FH, et al., eds. *Hypertension Primer (AHA).* Dallas, TX: American Heart Association, 1993:309.

184. Carvajal JA, Anderson WR, Weiss L, et al. Atheroembolism. An etiologic factor in renal insufficiency, gastrointestinal hemorrhages, and peripheral vascular diseases. *Arch Intern Med* 1967;119:593.

185. Eipper DF, Gifford RW Jr, Stewart B, et al. Abdominal bruits in renovascular hypertension Prevalence of atherosclerotic renal artery stenosis in patients with atherosclerosis elsewhere. *Am J Cardiol* 1990;88:46N.

186. Nally JV Jr, Olin JW, Lammert GK. Advances in noninvasive screening for renovascular disease. *Cleve Clin J Med* 1994;61:328.

187. Working Group on Renovascular Hypertension. Detection, evaluation, and treatment of renovascular hypertension. Final report. *Arch Intern Med* 1987;147:820.

188. Swales JD, Thurston H, Queiroz FP, et al. Sodium balance during the development of experimental hypertension. *J Lab Clin Med* 1972;80:539.

189. Gifford RW Jr. Evaluation of the hypertensive patient with emphasis on curable causes. *Milbank Mem Fund Q* 1969;47:170.

190. Ferguson RK. Cost and yield of the hypertensive evaluation. Experience of a community-based referral clinic. *Ann Intern Med* 1975;82:761.

191. Danielson M, Dammstrom B. The prevalence of secondary and curable hypertension. *Acta Med Scand* 1981;209:451.

192. Bech K, Hilden T. The frequency of secondary hypertension. *Acta Med Scand* 1975;197:65.

193. Lewin A, Blaufox MD, Castle H, et al. Apparent prevalence of curable hypertension in the Hypertension Detection and Follow-up Program. *Ann Intern Med* 1985;145:424.

194. Smithwick RH, Newton RC, Crocker DH, et al. Surgical management of renal hypertension. Combined experiences at the Massachusetts Memorial and the Peter Bent Brigham Hospitals. *Am J Surg* 1964;107:104.

195. Berglund G, Andersson O, Wilhelmsen L. Prevalence of primary and secondary hypertension: studies in a random population sample. *Br Med J* 1976;2:554.

196. Kennedy AC, Luke RG, Briggs JD, et al. Detection of renovascular hypertension. *Lancet* 1965;2:963.

197. Tucker RM, Labarthe DR. Frequency of surgical treatment for hypertension in adults at the Mayo Clinic from 1973 through 1975. *Mayo Clin Proc* 1977;52:549.

198. Ward R. Familial aggregation and genetic epidemiology of blood pressure. In: Laragh JH, Brenner HR, eds. *Hypertension: pathophysiology, diagnosis and management.* New York: Raven Press, 1990:81.

199. Davis BA, Crook JE, Vestal RE, et al. Prevalence of renovascular hypertension in patients with grade III or IV hypertensive retinopathy. *N Engl J Med* 1979;301:1273.

200. Canzanello VJ, Textor SC. Noninvasive diagnosis of renovascular disease. *Mayo Clin Proc* 1994;69:1172.

201. Derkx FH, Schalekamp MA. Renal artery stenosis and hypertension. *Lancet* 1994;344:237.

202. Svetkey LP, Helms MJ, Dunnick NR, et al. Clinical characteristics useful in screening for renovascular disease. *South Med J* 1990;83:743.

203. Keith TA. Renovascular hypertension in black patients. *Hypertension* 1982;4:438.

204. Anderson GH Jr, Blakeman N, Streeten DH. Prediction of renovascular hypertension. Comparison of clinical diagnostic indices. *Am J Hypertens* 1988;1:301.

205. Grim CE, Luft FC, Weinberger MH, et al. Sensitivity and specificity of screening tests for renal vascular hypertension. *Ann Intern Med* 1979;91:617.

206. Svetkey LP, Kadir S, Dunnick NR, et al. Similar prevalence of renovascular hypertension in selected blacks and whites. *Hypertension* 1991;17:678.

207. Vetrovec GW, Colley MJ, Landwehr DM, et al. High prevalence of renal artery stenosis in hypertensive patients with coronary artery disease. *J Am Coll Cardiol* 1984;3:518.

208. Hansen KJ, Edwards MS, Craven TE, et al. Prevalence of renovascular disease in the elderly: a population-based study. *J Vasc Surg* 2002;36:443.

209. Maxwell MH. Cooperative study of renovascular hypertension: current status. *Kidney Int* 1975;8(Suppl):S153.

210. Assendelft PM, Kooiker CJ, Mees EJ, et al. Renovascular hypertension in three children from one family. *J Clin Pathol* 1973;26:359.

211. Major P, Genest J, Cartier P, et al. Hereditary fibromuscular dysplasia with renovascular hypertension (letter). *Ann Intern Med* 1977;86:583.

212. Kaufman JJ. Renovascular hypertension: the UCLA experience. *J Urol* 1979;121:139–144.

213. Gifford RW Jr. Evaluation for renovascular hypertension and selection of patients for surgical treatment. In: Novick AC, Straffon RA, eds. *Vascular problems in urologic surgery.* Philadelphia: Saunders, 1982:139.

214. Ram CV. Diagnosis and management of hypertensive crises. In: Rippe JM, Irwin RS, Alpert JS, et al., eds. *Intensive care medicine.* Boston: Little Brown, 1991:228.

215. Diamond JR. Flash pulmonary edema and the diagnostic suspicion of occult renal artery stenosis. *Am J Kidney Dis* 1993;21:328.

216. Messina LM, Zelenock GB, Yao KA, et al. Renal revascularization for recurrent pulmonary edema in patients with poorly controlled hypertension and renal insufficiency: a distinct subgroup of patients with arteriosclerotic renal artery occlusive disease. *J Vasc Surg* 1992;15:73.

217. Pickering TG, Herman L, Devereux RB, et al. Recurrent pulmonary oedema in hypertension due to bilateral renal artery stenosis: treatment by angioplasty or surgical revascularisation. *Lancet* 1988;2:551.

218. Bloch MJ, Trost DW, Pickering TG, et al. Prevention of recurrent pulmonary edema in patients with bilateral renovascular disease through renal artery stent placement. *Am J Hypertens* 1999;12:1.

219. Ramirez G, Bugni W, Farber SM, et al. Incidence of renal artery stenosis in a population having cardiac catheterization. *South Med J* 1987;80:734.

220. Elkik F, Corvol P, Idatte JM, et al. Renal segmental infarction: a cause of reversible malignant hypertension. *J Hypertens* 1984;2:149.

221. Stanley JC, Graham LM. Renal artery fibrodysplasia and renovascular hypertension. In: Rutherford RB, ed. *Vascular Surgery.* Philadelphia: Saunders, 1984:1253.

222. Delin A, Fernstrom I, Swedenborg J. Intimal dissection of the renal artery following selective angiography. Report of two cases and review of the literature. *Vasa* 1979;8:78.

223. Toma H. Takayasu arteritis. In: Novick AC, Scoble J, Hamilton G, eds. *Renovascular disease.* London: Saunders, 1996:47.

224. Textor SC, Novick AC, Tarazi RC, et al. Critical perfusion pressure for renal function in patients with bilateral atherosclerotic renal vascular disease. *Ann Intern Med* 1985;102:308.

225. Hricik DE, Browning PJ, Kopelman R, et al. Captopril-induced functional renal insufficiency in patients with bilateral renal-artery stenoses or renal-artery stenosis in a solitary kidney. *N Engl J Med* 1983;308:373.

226. Wenting GJ, Tan-Tjiong HL, Derkx FH, et al. Splint renal function after captopril in unilateral renal artery stenosis. *Br Med J* 1984;288:886.

227. Wilcox CS. ACE inhibitors in the diagnosis of renovascular hypertension. *Hosp Pract* 1992;27:117.

228. Jackson B, Murphy BF, Johnston CI, et al. Renovascular hypertension: treatment with the oral angiotensin-converting enzyme inhibitor enalapril. *Am J Nephrol* 1986;6:182.

229. Wilcox CS. Use of angiotensin-converting-enzyme inhibitors for diagnosing renovascular hypertension. *Kidney Int* 1993;44:1379.

230. Kalra PA, Mamtora H, Holmes AM, et al. Renovascular disease and renal complications of angiotensin-converting enzyme inhibitor therapy. *Q J Med* 1990;77:1013.

231. van de Ven PJ, Beutler JJ, Kaatee R, et al. Angiotensin converting enzyme inhibitor-induced renal dysfunction in atherosclerotic renovascular disease. *Kidney Int* 1998;53:986.

232. Ram CV. Renovascular hypertension. *Cardiol Clin* 1988;6:483.

233. Ying CY, Tifft CP, Gavras H, et al. Renal revascularization in the azotemic hypertensive patient resistant to therapy. *N Engl J Med* 1984;311:1070.

234. Honari J, Ing TS. Renovascular hypertension. *Med Clin North Am* 1971;55:1429.

235. Hunt JC, Sheps SG, Harrison EG Jr, et al. Renal and renovascular hypertension. A reasoned approach to diagnosis and management. *Arch Intern Med* 1974;133:988.

236. Moser RJ Jr, Caldwell JR. Abdominal murmurs, an aid in the diagnosis of renal artery disease in hypertension. *Ann Intern Med* 1962;56:471.

237. Allen N, Mustian V. Origin and significance of vascular murmurs of the head and neck. *Medicine* 1962;41:227.

238. Gupta TC, Wiggers CJ. Basic hemodynamic changes produced by aortic coarctation of different degrees. *Circulation* 1951;3:17.

239. Rimmer JM, Gennari FJ. Atherosclerotic renovascular disease and progressive renal failure. *Ann Intern Med* 1993;118:712.

240. Kincaid-Smith P, McMichael J, Murphy EA. Clinical course and pathology of hypertension with papilledema (malignant hypertension). *Q J Med* 1958;27:117.

241. Zimbler MS, Pickering TG, Sos TA, et al. Proteinuria in renovascular hypertension and the effects of renal angioplasty. *Am J Cardiol* 1987;59:406.

242. Kumar A, Shapiro AP. Proteinuria and nephrotic syndrome induced by renin in patients with renal artery stenosis. *Arch Intern Med* 1980;140:1631.

243. Montoliu J, Botey A, Torras A, et al. Renin-induced massive proteinuria in man. *Clin Nephrol* 1979;11:267.

244. Chen R, Novick AC, Pohl M. Reversible renin mediated massive proteinuria successfully treated by nephrectomy. *J Urol* 1995;153:133.

245. Tegtmeyer CJ, Matsumoto AH, Angle JF. Percutaneous transluminal angioplasty in fibrous dysplasia in children. In: Novick AC, Scoble J, Hamilton G, eds. *Renovascular Disease.* Philadelphia: Saunders, 1996:363.

246. Bohrer MP, Deen WM, Robertson CR, et al. Mechanism of angiotensin II-induced proteinuria in the rat. *Am J Physiol* 1977;233:F13.

247. Gephardt GN, Tubbs RR, Novick AC, et al. Renal artery stenosis, nephrotic-range proteinuria, and focal and segmental glomerulosclerosis. *Cleve Clin Q* 1984;51:371.

248. Alkhunaizi AM, Chapman A. Renal artery stenosis and unilateral focal and segmental glomerulosclerosis. *Am J Kidney Dis* 1997;29:936.

249. Thadhani R, Pascual M, Nickeleit V, et al. Preliminary description of focal segmental glomerulosclerosis in patients with renovascular disease. *Lancet* 1996;347:231.

250. Novick AC, Pohl MA, Schreiber M, et al. Revascularization for preservation of renal function in patients with atherosclerotic renovascular disease. *J Urol* 1983;129:907.

251. Jacobson HR. Ischemic renal disease: an overlooked clinical entity? *Kidney Int* 1988;34:729.

252. Pohl MA. The ischemic kidney and hypertension. *Am J Kidney Dis* 1993;21(Suppl 2):22.

253. Anderson EA, Sinkey CA, Mark AL. Mental stress increases sympathetic nerve activity during sustained baroreceptor stimulation in humans. *Hypertension* 1991;17:III43.

254. Meyer P, Ecoiffier J, Alexandre JM, et al. Prognostic value of plasma renin activity in renovascular hypertension. *Circulation* 1967;36:570.

255. Gunnells JC Jr, McGuffin WL Jr, Johnsrude I, et al. Peripheral and renal venous plasma renin activity in hypertension. *Ann Intern Med* 1969;71:555.

256. Hussain RA, Gifford RW Jr, Stewart BH, et al. Differential renal venous renin activity in diagnosis of renovascular hypertension. Review of 29 cases. *Am J Cardiol* 1973;32:707.

257. Tucker RM, Sheps SG, Brennan LA. Saralasin infusion in renovascular hypertension: increased response rate in seated patients. *Mayo Clin Proc* 1980;55:99.

258. Weir MR. Calcium entry blockers. In: Izzo JR, Black HR, eds. *Hypertension primer.* Dallas: American Heart Association, 1993:311.

259. Arakawa K, Masaki Z, Osada Y, et al. Divided renal and peripheral venous renin as a means of predicting operative curability of renal hypertension. *Clin Sci Mol Med* 1973;45(Suppl 1):311s.

260. Morlin C, Lorelius LE, Wide L. Spontaneous variations in renal vein renin activity in man. *Clin Chim Acta* 1982;119:31.

261. Davis JO. The control of renin release. *Am J Med* 1973;55:333.

262. Weidmann P, Beretta-Piccoli C, Ziegler WH, et al. Age versus urinary sodium for judging renin, aldosterone, and catecholamine levels: studies in normal subjects and patients with essential hypertension. *Kidney Int* 1978;14:619.

263. Kaplan NM, Kem DC, Holland OB, et al. The intravenous furosemide test: a simple way to evaluate renin responsiveness. *Ann Intern Med* 1976;84:639.

264. Brunner HR, Laragh JH, Baer L, et al. Essential hypertension: renin and aldosterone, heart attack and stroke. *N Engl J Med* 1972;286:441.

265. Streeten DH, Anderson GH Jr, Bredenberg CE, et al. The diagnosis and treatment of renovascular hypertension. *Clin Invest Med* 1978;1:155.

266. Rosenthal JT, Libertino JA, Zinman LN, et al. Predictability of surgical cure of renovascular hypertension. *Ann Surg* 1981;193:448.

267. Laragh JH, Baer L, Brunner HR, et al. Renin, angiotensin and aldosterone system in pathogenesis and management of hypertensive vascular disease. *Am J Med* 1972;52:633.

268. Pickering TG, Sos TA, James GD, et al. Comparison of renal vein renin activity in hypertensive patients with stenosis of one or both renal arteries. *J Hypertens* 1985;3(Suppl 3):S291.

269. Muller FB, Sealey JE, Case DB, et al. The captopril test for identifying renovascular disease in hypertensive patients. *Am J Med* 1986;80:633.

270. Case DB, Laragh JH. Reactive hyperreninemia in renovascular hypertension after angiotensin blockade with saralasin or converting enzyme inhibitor. *Ann Intern Med* 1979;91:153.

271. Derkx FH, Tan-Tjiong HL, Wenting GJ, et al. Captopril test for the diagnosis of renal artery stenosis. In: Glorioso N, Laragh JH, Rapelli A, eds. *Renovascular hypertension.* New York: Raven Press, 1987:295.

272. Gosse P, Dupas JY, Reynaud P, et al. Captopril test in the detection of renovascular hypertension in a population with low prevalence of the disease. A prospective study. *Am J Hypertens* 1989;2:191.

273. Hansen PB, Garsdal P, Fruergaard P. The captopril test for identification of renovascular hypertension: value and immediate adverse effects. *J Intern Med* 1990;228:159.

274. Postma CT, van der Steen PH, Hoefnagels WH, et al. The captopril test in the detection of renovascular disease in hypertensive patients. *Ann Intern Med* 1990;150:625.

275. Svetkey LP, Himmelstein SI, Dunnick NR, et al. Prospective analysis of strategies for diagnosing renovascular hypertension. *Hypertension* 1989;14:247.

276. Thibonnier M, Sassano P, Joseph A, et al. Diagnostic value of a single dose of captopril in renin- and aldosterone-dependent, surgically-curable hypertension. *Cardiovasc Rev Rep* 1982;3:1659.

277. Elliott WJ, Martin WB, Murphy MB. Comparison of two noninvasive screening tests for renovascular hypertension. *Arch Intern Med* 1993;153:755.

278. Klassen PS, Svetkey LP. Diagnosis and management of renovascular hypertension. *Cardiol Rev* 2000;8:17.

279. Wilcox CS, Williams CM, Smith TB, et al. Diagnostic uses of angiotensin-converting enzyme inhibitors in renovascular hypertension. *Am J Hypertens* 1988;1:344S.

280. Wilcox CS, Smith TB, Frederickson ED, et al. The captopril glomerular filtration rate renogram in renovascular hypertension. *Clin Nucl Med* 1989;14:1.

281. Salvetti A, Arzilli F, Nuccorini A, et al. Acute response to captopril as a predictive test for surgery in renovascular hypertension. *Nephron* 1986;44[Suppl 1]:87.

282. Staessen J, Bulpitt C, Fagard R, et al. Long-term converting-enzyme inhibition as a guide to surgical curability of hypertension associated with renovascular disease. *Am J Cardiol* 1983;51:1317.

283. Staessen J, Wilms G, Baert A, et al. Blood pressure during long–term converting–enzyme inhibition predicts the curability of renovascular hypertension by angioplasty. *Am J Hypertens* 1988;1:208.

284. McAfee JG, Thomas FD, Grossman Z, et al. Diagnosis of angiotensinogenic hypertension: the complementary roles of renal scintigraphy and the saralasin infusion test. *J Nucl Med* 1977;18:669.

285. Case DB, Wallace JM, Keim HJ, et al. Usefulness and limitations of saralasin, a partial competitive agonist of angioten II, for evaluating the renin and sodium factors in hypertensive patients. *Am J Med* 1976;60:825.

286. Horne ML, Conklin VM, Keenan RE, et al. Angiotensin II profiling with saralasin: summary of Eaton collaborative study. *Kidney Int* 1979;(Suppl):S115.

287. Hollenberg NK, Williams GH, Adams DF, et al. Response to saralasin and angiotensin's role in essential and renal hypertension. *Medicine* 1979;58:115.

288. Abramowicz M. Saralasin for diagnosis of renovascular hypertension. *Med Lett* 1982;24:3.

289. Sealey JE, Buhler FR, Laragh JH, et al. The physiology of renin secretion in essential hypertension. Estimation of renin secretion rate and renal plasma flow from peripheral and renal vein renin levels. *Am J Med* 1973;55:391.

290. Woods JW, Michelakis AM. Renal vein renin in renovascular hypertension. *Arch Intern Med* 1968;122:392.

291. Stockigt JR, Collins RD, Noakes CA, et al. Renal-vein renin in various forms of renal hypertension. *Lancet* 1972;1:1194.

292. Vaughan ED Jr, Laragh JH. New concepts of the renin system and of vasoconstriction–volume mechanisms. Diagnosis and treatment of renovascular and renal hypertensions. *Urol Clin North Am* 1975;2:237.

293. Vaughan ED Jr. Renovascular hypertension. *Kidney Int* 1985;27:811.

294. Helmer OM, Judson WE. The presence of vasoconstrictor and vasopressor activity in renal vein plasma of patients with arterial hypertension. In: Skelton RF, ed. *Hypertension: Proceedings of the Council for High Blood Pressure Research.* New York: American Heart Association, 1960:38.

295. Rudnick MR, Maxwell MH. Diagnosis of renovascular hypertension: limitations of renin assays. In: Narins R, ed. *Controversies in nephrology and hypertension.* New York: Churchill Livingstone, 1984:123.

296. Pickering TG, Sos TA, Vaughan ED Jr, et al. Predictive value and changes of renin secretion in hypertensive patients with unilateral renovascular disease undergoing successful renal angioplasty. *Am J Med* 1984;76:398.

297. Pawsey CG, Vandongen R, Gordon RD. Renal venous renin ratio in the diagnosis of renovascular hypertension: measurement during active secretion of renin. *Med J Aust* 1971;1:121.

298. Maxwell MH, Marks LS, Lupu AN, et al. Predictive value of renin determinations in renal artery stenosis. *JAMA* 1977;238:2617.

299. Shambelan S, Glickman M, Stockigt JR. Selective renal-vein renin sampling in hypertensive patients with segmental renal lesions. *N Engl J Med* 1974;290:1153.

300. Strong CG, Hunt JC, Sheps SG, et al. Renal venous renin activity. Enhancement of sensitivity of lateralization by sodium depletion. *Am J Cardiol* 1971;27:602.

301. Juncos LI, Strong CG, Hunt JC. Prediction of results of surgery for renal and renovascular hypertension. *Arch Intern Med* 1974;134:655.

302. Melman A, Donohue JP, Weinberger MH, et al. Improved diagnostic accuracy of renal venous renin ratios with stimulation of renin release. *J Urol* 1977;117:145.

303. Aurell M, Delin K, Granerus G. Measures to increase the reliability in the diagnostics of renin dependent hypertension. *Acta Med Scand* 1981;646:58.

304. Michelakis AM, Simmons J. Effect of posture on renal vein renin activity in hypertension; its implications in the management of patients with renovascular hypertension. *JAMA* 1969;208:659.

305. Lyons DF, Streck WF, Kem DC, et al. Captopril stimulation of differential renins in renovascular hypertension. *Hypertension* 1983;5:615.

306. Thibonnier M, Joseph A, Sassano P, et al. Improved diagnosis of unilateral renal artery lesions after captopril administration. *JAMA* 1984;251:56.

307. Re R, Novelline R, Escourrou MT, et al. Inhibition of angiotensin-converting enzyme for diagnosis of renal-artery stenosis. *N Engl J Med* 1978;298:582.

308. Thind GS, Montojo PM, Johnson A, et al. Enhancement of renal venous renin ratios by intravenous hydralazine in renovascular hypertension. *Am J Cardiol* 1984;53:109.

309. Tucker RM, Strong CG, Brennan LA Jr, et al. Renovascular hypertension. Relationship of surgical curability to renin-angiotensin activity. *Mayo Clin Proc* 1978;53:373.

310. Maxwell MH, Gonick HC, Wiita R, et al. Use of the rapid-sequence intravenous pyelogram in the diagnosis of renovascular hypertension. *N Engl J Med* 1964;270:213.

311. Bookstein JJ, Abrams HL, Buenger RE, et al. Radiologic aspects of renovascular hypertension. 2. The role of urography in unilateral renovascular disease. *JAMA* 1972;220:1225.

312. Thornbury JR, Stanley JC, Fryback DG. Hypertensive urogram: a nondiscriminatory test for renovascular hypertension. *AJR Am J Roentgenol* 1982;138:43.

313. Havey RJ, Krumlovsky F, delGreco F, et al. Screening for renovascular hypertension. Is renal digital-subtraction angiography the preferred noninvasive test? *JAMA* 1985;254:388.

314. Burbank MK, Hunt JC, Tauze WN, et al. Radioisotopic renography. Diagnosis of renal arterial disease in hypertensive patients. *Circulation* 1963;27:328.

315. Maxwell MH, Lupu AN, Taplin GV. Radioisotope renogram in renal arterial hypertension. *J Urol* 1968;100:376.

316. Stewart BH, Haynie TP. Critical appraisal of the renogram in renovascular disease. *JAMA* 1962;180:454.

317. Chervu LR, Blaufox MD. Renal radiopharmaceuticals—an update. *Semin Nucl Med* 1982;12:224.

318. Textor SC, Tarazi RC, Novick AC, et al. Regulation of renal hemodynamics and glomerular filtration in patients with renovascular hypertension during converting enzyme inhibition with captopril. *Am J Med* 1984;76:29.

319. Sfakianakis GN, Bourgoignie JJ, Jaffe D, et al. Single-dose captopril scintigraphy in the diagnosis of renovascular hypertension. *J Nucl Med* 1987;28:1383.

320. Geyskes GG, Oei HY, Puylaert CB, et al. Renovascular hypertension identified by captopril-induced changes in the renogram. *Hypertension* 1987;9:451.

321. Fommei E, Ghione S, Palla L, et al. Renal scintigraphic captopril test in the diagnosis of renovascular hypertension. *Hypertension* 1987;10:212.

322. Dondi M, Franchi R, Levorato M, et al. Evaluation of hypertensive patients by means of captopril enhanced renal scintigraphy with technetium-99m DTPA. *J Nucl Med* 1989;30:615.

323. Nally JV Jr, Clarke HS Jr, Gupta BK, et al. Captopril renography in two kidney and one kidney Goldblatt hypertension in dogs. *J Nucl Med* 1987;28:1171.

324. Ploth DW. Angiotensin-dependent renal mechanisms in two-kidney, one-clip renal vascular hypertension. *Am J Physiol* 1983;245:F131.

325. Nally JV Jr, Clarke HS Jr, Grecos GP, et al. Effect of captopril on 99mTc-diethylenetriaminepentaacetic acid renograms in two-kidney, one clip hypertension. *Hypertension* 1986;8:685.

326. Huang WC, Navar LG. Effects of unclipping and converting enzyme inhibition on bilateral renal function in Goldblatt hypertensive rats. *Kidney Int* 1983;23:816.

327. Nally JV, Jr. Provocative captopril testing in the diagnosis of renovascular hypertension. *Urol Clin North Am* 1994;21:227.

328. Geyskes GG, Oei HY, Puylaert CB, et al. Renography with captopril. Changes in a patient with hypertension and unilateral renal artery stenosis. *Arch Intern Med* 1986;146:1705.

329. Erbsloh-Moller B, Dumas A, Roth D, et al. Furosemide-131I-hippuran renography after angiotensin-converting enzyme inhibition for the diagnosis of renovascular hypertension. *Am J Med* 1991;90:23.

330. Setaro JF, Saddler MC, Chen CC, et al. Simplified captopril renography in diagnosis and treatment of renal artery stenosis. *Hypertension* 1991;18:289.

331. Mann SJ, Pickering TG, Sos TA, et al. Captopril renography in the diagnosis of renal artery stenosis: accuracy and limitations. *Am J Med* 1991;90:30.

332. Fommei E, Ghione S, Hilson AJ, et al. Captopril radionuclide test in renovascular hypertension: a European multicentre study. European Multicentre Study Group. *Eur J Nucl Med* 1993;20:617.
333. Dondi M. Captopril renal scintigraphy with 99mTc-mercaptoacetyltriglycine (99mTc-MAG3) for detecting renal artery stenosis. *Am J Hypertens* 1991;4:737S.
334. Boner G, Morduchowicz G, Rotenberg Z, et al. Deterioration in renal function in patients with chronic renal failure after treatment with captopril. *Isr J Med Sci* 1985;21:892.
335. Nally JV Jr, Chen C, Fine E, et al. Diagnostic criteria of renovascular hypertension with captopril renography. A consensus statement. *Am J Hypertens* 1991;4:749S.
336. Kremer Hovinga TK, de Jong PE, Piers DA, et al. Diagnostic use of angiotensin converting enzyme inhibitors in radioisotope evaluation of unilateral renal artery stenosis. *J Nucl Med* 1989;30:605.
337. Taylor A Jr, Martin LG. The utility of 99mTc-mercaptoacetyltriglycine in captopril renography. *Am J Hypertens* 1991;4:731S.
338. Jafri RA, Britton KE, Nimmon CC, et al. Technetium-99m MAG3, a comparison with iodine-123 and iodine-131 orthoiodohippurate, in patients with renal disorders. *J Nucl Med* 1988;29:147.
339. Dunnick NR, Sfakianakis GN. Screening for renovascular hypertension. *Radiol Clin North Am* 1991;29:497.
340. Taylor A. Functional testing: ACEI renography. *Semin Nephrol* 2000;20:437.
341. Stewart BH, DeWeese MS, Conway J, et al. Renal hypertension. An appraisal of diagnostic studies and of direct operative treatment. *Arch Surg* 1962;85:617.
342. Thomas CS Jr, Brockman SK, Foster JH. Variability of the pressure gradient in renal artery stenosis. *Surg Gynecol Obstet* 1968;126:339.
343. Ramos F, Kotliar C, Alvarez D, et al. Renal function and outcome of PTRA and stenting for atherosclerotic renal artery stenosis. *Kidney Int* 2003;63:276.
344. Nahman NS Jr, Maniam P, Hernandez RA, Jr. et al. Renal artery pressure gradients in patients with angiographic evidence of atherosclerotic renal artery stenosis. *Am J Kidney Dis* 1994;24:695.
345. Vidt DG, Yutani FM, McCormack LJ, et al. Surgical treatment of unilateral renal vascular disease. Prognostic role of vascular changes in bilateral renal biopsies. *Am J Cardiol* 1972;30:827.
346. Geisinger MA, Pohl MA. Renal angiography. In: Jacobson HR, Striker GE, Klahr S, eds. *Principles and practice of Nephrology*. St. Louis: Mosby Year Book, 1965:55.
347. Hillman BJ. Digital radiology of the kidney. *Radiol Clin North Am* 1985;23:211.
348. Buonocore E, Meaney TF, Borkowski GP, et al. Digital subtraction angiography of the abdominal aorta and renal arteries. Comparison with conventional aortography. *Radiology* 1981;139:281.
349. Clark RA, Alexander ES. Digital subtraction angiography of the renal arteries. Prospective comparison with conventional arteriography. *Invest Radiol* 1983;18:6.
350. Zabbo A, Novick AC. Digital subtraction angiography for noninvasive imaging of the renal artery. *Urol Clin North Am* 1984;11:409.
351. Kim D, Edelman RR, Kent KC, et al. Abdominal aorta and renal artery stenosis: evaluation with MR angiography. *Radiology* 1990;174:727.
352. Debatin JF, Spritzer CE, Grist TM, et al. Imaging of the renal arteries: value of MR angiography. *AJR Am J Roentgenol* 1991;157:981.
353. Gedroyc W. Magnetic resonance angiography of the renal arteries. In: Novick A, Scoble J, Hamilton G, eds. *Renal vascular disease*. Philadelphia: Saunders, 1996:91.
354. Postma CT, Joosten FB, Rosenbusch G, et al. Magnetic resonance angiography has a high reliability in the detection of renal artery stenosis. *Am J Hypertens* 1997;10:957.
355. Marcos HB, Choyke PL. Magnetic resonance angiography of the kidney. *Semin Nephrol* 2000;20:450.
356. Olbricht CJ, Arlart IP. Magnetic resonance angiography—the procedure of choice to diagnose renal artery stenosis? *Nephrol Dial Transplant* 1998;13:1620.
357. Thornton MJ, Thornton F, O'Callaghan J, et al. Evaluation of dynamic gadolinium-enhanced breath–hold MR angiography in the diagnosis of renal artery stenosis. *AJR Am J Roentgenol* 1999;173:1279.
358. Wasser MN, Westenberg J, van dH V, et al. Hemodynamic significance of renal artery stenosis: digital subtraction angiography versus systolically gated three-dimensional phase-contrast MR angiography. *Radiology* 1997;202:333.
359. Vasbinder GB, Nelemans PJ, Kessels AG, et al. Diagnostic tests for renal artery stenosis in patients suspected of having renovascular hypertension: a meta-analysis. *Ann Intern Med* 2001;135:401.
360. Hawkins IF. Carbon dioxide digital subtraction arteriography. *AJR Am J Roentgenol* 1982;139:19.
361. Hawkins IF, Herrera MA. Carbon dioxide has promise as an arterial contrast agent. *Diagn Imag* 1985;7:82.
362. Hawkins IF, Kerns SR. Carbon dioxide subtraction angiography. In: Cope C, ed. *Current techniques in interventional radiology*. Philadelphia: Current Medicine, 1994:1.
363. Hawkins IF Jr, Mladinich CR, Storm B, et al. Short-term effects of selective renal arterial carbon dioxide administration on the dog kidney. *J Vasc Intervent Radiol* 1994;5:149.
364. Jenni R, Vieli A, Luscher TF, et al. Combined two-dimensional ultrasound Doppler technique. New possibilities for the screening of renovascular and parenchymatous hypertension? *Nephron* 1986;44(Suppl 1):2.
365. Strandness DE Jr. *Duplex scanning in vascular disorders*. New York: Raven Press, 1993.
366. Burns PN. The physical principles of Doppler and spectral analysis. *J Clin Ultrasound* 1987;15:567.
367. Strandness DE Jr. Duplex scanning in diagnosis of renovascular hypertension. *Surg Clin North Am* 1990;70:109.
368. Strandness DE Jr. Duplex ultrasound scanning. In: Novick A, Scoble J, Hamilton G, eds. *Renal vascular disease*. Philadelphia: Saunders, 1996:119.
369. Radermacher J, Mengel M, Ellis S, et al. The renal arterial resistance index and renal allograft survival. *N Engl J Med* 2003;349:115.
370. Radermacher J, Ellis S, Haller H. Renal resistance index and progression of renal disease. *Hypertension* 2002;39:699.
371. Radermacher J, Chavan A, Bleck J, et al. Use of doppler ultrasonography to predict the outcome of therapy for renal-artery stenosis. *N Engl J Med* 2001;344:410.
372. Rubin GD, Dake MD, Napel S, et al. Spiral CT of renal artery stenosis: comparison of three-dimensional rendering techniques. *Radiology* 1994;190:181.
373. Olbricht CJ, Paul K, Prokop M, et al. Minimally invasive diagnosis of renal artery stenosis by spiral computed tomography angiography. *Kidney Int* 1995;48:1332.
374. Elkohen M, Beregi JP, Deklunder G, et al. A prospective study of helical computed tomography angiography versus angiography for the detection of renal artery stenoses in hypertensive patients. *J Hypertens* 1996;14:525.
375. Scoble JE, Hamilton G. Atherosclerotic renovascular disease. *Br Med J* 1990;300:1670.
376. Kaylor WM, Novick AC, Ziegelbaum M, et al. Reversal of end stage renal failure with surgical revascularization in patients with atherosclerotic renal artery occlusion. *J Urol* 1989;141:486.
377. Hansen KJ. Prevalence of ischemic nephropathy in the atherosclerotic population. *Am J Kidney Dis* 1994;24:615.
378. Mailloux LU, Napolitano B, Bellucci AG, et al. Renal vascular disease causing end-stage renal disease, incidence, clinical correlates, and outcomes: a 20-year clinical experience. *Am J Kidney Dis* 1994;24:622.
379. Roche Z, Rutecki G, Cox J, et al. Reversible acute renal failure as an atypical presentation of ischemic nephropathy. *Am J Kidney Dis* 1993;22:662.
380. Hansen KJ, Thomason RB, Craven TE, et al. Surgical management of dialysis-dependent ischemic nephropathy. *J Vasc Surg* 1995;21:197.
381. Salmon P, Brown MA. Renal artery stenosis and peripheral vascular disease: implications for ACE inhibitor therapy [letter]. *Lancet* 1990;336:321.
382. Wilms G, Marchal G, Peene P, et al. The angiographic incidence of renal artery stenosis in the arteriosclerotic population. *Eur J Radiol* 1990;10:195.
383. Novick AC, Ziegelbaum M, Vidt DG, et al. Trends in surgical revascularization for renal artery disease. Ten years' experience. *JAMA* 1987;257:498.
384. Morris GC Jr, DeBakey ME, Cooley MJ. Surgical treatment of renal failure of renovascular origin. *JAMA* 1962;182:113.
385. Simon NM, del Greco F. Kidney function after renal revascularization for hypertension. *Circulation* 1964;29:376.
386. Appel RG, Bleyer AJ, Reavis S, et al. Renovascular disease in older patients beginning renal replacement therapy. *Kidney Int* 1995;48:171.
387. Ascer E, Gennaro M, Rogers D. Unilateral renal artery revascularization can salvage renal function and terminate dialysis in selected patients with uremia. *J Vasc Surg* 1993;18:1012.
388. Vidt DG, Eisele G, Gephardt GN, et al. Atheroembolic renal disease: association with renal arterial stenosis. *Cleve Clin J Med* 1989;56:407.
389. Bonelli FS, Macusic MA, Textor SC, et al. Renal artery angioplasty: technical results and clinical outcome in 320 patients. *Mayo Clin Proc* 1995;70:1041.
390. Cheung CM, Wright JR, Shurrab AE, et al. Epidemiology of renal dysfunction and patient outcome in atherosclerotic renal artery occlusion. *J Am Soc Nephrol* 2002;13:149.
391. Meyrier A. Vascular mechanisms of renal fibrosis. Vasculonephropathies and arterial hypertension. *Bull Acad Natl Med* 1999;183:33.
392. Wiggins RC, Fantone J, Phan SH. Mechanisms of vascular injury. In: Tisher CC, et al., eds. *Renal pathology with clinical and functional correlations*. Philadelphia: JB Lippincott, 1989:965.
393. Truong LD, Farhood A, Tasby J, et al. Experimental chronic renal ischemia: morphologic and immunologic studies. *Kidney Int* 1992;41:1676.
394. Textor SC, Wilcox CS. Ischemic nephropathy/azotemic renovascular disease. *Semin Nephrol* 2000;20:489.
395. Textor SC, Wilcox CS. Renal artery stenosis: a common, treatable cause of renal failure? *Annu Rev Med* 2001;52:421.
396. Heptinstall RH. *Pathology of the kidney*. Boston: Little, Brown, 1983.
397. Luke DJ, Curtis JJ. Nephrosclerosis. In: Schrier RW, Gottschalk CW, eds. *Diseases of the kidney*. Boston: Little, Brown, 1993:1433.
398. Chade AR, Rodriguez-Porcel M, Grande JP, et al. Distinct renal injury in early atherosclerosis and renovascular disease. *Circulation* 2002;106:1165.
399. Chade AR, Rodriguez-Porcel M, Grande JP, et al. Mechanisms of renal structural alterations in combined hypercholesterolemia and renal artery stenosis. *Arterioscler Thromb Vasc Biol* 2003;23:1295.
400. Hricik DE. Captopril-induced renal insufficiency and the role of sodium balance. *Ann Intern Med* 1985;103:222.

401. Abrahams HL, Cornell SH. Patterns of collateral flow and renal ischemia. *Radiology* 1965;84:1001.

402. Morris CG, Heider CF, Moyer JH. The protective effect of subfiltration arterial pressure on the kidney. *Surg Forum* 1956;6:623.

403. Zinman L, Libertino JA. Revascularization of the chronic totally occluded renal artery with restoration of renal function. *J Urol* 1977;118:517.

404. Schefft P, Novick AC, Stewart BH, et al. Renal revascularization in patients with total occlusion of the renal artery. *J Urol* 1980;124:184.

405. Baird RJ, Yendt ER, Firor WB. Anuria due to acute occlusion of the artery to a solitary kidney: Successful treatment by operative means. *N Engl J Med* 1965;272:1012.

406. Flye MW, Anderson RW, Fish JC, et al. Successful surgical treatment of anuria caused by renal artery occlusion. *Ann Surg* 1982;195:3463.

407. Kaufman JJ. Renal artery stenosis and azotemia. *Surg Gynecol Obstet* 1973;137:949.

408. Hallett JW Jr, Textor SC, Kos PB, et al. Advanced renovascular hypertension and renal insufficiency: trends in medical comorbidity and surgical approach from 1970 to 1993. *J Vasc Surg* 1995;21:750.

409. Sandy DT, Vidt, DG, Geisinger MA. Serum creatinine prior to angioplasty (PTRA): a predictor of clinical success in atherosclerotic disease [abstract]. *J Am Soc Nephrol* 1995;6:648.

410. Bedoya L, Ziegelbaum M, Vidt DG, et al. Baseline renal function and surgical revascularization in atherosclerotic renal arterial disease in the elderly. *Cleve Clin J Med* 1989;56:415.

411. Mercier C, Piquet P, Alimi Y, et al. Occlusive disease of the renal arteries and chronic renal failure: the limits of reconstructive surgery. *Ann Vasc Surg* 1990;4:166.

412. Chaikof EL, Smith RB, Salam AA, et al. Ischemic nephropathy and concomitant aortic disease: a ten-year experience. *J Vasc Surg* 1994;19:135, discussion 146.

413. Textor SC, McKusick MA, Schirger AA, et al. Atherosclerotic renovascular disease in patients with renal failure. *Adv Nephrol Necker Hosp* 1997;27:281.

414. Textor SC. Revascularization in atherosclerotic renal artery disease. *Kidney Int* 1998;53:799.

415. Dean RH, Lawson JD, Hollifield JW, et al. Revascularization of the poorly functioning kidney. *Surgery* 1979;85:44.

416. Libertino JA, Zinman L, Breslin DJ, et al. Renal artery revascularization. Restoration of renal function. *JAMA* 1980;244:1340.

417. Magilligan DJ Jr, DeWeese JA, May AG, et al. The occluded renal artery. *Surgery* 1975;78:730.

418. Morgan T, Wilson M, Johnston W, et al. Restoration of renal function by arterial surgery. *Lancet* 1974;1:653.

419. Sheil AG, Stokes GS, Tiller DJ, et al. Reversal of renal failure by revascularisation of kidneys with thrombosed renal arteries. *Lancet* 1973;2:865.

420. Smith SP Jr, Hamburger RJ, Donohue JP, et al. Occlusion of the artery to a solitary kidney. Restoration of renal function after prolonged anuria. *JAMA* 1974;230:1306.

421. Wasser WG, Krakoff LR, Haimov M, et al. Restoration of renal function after bilateral renal artery occlusion. *Arch Intern Med* 1981;141:1647.

422. Whitehouse WM Jr, Kazmers A, Zelenock GB, et al. Chronic total renal artery occlusion: effects of treatment on secondary hypertension and renal function. *Surgery* 1981;89:753.

423. Dean RH, Tribble RW, Hansen KJ, et al. Evolution of renal insufficiency in ischemic nephropathy. *Ann Surg* 1991;213:446, discussion 455.

424. U.S. Renal Data System. *Survival probabilities and causes of death: USRDS 1991 Annual Report.* Bethesda, MD: National Institutes of Health, 1991.

425. Fatica RA, Port FK, Young EW. Incidence trends and mortality in end-stage renal disease attributed to renovascular disease in the United States. *Am J Kidney Dis* 2001;37:1184.

426. Novick AC, Textor SC, Bodie B, et al. Revascularization to preserve renal function in patients with atherosclerotic renovascular disease. *Urol Clin North Am* 1984;11:427:477.

427. Eggers PW, Connerton R, McMullan M. The Medicare experience with end-stage renal disease: trends in incidence, prevalence, and survival. *Health Care Financing Rev* 1984;5:69.

428. Mailloux LU, Bellucci AG, Wilkes BM, et al. Mortality in dialysis patients: analysis of the causes of death. *Am J Kidney Dis* 1991;18:326.

429. Hylander B, Lundblad H, Kjellstrand CM. Changing patient characteristics in chronic hemodialysis. *Scand J Urol Nephrol* 1991;25:59.

430. Collins AJ, Hanson G, Umen A, et al. Changing risk factor demographics in end-stage renal disease patients entering hemodialysis and the impact on long-term mortality. *Am J Kidney Dis* 1990;15:422.

431. Shapiro FL, Umen A. Risk factors in hemodialysis patient survival. *Am Soc Artif Intern Organs* 1983;6:176.

432. Heptinstall RH. Renal biopsies in hypertension. *Br Heart J* 1954;16:133.

433. Hansen KJ, Cherr GS, Craven TE, et al. Management of ischemic nephropathy: dialysis-free survival after surgical repair. *J Vasc Surg* 2000;32:472.

434. Textor SC, Novick AC, Steinmuller DR, et al. Renal failure limiting antihypertensive therapy as an indication for renal revascularization. A case report. *Arch Intern Med* 1983;143:2208.

435. Toto RD, Mitchell HC, Lee HC, et al. Reversible renal insufficiency due to angiotensin converting enzyme inhibitors in hypertensive nephrosclerosis. *Ann Intern Med* 1991;115:513.

436. Martin PY, Gines P, Schrier RW. Nitric oxide as a mediator of hemodynamic abnormalities and sodium and water retention in cirrhosis. *N Engl J Med* 1998;339:533.

437. Coen G, Manni M, Giannoni MF, et al. Ischemic nephropathy in an elderly nephrologic and hypertensive population. *Am J Nephrol* 1998;18:221.

438. Chabova V, Schirger A, Stanson AW, et al. Outcomes of atherosclerotic renal artery stenosis managed without revascularization. *Mayo Clin Proc* 2000;75:437.

439. Webster J, Marshall F, Abdalla M, et al. Randomised comparison of percutaneous angioplasty vs continued medical therapy for hypertensive patients with atheromatous renal artery stenosis. Scottish and Newcastle Renal Artery Stenosis Collaborative Group. *J Hum Hypertens* 1998;12:329.

440. Uzzo RG, Novick AC, Goormastic M, et al. Medical versus surgical management of atherosclerotic renal artery stenosis. *Transplant Proc* 2002;34:723.

441. Cardiovascular Outcomes in Renal Atherosclerotic Lesions (CORAL) Study: 2005. Available at: http://www.coralclinicaltrial.org/ and NIH website: http://www.clinicaltrials.gov/ct/show/NCT00081731.

442. Pickering TG, Heptinstall RH. Nephrectomy and other treatment for hypertension in pyelonephritis. *Q J Med* 1953;21:1.

443. Smith HW. Unilateral nephrectomy in hypertensive disease. *J Urol* 1956;76:685.

444. Meares EM Jr, Gross DM. Hypertension owing to unilateral renal hypoplasia. *J Urol* 1972;108:197.

445. Freeman N. Thromboendarterectomy for hypertension due to renal artery occlusion. *JAMA* 1954;157:1077.

446. Jicha DL, Ehrenfeld WK. Surgical techniques for renal revascularization. In: Greenhalgh R, ed. *Vascular and endovascular surgical techniques.* London: Saunders, 1994:189.

447. Stoney RJ, Olofsson PA. Aortorenal arterial autografts: the last two decades. *Ann Vasc Surg* 1988;2:169.

448. Bergentz S, Weibull H. Renal endarterectomy. In: Novick AC, Scoble J, Hamilton G, eds. *Renovascular disease.* Philadelphia: Saunders, 1996:455.

449. Ernst CB, Stanley JC, Marshall FF, et al. Autogenous saphenous vein aortorenal grafts. A ten-year experience. *Arch Surg* 1972;105:855.

450. Novick AC. *Renal vascular disease.* Philadelphia: Saunders, 1996. Ref ID: 534.

451. Straffon R, Siegel DF. Saphenous vein bypass graft in the treatment of renovascular hypertension. *Urol Clin North Am* 1975;2:337.

452. Dubernard JM, Martin X, Gelet A, et al. Renal autotransplantation versus bypass techniques for renovascular hypertension. *Surgery* 1985;97:529.

453. Novick AC. Microvascular reconstruction of complex branch renal artery disease. *Urol Clin North Am* 1984;11:465.

454. Novick AC, Jackson CL, Straffon RA. The role of renal autotransplantation in complex urological reconstruction. *J Urol* 1990;143:452.

455. van Bockel JH, van den Akker PJ, Chang PC, et al. Extracorporeal renal artery reconstruction for renovascular hypertension. *J Vasc Surg* 1991;13:101, discussion 110.

456. Cormier JM, Fichelle JM, Laurian C, et al. Renal artery revascularization with polytetrafluoroethylene bypass graft. *Ann Vasc Surg* 1990;4:471.

457. Khauli RB, Novick AC, Coseriu GV. Renal revascularization with polytetrafluoroethylene grafts. *Cleve Clin Q* 1984;51:365.

458. Lagneau P, Michel JB, Charrat JM. Use of polytetrafluoroethylene grafts for renal bypass. *J Vasc Surg* 1987;5:738.

459. Brewster DC, Darling RC. Splenorenal arterial anastomosis for renovascular hypertension. *Ann Surg* 1979;189:353.

460. Khauli RB, Novick AC, Ziegelbaum M. Splenorenal bypass in the treatment of renal artery stenosis: experience with sixty-nine cases. *J Vasc Surg* 1985;2:547.

461. Chibaro EA, Libertino JA, Novick AC. Use of the hepatic circulation for renal revascularization. *Ann Surg* 1984;199:406.

462. Valentine RJ, Martin JD, Myers SI, et al. Asymptomatic celiac and superior mesenteric artery stenoses are more prevalent among patients with unsuspected renal artery stenoses. *J Vasc Surg* 1991;14:195.

463. Novick AC, Banowsky LH. Iliorenal saphenous vein bypass: an alternative for renal revascularization in patients with a surgically difficult aorta. *J Urol* 1979;122:243.

464. Novick AC. Ileorenal and mesenterorenal bypass. In: Novick AC, Streem SB, Pontes J, eds. *Stewart's operative urology.* Baltimore: Williams & Wilkins, 1989:279.

465. Khauli RB, Novick AC, Coseriu GV, et al. Superior mesenterorenal bypass for renal revascularization with infrarenal aortic occlusion. *J Urol* 1985;133:188.

466. Fry RE, Fry WJ. Supraceliac aortorenal bypass with saphenous vein for renovascular hypertension. *Surg Gynecol & Obstet* 1989;168:180.

467. Novick AC. Use of the thoracic aorta for renal revascularization. *Urol Clin North Am* 1994;21:355.

468. Novick AC, Stewart R. Use of the thoracic aorta for renal revascularization. *J Urol* 1990;143:77.

469. Darling RC III, Kreienberg PB, Chang BB, et al. Outcome of renal artery reconstruction: analysis of 687 procedures. *Ann Surg* 1999;230:524.

470. Shahian DM, Najafi H, Javid H, et al. Simultaneous aortic and renal artery reconstruction. *J Urol* 1980;115:1491.

471. Tarazi RY, Hertzer NR, Beven EG, et al. Simultaneous aortic reconstruction and renal revascularization: risk factors and late results in eighty-nine patients. *J Vasc Surg* 1987;5:707.

472. Hansen KJ, Starr SM, Sands RE, et al. Contemporary surgical management of renovascular disease. *J Vasc Surg* 1992;16:319, discussion 330.

473. Bredenberg CE, Sampson LN, Ray FS, et al. Changing patterns in surgery for chronic renal artery occlusive diseases. *J Vasc Surg* 1992;15:1018.

474. Libertino JA, Bosco PJ, Ying CY, et al. Renal revascularization to preserve and restore renal function. *J Urol* 1992;147:1485.

475. Hallett JW Jr, Fowl R, O'Brien PC, et al. Renovascular operations in patients with chronic renal insufficiency: do the benefits justify the risks? *J Vasc Surg* 1987;5:622.

476. Foster JH, Maxwell MH, Franklin SS, et al. Renovascular occlusive disease. Results of operative treatment. *JAMA* 1975;231:1043.

477. Pickering TG, Sos TA, Laragh JH. Role of balloon dilatation in the treatment of renovascular hypertension. *Am J Med* 1984;77:61.

478. Pickering TG, Laragh JH, Sos TA. Renovascular hypertension. In: Schrier RW, Gottschalk CW, eds. *Diseases of the kidney*. Boston: Little, Brown, 1993:1451.

479. Novick AC, Straffon RA, Stewart BH, et al. Diminished operative morbidity and mortality in renal revascularization. *JAMA* 1981;246:749.

480. Bergentz SE, Ericsson BF, Husberg B. Technique and complications in the surgical treatment of hypertension. *Acta Chir Scand* 1979;145:143.

481. Foster JH, Dean RH, Pinkerton JA, et al. Ten years experience with the surgical management of hypertension. *Ann Surg* 1973;177:755.

482. Lankford NS, Donohue JP, Grim CE, et al. Results of surgical treatment of renovascular hypertension. *J Urol* 1979;122:439.

483. Gruntzig A, Kuhlmann U, Vetter W, et al. Treatment of renovascular hypertension with percutaneous transluminal dilatation of a renal-artery stenosis. *Lancet* 1978;1:801.

484. Stanley JC. Renovascular hypertension: the surgical point of view. In: Schilfgaarde RV, ed. *Clinical aspects of renovascular hypertension*. Boston: Martinus Nijhoff, 1983:259.

485. Tegtmeyer CJ, Kellum CD, Ayers C. Percutaneous transluminal angioplasty of the renal artery. Results and long-term follow-up. *Radiology* 1984;153:77.

486. Thevenet A, Mary H, Boennec M. Results following surgical correction of renovascular. *J Cardiovasc Surg* 1980;21:517.

487. Lawrie GM, Morris GC Jr, Soussou ID, et al. Late results of reconstructive surgery for renovascular. *Ann Surg* 1980;191:528.

488. Steinbach F, Novick AC, Campbell S, et al. Long-term survival after surgical revascularization for atherosclerotic renal artery disease. *J Urol* 1997;158:38.

489. Starr DS, Lawrie GM, Morris GC Jr. Surgical treatment of renovascular hypertension. Long-term follow-up of 216 patients up to 20 years. *Arch Surg* 1980;115:494.

490. Bacharach JM, Childs MB, Olin JW. Preliminary patency experience with renal artery stents for atherosclerotic renal artery stenosis (abstract). Parmley, W. W. 23, 474A. 1994. New York, Elsevier Science. Abstracts of the Original Contributions presented at the 43rd Annual Scientific Session of the American College of Cardiology. Ref Type: Conference.

491. Dean RH, Krueger TC, Whiteneck JM, et al. Operative management of renovascular hypertension. Results after a follow-up of fifteen to twenty-three years. *J Vasc Surg* 1984;1:234.

492. Fry RE, Fry WJ. Renovascular hypertension in the patient with severe atherosclerosis. *Arch Surg* 1982;117:938.

493. Libertino JA. Renovascular hypertension. Changing concepts in management. *Postgrad Med* 1984;75:149.

494. Luft FC, Grim CE, Weinberger MH. Intervention in patients with renovascular hypertension and renal insufficiency. *J Urol* 1983;130:654.

495. Jamieson GG, Clarkson AR, Woodroffe AJ, et al. Reconstructive renal vascular surgery for chronic renal failure. *Br J Surg* 1984;71:338.

496. Hansen KJ, Ditesheim JA, Metropol SH, et al. Management of renovascular hypertension in the elderly population. *J Vasc Surg* 1989;10:266.

497. Marone LK, Clouse WD, Dorer DJ, et al. Preservation of renal function with surgical revascularization in patients with atherosclerotic renovascular disease. *J Vasc Surg* 2004;39:322.

498. Meyrier A, Buchet P, Simon P, et al. Atheromatous renal disease. *Am J Med* 988;85:139.

499. Diehl JT, Cali RF, Hertzer NR, et al. Complications of abdominal aortic reconstruction. An analysis of perioperative risk factors in 557 patients. *Ann Surg* 1983;197:49.

500. Franklin SS, Young JD Jr, Maxwell MH, et al. Operative morbidity and mortality in renovascular disease. *JAMA* 1975;231:1148.

501. Hertzer NR, Young JR, Kramer JR, et al. Routine coronary angiography prior to elective aortic reconstruction: results of selective myocardial revascularization in patients with peripheral vascular disease. *Arch Surg* 1979;114:1336.

502. Novick AC. Evaluation and preparation for surgical treatment of renal artery disease. *Ann Vasc Surg* 1988;2:150.

503. Dotter CT, Judkins MP. Transluminal treatment of arteriosclerotic obstruction. Description of a new technique and a preliminary report of its applications. *Circulation* 1964;30:654.

504. Hayes JM, Risius B, Novick AC, et al. Experience with percutaneous transluminal angioplasty for renal artery stenosis at the Cleveland Clinic. *J Urol* 1988;139:488.

505. Cicuto KP, McLean GK, Oleaga JA, et al. Renal artery stenosis: anatomic classification for percutaneous transluminal angioplasty. *AJR Am J Roentgenol* 1981;137:599.

506. Ramsay LE, Waller PC. Blood pressure response to percutaneous transluminal angioplasty for renovascular hypertension: an overview of published series. *BMJ* 1990;300:569.

507. Kuhlmann U, Greminger P, Gruntzig A, et al. Long-term experience in percutaneous transluminal dilatation of renal artery stenosis. *Am J Med* 1985;79:692.

508. Bell GM, Reid J, Buist TA. Percutaneous transluminal angioplasty improves blood pressure and renal function in renovascular hypertension. *Q J Med* 1987;63:393.

509. Maxwell MH, Bleifer KH, Franklin SS, et al. Cooperative study of renovascular hypertension. Demographic analysis of the study. *JAMA* 1972;220:1195.

510. Colapinto RF, Stronell RD, Harries-Jones EP, et al. Percutaneous transluminal dilatation of the renal artery: follow-up studies on renovascular hypertension. *AJR Am J Roentgenol* 1982;139:727.

511. Geyskes GG, Puylaert CB, Oei HY, et al. Follow up study of 70 patients with renal artery stenosis treated by percutaneous transluminal dilatation. *Br Med J* 1983;287:333.

512. Miller GA, Ford KK, Braun SD, et al. Percutaneous transluminal angioplasty vs. surgery for renovascular hypertension. *AJR Am J Roentgenol* 1985;144:447.

513. Martin LG, Price RB, Casarella WJ, et al. Percutaneous angioplasty in clinical management of renovascular hypertension: initial and long-term results. *Radiology* 1985;155:629.

514. Kaplan-Pavlohcic S, Koselj M, Obrez I, et al. Percutaneous transluminal renal angioplasty: follow up studies on renovascular hypertension. *Przegl Lek* 1985;42:342.

515. Brawn LA, Ramsay LE. Is "improvement" real with percutaneous transluminal angioplasty in the management of renovascular hypertension? *Lancet* 1987;2:1313.

516. Plouin PF, Chatellier G, Darne B, et al., for the Essai Multicentrique Medicaments vs. Angioplastie (EMMA) Study Group. Blood pressure outcome of angioplasty in atherosclerotic renal artery stenosis: a randomized trial. *Hypertension* 1998;31:823.

517. O'Donovan RM, Gutierrez OH, Izzo JL Jr. Preservation of renal function by percutaneous renal angioplasty in high-risk elderly patients: short-term outcome. *Nephron* 1992;60:187.

518. Pickering TG, Sos TA, Saddekni S, et al. Renal angioplasty in patients with azotemia and renovascular hypertension. *J Hypertens* 1986;4(Suppl 6):S667.

519. Sos TA. Angioplasty for the treatment of azotemia and renovascular hypertension in atherosclerotic renal artery disease. *Circulation* 1991;83:I162.

520. Paulsen D, Klow NE, Rogstad B, et al. Preservation of renal function by percutaneous transluminal angioplasty in ischaemic renal disease. *Nephrol Dial Transplant* 1999;14:1454.

521. Weibull H, Bergqvist D, Bergentz SE, et al. Percutaneous transluminal renal angioplasty versus surgical reconstruction of atherosclerotic renal artery stenosis: a prospective randomized study. *J Vasc Surg* 1993;18:841, discussion 850.

522. Dotter CT. Transluminally-placed coilspring endarterial tube grafts. Long-term patency in canine popliteal artery. *Invest Radiol* 1969;4:329.

523. Palmaz JC, Sibbitt RR, Reuter SR, et al. Expandable intraluminal graft: a preliminary study. Work in progress. *Radiology* 1985;156:73.

524. Rees CR, Palmaz JC, Becker GJ, et al. Palmaz stent in atherosclerotic stenoses involving the ostia of the renal arteries: preliminary report of a multicenter study. *Radiology* 1991;181:507.

525. Palmaz JC. Intravascular stents: tissue-stent interactions and design considerations. *AJR Am J Roentgenol* 1993;160:613.

526. Strecker EP, Liermann D, Barth KH, et al. Expandable tubular stents for treatment of arterial occlusive diseases: experimental and clinical results. Work in progress. *Radiology* 1990;175:97.

527. Trost D, Sos TA. Endovascular stents. In: Novick AC, Scoble J, Hamilton G, eds. *Renovascular disease*. Philadelphia: Saunders, 1996:403.

528. Dorros G, Prince C, Mathiak L. Stenting of a renal artery stenosis achieves better relief of the obstructive lesion than balloon angioplasty. *Catheter Cardiovasc Diagn* 1993;29:191.

529. Joffre F, Rousseau H, Bernadet P, et al. Midterm results of renal artery stenting. *Cardiovasc Intervent Radiol* 1992;15:313.

530. Kuhn FP, Kutkuhn B, Torsello G, et al. Renal artery stenosis: preliminary results of treatment with the Strecker stent. *Radiology* 1991;180:367.

531. van de Ven PJ, Kaatee R, Beutler JJ, et al. Arterial stenting and balloon angioplasty in ostial atherosclerotic renovascular disease: a randomised trial. *Lancet* 1999;353:282.

532. Leertouwer TC, Gussenhoven EJ, Bosch JL, et al. Stent placement for renal arterial stenosis: where do we stand? A meta-analysis. *Radiology* 2000;216:78.

533. Tuttle KR, Chouinard RF, Webber JT, et al. Treatment of atherosclerotic ostial renal artery stenosis with the intravascular stent. *Am J Kidney Dis* 1998;32:611.

534. Trost D, Sos T. Complications of renal angioplasty and stenting. *Semin Intervent Radiol* 1994;11(2):150.

535. Rees ER, Niblett R, Snead D. United States multicenter study of Palmaz-Schatz stents in the renal arteries. *CIRSE Annual Meeting and Postgraduate Course of the Cardiovascular and Interventional Radiological Society of Europe, Crete, June 1994, 1994.*

536. Olin JW, Graor RA, Bacharach JM. Renal artery stenting for control of congestive heart failure (abstract). In: Parmley WW, ed. *Abstracts of the Original Contributions presented at the 43rd Annual Scientific Session of the American College of Cardiology, March 13–17, 1994, Atlanta, GA.* New York: Elsevier Science, 1994:96A-Abstract # 96A.

537. Dorros G, Jaff M, Mathiak L, et al. Multicenter Palmaz stent renal artery stenosis revascularization registry report: four-year follow-up of 1,058 successful patients. *Catheter Cardiovasc Interv* 2002;55:182.

538. Isles CG, Robertson S, Hill D. Management of renovascular disease: a review of renal artery stenting in ten studies. *QJM* 1999;92:159.

539. Kennedy DJ, Colyer WR, Brewster PS, et al. Renal insufficiency as a predictor of adverse events and mortality after renal artery stent placement. *Am J Kidney Dis* 2003;42:926.

540. Novick AC. Renovascular hypertension in children. In: Kellerless P, Bellman, eds. *Clinical pediatric urology.* Philadelphia: Saunders, 1984.

541. Martinez A, Novick AC, Cunningham R, et al. Improved results of vascular reconstruction in pediatric and young adult patients with renovascular hypertension. *J Urol* 1990;144:717.

542. Novick AC. Percutaneous transluminal angioplasty and surgery of the renal artery. *Eur J Vasc Surg* 1994;8:1.

543. Shapiro AP, Perez-Stable E, Scheib ET, et al. Renal artery stenosis and hypertension. Observations on current status of therapy from a study of 115 patients. *Am J Med* 1969;47:175.

544. Pohl MA. Renovascular hypertension: an internist's point of view. In: Punzi HA, Flamenbaum W, eds. *Hypertension.* Mt. Kisco, NY: Futura, 1989:367.

545. Dean RH, Kieffer RW, Smith BM, et al. Renovascular hypertension: anatomic and renal function changes during drug therapy. *Arch Surg* 1989;116:1408.

546. Sheps SG, Osmundson PJ, Hunt JC, et al. Hypertension and renal artery stenosis. Serial observations on 54 patients treated medically. *Clin Pharmacol Ther* 1965;6:700.

547. Dustan HP, Page IH, Poutasse EF, et al. An evaluation of treatment of hypertension associated with occlusive renal arterial disease. *Circulation* 1963;27:1018.

548. Pickering TG. Medical management of renovascular hypertension. In: Kaplan NM, Brenner BM, Laragh JH, eds. *The kidney in hypertension.* New York: Raven Press, 1987.

549. Kaplan NM. Renal vascular hypertension. In: Kaplan NM, ed. *Clinical hypertension.* Baltimore: Williams & Wilkins, 1986:319.

550. Hollenberg NK. Treatment of renovascular hypertension: surgery, angioplasty, and medical therapy with converting enzyme inhibitors. *Am J Kidney Dis* 1987;10(Suppl 1):52.

551. Peart WS. Treatment of hypertension associated with renal artery stenosis. In: Engel A, Larsson T, eds. *Stroke: Thule International Symposium.* Stockholm: Nordiska Bokhandeins Forlag, 1967:237.

552. Kjellbo H, Lund N, Bergentz SE, et al. Renal artery stenosis. 3. Follow-up observations in operated and non-operated patients. *Scand J Urol Nephrol* 1970;4:49.

553. Owen K. Results of surgical treatment in comparison with medical treatment of renovascular hypertension. *Clin Sci Mol Med* 1973;45(Suppl 1):95.

554. Hunt JC, Strong CG. Renovascular hypertension: mechanisms, natural history and treatment. In: Laragh HD, ed. *Hypertension manual.* New York: York, 1976:5096.

555. Streeten DH, Anderson GH Jr. Outpatient experience with saralasin. *Kidney Int* 1979;(9) (Suppl):S44.

556. Buhler FR, Laragh JH, Vaughan ED Jr, et al. The antihypertensive action of propranolol. Specific antirenin responses in high and normal renin forms of essential, renal renovascular and malignant hypertension. In: Laragh HD, ed. *Hypertension manual.* New York: York, 1973:873.

557. Struder A, Luscher T, Griminger P, et al. Captopril in therapy—resistant, essential and renovascular hypertension. In: Brenner HT, Gross F, eds. *Recent advances in hypertensive therapy.* Amsterdam: Excerpta Medica, 1981:31.

558. Hollifield JW, Moore LC, Winn SD, et al. Angiotensin converting enzyme inhibition in renovascular hypertension. *Cardio Rev Rpts* 1982;3:673.

559. Case DB, Atlas SA, Marion RM, et al. Long-term efficacy of captopril in renovascular and essential hypertension. *Am J Cardiol* 1982;49:1440.

560. Prichard BN. Propranolol as an antihypertensive agent. *Am Heart J* 1970;79:128.

561. Vander AJ, Luciano JR. Neural and humoral control of renin release in salt depletion. *Circ Res* 1967;21(Suppl 2):69.

562. Nomura G, Kurosaki M, Takabatake T, et al. Reinnervation and renin release after unilateral renal denervation in the dog. *J Appl Physiol* 1972;33:649.

563. Bravo EL, Tarazi RC, Dustan HP. On the mechanism of suppressed plasma-renin activity during beta-adrenergic blockade with propranolol. *J Lab Clin Med* 1974;83:119.

564. Frishman WH. *Clinical pharmacology of the β–adrenoreceptor blocking drugs.* Norwalk, CT: Appleton–Century–Crofts, 1984.

565. Erdos EG. Angiotensin converting enzyme and the changes in our concepts through the years. *Hypertension* 1990;16:363.

566. Franklin SS, Smith RD. A comparison of enalapril plus hydrochlorothiazide with standard triple therapy in renovascular hypertension. *Nephron* 1986;44(Suppl 1):73.

567. Frishman WH. β–adrenergic blockers. *Med Clin North Am* 1988;72:37.

568. Salvetti A, Sassano P, Poli L, et al. The effect of beta-adrenergic blockade on patterns of urinary sodium excretion, blood pressure and plasma renin activity in patients with essential and renovascular hypertension. *Eur J Clin Invest* 1977;7:331.

569. Hollenberg NK. Renal hemodynamics in essential and renovascular hypertension. Influence of captopril. *Am J Med* 1984;76:22.

570. Hollenberg NK. Medical therapy of renovascular hypertension: efficacy and safety of captopril in 269 patients. *Cardio Rev Rpts* 1983;4:852.

571. Franklin SS, Smith RD. Comparison of effects of enalapril plus hydrochlorothiazide versus standard triple therapy on renal function in renovascular hypertension. *Am J Med* 1985;79:14.

572. Buhler FR, Laragh JH, Baer L, et al. Propranolol inhibition of renin secretion: a specific approach to diagnosis and treatment of renin-dependent hypertensive disease. *N Engl J Med* 1972;287:1209.

573. Case DB, Wallace JM, Keim HJ, et al. Possible role of renin in hypertension as suggested by renin-sodium profiling and inhibition of converting enzymes. *N Engl J Med* 1977;296:641.

574. Timmerman PB, Chiu AT, Herblin WR, et al. Angiotensin II receptor subtypes. *Am J Hypertens* 1992;5:406.

575. Keane WF. The role of lipids in renal disease: future challenges. *Kidney Int Suppl* 2000;75:S27.

576. Smith RD, Chin AT, Wong PC, et al. Pharmacology of non peptide angiotensin II receptor antagonists. *Ann Rev Pharmacol Toxicol* 1992;32:135.

577. Kon V, Fogo A, Ichikawa I. Bradykinin causes selective efferent arteriolar dilation during angiotensin I converting enzyme inhibition. *Kidney Int* 1993;44:545.

578. Mimran A, Jover B, Saladini D. Effect of losartan and enalapril in 1-kidney 1-clip sodium restricted rats. *J Am Soc Nephrol* 1994;5:546.

579. Epstein M. Calcium antagonists in the management of hypertension. In: Epstein M, ed. *Calcium antagonists in clinical medicine.* Philadelphia: Hanley & Belfus, 1992:49.

580. Bursztyn M, Grossman R, Rosenthal T. Nifedipine as a substitute for converting enzyme inhibitors in the treatment of renovascular hypertension. *Clin Exp Hypertens* 1985;A7:1187.

581. Triggle DJ. Calcium antagonists. In: Antonaccio MJ, ed. *Cardiovascular pharmacology.* New York: Raven Press, 1990:107.

582. Morris AD, Meredith PA, Reid JL. Pharmacokinetics of calcium antagonists: implications for therapy. In: Epstein M, ed. *Calcium antagonists in clinical medicine.* Philadelphia: Hanley & Belfus, 1992:49.

583. Churchill PG. Second messengers in renin secretion. *Am J Physiol* 1985;249:F175.

584. Hackenthal E, Paul M, Ganten D, et al. Morphology, physiology, and molecular biology of renin secretion. *Physiol Rev* 1990;70:1067.

585. Ribstein J, Mourad G, Mimran A. Contrasting acute effects of captopril and nifedipine on renal function in renovascular hypertension. *Am J Hypertens* 1988;1:239.

586. Miyamori I, Yasuhara S, Matsubara T, et al. Comparative effects of captopril and nifedipine on split renal function in renovascular hypertension. *Am J Hypertens* 1988;1:359.

587. Fiorentini C, Galli C, Tamborini G, et al. Hemodynamic and renin responses to nifedipine in renovascular hypertension. *Am Heart J* 1990;119:353.

588. Diamond JR, Cheung JY, Fang JS. Nifedipine-induced renal dysfunction. Alterations in renal hemodynamics. *Am J Med* 1984;77:905.

589. Lydtin H, Trenkwalder P. *Calcium antagonists: a critical review.* New York, Berlin: Springer-Verlag, 1990.

590. Piepho RW, Culbertson VL, Reid JL. Drug interactions with the calcium-entry blockers. *Circulation* 1987;75(Suppl V):V181.

591. Mathias CJ, Wilkinson A, Lewis PS, et al. Clonidine lowers blood pressure independently of renin suppression in patients with unilateral renal artery stenosis. *Chest* 1983;83:375S.

592. de Zeeuw D, Navis GJ, Donker AJ, et al. The angiotensin converting enzyme inhibitor enalapril and its effects on renal function. *J Hypertens* 1983;1:(Suppl 1):93.

593. Tillman DM, Malatino LS, Cumming AM, et al. Enalapril in hypertension with renal artery stenosis: long-term follow-up and effects on renal function. *J Hypertens* 1984;2(Suppl 2):S93.

594. Chrysant SG, Dunn M, Marples D, et al. Severe reversible azotemia from captopril therapy. Report of three cases and review of the literature. *Arch Intern Med* 1983;143:437.

595. Murphy BF, Whitworth JA, Kincaid-Smith P. Renal insufficiency with combinations of angiotensin converting enzyme inhibitors and diuretics. *Br Med J* 1984;288:844.

596. Hodsman GP, Brown JJ, Cumming AM, et al. Enalapril in treatment of hypertension with renal artery stenosis. Changes in blood pressure, renin, angiotensin I and II, renal function, and body composition. *Am J Med* 1984;77:52.

597. Postma CT, Hoefnagels WH, Barentsz JO, et al. Occlusion of unilateral stenosed renal arteries–relation to medical treatment. *J Hum Hypertens* 1989;3:185.

598. Williams PS, Hendy MS, Ackrill P. Captopril-induced acute renal artery thrombosis and persistent anuria in a patient with documented pre-existing renal artery stenosis and renal failure. *Postgrad Med J* 1984;60:561.

599. Hoefnagels WH, Thien T. Renal artery occlusion in patients with renovascular hypertension treated with captopril. *Br Med J Clin Res Ed* 1986;292:24.

600. Hannedouche T, Godin M, Fries D, et al. Acute renal thrombosis induced by angiotensin-converting enzyme inhibitors in patients with renovascular hypertension. *Nephron* 1991;57:230.
601. Murphy TP, Soares G, Kim M. Increase in utilization of percutaneous renal artery interventions by medicare beneficiaries, 1996–2000. *AJR Am J Roentgenol* 2004;183:561.
602. Basta LL, Williams C, Kioschos JM, et al. Regression of atherosclerotic stenosing lesions of the renal arteries and spontaneous cure of systemic hypertension through control of hyperlipidemia. *Am J Med* 1976;61:420.
603. Khong TK, Missouris CG, Belli AM, et al. Regression of atherosclerotic renal artery stenosis with aggressive lipid lowering therapy. *J Hum Hypertens* 2001;15:431.
604. Brown BG, Zhao XQ, Sacco DE, et al. Lipid lowering and plaque regression. New insights into prevention of plaque disruption and clinical events in coronary disease. *Circulation* 1993;87:1781.
605. Ost CR, Stenson S. Regression of peripheral atherosclerosis during therapy with high doses of nicotinic acid. *Scand J Clin Lab Invest* 1967;99:241.
606. Pearson TA, Marx HJ. The rapid reduction in cardiac events with lipid-lowering therapy: mechanisms and implications (editorial). *Am J Cardiol* 1993;72:1072.
607. Byington RP, Furberg CD, Crouse JR III, et al. Pravastatin, lipids, and atherosclerosis in the carotid arteries (PLAC-II). *Am J Cardiol* 1995;76: 54C.
608. de Groot E, Jukema JW, van Boven AJ, et al. Effect of pravastatin on progression and regression of coronary atherosclerosis and vessel wall changes in carotid and femoral arteries: a report from the Regression Growth Evaluation Statin Study. *Am J Cardiol* 1995;76:40C.
609. Duffield RG, Lewis B, Miller NE, et al. Treatment of hyperlipidaemia retards progression of symptomatic femoral atherosclerosis. A randomised controlled trial. *Lancet* 1983;2:639.
610. Martin EC, Mattern RF, Baer L, et al. Renal angioplasty for hypertension: predictive factors for long-term success. *AJR Am J Roentgenol* 1981;137: 921.
611. Hennequin LM, Joffre FG, Rousseau HP, et al. Renal artery stent placement: long-term results with the Wallstent endoprosthesis. *Radiology* 1994; 191:713.
612. Raynaud AC, Beyssen BM, Turmel-Rodrigues LE, et al. Renal artery stent placement: immediate and midterm technical and clinical results. *J Vasc Intervent Radiol* 1994;5:849.
613. Dorros G, Jaff M, Jain A, et al. Follow-up of primary Palmaz-Schatz stent placement for atherosclerotic renal artery stenosis. *Am J Cardiol* 1995;75: 1051.
614. van de Ven PJ, Beutler JJ, Kaatee R, et al. Transluminal vascular stent for ostial atherosclerotic renal artery stenosis. *Lancet* 1995;346:672.
615. Rundback JH, Jacobs JM. Percutaneous renal artery stent placement for hypertension and azotemia: pilot study. *Am J Kidney Dis* 1996;28:214.
616. Henry M, Amor M, Henry I, et al. Stent placement in the renal artery: three-year experience with the Palmaz stent. *J Vasc Intervent Radiol* 1996;7:343.
617. Blum U, Krumme B, Flugel P, et al. Treatment of ostial renal-artery stenoses with vascular endoprostheses after unsuccessful balloon angioplasty. *N Engl J Med* 1997;336:459.
618. Boisclair C, Therasse E, Oliva VL, et al. Treatment of renal angioplasty failure by percutaneous renal artery stenting with Palmaz stents: midterm technical and clinical results. *AJR Am J Roentgenol* 1997;168:245.
619. Harden PN, MacLeod MJ, Rodger RS, et al. Effect of renal-artery stenting on progression of renovascular renal failure. *Lancet* 1997;349:1133.

CHAPTER 53 ■ HYPERTENSION AND PREGNANCY

VERENA A. BRINER, MELISSA A. CADNAPAPHORNCHAI, AND ROBERT W. SCHRIER

In the Western world, hypertension, preeclampsia, and eclampsia are the most common causes of morbidity and mortality in the mother (1,2) and child (3). This chapter presents an overview of

- Physiologic changes in renal hemodynamics, blood pressure, and water metabolism in normal pregnancy
- Hypertensive disorders in pregnancy
- Pathophysiologic mechanisms in pregnancy-induced hypertension and preeclampsia and eclampsia
- Management of hypertensive disorders in pregnancy

PHYSIOLOGIC CHANGES IN SYSTEMIC AND RENAL HEMODYNAMICS AND WATER METABOLISM IN NORMAL PREGNANCY

Changes in Systemic Hemodynamics

Normal pregnancy is characterized by decreased systemic vascular resistance with decreased mean arterial pressure and increased cardiac output. In pregnant women, alterations in systemic hemodynamics are detectable by 6 weeks of gestation (4,5) (Figs. 53-1, 53-2). A decrease in peripheral vascular resistance occurs prior to blood volume expansion, thus supporting the conclusion that arterial vasodilation is the primary event and both the increase in cardiac output and volume expansion are secondary events (6) (Fig. 53-3). There are several mediators that may cause the early peripheral vasodilation in pregnancy. The plasma concentration of the vasodilating prostacyclin (PGI_2) and urinary excretion of its major metabolites are increased in pregnancy (7,8). Several hormones known to relax vascular smooth muscle such as estrogens, progesterone, and prolactin are increased in pregnancy; however, their administration does not cause hypotension. The mature placenta may act as an arteriovenous fistula. However, early in pregnancy when the vascular resistance falls and reaches the nadir, blood flow in the placenta and uterus is still rather small. Another vasodilating substance, is nitric oxide (NO). NO is a potent relaxant of vascular smooth muscle cells and also stimulates vasodilation in the presence of vasoconstricting peptides (9). In pregnant rats, plasma levels of NO (10,11) and plasma levels and urinary excretion of the second messenger of NO, cyclic guanosine monophosphate (cGMP), are increased (12–14). Upregulation of endothelial NO synthase in the resistance vessel has been documented in animal pregnancies (15). The physiologic decrease in blood pressure in pregnant spontaneously hypertensive rats has been shown to depend completely on NO release (16). The production of cGMP may result from stimu-lation of guanylate cyclase by NO but also by cytokines such as tumor necrosis factor-α (TNF-α).

Changes in Renal Hemodynamics

There are considerable alterations in renal hemodynamics during pregnancy. Some of these reflect cardiovascular changes such as peripheral vasodilation and an increase in cardiac output (4,5). An increase in fluid volumes and endocrine changes also occur. Renal blood flow (RBF) increases progressively until it peaks in the second trimester at about 180% of the preconception value (4,5,17–19). In parallel, glomerular filtration rate (GFR) rises beginning 4 weeks after conception (Fig. 53-1). Creatinine clearance is enhanced by about 50% in the first trimester and remains elevated until the last month of gestation (20,21). There is little change in creatinine production during pregnancy; therefore, changes in creatinine clearance result in a fall in plasma levels of creatinine on average to about 0.45 mg/dL as compared to 0.67 mg/dL in nonpregnant controls (22). Studies in rats suggest that the pregnancy-associated increase in GFR is due solely to renal vasodilation, with parallel relaxation of afferent and efferent arteriolar resistance leading to increased renal plasma flow (RPF) without change in glomerular blood pressure (23). The potent vasodilator responsible for the rise in GFR by 30% to 50% during pregnancy is not yet known. However, a major contribution to the increase in GFR may derive from enhanced NO production during pregnancy (24). Studies in rats demonstrate a reversal of glomerular hyperfiltration and renal vasodilation in pregnant rats during chronic inhibition of NO synthase (11).

After delivery, GFR returns to the pregestation range (18). Neither volume expansion, high-protein diet, nor unilateral nephrectomy has been shown to enhance GFR to the same level as occurs with pregnancy. Due to a lesser increase in GFR as compared to RBF, filtration fraction falls in early pregnancy. However, RBF decreases in the last weeks of gestation, and filtration fraction may rise. In pregnant rats with glomerulonephritis and superimposed pregnancy, GFR also increases (25). Pregnancy-induced changes in RBF and GFR also occur in women with hypertrophied single kidneys or transplant recipients (26,27) but may be attenuated in women with underlying renal insufficiency. In a study by Cunningham et al. only 50% of women with moderate and none of the women with severe chronic renal disease demonstrated any increase in GFR during pregnancy (28).

Urinary protein excretion may be increased in normal pregnancy to the upper limit of 300 mg/24 hours (29). The majority of normal pregnant women, however, will have a protein excretion of less than 150 mg/24 hours. Albumin excretion in nonpregnant women is less than 40 mg/24 hours. A rise in the ratio of urinary albumin to creatinine may demonstrate impaired glomerular permeability (30). This ratio method is accurate and avoids 24-hour urine collections.

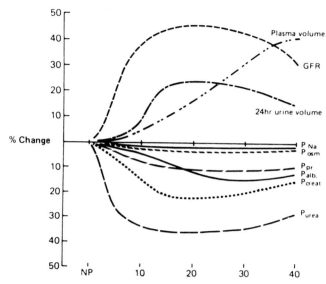

FIGURE 53-1. Physiologic hemodynamic and biochemical changes induced by pregnancy beginning at the nonpregnant (NP) state and through 40 weeks of pregnancy. In pregnant women, glomerular filtration rate (GFR) rises before blood volume expansion occurs. Increments and decrements of the various parameters are shown in percentage terms with reference to nonpregnant state. *GFR*, glomerular filtration rate; P_{alb}, plasma albumin; P_{creat}, plasma creatinine; P_{Na}, plasma sodium; P_{osm}, plasma osmolality; P_{pr}, plasma protein; P_{urea}, plasma urea. (From: Davison JM. Renal hemodynamics and volume homeostasis in pregnancy. *Scand J Clin Lab Invest* 1984;169(Suppl):15, with permission.)

Changes in Sodium and Water Homeostasis

Volume expansion is extraordinary during pregnancy and results in a total body water increase by 6 to 8 L (31). The mean plasma volume in pregnancy increases progressively from conception to term by almost 50% (32) (Fig. 53-1). The mechanism controlling volume expansion is poorly understood, but sodium retention is an important factor. An increase in GFR augments the filtered load of fluid and electrolytes; therefore, changes in tubular function are required to prevent urinary loss of these substances in the glomerular filtrate (33). The filtered sodium load increases from 20,000 to 30,000 mmol/day; however, due to increased sodium reabsorption in the proximal and distal renal tubules, sodium depletion is prevented. In fact, sodium retention during pregnancy totals nearly 1,000 mEq (32). This sodium retention may be induced or enhanced by estrogens, deoxycorticosterone, and aldosterone (33). It has been suggested that the increased aldosterone production in pregnancy exceeds the physiologic requirements. In nonpregnant humans, the continued administration of mineralocorticoids causes sodium retention of about 400 mEq of sodium; however, despite continuation of the hormone administration, no further sodium retention occurs. An adaptive mechanism known as mineralocorticoid escape thus prevents excessive sodium retention. Although basal plasma concentrations of aldosterone are high in pregnancy, changes in sodium intake, administration of diuretics, and changes in postural position lead to a similar pattern of changes in aldosterone production and plasma levels as occurs in normal nonpregnant humans (34). Thus, despite high levels of plasma aldosterone, adaptive mechanisms to various stimuli are qualitatively preserved in pregnancy.

Plasma osmolality decreases at 1 month after conception and plateaus at 10 to 12 weeks of pregnancy to levels about

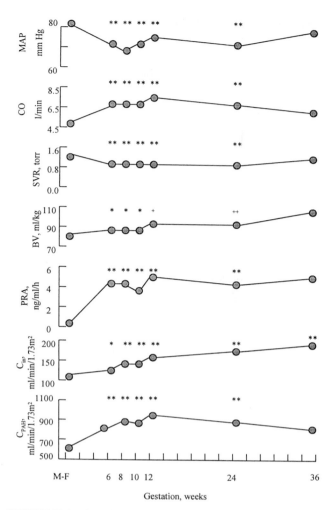

FIGURE 53-2. Physiologic hemodynamic alterations induced by pregnancy in women beginning at the midfollicular (M-F) phase of the menstrual cycle and through 36 weeks' pregnancy. Decreased mean arterial pressure (*MAP*), systemic vascular resistance (*SVR*), increased cardiac output (*CO*), blood volume (*BV*), plasma renin activity (*PRA*), inulin clearance (C_{in}), and paraaminohippurate clearance (C_{PAH}) are detectable by 6 weeks of gestation. $*p < 0.05$, $**p < 0.001$, $+p < 0.0001$. (From: Chapman AB, et al. Temporal relationships between hormonal and hemodynamic changes in early human pregnancy. *Kidney Int* 1998;54:2056, with permission.)

10 mOsm/kg below normal (35). Normally, a decrease of osmolality of this degree would cause inhibition of arginine vasopressin (AVP) secretion and a water diuresis. However, studies suggest that plasma AVP concentrations are either normal or increased in pregnancy as compared to nonpregnant controls (15,36). Furthermore, metabolic clearance of AVP in rats is increased in mid- to late pregnancy (37), coinciding with increased trophoblastic mass and hence increased levels of placental and plasma vasopressinase. Although once thought to be an *in vitro* phenomenon, abnormally high circulating vasopressinase activity can produce diabetes insipidus in human pregnancy (38).

Previous reports suggested that the threshold for vasopressin secretion and thirst is decreased in normal pregnancy and corresponds to the decrease in osmolality (39) (Fig. 53-4). Thus, gravidas maintain their new plasma osmolality, and neither fluid loading nor fluid restriction alters this "reset" osmolality. More recent results, however, suggest that pregnancy

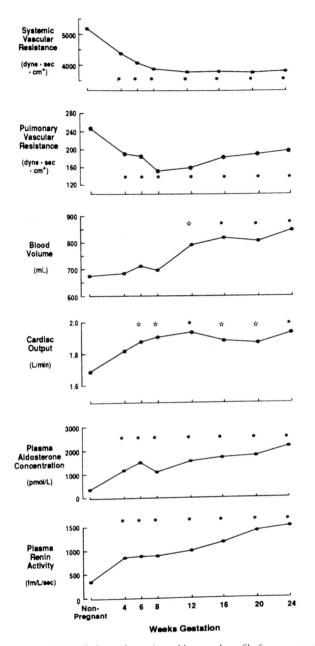

FIGURE 53-3. Early hemodynamic and humoral profile for pregnant baboons. A significant rise in cardiac output, plasma renin activity, and plasma aldosterone concentration occurs at 4 to 6 weeks of pregnancy and parallels a decrease in pulmonary and systemic vascular resistance. (From: Phippard AF, et al. Circulation adaptation to pregnancy: serial studies of hemodynamics, blood volume, renin and aldosterone in the baboon. *J Hypertens* 1986;4:773, with permission.)

is associated with increased expression of collecting duct aquaporin-2 water channels (36). As described in the "shuttle hypothesis" (40), circulating vasopressin binds to its V$_2$ receptor on the basolateral membrane of the principal cell of the renal collecting duct. This initiates cyclic adenosine monophosphate-mediated and protein kinase-mediated translocation of AQP2 water channels from cytosolic storage vesicles to the apical membrane, thus allowing reabsorption of water to occur. Upregulation of AQP2 water channels is evident in the first trimester of rat pregnancy and persists throughout pregnancy in association with hypoosmolality (36). Thus vasopressin re-

lease and AQP2 mediated with retention can explain the hypoosmolality of pregnancy.

Injection of estrogen or progesterone has failed to reduce plasma osmolality in nonpregnant rats (41). Although chronic NO synthase inhibition in pregnant rats returns systemic and renal hemodynamics to nonpregnant levels, hypoosmolality is maintained due to increased thirst (11). Alternatively, prolactin injection into rats (42) and human chorionic gonadotropin injection into nonpregnant women (but not men) may reduce the osmotic threshold (43). Although prolactin production is enhanced during lactation, serum osmolality increases after delivery in lactating mothers, suggesting little contribution to the reset osmolality of this hormone during pregnancy. In molar pregnancies, plasma osmolality and the threshold level for the release of vasopressin is reduced as long as human chorionic gonadotropin is increased (43). As noted previously, plasma osmolality may also be affected by changes in the metabolism of vasopressin (37,38).

Hormonal Changes in Pregnancy

Plasma concentrations of a number of hormones change substantially during pregnancy. Some of these hormones have effects on the kidney and the blood vessels to modulate hemodynamics. No individual hormone, however, is known to cause hemodynamic changes as large as those seen during pregnancy. In this section, we will discuss some of the hormones with rising blood concentrations during pregnancy that may contribute to the complex and diverse changes in salt and water homeostasis and hemodynamics associated with gestation.

Renin-Angiotensin-Aldosterone System

The renin-angiotensin-aldosterone (RAA) system has direct effects on vascular tone, and by causing sodium retention, may also increase plasma volume. The RAA system is stimulated in pregnancy, and most likely this is secondary to the peripheral arterial vasodilation (Fig. 53-3). Plasma renin concentration, renin substrate, and angiotensin II are increased throughout pregnancy, reaching peak levels close to term (44). In spite of increased angiotensin II levels, blood pressure declines during pregnancy. Vascular insensitivity to angiotensin II during normal pregnancy is maximal in the second trimester (45) (Fig. 53-5). Part of this loss of the vascular effect of angiotensin II may be the result of a decrease in angiotensin II receptors (46). In studies of pregnant baboons, the blood volume expansion occurs after stimulation of the RAA axis (6) (Fig. 53-3). If the blood volume expansion were primary, rather than secondary to the arterial vasodilation, suppression, not stimulation, of the RAA system would be expected. Basal renin substrate and plasma renin are both enhanced during pregnancy; these effects cannot be demonstrated in nonpregnant patients treated with progesterone and estrogens (47). Renin is produced in uteroplacental tissue (48), and that renin is indistinguishable from that found in the kidney. A role of uteroplacental renin in modulating uterine blood flow has been suggested (49). The administration of saralasin, an angiotensin II antagonist, or captopril, an angiotensin converting enzyme (ACE) inhibitor, attenuates uterine blood flow (50,51). The regulation of the RAA system in normal pregnancy, although it is activated, remains under similar control mechanisms as in the nonpregnant state, with activation and suppression occurring with sodium depletion and sodium loading, respectively (52).

As noted earlier, in normal pregnancy, vascular tone and blood pressure are resistant to an average dose of angiotensin II infusion (53) (Fig. 53-5). This angiotensin II refractoriness may be the result of mechanisms involving several intracellular pathways in vascular smooth muscle. The increase in prostacyclin

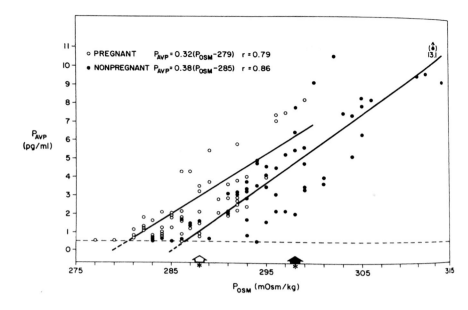

FIGURE 53-4. Relationship between plasma osmolality (P_{OSM}) and plasma vasopressin (P_{AVP}) during a 2-hour infusion of 5% saline in first trimester pregnant women (*open circles*) and 6 to 8 weeks' postpartum. The *arrow* indicates the thirst threshold, which is reduced during pregnancy. (From: Davison JM, et al. Altered osmotic threshold for vasopressin secretion and thirst in human pregnancies. *Am J Physiol* 1984;246:F105, with permission.)

concentrations during pregnancy stimulates adenylate cyclase to produce cyclic adenosine monophosphate (cAMP). An increase in cAMP attenuates the intracellular signaling of pressor hormones in vascular smooth muscle and inhibits vasoconstriction. The administration of a low dose of aspirin to block the production of the vasoconstricting prostaglandin thromboxane A_2 enhances the effects of prostacyclin and thus lessens angiotensin II-induced rise in blood pressure (54). In contrast, a dose of aspirin that also blocks prostacyclin production enhances the pressor effects of angiotensin II (54). Another cyclic nucleotide, cGMP, has effects similar to cAMP in smooth muscle. Plasma levels and urinary excretion of cGMP have been reported to be elevated or unchanged during pregnancy (12–14,55). There are also data to support the view that NO, a major stimulator of cGMP production, participates significantly in vasodilation in pregnancy. The peripheral arterial vasodilation during pregnancy stimulates the RAA system in a compensatory manner and thus explains why blood levels of renin, angiotensin, and aldosterone are elevated despite volume expansion during normal pregnancy. The rise in plasma aldosterone may counterbalance the increased amount of urinary sodium reaching the distal tubules as a result of the profound rise in GFR during pregnancy (56). Aldosterone thus may prevent excessive sodium loss and volume depletion during pregnancy. In addition to the RAA system, progesterone has also been shown to enhance aldosterone excretion (57). In nonpregnant humans, the administration of mineralocorticoids induces sodium retention with resultant water retention and a weight gain of about 2 to 3 kg. Continuation of the mineralocorticoid treatment does not cause any further sodium and water retention. This phenomenon is called the "mineralocorticoid escape" mechanism. As noted earlier, in spite of the increased basal concentration of aldosterone in pregnancy, there is a rise in plasma aldosterone levels in response to sodium restriction (58). These observations suggest a new set point in the RAA system during pregnancy. Plasma levels of the potent mineralocorticoid deoxycorticosterone also increase in pregnancy (59). It is suggested that this increment results mainly from the hydroxylation of progesterone (60).

Progesterone, Estriol, and Prolactin

Plasma progesterone, estriol, and prolactin concentrations markedly increase during pregnancy (61). The effects of progesterone are not restricted to the uteroplacental tissue. Progesterone and prolactin may both contribute to the rise in GFR during pregnancy (42,62). Independent of pregnancy, progesterone causes a natriuresis by a mechanism that in part is independent of the inhibition of aldosterone-induced sodium retention (63). Estrogen replacement therapy has been shown to promote vasodilation by decreasing plasma concentrations of renin (64), ACE (65), and endothelin-1 (66) and by increasing the ratio of NO to endothelin-1 (67). Vascular tone is most reduced during pregnancy when the concentrations of estrogen and progesterone are the highest (68). There is evidence that estrogens modulate NO during pregnancy. Pregnancy and estradiol administration cause an increase in the activity of calcium-dependent NO synthase in uterine artery and also in other tissues such as the kidney in guinea pigs (69). It has recently been suggested that estrogen mediates this effect via a mitogen-activated protein (MAP) kinase mechanism (70).

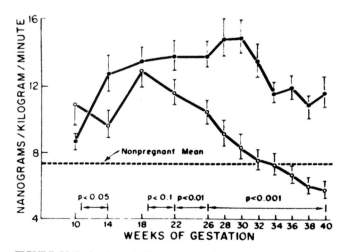

FIGURE 53-5. Angiotensin II response in 192 primigravidas. *Closed circles* demonstrate reduced sensitivity to angiotensin II and requirement of a greater dose to enhance diastolic blood pressure by 20 mm Hg compared with nonpregnant controls. *Open circles* demonstrate rising sensitivity to angiotensin II in women who develop pregnancy-induced hypertension. (From: Gant NF, et al. A study of angiotensin II pressor response throughout primigravid pregnancy. *J Clin Invest* 1973;52:2682, with permission.)

Calcium-independent NO synthase is not altered by pregnancy or female sex hormones. Progesterone does not significantly increase NO synthase (71). NO is therefore a vasodilator that has the potential to decrease vascular resistance, modulate renal hemodynamics (72), and antagonize vasoconstrictor-mediated smooth muscle cell contraction (73) in pregnancy.

Relaxin

There are several lines of evidence implicating the peptide hormone relaxin in the regulation of the altered renal hemodynamics and water metabolism in pregnancy (74). Relaxin is composed of two peptide chains that are connected by two interchain disulfide bonds, resembling the structure of insulin. Production of relaxin occurs in the corpus luteum of the ovary, the placenta, and the endometrium under the stimulation of human chorionic gonadotropin. Blood levels of relaxin rise in the first trimester of pregnancy (75), coincident with the pregnancy-associated rise in GFR and RPF. Circulating relaxin concentrations are also increased in the luteal phase of the menstrual cycle, when there is a transient 20% increase in GFR and RPF (76). Chronic administration of relaxin to nonpregnant rats results in elevations in GFR and RPF similar to the pregnant state (77); these effects appear to be mediated via NO. Moreover, relaxin administration in animals attenuates the renal vasoconstrictor response to angiotensin II infusion (77). Relaxin administration also increases water intake, reduces plasma osmolality, and alters the threshold for vasopressin release in rats (77,78). There seems to be an essential role of gelatinase in the relaxin-mediated renal effects of pregnancy and it is involved in the endothelial ET_B–NO pathway (79).

Endothelin 1

Endothelin-1 (ET-1) is an endothelium-derived peptide which acts as a potent vasoconstrictor through direct effects and via stimulation of the RAA and the sympathetic nervous system (reviewed in reference 80). ET-1 has complex effects on vascular tone. Although endothelin induces vasoconstriction in vascular smooth muscle cells via activation of ET_A receptors, activation of endothelial ET_B receptors is associated with transient hypotension and increased NO synthesis (81). Several studies have suggested a role for ET-1 in the regulation of blood pressure, renal and spiral artery hemodynamics in pregnancy. Urinary ET-1 excretion has been shown to be elevated in pregnancy (82). ET_B receptor antagonism produced a significant decrease in both GFR and RPF in pregnant rats (83). The magnitude of decline was greater in pregnant as compared to nonpregnant rats, suggesting a role for ET_B receptor activation in the maintenance of pregnancy-associated GFR and RPF elevations. Moreover, concomitant NO inhibition did not further decrease renal hemodynamics, implicating NO as a mediator of ET-1 action.

Adrenomedullin

Adrenomedullin is a 52-amino acid peptide that produces natriuresis and blood pressure reduction. Its concentration rises as pregnancy proceeds (84). Although adrenomedullin levels did not differ in preeclamptic patients, levels in the amniotic fluid and blood of the umbilical vein were several fold higher in eclampsia than in controls (85).

Pregnancy and Changes in Glucose Tolerance

Physiologic changes of the metabolic environment initially favor maternal fat deposition, and later fetal growth. By the eighth week of pregnancy, the fasting blood glucose level falls and reaches its nadir around the twelfth week. Postprandial blood glucose level rises to peak at around 30 weeks of ges-

tation. Fasting insulin level rises during pregnancy as does glucose-stimulated insulin secretion. Insulin sensitivity is reduced by about 50% during normal pregnancy while insulin requirement rises about threefold. This metabolic change is most prominent in the second and third trimester and resembles changes comparable to that in noninsulin-dependent diabetes mellitus. Insulin resistance in pregnancy appears to resolve immediately after delivery (86). Sex hormone binding globulin (SHBG) is a glycoprotein synthesized by the liver and binds circulating estrogens. Insulin inhibits the production of SHBG and therefore has been shown to be a marker of hyperinsulinemia and insulin resistance (87). Compared with controls, women who develops preeclampsia had significantly reduced first trimester SHBG levels (88). In addition, for every 100 nmol/L increase in SHBG there was a 31% reduction of the risk of preeclampsia (p <0.01). The independent association between SHBG levels and preeclampsia was seen in lean women, suggesting that in obesity SHBG is only one of the several contributing factors.

Insulin resistance leads to a variety of biochemical abnormalities. The capacity of the pancreatic β cells is important for compensation of impaired insulin sensitivity. About 5% of pregnancies are complicated by an abnormal glucose tolerance test and less than 5% of these develop gestational diabetes mellitus (89). Gestational diabetes is a harbinger of subsequent noninsulin-dependent type II diabetes mellitus (90), and type II is associated with a high rate of essential hypertension (91). Furthermore, it has been shown that pregnancy-induced hypertension and preeclampsia are more common in the presence of gestational diabetes (92). Even within the normal range, the level of plasma glucose elevation 1 hour following an oral glucose challenge is correlated with risk of preeclampsia (92). Hyperleptinemia has been suggested to play a role in insulin resistance. In pregnant women, leptin is synthesized in and secreted from placental trophoblasts into the maternal circulation at a considerable amount, with increases of 100% to 200% over prepregnancy values. Patients with preeclampsia exhibit serum leptin levels which are significantly higher than those of normal pregnant controls (93). Increased serum leptin concentration may be a marker of placental hypoxia in severe preeclampsia (94). TNF-α is another marker for insulin resistance (95) and circulating TNF-α levels correlate with microvascular permeability in preeclampsia (96). If evidence accumulates that pregnancy-induced hypertension and preeclampsia are at least partially mediated by insulin resistance, there may be a possibility to intervene with agents that enhance insulin sensitivity.

HYPERTENSIVE DISORDERS IN PREGNANCY

To understand gestational hypertension, it is important to know the physiologic changes in hemodynamics and blood pressure that occur during normal pregnancy. Soon after conception and during the first trimester of pregnancy, blood pressure decreases significantly despite increased plasma concentrations of angiotensin II. Decrements in diastolic blood pressure are in the range of 10 mm Hg (97). Women who are hypertensive before conception may demonstrate an even greater decrease in blood pressure (98). Subsequently in the second and third trimesters, blood pressure rises to reach near pregestation values at term (99). Thus, the definition of normal range of blood pressure differs in the pregnant from the nonpregnant state. The World Health Organization (100) classified hypertensive disorders of pregnancy in 1987 in a detailed manner, while the American College of Obstetricians and Gynecologists (101) and the National High Blood Pressure Education

Program Working Group (102) classified them in a more practical fashion and defined only four categories:

1. Chronic hypertension
2. Transient hypertension was changed to gestational hypertension in 2000 (102)
3. Preeclampsia and eclampsia
4. Preeclampsia and eclampsia superimposed on chronic hypertension

It is important to differentiate between these four disorders because prognosis and treatment vary. Despite the different classification of hypertensive disorders in pregnancy, hypertensive levels of blood pressure and increase in blood pressure thought to be critical for the development of preeclampsia are similar, namely systolic blood pressure $\geq$140 mm Hg and diastolic blood pressure $\geq$90 mm Hg, a rise in systolic blood pressure by $\geq$30 mm Hg or diastolic by $\geq$15 mm Hg. Early in pregnancy, blood pressure declines, with average values of 103 ± 11 mm Hg systolic and 56 ± 10 mm Hg diastolic in the first trimester (103); thus, before 20 weeks of gestation, a significant rise in blood pressure may still remain below designated preeclamptic levels and yet cause preeclampsia, especially when the increase in blood pressure occurs rapidly. A significant rise in blood pressure, especially in primiparas, is a suspicious sign of preeclampsia, and hospitalization should be considered. Although it may be difficult to make the diagnosis, overdiagnosing rather than underdiagnosing preeclampsia is preferred because the development of preeclampsia may be rapid and fulminant.

It may be very difficult to distinguish clinically between essential hypertension, secondary hypertension due to kidney disease, and pregnancy-induced hypertension or preeclampsia and combinations of these disorders. Preexisting hypertension may be suggested by microvascular changes in the retina. Preexisting renal disease may be suggested in women demonstrating reduced kidney size or proteinuria occurring without hypertension or occurring very early in pregnancy. However, glomerular diseases may occur in more than 20% of primipara pregnancies presenting with hypertension (104). Acceleration of renal diseases typically occurs during pregnancy in active lupus erythematosus. Pregnancy-associated changes in the thymus (105) and B-cell lymphopoiesis (106) may modulate autoantibody production and contribute to the flares observed in pregnant lupus patients.

Chronic Hypertension

Women with chronic hypertension have elevated blood pressures ($\geq$140/90 mm Hg) prior to pregnancy. Hypertension is usually well tolerated when diastolic blood pressure remains less than 100 mm Hg (102). In general, antihypertensive therapy should be continued during pregnancy. When hypertension is diagnosed during pregnancy and persists for more than 42 days after delivery, it is also termed chronic hypertension (102). Some drugs may have side effects that may require a change in medication during pregnancy. There may exist an underlying secondary cause for the hypertension such as renal parenchymal or renal vascular disease, hypercorticism, or hyperaldosteronism; however, the presence of primary essential hypertension is not unusual. Patients with preexisting hypertension demonstrate a decrease in blood pressure early in pregnancy to a similar or even greater degree than normotensive women (107). In the third trimester, blood pressure rises to levels approximating the nonpregnant state. If uric acid and antithrombin III levels (108) are normal in this state, it is likely that the patient still has chronic hypertension; thus weekly reexamination is indicated. Chronic hypertension is associated with adverse pregnancy outcome, regardless of superimposed

preeclampsia. It predisposes to preeclampsia by about a fivefold risk and small-for-gestational age babies by about a twofold risk (109,110). The risk for perinatal death also increases (111). Furthermore, women with chronic hypertension and proteinuria greater than 300 mg/24 hours before 26 weeks of gestation have a threefold increased risk of preterm delivery and small-for-gestational age babies as compared to women with chronic hypertension and no proteinuria (112). Chronically hypertensive African American women are more likely to develop preeclampsia (ca. 32%) than white women (ca. 15%)(113).

If blood pressure rises further in the third trimester and proteinuria and edema develop, it is suggestive of superimposed preeclampsia. The mechanism of inducing superimposed preeclampsia in women with chronic hypertension is not well known. Hypertension-induced vascular lesions and subsequent impairment of hemodynamics in the spiral arteries of the decidua and reduction of the perfusion of the uterus may result.

Gestational Hypertension

There are some women who demonstrate a mild to moderate rise in blood pressure to the hypertensive range in the third trimester, but without developing edema or proteinuria. This form of hypertension does not carry the perinatal and maternal morbidity of preeclampsia and does not progress to preeclampsia. Blood pressure normalizes within the first few days postpartum. Gestational hypertension has a high rate of recurrence in subsequent pregnancies (114,115), and it is believed that women of this group may develop essential hypertension later in life (116).

Preeclampsia and Eclampsia—Clinical Aspects

The syndrome of preeclampsia/eclampsia was recognized more than 100 years ago, when convulsions that occurred late in pregnancy and disappeared after delivery were reported. Later it was recognized that proteinuria and increased blood pressure frequently antedated these seizures associated with pregnancy (117). Circadian blood pressure measurements revealed a changing pattern in eclampsia demonstrating the highest pressure at midnight (118). Thus, it was suggested to classify this syndrome on arbitrary grounds of blood pressure levels and on the presence of proteinuria. It was hoped that these clinical criteria would allow recognition early in pregnancy of the group of women prone to subsequently develop preeclampsia and pregnancy-induced convulsion. However, although dramatically increased blood pressures may occur in women who progress to have convulsions, evaluation of blood pressure is only one component of the pathophysiology of eclampsia. For example, as many as 20% of pregnant women with eclampsia have blood pressure levels below 140/90 mm Hg just prior to the onset of convulsions (119,120), and up to 40% have little or no proteinuria (121). In 201 pregnant women, the blood pressure was measured within 1 hour of the onset of convulsion, and the mean diastolic pressure was 97 ± 14.6 mm Hg (119,122).

The diagnosis of preeclampsia is now based on criteria suggested by Chesley (123) and the National High Blood Pressure Education Program Working Group (102). These include: (1) proteinuria of $\geq$300 mg/day and often in the nephrotic range (124) associated with puffy edema; and (2) a rise in blood pressure of at least 15 mm Hg diastolic, 30 mm Hg systolic, or an increased mean blood pressure level of 20 mm Hg as compared to the levels before 20 weeks of pregnancy. In the absence of previous blood pressure measurements, blood pressure $\geq$140/90 mm Hg after 20 weeks of gestation is considered sufficient to fulfill the blood pressure criteria of preeclampsia (102). More recently, Redman and Jeffries (125) suggested that in addition to this rise in blood pressure, the diastolic blood pressure level first has to be less than 90 mm Hg. With this selection criterion, patients with chronic or essential hypertension could be excluded from those with real preeclampsia. A modest amount of edema develops very frequently in pregnancy; however, some women destined to develop preeclampsia may rapidly gain several kilograms before developing the critical stigmata of preeclampsia (126). Although nephrotic proteinuria in preeclampsia is associated with more severe lesions in the biopsy specimen, nephrotic proteinuria does not correlate with the severity of clinical findings when compared to preeclamptic women with proteinuria less than 3 g/day (104). Although the clinical features of preeclampsia and eclampsia are similar to the characteristics of malignant hypertension, there is usually no papilledema or retinal hemorrhages and no malignant nephrosclerosis in eclampsia. Thus, eclampsia is not pregnancy-induced malignant hypertension. The blood pressure level does not correlate as well with perinatal mortality as does the elevated uric acid concentration (127) and activation of the coagulation cascade (128). Thus, classification of preeclampsia on blood pressure alone may overemphasize the importance of hypertension in the pathophysiology and result in mismanagement of those women with preeclampsia without hypertension. There are no strict values and parameters for detecting women at risk of developing preeclampsia and eclampsia. There are, however, some rules of thumb that may be helpful. Patients with a significant rise in blood pressure, occurrence of proteinuria, or nausea and abdominal pain (129) or having headaches and feeling ill during the second trimester should be considered as developing preeclampsia. Patients with blood pressure ≥140/90 mm Hg and the new occurrence of proteinuria of 1+ or greater require hospitalization (1120).

Preeclamptic women may demonstrate abnormal left ventricular function (130), and visual disturbances such as blurred vision, scotomata, amaurosis, and cortical blindness also may occur (131). Pregnant women are at increased risk of thromboembolic accidents due to changes in the fibrinolytic activity and coagulation factors (132). All cases of perinatal death associated with preeclampsia/eclampsia have abnormal intravascular coagulation abnormalities suggesting activation of the coagulation cascade (128). Mild thrombocytopenia is the most commonly found hematologic disturbance associated with preeclampsia (133), and it often antedates the clinical disease (134). Bone marrow studies in women with preeclampsia show that increased peripheral consumption and platelet turnover cause the decreased number of circulating platelets (133). Platelets from humans with essential hypertension (135) or women with preeclampsia show an exaggerated calcium response to vasopressin (136). The activation and impaired calcium response of platelets antedate the increased vascular sensitivity of preeclampsia. In contrast to the vasopressin response, adenosine diphosphate-induced and serotonin-induced calcium rise in platelets is reduced in preeclampsia (137). A decrease of platelets below 100×10^9/L is an ominous sign (138) (Table 53-1) and is a cause for hospitalization.

Activation of the coagulation cascade and vasospasm are consistent early findings in preeclampsia and may cause reduced organ perfusion. Furthermore, fibrin thrombi are demonstrated in glomerulus (139), cerebral (140) and hepatic (141) capillaries of women suffering from eclampsia, and these thrombi may contribute to the impairment of microcirculation in the presence of enhanced vasoconstriction (142). Depending on the severity of occlusion of capillary lumens, renal, cerebral, or hepatic manifestations of eclampsia may dominate. At autopsy, severe cases of preeclampsia/eclampsia demonstrate features of disseminated intravascular coagulation (DIC). An increased level of fibrin degradation products (143) *in vivo* is

TABLE 53-1

OMINOUS SIGNS OF PREECLAMPSIA

Blood pressure ≥160 mm Hg systolic, ≥90 mm Hg diastolic
Proteinuria (occurrence for the first time) ≥2 g/24 hr
Serum creatinine (normal before pregnancy) ≥1.2 mg/dL
Platelet count ≤100,000/μL
Microangiopathic hemolytic anemia (haptoglobin ↓, schistocytes)
Liver enzymes ↑
Headache
Cerebral disturbances
Visual disturbances
Pulmonary edema
Epigastric pain

(From: National High Blood Pressure Education Program Working Group Report on High Blood Pressure in Pregnancy. *Am J Obstet Gynecol* 1990;163:1691, with permission.)

another sign of this coagulation disorder. By using sensitive assays, activation of the coagulation cascade can be demonstrated weeks to months before the clinical symptoms occur (144). A coagulation index based on the platelet count, factor VIII concentration, and serum fibrinolytic degradation products has been shown to correlate with the signs and symptoms of preeclampsia and also with perinatal death (128). Thrombocytopenia can occur weeks before clinical symptoms of preeclampsia and eclampsia are present (138) and even when there is no liver involvement (145). Spasm of the retinal arterioles is another prominent feature in patients with preeclampsia (146). The severity of spasm of retinal arteries correlates with the severity of glomerular lesions seen in kidney biopsies (146) (Fig. 53-6) and also with the occurrence of preeclampsia. Despite the capillary obstructions, intravascular coagulation is not necessarily the primary event that induces preeclampsia; however, DIC may be a major factor contributing to the impairment of organ perfusion and function.

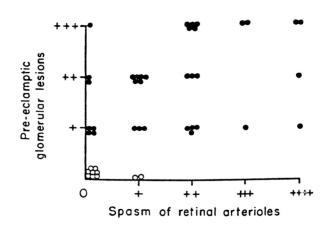

FIGURE 53-6. Funduscopic evaluation of retinal blood vessels demonstrates correlation of severity of spasm of retinal vessels and severity of preeclampsia-associated glomerular endotheliosis in kidney biopsies. Severe retinal arteriolar spasm was only seen in women with preeclampsia (*closed circles*) but not in hypertensive vascular disease (*open circles*). (From: Pollak VE, Nettles JB. The kidney in toxemia of pregnancy: a clinical and pathologic study based on renal biopsies. *Medicine* 1960;39:469, with permission.)

Genetic Factors Predisposing to the Development of Preeclampsia and Eclampsia

Genetic factors may predispose to the development of preeclampsia and eclampsia. Epidemiologic data suggest a familial tendency to preeclampsia (147). An analysis of the family history of patients with eclampsia demonstrated a fivefold increased risk in first-degree relatives and a twofold increased risk in second-degree relatives as compared to the general population (148). Chesley (149) suggests the existence of an autosomal-recessive gene defect that predisposes to preeclampsia. Studies of 26 Icelandic and 18 Australian families with a high rate of miscarriages, specifically 22 cases of eclampsia and 116 cases of preeclampsia, suggest that a dominant gene defect with low penetrance may be involved (150,151). A genome-wide scan of 72 Icelandic families, including 186 women with preeclampsia or eclampsia, suggests a maternal susceptibility locus for preeclampsia on chromosome 2p13 (152). In contrast, no linkage is found with angiotensinogen or endothelial NO synthase genes. Retrospective analysis of the records of 14 primigravidas giving birth to babies with trisomy 13 all demonstrated severe preeclampsia (153). In contrast, the first pregnancy was normal when the baby had trisomy 18 or trisomy 21. This may suggest a role for chromosome 13 in preeclampsia.

Incidence of Preeclampsia and Eclampsia

The incidence of eclampsia is quite similar in Western countries. In Great Britain, it is 4.9 per 10,000 pregnancies but may occur in up to 10% of primigravidas (119). In the United States, the incidence of eclampsia is 4.3 per 10,000 pregnancies (154). Analysis of regional incidences suggests that there has been a decline in incidence since introducing antihypertensive treatment. However, since then, no significant further decrease in incidence of eclampsia has occurred in the past 20 to 30 years (119,155,156). Douglas and Redman (119), Corkill (155), and Hibbard and Rosen (157) suggest that classic eclampsia presenting with high blood pressure and proteinuria may be prevented by screening and antenatal control. However, atypical presentation of eclampsia still has an unchanged incidence. In this regard, it is important to note that one-third of women have only mild or no hypertension before the onset of eclampsia, and therefore the diagnosis and treatment may be delayed. The incidence of preeclampsia is highest in primigravidas (156), especially in primigravidas older than 40 years (158) or younger than 20 years (98). Twin pregnancy increases the risk about five times (159). Women with preexisting hypertension (121); microangiopathy, such as diabetic angiopathy; moderate renal insufficiency due to pregestational renal disease (160); and patients who have had preeclampsia with proteinuria are at risk to develop preeclampsia (161) (Table 53-2).

Two-thirds of cases of eclampsia develop in women with the first pregnancy. In a multicenter study in Great Britain, 383 pregnancies were complicated by eclampsia, and 18% of cases were multiparous women with no previous history of preeclampsia (119). Eclampsia has not only been documented to occur antepartum but also during labor and up to 3 weeks' postpartum (162–164). In the British multicenter analysis (119), 38% of women had antepartum eclampsia, 18% intrapartum eclampsia, and 44% postpartum eclampsia. Preterm and antenatal eclampsia appear to be more dangerous to mother and child (119). Women with antepartum eclampsia are reported to have a higher incidence of abruptio placentae and *h*emolysis, *e*levated *l*iver enzyme levels and a *l*ow *p*latelet count (HELLP) syndrome (microangiopathic hemolytic anemia, elevated liver enzymes, and low platelets) as compared to those with postpartum eclampsia (165). Multiparous women who have preeclampsia will usually demonstrate a predisposing

TABLE 53-2

RISK FACTORS FOR DEVELOPING PREECLAMPSIA

Family history of preeclampsia, hypertension (159)
Diabetes mellitus, insulin resistance
Renal disease
Nulliparity (159)
Uric acid level ↑ (146)
β_2-microglobulin ↑ (381)
Platelet count ↓ (131)
Antithrombin III ↓ (105)
Blood pressure ↑ (99)
Plasma fibronectin ↑ (269)
Proteinuria new or ↑ (99)
Urinary calcium excretion ↓ (384)
Urinary 6-keto-prostaglandin $F_{1\alpha}$ ↓ (302)
Angiotensin II sensitivity test abnormal (47)
Rollover test abnormal (47,175)
Retroaortic left renal vein (370)

factor and will develop preeclampsia in about 70% of subsequent pregnancies (147). Patients with preeclampsia early in pregnancy very likely have underlying renal disease (165) or hydatidiform mole (166). Hydatidiform moles increase the risk of preeclampsia by about 10 times.

In patients with preeclampsia and eclampsia, total plasma volume is decreased as compared to pregnant women with normal pregnancies (167). There is a significant relationship between plasma volume at 38 weeks of gestation and birth weight of the neonate (32). Atrial natriuretic peptide (ANP) concentrations are increased in pregnancy-induced hypertension and may reflect a compensatory mechanism to attenuate blood pressure (168). There is good correlation of ANP levels and severity of hypertension and eclampsia. In this setting, ANP secretion is probably not stimulated by increased atrial pressure but rather by a different mechanism. Animal studies suggest that ANP is involved in the regulation of placental blood flow. Pregnant rats with hypertension may normalize impaired placental blood flow by increasing ANP concentrations (169). Hemoconcentration is a common finding in women with preeclampsia and eclampsia. Although fluid administration seems logical in such a situation, a state of increased afterload due to volume expansion may facilitate the development of pulmonary edema.

Preeclampsia usually becomes symptomatic after 20 weeks of gestation. In women who develop preeclampsia, blood pressure may rise early in the second trimester, although it may still be within the normal range. A characteristic finding in preeclampsia is the lability of blood pressure. In parallel to this lability, vascular resistance to the vasoconstricting effect of angiotensin II is lost by 14 to 16 weeks (45). The required dose of angiotensin II to increase diastolic blood pressure by 20 mm Hg decreases significantly (Fig. 53-5). Repetitive tests in preeclampsia-prone women will demonstrate that the increased sensitivity to angiotensin II-induced vasoconstriction antedates clinical symptoms and increases progressively (45). Wallukat et al. report that serum from a study of 25 preeclamptic patients contained stimulatory autoantibodies against the angiotensin-II type I receptor (170); it is believed that these autoantibodies may participate in the hypertension observed in preeclampsia. Despite the good correlation between changes in sensitivity to angiotensin II and the development of preeclampsia, the test is not practical as a screening method in large populations. The response of women with preeclampsia to other vasopressor hormones such as norepinephrine (171) or vasopressin (172) is less consistent. The rollover test, another test to screen for high-risk pregnant women, was introduced by Gant et al (173).

In this test, the pregnant woman is stabilized in the lateral position and her blood pressure recorded; thereafter, she is turned to the supine position, and the diastolic blood pressure is immediately measured. The test is considered positive when there is an increase of 20 mm Hg in the supine position. Women with a positive test have a twofold to fourfold increase in their rate of preeclampsia. A later evaluation of this test, however, demonstrated less optimistic predictive results (174).

Eclampsia

When preeclampsia progresses, nonspecific signs may occur such as hyperreflexia, restlessness, headaches (approximately 50%), epigastric pain (approximately 20%), and visual disturbances (approximately 20%) (119). However, whenever convulsions occur, the symptom complex is termed eclampsia. Some patients may have only minor systemic organ dysfunction and still demonstrate convulsions, while others are severely ill with progressive renal failure, microangiopathic hemolysis, and DIC without convulsions. Thus, some preeclamptic patients are equally or even more ill than some patients with overt eclampsia. Despite the improvement in treating eclampsia, maternal complications are high with a 1% to 2% mortality rate. More than one-third of eclamptic women have at least one major complication (119) (Table 53-3). Fetal outcome in the British multicenter eclampsia study demonstrated that 29% of 411 fetuses were small for their gestational age and there were 7.3% deaths. More recent data suggest that a convulsion is just one symptom of a broad range of signs that are the result of widespread endothelial cell damage (175). Therefore, the initial site of symptoms depends on the site of endothelial damage. On the other hand, the seizures of eclampsia may occur without other signs of preeclampsia but may still result from the same underlying endothelial injury mechanism.

Postmortem studies in women who have died from eclampsia have confirmed that eclampsia is a systemic disease. Fibrin deposition, petechial or gross hemorrhages, thrombosis, and fibrinoid necrosis were shown in blood vessels in several organs such as the brain, kidney, and liver (140). Reduced organ perfusion was the predominant anomaly. Evidence of vasoconstriction has been observed on funduscopic examination by demonstrating segmental narrowing and spasms of retinal arterioles (146). When using sensitive computed tomographic (CT) scanning equipment, nearly 50% of women with eclampsia demonstrate *in vivo* abnormal cerebral results (176) and some degree of edema (177). Eclampsia is a life-threatening complication of pregnancy, and urgent delivery is demanded. Even so, mortality is high in these patients (178). At necropsy, more than 50% of patients have cerebral hemorrhages as the lethal event (178). Although eclampsia is a disease of primigravidas, those who die tend to be older and multiparous (178). Placental abruption may occur in the setting of eclampsia and cause fetal death and contribute to the high mortality of the mother (179). Since the introduction of antihypertensive medications to lower blood pressure and magnesium sulfate to control convulsions, the frequency of developing overt eclampsia has decreased and is a rather rare complication in industrialized countries (180).

Renal Findings in Preeclampsia and Eclampsia

The majority of women with preeclampsia and eclampsia have mild to moderate impairment of kidney function as compared to normal pregnant women. As the creatinine clearance decreases, the rise in serum creatinine levels may still be less than 1 mg/dL, thus within the normal range for nonpregnant women. Characteristic changes in renal morphology occur in preeclampsia and eclampsia. The capillary wall in the glomerulus is thickened as a result of characteristic changes of glomerular endothelial swelling, termed *endotheliosis* (181,182). Glomerular endotheliosis has been observed in all primiparous women with preeclampsia (104). Narrowing of the glomerular capillaries frequently causes obliteration of the lumen. Deposits may be demonstrated in the mesangium that are consistent with fibrinogen. Deposition of immunoglobulin, most frequently IgM, in preeclamptic women (183) may reflect another underlying renal disease (104). In preeclampsia, the glomeruli are enlarged, and in severe cases, Bowman's capsule may be distended. Herniation of an enlarged glomerulus into the proximal tubule may occur in some cases (146). Glomerular epithelial cells may be enlarged with vacuolization and may contain hyaline deposits (184). There is, however, no glomerular crescent formation. Subendothelial depositions of fibrin and fibrinoid may be present and particularly prominent on electron microscopic examination (182,185). The glomerular basement membrane seems thickened and has a double contour (184). Electron microscopic examination has identified deposition of fibrils beneath the endothelial cells. The glomerular histology does not resemble findings of malignant hypertension but rather resembles the findings of hemolytic–uremic syndrome and DIC (186). Depending on the time point of performing a biopsy, the renal lesions may differ greatly. The subendothelial depositions resolve soon after delivery. Postdelivery, foam cells may be present in the glomerulus (184); it has been suggested that these are due to resolution of fibrinoid deposition. The changes in the basement membrane resolve after delivery, but this may take several weeks to months (187).

Gaber and Spargo (188) demonstrate focal glomerular sclerosis and suggest these findings are the result of an underlying renal disease, while Kincaid-Smith and Fairley (117) favor the idea that these renal changes are due to preeclampsia and eclampsia. Fisher et al. (104) observe that 74% of pregnant women with nephrosclerosis on renal biopsy later became hypertensive. Peyser and associates (189) show that 10 of 13 preeclamptic women with nephrosclerotic lesions became hypertensive within 2 to 7 years. Fisher et al. (104) report that on the basis of clinical findings the diagnosis of preeclampsia was made correctly in 54% of 176 pregnant women; however, the diagnosis was greater than 80% in primiparous women using the histology of renal biopsy as the "gold standard." Nochy et al. (183) biopsied 114 pregnant women after delivery and found that those women with clinical signs of preeclampsia also showed classic endotheliosis on renal biopsy. In addition,

TABLE 53-3

MAJOR MATERNAL COMPLICATIONS IN 382 CASES OF ECLAMPSIA

Complication	No. of patients
Death	7 (1.8%)
Persistent vegetative state	1 (<1%)
Cardiac arrest	6 (1.6%)
Cerebrovascular accident	7 (1.8%)
Adult respiratory distress syndrome	7 (1.8%)
Required ventilation	87 (23%)
Pulmonary embolism	5 (1.3%)
HELLP syndrome	27 (7%)
Disseminated intravascular coagulopathy (without HELLP)	33 (9%)
Renal failure	24 (6%)
Septicemia	2 (<1%)

HELLP, microangiopathic hemolytic anemia, elevated liver enzymes, and low platelets.
(From: Douglas KA, Redman CW. Eclampsia in the United Kingdom. *Br Med J* 1994;309:1395, with permission.)

patients with isolated pregnancy-induced hypertension, hyperuricemia, and no proteinuria also demonstrated the typical glomerular lesions of preeclampsia. The preeclamptic lesions could be superimposed in patients with preexisting nephropathy. Rarely, preeclampsia may cause acute tubular and cortical necrosis. Autopsy of seven infants born to mothers with preeclampsia or eclampsia demonstrated no lesions in the kidney (146).

After delivery, clinical pathology and laboratory abnormalities return to normal within days to weeks. However, organ function in some patients with preeclampsia and eclampsia may not recover immediately or recover incompletely due to severe tissue injury initiated during preeclamptic state. Proteinuria greatly resolves within 3 months (190). In most patients, nonspecific cerebral disorders resolve within weeks after delivery. In two patients suffering from eclampsia, Fredriksson and associates (191) demonstrated disseminated cerebral microvascular occlusion by CT and magnetic resonance imaging. These lesions disappeared completely without residua. In women without underlying disease, the long-term prognosis is excellent. The recurrence of the preeclampsia/eclampsia syndrome in subsequent pregnancies is 10 to 20 times less as compared to the risk for the first pregnancy (192). The remote prognosis of preeclampsia is a matter of debate. The discrepancy may in part be the result of different definitions of preeclampsia. Some cases of transient hypertension may have been misdiagnosed as preeclampsia. Some authors believe that in primiparous women the remote prognosis is identical to that of women with normal pregnancy (104,114,193). When the diagnosis was made on clinical and laboratory findings and confirmed by renal biopsy, the rate of later development of hypertension was identical to the expected rate of the overall population (104). In a more recent cohort study of 626, 272 births in Norway found that in preeclampsia a 1.2 fold higher long- term risk of all cause of death and eightfold risk of cardiovascular causes in preeclamptic women with a child of low birth weight (194). In contrast, a follow-up in 206 women who suffered from preeclampsia as a primigravida showed no increased incidence in hypertension more than 30 years later (114). Women who suffered from eclampsia with convulsions during the first pregnancy as long ago as 40 years did not demonstrate a different mortality rate in the follow-up period. In contrast, 64 women who developed eclampsia during the second or subsequent pregnancies more often had hypertension later in life and demonstrated an increased mortality rate as compared to controls without this complication (114) (Fig. 53-7). The best correlation of the occurrence of hypertension as a late complication of preeclampsia and eclampsia was seen with systolic blood pressure in the early phase of pregnancy (195). However, this higher systolic blood pressure during early pregnancy may have reflected an early sign of essential hypertension.

Microangiopathic Hemolytic Anemia, Elevated Liver Enzymes, and Low Platelets (HELLP Syndrome)

Hemolysis with red blood cell fragmentation, abnormal liver function, and thrombocytopenia have long been recognized as complications in preeclamptic women with hypertension (138,196), but these symptoms may occur in a great number of pregnant women without a rise in blood pressure (197). In 1982, Weinstein (190) described 29 women with these symptoms in association with preeclampsia or eclampsia and termed the disease the HELLP syndrome. The acronym HELLP stands for microangiopathic hemolytic anemia, elevated liver enzymes, and low platelets. While extremely high liver enzyme levels and thrombocytopenia of less than 100×10^9/L are usually demonstrated, these findings are not pathognomonic for the HELLP syndrome. These parameters may also be altered in patients with preeclampsia and eclampsia. The ratio

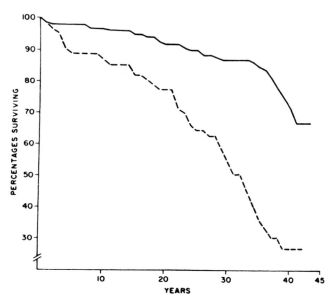

FIGURE 53-7. Survival of patients who had eclampsia as primigravidas (*solid line*) as compared to survival of women who had eclampsia as multigravidas (*dotted line*). Mortality of primigravidas was not different than matched controls. (From: Chesley LC, Annitto JE, Cosgrove RA. The remote prognosis of eclamptic women. *Am J Obstet Gynecol* 1976;124:446, with permission.)

of preeclampsia to HELLP syndrome is 1.2:1.0 when mild cases are included. Some authors consider the HELLP syndrome an early form of preeclampsia, while others believe it to be mild DIC that was misdiagnosed. Weinstein's clotting studies in these women were normal by measuring prothrombin time, partial thromboplastin time, and serum fibrinogen. Others suggest that hemolysis and low platelet counts reflect a low grade of intravascular coagulation, which is not detected by these insensitive tests (198). HELLP cases have been reported with the full signs of DIC (199). The syndrome may also develop during conservative management of patients with documented preeclampsia (190). The most reliable parameters to recognize microangiopathic hemolysis are schistocytes on peripheral smear, low plasma haptoglobin levels, reticulocytosis, and an increase in indirect plasma bilirubin (200). Serum concentration of total lactate dehydrogenase (LDH) is less frequently enhanced, while isoenzyme analysis has been shown to detect a rise in LDH_4 and LDH_5 early in the development of the syndrome. Liver enzymes and bilirubin are increased as well as serum uric acid levels. There are other liver diseases unique to pregnancy that may increase liver enzymes but are not associated with the HELLP syndrome, preeclampsia, or eclampsia (201). Classic hepatic lesions associated with the HELLP syndrome are periportal and/or focal parenchymal necrosis in which fibrin-like material can be seen.

Most common symptoms of the HELLP syndrome are nausea, headaches, right upper quadrant tenderness, or epigastric or right hypochondrial pain, which may easily be misdiagnosed as dyspepsia, gastroenteritis, hiatal hernia, viral hepatitis, or cholecystitis. None of these symptoms and signs is diagnostic for the HELLP syndrome. Regardless of the blood pressure, the patient requires hospitalization. Most often prompt delivery is indicated (102,141), although conservative management has been successful (197). In the absence of evidence of DIC, steroids may be given to accelerate fetal lung maturation; however, maternal and fetal conditions should be assessed continuously. Maternal mortality ranges between 1% and 20%, and fetal mortality is as high as 50% (190,197,198,200,202). Mothers are at risk for abruptio placentae, pulmonary edema, acute renal failure, and subcapsular liver hematomas, which may detach and eventually tear the capsule of the liver with liver rupture and intraabdominal bleeding (203). Hepatic failure may be caused by microemboli in the hepatic vasculature, leading to ischemia and tissue damage. Vasospasm causing endothelial injury may predispose to platelet aggregation and thrombocytopenia in the same manner as described for preeclampsia (198). The fetus may suffer perinatal distress and asphyxia; overall, however, neonatal survival is primarily dependent upon gestational age and birth weight at the time of delivery (204). The majority of these women have evidence of preeclampsia before delivery. Sibai (205) followed 59 women with the HELLP syndrome through 80 subsequent pregnancies. Only two patients (3.4%) had recurrence. In an analysis of this study, the syndrome developed in 62 of 206 (30%) cases a few hours to 6 days after parturition, and the remainder (70%) occurred before delivery (205).

PATHOPHYSIOLOGIC MECHANISMS IN PREGNANCY-INDUCED HYPERTENSION AND PREECLAMPSIA

The Role of Trophoblast and Spiral Arteries in the Development of Preeclampsia and Eclampsia

There is considerable evidence that preeclampsia/eclampsia is the result of impaired trophoblastic invasion and perfusion of the uterus. In normal pregnancies, trophoblastic invasion causes morphologic and functional changes in the spiral arteries but not the arcuate and radial arteries of the uterus (206). Invasive trophoblasts alter their adhesion molecule expression from epithelial to those of endothelial cells, a process of remodeling called "pseudovasculogenesis" (207). Yet little is known about the mechanism that promotes and controls this invasion of maternal tissue. A variety of cells such as natural killer (NK) cells, lymphocytes and macrophages are involved in the production of mediators in the decidua. Insulinlike growth factor, fibroblast and placental growth factor, vascular endothelial growth factor (VEGF), and cytokines such as TNF-α, transforming growth factor-β (TGF-β), epidermal growth factor, interleukin-1 (IL-1) and -6, tissue metalloproteinase inhibitors have been implicated in this process. During normal pregnancy, the spiral vessels increase their caliber markedly, lose muscular and elastic layers, and become low-resistance vessels that open into the intervillous space (207a). This process is completed by about 20 weeks of gestation (208). The changes extend through the decidua into the inner third of the myometrium (Fig. 53-8). Spiral arteries of women with preeclampsia do not demonstrate these structural changes (209), and trophoblast invasion is limited to the superficial decidua. Studies of trophoblast tissues show that cell differentiation and invasion in preeclamptic pregnancies are interrupted (210) and expression of adhesion molecules is abnormal (211). In addition, the lumens of many vessels are occluded by changes called acute atherosis and characterized by the presence of large foam cells, fibrinoid necrosis in the media of the vessel wall, and narrowed segments of the spiral arteries due to a lack of the physiologic adaptation (Fig. 53-8). Reduced spiral artery development and acute atherosis attenuate trophoblastic perfusion (212). Injection of ^{22}Na into the intervillous space is removed more slowly in women with preeclampsia than in women with normal pregnancy (213).

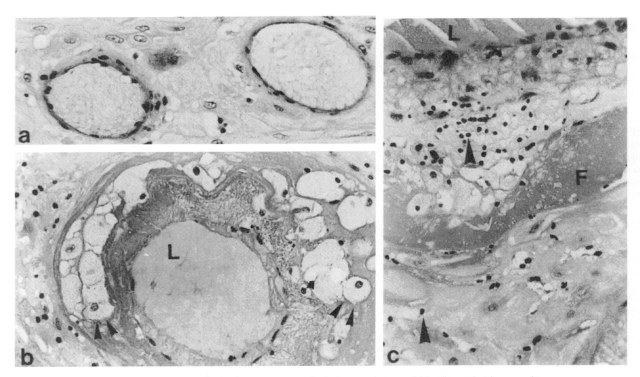

FIGURE 53-8. Acute decidual atherosis. **A:** Decidual tissue with normal blood vessel. Absence of inner elastic lamina and smooth muscle. **B,C:** Decidual arteriopathy. Acute atherosis characterized by thickening of the vessel wall. Accumulation of foamy macrophages (*double arrows*). **C:** Fibrin depositions (*F*) in the intima and sparse lymphocytic infiltrates (*arrows*) are observed. *L*, lumen of decidual vessel. (Hematoxylin and eosin ×350.) (Photographs courtesy of Dominique Gaeng, Pathology, University Hospitals, Bern, Switzerland.)

Women giving birth to small-for-gestational age babies have also demonstrated impaired trophoblast invasion (214). Vascular lesions in placentas derived from eclamptic patients are similar to vascular rejection in transplant grafts (215,216).

Other conditions that reduce trophoblast perfusion and predispose to preeclampsia independent of parity include increased placental mass as seen in twin pregnancies (159), trophoblastic tumors, hydatidiform moles (217), preexisting diabetes mellitus, collagen vascular diseases, and antecedent hypertension (206,209,218). Even without preeclampsia, diabetic women demonstrate atherosis in spiral arteries (206). This vasculopathy may lead to vascular thrombosis and vessel rupture with subsequent placental infarction, abruptio placentae, and retroplacental hemorrhage. The occurrence of preeclampsia in abdominal and molar pregnancies indicates that neither uterine nor fetal factors are required for the development of this syndrome. Experimental reduction of uterine perfusion by ligation of the abdominal aorta below the renal arteries causes the clinical picture of glomerular endotheliosis and preeclampsia in monkeys (219) and other mammals (220,221). In humans, those medical conditions that increase the risk of preeclampsia are all associated with microvascular diseases and thus the potential to reduce placental perfusion.

A number of other mediators such as hepatocyte growth factor (HGF), TGF-β, epidermal growth factor, and IL-1 have been shown to regulate trophoblast invasion. Thus, HGF knockout mice are lethal to the embryo due to abnormal placental development (222). The vascular endothelial growth factor (VEGF) plays a role in promoting angiogenesis. Its activity is modulated by the soluble fms-like tyrosine kinase 1 (sFlt 1), expressed on vascular endothelial cells. The sFlt 1 is a naturally occurring blocker of VEGF in patients with preeclampsia. The administration of sFlt 1 to rats has been shown to induce changes with albuminuria, hypertension and glomerular endotheliosis (223). In preeclamptic women sFlt 1 level increases as early as 13 weeks, several weeks before the onset of symptoms (preeclampsia 4382 pg/mL; control 1643 pg/mL p <0.001)(224). In contrast, the level of VEGF decreases before the onset of symptoms (225). Furthermore, VEGF knockout mice also demonstrate glomerular endotheliosis and proteinuria (226). However, sFlt 1 may play a critical role in some patients but does not induce alteration of clotting, suggesting additional factors contributing to the full picture of preeclampsia. Disturbance of the balanced interplay of these mediators may therefore impair trophoblast invasion. Under experimental conditions, fibrin deposition is initiated by injecting an extract from placental tissue into experimental animals; this results in fibrin deposition with hepatic lesions similar to those observed in eclampsia (227).

It is suggested that as a consequence of reduced uteroplacental blood flow, aberrant expression of genes occurs that may contribute to the pathophysiology of preeclampsia (228). In this context, it is interesting to note that preeclampsia/eclampsia is associated with a significant increase in embolic trophoblastic fragments in the venous circulation (229). These data further demonstrate the significance of trophoblasts in the induction of pregnancy-induced hypertension and preeclampsia and eclampsia.

Immunologic Factors Predisposing to Preeclampsia and Eclampsia

There is evidence that the maternal immune response may be changed from cellular responses toward humoral immunity (230). There is clinical evidence that in pregnancy cell-mediated immunity is weakened and humoral immunity is strengthened. The majority of women with rheumatoid arthritis, a cell-mediated disease, show remission of their symptoms

during pregnancy (231), while systemic lupus erythematosus, a disease resulting from excessive autoantibody production, may flare during gestation (232). The lack of human leukocyte antigens (HLA) on the syncytiotrophoblast and the presence of only the nonclassic HLA-G antigen on the cytotrophoblast cells preclude the fetal trophoblasts from playing a major part in currently recognized types of allogeneic immune reactions (233,234). The trophoblast produces a factor that inhibits T-cell proliferation and that may be a paracrine mechanism that contributes to fetal survival (235). Cytotoxicity, mediated by nonspecific NK cells, seems to be dampened by inhibition by the T_H1 helper cells, which produce cytokines such as interleukin-2 (IL-2) and interferon-γ (IFN-γ). In normal pregnancy, IL-2 levels are increased (236). On the other hand, activation of NK cells is enhanced in women with preeclampsia (237). In mice, the activation of these cells has been shown to result in fetal resorption (238).

Dudley et al. (238) further suggest that the regulation of cytokine production changes during normal pregnancy by a mechanism not resulting from specific fetal antigens. Nonspecific complement-mediated damage to the trophoblast may be inhibited by membrane-bound complement regulatory proteins, which protect the trophoblast from maternal complement-mediated damage arising from classic or alternate pathways and also systemic complement activation in response to microbial infections (239). However, pregnancy is not an immunodeficient state. Viral infections are not more common in pregnancy and are not more likely to become generalized as occurs in immunodeficient patients. The reason why falciparum malaria is more severe during the first pregnancy is not known (240) and why the resistance to the intracellular pathogens Listeria monocytogenes and Toxoplasma gondii is lowered is not known (241). Even more interesting is that women receiving malaria chemoprophylaxis during their first pregnancy have similar clinical course and prevalence of malaria infection of the placenta during the second pregnancy as do women not having received antimalaria medication during the first pregnancy (242). Current data do not suggest that pregnancy affects the course of human immunodeficiency virus infection in women (243). Immunologic tolerance between two genetically dissimilar tissues, maternal and fetal, is required for successful pregnancy. The current concept suggests that fetal trophoblast is not susceptible to attack by maternal T cells but suggests that other aspects of the immune system may be modulated during pregnancy as part of the maternal adaptations necessary for successful development of the fetus.

The thymus changes dramatically during pregnancy (105). In the cortex, the thymocytes die, and the medulla enlarges. Medullary epithelial cells become rearranged and proliferate to form the medullary epithelial rings. Estradiol is the most effective of the sex steroids at depleting immature CD4+ CD8+ thymocytes. Under experimental conditions, antithymocyte antibodies prevented implantation of the conceptus (244). Thus, cell death in the cortex may shut down the production of clones reactive with fetal antigens. However, the thymus is not necessary for a successful pregnancy (245). In addition to T cells, B cells are also affected by pregnancy. Estradiol pellets implanted in male or female mice demonstrated selective depression of B-cell precursors, and progesterone potentiated this effect (106,246).

That the etiology of preeclampsia/eclampsia has an immunologic component derives from the idea that normal mechanisms to protect fetoplacental tissue from rejection may be impaired (247). The following indirect evidence supports this hypothesis: (a) The risk to develop preeclampsia/eclampsia increases with a new partner, and (b) contraceptive methods that prevented exposure to sperm and seminal fluid prior to pregnancy enhance the risk of preeclampsia/eclampsia by 2.4-fold (248). Moreover, the risk of preeclampsia is reduced in the second pregnancy with the same partner but not with a new partner (249,250). The risk of preeclampsia in women whose partner had already a child with another women with eclampsia is twice as high as the risk with no family history of any side effect (251). However, the protective effects of previous pregnancy against preeclampsia is transient. When the inter birth interval was 10 years or more, the risk approximated that of nulliparous women (252). As suggested by Rebiller et al. (253), pregnancy-induced hypertension may be a problem not only of primi gravidity but also of primipaternity. The incidence of pregnancy-induced hypertension was 11.9% among primigravidas, 4.7% among same-paternity multigravidas, and 24% among new-paternity multigravidas. Furthermore, the overall incidence of pregnancy-induced hypertension of 11.9% decreased in their cohort to 3.3% in primigravidas who had more than 12 months of sexual contact with the same partner before conception. In pregnancies with artificial donor insemination, the incidence of preeclampsia/eclampsia is elevated twofold for primigravidas and ninefold for multigravidas (254). Five out of 10 women treated for infertility with oocyte implantation developed preeclampsia (255). In contrast, regular inoculation of the female genital tract with allogenic spermatozoa bearing histocompatibility antigens of the male reduces the incidence of subsequent preeclampsia (256). Thus, it is suggested that the dose of antigen presented by the trophoblast overwhelms the immune system of the mother, or factors responsible for placental immunoprotection may be produced in insufficient levels to produce an immunologic blockade to the fetal antigens. Recently it has been suggested that primipaternity in some cases may be a relevant risk factor rather than primiparity. In women with no history of preeclampsia a new father increased the risk of preeclampsia by 30% (257). In some patients with preeclampsia a new father was associated with a non-significant decrease in risk. First pregnancy may induce tolerance to the paternal antigen during the second pregnancy. Data from the Medical Birth Registry of Norway including more than 1.8 million births demonstrated that the risk of preeclampsia in the subsequent pregnancy was related to the time that had passed since the prior pregnancy ending with preeclampsia and not the change of the partner (258). The resulting vascular changes pathognomonic of preeclampsia caused a disruption of the balance between vasodilating and vasoconstricting mediators, thus resulting in impaired hemodynamics and hypoperfusion of the fetoplacental unit. Some mediator(s) are produced and released from the trophoblast and seem to cause activation or damage to the vascular endothelium in the circulation of the mother. Inhibin A and activin A are released from the preeclamptic placenta with subsequent rise in its blood level. In 71 patients of 1,496 nulliparous women preeclampsia developed. Still, the potential of this marker for identifying pre-symptomatic women at risk of developing the disease is less clear (259). During the first exposure to paternal antigens, the mother acquires protection for subsequent pregnancies. The role of the decidial NK cells are considered the endometrial memory of paternal antibodies. In experimental animals undergoing fetal resorption, immunization with allogeneic lymphocytes leads to enhanced fetoplacental survival and growth (260). Maternal immunity may also affect human pregnancy, since it has been shown that women with recurrent spontaneous abortion can deliver a healthy baby following immunization with paternal white blood cells (230).

T cells induce many of their effects by secretion of cytokines. Cytokines such as granulocyte–macrophage colony-stimulating factor (GMCSF) can enhance fetal growth, and cytokines such as TNF-α and IFN-γ can impair pregnancy (260). However, TNF-α and IFN-γ may also be required in the invasion of the trophoblast and development of the fetoplacental unit. Placentas from abortion-prone pregnancies induce predominantly TNF-α, IFN-γ, and IL-2 (230). These cytokines may be important for the remodeling of the uterus. Uteropla-

cental TNF-α production increases during gestation (261) but may be neutralized by a soluble TNF-α receptor produced by the trophoblast (262). Wegmann and associates (230) suggest that a decrease in the ratio of TNF-α to TNF-β receptor may initiate contraction and labor. The second pregnancy with the same partner would be less likely to stimulate the same immunologic processes because long-lived blocking immunoprotective factors were formed during the first pregnancy. Sufficient evidence therefore exists that some cases of preeclampsia may be the result of inadequate immunoprotection of the feto-placental unit.

Endothelial Dysfunction Prior To and During Preeclampsia and Eclampsia

Serum of preeclamptic women is cytotoxic. Moreover, there are several clinical and laboratory findings suggesting maternal endothelial dysfunction as an important component in the development of preeclampsia and eclampsia. The pathologic findings in tissue histology of women with preeclampsia/eclampsia are not the changes of blood vessel disruption typically occurring in patients with markedly elevated blood pressure. Rather, the most common findings are subendothelial necrosis and hemorrhages resembling ischemic injuries similar to patients with hypovolemic shock (201). As already discussed, the typical renal changes are swelling of glomerular endothelial cells, or glomeruloendotheliosis (263). No other form of hypertension demonstrates similar histologic findings except hemolytic–uremic syndrome, which preferentially presents with glomerular endothelial changes and fibrin thrombi (264). The increased rate of disappearance of Evans blue dye in preeclampsia is compatible with loss of endothelial cell integrity (265). *In vitro* studies also support the notion of endothelial damage as an important factor in the development of preeclampsia/eclampsia. Biochemical indicators of endothelial cell activation and injury are enhanced in the blood of women with preeclampsia/eclampsia. Serum from preeclamptic women added to the culture medium of human umbilical vein endothelial cells (HUVEC) enhanced ^{51}Cr release, an index of endothelial cell activation (266). In contrast, however, ^{51}Cr release induced with serum derived from the same women shortly after delivery was not different from controls (Fig. 53-9). When similar amounts

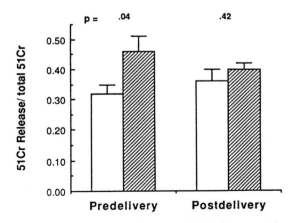

FIGURE 53-9. Cytotoxicity of serum derived from preeclamptic women (*hatched bars*) is enhanced compared to serum derived from healthy pregnant women (*open bars*) and causes increased ^{51}Cr release from prelabeled human endothelial cells. After delivery, ^{51}Cr release normalized and was not different from that in women with normal pregnancy. (From: Rodgers GM, Taylor RN, Roberts JM. Preeclampsia is associated with a serum factor cytotoxic to human endothelial cells. *Am J Obstet Gynecol* 1988;159:908, with permission.)

of serum from women with preeclampsia and normal pregnancy were added to HUVEC, ^{51}Cr release with the preeclamptic serum was not prevented, thus suggesting a toxic mediator in the serum rather than a deficiency of some factor(s) triggering this injury of endothelial cells. Recent studies suggest that the factor of preeclamptic serum that increases endothelial cell permeability acts by protein kinase C activation (267). Preeclampsia has histologic findings in common with hemolytic–uremic syndrome and thrombotic thrombocytopenic purpura, syndromes in which impairment of endothelial function has been suggested. The findings of unusually large von Willebrand multimers (268), cellular fibronectin (269) and thrombomodulin blood levels (270) in women with preeclampsia/eclampsia provide further biochemical evidence for disturbed endothelial cell function. An increase in endothelium-derived fibronectin levels predicted the development of gestation-induced hypertension 6 to 13 weeks before clinical abnormalities were obvious. On the other hand, women with transient hypertension had plasma fibronectin concentrations indistinguishable from those of normal controls (271) (Fig. 53-10).

Maternal Serum Markers of Preeclampsia and Eclampsia

Blood levels of a variety of substances have been shown to change during pregnancy and in preeclampsia and eclampsia. However, it is less clear whether these changes are the cause or solely the result of preeclampsia and eclampsia.

The fibronectins are a family of glycoproteins. In a longitudinal study, elevated fibronectin levels were measured at 2 to 3 months' gestation in women who develop preeclampsia (272). Adhesion molecules are receptors that modulate inflammatory responses and may be important in the placental bed during trophoblast invasion. Although intercellular adhesion molecule (ICAM) and vascular cell adhesion molecule (VCAM) are expressed in the deciduus (273) there seems no use of soluble forms of these molecules for prediction of subsequent preeclampsia (274). Endothelial dysfunction has been demonstrated in 10 of 43 women who eventually developed preeclampsia (275). Flow mediated dilation of the brachial artery was 3.58% versus 8.59% ($p <0.0001$). There was also a strong correlation between asymmetric dimethylarginine, the endogenous inhibitor of endothelial NO synthase. Still, it is not clear whether endothelial dysfunction is the cause or the consequence of preeclampsia.

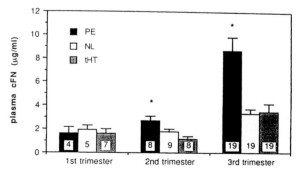

FIGURE 53-10. Prospective analysis of plasma levels of endothelium-derived fibronectin was performed throughout pregnancy. Average concentrations were determined for each trimester in the same group of patients. Fibronectin levels from women developing preeclampsia (PE) later in pregnancy were higher than in women with normal pregnancy (NL) or transient hypertension (tHT) during the second trimester. cFN, concentration of fibronectin. (From: Taylor RN, et al. High plasma cellular fibronectin levels correlate with biochemical and clinical features of pre-eclampsia but cannot be attributed to hypertension alone. *Am J Obstet Gynecol* 1991;165:895, with permission.)

Peroxidation Products During Preeclampsia and Eclampsia

In preeclamptic women, increased blood levels of lipid peroxidation products have been demonstrated and may contribute to the disorder by disruption of membrane lipids, inhibiting prostacyclin and NO production and stimulating endothelin synthesis (276–278) and platelet aggregation (279). Free radicals are produced during normal physiologic processes; however, their release is exaggerated during ischemia (280). These free radical species may induce endothelial cell toxicity and facilitate coagulation by oxidative conversion of unsaturated fatty acids to lipid peroxides (281). During normal pregnancy, free radical production is enhanced, and in preeclampsia, this process is even more exaggerated (282). High levels of oxygen free radicals correlated well with increased blood pressure levels (283). Superoxide anions scavenge NO and thus contribute to the removal of this very important vasodilator in the regulation of blood flow and hemodynamics (277). Increased endothelial NO synthase with decreased superoxide dismutase and increased nitrotyrosine immunostaining in the vasculature of women with preeclampsia is consistent with increased peroxynitrite formation (284). Free radicals may also be derived from activated monocytes, which have been demonstrated in the circulation of hypertensive pregnant women (285). Thromboxane synthesis in platelets is not affected by lipid peroxides. Lipofuscin, which derives from lipid peroxide, has been found more frequently in term placentas than in those less than 32 weeks of gestation. This finding suggests that peroxidation activity increases with gestation. When uncontrolled peroxidation occurs, membrane damage may be initiated. Under experimental conditions, elevation of circulating lipid peroxides or deprivation of vitamin E, an antioxidant, can reproduce the signs of endothelial cell dysfunction similar to those seen in preeclampsia and clinical signs and symptoms of typical preeclampsia (286). Reduced vitamin E levels have been observed in preeclamptic women (287). It is not known if the imbalance between lipid peroxides and vitamin E is a primary or secondary phenomenon; nevertheless, it may contribute to the impairment of endothelial cell function in preeclampsia.

Vasoactive Mediators in Preeclampsia and Eclampsia

The production and secretion of endothelin, a potent peptide hormone that may lead to sustained vasoconstriction, is stimulated in endothelial cells exposed to injuries, such as ischemia (286). The production of endothelin is also enhanced in preeclampsia and pregnancy-induced hypertension (288,290), and endothelin receptor sites are enhanced in the placenta of preeclamptic women (291). The production of another vasoconstrictor, platelet-derived growth factor (PDGF), is enhanced in the supernatant of human umbilical vein endothelial cells (HUVEC) incubated with medium supplemented with serum of preeclamptic women (292). In addition to the effect on vascular tone, PDGF is also mitogenic. Serum of preeclamptic women is selectively mitogenic for fibroblasts but not endothelial cells (293,294). Endothelium-dependent relaxation is impaired in arteries of women with preeclampsia as compared to arteries from normotensive pregnant women, while endothelium-independent vasodilation as assessed by sodium nitroprusside is not altered (295). Animal experiments suggest a major role of NO in the regulation of the physiologic decrease in blood pressure (16). Perfusion of rabbit arteries with serum from preeclamptic women but not from normal pregnant women increased the sensitivity of the vessel to angiotensin II and norepinephrine (296). As described previously, preeclamptic women have been shown to produce stimulatory autoantibodies against the angiotensin-ATI receptor (170). These autoantibodies may participate in the angiotensin II–induced exaggerated vasoconstriction in preeclampsia and contribute to impaired placental blood flow and infarction.

Prostaglandins in Preeclampsia and Eclampsia

Platelet activation (297) occurs in preeclampsia and enhances thromboxane release, which favors platelet aggregation, especially in the presence of factor VIII antigen (267), and stimulates uterine contraction (298). Platelet aggregation is followed by the release of thromboxane A_2 (TXA$_2$), serotonin, adenosine triphosphate (ATP), and adenosine diphosphate (ADP); the latter three of these are mediators that induce endothelium-dependent vasodilation. In the absence of the endothelium, paradoxical vasoconstriction and platelet aggregation occur (299). In the plasma and placenta of preeclamptic women, TXA$_2$ concentrations (212) are increased. Inhibition of the prostacyclin production (300) may be caused by endothelial cell injury and may antedate clinically overt disease (132). A multicenter prospective study has shown that reduced prostacyclin I_2 (PGI$_2$) production but not TXA$_2$ production occurs many months before the clinical onset of preeclampsia (302). Deficiency of PGI$_2$ results in an early increase in the vasoconstrictor to vasodilator ratio (TXA$_2$/PGI$_2$). Fitzgerald et al. (302) demonstrated reduced excretion of endothelium-derived prostacyclin metabolite, 6-keto-PGE$_{1\alpha}$, in pregnancy-induced hypertension. Furthermore, serial measurements of urinary 6-keto-PGE$_{1\alpha}$ could be used to predict the development of pregnancy-induced hypertension. In addition to the reduction in vasodilating prostaglandins, the synthesis of the vasoconstrictor TXA$_2$ is enhanced in pregnancy-induced hypertension (302) (Fig. 53-11). As discussed, the major sources of TXA$_2$ are activated or aggregated platelets.

Intravascular Coagulation in Preeclampsia and Eclampsia

Although the DIC associated with preeclampsia can rarely be demonstrated by measuring prothrombin time and partial thromboplastin time (199), more sensitive tests demonstrate abnormal results in a high percentage of preeclamptic women. For example, reduced concentrations of antithrombin III (108,132), an indicator of activation of coagulation, are a useful and sensitive indicator to differentiate preeclampsia from other causes of hypertension (108). Endothelial cells can attenuate the coagulation property by the ectoenzymes that rapidly metabolize platelet-derived ATP and ADP to adenosine, a strong inhibitor of platelet aggregation, and by endothelium-derived NO, which inhibits platelet adhesion. Fibrinolysis is stimulated by the release of plasminogen activator, which converts plasminogen to plasmin and thereafter splits fibrin into soluble degradation products. In normal pregnancy, fibrinolysis property is decreased, and in preeclampsia, this decrease is obvious much earlier (303). TNF-α has been shown to promote procoagulatory conditions (304), adhesion molecules, and secretion of other cytokines (305), which may perpetuate this process. To balance the coagulation process, endothelial cells may also release a plasminogen activator inhibitor (306). Changes in blood viscosity may contribute to the attenuation of the microvascular circulation in preeclampsia (307). In 50% of

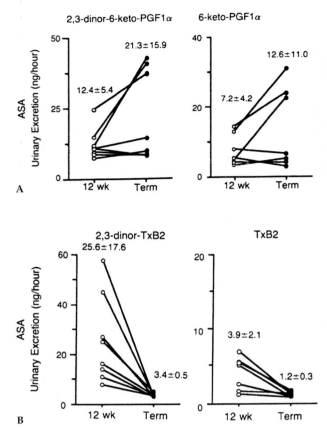

FIGURE 53-11. Effect of 60 mg/day of aspirin on prostaglandin excretion in pregnant women at risk for pregnancy-induced hypertension. **A:** Urinary excretion of 6-keto-prostaglandin F$_{1\alpha}$ (**right**) and its metabolite 2,3-dinor-6-keto-prostaglandin F$_{1\alpha}$ (**left**) did not change significantly in aspirin-treated and nontreated (not shown) women. **B:** Urinary excretion of the major thromboxane A$_2$ metabolite 2,3-dinor-thromboxane B$_2$, which largely derives from platelets, was reduced by 80% in women at risk for pregnancy-induced hypertension (**left**) and by 59% of mainly kidney-derived thromboxane B$_2$ excretion (**right**). (From: Benigni A, et al. Effect of low-dose aspirin on fetal and maternal generation of thromboxane by platelets in women at risk for pregnancy-induced hypertension. *N Engl J Med* 1989;321:357, with permission.)

women with preeclampsia and also in 15.4% of women with normal pregnancy, antiendothelial antibodies have been isolated, which have shown increased staining of renal cortical arterioles (308). The functional significance of this finding is not known yet. The rapid disappearance of cytotoxicity after delivery suggests a short half-life of the cytotoxic mediator(s) and makes it unlikely that antiendothelial antibodies induce endothelial injury because immunoglobulins have a half-life of days to weeks. The long duration of impaired organ function in some patients with preeclampsia and eclampsia compared to the short time of pathologic effects induced *in vitro* by serum derived from preeclamptic women may reflect severity of tissue injury initiated during the preeclamptic state.

Thrombocytopenia may be present in the newborn of a preeclamptic mother (309,310). This finding may suggest that a toxic, humoral factor is transferred transplacentally to the fetus. Clinically, the thrombocytopenia is generally no problem to the newborn (202). There seems, however, to be an association between the severity of hypertensive disorders in the mother and the thrombocytopenia in the newborn (311).

Conclusion

Preeclampsia is the result of very early events in pregnancy when angiogenesis is impaired. Narrowed spiral arteries and subsequent placental ischemia may be important in triggering the production of mediators that enter the maternal circulation to induce endothelial cell injury early in the development of preeclampsia and eclampsia. Many of the pathophysiologic changes of preeclampsia can be explained by derangement of endothelial cell function. Under physiologic conditions, endothelial cells produce substances to regulate tone of vascular smooth muscle cells to maintain adequate organ perfusion; endothelium-derived mediators inhibit coagulation; the endothelium produces growth factors, expresses adhesion molecules to capture blood cells such as leukocytes, produces extracellular matrix, and controls fluid and electrolyte transfer into the interstitial space (312). When endothelial cells are activated or injured, they may lose their normal responses and diminish the production of vasodilators and thus increase the sensitivity to normally circulating vasoconstrictors. In addition, endothelial cells may also demonstrate new activities such as synthesis of vasoconstrictor hormones, mitogens, and production of procoagulants to activate the coagulation cascade. Increased sensitivity to vasoconstrictor hormones, vasospasm, proteinuria, edema, activation of the coagulation cascade, and production of microthrombi may all be explained by endothelial dysfunction (Fig. 53-12). These processes impair maternal organ and placental perfusion. Placental perfusion is further impaired and the production of "trophotoxin(s)" sustained. A vicious cycle is thus established that often may be broken only by delivery of the fetus.

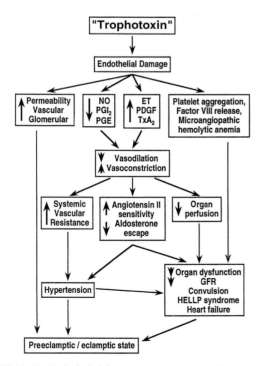

FIGURE 53-12. Endothelial damage attenuates vasodilation, enhances vasoconstriction, and promotes coagulation, which leads to the events characteristic for preeclampsia and eclampsia. *ET*, endothelin; *NO*, nitric oxide; *PDGF*, platelet-derived growth factor; *PGE*, prostaglandin E; *PGI$_2$*, prostacyclin; *TxA$_2$*, thromboxane A$_2$.

MANAGEMENT OF HYPERTENSIVE DISORDERS IN PREGNANCY

Although in most cases of pregnancy-induced hypertension the rise in blood pressure is transient, there is good reason to treat hypertension. Hypertension of the mother increases morbidity and mortality in both mother and child (110). In 24,000 women, increased perinatal mortality and increased risk of small-for-gestational age babies were demonstrated when the blood pressure of the mother increased to 125/75 mm Hg prior to the 32nd week of gestation and greater than 125/85 mm Hg thereafter (313). When mean arterial blood pressure was ≥90 mm Hg in the second trimester, there was greater risk of stillbirth, fetal growth retardation, and preeclampsia (111).

Treatment of Hypertension

The American College of Obstetricians and Gynecologists recommends treatment for acute hypertension with diastolic levels of ≥100 mm Hg (102). A lower threshold of diastolic blood pressure, namely ≥90 mm Hg, is believed by other experts to require therapy because many women may have diastolic blood pressure below 90 mm Hg during the second trimester and still develop symptoms of hypertension. In addition to the absolute level, the increase in blood pressure should also be considered important in the development of preeclampsia. Thus, diastolic blood pressure exceeding 75 mm Hg in the second trimester or 85 mm Hg in the third trimester may require surveillance at weekly intervals and may need treatment. Treating women with chronic or pregnancy-induced hypertension must take into account that antihypertensive drugs may have teratogenic effects, impair placental and uterine blood flow, or affect fetal development and organ function. Several groups also demonstrated that treating mild hypertension does not prevent the development of superimposed preeclampsia (314,315). In contrast, evidence strongly suggests that treating severe hypertension with antihypertensive medications may reduce the perinatal death rate and might prevent preeclampsia (316–318). Excessive reduction in blood pressure, however, has the risk of impairing maternal organ and fetal–placental perfusion and should therefore be avoided when antihypertensive medication is initiated. Blood pressure monitoring at weekly intervals is required when blood pressure is ≥130/80 mm Hg. Continuation of antihypertensive treatment after conception improves fetal growth and lowers perinatal mortality (167).

Diuretics

The use of diuretics in pregnancy is controversial. In contrast to women with normal pregnancy (319), preeclamptic women demonstrate contracted plasma volume (167). In addition, systemic vascular resistance is increased, and cardiac output may be normal or reduced (320). In a setting of reduced intravascular volume, as is seen in preeclampsia, it seems rather inappropriate to diminish plasma volume further with diuretic therapy. However, Collins et al. (321) conclude from the data of nine randomized trials, including more than 10,000 women, that preeclampsia could be prevented by therapy with diuretics. The incidence of stillbirths was reduced, and no increase in perinatal mortality was observed. Diuretics do not appear to affect fetal growth (322). Thus, if treatment of hypertension with diuretics has been initiated prior to pregnancy, this therapy probably does not require cessation if the patient becomes pregnant.

Agents Affecting the Adrenergic System

Central-acting adrenergic agonists, such as methyldopa and clonidine, have been most widely used and studied in pregnancy (323). Methyldopa given to pregnant women with essential hypertension has been demonstrated to reduce the number of midterm spontaneous abortions (324). No significant adverse maternal or fetal effects have been reported with methyldopa treatment (325). Children with intrauterine fetal exposure to methyldopa were followed for up to 7 years and did not show any adverse mental or physical effects (326). However, it has to be taken into account that methyldopa may cause somnolence. Methyldopa still remains the drug of choice for treating hypertension in pregnant women as recommended by the National Institutes of Health (NIH) working group (102).

Intrauterine growth retardation (327) and neonatal bradycardia have been reported with β-adrenergic antagonists (328). Attenuation of fetal growth seems to occur when the β-adrenergic antagonist propranolol is used for longer periods. By using oxprenolol, however, there was no difference in perinatal mortality in women with preeclampsia as compared to normotensive controls (329). In a prospective, randomized double-blind study of 120 women with preeclampsia, premature labor occurred in no patient treated with atenolol but in five women on placebo (330). Labetalol, a combined α- and β-adrenergic antagonist with more β-adrenergic antagonistic activity, has been found useful in treating both hypertension throughout pregnancy and an acute rise in blood pressure without affecting uteroplacental blood flow (315,331,332). The National High Blood Pressure Education Program Working Group has not recommended β-adrenergic antagonists as drugs of first choice in the treatment of hypertension during pregnancy, although they may be acceptable and safe agents for treating preexisting hypertension during pregnancy (102). Beta-adrenergic antagonists also cause less somnolence than methyldopa. They should however, whenever possible, be confined to short-term administration before the delivery. Pregnant patients with hypertension due to pheochromocytoma are at high risk of death. Immediate treatment with an α- and β-adrenergic blocker is warranted, and tumorectomy should be performed whenever possible during pregnancy (333).

Vasodilators

The vasodilator hydralazine is frequently used to treat hypertension in pregnancy. The drug seems quite safe; however, it may cause reflex tachycardia and a rise in cardiac output. Moreover, even used alone it may not be effective enough. Beta-adrenergic blockers prevent tachycardia and are efficient in reducing blood pressure when given in combination with vasodilators. In patients with essential hypertension, hydralazine may also be given with methyldopa during pregnancy. Hydralazine has been reported to induce neonatal thrombocytopenia (334). Vasodilators, like other smooth muscle relaxants, cause cessation of labor in a significant number of patients. Magnesium sulfate also suppresses myometrial and myocardial contractility.

Calcium Channel Blockers

Nifedipine has been used without major side effects in women with acute hypertension in pregnancy (335). Calcium channel blockers, however, may cause cessation of uterine contraction. When hypertensive ewes were treated with nicardipine, fetal acidemia was frequent, and 5 of 15 fetuses died within 1 hour after drug administration (336). Calcium channel blockers have teratogenic effects in rat studies when given in a pharmacologic dose 30 times the maximum recommended human dose. The drug is not recommended as first-line medication

throughout pregnancy; however, it may be used for short-term treatment during pregnancy (337).

Angiotensin-Converting Enzyme (ACE) Inhibitors and Angiotensin II Receptor (A II) Blockers

ACE inhibit the conversion of angiotensin I to angiotensin II and decrease bradykinin degradation. ACE inhibitors are effective in reducing blood pressure during pregnancy; however, in 22 women with essential hypertension, there were two miscarriages, and in four patients with preeclampsia, there were two stillbirths (338). Acute renal failure has been reported in neonates of women treated with ACE inhibitors (339). Additional reported fetal and neonatal complications of ACE inhibitor use in late pregnancy include oligohydramnios, intrauterine growth retardation, premature labor, bony malformations, limb contracture, persistent patent ductus arteriosus, prolonged hypotension, and neonatal death (340,341). Although retrospective studies of ACE inhibitor use at conception or during early pregnancy were not associated with adverse perinatal outcomes (342), ACE inhibitors should not be prescribed in pregnancy. There are limited reports of side effects of angiotensin II receptor blockers inducing fetal toxicity. Oligohydramnion, incomplete skull formation and oliguria occurred (343,344).

Treatment of Preeclampsia and Eclampsia

The preeclampsia/eclampsia syndrome is characterized by a phase of no or little clinical symptoms while biochemical markers in the maternal blood may already suggest alteration of endothelium function. However, it is not easy to predict the time point of the development of preeclampsia and eclampsia in these women. Bed rest has been recommended to prevent progression of the syndrome, but the beneficial effects have been questioned (345). Proteinuric preeclampsia requires hospitalization. Early delivery is often mandatory to remove the site of production of mediators that stimulate the progression of symptoms of preeclampsia and eclampsia. Conservative therapy (without delivery) of severe preeclampsia occurring in the second trimester may lead to a perinatal mortality of greater than 80% and a high rate of maternal morbidity (346). Interruption of the pregnancy therefore may be recommended in these settings (102). In contrast, isolated mild hypertension without other complicating factors can be followed on an ambulatory basis (347).

Antihypertensive Medication for Preeclampsia and Eclampsia

In hypertensive patients suffering from preeclampsia or eclampsia and especially in patients demonstrating intracerebral hemorrhage, blood pressure should be reduced rapidly. In this situation, blood pressure control is best by intravenous administration of drugs such as the vasodilator hydralazine (348). When there is no response, other drugs are necessary such as the α- and β-adrenergic blocker labetalol (348). Sublingual administration of the calcium channel blocker nifedipine has also been used successfully (349). Women with eclampsia receiving magnesium sulfate may have a precipitous fall in blood pressure. An interaction between nifedipine and magnesium sulfate has been reported to produce profound maternal muscle weakness. Treatment with intravenous sodium nitroprusside, another very potent vasodilator, may cause accumulation of cyanide (350) and should therefore be avoided, although a case report did not confirm this fear of intoxication (351). Reduction in systemic blood pressure may also affect uterine hemodynamics and lower uterine, placental, and subsequently fetal blood flow. It is not known if there is sufficient autoregulation of the uteroplacental vasculature to maintain sufficient perfusion. A number of antihypertensive agents are excreted in breast milk (352). Severe sustained hypertension postpartum requires treatment, and therefore breast-feeding is not recommended.

In the preeclampsia/eclampsia state with reduced intravascular volume, treatment with diuretics should be avoided unless signs and symptoms of pulmonary edema are present. Some observations indicate that volume expansion may improve peripheral vascular resistance and decrease blood pressure (353); however, pulmonary and cerebral edema may develop with this treatment. The significance of serotonin in the pathophysiologic events of preeclampsia is supported by the beneficial effect of receptor blockade with ketanserin. Attenuation of both blood pressure and platelet aggregation in preeclampsia has occurred with this medication (354).

Anticoagulation

The discovery of DIC, fibrin deposition, and thrombosis in preeclampsia and eclampsia suggests the possible treatment of these women with heparin (355). However, such a treatment may be deleterious in the presence of petechiae or overt bleeding and should therefore be omitted.

Anticonvulsant Therapy

Eclampsia by definition is associated with convulsions. Neither blood pressure level nor proteinuria is a good indicator of impending seizures. Chua and Redman (356) therefore suggest restricting anticonvulsant treatment to patients demonstrating overt convulsions. Magnesium sulfate has been used to prevent convulsions in women with peripartum hypertension and has been demonstrated to be superior to phenytoin as a prophylaxis against eclampsia (357). Evidence from the Magpie Trial has demonstrated in 10 out of 110 women a very important role of magnesium sulfate in preventing as well as controlling eclampsia (358). Although it is not an anticonvulsant or antihypertensive drug, magnesium sulfate inhibits calcium uptake in vascular smooth muscle cells, thereby lowering plasma endothelin-1 levels (359). Magnesium sulfate may also block the constrictor effect of endothelin, angiotensin II, and neuropeptide Y (360) and increase the production of cyclic guanosine monophosphate (cGMP), the second messenger of several vasodilators (361). Thus, attenuation or reversal of vasoconstriction (362) and improvement of cerebral perfusion may occur. Magnesium sulfate does reduce seizures in women with preeclampsia, however, does not improve electroencephalographic pathology (363) and overall mortality and morbidity (364). Therefore, its use in eclampsia is still somewhat a matter of debate. Other common anticonvulsants such as diazepam or distraneurin have been effective in treating eclampsia (365).

Epidural Anesthesia

In spite of antihypertensive medication and bed rest, there are still preeclamptic patients who are not responsive to this treatment. Lumbar epidural anesthesia blocks the abdominal sympathetic nerves and improves hypertension during preeclamptic labor. In preeclampsia, long-term epidural anesthesia for more than 3 weeks has been shown to improve the preeclamptic condition, with decreased blood pressure and increased platelet count and serum protein level (366). In addition, infants in the epidural group had a higher body weight of 2,240 ± 310 g compared to 1,590 ± 380 g in the control group treated with antihypertensives and bed rest.

Timing of Delivery

The therapy of eclampsia includes supportive care for the mother and the fetus and the need for a prompt decision regarding the time and mode of delivery. Delivery is always the best therapy for the mother with preeclampsia and eclampsia; however, this may not be the case for the baby. When the gestational age is between 25 and 30 weeks, fetal survival is a serious consideration. Thus, the delivery may be postponed in women with mild signs of preeclampsia and a premature fetus. Clinical and laboratory monitoring, however, are required in these cases. Deterioration in maternal condition with organ dysfunction (e.g., brain, kidney, liver) or fetal deterioration should be an indication for delivery. If maternal and fetal well-being remain stable, pregnancy should be continued, and spontaneous labor may be possible. Epidural anesthesia for cesarean section is a safe technique (367). With epidural anesthesia, peripheral vasodilation may cause a severe fall in blood pressure and diminished uteroplacental perfusion. This complication can be prevented with means such as volume expansion as used in nonpregnant patients with epidural anesthesia. General anesthesia is recommended when there is high risk of epidural hematoma with epidural anesthesia in patients with severe coagulation alterations (190,368,369). The risk of aspiration of gastric contents during intubation, however, is increased. Glucocorticoids may hasten fetal lung maturation; however, they have no effect on maternal outcome.

Prevention of Preeclampsia and Eclampsia

Since the mechanisms underlying preeclampsia are not well understood, prevention of this disorder focuses on intensive screening for women with high risk or early signs of preeclampsia and eclampsia. Taking into account that in experimental conditions impaired uterine blood flow may induce preeclampsia, there was great hope that ultrasound measurements of changes in placental and uterine circulation may predict the development of early preeclampsia (370,371). However the results of uterine arterial waveform by ultrasound and the risk of hypertension and eclampsia are conflicting. There are also many biochemical maternal serum parameters such as hyperuricemia, thrombocytopenia, increased liver enzymes, low levels of antithrombin III, and increases in β_2-microglobulin and fibronectin, that may be prodromal signs of preeclampsia; however, their absence does not exclude the syndrome (Table 53-2). Preeclampsia may progress rapidly to severe disease within days to weeks. Antenatal visits in primiparous women should be performed every 2 weeks (372), and when clinical or biochemical signs or symptoms of preeclampsia occur, hospitalization for more intensive monitoring or delivery can then be performed. While preeclampsia cannot be prevented, with this strategy the risk of severe maternal and fetal morbidity can be diminished.

A good indicator for monitoring the occurrence of preeclampsia is serum uric acid concentration (373). Normal pregnancy induces a 25% decrease in plasma uric acid concentration early in pregnancy (374). In the third trimester, uric acid levels may rise close to the normal range in healthy women but also in women with hypertensive disease without preeclampsia (146) (Fig. 53-13). In contrast, in preeclampsia, serum uric acid levels are consistently increased in the first trimester and subsequently continue to rise. Furthermore, there was a statistically significant correlation of the serum uric acid level with perinatal prognosis (373) and the severity of glomerular changes of preeclampsia and eclampsia (146) (Fig. 53-13). The mechanism of the hyperuricemia remains obscure. Renal insufficiency cannot be the responsible factor because many patients have no or little increase in serum creatinine levels. Plasma β_2-microglobulin levels also parallel the rise in uric acid concentrations in preeclampsia (375).

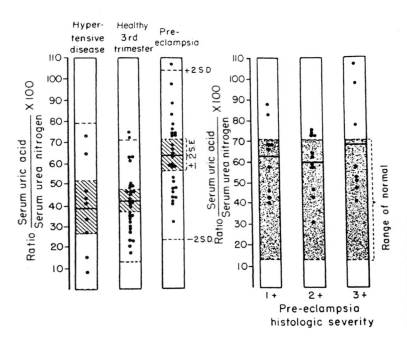

FIGURE 53-13. The diagram shows the distribution of serum uric acid in pregnant women. **Left three columns:** Uric acid levels do not differ in hypertensive compared to normotensive pregnant women, while preeclamptic patients demonstrate great increase in uric acid concentration. **Right three columns:** Severity score of glomerular histology ranging from mild (1+) to severe (3+) correlates with serum levels of uric acid. (From: Pollak VE, Nettles JB. The kidney in toxemia of pregnancy: a clinical and pathologic study based on renal biopsies. *Medicine* 1960;39:469, with permission.)

If endothelial cell injury were the cause of hypertension, proteinuria, and preeclampsia and eclampsia, one would expect that evidence of such injury would antedate these clinical disorders. As mentioned earlier, this is the case. Preventive means, therefore, need to start early in pregnancy, perhaps around 12 to 14 weeks of gestation. Screening tests to detect women who very likely will develop preeclampsia should be accurate, noninvasive, easy to perform, and inexpensive. So far the most reliable clinical test is the angiotensin II infusion test. However, it is not suitable as a routine method. A rise in blood pressure, proteinuria, or facial edema and rapid weight gain may be an early sign of the development of preeclampsia; however, these are not pathognomonic features of preeclampsia. Nevertheless, they are of concern for closer monitoring of the patient. Since preeclampsia and eclampsia are high-risk states for maternal and fetal morbidity, overdiagnosis of impending preeclampsia is preferable to underdiagnosis. If the condition is stable, weekly observations may be appropriate (102); however, if the disease progresses, more frequent visits are necessary, and hospitalization should be considered.

Antiplatelet Drugs

Activation and aggregation of platelets have been shown to occur in preeclampsia. The significance of platelets in preeclampsia has further been suggested by the finding of reduced numbers in this state (376). As discussed earlier, there is evidence that preeclampsia and eclampsia are associated with an imbalance in the ratio of vasoconstricting to vasodilating prostaglandins. Thus, it was believed that inhibition of the synthesis of vasoconstricting prostaglandins, for example, thromboxane, might shift the ratio toward the more physiologic range. Initial studies using platelet inhibitors such as aspirin or dipyridamole for prevention of preeclampsia showed promising results, including decreased incidence of proteinuric hypertension, preterm birth, infants small-for-gestational age, and perinatal death (377–379). However, a multicenter prospective study of women at risk for preeclampsia showed no benefit (380) However, women demonstrating a reduction in flow in the uterine artery measured by doppler may benefit of aspirin (381). Caritis et al. reported a significant decrease in urinary prostacyclin excretion and no change in urinary thromboxane excretion in 134 preeclamptic women as compared with 139 matched normotensive controls (382). This study suggests that prostacyclin deficiency, rather than increased thromboxane production, may contribute to the development of preeclampsia and thus may provide an explanation for the lack of efficacy of aspirin therapy in most of these patients.

Antioxidants

Oxidative stress has been implicated in the pathogenesis of preeclampsia. As noted previously, oxygen free radicals have been demonstrated to be increased in preeclampsia. Ascorbic acid is a scavenger of superoxide radicals and thus might potentially help preserve NO. Alphatocopherol and ascorbic acid also decrease low-density lipoprotein (LDL) oxidation. Therefore, it was suggested that antioxidant therapy with vitamins C and E could be beneficial in the prevention of preeclampsia. A double-blinded, randomized, placebo-controlled trial of vitamins C and E supplementation in 238 women at increased risk of preeclampsia demonstrated a decrease in the incidence of preeclampsia in the treated group (383). However, no differences in perinatal outcome were found. Further studies with large numbers of patients are needed before antioxidant supplementation can be recommended for prevention of preeclampsia. Other supplement of the nutrients such as calcium in 4,589 primiparae did not confirm earlier findings of a lower incidence of preeclampsia compared to controls (384).

References

1. Kaunitz AM, et al. Causes of maternal mortality in the United States. *Obstet Gynecol* 1985;65:605.
2. Augensen K, Bergsjo P. Maternal mortality in the Nordic countries, 1970–1979. *Acta Obstet Gynecol Scand* 1984;63:115.
3. Derham RJ, et al. Outcome of pregnancies complicated by severe hypertension and delivered before 34 weeks: stepwise logistic regression analysis of prognostic factors. *J Obstet Gynecol* 1989;96:1173.
4. Lees MM, et al. A study of cardiac output at rest throughout pregnancy. *J Obstet Gynaecol Br Commenw* 1967;74:319.
5. Chapman AB, et al. Temporal relationships between hormonal and hemodynamic changes in early human pregnancy. *Kidney Int* 1998;54:2056.
6. Phippard AF, et al. Circulation adaptation to pregnancy: serial studies of hemodynamics, blood volume, renin and aldosterone in the baboon. *J Hypertens* 1986;4:773.
7. Pedersen EG, et al. Pre-eclampsia: a state of prostaglandin deficiency? *Hypertension* 1983;5:105.

8. Gregoire I, et al. Prostanoid synthesis by isolated rat glomeruli: effect of oestrous cycle and pregnancy. *Clin Sci* 1987;l73:641.

9. Briner VA, Schrier RW. Peripheral arterial vasodilation hypothesis of sodium and water retention in pregnancy: implications for pathogenesis of preeclampsia—eclampsia. *Obstet Gynecol* 1991;77:632.

10. Conrad KP, et al. Identification of increased nitric oxide biosynthesis during pregnancy in rats. *FASEB J* 1993;7:566.

11. Cadnapaphornchai MA, Schrier RW. Chronic nitric oxide synthase inhibition reverses systemic vasodilation and glomerular hyperfiltration in pregnancy. *Am J Physiol Renal Physiol* 2001;280:F592.

12. Begum S, Yamasaki M, Mochizuki M. The role of nitric oxide metabolites during pregnancy. *Kobe J Med Sci* 1996;42:131.

13. Bocardo P, et al. Systemic and fetal—maternal nitric oxide synthesis in normal pregnancy and pre-eclampsia. *Br J Obstet Gynecol* 1996;103:879.

14. Conrad KP, Vernier KA. Plasma levels, urinary excretion, and metabolic production of cGMP during gestation in rats. *Am J Physiol* 1989;257:R847.

15. Xu DL, Martin PY, St. John J, et al. Upregulation of endothelial and neuronal constitutive nitric oxide synthase in pregnant rats. *Am J Physiol* 1996;271:R1739.

16. Ahokas RA, Mercer BM, Sibai MB. Enhanced endothelium-derived relaxing factor activity in pregnant, spontaneously hypertensive rats. *Am J Obstet Gynecol* 1991;164(Suppl):242.

17. Dunlop W. Serial changes in renal haemodynamics during normal human pregnancy. *Br J Obstet Gynecol* 1981;88:1.

18. Sims EA, Krantz KE. Serial studies of renal function during pregnancy and the puerperium in normal women. *J Clin Invest* 1958;37:1764.

19. Davison JM, Dunlop W. Renal hemodynamics and tubular function in normal human pregnancy. *Kidney Int* 1980;18:152.

20. Davison JM, Noble MC. Serial changes in 24 hour creatinine clearance during normal menstrual cycles and the first trimester of pregnancy. *Br J Obstet Gynecol* 1981;88:10.

21. Davison JM, Dunlop W, Ezimokhai M. 24-hour creatinine clearance during the third trimester of normal pregnancy. *Br J Obstet Gynecol* 1980;87:106.

22. Barron WM, Stamoutsos BA, Lindheimer MD. Role of volume in the regulation of vasopressin secretion during pregnancy. *J Clin Invest* 1984;73:923.

23. Baylis C. The mechanism of the increase in glomerular filtration rate in the 12-day pregnant rat. *J Physiol* 1980;305:405.

24. Conrad K, Colpoys MC. Evidence against the hypothesis that prostaglandins are the vasodepressor agents of pregnancy. *J Clin Invest* 1986;77:236.

25. Baylis C. Renal disease in gravid animal models. *Am J Kidney Dis* 1987;IX:350.

26. Davison JM. Change in renal function in early pregnancy in women with one kidney. *Yale J Biol Med* 1978;51:347.

27. Davison JM, Lind T, Uldall PR. Planned pregnancy in a renal transplant recipient. *Br J Obstet Gynecol* 1976;83:518.

28. Cunningham FG, et al. Chronic renal disease and pregnancy outcome. *Am J Obstet Gynecol* 1990;163:453.

29. Davison JM. The kidney in pregnancy: a review. *J R Soc Med* 1983;76:485.

30. Barrat M. Proteinuria. *Br Med J* 1983;287:1489.

31. Chesley LC. Weight changes and water balance in normal and toxic pregnancy. *Am J Obstet Gynecol* 1944;48:565.

32. Pirani BB, Campbell DA, MacGillvray I. Plasma volume in normal first pregnancy. *J Obstet Gynaecol Br Commenw* 1973;80:884.

33. Nolten WE, et al. Desoxycorticosterone in normal pregnancy: I. Sequential studies of the secondary patterns of desoxycorticosterone, aldosterone and cortisol. *Am J Obstet Gynecol* 1978;132:414.

34. Lindheimer MD, Weston PV. Effect of hypotonic expansion on sodium, water and urea excretion in late pregnancy: the influence of posture on these results. *J Clin Invest* 1969;48:947.

35. Davison JM, Vallotton MB, Lindheimer MD. Plasma osmolality and urinary concentration and dilution during and after pregnancy: evidence that lateral recumbency inhibits maximal urinary concentrating ability. *Br J Obstet Gynaecol* 1981;88:472.

36. Ohara M, et al. Upregulation of aquaporin 2 water channel expression in pregnant rats. *J Clin Invest* 1998;101:1076.

37. Davison JM, et al. Changes in the metabolic clearance of vasopressin and in plasma vasopressinase throughout human pregnancy. *J Clin Invest* 1989;83:1313.

38. Durr JA, et al. Diabetes insipidus due to abnormally high circulating vasopressinase activity in a pregnancy. *N Engl J Med* 1987;316:1070.

39. Davison JM, et al. Altered osmotic threshold for vasopressin secretion and thirst in human pregnancies. *Am J Physiol* 1984;246:F105.

40. Wade JB, Stetson DL, Lewis SA. ADH action: evidence for a membrane shuttle mechanism. *Ann NY Acad Sci* 1981;372:106.

41. Lindheimer MD, et al. Water homeostasis and vasopressin release during rodent and human gestation. *Am J Kidney Dis* 1987;9:270.

42. Walker J, Garland HO. Single nephron function during prolactin-induced pseudopregnancy in the rat. *J Endocrinol* 1985;107:127.

43. Davison JM, et al. Serial evaluation of vasopressin release and thirst in human pregnancy: role of human chorionic gonadotropin in the osmoregulatory changes of gestation. *J Clin Invest* 1988;81:798.

44. Weir RJ, et al. Plasma renin, renin substrate, angiotensin II and aldosterone in hypertensive diseases of pregnancy. *Lancet* 1973;I:291.

45. Gant NF, et al. A study of angiotensin II pressor response throughout primigravid pregnancy. *J Clin Invest* 1973;52:2682.

46. Baler PN, Broughton Pipkin F, Symonds EM. Platelet angiotensin II binding and plasma renin concentration, plasma renin substrate and plasma angiotensin II in human pregnancy. *Clin Sci* 1990;79:403.

47. Geelhoed GW, Vander AJ. Plasma renin activities during pregnancy and parturition. *J Clin Endocrinol Metab* 1968;28:412.

48. Johnson J, et al. The site of renin in the human uterus. *Histopathology* 1984;8:273.

49. Terragno NA, et al. Prostaglandins and the regulation of uterine blood flow in pregnancy. *Nature* 1974;249:57.

50. Rosenfeld CR, Gant NF. The chronically instrumented ewe: a model for studying vascular reactivity to angiotensin II in pregnancy. *J Clin Invest* 1981;67:486.

51. Ferris TF, Weir EK. The effect of captopril on uterine blood flow and prostaglandin synthesis in the rabbit. *J Clin Invest* 1983;71:809.

52. Bay WH, Ferris TF. Factors controlling plasma renin and aldosterone during pregnancy. *Hypertension* 1979;1:410.

53. Gant NF, et al. Control of vascular reactivity in pregnancy. *Am J Kidney Dis* 1987;9:303.

54. Sanchez-Ramos L, O'Sullivan MJ, Garrido-Calderon J. Effect of low-dose aspirin on angiotensin II pressor response in human pregnancy. *Am J Obstet Gynecol* 1987;156:193.

55. Conrad KP. Possible mechanisms for changes in renal hemodynamics during pregnancy: studies from animal models. *Am J Kidney Dis* 1987;IX:253.

56. Baylis C. Glomerular filtration and volume regulation in gravid animal models. *Clin Obstet Gynaecol* 1987;1:789.

57. Lindheimer MD, Del Greco F, Ehrlich EN. Postural effects on Na and steroid excretion and serum renin activity during pregnancy. *J Appl Physiol* 1973;35:343.

58. Becker RA, et al. Effects of positional change and sodium balance on the renin-angiotensin-aldosterone system, big renin and prostaglandins in normal pregnancy. *J Clin Endocrinol Metab* 1978;46:467.

59. Brown RD, Strott CA, Liddle GW. Plasma deoxycorticosterone in normal and abnormal pregnancy. *J Clin Endocrinol Metab* 1972;35:736.

60. Casey ML, MacDonald PC. Metabolism of deoxycorticosterone and deoxycorticosterone sulfate in men and women. *J Clin Invest* 1982;70:312.

61. Ledoux F, et al. Plasma progesterone and aldosterone in pregnancy. *Can Med Assoc J* 1975;112:943.

62. Atallah AN, et al. Progesterone increases glomerular filtration rate, urinary kallikrein excretion and uric acid clearance in normal women. *Braz J Med Biol Res* 1988;21:71.

63. Oparil S, Ehrlich EN, Lindheimer MD. Effect of progesterone on renal sodium handling in man: relation to aldosterone excretion and plasma renin activity. *Clin Sci Mol Med* 1975;49:139.

64. Schunkert H, et al. Effects of estrogen replacement therapy on the renin—angiotensin system in postmenopausal women. *Circulation* 1997;95:39.

65. Proudler AJ, et al. Hormone replacement therapy and serum angiotensin-converting enzyme activity in postmenopausal women. *Lancet* 1995;346:89.

66. Ylikorkala O, et al. Postmenopausal hormonal replacement decreases plasma levels of endothelin-1. *J Clin Endocrinol Metab* 1995;80:3384.

67. Best PJ, et al. The effect of estrogen replacement therapy on plasma nitric oxide and endothelin-1 levels in postmenopausal women. *Ann Intern Med* 1998;128:285.

68. Naden RP, Rosenfeld CR. Systemic and uterine responsiveness to angiotensin II and norepinephrine in estrogen-treated nonpregnant sheep. *Am J Obstet Gynecol* 1985;153:417.

69. Weiner CE, et al. In vitro release of endothelium-derived relaxing factor is increased during the guinea pig pregnancy. *Am J Obstet Gynecol* 1989;161:1599.

70. Chen Z, et al. Estrogen receptor alpha mediates the nongenomic activation of endothelial nitric oxide synthase by estrogen. *J Clin Invest* 1999;103:401.

71. Weiner CP, et al. Induction of calcium-dependent nitric oxide synthase by sex hormones. *Proc Natl Acad Sci USA* 1994;91:5212.

72. Romero JC, et al. Role of the endothelium-dependent relaxing factor nitric oxide on renal function. *J Am Soc Nephrol* 1992;2:1371.

73. Briner VA, Tsai P, Schrier RW. Bradykinin: potential for vascular constriction in the presence of endothelial injury. *Am J Physiol* 1993;264:F322.

74. Kakouris H, Eddie LW, Summers RJ. Relaxin: more than just a hormone of pregnancy. *Trends Biochem Sci* 1993;14:4.

75. Massicotte G, Parent A, St. Lous J. Blunted responses to vasoconstrictors in mesenteric vasculature but not in portal vein of spontaneous hypertensive rats treated with relaxin. *Proc Soc Exp Biol Med* 1989;190:254.

76. Stewart DR, et al. Relaxin in the peri-implantation period. *J Clin Endocrinol Metab* 1990;70:1771.

77. Danielson LA, et al. Relaxin is a potent renal vasodilator in conscious rats. *J Clin Invest* 1999;103:525.

78. Weisinger RS, et al. Relaxin alters the plasma osmolality-arginine vasopressin relationship in the rat. *J Endocrinol* 1993;137:505.

79. Jeyabalan A, et al. Essential role for vascular gelatinase activity in relaxin—induced renal vasodilation, hyperfiltration and reduced myogenic reactivity of small arteries. *Circ Res* 2003;93:1249.

80. Haynes WG, Webb DJ. Endothelin as a regulator of cardiovascular function in health and disease. *J Hypertens* 1998;16:1081.

81. Yanigisawa M, et al. A novel potent vasoconstrictor peptide produced by vascular endothelial cells. *Nature* 1988;332:411.

82. Tamas P, et al. Renal electrolyte and water handling in normal pregnancy: possible role of endothelin-1. *Eur J Obstet Gynecol Reprod Biol* 1994;55:89.

83. Conrad KP, et al. Endothelin mediates renal vasodilation and hyperfiltration during pregnancy in chronically instrumented conscious rats. *Am J Physiol* 1999;276:F767.

84. Minegishi T, et al. Adrenomedullin and atrial natriuretic peptide concentrations in normal pregnancy and preeclampsia. *Mol Hum Reprod* 1999;5:767.

85. Di Iorio R, et al. Adrenomedullin, a new vasoactive peptide, is increased in preeclampsia. *Hypertension* 1998;32:758

86. Ryan EA, O'Sullivan MJ, Skyler JS. Insulin action during pregnancy: studies with the euglycemic clamp technique. *Diabetes* 1985;34:380.

87. Linstedt G, et al. Low sex-hormone-binding globulin concentration as independent risk factor for development of NISSM. 12-year foul up of population study of women in Gotheburg, Sweden. *Diabetes* 1991;40:123.

88. Wolf M, et al. First trimester insulin resistance and subsequent preeclampsia: a prospective study. *J Clin Endo Metabol* 2002;87:1563.

89. Gabbe SG, et al. Management and outcome of class A diabetes mellitus. *Am J Obstet Gynecol* 1977;127:465.

90. UK Prospective Diabetes Study IV. Complications in newly diagnosed type 2 diabetes patients and their association with different clinical and biochemical risk factors. *Diabetes* 1995;13:1.

91. DeFronzo RA, Ferrannini E. Insulin resistance: a multifaceted syndrome responsible for NIDDM, obesity, hypertension, dyslipidemia and atherosclerotic cardiovascular disease. *Diabetes Care* 1991;14:173.

92. Joffe GM, et al. The relationship between abnormal glucose tolerance and hypertensive disorders of pregnancy in healthy nulliparous women. *Am J Obstet Gynecol* 1998;179:1032.

93. Laivuori H, et al. Leptin during and after preeclamptic or normal pregnancy: its relation to serum insulin and insulin sensitivity. *Metabolism* 2000;49:259.

94. Mise H, et al. Augmented placental production of leptin in preeclampsia: possible involvement of placental hypoxia. *J Clin Endocrinol Metab* 1998;83:3225.

95. Kirwan JP, et al. TNF-alpha is a predictor of insulin resistance in human pregnancy. *Diabetes* 2002;51:2207.

96. Anim-Nyame N, at al. Microvascular permeability is related to circulating levels of tumor necrosis factor-alpha in pre-eclampsia. *Cardiovasc Res* 2003;58:162.

97. Wilson M, et al. Blood pressure, the renin-aldosterone system and sex steroids throughout pregnancy. *Am J Med* 1980;68:97.

98. Chesley LC, Annatto JW. Pregnancy in the patient with hypertensive disease. *Am J Gynecol* 1947;53:372.

99. MacGillivray I, Rose GA, Rowe B. Blood pressure survey in pregnancy. *Clin Sci* 1969;37:395.

100. WHO Study Group. The hypertensive disorders of pregnancy. Geneva: World Health Organization, 1987:14. Technical Report Series No. 758.

101. American College of Obstetricians and Gynecologists. *Management of preeclampsia.* 1986. Washington, DC: Technical Bulletin No. 91.

102. National High Blood Pressure Education Program Working Group. Report on high blood pressure in pregnancy. *Am J Obstet Gynecol* 2000;183:S1.

103. Paller MS. Hypertension in pregnancy. *J Am Soc Nephrol* 1998;9:314.

104. Fisher KA, et al. Hypertension in pregnancy: clinical-pathological correlations and remote prognosis. *Medicine* 1981;60:267.

105. Clarke AG, Kendall MD. The thymus in pregnancy: the interplay of neural, endocrine and immune influence. *Immunol Today* 1994;15:545.

106. Kincade PW, et al. Pregnancy: a clue to normal regulation of B lymphopoiesis. *Immunol Today* 1994;15:539.

107. Browne FJ. Chronic hypertension in pregnancy. *Br Med J* 1947;2:283.

108. Weiner CP, et al. Antithrombin III activity in women with hypertension during pregnancy. *Obstet Gynecol* 1985;65:301.

109. Vanek M, et al. Chronic hypertension and the risk for adverse outcome after superimposed pre-eclampsia. *Int J Gynaecol Obstet* 2004;86:7.

110. Martikainen AM, Jeompmem KM, Saarolpslo SV. The effect of hypertension in pregnancy on fetal and neonatal condition. *Int J Gynecol Obstet* 1989;30:213.

111. Page EW, Christianson R. The impact of mean arterial blood pressure in middle trimester upon the outcome of pregnancy. *Am J Obstet Gynecol* 1976;125:740.

112. Sibai BM, et al. Risk factors for preeclampsia, abruptio placentae, and adverse neonatal outcomes among women with chronic hypertension. *N Engl J Med* 1998;339:667.

113. Rey E. Preeclampsia and neonatal outcome in chronic hypertension: comparison between white and black women.. *Etn Dis* 1997;7:5.

114. Chesley LC, Annitto JE, Cosgrove RA. The remote prognosis of eclamptic women. *Am J Obstet Gynecol* 1976;124:446.

115. Adams EM, MacGillivray I. Long-term effect of pre-eclampsia on blood pressure. *Lancet* 1961;II:1373.

116. Chesley LC, Sibai BM. Clinical significance of elevated mean arterial pressure in the second trimester. *Am J Obstet Gynecol* 1988;159:275.

117. Kincaid-Smith PS, Fairley KF. *The kidney and hypertension in pregnancy.* New York: Churchill Livingstone, 1993:1.

118. Miyamoto S, et al. Circadian rhythm of plasma atrial natriuretic peptide, aldosterone and blood pressure during third trimester in normal and preeclamptic pregnancies. *Am J Obstet Gynecol* 1988;158:393.

119. Douglas KA, Redman CW. Eclampsia in the United Kingdom. *Br Med J* 1994;309:1395.

120. Redman CW. Eclampsia still kills. *Br Med J* 1988;296:1209.

121. Sibai BM, et al. Eclampsia: I. Observations from 67 recent cases. *Obstet Gynecol* 1981;58:609.

122. Roberts JM, Redman CW. Pre-eclampsia: more than pregnancy-induced hypertension. *Lancet* 1993;341:1447.

123. Chesley L. Diagnostic criteria for preeclampsia. *Obstet Gynecol* 1985;65:423.

124. Fisher KA, et al. Nephrotic proteinuria with preeclampsia. *Am J Obstet Gynecol* 1977;129:643.

125. Redman CW, Jeffries M. Revised definition of preeclampsia. *Lancet* 1988;1:809.

126. Robertson EG. The natural history of edema during pregnancy. *J Obstet Gynaecol Br Commenw* 1971;78:520.

127. Redman CW, et al. Plasma-urate measurements in predicting fetal death in hypertensive pregnancy. *Lancet* 1976;II:1370.

128. Howie PW, et al. Use of coagulation tests to predict the clinical progress of pre-eclampsia. *Lancet* 1976;II:323.

129. Barry C, Fox R, Stirrat G. Upper abdominal pain in pregnancy may indicate preeclampsia. *Br Med J* 1994;308:1562.

130. Cunningham FG, et al. Peripartum heart failure: idiopathic cardiomyopathy or compounding events? *Obstet Gynecol* 1986;67:157.

131. Grimes DA, Ekbladh LE, McCartney WH. Cortical blindness as a complication of eclampsia. *Int J Gynecol Obstet* 1980;117:601.

132. deBoer K, et al. Enhanced thrombin generation in normal and hypertensive pregnancy. *Am J Obstet Gynecol* 1989;160:95.

133. Gibson B, et al. Thrombocytopenia in preeclampsia and eclampsia. *Semin Thromb Hemostat* 1982;8:234.

134. Redman CW. Platelets and the beginning of preeclampsia. *N Engl J Med* 1990;323:478.

135. Erne P, et al. Correlation of platelet calcium with blood pressure: effect of antihypertensive therapy. *N Engl J Med* 1984;310:1084.

136. Zemel MB, et al. Altered platelet calcium metabolism as an early predictor of increased peripheral vascular resistance and preeclampsia in urban black women. *N Engl J Med* 1990;323:434.

137. Barr SM, et al. Platelet intracellular free calcium concentration in normotensive and hypertensive pregnancies in the human. *Clin Sci* 1989;76:67.

138. Pritchard JA, Cunningham FG, Mason RA. Coagulation changes in eclampsia: their frequency and pathogenesis. *Am J Obstet Gynecol* 1976;124:855.

139. Morris RH, et al. Immunofluorescent studies of renal biopsies in the diagnosis of toxemia of pregnancy. *Obstet Gynecol* 1964;24:32.

140. McKay DG, et al. The pathologic anatomy of eclampsia, bilateral cortical necrosis, pituitary necrosis, and other acute fatal complications of pregnancy, and its possible relationship to the generalized Schwartzman phenomenon. *Am J Obstet Gynecol* 1953;66:507.

141. Rolfes DB, Ishak KG. Liver disease in toxemia of pregnancy. *Am J Gastroenterol* 1986;81:1138.

142. Saleh AA, et al. Preeclampsia, delivery and the hemostatic system. *Am J Obstet Gynecol* 1987;157:331.

143. Trofatter KF, et al. Use of fibrin D-dimer in screening for coagulation abnormalities in preeclampsia. *Obstet Gynecol* 1989;73:435.

144. Redman CW, et al. Factor-VIII consumption in preeclampsia. *Lancet* 1977;II:1249.

145. Schwartz ML, Brenner WE. Pregnancy-induced hypertension with life-threatening thrombocytopenia. *Am J Obstet Gynecol* 1983;146:756.

146. Pollak VE, Nettles JB. The kidney in toxemia of pregnancy: a clinical and pathologic study based on renal biopsies. *Medicine* 1960;39:469.

147. Sutherland A, et al. The incidence of severe pre-eclampsia amongst mothers and mothers-in-law of pre-eclamptics and controls. *Br J Obstet Gynecol* 1981;88:785.

148. Arngrimsson R, Bjornsson H, Geirsson R. Analysis of different inheritance patterns in preeclampsia/eclampsia syndrome. *Hypertens Pregnancy* 1995;14:27.

149. Chesley LC. Hypertension in pregnancy: definitions, familial factor, and remote prognosis. *Kidney Int* 1980;18:234.

150. Arngrimsson R, et al. Is genetic susceptibility for pre-eclampsia and eclampsia associated with implantation failure and fetal demise? [Letter]. *Lancet* 1994;I:1643.

151. Cooper D. Genetic control of susceptibility to eclampsia and miscarriage. *J Obstet Gynaecol* 1988;95:644.

152. Arngrimsson R, et al. A genome-wide scan reveals a maternal susceptibility locus for pre-eclampsia on chromosome 2p13. *Hum Mol Genet* 1999;8:1799.

153. Boyd PA, Lindenbaum RH, Redman C. Pre-eclampsia and trisomy 13: a possible association. *Lancet* 1987;II:425.
154. Saftlas AF, Olson DR, Franks AL, et al. Epidemiology of preeclampsia and eclampsia in the United States, 1979–1986. *Am J Obstet Gynecol* 1990;163:460.
155. Corkill TF. Experience of toxemia control in Australia and New Zealand. *Pathol Microbiol* 1961;24:428.
156. MacGillvray I. Some observations of the incidence of preeclampsia. *J Obstet Gynaecol Br Empire* 1958;65:536.
157. Hibbard BM, Rosen M. The management of severe preeclampsia and eclampsia. *Br J Anaesth* 1977;49:3.
158. Brassil MJ, et al. Obstetric outcome in first-time mothers aged 40 years and over. *Eur J Obstet Gynecol Reprod Biol* 1987;25:115.
159. Bulfin MJ, Lawler PE. Problems associated with toxemia in twin pregnancies. *Am J Obstet Gynecol* 1957;73:37.
160. Hou SH, Grossmann SD, Madias NE. Pregnancy in women with renal disease and moderate renal insufficiency. *Am J Med* 1985;78:185.
161. Nelson TR. A clinical study of pre-eclampsia. *J Obstet Gynaecol Br Empire* 1955;62:48.
162. Lao TT, et al. Labour-related eclampsia. *Eur J Obstet Gynecol Reprod Biol* 1987;26:97.
163. Brown DE, Cunningham FG, Pitchard JA. Convulsion in hypertensive, proteinuric primiparas more than 24 hours after delivery: eclampsia or some other cause? *J Reprod Med* 1987;32:499.
164. Samuels B. Postpartum eclampsia. *Obstet Gynecol* 1960;15:748.
165. Mattar F, Sibai BM. Eclampsia. VIII. Risk factors for maternal morbidity. *Am J Obstet Gynecol* 2000;182:307.
166. Chun D, et al. Clinical observations on some aspects of hydatidiform moles. *J Obstet Gynecol Br Commonw* 1964;71:180.
167. Gallery ED, Hunyor SN, Gyory AZ. Plasma volume contraction: a significant factor in both pregnancy-associated hypertension (pre-eclampsia) and chronic hypertension in pregnancy. *Q J Med* 1979;48:593.
168. Fievet P, et al. Atrial natriuretic factor in pregnancy-induced hypertension and preeclampsia: increased plasma concentrations possibly explaining these hypovolemic states with paradoxical hyporeninism. *Am J Hypertens* 1988;1:16.
169. Chemtob S, Potvin W, Varma DR. Selective increase in placental blood flow by atrial natriuretic peptide in hypertensive rats. *Am J Obstet Gynecol* 1989;160:477.
170. Wallukat G, et al. Patients with preeclampsia develop agonistic autoantibodies against the angiotensin AT1 receptor. *J Clin Invest* 1999;103:945.
171. Talledo OE, Chesley LC, Zuspan FP. Renin-angiotensin system in normal and toxemic pregnancies: III. Differential sensitivity to angiotensin II and norepinephrine in toxemia of pregnancy. *Am J Obstet Gynecol* 1968;100:218.
172. Dickmann WJ, Michel HL. Vascular renal effects of particular pituitary extracts in pregnant women. *Am J Obstet Gynecol* 1937;33:131.
173. Gant NF, et al. A clinical test useful for predicting the development of acute hypertension in pregnancy. *Am J Obstet Gynecol* 1974;120:1.
174. Kuntz WD. Supine pressor (roll-over) test: an evaluation. *Am J Obstet Gynecol* 1980;137:764.
175. Roberts JM. Preeclampsia: an endothelial cell disorder. *Am J Obstet Gynecol* 1989;161:1200.
176. Brown CE, Purdy P, Cunningham FG. Head computed tomographic scans in women with eclampsia. *Am J Obstet Gynecol* 1988;159:915.
177. Sheehan HL, Lynch JB. *Pathology of toxemia of pregnancy*. London: Churchill Livingstone, 1973.
178. Lopez-Llera M, Linares GR, Horta JL. Maternal mortality rate in eclampsia. *Am J Obstet Gynecol* 1976;124:149.
179. Lopez-Llera M, de la Luz Espinosa M, Arratia C. Eclampsia and placental abruptio: basic patterns, management and morbidity. *Int J Gynecol Obstet* 1988;27:335.
180. Pritchard JA, Pritchard SA. Standardized treatment of 154 consecutive cases of eclampsia. *Am J Obstet Gynecol* 1975;123:543.
181. Spargo B, McCartney CP, Winemiller R. Glomerular capillary endotheliosis in toxemia of pregnancy. *Arch Pathol* 1959;68:593.
182. Packham DK, et al. Morphometric analysis of preeclampsia in women biopsied in pregnancy and post-partum. *Kidney Int* 1988;34:704.
183. Nochy D, et al. Renal lesions in the hypertensive syndromes of pregnancy: immunomorphological and ultrastructural studies in 114 cases. *Clin Nephrol* 1980;13:155.
184. Kincaid-Smith P. Renal lesion of preeclampsia revisited. *Am J Kidney Dis* 1991;17:144.
185. Thomson D, et al. The renal lesions of toxaemia and abruptio placentae studied by light and electron microscopy. *J Obstet Gynaecol Br Commonw* 1972;79:311.
186. Gasser C, et al. Hämolytisch-urämisches syndrom: bilaterale nierenrindennekrosen bei akuten erworbenen hämolytischen anämie. *Schweiz Med Wochenschr* 1951;85:905.
187. Kincaid-Smith P. Participation of intravascular coagulation in the pathogenesis of glomerular and vascular lesions. *Kidney Int* 1975;7:242.
188. Gaber LW, Spargo BH. Pregnancy-induced nephropathy: the significance of focal segmental glomerulosclerosis. *Am J Kidney Dis* 1987;317:9.
189. Peyser MR, et al. Late follow-up in women with nephrosclerosis diagnosed at pregnancy. *Am J Obstet Gynecol* 1978;132:480.
190. Weinstein L. Syndrome of hemolysis, elevated liver enzymes and low platelet count. Of severe consequences of hypertension in pregnancy. *Am J Obstet Gynecol* 1982;142:159.
191. Fredriksson K, et al. Repeated cranial computed tomography and magnetic resonance imaging scan in two cases of eclampsia. *Stroke* 1989;20:547.
192. Chesley LC, Cooper DW. Genetics of hypertension in pregnancy: possible single gene control of pre-eclampsia and eclampsia in the descendants of eclamptic women. *Br J Obstet Gynecol* 1986;93:898.
193. Irgens HU, et al. Long term mortality of mothers and fathers after pre-eclampsia: Population based cohort study. *BMJ* 2001;323:1213.
194. Bryans OI Jr. The remote prognosis in toxemia of pregnancy. *Clin Obstet Gynecol* 1966;9:973.
195. Svensson A, Ahdersch B, Hansson L. Prediction of later hypertension following a hypertensive pregnancy. *J Hypertens* 1983;1:94.
196. Pritchard JA, et al. Intravascular hemolysis, thrombocytopenia and other hematologic abnormalities associated with severe toxemia of pregnancy. *N Engl J Med* 1954;250:89.
197. MacKenna J, Dover NL, Browne RG. Pre-eclampsia associated with hemolysis, elevated liver enzymes and low platelets: an obstetric emergency? *Obstet Gynecol* 1983;62:751.
198. Greer IA, Cameron AD, Walker JJ. HELLP syndrome: pathologic entity or technical inadequacy? *Am J Obstet Gynecol* 1985;152:113.
199. Van Dam PA, Renier M, Beakelandt M. Disseminated intravascular coagulation and the syndrome of hemolysis, elevated liver enzymes, and low platelets in severe preeclampsia. *Obstet Gynecol* 1989;73:97.
200. Poldre PA. Haptoglobin helps diagnose the HELLP syndrome. *Am J Obstet Gynecol* 1987;157:1267.
201. Schorr-Lesnick B, et al. Liver diseases unique to pregnancy. *Am J Gastroenterol* 1991;86:659.
202. Weinstein L. Preeclampsia/eclampsia with hemolysis, elevated liver enzymes, and thrombocytopenia. *Obstet Gynecol* 1985;66:657.
203. McKay DG. Hematologic evidence of DIC in eclampsia. *Obstet Gynecol Surv* 1972;27:399.
204. Magann EF, et al. Neonatal salvage by weeks gestation in pregnancies complicated by HELLP syndrome. *J Soc Gynecol Invest* 1994;1:206.
205. Sibai BM. The HELLP syndrome (hemolysis, elevated liver enzymes, and low platelets): much ado about nothing? *Am J Obstet Gynecol* 1990;162:311.
206. Robertson WB, et al. The placental bed biopsy: review from three European centers. *Am J Obstet Gynecol* 1986;155:401.
207. Zhou Y, et al. Preeclampsia is associated with failure of human cytotrophoblasts to mimic a vascular adhesion phenotype. One cause of defective endovascular invasion in this syndrom? *J Clin Invest* 1997;99:2152.
207a. Brosens I, Robertson WB, Dixon HG. The physiological response of the vessels of the placental bed to normal pregnancy. *J Pathol Bacteriol* 1967;93:569.
208. Pijnenborg R, et al. Review article: trophoblast invasion and the establishment of haemochorial placentation in man and laboratory animals. *Placenta* 1981;2:71.
209. Sheppard BL, Bonnar J. An ultrastructural study of uteroplacental spiral arteries in hypertensive and normotensive pregnancy and fetal growth retardation. *Br J Obstet Gynecol* 1981;88:695.
210. Damsky C, Sutherland A, Fisher S. Extracellular matrix: adhesive interaction in early mammalian embryogenesis, implantation and placentation. *FASEB J* 1994;7:1320.
211. Zhou Y, et al. Pre-eclampsia is associated with abnormal expression of adhesion molecules by invasive cytotrophoblasts. *J Clin Invest* 1993;91:950.
212. Lunell NO, et al. Uteroplacental blood flow in pregnancy induced hypertension. *Scand J Clin Lab Invest* 1984;169(Suppl):28.
213. Browne JC, Veall N. The maternal placental blood flow in normotensive and hypertensive women. *J Obstet Gynaecol Br Empire* 1953;60:141.
214. Gerretsen G, Huisjes HJ, Elema JD. Morphological changes of the spiral arteries in the placental bed in relation to pre-eclampsia and fetal growth retardation. *Br J Obstet Gynecol* 1981;88:876.
215. Laberrere CA. Acute atherosis: a histopathological hallmark of immune aggression? *Placenta* 1988;9:95.
216. Zeek PM, Assali NS. Vascular changes in the decidua associated with eclamptogenic toxemia. *Am J Clin Pathol* 1950;20:1099.
217. Page EW. The relation between hydatid moles, relative ischemia of the gravid uterus, and placental origin of eclampsia. *Am J Obstet Gynecol* 1939;37:291.
218. Kitzmiller JL, Watt N, Driscoll SG. Decidual arteriopathy in hypertension and diabetes in pregnancy: immunofluorescent studies. *Am J Obstet Gynecol* 1981;141:773.
219. Combs A, et al. Experimental preeclampsia produced by chronic constriction of the lower aorta: validation with longitudinal blood pressure measurements in conscious rhesus monkey. *Am J Obstet Gynecol* 1993;169:215.
220. Abitbol MM. Hemodynamic studies in experimental toxemia of the dog. *Obstet Gynecol* 1977;50:293.
221. Berger M, Cavanagh D. Toxemia of pregnancy: the hypertensive effect of acute experimental placental ischemia. *Am J Obstet Gynecol* 1963;87:293.
222. Uehara Y, et al. Placental defect and embryonic lethality in mice lacking hepatocyte growth factor/scatter factor. *Nature* 1995;373:702.

223. Maynard SE, et al. Excess placental soluble fms-like tyrosine kinase 1 (sFlt 1) may contribute to endothelial dysfunction, hypertension and protenuria in preeclampsia. *J Clin Invest* 2003;111:649.

224. Levine RJ, et al. Circulating angiogenic factors and the risk of preeclampsia. *N Engl J Med* 2004;350:672.

225. Thadhani R, et al. First trimester placental growth factor and soluble fms-like tyrosine kinase 1 and risk for preeclampsia. *J Clin Endocrinol Metab* 2004;89:770.

226. Eremina V, et al. Glomerular-specific alterations of VEGF-A expression lead to distinct congenital and acquired renal disease. *J Clin Invest* 2003;111:707.

227. Vassalli P, Morris RH, McCluskey RT. The pathogenic role of fibrin deposition in the glomerular lesions of toxemia of pregnancy. *J Exp Med* 1963;118:467.

228. Graham CH, et al. Role of oxygen in the regulation of trophoblast gene expression and invasion. *Placenta* 2000;21:443.)

229. Jaammeri KE, Koivuniemi AP, Carpen EO. Occurrence of trophoblasts in the blood of toxaemic patients. *Gynaecologia* 1965;160:315.

230. Wegmann TG, et al. Bidirectional cytokine interactions in the maternal-fetal relationship: is successful pregnancy a TH2 phenomenon? *Immunol Today* 1993;14:353.

231. DaSilva JA, Spector TD. The role of pregnancy in the course and etiology of rheumatoid arthritis. *Clin Rheumatol* 1992;11:189.

232. Varner W. Autoimmune disorders and pregnancy. *Semin Perinatol* 1991;15:238.

233. Billington WD. The normal fetomaternal immune relationship. *Clin Obstet Gynecol* 1992;6:417.

234. Kovats S, et al. A class I antigen, HLA-G, expressed in human trophoblasts. *Science* 1990;248:220.

235. Silver RK, et al. Soluble factors produced by isolated first-trimester chorionic villi directly inhibit proliferation of T cells. *Am J Obstet Gynecol* 1990;163:1914.

236. Favier R. Presence of elevated serum interleukin-2 levels in pregnant women. *N Engl J Med* 1990;322:270.

237. Varga P, et al. Natural lymphocyte cytotoxicity of women with different symptoms of toxemia. *Eur J Obstet Gynecol Reprod Biol* 1991;39:133.

238. Dudley DJ, et al. Adaptive immune responses during murine pregnancy: pregnancy-induced regulation of lymphokine production by activated T lymphocytes. *Am J Obstet Gynecol* 1993;168:155.

239. Holmes CH, Asimpson KL. Complement and pregnancy: new insights into the immunobiology of the fetomaternal relationship. *Clin Obstet Gynecol* 1992;6:439.

240. Bruce-Chwatt LJ. Malaria and pregnancy. *Br Med J* 1983;286:1457.

241. Luft BJ, Remington JS. Effect of pregnancy on augmentation of natural killer cell activity by Corynebacterium parvum and Toxoplasma gondii. *J Immunol* 1984;132:2375.

242. Greenwood AM, et al. Can malaria chemoprophylaxis be restricted to first pregnancies? *Transact R Soc Tropical Med Hygiene* 1994;88:681.

243. Brettle RP. Pregnancy and its effect on HIV/AIDS. *Clin Obstet Gynecol* 1992;6:125.

244. Kirby DR. Inhibition of egg implantation and induction of abortion in mice by heterologous immune serum. *Nature* 1967;216:1220.

245. Croy BA, Chapeau G. Evaluation of the pregnancy immunotrophism hypothesis by assessment of the reproductive performance of young adult mice of genotype scid/scid.bg/bg. *J Reprod Fertil* 1990;88:231.

246. Medina KL, Kincade PW. Pregnancy-related steroids are potential negative regulators of B lymphopoiesis. *Proc Natl Acad Sci USA* 1994;91:5382.

247. Beer AE, Need JA. Immunological aspects of pre-eclampsia–eclampsia. *Birth Defects* 1985;21:131.

248. Klonoff-Cohen HS, et al. An epidemiologic study of contraception and preeclampsia. *JAMA* 1989;262:3143.

249. Campbell D, MacGillvray I, Carr-Hill P. Pre-eclampsia in second pregnancy. *Br J Gynaecol* 1985;92:131.

250. Need J. Preeclampsia in pregnancy by different fathers. *Br Med J* 1975;1:548.

251. Esplin MS, et al. Paternal and maternal components of the predisposition to preeclampsia. *N Engl J Med* 2001;344:867.

252. Skjaerven R, et al. The interval between pregnancies and the risk of preeclmapsia. *N Engl J Med* 2002;346:33.

253. Robillard PY, et al. Association of pregnancy-induced hypertension with duration of sexual cohabitation before conception. *Lancet* 1994;344:973.

254. Need J, Bell B, Meffin E. Preeclampsia in pregnancy from donor insemination. *J Reprod Immunol* 1983;5:329.

255. Serhal P, Craft I. Immune basis for preeclampsia: evidence from oocyte recipients. *Lancet* 1987;1:744.

256. Marti JJ, Herman U. Immunogenosis: a new etiologic concept of "essential" EPH gestosis, with special reference of the primigravid patient. *Am J Obstet Gynecol* 1977;128:483.

257. Trogstad L, et al. Changing paternity and time since last pregnancy; the impact on eclampsia risk. *Int J Epidemiol* 2001;30:1317.

258. Skjaerven RS, Wilcox AJ, Lie RT. The interval between pregnancies and the risk of preeclampsia. *N Engl J Med* 2002;346:33.

259. Muttukrishna S, et al. Serum inhibin A and activin A are elevated prior to the onset of preeclampsia. *Hum Reprod* 2000;15:1640.

260. Chaouat G, et al. Control of fetal survival in CBAxDBA2 mice by lymphokine therapy. *J Reprod Fertil* 1990;89:447.

261. Chen HL, et al. Tumor necrosis factor alpha mRNA and protein are present in human placental and uterine cells at early and late stages of gestation. *Am J Pathol* 1991;139:327.

262. Austgulen R, et al. Expression of receptors for tumor necrosis factor in human placenta at term. *Acta Obstet Gynecol Scand* 1992;71:417.

263. McCartney CP. Pathological anatomy of acute hypertension of pregnancy. *Circulation* 1964;30(Suppl II):37.

264. Moake JL. Haemolytic—uremic syndrome: basic science. *Lancet* 1994;343:393.

265. Campbell DM, Campbell AJ. Evans blue disappearance rate in normal and preeclamptic pregnancy. *Clin Exp Hypertens* 1983;2:163.

266. Rodgers GM, Taylor RN, Roberts JM. Preeclampsia is associated with a serum factor cytotoxic to human endothelial cells. *Am J Obstet Gynecol* 1988;159:908.

267. Haller H, et al. Endothelial-cell permeability and protein kinase C in preeclampsia. *Lancet* 1998;351:945.

268. Scholtes MC, Gerretsen G, Haak HL. The factor VIII ratio in normal and pathologic pregnancy. *Eur J Obstet Gynecol Reprod Biol* 1983;16:89.

269. Lockwood CJ, Peters JH. Increased plasma levels of ED1+ cellular fibronectin precede the clinical signs of preeclampsia. *Am J Obstet Gynecol* 1990;162:358.

270. Boffa MC, et al. Predictive value of plasma thrombomodulin in preeclampsia and gestational hypertension. *Thromb Haemost* 1998;79:1092

271. Taylor RN, et al. High plasma cellular fibronectin levels correlate with biochemical and clinical features of preeclampsia but cannot be attributed to hypertension alone. *Am J Obstet Gynecol* 1991;165:895.

272. Chavarria ME, et al. Maternal plasma cellular fibronectin concentrations in normal and preeclamptic pregnancies: a longitudinal study for early prediction of preeclampsia. *Am J Obstet Gynecol* 2002;187:595.

273. Burrows TD, King A, Loke YW. Expression of adhesion molecules by endovascular trophoblast and decidual endothelial cells: implications for vascular invasion during implantation. *Placenta* 1994;15:21.

274. Airoldi L, et al. Soluble intercellular adhesion molecule-1 serum profil in physiologic and ppreeclamptic pregnancy. *Am J Reprod Immunoll* 1998;39:183.

275. Savvidou MD, et al. Endothelial dysfunction and raised plasma concentration of asymmetric dimethylargininge in pregnant women who subsequently develop pre-eclampsia. *Lancet* 2003;361:1511

276. Hubel CA, et al. Lipid peroxidation in pregnancy: new perspectives on preeclampsia. *Am J Obstet Gynecol* 1989;161:1025.

277. Gryglewski RJ, Palmer RM, Moncada S. Superoxide anions is involved in the breakdown of endothelium derived vascular relaxing factor. *Nature* 1986;320:454.

278. Lorentzen B, et al. Sera from preeclamptic women increase the content of triglycerides and reduce the release of prostacyclin in cultured endothelial cells. *Thromb Res* 1991;63:363.

279. Moncada S, et al. A lipid peroxide inhibits the enzyme in blood vessel microsomes that generates from prostaglandin endoperoxides the substance (prostaglandin X) which prevents platelet aggregation. *Prostaglandins* 1976;12:715.

280. Kloner RA, Przyklenk K, Whittaker P. Deleterious effects of oxygen radicals in ischemia/reperfusion: resolved and unresolved issues. *Circulation* 1989;80:1115.

281. Barrowcliffe TW, Gutteridge JM, Dormandy TL. The effect of fatty-acid auto-oxidation products on blood coagulation. *Thromb Diath Haemorrh* 1975;33:271.

282. Wickens D, et al. Free radical oxidation (peroxidation) products in plasma in normal and abnormal pregnancy. *Ann Clin Biochem* 1981;18:158.

283. Wickens D, et al. Lipid peroxide levels and lipid content of serum lipoprotein fractions of pregnant subjects with or without preeclampsia. *Clin Chim Acta* 1981;115:155.

284. Roggensack AM, Zhang Y, Davidge ST. Evidence for peroxynitrite formation in the vasculature of women with preeclampsia. *Hypertension* 1999;33:83.

285. Berge LN, Ostensen M, Revhaug A. Phagocytic activity in pre-eclampsia. *Acta Obstet Gynecol Scand* 1988;67:499.

286. Stamler FW. Fatal eclamptic disease of pregnant rats fed an anti-vitamin E stress diet. *Am J Pathol* 1959;35:1207.

287. Wang Y, et al. The imbalance between thromboxane and prostacyclin in pre-eclampsia is associated with an imbalance between lipid peroxides and vitamin E in maternal blood. *Am J Obstet Gynecol* 1991;165:1695.

288. Rakugi H, et al. Evidence for endothelin-1 release from resistance vessels of rats in response to hypoxia. *Biochem Biophys Res Commun* 1990;169:973.

289. Kamoi K, et al. Plasma endothelin-1 levels in patients with pregnancy-induced hypertension. *N Engl J Med* 1990;323:1486.

290. Taylor RN, et al. Women with preeclampsia have higher plasma endothelin levels than women with normal pregnancies. *J Clin Endocrinol Metab* 1990;71:1675.

291. Schiff E, et al. Endothelin-1 receptors on the human placenta and fetal membranes: evidence for different binding properties in preeclampsias. *Gynecol Endocrinol* 1993;7:67.

292. Taylor RN, et al. Preeclamptic sera stimulate increased platelet-derived growth factor mRNA and protein expression by cultured human endothelial cells. *Am J Reprod Immunol* 1991;25:105.

293. Musci TJ, et al. Mitogenic activity is increased in the sera of preeclamptic women before delivery. *Am J Obstet Gynecol* 1988;159:1446.
294. Taylor RN, Heilbron DC, Roberts JM. Growth factor activity in the blood of women destined to develop preeclampsia is elevated from early pregnancy. *Am J Obstet Gynecol* 1990;63:1839.
295. McCarthy AL, et al. Abnormal endothelial cell function of resistance arteries from women with preeclampsia. *Am J Obstet Gynecol* 1993;168:1323.
296. Tulenko T, et al. The in vitro effect on arterial wall function of serum from patients with pregnancy-induced hypertension. *Am J Obstet Gynecol* 1987;156:817.
297. Socol ML, et al. Platelet activation in preeclampsia. *Am J Obstet Gynecol* 1985;151:494.
298. Wilhelmsson L, Wikland M, Wiqvist N. PGH2, TxA2 and PGI2 have potent and differentiated actions on human uterine contractility. *Prostaglandins* 1981;21:277.
299. Vanhoutte PM. Endothelium and control of vascular function. *Hypertension* 1989;13:658.
300. Dadak C, et al. Reduced umbilical artery prostacyclin formation in complicated pregnancies. *Am J Obstet Gynecol* 1982;144:792.
301. Mills JL, et al. Prostacyclin and thromboxane changes predating clinical onset of preeclampsia. *JAMA* 1999;282:356.
302. Fitzgerald DJ, et al. Decreased prostacyclin biosynthesis preceding the clinical manifestation of pregnancy-induced hypertension. *Circulation* 1987;75:956.
303. Condie RG, Ogston D. Sequential studies on components of the haemostatic mechanism in pregnancy with particular reference to the development of preeclampsia. *Br J Obstet Gynecol* 1976;83:938.
304. van der Poll T, et al. Activation of coagulation after administration of tumor necrosis factor to normal subjects. *N Engl J Med* 1990;332:1622.
305. Estrada C, et al. Nitric oxide mediates tumor necrosis factor-alpha cytotoxicity in endothelial cells. *Biochem Biophys Res Comm* 1992;186:475.
306. deBoer K, et al. Placental-type plasminogen activator inhibitor in preeclampsia. *Am J Obstet Gynecol* 1988;158:518.
307. Zondervan HA, et al. Maternal whole blood viscosity in pregnancy hypertension. *Gynecol Obstet Invest* 1988;25:83.
308. Rappaport VJ, et al. Anti-vascular endothelial cell antibodies in severe preeclampsia. *Am J Obstet Gynecol* 1990;162:138.
309. Blereau RP. HELLP syndrome without hypertension. *South Med J* 1987;80:1068.
310. Pritchard JA, et al. How often does maternal preeclampsia–eclampsia incite thrombocytopenia in the fetus? *Obstet Gynecol* 1987;70:334.
311. Brazy JE, Grimm JK, Little VA. Neonatal manifestation of severe maternal hypertension occurring before the 36th week of pregnancy. *J Pediatr* 1982;100:265.
312. Briner VA, Lüscher TF. Role of vascular endothelial abnormalities in clinical medicine: atherosclerosis, hypertension, diabetes and endotoxemia. *Adv Intern Med* 1994;39:1.
313. Ferris TF. Hypertension in pregnancy. *Kidney* 1990;23:1.
314. Redman CW. Controlled trials of antihypertensive drugs in pregnancy. *Am J Kidney Dis* 1991;17:149.
315. Sibai BM, et al. A comparison of no medication versus methyldopa or labetalol in chronic hypertension during pregnancy. *Am J Obstet Gynecol* 1990;162:960.
316. Sibai MB, Anderson GD. Pregnancy outcome of intensive therapy in severe hypertension in first trimester. *Obstet Gynecol* 1986;67:517.
317. Redman CW. Treatment of hypertension in pregnancy. *Kidney Int* 1986;18:267.
318. Remuzzi G, Ruggenenti P. Prevention and treatment of pregnancy-associated hypertension: what have we learned in the last 10 years? *Am J Kidney Dis* 1991;XVIII:285.
319. Lund CJ, Donovan JC. Blood volume during pregnancy. *Am J Obstet Gynecol* 1967;98:394.
320. Clark SL, Cotton DB. Clinical indications for pulmonary artery catheterisation in the patient with severe pre-eclampsia. *Am J Obstet Gynecol* 1988;158:453.
321. Collins R, Yusuf S, Peto R. Overview of randomised trials of diuretics in pregnancy. *Br Med J* 1985;290:17.
322. Christianson R, Page EW. Diuretic drugs and pregnancy. *Obstet Gynecol* 1976;48:647.
323. Kincaid-Smith P, Bullen M, Mills J. Prolonged use of methyldopa in severe hypertension in pregnancy. *Br Med J* 1966;1:274.
324. Redman CW, et al. Fetal outcome in trial of antihypertensive treatment in pregnancy. *Lancet* 1976;II:753.
325. Redman CW, Berlin LG, Bonner J. Treatment of hypertension in pregnancy with methyldopa: blood pressure control and side effects. *Br J Obstet Gynecol* 1977;84:419.
326. Ounsted M, et al. Maternal hypertension with superimposed pre-eclampsia: effects on child development at years. *Br J Obstet Gynaecol* 1983;90:644.
327. Redmond GP. Propranolol and fetal growth retardation. *Semin Perinatol* 1982;6:142.
328. Buffers L, Kennedy S, Rubin P. Atenolol and fetal weight in chronic hypertension. *Clin Exp Hypertens* 1989;88:468(abst).
329. Gallery ED, et al. Randomized comparison of methyldopa and oxprenolol for treatment of hypertension in pregnancy. *Br Med J* 1979;1:1591.
330. Rubin PC, et al. Placebo-controlled trial of atenolol in treatment of pregnancy associated hypertension. *Lancet* 1983;I:431.
331. Nylund L, et al. Labetalol for the treatment of hypertension in pregnancy: pharmacokinetics and effects on the uteroplacental blood flow. *Acta Obstet Gynecol Scand* 1984;118:71.
332. Lamming GD, Symonds EB. Use of labetalol and methyldopa in pregnancy-induced hypertension. *Br J Clin Pharmacol* 1979;8:217S.
333. Fudge TL, McKinnon WM, Geary WL. Current surgical management of pheochromocytoma during pregnancy. *Arch Surg* 1980;115:1224.
334. Widerlöv E, Karlman I, Storsäter J. Hydralazine-induced neonatal thrombocytopenia. *N Engl J Med* 1980;301:1235.
335. Walters BN, Redman CW. Treatment of severe pregnancy-associated hypertension with the calcium antagonist nifedipine. *Br J Obstet Gynaecol* 1984;91:330.
336. Parisi VM, Salinas J, Stockmar EJ. Fetal vascular response to maternal nicardipine administration in the hypertensive ewe. *Am J Obstet Gynecol* 1989;161:1035.
337. Constantine G, et al. Nifedipine as a second line antihypertensive drug in pregnancy. *Br J Obstet Gynecol* 1987;94:1136.
338. Kreft-Jais C, et al. Angiotensin converting enzyme inhibitors during pregnancy: a summary of 22 treated patients given captopril and 9 given enalapril. *Br J Obstet Gynecol* 1988;95:420.
339. Schubiger G, Flury G, Nassberger J. Enalapril for pregnancy-induced hypertension: acute renal failure in a neonate. *Ann Intern Med* 1988;108:215.
340. Pryde PG, et al. Angiotensin converting enzyme inhibitor fetopathy. *J Am Soc Nephrol* 1993;3:1575.
341. Hanssens, SM, et al. Fetal and neonatal effects of treatment with angiotensin converting enzyme inhibitors. *Obstet Gynecol* 1991;78:128.
342. Nightingale FL. Warnings on the use of ACE inhibitor in the second and third trimester of pregnancy. *JAMA* 1991;267:244.
343. Nayar B, et al. Losartan inducet fetal toxicity. *Indin J Pediatr* 2003;70:923.
344. Saji H, et al. Losartan and fetal toxicity. *Lancet* 2001;357:363.
345. Bed rest and non-proteinuric hypertension in pregnancy. (Editorial). *Lancet* 1992;339:1023.
346. Sibai BM, et al. Maternal and perinatal outcome of conservative management of severe preeclampsia in midtrimester. *Am J Obstet Gynecol* 1985;152:32.
347. Tuffnell DJ, et al. Randomised controlled trial of day care for hypertension in pregnancy. *Lancet* 1992;339:224.
348. Mabie WC, et al. A comparative trial of labetalol and hydralazine in acute management of severe hypertension complicating pregnancy. *Obstet Gynecol* 1987;70:328.
349. Lindow SW, et al. The effect of sublingual nifedipine on uteroplacental blood flow in hypertensive pregnancy. *Br J Obstet Gynecol* 1988;95:1276.
350. Naulty J, Cefalo RC, Lewis PE. Fetal toxicity of nitroprusside in the pregnant ewe. *Am J Obstet Gynecol* 1981;139:708.
351. Shoemaker CT, Meyers M. Sodium nitroprusside for control of severe hypertensive disease of pregnancy: a case report and discussion of potential toxicity. *Am J Obstet Gynecol* 1984;149:171.
352. White WB. Management of hypertension during lactation. *Hypertension* 1984;6:297.
353. Gallery ED, Delprado W, Györy AZ. Antihypertensive effect of plasma volume expansion in pregnancy-associated hypertension. *Aust NZ J Med* 1981;11:20.
354. Weiner CP, Socol ML, Vaisrub N. Control of preeclamptic hypertension by ketanserin, a new serotonin receptor antagonist. *Am J Obstet Gynecol* 1984;149:496.
355. Bonnard J, Redman CW, Sheppard BL. Treatment of fetal growth retardation in utero with heparin and dipyridamole. *Eur J Obstet Gynecol Reprod Biol* 1975;5:123.
356. Chua S, Redman CW. Are prophylactic anticonvulsants required in severe preeclampsia? *Lancet* 1991;337:250.
357. Lucas MJ, Leveno KJ, Cunningham FG. A comparison of magnesium sulfate with phenytoin for prevention of eclampsia. *N Engl J Med* 1995;333:201.
358. The Magpie Trial Collaborative Group. Do women with pre-eclampsia, and their babies, benefit from magnesium sulfate? The Magpie Trial: a randomised placebo-controlled trial. *Lancet* 2002;359:1877.
359. Mastrogiannis DS, et al. Effect of magnesium sulfate on plasma endothelin-1 levels in normal and preeclamptic pregnancies. *Am J Obstet Gynecol* 1992;167:1554.
360. Kemp PA, et al. Magnesium sulphate reverses the carotid vasoconstriction caused by endothelin 1, angiotensin II and neuropeptide-Y, but not that caused by NG-nitro-L-arginine methyl ester, in conscious rats. *Clin Sci* 1993;85:175.
361. Barton JR, et al. Magnesium sulfate therapy in preeclampsia is associated with increased urinary cyclic guanosine phosphate excretion. *Am J Obstet Gynecol* 1992;167:931.
362. Belfort MA, Moise KJ Jr. Effect of magnesium sulfate on maternal brain blood flow in pre-eclampsia: a randomized, placebo-controlled study. *Am J Obstet Gynecol* 1992;167:661.
363. Sibai BM, et al. Effect of magnesium sulfate on electroencephalographic findings in preeclampsia–eclampsia. *Obstet Gynecol* 1984;64:261.
364. Sibai BM. Magnesium sulfate prophylaxis in preeclampsia: lessons learned from recent trials. *Am J Obstet Gynecol* 2004;190:1520.

365. Hutton JD, et al. Management of severe pre-eclampsia and eclampsia by UK consultants. *Br J Obstet Gynaecol* 1992;99:554.

366. Kanayama N, et al. A new treatment of severe preeclampsia by long-term epidural anesthesia. *J Hum Hypertension* 1999;13:167.

367. Shnider SM, Levinson G. Anesthesia for cesarean section. In: Shnider SM, Levinson G, eds. *Anesthesia for obstetrics,* 2nd ed. Baltimore: Williams & Wilkins, 1987:159.

368. Duffy BL. HELLP syndrome and the anaesthetist. *Anesthesia* 1988;43:223.

369. Brizgys RV, et al. The incidence and neonatal effects of maternal hypotension during epidural anesthesia for cesarean section. *Anesthesiology* 1987;67:782.

370. Campbell S, et al. Qualitative assessment of uteroplacental blood flow: early screening test for the high-risk pregnancies. *Obstet Gynecol* 1986;68:649.

371. Hanretty KP, Whittle MJ, Rubin PC. Doppler uteroplacental waveforms in pregnancy-induced hypertension: a re-appraisal. *Lancet* 1988;1:850.

372. Hall MH, Chng PK, MacGillivray I. Is routine antenatal care worth while? *Lancet* 1980;II:78.

373. Chesley LC, Williams LO. Renal glomerular and tubular function in relation to the hyperuricemia of pre-eclampsia and eclampsia. *Am J Obstet Gynecol* 1945;50:367.

374. Dunlop W, Davison JM. The effect of normal pregnancy upon the renal handling of uric acid. *Br J Obstet Gynecol* 1977;84:13.

375. Oian P, Monrad-Honsen HP, Maltau JM. Serum uric acid correlates with beta 2-microglobulin in pre-eclampsia. *Acta Obstet Gynecol* 1985;152:1038.

376. Redman CW, Bonnar J, Beilin L. Early platelet consumption in pre-eclampsia. *Br Med J* 1978;I:467.

377. Beaufils M, et al. Prevention of preeclampsia by early antiplatelet therapy. *Lancet* 1985;I:840.

378. Beaufils M, et al. Prospective controlled study of early antiplatelet therapy in prevention of preeclampsia. *Adv Nephrol* 1986;15:87.

379. Schiff E, et al. The use of aspirin to prevent pregnancy-induced hypertension and lower the ratio of thromboxane A2 to prostacyclin in relatively high risk pregnancies. *N Engl J Med* 1989;321:351.

380. CLASP Collaborative Group. CLASP: a randomised trial of low-dose aspirin for the prevention and treatment of pre-eclampsia among 9364 women. *Lancet* 1994;343:619.

381. Caritis S, et al. Low-dose aspirin to prevent preeclampsia in women at high risk. *N Engl J Med* 1998;338:701.

382. Coomarasamy A, et al. Aspirin for prevention of preeclampsia in women with historical risk factors: a systematic review. *Obst Gynecol* 2003;101:1319.

383. Chappell LC, et al. Effect of antioxidants on the occurrence of pre-eclampsia in women at increased risk: a randomised trial. *Lancet* 1999;354:810.

384. Levine RJ, et al. Trial of calcium to prevent preeclampsia. *N Engl J Med* 1997;337:69.

CHAPTER 54 ■ PATHOGENESIS AND TREATMENT OF HYPERTENSION IN THE DIABETIC PATIENT

RAYMOND O. ESTACIO AND ROBERT W. SCHRIER

INTRODUCTION

The prevalence of diagnosed diabetes in the United States continues to rise and has increased from 4.9% in 1990 (1) to 7.3% in 2000 (2). There were approximately 15 million U.S. adults aged 18 years or older who had a diagnosis of diabetes (6.3 million men and 8.7 million women) (2). In the United States, the prevalence of diabetes, specifically type 2, in African Americans, Native Americans, Asian Americans, and Hispanic Americans is two- to sixfold greater than white non-Hispanic American diabetic patients (3,4). Worldwide diabetes is expected to rise from 171 million in 2000 to an estimated 366 million by 2030 (5). This is alarming because diabetes places a tremendous burden on the current tenuous medical economy and, more importantly, its effects on human suffering. Epidemiologic data exist to suggest that the vascular complications associated with diabetes mellitus are substantially aggravated in the presence of hypertension which occurs in both type 1 and type 2 diabetes. Mortality among diabetic subjects is increased as much as fivefold when hypertension is present (6,7). Risks for cardiovascular disease (8–12), renal disease (13–17), retinopathy (18–20), and neuropathy (21) are also significantly increased when hypertension is found in association with diabetes.

One of the major differences between type 1 and type 2 diabetes is the onset of hypertension. The prevalence of hypertension in type 1 diabetes is similar to that of the general population until the onset of diabetic nephropathy (22). In comparison, nearly 50% of type 2 diabetic patients have hypertension at the time of diagnosis of their diabetes (23). Along with hypertension, type 2 diabetic patients often present with other potent risk factors for vascular disease, specifically obesity, hyperinsulinemia and abnormal lipid profiles which place them at a higher risk for cardiovascular disease. To compound the problem, the diagnosis of type 2 diabetes is often delayed resulting in prolonged exposure to these risk factors before any intervention is implemented (24). Thus it is paramount to identify these patients and aggressively treat them with interventions proven to decrease the morbidity and mortality. Recently, there have been a considerable number of prospective interventional studies demonstrating the effectiveness of treating hypertension in diabetes.

The purpose of this chapter is to review some of the potential pathogenic mechanisms by which hypertension develops in type 1 and type 2 diabetes and to provide an overview of recent clinical trials in order to guide the treatment of hypertension in diabetes.

Pathogenesis of Hypertension in Diabetes

Although not all diabetic patients will develop overt nephropathy leading to end-stage renal disease (ESRD), most patients who develop overt nephropathy and all patients who develop ESRD will have hypertension. In fact, the prevalence of hypertension increases with albuminuria stage. In type 1 diabetic patients, the prevalence of hypertension was 42%, 52%, and 79% in patients with normo-, micro- and overt albuminuria, respectively. The corresponding prevalences in type 2 diabetic patients were from 71%, 90%, and 93%, respectively (25). It is believed that there are several factors that contribute to the pathogenesis of hypertension in the diabetic patient. These include (a) genetic predisposition, (b) sodium retention, (c) metabolic factors such as insulin resistance that contribute to the genesis of hyperinsulinemia, and (d) accentuated neurohumoral responses. (Table 54-1).

Genetic Predisposition

It appears that genetics plays a significant role in the development of hypertension in both type 1 and type 2 diabetes. The notion of genetic susceptibility is supported by the difference of prevalence rates of hypertension in certain racial and ethnic groups such as in African Americans (63%) versus non-Hispanic whites (38%) and Hispanic whites (34%) (26), especially in type 2 diabetes. As mentioned earlier, the prevalence of hypertension increases in type 1 diabetes with increasing albuminuria stage. Thus it is not surprising to observe that the genetic susceptibility to hypertension in type 1 diabetes appears to be related to the progression of diabetic nephropathy (27–29). In a case-control study, Fagerudd et al., assessed the prevalence of hypertension among parents of type 1 diabetic patients with and without diabetic nephropathy. Arterial hypertension was present in 57% of parents of patients with diabetic nephropathy compared with 41% of parents of patients without diabetic nephropathy ($p = 0.034$) (29). In addition, the cumulative incidence of hypertension was higher among parents of patients with diabetic nephropathy, with a shift toward younger age at onset of hypertension in this group (29). The authors concluded that familial predisposition to essential hypertension increases the risk of diabetic nephropathy and may also contribute to the development of systemic hypertension in patients with type 1 diabetes and diabetic nephropathy. Other genetic associations that may increase the risk for the development of hypertension include increases in sodium-lithium (30–32) and sodium-hydrogen counter-transport (33) and insulin resistance (34–36).

Sodium Homeostasis

Diabetic patients are noted to have an increase in total body sodium which contributes to the development of hypertension. It appears that both hyperglycemia and hyperinsulinemia can independently contribute to this process. Sodium (Na^+) retention occurs as a characteristic alteration in both type 1 and type 2 diabetes, Weidmann et al. demonstrated that exchangeable total body Na^+ on average was increased by 10% when

TABLE 54-1

FACTORS INFLUENCING THE DEVELOPMENT OF HYPERTENSION IN DIABETES

	Factors
Genetic	African American race
	Predisposition Na^+/Li^+ Transport
	Insulin resistance
Electrolyte abnormalities	Increased vascular smooth muscle calcium
	Increased sodium retention
	Sodium/hydrogen cotransport
	Decreased magnesium
Neurohumoral	Renin-angiotensin-aldosterone system
	Plasma catecholamines
	Increased pressor response to norepinephrine
	Decreased β-receptor response

compared to healthy controls and hypertensive patients without diabetes (Fig. 54-1) (37). This abnormality which develops in the uncomplicated stage (no nephropathy) of both type 1 and type 2 diabetes differentiates diabetic from nondiabetic essential hypertensive subjects. This is further supported by Roland et al. who demonstrated a reduction of Na^+ excretion in diabetic patients versus nondiabetic patients when presented with a sodium load (38). Roland theorized this was secondary to enhance tubular absorption rather than impaired filtration as the glomerular filtration rate of the diabetic patients were higher than the nondiabetic patients.

Enhanced sodium reabsorption appears to occur by a number of mechanisms in diabetic patients. Hyperglycemia has been noted to increase total body sodium by enhancing the glucose–Na^+ cotransporter in the kidney (39). Na^+ retention is maintained as long as the hyperglycemia is not severe enough to induce an osmotic diuresis. DeFronzo et al. demonstrated that the administration of insulin in nondiabetic subjects resulted in a reduction in tubular Na^+ excretion in the absence of changes in the filtered load of glucose, glomerular filtration rate, renal blood flow, and plasma aldosterone concentration (40). DeFronzo suggested that insulin's effect was due to enhancement of Na^+ reabsorption in the diluting segment of the distal nephron. The mechanisms involve may include stimulation of the renal tubular Na^+-K^+ ATPase, Na^+-H^+ antiporter

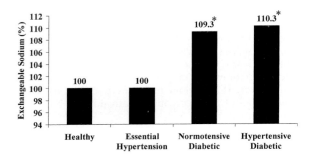

FIGURE 54-1. Comparison of exchangeable sodium after a sodium load in healthy nondiabetic patients, nondiabetic patients with essential hypertension, and diabetic patients without and with hypertension. *P<0.05. (From: Herman WH, Prior DE, Yassine MD, et al. Nephropathy in NIDDM is associated with cellular markers for hypertension. *Diabetes Care* 1993;16:815.)

and amplifying the action of aldosterone on Na^+ and K^+ transport (39).

It is clear once diabetic nephropathy occurs in either type 1 or type 2 diabetes, that one of the major mechanisms of hypertension is sodium retention. In subjects who were studied as inpatients receiving unrestricted sodium intake and in stable metabolic control, O'Hare et al. demonstrated that total exchangeable Na^+ was higher in diabetic patients with nephropathy than diabetic patients without nephropathy (41). Furthermore, the value for exchangeable Na^+ correlated with blood pressure only in diabetic patients with nephropathy ($r = 0.61$, $p < 0.01$). Thus, once diabetic nephropathy develops, hypertension becomes a consequence and a cause of further progression of renal disease in the diabetic patient (42,43).

Ion Transport Homeostasis

Electrolyte abnormalities associated with hypertension appear to involve not only alterations in ion transport of sodium but also in transport of calcium and magnesium. But what is not clear is whether the alterations occur prior to or a result of the milieu associated with the presence of diabetes and hypertension. One of the most studied disturbances in electrolyte abnormalities deal with sodium transport homeostasis. Sodium (Na^+)/lithium (Li^+) countertransport activity has been demonstrated to be strongly associated with the development of hypertension in the nondiabetic populations (44–47). Increased activity of Na^+/Li^+ CT strongly correlates with the development of hypertension in certain families (30–32).

In type 1 diabetic patients, Krolewski et al. demonstrated an association between the development of diabetic nephropathy and a predisposition to hypertension in subjects with an elevated maximal velocity of Na^+/Li^+ countertransport (30). In a review by Van Norren et al, Na^+/Li^+ countertransport activity was significantly higher in type 1 diabetic patients without nephropathy than in healthy control subjects (48). This prompted the authors to postulate that the etiology of the association is not clear but might be due to the association of Na^+/Li^+ countertransport activity with hypertension and hyperlipidemia, which are disorders frequently detected in diabetic patients.

In type 2 diabetes, it appears that insulin resistance may be associated with increased Na^+/Li^+ countertransport activity (49). Pinkney et al. measured Na^+/Li^+ countertransport activity in type 2 diabetic patients without nephropathy and found no correlation with fasting insulin levels ($r = 0.074$, $p = 0.28$), but did demonstrate a correlation between decreased insulin sensitivity and increased Na^+/Li^+ countertransport activity ($r = -0.37$, $p = 0.036$). Similar findings have been demonstrated by other investigators (50,51). Although the explanation for this association between increased Na^+/Li^+ countertransport activity and insulin resistance is not clear, it may be a marker or predictor for the development of hypertension and possibly diabetic nephropathy in insulin resistant, type 2 diabetes.

Another ion transport abnormality that has been studied is the sodium-hydrogen (Na^+/H^+) antiporter activity. Increased Na^+/H^+ antiporter activity has been shown to be increased in erythrocytes, leukocytes, and platelets from patients with essential hypertension and in lymphocytes and vascular smooth muscle cells from spontaneously hypertensive rat (52–54). In animal studies, induction of diabetes and increased blood glucose levels resulted in an increase in Na^+/H^+ antiporter activity which was then reversed with glycemic control (55). The mechanism by which this occurs appears to be via a glucose-induced protein kinase C–dependent mechanisms (56,57). The Na^+/H^+ antiporter has been shown to play a key role in the regulation of intracellular pH, cell volume, growth, differentiation, and contractility (58–61). Additionally, increased Na^+/H^+ antiporter activity may explain the relationship between intracellular Ca^{2+} metabolism in essential hypertension leading to enhanced vascular contractility (62).

As noted above, accumulation of intracellular Ca^{2+} has been implicated as major facilitator of hypertension in both diabetic and nondiabetic subjects. Acute intracellular calcium overload of vascular smooth muscle cells increases contractility leading to a rise in peripheral resistance resulting in essential hypertension (63). Results from diabetic animal models and from human subjects with diabetes reveal that intracellular calcium levels are increased in most tissues through various mechanisms and may play an essential role in the pathophysiology of diabetic complications (64).

Renin-Angiotensin-Aldosterone System

The renin-angiotensin-aldosterone system (RAAS) in diabetes has been examined by several investigators and has been implicated as a major contributor in the pathophysiology of the diabetic vascular complications. However, the role of RAAS in the pathogenesis of hypertension in the diabetic patient is not conclusive. In most studies, plasma renin activity (PRA) has not been found to be increased in hypertensive diabetic subjects (65,66). However, the "normal" PRA in an environment of elevated total body sodium and increased blood pressure, both known to suppress PRA, may infer inadequate suppression of RAAS in diabetic hypertension. Recent studies suggest that this may be the case (67,68). Price et al. compared the PRA response to the upright position on a low-salt diet and on a high-salt diet in hypertensive diabetic patients compared to healthy controls and hypertensive patients without diabetes. On the high-salt (200 mmol) diet, healthy subjects showed the expected PRA suppression (0.3 ± 0.1), but in patients with type 2 diabetes the PRA was less suppressed (1.2 ± 0.3 ng AI/mL/hour; $p = 0.003$) (68). The mechanism for this relative stimulation of the RAAS system has not been elucidated in the diabetic patient. Recently, Miller demonstrated that in healthy type 1 diabetic patients without complications during hyperglycemic conditions without glycosuria, mean arterial pressure (MAP), renal vascular resistance (RVR) and filtration fraction (FF) were significantly higher compared with the euglycemic phase (69). After the administration of losartan, an angiotensin II type 1 receptor blocker, a significant renal and peripheral vascular depressor effect was noted, with decreases in MAP, RVR, and FF in the hyperglycemic phase. During the euglycemic phase the responses to losartan were minimal. Miller suggested that moderate hyperglycemia, at least of a short duration, results in the activation of the circulating, and possibly the intrarenal, RAAS with resultant increases in blood pressure (69).

Additionally, a number of investigators have demonstrated that the diabetic vasculature is more sensitive to the pressor effects of angiotensin II (37,70). Weidmann et al. demonstrated that a lower infusion rate of angiotensin II was required in both normotensive and hypertensive type 2 diabetic patients to increase diastolic blood pressure by 20 mm Hg than in control subjects (37). The authors suggest that the increased sensitivity may be a reflection of disturbance in the RAAS feedback system. Drury et al. demonstrated a similar finding in type 1 diabetes (70).

Insulin Resistance and Hyperinsulinemia: Influence on Hypertension

There have been a number of studies demonstrating a clear relationship between insulin resistance, hyperinsulinemia and hypertension (71–74). Most recently, Ferrannini et al. demonstrated in 333 nondiabetic, normotensive, and nonobese patients that both decreased insulin sensitivity and increased fasting plasma insulin levels were independently associated with increases in blood pressure (73). The authors demonstrated that systolic blood pressure was 1.7 mm Hg and diastolic blood pressure was 2.3 mm Hg higher for each 10-unit increase in insulin resistance (i.e., a 10 μmol/min^{-1}/kg^{-1} decrement in the M value). Insulin resistance/hyperinsulinemia appears to contribute to the development of hypertension in several ways.

As already mentioned, insulin plays a role in Na^+ homeostasis by affecting the Na^+ transport systems and promoting Na^+ retention. Although insulin is considered to have direct vasodilatory effects in normotensive and nondiabetic subjects (75,76), possibly by inducing nitric oxide release (77), a number of studies have demonstrated that this response is blunted in obese (78), hypertensive (79,80) and diabetic subjects (81). In addition to the vasodilatory effects, insulin is also known to stimulate the sympathetic nervous system. Rowe et al. have demonstrated that the administration of insulin with subsequent stimulation of carbohydrate metabolism leads to the activation of the sympathetic nervous system and an increase in circulating norepinephrine levels (82), findings corroborated by other investigators (83–86). Thus, these studies suggest that insulin can affect the cardiovascular system by direct vasodilatory actions on the peripheral vasculature and an indirect effect on the sympathetic nervous system. These results suggest that an imbalance between these insulin effects favoring sympathetic stimulation may play a role in the pathogenesis of hypertension in diabetic patients. The mechanism by which insulin mediates its vasoactive effects through the sympathetic nervous system appears to be through beta-adrenergic receptors (87,88). Gros et al. demonstrated that insulin enhancement of vascular beta-adrenergic responsiveness resulting in vasodilation in normotensive animals is blunted in hypertensive animals (88).

Pathogenesis of Vascular Complications: Role of Hypertension and Diabetes

As we have already noted, the combination of hypertension and diabetes is associated with an increase in vascular complications. This next section will discuss the possible mechanisms by which this combination contributes to the pathogenesis of micro- and macrovascular diabetic complications. Although the mechanisms by which diabetes and hypertension cause vascular complications have not been completely defined, alterations in hemostasis and vascular endothelium function and structure appear to be involved (Table 54-2).

Hemostasis

Coagulation Abnormalities. Diabetes causes an imbalance between coagulation and fibrinolysis in favor of the procoagulant state. Specifically, diabetes is associated with an increase of procoagulant factors and impairment of fibrinolysis. Fibrinolysis is induced by plasmin which is mediated plasminogen activators. Plasminogen activator inhibitor-1 (PAI-1) produced by the liver and endothelial cells neutralizes the activity of the plasminogen activators leading to a decrease in fibrinolytic activity and a propensity for thrombosis (89). In this regard, PAI-1 levels have been noted to be elevated in both type 1 and type 2 diabetes (90,91) and in hypertension (92,93). The increased PAI-1 levels appear to be related not only to hyperinsulinemia but also to occur in conjunction with hyperglycemia and increased triglyceride levels (94). Other procoagulant factors that have

TABLE 54-2

FACTORS INFLUENCING THE PATHOGENESIS OF VASCULAR COMPLICATIONS
IN PATIENTS WITH HYPERTENSION IN DIABETES

	Diabetes	Hypertension
Hemostasis	Coagulation abnormalities Abnormal platelet aggregation and adhesion	Abnormal platelet aggregation and adhesion
Abnormal Vascular Endothelial Function and structure	Hypertrophy Impaired endothelium-mediated vasodilation	Hypertrophy Impaired endothelium-mediated vasodilation Leukocyte adherence

been noted to be increased in diabetes include endothelium-derived von Willebrand factor, factors VII and VIII, fibrinogen and thrombin-antithrombin complexes (95).

Platelet Abnormalities. Platelet adhesion and aggregation are enhanced in diabetic patients, further contributing to a procoagulant milieu in the diabetic individual (96). Increased platelet aggregation appears to be mediated by the high intracellular calcium and low magnesium reported to be present in diabetic and hypertensive subjects (96). Other abnormalities demonstrated in platelet function include an increase in the release of thromboglobulin and platelet factor 4, decreased levels of platelet-derived growth factor and serotonin, decreased platelet survival, increased platelet generation of vasoconstrictor prostanoids, reduced platelet generation of prostacyclin and other vasodilator prostanoids, and increased glycosylation of platelet proteins (97). Nitric oxide produced by platelets and endothelial tissue is decreased in diabetic and hypertensive states and thereby lead to an increase in platelet aggregation and adhesion to endothelial cells (98).

Vascular Endothelium Function and Structure. Both diabetes and hypertension have a number of functional and structural abnormalities in the vascular endothelium, which can precipitate the development of diabetic vascular complications. In the hyperglycemic state, protein kinase C can be activated and stimulate prostanoids, endothelin and angiotensin converting enzyme which can result in decreasing vascular relaxation (98,99). Hyperglycemia also increases endothelial cell collagen IV and fibronectin synthesis; increased activity of enzymes involved in collagen synthesis also may result in basement membrane thickening (100). Diabetes, specifically type 2 diabetes, is associated with lipid abnormalities which include higher triglyceride and very-low-density lipoproteins (VLDL) levels, lower high-density lipoprotein (HDL) levels, and increased levels of small dense low-density lipoprotein (LDL) particles (101). These specific lipid abnormalities have been associated with an increased risk for the development of vascular complications in the diabetic patient. Hyperinsulinemia may also mediate, through insulin-like growth factor-1 (IGF-1), their atherogenic effects on both vascular endothelial cells and vascular smooth muscle cells (VSMC) by increasing mitogenic signaling pathways and thymidine incorporation into DNA (96).

Panza et al. have demonstrated by strain-gauge plethysmography that nondiabetic patients with essential hypertension have impaired endothelium- mediated vasodilation (102). The primary mechanism by which hypertension affects endothelial function is by the elevation of shear stress resulting in structural changes which alter endothelial cell metabolism and even endothelial cell detachment (103). Hypertension also increases the accumulation of macrophages in the subendothelial space (104).

Treatment of Hypertension in Diabetes

It is clear that the combination of hypertension and diabetes increase the risk of micro- and macrovascular complications, and that blood pressure control as demonstrated in several trials can reduce the development and/or progression of these complications. A number of issues regarding blood pressure therapy need to be considered in the care of the diabetic patient: (a) when to start antihypertensive therapy, (b) the target of blood pressure level, and (c) the primary antihypertensive to be utilized. As opposed to glycemic control where increases in blood glucose levels can result in acute life-threatening complications such as diabetic ketoacidosis in type 1 diabetic patients or nonketotic hyperosmolar coma in type 2 diabetic patients, the deleterious effects of elevated blood pressure are often insidious. Currently, the consensus groups such as the Joint National Committee (JNC-7) on Prevention, Detection, Evaluation and Treatment of High Blood Pressure (104) and the American Diabetes Association (105) recommend that blood pressure control in diabetic patients be at or below 130/80 mm Hg with the use of an angiotensin converting enzyme inhibitor or an angiotensin receptor blocker as the initial antihypertensive agent.

Diabetic Nephropathy

Diabetic nephropathy is one of the leading causes of ESRD in the United States and occurs in approximately 30% to 35% of both type 1 and type 2 diabetic patients (106). In addition, diabetic nephropathy not only leads to ESRD but is also one of the strongest predictors of cardiovascular morbidity and mortality (107).

Normotensive Diabetic Patients with Normoalbuminuria

Data are sparse with regard to the treatment of normotensive diabetic patients with normal albuminuria levels. Three studies in type 1 diabetic patients with normal albuminuria levels and normotensive blood pressures have been published (107–108). Tuominen et al. evaluated the effects of lisinopril versus placebo on exercise-induced albuminuria, which is considered a predictor of microalbuminuria, in normotensive normoalbuminuric type 1 diabetic patients (108). A total of 26 patients with normoalbuminuria and an average blood pressure of approximately 118/81 mm Hg were randomized to lisinopril or placebo and followed over 2 years. Those randomized to lisinopril demonstrated a 40% decrease in exercise-induced urinary albumin excretion (UAE) rates in the first year ($p = 0.059$) and 66% decreased after the second year ($p < 0.01$), whereas exercise-induced UAE rates remained unchanged in the control group. Analyses of the systolic blood pressures (sBP) and diastolic blood pressures (dBP), however revealed significantly lower blood pressures in the lisinopril group at 2 years, 13 mm Hg ($p = 0.03$) and 9 mm Hg ($p = 0.052$), respectively. The authors concluded that lisinopril treatment reduces the exercise-induced UAE rate in normotensive normoalbuminuric type 1 diabetic patients and may have a protective effect against the development of microalbuminuria. Although not considered normotensive in the current guidelines, a multicenter study in Europe of type 1 diabetic patients with blood pressures <155/90 mm Hg were randomized to receive an angiotensin converting enzyme inhibitor (ACE-I), lisinopril, or placebo over a follow-up of 2 years (108). Although no difference was observed between those patients randomized to lisinopril versus placebo with regard to progression to microalbuminuria, those randomized to lisinopril had an overall lower urinary albumin excretion (UAE) rate (17.3%, $p = 0.05$) when adjusted for blood pressure and baseline UAE level. More recently, Kvetny et al. performed a randomized trial in normoalbuminuric type 1 diabetic patients with blood pressure <140/90 mm Hg and a mean blood pressure of about 90 mm Hg. Eighty-nine patients were randomized to perindopril versus placebo. After 36 months, the albumin/creatinine ratio (ACR) in the placebo group increased significantly to a value of 1.7 ± 1.1 mg/mmol ($p = 0.007$) versus the perindopril group whose ACR remained stable at 0.6 ± 0.2 mg/mmol. Although the group randomized to perindopril had lower mean blood pressures during the study, the difference was not statistically significant.

In type 2 diabetic patients, similar findings as in the type 1 diabetic studies were demonstrated by Ravid et al. (109). Randomization of patients with normoalbuminuria and a mean blood pressure <107 mm Hg to enalapril revealed a decrease in albumin excretion of 1.9 mg/24 hours at 2 years which was followed by a gradual increase of 4.2 mg/24 hours at 6 years. Whereas, those randomized to placebo had a larger increase in albumin excretion at 6 years (15.7 mg/24 hours, $p = 0.001$ for enalapril compared with placebo). The investigators also demonstrated lower incidence of microalbuminuria, absolute risk reduction of 12.5% (95% confidence interval [CI], 2% to 23%; $p = 0.042$), and a slower decline in creatinine clearance in the enalapril group ($p = 0.040$). Mean blood pressures in the treatment group were somewhat lower than those in the placebo group; this difference reached statistical significance during the fifth year of the study. Additionally, in the enalapril group, a significant correlation was found between the decrease in creatinine clearance and mean blood pressure ($r = 0.41$; $p = 0.05$), mean total plasma cholesterol level ($r = 0.42$, $p = 0.046$), and mean UAE ($r = 0.42$, $p = 0.044$). Therefore, it is difficult to discern whether the statistical benefit observed in the study was from the effect of the angiotensin converting enzyme inhibitor (ACE-I) and/or the effects associated with the decrease in blood pressure.

The results of the normotensive Appropriate Blood Pressure Control in Diabetes (ABCD) study evaluated the effects of intensive blood pressure control versus moderate blood pressure control with either enalapril or nisoldipine as the initial antihypertensive medication in 480 normotensive type 2 diabetic patients followed over a 5-year period (110). In a subanalysis of patients with normoalbuminuria at baseline, intensive blood pressure control (mean of 128/75 mm Hg) versus moderate

blood pressure control (mean of 137/81 mm Hg) resulted in a lower incidence of microalbuminuria independent of the use of an ACE-I or a calcium channel blocker (CCB). As a follow-up to the ABCD study, the Appropriate Blood Pressure Control in Diabetes Part 2 with Valsartan (ABCD-2V) study, 129 type 2 diabetic patients with a blood pressure <140/80 to 90 mm Hg without overt albuminuria were randomized to either intensive BP control (diastolic BP goal 75 mm Hg) utilizing an angiotensin II receptor blocker (ARB), Valsartan, versus moderate BP control (diastolic BP 80 to 90 mm Hg with placebo) (Estacio et al., presented at American Society of Hypertension, New York, 2004). The primary end point evaluated was the change in creatinine clearance, proportion of patients with doubling of serum creatinine and the change in UAE from baseline. The majority of the patients, >70%, had normoalbuminuria (<20 μg/min). The mean entrance BP was $126 \pm 8.8/84 \pm 2.4$ mm Hg with a follow-up period of 1.9 ± 1.0 years. During the follow-up period, the mean BP was $118 \pm 10.9/75 \pm 5.7$ for the intensive versus $124 \pm 10.9/80 \pm 6.5$ mm Hg for the moderate BP groups, $p < 0.001$. The study demonstrated that intensive blood pressure control led to a significant benefit in lowering UAE adjusting for baseline age, gender, race, duration of diabetes, hemoglobin A1cHbAc, and albuminuria status revealed a significant beneficial treatment effect ($p = 0.007$). The study suggests that even a lower blood pressure then 130/80 mm Hg with an ARB improved UAE in the early stages of nephropathy.

The data from these interventional studies suggest that treatment of blood pressure below the level of 130/80 mm Hg or even lower, as seen in the ABCD-2V study, may be beneficial with regard to progression to microalbuminuria. Does the type of antihypertensive medication matter? Although the EUCLID Study was not statistically significant for those with type 1 diabetic patients with normoalbuminuria, the 2-year follow-up period may have been inadequate to observe a difference. In the studies by Tuominen (108), Kvetny (110), and Ravid (111), an ACE-I was used against a placebo but, as noted above, statistically lower mean blood pressures were obtained in those patients randomized to the ACE-I. In the ABCD trial, intensive blood pressure control with either a dihydropyridine CCB or an ACE-I led to less progression to microalbuminuria (112). Although performed in hypertensive type 2 diabetic patients, the Bergamo Nephrologic Diabetes Complications Trial (BENEDICT) was designed to assess whether ACE-I and nondihydropyridine CCB, alone or in combination, would prevent microalbuminuria in subjects with normal UAE. Over 1,000 subjects were randomly assigned to receive at least 3 years of treatment with trandolapril (at a dose of 2 mg/day) plus verapamil (sustained-release formulation, 180 mg/day), trandolapril alone (2 mg/day), verapamil alone (sustained-release formulation, 240 mg/day), or placebo with a target blood pressure was 120/80 mm Hg. The study revealed that the use of trandolapril plus verapamil (5.6%, $p = 0.01$) or trandolapril alone (6%, $p = 0.01$) but not verapamil alone 11.9%, $p = 0.54$) decreased the incidence of microalbuminuria when compared to placebo. The data, while limited, suggest that the level at which the diagnosis of "hypertension" is made in diabetic patients may need to be redefined and that utilization of an agent that blocks RAAS would be most beneficial.

Patients with Microalbuminuria

Microalbuminuria may represent the "reversible" stage of diabetic nephropathy in which interventions can prevent the progression to overt nephropathy and inevitable renal failure. Thus, interventions at this stage may be crucial in preventing the progression to overt albuminuria.

In a type 1 diabetic study of six patients, Christensen et al. demonstrated the beneficial effect of treating patients with microalbuminuria with antihypertensive therapy utilizing a beta-blocker over a 5-year follow-up period (111). Subsequent studies in both type 1 and type 2 diabetes confirmed the effects of blood pressure control with various antihypertensive medications as monotherapy or in combination on slowing the progression to overt albuminuria (112–117). Angiotensin converting enzyme inhibitors consistently demonstrated beneficial effects with regard to retarding the progression of microalbuminuria when compared to placebo (118–124). As in the normotensive studies already cited, however, it is difficult to discern whether the blood pressure reduction, the specific properties of angiotensin converting enzyme inhibitors, or both result in the beneficial effects. Comparison studies evaluating the effects of angiotensin converting enzyme inhibitors with other antihypertensive medications on incipient diabetic nephropathy are few and are of short duration. A number of studies comparing the effects of CCBs with angiotensin converting enzyme inhibitors in patients with microalbuminuria have been performed but also are limited in size and study duration. When comparing "short-acting" CCBs to angiotensin converting inhibitors, angiotensin converting enzyme inhibitors demonstrated a clear advantage. In contrast, results of studies comparing angiotensin converting enzyme inhibitors to longer-acting formulations of CCBS are less clear (113,114). Similar findings were reported from the hypertensive ABCD study in which no difference was demonstrated between a long-acting CCB, nisoldipine, versus an angiotensin converting enzyme inhibitor, enalapril, with regard to the progression from microalbuminuria to overt albuminuria (115).

In a study of 590 hypertensive patients with type 2 diabetes and microalbuminuria, patients were randomized to receive irbesartan, at a dose of either placebo, 150 mg daily or 300 mg daily, and were followed for 2 years (116). The primary outcome was the time to the onset of diabetic nephropathy, defined by persistent albuminuria in overnight specimens, with a UAE rate that was greater than 200 μg/minute and at least 30% higher than the baseline level. Of the patients studied, 5.2% in the group that received 300 mg daily and 9.7% in the group that received 150 mg daily reached the primary end point, as compared with 14.9% in the placebo group (14.9%) (hazard ratios, 0.30 [p <0.001] and 0.61 [p = 0.081 for the two irbesartan groups, respectively]). The average blood pressure during the course of the study was slightly lower in the actively treated group, 144/83 mm Hg in the placebo group, 143/83 mm Hg in the 150 mg group, and 141/83 mm Hg in the 300 mg group (p = 0.004 for the comparison of systolic blood pressure between the placebo group and the combined irbesartan groups). In the Microalbuminuria Reduction with VALsartan (MARVAL) Study (117), valsartan was compared to amlodipine in patients with microalbuminuria. Although the follow-up period was only 24 weeks, the patients randomized to valsartan demonstrated a benefit with regard to lowering of UAE to 56% (95% CI 49.6–63.0) of baseline values as compared to 92% (95% CI 81.7–103.7) of baseline with amlodipine; there was a significant difference between the groups (p <0.001). Additionally, more patients regressed to normoalbuminuria with valsartan (29.9% vs. 14.5%; p = 0.001). Over the study period, BP reductions were similar between the two treatments (systolic/diastolic 11.2/6.6 mm Hg for valsartan, 11.6/6.5 mm Hg for amlodipine) and at no time point was there a between-group significant difference in BP values in either the hypertensive or the normotensive subgroup. Similar to trials with angiotensin converting enzyme inhibitors, ARBs at least compared to placebo demonstrated a benefit with regard to preventing or slowing the progression to overt nephropathy. Although the MARVAL study suggests that ARBs may be more efficacious than a dihydropyridine calcium channel blocker (CCB), more studies would be needed with a longer follow-up period when comparing to another agent.

Patients with Overt Nephropathy (Albuminuria)

In the study by Parving et al., antihypertensive treatment with metoprolol, hydralazine and furosemide or hydrochlorothiazide in type 1 diabetic patients with overt nephropathy led to an improvement in the rate of decline of the glomerular filtration rate over an 8-year period (118). During the study the mean treatment blood pressure was 129/84 mm Hg versus the pretreatment blood pressure of 143/96 mm Hg. Additionally, the investigators demonstrated a decrease in UAE of nearly 50% with treatment. Similar results were demonstrated with the use of a beta-blocker alone or in combination with hydralazine or furosemide (119). In 1993, Lewis et al. in a landmark study demonstrated the beneficial effects of an angiotensin converting enzyme inhibitor, captopril, versus placebo in decreasing the doubling of serum creatinine and the progression to death or ESRD in a group of type 1 diabetic patients with overt nephropathy and serum creatinine ≤2.5 mg/dL at baseline (120). These results confirmed earlier smaller reports demonstrating the beneficial effects of ACE-I versus placebo (121,122).

In type 2 diabetic patients with overt nephropathy, 2 studies utilizing ARBs, losartan (123) and irbesartan (124), demonstrated findings similar to those of Lewis's landmark study in type 1 diabetes. Both studies demonstrated that including an ARB in the antihypertensive regimen led to a decrease risk in the doubling of serum creatinine and progression to ESRD. In a study performed by Barnett et al., the use of an ARB, telmisartan, versus an ACE-I, enalapril, resulted in similar effects with regard to change in glomerular filtration rate and UAE over a 5-year follow-up period (125).

Studies comparing other antihypertensive medications with angiotensin converting enzyme inhibitors (ACE-I's) with regard to their effects on overt diabetic nephropathy have been conflicting (138–143). In a recent meta-regression analysis performed by Kasiske et al., including over 100 studies and nearly 2,500 patients, the effects of ACE-Is on diabetic nephropathy were compared to those of other antihypertensive medications (126). Whereas reductions in proteinuria from other antihypertensive agents could be entirely explained by changes in blood pressure, ACE-I's demonstrated an independent decrease proteinuria after adjusting for blood pressure, treatment duration, and the type of diabetes or stage of nephropathy, as well as study design (p <0.0001). Similar findings were demonstrated by Gansevoort et al. (127) and Weidmann et al. (128) in their meta-analyses comparing the effects of ACE-I's with other antihypertensive medications.

Two studies demonstrated no difference in the effects of an ACE-I with either a beta-blocker (129,130) and or a CCB (127) in hypertensive type 2 diabetic populations. In the United Kingdom Prospective Diabetic Study (UKPDS), no difference was demonstrated between the use of a beta-blocker, atenolol, with an ACE-I, captopril, with regard to urinary albumin concentrations (147). A slight difference in UAE was noted with tight blood pressure control (mean 144/82 mm Hg) versus less tight control (mean 154/87 mm Hg) at 6 years (p = 0.0085) but was not seen at 9 years (p = 0.33) (148). In addition, there was no difference in the occurrence of diabetic nephropathy in the UKPDS between the atenolol and captopril treated groups. In the hypertensive ABCD study, although treatment blood pressure for both the intensive (mean 132/78 mm Hg) and moderate (138/86 mm Hg) groups were lower than the UKPDS, no statistical difference was seen in treatment groups followed over 5 years on renal function as measured by creatinine clearance and UAE (127). ABCD Trial investigators also did not observe a difference with regard to the use of an ACE-I, enalapril, versus a CCB, nisoldipine, as the initial antihypertensive medication with regard to the renal outcomes. During the study, there was a steady decline in creatinine clearance of 5–6 mL/minute/1.73 m²/year in those patients who had diabetic nephropathy (UAE ≥300 mg/day) at baseline. These results for the overt albuminuria group were however limited by the relatively few patients with overt nephropathy at baseline.

Cardiovascular Disease

There have been a number of antihypertensive trials within the past few years confirming the advantage of BP control in diabetic populations with regard to cardiovascular events. As Haffner et al. demonstrated in a 7-year longitudinal study of type 2 diabetic subjects, the risk of developing a myocardial infarction for diabetic patients without a previous history of myocardial infarction is similar to that of nondiabetic patients with a previous myocardial infarction (131).

Two studies evaluating the treatment of isolated systolic hypertension in elderly diabetic patients with either diuretic therapy (132) or a long-acting CCA (133) demonstrated unequivocal advantage with active therapy than placebo with respect to cardiac disease. In both studies there were similar advantages with regard to overall cardiovascular disease and cardiovascular mortality in 5- and 2-year follow-up periods, respectively. In the UKPDS, tight blood pressure control demonstrated a clear advantage when compared to less tight control with regard to death related to diabetes and strokes (148). The result was independent of the use of captopril or atenolol although the lack of difference between the antihypertensive medications may have been due to inadequate dosing of captopril (147).

In the substudy of the Hypertension Optimal Treatment (HOT) study, 1,500 diabetic patients were randomized to three levels of diastolic blood pressure control (≤90 mm Hg vs. ≤85 mm Hg vs. ≤80 mm Hg) with felodipine (long-acting CCA) as the initial antihypertensive medication (134). Those randomized to ≤80 mm Hg when compared to <90 mm Hg demonstrated an advantage with regard to the cardiovascular mortality and total cardiovascular events. The investigators estimated that the ideal blood pressure was 138.5/82.6 mm Hg and found no evidence consistent with a J-curve. During the study, additional antihypertensive medications were added to achieve the blood pressure goals with 45% of patients in the ≤80 mm Hg group being on an ACE-I versus 35% in the ≤90 mm Hg group. Beta-blockers and diuretics were also utilized during the study, but as with the ACE-I, a statistical comparison with regard to the use of the specific antihypertensive medications was not reported across the treatment arms.

In the Heart Outcomes Prevention Evaluation (HOPE) study, subgroup analyses were performed on the 3577 diabetic patients enrolled in the study (81 type 1 and 3,496 type 2 diabetic patients) who were followed for nearly 5 years. Low-dose ramipril was compared to placebo as "add on" therapy to evaluate the effects on combined cardiovascular (myocardial infarction, strokes, and cardiovascular death) events (124). The study was stopped 6 months early after 4.5 years of follow-up by the Data Safety Monitoring Board because of a significant advantage of ramipril with regard to the primary outcome. During the study, there was a minor but statistically significant difference in the blood pressures between the ramipril group and placebo which the investigators postulated was too small to account for the difference seen between ramipril and placebo treatment arms.

In addition to the UKPDS, three additional trials have compared the effects of an ACE-I versus a CCB (135,136) or beta-blocker (137). In the ABCD Trial, the use of the ACE-I demonstrated an advantage with regard to the incidence of myocardial infarctions when compared to the CCB nisoldipine (153). The difference was independent of blood pressure,

smoking, total cholesterol, beta-blocker and past cardiovascular events. The investigators stressed that the study could not determine whether it was the beneficial cardiovascular effect of the ACE-I or a deleterious effect of the CCB or a combination of both. In another study, a similar result was obtained when a post hoc analysis revealed that fosinopril was associated with fewer cardiovascular events than amlodipine in a 2.8-year follow-up period (154). In the Captopril Prevention Project, the use of captopril was associated with less myocardial infarctions and total cardiovascular events in diabetic patients when compared to atenolol over a 5-year follow-up period (155). This result contrasts with the UKPDS findings which did not demonstrate a difference between the two antihypertensive medications (147). As stated earlier, the lack of difference seen in the UKPDS may be a result of the inadequate dosing of captopril during the study (25–50 mg twice a day [bid] rather than three times a day [tid]).

The Antihypertensive and Lipid-Lowering Treatment to Prevent Heart Attack Trial, or ALLHAT, was a study designed to determine whether treatment with a CCB, amlodipine, or ACE-I inhibitor, lisinopril, lowers the incidence of coronary heart disease (CHD) or other cardiovascular disease (CVD) events versus treatment with a diuretic, chlorthalidone (138). Initially the study also included doxazosin, alpha-blocker, but this arm was discontinued early because increased risk heart failure admissions (139). The main results compared the three remaining antihypertensive medications which also included over 11,000 type 2 diabetic patients with a mean follow-up period of 4.9 years. The primary outcome, fatal CHD or nonfatal myocardial infarction (MI), occurred in 2,956 participants, with no difference between treatments. In the diabetic population, amlodipine was associated with higher incidence of heart failure when compared with chlorthalidone (Risk Ratio [RR] 1.45, 95% CI 1.23–1.64). When comparing lisinopril to chlorthalidone in the diabetic patients, lisinopril was associated with a higher rate of combined CVD (CHD, stroke, angina, heart failure and peripheral artery disease) (RR 1.08, 95% CI 1.00–1.17) and, surprisingly, a higher incidence of heart failure (RR 1.22, 95% CI 1.05–1.42). The results of the ALLHAT study, in light of previously published studies, were surprising and some cited the difference in blood pressures, especially in the lisinopril group, as a specific factor contributing to the findings.

In the Losartan Intervention for Endpoint reduction in hypertension study (LIFE) substudy with diabetic patients, 1,195 patients with diabetes, hypertension, and signs of left ventricular hypertrophy (LVH) on electrocardiograms, a losartan-based versus a atenolol-based treatment was compared with follow-up period of least 4 years (mean 4.7 ± 1.1 years) (140). The study compared the effects of the drugs on the primary composite end point of cardiovascular morbidity and mortality (cardiovascular death, stroke, or MI). Both arms had similar blood pressures, 146/79 mm Hg in losartan patients and 148/79 mm Hg (19/11) in atenolol patients. The results revealed that losartan was associated with a lower risk in the primary endpoint (RR 0.76; 95% CI 0.58–0.98; $p = 0.031$), cardiovascular death (RR 0.63, 95% CI 0.42–0.95; $p = 0.028$) and all-cause mortality (RR 0.61, 95% CI 0.45-0.84, p = 0.002).

Summary

Hypertension unfortunately is a frequent partner with diabetes. The prediabetic and diabetic state, especially in type 2 diabetes, lends itself to the development of hypertension. Once hypertension is present, there are numerous mechanisms by which both diabetes and high blood pressure contribute to the development of the vascular complications. Fortunately, it appears that blood pressure control can stall or even prevent the development or progression of these complications, especially cardiovascular and renal disease. Review of the literature reveals that aggressive and early blood pressure control may be the key to antihypertensive therapy. In this regard, blood pressure therapy prior to the development of overt diabetic nephropathy or even microalbuminuria may be the most optimal strategy with regard to preventing ESRD. Although further studies are needed, results from studies evaluating the antihypertensive treatment of normotensive diabetic patients suggest that it may be even beneficial to treat normoalbuminuric patients with "normotensive" blood pressures below the current recommendations of 130/80 mm Hg. The ALLHAT study, although, demonstrated that a benefit with diuretic therapy with regard to cardiovascular outcomes, specifically heart failure, and inhibition of the RAAS with an ACE-I or ARB may have the added benefit of renal protection. Although we did not discuss the effects of combination antihypertensive therapy, it is clear that a majority of patients with diabetes, especially in the presence of even a mildly elevate UAE, will require at least two or even three antihypertensive medications. In the UKPDS, a study in which the target blood pressure were well above the current consensus guidelines of <130/80 mm Hg, 69% of patients required two antihypertensive medications and 29% of patients required more than two such medications (148).

References

1. Mokdad A, Ford E, Bowman B, et al. Diabetes trends in the United States, 1990 to 1998. *Diabetes Care* 2000;23:1278.
2. Gregg EW, Cadwell BL, Cheng YJ, et al. Trends in the prevalence and ratio of diagnosed to undiagnosed diabetes according to obesity levels in the U.S. *Diabetes Care* 2004;27(12):2806.
3. Harris MI. Non-insulin dependent diabetes in black and white Americans. *Diabetes Metab Rev* 1990;6:71.
4. Carter JS, Pugh JA, Monterosa A. Non-insulin dependent diabetes mellitus in minorities in the U.S. *Ann Intern Med* 1996;125:221.
5. Wild S, Roglic G, Green A, et al. Global prevalence of diabetes: estimates for the year 2000 and projections for 2030. *Diabetes Care* 2004;27(5):1047.
6. Dupree EA, Meyer MB. Role of risk factors in complications of diabetes mellitus. *Am J Epidemiol* 1980;112:200.
7. Nelson RG, Newman JM, Knowler WC, et al. Incidence of end-stage renal disease in NIDDM mellitus in Pima Indians. *Diabetologia* 1988;31(10):730.
8. Kannel WB, McGee DL. Diabetes and glucose tolerance as risk factors for cardiovascular disease. *Diabetes Care* 1979;2:120.
9. Krolewski AS, Kosinski DJ, Warram JH, et al. Magnitude and determinants of coronary artery disease in juvenile-onset, insulin-dependent diabetes mellitus. *Am J Cardiol* 1987;59(8):750.
10. Pyorala K. Diabetes and heart disease. In: Mogensen CE, ed. *Prevention and Treatment of Diabetic Late Complications*. New York: DeGruyter, 1989:151.
11. Fuller JH, Stevens LK. Epidemiology of hypertension in diabetic patients and implications for treatment. *Diabetes Care* 1991;14 (S4):8.
12. Satterfield S, Cutler J, Longford HG, et al. Trials of hypertension prevention: phase I design. *Ann Epidemiol* 1991;1:455.
13. Walker WG, Hermann J, Murphy R, et al. Elevated blood pressure and angiotensin II are associated with accelerated loss of renal function in diabetic nephropathy. *Trans Am Clin Climatol Assoc* 1985;97:94.
14. Christensen CH, Mogensen CE. The course of incipient diabetic nephropathy: studies of albumin excretion and blood pressure. *Diabetic Med* 1985;2:97.
15. Parving HH, Andersen AR, Smidt UM, et al. Diabetic nephropathy and arterial hypertension. *Diabetologia* 1983;24:10.
16. Christlieb AR, Warram JH, Krolewski AJ, et al. Hypertension: the major risk in juvenile-onset insulin dependent diabetes. *Diabetes* 1981;30:906.
17. Savage S, Schrier RW. Progressive renal insufficiency: the role of angiotensin converting enzyme inhibitors. *Adv Intern Med* 1992;37:85.
18. Knowler WC, Bennett PH, Ballantine EJ. Increased incidence of retinopathy in diabetes with elevated blood pressure. *N Engl J Med* 1980;301:645.
19. Ishihara M, Yukimura Y, Aizawa T, et al. High blood pressure as risk factor in diabetic retinopathy development in NIDDM patients. *Diabetes Care* 1987;10(1):20.
20. Klein R, Klein BE, Moss SE, et al. Is blood pressure a predictor of the incidence or progression of diabetic retinopathy? *Arch Intern Med,* 1989;149(11):2427.
21. Maser R. Epidemiological correlates of diabetic neuropathy. *Diabetes* 1989;38(11):1456.
22. Tester A, Eggerd M, Hermann JB. Diabetes and nephropathy: blood pressure in clinical diabetic patients and control population. *Arch Intern Med* 1989;149:1942.
23. Pell S, D'Anzo CA. Some aspects of hypertension in diabetes mellitus. *JAMA* 1967;202:104.
24. Harris M. Undiagnosed non-insulin dependent diabetes mellitus: clinical and public health issues. *Diabetes Care* 1993;16:642.
25. Tarnow L, Rossing P, Gall MA, et al. Prevalence of arterial hypertension in diabetic patients before and after the JNC-V. *Diabetes Care* 1994;17(11):1247.
26. National High Blood Pressure Education Program Working Group. National High Blood Pressure Education Program Working Group report on hypertension in diabetes. *Hypertension,* 1994;23:145.
27. Seaquist ER, Goetz FC, Rich S, et al. Familial clustering of diabetic kidney disease: evidence of genetic susceptibility to diabetic nephropathy. *N Engl J Med* 1989;320:1161.
28. Borch-Johnsen K, Norgaard K, Hommel E, et al. Is diabetic nephropathy an inherited complication? *Kidney Int,* 1992;41:719.
29. Fagerudd JA, Tarnow L, Jacobsen P, et al. Predisposition to essential hypertension and development of diabetic nephropathy in IDDM patients. *Diabetes* 1998;47(3):439.
30. Krolewski AS, Canessa H, Warram JH, et al. Predisposition to hypertension and susceptibility to renal disease in insulin-dependent diabetes mellitus. *N Engl J Med,* 1988;318:140.
31. Mangili R, Bending JJ, Scott GS, et al. Increased sodium-lithium counter transport activity in red cells of patients with insulin dependent diabetes and nephropathy. *N Engl J Med* 1988;318:146.
32. Crompton CH, Balfe JW, Balfe JA, et al. Sodium-lithium transport in adolescents with IDDM. *Diabetes Care* 1994;17:704.
33. Herman WH, Prior DE, Yassine MD, et al. Nephropathy in NIDDM is associated with cellular markers for hypertension. *Diabetes Care* 1993;16:815.
34. Forsblom CM, Ericksson JG, Ekstrand AV, et al. Insulin resistance and abnormal albumin excretion in nondiabetic first-degree relatives of patients with NIDDM. *Diabetologia* 1995;38:363.
35. Niskanen L, Laakso M. Insulin resistance is related to albuminuria in patients with type II (non–insulin-dependent) diabetes mellitus. *Metabolism* 1993;42:1541.
36. Rocchini AP. The relationship of sodium sensitivity to insulin resistance. *Am J Med Sci* 1994;307:S75.
37. Weidmann P, Beretta-Piccoli C, Trost BN. Pressor factors and responsiveness in hypertension accompanying diabetes mellitus. *Hypertension* 1985;7:II33.
38. Roland JM, O'Hare JP, Walters G, et al. Sodium retention in response to saline infusion in uncomplicated diabetes mellitus. *Diabetes Res* 1986;3:213.
39. Weidmann P, Ferrari P. Central role of sodium in hypertension in diabetic subjects. *Diabetes Care* 1991;14:220.
40. DeFronzo RA, Cooke CR, Andres R, et al. The effect of insulin on renal handling of sodium, potassium, calcium, and phosphate in man. *J Clin Invest.*
41. O'Hare JA, Ferriss JB, Brady D, et al. Exchangeable sodium and renin in hypertensive diabetic patients with and without nephropathy. *Hypertension* 1985;7:II43.
42. Weidmann P. Pathogenesis of hypertension associated with chronic renal failure. *Contrib Nephrol* 1984;41:47.
43. Preston RA, Singer I, Epstein M. Renal parenchymal hypertension: current concepts of pathogenesis and management. *Arch Intern Med.* 1996;156:602.
44. Rebbeck TR, Turner ST, Sing CF. Sodium-lithium countertransport genotype and the probability of hypertension in adults. *Hypertension* 1993;22:560.
45. Hilton PJ. Cellular sodium transport in essential hypertension. *N Engl J Med* 1986;314:222.
46. Rebbeck TR, Turner ST, Michels VV, et al. Genetic and environmental explanations for the distribution of sodium-lithium countertransport in pedigrees from Rochester, MN. *Am J Hum Genet* 1991;48:1092.
47. Krzesinski JM, Saint-Remy A, Du F, et al. Red blood cell Na-Li countertransport, hypertensive heredity, and cardiovascular risk in young adults. *Am J Hypertens* 1993;6(4):314.
48. Van Norren K, Thien T, Berden JH, et al. Relevance of erythrocyte Na+/Li+ countertransport measurement in essential hypertension, hyperlipidaemia and diabetic nephropathy: a critical review. *Eur J Clin Invest* 1998;28(5):339.
49. Pinkney JH, Denver AE, Foyle WJ, et al. Insulin resistance and not hyperinsulinaemia determines erythrocyte Na+/Li+ countertransport in non-insulin-dependent diabetes mellitus. *J Hum Hypertens* 1995;9:685.
50. Giordano M, Castellino P, Solini A, et al. Na+/Li+ and Na+/H+ countertransport activity in hypertensive non–insulin-dependent diabetic patients: role of insulin resistance and antihypertensive treatment. *Metabolism* 1997;46(11):1316.
51. Falkner B, Canessa M, Levison S, et al. Sodium-lithium countertransport is associated with insulin resistance and urinary albumin excretion in young African-Americans. *Am J Kidney Dis* 1997;29:45.
52. Ng LL, C Dudley C, Bomford J, et al. Leucocyte intracellular pH and Na+/H+ antiport activity in human hypertension. *J Hypertens* 1989;7:471.

53. Feig, PU, D'Occhio MA, Boylan JW. Lymphocyte membrane sodium-proton exchange in spontaneously hypertensive rats. *Hypertension* 1987;9:282.

54. Berk BC, Vallega G, Muslin AJ, et al. Spontaneously hypertensive rat vascular smooth muscle cells in culture exhibit increased growth and Na+/H+ exchange. *J Clin Invest* 1989;83:822.

55. Harris, RC, Brenner BM, Seifter JL. Sodium-hydrogen exchange and glucose transport in renal microvillus vesicles from rats with diabetes mellitus. *J Clin Invest* 1986;77:724.

56. Williams B, Schrier RW. Effect of elevated extracellular glucose concentrations on transmembrane calcium ion fluxes in cultured rat VSMC. *Kidney Int* 1993;44:344.

57. Williams B, Howard RL. Glucose-induced changes in Na+/H+ antiport activity and gene expression in cultured vascular smooth muscle cells. Role of protein kinase C. *J Clin Invest* 1994;93:2623.

58. Ober SS, Pardee AB. Intracellular pH is increased after transformation of Chinese hamster embryo fibroblasts. *Proc Natl Acad Sci USA* 1987;84:2766.

59. L'Allemain G, Paris S, Pouyssegur J. Growth factor activation and intracellular pH regulation in fibroblasts: evidence for a major role of the Na+/H+ antiport. *J Biol Chem* 1984;259:5809.

60. Grinstein S, Rotin D, Mason MJ. Na+/H + exchange and growth factor-induced cytosolic pH changes: role in cellular proliferation. *Biochim Biophys Acta* 1989;988:73.

61. Vallega GA, Canessa ML, Berk BC, et al. Vascular smooth muscle cell Na+/H+ exchanger kinetics and its activation by angiotensin II. *Am J Physiol* 1988;254:C751.

62. Aviv A, Livine A. The Na+/H+ antiport, cytosolic free Ca2+ and essential hypertension: a hypothesis. *Am J Hypertens* 1988;1:410.

63. Gonzalez JM, Suki WN. Cell calcium and arterial blood pressure. *Semin Nephrol* 1995;15:564.

64. Levy J, Gavin JR III, Sowers JR. Diabetes mellitus: a disease of abnormal cellular calcium metabolism? *Am J Med.* 1994;96:260.

65. Feldt-Rasmussen B, Mathiesen ER, Deckert T, et al. Central role for sodium in the pathogenesis of blood pressure changes independent of angiotensin, aldosterone and catecholamines in type 1 (insulin-dependent) diabetes mellitus. *Diabetologia* 1987;30:610.

66. Christlieb AR, Kaldany A, D'Elia JA. Plasma renin activity and hypertension in diabetes mellitus. *Diabetes* 1976;25:969.

67. De'Oliveira JM, Price DA, Fisher ND, et al. Autonomy of the renin system in type II diabetes mellitus: dietary sodium and renal hemodynamic responses to ACE inhibition. *Kidney Int* 1997;52:771.

68. Price DA, De'Oliveira JM, Fisher ND, et al. The state and responsiveness of the renin-angiotensin-aldosterone system in patients with type II diabetes mellitus. *Am J Hypertens* 1999;12:348.

69. Miller JA. Impact of hyperglycemia on the renin angiotensin system in early human type 1 diabetes mellitus. *J Am Soc Nephrol* 1999;10:1778.

70. Drury PL, Smith GM, Ferriss JB. Increased vasopressor responsiveness to angiotensin II in type 1 (insulin-dependent) diabetic patients without complications. *Diabetologia* 1984;27:174.

71. Ferrannini E, Buzzigoli G, Bonadonna R, et al. Insulin resistance in essential hypertension. *N Engl J Med.* 1987;317:350.

72. Manicardi V, Camellini L, Bellodi G, et al. Evidence for an association of high blood pressure and hyperinsulinemia in obese man. *J Clin Endocrinol Metab* 1986;62:1302.

73. Shimamoto K, Hirata A, Fukuoka M, et al. Insulin sensitivity and the effects of insulin on renal sodium handling and pressor systems in essential hypertensive patients. *Hypertension* 1994;23(Suppl I):I29.

74. Ferrannini E, Natali A, Capaldo B, et al. Insulin resistance, hyperinsulinemia, and blood pressure: role of age and obesity. European Group for the Study of Insulin Resistance (EGIR). *Hypertension.* 1997;30:1144.

75. Anderson EA, Hoffman RP, Balon TW, et al. Hyperinsulinemia produces both sympathetic neural activation and vasodilation in normal humans. *J Clin Invest* 1991;87:2246.

76. Lembo G, Rendina V, Iaccarino G, et al. Insulin reduces reflex forearm sympathetic vasoconstriction in healthy humans. *Hypertension* 1993;21:1015.

77. Steinberg HO, Brechtel G, Johnson A, et al. Insulin-mediated skeletal muscle vasodilation is nitric oxide dependent. A novel action of insulin to increase nitric oxide release. *J Clin Invest* 1994;94:1172.

78. Vollenweider P, Randin D, Tappy L, et al. Impaired insulin-induced sympathetic neural activation and vasodilation in skeletal muscle in obese humans. *J Clin Invest* 1994;93:2365.

79. Lembo G, Rendina V, Iaccarino G, et al. Insulin does not modulate reflex forearm sympathetic vasoconstriction in patients with essential hypertension. *J Hypertens Suppl.* 1993;11(Suppl 5):S272.

80. Laine H, Knuuti MJ, Ruotsalainen U, et al. Insulin resistance in essential hypertension is characterized by impaired insulin stimulation of blood flow in skeletal muscle. *J Hypertens* 1998;16:211.

81. Laakso M, Edelman SV, Brechtel G, et al. Impaired insulin-mediated skeletal muscle blood flow in patients with NIDDM. *Diabetes* 1992;41:1076.

82. Rowe JW, Young JB, Minaker KL, et al. Effect of insulin and glucose infusions on sympathetic nervous system activity in normal man. *Diabetes* 1981;30:219.

83. Elser M, Jennings G, Korner P, et al. Assessment of human sympathetic nervous system activity from measurements of norepinephrine turnover. *Hypertension* 1988;11:3.

84. Landsberg L, Dreiger DR. Obesity, metabolism and the sympathetic nervous system. *Am J Hypertens* 1989;2:1255.

85. Landsberg L, Young JB. Insulin-mediated glucose metabolism in the relationship between dietary intake and sympathetic nervous system activity. *Int J Obes* 1985;9(Suppl 2):63.

86. Berne C, Gafius J, Pollare T, et al. The sympathetic response to euglycemic.hyperinsulinemia: evidence from microelectrode nerve recordings in healthy subjects. *Diabetologia* 1992;35:873.

87. Lembo G, Iaccarino G, Vecchione C, et al. Insulin modulation of beta-adrenergic vasodilator pathway in human forearm. *Circulation* 1996;93:1403.

88. Gros R, Borkowski KR, Feldman RD. Human insulin-mediated enhancement of vascular beta-adrenergic responsiveness. *Hypertension* 1994;23:551.

89. Schneider DJ, Nordt TK, Sobel BE. Attenuated fibrinolysis and accelerated atherogenesis in type II diabetic patients. *Diabetes* 1993;42:1.

90. Ford I, Singh TP, Kitchen S, et al. Activation of coagulation in diabetes mellitus in relation to the presence of vascular complications. *Diabet Med* 1991;8:322.

91. Carmassi F, Morale M, Puccetti R, et al. Coagulation and fibrinolytic system impairment in insulin dependent diabetes mellitus. *Thromb Res* 1992;67:643.

92. Vukovich TC, Proidl S, Knöbl P, et al. The effect of insulin treatment on the balance between tissue plasminogen activator and plasminogen activator inhibitor-1 in type 2 diabetic patients. *Thromb Haemost* 1992;68:253.

93. Landin K, Tengborn L, Smith U. Elevated fibrinogen and plasminogen activator inhibitor (PAI-1) in hypertension are related to metabolic risk factors for cardiovascular disease. *J Intern Med* 1990;227:273.

94. Teger-Nilsson AC, Larsson PT, Hjemdahl P, et al. Fibrinogen and plasminogen activator inhibitor-1 levels in hypertension and coronary heart disease. Potential effects of beta-blockade. *Circulation* 1991;84:VI72.

95. Calles-Escandon J, Mirza SA, Sobel BE, et al. Induction of hyperinsulinemia combined with hyperglycemia and hypertriglyceridemia increases plasminogen activator inhibitor 1 in blood in normal human subjects. *Diabetes* 1998;47:290.

96. Sowers JR, Epstein M. Diabetes mellitus and associated hypertension, vascular disease, and nephropathy. An update. *Hypertension* 1995;26:869.

97. Epstein M. Diabetes and hypertension: the bad companions. *J Hypertens Suppl* 1997;15:S55.

98. Kaseta JR, Skafar DF, Ram JL, et al. Cardiovascular disease in the diabetic woman. *J Clin Endocrinol Metab* 1999;84:1835.

99. Tesfamariam B, Brown ML, Cohen RA. Elevated glucose impairs endothelium-dependent relaxation by activating protein kinase C. *J Clin Invest* 1001;87:1643.

100. Phillips GB, Jing TY, Resnick LM, et al. Sex hormones and hemostatic risk factors for coronary heart disease in men with hypertension. *J Hypertens* 1993;11:699.

101. Cagliero E, Roth T, Roy S, et al. Characteristics and mechanisms of high-glucose-induced overexpression of basement membrane components in cultured human endothelial cells. *Diabetes* 1991;40:102.

102. Siegel RD, Cupples A, Schaefer EJ, et al. Lipoproteins, apolipoproteins, and low-density lipoprotein size among diabetics in the Framingham offspring study. *Metabolism* 1996;45:1267.

103. Panza JA, Quyyumi AA, Brush JE Jr, et al. Abnormal endothelium-dependent vascular relaxation in patients with essential hypertension. *N Engl J Med* 1990;323:22.

104. Anderson PW, Hsueh WA. Hypertension and diabetic vascular complications. *Adv Intern Med* 1994;39:633.

105. Chobanian AV, Bakris GL, Black HR, et al. The Seventh Report of the Joint National Committee on Prevention, Detection, Evaluation, and Treatment of High Blood Pressure: the JNC 7 report. *JAMA* 2003;289(19):2560.

106. Hypertension Management in Adults with Diabetes. *Diabetes Care* 2004;27(90001):65S.

107. Estacio RO, Schrier RW. Diabetic nephropathy: pathogenesis, diagnosis, and prevention of progression. *Adv Intern Med* 2001;46:359.

108. Tuominen JA, Ebeling P, Koivisto VA. Long-term lisinopril therapy reduces exercise-induced albuminuria in normoalbuminuric normotensive IDDM patients. *Diabetes Care* 1998;21:1345.

109. Randomised placebo-controlled trial of lisinopril in normotensive patients with insulin-dependent diabetes and normoalbuminuria or microalbuminuria. The EUCLID Study Group. *Lancet* 1997;349:1787.

110. Kvetny J, Gregersen G, Pedersen RS. Randomized placebo-controlled trial of perindopril in normotensive, normoalbuminuric patients with type 1 diabetes mellitus. *QJM* 2001;94(2):89.

111. Ravid M, Brosh D, Levi Z, et al. Use of enalapril to attenuate decline in renal function in normotensive, normoalbuminuric patients with type 2 diabetes mellitus. A randomized, controlled trial. *Ann Intern Med* 1998;128:982.

112. Schrier RW. Anti-hypertensive therapy in the prevention of progression of nephropathy of type II diabetes. *American Society of Nephrology Meeting,* Miami, FL, 1999.

113. Christensen CK, Mogensen CE. Effect of antihypertensive treatment on progression of incipient diabetic nephropathy. *Hypertension* 1985;7:II109.

114. Gambardella S, Frontoni S, Grazia FM, et al. Efficacy of antihypertensive treatment with indapamide in patients with noninsulin-dependent diabetes and persistent microalbuminuria. *Am J Cardiol* 1990;65:46H.

115. Gambardella S, Frontoni S, Lala A, et al. Regression of microalbuminuria in type II diabetic, hypertensive patients after long-term indapamide treatment. *Am Heart J* 1991;122:1232.

116. Hommel E, Mathiesen E, Edsberg B, et al. Acute reduction of arterial blood pressure reduces urinary albumin excretion in type 1 (insulin-dependent) diabetic patients with incipient nephropathy. *Diabetologia* 1986;29:211.

117. Janka HU, Weitz T, Blumner E, et al. Hypertension and micro-albuminuria in diabetic patients taking indapamide. *J Hypertens Suppl* 1989;7:S316.

118. Marre M, Chatellier G, Leblanc H, et al. Prevention of diabetic nephropathy with enalapril in normotensive diabetics with microalbuminuria. *BMJ* 1988;297:1092.

119. Viberti G, Mogensen CE, Groop LC, et al. Effect of captopril on progression to clinical proteinuria in patients with insulin-dependent diabetes mellitus and microalbuminuria. European Microalbuminuria Captopril Study Group. *JAMA* 1994;271:275.

120. O'Donnell MJ, Rowe BR, Lawson N, et al. Placebo-controlled trial of lisinopril in normotensive diabetic patients with incipient nephropathy. *J Hum Hypertens* 1993;7:327.

121. Laffel LM, McGill JB, Gans DJ. The beneficial effect of angiotensin-converting enzyme inhibition with captopril on diabetic nephropathy in normotensive IDDM patients with microalbuminuria. North American Microalbuminuria Study Group. *Am J Med* 1995;99:497.

122. The Microalbuminuria Captopril Study Group: Captopril reduces the risk of nephropathy in IDDM patients with microalbuminuria. *Diabetologia* 1996;39:587.

123. Mathiesen ER, Hommel E, Hansen HP, et al. Randomised controlled trial of long term efficacy of captopril on preservation of kidney function in normotensive patients with insulin dependent diabetes and microalbuminuria. *BMJ* 1999;319:24.

124. Anonymous. Effects of ramipril on cardiovascular and microvascular outcomes in people with diabetes mellitus: results of the HOPE study and MICRO-HOPE substudy. Heart Outcomes Prevention Evaluation Study Investigators. *Lancet* 2000;355:253.

125. Bretzel RG. Effects of antihypertensive drugs on renal function in patients with diabetic nephropathy. *Am J Hypertens* 1997;10:208S.

126. Jungmann E, Malanyn M, Mortasawi N, et al. Effect of 1-year treatment with nitrendipine versus enalapril on urinary albumin and alpha 1-microglobulin excretion in microalbuminuric patients with type 1 diabetes mellitus. A randomized, single-blind comparative study. *Arzneimittelforschung* 1994;44:313.

127. Estacio RO, Jeffers BS, Gifford N, et al. Effect of blood pressure control on diabetic microvascular complications in patients with hypertension and type 2 diabetes. *Diabetes Care* 2000;23(Suppl 2):B54.

128. Parving HH, Lehnert H, Brochner-Mortensen J, et al. The effect of irbesartan on the development of diabetic nephropathy in patients with type 2 diabetes. *N Engl J Med* 2001;345(12):870.

129. Viberti G, Wheeldon NM. Microalbuminuria reduction with valsartan in patients with type 2 diabetes mellitus: a blood pressure-independent effect. *Circulation* 2002;106(6):672.

130. Parving HH, Andersen AR, Smidt UM, et al. Effect of antihypertensive treatment on kidney function in diabetic nephropathy. *Br Med J (Clin Res Ed)* 1987;294:1443.

131. Mogensen CE. Long-term antihypertensive treatment inhibiting progression of diabetic nephropathy. *Br Med J (Clin Res Ed)* 1982;285:685.

132. Lewis EJ, Hunsicker LG, Bain RP, et al. The effect of angiotensin-converting-enzyme inhibition on diabetic nephropathy. The Collaborative Study Group. *N Engl J Med* 1993;329:1456.

133. Taguma Y, Kitamoto Y, Futaki G, et al. Effect of captopril on heavy proteinuria in azotemic diabetics. *N Engl J Med* 1985;313:1617.

134. Björck S, Mulec H, Johnsen SA, et al. Renal protective effect of enalapril in diabetic nephropathy. *BMJ* 1992;304:339.

135. Brenner BM, Cooper ME, De Zeeuw D, et al. Effects of losartan on renal and cardiovascular outcomes in patients with type 2 diabetes and nephropathy. *N Engl J Med* 2001;345(12):861.

136. Lewis EJ, Hunsicker LG, Clarke WR, et al. Renoprotective effect of the angiotensin-receptor antagonist irbesartan in patients with nephropathy due to type 2 diabetes. *N Engl J Med* 2001;345(12):851.

137. Barnett AH, Bain SC, Bouter P, et al. Angiotensin-receptor blockade versus converting-enzyme inhibition in type 2 diabetes and nephropathy. *N Engl J Med* 2004;351(19):1952.

138. Bakris GL, Copley JB, Vicknair N, et al. Calcium channel blockers versus other antihypertensive therapies on progression of NIDDM associated nephropathy. *Kidney Int* 1996;50:1641.

139. Bakris GL, Weir MR, DeQuattro V, et al. Effects of an ACE inhibitor/calcium antagonist combination on proteinuria in diabetic nephropathy. *Kidney Int* 1998;54:1283.

140. Hansson L. Effects of angiotensin-converting enzyme inhibition versus conventional antihypertensive therapy on the glomerular filtration rate. *Cardiology* 1995;86(Suppl 1):30.

141. Murray KM. Calcium-channel blockers for treatment of diabetic nephropathy. *Clin Pharmacol Ther* 1991;10:862.

142. Nielsen FS, Rossing P, Gall MA, et al. Long-term effect of lisinopril and atenolol on kidney function in hypertensive NIDDM subjects with diabetic nephropathy. *Diabetes* 1997;46:1182.

143. Giordano M, Sanders LR, Castellino P, et al. Effect of alpha-adrenergic blockers, ACE inhibitors and calcium channel antagonists on renal function in hypertensive non–insulin-dependent diabetic patients. *Nephron* 1996;72:447.

144. Kasiske BL, Kalil RS, Ma JZ, et al. Effect of antihypertensive therapy on the kidney in patients with diabetes: a meta-regression analysis. *Ann Intern Med* 1993;118:129.

145. Gansevoort RT, Sluiter WJ, Hemmelder MH, et al. Antiproteinuric effect of blood-pressure-lowering agents: a meta-analysis of comparative trials. *Nephrol Dial Transplant* 1995;10:1963.

146. Weidmann P, Schneider M, Bohlen L. Therapeutic efficacy of different antihypertensive drugs in human diabetic nephropathy: an updated meta-analysis. *Nephrol Dial Transplant* 1995;10(Suppl 9):39.

147. UKPDS Study Group. Efficacy of atenolol and captopril in reducing risk of macrovascular and microvascular complications in type 2 diabetes: UKPDS 39. *BMJ* 1998;317:713.

148. UK Prospective Diabetes Study Group. Tight blood pressure control and risk of macrovascular and microvascular complications in type 2 diabetes: UKPDS 38. *BMJ* 1998;317:703.

149. Haffner SM, Lehto S, Ronnemaa T, et al. Mortality from coronary heart disease in subjects with type 2 diabetes and in nondiabetic subjects with and without prior myocardial infarction (see comments). *N Engl J Med* 1998;339:229.

150. Curb JD, Pressel SL, Cutler JA, et al. Effect of diuretic-based antihypertensive treatment on cardiovascular disease risk in older diabetic patients with isolated systolic hypertension. Systolic Hypertension in the Elderly Program Cooperative Research Group. *JAMA* 1996;276:1886.

151. Tuomilehto J, Rastenyte D, Birkenhager WH, et al. Effects of calcium-channel blockade in older patients with diabetes and systolic hypertension. Systolic Hypertension in Europe Trial Investigators. *N Engl J Med* 1999;340:677.

152. Hansson L, Zanchetti A, Carruthers SG, et al. Effects of intensive blood-pressure lowering and low-dose aspirin in patients with hypertension: principal results of the Hypertension Optimal Treatment (HOT) randomised trial. HOT Study Group. *Lancet* 1998;351:1755.

153. Estacio RO, Jeffers BW, Hiatt WR, et al. The effect of nisoldipine as compared with enalapril on cardiovascular outcomes in patients with non-insulin-dependent diabetes and hypertension. *N Engl J Med* 1998;338:645.

154. Tatti P, Pahor M, Byington RP, et al. Outcome results of the Fosinopril Versus Amlodipine Cardiovascular Events Randomized Trial (FACET) in patients with hypertension and NIDDM. *Diabetes Care* 1998;21:597.

155. Hansson L, Lindholm LH, Niskanen L, et al. Effect of angiotensin-converting-enzyme inhibition compared with conventional therapy on cardiovascular morbidity and mortality in hypertension: the Captopril Prevention Project (CAPPP) randomised trial. *Lancet* 1999;353:611.

156. Major outcomes in high-risk hypertensive patients randomized to angiotensin-converting enzyme inhibitor or calcium channel blocker vs diuretic: the Antihypertensive and Lipid-Lowering Treatment to Prevent Heart Attack Trial (ALLHAT). *JAMA* 2002;288(23):2981.

157. Major cardiovascular events in hypertensive patients randomized to doxazosin vs chlorthalidone: the antihypertensive and lipid-lowering treatment to prevent heart attack trial (ALLHAT). ALLHAT Collaborative Research Group. *JAMA* 2000;283(15):1967.

158. Lindholm LH, Ibsen H, Dahlof B, et al. Cardiovascular morbidity and mortality in patients with diabetes in the Losartan Intervention For Endpoint reduction in hypertension study (LIFE): a randomised trial against atenolol. *Lancet* 2002;359(9311):1004.

CHAPTER 55 ■ HYPERTENSION ASSOCIATED WITH ENDOCRINE DISORDERS

MYRON H. WEINBERGER

The frequency of secondary forms of hypertension in an unselected population of patients is unknown because the application of the requisite highly sensitive and specific screening and diagnostic tests in such individuals is expensive and not always risk-free. Moreover, no comprehensive surveys of unselected hypertensives have been performed using screening or diagnostic tests sensitive enough to establish the presence of the most common forms of potentially curable hypertension and thus to provide accurate estimates of the prevalence of these disorders. However, there are several clues that are helpful in identifying patients in whom the likelihood of a secondary form of hypertension is enhanced and in whom screening efforts are more likely to be productive. When the blood pressure elevation is noted at a young age, a secondary cause should be considered because primary ("essential") hypertension typically manifests in the fifth decade of life and later. A sudden onset of hypertension in an individual previously known to be normotensive or one in whom minimal antihypertensive therapy has previously been effective and who then becomes difficult to control despite probable compliance with treatment may be further clues to the presence of an identifiable form of hypertension. Severe hypertension and drug-resistant hypertension are also reasons to consider further evaluation. In addition, the various causes of secondary hypertension have specific findings that, when present, should trigger further assessment. This chapter considers the most common endocrine forms of secondary hypertension from the perspectives of relative frequency, pathophysiology, screening tests to establish their presence, diagnostic techniques to separate subtypes, and therapeutic approaches based on current information.

PRIMARY ALDOSTERONISM

Prevalence and Pathophysiology

Primary aldosteronism is probably the most recently recognized endogenous secondary form of hypertension, having been described initially in the mid-1950s. Based on the experience of several large referral centers, primary aldosteronism is second only to renal vascular hypertension in its prevalence as an identifiable and thus potentially curable form of hypertension (1,2).

Two recent studies in large groups of Italian (3) and Australian (4) hypertensive patients indicate a prevalence exceeding 9%. Several adrenal abnormalities capable of producing the syndrome of hyperaldosteronism have been identified and will be differentiated subsequently. To date, there have been no demographic or geographic bases for excluding the diagnoses. In brief, this group of disorders is characterized by anomalous, and generally autonomous, hypersecretion of aldosterone or other mineralocorticoids by the adrenal gland, leading to enhanced renal reabsorption of sodium in exchange for potassium and hydrogen ions. The enhanced sodium reabsorption produces extracellular fluid volume expansion and thus raises blood pressure. Despite continued excessive production of mineralocorticoids, the kidney ultimately "escapes" from continued and excessive sodium reabsorption (and volume expansion) by a combination of increases in perfusion pressure, renal blood flow, glomerular filtration, and the actions of natriuretic factors. Several studies have now identified increased levels of natriuretic peptide, presumably from the atrium, but also reportedly of adrenal origin, in patients with primary aldosteronism (5). These findings confirm a role for this peptide in the "escape" phenomenon. Although the sample sizes of the studies have been small, a suggestion has been made that patients with primary aldosteronism due to unilateral adenoma have higher plasma levels of natriuretic peptide than do those with bilateral (hyperplastic) adrenal disease.

Because of the mineralocorticoid-induced exchange of sodium for potassium and hydrogen ions, hypokalemia and metabolic alkalosis are commonly, but not invariably observed. Intracellular potassium depletion is typical and may produce carbohydrate intolerance, electrocardiographic abnormalities suggestive of left ventricular hypertrophy as well as arrhythmias, muscle weakness, and polyuria. Magnesium loss is also observed in primary aldosteronism, although not often evaluated, and contributes to muscle symptoms and arrhythmias. Renal cysts are commonly found in patients with primary aldosteronism as well as proteinuria. A recent report of renal nephrocalcinosis in a patient with primary aldosteronism suggests that the increased urinary calcium excretion and reduced citrate excretion may be related to stone formation (6). Proteinuria may reflect the glomerular hyperfiltration commonly seen in patients with primary aldosteronism. Accompanying the alkalosis, a decreased ionized calcium level is usually found, contributing to the muscle weakness and cramps and accounting for the occasional occurrence of tetany and a positive Chvostek's sign.

The blood pressure elevation in patients with primary aldosteronism is usually moderate or severe, and some studies have suggested that this syndrome is a common cause of malignant hypertension. While the hypertension is usually responsive to diuretic therapy and volume depletion, it is difficult to avoid worsening of the alkalosis, hypokalemia, hypomagnesemia, and decreased ionized calcium when diuretics are used, despite the use of potassium-sparing agents. The consideration of medical therapy will be discussed later. While several cases of primary aldosteronism during pregnancy have been observed, a recent report of the development of severe postpartum hypertension developing in two women confirms the masking effects of pregnancy, presumably attributable to the antialdosterone action of progesterone, on the clinical manifestations of this disorder (7).

Screening Tests

Measurement of serum potassium levels has traditionally been advocated as the most effective single screening test for primary aldosteronism. However, critical evaluation of the observations of several centers reporting studies in substantial numbers of patients with primary aldosteronism and with essential hypertension indicate that this may not be a very sensitive or specific screening test (1,2). One large study has recently reported normal plasma potassium levels in all patients with primary aldosteronism (3). Clues that would indicate a workup of a hypertensive patient for primary aldosteronism when the serum or plasma potassium levels are normal would be severe or refractory hypertension; onset of hypertension at a young age; or sudden increase in blood pressure in a previously normotensive or easily controlled hypertensive patient. At least 20% of patients with surgical confirmation of primary aldosteronism have been found to have serum (as opposed to plasma) levels of potassium that are within the normal range. Hemolysis of blood during venipuncture, which appears to be more common in patients with primary aldosteronism as is increased bruisability, may artifactually increase the potassium concentration. While the normal range for plasma potassium concentration may be as low as 3.5 mmol/L in some laboratories, serum potassium values rarely are below 4.0 mmol/L in normal subjects. Moreover, the majority of hypertensives manifesting hypokalemia have secondary aldosteronism from diuretic administration, the presence of renal vascular hypertension or other "high-renin" states leading to excessive stimulation of aldosterone production. Finally, when hypokalemia is found, repeat measurements, often after withdrawal of diuretics, and collection of 24-hour urine samples for measurement of sodium and potassium excretion have been advocated. This cumbersome and expensive series of screening maneuvers can be simplified by measuring plasma renin activity because in all cases of uncomplicated primary aldosteronism peripheral levels of renin are markedly suppressed by the elevated pressure, increased sodium balance, and expanded extracellular fluid volume associated with this syndrome. Thus the observation of "normal" or "elevated" plasma renin levels can effectively exclude primary aldosteronism when renal function is normal.

However, the finding of "low" or suppressed renin levels alone is not diagnostic of primary aldosteronism because as many as 40% of patients with "essential" hypertension may manifest suppressed plasma renin levels (e.g., the "low-renin essential hypertensive" subgroup). In addition, a variety of antihypertensive medications are known to influence renin levels. Most of these agents will raise renin, but antisympathetic drugs, acting centrally or peripherally, and β-adrenergic blocking agents can suppress plasma renin levels. Thus screening measurements of plasma renin activity should only be conducted when patients can safely be withdrawn from agents that are known to suppress renin release. Many of these, particularly the β-blocking drugs, have little or no effect on blood pressure in patients with primary aldosteronism.

We have found that the most sensitive and specific screening test for primary aldosteronism is the measurement of both plasma renin activity and plasma aldosterone concentration in peripheral venous blood obtained in ambulatory patients in whom agents that are known to suppress renin release have been withdrawn (8). Because renin is normally the primary stimulus to aldosterone production and in primary aldosteronism this relationship is essentially abolished, the sensitivity

of these measurements can be enhanced by expressing them as a ratio of aldosterone to renin (disregarding the units of measurement) with the lowest value for the latter being 0.7 in our hands. Although absolute values vary depending on the laboratory, in general, a ratio of 30 or more is a clear indication of primary aldosteronism and usually suggests a unilateral adenoma. A ratio between 15 and 30 is suggestive, and usually includes most patients with primary aldosteronism due to bilateral adrenal hyperplasia. In our hands, this measurement completely separates patients with primary aldosteronism from those with all forms of essential hypertension and, theoretically, can even be conducted in patients receiving antihypertensive medications that would be expected to stimulate renin release, such as diuretics, angiotensin-converting enzyme (ACE) inhibitors, calcium channel entry blockers, and other vasodilators. Because a few patients with primary aldosteronism appear to be exquisitely sensitive to angiotensin II, the finding of a normal aldosterone-to-renin ratio while receiving ACE inhibitors may require repeat sampling after withdrawal of the agents. However, like β-blockers, ACE inhibitors are usually not effective in reducing blood pressure in patients with uncomplicated primary aldosteronism. In our hands, this ratio is not only useful as a sensitive and specific screening test but also serves to differentiate the two most common forms of the syndrome (8). Two recent large studies confirm the utility of this screening test by estimating the prevalence of primary aldosteronism as 9% to 15% among "essential" hypertensive subjects (3,4).

Diagnosis

Traditionally, the diagnosis of primary aldosteronism has depended on the demonstration of excessive aldosterone production plus suppression of the normal stimulus, angiotensin II (renin). This has required the application of suppressive maneuvers to demonstrate hyperaldosteronism. These have included several days of a high-salt diet, often augmented by administration of intramuscular mineralocorticoids, such as deoxycorticosterone acetate (DOCA) to ensure sodium retention and volume expansion or the rapid intravenous administration of normal (0.9%) saline for the same purpose (1). Excessive aldosterone production is then based on measurement of one of several aldosterone metabolites in a 24-hour urine collection or, in the case of the saline infusion test, measurement of plasma aldosterone concentration (1). To complete the diagnostic approach it has been necessary to document suppressed renin levels, which traditionally has required a stimulatory maneuver such as several days of a low-sodium diet, often augmented with diuretic administration, or the use of intravenous or rapid diuretic-induced sodium and volume depletion to demonstrate the failure of the renin system to respond normally (1). Thus the diagnosis of primary aldosteronism requires not only evidence of excessive or inappropriate aldosterone production, but also its autonomy from the primary stimulus, renin.

Our recent observations, confirmed by several other groups, indicate that the diagnosis can be made simply by measurement of plasma renin and aldosterone levels in peripheral blood in an ambulant patient not receiving drugs known to interfere with the renin-angiotensin-aldosterone axis previously described (8). Not only is this approach easier to accomplish, it is also less expensive because it can be performed on an outpatient basis and is not subject to the inaccuracy that may accompany incomplete collection of urine or errors induced by alterations in aldosterone metabolism, since any one of the 13 metabolites found in urine may be normal or abnormal in specific patients (1,2). Finally, hypokalemia itself, common in primary aldosteronism, may alter the secretion and thus the urinary excretion of aldosterone, yielding false-negative results. After establishing the diagnosis of primary aldosteronism, the differentiation of several subtypes with important implications for treatment must be pursued.

Differentiation of Subtypes

The most common form of primary aldosteronism, accounting for 60% to 65% of cases in most series, is due to a unilateral adrenal adenoma. This form is most amenable to surgical intervention with a high rate of normalization of elevated blood pressure reported by most investigators. The adenomas are often small, frequently less than 1 cm in diameter, and thus localization techniques based on anatomy alone may not be effective. A recent report (9) of a group of 20 subjects with primary aldosteronism who were evaluated with magnetic resonance indicated a sensitivity of 60% with this technique, which is inadequate for use as a sole localizing procedure. In addition, several patients with apparent unilateral aldosteronism responsive to unilateral adrenalectomy have been found to have macro- and micronodular hyperplasia on microscopic examination. Yet long-lasting cure of hypertension has been produced by unilateral adrenalectomy (1). For these reasons, the use of adrenal venography, which may have substantial morbidity, computed tomography, magnetic resonance imaging, and isotopic scanning using a radioactive steroid precursor have been disappointing procedures, all fraught with unacceptably high rates of false-positive and false-negative results (1,10). The use of biochemical techniques or those based on the pathophysiology of primary aldosteronism have been of greater value in separating unilateral and bilateral forms of this syndrome.

Typically hyperaldosteronism resulting from a unilateral adrenal abnormality is modulated by adrenocorticotropic hormone (ACTH) but not by angiotensin II (11). Thus measurement of plasma aldosterone under conditions when the renin system would be relatively quiescent, such as early morning recumbency and again after activation of this system by upright posture for several hours, at noon, has been used to separate unilateral and bilateral forms (12). The rationale is that plasma levels in unilateral hyperaldosteronism would be expected to be higher early in the morning when the effect of ACTH is greater and to be relatively unresponsive to the increase in angiotensin II associated with assumption of the upright posture, producing lower values when plasma is sampled at noon. In contrast, normal subjects and those with bilateral forms of hyperaldosteronism would be more likely to have higher plasma aldosterone levels at noon compared to early morning levels. While this test has some usefulness, false-negative and false-positive results have been reported by several groups, including ours (10). This appears to be due to the fact that some of the adenomas have been reported to be angiotensin II responsive, accounting for the rise in plasma aldosterone levels with upright posture, and some patients with aldosteronism due to adrenal hyperplasia have demonstrated no increase or even a fall in plasma aldosterone levels when the noon value is compared to that obtained earlier during recumbency. Some investigators have advocated pharmacologic testing with a short-acting ACE inhibitor, captopril, based on the same pathophysiologic rationale. Again, false-positive and false-negative results have reduced the accuracy of this test.

Another biochemical measurement that has been helpful in the hands of some investigators has been the measurement of 18-hydroxycorticosterone in plasma or 18-oxocortisol in urine (13). Both of these steroids have been reported to be higher in patients with adenomas than in those with adrenal hyperplasia

in studies of small groups of patients from two laboratories. While encouraging, more extensive observations by a variety of investigators will be required to provide confirmation of these promising preliminary findings.

Adrenal venous blood sampling for the measurement of steroids is the most sensitive and specific way of separating unilateral and bilateral forms of this disorder (1,10). Nevertheless, while this technique is one that has been used for a long time, it has often been inconclusive or misleading. The reasons for previous failure have been both technical and physiological. Often the right adrenal vein cannot be located. In other situations, the adrenal venous drainage is multiple, or adrenal effluent may be diluted by blood from other sources such as the phrenic vein or left renal vein. In addition, steroid secretion is episodic, influenced by ACTH and perhaps other factors, thus potentially introducing another source of error. We have attempted to reduce these limitations by sampling adrenal venous blood during continuous infusion of ACTH and by measuring both aldosterone and cortisol in blood from the adrenals and the inferior vena cava (1,10). By expressing the observations as a ratio of aldosterone-to-cortisol, we can then correct for dilution of adrenal venous blood, minimize errors resulting from episodic secretion of steroids and, if one adrenal is not able to be sampled, infer the location of a unilateral lesion to that gland if the contralateral adrenal has an aldosterone-cortisol ratio that is lower than that in the inferior vena cava because extraadrenal sources of aldosterone have not been reported except in cases of metastatic malignancy (1). We have found that this technique has the highest accuracy (91%) in separating unilateral from bilateral disease (1,10), as recently confirmed by other investigators. We are most comfortable in making therapeutic recommendations when the adrenal venous data are corroborated by one of the anatomic or physiologic observations. An added benefit of localization, beyond determining whether a patient with primary aldosteronism is best treated with medication or with unilateral adrenalectomy, is the option of utilizing the less morbid dorsal (flank) or laparascopic approach in the latter case.

Molecular genetics has improved our recognition and understanding of a rare form of hyperaldosteronism which is remediable with dexamethasone (14). While several familial cases indicated a genetic basis for this syndrome, only with the ability to identify the aldosterone synthase gene and its mutations were the mysteries of this disorder elucidated. The most frequently encountered mutation of this type causes ACTH-responsive aldosterone production, accounting for the ability of glucocorticoid administration to provide persistent reduction in aldosterone production, relief of the syndrome of hyperaldosteronism, and a reduction in blood pressure with continued administration. However, long-term treatment with glucocorticoid may not be desirable in such patients. Evidence indicates that they can be treated with potassium-sparing diuretic combinations in most cases (15). An Australian group has recently reported another form of familial hyperaldosteronism not responsive to glucocorticoid administration (16). These families have revealed both adenomatous and bilateral forms of hyperaldosteronism, and future studies may elucidate the etiology of this interesting observation.

Two cases have been reported of primary aldosteronism resulting from bilateral solitary adrenal adenomas (1) which obviously produced confounding localization observations. When unilateral adrenalectomy with only transient improvement in the syndrome prompted reevaluation and exploration of the remaining adrenal the situation was clarified. Adrenal cortical carcinoma has been a rare cause of primary aldosteronism, but the malignant nature of the disease and the presence of excessive production of ketosteroids have usually been clues.

Treatment

When the evidence indicates that the patient has a unilateral source of hyperaldosteronism, adrenalectomy is almost uniformly effective in eliminating the hyperaldosteronism and its biochemical consequences and leads to normalization of blood pressure with no, or minimal amounts of, antihypertensive medication in over 70% of most reported cases (1). In some series, the normalization of blood pressure without medication has been reported to occur in a higher proportion of patients. The discrepancy between reports appears to be related to both the duration of disease before diagnosis and the duration of follow-up after surgery. While some patients demonstrate a reduction in blood pressure immediately after surgery, in others months may be required before the nadir in blood pressure is seen. In these latter patients, continued antihypertensive therapy may be required with trial withdrawal or reduction in doses after several months have elapsed. Extensive experience with the laparoscopic technique for adrenalectomy has now been described in the literature. However, some caveats are indicated. In one case, it took 4.5 hours to accomplish this procedure. Another report indicates recurrence of malignant adrenal tumor 6 months after removal of what was thought to have been a benign adrenal adenoma causing primary aldosteronism (17).

In bilateral disease, medical therapy is preferred. The aldosterone antagonist spironolactone is the most effective agent; however, doses as high as 800 mg per day may be required. Moreover, the side effects of spironolactone (e.g., painful gynecomastia) often lead to withdrawal of the agent. Eplerenone, a new mineralocoticoid receptor blocker, has not been extensively evaluated in primary aldsoteronism. Alternatively, potassium-sparing diuretics such as triamterene or amiloride combined with hydrochlorothiazide may be used with careful attention to the need for additional potassium and magnesium replacement (15). Calcium channel entry blockers have been reported to be effective in primary aldosteronism, but long-term experience in such patients is quite limited. There are scattered reports of the efficacy of ACE inhibitors, but these are largely anecdotal and unconfirmed.

For glucocorticoid-remediable hyperaldosteronism, glucocorticoids or potassium-sparing diuretics have been reported to be effective. There are few additional data regarding therapeutic responses to other agents in this rare disorder.

PHEOCHROMOCYTOMA

Prevalence and Pathophysiology

While pheochromocytoma is acknowledged to be less frequent than primary aldosteronism, its presence was often unsuspected and manifested by catastrophic outcomes during anesthesia and surgical procedures in the era before the availability of biochemical tests. In the past 30 years, it has become much easier to identify patients with this disorder, and the diagnosis is being considered in increasing numbers of hypertensive subjects. Unfortunately, because of the protean nature of the symptoms associated with pheochromocytoma, many more patients with hypertension not due to pheochromocytoma are evaluated for it in proportion to the few who are actually found to harbor tumors producing excessive catecholamines. In short, the symptoms and the diagnosis of pheochromocytoma are directly related to overproduction of catecholamines and thus must be differentiated from syndromes in which such overproduction results from physiologic or pharmacologic sources, frequently described as pseudopheochromocytoma (18).

The overwhelming majority (over 85% in most large series) of cases of pheochromocytoma result from adrenal medullary tumors. Extraadrenal pheochromocytomas are usually located below the diaphragm, typically in the periaortic area, and are more commonly malignant than the adrenal tumors, although malignancy can also be found in the latter. Cases of pheochromocytoma or paraganglioma have been reported in the urinary bladder, the heart, the brain, and the carotid body. Pheochromocytoma is included in several syndromes featuring multiple endocrine neoplasms (MEN type IIa) including thyroid and parathyroid tumors, MEN type IIb with ganglioneuromas, the von Hippel-Lindau syndrome (retinal angiomatosis, cerebellar hemangioblastoma), and other neuroectodermal abnormalities such as neurofibromas or "café-au-lait" skin lesions.

The symptoms of pheochromocytoma are generally nonspecific and may include headache, diaphoresis, pallor, tachycardia, anxiety or tremulousness, nausea, weakness, chest pain, dyspnea, fever, weight loss, and a variety of other systemic complaints. Sustained elevation of blood pressure is the most frequent finding, with about one-third of patients exhibiting episodic or paroxysmal hypertension and even normal blood pressure being observed in 10% to 15% of the subjects (19). A recent review from Italy of 284 patients with pheochromocytoma indicates paroxysmal hypertension in 67%, hypertensive crises in 59%, and normal blood pressure in 21% of the cases (20). Recent observations suggest that nocturnal hypertension can be found in those with apparent normotension during the daytime hours (21). Severe hypertension is common, and orthostatic hypotension has been reported to occur. Grade III or IV hypertensive retinopathy is observed in over 50% of patients with pheochromocytoma, presumably owing to the intense vasoconstriction that is the result of excessive catecholamine production. Raynaud's phenomenon and tremor are other findings observed in some patients. Rarely, an abdominal pheochromocytoma can be felt on deep palpation of the abdomen. However, the risk of precipitating a hypertensive crisis by manipulation of the tumor is reason not to be overly vigorous in such examination.

The majority of signs, symptoms, and findings associated with pheochromocytoma can be attributed to the effects of increased catecholamine production and the resultant stimulation of α- and β-adrenergic receptors. It is easy to understand why excessive release of catecholamines can raise blood pressure by inducing both vasoconstriction and an increase in cardiac output. Paroxysmal hypertension is also understandable given the variety of stimuli of catecholamine release, with an exaggerated response occurring in pheochromocytoma cases. Thus the episodic occurrence of headache, pallor, tremulousness, anxiety, and cardiovascular symptoms (e.g., tachycardia, arrhythmias, dyspnea, chest pain) can also be explained by the episodic release of catecholamines and the accompanying increase in blood pressure. It is more difficult to understand the reason for occasional reports of orthostatic hypotension or normotension (22) in these patients. Some have suggested that the intense vasoconstriction and elevated blood pressure induced by release of catecholamines can suppress baroreceptor reflex behavior. In addition, the vasoconstriction is also associated with a relatively contracted intravascular volume. Thus when the tumor is quiescent and vasorelaxation occurs, the gravitational effect of upright posture may not be adequately compensated for by the suppressed baroreceptor response and may be aggravated by the relative volume depletion. An additional explanation has been the vasodilatory effects of some catecholamines such as dopamine, which may be produced in preferential excess by some tumors. Finally, a variety of vasodilatory compounds have been identified that could be released in increased amounts to counter the catecholamine-induced vasoconstriction in an attempt to maintain pressure homeostasis, and thus could have a hypotensive effect when catecholamine release is abruptly diminished.

Pheochromocytoma has been identified in patients in whom it was not previously suspected when a paradoxical rise in blood pressure was observed following administration of a β-adrenergic blocking agent. This could even occur, theoretically, when β-blocker eyedrops are used because of the systemic absorption of these agents. The paradoxical rise in pressure occurs because of blockade of the β_2-receptor, typically associated with peripheral vascular vasodilation, leaving the vascular α-receptors, which are constrictor, unopposed.

Metabolic abnormalities are often seen in patients with pheochromocytoma. These include hyperglycemia and glucose intolerance as well as lipid abnormalities presumably related to the effects of catecholamines on glucose production (glycogenolysis) and/or uptake and α-adrenergic stimulation of triglyceride synthesis. Hypokalemia may occur because of catecholamine-induced shifts of potassium into skeletal muscle with β_2-receptor stimulation.

While unrecognized pheochromocytoma can be fatal, a high index of suspicion and the use of sensitive diagnostic tests provide a reasonable way of detecting most patients. One situation in which an unrecognized pheochromocytoma can be particularly catastrophic is in the pregnant patient (23). In this situation, high maternal and fetal mortality rates have been reported. Thus when hypertension or labile blood pressure is observed in pregnancy, it is important to rule out the presence of a pheochromocytoma. In patients in whom this has been recognized, surgical removal of the tumor has permitted the safe progression of the pregnancy to successful delivery.

A variety of factors, activities, and agents have been reported to trigger a paroxysm of blood pressure elevation or symptoms of pheochromocytoma in some patients. Such activities as defecation, sexual intercourse, bending over, Valsalva maneuver, coughing, sneezing, cigarette smoking, intake of red wine or hard cheeses (both of which contain tyramine), shaving, and a variety of invasive and surgical procedures have been incriminated. These and other normal stimuli of catecholamine production can trigger excessive release by a tumor and thus cause symptoms.

The presence of a pheochromocytoma can be mimicked by a variety of circumstances, frequently referred to as "pseudopheochromocytoma" (18). These events feature either excessive catecholamine production, excessive stimulation of adrenergic receptors, or both. Use of sympathomimetic agents (nasal sprays, cold remedies, diet aids, ephedrine and its congeners, amphetamines, and "street" drugs) or administration of drugs containing sympathomimetic substances, including agents such as imipramine and amitriptyline, to individuals receiving monoamine oxidase inhibitors, can produce symptoms suggestive of increased catecholamine production. Individuals undergoing addictive substance withdrawal also manifest evidence of a hyperadrenergic state. Further, abrupt or acute withdrawal from centrally acting α-adrenergic agonists such as clonidine, guanabenz, and guanfacine, particularly when used at higher doses, may precipitate a rebound hyperadrenergic response. Such exogenous causes of a hyperadrenergic state should be considered in the individual who presents with acute and/or severe symptoms suggestive of pheochromocytoma.

Screening Tests

The establishment of a diagnosis of pheochromocytoma requires a high index of suspicion because the symptoms and findings are not highly specific. The search for this disorder begins with studies to establish biochemical evidence of increased production of catecholamines. Before the advent of sensitive and specific screening and diagnostic tests, a variety of pharmacologic approaches were used, involving intravenous administration of substances known to stimulate catecholamine release (histamine, glucagon) or to block catecholamine-induced α-adrenergic stimulation (phentolamine). The stimulatory tests were fraught with catastrophic responses, including sudden death, in some patients with pheochromocytoma as well as false-positive responses in individuals in whom a tumor could not be found. The phentolamine test was also notoriously inaccurate, and thus these pharmacologic tests have been abandoned by most experts. The availability of sensitive and specific measurements of catecholamines and their metabolites in urine and in plasma has provided a safer, convenient, and reasonably accurate way to screen for the presence of a pheochromocytoma. However, these tests have also been fraught with inaccuracy for several reasons.

Plasma values for catecholamines can be in the normal range if the tumor releases catecholamines intermittently or can be elevated in patients without a pheochromocytoma for various reasons. The latter is not a major problem because additional screening or diagnostic tests can separate the false-positive responders from those harboring a tumor. A recent report of 35 patients with pheochromocytoma associated with von Hippel-Lindau disease or MEN-II indicates that plasma metanephrine and normetanephrine values had a sensitivity of 97% for the identification of tumors (24).

Urine studies are more frequently chosen to screen for pheochromocytoma. These can be influenced by several factors. The most obvious is the failure of the patient to collect a complete 24-hour sample. Some investigators have advocated "spot" urine samples, which may be influenced negatively by episodic secretion of catecholamines. Another source of error may be the choice of a specific metabolite for measurement that is not the major product of enzymatic action in a given patient. Thus it frequently becomes necessary to measure total catecholamines, norepinephrine, metanephrine, normetanephrine, vanillylmandelic acid, and/or homovanillic acid to be certain that the patient does not have a pheochromocytoma. The conventional techniques for screening for pheochromocytoma, therefore, may not be very useful. In addition, most antihypertensive drugs elevate catecholamines and thus may be a source of false-positive results. Exceptions to this are the centrally acting α-adrenergic agonists (clonidine, guanabenz, guanfacine) and reserpine when taken chronically.

We have developed a simple screening test that avoids many of these problems and has yielded a very high (over 98%) accuracy rate (25). We ask patients to collect the urine during the sleep period, discarding urine before retiring, saving any sample voided during the sleep period, and including the first sample upon arising. We then measure norepinephrine excretion in the sample by a specific radioenzymatic technique and express the results in units per hour, given the duration of the sleep period. This obviates the problems caused by incomplete 24-hour urine collection. In addition, since the period of sleep is a time of basal catecholamine release for normal subjects and hypertensives without pheochromocytoma, it becomes easier to identify even slight elevations in basal catecholamine production, which are invariably found in patients with pheochromocytoma. In our experience over the last 20 years with this approach, we have found the lowest value for a patient with pheochromocytoma to be seven times higher than the highest value for normal or essential hypertensive patients (25). These observations have recently been confirmed by other investigators, indicating that it has broad applicability. If elevated values are observed in hypertensives receiving antihypertensive medications, the study can be repeated after withdrawal of the offending drug(s). Obviously, the finding of elevated values in a patient ingesting one of the agents known to suppress catecholamine release would presumably indicate a positive screening result.

Diagnosis

Some investigators have advocated the use of plasma catecholamines as a screening test with the response of plasma catecholamines to oral administration of 0.3 mg of clonidine used as a diagnostic test. In untreated essential hypertensives with elevated plasma catecholamines, this dose of clonidine should reduce plasma levels by 50% after 3 hours. Many investigators have found this to be neither a sensitive nor a specific procedure and thus have abandoned its use (26,27). After documentation of an abnormal "sleep" urinary norepinephrine value or elevated 24-hour urine values for catecholamines or their metabolites, the next step is localization of the tumor. This is necessary for several reasons, including decisions regarding the therapeutic approach, which will be discussed subsequently. Fortunately, the majority of the tumors are located in the adrenal and are relatively large, usually greater than 2 cm in diameter. Thus computerized tomographic (CT) scanning will usually reveal the site of the tumor (28). The large Italian study (20) indicates a sensitivity of 99% for intraadrenal and 91% for extraadrenal tumors while the MIBG isotopic scan had a slightly lower (88.5%) sensitivity. Since hemorrhagic necrosis and subsequent calcification of parts of the tumor are not uncommon, they can sometimes be seen on a plain abdominal radiograph. The recent development of an isotopic product, labeled metaiodobenzylguanidine (MIBG), has provided another approach to localization of pheochromocytoma that is often useful when a lesion in the adrenal cannot be identified by computerized tomography or when extraadrenal or metastatic pheochromocytoma is suspected. Much less experience has been obtained with magnetic resonance imaging (MRI) and positron emission tomography (PET) scanning techniques. A recent study of 29 patients with pheochromocytoma compared the MIBG scan to the PET scan using fluorodeoxy-D-glucose and found the latter much more accurate (88% vs. 56%) (29). Rarely is it necessary to perform adrenal venography for the purpose of visualizing pheochromocytoma or, more commonly, to obtain venous blood samples for catecholamine content. The latter procedure may be required when other localizing techniques are not fruitful or when ectopic, multiple, or malignant pheochromocytoma is suspected.

Treatment

The preferred treatment of pheochromocytoma is surgical removal of the tumor (see below). Rarely, surgical intervention cannot be performed because of debility, relative or absolute contraindications, the presence of metastatic malignancy, or patient refusal. In such instances, treatment with effective doses of peripheral α-adrenergic blocking agents (vide infra) or metyrosine (Demser) can be useful. Recently several new, nonsurgical approaches to treatment have been reported. 131-I-MIBG has been used as radiotherapy in some cases of malignant tumors or tumors in areas not amenable to surgery (usually in the head and neck areas) alone (30) or in combination with chemotherapy (31).

The proper preparation of the patient for surgery is mandatory and must consider a variety of factors. First, the lesion must be localized so that the surgeon can minimize excessive exploration and manipulation of the tumor. Fortunately, the large size of most tumors makes it possible to identify them prior to surgery and thus permits the surgeon to go directly to the site and concentrate on ligation of the major blood supply of the tumor to reduce the amount of catecholamines introduced into the circulation. Another important requirement is for a period of 7 to 10 days of effective α-adrenergic blockade prior to surgery. This is not necessary for blood pressure or

arrhythmia control during the surgical procedure because intravenous administration of α- and β-adrenergic antagonists, respectively, can be used for that purpose, but rather to permit the contracted intravascular volume induced by the intense catecholamine-related vasoconstriction to expand before surgery is undertaken. Without such expansion of volume, the removal of a pheochromocytoma is associated with immediate vasodilation, which in the presence of a contracted extracellular fluid volume can produce rapid and irreversible shock and a state generally unresponsive to pressor agents. Effective α-adrenergic blockade can be assumed when the dose is titrated to a level at which the patient demonstrates a mild decrease in blood pressure on assumption of upright posture. Phenoxybenzamine (Dibenzyline), which chelates the α-receptor, may require a longer period of time to achieve effective doses than the use of the quinazoline class of α-blockers (prazosin, terazosin, and doxazosin). The doses of these agents required for effective α-blockade in pheochromocytoma are quite variable, ranging from 10 to 120 mg per day for phenoxybenzamine and as high as 40 mg per day for the quinazoline group. Beta-adrenergic blocking agents may also be required to decrease the tachycardia and arrhythmias during the preparatory phase. During the operative period, intravenous α-blockers (phentolamine) and short-acting parenteral β-blockers can be used. Several recent reports of successful removal of pheochromocytomas by the laparoscopic approach, occasionally utilizing laparoscopic ultrasound for localization, have been published (32,33). One such report described partial adrenal-sparing bilateral adrenalectomy (33).

Follow-up

Because multiple and malignant pheochromocytomas occur in about 10% of patients, it is prudent to evaluate catecholamine excretion periodically after removal of the tumor. If the patient becomes normotensive following surgery, assessment of urinary catecholamines at 6- to 12-month intervals is appropriate. Since familial pheochromocytoma is not uncommon, screening of family members with urinary catecholamine measurements is often pursued, and particular scrutiny should be given to any hypertensive family members.

CUSHING'S SYNDROME

Prevalence and Pathophysiology

Endogenous hypercortisolism is another endocrine form of hypertension that is potentially curable. The most frequent cause of this syndrome is exogenous steroid ingestion, but the signs and symptoms are the same for both. The typical observations are of truncal obesity with thin extremities because of the increased fat deposition in the abdomen and muscle wasting associated with the catabolic effects of glucocorticoids, increased cervical and dorsal fat pads manifesting as supraclavicular fullness and the "Dowager" or "buffalo" hump, increased facial fat distribution ("moon facies"), and increased capillary fragility often resulting in bruising of the skin, petechiae, and violaceous striae on the abdomen, inner thighs, and arms. The mechanisms responsible for the development of hypertension are not clear (34). There is some evidence that the renin-angiotensin system may play a role because glucocorticoids appear to increase the concentration of angiotensinogen, the renin substrate. In addition, high concentrations of glucocorticoids are capable of occupying the mineralocorticoid receptor of the kidney and inducing sodium and water retention and thus increasing extracellular fluid volume. Recent studies indicate that cortisol-induced hypertension is associated with sodium retention and volume expansion, but this is not believed to be the primary mechanism for the increase in blood pressure since it is not prevented by administration of the mineralocorticoid receptor antagonist, spironolactone (35). Additional observations indicate no increase in sympathetic nervous system activity but do suggest a suppression of nitric oxide activity (35). Carbohydrate intolerance and diabetes are frequently found in Cushing's syndrome and appear to be due to insulin resistance. Inappropriate elevation of leptin has been reported in Cushing's syndrome and may contribute to the abnormalities in glucose and lipid metabolism (36). Glucocorticoids also can inhibit osteoblastic activity and lead to osteoporosis and vertebral fractures.

The symptom complex can arise from either primarily pituitary or adrenal abnormalities. In about two-thirds of the cases, excessive ACTH production occurs due to a microadenoma of the pituitary, leading to sustained and excessive stimulation of the adrenals. In some patients, ectopic production of ACTH may stem from a carcinoma, often in the lung. Cushing's syndrome may also be a feature of the multiple endocrine adenomatosis (MEA, MEN) syndrome. Roughly 20% to 25% of patients with Cushing's syndrome are found to have a primary adrenal abnormality, typically an adenoma but also including adrenal carcinoma.

Screening Tests

The diagnosis of Cushing's syndrome requires a modestly high index of suspicion and demonstration of elevated or inappropriate glucocorticoid production. Since cortisol typically has an ACTH-driven diurnal rhythm, being higher in the morning than in the afternoon or evening, measurement of plasma cortisol in the morning and evening has been used as a screening technique. However, the sensitivity and specificity of this approach have been relatively poor because many factors can raise cortisol levels, including anxiety, venipuncture itself, estrogen administration, and others. Another long-used approach was to collect urine for the measurement of the major metabolites of cortisol, 17-hydroxycorticosteroids and 17-ketosteroids. However, these measurements can also be influenced by a variety of factors and are often elevated in simple obesity, a condition that mimics Cushing's syndrome because it is often associated with hypertension and carbohydrate intolerance. A single-dose dexamethasone suppression test can also be used as a screening procedure. Dexamethasone, 1 mg, is given orally at 11 PM, and plasma cortisol is measured at 8 AM the following morning. In normal individuals, plasma cortisol levels should be less than 5 μg/dL. The measurement of urinary excretion of free cortisol in a 24-hour sample appears to be the screening test with the highest sensitivity. A value greater than 100 μg/24 hours can be considered to be abnormal.

Diagnosis and Localization

After finding elevated urinary free cortisol excretion, the next step is to differentiate pituitary, adrenal, and ectopic etiologies. Plasma ACTH levels can separate primary adrenal disease from the other two sources. Typically, dexamethasone suppression tests can also separate pituitary and adrenal sources. There are two such tests. The first requires administration of 0.5 mg of dexamethasone every 6 hours for 2 days with collection of 24-hour urine samples for urinary free cortisol and 17-hydroxycorticosteroid excretion before and on the last day of dexamethasone. Plasma cortisol can also be measured on the morning following the last dose and should be less than 5 μg/dL. Urinary free cortisol should be less than

20 μg/24 hours, and 17 hydroxysteroid excretion less than 4 μg/24 hours. The high-dose dexamethasone test is then performed to separate pituitary and adrenal etiologies. Dexamethasone is given as 2 mg every 6 hours for eight doses, and a 24-hour urine collection is obtained on the second day. The majority of patients with pituitary Cushing's evidence have at least a 50% reduction from the pre-dexamethasone values, while in adrenal Cushing's, minimal change is seen in the overwhelming majority of patients. With ectopic ACTH syndromes, the suppression is less consistent, and steroid production is quite variable. Usually, marked wasting and elevated 17-ketosteroid excretion are seen in these patients.

Pituitary tumors are frequently detected by CT scan or magnetic resonance imaging (MRI). Adrenal tumors are also often visible on CT scan because they are usually larger than 1.5 to 2.0 cm in diameter. Occasionally, when the CT scan is not useful, iodocholesterol isotopic scanning may be helpful.

Treatment

When a pituitary adenoma is detected, surgical removal is usually curative, particularly when a microadenoma is found. In addition, such a lesion can usually be removed without requiring total hypophysectomy with its attendant hypopituitarism. Occasionally, irradiation of the pituitary is required if surgical removal is not feasible or yields incomplete results with a recurrence of Cushing's syndrome. When the lesion is localized in the adrenal, surgical removal is almost invariably curative except in the instance of adrenal carcinoma with metastases. Cushing's syndrome due to ectopic ACTH production is the least amenable to treatment because of the aggressive nature of the underlying malignancy, which has usually produced metastases by the time the metabolic abnormalities of Cushing's syndrome become manifest. A few reports of adrenalectomy by laparoscopic technique have now been reported for Cushing's syndrome (37).

HYPERTENSION ASSOCIATED WITH THYROID DISORDERS

Prevalence and Pathophysiology

Hypertension is encountered in both hyperthyroidism and hypothyroidism, although the mechanisms and manifestations appear to be different. In hypothyroidism, the major hemodynamic abnormality is an increase in peripheral vascular resistance, and cardiac output is usually reduced (38). This is often manifest as a primary elevation of diastolic pressure, although systolic elevation can also be seen. The increase in resistance is most likely the result of increased sympathetic nervous system activity or increased β-adrenergic responsiveness (39). Thyroid replacement therapy typically restores blood pressure to normal unless excessive doses are given. Since hypothyroidism may occur more frequently in older patients who often are more likely to have hypertension than younger individuals, residual blood pressure elevation may be seen despite adequate thyroid replacement therapy.

In hyperthyroidism, the dominant hemodynamic abnormality is an increase in cardiac output, and peripheral resistance may be normal (38). Thus a primary increase in systolic blood pressure is typically seen in hyperthyroidism. The mechanism most commonly invoked for the increase in cardiac output in hyperthyroidism is also related to the increased activity of the sympathetic nervous system (38). In this case, it appears to be related to increased β-adrenergic activity or responsiveness, particularly of cardiac β-receptors. Again, as with hypothyroidism, adequate treatment of the hyperthyroidism is usually associated with normalization of the elevated blood pressure except in those with background essential hypertension. It is unusual for hypertension to be the only presenting symptom of thyroid disease, but it can occur. This is particularly likely in older individuals in whom the symptoms of hypothyroidism may be subtle or masked by nonspecific complaints more frequently voiced by older patients such as constipation, coldness of the extremities, and the like. In older subjects, the "apathetic" form of hyperthyroidism is also more frequent, and thus hypertension may be the primary manifestation.

Screening Tests

Typically, measurements of circulating thyroxine (T_4) levels in plasma can establish the diagnosis of hyperthyroidism and, with thyroid-stimulating hormone (TSH) levels, of hypothyroidism. In some rare circumstances, T_4 levels may be normal in hyperthyroid individuals in whom the predominant production of triiodothyronine (T_3) may be excessive. Estrogen administration can be associated with increased plasma hormone binding proteins, and thus free hormone levels or assays that assess the unbound protein fraction ("uptake" assays) will provide a correct assessment of hormonal status. Since TSH is the dominant stimulus for thyroid hormone production it can be expected to be elevated in hypothyroidism in an attempt to increase thyroid hormone output from a diseased gland. TSH will be decreased in hyperthyroidism when the disorder is due to autonomous overproduction of thyroid hormone by the gland itself. Occasionally, hyperthyroidism is a disorder of excessive production of TSH, in which case both TSH and thyroid hormone levels will be elevated.

Diagnosis

The diagnosis of thyroid disorders after the abnormality is identified by the screening tests outlined above is based on determining the cause of the excessive or deficient thyroid hormone production. This is often simplified by the combination of T_4 (or T_3) and TSH measurements. When both are elevated, a pituitary or hypothalamic lesion is implied as the cause of hyperthyroidism. When hypothyroidism is accompanied by elevated TSH levels, primary thyroid deficiency is the usual cause. When hyperthyroidism occurs with low TSH levels, the lesion is usually in the thyroid itself, and an isotopic scan will reveal if it is due to diffuse overactivity or localized to one area of the thyroid, as with an adenoma or carcinoma, or to discrete multinodular lesions.

Treatment

The treatment of hypothyroidism is generally thyroid replacement therapy. In patients in myxedema coma, exquisite sensitivity to thyroid hormone is often encountered, and thus treatment is begun with very small doses, increased as tolerated based on the patient's cardiovascular and central nervous system responses. For most hypothyroid patients without myxedema, a small replacement dose of T_3 (0.1 mg per day) is initiated, with measurement of T_4 and TSH levels being performed after a period of 4 to 6 weeks. If abnormal, incremental increases or decreases in dose can be made. In some patients who are older and thus have decreased clearance of thyroid hormone, or those with cardiac disease or arrhythmias, a lower starting dose can be used.

In hyperthyroidism, several therapeutic options are available. Surgical removal of part or the entire gland is indicated only when malignancy is suspected, the patient is pregnant, or other treatment approaches have failed. Administration of radioactive iodine has become the preferred treatment for many patients. Both recurrent hyperthyroidism and hypothyroidism may occur with this approach. Continuing (lifelong) follow-up is necessary. Another option is for the use of antithyroid drugs such as methimazole and propylthiouracil, which inhibit thyroid hormone synthesis. After successful suppression of thyroid hormone production based on monitoring of thyroid function tests for a period of 4 to 6 months, it may be possible to taper the dose of antithyroid medication and, in some cases, withdraw it completely. In a substantial number of patients, recurrent hyperthyroidism may occur, but in others a state of normal thyroid function may be observed. Obviously, periodic monitoring of thyroid status will be required for these individuals as well. Often the initial clue to the recurrence of hyperthyroidism will be an increase in systolic blood pressure if this was observed before treatment was begun.

SUMMARY

Hypertension is often a manifestation of an underlying endocrinologic disorder. The initial medical contact for such a patient may be any of a variety of physicians with variable experience with such problems. A high index of suspicion coupled with an understanding of the pathophysiology, signs, and symptoms of the most frequent endocrine forms of hypertension as well as current information about effective screening tests for these disorders will enhance their identification. Definitive diagnostic tests and appropriate treatment will usually provide a means to relieve the hypertension and its sequelae in such individuals.

References

1. Weinberger MH, et al. Primary aldosteronism: diagnosis, localization, and treatment. *Ann Intern Med* 1979;90:386.
2. Gordon RD, et al. Evidence that primary aldosteronism may not be uncommon. *Clin Exp Pharmacol Physiol* 1993;20:296.
3. Fardella CE, et al. Primary hyperaldosteronism in essential hypertension: prevalence, biochemical profile and molecular biology. *J Clin Endocrinol Metab* 2000;85:1863.
4. Lim PO, et al. High prevalence of primary aldosteronism in the Tayside hypertension clinic population. *J Hum Hypertens* 2000;14:311.
5. Lee YJ, et al. Increased adrenal medullary atrial natriuretic polypeptide synthesis in patients with primary aldosteronism. *J Clin Endocrinol Metab* 1993;76:1357.
6. Kabadi UM. Renal calculi in primary hyperaldosteronism. *J Postgrad Med* 1995;41:17.
7. Nezu M, et al. Primary aldosteronism as a cause of severe postpartum hypertension in two women. *Am J Obstet Gynecol* 2000;182:745.
8. Weinberger MH, Fineberg NS. The diagnosis of primary aldosteronism and separation of two major subtypes. *Arch Intern Med* 1993;153:2125.
9. Sohaib SA, et al. Primary hyperaldosteronism (Conn syndrome): MR imaging findings. *Radiology* 2000;214:527.
10. Gleason PE, et al. Evaluation of diagnostic tests in the differential diagnosis of primary aldosteronism: unilateral adenoma versus bilateral micronodular hyperplasia. *J Urol* 1993;150:1365.
11. Kem DC, et al. Circadian rhythm of plasma aldosterone concentration in patients with primary aldosteronism. *J Clin Invest* 1973;52:2272.
12. Ganguly A, et al. Control of plasma aldosterone in primary aldosteronism: distinction between adenoma and hyperplasia. *J Clin Endocrinol Metab* 1973;37:765.
13. Ulick S, et al. The unique steroidogenesis of the aldosteronoma in the differential diagnosis of primary aldosteronism. *J Clin Endocrinol Metab* 1993;76:873.
14. Lifton RP, et al. A chimaeric 11 beta-hydroxylase/aldosterone synthase gene causes glucocorticoid-remediable aldosteronism and human hypertension. *Nature* 1992;355:262.

15. Ganguly A, Weinberger MH. Triamterene-thiazide combination: a practical alternative to spironolactone therapy for primary aldosteronism. *Clin Pharmacol Ther* 1981;30:246.
16. Stowasser M, et al. Familial hyperaldosteronism type II: five families with a new variety of primary aldosteronism. *Clin Exp Pharmacol Physiol* 1992;19:319.
17. Deckers S, et al. Peritoneal carcinomatosis following laparoscopic resection of an adrenocortical tumor causing primary hyperaldosteronism. *Horm Res* 1999;52:97.
18. Mann SJ. Severe paroxysmal hypertension (pseudopheochromocytoma): understanding the cause and treatment. *Arch Intern Med* 1999;159:670.
19. Orchard T, et al. Pheochromocytoma-continuing evolution of surgical therapy. *Surgery* 1993;114:1153.
20. Manelli M, et al. Pheochromocytoma in Italy: a multicentric retrospective study. *Eur J Endocrinol* 1999;141:619.
21. Ishiyama Y, et al. Pheochromocytoma associated with nocturnal hypertension. *Intern Med* 1993;32:781.
22. Smircic L, Suskovic T, Ferencic Z. Pheochromocytoma without hypertension. *J Intern Med* 1994;235:373.
23. Frier DT, Thompson NW. Pheochromocytoma and pregnancy: the epitome of high risk. *Surgery* 1993;114:1148.
24. Eisenhofer G, et al. Plasma normetanephrine and metanephrine for detecting pheochromocytoma in von Hippel-Lindau disease and multiple endocrine neoplasia type 2. *N Engl J Med* 1999;340:1872.
25. Ganguly A, et al. Diagnosis and localization of pheochromocytoma: detection by measurement of urinary norepinephrine during sleep, plasma norepinephrine concentration and computed axial tomography (CT-scan). *Am J Med* 1979;67:21.
26. Sjoberg RJ, Simcic KJ, Kidd GS. The clonidine suppression test for pheochromocytoma. *Arch Intern Med* 1992;152:1193.
27. Grossman E, et al. Glucagon and clonidine testing in the diagnosis of pheochromocytoma. *Hypertension* 1991;17:733.
28. Ganguly A, et al. Detection of adrenal tumors by computerized-tomography scan in endocrine hypertension. *Arch Intern Med* 1979;139:589.
29. Shulkin BL, et al. Pheochromocytomas: imaging with 2-(fluorine-18) fluoro-2-deoxy-D-glucose PET. *Radiology* 1999;212:35.
30. Troncone L, Rufini V. Nuclear medicine therapy of pheochromocytoma and paraganglioma. *Q J Nucl Med* 1999;43:344.
31. Sisson JC, et al. Treatment of malignant pheochromocytomas with 131-I metaiodobenzylguanidine and chemotherapy. *Am J Clin Oncol* 1999;22:364.
32. Brunt LM, et al. Laparoscopic ultrasound imaging of adrenal tumors during laparoscopic adrenalectomy. *Am J Surg* 1999;178:490.
33. Walther MM, et al. Laparoscopic partial adrenalectomy in patients with hereditary forms of pheochromocytoma. *J Urol* 2000;164:14.
34. Mantero F, Boscaro, M. Glucocorticoid-dependent hypertension. *J Steroid Biochem Mol Biol* 1992;43:409.
35. Kelly JJ, et al. Cortisol and hypertension. *Clin Exp Pharmacol Physiol* 1998;25(Suppl):S51.
36. Weise M, et al. Leptin secretion in Cushing's syndrome: preservation of diurnal rhythm and absent response to corticotropin-releasing hormone. *J Clin Endocrinol Metab* 1999;84:2075.
37. Pujol J, et al. Laparoscopic adrenalectomy. A review of 30 initial cases. *Surg Endosc* 1999;13:488.
38. Saito I, Saruta T. Hypertension in thyroid disorders. *Endocrinol Metab Clin North Am* 1994;23:379.
39. Bramnert M, et al. Decreased blood pressure response to infused noradrenaline in normotensive as compared to hypertensive patients with primary hypothyroidism. *Clin Endocrinol* 1994;40:317.

CHAPTER 56 ■ MALIGNANT HYPERTENSION AND OTHER HYPERTENSIVE CRISES

CHARLES R. NOLAN AND STUART L. LINAS

THE CLINICAL SPECTRUM OF SEVERE HYPERTENSION

The vast majority of hypertensive patients are asymptomatic for many years until complications due to atherosclerosis, cerebrovascular disease, or congestive heart failure develop. In a minority of patients this "benign" course is punctuated by a hypertensive crisis.

A *hypertensive crisis* is defined as the turning point in the course of an illness at which acute management of the elevated blood pressure plays a decisive role in the eventual outcome. The haste with which the elevated blood pressure must be controlled varies with each crisis. However, the crucial role of hypertension in the disease process must be identified and a plan for management of the blood pressure successfully implemented if the outcome is to be optimal. The absolute level of blood pressure is not the most important factor in determining the existence of a hypertensive crisis. In children, pregnant women, and other previously normotensive individuals in whom moderate hypertension develops suddenly, a hypertensive crisis can occur at a diastolic blood pressure normally well tolerated by adults with chronic hypertension. Furthermore, in adults with only mild to moderate hypertension, a crisis can occur when there is concomitant acute end-organ dysfunction involving the heart or brain. It has been estimated that of the 50 to 60 million hypertensive patients in the United States, approximately 1% will experience a hypertensive crisis during their lifetime (1). Moreover, the incidence of hypertensive crisis appears to be increasing over time. In the period from 1983 to 1992, the number of hospital admissions with malignant hypertension or accelerated hypertension as the primary diagnosis doubled, from approximately 16,000 to 32,000 (2). It has been postulated that this trend of increasing incidence of hypertensive crises may be explained at least in part by medical economics. Since a significant portion of the population lacks health insurance, the lack of a consistent health care provider may lead to inadequate treatment of patients with essential hypertension thereby increasing the number of patients at risk for development of a hypertensive crisis (3). The spectrum of hypertensive crises and other categories of severe hypertension are outlined in Table 56-1.

Malignant hypertension is a clinical syndrome characterized by marked elevation of blood pressure with widespread acute arteriolar injury. Funduscopy reveals *hypertensive neuroretinopathy* with striate (flame-shaped) hemorrhages, cotton-wool (soft) exudates, and often papilledema. Regardless of the degree of blood pressure elevation, malignant hypertension cannot be diagnosed in the absence of hypertensive neuroretinopathy (4). Some authors have defined *malignant hypertension* based on the presence of papilledema and have used the term *accelerated hypertension* when hemorrhages and cotton-

wool spots occur in the absence of papilledema (5). However, it is now accepted that the prognosis is the same in hypertensive patients with striate hemorrhages and cotton-wool spots whether or not papilledema is present (6,7). In this regard, the World Health Organization has recommended that accelerated hypertension and malignant hypertension be regarded as synonymous terms for the same disease (4). Hypertensive neuroretinopathy is thus an extremely important clinical finding that indicates the presence of a widespread hypertension-induced arteriolitis which may involve the central nervous system, heart, and kidneys. In patients with untreated malignant hypertension, there is a rapid and relentless progression to end-stage renal disease (ESRD) or death in less than 1 year. Mortality can result from hypertensive encephalopathy, intracerebral hemorrhage, congestive heart failure, and/or complications of uremia.

Hypertensive encephalopathy is a medical emergency in which cerebral malfunction is attributed to the severe elevation of blood pressure. It is one of the most serious complications of malignant hypertension. However, hypertensive encephalopathy can also occur in the absence of malignant hypertension (neuroretinopathy). Hypertensive encephalopathy can develop in the setting of severe hypertension of any cause, especially when acute blood pressure elevation occurs in previously normotensive individuals with eclampsia, acute glomerulonephritis, pheochromocytoma, or drug withdrawal hypertension. Clinical features include severe headache, blurred vision or blindness, nausea, vomiting, and mental confusion. If aggressive treatment is not initiated, stupor, convulsions, and death can ensue within hours. The *sine qua non* of hypertensive encephalopathy is the prompt and dramatic clinical response to antihypertensive therapy.

On occasion, hypertension that is not in the malignant phase (hypertensive neuroretinopathy is absent) may still qualify as a hypertensive crisis when acute end-organ dysfunction occurs in the presence of even moderate hypertension. The term *benign hypertension with acute complications* includes hypertension complicating acute pulmonary edema (acute diastolic dysfunction), acute myocardial infarction or unstable angina, acute aortic dissection, active bleeding, or central nervous system catastrophe (hypertensive encephalopathy, intracerebral or subarachnoid hemorrhage, or severe head trauma). In each case, control of the blood pressure is the cornerstone of successful therapy.

Catecholamine excess states such as pheochromocytoma crisis; monoamine oxidase inhibitor–tyramine interactions; use of sympathomimetic drugs (cocaine, amphetamines, phencyclidine, or high-dose phenylpropanolamine); and abrupt withdrawal of antihypertensive medications (clonidine, methyldopa, or guanabenz), can produce life-threatening hypertensive crises. The clinical presentation usually includes marked elevation of blood pressure with headache, diaphoresis, and

TABLE 56-1

THE CLINICAL SYNDROMES OF SEVERE HYPERTENSION

Hypertensive crises
  Malignant hypertension (hypertensive neuroretinopathy present)
  Hypertensive encephalopathy
  Benign hypertension with acute complications (acute organ system dysfunction but no hypertensive neuroretinopathy)
  Acute hypertensive heart failure (acute diastolic dysfunction with pulmonary edema)
  Atherosclerotic coronary vascular disease
    Acute myocardial infarction
    Unstable angina
  Acute aortic dissection
  Active bleeding including postoperative bleeding
  Central nervous system catastrophe
    Hypertensive encephalopathy
    Intracerebral hemorrhage
    Subarachnoid hemorrhage
    Severe head trauma
  Catecholamine excess states
    Pheochromocytoma crisis
    Monoamine oxidase inhibitor-tyramine interactions
    Antihypertensive drug withdrawal syndromes
    Phenylpropanolamine overdose
  Preeclampsia and eclampsia
  Poorly controlled hypertension in a patient requiring emergency surgery
  Severe postoperative hypertension
  Scleroderma renal crisis
  Miscellaneous hypertensive crises
    Severe hypertension complicating extensive burn injury
    High-dose cyclosporine in children after bone marrow transplantation
    Autonomic hyperreflexia in quadriplegic patients
    Severe hypertension with acute rejection or transplant renal artery stenosis in renal allograft recipients
    Hypoglycemia in patients receiving β-adrenergic receptor blockers

Benign hypertension with chronic stable complications (chronic end-organ dysfunction but no hypertensive neuroretinopathy)
  Chronic renal insufficiency due to primary renal parenchymal disease
  Chronic congestive heart failure with diastolic dysfunction
  Atherosclerotic coronary vascular disease
  Stable angina
  Previous myocardial infarction
  Chronic cerebrovascular disease
    Transient ischemic attacks
    Prior cerebrovascular accident

Severe uncomplicated hypertension (severe hypertension without hypertensive neuroretinopathy or end-organ dysfunction)

tachycardia. With the severe acute elevation of blood pressure a number of complications can occur, including hypertensive encephalopathy, intracerebral hemorrhage, and pulmonary edema due to acute left ventricular diastolic dysfunction. Thus, catecholamine-related hypertensive crises require prompt recognition and control of blood pressure to avert disaster.

Preeclampsia is a hypertensive disorder unique to pregnancy that usually presents after the 20th week of gestation with proteinuria, edema, and hypertension. Eclamptic seizures may ensue and without treatment may result in death. It is believed that eclampsia may be a subtype of hypertensive encephalopathy (8). Hypertensive disorders of pregnancy and their management are discussed in Chapter 53.

Poorly controlled hypertension in a patient requiring emergency surgery is a hypertensive crisis because of the increased cardiovascular risk that accompanies inadequate preoperative blood pressure control. Surgical manipulation of the carotid arteries or open-heart surgery (especially coronary artery bypass) is occasionally followed by severe hypertension in the immediate postoperative period. *Severe postoperative hypertension* represents a crisis requiring immediate blood pressure control because it can cause hypertensive encephalopathy or intracerebral hemorrhage, or jeopardize the integrity of vascular suture lines and thereby lead to postoperative hemorrhage.

In patients with progressive systemic sclerosis, *scleroderma renal crisis* can occur with sudden onset of hypertension that may enter the malignant phase. There is a rapid progression to ESRD within days to weeks unless the vicious cycle of hypertension, renal ischemia, and activation of the renin-angiotensin–aldosterone axis is interrupted.

Severe acute hypertension can also occur in patients with extensive burns or children receiving high-dose cyclosporine for allogeneic bone marrow transplantation. In quadriplegic patients, hypertensive crises may develop due to autonomic hyperreflexia resulting from stimulation of nerves below the level of the spinal cord injury. Hypertensive crises due to autonomic hyperreflexia can also develop in Guillain-Barré syndrome. Hypertensive crises may also complicate acute rejection or transplant renal artery stenosis in patients with renal allografts. In each of these conditions, a sudden increase in blood pressure may cause acute pulmonary edema, hypertensive encephalopathy, cerebrovascular accident, and/or death.

On the other hand, severe hypertension or the presence of hypertensive complications does not always imply the existence of a hypertensive crisis requiring immediate control of the blood pressure. Patients with benign hypertension (no hypertensive neuroretinopathy) and chronic stable end-organ dysfunction do not require emergent reduction of blood pressure, although a long-term lack of adequate blood pressure control often results in further deterioration of end-organ function. The term *benign hypertension with chronic stable complications* includes hypertension occurring in the setting of primary renal parenchymal disease with chronic kidney disease, chronic congestive heart failure, atherosclerotic coronary vascular disease (stable angina pectoris or prior myocardial infarction), or chronic cerebral vascular disease (prior transient ischemic attacks or cerebrovascular accident).

It is important to emphasize that the finding of severe hypertension does not always imply that a hypertensive crisis is present. In patients with severe hypertension that is not accompanied by acute end-organ dysfunction or evidence of malignant hypertension (hypertensive neuroretinopathy) eventual complications due to stroke, myocardial infarction, or congestive heart failure occur over a time frame of months to years rather than hours to days. Although long-term control of blood pressure can prevent these complications, a hypertensive crisis cannot be diagnosed, as there is no evidence that acute reduction of blood pressure results in any improvement in short-term or long-term prognosis. *Severe uncomplicated hypertension* is defined by a diastolic blood pressure higher than 115 mm Hg without evidence of malignant hypertension (no hypertensive neuroretinopathy) or signs of acute end-organ dysfunction. Although this is not a true hypertensive crisis as defined earlier, it is the most common presentation of severe hypertension. Severe uncomplicated hypertension is usually found in patients with chronic essential hypertension who are undiagnosed, undertreated, or not adherant with medical therapy. It is most often discovered incidentally in an otherwise asymptomatic patient. There is no evidence of hypertensive encephalopathy or other acute end-organ dysfunction. The fundi do not show striate hemorrhages, cotton-wool spots, or papilledema. Since the potential complications of severe uncomplicated hypertension develop with a time frame of months to years, the once common practice of abrupt reduction of blood pressure with oral antihypertensive agents prior to discharge from the acute care setting is no longer accepted as the standard of care (9–11). Instead, the goal of treatment should be the gradual reduction of blood pressure to normotensive levels over a few days in conjunction with frequent outpatient follow-up visits to modify the antihypertensive regimen and reinforce the importance of lifelong adherence with medical therapy. In the past this entity has been termed *urgent hypertension*. Use of the more descriptive term severe uncomplicated hypertension is preferable because there is no need for urgent reduction of blood pressure as would be required in patients with true hypertensive crises.

MALIGNANT HYPERTENSION

Historical Perspective

In 1914, Volhard and Fahr (12) introduced the descriptive terms *benign* and *malignant*, aimed at separating renal arteriosclerosis into two distinct types. The type without renal failure was called *benign nephrosclerosis* and was characterized pathologically by arteriosclerosis of the kidney. The type with renal failure was called *malignant nephrosclerosis* and was characterized by necrotizing arteriolitis with inflammatory changes in the glomeruli in addition to the arteriosclerosis seen in the benign form (13). Volhard later abandoned the concept of inflammatory changes and substituted prolonged ischemia secondary to vascular spasm as the cause of the renal lesion in the malignant type (14).

The prognostic importance of eyeground changes in hypertensive patients has long been recognized. *Albuminuric retinitis* was the term used by Liebreich in 1859 (15) to describe the retinal changes in some patients with advanced Bright's disease that were characterized by papilledema, ill-defined white exudates, a macular star, and linear hemorrhages. Volhard noted that the appearance of albuminuric retinitis was often the first

sign heralding a transition from the benign to the malignant type of nephrosclerosis (12,14).

In 1928, Keith et al. (16) coined the term *malignant hypertension* to describe a clinical syndrome characterized by severe hypertension with arteriolopathy manifested by papilledema, hemorrhages, and exudates (grade IV retinopathy). Virtually all of their patients died within 1 year of various combinations of brain, heart, and kidney failure. Interesting to note, at the time of presentation with severe hypertension and grade IV retinopathy, the majority of these patients had normal or only mildly impaired renal function.

By 1935, the concept had emerged that the clinical syndrome of malignant hypertension was not due to a single etiology but to a variety of different etiologies. Derow and Altschule (17) pointed out that malignant hypertension occurred in association with essential hypertension as well as secondary forms of hypertension such as chronic glomeulonephritis, chronic pyelonephritis, Cushing's syndrome, pheochromocytoma, renal artery stenosis, and polyarteritis nodosa.

Over the ensuing decades it was recognized that regardless of the underlying etiology of malignant hypertension, the relentless progression of the disease could be slowed or even reversed by reduction of blood pressure with any one of a number of treatments including sympathectomy (18,19), pyrogens (20), rice diet (21), excision of a unilaterally diseased kidney, adrenal resection in Cushing's syndrome (22), excision of a pheochromocytoma (23), and a variety of drugs that lower arterial pressure (24).

Untreated Prognosis and Natural History

A review of the survival statistics in the era before effective antihypertensive drugs became available reveals the reason why this disorder was called "malignant" hypertension. Keith et al. (5,16) described 81 patients with grade III or grade IV retinopathy in whom initial renal involvement was mild. Even in the absence of significant nephropathy, the short-term prognosis was grave. Their classic mortality curve is shown in Figure 56-1. They reported 1-year death rates in hypertensive patients catagorized on the basis of initial funduscopic findings. In group I (mild arteriolar narrowing or sclerosis of retinal vessels), the 1-year death rate was 10%; in group II (moderate sclerosis with increased light reflex and arteriovenous compression or localized arteriolar narrowing), 12%; in group III (retinal hemorrhages and exudates), 35%; and in group IV (hemorrhages and

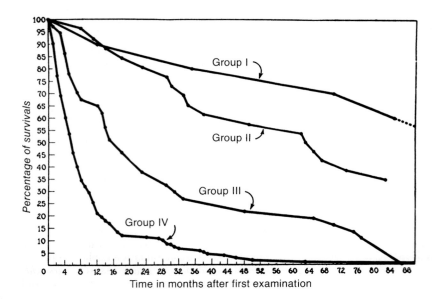

FIGURE 56-1. Survival curves based on the Keith and Wagener grade of hypertensive retinopathy. (From: Keith NM, Wagener HP, Barker NW. Some different types of essential hypertension: their course and prognosis. *Am J Med Sci* 1939;197:332, with permission.)

exudates plus papilledema), 80% 1-year mortality. Many other series of untreated hypertensive patients with severe retinopathy confirmed this dismal prognosis (25–29). The reported causes of death in untreated patients with malignant hypertension were similar in most series. Uremia was the most common cause of death, followed by congestive heart failure and cerebrovascular accident. Ellis (28) outlined four different clinical courses in patients with severe hypertension and hypertensive neuroretinopathy. In the *cerebral* type, patients died due to intracerebral hemorrhage or hypertensive encephalopathy. In the *cardiac* type, severe congestive heart failure with attacks of acute pulmonary edema dominated the clinical picture. With the *renal* type, death was the result of terminal uremia. In the combined type, patients died with manifestations of both congestive heart failure and uremia. Each type showed evidence of widespread vasculopathy and had a rapidly fatal course. In these series, the most important prognostic factor in untreated patients with malignant hypertension was the level of renal function at the time of diagnosis (25,26). Thus, the majority of untreated patients with malignant hypertension can be expected to die from uremia within 1 year. Congestive heart failure is often present. Some patients succumb earlier due to hypertensive encephalopathy or intracerebral hemorrhage at a time when renal involvement may not be pronounced.

Etiologies of Malignant Hypertension

Hypertension of virtually any etiology can enter a malignant phase (Table 56-2). Thus, malignant hypertension is not a single disease entity but rather a syndrome in which hypertension can be either primary (essential) or secondary to one of any number of different etiologies (17). Moreover, in the individual patient with malignant hypertension, on clinical grounds it is often difficult to distinguish whether the underlying hypertension is primary or secondary.

Malignant hypertension usually develops in patients with preexisting, poorly controlled, or undiagnosed hypertension. However, occasional patients have been described who experience an abrupt onset of so-called *de novo* malignant hypertension without a preceding phase of benign hypertension (27,29). The presence of de novo malignant hypertension almost always indicates an underlying secondary cause of hypertension (27).

Primary (Essential) Malignant Hypertension

In the era prior to the introduction of antihypertensive drugs, malignant hypertension evolved from underlying essential hypertension in more than 50% of patients (27,30). However, more recent series found a lower incidence of primary malignant hypertension, most likely reflecting prevention of malignant hypertension through effective control of blood pressure among patients with essential hypertension (31,32). In a series of patients collected between 1979 and 1985, primary malignant hypertension was found in only 20% (32). This observation may not apply to black patients, because among blacks, essential hypertension continues to represent the most common underlying etiology of malignant hypertension (33–35). Essential hypertension appears to be a rare cause of malignant hypertension in children. Secondary causes of hypertension such as chronic pyelonephritis, chronic glomerulonephritis, and renovascular hypertension are much more common in this younger age group (36).

Secondary Malignant Hypertension

The most common secondary cause of malignant hypertension is primary renal parenchymal disease. *Chronic glomerulonephritis* was reported to underlie the development of malignant hypertension in up to 20% of patients (30,32). Unless a history of an acute nephritic episode or long-standing hematuria or proteinuria is available, the underlying glomerulonephritis may be apparent only if a renal biopsy is performed (32). Recently, immunoglobulin A (IgA) nephropathy was reported as a frequent cause of malignant hypertension in series from Spain and Australia (32,37,38). In one series of 66 patients with IgA nephropathy, malignant hypertension developed in 10% (38).

Chronic pyelonephritis was reported as a cause of malignant hypertension in 9% to 16% of patients in recent series (31,32). In children, chronic atrophic pyelonephritis is the most frequent cause of malignant hypertension (39,40). Children with reflux nephropathy causing chronic atrophic pyelonephritis often present with either hypertensive encephalopathy or malignant hypertension (40).

In Australia, malignant hypertension complicates up to 7% of cases of *analgesic nephropathy* (41). Transient malignant hypertension responsive to volume expansion, an entity that is rare with other causes of malignant hypertension, can occur in the setting of analgesic nephropathy (41). It has been suggested that the salt-wasting state caused by tubulomedullary dysfunction contributes to the pathogenesis of malignant hypertension by causing severe volume depletion with activation of the renin-angiotensin axis (42).

Malignant hypertension is both an early and a late complication of *radiation nephritis* (25,44). In a series of patients with seminoma treated by radiotherapy to the posterior lymph nodes, acute radiation nephritis occurred in 13 patients with a latent period of 6 to 12 months. This was characterized by hypertension, anemia, albuminuria, and renal insufficiency. Hypertensive neuroretinopathy (striate hemorrhages, cotton-wool spots, and papilledema), indicating the development of malignant hypertension, occurred in five of these patients, three of whom died as a consequence of congestive heart failure, hypertensive encephalopathy, and uremia (44). In some patients, malignant hypertension developed as a late complication of radiotherapy with a latent period of 1.5 to 11.0 years, despite the absence of a history of prior acute radiation nephritis (44).

Congenital unilateral renal hypoplasia (Ask-Upmark kidney) is a rare cause of malignant hypertension in children and

TABLE 56-2

ETIOLOGIES OF MALIGNANT HYPERTENSION

Primary (essential) malignant hypertension[a]
Secondary malignant hypertension
  Chronic kidney disease
    Chronic glomerulonephritis[a]
    Chronic pyelonephritis[a]
    Analgesic nephropathy[a]
    Immunoglobulin A nephropathy[a]
    Acute glomerulonephritis
    Radiation nephritis
    Ask-Upmark kidney
  Renovascular hypertension[a]
  Oral contraceptives
  Renal cholesterol embolization
  Scleroderma renal crisis
  Antiphospholipid (anticardiolipin) antibody syndrome
  Chronic lead poisoning
  Endocrine hypertension
  Pheochromocytoma
  Aldosterone-producing adenoma
  Cushing's syndrome
  Congenital adrenal hyperplasia

[a] Most common underlying etiologies.

adolescents. This entity is characterized by unilateral renal hypoplasia with an enlarged and deformed renal pelvis that has one or more recesses that end blindly near the surface of the kidney. There is debate as to whether this represents a distinct clinicopathologic entity (43), or is simply the result of chronic pyelonephritis in a congenitally hypoplastic kidney (45).

Renovascular hypertension due to either fibromuscular dysplasia or atherosclerotic renal artery stenosis is a well-recognized cause of malignant hypertension. Its frequency, however, varies in different series. Some series in adult patients reported only a 3% to 4% incidence of underlying renovascular hypertension (25,27). A 10% incidence of renal artery stenosis was reported among children with severe hypertension (40). In contrast to these series, others found a very high incidence of underlying renovascular disease among patients with malignant hypertension (46). In a series of 123 patients with malignant hypertension, renovascular hypertension was found in 43% of white patients and 7% of black patients. The prevalence of renovascular hypertension was the same when the group with hemorrhages and exudates without papilledema was analyzed separately from the group with papilledema (46).

Although hypertension is usually mild to moderate in patients with *polyarteritis nodosa*, malignant hypertension has been reported (47). In polyarteritis, even in normotensive individuals, lesions indistinguishable from primary malignant nephrosclerosis may be seen in the interlobular arteries (proliferative endarteritis) and afferent arterioles (fibrinoid necrosis). However, the finding of healed and active lesions in larger medium-sized muscular arteries of the kidney (arcuate and larger arteries), mesentery, lungs, pancreas, and adrenals is unusual in primary malignant hypertension and suggests the diagnosis of polyarteritis nodosa (30).

In women of childbearing age, *oral contraceptives* may cause malignant hypertension (48–49). Some of the reported patients were normotensive prior to the initiation of oral contraceptives, although several patients had gestational hypertension during a prior pregnancy. In the absence of underlying renal disease, discontinuation of oral contraceptives is associated with an excellent long-term prognosis (49). However, a more recent series of women of childbearing age with malignant hypertension suggests that oral contraceptive use was not a common underlying etiology; instead a past history of pregnancy-induced hypertension was the most important risk factor (50).

Severe hypertension, which can enter the malignant phase, is a frequent complication of *atheroembolic renal disease* (cholesterol embolization) (51–54). In patients with severe aortic atherosclerotic disease undergoing aortic angiography, cardiac catheterization, or vascular surgery, evidence of cholesterol embolization may develop immediately after the procedure, with lower extremity livedo reticularis and purple toes, abdominal pain, eosinophilia, eosinophiluria, hypocomplementemia, and acute renal failure. Severe benign or malignant hypertension may develop acutely. Alternatively, the patient may present with malignant hypertension weeks to months after the inciting procedure, at a time when clinical signs of cholesterol embolization have entirely resolved.

Scleroderma renal crisis is the most acute and life-threatening manifestation of progressive systemic sclerosis. It is characterized by severe hypertension (sometimes malignant) with rapidly progressive renal failure (55,56). In one large series, scleroderma renal crisis occurred in 7% of white patients and 21% of black patients with progressive systemic sclerosis (57). The renal histology in scleroderma renal crisis is often virtually indistinguishable from that of primary malignant nephrosclerosis (58). However, in progressive systemic sclerosis, involvement of the renal vasculature, with proliferative endarteritis involving the interlobular arteries and fibrinoid necrosis of the afferent arterioles, may be a primary event that precedes either

hypertension or renal insufficiency (58). The renal ischemia that results from these lesions causes hypertension through activation of the renin–angiotensin system, leading to a vicious cycle of severe hypertension and renal ischemic injury. Scleroderma renal crisis was once a uniformly fatal complication of progressive systemic sclerosis. With the introduction of angiotensin-converting inhibitors as treatment, outcomes have improved significantly, though 39% to 50% of patients with scleroderma renal crisis continue to have poor outcomes, including permanent dialysis and death (56).

Patients with *antiphospholipid (anticardiolipin) antibody syndrome*, either primary or secondary to systemic lupus erythematosus, can develop malignant hypertension with renal insufficiency due to thrombotic microangiopathy even in the absence of overt lupus nephritis (59).

Malignant hypertension rarely complicates the course of immunoglobulin G (IgG) myeloma. Although the pathogenesis is not known, hyperviscosity has been implicated (60). Malignant hypertension may also develop in patients with immunotactoid glomerulopathy (Nolan, unpublished observation).

Patients with *chronic lead poisoning* can develop severe hypertension and the neuroretinopathy typical of malignant hypertension (17).

A number of endocrine disorders occasionally lead to secondary malignant hypertension. Malignant hypertension is a rare complication of *pheochromocytoma* (61). Although malignant hypertension secondary to *aldosterone-producing adenoma* is rare, occasional cases have been described (62). However, a diagnosis of primary hyperaldosteronism must be made with caution in patients with a history of malignant hypertension. Following successful treatment of malignant hypertension, plasma renin activity (PRA) rapidly returns to normal, whereas aldosterone secretion may remain elevated for up to a year. This observation has been attributed to persistent adrenal hyperplasia due to long-standing hyperreninemia with disordered feedback control (tertiary hyperaldosteronism) (63). During this period, hypokalemia, metabolic alkalosis, and hyperaldosteronism may persist, despite suppressed PRA, thereby mimicking primary hyperaldosteronism. These patients with tertiary hyperaldosteronism were found to have bilateral nodular adrenal hyperplasia at surgery (64,65). Although adrenalectomy alleviates hypokalemia in this setting, there is no improvement in blood pressure (64,65).

Cushing's syndrome with bilateral adrenal hyperplasia is most often associated with benign hypertension, although occasional cases of malignant hypertension have been reported (25,66). *Congenital adrenal hyperplasia* in patients with 11 β-hydroxylase deficiency (67) or 17 α-hydroxylase deficiency (68) can cause malignant hypertension.

Epidemiology of Malignant Hypertension

Incidence

Although malignant hypertension is often a complication of preexisting hypertension, the risk of its development in hypertensive patients is difficult to estimate. In early series the incidence of malignant hypertension among hypertensive patients was 1% to 7% (25,69). In the era of effective antihypertensive therapy for benign hypertension, the incidence of malignant hypertension appears to have declined to some extent. A review of death certificates in New York City between 1958 and 1974 revealed that the overall mortality due to malignant hypertension had declined by 78% from 2.25 deaths to 0.48 deaths/100,000 population/year (70). Although some of the decreased mortality was probably due to successful treatment of patients with malignant hypertension with antihypertensive drugs and dialysis, the authors speculated that the overall incidence of malignant hypertension had declined to less than 1% due to successful treatment of benign hypertension. However, despite recent advances in the treatment of essential hypertension, malignant hypertension is clearly not a disease that has vanished. In the United States, during the period from 1983 to 1992, the number of hospital admissions with malignant hypertension or accelerated hypertension as the primary diagnosis (International Classifcation of Diseases, ICD-9 Code 401.0) doubled from approximately 16,000 to 32,000. Moreover, the number of admissions in which one of these conditions was listed as a diagnosis tripled from approximately 23,000 to 75,000 (2). Reported experience in a multiracial population in England indicates that malignant hypertension is still common with a small proportion of hypertensive patients presenting with malignant hypertension each year (71). The incidence rate of malignant hypertension for the entire population was approximately one to two cases/100,000/year. Moreover, the incidence rate was not changed over the 24-year period from 1970 to 1993. Thus, despite the plethora of drugs available for the treatment of hypertension, failure to identify or adequately treat hypertension remains problematic and malignant hypertension undoubtedly will remain a clinical challenge for the foreseeable future (72,73).

Age

Malignant hypertension occurs more frequently in younger subjects. The mean age of patients with malignant hypertension ranges from 40 to 50 years, with 57% of patients between 30 and 50 years old (27). No difference has been found in the age at onset in men compared to women or whites compared to blacks (25–27,29,74). Pickering (45) suggests that the age dependency of malignant hypertension could be related to the increased frequency of secondary, more severe forms of hypertension in the young. Alternatively, it is possible that hypertension in patients destined to enter the malignant phase may be more rapidly progressive from the onset, so that the disease would be expected to occur predominantly in younger patients. Malignant hypertension is a rare development in patients beyond the age of 65 (27). The declining incidence of malignant hypertension in patients with essential hypertension relative to age is in marked contrast to the overall incidence of benign hypertension, which reaches a peak in the eighth decade (27). Patients over age 60 with malignant hypertension usually have underlying renovascular hypertension or primary renal parenchymal disease (75).

Gender

In most series of patients with malignant hypertension, males predominate over females by as much as 2 to 1 (25,26,29,30,69,74).

Race

Blacks have an increased incidence of essential hypertension compared to whites. Moreover, several studies demonstrate that blacks with essential hypertension also have an increased risk of developing malignant hypertension. In a population in which 31% of all hypertensive patients were black, 46% of 200 patients with malignant hypertension were found to be black (29). In a study of 135 pairs of black and white hypertensive patients matched for age and gender, 4.4% of the black patients had retinopathy consistent with malignant hypertension, whereas only 0.74% of the white patients had these funduscopic findings (76). The increased frequency of malignant hypertension among blacks may be due to the fact that they presented later in the course of essential hypertension, that antihypertensive therapy in blacks was inadequate to prevent the development of malignant hypertension, or that essential

hypertension may be a more aggressive and likely to enter the malignant phase in blacks than whites (77).

Preceding Duration of Benign Hypertension

Although there are occasional case reports in which the malignant phase appears to begin *de novo*, the majority of patients show evidence of a variable period of preceding benign hypertension before the onset of malignant hypertension. Among 77 patients with malignant hypertension, the documented duration of benign hypertension was 0 to 6 months in 4%, 6 months to 1 year in 10%, 1 to 2 years in 12%, 2 to 4 years in 23%, 4 to 6 years in 16%, 6 to 8 years in 17%, and 8 to 10 years in 4%. Only 14% had benign hypertension for more than 10 years prior to the onset of the malignant phase (25).

Smoking and Alcohol as Risk Factors

The risk of malignant hypertension is higher among hypertensive patients who smoke (78–80). In one series, 82% of the patients with malignant hypertension were smokers versus 50% of inpatients and 43% of outpatients with benign hypertension and 52% of normotensive control subjects (80). The relative risk for developing malignant hypertension was five times higher in hypertensive patients who smoked. Among patients with malignant hypertension, at initial presentation, renal insufficiency was also more common among smokers. The mean serum creatinine concentration for nonsmokers was 1.2 mg/dL, compared to 2.5 mg/dL for smokers. Moreover, of the 18 patients with a serum creatinine value over 2.8 mg/dL, 17 were smokers and one was a former smoker (80).

In contrast to the findings with regard to smoking risk, no significant difference has been found for the prevalence or quantity of alcohol consumption in groups of patients with benign or malignant hypertension (79).

Clinical Features of Malignant Hypertension

The clinical features of untreated malignant hypertension as outlined by Volhard and Fahr in 1914 (12) are still valid today: (a) elevation of diastolic blood pressure, usually fixed and severe; (b) funduscopic changes of hypertensive neuroretinopathy with striate hemorrhages, cotton-wool spots, and papilledema; (c) renal insufficiency; (d) rapid progression to a fatal outcome, usually due to uremia if inadequately treated; and (e) renal histology demonstrating malignant nephrosclerosis with fibrinoid necrosis of afferent arterioles and proliferative endarteritis of interlobular arteries.

Unless hypertensive neuroretinopathy is present, malignant hypertension cannot be diagnosed regardless of the height of the arterial blood pressure (4). However, the other clinical features need not be present initially to substantiate a diagnosis of malignant hypertension. There is no critical level of blood pressure that defines the presence of malignant hypertension. An acute increase in blood pressure in previously normotensive individuals can precipitate the malignant phase at a diastolic blood pressure as low as 100 to 110 mm Hg. Conversely, very high diastolic blood pressures may persist for many years in patients with essential hypertension without the development of malignant hypertension (81).

With untreated malignant hypertension, severe renal impairment inevitably occurs, although there may be minimal renal involvement at the time of presentation. In this regard, in patients dying early in the course of malignant hypertension due to cerebrovascular accident or congestive heart failure, histologic features of malignant neuphrosclerosis may be absent.

Some authors have distinguished *accelerated hypertension* (hemorrhages and cotton-wool spots) from *malignant hypertension* (hemorrhages, cotton-wool spots, and papilledema).

However, since the finding of striate hemorrhages and cotton-wool spots has the same prognostic significance whether or not papilledema is present (6,7), it has been recommended that accelerated hypertension and malignant hypertension be regarded as synonymous terms for a clinical syndrome in which there is widespread hypertension-induced acute arteriolar injury. The World Health Organization has recommended that the term *malignant hypertension* be used to describe this disease process (4). Use of the term *accelerated hypertension* should probably be abandoned because it is now commonly used to describe patients who have increasingly severe or resistant hypertension independent of the funduscopic findings that characterize true accelerated or malignant hypertension.

Presenting Symptoms

The most common presenting complaints in patients with malignant hypertension are headache, blurred vision, and weight loss (25–27). Less common presenting symptoms include dyspnea, fatigue, malaise, gastrointestinal complaints (nausea, vomiting, epigastric pain), polyuria, nocturia, and gross hematuria (26,27). In many series, the onset of symptoms was noted to be remarkably sudden, such that it could often be dated precisely (26,27,29). In contrast, an "asymptomatic" presentation of malignant hypertension is not uncommon, especially in young black males who deny any prior symptoms when they present in the end-stage of the hypertensive process with florid failure of the brain, heart, and kidneys.

Headache is the most frequent presenting complaint in patients with malignant hypertension. Unfortunately, headache is a nonspecific finding that also occurs frequently in patients with benign hypertension. Nonetheless, when patients with severe hypertension experience headaches of recent onset or the intensification of an existing headache pattern, malignant hypertension should be excluded (25).

In one large series, visual symptoms were present at initial diagnosis in 76% of patients and visual problems eventually developed in 90% (26). The most common complaints were blurred vision and decreased visual acuity. Sudden blindness occurred in 14% of patients. Scotoma, diplopia, and hemianopsia were also reported.

Weight loss is a very common symptom early in the course of malignant hypertension, and often occurs before the onset of anorexia or uremia (25,29,81). In many patients, at least a portion of the weight loss can be attributed to volume depletion resulting from a spontaneous natriuresis with the onset of malignant hypertension (42,82,83).

Level of Blood Pressure

There is apparently no absolute level of blood pressure above which malignant hypertension invariably occurs. In most series of patients with malignant hypertension, the average diastolic blood pressure is higher than 120 to 130 mm Hg (26,27). However, two series found considerable overlap of blood pressure levels in patients with benign and malignant hypertension (25,84) (Fig. 56-2).

Funduscopic Manifestations

Examination of the ocular fundus is of great importance in the assessment of patients with severe hypertension, especially with regard to prognosis (84–88). The description by Keith et al. (16) of the prognosis of hypertensive patients based on a grading system for hypertensive retinopathy was the landmark study in this field. They graded retinal findings in untreated hypertensive patients as follows: grade I—mild narrowing or sclerosis of arterioles; grade II—moderate sclerosis with an increased light reflex and arteriovenous compression; grade III—retinal hemorrhages and exudates; and grade IV—the findings in grade III plus papilledema. The presence of papilledema was associated with the worst prognosis and became synonymous with the term *malignant hypertension*. In subsequent years, the term *accelerated hypertension* was adopted to describe patients with grade III retinopathy (89).

The clinical utility of the Keith and Wagener classification, although widely accepted, has been questioned (6,57,87). It

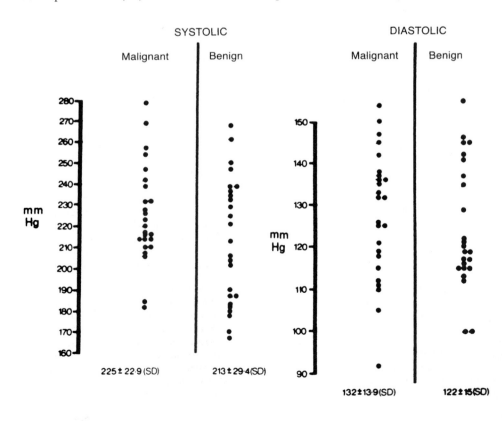

FIGURE 56-2. Systolic and diastolic blood pressures in patients with malignant hypertension compared with age- and gender-matched patients with severe benign hypertension. (From: Kincaid-Smith P. Malignant hypertension: mechanisms and management. *Pharmacol Ther* 1980;9:245, with permission.)

is extremely difficult to quantitate arteriolar narrowing (87). Moreover, there is observer bias such that patients with mild hypertension and questionable narrowing are inevitably placed in this group (87). Thus, the finding of grade I changes is of limited usefulness. There is also great interobserver variability with regard to the definition of arteriovenous crossing changes (90). Another objection to the Keith and Wagener classification is that it does not clearly distinguish between the retinal changes of benign and malignant hypertension (45). For example, the clinical significance of a large, ill-defined white exudate (cotton-wool spot) appearing in the fundus of a young man with severe hypertension is quite different from the clinical significance of a sharply defined, glistening, hard exudate in a 60-year-old patient with moderate hypertension. In the first example, the cotton-wool spot and the clinical circumstances suggest the onset of malignant hypertension. In the older patient, the retinal picture is consistent with retinal arteriosclerosis characteristic of benign hypertension (45). The therapeutic and prognostic implications of these two types of exudate are clearly different, although both would be assigned to grade III in the Keith and Wagener classification.

A number of authorities have recommended abandonment of the Keith and Wagener classification in favor of the hypertensive retinopathy classification initially proposed by Fishberg and Oppenheimer (86). This classification draws a distinction between *retinal arteriosclerosis with arteriosclerotic retinopathy*, which is characteristic of benign hypertension, and *hypertensive neuroretinopathy*, which defines the presence of malignant hypertension (Table 56-3). In essence, two different types of retinal disease occur in patients with hypertension: one that reflects changes induced by arteriolar narrowing (retinal arteriosclerosis); and one that represents acute retinal vascular injury induced by severe hypertension (hypertensive neuroretinopathy).

Retinal arteriosclerosis with or without arteriosclerotic retinopathy is seen in patients with long-standing benign hypertension from either primary or secondary causes. Retinal arteriosclerosis (arteriolosclerosis) is characterized histologically by the accumulation of hyaline material in arterioles. In the early stages, the material is deposited in the intima beneath the endothelium, while in older lesions deposits extend into the media and ultimately involve the entire vessel wall. Fundus-

copic changes reflecting retinal arteriosclerosis include irregularity of the lumen and focal narrowing, arteriovenous crossing changes, broadening of the light reflex, copper or silver wiring, perivasculitis (parallel white lines around blood column), and generalized arteriolar narrowing. Arteriosclerotic retinopathy, which results from this arteriosclerotic process, is manifested by the presence of hemorrhages and hard exudates. The hemorrhages are usually solitary, round or oval, and confined to the periphery of the fundus. They are caused by venous or arterial occlusion (87). Hard exudates may appear as multiple small white dots that give a powdery appearance to the retina, or they may appear as large glistening spots that are sharply defined from the adjacent retina. Arteriosclerotic retinopathy can also cause localized areas of retinal edema and hemorrhage due to occlusion of small branch veins. However, the principal findings of hypertensive neuroretinopathy, namely, striate hemorrhages, cotton-wool spots, and papilledema, are absent (Table 56-3).

The finding of retinal arteriosclerosis in hypertensive patients usually does not imply a poor prognosis. Even patients with severe arteriosclerotic retinopathy may live for many years before the development of morbid events due to coronary artery disease, congestive heart failure, or cerebrovascular accident. Furthermore, the presence of retinal arteriosclerosis in patients with essential hypertension is typically not associated with significant renal impairment. This observation is in sharp contrast to patients with hypertensive neuroretinopathy in whom renal impairment, if not already present, is imminent without treatment.

Furthermore, the finding of retinal arteriosclerosis in hypertensive patients is of no prognostic significance with regard to the risks of coronary atherosclerosis and cerebrovascular disease (85,87,88). As the arteries visualized with the ophthalmoscope are technically arterioles with a diameter less than 0.1 mm (87), hyaline arteriolosclerosis of the retinal vessels is a process that is entirely different from the atherosclerotic process that can affect larger muscular arteries. Thus, the finding of retinal arteriosclerotic changes is not predictive of the presence or absence of atherosclerotic disease of the coronary or cerebral vessels or other major arterial branches of the aorta (85). The prognostic significance of retinal changes in benign hypertension has also been questioned on the basis of the observation that normotensive control subjects between the ages of 40 and 60 have a high incidence of retinal arteriosclerosis, presumably reflecting age-related vascular changes (91).

In a study designed to assess the usefulness of ophthalmoscopy in mild to moderate hypertension, 25 patients with untreated essential hypertension were evaluated with direct ophthalmoscopy, assessment of fundus photographs, ambulatory blood pressure monitoring, estimation of left ventricular mass by electrocardiography and two-dimensional echocardiography, and measurement of urinary microalbumin excretion. No statistical relation was found between either clinic or ambulatory blood pressure readings and the severity of retinal arteriosclerosis as defined by the presence of arteriolar narrowing or arteriovenous crossing changes. Moreover, there was no independent relationship between retinal changes and age, measures of left ventricular mass, creatinine clearance, or urinary microalbumin excretion. Thus, the finding of retinal arteriosclerosis has little clinical utility in the evaluation of patients with mild to moderate hypertension (90).

The lack of clinical significance of retinal arteriosclerosis in hypertensive patients contrasts markedly with the importance and prognostic significance of the finding of hypertensive neuroretinopathy. The appearance of striate hemorrhages and cotton-wool spots with or without papilledema closely parallels the development of severe arteriolar damage (fibrinoid necrosis and proliferative endarteritis) in the circulation of other organs including the brain and kidneys. Hypertensive

---

TABLE 56-3

RETINAL CHANGES IN HYPERTENSION

Retinal arteriosclerosis and arteriosclerotic retinopathy
  Arteriolar narrowing (diffuse)
  Focal arteriolar narrowing
  Arteriovenous crossing changes
  Broadening of the light reflex
  Copper or silver wiring
  Perivasculitis
  Solitary round hemorrhages
  Hard exudates
  Central or branch venous occlusion

Hypertensive neuroretinopathy
  Generalized arteriolar narrowing
  Striate (flame-shaped) hemorrhages[a]
  Cotton-wool spots (soft exudates)[a]
  Bilateral papilledema[a]
  Macular star

[a]Features that distinguish hypertensive neuroretinopathy (characteristic of malignant hypertension) from retinal arteriosclerosis (characteristic of benign hypertension).

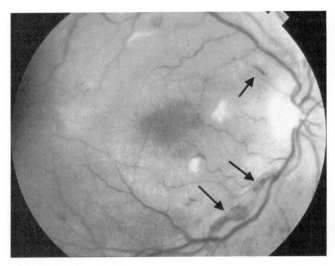

FIGURE 56-3. Striate hemorrhages (*arrows*) in the fundus of a 48-year-old white female with secondary malignant hypertension due to underlying immunoglobulin A nephropathy.

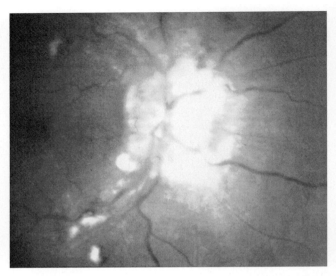

FIGURE 56-5. Papilledema in the fundus of an 18-year-old African American male with primary malignant hypertension. Cotton-wool spots are also apparent. This asymptomatic patient was incidentally noted to have severe hypertension during a routine dental examination.

neuroretinopathy is the clinical *sine qua non* of malignant hypertension and therefore signifies a far more ominous prognosis than does the finding of retinal arteriosclerosis in benign hypertension.

The appearance of small striate hemorrhages is often the first sign that malignant hypertension has developed. These hemorrhages are linear or flame-shaped and are most commonly observed in a radial arrangement around the optic disc (85,87) (Fig. 56-3). They arise from superficial capillaries in the nerve fiber bundles, which have high intravascular pressure because they are perfused directly by arterioles (85). The hemorrhages extend along nerve fibers parallel to the retinal surface. They often have a frayed distal border due to extravasation between nerve fiber bundles. Even when widespread, hemorrhages are rarely seen lateral to the macula in hypertensive neuroretinopathy. Striate hemorrhages often occur adjacent to cotton-wool spots (Fig. 56-4) and most likely arise from capillary microaneurysms at the margins of the spots. Since hemoglobin ab-

sorbs fluorescein, hemorrhages appear black with fluorescein angiography (85). Striate hemorrhages can usually be distinguished from the hemorrhages seen in retinal arteriosclerosis, which are solitary, round, and confined to the periphery of the fundus (87).

Cotton-wool spots are the most characteristic feature of malignant hypertension and are the result of ischemic infarction of nerve fiber bundles caused by arteriolar occlusion. They usually surround the optic disc and most commonly occur within three disc diameters of the optic disc (Figs. 56-4–56-6). Cotton-wool spots begin as grayish-white discoloration of the retina, but within 24 hours they become shiny white with fluffy margins. Red dots may be seen in the bed of the exudate (microaneurysms). Cotton-wool spots are not specific for

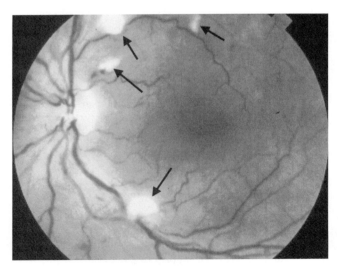

FIGURE 56-4. Cotton-wool spots (*arrows*) in the fundus of a 48-year-old white female with secondary malignant hypertension due to underlying immunoglobulin A nephropathy. Striate hemorrhages are also seen adjacent to some of the cotton-wool spots.

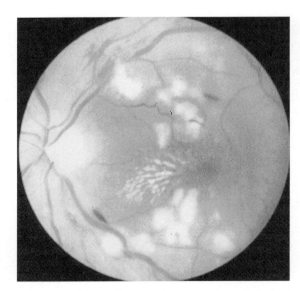

FIGURE 56-6. Full-blown hypertensive neuroretinopathy in fundus of a 30-year-old man with malignant hypertension demonstrating linear (striate) hemorrhages, cotton-wool spots, papilledema, and a star figure at the macula. (Photograph courtesy of Daniel J. Mayer, MD.)

hypertensive neuroretinopathy and can also be seen with diabetic retinopathy, retinal emboli, and central and branch retinal vein occlusion. However, differentiation of these disorders from malignant hypertension is usually not difficult.

Papilledema can occur in patients with hypertensive neuroretinopathy, but it is not invariably present. In malignant hypertension, papilledema is usually accompanied by striate hemorrhages and cotton-wool spots (Figs. 56-5 and 56-6). When papilledema occurs alone, the possibility of a primary intracranial process such as a tumor or cerebrovascular accident should be considered (45). However, lone bilateral papilledema has recently been described as a variant of hypertensive neuroretinopathy (92). Once intracerebral pathology has been excluded, these patients require aggressive treatment just as those with hypertensive neuroretinopathy accompanied by striate hemorrhages and cotton-wool spots.

A star figure at the macula represents hard exudates arranged in a radial fashion from the central fovea (Fig. 56-6). Although a star figure can occasionally be seen in arteriosclerotic retinopathy, it usually develops in conjunction with the florid retinal changes in malignant hypertension. In hypertensive neuroretinopathy the exudates form lines or sheets around the macula rather than the discrete dots around the macula that occur in arteriosclerotic retinopathy (45).

Hypertensive neuroretinopathy almost always precedes clinically apparent damage in other end organs but there are occasional reports of malignant nephrosclerosis appearing before the onset of hypertensive neuroretinopathy (93). It should also be noted that the findings of striate hemorrhages, cotton-wool spots, and papilledema are not specific for malignant hypertension. Funduscopic findings that are indistinguishable from those of hypertensive neuroretinopathy can occur with severe anemia, subacute bacterial endocarditis, systemic lupus erythematosus, polyarteritis, temporal arteritis, and scleroderma (45). In these disorders the retinopathy may develop even in the absence of hypertension. Central retinal vein occlusion can also mimic hypertensive neuroretinopathy but is usually unilateral, whereas hypertensive neuroretinopathy is almost always bilateral.

Severe hypertension can also affect the choroidal as well as the retinal circulation. Hypertensive choroidopathy can occur with malignant hypertension and is manifested by lesions known as acute *Elschnig's spots*, which are white areas of retinal pigment epithelial necrosis with overlying localized serous detachments of the retina (94) (Fig. 56-7). The serous retinal detachments may vary from one-third to six disc diameters. Fluorescein angiography reveals staining of the damaged pigment epithelium and leakage into the subretinal space (94). Although most patients with this hypertensive choroidopathy also have typical changes of hypertensive neuroretinopathy with striate hemorrhages and cotton-wool spots, if the elevation of blood pressure is relatively sudden, the changes of hypertensive choroidopathy may predominate (94).

As stated earlier, papilledema should not be regarded as an essential requirement for the diagnosis of malignant hypertension. By life table analysis, the 10-year survival rate for hypertensive patients was 46% in patients with hemorrhages and exudates and 48% when papilledema was also present (7). The lack of association between papilledema and the length of survival was confirmed using the Cox's proportional hazards model, which revealed associations between survival and age, smoking habit, initial serum creatinine concentration, and the level of blood pressure control achieved with therapy. No association was found with papilledema. When other covariates were controlled simultaneously, no association was found between the presence of papilledema and survival (Fig. 56-8). The failure of recent studies to find the previously reported difference in survival between grade III and grade IV retinopathy (5) may be due to the fact that the earlier study involved untreated

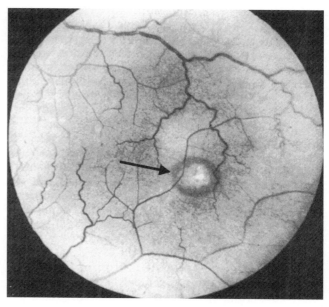

FIGURE 56-7. Hypertensive choroidopathy in malignant hypertension demonstrating focal serous detachment of the sensory retina with a whitish lesion at the level of the retinal pigment epithelium (acute Elschnig's spot). (From: de Venecia G, Jampol LM. The eye in accelerated hypertension: II. Localized serous detachments of the retina in patients. *Arch Ophthalmol* 1984;102:68, © 1984, American Medical Association, with permission.)

patients. Papilledema may be associated with a worse prognosis only when the hypertension is untreated or ineffectively treated (7).

There is no evidence to indicate that the apparent severity of hypertensive neuroretinopathy is predictive of a more severe hypertensive vasculopathy or more advanced end-organ

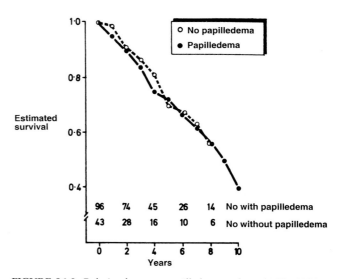

FIGURE 56-8. Relation between papilledema and survival in 139 hypertensive patients with bilateral retinal hemorrhages and exudates after controlling for age, gender, smoking habit, initial serum creatinine concentration, and initial and achieved blood pressure by multivariate analysis. Failure of papilledema to influence prognosis was confirmed by likelihood ratio test ($X = 0.89$, 1 df, $p = 0.34$). (From: McGregor E, et al. Retinal changes in malignant hypertension. *Br Med J* 1986;292:233, with permission.)

destruction. Papilledema is not always present even when there is severe malignant nephrosclerosis presenting as oliguric acute renal failure. In four series with a total of 25 patients presenting with malignant hypertension and acute renal failure, only 14 patients had papilledema. The other 11 patients had hemorrhages and cotton-wool spots but no papilledema (95–98). This lack of a difference in prognosis for patients with hypertensive neuroretinopathy whether or not it is accompanied by papilledema may be explained by the fact that cotton-wool spots and papilledema share a similar pathogenesis (*vide infra*) (99,100).

The diagnosis of malignant hypertension may be made in the setting of severe hypertension when only a single cotton-wool spot is observed. The approach to the treatment of hypertension in this setting should be just as aggressive as in patients with full-blown hypertensive neuroretinopathy with extensive striate hemorrhages, cotton-wool spots, and papilledema. Since the funduscopic findings in patients with malignant hypertension may sometimes be difficult to visualize, the evaluation of patients with severe hypertension should include a careful ophthalmologic examination after pupillary dilation with 1% tropicamide (101). Because the presence of even subtle hypertensive neuroretinopathy has important therapeutic and prognostic implications, if the retina cannot be adequately visualized, formal ophthalmologic evaluation with indirect ophthalmoscopy should be considered. Furthermore, retinal photographs provide permanent objective documentation of the presence of malignant hypertension.

Renal Manifestations

Malignant hypertension is a progressive systemic vasculopathy in which renal involvement is a secondary and relatively late development. Patients with malignant hypertension may present with a spectrum of renal involvement ranging from minimal albuminuria with normal renal function to ESRD indistinguishable from that seen in patients with primary renal parenchymal disease (25,27,74).

The first sign of renal involvement in malignant hypertension is often the abrupt appearance of proteinuria. About 20% of patients also have painless gross hematuria, while 50% have microhematuria (27). Pickering (45) regards the appearance of blood or more than a trace of protein in the urine of patients with essential hypertension to be an indication of the onset of malignant nephrosclerosis, as significant proteinuria and hematuria are rare in benign nephrosclerosis (27). However, recent reports suggest that nephrotic-range proteinuria can occasionally develop with severe benign nephrosclerosis (102,103).

Quantitation of 24-hour protein excretion in patients with malignant hypertension has revealed less than 2 g in one-third, between 2 and 4 g in one-third, and more than 4 g in one-third of patients (26). The level of protein excretion is of little value in the differentiation of primary (essential) malignant hypertension from malignant hypertension due to secondary causes (25,74).

Hematuria is a very important clinical finding in patients with essential hypertension. In the absence of primary renal parenchymal disease or a urologic source, the onset of hematuria is virtually diagnostic of malignant nephrosclerosis (45). In one series, hematuria was found in 100% of patients with malignant hypertension (74). However, the absence of hematuria does not exclude the diagnosis. Of interest is the fact that red blood cell casts were observed in patients with malignant hypertension who had no evidence of glomerulonephritis at renal biopsy (97).

Pyuria has been demonstrated in 75% of patients with malignant hypertension. However, the presence of pyuria does not differentiate between primary and secondary malignant hypertension (26).

Renal size is variable and depends on the duration of prior benign hypertension. In patients with primary (essential) malignant hypertension, the size of the kidneys may be normal to only slightly reduced. In fact, there may be little reduction in renal size even when patients develop terminal renal failure (25).

The clinical spectrum of renal involvement in malignant hypertension is variable. Four clinical renal syndromes have been described. Progressive subacute deterioration of renal function leading to ESRD occurs in some patients. In patients presenting with malignant hypertension and initially normal renal function, in the absence of adequate treatment, it is common to observe deterioration of renal function with progression to ESRD over a period of weeks to months. The second clinical renal syndrome observed in malignant hypertension is transient deterioration of renal function following the initial control of blood pressure. This well-described entity occurs in patients presenting with mild to moderate renal impairment. In the third clinical renal syndrome, patients with malignant hypertension present with established renal failure. The close similarity between the terminal stage of primary malignant nephrosclerosis and chronic nephritis with superimposed malignant hypertension has long been recognized. In this regard, it may not be possible to ascertain whether a patient presenting with severe hypertension, hypertensive neuroretinopathy, and renal failure has primary or secondary malignant hypertension (45). While a history of an acute nephritic episode or long-standing proteinuria or hematuria may suggest underlying primary renal parenchymal disease, the distinction between primary malignant nephrosclerosis and chronic nephritis often requires a renal biopsy (45,104). In the fourth clinical renal syndrome, patients with malignant hypertension present with oliguric acute renal failure. Cases of malignant hypertension have been described that were characterized by diastolic blood pressure higher than 130 mm Hg; advanced hypertensive neuroretinopathy; marked weight loss; and with an active urine sediment with proteinuria, hematuria, and red blood cell casts (97,98). Renal size was normal. There was often evidence of microangiopathic hemolytic anemia. Although the initial blood urea nitrogen (BUN) concentration was less than 60 mg/dL, in each case oliguric renal failure occurred and necessitated the initiation of dialysis within a few days of hospitalization. Despite dialytic therapy, the blood pressure was extremely difficult to control and each patient died. Renal histology revealed malignant nephrosclerosis with fibrinoid necrosis and proliferative endarteritis. The glomeruli were normal except for ischemic changes. Multifocal tubular necrosis was present and presumed to be secondary to ischemia. In most of these patients, the diagnosis of malignant hypertension was delayed because the patients were initially considered to have rapidly progressive glomerulonephritis or systemic vasculitis, which was treated with high-dose steroids. The diagnosis of malignant hypertension was not suspected until autopsy revealed malignant nephrosclerosis.

Neurologic Manifestations

Clarke and Murphy (105) detail the neurologic findings among 190 patients with malignant hypertension. Central nervous system involvement was present at some time during the course in 42% of patients. Of the 65 patients for whom a cause of death could be ascertained, 33 had a fatal neurologic event. Of the total deaths, 20% were due to a neurologic cause. Intracerebral hemorrhage occurred in 23 patients. Episodes of focal brain ischemia, presumed due to cerebral thrombosis, occurred in 35 patients. Generalized seizures occurred in 11 patients and focal seizures in 8. Bell's palsy occurred in seven patients. Primary subarachnoid hemorrhage occurred in 4 patients. The incidence of headache was comparable in patients with and those without neurologic complications. Thus, the presence of headache did not necessarily imply central nervous system involvement. In this series, hypertensive encephalopathy was found in only 1% of patients; however, other series reported a higher incidence (106). The clinical presentation, pathophysiology, and treatment of hypertensive encephalopathy are discussed in detail later in this chapter under Hypertensive Encephalopathy.

The cerebrospinal fluid (CSF) findings in patients with malignant hypertension are variable. Even among patients with papilledema, CSF pressure was greater than 200 mm of water in only 65% (26,105). In contrast, Pickering (107) found that patients with malignant hypertension had higher CSF pressures than did patients with benign hypertension and that there was a direct correlation between the level of blood pressure and the CSF pressure. Blood-stained or xanthochromic fluid was found only in patients with intracerebral or subarachnoid hemorrhage (105). Protein concentration was higher than 60 mg/dL in 69% of patients (range, 11 to 307 mg/dL). No pleocytosis was reported. Although Clarke and Murphy (105) report no complications from lumbar puncture, others report a 12% incidence of complications including severe headache, sudden blindness, coma, and death due to cerebellar herniation (26).

Gastrointestinal Manifestations

The most common gastrointestinal manifestations of malignant hypertension are nonspecific symptoms including nausea, vomiting, and epigastric pain. However, acute pancreatitis has been reported as a rare complication. In a series of 42 patients with malignant hypertension, severe acute pancreatitis that could not be attributed to gallstones or alcohol abuse developed in seven patients (108). All of the patients were black and were on maintenance hemodialysis for renal failure caused by malignant nephrosclerosis. The blood pressure remained poorly controlled while the patients were on dialysis. In another series reporting on the frequency of pancreatitis in a dialysis population, the majority of patients were found to have hypertensive nephrosclerosis as the cause of ESRD (109). It has been proposed that acute pancreatitis occurs with increased frequency in patients with malignant hypertension because of the use of hemodialysis. Although dialysis prevents death from uremia, if the blood pressure remains poorly controlled, hypertensive vasculopathy persists in other organs such as the pancreas. In this setting, the use of heparin for dialysis might lead to this complication by causing hemorrhage in inflamed pancreatic tissue (108).

Patients with malignant hypertension can present with an acute abdomen (110). Abdominal exploration revealed necrotic bowel with involvement of the distal ileum and ascending colon. Pathologic examination revealed fibrinoid necrosis and thrombotic occlusion of the small arteries of the bowel wall. Moreover, malignant hypertension may increase the risk of subsequent development of mesenteric ischemia in patients on chronic hemodialysis (111). Gastrointestinal hemorrhage can occur in patients with malignant hypertension due to hypertension-induced necrotizing mesenteric arteriolitis (112).

Hematologic Manifestations

A variety of hematologic findings have been observed in patients with malignant hypertension. Elevation of the erythrocyte sedimentation rate has been reported (25). The hemoglobin concentration at the time of presentation may correlate with the etiology of the malignant phase. A hemoglobin concentration higher than 12.5 g/dL is more often associated with primary malignant hypertension, while a lower value is more often associated with chronic glomerulonephritis or pyelonephritis (25,26).

There are numerous reports of microangiopathic hemolytic anemia in association with malignant hypertension. In one series of 24 patients with malignant hypertension, 16 were found to have evidence of microangiopathic hemolysis (113). Other significant abnormalities reported with malignant hypertension include thrombocytopenia, increased fibrin degradation products, increased factor VIII levels, increased fibrinogen, and increased urokinase sensitivity consistent with decreased fibrinolysis (114).

Cardiac Manifestations

Congestive heart failure can be a presenting feature of malignant hypertension. Moreover, heart failure, alone or in combination with uremia, was a common cause of death prior to the advent of effective antihypertensive drugs (26,27). Heart failure in patients with malignant hypertension is predominantly left-sided with pulmonary congestion resulting in orthopnea, paroxysmal nocturnal dyspnea, cardiac asthma, and recurrent episodes of acute pulmonary edema. Peripheral venous congestion with dependent edema or hepatic congestion may be minimal or absent even when death results from congestive heart failure. The management of acute pulmonary edema in patients with malignant hypertension is discussed later in this chapter under Acute Hypertensive Heart Failure.

Angina and acute myocardial infarction, though common with long-standing benign hypertension, are uncommon with malignant hypertension (25). Aortic dissection is also rare in patients with malignant hypertension (25).

Abnormalities of the Renin-Angiotensin-Aldosterone Axis

Evidence of activation of the renin-angiotensin-aldosterone axis is present in many, but not all, patients with malignant hypertension (63,115). Among 53 patients with malignant hypertension not secondary to renal artery stenosis, 55% had increased plasma renin activity (PRA) (116). Among 25 patients with malignant hypertension secondary to renal artery stenosis, PRA was consistently elevated (116).

Aldosterone secretion rate has been studied in patients with malignant hypertension (65). There was a marked increase in secretion rate in seven of eight patients with malignant hypertension (papilledema present), and in five of eight patients with accelerated hypertension (retinal hemorrhages without papilledema). The aldosterone secretion rate in these patients was often higher than that seen in patients with aldosterone-producing adenoma. Postmortem examination of the adrenal glands in seven patients with malignant hypertension revealed bilateral areas of focal nodular hyperplasia, especially in the zona glomerulosa (65). The renin-angiotensin axis was evaluated in a series of patients with malignant hypertension; the underlying disease was essential hypertension in 33 cases and chronic glomerulonephritis in 26 cases (117). Plasma renin activity was significantly higher in the group with essential hypertension than in the group with underlying chronic glomerulonephritis and angiotensin receptor blocker therapy induced a significant reduction of blood pressure only in the former group. These finding suggest that the renin-aldosterone system (RAS) plays a significant role in elevating blood pressure in primary malignant hypertension but may be less important in the pathogenesis of secondary malignant hypertension related to glomerulonephritis.

Of interest, in patients with malignant hypertension and elevated PRA and aldosterone secretion rate, there was often a transient period during therapy in which PRA returned to normal yet aldosterone secretion rate remained elevated. This

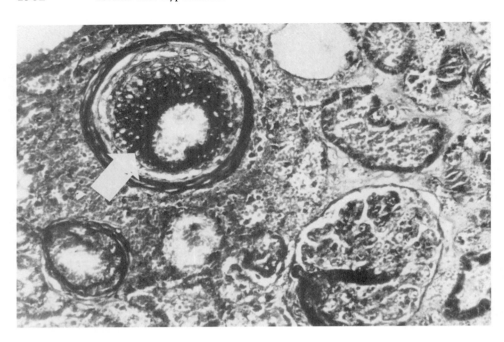

FIGURE 56-9. Fibrinoid necrosis in a large arteriole (*arrow*). Intimal onionskin formation is also present. (Trichrome stain.) (Photograph courtesy of Steve Guggenheim, MD.)

dissociation often persisted for months. The authors postulate that, with prolonged hyperreninemia, hyperplasia of the zona glomerulosa occurs. While renin levels quickly return to normal with therapy, persistent hyperplasia of the zona glomerulosa and a delay in resetting feedback control mechanisms lead to over secretion of aldosterone despite normal PRA (tertiary hyperaldosteronism) (63).

Electrolyte Abnormalities

Hypokalemic metabolic alkalosis was found in up to 50% of patients with malignant hypertension, presumably reflecting a state of hyperreninemia and secondary hyperaldosteronism (65). After effective therapy, aldosterone hypersecretion can persist long after volume depletion is corrected and renin levels have returned to normal. Thus, the findings of hypokalemia, increased urinary potassium losses, and aldosterone hypersecretion with suppressed PRA may mimic the findings of primary hyperaldosteronism (63).

Hyponatremia is not uncommon in patients with malignant hypertension, particularly when sodium restriction is instituted. Patients with malignant hypertension due to renal artery stenosis occasionally present with the striking hyponatremic hypertensive syndrome (118–120). The characteristic features of this syndrome include severe hypertension, hypertensive neuroretinopathy, polyuria, polydipsia, weight loss, and salt craving. Biochemical changes include hyponatremia, hypokalemia, and low total exchangeable sodium and potassium, with markedly elevated PRA, angiotensin II, aldosterone, and arginine vasopressin (AVP) levels. This syndrome may result from a vicious cycle of volume depletion with further activation of the renin–angiotensin axis as a result of a pressure-induced natriuresis from the contralateral kidney (119).

Pathologic Findings

Renal Pathology

With malignant nephrosclerosis, small pinpoint petechial hemorrhages may be present on the cortical surface, giving the kidney a peculiar flea-bitten appearance. The renal size varies de-

pending on the duration of preexisting benign hypertension or the presence of underlying primary renal parenchymal disease. When terminal renal failure occurs in patients with primary malignant hypertension, the kidneys may be normal in size (81). However, when secondary malignant hypertension is superimposed on primary renal disease, the kidneys may be small.

Fibrinoid necrosis of the afferent arterioles has traditionally been regarded as the hallmark of malignant nephrosclerosis (25,26) (Fig. 56-9). The characteristic finding is the deposition in the arteriolar wall of a granular material that appears bright pink with hematoxylin and eosin stain. On trichrome staining, this granular material is deep red. This fibrinoid material is usually found in the media, but it may also be present in the intima. Histochemical and immunofluorescent techniques have identified this material as fibrin. Within the media, muscle fibers cannot be identified and cell nuclei are lost or fragmented. Whole or fragmented erythrocytes may be extravasated into the arteriolar wall. The hemorrhages that occur may account for the petechiae observed on the cortical surface. The arteriolar lumen may be reduced in size as a result of wall thickening and intraluminal fibrin thrombi. Infrequently, polymorphonuclear leukocytes and monocytes may infiltrate the arterioles, giving the appearance of necrotizing arteriolitis.

The interlobular arteries reveal characteristic lesions variously referred to as *proliferative endarteritis, productive endarteritis, endarteritis fibrosa,* or the onionskin lesion. The typical finding is intimal thickening that causes moderate to severe luminal narrowing. In severely affected vessels, the luminal diameter may be reduced to the size of a single red blood cell. Occasionally, there is complete obliteration of the lumen by a fibrin thrombus.

Traditionally, three patterns of intimal thickening in malignant nephrosclerosis have been described (121). The *onionskin* pattern consists of pale layers of elongated, concentrically arranged, myointimal cells. Delicate connective tissue fibrils give rise to a lamellated appearance (Fig. 56-10). The media often appears as an attenuated layer stretched around the expanded intima. *Mucinous* intimal thickening consists of a scarcely cellular lesion containing a lucent, faintly basophilic-staining amorphous material (Fig. 56-11). In *fibrous* intimal thickening, there are hyaline deposits, reduplicated bands of

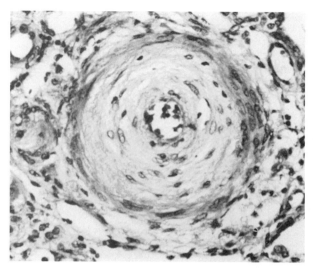

FIGURE 56-10. Onionskin lesion consisting of pale layers of elongated, concentrically arranged myointimal cells and delicate connective tissue fibrils that produce a lamellated appearance. The media is attenuated and stretched around the thickened intima. (Hematoxylin and eosin stain ×350.) (From: Sinclair RA, Antonovych TT, Mostofi FK. Renal proliferative arteriopathies and associated glomerular changes: a light and electron microscopic study. *Hum Pathol* 1976;7:565, with permission.)

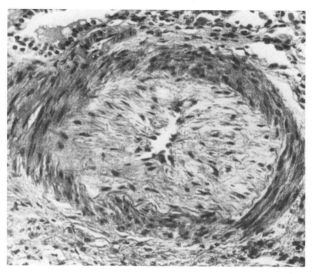

FIGURE 56-12. Fibrous intimal thickening. The lesion consists of a thick layer of connective tissue, which stains for collagen and elastin. (Hematoxylin and eosin stain ×300.) (From: Sinclair RA, Antonovych TT, Mostofi FK. Renal proliferative arteriopathies and associated glomerular changes: a light and electron microscopic study. *Hum Pathol* 1976;7:565, with permission.)

elastica, and coarse layers of pale connective tissue with the staining properties of collagen (Fig. 56-12). In rare cases, fibrinoid necrosis may also be apparent in the interlobular arteries (121).

The renal histology in blacks with malignant hypertension may be somewhat different (34,35). Although fibrinoid necrosis of the afferent arterioles is not found, there is instead a marked degree of arteriolar hyalinization. In addition, there is a prominent and characteristic finding in the larger arterioles

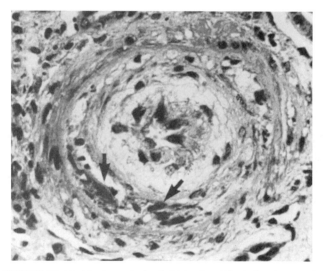

FIGURE 56-11. Mucinous intimal thickening. The lesion is sparsely cellular and consists mainly of a lucent, faintly basophilic-staining amorphous material. There are small foci of fibrinoid necrosis (*arrows*) deep within the intima. (Hematoxylin and eosin stain ×350.) (From: Sinclair RA, Antonovych TT, Mostofi FK. Renal proliferative arteriopathies and associated glomerular changes: a light and electron microscopic study. *Hum Pathol* 1976;7:565, with permission.)

and interlobular arteries known as *musculomucoid intimal hyperplasia* (34,35,122) (Fig. 56-13). The arterial walls are thickened due to the presence of hyperplastic smooth muscle cells. A small amount of myxoid material, which stains light blue with hematoxylin and eosin, is observed between the cells. With periodic acid-Schiff staining this material resembles basement membrane. Staining for acid mucopolysaccharide suggests the presence of chondroitin sulfate and possibly hyaluronic acid.

By electron microscopy, in each of the above-mentioned types of intimal thickening, the most abundant cellular element is a modified smooth muscle cell called a *myointimal cell.* In these cells there are smooth musclelike ultrastructural features including cytoplasmic myofilaments and abundant rough endoplasmic reticulum (121,123). In the pure onionskin variant, the intercellular space is occupied by multiple strands of nonperiodic fibrils with the ultrastructural features of basement membrane (121). In the mucinous variant, broad electron-lucent zones with scattered finely granular material are found in the intercellular space (123). With the fibrous variant, numerous bundles of collagen, recognizable by characteristic banding, are dispersed between the myointimal cells (123).

There are no characteristic changes in the arcuate and larger renal arteries in malignant hypertension. However, fibrous thickening and elastic reduplication may be found if longstanding benign hypertension is also present.

In large autopsy series from the pretreatment era, focal and segmental fibrinoid necrosis was the typical glomerular finding (30,124,125). Glomerular lesions often occurred in continuity with a necrotic afferent arteriole. Glomerular crescent formation and segmental proliferation in areas of necrosis were also found. Rupture of these necrotic capillaries gave rise to hemorrhage into the glomerular or tubular space, accounting for some of the petechiae seen grossly. The occurrence of this necrotizing glomerulonephritis led Volhard and Fahr (12) to propose that malignant nephrosclerosis was due to arteriosclerosis with superimposed exogenous nephritis. However, even in cases of terminal uremia, the percentage of involved glomeruli was typically only 5% to 30% (30,124,125). Thus, the focal and segmental nature of the glomerular lesion in primary malignant

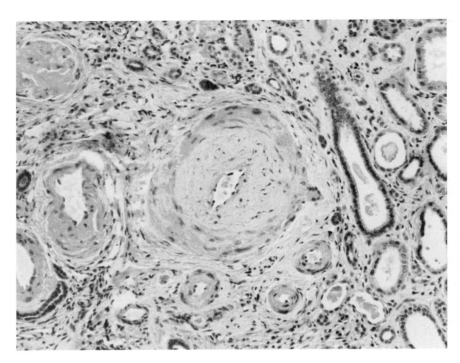

FIGURE 56-13. Musculomucoid intimal hyperplasia of an interlobular artery. The arterial walls are thickened by hyperplastic smooth muscle cells. A small amount of myxoid material is seen between the smooth muscle cells. (Hematoxylin and eosin stain ×170.) (From: Pitcock JA, et al. Malignant hypertension in blacks: malignant intrarenal arterial disease as observed by light and electron microscopy. *Hum Pathol* 1976;7:333, with permission.)

hypertension can be used to distinguish this entity from chronic glomerulonephritis with superimposed malignant nephrosclerosis, in which glomerular involvement is diffuse and global (124).

The focal and segmental necrotizing lesions that were originally described in autopsy cases of untreated malignant hypertension are now rarely seen in tissue obtained at renal biopsy in treated patients (35,126). This observation might be due to the sampling error inherent in closed renal biopsy. Alternatively, these lesions may resolve rapidly with initiation of antihypertensive therapy, and may thus not be apparent if renal biopsy is performed following adequate control of blood pressure.

In patients who have received antihypertensive therapy, as well as blacks with treated or untreated malignant hypertension, the most characteristic glomerular lesion in malignant nephrosclerosis is accelerated glomerular obsolescence secondary to the intense ischemia produced by the obliterative arterial lesions (35,126). The earliest glomerular changes consist of thickening and wrinkling of the basement membrane (35,126) (Fig. 56-14). Later, there is shrinkage of the tuft such that it does not fill Bowman's space. There is laminar reduplication of Bowman's capsule around the shrunken glomerulus (121). The end stage is the obsolescent glomerulus, which is an avascular, wrinkled glomerular tuft surrounded by a

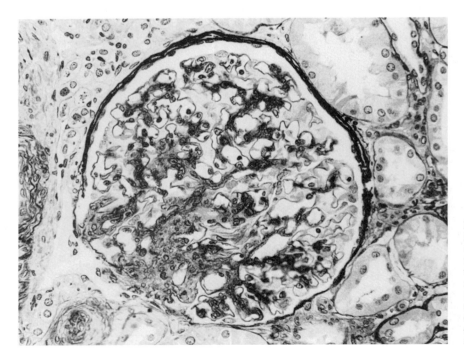

FIGURE 56-14. The earliest ischemic glomerular change in malignant hypertension consists of some basement membrane wrinkling, particularly in areas adjacent to the mesangium, with a slight increase in mesangial matrix. (Periodic acid–silver methenamine stain ×250.) (From: Pitcock JA, et al. Malignant hypertension in blacks: malignant intrarenal arterial disease as observed by light and electron microscopy. *Hum Pathol* 1976; 7:333, with permission.)

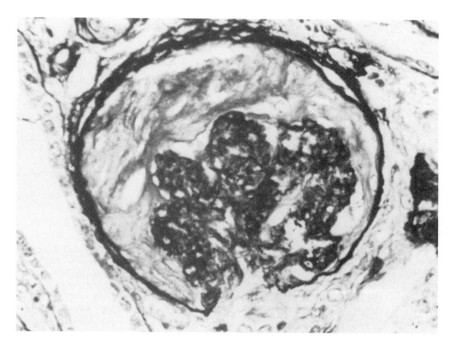

FIGURE 56-15. Glomerular obsolescence in malignant hypertension. The collapsed, avascular glomerular tuft consists predominantly of markedly convoluted basement membranes. The sclerosed tuft is partially enclosed within a collar of hyaline material filling Bowman's space. (Periodic acid–silver methenamine stain ×485.) (From: Sinclair RA, Antonovych TT, Mostofi FK. Renal proliferative arteriopathies and associated glomerular changes: a light and electron microscopic study. *Hum Pathol* 1976;7:565, with permission.)

collagenous scar that fills Bowman's space (Fig. 56-15). Focal segmental glomerulosclerosis may occur in primary malignant hypertension either as the result of glomerular hyperfiltration or fibrinoid necrosis, and may contribute to renal dysfunction. In an autopsy series of 38 black South Africans with primary malignant hypertension, mucoid intimal hyperplasia was present in all sections while fibrinoid necrosis was seen in 76%. Glomerulosclerosis was present in 38 cases, and was axially distributed in 18%, segmental in 58% and global in 24% of sections. Cases with segmental sclerosis tended to have the highest proteinuria, while those with glomerulosclerosis had the highest serum creatinine levels (127).

By electron microscopy, the lamina densa of the glomerular capillary basement membrane is thickened and wrinkled (126) (Fig. 56-16). Eventually, the entire basement membrane becomes thickened. These glomerular changes are not specific for malignant nephrosclerosis as they also can occur in scleroderma renal crisis, hemolytic–uremic syndrome, and even severe benign nephrosclerosis. However, the glomerular changes in malignant nephrosclerosis differ from the simple ischemic obsolescence observed in benign hypertension. In addition to the wrinkled basement membrane observed in benign nephrosclerosis, there is constriction of the glomerular vascular bed in malignant nephrosclerosis due to the deposition of a

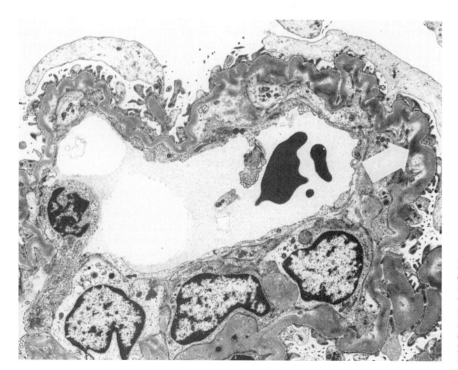

FIGURE 56-16. Accelerated glomerular obsolescence in malignant hypertension. The glomerular capillaries show striking basement membrane wrinkling (*arrow*) and some reduplication of the inner basement membrane. (Uranyl acetate and lead citrate ×4,250.) (From: Jones DB. Arterial and glomerular lesions associated with severe hypertension: light and electron microscopic studies. *Lab Invest* 1974;31:303, with permission.)

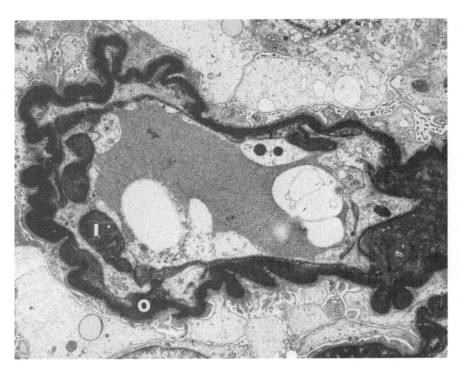

FIGURE 56-17. Accelerated glomerular obsolescence in malignant hypertension. The outer basement membrane (*O*) is thickened and wrinkled. There is a reduplicated inner basement membrane (*I*) with the capillary lumen still patent. (Uranyl acetate and lead citrate stain ×4,250.) (From: Jones DB. Arterial and glomerular lesions associated with severe hypertension: light and electron microscopic studies. *Lab Invest* 1974;31:303, with permission.)

new subendothelial layer of basement membrane material inside the original basement membrane (126) (Fig. 56-17). The new capillary lumen formed by this process is smaller, resulting in decreased blood volume in the ischemic glomerulus.

In malignant nephrosclerosis, the tubules may be atrophied and focally destroyed in areas supplied by severely narrowed arteries. Occasional tubules may be dilated and filled with eosinophilic cast material (30,125). In the interstitium in these areas, there may be a fine reticular fibrosis and chronic inflammatory cells. In malignant hypertension, as in primary renal parenchymal diseases, renal insufficiency appears to correlate best with the degree of tubular atrophy (35).

Immunofluorescence microscopy in patients with malignant nephrosclerosis has demonstrated deposition of gamma globulin, fibrinogen, albumin, and sometimes complement components in the walls of arterioles demonstrating fibrinoid necrosis by light microscopy (128). Some of the glomeruli, especially those with focal necrosis, may contain gamma globulin, albumin, and complement. Fibrinogen may be found diffusely along capillary basement membranes. Fibrinogen may also be found in the intima of interlobular arteries that by light microscopy show cellular or mucinous thickening (125).

Striking juxtaglomerular hyperplasia has been reported in patients with malignant hypertension (126,129,130). This ultrastructural finding is consistent with the hyperreninemic state often noted clinically (129).

Effective antihypertensive therapy may alter the pathology of malignant nephrosclerosis (130–132). Within days, there may be resolution of fibrinoid necrosis, which leaves behind residual hyaline deposits in the arteriolar wall. In contrast to benign nephrosclerosis in which arteriolar hyaline change is often subendothelial, in treated malignant hypertension the hyaline material may be present throughout the entire vessel wall. Fibrosis of the arterioles with collagen replacement of the arteriolar muscle and elastica may also occur. Within several weeks after initiation of therapy, the glomerular segmental fibrinoid necrosis may also resolve, leaving behind an area of hyaline deposition that can mimic focal segmental glomerulosclerosis (FSGS). Furthermore, with treatment, in the intima of the interlobular arteries there may be an evolution from

cellular hyperplasia to a more fibrous form of intimal thickening. A newly formed internal elastic lamina often separates this new collagen from the narrowed lumen. Heptinstall has postulated that the cellular lesion is an early finding implying active disease, whereas the acellular fibrotic lesion is a later process often reflecting a response to treatment (125). These modifications in the interlobular arteries that occur following treatment may not be accompanied by any increase in the caliber of the lumen. Severely narrowed interlobular arteries often do not improve and the renal parenchyma distal to these arteries undergoes severe ischemic atrophy and scarring (131). However, the nephrons supplied by interlobular arteries of normal caliber may undergo substantial hypertrophy following treatment of malignant hypertension. These histologic changes may explain the improvement in renal function that sometimes occurs in some patients following institution of antihypertensive therapy with resolution of malignant hypertension.

In summary, although fibrinoid necrosis was the hallmark of malignant nephrosclerosis in untreated patients at autopsy, it is now rarely observed. In treated patients with malignant hypertension or blacks with untreated malignant hypertension, closed renal biopsy most often reveals marked intimal hyperplasia of the interlobular arteries in association with accelerated glomerular obsolescence (34,35,126).

Renal Pathology in Secondary Malignant Hypertension

A variety of primary renal parenchymal diseases can cause secondary malignant hypertension. Although it is often impossible to differentiate primary (essential) malignant hypertension from secondary malignant hypertension by clinical criteria, this distinction can usually be made by renal biopsy.

Malignant hypertension can develop during the course of chronic glomerulonephritis. When glomerulonephritis causes malignant hypertension, there is usually evidence of diffuse glomerular disease in addition to the vascular lesions seen in malignant nephrosclerosis. In contrast to the focal and segmental glomerular lesions seen in primary malignant hypertension, in secondary malignant hypertension due to chronic glomerulonephritis, diffuse and global changes usually involve more than 90% of glomeruli (125,133).

Chronic pyelonephritis can also cause secondary malignant hypertension. The pyelonephritic process can be unilateral or bilateral. There is coarse irregular scarring of the kidney(s), as well as difference in the size and shape of the two kidneys (25). The cortex is affected in a patchy fashion with alternating areas of scarred and normal-appearing tissue. Histologically, alternating areas of sharply demarcated normal and scarred parenchyma are observed (30). In scarred areas, there are dilated, colloid-filled tubules, crowded hyalinized glomeruli, and periglomerular fibrosis. In the interstitium there is severe fibrosis with a chronic inflammatory infiltrate. Vascular lesions indistinguishable from malignant nephrosclerosis may be seen in scarred areas, even in normotensive subjects with chronic pyelonephritis. However, with superimposed malignant hypertension, vascular lesions of malignant hypertension are found in unscarred areas of the kidney (30,134). Moreover, in unilateral pyelonephritis with superimposed malignant hypertension, histologic findings of malignant nephrosclerosis occur in the contralateral kidney (30).

In the microscopic form of polyarteritis nodosa (PAN), fibrinoid necrosis of the afferent arterioles and proliferative endarteritis of the interlobular arteries can occur in the absence of malignant hypertension. However, malignant nephrosclerosis and PAN can usually be differentiated histologically. In PAN, there is usually diffuse glomerular involvement as well as an active cellular infiltrate in the necrotic vascular and glomerular lesions. In addition, there are often healed and active necrotizing lesions typical of PAN in larger medium-sized muscular arteries of the kidney, mesentery, pancreas, and adrenals. Involvement of vessels of this size in primary malignant hypertension is rarely observed (30).

In scleroderma renal crisis, changes in the renal vessels may be virtually identical to primary malignant hypertension (58). The characteristic extrarenal manifestations of progressive systemic sclerosis must be used to differentiate these two entities.

Distribution of Vascular Lesions

Malignant hypertension is a diffuse hypertension-induced vasculopathy and in its terminal stages, widespread arterial and arteriolar lesions are found in a variety of organs (25,135). These vascular changes are similar to those seen in the kidney, namely, proliferative endarteritis of small arteries and fibrinoid necrosis of arterioles. The vascular beds of the pancreas, gastrointestinal tract, and liver are most frequently involved (136). Similar vascular lesions have also been observed in the retina (137), brain (137), myocardium (136), prostate (25), and skeletal muscle (135). The pathologic changes in the various organs and tissues are secondary to ischemia caused by these obliterative vascular changes.

Ophthalmic Pathology

In patients with malignant hypertension, thickening and hyalinization of the walls of the arterioles and capillaries of the retina and choroid are invariably present (137). Fibrinoid necrosis may also be found in some patients. Fibrin thrombi may be present in arterioles. Microaneurysms at or near the occluded segments of capillaries also occur. Small ischemic infarcts of the retina (cytoid bodies), corresponding to the cotton-wool spots seen clinically, are present in most patients (137). These infarcts are located in the nerve fiber and ganglion cell layers of the retina in the vicinity of vascular lesions. The arterioles supplying the optic nerve are thickened and hyalinized to varying degrees and fibrinoid necrosis may be present (137).

Cardiac Pathology

Left ventricular hypertrophy with normal chamber size is the predominant finding in most patients with malignant hypertension (25,26). Significant coronary atherosclerosis is a rare finding in these patients (25,26).

Pulmonary Pathology

In the era before effective antihypertensive therapy, uremic edema of the lung was frequently found in fatal cases of malignant hypertension (138). Gross examination of the lungs revealed widespread gelatinous consolidation that was most intense in the perihilar region.

Adrenal Pathology

Fibrinoid necrosis of the small arterioles of the adrenal glands is observed in up to 50% of fatal cases of malignant hypertension (25). The adrenals are often enlarged with multiple macroscopic nodules. This adrenal hyperplasia reflects sustained activation of the renin-angiotensin-aldosterone axis (65).

Gastrointestinal Pathology

Significant involvement of the mesenteric arterioles is a frequent finding in patients with malignant hypertension (136). In addition, among 100 patients with malignant hypertension, 60% had proliferative endarteritis of the pancreatic arterioles (139). Pancreatic lesions including infarcts associated with arterial thrombosis, focal parenchymal necrosis, and foci of atrophy and fibrosis are frequently found.

Pathophysiology

On the basis of the clinical presentation, natural history, and renal pathology, it can be concluded that benign and malignant hypertension are distinct clinicopathologic entities rather than a spectrum of the same disease. However, the mechanisms that initiate the transition from benign to malignant hypertension are not entirely clear. The primary function of the microcirculation is to ensure that the cardiac output is distributed to a variety of tissues that vary widely in metabolic requirements. The arterioles control the blood flow to the capillary network through the process of autoregulation. Thus, it is not surprising that the arterioles are the major target of the acute vascular damage in malignant hypertension. However, the central question is whether severe hypertension alone is sufficient to cause the vascular injury characteristic of malignant hypertension, or whether additional cofactors are required.

Role of Increased Blood Pressure Per Se (the Pressure Hypothesis)

According to the pressure hypothesis, the development of fibrinoid necrosis and proliferative endarteritis is a direct consequence of the mechanical stress placed on vessel walls by severe hypertension (45,104,125,140,141). Several lines of evidence support the hypothesis that severe hypertension is the fundamental pathogenic process in malignant hypertension. In this regard, although there are numerous diverse etiologies of malignant hypertension, the process is reversible given adequate blood pressure control (22). Moreover, the transition from benign to malignant hypertension is usually accompanied by a dramatic rise in blood pressure (45). In addition, the occurrence of fibrinoid necrosis tends to correlate with the height of the arterial pressure (125).

Another finding supporting the crucial role of severe hypertension in the development of the vascular lesions of malignant hypertension is the absence of these lesions in vascular beds protected from the elevated blood pressure. In the two-kidney, two-clip model of malignant hypertension in the dog, vascular necrosis occurs in mesenteric arterioles and other vessels exposed to the high pressure, but not in renal arterioles protected from the high perfusion pressure (142). Likewise, in rats with two-kidney, one-clip malignant hypertension, vascular necrotic lesions develop in the nonclipped kidney and the systemic circulation but not in the clipped kidney (143). One report described patients with unilateral renal artery stenosis and malignant hypertension in whom arteriolar necrosis occurred in the contralateral kidney but not in the stenotic kidney (144).

A number of experimental models of malignant hypertension lend support to the pressure hypothesis. Brief overdistention of the arteriolar system by forceful injection of saline solution into the aorta results in a sudden increase in mean arterial pressure of 80 to 90 mm Hg accompanied by the development of fibrinoid necrosis in the interlobular arteries and afferent arterioles of the kidney (145). Fibrinoid necrosis does not develop if the kidney is protected from the sudden rise in pressure.

In studies that utilize windows in the skull and abdominal wall to view the microcirculation in rats with one-kidney, one-clip malignant hypertension, cerebral and mesenteric arterioles develop focal constrictions and dilations giving rise to a string of beads or sausage-string pattern (146). Intravenous injection of trypan blue results in patchy leakage of dye in dilated regions but not in constricted regions. The dilated regions are the sites of fibrinoid necrosis (147).

The sausage-string pattern develops rapidly in mesenteric arterioles in the rat when the blood pressure is increased acutely with angiotensin or norepinephrine. When colloidal carbon particles are injected, carbon deposits in the walls of dilated segments but not constricted segments, thereby suggesting that the abnormal vascular pattern is the direct result of the elevated blood pressure and that the dilated segments represent the earliest sites of vascular damage as manifested by increased permeability to plasma proteins (148).

The extent of carbon deposition is related to the height of the arterial pressure rather than to the type of pressor substance infused (angiotensin, norepinephrine, or renal extract) (147). If the increase in blood pressure is prevented by the administration of hydralazine, the sausage-string pattern fails to develop and carbon is not deposited in the vascular walls. Thus, the abnormal permeability in dilated segments appears to be the result of hypertension-induced structural damage to the vessel wall. These studies do not support the concept of a direct vasculotoxic effect of angiotensin or norepinephrine independent of a pressor effect.

These sausage-string lesions have been evaluated using electron microscopy (148). In dilated segments, breaks in the endothelium are observed as a result of disruption of intracellular junctions or destruction of the cell body. These lesions give rise to gaps in the endothelium that are permeable to intravenously injected colloidal carbon particles. Amorphous deposits consisting of plasma, carbon particles, and fibrinlike material deposit in the media. The vascular lesions do not appear to be caused simply by a direct vasculotoxic effect of angiotensin because identical results have been reported with deoxycorticosterone acetate (DOCA)-salt hypertension, a model in which angiotensin levels are suppressed (149).

Based on these experiments, it has been concluded that the mechanical stress of severe hypertension is the principal cause of fibrinoid necrosis in malignant hypertension. Moreover, all of the vascular changes can be attributed to the indirect pressor effect of the infused substances rather than to any direct effect of these substances on vascular permeability. The following mechanism for the development of fibrinoid necrosis has been proposed (147,148,150). With mild to moderate elevations in blood pressure, the initial hemodynamic response is arterial and arteriolar vasoconstriction. This autoregulatory process maintains tissue perfusion at a relatively constant level and prevents the elevated pressure from being transmitted to the smaller, more distal vessels. With increasingly severe hypertension, however, autoregulation eventually fails such that hypertension is transmitted to more distal vessels. The resulting rise in downstream perfusion pressure damages the arterioles and capillaries. Because smooth muscle may not be uniformly distributed along arterioles, when the arterial pressure is sufficiently increased by whatever means, local areas of the arterial wall are unable to withstand the mechanical stress and become forcibly dilated (sausage-string pattern). By the law of Laplace, as the radius increases in dilated segments, wall tension increases proportionately. As a consequence, the endothelium becomes stretched, damaged, and abnormally permeable. Disruption of the vascular endothelium then allows extravasation of plasma proteins and fibrinogen into the vessel wall, compressing and destroying smooth muscle. Local fibrinogen deposition occurs, producing fibrinoid necrosis and obliteration of the vascular lumen.

The Vasculotoxic Hypothesis

The major criticism of the pressure hypothesis is that there is substantial overlap between the levels of blood pressure observed in patients with benign hypertension and those with malignant hypertension (25,84). Moreover, occasional patients tolerate severe diastolic hypertension for long periods without developing malignant hypertension (81). The abrupt change from an asymptomatic patient with severe hypertension to a critically ill patient with a multisystem disease suggests that factors in addition to blood pressure may contribute to the transition from benign to malignant hypertension (41). According to the vasculotoxic theory, severe hypertension is necessary but not sufficient to cause malignant hypertension.

The vasculotoxic theory proposes that humoral factors interact with the hypertension-induced hemodynamic stress to cause the vascular damage observed in malignant hypertension. Based on his classic dog model of renovascular hypertension, Goldblatt (142) believed that renal failure was a necessary cofactor for the development of malignant hypertension. He proposed that a vasculotoxic factor accumulated in severe renal disease. However, it has subsequently been demonstrated in both humans and experimental animals that malignant hypertension can develop in the absence of uremia and even before the vascular lesions of malignant nephrosclerosis develop in the kidney (16,28).

It has been suggested that vascular permeability factors such as renin, angiotensin, catecholamines, and vasopressin may cause vascular damage independent of their pressor effects. For example, administration of rat kidney extracts to nephrectomized rats produces a lethal syndrome characterized by large pleural effusions, ascites, edema of the pancreas, and the arteriolar fibrinoid necrosis characteristic of malignant hypertension (152). To explain these findings, the presence of a vascular permeability factor of renal origin has been postulated.

There is convincing evidence that angiotensin II does have a direct effect on the vascular endothelium to increase permeability (153). The injection of 100 pg of angiotensin II into a segment of rabbit abdominal aorta isolated between two ligatures causes a diffuse increase in permeability of the aortic endothelium as evidenced by extravasation of intravenously injected Evans blue dye. Areas of the aorta not exposed to angiotensin II do not show any increase in permeability. Injections of Ringer's solution (vehicle) produce no blue staining of the aortic endothelium. Evaluation of the areas exposed to angiotensin II by electron microscopy reveals rounding and shortening of the endothelial cells with widening of spaces between endothelial cells.

Studies of dermal capillary permeability in response to vasoactive agents have confirmed the fact that there appears to be a direct effect of angiotensin II on vascular endothelium (153). When norepinephrine or angiotensin I is injected into the dermis, there is no extravasation of Evans blue dye. However, when angiotensin II is injected in low concentrations, there is severe capillary leak. The increased permeability can be prevented by simultaneous administration of angiotensin II receptor antagonists but not by antihistamines. Angiotensin II appears to increase vascular permeability independent of any pressor effect by causing contraction of endothelial cells (153).

Role of the Renin-Angiotensin Axis

In patients with malignant hypertension there is often evidence of activation of the renin-angiotensin system (65,115). At the time of presentation, some but not all patients have increased PRA (63). Hyperplasia of the juxtaglomerular apparatus is often present. The adrenal glands frequently reveal hyperplasia and nodularity of the zona glomerulosa (65).

In patients with malignant hypertension, activation of the renin-angiotensin system may be primary or secondary. For example, activation of the renin-angiotensin system could be a critical step in the transition from benign to malignant hypertension through either direct (vasculotoxic) or indirect (hemodynamic) effects on the vasculature. Conversely, hyperreninemia may be a secondary phenomenon occurring in response to renal ischemia caused by the arteriolar lesions of malignant hypertension. These two processes are not mutually exclusive. In fact, both may occur simultaneously, resulting in a vicious cycle of hypertension-induced vascular damage causing renal ischemia, which leads to enhanced renin release that may exacerbate the hypertension.

In a two-kidney, one-clip model of renovascular hypertension in the rat, there is onset of malignant hypertension after 3 to 5 weeks (154). The sequence of events following the application of a sufficiently small clip to one renal artery has been well characterized. Initially there is evidence of activation of the renin-angiotensin system with a resulting increase in blood pressure. When the systolic blood pressure surpasses a critical level of 180 to 190 mm Hg, spontaneous natriuresis and diuresis occur. Water intake increases, but weight loss and hyponatremia ensue. Eventually, renal function deteriorates, and the histologic findings of malignant nephrosclerosis become apparent in the contralateral kidney. The rats eventually die due to renal failure, heart failure, or cerebral hemorrhage. In this model of malignant hypertension, it is apparent that a vicious cycle develops following activation of the renin-angiotensin system. Renal ischemia results in activation of the renin-angiotensin system with the development of hypertension. The sudden, severe hypertension causes natriuresis, diuresis, and volume depletion. Volume depletion further stimulates the renin-angiotensin system. As the gain on this cycle increases, hypertension-induced vascular damage or the direct vasculotoxic effect of angiotensin induces vascular damage and deterioration of renal function. Volume depletion is pivotal in the pathogenesis of malignant hypertension in this model. Rats with malignant hypertension, given a choice of deionized water or normal saline, exhibit compulsive saline drinking (155). During the first 24 hours of saline drinking, there is a marked decrease in blood pressure and an increase in body weight. Moreover, there is correction of the abnormal levels of hematocrit, serum sodium, renin, and angiotensin II. With continued saline drinking for 2 to 7 days, the blood pressure increases to the previous high levels, but signs of malignant hypertension do not recur. If saline is withdrawn at this time, within 2 days the cycle of volume depletion, activation of the renin-angiotensin system, and malignant hypertension recurs. Thus, the patho-

genesis of malignant hypertension in this model appears to be critically dependent on spontaneous natriuresis, volume depletion, and activation of the renin-angiotensin system.

The unclipped kidney is clearly the source of the spontaneous natriuresis and diuresis in the two-kidney, one-clip model. In the one-kidney, one-clip rat model, there is no phase of renal salt loss (156). Likewise, in rats with two-kidney, two-clip hypertension, the phase of salt loss does not occur. However, if one clip is removed, there is an immediate onset of a salt-losing state associated with development of the syndrome of malignant hypertension with fibrinoid necrosis in the unclipped kidney.

In the stroke-prone spontaneously hypertensive rat (SHR-SP) model of malignant hypertension, life-long treatment with an antihypertensive dose of the converting enzyme inhibitor ramipril completely prevents the renal arteriolar neointimal proliferation and sclerosis, fibrinoid necrosis, glomerulopathy and tubular-interstitial fibrosis observed in placebo-treated animals (157). The nephroprotective effect of ramipril was associated with a dose-dependent inhibition of plasma and renal tissue angiotensin-converting enzyme activities. Although there was some subtle evidence of nephroprotection with a lower non-antihypertensive dose of ramipril, prevention of hypertension with high-dose ramipril was also required to completely prevent the development of malignant nephrosclerosis in the SHR-SP model.

Over the last decade, polymorphisms in the genes regulating the RAS system have been identified. These include the 287 base pair sequence deletion (D) insertion (I) polymorphism of the angiotensin-converting enzyme (ACE) gene and the methionine (M) to threonine (T) point mutation polymorphism in the angiotensinogen gene (AGT). Genotypes with respect to ACE I/D and AGT M/T loci were evaluated in a series of 42 patients with malignant hypertension, 42 patients with nonmalignant hypertension and 85 normotensive controls (158). The frequency of the DD genotype was significantly increased in patients with malignant hypertension (43%) compared with patients with nonmalignant hypertension (14%) and normotensive control subjects (18%). The frequency distribution of AGT M/T genotype did not differ between groups. These data suggest that ACE gene polymorphism is a significant risk factor for initiation of malignant hypertension.

Whereas activation of the renin-angiotensin system may be crucial in the development of the malignant phase in some experimental models and some patients with malignant hypertension, the clinical and pathologic features of malignant hypertension sometimes occurs in the absence of activation of the systemic renin-angiotensin system (63). For example, widespread necrotizing arteriolar disease occurs with hypertension caused by bilateral nephrectomy in experimental animals. On the other hand, there is emerging evidence from transgenic animals of activation of a local paracrine renin-angiotensin system in the pathogenesis of the vascular injury in malignant hypertension. Animal models provide pathological, pharmacologic, and genetic evidence supporting the hypothesis that intrarenal generation of AII and exposure of the microcirculation to elevated blood pressure cooperate in causing tissue damage in malignant hypetension (159).

Elevated levels of angiotensin II in malignant hypertension may contribute to renal injury by mediating renal inflammation independent of any blood pressure effect. In a solvent-treated two-kidney/one-clip rat model of malignant hypertension, low-dose angiotensin receptor blockade with valsartan does not prevent an increase in blood pressure but prevents the development of lethal malignant hypertension (160). In nonclipped kidneys of solvent-treated renovascular hypertensive rats, there was a prominent interstitial infiltrate of macrophages and increased expression of monocyte chemoattractant protein-1. These changes were completely prevented by low-dose valsartan. These finding suggest that reduction of AII-induced inflammation in the kidney may contribute to the protective effects of valsartan in this model of malignant hypertension.

In summary, neither hypersecretion of renin nor the presence of kidneys appears to be required for the development of malignant hypertension. On the other hand, a high concentration of angiotensin II can be an aggravating factor or in some circumstances, can actually trigger the onset of malignant hypertension. Moreover, activation of the renin-angiotensin system by renal ischemia may contribute to the vicious cycle of severe hypertension and renal injury observed in malignant hypertension.

Role of Volume Depletion

In several experimental models, spontaneous natriuresis appears to be the initiating event in the transition from benign to malignant hypertension (154,155,161,162). In patients with malignant hypertension, an abrupt onset of weight loss early in the course of the disease has been reported (16,25,27). In the series of Kincaid-Smith et al. (25), the onset of malignant hypertension often appeared suddenly. Despite minor increases in blood pressure, the patients became suddenly ill with weakness, wasting, and profound weight loss. The rapidity of the weight loss could only be explained by natriuresis-induced volume depletion and may be the human counterpart of the rat two-kidney, one-clip model of malignant hypertension in which spontaneous natriuresis is the inciting event (154,155). In patients with analgesic nephropathy, volume depletion often accompanies malignant hypertension, whereas restoration of normal volume status leads to lowering of blood pressure and resolution of malignant hypertension (42).

In summary, it appears that volume depletion due to spontaneous natriuresis is often associated with the transition from the benign to the malignant phase of hypertension in both experimental and human malignant hypertension. The mechanism of the spontaneous salt wasting is not known. In the isolated, perfused kidney, an acute increase in arterial perfusion pressure results in increased urine flow rate and sodium excretion. Because glomerular filtration rate and renal blood flow remain unchanged, the natriuresis has been attributed to inhibition of tubular sodium resorption by elevated blood pressure.

Role of Localized Intravascular Coagulation

Evidence of microangiopathic hemolytic anemia and disorders of coagulation and fibrinolysis has been reported in experimental models of malignant hypertension (163). This anemia is characterized by red cell fragmentation and hemoglobinuria with iron deposition in the renal tubules.

Localized intravascular coagulation has been proposed to play an important role in the pathogenesis of malignant hypertension. Severe hypertension, perhaps augmented by vasculotoxic factors, injures arteriolar walls. This injury leads to increased endothelial permeability to fibrinogen and other plasma proteins. The clotting cascade is activated by tissue thromboplastin and fibrin that is deposited in the vessel wall and lumen. Platelets are deposited, and microangiopathic hemolytic anemia is produced by fragmentation of red cells as they traverse intravascular fibrin strands. The lysis of platelets and red cells produces adenine diphosphate and thromboplastin, which aggravate intravascular coagulation and produce a vicious cycle of hemolysis and fibrin deposition. Tissue ischemia is produced by a combination of intravascular fibrin deposition and arteriolar wall thickening that constrict the vessel lumen.

In this scheme, intravascular coagulation is the consequence of hypertension-induced vascular injury. It has also been postulated that the coagulation abnormalities may be the primary event that incites the development of malignant hypertension (114). This theory is based on the observation that renal vascular lesions identical to those in primary malignant nephrosclerosis can occur with idiopathic postpartum renal failure and the hemolytic–uremic syndrome. In these disorders, abnormalities of coagulation and fibrinoid necrosis often precede the development of hypertension (164).

To investigate the hypothesis that abnormalities of thrombogenesis and endothelial damage/dysfunction are greater in malignant hypertension compared with uncomplicated nonmalignant essential hypertension, Lip et al. measured markers of endothelial function (von Willebrand factor), platelet activation (soluble P-selectin) and fibrinogen in 18 consecutive patients with malignant hypertension, 50 patients with untreated essential hypertension and 34 healthy controls (165). Mean plasma fibrinogen and von Willebrand factor levels were highest in patients with malignant hypertension, intermediate in the nonmalignant hypertension group and lowest in the normotensive controls. Soluble P-selectin levels were higher in both hypertensive groups than in normotensive controls. These data suggest that endothelial damage (elevated von Willebrand factor) and platelet activation may be involved in the pathogenesis of malignant hypertenson.

Role of Prostacyclin

Abnormal prostacyclin (prostaglandin I_2 [PGI_2]) metabolism has been postulated to play a role in the pathogenesis of malignant hypertension in cigarette smokers and women taking oral contraceptives (50). Enhanced PGI_2 synthesis by vessel walls may be a protective mechanism that limits the vascular injury caused by hypertension (167). For example, PGI_2 may limit the extent of thrombus formation at sites of endothelial injury. Both oral contraceptives (166) and cigarette smoking (168) are associated with lower concentrations of 6-keto-prostaglandin $F_{1\alpha}$, a stable metabolite of PGI_2. Impaired vessel wall synthesis of PGI_2 may thus predispose to the development of malignant hypertension (50). Moreover, absence of the protective effect of PGI_2 could amplify the vascular endothelial injury caused by severe hypertension.

Role of Intracellular Calcium

Increased availability of free calcium in vascular smooth muscle may be important in the pathogenesis of hypertension. Moreover, it has been suggested that an excess of cytosolic calcium may be a crucial step in the development of malignant hypertension and that this deleterious calcium overload may be activated or inhibited independent of the arterial blood pressure (169). Dahl salt-sensitive rats on a high-salt diet develop fulminant hypertension with a necrotizing vasculitis in the kidney. However, treatment with nifedipine, which inhibits calcium influx via activated membrane calcium channels, prevents the rise in blood pressure and the occurrence of necrotizing vascular lesions. A similar protective effect has been described with nisoldipine and nitrendipine but not with captopril (169).

The stroke-prone spontaneously hypertensive rat is another experimental model of malignant hypertension that mimics the renal and vascular changes seen in primary malignant hypertension in humans (170). In salt-loaded stroke-prone spontaneously hypertensive rats, treatment with either nimodipine or parathyroidectomy dramatically reduces vascular injury and mortality despite an insignificant effect on the level of blood pressure. Since hypertension-induced vascular injury can be prevented by manipulation of calcium influx into cells, it has been postulated that vascular injury in malignant hypertension is mediated by intracellular calcium overload in vascular smooth muscle cells (169).

Role of Dietary Potassium

In Dahl salt-sensitive rats on a high-salt diet, supplementation of dietary potassium intake can prevent the hypertension-induced intimal thickening of the interlobular arteries without a concomitant reduction in blood pressure (171). In addition, in the stroke-prone spontaneously hypertensive rat model of malignant hypertension, a high-potassium diet prevented the intimal thickening of mesenteric and cerebral arteries, independent of an effect on blood pressure (172).

It has been suggested that the low-potassium diet characteristically consumed by African Americans in the southern United States may exacerbate the hypertension-induced endothelial injury in the interlobular arteries, leading to the development of pronounced musculomucoid intimal hyperplasia (malignant nephrosclerosis) (173). Low dietary potassium intake may, at least in part, explain the high frequency of ESRD due to hypertension among African Americans.

Role of the Kallikrein-Kinin System

In addition to enhanced activity of vasopressor hormones, decreased activity of vasodilator hormone systems may be involved in the pathogenesis of malignant hypertension. Kinins are potent vasodilators that exert a marked influence on renal salt and water excretion. Plasma levels of kininogen are markedly decreased in patients with malignant hypertension compared with either patients with benign hypertension or normotensive control subjects (174). Urinary kallikrein excretion is also significantly decreased in patients with malignant hypertension, particularly those with primary (essential) malignant hypertension (175). Decreased urinary kallikrein could be indicative of depressed activity of the renal kallikrein-kinin system, which may be a risk factor for development of malignant hypertension in individuals with essential hypertension.

Role of Endothelium-Derived Relaxing Factors and Endothelin

Hypertension is associated with various functional changes of the vascular endothelium including decreased formation of nitric oxide, the endothelium-derived relaxing factor (EDRF), and increased release of contracting factors such as endothelin. This dysfunction of the hypertensive endothelial organ may contribute to the elevation of peripheral resistance and the development of hypertensive complications in the cerebral, coronary, or renal circulation (176,177).

Plasma immunoreactive endothelin-1 (ET-1) levels have been measured in various rat models of hypertension (178). Endothelin-1 levels are not increased in the prehypertensive and benign hypertension phases in spontaneously hypertensive rats compared to normotensive Wistar-Kyoto rats. In contrast, treatment of spontaneously hypertensive rats (SHR) with DOCA and salt results in the development of malignant hypertension with renal insufficiency and increased plasma ET-1 levels. However, ET-1 levels do not increase in Wistar-Kyoto rats treated with DOCA-salt. In the DOCA-salt-treated SHR model of malignant hypertension, treatment with combined endothelin type A/type B receptor antagonists not only reduced blood pressure but also prevented mesangial hypercellularity, glomerular sclerotic changes, and tubulo-interstitial damage (179). Reduction of blood pressure with hydralazine alone was less effective in preventing DOCA–salt-induced renal structural injury in this model.

The ability of endothelin receptor blockade to prevent or to treat established cerebral and renal injury has recently been investigated in the salt-loaded, SHR-stroke prone model of malignant hypertension using an endothelin receptor subtype-A antagonist (180). Initiation of endothelin receptor blocker treatment at the start of salt loading prolonged survival and completely prevented the development of cerebral edema and reduced blood pressure and proteinuria in a dose-dependent fashion. However, delaying treatment until after the onset of cerebral edema failed to prolong survival. These data suggest that in the SHR-stroke prone model the endothelin A receptor participates actively in the development of increased blood pressure and initiation of target-organ damage but has a minimal role in the pathogenesis of established malignant hypertension and the progression of target-organ damage.

Role of Oxidate Stress

Oxidative stress has been implicated in the pathogenesis of hypertension. In the stroke-prone spontaneously hypertensive (SP-SHR) rat model of malignant hypertension treatment with the superoxide dismutase mimetic, tempol prevented the progression of hypertension (181). Tempol reduced the media:lumen ratio compared to controls. Moreover vascular superoxide anion levels were lower and plasma total antioxidant levels were higher in the tempol-treated group. These data suggest that oxidative stress may play an important role in the vascular damage associated with malignant hypertension in the SP-SHR.

Development of Fibrinoid Necrosis and Proliferative Endarteritis

In experimental models of malignant hypertension, vascular damage from either the mechanical stress of hypertension or vasculotoxic hormones leads to endothelial injury that is manifested by the sausage-string pattern and accompanied by seepage of plasma proteins including fibrinogen into the vessel wall. Contact of plasma constituents with smooth muscle cells activates the coagulation cascade, and fibrin is deposited in the wall. Fibrin deposits cause necrosis of smooth muscle cells and the development of fibrinoid necrosis.

Proliferative endarteritis occurs when the vascular smooth muscle cells undergo a phenotypic change from the normal contractile phenotype to the proliferative–secretory phenotype that was predominant during embryologic development. It has been proposed that the sudden severe elevation of blood pressure produces forced vasodilation of the interlobular arteries with denudation of the vascular endothelium, resulting in the attachment of platelets at the sites of endothelial injury with synthesis and release of platelet-derived growth factor (PDGF) (182,183). PDGF stimulates chemotaxis of medial smooth muscle cells to the intima, where they proliferate and secrete mucopolysaccharide and later collagen and other extracellular matrix components, resulting in the lesions characteristic of proliferative endarteritis or musculomucoid intimal hyperplasia.

Summary of Pathophysiology

Based on the foregoing discussion, it is clear that the exact pathophysiologic mechanism underlying the transition from benign to malignant hypertension is not fully understood. Undoubtedly, a marked increase in blood pressure is pivotal. Severe hypertension is the common element in malignant hypertension in humans and in each of the animal models of malignant hypertension. Moreover, reduction of the blood pressure leads to a resolution of the malignant phase regardless of the underlying etiology. Thus, a significant elevation of the blood pressure is necessary for the development and progression of malignant hypertension. The major issue is whether the mechanical stress of severe hypertension alone is *sufficient* to cause the transition from benign to malignant hypertension. Because there is considerable overlap in the levels of blood pressure seen in patients with benign and those with malignant hypertension, it is likely that severe hypertension alone is *not sufficient* to cause the malignant hypertension in all patients and that additional factor(s) probably participate. These cofactors are not necessarily the same in every case. For example, activation of the renin-angiotensin axis may be important in some patients but not in others. In some patients, perhaps catecholamines, or activation of the clotting cascade interact with hemodynamic stress to induce malignant hypertension.

The vicious cycle of malignant hypertension is best demonstrated in the kidneys but applies equally well to the vascular beds of the pancreas, gastrointestinal tract, retina, and brain (Fig. 56-18). In this scheme, severe hypertension is central. Hypertension may be either essential or secondary to any one of a variety of disorders. The interaction between the level of blood pressure and the adaptive capacity of the vasculature may be important. Chronic hypertension results in thickening and remodeling of arterial walls, which may be an adaptive mechanism to prevent vascular damage from mechanical stress (184). However, when the blood pressure rises to a level or at a rate that is excessive, these adaptive mechanisms may

be overwhelmed, resulting in vascular damage. As a result of the mechanical stress of increased transmural pressure, focal segments of the vascular system become dilated, producing the sausage-string pattern. Other hormonal factors may act synergistically with hypertension to damage the arterial vasculature. For example, spontaneous natriuresis at some critical level of blood pressure may result in volume depletion with activation of the renin-angiotensin, vasopressin, or catecholamine systems, which further elevates blood pressure. In addition, these hormones may be directly vasculotoxic. Fibrinogen and other plasma proteins may permeate the damaged vascular wall and activate the intrinsic clotting system, causing deposition of fibrin in the vessel wall and lumen, leading to fibrinoid necrosis. The onset of localized intravascular coagulation may cause a cycle in which red blood cells and platelets are disrupted on intravascular strands, with release of adenine diphosphate and thromboplastin with further activation of the clotting cascade. Platelet adherence to damaged endothelium with release of PDGF leads to myointimal proliferation in the

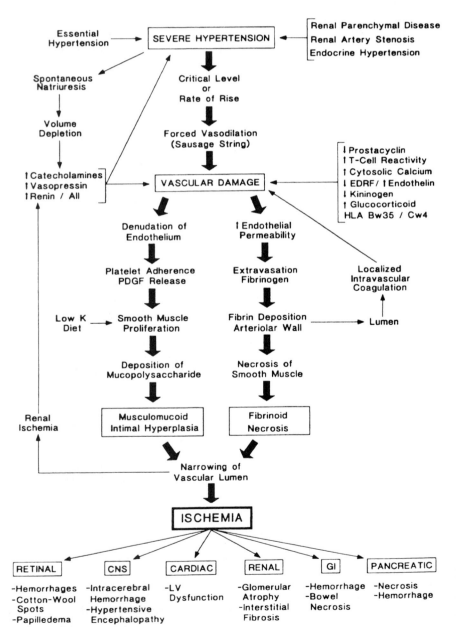

FIGURE 56-18. Pathophysiology of malignant hypertension. *AII*, angiotensin II; *EDRF*, endothelium-derived relaxing factor; *PDGF*, platelet-derived growth factor; *LV*, left ventricular.

interlobular arteries, which results in proliferative endarteritis. The wall thickening and luminal narrowing in the interlobular arteries and afferent arterioles result in glomerular ischemia, accelerated glomerular obsolescence, and renal insufficiency. Renal ischemia may lead to increased activation of the renin-angiotensin system, which may cause further increases in blood pressure, vascular damage, and pressure-induced natriuresis, such that a vicious cycle of hypertension, vascular damage, and renal insufficiency develops.

Other factors, although less certain, may also be important in the development of malignant hypertension. Low dietary potassium may predispose to hypertensive arterial injury in black patients with severe hypertension. Abnormalities in membrane sodium transport and cytosolic calcium may mediate hypertension-induced vascular injury. Cigarette smoking or oral contraceptives may decrease prostacyclin production and inhibit repair of hypertensive vascular damage. Abnormalities in the kallikrein-kinin system may also be important in some cases.

Unfortunately, the chain of pathogenetic processes leading to fibrinoid necrosis and neointimal proliferation have not yet been well studied at the molecular level to accurately assess the role of cytokines and growth factors in the development of these vascular lesions in the systemic and renal vasculature (185).

Pathophysiology of Hypertensive Neuroretinopathy

Retinal arteriolar vasculopathy in malignant hypertension leads to obliteration or rupture of vessels, resulting in striate hemorrhages, cotton-wool spots, and papilledema. Hypertensive neuroretinopathy is not simply the result of renal failure as hypertensive neuroretinopathy can clearly occur in malignant hypertension prior to the onset of clinically significant renal disease (86). It also appears that hypertensive neuroretinopathy often occurs in the absence of increased intracranial pressure (86).

The retinal circulation is under autoregulatory control and does not have a sympathetic nerve supply. As the systemic blood pressure increases, if autoregulation is intact, the retinal arterioles constrict to keep the retinal blood flow constant. The appearance of hypertensive neuroretinopathy implies that autoregulation has failed (85).

Striate hemorrhages result from bleeding from superficial capillaries in the nerve fiber bundles near the optic disc. These capillaries originate from arterioles, so that when autoregulation fails, the high systemic pressure is transmitted directly to the capillaries. This leads to breaks in the continuity of the capillary endothelium with subsequent hemorrhage (85).

Cotton-wool spots result from ischemic infarction of nerve fiber bundles due to arteriolar occlusion (85). Fluorescein angiography demonstrates that cotton-wool spots are areas of retinal nonperfusion (186). Embolization of pig retina with glass beads produces immediate intracellular edema followed by accumulation of mitochondria and other subcellular organelles in the ischemic nerve fibers (187). It has been postulated that the normal axoplasmic flow of subcellular organelles is disrupted by ischemia such that accumulation of organelles in ischemic nerve fiber bundles results in a visible white patch (100). Cotton-wool spots tend to distribute around the optic disc because the nerve fiber bundles are most dense in this region.

The pathogenesis of papilledema in malignant hypertension has been controversial. Pickering (107) maintained that papilledema results from increased intracranial pressure. However, intracranial pressure is not always increased in malignant hypertension (86). Papilledema has been produced in rhesus monkeys by occlusion of the long posterior ciliary artery, which supplies the optic disc (188). Thus papilledema, like cotton-wool spots, most likely results from ischemia of nerve fibers in the optic disc (99,189).

Treatment

Malignant hypertension must be treated expeditiously in order to prevent complications such as hypertensive encephalopathy, intracerebral hemorrhage, acute pulmonary edema, and renal failure. The hypertensive patient with hypertensive neuroretinopathy (hemorrhages, cotton-wool spots with or without papilledema) should be hospitalized for intensive medical therapy. Initiation of appropriate therapy should not be delayed pending extensive laboratory and roentgenographic examinations aimed at defining a potential underlying etiology. The workup for secondary causes should be deferred until the blood pressure has been controlled and the patient stabilized.

The traditional approach to patients with malignant hypertension has been the initiation of therapy with rapid-acting parenteral hypotensive agents such as sodium nitroprusside, trimethaphan, and diazoxide (190). In Table 56-4 are listed the settings in which the use of parenteral antihypertensive agents is recommended for the initial management of malignant hypertension. In general, parenteral therapy should be utilized in patients who have evidence of acute end-organ damage or who are unable to tolerate oral medications. The management of patients with acute hypertensive heart failure, hypertensive encephalopathy, or intracerebral hemorrhage is discussed later in separate sections on each of these topics.

The drug of choice for the management of patients with malignant hypertension requiring parenteral therapy is sodium nitroprusside (191). Preliminary studies suggest that the dopamine receptor (DA_1 selective) agonist fenoldopam may also be useful for parenteral treatment of malignant hypertension (3,192). Trimethaphan is an alternative, but a number of significant adverse effects limit its usefulness. Diazoxide, employed in mini-bolus fashion, may be advantageous in selected patients for whom monitoring in an intensive care unit is not available. Mini-bolus injections of labetalol have also been used for the treatment of malignant hypertension (191).

There are no absolute guidelines for the blood pressure goal during parenteral therapy. The theoretic risks of rapid reduction of blood pressure are discussed later in the section on the controversy over gradual versus rapid reduction of blood pressure. As a general rule, it is safe to initially reduce the mean arterial pressure by 20% or to a level of 160 to 170 mm Hg systolic and 100 to 110 mm Hg diastolic (193). During the reduction of blood pressure with parenteral antihypertensives, the patient should be monitored closely for evidence of cerebral or myocardial hypoperfusion. The use of a short-acting agent

TABLE 56-4

INDICATIONS FOR PARENTERAL THERAPY IN MALIGNANT HYPERTENSION

Patients unable to tolerate oral therapy due to intractable vomiting
Hypertensive encephalopathy
Rapidly failing vision
Intracerebral hemorrhage
Acute pulmonary edema
Acute myocardial infarction
Rapid deterioration of renal function
Acute pancreatitis
Gastrointestinal hemorrhage
Acute abdomen secondary to mesenteric vasculitis

such as sodium nitroprusside or fenoldopam has obvious advantages because the blood pressure can be stabilized quickly at a higher level if complications develop during rapid blood pressure reduction. If there is no evidence of vital organ hypoperfusion following this initial reduction of blood pressure, the diastolic blood pressure can gradually be lowered to 90 mm Hg over a period of 12 to 36 hours.

Oral antihypertensive agents should be initiated as soon as possible so that the duration of parenteral therapy can be minimized. However, a common error in the management of patients with malignant hypertension is the abrupt discontinuation of parenteral therapy immediately after oral therapy has been initiated. With this approach, severe rebound hypertension often develops before the oral antihypertensive regimen becomes effective. Ideally, oral antihypertensives should be initiated as soon as the patient has been stabilized and is able to tolerate medications by mouth. The nitroprusside infusion should be continued until the oral agents have taken effect and have been titrated to an effective dose. The nitroprusside or fenoldopam infusion can then be weaned as the oral regimen is gradually increased.

Although other agents may be effective in the long-term management of patients with malignant hypertension, the cornerstone of initial oral therapy should be an arteriolar vasodilator such as hydralazine, sustained-release nifedipine, or minoxidil. Vasodilators may reflexively activate the adrenergic system and cause tachycardia with an increase in cardiac output, which may blunt the hypotensive response. Therefore, treatment with β-adrenergic blockers is usually also required. Direct-acting vasodilators also cause renal salt and water retention, fluid overload, and the development of pseudotolerance to the hypotensive effect of the drug. Thus, although diuretics may not be required for the initial management of patients with malignant hypertension (vide infra), they are usually required as a part of the long-term maintenance antihypertensive regimen. The regimen that follows has proved to be generally effective in the conversion from parenteral to oral therapy. After the blood pressure has been controlled with sodium nitroprusside and while the infusion is continued, hydralazine (50 mg) and propranolol (40 mg) are administered orally. As the oral agents become effective and the blood pressure declines, the nitroprusside infusion is tapered. Brief interruption of the infusion can be used to assess the hypotensive response to oral agents. If after 6 to 8 hours the diastolic blood pressure remains higher than 100 mm Hg, a second dose of hydralazine (100 mg) should be given. The propranolol dose is increased as needed to maintain adequate β-blockade (heart rate, 60 to 80 beats/minute). The usual dose of propranolol is 80 to 120 mg administered twice daily, but larger doses occasionally may be required. If the blood pressure is not controlled with hydralazine at a dose of 100 mg twice daily, minoxidil should be substituted for hydralazine. The starting dose of minoxidil (2.5 mg) is increased by 2.5 to 5.0 mg every 6 to 8 hours until the blood pressure is adequately controlled. The usual effective dose is 5 to 10 mg twice daily. Treatment with a beta-blocker is recommended as for hydralazine. As the blood pressure is brought under control with oral agents, the sodium nitroprusside infusion is gradually weaned. When the convalescing patient is mobilized, upright blood pressure should be carefully monitored to avoid significant orthostatic hypotension. A diuretic, usually furosemide at a starting dose of 40 mg twice daily, is added to either the hydralazine or the minoxidil regimen when it becomes evident that salt and water retention is beginning to occur.

Volume Status and the Role of Diuretics

It has traditionally been taught that patients with malignant hypertension require potent parenteral diuretic therapy during the initial phase of treatment with parenteral vasodilators (190). However, there is now evidence suggesting that routine parenteral diuretic therapy during the acute phase of treatment for malignant hypertension may actually be deleterious (41). Overdiuresis may result in deterioration of renal function due to superimposed prerenal azotemia. Moreover, volume depletion may activate the renin-angiotensin axis and other pressor hormone systems.

Even patients with malignant hypertension and pulmonary edema may not have an increase in total body salt and water content. Pulmonary congestion in this setting may result from an increase in left ventricular filling pressure due to a decrease in the compliance of the left ventricle (diastolic dysfunction) rather than an increase in left ventricular volume per se. With severe hypertension, the ventricle may become noncompliant due to the excessive workload imposed by the elevated systemic vascular resistance. As a result, left ventricular end-diastolic pressure (LVEDP) increases dramatically even though left ventricular end-diastolic volume may be near normal. With vasodilator therapy, the systemic vascular resistance decreases, left ventricular compliance improves, LVEDP decreases, and left ventricular end-diastolic volume may actually increase (194). Despite the increase in left ventricular end-diastolic volume, pulmonary congestion improves because of the reduction in pulmonary capillary pressure. Thus, even in patients with malignant hypertension complicated by pulmonary edema, afterload reduction rather than vigorous diuretic therapy should be the mainstay of initial therapy.

Some patients with malignant hypertension may actually benefit from a cautious trial of volume expansion. Intravascular volume depletion in patients with malignant hypertension should be considered in patients with exquisite sensitivity to vasodilator therapy manifest by a precipitous drop in blood pressure at relatively low infusion rates. Patients with malignant hypertension due to analgesic nephropathy are particularly prone to be severely volume-depleted at presentation due to the presence of chronic interstitial damage with a salt-wasting nephropathy (41,42).

In summary, the need for diuretic therapy during the initial phase of treatment for malignant hypertension depends on an assessment of volume status. Unless obvious fluid overload is present, diuretics should not be given initially. Although vasodilator therapy will eventually result in salt and water retention by the kidney, an increase in total-body sodium content cannot occur unless the patient is given sodium. Thus, in the initial phase of treatment, patients should be placed on a no-added salt diet with close monitoring of intravenous fluid administration. Nonetheless, during subsequent long-term treatment with oral vasodilators, the use of diuretics is usually mandatory in order to prevent fluid retention and maintain adequate blood pressure control.

Management of Malignant Hypertension Complicated by Renal Insufficiency

All patients with malignant hypertension should receive aggressive antihypertensive therapy to prevent further renal damage, regardless of the degree of renal impairment. Control of blood pressure in patients with malignant hypertension and renal insufficiency occasionally precipitates oliguric acute renal failure, especially when the initial glomerular filtration rate is less than 20 mL/minute. However, this is not a contraindication to aggressive antihypertensive therapy aimed at normalization of the blood pressure. Control of hypertension protects other vital organs such as the brain and heart whose function cannot be replaced. Moreover, with tight blood pressure control, even patients who appear to have ESRD due to malignant nephrosclerosis have recovered renal function (95,97,195–205).

In patients in whom aggressive control of hypertension precipitates the need for dialysis, dialysis is utilized to control serum chemistry values, treat uremia, and correct fluid overload. However, since dialysis alone rarely results in adequate control of blood pressure in patients with malignant hypertension, concomitant antihypertensive drug therapy is almost always required. A regimen with minoxidil and propranolol has proved to be particularly efficacious in this setting (95,96,200,203,206,207).

Role of Nephrectomy

In the past, the use of bilateral nephrectomy to control severe hypertension in patients with malignant hypertension and azotemia was advocated (208–210). In many patients with malignant hypertension and uremia accompanied by encephalopathy, bilateral nephrectomy was lifesaving. In 1972, Lazarus and associates (209) proposed a role for urgent bilateral nephrectomy in patients with malignant hypertension who had life-threatening complications such as cerebrovascular accident, rapidly progressive congestive heart failure, or encephalopathy. The authors suggested that nephrectomy might be of value if performed early, even before the development of ESRD. Patients with serum creatinine levels as low as 7.0 mg/dL were sometimes nephrectomized.

However, following the introduction of minoxidil, the role of nephrectomy in the management of malignant hypertension with azotemia was questioned (211). Eleven patients with malignant hypertension who had been refractory to maximal doses of conventional antihypertensive agents were reported. Seven of these patients had advanced renal failure and were candidates for nephrectomy to control blood pressure. Institution of a regimen of minoxidil combined with diuretics or dialysis to control fluid retention and propranolol to control reflex tachycardia resulted in blood pressure reduction to normotensive levels in all patients with remarkably few side effects (207). Even in patients with renal failure requiring dialysis, hypertension can usually be controlled with minoxidil (202,206,207,211). Given the proven efficacy of minoxidil, bilateral nephrectomy is rarely, if ever, indicated to control refractory hypertension. Nephrectomy should clearly be a last resort as delayed recovery of renal function is possible in many cases.

In summary, the long-term management of patients with ESRD secondary to malignant hypertension should include vigorous antihypertensive therapy with the goal of sustained normotension. Dramatic recovery of renal function may occasionally occur. Even if renal function fails to recover, adequate control of blood pressure is essential to prevent other potentially fatal complications of malignant hypertension such as hypertensive encephalopathy, intracerebral hemorrhage, congestive heart failure, and hemorrhagic pancreatitis.

Initial Oral Therapy

While many patients with malignant hypertension require prompt treatment with parenteral antihypertensive agents, some patients may not yet have evidence of cerebral or cardiac complications, or rapidly deteriorating renal function and therefore do not require instantaneous control of the blood pressure (41,190,212,213). These patients may be safely managed with an intensive oral regimen designed to bring the blood pressure under control over a period of 12 to 24 hours.

In patients with malignant hypertension, a multidrug oral regimen is often required to achieve adequate blood pressure control. The most useful combinations include a diuretic, a β-adrenergic blocker, and an arteriolar vasodilator. Minoxidil appears to be particularly well suited for the initial management of malignant hypertension that requires prompt but not immediate blood pressure reduction (212,214–216). Alpert and Bauer (216) describe the use of a triple regimen of furosemide, propranolol, and minoxidil in nine patients with

a diastolic blood pressure higher than 120 mm Hg. Seven of these patients had malignant hypertension. Furosemide (40 mg) and propranolol (40 mg) were given initially by mouth. Two hours later, if the diastolic pressure was higher than 120 mm Hg, a loading dose of minoxidil (20 mg) was administered. If the diastolic pressure was still over 100 mm Hg 4 hours after the loading dose, a booster dose of minoxidil was given. The amount of the booster dose was estimated based on the magnitude of the response to the loading dose. Maintenance therapy with minoxidil was begun with one-half the sum of the loading and booster doses given twice daily, with adjustment of beta-blocker and diuretic doses as necessary for control of heart rate and fluid balance. Following the booster dose of minoxidil, a sustained decrease in blood pressure was seen in all patients. No overshoot hypotension or other adverse effects were encountered. During long-term therapy, the physicians were able to substitute hydralazine for minoxidil in five patients. However, the remaining four patients required chronic minoxidil therapy for adequate blood pressure control (212,216).

Initial oral therapy with sustained-release nifedipine recently was shown to be effective in the management of malignant hypertension in black patients who did not require parenteral therapy for hypertensive encephalopathy or acute pulmonary edema (213). No precipitous decreases in blood pressure or neurologic complications were encountered. However, despite adequate control of blood pressure during the first 24 hours with sustained-released nifedipine, all patients eventually required one or more additional drugs for long-term blood pressure control. Although treatment with sublingual or oral nifedipine capsules has also been recommended for the initial management of malignant hypertension (217,218), the sustained-release nifedipine preparation is preferable because there appears to be less risk of overshoot hypotension (213).

The angiotensin-converting enzyme inhibitors have also been reported to be effective in the treatment of malignant hypertension. However, angiotensin-converting enzyme inhibitors can produce profound hypotension in volume-depleted patients, so they should be used with caution during the initial phase of treatment. Moreover, they may not always be effective in the acute management of malignant hypertension (219).

Oral loading regimens with clonidine have been advocated in severe uncomplicated (urgent) hypertension (220). However, there is limited information on the use of oral clonidine loading in the initial management of malignant hypertension. Clonidine loading can cause significant sedation, which may interfere with the assessment of potential neurologic complications during acute blood pressure reduction. Moreover, common side effects such as sedation and dry mouth can have a negative impact on compliance in patients treated with clonidine for the long term. Thus, oral clonidine loading regimens are not indicated for the initial management of malignant hypertension.

Long-Term Management

After the immediate crisis has resolved and the blood pressure has been brought under control with parenteral therapy, oral therapy, or both, lifelong surveillance of the blood pressure is essential. Close follow-up and aggressive treatment are mandatory because noncompliance or inadequate therapy may have devastating consequences. If blood pressure control becomes inadequate, malignant hypertension may recur even after years of successful antihypertensive therapy. In a study of the quality of care provided to patients with a history of malignant hypertension who subsequently died, only 27% of patients had an average treated diastolic blood pressure of less than 110 mm Hg (221). Thus, meticulous long-term treatment of hypertension is imperative in patients with a history of malignant hypertension. Triple therapy with a diuretic, a beta-blocker, and

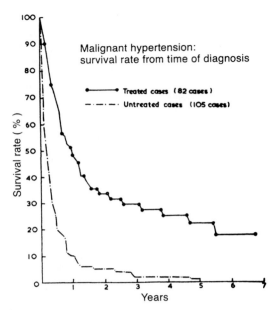

FIGURE 56-19. Survival in patients with malignant hypertension. Treated patients received ganglionic blocking agents. Untreated patients are historical controls from the pretreatment era. (From: Harington M, Kincaid-Smith P, McMichael J. Results of treatment in malignant hypertension: a seven-year experience in 94 cases. *Br Med J* 1959;2:969, with permission.)

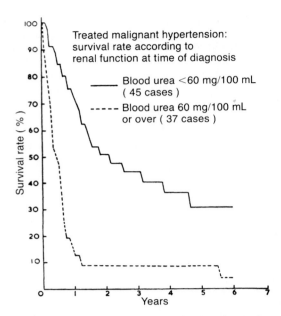

FIGURE 56-20. Survival in treated patients with malignant hypertension according to the level of renal function at the time of initial presentation. (From: Harington M, Kincaid-Smith P, McMichael J. Results of treatment in malignant hypertension: a seven-year experience in 94 cases. *Br Med J* 1959;2:969, with permission.)

a vasodilator is often required to achieve satisfactory blood pressure control.

Response to Therapy

In the absence of adequate blood pressure control, malignant hypertension has a uniformly poor prognosis. Without treatment, the 1-year mortality rate approaches 80% to 90%, and uremia is the most common cause of death (25,26). However, since the introduction of potent antihypertensive agents, studies have shown that with control of blood pressure, dialysis-free survival can be substantially prolonged (130) (Fig. 56-19).

In a more recent series of treated patients collected between 1979 and 1985, the 1-year and 5-year survival rates were 94% and 75%, respectively. The rates for renal survival, defined as patients surviving with native renal function, were 66% at 1 year and 51% at 5 years (32). In another series collected between 1980 and 1989, the 5-year survival was 74% (221). Median survival time was found to be significantly shorter in black patients compared to white or Asian patients (221). The poorer prognosis for black patients could be explained by their late presentation with severe hypertension and the higher prevalence of renal impairment at presentation. The improved patient survival in recent years has been attributed to a decrease in uremic deaths due to not only the availability of dialysis but also the prevention of ESRD because of adequate blood pressure control (28,29). Nonetheless, malignant hypertension remains a disease with a poor overall prognosis associated with a substantial risk of progression to death or chronic renal failure (221).

Prognostic Importance of Renal Function at the Time of Diagnosis

Numerous series have documented the prognostic significance of the level of renal function at the time of the initial presentation with malignant hypertension. In the early studies of the response of malignant hypertension to antihypertensive therapy, those patients with an initial blood urea level higher than 60 mg/dL (BUN greater than 30 mg/dL) had a 13% 1-year survival rate, compared with a 73% 1-year survival rate among those with an initial blood urea less than 60 mg/dL (130) (Fig. 56-20). Thus, with antihypertensive therapy, renal function tended to remain normal in patients with good renal function at presentation. In contrast, despite blood pressure control, renal function often deteriorated in patients with renal insufficiency at presentation. It was concluded that hypotensive therapy did not halt the progression of established renal insufficiency, and that a good long-term prognosis could be anticipated only in patients with nonuremic malignant hypertension.

Based on the experience between 1950 and 1965, most published series concluded that aggressive treatment of malignant hypertension in patients with renal insufficiency often resulted in worsening of renal function and sometimes even precipitated ESRD. As recently as the mid-1960s, it was routinely stated that azotemic patients with malignant hypertension should be managed conservatively, and that if the BUN was higher than 60 mg/dL, no antihypertensive therapy should be undertaken (222). Woods and Blythe were the first to report that treatment of hypertension prolonged survival in patients with malignant hypertension and severe renal insufficiency (223,224). Subsequent studies demonstrated that aggressive antihypertensive therapy could result in substantial improvement in renal function (225,226). The crucial factor in determining the risk of progression to ESRD appeared to be the adequacy of long-term blood pressure control.

There may be two distinct groups of patients with malignant hypertension and renal insufficiency (225). In one group, malignant hypertension is secondary to underlying renal parenchymal disease. Renal biopsy reveals evidence of primary glomerulonephritis with superimposed vascular changes of malignant nephrosclerosis. In this group, initial control of blood pressure may result in a temporary stabilization of renal function. However, despite adequate blood pressure control, eventually the underlying renal disease slowly progresses to end-stage. In the other group, primary (essential) malignant hypertension is present and renal biopsy reveals only malignant nephrosclerosis with ischemic glomeruli. In these patients, intensive antihypertensive therapy may result in an improvement in renal function, especially if initial renal impairment is mild to moderate. Even in patients with severe renal impairment, recovery of renal function sometimes occurs during sustained normotension. However, many months of therapy may be required before recovery of renal function is apparent, presumably reflecting the time required for resolution of the vascular lesions (205).

Recently, the observation has been made that the combined length of the two kidneys at presentation (combined renal length) as determined by ultrasonography is predictive of the chance for recovery of renal function in patients with malignant hypertension and severe renal failure (227). The mean combined renal length was 20.2 cm in the group that recovered renal function and 14.2 cm in the group with persistent renal failure despite strict blood pressure control.

Despite the prognostic significance of the initial level of renal function in patients with malignant hypertension (32), a number of recent reports describe dramatic recovery of renal function in patients with presumed ESRD due to malignant nephrosclerosis, even after maintenance hemodialysis for months to years. Recovery of renal function in these cases has been attributed to strict control of blood pressure. These reports challenged the notion that established renal failure in malignant hypertension is irreversible (95,96,195–205). In the majority of these reports, recovery of renal function was associated with the use of the potent peripheral vasodilator minoxidil in combination with a β-adrenergic blocking drug and dialysis. Often patients who had refractory hypertension or disabling side effects while taking maximal doses of conventional antihypertensive agents eventually became normotensive with minimal side effects after the initiation of this regimen (206,207). Recovery of renal function with strict control of blood pressure has been reported up to 26 months after the initiation of maintenance hemodialysis (96). In most of the reports describing the recovery of renal function after prolonged maintenance dialysis, the initial clinical presentation was that of oliguric acute renal failure (200). In the largest reported series, 12 out of 54 patients with primary malignant hypertension requiring dialysis recovered sufficient renal function to allow withdrawal of dialysis (228). Substantially delayed recovery of renal function following initiation of dialysis for malignant nephrosclerosis is thus a distinct possibility and should be considered in such patients before long-term strategies such as renal transplantation are contemplated (205). In the modern treatment era it appears that the severity of malignant hypertension and the magnitude of renal impairment at presentation do not always predict outcome (229). Instead, the best predictor of long-term renal function seems to be the adequacy of the blood pressure control obtained during follow-up.

In patients with malignant hypertension who progressed to ESRD and were treated with long-term dialysis, the survival rates at 1, 5, and 8 years were 87%, 82%, and 50%, respectively. This was not different from age-matched controls with other causes of renal failure admitted to the same dialysis unit (230). One study found that the chance of recovery of renal function was better for patients with primary malignant hypertension treated with continuous ambulatory peritoneal dialysis compared with conventional hemodialysis (231).

Mechanism of Recovery of Renal Function

The mechanism of recovery after prolonged renal failure in malignant hypertension is uncertain. Extensive tubular damage resembling acute tubular necrosis has been reported in patients with oliguric acute renal failure (97,200). This tubular damage is thought to result from ischemia caused by the obliterative vascular lesions of malignant nephrosclerosis. In this regard, it has been postulated that the mechanism of recovery is the resolution of tubular necrosis (200). However, it is not clear why the need for dialysis often persists well beyond the usual time frame for resolution of ischemia-induced acute tubular necrosis.

Kincaid-Smith postulated that the initial loss of renal function results from glomerular ischemia due to narrowing of the interlobular arteries by proliferative endarteritis (41). Although endarteritis may be arrested by adequate blood pressure control, narrowing of the arterioles may persist. Therefore, improvement in renal function may not result from the resolution of arteriolar lesions, but rather from hyperfiltration by the remaining nephrons supplied by patent interlobular arteries. Regardless of the mechanism, it is clear that recovery of renal function is critically dependent on sustained normalization of blood pressure.

Reversal of Hypertensive Neuroretinopathy

The funduscopic changes associated with hypertensive neuroretinopathy are reversible with control of blood pressure (85,232). Striate hemorrhages cease to form as soon as the blood pressure is controlled. Clearance of existing hemorrhages takes 2 to 8 weeks. Cotton-wool spots may continue to form for several days after the blood pressure is controlled. The cellular (axonal) debris that comprises the cotton-wool spots is cleared away within 2 to 12 weeks. Hard exudates clear more slowly. A macular star may require more than a year to resolve completely. Papilledema often continues to increase during the first few days of treatment. However, in the majority of patients, it resolves slowly over several weeks. In contrast, the changes reflecting retinal arteriolosclerosis such as arteriolar narrowing, arteriovenous crossing defects, and changes in the light reflexes usually persist despite adequate blood pressure control (232).

Evaluation for Secondary Causes

The various secondary causes of malignant hypertension were discussed previously in the section on etiologies of malignant hypertension. Whereas less than 5% of patients with benign hypertension have an underlying secondary cause of hypertension, malignant hypertension may be associated with a secondary cause in up to 50% of patients. For example, among patients with benign hypertension, the incidence of renovascular hypertension was less than 0.5% (233). In contrast, there is a substantial incidence of renovascular hypertension (43% in whites, 7% in blacks) among patients with malignant hypertension (46). Thus, after malignant hypertension has been treated successfully, the possibility of underlying renovascular hypertension should be investigated. Noninvasive screening tests such as rapid sequence intravenous pyelography and radionuclide renal scans are of little value because of the high frequency of false-positive and false-negative results (233). Renal arteriography is the procedure of choice to exclude the possibility of anatomic renal artery stenosis. The diagnosis and treatment of renovascular hypertension is discussed in detail in Chapter 52.

Pheochromocytoma is a rare cause of malignant hypertension. However, given the likelihood of surgical cure or amelioration of hypertension, pheochromocytoma should be considered if symptoms consistent with catecholamine excess persist following control of blood pressure. The approach to the diagnosis of pheochromocytoma is discussed in Chapter 55.

Primary hyperaldosteronism due to an adrenal aldosterone-producing adenoma is an extremely rare cause of malignant hypertension. However, the biochemical abnormalities in patients with treated malignant hypertension may mimic those of primary hyperaldosteronism. Long after the malignant phase has resolved, hypokalemia with inappropriate urinary potassium wasting, increased aldosterone secretion, and suppressed PRA may persist. This phenomenon may represent a form of tertiary hyperaldosteronism (63). With sustained treatment of hypertension, this hyperaldosteronism eventually resolves. Because primary hyperaldosteronism is an unusual cause of malignant hypertension, an evaluation for primary hyperaldosteronism should not be undertaken unless these abnormalities persist for more than a year after malignant hypertension has resolved.

The role of renal biopsy in the diagnosis of possible underlying primary renal parenchymal disease in patients with malignant hypertension is controversial. In patients presenting with malignant hypertension and renal failure, it may not be possible on clinical grounds to distinguish primary malignant hypertension from chronic glomerulonephritis or chronic interstitial nephritis with superimposed malignant nephrosclerosis. A renal biopsy may be required to make this distinction. When the kidneys appear small by ultrasonography, a biopsy is not indicated because it is unlikely that the results of the biopsy will alter therapy. In contrast, when the kidneys are normal in size, a renal biopsy may provide useful information. If primary malignant nephrosclerosis with ischemic but viable glomeruli is found, then intensive antihypertensive therapy may be associated with the eventual recovery of renal function, even after months of maintenance dialysis. Conversely, the finding of chronic glomerulonephritis or chronic interstitial nephritis with superimposed malignant nephrosclerosis suggests a less favorable long-term outcome.

Malignant hypertension can mimic acute glomerulonephritis or vasculitis. Patients can present with severe hypertension and oliguric acute renal failure with a nephritic urinary sediment (97). In this setting, diagnostic renal biopsy is essential since acute glomerulonephritis or vasculitis may require specific therapy in addition to antihypertensive treatment.

Since uremia and severe hypertension predispose to serious hemorrhagic complications after renal biopsy, it is prudent to manage the patient with dialysis and blood pressure control for 1 to 3 weeks prior to performance of a percutaneous renal biopsy. Unfortunately, this delay in obtaining tissue may make the diagnosis of malignant nephrosclerosis more difficult because the lesions of fibrinoid necrosis may heal rapidly with the institution of antihypertensive treatment, leaving a residual hyaline or fibrous scar (130,132). Moreover, given the sampling error inherent in closed renal biopsy, the patchy lesions of malignant nephrosclerosis might be missed. Thus, the diagnosis of malignant nephrosclerosis is often made on the basis of the findings of accelerated glomerular obsolescence and marked intimal hyperplasia of the arterioles (126).

Unilateral renal disease from atrophic pyelonephritis occasionally causes malignant hypertension in both children and adults (22,39,40). However, the experience with unilateral nephrectomy for hypertension control has been disappointing (234). In children, cure of malignant hypertension has been reported after partial nephrectomy of a scarred segment if high renin values are documented on segmental renal vein catheterization (235,236).

Benign Versus Malignant Hypertension

Since the original description by Volhard and Fahr (12), two forms of essential hypertension have been recognized, benign and malignant. It is worth emphasizing that these two forms of hypertension should be conceptualized as distinct clinical and pathologic entities. In benign hypertension there is usually a long asymptomatic phase, with death resulting from complications of cerebrovascular disease, atherosclerotic disease, or congestive heart failure, rather than renal disease (29). In benign essential hypertension (i.e., without underlying primary renal disease or superimposition of malignant hypertension), ESRD seldom occurs (81,93,125,237,238). In contrast, malignant hypertension left untreated, uniformly progresses to ESRD.

There is much controversy in the field of hypertension regarding the frequency with which benign hypertension (benign arteriolar nephrosclerosis), in the absence of occult primary renal disease or superimposed malignant hypertension, causes ESRD. Recent reviews suggest that the number of patients reaching ESRD attributable to benign nephrosclerosis might have been significantly overestimated (239,240). Goldring and Chasis (93) extensively evaluated renal function in a large group of patients with essential hypertension in the pre-antihypertensive treatment era. Most patients with long-standing essential hypertension had anatomic lesions in kidneys consistent with hyaline arteriolar nephrosclerosis. Moreover, the majority had demonstrable renal abnormalities including abnormal urinalysis with hyaline and granular casts, low-grade proteinuria (less than 1 g/day), decreased tubular maximum for para-aminohippurate, decreased renal blood flow, normal to slightly decreased glomerular filtration rate, and increased filtration fraction. However, they found that ESRD rarely occurred in patients with benign hypertension. Among 150 hypertensive patients with ESRD, only one was found to have benign nephrosclerosis as the sole underlying etiology (93). These authors concluded that in patients with benign hypertension, functional failure occurred earlier in the heart and brain than in the kidney and that death from renal failure without superimposed malignant hypertension was a rare event.

In contrast to these early reports, which were based principally on renal histologic findings at autopsy, in more recent series, "hypertensive nephrosclerosis" is listed as a common cause of ESRD, especially among African American patients. For example, blacks have a four- to eightfold elevation in the risk of hypertension-induced ESRD compared to whites (241,242). The studies suggest that much of the excess risk of ESRD among blacks can be explained by an extraordinarily high rate of renal failure from hypertensive nephrosclerosis. On a national scale, an estimated 29% of blacks with ESRD have hypertension as the primary cause (241). However, in these recent studies, classification of the causes of ESRD was based on clinical rather than histologic evidence. Furthermore, in these studies it was not clear whether the term *hypertensive nephrosclerosis* refers to benign or malignant nephrosclerosis. In the few available studies detailing the pathologic findings in blacks with ESRD due to hypertension, the characteristic findings have been those of malignant nephrosclerosis, namely, musculomucoid intimal hyperplasia of the interlobular arteries and accelerated glomerular obsolescence (35,173). Moreover, there appears to be a racial bias with regard to the diagnosis of hypertensive nephrosclerosis. In a recent survey, nephrologists were asked to review identical case histories of patients with ESRD in which only the race of the patient was randomly assigned as either black or white. It was found that black patients were twice as likely as white patients to be labeled as having ESRD secondary to hypertensive nephrosclerosis (243).

The relationship between essential hypertension and ESRD remains circumstantial despite the fact that these syndromes have long been associated in the medical literature (240). Nephrologists credit essential hypertension as the cause of ESRD in 25% of patients initiating Medicare-supported renal replacement therapy. Surprisingly, the widely held notion that benign hypertension with benign nephrosclerosis is a common cause of ESRD is difficult to support (81,239,240,244). In contrast to the large body of literature relating mild to moderate benign hypertension to excessive cardiovascular morbidity, there is a dearth of information available regarding the corresponding risk of significant renal disease (244). In available studies, serum creatinine levels infrequently increase in patients with long-standing mild to moderate hypertension. An analysis of the data from three recent large clinical trials in patients with essential hypertension revealed that advanced renal failure developed in less than 1% of 10,000 patients during the 4 to 6 years of follow-up (89,245–247). Moreover, a very low incidence of clinically significant deterioration of renal function was also noted in the Hypertension Detection and Follow-up Program (248). Another study of untreated patients with mild to moderate essential hypertension found only minor declines in glomerular filtration rate (1.6%/year) and renal blood flow (2.1%/year), which did not differ from the renal function decline associated with aging in normotensive individuals (249). Even severe untreated hypertension (diastolic blood pressure, 120 to 150 mm Hg), in the absence of a malignant hypertension (hypertensive neuroretinopathy), caused only a minor decrement in glomerular filtration rate (1.7%/year) (249). Thus, hypertensive nephrosclerosis is commonly reported to Medicare as the cause of ESRD despite the fact that the risk of progressive renal dysfunction in clinical studies of patients with essential hypertension appears to be very low. This paradox could possibly be explained by the fact that the number of patients with essential hypertension is so large that even the small percentage at risk constitutes a relatively large number of patients who eventually develop ESRD. Long-term follow-up data from the Multiple Risk Factor Intervention Trial (MRFIT), in which over 322,000 men were screened for possible entry, support this hypothesis (250). A direct correlation was found between the initial blood pressure and the risk of development of ESRD from any cause at 16-year follow-up. Nonetheless, the age-adjusted rate of ERSD in this group was only 0.34% at 16 years.

Patients classified as having hypertensive ESRD typically present with advanced disease, making the processes that initiated the renal disease difficult to discern. It has been proposed that many patients classified as having hypertensive nephrosclerosis actually have intrinsic renal parenchymal disease (often IgA nephropathy), unrecognized renal artery stenosis with ischemic nephropathy, unrecognized episodes of malignant hypertension, or primary renal microvascular disease (239,240). At least among white patients with hypertension and renal impairment, if renal artery stenosis and malignant hypertension have been excluded, the most likely diagnosis is underlying primary renal parenchymal disease rather than benign nephrosclerosis (81,251).

In contrast to these studies, a provocative study found that mild to moderate benign hypertension did cause renal insufficiency that progressed despite adequate blood pressure control (252). However, since renal biopsies were not performed, the data do not exclude the possibility of occult primary renal parenchymal disease in patients demonstrating progressive renal insufficiency (253).

In summary, while it is clear that malignant hypertension is a frequent cause of ESRD, especially among blacks, there remains considerable controversy regarding the commonly held belief that benign hypertension *per se* commonly causes ESRD. The critical issue that has yet to be resolved is why blacks constitute a disproportionately high percentage of patients with ESRD in the United States (241). Epidemiologic studies suggest that essential hypertension occurs more frequently in blacks and is associated with more severe cardiovascular end-organ damage for any given level of blood pressure (254). In angiographic studies of patients with mild to moderate essential hypertension and normal renal function, blacks tended to have more severe angiographic evidence of nephrosclerosis than did whites (255). Tobian postulates that the low-potassium

diet characteristically consumed by blacks in the United States (30 mmol/day versus 65 mmol/day in the general population) accelerates the intimal thickening of the renal vasculature that occurs due to hypertensive damage. He proposes that this might account for the increased risk of progressive renal insufficiency due to hypertension among blacks (173).

There are several other plausible explanations for the high frequency with which hypertensive nephrosclerosis is reported as a cause of ESRD in the black population. Since most of the available data are based on clinical diagnoses, there may be a tendency on the part of physicians to identify hypertension as the cause of ESRD given the known high prevalence of hypertension in blacks, even when a primary renal parenchymal disease cannot be excluded on clinical grounds (244). Another possibility is that blacks with essential hypertension tend to develop more severe benign nephrosclerosis, which, unlike benign nephrosclerosis in whites, more often results in progressive renal insufficiency and ESRD (240). Results from the African American Study of Kidney Disease (AASK) Trial indicate that benign nephrosclerosis can be accurately diagnosed in black patients with hypertension and renal insufficiency. A renal biopsy was performed in 39 nondiabetic black patients with chronic renal failure who did not have marked proteinuria (urine protein to creatinine ratio less than 2.0). Only changes compatible with benign nephrosclerosis were seen in 38 patients. The remaining patient most likely had primary focal segmental glomerulosclerosis (256). It is possible that genetic factors may increase the susceptibility of blacks to renal damage induced by benign hypertension. Animal studies in which genetically different but histocompatible kidneys were exposed to the same blood pressure in an individual host have clearly demonstrated that some kidneys are more sensitive than others to hypertension-induced renal damage (257). Finally, it is possible that recurrent bouts of unrecognized or inadequately treated malignant hypertension are an underestimated cause of the high incidence of ESRD in minority populations. In this regard, a recent study of 100 patients admitted to an inner-city hospital with a diagnosis of hypertensive emergency showed that two-thirds had malignant hypertension based on funduscopic findings (258). These patients were predominantly young, male, black, or Hispanic individuals of lower socioeconomic status. At least 93% of these patients had been previously diagnosed as hypertensive, and at least 83% were aware of their diagnosis of hypertension. At least 87% were known to have received prior pharmacologic treatment for hypertension. However, no source of regular health care could be documented in 60% of patients. More than 50% were noted to have stopped their antihypertensive medications more than 30 days prior to admission and only 24% had taken any medication on the day of admission. If the overrepresentation of young blacks with ESRD is due to undiagnosed or inadequately treated malignant hypertension, this would have tremendous public health implications given that because malignant hypertension is clearly preventable, and even significant renal dysfunction is potentially reversible with tight control of blood pressure.

HYPERTENSIVE ENCEPHALOPATHY

Most of the deleterious effects of hypertension on the brain are the result of long-standing mild to moderate elevations of blood pressure, including atherothrombotic infarction, lacunar infarction, and intracerebral hemorrhage. Occasionally, severe acute hypertension can produce dramatic and life-threatening cerebral complications. Hypertensive encephalopathy is an acute cerebral syndrome that develops in association with a sudden, sustained elevation of blood pressure (106). It can occur with malignant hypertension or severe hypertension that is not accompanied by hypertensive neuroretinopathy. Hypertensive encephalopathy is a medical emergency that demands prompt diagnosis and rapid control of blood pressure to prevent irreversible brain damage or death. The clinical *sine qua non* of hypertensive encephalopathy is the prompt resolution of symptoms when the blood pressure is brought under control.

Clinical Presentation

The diagnosis of hypertensive encephalopathy is usually made on clinical grounds. The appearance of cerebral symptoms usually follows the sudden onset of hypertension in previously normotensive individuals or an abrupt increase in blood pressure in patients with chronic hypertension. The abrupt blood pressure elevation usually occurs 12 to 48 hours before the onset of symptoms, although this is often difficult to document. Symptoms may appear at lower levels of blood pressure in previously normotensive individuals compared to those with chronic hypertension. For example, in children with acute glomerulonephritis or pregnant women with eclampsia, hypertensive encephalopathy may occur when the blood pressure is no higher than 160/100 mm Hg (259). However, the syndrome rarely occurs in chronically hypertensive individuals at pressures less than 200/120 mm Hg and may not occur until the blood pressure is more than 250/150 mm Hg.

The initial symptom of hypertensive encephalopathy is usually a severe, generalized headache that increases steadily in severity (260). Unfortunately, headache is a nonspecific symptom, and even among patients with malignant hypertension, it does not necessarily imply central nervous system damage (105). Weakness, nausea, and vomiting (sometimes projectile) are often present. Neck stiffness is an occasional finding. Loss of vision is another common feature. Visual loss may be caused by the retinal edema and hemorrhages that accompany hypertensive neuroretinopathy or as the result of cortical (occipital) blindness (261). Denial of visual loss or loss of vision in the presence of a normal light reflex suggests cortical blindness.

Altered mental status is a prominent clinical feature of hypertensive encephalopathy. Apathy, somnolence, and confusion are the initial manifestations that usually appear several hours to days after the onset of headache. If treatment is not instituted, coma and death can occur. Recurrent seizures are common, and they can be either focal or generalized.

There are numerous reports of transient focal neurologic disturbances in patients with hypertensive encephalopathy including fleeting paresthesias and numbness in the extremities, transient paralysis, and aphasia (106,261). Thus, the presence of focal neurologic deficit in a patient with severe hypertension does not necessarily exclude the diagnosis of hypertensive encephalopathy.

Hypertensive neuroretinopathy (striate hemorrhages, cotton-wool spots, and papilledema) is present when hypertensive encephalopathy occurs in patients with malignant hypertension. However, it may be absent when hypertensive encephalopathy develops in the setting of acute glomerulonephritis, eclampsia, monoamine oxidase inhibitor–tyramine interactions, antihypertensive drug withdrawal syndromes, or pheochromocytoma (259,261,262).

Many authors have cautioned that lumbar puncture should be avoided in patients with suspected hypertensive encephalopathy because of the risk of cerebellar herniation (26,263). When performed, lumbar puncture has revealed elevated CSF pressure in most patients ranging from 230 to 560 mm of water (137,261). CSF protein concentration is usually moderately elevated (48 to 90 mg/dL) but may be normal. The cell count is usually normal (137,261), but neu-

trophilic pleocytosis has also been reported in hypertensive encephalopathy (264).

Computerized tomography and magnetic resonance imaging (MRI) reveal characteristic findings in hypertensive encephalopathy (260,263,265,266). Abnormalities on imaging include areas of low white-matter attenuation on computerized tomography scans and T1-weighted hypointense and T2-weighted hyperintense areas on MRI (267,268). These changes probably represent cerebral edema with increased water in the white matter. The most common location of the white-matter abnormalities on neuroimaging is the posterior regions of the cerebral hemispheres. The multifocal abnormalities include both hemispheres and tend to be symmetric (266). Commonly involved areas in descending order of frequency include the occipital lobes, the posterior parietal lobes, and the posterior temporal lobes. The pons, the thalamus, and the cerebellum are occasionally involved. The term *reversible posterior leukoencephalopathy syndrome* has been coined to describe patients with these typical radiographic findings and a reversible syndrome of headache, altered mental status, seizures, and loss of vision (266). A reversible hypertensive brainstem encephalopathy with predominant involvement of the brainstem and relative sparing of supratentorial regions has also been reported (269).

Etiologies

Although hypertensive encephalopathy can complicate malignant hypertension, not all patients with hypertensive encephalopathy have malignant hypertension. In fact, it most commonly occurs in previously normotensive individuals who experience sudden, severe hypertension (Table 56-5). The reported causes of hypertensive encephalopathy include acute glomerulonephritis (260,261,269), eclampsia (270, 271), renovascular hypertension (259), postcoronary artery bypass hypertension (272), clonidine withdrawal (273), monoamine oxidase inhibitor–tyramine interactions (274), pheochromocytoma (275), phencyclidine (PCP) poisoning (276), licorice ingestion (277), phenylpropanolamine overdose (278,279), acute renal artery occlusion (261), acute lead poisoning (261), immunosuppressive therapy with cyclosporine or tacrolimus for kidney, liver, or bone marrow transplantation (266,280,281),

TABLE 56-5

ETIOLOGIES OF HYPERTENSIVE ENCEPHALOPATHY

Malignant hypertension of any etiology
Acute glomerulonephritis
Eclampsia
Renovascular hypertension
Postcoronary artery bypass hypertension
Abrupt withdrawal of antihypertensive therapy
Monoamine oxidase inhibitor-tyramine interactions
Pheochromocytoma
Phencyclidine (PCP) poisoning
Phenylpropanolamine overdose
Recombinant erythropoietin therapy in dialysis patients
Scorpion envenomation, especially in children
Cocaine hydrochloride or alkaloidal (crack) cocaine
Acute renal artery occlusion
Acute lead poisoning in children
Cyclosporine-induced or tacrolimus-induced hypertension
Transplant renal artery stenosis or acute rejection
Femoral lengthening procedures
Acute or chronic spinal cord injuries

chemotherapy for acute leukemia in children (282), transplant renal artery stenosis or acute rejection (283,284), and femoral lengthening procedures in children (285). The preeclampsia–eclampsia syndrome has been hypothesized to reflect a subtype of hypertensive encephalopathy accompanied by impaired cerebral autoregulation and endothelial dysfunction (8,262,266,270, 271). The clinical and radiographic findings in patients with cyclosporine-induced neurotoxicity have been found to be identical to those seen in hypertensive encephalopathy (281). The only major factor found to be associated with the neurotoxic effect of cyclosporine in all patients was hypertension. Subcortical edema, affecting the posterior regions of the brain, tends to resolve following reduction in blood pressure, with or without concomitant reduction in cyclosporine dose. Hypertensive encephalopathy may also occur in patients with acute or chronic spinal cord injuries if there is autonomic hyperreflexia due to bowel or bladder distention (286,287). Acute elevation of blood pressure during recombinant human erythropoietin therapy occasionally results in hypertensive encephalopathy and seizures (288). This complication is unrelated to the extent or rate of increase in hematocrit, but is associated with a rapid increase in blood pressure and may occur in previously normotensive patients. Scorpion envenomization results in stimulation of the autonomic nervous system and adrenals and in children can lead to severe hypertension and a clinical picture consistent with hypertensive encephalopathy (289). Cocaine use can also induce a sudden increase in blood pressure accompanied by hypertensive encephalopathy (290).

Pathogenesis

The breakthrough theory of autoregulation originally proposed by Lassen and Angoli (291) is the generally accepted view of the pathogenesis of hypertensive encephalopathy (Fig. 56-21). Under normal circumstances, there is autoregulation of the cerebral microcirculation such that over a wide range of perfusion pressures, cerebral blood flow remains con-

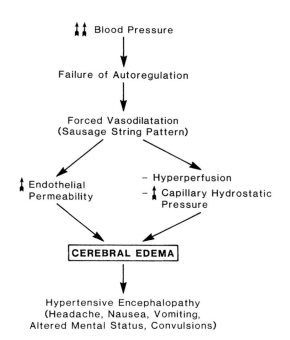

FIGURE 56-21. The breakthrough theory of hypertensive encephalopathy.

stant. It has been proposed that in the setting of a sudden, severe increase in blood pressure, autoregulatory vasoconstriction fails, and there is forced vasodilation. The dilation is initially segmental (sausage-string pattern), but eventually becomes diffuse. The endothelium in the dilated segments becomes abnormally permeable, and there is extravasation of plasma components with the development of cerebral edema. This theory may explain the clinical observation that hypertensive encephalopathy develops at a much lower blood pressure in previously normotensive individuals than it does in those with chronic hypertension. With long-standing hypertension, structural changes and remodeling of the cerebral arterioles may lead to a shift in the autoregulatory curve such that much higher perfusion pressures can be tolerated before forced vasodilation and breakthrough of autoregulation occur (292,293).

Strandgaard and co-workers (294) report studies on the regulation of cerebral blood flow in baboons with acute hypertension. Cerebral blood flow was measured using the xenon washout technique as the blood pressure was gradually increased during angiotensin II infusion. Cerebral blood flow remained constant up to a mean arterial pressure of 120 to 139 mm Hg by virtue of an increase in cerebrovascular resistance (intact autoregulation). However, at this level of mean arterial pressure, cerebrovascular resistance reached a maximum. At higher mean arterial pressures, cerebral blood flow increased significantly as cerebrovascular resistance decreased, consistent with a breakthrough of autoregulation. There was no evidence of spasm or decreased cerebral blood flow (overregulation) in response to severe hypertension.

Hypertensive-induced damage to the blood-brain barrier develops within minutes of a sudden, marked increase in blood pressure (296). The injury is most likely due to overstretching of vessels rather than from spasm and ischemia, as hypoxic injury to the blood-brain barrier would require several hours to develop (295). In a rat model of hypertensive encephalopathy due to one-kidney, one-clip renovascular hypertension, the sausage-string pattern develops in pial vessels in response to severe hypertension. Injection of colloidal carbon particles demonstrates that there is increased vascular permeability in the dilated segments (148).

Structural damage to the blood-brain barrier may not be required for the formation of cerebral edema in response to sudden hypertension. Cerebral arterioles and capillaries become abnormally permeable to protein-bound dyes within seconds after induction of severe hypertension (297). Pinocytotic vessels transport these large molecular markers through the structural components of the blood-brain barrier during periods of acute hypertension. The passage of protein molecules by pinocytosis may result in the extravascular accumulation of protein-rich fluid (cerebral edema).

Treatment

The treatment of choice for hypertensive encephalopathy is prompt reduction of blood pressure. When the diagnosis of hypertensive encephalopathy seems likely, antihypertensive therapy should be initiated prior to obtaining the results of time-consuming laboratory and radiologic examinations. The goal of therapy, especially in the previously normotensive patient with acute hypertension, should be the reduction of blood pressure to normal or near-normal levels as quickly as possible (259). Although cerebral blood flow could theoretically be jeopardized by failure of autoregulation during rapid reduction of blood pressure in patients with chronic hypertension (292,293), clinical experience has shown that the prompt reduction of blood pressure with the avoidance of frank hypotension is beneficial in patients with hypertensive encephalopathy

(259). Of the conditions in the differential diagnosis of hypertension with acute cerebral dysfunction, only cerebral infarction might be adversely affected by the abrupt reduction of blood pressure (298). Pharmacologic agents that have a rapid onset and short duration of action such as sodium nitroprusside or possibly fenoldopam should be utilized so that the blood pressure can be carefully titrated with close monitoring of the patient's neurologic status. The clinical *sine qua non* of hypertensive encephalopathy is a prompt clinical response to blood pressure reduction. Conversely, when antihypertensive therapy is associated with the development of new or progressive neurologic deficits, other diagnoses should be considered, and the blood pressure should be stabilized at a higher level.

In women with eclampsia, convulsions and other neurologic manifestations occur and are indistinguishable from those observed in nonpregnant individuals with hypertensive encephalopathy, except that in eclampsia they occur at a lower level of blood pressure (271). Eclampsia is associated with extreme risk to both the mother and the fetus. Although delivery of the fetus is the definitive cure in most cases, rapid control of the blood pressure and encephalopathic manifestations is essential before the induction of labor or performance of a cesarean section (262,270).

ACUTE HYPERTENSIVE HEART FAILURE

Both malignant hypertension and severe benign hypertension can be complicated by acute pulmonary edema. Acute fulminant pulmonary edema was a frequent cause of death among patients with malignant hypertension in the preantihypertensive treatment era (25,30). However, with the advent of effective antihypertensive therapy, the prognosis for hypertensive patients with left ventricular failure has improved dramatically.

Traditionally, congestive heart failure has been equated with systolic dysfunction in which there is an inability of the myofibrils to shorten against a load such that the left ventricle loses its ability to eject blood into the high-pressure aorta. The end result is a dilated, poorly contractile left ventricle with a low ejection fraction and a reduced cardiac output. However, in recent years, there has been increasing recognition that hypertension very frequently causes abnormalities in the diastolic function of the left ventricle that result in symptoms of congestive heart failure despite the presence of a normal ejection fraction and normal cardiac output (299–302). Diastolic dysfunction implies that the ventricle cannot fill normally at low filling pressures. Ventricular filling is slow, delayed, or incomplete unless the atrial pressure increases (299,301). A compensatory increase in filling pressure occurs and is sufficient to maintain normal systolic function but at the expense of pulmonary and systemic venous congestion. Thus, signs and symptoms of pulmonary or systemic venous congestion are not always the result of systolic dysfunction; instead, they may result from isolated abnormalities of the diastolic properties of the left ventricle. The treatment of hypertension-associated heart failure varies depending on whether the diastolic dysfunction manifests as chronic congestive heart failure or a hypertensive crisis with acute pulmonary edema.

Hypertensive patients with chronic congestive heart failure manifested by dyspnea and symptoms of pulmonary and systemic venous congestion are not infrequently found to have isolated diastolic dysfunction as defined by echocardiographic or radionuclide evaluation of diastolic filling (300,302,303). Thus, in patients with hypertension, left ventricular hypertrophy, and evidence of congestive heart failure, the possibility of hypertensive cardiomyopathy with chronic diastolic dysfunc-

tion should be considered. The left ventricular hypertrophy that develops in response to chronic systemic hypertension may cause abnormal myocardial relaxation and increased left ventricular chamber stiffness, which lead to the impairment in diastolic filling that characterizes diastolic dysfunction. In clinical practice the presence of dyspnea, pulmonary rales, and radiographic evidence of pulmonary venous congestion, despite a normal ejection fraction, should suggest the possibility of diastolic dysfunction (299). Traditional treatment for congestive heart failure with digitalis and arterial vasodilators may be deleterious in patients with isolated diastolic dysfunction due to hypertensive heart disease (303). This type of chronic diastolic dysfunction in hypertensive patients is best managed with beta-blockers, calcium channel blockers, or both. These drugs decrease heart rate and improve the balance between myocardial oxygen supply and demand and thus may improve myocardial relaxation and overall diastolic function. Classes of drugs that are associated with regression of left ventricular hypertrophy such as angiotensin-converting enzyme inhibitors, nondihydropyridine calcium channel blockers, beta-blockers, and centrally acting α-adrenergic agonists may result in an improvement in diastolic function as the hypertrophy regresses (304). Diuretics and salt restriction may be used to treat congestive symptoms but care should be taken to avoid excessive preload reduction that may compromise systolic function (299). Venodilation and preload reduction with nitrates may also improve symptoms of pulmonary congestion (299).

Isolated diastolic dysfunction is also the pathophysiologic process that underlies the development of acute pulmonary edema in patients with either malignant hypertension or severe benign hypertension. However, in the setting of *acute hypertensive heart failure*, the proximate cause of the left ventricular diastolic dysfunction is the markedly increased workload imposed on the heart by a pronounced increase in systemic vascular resistance (194,305). Hypertension complicated by acute pulmonary edema represents a crisis requiring immediate control of blood pressure with potent peripheral vasodilators, such as sodium nitroprusside, in order to quickly reduce the high systemic vascular resistance that underlies this disorder.

The hemodynamic derangements in acute hypertensive heart failure were characterized in a study comparing five patients with severe long-standing essential hypertension complicated by acute pulmonary edema with a control group of five patients of similar age who had long-standing hypertension of similar severity but who had no history of congestive heart failure (194,305). The subjects in both groups had electrocardiographic evidence of left ventricular hypertrophy and chest radiographic evidence of cardiomegaly with left ventricular prominence. However, pulmonary venous engorgement was evident only in the group with heart failure. The hemodynamic findings in the two groups of severely hypertensive patients are displayed in Figure 56-22. The mean arterial pressure, heart rate, cardiac index, and stroke work index were the same in both groups. The left ventricular end-diastolic volume was similarly elevated in both groups. In fact, the only hemodynamic difference between the two groups was a significant elevation of left ventricular filling pressure (pulmonary capillary wedge pressure) in the patients with acute hypertensive heart failure. Thus in this small series of patients with acute hypertensive heart failure, systolic function was normal as evidenced by the normal resting cardiac index. The finding of elevated left ventricular end-diastolic pressure (LVEDP) despite normal ejection fractions and cardiac indices implies the presence of isolated diastolic dysfunction. The increase in LVEDP was not the result of volume overload because the left ventricular end-diastolic volume was the same in both groups (Fig. 56-22). The increase in left ventricular filling pressure despite a similar end-diastolic volume can only be explained on the basis of a decrease in left ventricular compliance in the patients with acute

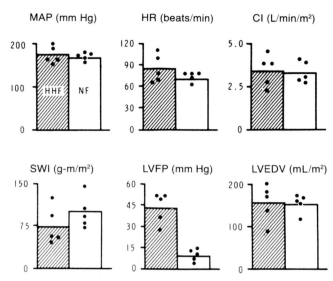

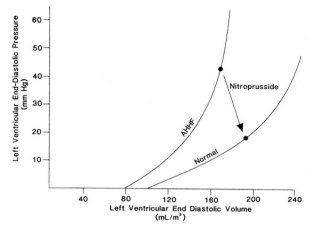

FIGURE 56-23. Schematic representation of the left ventricular end-diastolic pressure–volume relationship in a patient with acute hypertensive heart failure (AHHF) treated with sodium nitroprusside. In AHHF, the pressure–volume curve is shifted up and to the left, reflecting a decrease in left ventricular (LV) compliance. A higher than normal left ventricular end-diastolic pressure (LVEDP) is required to achieve any level of left ventricular end-diastolic volume (LVEDV). Normal LV systolic function is maintained but at the expense of a very high wedge pressure, which results in acute pulmonary edema. Treatment with sodium nitroprusside causes a reduction in the high systemic vascular resistance with a concomitant decrease in impedance to LV ejection. As a result, LV compliance improves. Pulmonary edema resolves due to a reduction in LVEDP despite the fact that LVEDV actually increases during sodium nitroprusside infusion.

FIGURE 56-22. Pretreatment hemodynamics in patients with acute hypertensive heart failure (HHF) and those with severe hypertension but without heart failure (NF). *CI,* cardiac index; *HR,* heart rate; *LVEDV,* left ventricular end-diastolic volume; *LVFP,* left ventricular filling pressure; *MAP,* mean arterial pressure; *SWI,* stroke work index. The MAP, HR, SWI, and LVEDV were the same in both groups. The only difference between the groups was a significant elevation of LVFP in the patients with HHF. These findings suggest a decrease in left ventricular compliance in the patients with HHF, as the LVFP was significantly increased even though the LVEDV was the same as in patients without heart failure. (From: Cohn JN, Rodriguera E, Guiha NH. Hypertensive heart disease. In: Onesti O, Kim KE, Moyer JH, eds. *Hypertension: mechanisms and management.* New York: Grune & Stratton, 1973, with permission.)

hypertensive heart failure (194,305). The importance of decreased left ventricular compliance in the pathogenesis of acute hypertensive heart failure was confirmed by the hemodynamic responses to vasodilator therapy (194,305). Sodium nitroprusside infusion resulted in prompt relief of congestive symptoms in the patients with acute hypertensive heart failure with a dramatic decrease in LVEDP from a mean of 43 to 18 mm Hg. The decrease in left ventricular filling pressure was not due to venodilation and decreased venous return because the left ventricular end-diastolic volume actually increased during sodium nitroprusside infusion. Thus the benefit of sodium nitroprusside therapy was mediated through a decrease in systemic vascular resistance, which led to improvement in left ventricular compliance. The signs and symptoms of pulmonary congestion improved because there was a reduction in LVEDP. This reduction in wedge pressure occurred despite an increase in left ventricular volume because of simultaneous improvement in ventricular compliance.

A schematic representation of the changes in the left ventricular end-diastolic pressure–volume relationship in patients with acute hypertensive heart failure treated with sodium nitroprusside is displayed in Figure 56-23. The diastolic pressure–volume relationship is considered to be an index of left ventricular compliance. In acute hypertensive heart failure, the pressure–volume curve is shifted up and to the left, reflecting a decrease in compliance such that a higher LVEDP is required to achieve any given level of left ventricular end-diastolic volume. Normal systolic function is maintained but at the expense of a very high wedge pressure that results in acute pulmonary edema. Treatment with sodium nitroprusside causes a reduction in the high systemic vascular resistance. The concomitant decrease in impedance to left ventricular ejection results in an

improvement in compliance such that a lower filling pressure is required to maintain systolic function. Symptoms of pulmonary edema resolve as a result of the reduction in LVEDP despite the fact that the left ventricular end-diastolic volume actually increases during sodium nitroprusside infusion.

Compliance is only one index of diastolic performance. Aortic cross-clamp experiments in a canine model have been used to study the effects of acute increases in systemic vascular resistance (afterload) on other indices of left ventricular diastolic function (306). During acute cross-clamping, the isovolumic relaxation rate and early diastolic filling rate are inversely proportional to the left ventricular systolic pressure. Thus, an acute increase in systolic load results in instantaneous changes in left ventricular diastolic function. The authors postulate that in patients with severe hypertension complicated by acute pulmonary edema, an acute increase in left ventricular systolic load due to increased systemic vascular resistance may lead to abnormal myocardial relaxation and diastolic filling, resulting in an elevation of left ventricular filling pressure and pulmonary congestion.

It is not clear why heart failure does not develop in some patients with long-standing severe hypertension, while it develops as a relatively early complication of hypertension in other patients. The rate of rise of blood pressure may be important. Sudden worsening of preexisting hypertension, as occurs in patients with malignant hypertension superimposed on chronic essential hypertension, may precipitate heart failure. Moreover, acute hypertension in previously normotensive patients, as occurs in the setting of preeclampsia or acute glomerulonephritis, may cause left ventricular failure even though the blood pressure is only modestly elevated. In contrast, more severe hypertension, which develops gradually, may be tolerated for years without cardiac decompensation.

It is possible that with longstanding hypertension, the development of left ventricular hypertrophy may be a compensatory mechanism that serves to decrease left ventricular wall stress in the face of the increased impedance to left ventricular ejection (194). However, when the onset of hypertension is abrupt or there is a sudden worsening of chronic hypertension, compensatory mechanisms may not be fully developed. Under these circumstances, precipitous left ventricular diastolic dysfunction with pulmonary and systemic venous congestion may occur (194).

In summary, available evidence suggests that acute hypertensive heart failure results from a primary increase in systemic vascular resistance, which causes an increase in aortic impedance or resistance to left ventricular ejection. Systolic dysfunction (low cardiac output) does not occur because there is an increase in left ventricular wall tension that is sufficient to overcome the impedance to ejection. However, acute pulmonary edema develops because abnormalities of diastolic function such as delayed myocardial relaxation, decreased early diastolic filling, and reduced left ventricular compliance result in an increase in LVEDP that is transmitted to the pulmonary capillaries, resulting in transudation of fluid into alveoli (194,306).

These pathophysiologic mechanisms have important therapeutic implications in the treatment of hypertensive patients with acute pulmonary edema. Since the proximate cause of the impaired diastolic performance in acute hypertensive heart failure is the contraction load imposed on the ventricle by the increase in systemic vascular resistance, potent peripheral vasodilators are clearly the treatment of choice (194,305). However, it is important to distinguish patients in whom acute pulmonary edema is secondary to severe hypertension (acute diastolic dysfunction) from those in whom hypertension is a reflex response to acute respiratory distress during an exacerbation of heart failure due to chronic *systolic* dysfunction. A history of chronic hypertension, diastolic blood pressure over 120 to 130 mm Hg, funduscopic changes of hypertensive neuroretinopathy, and most important, failure of the hypertension to respond rapidly to the administration of oxygen, potent diuretics, and morphine are findings that should suggest that severe hypertension may be the proximate cause of acute pulmonary edema. Furthermore, even in patients with suspected reflex hypertension, if hypertension persists after institution of therapy with preload reducing agents, treatment with a parenteral antihypertensive agent is indicated.

Sodium nitroprusside is the preferred drug for the management of acute hypertensive heart failure because it reduces both preload and afterload. There is no absolute blood pressure goal. The dose of sodium nitroprusside should be increased until signs and symptoms of pulmonary congestion subside or the arterial pressure falls to hypotensive levels. However, it is rarely necessary to lower the blood pressure to hypotensive levels since a reduction to levels still within the hypertensive range is usually associated with a dramatic improvement in symptoms. Although hemodynamic monitoring is not always required, it is essential in patients in whom concomitant myocardial ischemia or compromised cardiac output is suspected. Recent evidence suggests that nitric oxide (NO) donors such as sodium nitroprusside and nitroglycerin may directly modulate diastolic relaxation in patients with a hypertrophied myocardium (307). Intracoronary infusion of nitroglycerin or sodium nitroprusside was found to cause a marked fall in LVEDP with only a slight change in left ventricular peak systolic pressure (afterload), which is consistent with a direct beneficial effect of NO donors on diastolic function.

After the acute episode of hypertension with acute pulmonary edema has resolved, oral therapy can be substituted as the sodium nitroprusside infusion is weaned. Unfortunately, guidelines for long-term antihypertensive treatment in patients with a history of acute hypertensive heart failure are not well defined. Despite the fact that direct-acting vasodilators may sustain or even promote left ventricular hypertrophy, in some patients with severe or resistant hypertension, adequate blood pressure control may require use of hydralazine or minoxidil in conjunction with beta-blockers to control reflex tachycardia and use of diuretics to prevent reflex salt and water retention. Nonetheless, as in the treatment of hypertensive patients with chronic symptoms of congestive heart failure due to diastolic dysfunction, agents such as beta-blockers and calcium channel blockers, which not only decrease blood pressure but also improve diastolic function, may represent the most logical first-line therapy. Moreover, control of blood pressure with beta-blockers, calcium channel blockers, converting enzyme inhibitors, or central α-adrenergic agonists may lead to a regression of left ventricular hypertrophy (304). However, it has not been demonstrated that regression of left ventricular hypertrophy leads to a long-term improvement in diastolic function, congestive symptoms, or prognosis. Furthermore, it is conceivable that regression of left ventricular hypertrophy might predispose to subsequent episodes of acute hypertensive heart failure if severe hypertension suddenly recurs.

HYPERTENSION COMPLICATING CEREBROVASCULAR ACCIDENT

The importance of hypertension as a risk factor for cerebrovascular accident is well established. The Framingham Study shows that regardless of gender or age, hypertension is associated with an increased incidence of ischemic and hemorrhagic stroke (308). Several prospective, randomized clinical trials demonstrate that long-term antihypertensive drug therapy results in a significant reduction in morbidity and mortality from cerebrovascular accident (309). Despite the proven benefits of blood pressure control in the prevention of stroke, the role of treatment of hypertension in the acute phase of stroke remains controversial. Whether antihypertensive therapy is indicated depends not only on the magnitude of the blood pressure elevation, but also on the type of cerebrovascular accident. It should be emphasized that the management of hypertension accompanying cerebral infarction is different from that for hypertension complicating either intracerebral hemorrhage or subarachnoid hemorrhage.

Cerebral Infarction

In the cerebral circulation, the sites of predilection for atherosclerosis are the bifurcations of the common carotid arteries, the carotid siphons, the origins of the vertebral and basilar arteries, the circle of Willis, and the proximal parts of the cerebral arteries (310). Cerebral infarction can result from partial or complete occlusion of an artery by a plaque or embolization of atherothrombotic debris from a plaque. The atherothromboembolic infarcts produced by one of these mechanisms typically involve the cerebral or cerebellar cortex or the pons (310). In contrast, hypertension-induced lipohyalinosis of the small penetrating cerebral end arteries is the principal cause of the small, deep lacunar infarcts that occur in the basal ganglia, pons, thalamus, cerebellum, and deep hemispheric white matter (310).

Hypertension is common in the setting of acute cerebral infarction. In a series of 334 consecutive patients admitted for acute stroke, the blood pressure was elevated in 84% of the patients on the day of admission. Even without specific antihypertensive treatment, the blood pressure decreased spontaneously by an average of 20 mm Hg systolic and 10 mm Hg diastolic in the 10 days following the acute event (311).

This early elevation in blood pressure most likely represents a physiologic response to brain ischemia. Decreases in blood pressure accompany recovery of brain function.

Because of the known benefits of antihypertensive therapy with regard to stroke prevention, it has been assumed that reduction in blood pressure would benefit patients with acute cerebral infarction. Unfortunately, because treatment of hypertension in this setting has never been evaluated in a prospective, randomized trial, there are no good data to guide management. Moreover, there is no evidence to suggest that rapid reduction of blood pressure is beneficial. In fact, several cases have been reported in which worsening of the patient's neurologic status was apparently precipitated by emergency treatment of hypertension (312,313). The rationale for not treating hypertension in acute ischemic strokes is based on concerns regarding impairment in autoregulation of cerebral blood flow in this setting (313–315). In normal individuals, cerebral blood flow is maintained constant at mean arterial pressures ranging between 60 and 120 mm Hg. However, in patients with chronic hypertension as well as older adult patients, the curve is shifted such that the lower limit of autoregulation occurs at a higher mean arterial pressure. Furthermore, there is evidence that local autoregulation of cerebral blood flow is disturbed in the so-called ischemic penumbra that surrounds an area of acute infarction (314). Without intact autoregulation, the regional blood flow becomes critically dependent on the perfusion pressure. Thus, to some extent, the presence of hypertension may be beneficial in the setting of acute cerebral infarction, whereas reduction of blood pressure may cause a regional decrease in blood flow with extension of the infarct.

Because there is no evidence that mild to moderate hypertension has a deleterious effect on the outcome of cerebral infarction during the acute stage, it is probably wise to allow the blood pressure to seek its own level during the first few days to weeks after the event. In most cases, the hypertension tends to resolve spontaneously over the first week without specific therapy (311). On the other hand, if hypertension persists for more than 3 weeks in a patient with a completed stroke, gradual reduction of blood pressure into the normal range can be accomplished safely (316). The goal of long-term antihypertensive treatment in hypertensive stroke survivors is the prevention of stroke recurrence. The benefits of antihypertensive therapy in secondary stroke prevention are uncertain, but large clinical trials are in progress that should provide helpful guidelines for clinical practice.

Although benign neglect of mild to moderate hypertension is prudent in the setting of acute cerebral infarction, there may be certain indications for active treatment of hypertension. When the diastolic blood pressure is sustained more than 130 mm Hg, many authorities recommend cautious reduction of the systolic blood pressure to 160 to 170 mm Hg and diastolic to 100 to 110 mm Hg with a short-acting parenteral agent such as sodium nitroprusside (293,313,317–319). Stroke accompanied by other hypertensive crises such as acute myocardial ischemia or left ventricular dysfunction with acute pulmonary edema is also an indication for cautious blood pressure reduction (313,318). Stroke due to carotid occlusion caused by aortic dissection mandates aggressive blood pressure reduction to prevent propagation of the dissection (313,318). In some patients with severe hypertension, it may be impossible to distinguish between hypertensive encephalopathy and cerebral infarction on clinical grounds. Since rapid lowering of the blood pressure may be lifesaving in the patient with hypertensive encephalopathy, a cautious diagnostic trial of blood pressure reduction with a short-acting parenteral antihypertensive agent, such as sodium nitroprusside, may be indicated (318). In patients who have suffered a stroke and require anticoagulation therapy, moderate control of severe hypertension into the 160 to 170 mm Hg systolic and 100 to 110 mm Hg diastolic range may

also be prudent. In the severely hypertensive patient with progressing stroke in whom continued deterioration is believed to be secondary to concomitant cerebral edema, cautious blood pressure reduction may be warranted. Appropriate management of such patients may require continuous intracranial as well as intraarterial pressure monitoring so that cerebral perfusion pressure can be optimized (318).

In a recent study, sodium nitroprusside, given at a dose that reduced mean arterial pressure by 10 mm Hg, significantly inhibited platelet aggregation and adhesion molecule expression and improved regional cerebral blood flow in patients with acute ischemic stroke (320). These findings were attributed to beneficial effects of nitric oxide on platelet function and local vasodilation in the area of the ischemic penumbra.

In the setting of acute cerebral infarction, hypertension tends to be very labile and exquisitely sensitive to hypotensive therapy. Even modest doses of oral antihypertensive agents may cause profound and devastating overshoot hypotension (312). Antihypertensive treatment, when indicated, should be initiated with extreme caution using small doses of short-acting agents such as sodium nitroprusside. Use of oral or sublingual nifedipine may be associated with overshoot hypotension resulting in extension of the infarct and is contraindicated for the treatment of hypertension accompanying acute cerebral infarction. Oral clonidine loading is also contraindicated because it may induce overshoot hypotension or lead to sedation, which will interfere with assessment of mental status. It had been proposed that there the calcium channel blocker nimodipine, which is a cerebral vasodilator, might theoretically minimize arterial spasm and therefore improve cerebral ischemia. However, a large controlled clinical trial demonstrated no improvement in outcome in patients with thrombotic stroke treated with nimodipine when compared to placebo treatment (321).

Intracerebral Hemorrhage

Hypertension is a major risk factor for intracerebral hemorrhage. The small-diameter, penetrating cerebral end arteries are especially vulnerable to the deleterious effects of hypertension because they arise directly from the main arterial trunks (310). The most common sites of hypertension-associated hemorrhage include the basal ganglia, pons, thalamus, cerebellum, and deep hemispheric white matter (322). Lacunar infarcts arise from the same vessels and are similarly distributed.

Hypertensive hemorrhage most often occurs in patients older than 50 years of age. Intracerebral hemorrhage characteristically begins abruptly with headache and vomiting followed by steadily increasing focal neurologic deficits and alteration of consciousness (322). More than 90% of hemorrhages rupture through brain parenchyma into the ventricles, producing a bloody CSF (322). Patients presenting with acute intracerebral hemorrhage invariably have elevated blood pressure. In fact, the finding of a normal or low blood pressure makes the diagnosis of intracerebral hemorrhage unlikely (322). In contrast to cerebral infarction, the blood pressure does not tend to decrease spontaneously during the first week after the event (311). Once the hemorrhage has occurred, the patient's condition worsens steadily over a period of minutes to days until either the neurologic deficit stabilizes, or the patient dies (322). When death occurs, it is most often due to herniation caused by the expanding hematoma and surrounding edema.

Small hemorrhages, which may be clinically indistinguishable from cerebral infarction, probably require no specific therapy (310). The issue of treatment of hypertension in the setting of a large (greater than 3 cm) intracerebral hemorrhage is controversial. There is almost always a rise in intracranial pressure accompanied by a reflex increase in systemic blood pressure (311). Because cerebral perfusion pressure is a function of the difference between systemic arterial pressure and intracranial pressure, reduction of blood pressure may compromise cerebral perfusion. Furthermore, the hematoma impairs the local autoregulatory response in the surrounding area of marginal ischemia (313). Because there is no good evidence that persistent hypertension promotes further bleeding, some authorities strongly advise against treating hypertension in patients with intracerebral hemorrhage (1,312,315). On the other hand, cerebral vasogenic edema may develop as a consequence of an abrupt, severe increase in blood pressure (310), and treatment of hypertension may be beneficial by virtue of a reduction in cerebral edema and intracranial pressure. Thus, in deciding to treat hypertension, a precarious balance must be struck between prevention of cerebral edema on the one hand, and deleterious reduction of cerebral blood flow on the other. In a study of eight patients with intracerebral hemorrhage treated with trimethaphan, cerebral blood flow measurements revealed that the cerebral autoregulation curve was intact but shifted such that the lower limit of autoregulation was at 80% of the initial level of blood pressure (323). Thus, a 20% decrease in mean arterial pressure should be considered the maximal reduction of blood pressure during the acute stage. Active treatment of the blood pressure should only be undertaken in the intensive care environment where intracranial pressure and intraarterial pressure can be closely monitored (310,324).

The drug of choice for the management of hypertension in the setting of intracerebral hemorrhage is a matter of debate. Sodium nitroprusside has traditionally been regarded as the best agent because its brief duration of action allows for rapid titration with avoidance of the catastrophic consequence of sustained overshoot hypotension (1,319). However, concern has been expressed that because sodium nitroprusside causes an increase in venous capacitance as well as cerebral arterial vasodilation, the resulting increase in cerebral blood volume may cause a further elevation of intracranial pressure (325–327). Other cerebral vasodilators such as intravenous nitroglycerin, hydralazine, or calcium channel blockers also can cause potentially deleterious elevations of intracranial pressure in patients with compromised intracranial compliance due to intracranial disease (327). Because labetalol and urapidil (a postsynaptic α-receptor blocker) may not alter intracranial pressure, they have been recommended for treatment of hypertension in patients undergoing neurosurgery (327). Unfortunately, these agents have the potential to cause overshoot hypotension, which may be difficult to quickly reverse. Thus, despite the theoretic risk of elevation of intracranial pressure, sodium nitroprusside remains the treatment of choice when severe hypertension must be treated in the patient with intracerebral hemorrhage because its brief duration of action allows for cautious, graded blood pressure reduction, which can be quickly reversed if the patient's neurologic status deteriorates or a further increase in intracranial pressure occurs. Of interest, some patients with cerebral infarction or hemorrhage have extreme elevations of catecholamine levels that may render hypertension refractory to sodium nitroprusside in the absence of concomitant beta-blocker therapy (328).

Cerebellar hemorrhage represents a neurosurgical emergency requiring prompt diagnosis and treatment (329). Typically, patients complain of the sudden onset of dizziness, nausea, vomiting, headache, and difficulty walking. Truncal ataxia, nystagmus, and ipsilateral sixth nerve paresis may be present (329). If the process continues unchecked, brainstem compression or herniation produces progressive stupor and coma. The untreated mortality is extremely high. The diagnosis can usually be confirmed by computerized tomography. Treatment consists of emergency suboccipital craniotomy with evacuation of the hematoma (329).

Subarachnoid Hemorrhage

Subarachnoid hemorrhage (SAH) accounts for less than 10% of all cerebrovascular accidents. Rupture of a congenital aneurysm is the most common cause. Rupture is heralded by the sudden onset of a profound headache and is often followed by brief syncope. If the mass of the hemorrhage is large, patients rapidly become comatose. As the hemorrhage diffuses throughout the subarachnoid space, the patient may awaken and experience headache, nausea, vomiting, and seizures. Within 24 hours, nuchal rigidity and other meningeal signs develop. Initially, neurologic findings are nonfocal. Computerized tomography can be used to confirm the diagnosis.

Recurrent hemorrhage is a potential complication associated with a high mortality. Whether treatment of hypertension after SAH reduces the risk of recurrent bleeding or improves prognosis is uncertain. In the setting of elevated intracranial pressure or cerebral arterial vasospasm, hypertension may actually be protective because it helps to maintain cerebral perfusion pressure. Thus, reduction of the blood pressure could conceivably result in aggravation of cerebral vasospasm and ischemia.

Early surgical repair of the aneurysm has reduced the incidence of rebleeding in patients with SAH. In fact, delayed cerebral ischemia due to cerebral arterial vasospasm has been found to be the most important cause of morbidity and mortality in patients who survive the initial hemorrhage (330,331). Vasospasm, which is probably caused by the irritating effects of blood in the subarachnoid space closely opposed to the large arteries, usually develops 4 to 12 days after the acute hemorrhage. Symptoms include a gradual deterioration of the level of consciousness, accompanied by focal neurologic deficits.

Surgical clipping of the aneurysm is usually undertaken as soon as possible to prevent rebleeding (331,332). There is conflicting evidence as to whether or not postoperative treatment with intravascular volume expansion, in conjunction with deliberate induction of arterial hypertension using dopamine or dobutamine, may be an effective means of reversing the ischemic neurologic deficits caused by cerebral vasospasm (333,334).

Nimodipine, a 1,4-dihydropyridine calcium channel blocker, has been approved for the prevention and treatment of delayed cerebral ischemia caused by subarachnoid hemorrhage from ruptured congenital aneurysms. Nimodipine is highly lipid-soluble and readily crosses the blood-brain barrier (335). It dilates cerebral blood vessels at concentrations lower than those required for dilation of the peripheral vasculature (335). Thus, it may dilate intracerebral vessels at doses that do not result in a significant reduction in mean arterial pressure. Furthermore, inhibition of calcium uptake by neurons may also protect against ischemic injury at the cellular level, independent of an effect on cerebral blood flow (335). Nimodipine has been shown, in randomized, placebo-controlled trials, to reduce the severity of neurologic deficits resulting from vasospasm in patients who have had a recent subarachnoid hemorrhage (336,337). The recommended dosage is 60 mg orally every 4 hours for 21 consecutive days beginning within 96 hours of the subarachnoid hemorrhage. The liquid content of the capsules can be given through a nasogastric tube in unconscious patients. The optimal timing of surgery in nimodipine-treated patients has not yet been defined.

Hypertension Complicating Severe Head Trauma

Systemic hypertension can contribute to the increase in intracranial pressure that often accompanies traumatic head injury (338). In patients with severe head injury, the degree of intracranial hypertension correlates with mortality. If the intracranial pressure is less than 20 mm Hg, mortality is about 20%. However, if the intracranial pressure exceeds 40 mm Hg, mortality is more than 80% (339). The primary danger of intracranial hypertension is a compromise of cerebral blood flow with secondary ischemic injury. Severe, uncontrolled intracranial hypertension can result in rapid brain death due to global cerebral ischemia. The minimum cerebral perfusion pressure (mean arterial pressure minus intracranial pressure) necessary to prevent secondary cerebral ischemia is 50 mm Hg (338).

A major goal of treatment in the patient with a head injury is to maintain intracranial pressure at levels less than 30 mm Hg. However, effective treatment requires measurement of intracranial pressure with a device such as a ventricular catheter, subarachnoid bolt, or epidural transducer. Major treatments for reducing elevated intracranial pressure include hyperventilation, osmotic diuretics, removal of CSF, corticosteroids, high-dose barbiturates, and control of arterial blood pressure (338). Autoregulation of cerebral blood flow is impaired in patients with severe head injury such that changes in mean arterial pressure will cause parallel changes in intracranial pressure through alterations in cerebral blood volume. Moreover, severe hypertension may cause a breakthrough of cerebral autoregulation, leading to cerebral edema in a manner analogous to hypertensive encephalopathy. On the other hand, some increase in blood pressure may be beneficial with regard to maintenance of cerebral perfusion pressure in the patient with increased intracranial pressure. Therefore, rational treatment of hypertension in the setting of severe head trauma requires continuous monitoring of mean arterial pressure, intracranial pressure, pulmonary capillary wedge pressure, and cardiac output. Frequent neurologic examinations must be performed to assess response to therapy. The choice of antihypertensive agent is also important. Vasodilators, when used alone, tend to be relatively ineffective so the patient should also be pretreated with β-adrenergic receptor blockers. Vasodilators such as sodium nitroprusside and intravenous nitroglycerin are the treatments of choice (338). If an increase in intracranial pressure accompanied by compromise of cerebral perfusion pressure occurs with vasodilator therapy, intravenous labetalol may be a suitable alternative. Diuretics should be avoided because a decrease in intravascular volume reduces cardiac output and increases sympathetic tone.

HYPERTENSION COMPLICATING ACUTE MYOCARDIAL INFARCTION

Transient systemic hypertension is a frequent occurrence during the early stages of acute myocardial infarction, even among previously normotensive patients. This postinfarction hypertension has been attributed to a hyperadrenergic state resulting from release of catecholamines from infarcted myocardium or to an increase in sympathetic tone in response to stress, pain, or anxiety. Serial measurements of plasma epinephrine and norepinephrine in patients with acute myocardial infarction have revealed a significant direct correlation between plasma catecholamine levels and systolic blood pressure (340). A cardiogenic hypertensive chemoreflex has been described. Injection of serotonin into the left atrium or branches of the proximal left coronary artery in dogs produces an intense pressor response that is dependent on vagal afferent impulses to the central nervous system and is blocked by the α-adrenergic blocking agent phentolamine. By histologic examination, a small structure resembling a chemoreceptor has been identified. This chemoreceptor receives its blood supply from the left coronary artery (341). It has been postulated that in the setting of acute myocardial infarction, platelet deposition in stenosed vessels results in the release of serotonin with activation of this chemoreceptor. The chemoreceptor reflex results in increased sympathetic tone and systemic hypertension (340).

In most patients, hypertension is a transient finding early in the course of acute myocardial infarction that resolves without specific therapy other than pain control and sedation. The short-term changes in blood pressure in untreated patients with acute myocardial infarction have been well characterized (342). During the first hour of hospitalization the mean systolic blood pressure averages 150 ± 30.7 mm Hg, and systolic pressure of at least 160 mm Hg is present in 30% of patients. The mean diastolic blood pressure averages 92 ± 18.7, and diastolic pressure of at least 100 mm Hg is present in 42% of patients. Overall, 45% of patients have a blood pressure of at least 140/90 mm Hg and 32% have a blood pressure of a least 160/100 mm Hg during the first hour of hospitalization. However, during the subsequent 6 hours, the blood pressure spontaneously normalizes in the majority of patients. By the sixth hour of hospitalization systolic pressure falls to 130 ± 24 mm Hg, and diastolic pressure decreases to 81 ± 15.5 mm Hg. Among the patients with an initial blood pressure of at least 140/90 mm Hg, only 25% are still hypertensive by 6 hours. Patients with an initial blood pressure of at least 160/100 mm Hg demonstrate a similar decrease in blood pressure, such that it remains above this level at 6 hours in only 20%. No difference was found in the clinical course of the patients with and those without hypertension (342). Based on this study it was concluded that in early, uncomplicated acute myocardial infarction, no specific therapy of hypertension is indicated other than attention to relief of pain and adequate sedation (342).

In contrast, a number of studies indicate that hypertension in the setting of acute myocardial infarction signifies a less favorable prognosis. In a study of 143 patients with acute myocardial infarction, high systolic blood pressure on admission indicated a worse prognosis for 2-year survival (343). In another study of 106 patients with acute myocardial infarction who had systolic blood pressure of at least 170 mm Hg that persisted for at least 30 minutes, the blood pressure fell spontaneously to less than 150 mm Hg within 72 hours in all patients (344). No antihypertensive therapy was employed. The control group consisted of 106 patients with acute myocardial infarction who had a systolic pressure of 120 to 150 mm Hg and a diastolic pressure of 100 mm Hg or lower. Mean peak aspartate aminotransferase (AST) levels were significantly higher in the systolic hypertension group than in the normotensive group. The duration of systolic blood pressure of at least 170 mm Hg before return to normotension correlated with the mean peak AST level and presumably infarct size. The overall mortality, incidence of major arrhythmias, and incidence of cardiac failure were higher in the hypertensive group.

Postinfarction hypertension may be the most important risk factor for cardiac rupture (345). Although the incidence of chronic hypertension prior to acute myocardial infarction was similar in patients with and those without rupture, 40% of the patients with cardiac rupture had postinfarction hypertension (diastolic pressure ≥ 90 mm Hg) compared with 15% of patients without cardiac rupture.

A major objective of therapy in acute myocardial infarction is to minimize myocardial infarct size. The extent of ischemic damage is dependent on the balance between myocardial oxygen supply and demand. In experimental models, factors that increase myocardial oxygen demand increased infarct size. Conversely, infarct size was minimized by reducing myocardial oxygen consumption (346). Heart rate, wall tension, and myocardial contractility are the major determinants of myocardial oxygen consumption.

Treatment with β-adrenergic receptor blockers leads to a reduction in myocardial oxygen demand through a reduction in heart rate, systemic vascular resistance, and myocardial contractility. In addition, beta-blockers counter the excess production of catecholamines commonly seen in patients with acute myocardial infarction. They also have antiarrhythmic properties. When given intravenously within the first few hours after the acute event, beta-blockers can reduce both infarct size and early in-hospital mortality (347,348). Intravenous beta-blocker therapy should be considered in all patients with acute myocardial infarction unless contraindications such as severe bradycardia, heart block, systemic hypotension, severe left ventricular systolic dysfunction, and reactive airways disease are present (347). The presence of mild to moderate left ventricular systolic dysfunction should not necessarily be considered a contraindication to acute or chronic treatment with beta-blockers. Several of the larger trials did include high-risk patients with a history of compensated heart failure or with acute signs suggesting mild left ventricular dysfunction. These trials indicated that beta-blocker treatment was well tolerated by patients with left ventricular dysfunction, both in the acute phase of myocardial infarction and during long-term treatment (349). Long-term trials showed a marked (43% to 47%) reduction in the likelihood of sudden death among patients with left ventricular dysfunction treated with beta-blockers (349).

In patients with acute myocardial infarction who have relative contraindications to β-blockade such as evidence of severe left ventricular dysfunction, obstructive airways disease, and bradycardia, dose titration with intravenous esmolol may be a safe alternative (350). Moreover, the ability to tolerate esmolol infusion is a good predictor of subsequent outcome with oral beta-blocker therapy (350).

Secondary prevention trials showed that chronic beta-blocker treatment after myocardial infarction reduces both nonfatal reinfarction rate and long-term mortality (347,351). Impressive effects on morbidity and mortality have been obtained with propranolol, timolol, and metoprolol, whereas beta-blockers with intrinsic sympathomimetic activity are less effective (347). Recent studies also suggest that treatment with converting enzyme inhibitors, started within 24 hours of the onset of acute myocardial infarction, may be beneficial in patients with a history of hypertension in that they decrease the risk of severe congestive heart failure and reduce 1-year mortality rate (352).

During the first few days after an acute myocardial infarction, the systemic arterial pressure is the most important determinant of LVEDP (353). Accordingly, it has been proposed that in the setting of postinfarction hypertension, reduction of the blood pressure with arteriolar vasodilators might prevent extension of ischemia by reducing LVEDP, wall tension, and myocardial oxygen demand. Studies of vasodilator therapy with intravenous nitroglycerin, sodium nitroprusside, or trimethaphan in patients with hypertension complicating acute myocardial infarction demonstrate improved cardiac performance with decreased LVEDP and stable or increased cardiac output, findings that should be associated with a reduction in myocardial oxygen demand (354,355). Moreover, intravenous nitroglycerin has been shown to cause reversal of the restrictive left ventricular diastolic filling pattern on pulsed-wave Doppler in patients with acute anterior wall myocardial infarction (356).

In the setting of acute myocardial infarction, patients with a blood pressure higher than 160/100 mm Hg that lasts longer than 1 hour and is unresponsive to intravenous beta-blocker therapy should be considered candidates for treatment with parenteral vasodilators to decrease systemic vascular resistance, afterload, and myocardial oxygen demand. Because systemic hemodynamics can change rapidly in the setting of acute myocardial infarction, the use of agents with a short duration of

action is recommended. Intravenous nitroglycerin and sodium nitroprusside are preferred in this setting. Nitroglycerin has theoretic advantages as a vasodilator in the setting of acute myocardial infarction because it dilates intercoronary collaterals and improves blood flow to the ischemic myocardium (357–359). Diazoxide and hydralazine are contraindicated because their use may result in reflex activation of the adrenergic system, resulting in increases in heart rate, cardiac output, and myocardial oxygen demand.

Acute reduction of blood pressure in patients with acute myocardial infarction necessitates careful monitoring of filling pressure and cardiac output. Definition of an arbitrary blood pressure goal is impossible. The blood pressure should be gradually reduced over a period of 10 to 15 minutes with frequent checks of systemic hemodynamics. The goal of therapy should be the reduction of system vascular resistance such that LVEDP is reduced to the range of 15 to 18 mm Hg without reflex tachycardia or compromise of cardiac output (360). The blood pressure may be reduced to normotensive levels as long as cardiac output remains stable or increases, the heart rate does not increase, and there is no evidence of increased myocardial ischemia (pain or increased ischemic changes on electrocardiogram). Vasodilator therapy can usually be weaned within 24 hours as the hypertension resolves.

Despite the fact that afterload reduction can improve myocardial performance and decrease myocardial oxygen demands, it should be undertaken with great caution. Myocardial blood flow is critically dependent on coronary perfusion pressure, and overshoot hypotension can worsen ischemia and extend the infarct. Afterload reduction should be restricted to patients with increased LVEDP (wedge pressure $\geq$15 mm Hg) (360). The use of vasodilator therapy in patients with a normal or reduced filling pressure can cause a decrease in cardiac output and reflex tachycardia, which can worsen myocardial ischemia (360).

Aortic Dissection

Acute aortic dissection is a hypertensive crisis requiring immediate antihypertensive therapy aimed at halting the progression of the dissecting hematoma. Patients with acute aortic dissection should be stabilized with intensive antihypertensive therapy to prevent life-threatening complications.

A small intimal tear usually initiates aortic dissection. In 60% to 65% of patients, the intimal tear arises in the ascending aorta within a few centimeters of the aortic valve. In 30% to 35%, it begins in the descending thoracic aorta just distal to the origin of the left subclavian artery, while in 5% to 10% the dissection originates in the transverse aortic arch (361). The most clinically useful classification of aortic dissection is based on the presence or absence of involvement of the ascending aorta regardless of the site of the original intimal tear (362,363) (Fig. 56-24). Proximal dissections include all dissections that involve the ascending aorta, including those that begin in the descending aorta and propagate retrograde into the ascending aorta. Distal dissections involve only the descending aorta. In general, the type of dissection, proximal or distal, defines whether management should be accomplished with drug therapy plus surgery or intensive medical therapy alone.

Degenerative changes in the aortic media underlie most cases of aortic dissection. This medial degeneration is believed to be the result of chronic stress on the aortic wall. Chronic hypertension is the most important risk factor for the development of aortic dissection (364). Typical patients with aortic dissection are 60- to 80-year-old men with a long history of essential hypertension. Less common factors predisposing to aortic dissection include Marfan's syndrome, Ehlers-Danlos syndrome, bicuspid aortic valve, coarctation of the aorta, and

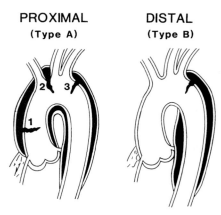

PROXIMAL (Type A)   **DISTAL** (Type B)

FIGURE 56-24. Classification of aortic dissection based on the presence or absence of involvement of the ascending aorta. The dissection is defined as proximal if there is involvement of the ascending aorta. The primary intimal tear in proximal dissection may arise in the ascending aorta (1), transverse aortic arch (2), or descending aorta (3). In distal dissections, the process is confined to the descending aorta; the ascending aorta is not involved. The primary intimal tear occurs most commonly just distal to the origin of the left subclavian artery. Proximal dissections account for approximately 67% and distal dissections 43% of all acute aortic dissections. (Adapted from: Wheat MW Jr. Acute dissecting aneurysms of the aorta: diagnosis and treatment, 1979. *Am Heart J* 1980;99:373.)

pregnancy (365). Patients with Marfan's syndrome and aortic dissection often have a family history of dissection. There may also be an association between Marfan's syndrome and dissection that occurs in the third trimester of pregnancy.

Following the initial intimal tear, a column of blood driven by the force of arterial pressure enters the aortic wall and destroys the media while stripping the intima for a variable distance along the length of the aorta. The extent of propagation of the dissecting hematoma is determined by several mechanical factors, including the systolic blood pressure, velocity of shearing forces, turbulence of blood flow, and the steepness of the pulse wave (contractility) (361). Experimental evidence suggests that the two most important factors are the blood pressure and the steepness of the pulse wave (366,367). Without treatment, acute aortic dissection is almost always fatal. In a review of survival in untreated patients, one-fourth died within 24 hours, one-half died within 1 month, and more than 90% died within 1 year. The three major complications of aortic dissection are rupture of the aorta, occlusion of major arterial branches arising from the aorta, and acute aortic insufficiency (361). The most frequent mechanism of death is through-and-through rupture of the weakened aortic adventitia (361). The most common site of rupture is the ascending aorta. Because the parietal pericardium is attached to the aorta just proximal to the origin of the innominate artery, rupture of any portion of the ascending aorta leads to hemopericardium and pericardial tamponade. Rupture of the aortic arch causes hemorrhage into the mediastinum. Rupture of the descending thoracic aorta leads to hemorrhage into the left pleural space. Retroperitoneal hemorrhage results from rupture of the abdominal aorta.

The clinical features of acute aortic dissection have been extensively reviewed (363,365,368). Men predominate over women by a ratio of 3:1. The peak incidence is in the sixth and seventh decades. The pain is usually cataclysmic in onset and maximal at its inception in contrast to the crescendo nature of pain seen with acute myocardial infarction. The pain is often described as tearing, ripping, or stabbing. Another characteristic of the pain is its tendency to migrate from the point of origin along the path followed by the dissecting hematoma.

The location of the pain is suggestive of the site of origin. Pain felt maximally in the anterior thorax is more frequently due to proximal dissection, whereas pain felt maximally in the interscapular area is more common in distal dissections. Vasovagal symptoms such as diaphoresis, apprehension, nausea, and vomiting are common. Less common presenting symptoms include syncope (usually due to cardiac tamponade) and acute pulmonary edema (secondary to acute aortic insufficiency). In proximal dissections, stroke or altered consciousness can occur due to extension of the dissection into the carotid arteries with diminished carotid blood flow. Occlusion of coronary ostia can lead to acute myocardial infarction. Horner's syndrome can occur if there is compression of the superior cervical sympathetic ganglion. Vocal cord paralysis accompanies compression of the left recurrent laryngeal nerve. Involvement of the descending aorta can lead to mesenteric ischemia, renal insufficiency, lower extremity ischemia or pulse deficits, and focal neurologic abnormalities due to spinal artery occlusion with spinal cord ischemia. Occlusion of renal artery ostia may be signaled by the development of severe hypertension due to renin release from the ischemic kidney (363).

Although the majority of patients with aortic dissection have evidence of long-standing hypertension, the blood pressure can fall such that hypertension is absent at the time of presentation. In one study, at presentation, 56% of patients with distal dissections were hypertensive compared with 9% of patients with proximal dissections (364). True hypotension, which is more common with proximal dissections, is attributable to rupture of the dissected aorta with cardiac tamponade or hemorrhage into the pleural space or retroperitoneum (364). Pseudohypotension can be caused by compromise of flow through either or both subclavian arteries (364). Significant variation in blood pressure between the two arms is not uncommon.

Acute aortic insufficiency can develop with proximal dissection due to dilation of the aortic root or widening of the annulus by the dissecting hematoma so that the valve leaflets fail to oppose during diastole (363). In contrast to the finding in primary aortic valve disease, the murmur of aortic insufficiency is most commonly heard along the right sternal border. Moreover, the murmur may be quite short due to rapid ventricular filling with early equilibration of aortic and left ventricular diastolic pressures.

Although the chest roentgenogram may show widening of the mediastinum, this sign is present in only 40% to 50% of patients (361). The mediastinum bulges to the right with involvement of the ascending aorta and to the left with involvement of the descending thoracic aorta. At the aortic knob, more than 1 cm of separation of intimal calcification from the adventitial border, the so-called calcium sign, is highly suggestive but not diagnostic of aortic dissection (363). A left pleural effusion due to hemothorax can also occur.

In the past decade there has been a dramatic shift away from invasive diagnosis of aortic dissection with aortography to the use of noninvasive diagnostic modalities such as transesophageal echocardiography (TEE) or MRI (368). Imaging modalities are used to confirm the diagnosis and identify the presence or absence of involvement of the ascending aorta thereby defining the dissection as proximal or distal. Additional diagnostic information available from these studies includes the extent of the dissection and the sites of entry and reentry, presence of thrombus in the false lumen, presence of aortic insufficiency or pericardial effusion, and involvement of the coronary arteries or other arterial trunks. These data are crucial in deciding between medical and surgical therapy and for planning surgical intervention.

TEE has rapidly become the preferred imaging technique for evaluation of suspected aortic dissection (369). Although it requires esophageal intubation, TEE can easily be performed in the emergency room to provide an accurate diagnosis within minutes. In a study designed to assess the comparative diagnostic value of TEE and retrograde aortography, TEE actually had better sensitivity (98% vs. 88%) and negative predictive value (97% vs. 85%) than did aortography (370). The superior sensitivity of TEE was due to the ability to identify noncommunicating dissection (dissection without an apparent intimal tear). However, angiography was more accurate in assessing the site of entry of the dissection (97% vs. 78%). There were no significant differences between the techniques with regard to assessing secondary tears, aortic regurgitation, coronary dissection, or extension of the dissection. Biplane and multiplane TEE are widely used since they permit visualization of the ascending aorta in multiple imaging planes (371). Thus, either TEE or aortography is adequate to diagnose aortic dissection and plan surgical intervention.

MRI also provides an accurate noninvasive technique for evaluating the thoracic aorta in patients with suspected dissection (372). The main disadvantages are that it is difficult to closely monitor the patient during prolonged scanning and that MRI is not readily available on an emergency basis at many institutions. However, MRI may be quite useful for long-term follow-up of patients with aortic dissection.

Treatment of Acute Aortic Dissection

Intensive medical therapy should be instituted immediately in patients with suspected acute dissection, preferably even before definitive diagnostic procedures are undertaken. The initial therapeutic goal is the elimination of pain (which correlates with a halting of the dissection process) and reduction of systolic blood pressure to the 100 to 120 mm Hg range or the lowest level compatible with maintenance of adequate renal, cardiac, and cerebral perfusion. Even in the absence of hypertension, therapy should be instituted. Antihypertensive therapy should be designed not only to lower blood pressure but also to decrease the steepness of the pulse wave. The most commonly used treatment regimen consists of an intravenous β-adrenergic blocking drug such as propranolol, metoprolol, or esmolol in combination with sodium nitroprusside (363,364,373). Beta-blockade should be initiated prior to nitroprusside in order to prevent an adrenergic-mediated reflex increase in cardiac contractility that could further propagate the dissection. After an initial test dose of 0.5 mg, propranolol is administered in 1-mg increments over 5 minutes until there is adequate β-blockade as evidenced by a pulse rate of approximately 60 beats/minute (365). However, the total dose should not exceed 0.15 mg/kg. Subsequent propranolol doses should be given every 4 to 6 hours to maintain β-blockade (374). Pretreatment with intravenous esmolol or metoprolol is also acceptable (374). In patients with bronchospasm, metoprolol can be administered in loading doses of 1 mg every 5 minutes followed by 5- to 15-mg maintenance doses every 4 to 6 hours as necessary. After pretreatment with beta-blocker, sodium nitroprusside is administered to lower the systolic blood pressure into the 100- to 120-mm Hg range.

Trimethaphan has been considered by some to be the preferred drug for the treatment of acute aortic dissection (361,375). In animal models, doses of propranolol much larger than those necessary to produce bradycardia are required to prevent the reflex increase in contractility associated with the use of sodium nitroprusside (375). In contrast, trimethaphan is not associated with reflex increases in heart rate or contractility because it blocks the adrenergic system. Unfortunately, the prolonged use of trimethaphan is limited by its sympathoplegic side effects as well as the rapid development of tachyphylaxis (363).

Labetalol, by virtue of its combined α_1- and β-blocking properties, may be useful in the management of acute dissection. However, its long duration of hypotensive action may not be desirable in critically ill patients with acute aortic dissection who may require urgent surgical intervention. Selective arteriolar vasodilators such as diazoxide, hydralazine, and minoxidil, which activate the adrenergic system, are contraindicated in acute aortic dissection.

After the blood pressure is controlled and the patient is pain-free, TEE or angiography should be performed. When one is deciding between medical and surgical therapy, the most important diagnostic finding is involvement of the ascending aorta. Collective results from long-term follow-up studies indicate that surgical therapy is superior to medical therapy alone in patients with proximal dissections (361,376). Operative mortality for proximal dissections at experienced centers varies from 7% to 20%, which is well below the more than 50% mortality with medical therapy alone. Conversely, in patients with distal dissections, intensive drug therapy leads to an 80% survival rate compared with only 50% in surgically treated patients (361).

Surgical therapy is advantageous in patients with proximal dissection because progression of the dissecting hematoma can result in devastating consequences including neurologic compromise, acute aortic insufficiency, and aortic rupture with cardiac tamponade. Surgical therapy involves excision of the intimal tear, obliteration of proximal entry into the false lumen, and reconstitution of the aorta with interposition of a synthetic vascular graft (377). In patients with aortic insufficiency, restoration of aortic valve competence can be accomplished by resuspension of the native aortic valve or by aortic valve replacement.

There are a number of explanations for the advantage of medical therapy over surgical therapy for acute distal dissection. These patients are generally at greater surgical risk because they are older and have a higher incidence of advanced atherosclerosis and coexistent cardiopulmonary disease (365, 377). A major complication of surgery for distal dissections is spinal cord ischemia and resultant paralysis. Moreover, the risk of life-threatening complications such as cardiac tamponade, aortic insufficiency, and cerebrovascular accident is less than that with proximal dissections. Although medical therapy is generally the treatment of choice in distal dissections, there are situations in which surgery is required. These include inability to control blood pressure, inability to control pain (which implies continued propagation), compromise or occlusion of a major branch of the aorta, or the development of a saccular aortic aneurysm during long-term medical therapy. There is also general agreement that acute distal dissection in patients with Marfan's syndrome should be managed surgically (363).

Long-Term Medical Management of Aortic Dissection

After diagnosis by TEE or aortography, patients with uncomplicated distal dissection should be continued on propranolol and nitroprusside or trimethaphan infusions. A transition to oral antihypertensive therapy should be initiated after the blood pressure has stabilized and clinical evidence of progression or complications of dissection have subsided. Survivors of surgical intervention should also receive long-term medical therapy. The preferred antihypertensive agents for the long-term management of patients with aortic dissection are those that have a negative inotropic effect such as beta-blockers without intrinsic sympathomimetic activity, verapamil, diltiazem, labetalol, methyldopa, and reserpine. Vasodilators such as prazosin, hydralazine, and minoxidil, which cause a reflex increase in sympathetic tone, should be avoided. Nifedipine and isradipine can cause a reflex increase in heart rate and cardiac output and should probably be avoided or used only in combination with a beta-blocker (374). Converting enzyme inhibitors may also be useful for long-term medical management of aortic dissection (374). The objective of therapy should be to maintain the systolic blood pressure below 130 mm Hg. Even patients without hypertension should be given β-adrenergic blocking drugs postoperatively if at all possible (363).

Reoperation may be required for late complications including progressive aortic insufficiency, localized saccular aneurysm formation, and recurrent dissection (363). The 10-year actuarial survival rate of patients who leave the hospital is approximately 60% (376). In a long-term study of surgically treated survivors of aortic dissection, 29% of all late deaths were due to the development and eventual rupture of a localized saccular aneurysm (378). Thus, close lifelong monitoring of treated survivors of aortic dissection is required. It may be useful to perform a baseline thoracic MRI prior to discharge with follow-up examinations at 6 months and 1 year. Subsequent follow-up studies are usually performed every 1 to 2 years.

HYPERTENSIVE CRISES IN THE PATIENT REQUIRING SURGERY

Poorly Controlled Hypertension in the Patient Requiring Surgery

In the preoperative setting, the goals of blood pressure management include: (a) assessment of the perioperative risks of acute or chronic hypertension; (b) modification of the risk to minimize perioperative cardiac complications; and (c) sometimes the substitution of alternative antihypertensive agents for the patient's chronic oral antihypertensives during the perioperative period (379). Hypertension in the preoperative patient is a common problem. In a series of 1,000 patients over the age of 40 presenting for surgery, 28% were hypertensive (380). However, studies of perioperative cardiac risk have demonstrated that mild to moderate hypertension is not an independent risk factor for the development of postoperative myocardial infarction, pulmonary edema, ventricular tachycardia, or cardiac death (380,381). On the other hand, one study that evaluated intraoperative systemic hemodynamics in patients with either preoperative normotension, adequately treated hypertension, or inadequately treated hypertension demonstrated the benefits of preoperative control of blood pressure (382). During anesthesia, cardiac output decreased by 30% in all three groups. Normotensives and adequately treated hypertensives had only minor changes in systemic vascular resistance resulting in modest decreases in mean arterial pressure of 23% and 33%, respectively. In contrast, the inadequately treated hypertensives experienced, on average, a 27% decrease in systemic vascular resistance which, coupled with the declines in cardiac output, resulted in reduction of mean arterial pressure by 45% during anesthesia. Electrocardiographic changes consistent with myocardial ischemia were commonly observed in the latter group. Hypertensive patients can develop wide swings in blood pressure intraoperatively, which increase the risk of postoperative cardiac and renal complications (383). Thus, while mild to moderate hypertension with diastolic blood pressure under 110 mm Hg may not be an independent risk factor for adverse cardiac outcomes, it may predispose to the development of intraoperative hypotension or hypertension which in turn increases the risk of postoperative complications (379).

Poor control of preoperative hypertension, with a diastolic blood pressure higher than 110 mm Hg, is a relative contraindication to elective surgery. In patients with a diastolic blood pressure higher than 110 mm Hg, perioperative morbidity and mortality are increased due to a high incidence of intraoperative hypotension accompanied by myocardial ischemia and postoperative acute renal failure (384).

However, it should be noted that these data were collected in patients hospitalized for preoperative evaluation in which multiple blood pressure readings were available to document persistently poor preoperative blood pressure control. It is not clear whether these criteria should be applied to patients presenting for outpatient surgery who are found to have a diastolic blood pressure over 110 mm Hg. The finding of elevated blood pressure in this circumstance may not necessarily be reflective of long-term inadequate blood pressure control. In this setting, if there is no history of long-standing inadequate blood pressure control and if the blood pressure responds satisfactorily to sedation, sublingual nifedipine, or mini-bolus labetalol, it may be possible to proceed with elective outpatient surgery (385).

Malignant hypertension clearly represents an excessive surgical risk, and all but lifesaving emergency surgery should be deferred until the blood pressure can be controlled and organ function stabilized (385).

Some authorities believe that mild to moderate, uncomplicated, preoperative hypertension (diastolic blood pressure $\leq$110 mm Hg) does not significantly increase the risk of surgery and is therefore not a reason to postpone elective surgery (384,386,387). However, patients with mild to moderate hypertension and a preexisting complication such as ischemic heart disease, cerebrovascular disease, congestive heart failure, or chronic renal insufficiency represent a subgroup with a significantly increased perioperative risk (384). In these patients, adequate preoperative control of blood pressure is imperative (388). Even though the blood pressure in patients with severe or complicated hypertension can usually be controlled within hours using aggressive parenteral therapy, such precipitous control of hypertension carries the risk of significant complications such as hypovolemia, electrolyte abnormalities, and marked intraoperative and postoperative blood pressure lability. These risks predispose to myocardial ischemia, cerebrovascular accidents, and acute renal failure (386). In these high-risk groups, if possible, elective surgery should be postponed and blood pressure brought under control for a few weeks before surgery (386). Ideally, sustained adequate preoperative blood pressure control should be the aim in all hypertensive patients (386,388).

In patients with adequately treated hypertension, antihypertensive and antianginal medications should be continued up to and including the morning of surgery. Such treatment decreases intraoperative blood pressure lability and protects against the hypertensive response associated with endotracheal intubation and other noxious stimuli during surgery (388,389). Oral administration of blood pressure medications with a small amount of water (15 to 20 mL) a few hours before surgery does not increase the risk of gastric aspiration during anesthesia induction (386). Since hypovolemia increases the risk of intraoperative hypotension and postoperative acute renal failure, diuretics should be withheld for 1 to 2 days preoperatively except in patients with overt heart failure or fluid overload. Adequate potassium supplementation should be provided to correct hypokalemia well in advance of surgery. Drugs such as clonidine, which carry the potential for withdrawal reactions or hypertensive rebound during the postoperative period, may be electively tapered and replaced with other medications over 1 to 2 weeks preoperatively. Alternatively, the clonidine transdermal therapeutic system has been recommended for the perioperative management of patients receiving long-term centrally acting α_2-agonist therapy (390).

Theoretically, β-adrenergic blockers could cause hemodynamic instability in the setting of surgical stress, blood loss, and the myocardial depression caused by anesthetics. However, studies have shown that elective withdrawal of beta-blockers preoperatively not only is unnecessary but also may be deleterious in patients with underlying coronary artery disease. Continuation of beta-blockers until a few hours before general anesthesia does not appear to impair hemodynamic function (391). Furthermore, patients pretreated with beta-blockers have less hypertension, tachycardia, myocardial ischemia, and dysrhythmias during endotracheal intubation than do patients who do not receive beta-blockers (392).

The use of converting enzyme inhibitors in the preoperative management of the hypertensive patient is controversial (393). The current consensus is that patients receiving chronic therapy with a converting enzyme inhibitor should continue the drug up until surgery and then restart therapy as soon as possible postoperatively. However, given the physiologic role of the renin-angiotensin system in patients subjected to a hypovolemic insult intraoperatively, concern has been raised regarding the risk of intraoperative hemodynamic instability in patients undergoing extensive surgical procedures involving large amounts of blood loss or fluid shifts (394). In contrast, there are data that suggest that converting enzyme inhibitors may be beneficial in patients undergoing coronary artery bypass surgery. Comparison of systemic hemodynamics and renal function in patients pretreated with either captopril or placebo showed that renal plasma flow, glomerular filtration rate, and urinary sodium excretion were higher in patients treated with captopril (395).

The choice of anesthetic technique in the hypertensive patient should be individualized (386,389). For peripheral procedures, regional nerve block involves minimal physiologic stress and may be the procedure of choice. Although spinal anesthesia for lower extremity and certain abdominal procedures minimizes myocardial depression and is not associated with sympathetic discharge during endotracheal intubation, the concomitant sympathetic blockade is not quickly reversible and may lead to cardiovascular collapse in high-risk hypertensive patients (386). For general anesthesia, most of the commonly used anesthetics are acceptable for use in the hypertensive patient. However, drugs such as ketamine that provoke hypertensive responses should be avoided. During anesthesia there are often wide and rapid fluctuations in blood pressure that require close monitoring, often by the direct intraarterial method (386). Continuous electrocardiographic monitoring is essential to monitor for evidence of myocardial ischemia. Accurate measurement of urine output is a helpful indirect measure of the adequacy of renal perfusion. Patients with severe hypertension undergoing upper abdominal or thoracic surgery may require central venous pressure monitoring as a guide to fluid replacement. Monitoring of cardiac output and wedge pressure should be considered in patients with a history of left ventricular failure or ischemic heart disease or those undergoing major thoracic or cardiovascular procedures (386).

The hypertensive surge during endotracheal intubation can be managed with infusion of sodium nitroprusside, esmolol, or minibolus labetalol (389,396,397). In complicated patients with a history of cardiovascular disease or congestive heart failure, intraoperative and postoperative hypertension should be managed with short-acting agents such as sodium nitroprusside or possibly fenoldopam until the preoperative oral antihypertensive regimen can be resumed (3). Given the benefits of intravenous nitroglycerin with regard to coronary vasospasm and the collateral circulation, it may be a useful agent for the management of perioperative hypertension in patients with coronary artery disease undergoing either noncardiac surgery or coronary artery bypass surgery (398). In postoperative patients, trimethaphan is contraindicated because of the risk of bowel and bladder atony.

In uncomplicated patients, intermittent intravenous labetalol injections may be useful in the management of mild to moderate postoperative hypertension (399,400). However, tachycardia and paradoxical hypertension may occur in the setting of volume depletion in patients with chronic hypertension. Therefore, physiologic tachycardia in response to volume depletion should always be excluded prior to parenteral administration of any beta-blocker. Parenteral agents such as furosemide, beta-blockers, and hydralazine, or oral antihypertensive agents given by nasogastric tube have also been recommended for the management of uncomplicated postoperative hypertension until oral therapy can be resumed. Newer agents such as nicardipine and fenoldopam may offer potential advantages over older agents in the treatment of perioperative hypertension (401). However, the cost–benefit ratio of these newer agents must also be considered. Despite the fact that perioperative hypertension is aggressively treated, there are no long-term, large-scale study data indicating that aggressive treatment affects long-term patient outcome (401).

Many patients with long-standing severe hypertension require much smaller doses of antihypertensive medications in the early postoperative course. Thus, the preoperative regimen should not be automatically restarted. Routine measurements of supine and standing blood pressure should be utilized as a guide to dosage adjustments during the postoperative recovery period. In most instances, the requirement for antihypertensive medications will gradually increase over a few days to weeks to eventually equal the preoperative regimen.

Postcoronary Bypass Hypertension

Paroxysmal hypertension in the immediate postoperative period is a frequent and serious complication of cardiac surgery. It is the most common complication of coronary artery bypass surgery, occurring in 30% to 50% of patients (401). Postbypass hypertension is mediated by increases in systemic vascular resistance. The heightened systemic vascular resistance increases cardiac work and myocardial oxygen demand. The accompanying increase in LVEDP impairs subendocardial perfusion and can cause myocardial ischemia in patients with limited coronary reserve. The acute increase in afterload can also impair cardiac performance and precipitate acute pulmonary edema. In addition, hypertension increases the incidence and severity of postoperative bleeding in recently heparinized patients. Therefore, postbypass hypertension should be diagnosed and rapidly treated.

There are numerous precipitating factors for hypertension in the postoperative setting including emergence from anesthesia, tracheal or nasopharyngeal irritation from the endotracheal tube, pain, hypothermia with shivering, ventilator asynchrony, hypoxemia, hypercarbia, myocardial ischemia, and withdrawal phenomena resulting from preoperative discontinuation of antihypertensive medications (401). Hypervolemia, though often cited as a mechanism of postoperative hypertension, is a rare cause of hypertension in this setting except in patients with renal failure (401). Marked sympathetic overreaction to hypovolemia is a common, often unrecognized, cause of severe postoperative hypertension and impaired tissue perfusion (403,404).

Hypertension after myocardial revascularization occurs as often in previously normotensive patients as in those with chronic hypertension (405). The increase in blood pressure usually occurs during the first 4 hours after surgery and tends to resolve 6 to 12 hours postoperatively. The hypertension, which results from a rise in systemic vascular resistance without a change in cardiac output, may be related to an increase in sympathetic tone due to activation of pressor reflexes from the heart, great vessels, or coronary arteries (401,405).

The initial management of postbypass hypertension should include attempts to ameliorate the reversible causes of hypertension previously mentioned. Hypertension resulting from pain and anxiety should be managed with analgesics or sedatives. Hypothermia should be treated with warming blankets; intravenous fluids should be preheated to 37°C. Patients with paradoxical hypertension in response to volume depletion are exquisitely sensitive to vasodilator therapy and may develop precipitous hypotension even with low-dose infusions of sodium nitroprusside or nitroglycerin. Hypertension in this setting should be treated using careful volume expansion with crystalloid or transfusion as required (403). If these general measures fail to control the blood pressure, further therapy should be guided by measurement of systemic hemodynamics. Parenterally administered vasodilators are the treatment of choice for postbypass hypertension. Sodium nitroprusside or intravenous nitroglycerin can be utilized to provide controlled reduction in the systemic vascular resistance and blood pressure. Intravenous nitroglycerin is as effective for hypertension in this setting as is sodium nitroprusside (398). Nitroglycerin may be the preferred drug because it dilates intercoronary collaterals and causes less intrapulmonary shunting than does sodium nitroprusside. Moreover, sustained infusion of even low-dose sodium nitroprusside may result in cyanide toxicity, which should be considered in the differential diagnosis in postcoronary bypass graft patients who develop unexplained neurologic, cardiac, or pulmonary complications (406). Recent studies suggest that fenoldopam may be useful for the management of hypertension following bypass surgery (407,408). Postbypass hypertension is usually transient and resolves over 6 to 12 hours, after which the vasodilator can be weaned. The hypertension does not usually recur after the initial episode in the immediate postoperative period (405).

An intravenous beta-blocker is occasionally recommended for control of hypertension in patients with tachycardia prior to surgery. However, beta-blockers are generally not indicated in the setting of postbypass hypertension because the hypertension is usually secondary to increased systemic vascular resistance rather than to increased cardiac output (402,405). Moreover, the tachycardia may be a physiologic response to volume depletion. Beta-blocker therapy may be detrimental as these agents compromise cardiac output and increase systemic vascular resistance. In this regard, labetalol has been shown to cause a significant reduction in cardiac index in patients with hypertension following bypass surgery (409).

Postcarotid Endarterectomy Hypertension

Hypertension in the immediate postoperative period is extremely common after carotid endarterectomy. In one large series, 58% of patients had postcarotid endarterectomy hypertension as defined by an increase in systolic blood pressure of more than 35 mm Hg or systolic blood pressure requiring treatment with sodium nitroprusside (410). A history of hypertension, especially with poor control of hypertension preoperatively, dramatically increases the risk of postoperative hypertension (411,412). Severe postoperative hypertension following carotid endarterectomy is associated with an increased incidence of stroke with focal neurologic deficits, intracerebral hemorrhage, and increased postoperative mortality (411–414).

The mechanism of postcarotid endarterectomy hypertension is poorly understood. The incidence of hypertension is the same whether or not the carotid sinus nerves are preserved (411). A mechanism for the development of postoperative hemorrhage due to hypertension has been proposed (413). In patients with high-grade carotid artery stenosis, the distal cerebral bed has been protected from systemic hypertension by the stenosis. Following removal of the obstructing lesion, a relative increase in perfusion pressure occurs in the previously protected arteriocapillary bed. Especially in the setting of postop-

erative hypertension, cerebral autoregulation may fail such that there is overperfusion and rupture resulting in hemorrhagic infarction.

Because poor preoperative blood pressure control increases the risk of postoperative hypertension, strict blood pressure control is mandatory prior to elective carotid endarterectomy. Furthermore, intraarterial blood pressure should be monitored intraoperatively and in the immediate postoperative period. Ideally, the patient should be awake and extubated prior to reaching the recovery room so that serial neurologic examinations can be used to assess the development of focal deficits. When the systolic blood pressure exceeds 200 mm Hg, an intravenous infusion of sodium nitroprusside should be initiated to maintain systolic blood pressure between 160 and 200 mm Hg (411). The use of a short-acting parenteral agent is imperative to avoid overshoot hypotension and cerebral hypoperfusion.

Hypertensive Crises After Repair of Aortic Coarctation

During the first week after repair of coarctation of the aorta, severe systemic hypertension frequently develops (415). This so-called paradoxical hypertension usually resolves spontaneously if the repair has been satisfactory. There are two distinct phases to the paradoxical hypertensive response: an acute rise in systolic blood pressure on the first postoperative day and a later rise in the diastolic pressure during the second through fourth postoperative days (415,416). The immediate postoperative increase in systolic blood pressure lasts 8 to 12 hours and is similar in mechanism to the postmyocardial revascularization hypertension previously described. The second phase of hypertension, which is accompanied by abdominal pain and signs of an acute abdomen, causes considerable morbidity and mortality due to the development of mesenteric endarteritis (417).

After repair of coarctation, the decline in blood pressure in the upper body results in baroreceptor activation. The release of the sympathetic axis from tonic baroreceptor inhibition results in "vasomotor storm" with markedly increased heart rate and blood pressure. The renin-angiotensin axis may also be activated by the increase in sympathetic tone, and angiotensin-mediated vasoconstriction may account for part of the pressor response (415). The mesenteric vessels that had been exposed to the low pressure distal to the coarctation are suddenly exposed to severe hypertension. This may cause endarteritis and vascular necrosis with intestinal ischemia and infarction.

Prophylactic oral propranolol, at a dosage of 1.5 mg/kg/day in divided doses for 2 weeks before surgery, can prevent paradoxical postcoarctectomy hypertension (415). Sodium nitroprusside and parenteral beta-blockers have also been used successfully to treat postcoarctectomy hypertension. The goal of therapy should be to maintain systolic blood pressure in the range of 120 to 150 mm Hg. As soon as possible, oral propranolol should be instituted as the sodium nitroprusside infusion is weaned (418).

Hypertension Complicating Postoperative Bleeding

Hypertension in the postoperative period can result in severe and intractable bleeding from vascular suture lines. Hypertension can also aggravate bleeding in the setting of severe epistaxis, and tracheal, gastrointestinal, or urinary tract hemorrhage. Retroperitoneal hemorrhage after closed renal biopsy can be exacerbated by hypertension. In each situation, control of the blood pressure is required for normal hemostasis.

Sodium nitroprusside should be utilized for immediate and precise control of the blood pressure.

CATECHOLAMINE-RELATED HYPERTENSIVE CRISES

Hypertensive Crises with Pheochromocytoma

The diagnosis and treatment of pheochromocytoma are discussed in detail in Chapter 55. The comments here are restricted to treatment of hypertensive crises in patients with pheochromocytoma, with emphasis on the perioperative management of hypertension. In the majority of patients, pheochromocytoma causes sustained hypertension that occasionally enters the malignant phase. In roughly 30% of patients, paroxysmal hypertension is present. Paroxysms usually occur spontaneously and consist of severe hypertension, headache, profuse diaphoresis, pallor of the face, coldness of the hands and feet, palpitations, and abdominal discomfort. Marked elevation of blood pressure can lead to intracerebral hemorrhage, hypertensive encephalopathy, or acute pulmonary edema (419). Prompt reduction of blood pressure is mandatory to prevent these life-threatening complications. Although the nonselective α-adrenergic receptor blocker phentolamine is often cited as the treatment of choice for pheochromocytoma-related hypertensive crises, sodium nitroprusside is equally effective (420,421). Phentolamine is given in 5- to 10-mg intravenous boluses every 5 minutes as necessary to control blood pressure. Given its short duration of action, a continuous infusion of phentolamine can also be utilized. After the blood pressure has been controlled with sodium nitroprusside or phentolamine, intravenous β-adrenergic receptor blockers such as esmolol and propranolol can be used to control tachycardia or arrhythmias. After resolution of the hypertensive crisis, oral antihypertensive agents should be instituted as the parenteral agents are weaned.

Skillful preoperative management of blood pressure and volume status is clearly a prerequisite to successful surgical intervention (420–422). Usually, the nonselective α-blocker phenoxybenzamine is administered for 1 to 2 weeks prior to elective surgery. The initial dose of 10 mg twice daily is increased every other day until normotension, accompanied by moderate (15 mm Hg) asymptomatic orthostatic hypertension, has been attained and paroxysms are well controlled (421,422). The last dose of phenoxybenzamine is usually administered at 10 PM on the evening before surgery. After adequate α-blockade has been achieved, oral beta-blocker therapy can be initiated if needed to control tachycardia. Oral or intravenous beta-blockers should *never* be administered before adequate α-adrenergic blockade has been achieved. Administration of a beta-blocker to patients with catecholamine-secreting tumors can lead to severe hypertension with acute pulmonary edema as the result of intense α-adrenergic-mediated vasoconstriction that is no longer opposed by β-adrenergic vasodilatory stimuli. Prazosin, a selective α_1-antagonist, has been used for preoperative management of hypertension (423). However, hypertensive crises responsive to low-dose phenoxybenzamine have been observed in patients receiving apparently adequate α-blockade with prazosin (424). Labetalol has also been advocated for the preoperative management of hypertension in patients with pheochromocytoma (425). However, hypertensive crises precipitated by the use of labetalol have been reported (426). The paradoxical increase in blood pressure is due to the fact that labetalol exhibits more potent β-blockade that α-blockade.

Careful attention to volume status is imperative in the preoperative period (421,422). Alleviation of the chronic state of catecholamine-induced vasoconstriction by α-blockade results in increases in both arterial and venous capacitance. Preoperative volume expansion guided by measurements of central venous pressure or pulmonary capillary wedge pressure has been advocated to reduce the severity of intraoperative hypotension (422). However, other authors maintain that a high-salt diet or infusions of crystalloid are usually not necessary in the majority of patients during the preoperative period because treatment with α-adrenergic blockade for 1 to 2 weeks alleviates the chronic state of vasoconstriction and allows for spontaneous restoration of normal plasma volume (420). Moreover, caution has been advised if intravenous fluids are administered during the preoperative period because pulmonary edema can occur if an underlying catecholamine-induced cardiomyopathy is present (420).

Cardiac status should be evaluated carefully in the preoperative period. Approximately 25% of patients with catecholamine-secreting tumors have some degree of cardiomyopathy with biventricular dysfunction caused either by a direct toxic effect of catecholamines on the myocardium or indirectly by chronic hypertension (420). This catecholamine-induced cardiomyopathy is associated with an increased risk of sudden death from arrhythmias, as well as increased surgical risk. Thus, preoperative evaluation should include echocardiography to assess ventricular function. The cardiomyopathy is usually reversible with adequate preoperative chronic adrenergic blockade. Surgical intervention should generally be deferred until serial echocardiograms confirm that ventricular function has improved in response to treatment with adrenergic blocking drugs.

During surgery, rapid and wide fluctuation in blood pressure should be anticipated (421). Adequate premedication should be used to minimize the risk of sympathetic activation during endotracheal intubation and induction of anesthesia. Diazepam and short-acting barbiturates are the agents of choice for premedication (421). Droperidol, phenothiazines, and morphine are contraindicated because they can cause catecholamine release. Atropine should be avoided because its vagolytic effect results in tachycardia in the setting of high-circulating catecholamine levels.

Careful intraoperative monitoring of intraarterial blood pressure, cardiac output, pulmonary capillary wedge pressure, and systemic vascular resistance is required to manage rapid swings in blood pressure (421). Despite adequate preoperative α-blockade with phenoxybenzamine, severe hypertension can occur during intubation or intraoperatively due to catecholamine release during tumor manipulation. Though intermittent bolus phentolamine has been advocated in this setting, prolonged α-blockade may predispose to significant hypotension following tumor devascularization (421). Therefore, sodium nitroprusside, with its immediate onset and short duration of action, is the agent of choice for controlling acute hypertension during pheochromocytoma surgery (421). Infusions of esmolol, propranolol, or lidocaine can be used for short-term control of arrhythmias (420,421).

At the opposite end of the spectrum, severe intraoperative hypotension can occur. Hypotension or even frank shock can supervene following isolation of tumor venous drainage from the circulation, with a resultant abrupt decrease in circulating catecholamine levels. This hypotension is caused by a precipitous reduction in vascular tone, which can be aggravated further by operative blood loss, downregulation of adrenergic receptors in response to chronic increases in catecholamines, α-adrenergic blockade, or impaired heart rate response resulting from β-adrenergic blocking drugs (421). Volume expansion with crystalloid, colloid, or blood as needed is the recommended treatment for intraoperative hypotension. Volume repletion should be guided by measurements of pulmonary capillary wedge pressure and cardiac output. Pressors should only be employed when hypotension is unresponsive to adequate volume repletion (421). The risk of hypotension due to hypovolemia extends into the postoperative period during which close monitoring of volume status is essential. In the postoperative period, required volume replacement not uncommonly exceeds measured fluid losses (421).

Hypertensive Crises Secondary to Withdrawal of Antihypertensive Therapy

Abrupt discontinuation of high doses of centrally acting antihypertensive agents such as clonidine (273,427), methyldopa (428), and guanabenz (427,429) can produce a withdrawal syndrome characterized by sympathetic overactivity (430). Symptoms consisting of headache, nausea, restlessness, agitation, insomnia, and tremor usually begin 12 to 72 hours after discontinuation of the drug. Occasionally, this withdrawal syndrome is accompanied by a rapid increase in blood pressure to above pretreatment levels (overshoot hypertension) (431). The abrupt rise in blood pressure can precipitate a hypertensive crisis with hypertensive encephalopathy or acute pulmonary edema.

The symptoms that develop following cessation of centrally acting α-receptor agonists are suggestive of sympathetic overactivity. It has been postulated that the syndrome may be related to excessive circulating catecholamine levels (430). Because the antihypertensive action of central α-agonists is due to a reduction in catecholamine release from nerve terminals, abrupt discontinuation may provoke a sudden catecholamine surge. Increased plasma and urine catecholamine levels have been found after abrupt discontinuation of high-dose clonidine (273). The renin-angiotensin system may also be involved in withdrawal phenomenon. As clonidine and methyldopa suppress plasma renin activity (PRA), it is possible that a rebound increase in PRA and angiotensin II could mediate the hypertensive overshoot following drug withdrawal (432).

In general, withdrawal symptoms or rebound hypertension occur only after cessation of large doses of drugs. Withdrawal symptoms rarely appear after discontinuation of clonidine in doses less than 1.2 mg/day (433). The average dose of guanabenz in the reported cases of withdrawal syndrome was 48 mg/day (429). However, the withdrawal syndrome can occasionally be precipitated by cessation of lower doses of drugs. This is especially apt to occur in patients with underlying renal insufficiency or renovascular hypertension (432). Patients treated with beta-blockers may be predisposed to develop severe hypertension during withdrawal of centrally acting α-agonists (434). Beta-adrenergic receptor blockade inhibits the vasodilatory effect of β_2-receptors on the peripheral vasculature, leaving vasoconstrictor α_1-receptors unopposed.

Treatment of antihypertensive drug withdrawal syndromes should be individualized. In patients with generalized symptoms of sympathetic overactivity but without excessive blood pressure elevation, reinstitution of the previously administered drug is usually all that is required (430). However, if the withdrawal syndrome is associated with severe hypertension, hypertensive encephalopathy, or acute pulmonary edema, rapid control of blood pressure with parenteral antihypertensive agents is imperative. Sodium nitroprusside or phentolamine should be used for the management of these hypertensive crises. After the blood pressure is controlled with parenteral agents, oral clonidine, guanabenz, or methyldopa should be restarted. The offending drug should then be gradually withdrawn with close monitoring for withdrawal symptoms and rebound hypertension. Another oral antihypertensive regimen, preferably without a beta-blocker, should be initiated simultaneously.

Hypertensive Crises Secondary to Monoamine Oxidase Inhibitor Interactions

Severe paroxysmal hypertension complicated by intracerebral or subarachnoid hemorrhage, hypertensive encephalopathy, or acute pulmonary edema can occur in patients receiving monoamine oxidase (MAO) inhibitors after ingestion of certain foods or drugs (274,435). The three major MAO inhibitors available in the United States are the antidepressant drugs tranylcypromine (Parnate), phenelzine (Nardil), and isocarboxazid (Marplan).

Although catechol O-methyltransferase is important in the metabolism of circulating catecholamines, MAO is required for the degradation of intracellular amines including epinephrine, norepinephrine, and dopamine (436). Since MAO normally limits intracellular amine accumulation, MAO inhibitors cause an increase in the quantity of amines within storage granules. The amino acid tyramine releases these stores of catecholamines from nerve endings, causing a profound pressor response. Certain foods contain substantial amounts of tyramine including natural or aged cheeses, Chianti wines, champagne, imported beers, pickled herring, chicken liver, yeast, soy sauce, fermented sausage, coffee, avocado, banana, chocolate, overripe or spoiled food, and aged fish or meat (salami, pepperoni, and bologna) (435,437). As a result of hepatic and intestinal MAO-inhibition, tyramine escapes oxidative degradation and causes release of norepinephrine from nerve endings. Sympathomimetic amines in nonprescription cold remedies such a phenylpropanolamine can also provoke neurotransmitter release. A hyperadrenergic state resembling pheochromocytoma then ensues.

In a large series of patients treated with MAO inhibitors, symptoms typically began within 10 minutes to 2 hours after ingestion of the offending food or drug. Symptoms include sudden onset of severe pounding headache, palpitations, throbbing vessels in the neck, flushing or pallor, profuse diaphoresis, nausea, vomiting, and extreme prostration. Abrupt onset of marked hypertension is a characteristic finding. The mean increase in blood pressure is 55 mm Hg systolic and 30 mm Hg diastolic. Complications include intracerebral hemorrhage, subarachnoid hemorrhage, hypertensive encephalopathy, and acute pulmonary edema. The duration of the attacks varies from 10 minutes to 6 hours (435).

Either sodium nitroprusside or phentolamine can be used to manage this type of hypertensive crisis. Because most patients are normotensive prior to the onset of the hypertensive crisis, the goal of treatment should be the normalization of blood pressure. Intravenous beta-blockers may also be required for control of heart rate and tachyarrhythmias. Because hypertensive crisis with MAO inhibitor–tyramine interactions is usually self-limited, the nitroprusside or phentolamine infusion can be weaned without institution of an oral antihypertensive agent.

Hypertensive Crises Due to Nonprescription Sympathomimetic Amines

Phenylpropanolamine, phenylephrine, ephedrine, and pseudoephedrine are sympathomimetic amines available in a wide variety of over-the-counter drug preparations that are marketed as nasal decongestants, appetite suppressants, or stimulants. However, toxic effects can result from overdose (278,279,438). Moreover, there may be substantial abuse potential for use as amphetamine substitutes (279). A recent study in healthy, normotensive subjects found that 150 mg of phenylpropanolamine (the amount contained in a double dose of an over-the-counter appetite suppressant) substantially elevated blood pressure (439). Review of adverse drug effect case reports suggests that overdose of phenylpropanolamine can cause a significant increase in blood pressure that can be complicated by severe headache, hypertensive encephalopathy, intracerebral hemorrhage, seizures, and even death (278). Given the majority of serious adverse events, the FDA has recently banned the use of phenylpropanolamine in over-the-counter medications (440). In patients who present with hypertensive encephalopathy of unknown origin, the possibility of recent ingestion of over-the-counter sympathomimetic amines should be investigated. Hypertensive crises secondary to sympathomimetic amines should be treated with a rapid-acting agent such as sodium nitroprusside or phentolamine. This is generally the only treatment required because these drugs are rapidly eliminated and the duration of the toxic reaction is usually less than 6 hours (279).

AUTONOMIC HYPERREFLEXIA FOLLOWING SPINAL CORD INJURY

Autonomic hyperreflexia (or autonomic dysreflexia) is an acute medical emergency that occurs in quadriplegics and paraplegics whose spinal cord lesion lies above the greater splanchnic outflow from the thoracolumbar preganglionic sympathetic neurons (lesions at T-6 or above) (287,441–444). This potentially life-threatening syndrome results from interruption of normal feedback mechanisms in the sympathetic pathway (441). Attacks of autonomic hyperreflexia usually begin at 4 to 6 months after the injury and can recur episodically for the rest of the patient's life (444). Autonomic hyperreflexia develops in 50% to 80% of patients with spinal cord injury (287,444). Hypertensive crises, presumably due to autonomic hyperreflexia, have also been reported in patients with Guillain-Barré syndrome (445). Noxious stimuli arising below the level of the injury, most commonly due to distention of the bladder or bowel, trigger a response mediated by the sympathetic nervous system (442). Afferent impulses from nerves below the level of the cord lesion cause excess stimulation of preganglionic sympathetic neurons. The result is reflex sympathetic outflow via the splanchnic nerves with profound vasoconstriction in the visceral arteries of the splanchnic bed leading to a sudden increase in blood pressure. The elevated blood pressure stimulates baroreceptors in the carotids and aortic arch and signals are sent to the vasomotor center in the brainstem. Parasympathetic efferent impulses from the brainstem via the tenth cranial nerve cause bradycardia, which may be transient. However, in patients with spinal cord lesions above the major splanchnic sympathetic outflow, descending inhibitory feedback is blocked so that reflex vasoconstriction of the peripheral and splanchnic vasculature continues unabated. The end-result is a sudden increase in blood pressure, often reaching systolic pressures over 250 mm Hg. It is important to note that the normal resting systolic blood pressure in patients with spinal cord injury is often 80 to 90 mm Hg, and a systolic blood pressure of 130 mm Hg may be a sign of autonomic hyperreflexia. The most common symptom during a paroxysm of autonomic hyperreflexia is severe headache, but the sudden increase in blood pressure may trigger a hypertensive crisis with seizures, cortical blindness, hypertensive encephalopathy, intracerebral hemorrhage, or acute hypertensive heart failure. Additional symptoms and signs include feelings of doom, facial flushing, nasal congestion, diaphoresis and piloerection above the level of the

cord lesion, and cool clammy skin below the level of injury. Bradycardia is present in only 50% of cases. Educating patients about dysreflexia is an important part of the initial rehabilitation from spinal cord injury. Most patients can recognize the occurrence of their specific pattern of signs and symptoms of dysreflexia.

Autonomic hyperreflexia can be triggered by any noxious stimulus in the dermatomes, muscles, or viscera supplied by nerves below the level of the cord injury. Stimuli related to distention of a hollow viscus are particularly effective in eliciting this response (441–444). Bladder distention and fecal impaction are the most frequent inciting stimuli (286). Urinary tract instrumentation, gynecologic instrumentation, or labor and delivery may also provoke an attack. Spinal cord injury patients undergoing abdominal or bladder surgery are also at high risk. In addition, a variety of medical problems including pressure sores, occult fractures, deep venous thrombosis, and heterotopic ossification may cause symptoms of dysreflexia. Patients at risk should be cautioned about the use of over-the-counter sympathomimetic medications, such as decongestants and appetite suppressants, which may also provoke an attack.

Autonomic hyperreflexia is best managed by prevention. If routine bowel or bladder care (bladder catheterization or bowel programs) trigger an attack, local anesthesia with Xylocaine lubricant may be used. Individuals with frequently occurring symptoms may benefit from prophylactic treatment with nifedipine or phenoxybenzamine. Drug regimens should only be implemented after a thorough search for potentially underlying correctable causes. Management of hypertensive crises due to autonomic hyperreflexia requires prompt recognition with correction of precipitating causes. Failure to recognize autonomic hyperreflexia or misdiagnosis can lead to substantial morbidity. Any spinal cord injury patient presenting with an emergency or strange symptoms should be suspected of having autonomic dysreflexia until proven otherwise (443,444). The severe hypertension must be treated expeditiously to avoid such complications as retinal hemorrhage, seizures, hypertensive encephalopathy, or intracerebral hemorrhage. During an acute episode, the patient should be brought to a sitting position with legs dangling to take advantage of the natural orthostasis that occurs with spinal cord injury. The bladder should be checked for distention by immediate catheterization. If bladder distention is not found, rectal examination should be performed to exclude fecal impaction. If these measures fail, medication to blunt the sympathetic response should be administered. Transdermal nitroglycerin may break the hypertensive reflex and this agent can be removed when the blood pressure normalizes. Oral clonidine or nifedipine may also be useful alternatives. Once the autonomic reflex is broken, long-term antihypertensive drug therapy is seldom needed. Occasionally, development of a hypertensive crisis with encephalopathy or seizures may necessitate treatment with parenteral antihypertensive agents such as diazoxide, trimethaphan, nitroprusside, or fenoldopam. Nitroprusside is particularly useful for management of intraoperative hypertension in patients with spinal cord injury.

MISCELLANEOUS HYPERTENSIVE CRISES

Hypertensive crises have been reported in a wide variety of clinical settings. Patients with extensive second- or third-degree burns may develop hypertensive crises 3 to 4 days after hospitalization (446). Hypertensive crises have been reported as idiosyncratic reactions to a number of drugs including amphotericin B (447), lithium (intoxication) (448), amitriptyline

(449), and metrizamide (450). Severe hypertension with hypertensive encephalopathy has been reported to occur in a dose-related fashion in children treated with high-dose cyclosporine for allogenic bone marrow transplantation (280,281). Hypertensive crises can also complicate the use of illicit drugs including cocaine hydrochloride or alkaloidal (crack) cocaine (451,452), and phencyclidine hydrochloride (PCP) (276).

In each of these conditions sudden elevation of blood pressure in previously normotensive individuals can cause hypertensive encephalopathy, intracerebral hemorrhage, or acute pulmonary edema. Sodium nitroprusside is the treatment of choice for the management of hypertension in these diverse settings.

Hypertensive crises have been reported in patients with insulin-induced hypoglycemia who are concomitantly treated with beta-blockers (453). It has been postulated that epinephrine release induced by hypoglycemia, in the presence of vascular β_2-receptor blockade by propranolol, causes severe hypertensive reactions due to unopposed α_1-receptor-mediated vasoconstriction.

Hypertensive crises may develop in renal allograft recipients due to acute rejection, high-dose glucocorticoid treatment, or transplant renal artery stenosis (283,284,454). Refractory hypertension complicated by hypertensive encephalopathy can also occur in patients with chronic allograft rejection who have returned to dialysis. This complication tends to develop during tapering of immunosuppressive therapy and may be caused by superimposed acute allograft rejection. Allograft nephrectomy may be indicated for the long-term control of blood pressure in this setting.

THE CONTROVERSY OVER GRADUAL VERSUS RAPID REDUCTION OF BLOOD PRESSURE

Over the last several years, some authors have cautioned against rapid lowering of blood pressure in patients with hypertensive crises and have recommended a more gradual reduction of blood pressure (319,455–457). The case for gradual reduction of blood pressure is based largely on the finding of altered autoregulation of cerebral blood flow in hypertensive patients and scattered case reports of serious neurologic sequelae resulting from overly aggressive reduction of blood pressure in patients with severe hypertension or hypertensive crises (294,458–464).

In both hypertensive and normotensive individuals, cerebral blood flow is maintained constant, at approximately 50 mL/minute/100 g of brain tissue, over a wide range of perfusion pressures, by virtue of various intrinsic and neurohumoral autoregulatory mechanisms. The lower limit of cerebral blood flow autoregulation is the blood pressure below which autoregulatory vasodilation becomes maximal and cerebral blood flow decreases. In normotensive subjects, the lower limit of autoregulation is a mean arterial pressure of 60 to 70 mm Hg. In chronically hypertensive patients, the lower limit of autoregulation is shifted so that autoregulation fails and cerebral blood flow decreases at a higher blood pressure than in normotensive individuals (292,293). This effect may be the result of hypertension-induced changes in the cerebral arterioles. In animal models, chronic hypertension causes hypertrophy of the walls of cerebral vessels with a reduction in internal diameter. Moreover, during chronic hypertension, cerebral arterioles undergo structural remodeling, which results in a smaller external diameter and encroachment on the vascular lumen (184).

On the one hand, these structural changes are protective in that the thickened cerebral arterioles are able to maintain constant cerebral blood flow at a higher perfusion pressure than would be tolerated by normotensive individuals. In this regard, in chronically hypertensive individuals, the mean arterial pressure at which autoregulatory vasoconstriction gives way to pressure-induced forced vasodilation and hyperperfusion, that is, the upper limit of cerebral blood flow autoregulation, is shifted to a higher level compared to the upper limit in normotensive individuals (see discussion of breakthrough theory in the above section on hypertensive encephalopathy) (292,293). However, as a consequence of these structural changes, the arterioles are not able to dilate fully at low mean arterial pressures, which could predispose hypertensive patients to cerebral ischemia if the blood pressure is lowered excessively.

Fortunately, with long-term control of blood pressure these changes in cerebral arterioles appear to be at least partially reversible given the observation that patients with previously severe but adequately treated hypertension have a lower limit of autoregulation, which is shifted toward the range for normotensive subjects (465) (Table 56-6).

The upward shift in the autoregulatory curve in patients with chronic hypertension is one of the major arguments put forward by those who favor gradual reduction of blood pressure in patients with hypertensive crises (319,456). However, the clinical importance and therapeutic implications of this shift in the autoregulatory curve may have been overemphasized. The demonstration of hypertensive adaptation of cerebral autoregulation should not be interpreted to mean that acute reduction of blood pressure in hypertensive crises is

TABLE 56-6

AUTOREGULATION OF CEREBRAL BLOOD FLOW DURING TRIMETHAPHAN-INDUCED HYPOTENSION[a]

Group	MAP (mmHg)			Percent of resting MAP %	
	Resting level	Autoregulation	Tolerated MAP	Autoregulation	Tolerated
Uncontrolled severe hypertensives ($N = 13$)	145 ± 17	$113 \pm 17^{b,c}$	65 ± 10^{b}	79 ± 10	45 ± 6
Controlled hypertensives ($N = 9$)	116 ± 18	96 ± 17	53 ± 18	72 ± 29	46 ± 16
Normotensives ($N = 10$)	98 ± 10	73 ± 9	43 ± 8	74 ± 12	45 ± 12

MAP, mean arterial pressure.
[a]Values given as mean $\pm$ SD.
[b]$p < 0.01$ for difference between normotensives and uncontrolled hypertensives.
[c]$p < 0.01$ for difference between controlled and uncontrolled hypertensives.
(Adapted from: Gifford RW Jr. Effect of reducing elevated blood pressure on cerebral circulation. *Hypertension* 1983;5[Suppl III]:III-17, with permission.)

unwise (293). In the various hypertensive crises in which rapid reduction of blood pressure is indicated (vide supra), the proven benefits of acute reduction of blood pressure (i.e., decreased risk of intracerebral hemorrhage, hypertensive encephalopathy, or acute pulmonary edema) clearly outweigh the theoretic risk of blood pressure reduction (i.e., possible cerebral ischemia).

In practice, moderate, controlled reduction of blood pressure in hypertensive crises rarely causes cerebral ischemia (293). This clinical observation may be explained by the fact that even though the autoregulatory curve is shifted toward a higher blood pressure in chronically hypertensive patients, there is still a considerable difference between the presenting blood pressure and the lower limit of autoregulation (Table 56-6). Strandgaard (465) has studied the autoregulation of cerebral blood flow during controlled hypotension produced with trimethaphan and a 25-degree head-up tilt in 13 patients with untreated or ineffectively treated hypertension. At least eight of these patients had grade III or grade IV changes on funduscopy consistent with the diagnosis of malignant hypertension. The control groups included 9 patients who had been severely hypertensive in the past but whose blood pressure was effectively controlled at the time of the study, and 10 normotensive subjects. Baseline mean arterial pressures in the three groups were 145 ± 17, 116 ± 18, and 98 ± 10 mm Hg, respectively (Table 56-6). The lower limit of mean arterial pressure at which autoregulation of cerebral blood flow failed was 113 ± 17 mm Hg in uncontrolled hypertensives, 96 ± 17 mm Hg in controlled hypertensives, and 73 ± 9 mm Hg in normotensive individuals. Although the absolute level at which autoregulation failed differed substantially in the three groups, the percentage reduction of mean arterial pressure at which autoregulation failed was similar. The mean arterial pressure at the lower limit of autoregulation was 79% ± 10% of the resting mean arterial pressure in the uncontrolled hypertensives, 72% ± 29% in the controlled hypertensive group, and 74% ± 12% in the normotensive group. Thus, a reduction in mean arterial pressure of approximately 20% to 25% from the baseline level was required in each group to reach the lower limit of autoregulation. Therefore, even in uncontrolled hypertensive patients, there was a considerable safety margin before the limit of autoregulation was reached. Another important observation from this study was that symptoms of cerebral hypoperfusion did not occur until the blood pressure was reduced substantially below the lower limit of autoregulation (465). Studies have shown that with normal cerebral blood flow, oxygen extraction is not maximal because oxygen saturation in the jugular venous blood at rest is normally 60% to 70%. Thus, even when the mean arterial pressure is reduced below the lower limit of autoregulation, cerebral metabolism can be maintained and ischemia prevented by increasing oxygen extraction from the blood (293). The lowest tolerated blood pressure, which was defined as the level at which mild symptoms of brain hypoperfusion were encountered (yawning, nausea, and hyperventilation with hypocapnia), was 65 ± 10 mm Hg in patients with uncontrolled hypertension, 53 ± 18 mm Hg in patients with controlled hypertension, and 43 ± 8 mm Hg in normotensive subjects. These values were 45% ± 6%, 46% ± 16%, and 45% ± 12% of the resting baseline mean arterial pressures, respectively. Thus, symptoms of cerebral hypoperfusion did not occur until the mean arterial pressure was reduced by an average of 55% from the resting level (Table 56-6).

In summary, with regard to the shift in cerebral autoregulation in chronically hypertensive patients, there is a therapeutic threshold above which the blood pressure can be reduced safely in patients with hypertensive crises who require immediate control of hypertension. Strandgaard concludes that the upward shift in cerebral autoregulation should not be taken as a warning against aggressive antihypertensive therapy in hypertensive crises. It merely implies that the initial treatment should be aimed at partial reduction but not complete normalization of blood pressure (465,466).

The second argument used to support the recommendation for gradual reduction of blood pressure is based on case reports of the occurrence of acute neurologic sequelae during rapid blood pressure reduction in the treatment of severe hypertension or hypertensive crises (394,458–464).

Franklin reviews 19 reported cases of neurologic complications following aggressive antihypertensive therapy (193). The average age of the patients was 36 years. All had evidence of severe antecedent hypertension with an average mean arterial pressure of 188 ± 19 mm Hg. Malignant hypertension, based on the finding of hypertensive neuroretinopathy, was present in 79% and hypertensive encephalopathy was present in 53% of these patients. Aggressive antihypertensive treatment resulted in a reduction of mean arterial pressure to 84 ± 18 mm Hg. This represented a 56% decrease from the baseline blood pressure level, a level clearly below the predicted autoregulatory range for hypertensive patients. The time course of blood pressure reduction was within minutes in 26% and over hours in 74% of patients. However, the most critical factor in the development of neurologic sequelae was the long duration of drug-induced overshoot hypotension, which varied from a period of hours to days. Neurologic complications consisted of permanent blindness in 47%, coma in 32%, pyramidal tract signs in 32%, residual neurologic deficits after therapy in 58%, and death in three patients. The majority of these patients (80%) had received a large intravenous bolus of diazoxide. Three patients received no parenteral agents but had sustained hypotension induced with multiple oral agents. Franklin concludes that rather than the rapidity with which blood pressure was reduced, the duration of excessive hypotension was the factor that correlated best with the development of neurologic complications.

In summary, the data suggest that in the treatment of patients with hypertensive crises who require prompt control of blood pressure, potent parenteral agents can be used safely if excessive lowering of blood pressure is avoided. The studies of Strandgaard suggest that autoregulation of cerebral blood flow can be maintained in hypertensive patients as long as the mean arterial pressure is not reduced below 120 mm Hg (465,466). This value is two standard deviations above the average mean arterial pressure at which patients in the reported series developed neurologic sequelae.

In general, an initial blood pressure reduction to 160 to 170 mm Hg systolic and 100 to 110 mm Hg diastolic or to a mean arterial pressure of 120 to 130 mm Hg can be safely accomplished in patients who require immediate control of blood pressure in the setting of hypertensive crises (193). Alternatively, the initial antihypertensive therapy can be individualized based on the pretreatment level of blood pressure. In the individual patient, reduction of the mean arterial pressure by 20% should be the initial therapeutic goal. At this level, the blood pressure should still be above the predicted autoregulatory lower limit. Once this goal is obtained, the patient should be carefully evaluated for evidence of cerebral hypoperfusion. Further reduction of blood pressure can then be undertaken if necessary in a controlled fashion based on the overall status of the patient. In previously normotensive individuals in whom acute hypertensive crises develop, such as patients with acute glomerulonephritis complicated by hypertensive encephalopathy, eclampsia, and autonomic hyperreflexia, the autoregulatory curve may not yet be shifted and the initial goal of therapy will often be normalization of the blood pressure.

The use of potent parenteral agents with a rapid onset and short duration of action, such as sodium nitroprusside, has obvious advantages. If overshoot hypotension or neurologic sequelae develop, they can be quickly reversed by allowing the blood pressure to stabilize at a higher level. Agents with a long duration of action all have an inherent disadvantage in that excessive reduction of blood pressure cannot be easily reversed. Thus, diazoxide, labetalol, minoxidil, hydralazine, converting enzyme inhibitors, calcium channel blockers, and central α-agonists should be used with extreme caution in patients requiring rapid blood pressure reduction in order to avoid prolonged overshoot hypotension.

Although in the great majority of hypertensive patients, cautious blood pressure reduction can be undertaken without a significant risk of causing cerebral hypoperfusion, it should be noted that there is one clinical setting in which there is a significant risk of causing cerebral ischemia even with moderate blood pressure reduction. In patients with acute cerebral infarction, because of failure of autoregulation in the surrounding marginally ischemic zone, even moderate blood pressure reduction can be detrimental. Therefore, in acute cerebral infarction, the aforementioned considerations regarding the general safety of acute blood pressure reduction do not apply. The management of hypertension complicating acute cerebral infarction has been outlined in the section entitled Hypertension Complicating Cerebrovascular Accident.

PHARMACOLOGY OF DRUGS USEFUL IN THE TREATMENT OF HYPERTENSIVE CRISES

Sodium Nitroprusside

In 1929, intravenous administration of the color indicator sodium nitroprusside was reported to lower blood pressure (467). Nonetheless, concern that the hypotensive action of the drug was related to the release of cyanide led to a delay in the introduction of the drug. In 1955, intravenous infusion of sodium nitroprusside was shown to be a safe and effective method for achieving short-term blood pressure control (468). However, it was not until 1974 that sodium nitroprusside (Nipride) was approved for clinical use. Over the last 25 years, it has remained the drug of choice for the management of virtually all hypertensive crises. Sodium nitroprusside is useful for the management of hypertensive crises due to malignant hypertension, pheochromocytoma, and other catecholamine-related hypertensive crises, hypertensive encephalopathy, acute pulmonary edema, intracerebral hemorrhage, aortic dissection (in combination with propranolol), and perioperative hypertension (360,469).

Mechanism of Action

Sodium nitroprusside is a potent intravenous hypotensive agent with an immediate onset and brief duration of action. The site of action is the vascular smooth muscle. It has no direct effect on the myocardium, although it may indirectly affect cardiac performance through alterations in systemic hemodynamics. In therapeutic doses it has no effect on duodenal or uterine smooth muscle (468). It has no direct central nervous system effect. Sodium nitroprusside causes vasodilation of both arteriolar resistance vessels and venous capacitance vessels. Its hypotensive action is the result of a decrease in systemic vascular resistance. Venodilation results in a decrease in venous return; hence preload is reduced. The combined decrease in preload and afterload reduces left ventricular wall tension and myocardial oxygen demand.

The net effect of sodium nitroprusside on cardiac output and heart rate depends on the intrinsic state of the myocardium (436,469). In the absence of congestive heart failure, venodilation and preload reduction can result in a small decrease in cardiac output with a reflex increase in sympathetic tone and

heart rate (470–472). In contrast, in patients with left ventricular dysfunction and elevated left ventricular end-diastolic volume or pressure, sodium nitroprusside causes an increase in stroke volume and cardiac output as the result of a reduction in afterload and impedance to left ventricular ejection. There is usually a reduction in heart rate as the result of improved cardiac performance (470–472).

The cellular mechanism of action of nitroprusside has been well defined (473,474). Nitroprusside is an iron coordination complex with five cyanide moieties and a nitroso group. The action of sodium nitroprusside, as well as that of other nitrogen oxide-containing vasodilators, is mediated by a reaction with cysteine to form nitrosocysteine and other short-acting S-nitrosothiols. Nitrosocysteine, a potent activator of guanylate cyclase, causes cyclic guanosine monophosphate accumulation and relaxation of vascular smooth muscle (473,474).

Pharmacokinetics

The hypotensive effect of sodium nitroprusside appears within seconds and is immediately reversible when the infusion is stopped. It is rapidly metabolized, with a reported half-life of 3 to 4 minutes. Cyanide is formed, as a short-lived intermediate product, by direct combination of sodium nitroprusside with sulfhydryl groups in red cells and tissues (468). The cyanide groups are rapidly converted to thiocyanate by the liver in a reaction in which thiosulfate acts as a sulfur donor. Thiocyanate is excreted unchanged by the kidney with a half-life of 1 week in patients with normal renal function (469).

Dosage and Administration

The contents of a 50-mg sodium nitroprusside vial should be dissolved in 2 mL of dextrose in water. No other diluent should be used. The stock solution is diluted in 250 mL of dextrose in water to yield a concentration of 200 μg/mL. The container is immediately wrapped in aluminum foil to prevent decomposition on exposure to light. A small portion of the tubing can be left uncovered to observe the solution for color changes during administration. The freshly prepared solution has a faint brownish tint. The nitroprusside molecule reacts with a wide variety of organic and inorganic substances to yield highly colored reaction products. Therefore, the infusion fluid should not be used as a vehicle for the delivery of other drugs. If a color change occurs, the solution should be replaced. Regardless, the solution should be changed every 24 hours.

In patients who are not taking other antihypertensive agents, the average effective dose is 3.0 μg/kg/minute (range, 0.5 to 10.0 μg/kg/minute). The initial infusion rate should be 0.5 μg/kg/minute. The flow rate should be increased in increments of 1 μg/kg/minute every 2 to 3 minutes until the desired hypotensive response is obtained. The solution should be administered by infusion pump or microdrip regulator to allow for precise measurement of flow rate. The blood pressure should be monitored every 30 to 60 seconds during the initial titration and every 15 minutes thereafter. To avoid excessive accumulation of thiocyanate and the risk of cyanide toxicity, the infusion rate should not be increased above 10 μg/kg/minute. Sodium nitroprusside failures are extremely rare, and tachyphylaxis does not occur. Concomitant oral antihypertensive agents should be initiated as soon as possible and the sodium nitroprusside infusion weaned as it becomes effective.

Adequate facilities, equipment, and personnel must be available for close monitoring of blood pressure during sodium nitroprusside administration. Auscultatory or oscillometric pressure is usually adequate, so that intraarterial pressure monitoring is not routinely required (469). However, in hypertensive patients with acute myocardial infarction or acute pulmonary edema, hemodynamic monitoring may be required for assessment of left ventricular filling pressure and cardiac output (469).

Adverse Effects

Nitroprusside is the most effective parenteral agent for the management of hypertensive crises. When properly administered in an intensive care unit setting, it is very safe and clinically significant adverse reactions are uncommon. Overshoot hypotension can result from accidental bolus infusion, faulty infusion equipment, or failure to frequently monitor the blood pressure. However, the hypotensive action is evanescent and hypotension can be reversed easily by slowing or discontinuing the infusion.

The most frequent side effects include anorexia, nausea, vomiting, abdominal cramps, diaphoresis, headache, apprehension, restlessness, and palpitations. Most of these adverse reactions result from rapid blood pressure reduction per se and they usually disappear if the infusion is slowed.

Thiocyanate accumulation and toxicity can occur when a high-dose or prolonged infusion is required, especially in the setting of renal insufficiency. When these factors are present, thiocyanate levels should be monitored and the infusion reduced or discontinued if the plasma level exceeds 10 mg/dL. Thiocyanate toxicity is rare in patients with normal renal function requiring less than 3 μg/kg/minute for less than 72 hours. Symptoms of thiocyanate toxicity include fatigue, anorexia, weakness, tinnitus, blurred vision, and disorientation, which may progress to frank organic psychosis with hallucinations. Seizures have also been reported. Treatment consists of discontinuing the infusion. Thiocyanate is also efficiently removed by both peritoneal dialysis and hemodialysis (469).

Cyanide poisoning is a very rare complication of sodium nitroprusside use. Since hepatic clearance of cyanide may be deficient in patients with severe liver disease (360) and in rare conditions such as Leber's optic atrophy or tobacco amblyopia (475), the use of sodium nitroprusside is contraindicated in these settings. Most of the reported deaths from cyanide poisoning occurred when very high doses of nitroprusside (20 μg/kg/minute) were required for the control of refractory hypertension or in normotensive patients in whom very large doses were used to induce deliberate surgical hypotension (476,477). The cyanide ion combines with cytochrome c and inhibits aerobic metabolism so that lactic acidosis results. Cyanide toxicity most often occurs within the first 6 to 8 hours of therapy. Cyanide toxicity should be considered if there appears to be increased tolerance to the drug. Tachyphylaxis and an increased anion gap metabolic acidosis are the most reliable early signs of cyanide toxicity. Other signs include the smell of bitter almonds on the breath, anxiety, headache, stiffness of the lower jaw, dyspnea, and widely dilated pupils. Coma, seizures, and death may follow. Occult cyanide toxicity has been reported in patients who are treated with prolonged low-dose infusion of sodium nitroprusside following cardiac surgery (406). Treatment of cyanide toxicity consists of amyl nitrite inhalation, and sodium nitrite, thiosulfate, and hydroxocobalamin infusions (360,478).

The safe use of sodium nitroprusside during pregnancy has not been established. In animals, nitroprusside readily crosses the placenta. In a study of eight normotensive gravid ewes, five required high doses of nitroprusside (mean, 25 μg/kg/minute) to reduce blood pressure by 20% for 1 hour (479). Among these five animals, a marked accumulation of maternal cyanide occurred. Fetal blood levels of cyanide were even higher and all of these fetuses died. However, in the other three ewes, hypotension was achieved with low doses of sodium nitroprusside (less than 1 μg/kg/minute). In this group, all of the fetuses survived and umbilical cord blood cyanide levels were low.

When sodium nitroprusside was used to achieve normotension for 50 minutes in ewes with norepinephrine-induced hypertension, the mean infusion rate required to control blood pressure was only 2.3 μg/kg/minute, and no fetal or maternal deaths occurred (480). Neither maternal nor fetal blood samples contained more than 50 μg/L of cyanide (toxic levels in humans, 5,000 μg/L).

There are some reports on the safe use of sodium nitroprusside for hypertensive crises in pregnant women (481–483). It has been recommended that the use of sodium nitroprusside for hypertensive crises during pregnancy be restricted to patients who are unresponsive to intravenous hydralazine or diazoxide (484). When nitroprusside is required, it should only be used briefly to manage the acute crisis, and delivery should be performed as quickly as possible.

In summary, sodium nitroprusside has several characteristics that make it nearly the ideal drug for the short-term management of hypertensive crises. These include rapid onset of action, immediate reversibility, specific effects on resistance and capacitance vessels with no direct effect on the myocardium or central nervous system, lack of tachyphylaxis, and high potency. It is also a very safe drug when used appropriately. It is the most useful and consistently effective drug available for parenteral use in the treatment of hypertensive crises.

Fenoldopam

Fenoldopam is a selective dopamine receptor (DA$_1$) agonist. Recent studies have shown that intravenous fenoldopam, when used in the setting of hypertensive crises or perioperative hypertension, can safely lower blood pressure while maintaining or improving renal function (3,485). Fenoldopam, a benazepine derivative of dopamine, was initially developed as an oral agent for the treatment of hypertension, renal insufficiency, and congestive heart failure. However, it was eventually withdrawn from development because of poor oral bioavailability. When subsequent studies demonstrated that intravenous fenoldopam exhibited a short-half life and predictable pharmacokinetics and dose-response characteristics, it was subsequently evaluated as a potential alternative to sodium nitroprusside for parenteral treatment of hypertension. Intravenous fenoldopam mesylate (Corlopam) was approved by the Food and Drug Administration in 1997 for use in hypertension when oral therapy is not feasible or possible and for use in patients with severe hypertension, with or without target-organ damage (3).

Pharmacology and Pharmacokinetics

Fenoldopam selectively binds to DA$_1$ receptors and functions as a dopamine agonist. It does not bind to DA$_2$ receptors or β-adrenergic receptors. Fenoldopam is also an α-adrenergic receptor antagonist with greater activity at α_2 than α_1 receptors. However, this activity is observed only at higher concentrations than those required for activation of DA$_1$ receptors and it is unlikely that α-adrenoreceptor antagonism contributes to the hemodynamic and renal effects of therapeutic doses of fenoldopam. Peripheral DA$_1$ receptors are located postsynaptically in the systemic and renal vasculature, and at various sites in the nephron and gastrointestinal tract. These receptors mediate systemic, renal, and mesenteric vasodilation. Fenoldopam exerts its hypotensive effect by decreasing systemic vascular resistance. Unlike sodium nitroprusside, it also increases renal blood flow and causes a natriuresis and diuresis. It is six times as potent as dopamine in causing renal vasodilation. In patients with severe hypertension, intravenous infusion of fenoldopam significantly increases renal blood flow, and decreases renal vascular resistance with a significant increase in creatinine clearance, urine flow rate, and sodium excretion (486). Because of its selective receptor binding characteristics, fenoldopam exhibits minimal adrenergic effects. Although DA$_1$ receptors are present in the central nervous system (CNS), fenoldopam does not have any direct CNS effect because it does not cross the blood-brain barrier. Fenoldopam is metabolized in the liver to a variety of nontoxic methyl, sulfate, and glucuronide metabolites. There are two principal inactive metabolites, 7- and 8-methoxy-fenoldopam, that are eliminated by the kidney (80%) and in the feces (20%). Less than 1% is excreted unchanged in the urine; therefore dosage adjustment is not required in the setting of renal insufficiency. Moreover, pharmacokinetic parameters do not appear to be significantly altered in the setting of hepatic insufficiency (486). Fenoldopam is not metabolized by the cytochrome P 450 system and has no major drug-drug interactions although concomitant acetaminophen administration may increase fenoldopam levels by 30% to 70%. Following intravenous administration, the onset of action is within 10 minutes, and the half-life is 9.8 minutes. There is no evidence of rebound hypertension after stopping the infusion. The volume of distribution is 0.6 L/kg.

Dosage and Administration

Fenoldopam is available in 5-mL ampules at a concentration of 10 mg/mL. Following dilution, the solution, which is light stable, can be used for up to 24 hours. For the treatment of severe hypertension or hypertensive crises, fenoldopam is administered by continuous infusion with an initial dose of 0.1 μg/kg/minute. The infusion may be increased in increments of 0.1 μg/kg/minute every 20 minutes until the target blood pressure is achieved. The maximum recommended dosage is 1.7 μg/kg/minute. The average infusion rate required is 0.25 to 0.5 μg/kg/minute. Mean plasma fenoldopam levels after a 2-hour infusion at 0.5 μg/kg/minute is between 13 to 50 ng/mL. When the desired response has been achieved, fenoldopam infusion may be discontinued gradually or abruptly, as rebound elevation of blood pressure has not been observed. Oral antihypertensive medications may be started as the fenoldopam infusion is weaned.

Adverse Effects

Adverse events attributed to fenoldopam in the treatment of hypertensive emergencies and urgencies were generally mild, occurred within the first 24 hours, and were related to the vasodilatory action of the drug (486). Headache was reported in 11% to 36% of patients, flushing in 7% to 11%, nausea in 20%, and dizziness in 10%. Asymptomatic ST-segment abnormalities occurred in 6% to 33% of patients. The etiology of these nonspecific ST- and T-wave abnormalities, which are similar to those seen with the use of other vasodilators, is unknown. They appear to be a benign phenomenon related to blood pressure lowering with alterations in myocardial repolarization rather than an indication of subclinical myocardial ischemia (486). Less frequently reported adverse events included palpitations, transient hypotension, asthenia, and sinus bradycardia. Fenoldopam, unlike sodium nitroprusside produced a reversible, dose-related increase in intraocular pressure and should be used with caution in patients with glaucoma. In comparative trials, the adverse event profiles of fenoldopam and sodium nitroprusside were generally similar, although fenoldopam may be associated with a lower incidence of transient hypotension than sodium nitroprusside.

Use for Treatment of Hypertensive Crises

Fenoldopam has been compared mostly with sodium nitroprusside in patients with acute severe hypertension (either severe uncomplicated hypertension or true hypertensive crises) (485,487,488). Treatment with fenoldopam or sodium nitroprusside reduced mean diastolic blood pressure to a similar extent and to goal levels in most patients (486). The time to

achievement of goal blood pressure was similar to that with sodium nitroprusside. There was no evidence of rebound hypertension following cessation of either drug. There was no evidence of tolerance to the antihypertensive effect of either drug during maintenance infusion. In patients with hypertension following noncardiac surgery or coronary artery bypass grafting, fenoldopam and sodium nitroprusside were equally efficacious in lowering blood pressure (489,490).

The efficacy, safety and cost of sodium nitroprusside versus fenoldopam has been compared in a retrospective analysis of consecutive patients with hypertensive crises admitted to a level-1 trauma center and treated with nitroprusside ($N = 21$) or fenoldopam ($N = 22$) (488). Neither the mean pretreatment mean arterial pressure (nitroprusside 168 $\pm$ 19; fenoldopam 163 $\pm$ 9; $p = 0.45$), time to reach MAP goal (3.6, range 0.4 to 30 hours vs. 4.0, range 1 to 22 hours; $p = 0.5$), nor the duration of infusion (18, range 0.7 to 113 hours vs. 18, range 3 to 74 hours; $p = 0.45$) differed between the treatment groups. Time to imitation of oral antihypertensive therapy was similar between nitroprusside (4.5, range 0.5 to 22 hours) and fenoldopam (6.5, range 1 to 100 hours) treated patients, $p = 0.45$. Change in creatinine clearance and the incidence of tachycardia did not differ between the two groups. No symptoms of cyanide toxicity were detected in nitroprusside-treated patients. Cost of therapy was less with nitroprusside (2.66, range $1.68 to $3.48) than with fenoldopam (567, range $199 to $6,675 dollars). Thus, treatment of hypertensive crises with fenoldopam appears to result in patient outcomes equal to those with nitroprusside but at substantially higher cost.

Additional studies are needed to compare fenoldopam and sodium nitroprusside in the treatment of true hypertensive crises. Because fenoldopam preferentially dilates the renal vasculature, it has theoretical advantages in the treatment of patients with severe hypertension associated with renal impairment. Moreover, fenoldopam is not associated with the risk of toxicity from thiocyanate accumulation or cyanide. It is possible that it may also offer advantages in patients in whom cross clamping of the aorta above the level of the renal arteries is required.

Diazoxide

Diazoxide (Hyperstat) is structurally related to the thiazide diuretics, but its pharmacologic effect is a direct relaxation of smooth muscle (arteriolar, uterine, and gastrointestinal). The major role of diazoxide is in the treatment of malignant hypertension or hypertensive encephalopathy in situations in which administration of sodium nitroprusside is not feasible. It is also useful in the management of acute obstetric hypertensive emergencies refractory to hydralazine (491–494).

Diazoxide lowers blood pressure by relaxing arteriolar smooth muscle and reducing systemic vascular resistance. It has no effect on venous capacitance vessels. Although it has no direct cardiac effect, it does produce reflex sympathetic activation. Heart rate increases and the cardiac output may double (470). In patients with preexisting atherosclerotic disease, diazoxide may cause myocardial ischemia as a result of the increase in myocardial oxygen demand (495). Moreover, given the reflex increase in heart rate and contractility, use of diazoxide is contraindicated in patients with aortic dissection.

Diazoxide, like other arterial vasodilators, causes avid renal salt and water retention (496). With prolonged use, fluid retention can cause pseudotolerance. This has led to the recommendation that loop diuretics be given concomitantly with diazoxide. However, routine use of diuretics at the initiation of diazoxide therapy is not recommended. Because patients with malignant hypertension may be volume-depleted, the combined use of furosemide and diazoxide can lead to overshoot hypotension. Unless there is obvious fluid overload, diuretic use should be avoided.

Following a bolus injection of 50 mg of diazoxide, a hypotensive response begins within 1 minute and reaches a peak within 5 minutes. The bolus dose can then be titrated to as high as 300 mg depending on the blood pressure response. Thereafter, the duration of the hypotensive effect ranges from 4 to 20 hours. This rapid onset and long duration of action may be an advantage. Continuous infusion is not required and once the desired blood pressure has been achieved, continuous blood pressure monitoring is not required. The long half-life results from extensive protein binding of the drug. Approximately 50% of the drug is eliminated unchanged by the kidney, while the other 50% undergoes hepatic metabolism. The hypotensive response to diazoxide is increased in uremia because the drug is displaced from plasma protein-binding sites. Thus, in uremic patients the dose of diazoxide should be reduced (497).

Diazoxide activates ATP-sensitive K^+ channels, which hyperpolarizes smooth muscle cells and leads to vasodilation (498). It has a generalized effect on smooth muscle, as myometrium and gastrointestinal smooth muscle are also affected.

Although administration of a single large bolus infusion has been recommended in the past, it is now known that diazoxide is effective in more than 90% of patients when it is administered as a series of small injections rather than a single large bolus injection (499,500). In the past, diazoxide was administered as a 300-mg bolus over 15 seconds, given the belief that a large bolus was necessary to saturate plasma protein-binding sites so that a sufficient quantity of free drug would be available to interact with vascular smooth muscle (496). The sustained hypotensive effect was thought to be caused by irreversible binding to vascular receptors. Unfortunately, this large bolus injection technique was often associated with a significant risk of severe, sustained overshoot hypotension (457,458,463). Since the total plasma diazoxide concentration can be directly correlated with its hypotensive action independent of the rate of administration, use of the large (300 mg) single bolus injection technique is no longer recommended (499,500).

Through the use of multiple small injections of diazoxide, the blood pressure can be more carefully titrated. In the mini-bolus technique, 50 to 100 mg is rapidly injected over 15 to 30 seconds every 10 to 15 minutes until the desired hypotensive response is obtained. The hypotensive action lasts 4 to 20 hours. Repeated small bolus injections of 50 to 100 mg every 4 to 6 hours can then be utilized to maintain the hypotensive response. Most patients respond after total doses of 150 to 450 mg, although some require 600 mg or more (499,500). Slow continuous infusion of diazoxide at 15 mg/minute for 20 to 30 minutes (5 mg/kg total dose) also can be safe and effective treatment for severe hypertension (491). The diazoxide solution is very alkaline (pH 11.6), and extravasation can cause severe local pain and cellulitis.

Although myocardial infarction, angina, arrhythmias, electrocardiographic abnormalities, strokes, seizures, and coma have all been reported with diazoxide use, most of these adverse events occurred in patients with precipitous hypotension induced by the rapid administration of a 300-mg bolus, especially in patients with underlying cardiovascular and cerebrovascular disease. Precipitous hypotension is more likely to occur in patients who are volume-depleted due to prior diuretic administration or who are receiving other antihypertensive agents. Diazoxide is contraindicated in patients with acute myocardial infarction or aortic dissection (501). Because diazoxide can precipitate cerebral ischemia, it is contraindicated in patients with cerebrovascular disease or intracerebral hemorrhage (190).

Diazoxide causes hyperglycemia by inhibiting insulin release from pancreatic islet cells (502). The hyperglycemia is usually mild and rarely requires therapy but the blood glucose concentration should be closely monitored in patients with renal insufficiency or type II diabetes mellitus. Failure to recognize and treat hyperglycemia can lead to diabetic ketoacidosis and nonketotic hyperosmolar coma (503).

The use of diazoxide to treat pregnancy-related hypertensive crises is controversial, but has been recommended as an alternative to hydralazine (504,505). Since diazoxide relaxes uterine smooth muscle, uterine hypotonia and cessation of labor can occur. However, this effect can be overcome with oxytocin. The drug crosses the placenta and can cause neonatal hyperglycemia and hyperbilirubinemia (506). Overshoot hypotension, which may compromise uteroplacental blood flow and result in fetal bradycardia, is usually reversible with fluid administration (491).

Trimethaphan

Trimethaphan camsylate (Arfonad) is a potent parenteral ganglionic blocking agent that is utilized infrequently now that other parenteral agents with fewer side effects have become available. However, some authors consider it to be the drug of choice for the management of acute aortic dissection (376). Moreover, it has been used for the management of hypertensive encephalopathy, subarachnoid hemorrhage, and hypertension complicated by acute pulmonary edema. It is also useful in the management of autonomic hyperreflexia in patients with spinal cord injuries.

The antihypertensive effect of trimethaphan is produced by ganglionic blockade. It blocks both sympathetic and parasympathetic autonomic ganglionic transmission by occupying postsynaptic receptor sites, thereby preventing binding of acetylcholine liberated from presynaptic terminals (436). The sympathetic blockade causes dilation of arteriolar resistance vessels. In addition, there is venodilation so that venous return and preload are reduced. Unlike nitroprusside and other peripheral vasodilators that can cause reflex sympathetic stimulation, trimethaphan blocks sympathetic reflexes so that peripheral vasodilation is not accompanied by a reflex increase in inotropy or chronotropy. Therefore, trimethaphan does not cause an increase in cardiac output in patients with normal left ventricular function, because preload is reduced and sympathetic reflexes are blocked.

The onset of action of trimethaphan occurs within minutes. After the infusion is stopped, the duration of the hypotensive effect is 5 to 15 minutes. The metabolic fate of trimethaphan is unclear. The relatively brief duration of action is believed to be due to destruction of trimethaphan by cholinesterase (507).

Tachyphylaxis often develops after 24 to 48 hours so that the dose may have to be increased to maintain the hypotensive response. In addition, pseudotolerance can be caused by renal salt and water retention. In this circumstance, responsiveness can be reestablished with parenteral diuretic administration.

Most of the side effects of trimethaphan are those expected of parasympathetic blockade. Blurred vision results from paralysis of accommodation and mydriasis. The use of trimethaphan is contraindicated in patients with glaucoma. Paralytic ileus results from decreased tone and mobility of the gastrointestinal tract. Thus, it should not be used for the postoperative management of hypertension. Urinary retention occurs with use of trimethaphan for more than 48 hours. Despite bladder distention, patients experience no urge to void. Thus, a bladder catheter is required in most patients. Ganglionic blockade results in inactivation of pupillary reflexes. This can cause confusion in the evaluation of comatose patients with hypertensive encephalopathy, head injury, or intracerebral hemorrhage. Since hypoventilation and respiratory arrests were associated with the curare-like action at the neuromuscular junction, trimethaphan is contraindicated in patients with respiratory insufficiency (508). Use of trimethaphan during pregnancy can lead to meconium ileus in the newborn (509).

Intravenous Nitroglycerin

Intravenous nitroglycerin is particularly useful for the management of hypertension complicating acute myocardial infarction and hypertension occurring after coronary artery bypass. Nitroglycerin causes relaxation of vascular smooth muscle. The predominant effect at lower doses is venodilation. At higher doses, both venous and arterial dilation occur in a dose-dependent fashion (510). As with nitroprusside, the effects of intravenous nitroglycerin on stroke volume and cardiac output vary, depending on the presence or absence of left ventricular dysfunction. In patients without heart failure, the reduction in preload usually predominates and stroke volume falls. In contrast, in patients with left ventricular systolic dysfunction, the decrease in afterload results in a decrease in the impedance to left ventricular ejection such that stroke volume is maintained despite a reduction in preload.

For the treatment of hypertension complicating acute myocardial infarction or postcardiac bypass hypertension, nitroglycerin may have an advantage over sodium nitroprusside (358). In a study of 10 patients with acute myocardial infarction treated with nitroprusside at a rate that lowered the mean arterial pressure by 25 mm Hg, all of the patients showed an increase in ST segment elevation by precordial mapping, suggesting a worsening of regional myocardial ischemia (511). In five patients, subsequent use of sublingual nitroglycerin reduced mean arterial pressure by 14 mm Hg. However, there was a concomitant decrease in ST segment elevation, suggesting an improvement in regional ischemia.

Nitroglycerin and nitroprusside have different effects on regional myocardial blood flow (357,359). Although both drugs dilate coronary vessels, nitroglycerin has a predominant effect on large coronary conductance arteries, including intercoronary collaterals, and relatively little effect on small resistance arterioles. This phenomenon is explained by the fact that coronary resistance vessels less than 100 microns in diameter cannot convert nitrates to nitric oxide such that there is preferential dilation of the larger epicardial collateral vessels (512). In contrast, sodium nitroprusside predominantly dilates the resistance vessels and has less effect on intercoronary collaterals. In the setting of regional myocardial ischemia, resistance vessels in the ischemic region are already maximally dilated. Thus, sodium nitroprusside may dilate resistance vessels in nonischemic areas and shunt blood away from ischemic areas (coronary steal). Nitroglycerin, by predominantly dilating conductance vessels, improves blood flow to the ischemic region. Given the potentially deleterious effect of nitroprusside on regional myocardial blood flow, it has been recommended that intravenous nitroglycerin be used in preference to nitroprusside for the treatment of hypertension with left ventricular dysfunction in association with acute myocardial infarction (358).

Nitrates produce vasodilation through the formation of nitric oxide (endothelium-derived relaxing factor), which activates guanylate cyclase (513). There appears to be tight coupling between the cyclic guanosine monophosphate (cGMP) production and smooth muscle relaxation. A cGMP-dependent protein kinase is stimulated, resulting in alterations in the phosphorylation of various proteins in smooth muscle. Dephosphorylation of the light chain of myosin leads to smooth muscle relaxation (514).

Intravenous nitroglycerin has a rapid onset and brief duration of action with a half-life of 1 to 4 minutes. It is metabolized in the liver by a glutathione-dependent organic nitrate reductase. Intravenous nitroglycerin is supplied in 10-mL bottles containing 50 mg, which should be diluted in 5% dextrose in water or 0.9% sodium chloride. Usually one bottle is diluted in a 250 mL volume to yield a final concentration of 200 μg/mL. Nitroglycerin interacts with many types of plastic. Thus, the drug should be diluted only in glass parenteral solution bottles. Special infusion sets that have been developed absorb fewer nitroglycerins than standard polyvinyl chloride tubing. The initial infusion rate should not exceed 5 μg/minute. The dose is titrated in 5 μg/minute increments every 3 to 5 minutes until the desired hypotensive response is achieved. There is no standard optimal dose of nitroglycerin. There tends to be great variability in response from patient to patient. Blood pressure should be monitored every 30 seconds during the titration phase and every 15 minutes thereafter. As with nitroprusside, close monitoring in an intensive care unit setting is required. In the setting of acute myocardial infarction, monitoring of cardiac output and left ventricular filling pressure is essential.

Intravenous nitroglycerin has also been recommended for the management of the potentially dangerous posttreatment hypertensive response that inevitably follows electroconvulsive therapy (515).

Labetalol

Intravenous labetalol may be of value in a variety of hypertensive crises including malignant hypertension (192), hypertensive encephalopathy (192,516), aortic dissection (517), and hypertensive crises during pregnancy (517).

Labetalol has selective α_1- and nonselective β-blocking properties (518,519). The ratio of β- to α-blocking potency is 7:1 for intravenous labetalol. The acute antihypertensive effect after intravenous administration appears to be caused by a decrease in systemic vascular resistance without an appreciable change in cardiac output (519). However, when used in the treatment of hypertension following open heart surgery, labetalol causes a significant reduction in cardiac output (409). The β-blocking effect offsets the baroreceptor-mediated sympathetic response to hypotension. Thus, heart rate remains unchanged or decreases slightly.

After intravenous injection, the full antihypertensive effect occurs within 5 to 10 minutes, and the blood pressure gradually rises to pretreatment levels over 16 to 18 hours. The duration of action, defined as the time from the last injection until the diastolic blood pressure rises 10 mm Hg above the nadir pressure, ranges from 2.0 to 6.5 hours (192). The major route of elimination is via glycuronide conjugation in the liver. Thus, the labetalol dose must be decreased in patients with liver dysfunction but need not be modified in patients with renal failure.

Labetalol is supplied in 20-mL ampules containing 100 mg of drug. It is usually administered by repeated mini-bolus injections through an intravenous line. The initial dose is 20 mg (4 mL) injected slowly over a 2-minute period. The maximum hypotensive response usually occurs within 5 minutes of the injection. If the desired hypotensive response is not obtained after 10 minutes, a 40-mg bolus is administered over 2 minutes. Additional injections of 40 to 80 mg can be given at 10-minute intervals until the desired hypotensive response is obtained or the maximum total dose of 300 mg has been given.

Labetalol can also be given by continuous infusion. The contents of two ampules (200 mg, 40 mL) are added to 160 mL of diluent to yield a volume of 200 mL with a final concentration of 1 mg/mL. The infusion is begun at 2 mg/minute. The infusion is continued until the desired response is obtained and then discontinued. Again, the maximum total dose of 300 mg should not be exceeded.

After the blood pressure is controlled with either the mini-bolus or the continuous infusion technique, oral therapy can be initiated with labetalol as soon as the supine diastolic pressure increases by 10 mm Hg above the minimum obtained with parenteral therapy. The initial oral dose is 200 mg. Thereafter the oral dose is titrated beginning at 200 mg twice daily and increased to 600 mg twice daily as required. The addition of a diuretic often enhances the long-term blood pressure response.

As with other parenteral antihypertensive agents, intravenous labetalol can cause precipitous hypotension, which can result in cerebral ischemia. Exaggerated hypotensive responses are usually reported when the initial injection is large (1.5 to 2.0 mg/kg); however, overshoot hypotension can also develop with either the mini-bolus or the continuous infusion technique. Chronically hypertensive patients sometimes develop paradoxical hypertension in response to volume depletion (403,404). In this setting treatment with labetalol can cause sustained overshoot hypotension. Before labetalol is used to treat a patient with hypertension and tachycardia, the possibility of physiologic tachycardia due to volume depletion should be considered.

Other side effects of labetalol are related to its nonselective β-blocking properties. It should be avoided in patients with severe sinus bradycardia, heart block greater than first degree, bronchial asthma, or congestive heart failure.

Oral labetalol has been used safely for pregnancies complicated by pregnancy-induced hypertension (520). However, intravenous labetalol should be used with caution because it has been associated with evidence of neonatal β-adrenergic blockade such as hypoglycemia, bradycardia, and hypotension (521).

Labetalol can cause a significant reduction in cardiac index when used in the setting of hypertension after open-heart surgery (409). The hypotensive action of the drug in this setting appears to result from a decrease in cardiac output rather than from a decrease in systemic vascular resistance. Thus, labetalol should be avoided after open-heart surgery, a setting in which nitroglycerin or sodium nitroprusside is preferred for management of hypertension.

Although there are reports of preoperative management of pheochromocytoma with labetalol (425,522), β-blockade can result in exacerbation of hypertension if α-blockade is incomplete. In this regard, there have been reports of paradoxical hypertension when labetalol was used to treat pheochromocytoma (426,523). Therefore, routine use of labetalol for the preoperative management of pheochromocytoma is not recommended.

Although intravenous labetalol has been recommended as an effective agent for the treatment of severe acute hypertension in patients with chronic renal failure (524), life-threatening hyperkalemia has been reported in patients with renal failure that received intravenous labetalol for the treatment of hypertensive crises (525,526). Beta-adrenergic stimulation is known to shift potassium into cells and β-agonists have been proposed as acute therapy for hyperkalemia in dialysis patients. Conversely, hyperkalemia may be caused by nonselective beta-blockers through inhibition of Na-K-ATPase with decreased cellular uptake of potassium, independent of effects on insulin or aldosterone (527). Thus, labetalol and other nonselective beta-blockers should probably be avoided for the acute management of postoperative hypertension and other hypertensive crises in patients with renal failure.

In summary, although intravenous labetalol has been used to treat a variety of hypertensive crises, its long duration of action and beta-blocking properties are potential disadvantages. For this reason, sodium nitroprusside usually represents a more logical choice for the acute management of patients with hypertensive crises requiring parenteral therapy.

Phentolamine

Phentolamine is useful in the management of catecholamine-related hypertensive crises including pheochromocytoma, MAO inhibitor–tyramine interactions, and clonidine, methyldopa, or guanabenz withdrawal reactions. It is not consistently effective in other hypertensive crises. In fact, phentolamine has largely been replaced by sodium nitroprusside in the management of catecholamine-related hypertensive crises.

Phentolamine is a nonselective α-adrenergic blocking agent that competitively inhibits the effect of norepinephrine on vascular smooth muscle α_1-receptors. It does not have β-blocking activity and therefore does not block the cardiac effects associated with β_1-receptor activation by catecholamines. Phentolamine produces dilation of both arteriolar resistance vessels and venous capacitance vessels (436,528).

The intravenous injection of 1 to 5 mg produces a hypotensive effect within 2 to 3 minutes; however, the duration of action may be only 15 to 30 minutes, so that frequent dosing is required to control blood pressure. Phentolamine is supplied in ampules containing 5 mg. The initial dose should be 1 mg. Subsequent boluses of 1 to 5 mg are administered up to a total dose of 20 to 30 mg or until the blood pressure is controlled. After the desired blood pressure is achieved, intermittent injections are given as necessary to maintain the response.

Side effects due to phentolamine are common. Tachycardia and arrhythmias can occur due to β-adrenergic cardiac stimuli that are not blocked by phentolamine. Gastrointestinal side effects include abdominal pain, nausea, vomiting, and diarrhea. Exacerbation of peptic ulcer disease can occur, so phentolamine should be used with caution in patients with a history of gastritis or peptic ulcer disease (436).

Hydralazine

In the past, parenteral hydralazine was often used for the treatment of hypertensive crises. Most obstetricians still consider hydralazine to be the drug of choice for the management of hypertensive crises during pregnancy (484). However, aside from its use during pregnancy, hydralazine has largely been replaced by other agents in the treatment of hypertensive crises.

The hypotensive response to either intramuscular or intravenous hydralazine is unpredictable. The onset of action occurs 10 to 30 minutes after a parenteral dose. The duration of action is 3 to 9 hours. The dose and frequency of administration needed to control the blood pressure are highly variable (472). Profound and sustained hypotension can occur with an intravenous dose as low as 10 mg. Hydralazine is a direct-acting arteriolar vasodilator. It causes reflex activation of the adrenergic nervous system (472). Because venous capacitance vessels are not affected, venous return is maintained. In association with activation of the adrenergic system, there are increases in heart rate and stroke volume (472). Hydralazine is contraindicated in the treatment of aortic dissection because the increase in myocardial contractility can result in propagation of the dissection. It is also contraindicated in patients with ischemic heart disease because the increased myocardial oxygen demand can precipitate angina or myocardial infarction.

Parenteral hydralazine is still used in acute hypertensive crises of pregnancy. In the majority of patients, hydralazine reduces the blood pressure to acceptable levels and is well tolerated by both mother and fetus, despite reflex activation of the adrenergic system (484). Dosing guidelines for the use of parenteral hydralazine during pregnancy are well established

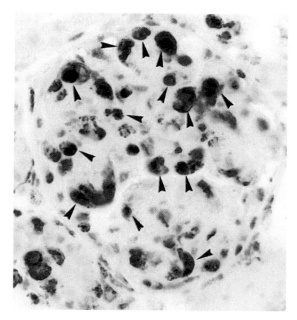

COLOR FIGURE 60-6. A rat glomerulus demonstrating hypercellularity from an animal with induced anti-glomerular basement membrane nephritis. Double immunostaining demonstrated that numerous glomerular macrophages (*arrows*; ED-1 positive [*brown*]) were proliferating (proliferating cell nuclear antigen positive [*blue/black*]) and contributing to the glomerular hypercellularity. (Periodic acid-Schiff, magnification ×400.)

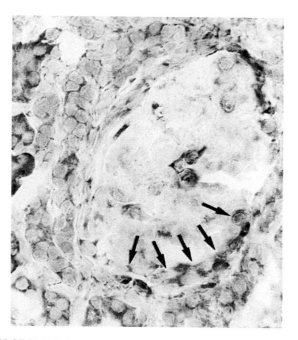

COLOR FIGURE 60-10. *In situ* hybridization demonstrating intercellular adhesion molecule-1 (ICAM-1) messenger RNA (mRNA) expression in a crescent from a rat with anti–glomerular basement membrane nephritis (*arrows*). The ICAM-1 mRNA has been depicted using *in situ* hybridization histochemistry. (Magnification ×400.)

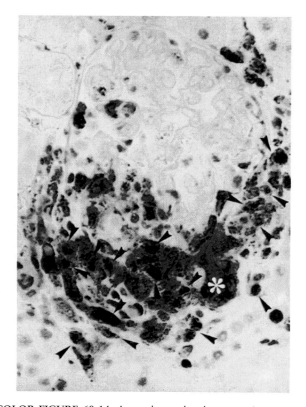

COLOR FIGURE 60-14. A rat glomerulus demonstrating an extensive crescent from an animal with anti-glomerular basement membrane nephritis. Macrophages are demonstrated using the ED-1 monoclonal antibody (*brown*), and the proliferating cell nuclear antigen antibody (*blue*) has been used to demonstrate proliferating cells. Proliferating macrophages are indicated by *arrowheads* and mononuclear giant cells by the *asterisk*. (Periodic acid-Schiff, magnification ×400.)

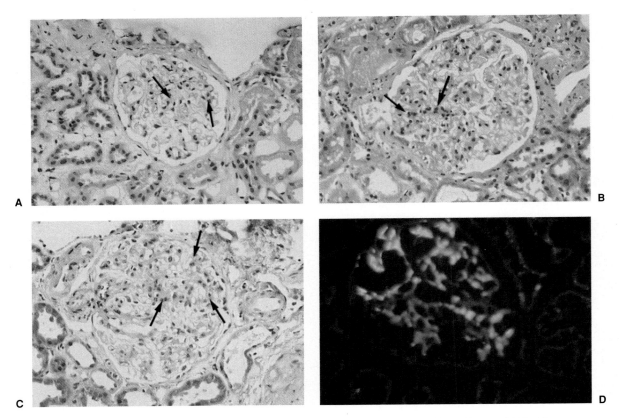

COLOR FIGURE 65-2. Histologic characteristics of mesangial glomerulonephropathy (World Health Organization Class II) in a patient with systemic lupus erythematosus. **A:** A normal glomerulus for comparison. Note the number and distribution of mesangial cells (*arrows*). (Hematoxylin and eosin, magnification ×200.) **B:** An early mesangial nephropathy displaying a subtle increase of mesangial cells (*arrows*). Compare with the normal glomerulus in **A**. (Hematoxylin and eosin, magnification ×200.) **C:** Another glomerulus from the same patient as in **B** but with a segmental accentuation of mesangial cells (*arrows*). This would be classified as a World Health Organization Class IIb lesion. (Hematoxylin and eosin, magnification ×200.) **D:** The mesangial matrix is accentuated by immunofluorescent deposits of IgG. This is an immunofluorescence analysis of the biopsy material shown in **B**. (Anti-IgG, magnification ×200.)

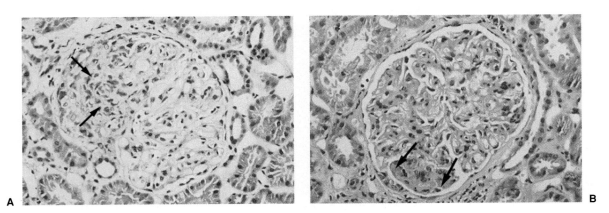

COLOR FIGURE 65-4. Histologic characteristics of focal proliferative glomerulonephritis (World Health Organization Class III) in a patient with systemic lupus erythematosus. **A:** Approximately one-half of this glomerular tuft is involved by mesangial proliferation (*arrows*), which at medium power is discernible as a segmental lesion. (Hematoxylin and eosin, magnification ×200.) **B:** Another glomerulus from the same patient. Here there is a mild global increase of mesangial cells and a segmental lesion with a suggestion of early tuft necrosis (*arrows*). (Hematoxylin and eosin, magnification ×200.) Less than half of the glomeruli in this biopsy demonstrated segmental lesions.

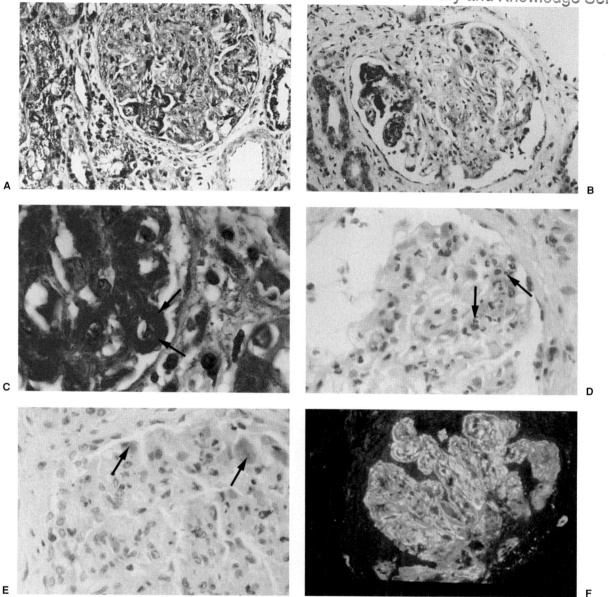

COLOR FIGURE 65-5. Histologic characteristics of diffuse proliferative glomerulonephritis (World Health Organization Class IV) in a patient with systemic lupus erythematosus. This plate also shows examples of the abnormalities used in the scoring of the activity index (Table 65-4). **A:** The majority of glomeruli in this case were involved by a global proliferation of mesangial cells and varying indicators of acute activity. (Trichrome, magnification ×200.) **B:** This trichrome stain accentuates the intracapillary thrombi present in the same biopsy as **A. C:** Subendothelial deposits are seen within the capillary loop (*arrows*). The resultant thickening of the membrane contour is the source of the descriptive term "wire loop." (Trichrome, magnification ×800.) **D:** Multiple neutrophils are apparent within the mesangium and capillary lumens (*arrows*). (Hematoxylin and eosin, magnification ×400.) **E:** Hematoxylin bodies (*arrows*) are not often seen in biopsy material. They are the result of altered nuclear DNA and are considered pathognomonic of lupus nephritis. Notice also the neutrophilic infiltrates and cellular proliferation, both features of an active lesion. (Hematoxylin and eosin, magnification ×400.) **F:** Extensive glomerular deposition of immunoglobulin demonstrated by immunofluorescent staining for IgG. Compare the distribution and intensity of staining with the immunofluorescence analysis of mesangial nephropathy shown in Figure 65-2D. (From: Kotzin BL, O'Dell JR. Systemic lupus erythematosus. In: Frank MM, et al, eds. *Samter's Immunologic Diseases,* 5th ed. Boston: Little, Brown; 1994, with permission.)

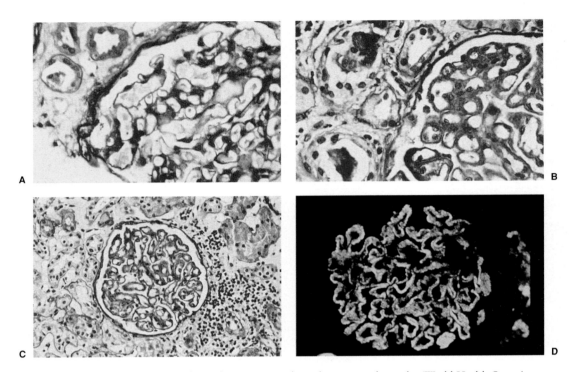

COLOR FIGURE 65-7. Histologic characteristics of membranous nephropathy (World Health Organization Class V) in a patient with systemic lupus erythematosus. **A:** Normal glomerulus for comparison. Notice the thin, delicate profile of the basement membranes. (Periodic acid–Schiff, magnification ×400.) **B:** Membranous nephropathy with thickened basement membranes. (Periodic acid–Schiff, magnification ×400.) Compare with the normal glomerulus in **A. C:** The thickened, rigid-appearing basement membranes of advanced membranous nephropathy are obvious even at medium power. (Periodic acid–Schiff, magnification ×200.) Lymphocytes are seen in the interstitium, and there is a hint of tubular dropout, an indicator that this is a chronic lesion. **D:** Immunofluorescence study of the same patient illustrated in **C.** The membranes are highlighted by fluorescent deposits of IgG. (Anti-IgG, magnification ×200.)

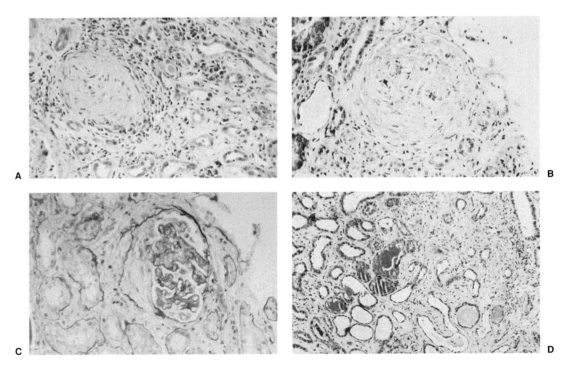

COLOR FIGURE 65-9. Examples of histologic features utilized in the chronicity index. **A:** An obsolescent glomerulus is surrounded by small strophic tubules. (Hematoxylin and eosin, magnification ×200.) **B:** The residuum of a glomerulus is barely visible in this example of a fibrous crescent. (Trichrome, magnification ×200.) **C:** A shrunken glomerular tuft is displaced by a fibrous crescent. **D:** Simplified, dilated tubules in a fibrotic stroma. (Hematoxylin and eosin, magnification ×200.)

(529). Because maternal hypertension helps to maintain placental perfusion, there is concern that aggressive treatment aimed at normalization of blood pressure might further compromise placental perfusion to the detriment of the fetus. Therefore, hydralazine treatment is usually instituted only if the diastolic blood pressure is more than 110 mm Hg and the goal of therapy is a diastolic pressure in the 90 to 100 mm Hg range. After an initial intravenous dose of 5 mg, additional 5- to 10-mg doses are administered every 15 to 20 minutes until the desired response is obtained. Because preeclampsia is associated with intravascular volume depletion, it is important to initiate therapy with a low dose to avoid overshoot hypotension. Intramuscular injection of hydralazine is unsatisfactory because the onset of action and magnitude of response are unpredictable.

Calcium Channel Blockers

Intravenous *nicardipine* has been reported to be effective in the acute treatment of severe hypertension in both adults and children (530–532). It may be useful in the management of postoperative hypertension in both cardiac and noncardiac patients (532). Intravenous nicardipine is also effective in preventing circulatory responses to laryngoscopy and tracheal intubation in hypertensive patients (533). Safe use of nicardipine in preeclamptic patients has also been reported (534).

Nicardipine is a dihydropyridine calcium channel blocker that inhibits the transmembrane influx of calcium into vascular smooth muscle, resulting in vasodilation with a decrease in systemic vascular resistance. The effect on heart rate is dependent on the intrinsic state of the myocardium. In patients with intact systolic function, reflex increases in heart rate may occur in response to blood pressure reduction. In patients with impaired left ventricular function, cardiac output may increase in response to afterload reduction.

Compared to other parenteral medications available for the treatment of hypertensive crises, the pharmacokinetic properties of nicardipine (as well as other calcium channel blockers) are unfavorable. The currently available dihydropyridine calcium channel blockers have very long half-lives. The β–half-life of nicardipine is 40 minutes, whereas its γ–half-life is approximately 13 hours. Because about 14% of the drug is eliminated during the γ-phase, the hypotensive effect is prolonged. Discontinuation of the infusion is followed by a 50% reduction in the hypotensive action within 30 minutes but a gradually decreasing antihypertensive effect may last for about 50 hours. Thus, nicardipine may not be the best choice for true hypertensive crises in which moment-to-moment titration of the blood pressure is the desired therapeutic goal.

In the past, *nimodipine* had been recommended for the treatment of patients undergoing cardiac valve replacement to decrease the incidence of postoperative neurologic sequelae by increasing cerebral blood flow and protecting against anoxic brain-cell damage. However, a recent placebo controlled trial of oral nimodipine following cardiac valve replacement was terminated prematurely because of a lack of evidence of benefit of nimodipine and an unexpected increase in the death rate of patients treated with nimodipine compared to placebo (535). The higher mortality rate was attributed to an increase risk of major bleeding in patients treated with nimodipine. Excess bleeding in patients treated with calcium channel blocker may be explained by the combination of vasodilation and the antiplatelet action of calcium antagonists.

The clinical use of nifedipine for severe uncomplicated hypertension and hypertensive crises has been reviewed (218,536,537). Nifedipine produces a prompt fall in systemic arterial pressure after a single oral dose. The antihypertensive effect results from arteriolar vasodilation with a decrease in systemic vascular resistance. Nifedipine produces a prompt reduction in systolic, diastolic, and mean arterial pressures of about 25% below the baseline value in most patients (537).

Nifedipine is usually administered as a 10-mg sublingual, buccal, or oral dose. The onset of action occurs 5 to 10 minutes after sublingual or buccal administration of the liquid drug, which has been squeezed or aspirated with a needle and syringe from the capsule. With oral administration of the intact capsule, the onset of action occurs at 15 to 20 minutes. A recent study showed that absorption of nifedipine from the oral mucosa is negligible and that most absorption occurs in the stomach (538). The rapid onset of action when the liquid is administered by the sublingual route is explained by the absorption of swallowed liquid from the stomach. The lag in onset of action when the intact capsule is swallowed is due to the time required for dissolution of the capsule. The most reliable method of administration of the drug may be to bite and swallow the capsule (538). The peak effect occurs in 20 to 30 minutes. The duration of action is 4 to 6 hours regardless of the route of administration (218,538).

The major acute side effects of nifedipine include a burning sensation in the face and legs, facial flushing, headache, and palpitations. Overshoot hypotension has been observed, especially in hypovolemic patients or patients pretreated with diuretics (539,540). Exaggerated hypotension can cause myocardial ischemia in patients with underlying coronary atherosclerosis (539,541).

Sublingual or oral nifedipine may be useful in the management of patients with malignant hypertension who do not have an absolute indication for parenteral antihypertensive therapy. Extended-release nifedipine may also be useful in this setting (213). However, in patients with hypertensive crises requiring careful titration of the hypotensive response, the prolonged duration of action and the potential risk of overshoot hypotension with nifedipine are major disadvantages. Sodium nitroprusside is clearly preferable for the management of true hypertensive crises. The role of nifedipine in the acute treatment of severe uncomplicated hypertension in the emergency room setting prior to discharge is discussed in the section entitled Severe Uncomplicated Hypertension.

Minoxidil

Minoxidil is a potent antihypertensive agent that is available only for oral use. In combination with a potent diuretic and a beta-blocker, it is very useful in the control of hypertension refractory to conventional antihypertensive regimens. The efficacy of a triple-drug regimen with minoxidil in the management of the patient with malignant hypertension and azotemia has already been discussed. Minoxidil is often employed for the long-term control of blood pressure in patients with malignant hypertension after initial control of the blood pressure with parenteral medications. Furthermore, in patients with malignant hypertension not requiring immediate blood pressure reduction, an oral triple-drug regimen consisting of minoxidil, a beta-blocker, and a loop diuretic can effectively control the blood pressure over a period of hours to days and thereby eliminate the need for parenteral antihypertensive therapy (see Treatment subsection under Malignant Hypertension earlier in this chapter).

Minoxidil is a direct-acting arteriolar vasodilator. Its antihypertensive effect results from a decrease in systemic vascular resistance (542). It has no effect on venous capacitance vessels. The hypotensive response to minoxidil is accompanied by a baroreceptor-mediated reflex increase in sympathetic tone, which results in an increase in heart rate, contractility, and cardiac output. Unopposed, the cardiac output may increase threefold to fourfold and attenuate the fall in blood pressure (542,543). The resulting increase in myocardial oxygen demand may precipitate ischemia in patients with limited coronary reserve. For this reason minoxidil is usually given concomitantly with a β-adrenergic blocking drug.

As with other peripheral vasodilators, minoxidil induces profound renal salt and water retention (542). This fluid retention is probably related to the hypotensive effect of the drug. A similar antinatriuresis occurs with both hydralazine and diazoxide. Minoxidil causes more fluid retention because it is a more potent arteriolar vasodilator. Several factors enhance renal salt and water retention (543). Decreased peritubular capillary pressure is a potent stimulus for salt and water reabsorption in the proximal tubule. Increased adrenergic tone also enhances proximal tubular salt and water reabsorption. Like other vasodilators, minoxidil increases renin release, which leads to increased aldosterone production and enhanced distal tubular sodium reabsorption (543). Pseudotachyphylaxis to the original hypotensive effect of minoxidil can occur if either β-blockade or diuretic therapy is inadequate.

The serum half-life of minoxidil is 4.5 hours; however, the duration of action is longer than the half-life would predict (543). After oral administration, the antihypertensive effect begins within 30 to 60 minutes, reaches a maximum in 2 to 4 hours, and slowly abates over the next 12 to 18 hours. The prolonged hypotensive effect is probably due to persistent binding of minoxidil at the site of action in vascular smooth muscle. About 15% of the parent compound is excreted in the urine, while the remainder is metabolized in the liver by glucuronide conjugation (543).

Although the serum half-life is 4 hours, the persistent hypotensive effect allows for a twice-daily dosing schedule. Prior to the initiation of minoxidil, all other antihypertensives except diuretics and beta-blockers should be discontinued. Minoxidil is started at a dose of 2.5 mg twice daily and increased in 5-mg/day increments every 2 to 3 days until the desired response is obtained. The usual effective dose is 10 to 40 mg/day. The doses of loop diuretic and beta-blocker are titrated to maintain dry weight and prevent tachycardia, respectively.

When more rapid control of arterial pressure is required, incremental changes in minoxidil dosage can be made every 6 hours. The initial 2.5-mg dose is doubled every 6 hours up to a maximum dose of 20 mg, or until the desired response is obtained. The effective dose should then be administered every 12 hours and the dose of diuretic and beta-blocker titrated as necessary (543).

The dose of beta-blocker required to prevent reflex tachycardia in patients treated with minoxidil is often in excess of the usual β-blocking dose. This is because the sympathetic nervous system is activated by minoxidil and beta-blockers compete with catecholamines for receptor binding (543). The starting dose of beta-blocker should be propranolol at 160 mg/day or an equivalent. The dose is then titrated to maintain resting heart rate at 70 to 80 beats/minute.

In general, thiazide diuretics are not potent enough to counteract minoxidil-induced antinatriuresis, especially if renal insufficiency is present. The starting dose of furosemide is 40 mg twice daily. However, a dose of 300 to 400 mg/day may be required to prevent fluid retention and maintain dry weight.

The most common side effects of minoxidil are related to its pharmacologic properties. Fluid retention can lead to weight gain, edema, anasarca, congestive heart failure, and pericardial effusion. With inadequate β-blockade, reflex sympathetic stimulation can lead to angina or myocardial infarction in patients with underlying coronary disease. Electrocardiographic changes following the initiation of minoxidil have been reported. In more than 90% of patients flattening or inversion of T waves develops (543). Although often marked, these changes do not necessarily indicate myocardial ischemia, and they usually resolve with continued therapy (542,543).

Pericardial effusion has been reported with minoxidil treatment; however, progression to cardiac tamponade is rare. The cause of the effusion is unknown, but it occurs most commonly in patients with renal failure, collagen vascular diseases, or inadequate diuretic therapy. A hemodynamically insignificant effusion is not necessarily a reason to discontinue minoxidil, but the patient should be treated aggressively with diuretics and followed closely for signs of tamponade (542,543). Patients on dialysis should have a trial of intensive daily dialysis to achieve and maintain dry weight.

Reversible hypertrichosis of the face, back, and arms occurs in almost all patients taking minoxidil and is the most frequent reason for discontinuation of the drug, especially among female patients. Calcium thioglycolate depilatory agents and shaving are used to control this cosmetic side effect.

Triple therapy with minoxidil, a beta-blocker, and a loop diuretic is often dramatically effective in the long-term management of malignant hypertension, even when conventional antihypertensive regimens are unsuccessful or produce intolerable side effects (202,206,207,544).

Angiotensin Converting Enzyme Inhibitors

Captopril has been used successfully in the treatment of hypertensive crises. Both oral and sublingual routes of administration have been described (545,546). Angiotensin converting enzyme inhibitors are clearly the treatment of choice for scleroderma renal crisis (55).

Unfortunately, first-dose hypotension has been reported as a significant risk in the treatment of hypertensive crises with converting enzyme inhibitors. Hypotension is most likely to occur in patients with high levels of angiotensin II, underlying renovascular hypertension, or intravascular volume depletion resulting from spontaneous natriuresis in malignant hypertension or from prior diuretic treatment. In addition, the use of converting enzyme inhibitors in the initial management of patients with renal insufficiency can lead to confusion if the renal dysfunction persists or worsens. Use of converting enzyme inhibitors is contraindicated in pregnancy because they can cause acute renal failure in the neonate (547).

Although malignant hypertension is often characterized by high PRA, this is not invariably the case. Therefore, converting enzyme inhibitors may not be effective in all patients with malignant hypertension. Moreover, whereas angiotensin-converting enzyme inhibitors may be useful in the long-term management of patients with malignant hypertension, captopril has not been shown to be superior to other antihypertensive agents in preventing the recurrence of malignant hypertension (219).

Thus, although angiotensin-converting enzyme inhibitors may be useful in the long-term management of hypertension in patients with a history of malignant hypertension or other hypertensive crises, converting enzyme inhibitors are not usually recommended for the initial management of hypertensive crises except in patients with scleroderma renal crisis.

Methyldopa

In the past, parenteral methyldopa was often recommended for the treatment of hypertensive crises. However, it has several disadvantages including a delayed onset of action, unpredictable hypotensive effect, and central nervous system sedation. More rapidly acting and predictable parenteral agents such as sodium nitroprusside and diazoxide have largely replaced methyldopa.

Reserpine

Intramuscular reserpine in a dose of 1 to 5 mg was widely used in the past for the treatment of hypertension complicating acute pulmonary edema, pheochromocytoma, toxemia of pregnancy, and aortic dissection (548). However, with the advent of more reliable agents with fewer side effects, the use of reserpine for the management of hypertensive crises can no longer be recommended (2190).

Clonidine

Oral clonidine loading has been recommended for the management of severe hypertension that is *not* accompanied by evidence of end-organ dysfunction (220). However, oral clonidine loading is *not* recommended for the management of the true hypertensive crises outlined in Table 56-1. Thus, if hypertension is accompanied by hypertensive neuroretinopathy (malignant hypertension), hypertensive encephalopathy, congestive heart failure, acute myocardial infarction, aortic dissection, or central nervous system catastrophe, oral clonidine loading is not recommended (220). In patients with hypertensive encephalopathy or another central nervous system catastrophe, clonidine can cause sedation, which would interfere with the assessment of mental status. Moreover, the relatively long duration of action represents a disadvantage in the treatment of hypertensive crises requiring moment-to-moment titration of blood pressure. The oral clonidine loading regimen was described specifically for the management of severe hypertension that is not associated with end-organ dysfunction, an entity known as *urgent hypertension* or severe uncomplicated hypertension (220). There has been an unfortunate tendency to utilize this type of regimen for the treatment of true hypertensive crises in which potent parenteral medications described earlier are clearly indicated. Use of oral clonidine loading in the outpatient setting for the management of severe uncomplicated hypertension is discussed in the next section.

SEVERE UNCOMPLICATED HYPERTENSION

The benefits of acute reduction of blood pressure in the setting of true hypertensive crises are obvious. Fortunately, hypertensive crises are relatively rare events that never affect the vast majority of hypertensive patients. Another type of presentation that is more common than true hypertensive crisis is the patient who presents with severe hypertension (diastolic blood pressure greater than 115 mm Hg) in the absence of the hypertensive neuroretinopathy or other acute end-organ damage that would signify a true crisis. This entity, which is known as *severe uncomplicated hypertension*, is very common in the emergency department setting. In a recent study of severe uncomplicated hypertension treated in an emergency room, 60% of the patients were entirely asymptomatic and had presented for prescription refills or routine blood pressure checks, or were found to have elevated blood pressure during routine examinations. The other 40% presented with nonspecific symptoms such as headache, dizziness, and weakness in the absence of evidence of acute end-organ dysfunction (549).

In the past, this entity has been referred to as *urgent hypertension,* reflecting the widely accepted notion that acute reduction of blood pressure, over a few hours prior to discharge from the emergency room, was essential to minimize the risk of short-term complications from the severe hypertension (220,550). Commonly used treatment regimens include oral clonidine loading, or sublingual nifedipine given to acutely reduce the blood pressure prior to initiation of a maintenance antihypertensive regimen (220,549,550).

In recent years, however, the urgency of treatment in patients with severe uncomplicated hypertension has been questioned (9,11,551). While it is clear that in comparison to patients with mild or moderate hypertension, patients with severe uncom-

plicated hypertension are at increased long-term risk of cardiovascular complications (552), they are generally not in any immediate danger of an untoward event (10). The argument supporting the acute reduction of blood pressure is based on the following assumptions: (a) It is important to reduce blood pressure immediately to avoid complications; (b) oral antihypertensive loading prior to initiation of maintenance therapy produces improved immediate and long-term blood pressure control; and (c) there are no adverse consequences of this form of treatment (9). Two studies provided some useful information regarding the need to reduce blood pressure immediately with the aim of preventing hypertensive complications. In the Veterans Administration Cooperative Study of patients with severe hypertension (552), there were 70 untreated patients who had no evidence of malignant hypertension or significant end-organ dysfunction despite the presence of diastolic blood pressures averaging 121 mm Hg. Among these patients, 27 experienced morbid events at an average of 11 ± 8 months into follow-up. The earliest morbid event occurred after 2 months. Likewise, a similar study in Baltimore showed that among 42 untreated patients with severe but uncomplicated hypertension, 19 patients experienced morbid events (congestive heart failure, onset of malignant hypertension, cerebrovascular accident, or evidence of declining renal function) at a mean of 12 ± 7 months into follow-up. The earliest morbid event occurred at 2 months (553). These data suggest that patients who have severe but uncomplicated hypertension need not be exposed to the risk of "urgent" blood pressure reduction in the emergency room setting because hypertensive complications tend to occur over a matter of months to years rather than hours to days.

Another study addressed the question of whether antihypertensive loading prior to the initiation of maintenance therapy improves or hastens blood pressure control (11). Sixty-four asymptomatic patients with severe hypertension were randomized to treatment with hourly doses of clonidine followed by clonidine and thiazide diuretic maintenance therapy, or an initial dose of clonidine followed by hourly placebo and then subsequent maintenance therapy, or initiation of maintenance therapy without prior antihypertensive loading. There was no difference between the first two groups with regard to the time required to achieve acceptable blood pressure control during loading therapy. Furthermore, there were no differences between the three groups with regard to adequacy of blood pressure control at 24 hours or 1 week. The authors conclude that sustained blood pressure control resulted solely from maintenance therapy and that the time to adequate control and eventual level of blood pressure were independent of the administration of an initial loading dose. They suggest that the common practice of acute oral antihypertensive loading to treat severe, asymptomatic hypertension should be reconsidered (11). In this regard, a recent study of 32 patients with severe uncomplicated hypertension found that a significant decrease in blood pressure frequently occurred in the emergency department even before pharmacologic intervention was initiated. The mean arterial pressure decreased by 6% without treatment within 1 hour after the initial blood pressure reading (554). The authors suggest that given a short period of observation, many patients with severe uncomplicated hypertension will experience a decrease in blood pressure to mildly or moderately hypertensive levels, which would clearly make acute blood pressure reduction with an antihypertensive loading regimen unnecessary.

Although generally safe, the oral antihypertensive loading regimens occasionally cause significant adverse effects. Sublingual nifedipine can produce severe headache and profound overshoot hypotension (540). The marked blood pressure reduction can exacerbate underlying ischemic heart disease, resulting in angina or myocardial infarction (539,541). It has even been suggested that a moratorium be placed on the use of sublingual nifedipine for the treatment of severe uncomplicated hypertension (555). Loading doses of clonidine cause sedation in 60% of patients and some of these patients are difficult to awaken and require assistance in returning home (549). Furthermore, the recommended conversion from the oral loading dose to a twice-daily dose of clonidine (220) may represent special problems in the treatment of patients with severe uncomplicated hypertension. Clonidine produces a number of common side effects including dry mouth, drowsiness, and constipation, which may interfere with long-term compliance with medical therapy. The risk of hypertensive rebound on abrupt discontinuation of clonidine (427) should also be considered since many patients with this form of hypertension are noncompliant with medical therapy (11).

While the acute reduction of blood pressure in patients with severe uncomplicated hypertension with sublingual nifedipine or oral clonidine loading regimens has become the de facto standard of care in the acute care setting, this practice is often an emotional response on the part of the treating physician to the dramatic elevation of blood pressure (10). This aggressive approach may also be motivated by fear of medicolegal repercussions in the unlikely event that an untoward hypertensive complication occurs shortly after the emergency room visit (10). Although observing and documenting the dramatic fall in blood pressure prior to discharge is a satisfying therapeutic maneuver, there is no scientific basis for this approach and it is unclear if even the small but definite risks of acute blood pressure reduction are justified. There is, at present, no literature to support the notion of an absolute level of blood pressure above which the acute reduction of blood pressure is mandatory before the patient can be discharged from the acute care setting. For asymptomatic patients with severe uncomplicated hypertension, acute reduction of blood pressure in the emergency room is often counterproductive because it can produce untoward symptoms that render the patient less likely to comply with long-term drug therapy. Because the available data suggest that the risks to the patient are not immediate, therapeutic intervention should focus on tailoring an effective, well-tolerated maintenance antihypertensive regimen with emphasis on patient education to enhance long-term compliance (11). Therefore, oral antihypertensive loading in this setting is of little value. If the patient has simply run out of medications, reinstitution of the previous regimen should suffice. If the patient is thought to be compliant with an existing drug regimen, a sensible change in therapy such as an increase in a suboptimal dosage of an existing drug or the addition of a drug of another class is appropriate. Addition of a low dose of a thiazide diuretic as a second-step agent to existing monotherapy with converting enzyme inhibitor, calcium channel blocker, beta-blocker, or central α_2-agonist is often efficacious (390). Another essential goal of the intervention should be to arrange for suitable outpatient follow-up within a few days. Gradual reduction of blood pressure to normotensive levels over the next few days to a week should be accomplished in conjunction with frequent outpatient follow-up visits to modify drug regimens and reinforce the importance of lifelong compliance with therapy. Though less dramatic than acute reduction of blood pressure in the emergency room, this type of approach to the treatment of this chronic disease is more likely to prevent long-term hypertensive complications as well as recurrent episodes of severe uncomplicated hypertension.

Finally, an important entity that can masquerade as severe uncomplicated hypertension deserves special mention. *Pseudohypertension* is a condition in which indirect measurement of arterial pressure using a cuff sphygmomanometer is artificially high in comparison to direct intraarterial pressure measurements (556). Failure to recognize pseudohypertension can result in unwarranted and sometimes frankly dangerous treatment. Pseudohypertension can result from Mönckeberg's medial calcification, advanced atherosclerosis with widespread calcification of intimal plaques, or azotemic arteriopathy (metastatic vascular calcification in patients with ESRD) (556). In these entities, stiffening of the arterial wall may prevent its collapse by externally applied pressure, resulting in artificially high indirect blood pressure readings affecting both systolic and diastolic measurements. Pseudohypertension should be suspected in the patient with severe hypertension in the absence of significant target-organ damage. The presence of a positive *Osler's maneuver*, in which the radial or brachial artery remains clearly palpable despite being made pulseless by proximal inflation of a cuff above systolic blood pressure, is an important physical examination finding that should suggest the diagnosis (557). Roentgenograms of the extremities will often reveal calcified vessels (556). However, the diagnosis can only be made definitively by direct measurement of intraarterial pressure. If unrecognized, pseudohypertension may result in unwarranted treatment. Patients with pseudohypertension are often older adults and therefore may have critical limitation of blood flow to the brain or heart such that inappropriate blood pressure reduction may precipitate life-threatening ischemic events (556).

References

1. Calhoun D, Oparil S. Treatment of hypertensive crises. *N Engl J Med* 1990; 323:1177.
2. National Center for Health Statistics. *Vital and health statistics: detailed diagnoses and procedures for patients discharged from short-stay hospitals: United States, 1983—1990.* National Health Survey. Hyattsville, MD: Department of Health and Human Services, 1985-1993.
3. Oparil S, et al. Fenoldopam: a new parenteral antihypertensive. Consensus roundtable on the management of hypertensive crises. *Am J Hypertens* 1999;12:653.
4. World Health Organization. Arterial hypertension-report of a WHO expert committee. *WHO Tech Rep Ser* 1978;628:7.
5. Keith NM, Wagener HP, Barker NW. Some different types of essential hypertension: their course and prognosis. *Am J Med Sci* 1939;197:332.
6. Ahmed ME, et al. Lack of difference between malignant and accelerated hypertension. *Br Med J* 1986;292:235.
7. McGregor E, et al. Retinal changes in malignant hypertension. *Br Med J* 1986;292:233.
8. Zunker P, et al. Cerebral hemodynamics in pre-eclampsia/eclampsia syndrome. *Ultrasound Obstet Gynecol* 1995;6:411.
9. Fagan TC. Acute reduction of blood pressure in asymptomatic patients with severe hypertension. An idea whose time has come-and gone. *Arch Intern Med* 1989;149:2169.
10. Ferguson RK, Vlasses PH. Hypertensive emergencies and urgencies. *JAMA* 1986;255:1607.
11. Zeller KR, Kuhnert LV, Matthews C. Rapid reduction of severe asymptomatic hypertension. *Arch Intern Med* 1989;149:2186.
12. Volhard F, Fahr T. *Die brightische neirenkrankheit, klinik pathologie und atlas.* Berlin: Julius Springer, 1914.
13. Fahr TS. Ueber die beziehungen von arteriolensklerose, hypertonie und herzhypertrophie. *Virchows Arch A Pathol Anat Histol* 1922;239:41.
14. Volhard F. Der arterielle hochdruck. *Verh Dt Ges Inn Med* 1923;35:134.
15. Leibreich R. Ophthalmoskopischer befund bei morbus Brightii. *Albrecht Graefes Arch Ophthalmol* 1859;5:256.
16. Keith NM, Wagener HP, Kernohan JW. The syndrome of malignant hypertension. *Arch Intern Med* 1928;41:141.
17. Derow HA, Altschule MD. Malignant hypertension. *N Engl J Med* 1935; 213:951.
18. Hollenhorst RW, Wagener HP. The ocular fundi in relation to operations for hypertensive cardiovascular disease. *Am J Med* 1949;218:225.
19. Woods WW, Peet MM. The surgical treatment of hypertension II. Comparison of mortality following operations with that of the Wagener-Keith medically treated control series. *JAMA* 1941;117:1508.
20. Page IH, Taylor RD. Pyrogens in the treatment of malignant hypertension. *Mod Concepts Cardiovasc Dis* 1949;18:51.
21. Kempner W. Treatment of hypertensive vascular disease with rice diet. *Am J Med* 1948;4:545.
22. Pickering G. Reversibility of malignant hypertension. Follow-up of three cases. *Lancet* 1971;1:413.
23. Hamilton M, et al. Pheochromocytoma. *Br Heart J* 1953;15:241.
24. Smirk FH, Alstad KS. Treatment of arterial hypertension by penta- and hexamethonium salts. *Br Med J* 1951;1:1217.
25. Kincaid-Smith P, McMichael I, Murphy EA. The clinical course and pathology of hypertension with papilloedema (malignant hypertension). *Q J Med* 1958;27:117.

26. Schottstaedt MF, Sokolow M. The natural history and course of hypertension with papilledema (malignant hypertension). *Am Heart J* 1953;45:331.
27. Milliez P, et al. The natural course of malignant hypertension. In: Bock KD, Cottier P, eds. *Essential hypertension: an international symposium.* Berlin: Springer-Verlag, 1960:214.
28. Ellis LB. The clinical course of malignant hypertension. *Med Clin North Am* 1932;15:1025.
29. Perera GA. The accelerated form of hypertension-a unique entity? *Trans Assoc Am Physicians* 1958;71:62.
30. Heptinstall RH. Malignant hypertension: a study of fifty-one cases. *J Pathol Bacteriol* 1953;65:423.
31. Gudbrandsson T, et al. Malignant hypertension-improving prognosis in a rare disease. *Acta Med Scand* 1979;206:495.
32. Yu SH, Whitworth JA, Kincaid-Smith PS. Malignant hypertension: aetiology and outcome in 83 patients. *Clin Exp Hypertens (A)* 1986;8:1211.
33. Milne FJ, James SH, Veriava Y. Malignant hypertension and its renal complications in black South Africans. *S Afr Med J* 1989;76:164.
34. Muirhead EE, Pitcock JA. Histopathology of severe renal vascular damage in blacks. *Clin Cardiol* 1989;12:IV.
35. Pitcock JA, et al. Malignant hypertension in blacks. Malignant intrarenal arterial disease as observed by light and electron microscopy. *Hum Pathol* 1976;7:33.
36. Kumar P, et al. Malignant hypertension in children in India. *Nephrol Dialysis Transplant* 1996;11:1261.
37. Perez-Fontan M, et al. Idiopathic IgA nephropathy presenting as malignant hypertension. *Am J Nephrol* 1986;6:482.
38. Subias R, et al. Malignant or accelerated hypertension in IgA nephropathy. *Clin Nephrol* 1987;27:1.
39. Holland NH, Kotchen T, Bhathens D. Hypertension in children with chronic pyelonephritis. *Kidney Int* 1975;8:S-234.
40. Still JL, Cottom D. Severe hypertension in childhood. *Arch Dis Child* 1967;42:34.
41. Kincaid-Smith P. Malignant hypertension: mechanisms and management. *Pharmacol Ther* 1980;9:245.
42. Nanra RS, et al. Analgesic nephropathy: etiology, clinical syndrome, and clinicopathologic correlations in Australia. *Kidney Int* 1978;13:79.
43. Zezulka AV, Arkell DG, Beevers DG. The association of hypertension, the Ask-Upmark kidney and other congenital abnormalities. *J Urol* 1986;135:1000.
44. Luxton RW. Radiation nephritis. *Q J Med* 1953;22:215.
45. Pickering GW. *High blood pressure,* 2nd ed. New York: Grune & Stratton, 1968.
46. Davis BA, et al. Prevalence of renovascular hypertension in patients with grade III or IV hypertensive retinopathy. *N Engl J Med* 1979;301:1273.
47. Thel MC, Mannon RB, Allen NB. Hyperrenin—hyperaldosterone-dependent malignant hypertension in polyarteritis nodosa. *South Med J* 1993;86:1400.
48. Lim KG, et al. Malignant hypertension in women of childbearing age and its relation to the contraceptive pill. *Br Med J* 1987;294:1057.
49. Petitti DB, Klatsky AL. Malignant hypertension in women aged 15 to 44 and its relation to cigarette smoking and oral contraceptives. *Am J Cardiol* 1983;52:297.
50. Lip GY, Beevers M, Beevers DG. Malignant hypertension in young women is related to previous hypertension in pregnancy, not oral contraception. *Q J Med* 1997;90:571.
51. Dalakos TG, et al. "Malignant" hypertension resulting from atheromatous embolization predominantly of one kidney. *Am J Med* 1974;57:135.
52. Jones DB, Iannaccone PM. Atheromatous emboli in renal biopsies. *Am J Pathol* 1975;78:261.
53. Ritz E, et al. Acute renal failure, hypertension and skin necrosis in a patient with streptokinase therapy. *Am J Nephrol* 1984;4:193.
54. Rosansky SJ. Multiple cholesterol emboli syndrome. *South Med J* 1982;75:677.
55. Steen VD. Scleroderma renal crisis. *Rheum Dis Clin North Am* 2003;29:315.
56. Rhew EY, Barr WG. Scleroderma renal crisis: new insights and developments. *Curr Rheum Report* 2004;6:129.
57. Traub YM, et al. Hypertension and renal failure (scleroderma renal crisis) in progressive systemic sclerosis. *Medicine* 1983;62:335.
58. Cannon PJ, et al. The relationship of hypertension and renal failure in scleroderma (progressive systemic sclerosis) to structural and functional abnormalities of the renal cortical circulation. *Medicine* 1974;53:1.
59. Cacoub P, et al. Malignant hypertension in antiphospholipid syndrome without overt lupus nephritis. *Clin Exp Rheumatol* 1993;11:479.
60. Rubio-Garcia R, et al. IgG myeloma with hyperviscosity presenting as malignant hypertension. *Am J Med* 1989;87:119.
61. Harrison TS, Birbari A, Seaton JF. Malignant hypertension in pheochromocytoma: correlation with plasma renin activity. *Johns Hopkins Med J* 1972;130:329.
62. Zarifis J, et al. Malignant hypertension in association with primary aldosteronism. *Blood Pressure* 1996;5:250.
63. McAllister RG, et al. Malignant hypertension: effect of therapy on renin and aldosterone. *Circ Res* 1971;28(Suppl II):II-160.
64. Conn JW. Aldosteronism in man. Some clinical and climatological aspects. *JAMA* 1963;183:871.
65. Laragh JH, et al. Aldosterone secretion and primary and malignant hypertension. *J Clin Invest* 1960;39:1091.
66. Soule SG, et al. Cushing's syndrome—a reversible cause of malignant hypertension. *S Afr Med J* 1993;83:800.
67. Hague WM, Honour JW. Malignant hypertension in congenital adrenal hyperplasia due to 11-β hydroxylase deficiency. *Clin Endocrinol* 1983;18:505.
68. Morimoto I, et al. An autopsy case of 17α-hydroxylase deficiency with malignant hypertension. *J Clin Endocrinol Metab* 1983;56:915.
69. Perera GA. Hypertensive vascular disease; description and natural history. *J Chronic Dis* 1955;1:33.
70. Lee TH, Alderman MH. Malignant hypertension. Declining mortality rate in New York City, 1958 to 1974. *NY State Med J* 1978;78:1389.
71. Lip GY, Beevers M, Beevers G. The failure of malignant hypertension to decline: a survey of 24 years' experience in a multiracial population in England. *J Hypertens* 1994;12:1297.
72. Beutler JJ, Koomans HA. Malignant hypertension: still a challenge. *Nephrol Dial Transplant* 1997;12:2019.
73. Edmunds E, Beevers DG, Lip GY. What has happened to malignant hypertension? A disease no longer vanishing. *J Hypertens* 2000;14:159.
74. Jhetam D, et al. The malignant phase of essential hypertension in Johannesburg blacks. *S Afr Med J* 1982;61:899.
75. Grim CE. Emergency treatment of severe or malignant hypertension. *Geriatrics* 1980;35:57.
76. Munro-Faure AD, et al. Comparison of black and white patients attending hypertension clinics in England. *Br Med J* 1979;1:1044.
77. Patel R, Ansari A, Grim CE. Prognosis and predisposing factors for essential malignant hypertension in predominantly black patients. *Am J Cardiol* 1990;66:868.
78. Bloxham CA, Beevers DF, Walker JM. Malignant hypertension and cigarette smoking. *Br J Med* 1979;1:581.
79. Elliot JM, Simpson FO. Cigarettes and accelerated hypertension. *NZ Med J* 1980;91:447.
80. Isles C, et al. Excess smoking in malignant-phase hypertension. *Br Med J* 1979;1:579.
81. Kincaid-Smith P. *The kidney: a clinicopathologic study.* Oxford: Blackwell, 1975:205.
82. Barraclough MA. Sodium and water depletion with acute malignant hypertension. *Am J Med* 1966;40:265.
83. Gill JR, et al. Hyperaldosteronism and renal sodium loss reversed by drug treatment for malignant hypertension. *N Engl J Med* 1964;270:1088.
84. Bevan AT, Honour AI, Stott FH. Direct arterial pressure recording in unrestricted man. *Clin Sci* 1969;36:329.
85. Dollery CT. Hypertensive retinopathy. In: Genest J, et al., eds. *Hypertension: pathophysiology and treatment.* New York: McGraw-Hill, 1983: 723.
86. Fishberg AM, Oppenheimer BS. The differentiation and significance of certain ophthalmoscopic pictures in hypertensive diseases. *Arch Intern Med* 1930;46:901.
87. Kirkendall WM. Retinal changes of hypertension. In: Mausolf FA, ed., *The eye in systemic disease.* St. Louis: Mosby, 1975:212.
88. Scheie HG. Evaluation of ophthalmoscopic changes of hypertension and arteriolar sclerosis. *Arch Ophthalmol* 1953;49:117.
89. Bulpitt CJ. Prognosis of treated hypertension 1951–1981. *Br J Clin Pharmacol* 1982;13:73.
90. Dimmitt SB, et al. Usefulness of ophthalmoscopy in mild to moderate hypertension. *Lancet* 1989;1:1103.
91. Van Buchem FSP, Heuvel-Aghina JW, Heuvel JE. Hypertension and changes of the fundus oculi. *Acta Med Scand* 1964;176:539.
92. Lip GY, et al. Severe hypertension with lone bilateral papilledema: a variant of malignant hypertension. *Blood Pressure* 1995;4:339.
93. Goldring W, Chasis H. *Hypertension and hypertensive disease.* New York: The Commonwealth Fund, 1944.
94. De Venecia G, Jampol LM. The eye in accelerated hypertension. II. Localized serous detachments of the retina in patients. *Arch Ophthalmol* 1984;102:68.
95. Cordingley FT, et al. Reversible renal failure in malignant hypertension. *Clin Nephrol* 1980;14:98.
96. Mamdani BH, et al. Recovery from prolonged renal failure in patients with accelerated hypertension. *N Engl J Med* 1974;291:1343.
97. Mattern WD, Sommers SC, Kassirer JP. Oliguric acute renal failure in malignant hypertension. *Am J Med* 1972;52:187.
98. Sevitt LH, Evans DJ, Wrong OM. Acute oliguric renal failure due to accelerated (malignant) hypertension. *Q J Med* 1971;40:127.
99. McLeod D, Marshall J, Kohner EM. Role of axoplasmic transport in the pathophysiology of ischaemic disc swelling. *Br J Ophthalmol* 1980;64:247.
100. McLeod D, et al. The role of axoplasmic transport in the pathogenesis of retinal cotton-wool spots. *Br J Ophthalmol* 1977;61:177.
101. Steinmann WC, Millstein ME, Sinclair SH. Pupillary dilation with tropicamide 1% for funduscopic screening. *Ann Intern Med* 1987;107:181.
102. Mujais SK, et al. Marked proteinuria in hypertensive nephrosclerosis. *Am J Nephrol* 1985;5:190.
103. Narvarte J, et al. Proteinuria in hypertension. *Am J Kidney Dis* 1987;10:408.
104. Fishberg AM. *Hypertension and nephritis,* 5th ed. Philadelphia: Lea & Febiger, 1954.

105. Clarke E, Murphy EA. Neurological manifestations of malignant hypertension. Br Med J 1956;2:1319.

106. Oppenheimer BS, Fishberg AM. Hypertensive encephalopathy. Arch Intern Med 1928;41:264.

107. Pickering GW. The cerebrospinal fluid pressure in arterial hypertension. Clin Sci 1934;1:397.

108. Barcenas CG, Gonzalez-Molina M, Hull AR. Association between acute pancreatitis and malignant hypertension with renal failure. Arch Intern Med 1978;138:1254.

109. Avram MM. High prevalence of pancreatic disease in chronic renal failure. Nephron 1977;18:68.

110. Guerra C, et al. Acute abdominal symptoms in malignant hypertension: clinical presentation in five cases. Clin Exp Hypertens 2001;23:461.

111. Erdberg A, et al. Malignant hypertension: a possible precursor to the future development of mesenteric ischaemia in chronically haemodialyzed patients. Nephrol Dial Transplant 1992;7:541.

112. Shin MS, Ho KJ. Malignant hypertension as a cause of massive intestinal bleeding. Am J Surg 1977;133:742.

113. Linton AL, et al. Microangiopathic haemolytic anaemia and the pathogenesis of malignant hypertension. Lancet 1969;1:1277.

114. Gavras H, et al. Abnormalities of coagulation and the development of malignant phase hypertension. Kidney Int 1975;8-S-252.

115. Beevers DG, et al. The clinical value of renin and angiotensin estimations. Kidney Int 1975;8-S-181.

116. Brown JJ, et al. Plasma renin concentration in human hypertension. III: Renin in relation to complications of hypertension. Br Med J 1966;1:505.

117. Kawazoe N, et al. Pathophysiology in malignant hypertension: with special reference to the renin-angiotensin system. Clin Cardiol 1987;10:513.

118. Agarwal M, et al. Hyponatremic-hypertensive syndrome with renal ischemia: an underrecognized disorder. Hypertension 1999;33:1020.

119. Atkinson AB, et al. Hyponatremic hypertensive syndrome with renal-artery occlusion corrected by captopril. Lancet 1979;2:606.

120. Heslop H, et al. Hyponatraemic—hypertensive syndrome due to unilateral renal ischaemia in women who smoke heavily. NZ Med J 1985;98:739.

121. Sinclair RA, Antonovych TT, Mostofi FK. Renal proliferative arteriopathies and associated glomerular changes. A light and electron microscopic study. Hum Pathol 1976;7:565.

122. Kadiri S, Thomas JO. Kidney histology and clinical correlates in malignant hypertension. East Afr Med J 1993;70(2):112.

123. Hsu HC, Churg J. The ultrastructure of mucoid "onionskin" intimal lesions in malignant nephrosclerosis. Am J Pathol 1980;99:67.

124. Heptinstall RH. Pathology of the kidney, 4th ed. Boston: Little, Brown, 1992.

125. Heptinstall RH. Renal biopsies in hypertension. Br Heart J 1954;16:133.

126. Jones DB. Arterial and glomerular lesions associated with severe hypertension. Light and electron microscopic studies. Lab Invest 1974;31:303.

127. Kadiri S, Thomas JO. Focal segmental glomerulosclerosis in malignant hypertension. S Afr Med J 2002;4:303.

128. Paronetto F. Immunocytochemical observations on the vascular necrosis and renal glomerular lesions of malignant nephrosclerosis. Am J Pathol 1965;46:901.

129. McLaren K, MacDonald MK. Histological and ultrastructural studies of the human juxtaglomerular apparatus in benign and malignant hypertension. J Pathol 1983;139:41.

130. Harrington M, Kincaid-Smith P, McMichael J. Results of treatment in malignant hypertension. A seven-year experience in 94 cases. Br Med J 1959;2:969.

131. Kincaid-Smith P. Renal pathology in hypertension and the effects of treatment. Br J Clin Pharmacol 1982;13:107.

132. McCormack LJ, et al. Effects of antihypertensive treatment on the evolution of the renal lesions in malignant nephrosclerosis. Am J Pathol 1958;34:1011.

133. Horn H, Klemperer P, Steinberg MF. Vascular phase of chronic diffuse glomerulonephritis. Arch Intern Med 1942;70:260.

134. Weiss S, Parker F Jr. Pyelonephritis: its relation to vascular lesions and to arterial hypertension. Medicine (Baltimore) 1939;18:221.

135. Wagener HP, Keith NM. Diffuse arteriolar disease with hypertension and the associated retinal lesions. Medicine (Baltimore) 1939;18:317.

136. Keith NM, et al. Pathologic studies of the arterial system in severe hypertension. Proc Staff Meet Mayo Clin 1939;14:209.

137. Chester EM, et al. Hypertensive encephalopathy: a clinicopathologic study of 20 cases. Neurology 1978;28:928.

138. Doniach I. Uremic edema of the lungs. Am J Roentgenol 1947;58:620.

139. Hranilovich GT, Baggenstoss AH. Lesions of the pancreas in malignant hypertension. Arch Pathol 1953;55:443.

140. Beilin LJ, Goldby FS. High arterial pressure versus humoral factors in the pathogenesis of the vascular lesions of malignant hypertension. The case for pressure alone. Clin Sci Mol Med 1977;52:111.

141. Byrom FB. The pathogenesis of hypertensive encephalopathy and its relation to the malignant phase of hypertension. Experimental evidence from the hypertensive rat. Lancet 1954;2:201.

142. Goldblatt H. Studies on experimental hypertension. VII. The production of the malignant phase of hypertension. J Exp Med 1938;67:809.

143. Wilson C, Byrom FB. The vicious circle in chronic Bright's disease. Experimental evidence from the hypertensive rat. Q J Med 1941;10:65.

144. Saphir O, Ballinger J. Hypertension (Goldblatt) and unilateral malignant nephrosclerosis. Arch Intern Med 1940;66:541.

145. Byrom FB, Dodson LF. The causation of acute arterial necrosis in hypertensive disease. J Pathol Bacteriol 1948;60:357.

146. Byrom FB. Tension and the artery: the experimental elucidation of pseudouraemia and malignant nephrosclerosis. Clin Sci Mol Med 1976;51:3s.

147. Byrom FB. The evolution of acute hypertensive arterial disease. Prog Cardiovasc Dis 1974;17:31.

148. Giese J. Acute hypertensive vascular disease. 2. Studies on vascular reaction patterns and permeability changes by means of vital microscopy colloidal tracer technique. Acta Pathol Microbiol Scand 1964;62:497.

149. Goldby FS, Beilin LJ. Relationship between arterial pressure and the permeability of arterioles to carbon particles in acute hypertension in the rat. Cardiovasc Res 1972;6:384.

150. Goldby FS, Beilin LJ. How an acute rise in arterial pressure damages arterioles. Electron microscopic changes during angiotensin infusion. Cardiovasc Res 1972;6:569.

151. Goldby FS. The arteriolar lesions of steroid hypertension in rats. Clin Sci Mol Med 1976;51:31s.

152. Asscher AW, Anson SG. A vascular permeability factor of renal origin. Nature 1963;198:1097.

153. Robertson AL, Khairallah PA. Effects of angiotensin II and some analogues on vascular permeability in the rabbit. Circ Res 1972;31:923.

154. Möhring J, et al. Studies on the pathogenesis of the malignant course of renal hypertension in rats. Kidney Int 1975;8-S-174.

155. Möhring J, et al. Effects of saline drinking on malignant course of renal hypertension in rats. Am J Physiol 1976;230:849.

156. Gross R, et al. Salt loss as a possible mechanism eliciting an acute malignant phase in renal hypertensive rats. Clin Exp Pharmacol Physiol 1975;2:323.

157. Linz W, et al. Nephroprotection by long-term ACE inhibition with ramipril in spontaneously hypertensive stroke prone rats. Kidney Int 1998;54:2037.

158. Stefansson B, et al. Angiotensin-converting enzyme gene I/D polymorphism in malignant hypertension. Blood Pressure 2000;9:104.

159. Fleming S. Malignant hypertension—the role of the paracrine renin-angiotensin system. J Pathol 2000;192:135.

160. Hilgers KF, et al. Angiotensin II type 1 receptor blockade prevents lethal malignant hypertension: relation to kidney inflammation. Circulation 2001;104:1436.

161. Gavras H, et al. Malignant hypertension resulting from deoxycorticosterone acetate and salt excess. Role of renin and sodium in vascular changes. Circ Res 1975;36:300.

162. Dzau VJ, et al. Sequential renal hemodynamics in experimental benign and malignant hypertension. Hypertension 1981;3(Suppl I):I-63.

163. Venkatachalam MA, Jones DB, Nelson DA. Microangiopathic hemolytic anemia in rats with malignant hypertension. Blood 1968;32:278.

164. Bohle A, et al. Primary malignant nephrosclerosis. Clin Sci Mol Med 1976;51(Suppl):23s.

165. Lip GY, et al. A cross-sectional, diurnal, and followup study of platelet activation and endothelial dysfunction in malignant phase hypertension. Am J Hypertens 2001;14:823.

166. Roy L, Mehta J, Mehta P. Increased plasma concentrations of prostacyclin metabolite 6-keto-PGF$_{1\alpha}$ in essential hypertension. Am J Cardiol 1983;51:464.

167. Ylikorkala O, Puolakka J, Viinikka L. Oestrogen containing oral contraceptives decrease prostacyclin production. Lancet 1981;1:42.

168. Mehta P, Metha J. Effects of smoking on platelets and on plasma thromboxane–prostacyclin balance in man. Prostaglandins Lenkot Med 1982;9:141.

169. Kazda S, Garthoff B, Luckhaus G. Calcium and malignant hypertension in animal experiment: effects of experimental manipulation of calcium influx. Am J Nephrol 1986;6(Suppl 1):145.

170. Ogata J, et al. Stroke-prone spontaneously hypertensive rats as an experimental model of malignant hypertension. A pathologic study. Virchows Arch (A) 1982;394:185.

171. Tobian L, et al. Potassium protection against lesions of the renal tubules, arteries, and glomeruli and nephron loss in salt-loaded hypertensive Dahl S rats. Hypertension 1984;6(Suppl I):I-170.

172. Tobian L, et al. Potassium reduces cerebral hemorrhage and death rate in hypertensive rats, even when blood pressure is not lowered. Hypertension 1985;7(Suppl I):I-110.

173. Tobian L. Hypothesis: low dietary k may lead to renal failure in blacks with hypertension and severe intimal thickening. Am J Med Sci 1988;295:384.

174. Ribeiro AB, et al. Malignant hypertension: a syndrome accompanied by plasmatic diminution of low and high molecular weight kininogens. Hypertension 1983;5(Suppl V):V-158.

175. Lilme E, et al. Urinary kallikrein excretion is low in malignant hypertension. J Hypertens 1992;10(8):869.

176. Luscher TF, et al. Endothelium-derived relaxing and contracting factors: perspectives in nephrology. Kidney Int 1991;39:575.

177. Shichiri M, et al. Plasma endothelin levels in hypertension and chronic renal failure. Hypertension 1990;15:493.

178. Kohno M, et al. Plasma immunoreactive endothelin-1 in experimental malignant hypertension. *Hypertension* 1991;18:93.
179. Kohno M, et al. Renoprotective effects of combined endothelin type A/type B receptor antagonists in experimental malignant hypertension. *Metabolism* 1997;46:1032.
180. Blezer EL, et al. Early-onset but not late-onset endothelin-A-receptor blockade can modulate hypertension, cerebral edema, and proteinuria in stroke-prone hypertensive rats. *Hypertension* 1999;33:137.
181. Park JB, et al. Chronic treatment with a superoxide dismutase mimetic prevents vascular remodeling and progression of hypertension in salt-loaded stroke-prone spontaneously hypertensive rats. *Am J Hypertens* 2002;15:78.
182. Schwartz SM, Campbell GR, Campbell JH. Replication of smooth muscle cells in vascular disease. *Circ Res* 1986;58:427.
183. Ohamura M, et al. Platelet-derived growth factor gene expression in the kidney in malignant hypertension. *Blood Pressure* 1992;3(Suppl):17.
184. Baumbach GL, Heistad DD. Remodeling of cerebral arterioles in chronic hypertension. *Hypertension* 1989;13:968.
185. Gustafson F. Hypertensive arteriolar necrosis revisited. *Blood Pressure* 1997;6:71.
186. Hodge JV, Dollery CT. Retinal soft exudates. A clinical study by colour and fluorescence photography. *Q J Med* 1964;33:117.
187. Shakib M, Ashton N. Ultrastructural changes in focal retinal ischaemia. *Br J Ophthalmol* 1966;50:325.
188. Hayreh SS, Baines JA. Occlusion of the posterior ciliary artery III. Effects on the optic nerve head. *Br J Ophthalmol* 1972;56:754.
189. Hayreh S, Servais GE, Virdi PS. Fundus lesions in malignant hypertension V. Hypertensive optic neuropathy. *Ophthalmology* 1986;93:74.
190. American Medical Association Committee on Hypertension. The treatment of malignant hypertension and hypertensive emergencies. *JAMA* 1974;228:1673.
191. Vaughn CJ, Delanty. Hypertensive emergencies. *Lancet* 2000;356:411.
192. Devlin JW, et al. Fenoldopam versus nitroprusside for the treatment of hypertensive emergency. *Ann Pharmacother* 2004;38:755.
193. Franklin SS. Hypertensive emergencies: the case for more rapid lowering of blood pressure. In: Narins RG, ed. *Controversies in nephrology and hypertension*. New York: Churchill-Livingstone, 1984:241.
194. Cohn JN, Rodriguera E, Guiha NH. Hypertensive heart disease. In: Onesti O, Kim KE, Moyer JH, eds. *Hypertension: mechanisms and management*. New York: Grune & Stratton, 1973:191.
195. Adelman RD, Russo J. Malignant hypertension: recovery of renal function after treatment with antihypertensive medications and hemodialysis. *J Pediatr* 1981;98:766.
196. Bacon BR, Ricanati ES. Severe and prolonged renal insufficiency. Reversal in a patient with malignant hypertension. *JAMA* 1978;239:1159.
197. Barcenas CG, et al. Recovery from malignant hypertension with anuria after prolonged hemodialysis. *South J Med* 1976;69:1230.
198. Bischel MD, Gans DS, Barbour BH. Bilateral nephrectomy for hypertension. *Ann Intern Med* 1972;77:656.
199. Dichoso CC, Minuth AN, Eknoyan G. Malignant hypertension. Recovery of kidney function after renal allograft failure. *Arch Intern Med* 1975;135:300.
200. Isles CG, McLay A, Boulton Jones JM. Recovery in malignant hypertension presenting as acute renal failure. *Q J Med* 1984;53:439.
201. Luft FC, et al. Minoxidil treatment of malignant hypertension. Recovery of renal function. *JAMA* 1978;240:1985.
202. Mehta PK, et al. Severe hypertension. Treatment with minoxidil. *JAMA* 1975;233:249.
203. Mitchell HC, Graham RM, Pettinger WA. Renal function during long-term treatment of hypertension with minoxidil. *Ann Intern Med* 1980;93:676.
204. Wauters JP, Brunner HR. Discontinuation of chronic haemodialysis after control of arterial hypertension: long term follow-up. *Proc Eur Dialysis Transplant Assoc* 1982;19:182.
205. Yaqoob M, McClelland P, Ahmad R. Delayed recovery of renal function in patients with acute renal failure due to accelerated hypertension. *Postgrad Med J* 1991;67:829.
206. Limas CJ, Freis ED. Minoxidil in severe hypertension with renal failure. Effect of its addition to conventional antihypertensive drugs. *Am J Cardiol* 1973;31:355.
207. Pettinger WA, Mitchell HC. Minoxidil-an alternative to nephrectomy for refractory hypertension. *N Engl J Med* 1973;289:167.
208. Donohue JP, et al. Bilateral nephrectomy: its role in management of the malignant hypertension of end-stage renal disease. *J Urol* 1971;106:488.
209. Lazarus JM, et al. Urgent bilateral nephrectomy for severe hypertension. *Ann Intern Med* 1972;76:733.
210. Mahony JF, et al. Bilateral nephrectomy for malignant hypertension. *Lancet* 1972;1:1036.
211. Mroczek WJ. Malignant hypertension: kidneys too good to be extirpated. *Ann Intern Med* 1974;80:754.
212. Alpert MA, Bauer JH. Rapid control of severe hypertension with minoxidil. *Arch Intern Med* 1982;142:2099.
213. Isles CG, Johnson AO, Milne FJ. Slow release nifedipine and atenolol as initial treatment in blacks with malignant hypertension. *Br J Clin Pharmacol* 1986;21:377.
214. Alpert MA, Bauer JH. Hypertensive emergencies: recognition and pathogenesis. *Cardiovasc Rev Rep* 1985;6:407.
215. O'Malley K, McNay JL. A method for achieving blood pressure control expeditiously with oral minoxidil. *Clin Pharmacol Ther* 1975;18:39.
216. Alpert MA, Bauer JH. Hypertensive emergencies: management. *Cardiovasc Rev Rep* 1985;6:602.
217. Bertel O, Conen LD. Treatment of hypertensive emergencies with the calcium channel blocker nifedipine. *Am J Med* 1985;79(Suppl 4A):31.
218. Frishman WH, et al. Calcium entry blockers for the treatment of severe hypertension and hypertensive crisis. *Am J Med* 1984;77(Suppl 2B):35.
219. Ferguson RK, Vlasses PH, Rotmensch HH. Clinical applications of angiotensin-converting enzyme inhibitors. *Am J Med* 1984;77:690.
220. Anderson RJ, et al. Oral clonidine loading in hypertensive urgencies. *JAMA* 1981;246:848.
221. Lip GY, Beevers M, Beevers DG. Complications and survival of 315 patients with malignant-phase hypertension. *J Hypertens* 1995;13:915.
222. Langford HG, Bonar JR. Treatment of the uremic hypertensive patient. *Modern Treat* 1966;3:62.
223. Woods JW, Blythe WB. Management of malignant hypertension complicated by renal insufficiency. *N Engl J Med* 1967;277:57.
224. Woods JW, Blythe WB, Huffines WD. Management of malignant hypertension complicated by renal insufficiency. A follow-up study. *N Engl J Med* 1974;291:10.
225. Mroczek WJ, et al. The value of aggressive therapy in the hypertensive patient with azotemia. *Circulation* 1969;40:893.
226. Herlitz H, Gudbrandsson T, Hansson L. Renal function as an indicator of prognosis in malignant essential hypertension. *Scand J Urol Nephrol* 1982;16:51.
227. Nicholson GD. Long-term survival after recovery from malignant nephrosclerosis. *Am J Hypertens* 1988;1:73.
228. James JF, et al. Partial recovery of renal function in black patients with apparent end-stage renal failure due to primary malignant hypertension. *Nephron* 1995;71:29.
229. Lip GY, Beevers M, Beevers DG. Does renal function improve after a diagnosis of malignant hypertension?. *J Hypertens* 1997;15:1309.
230. De Lima JJ, et al. Outcome of patients with malignant hypertension and end-stage renal disease treated by long-term hemodialysis. *Cardiology* 1999;92:93.
231. Katz IJ, et al. Recovery of renal function in Black South Africans with malignant hypertension: superiority of continuous ambulatory peritoneal dialysis over hemodialysis. *Peritoneal Dialysis Int* 2001;21:581.
232. Bock KD. Regression of retinal vascular changes by antihypertensive therapy. *Hypertension* 1984;6(Suppl III):III-158.
233. Working Group on Renovascular Hypertension. Detection, evaluation, and treatment of renovascular hypertension. *Arch Intern Med* 1987;147:820.
234. Smith HW. Unilateral nephrectomy in hypertensive disease. *J Urol* 1956;76:685.
235. Javadpour N, et al. Segmental renal vein renin assay and segmental nephrectomy for correction of renal hypertension. *J Urol* 1976;115:580.
236. Poutasse EF, et al. Malignant hypertension in children secondary to chronic pyelonephritis: laboratory and radiologic indications for partial or total nephrectomy. *J Urol* 1978;119:264.
237. Kimmelstiel P, Wilson C. Benign and malignant hypertension and nephrosclerosis. *Am J Pathol* 1936;12:45.
238. Beevers DG, Lip GY. Does non-malignant hypertension cause renal damage? A clinician's view. *J Hum Hypertens* 1996;10:695.
239. Shirley D, et al. Clinical documentation of end-stage renal disease due to hypertension. *Am J Kidney Dis* 1994;23:655.
240. Freedman BI, Iskander SS, Appel RG. The link between hypertension and nephrosclerosis. *Am J Kidney Dis* 1995;25:207.
241. Rostand SG, et al. Racial differences in the incidence of treatment for end-stage renal disease. *N Engl J Med* 1982;306:1276.
242. Perneger TV, et al. Projections of hypertension-related renal disease in middle-aged residents of the United States. *JAMA* 1993;269:1272.
243. Perneger TV, et al. Diagnosis of hypertensive end-stage renal disease: effect of patient's race. *Am J Epidemiol* 1995;141:10.
244. Whelton PK, Klag MJ. Hypertension as risk factor for renal disease. Review of clinical and epidemiological evidence. *Hypertension* 1989;13(Suppl I):I-19.
245. Bulpitt CJ, et al. The survival of treated hypertensive patients and their causes of death: a report from the DHSS Hypertensive Care Computing Project (DHCCP). *J Hypertens* 1986;4:93.
246. Isles CG, et al. Mortality in patients of the Glasgow Blood Pressure Clinic. *J Hypertens* 1986;4:141.
247. Labeeuw M, et al. Renal failure in essential hypertension. *Contrib Nephrol* 1989;71:90.
248. Shulman NB, et al. Prognostic value of serum creatinine and effect of treatment of hypertension on renal function. Results from the Hypertension Detection and Follow-up Program. *Hypertension* 1989;13 (Suppl I):I-80.
249. Reubi FC. The late effects of hypotensive drug therapy on renal functions of patients with essential hypertension. In: Bock KD, Cottier P, eds. *Essential hypertension: an international symposium*. Berlin: Springer, 1960:317.
250. Klag MJ, et al. Blood pressure and end-stage renal disease in men. *N Engl J Med* 1996;334:13.

251. Kincaid-Smith P, Whitworth JA. Pathogenesis of hypertension in chronic renal disease. *Semin Nephrol* 1988;8:155.
252. Rostand SG, et al. Renal insufficiency in treated essential hypertension. *N Engl J Med* 1989;320:684.
253. Klahr S. The kidney in hypertension-villain and victim. *N Engl J Med* 1989;320:731.
254. Entwisle G, et al. Target organ damage in black hypertensives. *Circulation* 1977;55:792.
255. Levy SB, et al. Renal vasculature in essential hypertension: racial differences. *Ann Intern Med* 1978;88:12.
256. Fogo A, et al. Accuracy of the diagnosis of hypertensive nephrosclerosis in African Americans: a report from the African American Study of Kidney Disease (AASK) Trial. *Kidney Int* 1997;51:244.
257. Churchill PC, et al. Genetic susceptibility to hypertension-induced renal damage in the rat. Evidence based on kidney-specific genome transfer. *J Clin Invest* 1997;100:1373.
258. Bennett NM, Shea S. Hypertensive emergency: case criteria, sociodemographic profile, and previous care of 100 cases. *Am J Public Health* 1988;78:636.
259. Gifford RW Jr, Westbrook E. Hypertensive encephalopathy: Mechanisms, clinical features, and treatment. *Prog Cardiovasc Dis* 1974;17:115.
260. Dinsdale HB. Hypertensive encephalopathy. *Neurol Clin* 1983;1:3.
261. Jellinek EH, et al. Hypertensive encephalopathy with cortical disorders of vision. *Q J Med* 1964;33:239.
262. Donaldson JO. Neurologic emergencies in pregnancy. *Obstet Gynecol Clin North Am* 1991;18:199.
263. Dinsdale HB. Hypertensive encephalopathy. *Stroke* 1982;13:717.
264. McDonald CK, Waters ML, Griffin FM Jr. Case report: neutrophilic CSF pleocytosis in hypertensive encephalopathy. *Am J Med Sci* 1993;306:167.
265. Schwartz RB, et al. Hypertensive encephalopathy: findings on CT, MR imaging, and SPECT imaging in 14 cases. *Am J Roentgenol* 1992;159:379.
266. Hinchey J, et al. A reversible posterior leukoencephalopathy syndrome. *N Engl J Med* 1996;334:494.
267. Weingarten K, et al. Acute hypertensive encephalopathy: finding on spin-echo and gradient-echo MR imaging. *Am J Roentgenol* 1994;162:665.
268. Marra TR, Shah M, Mikus MA. Transient cortical blindness due to hypertensive encephalopathy. Magnetic resonance imaging correlation. *J Clin Neuroophthalmol* 1993;13:35.
269. Thambisetty M, Biousse V, Newman NJ. Hypertensive brainstem encephalopathy: clinical and radiographic findings. *J Neurological Sci* 2003;208:93.
270. Usta IM, Sibai BM. Emergent management of puerperal eclampsia. *Obstet Gynecol Clin North Am* 1995;22:315.
271. Mabie WC. Management of acute severe hypertension and encephalopathy. *Clin Obstet Gynecol* 1999;42:19.
272. Conomy JP. Impact of arterial hypertension on the brain. *Postgrad Med J* 1980;68:86.
273. Reid JL, et al. Clonidine withdrawal hypertension. Changes in blood-pressure and plasma and urinary noradrenaline. *Lancet* 1977;1:1171.
274. Glazener FS, et al. Pargyline, cheese, and acute hypertension. *JAMA* 1964;188:754.
275. Graham JB. Pheochromocytoma and hypertension. An analysis of 207 cases. *Int Abstr Surg/Surg Gynecol Obstet* 1951;92(Suppl):105.
276. Eastman JW, Cohen SN. Hypertensive crisis and death associated with phencyclidine poisoning. *JAMA* 1975;231:1270.
277. Russo S, et al. Low doses of liquorice can induce hypertensive encephalopathy. *Am J Nephrol* 2000;20:145.
278. Lake CR, et al. Adverse drug effects attributed to phenylpropanolamine: a review of 142 case reports. *Am J Med* 1990;89:195.
279. Pentel P. Toxicity of over-the-counter stimulants. *JAMA* 1984;252:1898.
280. Joss DV, et al. Hypertension and convulsions in children receiving cyclosporin A. *Lancet* 1982;1:906.
281. Schwartz RB, et al. Cyclosporine neurotoxicity and its relationship to hypertensive encephalopathy: CT and MR findings in 16 cases. *Am J Roentgenol* 1995;165:627.
282. Cooney MJ, et al. Hypertensive encephalopathy: complication in children treated for myeloproliferative disorders-report of three cases. *Radiology* 2000;214:711.
283. McGonigle RJ, et al. Hypertensive encephalopathy complicating transplant renal artery stenosis. *Postgrad Med J* 1984;60:356.
284. Tejani A. Post-transplant hypertension and hypertensive encephalopathy in renal allograft recipients. *Nephron* 1983;34:73.
285. Miller A, Rosman MA. Hypertensive encephalopathy as a complication of femoral lengthening. *Can Med Assoc J* 1981;124:296.
286. Erickson RP. Autonomic hyperreflexia: pathophysiology and medical management. *Arch Phys Med Rehabil* 1980;61:431.
287. Naftchi NE, et al. Hypertensive crises in quadriplegic patients. *Circulation* 1978;57:336.
288. Beccari M. Seizures in dialysis patients treated with recombinant erythropoietin. Review of the literature and guidelines for prevention. *Int J Artificial Organs* 1994;17:5.
289. Gueron M, Ilia R, Sofer S. The cardiovascular system after scorpion envenomation. A review. *J Toxicol Clin Toxicol* 1992;30:245.
290. Grewal RP, Miller BL. Cocaine induced hypertensive encephalopathy. *Acta Neurol* 1991;13:279.
291. Lassen NA, Angoli A. The upper limit of autoregulation of cerebral blood flow-on the pathogenesis of hypertensive encephalopathy. *Scand J Lab Clin Invest* 1972;30:113.
292. Strandgaard S, et al. Autoregulation of brain circulation in severe arterial hypertension. *Br Med J* 1973;1:507.
293. Strandgaard S, Paulson OB. Cerebral blood flow and its pathophysiology in hypertension. *Am J Hypertens* 1989;2:486.
294. Strandgaard S, et al. Studies on the cerebral circulation of the baboon in acutely induced hypertension. *Stroke* 1976;7:287.
295. Smeda JS, Payne GW. Alterations in autoregulation and myogenic function in the cerebrovasculature of Dahl salt-sensitive rats. *Stroke* 2003;34:1484.
296. Johansson B, et al. The effect of acute arterial hypertension on the blood-brain barrier to protein tracers. *Acta Neuropathol (Berlin)* 1970;16:117.
297. Nag S, Roberston DM, Dinsdale HB. Cerebral cortical changes in acute experimental hypertension. An ultrastructural study. *Lab Invest* 1977;36:150.
298. Cressman MD, Gifford RW. Hypertension and stroke. *J Am Coll Cardiol* 1983;1:521.
299. Stauffer JC, Gaasch WH. Recognition and treatment of left ventricular diastolic dysfunction. *Prog Cardiovasc Dis* 1990;32:319.
300. Dougherty AH, et al. Congestive heart failure with normal systolic function. *Am J Cardiol* 1984;54:778.
301. Little WC, Downes TR. Clinical evaluation of left ventricular diastolic performance. *Prog Cardiovasc Dis* 1990;32:273.
302. Soufer R, et al. Intact systolic left ventricular function in clinical congestive heart failure. *Am J Cardiol* 1985;55:1032.
303. Topol EJ, Trailld TA, Fortuin NJ. Hypertensive hypertrophic cardiomyopathy of the elderly. *N Engl J Med* 1985;312:277.
304. Weber JR. Left ventricular hypertrophy: its prime importance as a controllable risk factor. *Am Heart J* 1988;116:272.
305. Rodriguera E, Guiha N, Cohn JN. Left ventricular function in hypertensive heart failure (HHF). *Circulation* 1971;44(Suppl II):II-129.
306. Zile MR, Gaasch WH. Mechanical loads and the isovolumic and filling indices of left ventricular relaxation. *Prog Cardiovasc Dis* 1990;32:333.
307. Matter CM, et al. Effect of NO donors on diastolic function in patients with severe pressure-overload hypertrophy. *Circulation* 1999;99:2396.
308. Kannel WB, et al. Epidemiologic assessment of the role of blood pressure in stroke. The Framingham Study. *JAMA* 1970;214:301.
309. Cutler JA, MacMahon SW, Furberg CD. Controlled clinical trials of drug treatment for hypertension. A review. *Hypertension* 1989;13(Suppl I):I-36.
310. Phillips S. Pathogenesis, diagnosis, and treatment of hypertension-associated stroke. *Am J Hypertens* 1989;2:493.
311. Wallace JD, Levy LL. Blood pressure after stroke. *JAMA* 1981;246:2177.
312. Britton M, de Faire U, Helmers C. Hazards of therapy for excessive hypertension in acute stroke. *Acta Med Scand* 1980;207:253.
313. Lavin P. Management of hypertension in patients with acute stroke. *Arch Intern Med* 1986;146:66.
314. Meyer JS, et al. Impaired neurogenic cerebrovascular control and dysautoregulation after stroke. *Stroke* 1973;4:169.
315. Yatsu FM, Zivin J. Hypertension in acute ischemic stroke. Not to treat. *Arch Neurol* 1985;42:999.
316. Harmsen P, Kjaerulff J, Skinhoj E. Acute controlled hypotension and EEG in patients with hypertension and cerebrovascular disease. *J Neurol Neurosurg Psychiatry* 1971;34:300.
317. O'Connell JE, Gray CS. Treatment of post-stroke hypertension. A practical guide. *Drugs Aging* 1996;8:408.
318. Spence JD, Del Maestro RF. Hypertension in acute ischemic strokes—treat. *Arch Neurol* 1985;42:1000.
319. Ledingham JG. Management of hypertensive crises. *Hypertension* 1983;5(Suppl III):III-114.
320. Butterworth RJ, et al. Pathophysiologic assessment of nitric oxide (given as sodium nitroprusside) in acute ischaemic stroke. *Cerebrovasc Dis* 1998;8:158.
321. Trust Study Group. Randomized, double-blind placebo-controlled trial of nimodipine in acute stroke. *Lancet* 1990;336:1205.
322. Cuneo RA, Caronna JJ. The neurologic complications of hypertension. *Med Clin North Am* 1977;61:565.
323. Kaneko T, et al. Lower limit of blood pressure in treatment of acute hypertensive intracranial hemorrhage. *J Cereb Blood Flow Metab* 1983;3(Suppl 1):S51.
324. Caplan LR. Intracerebral hemorrhage. *Lancet* 1992;339:656.
325. Candia GJ, et al. Effect of intravenous sodium nitroprusside on cerebral blood flow and metabolism. *Neurosurgery* 1978;3:50.
326. Strandgaard S, Paulson OB. Cerebral autoregulation. *Stroke* 1984;15:413.
327. Van Aken H, et al. Treatment of intraoperative hypertensive emergencies in patients with intracranial disease. *Am J Cardiol* 1989;63:43C.
328. Feibel JH, Baldwin CA, Joynt RJ. Catecholamine-associated refractory hypertension following acute intracranial hemorrhage: control with propranolol. *Ann Neurol* 1981;9:340.
329. Heros RC. Cerebellar hemorrhage and infarction. *Stroke* 1982;13:106.
330. Heros RC, Zervas NT, Varsos V. Cerebral vasospasm after subarachnoid hemorrhage: an update. *Ann Neurol* 1983;14:599.
331. Weir B, MacDonald L. Cerebral vasospasm. *Clin Neurosurg* 1993;40:40.
332. Plets C. Arterial hypertension in neurosurgical emergencies. *Am J Cardiol* 1989;63:41C.

333. Ullman JS, Bederson JB. Hypertensive, hypervolemic, hemodilution therapy for aneurysmal subarachnoid hemorrhage. Is it efficacious? Yes. *Controvers Crit Care Med* 1996;12:697.

334. Oropello JM, Weiner L, Benjamin E. Hypertensive, hypervolemic, hemodilution therapy for aneurysmal subarachnoid hemorrhage. Is it efficacious? No. *Controvers Crit Care Med* 1996;12:709.

335. Langley MS, Sorkin EM. Nimodipine. A review of its pharmacodynamic and pharmacokinetic properties, and therapeutic potential in cerebrovascular disease. *Drugs* 1989;37:669.

336. Öhman J, Servo A, Heiskanen O. Long-term effects of nimodipine on cerebral infarcts and outcome after aneurysmal subarachnoid hemorrhage and surgery. *J Neurosurg* 1991;74:8.

337. Pickard JD, et al. Effect of oral nimodipine on cerebral infarction and outcome after subarachnoid haemorrhage: British aneurysm nimodipine trial. *Br Med J* 1989;298:636.

338. Fink ME. Emergency management of the head-injured patient. *Emerg Med Clin North Am* 1987;5:783.

339. Miller JD, et al. Significance of intracranial hypertension in severe head injury. *J Neurosurg* 1977;47:503.

340. Siggers DC, Salter C, Fluck DC. Serial plasma adrenaline and noradrenaline levels in myocardial infarction using a new double isotope technique. *Br Heart J* 1971;33:878.

341. James TN, Isobe JH, Urthaler F. Analysis of components in a cardiogenic hypertensive chemoreflex. *Circulation* 1975;52:179.

342. Gibson TC. Blood pressure levels in acute myocardial infarction. *Am Heart J* 1978;96:475.

343. Luria MH, et al. Acute myocardial infarction: prognosis after recovery. *Ann Intern Med* 1976;85:561.

344. Fox KM, et al. Prognostic significance of acute systolic hypertension after myocardial infarction. *Br Med J* 1975;3:128.

345. Naeim F, de La Maza LM, Robbins SL. Cardiac rupture during myocardial infarction. *Circulation* 1972;45:1231.

346. Franciosa JA, Notargiacomo AV, Cohn JN. Comparative haemodynamic and metabolic effects of vasodilator and inotropic agents in experimental myocardial infarction. *Cardiovasc Res* 1978;12:294.

347. Hjalmarson A, Olsson G. Myocardial infarction. Effects of beta-blockade. *Circulation* 1991;84(Suppl 6):VI101.

348. ISIS-1 (First International Study of Infarct Survival) Collaborative Group. Randomized trial of intravenous atenolol among 16,027 cases of suspected acute myocardial infarction: ISIS-1. *Lancet* 1986;2:57.

349. Held P. Effects of beta blockers on ventricular dysfunction after myocardial infarction: tolerability and survival effects. *Am J Cardiol* 1993;71:39C.

350. Mooss AN, Hilleman DE, Mohiuddin SM. Safety of esmolol in patients with acute myocardial infarction treated with thrombolytic therapy who had relative contraindications to beta-blocker therapy. *Ann Pharmacother* 1994;28:701.

351. Goldman L, Sia ST, Cook EF. Costs and effectiveness of routine therapy with long-term beta-adrenergic antagonists after acute myocardial infarction. *N Engl J Med* 1988;319:152.

352. Borghi C, et al. Effects of the administration of angiotensin-converting enzyme inhibitor during the acute phase of myocardial infarction in patients with arterial hypertension. SMILE Study Investigators. Survival of Myocardial Infarction Long-term Evaluation. *Am J Hypertens* 1999;12:665.

353. Franciosa JA, et al. Arterial pressure as a determinant of left ventricular filling pressure after acute myocardial infarction. *Am J Cardiol* 1974;34:506.

354. Armstrong PW, et al. Vasodilator therapy in acute myocardial infarction. A comparison of sodium nitroprusside and nitroglycerin. *Circulation* 1975;52:1118.

355. Shell WE, Sobel BE. Protection of jeopardized ischemic myocardium by reduction of ventricular afterload. *N Engl J Med* 1974;291:481.

356. Garadah T, et al. Impact of intravenous nitroglycerin on pulsed Doppler indexes of left ventricular filling in acute anterior myocardial infarction. *Am Heart J* 1998;136:812.

357. Capurro NL, Kent KM, Epstein SE. Comparison of nitroglycerin-, nitroprusside-, and phentolamine-induced changes in coronary collateral function in dogs. *J Clin Invest* 1977;60:295.

358. Flaherty JT. Comparison of intravenous nitroglycerin and sodium nitroprusside in acute myocardial infarction. *Am J Med* 1983;74[Suppl 6B]:53.

359. Mann T, et al. Effect of nitroprusside on regional myocardial blood flow in coronary artery disease. *Circulation* 1978;57:732.

360. Cohn JN, Burke LP. Nitroprusside. *Ann Intern Med* 1979;91:752.

361. Wheat MW. Acute dissecting aneurysms of the aorta: diagnosis and treatment-1979. *Am Heart J* 1980;99:373.

362. Daily PO, et al. Management of acute aortic dissections. *Ann Thorac Surg* 1970;10:237.

363. DeSanctis RW, et al. Aortic dissection. *N Engl J Med* 1987;317:1060.

364. Slater EE, DeSanctis RW. The clinical recognition of dissecting aortic aneurysm. *Am J Med* 1976;60:625.

365. Slater EE, DeSanctis RW. Dissection of the aorta. *Med Clin North Am* 1979;63:141.

366. Moran JF, Derkac WM, Conkle DM. Pharmacologic control of acute aortic dissection in hypertensive dogs. *Surg Forum* 1978;29:231.

367. Prokop EK, Palmer RF, Wheat MW. Hydrodynamic forces in dissecting aneurysms. In vitro studies in a tygon model and in dog aortas. *Circ Res* 1970;27:121.

368. Spittell PC, et al. Clinical features and differential diagnosis of aortic dissection: experience with 236 cases (1980 through 1990). *Mayo Clin Proc* 1993;58:642.

369. Cigarroa JE, et al. Diagnostic imaging in the evaluation of suspected aortic dissection. *N Engl J Med* 1993;328:35.

370. Chirillo F, et al. Comparative diagnostic value of transesophageal echocardiography and retrograde aortography in the evaluation of thoracic aortic dissection. *Am J Cardiol* 1994;74:590.

371. Keren A, et al. Accuracy of biplane and multiplane transesophageal echocardiography in diagnosis of acute aortic dissection and intramural hematoma. *J Am Coll Cardiol* 1996;28:627.

372. Nienaber CA, et al. Diagnosis of thoracic aortic dissection: magnetic resonance imaging versus transesophageal echocardiography. *Circulation* 1992;85:434.

373. Crawford ES. The diagnosis and management of aortic dissection. *JAMA* 1990;264:2537.

374. Eagle KA, DeSanctis KC. Aortic dissection. *Curr Probl Cardiol* 1989;14:229.

375. Palmer RF, Lasseter KC. Nitroprusside and aortic dissection. *N Engl J Med* 1976;294:1403.

376. Doroghazi RM, et al. Long-term survival of patients with treated aortic dissection. *J Am Coll Cardiol* 1984;3:1026.

377. Rosenborough G, et al. Twenty-year experience with acute distal aortic dissections. *J Vasc Surg* 2004;40:235.

378. DeBakey ME, et al. Dissection and dissecting aneurysms of the aorta: twenty-year follow-up of five hundred twenty-seven patients treated surgically. *Surgery* 1982;92:1118.

379. Neely CF. Postoperative hypertension. In Goldmann DR, Brown FH, Guarnieri DM, eds. *Perioperative medicine: the medical care of the surgical patient.* New York: McGraw-Hill, 1994:531.

380. Goldman L, et al. Multifactorial index of cardiac risk in noncardiac surgical procedures. *N Engl J Med* 1977;297:845.

381. Detsky AL, et al. Predicting cardiac complications in patients undergoing non-cardiac surgery. *J Gen Intern Med* 1986;1:211.

382. Prys-Roberts C, Meloche R, Foëx P. Studies on anaesthesia in relation to hypertension. I: Cardiovascular responses of treated and untreated patients. *Br J Anaesth* 1971;43:122.

383. Charlson ME, et al. Preoperative characteristics predicting intraoperative hypotension and hypertension among hypertensives and diabetics undergoing noncardiac surgery. *Ann Surg* 1990;212:66.

384. Goldman L, Caldera DL. Risks of general anesthesia and elective operation in the hypertensive patient. *Anesthesiology* 1979;50:285.

385. Adler AG, Leahy JJ, Cressman MD. Management of perioperative hypertension using sublingual nifedipine. *Arch Intern Med* 1986;146:1927.

386. Martin DE, Kammerer WS. The hypertensive surgical patient. Controversies in management. *Surg Clin North Am* 1983;63:1017.

387. Breslin DJ, Swinton NW. Elective surgery in hypertensive patients-preoperative considerations. *Surg Clin North Am* 1970;50:585.

388. Prys-Roberts C. Hypertension and anesthesia-fifty years on. *Anesthesiology* 1979;50:281.

389. Prys-Roberts C, Meloche R. Management of anesthesia in patients with hypertension or ischemic heart disease. *Int Anesthesiol Clin* 1980;18:181.

390. Joint National Committee on Detection, Evaluation and Treatment of High Blood Pressure: the sixth report of the Joint National Committee on Detection, Evaluation, and Treatment of High Blood Pressure (JCN VI). *Arch Intern Med* 1997;157:2413.

391. Kopriva CJ, Brown AC, Pappas G. Hemodynamics during general anesthesia in patients receiving propranolol. *Anesthesiology* 1978;48:28.

392. Prys-Roberts C, et al. Studies on anaesthesia in relation to hypertension V. Adrenergic beta-receptor blockade. *Br J Anaesth* 1973;45:671.

393. Mirenda JV, Grissom TE. Anesthetic implications of the renin-angiotensin system and angiotensin-converting enzyme inhibitors. *Anesth Analg* 1991;72:667.

394. Zerbe RL, Feurestein G, Kopin IJ. Effect of captopril on cardiovascular, sympathetic and vasopressin responses to hemorrhage. *Eur J Pharmacol* 1981;72:391.

395. Colson P, et al. Effect of angiotensin converting enzyme inhibition on blood pressure and renal function during open heart surgery. *Anesthesiology* 1990;72:23.

396. Cucchiara RF, et al. Evaluation of esmolol in controlling increases in heart rate and blood pressure during endotracheal intubation in patients undergoing carotid surgery. *Anesthesiology* 1986;65:528.

397. Leslie JB, et al. Attenuation of the hemodynamic responses to endotracheal intubation with preinduction intravenous labetalol. *J Clin Anesth* 1989;1:194.

398. Flaherty JT, et al. Comparison of intravenous nitroglycerin and sodium nitroprusside for the treatment of acute hypertension developing after coronary artery bypass surgery. *Circulation* 1982;65:1072.

399. Dimich I, et al. Comparative hemodynamic effects of labetalol and hydralazine in the treatment of postoperative hypertension. *J Clin Anesth* 1989;1:201.

400. Orlowski JP, et al. The hemodynamic effects of intravenous labetalol for postoperative hypertension. *Clev Clin J Med* 1989;56:29.

401. Goldberg ME, et al. Perioperative hypertension. *Pharmacotherapy* 1998;18:911.

402. Estafanous FG, Tarazi RC. Systemic arterial hypertension associated with cardiac surgery. *Am J Cardiol* 1980;46:685.

403. Cohn JN. Paroxysmal hypertension and hypovolemia. *N Engl J Med* 1966;275:643.

404. Hanson EL, et al. Comparison of patients with coronary artery or valve disease: intraoperative differences in blood volume and observations of vasomotor response. *Ann Thorac Surg* 1976;22:343.

405. Fouad FM, Estafanous FG, Tarazi RC. Hemodynamic of postmyocardial revascularization hypertension. *Am J Cardiol* 1978;41:564.

406. Patel CV, et al. Use of sodium nitroprusside in post-coronary bypass surgery. A plea for conservatism. *Chest* 1986;89:663.

407. Gombotz H, et al. DA1-receptor stimulation with fenoldopam in the treatment of postcardiac surgical hypertension. *Acta Anesthesiol Scand* 1998;42:834.

408. Hill AJ, Feneck RO, Walesby RK. A comparison of fenoldopam and nitroprusside in the control of hypertension following coronary artery surgery. *J Cardiothorac Vasc Anesth* 1993;7:279.

409. Meretoja OA, et al. Combined alpha- and beta-blockade with labetalol in post-open heart surgery hypertension. Reversal of hemodynamic deterioration with glucagon. *Chest* 1980;78:810.

410. Skydell JL, et al. Incidence and mechanism of post-carotid endarterectomy hypertension. *Arch Surg* 1987;122:1153.

411. Towne JB, Bernhard VM. The relationship of postoperative hypertension to complications following carotid endarterectomy. *Surgery* 1980;88:575.

412. Wong JH, Findlay JN, Suarez-Almazor ME. Hemodynamic instability after carotid endarterectomy: risk factors and associations with operative complications. *Neurosurgery* 1997;41:35.

413. Naylor AR, et al. Seizures after carotid endarterectomy: hyperperfusion, dysautoregulation or hypertensive encephalopathy?. *Eur J Vasc Endovasc Surg* 2003;26:39.

414. Ouriel K, et al. Intracerebral hemorrhage after carotic endarterectomy: incidence, contribution to neurologic morbidity, and predictive factors. *J Vasc Surg* 1999;29:82.

415. Gidding SS, et al. Therapeutic effect of propranolol on paradoxical hypertension after repair of coarctation of the aorta. *N Engl J Med* 1985;312:1224.

416. Sealy WC. Coarctation of the aorta and hypertension. *Ann Thorac Surg* 1967;3:15.

417. Verska JJ, DeQuattro V, Woolley MM. Coarctation of the aorta: the abdominal pain syndrome and paradoxical hypertension. *J Thorac Cardiovasc Surg* 1969;58:746.

418. Will RJ, et al. Sodium nitroprusside and propranolol therapy for management of postcoarctectomy hypertension. *J Thorac Cardiovasc Surg* 1978;75:722.

419. Ram CV. Pheochromocytoma. *Cardiol Clin* 1988;6:517.

420. Hull CJ. Phaeochromocytoma. Diagnosis, preoperative preparation, and anaesthetic management. *Br J Anaesth* 1956;58:1453.

421. Shapiro B, Fig LM. Management of pheochromocytoma. *Endocrinol Metab Clin North Am* 1989;18:443.

422. Pinaud M, et al. Preoperative acute volume loading in patients with pheochromocytoma. *Crit Care Med* 1985;13:460.

423. Cubeddu LX, et al. Prazosin and propranolol in preoperative management of pheochromocytoma. *Clin Pharmacol Ther* 1982;32:156.

424. Knapp HR, Fitzgerald GA. Hypertensive crisis in prazosin-treated pheochromocytoma. *South Med J* 1984;77:535.

425. Rosei EA, et al. Treatment of pheochromocytoma and of clonidine withdrawal hypertension with labetalol. *Br J Clin Pharmacol* 1976;3(Suppl):809.

426. Navaratnarajah M, White DC. Labetalol and pheochromocytoma. *Br J Anaesth* 1984;56:1179.

427. Houston MC. Abrupt cessation of treatment in hypertension: consideration of clinical features, mechanisms, prevention and management of the discontinuation syndrome. *Am Heart J* 1981;102:415.

428. Burden AC, Alexander CP. Rebound hypertension after acute methyldopa withdrawal. *Br Med J* 1976;1:1056.

429. Ram CV, et al. Withdrawal syndrome following cessation of guanabenz therapy. *J Clin Pharmacol* 1979;19:148.

430. Garbus SB, et al. The abrupt discontinuation of antihypertensive treatment. *J Clin Pharmacol* 1979;19:476.

431. Neusy AJ, Lowenstein J. Blood pressure and blood pressure variability following withdrawal of propranolol and clonidine. *J Clin Pharmacol* 1989;29:18.

432. Strauss FG, et al. Withdrawal of antihypertensive therapy. Hypertensive crises in renovascular hypertension. *JAMA* 1977;238:1734.

433. Hoobler SW, Kashima T. Central nervous system actions of clonidine in hypertension. *Mayo Clin Proc* 1977;52:395.

434. Bailey RR, Neale TJ. Rapid clonidine withdrawal with blood pressure overshoot exaggerated by beta-blockade. *Br Med J* 1976;1:942.

435. Blackwell B, et al. Hypertensive interactions between monoamine oxidase inhibitors and foodstuffs. *Br J Psychiatry* 1967;113:349.

436. Tailor SA, et al. Hypertensive episode associated with phenelzine and tap beer—a reanalysis of the role of pressor amines in beer. *J Clin Pharmacol* 1994;14:5.

437. Food interaction with MAO inhibitors. *Med Lett Drugs Ther* 1989;31:11.

438. Lefebvre H, Richard R, Noblet C, et al. Life-threatening pseudophaechromocytoma after toloxatone, terbutaline, and phenylephrine. *Lancet* 1993;341:555.

439. Lake CR, et al. Transient hypertension after two phenylpropanolamine diet aids and the effects of caffeine: a placebo-controlled follow-up study. *Am J Med* 1989;86:427.

440. SoRelle R. FDA wayns of stroke risk associated with phenylpropanolamine cold remedies and drugs removed from store shelves. *Circulation* 2000;102:E9041.

441. Teasell RW, et al. Cardiovascular consequences of loss of supraspinal control of sympathetic nervous system after spinal cord injury. *Arch Physical Med Rehab* 2000;81:506.

442. Frost F. Pitfalls in managing routine medical problems of patients with spinal cord injury. *Clev Clin J Med* 199764:302.

443. McGuire TJ, Kumar VN. Autonomic dysreflexia in the spinal cord injured. *Postgrad Med* 1986;80:81.

444. Lindan R, et al. Incidence and clinical features of autonomic dysreflexia in patients with spinal cord injury. *Paraplegia* 1980;18:285.

445. Davidson DL, Jellinek EH. Hypertension and papilloedema in the Guillain-Barré syndrome. *J Neurol Neurosurg Psychiatry* 1977;40:144.

446. Brizio-Molteni L, et al. Incidence of post-burn hypertensive crisis in patients admitted to two burn centers and a community hospital in the United States. *Scand J Plast Reconstr Surg* 1979;13:21.

447. Dukes CS, Perfect JR. Amphotericin B-induced malignant hypertensive episodes. *J Infect Dis* 1990;161:588.

448. Michaeli J, et al. Severe hypertension and lithium intoxication. *JAMA* 1984;251:1680.

449. Dunn FG. Malignant hypertension associated with the use of amitriptyline hydrochloride. *South Med J* 1982;75:1124.

450. Rodman MD, White WB. Accelerated hypertension associated with the central nervous system toxicity of metrizamide. *Drug Intell Clin Pharmacol* 1986;20:62.

451. Grannis FW, et al. Acute aortic dissection associated with cocaine abuse. *Clin Cardiol* 1988;11:572.

452. Levine SR, et al. A comparative study of the cerebrovascular complications of cocaine:alkaloidal versus hydrochloride-a review. *Neurology* 1991;41:1173.

453. Mann SJ, Krakoff LR. Hypertensive crisis caused by hypoglycemia and propranolol. *Arch Intern Med* 1984;144:2427.

454. Schramek A, et al. Hypertensive crisis, erythrocytosis, and uraemia due to renal-artery stenosis of kidney transplants. *Lancet* 1975;1:70.

455. Barry DI. Cerebrovascular aspects of antihypertensive treatment. *Am J Cardiol* 1989;63:14C.

456. Hurtig HI. Hypertensive emergencies: the case for gradual reduction of blood pressure. In: Narins RG, ed. *Controversies in nephrology and hypertension.* New York: Churchill-Livingstone, 1984.

457. Ledingham JG, Rajagopalan B. Cerebral complications in the treatment of accelerated hypertension. *Q J Med* 1979;48:25.

458. Cove DH, et al. Blindness after treatment for malignant hypertension. *Br Med J* 1979;2:245.

459. Graham DI. Ischaemic brain damage of cerebral perfusion failure type after treatment of severe hypertension. *Br Med J* 1975;4:739.

460. Haas DC, et al. Death from cerebral hypoperfusion during nitroprusside treatment of acute angiotensin-dependent hypertension. *Am J Med* 1983;75:1071.

461. Hankey GJ, Gubbay SS. Focal cerebral ischemia and infarction due to antihypertensive therapy. *Med J Aust* 1987;146:412.

462. Hulse JA, Taylor DS, Dillon MJ. Blindness and paraplegia in severe childhood hypertension. *Lancet* 1979;2:553.

463. Kumar KG, et al. Side effects of diazoxide. *JAMA* 1976;235:275.

464. Pryor JS, Davies PD, Hamilton DV. Blindness and malignant hypertension. *Lancet* 1979;2:803.

465. Strandgaard S. Autoregulation of cerebral blood flow in hypertensive patients. The modifying influence of prolonged antihypertensive treatment on the tolerance to acute, drug-induced hypotension. *Circulation* 1976;53:720.

466. Strandgaard S. Cerebral blood flow in hypertension. *Acta Med Scand* 1983;678(Suppl):11.

467. Johnson CC. The toxicity and actions of sodium nitroprusside. *Arch Int Pharmacol Ther* 1929;35:480.

468. Page IH, et al. Cardiovascular actions of sodium nitroprusside in animals and hypertensive patients. *Circulation* 1955;11:188.

469. Palmer RF, Lasseter KC. Sodium nitroprusside. *N Engl J Med* 1975;292:294.

470. Bhatia SK, Frohlich ED. Hemodynamic comparison of agents useful in hypertensive emergencies. *Am Heart J* 1973;85:367.

471. Chen RY, et al. Baroreceptor control of heart rate in humans during nitroprusside-induced hypotension. *Am J Physiol* 1982;243:R18.

472. Tarazi RC, et al. Vasodilating drugs: contrasting haemodynamic effects. *Clin Sci Mol Med* 1976;51:575s.

473. Gruetter CA, et al. Relationship between cyclic guanoxine 3':5'-monophosphate formation and relaxation of coronary arterial smooth muscle by glyceryl trinitrate, nitroprusside, nitrite and nitric oxide: effects of methylene blue and methemoglobin. *J Pharmacol Exp Ther* 1981;219:181.

474. Ignarro IJ, et al. Mechanism of vascular smooth muscle relaxation by organic nitrates, nitrites, nitroprusside and nitric oxide: evidence for the involvement of s-nitrosothiols as active intermediates. *J Pharmacol Exp Ther* 1981;218:739.

475. Wilson J. Leber's hereditary optic atrophy: a possible defect of cyanide metabolism. *Clin Sci* 1965;29:505.

476. Cole P. The safe use of sodium nitroprusside. *Anesthesia* 1978;33:473.

477. Davies DW, et al. A sudden death associated with the use of sodium nitroprusside for induction of hypotension during anaesthesia. *Can Anaesth Soc J* 1975;22:547.

478. Cottrell JE, et al. Prevention of nitroprusside-induced cyanide toxicity with hydroxocobalamin. *N Engl J Med* 1978;298:809.

479. Naulty J, Cefalo RC, Lewis PE. Fetal toxicity of nitroprusside in the pregnant ewe. *Am J Obstet Gynecol* 1981;139:708.

480. Ellis SC, et al. Fetal and maternal effects of sodium nitroprusside used to counteract hypertension in gravid ewes. *Am J Obstet Gynecol* 1982;143:766.

481. Donchin Y, et al. Sodium nitroprusside for aneurysm surgery in pregnancy. *Br J Anaesth* 1978;50:849.

482. Rigg D, McDonogh A. Use of sodium nitroprusside for deliberate hypotension during pregnancy. *Br J Anaesth* 1981;53:985.

483. Stempel JE, et al. Use of sodium nitroprusside in complications of gestational hypertension. *Obstet Gynecol* 1982;60:533.

484. Berkowitz RL. The management of hypertensive crises during pregnancy. In: Berkowitz RL, ed. *Critical care of the obstetric patient.* New York: Churchill Livingstone, 1983:299.

485. Tumlin JA, et al. Fenoldopam, a dopamine agonist, for hypertensive emergency: a multicenter randomized trial. *Academic Emerg Med* 2000;7: 653.

486. Brogden RN, Markham A. Fenoldopam: a review of its pharmacodynamic and pharmacokinetic properties and intravenous clinical potential in the management of hypertensive urgencies and urgencies. *Drugs* 1997;54: 634.

487. Bodmann KF, et al. Hemodynamic profile of intravenous fenoldopam in patients with hypertensive crises. *Clin Invest* 1993;72:60.

488. Devlin JW, et al. Fenoldopam versus nitroprusside for treatment of hypertensive emergencies. *Ann Pharmacother* 2004;38:755.

489. Goldberg ME, et al. Fenoldopam infusion for the treatment of postoperative hypertension. *J Clin Anesth* 1993;5:386.

490. Hill AJ, Feneck RO, Walesby RK. A comparison of fenoldopam and nitroprusside in the control of hypertension following coronary artery surgery. *J Cardiothorac Vasc Anesth* 1993;7:279.

491. Huysmans FT, Thein T, Koene RA. Acute treatment of hypertension with slow infusion of diazoxide. *Arch Intern Med* 1983;143:882.

492. Michael CA. The control of hypertension in labour. *Aust NZ J Obstet Gynecol* 1972;12:48.

493. Pennington JC, Picker RH. Diazoxide and the treatment of the acute hypertensive emergency in obstetrics. *Med J Aust* 1972;2:1051.

494. Sankar D, Moodley J. Low-dose diazoxide in the emergency management of severe hypertension in pregnancy. *S Afr Med J* 1984;65:279.

495. Moser M. Diazoxide-an effective vasodilator in accelerated hypertension. *Am Heart J* 1974;87:791.

496. Koch-Weser J. Vasodilator drugs in the treatment of hypertension. *Arch Intern Med* 1974;133:1017.

497. O'Malley K, et al. Decreased plasma protein binding of diazoxide in uremia. *Clin Pharmacol Ther* 1975;18:53.

498. Standen NB, et al. Hyperpolarizing vasodilators activate ATP-sensitive K+ channels in arterial smooth muscle. *Science* 1989;245:177.

499. Ram CV, Kaplan NM. Individual titration of diazoxide dosage in the treatment of severe hypertension. *Am J Cardiol* 1979;43:627.

500. Velasco M, et al. A new technique for safe and effective control of hypertension with intravenous diazoxide. *Curr Ther Res* 1976;19:185.

501. O'Brien KP, Grigor RR, Taylor PM. Intravenous diazoxide in treatment of hypertension associated with recent myocardial infarction. *Br Med J* 1975;4:74.

502. Greenwood RH, Mahler RF, Hales CN. Improvement in insulin secretion in diabetes after diazoxide. *Lancet* 1976;1:444.

503. Charles MA, Danforth E. Nonketoacidotic hyperglycemia and coma during intravenous diazoxide therapy in uremia. *Diabetes* 1971;20:501.

504. Morris JA, et al. The management of severe preeclampsia and eclampsia with intravenous diazoxide. *Obstet Gynecol* 1977;49:675.

505. Neuman J, et al. Diazoxide for the acute control of severe hypertension complicating pregnancy: a pilot study. *Obstet Gynecol* 1979;53[Suppl]:50S.

506. Milsap RL, Auld PA. Neonatal hyperglycemia following maternal diazoxide administration. *JAMA* 1980;243:144.

507. Tewfik GI. Trimethaphan. Its effect on the pseudo-cholinesterase level of man. *Anaesthesia* 1957;12:326.

508. Dale RC, Schroeder ET. Respiratory paralysis during treatment of hypertension with trimethaphan camsylate. *Arch Intern Med* 1976;136: 816.

509. Hallum JL, Hatchuel WL. Congenital paralytic ileus in a premature baby as a complication of hexamethonium bromide therapy for toxaemia of pregnancy. *Arch Dis Child* 1954;29:354.

510. Flaherty JT, et al. Intravenous nitroglycerin in acute myocardial infarction. *Circulation* 1975;51:132.

511. Chiariello M, et al. Comparison between the effects of nitroprusside and nitroglycerin on ischemic injury during acute myocardial infarction. *Circulation* 1976;54:766.

512. Harrison DG, Bates JN. The nitrovasodilators. New ideas about old drugs. *Circulation* 1993;87:1461.

513. Zelis R. Mechanisms of vasodilation. *Am J Med* 1983;74 (Suppl 6B):3.

514. Waldman SA, Murad F. Cyclic GMP synthesis and function. *Pharmacol Rev* 1987;39:163.

515. Nurenberg JR. Intravenous nitroglycerine in the management of post-treatment hypertension during electroconvulsive therapy. *J Nerv Ment Dis* 1991;179:292.

516. Cressman MD, et al. Intravenous labetalol in the management of severe hypertension and hypertensive emergencies. *Am Heart J* 1984;107: 980.

517. Cumming AM, Davies DL. Intravenous labetalol in hypertensive emergency. *Lancet* 1979;1:929.

518. MacCarthy EP, Bloomfield SS. Labetalol: a review of its pharmacology, pharmacokinetics, clinical uses and adverse effects. *Pharmacotherapy* 1983;3:193.

519. Mehta J, et al. Systemic, pulmonary, and coronary hemodynamic effects of labetalol in hypertensive subjects. *Am J Med* 1983;75(Suppl 4A):32.

520. Mahmoud TZ, Bjornsson S, Calder AA. Labetalol therapy in pregnancy induced hypertension: the effects on fetoplacental circulation and fetal outcome. *Eur J Obstet Gynecol Reprod Biol* 1993;50:109.

521. Klarr JM, Bhatt-Mehta V, Donn SM. Neonatal adrenergic blockade following single dose maternal labetalol administration. *Am J Perinatol* 1994;11:91.

522. Reach G, et al. Effect of labetalol on blood pressure and plasma catecholamine concentrations in patients with phaechromocytoma. *Br Med J* 1980;280:1300.

523. Briggs RS, Birtwell AJ, Pohl JE. Hypertensive response to labetalol in pheochromocytoma. *Lancet* 1978;1:1045.

524. Heyka RJ, Vidt DG. Control of hypertension in patients with chronic renal failure. *Clev Clin J Med* 1989;56:65.

525. Arthur S, Greenberg A. Hyperkalemia associated with intravenous labetalol therapy for acute hypertension in renal transplant patients. *Clin Nephrol* 1990;33:269.

526. Hamad A, et al. Life-threatening hyperkalemia after intravenous labetalol injection for hypertensive emergency in hemodialysis patients. *Am J Nephrol* 2001;21:241

527. Rosa RM, et al. Adrenergic modulation of extrarenal potassium disposal. *N Engl J Med* 1980;302:431.

528. Das PK, Parratt JR. Myocardial and haemodynamic effects of phentolamine. *Br J Pharmacol* 1971;41:437.

529. Cunningham FG, et al., eds. Hypertensive disorders of pregnancy. In: *Williams obstetrics,* 19th ed. Norwalk, CT: Appleton & Lange, 1993: 763.

530. Neutel JM, Smith DH, Wallin D. A comparison of intravenous nicardipine and sodium nitroprusside in the immediate treatment of severe hypertension. *Am J Hypertens* 1994;7:623.

531. Treluyer JM, et al. Intravenous nicardipine in hypertensive children. *Eur J Pediatr* 1993;152:712.

532. Halpern NA, et al. Postoperative hypertension: a multicenter, prospective, randomized comparison between intravenous nicardipine and sodium nitroprusside. *Crit Care Med* 1992;20:1637.

533. Omote K, et al. Effects of nicardipine on the circulatory responses to tracheal intubation in normotensive and hypertensive patients. *Anaesthesia* 1992;47:24.

534. Carbonne B, et al. Nicardipine treatment of hypertension during pregnancy. *Obstet Gynecol* 1993;81:908.

535. Legault C, et al. Nimodipine neuroprotection in cardiac valve replacement. Report of early termination of a trial. *Stroke* 1995;27:593.

536. Houston MC. Treatment of hypertensive urgencies and emergencies with nifedipine. *Am Heart J* 1986;111:963.

537. Sorkin EM, Clissold SP, Brogden RN. Nifedipine: a review of its pharmacodynamic and pharmacokinetic properties, and therapeutic efficacy, in ischaemic heart disease, hypertension and related cardiovascular disorders. *Drugs* 1985;30:182.

538. McAllister RG. Kinetics and dynamics of nifedipine after oral and sublingual doses. *Am J Med* 1986;81(Suppl 6A):2.

539. O'Mailia JJ, Sander GE, Giles TD. Nifedipine-associated myocardial ischemia or infarction in the treatment of hypertensive urgencies. *Ann Intern Med* 1987;107:185.

540. Wachter RM. Symptomatic hypotension induced by nifedipine in the acute treatment of severe hypertension. *Arch Intern Med* 1987;147:556.

541. Shelligar VR, Loungani R. Adverse effects of sublingual nifedipine in acute myocardial infarction. *Crit Care Med* 1989;17:196.

542. Linas SL, Nies AS. Minoxidil. *Ann Intern Med* 1981;94:61.

543. Campese VM. Minoxidil: a review of its pharmacological properties and therapeutic use. *Drugs* 1981;22:257.

544. Bennett WM, et al. Efficacy of minoxidil in the treatment of severe hypertension in systemic disorders. *J Cardiovasc Pharmacol* 1980;2(Suppl 2):S142.

545. Biollaz J, Waeber B, Brunner HR. Hypertensive crisis treated with orally administered captopril. *Eur J Clin Pharmacol* 1983;25:145.

546. Case DB, et al. Acute and chronic treatment of severe and malignant hypertension with the oral angiotensin-converting enzyme inhibitor captopril. *Circulation* 1981;64:765.

547. Schubiger G, Flury G, Nussberger J. Enalapril for pregnancy-induced hypertension:acute renal failure in a neonate. *Ann Intern Med* 1988;108: 215.

548. Hughes WM, Moyer JH, Daechner WC Jr. Parenteral reserpine in treatment of hypertensive emergencies. *Arch Intern Med* 1955;95:536.

549. Jaker M, et al. Oral nifedipine vs oral clonidine in the treatment of urgent hypertension. *Arch Intern Med* 1989;149:260.

550. Houston MC. Treatment of severe hypertension and hypertensive crises with nifedipine. *West J Med* 1987;146:701.

551. Ferguson RK, Vlasses PH. How urgent is "urgent" hypertension? *Arch Intern Med* 1989;149:257.

552. Veterans Administration Cooperative Study Group on Antihypertensive Agents. Effects of treatment on morbidity in hypertension. Results in patients with diastolic blood pressures averaging 115 through 129 mm Hg. *JAMA* 1967;202:1028.

553. Wolff FW, Lindeman RD. Effects of treatment in hypertension. Results of a controlled study. *J Chronic Dis* 1966;19:227.

554. Lebby T, et al. Blood pressure decrease prior to initiating pharmacological therapy in nonemergent hypertension. *Am J Emerg Med* 1990;8: 27.

555. Grossman E, et al. Should a moratorium be placed on sublingual nifedipine capsules for hypertensive emergencies or pseudoemergencies? *JAMA* 1996;276:1328.

556. Oster JR, Materson BJ. Pseudohypertension: a diagnostic dilemma. *J Clin Hypertens* 1986;4:307.

557. Messerli FH, Ventura HO, Amodeo C. Osler's maneuver and pseudohypertension. *N Engl J Med* 1985;312:1548.

SECTION IX: GLOMERULAR, INTERSTITIAL, AND VASCULAR RENAL DISEASES

CHAPTER 57 ■ MECHANISMS OF TISSUE INJURY AND REPAIR IN RENAL DISEASES

STEPHAN SEGERER, MATTHIAS KRETZLER, FRANK STRUTZ, AND DETLEF SCHLÖNDORFF

INTRODUCTION

In order to consider "the mechanisms of tissue injury and repair" for "glomerular, interstitial and vascular renal diseases," the general stage has to be set. This will involve a brief description of inflammation as well as factors contributing either to repair, with resolution and maintenance of overall function, or to persistent tissue injury with progressive fibrosis, and loss of function. The overall goal of the inflammatory process is to eliminate the original insult, to clear up the battlefield by removing cell and matrix debris, and to repair the lost tissue components. Ideally this results in a reconstitution of the original tissue architecture and function.

Complete healing requires maintanance of the tissue microarchiteture. It can only be achieved when the extracellular matrix (ECM)—predominantly the basement membranes—remain intact, as a scaffold on which the tissue can regenerate. Once this scaffold is severely damaged or lost, the original architecture can not be reestablished, and the damaged tissue will be replaced by fibrous scar tissue. This involves the interaction of infiltrating leukocytes and perhaps bone marrow–derived fibrocytes, activation of fibroblasts and epithelial-mesenchymal transition. The latter can occur when epithelial cells have lost their basement membrane, allowing them to migrate out beyond their normal environment and boundaries. Eventually it will result in a local distortion of the parenchymal architecture and a loss of function, setting the stage for a progressive process.

A GENERAL SCHEME OF TISSUE INJURY AND REPAIR

Cell Injury

Differentiated cell function depends on a specific functional and anatomical environment. Cells can adapt to stress within certain limits (1). If the adaptive capacity of the cell is exceeded, injury becomes irreversible and cell death occurs. Cell death follows two major patterns, with some overlap (i.e., necrosis and apoptosis).

Necrosis is characterized by cellular swelling, protein denaturation, organellar swelling and breakdown with release of proinflammatory products, which result in inflammation.

Apoptosis in contrast is a controlled and programmed form of cell death and removal, with intracellular organized breakdown of proteins, RNA and DNA, and rapid uptake of residual particles (apoptotic bodies) by phagocytic cells. The uptake of apoptotic particles initiates an anti-inflammatory program, since apoptosis does generally not result in inflammation (1).

In the kidney the general type of cellular stress and injury are of the same types as in other organs. However, because of the intricate anatomical and functional arrangements of the kidney, these injury responses may result in nephron segment specific responses, that may spread from the original site to involve "downstream" injury. The causes of injury involved in renal diseases are based on immunologic reactions (immune complexes [ICs] or immune cells), oxygen deprivation (local hypoxia as well as ischemia), chemical agents (ranging from drugs to endogenous substances in high concentrations, e.g., glucose), and genetic defects. The cellular responses to stress are dependent on the type, the severity and duration of injury (2). The systems that are generally most vulnerable to injury are membrane organization, adenosine triphosphate (ATP) generation, maintenance of calcium homeostasis, protein synthesis, and the integrity of the genetic apparatus (1,3,4).

Repair Involves Inflammation in the Postembryonic State

Irrespective of the initial insult to the tissue, an inflammatory response will ensue (5–8). Only in the embryo can loss of tissue be repaired without inflammation, scarring, or fibrosis (5,6). After birth repair is always associated with an inflammatory process, irrespective of the eventual outcome, such as healing, or limited or progressive fibrosis. Overall, inflammation follows a rather uniform scenario involving the local release or generation of soluble factors, an increase in local vascular permeability, activation of endothelial cells, and the emigration of leukocytes (9). The term *leukocyte* is used here in a generic way, referring to all types of circulating inflammatory cells. Inflammation is closely related to tissue repair with regeneration of parenchymal cells and filling of tissue defects with fibrous tissue, that is, scar formation. The inflammatory response therefore represents a two-edged sword: beneficial in terms of the repair process to injury; detrimental when proceeding in an uncontrolled manner, leading to progressive fibrosis with loss of function.

Soluble Mediators Are Involved in Inflammation and Tissue Repair

The major classes of soluble mediators generated at sites of renal tissue injury and involved in leukocyte migration, activation and tissue repair include the cytokines (especially the chemokines and growth factors), as well as lipid mediators, such as prostaglandins (PGs), leukotrienes (LTs), lipoxins (LXs), and platelet activating factor (PAF). The previous edition of this chapter includes an excellent review of the subject in the context of the kidney.

Cytokines

Cytokines are a large group of polypeptide molecules, predominantly generated and released by leukocytes, but also in a more restricted manner by other cells (9–11). Cytokine production requires cell stimulation and is tightly regulated. Specific cytokines in turn will activate synthesis of other cytokines by the same cell (autocrine), by adjacent cells (paracrine), or even by distant cells (endocrine). Thus they act in a network fashion. Cytokines also include growth factors such as vascular endothelial growth factor (VEGF), platelet derived growth factor (PDGF), fibroblast growth factor (FGF), epidermal growth factor (EGF), connective tissue growth factor (CTGF), tumor growth factor-β (TGF-β), and insulin-like growth factor 1 (IGF-1). The effects of the various cytokines on leukocytes, fibroblasts, endothelial, epithelial and vascular smooth muscle cells, is generally termed pleiotropic, that is, it can vary depending on the cell type and the general context. Thus depending on their state of "preconditioning" by other mediators or cytokines, by extracellular-matrix components, or by neighboring cells the response can be very different.

The major groups of cytokines (excluding general growth factors) are:

Cytokines involved in regulating growth, differentiation, and activation, for example, IL-2 for lymphocytes and macrophage colony stimulating factor (M-CSF) for monocytes

Cytokines involved in a direct response to tissue injury as part of innate immunity (e.g., TNF, IL-1)

Cytokines that activate inflammatory cells, that is, monocyte/macrophages (e.g., interferon-γ [IFN-γ], interleukin-12 [IL-12])

Cytokines that stimulate the growth and development of the various hematopoetic cell lines (e.g., M-CSF, granulocyte macrophage colony stimulating factor (GM-CSF), interleukin-3 [IL-3])

Chemotactic cytokines, the chemokines (Table 57-1)

Obviously considerable overlap exists between these groups and their function. The complexity and pleiotropic aspects of cytokine action are probably best illustrated by the TGF-β members, namely, TGF-β1, 2, and 3. They may require pre-activation, release from matrix, can be pro- and antiproliferative, pro-apoptotic, cause epithelial-mesenchymal transition (EMT), act in a profibrotic manner by stimulating the formation of matrix components and inhibiting metalloproteinases, or can even act in an anti-inflammatory and antifibrotic manner (12,13). Thus the effects of TGF-β will vary depending on the specific isoform, and the local anatomical and cytokine context. Furthermore, studies of TGF-β by messenger RNA (mRNA) determination, immunohistology, or enzyme-linked immunosorbent assay (ELISA) may not at all reflect its actual activity. Therefore the common notion of TGF-β as the major profibrotic cytokine is a vast oversimplification (12–14). We will discuss the cytokines in further detail in the context of the specific renal diseases.

TABLE 57-1

CHEMOKINE RECEPTOR, CHEMOKINE LIGANDS, AND THE CORRESPONDING CHEMOKINE RECEPTOR EXPRESSING CELL TYPES

Chemokine receptor	Chemokine ligands	Chemokine receptor-positive cells
CCR1	CCL3, CCL5, CCL7, CCL8, CCL13, CCL14, CCL15, CCL23	Monocytes, dendritic cells (immature), T cells, neutrophils, mesangial cells, NK cells
CCR2	CCL2, CCL7, CCL8, CCL13	Monocytes, dendritic cells (immature), basophiles, NK cells, B and T cells
CCR3	CCL5, CCL7, CCL8, CCL11, CCL13–CCL15	T cells, NK cells, fibroblasts
CCR4	CCL17, CCL22	Eosinophiles, basophiles, T cells (TH2), dendritic cells, NK cells
CCR5	CCL3, CCL4, CCL5, CCL8, CCL11, CCL13, CCL14	Monocytes, dendritic cells (immature), T cells (TH1), basophiles, B cells
CCR6	CCL20	T cells, B cells, dendritic cells (immature)
CCR7	CCL19, CCL21	Dendritic cells (mature), T cells, B cells
CCR8	CCL1, CCL16	Dendritic cells (mature), T cells, B cells, thymocytes
CCR9	CCL25	T cells, thymocytes
CCR10	CCL27, CCL28	T cells, thymocytes
CXCR1	CXCL5, CXCL6, CXCL8	Neutrophiles, monocytes, astrocytes, endothelial cells
CXCR2	CXCL1, CXCL2, CXCL3, CXCL5, CXCL7, CXCL8	Neutrophiles, monocytes, eosinophils, endothelial cells
CXCR3	CXCL9, CXCL10, CXCL11	T cells (TH1), B cells, NK cells
CXCR4	CXCL12	T cells, dendritic cells, monocytes, B cells, neutrophils, platelets, astrocytes, thymocytes, endothelial cells
CXCR5	CXCL13	T cells, B cells, astrocytes
CXCR6	CXCL16	T cells
CX3CR1	CX3CL1	T cells, monocytes, NK cells, neurones, microglia
XCR1	XCL1, XCL2	T cells, NK cells

Chemokines

Chemokines are members of a large family of *chemo*tactic cyto*kines*, which play pivotal roles during the recruitment of subpopulations of inflammatory cells (15–19). In addition to cell positioning (e.g., during inflammation, lymphopoiesis and, immunregulation), chemokines can activate effector functions of leukocytes (including fibrotic processes), influence hematopoiesis and the release of stem-cells from the bone marrow, modulate angiogenesis, and even play roles during carcinogenesis and metastasis (18,20,21). Over 40 chemokines and 19 corresponding chemokine receptors have been described to date (15,22). Chemokines are subclassified into four groups (CC, CXC, CX3C, and C chemokines), according to a shared structural motif of conserved cysteine residues. The CC and CXC chemokines represent the vast majority of chemokines. CX3CL1/Fraktalkine combines the functions of a chemokine and an adhesion molecule. It can be directly tethered to the cell membrane via a transmembrane segment (a long mucin stalk), and it can induce chemotaxis and leukocyte arrest on endothelial cells. Furthermore it can be released by proteases and become a soluble chemokine (23). Chemokine functions are mediated through seven transmembrane spanning serpentine Gi/Go-protein coupled receptors, which are sensitive to pertussis toxin (Table 57-1). The specificities can overlap as some chemokines bind to multiple receptors, and some receptors can bind multiple chemokines.

Upon appropriate stimulation, essentially all cell types appear capable of expressing chemokines (24). The production occurs in a cell- and stimulus-specific manner. Various substances that is cytokines, ICs, growth factors, serum proteins, and even chemokines themselves are capable of inducing chemokine expression. A common denominator for the stimulation may be the generation of reactive oxygen species, and subsequent activation of transcription factors, such as NF-κB (25). In general, proinflammatory cytokines such as TNF, IL-1β, IFN-γ, and LPS, especially in combination, rapidly (within hours) induce CCL2/MCP-1, CXCL8/IL-8, and CXCL10/IP–10, whereas the induction of CCL5/RANTES is usually slower (12 to 48 hours). ICs induce upregulation of CCL2/MCP-1, CCL5/RANTES, CXCL8/IL–8, and CXCL10/IP-10 expression. Growth factors such as PDGF and bFGF can induce CCL2/MCP-1 and CCL5/RANTES expression. This may relate to the macrophage influx seen during proliferative responses in tissue repair, regeneration, and remodeling (14–21).

The role of two chemokine binding proteins DARC and D6 during inflammation is still under investigaion (26–28). Both proteins bind multiple chemokines but do not signal. It is possible that these proteins are involved in the transendothelial transport, positioning, and presentation of chemokines on vascular and lymphatic vessels and even angiogenesis. Therefore these proteins might be doorkeepers for the migration of inflammatory cells both into, as well as out of specific tissues. Furthermore, Duffy antigen/receptor for chemokines (DARC) on erythrocytes may serve as a sink or even reservoir of chemokines in the circulation.

Lipid Mediators

The lipid mediators, the eicosanoids prostaglandins (PGs), LTs, and LXs, and the phopholipid derivative PAF play considerable roles in inflammation.

Prostaglandins (PGs) belong to the oldest known class of lipid mediators of inflammation. With the molecular characterization of two forms of cyclooxygenases (i.e., COX1 and COX2) and the cloning of multiple prostaglandin receptors, with different signaling cascades and functional effects, the role

of postaglandins in physiology and pathophysiology has undergone a renaissance (Fig. 57-1 [29,30]). The stimuli for the activation of phospholipases and subsequent eicosanoid production include mechanical or hypoxic cell stress, proinflammatory cytokines and growth factors and vasoactive peptides (e.g., angiotensin II, etc.). The type of prostaglandin generated depends predominantely on the cell type. While cycloxygenases will generate the intermediate endoperoxides irrespective of cell type, the subsequent conversion to the specific prostaglandins (e.g., prostacyclin, PGI2, thromboxane, PGE2, PGF2α, or PGD2) depends on the cell-specific expression of isomerases and synthetases (29,30).

The leukotrienes (LTs) are also generated from arachidonic acid. The leukocyte-restricted 5-lipoxygenase generates leukotriene A4 (LTA4) which can be converted to LTB4 by the LTA4-hydrolase or to the cysteinyl leukotrienes LTC4, LTD4, and LTE4 (30). LTs and PGs act through a variety of G-protein coupled receptors that are also expressed in a cell-specific manner. Although the chemotactic activity of LTB4 was known for a long time, new roles for LTB4 and PGD2 in T cell trafficking have been identified recently (31). This depends on the expression of the LTB4 receptor BLT and the PGD2 receptor DP-2 on specific T-cell subsets. DP-2 is present on a small fraction of CD8-positive T cells producing IL-4 and IL-13. This may be of special interest for progressive tissue injury, as IL-13 production favors fibrosis, at least in liver and lung (32,33). LTB4 converts rolling of specific T cell subsets to firm adhesion on endothelial cells, an effect mediated by BLT-1 receptor activation of integrins (30,34).

The generation of the LIPOXINS (LXs), which are also arachidonate derivatives, involves the interaction of neutrophils and platelets (35). The neutrophil 5-lipoxygenase generates LTA4, which can be converted by adjacent platelets via 12-lipoxygenase to lipoxin A4 (LXA4) and B4 (LXB4). LXA4 causes vasodilation and antagonizes the vasoconstrictor effect of the cysteinyl-leukotriene LTC4. Furthermore, it decreases chemotaxis and adhesion of neutrophils while enhancing that of monocytes. It has been suggested that the lipoxins are the natural brake for actions of leukotrienes thereby limiting the local inflammatory process (35).

Platelet activating factor (PAF) is another but less cell-type specific lipid mediator of inflammation (36). PAF received its name from the original observation that it aggregated and degranulated platelets. Chemically it is an ether-phospholipid, that is, 1-alkyl, 2-acetyl glycerophosphocholine. It is generated from membrane phosphocholine lipids with an ether bond in position one, by the action of phospholipase A2 (releasing arachidonic acid at the same time), followed by acetylation in position 2. PAF is inactivated by acetylhydrolases assuring a tightly regulated system. PAF is a very potent vasoactive agent, activator of leukocyte adhesion, including selectin activation, chemotaxis, leukocyte degranulation, and oxidative burst. PAF may also be part of local amplification loops as it can in turn stimulate the synthesis of cytokines, chemokines, and eicosanoids by the infiltrating leukocytes (36). Thus there is an intricate connection between the lipid and peptide mediators of inflammation.

Complement

The complement cascade is composed of a large number of effector and regulatory proteins (37). The activation of the complement cascade can be mediated through the classical, the alternative, and the lectin pathway. The progression down the cascade involves the proteolytic cleavage and subsequent activation of complement components (37). C5b plays a role in the activation of downstream complement events, while C5a acts as a potent chemoattractant for monocytes and neutrophils,

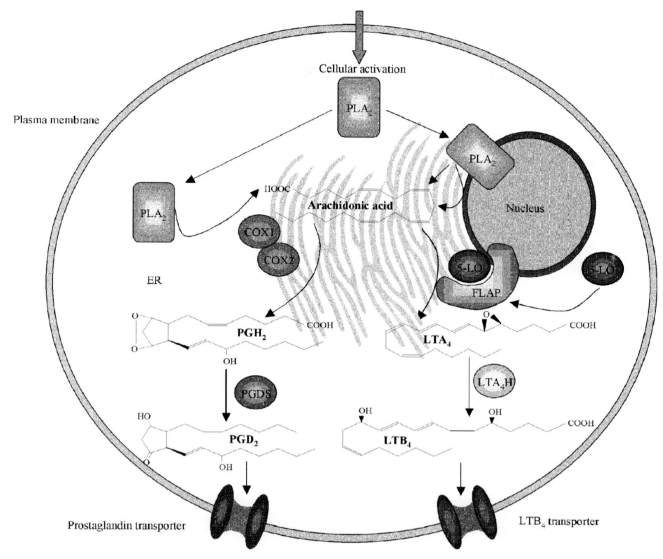

FIGURE 57-1. Schematic scheme of the synthesis of lipid mediators. Cell activation by various stimuli (e.g., trauma, cytokines, etc.) triggers the translocation of cytosolic phospholipase A2 (PLA2) to the nuclear membrane as well as to the endoplasmatic reticulum (ER), leading to the release of arachidonic acid. 5-Lipoxygenase (5-LO) leads to the production of leukotrienes (LTs, *right*, 5-LO activating protein: FLAP, LTA4 hydrolase: LTA4H). COX lead to the production of 4PGH2 which is converted to PGD2 via PGD synthase. (Modified from: Luster AD, Tager AM T-cell trafficking in asthma: lipid mediators grease the way. *Nat Rev Immunol* 2004;4:711.)

increases vascular permeability, upregulates adhesion molecules, and propagates contraction of smooth muscle cells (38). The classical pathway is initiated when immunoglobulins (e.g., immunoglobulin G 1–3 [IgG1–3] or immunoglobulin M [IgM]) bind their respective antigen leading to the formation of the C3 convertase (C4b2b). A C3 convertase can also be formed through the alternative pathway by fragments of C3 and factor B (C3bBb). Basement membrane fragments or bacterial cell wall components can activate the alternative pathway (37,39). The third pathway, the lectin pathway, is triggered by distinct carbohydrates and involves the mannose-binding lectin and the MBL-associated serine protease (37,39). All three pathways converge upon the generation of C3 convertase, which cleaves C3 into C3a and C3b. C3b promotes the first step in the activation of the terminal complement complex, as it associates with either the classical or alternative C3 convertase to generate a C5 convertase. C5 convertase cleaves C5 into C5a and C5b, which directs formation of the membrane-attack complex

composed of C6, C7, C8, and C9. C5a is a ligand for a seven-transmembrane-segment G protein coupled receptor, which is abundantly expressed by neutrophils, mast cells, basophils, endothelial cells, and monocyte/macrophages (39).

NO and Vasoactive Substances

Nitric oxide (NO) is generated by three isoforms of NO synthase, the neuronal nNOS, the inducible iNOS, and the constitutive endothelial eNOS (40). The latter is predominantly present on endothelial cells and can be activated by shear stress, bradykinin, and thrombin. The iNOS is expressed on endothelial smooth muscle cells and on macrophages. It can be induced by inflammatory mediators such as IL-1, TNF, IFN-γ, and endotoxin. NO's role in inflammation includes vasodilatation, antagonizing platelet activation, reducing leukocyte recruitment, decreasing proinflammatory cytokine and chemokine production, and acting as a microbicidal agent (40). With lack of appropriate co-factors the NO synthetase can, however, become a major source of reactive oxygen species and as such turn into a perpetuator of tissue injury (40).

Finally it should be briefly noted that the renin-angiotensin system also has an immune modulator activity that appears to be independent of its vasoactive properties (41). This "inflammatory" aspect of angiotensin may also play a role in progressive disease processes (24).

Vascular Changes Set the Stage for Leukocyte Extravasation

Acute inflammation is short in duration (hours, a few days) and is initially characterized by a predominant influx of neutrophils followed by monocytes/macrophages (42–44). The extravasation of leukocytes occurs through the specialized endothelia of postcapillary venules (Fig. 57-2). Only in the special cases of the pulmonary alveolar and renal glomerular microcirculation can leukocytes also leave the bloodstream through capillaries. The reasons for this restriction to these special microvascular anatomic sites most likely involve the high velocity of blood flow with high shear stress forces in other vascular beds, as well as differences in the expression of adhesion molecules on the various endothelia. Of note is the absolute prerequisite that

both the leukocytes and the endothelial cells be activated in order for their normally brief encounters to be of consequence and result in leukocyte adhesion and extravasation (Fig. 57-2). During acute inflammation arteriolar vasodilatation leads to an expansion of the capillary bed, which together with an increase in vascular permeability results in extravasation of fluid into the extracellular space. The blood viscosity increases and the blood flow slows, ultimately resulting in stasis. Leakiness of the microvasculature is mediated through endothelial cell contraction (by histamines, bradykinin, LTs resulting in gaps in venules), endothelial cell retraction (mediated by cytokines, e.g., TNF, IL-1 which results in reorganization of the cytoskeleton), and endothelial cell injury (45,46).

Leukocyte Extravasation

Vascular dilatation, increased permeability and slowing of flow allows the margination of leukocytes. This is followed by a cascade of events involving rolling, activation, firm adhesion and transmigration of leukocytes on the activated endothelium (Fig. 57-2 [34,42–47]). After extravasation leukocytes follow various chemotactic gradients, mostly in a haptotactic, that is, matrix bound manner, toward the site of tissue injury. Leukocyte extravasation is mediated through the interaction of adhesion molecules with their respective counter-receptors, in

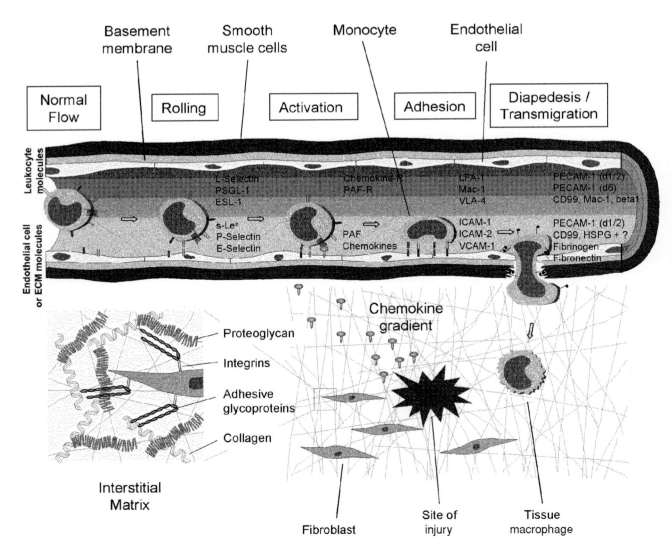

FIGURE 57-2. Extravasation cascade of inflammatory cells.

concert with activation by lipid mediators, chemokines, and cytokines, which can activate integrins and regulate the expression of adhesion molecules.

Selectins and Their Ligands Establish the Initial Contact Between Leukocytes and Endothelial Cells

The decrease in shear stress forces allows the low-affinity contact between the first class of adhesion molecules, the selectins, and their carbohydrate ligands (see Table 57-2). Selectins are expressed on leukocytes and endothelial cells (34,48–50). At present three members of the selectin family are known. Their adhesive character is determined by amino-terminal lectin domains. Following the lectin domain is an epidermal growth factor (EGF) domain, a variable number of complement regulatory domain sequences, and a single transmembrane sequence with a cytoplasmic tail. The number of complement regulatory domains varies on the different selectins. The exact function of the complement regulatory elements remains unknown, but altering them results in different binding characteristics. On leukocytes the L-selectin is concentrated on cell projections allowing the early contact with their counterparts on the endothelial surface. Leukocyte L-selectin is expressed

TABLE 57-2

ADHESION MOLECULES, THE CORRESPONDING LIGANDS AND THE MAJOR FUNCTION IN CELL RECRUITMENT

Adhesion molecule	Ligand	Function
Selectins		
L-Selectin (CD62L, on leukocytes)	MadCAM-1 (mucosal addressin cell adhesion molecule, HEVs of Peyer plaques) CD34 (endothelium) GlyCAM-1 (endothelium) Podocalyxin Mannose receptor	Rolling of neutrophils and monocytes
P Selectin (CD62P, on platelets and endothelium)	PSGL-1 Sialyl Lewis X modified proteins	Rolling of neutrophils, monocytes, and lymphocytes
E-Selectin (CD62E on endothelium)	Sialyl Lewis X modified proteins (on leukocytes)	Rolling and adhesion of neutrophils, monocytes, and T cells
Integrins		
VLA-4 ($\alpha 4\beta 1$)	VCAM-1 Fibronectin (CS-1)	Adhesion of monocytes, lymphocytes, and eosinophils
LFA-1 (CD11a/CD18)	ICAM-1 ICAM-2 ICAM-3	Adhesion and arrest of monocytes, lymphocytes, and neutrophils
MAC-1 (CD11b/CD18)	ICAM-1 C3bi Fibrinogen Factor X	
CD11c/CD18 (p150,95)	Fibrinogen ICAM-1	
CD11d/CD18	Unknown	
$\alpha 4\beta 7$	MadCAM-1 VCAM-1	
Adhesion molecules of the immunoglobulin superfamily		
ICAM-1 (on endothelium, mesangial cells, epithelial cells, and leukocytes)	CD11a/CD18, CD11b/CD18 CD11c/CD18 CD43 Fibrinogen Hyaluronic acid	
ICAM-2 (on endothelium, leukocytes)	CD11a/CD18 DC-SIGN (CD209)	
ICAM-3 (leukocytes)	DC-SIGN (CD209)	
VCAM-1 (parietal epithelial cells, endothelium, epithelial cells, mesangial cells)	VLA-4	
PECAM-1 (CD31, on leukocytes, endothelium)	PECAM-1 (CD31) $\alpha 5\beta 3$ CD38	
Others		
CD44	Hyaluronic acid	Rolling

constitutively, while E-selectin surface expression on endothelial cells requires *de novo* synthesis after prestimulation by inflammatory mediators. P-selectin is stored in platelets, and in Weibel-Palade bodies in endothelial cells, and is rapidly distributed to the surface upon stimulation. With continued stimulation P-selectin can be present constantly on the endothelium in areas of chronic inflammation.

Similarly to the expression of selectins, their counterpart glycoproteins are also regulated. The regulation involves mostly alterations in the "sticky" sugar coating. In the case of the L-selectin ligand CD34 on endothelial cells, the proper decoration of the protein backbone with the Sialyl-Lewis carbohydrates has to occur by stimulation of the respective enzymes, for example, fucosyl- and sialyl-transferases. Even the major P-selectin glycoprotein ligand-1 (PSGL-1), which is constitutively present on neutrophils and T-cells, may require some change in its carbohydrate decoration to allow for optimal interactions with P-selectin. So already the initial adhesion contact allows for a fine tuning by combining constitutive and regulated expression with rapid surface transfer of the molecules, and modification of their sugar moieties (34,48–50).

The tethering of leukocytes on the endothelium, termed rolling, by itself would be inconsequential, as the binding forces between the selectins and their ligands are too weak, and will only result in short lasting leukocyte-endothelial contact without firm adhesion. Only if the endothelial cell presents leukocyte-activating molecules (e.g., chemokines, LTB4 or PAF) on its surface for the respective receptor on the passing leukocytes, will this brief encounter be converted to firm adhesion of the leukocyte (42–44,46).

Integrins and Their Counterparts of the Immunoglobulin Superfamily Mediate Firm Leukocyte-Endothelial Adhesion

Before the next crucial step, that is, firm adhesion can occur, the involved adhesion molecules, the integrins on the leukocytes need to be activated to a status of high affinity. Integrins are a family of cell surface molecules that are involved in attachment of cells to their extracellular matrix and also in cell–cell binding (9,46). They are heterodimeric receptors consisting of paired α- and β-chains (Table 57-2). The β-chain determines the type of integrin. Different types of leukocytes can express essentially two types of $\beta2$-integrins. The $\beta2$ (CD18) can be paired with either αL (CD11a) or αM (CD11b), resulting in CD11a/CD18 (or LFA-1) or CD11b/CD18 (or Mac-1), respectively. In addition, many leukocyte types express the $\beta1$ integrin $\alpha4\beta1$ or very late antigen 4 (VLA-4). Under basal conditions the integrins on leukocytes are in a low-affinity binding state. Upon activation by inflammatory mediators the strength of their interaction with endothelial ligands is enhanced by conformational changes and by increasing their density on the binding surface, via clustering at the site of leukocyte-endothelial contact. The activation of the different types of leukocytes occurs predominantly by soluble mediators of inflammation, which may, however, be presented in a membrane-bound form by the endothelial cell surface. Most of the respective receptors on leukocytes belong to the serpentine, seven transmembrane spanning, G protein-coupled receptors (9,46). The predominant class of mediators include the chemokines, LTB4, PAF, complement C5a, and formylated peptides of bacterial origin (e.g., FMLP). The endogenous mediators such as chemokines, LTB4, and PAF are locally produced by the cells of the injured tissue—be they parenchymal or endothelial—and reach the vascular endothelial luminal surface either by transcytosis or by diffusion (9,46). On the endothelial surface they present themselves to the rolling leukocytes bound to proteoglycans,

which serve as lampposts for presentation to the specific leukocyte receptors. Different types of leukocytes are activated by different types of chemokines and also use different molecules for rolling and firm adhesion. Not only are the integrins regulated, but also the endothelial integrin counterparts, members of the immunoglobulin family ICAM-1, VCAM-1, PECAM can be modified by cytokines (9,46).

Leukocyte-Endothelial Transmigration

Firm adhesion is followed by diapedesis of leukocytes at the specialized endothelial-endothelial junctions, a step involving yet another group of adhesion molecules (9,46). During the transmigration of leukocytes the adherens junctions of adjacent endothelial cells have to disorganize temporarily to allow the squeezing through of the leukocytes (42–45,47,51,52). Within minutes, however, the junctions are reformed and during the whole process a tight seal seems to form between the endothelial cells and the transmigrating leukocytes as demonstrated by the maintenance of electrical resistance during the entire process. In contrast to the heterophilic interactions between integrins and VCAM, ICAM, and PECAM during leukocyte adhesion to the endothelium, the molecules involved during transmigration engage in homophilic interactions. Thus PECAM-1/CD31 and CD99 on endothelial cells engage PECAM-1 and CD99, respectively on leukocytes. Blocking PECAM-1 *in vitro* or *in vivo* will inhibit diapedesis. CD99, a highly glycosylated protein seems to be involved in the homophilic interactions required for the transmigration process at a step distal to PECAM-1. Blockage of CD99 will also decrease leukocyte transmigration and blocking both PECAM-1 and CD99 results in additive inhibition (52). Furthermore, components of the endothelial-endothelial junctions, such as junctional adhesion molecules (JAMs) and cadherins are involved in the leukocyte transmigration (45,51). While it is generally accepted that the predominant site of leukocyte emigration is between endothelial cells, there is also some evidence that under certain conditions leukocytes can actually migrate through endothelial cell bodies. In the case of fenestrated endothelia, as present in the glomerulus and in vasa recta in the kidney, the possibility of leukocytes migrating across these fenestrae exists, though we are not aware of any evidence in favor or against this possibility.

Leukocyte Migration Through the Extracellular Matrix (ECM)

Once the leukocyte has transmigrated the endothelial layer, which is a matter of seconds or minutes, it will get arrested on the underlying basement membrane. The molecules and mechanisms involved in the crossing of basement membranes by leukocytes are much less understood, but may also involve interaction of adhesion molecules such as integrins on leukocytes with ligands consisting of matrix components (53,54). In addition, local activation of matrix metalloproteinases (MMPs) may allow the leukocyte to "eat" its way across the basement membrane. Similar considerations apply to the subsequent migration of leukocytes through the ECM toward the site of tissue injury. Subgroups of inflammatory cells use different (but at times overlapping) combinations of mediators that may be generated at different times (53–55). The type of recruited cell therefore not only depends on the type and the site of injury, but also on the duration of the process. Neutrophils predominate early (within the first 24 hours) and are replaced by monocytes/macrophages which may be explained by the pattern of chemotactic factors and adhesion molecules generated with a different time points. The short-lived neutrophils undergo apoptosis within 2 days after exiting the bloodstream, whereas monocytes persist for long periods.

Having left the bloodstream, leukocytes follow gradients of chemotactic substances toward the site of tissue injury. During the migration through the extracellular space the chemokines may be matrix bound (a process termed haptotaxis) or exist as a diffusible gradient (chemotaxis) (15–19). Having reached the site of injury, leukocytes frequently engage in an amplification loop, that is, they release further mediators such as cytokines, chemokines, reactive oxygen species (ROS), NO, and lipid mediators (53–55).

Leukocyte Activation at the Site of Tissue Injury

Once at the site of tissue injury the leukocytes will start the repair process by ingesting, and processing the inciting agents, be they infectious, immune complexes (ICs), or remnants of cells and matrix. Phagocytosis and release of degradative enzymes are early events after recruitment of leukocytes to the site of injury (53–55) (Fig. 57-3). Phagocytosis involves recognition and attachment (facilitated by opsonins), engulfment, and degradation of the ingested material. The most important opsonins are IgG, complement split products (C3b), and carbohydrate binding lectins (collectins). Activation of leukocytes further involves receptors for chemokines and cytokines, receptors for pathogen-associated molecular patterns (i.e., toll-like receptors), and scavenger receptors (53–55). Activated leukocytes will generate an oxidative burst, degranulate and discharge lysosomal enzymes, release and activate various enzymes such as phospholipases and MMPs. The released enzymes include elastase, collagenases, cathepsin, and other proteases, which can degrade ECM components as well as generate vasoactive or pro-inflammarory peptides from precursors (e.g. components of the complement, kinin, or coagulation systems). The action of the proteases on the matrix will help in removing damaged matrix and thus clear the way for the repair process. If, however, this process becomes extensive, it could also remove the extracellular scaffold itself, for example, the basement membrane that is required to reestablish the original tissue architecture. This could create gaps allowing epithelial cells to migrate out of their normal cellular organisation and open up the possibility for epithelial-mesenchymal transition (EMT), which could contribute to fibrosis and loss of functional units (56).

In this context the special roles of infiltrating macrophages has to be considered. The activated macrophage can exist in multiple forms, depending on the surrounding milieu, interacting cells, and on its mode of activation (7,54,57,58). It can develop into a major source of growth factors (e.g., PDGF, FGF, TGF-β) that are required for tissue regeneration. Some of these, for example, VEGF, PDGF are angiogenic and favor neovascularization, others may favor matrix deposition. Upon exposure to IL-4 and especially IL-13 macrophages can develop into a profibrotic phenotype, that, at least in lung and liver, may be TGF-β independent (32,33). Alternatively, the macrophage may evolve to generate a cytokine profile favoring a T helper type 2 (TH2) immune response (leading to a humoral response) or develop into dendritic cells (7,54,57). Specific circulating monocyte-like precursor cells, also termed fibrocytes, may not only become a source of profibrotic cytokines such as TGF-β, but may actually become themselves a major source of matrix components for example collagen I (59–61).

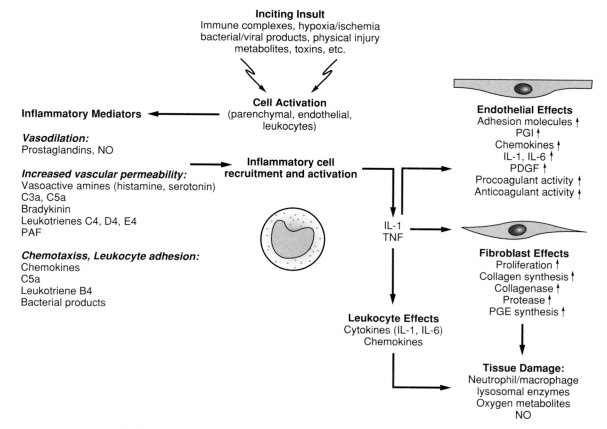

FIGURE 57-3. Scematic scheme of cellular activation, resulting in tissue damage.

In general, the myofibroblast has been considered as the major collagen-producing cell in fibrosis. In this scheme the myofibroblasts arise from activation (predominantly by TGF-β of macrophage or parenchymal origin) of interstitial fibroblasts or by transition of parenchymal epithelia to cells with mesenchymal characteristics (56). This epithelial-mesenchymal transition could result in the emigration from the organized epithelial layer into the interstitial space, provided the basement membrane loses its integrity. There they become myofibroblasts and a major source of excess collagen and hence fibrosis. Lately evidence for a different origin of excess collagen formation has been generated in models of pulmonary and liver fibrosis (59–61). Here the collagen-producing cells were of bone marrow origin and probably represent so-called "fibrocytes." These fibrocytes had been identified earlier as a unique cell population, that circulates in low number in the peripheral blood (61). They express the chemokine receptors CXCR4 and CCR7, and migrate in response to the corresponding chemokines CXCL12/SDF-1 and CCL21/SLC (59). Potentially the latter chemokines, generated at the site of tissue injury by the infiltrating macrophages, could attract the fibrocytes and involve them in the fibrotic process. Whether this mechanism is universal or specific to some forms of lung and liver injury remains to be evaluated. Reevaluation of the potential source of myofibroblasts, that is, local parenchymal versus bone marrow, in progressive fibrosis obviously might also have considerable therapeutic implications.

TGF-β1 or -2, either released and activated by the macrophage themselves, or released from its binding to ECM by proteases, can cause epithelial-mesenchymal transition; fibroblast activation; generation of matrix components and inhibition of their breakdown by MMPs (11–14); local immunsuppression; apoptosis, etc. TGF-β3 may have opposite effects, but in the adult tissue is only present in low amounts (5). The uptake of apoptotic bodies is a major function of macrophages in the repair of tissue injury (62–64). It represents a very important function, since nonremoval of apoptotic bodies will result in the generation of proinflammatory components and thus exacerbate inflammation. By contrast, the normal uptake and removal of apoptotic cells by macrophages alters their phenotype to an immuno-inhibitory, antiinflammatory one, which will produce less CXCL8/IL-8 and other chemokines, less TNF and IL-1β, and secrete more NO, TGF-β, and PGE2. The latter will further inhibit local chemokine and cytokine generation in an auto- and paracrine manner. Furthermore, upon uptake of apoptotic cells macrophages will suppress local T-cell proliferation, interrupting a vicious cycle of mutual stimulation (62–64). In this context it should be pointed out that once macrophages and T cells have reached the site of tissue injury, they engage in a dialogue. Initially the macrophage activates the lymphocyte, which in turn release proinflammatory mediators (7,54,57). The uptake of the apoptotic bodies will interrupt this vicious cycle as outlined above.

Because of the functional plasticity and the multiple and dynamic phenotypes of the macrophage, it has been questioned recently if indentification of the various macrophage activation states can be achieved. Defining macrophage subsets by surface or functional phenotype during an inflammatory episode might be akin to defining chameleons by their color display at a given moment (57).

Role of Heparan Sulfate Proteoglycans (HSPG) in Inflammatory Cell Recruitment

HSPGs play multiple roles in the process of leukocyte adhesion, and in endothelial and extracellular matrix transmigration (65,66). Proteoglycans consist of a core protein of varying size (molecular weight [MW] = 11,000 to 220,000) to which one or more (up to 100) sulfated carbohydrate glycosaminoglycans (GAGs) are attached. Proteoglycans are named according to the principal repeating disaccharides (e.g., heparan sulfate, chondroitin sulfate), which are heavily negatively charged and bind to other matrix and cell membrane components. The HSPGs are extremely versatile and diverse as their side chains can be enzymatically modified by N-deacetylases, N- and O-sulfotransferases, and epimerases. This occurs in a cell-specific manner and can be modified by inflammatory mediators. Proteins that can bind to HSPGs include chemokines, growth factors, adhesion molecules such as selectins, integrins, PECAM, enzymes, enzyme inhibitors and ECM proteins (fibronectin, collagens, laminin, fibrillin, thrombospondin, vitronectin). The functional consequences of the binding of the ligand to the HSPGs are: (a) immobilization resulting in a high local concentration of the ligand; (b) conformational changes of both the HSPG and the ligand with functional consequences; (c) oligomerization of the ligands, which, in the case of cytokines and chemokines, allows dimerization and thus receptor signaling; and (d) storage and protection from degradation of the ligands.

During inflammation the surface binding of for example chemokines to HSPGs on endothelial cells and ECM allows for the establishment of a gradient for the leukocytes to follow. Endothelial and leukocyte surface HSPGs are directly involved in cell–cell interaction via for example selectins and β2 integrins. Activated endothelial cells and leukocytes exert heparanase activity, which facilitates leukocyte transmigration by degrading HSPGs (e.g., the ECM). Furthermore, the haparanase may release bound chemokines and growth factors (e.g., TGF-β, EGF, FGF, PDGF, VEGF).

The HSPGs syndecan-1, -3, and -4 and glypican are differentially expressed on different endothelial cells. In the kidney only syndecan-1 and 4 have been identified (66). Beta glycans contain heparan sulfate and chondroitin sulfate chains. They bind TGF-β and are present in the interstitial space and on micro-vascular endothelium. CD44, the cell-surface receptor for hyaluronic acid, is expressed on restricted endothelial cells and on mesangial cells. Hyaluronic acid (HA) is a polysaccharide of the GAG family and is found in the ECM of many tissues. HA exists in a glycosylated and nonglycosylated form, and in numerous isoforms. Both CD44 and HA play roles in inflammation, including cell proliferation.

Outcome of Tissue Injury, Inflammation, and Repair

As long as the inflammatory response is short-lived and the injury locally limited with minimal disruption of the underlying tissue architecture, the repair process will restore almost normal histology and function. Obviously this requires that no new insults occur, that production of pro-inflammatory mediators ceases, or that their action becomes neutralized, and that leukocytes accumulated at the site of tissue injury disappear by either undergoing apoptosis locally or by leaving the site via blood or lymphatic vessels (reverse migration) (42–44,55,62). Furthermore, the extracellular matrix scaffold has to be remodeled to its original form and the parenchymal cells have to replace the lost ones in the original pattern. Unfortunately this scenario is the exception rather than the rule. Under most conditions there is enough disruption of the original intricate tissue structure, so that repair can only occur in an incomplete manner, that is with scar-fibrosis formation. As the tissue structure based on the ECM scaffold and the specific cell-cell organization is lost, it will be replaced by an amorphous fibrous tissue. The fibrotic process involves a similar set of players as the initial inflammation, that is, leukocytes, mediators of inflammation including cytokines, chemokines, etc. However, these now fulfill different functions, for example, the leukocytes inducing EMT and fibroblast formation with deposition of excess extracellular fibrous matrix. As capillary blood supply may also be lost due to tissue injury, the area of repair may become chronically hypoxic and thus susceptible to progressive inflammation, unless adequate neovascularization occurs. Thus, in tissues with high oxygen demands such as the kidney, scar formation and fibrosis may predispose to smoldering hypoxic-ischemic damage resulting in chronic inflammation and progressive fibrosis with loss of function (67). In this process the persistence of macrophages and lymphocytes play a major role through the production of proinflammatory, profibrotic cytokines (see above). Under many circumstances, including progressive renal diseases, it remains unclear what causes the local retention, proliferation, and activation of macrophages and lymphocytes. Factors that could contribute are cytokines and other mediators released by "stressed" parenchymal-epithelial or even endothelial cells. The stress may include chronic hypoxia (see above [68]), "overwork" by the remaining parenchymal cells with generation of metabolic mediators, including ROS. During these processes hidden antigens could be "unmasked" or neo-antigens generated resulting in de novo local autoimmune processes with progressive inflammation, fibrosis, and loss of function.

Tissue Injury and Repair in the Kidney

Anatomical and Functional Specificities

The Glomerular and Peritubular Vasculature is Arranged in Sequence. Essentially the renal microvasculature is organized in two capillary beds in sequence, that is, the glomerular capillary convolute and the peritubular capillary network. This sequential organization allows for an exquisite balance of the glomerular filtration with the tubular re-absorption, that is, the maintenance of glomerular tubular balance. The downside of this physiologically extremely dynamic adaptive and fine-tuned system is its vulnerability to upstream interference with blood flow, that is, a decrease in preglomerular or glomerular blood flow will inevitably jeopardize the downstream peritubular blood flow. This is especially pertinent as there is essentially no collateral blood supply for the postglomerular microcirculation. Thus any acute or chronic glomerular injury, with a decrease in glomerular blood flow, will be associated with an obligatory reduction in peritubular blood flow which, depending on the degree of hypoxia, will entail tubulointerstitial injury and tissue remodeling.

Another consequence of these sequential capillary beds is that there are two potential sites for leukocyte extravasation during inflammatory renal disease, the glomerulus or the tubulointerstitium. However, as the peritubular circulation is downstream of the glomerular circulation, inflammation, or at least some mediators involved, may spill over during glomerular inflammation from the glomerular vascular convolute into the peritubular microcirculation and thus contribute to the frequently observed intersititial inflammatory reaction in glomerulonephritis.

Glomerular and Tubular Functions Are Organized in Sequence. The downstream position of the tubulus in respect to the the glomerulus does not only apply to the blood flow but also to the ultrafiltrate. While this is part of the elegant homeostatic system of kidney function in health, in disease it may become another avenue for spreading a primarily glomerular disease to the tubulointerstitial compartment. Due to the increased glomerular capillary permeabllity and loss of permse-

lectivity in glomerular diseases, the tubular epithelial cells will be exposed to an abnormal ultrafiltrate, and thereby to a variety of potentially noxious substances, which may in turn set off tubular epithelial injury with secondary peritubular inflammation. Thus the dual downstream position of the tubulointerstitium, that is, in terms of blood and utlrafiltration flow, which in health ensures an exquisite functional tuning of the glomerular-tubular balance, may become the Achilles tendon in disease with secondary injury to the tubulointerstitium in primary glomerular processes.

Obviously the reverse would not be true, as primary insults to the tubulointerstitium would not reach the glomerulus. Indeed in most forms of primary tubulointerstitial renal diseases the glomerular architecture is preserved until far advanced interstitial fibrosis occurs. Thus the concept of the nephron as a functional unit may not only apply to renal physiology, but also to the pathophysiology of renal disease. The glomerulus itself should also be regarded as a functional unit with each individual constituent, that is, endothothelial, mesangial, and epithelial cells and their extracellular matrix representing an integral part of normal function. Damage to one will influence the other in part through direct cell–cell connections (e.g., gap junctions), soluble mediators such as chemokines, cytokines, growth factors, changes in matrix and basement membrane composition.

The Glomerulus as the Site of the Primary Insult

Glomerular Injury in Human Kidney Diseases. From a pathogenetic standpoint human glomerular diseases can be broadly divided into those

1. Without glomerular inflammation or deposition of immunoglobulins (e.g., minimal change disease, idiopathic focal, and segmental glomerulosclerosis [FSGS]).
2. With deposition of immunoglobulins, but without relevant glomerular inflammation, most likely due to the localization of the immunoglobulins (e.g., membranous nephropathy)
3. With deposition of immunoglobulins leading to increased cellularity (proliferative glomerulonephrities, e.g., lupus nephritis, IgA nephropathy, anti-GBM, postinfectious GN)
4. With severe glomerular injury and inflammation, but without deposition of immunoglobulins (e.g., pauci immune glomerulonephritis).

This is of course an oversimplification, as some glomerular lesions are not included in this system (e.g. diabetes or amyloidosis), but it helps to separate broad glomerular disease entities (69). The podocyte seems to be the major target in the first and second group, which therefore will be described below (69). This will be followed by diseases of the third group, in which ICs lead to activation of intrinsic renal cells (via Fc receptors and complement products) resulting in inflammatory cell recruitment. For space reasons we will not describe the injury process in pauci-immune crescentic GN, diabetic nephropathy, and renal involvement in paraproteinemia. For these entities please refer to Chapters 60, 73, and 75 in this book.

Podocytes in Injury. Glomerular podocytes are highly specialized cells covering the outer aspect of the GBM with interdigitating foot processes. Foot processes intervene with slit diaphragms, a crucial element for the selective glomerular permeability. Injury to podocytes leads to proteinuria, a hallmark of most glomerular diseases. Recent studies implicate a loss of podocytes as a driving force of progressive glomerular disease (70). Podocytes can be lost via apoptosis or detachment from the GBM, and can be recovered in urine of mouse and human (70,71).

Damage to the Glomerular Filtration Barrier Results in Proteinuria. Podocytes maintain the large filtration surface through the slit membranes and are responsible for 40% of the hydraulic resistance of the glomerular filtration barrier. During proteinuric diseases, the ultrafiltration coefficient (Kf) and thus the GFR are often lowered (for a detailed review see Deen et al. [72]). Proteinuria may be caused by defects of the podocytes, the GBM, the endothelial cells, and/or by alterations of the negatively charged proteins present on all three components of the glomerular filtration barrier. However, it is still a matter of debate whether the size selectivity of the glomerular filtration barrier is disturbed in proteinuria and whether the glomerular filtration barrier interacts with proteins by virtue of charge characteristics or its gel filtration properties (73).

Our understanding of the function and failure of the filtration barrier has been greatly improved by studies showing the essential role of slit diaphragm molecules, including ZO-1 (74), nephrin (75), CD2AP (76), FAT (77), Neph1 (77), Densin (78), and P-cadherin (79) in human or murine hereditary glomerular diseases. This was first shown for nephrin in the congenital nephrotic syndrome of the Finnish type (75), followed by the identification of mutations in the gene for podocin in autosomal-recessive (80) and alpha-actinin-4 in a autosomal-dominant FSGS (81). Several studies could also demonstrate the regulation of these molecules in acquired glomerular diseases (82). The molecular interaction and intrinsic signaling properties of the various molecules involved have been reviewed recently (83).

Glomerular Basement Membrane Alteration in Proteinuria. During glomerulogenesis, the GBM is generated by glomerular endothelial and epithelial cells as two separate layers and fused together to produce the mature GBM. The podocyte continues to add and assemble matrix molecules to the GBM, maintaining a hydrated meshwork consisting of collagen IV, laminin, entactin, agrin, and perlecan (84). The flexibility and dynamic of mature GBM requires a constant turnover. To achieve this, podocytes not only produce GBM components, but also secrete matrix-modifying enzymes (85,86).

The relevance of the GBM composition for podocyte architecture is exemplified by foot process fusion and proteinuria in the laminin beta 2-chain–deficient mouse (87). Alpha 5-, beta 2-, and gamma 1-laminin chains are assembled to form the GBM-specific heterotrimeric laminin 11 (88). The lack of a single laminin monomer is sufficient to cause severe disruption in the filtration barrier, leading to a nephrotic phenotype.

Specific matrix receptors anchor the podocyte foot processes by binding to their ligands in the GBM (88,89). Initial studies concentrated on a specific integrin heterodimer, consisting of alpha3-/beta 1-integrins, found at the "sole" of podocyte foot processes facing the GBM (90,91). Alpha3-/beta 1-integrins have been described to bind to collagen IV alpha 3-, 4-, and 5-chains, fibronectin, laminin, and entactin/nidogen, in the GBM (92). A series of experimental and genetic studies indicate an involvement of integrin-mediated podocyte matrix interaction in failure of the filtration barrier (89,90,93). Genetic evidence for the requirement of alpha 3-integrins for an intact filtration barrier was generated with the alpha 3-integrin knockout mouse, exhibiting an immature GBM and foot process effacement at birth (94). These findings led to the hypothesis that changes in podocyte integrins could result in proteinuria by interfering with the dynamic of foot process anchoring in the GBM. Integrin signaling via focal adhesion kinase (FAK) und integrin linked kinase (ILK) has also been shown to be activated in podocyte damage, in vitro and in vivo (95–97).

The expression of a second matrix receptor in podocytes, the dystroglycan complex, is negatively correlated with proteinuria in animal models (98) and in minimal-change disease in humans (99). Both integrins and dystroglycans are coupled via adapter molecules to the podocyte cytoskeleton. A series of studies have shown an association of altered GBM, loss of slit membranes, and proteinuria with rearranged cytoskeletal proteins. Systematic ultrastructural and immunohistochemical analysis detected a rearrangement of cytoskeletal proteins (F-actin and alpha-actinin) in response to foot process effacement in anti-GBM antibody-induced Masugi nephritis (100) and in puromycin nephrosis (PAN) in rats (101).

Cytoskeletal Alterations in Podocyte Damage. The integrity of the foot process is crucial for establishing stability between the cell–cell and the cell–matrix contact of podocytes. Foot process effacement, also referred to as process simplification, retraction, or fusion, is initiated at the cytoskeleton of the podocyte and results in the alteration of the cell–cell contacts at the slit diaphragm and in a mobilization of the cell matrix contacts (102,103). It is accompanied by an increase in microfilament density forming a mat of intercrossing stress fibers at the sole of the foot process (104,105). Podocyte damage models, by polycations such as protamine sulfate or the cytotoxic antibiotic puromycin, cause foot process effacement and proteinuria in rats in vivo (103,106) and allow the study of cytoskeletal responses in podocyte damage in vitro (79). Kerjaschki et al. blocked actin dynamics via calcium depletion, low temperature, or cytochalasin B and reduced proteinuria by 50% in the protamine sulfate perfused kidney (105). In contrast, interference with microtubular function with colchicine or vinblastine did not alter foot process dynamics (105).

Alpha-actinin-4 is widely expressed in podocyte foot processes, colocalizing with actin stress fibers (107) and is increased in podocyte damage in vivo (100,108). Mutations of ACTN4, encoding alpha-actinin-4, were found to cause a late-onset autosomal-dominant focal segmental glomerulosclerosis in humans (81). Initial functional experiments are consistent with an increased F-actin bundling by mutant alpha-actinin-4. Smoyer et al. evaluated the regulation of hsp27, a chaperone protecting cytoskeletal integrity in oxidative stress in podocyte failure (109). After puromycin-induced nephrosis, an increase of both total hsp27 and phosphorylated hsp27 was found (110). Hsp27 was shown to regulate the morphologic and actin cytoskeletal response of cultured podocytes to puromycin-induced injury (111).

Cytokines and Chemokines in Podocyte Damage. Podocytes may be the target of systemically produced cytokines and chemokines or might be the source of inflammatory mediators. As the development of nephrotic syndrome is associated with allergic reactions in some cases, TH2-inflammatory mediators may play a central role in podocyte failure (112). Podocytes from patients with minimal change nephropathy and undifferentiated rat podocytes express the TH-2 cytokine receptors for IL4 (IL-4R) and IL-13 (IL-13R2) (113). The respective ligands (IL-4 and IL-13) decrease transepithelial electrical resistance in vitro (113,114). Both cytokines also activate basolateral proton secretion, secretion of the lysosomal proteinase procathepsin L and induce the redistribution of the small GTPases, Rab5b and Rab7, in vitro. IL-4 decreases podocyte survival, changes the pattern of the tight junction protein ZO-1 (115), and inhibits the release of the glomerular endothelial survival factor VEGF (116,117). However, conclusive in vivo evidence of a pathogenic role of this pathway is still lacking.

In a subpopulation of patients with primary FSGS massive proteinuria can already reappear hours after renal transplantation. A soluble factor seems to mediate the filtration barrier failure, as plasmapheresis can effectively lower proteinuria and plasma from these patients is able to induce proteinuria in rats. Using an in vitro assay of glomerular permeability, studies are under way to uncover the molecular identity of the so far elusive "proteinuria factor" (117).

The expression of functional active chemokine receptors CCR4, CCR8, CCR9, CCR10, CXCR1, CXCR3, CXCR4, and CXCR5 has been described in human differentiated podocytes *in vitro*. Ligands of these chemokine receptors increased intracellular calcium and stimulated the generation of superoxide anion in podocytes, making podocytes a target for chemokine induced inflammatory response (118). The significance of these findings obtained in cell culture for the *in vivo* situation remains to be established, as so far there is only scanty evidence for the expression of these chemokine receptors on podocytes *in situ* in the kidney. Concerning the chemokine ligands, expression of CXCL8/IL-8, a ligand for the CXCR1/CXCR2 receptor, might represent an autocrine activation of podocytes (118). CXCL8/IL-8 has been incriminated in minimal change nephropathy and complement-mediated glomerular injury (119). A neutralizing antibody against CXCL8/IL-8 prevented podocyte foot process retraction and proteinuria in an acute immune complex-mediated glomerulonephritis, supporting a role for CXCL8/IL-8 for the development of proteinuria (120).

A chemokine-based mesangium-podocyte cross-talk has been detected with CCR7 expression on mesangial cells and CCL21/SLC production by podocytes (121). Activation of the mesangial receptor resulted in migration, proliferation, and inhibition of Fas/CD95-mediated apoptosis of mesangial cells. Besides CXCL8/IL-8 and CCL21/SLC, undifferentiated rat podocytes have been shown to release CCL2/MCP-1, further supporting the notion of the inflammatory potential of activated podocytes (122).

Generation of Reactive Oxygen Species as a Key Mechanism for Podocyte Injury. Reactive oxygen species (ROS) appear to mediate damage to podocytes induced by toxins, antibodies, complement factors, and mechanical stress. The reactive oxygen product hydrogen peroxide (H_2O_2) acts either directly or serves as a source of hypochloride. It is formed in the presence of chloride and myeloperoxidase, an enzyme secreted by polymorphonuclear leukocytes (123). The glomerular toxicity of H_2O_2 has been directly demonstrated in studies of intraarterial infusion of H_2O_2, which caused derangements in glomerular permselectivity without structural or hemodynamic changes of the glomerulus. H_2O_2-induced proteinuria was inhibited by pretreatment with catalase or deferroxamine, suggesting that iron-dependent metabolites of hydrogen peroxide mediate the effects of H_2O_2 (124). In more physiologic experimental setings overproduction of ROS has been detected in several glomerular diseases, including puromycin nephrosis (125), Heyman nephritis, a model of membranous nephropathy (126), and the Mpv 17 (–/–) mouse, a model for steroid-resistant focal segmental sclerosis (127). In these glomerular diseases, pretreatment of animals with ROS scavengers prevented foot process effacement and proteinuria (125,127). In puromycin nephrosis, phosphatidylcholine bound superoxide dismutase decreased proteinuria to the control level, improved podocyte density, and stabilized alpha 3-integrin expression (128). In biopsies of patients with membranous nephropathy, Grone et al. demonstrated oxidatively modified proteins in podocytes, mesangial cells, and basal membranes (129). In addition, an increase in glomerular xanthine oxidase activity due to a conversion of xanthine dehydrogenase to the oxidase form has been shown to be responsible for ROS production (130). Podocytes seem to be not only the target but also to be the source of ROS. In Heymann nephritis in rats sublytic complement C5b-9 attack complex on podocytes can cause upregulation and membrane translocation of the NADPH oxidoreductase enzyme complex. ROS are produced locally, reach the GBM matrix, initiate lipid peroxidation, and result in subsequent degradation of GBM collagen IV, leading to proteinuria (131).

Podocyte depletion is a crucial hallmark of glomerulosclerosis, considered a central problem in the progression of renal diseases (132). Experimentally sequential administration of PAN reduces glomerular podocyte numbers, most likely via apoptosis. The segment of the glomerulus lacking podocytes then develops glomerulosclerosis (70).

Recently, the molecular pathogenesis of membranous nephropathy could be defined for a group of patients with perinatal membranous GN (MGN). This study for the first time elegantly demonstrated, that the principle of the Heyman nephritis model can indeed be applied to human membranous nephritis. In Heyman's nephritis injection of antibodies directed against megalin, which is found on the sole of the rat podocyte foot process, causes the typical histologic picture of MGN (133). In humans, however, megalin is not expressed in podocytes and the antigen of MGN remained elusive. A case of perinatal MGN allowed the identification of neutral endopeptidase (NEP) as the podocyte antigen for immuncomplex formation. In a series of studies, the generation of anti-NEP antibodies was demonstrated in NEP deficient mothers, after immunization against the placental expressed fetal antigen. The transplacental transmission of maternal anti-NEP1 antibodies caused the typical histological and clinical picture of MGN, with subepithelial deposition along the GBM and nephrotic range proteinuria in the newborn. With the disappearance of the maternal antibodies after birth, all patients identified underwent spontaneous remission of proteinuria (134,135). These findings are a proof of principle, that MGN can be initiated by antibodies against renal antigens in humans. However, in adult-onset MGN no NEP-1 antibodies could be detected in these studies, so that antigens responsible for most cases of human MGN still remain to be determined.

From Podocyte Damage to Progressive Nephron Loss

Classic Focal-Segmental Glomerulosclerosis (FSGS). A sequence of glomerular alterations was established in models with glomerular hypertension and hyperfiltration, from which a working hypothesis for podocyte damage and loss was derived. Alterations of the filtration barrier consist of podocyte cell hypertrophy, foot process effacement, cell body attenuation, pseudocyst formation, cytoplasmic overload with reabsorption droplets, and, finally, detachment from the GBM (136,137). Cell-body attenuation and pseudocyst formation may result directly from mechanical overextension (138). After podocyte loss from a capillary loop, compensatory hypertrophy of the remaining cells results in further acceleration of podocyte damage. If podocyte loss per glomerulus reaches a threshold, progression to segmental or global glomerulosclerosis follows (70).

Collapsing FSGS. In HIV-infected patients, a distinctly different kind of glomerulopathy is found with proliferation of dedifferentiated podocytes and collapse of the glomerular tuft, termed collapsing glomerulosclerosis (139). The dedifferentiated podocytes have lost the foot process architecture including most components of the cytoskeleton, the expression of several podocyte-specific proteins including WT-1, and synaptopodin (140,141). Podocyte proliferation can obstruct the entire Bowman's space and this is paralleled by a collapse of the glomerular tuft, resulting in a "collapsing" glomerulosclerosis.

The glomerular damage can progress to loss of the respective nephron by damage to the glomerulus itself and the downstream tubular system (see below).

In summary, podocytes are, as a consequence of their highly specialized function, the most vulnerable element of the filtration barrier. They can be injured by a wide variety of mechanisms, ranging from genetic defects to soluble mediators (some of them as yet to be determined), ICs, mechanical stretch, or complement activation. Oxidative stress appears to be a common denominator for many types of podocyte damage. Interference with any of the three essential functional elements of the podocyte (slit diaphragm, the podocyte cytoskeleton, and the cell-matrix interaction), results in proteinuria, a key progression factor of tubulo-interstitial damage in animal models and human disease.

Glomerular Injury Due to Deposition of Immunoglobulins

The Thy 1.1 Nephropathy as a Model of Glomerular Injury and Repair. One of the most commonly studied rodent models of glomerular injury and repair is the Thy 1.1 nephropathy in rats. Only in rats is the Thy 1.1 antigen restricted to mesangial cells. Therefore the injection of an antibody against this antigen results in rats in complement mediated mesangial cell lysis. The mesangiolytic phase of anti-Thy 1.1 nephropathy is complement dependent, and therefore complement depletion prevents the injury process. Consistently, the blockade of the complement inhibitor CRRY increased the severity of glomerular injury. The subsequent repair process involves a phase with increased mesangial cell numbers ("proliferative GN"). The hypercellularity is due to proliferation of mesangial cells, the recruitment of bone marrow derived mesangial cell precursors, and inflammatory cell influx. As long as the scaffolding, that is the basement membrane, is preserved this results in complete healing, without loss of function or glomerular scarring. Increased cell numbers are cleared in part via an increased rate of apoptosis.

Platelet derived growth factors have received a lot of attention in the Thy 1.1 model. The PDGF family consists of dimers of PDGF-A chain and-B chain (forming PDGF AA, AB, and BB). PDGF-A binds to PDGFRα chain, while PDGF-B binds both PDGFRα and PDGFRβ chains (forming the receptor dimers). Two additional chains PDGF-C and PDGF-D (forming PDGF CC and PDGF DD) have recently been described. PDGF-B is essential for the development of the glomerulus as both PDGF-B and PDGFRβ deficient mice do not form glomerular tufts as they lack mesangial cells and die perinatally (142,143). PDGFRβ is constitutively expressed by mesangial cells, and activation through PDGF BB leads to cell proliferation and increased production of extracellular matrix, both *in vitro* and *in vivo* (144). Antagonizing PDGF BB in the Thy 1.1 model using various approaches reduced mesangial cell accumulation and matrix expansion. Furthermore PDGF seems to be involved in the recruitment of bone marrow progenitor cells into the glomerulus during Thy 1.1 nephropathy (145–147).

During Thy 1.1 nephropathy vascular endothelial growth factor VEGF is expressed by glomerular epithelial cells, mesangial cells, and infiltrating leukocytes. Treatment with VEGF significantly enhanced endothelial cell proliferation and capillary repair by increasing endothelial cell proliferation and the number of glomerular capillaries (148). Using morphologic methods, a role for capillary growth (nonsprouting angiogenesis) has been suggested to be important in the recovery phase (149).

Induction of various chemokines (e.g., CCL2/MCP-1) has been described, which correlates with the recruitment of macrophages during Thy 1.1 nephropathy. Treatment with chemokine blocking agents reduced the macrophage influx.

During the Thy 1.1 nephropathy a co-activation of the arachidonic acid cyclooxygenase pathway synthesis of prostaglandins (PG) and thromboxane (mainly TXA$_2$) and of lipoxygenase pathways toward synthesis of hydroxyeicosatetraenoic acids (HETEs) and leukotrienes (LTs) has been demonstrated. Blockade of TXA$_2$ lead to increased production of prostaglandins with beneficial effects, the blockade of TXB$_2$ prevented the fall in GFR (150).

An increased rate of apoptosis clears the increased cell number and finally results in resolution of the injury process (151).

In summary the "one-shot" Thy 1.1 injection into rats is a good model of glomerular injury with full repair. Accordingly the predictions outlined in the general part are fulfilled in this model: with complement mediated cell lysis, generation of the various mediators, activation and proliferation of mesangial cells, activation of adhesion molecules, monocyte influx, matrix remodelling and cellular repopulation (due to space limitations only some of which have been described above, for further details refer to (151–153)). Unfortunately, the Thy 1.1 model does not reflect any particular human disease, perhaps with the exception of mesangiolysis that can sometimes be seen during thrombotic microangiopathy. The healing phase of Thy 1.1 injury with mesangial expansion, though self-limited in the model, may serve to some extent as a model of mesangial proliferative diseases, such as IgA nephropathy.

General Mechanisms of Immune-Injury to Glomeruli in Humans. The etiologic agents in human glomerulonephritis are mainly unknown with a few exceptions (e.g., beta streptococci in poststreptococcal GN, or hepatitis C virus in cryoglobulinemic membranoproliferative glomerulonephritis). In the most common forms of human glomerular diseases the primary insult to glomeruli is the deposition of ICs (either formed *in situ* or deposited from the circulation). Antigens for *in situ* binding of immunoglobulins can be intrinsic glomerular proteins (e.g. anti-GBM), or antigens planted in the glomerulus. Self (e.g., DNA-nucleosome complexes in systemic lupus), and non-self antigens might become localized to glomeruli through charge affinity, passive trapping, or local precipitation (as it is likely in hepatitis C associated cryoglobulinemia).

Immune complexes (Ics) can be found in the mesangium (as in IgA nephropathy, lupus nephritis, and postinfectious GN), along the glomerular basement membrane (as in anti-GBM disease), in the subendothelium (in systemic lupus erythematodes [SLE], membranoproliferative glomerulonephritis [MPGN]), and in the subepithelial area (as in membranous nephropathy, and postinfectious GN) (154,155). The response to injury depends on the site of IC deposition, for example, mesangial deposits mainly lead to mesangial cell proliferation, and subendothelial deposits predominantly result in inflammatory cell recruitment. Only when circulating inflammatory cells can be activated through the contact with immunoglobulins, or with soluble products released by intrinsic renal cells, a strong inflammatory response can result. This is the case in subendothelial, mesangial, or membrane deposits. ICs on the outer surface of the glomerular basement membrane (as in membranous nephropathy) do not seem to provoke glomerular inflammation. It is generally thought that circulating cells do not get in contact with the site of subepithelial immunoglobulin and complement deposition. Besides the site of deposition the response depends on the properties of the deposited immunoglobulins with more severe injury caused by complement-fixing IgG subtypes (e.g., IgG1 and IgG3). Additionally, the *in situ* formation with complement activation may cause more severe injury as compared to trapped ICs.

Glomerular Injury Mediated by ICs. ICs can initiate multiple inflammatory pathways in intrinsic renal cells (e.g., the release of cytokines, growth factors, chemokines, prostaglandins etc.), leading to inflammatory cell recruitment. Disease models, which have been used most extensively for studies on immune mediated glomerular injury (IC-GN) are rodent models of nephrotoxic nephritis (NTN), repeated injections of foreign antigens (e.g., horse appoferritin injection into mice) and lupus-prone mouse strains (e.g., NZBXNZW-F1, MRL-Fas[lpr]). These models mimic IC-GN in humans to some extent and allow detailed studies on the response to injury.

The Role of Complement in IC-GN. Complement activation is a main factor mediating tissue injury after IC deposition (37). The activation of complement can lead to activation of intrinsic glomerular cells (endothelial cells, mesangial cells and podocytes) through formation of sublytic doses of the C5-9 membrane attack complex. Additionally, it can be involved in leukocyte recruitment through the release of chemotactic C5a and C3a. Sublytic quantities of C5b-9 result in cell activation with production of oxidants, chemokines, proteases, and up-regulation of adhesion molecules (which might be more important for cell recruitment than C5a/C3a) (156).

NTN was significantly ameliorated in mice transgenic for the complement inhibitor CRRY (a rodent homolog of the human complement receptor 1) as well as in mice deficient in the complement components C3 and C4. Treatment of MRL-Fas^{lpr} mice with recombinant CRRY reduced glomerular injury and proteinuria (157). Although glomerular injury was reduced by complement inhibition, circulating IC levels were markedly higher in complement-inhibited animals, indicating a role of complement in immune complex handling. A monoclonal antibody against C5 ameliorated glomerulonephritis and prolonged survival in lupus mice (NZB/W-F1) (158). Deposition of complement C3 has long been used as a diagnostic marker in renal biopsies in human glomerular diseases (e.g., lupus nephritis, MPGN, and postinfectious GN).

It should be mentioned that it becomes increasingly apparent that the deposition of ICs or complement are not sufficient to cause injury when animals are deficient in downstream pathways. For example, deficiency in IL-12 protected from glomerular injury in a lupus nephritis model although the amount of deposited ICs was the same as in wild-type animals (159). Similar results have been obtained in mice deficient in CCL2/MCP-1, CCR2, IFN-γ, and Fc receptors (160).

The Role of Cytokines in IC-GN. In the general part some of the most important cytokines, chemokines and growth factors involved in renal inflammation have been introduced. A comprehensive review of the existing literature goes beyond the scope of this chapter, but some aspects should be discussed herein. The most widely studied cytokines are proinflammatory substances (IFN-γ, IL-1, TNF-α, IL-6), anti-inflammatory cytokines (IL-4, IL-10, IL-13) and growth factors (e.g., PDGF, see under The Thy 1.1 Nephropathy as a Model of Glomerular Injury and Repair).

In response to ICs mesangial cells in culture produce a variety of proinflammatory cytokines including IL-1, IL-6, and TNF-α. These mediators can activate glomerular cells in an autocrine (e.g., mesangial cells), as well as a paracrine way (e.g., endothelial cells produce IL-6 in response to IL-1 and TNF-α). Gene profiling by oligonucleotide microarrays in NTN demonstrated an early induction of IL-1 and IL-6, TNF-α was increased during the entire disease process (161).

Type I interferons (IFN), consisting of IFN-α and -β, have antiviral activity, whereas the Type II interferon (IFN-γ), has a multitude of immunoregulatory functions (162). The production of IFN-γ by T cells can be triggered via T cell receptor activation. IFN-γ activates macrophages, and increases macrophage cytotoxicity by increasing oxidative burst and the production of other oxidants such as nitric oxide (162). IFN-γ is a key cytokine that controls antibody production. It plays a key role in lupus models (MRL/*lpr* mice, NZB × NZW mice) which has been demonstrated by increased expression during the disease course, exacerbation through the treatment with IFN-γ, and amelioration of disease by the inactivation of IFN-γ (163,164). Studies of IFN-γ deficient mice demonstrated that this cytokine is necessary for autoantibody production in MRL/*lpr* mice. IFN-$\gamma^{+/-}$ MRL/*lpr* mice are protected from glomerulonephritis despite intact autoantibody production and IC deposition (165). By transfer of IFN-$\gamma^{+/+}$ monocyte/

macrophages into IFN-$\gamma^{/-}$ mice it could be demonstrated that IFN-γ production by infiltrating macrophages is responsible for adhesion molecule up-regulation, macrophage accumulation, and renal inflammation, in the absence of autoantibody deposits (163).

In an anti-GBM model induced by the immunization with alpha3-alpha5(IV)NC1 heterodimers IFN-$\gamma^{-/-}$ mice developed a more severe form of glomerular injury as compared to the wild-type counterparts. This implies that depending on the context of the immune response IFN-γ has different effects (166).

Using the lupus model of MRL-Fas^{lpr} in mice deficient in type I IFN receptor, type II receptor, or both, demonstrated an amelioration of the disease in IFN II receptor deficient animals, but an unexpected worsening in IFN I receptor deficient animals. Double knockouts demonstrated a phenotype intermediate between wild-type and IFN RII deficient mice (167). In renal biopsies from patients with lupus nephritis IFN-γ expression correlated with the activity index (168). Therefore IFN-γ seems to play a key role in IC mediated diseases, both mediating antibody production as well as local inflammation.

Besides resident cells TNF-α is released by infiltrating monocytes/macrophages in response to ICs. TNF-α can reduce glomerular blood flow and filtration rate, and propagates formation of capillary thrombi and recruitment of inflammatory cells (169). The expression can be amplified by IL-1. Bioactivity of TNF might be regulated through soluble TNF-binding proteins (e.g., TNF receptor released by proteolytic cleavage). Administration of soluble TNF receptors to rats with NTN reduced glomerular injury and prevented crescent formation.

IL-1β is a pluripotent, proinflammatory cytokine that orchestrates inflammatory cells, augments T-cell responses, increases expression of vascular adhesion molecules, and induces proinflammatory cytokines, and chemokines (170). The resulting inflammatory reaction is dependent on the balance between IL-1 and the IL-1 receptor antagonist (171,172). Treatment with anti IL-1β antibodies decreased proteinuria in NTN. Bone marrow tranplantation from IL-1β knockout animals into wild-type mice clearly demonstrated that leukocyte- and not renal cell–derived IL-1β was involved in the induction of TNF and in glomerular injury. Absence of IL-1RI on leukocytes had no beneficial effect, whereas the absence of renal cell IL-1RI decreased glomerular TNF expression and glomerular injury (173).

It is thought that the inflammatory response after activation of intrinsic glomerular cells is switched off via the induction of antiinflammatory cytokines (e.g., IL-4, IL-10, IL-13). Treatment with IL-4 reduced albuminuria, and macrophage recruitment in NTN. The expression of IL-4 messenger RNA (mRNA) progressively increased during NTN in rats (172). Consistently, NTN induced in IL-4 deficient mice lead to increased macrophage recruitment and decreased renal function as compared to wild-type animals (174). The beneficial effect of IL-4 might be mediated in part by a downregulation of proinflammatory mediators by macrophages. Similar to the situation described for IL-4, the treatment with IL-10 was of significant benefit in NTN and genetic deficiency of IL-10 increased disease severity of NTN. IL-10 immunoreactivity was also significantly increased in renal biopsies from patients with IgA nephropathy. Treatment with FK506 of lupus mice (NZBXNZW-F1) resulted in a suppression of proinflammatory IL-2, IFN-γ, while the anti-inflammatory IL-4 and IL-10 cytokines were not changed significantly. Beneficial effects were demonstrated by increased survival, decreased IC deposits, and decreased proteinuria (175).

These are just some recent examples of how the roles of cytokines (pro vs. anti-inflammatory) and their sources (intrisic cells vs. infiltrating cells) become increasingly apparent through the use of genetically engineered mice (for further details on cytokines in glomerular injury see (171,176–181)).

The Role of Chemokines and Chemokine Receptors in IC-GN. The role of chemokines and chemokine receptors in renal disease has extensively been reviewed (24,182–184). Immunoglobulins or ICs can stimulate chemokine production by intrinsic glomerular cells via Fc receptors. Chemokine release by intrinsic glomerular cells is an important early event in the recruitment of inflammatory cells to the glomerular tuft (24). In mouse models of lupus nephritis the induction of chemokines appears earlier in the time course than the inflammatory cell recruitment, and in reversible models the reduction of inflammatory cells follows downregulation of chemokine expression (185). A variety of chemokines (e.g., CCL2/MCP-1, CCL3/MIP-1α, CCL4/MIP-1β, CCL5/RANTES, CCL7/MCP-3, CCL22/MDC, CXCL1/MIP-2, CXCL4/PF4, CCL21/TCA3, CX3CL1/fractalkine, CXCL10/IP-10) are upregulated in nephritic glomeruli, both in rodents (e.g., NTN, appoferritin induced IC-GN), as well as in human glomerulonephritis (e.g., lupus nephritis) (24,186). Deficiency in either CCL2/MCP-1 or the corresponding receptor CCR2 ameliorates renal injury and proteinuria in the MRL-Fas[lpr] lupus model, although the amount of glomerular ICs is not different to wild-type mice (160). A large number of studies illustrate a potential benefit of chemokine blockade (e.g., blockade of CCL2/MCP-1, CCL22/MDC (186) or growth-related oncogene protein-alpha (GRO-α) reduced the glomerular macrophage accumulation), although some studies also demonstrated negative results (implying regulatory roles during some disease phases) (187). In human lupus nephritis the accumulation of macrophages in glomeruli is associated with CCL2/MCP-1 expression in this compartment and with an increased excretion of CCL2/MCP-1 in the urine. Furthermore, a CCL2/MCP-1 polymorphism predisposes to the development of SLE and these patients are at higher risk of developing lupus nephritis (188).

The Role of Prostaglandins in IC-GN. Proinflammatory cytokines (e.g., IL-1β, TNF-α) and even IC can induce the release of PGs (e.g., PGE2) by mesangial cells. Induction of COX-2 as well as PLA2 has been demonstrated *in vitro*. In various models (e.g., NZB/W lupus, NTN) a protective effect of PGE1 and PGI2 (probably due to the vasodilatory, and antiplatelet effects as well as suppressive effects on cyto- and chemokine generation) has been suggested. The expression of adhesion molecules is also influenced by prostaglandins. For example, intraglomerular expression of ICAM-1 was suppressed by PGI2 in NTN in rats, which resulted in decreased macrophage recruitment. Furthermore, PGI2 is involved in ECM turnover through the regulation of metalloproteinases like MMP-9 and MMP-2 (by mesangial cells). On the other hand TXA$_2$ with its pro-aggregatory, vasoconstrictive and chemotactic actions is thought to have a negative impact. TXA$_2$ was significantly increased in glomeruli isolated from NTN mice and it retards the clearance of aggregated proteins in nephritic glomeruli via a decreased uptake by mesangial cells.

Cyclooxygenase (COX) exists in two isoforms, COX-1 and COX-2, with specific functions in different segments of the nephron (189). COX-2 deficient mice develop fatal nephropathy, which implies that COX-2 plays an important role during nephrogenesis (190). An increased production of prostaglandins and thromboxane has been demonstrated in human glomerulonephritis (e.g., lupus nephritis). Upregulation of COX-2 was found in human glomeruli during active lupus nephritis, as compared to normal controls. The expression was localized mainly to glomerular macrophages and to a lesser extent to mesangial cells. In contrast the expression of COX-1 did not change during lupus nephritis.

In summary, expression of cyclooxygenase (particularly COX-2) is induced during glomerular injury and a complex interaction between the prostaglandin system and other pathways like the chemokines, angiotensin and the adhesion molecules exists during glomerular inflammation (reviewed in [24,191,192]).

The Role of Leukotrines and Lipoxins in IC-GN. Both leukotrienes (LTs) and lipoxins (LXs) are lipoxygenase products of arachidonic acid. While LTs are proinflammatory, LXs antagonize many leukotriene effects, attenuate neutrophil recruitment, and might promote resolution of inflammation. Mesangial cells proliferate and contract in response to LT C4 and LT D4 (193,194). Intrarenal infusion of LT B4 into rats with NTN lead to increased polymorphonuclear cell recruitment and decreased GFR (195). Treatment of rats with NTN with an LT B4 receptor antagonist reduced proteinuria, glomerular monocytes/macrophage accumulation, and the number of crescents (196). A 5-lipoxygenase inhibitor given to rats with NTN also resulted in a significant reduction in proteinuria (197).

The lipoxin LX A4 inhibits both PDGF and LT D4 stimulated proliferation of mesangial cells (193). LXs are produced in large amounts during NTN. A decreased production of LXs (LX A4) was found during NTN in p-selectin deficient mice, resulting in an increased recruitment of inflammatory cells. It has been proposed that lipoxins might be important during the resolution phase of glomerular inflammation.

The Role of PAF in IC-GN. PAF is produced in large amounts by cytokine activated mesangial cells. Exposure of mesangial cells to PAF resulted in the expression of TGF-β, leading to an induction of fibronectin and type IV collagen expression (198). In the lupus model of NZB/W mice urinary PAF excretion correlated with proteinuria and a PAF receptor antagonist delayed the onset of proteinuria and prolonged survival (199). In NTN in rats, treatment with PAF antagonists also reduced urinary protein excretion, but did not result in a histopathological improvement. Thus PAF may be part of the proinflammatory mediators in IC-GN.

The Role of Adhesion Molecules in IC-GN. P-selectin is present on platelets and endothelial cells. It is not expressed by normal glomerular endothelium, but is upregulated during glomerular inflammation (in animal models and humans) (200). Blockade of P-selectin during NTN in mice reduced glomerular neutrophil influx (201). Administration of a P- and L-selectin antagonist (fucoidan F7) on the other hand did not change the number of glomerular leukocytes (7). The genetic deficiency in P-selectin resulted in an increased number of glomerular neutrophils (likely due to decreased lipoxin expression) indicating the complexity of the system. E-selectin although not expressed by normal glomerular endothelium has been described to be upregulated in humans with acute GN, lupus nephritis and IgA nephropathy. Little is known about the corresponding mucin ligands. ICAM-1 is only weakly expressed in the normal glomerulus (by endothelial and mesangial cells), but is induced during NTN as well as in human IgA nephropathy and human proliferative lupus nephritis. ICAM-1 blockade (or blockade of the counterreceptor LFA-1) reduced macrophage accumulation in NTN in rats (7). It is important to note that ICAM-1 can also be expressed in the absence of a glomerular infiltrate, for example, during minimal change and membranous disease. Thus expression of the adhesion molecule alone is insufficient for glomerular leukocyte recruitment, as to be expected.

VCAM-1 expression has not been detected on normal human glomerular endothelium, but has been shown to be present in glomeruli from MRL-Fas[lpr] mice. In rats with NTN the blockade of VCAM-1 or the ligand VLA-4 had no beneficial effect. Further studies are clearly needed to define the role of the different combinations of adhesion molecules and soluble mediators in the different renal compartments.

HSPGs are expressed on both endothelial cells as well as in the ECM and modulate inflammatory cell behaviour. During human lupus nephritis a decreased staining of glomerular GBM heparan sulfate correlated with Ig deposits and albuminuria, indicating a role in proteinuria (e.g., via decrease in sulfate-related anionic sites). The significance of the HSPG for chemokine and cytokine binding and presentation was discussed above in the general introduction. Inflammatory cells release elastase and heparanase which might mediate the decrease in heparan sulfate staining in glomeruli with proliferative GN (66). Urinary excretion of GAGs and heparan sulfate was found to be increased in patients with lupus nephritis (202). The exploration of the GAG system in GN is currently under investigation (for details see [66]).

The Role of Inflammatory Cells in IC-GN. As described above, recruitment of inflammatory cells depends on the interplay between induction and activation of adhesion molecules by proinflammatory cytokines and chemotactic factors. Neutrophils and macrophages are the predominant intraglomerular cell types in human glomerulonephritis. Neutrophil recruitment is thought to be an early and short lived (days) event, for example, in postinfectious GN (203). The appearance of macrophages follows closely and in an overlapping manner but persists unless remission ensues. Having reached the site of IC deposition, neutrophils and macrophages ingest ICs, and undergo a respiratory burst. Furthermore, activated neutrophils release serine proteases, such as elastase and cathepsin G, which by degrading the extracellular scaffold of the glomerular tuft, may lead to irreversible injury. Consistent with this scheme elastase inhibitors suppressed glomerular injury in NTN.

Monocytes/macrophages are a prominent feature in the glomerular tuft of lupus nephritis and MPGN (particularly in association with cryoglobulins). An association between glomerular macrophages and chemokine expression (e.g., CCL2/MCP-1) has been described in mouse and human. Macrophages can be both targets as well as the source for chemokines (leading to secondary waves of cell recruitment). Using bone marrow transplantation experiments it could be demonstrated that cytokines that activate macrophages come from different sources, for example, TNF-α is mainly produced by intrinsic renal cells, whereas IFN-γ is produced by intrinsic as well as infiltrating cells. The increase in number of macrophages in glomeruli results from recruitment, and to some extent also local proliferation (also demonstrated in human biopsies). In NTN macrophages mediate glomerular injury while depletion of macrophages (e.g., by radiation, by antisera), reduces injury, and results in decreased proteinuria. Macrophage effector mechanisms involved in glomerular injury are the production of oxygen radicals, PAF, coagulation products, and nitric oxide (204). Macrophages release various cytokines which lead to mesangial cell proliferation, for example, PDGF, FGF-2, and IL-1 (205). Still little is known about the macrophage phenotype during different phases of glomerular diseases. It is important to recall that the major goal of macrophages during glomerular inflammation is the removal of injurious products such as ICs. Interference with macrophage infiltration during an early phase of disease induction may therefore also have an untoward downside.

In summary, during recent years the various pathways involved in IC-GN have been described in further detail. Many of the injury processes mentioned in the general part of this chapter have been demonstrated in models of glomerular injury. Intrinsic glomerular cells (mesangial cells, endothelial cells), and/or their adjacent basement membrane or matrix are the *primary* site of the immune-deposits (Fig. 57-4). The deposition of ICs in glomeruli results in intrinsic glomerular cell activation (e.g., via Fc receptors and complement). The cells proliferate, and produce inflammatory mediators and extracellular matrix. Additionally, ICs might contain antigens or nucleic acids (RNA, DNA) from infectious particles, which could activate intrinsic renal cells via pattern recognition receptors (e.g., the toll-like receptors, TLRs) (155). *Secondary* injury results from free radicals, soluble mediators, and proteases released by recruited inflammatory cells (mainly neutrophils and macrophages). The soluble factors, for example, cytokines, growth factors, chemokines, eicosanoids, complement components further propagate the recruitment of inflammatory cells. They are filtered into the ultrafiltrate because of loss of permselectivity and thereby reach tubular cells; they also leave the glomerulus via the bloodstream to reach the peritubular vessels. Thus the inflammatory mediators generated in the glomerulus would activate podocytes and tubular epithelial cells via the ultrafiltrate and the peritubular circulation via the bloodstream thereby propagating tubulo-interstitial injury during a primary glomerular inflammation.

The Tubulointerstitium During Primary Insult and Progressive Disease

Significance of Fibrosis. Chronic progressive renal disease is characterized by the triad of glomerulosclerosis, tubular atrophy, and tubulointerstitial fibrosis. Fibrosis is the eventual consequence of persistent inflammation. The involvement of the tubulointerstitium may be at least as important as that of the glomeruli for the progression and hence prognosis of any renal disease. This may not be too surprising in view of the interconnection between glomeruli and tubules (see Introduction) and the fact that tubules and interstitium occupy more than 90% of kidney volume (206).

The exact mechanisms whereby increasing fibrosis leads to deterioration of renal function remain to be clarified. A number of theories exist, including the proposals that loss of postglomerular capillaries (207), formation of nonfiltering atubular glomeruli (208), and tubular atrophy (209) contribute to the loss of renal function. A morphometric analysis by Bohle et al. of biopsies from patients with a variable degree of impaired renal function demonstrated a robust correlation between reduced number and area of postglomerular capillaries and the rise in the serum creatinine (210). Recently Kang et al. confirmed a loss of microvasculature in progressive renal disease (207). This loss may be due to sclerosis of glomeruli with loss of downstream circulation, a lack of nutrients and growth factors, such as VEGF, and a predominance of factors such as thrombospondin-1 that promote endothelial cell apoptosis.

A second mechanism by which fibrosis may result in decreased renal function is the formation of atubular glomeruli. In 1939, Oliver described some glomeruli without attached tubules in patients with glomerulopathies, leading him to coin the term *atubular glomeruli* (211). Since no ultrafiltration can occur in atubular glomeruli, overall filtration rate is reduced (212). Marcussen and co-workers expanded this observation to document that atubular glomeruli are characterized by a reduced number of glomerular capillaries and a smaller size than their normal counterparts (212). The number of atubular glomeruli was lowest in diabetic nephropathy (8.8%) and highest in chronic pyelonephritis (50%) and renal artery stenosis (52%) (213–215). All studies on atubular glomeruli concurred that there was a good correlation between the number of glomeruli deprived of tubular connection and the degree of interstitial fibrosis.

Atrophic tubules may be the result of decreased ultrafiltrate containing various nutrients, hypoxia, and tubular toxicity by abnormal constituents of the ultrafiltrate such as free iron

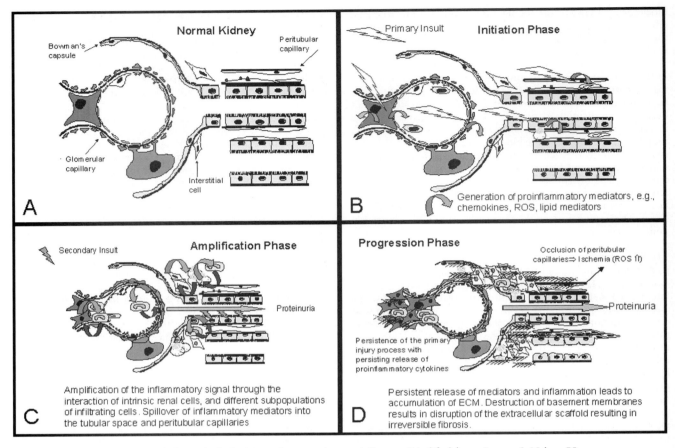

FIGURE 57-4. Hypothetical scheme of progressive renal diseases (Modified from: Segerer S, Nelson PJ, Schlondorff D. Chemokines, chemokine receptors, and renal disease: from basic science to pathophysiologic and therapeutic studies. *J Am Soc Nephrol* 2000;11:152.)

(released from transferrin–iron complexes) or even proteinuria itself (216–219). Apoptosis was shown to contribute directly to the decline in renal function in polycystic kidney disease (220), in a transgenic mouse model of interstitial fibrosis (221) as well as in a mouse model of chronic toxic nephropathy (222).

Renal Fibrogenesis. The development of tubulointerstitial fibrosis follows the general scheme outlined in the introduction to tissue injury and repair (see under A General Scheme of Tissue injury and Repair). It involves the generation of soluble mediators at the site of tissue injury, the extravasation of leukocytes across the endothelium, and subsequent secretion of various mediators by infiltrating leukocytes and tubulointerstitial cells, which results in the activation of profibrotic cells. The latter may then, through local disturbance in anatomical, hemodynamic and metabolic balances, initiate a vicious cycle of cell stress leading to generation of proinflammatory and profibrotic mediators, leukocyte infiltration and eventually fibrosis.

Induction and Development of the Inflammatory Response. Essentially all forms of interstitial fibrosis are associated with an inflammatory infiltrate. What are the factors involved in the formation of this interstitial infiltrate in tubulointerstitial and glomerular diseases? While a small number of interstitial macrophages may originate from *in situ* proliferation of resident interstitial macrophages, most of these cells migrate from the circulation through the postcapillary venules and peritubular capillaries into the interstitial space following gradients of chemoattractant and chemokinetic molecules as described

above. All types of renal cells can generate such soluble mediators, and especially chemokines, when appropriately stressed (24). In tubulointerstitial fibrosis, stimuli for tubular cells include: hypoxia, ischemia, infectious agents, exogenous (e.g., antibiotics, xenobiotics) and endogenous toxins (e.g. altered lipids, high glucose, paraproteins) or genetic factors, for example, in cystic renal diseases. In glomerular diseases, the loss of permselectivity exposes tubular cells to proteins normally not filtered, such as complement components, proinflammatory cytokines, and albumin in high concentrations. All of the above have been shown to induce chemokine production by tubular epithelial cells (24). The significance of proteinuria for progressive tubulointerstitial fibrosis derives from clinical studies showing that patients with a higher degree of proteinuria have a more rapid decline in renal function (223). Table 57-3 gives an overview of the factors involved. The majority of these has been discussed in the general introduction and in more detail elsewhere (224).

Recently, Johnson et al. suggested that uric acid may also play an important role in the promotion of interstitial infiltrates and progression of disease (225). Uric acid may be proinflammatory due to stimulation of synthesis of CCL2/MCP-1 in vascular smooth muscle cells (226) and of IL-1β, IL-6, and TNF-α in mononuclear cells (227). In the remnant kidney model, rats with experimentally induced hyperuricemia had higher scores of glomerulosclerosis and interstitial fibrosis compared to the normouricemic remnant kidney controls (207).

The potential role of the tubular epithelial cell in the formation of secondary interstitial inflammation is reviewed in detail elsewhere (224). In addition to epithelial cells, involvement

TABLE 57-3

FACTORS INVOLVED IN THE FORMATION OF TUBULOINTERSTITIAL INFILTRATES

Proteinuria
Immune deposits
Chemokines
Cytokines
Calcium phosphate
Metabolic acidosis
Uric acid
Lipids
Hypoxia
Reactive oxygen species

TABLE 57-4

PROFIBROTIC FACTORS INVOLVED IN RENAL FIBROGENESIS

Angiotensin II
TGF-β1
CTGF
PDGF
FGF-2
EGF
ET-1
Mast cell tryptase

of the endothelium has to be considered in mediating the interstitial infiltrate since all infiltrating cells have to transmigrate this barrier (see under Leukocyte-Endothelial Transmigration). However, knowledge about endothelial changes during the early phase of fibrogenesis is surprisingly limited. In acute renal failure de Greef et al. recently observed that endothelial cells of the vasa recta displayed *de novo* expression of the co-stimulatory molecule B7-1 starting 2 hours after reperfusion. Blocking this molecule by neutralizing antibodies completely prevented reperfusion injury (228). Similar observations have been made with other adhesion molecules. It remains to be established how these findings relate to renal fibrogenesis in chronic kidney disease.

The Inflammatory Infiltrate. This phase is characterized mainly by the influx of mononuclear cells. In almost all forms of primary or secondary glomerular disease, interstitial infiltrates have been described (229). Infiltrating mononuclear cells are composed of monocytes/macrophages and lymphocytes, particularly T-lymphocytes (230). The degree of interstitial infiltrate correlates with renal function in several forms of immune-mediated renal disease, including lupus nephritis and membranous glomerulonephritis (231). The number of tissue CD4-positive T cells in particular displays a close correlation with renal function (230) as does the number of CD3 T cells bearing the chemokine receptors CCR5 and CXCR3 (232,233).

While a role for macrophages in tissue damage, including renal diseases, has been established, a correlation of CD14 positive monocytes/macrophages with histological damage is less clear (234). Of interest are observations by Kondo et al. showing a good correlation between the number of infiltrating mast cells and the degree of interstitial fibrosis, pointing to the mast cell as a potentially underestimated player in progressive fibrosis (235).

Profibrotic Cytokines. The phase of inflammatory matrix synthesis is characterized by the stimulation of fibroblasts by cytokines from infiltrating inflammatory cells as well as from resident renal cells. Table 57-4 gives an overview over the most important profibrotic cytokines, which will be discussed briefly (see Cytokines).

One of the most relevant cytokines from a clinical point of view is angiotensin II. A wealth of data supports a beneficial role of blocking the renin-angiotensin system in the progression of experimental and human renal disease (summarized in [206]). Mice deficient in angiotensin II or its type I receptor develop less severe interstitial scarring compared to wild-type mice in the unilateral ureteral obstruction (UUO) model (236) and anti-GBM disease (237). Pharmacologic blockade of the angiotensin system decreased TGF-β levels in patients

with chronic allograft nephropathy and diabetes mellitus, thus preserving renal function (238,239). Angiotensin II can induce TGF-β synthesis in tubular epithelial cells and fibroblasts. However, at least some of the effects of angiotensin II are independent of TGF-β1 as was recently demonstrated by Ma et al. in mice lacking integrin beta6, which is required for activation of latent TGF-β (240). It induces hypertrophy in tubular epithelial cells, which is at least in part dependent on connective tissue growth factor (CTGF) expression (241). Angiotensin II can induce tubular hypertrophy and collagen expression *in vitro* in interstitial fibroblasts (242) and tubular epithelial cells (243).

TGF-β is currently viewed as the key cytokine in renal fibrogenesis though not all effects in renal fibrogenesis can be tracked to TGF-β (see under Cytokines about the pleotrophic effects of the TGF-β). *In vitro* it mediates chemotaxis for fibroblasts, transition of fibroblasts to myofibroblasts, and the synthesis of extracellular matrix proteins such as fibronectin and collagen type I. However TGF-β also has major functions in immune regulation and induction of apoptosis. Deficiency of TGF-β by genetic manipulation leads to a severe form of autoimmune-like wasting disease. Therefore TGF-β's role has to be viewed in the special circumstances and cannot simply be considered as universally profibrotic.

Evidence for the particular role of TGF-β in renal disease comes from studies using TGF-β transgenic mice, which develop glomerulosclerosis and interstitial fibrosis (244). Three isoforms have been described in humans and at least two have profibrotic effects on cultured rat tubular cells and fibroblats (245). Increased expression of TGF-β1 is documented in numerous models of renal, pulmonary, and hepatic fibrosis (246–252). TGF-β1 is predominantly produced by infiltrating inflammatory mononuclear cells and to some extent also by resident renal cells (see under Cytokines about difficulties in evaluating TGF-β by immunohistology). *In vitro*, TGF-β1 formation can be induced by angiotensin II, ET-1, glucose, insulin-like growth factor-1 (IGF-1), atrial natriuretic factor, PAF, thromboxane, and certain drugs such as cyclosporine A (206). In addition, autoinduction of TGF-β1 may occur. Secreted TGF-β requires extracellular activation to release the active 25 kD dimer (253). This activation is mainly performed by thrombospondin-1, though other mechanisms may play a role as well (254). Thus, upregulation of thrombospondin-1 expression is required in addition to increased TGF-β1 secretion. Active TGF-β binds to the type II receptor, which subsequently activates the type I receptor. The receptor complex then activates cytoplasmic proteins of the SMAD family by phosphorylation (255). Most cells express the TGF-β receptors indicating that receptor availability is not rate-limiting. However, even the active form of TGF-β1 may be modified by binding to extracellular matrix or to individual matrix molecules including the proteoglycans decorin and biglycan. Schaefer et al. found significantly increased interstitial matrix deposition in mice deficient in decorin expression

(256). These findings were extended, when the effects of decorin (and biglycan) were shown to be mediated by induction of fibrillin-1 expression (257).

Effects of TGF-β can also be mediated indirectly by a downstream mediator, that is, CTGF (258). CTGF was originally isolated from endothelial cells. Its expression is upregulated in human interstitial fibrosis, and it may mediate TGF-β induced collagen synthesis (258,259). Furthermore, increased expression has been described in models of diabetic nephropathy and UUO (260,261). Both cytokines may have synergistic effects. In a model of skin fibrosis only combined injections of CTGF and TGF-β1 resulted in persistent scarring (262). The receptor and signaling events induced by CTGF are still unclear and further studies are necessary to define the role of CTGF in renal fibrogenesis.

Very recently, IL-13 has attracted attention as a chemotactic and growth factor for fibroblasts that also promotes collagen type I synthesis (263–265). In models of liver and lung fibrosis the effects of IL-13 were largely independent of TGFβ (33). It remains to be seen, whether this effect of IL-13 also applies to fibrosis in the kidney.

The role of EGF in renal fibrogenesis is still controversial. Whereas Chevalier and co-workers described an attenuation of renal fibrosis in the UUO model after administration of EGF (266), a study by Terzi et al. using transgenic mice expressing a dominant negative form of the EGF receptor came to the opposite conclusion—that EGF was a strong profibrotic cytokine (267). The latter assumption is also supported by some *in vitro* data (268).

Endothelin-1 (ET-1) may also have a role in renal fibrosis. Three different isoforms and two types of receptors have been described. Type A receptors are expressed mainly on vascular smooth muscle cells and type B receptors on endothelial cells. Besides its induction of TGF-β1, ET-1 may directly stimulate matrix synthesis and decrease collagenase activity. Transgenic mice overexpressing human ET-1 did not have hypertension, but displayed severe interstitial fibrosis and tubular cysts (269). Furthermore, addition of ET-1 type A receptor blockers decreased the severity of tubulointerstitial fibrosis in models of chronic transplant nephropathy (270) and lupus nephritis (271).

Fibroblast Proliferation and Activation. Once inflammatory cells have infiltrated the tubulointerstitial space, one begins to see activation and proliferation of fibroblasts. While a number of studies in human glomerular disease describe a good correlation between the number of α-smooth muscle positive interstitial cells and renal function, these studies probably do not sample the universe of the entire fibroblast participation (272). Fibroblast activation is uneven and the pool of fibroblasts engaged in fibrogenesis is heterogenous in relation to their cellular characteristics and biochemical synthetic profiles (273,274). Immunohistochemical profiles in normal human kidney suggest that a subpopulation of interstitial fibroblasts may constitutively express α-smooth muscle actin, as well as the PDGF receptor α-chain (275). For most fibroblasts, activation is required in order to express α-smooth muscle actin, which is normally confined to vascular smooth muscle cells, hence the name myofibroblasts. It is currently unclear if the increase in number of α-smooth muscle actin-positive cells is the result of proliferation of smooth muscle cells or of fibroblasts, constitutively expressing this protein; or of *de novo* expression by formerly non-expressing cells. Furthermore, for perhaps the majority of fibroblasts, activation is not associated with *de novo* expression of α-smooth muscle actin (274). The degree of change in phenotype in the transition from fibroblast to myofibroblast may be underappreciated since expression of α-smooth muscle actin is not the only biochemical change to occur (276). For example, Rodemann and Muller demonstrated that fibroblasts from fi-

brotic kidneys expressed a number of proteins not detectable in their counterparts derived from normal kidneys (277). Even so-called myofibroblasts may exhibit a higher degree of variability and complexity due to different levels of α-smooth muscle actin expression (278). These studies support the notion that fibroblasts from kidneys with interstitial fibrosis may differ from fibroblasts from normal kidneys. Thus the origin and even the significance of myofibroblasts for excess collagen production, and for interstitial fibrosis remain to be fully clarified.

Based on a classic paper by Cohnheim in 1867 (279) it had been thought that fibroblasts derived from migrating leukocytes. However in 1970 Ross performed a study in rats which indicated that tissue fibroblasts were probably of local origin (280). Recently, the concept of bone marrow derived cells populating the renal interstitium has returned (281). Abe et al. demonstrated that collagen-producing fibrocytes can be derived from a CD14 positive enriched cell population within the blood, confirming Cohnheim's postulate from over 130 years ago (61). A number of studies have confirmed the existence of bone marrow–derived fibrocytic cells within the interstitium (282) and the transition of bone marrow cells to tubular epithelium (283). In fibrosing models of lung disease, recent studies have emphasized the role of circulating cells of hematopoietic origin as the major source of collagen production in pulmonary fibroblasts (59,60,284). These cells were attracted to the lung in response to the chemokine CXCL12/SDF-1. At present, it is unclear if these findings apply to other organs as well.

Evidence using genetically tagged fibroblasts and tubular epithelial cells indicates that fibroblasts derived from bone marrow comprise about 12% of the resident interstitial population in normal murine kidneys (281). During interstitial disease this percentage did not change compared to an increase up to 36% of cells producing extracellular matrix that were derived from tubular epithelial cells by EMT. Though many studies demonstrated the possible contribution of EMT to renal fibrogenesis, fibroblasts may still be the predominant cells producing extracellular matrix in the diseased kidney. Fibroblasts become activated by cytokines, mostly derived from infiltrating macrophages. One of the major mitogens for fibroblasts is PDGF. It is secreted mainly by macrophages (285) and exists in at least four isoforms (286). Application of recombinant PDGF-BB to rats resulted in the influx of macrophages and the formation of myofibroblasts (287). Furthermore, increased expression of the PDGF receptor B subunit has been described in human kidney disease (288). Recently, a novel form of PDGF that is PDGF-C was found in glomerular and interstitial scars in several rat models (289). In human renal biopsies Eitner et al. described upregulated expression of PDGF-C in podocytes and interstitial cells (290). Hudkins et al. injected it into mice to further analyze the functions of PDGF-B, -C, and –D (286). Mice overexpressing PDGF-D after injection of adenovirus constructs showed a severe mesangial proliferation, but only mild changes within the tubulointerstitium and overexpression of the other PDGF isoforms resulted in even more discrete interstitial changes. Final conclusions on the role of the PDGF isoforms in renal fibrosis will require further studies.

Another important mitogen for renal fibroblasts is bFGF-2. Due to different translation start sites, five different isoforms of bFGF or FGF-2 can be distinguished of which only the 18 kD isoform gets secreted. The effects of bFGF are mediated by four different high affinity receptors. Additionally, various heparan sulfate proteoglycans serve as low-affinity receptors. The particular significance of bFGF for fibrogenesis is underlined by a seminal paper by Whitby and Ferguson who examined the differences between fetal (scarless) and neonatal (scarring) wound healing (see introduction) and found no bFGF in fetal wounds, whereas the cytokine was abundantly present in healing after birth (291). Infusion of rats with high doses of bFGF results in glomerulosclerosis and interstitial fibrosis (292).

In vitro bFGF induced proliferation of primary cortical fibroblasts and promotes the expression of α-smooth muscle actin, but had only marginal effects on the synthesis of extracellular matrix proteins (293). *In vivo* many of the above cytokines may be involved in a concerted action during tissue repair and fibrosis, so that most likely no single profibrotic "master-cytokine" exists.

Epithelial-Mesenchymal Transition (EMT). EMT was first demonstrated in a murine model of anti-tubular basement membrane disease by cloning of a specific fibroblast marker, named fibroblast specific protein-1 (FSP-1), a member of the S100 family (294). Its expression is constitutive in tissue fibroblasts under physiologic conditions (294) and its promoter contains a *cis*-acting element (FTS-1) highly specific for fibroblasts (295,296). In mouse models of chronic progressive renal disease FSP-1 expression was robustly upregulated in the tubulointerstitium. The initial staining pattern followed the distribution of collagen-producing cells in a rabbit model of anti-GBM disease (297). In addition, *de novo* expression of the fibroblast-specific protein could be detected in tubular epithelial cells suggesting their transition to a mesenchymal phenotype (298). This phenomenon had been described in a number of organs (reviewed in 299). Moreover, EMT plays a central role in embryogenesis, tumor formation, and in the diseased kidney which replicates the renal developmental programs (300). Ng and co-workers described the *de novo* expression of α-smooth muscle actin in tubular epithelial cells starting at day 21 after 5/6 nephrectomy (301). Tubular epithelial cells lost their apical-basal polarity and seemed to migrate into the interstitium, as demonstrated by electron microscopy (Fig. 57-5). Of particular interest, and consistent with the general principles of tissue repair outlined initially, loss of epithelial characteristics occurred exclusively in areas where the basement membrane was disrupted.

What causes the plasticity of EMT? Various cytokines can induce the expression of FSP-1 in tubular epithelial cells *in vitro*. These include TGF-β and epidermal growth factor (EGF) (268,302). The group of Strutz described the effects of FGF-2 on four aspects of EMT: expression of epithelial and/or mesenchymal cell markers, cell motility, secretion of MMPs and matrix synthesis in two murine epithelial cell lines. FGF-2 had similar effects as EGF, but its main effect was the potentiation of the induction of EMT by TGF-β1 (303). Only TGF-β1 induced matrix synthesis, whereas all cytokines resulted in expression of mesenchymal markers, cell motility and MMP-2 and -9 secretion. *In vivo*, the stimulation by cytokines is probably not sufficient to induce EMT, and changes in extracellular matrix may also be required (304). For example, disrupting the tubular epithelial membrane by inhibition of collagen type IV assembly with soluble α1NC1-domains resulted in EMT conversion (304). Conversely, the tubular basement membrane did have a stabilizing function on the epithelial phenotype. These *in vitro* studies confirmed the aforementioned *in vivo* study by Ng et al. that complete transition to a mesenchymal cell can only be observed when the tubular basement membrane is disrupted (301). This concept is further corroborated by a study of Yang et al. in the UUO model of progressive fibrosis, where experimentally decreasing the activity of MMP-9 led to less degradation of type IV collagen and basement membrane, associated with less staining for α-smooth muscle actin in tubular epithelial cells, interpreted as less EMT (305). Changes in the basement membrane occur in progressive kidney disease, particularly in diabetic nephropathy (306). Such changes in the structure and the composition of the basement membrane could also promote EMT (300).

The signal transduction mechanisms of EMT point toward activation of integrin-linked kinase (307) and of the RhoA/Rho-associated coiled-coil kinase (ROCK) (308) pathways as important factors resulting eventually in the loss of the adhesion molecule E-cadherin. E-cadherin is important for the maintenance of the epithelial-epithelial adhesion and epithelial phenotype in the context of an organized tubular structure (300). Figure 57-4 illustrates the mechanisms involved in EMT schematically.

Postinflammatory Repair and Progression. The phase of postinflammatory matrix synthesis distinguishes tissue fibrogenesis from typical wound healing where resolution is expected. In this phase, the primary inflammatory process, be it in the glomerulus, the interstitium, or the vasculature, has subsided, yet interstitial inflammation may persist in a few areas. Several hypotheses about smoldering fibrosis have been entertained: First, stimulation by the remaining interstitial infiltrate is strong enough to result in continuous fibroblast activation. Second, autocrine loops in activated fibroblast may result in autonomous stimulation of these cells. Roles for IL-1, FGF-2 and TGF-β1 have been postulated in this context (293,309). A third mechanism postulates the interaction between secreted PDGF, TGF-β and tubular epithelial cells and fibroblasts (310–312). However, the existence of autocrine loops has only been described *in vitro* and their existence *in vivo* remains to be determined. Furthermore these schemes imply a persistent stimulation of one cell type or another, which in turn indicates continued cell stress and injury as the basis for the fibrosis.

In addition to persistent proteinuria another stimulus could be the aforementioned reductions in number of interstitial capillaries leading to hypoxia, which in turn may induce matrix formation (313). Hypoxia is a potent regulator of a number of genes, to a large extent mediated by the transcription factor: hypoxia induced factor 1 (HIF 1). The most prominent HIF-1 induced gene in the kidney is erythropoietin (314). In a model of progressive renal failure the expression of HIF-1α correlated

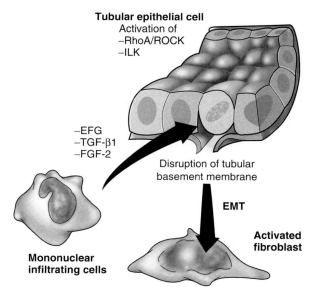

Tubular epithelial cell
Activation of
–RhoA/ROCK
–ILK

–EFG
–TGF-β1
–FGF-2

Disruption of tubular
basement membrane

EMT

**Activated
fibroblast**

**Mononuclear
infiltrating cells**

FIGURE 57-5. Hypothetical scheme of EMT in renal fibrogenesis. Stimulation of tubular epithelial cells by cytokines such as EGF, FGF-2, and TGF-β1, secreted mainly by infiltrating mononuclear cells, results in a partial loss of epithelial and de novo expression of mesenchymal proteins (transitional cell). If there is complete disruption of the tubular basement membrane, complete transition to an activated fibroblast ensues with synthesis of extracellular matrix proteins. (Modified from: Strutz F, Neilson EG. New insights into mechanisms of fibrosis in immune renal injury. *Springer Semin Immunopathol* 2003;24:459.)

closely with the number of peritublar capillaries (315). Moreover, Manotham et al. showed that the number of capillaries was reduced 4 and 7 days after induction of the remnant kidney model (316). This reduction was subsequently followed by the development of interstitial fibrosis. Similar findings were obtained in a rat model of progressive glomerular disease (317). Synthesis and secretion of ET-1 and TGF-β1 in proximal tubular epithelial cells could be stimulated by hypoxia (318,319). Moreover, hypoxia induced the synthesis of collagen type I but not of type IV in tubular epithelial cells (319). Hypoxia may also promote apoptosis of tubular epithelial cells through an upregulation of HIF-1 and Bax (320). Finally, hypoxia may induce EMT in cultured tubular epithelial cells (321). Hypoxia may also induce the formation of proinflammatory mediators, including eicosanoids, PAF, cytokines, and chemokines via generation of free radicals by any of the cell type stressed. All of the above factors could contribute to a persistent inflammatory infiltrate, either by influx or persistence of leukocytes, their activation perpetuating the vicious cycle of inflammation, fibrosis, hypoxia, and loss of functional nephrons.

Reversibility of Fibrosis. A central question in renal fibrogenesis concerns the potential reversibility of fibrotic lesions. In order to achieve this, the imbalance between matrix synthesis and degradation would have to be corrected. Until very recently, fibrotic lesions were thought to be irreversible. However, work by Fogo et al. demonstrated potential reversibility of mild focal segmental glomerulosclerosis in an animal study by treatment with an angiotensin receptor blocker (322). Similar results were obtained by Boffa et al. in a model of nitric oxide deficient hypertensive rats (323), by Adamczak et al. in the 5/6th nephrectomy model (324) and by Koo et al. in a model of reversible UUO (325).

In recent studies the role of bone morphogenetic protein (BMP)-7 in renal fibrosis was studied. Generation of BMP-7-deficient mice demonstrated changes of bone formation, lens development, and surprisingly also severe impairment of renal development resulting in death from renal failure a few days after birth (326,327). Morphologically, kidneys were hypoplastic and displayed dilated collecting ducts separated by stromal cells and extracellular matrix (326). BMP-7 expression begins at day 11.5 of mouse development in the ureteric bud as well as in the condensing mesenchyme, where it acts as an important cell survival factor (328). BMP-7 expression, unlike other morphogens, persists postnatally, particularly in distal and medullary collecting tubules where it may function as a cellular differentiation factor (329). BMP-7 effects are mediated via Alk 3 and Alk 6 receptors. Therapeutically, BMP-7 was first tested in acute renal failure. Vukicevic and co-workers were able to demonstrate that administration of BMP-7 (formerly known as OP-1 ["osteogenic protein]) reduced the severity of acute renal failure (330). Hruska and co-workers administered BMP-7 to animals with UUO demonstrating a delay of the loss of renal function by 5 days (331). Interestingly, in that study BMP-7 was more effective than the ACE-inhibitor enalapril. Similarly, a positive effect on renal fibrogenesis by BMP-7 was demonstrated in a model of Alport's disease. However, therapy was initiated at an early time point in that study. In order to resemble the clinical situation more closely, BMP-7 application was delayed in nephrotoxic serum nephritis. This delayed treatment not only prevented progression, but even resulted in regression of fibrotic changes and tubular atrophy (332). Zeisberg et al. demonstrated that BMP-7 counteracted the effects of TGF-β1, particularly on EMT of tubular epithelial cells. *In vivo*, placebo treated animals displayed expression of FSP-1, and a simultaneous downregulation of E-cadherin in tubular epithelial cells, indicating EMT. These changes were prevented in BMP-7 treated mice. Similar results were recently obtained by Wang et al. in a model of diabetic nephropathy (329). Con-

versely, Ikeda et al. applied BMP-7 to rats undergoing protein overload proteinuria and found only modest effects on the disease course, possibly due to the fact that tubular atrophy and EMT are not prominent features in that model (333). At the present stage, BMP-7 represents one of the most exciting strategies to prevent progression and possibly even reverse fibrosis.

What is the situation in humans regarding reversibility of fibrotic lesions? Fioretto et al. demonstrated that regression of early diabetic sclerotic changes is possible in principle (334). Type 1 diabetics who underwent pancreas transplantation with some degree of renal involvement at that point were observed for a period of 10 years. Renal biopsies were taken at 0, 5, and 10 years after pancreas transplantation. Whereas after 5 years there was a tendency for deterioration of sclerotic changes in the glomeruli, a definite reduction of mesangial matrix score was noted 10 years after the normalization of glucose levels. Although this study was performed in only a small number of patients with early diabetic changes and the tubulointerstitial space was not evaluated, it demonstrates two things: First, early sclerotic changes are potentially reversible even in humans and second, regression of sclerotic changes may require a very long time period, at least in diabetes. Reversibility of fibrotic lesions has also been described in other organs, particularly liver (335) and heart (336). Thus, the former paradigm of irreversibility of fibrotic lesions may not be true. However, the majority of studies showing reversibility have been performed in mild fibrotic lesions, where the underlying architectural scaffolding was intact and thus full restoration still a possibility. It remains to be seen if severe and long-lasting fibrosis with distortion of basic nephron architecture is truely reversible or if there may be a point of no return. Finally, not all fibrotic processes may be equal, so that the degree of reversibility may also depend on the underlying disease.

ACKNOWLEDGMENTS

S. Segerer is supported by a grant of the Else Körner-Fresenius Stiftung, Bad Homburg an der Höhe. Figures were designed by H. Meier.

References

1. Mitchell RN, Cotran RS. Cell injury, adaptation, and death. In: Kumar V, Cotran RS, Robbins SL, eds. *Cell injury, adaptation, and death,* 7th ed. Philadelphia: Saunders, 2003:3.
2. *Cellular adaptations, cell injury, and cell death,* 7th ed. Philadelphia: Elsevier Saunders, 2004.
3. Vaziri ND. Roles of oxidative stress and antioxidant therapy in chronic kidney disease and hypertension. *Curr Opin Nephrol Hypertens* 2004;13:93.
4. Vaziri ND. Oxidative stress in uremia: nature, mechanisms, and potential consequences. *Semin Nephrol* 2004;24:469.
5. Ferguson MW, O'Kane S. Scar-free healing: from embryonic mechanisms to adult therapeutic intervention. *Philos Trans R Soc Lond B Biol Sci* 2004; 359:839.
6. Martin P, Parkhurst SM. Parallels between tissue repair and embryo morphogenesis. *Development* 2004;131:3021.
7. Kluth DC, Erwig LP, Rees AJ. Multiple facets of macrophages in renal injury. *Kidney Int* 2004;66:542.
8. Wilson HM, Walbaum D, Rees AJ. Macrophages and the kidney. *Curr Opin Nephrol Hypertens* 2004;13:285.
9. Kofler S, Nickel T, Weis M. The role of cytokines in cardiovascular diseases. Focus on endothelial response to inflammation. *Clin Sci (Lond)* 2004.
10. Pestka S, Krause CD, Walter MR. Interferons, interferon-like cytokines, and their receptors. *Immunol Rev* 2004;202:8.
11. Johnson RJ. Cytokines, growth factors and renal injury: where do we go now? *Kidney Int Suppl* 1997;63:S2.
12. Massague J. How cells read TGF-beta signals. *Nat Rev Mol Cell Biol* 2000;1:169.
13. Roberts AB. The ever-increasing complexity of TGF-beta signaling. *Cytokine Growth Factor Rev* 2002;13:3.
14. Bottinger EP, Bitzer M. TGF-beta signaling in renal disease. *J Am Soc Nephrol* 2002;13:2600.

15. Murphy PM. International Union of Pharmacology. XXX. Update on chemokine receptor nomenclature. *Pharmacol Rev* 2002;54:227.
16. Luster AD. The role of chemokines in linking innate and adaptive immunity. *Curr Opin Immunol* 2002;14:129.
17. Luster AD. Chemokines—chemotactic cytokines that mediate inflammation. *N Engl J Med* 1998;338:436.
18. Baggiolini M. Chemokines in pathology and medicine. *J Intern Med* 2001;250:91.
19. Baggiolini M. Chemokines and leukocyte traffic. *Nature* 1998;392:565.
20. Campbell JJ, Butcher EC. Chemokines in tissue-specific and micro-environment-specific lymphocyte homing. *Curr Opin Immunol* 2000;12:336.
21. Murphy PM. Chemokines and the molecular basis of cancer metastasis. *N Engl J Med* 2001;345:833.
22. Murphy PM, Baggiolini M, Charo IF, et al. International union of pharmacology. XXII. Nomenclature for chemokine receptors. *Pharmacol Rev* 2000;52:145.
23. Fong AM, Robinson LA, Steeber DA, et al. Fractalkine and CX3CR1 mediate a novel mechanism of leukocyte capture, firm adhesion, and activation under physiologic flow. *J Exp Med* 1998;188:1413.
24. Segerer S, Nelson PJ, Schlondorff D. Chemokines, chemokine receptors, and renal disease: from basic science to pathophysiologic and therapeutic studies. *J Am Soc Nephrol* 2000;11:152.
25. Guijarro C, Kim Y, Kasiske BL, et al. Central role of the transcription factor nuclear factor-kappa B in mesangial cell production of chemokines. *Contrib Nephrol* 1997;120:210.
26. Rot A, von Andrian UH. Chemokines in innate and adaptive host defense: basic chemokinese grammar for immune cells. *Annu Rev Immunol* 2004;22:891.
27. Nibbs R, Graham G, Rot A. Chemokines on the move: control by the chemokine "interceptors" Duffy blood group antigen and D6. *Semin Immunol* 2003;15:287.
28. Weber M, Blair E, Simpson CV, et al. The chemokine receptor D6 constitutively traffics to and from the cell surface to internalise and degrade chemokines. *Mol Biol Cell* 2004.
29. Breyer MD. Beyond cyclooxygenase. *Kidney Int* 2002;62:1898.
30. Funk CD. Prostaglandins and leukotrienes: advances in eicosanoid biology. *Science* 2001;294:1871.
31. Luster AD, Tager AM. T-cell trafficking in asthma: lipid mediators grease the way. *Nat Rev Immunol* 2004;4:711.
32. Kolodsick JE, Toews GB, Jakubzick C, et al. Protection from fluorescein isothiocyanate-induced fibrosis in IL-13-deficient, but not IL-4-deficient, mice results from impaired collagen synthesis by fibroblasts. *J Immunol* 2004;172:4068.
33. Kaviratne M, Hesse M, Leusink M, et al. IL-13 activates a mechanism of tissue fibrosis that is completely TGF-beta independent. *J Immunol* 2004;173:4020.
34. Imhof BA, Aurrand-Lions M. Adhesion mechanisms regulating the migration of monocytes. *Nat Rev Immunol* 2004;4:432.
35. Kieran NE, Maderna P, Godson C. Lipoxins: potential anti-inflammatory, proresolution, and antifibrotic mediators in renal disease. *Kidney Int* 2004;65:1145.
36. Prescott SM, Zimmerman GA, Stafforini DM, et al. Platelet-activating factor and related lipid mediators. *Annu Rev Biochem* 2000;69:419.
37. Quigg RJ. Complement and autoimmune glomerular diseases. *Curr Dir Autoimmun* 2004;7:165.
38. Gasque P. Complement: a unique innate immune sensor for danger signals. *Mol Immunol* 2004;41:1089.
39. Bohana-Kashtan O, Ziporen L, Donin N, et al. Cell signals transduced by complement. *Mol Immunol* 2004;41:583.
40. Coleman JW. Nitric oxide: a regulator of mast cell activation and mast cell-mediated inflammation. *Clin Exp Immunol* 2002;129:4.
41. Oliver JA. Unexpected news in renal fibrosis. *J Clin Invest* 2002;110:1763.
42. Muller WA. Leukocyte-endothelial cell interactions in the inflammatory response. *Lab Invest* 2002;82:521.
43. Muller WA. New mechanisms and pathways for monocyte recruitment. *J Exp Med* 2001;194:F47.
44. Muller WA. Leukocyte-endothelial-cell interactions in leukocyte transmigration and the inflammatory response. *Trends Immunol* 2003;24:327.
45. Dejana E. Endothelial cell-cell junctions: happy together. *Nat Rev Mol Cell Biol* 2004;5:261.
46. Cotran RS, Mayadas-Norton T. Endothelial adhesion molecules in health and disease. *Pathol Biol (Paris)* 1998;46:164.
47. Alon R, Luscinskas FW. Crawling and INTEGRating apical cues. *Nat Immunol* 2004;5:351.
48. Ley K, Kansas GS. Selectins in T-cell recruitment to non-lymphoid tissues and sites of inflammation. *Nat Rev Immunol* 2004;4:325.
49. Ley K. The role of selectins in inflammation and disease. *Trends Mol Med* 2003;9:263.
50. Tam FW. Role of selectins in glomerulonephritis. *Clin Exp Immunol* 2002;129:1.
51. Aurrand-Lions M, Johnson-Leger C, Imhof BA. The last molecular fortress in leukocyte trans-endothelial migration. *Nat Immunol* 2002;3:116.
52. Schenkel AR, Mamdouh Z, Muller WA. Locomotion of monocytes on endothelium is a critical step during extravasation. *Nat Immunol* 2004;5:393.
53. Jaeschke H, Smith CW. Mechanisms of neutrophil-induced parenchymal cell injury. *J Leukoc Biol* 1997;61:647.
54. Eardley K, Cockwell P. Macrophages and progressive tubulointerstitial disease. *Kidney Int* 2005;68:437.
55. Mitchell RN, Cotran RS. Acute and chronic inflammation. In: Kumar V, Cotran RS, Robbins SL, eds. *Acute and chronic inflammation,* 7th ed. Philadelphia: Saunders, 2003:33.
56. Kalluri R, Neilson EG. Epithelial-mesenchymal transition and its implications for fibrosis. *J Clin Invest* 2003;112:1776.
57. Stout RD, Suttles J. Functional plasticity of macrophages: reversible adaptation to changing microenvironments. *J Leukoc Biol* 2004;76:509.
58. Nikolic-Paterson DJ. A role for macrophages in mediating tubular cell apoptosis? *Kidney Int* 2003;63:1582.
59. Phillips RJ, Burdick MD, Hong K, et al. Circulating fibrocytes traffic to the lungs in response to CXCL12 and mediate fibrosis. *J Clin Invest* 2004;114:438.
60. Hashimoto N, Jin H, Liu T, et al. Bone marrow-derived progenitor cells in pulmonary fibrosis. *J Clin Invest* 2004;113:243.
61. Abe R, Donnelly SC, Peng T, et al. Peripheral blood fibrocytes: differentiation pathway and migration to wound sites. *J Immunol* 2001;166:7556.
62. Savill J, Mooney A, Hughes J. What role does apoptosis play in progression of renal disease? *Curr Opin Nephrol Hypertens* 1996;5:369.
63. Ellis RE, Yuan JY, Horvitz HR. Mechanisms and functions of cell death. *Annu Rev Cell Biol.* 1991;7:663.
64. Savill J, Fadok V. Corpse clearance defines the meaning of cell death. *Nature* 2000;407:784.
65. Gotte M. Syndecans in inflammation. *Faseb J* 2003;17:575.
66. Rops AL, van der Vlag J, Lensen JF, et al. Heparan sulfate proteoglycans in glomerular inflammation. *Kidney Int.* 2004;65:768.
67. Fine LG, Norman JT. The breathing kidney. *J Am Soc Nephrol* 2002;13:1974.
68. Manalo DJ, Rowan A, Lavoie T, et al. Transcriptional regulation of vascular endothelial cell responses to hypoxia by HIF-1. *Blood* 2004.
69. Couser WG. Pathogenesis of glomerular damage in glomerulonephritis. *Nephrol Dial Transplant* 1998;13(Suppl 1):10.
70. Kim YH, Goyal M, Kurnit D, et al. Podocyte depletion and glomerulosclerosis have a direct relationship in the PAN-treated rat. *Kidney Int* 2001;60:957.
71. Vogelmann SU, Nelson WJ, Myers BD, et al. Urinary excretion of viable podocytes in health and renal disease. *Am J Physiol Renal Physiol* 2003;285:F40.
72. Deen WM, Lazzara MJ, Myers BD. Structural determinants of glomerular permeability. *Am J Physiol Renal Physiol* 2001;281:F579.
73. Smithies O. Why the kidney glomerulus does not clog: a gel permeation/diffusion hypothesis of renal function. *Proc Natl Acad Sci USA* 2003;100:4108.
74. Schnabel E, Anderson JM, Farquhar MG. The tight junction protein ZO-1 is concentrated along slit diaphragms of the glomerular epithelium. *J Cell Biol* 1990;111:1255.
75. Kestilä M, Lenkkeri U, Männikkö M, et al. Positionally cloned gene for a noval glomerular protein-nephrin- is mutated in congenital nephrotic syndrome. *Mol Cell* 1998;1:575.
76. Shih NY, Li J, Karpitskii V, et al. Congenital nephrotic syndrome in mice lacking CD2-associated protein. *Science* 1999;286:312.
77. Inoue T, Yaoita E, Kurihara H, et al. FAT is a component of glomerular slit diaphragms. *Kidney Int* 2001;59:1003.
78. Ahola H, Heikkila E, Astrom E, et al. A novel protein, densin, expressed by glomerular podocytes. *J Am Soc Nephrol* 2003;14:1731.
79. Reiser J, Kriz W, Kretzler M, et al. The glomerular slit diaphragm is a modified adherens junction. *J Am Soc Nephrol* 2000;11:1.
80. Boute N, Gribouval O, Roselli S, et al. NPHS2, encoding the glomerular protein podocin, is mutated in autosomal recessive steroid-resistant nephrotic syndrome. *Nature Genetics* 2000;24:349.
81. Kaplan J, Kim S, North K, et al. Mutations in ACTN4, encoding alpha-actinin-4, cause familial focal segmental glomerulosclerosis. *Nat Genet* 2000;24:251.
82. Schmid H, Henger A, Cohen CD, et al. Gene expression profiles of podocyte-associated molecules as diagnostic markers in acquired proteinuric diseases. *J Am Soc Nephrol* 2003;14:2958.
83. Benzing T. Signaling at the slit diaphragm. *J Am Soc Nephrol* 2004;15:1382.
84. Miner JH. Renal basement membrane components. *Kidney Int* 1999;56:2016.
85. Martin J, Steadman R, Knowlden J, et al. Differential regulation of matrix metalloproteinases and their inhibitors in human glomerular epithelial cells in vitro. *J Am Soc Nephrol* 1998;9:1629.
86. McMillan JI, Riordan JW, Couser WG, et al. Characterization of a glomerular epithelial cell metalloproteinase as matrix metalloproteinase-9 with enhanced expression in a model of membranous nephropathy. *J Clin Invest* 1996;97:1094.
87. Noakes PG, Miner JH, Gautam M, et al. The renal glomerulus of mice lacking s-laminin/laminin beta 2: nephrosis despite molecular compensation by laminin beta 1. *Nat Genet* 1995;10:400.
88. Kreidberg JA, Symons JM. Integrins in kidney development, function, and disease. *Am J Physiol Renal Physiol* 2000;279:F233.
89. Adler S. Characterization of glomerular epithelial cell matrix receptors. *Am J Pathol* 1992;141:571.

90. Adler S. Integrin receptors in the glomerulus: potential role in glomerular injury. *Am J Physiol* 1992;262:F697.

91. Korhonen M, Ylanne J, Laitinen L, et al. The alpha 1-alpha 6 subunits of integrins are characteristically expressed in distinct segments of developing and adult human nephron. *J Cell Biol* 1990;111:1245.

92. Dedhar S, Jewell K, Rojiani M, et al. The receptor for the basement membrane glycoprotein entactin is the integrin alpha 3/beta 1. *J Biol Chem* 1992;267:18908.

93. O'Meara YM, Natori Y, Minto AW, et al. Nephrotoxic antiserum identifies a beta 1-integrin on rat glomerular epithelial cells. *Am J Physiol* 1992;262:F1083.

94. Kreidberg JA, Donovan MJ, Goldstein SL, et al. Alpha 3 beta 1 integrin has a crucial role in kidney and lung organogenesis. *Development* 1996;122:3537.

95. Kretzler M, Teixeira VP, Unschuld PG, et al. Integrin-linked kinase as a candidate downstream effector in proteinuria. *Faseb J* 2001;15:1843.

96. Cybulsky AV, McTavish AJ. Extracellular matrix is required for MAP kinase activation and proliferation of rat glomerular epithelial cells. *Biochem Biophys Res Commun* 1997;231:160.

97. Bijian K, Takano T, Papillon J, et al. Extracellular matrix regulates glomerular epithelial cell survival and proliferation. *Am J Physiol Renal Physiol* 2004;286:F255.

98. Raats CJ, van den Born J, Bakker MA, et al. Expression of agrin, dystroglycan, and utrophin in normal renal tissue and in experimental glomerulopathies. *Am J Pathol* 2000;156:1749.

99. Regele HM, Fillipovic E, Langer B, et al. Glomerular expression of dystroglycans is reduced in minimal change nephrosis but not in focal segmental glomerulosclerosis. *J Am Soc Nephrol* 2000;11:403.

100. Shirato I, Hosser H, Kimura K, et al. The development of focal segmental glomerulosclerosis in masugi nephritis is based on progressive podocyte damage. *Virchows Arch* 1996;429:255.

101. Whiteside CI, Cameron R, Munk S, et al. Podocytic cytoskeletal disaggregation and basement-membrane detachment in puromycin aminonucleoside nephrosis. *Am J Pathol* 1993;142:1641.

102. Andrews PM. Scanning electron microscopy of the nephrotic kidney. *Virchows Arch B Cell Pathol* 1975;17:195.

103. Farquhar MG, Vernier RL, Good RA. An electron microscopic study of the glomerulus in nephrosis, glomerulonephritis and lupus erythematosus. *J Exp Med* 1957;106:649.

104. Fries JW, Sandstrom DJ, Meyer TW, et al. Glomerular hypertrophy and epithelial cell injury modulate progressive glomerulosclerosis in the rat. *Lab Invest* 1989;60:205.

105. Kerjaschki D. Polycation-induced dislocation of slit diaphragms and formation of cell junctions in rat kidney glomeruli: effects of low temperature, divalent cations, colchicine, and cytochalasin B. *Lab Invest* 1978;39:430.

106. Kanwar YS, Rosenzweig LJ. Altered glomerular permeability as a result of focal detachment of the visceral epithelium. *Kidney Int* 1982;21:565.

107. Lachapelle M, Bendayan M. Contractile proteins in podocytes: immunocytochemical localization of actin and alpha-actinin in normal and nephrotic rat kidneys. *Virchows Arch B Cell Pathol Incl Mol Pathol* 1991;60:105.

108. Smoyer WE, Mundel P, Gupta A, et al. Podocyte alpha-actinin induction precedes foot process effacement in experimental nephrotic syndrome. *Am J Physiol* 1997;273:F150.

109. Smoyer WE, Gupta A, Mundel P, et al. Altered expression of glomerular heat shock protein 27 in experimental nephrotic syndrome. *J Clin Invest* 1996;97:2697.

110. Mehlen P, Briolay J, Smith L, et al. Analysis of the resistance to heat and hydrogen peroxide stresses in COS cells transiently expressing wild type or deletion mutants of the Drosophila 27-kDa heat-shock protein. *Eur J Biochem* 1993;215:277.

111. Smoyer WE, Ransom RF. Hsp27 regulates podocyte cytoskeletal changes in an in vitro model of podocyte process retraction. *Faseb J* 2002;16:315.

112. Meadow SR, Sarsfield JK. Steroid-responsive and nephrotic syndrome and allergy: clinical studies. *Arch Dis Child* 1981;56:509.

113. Van Den Berg JG, Aten J, Chand MA, et al. Interleukin-4 and interleukin-13 act on glomerular visceral epithelial cells. *J Am Soc Nephrol* 2000;11:413.

114. Van Den Berg JG, Aten J, Annink C, et al. Interleukin-4 and -13 promote basolateral secretion of H(+) and cathepsin L by glomerular epithelial cells. *Am J Physiol Renal Physiol* 2002;282:F26.

115. Coers W, Vos JT, Van der Meide PH, et al. Interferon-gamma (IFN-gamma) and IL-4 expressed during mercury-induced membranous nephropathy are toxic for cultured podocytes. *Clin Exp Immunol* 1995;102:297.

116. Parry RG, Gillespie KM, Mathieson PW. Effects of type 2 cytokines on glomerular epithelial cells. *Exp Nephrol* 2001;9:275.

117. Savin VJ, McCarthy ET, Sharma M. Permeability factors in focal segmental glomerulosclerosis. *Semin Nephrol* 2003;23:147.

118. Huber TB, Reinhardt HC, Exner M, et al. Expression of functional CCR and CXCR chemokine receptors in podocytes. *J Immunol* 2002;168:6244.

119. Garin EH, Blanchard DK, Matsushima K, et al. IL-8 production by peripheral blood mononuclear cells in nephrotic patients. *Kidney Int* 1994;45:1311.

120. Wada T, Tomosugi N, Naito T, et al. Prevention of proteinuria by the administration of anti-interleukin 8 antibody in experimental acute immune complex-induced glomerulonephritis. *J Exp Med* 1994;180:1135.

121. Banas B, Wornle M, Berger T, et al. Roles of SLC/CCL21 and CCR7 in human kidney for mesangial proliferation, migration, apoptosis, and tissue homeostasis. *J Immunol* 2002;168:4301.

122. Natori Y, Nishimura T, Yamabe H, et al. Production of monocyte chemoattractant protein-1 by cultured glomerular epithelial cells: inhibition by dexamethasone. *Exp Nephrol* 1997;5:318.

123. Malle E, Buch T, Grone HJ. Myeloperoxidase in kidney disease. *Kidney Int* 2003;64:1956.

124. Yoshioka T, Ichikawa I, Fogo A. Reactive oxygen metabolites cause massive, reversible proteinuria and glomerular sieving defect without apparent ultrastructural abnormality. *J Am Soc Nephrol* 1991;2:902.

125. Ricardo SD, Bertram JF, Ryan GB. Antioxidants protect podocyte foot processes in puromycin aminonucleoside-treated rats. *J Am Soc Nephrol* 1994;4:1974.

126. Neale TJ, Ullrich R, Ojha P, et al. Reactive oxygen species and neutrophil respiratory burst cytochrome b558 are produced by kidney glomerular cells in passive Heymann nephritis. *Proc Natl Acad Sci USA* 1993;90:3645.

127. Binder CJ, Weiher H, Exner M, et al. Glomerular overproduction of oxygen radicals in mpv17 gene-inactivated mice causes podocyte foot process flattening and proteinuria: a model of steroid-resistant nephrosis sensitive to RadicalScavenger therapy. *Am J Pathol* 1999;154:1067.

128. Kojima K, Matsui K, Nagase M. Protection of alpha(3) integrin-mediated podocyte shape by superoxide dismutase in the puromycin aminonucleoside nephrosis rat. *Am J Kidney Dis* 2000;35:1175.

129. Grone HJ, Walli AK, Grone EF. The role of oxidatively modified lipoproteins in lipid nephropathy. *Contrib Nephrol* 1997;120:160.

130. Gwinner W, Plasger J, Brandes RP, et al. Role of xanthine oxidase in passive Heymann nephritis in rats. *J Am Soc Nephrol* 1999;10:538.

131. Kerjaschki D, Neale TJ. Molecular mechanisms of glomerular injury in rat experimental membranous nephropathy (Heymann nephritis). *J Am Soc Nephrol* 1996;7:2518.

132. Kriz W, Lemley KV. The role of the podocyte in glomerulosclerosis. *Curr Opin Nephrol Hypertens* 1999;8:489.

133. Farquhar MG, Saito A, Kerjaschki D, et al. The Heymann nephritis antigenic complex: megalin (gp330) and RAP. *J Am Soc Nephrol* 1995;6:35.

134. Debiec H, Guigonis V, Mougenot B, et al. Antenatal membranous glomerulonephritis due to anti-neutral endopeptidase antibodies. *N Engl J Med* 2002;346:2053.

135. Debiec H, Nauta J, Coulet F, et al. Role of truncating mutations in MME gene in fetomaternal alloimmunisation and antenatal glomerulopathies. *Lancet* 2004;364:1252.

136. Kerjaschki D. Caught flat-footed: podocyte damage and the molecular bases of focal glomerulosclerosis. *J Clin Invest* 2001;108:1583.

137. Kriz W. Progressive renal failure—inability of podocytes to replicate and the consequences for development of glomerulosclerosis. *Nephrol Dial Transplant* 1996;11:1738.

138. Nagata M, Schaerer K, Kriz W. Glomerular damage after uninephrektomy in young rats. II Mechanical stress on podocytes as a pathway to sclerosis. *Kidney Int* 1992;42:148.

139. D'Agati V, Appel GB. Renal pathology of human immunodeficiency virus infection. *Semin Nephrol* 1998;18:406.

140. Bariety J, Nochy D, Mandet C, et al. Podocytes undergo phenotypic changes and express macrophagic-associated markers in idiopathic collapsing glomerulopathy. *Kidney Int* 1998;53:918.

141. Barisoni L, Kriz W, Mundel P, et al. The dysregulated podocyte phenotype: a novel concept in the pathogenesis of collapsing idiopathic focal segmental glomerulosclerosis and HIV-associated nephropathy. *J Am Soc Nephrol* 1999;10:51.

142. Leveen P, Pekny M, Gebre-Medhin S, et al. Mice deficient for PDGF B show renal, cardiovascular, and hematological abnormalities. *Genes Dev* 1994;8:1875.

143. Soriano P. Abnormal kidney development and hematological disorders in PDGF beta-receptor mutant mice. *Genes Dev* 1994;8:1888.

144. Floege J, Eitner F, Van Roeyen C, et al. PDGF-D and renal disease: yet another one of those growth factors? *J Am Soc Nephrol* 2003;14:2690.

145. Ito T, Suzuki A, Imai E, et al. Bone marrow is a reservoir of repopulating mesangial cells during glomerular remodeling. *J Am Soc Nephrol* 2001;12:2625.

146. Rookmaaker MB, Smits AM, Tolboom H, et al. Bone-marrow-derived cells contribute to glomerular endothelial repair in experimental glomerulonephritis. *Am J Pathol* 2003;163:553.

147. Suzuki A, Iwatani H, Ito T, et al. Platelet-derived growth factor plays a critical role to convert bone marrow cells into glomerular mesangial-like cells. *Kidney Int* 2004;65:15.

148. Masuda Y, Shimizu A, Mori T, et al. Vascular endothelial growth factor enhances glomerular capillary repair and accelerates resolution of experimentally induced glomerulonephritis. *Am J Pathol* 2001;159:599.

149. Notoya M, Shinosaki T, Kobayashi T, et al. Intussusceptive capillary growth is required for glomerular repair in rat Thy-1.1 nephritis. *Kidney Int* 2003;63:1365.

150. Stahl RA, Thaiss F, Kahf S, et al. Immune—mediated mesangial cell injury—biosynthesis and function of prostanoids. *Kidney Int* 1990;38:273.

151. Roos A, Sato T, Maier H, et al. Induction of renal cell apoptosis by antibodies and complement. *Exp Nephrol* 2001;9:65.

152. Ikezumi Y, Kanno K, Karasawa T, et al. The role of lymphocytes in the experimental progressive glomerulonephritis. *Kidney Int* 2004;66:1036.

153. Jefferson JA, Johnson RJ. Experimental mesangial proliferative glomerulonephritis (the anti-Thy-1.1 model). *J Nephrol* 1999;12:297.
154. Couser WG, Johnson RJ. Mechanisms of progressive renal disease in glomerulonephritis. *Am J Kidney Dis* 1994;23:193.
155. Schlondorff D, Segerer S. Pathogenesis of glomerulonephritis, a perspective from the last 30 years. *J Nephrol* 1999;12(Suppl 2):S131.
156. Couser WG. Complement inhibitors and glomerulonephritis: are we there yet? *J Am Soc Nephrol* 2003;14:815.
157. Bao L, Haas M, Kraus DM, et al. Administration of a soluble recombinant complement C3 inhibitor protects against renal disease in MRL/lpr mice. *J Am Soc Nephrol* 2003;14:670.
158. Wang Y, Hu Q, Madri JA, et al. Amelioration of lupus-like autoimmune disease in NZB/WF1 mice after treatment with a blocking monoclonal antibody specific for complement component C5. *Proc Natl Acad Sci USA* 1996;93:8563.
159. Calvani N, Satoh M, Croker BP, et al. Nephritogenic autoantibodies but absence of nephritis in Il-12p35-deficient mice with pristane-induced lupus. *Kidney Int* 2003;64:897.
160. Tesch GH, Maifert S, Schwarting A, et al. Monocyte chemoattractant protein 1-dependent leukocytic infiltrates are responsible for autoimmune disease in MRL-Fas(lpr) mice. *J Exp Med* 1999;190:1813.
161. Kim JH, Ha IS, Hwang CI, et al. Gene expression profiling of anti-GBM glomerulonephritis model: the role of NF-kappaB in immune complex kidney disease. *Kidney Int* 2004;66:1826.
162. Ellis TN, Beaman BL. Interferon-gamma activation of polymorphonuclear neutrophil function. *Immunology* 2004;112:2.
163. Carvalho-Pinto CE, Garcia MI, Mellado M, et al. Autocrine production of IFN-gamma by macrophages controls their recruitment to kidney and the development of glomerulonephritis in MRL/lpr mice. *J Immunol* 2002;169:1058.
164. Seery JP. IFN-gamma transgenic mice: clues to the pathogenesis of systemic lupus erythematosus? *Arthritis Res* 2000;2:437.
165. Balomenos D, Rumold R, Theofilopoulos AN. Interferon-gamma is required for lupus-like disease and lymphoaccumulation in MRL-lpr mice. *J Clin Invest* 1998;101:364.
166. Kitching AR, Turner AL, Semple T, et al. Experimental autoimmune antiglomerular basement membrane glomerulonephritis: a protective role for IFN-gamma. *J Am Soc Nephrol* 2004;15:1764.
167. Hron JD, Peng SL. Type I IFN protects against murine lupus. *J Immunol* 2004;173:2134.
168. Uhm WS, Na K, Song GW, et al. Cytokine balance in kidney tissue from lupus nephritis patients. *Rheumatology (Oxford)* 2003;42:935.
169. Baud L, Ardaillou R. Tumor necrosis factor in renal injury. *Miner Electrolyte Metab* 1995;21:336.
170. Basu A, Krady JK, Levison SW. Interleukin-1: a master regulator of neuroinflammation. *J Neurosci Res* 2004;78:151.
171. Rantala I, Mustonen J, Hurme M, et al. Pathogenetic aspects of IgA nephropathy. *Nephron* 2001;88:193.
172. Baud L, Fouqueray B, Bellocq A. Switching off renal inflammation by antiinflammatory mediators: the facts, the promise and the hope. *Kidney Int* 1998;53:1118.
173. Timoshanko JR, Kitching AR, Iwakura Y, et al. Leukocyte-derived interleukin-1beta interacts with renal interleukin-1 receptor I to promote renal tumor necrosis factor and glomerular injury in murine crescentic glomerulonephritis. *Am J Pathol* 2004;164:1967.
174. Kitching AR, Tipping PG, Mutch DA, et al. Interleukin-4 deficiency enhances Th1 responses and crescentic glomerulonephritis in mice. *Kidney Int* 1998;53:112.
175. Sugiyama M, Funauchi M, Yamagata T, et al. Predominant inhibition of Th1 cytokines in New Zealand black/white F1 mice treated with FK506. *Scand J Rheumatol* 2004;33:108.
176. Haas CS, Schocklmann HO, Lang S, et al. Regulatory mechanism in glomerular mesangial cell proliferation. *J Nephrol* 1999;12:405.
177. Kluth DC, Rees AJ. New approaches to modify glomerular inflammation. *J Nephrol* 1999;12:66.
178. Schena FP. Cytokine network and resident renal cells in glomerular diseases. *Nephrol Dial Transplant* 1999;14(Suppl 1):22.
179. Baud L, Fouqueray B, Bellocq A. Cytokines and hormones with antiinflammatory effects: new tools for therapeutic intervention. *Curr Opin Nephrol Hypertens* 2001;10:49.
180. Isaka Y, Akagi Y, Ando Y, et al. Cytokines and glomerulosclerosis. *Nephrol Dial Transplant* 1999;14(Suppl 1):30.
181. Ortiz A, Gomez-Chiarri M, Alonso J, et al. The potential role of inflammatory and fibrogenic cytokines in the glomerular diseases. *J Lipid Mediat Cell Signal* 1994;9:55.
182. Anders HJ, Vielhauer V, Schlondorff D. Chemokines and chemokine receptors are involved in the resolution or progression of renal disease. *Kidney Int* 2003;63:401.
183. Anders HJ, Vielhauer V, Schlondorff D. Current paradigms about chemokines as therapeutic targets. *Nephrol Dial Transplant* 2004;
184. Segerer S, Alpers CE. Chemokines and chemokine receptors in renal pathology. *Curr Opin Nephrol Hypertens* 2003;12:243.
185. Perez de Lema G, Maier H, Nieto E, et al. Chemokine expression precedes inflammatory cell infiltration and chemokine receptor and cytokine expression during the initiation of murine lupus nephritis. *J Am Soc Nephrol* 2001;12:1369.
186. Garcia GE, Xia Y, Harrison J, et al. Mononuclear cell-infiltrate inhibition by blocking macrophage-derived chemokine results in attenuation of developing crescentic glomerulonephritis. *Am J Pathol* 2003;162:1061.
187. Anders HJ, Frink M, Linde Y, et al. CC Chemokine Ligand 5/RANTES Chemokine antagonists aggravate glomerulonephritis despite reduction of glomerular leukocyte infiltration. *J Immunol* 2003;170:5658.
188. Tucci M, Barnes EV, Sobel ES, et al. Strong association of a functional polymorphism in the monocyte chemoattractant protein 1 promoter gene with lupus nephritis. *Arthritis Rheum* 2004;50:1842.
189. Perazella MA. COX-2 selective inhibitors: analysis of the renal effects. *Expert Opin Drug Saf* 2002;1:53.
190. Morham SG, Langenbach R, Loftin CD, et al. Prostaglandin synthase 2 gene disruption causes severe renal pathology in the mouse. *Cell* 1995;83:473.
191. Montero A, Badr KF. 15-Lipoxygenase in glomerular inflammation. *Exp Nephrol* 2000;8:14.
192. Jensen BL, Stubbe J, Madsen K, et al. The renin-angiotensin system in kidney development: role of COX-2 and adrenal steroids. *Acta Physiol Scand* 2004;181:549.
193. McMahon B, Mitchell D, Shattock R, et al. Lipoxin, leukotriene, and PDGF receptors cross-talk to regulate mesangial cell proliferation. *Faseb J* 2002;16:1817.
194. Clarkson MR, McGinty A, Godson C, et al. Leukotrienes and lipoxins: lipoxygenase-derived modulators of leukocyte recruitment and vascular tone in glomerulonephritis. *Nephrol Dial Transplant* 1998;13:3043.
195. Yared A, Albrightson-Winslow C, Griswold D, et al. Functional significance of leukotriene B4 in normal and glomerulonephritic kidneys. *J Am Soc Nephrol* 1991;2:45.
196. Suzuki S, Kuroda T, Kazama JI, et al. The leukotriene B4 receptor antagonist ONO-4057 inhibits nephrotoxic serum nephritis in WKY rats. *J Am Soc Nephrol* 1999;10:264.
197. Petric R, Ford-Hutchinson A. Inhibition of leukotriene biosynthesis improves renal function in experimental glomerulonephritis. *J Lipid Mediat Cell Signal* 1995;11:231.
198. Ruiz-Ortega M, Largo R, Bustos C, et al. Platelet-activating factor stimulates gene expression and synthesis of matrix proteins in cultured rat and human mesangial cells: role of TGF-beta. *J Am Soc Nephrol* 1997;8:1266.
199. Morigi M, Macconi D, Riccardi E, et al. Platelet-activating factor receptor blocking reduces proteinuria and improves survival in lupus autoimmune mice. *J Pharmacol Exp Ther* 1991;258:601.
200. Adler S, Brady HR. Cell adhesion molecules and the glomerulopathies. *Am J Med* 1999;107:371.
201. Tipping PG, Huang XR, Berndt MC, et al. A role for P selectin in complement-independent neutrophil-mediated glomerular injury. *Kidney Int* 1994;46:79.
202. Parildar Z, Uslu R, Tanyalcin T, et al. The urinary excretion of glycosaminoglycans and heparan sulphate in lupus nephritis. *Clin Rheumatol* 2002;21:284.
203. Ruiz P, Soares MF. Acute postinfectious glomerulonephritis: an immune response gone bad? *Hum Pathol* 2003;34:1.
204. Cattell V. Macrophages in acute glomerular inflammation. *Kidney Int* 1994;45:945.
205. Nikolic-Paterson DJ, Atkins RC. The role of macrophages in glomerulonephritis. *Nephrol Dial Transplant* 2001;16(Suppl 5):3.
206. Eddy AA. Molecular basis of renal fibrosis. *Pediatr Nephrol* 2000;15:290.
207. Kang DH, Kanellis J, Hugo C, et al. Role of the microvascular endothelium in progressive renal disease. *J Am Soc Nephrol* 2002;13:806.
208. Marcussen N. Atubular glomeruli in chronic renal disease. *Curr Top Pathol* 1995;88:145.
209. Strutz F, Müller GA. Mechanisms of renal fibrogenesis. In: Neilson EG, Couser WC, ed. *Mechanisms of renal fibrogenesis*. Philadelphia, New York: Lippincott, Williams & Wilkins, 2001:73.
210. Bohle A, Gise HV, Mackensen-Haen S, et al. The obliteration of the postglomerular capillaries and its influence upon the function of both glomeruli and tubuli. *Klin Wochenschr* 1981;59:1043.
211. Oliver J. *Architecture of the kidney in chronic Bright's disease*. New York: Hoeber, 1939.
212. Marcussen N. Biology of disease. Atubular glomeruli and the structural basis for chronic renal failure. *Lab Invest* 1992;66:265.
213. Marcussen N, Olsen TS. Atubular glomeruli in patients with chronic pyelonephritis. *Lab Invest* 1990;62:467.
214. Marcussen N. Atubular glomeruli in renal artery stenosis. *Lab Invest* 1991;65:558.
215. Marcussen N, Nyengaard JR, Christensen S. Compensatory growth of glomeruli is accompanied by an increased number of glomerular capillaries. *Lab Invest* 1994;70:868.
216. Olbricht CJ, Cannon JK, Tisher CC. Cathepsin B and L in nephron segments of rats with puromycin aminonucleoside nephrosis. *Kidney Int* 1987;32:354.
217. Maack T, Park CH, Camargo MJ. Renal filtration, transport, and metabolism of proteins. In: Seldin DW, Giebisch G, eds., *Renal filtration, transport, and metabolism of proteins*, New York: Raven Press, 1985:1773.
218. Alfrey AC, Fromment DH, Hammond WS. Role of iron in tubulointerstitial injury in nephrotoxic serum nephritis. *Kidney Int* 1989;36:753.
219. Howard RL, Buddington B, Alfrey AC. Urinary albumin, transferrin and iron excretion in diabetic patients. *Kidney Int* 1991;40:923.

220. Woo D. Apoptosis and loss of renal tissue in polycystic kidney disease. *N Engl J Med* 1995;333:18.
221. Hocher B, Rohmeiss P, Thone-Reineke C, et al. Apoptosis in kidneys of endothelin-1 transgenic mice. *J Cardiovasc Pharmacol* 1998;31:S554.
222. Strutz F, Heeg M, Renziehausen A, et al. Possible mechanisms of tubular atrophy. *J Am Soc Nephrol* 2000;11:538A (abstr).
223. D'Amico G. The clinical role of proteinuria. *Am J Kid Dis* 1991;17:48.
224. Strutz F, Neilson EG. New insights into mechanisms of fibrosis in immune renal injury. *Springer Semin Immunopathol* 2003;24:459.
225. Johnson RJ, Kang DH, Feig D, et al. Is there a pathogenetic role for uric acid in hypertension and cardiovascular and renal disease? *Hypertension* 2003;41:1183.
226. Kanellis J, Watanabe S, Li JH, et al. Uric acid stimulates monocyte chemoattractant protein-1 production in vascular smooth muscle cells via mitogen-activated protein kinase and cyclooxygenase-2. *Hypertension* 2003;41:1287.
227. Netea MG, Kullberg BJ, Blok WL, et al. The role of hyperuricemia in the increased cytokine production after lipopolysaccharide challenge in neutropenic mice. *Blood* 1997;89:577.
228. De Greef KE, Ysebaert DK, Dauwe S, et al. Anti-B7-1 blocks mononuclear cell adherence in vasa recta after ischemia. *Kidney Int* 2001;60:1415.
229. Strutz F, Caron R, Tomaszewski J, et al. Transdifferentiation: a new concept in renal fibrogenesis. *J Am Soc Nephrol* 1994;5:819 (abstr).
230. Müller GA, Markovic-Lipkovski J, Frank J, et al. The role of interstitial cells in the progression of renal diseases. *J Am Soc Nephrol* 1992;2:S198.
231. Alexopoulos E, Seron D, Hartley RB, et al. Lupus nephritis: correlation of interstitial cells with glomerular function. *Kidney Int* 1990;37:100.
232. Segerer S, Mack M, Regele H, et al. Expression of the C-C chemokine receptor 5 in human kidney diseases. *Kidney Int* 1999;56:52.
233. Segerer S, Banas B, Wornle M, et al. CXCR3 is involved in tubulointerstitial injury in human glomerulonephritis. *Am J Pathol* 2004;164:635.
234. Eddy AA. Interstitial macrophages as mediators of renal fibrosis. *Exp Nephrol* 1995;3:76.
235. Kondo S, Kagami S, Kido H, et al. Role of mast cell tryptase in renal interstitial fibrosis. *J Am Soc Nephrol* 2001;12:1668.
236. Fern RJ, Yesko CM, Thornhill BA, et al. Reduced angiotensinogen expression attenuates renal interstitial fibrosis in obstructive nephropathy in mice. *J Clin Invest* 1999;103:39.
237. Hisada Y, Sugaya T, Tanaka S, et al. An essential role of angiotensin II receptor type 1a in recipient kidney, not in transplanted peripheral blood leukocytes, in progressive immune-mediated renal injury. *Lab Invest* 2001;81:1243.
238. Campistol JM, Inigo P, Jimenez W, et al. Losartan decreases plasma levels of TGF-beta1 in transplant patients with chronic allograft nephropathy. *Kidney Int* 1999;56:714.
239. Sharma K, Eltayeb BO, McGowan TA, et al. Captopril-induced reduction of serum levels of transforming growth factor-beta1 correlates with long-term renoprotection in insulin- dependent diabetic patients. *Am J Kidney Dis* 1999;34:818.
240. Ma LJ, Yang H, Gaspert A, et al. Transforming growth factor-beta-dependent and -independent pathways of induction of tubulointerstitial fibrosis in beta6(-/-) mice. *Am J Pathol* 2003;163:1261.
241. Liu BC, Sun J, Chen Q, et al. Role of connective tissue growth factor in mediating hypertrophy of human proximal tubular cells induced by angiotensin II. *J Nephrol* 2003;23:429.
242. Ruiz-Ortega M, Egido J. Angiotensin II modulates cell growth-related events and synthesis of matrix proteins in renal interstitial fibroblasts. *Kidney Int* 1997;52:1497.
243. Wolf G, Kalluri R, Ziyadeh FN, et al. Angiotensin II induces alpha3(IV) collagen expression in cultured murine proximal tubular cells. *Proc Assoc Am Physicians* 1999;111:357.
244. Kopp JB, Factor VM, Mozes M, et al. Transgenic mice with increased plasma levels of TGF-beta 1 develop progressive renal disease. *Lab Invest* 1996;74:991.
245. Yu L, Border WA, Huang Y, et al. TGF-beta isoforms in renal fibrogenesis. *Kidney Int* 2003;64:844.
246. Border WA, Noble NA. Transforming growth factor beta in tissue fibrosis. *N Engl J Med* 1994;331:1286.
247. Yamamoto T, Noble NA, Miller DE, et al. Sustained expression of TGF-b1 underlies development of progressive kidney fibrosis. *Kidney Int* 1994;45:916.
248. Eddy AA. Experimental insights into the tubulointerstitial disease accompanying primary glomerular lesions. *J Am Soc Nephrol* 1994;5:1273.
249. Eddy AA. Protein restriction reduces transforming growth factor β and interstitial fibrosis in chronic purine aminonucleoside nephrosis. *Am J Physiol* 1994;266:F884.
250. Downer G, Phan SH, Wiggins RC. Analysis of renal fibrosis in a rabbit model of crescentic nephritis. *J Clin Invest* 1988;82:998.
251. Hamaguchi A, Kim S, Ohta K, et al. Transforming growth factor-β1 expression and phenotypic modulation in the kidney of hypertensive rats. *Hypertension* 1995;26:199.
252. Kaneto H, Morrissey J, Klahr S. Increased expression of TGF-b1 mRNA in the obstructed kidney of rats with unilateral ureteral ligation. *Kidney Int* 1993;44:313.
253. Taipale J, Keski-Oja J. Growth factors in the extracellular matrix. *FASEB J* 1997;11:51.

254. Crawford SE, Stellmach V, Murphy-Ullrich JE, et al. Thrombospondin-1 is a major activator of TGF-beta1 in vivo. *Cell* 1998;93:1159.
255. Schiffer M, von Gersdorff G, Bitzer M, et al. Smad proteins and transforming growth factor-beta signaling. *Kidney Int* 2000;58(Suppl 77):S45.
256. Schaefer L, Macakova K, Raslik I, et al. Absence of decorin adversely influences tubulointerstitial fibrosis of the obstructed kidney by enhanced apoptosis and increased inflammatory reaction. *Am J Pathol* 2002;160:1181.
257. Schaefer L, Mihalik D, Babelova A, et al. Regulation of fibrillin-1 by biglycan and decorin is important for tissue preservation in the kidney during pressure-induced injury. *Am J Pathol* 2004;165:383.
258. Duncan MR, Frazier KS, Abramson S, et al. Connective tissue growth factor mediates transforming growth factor beta-induced collagen synthesis: down-regulation by cAMP. *FASEB J* 1999;13:1774.
259. Ito Y, Aten J, Bende RJ, et al. Expression of connective tissue growth factor in human renal fibrosis. *Kidney Int* 1998;53:853.
260. Riser BL, Denichilo M, Cortes P, et al. Regulation of connective tissue growth factor activity in cultured rat mesangial cells and its expression in experimental diabetic glomerulosclerosis. *J Am Soc Nephrol* 2000;11: 25.
261. Yokoi H, Sugawara A, Mukoyama M, et al. Role of connective tissue growth factor in profibrotic action of transforming growth factor-beta: a potential target for preventing renal fibrosis. *Am J Kidney Dis* 2001;38:S134.
262. Mori T, Kawara S, Shinozaki M, et al. Role and interaction of connective tissue growth factor with transforming growth factor-beta in persistent fibrosis: A mouse fibrosis model. *J Cell Physiol* 1999;181:153.
263. Kohyama T, Liu X, Wen FQ, et al. IL-4 and IL-13 induce chemotaxis of human foreskin fibroblasts, but not human fetal lung fibroblasts. *Inflammation* 2004;28:33.
264. Ingram JL, Rice AB, Geisenhoffer K, et al. IL-13 and IL-1beta promote lung fibroblast growth through coordinated up-regulation of PDGF-AA and PDGF-Ralpha. *FASEB J* 2004;18:1132.
265. Jinnin M, Ihn H, Yamane K, et al. Interleukin-13 stimulates the transcription of the human alpha2(I) collagen gene in human dermal fibroblasts. *J Biol Chem* 2004;279:41783.
266. Chevalier RL, Goyal S, Wolstenholme JT, et al. Obstructive nephropathy in the neonatal rat is attenuated by epidermal growth factor. *Kidney Int* 1998;54:38.
267. Terzi F, Burtin M, Hekmati M, et al. Targeted expression of a dominant-negative EGF-R in the kidney reduces tubulo-interstitial lesions after renal injury. *J Clin Invest* 2000;106:225.
268. Okada H, Danoff TM, Kalluri R, et al. Early role of Fsp1 in epithelial-mesenchymal transformation. *Am J Physiol* 1997;273:F563.
269. Hocher B, Thone-Reineke C, Rohmeiss P, et al. Endothelin-1 transgenic mice develop glomerulosclerosis, interstitial fibrosis, and renal cysts but not hypertension. *J Clin Invest* 1997;99:1380.
270. Orth SR, Odoni G, Amann K, et al. The ET(A) receptor blocker LU 135252 prevents chronic transplant nephropathy in the "Fisher to Lewis" model. *J Am Soc Nephrol* 1999;10:387.
271. Nakamura T, Ebihara I, Tomino Y, et al. Effect of a specific endothelin A receptor antagonist on murine lupus nephritis. *Kidney Int* 1995;47:481.
272. Hewitson TD, Becker GJ. Interstitial myofibroblasts in IgA glomerulonephritis. *Am J Nephrol* 1995;15:111.
273. Müller GA, Strutz F. Renal fibroblast heterogeneity. *Kidney Int* 1995; 48(Suppl 50):S33.
274. Okada H, Ban S, Nagao S, et al. Progressive renal fibrosis in murine polycystic kidney disease: an immunohistochemical observation. *Kidney Int* 2000;58:587.
275. Alpers CE, Davis CL, Barr D, et al. Identification of platelet-derived growth factor A and B chains in human renal vascular rejection. *Am J Pathol* 1996;148:439.
276. Grinnell F. Fibroblasts, myofibroblasts, and wound contraction. *J Cell Biol* 1994;124:401.
277. Rodemann HP, Müller GA. Characterization of human renal fibroblasts in health and disease: II. In vitro growth, differentiation, and collagen synthesis of fibroblasts from kidneys with interstitial fibrosis. *Am J Kidney Dis* 1991;17:684.
278. Ru Y, Eyden B, Curry A, et al. Actin filaments in human renal tubulo-interstitial fibrosis: significance for the concept of epithelial-myofibroblast transformation. *J Submicrosc Cytol Pathol* 2003;35:221.
279. Cohnheim J. Über Entzündung und Eiterung. *Virchows Arch* 1867;40:1.
280. Ross R, Everett NB, Tyler R. Wound healing and collagen formation. VI. The origin of the wound. Fibroblast studied in parabiosis. *J Cell Biol* 1970;44:645.
281. Iwano M, Plieth D, Danoff TM, et al. Evidence that fibroblasts derive from epithelium during tissue fibrosis. *J Clin Invest* 2002;110:341.
282. Grimm PC, Nickerson P, Jeffery J, et al. Neointimal and tubulointerstitial infiltration by recipient mesenchymal cells in chronic renal-allograft rejection. *N Engl J Med* 2001;345:93.
283. Poulsom R, Forbes SJ, Hodivala-Dilke K, et al. Bone marrow contributes to renal parenchymal turnover and regeneration. *J Pathol* 2001;195:229.
284. Garantziotis S, Steele MP, Schwartz DA. Pulmonary fibrosis: thinking outside of the lung. *J Clin Invest* 2004;114:319.
285. Kovacs EJ. Fibrogenic cytokines: the role of immune mediators in the development of scar tissue. *Immunol Today* 1991;12:17.
286. Hudkins KL, Gilbertson DG, Carling M, et al. Exogenous PDGF-D is a

potent mesangial cell mitogen and causes a severe mesangial proliferative glomerulopathy. *J Am Soc Nephrol* 2004;15:286.

287. Tang WW, Ulich TR, Lacey DL, et al. Platelet-derived growth factor-BB induces renal tubulointerstitial myofibroblast formation and tubulointerstitial fibrosis. *Am J Pathol* 1996;148:1169.

288. Gesualdo L, Di Paolo S, Milani S, et al. Expression of platelet-derived growth factor receptors in normal and diseased human kidney. An immunohistochemistry and in situ hybridization study. *J Clin Invest* 1994;94:50.

289. Eitner F, Ostendorf T, Van Roeyen C, et al. Expression of a novel PDGF Isoform, PDGF-C, in normal and diseased rat kidney. *J Am Soc Nephrol* 2002;13:910.

290. Eitner F, Ostendorf T, Kretzler M, et al. PDGF-C expression in the developing and normal adult human kidney and in glomerular diseases. *J Am Soc Nephrol* 2003;14:1145.

291. Whitby DJ, Ferguson MW. The extracellular matrix of lip wounds in fetal, neonatal, and adult mice. *Development* 1991;112:651.

292. Kriz W, Hähnel B, Rösener S, et al. Long-term treatment of rats with FGF-2 results in focal segmental glomerulosclerosis. *Kidney Int* 1995;48:1435.

293. Strutz F, Zeisberg M, Hemmerlein B, et al. Basic fibroblast growth factor expression is increased in human renal fibrogenesis and may mediate autocrine fibroblast proliferation. *Kidney Int* 2000;57:1521.

294. Strutz F, Okada H, Lo CW, et al. Identification and characterization of fibroblast-specific protein 1 (FSP1). *J Cell Biol* 1995;130:393.

295. Okada H, Danoff TM, Fischer A, et al. Identification of a novel cis-acting element for fibroblast-specific transcription of the FSP1 gene. *Am J Physiol* 1998;275:F306.

296. Iwano M, Fischer A, Okada H, et al. Conditional abatement of tissue fibrosis using nucleoside analogs to selectively corrupt dna replication in transgenic fibroblasts. *Mol Ther* 2001;3:149.

297. Wiggins R, Goyal M, Merritt S, et al. Vascular adventitial cell expression of collagen I messenger ribonucleic acid in anti-glomerular basement membrane antibody-induced crescentic nephritis in the rabbit. A cellular source for interstitial collagen synthesis in inflammatory renal disease. *Lab Invest* 1993;68:557.

298. Strutz F, Müller GA, Neilson EG. Transdifferentiation: a new angle on renal fibrosis. *Exp Nephrol* 1996;4:267.

299. Hay ED, Zuk A. Transformations between epithelium and mesenchyme: normal, pathological, and experimentally induced. *Am J Kidney Dis* 1995;26:678.

300. Zeisberg M, Kalluri R. The role of epithelial-to-mesenchymal transition in renal fibrosis. *J Mol Med* 2004;82:175.

301. Ng YY, Huang TP, Yang WC, et al. Tubular epithelial-myofibroblast transdifferentiation in progressive tubulointerstitial fibrosis in 5/6 nephrectomized rats. *Kidney Int* 1998;54:864.

302. Fan JM, Ng YY, Hill PA, et al. Transforming growth factor-beta regulates tubular epithelial-myofibroblast transdifferentiation in vitro. *Kidney Int* 1999;56:1455.

303. Strutz F, Zeisberg M, Ziyadeh FN, et al. Role of basic fibroblast growth factor-2 in epithelial-mesenchymal transformation. *Kidney Int* 2002;61:1714.

304. Zeisberg M, Maeshima Y, Mosterman B, et al. Renal fibrosis. Extracellular matrix microenvironment regulates migratory behavior of activated tubular epithelial cells. *Am J Pathol* 2002;160:2001.

305. Yang J, Shultz RW, Mars WM, et al. Disruption of tissue-type plasminogen activator gene in mice reduces renal interstitial fibrosis in obstructive nephropathy. *J Clin Invest* 2002;110:1525.

306. Brito PL, Fioretto P, Drummond K, et al. Proximal tubular basement membrane width in insulin-dependent diabetes mellitus. *Kidney Int* 1998;53:754.

307. Li Y, Yang J, Dai C, et al. Role for integrin-linked kinase in mediating tubular epithelial to mesenchymal transition and renal interstitial fibrogenesis. *J Clin Invest* 2003;112:503.

308. Tian YC, Fraser D, Attisano L, et al. TGF-beta1-mediated alterations of renal proximal tubular epithelial cell phenotype. *Am J Physiol Renal Physiol* 2003;285:F130.

309. Lonnemann G, Shapiro L, Engler-Blum G, et al. Cytokines in human renal interstitial fibrosis. I. IL-1 is an autocrine growth factor for cultured fibrosis-derived kidney fibroblasts. *Kidney Int* 1995;47:837.

310. Frank J, Engler-Blum G, Müller GA. Characterization of a monoclonal antibody (TN20) specific for cultured human renal fibroblasts. *J Am Soc Nephrol* 1993;4:651A.

311. Johnson DW, Saunders HJ, Baxter RC, et al. Paracrine stimulation of human renal fibroblasts by proximal tubule cells. *Kidney Int* 1998;54:747.

312. Phillips AO, Topley N, Morrisey K, et al. Basic fibroblast growth factor stimulates the release of preformed transforming growth factor beta 1 from human proximal tubular cells in the absence of de novo gene transcription or mRNA translation. *Lab Invest* 1997;76:591.

313. Fine LG, Orphanides C, Norman JT. Progressive renal disease: the chronic hypoxia hypothesis. *Kidney Int* 1998;53(Suppl 65):S74.

314. Fisher JW. Erythropoietin: physiologic and pharmacologic aspects. *Proc Soc Exp Biol Med* 1997;216:358.

315. Kairaitis LK, Wang Y, Gassmann M, et al. HIF-1α expression follows microvascular loss in advanced murine Adriamycin nephrosis. *Am J Physiol Renal Physiol* 2004;288:F198.

316. Manotham K, Tanaka T, Matsumoto M, et al. Evidence of tubular hypoxia in the early phase in the remnant kidney model. *J Am Soc Nephrol* 2004;15:1277.

317. Matsumoto M, Tanaka T, Yamamoto T, et al. Hypoperfusion of peritubular capillaries induces chronic hypoxia before progression of tubulointerstitial injury in a progressive model of rat glomerulonephritis. *J Am Soc Nephrol* 2004;15:1574.

318. Ong AC, Jowett TP, Firth JD, et al. An endothelin-1 mediated autocrine growth loop involved in human renal tubular regeneration. *Kidney Int* 1995;48:390.

319. Orphanides C, Fine LG, Norman JT. Hypoxia stimulates proximal tubular cell matrix production via a TGF- beta1-independent mechanism. *Kidney Int* 1997;52:637.

320. Tanaka T, Hanafusa N, Ingelfinger JR, et al. Hypoxia induces apoptosis in SV40-immortalized rat proximal tubular cells through the mitochondrial pathways, devoid of HIF1-mediated upregulation of Bax. *Biochem Biophys Res Commun* 2003;309:222.

321. Manotham K, Tanaka T, Matsumoto M, et al. Transdifferentiation of cultured tubular cells induced by hypoxia. *Kidney Int* 2004;65:871.

322. Ma LJ, Nakamura S, Whitsitt JS, et al. Regression of sclerosis in aging by an angiotensin inhibition-induced decrease in PAI-1. *Kidney Int* 2000;58:2425.

323. Boffa JJ, Lu Y, Placier S, et al. Regression of renal vascular and glomerular fibrosis: role of angiotensin II receptor antagonism and matrix metalloproteinases. *J Am Soc Nephrol* 2003;14:1132.

324. Adamczak M, Gross ML, Krtil J, et al. Reversal of glomerulosclerosis after high-dose enalapril treatment in subtotally nephrectomized rats. *J Am Soc Nephrol* 2003;14:2833.

325. Koo JW, Kim Y, Rozen S, et al. Enalapril accelerates remodeling of the renal interstitium after release of unilateral ureteral obstruction in rats. *J Nephrol* 2003;16:203.

326. Luo G, Hofmann C, Bronckers AL, et al. BMP-7 is an inducer of nephrogenesis, and is also required for eye development and skeletal patterning. *Genes Dev* 1995;9:2808.

327. Karsenty G, Luo G, Hofmann C, et al. BMP 7 is required for nephrogenesis, eye development, and skeletal patterning. *Ann NY Acad Sci* 1996;785:98.

328. Vukicevic S, Kopp JB, Luyten FP, et al. Induction of nephrogenic mesenchyme by osteogenic protein 1 (bone morphogenetic protein 7). *Proc Natl Acad Sci USA* 1996;93:9021.

329. Wang S, Hirschberg R. BMP7 antagonizes TGF-beta -dependent fibrogenesis in mesangial cells. *Am J Physiol Renal Physiol* 2003;284:F1006.

330. Vukicevic S, Basic V, Rogic D, et al. Osteogenic protein-1 (bone morphogenetic protein-7) reduces severity of injury after ischemic acute renal failure in rat. *J Clin Invest* 1998;102:202.

331. Hruska KA, Guo G, Wozniak M, et al. Osteogenic protein-1 prevents renal fibrogenesis associated with ureteral obstruction. *Am J Physiol Renal Physiol* 2000;279:F130.

332. Zeisberg M, Hanai J, Sugimoto H, et al. BMP-7 counteracts TGF-beta1-induced epithelial-to-mesenchymal transition and reverses chronic renal injury. *Nat Med* 2003;9:964.

333. Ikeda Y, Jung YO, Kim H, et al. Exogenous bone morphogenetic protein-7 fails to attenuate renal fibrosis in rats with overload proteinuria. *Nephron Exp Nephrol* 2004;97:e123.

334. Fioretto P, Steffes MW, Sutherland DE, et al. Reversal of lesions of diabetic nephropathy after pancreas transplantation. *N Engl J Med* 1998;339:69.

335. Hammel P, Couvelard A, O'Toole D, et al. Regression of liver fibrosis after biliary drainage in patients with chronic pancreatitis and stenosis of the common bile duct. *N Engl J Med* 2001;344:418.

336. Miric G, Dallemagne C, Endre Z, et al. Reversal of cardiac and renal fibrosis by pirfenidone and spironolactone in streptozotocin-diabetic rats. *Br J Pharmacol* 2001;133:687.

CHAPTER 58 ■ ACUTE POSTSTREPTOCCAL GLOMERULONEPHRITIS AND OTHER BACTERIAL INFECTION-RELATED GLOMERULONEPHRITIS

SIDNEY KOBRIN AND MICHAEL P. MADAIO

Acute glomerulonephritis is characterized by the sudden appearance of hematuria, proteinuria, and red blood cell casts. The differential diagnosis of this syndrome is listed in Table 58-1(1). The initial diagnostic approach includes clinical evaluation and serologic determinations. Pathologic evaluation is very useful in confirming the diagnosis and defining the extent of inflammation and fibrosis. This chapter will consider glomerulonephritis associated with bacterial infections. Glomerular disease that accompanies infection with other organisms is covered in subsequent chapters. Acute poststreptococcal glomerulonephritis is the prototype, and it is distinguished from the other causes of acute glomerulonephritis by its typical serologic, histologic, and chronological features. A link between streptococci and acute glomerulonephritis can be traced to epidemics of scarlet fever in the 18th century (reviewed in [2]). During the earlier part of the 20th century, it was recognized that infection with β-hemolytic streptococci could lead to glomerulonephritis (2–5). Since this discovery, the clinical, serologic, and histologic features of the disease have been carefully documented, and there has been considerable progress in identifying the pathogenic mechanisms that participate in this disease. These features will be the focus of the initial discussion; consideration of other bacterial infections that may lead to acute glomerulonephritis will follow.

ACUTE POSTSTREPTOCOCCAL GLOMERULONEPHRITIS (APSGN)

Epidemiology and Incidence

APSGN may occur sporadically or in epidemic form. Although the sporadic form is more common, information obtained about the disease through analysis of epidemics has been particularly revealing (6–24). It affects children more than adults, with the peak age incidence from 2 to 6 years (Table 58-2). Approximately 5% of cases are found among children younger than 2 years, and 5 to 10% of patients with the disease are older than 40. Spread among family members is common, and nephritogenic streptococci have also been isolated from household pets with scabies (25). Males more often have clinical evidence of nephritis, although females are more likely to have subclinical disease (14,26). Patients with subclinical nephritis outnumber those of overt nephritis by a ratio ranging from 4:1 to 10:1 (2). This is consistent with pathologic review of biopsy specimens (nonepidemic form), where evidence of healed disease is greater than anticipated from the clinical diagnosis (27). In more temperate zones, APSGN occurs more commonly in winter months, and most often after pharyngitis,

whereas in the tropics, skin infection (i.e., impetigo) during the summer is usually the initiating event (28). Cyclical outbreaks of epidemic forms have been reported by Rodriguez-Iturbe and others, although the reason for these cycles has not been fully explained (20,29,30).

APSGN follows infection with only certain groups of streptococci, and these strains are designated nephritogenic. Group A streptococci are responsible for the vast majority of cases, and among them certain types predominate (2). Occasionally non–group A streptococci have been linked to glomerulonephritis (31,32). "Nephritogenic" group A streptococci have been characterized serologically by their cell wall proteins, termed M and T proteins, and the known nephritogenic strains include the M types: 1, 2, 3, 4, 12, 18, 25, 49, 55, 57, 59, 60, and 61 (2,33–39). The risk of nephritis following infection with nephritogenic strains depends on the location of infection. For example, with type-49 streptococci, the risk of nephritis is five times greater with skin infections than with pharyngitis (28). Nephritis following pyoderma with types 47, 55, 57, and 60 is also common (2,14). Many cases have also been associated with strains that do not have an M or a T type designation. Nevertheless, the identification of nephritogenic strains suggests that factors unique to these strains are responsible for nephritis (see below). However, it should be emphasized that host factors are also important, because only a minority (approximately 10%) of patients infected with nephritogenic strains develop overt disease. ASPGN has been reported following renal transplantation, although these patients are at no greater risk for the disease (40).

Pathology

Most commonly there is diffuse glomerulonephritis, although the severity of involvement usually varies among glomeruli and within segments of individual glomeruli (40–44). On light microscopy, there is cellular infiltration and glomerular cellular proliferation (45) (Fig. 58-1). The predominant cell types depend on the timing of the biopsy. Within the first 2 weeks of disease, neutrophils, eosinophils, lymphocytes, and monocytes are present in the capillary lumen and in the mesangium, and endothelial and mesangial cell proliferation is prominent (2,35,46). CD4 T cells usually exceed CD8 cells early on, whereas later CD8 cells predominate. Periglomerular accumulation of T cells may also be observed (47). Occlusion of capillary lumen is not unusual, and mesangial expansion is typical (44). Intracapillary fibrin thrombi and deposits and/or necrosis are observed in some cases. This pattern characterizes the so-called exudative phase. During this period, intermittent thickening of capillary walls, corresponding to large

TABLE 58-1

MAJOR CAUSES OF ACUTE NEPHRITIS

Low serum complement level[a]	Normal serum complement level
Systemic diseases	**Systemic diseases**
Systemic lupus erythematosus (focal ~75%, diffuse ~90%)[a]	Polyarteritis nodosa
Cryoglobulinemia (~85%)	Wegener's granulomatosis
Subacute bacterial endocarditis (~90%)	Hypersensitivity vasculitis
"Shunt" nephritis (~90%)	Henoch-Schönlein purpura
	Goodpasture's syndrome
	Visceral abscess
Renal diseases	**Renal diseases**
Acute poststreptococcal glomerulonephritis (~90%)	IgG-IgA nephropathy
Membranoproliferative glomerulonephritis	Idiopathic RPGN (rapidly progressive glomerulonephritis)
Type I (~50%–80%)[b]	Anti-GBM disease
Type II (~80%–90%)	Pauci-immune[c] (no immune deposits)
	Immune-deposit disease

Normal serum complement levels indicate that production of complement components is keeping up with consumption; it does not exclude participation of complement in the inflammatory process. Repeat measurements useful (2–3 × 1 week apart). Consistently normal serum levels are useful in narrowing the diagnostic possibilities.
[a]Percentages indicate the approximate frequencies of depressed C3 or hemolytic complement levels during the course of disease.
[b]Most common pathologic findings associated with hepatitis C infection.
[c]Pauci-immune indicates lack of significant glomerular deposition of immunoglobulin by direct immunofluorescence. Many patients have circulating ANCA.
(Reprinted with permission from: Madaio MP, Harrington JT. The diagnosis of glomerular diseases: acute glomerulonephritis and the nephrotic syndrome. *Arch Intern Med* 2001;161.)

subepithelial immune deposits, are often observed (i.e., by trichrome staining). Focal capsular adhesions or segmental crescents are relatively common. Abundant crescent formation is unusual, although it is occasionally observed in more severe situations (2,48). Over 4 to 6 weeks, polymorphonuclear neutrophils (PMNs) are no longer present, and hypercellularity with mononuclear cells (mesangial cells and/or infiltrating monocytes) predominates. During this latter phase, capillary lumens are usually patent. Glomerular hypercellularity usually slowly resolves, although mesangial hypercellularity may persist for months. Extraglomerular abnormalities are usually not as prominent during either phase, however interstitial edema, tubular necrosis, scattered mononuclear interstitial infiltrates, and/or mild arteriolitis has been observed (49). Severe vasculitis has been reported but is unusual (50–52).

By immunofluorescence microscopy, deposits of immunoglobulin G (IgG) and C3 are distributed in a diffuse granular pattern within the mesangium and capillary walls (25,44, 53–55). C3 is invariably present, whereas the quantity of IgG depends on the timing of the biopsy, and it is not uncommon to see only C3 deposits very early or late in disease. IgM is often present early in disease but may also be observed in smaller amounts later on. Significant amounts of IgA suggest an alternative diagnosis (e.g., IgA nephropathy or Henoch-Schönlein purpura). C1q and C4 are not usually detected; however, properdin and terminal complement components (C5b-9) are often present and distributed in a granular pattern. Fibrin deposits are occasionally detected in more severe cases. Different patterns of immune deposition have been observed, however they are likely related to the timing of renal biopsy. Early in the disease (the first few weeks), the fine granular appearance of immune deposits often gives a "starry-sky-like" appearance; this pattern is associated with glomerular hypercellularity (53–55). With resolution of the disease (i.e., 4–6 weeks after onset), the immune deposits take on a more mesangial pattern, prior to disappearing. C3 may be present in the absence of detectable Ig, either very early in the disease (less than 2 weeks) or with disease resolution (i.e., with resolution of the IgG deposits). In about one-fourth of cases, the deposits are large, and they aggregate in a "rope" of "garland-like" pattern, and this pattern may be associated with persistent mesangial hypercellularity on light microscopy. When these type deposits are present, they may last for months, and they may be associated with persistence of heavy proteinuria and development glomerulosclerosis (53–56). By contrast, transition to a more mesangial pattern (IF) is usually associated with clinical and pathologic resolution. Occasionally immune deposits in small vessels occur in the setting of vasculitis.

Dome-shaped subepithelial electron-dense deposits that resemble camel "humps" are the most characteristic feature on electron microscopy (46). These humps contain Ig, are most abundant within the first month, and are frequently observed near epithelial slit pores (10,42,54,57). They have been associated with heavy proteinuria, and they usually resolve within 4 to 8 weeks. In later stages of the disease, they may be absent; however, remnant electron-lucent areas are occasionally

TABLE 58-2

GENERAL CHARACTERISTICS OF APSGN

Age:	Children > adults (5% <2 yr; 5%–10% >40 yr)
Sex:	Male > Female

Clinical manifestations: subclinical 4–10 × >overt nephritis
Site of infection: pharynx (temperate zones), skin (tropics)

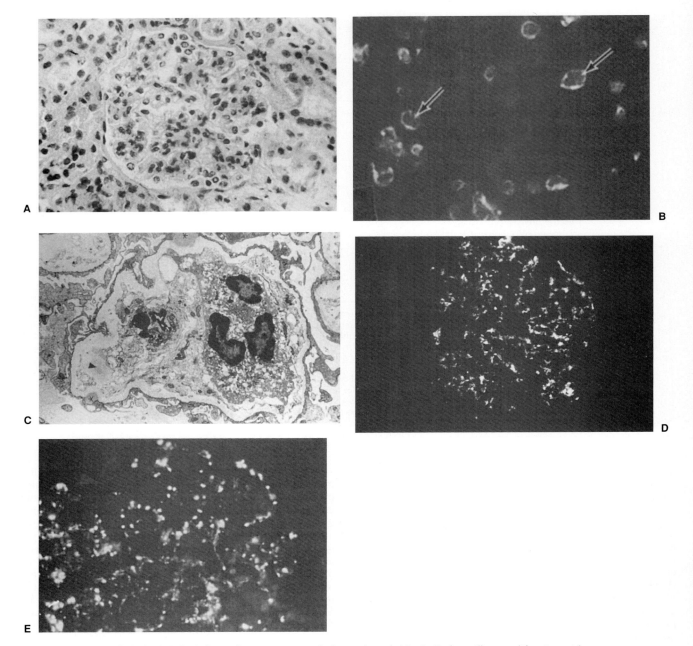

FIGURE 58-1. Pathology of poststreptococcal glomerulonephritis. **A:** Endocapillary proliferation with increased number of messangial cells and glomerular infiltration with neutrophils (PMN). Biopsy specimen taken 10 days after the beginning of symptoms. (Hematoxylin & eosin ×500.) **B:** Intraglomerular cells reactive with OKM1 monoclonal antibody (*arrows*) in a biopsy specimen obtained 14 days after the initial symptoms. Monocytes and neutrophils are recognized by the antibody, and reactivity with antihuman lactoferrin (which identifies PMN) in serial sections was use to define glomerular moncyte infiltration. **C:** Glomerular capillary loop with polymorphonuclear leukocytes in the lumen. Electron-dense deposits are present in subepithelial ("humps") (*) and subendothelial (◁) locations. (×12,000). **D:** C3 deposits (+1) in the glomerular basement membranes and mesangium. (FITC-labeled antihuman ×500.) **E:** Glomerular deposition of the membrane attack complex of complement in a biopsy specimen obtained 16 days after onset identified with monoclonal poly-C9 antibody, which recognizes a neoantingen on C9. Pattern and localization of deposits is similar to the one found for C3 and C5. (B and E reproduced with permission from: Parra G, et al. Cell populations and membrane attack complex in glomeruli of patients with poststreptococcal glomerulonephritis: identification using monoclonal antibodies by indirect immunofluorescence. *Clin Immunol Immunopathol* 1984;33:324.)

observed and provide diagnostic clues (58). Subendothelial, mesangial, and intramembranous deposits (along with smaller subepithelial deposits) are often present in variable amounts, and they usually persist after resolution of subepithelial deposits (humps) (58). Patients with large subendothelial deposits, without mesangial deposits, were found to have more proteinuria and edema (59). Large intramembranous deposits are associated with the garland-like pattern of immune deposits on immunofluorescence described previously (54). The basement membrane itself is usually of normal diameter, although thickening has occasionally been observed (49). Cellular infiltration and proliferation depends upon timing of the biopsy, as described above in the description of light microscopic changes.

Pathophysiology

The association with streptococcal infections has largely stimulated investigation of the pathogenesis of this disease. However, since only certain strains of streptococci are "nephritogenic," leading to the notion that there are unique properties of these strains. Furthermore, not all individuals infected with nephritogenic streptococci (i.e., as detected during epidemics of nephritis) develop disease, suggesting that host factors are also important for disease expression. Based on these observations, a number of theories pertaining to pathogenesis have emerged. For disease expression, the susceptible host must both be infected with a nephritogenic strain and mount a pathogenic immune response. With regard to the former, recent analysis of nephritogenic streptococci and their products has provided novel insights, although differences of opinion pertaining to the precise sequence of events leading to immune deposit formation and inflammation persist. Three major pathogenic theories have emerged, and they will be considered briefly.

A popular theory that originated in the 1960s invokes deposition of streptococcal antigens within glomeruli (60,61). Accordingly, nephritogenic streptococci produce proteins with unique antigenic determinants that, in addition to eliciting a potent antibody response, have a particular affinity for sites within the normal glomerulus. Following release into circulation, streptococcal protein fragments encounter ligands within glomeruli and lodge there, affixed to sites for which they have intrinsic affinity. Once glomerular-bound, they activate complement directly by attracting properdin, leading to stimulation of the alternate complement pathway. At the same time, the glomerular-bound streptococcal proteins serve as planted antigens for immune complex formation with circulating antistreptococcal antibodies. Immune complex formation leads to additional complement fixation that, in turn, leads to the recruitment of additional inflammatory mediators and cells. As importantly, the glomerular bound antibodies engage Fc receptor on circulating cells, which further enhances cellular infiltration, including mononuclear cells.

In support of this hypothesis, a number of candidate proteins have been identified that meet most of these criteria. A relatively small complex of intracellular anionic proteins, termed endostreptosins, have been isolated from nephritogenic streptococci by Lange, Treser, Yoshizawa and co-workers (36,61–64). Antibodies specific for these proteins react with glomeruli of patients with nephritis (presumably containing this antigen), and elevated antibody titers are present in patients with active disease. Administration of endostreptosin to rats resulted in glomerular localization of antigen for the first four days after injection, and this was followed by deposition of IgG and complement (65). This particular antigen complex is not unique to nephritogenic streptococci, however, and elevated antibody titers have been found in patients with streptococci

cal infections that do not develop nephritis, raising questions about its pathogenic relevance. Nevertheless, this is not surprising since *both* a nephritigenic antigen *and* a pathogenic immune response are necessary for disease expression. Treser et al. provide further insights (66). They isolated a potentially relevant antigen from this complex, termed PA-Ag (for preabsorbing antigen), with a molecular weight of 43,000 and pI of 4.7. Antibodies to PA-Ag were present in 30 of 31 patients with APSGN, whereas they were only detected in 1 of 36 individuals with uncomplicated group A streptococcal upper respiratory infections. Particularly noteworthy, PA-Ag, and not other streptococcal components were detected in glomeruli of patients with APSGN. Furthermore, PA-Ag was capable of activating the alternate complement pathway, suggesting that it is involved in the pathogenesis of this disease. In a series of elegant studies, Oda, Yoshizawa, and co-workers recently extended these observations (67,68). They isolated an antigen termed nephritis associated plasmin receptor (NAPlr) that binds to plasmin and extends its proteolytic activity. Both plasmin and the receptor (NAPlr) were present in biopsy specimens of ASPGN patients but not in other disease samples. This lead the investigators to postulate that when released into the circulation from nephritogenic strains, NAPlr binds to glomeruli. Thereafter it engages circulating plasmin, which, in turn, initiates nephritis by activating metalloproteinases and recruiting cells, and then by serving as a planted antigen for subsequent immune complex formation.

Zabriski and co-workers have also identified disease related protein (or set of proteins) (69,70). They described an extracellular, 46 kD protein, termed nephritis strain-associated protein (NKAP), isolated from strains derived from patients with APSGN, the secreted protein was not usually produced by other strains. Anti-NKAP antibodies were identified both in sera and 18 of 21 renal biopsies of APSGN patients (71). Although NKAP was initially thought to be streptokinase, subsequent evidence has proved that this is not the case (37,71,72). Peake and co-workers isolated a protein with similar properties that was capable of both activating complement and binding to normal human glomeruli (73). Poon-King et al. identified yet another closely related protein (with similar properties as NKAP (74), initially termed nephritis plasmin binding protein (NPBP). Subsequently, sequence analysis of NPBP demonstrated sequence homology with streptococcal pyrogenic exotoxin B precursor (SPEB, previously termed zymogen). Since plasmin is capable of binding to glomerular-bound NPBP, this could account for activation of the complement cascade and initiation of inflammation, observed prior to the deposition of IgG early in disease. In support of this conclusion, sera from ASPGN patients has been observed to have anti-SPEB antibodies, and the SPEB antigen was demonstrated in glomerular lesions (75).

There has been support for other nephritogenic proteins, and there may not be a single species. Vogt et al. identified a cationic proteinase produced by nephritogenic streptococci, related to an erythrogenic toxin (76). Serum antibodies to this protein are present in many patients with APSGN but not other forms of nephritis. Bergy and Stinson described a soluble heparin-inhabitable basement membrane binding protein derived from a nephritogenic strain that also bound to tissue sections (77), and Glurich et al. identified streptococcal-derived proteins that bind to rabbit kidney *in vitro* and *in vivo* (78). Streptokinase has also been implicated by its capacity to induce nephritis in normal mice (78–80). Of potential clinical relevance, streptokinase activated complement directly within the kidney prior to antibody deposition, in a manner analogous to previous observations of glomerular complement activity patients in the early stages of APSGN. Although these and other proteins have not been as extensively studied as those described previously, it is likely that different proteins are involved in different patients, with host factors contributing to disease expression.

Another hypothesis, initially raised by McIntosh and co-workers, invokes alteration of normal IgG by streptococcal enzymes as the initial event. This has two effects. The altered IgG is recognized as a "foreign" antigen and elicits an antibody response. It also acquires affinity for glomeruli (e.g., it becomes more cationic) and deposits therein (81). Once deposited, this altered and relatively cationic IgG serves as a fixed or "planted"' glomerular antigen for the subsequent binding of anti-IgG. In support of this hypothesis, Fc receptors are present on streptococci (82,83). Furthermore, neuraminidase-producing streptococci are capable of desialation of Ig (making it more cationic) (84,85). Therefore streptococci have the capacity to engage IgG and render it pathogenic. Furthermore, elevated levels of both serum rheumatoid factor, neuraminidase activity, and free sialic acid are often present in patients with acute poststreptococcal GN, and anti-Ig antibodies have been eluted from the kidney of a patient with this disease (84,85).

Although neuraminades may effect neutrophil activity locally (86), neuraminidase-producing streptococci are not unique to patients with acute poststreptococcal glomerulonephritis, and rheumatoid factor activity is present in many individuals with streptococcal infection who do not develop glomerulonephritis.

The possibility of antigenic mimicry, between nephritogenic streptococci and normal glomerular antigens, has also been considered (reviewed in [36]). This hypothesis invokes the production of antibodies against streptococcal membrane proteins that share structural determinants with glomerular antigens. Early reports demonstrated that soluble glycoprotein derived from nephritogenic strains of streptococci induced nephritis in animals, and disease could be transferred to normal animals using antiserum from the diseased animals (87-89). Subsequently, antibodies against streptococcal cell membranes, derived from nephritis patients, were observed to cross-react with glomeruli (36). Furthermore, homologies between M proteins derived from nephritogenic strains and basement membrane antigens are consistent with this notion (90). Antibodies produced against a tetrapeptide (Ile-Arg-Leu-Arg) derived from the M-1 protein of a nephritogenic strain were found to cross-react with normal glomerular antigens in vitro (91,92). However, although the tetrapeptide shares homology with the cytoskeletal filament protein, vimentin, the pathogenic relevance of this cross-reaction is unclear (91). Similarly, antibodies to other extracellular antigens, including laminin, heparin sulfate, and type IV collagen have been detected in serum from patients with APSGN (93–95). It is tempting to speculate that different antibody-antigen interactions are responsible for glomerular deposits at different sites within glomeruli.

Other factors may also contribute to disease susceptibility. Outbreaks among families were first noted by Wells (96). This was confirmed by Dodge et al. and later by Rodriguez-Iturbe and co-workers; they observed that the familial incidence of disease during epidemics was higher that the attack rate in the population at large (26,41). Unfortunately genetic studies have thus far failed to support linkage (as opposed to rheumatic fever where genetic linkage has been found [97]). T cells, monocytes, platelets and endogenous glomerular cells (along with cytokines and chemokines produced by these cells) have been detected within APSGN lesions. They participate in the local inflammatory response, and along with upregulation of adhesion molecules (47,54,98–100), they influence the severity of disease. Additionally, streptococcal cell wall proteins and exotoxins may serve as superantigens to engage larger populations of T and B cells in the process.. The contribution of both infectious and host factors likely influence the specific characteristics and severity of disease. The reader is referred to Chapter 57

for a more general discussion of the role of these individual participants in glomerulonephritis.

Clinical Manifestations

Although not diagnostic, the symptoms of the disease are quite characteristic. However most patients present with only a few of the features of the *acute nephritic syndrome* (101). Typical presentations include edema, gross hematuria, and back pain, although the actual incidence of symptoms varies somewhat among reports (Table 58-3) (9,10,12–14,20,23,25,41,102). Anasarca is more common among young children (2). Occasionally, patients with gross hematuria will complain of dysuria. Transient oliguria is present in approximately one-half of the patients, but anuria is rare (2). Hypertension is found in 60% to 80% of patients at initial presentation, although hypertensive encephalopathy is unusual. Nevertheless, if untreated it may be associated with seizures (2,10). In others, encephalopathy may occur in the absence of significant hypertension, and this may be due to cerebral vasculitis (103). Some patients present with signs and symptoms of congestive heart failure; however, the coexistence of rheumatic fever is rare (14). Hypertension and heart failure are mostly due to sodium retention, and the renin-angiotensin system is typically suppressed (2). Decreased glomerular filtration rate may also contribute to sodium retention (14). Rapidly progressive glomerulonephritis with acute renal failure is unusual but has been well documented. (104). Hypertension and heart failure usually resolve after diuresis. Generalized symptoms, including anorexia, malaise, nausea, and vomiting are common at initial presentation, whereas arthralgias and skin rashes are uncommon. When the latter symptoms are observed, other causes of glomerulonephritis should also be considered (i.e., lupus, vasculitis). Backache in the lumbar region has been attributed to intrarenal edema with stretching of the renal capsule.

Children are more frequently affected than adults, although the disease can occur at any age, and it may be overlooked in the elderly (2,14,20,26,30). During epidemics, most infected with nephritogenic strains develop only subclinical evidence of nephritis (i.e., abnormal urinalysis; see above) (26,28,41,105),

---

TABLE 58-3

CLINICAL AND LABORATORY MANIFESTATIONS OF APSGN

Clinical	
Edema	85%
Gross hematuria	30%
Back pain	5%
Oliguria (transient)	50%
Hypertension	60%–80%
Nephrotic syndrome	5%
Laboratory	
Urinalysis: proteinuria, hematuria, casts	100%
Nephrotic range proteinuria	10%
Serum creatinine ≥2 mg/dL	25%
Streptococcal antibody profile (streptozyme)	
in patients with pharyngitis	>95%
in patients with skin infections	80%
false positive rate	5%
Early Abic Rx prevents antibody response	
C3, C4, and/or CH50 depressed in	>90%
Hypergammaglobulinemia	90%
Cryoglobulinemia	75%

indicating that the disease may go unrecognized. Nephrotic syndrome occurs in 5% to 10% of children, but it is more frequently observed in adults (20%) (2). It may occur either at initial presentation or later in the course, with improvement of glomerular filtration rate (GFR). Rapidly progressive glomerulonephritis with acute renal failure occurs in fewer than 2% of children, and it is slightly more common in adults. In children, the clinical symptoms of acute glomerulonephritis usually resolve within 1 to 2 weeks; in adults, resolution may be more prolonged, and there is a higher incidence of progressive renal disease (see below).

The latent period between streptococcal infection and nephritis depends on the site of infection. Following pharyngitis, it is usually 1 to 3 weeks, whereas after skin infection, it is more prolonged at 3 to 6 weeks (14). Shorter latent periods of days (i.e., hematuria following upper respiratory infection) suggest an alternative diagnosis (i.e., IgA nephropathy). The preceding infection may be accompanied by severe symptoms (i.e., fever, pharyngitis), or be relatively asymptomatic. In many cases, it is not possible to identify an antecedent infection with certainty. Regional lymphadenopathy may be present, even after other symptoms and signs of the primary infection have resolved, and their presence should provide clues to the diagnosis. Typically the acute nephritic syndrome lasts 4 to 7 days, however it may be more prolonged in adults, especially in those presenting with rapidly progressive glomerulonephritis (RPGN) and crescentic glomerulonephritis (23). Coincident rheumatic fever is unusual (106), as is coincident arthritis (107), however glomerulonephritis may be associated with infections at other sites. Recurrent episodes are uncommon, however repeated bouts of hematuria may occur during the initial episode. Although de novo disease involving transplanted kidneys is usual, it may be associated with deterioration of graft function (108). Extrarenal manifestations are uncommon but include arthritis and choroiditis (109).

Laboratory Findings and Diagnosis

The urinalysis is always abnormal (see Table 58-3). Hematuria and proteinuria are invariably present, and casts are common. Red blood cell casts are frequently detected in a freshly voided specimen, and dysmorphic red blood cells indicative of glomerular hematuria are usually detected by phase-contrast microscopy. Renal tubular cells and casts, granular and/or pigmented casts, and white blood cells are also commonly found. White blood cell casts are occasionally observed in patients with severe exudative glomerulonephritis. Proteinuria is characteristic; however, nephrotic syndrome occurs in only 5% of patients at initial presentation (43,110). Occasionally in patients with severe disease at onset, there may be a transient increase in proteinuria to the nephrotic range with improvement in the glomerular filtration rate associated as the disease resolves.

The GFR is reduced and the serum creatinine is usually elevated, but the serum creatinine may remain within the upper limits of the normal laboratory range. Approximately 25% of patients have a serum creatinine greater than 2 mg/dL (2). The GFR, when measured, is almost always depressed in the initial stages of the disease, and it returns toward normal with disease resolution. Anemia may be present during the acute illness and early recovery period (111).

Throat cultures are frequently positive in affected individuals with pharyngitis. In the first 2 weeks of active nephritis the C3 and CH50 levels are significantly depressed in more than 90% of patients (2,101,112–114). The C4 and C2 levels are usually normal or only mildly decreased; marked depression suggests another diagnosis. Properdin levels are decreased in over 50% of patients and reflect activation of the alternate

pathway of complement activation (115). Elevation of plasma levels of C5b–9 levels reflect the contribution of the membrane attack complex to pathogenesis (116). In most cases, the serum complement levels return to normal by 4 weeks; however, occasionally, it may take as long as 3 months (117). In patients with insidious and/or prolonged symptoms prior to visiting their physician, complement levels may have returned to normal at the time of initial presentation. The level of reduction of complement levels does not have prognostic significance. Persistent hypocomplementemia, however, is unusual and suggests another diagnosis (114). C3 nephritic factor may be present in low amounts, but marked and/or persistent elevations are more typical of membranoproliferative glomerulonephritis (101). Hypergammaglobulinemia is present in 90% of the patients, and polyclonal cryoglobulinemia (containing both IgG and IgM) is present in 75% of individuals with overt nephritis (2,118). Rheumatoid factor activity is found in about a third of patients early in the course of disease (2).

Antibodies to extracellular products of streptococci, as measured in the streptozyme test, are positive in more than 95% of patients with pharyngitis and 80% of patients with skin infections (2,14,39,119). These include anti-streptolysin (ASO), anti-hyaluronidase (AHase), anti-streptokinase (ASKase), anti-nicotinamide-adenine dinucleotidase (anti-NAD), and anti-DNAse B antibodies. The ASO, anti-DNAse B, anti-NAD, and AHase are more commonly positive after pharyngeal infections, whereas anti-DNAase B and AHase are more often positive following skin infections (120–122). Overall, these tests are relatively specific for streptococcal infections, with a 5% false-positive rate. However, since the incidence of streptococcal infections in the general population is relatively high (especially in young children), they may be elevated in patients with unrelated streptococcal infection and glomerulonephritis. Antibodies to nephritogenic streptococcal antigens may prove to be of diagnostic significance, but they require further evaluation (2,119) (123). Overall, antibody titers are generally elevated at 1 week, peak at 1 month, and fall toward their preinfection level after many months (124,125). An increasing antibody titer is indicative of recent infection. Antibodies against M proteins are type-specific and confer strain-specific immunity (38). They are detectable at 4 weeks following infection and persist for years, however the antibody levels (to M proteins) are unrelated to the severity of disease. Early treatment with antibiotic therapy often prevents the antibody response to both extracellular products and M proteins. Negative results in a patient who previously received antibiotics, therefore, do not exclude the diagnosis.

Natural History and Prognosis

In general, the overall prognosis is very good, as less than 0.5% die of the initial disease and, fewer than 2% of patients die or develop end-stage renal disease (6,8,11,15–17,20,21,24,43,126,127). Both the natural history of this particular disease and management of its complications contribute to the excellent outcome. Children have a better prognosis than adults, and patients older than 40 years with rapidly progressive renal failure and crescentic glomerulonephritis have a worse prognosis (11,20,30). Patients with RPGN associated with post-streptococcal disease have a better prognosis than other forms of RPGN; recovery after short-term dialysis dependence is not atypical, although renal function may not return completely to normal. There appears to be no difference in outcome with either epidemic or sporadic forms, although conclusions regarding prognosis are largely derived from well-documented epidemics in children. By contrast, opinion for less favorable outcomes come from smaller series of sporadic cases in adults (2). Persistent urinary and histologic abnormalities are common in both adults and children and may persist for years (11,19,128). The persistence of proteinuria at 3 and 10 years is approximately 15% and 2%, respectively (128). In most large series of well-documented cases, these abnormalities eventually resolve, and the incidence of chronic renal failure is low.

Patients with prolonged nephrotic syndrome or persistence of heavy proteinuria have a worse prognosis, and this is often associated with an evolution to a "garland"-like pattern of immune deposits with disease progression (21,53–55). In one series of adults with APSGN, a larger percentage of patients developed persistent hypertension and/or end-stage renal disease years after the initial episode of acute of acute glomerulonephritis (43,129). It was unclear, however, whether progressive renal failure was due to nephrosclerosis associated with poorly controlled hypertension or progressive glomerular scarring. As previously discussed, most studies of patients with APSGN have not confirmed this pessimistic outlook, and it is likely that selection of patients for follow-up influenced the results in the one series (2). Nevertheless, the results are consistent with the notion that a small group of patients with residual damage may develop progressive renal insufficiency.

Treatment and Prevention

The therapy for patients with acute post-streptococcal glomerulonephritis is symptomatic and dependent on the clinical severity of the illness. The major aims of therapy of acute nephritis are control of blood pressure and treatment of volume overload. During the acute phase of the disease, salt and water should be restricted. If significant edema and/or hypertension develop, diuretics should be administered. Furosemide usually provides a prompt diuresis, with reduction of blood pressure. For hypertension uncontrolled by diuretics, vasodilators (i.e., calcium channel blockers or angiotensin converting enzyme [ACE] inhibitors) are usually effective. Intravenous agents may be required for management of rare cases of either severe or malignant hypertension. The serum potassium should be monitored and treated appropriately. Dialysis may be necessary to treat uremia. Restriction of physical activity is appropriate during the first few days of the illness but is unnecessary once the patient feels well. The most acute phase of the illness usually resolves within a week, and most patients undergo spontaneous diuresis after that interval.

Steroids, immunosuppressive agents, and/or plasmapheresis are generally not indicated. In patients with rapidly progressive renal failure, however, a renal biopsy may be indicated. If crescents are present in over 30% of glomeruli, we recommend treatment with a short course of intravenous pulse steroid therapy (500 mg to 1 g per 1.73 M^2 of intravenous Solu-Medrol [Upjohn] daily, for 3 to 5 successive days). Although there are no controlled trials of this therapy in patients with acute poststreptococcal glomerulonephritis, it has been beneficial in patients with rapidly progressive glomerulonephritis associated with other diseases (see Chapter 60). We do not recommend more prolonged treatment with steroids or other immunosuppressive therapy. Long term antihypertensive therapy in patients with hypertension and chronic renal insufficiency is essential to prevent the development of renal failure, and angiotensin converting enzyme inhibitors are the drugs of choice for this purpose.

Specific therapy for streptococcal infections is an essential part of the therapeutic regimen. This includes treatment of both the patient (if infected) and any infected family member or close personal contact. Throat cultures should be performed on all these individuals, and treatment with penicillin (oral penicillin G 250 mg four times a day [qid] for 7 to 10 days) or erythromycin (250 mg qid for 7 to 10 days) in patients allergic to penicillin, is indicated to prevent both the development of

nephritis in carriers and the spread of nephritogenic strains to others. Whether or not early treatment of infected patients prevents nephritis is not known. For patients with skin infections, attention to personal hygiene is also essential. In epidemics, empirical prophylactic treatment of patients at risk, including close contacts and family members is recommended (130).

BACTERIAL ENDOCARDITIS

Epidemiologic Patterns

The precise incidence of glomerulonephritis in patients with bacterial endocarditis is unclear because prospective analysis of renal tissue in a large cohort of patients has never been conducted. Investigations to define the incidence of this complication have the typical limitations of retrospective studies or/and lacked histologic confirmation (131,132). Autopsy studies are difficult to interpret, as the presence of azotemia in patients with endocarditis may be associated with higher mortality rates, thereby overestimating the incidence of glomerulonephritis. Conversely effective antibiotic therapy may underestimate the frequency of this problem. Rates derived from renal biopsy studies often exaggerate the severity and underestimate the prevalence of glomerulonephritis, because biopsy is usually performed in patients with the most significant renal dysfunction. By contrast, studies that depend solely on urinalysis for diagnosis overestimate the prevalence of disease, because hematuria and leukocyturia may be due to either tubulointerstitial nephritis or embolic disease. Furthermore, advances in early, more effective therapies, and changes in the most common causative organisms have led to changes in the incidence of glomerulonephritis over recent years.

Despite these limitations, two trends have emerged. The overall incidence of glomerulonephritis associated with *Streptococcus viridans*–induced endocarditis has declined in the antibiotic era. Coincident with this decline has been the rise in glomerulonephritis associated with acute bacterial endocarditis, particularly involving *Staphylococcus aureus*. While *S. viridans* and *S. aureus* remain the most common causes of glomerulonephritis associated with subacute and acute endocarditis, respectively, isolated reports of other organisms such as Gram-positive and Gram-negative bacteria, *Coxiella burnetti*, and fungi have also been linked to glomerulonephritis associated with endocarditis. Several new associations between bacterial endocarditis and glomerulonephritis have been reported in recent years, including endocarditis due to *Bartonella henselae*, Brucellosis, and Actinobacillus (131,132). A heightened index of suspicion as well as better culture techniques to identify fastidious organisms may explain the emergence of these associations. The evolutionary trend regarding *S. viridans* and *S. aureus* is briefly reviewed below.

In the preantibiotic era, glomerulonephritis was documented in as many as 82% of patients dying from subacute bacterial endocarditis (SBE) (133–136). Following the availability of antibiotics, the prevalence of postmortem documentation of glomerulonephritis in patients dying from subacute bacterial endocarditis decreased precipitously to 25% (132–136). Early studies also suggested that glomerulonephritis occurred less frequently in patients with acute bacterial endocarditis; estimates of glomerulonephritis in the antibiotic era ranged from 36% of patients with fatal acute bacterial endocarditis to 82% of patients with fatal subacute bacterial endocarditis (133). It was assumed that the higher incidence of glomerulonephritis in subacute disease was due to differences in the virulence of the causative organisms. Investigators reasoned that infection with less virulent organisms led to a more indolent and prolonged course, resulting in a greater antibody response that lead to a higher incidence of immunologically mediated events (129,132,137–139). More recent studies, however, indicated that acute endocarditis is responsible for a greater proportion of endocarditis-associated glomerulonephritis than what was originally reported, suggesting that either strain or host dependent factors were also operative. In this regard an autopsy series reported by Neugarten et al. found that *S. aureus* caused a disproportionate frequency of glomerulonephritis due to acute bacterial endocarditis (132).

Several factors may account for the changing epidemiologic pattern. *S. viridans*–associated subacute bacterial endocarditis has become much less common, due to both the declining occurrence of rheumatic fever in the United States as well as the successful implementation of prophylactic antibiotic regimens in patients with known valvular lesions. In addition, earlier recognition of endocarditis, with institution of more effective antibiotic and/or surgical therapy has led to a shorter duration of infection and associated complications (136).

Coincident with this decline, there has been an increase in acute endocarditis in intravenous drug abusers. This is often due to *S. aureus* bacteremia leading to infection of normal heart valves, and clinical evidence of glomerulonephritis has been found in 40% to 78% of patients with *S. aureus* acute bacterial endocarditis (132,140,141). Particularly noteworthy, the mean duration of clinical illness prior to the onset of glomerulonephritis is less than 10 days, and many patients are treated with antibiotics during the prodromal period. This suggests that either intrinsic properties related to the causative organism, the immune response or both, predispose these individuals to this form of glomerulonephritis.

Pathologic Features

Although, like ASPGN, many features have been reported, a few typical patterns are more common. In general, the pathology can be divided into subacute and acute forms. Glomerular changes occurring with subacute endocarditis (e.g., due to *S. viridans*) are usually less severe. The lesions are typically focal and segmental, with increased cellularity in the mesangial and endothelial portions of the tuft (133,142). Polymorphonuclear cells (PMN) and macrophage infiltration contribute to the hypercellularity, along with endogenous cell proliferation. The capillary walls are thin and single contoured. By contrast, patients with the more acute form of the disease (e.g., due to *S. aureus*) typically have more severe disease with diffuse proliferative glomerulonephritis. The hypercellularity involves mesangial and endothelial cells along with infiltration of neutrophils and monocytes (131). Double contours of capillary walls may be present to varying degrees. Epithelial and fibroepithelial crescents, both partial and circumferential, may also be seen (132,143). Rarely, features more typical of membranoproliferative glomerulonephritis have been reported (132,144,145).

The interstitium is often edematous and infiltrated by mononuclear leukocytes (131,132,136,146). These changes may be either immune-mediated or related to infection. Alternatively, interstitial disease due to antibiotics (i.e., hypersensitivity) may complicate the situation (131,147). One or all of these features may be present in an individual patient, and the precise cause(s) may be difficult to reconcile. Histologic evidence of renal embolization has been reported in 30% to 60% of patients with fatal bacterial endocarditis and should be considered in patients with unexplained renal failure, although (148) clinical manifestations of renal embolization are infrequent (132).

By direct immunofluorescence, granular mesangial and subendothelial capillary wall deposits of IgG and/or IgM, and complement (C3 predominantly, C1q less frequently) are observed in all glomeruli in patients with either focal or diffuse

glomerulonephritis (131,146,149). Extraglomerular deposits are infrequent. By electron microscopy, subendothelial and mesangial deposits are usually present, although the quantity of deposits varies (146,149). By contrast, patients with acute *S. aureus* endocarditis often have subepithelial and intramembranous deposits 4 (149).

Clinical Features

The clinical manifestations depend on the duration and severity of disease. Microscopic hematuria, pyuria, and proteinuria are the most frequently detected abnormalities in patients with focal glomerulonephritis, however, these features may be absent despite histologic evidence of active disease (132,146). Less commonly, heavy proteinuria, hypertension, and renal dysfunction develop, and advanced renal failure leading to uremia may result. This latter scenario is more prevalent when bacteriologic cure is not achieved (132,146,150–152).

Microscopic hematuria and proteinuria are always present in patients with diffuse glomerulonephritis, and the nephrotic syndrome is not uncommon (i.e., ~15%) (132). Gross hematuria may be observed in patients with diffuse glomerulonephritis, although its appearance should raise suspicion of other conditions, such as either renal infarction or drug-induced interstitial nephritis (153). Pyuria occurs in approximately two-thirds of patients, and 15% to 30% of them have positive urine cultures (154,155). Unlike other forms of postinfectious glomerulonephritis, hypertension occurs infrequently (perhaps due to cardiac involvement) (132,156). Reduced GFR is variable, although it may occasionally be the presenting manifestation (148).

In the preantibiotic era, uremia contributed to the death of 5% to 10% of patients. With the advent of antibiotic therapy, mortality has fallen to less than 5% (156). With successful therapy, GFR typically is at its nadir prior to or shortly after the commencement of antibiotic therapy, and it usually improves with eradication of the infection (132). However, patients with advanced renal dysfunction at presentation, may have further deterioration of the GFR, requiring dialysis. The mortality rate is high in this population, and this is most likely related to the combination of severe infection and uremia.

Laboratory Findings

Although there are no pathognomonic findings, many serologic abnormalities are often present in patients with bacterial endocarditis. Rheumatoid factor is variable (i.e., detected in 10% to 70% of patients, depending on the series), however correlation between rheumatoid factor activity and the presence of glomerulonephritis is uncertain (157,158). Although the levels vary considerably, circulating immune complexes are found in 90% of patients with endocarditis, and high levels have been associated with a more indolent course, right sided lesions, and less virulent organisms (132,159–162). While mixed cryoglobulins are present in the serum of up to 95% of patients with endocarditis, there is no correlation between the levels of the cryoglobulins and the presence of glomerulonephritis (141,160). Recently, high titers of antineutrophil cytoplasmic antibody (ANCA) were found in a few patients with bacterial endocarditis-associated vasculitis and glomerulonephritis (163–165). Thus, endocarditis should be excluded in ANCA-positive patients, where either infection is suspected or manifestations of vasculitis are atypical.

Hypocomplementemia (depressed C3, C4 levels) is a frequent, but not invariable or specific, indicator of glomerulonephritis during the course of bacterial endocarditis (140, 150,151,156,160,161). In patients with acute bacterial endocarditis with diffuse glomerulonephritis, the serum complement levels were depressed in 68%. By contrast, hypocomplementemia has been documented more frequently in patients with diffuse glomerulonephritis associated with subacute bacterial endocarditis (~90%), whereas 60% of those with focal glomerulonephritis had reduced levels (132). Typically C4 and C1q levels are significantly depressed, invoking activation of the classic pathway (140,161). Nevertheless, there have also been reports of primarily alternative pathway activation, particularly in patients with *S. aureus* endocarditis and glomerulonephritis (132). Based on these observations, it was suggested that *S. aureus* bacterial wall antigens may be capable of direct activation of the alternative complement pathway, as described previously for nephritogenic streptococci. In this manner direct activation of complement by *S. aureus* (localized within glomeruli) may lead to glomerulonephritis soon after the onset of clinical endocarditis, without significant glomerular IgG deposition (132,166). Normalization of complement levels usually occurs with bacteriologic cure and resolution of glomerulonephritis. By contrast, persistent hypocomplementemia suggests failure to control infection, which in turn may lead to progressive renal failure (167). Therefore, in patients who initially manifest hypocomplementemia, serial complement determinations may serve as a guide to the activity of glomerulonephritis (132,167).

Differential Diagnosis

In addition to glomerulonephritis, several other renal abnormalities can occur in patients with endocarditis. These considerations are especially important in patients with deteriorating renal function. Embolization of valvular vegetations to the kidney can result in infarction, producing the gross pathologic appearance of "flea-bitten" kidneys (168). The clinical presentation is gross hematuria, sometimes associated with flank pain. Septic emboli may lead to renal abscesses, and endocarditis should always be considered in patients with multiple renal abscesses. Alternatively, septicemia, with or without hypotension, can result in acute tubular necrosis. Thus in patients with endocarditis and acute renal failure, distinguishing glomerulonephritis from other causes may be difficult. Nevertheless, the presence of heavy proteinuria, red blood cell casts, and dysmorphic red blood cells suggests glomerulonephritis. Alternatively, temporal relationship of therapy, the presence of fever, rash and eosinophilia, or eosinophiluria in a patient with sterile pyuria should raise the possibility of hypersensitivity interstitial nephritis. Occasionally, renal biopsy is necessary to distinguish glomerulonephritis and acute hypersensitivity interstitial nephritis.

Treatment and Outcome

Eradication of infection with antibiotic and valve replacement (when appropriate) remain the mainstays of therapy. With control of infection, the urinary abnormalities and mild to moderate degrees of renal insufficiency usually resolve (167). Proteinuria and microscopic hematuria can persist for months and rarely for years after bacteriologic cure. The outcome of patients with severe renal dysfunction is variable, ranging from continued improvement over weeks to months in some, to persistent and progressive renal failure requiring dialysis in others, despite bacteriologic cure. Patients with a high proportion of glomerular crescents in renal biopsy specimens are more likely to have irreversible disease or progressive renal insufficiency (132,167).

The role of immunosuppressive therapy in patients with progressive renal insufficiency, despite optimal antibiotic and surgical treatment, remains controversial. Anecdotal case reports suggested that plasmapharesis, corticosteroids and cytotoxic agents, alone or in combination, may be useful in this situation (143,159,169–173). However, in addition to the usual adverse effects of these agents, this therapy poses the risk of exacerbating the underlying infectious process. Therefore,

these agents should only be considered under very specific circumstances. In our opinion, there should be clinical and laboratory evidence of bacteriologic cure, and histologic evidence of acute glomerulonephritis with the absence of overwhelming, severe chronic changes.

Conlon et al recently evaluated the risk of developing renal failure in 204 consecutive episodes of bacterial endocarditis (174). One third developed an elevated serum creatinine (≥2 mg/dL), and there was a fivefold increase in mortality in this subgroup. Factors associated with an increased risk of acute renal failure included: increased age, hypertension, thrombocytopenia, *S. aureus* infection, and prosthetic valve involvement. Although renal biopsies were not performed in the majority of patients in this retrospective analysis (i.e., the cause of renal failure was not determined), it is likely that glomerulonephritis leading to renal failure contributed to their poor outcome.

Shunt Nephritis

Epidemiologic Patterns

Surgically implanted ventriculoatrial, ventriculojugular, and ventriculovenal caval shunts have been commonly used to treat hydrocephalus (175). Overall, infection occurs in 6% to 27% of patients with these ventriculovascular shunts (175). The most common organism isolated is *Staphylococcus epidermidis*, accounting for 75% of infections (131,176). Other organisms that have been isolated include *S. aureus*, diphtheroids, *Listeria monocytogenes*, *Peptococcus* species, *Serratia* species, *Bacillus subtilis*, *Corynebacterium bovis*, *Gemella morbillorum*, *Propionibacterium acnes*, and a variety of fungi (177–186). It has been estimated that glomerulonephritis occurs in 1% to 4% of patients with infected shunts (177). In recent years, ventriculovascular shunts have been virtually abandoned and replaced by ventriculoperitoneal shunts. The latter devices are more resistant to colonization and infection, and associated glomerulonephritis is rare (187,188). The majority of cases of shunt nephritis have been reported in children, but rare cases have been documented in adults (175,179,184).

Clinical Manifestations

Symptoms of glomerulonephritis may develop within weeks to years after the shunt placement. Fever is present in nearly all patients with nephritis (175). Arthralgias, malaise, and weight loss are common and suggest infection (142,175). Clinical examination may reveal the presence of purpura, lymphadenopathy, and hepatosplenomegaly, and anemia is often present (131,142). Hematuria is universal, with gross hematuria present in half of the reported cases, and the nephrotic syndrome develops in 30% of patients (175). At initial presentation one-half of the patients have mild to moderate renal dysfunction, one-fourth have normal renal function, while the remainder have severe renal insufficiency (131,175). Hypertension is uncommon.

Laboratory Findings

Nondiagnostic abnormalities are characteristic. Hyperglobulinemia, cryoglobulinemia (associated with elevated rheumatoid factor titers), and raised plasma immune complex levels are usually present, suggesting an immunologic basis for this disorder (175,179,182). Hypocomplementemia, with reduced levels of both C3 and C4, is usually present with shunt nephritis, whereas patients with uncomplicated shunt infection usually have normal complement levels (189). The serum complement levels normalize with successful treatment of the underlying infection and resolution of the glomerulonephritis, and therefore serial determinations of serum complement may be a useful monitor of the activity of glomerulonephritis. Persistently depressed levels suggest either inadequate therapy or another cause of glomerulonephritis (190).

Blood and cerebrospinal fluid cultures are often positive. However, sometimes the organisms are difficult to grow, and identification of bacteria may be possible only by culture of material from the removed shunt.

Pathologic Features

The glomerular lesions are similar to membranoproliferative glomerulonephritis type I, with endocapillary proliferation, double-contoured capillary walls, and lobular accentuation. A few crescents are occasionally observed (142,149,175). Rarely, diffuse proliferative changes similar to post-infectious glomerulonephritis may be present (191). Granular IgM, IgG, and C3 deposits are usually observed by immunofluorescence, and bacterial antigens have been detected within these deposits. Electron microscopy typically demonstrates subendothelial and mesangial electron dense deposits.

Treatment and Outcome

Because antibiotic therapy alone is usually unsuccessful, treatment should include prompt removal of the infected shunt. Full recovery of renal function has been reported in two-thirds of patients after successful eradication of infection (176,178,189,192). The remaining third, however, demonstrate persistent azotemia and urinary abnormalities (131,175). Rarely, progression to end-stage renal disease has been reported (175). Immunosuppressive therapy has not been reported to be successful in these patients (181).

Visceral Sepsis-Associated Glomerulonephritis

Epidemiologic Patterns

Subacute or chronic infections including intrathoracic and intraabdominal abscesses, osteomyelitis, dental and maxillary sinus abscesses, septic abortions, and aortofemoral bypass graft infections have all been associated with glomerulonephritis (193–196). Glomerulonephritis has also been reported coincident with tuberculosis, pneumococcal pneumonia, *Campylobacter (Helicobacter) jejuni* enteritis, *Salmonella-Schistosoma mansoni* infections, and typhoid fever (193–196).

Clinical Manifestations

Many affected patients have signs and symptoms consequent to the underlying infectious process. They are often severely ill with high fever and weight loss. The interval between the onset of infection and diagnosis of glomerulonephritis varies from 2 weeks to 3 years (193). Rarely, patients present with glomerulonephritis as the initial manifestation of their illness. Common extrarenal manifestations include purpura (usually lower extremities) and arthralgias in approximately one-third of patients, and these phenomena are usually related to circulating cryoglobulins (193,197). Renal manifestations include hematuria, proteinuria, and acute renal failure. Similar to the situation described for glomerulonephritis associated with endocarditis, other causes of impaired renal dysfunction may be present in these patients. However, the presence of proteinuria and hematuria, especially dysmorphic red blood cells and red blood cell casts, usually distinguishes glomerulonephritis from other causes of acute renal failure. Approximately 50% of patients are oliguric and hypertensive (193,197).

Laboratory Findings

Blood cultures are frequently negative, and this has been attributed to the antecedent administration of antibiotics in many cases. Mixed cryoglobulins are usually present at the time of diagnosis and disappear with eradication of the underlying infection (193,197). The serum C3, C4, and CH50 levels are typically normal, unless there is an associated endovasculitis; C3 nephritic factor has occasionally been identified (1,142,198). Circulating immune complexes may be present in some patients. Rheumatoid factor is usually absent (198).

Pathologic Features

Proliferative glomerulonephritis is typical. However, a diverse group of lesions have been reported. These include mesangial proliferative glomerulonephritis, membranoproliferative glomerulonephritis, and diffuse proliferative glomerulonephritis; on occasion crescents are present (142,194,198). Immune deposits consisting primarily of C3 are the most consistent feature on immunofluorescence studies, although IgG and IgM may also be observed in mesangial, subendothelial, or subepithelial locations. While electron microscopic studies have not been commonly reported, electron-dense deposits in the mesangium as well as the occasional presence of subepithelial humps have been observed (131).

Treatment and Outcome

Complete remission of glomerulonephritis is usually achievable with early and complete eradication of the underlying infection (194,196,198). However, delayed and unsuccessful treatment may result in irreversible loss of renal function (198).

Methicillin-Resistant Staphylococcus-Associated-Glomerulonephritis

In 1995, Koyama et al. described 10 cases of glomerulonephritis following methicillin-resistant Staphylococcus aureus (MRSA) infection (199). Subsequently, several case series and reports have confirmed this association. MRSA-associated glomerulonephritis differs from staphylococcal endocarditis induced glomerulonephritis and staphylococcus associated shunt nephritis (200,201) in that serum complement levels are usually normal (albeit the lower limits of normal); there is polyclonal elevation of serum IgA and IgG levels; and IgA is often present within glomerular deposits along with IgG and C3 (202).

In a review of 26 patients with MRSA associated glomerulonephritis, Kobayashi et al. reported that the glomerulonephritis presented an average of 5.4 weeks following the onset of severe MRSA related infection. Approximately 50% of these infections were associated with pleural or abdominal abscesses. The renal presentation was usually that of either RPGN and/or the nephrotic syndrome (200). Thirty percent of patients had leukocytoclastic vasculitis and thrombocytosis was seen in 77%. Renal pathology showed a variety of types of mesangial and/or endocapillary proliferative glomerulonephritis with varying degrees of crescent formation. Immunofluorescence revealed glomerular deposits of IgA, IgG, and C3. There were electron-dense deposits in the glomerular basement membrane, mesangium and capillary walls. S. aureus antigens and staphylococcal enterotoxins were not demonstrable.

MRSA-associated glomerulonephritis appears to improve in the majority of cases where antibiotic therapy successfully eradicates the MRSA infection (203). However, some patients do not respond to antibiotic therapy and progress to end-stage renal disease (204). In two cases, corticosteroids were administered following apparent successful treatment of the underlying

MRSA infection (203). In these patients, relapse of the infection occurred, and they later died from sepsis. Therefore, great caution should be exercised before initiating immunosuppressive therapy. In cases refractory to antibiotic therapy, hemoperfusion with polymyxin B–immobilized fiber may be a useful therapy to reduce proteinuria (205).

Recently, isolated case reports have described MRSA infections associated with amyloid A renal amyloidosis, Henoch-Schönlein purpura, IgA nephropathy, and an IgA-dominant acute glomerulonephritis complicating diabetic nephropathy (206–208). These findings underscore the importance of renal biopsy in distinguishing the underlying cause of disease.

Syphilitic Glomerulopathy

Epidemiologic Patterns

Nephrotic syndrome is more common with congenital syphilis (up to 8% of patients) than in secondary forms (<1%) (206–208). Since the advent of mass screening and treatment campaigns, these forms of syphilis are now seen less commonly in developed countries.

Pathologic Features

The most common lesion identified on light microscopy resembles membranous nephropathy (209). In some patients, mild mesangial and endothelial cell proliferation, associated with mesangial deposits of IgG and IgM, may also be present (142). Electron microscopy usually consists of variable thickening of the basement membrane with subepithelial and occasional subendothelial dense deposits. Rarely, the histology resembles lesions associated with APSGN. Treponemal antigen and antitreponemal antibody have been identified within glomeruli of affected patients, which supports their role in the pathogenesis of nephritis (210).

Clinical Manifestations

Affected children with congenital syphilis usually present at the ages of 1 to 4 months with edema and hypertension (209,211,212). Rash and hepatosplenomegaly are common, and the typical radiologic findings associated with congenital syphilis are usually present. Adults most often present with features of the nephrotic syndrome during active secondary syphilis (212). Rarely, acute glomerulonephritis is the principal manifestation of renal involvement.

Laboratory Findings

Positive results on serologic testing for syphilis in the appropriate clinical setting, in association with renal histologic findings, support the diagnosis. Serum complement levels (C3 and C4) are depressed in congenital syphilis, but they are usually normal in adults with secondary syphilis and nephropathy (142). Circulating immune complexes are frequently present during the active stage of syphilitic nephropathy and disappear following successful treatment.

Treatment

Penicillin is the treatment of choice (142). For congenital syphilis, aqueous crystalline penicillin G, 50,000 units/kg/day, is given intravenously in divided doses for 10 days, or penicillin G procaine, 50,000 units/kg/day, is given intramuscularly for 10 days. For secondary syphilis, penicillin benzathine, 2.4 million units, is given intramuscularly (one dose) or penicillin G procaine, 600,000 units/day, is given intramuscularly for 8 days. Proteinuria subsides within 6 weeks of successful therapy in most patients.

References

1. Madaio MP, Harrington JT. The diagnosis of glomerular diseases: acute glomerulonephritis and the nephrotic syndrome. *Arch Intern Med* 2001;161(1):25.
2. Rodriguez-Iturbe B. Acute poststreptococcal glomerulonephritis. In: Schrier R, ed. *Diseases of the kidney*. Boston: Little Brown, 1993:1929.
3. Rammelkamp CH, Weaver RS. Acute glomerulonephritis. The significance of variations in the incidence of disease. *J Clin Invest* 1953;32:345.
4. Rammelkamp CH. Acute hemorrhagic glomerulonephritis. In: McCarty M (ed.). *Streptococcal infections*. New York: Columbia University Press, 1954.
5. Stetson CA, Rammelkamp CH, Krause RM. Epidemic acute nephritis: studies on etiology, natural history and prevention. *Medicine* 1955;34:431.
6. Drachman R, Aladjem M, Vardy PA. Natural history of an acute glomerulonephritis epidemic in children. An 11 to 12 year follow up. *J Med Sci* 1986;18:603.
7. Dodge WF, Spargo BH, Bass JA, et al. The relationship between the clinical and pathologic features of poststreptococcal glomerulonephritis. A study of the early natural history. *Medicine (Baltimore)* 1968;47(3):227.
8. Garcia R, Rubio L, Rodriguez-Iturbe B. Long-term prognosis of epidemic poststreptococcal glomerulonephritis in Maracaibo: follow-up studies 11-12 years after the acute episode. *Clin Nephrol* 1981;15(6):291.
9. Kaplan EL, Anthony BF, Chapman SS, et al. Epidemic acute glomerulonephritis associated with type 49 streptococcal pyoderma. I. Clinical and laboratory findings. *Am J Med* 1970;48(1):9.
10. Lewy JE, Salinas-Madrigal L, Herdson PB, et al. Clinico-pathologic correlations in acute poststreptococcal glomerulonephritis. A correlation between renal functions, morphologic damage and clinical course of 46 children with acute poststreptococcal glomerulonephritis. *Medicine (Baltimore)* 1971;50(6):453.
11. Lien JW, Mathew TH, Meadows R. Acute post-streptococcal glomerulonephritis in adults: a long-term study. *Q J Med* 1979;48(189):99.
12. Poon-King T, Mohammed I, Cox R, et al. Recurrent epidemic nephritis in South Trinidad. *N Engl J Med* 1967;277(14):728.
13. Morgan AG, Shah DJ, Williams W, et al. Proteinuria and glomerular disease in Jamaica. *Clin Nephrol* 1984;21(4):205.
14. Nissenson AR, Baraff LJ, Fine RN, et al. Poststreptococcal acute glomerulonephritis: fact and controversy. *Ann Intern Med* 1979;91(1):76.
15. Nissenson AR, Mayon-White R, Potter EV, et al. Continued absence of clinical renal disease seven to 12 years after poststreptococcal acute glomerulonephritis in Trinidad. *Am J Med* 1979;67(2):255.
16. Potter EV, Lipschultz SA, Abidh S, et al. Twelve to seventeen-year follow-up of patients with poststreptococcal acute glomerulonephritis in Trinidad. *N Engl J Med* 1982;307(12):725.
17. Potter EV, Abidh S, Sharrett AR, et al. Clinical healing two to six years after poststreptococcal glomerulonephritis in Trinidad. *N Engl J Med* 1978;298(14):767.
18. Richter ED. Epidemic nephritis. *N Engl J Med* 1967;277:763.
19. Berrios X, Lagomarsino E, Solar E, et al. Post-streptococcal acute glomerulonephritis in Chile—20 years of experience. *Pediatr Nephrol* 2004;19(3):306.
20. Rodriguez-Iturbe B, Garcia R, Rubio L. Epidemic glomerulonephritis in Maracaibo. Evidence for progression to chronicity. *Clin Nephrol* 1976;15:283.
21. Sorger K, Gessler M, Hubner FK, et al. Follow-up studies of three subtypes of acute postinfectious glomerulonephritis ascertained by renal biopsy. *Clin Nephrol* 1987;27(3):111.
22. Schacht RG, Gluck MC, Gallo GR. Progression to uremia after remission of acute poststrepococcal glomerulonephritis. *N Engl J Med* 1976;295:977.
23. Washio M, Oh Y, Okuda S. Clinicopathological study of poststreptococcal glomerulonephritis in the elderly. *Clin Nephrol* 1994;41:265.
24. Vogl W, Renkre M, Eichberger-Mayer D. Long-term prognosis for endocapillary glomerulonephritis of poststreptococcal type in children and Adults. *Nephron* 1986;44:58.
25. Svartman M, Potter EV, Finklea JF. Epidemic scabies and acute glomerulonephritis. *Lancet* 1972:249.
26. Rodriguez-Iturbe B, Rubio L, Garcia R. Attack rate of poststreptococcal nephritis in families. A prospective study. *Lancet* 1981;1(8217):401.
27. Haas M. Incidental healed postinfectious glomerulonephritis: a study of 1012 renal biopsy specimens examined by electron microscopy. *Hum Pathol* 2003;34(1):3.
28. Anthony BF, Kaplan EL, Wannamaker LW. Attack rates of acute nephritis after type 49 streptococcal infection of the skin and respiratory tract. *J Clin Invest* 1969;48:1697.
29. Muscatello DJ, O'Grady KA, Neville K, et al. Acute poststreptococcal glomerulonephritis: public health implications of recent clusters in New South Wales and epidemiology of hospital admissions. *Epidemiol Infect* 2001;126(3):365.

30. Rodriguez-Iturbe B. Epidemic poststreptococcal glomerulonephritis (clinical conference). *Kidney Int* 1984;25(1):129.

31. Barnham M, Thornton TJ, Lange K. Nephritis caused by Streptococcus zooepidemicus (Lancefield group C). *Lancet* 1983;1(8331):945.

32. Pruksakorn S, Sittisombut N, Phornphutkul C, et al. Epidemiological analysis of non-M-typeable group A Streptococcus isolates from a Thai population in northern Thailand. *J Clin Microbiol* 2000;38(3):1250.

33. Nicholson ML, Ferdinand L, Sampson JS, et al. Analysis of immunoreactivity to a Streptococcus equi subsp. zooepidemicus M-like protein to confirm an outbreak of poststreptococcal glomerulonephritis, and sequences of M-like proteins from isolates obtained from different host species. *J Clin Microbiol* 2000;38(11):4126.

34. Brandt ER, Yarwood PJ, McMillan DJ, et al. Antibody levels to the class I and II epitopes of the M protein and myosin are related to group A streptococcal exposure in endemic populations. *Int Immunol* 2001;13(10):1335.

35. Brenner RM, Peterson J. Postinfectious glomerulonephritis. *Nephrology Rounds* 2000;3:1.

36. Lange CF. Antigenicity of kidney glomeruli: evaluations by antistreptococcal cell membrane antisera. *Transplant Proc* 1980;12(3)(Suppl 1):82.

37. Ohkuni H, Todome Y, Yoshimura K, et al. Detection of nephritis strain-associated streptokinase by monoclonal antibodies. *J Med Microbiol* 1991;35(1):60.

38. Stollerman GH. Streptococcal immunology: protection versus injury (editorial). *Ann Intern Med* 1978;88(3):422.

39. Stollerman GH, Lewis A, Schultz I. Relationship of immune response to group A streptococci to the course of acute and chronic recurrent rheumatic fever. *Am J Med* 1956;20:163.

40. Sorof JM, Weidner N, Potter D, et al. Acute post-streptococcal glomerulonephritis in a renal allograft. *Pediatr Nephrol* 1995;9(3):317.

41. Dodge WF, Spargo BH, Travis LB, et al. Poststreptococcal glomerulonephritis. A prospective study in children. *N Engl J Med* 1972;286(6):273.

42. Fish AJ, Herdman RC, Michael AF, et al. Epidemic acute glomerulonephritis associated with type 49 streptococcal pyoderma. II. Correlative study of light, immunofluorescent and electron microscopic findings. *Am J Med* 1970;48(1):28.

43. Baldwin DS, Gluck MC, Schacht RG, et al. The long-term course of poststreptococcal glomerulonephritis. *Ann Intern Med* 1974;80(3):342.

44. Feldman H, Mardiney MR, Shuler SE. Immunology and morphology of acute post-streptococcal glomerulonephritis. *J Clin Invest* 1965;40:283.

45. Oda T, Yoshizawa N, Takeuchi A, et al. Glomerular proliferating cell kinetics in acute post-streptococcal glomerulonephritis (APSGN). *J Pathol* 1997;183(3):359.

46. Kimmelstiel P. The hump-a lesion of acute glomerulonephritis. *Bull Pathol* 1965;6:187.

47. Parra G, Platt JL, Falk RJ, et al. Cell populations and membrane attack complex in glomeruli of patients with post-streptococcal glomerulonephritis: identification using monoclonal antibodies by indirect immunofluorescence. *Clin Immunol Immunopathol* 1984;33(3):324.

48. Gruppe WE. Case records: 6-1975. *N Engl J Med* 1975;292:307.

49. Earle DP, Jennings RB. Studies of poststreptococcal nephritis and other glomerular diseases. *Ann Intern Med* 1959;51:851.

50. Ingelfinger JR, McCluskey RT, Schneeberger EE, et al. Necrotizing arteritis in acute poststreptococcal glomerulonephritis: report of a recovered case. *J Pediatr* 1977;91(2):228.

51. Fordham CC 3rd, Epstein FH, Huffines WD, et al. Polyarteritis and acute post-streptococcal glomerulonephritis. *Ann Intern Med* 1964;61:89.

52. Bodaghi E, Kheradpir KM, Maddah M. Vasculitis in acute streptococcal glomerulonephritis. *Int J Pediatr Nephrol* 1987;8(2):69.

53. Sorger K, Balun J, Hubner FK, et al. The garland type of acute postinfectious glomerulonephritis: morphological characteristics and follow-up studies. *Clin Nephrol* 1983;20(1):17.

54. Sorger K, Gessler U, Hubner FK, et al. Subtypes of acute postinfectious glomerulonephritis. Synopsis of clinical and pathological features. *Clin Nephrol* 1982;17(3):114.

55. Sorger K. Postinfectious glomerulonephritis. Subtypes, clinico-pathological correlations, and follow-up studies. *Veroff Pathol* 1986;125:1.

56. Freedman P, Peters JH, Kark RM. Localization of gamma-globulin in the diseased kidney. *Arch Intern Med* 1960;105:524.

57. Seegal BC, Andres JA, Hsu KC. Studies on the pathogenesis of acute and progressive glomerulonephritis in man by immunofluorescence and immunoferritin techniques. *Fed Proc* 1965;24:100.

58. Tornroth T. The fate of subepithelial deposits in acute poststreptococcal glomerulonephritis. *Lab Invest* 1976;35(5):461.

59. West CD, McAdams AJ. Glomerular deposits and hypoalbuminemia in acute post-streptococcal glomerulonephritis. *Pediatr Nephrol* 1998;12(6):471.

60. Zabriskie JB. The role of streptococci in human glomerulonephritis. *J Exp Med* 1971;134(3)(Suppl):180s.

61. Treser G, Semar M, McVicar M, et al. Antigenic streptococcal components in acute glomerulonephritis. *Science* 1969;163(868):676.

62. Yoshizawa N, Treser G, Sagel I. Demonstration of antigenic sites in glomeruli of patients with acute PO streptococcal glomerulonephritis by immunofluorescein and immunoferritin technics. *Am J Pathol* 1972;70:131.

63. Treser G, Semar M, Ty A, et al. Partial characterization of antigenic streptococcal plasma membrane components in acute glomerulonephritis. *J Clin Invest* 1970;49(4):762.

64. Lange K, Ahmed U, Kleinberger H, et al. A hitherto unknown streptococcal antigen and its probable relation to acute poststreptococcal glomerulonephritis. *Clin Nephrol* 1976;5(5):207.

65. Cronin WJ, Lange K. Immunologic evidence for the in situ deposition of a cytoplasmic streptococcal antigen (endostreptosin) on the glomerular basement membrane in rats. *Clin Nephrol* 1990;34(4):143.

66. Yoshizawa N, Oshima S, Sagel I, et al. Role of a streptococcal antigen in the pathogenesis of acute poststreptococcal glomerulonephritis. Characterization of the antigen and a proposed mechanism for the disease. *J Immunol* 1992;148(10):3110.

67. Oda T, Yamakami K, Omasu F, et al. Glomerular plasmin-like activity in relation to nephritis-associated plasmin receptor in acute poststreptococcal glomerulonephritis. *J Am Soc Nephrol* 2005;16(1):247.

68. Yoshizawa N, Yamakami K, Fujino M, et al. Nephritis-associated plasmin receptor and acute poststreptococcal glomerulonephritis: characterization of the antigen and associated immune response. *J Am Soc Nephrol* 2004;15(7):178.

69. Villarreal H Jr, Fischetti VA, van de Rijn I, et al. The occurrence of a protein in the extracellular products of streptococci isolated from patients with acute glomerulonephritis. *J Exp Med* 1979;149(2):459.

70. Johnston KH, Zabriskie JB. Purification and partial characterization of the nephritis strain- associated protein from Streptococcus pyogenes, group A. *J Exp Med* 1986;163(3):697.

71. Mezzano S, Burgos E, Mahabir R, et al. Failure to detect unique reactivity to streptococcal streptokinase in either the sera or renal biopsy specimens of patients with acute poststreptococcal glomerulonephritis. *Clin Nephrol* 1992;38(6):305.

72. Ohkuni H, Todome Y, Suzuki H, et al. Immunochemical studies and complete amino acid sequence of the streptokinase from Streptococcus pyogenes (group A) M type 12 strain A374. *Infect Immun* 1992;60(1):278.

73. Peake PW, Pussell BA, Karplus TE, et al. Post-streptococcal glomerulonephritis: studies on the interaction between nephritis strain-associated protein (NSAP), complement and the glomerulus. *Apmis* 1991;99(5):460.

74. Poon-King R, Bannan J, Viteri A, et al. Identification of an extracellular plasmin binding protein from nephritogenic streptococci. *J Exp Med* 1993;178(2):759.

75. Cu GA, Mezzano S, Bannan JD, et al. Immunohistochemical and serological evidence for the role of streptococcal proteinase in acute post-streptococcal glomerulonephritis. *Kidney Int* 1998;54(3):819.

76. Vogt A, Batsford S, Rodriguez-Iturbe B, et al. Cationic antigens in post-streptococcal glomerulonephritis. *Clin Nephrol* 1983;20(6):271.

77. Bergey EJ, Stinson MW. Heparin-inhibitable basement membrane-binding protein of Streptococcus pyogenes. *Infect Immun* 1988;56(7):1715.

78. Glurich I, Winters B, Albini B, et al. Identification of Streptococcus pyogenes proteins that bind to rabbit kidney in vitro and in vivo. *Microb Pathog* 1991;10(3):209.

79. Nordstrand A, Norgren M, Holm SE. An experimental model for acute post-streptococcal glomerulonephritis in mice. *Adv Exp Med Biol* 1997;418:809.

80. Nordstrand A, Norgren M, Ferretti JJ, et al. Streptokinase as a mediator of acute post-streptococcal glomerulonephritis in an experimental mouse model. *Infect Immun* 1998;66(1):315.

81. McIntosh RM, Kaufman DB, McIntosh JR, et al. Glomerular lesions produced by autologous serum and autologous IgG modified by treatment with a culture of a -haemolytic streptococcus. *J Med Microbiol* 1972;5(1):1.

82. Kronvall G. A surface component in group A, C, and G streptococci with non-immune reactivity for immunoglobulin G. *J Immunol* 1973;111(5):1401.

83. Grubb A, Grubb R, Christensen P, et al. Isolation and some properties of an IgG Fc-binding protein from group A streptococci type 15. *Int Arch Allergy Appl Immunol* 1982;67(4):369.

84. Mosquera J, Rodriguez-Iturbe B. Extracellular neuraminidase production of Streptococci associated with acute nephritis. *Clin Nephrol* 1984;21:21.

85. Mosquera J, Katiyar V, Coello J. Neuraminidase production by Streptococci from patients with glomerulonephritis. *J Infect Dis* 1985;151:259.

86. Marin C, Mosquera J, Rodriguez-Iturbe B. Histological evidence of neuraminidase involvement in acute nephritis: desialized leukocytes infiltrate the kidney in acute post-streptococcal glomerulonephritis. *Clin Nephrol* 1997;47(4):217.

87. Markowitz AS, Horn D, Aseron C, et al. Streptococcal related glomerulonephritis. 3. Glomerulonephritis in rhesus monkeys immunologically induced both actively and passively with a soluble fraction from nephritogenic streptococcal protoplasmic membranes. *J Immunol* 1971;107(2):504.

88. Markowitz AS, Clasen R, Nidus BD, et al. Streptococcal related glomerulonephritis. II. Glomerulonephritis in rhesus monkeys immunologically induced both actively and passively with a soluble fraction from human glomeruli. *J Immunol* 1967;98(1):161.

89. Becker C, Murphy G. The experimental induction of glomerulonephritis like that in man by infection with Group A Streptococci. *J Exp Med* 1967;127:1.

90. Khandke KM, Fairwell T, Manjula BN. Difference in the structural features of streptococcal M proteins from nephritogenic and rheumatogenic serotypes. *J Exp Med* 1987;166(1):151.

91. Kraus W, Beachey EH. Renal autoimmune epitope of group A streptococci specified by M protein tetrapeptide Ile-Arg-Leu-Arg. *Proc Natl Acad Sci USA* 1988;85(12):4516.

92. Kraus W, Ohyama K, Snyder DS, et al. Autoimmune sequence of streptococcal M protein shared with the intermediate filament protein, vimentin. *J Exp Med* 1989;169(2):481.
93. Kefalides NA, Ohno N, Wilson CB, et al. Identification of antigenic epitopes in type IV collagen by use of synthetic peptides. *Kidney Int* 1993;43(1):94.
94. Kefalides NA, Pegg MT, Ohno N, et al. Antibodies to basement membrane collagen and to laminin are present in sera from patients with poststreptococcal glomerulonephritis. *J Exp Med* 1986;163(3):588.
95. Fillit H, Damle SP, Gregory JD, et al. Sera from patients with poststreptococcal glomerulonephritis contain antibodies to glomerular heparan sulfate proteoglycan. *J Exp Med* 1985;161(2):277.
96. Wells WC. Observations on the dropsy which succeeds scarlet fever. *Trans Soc Imp Chir Knowledge* 1812;3:167.
97. Layrisse Z, Rodriguez-Iturbe B, Garcia-Ramirez R, et al. Family studies of the HLA system in acute post-streptococcal glomerulonephritis. *Hum Immunol* 1983;7(3):177.
98. Reid HF, Read SE, Zabriskie JB, et al. Suppression of cellular reactivity to group A streptococcal antigens in patients with acute poststreptococcal glomerulonephritis. *J Infect Dis* 1984;149(6):841.
99. Fillit HM, Read SE, Sherman RL, et al. Cellular reactivity to altered glomerular basement membrane in glomerulonephritis. *N Engl J Med* 1978;298(16):861.
100. Rastaldi MP, Ferrario F, Yang L, et al. Adhesion molecules expression in noncrescentic acute post-streptococcal glomerulonephritis. *J Am Soc Nephrol* 1996;7(11):2419.
101. Madaio MP, Harrington JT. Current concepts. The diagnosis of acute glomerulonephritis. *N Engl J Med* 1983;309(21):1299.
102. Jennings RB, Earle DP. Post-streptococcal glomerulonephritis: histopathologic and early clinical latent phases. *J Clin Invest* 1961;40:1525.
103. Rovang RD, Zawada ET Jr, Santella RN, et al. Cerebral vasculitis associated with acute post-streptococcal glomerulonephritis. *Am J Nephrol* 1997;17(1):89.
104. Couser WG, Johnson RJ, Alpers CE. Postinfectious glomerulonephritis. In: Neilson EG, Couser WG, eds. *Immunologic renal diseases,* 2nd ed. Philadelphia: Lippincott, Williams & Wilkins, 2001:899.
105. Sagel I, Treser G, Ty A, et al. Occurrence and nature of glomerular lesions after group A streptococci infections in children. *Ann Intern Med* 1973;79(4):492.
106. Akasheh MS, al-Lozi M, Affarah HB, et al. Rapidly progressive glomerulonephritis complicating acute rheumatic fever. *Postgrad Med J* 1995;71(839):553.
107. Niewold TB, Ghosh AK. Post-streptococcal reactive arthritis and glomerulonephritis in an adult. *Clin Rheumatol* 2003;22(4–5):350.
108. Moroni G, Papaccioli D, Banfi G, et al. Acute post-bacterial glomerulonephritis in renal transplant patients: description of three cases and review of the literature. *Am J Transplant* 2004;4(1):132.
109. Besada E, Frauens BJ, Schatz S. Choroiditis, pigment epithelial detachment, and cystoid macular edema as complications of poststreptococcal syndrome. *Optom Vis Sci* 2004;81(8):578.
110. Hinglais N, Garcia-Torres R, Kleinknecht D. Long-term prognosis in acute glomerulonephritis. The predictive value of early clinical and pathological features observed in 65 patients. *Am J Med* 1974;56(1):52.
111. Becker A, Gonzalez E, Vial S, et al. Anemia associated with acute post streptococcal glomerulonephritis. *Rev Med Chil* 1994;122(11):1276.
112. Sjoholm AG. Complement components and complement activation in acute poststreptococcal glomerulonephritis. *Int Arch Allergy Appl Immunol* 1979;58(3):274.
113. Lewis EJ, Carpenter CB, Schur PH. Serum complement component levels in human glomerulonephritis. *Ann Intern Med* 1971;75(4):555.
114. Cameron JS, Vick RM, Ogg CS, et al. Plasma C3 and C4 concentrations in management of glomerulonephritis. *Br Med J* 1973;3(882):668.
115. McLean RH, Michael AF. Properdin and C3 proactivator: alternate pathway components in human glomerulonephritis. *J Clin Invest* 1973;52(3):634.
116. Matsell DG, Roy SD, Tamerius JD, et al. Plasma terminal complement complexes in acute poststreptococcal glomerulonephritis. *Am J Kidney Dis* 1991;17(3):311.
117. Williams DG, Peters DK, Fallows J, et al. Studies of serum complement in the hypocomplementaemic nephritides. *Clin Exp Immunol* 1974;18(3):391.
118. McIntosh RM, Griswold WR, Chernack WB, et al. Cryoglobulins. III. Further studies on the nature, incidence, clinical, diagnostic, prognostic, and immunopathologic significance of cryoproteins in renal disease. *Q J Med* 1975;44(174):285.
119. Zaum R, Vogt A, Rodriguez-Iturbe B. Analysis of the immune response to streoriciceal proteinase in poststrepococcal disease. Xth Lancefield International Symposium on Streoticicceal Diseases, Cologne, Germany, 1987: 88.
120. Wannamaker LW. Differences between streptococcal infections of the throat and of the skin (second of two parts). *N Engl J Med* 1970;282(2):78.
121. Bisno AL, Nelson KE, Waytz P, et al. Factors influencing serum antibody responses in streptococcal pyoderma. *J Lab Clin Med* 1973;81(3):410.
122. Dillon HC Jr, Reeves MS. Streptococcal immune responses in nephritis after skin infections. *Am J Med* 1974;56(3):333.
123. Okada K, Katano T, Kamogashira T, et al. Streptokinase gene vari-

124. McCarty M. The antibody response in streptococcal infections. In: McCarty M (ed): *Streptococcal infections.* New York: Columbia University Press, 1954.
125. Lyttle JD, Seegal D, Loeb E. The serum antistreptolysin titer in acute glomerulonephritis. *J Clin Invest* 1938;17:632.
126. Perlman LV, Herdman RC, Kleinman H, et al. Poststreptococcal glomerulonephritis. A ten-year follow-up of an epidemic. *JAMA* 1965;194(1):63.
127. Kasahara T, Hayakawa H, Okubo S, et al. Prognosis of acute poststreptococcal glomerulonephritis (APSGN) is excellent in children, when adequately diagnosed. *Pediatr Int* 2001;43(4):364.
128. Buzio C, Allegri L, Mutti A, et al. Significance of albuminuria in the follow-up of acute poststreptococcal glomerulonephritis. *Clin Nephrol* 1994;41(5):259.
129. Baldwin DS. Chronic glomerulonephritis: nonimmunologic mechanisms of progressive glomerular damage. *Kidney Int* 1982;21(1):109.
130. Zoch-Zwierz W, Wasilewska A, Biernacka A, et al. [The course of poststreptococcal glomerulonephritis depending on methods of treatment for the preceding respiratory tract infection]. *Wiad Lek* 2001;54(1–2):56.
131. Alder SG, Cohen AH. *Glomerulonephritis with bacterial endocarditis.* Boston: Little Brown, 1993.
132. Neugarten J, Baldwin DS. Glomerulonephritis in bacterial endocarditis. *Am J Med* 1984;77(2):297.
133. Bell EJ. The glomerular lesion associated with endocarditis. *Am J Pathol* 1932;8:639.
134. Baehr G, Glosbe. Glomerular lesion of subacute bacterial endocarditis. *J Exp Med* 1912;15:330.
135. Keefer CS. Subacute bacterial endocarditis: Active cases without bacteremia. *Ann Intern Med* 1937–1938;11:714.
136. Spain DM, King DW. The effect of penicillin on the renal lesion of subacute bacterial endocarditis. *Ann Intern Med* 36:1086.
137. Libman E. Characterization of various forms of glomerulonephritis. *JAMA* 1923;80:813.
138. Glassock RJ. Secondary glomerular diseases. In: Brenner BM, Rector FC, eds. *The kidney.* Boston: Little Brown, 1992:1493.
139. Pankey GA. Acute bacterial endocarditis at the University of Minnesota Hospitals, 1939–1959. *Am Heart J* 1962;64:583.
140. O'Connor DT, Weisman MH, et al. Activation of the alternate complement pathway in Staph. aureus infective endocarditis and its relationship to thrombocytopenia, coagulation abnormalities, and acute glomerulonephritis. *Clin Exp Immunol* 1978;34(2):179.
141. Hurwitz D, Quismorio FP, Friou GJ. Cryoglobulinaemia in patients with infectious endocarditis. *Clin Exp Immunol* 1975;19(1):131.
142. Madaio MP. Postinfectious glomerulonephritis. In: Jacobson HR, Striker GE, Klahr S, eds. *The principles and practice of nephrology* 2nd ed. St. Louis: Mosby, 1995:122.
143. Kannan S, Mattoo TK. Diffuse crescentic glomerulonephritis in bacterial endocarditis. *Pediatr Nephrol* 2001;16(5):423.
144. Neufeld GK, Branson CG, Marshall LW, et al. Infective endocarditis as a complication of heroin use. *South Med J* 1976;69(9):1148.
145. Spitzer RE, Stitzel AE, Urmson JR. Is glomerulonephritis after bacterial sepsis always benign? *Lancet* 1978;1(8069):871.
146. Morel-Maroger L, Sraer JD, Herreman G, et al. Kidney in subacute endocarditis. Pathological and immunofluorescence findings. *Arch Pathol* 1972;94(3):205.
147. Colvin RB, Fang LS. Interstitial nephritis. In: Tisher CC, Brenner BM, eds. *Renal pathology with functional correlations.* Philadelphia: Lippincott, 1989.
148. Lerner PI, Weinstein L. Infective endocarditis in the antibiotic era. *N Engl J Med* 1966;274(7):388.
149. Gutman RA, Striker GE, Gilliland BC, et al. The immune complex glomerulonephritis of bacterial endocarditis. *Medicine (Baltimore)* 1972;51(1):1.
150. Boulton-Jones JM, Sissons JG, Evans DJ, et al. Renal lesions of subacute infective endocarditis. *Br Med J* 1974;2(909):11.
151. Boyarsky S, Burnett JM, Barker WH. Renal failure in embolic glomerulonephritis as a complication of subacute bacterial endocarditis. *Bull Johns Hopkins Hosp* 1949;84:207.
152. Williams RC Jr, Kunkel HG. Rheumatoid factor, complement, and conglutinin aberrations in patients with subacute bacterial endocarditis. *J Clin Invest* 1962;41:666.
153. Glassock RJ. Clinical aspects of acute, rapidly progressive and chronic glomerulonephritis. In: Earley LE, Gottschalk CW, eds. *Diseases of the kidney.* Boston: Little Brown, 1979:691.
154. Lee BK, Crossley K, Gerding DN. The association between Staphylococcus aureus bacteremia and bacteriuria. *Am J Med* 1978;65(2):303.
155. Musher DM, McKenzie SO. Infections due to Staphylococcus aureus. *Medicine (Baltimore)* 1977;56(5):383.
156. Gorlin R, Favour CB, Emery FJ. Long-term follow-up study of penicillin-treated subacute bacterial endocarditis. *N Engl J Med* 1950;242(26):995.
157. Pelletier LL Jr, Petersdorf RG. Infective endocarditis: a review of 125 cases from the University of Washington Hospitals, 1963–72. *Medicine (Baltimore)* 1977;56(4):287.
158. Sheagren JN, Tuazon CU, Griffin C, Padmore N. Rheumatoid factor in acute bacterial endocarditis. *Arthritis Rheum* 1976;19(5):887.

able region classification in streptococci: lack of correlation with poststreptococcal glomerulonephritis. *Clin Nephrol* 1995;44(1):8.

159. Bayer AS, Theofilopoulos AN. Immunopathogenetic aspects of infective endocarditis. *Chest* 1990;97(1):204.
160. Cabane J, Godeau P, Herreman G, et al. Fate of circulating immune complexes in infective endocarditis. *Am J Med* 1979;66(2):277.
161. Kauffmann RH, Thompson J, Valentijn RM, et al. The clinical implications and the pathogenetic significance of circulating immune complexes in infective endocarditis. *Am J Med* 1981;71(1):17.
162. Hooper DC, Bayer AS, Karchmer AW, et al. Circulating immune complexes in prosthetic valve endocarditis. *Arch Intern Med* 1983;143(11):2081.
163. Angangco R, Thiru S, Oliveira DB. Pauci-immune glomerulonephritis associated with bacterial infection. *Nephrol Dial Transplant* 1993;8(8):754.
164. Soto A, Jorgensen C, Oksman F, et al. Endocarditis associated with ANCA. *Clin Exp Rheumatol* 1994;12(2):203.
165. Subra JF, Michelet C, Laporte J, et al. The presence of cytoplasmic antineutrophil cytoplasmic antibodies (C-ANCA) in the course of subacute bacterial endocarditis with glomerular involvement, coincidence or association? *Clin Nephrol* 1998;49(1):15.
166. Pertschuk LP, Woda BA, Vuletin JC, et al. Glomerulonephritis due to Staphylococcus aureus antigen. *Am J Clin Pathol* 1976;65(3):301.
167. Neugarten J, Gallo GR, Baldwin DS. Glomerulonephritis in bacterial endocarditis. *Am J Kidney Dis* 1984;3(5):371.
168. Horder TJ. Infective endocarditis with an analysis of 150 cases with special reference to the chronic form of the disease. *Q J Med* 1909;2:289.
169. McKinsey DS, McMurray TI, Flynn JM. Immune complex glomerulonephritis associated with Staphylococcus aureus bacteremia: response to corticosteroid therapy. *Rev Infect Dis* 1990;12(1):125.
170. McKenzie PE, Taylor AE, Woodroffe AJ, et al. Plasmapheresis in glomerulonephritis. *Clin Nephrol* 1979;12(3):97.
171. Rovzar MA, Logan JL, Ogden DA, et al. Immunosuppressive therapy and plasmapheresis in rapidly progressive glomerulonephritis associated with bacterial endocarditis. *Am J Kidney Dis* 1986;7(5):428.
172. Daimon S, Mizuno Y, Fujii S, et al. Infective endocarditis-induced crescentic glomerulonephritis dramatically improved by plasmapheresis. *Am J Kidney Dis* 1998;32(2):309.
173. Le Moing V, Lacassin F, Delahousse M, et al. Use of corticosteroids in glomerulonephritis related to infective endocarditis: three cases and review. *Clin Infect Dis* 1999;28(5):1057.
174. Conlon PJ, Jefferies F, Krigman HR, et al. Predictors of prognosis and risk of acute renal failure in bacterial endocarditis. *Clin Nephrol* 1998;49(2):96.
175. Arze RS, Rashid H, Morley R, et al. Shunt nephritis: report of two cases and review of the literature. *Clin Nephrol* 1983;19(1):48.
176. Moncrieff MW, Glasgow EF, Arthur LJ, et al. Glomerulonephritis associated with Staphylococcus albus in a Spitz Holter valve. *Arch Dis Child* 1973;48(1):69.
177. Schoenbaum SC, Gardner P, Shillito J. Infections of cerebrospinal fluid shunts: epidemiology, clinical manifestations, and therapy. *J Infect Dis* 1975;131(5):543.
178. Caron C, Luneau C, Gervais MH, et al. Shunt glomerulonephritis: clinical and histopathological manifestations. *Can Med Assoc J* 1979;120(5):557.
179. Bolton WK, Sande MA, Normansell DE, et al. Ventriculojugular shunt nephritis with Corynebacterium bovis. Successful therapy with antibiotics. *Am J Med* 1975;59(3):417.
180. Forrest JW Jr, John F, Mills LR, et al. Immune complex glomerulonephritis associated with Klebsiella pneumoniae infection. *Clin Nephrol* 1977;7(2):76.
181. Stickler GB, Shin MH, Burke EC, et al. Diffuse glomerulonephritis associated with infected ventriculoatrial shunt. *N Engl J Med* 1968;279(20):1077.
182. Strife CF, McDonald BM, Ruley EJ, et al. Shunt nephritis: the nature of the serum cryoglobulins and their relation to the complement profile. *J Pediatr* 1976;88(3):403.
183. Peeters W, Mussche M, Becaus I, et al. Shunt nephritis. *Clin Nephrol* 1978;9(3):122.
184. Pereria BJ, et al. Shunt nephritis associated with Staphylococcus aureus septicaemia. *J Assoc Phys Ind* 1987;35:796.
185. Nagashima T, Hirata D, Yamamoto H, et al. Antineutrophil cytoplasmic autoantibody specific for proteinase 3 in a patient with shunt nephritis induced by Gemella morbillorum. *Am J Kidney Dis* 2001;37(5):E38.
186. Balogun RA, Palmisano J, Kaplan AA, et al. Shunt nephritis from Propionibacterium acnes in a solitary kidney. *Am J Kidney Dis* 2001;38(4):E18.

187. Dobrin RS, Day NK, Quie PG, et al. The role of complement, immunoglobulin and bacterial antigen in coagulase-negative staphylococcal shunt nephritis. *Am J Med* 1975;59(5):660.
188. Noe HN, Roy S 3rd. Shunt nephritis. *J Urol* 1981;125(5):731.
189. Levy M, Gubler MC, Habib R. Pathology and immunopathology of shunt nephritis in children: Report of 10 cases. In: Zurukzoglu W, ed. *Proceedings 8th International Congress of Nephrology*. Basel: Krager, 1981.
190. Wyatt RJ, Walsh JW, Holland NH. Shunt nephritis. Role of the complement system in its pathogenesis and management. *J Neurosurg* 1981;55(1):99.
191. Toth T, Redl J, Beregi E. Shunt nephritis with crescent formation. *Int J Pediatr Nephrol* 1987;8(4):231.
192. Yeh BP, Young HF, Schatzki PF, et al. Immune complex disease associated with an infected ventriculojugular shunt: a curable form of glomerulonephritis. *South Med J* 1977;70(9):1141.
193. Beaufils M, Morel-Maroger L, Sraer JD, et al. Acute renal failure of glomerular origin during visceral abscesses. *N Engl J Med* 1976;295(4):185.
194. Boulton-Jones JM, Davidson AM. Persistent infection as a cause of renal disease in patients submitted to renal biopsy. A report from the glomerulonephritis registry of the United Kingdom MRC. *Q J Med* 1986;58(58):123.
195. Whitworth JA, Morel-Maroger L, Mignon F, et al. The significance of extracapillary proliferation. Clinicopathological review of 60 patients. *Nephron* 1976;16(1):1.
196. Boonshaft B, Maher JF, Schreiner GE. Nephrotic syndrome associated with osteomyelitis without secondary amyloidosis. *Arch Intern Med* 1970;125(2):322.
197. Beaufils M. Glomerular disease complicating abdominal sepsis. *Kidney Int* 1981;19(4):609.
198. Beaufils M, Gibert C, Morel-Maroger L, et al. Glomerulonephritis in severe bacterial infections with and without endocarditis. *Adv Nephrol Necker Hosp* 1977;7:217.
199. Koyama A, Kobayashi M, Yamaguchi N, et al. Glomerulonephritis associated with MRSA infection: a possible role of bacterial superantigen. *Kidney Int* 1995;47(1):207.
200. Kobayashi M, Koyama A. Methicillin-resistant Staphylococcus aureus (MRSA) infection in glomerulonephritis—a novel hazard emerging on the horizon. *Nephrol Dial Transplant* 1998;13(12):2999.
201. Yoh K, Kobayashi M, Yamaguchi N, et al. Cytokines and T-cell responses in superantigen-related glomerulonephritis following methicillin-resistant Staphylococcus aureus infection. *Nephrol Dial Transplant* 2000;15(8):1170.
202. Grcevska L, Polenakovic M. Garland pattern post-streptococcal glomerulonephritis (PSGN, clinical characteristics and follow-up [letter]. *Clin Nephrol* 1996;46(6):413.
203. Nagaba Y, Hiki Y, Aoyama T, et al. Effective antibiotic treatment of methicillin-resistant Staphylococcus aureus-associated glomerulonephritis. *Nephron* 2002;92(2):297.
204. Yamashita Y, Tanase T, Terada Y, et al. Glomerulonephritis after methicillin-resistant Staphylococcus aureus infection resulting in end-stage renal failure. *Intern Med* 2001;40(5):424.
205. Nakamura T, Ushiyama C, Suzuki Y, et al. Hemoperfusion with polymyxin B-immobilized fiber in septic patients with methicillin-resistant Staphylococcus aureus-associated glomerulonephritis. *Nephron Clin Pract* 2003;94(2):c33.
206. Yokota N, Morita H, Iwaski S, et al. Reversible nephrotic syndrome in a patient with amyloid A amyloidosis of the kidney following methicillin-resistant Staphylococcus aureus infection. *Nephron* 2001;87(2):177.
207. Pola E, Logroscino G, De Santis V, et al. Onset of Berger disease after Staphylococcus aureus infection: septic arthritis after anterior cruciate ligament reconstruction. *Arthroscopy* 2003;19(4):E29.
208. Hirayama K, Kobayashi M, Kondoh M, et al. Henoch-Schonlein purpura nephritis associated with methicillin-resistant Staphylococcus aureus infection. *Nephrol Dial Transplant* 1998;13(10):2703.
209. Kleinknecht C, Levy M, Gagnadoux MF, et al. Membranous glomerulonephritis with extra-renal disorders in children. *Medicine (Baltimore)* 1979;58(3):219.
210. O'Regan S, Fong JS, de Chadarevian JP, et al. Treponemal antigens in congenital and acquired syphilitic nephritis: demonstration by immunofluorescence studies. *Ann Intern Med* 1976;85(3):325.
211. Pollner P. Nephrotic syndrome associated with congenital syphilis. *JAMA* 1966;198(3):263.
212. Choubrac P, Barbanel C, Haas C, et al. (Glomerulonephritis and secondary syphilis). *Ann Med Interne (Paris)* 1977;128(5).

CHAPTER 59 ■ VIRAL GLOMERULAR DISEASES

PAUL L. KIMMEL AND JACK MOORE, JR.

There are few citations regarding renal disease associated with viral illness in the classic renal texts of the 1970s. Wilson and Dixon (1) outlined renal diseases associated with hepatitis B virus (HBV) (polyarteritis nodosa [PAN], membranous nephropathy [MN], and membranoproliferative [mesangiocapillary] glomerulonephritis [MPGN]), measles, oncornavirus, Coxsackie B virus, dengue, mumps, varicella, and Epstein-Barr virus infections in humans and animals. The pathogenic link between these viral infections and renal disease, however, often had not been directly established.

An association between HBV and human renal disease was noted in the 1970s, shortly after the characterization of the Australia or hepatitis-associated antigen (HAA) in 1964 (2), and the later identification of the virus. A serum sickness-like disease, associated with HBV infection, characterized by arthritis, proteinuria and hematuria, renal insufficiency, and hypocomplementemia (3,4), was presumptively identified as an immune complex-mediated disease. Immune complex mechanisms, immunodeficiency, and the chronicity of viral infections were thought to be the most important factors in mediating the pathogenesis of renal disease (5). Lack of proper reagents to document the presence of viral antigens in renal tissue and lack of epidemiologic and pathologic screening studies in appropriate populations to link viral infections to glomerular disease were impediments to establishing direct diagnostic associations (5). These latter authors (5) posed the question of how much renal disease was intimately related to the viral infections themselves and suggested that the host response, in particular interferon (IFN) production, might exacerbate nephropathy. Since that time, IFNs have been recognized as not only a component of the host response to viral infection but also a possible treatment for viral illnesses.

In a symposium published in 1990, human renal diseases were directly linked with HBV, human immunodeficiency virus (HIV), hantavirus, yellow fever, mumps, and BK papovavirus infections (6) (Table 59-1). Measles virus and varicella were indirectly associated with the pathogenesis of human renal disease (6). Although its contribution to renal interstitial disease was recognized, the role of cytomegalovirus (CMV) infection in the pathogenesis of glomerular disease, and in particular immunoglobulin A (IgA) nephropathy, was unclear (7). Of note, the virus associated with non-A, non-B hepatitis had not been isolated; therefore, there were no reports of hepatitis C virus (HCV)–associated renal disease. By 1990, the pathogenic mechanisms putatively involved in the development of immune complex renal disease associated with viral infection had been elaborated and partially delineated. In his paper on this subject, Glassock (8) outlined several etiologic possibilities for the pathogenesis of renal diseases associated with viral illnesses, as summarized in Table 59-2.

Pathways by which viruses may cause immunologic renal disease can be broadly classified into circulating and in situ mechanisms. The former mechanisms may involve circulating viral antigens, either deposited in the kidney alone or, classi-cally, bound to antiviral antibodies. Alternatively, circulating endogenous antigens, induced by viral changes in membrane proteins, may be shed into the circulation and induce a host antibody response. Such processes may account for the failure to detect viral antigens in renal tissue of patients with clinically diagnosed viral-associated renal diseases.

The role of *in situ* pathogenic mechanisms of immune complex-mediated nephropathy, originally outlined in models of lupus nephritis and MN (9), has been considered for renal diseases related to viral illnesses. *In situ* processes may be critical in the pathogenesis of renal diseases previously thought to be unassociated with viral infections (10–14). Mechanisms of nephropathogenesis may include viral gene expression in renal tissue or viral antigen binding to renal cells, which induces a secondary host humoral-mediated or cell-mediated immune response. These may include the synthesis of new host proteins, such as cytokines and chemokines (13,15–22) which may initiate or amplify local immune responses.

In clinical settings, it is often difficult to prove a pathogenic relationship between the renal disease and the postulated causative infectious agent in glomerulonephritides associated with viral illnesses. Clinical criteria to establish causality include the demonstration of improvement in renal disease simultaneously with clearance of the suspected antigen or the recurrence of glomerulonephritis after antigenic rechallenge or reinfection with a particular virus. Detection of specific immune complexes in the circulation supports an association, but to establish a diagnostic causal linkage with glomerulonephritis, viral antigens and host antibodies must be identified in the mesangium or glomerular capillaries in higher concentration than in the circulation (8,12,13).

Our expertise as diagnosticians has certainly advanced compared to our relatively limited capability only three decades ago. Better understanding of the etiology and pathogenesis of renal disease depends on precise identification of clinical syndromes and infective agents, improved serologic diagnosis (which requires knowledge of viral structure and immune response), epidemiologic characterization of infected populations (which is dependent on proper screening studies), and ultimately, rigorous virologic and molecular analysis of pathologic tissue (Table 59-3). Understanding these factors is critical to permit the development of rational and effective treatments. Current technology permits us to move beyond the association of viral illnesses solely with immune complex mechanisms.

The present armamentarium of tools used to address diagnostic issues is vast, and includes classic histochemical methods as well as molecular biologic approaches. Microdissection and the polymerase chain reaction (PCR) can be used to detect and amplify viral nucleic acid sequences in tissue (23–25). In situ hybridization techniques and in situ PCR technology are used to localize viral sequences in pathologic tissue (26–28), and the development of transgenic animal models has added a wealth of information to the study of renal diseases (28–31) (Table 59-4).

TABLE 59-1

VIRAL INFECTIONS MEDIATING RENAL DISEASE

Hepatitis B virus
Hepatitis C virus
Human immunodeficiency virus
Cytomegalovirus
Hantavirus
BK papovavirus
JC virus
Yellow fever
Mumps
Measles
Varicella
Others

The expression of renal disease associated with viral infection is likely to be affected by the host response (Table 59-5). Factors that may modulate expression of renal disease include the patient's age, gender, genetic background, and immunologic responsiveness (including the extent and duration of humoral as compared to cell-mediated responses). A humoral response resulting in the development of cryoprecipitable immune reactants, a characteristic of the response to viral infections (32–36), may have late sequelae that seem unrelated to the original viral illness. Socioeconomic status and access to care may also ultimately modify organ responses to viral infections. An important question to be considered is whether a virus of interest infects renal cells. The expression of viral proteins or abnormal host proteins in the kidney may result in the development of renal disease through various pathways. Viral proteins may engender cell death through necrosis or apoptosis, or may cause cell dysfunction (13,16,17,37,38–41). Alternatively, such proteins might increase the propensity to develop circulating or *in situ* immune-mediated pathogenic mechanisms or might lead to increased matrix synthesis and/or decreased matrix degradation (13,16,18,19). Selected viral or host proteins could in-

TABLE 59-2

PATHOGENESIS OF IMMUNE COMPLEX NEPHROPATHY IN VIRAL DISEASES

Circulating immune complex disease involving viral antigens and host antiviral antibody
Circulating immune complex disease involving endogenous antigens released by viral-induced injury to cells and host-autoantibody
In situ immune complex disease involving viral antigen binding to glomerular structures and host antiviral antibody or cell-mediated immunity
Autoimmune reactions to host glomerular structures induced by viruses (e.g., induction of self-reactive T or B cells, release of sequestered antigen, "molecular-mimicry," or activation of idiotype–antiidiotype networks involving "peptidic self")
Virus induced activation of cytokines and/or cell adhesion molecules
Direct cytopathogenic effect of virus on glomerular cells

(From: Glassock RJ. Immune complex-induced glomerular injury in viral diseases: an overview. *Kidney Int* 1991;40(Suppl 35):S-5, with permission.)

TABLE 59-3

STEPS INVOLVED IN ELUCIDATING PATHOGENIC MECHANISMS OF VIRAL-INDUCED NEPHROPATHY

1. Identification of clinical syndromes and infective agents
2. Serologic diagnosis—dependent on knowledge of viral structure and immune response
3. Epidemiologic characterization of infected populations by proper screening studies
4. Virologic, immunologic, and molecular analysis of pathologic tissues

duce the synthesis of cytokines, chemokines, growth factors, or adhesion molecules, which may result in the development or worsening of nephropathy (11,13,16–22). Finally, some renal diseases seen in patients with viral infections may be related to treatment.

Cryoglobulins, which are part of the spectrum of the host response to viral infection, are immunoglobulins that precipitate in the cold (32–34,36,42–44). Cryoglobulins are classified, according to Brouet et al. (33), into three types. Type I cryoglobulinemia is characterized by a monoclonal immunoglobulin, usually IgM, and is usually associated with either myeloma or Waldenström's macroglobulinemia. Mixed cryoglobulinemia (types II and III) is defined by the presence of cryoprecipitable circulating immune complexes of at least two different immunoglobulin classes. One of the immunoglobulins must be polyclonal. Type II cryoglobulinemia usually consists of a monoclonal IgM-κ with rheumatoid factor activity, and a polyclonal IgG. Type III cryoglobulinemia consists of more than one polyclonal immunoglobulin, of which one, usually IgM, has rheumatoid factor activity. Both forms of mixed cryoglobulinemia have been associated with a variety of illnesses eliciting an immune response (e.g., viral, bacterial, parasitic, spirochetal, and fungal infections and lymphoproliferative disorders) (32). Until a little more than a decade ago, many cases were termed "essential" since no underlying cause could be identified. Since the availability of serologic testing to diagnose HCV infection, many cases are now thought to be the result of HCV infection (45–47). The syndrome of mixed cryoglobulinemia includes weakness, palpable purpura (a physical finding suggestive of vasculitis), Raynaud's phenomenon, leg ulcers, arthritis, peripheral neuropathy, and liver function test abnormalities. Renal disease associated with cryoglobulinemia has long been recognized (48) and occurs in approximately half the cases of cryoglobulinemia (49–51). MPGN is the classic expression of cryoglobulinemia-associated renal disease (52), characterized by glomerular endocapillary proliferation, intraluminal thrombi, double-contoured thickening of the glomerular basement membrane, small- and medium-sized vessel vasculitis, and glomerular and interstitial mononuclear cell infiltration.

The pathophysiology of renal disease associated with mixed cryoglobulinemia remains incompletely delineated, since no correlation has been found between the quantity of cryoglobulins in serum and the presence and severity of renal disease. It has been postulated that the renal lesions could result from

TABLE 59-4

VIRUS HUNTING IN THE KIDNEY

Microdissection and the polymerase chain reaction (PCR)
In situ hybridization/PCR techniques
Transgenic animal models

TABLE 59-5

INFLAMMATORY VIRAL RENAL DISEASE

Host factors
  Age
  Gender
  Genetic background
  Immune status
  Socioeconomic status
  Access to care
Immunologic factors
  Classic immune complex disease
  Host antiviral antibody reactive with viral antigens
  Host antibody reactive with circulating endogenous
    antigens induced by viral changes in host membrane
    proteins shed into the circulation
  In situ mechanisms of nephropathogenesis
  Viral gene expression in renal tissue
  Abnormal host protein expression in renal tissue
  Viral antigen binding to renal cells with subsequent host
    antibody- or cell-mediated immune response
  Host chemokine and cytokine expression

the interaction of antibodies either with circulating antigens deposited in the kidney or with renal structural antigens. Support for the latter hypothesis includes the observation that solubilized mixed cryoglobulins from patients with cryoglobulinemia and renal disease resulted in the development of MPGN when injected into mice. The IgM monoclonal component of these cryoglobulins was found to be deposited in glomeruli, suggesting *in situ* immune complex formation. Subsequently, a candidate antigen in kidney tissue was identified as alpha-enolase, a glycolytic enzyme present on renal tubular cell membranes that functions to catalyze the dehydration of 2-phosphoglycerate to phosphoenolpyruvate (53). Subsequent studies will be necessary to elucidate more completely the role of the interaction between cryoglobulins and structural antigens in the kidney in the pathophysiology of renal disease associated with cryoglobulinemia.

Current diagnostic and investigative technologies will allow us to use renal diseases caused by viruses as models to answer questions about and elucidate pathogenic mechanisms regarding nephropathies associated with viral infections, as well as disorders not previously linked with viral infections. Such tools will ultimately allow us to understand the complex and probably multiple reasons that some viruses are nephropathogenic while others are not.

HEPATITIS B VIRUS–ASSOCIATED GLOMERULONEPHRITIS

Glomerular disease resulting from HBV infection has been said to be the prototype of viral-induced glomerular injury (3). Much of the information known about injury associated with HCV infection and human immunodeficiency virus (HIV) infection has resulted directly from the information gleaned from the study of HBV infection.

HBV infection is one of the most common infectious disorders in the world. It has been estimated that the incidence of infection is greater than 50 million persons per year and that the prevalence may exceed 1 billion persons (54). Infection results in transient and minor illness in most persons, who become free of virus after a period of several weeks. A minority of patients develop chronic sequelae of HBV infection,

including chronic hepatitis, cirrhosis, and hepatocellular carcinoma. A few patients develop complications related to the presence of circulating HBV-associated antigens in the circulation and the antibody response(s) that they evoke. The circulating immune complexes give rise to a variety of disorders reminiscent of those seen with serum sickness, including several different forms of glomerulonephritis, as well as a number of vasculitic disorders. Other patients may develop complications from the deposition of HBV-associated antigens in tissues, leading to antibody binding and injury from immune mechanisms. Either circulating or deposited antigens may evoke a wide array of responses independent of classically defined immune mechanisms. The heterogeneity of responses associated with HBV infection is not consistent with a simplistic view of the mechanism of injury. Unfortunately, investigators have focused largely on descriptive studies. There are few studies that delineate pathogenesis and even fewer that address the issue of treatment strategies for HBV-related renal disorders.

The HBV is a DNA virus of the hepadnavirus family, and infection is restricted to humans and nonhuman primates. It is depicted schematically in Figure 59-1 (55). The complete virus is known as the Dane particle, a 42-nm spherical structure consisting of an envelope of viral-encoded proteins and lipid components derived from the host. The envelope contains the hepatitis B surface antigen (HBsAg), against which neutralizing antibody (HBsAb) is directed. The inner core of the virion contains the hepatitis core antigen (HBcAg), viral DNA, and the DNA polymerase protein. The virus also produces 22-nm dimorphic spherical and filamentous particles that are composed of envelope proteins only. Since these particles do not contain the HBV genome, they are noninfectious. They are the most abundant forms of virus particles in the circulation, and are present in the circulation in concentrations several logs greater than intact viruses. The genome of HBV is semicircular, partially double-stranded DNA approximately 3,200 base pairs in length. HBV is classified into seven genotypes (A to G) based upon differences in the complete nucleotide sequence. The clinical significance of the genotypes is not yet clearly delineated (56).

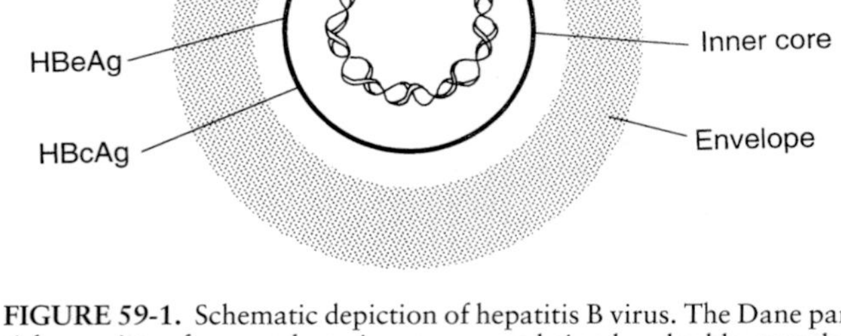

Dane Particle

42 nm

FIGURE 59-1. Schematic depiction of hepatitis B virus. The Dane particle consists of an envelope, inner core, and circular, double-stranded DNA. Several of the viral proteins may be found in the circulation of infected patients. Antibodies directed against all the depicted viral antigens may be found in the patient's circulation at different stages of the infection. *HBcAg*, hepatitis B virus core antigen; *HBeAg*, hepatitis B virus e antigen; *HBsAg*, hepatitis B virus surface antigen; *HBV*, hepatitis B virus; *viral DNA*, double-stranded HBV DNA.

Patients infected with HBV express three antigenic proteins to which antibodies may be formed: HBcA, giving rise to anti-HBcAg (HBcAb); hepatitis B e antigen (HBeAg), against which anti-HBeAg is formed (HBeAb); and HBsAg, which evokes generation of anti-HBsAg (HBsAb). If the patient is immunocompetent, generation of antigen-specific antibody results in clearance of the antigen and resolution of infection. Circulating antibody becomes a marker of previous infection. If infection is prolonged, so that antigenemia is chronic, immune complexes may form and be detected in the circulation. The pathogenicity of the immune complexes depends in part on their size and electrical charge and the physicochemical factors that result in lattice formation (57).

The molecular biology and immunology of the HBV have been extensively reviewed (56–59). There are four open reading frames that encode the envelope, core/pre-core, polymerase, and X proteins. Envelope proteins include the large (L), middle (M), and small (S) envelope proteins. The M and S envelope proteins are found in all forms of viral and subviral particles. The L envelope protein is found predominantly in complete virions. Proteins encoded by the core/pre-core reading frames include a precore polypeptide which is posttranslationally modified into a soluble protein, HBeAg. Further translation produces the core protein (HBcAg). The open reading frame encoding the polymerase overlaps with the core, envelope, and X reading frames. The polymerase protein consists of a protein primer, a spacer, a reverse transcriptase/DNA polymerase, and an RNAase H domain. The X protein, which is not essential for viral replication, is a transcriptional transactivator of many promoters including HBV and cellular oncogenes. The HBx protein has been implicated in hepatocarcinogenesis.

The HBsAg has a molecular weight of 3.5 to 4.4 million daltons, with its antigenic determinants expressed on peptides that are considerably smaller (22,000 to 49,000 daltons) (60). The inner core of HBV contains HBcAg, which consists of multiple copies of a 22-kd molecular weight protein (p22). HBcAg is not found in the circulation. HBeAg is a 15-kd protein that can be released from the core antigen by treatment with proteolytic enzymes. The HBeAg can circulate in a variety of forms: as a 30-kd dimer bound to albumin or as a hexamer bound to specific immunoglobulin G (IgG) antibodies (anti-HBeAb). HBeAg-IgG is a large complex, with a molecular weight of 240,000 to 540,000 daltons and a cationic isoelectric point. There is substantial evidence implicating the albumin-bound "small" HBeAg and IgG-associated "large" HBeAg in the pathogenesis of glomerular disease. The presence of any form of the HBeAg in the circulation correlates with the presence of the intact virus in the circulation and is indicative of infectivity. The presence of HBeAb connotes viral clearance and subsequent immunity.

The prevalence of chronic HBV infection, particularly as assessed by chronic HBsAg antigenemia, varies widely according to geographic area. It varies from 0.1% to 2.0% in low-prevalence areas (United States and Canada, Western Europe, Australia and New Zealand), to 3% to 5% in intermediate-prevalence areas (Mediterranean countries, Japan, Central Asia, Middle East, and Latin and South America), to 10% to 20% in high-prevalence areas (southeast Asia, China, and sub-Saharan Africa (54,61).

The etiology of the infection also varies according to the area of study. In adults, the transmission of infection is often horizontal and is frequently accompanied by an episode of clinically apparent infection. Since blood transfusions in developed countries are an increasingly uncommon cause of HBV infection, infection in adults often results from the communal use of needles among intravenous drug users or as a sexually transmitted disease. Conversely, HBV infection in children is more often transmitted in a vertical pattern, passing from mother to child. It has usually been thought that such children are asymp-

tomatic and have no history of overt hepatitis (62). Bhimma et al. examined the HBV status and measured proteinuria in family members and household contacts of index children with HBV-associated MN. These investigators found that 37% of the subjects were HBV carriers, and 27% had abnormal proteinuria. The prevalence of proteinuria was much higher than in community-based control subjects, although it was not dependent upon carriage of HBV (63).

There are several defined renal clinicopathologic disorders associated with HBV infection, including a number of different forms of glomerular disease and a variety of serum sickness-like and vasculitic illnesses. Although these disorders are not uncommon, they do not occur or are not detected with a frequency commensurate with the prevalence of HBV infection in the population. Therefore, they probably do not result from HBV infection alone, but from a combination of the infection and the immunologic responses of the host.

HBV infection has been thought to result in glomerular disease through immune complex mechanisms since the early descriptions of HBV-associated renal disease. At least one of these mechanisms involves deposition of an antigen in renal tissue, followed by binding of a strategically placed antibody, which results in complement fixation and immunologic injury. Alternatively, circulating immune complexes composed of HBV antigens and antibodies may deposit in glomeruli and result in nephropathy. Current concepts regarding the pathogenesis of HBV-associated nephropathy, however, are considerably more complex. While it is clear that HBV results in renal damage through circulating immune complex mechanisms in certain instances, there are other pathogenic pathways that remain incompletely understood. In addition to immune complex deposition, other potential pathways include a direct cytopathic effect induced by the virus, viral-induced specific effector mechanisms (specific T cell or antibody) which damage the kidney, or renal injury mediated through viral-induced cytokines or other mediators (64). While we have long been aware of the association between HBV infection and renal disease, our understanding of the pathophysiology of this relationship is still inadequate.

Several glomerular diseases have been associated with HBV infection. In most reports, MN has been the most frequent pathologic lesion encountered in patients with HBV infection and renal disease. MPGN has been noted less frequently, as has IgA nephropathy. Two other disorders with renal manifestations are closely associated with HBV: PAN and cryoglobulinemia.

Hepatitis B Virus and Membranous Nephropathy, Membranoproliferative Glomerulonephritis, and Immunoglobulin A Nephropathy

MN was the first renal disorder to be associated with HBV. Combes and co-workers (65) reported a 53-year-old man who presented with nephrotic syndrome 18 months after receiving a blood transfusion. Four months after the transfusion, he developed jaundice, and circulating Australia antigen was detected. Nearly 2 years later, this man was found to have proteinuria and underwent renal biopsy. The biopsy revealed diffusely thickened glomerular capillary basement membranes and mesangial hypercellularity, with ultrastructural changes typical of MN. The authors demonstrated staining for the Australia antigen with indirect immunofluorescence using guinea pig antibody reactive against commercially obtained Australia antigen and rabbit anti-guinea pig antibody. They concluded that these findings were highly suggestive that the renal disease was caused by deposition of Australia antigen-containing immune complexes in the kidney, although they were not able to elute such complexes from renal tissue.

Subsequently Kneiser et al. (66) reported three patients with chronic HBV infection, each of whom had a different form of glomerulopathy (i.e., MPGN, focal glomerulosclerosis, and MN). HBsAg was detected in each patient's renal tissue by indirect immunofluorescence using rabbit anti-HBsAg and guinea pig anti-rabbit globulin. The authors emphasized the similarities between the morphologic findings in their patients and those in the studies of circulating immune complex induction of glomerulonephritis performed by Oldstone and Dixon (67). That HBV MN was a circulating immune complex disease was supported by the studies of Kohler et al. (68), who reported a 42-year-old man with chronic active hepatitis and MN. HBsAg was detected by indirect immunofluorescence in glomerular capillary walls. The patient's serum contained 10 mg/dL of cryoprecipitate composed of antibody directed against HBsAg as well as the HBsAg. The demonstration of HBsAg in renal tissue, as well as the detection of circulating immune complexes containing both antigen and its antibody, was convincing evidence of the pathogenic role of circulating immune complexes in HBV MN. The concept that circulating immune complexes, consisting of the HBsAg and its antibody, could localize in glomeruli and result in disease became a well-accepted paradigm.

Subsequently, however, Couser and Salant (9) proposed that immune complexes could be formed in situ, offering a mechanism for immune complex injuries that did not require them to be in the circulation. Simultaneously, the complexity of the structure of the HBV became more apparent (9). It seemed obvious that at least some of the components of the HBV, because of their size or charge, would not be able to traverse the glomerular capillary basement membrane to localize in the subepithelial space. It was more likely, and consistent with the hypothesis of *in situ* immune complex formation, that an alternative potential mechanism of HBV-associated glomerular injury was the deposition of HBV-associated antigen in the glomerular capillary, followed by antibody deposition. A second mechanism might involve the formation of new antigens from renal tissue damaged by HBV. These alternative hypotheses for the pathogenesis of HBV-associated glomerular disease served to address two areas of concern. First, the subepithelial location of immune deposits thought to be HBV antigens and accompanying antibodies in renal biopsy material seemed improbable because the deposits were too large. Second, circulating immune complexes could not be found in the majority of specimens (69–71).

The clinical manifestations of HBV-associated MN have been reported in several large, older series (72–75). In most reports, the diagnosis of HBV-associated MN was based on one or more of the following criteria: persistent HBV-associated antigenemia, absence of evidence of other causes of glomerulonephritis, and detection of at least one HBV antigen in renal tissue. The majority of patients reported were seropositive for at least one HBV-associated antigen, usually HBsAg. Inclusion of patients without other glomerular diseases was determined on clinical grounds.

The detection of HBV-associated antigens in renal tissue was more problematic. Many cases reported as HBV-associated MN did not have any HBV-associated antigen detected in renal tissue, and few investigators reported elution of immune complexes or HBV antigen-specific antibody from renal tissue. Thus, the clinical criterion used to define HBV-associated nephropathies in many early clinical studies was, in fact, simply the occurrence of renal abnormalities in a patient with HBV infection. For example, Lai et al. (72) reported 25 patients with MN from a cohort of 74 patients with HBsAg antigenemia and a variety of different forms of glomerulonephritis, of which MN was the most common (35%). All biopsies revealed the ultrastructural changes typical of MN. The investigators attempted to detect HBsAg, HBcAg, and HBeAg using immunoperoxidase techniques with polyclonal monospecific rabbit antihuman antisera on paraffin sections of renal tissue, or with indirect immunofluorescence with the same antisera on frozen sections of renal tissue. They were only able to detect renal tissue HBcAg in three patients, HBsAg in two patients, and both renal tissue HBcAg and HBsAg in two patients. Given the inability of the investigators to detect HBV-associated antigens in renal tissue, this study could be interpreted as simply a description of patients with HBV-associated antigenemia with incidental MN. Other studies were similar. Lee and others (74) reported 87 patients with chronic HBsAg antigenemia who had glomerular disease. Twenty-nine patients had MPGN, and 18 had MN. These 47 patients were said to have HBV-associated glomerulonephritis. However, the authors could not detect HBsAg in the six biopsy samples tested and did not test for other HBV-associated antigens.

Moreover, while HBV-associated antigens were absent from the tissue of many of the HBsAg-positive patients thought to have HBV-associated renal disease, HBsAg was reported in glomerular deposits in patients seronegative for HBsAg, leading to further confusion about the importance that HBV-associated antigens might play in the pathogenesis of glomerular injury (75,76).

In virtually all reports in which HBsAg was detected in renal tissue, it was detected by indirect immunofluorescence. This technique involved raising antibody to the HBsAg or other HBV-associated antigens in rabbits and layering the immunoglobulin on the renal tissue of interest. Then, anti-rabbit antibody was used to detect whether binding of the anti-HBV antibody by renal tissue had occurred. The specificity of staining in this technique should be confirmed by using anti-rabbit antisera as a control. However, so few studies of putative HBV MN had detectable renal tissue HBV-associated antigens determined by rigorous criteria that Magiore and co-workers (77) questioned the specificity of staining for HBV-associated antigens in renal tissue. These investigators systematically examined the problem of antibody specificity and determined that endogenous immunoglobulin M (IgM) antibody in glomerular tissue had antiimmunoglobulin activity that resulted in false-positive staining for HBsAg. They demonstrated improved specificity with the use of fluoresceinated F(ab')$_2$ probes prepared from commercial rabbit antisera. They performed studies that clearly demonstrated that methods that did not use F(ab') probes to detect HBV-associated antigens in renal tissue resulted in false-positive staining for these antigens. Thus, much of the clinical literature, including reports of patient material identified as HBV-associated glomerulonephritis, which had been published prior to the Magiore report, was of limited heuristic value.

Subsequently, Hiroshi et al. (78) devised a method of detecting HBV antigens in renal tissue that abrogated the problem of false-positive staining. At the same time, these authors demonstrated that the principal HBV antigen involved in HBV MN was the HBeAg, rather than the HBsAg. They immunized BALB/c mice with plasma containing HBeAg and high titers of HBsAg. Spleen cells were harvested and fused with mouse myeloma cells. Subsequently, clones yielding anti-HBe were grown in ascitic mice, and the resultant gamma globulin fraction was precipitated with acid. This monoclonal antibody was digested with pepsin to obtain F(ab')$_2$ fragments, which were then conjugated with fluorescein isothiocyanate and used to stain tissue. These monoclonal antibody fragments were shown to be quite specific by blocking and inhibition studies. Immune deposits in the glomeruli of 10 of 16 patients with MN, seropositive for HBsAg, were positive for HBeAg. None of the deposits was positive for HBsAg or HBcAg. Moreover, of the 10 patients with glomerular deposits of HBeAg, nine were seropositive for HBeAg, and the one that was not had circulating anti-HBeAb. These studies confirmed that previous studies using conventional immunofluorescence were flawed. They also demonstrated that HBeAg, not HBsAg, was the principal antigen associated with HBV MN.

HBeAg had previously been found to be a part of the HBV capsid and to exist in both small and large forms (79). Subsequently, its participation in the pathogenesis of HBV-associated renal disease was reported by Takekoshi et al. (80). These investigators studied two children seropositive for both HBsAg and HBeAg who developed nephrotic syndrome, in both of whom renal biopsy revealed MN. The authors detected two forms of HBeAg in the serum: a small form, and a larger form bound to IgG. They also detected HBeAg in the same pattern as IgG in renal tissue, which did not stain for other HBV antigens. Through an elegant series of blocking and inhibition studies, the authors ensured the specificity of the detection of HBeAg. This reemphasized the importance of HBeAg in the pathogenesis of HBV-associated MN. These investigators also helped to delineate the relationship between the nature of the HBV-associated antigen and the propensity to develop glomerular disease. They noted that the molecular weight of HBeAg, even if bound to IgG, was substantially less than that of HBsAg and concluded that HBeAg, because of its size, was far more likely to localize in the subepithelial space than the very large HBsAg.

Subsequently, Lai and co-workers (81) studied 21 patients with adult-onset HBV MN. These patients had persistent HBsAg antigenemia and proteinuria greater than 1 g/day. The diagnosis of HBV-associated glomerulonephritis was restricted to only those patients with glomerular capillary deposition of a HBV antigen detected by F(ab) monoclonal antibody fragments. None of the patients had a history of hepatitis, although there was either historical or serologic evidence of HBV infection in some relative in the majority of their families. There were 17 males and 4 females, with a mean age of 30 years (range, 15 to 53 years). Twelve had nephrotic syndrome, 7 had asymptomatic proteinuria, and 2 had chronic renal failure. The duration of symptoms ranged from 1 to 36 months. Mean protein excretion was 4.1 g/day (range, 1.0 to 12.5 g/day). One-fourth of the patients had some impairment of renal function, while one-third were hypertensive at the time of presentation. All biopsy specimens revealed electron microscopic subepithelial electron-dense deposits, although virus-like particles were seen in only one specimen. The investigators searched for HBV-associated antigens with indirect and direct immunofluorescence using F(ab')₂ fragments of murine monoclonal and polyclonal antibodies and immunoperoxidase techniques. Sixteen of the patients had granular deposits of HBeAg detected in capillary walls. The other five patients had an HBV-associated antigen in biopsy tissue, although the specificity of the polyclonal antibody resulted in some crossreactivity between HBcAg and HBeAg. Polyclonal antibodies had previously been shown to be less specific than monoclonal antibodies when used to detect HBV-associated antigens in kidney tissue (82). This was the first study to describe patients with HBV-associated MN in which diagnostic criteria restricted entry to only those patients with specifically detected HBV-associated antigen(s) in the appropriate anatomic location in renal tissue.

Using these more restrictive diagnostic criteria, Lai and co-workers (83) subsequently reported a large series of patients with HBV-associated glomerular disease. They studied 100 consecutive patients who presented from 1985 to 1992 with primary glomerulonephritis who were HBsAg seropositive. Thirty-nine patients had at least one HBV-associated antigen in renal tissue as detected by monoclonal antibodies. Of these 39, HBsAg was detected in renal tissue in 21, HBcAg in 2, and HBeAg in 27. The glomerular pathologic descriptions

TABLE 59-6

HEPATITIS B VIRUS-ASSOCIATED GLOMERULOPATHIES: TISSUE IMMUNOREACTANT DIAGNOSES

Tissue immunoreactant	Pathology
HBeAg	MN; mixed lesions
HBsAg	IgA nephropathy; MN; mixed lesions
HBcAb	MN; IgA nephropathy[a]

[a]Two patients only.

were heterogeneous and are depicted in Table 59-6. Of the 21 patients with glomerular HBsAg, MPGN with immunofluorescent features characteristic of IgA nephropathy was the most common lesion, with MN a distant second. Several patients had combination lesions, such as MN and IgA nephropathy, or MN and MPGN. There were two patients with glomerular HBcAg: 1 with MN and 1 with IgA nephropathy. Twenty-seven patients had glomerular HBeAg, of whom 15 had MN, 1 had IgA nephropathy, and 2 had MPGN. The remainder had combinations of lesions, such as MN–IgA nephropathy and MN–MPGN.

This study is notable for several reasons. First, it is the largest description of patients with HBV-associated glomerulonephritis in which the essential diagnostic criterion is detection of HBV-associated antigens in glomerular tissue by the use of monoclonal antibodies. Second, it clearly demonstrates that HBV-associated glomerulonephritis has diverse morphologic presentations, although three lesions appear to be most common. They include MN, MPGN, and IgA nephropathy. The previously widely accepted concept that most HBV-associated glomerulonephritis is MN has been changed because it is now clear that HBsAg is most commonly associated with mesangial proliferative lesions, while HBeAg is most commonly detected in cases of MN. Third, the study underscores the relative infrequency with which the HBcAg is associated with glomerulopathy. Finally, the study demonstrates that combination lesions, such as MN–IgA nephropathy or MN–MPGN, are not uncommon.

Lai and co-workers extended these observations using molecular biologic techniques to corroborate their findings with monoclonal antibodies. They used in situ hybridization and PCR techniques to probe for HBV DNA and RNA in renal biopsy tissue from 40 chronic HBV carriers with a variety of morphologic presentations, including MN, MPGN, and IgA nephropathy. They found HBV DNA to be located mainly in the cytoplasm of proximal tubular cells rather than glomeruli. HBcAg RNA was found in the nuclei and cytoplasm of both glomerular and tubular cells in 56%, 20%, and 36% of renal biopsies showing MN, MPGN, and IgA nephropathy, respectively. These findings, in which viral transcripts were found in renal cells, support even more strongly an etiologic role for HBV in the pathogenesis of renal disease (84). Similar data were provided by He et al. in a study of children (85).

The availability and use of monoclonal antibodies and molecular techniques to detect HBV-associated antigens in renal tissue has allowed investigators to be more confident that the glomerulonephritis seen in patients with HBV is really HBV-associated glomerulonephritis. Moreover, it has allowed investigators to define clinical populations more precisely. This led to the ability to observe not only the natural history of HBV-associated glomerulonephritis but also, in certain instances, patients' responses to therapy. Multiple studies in the era before precise definition of HBV-associated glomerulonephritis was possible suggested that the nephrotic syndrome usually remitted in 30% to 60% of patients, while the remainder had a more indolent course. Lai and co-workers (72) had previously noted that, in a study of 69 patients with HBV-associated glomerular disease, 14% had progressive renal failure, although none reached end-stage renal disease (ESRD).

In one large clinical study with follow-up that defined patients with HBV MN more precisely, Lin (86) studied 34 children (25 boys, 9 girls) with HBV-associated MN, in whom F(ab') fragments of monoclonal antibodies were used to detect HBeAg in the glomeruli from 30 (88%). All but 4 children had nephrotic syndrome, and all were seropositive for HBsAg; all but 2 were seropositive for HBeAg. Many patients were hypocomplementemic during the first 6 months of their renal illness, although serum complement concentrations became normal in most after several months, independent of whether the renal disease remitted. Serum levels of circulating IgM and HBsAg immune complexes were elevated initially but returned to values not different from those of seropositive controls without renal disease on remission of proteinuria. Four patients progressed morphologically, with the MN lesion having changed from stage I or II to stage III. One child had impaired renal function. Ito and others (87), in an earlier report in which serial renal biopsies of 6 children with HBeAg-associated MN were described, noted regression of the pathologic features of MN and regression of proteinuria in 2 patients who seroconverted from HBeAg-positive to HBeAb-positive. Second biopsies confirmed the absence of HBeAg in patients in whose kidney it had previously been detected, as well as resolution of deposits in glomerular basement membranes. The suggestion that seroconversion from antigen positivity could result in resolution of glomerular disease had previously been made by Knecht and Chisari (88), who reported a patient who was seropositive for HBsAg and had HBV-associated MPGN. The patient's nephrotic syndrome resolved in conjunction with loss of HBsAg seropositivity.

There are no large-scale follow-up studies in adults in whom HBV MN has been properly defined. At present it appears that HBV-associated renal disease has a varied natural history, although so few precisely defined patients have been longitudinally studied that generalizations about natural history are of limited value. Progression to ESRD does, however, appear to be uncommon, at least as is reflected in the literature. Seroconversion from HBV antigen positivity may be associated with a more favorable renal prognosis, although there are limited data to support a more definitive statement about seroconversion.

Treatment

The treatment of HBV MN has been the subject of largely anecdotal reports because there are virtually no adequately designed prospective controlled trials. In parallel with the enthusiasm afforded corticosteroids (CS) in the treatment of idiopathic MN, some patients with HBV infection have been treated with CS in attempts to induce remission of their renal disease, usually the nephrotic syndrome. In the previously mentioned study by Lin (86), 32 patients were treated with CS. One had an early response, while 11 had persistent nephrotic syndrome. Thirteen patients responded but had frequent relapses. Four patients sustained complete remission months after completion of the CS regimen, without clearing HBsAg or HBeAg from the circulation.

Following this study, Lin (89) extended his observations in this same cohort and demonstrated that treatment with CS might be harmful. He harvested macrophages, B cells, and T cells from some of these patients and performed Southern blot hybridization using EcoRI digestion of an HBV-plasmid clone, pTWL1 (90). In one patient who had not received CS, HBV DNA was found in macrophages, T cells, and B cells. Six months later, the HBV DNA was no longer detectable. In a patient who had received CS, cellular HBV DNA was detectable 3 years later. Moreover, dexamethasone was able to stimulate production of both HBsAg and HBeAg from peripheral blood mononuclear cells. Lai et al. (91) had observed a similar effect of CS therapy to enhance viral replication in a study of eight patients with HBV-associated MN. HBV DNA was determined in serum by dot blot hybridization using an oligonucleotide probe (92). Five of the six patients treated with CS and studied by this technique had an increase in serum HBV DNA, which decreased when CS therapy was discontinued. No favorable effect of CS was noted on any renal parameter when compared to control patients treated with diuretics alone.

The unsatisfactory results of treatment with CS prompted a search for more effective regimens. Scullard et al. (93) reported the disappearance of HBcAg, HBeAg, and HBsAg from the sera and livers of patients treated with IFN and the antiviral agent adenine arabinoside. This prompted a few reports of treatment of patients with HBV-associated glomerular disease with IFN. Garcia and co-workers (94) treated two patients, one adult and one child, both of whom had MN associated with seropositivity for HBsAg, with leukocyte IFN. The adult was treated for 4 weeks, with a rapid fall in DNA polymerase activity, loss of HBsAg and HBeAg, development of HBeAb, and resolution of nephrotic syndrome. However, despite the continued absence of HBV antigens, the adult patient's nephrotic syndrome recrudesced 7 months after the IFN was stopped. The child had a relapsing course, accompanied by a fall in DNA polymerase activity but no change in his HBV antigen status. After several courses of IFN, the child's nephrotic syndrome remitted, although he remained seropositive. This experience prompted Lisker-Melman and co-workers (95) to prospectively administer recombinant human IFN to five patients seropositive for HBsAg, HBeAg, HBV DNA, and DNA polymerase who had MN (four patients) or MPGN (one patient). Patients were treated with 5 million units of IFN subcutaneously daily for 4 months. Serum levels of HBV DNA and DNA polymerase activity decreased in all five patients, and four became negative for both these markers as well as for HBeAg; three of the four became seropositive for HBeAb. Urine protein levels fell from a mean of 7.9 g/day to 2.5, 2.8, and 1.0 g/day 4, 8, and 12 months after therapy, respectively. Unfortunately, side effects, although transient, were extremely common.

Jonas et al. (96) reported their experience with a 7-year-old child who they treated with IFN. Although the girl had resolution of her nephrotic syndrome, she had seroconverted from HBeAg to HBeAb a short time before receiving the IFN. Therefore, the response may have been unrelated to the treatment. Esteban and co-workers (97) treated a 9-year-old boy with HBV MN with adenine arabinoside for 6 weeks. This was associated with a prompt fall in urinary protein excretion, conversion of HBeAg to HBeAb, and disappearance of HBV DNA from serum. The patient was entirely well after 11 months of follow-up.

Lin (98) reported his experience with the treatment of HBV-associated MN in children with recombinant IFN. In this prospective, controlled, open-labeled trial, 40 children who had HBV-associated MN diagnosed by strict criteria were randomly assigned to receive either subcutaneous recombinant IFN or supportive therapy alone. All patients had undergone a 2-month trial of CS and had not responded and all had heavy proteinuria. All patients had normal serum creatinine concentrations, and none was hypertensive. Group 1 patients received 5 million units of IFN subcutaneously three times weekly for 1 year. Group 2 patients received only supportive therapy. The mean age of the patients was 6.2 and 6.8 years, and the mean protein excretion was 4.1 and 4.0 g/24 hours in groups 1 and 2, respectively. All patients were seropositive for both HBeAg and HBsAg at the start of the trial.

Two months after IFN therapy was begun, heavy proteinuria disappeared in 16 of 20 (80%) patients in group 1, while 4 patients (20%) had only light proteinuria. By the end of the third month, all 20 patients in this treatment group were free of proteinuria. At both 1 and 2 years after the start of the trial, no patients had relapsed with proteinuria. Conversely, after 2 months of supportive therapy, 12 of 20 (60%) patients in group 2 continued to have heavy proteinuria, while 8 of 20 (40%) continued to have light proteinuria, which increased during upper respiratory infections. By the end of the third month, 50% of the patients continued with heavy proteinuria, and 50% had light proteinuria, which increased concomitant with respiratory infections. By the end of the first year of the trial, 6 of 20 (30%) patients in group 2 persisted with heavy proteinuria, 12 of 20 (60%) had light proteinuria with frequent relapses, while only 2 of 20 (10%) were free of proteinuria. By the end of the second year, 3 of 20 (15%) and 10 of 20 (50%) patients in group 2 had heavy and periodically relapsing light proteinuria, respectively. Only 7 of 20 (35%) patients were free of proteinuria.

Even more striking was the effect of treatment with IFN on the rate of HBV-associated antigen seroconversion. After 2 years, 11 of 20 patients in group 1 had HBeAg and HBsAg seroconversion. Five of 20 were HBeAb-positive, while 4 of 20 persisted with both HBsAg and HBeAg. Conversely, in the group 2 patients, all patients remained seropositive for both HBsAg and HBeAg after 2 years. No patient in either group developed renal dysfunction over the time course of the study.

The side effects of IFN were significant. All patients developed flulike symptoms and fever. Fever generally remitted after 3 weeks of therapy. There was no leukopenia. Late side effects included anxiety, depression, and suicidal ideation, the latter two symptoms affecting nearly 20% of the patients. All adverse psychiatric effects disappeared with reduction in the dose of IFN. No hematologic, infectious, or autoimmune complications were noted.

Lin (98) interpreted these results cautiously and suggested that children with HBV-associated MN with heavy proteinuria persistent for more than 2 months should be considered for therapy with IFN. Not only did such therapy appear to exert an extremely salutary effect on the duration of proteinuria, but it also was associated with a significant rate of seroconversion from HBV-associated antigenemia. It is possible that proteinuria would eventually resolve in untreated patients, as that trend was apparent in the untreated group. Nonetheless, the persistence of HBV-associated antigenemia in this group for at least 2 years may represent a marker of impaired immunoregulation and may be a risk factor for progressive renal dysfunction.

Information about treating adults with HBV infection and renal disease with IFN is more limited. Conjeevaram et al. (99) reported the results of a 4-month trial of IFN in 15 patients with HBV MN and MPGN. Eight patients had a long-term serologic response, with loss of HBeAg and HBV DNA. Seven of the eight responding patients showed gradual but marked improvement in proteinuria. The seven nonresponding patients had continued evidence of active liver and renal disease. Chung et al. (100) reported the results of therapy with IFN in eight adults with a variety of different forms of HBV-associated GN. One of the eight was only treated for 2 months because of side effects. The response of serologic markers of HBV infection to IFN was variable, while proteinuria diminished in only two patients. The results of these two relatively small cohorts of patients suggested that prolonged IFN therapy represented a promising, albeit not entirely proven, therapeutic option for patients with HBV-associated MN. Its cost, however, given the dose and length of treatment that appear to be necessary, may

be prohibitive. Side effects and risks associated with such therapy may exceed its benefits.

Recently there have been reports about the use of the agent lamivudine in the treatment of HBV-associated MN. Lamivudine is a cytosine analog which, after triphosphorylation, is incorporated into the viral DNA by hepatitis B virus polymerase, resulting in DNA chain termination. Connor et al. reported on a six-year-old male with HBV-associated MN with nephritic syndrome who was treated with oral lamivudine. After two months of treatment, his nephritic syndrome had resolved, and all immunologic markers of HBV infection had disappeared. He was treated for a total of 12 months, and after nearly a year of observation, remained completely well (101). Filler et al. reported a 15-year-old Vietnamese female with HBV-associated MN who received lamivudine for a total of slightly over 13 months. After two months of treatment, the nephrotic syndrome and markers of viral infection disappeared, but ultimately she sustained a relapse of both her MN and evidence of active viral infection (102). Although such reports are preliminary, it is intriguing that the toxicity of lamivudine appears to be remarkably less than that of INF. The oral agent is relatively well tolerated, and undoubtedly will be incorporated into future clinical trials, Moreover, a number of other promising new antiviral agents, including adefovir, dipivoxil, emtricitabine (FTC), entecavir, beta-L-thymidine, and clevudine are being evaluated in clinical trials of treatment of chronic HBV infection. To our knowledge, none of these agents has yet been tested in a trial of patients with HBV-associated MN.

At present the appropriate therapy for patients with HBV MN, particularly in adults, remains unknown. CS generally should not be used because they promote viral replication. Clinical experience with the use of antiviral agents in conjunction with IFN is so limited that firm recommendations regarding the use of these agents in HBV-associated glomerular diseases are not possible. At present, there are still no data from well-designed, controlled trials regarding the use of newer antiviral or immunosuppressant therapies in patients with renal disease associated with HBV infection. There continues to be a need for properly designed, long-term, prospective trials of patients adequately stratified for clinical, immunologic, virologic, and histologic variables to determine whether antiviral agents in conjunction with immunomodulators are efficacious in these disorders.

Another issue that needs to be examined is the true incidence and prevalence of HBV-associated glomerular disease. Multiple studies have been performed in the Far East, an area in which HBV infection is endemic, with a carrier rate in the general population of nearly 15%. There are no data of which we are aware regarding the incidence and prevalence of HBV-associated renal disease in areas of the world where HBV infection is not endemic. Properly designed epidemiologic studies would permit assessment of the scope of the problem and assist in the development of well-designed natural history and intervention trials.

We must also determine whether the use of molecular biologic tools such as in situ DNA hybridization and PCR will actually improve our ability to understand the pathophysiology of HBV-associated renal disease. For example, Lin (103) studied 14 children with biopsy-proven HBV MN, diagnosed according to strict criteria, of whom eight had follow-up biopsies. He used in situ DNA hybridization and determined that seven of eight patients demonstrated HBV DNA in glomerular and tubular cells within 6 months of onset of disease. In contrast, only three of 14 patients had HBV DNA in tubular epithelia, and none in glomeruli, when samples were taken more than 6 months after the onset of the illness. Finally, he found that patients with progressive disease continued to have detectable HBV DNA in the kidney, while those with nonprogressive disease no longer had detectable HBV DNA.

PCR technology allows detection of attamole quantities of nucleic acid in renal tissue and has been used to advance hypotheses about the progression of renal disease (104). Clearly, further advances in our understanding of HBV-associated glomerular disease will require innovative thought to generate hypotheses that are testable using the techniques of molecular biology.

Finally, it may be essential to examine more carefully the role of preventive strategies that may be capable of reducing not only the rate of infection with HBV, but also the incidence of HBV-associated MN. Lee et al demonstrated that mass immunization against HBV reduced the HBV carriage rate in children from about 10% to 0.9% (105). Sun et al. (106) reported that the incidence rate of HBV-associated MN was remarkably reduced in children after mass immunization against HBV was begun in China in 1992. In their retrospective study, the investigators found only 6 cases of HBV-associated MN in 231 vaccinated children (2.6%), compared to 40 cases in 381 unvaccinated children (10.5%). Unfortunately, vaccination did not eradicate the occurrence of HBV-MN in some children, who had serologic evidence of either incomplete vaccination or vaccine failure. Finally, government health officials in Durban, South Africa reported that vaccination against HBV reduced incidence rates of HBV-associated MN in children from 0.33 per 10^5 population to 0.03 per 10^5 population within a decade (107). These data, obtained from areas endemic for HBV infection, underscore the possibility that wide spread immunization policies may represent a real opportunity to reduce the rate of HBV infection and its associated diseases.

HEPATITIS B VIRUS AND POLYARTERITIS NODOSA

Classic PAN is a form of vasculitis in which small- to medium-sized vessels are affected (50). A similar form of vasculitis can affect smaller vessels, including arterioles and capillaries, in which case the term microscopic polyangitis is used (108). PAN is a classic multisystem disease that affects a number of different organ systems. In its untreated state, PAN carries a high mortality. Fortunately, CS and cyclophosphamide have been shown to be effective, and complete remission is common in patients in whom the disorder is diagnosed early. The diagnosis of PAN is made using 10 objective criteria, one of which includes a tissue diagnosis (50,108–110). These criteria are listed in Table 59-7.

TABLE 59-7

CRITERIA FOR THE DIAGNOSIS OF POLYARTERITIS NODOSA[a]

Livedo reticularis
Testicular pain and/or tenderness
Myalgias or muscle weakness
Mono- or polyneuropathy
Diastolic blood pressure >90 mm Hg
Elevated blood urea nitrogen and/or creatinine
Hepatitis B virus in sera (antigen or antibody)
Arteriographic abnormality
Biopsy of small or medium artery with polymorphonuclear neutrophil leukocytes

[a]Three of 10 criteria should be present for diagnosis.
(Modified from: Conn DL. Polyarteritis. In: Klippel JH, Dieppe PA, eds. *Rheumatology*. St. Louis: Mosby, 1994, with permission.)

Although the pathogenesis of PAN remains unclear, a small proportion of cases appear to be causally linked to HBV infection. The mechanism that is best supported in the literature is one in which disease results from circulating immune complexes that contain an HBV-associated antigen and complement-activating immunoglobulin. These immune complexes deposit in vascular tissue and result in destructive inflammation. It is not yet clear why certain vessels appear to be affected more than others, nor why only a minority of patients with circulating immune complexes develop injury. The paradigm of the pathogenic role of HBV-associated immune complexes in PAN is that of serum sickness, in which there is sustained, usually foreign, antigenemia, which evokes host antibody formation. Subsequently, circulating immune complexes form, deposit in target tissues, and activate the complement cascade. There are substantial data to support this paradigm, both in laboratory animals (111), as well as in humans. Lawley and co-workers (112) reported their experience with 12 patients who had received prolonged courses of intravenous horse antithymocyte globulin for bone marrow failure. Eleven patients developed circulating immune complexes concomitant with the development of clinical signs and symptoms of serum sickness, although no mention was made of renal abnormalities. Both C4 and C3 levels fell precipitously as immune complexes appeared in sera. Biopsy of skin lesions in five patients revealed immune deposits in the blood vessels of three patients.

The circulating immune complex mechanism has traditionally been proposed to explain the relationship between HBV infection and PAN. The first association between hepatitis and vasculitis was noted by Paull (113), who reported four army officers who developed hepatitis and fatal vasculitis after yellow fever immunization. The link between HBV infection and PAN was first suggested by Gocke and others (114), who detected immune complexes by immunofluorescence in inflamed vessel walls in a patient with vasculitis. The immune complexes were shown to consist of the Australia antigen, IgG, and C3. This finding was taken as evidence that Australia antigen-containing immune complexes could be pathogenic.

Subsequently, Alpert et al. (115) reported 18 patients with acute viral hepatitis who had arthritis, arthralgias, or urticaria. None, however, had renal disease. Nine patients were extensively evaluated and found to have depressed concentrations of both total hemolytic complement (CH50) and C4. Serum complement concentrations were lowest when hepatitis-associated antigen titers were at a maximum level. Moreover, joint and skin symptoms correlated with depressed levels of complement. Wands et al. (116) later extended the observations of this group of investigators and found that the circulating immune complexes in cryoprecipitates from six patients with arthritis and acute viral hepatitis contained HBsAg, IgG, and IgM. The IgG subtypes were complement fixing. HBsAg and anti-HBs were concentrated several fold higher in the cryoprecipitates than in serum. The immune complexes were able to activate complement in patients with active arthritis, whereas cryoprecipitates from patients with uncomplicated acute hepatitis were unable to activate complement. These investigators concluded that the presence of complement-activating immune complexes were pathogenic in the arthritis of HBV infection.

Trepo et al. (117) investigated the circulating immune complexes found in the sera of 55 patients with histologically proven PAN, of whom 23 had active disease. Few clinical details were reported, nor was there information about renal involvement. They found HBsAg seropositivity in 30 of 55 patients (54.5%) and HBsAb in 13 of 45 (28%). Five of 45 patients (11%) had both. The Trepo group detected a variety of different particles, including the 42-nm Dane particle and 20-nm spherical and filamentous particles associated with HBsAg, in HBsAg-positive sera by electron microscopic examination. No particles were detected in sera containing HBsAb.

These investigators demonstrated the presence of coexistent HBsAg and HBsAb in the sera of 4 of 23 (17.3%) patients with active vasculitis and could not demonstrate such findings in patients with quiescent vasculitis or liver disease alone. They were concerned that they could not demonstrate HBsAg/HBsAb immune complexes in a higher proportion of cases of active vasculitis and speculated that their immune complex detection methods were not sufficiently sensitive.

The concept that immune complexes were pathogenic in PAN was supported by the work of Michalak (118), who reported an autopsy series of seven cases of PAN in HBsAg-seropositive subjects. Six of the seven had glomerulonephritis, although no clinical details were given. Michalak was able to detect HBsAg, IgG, and C1q in vascular lesions and, on elution of these complexes from vascular tissue, found that the complexes contained HBsAg and immunoglobulin fragments when they were dissociated with sodium thiocyanate and ammonium sulfate. He also noted that the amount of HBsAg immune complexes was largest in the vascular lesions with the greatest degree of acute inflammation and absent from healed vascular lesions. He interpreted these findings as supporting a role for HBsAg-containing immune complexes in the pathogenesis of PAN.

Gupta and Kohler (119) investigated the nature of circulating immune complexes in sera obtained from five patients with arteritis and three patients with venulitis, all of whom were thought to have vasculitis associated with HBV infection (119). Using a variety of techniques to dissociate the immune complexes, they determined that the immune complexes in both cohorts of patients contained several different antigen moieties of HBsAg, ranging in molecular weight from 23 to 97 kd. The antigen components in the immune complexes were identical in all patients; however, the antibody composition of the complexes differed among patients. This led the authors to conclude that while the antigenic components in different patients with HBV-associated PAN were the same, individual patients' antibody responses were different and might determine the degree of injury to vessel walls and expression of disease.

In 1976 Sergent and co-workers (120) reported nine patients with systemic vasculitis and HBsAg antigenemia. The patients ranged from 26 to 63 years of age; all were white. All were seropositive for HBsAg, including three patients who were thought to have been infected through blood transfusions and three through venereal transmission. In all cases, the vasculitis followed either exposure to the hepatitis virus or overt hepatitis. No test was performed to determine whether any patient had circulating immune complexes, although in the two patients in whom complement concentrations were measured, the complement was depressed in one. Although this report is rich in clinical detail, it is of limited use in advancing our understanding of the causal relationship, if any, between HBV infection and PAN.

Adu and others (121) reported a large series of patients with polyarteritis in the first study to provide detailed information about renal involvement in a large cohort. The majority of the 43 patients studied, however, had microscopic polyangiitis rather than classic PAN. No information about HBV status was provided.

McMahon et al. (122) provided compelling evidence of the strong relationship between HBV infection and PAN in their report of 13 patients with PAN and HBV infection. All patients were Yupik Eskimos from an area of Alaska hyperendemic for HBV infection. All patients were seropositive for both HBsAg and HBeAg at diagnosis, and in eight patients clinical and/or serologic evidence indicated that the PAN had followed recent HBV infection. In the 10 patients in whom components of the complement system were measured, 4 had depressed levels of C3 or C4, while such levels were normal in the remaining 6.

Our understanding of the pathogenesis of certain forms of systemic vasculitis, including Wegener's granulomatosis, PAN, and the form of rapidly progressive glomerulonephritis known as pauci-immune glomerulonephritis, has increased with the discovery of antineutrophil cytoplasmic antibodies (ANCA) (50,123). There are two forms of ANCA, both of which can be detected by indirect immunofluorescence of polymorphonuclear leukocytes fixed in absolute alcohol, as well as by enzyme-linked immunosorbent assay (ELISA). Cytoplasmic ANCA (c-ANCA) is directed against proteinase 3, a constituent of primary granules. Perinuclear ANCA (p-ANCA) is directed against myeloperoxidase. The spectrum of renal disorders associated with ANCA has been extensively reviewed (50,124). There was little information as to whether ANCA participated in the pathogenesis of HBV-associated PAN (125,126) until the studies of Guillevin et al. (127), who studied 28 patients with HBV-associated PAN, in whom they tested sera for the presence of ANCA. Sera from 11 men and women with biopsy-proven, active PAN, all of whom had either HBsAg or HBeAg in sera or tissue, were tested for ANCA by indirect immunofluorescence and ELISA. Three of 28 (10.7%) were positive for ANCA by immunofluorescence, while 2 of 18 (11.1%) were positive by ELISA; these latter 2 were determined to have ANCA directed against myeloperoxidase. The authors concluded that ANCA is uncommon in HBV-associated PAN.

There are very few reports of treatment of HBV-associated PAN (128,129). While CS and cyclophosphamide have long been considered the most effective form of therapy for idiopathic PAN, the use of CS in HBV-associated PAN has been considered ill-advised because of the known deleterious effect of CS on the ability to resolve HBV infection. There is an absence of well-designed and powered randomized controlled therapeutic trials.

Nonetheless, a prospective study using sequential therapy with CS, the antiviral agent vidarabine, and plasma exchange shows promising results. Guillevin (130) chose to use CS to control severe life-threatening aspects of PAN, followed by vidarabine to induce HBeAg/HBeAb seroconversion, with concomitant plasma exchange to remove immune complexes. He initially studied 33 patients with HBV-associated PAN, all of whom had histopathologic or arteriographic evidence of active vasculitis, were seropositive for HBsAg and HBeAg, had no detectable HBV-associated antibodies, and had evidence of active replication of HBV as measured by HBV DNA or DNA polymerase activity in sera. Seventeen men and 16 women with a mean age of 50.9 ± 17.5 years were studied. Two patients had glomerulonephritis, and six had renal insufficiency. Seven patients had renal artery microaneurysms, and nine had renal infarction detected angiographically. No renal biopsies were performed. Remission was defined as stabilization or improvement of clinical symptoms and normalization of laboratory abnormalities while on therapy. Control of disease was defined as improvement in the patient's overall condition, absence of new or improvement of existing symptoms, and normalization of the erythrocyte sedimentation rate. Complete recovery was considered to have occurred when the criteria defined for control of disease were met and maintained for at least 18 months after discontinuation of all treatment. Clearance of HBV antigenemia was not a treatment-dependent outcome.

On entry into the study, all patients were initially treated with 1 mg per kg per day of prednisone for 1 week; prednisone was rapidly withdrawn over the second week. Immediately thereafter, vidarabine was administered by continuous intravenous infusion at a dosage of 15 mg per kg per day for the first week and 7.5 mg/kg/day for the next 2 weeks. Plasma exchange was initiated at entry into the study and was performed three times each week for the first 2 weeks, followed by 14 exchanges over the ensuing 3 weeks, while the patients continued therapy with vidarabine. Following completion of vidarabine therapy, plasma exchanges were performed three times weekly for 3 weeks and then twice weekly for 2 weeks. Exchanges could then be performed once or twice weekly thereafter, depending on the clinical situation. IFN, given at a dose of 3 million units thrice weekly, could be administered to those patients who did not develop HBeAb or who could not tolerate vidarabine.

No side effects of CS therapy were noted. Three patients developed transient thrombocytopenia during vidarabine therapy. IFN was given to four patients. The mean number of plasma exchanges performed was 23 (range, 6 to 34). No serious complications of therapy were noted.

Six months after entry into the study, 26 patients (78%) were controlled, while 4 (12.1%) and 3 (9.1%) were either uncontrolled or dead, respectively. After 5 years of observation, 1 patient remained in remission, while 24 (72.7%) had made a complete recovery. Eight patients (24.2%) had died. Only 1 patient died of renal causes. Seroconversion to HBsAb and HBeAb occurred in 15 (45.4%) and 6 patients (18.1%), respectively. Most patients who seroconverted did so after the first several months following the end of therapy.

Subsequently, Guillevin et al. (131) reported the results of their nonrandomized prospective trial of IFN and plasma exchange in HBV-associated PAN. Their cumulative clinical experience included 41 patients, many of whom were included in the earlier study (130). Thirty-five patients were treated with vidarabine, while six were treated with INF. All patients received plasma exchange therapy. More than half of the patients no longer expressed serologic evidence of HBV replication after therapy. Thirty-three of 41 patients (80.5%) were considered cured, while 8 patients died during the study period. None of these deaths were attributed to the treatment protocol. Only one-third of the patients had clinical renal disease, and few details are available to permit determination of the effect of treatment on renal parameters.

Case reports have also documented a salutary effect of treatment of vasculitis associated with HBV infection with lamivudine, but details regarding renal parameters are incomplete (132–136). Guillevin and his colleagues reported on the use of lamivudine combined with short-course CS and plasma exchange in the treatment of HBV-associated PAN (137). In a multicenter, prospective, observational trial, 10 patients (8 men, 2 women) with previously untreated HBV-related PAN were treated with prednisone (1 mg/kg/day) for 1 week, which was then tapered and withdrawn within 1 week. Then, lamivudine (100 mg/day) was started for a maximum of 6 months. Plasma exchanges were performed on a tapering schedule until HBeAg to HBeAb seroconversion was obtained or until 2–3 months of clinical recovery was sustained. The primary trial endpoint was clinical recovery from HBV-PAN at 6 months. The secondary end point was loss of detectable serum HBeAg and HBV DNA, and HBeAg to HBeAb seroconversion at 9 months. One death, from catheter–related sepsis, occurred. By six months, all nine survivors had achieved clinical recovery and by nine months, six of nine had seroconverted. The investigators concluded that a strategy of short-term steroid therapy followed by lamivudine and plasma exchanges not only led to recovery from HBV-PAN, but also because of its oral administration and good safety profile, lamivudine should be considered the antiviral agent of choice to treat HBV-related PAN. Unfortunately, as in previous reports, few details are available regarding kidney disease in these patients, and it is difficult to assess the effects of the treatment on kidney outcomes (137).

Nonetheless, the results of these studies are quite encouraging and offer promise that more effective and less complicated therapeutic regimens for HBV-associated PAN may be developed. The response of patients to plasma exchange certainly suggests that circulating immune complexes are involved in the pathogenesis of the disease. Often, however, whether immune complexes were measured is not reported. Moreover, the response to plasma exchange should not be used as conclusive evidence that immune complexes are the sole mechanism underlying the pathogenesis of the disease (138,139). Plasma exchange may exert salutary effects on disease through a variety of mechanisms in addition to removing complexes from sera. For example, the effects, if any, of plasma exchange on immunomodulators such as cytokines have not been extensively evaluated.

Therefore, although there is an extensive literature that relates PAN to HBV infection, our understanding of this disorder remains rather limited. The same sophisticated diagnostic maneuvers that are being used in other forms of renal disease associated with viral infections should be applied to a cohort of patients with this disorder. The field requires implementation of well-designed and powered randomized controlled therapeutic trials of antiviral therapies, immunosuppressants, and plasma exchange in patients in whom virologic and immune parameters, as well as side effects, are carefully delineated. Inclusion of patients with clinically important kidney disease in such studies may permit inferences regarding the specific effects of treatment on renal outcomes. It seems likely that safe and effective therapy will depend on the outcome of such studies.

HEPATITIS B VIRUS AND CRYOGLOBULINEMIA

Although an association between cryoglobulinemia and acute and chronic liver diseases had been noted (140), cryoglobulinemia was first associated with HBV infection by two groups in 1976 (141) and 1977 (142,143). Two-thirds of patients with essential mixed cryoglobulinemia had abnormal liver function tests, and the majority had circulating antibodies reactive with HBsAg. Almost three-fourths of patients had detectable HBsAg or anti-HBsAb in the cryoprecipitates (142). Approximately half the patients had glomerulonephritis (143). Renal histologic data and the relationship of renal disease to the antibody status and composition of the cryoprecipitate were not presented in these studies. The generalizability of these findings, furthermore, has been disputed (144,145). Speculation centered on whether differences between populations (146), consequences of hepatic dysfunction, or other etiologic agents might be confounding factors that would explain the disparate findings (147). It has even been conjectured that HBV infection in patients with essential mixed cryoglobulinemia might have been a result of transfusions received as therapy for symptoms of the cryoglobulinemia (148). Rarely has the renal disease been fully delineated in studies of patients with cryoglobulinemia in the setting of HBV infection (i.e., shown to be definitively related to the HBV infection), or the components of the cryoprecipitate shown to be reactive with HBV antigens.

Contemporary studies should focus on the incidence and prevalence of the complication in HBV-infected patients who have not been exposed to HCV. Recently, for example, Ferri et al. reported on 231 patients with mixed cryoglobulinemia. Using sophisticated serologic and virologic assessment, the investigators found that HBV infection was likely to be causative in only four patients in the entire cohort, whereas evidence of hepatitis C infection was evident in more than 92% of patients (149).

Reports of patients with cryoglobulinemia often do not distinguish between essential and secondary forms of the disease, and treatment trials of therapy in patients with hepatic disease often do not distinguish patients with cryoglobulinemia and/or renal disease for separate analysis (150,151). Various regimens have been used to treat such patients, with therapy most often directed at the underlying viral illness. There are no adequate trials limited specifically to patients with HBV infection and cryoglobulinemia that have been prospective, well designed, and properly controlled. In addition, many patients are often infected with other viruses, potentially confounding analytic strategies. Although immunosuppressive therapies consisting of CS, cytotoxic drugs, and plasmapheresis have been employed to treat essential mixed cryoglobulinemia (150,151), recommendations for the use of such therapy in patients with HBV infection, cryoglobulinemia, and glomerulonephritis cannot be easily made. There is a need for properly designed and conducted clinical trials including surveillance of virologic outcome in addition to renal parameters, with stratification of clinical, immunologic, and histologic variables to determine which therapies may be effective in this disorder. In individual cases, the possible benefits of a specific therapy must be balanced by any conceivable risks, including exacerbation of viral replication. Plasma exchange is likely to be the least harmful therapy, but its efficacy is unknown in this specific population of patients (152).

HEPATITIS C VIRUS–ASSOCIATED GLOMERULONEPHRITIS

The identification of a syndrome of non-A, non-B hepatitis was dependent on serologic identification of hepatitis A virus (153) and HBV (154). HCV, cloned in 1989 (155), has been recognized as the major cause of non-A, non-B hepatitis (156,157). HCV is a single-stranded RNA virus (158,159) in the Flaviviridae family. It is a 50- to 65-nm particle, composed of a lipid envelope, several glycoproteins, and single-stranded RNA in the nucleus. The recombinant immunoblot assay (RIBA) is directed against the C 22 antigen. Alternatively, second or third generation immunoassays (EIAII or EIAIII) that detect a number of different capsular and core antigens are available. HCV infection is characterized by persistent, prolonged viremia in the face of an ongoing immune response, which promotes the development of immune complex disorders. Resolution of viremia is uncommon, but patients may note few or no clinical symptoms. Infection is transmitted through transfusion of blood products, intravenous drug use, and sexual and maternal–infant routes. Infection with HCV may culminate in chronic active hepatitis, cirrhosis, or hepatocellular carcinoma.

Studies using the first-generation EIA documented that a clinically significant proportion of patients with ESRD treated with hemodialysis in Europe and the United States had been exposed to HCV. Subsequent studies confirmed a 10% to 40% prevalence of HCV infection, depending on the center, and suggested the prevalence of infection may be even higher if second-generation assays or the detection of HCV RNA are used as the gold standard (160–162). The prevalence of HCV infection in patients treated for ESRD with hemodialysis outside the United States may be greater. The incidence and prevalence of HCV infection in dialysis patients is stable or declining (162,163) and the latest data suggest a prevalence of about 8-10% (163,164). Curiously, one report suggested the viral burden may be higher in males undergoing hemodialysis compared with females undergoing hemodialysis (165). The reasons for this difference are unknown but may include behavioral and risk factors that differ between the sexes or differences related to sex hormones. The mechanisms involved in transmission in dialysis units are unknown, but transfusion-related or dialysis-related processes may be involved, since a relatively lower proportion of patients on continuous ambulatory peritoneal dialysis may be infected (160,163,166). These findings are important because of uncertainty whether HCV infection in ESRD

settings is solely treatment-related or whether HCV seropositivity represents an association with or is the cause of the renal disease. In a study assessing the prevalence of exposure to HCV infection in patients with chronic renal insufficiency, 7.9% of patients with renal disease in a Spanish cohort were infected with HCV, compared with a significantly lower proportion of patients (1.03%) who were healthy blood donors (167). There was also a higher prevalence of HCV seropositivity in patients with chronic glomerulonephritis compared with patients with other renal diseases. The high prevalence of HCV seropositivity in patients with renal disease, and more specifically, glomerulonephritis, suggests the infection might be a causal factor in the pathogenesis of nephropathy. Alternatively, patients with renal disease may acquire infection because of altered immune function related to renal insufficiency (168–170) or other factors, such as the use of intravenous drugs, that could be associated with both conditions (167).

There is a high prevalence of circulating, cryoprecipitable HCV RNA and/or antibodies in patients with mixed cryoglobulinemia (46,163,171–178). A study based in research centers in France demonstrated 56% of HCV-infected patients had mixed cryoglobulinemia (179). Interestingly, serologic and PCR analyses for HCV antibodies and RNA showed the PCR to be a much more sensitive test (175). In some patients, it is possible that the immune response comprises antibodies not detected by currently employed immunoassays. Misiani et al. (180), however, showed the vast majority of patients with cryoglobulinemia had HCV antibodies detected. In an autopsy study, a relatively large proportion of patients with HCV infection had various glomerular diseases (57.4%), although almost one-fourth had minimal abnormalities (181). Renal disease severely affected prognosis, increasing mortality risk. Ferri et al demonstrated that HCV RNA could be detected in the sera of 86% of patients with cryoglobulinemia (172). These findings were soon corroborated by Agnello el al. (175). A recent review by Ferri et al. (149) showed HCV infection in 92% of cases, while HBV infection was present in only 1.8% of cases with mixed cryoglobulinemia.

Beddhu et al described 17 patients with renal disease and cryoglobulinemia. Eleven of the patients were seropositive for HCV, and three additional patients had clinical abnormalities consistent with a connective tissue disorder. Only three patients had no demonstrable systemic illness. Eleven patients, some HCV negative, had MPGN on renal biopsy. Patients presented with a wide array of renal findings, including nephritic syndrome, inflammatory urinary sediments, renal failure, and hypertension (182). Differences in epidemiologic factors and viral strains in the studies may, in part, explain discrepancies in the proportion of patients with cryoglobulinemia and HCV infection detected in different investigations. Recent work has expanded our understanding of the pathogenesis and clinical consequences of the syndrome (45,183).

Several studies have also demonstrated an association of HCV infection and MPGN (180–196), independent of cryoglobulinemia. Evidence suggesting the viral infection is directly linked to glomerulonephritis comes from the work of Johnson et al. (191), who demonstrated antibody directed against HCV peptides and HCV RNA, determined by immunoblot and PCR respectively, in the cryoprecipitates of all eight patients they studied with MPGN and HCV infection.

The overwhelming majority of the patients studied by the Johnson group had microscopic hematuria, edema, renal insufficiency, hypertension, and normochromic normocytic anemia (191). Half had hepatomegaly. All patients had hypoalbuminemia, abnormally elevated serum aminotransferase concentrations, diminished total hemolytic complement levels, and increased rheumatoid factor activity. Most patients had low levels of C3 and C4. All patients had proteinuria; the majority had more than 3.5 g/day. Urinalysis revealed red blood cell casts in over one-third of patients. Approximately two-thirds of patients had cryoglobulinemia and circulating immune complexes. Most patients had circulating IgG reactive with non-structural HCV antigens, and all had antibodies to HCVc, the nucleocapsid core antigen. Anti-HCVc and anti-c33-c (a nonstructural protein) IgG antibodies were present in the cryo-precipitates of all three patients studied. Serum and cryopre-cipitates also contained IgM antibodies reactive with HCVc antigen (191,192). Typically the renal disease is indolent (197).

Renal biopsies in all eight patients showed MPGN, with a lobular increase in glomerular cellularity, and interstitial mononuclear infiltration. Immunofluorescence demonstrated glomerular capillary IgM, IgG, and C3. IgA and C1q were present in the minority of cases. Electron microscopy demonstrated interposition of mesangial cells with subendothelial, mesangial, and rare intramembranous deposits. Immunotactoid structures were present in several patients. Of note, HCV antigens and anti-HCV immunoglobulins were not identified in renal tissue in a characteristic anatomic distribution in this study. Therefore, although the evidence linking the renal disease to the virus is circumstantially strong, direct causal association between HCV antigens and the occurrence of MPGN remains to be demonstrated (198). Further work by Johnson's group (192) demonstrated that patients with HCV infection exhibit a spectrum of clinical renal syndromes, including asymptomatic urinary abnormalities, such as hematuria and proteinuria, variable levels of renal insufficiency, and the nephrotic syndrome (199) (Table 59-8). A spectrum of histologic changes, including MPGN, MN (200–204), vasculitis, and proliferative glomerulonephritis (163,192) have been noted in HCV-infected patients with renal disease. The majority of patients were white and male. More than half of the patients had cryoglobulinemia, often with characteristic symptoms. The majority had abnormal transaminase levels and hypoalbuminemia, as well as longstanding HCV infection, but only approximately 20% had physical signs of hepatic disease. Hypocomplementemia (CH50, C4) and the presence of rheumatoid factors may be noted in most patients. Low C3 levels were noted in almost half of the patients (199). Renal disease may be present, however, in the absence of clinical signs and symptoms of the HCV infection or cryoglobulinemia. Rapidly progressive glomerulonephritis (205), IgA nephropathy (206), and thrombotic microangiopathic diseases (207) have also been reported in HCV-infected patients (208,209) but the etiologic relationships are less clear in these cases. The spectrum of disease has also been reported in Japan (210,211).

A proliferative glomerulopathy with pathologic features similar to MPGN has been noted in HCV-infected patients after liver (189) and renal (192,212,213) transplantation. The relationship of this lesion to chronic transplant allograft nephropathy remains unclear (214). Cosio et al. measured serum antibodies to HCV in patients with native kidney disease and compared the results to those found in patients with acute and chronic transplant allograft nephropathy. Native renal diseases included focal segmental sclerosis, diabetic nephropathy, MN, and MPGN. HCV serologies were negative in all patients with native renal disease without a history of intravenous drug abuse. Of the patients with acute and chronic transplant allograft nephropathy, 29% and 33%, respectively, had detectable HCV antibodies. The authors concluded that there was an association between HCV infection and certain forms of allograft nephropathy (215).

Cruzado and co-workers studied six HCV-infected renal allograft recipients with proteinuria and hematuria. All had circulating immune complexes and cryoglobulins. In all six patients, the cryoglobulins were type II IgG polyclonal–IgMk monoclonal. Renal tissue demonstrated features of a proliferative lesion, in which IgM was deposited diffusely. HCV RNA was found in higher concentrations than in serum, leading the authors to conclude that the infection might be the etiology of the glomerular lesions (216). Conversely, Morales et al. reported 15 patients with HCV infection who developed de novo allograft MN 2 years after transplantation. There was a 10-fold higher incidence in the development of MN in allografts of HCV-positive patients than in HCV-negative patients. In the majority of patients, renal function declined until dialysis had to be instituted (217).

Kendrick and others studied 197 liver transplant recipients, of whom 91 were HCV-infected. The other 106 were uninfected with HCV. Four of 10 HCV-infected patients who developed proteinuria had MPGN on renal biopsy, while none of seven HCV-uninfected patients with proteinuria had MPGN. Several patients received treatment with INF, which appeared to stabilize proteinuria, but did not reverse the renal dysfunction (218).

Pathology

MPGN type I is the most common pathologic lesion identified in clinicopathologic studies of patients with HCV infection and renal disease (187–199,219,220). Increased glomerular cellularity and double-contoured glomerular basement membranes are hallmarks of the disease. Mesangial proliferation and sclerosis may be seen. Mesangial and glomerular capillary deposition of IgM, IgG, and C3 are often present. Subendothelial deposits are seen on electron microscopic examination in MPGN type I, but occasionally mesangial and subepithelial electron-dense deposits may also be noted. Ultrastructural features of cryoglobulins, including granular, fibrillar, and immunotactoid structures may be seen within the subendothelial space. Glomerular findings are often accompanied by tubulointerstitial inflammation and fibrosis. Small- and medium-sized renal vasculitis may be present. More rarely, subepithelial electron-dense deposits (characterizing MPGN type III) are present. Viral genome or gene products have not usually been identified in glomeruli in studies. In one study of a patient with diffuse proliferative glomerulonephritis, however, viruslike particles, similar to those seen in sera of patients with non-A, non-B hepatitis, were found in the mesangium (201). Microtubular inclusions in endothelial cells were noted as well. Since the HIV status of this patient was not reported, the significance of these ultrastructural findings is unclear.

Johnson et al. (192) and others (200–204) have also noted several patients with MN in the presence of HCV infection. A causal relationship between the viral infection and the renal disease has not been established, but the renal disease is a possible consequence of a secondary immune response (40,41,198). Such patients have typical pathologic findings, and no evidence of hypocomplementemia, rheumatoid factor activity, or

---

TABLE 59-8

GLOMERULAR SYNDROMES ASSOCIATED WITH HEPATITIS C VIRUS INFECTION

Hepatitis C virus-associated immune complex disease
  Membranoproliferative glomerulonephritis
    With cryoglobulinemia
    Without cryoglobulinemia
  Vasculitis
  Proliferative glomerulonephritis
  Membranous glomerulopathy
  Transplant nephropathy?

cryoglobulinemia (194,199). HCV infection has also been associated with fibrillary glomerulonephritis and immunotactoid glomerulopathy (191,192,220–222). The clinical presentation is indistinguishable from other forms of glomerulonephritis. Renal biopsy is required for diagnosis.

Pathogenesis

Glomerular deposition of circulating immune complexes likely plays a role in the pathogenesis of the renal diseases associated with HCV infection (1,8–12). Immune-mediated renal disease may be facilitated because of the persistent viremia and ongoing antibody response seen in HCV-infected patients. Glomerulonephritis associated with HCV-induced cryoglobulinemia has been linked to IgM kappa rheumatoid factors (195,223). Specific immunochemical or physicochemical characteristics may be associated with nephropathogenicity. The generation of idiotypic antibodies may be important in the development of renal disease because of physicochemical characteristics (1,9–12) or directly through immune dysregulation (1,8,12,13), or it may only reflect the immune dysregulation noted in a chronic viral illness (8,12,13). HCV proteins (224) and genetic material (201) have been demonstrated in tissue of patients with MN associated with HCV infection and cryoglobulinemic membranoproliferative glomerulonephritis (225). A study demonstrated the presence of HCV RNA in renal biopsies in patients with HCV infection, and none in the absence of HCV infection (226). Interestingly, *in situ* hybridization localized HCV RNA to tubular epithelial cells and tubulointerstitial blood vessels. Few studies have assessed molecular evidence for virologic involvement in the pathogenesis of glomerular disease (198). The small study sizes, difficulty in localization of nucleic acid in distinct or specific compartments in diseases linked to HCV infection (226), and lack of definitive evaluations in large control populations, render determination of a pathogenic link from these studies problematic.

Treatment

IFN-α has been used for the treatment of "essential" mixed cryoglobulinemia (227–229), HCV infection (230,231), and cryoglobulinemia associated with HCV infection (232–235). Treatment may result in suppression of viremia and improvement in parameters of hepatic disease, but disease markers often recur in patients after discontinuation of therapy. In uncontrolled studies, Johnson et al. (199) treated 17 patients with MPGN with and without cryoglobulinemia with IFN-α. Patients had decreased urinary protein excretion and normalization of liver function test abnormalities during treatment with IFN-α of up to 6 months' duration. There was no significant change, however, in renal function noted in this study. Loss of circulating HCV RNA during therapy may be a favorable prognostic sign. Viremia and signs of renal disease, however, often recurred after cessation of therapy. Several other studies of HCV-infected patients with MPGN (236,237) show improvement in parameters of renal disease, perhaps in association with use of higher doses of INF (236). Relapses may have been less frequent when higher doses of INF were used (163,164). In a Japanese study, glucocorticoid therapy was associated with improvement in renal function parameters, while there was no effect of therapy with INF-α (210). Steroid therapy, however, was associated with an increase in circulating titers of HCV RNA.

Side effects of therapy with IFN-α include a flulike syndrome in the majority of patients, but the occurrence of erythema multiforme and worsening neuropathy often necessitates discontinuation of treatment. It is unclear whether progressive renal insufficiency, which may occur during therapy, represents a side effect of treatment (238–243) or progression of the underlying nephropathy. Because of the unknown natural history of HCV-related renal disease, the heterogeneous long-term response to treatment, the lack of prognostic determinants, and the often transitory nature of improvement in renal and hepatic disease markers, this costly therapy must be considered on an individual basis, the risks and benefits being carefully weighed for each patient.

The sustained response of HCV infection to therapy with INF has been disappointing, leading to the development of regimens including the addition of ribavirin to INF (163) and the use of pegylated INF therapy (163). Three randomized controlled trials demonstrated the superiority of pegylated INF compared with therapy with INF (163,244–246). Trials have also used the combination of ribavirin and pegylated INF, compared with pegylated INF alone and combinations using INF in HCV-infected patients (163,247–249). Therapy with ribavirin has been associated with a dose-related occurrence of hemolysis, and the drug is cleared by the kidneys. Combination therapy may also result in infectious and autoimmune complications, as well as rarely being associated with nephrotoxicity (163). These regimens have often not been well studied in patients with coexisting renal disease, in part because of their exclusion in clinical trials (163).

Classically, therapy for cryoglobulinemic renal disease has included oral and intravenous CS, with or without plasmapheresis, and supplemental immunosuppression with cytotoxic drugs, such as cyclophosphamide (49,50,151,192,250). Nafomostat mesilate, an inhibitor of complement serine proteases, has been used to treat patients with immune complex-mediated glomerulonephritis, including essential mixed cryoglobulinemia, with a resultant decrease in proteinuria (251). INF has been used in treatment of HCV-associated renal diseases, cryoglobulinemia, and vasculitis, but it has shortcomings (163,164,235,238–243,252–258). Casato and co-workers reported a response rate of 62% in patients with cryoglobulinemia treated with INF, but the relapse rate was high. Only 10% of patients experienced a long-term remission (259). INF has also been associated with the appearance or worsening of nephropathy in treated patients (238–243,260–264). Addition of ribavirin has been considered for patients with HCV-associated cryoglobulinemia and vasculitis (44,265–269). Rossi et al. (270) treated three patients with cryoglobulinemia and glomerulonephritis in the setting of HCV infection with ribavirin 15 mg/kg/day, adjusted according to the level of hemoglobin, and added IFN-α2b after 4 weeks. Treatment with ribivarin for four weeks was not associated with clinical change in renal parameters. Level of urinary protein excretion decreased and creatinine clearance increased, and either normalized or approached normal levels in all three patients. Similar cases were described by Misiani et al. (271), Garini et al. (272), Loustad-Ratti et al. (273), and Sabry et al. (274). Rituximab has recently been suggested as an additional treatment for HCV-associated cryoglobulinemia (275–277). Rocatello et al. (277) treated six patients with HCV infection and type-II mixed cryoglobulinemia with rituximab, with improvement in levels of cryocrit and urinary protein excretion. Alric et al. (278) reported on 25 patients with nephrotic syndrome due to HCV-associated membranoproliferative glomerulonephritis and HCV infection. All patients initially received therapy with CS. They tested the effects of standard or pegylated interferon alfa and ribavirin in 18 patients compared with therapy with prednisone, furosemide and plasmapheresis alone in 7 patients with cryoglobulinemia and MPGN or mesangial proliferative glomerulonephritis associated with HCV infection in a nonrandomized study. In the group treated with antivirals, 12 patients were responders and 6 did not respond. Urinary protein excretion decreased in "responder" patients treated with antiviral therapy, but there was no decrease in level of serum creatinine concentration in any of the groups. These patients also had a reduction in cryoglobulin levels compared with pretreatment values.

Infliximab has also been used to treat refractory vasculitis in patients with HCV infection and mixed cryoglobulinemia (279). D'Amico has suggested antiviral therapy using pegylated interferon and ribavirin for 48 weeks, adding steroids and cyclophosphamide in the face of severe symptoms, and plasmapheresis as necessary (163), but such treatment has not been validated in well-controlled randomized trials.

End-Stage Renal Disease

Relatively few studies have assessed the use of INF in ESRD patients infected with HCV (163). The sustained virologic response in HCV infected patients treated with dialysis has been about 40%, which is higher than that obtained in patients in clinical trials in the absence of renal disease (163). This response, however, has been associated with high rates of serious adverse events, dose modification, and early withdrawal from studies (163). It is possible such findings relate to the diminished clearance of INF in ESRD patients (163). The recommendation of a workshop held in 2002 was that therapy with INF in ESRD dialysis patients is controversial, and should be reserved for patients with severe liver disease, minimal comorbidity, and a reasonable prognosis, especially if renal transplantation is being considered (163), and others have endorsed similar strategies (280). Ribavirin is relatively contraindicated in ESRD patients treated with dialysis because of the occurrence of hemolytic anemia, but dosage adjustment schemes and use of erythropoietin have been attempted to facilitate treatment in patients with renal disease(163,269,281–285).

Interferon is generally contraindicated in patients who have had renal transplantation, because of the possible increased risk of graft rejection (163), but some studies have evaluated outcomes in such patients (212,286,287).

Long-term survival for HCV-infected ESRD patients is shortened compared with uninfected patients (163,288,289). Recipients of donor hepatitis C virus infected kidneys have worsened survival, although the mechanisms underlying the finding are unknown and may relate in part to selection biases (163,290). Type of immunosuppression may affect outcomes (163,291).

Conclusions

Relatively few well-designed and controlled trials have been available to guide clinical practice in treating patients with HCV infection and renal disease. The long-term effects of steroid and immunosuppressive treatment on the viral infection, which may be associated with increased viremia (199), may be a critical factor in determining the treatment options in patients with severe, acute illness. There is a need for properly designed and conducted clinical trials of combination therapy with immunosuppressants, plasmapheresis, and antiviral medications such as ribavirin (292,293) and immunologic therapies such as rituximab (275–277), including surveillance of virologic outcome in addition to renal parameters, with stratification of clinical, immunologic, and histologic variables to determine which therapies and drug doses may be effective in patients with various HCV-associated renal diseases. Care-

fully controlled studies of treatment of patients with HCV infection and acute and chronic kidney disease, evaluating outcomes such as viremia, viral burden, renal functional parameters, and morbidity and mortality, may clarify which patients may respond to a specific therapy with the fewest complications.

HUMAN IMMUNODEFICIENCY VIRUS–ASSOCIATED RENAL DISEASES

Since the beginning of the epidemic, a spectrum of renal diseases has been associated with acquired immunodeficiency syndrome (AIDS) and HIV infection (17,294–299). Several well-defined clinicopathologic disorders have been reported in patients with HIV infection, including a number of different forms of glomerular diseases and a variety of immune complex and vasculitic illnesses (17,294–299). These disorders do not occur or are not detected with a frequency commensurate with the prevalence of HIV infection, affecting at most 10% of the population at risk, in the era before highly active antiretroviral drug therapy (HAART) (294,298–300). Therefore, the renal diseases probably do not result from HIV infection alone, but from a combination of the infection and the immunologic responses of the host (17,295,298–301). Renal complications affect specific subsets of the HIV-infected population, primarily male African American patients in the United States (294–305), suggesting that a host response or genetic component may be associated with the incidence of the disease (294–305). Factors linked to socioeconomic status may also be related to disease pathogenesis (305).

The common renal syndromes in HIV-infected patients include asymptomatic urinary abnormalities, acute renal failure, chronic renal insufficiency, and nephrotic range proteinuria associated with focal glomerulosclerosis, the classic HIV-associated nephropathy (HIVAN) (294–300,302,303,306), and various proliferative glomerulonephritides, which may be termed HIV-associated immune complex disease (HIVICD) (294,295,297–299,302,303,307–320) (Table 59-9). Over the past decade it has become clear that there are four syndromes of chronic renal disease intimately associated with HIV infection. These are HIVAN, HIVICD, including HIV-associated IgA nephropathy, and HIV-associated thrombotic microangiopathy (17,295,298,299). Other renal diseases in HIV-infected patients, including cryoglobulinemia and vasculitis, may be related to host responses to the infection, or

TABLE 59-9

GLOMERULAR SYNDROMES ASSOCIATED WITH HUMAN IMMUNODEFICIENCY VIRUS INFECTION

HIV focal glomerulosclerosis (classic HIV-associated nephropathy)
HIV mesangial hyperplasia
HIV-associated immune complex disease
IgA nephropathy
Idiotypic
Other mechanisms
Immune complex proliferative glomerulonephritis
Postinfectious
Lupus-like
Mixed immune complex–sclerotic

infections complicating the immunodeficiency state. Additionally, treatment effects may be associated with adverse renal outcomes (298–321).

CLASSIC HUMAN IMMUNODEFICIENCY VIRUS–ASSOCIATED NEPHROPATHY

Epidemiology and Clinical Features

Classic HIVAN is the most commonly reported chronic renal disease associated with HIV infection (17,294–300,322,323). This may be due in part to its association with the nephrotic syndrome and the reluctance of performing biopsies in patients with HIV infection and mild urinary abnormalities. The disease disproportionately affects men of African heritage (294,296–300,302,305,322,323), which may also account for the relative frequency of HIVAN reported in biopsy series from Europe and the United States. Clinical highlights of the disease are nephrotic range proteinuria and renal insufficiency. In most reports, hypertension and edema are relatively uncommon. This may be a consequence of the stage of disease or the presence of malnutrition in patients. The kidneys are large and echogenic on ultrasonic examination (294,296,297,302,303,322,323).

Pathology

HIVAN has been termed a "pan nephropathy" because of characteristic involvement of the glomeruli, tubules, and interstitium (324). Glomerular capillary wall collapse of varying severity is often noted (296–299,324,325). Mesangial hyperplasia and other abnormalities may be an early stage of the nephropathy (294), or this histologic variant may differentially involve children. Glomerular visceral epithelial cells are characteristically abnormal, exhibiting hyperplasia, hypertrophy, and vacuolation. Varying degrees of segmental or diffuse and global increased mesangial matrix are seen, as well as obsolescent glomeruli (17). Tubular cells show marked degenerative changes, flattening, simplification, brush-border abnormalities, and necrosis. Microcystic tubular dilation and hypertrophy are common. The interstitium shows immune cell infiltration of mononuclear cells, primarily macrophages and T-lymphocytes (17,325,326). Interestingly, T-lymphocytes are more prevalent than B-lymphocytes (326). Interstitial fibrosis and edema of the interstitium are common. Results of immunofluorescent evaluations are variable and nondiagnostic. Electron microscopy shows glomerular epithelial cell foot process effacement, wrinkling, and abnormalities of glomerular basement membrane structure (294,325). Tubular reticular structures are common, but not pathognomonic. They are found in glomerular and peritubular capillary endothelial cells and are probably a concomitant of the action of IFN-α.

Although the individual features of HIV focal glomerulosclerosis are not specific, the concomitant findings of glomerular collapse, glomerular and tubular epithelial cell abnormalities, increased mesangial matrix, renal tubular atrophy or microcystic dilation, and interstitial immune cell infiltration, in combination with tubular reticular structures are virtually diagnostic of classic HIVAN (17,299,324,325). The clinicopathologic characteristics of HIVAN have been compared to those of the collapsing variant of focal segmental glomerulosclerosis in the absence of HIV infection and found to be similar (327). Although it can be suspected on clinical grounds, the diagnosis of HIVAN cannot be made reliably in the absence of a biopsy, since other diseases such as diabetic nephropathy and HIV-associated immune complex renal disease can have similar presentations and features.

Pathogenesis

Although early in the epidemic, HIVAN was thought by some to be an epiphenomenon, or a complication secondary to intravenous drug use in patients, several lines of evidence suggest the renal disease is intimately related to infection with HIV (17,294,295,299,322,323). The development of classic HIVAN in the infant children of mothers with HIV infection (328) and the development of renal disease reminiscent of HIVAN in transgenic murine models (29,296,329–332) and in primates infected with simian immunodeficiency virus (SIV) (333–335) underscore the pathogenic relationship between the virus and the renal disease. Expression of HIV proteins within renal tissue appears to be a prerequisite for the development of renal disease (16,17,29,295,296,299,322,323,329,330). HIV proteins may affect renal cell biologic responses in diverse ways (299). HIV peptides are toxic to many cell types (16,17). Apoptosis of renal cells secondary to exposure to HIV peptides or as a result of their expression within renal tissue is a probable cause of renal disease and a matter of current research interest (16,17,295,296,299,322,323,329,330,336,337).

Abnormal proliferation and dedifferentiation of podocytes may be related to HIV infection of renal tissue and the expression of Nef (299,338) on signal transduction pathways (338) and cyclin biology (338,339). Stat3 and MAPK1,2 phosphorylation were increased in podocytes from kidneys of patients with HIVAN, compared to those of uninfected patients with focal segmental glomerulosclerosis (FGS) and other renal diseases, as well as kidneys from HIV-infected patients in the absence of renal disease, implicating these pathways in HIVAN pathogenesis, however other mediators are involved (338). Kajiyama et al. showed, in HIV-1 transgenic mice, that Nef is not necessary for induction of renal disease, but may rather potentiate nephropathy dependent on the expression of other HIV-1 gene products (340). Dickie et al. showed, in transgenic mice with mutations in either or both nef and vpr accessory genes, that proteinuria and FGS developed only in animals carrying the vpr gene. In animals encoding Tat and Vpr, Vpr protein was localized by immunostaining in glomerular and tubular epithelium. Breeding experiments produced mice with increased severity of nephropathy without increase of Vpr expression, leading the authors to conclude multiple genes must contribute to the development of renal disease in HIV-1 transgenic mice (341).

Inhibition of cyclin-dependent kinase improved urinary and histopathologic parameters of nephropathy in HIV-1 transgenic mice (342,343). Dysregulation of podocyte biology may be an important mediator of the development of HIVAN, and abnormal expression of glomerular epithelial cell proteins is associated with the disease (16,299,322–345). Podocan expression was increased in podocytes of HIV-1 transgenic mice compared with controls (346). Increased expression of transforming growth factor-β, perhaps as a result of viral infection, is also a possible mediator of nephropathy (347–350). Interestingly, expression of transforming growth factor beta has been linked to apoptosis of podocytes (350).

We compared tissue levels of transforming growth factor-β and chemokines from biopsies of patients with HIV-associated nephropathy, HIV-associated glomerulonephritis and idiopathic focal glomerulosclerosis without HIV infection (299,351). Transforming growth factor-beta, monocyte chemoattractant protein-1 (MCP-1) and RANTES levels were increased in renal glomerular and interstitial tissue from patients with HIV infection, regardless of the type or presence of renal disease, suggesting chemokine expression might be a nonspecific response. Renal chemokine expression could act to interfere with local HIV infection by engaging renal chemokine receptors. These data are also consistent with renal deposition of circulating chemokines. In contrast, proteins associated with antigen presentation and response to infection, such as MHC-Class II proteins, interferon-α, and interferon-γ receptor protein were specifically increased in glomerular and interstitial tissue of biopsies of patients with HIV-associated nephropathy, compared with uninfected control tissue with and without renal disease, or renal diseases in the setting of HIV infection. The findings suggest genetic susceptibility, host responses, and a immunologically activated microenvironment may be critical to disease pathogenesis. High levels of tissue interferon-α are consistent with the pathologic feature of tubuloreticular inclusions (299). The pathogenesis of HIVAN is probably a concomitant of relationships between renal cellular infection and immune cell infiltration, effects on renal and infiltrating cellular cytokine, growth factor, and chemokine responses, and host factors. In addition, clinical and animal studies suggest an important role for genetic susceptibility in association with the development of nephropathy (301,352). Socioeconomic status, including access to antiretroviral medications may also be an important determinant of outcome (298,299,353).

Many of these processes depend on the presence of productive infection of renal cells by HIV. We showed that HIV DNA was present in renal tissue of patients with and without nephropathy (23). Detection of HIV RNA in renal tissue of patients with HIVAN has recently been confirmed (322–356). Renal cells can be infected by HIV *in vivo* (16,295,296,354,355,357). Tubular and glomerular epithelial cells can be infected by HIV *in vitro* (337,358), but in some studies mesangial cells could not (359). Infection of the glomerular epithelial cell and subsequent podocyte injury may be critical to the pathogenesis of HIVAN (16,299, 322,323,330,344). The infiltration of immune cells in renal tissue may be associated with progressive nephropathogenesis (326). Preliminary evidence suggests chemokine receptors are not present on renal cells from biopsy tissue (360–362), although they may be expressed in pathologic states in inflammatory cells in renal tissue (360), and may be detected by molecular techniques *in vitro* (337). Differential expression of chemokine receptors in renal tissue in different HIV-infected populations could be associated with different patterns of susceptibility to renal disease. The role of expression of CD4 and coreceptors for HIV infection in renal cells must be further investigated.

Prognosis and Treatment

Treatment studies have sharpened our understanding of the pathogenesis of HIV-associated diseases. In the era before widespread availability of antiretroviral therapy, HIVAN was characterized as a disease with an extremely rapid progression to its end stage (294,363,364). Several anecdotal studies suggested antiretroviral therapy improved the course of HIVAN (reviewed in [16,363,364]). Four therapeutic approaches have been used in patients with HIVAN. Limited data suggested cyclosporine ameliorated the course of the renal disease (363), but few patients have been assessed with this therapy. In addition, concern has been raised regarding the risk/benefit ratio of immunosuppression in patients with HIV infection. Several of these reports are difficult to evaluate since treated patients were not always evaluated with renal biopsies. Individual case reports (17,363–367) have suggested glucocorticoids may be effective in slowing the progression of HIVAN. A case series

of patients with HIV infection and renal disease, treated with steroids, showed impressive diminution in urinary protein excretion and improvement in renal function (368). These studies, unfortunately, were not performed in a randomized controlled manner. In addition, there was a relatively high frequency of side effects such as psychosis, gastrointestinal bleeding, and infections (368). Finally, since survival analyses were not conducted in this series, the long-term effects of such treatments were poorly understood. More recently, Eustace et al. (369) found a salutary effect of treatment of patients with HIVAN with CS. Almost a quarter of patients maintained sufficient renal function to remain independent of need for renal replacement therapy for up to a year, in contradistinction to previous findings. Patients treated with CS, however, had longer hospital stays. Concurrent therapy with antiretroviral drugs and drugs which inhibit the renin-angiotensin system, as a result of advances in therapeutics, may have influenced outcomes in this uncontrolled study.

The angiotensin-converting enzyme (ACE) inhibitors, captopril and fosinopril, have been used in patients with HIVAN both to decrease urinary protein excretion and to halt progression of disease. Therapy with captopril increased length of time before death or start of dialysis in a case-control study (17,363,364). Nine patients with HIVAN were treated with captopril. Their course was compared to age, race, gender, CD4 count, and serum creatinine concentration versus matched control patients untreated with ACE inhibitors. All patients in both groups had HIVAN evaluated on renal biopsy. Renal survival was longer in patients treated with captopril. In another study, HIV-infected patients with proteinuria were treated with fosinopril (370). Patients who refused fosinopril treatment had an increase in serum creatinine concentration compared with those treated with fosinopril. These studies suggest a therapeutic effect of ACE inhibitors in patients with HIVAN. Neither of these studies was randomized or placebo-controlled. Wei et al. recently reported long-term results in the patients treated with fosiniopril, suggesting excellent outcomes (371). Twenty-eight patients were treated with fosinopril, compared to 16 in an untreated comparison group, in this nonrandomized, non–time-controlled study. Mean renal survival was 479.5 days in treated patients compared with 146.5 days in the comparison group. All patients untreated with ACE inhibition went on to ESRD, compared with one patient in the fosinopril group during a more than five year observation period. The authors however could not show an independent effect of treatment with antiretroviral drugs in this small uncontrolled study. Once again, the influence of change in clinical practice, especially regarding the use of antiretroviral drugs and HAART must be considered as potential confounding factors.

These findings were corroborated in studies of Bird et al. (372), who showed administration of captopril to HIV-transgenic mice that exhibited characteristics of HIVAN was associated with improvement of several renal functional parameters, such as urinary protein excretion, azotemia, and histologic abnormalities, despite the expression of HIV genes. A likely mechanism underlying the action of these drugs is the decrease in the expression of transforming growth factor beta afforded by ACE inhibitors (347,363,364,372).

Studies of treatment with antiretroviral drugs before the HAART era were inconclusive, because of small size and lack of definitive controls (298,299), but often showed beneficial effects on the nephropathy, as well as morbidity and mortality (298,299,322,323,354,373). Recent uncontrolled studies have suggested improved outcomes in patients with HIV infection and renal disease treated with HAART (374–376). Interpretation of the findings is often difficult because biopsies are often not performed in all patients reported. In patients treated with captopril, use of antiretrovirals was independently associated with improved renal survival (364).

A case report detailed improvement in the nephrotic syndrome in a child treated with HAART (377). Two cases of patients with HIVAN complicating early stages of infection demonstrate treating patients with HIV-associated nephropathy with HAART may cause resolution of both functional and pathologic abnormalities (354,378), although productive infection of kidney tissue may continue (354). Recent work in an uncontrolled observational cohort of patients with HIV infection and renal disease who underwent renal biopsy suggests treatment with antiretroviral drugs was associated with improved outcomes in patients with HIVAN (353). Such data also bolster evidence for the causal relationship between viral infection and nephropathy.

ACE inhibitors represent a safe, possibly effective long-term therapy for patients with HIVAN. Because there is evidence that treatment with both HAART and ACE inhibitors is associated with improved outcomes in patients with HIVAN, the field requires implementation of well-designed and powered randomized controlled therapeutic trials of antiviral therapies and ACE inhibitors in patients stratified for age, gender, and histologic parameters, in whom virologic and immune parameters, as well as side effects, are carefully delineated. In some patients treated with both ACE inhibitors and HAART, in whom the disease progresses, consideration may be given to the use of CS. The role of treatment with CS, however, is unclear and awaits the performance of controlled clinical trials to determine its utility and safety. The development of renal disease in a patient with HIV infection may be an indication for HAART, regardless of stage of the viral illness, unless it is specifically contraindicated (298,299,322). Because not all renal disease in HIV infected patients is HIVAN, consideration should be given to performing a renal biopsy if the diagnosis is unclear (298,299,353).

Initial reports indicated survival of HIV infected patients with ESRD treated with dialysis was poor (299,379). While the initial growth of HIV infection in the U.S. ESRD program was quite high, recently the incidence has stabilized at 1.25% to 1.5% (298,299,380). The prevalence of HIV infected patients in the ESRD program has increased dramatically, from 0.45% in 1995 to 0.83% in 2000, in part because of the improved survival of patients with HIV infection (380–382). It is possible that trends in both incidence and prevalence of ESRD since 1996 have been affected by the availability of HAART in the US (299,380). HIV infection in the ESRD program is more common in men (380). Outcomes for patients treated with peritoneal and hemodialysis have been equivalent (383,384). In contrast, very few HIV-infected children have been treated for ESRD, and only 50% are male (385). Survival of children was better than for HIV-infected adults with ESRD (385). Girls with HIV infection and ESRD have better survival than boys (385).

Recent studies have concentrated on treatment of HIV infected patients with ESRD with renal transplantation (298,299,386,387–390). Consideration for such experimental treatment currently requires patients to be treated with HAART and have undetectable viral loads (298,299).

HUMAN IMMUNODEFICIENCY VIRUS–ASSOCIATED GLOMERULONEPHRITIS

Less common than classic HIVAN, HIVICD (13,298,299,312, 317) comprises proliferative glomerulonephritis, renal insufficiency, and proteinuria. Circulating immune complexes composed of immunoglobulins, characteristically IgG or IgA, reactive with specific HIV antigens such as p24, gp41, and gp120 are present, and identical complexes may be eluted in higher titer from renal tissue. HIV peptides may also be demon-

strated intracellularly in eluted glomerular tissue by laser-enhanced microscopy (317). Three main types of clinically distinguishable HIV-associated immune complex renal disease may be delineated: HIV-associated immune glomerulonephritis, a mixed sclerotic–immune complex nephropathy (319), and HIV-associated IgA nephropathy (17,23,295,298,299,312). Mesangial hyperplasia may also be a glomerulopathy associated with HIV infection (294,328,365,391), but it is most often considered a part of the spectrum of FGS. A "lupus-like" appearance to the glomerulonephritis has also been noted in a subset of cases (319,392)

HUMAN IMMUNODEFICIENCY VIRUS IMMUNE COMPLEX–MEDIATED RENAL DISEASE

Circulating immune complexes, often identifiable as HIV-related, are common in HIV-infected patients at all stages of the disease (393–398). MPGN, diffuse proliferative glomerulonephritis, immunotactoid glomerulopathy, and MN have been reported in patients with HIV infection (202,294,297, 302,303,307–309,317–319,325,399–407). In several studies of HIV-infected patients with nephrotic range proteinuria, more than one-fourth had glomerulonephritis as opposed to HIV-associated focal glomerulosclerosis (13,23,353,408).

Epidemiology

Of 28 patients with HIV infection and nephrotic range proteinuria who underwent evaluation in our series (23), 28.6% had a form of proliferative glomerulonephritis; 87.5% of the latter were African American. In subsequent studies, 40% of patients with HIV infection and renal disease who underwent renal biopsy had findings consistent with an immune-mediated glomerular disease (13). Excluding patients with IgA nephropathy, 30% of patients with renal abnormalities and HIV infection evaluated by renal biopsy had a type of proliferative glomerulonephritis. Nochy and co-workers (319) describe a population of European, Caribbean, and African patients with HIV infection and renal disease evaluated in Paris. Approximately 37% of patients had immune complex glomerulonephritis. Twenty-one percent of black patients had immune complex renal disease. Interestingly, only one black patient in that series had immune complex glomerulonephritis alone; the remainder had mixed focal glomerulosclerosis and immune complex nephropathy. Approximately half of the white patients had immune complex glomerulonephritis, commonly with a variable tubulointerstitial nephritis. The majority of these patients were homosexual. Only one of the white patients, an intravenous drug user, had the "mixed" nephropathy. Three other European studies from the United Kingdom and Italy emphasize a high proportion of patients with nephrotic syndrome in the setting of HIV infection have glomerulonephritis (400–402). A study from Thailand of HIV infected patients with renal disease reported a diverse set of glomerulonephridites, but no cases of classic HIVAN (407). While in general, patients of African heritage are more likely to have HIVAN, European and Asian populations more often appear to have glomerulonephritis. HIVICD did occur in patients of African heritage in the European studies (319,400,401). In the large Italian study (402), although there were a variety of glomerulonephritides delineated, no patient of Italian heritage had HIVAN. In a recent U.S. multicenter study in which 89 patients with HIV infection and renal disease underwent renal biopsy, 14.6% had immune complex glomerulonephritis, 9% had MN, 5.6% had MPGN, and 1.1% had IgA nephropathy and MCD (353).

Clinical Features

All patients we studied with HIVICD were African Americans with renal failure and proteinuria (13,317). Three had proliferative glomerulonephritis, crescentic and sclerotic changes, marked renal insufficiency, and nephrotic proteinuria. One had a clinical constellation consistent with postinfectious glomerulonephritis, with mild renal insufficiency. Most patients were homosexual, but one patient was thought to have acquired HIV infection through heterosexual transmission. Clinical stage of HIV infection was not related to the occurrence of disease (317,319). The patients with HIVICD usually had mild hypertension, in contrast to those with HIVAN. All patients had proteinuria, often in the nephrotic range. Hematuria was not an invariable finding. Red blood cell and granular casts were variably present on urinalysis. Renal insufficiency and hypocomplementemia to a variable degree were encountered. All patients in our series had circulating immune complexes composed of immunoglobulins reactive with HIV proteins, which, in most cases, were eluted from renal tissue in higher titers than in the plasma. Circulating immune complexes were isolated in all four patients, composed of IgA-p24, IgG-gp120, and IgG-p24. Identical complexes were eluted from renal tissue in the first three cases; only p24 and complement were eluted from the fourth. Eluted antibodies reacted with the HIV antigens isolated from the circulating immune complexes. We were not able to demonstrate cryoprecipitation in any case.

Renal Pathology

Nochy and co-workers (319) describe several subtypes of HIV-associated immune complex glomerulonephritis. These include a diffuse exudative endocapillary proliferative form termed "postinfectious;" a second type that resembles lupus nephritis with diffuse endocapillary proliferative changes, wire loops, hyaline thrombi in capillary lumina, and mesangial, intracapillary, and subepithelial deposits of immunoglobulin, C3, and C1q; and a "mixed" type with features of both focal glomerulosclerosis and immune complex nephropathy. Two of the patients in our series might be considered of the mixed type (317). We found a spectrum of pathologic changes, including variable degrees of mesangial expansion, segmental increase of mesangial cells and matrix, and segmental or diffuse proliferation of glomerular tufts. Increased cellularity with lobular transformation, segmental condensation or simplification of the glomerular tuft, and segmental or global proliferative and sclerosing changes were seen. Visceral epithelial cells were often prominent, and fibrocellular crescents were often present. Microcystic tubular dilation and atrophy and interstitial fibrosis or edema were often noted. Biopsies were characterized by interstitial infiltration with mononuclear cells, primarily macrophages and lymphocytes, and occasionally plasma cells, polymorphonuclear leukocytes, and eosinophils. Occasionally, infiltrating cells disrupted the tubular basement membrane. The proportion of interstitial macrophages was higher in tissue from patients with classic HIVAN compared with tissue from patients with HIVICD. On the other hand, interstitial tissue from biopsies of patients with HIVICD had a higher percentage of B cells compared with HIVAN tissue (326). Such findings are consistent with different populations of infiltrating immune cells causing different histologic types of disease or different tissue chemokine profiles in different nephropathies

caused by the same virus, which attract different cell types to the site of injury.

Immunofluorescence microscopy demonstrated intramembranous and mesangial deposits of immunoglobulins and complement (317). Electron microscopy usually reveals subendothelial, intramembranous, and mesangial electron-dense deposits. Electron-dense deposits are found within mesangial cells, and glomerular capillaries occasionally exhibit both subepithelial and subendothelial deposits. Foot processes of visceral epithelial cells are approximated. Tubular reticular structures can be detected in endothelial cells.

Diagnosis

Renal biopsy is important in determining the histologic diagnosis in patients with HIV infection and renal disease, including those who present with nephrotic range proteinuria (13,23,317,353), and is the only definitive way to diagnose HIVICD. Several of the patients in our series were thought to have HIVAN before biopsy. Renal biopsy must show histologic evidence of glomerular inflammation, with immunofluorescent microscopy confirming deposition of immunoglobulin and complement and electron microscopy demonstrating mesangial or capillary deposits. More precise diagnosis may be achieved by identifying HIV protein–immunoglobulin complexes in glomerular capillaries or the mesangium in higher titer than in the circulation, although such studies are often primarily research techniques. The role of specific therapeutic interventions could be evaluated in controlled trials in HIV-infected patients with renal disease with defined clinical and histologic parameters.

An interesting subgroup is comprised of patients coinfected with HCV and HIV who have renal disease (35,186,409–411). The majority of reported cases were intravenous drug users who had glomerulonephritis, typically MPGN, rather than HIVAN. MN and immunotactoid and fibrillary glomerulonephritis have also been reported (35,202,405). HCV RNA was detected in renal tissue in half of the patients evaluated in the study by Stokes et al. (409). Etiologic relationships between the immune complexes, the inciting antigen, and the renal disease have not often been reported. Renal biopsy is necessary to make a clinical diagnosis.

Prognosis and Treatment

Prognosis depends, in part, on renal functional status and histologic findings. All patients we evaluated with findings of "mixed" disease progressed to ESRD. Another patient with mild urinary abnormalities and well-preserved renal function had relatively stable renal function for almost 2 years while the viral illness progressed. Antiretroviral therapy had been instituted in some patients with HIVICD without obvious effect. Its role in the treatment of HIV-related glomerulonephritis must be studied rigorously. One patient with advanced renal insufficiency and nephrotic range proteinuria treated with steroids had transient improvement in renal function of several months' duration but later progressed to ESRD (317). Patients in other studies have had variable outcomes, but follow-up has usually not been extensive. Patients with glomerulonephritis and HCV and HIV infection appear to have a variable, but worse outcome than patients with HCV-associated glomerulonephritis (353,409,410). In a recent U.S. multicenter observational study, patients with renal diseases other than HIVAN had a longer course until the development of ESRD (731 ± 642 compared with 254 ± 331 days) and had better overall survival (353). No differential effect of treatment with antiretroviral drugs was noted in the group of patients without HIVAN.

HUMAN IMMUNODEFICIENCY VIRUS-ASSOCIATED IMMUNOGLOBULIN A NEPHROPATHY

IgA nephropathy has been described in several patients with HIV infection. IgA antibodies directed against HIV antigens are part of the early response to HIV infection (412–416). Circulating antigen–antibody complexes containing IgA are often present in HIV-infected patients. Rather than being the chance association of two unrelated diseases, it appears that the renal disease is intimately associated with the viral infection. In HIV-associated IgA nephropathy, we detected idiotypic IgA immunoglobulins directed against anti-HIV antigen–antibody complexes, which were identical to those found in renal tissue (312). Immunochemical analysis revealed circulating, idiotypic IgA antibodies, bound to IgG-gp41 and IgM-p24 complexes (312). Identical immune complexes were eluted from biopsied tissue, in higher concentration than the circulating immune complex. In addition, HIV gene sequences were amplified by PCR from renal tissue. These data are similar to findings in IgA nephropathy in non-HIV-infected populations (417), suggesting immune mediation and a genetic predisposition to a particular pathologic outcome.

Epidemiology and Clinical Features

Almost all patients with HIV IgA nephropathy reported are white or Hispanic (310–316). Hsieh and others reported a black patient with HIV infection and crescentic IgA nephropathy (320). Two Southeast Asian patients with HIV infection and IgA nephropathy have been reported (407). Most patients are homosexual men, although the disease has also been reported in boys. Patients have hematuria and proteinuria, sometimes in the nephrotic range. Red cell casts are usually noted. Renal insufficiency is common but is often stable and can improve. Serum IgA levels are increased, but this is a common finding in HIV-infected patients in the absence of renal disease. Occasional patients have hypertension. Katz et al. (311) evaluated three white homosexual men and a Hispanic boy with HIV infection and IgA nephropathy. All patients had circulating immune complexes composed of immunoglobulins, including IgA reactive with various HIV antigens and IgA rheumatoid factors (311). We demonstrated the presence of circulating immune complexes composed of idiotypic IgA antibodies directed against IgG or IgM antibodies reactive with HIV peptides in two patients (312). The IgA antiimmunoglobulin response in both patients was specific both for types of immunoglobulin and for immunoglobulin reactive with specific HIV antigens. The anti-HIV antigen response was also both viral peptide-specific and patient-specific. Cryoprecipitation was demonstrated in one case.

The low reported prevalence of IgA nephropathy in HIV-infected patients may be related to a true low incidence of the disease (312,418), perhaps related to host and genetic background in infected patients (312,417–419). Alternatively, the low prevalence may reflect the reluctance to perform renal biopsies in patients with urinary abnormalities and mild renal insufficiency, in the absence of perceived effective treatment, and in the presence of a disease that is thought to be more linked to survival than the nephropathy (312). A study from France, however, suggests almost 8% of postmortem cases show mesangial deposition of IgA (420). In a recent U.S. multicenter study in which 89 patients with HIV infection and renal disease underwent renal biopsy, only 1.1% had IgA nephropathy (353).

Renal Pathology

Light microscopy usually shows diffuse or segmental increase in mesangial matrix, with segmental proliferative changes. Rarely, thrombi are seen in glomerular capillaries, and areas of segmental sclerosis may be noted. Occasionally fibrocellular crescents are seen (311,312,316,320). IgA is the predominant immunoglobulin in the mesangium and in glomerular capillary walls, along with C3, IgM, and less often IgG. Electron microscopy shows increased mesangial matrix with mesangial and peripheral (intramembranous, subepithelial) electron-dense deposits. Tubular reticular structures may be noted in glomerular endothelial cells. Nuclear bodies may be seen in interstitial cells (311).

Prognosis and Treatment

Jindal et al. (316) used steroid therapy in a patient with renal insufficiency and IgA nephropathy before the HIV infection was diagnosed. The level of serum creatinine decreased, suggesting a beneficial clinical response may have been related to this treatment. Most patients, however, have had mild, nonprogressive renal insufficiency, and there are few data regarding treatment. The effects of CS and antiretroviral therapy on the natural history of the disease are unknown. A patient with HIV infection treated with didanosine, and IgA nephropathy with urinary protein excretion of 12 g/day was given captopril. Over 3.5 months, urinary protein excretion decreased to 0.5 g/day, associated with an increase of circulating levels of serum protein and albumin (421). Prospective, controlled studies are necessary to evaluate the role of inhibition of the renin-angiotensin system and the use of HAART in HIV infected patients with IgA nephropathy.

HUMAN IMMUNODEFICIENCY VIRUS–ASSOCIATED THROMBOTIC MICROANGIOPATHIES

Both thrombotic thrombocytopenic purpura (TTP) and hemolytic–uremic syndrome (HUS) have been reported in patients with HIV infection (422–431). A French study suggests the thrombotic microangiopathies are a common cause for acute renal failure in HIV-infected patients (423). Evidence suggests the disease can be caused in animal models by retroviral infection (431,432), and that the virus might mediate dysfunction of endothelial cells (431,433–437). The diseases manifest their common presentations, but because of the protean manifestations of HIV infection, may prove difficult to diagnose. Abnormalities of the peripheral blood smear remain the criterion for making the diagnosis (422). Although a variety of different therapeutic approaches have been employed (298,299,431,438), plasmapheresis remains the safest and perhaps the most effective treatment for HIV-infected patients with TTP. The potential therapeutic role of antiretroviral therapy in such cases, while attractive on theoretical grounds, has not been tested adequately in well-designed clinical studies (439,440). Few studies exist on the treatment of HUS in the setting of HIV infection. Randomized controlled trials of therapy in patients with HIV infection and the thrombotic microangiopathies have been lacking (298,299,431).

RENAL DISEASE RELATED TO TREATMENT

The host response to ongoing viremia may include continued antibody synthesis, cell-mediated immune responses, and cellular antiviral responses. Therapy with IFN-α has been associated with a variety of renal disorders. We studied an HIV-infected patient treated with IFN-α who developed MPGN. An IFN-α-immunoglobulin immune complex was identified in the circulation and in higher titer in renal eluates, demonstrating that glomerulonephritis in HIV-infected patients may be secondary to a host response to treatment (239). Distinguishing the progression of disease from iatrogenic effects may be an important clinical dilemma in patients treated with this immunomodulator who develop increased renal insufficiency. The extent of renal disease related to therapy with IFN-α in patients with HIV, HBV, or HCV infection, however, is unknown.

The newer antiretroviral drugs, especially the protease inhibitors, in particular indinavir (321,363,441,442) and to a lesser extent, ritonavir (363,443) may cause reversible nephropathy by several mechanisms (299,321,441,444–446). It is important to distinguish such effects from the progression of the underlying renal disease. Rhabdomyolysis may be an increasingly common cause of acute renal failure as patients with lipodystrophy induced by antiretroviral therapy are treated with statins (299,447–450). Adefovir, cidofovir, abacavir and tenofovir have all been associated with the development of tubular injury (299,451–455).

RENAL DISEASE INDIRECTLY ASSOCIATED WITH VIRAL INFECTION

Glomerular diseases may occur in HIV-infected patients that are unrelated to the viral infection, are related to coinfections, or reflect the immune dysregulation seen in HIV infection (13,16,17,294,297,456,457). A patient with glomerulonephritis and HIV infection exhibited characteristics of poststreptococcal glomerulonephritis (456). The biopsy, however, showed tubular reticular structures, which are a hallmark of HIV-associated renal diseases. Therefore, this patient may have had two different glomerular diseases, or the electron microscopic findings may have been nonspecific. The slow resolution of the renal disease in this case may reflect the disordered immunoregulation seen in HIV-infected patients, compared with immunologically normal hosts who develop glomerulonephritis after streptococcal infections. We evaluated a white man with nephrotic syndrome in the presence of HIV and HBV infection. The renal biopsy was suggestive of MN secondary to HBV infection, rather than an HIV-associated glomerulopathy (399). The association of these two diseases was confirmed when the proteinuria remitted concurrently with the clearance of HBeAg from the patient's circulation (458). There are a paucity of well-described cases of lupus nephritis in the setting of HIV infection (392,459). It is possible that the disordered immunoregulation associated with the viral infection mediates altered renal outcomes in such patients.

CRYOGLOBULINEMIA AND VASCULITIS

Occasionally patients with vasculitis and/or cryoglobulinemia in the presence of HIV infection have been reported (460–466), although the extent of renal involvement in such patients is often unclear. A report outlined 16 HIV-infected patients with large vessel disease (467). Another study of HCV-infected patients linked the presence of cryoglobulinemia to vasculitis and coexisting HIV infection (179). Coinfection with HBV and HCV make the pathogenesis of this disorder difficult to assess, in light of the abnormal immunoregulation present in HIV infection, in the absence of rigorous, precise identification of tissue-deposited immunoreactants (468).

Antibodies reactive with HIV p24 have occasionally been noted in patients with autoimmune diseases (469). Sera from several patients with essential cryoglobulinemia reacted with human T-cell lymphotrophic virus type I proteins, and reverse transcriptase activity was found in several patients as well (469). None of the sera reacted with HIV-1 peptides. The significance of these findings is unclear, but it is possible that these antibodies may only be cross-reactive with the retroviral proteins or be directed against endogenous proteins, coded by retroviral-like sequences in the human genome or sharing homology with retroviral proteins (469–471). Vasculitis and cryoglobulinemia, however, appear to be relatively rare compared with the prevalence of HIV infection. It is also frequently difficult, in the absence of intensive immunologic analysis, to assess whether the cryoglobulinemia is associated with HIV or other coexistent infections. Renal vasculitis has not been an important clinical finding in such patients. In a patient with HIV and HBV infection, cryoglobulinemia and proliferative glomerulonephritis were evaluated. Two circulating immune complexes were detected in this patient. One was composed of an IgG–HIV p24 complex, the other a cryoprecipitable IgA–IgG complex. Interestingly, the HIV peptide complex was not implicated in the pathogenesis of the nephropathy (13). This case illustrates the importance of a careful immunochemical evaluation in establishing a precise diagnosis of the renal disease in HIV-infected patients.

MECHANISTIC POSSIBILITIES IN THE PATHOGENESIS OF HUMAN IMMUNODEFICIENCY VIRUS-ASSOCIATED IMMUNE COMPLEX DISEASE

The pathogenesis of HIVICD is largely unknown; however, in our studies, the overwhelming majority of HIV-infected patients with renal disease show the presence of HIV genome in the kidney (13,23,317). Cohen et al. (472) also demonstrated proviral HIV DNA in tubular and glomerular epithelial cells in biopsies and autopsy tissue from HIV-infected patients with immune complex glomerulonephritis using in vitro DNA hybridization techniques. They also found such renal tissue markers in patients with AIDS without clinically obvious renal disease. However, they were unable to demonstrate the presence of either HIV core or envelope protein antigens in glomerular deposits in their patients with immune complex glomerulonephritis. Interestingly, we also demonstrated the presence of HIV genome in autopsy tissue of patients without the presence of renal lesions (13). Such findings suggest the presence of HIV genomic material in the kidney is not alone sufficient to induce nephropathy. Triggering and facilitating mechanisms seem likely, therefore, to be associated with mechanisms that cause nephropathy. Understanding the pathogenesis of such renal disease and the nature of such mechanisms might lead to preventive or ameliorative strategies.

The role of cellular incorporation of HIV genome products in the development of renal disease, contrasted with circulating immune mechanisms, is unknown. The development of glomerulonephritis may be dependent on the renal parenchymal incorporation of HIV antigens, although renal cellular HIV infection may not be a sufficient condition for disease expression. Evidence suggests HIV may infect renal tissue, specifically glomerular epithelial cells (322,323,337,354–356,472) and mesangial cells *in vitro* (357,473). The tubular epithelium may also be a target for infection (337,358). Tubular cells can be infected by HIV *in vitro* (358).

It is possible that renal cellular viral infection itself, by the expression of viral antigens or alteration of renal cellular proteins, might lead to subsequent attachment of circulating anti-HIV antibodies or complexes to an implanted or transformed antigen. Alternatively, such findings may be the result of deposition of circulating immune complexes in renal tissue, which subsequently initiate an inflammatory response. Analysis of pathologic tissue cannot differentiate definitively between these two pathogenic mechanisms. The pathogenic significance of a positive PCR remains to be established.

Similarly, the role of genetic and host responses may be crucial in determining renal pathologic outcomes. It is of interest that a substantial proportion of the polyclonal immunoglobulin response in HIV-infected patients is composed of IgA, and that IgA-containing immune complexes are prevalent in patients with HIV infection and AIDS (412–416). These immune responses may partially explain the prevalence of IgA nephropathy seen in HIV-infected patients. It is possible that certain specific immune responses, perhaps related to specific modes of antigen presentation, or specific circulating immune complexes are more likely to provoke an ongoing renal inflammatory response. Finally, the role of concurrent or intercurrent viral infection in affecting renal responses remains to be determined.

Since HIVICD is characterized by a dense interstitial infiltrate (13,23,312,317,325,326) that aids in the identification of its HIV-associated nature, immune cell infiltration in renal tissue may be important in its pathogenesis. Because different cell populations characterize different nephropathies, the immune cell population may also have an important effect on histologic outcome. Alternatively, different pathogenic processes may elicit different infiltrating cells. Cytokines and growth factors, which are products of immune cells, may also enhance nephropathogenicity. IFNs are expressed in response to viral infections (474). Treatment with IFNs has been associated with reversible nephropathy, including interstitial nephritis and glomerulonephritis (239,240–243,475–478). Several cytokines and growth factors can modulate the growth and function of mesangial cells in culture, including platelet-derived growth factor, epidermal growth factor, interleukin-1 (IL-1), tumor necrosis factor, and transforming growth factor-β (21,479–488). A role for cytokines and growth factors in the activation of latent HIV-1 virus has also been suggested (489–495). In addition, HIV-1 proteins may have cytotoxic or other effects on renal cells that could enhance nephropathogenicity. The HIV protein gp120 is cytotoxic, causing death of astrocytes in human brain cultures *in vitro* and inducing cellular IFN-α and IFN-γ, tumor necrosis factor-α, IgG, IL-1, and IL-6 production (496–498). The HIV-1 *trans*-activator protein Tat has variable stimulatory or inhibitory effects on cell proliferation (499–502). gp120 and gp120-anti-gp120 antigen–antibody complexes are immunomodulatory (498,503,504). Therefore, HIV peptides and antibodies directed against them may modulate renal cellular function, leading to susceptibility to immune complex renal disease.

CYTOMEGALOVIRUS (CMV) INFECTION AND GLOMERULONEPHRITIS

CMV infection has been associated with transplant glomerulopathy and chronic allograft nephropathy (505–511) and

acute rejection (511,512), although this notion is still a controversial area of research and vigorously disputed (513–518). The lesion may be associated with vascular rejection (512,513,515,519). A case report demonstrated the presence of immunotactoid glomerulopathy with renal failure in a renal transplant patient who simultaneously had CMV viremia (520). The glomerular lesion and renal dysfunction resolved concurrently with successful treatment of the CMV infection, circumstantially suggesting an association between the viral disease and the glomerulopathy.

Controversy also exists regarding whether CMV infection is intimately associated with glomerulonephritis in general and specifically with IgA nephropathy (417,521,522). A report implicated CMV infection in the development of recurrence of glomerulonephritis in a patient with preexisting MPGN (522) by virtue of improvement after treatment with ganciclovir. No evidence of CMV renal infection, however, was reported. Detwiler et al. reported a necrotizing, crescentic glomerulonephritis in a patient who received a renal transplant (523). Interestingly, although there was little evidence of immune-complex mediated mechanistic processes, CMV was detected in renal tissue by immunochemistry and *in situ* hybridization techniques. In this case, ganciclovir therapy also ameliorated signs of renal disease.

CMV can infect and replicate in human mesangial cells (524), and CMV infection in mice is associated with glomerulonephritis (525). In animal models, IgA nephropathy may result from various viral infections (417). Ozawa and Stewart (526) described a patient with hematuria and proteinuria, with normal renal function, who died of gastrointestinal hemorrhage while being treated with CS. Autopsy revealed focal proliferative mesangial hypercellularity. IgG, IgA, C3, and C4, as well as CMV antigens, localized by guinea pig anti-CMV antiserum, were present in a granular pattern within the mesangium (526). IgG antibody reactive with CMV was detected in renal eluates in lower titer than in the circulation. The authors interpreted these findings as consistent with a CMV immune-mediated glomerulonephritis. Gregory and co-workers (7) consistently detected CMV antigens in tissue from patients with IgA nephropathy using indirect immunofluorescence techniques, employing polyclonal antihuman CMV antibodies (7). Waldo and others (527) suggested these results may have been nonspecific, and other investigators have been unable to confirm the positive results (528,529). Ortmanns et al. described a patient with IgA nephropathy who was treated with immunosuppressive drugs who subsequently developed CMV infection (530). Renal function improved after immunosuppression was discontinued and therapy with ganciclovir initiated. After discontinuation of ganciclovir, renal function worsened. Renal function improved after reinstitution of ganciclovir. The authors interpreted these findings as evidence for an important role of CMV in the pathogenesis of IgA nephropathy, but it is also possible that two distinct renal pathogenic mechanistic processes occurred simultaneously. Lai et al. (531), using monoclonal antibodies directed against CMV antigens in indirect immunofluorescence studies, were unable to detect CMV peptides in tissue from patients with IgA nephropathy. They suggested the conflicting findings might be based on differential antibody specificity and the positive findings were artifactual.

Studies have investigated whether the CMV genome may be found in renal tissue of patients with IgA nephropathy. Okamura and co-workers (532) and Kanahara co-workers (533) were unable to detect CMV DNA in renal tissue from patients with IgA nephropathy. Smith et al. (534) were also unable to confirm the presence of CMV antigens in a large proportion of renal tissue from patients with IgA nephropathy using immunochemical techniques. Similarly, they were unable to localize CMV DNA in such tissue using in situ DNA hybridization. Bene et al. (535), using monoclonal antibodies directed against CMV antigens, were unable to detect CMV peptides and, using PCR technology, were able to detect CMV genome in only 1 of 14 samples of renal tissue from patients with IgA nephropathy. The authors concluded that CMV infection was not associated with IgA nephropathy. Telenti and co-workers (536) failed to show CMV DNA in renal tissue from 10 patients with IgA nephropathy.

Muller et al. (537,538), however, detected CMV DNA by PCR in renal tissue from 74% of 19 biopsies of patients with IgA nephropathy. Immunohistochemical examination of tissue for CMV antigens was positive in only 2 of 17 evaluations. CMV antigens were detected in a mesangial distribution. The CMV genome, however, was also detected in 4 of 18 (22%) samples of frozen tissue from normal kidneys, although the difference between the proportions of positive detections was statistically significantly different in the two groups. CMV genome was not amplified from samples of kidneys from patients with focal glomerulosclerosis (537). In addition, detection of the CMV genome was less common (only 1 of 17, or 6%) in paraffin-embedded sections in contrast to frozen material. However, only a few specimens were assessed in tandem using the two preparations from individual patients. These results are in accordance with the notion that CMV infection is associated with the pathogenesis of IgA nephropathy but do not establish a causal relationship. Alternatively, the host immune response to CMV infection may culminate in the development of IgA nephropathy in selected patients.

Kadereit et al. (539) showed, in an early study, that CMV genome could be detected in 40% of renal biopsies of patients who had circulating antibodies directed against CMV, indicating prior exposure to the virus. However, 30% of seronegative patients also had a positive PCR evaluation in renal tissue, suggesting the technique is more sensitive than serologic assessments. A seronegative control without kidney disease also had a positive PCR determination. All negative genomic controls had negative PCR evaluations. There was no correlation of a positive PCR result with type of nephropathy. Such data suggest the finding of a positive CMV PCR may be relatively common in renal tissue of patients with and without renal disease, reflecting the high prevalence of CMV infection. Park et al. (540), however, used the PCR technique to amplify CMV DNA from renal tissue from patients with IgA nephropathy and tissue from both patients with other glomerulonephritides and normal renal tissue as controls. These investigators were able to amplify CMV gene products from 60% of paraffin-embedded renal biopsy tissue from patients with IgA nephropathy, but CMV DNA was also detected in 71% of control tissue from patients with other forms of glomerulonephritis. They were unable to demonstrate CMV antigen, however, by immunologic techniques in renal tissue from patients with IgA nephropathy. These results suggest that the presence of CMV genome in renal tissue from patients with IgA nephropathy is not specific and that renal cellular infection with CMV may be associated with glomerulonephritis. This association may not, however, be one of cause and effect.

PCR results are likely to be more sensitive (13,23,24) but also are dependent on the primers and probes used and the technique employed (541) and are subject to contamination. In addition, material may be present during PCR that may inhibit the reaction, leading to false-negative results. Therefore, in addition to scrupulous technique, it is important that positive and negative controls, from the same laboratory, be simultaneously assessed in this type of study to allow valid conclusions to be drawn from the data. Geographic variations, considering the genetic predispositions to development of IgA nephropathy and differences in rates of endemic viral infections and strain differences worldwide, should also be considered when analyzing such results. Ultimately, the demonstration of specific viral peptides and antiviral antibodies in characteristic anatomic lo-

cations will be necessary to validate a causal association between CMV infection and glomerulonephritis.

HANTAVIRUS INFECTION AND THE KIDNEY

The hantaviruses are a group of single-stranded RNA viruses of the Bunyaviridae family (542). Although hantavirus is endemic in Korea and other parts of Asia, cases have been noted in Western Europe, and exposure to hantavirus infection has been documented in inner city populations in the United States (543). Since a greater proportion of patients in Baltimore, Maryland with renal disease and hypertension had antibodies to hantavirus compared with control groups of patients seen in an emergency setting and in a sexually transmitted disease clinic, some have speculated on an association between exposure to hantavirus and the pathogenesis of chronic renal disease in the United States (543). Such preliminary results were confirmed in a study of biopsy-proved cases of acute and chronic renal disease (544). Three percent of patients with congenital renal disease had serologic evidence of exposure to hantavirus, while more than one-fourth of a group of patients with various acute and chronic renal diseases had antibodies against hantavirus. Patients with tubulointerstitial nephritis, necrotizing glomerulonephritis, and IgA nephropathy were most likely to have had antibodies directed against hantavirus. The pathogenic mechanisms underlying these associations remain to be clarified. Studies suggest chronic alterations in kidney function, including glomerular filtration, glomerular permeability and tubular function may occur after viral infection (545–548).

Hantavirus infections have been associated with acute renal failure, including nephropathia epidemica, associated with Puumala virus infection, and the more severe hemorrhagic fever with renal syndrome, in those infected with Hantaan virus. Infection with the Seoul virus has been associated with a less severe form of hemorrhagic fever with renal syndrome (549). Characteristic clinical signs of hemorrhagic fever with renal syndrome include fever, hemorrhagic manifestations, and renal failure. The disease is divided into five phases: febrile, hypotensive, oliguric, diuretic, and convalescent. In many cases, renal function returns to normal, but often over a period of months. The renal disease is often characterized by tubular, rather than glomerular disorders. Pathologic findings of hemorrhage in medullary interstitium, inflammatory cell infiltration, and glomerular epithelial cell and basement membrane abnormalities are encountered. Tubular lesions such as sloughing and necrosis of epithelial cells are common, but glomerular abnormalities are not. The pathogenic contributions of vasodilation, microcirculatory abnormalities, platelet dysfunction, and disseminated intravascular coagulation to the pathologic findings are unclear. Immune complex-mediated mechanisms have been thought to be important because they may be detected in the circulation and glomeruli (542,549). Complement activation has been noted concurrently with high levels of immune complex detection and peak vascular injury. Treatment of the renal disease consists of supportive measures and appropriate renal replacement therapy. Several reviews have considered this area (550,551), while the number of case reports and series describing specific aspects of the disease has burgeoned.

In a large series of patients from Finland with nephropathia epidemica diagnosed serologically, tubular and interstitial abnormalities were most common, although in 20 of 53 patients who had glomeruli for analysis, abnormalities such as mesangial hypercellularity were noted (552). Half these glomeruli had negative immunofluorescent evaluations. In the other half, a variety of immunoreactants, including complement, were noted in a granular mesangial distribution, with patterns ranging from focal and segmental to diffuse and global. In one case, the diagnosis of IgA nephropathy was made. Although rare case reports of glomerulonephritis in patients with hantavirus infection exist (546,553,554), it is not clear whether the glomerulonephritis was directly related to the viral infection or represented the occurrence of two distinct diseases.

EPSTEIN-BARR VIRUS INFECTION

Rare cases of renal disease have been reported in patients with Epstein-Barr virus (EBV) infection (555–567). Several cases of immune complex renal disease with glomerular ultrastructural abnormalities have been reported in association with EBV infection (555–557,559,560,562,563) including a case of IgA nephropathy (558) and diverse types of glomerular abnormalities (555,565). Causal links cannot as yet be conclusively established between the glomerulonephritis and the viral illness, however, using strict criteria (8,10,13). The majority of cases of acute renal failure in the setting of EBV infection have been either due to rhabdomyolysis or interstitial nephritis (563–568), although a case of renal lymphoma associated with EBV infection has been reported (569). An elegant study suggests EBV infection is characteristic of renal tissue of patients with chronic interstitial nephritis (570). The role of EBV infection in modifying outcomes in renal transplantation is unclear (511,571,572).

POLYOMAVIRUS INFECTIONS

JC and BK viruses are double-stranded DNA viruses of the Polyomavirus family that have been associated with interstitial renal disease in renal transplant patients (573,574). BK virus, which has a seroprevalence of 60% to 80% in different populations, has a high degree of homology with simian virus 40 (SV40), as does JC virus. The role of BK virus in mediating renal disease in the absence of immunosuppression or preexisting nephropathy is unclear (575,576). One early study attempted to implicate BK-associated immune complexes with various immune-complex glomerular diseases (576). A recent study suggested BK virus infects glomerular epithelial cells in transplant patients (577). Renal tissue shows renal tubular abnormalities and interstitial infiltration (578). Treatment involves curtailing immunosuppression, but this may lead to rejection. Better transplant kidney function was associated with less virus detected in a study involving the use of protocol transplant biopsies (578). Quantitative PCR may allow more precise diagnosis of BK virus allograft nephropathy (579). Recently patients with BK nephropathy have been treated with cidofovir (580), although the drug can exhibit nephrotoxicity.

Recent preliminary data suggest SV40, a simian Polyomavirus, can be detected more commonly from cells of urine of patients with renal disease, compared to those of normal controls (581). A role for SV40 in the pathogenesis of focal glomerulosclerosis was suggested. Further work has tested such hypotheses (582). Such data, although associative, provide a basis for investigation of the role of SV40 in the initiation or mediation of renal disease.

PARVOVIRUS INFECTIONS

Parvovirus B19 is a single-stranded DNA virus that is a member of the Parvoviridae family. It is the only virus of this family to infect humans. Its seroprevalence ranges between 40% and 60% in adults in developed countries. It has been associated with glomerulonephritis in patients with diagnoses such as sickle cell disease (583,584) and vasculitis (585,586),

as well as a variety of other glomerulonephridites (35,587–593) including Henoch-Schönlein purpura (594,595). Mesangioproliferative glomerulonephritis, mesangiocapillary proliferative glomerulonephritis, and acute endocapillary proliferative glomerulonephritis have all been reported associated with parvovirus infection. Patients may have hypocomplementemia (590,591). Histologic studies have linked the presence of viral protein (590,592) and genome (588,592,594) to the renal disease with varying assessments of control tissue, but causality has not been definitively proved.

Viral DNA was detected in a higher proportion of tissue from patients with focal glomerulosclerosis compared with tissue from patients with other glomerular diseases or normal tissue (596). Viral DNA, however, was not detected by *in situ* hybridization. Parvovirus B19 has since been linked to the presence of collapsing glomerulopathy by several investigators (35,597–600). Moudgil et al. showed parvovirus B19 DNA could be detected in renal tissue from patients with collapsing glomerulopathy with higher frequency (78.3%) than from tissue from patients with HIV-associated nephropathy or focal glomerulosclerosis (599). Viral genome was detected in glomerular epithelial cells and tubular cells, suggesting a possible pathogenic pathway for the development of the disease. The investigators speculated host factors could be critical in determining disease expression.

Finally, parvovirus infection has been associated with anemia and renal dysfunction in patients who received kidney transplants (507,598,601–603). Murer et al. reported four cases of thrombotic microangiopathy in renal allografts associated with parvovirus infection (604). The role of this virus in mediating the initiation and progression of various forms of chronic renal diseases deserves further study.

CONCLUSION

Renal disease occurs in patients with HBV, HCV, and HIV and other viral infections, and is often immune complex mediated. Viral-associated glomerulonephritis comprises a spectrum of proliferative glomerulonephritis to MN, likely reflecting differential deposition of antibody and antigen–antibody complexes, *in situ* immune mechanisms, and variation in host responses and genetic background. The role of the association of viral infection in the pathogenesis of focal segmental glomerulosclerosis is under active investigation. Infection of glomerular epithelial cells by particular viruses may contribute to the pathogenesis of focal segmental glomerulosclerosis. Differences in expression of renal disease may vary with the nephropathogenicity of specific viral peptides and the physicochemical characteristics of the associated immune complexes, the anatomic location of their deposition, and systemic and local clearance rates. Diagnosis and therefore the true prevalence of viral-related glomerulonephritis will depend on the specificity and sensitivity of the tests employed in the diagnosis. The demonstration of both viral antigens and host antibody in the mesangium and in glomerular capillaries and the isolation of identical viral immune complexes from distinct renal anatomic areas, in higher titers than the circulation, remain the gold standard for diagnostic purposes. Immunochemical and molecular biologic evaluations will prove increasingly important for our understanding the pathogenesis of viral and nonviral renal diseases in animal models and in human tissue.

References

1. Wilson CB, Dixon FJ. The renal response to immunological injury. In: Brenner BM, Rector FC, eds. *The kidney,* 2nd ed. Philadelphia: Saunders, 1981:1237.

2. Blumberg BS, Alter HJ, Vinich S. A "new" antigen in leukemia serum. *JAMA* 1964;191:101.
3. Kohler PF. Clinical immune complex disease: manifestations in systemic lupus erythematosus and hepatitis B virus infection. *Medicine* 1973;52:419.
4. Ozawa T, et al. Acute immune complex disease associated with hepatitis. Etiopathogenic and immunopathologic studies of the renal lesion. *Arch Pathol Lab Med* 1976;100:484.
5. Ronco P, Verroust P, Morel-Maroger L. Viruses and glomerulonephritis. *Nephron* 1982;31:97.
6. Vas SI. Primary and secondary role of viruses in chronic renal failure. *Kidney Int* 1991;40(Suppl 35):S-2.
7. Gregory MC, Hammond ME, Brewer ED. Renal deposition of cytomegalovirus antigen in immunoglobulin-A nephropathy. *Lancet* 1988;1:11.
8. Glassock RJ. Immune complex-induced glomerular injury in viral diseases: an overview. *Kidney Int* 1991;40(Suppl 35):S-5.
9. Couser WG, Salant DJ. In situ immune complex formation and glomerular injury. *Kidney Int* 1980;17:1.
10. Couser WG. Mechanisms of glomerular injury in immune-complex disease. *Kidney Int* 1985;28:569.
11. Couser WG. Mediation of immune glomerular injury. *J Am Soc Nephrol* 1990;1:13.
12. Wilson CB. The renal response to immunologic injury. In: Brenner BM, Rector FC, eds. *The kidney*, 4th ed. Philadelphia: Saunders, 1991.
13. Kimmel PL, Phillips TM. Immune complex glomerulonephritis associated with HIV infection. In: Kimmel PL, Berns JS, eds. *Renal and urologic aspects of HIV infection*. New York: Churchill Livingstone, 1995:77.
14. Quigg RJ. Complement and autoimmune glomerular diseases. *Curr Dir Autoimmun* 2004;7:165.
15. Segerer S, Nelson PJ, Schlondorff D. Chemokines, chemokine receptors, and renal disease: from basic science to pathophysiologic and therapeutic studies. *J Am Soc Nephrol* 2000;11:152.
16. Kimmel PL. HIV-associated nephropathy: virologic issues related to renal sclerosis. *Nephrol Dial Transplant* 2003;18(Suppl 6):vi59.
17. Kimmel PL. Clinical and immunopathogenic aspects of HIV-associated renal diseases. In: Nielson EG, Couser W, eds. *Immunologic renal disease*, 2nd ed. New York: Lippincott, 2001:1203.
18. Strutz F, Neilson EG. New insights into mechanisms of fibrosis in immune renal injury. *Springer Semin Immunopathol* 2003;24:459.
19. Yokoyama H, Wada T, Furuichi K. Chemokines in renal fibrosis. *Contrib Nephrol* 2003;139:66.
20. Segerer S, Alpers CE. Chemokines and chemokine receptors in renal pathology. *Curr Opin Nephrol Hypertens* 2003;12:243.
21. Anders HJ, Vielhauer V, Schlondorff D. Chemokines and chemokine receptors are involved in the resolution or progression of renal disease. *Kidney Int* 2003;63:401.
22. Segerer S. The role of chemokines and chemokine receptors in progressive renal disease. *Am J Kidney Dis* 2003;41(3 Suppl 1):S15.
23. Kimmel PL, et al. Viral DNA in micro-dissected renal biopsies of HIV-infected patients with nephrotic syndrome. *Kidney Int* 1993;43:1347.
24. Cohen CD, Kretzler M. Gene expression analysis in microdissected renal tissue. Current challenges and strategies. *Nephron* 2002;92:522.
25. Alcorta DA, et al. Future molecular approaches to the diagnosis and treatment of glomerular disease. *Semin Nephrol* 2000;20:20.
26. Embretson J, et al. Massive covert infection of helper T lymphocytes and macrophages by HIV during incubation of AIDS. *Nature* 1993;362:359.
27. Barnes JL, Milani S. In situ hybridization in the study of the kidney and renal diseases. *Semin Nephrol* 1995;15:9.
28. Grandaliano G, Chodhury GG, Abboud HE. Transgenic animal models as a tool in the diagnosis of kidney diseases. *Semin Nephrol* 1995;15:43.
29. Kopp JB, et al. Progressive glomerulosclerosis and enhanced renal accumulation of basement membrane components in mice transgenic for human immunodeficiency virus type 1 genes. *Proc Natl Acad Sci USA* 1992;89:1577.
30. Hanafusa N, et al. Contribution of genetically engineered animals to the analyses of complement in the pathogenesis of nephritis. *Nephrol Dial Transplant* 2002;17(Suppl 9):34.
31. Kopp JB. Gene expression in kidney using transgenic approaches. *Exp Nephrol* 1997;5:157.
32. Clinicopathological Conference. A 57-year-old woman with recurrent skin lesions, arthritis and renal dysfunction. Case 11-1989. *N Engl J Med* 1989;320:718.
33. Brouet JC, et al. Biologic and clinical significance of cryoglobulins. *Am J Med* 1974;57:775.
34. Dispenzieri A, Gorevic PD. Cryoglobulinemia. *Hematol Oncol Clin North Am* 1999;13:1315.
35. di Belgiojoso GB, Ferrario F, Landrianni N. Virus-related glomerular diseases: Histological and clinical aspects. *J Nephrol* 2002;15:469.
36. Ferri C, Zignego AL, Pileri SA. Cryoglobulins. *J Clin Pathol* 2002;55:4.
37. Hilleman MR. Strategies and mechanisms for host and pathogen survival in acute and persistent viral infections. *Proc Natl Acad Sci USA* 2004;101(Suppl 2):14560.
38. Dlamini Z, Mbita Z, Zungu M. Genealogy, expression and molecular mechanisms in apotosis. *Pharmacol Ther* 2004;101:1.
39. Lisowaska A, Witkowski JM. Viral strategies in modulation of NF-kappa B activity. *Arch Immunol Ther Exp* 2003;51:367.
40. Irusta PM, Chen YB, Hardwick JM. Viral modulators of cell death provide new links to old pathways. *Curr Opin Cell Biol* 2003;15:700.
41. Clemens MJ. Interferons and apotosis. *J Interferon Cytokine Res* 2003;23:277.
42. Cacoub P, et al. Cryoglobulinemia vasculitis. *Curr Opin Rheumatol* 2002;14:29.
43. Dammacco F, et al. The cryoglobulins: An overview. *Eur J Clin Invest* 2001;31:628.
44. Ramos-Casals M, et al. Mixed cryoglobulinemia: new concepts. *Lupus* 2000;9:83.
45. Ferri C, et al. HCV-related cryoglobulinemic vasculitis: An update on its etiopathogenesis and therapeutic strategies. *Clin Exp Rheumatol* 2003;21(6 Suppl 32):S78.
46. Schott P, Hartmann H, Ramadori G. Hepatitis C virus-associated mixed cryoglobulinemia. Clinical manifestations, histopathological changes, mechanisms of cryoprecipitation and options of treatment. *Histol Histopathol* 2001;16:1275.
47. Trendelenburg M, Schifferli JA. Cryoglobulins in chronic hepatitis C virus infection. *Clin Exp Immunol* 2003;133:153.
48. Meltzer M, et al. Cryoglobulinemia—a clinical and laboratory study. II. Cryoglobulins with rheumatoid factor activity. *Am J Med* 1966;40:837.
49. Gorevic PD, et al. Mixed cryoglobulinemia: clinical aspects and long-term follow-up of 40 patients. *Am J Med* 1980;69:287.
50. Jennette JC, Falk RJ. Small vessel vasculitis. *N Engl J Med* 1997;337:1512.
51. Beddhu S, Bastacky S, Johnson J. The clinical and morphologic spectrum of renal cryoglobulinemia. *Medicine* 2002;81:398.
52. D'Amico G, et al. Renal involvement in essential mixed cryoglobulinemia. *Kidney Int* 1989;35:1004.
53. Migliorini P, et al. Mechanisms of renal damage in mixed cryoglobulinemic nephritis. *Nephrol Dial Transplant* 2001;16(Suppl 6):58.
54. Levy M, Chen N. Worldwide perspective of hepatitis B-associated glomerulonephritis in the 80s. *Kidney Int* 1991;40(Suppl 35):S24.
55. Sherker AH, Robinson WS. Hepatitis B and Hepatitis D. In: Hoeprich PD, Colin Hordan M, Ronald AR, eds. *Infectious diseases*, 5th ed. Philadelphia: Lippincott, 1994:801.
56. Scaglioni P, Melegari M, Wands J. Recent advances in the molecular biology of hepatitis B virus. *Baillieres Clin Gastroenterol* 1996;10:207.
57. Mannik M, Agodoa LY, David KA. Rearrangement of immune complexes in glomeruli leads to persistence and development of electron-dense deposits. *J Exp Med* 1983;157:1516.
58. Tiollais P, Pourcel C, Dejean A. The hepatitis B virus. *Nature* 1985;317:489.
59. Seeger C, Mason WS. Hepatitis B virus biology. *Microbiol Mol Biol Rev* 2000;64:51.
60. Takekoshi Y, et al. Immunopathogenetic mechanisms of hepatitis B virus-related glomerulopathy. *Kidney Int* 1991;40(Suppl 35):S34.
61. Maynard J, Hepatitis B. Global importance and need for control. *Vaccine* 1990;8(Suppl):S18.
62. Lai KN, Lai FM. Clinical features and the natural course of hepatitis B virus-related glomerulopathy in adults. *Kidney Int* 1991;40(Suppl 35):S40.
63. Bhimma R, et al. HBV and proteinuria in relatives and contacts of children with hepatitis B virus-associated membranous nephropathy. *Kidney Int* 1999;55:2440.
64. Bhimma, R, Coovadia HM. Hepatitis B virus-associated nephropathy. *Am J Nephrol* 2004;24:198.
65. Combes B, et al. Glomerulonephritis with deposition of Australia-antigen antibody complexes in glomerular basement membrane. *Lancet* 1971;ii:234.
66. Kneiser MR, et al. Pathogenesis of renal disease associated with viral hepatitis. *Arch Pathol* 1974;97:193.
67. Oldstone MD, Dixon FJ. Pathogenesis of chronic disease associated with persistent lymphocytic choriomeningitis viral infection. *J Exp Med* 1969;119:483.
68. Kohler PF, et al. Chronic membranous glomerulonephritis caused by hepatitis B antigen—antibody immune complexes. *Ann Intern Med* 1974;81:443.
69. Austin HA, et al. Membranous nephropathy (NIH conference). *Ann Intern Med* 1992;116:672.
70. Kerjaschki D. Molecular pathogenesis of membranous nephropathy. *Kidney Int* 1992;41:1090.
71. Johnson RJ, Couser WG. Hepatitis B infection and renal disease: clinical, immunopathogenetic and therapeutic considerations. *Kidney Int* 1990;37:663.
72. Lai KN, et al. The clinico-pathologic features of hepatitis B virus-associated glomerulonephritis. *Q J Med* 1987;240:323.
73. Venkataseshan VS, et al. Hepatitis-B-associated glomerulonephritis: pathology, pathogenesis, and clinical course. *Medicine* 1990;69:200.
74. Lee HS, et al. A renal biopsy study of hepatitis B virus-associated nephropathy in Korea. *Kidney Int* 1988;34:537.
75. Nagy J, et al. The role of hepatitis B surface antigen in the pathogenesis of glomerulopathies. *Clin Nephrol* 1979;12:109.
76. Brzosko WJ, et al. Glomerulonephritis associated with hepatitis B surface antigen immune complexes in children. *Lancet* 1974;2:477.
77. Magiore W, et al. HBsAg glomerular deposits in glomerulonephritis: fact or artifact? *Kidney Int* 1981;19:579.
78. Hiroshi H, et al. Deposition of hepatitis E antigen in membranous glomerulonephritis: identification by F (ab')$_2$ fragments of monoclonal antibody. *Kidney Int* 1984;26:338.
79. Takahashi K, et al. Demonstration of hepatitis E antigen in the core of Dane particles. *J Immunol* 1979;122:275.

80. Takekoshi Y, et al. Free "small" and IgG-associated "large" hepatitis E antigen in the serum and glomerular capillary walls of two patients with membranous glomerulonephritis. *N Engl J Med* 1979;300:814.
81. Lai KN, et al. Membranous nephropathy related to hepatitis B virus in adults. *N Engl J Med* 1991;324:1457.
82. Lai KN, Lai FM, Tam JS. Comparison of polyclonal and monoclonal antibodies in determination of glomerular deposits of hepatitis B virus antigens in hepatitis B virus-associated glomerulonephritides. *Am J Clin Pathol* 1989;92:159.
83. Lai FM, et al. Primary glomerulonephritis with detectable glomerular hepatitis B virus antigens. *Am J Surg Pathol* 1994;18:175.
84. Lai KN, et al. Detection of hepatitis B virus DNA and RNA in kidneys of HBV-related glomerulonephritis. *Kidney Int* 1996;50:1965.
85. He XY, et al. In situ hybridization of hepatitis B DNA in hepatitis B-associated glomerulonephritis. *Pediatr Nephrol* 1998;12:117.
86. Lin CY. Hepatitis B virus-associated membranous nephropathy: clinical features, immunological profiles, and outcome. *Nephron* 1990;57:37.
87. Ito H, et al. Hepatitis B e antigen-mediated membranous glomerulonephritis: correlation of ultrastructural changes with HBeAg in the serum and glomeruli. *Lab Invest* 1981;44:214.
88. Knecht GL, Chisari FV. Reversibility of hepatitis B virus induced glomerulonephritis and chronic active hepatitis after spontaneous clearance of serum hepatitis B surface antigen. *Gastroenterology* 1978;75:1152.
89. Lin CY. Clinical features and natural course of HBV-related glomerulopathy in children. *Kidney Int* 1991;40(Suppl 35):S46.
90. Lo SJ. Characterization of restriction endonuclease maps of hepatitis viral DNAs. *Biochem Biophys Res Commun* 1985;129:797.
91. Lai KN, et al. The therapeutic dilemma of the usage of corticosteroid in patients with membranous nephropathy and persistent hepatitis B virus surface antigenemia. *Nephron* 1990;54:12.
92. Lin HJ, Wu PC, Lai CL. An oligonucleotide probe for the detection of hepatitis B virus DNA in serum. *J Virol Methods* 1987;15:139.
93. Scullard GH, Pollard RB, Smith JL. Antiviral treatment of chronic hepatitis B infection. I. Changes in viral markers with interferon combined with adenine arabinoside. *J Infect Dis* 1981;143:772.
94. Garcia G, et al. Preliminary observation of hepatitis B-associated membranous glomerulonephritis treated with leukocyte interferon. *Hepatology* 1985;5:317.
95. Lisker-Melman M, et al. Glomerulonephritis caused by chronic hepatitis B virus infection: treatment with recombinant human alpha-interferon. *Ann Intern Med* 1989;111:479.
96. Jonas MM, Ragin L, Silva MO. Membranous glomerulonephritis and chronic persistent hepatitis B in a child: treatment with recombinant interferon alfa. *J Pediatr* 1991;119:818.
97. Esteban R, et al. Hepatitis B-associated membranous glomerulonephritis treated with adenine arabinoside monophosphate. *Hepatology* 1986;6:762.
98. Lin CY. Treatment of hepatitis B virus-associated membranous nephropathy with recombinant alpha-interferon. *Kidney Int* 1995;47:225.
99. Conjeevaram HS, et al. Long-term outcome of hepatitis B virus-related glomerulonephritis after therapy with interferon-alfa. *Gastroenterology* 1995;109:540.
100. Chung DR, et al. Treatment of hepatitis B virus-associated glomerulonephritis with recombinant human alpha interferon. *Am J Nephrol* 1997;17:112.
101. Connor FL, et al. HBV associated nephrotic syndrome: resolution with oral lamivudine. *Arch Dis Child* 2003;88:446.
102. Filler G, et al. Another case of HBV associated membranous glomerulonephritis resolving on lamivudine. *Arch Dis Child* 2003;88:460.
103. Lin CY. Hepatitis B virus deoxyribonucleic acid in kidney cells probably leading to viral pathogenesis among hepatitis B virus associated membranous nephropathy patients. *Nephron* 1993;63:58.
104. Carome MA, et al. Human glomeruli express TIMP-1 mRNA and TIMP-2 protein and mRNA. *Am J Physiol* 1993;264:F923.
105. Lee C, Ko Y. Hepatitis B vaccination and hepatocellular carcinoma in Taiwan. *Pediatrics* 1997;99:351.
106. Sun L, et al. Effect of hepatitis B vaccine immunization on HBV associated nephritis in children. *Zhonghua Er Ke Za Zhi* 2003;41:666.
107. The People of South Africa. Population Census, 1996. *Statistics South Africa* 1998;4.
108. Jennette JC, Thomas B, Falk RJ. Microscopic polyangitis (microscopic polyarteritis). *Semin Diagn Pathol* 2001;18:3.
109. Jennette JC, et al. Nomenclature of systemic vasculitides. Proposal of an international conference. *Arthritis Rheum* 1994;37:187.
110. Conn DL. Polyarteritis. In: Klippel JH, Dieppe PA, eds. *Rheumatology*. St. Louis: Mosby, 1994.
111. Dixon FJ, Feldman JD, Vazquez JJ. Experimental glomerulonephritis: the pathogenesis of a laboratory model resembling the spectrum of human glomerulonephritis. *J Exp Med* 1961;113:899.
112. Lawley TJ, et al. A prospective clinical and immunologic analysis of patients with serum sickness. *N Engl J Med* 1984;311:1407.
113. Paull R. Periarteritis nodosa (panarteritis nodosa) with report of four proven cases. *Cal Med* 1947;67:309.
114. Gocke DJ, Hsu K, Morgan C. Association between polyarteritis and Australia antigen. *Lancet* 1970;ii:1149.
115. Alpert E, Isselbacher KJ, Schur PH. The pathogenesis of arthritis associated with viral hepatitis. *N Engl J Med* 1971;285:185.
116. Wands JR, et al. The pathogenesis of arthritis associated with acute hepatitis-B surface antigen-positive hepatitis. *J Clin Invest* 1975;55:930.
117. Trepo CG, et al. The role of circulating hepatitis B antigen/antibody immune complexes in the pathogenesis of vascular and hepatic manifestations in polyarteritis nodosa. *J Clin Pathol* 1974;27:863.
118. Michalak T. Immune complexes of hepatitis B surface antigen in the pathogenesis of periarteritis nodosa. *Am J Pathol* 1978;90:619.
119. Gupta RC, Kohler PF. Identification of HBsAg determinants in immune complexes from hepatitis B virus-associated vasculitis. *J Immunol* 1984;132:1223.
120. Sergent JS, et al. Vasculitis with hepatitis B antigenemia. *Medicine* 1976;55:1.
121. Adu D, et al. Polyarteritis and the kidney. *Q J Med* 1987;62:221.
122. McMahon BJ, et al. Hepatitis B-associated polyarteritis nodosa in Alaskan Eskimos: clinical and epidemiologic features and long-term follow-up. *Hepatology* 1989;9:97.
123. Savage CO, et al. Prospective study of radioimmunoassay for antibodies against neutrophil cytoplasm in diagnosis of systemic vasculitis. *Lancet* 1987;i:1389.
124. Jennette JC, Falk RJ. Antineutrophil cytoplasmic autoantibodies and associated diseases: a review. *Am J Kidney Dis* 1990;15:517.
125. Harper L, Savage CO. Pathogenesis of ANCA-associated systemic vasculitis. *J Pathol* 2000;190:349.
126. Kallenberg GC, Tervaert JW. What is new with anti-neutrophil cytoplasmic antibodies: diagnostic, pathogenetic and therapeutic implications. *Curr Opin Nephrol Hypertens* 1999;8:307.
127. Guillevin L, et al. Antineutrophil cytoplasmic antibodies in systemic polyarteritis nodosa with and without hepatitis B virus infection and Churg-Strauss syndrome—62 patients. *J Rheumatol* 1993;20:1345.
128. Han SH. Extraheaptic manifestations of chronic hepatitis B. *Clin Liver Dis* 2004;8:403.
129. Guillevin L. Treatment of classic polyarteritis nodosa in 1999. *Nephrol Dial Transplant* 1999;14:2077.
130. Guillevin L. Treatment of polyarteritis nodosa related to hepatitis B virus with short term steroid therapy associated with antiviral agents and plasma exchanges. A prospective trial in 33 patients. *J Rheumatol* 1993;20:289.
131. Guillevin L, et al. Polyarteritis nodosa related to hepatitis B virus: a prospective study with long-term observation of 41 patients. *Medicine* 1995;74:238.
132. Gupta S, Piraka C, Jaffe M. Lamivudine in the treatment of polyarteritis nodosa associated with acute hepatitis B. *N Engl J Med* 2001;344:1645.
133. Sawabe T, et al. Remission of hepatitis B virus-related vasculitis with lamivudine. *Ann Intern Med* 2004;140:672.
134. Lau CF, et al. Hepatitis B associated fulminant polyarteritis nodosa: successful treatment with pulse cyclophosphamide, prednisolone and lamivudine. *Eur J Gastroenterol Hepatol* 2002;14:563.
135. Bedani PL, et al. HBV-related cutaneous periarteritis nodosa in a patient 16 years after renal transplantation: efficacy of lamivudine. *J Nephrol* 2001;14:428.
136. Erhardt A, et al. Successful treatment of hepatitis B virus associated polyarteritis nodosa with a combination of prednisolone, alpha-interferon and lamivudine. *J Hepatol* 2000;33:677.
137. Guillevin L, et al. Short-term corticosteroids then lamivudine and plasma exchanges to treat hepatitis B virus-related polyarteritis nodosa. *Arthritis Rheum* 2004;15;51:482.
138. Deeren DH, et al. Treatment of hepatitis B virus-related polyarteritis nodosa: two case reports and a review of the literature. *Clin Rheumatol* 2004;23:172.
139. Deleaval P, et al. Life-threatening complications of hepatitis B virus-related polyarteritis nodosa developing despite interferon-alpha2b therapy: successful treatment with a combination of interferon, lamivudine, plasma exchanges and steroids. *Clin Rheumatol* 2001;20:290.
140. Florin-Christensen A, Roux ME, Arana RM. Cryoglobulins in acute and chronic liver diseases. *Clin Exp Immunol* 1974;16:599.
141. McIntosh RM, Koss MN, Gocke DJ. The nature and incidence of cryoproteins in hepatitis B antigen positive patients. *Q J Med* 1976;177:23.
142. Levo Y, et al. Association between hepatitis B virus and essential mixed cryoglobulinemia. *N Engl J Med* 1977;296:1501.
143. Levo Y, et al. Mixed cryoglobulinemia—an immune complex disease often associated with hepatitis B virus. *Trans Assoc Am Phys* 1977;90:167.
144. Dienstag JL, Wands JR, Isselbacher KJ. Hepatitis B and essential mixed cryoglobulinemia. *N Engl J Med* 1977;297:946.
145. Galli M, et al. Hepatitis B virus and essential mixed cryoglobulinemia. *Lancet* 1980;1:1093.
146. Clinicopathological Conference. A 57-year-old man with hepatic cirrhosis, cryoglobulinemia and impaired renal function. Case 51-1990. *N Engl J Med* 1990;323:1756.
147. Galli M, et al. Cryoglobulinaemia and serological markers of hepatitis viruses. *Lancet* 1991;338:104.
148. Baker AL. Cryoglobulinemia and hepatotrophic viruses. *Hepatology* 1993;18:698.
149. Ferri C, et al. Mixed cryoglobulinemia: demographic, clinical, and serologic features and survival in 231 patients. *Semin Arthritis Rheum* 2004;33:355.
150. Perez GO, Pardo V, Fletcher MA. Renal involvement in essential mixed cryoglobulinemia. *Am J Kidney Dis* 1987;10:276.

151. Frankel AH, et al. Type II essential mixed cryoglobulinaemia: presentation, treatment and outcome in 13 patients. *Q J Med* 1992;82:101.
152. Ferri C, et al. Treatment of renal involvement in mixed cryoglobulinemia with prolonged plasma exchange. *Nephron* 1986;43:246.
153. Feinstone SM, Kapikian AZ, Purcell RH. Hepatitis A: detection by immune electron microscopy of a virus-like antigen associated with acute illness. *Science* 1973;182:1026.
154. Feinstone SM, et al. Transfusion-associated hepatitis not due to viral hepatitis type A or B. *N Engl J Med* 1975;292:767.
155. Choo QL, et al. Isolation of a cDNA clone derived from a blood-borne non-A, non-B viral hepatitis genome. *Science* 1989;244:359.
156. Aach RD, et al. Hepatitis C virus infection in post-transfusion hepatitis: an analysis with first and second-generation assays. *N Engl J Med* 1991;325:1325.
157. Alter HJ, et al. Detection of antibody to hepatitis C virus in prospectively followed transfusion recipients with acute and chronic non-A, non-B hepatitis. *N Engl J Med* 1989;321:1494.
158. Houghton M, et al. Molecular biology of the hepatitis C viruses: implications for diagnosis, development and control of viral disease. *Hepatology* 1991;14:381.
159. Stehman-Breen C, Johnson RJ. Hepatitis C virus-associated glomerulonephritis. *Adv Intern Med* 1998;43:79.
160. Roth D. Hepatitis C virus: the nephrologist's perspective. *Am J Kidney Dis* 1995;25:3.
161. Pereira BJ, Levey AS. Hepatitis C virus infection in dialysis and renal transplantation. *Kidney Int* 1997;51:981.
162. Murthy BV, Pereira BJ. A 1990s perspective of hepatitis C, human immunodeficiency virus and tuberculosis infections in hemodialysis patients. *Semin Nephrol* 1997;17:346.
163. Meyers CM, et al. Hepatitis C and renal disease: an update. *Am J Kidney Dis* 2003;42:631–657.
164. Diego JM, Roth D. Treatment of hepatitis C infection in patients with renal disease. *Curr Opin Nephrol Hypertens* 1998;7:557.
165. DuBois DB. Quantitation of hepatitis C viral RNA in sera of hemodialysis patients: gender-related differences in viral load. *Am J Kidney Dis* 1994;24:795.
166. Natov SN, Periera BJ. Hepatitis C in dialysis patients. *Adv Renal Replace Ther* 1996;3:275.
167. Garcia-Valdecasas J, et al. Epidemiology of renal disease in patients with hepatitis C virus infection. *J Am Soc Nephrol* 1994;5:186.
168. Dobbelstein H. Immune system in uremia. *Nephron* 1979;17:409.
169. Kay NE, Raij LR. Immune abnormalities in renal failure and hemodialysis. *Blood Purification* 1986;4:120.
170. Haag-Weber M, Horl WH. Uremia and infection: mechanism of impaired cellular host defense. *Nephron* 1993;63:125.
171. Ferri C, et al. Antibodies against hepatitis C virus in mixed cryoglobulinemia patients. *Infection* 1991;19:417.
172. Ferri C, et al. Association between hepatitis C virus and mixed cryoglobulinemia. *Clin Exp Rheumatol* 1991;9:621.
173. Ferri C, et al. Hepatitis C virus antibodies in mixed cryoglobulinemia. *Clin Exp Rheumatol* 1991;9:95.
174. Pechere-Bertschi A, et al. Hepatitis C: a possible etiology for cryoglobulinaemia Type II. *Clin Exp Immunol* 1992;89:419.
175. Agnello V, Chung RT, Kaplan LM. A role for hepatitis C virus infection in Type II cryoglobulinemia. *N Engl J Med* 1992;327:1490.
176. Marcellin P, et al. Cryoglobulinemia with vasculitis associated with hepatitis C virus infection. *Gastroenterology* 1993;104:272.
177. Levey JM, et al. Mixed cryoglobulinemia in chronic hepatitis C infection. *Medicine* 1994;73:53.
178. Cacoub P, et al. Mixed cryoglobulinemia and hepatitis C virus. *Am J Med* 1994;96:124.
179. Cacoub P, et al. Extrahepatic manifestations associated with hepatitis C virus infection. A prospective multicenter study of 321 patients. *Medicine* 2000;79:47.
180. Misiani R, et al. Hepatitis C virus infection in patients with essential mixed cryoglobulinemia. *Ann Intern Med* 1992;117:573.
181. Arase Y, et al. Glomerulonephritis in autopsy cases with hepatitis C virus infection. *Intern Med* 1998;37:836.
182. Beddhu S, Bastacky S, Johnson J. The clinical and morphologic spectrum of renal cryoglobulinemia. *Medicine* 2002;81:398.
183. Agnello V, De Rosa FG. Extrahepatic disease manifestations of HCV infection: Some current issues. *J Hepatol* 2004;40:341.
184. Pascual M, et al. Hepatitis C virus in patients with cryoglobulinemia Type II. *J Infect Dis* 1990;162:669.
185. Horikoshi S, et al. Diffuse proliferative glomerulonephritis with hepatitis C virus-like particles in paramesangial dense deposits in a patient with chronic hepatitis C virus. *Nephron* 1993;64:462.
186. Gonzalo A, et al. Membranoproliferative glomerulonephritis and hepatitis C virus infection. *Nephron* 1993;63:475.
187. Doutrelpont JM, et al. Hepatitis C infection and membranoproliferative glomerulonephritis. *Lancet* 1993;341:317.
188. Harle JR, et al. Membranoproliferative glomerulonephritis and hepatitis C infection. *Lancet* 1993;341:904.
189. Bursten DM, Rodby RA. Membranoproliferative glomerulonephritis associated with hepatitis C virus infection. *J Am Soc Nephrol* 1993;4:1288.

190. Pasquariello A, et al. Cryoglobulinemic membranoproliferative glomerulonephritis and hepatitis C virus infection. *Am J Nephrol* 1993;13:300.
191. Johnson RJ, et al. Membranoproliferative glomerulonephritis associated with hepatitis C virus infection. *N Engl J Med* 1993;328:465.
192. Johnson RJ, et al. Renal manifestations of hepatitis C virus infection. *Kidney Int* 1994;46:1255.
193. Fornasieri A, D'Amico G. Type II mixed cryoglobulinemia, hepatitis C virus infection and glomerulonephritis. *Nephrol Dial Transplant* 1996;11[Suppl 4]:25.
194. Stehman-Breen C, et al. Hepatitis C virus-associated glomerulonephritis. *Curr Opin Nephrol Hypertens* 1995;4:287.
195. D'Amico G, Fornasieri A. Cryoglobulinemic glomerulonephritis: a membranoproliferative glomerulonephritis induced by hepatitis C virus. *Am J Kidney Dis* 1995;25:361.
196. Sinico RA, Fornasieri A, D'Amico G. Renal manifestations associated with hepatitis C virus. *Ann Intern Med* 2000;151:41.
197. Tarantino A, et al. Long-term predictors of survival in essential mixed cryoglobulinemic glomerulonephritis. *Kidney Int* 1995;47:618.
198. Hoch B, Juknevicius I, Liapis H. Glomerular injury associated with hepatitis C infection: a correlation with blood and tissue HCV-PCR. *Semin Diagn Pathol* 2002;19:175.
199. Johnson RJ, et al. Hepatitis C virus-associated glomerulonephritis. Effect of α-interferon therapy. *Kidney Int* 1994;46:1700.
200. Rollino C, et al. Hepatitis C virus infection and membranous glomerulonephritis. *Nephron* 1991;59:319.
201. Davida R, et al. Membranous glomerulonephritis in association with hepatitis C virus infection. *Am J Kidney Dis* 1993;22:452.
202. Gonzalo A, et al. Membranous nephropathy associated with hepatitis C virus infection and human immunodeficiency virus disease. *Nephron* 1994;67:248.
203. Romas E, et al. Membranous glomerulonephritis associated with hepatitis C virus infection in an adolescent. *Pathology* 1994;26:399.
204. Uchiyama-Tanaka Y, et al. Membranous glomerulonephritis associated with hepatitis C virus infection: case report and literature review. *Clin Nephrol* 2004;61:144.
205. Usulan C, et al. Rapidly progressive glomerulonephritis associated with hepatitis C virus infection. *Clin Nephrol* 1998;49:129.
206. Gonzalo A, et al. IgA nephropathy associated with hepatitis C virus infection. *Nephron* 1995;69:354.
207. Hertzenberg AM, et al. Thrombotic microangiopathy associated with cryoglobulinemic membranoproliferative glomerulonephritis. *Am J Kidney Dis* 1998;31:521.
208. Pouteil-Noble C, et al. Glomerular disease associated with hepatitis C virus infection in native kidneys. *Nephrol Dial Transplant* 2000;15(Suppl 8):S28.
209. Fabrizi F, et al. Hepatitis C virus infection and acute or chronic glomerulonephritis: an epidemiological and clinical appraisal. *Nephrol Dial Transplant* 1998;13:1991.
210. Komatsuda A, et al. Clinicopathological analysis and therapy in hepatitis C virus-associated nephropathy. *Intern Med* 1996;35:529.
211. Yamabe H, et al. Hepatitis C virus infection and membranoproliferative glomerulonephritis in Japan. *J Am Soc Nephrol* 1995;6:220.
212. Morales JM. Hepatitis C virus infection and renal disease after renal transplantation. *Transplant Proc* 2004;36:760.
213. Cruzado JM, et al. Hepatitis C virus infection and de novo glomerular lesions in renal allografts. *Am J Transplant* 2001;1:171.
214. Habib R, Broyer M. Clinical significance of allograft glomerulopathy. *Kidney Int* 1993;44:S95.
215. Cosio FG, et al. Prevalence of hepatitis C in patients with idiopathic glomerulopathies in native and transplant kidneys. *Am J Kidney Dis* 1996;28:752.
216. Cruzado JM, et al. Hepatitis C virus-associated membranoproliferative glomerulonephritis in renal allografts. *J Am Soc Nephrol* 1996;7:2469.
217. Morales JM, et al. Membranous glomerulonephritis associated with hepatitis C virus infection in renal transplant patients. *Transplantation* 1997;63:1634.
218. Kendrick EA, et al. Renal disease in hepatitis C-positive liver transplant recipients. *Transplantation* 1997:63:1287.
219. Donnadio JV Jr, Holley KE. Membranoproliferative glomerulonephritis. *Semin Nephrol* 1982;2:214.
220. Rennke HG. Secondary membranoproliferative glomerulonephritis. *Kidney Int* 1995;47:643.
221. Coroneos E, Truong L, Olivero J. Fibrillary glomerulonephritis associated with hepatitis C viral infection. *Am J Kidney Dis* 1997;29:132.
222. Markowitz GS, et al. Hepatitis C viral infection is associated with fibrillary glomerulonephritis and immunotactoid glomerulopathy. *J Am Soc Nephrol* 1998;9:2244.
223. D'Amico G, Fornasieri A. Type II mixed cryoglobulinemia, hepatitis C infection, and glomerulonephritis. *Nephrol Dial Transplant* 1996;11(Suppl 4):25.
224. Okada K, et al. Detection of hepatitis C virus core protein in the glomeruli of patients with membranous glomerulonephritis. *Clin Nephrol* 1996;45:71.
225. Sansonno D, et al. Hepatitis C virus-related proteins in kidney tissue from hepatitis C virus infected patients with cryoglobulinemic membranoproliferative glomerulonephritis. *Hepatology* 1997;25:1237.
226. Rodriguez-Inigo E, et al. Hepatitis C virus RNA in kidney biopsies from infected patients with renal diseases. *J Viral Hepatitis* 2000;7:23.

227. Bonomo L, et al. Treatment of idiopathic mixed cryoglobulinemia with alpha interferon. *Am J Med* 1987;83:554.
228. Ferri C, et al. Alpha interferon in the treatment of mixed cryoglobulinemia patients. *Eur J Cancer* 1991;27:S81.
229. Ferri C, et al. Interferon-α in mixed cryoglobulinemia patients. A randomized, crossover-controlled trial. *Blood* 1993;81:1132.
230. Davis GL, et al. Treatment of chronic hepatitis C with recombinant interferon alfa. *N Engl J Med* 1989;321:1501.
231. DiBisceglie AM, Hoofnagle JH. Recombinant interferon alfa therapy for chronic hepatitis C. *N Engl J Med* 1989;321:1506.
232. Knox TA, Kaplan MM, Berkman EM. Mixed cryoglobulinemia responsive to interferon-α. *Am J Med* 1991;91:554.
233. Durand JM, et al. Effect of interferon-α2b on cryoglobulinemia related to hepatitis C virus infection. *J Infect Dis* 1992;165:778.
234. Taillan B, et al. Low dose interferon-α for mixed cryoglobulinemia associated with hepatitis C virus. *Am J Med* 1991;93:476.
235. Misiani R, et al. Interferon alpha-2a therapy in cryoglobulinemia associated with hepatitis C virus. *N Engl J Med* 1994;330:751.
236. Sarac E, Bastacky S, Johnson JP. Response to high dose INF-α after failure of standard therapy in MPGN associated with hepatitis C virus infection. *Am J Kidney Dis* 1997;30:113.
237. Yamabe H, et al. Membranoproliferative glomerulonephritis associated with hepatitis C virus infection responsive to interferon-α. *Am J Kidney Dis* 1995;25:67.
238. Roy V, Newland AC. Raynaud's phenomenon and cryoglobulinemia associated with the use of recombinant interferon alpha. *Lancet* 1988;1:944.
239. Kimmel PL, Abraham AA, Phillips TM. Membranoproliferative glomerulonephritis in a patient treated with interferon alpha for HIV infection. *Am J Kidney Dis* 1994;24:858.
240. Averbusch SD, et al. Acute interstitial nephritis with the nephrotic syndrome following recombinant leukocyte a interferon therapy for mycosis fungoides. *N Engl J Med* 1984;310:32.
241. Lederer E, Truong L. Unusual glomerular lesion in a patient receiving long-term interferon alpha. *Am J Kidney Dis* 1992;20:516.
242. Phillips TM. Interferon-alpha induces renal dysfunction and injury. *Curr Opin Nephrol Dial* 1996;5:380.
243. Endo M, et al. Appearance of nephrotic syndrome following interferon-α therapy in a patient with hepatitis B virus and hepatitis C virus coinfection. *Am J Nephrol* 1998;18:439.
244. Heathcote EJ, et al. Peginterferon alfa-2a in patients with chronic hepatitis C and cirrhosis. *N Engl J Med* 2000;343:1673.
245. Zeuzem S, et al. Peginterferon alfa-2a in patients with chronic hepatitis C. *N Engl J Med* 2000;343:1666.
246. Lindsay KL, et al. A randomized, double-blind trial comparing pegylated interferon alfa-2b to interferon alfa-2b as initial treatment for chronic hepatitis C. *Hepatology* 2001;34:395.
247. Shepherd J, et al. Pegylated interferon alpha-2a and –2b in combination with ribavirin in the treatment of chronic hepatitis C: a systematic review and economic evaluation. *Health Technol Assess* 2004;8:1.
248. Manns MP, et al. Peginterferon alfa-2b plus ribavirin compared with interferon alfa-2b plus ribavirin for initial treatment of chronic hepatitis C: a randomised trial. *Lancet* 2001;358:958.
249. Fried MW, et al. Peginterferon alfa-2a plus ribavirin for chronic hepatitis C virus infection. *N Engl J Med* 2002;347:975.
250. Geltner D. Therapeutic approaches in mixed cryoglobulinemia. *Springer Semin Immunopathol* 1988;10:119.
251. Miyata T, et al. Effectiveness of nafomostat mesilate on glomerulonephritis in immune-complex diseases. *Lancet* 1993;341:1353.
252. Guillevin L, Lhote F, Gherardi R. The spectrum and treatment of virus-associated vasculitides. *Curr Opin Rheumatol* 1997;9:3.
253. Daghestani L, Pomeroy C. Renal manifestations of hepatitis C infection. *Am J Med* 1999;106:347.
254. Gross WL. New concepts in treatment protocols for severe systemic vasculitis. *Curr Opin Rheumatol* 1999;11:41.
255. Gilli P, et al. Effect of human leukocyte alpha interferon on cryoglobulinaemic membranoproliferative glomerulonephritis associated with hepatitis C virus infection. *Nephrol Dial Transplant* 1996;11:526.
256. Polzien F, et al. Interferon-alpha treatment of hepatitis C virus-associated mixed cryoglobulinemia. *J Hepatol* 1997;27:63.
257. Cresta P, et al. Response to interferon alpha treatment and disappearance of cryoglobulinaemia in patients infected by hepatitis C virus. *Gut* 1999;45:122.
258. Dammacco F, et al. Natural interferon alpha versus its combination with 6-methyl-prednisolone in the therapy of type II mixed cryoglobulinemia: a long-term, randomized controlled study. *Blood* 1994;84:3336.
259. Casato M, et al. Predictors of long-term response to high-dose interferon therapy in type II cryoglobulinemia associated with hepatitis C virus infection. *Blood* 1997;90:3865.
260. Gordon AC, Adgar JD, Finch RG. Acute exacerbation of vasculitis during interferon-alpha therapy for hepatitis C-associated cryoglobulinemia. *J Infect* 1998;36:229.
261. Ohta S, et al. Exacerbation of glomerulonephritis in subjects with chronic hepatitis C virus infection after interferon therapy. *Am J Kidney Dis* 1999;33:1040.
262. Suzuki T, et al. Progressive renal failure and blindness due to retinal hemorrhage after interferon therapy for hepatitis C virus-associated membranoproliferative glomerulonephritis. *Intern Med* 2001;40:708.
263. Dizer U, et al. Minimal change disease in a patient receiving IFN-alpha therapy for chronic hepatitis C virus infection. *J Interferon Cytokine Res* 2003;23:51.
264. Gordon A, et al. Combination pegylated interferon and ribavirin therapy precipitating acute renal failure and exacerbating IgA nephropathy. *Nephrol Dial Transplant* 2004;19:2155.
265. Jefferson JA, Johnson RJ. Treatment of hepatitis C-associated glomerular disease. *Semin Nephrol* 2000;20:286.
266. Zuckerman E, et al. Treatment of refractory, symptomatic, hepatitis C virus related mixed cryoglobulinemia with ribavirin and interferon-alpha. *J Rheumatol* 2000;27:2172.
267. Calleja JL, et al. Sustained response to interferon-alpha or to interferon-alpha plus ribavirin in hepatitis C virus-associated symptomatic mixed cryoglobulinaemia. *Aliment Pharmacol Ther* 1999;13:1179.
268. Cacoub P, et al. Interferon-alpha and ribavirin treatment in patients with hepatitis C virus-related systemic vasculitis. *Arthritis Rheum* 2002;46:3317.
269. Bruchfield A, et al. Interferon and ribavirin treatment in patients with hepatitis C-associated renal disease and renal insufficiency. *Nephrol Dial Transplant* 2003;18:1573.
270. Rossi P, et al. Hepatitis C virus-associated cryoglobulinemic glomerulonephritis: long-term remission after antiretroviral therapy. *Kidney Int* 2003;63:2236.
271. Misiani R, et al. Successful treatment of HCV-associated cryoglobulinemic glomerulonephritis with a combination of interferon-α and ribavirin. *Nephrol Dial Transplant* 1999;14:1558.
272. Garini G, et al. Interferon-α in combination with ribavirin as initial treatment for hepatitis C virus-associated cryoglobulinemic membranoproliferative glomerulonephritis. *Am J Kidney Dis* 2001;38:1.
273. Loustad-Ratti V, et al. Interferon alpha and ribavirin for membranoproliferative glomerulonephritis and hepatitis C infection. *Am J Med* 2002;113:516.
274. Sabry AA, et al. Effect of combination therapy (ribavirin and interferon) in HCV-related glomerulopathy. *Nephrol Dial Transplant* 2002;17:1924.
275. Sansonno D, et al. Treatment of mixed cryoglobulinemia resistant to interferon-alpha with an anti-CD 20 monoclonal antibody. *Blood* 2003;101:3818.
276. Lamprecht P, et al. Rituximab induces remission in refractory HCV associated cryoglobulinaemic vasculitis. *Ann Rheum Dis* 2003;62:1230.
277. Roccatello D, et al. Long-term effects of anti-CD 20 monoclonal antibody treatment of cryoglobulinaemic glomerulonephritis. *Nephrol Dial Transplant* 2004;19:3054.
278. Alric L, et al. Influence of antiviral therapy in hepatitis C virus-associated cryoglobulinemic MPGN. *Am J Kidney Dis* 2004;43:617.
279. Chandresis MO, et al. Infliximab in the treatment of refractory vasculitis secondary to hepatitis C-associated mixed cryoglobulinemia. *Rheumatology* 2002;41:1126.
280. Poordad FF, Fabrizi F, Martin P. Hepatitis C infection associated with renal disease and chronic renal failure. *Semin Liver Dis* 2004;24(Suppl 2):69.
281. Maeda Y, et al. Dosage adjustment of ribavirin based on renal function in Japanese patients with chronic hepatitis C. *Ther Drug Monit* 2004;26:9.
282. Tan AC, et al. Safety of interferon and ribavirin therapy in haemodialysis patients with chronic hepatitis C: results of a pilot study. *Nephrol Dial Transplant* 2001;16:193.
283. Kamar N, et al. Ribavirin pharmacokinetics in renal and liver transplant patients: evidence that it depends on renal function. *Am J Kidney Dis* 2004;43:140.
284. Tang S, et al. Successful treatment of hepatitis C after kidney transplantation with combined interferon alpha-2b and ribavirin. *J Hepatol* 2003;39:875.
285. Kamar N, et al. Long-term ribavirin therapy in hepatitis C virus-positive renal transplant patients: effects on renal function and liver histology. *Am J Kidney Dis* 2003;42:184.
286. Shu KH, et al. Ultralow-dose alpha interferon plus ribavirin for the treatment of active hepatitis C in renal transplant recipients. *Transplantation* 2004;77:1894.
287. Chan SE, Schwartz JM, Rosen HR. Treatment of hepatitis C in solid organ transplantation. *Drugs* 2004;64:489.
288. Mathurin P, et al. Impact of hepatitis B and C virus on kidney transplantation outcome. *Hepatology* 1999;29:257.
289. Batty DS Jr, et al. Hepatitis C virus seropositivity at the time of renal transplantation in the United States: associated factors and patient survival. *Am J Transplant* 2001;1:179.
290. Bucci JR, et al. Donor hepatitis C seropositivity: clinical correlates and effect on early graft and patient survival in adult cadaveric kidney transplantation. *J Am Soc Nephrol* 2002;13:2974.
291. Abbott KC, et al. Hepatitis C and renal transplantation in the era of modern immunosuppression. *J Am Soc Nephrol* 2003;14:2908.
292. Lunel F, Cacoub P. Treatment of autoimmune and extrahepatic manifestations of hepatitis C virus infection. *J Hepatol* 1999;31(Suppl 1):210.
293. Pol S, et al. Treatment of chronic hepatitis C in special groups. *J Hepatol* 1999;31(Suppl 1):205.
294. Bourgoignie JJ. Renal complications of human immunodeficiency virus type I. *Kidney Int* 1990;37:1571.

295. Kimmel PL. The nephropathies of HIV infection: pathogenesis and treatment. *Curr Opin Nephrol Hypertens* 2000;9:117.
296. Klotman PE. HIV-associated nephropathy. *Kidney Int* 1999;56:1161.
297. D'Agati V, Appel GB. HIV infection and the kidney. *J Am Soc Nephrol* 1997;8:138.
298. Weiner NJ, Goodman JW, Kimmel PL. The HIV-associated renal diseases: current insight into pathogenesis and treatment. *Kidney Int* 2003;63:1618.
299. Kimmel PL, Barisoni L, Kopp JB. Pathogenesis and treatment of HIV-associated renal diseases: lessons from clinical and animal studies, molecular pathogenic correlations and genetic investigations. *Ann Intern Med* 2003;139:214.
300. Kopp JB, Winkler C. HIV-associated nephropathy in African-Americans. *Kidney Int Suppl* 2003;S43.
301. Freedman BI, et al. Familial clustering of end stage renal disease in blacks with HIV-associated nephropathy. *Am J Kidney Dis* 1999;34:254.
302. Glassock RJ, et al. HIV infection and the kidney. *Ann Intern Med* 1990;112:35.
303. Seney FD Jr, Burns DK, Silva FG. AIDS and the kidney. *Am J Kidney Dis* 1990;16:1.
304. Bourgoignie JJ, et al. Race, a co-factor in HIV-1 associated nephropathy. *Transplant Proc* 1989;21:3899.
305. Cantor ES, Kimmel PL, Bosch JP. Effect of race on the expression of AIDS associated nephropathy. *Arch Intern Med* 1991;151:125.
306. Rao TK, et al. Associated focal and segmental glomerulosclerosis in the acquired immunodeficiency syndrome. *N Engl J Med* 1984;310:669.
307. Gardenswartz MH, et al. Renal disease in patients with AIDS: a clinicopathologic study. *Clin Nephrol* 1984;21:197.
308. Vaziri ND, et al. Spectrum of renal abnormalities in acquired immunodeficiency syndrome. *J Natl Med Assoc* 1985;77:369.
309. Kenneth KK, Factor SM. Membranoproliferative glomerulonephritis and plexogenic pulmonary arteriopathy in a homosexual man with acquired immunodeficiency syndrome. *Hum Pathol* 1987;18:1293.
310. Kenouch S, et al. Mesangial IgA deposits in two patients with AIDS-related complex. *Nephron* 1990;54:338.
311. Katz A, et al. IgA nephritis in HIV-positive patients: a new HIV-associated nephropathy? *Clin Nephrol* 1992;38:61.
312. Kimmel PL, et al. Idiotypic IgA nephropathy in patients with HIV infection. *N Engl J Med* 1992;327:702.
313. Schoeneman MJ, et al. IgA nephritis in a child with human immunodeficiency virus: a unique form of human immunodeficiency virus-associated nephropathy? *Pediatr Nephrol* 1992;6:46.
314. Kenouch S, et al. Mesangial IgA deposits in two patients with AIDS related complex. *Nephron* 1990;54:338.
315. Trachtman H, et al. IgA nephropathy in a child with human immunodeficiency virus type 1 infection. *Pediatr Nephrol* 1991;5:724.
316. Jindal KK, et al. Crescentic IgA nephropathy as a manifestation of human immunodeficiency virus infection. *Am J Nephrol* 1991;11:147.
317. Kimmel PL, et al. HIV-associated immune mediated renal disease. *Kidney Int* 1993;44:1022.
318. Butcher-Ortiz C. The spectrum of kidney diseases in patients with human immunodeficiency. *Curr Opin Nephrol Hypertens* 1993;2:355.
319. Nochy D, et al. Renal disease associated with HIV infection: a multicentric study of 60 patients from Paris hospitals. *Nephrol Dial Transplant* 1993;8:11.
320. Hsieh WS, et al. Crescentic IgA nephropathy and acute renal failure in an HIV-positive patient with enteric *Salmonella* infection. *Nephrol Dial Transplant* 1996;11:2320.
321. Daugas E, Rougier JP, Hills GS. HAART-related nephropathies in HIV-infected patients. *Kidney Int* 2005;67:393.
322. Herman ES, Klotman PE. HIV-associated nephropathy: epidemiology, pathogenesis and treatment. *Semin Nephrol* 2003;23:200.
323. Ross MJ, Klotman PE. Recent progress in HIV-associated nephropathy. *J Am Soc Nephrol* 2002;13:2997.
324. Cohen AH, Nast CC. HIV-associated nephropathy. A unique combined glomerular, tubular and interstitial lesion. *Mod Pathol* 1988;1:87.
325. D'Agati V, Appel GB. Renal pathology of human immunodeficiency virus infection. *Semin Nephrol* 1998;18:378.
326. Bodi I, Abraham AA, Kimmel PL. Macrophages in HIV-associated kidney diseases. *Am J Kidney Dis* 1994;24:762.
327. Laurinavicius A, Horowitz S, Rennke HG. Collapsing glomerulopathy in HIV and non-HIV patients: a clinicopathological study. *Kidney Int* 1999;56:2203.
328. Strauss J, et al. Renal disease in children with the acquired immunodeficiency syndrome. *N Engl J Med* 1989;321:625.
329. Bruggeman LA, et al. Nephropathy in human immunodeficiency virus-1 transgenic mice is due to renal transgene expression. *J Clin Invest* 1997;100:84.
330. Barisoni L, et al. HIV-1 induces renal epithelial dedifferentiation in a transgenic model of HIV-associated nephropathy. *Kidney Int* 2000;58:173.
331. Reid W, et al. An HIV-1 transgenic rat that develops HIV-related pathology and immunologic dysfunction. *Proc Natl Acad Sci USA* 2001;98:9271.
332. Ray PE, et al. A novel HIV-1 transgenic rat model of childhood HIV-1-associated nephropathy. *Kidney Int* 2003;63:2242.
333. Alpers CE, et al. Focal segmental glomerulosclerosis in primates infected with a simian immunodeficiency virus. *AIDS Res Hum Retrovirus* 1997;13:413.
334. Gattone VH 2nd, et al. SIV-associated nephropathy in rhesus macaques infected with lymphocyte-tropic SIVmac239. *AIDS Res Hum Retrovirus* 1998;14:1163.
335. Stephens EB, et al. Simian-human immunodeficiency virus-associated nephropathy in macaques. *AIDS Res Hum Retroviruses* 2000;16:1295.
336. Bodi I, Abraham AA, Kimmel PL. Apoptosis in human immunodeficiency virus-associated nephropathy. *Am J Kidney Dis* 1995;26:286.
337. Conaldi PG, et al. HIV-1 kills renal tubular epithelial cells in vitro by triggering an apoptotic pathway involving caspase action and Fas upregulation. *J Clin Invest* 1998;102:2041.
338. He JC, et al. Nef stimulated proliferation of glomerular podocytes through activation of Src-dependent Stat3 and MAPK1,2 pathways. *J Clin Invest* 2004;114:643.
339. Sunamoto M, et al. Critical role for Nef in HIV-1-induced podocyte dedifferentiation. *Kidney Int* 2003;64:1695.
340. Kajiyama W, et al. Glomerulosclerosis and viral gene expression in HIV-transgenic mice: role of nef. *Kidney Int* 2000;58:1148.
341. Dickie P, et al. Focal glomerulosclerosis in proviral and c-fms transgenic mice links Vpr expression to HIV-associated nephropathy. *Virology* 2004;322:69.
342. Nelson PJ, et al. Amelioration of nephropathy in mice expressing HIV-1 genes by the cyclin-dependent kinase inhibitor flavopiridol. *J Antimicrob Chemother* 2003;51:921.
343. Gherardi D, et al. Reversal of collapsing glomerulopathy in mice with the cyclin-dependent kinase inhibitor CYC202. *J Am Soc Nephrol* 2004;15:1212.
344. Barisoni L, et al. The dysregulated podocyte phenotype: a novel concept in the pathogenesis of collapsing idiopathic focal segmental glomerulosclerosis and HIV-associated nephropathy. *J Am Soc Nephrol* 1999;10:51.
345. Yang Y, Gubler MC, Beaufils H. Dysregulation of podocyte phenotype in idiopathic collapsing glomerulopathy and HIV-associated nephropathy. *Nephron* 2002;91:416.
346. Ross MD, et al. Podocan, a novel small leucine-rich repeat protein expressed in the sclerotic glomerular lesion of experimental HIV-associated nephropathy. *J Biol Chem* 2003;278:33248.
347. Bodi I, et al. Renal TGF-beta in HIV-associated kidney diseases. *Kidney Int* 1997;51:1568.
348. Yamamoto T, et al. Increased levels of transforming growth factor-beta in HIV-associated nephropathy. *Kidney Int* 1999;55:579.
349. Shukla RR, Kumar A, Kimmel PL. Transforming growth factor-b increases the expression of HIV-1 gene in transfected human mesangial cells. *Kidney Int* 1993;44:1022.
350. Schiffer M, et al. Apoptosis in podocytes induced by TGF-beta and Smad-7. *J Clin Invest* 2001;108:807.
351. Kimmel PL, et al. Upregulation of MHC class II, interferon-alpha and interferon-gamma receptor protein expression in HIV-associated nephropathy. *Nephrol Dial Transplant* 2003;18:285.
352. Gharavi AG, et al. Mapping a locus for susceptibility to HIV-1-associated nephropathy to mouse chromosome 3. *Proc Natl Acad Sci USA* 2004;101:2488.
353. Szczech LA, et al. The clinical epidemiology and course of the spectrum of renal diseases associated with HIV infection. *Kidney Int* 2004;66:1145.
354. Winston JA, et al. Nephropathy and establishment of a renal reservoir of HIV type 1 during primary infection. *N Engl J Med* 2001;344:1979.
355. Marras D, et al. Replication and compartmentalization of HIV-1 in kidney epithelium of patients with HIV-associated nephropathy. *Nat Med* 2002;8:522.
356. Bruggeman LA, et al. Renal epithelium is a previously unrecognized site of HIV-1 infection. *J Am Soc Nephrol* 2000;11:2079.
357. Green DF, Resnick L, Bourgoignie JJ. HIV infects glomerular endothelial and mesangial, but not epithelial cells in vitro. *Kidney Int* 1992;41:956.
358. Ray PE, et al. Infection of primary renal epithelial cells with HIV-1 from children with HIV-associated nephropathy. *Kidney Int* 1998;53:1217.
359. Alpers CE, McClure J, Bursten SL. Human mesangial cells are resistant to productive infection by multiple strains of human immunodeficiency virus types 1 and 2. *Am J Kidney Dis* 1992;19:126.
360. Eitner F, et al. Chemokine receptor CCR5 and CXCR4 expression and HIV-1 detection in HIV-associated kidney disease. *J Am Soc Nephrol* 2000;11:856.
361. Segerer S, et al. Expression of the C-C chemokine receptor 5 in human kidney diseases. *Kidney Int* 1999;56:52.
362. Eitner F, et al. Chemokine receptor (CCR5) expression in human kidneys and in the HIV-infected macaque. *Kidney Int* 1998;54:1945.
363. Kimmel PL, Bosch JP, Vassalotti JA. Treatment of human immunodeficiency virus-associated nephropathy. *Semin Nephrol* 1998;18:446.
364. Kimmel PL, Mishkin GJ, Umana WO. Captopril and renal survival in patients with HIV associated nephropathy. *Am J Kidney Dis* 1996;28:202.
365. Appel RG, Neill J. A steroid-responsive nephrotic syndrome in a patient with human immunodeficiency virus infection. *Ann Intern Med* 1990;113:892.
366. Briggs WA, et al. Clinicopathologic correlates of prednisone treatment of human immunodeficiency virus-associated nephropathy. *Am J Kidney Dis* 1996;28:618.
367. Watterson MK, Detwiler RK, Bolin JP. Clinical response to prolonged corticosteroids in a patient with human immunodeficiency virus-associated nephropathy. *Am J Kidney Dis* 1997;29:624.

368. Smith MC, et al. Prednisone improves renal function and proteinuria in human immunodeficiency virus-associated nephropathy. *Am J Med* 1996;101:41.

369. Eustace JA, et al. Cohort study of the treatment of severe HIV-associated nephropathy with corticosteroids. *Kidney Int* 2000;58:1253.

370. Burns GC, et al. Effect of angiotensin-converting enzyme inhibition in HIV-associated nephropathy. *J Am Soc Nephrol* 1998;8:1140.

371. Wei A, et al. Long-term renal survival in HIV-associated nephropathy with angiotensin-converting enzyme inhibition. *Kidney Int* 2003;64:1462.

372. Bird JE, et al. Captopril prevents nephropathy in HIV-transgenic mice. *J Am Soc Nephrol* 1998: 9:1441.

373. Burns GC, Klotman PE. Treatment of HIV-associated nephropathy. *Semin Nephrol* 2000;20:293.

374. Szczech LA, et al, Protease inhibitors are associated with a slowed progression of HIV-related renal diseases. *Clin Nephrol* 2002;57:336.

375. Cosgrove CJ, Abu-Alfa AK, Perazella MA. Observations on HIV-associated renal disease in the era of highly active antiretroviral therapy. *Am J Med Sci* 2002;323:102.

376. Kirchner JT. Resolution of renal failure after initiation of HAART: 3 cases and a discussion of the literature. *AIDS Read* 2002;12:103.

377. Viani RM, et al. Resolution of HIV-associated nephrotic syndrome with highly active antiretroviral therapy delivered by gastrostomy tube. *Pediatrics* 1999;104:1394.

378. Wali RK, et al. HIV-1-associated nephropathy and response to highly-active antiretroviral therapy. *Lancet* 1998;352:783.

379. Rao TK, Friedman EA, Nicastri AD. The types of renal disease in the acquired immunodeficiency syndrome. *N Engl J Med* 1987;316:1062.

380. Eggers PW, Kimmel PL. Is there an epidemic of HIV infection in the US ESRD program? *J Am Soc Nephrol* 2004;15:2477.

381. Ahuja TS, Grady J, Khan S. Changing trends in the survival of dialysis patients with human immunodeficiency virus in the United States. *J Am Soc Nephrol* 2002;13:1889.

382. Ahuja TS, O'Brien WA. Special issues in the management of patients with ESRD and HIV infection. *Am J Kidney Dis* 2003;41:279.

383. Kimmel PL, et al. Continuous ambulatory peritoneal dialysis and survival of HIV infected patients with end-stage renal disease. *Kidney Int* 1993;44:373.

384. Ahuja TS, et al. Is dialysis modality a factor in survival of patients with ESRD and HIV-associated nephropathy? *Am J Kidney Dis* 2003;41:1060.

385. Ahuja TS, et al. HIV-associated nephropathy and end-stage renal disease in children in the United States. *Pediatr Nephrol* 2004;19:808.

386. Gow PJ, Pillay D, Mutimer D. Solid organ transplantation in patients with HIV infection. *Transplantation* 2001;72:1777.

387. Roland ME, Stock PG. Review of solid-organ transplantation in HIV-infected patients. *Transplantation* 2003;75:425.

388. Abbott KC, et al. Human immunodeficiency virus infection and kidney transplantation in the era of highly active antiretroviral therapy and modern immunosuppression. *J Am Soc Nephrol* 2004;15:1633.

389. Sayegh SE, et al. Solid organ transplantation in HIV-infected recipients. *Pediatr Transplant* 2004;8:214.

390. Pelletier SJ, et al. Review of transplantation in HIV patients during the HAART era. *Clin Transpl* 2004;18:63.

391. Bourgoignie JJ, et al. The clinical spectrum of renal disease associated with human immunodeficiency virus. *Am J Kidney Dis* 1988;12:131.

392. Tabechian D, et al. Lupus-like nephritis in an HIV-positive patient: report of a case and review of the literature. *Clin Nephrol* 2003;60:187.

393. McDougal SJ, et al. Immune complexes in the acquired immunodeficiency syndrome: relationship to disease manifestation, risk group, and immunologic defect. *J Clin Immunol* 1985;5:130.

394. Morrow WJ, et al. Circulating immune complexes in patients with the acquired immunodeficiency syndrome contain the AIDS-associated retrovirus. *Clin Immunol Immunopathol* 1986;40:515.

395. McDougal JS, et al. Antibody response to human immunodeficiency virus in homosexual men. *J Clin Invest* 1987;80:316.

396. Nishanian P, et al. A simple method for improved assay demonstrates that HIV p24 antigen is present as immune complexes in most sera from HIV-infected individuals. *J Infect Dis* 1990;162:21.

397. McHugh TM, et al. Relation of circulating levels of human immunodeficiency virus antigen, antibody to p24, and HIV-containing immune complexes in HIV-infected patients. *J Infect Dis* 1988;158:1088.

398. Portera M, et al. Free and antibody-complexed antigen and antibody profile in apparently healthy HIV seropositive individuals and in AIDS patients. *J Med Virol* 1990;30:30.

399. Guerra IL, et al. Nephrotic syndrome associated with chronic persistent hepatitis B in an HIV antibody positive patient. *Am J Kidney Dis* 1987;10:385.

400. Connolly JO, Weston CE, Hendry BM. HIV-associated renal disease in London hospitals. *Q J Med* 1995;88:627.

401. Williams DI, et al. Presentation, pathology and outcome of HIV associated renal disease in a specialist centre for HIV/AIDS. *Sex Transm Infect* 1998;74:179.

402. Casanova S, et al. Pattern of glomerular involvement in human immunodeficiency virus-infected patients: an Italian study. *Am J Kidney Dis* 1995;26:446.

403. Martin JL, Thomas D, Colindres RE. Immunotactoid glomerulopathy in an HIV-positive African-American man. *Am J Kidney Dis* 2003;42:E6.

404. Chidambaram M, et al. Type I membranoproliferative glomerulonephritis

405. Haas M, et al. Fibrillary/immunotactoid glomerulonephritis in HIV-positive patients; A report of three cases. *Nephrol Dial Transplant* 2000;15:1679.

406. Rivera M, et al. The heterogeniety of glomerulonephritis associated with HIV. *Nephrol Dial Transplant* 1999;14:244.

407. Praditpornsilpa K, Napathorn S, Yenrudi S, et al. Renal pathology and HIV infection in Thailand. *Am J Kidney Dis* 1999;33:282.

408. Winston JA, Klotman ME, Klotman PE. HIV-associated nephropathy is a late, not early, manifestation of HIV-1 infection. *Kidney Int* 1999;55:1036.

409. Stokes MB, et al. Immune complex glomerulonephritis in patients coinfected with HIV and hepatitis C virus. *Am J Kidney Dis* 1997;29:514.

410. Cheng JT, et al. Hepatitis C virus-associated glomerular disease in patients with human immunodeficiency virus coinfection. *J Am Soc Nephrol* 1999;10:1566.

411. Morales E, et al. Hepatitis C virus-associated cryoglobulinemic membranoproliferative glomerulonephritis in patients infected by HIV. *Nephrol Dial Transplant* 1997;12:1980.

412. Fling J, et al. The relationship of serum IgA concentration to human immunodeficiency virus infection: a cross-sectional study of HIV-positive individuals detected by screening in the United States Air Force. *J Allergy Clin Immunol* 1988;82:965.

413. Procaccia S, et al. IgM, IgG and IgA rheumatoid factors and circulating immune complexes in patients with AIDS and AIDS related complex with serological abnormalities. *Clin Exp Immunol* 1987;67:236.

414. Jackson S, Dawson LM, Kotler DP. IgA1 is the major immunoglobulin component of immune complexes in the acquired immunodeficiency syndrome. *Clin Immunol* 1988;8:64.

415. Jackson S, et al. Occurrence of polymeric IgA1 rheumatoid factor in the acquired immunodeficiency syndrome. *Clin Immunol* 1988;8:390.

416. Lightfoote MM, et al. Circulating IgA immune complexes in AIDS. *Immunol Invest* 1985;14:341.

417. Emancipator SN. Immunoregulatory factors in the pathogenesis of IgA nephropathy. *Kidney Int* 1990;38:388.

418. Bourgoignie JJ, Pardo V. HIV-associated nephropathies. *N Engl J Med* 1993;327:729.

419. Jennette JC, Wall SD, Wilkman AS. Low incidence of IgA nephropathy in blacks. *Kidney Int* 1985;28:944.

420. Beaufils H, et al. HIV-associated IgA nephropathy—a post mortem study. *Nephrol Dial Transplant* 1995;10:35.

421. Gorriz JL, et al. IgA nephropathy associated with human immunodeficiency virus infection: antiproteinuric effect of captopril. *Nephrol Dial Transplant* 1997;12:2796.

422. Berns JS. Hemolytic uremic syndrome and thrombotic thrombocytopenic purpura associated with HIV infection. In: Kimmel PL, Berns JS, Stein JH, eds. *Renal and urologic aspects of HIV infection.* New York: Churchill Livingstone, 1995:111.

423. Peraldi MN, et al. Acute renal failure in the course of HIV infection: a single-institution retrospective study of ninety-two patients and sixty renal biopsies. *Nephrol Dial Transplant* 1999;14:1578.

424. Sutor GC, Scmidt RE, Albrecht H. Thrombotic microangiopathies and HIV infection: report of two typical cases, features of HUS and TTP, and review of the literature. *Infection* 1999;27:12.

425. de man AM, Smulders YM, Roozendaal KJ, et al. HIV-related thrombotic thrombocytopenic purpura: report of two cases and review of the literature. *Neth J Med* 1997;51:103.

426. Gadallah MF, et al. Disparate prognosis of thrombotic microangiopathy in HIV-infected patients with and without AIDS. *Am J Nephrol* 1996;16:446.

427. Jokela J, Flynn T, Henry K. Thrombotic thrombocytopenic purpura in a human immunodeficiency virus-seropositive homosexual man. *Am J Hematol* 1987;25:341.

428. Ucar A, et al. Thrombotic microangiopathy and retroviral infections: A 13 year experience. *Am J Hematol* 1994;45:304.

429. Badesha PS, Saklayen MG. Hemolytic uremic syndrome as a presenting form of HIV infection. *Nephron* 1996;72:472.

430. Charasse C, et al. Thrombotic thrombocytopenic purpura with the acquired immunodeficiency syndrome: a pathologically documented report. *Am J Kidney Dis* 1991;17:80.

431. Alpers CE. Light at the end of the TUNEL: HIV-associated thrombotic microangiopathy. *Kidney Int* 2003;63:385.

432. Eitner F, et al. Thrombotic microangiopathy in the HIV-2 infected macaque. *Am J Pathol* 1999;155:649.

433. Mitra D, et al. Thrombotic thrombocytopenic purpura and sporadic hemolytic uremic syndrome plasmas induce apoptosis in restricted lineages of human microvascular endothelial cells. *Blood* 1997;89:1224.

434. Mitra D, et al. Role of caspases 1 and 3 and Bcl-2-related molecules in endothelial cell apoptosis associated with thrombotic microangiopathies. *Am J Hematol* 1998;59:279.

435. Del Arco A, et al. Thrombotic thrombocytopenic purpura associated with human immunodeficiency virus infection: Demonstration of p24 antigen in endothelial cells. *Clin Infect Dis* 1993;17:360.

436. Lafrenie RM, et al. HIV-1-tat modulates the function of monocytes and alters their interactions with microvessel endothelial cells. *J Immunol* 1996;156:1638.

in an HIV-infected individual without hepatitis C coinfection. *Clin Nephrol* 2002;57:154.

437. Sahud MA, et al. Von Willebrand factor-cleaving protease in a patient with human immunodeficiency syndrome-associated thrombotic thrombocytopenic purpura. *Br J Haematol* 2002;116:909.

438. Bottieau E, Colebunders R, Bosmans JL. Favourable outcome of haemolytic uraemic syndrome in an HIV-infected patient treated only with prednisone. *J Infect* 2000;41:108.

439. Salem G, Terebelo H, Raman S. Human immunodeficiency virus associated with thrombotic thrombocytopenic purpura: successful treatment with zidovudine. *South Med J* 1991;84:493.

440. Gruszecki AC, et al. Management of a patient with HIV infection-induced anemia and thrombocytopenia who presented with thrombotic thrombocytopenic purpura. *Am J Hematol* 2002;69:228.

441. Kopp JB, et al. Crystalluria and urinary tract abnormalities associated with indinavir. *Ann Intern Med* 1997;127:119.

442. Jaradat M, et al. Acute tubulointerstitial nephritis attributable to indinavir therapy. *Am J Kidney Dis* 2000;35:E16.

443. Benveniste O, et al. Two episodes of acute renal failure, rhadomyolysis, and severe hepatitis in an AIDS patient successively treated with ritonavir and indinavir. *Clin Infect Dis* 1999;28:1180.

444. Olyaei AJ, deMattos AM, Bennet WM. Renal toxicity of protease inhibitors. *Curr Opin Nephrol Hypertens* 2000;9:473.

445. Izzedine H, Launay-Vacher V, Deray G. Antiretroviral drugs and the kidney: Dosage adjustment and renal tolerance. *Curr Pharm Des* 2004;10: 4071.

446. Izzedine H, et al. Antiretroviral and immunosuppressive drug-drug interactions: An update. *Kidney Int* 2004;66:532.

447. Joshi MK, Liu HH. Acute rhabdomyolyis and renal failure in HIV-infected patients: risk factors, presentation and pathophysiology. *AIDS Patient Care STDS* 2000;14:541.

448. Hare CB, et al. Simvastatin-nelfinavir interaction implicated in rhabdomyolysis and death. *Clin Infect Dis* 2002;35:e111.

449. Cheng CH, et al. Rhabdomyolysis due to probable interaction between simvastatin and ritonavir. *Am J Health Syst Pharm* 2002;59:728.

450. Mastroianni CM, et al. Rhabdomyolysis after cerivastatin-gemfibrozil therapy in an HIV-infected patient with protease inhibitor-related hyperlipidemia. *AIDS* 2001;15:820.

451. Verhelst D, et al. Fanconi syndrome and renal failure induced by tenofovir. *Am J Kidney Dis* 2002;40:1331.

452. Rifkin BS, Perazella MA. Tenofovir-associated nephrotoxicity: Fanconi syndrome and renal failure. *Am J Med Sci* 2004;117:282.

453. James CW, et al. Tenofovir-related nephrotoxicity: Case report and review of the literature. *Pharmacotherapy* 2004;24:415.

454. Coca S, Perazella MA. Rapid communication: acute renal failure associated with tenofovir: evidence of drug-induced nephrotoxicity. *Am J Med Sci* 2002;324:342.

455. Perazalla MA. Acute renal failure in HIV-infected patients: a brief review of common causes. *Am J Med Sci* 2000;319:385.

456. Korbet SM, Schwartz MM. Human immunodeficiency virus infection and nephrotic syndrome. *Am J Kidney Dis* 1992;20:97.

457. Enriquez R, et al. Postinfectious diffuse proliferative glomerulonephritis and acute renal failure in an HIV patient. *Clin Nephrol* 2004;61:278.

458. Schectman JM, Kimmel PL. Remission of hepatitis B-associated membranous glomerulonephritis in human immunodeficiency virus infection. *Am J Kidney Dis* 1991;17:716.

459. Chang BJ, et al. Renal manifestations of concurrent systemic lupus erythematosus and HIV infection. *Am J Kidney Dis* 1999;33:441.

460. Taillan B, et al. Cryoglobulinemia related to hepatitis C virus infection in patients with the human immunodeficiency virus infection. *Clin Exp Rheumatol* 1993;11:350.

461. Stricker RB, et al. Mononeuritis multiplex associated with cryoglobulinemia in HIV infection. *Neurology* 1992;42:2103.

462. Gherardi R, et al. The spectrum of vasculitis in human immunodeficiency virus-infected patients. *Arthritis Rheum* 1993;36:1164.

463. Font C, et al. Polyarteritis nodosa in human immunodeficiency virus infection: report of four cases and review of the literature. *Br J Rheumatol* 1996;35:796.

464. Chertow GM, et al. Renal vasculitis with HIV seropositivity: potential manifestation of cytomegalovirus infection. *Am J Kidney Dis* 1997;30: 428.

465. Guillevin L. Virus-induced systemic vasculitides: new therapeutic approaches. *Clin Dev Immunol* 2004;11:227.

466. Chetty R. Vasculitides associated with HIV infection. *J Clin Pathol* 2001;54:275.

467. Chetty R, Batitang S, Nair R. Large artery vasculopathy in HIV-positive patients: another vasculitic enigma. *Hum Pathol* 2000;31:374.

468. Gisselbrecht M, et al. HIV-related vasculitis: clinical presentation of a therapeutic approach to 8 cases. *Ann Med Interne* 1998;149:398.

469. Perl A, et al. Antibodies to retroviral proteins and reverse transcriptase activity in patients with essential cryoglobulinemia. *Arthritis Rheum* 1991;34:1313.

470. Shih A, Misra R, Rush MG. Detection of multiple, novel reverse transcriptase coding sequences in human nucleic acids: relation to primate retroviruses. *J Virol* 1989;63:64.

471. Query CC, Keene JD. A human autoimmune protein associated with U1 RNA contains a region of homology that is cross-reactive with retroviral p30 r gag antigen. *Cell* 1987;51:211.

472. Cohen AH, et al. Demonstration of human immunodeficiency virus in renal epithelium in HIV-associated nephropathy. *Mod Pathol* 1989;2:125.

473. Shukla RR, Kumar A, Kimmel PL. Transforming growth factor-β increases the expression of HIV-1 gene in transfected human mesangial cells. *Kidney Int* 1993;44:1022.

474. Schattner A. Interferons and autoimmunity. *Am J Med Sci* 1988;295:532.

475. Nassar GM, et al. Reversible renal failure in a patient with the hypereosinophilia syndrome during therapy with alpha interferon. *Am J Kidney Dis* 1998;31:121.

476. Gotsman I, et al. Beta-interferon-induced nephrotic syndrome in a patient with multiple sclerosis. *Clin Nephrol* 2000;54.

477. Nakao K, et al. Minimal change nephrotic syndrome developing during postoperative interferon-beta therapy for malignant melanoma. *Nephron* 2002;90:498.

478. Tola MR, et al. Recurrent nephrotic syndrome in a patient with multiple sclerosis treated with interferon beta-1a. *J Neurol* 2003;250:768.

479. Kujubu DA, Fine LG. Polypeptide growth factors and renal disease. *Am J Kidney Dis* 1989;14:61.

480. Wardle EN. Cytokine growth factors and glomerulonephritis. *Nephron* 1991;57:257.

481. Border WA, Ruoslahti E. TGF-β in disease: the dark side of tissue repair. *J Clin Invest* 1992;90:1.

482. Sharma K, Ziyadeh F. The transforming growth factor-β (TGF-β) system and the kidney. *Semin Nephrol* 1993;13:116.

483. Floege J, et al. PDGF-D and renal disease: yet another of those growth factors? *J Am Soc Nephrol* 2003;14:2690.

484. Cooper ME, Thomas MC. Interactions between growth factors in the kidney: implications for progressive renal injury. *Kidney Int* 2003;63:1584.

485. Iwano M, Neilson EG. Mechanisms of tubulointerstitial fibrosis. *Curr Opin Nephrol Hypertens* 2004;13:279.

486. Tamaki K, Okuda S. Role of TGF-beta in the progression of renal fibrosis. *Contrib Nephrol* 2003;139:44.

487. Hugo C. The thrombospondin 1-TGF-beta axis in fibrotic renal disease. *Nephrol Dial Transplant* 2003;18:1241.

488. Schnaper HW, et al. TGF-beta signal transduction and mesangial cell fibrosis. *Am J Physiol Renal Physiol* 2003;284:F243.

489. Greene WC. Molecular biology of HIV type I infection. *N Engl J Med* 1991;324:308.

490. Bednarik DP, Folks TM. Mechanism of HIV-1 latency. *AIDS* 1992;6:3.

491. Breen EC. Pro- and antinflammatory cytokines in human immunodeficiency virus infection and acquired immunodeficiency syndrome. *Pharmacol Ther* 2002;95:295.

492. Gougeon ML, et al. HIV, cytokines and programmed cell death. A subtle interplay. *Ann NY Acad Sci* 2000;926:30.

493. DeVico AL, Gallo RC. Control of HIV-1 infection by soluble factors of the immune response. *Nat Rev Microbiol* 2004;2:401.

494. Kedzierska K, Crowe SM. Cytokines and HIV-1: interactions and clinical implications. *Antivir Chem Chemother* 2001;12:133.

495. Poli G. Cytokines and the human immunodeficiency virus: from bench to bedside. *Eur J Clin Invest* 1999: 29:723.

496. Pullium L, et al. HIV-1 envelope gp 120 alters astrocytes in human brain cultures. *AIDS Res Hum Retrovirus* 1993;9:439.

497. Capobianchi MR, et al. Coordinate induction of interferon α and γ by recombinant HIV-1 glycoprotein 120. *AIDS Res Hum Retrovirus* 1993;9: 957.

498. Becker Y. HIV-1 induced AIDS is an allergy and the allergen is the shed gp120 – a review, hypothesis and implications. *Virus Genes* 2004;28:319.

499. Ensoli B, et al. Tat protein of HIV-1 stimulates growth of cells derived from Kaposi sarcoma lesions of AIDS patients. *Nature* 1990;345:84.

500. Viscidi RR, et al. Inhibition of antigen-induced lymphocyte proliferation by Tat protein from HIV-1. *Science* 1989;246:1606.

501. Gatignol A, Jeang KT. Tat as a transcriptional activator and a potential therapeutic target for HIV-1. *Adv Pharmacol* 2000;48:209.

502. Watson K, Edwards RJ. HIV-1-trans-activating (Tat) protein: both a target and a tool in therapeutic approaches. *Biochem Pharmacol* 1999;58:1521.

503. Pantaleo G, Graziosi C, Fauci AS. New concepts in the pathogenesis of HIV infection. *N Engl J Med* 1993;328:327.

504. Banda NK. Cross-linking CD4 by HIV gp120 primes T cells for activation-induced apoptosis. *J Exp Med* 1992;176:1099.

505. Richardson WP. Glomerulopathy associated with cytomegalovirus viremia in renal allografts. *N Engl J Med* 1980;305:57.

506. Lopez-Rocafort L, Brennan DC. Current review of cytomegalovirus in renal transplantation. *Minerva Urol Nefrol* 2001;53:145.

507. Cainelli F, Vento S. Infections and solid organ transplant rejection: a cause and effect relationship? *Lancet Infect Dis* 2002;2:539.

508. Soderberg-Naucler C, Emery VC. Viral infections and their impact on chronic allograft dysfunction. *Transplantation* 2001;71(Suppl 11):SS24.

509. Griffiths PD. Cytomegalovirus therapy: current constraints and future opportunities. *Curr Opin Infect Dis* 2002;14:765.

510. Sola R, et al. Significance of cytomegalovirus infection in renal transplantation. *Transplant Proc* 2003;35:1753.

511. Aiello FB, et al. Acute rejection and graft survival in renal transplanted patients. *Mod Pathol* 2004;17:189.

512. Sageda S, et al. The impact of cytomegalovirus infection and disease on rejection episodes in renal allograft recipients. *Am J Transplant* 2002;2: 850.

513. Herrera GA. Cytomegalovirus glomerulopathy: a controversial lesion. *Kidney Int* 1986;29:725.
514. Battegay EJ, et al. Cytomegalovirus and the kidney. *Clin Nephrol* 1988;30:239.
515. Boyce NW, et al. Cytomegalovirus infection complicating renal transplantation and its relationship to acute transplant glomerulopathy. *Transplantation* 1988;45:707.
516. Birk PE, Chavers BM. Does cytomegalovirus cause glomerular injury in renal allograft recipients? *J Am Soc Nephrol* 1997;8:1801.
517. Helantera I, et al. The impact of cytomegalovirus infections and acute rejection episodes on the development of vascular changes in 6-month protocol biopsy specimens of cadaveric kidney allograft recipients. *Transplantation* 2003;75:1858.
518. Kashyap R, et al. The clinical significance of cytomegaloviral inclusions in the allograft kidney. *Transplantation* 1999;67:98.
519. Sissons JG, Sinclair JH, Borysiewicz LK. Pathogenesis of human cytomegalovirus disease and the kidney. *Kidney Int* 1991;40:S8.
520. Rao KV, et al. De novo immunotactoid glomerulopathy of the renal allograft: possible association with cytomegalovirus infection. *Am J Kidney Dis* 1994;24:97.
521. Galla JH. IgA nephropathy. *Kidney Int* 1995;47:377.
522. Andresdottir MB, et al. Type I membranoproliferative glomerulonephritis in a renal allograft: a recurrence induced by a cytomegalovirus infection? *Am J Kidney Dis* 2000;35:E6.
523. Detwiler RK, et al. Cytomegalovirus-induced necrotizing and crescentic glomerulonephritis in a renal transplant patient. *Am J Kidney Dis* 1998;32:820.
524. Heiren MH, van der Woude FJ, Balfour HH Jr. Cytomegalovirus replicates efficiently in human kidney mesangial cells. *Proc Natl Acad Sci USA* 1988;85:1642.
525. Wehner RW, Smith RD. Progressive cytomegalovirus glomerulonephritis. An experimental model. *Am J Pathol* 1983;112:313.
526. Ozawa T, Stewart JA. Immune complex glomerulonephritis associated with cytomegalovirus infection. *Am J Clin Pathol* 1979;72:103.
527. Waldo FB, et al. Non-specific mesangial staining with antibodies against cytomegalovirus in immunoglobulin-A nephropathy. *Lancet* 1989;1:129.
528. Sato M, et al. Cytomegalovirus and IgA nephropathy. *Lancet* 1988;2:1251.
529. Dueymes M, et al. Mesangial staining with cytomegalovirus antibodies in IgA nephropathy. *Lancet* 1988;1:619.
530. Ortmanns A, et al. Remission of IgA nephropathy following treatment of cytomegalovirus infection with ganciclovir. *Clin Nephrol* 1998;49:379.
531. Lai FM, Tam JS, Lai KN. Cytomegalovirus antigens in IgA nephropathy: facts or artefact? *Nephron* 1990;55:87.
532. Okamura M, et al. Failure to detect cytomegalovirus-DNA in IgA nephropathy by in-situ hybridization. *Lancet* 1989;1:265.
533. Kanahara K, et al. In situ hybridization analysis of cytomegalovirus and adenovirus DNA in immunoglobulin A nephropathy. *Nephron* 1992;62:166.
534. Smith SM, Wheeher C, Hoy W. Viral antigens in IgA nephropathy. *Clin Nephrol* 1991;36:152.
535. Bene MC, Tang J, Faure GC. Absence of CMV DNA in kidneys in IgA nephropathy. *Lancet* 1990;336:868.
536. Telenti A, Donadio JV, Smith TF. Failure to detect cytomegalovirus DNA in IgA nephropathy by polymerase chain reaction. *J Am Soc Nephrol* 1990;1:841.
537. Muller GA, et al. Detection of human cytomegalovirus-DNA in IgA nephropathy. *Nephron* 1991;57:383.
538. Muller GA, et al. Human cytomegalovirus in immunoglobulin A nephropathy: detection by polymerase chain reaction. *Nephron* 1993;59:389.
539. Kadereit S, et al. Polymerase chain reaction detection of cytomegalovirus genome in renal biopsies. *Kidney Int* 1992;42:1012.
540. Park JS, et al. Cytomegalovirus is not specifically associated with immunoglobulin A nephropathy. *J Am Soc Nephrol* 1994;4:1623.
541. Rodriguez ER, et al. Human immunodeficiency virus in cardiac myocytes and dendritic cells individually microdissected from right ventricular endomyocardial biopsy tissue: detection by multiplex, nested, polymerase chain reaction. *Am J Cardiol* 1991;68:1511.
542. Cosgriff TM, Lewis RM. Mechanisms of disease in hemorrhagic fever with renal syndrome. *Kidney Int* 1991;40(Suppl 35):S72.
543. Glass GE, et al. Infection with a ratborne hantavirus in U.S. residents is consistently associated with hypertensive renal disease. *J Infect Dis* 1993;167:614.
544. Patnaik M, Velosa JA, Peter JB. Hantavirus-specific IgG, IgM, and IgA in acute and chronic renal disease versus congenital renal disease in the United States. *Am J Kidney Dis* 1999;33:734.
545. Ala-Houla I, et al. Increased glomerular permeability in patients with nephropathia epidemica caused by Puumala hantavirus. *Nephrol Dial Transplant* 2002;17:246.
546. Mustonen J, et al. Mesangiocapillary glomerulonephritis caused by Puumala hantavirus infection. *Nephron* 2001;89:402.
547. Makela S, et al. Renal function and blood pressure five years after Puumala virus-induced nephropathy. *Kidney Int* 2000;58:1711.
548. George J, et al. Hantavirus seropositivity in Israeli patients with renal failure. *Viral Immunol* 1998;11:103.
549. Cosgriff TM. Hemorrhagic fever with renal syndrome. *Ann Intern Med* 1989;110:313.
550. Peters CJ, Simpson GL, Levy H. Spectrum of hantavirus infection: hemorrhagic fever with renal syndrome and hantavirus pulmonary syndrome. *Ann Rev Med* 1999;50:531.
551. Settergren B, et al. Pathogenetic and clinical aspects of the renal involvement in hemorrhagic fever with renal syndrome. *Renal Fail* 1997;19:1.
552. Mustonen J, et al. Renal biopsy findings and clinicopathologic correlations in nephropathia epidemica. *Clin Nephrol* 1994;41:121.
553. Grcevska L, et al. Differential pathohistological presentations of acute renal involvement in Hantaan virus infection: report of two cases. *Clin Nephrol* 1991;34:197.
554. van Ypersele de Strihou C, Mery JP. Hantavirus-related acute interstitial nephritis in Western Europe. Expansion of a world-wide zoonosis. *Q J Med* 1989;73:941.
555. Mayer HB, et al. Epstein-Barr virus-induced infectious mononucleosis complicated by acute renal failure. *Clin Infect Dis* 1996;22:1009.
556. Wallace M, Leet G, Rothwell P. Immune complex-mediated glomerulonephritis with infectious mononucleosis. *Aust NZ J Med* 1974;4:192.
557. Andres GA, et al. Immune deposit nephritis in infectious mononucleosis. *Int Arch Allergy Appl Immunol* 1976;54:136.
558. Woodroffe AJ, et al. Nephritis in infectious mononucleosis. *Q J Med* 1974;43:451.
559. Kano K, et al. Glomerulonephritis in a patient with chronic active Epstein-Barr virus infection. *Pediatr Nephrol* 2005;20:89.
560. Andresdottir MB, et al. Primary Epstein-Barr virus infection and recurrent type 1 membranoproliferative glomerulonephritis after renal transplantation. *Nephrol Dial Transplant* 2000;15:1235.
561. Iwama H, et al. Epstein-Barr virus detection in kidney biopsy specimens correlates with glomerular mesangial injury. *Am J Kidney Dis* 1998;32:785.
562. Lande MB, et al. Immune complex disease associated with Epstein-Barr virus infectious mononucleosis. *Pediatr Nephrol* 1998;12:651.
563. Joh K, et al. Epstein-Barr virus genome-positive tubulointerstitial nephritis associated with immune complex-mediated glomerulonephritis in chronic active EB virus infection. *Virchows Arch* 1998;432:567.
564. Verma N, et al. Acute interstitial nephritis secondary to infectious mononucleosis. *Clin Nephrol* 2002;58:151.
565. Okada H, et al. An atypical pattern of Epstein-Barr virus infection in a case with tubulointerstitial nephritis. *Nephron* 2002;92:440.
566. Cataudella JA, Young ID, Iliescu EA. Epstein-Barr virus-associated acute interstitial nephritis: infection or immunologic phenomenon. *Nephron* 2002;92:437.
567. Stratta P, et al. Primary Epstein-Barr virus infection associated with renal flare-up of HCV-related cryoglobulinemia. *Nephrol Dial Transplant* 2000;15:1874.
568. Tsai JD, et al. Epstein-Barr virus-associated acute renal failure: diagnosis, treatment and follow-up. *Pediatr Nephrol* 2003;18:667.
569. Merchant SH, et al. Epstein-Barr virus-associated intravascular large T-cell lymphoma presenting as acute renal failure in a patient with acquired immunodeficiency syndrome. *Hum Pathol* 2003;950.
570. Becker JL, et al. Epstein-Barr virus infection of renal proximal tubule cells: possible role in chronic interstitial nephritis. *J Clin Invest* 1999;104:1673.
571. Arias LF, et al. Epstein-Barr virus latency in kidney specimens from transplant recipients. *Nephrol Dial Transplant* 2003;18:2638.
572. Babel N, et al. Association between Epstein-Barr virus infection and late acute transplant rejection in long-term transplant patients. *Transplantation* 2001;27:736.
573. Nickeleit V, et al. Testing for Polyomavirus type BK DNA in plasma to identify renal allograft recipients with viral nephropathy. *N Engl J Med* 2000;342:1309.
574. Randhawa PS, Demetris AJ. Nephropathy due to Polyomavirus type BK. *N Engl J Med* 2000;342:1361.
575. Nickeleit V, et al. BK-virus nephropathy in renal transplants-tubular necrosis, MHC-class II expression and rejection in a puzzling game. *Nephrol Dial Transplant* 2000;15:324.
576. Donini U, et al. BK papovavirus immune complexes in glomerulonephritis. *Proc Eur Dial Transplant Assoc* 1980;17:637.
577. Celik B, Randhawa PS. Glomerular changes in BK virus nephropathy. *Hum Pathol* 2004;35:367.
578. Buehrig CK, et al. Influence of surveillance renal allograft biopsy on diagnosis and prognosis of polyomavirus-associated nephropathy. *Kidney Int* 2003;64:665.
579. Randhawa PS, et al. Quantitation of viral DNA in renal allograft tissue from patients with BK virus nephropathy. *Transplantation* 2002;74:485.
580. Kadambi PV, et al. Treatment of refractory BK virus-associated nephropathy with cidofovir. *Am J Transplant* 2003;3:186.
581. Li RM, et al. Molecular identification of SV40 infection in human subjects and possible association with kidney disease. *Am J Kidney Dis* 2000;13:2320.
582. Galdenzi C, et al. Is the simian virus SV40 associated with idiopathic focal segmental glomerulosclerosis in humans? *J Nephrol* 2003;16:350.
583. Wierenga KJ, et al. Glomerulonephritis after human parvovirus infection in homozygous sickle-cell disease. *Lancet* 1995;346:475.
584. Tolaymat A, et al. Parvovirus glomerulonephritis in a patient with sickle cell disease. *Pediatr Nephrol* 1999;13:340.
585. Finkel TH, et al. Chronic parvovirus B19 infection and systemic necrotising vasculitis: opportunistic infection or aetiological agent? *Lancet* 1994;343:1255.

586. Chakravarty K, Merry P. Systemic vasculitis and atypical infections: report of two cases. *Postgrad Med J* 1999;75:544.
587. Ohtomo Y, et al. Nephrotic syndrome associated with human parvovirus B19 infection. *Pediatr Nephrol* 2003;18:280.
588. Iwafuchi Y, et al. Acute endocapillary proliferative glomerulonephritis associated with human parvovirus B19 infection. *Clin Nephrol* 2002;57:246.
589. Mori Y, et al. Association of parvovirus B19 infection with acute glomerulonephritis in healthy adults: case report and review of the literature. *Clin Nephrol* 2002;57:69.
590. Takeda S, et al. Renal involvement induced by human parvovirus B19 infection. *Nephron* 2001;89:280.
591. Komatsuda A, et al. Endocapillary proliferative glomerulonephritis in a patient with parvovirus B19 infection. *Am J Kidney Dis* 2000;36:851.
592. Nakazawa T, et al. Acute glomerulonephritis after human parvovirus B19 infection. *Am J Kidney Dis* 2000;35:E31.
593. Scmid ML, McWhinney PH, Will EJ. Parvovirus B19 and glomerulonephritis in a healthy adult. *Ann Intern Med* 2000;132:682.
594. Cioc AM, et al. Parvovirus B19 associated adult Henoch Schonlein purpura. *J Cutan Pathol* 2002;29:602.
595. Diaz F, Collazos J. Glomerulonephritis and Henoch-Schoenlein purpura associated with acute parvovirus B19 infection. *Clin Nephrol* 2000;53:237.
596. Tanawattanacharoen S, et al. Parvovirus B19 DNA in kidney tissue of patients with focal segmental glomerulosclerosis. *Am J Kidney Dis* 2000;35:1166.
597. Coventry S, Shoemaker LR. Collapsing glomerulopathy in a 16 year old girl with pulmonary tuberculosis: the role of systemic inflammatory mediators. *Pediatr Dev Pathol* 2004;7:166.
598. Schwimmer JA, et al. Collapsing glomerulopathy. *Semin Nephrol* 2003;23:209.
599. Moudgil A, et al. Association of parvovirus B19 infection with idiopathic collapsing glomerulopathy. *Kidney Int* 2001;59:2126.
600. Avila-Casado MC, et al. Familial collapsing glomerulopathy: clinical, pathological and immunogenetic features. *Kidney Int* 2003;63:233.
601. Moudgil A, et al. Parvovirus B19 infection-related complications in renal transplant recipients: Treatment with intravenous immunoglobulin. *Transplantation* 1997;64:1847.
602. Liefeldt L, et al. Eradication of parvovirus B19 infection after renal transplantation requires reduction of immunosuppression and high-dose immunoglobulin therapy. *Nephrol Dial Transplant* 2002;17:1840.
603. Cavallo R, et al. B19 virus infection in renal transplant recipients. *J Clin Virol* 2003;26:361.
604. Murer L, et al. Thrombotic microangiopathy associated with parvovirus B19 infection after renal transplantation. *J Am Soc Nephrol* 2000;11:1132.

CHAPTER 60 ■ RAPIDLY PROGRESSIVE GLOMERULONEPHRITIS

PETER G. KERR, DAVID J. NIKOLIC-PATERSON, AND ROBERT C. ATKINS

Rapidly progressive glomerulonephritis (RPGN) is one of the most calamitous of nephrologic conditions, and patients can progress from normal renal function to end-stage renal failure within weeks. RPGN is a syndrome and consists clinically of sudden and relentless deterioration in renal function associated with the pathologic finding on renal biopsy of extensive crescent formation involving most glomeruli.

Many types of glomerulonephritis can exhibit crescent formation and sometimes renal failure. These types are listed in Table 60-1 and include both primary glomerular disease and systemic disease with a glomerular component. Consequently, the definition of RPGN has been difficult, and the terminology has varied over the years, incorporating either the clinical or pathologic components, or both.

Crescents were first described by Langhans (1) over 100 years ago (Fig. 60-1). Volhard and Fahr (2) used the term *extra-capillary glomerulonephritis* in 1914 because of the glomerular crescents surrounding the capillary tuft, and Lohlein (3) called this type of glomerulonephritis a *stormy course* because of the renal failure that led to death. Ellis (4) coined the phrase *rapidly progressive type 1,* but the disease has also since been referred to as *malignant* (5), *acute necrotizing* (6), *acute anuric* (7), *proliferative, with crescents* (8), and *nonstreptococcal rapidly progressive glomerulonephritis* (9). The most commonly used synonym for RPGN today is *idiopathic crescentic glomerulonephritis* (10).

Therefore, in this chapter, *RPGN* is used to describe this relatively rare syndrome, consisting clinically of an acute glomerulonephritis, with a rapid and progressive deterioration in renal function, and pathologically of extensive crescent formation involving most of the glomeruli in the absence of another type of primary glomerulonephritis or systemic disease. In spite of these restrictions, RPGN is still a heterogeneous entity and can be divided further on immunopathogenetic criteria into subgroups with different prognoses and responses to treatment. RPGN is traditionally divided into three entities: antiglomerular basement membrane disease (anti-GBM, so-called Goodpasture's syndrome), immune GN, and the previously named pauci-immune group that we now know to be varieties of vasculitis, usually antineutrophil cytoplasmic antibody (ANCA) positive.

PATHOLOGY

Crescents

The pathognomonic feature of RPGN is the presence of crescents in Bowman's space (Figs. 60-2 and 60-3). A glomerular crescent may be defined as an aggregation of cells, at least two layers deep, in Bowman's space that may encroach on and destroy the capillary tuft. There is no agreement on the extent of crescent formation required for the diagnosis of RPGN to

be made. Studies vary from 20% of glomeruli involved (11) to more than 80% (12). Neild et al. (13), in an extensive review of the Guy's Hospital experience, introduced the concept of the importance of the degree of the glomerular circumferential involvement. They defined the pathologic criteria for RPGN as greater than 60% of circumferential involvement of more than 60% of glomeruli. In general, those patients with the most rapid progression and most severe renal failure have a greater number of glomerular crescents (12,14).

Crescents are composed of cells and fibrous connective tissue. During the acute phase, crescents are predominantly cellular (Fig. 60-3), whereas chronicity is typified by progressive fibrosis and eventually sclerosis of the crescent (Fig. 60-4). Early crescents are composed of large, pale-staining, elongated cells with occasional mitoses evident (Figs. 60-2 and 60-3). It was traditionally held that these cells were derived from proliferated epithelial cells, and the term *epithelial crescent* was used (9,10,15). However, studies using monoclonal antibodies as specific markers have shown that the major identifiable cell type in crescents is of macrophage origin (16). Consistent with these data, tissue culture studies of glomeruli isolated from patients with RPGN produced predominant outgrowths of macrophages (17–19) (Fig. 60-5). A cellular crescent also frequently contains erythrocytes, polymorphonuclear leukocytes, and deposits of fibrin (Fig. 60-3). Over time, progression from a cellular to a sclerosed, fibrous crescent is seen as acute infiltrating leukocytes and epithelial cells are lost through apoptosis or migration out of the crescent and are replaced by myofibroblasts and fibroblasts, which secrete matrix and contribute to fibrosis and eventual sclerosis of the crescent (see Pathogenesis, below). RPGN frequently is a nonuniform process, and various degrees and stages of crescent formation may be seen in different glomeruli from the same biopsy.

Glomerular Tuft

Most patients also have glomerular tuft involvement, which may consist of focal and segmental necrosis of glomerular capillaries, fibrin deposition, cellular infiltration, and cellular proliferation (Fig. 60-3). In cases of extensive crescent formation, the glomerular tuft can be almost completely compressed and ischemic changes may be evident. In less severely damaged glomeruli, there may be proliferation of resident kidney cells (endothelial and mesangial cells) and accumulation of leukocytes (macrophages, polymorphs, and lymphocytes). Multinucleated giant cells also have been found (20). Cells in the tuft may proliferate, become activated, release proinflammatory cytokines, and mediate thrombosis, tissue damage, and fibrosis (see Pathogenesis below) (Fig. 60-6).

The advent of monoclonal antibodies (21) enabled specific identification of individual antigens on both leukocytes and intrinsic glomerular cells (22–26), making it possible to assess

TABLE 60-1

TYPES OF GLOMERULONEPHRITIS THAT CAN BE
ASSOCIATED WITH RAPID DETERIORATION IN
RENAL FUNCTION AND GLOMERULAR CRESCENT
FORMATION

Primary Renal Diseases
  RPGN—anti-GBM without lung involvement
  RPGN—immune complex deposition
  RPGN—without immune deposits (>80% ANCA positive)
  Membranoproliferative glomerulonephritis
  Membranous nephropathy
  Immunoglobulin A disease
  Hereditary nephritis

Systemic Diseases
  Goodpasture's syndrome
  Postinfectious
  Poststreptococcal (Chapter 58)
  Endocarditis (Chapter 58)
  Shunt nephritis (Chapter 58)
  Abscess (Chapter 58)
  Henoch-Schönlein disease (Chapter 61)
  Lupus nephritis (Chapter 65)
  Polyarteritis (Chapter 68)
  Wegener's granulomatosis (Chapter 68)
  Cryoglobulinemia (Chapter 69)
  Scleroderma (Chapter 66)
  Relapsing polychondritis
  Malignancy
  Malignant hypertension (Chapter 56)

ANCA, antineutrophil cytoplasmic antibody; *anti-GBM*,
antiglomerular basement membrane disease; *RPGN*, rapidly
progressive glomerulonephritis.

the number of individual glomerular cell types and infiltrating leukocytes *in situ*. Glomeruli from patients with RPGN have increased numbers of macrophages and polymorphonuclear leukocytes (27–34). Intraglomerular T cells have been demonstrated in glomeruli of patients with crescentic glomerulonephritis (29–34). Such T cells are functionally active, as

demonstrated by their association with activated monocytes and fibrin, the other components of cell-mediated immunity (35), and their expression of receptors for interleukin-2 (IL-2R), denoting immune activation (3,32).

Interstitial Infiltrate

In most renal biopsies of patients with RPGN, there is a prominent interstitial inflammatory cell infiltrate (10). It usually is widespread throughout the interstitium but often is most marked surrounding Bowman's capsule (Figs. 60-2 through 60-4). The interstitial changes in RPGN may well relate more to the outcome of the disease than do the glomerular changes (28). It has been shown that there is a highly significant correlation between the degree of interstitial mononuclear cell infiltration and impairment of renal function, whereas there is minimal correlation between glomerular cell numbers and renal function (28). All these findings suggest that the interstitial mononuclear cell infiltrate is a very important component of the renal response to glomerular injury (36,37).

The composition of the interstitial leukocytic infiltrate in RPGN has been evaluated (28,29). Hooke et al. (28) compared the interstitial cell infiltrate in 14 patients with RPGN with 84 other types of glomerulonephritis. This study found that the interstitial leukocyte numbers were greater in the RPGN group of patients, that the T lymphocyte was the major cell involved (64%), and that the CD4+/CD8+ ratio was 1.0, which was the same as in other glomerulonephritides and in normal biopsies. The other interstitial mononuclear cells were monocytes (22%), B cells (10%), and granulocytes (2%). A typical interstitial leukocytic infiltrate stained by the monoclonal antibody PHM1, which recognizes a cell membrane antigen that is present on all human leukocytes (38), is shown in Figure 60-7. A further study demonstrated IL-2R expression by a high proportion of the interstitial mononuclear cells in RPGN, indicating an activated phenotype (3). Stachura et al. (29) published similar interstitial findings in 16 patients with RPGN. They found that the mononuclear interstitial infiltrate consisted mainly of T lymphocytes (80%) and monocytes (19%) and very small numbers of B cells and natural killer cells. Most of the T lymphocytes, both in the interstitium as well as in glomeruli, were of the helper (CD4+) phenotype in normal patients as

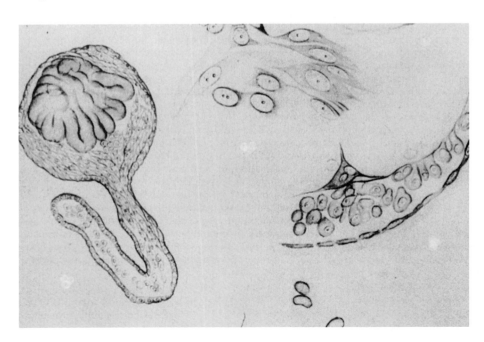

FIGURE 60-1. Reproduction of drawings from Langhans's paper, published over 100 years ago, which first described crescents in Bowman's space and inferred an epithelial cell origin. (From: Langhans, T. Uber die vernaderungen der glomeruli bei der nephritis nebst einigen Bemerkungen uber die Entsehung der Fibrinzylinder. *Arch Pathol Physiol Klin Med* 1879;76:85.)

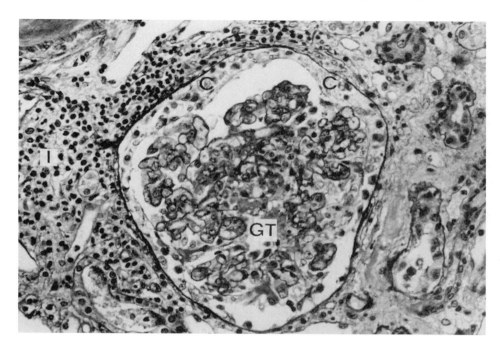

FIGURE 60-2. A small cellular crescent (C) surrounding a glomerular tuft (GT) from a 67-year-old patient with rapidly progressive glomerulonephritis. The glomerulus shows some mesangial and endothelial cell proliferation. There is a pronounced interstitial cellular infiltrate (I). (Silver-Masson trichrome, magnification ×400.)

well as in patients with RPGN. These studies clearly support a role for cellular immunity in RPGN.

Immune Deposits

The nature of the immune deposits (immunoglobulin and complement) in crescentic glomerulonephritis, as detected by immunofluorescence or an immunoperoxidase technique, depends on the underlying type of glomerulonephritis. The three patterns are (a) linear GBM deposition of immunoglobulins (anti-GBM antibody), with or without complement (C3); (Fig. 60-8A); (b) granular deposition of immunoglobulin and complement along capillary loops and mesangium, suggesting

an immune complex disease (Fig. 60-8B); and (c) no or very scanty immunoglobulin or complement deposition—so-called pauci-immune RPGN (Fig. 60-8C). The proportion of cases in each individual group varies markedly from one series to another (12,13,39–45). In very general terms, however, approximately 30% of cases of RPGN account for each category of immunopathogenesis, although more recent studies indicate higher numbers of the pauci-immune group. In addition, there seems to be a great geographic variation. In the United States and Australia, anti-GBM disease is relatively common, whereas in Europe it is uncommon. In a series of 195 biopsies from patients from various disease areas and containing more than 50% crescents, 11% of the patients had anti-GBM disease, 29% had immune complex glomerulonephritis, and 60%

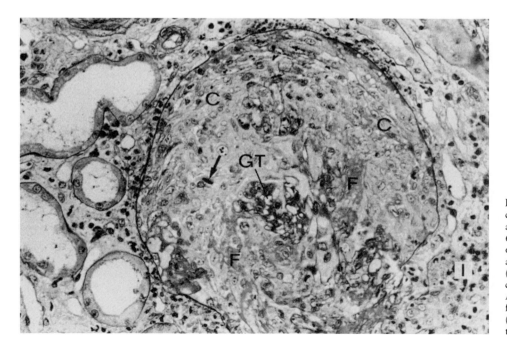

FIGURE 60-3. An extensive cellular crescent (C) from the same biopsy as that shown in Figures 60-2 and 60-7B. There is virtual obliteration of the glomerular tuft (GT). There are large areas of fibrin deposition (F) in the crescent. A mitotic figure can be seen in the crescent (arrow). An interstitial mononuclear cell infiltrate (I) surrounds the glomerulus. (Silver-Masson trichrome, magnification ×400.)

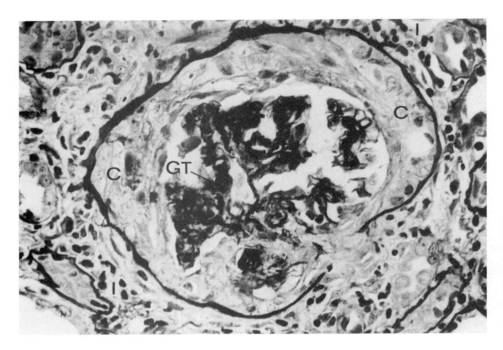

FIGURE 60-4. A glomerulus showing a fibrocellular crescent (C) surrounding the glomerular tuft (GT) from a patient with rapidly progressive glomerulonephritis, 90% crescent formation, and no immunoglobulin deposition. Interstitial infiltration with mononuclear cells is present (I). The patient is the same as in Figure 60-6. (Silver-Masson trichrome, magnification ×400.)

had pauci-immune glomerulonephritis (46). Fibrin/fibrinogen deposition usually is detected in both the crescent and the capillary tuft.

Electron microscopy confirms the presence or absence of mesangial or capillary loop immune deposits in immune complex crescentic glomerulonephritis. Collapse of the capillary wall and necrosis of glomerular cells in the tuft frequently are seen (9,15,47–49), and ruptures in the capillary loops are common and may be important in crescent formation (50). Electron microscopy also commonly demonstrates macrophages, epithelioid cells, and epithelial cells in the crescent (47,50), although this technique is not well suited to the determination of the relative proportion of each of these cell types in the crescent. Fibrin normally is seen between the cells of the crescent and,

as the crescent evolves, basement membrane material and collagen fibers also may be seen. The electron micrograph shown in Figure 60-9 illustrates many of these features in a crescent from a patient with RPGN.

PATHOGENESIS

Our current understanding of the immunopathogenesis of this disease has come largely from examination of glomerular immune deposition and immune cell participation in patients and the study of experimentally induced RPGN in animals. More recent studies also have indicated that progressive tubulointerstitial injury is a prominent feature of RPGN (51,52).

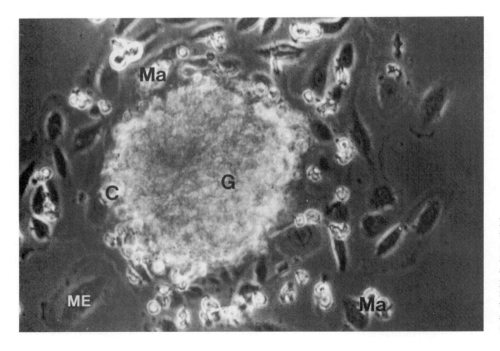

FIGURE 60-5. Phase-contrast photomicrograph of an isolated glomerulus (G) in tissue culture from a patient with rapidly progressive glomerulonephritis and 100% crescent formation. A large population of macrophages (Ma) is seen in the crescent (C) and egressing into the culture. Mesangial cells (ME) also are present in the culture outgrowth. (Magnification ×150.)

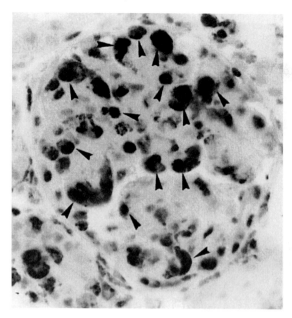

FIGURE 60-6. A rat glomerulus demonstrating hypercellularity from an animal with induced anti-glomerular basement membrane nephritis. Double immunostaining demonstrated that numerous glomerular macrophages (*arrows*; ED-1 positive [*brown*]) were proliferating (proliferating cell nuclear antigen positive [*blue/black*]) and contributing to the glomerular hypercellularity. (Periodic acid-Schiff, magnification ×400.) (See Color Plate.)

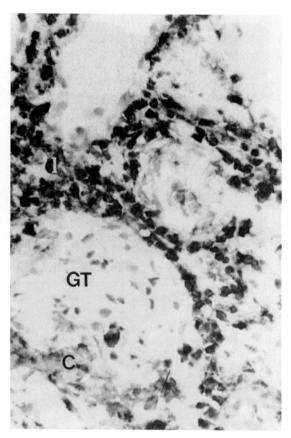

FIGURE 60-7. A cryostat section of a biopsy from the patient with rapidly progressive glomerulonephritis in Figure 60-4. Leukocytes are identified by the monoclonal antibody PHM1 (91) and a four-layer peroxidase anti-peroxidase technique giving black staining. The total infiltrating leukocyte population is identified by PHM1 as it recognizes a leukocyte common antigen. Large numbers of interstitial leukocytes (l) can be seen, particularly surrounding the glomerulus (GT). There also are mononuclear leukocytes identified in the glomerular tuft (GT). Many cells in the crescent (C) also are stained. (Magnification ×125; courtesy of Dr. D. Hooke.)

The histologic pattern and clinical course of the entity of RPGN resulting from several underlying immunopathogenetic mechanisms is discussed. However, it is likely that these mechanisms can coexist and perhaps may be variations in a spectrum of disease (40,46,53,54).

Glomerular Deposition of Anti–Glomerular Basement Membrane Antibody

The pattern of immunoglobulin deposition in the glomerulus separates this condition from the immune complex group (see above discussion). In approximately one-fifth of all patients with RPGN, linear deposition of immunoglobulin (predominantly immunoglobulin G [IgG]) along the GBM is detected. In these patients, anti-GBM antibody also usually is detected in the circulation, particularly if a sensitive and specific radioimmunoassay is used to detect the antibody (55). In some patients, this antibody also reacts with the pulmonary basement membrane and results in pulmonary hemorrhage (56), thus producing Goodpasture's syndrome. The anti-GBM antibody also can cross-react with renal tubular basement membrane, and this has been linked to a more severe interstitial component (57). The "Goodpasture antigen" has now been identified in the noncollagenous globular domain, termed NC1, of type IV collagen. More specifically, more than 90% of patients have antibodies to the $\alpha3$ (IV) chains of the type IV collagen (58,59). The molecular organization of the autoantigen in the native alpha3alpha4alpha5(IV) collagen network of the GBM has recently been described (60).

Rapidly progressive glomerulonephritis caused by anti-GBM antibody can be induced in animals, notably in sheep, by the repeated injection of particulate heterologous (e.g., rabbit) or homologous (i.e., sheep) GBM in complete Freund's adjuvant, causing Steblay's nephritis (61). If serum from sheep with anti-GBM glomerulonephritis (induced by rabbit GBM) is injected intravenously into rabbits, then the anti-GBM antibody fixes to the rabbit GBM, inducing proteinuria (heterologous phase of nephrotoxic nephritis). With the development 5 to 6 days later of a rabbit antibody response to the sheep antibody on the rabbit GBM, a rapidly progressive crescentic glomerulonephritis develops (autologous phase of nephrotoxic nephritis) (62). This type of passive transfer of anti-GBM serum can be used to induce a rat model of accelerated anti-GBM nephritis with resultant disease that closely mimics human Goodpasture's syndrome, complete with pulmonary hemorrhage (63,64).

Evidence that human anti-GBM antibodies are pathogenic comes from studies in which anti-GBM antibodies, eluted from human kidneys, induced acute glomerulonephritis upon transfer into monkeys (65). Using mice that have been genetically modified to only produce human immunoglobulins (XenoMouse II), Meyers et al. (66) demonstrated that immunization with $\alpha3$(IV)NC1 collagen leads to the production of human anti-GBM autoantibodies that, when transferred to a normal XenoMouse, induced proteinuria and proliferative glomerulonephritis. However, while these studies provide clear evidence that anti-GBM antibodies are pathogenic, there is also

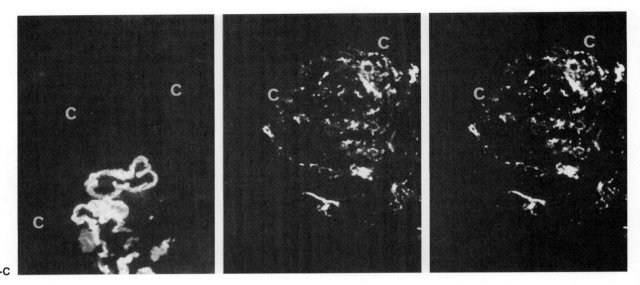

FIGURE 60-8. Immunofluorescence micrographs of renal biopsies from three different patients with rapidly progressive glomerulonephritis (RPGN) demonstrate the three underlying immunopathogenetic mechanisms. The crescents (C) are identified. **A:** Linear pattern of immunoglobulin G (IgG) deposition along the glomerular basement membrane of a patient with anti–glomerular basement membrane RPGN. **B:** Granular fluorescence of IgG along the capillary loops of the same patient with RPGN as in Figures 60-2 and 60-3, due to immune complex deposition. **C:** No definite immunoglobulin deposition is seen in the capillary tuft, but some deposits of C3 are evident on the visceral layer of Bowman's capsule in a patient with idiopathic or no-immune-deposit RPGN.

a critical role for cell-mediated immunity in disease pathogenesis (see below).

Glomerular Immune Complex Deposition

A granular deposition of immunoglobulin and complement along the capillary loops and in the mesangium is seen in approximately one-third of patients with RPGN. This pattern strongly suggests an immune complex pathogenesis, although circulating immune complexes are not commonly detected in these patients. The actual antigens involved are not known. The possibility of a viral etiology has been suggested by the demonstration of type IV nuclear bodies in the kidneys of some patients with crescentic glomerulonephritis (67). RPGN due to deposition of immune complexes can be induced in animals, especially the rabbit, by the daily intravenous injection of bovine serum albumin (BSA) in a dose according to the animal's antibody response to the BSA (chronic serum sickness). Immune complexes of BSA–anti-BSA can be detected in large amounts in the circulation and deposit in the glomerular capillary loops and mesangium (68). RPGN of this type may, in some cases,

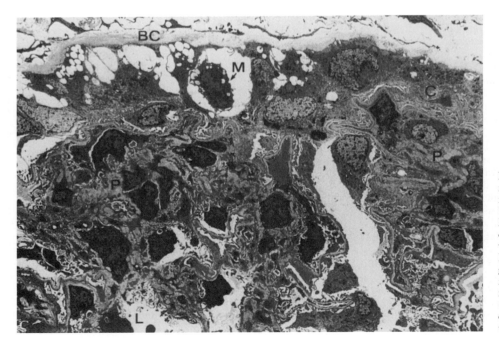

FIGURE 60-9. Transmission electron micrograph of part of a glomerulus from a renal biopsy of a 12-year-old boy with rapidly progressive glomerulonephritis, illustrating an early crescent (C) adjacent to the urinary space in which a macrophage (M) can be seen. Bowman's capsule (BC) surrounds the glomerulus. Some capillary loops (L) remain patent, but there are areas of marked endocapillary cell proliferation (P), one of which is adjacent to the early crescent. (Magnification ×3,000; courtesy of Prof. E. F. Glasgow.)

simply represent the severe end of the spectrum of common forms of glomerulonephritis (e.g., crescentic immunoglobulin A [IgA] nephropathy).

Minimal or Absent Glomerular Immune Deposits

In many patients with RPGN, significant immune deposits are not detected in the glomeruli (11). Hence, it has been difficult to incriminate humoral immune mechanisms in these patients. However, over 80% of these patients have circulating ANCA (43,46,68,69) and it appears that these patients have renal vasculitis, with or without systemic clinical manifestations (70) (see below).

Anti-neutrophil cytoplasmic antibodies (ANCA), first described by Davies et al. in 1982 (71) are a marker for "idiopathic" glomerulonephritis when it occurs with no evidence of extrarenal disease and in glomerulonephritis associated with systemic necrotizing arteritides, including microscopic polyangiitis and Wegener's granulomatosis (43,46,72–76).

Anti-neutrophil cytoplasmic antibodies have been detected in approximately 80% of patients with pauci-immune crescentic glomerulonephritis in one center (43,46,73). Jayne et al. (77) found that the sera of 28% of 889 consecutive patients with suspected RPGN were positive for ANCA. Tervaert et al. (78) reviewed 35 consecutive patients with crescentic glomerulonephritis without glomerular immunoglobulin deposition and concluded that both vasculitis-associated and idiopathic crescentic glomerulonephritis were specifically associated with ANCAs to myeloid lysosomal enzymes. Thus, it appears likely that idiopathic crescentic RPGN without glomerular immune deposits is part of the spectrum of the vasculitides. Although there are obviously ANCAs to various antigens (46,77,78), it may be that c-ANCA (cytoplasmic staining to a serine proteinase) occurs predominantly in Wegener's granulomatosis and p-ANCA (with perinuclear staining predominantly to myeloperoxidase) is found in patients with so-called microscopic polyarteritis (or polyangiitis) with crescentic glomerulonephritis but little or no systemic disease (79). Both of these conditions predominantly involve small-caliber arteries/arterioles. True polyarteritis nodosa is a disease of medium-sized arteries not commonly associated with glomerulonephritis, and is more commonly ANCA-negative.

The potential role of ANCAs in disease pathogenesis has been a controversial subject. However, recent studies in animal models have provided convincing evidence that ANCA are indeed pathogenic (80). Immunization of rats with myeloperoxidase (MPO) induces autoantibodies to rat and human MPO that aggravate renal injury induced by anti-GBM antibodies or by renal artery perfusion with a neutrophil lysosomal extract and hydrogen peroxide (81,82). Definitive experimental evidence that ANCAs are pathogenic has come from a recent study in which MPO gene deficient mice were immunized with mouse MPO. Purified anti-MPO IgG was transferred into immunodeficient (*Rag2–/–*) or normal mice, resulting in focal necrotizing and crescentic glomerulonephritis with a paucity of glomerular Ig deposition (83).

Immunoglobulin Receptors

Receptors for the Fc portion of immunoglobulin G (FcRγ) play an important role in the pathogenesis of experimental anti-GBM glomerulonephritis. There are both activating and inhibitory Fc receptors for IgG. Human and mouse share two activating Fc receptors (FcγRI, FcγRIIIa) and a single inhibitor receptor FcγRIIb (84). The two activating Fcγ receptors re-

quire a common FcRγ chain for their cell-surface assembly and signaling functions. Thus, mice deficient for FcRγ chain lack functional FcγI and FcγRIIIa receptors and these mice are completely protected from fatal, acute anti-GBM glomerulonephritis (85). Subsequent studies have confirmed that deletion of both FcRγI and III gives protection from crescentic anti-GBM glomerulonephritis, but there is debate as to the relative contribution of FcRγI versus FcRγIII (86,87). In addition to FcR promoting renal injury, it has been shown that the inhibitory FcγIIB is protective. Deletion of FcγIIB makes mice susceptible to the spontaneous autoimmune glomerulonephritis depending on the background strain (88). Furthermore, immunization of FcRγIIB deficient mice with collagen type IV leads to Goodpasture's syndrome with linear deposition of IgG along the glomerular and tubular basement membranes, massive pulmonary hemorrhage with neutrophil and macrophage infiltration and crescentic glomerulonephritis (89).

Cell-Mediated Immunity—T Cells

Prominent T-cell and macrophage accumulation and activation in glomeruli, crescents, and the tubulointerstitium are striking features in RPGN suggesting that cellular immunity plays a central role in the pathogenesis of these diseases. Indeed, the immunopathologic features of RPGN show marked similarities to delayed-type hypersensitivity (DTH) reactions, which include local accumulation of T cells and macrophages, multi-nucleated giant cell formation, and fibrin deposition – even in the absence of immunoglobulin deposition (3,11,16,20,28,29,31,34,57,90–94).

The role of T cells in RPGN was first suggested by studies performed in 1970 (95) in which lymphocytes from patients with RPGN showed *in vitro* delayed-type hypersensitivity (DTH) responses in the presence of GBM. More recently, it has been shown that the Goodpasture antigen is expressed in normal human thymus. In Goodpasture's disease, limiting dilution analysis identified increased frequencies of CD4+ T cells reactive with alpha3(IV)NC1 in patients with acute disease, which reduced during the recovery phase. Indeed, this loss of autoreactive CD4+ T cells may explain why recurrences of this disease are infrequent (96).

Detailed time course studies in a rat model of anti-GBM glomerulonephritis that shares many features of human RPGN has shown that immune-activated T cells are exclusively localized to the areas of histologic damage, appearing to play a role in Bowman's capsular rupture, glomerular crescent fibrosis, tubulointerstitial fibrosis, and pulmonary fibrosis (63,64,97,98). Quantitative analysis showed that the number of interstitial T cells, particularly activated T cells, correlates significantly with the severity of proteinuria and renal impairment (63), suggestive of a pathogenic role for T cells in the mediation of the disease.

There is now strong evidence that T cells play a key role in the pathogenesis of crescentic glomerulonephritis. Bhan et al. (99) demonstrated that transfer of sensitized T cells into rats with planted heterologous anti-GBM globulin results in proliferative glomerulonephritis. Bolton et al. (100) induced a similar glomerular injury in chickens after transfer of T cells sensitized to GBM. Rennke et al (101) induced a granulomatous nephritis with glomerular crescent formation in the rat with sensitized T cells. These examples of glomerular injury occurred in the absence of antibody deposition.

Antibody-based depletion of either CD8+ or CD4+ T cells with monoclonal antibodies resulted in prevention of macrophage accumulation, proteinuria and crescent formation in different rat models of passive anti-GBM glomerulonephritis (102,103). While T cell depletion is a useful experimental tool, it has little clinical applicability. Therefore, efforts have been made to block T cell activation in order to prevent or suppress the renal cellular immune response. The induction of autoantibody formation and crescentic glomerulonephritis in Wistar-Kyoto (WKY) rats immunized with rat GBM can be prevented by administration of CTLA4-Ig which blocks the CD28-CD80 and CD28-CD86 co-stimulation interactions involved in T cell activation (104,105). Furthermore, blockade of only the CD28-CD80 interaction substantially prevented T cell and macrophage infiltration, proteinuria, glomerular lesions and renal failure without affecting production and glomerular deposition of anti-GBM antibodies, demonstrating that T cell activation is essential for disease development in this model (105).

Blockade of another T cell co-stimulation interaction, CD40-CD154, can also prevent the induction of autoimmune anti-GBM glomerulonephritis in WKY rats. Delaying the anti-CD154 antibody treatment to 1 week after GBM immunization still provided moderate protection, but delaying treatment for two weeks had no significant effect upon disease development (106).

The most direct demonstration of T cell dependent RPGN comes from studies in which CD4+ antigen-specific T cell lines were derived from WKY rats after immunization with a recombinant form of the glomerular basement membrane (GBM) antigen, Col4α3NC1. Adoptive transfer of these CD4+ T cells to normal rats induced severe proteinuria with glomerular crescent formation in 5 of 11 animals in the complete absence of antibody or C3 deposition (107). Furthermore, immunization of WKY rats with a single peptide from Col4αa3NC1 has been shown to induce severe anti-GBM glomerulonephritis featuring nearly 100% of glomeruli with crescentic lesions or tuft necrosis in the complete absence of glomerular antibody deposition (108).

The mechanisms by which T cells coordinate the immune response in RPGN have been investigated. In the current paradigm of helper T-cell function, the role of a dominant type 1 helper T-cell (Th1) response in RPGN has been postulated, and the evidence for this was reviewed by Holdsworth et al. (109). While severe renal injury can be induced by passive transfer of anti-GBM antibodies to sensitized C57BL/6J (Th1-biased) and BALB/c (Th2-biased) mice, glomerular leukocyte infiltration and crescent formation was only seen in the Th1-biased strain (110). Augmentation of the Th1 response by the administration of interleukin (IL)-12, or via IL-4 gene knockout, enhanced crescent formation in anti-GBM glomerulonephritis in C57BL/6J mice (111,112), whereas antagonism of the Th1 response through IL-12 blockade (111) or IL-4 plus IL-10 administration diminished crescent formation (113). The situation is less clearly defined in larger rodents and in humans. Anti-Th1 therapy with IL-10 was studied in an accelerated model of anti-GBM disease in Sprague-Dawley rats (114). Administration of IL-10 after priming, but before disease initiation, failed to prevent crescent formation or renal injury despite inhibiting a skin DTH response to the same antigen (114). The systemic humoral immune response was enhanced by treatment, and this may have contributed to renal injury and crescent formation.

Immunohistochemical evaluation of human biopsy specimens from patients with RPGN supports a role for cell-mediated immunity, although the Th1/Th2 orientation of T cells promoting the response has been difficult to identify. Peripheral T cells specifically reactive with potentially nephritogenic GBM antigens have been identified, but not classified as either Th1 or Th2 (115,116). The immunoglobulin subclasses of potentially pathogenic antibodies produced by patients with RPGN have been studied to look for Th1 (IgG3) or Th2 (IgG4) bias, but no clear consensus has emerged (117,118). Identification of regulatory CD25+ T cells that can suppress the T cell response to the Goodpasture antigen in human anti-GBM dis-

ease raises the possibility that T cell may also play an important immunoregulatory role in RPGN (119).

Cell-Mediated Immunity—Macrophages

After the original discovery that large numbers of macrophages could be identified in glomerular cultures from patients with RPGN (120), immunohistochemistry-based studies showed the macrophage to be the major cell type found in crescentic glomeruli in biopsy tissue obtained from patients with this disease (16,17,92,121). Analysis of these biopsies also revealed marked accumulation of macrophages in areas of tubulointerstitial damage (28,122). Activation of the renal macrophage infiltrate has been demonstrated by macrophage production of cytokines such as IL-1, tumor necrosis factor-α (TNF-α) and macrophage migration inhibitory factor (MIF) (123–126), gene transcription of inducible nitric oxide (iNOS) (127) and matrix metalloproteinase-12 (MMP-12) (128), and expression of activation antigens MRP8/14 and CD86 (129,130).

Despite the fact that most studies examining the role of macrophages in RPGN have focused on mediation of renal injury, it is important to remember that macrophages are highly heterogeneous cells and can perform many different functions. Macrophages can efficiently process and present antigens to T cells and modulate the nature (Th1/Th2) of the immune response through their profile of cytokine secretion. Upon activation, macrophages have the potential to cause tissue damage by the secretion a wide array of pro-inflammatory cytokines (i.e., IL-1, TNF-α, MIF), oxidants (i.e., reactive oxygen species, nitric oxide), proteases (i.e., MMP-12, elastase), growth factors (platelet-derived growth factor [PDGF]), fibroblast growth factor-2 (FGF-2), and transforming growth factor-β1 [(TGF-β1)] and expression of procoagulant activity. Indeed, macrophages can be activated to produce these mediators via T cell-derived cytokines (i.e., IL-1, TNF-α, interferon-γ [IFN-γ]) or via T cell-independent mechanisms (i.e., immune complexes, complement, cytokines produced by intrinsic renal cells, endotoxin). The potentially beneficial aspect to renal macrophage infiltration is the removal of microorganisms via the innate immune response and promoting tissue repair through the production of antiinflammatory molecules, phagocytosis of apoptotic cells, removal of immune complexes and fibrin, matrix remodelling and enhancing vascularization.

Depletion strategies have been used to examine the pathogenic role of macrophages in experimental RPGN. Methods such as X-irradiation (131), antimacrophage serum (132), and nitrogen mustard treatment (133) have been used to induce systemic monocyte/macrophage depletion in animal models of anti-GBM glomerulonephritis, resulting in a significant reduction of kidney macrophage infiltration and abrogation of renal injury.

Direct evidence of macrophage-mediated renal injury has come from adoptive transfer studies. Early studies in a rabbit model of anti-GBM disease showed that transferred peritoneal macrophages can be recruited into the glomeruli of animals in which anti-GBM antibody is deposited, resulting in mild proteinuria in some animals (133). In recent studies, we have used adoptive transfer in the rat to demonstrate that macrophages recruited to the glomerulus directly induce moderate proteinuria and mesangial cell proliferation in acute anti-GBM disease (134). Activation of bone marrow-derived macrophages with IFN-γ prior to transfer augmented macrophage-mediated renal injury in rat anti-GBM disease, whereas treatment with glucocorticoids prevented macrophage activation and inhibited renal injury (135). Furthermore, macrophage-mediated renal injury in this model was shown to be dependent upon signaling through the c-Jun amino terminal kinase (JNK) pathway, with *in vitro* studies identifying a role for JNK signaling in macrophage production of TNF-α, monocyte chemoattractant protein-1 (MCP-1), and nitric oxide (136).

An alternative to systemic monocyte/macrophage depletion is to prevent circulating monocytes from entering the kidney. Two chemotactic factors which are relatively specific for monocytes, MCP-1 and osteopontin (OPN), have been extensively studied in RPGN. Increased renal MCP-1 production is associated with glomerular and interstitial macrophage accumulation in human RPGN (137,138). Similarly, the induction of tubular OPN expression is tightly associated with interstitial macrophage accumulation (139,140). Antibody-based neutralization of MCP-1 inhibits glomerular macrophage accumulation and the induction of proteinuria and glomerular lesions in anti-GBM glomerulonephritis (141–143). In contrast, Tesch et al. (144) found that glomerular macrophage accumulation was unaffected in anti-GBM glomerulonephritis in MCP-1 gene deficient mice, but that interstitial macrophage accumulation and tubular damage were attenuated. Antibody-based blockade of OPN has also been shown to prevent glomerular and interstitial macrophage accumulation in rat anti-GBM glomerulonephritis with a consequent reduction in proteinuria and histologic damage (145). A role for macrophages in mediating progressive renal injury in RPGN has come from studies in which administration of neutralizing antibodies to MCP-1 or OPN in established anti-GBM disease were shown to suppress disease progression (143,145).

Adhesion Molecules

Adhesion molecules play a critical role in facilitating leukocyte attachment to the endothelium and their subsequent migration into sites of inflammation (146). Studies of human RPGN have identified upregulation of intracellular adhesion molecule-1 (ICAM-1; CD54) and vascular adhesion molecule-1 (VCAM-1; CD106) in endothelium, mesangial cells and tubules which is associated with T cell and macrophage accumulation (147–149).

Upregulation of selectin expression in the glomerular endothelium is a very early event following the deposition of anti-GBM antibodies in rat RPGN. Antibody-based blocking studies have shown a pathogenic role for P-selectin in the early, transient glomerular neutrophil accumulation and induction of proteinuria following administration of anti-GBM antibodies to experimental animals (150). Endothelial ICAM-1 expression is also upregulated rapidly following administration of anti-GBM antisera in rats, with co-localization of leukocyte function associated antigen one (LFA-1) and ICAM-1 at sites of monocyte adhesion to activated endothelium in the glomerulus and interstitium identified using immuno-electron microscopy (151,152). Up-regulation of tubular ICAM-1 expression during development of this disease model is associated with macrophage accumulation and tubular necrosis (152) (see Fig. 60-10). The pathological role of the ICAM-1/LFA-1 interaction was demonstrated by the ability of neutralizing anti-ICAM-1 plus anti-LFA-1 antibodies to abrogate leukocyte infiltration, proteinuria and histologic damage in rat anti-GBM glomerulonephritis (153,154). Consistent with these findings, ICAM-1 gene deficient mice are largely protected from the induction of anti-GBM glomerulonephritis, with reduced macrophage accumulation, proteinuria, and histological damage (155). In contrast, anti-VCAM-1 antibody treatment had no effect upon the development of anti-GBM glomerulonephritis in WKY rats. However, blockade of the VCAM-1 ligand, very late activation antigen-4 (VLA-4; CD29/49d) in this model protects against proteinuria and crescent formation without affecting glomerular macrophage recruitment (156). Furthermore, commencing anti-VLA-4 antibody treatment in

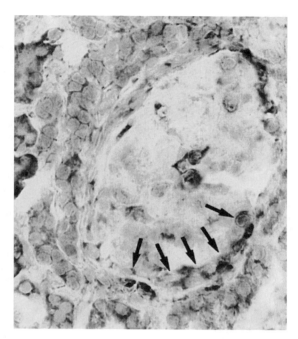

FIGURE 60-10. *In situ* hybridization demonstrating intercellular adhesion molecule-1 (ICAM-1) messenger RNA (mRNA) expression in a crescent from a rat with anti–glomerular basement membrane nephritis (*arrows*). The ICAM-1 mRNA has been depicted using *in situ* hybridization histochemistry. (Magnification ×400.) (See Color Plate.)

established disease was shown to attenuate disease progression (157).

Cytokines

Interleukin-1 is a classic proinflammatory cytokine. Renal production of IL-1 activity was first described in cultured glomeruli from patients with RPGN (123). Subsequent studies have identified IL-1 gene and protein expression in infiltrating macrophages as well as intrinsic renal cells in human and experimental RPGN (124,158,159). Blockade of IL-1 activity in the acute, neutrophil-mediated phase of rat anti-GBM glomerulonephritis has produced variable results (160–164). However, longer periods of IL-1 blockade have been shown to suppress disease. Treatment with the IL-1 receptor antagonist (IL-1ra) during the first 14 days of rat anti-GBM glomerulonephritis suppressed glomerular macrophage accumulation and proteinuria, and prevented glomerular crescent formation and a loss of renal function (160). This effect was attributed to preventing upregulation of leukocyte adhesion molecules ICAM-1, OPN, and CD44 (165–167). Furthermore, delaying IL-1ra treatment until crescentic disease was already established was shown to halt disease progression and return renal function to normal (168), demonstrating the therapeutic potential for IL-1 blockade in RPGN.

Tumour necrosis factor-α (TNF-α) is another classic proinflammatory cytokine that plays an important role in RPGN. Upregulation of TNF-α has been described in human RPGN (124,125,158), and administration of a neutralizing anti-TNF-α antibody was shown to reduce renal injury in acute anti-GBM disease in the rat (161,163,164,169). In longer-term studies, administration of a soluble TNF receptor in rat anti-GBM glomerulonephritis produced a 55% to 70% inhibition in macrophage accumulation, 34% reduction in proteinuria, prevented a loss of renal function and abrogated glomerular crescent formation (170). Furthermore, delayed administration of a soluble TNF-α receptor in established anti-GBM disease in WKY rats significantly reduced albuminuria and glomerular inflammation, including the prevalence of crescent formation. (171). The success of these studies in experimental RPGN has led to clinical trials in vasculitis (see Experimental Approaches to Treatment, below).

One of the earliest described cytokines is macrophage migration inhibitory factor (MIF) which plays a key role in the DTH reaction (172). MIF has proinflammatory actions as well as being a counter-regulatory of glucocorticoids (172). Blood lymphocytes from patients with RPGN produce MIF activity *in vitro* in the presence of GBM (95). More recently, an *in situ* hybridization and immunohistochemistry study identified increased MIF expression in human RPGN. The prominent T cell and macrophage infiltrates in human crescentic glomerulonephritis were largely restricted to areas of MIF upregulation and contributed to glomerular hypercellularity, glomerular focal and segmental lesions, crescent formation, tubulitis and granulomatous lesions (126). In addition, increased urinary MIF excretion has been identified in patients with crescentic glomerulonephritis and was found to correlate with renal dysfunction, histological damage and leukocytic infiltration (173).

Production of MIF-like bioactivity has been described in rat anti-GBM disease (174). More recently, increased MIF messenger RNA (mRNA) and protein expression has been quantified and localized in rat crescentic anti-GBM glomerulonephritis (175). Anti-MIF antibody treatment in this model attenuated leukocyte infiltration, reduced proteinuria, prevented renal dysfunction, reduced proteinuria, and markedly reduced histological damage, including glomerular crescent formation (176). Furthermore, delayed anti-MIF treatment was able to partially reverse established crescentic disease (177), demonstrating the therapeutic potential of this strategy. Using a different approach to demonstrate the pathologic effects of MIF, Sasaki et al. (178) induced transgenic overexpression of MIF in mouse podocytes that resulted in glomerulosclerosis and renal failure.

Signaling Pathways

An alternative approach to blocking individual cytokines or growth factors that mediate renal inflammation or fibrosis is to target common intracellular signalling pathways by which these factors exert their actions. Engagement of a wide range of cell surface receptors (i.e., IL-1 and TNF-α receptors, Toll-like receptors [TLR], T cell receptor, CD40) can lead to activation of the nuclear factor-kappaB (NF-κB) signaling pathway, resulting in inflammation, immune regulation, survival, and cell proliferation responses (179). Activation of the NF-κB pathway has been demonstrated in human and experimental RPGN (180–182). Efforts to block NF-κB signaling have suffered from a lack of specific reagents. However, gene therapy of rat anti-GBM disease using a specific NF-κB decoy, substantially inhibited proteinuria and histologic damage in association with a significant reduction in leukocytic infiltration, renal expression of cytokines, and leukocyte adhesion molecules (183). Further evidence that NF-κB signaling may promote renal injury comes from a study in which administration of unmethylated CpG oligonucleotides (common in bacteria and viruses but not in mammalian cells), that bind to and activate TLR9, caused increased macrophage accumulation, worse proteinuria, and more severe histologic lesions in a mouse model of immune-complex glomerulonephritis (184).

Cellular stresses (i.e., reactive oxidative species, nitric oxide, ultraviolet [UV] light, and osmotic stress) and cytokines and growth factors (i.e., IL-1, TNF-α, angiotensin II, TGF-β1) all induce signaling through the p38 and c-Jun NH2-terminal

kinase (JNK) mitogen-activated protein kinase (MAPK) pathways (185). A marked increase in p38 MAPK activity has been described in human RPGN, although the individual cell types involved in p38 MAPK signaling is controversial (186,187). Stambe et al. (190,191) identified p38 MAPK activation in infiltrating macrophages as well as many intrinsic renal cells including podocytes and tubular epithelial cells, and found a significant correlation between the number of cells with phosphorylation (activation) of p38 MAPK and the degree of renal dysfunction and histologic damage. Administration of small molecule inhibitors of p38 MAPK have been shown to inhibit the development of renal injury in rat models of anti-GBM glomerulonephritis (189,190). Specifically, upregulation of P-selectin gene expression and the transient glomerular neutrophil influx that follows the deposition of anti-GBM antibodies was shown to be dependent upon p38 MAPK signaling (190).

Increased signaling through the JNK pathway has also been described in rat crescentic anti-GBM glomerulonephritis (181,191). *In vitro* studies suggest that blocking JNK signaling may be beneficial in RPGN, but no specific blocking studies in disease models have yet been reported.

Glucocorticoids are a mainstay treatment of RPGN. One of the beneficial effects of glucocorticoids may derive from their ability to inhibit signaling through the NF-κB and JNK signaling pathways (181,192,193). Furthermore, JNK can inhibit glucocorticoid receptor-mediated transcriptional activation by directly phosphorylating the glucocorticoid receptor (194). Thus, development of specific pharmacologic inhibitors of NF-κB and JNK signaling pathways may provide more effective treatment with fewer side effects than with current glucocorticoid therapy.

Bone morphogenic protein-7 (BMP7), a member of the TGF-β1 superfamily, can block TGF-β1-induced fibrosis (195). Administration of recombinant human BMP7 protein in a mouse model of anti-GBM glomerulonephritis beginning one week after disease induction prevented disease progression and delaying BMP7 treatment until week 3, after disease induction was still able to substantially protect the animals from end-stage renal disease and reverse disease pathology (196). Thus, antagonism of TGF-β1-induced cell signaling is another approach with therapeutic potential in RPGN.

THE MECHANISM OF CRESCENT FORMATION

The composition of cellular crescents and the mechanisms by which these arise has been an issue of debate for many years. Despite this, however, there is general agreement that cellular crescents can undergo fibrous organization by progressing through a fibrocellular stage to become a fibrous crescent (197). Cellular crescents can resolve as seen in cases of poststreptococcal crescentic glomerulonephritis and flares of crescentic IgA nephropathy. The key issue as to whether cellular crescents can resolve or progress may center on whether Bowman's capsule remains intact or becomes ruptured.

Epithelial Cells in Crescent Formation

The initial histologic studies describing crescent formation were done over 100 years ago by Langhans (1), and his sketches are reproduced in Figure 60-1. Since then, the cellular crescent traditionally has been considered to be composed of proliferated epithelial cells. This belief has been based primarily on light and ultrastructural studies of cells of the crescents

(8,9,15,198). Analysis of crescents by immunohistochemistry has identified monocyte/macrophages and epithelial cells as the predominant cell types involved, with fibroblasts present with the development of fibrous organization. However, the relative proportion of macrophages to epithelial cells varies widely in the different studies reported (16,50,199,200). Although this variation may simply reflect the highly heterogenous nature of crescents within individual biopsies and the heterogenous nature of the patient groups exhibiting glomerular crescent formation, there may also be an important mechanistic reason. A study by Boucher et al. (92) found that cellular crescents contained 55% to 95% epithelial cells and 15% to 35% mononuclear leukocytes when Bowman's capsule remained intact, whereas macrophages and T cells were the dominant population in crescents when Bowman's capsule was ruptured. Thus, the integrity of Bowman's capsule may have a profound influence on crescent composition and progression to fibrous organization—a factor not examined in most human studies.

Recent studies in mouse anti-GBM glomerulonephritis have identified early cellular crescents containing epithelial cells which lack any detectable infiltration of F4/80+ macrophages, indicating an epithelial origin of the early cellular crescents (201,202). The presence of F4/80+ macrophages was only seen in crescents at a later stage when Bowman's capsule became ruptured enabling migration into Bowman's space of the prominent periglomerular F4/80+ macrophage infiltrate. In this model, podocyte bridges between the glomerular tuft and Bowman's capsule have been proposed as the first step in the process of crescent formation (202). The use of genetic markers demonstrated that many of the epithelial cells seen in these crescents were of podocyte origin that had dedifferentiated and lost their characteristic podocyte markers upon detachment from the GBM (203). While this is an appealing hypothesis, a note of caution is warranted in that glomerular macrophages are phenotypically heterogeneous and, in particular, mouse glomerular macrophages do not express the F4/80 antigen (204). Furthermore, macrophages in early cellular crescents have been identified in mouse anti-GBM glomerulonephritis using alternative markers (110,204).

Mononuclear Cells in Crescent Formation

The first direct demonstration that mononuclear phagocytes are involved in crescent formation came from studies in which large numbers of highly motile cells which phagocytosed latex and yeast particles, and had ultrastructural characteristics of macrophages, were observed in the outgrowth from cultured glomeruli that had been isolated from patients with RPGN (120). These macrophage outgrowths were predominantly from crescents, with much smaller macrophage outgrowths detected in other types of non-crescentic glomerulonephritis (18).

To identify the cell types present in glomerular crescents in patients with RPGN, we developed specific monoclonal antibodies to human epithelial cells and to macrophages and monocytes (23,38,205). To assess the cell types present in the different stages of the evolution of the crescent, 12 patients with RPGN, 9 with cellular, and 3 with sclerosed crescents, were examined (16). Cellular crescents consisted of 35% macrophages, 12% polymorphonuclear leukocytes, and 10% epithelial cells. Sclerosed crescents contained few macrophages (5%) but similar proportions of polymorphonuclear leukocytes (11%) and epithelial cells (12%). Many of the crescent cells were unlabeled, but they were probably fibroblasts because of their morphologic appearance and the expression of surface fibronectin. Figure 60-11 demonstrates the complementary staining of epithelial cells and macrophages in the glomerular tuft as well as the crescent in the renal biopsy of a patient with RPGN. The presence of large numbers of macrophages in crescents was confirmed by the unique study of Schiffer and Michael (206). Crescentic glomerulonephritis developed in two human female kidney grafts that had been transplanted into male recipients. As demonstrated by the presence of Y-body positivity, 35% of cells in the crescents were infiltrating leukocytes from the recipient.

The accumulation of macrophages within crescents is thought to be part of a DTH-like reaction. The components of the DTH reaction (T-cell infiltration and activation, macrophage accumulation, procoagulant activity and fibrin deposition), as well as local production of MIF, have all been documented in RPGN (3,16,31,32,90,95,96,120,126). The presence of humoral immune reactants, such as immunoglobulin and complement, are not necessary for crescent formation (11). The presence of DTH reactants has also been characterized in ANCA-associated RPGN (94).

Animal studies provide strong support for a pivotal role of macrophages in crescent formation. In early studies, Kondo et al. (207) performed a morphologic evaluation of a rabbit model of anti-GBM glomerulonephritis in which large numbers of clear cells in the crescent and glomerular tuft, with the features of monocytes, were described. Further morphologic support came from studies on serial renal biopsies of animals developing crescentic nephritis (208). The initial event of crescent formation was shown to be the deposition of fibrin within Bowman's space. This was followed by an influx of mononuclear cells into Bowman's space, where they phagocytosed fibrin. Epithelioid and giant cell transformation then occurred. These morphologic observations suggest that crescent formation is a result of the transformation of infiltrating macrophages (Fig. 60-12). In Figure 60-13, a scanning electron micrograph of an isolated glomerulus in tissue culture from a rabbit with nephrotoxic nephritis, with illustrated macrophages in the crescent.

In experimental RPGN induced by either anti-GBM antibodies (209) or immune complexes (68), enzyme histochemistry has demonstrated that most crescentic cells have an enzymatic profile consistent with a macrophage origin. Cattell and Arlidge (210) using irradiation to induce leukocyte depletion, also suggested that the crescents originate from circulating leukocytes. Furthermore, in an ultrastructural analysis of crescent formation in both rats and rabbits with nephrotoxic nephritis, Clarke et al. (211) concluded that the crescent cells evolve predominantly from circulating macrophages.

As discussed earlier, a variety of strategies have been used to inhibit T cell and macrophage accumulation activation and thus prevent renal injury in experimental models of RPGN (see Pathogenesis). In particular, delaying treatments that target T cell co-activation molecules (CD28-CD80/86 interaction), cytokines (IL-1, TNF-α, or MIF), adhesion molecules (VLA-4) or chemokines (OPN and MCP-1) until crescentic disease is already established has been successful in suppressing further crescent formation and disease progression (104,143, 145,157,168,171,177).

Parietal epithelial cells may be important in attracting macrophages into Bowman's space via the secretion of chemotactic molecules and expression of leukocyte adhesion molecules (Fig. 60-10). Parietal epithelial cells are induced to express, or upregulate, a variety of molecules involved in glomerular macrophage and T cell accumulation, including chemotactic molecules (MCP-1, OPN, MIF) and leukocyte adhesion molecules (ICAM-1, VCAM-1, CD44) (143,156,165,175, 212,213). A common feature of these chemotactic and adhesion molecules is that they can be induced by the cytokine IL-1. Indeed, one of the reasons for the success of IL-1 blockade in established crescentic anti-GBM disease is the suppression of glomerular expression of ICAM-1, OPN, and CD44 by intrinsic glomerular cells (165–168).

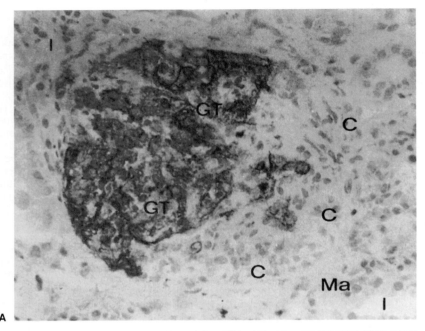

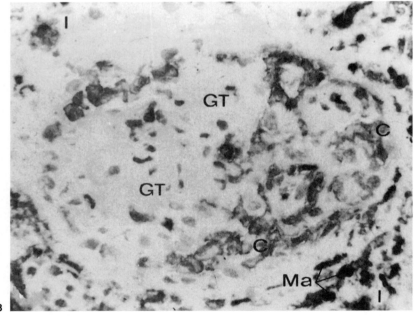

FIGURE 60-11. Serial cryostat sections from the renal biopsy of a patient with rapidly progressive glomerulonephritis, with immunohistochemical labeling of monoclonal antibodies by the four-layer peroxidase antiperoxidase technique (23). In both **A** and **B,** the glomerular tuft (GT) has been compressed into the left half of Bowman's space by the crescent (C), which occupies the right half. **A:** The epithelial cells of the glomerulus (GT) are stained using the antiglomerular epithelial cell marker PHM5. This labels all the epithelial cells in the compressed glomerular tuft (GT), but virtually none of the cells of the crescent (C). **B:** Macrophages (Ma) are stained using monoclonal antibody FMC32 recognizing monocyte/macrophages. Over 90% of the cells in the crescent are stained together with many macrophages (Ma) in the interstitium (I) surrounding the glomerulus. (Hematoxylin and eosin, magnification ×250.)

Local proliferation is another mechanism of macrophage accumulation during crescent formation within Bowman's space (Fig. 60-14). In rat anti-GBM glomerulonephritis, greater than 50% of glomeruli develop crescent formation by day 21 with macrophages accounting for 50% to 80% of total crescent cells (214). A striking finding was that over half of the macrophages within crescents were proliferating on the basis of PCNA expression, bromodeoxyuridine incorporation and the presence of macrophage mitotic figures, which was a higher level of macrophage proliferation than that present in the glomerular tuft (214). Marked macrophage proliferation within crescents has been confirmed in studies of human RPGN (93). Furthermore, expression of macrophage colony-stimulating factor (M-CSF) within crescents suggests that local M-CSF production drives the local macrophage proliferation within Bowman's space (122).

Yet another mechanism by which macrophages and T cell may enter Bowman's capsule during crescent formation is through ruptures in Bowman's capsule. Boucher et al. (92) demonstrated that epithelial cells were present in greater numbers than macrophages in cellular crescents when Bowman's capsule was intact, but that this pattern was reversed with rupture of Bowman's capsule. Periglomerular infiltration of macrophages and T cells is a prominent feature in both human (31,92,215,216) and experimental crescentic glomerulonephritis (63,97,101). Indeed, it may be case that the periglomerular infiltrate may actually mediate rupture of Bowman's capsule. In a study of rat anti-GBM glomerulonephritis, 25% to 52% of glomerular cross-sections exhibiting Bowman's capsule rupture had no evidence of crescent formation, whereas focal periglomerular accumulation of immune activated (IL-2R$^+$) CD4$^+$ T-cells and macrophages were invariably present

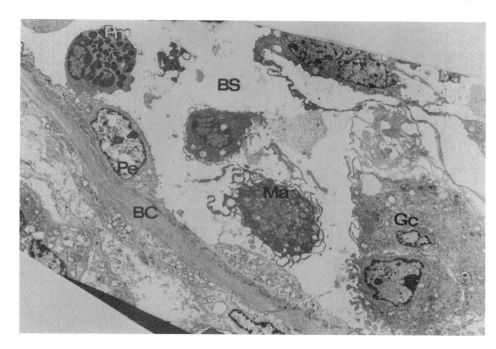

FIGURE 60-12. Transmission electron micrograph depicting a glomerulus from a rabbit with nephrotoxic nephritis at day 10 of the disease (i.e., the stage of early crescent formation). Bowman's space (BS), bounded on one side by Bowman's capsule (BC) and a parietal epithelial cell (Pe), contains a number of exudative macrophages (Ma) and a polymorphonuclear leukocyte (Pm). A macrophage that has undergone giant cell (Gc) transformation can be seen. (Magnification ×4,800; courtesy of Prof. E. F. Glasgow.)

at the site of Bowman's capsule rupture (97). Disruption of Bowman's capsule facilitated the entry of periglomerular fibroblasts, macrophages and activated (IL-2R⁺) T-cells into Bowman's space and the development of glomerular fibrosis (97).

Deposition of Fibrin in Crescent Formation

The experiments of Vassalli and McCluskey (217) provided the first evidence that the presence of fibrin in Bowman's space is an important stimulus for crescent formation. A causal link between fibrin deposition and macrophage migration into Bowman's space was provided by studies in which defibrination of animals with ancrod prevented crescent formation in rabbit anti-GBM glomerulonephritis, despite the inflammatory re-

action and macrophage accumulation in the glomerular tuft being unaltered (218). This finding is in accord with the observation in humans that fibrin is most commonly found in freshly formed crescents and tends to disappear as the crescents become sclerotic (45). In addition, we demonstrated that macrophages in the crescent in human RPGN have tissue factor expressed on their surface, as recognized by a specific monoclonal antibody, and that these macrophages are associated with fibrin deposition (90). Fibrin deposition is also present in crescents in ANCA-associated RPGN (94).

The importance of fibrin deposition in the progression of rabbit crescentic anti-GBM disease has been demonstrated by Zoja et al. (219). Recombinant plasminogen activator, which causes lysis of fibrin clots by activating plasminogen to plasmin, reduced glomerular fibrin deposition and crescent formation together with prevention of renal failure. Consistent with this

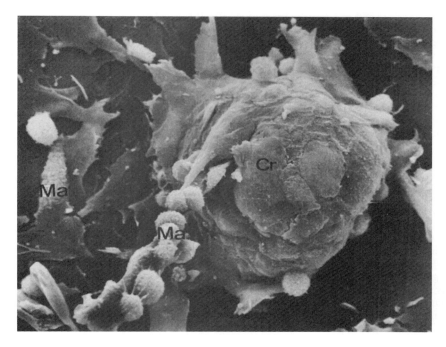

FIGURE 60-13. Scanning electron micrograph of a nephrotoxic glomerulus in tissue culture. The glomerulus itself is covered by a cellular crescent (Cr) from which macrophages (Ma) are emerging. (Courtesy of Prof. E. F. Glasgow.)

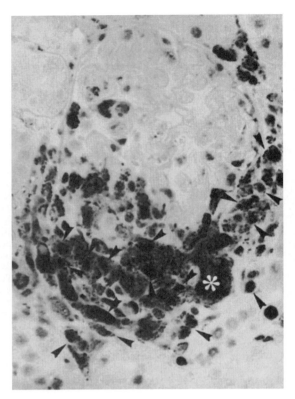

FIGURE 60-14. A rat glomerulus demonstrating an extensive crescent from an animal with anti-glomerular basement membrane nephritis. Macrophages are demonstrated using the ED-1 monoclonal antibody (*brown*), and the proliferating cell nuclear antigen antibody (*blue*) has been used to demonstrate proliferating cells. Proliferating macrophages are indicated by *arrowheads* and mononuclear giant cells by the *asterisk*. (Periodic acid-Schiff, magnification ×400.) (See Color Plate.)

finding, mice deficient for the fibrinogen gene develop a less severe anti-GBM glomerulonephritis compared to wild-type mice with a significant reduction in glomerular crescent formation (220).

Macrophages have been shown to be responsible for the glomerular fibrin deposition and express augmented procoagulant activity in rabbit anti-GBM disease (221). Furthermore, blockade of tissue factor, using either neutralizing antibodies or recombinant tissue factor pathway inhibitor, have been shown to inhibit renal injury in rabbit anti-GBM glomerulonephritis (222). In addition, an important role for thrombin in mediating fibrin deposition and consequent renal injury and glomerular crescent formation has been demonstrated in a mouse model of anti-GBM glomerulonephritis using hirudin as a selective thrombin antagonist and mice deficient in protease-activated receptor (PAR)-1—a cellular receptor for thrombin (223).

Fibroblasts in Crescent Formation

Cellular crescents can undergo a process of fibrous organization which involves a fibrocellular stage characterized by the presence of fibroblasts and collagen deposition within Bowman's space followed by a fibrous stage in which progressive collagen deposition within Bowman's space and a loss of cells leads to scar formation (197). At this stage, the glomerular tuft is often substantially compressed with capillary obliteration.

The entry of fibroblasts into Bowman's space is generally accepted as the key event in determining fibrous organization of cellular crescents. There are at least four possible ori-

gins of the fibroblasts that accumulate in fibrocellular crescents. First, the major source of these cells is probably from the periglomerular area. As discussed above (see Mononuclear Cells in Crescent Formation), rupture of Bowman's capsule is an important determinant of crescent composition. Fibroblast accumulation and upregulation of collagen mRNA levels in the periglomerular area is a very early event in experimental anti-GBM glomerulonephritis (224), and a number of studies have suggested that periglomerular fibroblasts enter Bowman's space via ruptures in Bowman's capsule to induce fibrous organization of cellular crescents (97,225,226). Second, glomerular mesangial cells can differentiate into α-smooth muscle actin (SMA)—expressing motile cells with a myofibroblast-like phenotype (227). These mesangial-derived SMA+ myofibroblasts could easily migrate into Bowman's space and promote fibrosis. Third, epithelial-mesenchymal transdifferentiation of parietal epithelial cells into SMA+ myofibroblasts has been described in crescents using immunohistochemistry and electron microscopy in rat anti-GBM glomerulonephritis (228). Fourth, a circulating fibrocyte population has been described which has been shown to migrate into sites of tissue damage and promote tissue fibrosis (229,230). Such a cell type has the potential to contribute to the development of fibrocellular crescents, but no studies to date have provided evidence to support this possibility. Irrespective of the origin of the SMA+ myofibroblast-like cells that enter cellular crescents, the high level of cell proliferation evident in this population is likely to make an important contribution to the ongoing accumulation of these cells (214,228). The production of growth factors such as PDGF, FGF-2, and TGF-β1 within crescents is likely to promote myofibroblast proliferation and matrix deposition (228,231,232).

CLINICAL FEATURES

Rapidly progressive glomerulonephritis is an uncommon disease, comprising approximately 2% of all cases of glomerulonephritis, although the reported incidence varies from 1.5% to 5% (12,42,57,233). In population terms, a German study reported a calculated annual incidence of RPGN of 0.7 per 100,000 population (234). A recent French report noted an increasing incidence of crescentic nephritis, with incidence rates for the 60 to 79 year age group increasing from 5 per million prior to 1985 to 27 per million since 1996 (235). Similarly, a Chinese report of over 10,000 renal biopsies noted an increase from 0.5% of all biopsies to 2.2% when comparing the 1980's to the 1990's (233). The disease is predominantly seen in the third to sixth decade, with a reported median age ranging from 39 to 58 years (9–13,236,237). Occurrence in childhood is very rare (235,238–240). Patients with RPGN associated with anti-GBM antibody or endocapillary cell proliferation tend to be younger than those with ANCA-positive RPGN (14). In contrast, severe crescentic glomerulonephritis of poststreptococcal etiology is most frequent in children (10,238) whereas crescentic disease in the elderly is not infrequently associated with systemic vasculitis, particularly with microscopic polyangiitis (10,241–243). Men are more commonly affected than women (2:1) (10–14) and this ratio is higher in patients with anti-GBM disease. There is a genetic predisposition to RPGN in that there is a susceptibility to anti-GBM antibody synthesis in patients who are human leukocyte antigen (HLA)-DR2 (244,245) The resultant glomerulonephritis is reported to be more severe when it is associated with HLA-B7 (244).

Despite the varying underlying immunopathogenetic mechanisms of RPGN, the clinical features are remarkably similar in all three subgroups (Table 60-2). It is not possible to reliably predict on clinical grounds which immunopathologic group the patient belongs to (anti-GBM, immune, or ANCA positive). Indeed, the signs and symptoms depend more on the stage of

TABLE 60-2

CLINICAL FEATURES OF RAPIDLY PROGRESSIVE GLOMERULONEPHRITIS

Median age: fifth and sixth decades	
Sex: M/F = 2:1	
Prodromal illness: common (upper respiratory infection, "flulike" illness, fever)	
Presenting features:	Percent of patients:
Nonspecific symptoms of malaise, lethargy	>90
Symptoms of renal failure	60
Oliguria	>60
Edema	60–70
Macroscopic hematuria	20–30
Nephrotic syndrome	10–30
Acute nephritic syndrome	10–20
Hypertension	10–20

the disease at presentation. Usually, the onset is insidious, and patients present with nonspecific symptoms for several weeks (7,9,12,79,236,237,243,246–250).

These symptoms include malaise, lethargy, weakness, anorexia, and nausea. At presentation, many have symptoms of renal failure. Most patients with advanced disease are oliguric, and some are anuric. Occasionally, the onset is very acute, with features of an acute nephritic syndrome, and advanced renal failure develops over a few days. Macroscopic hematuria is not uncommon, and microscopic hematuria is invariable. Edema is seen in most patients, and the nephrotic syndrome is seen in 10% to 45% (9,12,237,251). Hypertension may be present in up to 60% (251), but is mild when not due to sodium and water retention (14). In approximately 50% of patients, an upper respiratory or influenza-like illness precedes the other symptoms; however, only rarely has a specific viral etiology been established. Aronson and Phillips (252) found evidence of infection with coxsackie virus B5 in six patients with acute oliguric renal failure, and an outbreak of influenza A2 has been associated with RPGN with anti-GBM antibody (253). A greater than expected association with exposure to hydrocarbon solvents also has been reported, especially for anti-GBM disease (254) and other researchers have noticed an increased association with myocardial infarction (11), malignancy (11,255), and membranous glomerulonephritis.

By contrast, patients with crescentic glomerulonephritis associated with vasculitis may have prominent systemic symptoms, such as recurring fever, purpuric skin rash, arthritis/arthralgia, mucosal ulceration, and respiratory symptoms, including dyspnea and hemoptysis (79,256). Similarly, patients with crescentic glomerulonephritis associated with systemic illnesses such as scleroderma, systemic lupus erythematosus (SLE), endocarditis, cryoglobulinemia, or Schönlein-Henoch syndrome may have the systemic features of these diseases.

Frank hemoptysis suggests Goodpasture's syndrome (glomerulonephritis and pulmonary hemorrhage associated with anti-GBM antibody), but this also can be a prominent feature of systemic vasculitis (56). Goodpasture's syndrome is the combination of hematuria, hemoptysis, and (acute) renal failure, but is not specific for anti-GBM disease and is relatively common in the vasculitides, especially Wegener's granulomatosis (234). Indeed, in one study of patients with pulmonary-renal syndrome, 54% had ANCA disease, 7% had ANCA and anti-GBM antibodies, and only 6% had anti-GBM alone (257). Thus, presenting symptoms may be relatively nonspecific and variable and, apart from a rapid deterioration in renal function, provide little to alert the clinician to the seriousness of this relatively rare disease.

LABORATORY FINDINGS

The laboratory findings are summarized in Table 60-3.

Nondiscriminatory Findings

Microscopic hematuria is invariable, the red cells being dysmorphic, indicating a glomerular lesion (258). Red cell, granular, and leukocyte casts are frequent, although the urinary sediment correlates poorly with the severity of disease.

Proteinuria is always present, although in the nephrotic range in only 10% to 45% (9,12,237,251). More severe disease is less likely to be associated with heavy proteinuria, which simply reflects the low glomerular filtration rate. Fibrin degradation products may be elevated in both the serum and the urine (259–261).

Most patients have elevated serum creatinine and blood urea nitrogen levels at presentation and often are in severe renal failure, with a serum creatinine elevated to more than 5.0 mg/dL and a creatinine clearance that is less than 10% of normal. The degree of renal failure at presentation depends on the chronicity and severity of the renal lesion. However,

TABLE 60-3

LABORATORY FEATURES OF RAPIDLY PROGRESSIVE GLOMERULONEPHRITIS

Urine:	Microscopic hematuria (dysmorphic): 100% of patients
	Casts (red cell, granular, leukocyte): common
	Proteinuria: 100% (>3 g/24 hr: 10%–30%)
Renal function:	Impaired: 100%
	Creatinine clearance <20 mL/min: (30%)
Normal renal size	
Normocytic normochromic anemia	
Erythrocyte sedimentation rate: moderate rise (<100 mm first hour)	
Circulating antiglomerular basement membrane antibody (30%)	
Circulating immune complexes (10%–15%)	
Serum complement components: normal	
Anti-DNA antibody: negative	
Antistreptolysin 0 titer: no rise	
Antineutrophil cytoplasmic antibody (80% if absent glomerular immune deposits)	

TABLE 60-4

PROGNOSIS OF RAPIDLY PROGRESSIVE GLOMERULONEPHRITIS ACCORDING TO URINE OUTPUT AT PRESENTATION

	No. of patients	Percentage of patients with renal function at 12 months		
		All patients (%)	Nonoliguric (%)	Oliguric (%)
Whitworth, 1976 (12)	60	72	87	53
Morrin, 1978 (14)	29	31	59	20
Neild, 1983 (13)	19	52	100	10
Heilman, 1987 (199)	24	40	78	22
Weighted mean		54	81	34

as discussed in the following section, most untreated patients progress to end-stage renal failure within several weeks or months.

A normochromic normocytic anemia frequently is observed and often is more profound than expected from the degree of renal failure. In patients with lung hemorrhage, especially those with anti-GBM disease, anemia may be severe, and these two factors contribute to poor tissue oxygenation. Lung hemorrhage frequently is associated with an increased diffusing capacity for carbon monoxide (262). The erythrocyte sedimentation rate usually is elevated; however, if it is very high (>100 mm in the first hour), an underlying systemic disease such as vasculitis should be suspected.

Findings Specific to Rapidly Progressive Glomerulonephritis

Serum complement levels typically are not depressed (9,44, 263). Circulating immune complexes are present in 20% to 30% of patients with immune deposits in glomeruli, suggesting an immune complex etiology for their disease (264,265). However, circulating immune complexes also have been described in sera of patients with no glomerular immune deposits (3,266,267) and probably are of little clinical value. The presence of ANCA suggests the vasculitic group (43,46,69,268). In the group of patients with RPGN who have linear deposition of antibody along the GBM, circulating anti-GBM antibody usually is detected (269–271), particularly if a specific and sensitive radioimmunoassay is used (55,272,273). About a quarter of patients with anti-GBM antibodies also have detectable ANCA antibodies (274).

Findings Related to an Underlying Condition

The presence of circulating cryoglobulin has been reported in some patients (266,272,275), particularly in association with hepatitis C (276). Anti-DNA antibodies usually are not found outside of those patients with SLE. Hypocomplementemia may be seen in the crescentic glomerulonephritis of both poststreptococcal glomerulonephritis and SLE.

NATURAL HISTORY

As mentioned previously, most patients have severe renal failure at the time of presentation, reflecting extensive glomerular damage. Thus prognosis already is predetermined, at least in part, by the degree of irreversible renal damage.

In several reported series of patients with RPGN (9,44,251, 277), the authors have attempted to determine prognostic factors and the effect of treatment. These series are not strictly comparable because there are variations in the criteria for diagnosis—the underlying immunopathogenetic processes, the extent of crescent formation (>30% crescents, >50% crescents, or >80% crescents), and the inclusion or exclusion of clinically suspected microscopic vasculitis or Goodpasture's syndrome. Moreover, a valid life table analysis of persistence of renal function and survival of patients rarely has been undertaken. However, a synthesis of these reports indicates that approximately 20% of patients present with permanent end-stage renal failure. Approximately 50% progress to end-stage renal failure by 1 year, and 75% by 2 years, although these results are better in ANCA disease, with up to 90% of patients in remission at 1 year (278) (Table 60-4). A variety of patterns of deterioration or improvement in renal function are seen. Some patients show spontaneous rapid improvement in renal function soon after presentation. In a few patients, this improvement is sustained, and in others it is temporary, with the patients drifting into renal failure within months. Other patients show progressive decline in renal function after presentation, whereas others maintain stable renal function. These variable patterns of outcome probably reflect a number of factors, including the persistence or loss of the causative factors, the degree of initial renal damage, the severity of the scarring process that subsequently evolves (e.g., fibrosis of crescents and interstitial fibrosis), and the development or absence of vascular damage and hypertension. These patterns also may be altered by the various therapeutic measures used in this disease.

Urine Output at Presentation

It has become evident that the presence of oliguria at presentation of RPGN is associated with a significantly poorer outcome than is seen in patients who have maintained good urine output. Table 60-4 summarizes the results from four series of patients with RPGN (12–14,277) and the persistence of renal function at 12 months, in patients who presented with or without oliguria, is listed. Although there is a wide variation, each series shows a significant difference in survival between oliguric and nonoliguric patients. Temporary or sustained recovery of renal function was seen in only 34% of patients who were oliguric at presentation. On the other hand, 81% of nonoliguric patients were alive at 12 months with adequate renal function.

Patients who are anuric at presentation are less likely to recover renal function. The poor outcome associated with oligoanuria reflects the degree of crescent formation, as in 80% of oligoanuric patients, more than 80% of the glomeruli are involved (13,239,279).

TABLE 60-5

IMPROVEMENT IN RENAL FUNCTION FOLLOWING RAPIDLY PROGRESSIVE GLOMERULONEPHRITIS ACCORDING TO THE EXTENT OF CRESCENT FORMATION

	100%	90–99%	80–89%	70–79%	60–69%
Number of patients (total 200)	66	43	36	35	20
Number of patients with improvement in renal function	10	14	18	20	11
Percentage	15%	32%	50%	56%	55%

(Adapted from Neild GH, et al. Rapidly progressive glomerulonephritis with extensive glomerular crescent formation. *Q J Med* 1983;207:395, with permission.)

Extent of Crescent Formation

Several studies have shown a positive correlation between the percentage of glomeruli affected by crescent formation and the severity of initial and subsequent renal failure (11–14,90, 236,243,273,280).

In two studies, all patients with crescents in 100% of the glomeruli progressed rapidly to end-stage renal failure (14, 239), whereas other authors have reported the recovery of renal function in less than 10% of such patients (281,282). Habib (239,283) found a similar incidence of end-stage renal failure in patients with more than 80% crescents. Morrin et al. (14) found that 39% of patients with more than 80% crescents showed some recovery of renal function, compared with 90% of patients with less than 60% crescents. Neild et al. (13) reviewed 11 published series of RPGN, totaling 200 patients, and confirmed the findings that the more extensive the crescent formation, the less there is a chance of recovery of renal function (Table 60-5).

The development of crescents in other forms of primary glomerulonephritis (e.g., membranoproliferative glomerulonephritis) and in glomerulonephritis of a systemic disease also is associated with a poor outcome. However, in the setting of IgA nephropathy with synpharyngitic hematuria, crescents may not be indicative of a poor prognosis (284).

Changes in the Glomerular Tuft

Endocapillary cell proliferation (glomerular hypercellularity) has been reported as a good prognostic feature compared with normocellularity of the glomerular tuft (13,14,27,237). Morrin et al. (14) reported recovery of renal function in only 30% of patients with RPGN who had normal glomerular tuft cellularity, compared with 50% of patients with hypercellular glomerular tufts.

Glomerular tuft necrosis is thought to be a poor prognostic feature (14,237,285). This notion is supported by the observation that in the microscopic form of polyarteritis, where segmental or diffuse tuft necrosis is very prominent, severe renal failure may be present with minimal crescent formation. Global glomerular sclerosis and breaks in Bowman's capsule also are poor prognostic features (286).

Interstitial Fibrosis and Tubular Atrophy

It has been reported that the extent of interstitial fibrosis correlates with the severity of initial and ultimate renal dysfunction (237,240,286). Striker et al. (237) found that if interstitial fibrosis involved more than 30% of the biopsy tissue, then recovery of renal function was unusual, and the patients often were anuric at presentation.

Immunopathogenesis and Outcome

The group of patients with ANCA-positive RPGN seems to have the best prognosis (11), although this has not been the experience of all authors (12). Granular immune deposits also have been reported as indicative of a better prognosis (14). On the other hand, other authors reported a poor prognosis for patients with granular immune deposits (12). This conflict of findings may reflect the inclusion, in some series, of patients with poststreptococcal crescentic glomerulonephritis. The group with RPGN associated with anti-GBM antibody has the worst prognosis (13,14,20,234). The reason for this occurrence is not clear. The chronicity of the immune insult may explain the worse prognosis. Urine protein excretion, degree of interstitial cellular infiltration, and age show a weak correlation with outcome (277). A summary of the factors determining the outcome of RPGN is outlined in Table 60-6.

TREATMENT

Many therapeutic regimens have been used in the treatment of RPGN, and the relative benefits of these regimens are very much in dispute. Because of the rarity of RPGN, there have been very few controlled trials comparing either one treatment regimen with another or with no treatment. Many studies have simply assessed outcome compared with historical controls. This is not a valid comparison, particularly given the advances made in the minimization of progression of renal disease with less specific therapy, such as control of hypertension, use of angiotensin-converting enzyme inhibitors, diet, and the more successful management of renal failure, including temporary dialysis. In addition, many of the therapies used to treat RPGN have the potential to induce serious complications, including sepsis, hemorrhage, sterility, and malignancy.

Few controlled trials have been performed and therapy has been largely empirical. Further evaluation of the various therapies should, therefore, continue. It also must be said that several authors have noted spectacular recovery from RPGN in an appreciable number of patients given immunosuppressive and anticoagulant agents, in whom the expected recovery rate would be nil (e.g., advanced renal failure with 100% crescents). These observations coupled with our understanding of the immunopathogenesis of RPGN have been sufficient evidence for

TABLE 60-6

FACTORS DETERMINING THE OUTCOME OF RAPIDLY PROGRESSIVE GLOMERULONEPHRITIS

Factors	Poorer prognosis	Better prognosis
Urine output at presentation	Oliguric	Nonoliguric
Extent of crescent formation	>80%	50–80%
The glomerulus	Fibrinoid necrosis	Endocapillary cell proliferation
Glomerular immune deposits	Linear deposition (antiglomerular basement membrane)	Granular deposition (immune complex) or no immune reactants
Interstitium	Interstitial fibrosis and tubular atrophy	

many renal physicians routinely to use this therapy for such patients.

Corticosteroids

Because of their antiinflammatory properties, corticosteroids are frequently used in the treatment of RPGN. There are very few published data on the use of corticosteroids alone in experimental crescentic glomerulonephritis. However, several reports have demonstrated marked improvement in renal function with intravenous methylprednisolone (287–289). Holdsworth and Bellomo (290) and Tipping and Holdsworth (291) have shown that glomerular injury induced by macrophages in rabbits can be reduced substantially by corticosteroids, whereas injury induced by polymorphonuclear leukocytes is unaffected. As discussed earlier, both polymorphonuclear leukocytes and macrophages are thought to be injurious in crescentic glomerulonephritis. More recent data suggest that corticosteroids inhibit the activation of NF-κB, an important transcription protein in the immune response, resulting in inhibition of inflammatory cytokine production (292).

There is no evidence that oral steroids alone are of benefit in nonvasculitic RPGN (7,243,281,293). Their use is usually in conjunction with immunosuppressive agents. The lack of benefit from steroids alone is strikingly different from their often dramatic effect in necrotizing (ANCA positive) crescentic glomerulonephritis associated with vasculitis (263,294,295). In the latter condition, corticosteroids alone offer a remission rate similar to that obtained with other therapy (see below), but a threefold higher relapse rate (296). However, several reports indicate that high-dose intravenous "pulse" methylprednisolone therapy, given daily or on alternate days for three to six doses, can lead to dramatic and sustained improvement in renal function in nonvasculitic RPGN (11,280,296–302). Bolton et al. (297,303) found this benefit only in patients with RPGN that was not caused by anti-GBM antibody. All these investigators have commented on the low incidence of side effects of intravenous pulse steroid therapy. There is some evidence that intravenous methylprednisolone has a distinct effect of decreasing superoxide production by neutrophils from patients with ANCA-positive crescentic glomerulonephritis (304).

Cytotoxic Agents

Immunosuppression with either azathioprine or cyclophosphamide (or occasionally chlorambucil) is commonly used in the treatment of crescentic glomerulonephritis, again usually in combination with steroids and, more recently, plasma exchange.

There appears to be little or no evidence to support the use of either cyclophosphamide or azathioprine as single treatments. Several authors have reported substantial benefit from the combination of cyclophosphamide with anticoagulation, steroids, and antiplatelet drugs, whereas others have been unable to demonstrate benefit (282,285,305,306). There are very few controlled data to support the use of cyclophosphamide (or azathioprine) in RPGN, although most clinicians believe they are necessary components of the treatment. The use of intravenous cyclophosphamide in the treatment of RPGN has only rarely been reported (307,308) and has not demonstrated any advantage over daily oral dosing, unlike its use in lupus nephritis. In the vasculitic subgroup, intravenous cyclophosphamide, given as a monthly pulse dose, was as effective as a daily oral dose and had fewer side effects in one study (309), but another retrospective study of patients specifically with Wegener's granulomatosus with renal involvement suggested a worse outcome with monthly intravenous pulses of cyclophosphamide (310). Given the paucity of data, it is difficult to make recommendations regarding oral versus IV-pulse cyclophosphamide use in RPGN.

Anticoagulants

For a number of years, it has been appreciated that glomerular fibrin deposition is prominent in crescentic glomerulonephritis, in the glomerular tuft, and especially in Bowman's space and the crescent (10,242,264). The role of the coagulation process in development of the crescent in experimental glomerulonephritis has already been discussed. Several studies in experimental glomerulonephritis have shown that anticoagulation with heparin, before the onset of the glomerular injury, can reduce the formation of crescents and severity of renal failure, although enormous doses of heparin were required (311–313). Some authors have failed to demonstrate a significant benefit of this approach (314,315). Anticoagulation with warfarin also has been shown to reduce, to a smaller degree, crescent formation (217,316). It has been suggested that the pathogenetic mechanisms occurring locally in the glomerulus are capable of producing local coagulation, overriding the effects of circulating anticoagulants. This occurrence could possibly result from a failure of heparin, a highly charged molecule, to penetrate the mesangium and Bowman's space. Another explanation for the relative ineffectiveness of heparin is that the fibrin deposition results from thrombin-independent mechanisms, as discussed previously.

Anticoagulation with heparin for human RPGN was first reported by Kincaid-Smith et al. in 1968 (317). The subsequent use of heparin in this disease usually has been in combination with one or more other drugs, including steroids, immunosuppressives, and antiplatelet agents (49,285,305,318–320). It therefore has been difficult to determine the relative benefit of the anticoagulation, and even now there is still no clear-cut evidence that use of these agents is beneficial.

Antiplatelet Age

Platelets are potential mediators of glomerular injury, particularly through the release of vasoactive amines. However, little direct evidence exists that they are involved in crescentic glomerulonephritis, although a role in the coagulation process in the glomerulus has not been excluded (318,321,322). Antiplatelet agents, such as dipyridamole and sulfinpyrazone, have been used in the disease as part of a "cocktail," with no proven benefit.

Plasma Exchange

Since the demonstration of the definite benefit of plasma exchange for patients with Goodpasture's syndrome (75,323–326), the technique has been used widely in a variety of types of glomerulonephritis, including RPGN (241,267,268,279, 327–332), usually in conjunction with immunosuppression, although not always with success (333). Glockner et al. (334) reported in 1988 a randomized study of plasma exchange in 26 patients with RPGN, also given steroids and immunosuppression, and were unable to demonstrate a difference in outcome of renal function after 8 weeks. Another randomized study from the Canadian Apheresis Study Group failed to demonstrate any additional benefit of plasma exchange over prednisolone and azathioprine out to 12 months in 32 patients with idiopathic crescentic nephritis (335). In the latter study, there may have been a benefit of plasma exchange in dialysis-dependent patients, but numbers were too small. On the other hand, several prominent groups have reported on the additional benefits of plasma exchange in severe ANCA-positive crescentic nephritis (336,337). The best results appear to be in those who were dialysis dependent at presentation but still were not dramatically better than those obtained with steroids and cyclophosphamide without plasma exchange (337). A reanalysis of two French studies designed to assess the value of plasma exchange in systemic vasculitis demonstrated no additional benefit of plasma exchange in those patients with renal involvement (338). A more recent randomized study compared six treatments of either plasma exchange or immunoadsorption in a total of 44 patients with RPGN (339). All patients also received corticosteroids and cyclophosphamide. There was no difference in outcome with these two treatment modalities. However, in the study, 6 of 6 dialysis-dependent anti-GBM patients remained on dialysis, whereas 7 of 10 non–anti-GBM patients who were initially dialysis dependent improved to become dialysis independent (339). Earlier data from the Hammersmith group had suggested that unless pulmonary hemorrhage was present, treatment of patients with anti-GBM disease and a serum creatinine over 600 μmol/L (6.8 mg/dL) with plasma exchange was futile (337). This then creates a paradoxical situation: Plasma exchange is of most value in anti-GBM disease when the creatinine is less than 600 μmol/L, but in vasculitis and probably immune-RPGN, the best results with plasma exchange appear to be in those who are dialysis dependent at presentation. The reason for this difference is not clear.

Experimental Approaches to Treatment

The most commonly used alternative agent is mycophenolate mofetil. This agent is gathering favor as an alternative to cyclophosphamide, especially in the maintenance phase of management. In Class IV lupus nephritis (see Chapter 65), mycophenolate is gaining a defined role based on several trials of its use either as induction (340) or maintenance therapy (341). However, in vasculitis, there are as yet anecdotal reports only. As an example, one report detailed 14 patients with Wegener's granulomatosis who had all received induction therapy with cyclophosphamide and glucocorticoids and then received mycophenolate as maintenance therapy with excellent results (342). Another approach, particularly applied in vasculitis is the use of anti-TNF-alpha therapies. The soluble p75 TNF receptor etanercept has been used with some success in vasculitis, although there have been reports of a high relapse rate. Curiously, there are also reports of etanercept induced vasculitis, including RPGN (343). Infliximab, a humanized anti-TNF chimeric antibody, has also been used with success to treat difficult cases of ANCA positive vasculitis with a reported relapse rate of 20%. There was some concern over a high rate of infection with encapsulated organisms (344). Other agents that remain at an early phase of development include leflunomide, interleukin-1 receptor antagonist, and the antibodies Mabthera and CAMPATH II.

Renal Transplantation

Successful transplantation is possible in patients with RPGN (234,345). The disease can recur in the allograft (236,345,346), but at least for anti-GBM disease, this is unusual if transplantation is delayed until the circulating anti-GBM antibody has disappeared. The transplantation of a normal kidney into a patient with Alport's syndrome potentially incites an antibody response to the normal glomerular basement membrane. Although linear IgG may be seen in the glomeruli of as many as 30% of these transplants, crescents are not common and the course is most often benign (347). Recurrent ANCA-positive vasculitis is reported to occur in approximately 20% of cases in the setting of a positive ANCA titer at the time of transplantation (348). De novo RPGN occurring in a renal transplant also has been described (349).

Factors To Be Considered in the Treatment of Rapidly Progressive Glomerulonephritis

The simple diagnosis of RPGN alone is not sufficient to determine the type of treatment. Several other factors are likely to be relevant to the potential benefit, or not, of treatment.

1. The acute or chronic nature of the glomerular lesion is significant. The presence of acute cellular crescents with extensive fibrin deposition is more indicative of a likely positive response to immunosuppression than disease in which crescents are undergoing fibrosis and in which glomerulosclerosis and interstitial fibrosis are prominent.
2. The presence of segmental glomerular capillary loop necrosis should raise the possibility of an underlying vasculitis and thus a greater chance of a response to immunosuppression. Similarly, the presence of systemic symptoms other than those of renal failure should suggest the possibility of vasculitis.
3. Immunosuppression, anticoagulation, and the use of plasma exchange all have the potential for inducing severe and occasionally fatal side effects (350–352). It could be argued

that the patient particularly at risk from these side effects (e.g., the elderly, infected, or patients with peptic ulceration) is better treated by aggressive control of hypertension and renal failure rather than by immunosuppression. If immunosuppression is to be successful, early diagnosis of RPGN is essential before irreparable damage has occurred. Early diagnosis depends on urinalysis and assessment of renal function in any patient presenting to a general practitioner with persistent nonspecific symptoms (353).

The authors' approach to the treatment of RPGN is to treat all patients, unless renal biopsy shows an end-stage kidney, with a trial of immunosuppression, consisting of corticosteroids and cyclophosphamide, without anticoagulation. Pulse methylprednisolone is given intravenously (1 g) on each of 3 successive days. This is followed by oral prednisolone at a dosage of 60 mg/day for 4 to 6 weeks, which is then reduced gradually to a maintenance dose of 10 to 15 mg/day and sustained for 6 months to 1 year, depending on the clinical progress. Oral cyclophosphamide is used at 2 to 3 mg/kg of body weight, usually for 3 to 6 months. Monthly pulses of cyclophosphamide are used routinely in lupus nephritis and occasionally in ANCA-positive vasculitis. Anticoagulation with heparin is not used routinely, nor is dipyridamole or other antiplatelet agents. Plasma exchange is always used for anti-GBM disease, typically as 3- to 4-L exchanges every other day for six exchanges. Short-term plasma exchange also may be considered in other forms of severe RPGN in patients who are refractory or become dialysis dependent, especially in ANCA-positive forms of the disease.

Failure of response to these measures leads to an early rather than late cessation of therapy to minimize complications. Maintenance dialysis remains the alternative for those patients who are not treated or are not responding to treatment.

References

1. Langhans, T. Uber die vernaderungen der glomeruli bei der nephritis nebst einigen Bemerkungen uber die Entshehung der Fibrinzylinder. *Arch Pathol Physiol Klin Med* 1879;76:85.
2. Volhard F, Fahr T. Die Brightsche Nierenkranheit. *Springer* 1914:115.
3. Li HL, et al. Activated (IL-2R+) intraglomerular mononuclear cells in crescentic glomerulonephritis. *Kidney Int* 1991;39:793.
4. Ellis, A. Natural history of Bright's Disease. Clinical, histological and experimental observations. *Lancet* 1942;1:1.
5. Hamburger J. Les glomerulonephritis malignes. *Entretiens de Bichat*. Paris: Expansion, 1956.
6. Bialestock DA. Acute necrotizing glomerulitis: the clinical features and pathology in nine cases. *Aust Ann Med* 1959;8:281.
7. Berlyne GM, De Baker SB. Acute Anuric Glomerulonephritis. *Q J Med* 1964;33:105.
8. Pollack V. Defibrination with ancrod in glomerulonephritis. Effect on clinical and histologic findings and on blood coagulation. *Am J Nephrol* 1982;2:195.
9. Bacani RA, et al. Rapidly progressive (nonstreptococcal) glomerulonephritis. *Ann Intern Med* 1968;69:463.
10. Heptinstall R. Pathology of the kidney In: *Pathology of the kidney*. Boston: Little, Brown; 1983:443.
11. Stilmant MM, et al. Crescentic glomerulonephritis without immune deposits: clinicopathologic features. *Kidney Int* 1979;15:184.
12. Whitworth JA, et al. The significance of extracapillary proliferation. Clinicopathological review of 60 patients. *Nephron* 1976;16:1.
13. Neild GH, et al. Rapidly progressive glomerulonephritis with extensive glomerular crescent formation. *Q J Med* 1983;52:395.
14. Morrin PA, et al. Rapidly progressive glomerulonephritis. A clinical and pathologic study. *Am J Med* 1978;65:446.
15. Morita T, Suzuki Y, Churg J. Structure and development of the glomerular crescent. *Am J Pathol* 1973;72:349.
16. Hancock WW, Atkins RC. Cellular composition of crescents in human rapidly progressive glomerulonephritis identified using monoclonal antibodies. *Am J Nephrol* 1984;4:177.
17. Kincaid-Smith P, d'Apice A, Atkins RC. Glomerular cells in glomerulonephritis. In: *Progress in glomerulonephritis*. New York: Wiley; 1979.
18. Atkins RC, et al. Tissue culture of isolated glomeruli from patients with glomerulonephritis. *Kidney Int* 1980;17:515.
19. Becker G, Atkins RC, Kincaid-Smith P. The cellular participants in human glomerulonephritis. In: *Proceedings of the Second Asian Pacific Congress of Nephrology*, 1984.
20. Kalowski S, et al. Multinucleated giant cells in antiglomerular basement membrane antibody-induced glomerulonephritis. *Nephron* 1976;16:415.
21. Kohler G, Milstein C. Continuous cultures of fused cells secreting antibody of predefined specificity. *Nature* 1975;256:495.
22. Atkins RC, et al. Cellular immune mechanisms in human glomerulonephritis: the role of mononuclear leucocytes. *Springer Semin Immunopathol* 1982;5:269.
23. Hancock WW, Atkins RC. Monoclonal antibodies to human glomerular cells: a marker for glomerular epithelial cells. *Nephron* 1983;33:83.
24. Hancock WW, et al. Production of monoclonal antibodies to fibronectin, type IV collagen and other antigens of the human glomerulus. *Pathology* 1984;16:197.
25. Muller GA, Muller C. Characterisation of renal antigens on distinct parts of the human nephron by monoclonal antibodies. *Klin Wochenschr* 1983;61:893.
26. Striker G. Monolocal antibodies as probes of normal and abnormal renal structure. In: *International Society of Nephrology*. New York: Springer, 1984.
27. Atkins R. Macrophage identification in human and experimental glomerulonephritis. In *VIIIth International Congress of Nephrology*. Karger, 1981
28. Hooke DH, Gee DC, Atkins RC. Leukocyte analysis using monoclonal antibodies in human glomerulonephritis. *Kidney Int* 1987;31:964.
29. Stachura I, Si L, Whiteside TL. Mononuclear-cell subsets in human idiopathic crescentic glomerulonephritis (ICGN): analysis in tissue sections with monoclonal antibodies. *J Clin Immunol* 1984;4:202.
30. Bolton WK, et al. T-cells and macrophages in rapidly progressive glomerulonephritis: clinicopathologic correlations. *Kidney Int* 1987;32:869.
31. Hooke DH, et al. Monoclonal antibody analysis of glomerular hypercellularity in human glomerulonephritis. *Clin Nephrol* 1984;22:163.
32. Li HL, et al. Mononuclear cell activation and decreased renal function in IgA nephropathy with crescents. *Kidney Int* 1990;37:1552.
33. Muller GA, et al. Renal, major histocompatibility complex antigens and cellular components in rapidly progressive glomerulonephritis identified by monoclonal antibodies. *Nephron* 1988;49:132.
34. Nolasco FE, et al. Intraglomerular T cells and monocytes in nephritis: study with monoclonal antibodies. *Kidney Int* 1987;31:1160.
35. Neale TJ, et al. Participation of cell-mediated immunity in deposition of fibrin in glomerulonephritis. *Lancet* 1988;2:421.
36. Nikolic-Paterson DJ, Atkins RC. The role of macrophages in glomerulonephritis. *Nephrol Dial Transplant* 2001;16(Suppl 5):3.
37. Atkins RC, Lan HY, Paterson DJ. Pathogenic mechanisms of interstitial leucocyte infiltration in glomerulonephritis. In: *Issues in nephrosciences*. Milan: Wichtig, 1991.
38. Becker GJ, et al. Monoclonal antibodies to human macrophage and leucocyte common antigens. *Pathology* 1981;13:669.
39. Gartner HV, Wehner H, Bohle A. (The immunohistological findings in various forms of glomerulonephritis: a comparative investigation based on 335 renal biopsies. Part II: Minimal proliferating intercapillary glomerulonephritis (with nephrotic syndrome), focal sclerosing, epi-extra-perimembranous, membranoproliferative and extracapillary (rapidly progressive) glomerulonephritis (author's transl). *Pathol Res Pract* 1978;162:198.
40. Couser WG. Rapidly progressive glomerulonephritis: classification, pathogenetic mechanisms, and therapy. *Am J Kidney Dis* 1988;11:449.
41. Berger J, Yaneva J, Hinglais N. *Immunohistochemistry of glomerulonephritis: advances in nephrology*. Chicago: Year Book, 1971.
42. Dash SC, et al. Spectrum of rapidly progressive (crescentic) glomerulonephritis in northern India. *Nephron* 1982;30:45.
43. Jennette JC, Falk RJ. Antineutrophil cytoplasmic autoantibodies and associated diseases: a review. *Am J Kidney Dis* 1990;15:517.
44. Lewis EJ, et al. An immunopathologic study of rapidly progressive glomerulonephritis in the adult. *Hum Pathol* 1971;2:185.
45. Nagai T, Tamura T, Kawai C. Immunohistologic findings in the glomerular crescents in various renal diseases. *Jpn Circ J* 1979;43:83.
46. Jennette JC. The pathology of vasculitis involving the kidney. *Am J Kidney Dis* 1994;24:130.
47. Bohman SO, Olsen S, Peterson VP. Glomerular ultrastructure in extracapillary glomerulonephritis. *Acta Pathol Microbiol Scand (A)* 1974;(Suppl 249):29.
48. Farquhar MG, Vernier RL, Good RA. An electron microscope study of the glomerulus in nephrosis, glomerulonephritis, and lupus erythematosus. *J Exp Med* 1957;106:649.
49. Suc JM, et al. The use of heparin in the treatment of idiopathic rapidly progressive glomerulonephritis. *Clin Nephrol* 1976;5:9.
50. Magil AB, Wadsworth LD. Monocyte involvement in glomerular crescents: a histochemical and ultrastructural study. *Lab Invest* 1982;47:160.
51. Lan HY, Atkins RC. Glomerulonephritis and its progression. *Asian Nephrology*. London: Oxford University Press; 1994.
52. Cameron JS. Tubular and interstitial factors in the progression of glomerulonephritis. *Paediatr. Nephrol* 1992;6:292.
53. Bruijn JA, Hoedemaeker PJ, Fleuren GJ. Pathogenesis of anti-basement membrane glomerulopathy and immune-complex glomerulonephritis: dichotomy dissolved. *Lab Invest* 1989;61:480.

54. Pusey CD, Lockwood CM. Autoimmunity in rapidly progressive glomerulonephritis. *Kidney Int* 1989;35:929.

55. Holdsworth SR, Wischusen NJ, Dowling JP. A radioimmunoassay for the detection of circulating anti-glomerular basement membrane antibodies. *Aust N Z J Med* 1983;13:15.

56. Holdsworth S, et al. The clinical spectrum of acute glomerulonephritis and lung haemorrhage (Goodpasture's syndrome). *Q J Med* 1985;55:75.

57. Andres G, et al. Histology of human tubulo-interstitial nephritis associated with antibodies to renal basement membranes. *Kidney Int* 1978;13:480.

58. Hellmark T, Johansson C, Wieslander J. Characterization of anti-GBM antibodies involved in Goodpasture's syndrome. *Kidney Int* 1994;46:823.

59. Butkowski, RJ, et al. Characterization of type IV collagen NC1 monomers and Goodpasture antigen in human renal basement membranes. *J Lab Clin Med* 1990;115:365.

60. Borza DB, Neilson EG, Hudson BG. Pathogenesis of Goodpasture syndrome: a molecular perspective. *Semin Nephrol* 2003;23:522.

61. Steblay RW. Glomerulonephritis induced in sheep by injections of heterologous glomerular basement membrane and Freund's complete adjuvant. *J Exp Med* 1962;116:253.

62. Masugi M. Uber die experimentalle glomerulonephritis durch das spezifische antinieren serum. Ein beitrag der diffusen glomrulonephritis. *Beitr Pathol Anat* 1934;92:429.

63. Lan HY, Paterson DJ, Atkins RC. Initiation and evolution of interstitial leukocytic infiltration in experimental glomerulonephritis. *Kidney Int* 1991;40:425.

64. Lan HY, et al. Leukocyte involvement in the pathogenesis of pulmonary injury in experimental Goodpasture's syndrome. *Lab Invest* 1991;64:330.

65. Lerner RA, Glassock RJ, Dixon FJ. The role of anti-glomerular basement membrane antibody in the pathogenesis of human glomerulonephritis. *J Exp Med* 1967;126:989.

66. Meyers KE, et al. Human antiglomerular basement membrane autoantibody disease in XenoMouse II. *Kidney Int* 2002;61:1666.

67. Graham AR, Payne CM, Nagle RB. A quantitative light- and electron-microscopic study of type IV nuclear bodies in crescentic glomerulonephritis. *Am J Pathol* 1981;102:359.

68. Becker GJ, et al. Involvement of the macrophage in experimental chronic immune complex glomerulonephritis. *Nephron* 1982;32:227.

69. Jennette JC, Falk RJ. Diagnosis and management of glomerulonephritis and vasculitis presenting as acute renal failure. *Med Clin North Am* 1990;74:893.

70. Salant DJ. Immunopathogenesis of crescentic glomerulonephritis and lung purpura. *Kidney Int* 1987;32:408.

71. Davies DJ, et al. Segmental necrotising glomerulonephritis with antineutrophil antibody: possible arbovirus aetiology? *Br Med J (Clin Res Ed)* 1982;285:606.

72. Andrassy K, et al. Diagnostic significance of anticytoplasmatic antibodies (ACPA/ANCA) in detection of Wegener's granulomatosis and other forms of vasculitis. *Nephron* 1988;9:257.

73. Falk RJ, Jennette JC. Anti-neutrophil cytoplasmic autoantibodies with specificity for myeloperoxidase in patients with systemic vasculitis and idiopathic necrotizing and crescentic glomerulonephritis. *N Engl J Med* 1988;318:1651.

74. Hall JB, et al. Vasculitis and glomerulonephritis: a subgroup with an antineutrophil cytoplasmic antibody. *Aust N Z J Med* 1984;14:277.

75. Lockwood CM, et al. Association of alkaline phosphatase with an autoantigen recognised by circulating anti-neutrophil antibodies in systemic vasculitis. *Lancet* 1987;1:716.

76. Walters MD, et al. Antineutrophil cytoplasm antibody in crescentic glomerulonephritis. *Arch Dis Child* 1988;63:814.

77. Jayne DR, et al. Autoantibodies to GBM and neutrophil cytoplasm in rapidly progressive glomerulonephritis. *Kidney Int* 1990;37:965.

78. Tervaert JW, et al. Autoantibodies against myeloid lysosomal enzymes in crescentic glomerulonephritis. *Kidney Int* 1990;37:799.

79. Robinson AJ. Antineutrophil cytoplasmic antibodies (ANCA) and the systemic necrotizing vasculitides. *Nephrol Dial Transplant* 1994;9:119.

80. Falk RJ, Jennette JC. ANCA are pathogenic—oh yes they are! *J Am Soc Nephrol* 2002;13:1977.

81. Heeringa P, et al. Autoantibodies to myeloperoxidase aggravate mild antiglomerular-basement-membrane-mediated glomerular injury in the rat. *Am J Pathol* 1996;149:1695.

82. Heeringa P, et al. Expression of iNOS, eNOS, and peroxynitrite-modified proteins in experimental anti-myeloperoxidase associated crescentic glomerulonephritis. *Kidney Int* 1998;53:382.

83. Xiao H, et al. Antineutrophil cytoplasmic autoantibodies specific for myeloperoxidase cause glomerulonephritis and vasculitis in mice. *J Clin Invest* 2002;110:955.

84. Hogarth PM. Fc receptors are major mediators of antibody based inflammation in autoimmunity. *Curr Opin Immunol* 2002;14:798.

85. Park SY, et al. Resistance of Fc receptor- deficient mice to fatal glomerulonephritis. *J Clin Invest* 1998;102:1229.

86. Tarzi RM, et al. Nephrotoxic nephritis is mediated by Fcgamma receptors on circulating leukocytes and not intrinsic renal cells. *Kidney Int* 2002;62:2087.

87. Fujii T, et al. Predominant role of FcgammaRIII in the induction of accelerated nephrotoxic glomerulonephritis. *Kidney Int* 2003;64:1406.

88. Bolland S, Ravetch JV. Spontaneous autoimmune disease in Fc(gamma)-RIIB-deficient mice results from strain-specific epistasis. *Immunity* 2003;13:277.

89. Nakamura A, et al. Fcgamma receptor IIB-deficient mice develop Goodpasture's syndrome upon immunization with type IV collagen: a novel murine model for autoimmune glomerular basement membrane disease. *J Exp Med* 2000;191:899.

90. Hancock W, Atkins R. Activation of coagulation pathways and fibrin deposition in human glomerulonephritis. *Semin Nephrol* 1985;5:69.

91. Atkins RC, Holdsworth SR. Cellular mechanisms of immune glomerular injury. *Cellular Mechanisms of Injury in GN*. New York: Churchill Livingstone; 1988.

92. Boucher A, et al. Relationship between the integrity of Bowman's capsule and the composition of cellular crescents in human crescentic glomerulonephritis. *Lab Invest* 1987;56:526.

93. Yang N, et al. Local macrophage proliferation in human glomerulonephritis. *Kidney Int* 1998;54:143.

94. Cunningham MA, et al. Prominence of cell-mediated immunity effectors in "pauci-immune" glomerulonephritis. *J Am Soc Nephrol* 1999;10:499.

95. Rocklin RE, Lewis EJ, David JR. In vitro evidence for cellular hypersensitivity to glomerular-basement-membrane antigens in human glomerulonephritis. *N Engl J Med* 1970;283:497.

96. Salama AD, et al. In Goodpasture's disease, CD4(+) T cells escape thymic deletion and are reactive with the autoantigen alpha3(IV)NC1. *J Am Soc Nephrol* 2001;12:1908.

97. Lan HY, Nikolic-Paterson DJ, Atkins RC. Involvement of activated periglomerular leukocytes in the rupture of Bowman's capsule and glomerular crescent progression in experimental glomerulonephritis. *Lab Invest* 1992;67:743.

98. Lan HY, et al. Local macrophage proliferation in the progression of glomerular and tubulointerstitial injury in rat anti-GBM glomerulonephritis. *Kidney Int* 1995;48:753.

99. Bhan AK, et al. Evidence for a pathogenic role of a cell-mediated immune mechanism in experimental glomerulonephritis. *J Exp Med* 1978;148:246.

100. Bolton WK, Tucker FL, Sturgill BC. New avian model of experimental glomerulonephritis consistent with mediation by cellular immunity. Nonhumorally mediated glomerulonephritis in chickens. *J Clin Invest* 1984;73:1263.

101. Rennke HG, Klein PS, Mendrick DL. Cell mediated immunity (CMI) in hapten induced interstitial nephritis and glomerular crescent formation in the rat. *Kidney Int* 1990;37:428.

102. Kawasaki K, et al. Depletion of CD8 positive cells in nephrotoxic serum nephritis of WKY rats. *Kidney Int* 1992;41:1517.

103. Huang XR, Holdsworth SR, Tipping PG. Evidence for delayed-type hypersensitivity mechanisms in glomerular crescent formation. *Kidney Int* 1994;46:69.

104. Nishikawa K, et al. Effect of CTLA-4 chimeric protein on rat autoimmune anti-glomerular basement membrane glomerulonephritis. *Eur J Immunol* 1994;24:1249.

105. Reynolds J, et al. CD28-B7 blockade prevents the development of experimental autoimmune glomerulonephritis. *J Clin Invest* 2000;105:643.

106. Reynolds J, et al. Blockade of the CD154-CD40 costimulatory pathway prevents the development of experimental autoimmune glomerulonephritis. *Kidney Int* 2004;66:1444.

107. Wu J, et al. CD4(+) T cells specific to a glomerular basement membrane antigen mediate glomerulonephritis. *J Clin Invest* 2002;109:517.

108. Wu J, et al. T-cell epitope of alpha3 chain of type IV collagen induces severe glomerulonephritis. *Kidney Int* 2003;64:1292.

109. Holdsworth SR, Kitching AR, Tipping PG. Th1 and Th2 T helper cell subsets affect patterns of injury and outcomes in glomerulonephritis. *Kidney Int* 1999;55:1198.

110. Huang XR, et al. Th1 responsiveness to nephritogenic antigens determines susceptibility to crescentic glomerulonephritis in mice. *Kidney Int* 1997;51:94.

111. Kitching AR, Tipping PG, Holdsworth SR. IL-12 directs severe renal injury, crescent formation and Th1 responses in murine glomerulonephritis. *Eur J Immunol* 1999;29:1.

112. Kitching AR, et al. Interleukin-4 deficiency enhances Th1 responses and crescentic glomerulonephritis in mice. *Kidney Int* 1998;53:112.

113. Kitching AR, et al. Interleukin-4 and interleukin-10 attenuate established crescentic glomerulonephritis in mice. *Kidney Int* 1997;52:52.

114. Chadban SJ, et al. Effect of interleukin-10 treatment on crescentic glomerulonephritis in rats. *Kidney Int* 1997;51:1809.

115. Merkel F, et al. Autoreactive T-cells in Goodpasture's syndrome recognize the N-terminal NC1 domain on alpha 3 type IV collagen. *Kidney Int* 1996;49:1127.

116. Derry CJ, et al. Analysis of T cell responses to the autoantigen in Goodpasture's disease. *Clin Exp Immunol* 1995;100:262.

117. Weber M, et al. IgG subclass distribution of autoantibodies to glomerular basement membrane in Goodpasture's syndrome compared to other autoantibodies. *Nephron* 1988;49:54.

118. Segelmark M, Butkowski R, Wieslander J. Antigen restriction and IgG subclasses among anti-GBM autoantibodies. *Nephrol Dial Transplant* 1990;5:991.

119. Salama, AD, et al. Regulation by CD25+ lymphocytes of autoantigen-specific T-cell responses in Goodpasture's (anti-GBM) disease. *Kidney Int* 64:1685.

120. Atkins RC, et al. The macrophagen in human rapidly progressive glomerulonephritis. *Lancet* 1976;1:830.
121. McCluskey RT, Bhan AK. Cell-mediated mechanisms in renal diseases. *Kidney Int Suppl* 1982;11:S6.
122. Isbel NM, et al. Local macrophage proliferation correlates with increased renal M-CSF expression in human glomerulonephritis. *Nephrol Dial Transplant* 2001;16:1638.
123. Matsumoto K, Dowling J, Atkins RC. Production of interleukin 1 in glomerular cell cultures from patients with rapidly progressive crescentic glomerulonephritis. *Am J Nephrol* 1988;8:463.
124. Takemura T, et al. Cellular localization of inflammatory cytokines in human glomerulonephritis. *Virchows Arch* 1994;424:459.
125. Ma L, et al. Intercellular adhesion molecule-1 and tumour necrosis factor-alpha in human glomerulonephritis. *Nephrology* 1996;3:329.
126. Lan HY, et al. Expression of macrophage migration inhibitory factor in human glomerulonephritis. *Kidney Int* 2000;57:499.
127. Kashem A, et al. Expression of inducible-NOS in human glomerulonephritis: the possible source is infiltrating monocytes/macrophages. *Kidney Int* 1996;50:392.
128. Kaneko Y, et al. Macrophage metalloelastase as a major factor for glomerular injury in anti-glomerular basement membrane nephritis. *J Immunol* 2003;170:3377.
129. Frosch M, et al. Expression of MRP8 and MRP14 by macrophages is a marker for severe forms of glomerulonephritis. *J Leukoc Biol* 2004;75:198.
130. Wu Q, et al. Costimulatory molecules CD80 and CD86 in human crescentic glomerulonephritis. *Am J Kidney Dis* 2003;41:950.
131. Schreiner GF, et al. A mononuclear cell component in experimental immunological glomerulonephritis. *J Exp Med* 1978;47:369.
132. Holdsworth SR, Neale TJ, Wilson CB. Abrogation of macrophage-dependent injury in experimental glomerulonephritis in the rabbit. Use of an antimacrophage serum. *J Clin Invest* 1981;68:686.
133. Holdsworth SR, Neale TJ. Macrophage-induced glomerular injury. Cell transfer studies in passive autologous antiglomerular basement membrane antibody-initiated experimental glomerulonephritis. *Lab Invest* 1984;51:172.
134. Ikezumi Y, et al. Adoptive transfer studies demonstrate that macrophages can induce proteinuria and mesangial cell proliferation. *Kidney Int* 2003;63:83.
135. Ikezumi Y, Atkins RC, Nikolic-Paterson DJ. Interferon-gamma augments acute macrophage-mediated renal injury via a glucocorticoid-sensitive mechanism. *J Am Soc Nephrol* 2003;14:888.
136. Ikezumi Y, et al. Macrophage-mediated renal injury is dependent on signaling via the JNK pathway. *J Am Soc Nephrol* 2004;15:1775.
137. Rovin BH, Doe N, Tan LC. Monocyte chemoattractant protein-1 levels in patients with glomerular disease. *Am J Kidney Dis* 1996;27:640.
138. Segerer S, et al. Expression of the chemokine monocyte chemoattractant protein-1 and its receptor chemokine receptor 2 in human crescentic glomerulonephritis. *J Am Soc Nephrol* 2000;11:2231.
139. Hudkins KL, et al. Osteopontin expression in human crescentic glomerulonephritis. *Kidney Int* 2000;57:105.
140. Okada H, et al. Tubular osteopontin expression in human glomerulonephritis and renal vasculitis. *Am J Kidney Dis* 2000;36:498.
141. Tang WW, Qi M, Warren JS. Monocyte chemoattractant protein 1 mediates glomerular macrophage infiltration in anti-GBM Ab GN. *Kidney Int* 1996;50:665.
142. Wada T, et al. Intervention of crescentic glomerulonephritis by antibodies to monocyte chemotactic and activating factor (MCAF/MCP-1). *FASEB J* 1996;10:1418.
143. Lloyd CM, et al. RANTES and monocyte chemoattractant protein-1 (MCP-1) play an important role in the inflammatory phase of crescentic nephritis, but only MCP-1 is involved in crescent formation and interstitial fibrosis. *J Exp Med* 1997;185:1371.
144. Tesch GH, et al. Monocyte chemoattractant protein-1 promotes macrophage-mediated tubular injury, but not glomerular injury, in nephrotoxic serum nephritis. *J Clin Invest* 1999;103:73.
145. Yu XQ, et al. A functional role for osteopontin in experimental crescentic glomerulonephritis in the rat. *Proc Assoc Am Physicians* 1998;110:50.
146. Zen K, Parkos CA. Leukocyte-epithelial interactions. *Curr Opin Cell Biol* 2003;15:557.
147. Lhotta, K, et al. Renal expression of intercellular adhesion molecule-1 in different forms of glomerulonephritis. *Clin Sci (Lond)* 1991;81:4770.
148. Muller GA, Markovic-Lipkovski J, Muller CA. Intercellular adhesion molecule-1 expression in human kidneys with glomerulonephritis. *Clin Nephrol* 1991;36:203.
149. Seron D, Cameron JS, Haskard DO. Expression of VCAM-1 in the normal and diseased kidney. *Nephrol Dial Transplant* 1991;6:917.
150. Tipping PG, et al. A role for P selectin in complement-independent neutrophil-mediated glomerular injury. *Kidney Int* 1994;46:79.
151. Hill PA, et al. The ICAM-1/LFA-1 interaction in glomerular leukocytic accumulation in anti-GBM glomerulonephritis. *Kidney Int* 1994;45:700.
152. Hill PA, et al. ICAM-1 directs migration and localization of interstitial leukocytes in experimental glomerulonephritis. *Kidney Int* 1994;45:32.
153. Nishikawa K, et al. Antibodies to intercellular adhesion molecule 1/lymphocyte function-associated antigen 1 prevent crescent formation in rat autoimmune glomerulonephritis. *J Exp Med* 1993;177:667.
154. Kawasaki K, et al. Antibodies against intercellular adhesion molecule-1 and lymphocyte function-associated antigen-1 prevent glomerular injury in rat experimental crescentic glomerulonephritis. *J Immunol* 1993;150:1074.
155. Janssen U, et al. Improved survival and amelioration of nephrotoxic nephritis in intercellular adhesion molecule-1 knockout mice. *J Am Soc Nephrol* 1998;9:1805.
156. Allen AR, et al. Endothelial expression of VCAM-1 in experimental crescentic nephritis and effect of antibodies to very late antigen-4 or VCAM-1 on glomerular injury. *J Immunol* 1999;162:5519.
157. Khan SB, et al. Blocking VLA-4 prevents progression of experimental crescentic glomerulonephritis. *Nephron Exp Nephrol* 2003;95:e100.
158. Noronha IL, et al. In situ production of TNF-alpha, IL-1 beta and IL-2R in ANCA-positive glomerulonephritis. *Kidney Int* 1993;43:682.
159. Tesch GH, et al. Intrinsic renal cells are the major source of interleukin-1 beta synthesis in normal and diseased rat kidney. *Nephrol Dial Transplant* 1997;12:1109.
160. Lan HY, et al. Suppression of experimental crescentic glomerulonephritis by the interleukin-1 receptor antagonist. *Kidney Int* 1993;43:479.
161. Mulligan MS, et al. Requirements for leukocyte adhesion molecules in nephrotoxic nephritis. *J Clin Invest* 1993;91:577.
162. Tang WW, et al. Interleukin-1 receptor antagonist ameliorates experimental anti-glomerular basement membrane antibody-associated glomerulonephritis. *J Clin Invest* 1994;93:273.
163. Karkar AM, et al. Modulation of antibody-mediated glomerular injury in vivo by IL-1ra, soluble IL-1 receptor, and soluble TNF receptor. *Kidney Int* 1995;48:1738.
164. Karkar, AM, et al. Passive immunization against tumour necrosis factor-alpha (TNF-alpha) and IL-1 beta protects from LPS enhancing glomerular injury in nephrotoxic nephritis in rats. *Clin Exp Immunol* 1992;90:312.
165. Nikolic-Paterson DJ, et al. Suppression of experimental glomerulonephritis by the interleukin-1 receptor antagonist: inhibition of intercellular adhesion molecule-1 expression. *J Am Soc Nephrol* 1994;4:1695.
166. Yu XQ, et al. IL-1 up-regulates osteopontin expression in experimental crescentic glomerulonephritis in the rat. *Am J Pathol* 1999;154:833.
167. Takazoe K, et al. Interleukin-1 induces renal CD44 expression in vivo and in vitro: role of the transcription factor Egr-1. *Nephrology* 2002;7:136.
168. Lan HY, et al. Interleukin-1 receptor antagonist halts the progression of established crescentic glomerulonephritis in the rat. *Kidney Int* 1995;47:1303.
169. Hruby ZW, et al. Antiserum against tumor necrosis factor-alpha and a protease inhibitor reduce immune glomerular injury. *Kidney Int* 1991;40:43.
170. Lan HY, et al. TNF-alpha up-regulates renal MIF expression in rat crescentic glomerulonephritis. *Mol Med* 1997;3:136.
171. Karkar AM, Smith J, Pusey CD. Prevention and treatment of experimental crescentic glomerulonephritis by blocking tumour necrosis factor-alpha. *Nephrol Dial Transplant* 2001;16:518.
172. Calandra T, Bucala R. Macrophage migration inhibitory factor (MIF): a glucocorticoid counter-regulator within the immune system. *Crit Rev Immunol* 1997;17:77.
173. Brown FG, et al. Urine macrophage migration inhibitory factor reflects the severity of renal injury in human glomerulonephritis. *J Am Soc Nephrol* 2002;13(Suppl 1):S7.
174. Boyce NW, Tipping PG, Holdsworth SR. Lymphokine (MIF) production by glomerular T-lymphocytes in experimental glomerulonephritis. *Kidney Int* 1986;30:673.
175. Lan HY, et al. De Novo renal expression of macrophage migration inhibitory factor during the development of rat crescentic glomerulonephritis. *Am J Pathol* 1996;149:1119.
176. Lan HY, et al. The pathogenic role of macrophage migration inhibitory factor in immunologically induced kidney disease in the rat. *J Exp Med 199* 1997;185:1455.
177. Yang N, et al. Reversal of established rat crescentic glomerulonephritis by blockade of macrophage migration inhibitory factor (MIF): potential role of MIF in regulating glucocorticoid production. *Mol Med* 1998;4:413.
178. Sasaki S, et al. Transgene of MIF induces podocyte injury and progressive mesangial sclerosis in the mouse kidney. *Kidney Int* 2004;65:469.
179. Bonizzi G, Karin M. The two NF-kappaB activation pathways and their role in innate and adaptive immunity. *Trends Immunol* 2004;25:280.
180. Sakurai H, et al. Activation of transcription factor NF-kappa B in experimental glomerulonephritis in rats. *Biochim Biophys Acta* 1996;1316:132.
181. Seto M, et al. Effects of prednisolone on glomerular signal transduction cascades in experimental glomerulonephritis. *J Am Soc Nephrol* 1998;9:1367.
182. Hernandez-Presa MA, Gomez-Guerrero C, Egido J. In situ non-radioactive detection of nuclear factors in paraffin sections by Southwestern histochemistry. *Kidney Int* 1999;55:209.
183. Tomita N, et al. In vivo administration of a nuclear transcription factor-kappaB decoy suppresses experimental crescentic glomerulonephritis. *J Am Soc Nephrol* 2000;11:1244.
184. Anders HJ, et al. Bacterial CpG-DNA aggravates immune complex glomerulonephritis: role of TLR9-mediated expression of chemokines and chemokine receptors. *J Am Soc Nephrol* 2003;14:317.
185. Dong C, Davis RJ, Flavell RA. MAP kinases in the immune response. *Annu Rev Immunol* 2002;20:55.
186. Stambe C, et al. p38 Mitogen-activated protein kinase activation and cell localization in human glomerulonephritis: correlation with renal injury. *J Am Soc Nephrol* 2004;15:326.

187. Sakai N, et al. p38 MAPK phosphorylation and NF-kappa B activation in human crescentic glomerulonephritis. *Nephrol Dial Transplant* 2002;17: 998.
188. Masaki T, et al. Activation of the extracellular-signal regulated protein kinase pathway in human glomerulopathies. *J Am Soc Nephrol* 2004;15: 1835.
189. Wada T, et al. Involvement of p38 mitogen-activated protein kinase followed by chemokine expression in crescentic glomerulonephritis. *Am J Kidney Dis* 2001;38:1169.
190. Stambe C, et al. Blockade of p38alpha MAPK ameliorates acute inflammatory renal injury in rat anti-GBM glomerulonephritis. *J Am Soc Nephrol* 2003;14:338.
191. Stambe C, et al. Activation and cellular localization of the p38 and JNK MAPK pathways in rat crescentic glomerulonephritis. *Kidney Int* 2003;64:2121.
192. Swantek JL, Cobb MH, Geppert TD. Jun N-terminal kinase/stress-activated protein kinase (JNK/SAPK) is required for lipopolysaccharide stimulation of tumor necrosis factor alpha (TNF-alpha) translation: glucocorticoids inhibit TNF-alpha translation by blocking JNK/SAPK. *Mol Cell Biol* 1997;17:6274.
193. Hermoso MA, Cidlowski JA. Putting the brake on inflammatory responses: the role of glucocorticoids. *IUBMB Life* 2003;55:497.
194. Rogatsky I, Logan SK, Garabedian MJ. Antagonism of glucocorticoid receptor transcriptional activation by the c-Jun N-terminal kinase. *Proc Natl Acad Sci USA*. 1998;95:2050.
195. Wang S, Hirschberg R. Bone morphogenetic protein-7 signals opposing transforming growth factor beta in mesangial cells. *J Biol Chem* 2004;279:23200.
196. Zeisberg M, et al. BMP-7 counteracts TGF-beta1-induced epithelial-to-mesenchymal transition and reverses chronic renal injury. *Nat Med* 2003;9:964.
197. Atkins, RC, et al. Modulators of crescentic glomerulonephritis. *J Am Soc Nephrol* 1996;7:2271.
198. Olsen S. Extracapillary glomerulonephritis. A semiquantitative lightmicroscopical study of 59 patients. *Acta Pathol Microbiol Scand (A)* 1974;(Suppl 249):7.
199. Jennette JC, Hipp CG. The epithelial antigen phenotype of glomerular crescent cells. *Am J Clin Pathol* 1986;86:274.
200. Guettier C, et al. Immunohistochemical demonstration of parietal epithelial cells and macrophages in human proliferative extra-capillary lesions. *Virchows Arch A Pathol Anat Histopathol* 1986;409:739.
201. Ophascharoensuk V, et al. Role of intrinsic renal cells versus infiltrating cells in glomerular crescent formation. *Kidney Int* 1998;54:416.
202. Le Hir M, et al. Podocyte bridges between the tuft and Bowman's capsule: an early event in experimental crescentic glomerulonephritis. *J Am Soc Nephrol* 2001;12:2060.
203. Moeller MJ, et al. Podocytes populate cellular crescents in a murine model of inflammatory glomerulonephritis. *J Am Soc Nephrol* 2004;15: 61.
204. Masaki T, et al. Heterogeneity of antigen expression explains controversy over glomerular macrophage accumulation in mouse glomerulonephritis. *Nephrol Dial Transplant* 2003;18:178.
205. Hancock HW, Zola H, Atkins RC. Antigenic heterogeneity of human mononuclear phagocytes: immunohistologic analysis using monoclonal antibodies. *Blood* 1983;62:1271.
206. Schiffer MS, Michael AF. Renal cell turnover studied by Y chromosome (Y body) staining of the transplanted human kidney. *J Lab Clin Med* 1978;92:841.
207. Kondo Y, Shigematsu H, Kobayashi Y. Cellular aspects of rabbit Masugi nephritis. II. Progressive glomerular injuries with crescent formation. *Lab Invest* 1972;27:620.
208. Thomson NM, et al. The macrophage in the development of experimental crescentic glomerulonephritis. Studies using tissue culture and electron microscopy. *Am J Pathol* 1979;94:223.
209. Holdsworth SR, et al. Histochemistry of glomerular cells in animal models of crescentic glomerulonephritis. *Pathology* 1980;12:339.
210. Cattell V, Arlidge S. The origin of proliferating cells in the glomerulus and Bowman's capsule in nephrotoxic serum nephritis: effects of unilateral renal irradiation. *Br J Exp Pathol* 1981;62:669.
211. Clarke BE, et al. Macrophages and glomerular crescent formation. Studies with rat nephrotoxic nephritis. *Pathology* 1983;15:75.
212. Lan H, et al. De novo glomerular osteopontin expression in rat crescentic glomerulonephritis. *Kidney Int* 1998;53:136.
213. Nikolic-Paterson DJ, et al. D novo CD44 expression by proliferating mesangial cells in rat anti-Thy-1 nephritis. *J Am Soc Nephrol* 1996;7:1006.
214. Lan HY, et al. Local macrophage proliferation in the pathogenesis of glomerular crescent formation in rat anti-glomerular basement membrane (GBM) glomerulonephritis. *Clin Exp Immunol* 1997;110:233.
215. D'Amico G. Role of interstitial infiltration of leukocytes in glomerular diseases. *Nephrol Dial Transplant* 1988;3:596.
216. Markovic-Lipkovski J, et al. Association of glomerular and interstitial mononuclear leukocytes with different forms of glomerulonephritis. *Nephrol Dial Transplant* 1990;5:10.
217. Vassalli P, McCluskey RT. The pathogenic role of the coagulation process in rabbit Masugi nephritis. *Am J Pathol* 1964;45:653.
218. Holdsworth SR, et al. The effect of defibrination on macrophage participa-

219. Zoja C, et al. Tissue plasminogen activator therapy of rabbit nephrotoxic nephritis. *Lab Invest* 1990;62:34.
220. Drew AF, et al. Crescentic glomerulonephritis is diminished in fibrinogen-deficient mice. *Am J Physiol Renal Physiol* 2001;281:F1157.
221. Tipping PG, Lowe MG, Holdsworth SR. Glomerular macrophages express augmented procoagulant activity in experimental fibrin-related glomerulonephritis in rabbits. *J Clin Invest* 1988;82:1253.
222. Erlich JH, et al. Renal expression of tissue factor pathway inhibitor and evidence for a role in crescentic glomerulonephritis in rabbits. *J Clin Invest* 1996;98:325.
223. Cunningham MA, et al. Protease-activated receptor 1 mediates thrombin-dependent, cell-mediated renal inflammation in crescentic glomerulonephritis. *J Exp Med* 2000;191:455.
224. Merritt SE, et al. Analysis of alpha 1 (I) procollagen alpha 1 (IV) collagen, and beta-actin mRNA in glomerulus and cortex of rabbits with experimental anti-glomerular basement membrane disease. Evidence for early extraglomerular collagen biosynthesis. *Lab Invest* 1990;63:762.
225. Morel-Maroger Striker L, et al. The composition of glomerulosclerosis. I. Studies in focal sclerosis, crescentic glomerulonephritis, and membranoproliferative glomerulonephritis. *Lab Invest* 1984;51:181.
226. Silva FG, Hoyer JR, Pirani CL. Sequential studies of glomerular crescent formation in rats with antiglomerular basement membrane-induced glomerulonephritis and the role of coagulation factors. *Lab Invest* 1984;51:404.
227. Johnson RJ, et al. The activated mesangial cell: a glomerular "myofibroblast?" *J Am Soc Nephrol* 1992;2:S190.
228. Ng YY, et al. Glomerular epithelial-myofibroblast transdifferentiation in the evolution of glomerular crescent formation. *Nephrol Dial Transplant* 1999;14:2860.
229. Abe R, et al. Peripheral blood fibrocytes: differentiation pathway and migration to wound sites. *J Immunol* 2001;166:7556.
230. Phillips RJ, et al. Circulating fibrocytes traffic to the lungs in response to CXCL12 and mediate fibrosis. *J Clin Invest* 2004;114:438.
231. Ng YY, et al. Expression of basic fibroblast growth factor and its receptor in the progression of rat crescentic glomerulonephritis. *Nephrology* 1995;1:569.
232. Fujigaki Y, et al. Cytokines and cell cycle regulation in the fibrous progression of crescent formation in antiglomerular basement membrane nephritis of WKY rats. *Virchows Arch* 2001;439:35.
233. Chen H, et al. Pathological demography of native patients in a nephrology center in China. *Chin Med J (Engl)* 2003;116:1377.
234. Andrassy K, et al. Rapidly progressive glomerulonephritis: analysis of prevalence and clinical course. *Nephron* 1991;59:206.
235. Simon P, et al. Epidemiologic data of primary glomerular diseases in western France. *Kidney Int* 2004;66:905.
236. Mathew TH, Kincaid-Smith P. Severe fibrin and crescent glomerulonephritis: clinical and morphological aspects of 33 patients. *Perspect Nephrol Hypertens* 1973;1 Pt 2:727.
237. Striker GE, et al. Renal failure, glomerulonephritis and glomerular epithelial cell hyperplasia. *Perspect Nephrol Hypertens* 1973;1 Pt 2:657.
238. Anand SK, et al. Extracapillary proliferative glomerulonephritis in children. *Pediatrics* 1975;56:434.
239. Habib R. Classification anatomique des nephropathies glomerularies. *Paediat Fort* 1970;81.
240. Group SPNS. A clinicopathologic study of crescent glomerulonephritis in 50 children. *Kidney Int* 1985;450.
241. Asaba H, et al. Clinical trial of plasma exchange with a membrane filter in treatment of crescentic glomerulonephritis. *Clin Nephrol* 1980;14:60.
242. Davson J, Platt RA. A clinical and pathological study of renal disease: I. Nephritis. *Q J Med* 1949;149.
243. Harrison CV, Loughridge LW, Milne MD. Acute oliguric renal failure in acute glomerulonephritis and polyarteritis nodosa. *Q J Med* 1964;33: 39.
244. Rees AJ, et al. The influence of HLA-linked genes on the severity of anti-GBM antibody-mediated nephritis. *Kidney Int* 1984;26:445.
245. Kelly PT, Haponik EF. Goodpasture syndrome: molecular and clinical advances. *Medicine (Baltimore)* 1994;73:171.
246. Cameron JS, Ogg CS. Rapidly progressive glomerulonephritis with extensive crescents. *Perspect Nephrol Hypertens* 1973;1 Pt 2:735.
247. Forland M, et al. Clinical and renal biopsy observations in oliguric glomerulonephritis. *J Chronic Dis* 1966;19:163.
248. Lawrence JR. Glomerulonephritis with fibrin and crescent formation. *Perspect Nephrol Hypertens* 1973;1 Pt 2:739.
249. Proesmans W. Proliferative glomerulonephritis with crescents. In: *2nd International Symp Paediatr Nephrol*. Paris, 1971:91.
250. Rosen S. Crescenteric glomerulonephritis: occurrence, mechanisms, and prognosis. *Pathol Annu* 1975;10:37.
251. Tang Z, et al. Clinical spectrum of diffuse crescentic glomerulonephritis in Chinese patients. *Chin Med J (Engl)* 2003;116:1737.
252. Aronson MD, Phillips CA. Coxsackievirus B5 infections in acute oliguric renal failure. *J Infect Dis* 1975;132:303.
253. Wilson CB, Smith RC. Goodpasture's syndrome associated with influenza A2 virus infection. *Ann Intern Med* 1972;76:91.
254. Hotz P. Occupational hydrocarbon exposure and chronic nephropathy. *Toxicology* 1994;90:163.

255. Hopper J, Biava C, Naughton C. Glomerular extracapillary proliferation (crescentic glomerulonephritis) associated with non-renal malignancies. *Kidney Int* 1976;554.

256. Kallenberg CG, et al. Anti-neutrophil cytoplasmic antibodies: current diagnostic and pathophysiological potential. *Kidney Int* 1994;46:1.

257. Niles JL, et al. The syndrome of lung hemorrhage and nephritis is usually an ANCA-associated condition. *Arch Intern Med* 1996;156:440.

258. Birch DF, et al. Urinary erythrocyte morphology in the diagnosis of glomerular hematuria. *Clin Nephrol* 1983;20:78.

259. Chirawong P, Nanra RS, Kincaid-Smith P. Degradation products and the role of coagulation in "persistent" glomerulonephritis. *Ann Intern Med* 1971;74:853.

260. Dotremont G, et al. Urinary excretion of fibrinogen-fibrin-related antigen in glomerulonephritis: effect of indomethacin. *Perspect Nephrol Hypertens* 1973;1 Pt 2:829.

261. Katmitsuji H, Tani K, Taniguchi A. Urinary fibrin-fibrinogen degradation products and intraglomerular fibrin-fibrinogen deposition in various renal diseases. *Thromb Res* 1981;285.

262. Ewan PW, et al. Detection of intrapulmonary hemorrhage with carbon monoxide uptake. Application in Goodpasture's syndrome. *N Engl J Med.* 1976;295:1391.

263. Falk RJ, et al. Clinical course of anti-neutrophil cytoplasmic autoantibody-associated glomerulonephritis and systemic vasculitis. The Glomerular Disease Collaborative Network. *Ann Intern Med* 1990;113:656.

264. Cairns S. The significance of circulating immune complexes in idiopathic glomerulonephritis. *Kidney Int* 1979;911.

265. Lockwood CM, et al. Plasma-exchange and immunosuppression in the treatment of fulminating immune-complex crescentic nephritis. *Lancet* 1977;1:63.

266. Woodroofe A. Detection of circulating immune complexes in glomerulonephritis. *Kidney Int* 1977;268.

267. Stachura I, Whiteside TL, Kelly RH. Circulating and deposited immune complexes in patients with glomerular disease: immunopathologic correlations. *Am J Pathol* 1981;103:21.

268. Russ G, d'Apice AJ. Plasma exchange and immunosuppression in crescentic glomerulonephritis. In: *8th International Congress of Nephrology.* Basel: Karger; 1981.

269. Jordan SC. Treatment of systemic and renal-limited vasculitic disorders with pooled human intravenous immune globulin. *J Clin Immunol* 1995;15:76S.

270. Mahieu P, Lambert PH, Miescher PA. Detection of anti-glomerular basement membrane antibodies by radioimmunological technique. Clinical application in human nephropathies. *J Clin Invest* 1974;54:128.

271. Macanovic M, Evans DJ, Peters DK. Allergic response to glomerular basement membrane in patients with glomerulonephritis. *Lancet* 1972;2:207.

272. McIntosh RM, et al. Cryoglobulins. III. Further studies on the nature, incidence, clinical, diagnostic, prognostic, and immunopathologic significance of cryoproteins in renal disease. *Q J Med* 1975;44:285.

273. Wilson C, Marquardt H, Dixon FJ. Radioimmunoassay for circulating antiglomerular basement membrane antibody. *Kidney Int* 1974.

274. Jennette JC. Rapidly progressive crescentic glomerulonephritis. *Kidney Int* 2003;63:1164.

275. Adam C, Morel-Maroger L, Richet G. Cryoglobulins in glomerulonephritis not related to systemic disease. *Kidney Int* 1973;3:334.

276. Johnson RJ, et al. Membranoproliferative glomerulonephritis associated with hepatitis C virus infection. *N Engl J Med* 1993;328:465.

277. Heilman RL, et al. Analysis of risk factors for patient and renal survival in crescentic glomerulonephritis. *Am J Kidney Dis* 1987;9:98.

278. Jayne D. Update on the European Vasculitis Study Group trials. *Curr Opin Rheumatol* 2001;13:48.

279. Hind CR, et al. Prognosis after immunosuppression of patients with crescentic nephritis requiring dialysis. *Lancet* 1983;1:263.

280. O'Neil W, Etheridge WB, Bloomer HA. A high dose corticosteroids: Their use in treating idiopathic rapidly progressive glomerulonephritis. *Arch Intern Med* 1979;139:514.

281. Nakamoto S, et al. Treatment of oliguric glomerulonephritis with dialysis and steroids. *Ann Intern Med* 1965;63:359.

282. Nakamoto Y. Combined anticoagulant and immunosuppressive treatment in rapidly progressive glomerulonephritis: A long term follow up study. *Jpn J Med* 1979;18:210.

283. Habib R. Contribution of immunofluorescent microscopy to classification of glomerular diseases. In: Kincaid-Smith PA, d'Apice AJ, Atkins RC, eds. *Progress in glomerulonephritis.* New York: Wiley, 1979.

284. Alamartine E, Laurent-Pilonchery B, Berthoux F. Glomerular crescents and IgA glomerulonephritis. Nosological and prognostic problems. *Ann Med Interne (Paris)* 1993;144:317.

285. Brown CB, et al. Combined immunosuppression and anticoagulation in rapidly progressive glomerulonephritis. *Lancet* 1974;2:1166.

286. Muller GA, Seipel L, Risler T. Treatment of non anti-GBM-antibody mediated, rapidly progressive glomerulonephritis by plasmapheresis and immunosuppression. *Klin Wochenschr* 1986;64:231.

287. Ballerman BJ. Regulation of bovine glomerular endothelial cell growth in vitro. *Am J Physiol* 1988;256.

288. Pendergraft WF, et al. ANCA antigens, proteinase 3 and myeloperoxidase, are not expressed in endothelial cells. *Kidney Int* 2000;57:1981.

289. Kobayashi Y, et al. Effect of methylprednisolone on progressive Masugi nephritis in the rabbit. I. Suppression of antibody production and crescent formation. *Virchows Arch B Cell Pathol Incl Mol Pathol* 1980;35:45.

290. Holdsworth SR, Bellomo R. Differential effects of steroids on leukocyte-mediated glomerulonephritis in the rabbit. *Kidney Int* 1984;26:162.

291. Tipping PG, Holdsworth SR. The mechanism of action of corticosteroids on glomerular injury in acute serum sickness in rabbits. *Clin Exp Immunol* 1985;59:555.

292. Karin M. The NF-kappa B activation pathway: its regulation and role in inflammation and cell survival. *Cancer J Sci Am* 1998;4(Suppl 1):S92.

293. Cameron JS. Immunosuppressant agents in the treatment of glomerulonephritis. 2. Cytotoxic drugs. *J R Coll Physicians Lond* 1971;5:301.

294. Cohen RD, Conn DL, Ilstrup DM. Clinical features, prognosis, and response to treatment in polyarteritis. *Mayo Clin Proc* 1980;55:146.

295. Pirofsky B, Bardana EJ Jr. Immunosuppressive therapy in rheumatic disease. *Med Clin North Am* 1977;61:419.

296. Nachman PH, et al. Treatment response and relapse in antineutrophil cytoplasmic autoantibody-associated microscopic polyangiitis and glomerulonephritis. *J Am Soc Nephrol* 1996;7:33.

297. Bolton WK, Couser WG. Intravenous pulse methylprednisolone therapy of acute crescentic rapidly progressive glomerulonephritis. *Am J Med* 1979;66:495.

298. Cole BR, et al. "Pulse" methylprednisolone therapy in the treatment of severe glomerulonephritis. *J Pediatr* 1976;88:307.

299. Ferraris JR, et al. "Pulse' methylprednisolone therapy in the treatment of acute crescentic glomerulonephritis. *Nephron* 1983;34:207.

300. Stevens ME, McConnell M, Bone JM. Aggressive treatment with pulse methylprednisolone or plasma exchange is justified in rapidly progressive glomerulonephritis. *Proc Eur Dial Transplant Assoc* 1983;19:724.

301. Wing EJ, et al. Infectious complications with plasmapheresis in rapidly progressive glomerulonephritis. *JAMA* 1980;244:2423.

302. Takeda S, et al. Effects of methylprednisolone pulse therapy in the insidious type of crescentic glomerulonephritis. *Nippon Jinzo Gakkai Shi* 1997;39:490.

303. Bolton W, Sturgill B. Pulse methylprednisolone therapy of rapidly progressive glomerulonephritis—10 years experience. *Kidney Int* 1985;180.

304. Macconi D, et al. Methylprednisolone normalizes superoxide anion production by polymorphs from patients with ANCA-positive vasculitides. *Kidney Int* 1993;44:215.

305. Cameron JS, et al. Letter: Combined immunosuppression and anticoagulation in rapidly progressive glomerulonephritis. *Lancet* 1975;2:923.

306. Neild GH, et al. Relapsing polychondritis with crescentic glomerulonephritis. *Br Med J* 1978;1:743.

307. Tietjen DP, Moore WJ. Treatment of rapidly progressive glomerulonephritis due to Behçet's syndrome with intravenous cyclophosphamide. *Nephron* 1990;55:69.

308. Kunis CL, et al. Intravenous "pulse" cyclophosphamide therapy of crescentic glomerulonephritis. *Clin Nephrol* 1992;37:1.

309. Haubitz M, et al. Intravenous pulse administration of cyclophosphamide versus daily oral treatment in patients with antineutrophil cytoplasmic antibody-associated vasculitis and renal involvement: a prospective, randomized study. *Arthritis Rheum* 1998;41:1835.

310. Aasarod K, et al. Wegener's granulomatosis: clinical course in 108 patients with renal involvement. *Nephrol Dial Transplant* 2000;15:611.

311. Halpern B, et al. Protective action of heparin in experimental immune nephritis. *Nature* 1965;205:257.

312. Kleinerman J. Effects of heparin on experimental nephritis in rabbits. *Lab Invest* 1954;3:495.

313. Thomson NE. Defibrination with ancrod in experimental chronic immune complex nephritis. *Clin. Exp. Immunol* 1975;20:527.

314. Border WA, Wilson CB, Dixon FJ. Failure of heparin to affect two types of experimental glomerulonephritis in rabbits. *Kidney Int* 1975;8:140.

315. Bone JM, et al. Heparin therapy in anti-basement membrane nephritis. *Kidney Int* 1975;72.

316. Borrero J, et al. Masugi nephritis: the renal lesion and the coagulation processes. *Clin Nephrol* 1972;1:86.

317. Kincaid-Smith P, Saker BM, Fairley KF. Anticoagulants in "irreversible" acute renal failure. *Lancet* 1968;2:1360.

318. Cameron JS. Platelets and glomerulonephritis. *Nephron* 1977;18:253.

319. Cameron JS. The natural history of glomerulonephritis. In: *Progress in glomerulonephritis.* New York: Wiley; 1979

320. Herdman RC, et al. Anticoagulants in renal disease in children. *Am J Dis Child* 1970;119:27.

321. George CR, Clark WF, Cameron JS. The role of platelets in glomerulonephritis. *Adv Nephrol Necker Hosp* 1975;5:19.

322. Parbtani A, Cameron JS. Platelet and plasma serotonin concentration in glomerulonephritis I. *Thromb Res* 1979;15:109.

323. Kincaid-Smith P, d'Apice AJ. Plasmapheresis in rapidly progressive glomerulonephritis. *Am J Med* 1978;65:564.

324. Lang CH, et al. Goodpasture syndrome treated with immunosuppression and plasma exchange. *Arch Intern Med* 1977;137:1076.

325. Savage CO, et al. Antiglomerular basement membrane antibody mediated disease in the British Isles 1980-4. *Br Med J (Clin Res Ed)* 1986;292:301.

326. Walker RG, et al. Plasmapheresis in Goodpasture's syndrome with renal failure. *Med J Aust* 1977;1:875.

327. Becker GJ, et al. Plasmapheresis in the treatment of glomerulonephritis. *Med J Aust* 1977;2:693.

328. Cole E. Plasma exchange in rapidly progressive glomerulonephritis. *Prog Clin Biol Res* 1990;337:257.
329. Harmer D, et al. Plasmapheresis in fulminating crescentic nephritis. *Lancet* 1979;1:679.
330. Heaf JG, Jorgensen F, Nielsen LP. Treatment and prognosis of extracapillary glomerulonephritis. *Nephron* 1983;35:217.
331. Rifle G, et al. Treatment of idiopathic acute crescentic glomerulonephritis by immunodepression and plasma-exchanges. A prospective randomised study. *Proc Eur Dial Transplant Assoc* 1981;18:493.
332. Warren SE, et al. Recovery from rapidly progressive glomerulonephritis. Improvement after plasmapheresis and immunosuppression. *Arch Intern Med* 1981;141:175.
333. Swainson CP, et al. Plasma exchange in severe glomerulonephritis—who benefits? *Proc Eur Dial Transplant Assoc* 1983;19:732.
334. Glockner WM, et al. Plasma exchange and immunosuppression in rapidly progressive glomerulonephritis: a controlled, multi-center study. *Clin Nephrol* 1988;29:1.
335. Cole E, et al. A prospective randomized trial of plasma exchange as additive therapy in idiopathic crescentic glomerulonephritis. The Canadian Apheresis Study Group. *Am J Kidney Dis* 1992;20:261.
336. Frasca GM, et al. Plasma exchange treatment in rapidly progressive glomerulonephritis associated with anti-neutrophil cytoplasmic autoantibodies. *Int J Artif Organs* 1992;15:181.
337. Pusey CD, et al. Plasma exchange in focal necrotizing glomerulonephritis without anti-GBM antibodies. *Kidney Int* 1991;40:757.
338. Guillevin L, et al. Treatment of glomerulonephritis in microscopic polyangiitis and Churg-Strauss syndrome. Indications of plasma exchanges, Meta-analysis of 2 randomized studies on 140 patients, 32 with glomerulonephritis. *Ann Med Interne (Paris)* 1997;148:198.
339. Stegmayr BG, et al. Plasma exchange or immunoadsorption in patients with rapidly progressive crescentic glomerulonephritis. A Swedish multi-center study. *Int J Artif Organs* 1999;22:81.
340. Chan TM, et al. Efficacy of mycophenolate mofetil in patients with diffuse proliferative lupus nephritis. Hong Kong-Guangzhou Nephrology Study Group. *N Engl J Med* 2000;343:1156.
341. Contreras G, et al. Sequential therapies for proliferative lupus nephritis. *N Engl J Med* 2004;350:971.
342. Langford CA, Talar-Williams C, Sneller MC. Mycophenolate mofetil for remission maintenance in the treatment of Wegener's granulomatosis. *Arthritis Rheum* 2004;51:278.
343. Jarrett SJ, et al. Anti-tumor necrosis factor-alpha therapy-induced vasculitis: case series. *J Rheumatol* 2003;30:2287.
344. Booth A, et al. Prospective study of TNF alpha blockade with infliximab in anti-neutrophil cytoplasmic antibody-associated systemic vasculitis. *J Am Soc Nephrol* 2004;15:717.
345. Dixon FJ, McPhaul JJ, Lerner RA. The contribution of kidney transplantation o the study of glomerulonephritis—the recurrence of glomerulonephritis in renal transplants. *Transplant Proc* 1969;1:194.
346. Halgrimson CG, et al. Goodpasture's syndrome. Treatment with nephrectomy and renal transplantation. *Arch Surg* 1971;103:283.
347. Peten E, et al. Outcome of thirty patients with Alport's syndrome after renal transplantation. *Transplantation* 1991;52:823.
348. Nachman PH, et al. Recurrent ANCA-associated small vessel vasculitis after transplantation: a pooled analysis. *Kidney Int* 1999;56:1544.
349. Ihle BU, et al. De novo crescentic glomerulonephritis in a renal transplant. *Transplant Proc* 1983;15:2147.
350. Johnson JP, et al. Therapy of anti-glomerular basement membrane antibody disease: analysis of prognostic significance of clinical, pathologic and treatment factors. *Medicine (Baltimore)* 1985;64:219.
351. Rondeau E, et al. Plasma exchange and immunosuppression for rapidly progressive glomerulonephritis: prognosis and complications. *Nephrol Dial Transplant* 1989;4:196.
352. Mokrzycki MH, Kaplan AA. Therapeutic plasma exchange: complications and management. *Am J Kidney Dis* 1994;23:817.
353. Cassidy MJ, et al. Towards a more rapid diagnosis of rapidly progressive glomerulonephritis. *BMJ* 1990;301:329.

CHAPTER 61 ■ IMMUNOGLOBULIN A NEPHROPATHY AND HENOCH-SCHÖNLEIN PURPURA

RANDALL JAMES FAULL AND ANTHONY R. CLARKSON

Immunoglobulin A (IgA) nephropathy is the most common form of primary glomerulonephritis, and is a major contributor to the worldwide burden of end-stage renal failure. It is characterized pathologically by proliferation of the glomerular mesangium and mesangial deposition of IgA molecules, and clinically by wide variations in its presentation and prognosis. Its recognition as a distinct disease in its own right dates to the first description of the typical mesangial IgA immunofluorescence by Berger in 1968 (1). Despite considerable effort, elucidation of its etiology as well as satisfactory treatments have both remained largely elusive.

Henoch-Schönlein purpura (HSP) is a small vessel vasculitis that exhibits identical renal histopathologic appearances to IgA nephropathy, but with additional systemic features that readily identify it as a syndrome in its own right. It will be discussed in more detail at the end of this chapter.

IgA NEPHROPATHY

Incidence and Prognosis

The reported incidence and prevalence of IgA nephropathy varies widely, and is dependent to an important degree on variations in renal biopsy policies between different countries. Studies from Europe have estimated the incidence to be 15 to 40 new cases per million population per year. The incidence is higher in Japan, where routine screening for urinary abnormalities is performed in all school-aged children. Prevalence rates, expressed as a percentage of renal biopsy diagnoses, are reported to be 20% to 40% in Asia, Australia, Finland and Southern Europe, but as low as 2% to 10% in the United States. While the local enthusiasm for detecting asymptomatic urinary abnormalities and then biopsying those individuals undoubtedly contributes greatly to these variations, there also appear to be important differences in susceptibility across different ethnic groups (2–4). For example, it is less common in African Americans, black South Africans, and New Zealand Polynesians than in Caucasians of European origin. Subclinical disease without urinary abnormalities may also be much more common than these figures indicate. For example, a recent study of renal allografts in Japan revealed mesangial IgA deposition in 16% (82 out of 510), and 19 of those had mesangial proliferation (5). Two separate studies have found IgA mesangial deposition in 2% and 4.8% of unselected autopsy series (6,7).

Uncertainties about true incidence and different approaches to individuals with asymptomatic urinary abnormalities also affect estimations of prognosis. Centers that trouble to diagnose milder cases will naturally observe a more benign disease course. Undoubtedly the majority of sufferers of IgA nephropathy do have a benign disease that does not lead to progressive renal dysfunction, and in some all signs of disease resolve with time. However, the significant majority have persistent urinary abnormalities (microscopic hematuria +/− proteinuria), and 20% to 40% will eventually progress to end-stage renal failure (8–11). The combination of relative frequency of the disease and a high proportion with poor prognosis means that IgA nephropathy is a major contributor to the number of individuals who require end-stage renal failure replacement therapy. For example, according to the Australian and New Zealand dialysis and transplant registry, 7.0% of patients diagnosed with end-stage renal failure in 2002 had biopsy proven IgA nephropathy (12). For some, the renal demise will be relatively rapid (months to several years), because of more aggressive disease and/or late presentation, whereas others can take decades from first presentation. It will be clear in the later discussion about treatment that estimating an individual's prognosis is crucial when considering active intervention.

Clinical Presentation

The variability of presentations and subsequent course is a feature of IgA nephropathy, and a list of the wide range of initial manifestations is shown in Table 61-1. There is an approximately 3:1 male preponderance.

Macroscopic Hematuria

The most characteristic and, at least to the patient, most dramatic presentation of IgA nephropathy is with episodic macroscopic hematuria in a young adult. Approximately one-third of diagnoses of IgA nephropathy occur as a result of such a presentation. There is a highly characteristic close temporal relationship between its onset and an upper respiratory tract infection, especially pharyngitis or tonsillitis, the hematuria coinciding with or occurring within 1 to 2 days of the sore throat. This has led to wide use of the term "synpharyngitic hematuria," and the timing differentiates it from the 2 to 3 week gap between infection and macroscopic hematuria in postinfectious glomerulonephritis. Less frequently, such hematuria also accompanies infections of other mucosal surfaces (e.g., gastroenteritis and urinary tract infections). The hematuria is painless but often associated with systemic symptoms such as fever, malaise, fatigue, diffuse muscle aches, and abdominal and dull loin pain. It is usually short-lived, lasting 1 to 5 days, and its disappearance coincides with resolution of the systemic symptoms. Occasionally there is associated transient acute renal impairment.

Differentiation from other causes of macroscopic hematuria is important, because frequent and unnecessary radiographic and urologic investigations may ensue if the true cause is not recognized. Of paramount importance is examination of the centrifuged urinary sediment, which displays dysmorphic red

TABLE 61-1

PATTERNS OF CLINICAL PRESENTATION OF IgA NEPHROPATHY

Common
Synpharyngitic macroscopic hematuria +/− loin pain
Microscopic hematuria, usually with proteinuria
Hypertension
Chronic renal failure
Henoch-Schönlein purpura
Uncommon
Malignant hypertension
Acute nephritic syndrome
Acute renal failure
Nephrotic syndrome

blood cells (of glomerular origin), plus granular and red cell casts. Under these circumstances, renal biopsy is the appropriate first diagnostic procedure. The urinary abnormalities of microscopic hematuria +/− proteinuria persist in between episodes of macroscopic hematuria.

Macroscopic hematuria due to IgA nephropathy occurs far more frequently in children and young adults than in middle-aged or elderly patients, in whom such a symptom should raise the suspicion of urinary tract malignancy or stones. Almost universally the episodes stop by the age of 40 or younger, even though mucosal infections still occur and the underlying disease process continues. The reason for resolution of these episodes with age is unclear.

Asymptomatic Hematuria and Proteinuria

At least another third of diagnoses of IgA nephropathy are made following investigation of incidentally discovered microscopic hematuria, usually accompanied by proteinuria. This can occur at any age, and is typical in the older patient. Again, local attitudes to screening and investigating asymptomatic urinary abnormalities dictate the frequency of such presentations. A common source of such referrals is medical examinations performed for work or life insurance purposes.

Proteinuria and Nephrotic Syndrome

Proteinuria in the absence of hematuria is distinctly uncommon in IgA nephropathy. Nephrotic-range proteinuria is also uncommon, but can occur in the presence of either very active acute disease or advanced disease with considerable scarring. At times, both IgA nephropathy and minimal change disease occur together, which may simply be chance association of two relatively common disorders. It is important to recognize this possibility, as the nephrotic syndrome should be treated as for minimal change disease in isolation, with a similar expectation of response (13).

Hypertension and Malignant Hypertension

An important (and in our experience, increasing) proportion of patients with IgA nephropathy are detected during investigation of newly diagnosed hypertension, and it is one of the major causes of secondary hypertension in young adults. The more widespread use of blood pressure screening programs than urine screening programs may account for this increase. The more dramatic presentation of malignant hypertension is also well recognized, and the renal biopsy findings will often include evidence of severe and long-standing glomerular disease.

Acute Renal Failure

Acute renal failure is an uncommon feature of *de novo* IgA nephropathy. As described above, it may occur during episodes of macroscopic hematuria, possibly as a result of tubular obstruction by red blood cells. Such episodes resolve without specific therapy apart from occasional resort to temporary dialysis (14). Rapidly progressive renal failure can also occur as a result of acute necrotizing, crescentic glomerular injury. It is important to recognize this severe manifestation of the disease, as it is perhaps the strongest indication for aggressive therapeutic intervention.

Chronic Renal Failure

The precise proportion of patients with IgA nephropathy who have chronic, established renal failure at presentation is clouded by the fact that many who come to our attention late in the course of renal disease do not have a renal biopsy performed. Undoubtedly many of those with end or near-end-stage renal failure with small kidneys had unrecognized IgA nephropathy for years or decades. The lack of a reliable peripheral diagnostic marker of IgA nephropathy is an obvious deficit. We have on several occasions made a presumptive, retrospective diagnosis in renal transplant recipients with a failing graft where a transplant biopsy showed recurrent IgA nephropathy.

Disease Associations

The literature is replete with descriptions of associations of diseases with IgA nephropathy, although it is likely that many of these are chance associations. Some of the important and more established associations are shown in Table 61-2.

Deposition of IgA in the mesangium is relatively common and long-recognised in chronic liver disease, particularly alcoholic cirrhosis (15–17), although more overt renal disease is less common. Impaired clearance of IgA by the damaged liver cells is thought to account for this observation. In contrast, despite high levels of circulating IgA in IgA paraproteinemias, there have only been very occasional reported associations with IgA nephropathy (18,19). Likewise, there is a polyclonal increase in IgA levels in human immunodeficiency virus/acquired immune deficiency syndrome (AIDS), but no clear increase in the incidence of IgA nephropathy in association (20). These observations support the current view of the pathogenesis of IgA nephropathy, that it is alterations in the structure of the IgA molecule rather than the serum levels that lead to disease (see below).

Clinical Course

The clinical course of IgA nephropathy may be very clear at the time of diagnosis, in that those presenting late in the course of the disease may already have established renal impairment

TABLE 61-2

DISEASE ASSOCIATIONS WITH IgA NEPHROPATHY

Henoch-Schönlein purpura
Liver disease (alcoholic)
Inflammatory bowel disease
Celiac disease
Dermatitis herpetiformis

or even end-stage renal failure. Others usually follow one of several patterns of disease behavior, although precise estimates of the frequency of each pattern is not possible due to wide variations in screening and diagnosis approaches (discussed above). The patterns are: resolution of mild disease, ongoing mild disease without progressive renal failure, slowly progressive renal failure, and rapidly progressive renal failure. Hypertension is a frequent association, and is invariable and often severe in those with progressive disease. It is reasonable to assume that there is a large body of individuals with benign, asymptomatic disease with good prognosis who are never recognised. Pooling of data from a number of clinical studies has given useful information about the natural history of the disease and predicting its prognosis (8–11).

An important minority, perhaps 15% of those diagnosed, will have mild disease at presentation (i.e., normal renal function, minimal proteinuria and hematuria) and with time undergo spontaneous resolution of all signs of the problem. Associated disappearance of mesangial IgA is suggested by a study of repeated biopsies (21). Approximately 50% of patients diagnosed with IgA nephropathy have persistent but benign disease. Typical is a pattern of ongoing low-grade microscopic hematuria, low levels of or absent proteinuria, normal renal function, and normotension or mild, easily controlled hypertension. Such individuals should be monitored regularly, but longish intervals are reasonable as significant changes in their disease status will be measured in years or even decades. Both of these groups of patients do not require specific treatment for the IgA nephropathy—the challenge is predicting at the time of diagnosis those who will have benign disease.

Most of the remaining patients will have slowly progressive renal impairment, over years to decades, eventually leading to end-stage renal failure if lifespan permits. A more malignant course, measured in months, to severe renal failure is uncommon but well recognized. Frank crescentic disease on diagnostic renal biopsy predicts a rapidly progressive course. Specific and nonspecific (e.g., control of hypertension) treatment needs to target individuals with or at high risk of progressive disease.

Clinical and histologic features can be used to generate meaningful prognostic information (8–11,22,23). Hypertension, persistent proteinuria of >1g per 24 hours, and impaired renal function at time of diagnosis, are consistent and strong clinical predictors of poor renal survival. Histologically, glomerular sclerosis, tubular atrophy, interstitial fibrosis, and hypertensive vascular changes all correlate with poor outcome. Episodic macroscopic hematuria, initially thought to be a poor prognostic sign (24), is now considered more likely to indicate a benign prognosis. The lead-time bias following early and more likely diagnosis because of the dramatic clinical presentation probably accounts for this skewing to milder disease. Individuals with persistent normal blood pressure and proteinuria of <0.2 g per 24 hours have a negligible risk of progression (10). However, presentation with isolated microscopic hematuria may not be a reliable sign of good long term outcome. A study in Hong Kong patients found that 44% of 72 patients presenting with microscopic hematuria and minimal proteinuria (<0.4g per 24 hours) developed proteinuria >1gm per 24 hours, hypertension, or renal impairment over 7 years (25). In 14% the hematuria resolved.

Diagnosis and Laboratory Features

While clinical suspicion based on presenting features (e.g., synpharyngitic hematuria) will often lead to the correct diagnosis of IgA nephropathy, a renal biopsy is an absolute requirement for confirmation. No other investigation has been proven to reliably distinguish IgA nephropathy from other renal diseases. This is frustrating because it means that a renal biopsy still is required for diagnosis—a procedure often judged unnecessary in a person with just microscopic hematuria. In the latter situation, glomerular-type hematuria usually is due either to mild IgA nephropathy or to thin basement membrane nephropathy.

Most accounts describe an elevation of serum IgA concentrations in up to 50% of cases, which has no diagnostic power (14). Neither, despite the original claims (26), has the detection of elevated plasma IgA–fibronectin complexes (27). An elevated serum IgA/C3 ratio in combination with elevated serum IgA level improves the diagnostic accuracy, but cannot supplant the histopathology (28).

Pathology

The histopathologic diagnosis of IgA nephropathy is usually clear and straightforward, with little opportunity to consider a differential diagnosis. The key is the immunohistochemical identification of IgA deposition in the glomerular mesangium. It is an excellent example of the strength of clinicopathologic correlation and of the power of the combination of light microscopy, immunohistochemistry, and electron microscopy. Histologic classifications have been proposed but are not widely used, and, apart from in advanced disease with significant scarring, have limited prognostic value (29–31). The histologic features are illustrated in Figure 61-1.

Light Microscopy

The light microscopic hallmark of IgA nephropathy is focal or diffuse expansion of mesangial regions with cells and matrix. In their mildest forms, the mesangial changes may be quite focal as well as segmental. Appreciable numbers of glomerular tufts may appear to be normal and, even in those affected, the mesangial cells and matrix changes may be quite marginal. Classically, however, the disease is diffuse, although the tuft changes may be segmental or global in distribution. As a result of mesangial proliferation, the tuft stalk expands and becomes accentuated, often markedly so, an appearance described as *arborization*.

Capillary loops usually are patent, with a normal configuration of capillary walls. However, in more florid disease, mesangial proliferative activity results in the matrix extending peripherally and circumferentially in the capillary walls, resulting in double-contouring or "tram-line" effect, usually with lumen narrowing.

In active disease, there may be tuft necrosis associated with an exudate of fibrin and infiltration of neutrophils, some of which may show karyorrhexis. This occurrence is associated with crescent formation.

In long-standing disease, areas of segmental tuft collapse and sclerosis, sometimes with overlying hyalinosis, are seen, which usually are associated with broad synechiae. In progressive disease, the end result is total glomerular obsolescence and sclerosis. The presence in one biopsy of all the lesions described is not infrequent.

Proportional to the degree of glomerular damage, there may be tubulointerstitial disease. When active glomerular disease is present, there often is interstitial edema associated with mild to moderate infiltrate of mononuclear cells and scattered neutrophils. Secondary tubular damage also may be evident. Interstitial scarring and tubular atrophy are features of advanced disease and correlate best with long-term outcome. Hypertensive changes complicate advanced cases, and related vascular lesions become evident.

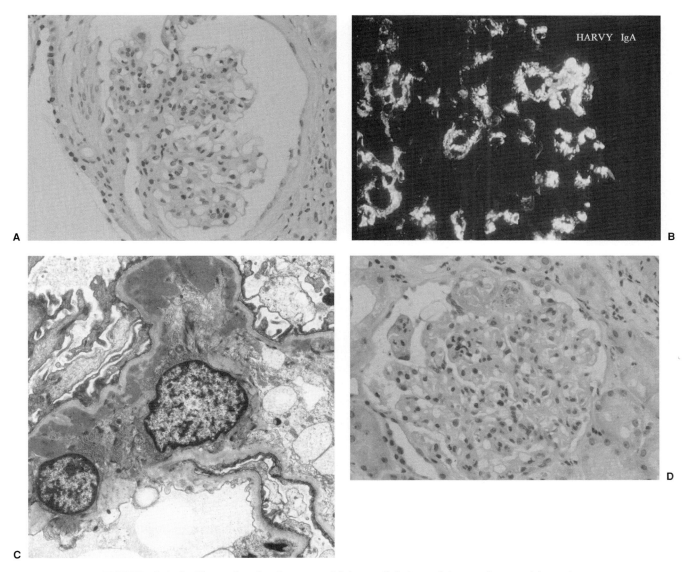

FIGURE 61-1. A: Glomerulus showing mesangial hypercellularity and increased mesangial matrix. (Hematoxylin and eosin stain, magnification, ×200.) B: Glomerulus, with brightly fluorescing mesangial deposits of IgA. (Fluorescinated anti-human IgA, magnification 200x). C: Electron micrograph of glomerular mesangium showing multiple mesangial electron dense deposits typical of IgA nephropathy. (Magnification ×3,000.) D: Glomerulus showing an acute lesion with segmental fibrinoid change and karryorhectic debris. (Hematoxylin and eosin, magnification ×200.) (*continued*)

Immunohistochemistry

Mesangial expansion is not specific to IgA nephropathy, and can be seen in other glomerular diseases including diabetic nephropathy and focal segmental glomerulosclerosis. A definitive diagnosis can be made only with the aid of immunofluorescent or immunoperoxidase techniques applied to renal tissue. Granular deposition of IgA and usually C3 is present predominantly in the mesangium, even in apparently normal or minimally affected glomeruli. In addition, there may be variable deposits of immunoglobulin G (IgG), immunoglobulin M (IgM), or both, frequently fluorescing with lesser intensity. C1q and C4 are found rarely.

Capillary loop fluorescence for IgA is observed most commonly when active disease is present. Such cases also may show mesangial and capillary wall fibrinogen; the latter also is present in crescents. IgM also is present in areas of sclerosis. Walls of small and medium-sized blood vessels may contain abundant granular C3, particularly if the patient is hypertensive.

Electron Microscopy

There is a varying degree of expansion and proliferation of both mesangial cells and matrix, and electron-dense deposits of differing sizes and amounts are present in the matrix. Not infrequently, the deposits are particularly evident in perimesangial regions or even localized to this site. Corresponding to the segmental nature of the disease process, the distribution and amount of deposits may be quite patchy. Some mesangial sites may be distinctly free of deposits, yet others in the same glomerulus may be packed with them. The deposits usually are solid and homogeneous.

Nephrotic syndrome with the clinical and pathologic features of minimal-change disease also has been noted in patients with IgA nephropathy (13). Occasionally, glomerular basement

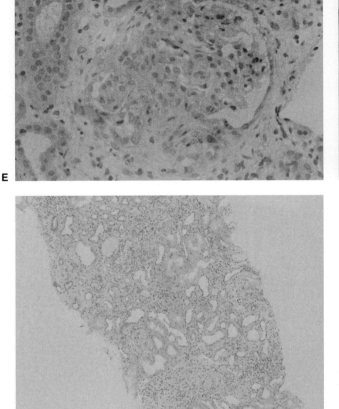

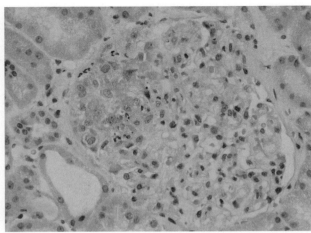

FIGURE 61-1. (*Continued*) **E:** Glomerulus showing an acute lesion with segmental crescent. (Hematoxylin and eosin, magnification ×200.) **F:** Sclerosing glomerulus with mesangial proliferation. (Hematoxylin and eosin, magnification ×200.) **G:** Low-power view of advanced IgA nephropathy, showing tubular dropout, interstitial fibrosis and chronic inflammatory interstitial infiltrate. (Hematoxylin and eosin, magnification ×40.) All photographs courtesy of Dr. James Nolan.

membranes are uniformly thin and this observation probably signifies the presence together of two common conditions, IgA nephropathy and thin basement membrane nephropathy. However, one study of IgA nephropathy biopsies (32) describes 40% with thin glomerular basement membranes, so perhaps mesangial IgA deposits interfere in some way with normal glomerular basement membrane synthesis. This association, however, does not have any obvious prognostic implications.

Pathogenesis

The cause (or causes) of IgA nephropathy has been frustratingly elusive. Its frequent recurrence following renal transplantation (33–36), and documented resolution of IgA mesangial deposits in renal allografts (37,38), point to problems in the host's IgA immune system rather than the kidney itself. While it is accepted that the initiating event in the renal disease is the mesangial deposition of IgA, there is considerable variability in the subsequent events. These range from little or no renal disease, through continued deposition of IgA but minimal glomerular inflammation without renal impairment, to continued deposition and progressive renal failure. With the possible exception of capillary loop IgA deposition, which may indicate a poor prognosis, the extent and site of deposition bears no relationship with prognosis. This heterogeneity suggests that IgA nephropathy is more than just a simple disease caused by a single, defined abnormality.

Immunobiology of Immunoglobulin A

A working knowledge of the immunobiology of IgA is important to understand the pathogenesis of IgA nephropathy (39–41). IgA is the major immunoglobulin in mucosal secretions but is present in relatively low concentrations in serum. Its predominant function is in mucosal defense, where polymeric IgA binds and neutralizes microbes and toxins.

Two subclasses exist in humans, IgA1 and IgA2, both of which occur in monomeric (mIgA) and polymeric (pIgA) forms. IgA1 appears very late in the evolutionary chain, being present only in chimpanzees, orangutans, and humans. Plasma cells in the gastrointestinal tract and respiratory tract produce both IgA1 and IgA2 that is found in mucosal secretions at these sites. In the bone marrow, lymph nodes, and spleen, the plasma cells predominantly produce IgA1 that is expressed in the serum. The IgA that is found in the serum is 90% monomeric, whereas that found in mucosal secretions is virtually all polymeric. IgA1 accounts for 90% of serum IgA, whereas IgA2 comprises 60% of IgA in secretions (Table 61-3). Polymeric IgA (which is usually a dimer) contains a bridging or joining polypeptide—the J chain—that is linked to the heavy chain during the formation of the multimers within the plasma cell. IgM also exists as polymers linked by J chains.

IgA1 possesses an 18 amino acid hinge region situated between the CHI and CH2 domains of the heavy chain. This is absent in IgA2, and is the main structural difference between the two subclasses. The hinge region consists of an unusual repeating sequence of proline, serine, and threonine residues, and carries multiple O-linked carbohydrate side chains connected

TABLE 61-3

PROPERTIES OF NORMAL HUMAN IgA

	Serum	Mucosal
Concentration	Low	High
Size	Mostly monomeric	Mostly polymeric
Subclass	Mostly IgA1 (90%)	IgA1 (40%) and IgA2 (60%)
Source	Bone marrow	Mucosal plasma cells

to the serines and threonines. The grouping of O-linked sugars in the IgA1 molecule increases its size significantly and confers to it a highly negative charge because of sialylation of the sugars. Such O-linked sugars are uncommon on circulating proteins. The glycosylation pattern varies, so that an array of different IgA1 O-glycoforms is found in the serum at any time.

Plasma cells that produce IgA are mainly located at mucosal immune sites, and the IgA is rapidly transported across the adjacent epithelial cells into the external secretions. Very little gets into the blood. Secretion of the multimeric IgA across the mucosa depends on the acquisition of secretory component (SC), which is a portion of the polymeric immunoglobulin receptor expressed at the basolateral surface of epithelial cells. Secretory IgA (sIgA) is more stable at these sites than serum IgA, which is readily degraded. The IgA found in the serum is predominantly produced in the bone marrow. Regulation of IgA production is broadly under T lymphocyte control. It is of interest that, in contrast to IgG, interleukin 10 and transforming growth factor-β both stimulate B lymphocyte production of IgA (42).

The liver has an important role in the clearance of IgA and IgA-containing immune complexes. IgA-binding receptors present in the liver are the hepatocyte asialoglycoprotein receptor and the Fcα receptor CD89 on Kupffer cells (43–45). The asialoglycoprotein receptor recognizes the terminal galactose and galactosamine carbohydrate residues of the IgA molecule (46). Macrophages and neutrophils also express CD89 and are able to remove and catabolize IgA. Expression of CD89 by these cells is decreased in patients with IgA nephropathy, which potentially compromises this clearance pathway (47).

Animal Models of IgA Nephropathy

Many animal models of IgA nephropathy have been developed, but they have added little to the understanding of the human disease. In mice, the deposition in mesangia of immunoglobulins, and specifically IgA and IgG, occurs naturally in many breeds, so that results of experimentally induced diseases must be interpreted against this background. More important, perhaps, is the understanding that IgA1 as a protective immunoglobulin appears very late in the evolutionary chain, with only humanoids possessing this subclass of IgA. In other animals the IgA is structurally more like human IgA2 and does not have the hinge region characteristic of IgA1. It is likely, therefore, that if abnormally glycosylated IgA1 plays a significant role in the pathogenesis of the human diseases (see below), then most animal models do not represent what occurs in humans.

Production of IgA in IgA Nephropathy

Much circumstantial evidence points to the probability that there exists a defect in mucosal immunity in IgA nephropathy. The most easily recognizable and dramatic symptom of macroscopic hematuria coincides with infections of mucosal

surfaces. It is likely that the site of the immune response is important, not the antigen. Increased IgA antibodies against a variety of antigens have been described, but none is ubiquitous, and the finding of such antigens in the glomerular deposits has not been established. IgA nephropathy also occurs in association with diseases with known mucosal defects such as celiac disease (48).

Approximately one-third to one-half of patients with IgA nephropathy have elevated serum levels of IgA, and this elevation is restricted to IgA1 (49,50). In patients with IgA nephropathy, there is increased production of IgA in response to viral and bacterial vaccines and tetanus toxoid, compared with control subjects without IgA nephropathy (50–52). Overproduction (overresponse) of these and recall antigens is restricted to the IgA1 subclass.

Elevated serum IgA by itself is insufficient to cause the disease (18–20). A key appears to be the increased levels of specifically polymeric IgA (51), including pIgA against mucosal antigens (52,53). This macromolecular IgA, which is normally predominantly found in mucosal secretions, is likely to be more prone to trapping within the glomerular mesangium.

It is not, however, a simple case of elevated mucosal production of polymeric IgA1 which then spills over into the systemic circulation. Both mucosal IgA plasma cells and polymeric IgA levels are normal or even decreased, whereas bone marrow IgA plasma cells numbers are increased in IgA nephropathy (54–57). This points to a defect leading to relative overproduction of polymeric IgA1 in systemic sites such as the bone marrow.

Clearance of IgA in IgA Nephropathy

The liver clearance of IgA is reduced in IgA nephropathy, although there is no clear evidence for a specific liver cell defect (58,59). It is also known that liver disease, where IgA clearance is impaired, is associated with mesangial IgA deposition, but not necessarily clinical disease (15–17). The overproduction of pathogenic polymeric IgA1 may either overwhelm the normal clearance mechanisms, or be of a form that resists the normal clearance pathways.

Mesangial Deposition of Abnormally Glycosylated IgA

The mesangial IgA found in IgA nephropathy is not necessarily fixed. It is known that it clears when disease remission occurs or when such kidneys are inadvertently transplanted into individuals without IgA nephropathy.

A consistent finding, though, is that it is IgA1 that is deposited in the mesangium in clinical disease (60–62). Several studies have found that the mesangial IgA1 in IgA nephropathy is abnormally glycosylated, and that the same abnormal IgA is increased in the serum in patients with disease (63–67). The difference between the IgA1 molecule in healthy people and patients with IgA nephropathy resides in the O-glycosylation of residues in the hinge region. A normal variant exists with terminal N-acetylgalactosamine or sialylated N-acetylgalactosamine and reduced galactosylation and sialylation, but this is rare in normal serum. It is uniquely more common in IgA nephropathy patients (68,69). The altered O-galactosylation in IgA nephropathy may result from a B-cell–restricted downregulation of β1-3 galactosyltransferase activity (70), which limits the addition of D-galactose to GalNAc, rather than any aberration of the nucleotide sequence of the IgA$_1$ hinge region, which is similar in structure and sequence to the hinge region found in healthy people (71,72).

These variant IgA1 molecules are more likely to self-aggregate, and form antigen-antibody complexes with IgG antibodies directed against IgA1 hinge epitopes (68,73). IgA1 from patients with IgA nephropathy persists longer in the circulation than that from normal controls when injected into mice

(74). Liver clearance is reduced, perhaps because the polyclonal IgA1 is unable to pass through endothelial fenestrae in the liver to reach the hepatocytes (75). The net effect of this structural alteration is to increase serum levels of polyclonal IgA1 that is more prone to mesangial deposition and/or is more resistant to clearance from the mesangium.

It remains unclear whether there is a specific receptor on mesangial cells for IgA1. Indeed, the possibility exists that there is no necessity for a specific IgA receptor on mesangial cells because the altered molecule may bind nonspecifically to mesangial structures. However, it appears most likely that mesangial cells express at least one receptor that differs from the known IgA receptors (CD89, asialoglycoprotein receptor, polymeric immunoglobulin receptor (76)). Candidates include the transferring receptor (CD71), an asialoglycoprotein receptor, an Fc α/μ receptor, and a novel Fcα receptor (77–81). Irrespective of the presence or otherwise of a specific receptor, mesangial cells are capable of endocytosis and catabolism of IgA and are therefore likely to contribute actively to its clearance (79, 82).

Events After Mesangial Deposition of IgA

There is no doubt that the IgA1 deposited in the mesangium incites an inflammatory reaction, at least in those patients with clinical disease, and the classic mediators of inflammation such as complement, cytokines, leucocytes, platelets, and coagulation/fibrinolysis are involved. The mechanisms of crescentic disease are similar to those in other crescentic glomerular diseases. Acute lesions, although visually impressive, often are self-limiting. Much more important in the long term is the development of increased mesangial matrix, glomerulosclerosis, interstitial scarring, and hypertensive vascular disease.

Polymeric, but not monomeric, IgA molecules initiate an inflammatory glomerulonephritis in a rat model of acute nephritis (83,84). Interactions with IgA complexes and mesangial cells induces a proinflammatory and prosclerotic response, including mesangial cell proliferation and production of cytokines (e.g., interleukin-6, platelet-derived growth factor [PDGF], and transforming growth factor [TGF]-β) and matrix proteins (85–88). The altered glycosylation structure of the variant IgA1 molecules deposited in the mesangium may also specifically predispose to the pathogenic mesangial responses that follow (89).

The mechanisms of the subsequent inflammation and scarring in the glomerulus and interstitium in IgA nephropathy are probably not significantly different from other inflammatory glomerular diseases. Resolution or progression of the disease process may depend on the presence or otherwise of critical glomerular podocyte damage (90,91).

Genetics of IgA Nephropathy

The genetic makeup of the individual may dictate the initiation, progression, or resolution of IgA nephropathy. In support of a genetic predisposition are the apparent racial differences in prevalence of IgA nephropathy, and instances of occurrence in first-degree relatives (with many others having similar immune abnormalities *in vitro*) (92–94). On the other hand, more than 90% of cases of IgA nephropathy occur sporadically. Results of genetic studies, however, in general have been disappointing and associations reported are inconsistent. Associations have been described with DR4 (95,96) and, also on chromosome 6, with complement genes (C4A and C4B null phenotypes (93), and with the immunoglobulin "switch region" on chromosome 14 (97). A disease susceptibility gene has been localized to a region on chromosome 6 (98). Polymorphisms of genes encoding cytokines (TNF-α, interferon-γ, interleukin-4) have also been associated with development or progression of disease (99–101).

Progression of disease has also been associated with a deletion polymorphism of the angiotensin-converting enzyme (ACE) that increases serum and tissue ACE levels (94). However, further studies have not supported the proposal that this polymorphism in isolation is a significant factor in disease progression (102,103).

Summary of Pathogenesis

Current opinion about the pathogenesis of IgA nephropathy centers around the presence of excess serum levels of abnormally glycosylated immunoglobulin A molecules. These aggregate into polymeric IgA, which is less efficiently cleared by the liver and is prone to trapping in the glomerular mesangium. Evidence points to the bone marrow as the source of the abnormal IgA molecules rather than the mucosa. Ill-defined genetic influences may predispose individuals to development of this disease.

Treatment

There is no known cure for IgA nephropathy despite studies of many possible treatments. Current options mainly aim to control disease progression, and in general these do not differ significantly from recommended strategies for other progressive renal diseases. Establishing efficacy of a specific treatment for a disease such as IgA nephropathy is difficult where the majority of sufferers have a benign course, predicting those with unfavorable outcome is often difficult, and the time course of progression may be measured in decades. For the same reasons, it is difficult to establish a satisfactory risk versus benefit profile for proposed interventions such as immunosuppressive therapy. Relevant to this is the observation that IgA nephropathy frequently recurs in renal transplants despite the use of corticosteroids, azathioprine, mycophenolate mofetil, cyclosporine, and tacrolimus. For these reasons, treatments frequently have been used only in those with a known poor prognosis, that is, those patients who already have consistent proteinuria, hypertension, and impairment of renal function. A disappointingly small number of randomized controlled trials have been conducted of treatment of this common and important condition (104).

"Good prognosis" disease (i.e., minimal or no proteinuria, normal blood pressure, normal renal function, little or no scarring on renal biopsy) requires no more than regular observation. Hypertension commonly develops with time and should be managed aggressively (aim for <135/85 mm Hg).

The dramatic presenting symptom of synpharyngitic hematuria has prompted popularization of tonsillectomy as a treatment option, particularly in Japan and some parts of Europe. Results from studies have been conflicting (105–107), and prospective randomized studies are needed before it can be recommended. Supportive therapy, including analgesia as required, is all that is required for acute episodes of macroscopic hematuria, as well as any clinically indicated search for an alternative cause (e.g., urinary tract infection, renal calculi, malignancy).

An early controlled trial of phenytoin, which reduces serum IgA levels, failed to show any benefit (108). There is also no benefit in other methods to reduce antigen or antibody load, such as dietary restrictions or prophylactic antibiotics.

An array of studies, of varying quality, have examined combinations of immunosuppressive agents for treatment of IgA nephropathy. Results to this point have not been sufficiently clearcut to routinely recommend such an approach, except perhaps in the relatively uncommon cases of crescentic, rapidly progressive disease or in cases with nephrotic syndrome due to concurrent minimal change disease. In the latter the proteinuria typically responds to standard treatment for isolated minimal change disease.

In a randomized trial, corticosteroids alone (intravenous methylprednisolone 1g per day for 3 consecutive days at beginning of months 1, 3, and 5, plus oral prednisolone 0.5 mg per/kg alternate days for 6 months) in IgA nephropathy patients with significant but subnephrotic proteinuria (1.0 to 3.5 g per day) reduced proteinuria by approximately 50% and reduced the risk of a 50% increase in serum creatinine by 50% at 5 years (109). Three other small trials of corticosteroids alone showed a reduction in proteinuria and some improvement in histologic parameters, but without effect on renal function (110–112). A small trial of 2 years of corticosteroids plus azathioprine in children with early disease modestly reduced proteinuria but had no effect on renal function (113). A more recent randomized, prospective trial of prednisolone and cytotoxic agents (oral cyclophosphamide and then azathioprine) in patients with progressive IgA nephropathy and controlled hypertension showed a significant preservation of renal function compared to controls out to 5 years. Proteinuria was also reduced (114). Corticosteroids +/- cytotoxic agents may be cautiously recommended in poor prognosis disease (heavy proteinuria, early but progressive renal impairment), taking into account the risk of important side effects.

Other immunosuppressive drugs such as cyclosporine (115) and mycophenolate (116) also have been used, but the high incidence of recurrence in renal transplants casts doubt on their efficacy.

The risk/benefit equation shifts toward aggressive treatment in the setting of rapidly progressive, crescentic IgA nephropathy, where there is likely to be a rapid decline to end-stage renal failure without intervention. The treatment that is usually used (plasmapheresis, prednisolone, cyclophosphamide) is similar to that for other forms of rapidly progressive, crescentic renal disease. There is a lack of good quality, randomized trials. Small studies show an early response to treatment but a disappointing longer term outlook (117,118).

An alternative approach adopted with some enthusiasm in parts of the world has been the use of fish oil/omega-3 fatty acids for treatment, particularly of progressive IgA nephropathy (119). In the largest controlled study, it slowed progression into renal failure in poor prognosis treated patients compared with controls (120), and this effect has been long-lasting (121). A later study showed no benefit of high doses of fish oil over low doses (122). This study has been criticized because of the relatively rapid progression of disease in the control group, and other studies have not shown such benefit (104,123,124,125). There remains insufficient evidence to routinely recommend this approach.

There do not appear to be substantive differences in the mechanisms of progressive renal impairment in established IgA nephropathy compared to other glomerular diseases, and so it is not at all surprising to find that similar approaches to delaying disease progression have been studied and used extensively in this condition. It has long been established that control of hypertension is crucial to delaying progression of renal impairment in glomerular diseases. More recently, seminal studies, first in diabetic nephropathy and then in other renal conditions, have shown important and specific advantages of blood pressure control with angiotensin-converting enzyme (ACE) inhibitors (126). Comparable advantages exist with angiotensin II receptor (AIIR) blockers, and the most recent evidence suggests that there is a synergistic advantage in using both. Experimental evidence indicates that such agents reduce glomerular capillary hypertension, decrease proteinuria, and protect against hyperfiltration injury. An established aim of strategies to delay progression is now the targeting of proteinuria in addition to hypertension, and trial evidence supports the notion that incremental reductions in proteinuria are associated with improvements in renal prognosis.

Few studies to date have specifically examined the role of ACE inhibitors or AIIR antagonists in progressive IgA nephropathy, and much of the evidence favoring their use in this condition is based on studies of other proteinuric glomerular diseases (e.g., diabetic nephropathy) (127). Some studies have shown a reduction in proteinuria with ACE inhibition without improvement in renal function (128,129), although 2 more recent studies found that it delayed progression as well (130,131). AIIR blockers cause comparable proteinuria reduction in IgA nephropathy (132). The combination of both ACE inhibitor and AIIR blocker synergistically reduces proteinuria in IgA nephropathy, and there is now evidence that this confers additional benefit in delaying progression of renal impairment (133–135). Despite the relative paucity of specific data, blockade of the renin-angiotensin system is recommended where there is significant proteinuria (>1 g per 24 hours).

Transplantation for IgA Nephropathy

Although kidney transplantation should be offered to all patients with IgA nephropathy provided there is no other contraindication, they should be made aware of the possibility of disease recurrence, the risk of which is approximately 45% (33,34). Those who already have lost a graft because of recurrent disease may be at high risk for repeated graft loss, but experience is too limited for this to be an absolute contraindication to repeat transplantation (35,36). Despite the risk of recurrence, the prognosis of transplants for this group is comparable with that of patients with other causes of end-stage renal failure.

Recurrent disease has been considered to be mild and usually of little clinical significance (136,137). However, other studies challenge this concept (33,35). In one of these, 17 of 29 grafts had recurrent IgA deposits and 5 of those 17 affected had clinical and histologic evidence of recurrent IgA disease, with failing grafts (33). In our series of 81 grafts in 76 patients, the mean time from transplantation to the onset of clinical disease (microhematuria) was 4.8 years (36). In those with more severe recurrent disease causing graft loss, the mean time from transplantation to graft loss was 4.6 years. It is suggested that graft loss due to recurrent IgA nephropathy is underreported, and unless immunofluorescence studies are performed on transplant biopsies and nephrectomies, losses will be attributed to chronic rejection or transplant glomerulopathy rather than recurrent disease.

HENOCH-SCHÖNLEIN PURPURA

The almost identical renal immunopathologic features of Henoch-Schönlein purpura (HSP) and IgA nephropathy questions the separate identity of these conditions. Historically, HSP is a much older disease than IgA nephropathy, as it is a clinical syndrome readily recognized because of the overt purpuric rash, arthritis, gut manifestations, and glomerulonephritis. Whereas Schönlein (138) in 1837 associated the purpura and arthritis, and Henoch in 1874 (139) recognized the gastrointestinal and renal manifestations, the first clinical description of the disease was probably by Heberden in 1806 (140). Until the 1970s, most accounts of HSP were descriptive but, once again, the advent of immunofluorescence technology allowed exploration of possible immunopathogenetic mechanisms. As with IgA nephropathy, positive IgA immunofluorescence occurs in the glomerular mesangium, skin (especially in purpuric lesions) (141), and other organs.

Although the clinical features, incidence, and age of onset tend to vary, the many similarities of these two conditions suggest that they may represent a spectrum of the same systemic disease (142,143). HSP is most prevalent in the first decade of life, and much more common in children than in adults. In children it is frequently a transient disease without long-term consequences. The prevalence of glomerular disease in patients with HSP, especially in children, varies from 20% to 100% (144), depending on how carefully evidence for it is sought. When glomerular disease occurs in HSP, frank nephritic or nephrotic syndrome, or acute renal failure due to crescentic disease, are more common than in IgA nephropathy. The natural history of HSP is less well defined than IgA nephropathy, and is confounded by the fact that many patients have elements of the syndrome without clinical glomerulonephritis. Complete recovery occurs in 94% and 89% of children and adults, respectively, and the renal disease may be more likely to be severe and progressive in adults than in children (145). Progression to end-stage renal failure is well described, and like IgA nephropathy, can occur relatively rapidly or over decades. The nonrenal features of the syndrome are transient although recurrent in approximately one-third of patients. The renal disease resolves in most but persists in an important minority.

The characteristic purpuric rash, joint, and gastrointestinal involvement usually make the syndrome of HSP clearly identifiable in children and adults. It commonly occurs soon after an upper respiratory tract infection. In one series, the relative frequency of the major symptoms in children was purpura (100%); arthritis (82%); abdominal pain (63%); renal disease (40%); and gastrointestinal bleeding (33%) (146). The rash is distributed symmetrically over the arms and legs. Pain in multiple large joints (typically knees and ankles) without frank arthritis or permanent damage is typical, and the abdominal pain may be severe, disabling, and accompanied by visible rectal bleeding. Although these symptoms may cause much acute morbidity, recovery is usual. Renal involvement usually is apparent within 4 weeks of diagnosis, although it can develop much later. As with IgA nephropathy, intermittent macroscopic hematuria or persisting microscopic hematuria are the most common findings. Likewise, more severe cases have significant proteinuria, nephrotic syndrome, hypertension, and renal impairment, and synpharyngitic hematuria is typical.

In patients with HSP, most clinical features are a reflection of a systemic leukocytoclastic vasculitis, characteristically affecting the skin, gastrointestinal tract, and joints. It is a disease of the small blood vessels, particularly the postcapillary venules, and is probably the result of immune complex deposition, with activation of complement and consequent leukotaxis. Neutrophils attracted to the site frequently undergo karyorrhexis. There is variable endothelial cell proliferation, mural fibrin, and, in severe cases, fibrinoid necrosis. These changes are more common in the glomerulus in HSP than in IgA nephropathy. In severe cases, there may be cutaneous infarction with ulcer formation. Deposits of C3, frequently associated with IgA and IgM, may be found in blood vessel walls. Electron-dense deposits and fibrin have been demonstrated in early lesions.

Studies of HSP are much more limited than IgA nephropathy, but similar aberrations exist in the control of IgA production. As with IgA nephropathy, the IgA in the mesangial deposits of HSP is of the IgA1 subclass, and there are circulating IgA1-containing immune complexes or immune aggregates (147–149). The circulating IgA1 immune complexes are larger in HSP than IgA nephropathy, and levels of plasma IgE are increased (142). HSP has been associated with hypersensitivity reactions (150). Like IgA nephropathy, abnormally glycosylated IgA is more abundant in individuals with HSP and glomerulonephritis (151).

Most patients with the acute syndrome neither require nor receive specific therapy. Corticosteroids may speed resolution of the arthritis and abdominal pain, but do not appear to prevent recurrent disease (146). Specific treatment of the renal disease should be considered only in patients with marked proteinuria and/or impaired renal function during the acute episode. Aggressive corticosteroid therapy may be beneficial in patients with crescentic nephritis (152). Limited data from uncontrolled studies support a role for plasmapheresis in aggressive acute disease (153). There is no specific controlled data for treatment of non-acute, progressive HSP renal disease, but the similarities to IgA nephropathy suggest that an identical approach is reasonable. Renal transplantation is a valid option should end-stage renal failure result, although recurrence of HSP nephritis in the graft is not uncommon (154). Most recurrences are subclinical, but it leads to graft loss in approximately 10%.

References

1. Berger J, Hinglais N. Les depots intercapillaires d'IgA-IgG. *J Urol* 1968;74:694.
2. D'Amico G. The commonest glomerulonephritis in the world: IgA nephropathy. *Q J Med* 1987;64:709.
3. Levy M, Berger J. Worldwide perspective of IgA nephropathy. *Am J Kidney Dis* 1988;12:340.
4. Julian BA, Waldo FB, Rifai A, et al. IgA nephropathy, the most common glomerulonephritis worldwide: a neglected disease in the United States? *Am J Med* 1988;84:129.
5. Suzuki K, Honda K, Tanabe K, et al. Incidence of latent mesangial IgA deposition in renal allograft donors in Japan. *Kidney Int* 2003;63:2286.
6. Sinniah R. Occurrence of mesangial IgA and IgM deposits in a control necropsy population. *J Clin Pathol* 1983;36:276.
7. Waldherr R, Rambausek M, Duncker WD, et al. Frequency of mesangial IgA deposits in a non-selected autopsy series. *Nephrol Dial Transplant* 1989;4:943.
8. D'Amico G. Natural history of IgA nephropathy: role of clinical and histologic prognostic factors. *Am J Kidney Dis* 2000;36:227.
9. Ibels LS, Gyory AZ. IgA nephropathy: analysis of the natural history, important factors in the progression of renal disease, and a review of the literature. *Medicine (Baltimore)* 1994;73:79.
10. Bartosik L, Lajoie G, Sugar L, et al. Predicting progression in IgA nephropathy. *Am J Kidney Dis* 2001;38:728.
11. Geddes CC, Rauta V, Gronhagen-Riska C, et al. A tricontinental view of IgA nephropathy. *Nephrol Dial Transplant* 2003;18:1541.
12. ANZDATA Registry Report 2003, Australia and New Zealand Dialysis and Transplant Registry, Adelaide, South Australia.
13. Mustonen J, Pasternack A, Rantala I. The nephrotic syndrome in IgA glomerulonephritis: response to corticosteroid therapy. *Clin Nephrol* 1983;20:172.
14. Clarkson AR, Seymour AE, Thompson A, et al. IgA nephropathy: a syndrome of uniform morphology, diverse clinical features and uncertain prognosis. *Clin Nephrol* 1977;8:459.
15. Berger J, Yaneva H, Nabarra B, et al. Glomerular changes in patients with cirrhosis of the liver. *Adv Nephrol* 1978;7:3.
16. Callard P, Feldmann D, Prandi D, et al. Immune complex type glomerulonephritis in cirrhosis of the liver. *Am J Pathol* 1975;80:329.
17. Nochy D, Callard P, Bellon B, et al. Association of overt glomerulonephritis and liver disease: a study of 34 patients. *Clin Nephrol* 1976;6:422.
18. Dosa S, Cairns SA, Mallick NP, et al. Relapsing Henoch-Schönlein syndrome with renal involvement in a patient with an IgA monoclonal gammopathy. *Nephron* 1980;26:145.
19. van der Helm-van Mil AH, Smith AC, Pouria S, et al. Immunoglobulin A multiple myeloma presenting with Henoch-Schonlein purpura associated with reduced sialylation of IgA1. *Br J Haematol* 2003;122:915.
20. Cohen AH. Human immunodeficiency virus and IgA nephropathy. *Nephrology* 1997;3:51.
21. Hotta O, Furuta T, Chiba S, et al. Regression of IgA nephropathy: a repeat biopsy study. *Am J Kidney Dis* 2002;39:493.
22. Alamartine E, Sabatier JC, Guerinc C, et al. Prognostic factors in mesangial IgA glomerulonephritis: an extensive study with univariate and multivariate analyses. *Am J Kidney Dis* 1991;18:12.
23. Radford MG Jr, Donadio JV, Bergstralh EJ, et al. Predicting renal outcome in IgA nephropathy. *J Am Soc Nephrol* 1997;8:199.
24. Bennett WM, Kincaid-Smith PS. Macroscopic hematuria in mesangial IgA nephropathy: correlation with glomerular crescents and renal dysfunction. *Kidney Int* 1983;23:393.
25. Szeto CC, Lai FM, To KF, et al. Natural history of immunoglobulin A nephropathy presenting with hematuria and minimal proteinuria. *Am J Med* 2001;110:434.
26. Cederholm B, Wieslander J, Bygren P, et al. Circulating complexes containing IgA antifibronectin in patients with primary IgA nephropathy. *Proc Natl Acad Sci USA* 1988;85:4865.
27. Davin JC, Li Vecchi M, Nagy J, et al. Evidence that the interaction between circulating IgA and fibronectin is a normal process enhanced in primary IgA nephropathy. *J Clin Immunol* 1991;11:78.

28. Maeda A, Gohda T, Funabiki K, et al. Significance of serum IgA and serum IgA/C3 ratio in diagnostic analysis of patients with IgA nephropathy. *J Clin Lab Anal* 2003;17:73.

29. Lee SM, Rao VM, Franklin WA, et al. IgA nephropathy: morphological predictors of progressive renal disease. *Hum Pathol* 1982;13:314.

30. Haas M. Histologic subclassification of IgA nephropathy: a clinicopathologic study of 244 cases. *Am J Kidney Dis* 1997;29:829.

31. Feehally J. Predicting prognosis in IgA nephropathy. *Am J Kidney Dis* 2001;38:881.

32. Berthoux FC, Laurent B, Koller J, et al. Primary IgA glomerulonephritis with thin glomerular basement membrane: a peculiar pathologic marker versus thin membrane nephropathy association. *Contrib Nephrol* 1995;111:1.

33. Odum J, Peh CA, Clarkson AR, et al. Recurrent mesangial IgA nephritis following renal transplantation. *Nephrol Dial Transplant* 1994;9:309.

34. Ohmacht C, Kleim V, Burg M, et al. Recurrent immunoglobulin A nephropathy after renal transplantation. *Transplantation* 1997;64:1493.

35. Floege J, Burg M, Kliem V. Recurrent IgA nephropathy after kidney transplantation: not a benign condition. *Nephrol Dial Transplant* 1998;13:1933.

36. Clarkson AR, Elias TJ, Faull RJ, et al. Immunoglobulin A nephropathy and renal transplantation. *Transplant Rev* 1999;13:174.

37. Sanfilippo F, Croker BP, Bollinger RR. Fate of four cadaveric renal allografts with mesangial IgA deposits. *Transplantation* 1982;33:370.

38. Silva FG, Chander P, Pirani CL, et al. Disappearance of mesangial IgA deposits after renal allograft transplantation. *Transplantation* 1982;33:214.

39. Kerr MA. The structure and function of human IgA. *Biochem J* 1990;271:285.

40. Johansen FE, Braathen R, Brandtzaeg P. Role of J chain in secretory immunoglobulin formation. *Scand J Immunol* 2000;52:240.

41. Barratt J, Feehally J, Smith AC. Pathogenesis of IgA nephropathy. *Semin Nephrol* 2004;24:197.

42. Defrance T, Vanbervliet B, Briere F, et al. Interleukin 10 and transforming growth factor beta cooperate to induce anti-CD40-activated naïve human B cells to secrete immunoglobulin A. *J Exp Med* 1992;175:671.

43. Van Egmond M, van Garderen E, van Spriel AB, et al. FcalphaRI-positive liver Kupffer cells: reappraisal of the function of immunoglobulin A in immunity. *Nat Med* 2000;6:680.

44. Rifai A, Schena FP, Montinaro V, et al. Clearance kinetics and fate of macromolecular IgA in patients with IgA nephropathy. *Lab Invest* 1989;61:381.

45. Rifai A, Fadden K, Morrison SL, et al. The N-glycans determine the differential blood clearance of and hepatic uptake of human immunoglobulin (Ig)A1 and IgA2 isotypes. *J Exp Med* 2000;191:2171.

46. Stockert RJ, Kressner MS, Collins JC, et al. IgA interaction with the asialoglycoprotein receptor. *Proc Natl Acad Sci USA* 1982;79:6229.

47. Grossetete B, Launay P, Lehuen A, et al. Down-regulation of Fc alpha receptors on blood cells of IgA nephropathy patients: evidence for a negative regulatory role of serum IgA. *Kidney Int* 1998;53:1321.

48. Helin H, Mustonen J, Reunala T, et al. IgA nephropathy associated with celiac disease and dermatitis herpetiformis. *Arch Pathol Lab Med* 1983;107:324.

49. Layward L, Allen AC, Hattersley JM, et al. Elevation of IgA in IgA nephropathy is localized in the serum and not saliva and is restricted to the IgA1 subclass. *Nephrol Dial Transplant* 1993;8:25.

50. Van den Wall Bake AW, Beyer WE, Evers-Schouten JH, et al. Humoral immune responses to influenza vaccination in patients with primary IgA nephropathy. An analysis of isotype distribution and size of the influenza-specific antibodies. *J Clin Invest* 1989;84:1070.

51. Layward L, Allen AC, Harper SJ, et al. Increased and prolonged production of specific polymeric IgA after systemic immunization with tetanus toxoid in IgA nephropathy. *Clin Exp Immunol* 1992;88:394.

52. Leinikki PO, Mustonen J, Pasternack A. Immune responses to oral polio vaccine in patients with IgA glomerulonephritis. *Clin Exp Immunol* 1987;68:33.

53. Barratt J, Bailey EM, Buck KS, et al. Exaggerated systemic antibody response to mucosal Helicobacter pylori infection in IgA nephropathy. *Am J Kidney Dis* 1999;33:1049.

54. Westberg NG, Baklien K, Schmekel B, et al. Quantitation of immunoglobulin-producing cells in small intestinal mucosa of patients with IgA nephropathy. *Clin Immunol Immunopathol* 1983;26:442.

55. Harper SJ, Pringle JH, Wicks AC, et al. Expression of J chain mRNA in duodenal IgA plasma cells in IgA nephropathy. *Kidney Int* 1994;45:836.

56. De Fijter JW, Eijgenraam JW, Braam CA, et al. Deficient IgA1 immune response to nasal cholera toxin subunit B in IgA nephropathy. *Kidney Int* 1996;50:952.

57. Van den Wall Bake AW, Daha MR, Evers-Schouten J, et al. Serum IgA and the production of IgA by peripheral blood and bone marrow lymphocytes in patients with primary IgA nephropathy: evidence for the bone marrow as the source of mesangial IgA. *Am J Kidney Dis* 1988;12:410.

58. Roccatello D, Picciotto G, Coppo R, et al. The fate of aggregated immunoglobulin A injected in IgA nephropathy patients and healthy controls. *Am J Kidney Dis* 1991;18:20.

59. Roccatello D, Picchiotto G, Torchio M, et al. Removal systems of immunoglobulin A and immunoglobulin A containing complexes in IgA nephropathy and cirrhosis patients: the role of asialoglycoprotein receptors. *Lab Invest* 1993;69:714.

60. Lomax-Smith JD, Zabrowarny L, Howarth G, et al. The immunochemical characterisation of mesangial IgA deposits. *Am J Pathol* 1983;113:359.

61. Tomino Y, Sakai H, Miura H, et al. Detection of polymeric IgA in glomeruli from patients with IgA nephropathy. *Clin Exp Immunol* 1982;49:419.

62. Hisano S, Matsushita M, Fujita T, et al. Mesangial IgA2 deposits and lectin pathway-mediated complement activation in IgA glomerulonephritis. *Am J Kidney Dis* 2001;38:1082.

63. Mestecky J, Tomana M, Crowley-Nowick PA, et al. Defective galactosylation and clearance of IgA1 molecules as a possible etiopathogenic factor in IgA nephropathy. *Contrib Nephrol* 1993;104:172.

64. Tomana M, Matousovic K, Julian BA, et al. Galactose-deficient IgA1 in sera of IgA nephropathy patients is present in complexes with IgG. *Kidney Int* 1997;52:509.

65. Hiki Y, Tanaka A, Kokubo T, et al. Analyses of IgA1 hinge glycopeptides in IgA nephropathy by matrix-assisted laser desorption/ionization time-of-flight mass spectrometry. *J Am Soc Nephrol* 1998;9:577.

66. Hiki Y, Odani H, Takahashi M, et al. Mass spectrometry proves under-O-glycosylation of glomerular IgA1 in IgA nephropathy. *Kidney Int* 2001;59:1077.

67. Allen AC, Bailey EM, Brenchley PE, et al. Mesangial IgA1 in IgA nephropathy exhibits aberrant O-glycosylation: observations in three patients. *Kidney Int* 2001;60:969.

68. Tomana M, Novak J, Julian BA, et al. Circulating immune complexes in IgA nephropathy consist of IgA1 with galactose-deficient hinge region and antiglycan antibodies. *J Clin Invest* 1999;104:73.

69. Allen AC, Harper SJ, Feehally J. Galactosylation of N- and O-linked carbohydrate moieties of IgA1 and IgG in IgA nephropathy. *Clin Exp Immunol* 1995;100:470.

70. Allen AC, Topham PS, Harper SJ, et al. Leukocyte β1-3 galactosyltransferase activity in IgA nephropathy. *Nephrol Dial Transplant* 1997;12:701.

71. Kokubo T, Hiki Y, Iwase H. Exposed peptide core of IgA1 hinge region in IgA nephropathy. *Nephrol Dial Transplant* 1999;14:81.

72. Greer MR, Barratt J, Harper SJ, et al. The nucleotide sequence of the IgA1 hinge region in IgA nephropathy. *Nephrol Dial Transplant* 1998;13:1980.

73. Kokubo T, Hiki Y, Iwase H, et al. Protective role of IgA1 glycans against IgA1 self-aggregation and adhesion to extracellular matrix proteins. *J Am Soc Nephrol* 1998;9:2048.

74. Mestecky J, Hashim OH, Tomana M. Alterations in the IgA carbohydrate chains influence the cellular distribution of IgA1. *Contrib Nephrol* 1995;111:66.

75. Novak J, Julian BA, Tomana M, et al. Progress in molecular and genetic studies of IgA nephropathy. *J Clin Immunol* 2001;21:310.

76. Monteiro RC, Van De Winkel JG. IgA Fc receptors. *Annu Rev Immunol* 2003;21:177.

77. Moura IC, Centelles MN, Arcos-Fajardo M, et al. Identification of the transferrin receptor as a novel immunoglobulin (Ig)A1 receptor and its enhanced expression on mesangial cells in IgA nephropathy. *J Exp Med* 2001;194:417.

78. Haddad E, Moura IC, Arcos-Fajardo M, et al. Enhanced expression of the CD71 mesangial IgA1 receptor in Berger disease and Henoch-Schonlein nephritis: association between CD71 expression and IgA deposits. *J Am Soc Nephrol* 2003;14:327.

79. Gomez-Guerrero C, Duque N, Egido J. Mesangial cells possess an asialoglycoprotein receptor with affinity for human immunoglobulin A. *J Am Soc Nephrol* 1998;9:568.

80. McDonald KJ, Cameron AJ, Allen JM, et al. Expression of Fcαμ receptor by human mesangial cells: a candidate receptor for immune complex deposition in IgA nephropathy. *Biochem Biophys Res Commun* 2002;290:438.

81. Barratt J, Greer MR, Pawluczyk IZ, et al. Identification of a novel Fcα receptor expressed by human mesangial cells. *Kidney Int* 2000;57:1936.

82. Gomez-Guerrero C, Lopez-Armada MJ, Gonzalez E, et al. Soluble IgA and IgG aggregates are catabolized by cultured rat mesangial cells and induce production of TNF-alpha and IL-6, and proliferation. *J Immunol* 1994;153:5247.

83. Stad RK, Bruijn JA, van Gijlswijk DJ, et al. An acute model for IgA-mediated glomerular inflammation in rats induced by monoclonal polymeric rat IgA antibodies. *Clin Exp Immunol* 1993;92:514.

84. Van Dixhoorn MG, Sato T, Muizert Y, et al. Combined glomerular deposition of polymeric rat IgA and IgG aggravates renal inflammation. *Kidney Int* 2000;58:90.

85. Fujii K, Muller KD, Clarkson AR, et al. The effect of IgA immune complexes on the proliferation of cultured human mesangial cells. *Am J Kidney Dis* 1990;16:207.

86. Chen A, Chen WP, Sheu LF, et al. Pathogenesis of IgA nephropathy: in vitro activation of human mesangial cells by IgA immune complex leads to cytokine secretion. *J Pathol* 1994;173:119.

87. Niemir ZI, Stein H, Noronha IL, et al. PDGF and TGF-beta contribute to the natural course of human IgA glomerulonephritis. *Kidney Int* 1995;48:1530.

88. Monteiro RC, Moura IC, Launay P, et al. Pathogenic significance of IgA receptor interactions in IgA nephropathy. *Trends Mol Biol* 2002;8:464.

89. Amore A, Cirina P, Conti G, et al. Glycosylation of circulating IgA in patients with IgA nephropathy modulates proliferation and apoptosis of mesangial cells. *J Am Soc Nephrol* 2001;12:1862.

90. Kriz W, Gretz N, Lemley KV. Progression of glomerular diseases: is the podocyte the culprit? *Kidney Int* 1998;54:687.

91. Floege J. Glomerular remodelling: novel therapeutic approaches derived from the apparently chaotic growth factor network. *Nephron* 2002;91:582.

92. Tolkoff-Rubin NE, Cosimi AB, Fuller T, et al. IgA nephropathy in HLA-identical siblings. *Transplantation* 1978;26:430.

93. Julian BA, Quiggins PA, Thompson JS, et al. Familial IgA nephropathy: evidence for an inherited mechanism of disease. *N Engl J Med* 1985;312:202.

94. Hsu SI, Ramirez SB, Winn MP, et al. Evidence for genetic factors in the development and progression of IgA nephropathy. *Kidney Int* 2000;57:1818.

95. Hiki Y, Kobayashi Y, Tateno S, et al. Strong association of HLA-DR4 with benign IgA nephropathy. *Nephron* 1982;32:222.

96. Kashiwabara H, Shishioo H, Tomura S, et al. Strong association between IgA nephropathy and HLA-DR4 antigen. *Kidney Int* 1982;22:377.

97. Demaine AG, Rambausek M, Knight JF, et al. Relationship of mesangial IgA glomerulonephritis to polymorphism of immunoglobulin heavy chain switch region. *J Clin Invest* 1988;81:611.

98. Gharavi AG, Yan Y, Scolari F, et al. IgA nephropathy, the most common form of glomerulonephritis, is linked to 6q22-23. *Nat Genet* 2000;26:354.

99. Syrjanen J, Hurme M, Lehtimaki T, et al. Polymorphism of the cytokine genes and IgA nephropathy. *Kidney Int* 2002;61:1079.

100. Shu KH, Lee SH, Cheng CH, et al. Impact of interleukin-1 receptor antagonist and tumor necrosis factor-alpha gene polymorphism on IgA nephropathy. *Kidney Int* 2000;58:783.

101. Masutani K, Miyake K, Nakashima H, et al. Impact of interferon-γ and interleukin-4 gene polymorphisms on development and progression of IgA nephropathy in Japanese patients. *Am J Kidney Dis* 2003;41:371.

102. Schena FP, D'Altri C, Cerullo G, et al. ACE gene polymorphism and IgA nephropathy: an ethnically homogeneous study and a meta-analysis. *Kidney Int* 2001;60:732.

103. Yoon HJ, Kim H, Kim HL, et al. Interdependent effect of angiotensin-converting enzyme and platelet activating factor acetylhydrolase gene polymorphisms on the progression of immunoglobulin A nephropathy. *Clin Genet* 2002;62:128.

104. Strippoli GF, Manno C, Schena FP. An "evidence-based" survey of therapeutic options for IgA nephropathy: assessment and criticism. *Am J Kidney Dis* 2003;41:1129.

105. Hotta OF, Miyazaka M, Furuta T, et al. Tonsillectomy and steroid pulse therapy significantly impacts on clinical remission in patients with IgA nephropathy. *Am J Kidney Dis* 2001;38:736.

106. Rasche FM, Schwarz A, Keller F. Tonsillectomy does not prevent a progressive course in IgA nephropathy. *Clin Nephrol* 1999;51:147.

107. Xie Y, Nishi S, Ueno M, et al. The efficacy of tonsillectomy on long-term renal survival in patients with IgA nephropathy. *Kidney Int* 2003;63:1861.

108. Clarkson AR, Seymour AE, Woodroffe AJ, et al. Controlled trial of phenytoin therapy in IgA nephropathy. *Clin Nephrol* 1980;13:215.

109. Pozzi C, Bolasco PG, Fogazzi GB, et al. Corticosteroids in IgA nephropathy: a randomised controlled trial. *Lancet* 1999;13:883.

110. Lai KN, Fai FM, Ho CP, et al. Corticosteroid therapy in IgA nephropathy with nephrotic syndrome: a long-term controlled trial. *Clin Nephrol* 1986;26:174.

111. Shoji T, Nakanishi I, Suzuki A, et al. Early treatment with corticosteroids ameliorates proteinuria, proliferative lesions, and mesangial phenotypic modulation in adult diffuse proliferative IgA nephropathy. *Am J Kidney Dis* 2000;35:194.

112. Kuriki M, Asahi K, Asano K, et al. Steroid therapy reduces mesangial matrix accumulation in advanced IgA nephropathy. *Nephrol Dial Transplant* 2003;18:1311.

113. Yoshikawa H, Ito H, Sakai T, et al. A controlled trial of combined therapy for newly diagnosed severe childhood IgA nephropathy. *J Am Soc Nephrol* 1999;10:101.

114. Ballardie FW, Roberts IS. Controlled prospective trial of prednisolone and cytotoxics in progressive IgA nephropathy. *J Am Soc Nephrol* 2002;13:142.

115. Lai KN, Lai FM, Li PT, et al. Cyclosporin treatment of IgA nephropathy: a short term controlled trial. *Br Med J* 1987;295:1165.

116. Nowack R, Brick R, Van Der Woode FJ. Mycophenolate mofetil for systemic vasculitis and IgA nephropathy. *Lancet* 1997;349:774.

117. Roccatello D, Ferro G, Cesano D, et al. Steroid and cyclophosphamide in IgA nephropathy. *Nephrol Dial Transplant* 2000;15:833.

118. Tumlin JA, Lohavichan V, Hennigar R. Crescentic, proliferative IgA nephropathy: clinical and histologic response to methylprednisolone and intravenous cyclophosphamide. *Nephrol Dial Transplant* 2003;18:1321.

119. Donadio JV, Grande JP. The role of fish oil/omega-3 fatty acids in the treatment of IgA nephropathy. *Semin Nephrol* 2004;24:225.

120. Donadio JV, Bergstralh EJ, Offord KP, et al. A controlled trial of fish oil in IgA nephropathy. *N Engl J Med* 1994;331:1194.

121. Donadio JV, Grande JP, Bergstralh EJ, et al. The long term outcome of patients with IgA nephropathy treated with fish-oil in a controlled trial. *J Am Soc Nephrol* 1999;10:1772.

122. Donadio JV, Larson TS, Bergstralh EJ, et al. A randomised trial of high-dose compared with low-dose omega-3 fatty acids in severe IgA nephropathy. *J Am Soc Nephrol* 2001;12:791.

123. Bennett WM, Walker RG, Kincaid-Smith P. Treatment of IgA nephropathy with eicosapentaenoic acid (EPA): a two-year prospective trial. *Clin Nephrol* 1989;31:128.

124. Pettersson EE, Rekola S, Berglund L, et al. Treatment of IgA nephropathy with omega-3 polyunsaturated fatty acids: a prospective double-blind randomized study. *Clin Nephrol* 1994;41:183.

125. Dillon JJ. Fish oil therapy for IgA nephropathy:efficacy and interstudy variability. *J Am Soc Nephrol* 1997;8:1739.

126. Jafar TH, Schmid CH, Landa M, et al. Angiotensin-converting enzyme inhibitors and progression of nondiabetic renal disease. A meta-analysis of patient-level data. *Ann Intern Med* 2001;135:73.

127. Dillon JJ. Angiotensin-converting enzyme inhibitors and angiotensin receptor blockers for IgA nephropathy. *Semin Nephrol* 2004;24:218.

128. Maschio G, Cagnoli L, Claroni F, et al. ACE inhibition reduces proteinuria in normotensive patients with IgA nephropathy: a multicentre, randomized, placebo-controlled study. *Nephrol Dial Transplant* 1994;9:265.

129. Bannister KM, Weaver A, Clarkson AR, et al. Effect of angiotensin-converting enzyme and calcium channel inhibition on progression of IgA nephropathy. *Contrib Nephrol* 1995;111:184.

130. Ruggenenti P, Perna A, Gherardi G, et al. Chronic proteinuric nephropathies: outcomes and response to treatment in a prospective cohort of 352 patients with different patterns of renal injury. *Am J Kidney Dis* 2000;35:1155.

131. Praga M, Gutierrez E, Gonzalez E, et al. Treatment of IgA nephropathy with ACE inhibitors: a randomized and controlled trial. *J Am Soc Nephrol* 2003;14:1578.

132. Perico N, Remuzzi A, Sangalli F, et al. The antiproteinuric effect of angiotensin antagonism in human IgA nephropathy is potentiated by indomethacin. *J Am Soc Nephrol* 1998;2:2308.

133. Russo D, Minutolo R, Pisani A, et al. Coadministration of losartan and enalapril exerts additive antiproteinuric effect in IgA nephropathy. *Am J Kidney Dis* 2001;38:18.

134. Campbell R, Sangalli F, Perticucci E, et al. Effects of combined ACE inhibitor and angiotensin II antagonist treatment in human chronic nephropathies. *Kidney Int* 2003;63:1094.

135. Nakao N, Yoshimura A, Morita H, et al. Combination treatment of angiotensin-II receptor blocker and angiotensin-converting-enzyme inhibitor in non-diabetic renal disease (COOPERATE): a randomized controlled trial. *Lancet* 2003;361:117.

136. Berger J, Noel LH, Nabarra B, et al. Recurrence of mesangial IgA nephropathy after renal transplantation. *Contrib Nephrol* 1984;40:195.

137. Briganti EM, Russ GR, McNeil JJ, et al. Risk of renal allograft loss from recurrent glomerulonephritis. *N Engl J Med* 2002;347:103.

138. Schönlein H. *Alleg Spec Pathol Ther* 1837;2:48.

139. Henoch E. *Berl Klin Wochenschr* 1874;11:641.

140. Heberden W. *Commentaries on the history and cure of diseases.* London, 1806:396.

141. Baart de la Faille-Kuyper EH, Kater L, Kooiker CJ, et al. IgA deposits in cutaneous blood vessel walls and mesangium in Henoch Schönlein syndrome. *Lancet* 1973;1:892.

142. Davin JC, Ten Berge IJ, Weening JJ. What is the difference between IgA nephropathy and Henoch-Schonlein purpura nephritis? *Kidney Int* 2001;59:823.

143. Rai A, Nast C, Adler S. Henoch-Schonlein purpura nephritis. *J Am Soc Nephrol* 1999;10:2637.

144. Meadow SR. The prognosis of Henoch-Schönlein nephritis. *Clin Nephrol* 1978;9:87.

145. Blanco R, Martinez-Taboada VM, Rodriguez-Valverde V, et al. Henoch-Schonlein purpura in adulthood and childhood: two different expressions of the same syndrome. *Arthritis Rheum* 1997;40:859.

146. Saulsbury, FT. Henoch-Schonlein purpura in children. Report of 100 patients and review of the literature. *Medicine (Baltimore)* 1999;78:395.

147. Coppo R, Basolo B, Martina G, et al. Circulating immune complexes containing IgA IgG and IgM in patients with primary IgA nephropathy and with Henoch-Schönlein nephritis: correlation with clinical and histologic signs of activity. *Clin Nephrol* 1982;18:230.

148. Woodroffe AJ, Gormly AA, McKenzie PE, et al. Immunologic studies in IgA nephropathy. *Kidney Int* 1980;18:366.

149. Levinsky RJ, Barratt TM. IgA immune complexes in Henoch-Schönlein purpura. *Lancet* 1979;2:1100.

150. McCombs RP, Patterson JF, MacMahon HE, et al. Syndromes associated with "allergic" vasculitis. *N Engl J Med* 1956;255:251.

151. Allen AC, Willis FR, Beattie TJ, et al. Abnormal IgA glycosylation in Henoch-Schonlein purpura restricted to patients with clinical nephritis. *Nephrol Dial Transplant* 1998;13:930.

152. Niaudet P, Habib R. Methylprednisolone pulse therapy in the treatment of severe forms of Schönlein-Henoch purpura nephritis. *Pediatr Nephrol* 1998;12:238.

153. Hattori M, Ito K, Konomoto T, et al. Plasmapheresis as the sole therapy for rapidly progressive Henoch-Schönlein purpura nephritis in children. *Am J Kidney Dis* 1999;33:427.

154. Meulders Q, Pirson Y, Cosyns JP, et al. Course of Henoch-Schönlein nephritis after renal transplantation. Report of ten patients and review of the literature. *Transplantation* 1994;58:1179.

CHAPTER 62 ■

MEMBRANOPROLIFERATIVE GLOMERULONEPHRITIS

GIOVANNI BARBIANO DI BELGIOJOSO AND FRANCO FERRARIO

The term *membranoproliferative glomerulonephritis* (MPGN), or *mesangiocapillary glomerulonephritis* (GN), refers to the histopathologic entity characterized by (a) intense glomerular hypercellularity, accompanied by increase of mesangial matrix (1–4); (b) thickening of the peripheral capillary walls by subendothelial deposits (type I) or dense intramembranous deposits (type II) (5); and (c) mesangial interposition into the capillary walls with apparent splitting of the glomerular basement membrane (GBM) (1,2,6–9). The designation MPGN is used by most authors throughout the world, but *mesangiocapillary glomerulonephritis* is an equally acceptable term (10) that emphasizes the importance of peripheral capillary wall thickening and interposition of mesangial cellular and fibrillary material. Other descriptive names have been used over the years: hypocomplementemic chronic glomerulonephritis (6,11–13), chronic lobular glomerulonephritis (7,14), and mixed membranous and proliferative glomerulonephritis (15). As already mentioned, on the basis of capillary wall lesions, all authors have subtyped MPGN into types I, and II; some also include a type III. Type II, or dense intramembranous deposit disease, historically included in the MPGN group, is considered by several authors to be a separate disease entity because of its peculiar ultrastructural aspect and pathogenetic mechanisms (16–21).

Membranoproliferative glomerulonephritis designates a morphologic pattern that occurs, in most cases, in the absence of underlying diseases (idiopathic MPGN). It can be observed in association with a variety of systemic, neoplastic and infectious disorders; the secondary forms of MPGN are listed in Table 62-1. Therefore, MPGN is a term that indicates a morphologic pattern that must be integrated into an etiologic context whenever possible, and underlying systemic conditions must be excluded.

Epidemiologic data indicate that MPGN is a rare disease (4% to 5% among the histologically proven primary glomerulonephritides) and that its incidence has decreased in the developed countries of the world since the early 1980s (22–30). In fact, from epidemiologic studies of primary glomerulonephritis in France, Italy, and Spain, among adult and pediatric, rural and urban populations, the incidence of type I MPGN fell from 18% to 20% in early 1970s to approximately 12% in 1980, to 6% to 8% in 1990 and still lower since the mid-1990s. Similar reduction was noted in Japan (31). Frequency of MPGN, as reported by the Italian Registry of renal biopsy was, during the years 1996 to 2000, 6.2% for males and 8.0% for females (32). Jungers et al. found that in the Paris area, the annual incidence of type I MPGN among 1,003 cases of primary glomerulonephritis, for the 1987 to 1991 period, was 5.8% (33). The decrease of annual incidence of MPGN was confirmed by Simon et al. (34) after a 27-year follow-up in a study carried out from January 1976 to December 2002 in a region located in western France.

The relative frequency of type I MPGN as a cause of unexplained adult nephrotic syndrome in a large series of primary glomerulonephritis studied in Chicago (35) declined from the 1976 to 1979 period to the 1995 to 1997 period (6% to 2%). By contrast, the incidence of type II MPGN has remained unchanged. In still developing countries MPGN has not decreased in frequency (36,37). Other etiologic factors in MPGN such as age, sex, mode of presentation, also have not changed during the periods studied (25). The reductions in incidence in industrialized countries have multiple explanations. Improved hygienic and environmental factors in the past few decades have been postulated, with a decline of bacterial infections due to greater use of antibacterials. It has also been suggested that many cases of apparently idiopathic MPGN were due to hepatitis C virus (HCV) infections, with or without cryoglobulinemia that had been misdiagnosed. More careful screening for HCV led to a decline in HCV infection in the general population and subsequently in MPGN (38). Overall, a more precise diagnosis of underlying disease also may have contributed to the decline of "idiopathic" MPGN. The reduction in the frequency of MPGN also may depend partly on the overall increase in the age of biopsy population from the earlier to the later periods of study, because MPGN has a relative higher frequency in younger patients (35). The classical hypothesis that elevated incidence of bacterial infections in developing countries correlates with higher frequency of MPGN as well as other proliferative glomerulopathies has been recently questioned by Johnson et al. (39), following the striking finding of the lack of evidence for such active infections in cases of MPGN in Peru (36). The authors suggest that MPGN might result from an aberrant immune response to an innocuous antigen rather than a strong immune response to a virulent infective agent. Therefore an imbalance of immune system, induced by hygiene and other environmental factors, may underlie the pathogenesis of MPGN as well as other glomerular diseases. According to these authors, the type of immune response, as revealed by Th1/Th2 balance, may be more relevant in determining the variant of glomerulonephritis and in particular MPGN rather than the presence of specific antigen (39,40). This idea will be developed later in this chapter.

Membranoproliferative glomerulonephritis still presents many challenging issues for investigators, and the following items are still debated: (a) the relationships between immune complexes and mesangial interposition or complement abnormalities in the development of the lesion; (b) the precise nature of the dense deposit in type II MPGN and their connection with complement activation; (c) the nosologic definition and pathogenesis of type III MPGN; (d) the role HCV infection in noncryoglobulinemic MPGN and the involvement of HCV antigen in mediating the immune complex glomerular lesion; (e) the nature of spontaneous clinical remissions which occur

TABLE 62-1

MEMBRANOPROLIFERATIVE ASSOCIATED DISORDERS

Systemic immune disorders
    Systemic lupus erythematosus
    Sjögren's syndrome
    Hereditary complement and immunoglobulin deficiencies
    Rheumatoid arthritis
    Autoimmune tyroiditis
Neoplastic diseases
    Light-chain disease and plasma cell dyscrasia
    Leukemia and lymphomas
    Nephroblastoma
    Melanoma
Infectious diseases
    Bacterial
        Subacute endocarditis
        Visceral abscesses and infected shunts
    Viral
        Hepatitis C virus, with or without cryoglobulinemia
        Hepatitis B virus
        Human immunodeficiency virus
        Cocksackie, EBV
    Other
        Malaria, schistosomiasis, candida
Chronic liver disease
    Chronic active hepatitis
    Liver cirrhosis
    α1-antitrypsin deficiency
Miscellaneous
    Partial lipodystrophy
    Sarcoidosis
    Sickle cell disease
    Portosystemic shunt
    Transplant glomerulopathy

in all types of MPGN independent of therapy; and (f) the lack of proven effective therapy.

PATHOLOGY

Membranoproliferative glomerulonephritis is a histologically distinct entity characterized by intense glomerular hypercellularity mainly due to mesangial proliferation involving both cells and matrix and thickening of peripheral capillary wall with "double contour" appearance (2,7,9,21,41–43). Since the early 1980s, several forms or variant of so called MPGN have been described. Two major morphologic categories have been identified referred by the majority of authors as type I and type II (2,8,9,16–18,43–54).

Type I is characterized by the presence of numerous glomerular subendothelial deposits, marked involvement of the mesangium and extension of the mesangium into the glomerular capillary walls. In type II, homogeneous dense deposits in many renal basement membranes (glomerular, tubular, and arteriolar) are typical. At the glomerular level the dense deposits are clearly intramembranous, and very rarely the mesangium extended into the capillary walls with "double contour" appearance. In the past, type II was considered a MPGN because its morphological alterations on light microscopy were extremely similar to those of type I MPGN (5,18,55–57). In spite of many morphologic and clinical similarities, in particu-

lar with regards to the presence in both diseases of hypocomplementemia, there are sufficient differences from histologic and immunologic points of view to suggest that type II form is a separate and distinct entity and should not be considered a subtype of MPGN (20,48,58,59). Further variations or types of the membranoproliferative pattern have been noted by a number of investigators. A type with many of the features of MPGN type I, but with the added presence of numerous electron-dense deposits on the subepithelial side of the glomerular capillary basement membranes, was designated "type III" by Burkholder et al. (15). In this pattern, some glomerular capillaries were indistinguishable from those type I MPGN, whereas other segments of the glomerular tuft showed changes similar to those as classic membranous glomerulonephritis. Although this terminology did not find much favor, the issue is now complicated by the use of the term "type III" to designate a form of MPGN described by two other groups of workers (15,60,61). This form is characterized by the simultaneous presence of subendothelial and subepithelial deposits associated with lamination and disruption of the lamina densa of the GBM at electron microscopy (62–65). However, many reports (47–48) and recent personal data from a multicenter study of Italian Group of Renal Immunopathology, based on retrospective clinicohistologic analysis of 368 cases of idiopathic MPGN, suggest that these features are insufficient to warrant a separate entity, because epimembranous deposits are found in 20% of both types of MPGN and their number vary in repeat biopsies (66). Moreover the complement abnormalities, immunohistologic features, and clinical presentation and course of type III MPGN are similar to those in type I, and thus these two forms should be considered variants of the same disease rather than separate entities (64,66). Finally, there is some doubt over whether MPGN in all its subtypes should be considered a homogeneous and distinct histologic entity. The list of various forms of diseases associated with a membranoproliferative pattern is constantly growing. In fact, these patterns (especially type I) can occur as an idiopathic (primary), apparently isolated disease or can be associated with or stem from a wide variety of well-defined disease states, such as bacterial endocarditis, sickle cell disease, hepatitis B or C infection, cryoglobulinemia, and systemic lupus erythematosus (SLE). Although the etiologic and pathogenetic mechanisms might not be identical in all patients, most authors believe that MPGN is likely a result of chronic antigenemia. Moreover in a primary, apparently isolated (idiopathic) MPGN, several morphologic variants have been described because of heterogeneous intensity and distribution of the main basic histologic lesions; these possibly are the expression of different morphogenetic/pathogenetic mechanisms (66–69).

Type I Membranoproliferative Glomerulonephritis (Subendothelial Deposits)

Light Microscopy

By light microscopy, the most common form is the "classic" pattern characterized by widespread and massive mesangial proliferation and mesangial matrix expansion (1,2,4,7–9,21,41,44–50,70–72) (Fig. 62-1). The hypercellularity is usually global involving all portions of each glomerular tuft to approximately the same degree. Mesangial expansion is due to cellular proliferation, matrix growth, and to the presence of immunodeposits. Sometimes the increase in cells in the mesangial regions and the amount of mesangial matrix creates a much larger mesangial or centrilobular area, with the lobules assuming a club shape (lobular pattern) (Fig. 62-2).

There is marked diffuse thickening of the glomerular capillary walls; the thickening can be more prominent in some

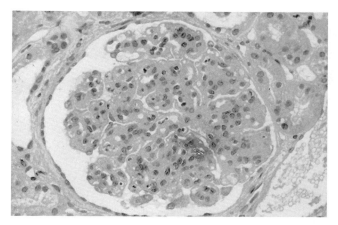

FIGURE 62-1. Type I membranoproliferative glomerulonephritis, classical pattern: widespread and massive mesangial proliferation, mesangial matrix expansion, and diffuse glomerular basement membrane thickening with "double-contour" appearance. (Trichrome, magnification, ×250.)

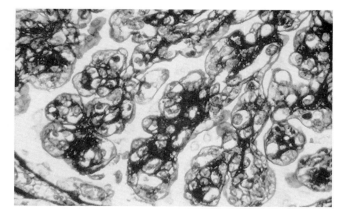

FIGURE 62-3. Type I membranoproliferative glomerulonephritis, note diffuse glomerular basement membrane thickening with clear "double-contour" appearance. (Silver stain, magnification ×400.)

glomeruli and in some capillary loops than in others. Periodic acid-Schiff (PAS) and silver methenamine stains show that the thickened glomerular capillary walls often have two basement membranes with a clear or nonargyrophilic region between them. This double contour is sometimes termed *tram-tracking, splitting,* or *duplication* of the GBM (Fig. 62-3). In some capillaries, the replication of basement membranes is very complex, resulting in multiple laminations. The double contour is created by the outward migration of mesangial cells along the inside of the capillary walls. Because mesangial cells produce basement membrane-like material, the cytoplasm of these cells is covered on the outside by the original basement membrane and on the inside by the newly formed "membrane." Both the membranes stain positively with silver and so give rise to the double-contour appearance. Capillary lumina usually are narrowed as a result of mesangial expansion, endothelial cell proliferation, and accumulation of subendothelial deposits. Using trichrome staining, large subendothelial deposits sometimes may be identified, although they are better demonstrated using immunofluorescence and electron microscopy. Mesangial deposits are rare and usually small. In type I MPGN, in addi-

tion to subendothelial deposits, many authors have described morphologic evidence of subepithelial deposits resembling to "humps" (2,3,41,43,47,48,66,69,72). In some cases mesangial matrix expansion and sclerosis is particularly evident giving a pattern of nodular glomerulosclerosis (Fig. 62-4).

Personal experience and the descriptions of other investigators (66,73–76) suggest that a true "nodular" pattern should be distinguished from lobular form of classical pattern. The lesions are mainly characterized by massive centrolobular sclerosis, always associated with microaneurysmal dilatation of glomerular capillaries, probably due to a mesangiolytic process with disruption of anchoring points at which peripheral capillary loop basement membrane attaches to mesangial stalks (Fig. 62-5). This process could be similar to that described in other nephropathies with nodular lesions as in diabetic glomerulosclerosis and light chain deposition disease (77–82). The morphogenetic mechanism of nodule formation with concentric enlargement of the mesangial matrix, strictly associated with microaneurysmal dilatation, suggests that the nodular pattern is not the late sclerotic stage of classical form but a different morphologic variant of type I MPGN, probably associated with more severe mesangial damage with consequent mesangiolysis or more severe vascular damage (66). Moreover, a morphologic transformation from classical to nodular

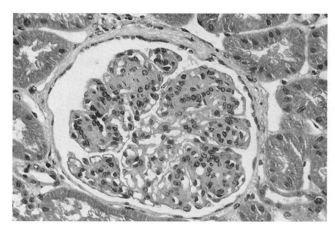

FIGURE 62-2. Type I membranoproliferative glomerulonephritis, lobular pattern: marked mesangial proliferation with mesangial matrix expansion and pronounced lobulation of the glomerular tuft. (Trichrome, magnification ×250.)

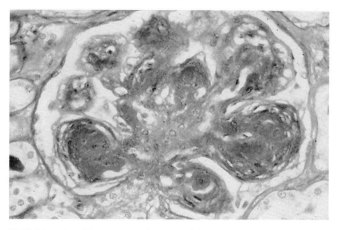

FIGURE 62-4. Type I membranoproliferative glomerulonephritis, nodular pattern: marked mesangial matrix expansion and sclerosis with large acellular nodule formation. (Trichrome, magnification ×250.)

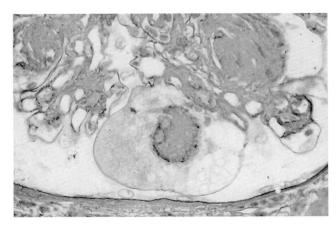

FIGURE 62-5. Type I membranoproliferative glomerulonephritis, nodular pattern: nodules of glomerulosclerosis associated with microaneurysmatic dilatation of glomerular basement membrane. (Silver stain, magnification ×400.)

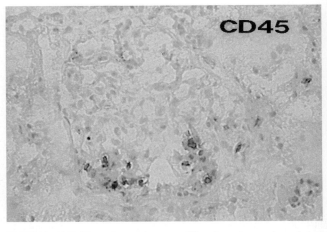

FIGURE 62-7. Type I membranoproliferative glomerulonephritis, exudative pattern: intraglomerular accumulation of monocyte-macrophages. (CD68, immunoperoxidase, magnification ×250.)

pattern has been described only rarely in studies using serial biopsies (66,68,83,84). Monga et al. suggested the possibility of double or superimposed glomerulopathies, such as describing diabetic nodular glomerulosclerosis associated with MPGN (85).

Although a moderate infiltration of neutrophils and monocytes is often present in the classical form of type I MPGN, the infiltration of inflammatory cells, mainly monocytes, is marked in approximately 20% of cases (4,86–89) (Fig. 62-6). Immunohistochemical methods, using specific antibody against monocyte-macrophages (CD68) confirm the prevalence of these cells in the glomerular tuft (Fig. 62-7). In this morphologic form, there is a marked and clearly visible "double contour" aspect of the thickened basement membrane, mainly due to the subendothelial interposition of the infiltrating inflammatory cells rather than to mesangial interposition (Fig. 62-8). This variant of "exudative" glomerulonephritis closely resembles the morphologic pattern of secondary forms of diffuse lupus nephritis, of cryoglobulinemic nephritis and some nephritis associated with other infectious diseases (88–94). Although subepithelial deposits are common in these cases the chronic clinical course, with persistent hypocomplementemia, and the immunohistologic feature of diffuse subendothelial deposition

of C3, sharply differentiate this type of glomerulonephritis from the acute postinfectious nephritides, and characterize this morphologic entity as a variant of idiopathic MPGN (95,96).

Many reports of focal and segmental forms confirm the heterogeneity of morphologic lesions in type I MPGN (41,65,68,71,84,97,98)(Fig. 62-9). In these cases, only some glomeruli show lesions whereas others do not, and membranoproliferative alterations frequently are restricted to a segment of the glomerular tuft. The question of whether the focal form is a stage of less marked damage during the natural course of the disease, or is a separate entity, and thus an expression of less aggressive disease, is still open to debate. Some studies on repeat biopsies have demonstrated morphologic transformation from the focal to diffuse pattern and vice versa. Taguchi and Bohle (83) have described sequential biopsies from 33 patients with MPGN (types I and II). Twenty-four of 25 patients with diffuse forms of MPGN maintained that pattern on subsequent biopsies, whereas 4 of 6 patients with a focal MPGN pattern showed signs of a diffuse form on second biopsy. Two patients who had no histologic findings of MPGN on initial biopsy (one had focal MPGN and other had mild mesangial proliferative glomerulonephritis with small crescents) later showed evidence of a diffuse form of MPGN

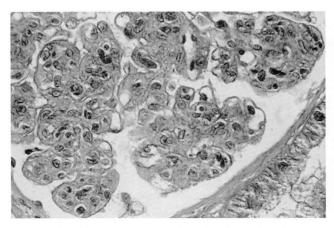

FIGURE 62-6. Type I membranoproliferative glomerulonephritis, exudative pattern: marked endocapillary hypercellularity mainly due to intracapillary infiltration of inflammatory cells. (Trichrome, magnification ×250.)

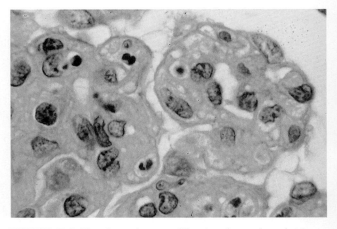

FIGURE 62-8. Type I membranoproliferative glomerulonephritis, exudative pattern: clearly visible "double contour" aspect of thickened glomerular basement membrane with subendothelial interposition of infiltrating inflammatory cells. (Trichrome, magnification ×1,000.)

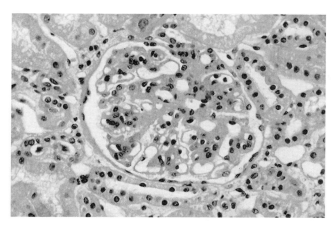

FIGURE 62-9. Type I membranoproliferative glomerulonephritis, focal segmental pattern: mesangial proliferation, mesangial matrix expansion, and glomerular basement membrane thickening are restricted to segmental part of the tuft. (Trichrome, magnification ×250.)

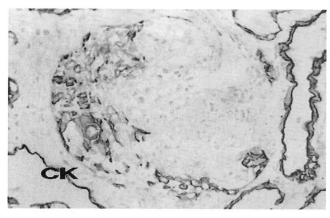

FIGURE 62-11. Type I membranoproliferative glomerulonephritis, extracapillary pattern: crescent formation strongly positive for a cytokeratins. (Cytokeratin, immunoperoxidase, magnification ×250.)

on subsequent biopsy. Our experience that the subendothelial deposits of C3 detected by immunofluorescence often are diffuse in each glomerulus supports the hypothesis that focal and segmental form could be stages of less marked damage during the natural course of the classical pattern (66–84).

Crescents also may be present in approximately 15% of patients with MPGN (8,48,99–103). These crescents may be small and segmental, or larger and circumferential, affecting most of the glomeruli (Fig. 62-10). These crescentic forms present some morphologica features that are totally different from necrotizing-extracapillary lesions typical of anti-neutrophil cytoplasmic antibody (ANCA)–associated renal vasculitis (104). The membranoproliferative crescentic patterns has minimal intraglomerular leukocyte infiltration, usually which is massive in vasculitis, and vascular cell adhesion molecule-1 is completely negative in the glomerular tuft in MPGN. Moreover, almost all cells in the crescent are positive for cytokeratins (Fig. 62-11) and their positivity for proliferating cell nuclear antigen suggests widespread proliferation of the parietal epithelial cells of Bowman's capsule (Fig. 62-12). Necrotizing glomerular lesions usually are not detected by light microscopy, whereas intraglomerular proliferation always is

present. In addition, immunofluorescence demonstrates fibrinogen positivity only in the crescents. All these features suggest that membranoproliferative crescentic nephritis is based on a different pathogenetic/morphogenetic mechanism than necrotizing-crescentic forms typical of primary renal vasculitis (104), in which necrosis of the glomerular tufts induces a marked inflammatory reaction with massive accumulation of monocytes and macrophages.

Our experience in a reevaluation of 41 cases of "idiopathic" crescentic glomerulonephritis, (104) and some previous ultrastructural studies (105–107), suggest that in crescentic forms of MPGN, the pathogenetic mechanism is segmental disruption of the GBM with escape of cells and fibrin through these gaps and subsequent epithelial cell proliferation and formation of circumferential crescents in an intact Bowman's capsule, leading to compression of glomerular tuft. The poor response of these patients to the same therapeutic regimen that improves necrotizing crescentic vasculitis lends support to this hypothesis (99,102,104).

Tubulointerstitial Lesions

Only since the mid-1990s has research on renal diseases concentrated on the presence and prognostic value of tubulointerstitial lesions in primary or secondary glomerulonephritis (108). Recent studies have demonstrated that the degree of

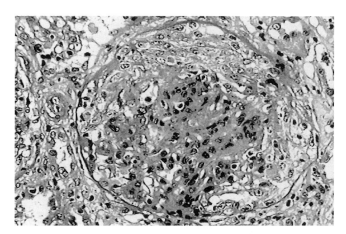

FIGURE 62-10. Type I membranoproliferative glomerulonephritis, extracapillary pattern: circumferential cellular crescent totally filling the Bowman's space, leading to compression of glomerular tuft. (Trichrome, magnification ×250.)

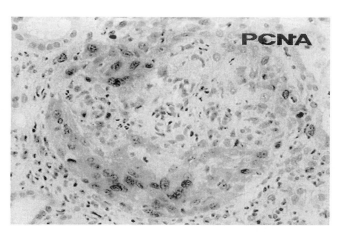

FIGURE 62-12. Type I membranoproliferative glomerulonephritis, extracapillary pattern: most crescent cells are positive for proliferative cell nuclear antigen. (Immunoperoxidase, magnification ×250.)

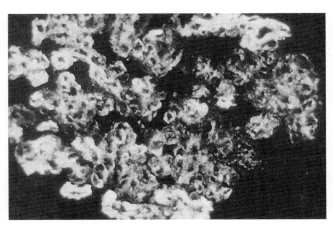

FIGURE 62-13. Type I membranoproliferative glomerulonephritis, immunofluorescence demonstrates diffuse and intense mesangial and parietal deposits. (Anti-C3, magnification ×250.)

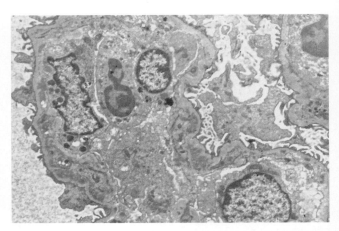

FIGURE 62-15. Type I membranoproliferative glomerulonephritis, electron micrograph of a part of a glomerulus shows subendothelial electron-dense deposits, double contour appearance of the glomerular basement membrane and some inflammatory cells. (Magnification ×3,600; courtesy of Dr. E. Schiaffino, Department of Pathology, San Carlo Hospital, Milan.)

tubulointerstitial lesions rather than glomerular changes determines renal outcome (107–112). The same correlation between the severity of interstitial changes and renal function also has been described in type I MPGN (113–117); it is becoming an accepted hypothesis that some factors produced during glomerular inflammatory process may induce reactive changes in the tubular cells, favor the passage of macromolecules into the interstitium, and finally trigger a T-cell-mediated immune reaction that can progress as an independent phenomenon. This T-lymphocytes and monocytes interstitial infiltration, which can be found early in the course of this disease, can stimulate proliferation of fibroblasts with resultant fibrosis and consequent impairment of renal function (108–112,118).

Immunofluorescence Findings

Immunofluorescence staining shows some variability in composition and distribution of deposits, confirming the heterogeneity of the pathogenetic mechanisms in patients with type I MPGN (2,41,46,71,119–124). There is almost always granular staining for C3 with two major patterns of deposition: one pattern is characterized by diffuse and regular deposits along the internal side of GBM associated with mesangial deposits (Fig. 62-13); the other pattern consists of deposits along the GBM outlining a lobulated tuft, but none in the mesangial stalk (Fig. 62-14). The latter pattern is associated mainly with

lobular or nodular lesions seen by light microscopy (71,125). Early components of complement activation (C4 and C1q) are present in approximately 50% of cases, whereas properdin is almost always present (9,46,119,121,124). In two-thirds of cases, glomerular structures stain positive for immunoglobulins (Immunoglobulin G [IgG] and immunoglobulin M [IgM]) in a manner similar to that for C3, although usually with less intensity (9,46,121,123). IgA usually is absent; when present, it is extremely important to determine if it is the predominant antiserum so that an MPGN secondary to IgA nephritis (Berger's disease, liver diseases) can be diagnosed (126,127). Rarely, C3 deposits are present in Bowman's capsule and the tubular basement membrane (128).

Electron Microscopy Findings

Electron microscopy in type I MPGN helps clarify light microscopy observations, showing increased mesangial cells and matrix, widespread subendothelial electron-dense deposits, and thickened basement membranes with the double-contour appearance (2,9,21,41,43,45,46,129–131) (Fig. 62-15). Usually, a diffuse increase in the number of mesangial cells is accompanied by a proportional increase in the amount of mesangial matrix, but in some cases (focal forms), the degree of mesangial proliferation varies between glomeruli, being different even in individual segments of a given glomerulus. Mesangial deposits usually are scarce and rarely abundant. The double-contoured GBM lesion consists of a normal native basement membrane with a new basement membrane-like material formed beneath the endothelium. This thickened capillary wall also is composed of interposed mesangial cells and electron-dense immunodeposits. The deposits, usually described as "subendothelial," range from small and segmental to large and diffuse (Fig. 62-16).

In more exudative forms, the double contour aspect of the thickened basement membrane is due mainly to the subendothelial interposition of infiltrating inflammatory cells rather than to mesangial interposition (23–66). This variant of MPGN closely resembles the morphologic pattern of the secondary forms of cryoglobulinemic glomerulonephritis (93,132,133). To distinguish the two forms it is important to perform ultrastructural studies at high magnification to exclude the deposits that have the typical structure seen in cryoglobulinemia (93,132,133). In approximately 30% of cases, glomerular

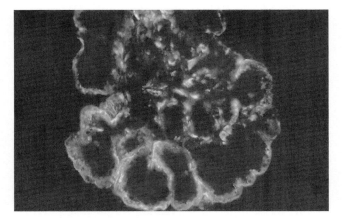

FIGURE 62-14. Type I membranoproliferative glomerulonephritis, immunofluorescence shows granular staining of the capillary wall with peripheral lobular accentuation. (Anti-C3, magnification ×250.)

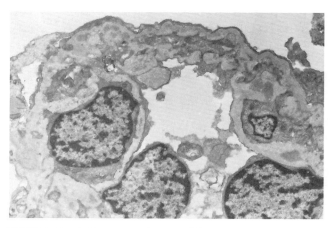

FIGURE 62-16. Type I membranoproliferative glomerulonephritis, electron micrograph of a capillary wall shows thickened glomerular basement membrane (GBM), subendothelial electron-dense deposits and double-contour appearance of GBM. (Magnification ×6,000; courtesy of Dr. E. Schiaffino, Department of Pathology, San Carlo Hospital, Milan.)

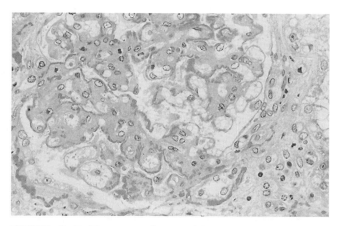

FIGURE 62-17. Type II membranoproliferative glomerulonephritis, with diffuse dense intramembranous deposits. Similar deposits are present in the basal lamina of Bowman's capsule. (Thricrome, magnification ×250.)

subepithelial deposits quite similar to the "humps" typical of acute postinfectious glomerulonephritis are present (2,71,130,131). Subepithelial deposits can be small and isolated or diffuse and abundant emphasizing that a clear separation between type I and type III of MPGN is problematic. The endothelial cells may be increased and swelling and the foot processes of visceral epithelial cells may be diffusely effaced.

Type II Membranoproliferative Glomerulonephritis (Dense-Deposit Disease)

In 1963, Berger and Galle (5) described a particular basement membrane lesion characterized by dense intramembranous deposits, mainly apparent on electron microscopy, in some patients with a membranoproliferative pattern of disease. Since the first description, this pattern of nephritis has been considered by many researches to be a variant of MPGN because in many cases it presents histologically with intense mesangial proliferation, frequent lobular accentuation of the tuft, and glomerular capillary wall thickening (16–20,44,50,56,57,59,134–139). Moreover, types I and II MPGN show clinical similarities, in particular the presence in both diseases of hypocomplementemia. However, many authors have stressed the morphologic differences on light, immunofluorescent, and electron microscopy between types I and II MPGN, suggesting that the latter form should clearly be designated as a separate disease entity (18,20,51,57,58,135,136).

Light Microscopy

The characteristic lesion of type II MPGN is thickened GBM due to irregular intramembranous deposits that are ribbon-like, brightly eosinophilic, and sometimes refractile (Figs. 62-17 and 62-18). They are intensely PAS positive and appear fuchsinophilic with trichrome stain. The glomerular intramembranous deposits vary greatly in size and number, and it is this feature that determines the extent of the glomerular capillary wall thickening. Although some authors believe that dense deposit disease can be diagnosed by light microscopy, in some cases electron microscopy may be needed to establish the presence of deposits with certainty. In some biopsies, PAS- and trichrome-positive mesangial deposits are evident, although it

is often difficult to be sure that these represent bona fide mesangial deposits. Electron microscopy often reveals mesangial deposits that cannot be identified by light microscopy. Deposits also are noted in the basal lamina of Bowman's capsule and the basement membranes of both proximal and distal tubules; the extent of this extraglomerular involvement is quite variable (140–142). Discrete glomerular subepithelial electron-dense deposits similar to the subepithelial humps noted in classical acute postinfectious (poststreptococcal) glomerulonephritis may be seen in dense deposit disease (16,41,47). Rarely, spikes of GBM-like material (as seen in membranous glomerulonephritis) may be noted around the subepithelial humps. Electron dense deposits may be occasionally identified in same arterioles (16,143).

In addition to characteristic and variable capillary wall lesions, the glomeruli show, as in type I MPGN, a great range of mesangial involvement, from minimal to diffuse, proliferative lesions and a diffuse crescentic pattern (21,41,51–53,135,140). Recent International Collaborative Study Group on Dense Deposit Disease (DDD) organized by Renal Pathology Society, confirmed the variability of morphologic lesions in the largest collected series of DDD to date (unpublished data). Five patterns emerged from the review of 71 cases: classical DDD (MPGN features) 25%; focal proliferative DDD 45%;

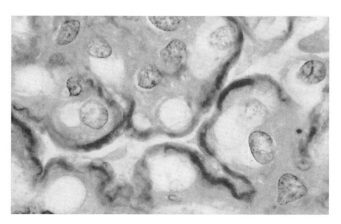

FIGURE 62-18. Type II membranoproliferative glomerulonephritis, showing overt dense intramembranous deposits. (Trichrome, magnification ×1,000.)

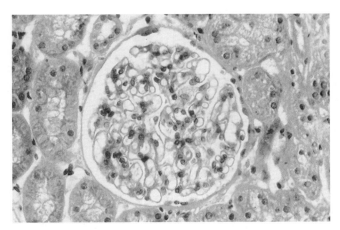

FIGURE 62-19. Type II membranoproliferative glomerulonephritis, with minimal mesangial proliferation and segmental thickening of the capillary walls. (Trichrome, magnification ×250.)

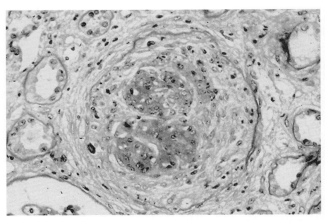

FIGURE 62-21. Type II membranoproliferative glomerulonephritis, the circumferential cellular crescent completely fills the Bowman's space. (Trichrome, magnification ×250.)

crescentic DDD 40%; acute proliferative and exudative DDD 13%; and atypical DDD (interrupted and markedly thick dense deposits) 3%. There were differences between the American and European Centers. Only one case of crescentic DDD and no cases of atypical DDD were seen in the European Centers. Crescentic DDD accounted for 35% of North American cases.

An inconsistent degree of mesangial proliferation may be seen with a picture of quite normal glomeruli but with some glomerular capillary wall thickening (Fig. 62-19). Other renal biopsies show a more pronounced glomerular tuft hypercellularity with a diffuse proliferative glomerulonephritis (Fig. 62-20). Leukocytes may be more common when the lesions are diffuse than when they are focal and segmental. Glomeruli may show areas of marked endothelial swelling that cause narrowing of the capillary lumina. The mesangium may display differing degrees of matrix proliferation (mesangial sclerosis), and, at the end of the spectrum, there are sclerotic nodules with an accentuated lobular pattern (so-called lobular glomerulonephritis). We have never seen a "true" nodular pattern in our cases of type II MPGN. Crescents may be present in a large or small numbers and with diffuse and circumferential extracapillary proliferation (51,135) (Fig. 62-21). By contrast, we have never seen focal and segmental necrotizing lesion occasionally noted

by Siblay and Kim (135). There may be interstitial inflammation, mostly caused by chronic inflammatory cells. Foam cells are sometimes present, indicative of the nephrotic syndrome. Interstitial fibrosis appears as renal failure develops. As in all other forms of glomerulonephritis, the *tubulo-interstitial lesion* may play a crucial role in the progression of the disease.

Immunofluorescence Findings

The characteristic immunohistologic finding in type II MPGN is intense staining for C3 along the glomerular capillary walls and in the glomerular mesangial regions (16,17,19,21,41,44, 51,52,119,135–137,139). The immunohistologic pattern has been variously described as linear, pseudolinear, ribbonlike, granular, or nodular. Moreover, the intensity on distribution of deposits varies considerably. The most common finding is C3 along the capillary walls in a double-contour linear configuration giving a "railroad track" appearance and ring-shaped mesangial linear deposition (19,119,135) (Fig. 62-22). Granular staining, distinct from the linear deposits and the mesangial rings, are also frequently found in the mesangium. C3 also is frequently present in Bowman's capsule and along tubular basement membranes (119,141,142) (Fig. 62-22). The early components of complement (C4 and C1q) are noted rarely (144). Deposition of immunoglobulins is rare and tends to be focal,

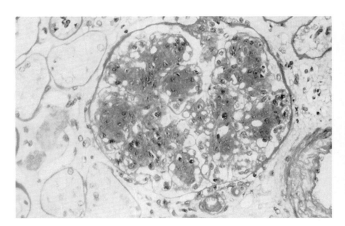

FIGURE 62-20. Type II membranoproliferative glomerulonephritis, showing pronounced glomerular tuft hypercellularity with a diffuse proliferative pattern. (Trichrome, magnification ×250.)

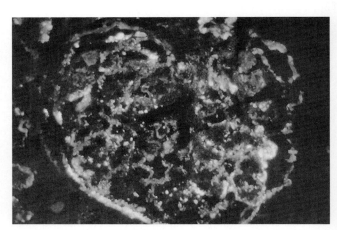

FIGURE 62-22. Type II membranoproliferative glomerulonephritis, immunofluorescence shows linear staining of the peripheral capillary wall, Bowman's capsule and tubular basement membranes. Note bright granules in mesangium. (Anti-C3, magnification ×250.)

segmental, and less intense than that of complement components (19,119).

Many studies using various staining methods showed major differences in the pattern and composition of the deposits between dense deposit disease and type I MPGN, providing valuable information for making the histologic diagnosis and understanding the morphogenesis of type II MPGN. Some investigators demonstrated that dense deposits stain brightly with thioflavine-T (18,145). Muda et al. (54) in an ultrastructural histochemical investigations, demonstrated that the dense deposits have a higher affinity for osmium than the lamina densa of normal basement membranes, and that the electron density is strictly osmium dependent, suggesting the presence of a lipid component. Nevins (146) and Galle and Mahieu (57) suggested that the dense deposit basement membrane changes are characterized by the accumulation of a glycoprotein membrane material that contains large amount of sialic acid. Further studies are warranted to determine the exact chemical composition of the dense deposit material.

Electron Microscopy Findings

There is generally good agreement that confirmation of the diagnosis of dense deposit disease requires electron microscopy examination (5,16–18,41,44,57). The characteristic lesion is a basement membrane thickening due to the presence of electron-dense material within the lamina densa (Fig. 62-23). Distribution can be segmental, discontinuous, or diffuse. The electron dense deposits do not show a particular substructure and are different from the fine granular deposits that characterize the various forms of immunocomplex glomerulonephritis, and therefore they can be clearly differentiated from the deposits seen in type I MPGN.

Similar electron-dense material usually is present in the mesangial area. These deposits may be well circumscribed and correspond to the mesangial rings made on immunofluorescence. Electron-dense deposits usually are noted along the basal lamina of Bowman's capsule, along the tubular basement membranes and in capillaries, arterioles and small arteries (16,136). More frequently than in type I MPGN, humplike subepithelial deposits are noted (16,44,136,143). Other changes seen on electron microscopy include mesangial proliferation and mesangial matrix expansion, with great variability in intensity and diffusion of these lesions.

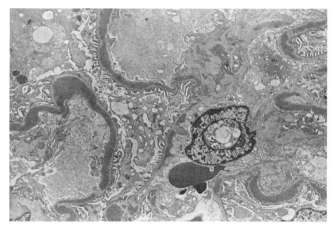

FIGURE 62-23. Type II membranoproliferative glomerulonephritis, electron micrograph of a part of a glomerulus shows the thickened capillary basement membranes; a homogeneous electron-dense material replaces the lamina densa with a diffuse distribution. (Magnification ×2,800; courtesy of Dr. E. Schiaffino, Department of Pathology, San Carlo Hospital, Milan).

The presence of dense-deposits in other organ system (e.g., brain, heart, lung, liver, adrenal glands, or pancreas) has not been reported. Eye fundus lesions, described by Duvall-Young et al. (147) and others (148), are described later in this chapter.

Type III Membranoproliferative Glomerulonephritis

Burkholder et al. (15) discussed a type of MPGN they termed *mixed membranous and proliferative glomerulonephritis*. This pattern had some of the features of typical type I MPGN, such as thickening of the glomerular capillary walls, double contours, mesangial interposition, and subendothelial deposits. In addition, however, there were silver-positive spikes along the GBM and trichrome-positive subepithelial humps such as seen in stage II membranous glomerulonephritis. Ultrastructural studies confirmed the presence of glomerular electron-dense deposits, and immunofluorescent staining showed a heavy granular pattern along the glomerular capillary walls and mesangium for C3 and sometimes for IgG and IgM. The clinical features were similar to those of type I MPGN and DDD; the serum C3 level was depressed in two of five patients.

Anders et al. (62) and Strife et al. (63), using mainly electron microscopy, characterized another variant that they also designated type III MPGN. The lamina densa was disrupted often with thickening and expansion of the basement membrane and layering by a silver-negative basement membrane material. There were glomerular subendothelial and subepithelial deposits that were contiguous or connect through the lamina densa of GBM (3,62,63,129). The controversy over whether type III should be recognized as an established and distinct clinico-pathologic entity or a simple variant of type I MPGN remains open. Jackson et al. (64) concluded that "despite some differences, type I and III should be considered variants of the same disease, rather than separate diseases."

ASSOCIATION WITH OTHER DISORDERS: DIFFERENTIAL DIAGNOSIS

Morphologic lesions referred to as MPGN have been described in numerous forms with recognizable etiologic agents or as occurring in association with other diseases. Usually the clinical features and specific laboratory findings allow the clinician and pathologist to propose a precise differential diagnosis. Moreover, many forms of MPGN associated with systemic diseases show peculiar histologic, immunohistologic and ultrastructural features that allow a clear morphologic differentiation from the "idiopathic" form.

Mixed Cryoglobulinemia (MC)

Cryoglobulinemia is a pathologic condition in which the blood contains immunoglobulins that precipitate reversibly at cold temperatures. According to the widely used classification, there are three types of cryoglobulinemia (93,149). In type I cryoglobulinemia, the cryoprecipitable immunoglobulin is a single monoclonal immunoglobulin, usually a myeloma protein or a macroglobulin (Waldenström's macroglobulinemia). In type II MC, a monoclonal immunoglobulin (usually an IgM) is bound to a polyclonal IgG and acts as an anti-IgG rheumatoid factor, whereas in type III, the anti-IgG rheumatoid factor is a polyclonal immunoglobulin. Both types of MC are frequently associated with a single monoclonal immunoglobulin, usually a myelomatous protein. Although the glomerular lesions are variable and nonspecific in the few cases of type III MC, a particularly well-characterized pattern of glomerular involvement called "cryoglobulinemia glomerulonephritis" has been described in type II MC, in which the monoclonal rheumatoid factor usually is an IgM-k (93,94,150–154).

The glomerular pattern of cryoglobulinemic glomerulonephritis is characterized by massive endocapillary hypercellularity due to an infiltration of leukocytes, mainly monocytes (4,104,154,155). Immunohistochemical analysis with monoclonal antibodies confirms this massive accumulation of monocytes, which is more impressive than in idiopathic MPGN (88).

Another typical morphologic feature is the frequent and sometimes massive presence of amorphous, eosinophilic, PAS-positive deposits totally filling the capillary lumina with aspect of "intraluminal thrombi" (93,94,152,153,156,157). Thickening of GBM, with a double-contoured appearance, is more diffuse and evident than in SLE and idiopathic MPGN, and is due mainly to peripheral interposition of monocytes (93,94,155). In spite of the intense intracapillary proliferation and exudation, extracapillary proliferation is an uncommon finding. In at least one-third of patients with MC, vasculitis of small and medium-sized arteries is found (94,151,152,158).

Immunohistologic features follow a predictable pattern, and the pattern of deposition or the identity of the prevailing immunoreactants is particularly important in the differential diagnosis (152,158–160). The pattern is characterized by large deposits in capillary lumina as intraluminal thrombi and diffuse granular staining of peripheral capillary walls (subendothelial deposits). IgM and IgG are the prevailing immunoreactants, suggesting that the deposits are locally trapped or precipitated cryoglobulins.

Electron-dense deposits can be found in the capillary walls and lumina (thrombi). Sometimes they are amorphous, immune complex–like deposits, but often they show a typical and peculiar fibrillar or crystalloid structure, identical to that seen in the *in vitro* cryoprecipitate of the same patients (93,152,155,156,158,161–164). Ultrastructural examination confirms the massive infiltration of monocytes in the capillary lumina and in the double contour of thickened GBM (4,154,164).

Systemic Lupus Erythematosus (SLE)

Renal morphologic features similar to those of idiopathic MPGN, with marked and homogeneous mesangial proliferation and diffuse double-contoured appearance of thickened capillary walls, are uncommon in SLE. According to new SLE nephritis International Society of Nephrology/Renal Pathology Society (ISN/RPS) classification, the differential diagnosis should be posed with class IV global diffuse lupus nephritis (90). Class IV-G is characterized by diffuse and global endocapillary, mesangial, and frequent extracapillary proliferation (165).

Many active lesions, usually absent in type I MPGN, may be present in class IV-G: widespread wire-loops, capillary loop necrosis, karyorrhexis, and hematoxylin bodies (167–169).

The immunohistologic pattern in class IV-G lupus glomerulonephritis is characterized by massive parietal deposits mimicking the wire-loop seen at light microscopy (170). IgG is found in all patients and IgM in approximately 60% of cases, whereas IgA is rare. (170,171). Of the complement components, C3 is the most frequent, followed by C1q which usually stains very intensively. The intense positivity for C1q in SLE nephritis is an important feature in the differential diagnosis with regard to other forms of MPGN (172). Finally, ultrastruc-

tural evidence of deposits simultaneously located in the mesangial, subendothelial, intramembranous, and subepithelial sites is considered suggestive for SLE-associated glomerulonephritis (89,166,173,174).

Light-Chain Disease

The appearance of glomerular lesions occurring in light-chain disease may be variable but the most common feature is characterized by massive mesangial nodules similar to those seen in the nodular form of type I MPGN (80, 81,175–178). The staining characteristics of the glomerular nodules, however, are different in the two diseases: those in light-chain disease are more PAS positive, and negative on silver stain. Moreover, the constant presence in light-chain disease of tubular basement membrane, vascular, and interstitial deposits frequently is sufficient to trigger the suspicion that the underlying cause of the nephropathy is systemic deposition of immunoglobulin fragments. Immunofluorescence allows a further differentiation, with a strong staining for K light chains in glomeruli, tubular basement membrane, vessels and interstitium (175,176,179,180). Finally, electron microscopy shows typical fine granular deposits of extremely electron-dense material distributed through mesangial area and along GBM (181–183).

Light-chain nephropathy occasionally may resemble type II MPGN, although the electron-dense deposits of light chain nephropathy tend to be more coarsely granular and subendothelial in location, and do not stain for C3 by immunofluorescence.

Liver Disease

A pattern of membranoproliferative glomerulonephritis in liver disease has been described by many authors (127,184). The morphologic picture often is indistinguishable from the glomerular lesions of classical type I MPGN. The prevalent and intense positivity for IgA in the mesangium and capillary walls is the most important characteristic finding.

CLINICAL MANIFESTATIONS OF IDIOPATHIC MEMBRANOPROLIFERATIVE GLOMERULONEPHRITIS

Since the mid-1960s, the clinical and laboratory features of MPGN have been described in a number of clinical studies and reviews (1,2,6–8,10,11,15,16,44,67,71,185). Idiopathic MPGN affects children and adolescents more frequently than adults, and rarely occurs before 5 years of age and after the sixth decade (17,186). Type II MPGN is more frequent at younger ages. Sex predominance varies in single reports, but in the cumulative experience, both sexes are equally affected. The disease is more common among whites than among black and Asian populations. Familial cases of both type I and type II have been reported, which argues in favor of genetic factors being involved in their origin (187,188). Tissue typing studies showed that the extended haplotype on chromosome 6q, human leukocyte antigen (HLA)-B8, DR3, SC01, GL02, is found in 13% of patients with MPGN types I and III and in 1% of control haplotypes (189). However, this haplotype is not specific for MPGN and also is associated with SLE, gluten-sensitive enteropathy, and type I diabetes mellitus. Type II MPGN is much less common than type I. In series with consecutive patients of both types, type II usually represents 10% to 20% of total cases and type I most of the rest; approximately 5% of cases have type III.

In type I MPGN, the clinical presentation is nephrotic syndrome for 60% or more of cases, usually accompanied by microscopic hematuria. Acute nephritic syndrome may be the presenting feature in 15% to 20% of cases, recurrent macroscopic hematuria occasionally is seen. The remainder present with asymptomatic microscopic hematuria or proteinuria. These clinical types and symptoms often overlap. Two children with few urinary abnormalities and hypocomplementemia were described with typical type I MPGN at renal biopsy; the clinical picture remained unchanged for many years (190). The onset of disease can be preceded, especially in children, by an infectious episode in the upper respiratory tract, more commonly in type II. Hypertension increases in frequency during the course of disease, even before the onset of a reduction in glomerular filtration rate (GFR). On initial diagnosis, hypertension is present in 30% of cases, and renal insufficiency in 20%. Renal symptoms at presentation may be accompanied in approximately 25% of cases by fatigue, weight loss, pallor, lack of appetite. A moderate degree of anemia (hemoglobin between 8 and 10 g/dL), which is out of proportion of the degree of renal function impairment, is present in 25% to 40% of cases. It may be caused by increased hemolysis, related to complement activation on red blood cells surface.

The presenting syndrome in type II MPGN is similar to that in type I, but acute nephritic syndrome or recurrent macroscopic hematuria are more common. Some authors (50) report a reversal of acute nephritic episodes in type II MPGN, most often occurring during the onset of disease, but this observation has not been confirmed by others (9). More recently, ocular alterations have been demonstrated in type II MPGN. Autopsy studies have shown dense deposit material using PAS staining of the wall of choroidal blood vessels and Bruch's membrane (147). These patients had been diagnosed with dense deposit disease by renal biopsy 2 years earlier. These deposits were confirmed by electron microscopy, and were similar to those seen in renal tissue, they were localized in the basement membrane of the ciliary epithelium, the capillaries and along the inner collagenous layer of Bruch's membrane. The high frequency of eye abnormalities has been confirmed by several clinical studies with fundal examination by ophthalmoscopy and fluorescein angiography. The ophthalmoscopically examined lesion resembles basal laminar drusen and worsens in extension and number with the duration of disease (191, 192). Michielsen et al. (193) found diffuse retinal pigment alterations in 11 out of 12 patients with type II MPGN and 4 of these patients also had disciform macular detachment and choroidal neovascularization. Subretinal neovascularization is therefore a complication of dense deposit disease (194). Type I MPGN is not associated with fundus lesions.

The clinical presentation and course of type III MPGN are similar to those of the other types, except that the patients tend to be older, the disease has more insidious onset, complement abnormalities are different from type I (62,195), the outcome may be more serious, and clinical and laboratory manifestations less responsive to steroids.

LABORATORY FINDINGS

Membranoproliferative glomerulonephritis exhibits a distinctive laboratory feature that is unique among the primary glomerular diseases. This is the frequent finding of an abnormal serum complement profile. The abnormality in type I consists of a reduction of serum C3 in 60% to 70% of cases, and, more rarely, of C4 at time of diagnosis; hypocomplementemia is more pronounced during follow-up, but normalizes with time in some patients. Nevertheless, normal values throughout an entire course of observation can be seen. C3 is more frequently (60% to 70% of cases) and severely reduced in type II than type I, but the differences are less pronounced than formerly believed. Adults and children have similar complement profiles. Most patients with type III MPGN exhibit a depression of C3, but C4 is almost always normal (64). The C3 nephritic factor of amplification loop (NFa), an IgG autoantibody to a C3 convertase (C3b,Bb), isolated from sera of patients with type II disease, is found in 80% of cases in this form and was initially believed to be characteristic of type II MPGN. However, it can also be found in few patients with type I disease. This factor is a conformational autoantibody that binds to C3b,Bb, the C3 convertase of alternate pathway that normally cleaves C3 into C3a and C3b. Binding of this autoantibody protects C3b,Bb from enzymatic inactivation and stabilizes the convertase, thereby allowing continued C3 breakdown and increasing C3 consumption.

It therefore is responsible for the persistent depression of C3. Thus, membrane-bound C3/C5 convertase does not form, and activation of the terminal pathway does not occur. C3NFa is more common in children with type II MPGN than in adults, is a fast activator, with a molecular weight of 240 kd. Another autoantibody against the terminal complement components in patients with type I MPGN has been observed (196–199). This terminal nephritic factor (NFt), an autoantibody against C3b,Bb,P, is a slow activator of the terminal components C5b,6,7,8, providing a binding site for C3b. It is found in type I (approximately 20% of cases), rarely in type II, and in approximately 70% of type III (199). NFt is properdin dependent and has a molecular weight of 980 kd and its presence in sera is associated with reduced concentrations of C3 and terminal complex C5b,6,7,8,9. Finally, a nephritogenic factor (NFc), which causes C4 activation, is found in sera of 15% of patients with type I MPGN. This autoantibody affects classical pathway C3 convertase, stabilizes C4b,2a and increases the classical pathway activation in the presence of circulating immune complexes (200). In about half of patients with type I MPGN the terminal C5b-9 complement complex (TCC) levels were found to accumulate in plasma and urine. TCC was also found in glomerular deposits. Increased TCC was associated with acute phase hypocomplementemia, with a lower response to steroids and poor long-term prognosis (201). Vitronectin and clusterin, which are both regulatory proteins for TCC, are also involved (202) and play a role in reducing the formation of TCC in glomerular tissue.

Circulating immune complexes are found in both types I and II MPGN, more frequently in type I (60% to 70% of cases) than type II (30% to 40%) (203). Serial measurements of circulating immune complexes have shown that the complexes are found intermittently, transiently, with wide variations over time (204).

In routine laboratory investigations, patients with MPGN show the aforementioned anemia, which is of the normochromic normocytic type. When present, all laboratory features of nephrotic syndrome, (e.g., hypoalbuminemia, lipid abnormalities) are detectable. Obviously, the urinalysis reveals various degrees of glomerular nonselective proteinuria on electrophoretic examination and dysmorphic erythrocytes and red cell casts in the urinary sediment.

Other laboratory investigations in all patients with a histological diagnosis of MPGN must be geared toward a complete search for the underlying disease. This procedure is mandatory before a patient is categorized as affected by a primary or idiopathic MPGN because of the frequent association of MPGN with systemic disease, including a chronic bacterial or viral infection. These investigations include testing for antinuclear and anti-DNA antibodies, cryoglobulins, serum and urine protein immunoelectrophoresis or immunofixation for paraproteins,

ANCA, serology for hepatitis B and C, hepatic enzymes, and screening studies for malignancies, especially in older patients. Moreover, blood cultures for a possible bacterial infection should be performed. Screening for HCV antibody or HCV RNA by polymerase chain reaction is important. If an MC related to HCV accompanies a MPGN, C4 will be severely depressed, unlike the primary form of MPGN, in which C3 is often decreased to a greater extent than C4. The relation between HCV and MPGN is discussed later in this chapter.

PATHOGENESIS

The pathogenesis of all types of MPGN remains incompletely understood. Type I MPGN has many features that suggest an immune complex-mediated disorder. In favor of this hypothesis is the frequent detection of circulating immune complexes (203,204), the subendothelial presence of immunoglobulins and complement components in glomeruli by direct immunofluorescence (2,9,16,17,44,48,119), the evidence in serum of activation of the classical complement pathway (6,205–207), the analogy with experimental models induced by immune complexes, and the similarity between MPGN and human diseases caused by immune deposits such as chronic bacteremic or viremic states and SLE, whose antigen is well known (208,209). In type I MPGN, unlike type III or II, the constant presence of subendothelial deposits during hypocomplementemic accords with the hypothesis of nephritis arising from immune complexes deposition. Deposition of circulating immune complexes is the predominant nephritogenic agent in type I MPGN, with evidence for classical pathway activation, even though other nephritic factors may be present in some patients. In a few severely hypocomplementemia patients with type I disease, paramesangial deposits were observed that correlated with the hypocomplementemia, which is in agreement with the presence in serum of native convertase in excess and of circulating nephritic factors (210,211).

However, because many patients with circulating immune complexes do not acquire MPGN, additional factors, such as type of antigen, type and charge on the antibody, size of the complexes, their ability to dissociate and reassociate, and local glomerular factors must play a role. In addition, mechanisms of immune complexes clearance can be defective. Other glomerular complexes are formed *in situ*, depending on the antigenic stimulus and antibody response.

Moreover, in type I MPGN, besides the classical pathway of complement activation (low C4, C2, C1q, B, C3), terminal (low C3, C5, C8, C9) and alternate pathway activation (low C3) also sometimes are observed. Therefore three patterns of complement activation are seen in type I MPGN. In fact, in type I MPGN, besides the classical immune complex mechanism, both NFa and NFt are involved. In some cases, the C1 bypass, which reacts with C1, properdin and factor B, also is found.

Complement abnormalities may be relevant to disease's pathogenesis, because frequent defects of complement components in type I MPGN are observed. These primary defects include inherited partial deficiencies of C3, C3 factor B, C6, and C7, and structural abnormalities in C3 and C7 (212–216). A membranoproliferative glomerulonephritis was described in a 10-year-old female patient with an inherited C4 deficiency. Focal MPGN was observed at renal biopsy with electron-dense deposits in paramesangium and subepithelial regions and isolated C3 deposits along GBM and mesangial areas (217). Such deficiencies, related to a defect in a structural or regulatory gene, could play a permissive role by interfering with the clearance and solubilization of antigen–antibody complexes after a

viral or bacterial infection, leading to increased glomerular deposition and development of MPGN. For example, in Finnish Landrace lambs (218), which are C3 deficient, type I MPGN develops, with a predominant C3 glomerular deposition as an early lesion and subsequent deposition of immunoglobulins and development of a more generalized immune complex disease. A mixture of different types of MPGN can be observed in the same family. Berry et al. (219) described two siblings, a brother who had type III disease and a sister with type I; in a second family, two brothers had type I disease. In conclusion, even though the complement profile in type I MPGN may sometimes indicate the presence of a nephritic factor, circulating immune complexes appear to be basic to pathogenesis (210).

The mechanisms of capillary wall injury can be divided into two phases. A first "active" phase, the more proximal layers of the glomerular capillary walls are involved directly, by complement cytolytic activity and by accumulation and infiltration of inflammatory cells, in particular neutrophils and monocytes (220). Such cells in MPGN show an increased expression of some surface adhesion molecules, which interfere with intercellular adhesion molecule-1, which is expressed in endothelial and mesangial cells. The second injury phase, results in expansion of mesangial matrix and duplication of basement membrane. During the second phase tissue repair with thickening of the peripheral capillary wall, the characteristic double-contoured basement membrane and expansion of the mesangium are the prevailing features (220).

Type II MPGN is a unique lesion with no experimental analog and many factors differentiate the disease from the other histologic variants of MPGN (26,51), including the presence of peculiar and specific intramembranous deposits, the absence of immunoglobulins in glomerular deposits, the more frequent and persistent reduction of C3, the evidence of NFa in serum, the occasional association of partial lipodystrophy, and the recurrence of the disease in a transplanted kidney (16,17,44,56,137,221,222). Type II MPGN is considered to be associated with the alternative pathway of complement activation, with the amplification loop mechanism being operative.

Factor H deficiency and dysfunction have been described in type II MPGN (210). Factor H, a β1-globulin located on the gene cluster on chromosome 1, is a regulatory protein of complement activation. It inhibits C3/C5 convertase activation of C3 by cleaving Bb from C3,Bb. Factor H dysfunction leads to accumulation of alternative pathway convertase C3b,Bb and C3 consumption. Factor H also serves as a cofactor for the C3b-cleaving enzyme, factor I. Homozygous factor H deficiency was associated with type II or type I MPGN (223). In the same series other patients with homozygous or heterozygous factor H deficiency presented with typical or atypical hemolytic-uremic syndrome (223). This report confirms that glomerular lesions in MPGN are secondary to uncontrolled C3 alternative pathway activation.

Partial lipodystrophy is a rare disease, characterized by a symmetric loss of facial fat and of the disappearance, in some cases, of fat from the arms and upper part of trunk. These patients have hypocomplementemia, circulating serum Nfa and activation of the alternative pathway of complement, and a type II MPGN develops in some of them. In this disease, hypocomplementemia precedes the onset of nephritis. This suggests that additional factors also may be involved, such as circulating immune complexes. NFa also is involved in damage to adipocytes; adipocytes produce a protein (adipsin) that is identical to factor D of alternative pathway of complement activation. The pattern of damage is related to the amount of factor D produced by the adipocyte (186). More rarely, types I and III are associated with partial lipodystrophy.

Whether type II MPGN has the same genetic predisposition as type I is uncertain. Power et al (188) described the incidence of C3 nephritic factor, partial lipodystrophy and type II MPGN in members of two generations of a single family. This suggests that the pathogeneses of these conditions may be linked and that genetically determined factors may, in some circumstances, contribute to disease susceptibility.

Biochemical analysis of membranes containing dense deposits in type II MPGN showed an accumulation of a biochemically modified glycoprotein membrane substance that had increased sialic acid and decreased cysteine (57). GBM containing dense material lose its endothelial antigens (57), and has decreased antigenic binding sites. It has been reported (146) that dense deposits had a selective reactivity for certain lectins, indicating the presence of an appreciable amount of internally linked N-acetylglucosamine. The Cincinnati group (224) identified the mesangial deposits in type II MPGN as paramesangial (granules at the base of the capillary tuft) and, more importantly, demonstrated that their presence correlates closely with hypocomplementemia. Such deposits more likely result from circulating convertase stabilized by the NFa. More recently the same investigators (225) observed that paramesangial deposits, present only during hypocomplementemia, in type II MPGN are composed only of C3c, which can be formed from a circulating complement breakdown product, induced by NF. The C3c deposits are devoid of properdin, while C5 is present in only small amounts. These observations suggest that NF has a role in the pathogenesis of type II MPGN, the C3 level having a possible prognostic significance.

The pathogenesis of type III MPGN is uncertain. The general absence of IgG and C4 from the glomerular deposits and the aforementioned changes in the complement profile, together with the lack of classical pathway of activation, tends to rule out an origin from circulating immune complexes. Type III MPGN is a consequence of the formation of the NFt autoantibody, a slow acting, properdin-dependent antibody at the terminal pathway. Late terminal components are activated to a greater extent than in other types (197,198). Hypocomplementemia is therefore due to circulating nephritic factor which stabilizes the convertase, C3b, Bb, P. Hypocomplementemia was found to be correlated with the presence of subendothelial and subepithelial deposits, but if the patient becomes normocomplementemic during the course of disease, the deposits slowly disappear. The first deposits to disappear are subendothelial, followed by paramesangial deposits. Much later, the "type III lesions" (i.e., association of subendothelial deposits and interruptions of lamina densa) also disappear (211). In type III subendothelial deposits are present only in half of the cases in hypocomplementemic patients and are absent in normocomplementemic patients. This could depend on a less complete rearrangement of the deposited material than in type I, because of the absence of IgG (62). Paramesangial subepithelial deposits are a hallmark of type III MPGN, they are correlated with elevated circulating levels of the convertase C3b. These deposits, in type III MPGN, differ from those in type II in that they can persist for up to a year after NFt has disappeared and hypocomplementemia resolved (210,211). Remission of type III MPGN, eventually induced by steroids, is coincident with normocomplementemia and absence of type III lesion and deposits. On the other hand type III lesion can be absent at the onset of disease, when severe hypocomplementemia is observed; the histologic lesions can develop later in the course of disease.

In conclusion, abnormal circulating levels of the convertase, stabilized by the nephritic factors, are closely associated with glomerular deposits and therefore are nephritogenic (211). The elimination of nephritic factors, and consequent normalization of serum C3 level, is the primary goal of the therapy of types II and III MPGN.

Hepatitis C Virus and Membranoproliferative Glomerulonephritis

Various studies have demonstrated an association between HCV infection and MPGN. Occult chronic infection with HCV in apparent primary MPGN is thought to be more common than previously detected (38,226–228). Two-thirds of HCV-related MPGN cases had cryoglobulinemia and circulating immune complexes. The MPGN was type I and type III. The real prevalence of noncryoglobulinemic MPGN, compared with the more frequent cryo-mediated GNMP, is still debated. Patients with MC and MPGN have HCV antibodies of the IgG type that stimulate the production of cryoprecipitable IgM-k anti IgG. The production of glomerular lesions is related to cryoglobulin formation. The hypothesis that HCV antigen-containing immune complexes without IgM-k also can be responsible for noncryoglobulinemic MPGN is controversial. Some patients apparently without systemic manifestations exhibit symptoms of cryoglobulinemia later in the course of disease.

The explanation for the finding of noncryoglobulinemic MPGN associated with HCV infection, at least in some geographic areas such as the United States and northern Japan, is that the production of cryoglobulins might not reach a level detectable by standard laboratory technique. In addition, patients could produce antibodies of the "rheumatoid factor" type but that could be without the ability to induce immune complexes precipitable by cold. Finally, these patients can have an immune complex–mediated MPGN without detectable circulating cryoglobulins (220,229) although the cryoglobulins may be detected after a few months of disease.

Nevertheless, the prevalence of HCV antibody in patients with apparent "idiopathic" MPGN in many series is low, and comparable to the prevalence in the general population (230–238). In conclusion, HCV infection induces glomerular damage mainly through endogenous production of cryoprecipitable IgM-k anti-IgG antibody. Nevertheless, the induction of an immune complex mediated GN without IgM-k is a possible event (238–240).

Cellular Immune Function

Cellular immune function in patients with idiopathic MPGN has been investigated with inconclusive results (241,242). Prominent cell-mediated immunity and related immune response have been recently studied in single glomerular diseases. Human immune response leading to different patterns of injury can be directed by two specific subsets of T helper cells, which involve cell-mediated effector mechanisms and promote antibody production and antibody mediated effector mechanisms. Th1 or Th2 predominance of nephritogenic immune response is relevant for the single histopathologic patterns and outcomes of glomerular diseases. Evidence that Th1 predominant immune response is associated with MPGN has been reported a few years ago (243). Th1 or Th2 predominance can also be evaluated by IgG subtypes involvement or cytokine production (40). Elevated serum IgG3 values in patients with MPGN, in parallel with IgG3 glomerular deposits, are in agreement with a prevalent Th1 pattern in MPGN (244). Moreover, in the same patients, high levels of serum cytokines IL-2 and IL2-R also suggest that Th1 pattern has an important role in the pathogenetic mechanism of MPGN (244). Accordingly, the principal function of CD4+ cells expressing Th1 phenotype is the complement-fixing antibody, while IgG3 subclasses are strong initiators of complement activation. As already mentioned, prevailing Th1/Th2 balance directs the nephritogenic immune response and may be driven by hygiene and other environmental factors (hygiene hypothesis) (39). This could explain the divergent prevalence of MPGN in different geographic areas worldwide and changes in epidemiology according to improved socioeconomic status.

Role of Platelets

Evidence of platelet involvement in the pathogenesis of MPGN has been found in experimental and clinical studies (245). Platelets may participate in the glomerular damage in models of experimental MPGN, together with other mediators (246). Selective platelet consumption and reduced survival have been detected in most patients with MPGN. Platelets contain a potent mitogenic factor, platelet-derived growth factor (PDGF), that recruits and mitogenically stimulates mesenchymal cells (247). Platelet-derived growth factor and the platelet-specific protein factor-4 have chemotactic activity for neutrophils and monocytes (248). Activated platelets also release transforming growth factor-β, which plays a predominant role in the evolution of glomerular lesions to sclerosis by stimulating matrix protein deposition and inhibiting their reabsorption. George et al. (249) found selective platelet consumption in patients with different types of glomerulonephritis, including MPGN. Donadio et al (250) provided evidence for decreased platelet survival in 70% of patients with MPGN, with a favorable effect of antiplatelet agents (dipyridamole and aspirin). Whether platelet activation and consumption can cause direct endothelial damage through tissue deposition or release of mitogenic proteins is unknown. The true role and importance of platelet activation in initiation and progression of injury remain unknown.

NATURAL HISTORY AND PROGNOSIS

The clinical course of MPGN appears to be comparable for all types of MPGN, and variations in the clinical severity of the disease can occur with prolonged remissions, either spontaneous or after various forms of treatment (186,251,252). Clinical remissions also were correlated with a regression of the histologic lesions (248,253,254). Episodes of acute deterioration of renal function or rapid variations of proteinuria can occur without any obvious triggering events. Moreover, the disease can remain stable for years, despite persistent proteinuria. Clinical remissions have been reported in 7% to 10% of patients in older series and persistent proteinuria in 30% to 40% of cases. Chronic renal insufficiency in 10% to 15%, and uremia with need for replacement therapy is observed in 40% to 45%. The mean renal survival rate is approximately 50% at 10 years (47,131,251,255). Droz et al. (251) reported a survival rate at 10 years of 60% for "pure" MPGN, and of 36% for the lobular form. Pediatric series have a better prognosis (256,257).

Type II MPGN does not show a different clinical course, even though clinical remissions are uncommon (16,48) and loss of renal function is somewhat faster than for type I. The mortality rate is 50% at 10 years from diagnosis for children (16) and at 8 years for a series of children and adults (48). More prolonged courses are reported by others (50). Children with type II MPGN had a slightly better prognosis in some studies, but longer follow-up series did not show any difference in outcome from that of the adult population (48,258). In four long-term follow-up studies, similar patient survival or renal failure rates were found for all the morphologic groups of MPGN (2,44,47,50). A comparison between clinical course in type I and type III MPGN was performed recently by the Cincinnati group (195). Twenty-one children with types I and 25 with type III MPGN, with similar clinical characteristics at

onset and both treated with alternate day steroids, were followed for a period of at least 5 years. Patients with type I disease had a lower initial mean GFR. The frequency of complications of therapy did not differ between the two groups. Ninety percent of patients with type I and less than 50% of those with type III disease normalized their serum C3 levels after 1 year; this difference was statistically significant. After 3 years, 95% of patients with type I and 67% of those with type III had normalized their complement level. A disease relapse at 3 years occurred in six patients of type III and in none of the patients with type I disease. At last follow-up, a slight improvement in mean GFR was observed for the patients with type I disease, whereas a 25% decrease in mean GFR was seen in patients with type III. Residual urinary abnormalities were significantly more frequent in patients with type III than type I MPGN.

Two large, multicenter series of type I MPGN, 220 patients in a German study (113) and in an Italian study (66,259), reported similar data for clinical courses after a mean follow-up of 83 months from the apparent onset: 30% to 40% of patients maintained normal renal function with persistent urinary abnormalities, 25% to 30% had chronic renal insufficiency, and 25% had end-stage renal disease with replacement therapy. In the German study, there was a high mortality rate (23%). The calculated actuarial renal survival rates at 10 years from renal biopsy were 64% for the German and 60% for the Italian population. The Italian study also showed no difference in renal survival compared with 28 patients with type II MPGN. In both series, there was a mixed cohort of treated and untreated patients.

Clinicopathologic Correlations

Many clinical and histological studies have tried to identify clinical or histologic parameters that were correlated with a worse prognosis (2,47,48,50,255,256). Factors at onset of disease that adversely influenced the progression to end-stage renal disease were hypertension, early impaired renal function, and the nephrotic syndrome; among the histologic parameters, epithelial crescents and interstitial damage indicated a poor prognosis (113). Other reports did not indicate persistent nephrotic syndrome as a poor prognostic sign (113,251). There is more agreement about renal impairment at presentation, with most patients with early azotemia progressing to advanced renal failure (2,9,49,113,255,256). Hypertension is also a commonly reported bad prognostic index (9,113,252), and many investigators have found that epithelial crescents in more than 40% of glomeruli was associated with an adverse outcome (47,48,260,261). Macroscopic hematuria was found by some authors to have a bad prognosis (2,262), but this was not confirmed by others (255). Serum complement levels, presence of C3 nephritic factor, or detection of circulating immune complexes had no influence on prognosis (2,56,204–207,262–265). In the Italian study multivariate analysis showed that reduced GFR, severe proteinuria, and hypertension at presentation were significant independent risk factors. The German study did not report nephrotic syndrome as an adverse factor but gave similar results for the other clinical parameters (113). Among the histologic data, surprisingly, glomerular sclerosis was not significantly correlated with prognosis in either study, whereas interstitial infiltration and fibrosis were indicators of adverse outcome in both series. Interstitial damage also is related to a worse prognosis in other glomerular diseases, such as focal glomerulosclerosis (266), membranous nephropathy (267), and IgA nephropathy (268,269). This observation points to the role of a cell-mediated mechanism of interstitial damage, possibly responsible for the progression of disease (118,270). Whether this interstitial damage is dependent on concomitant glomerular involvement is controversial (66, 117). Arteriolar hyalinosis correlated with a worse prognosis in the Italian study, but was not evaluated in the German report. Moreover, in the two studies, renal survival was compared in subgroups with glomerular changes of different severity. In both series, the subgroup with epithelial crescents had poor survival rates; in the Italian study, the nodular variant had a significantly worse prognosis. Although the nodular pattern is considered a distinct entity by some (271), it was not considered as a separate subgroup in the German study (113).

Pregnancy

During pregnancy, proteinuria can increase because of the hemodynamic features of pregnancy. When the patient is in renal failure, spontaneous abortion in early pregnancy is more frequent (272). Rapid deterioration of renal function has been described in patients with MPGN and renal insufficiency who became pregnant. The renal function that can be adversely influenced by pregnancy has been estimated at approximately 50 mL/minute GFR or less (273).The morphologic counterparts of such deterioration is fibrinoid thrombi in the capillary lumina and crescent formation, with subsequent focal sclerosis (274). Fairley (275) observed the deterioration of renal function in a patient with MPGN whose repeat biopsy had shown crescents. Preexisting hypertension is a factor that predisposes to a higher risk of preeclampsia. The outcome for the fetus in preexisting hypertension is worse, with a fetal loss rate of 25% (276). Overall, pregnant women with MPGN have a higher risk of development of nephrotic syndrome and a higher incidence of preterm and small-for-gestational-age infants, especially if they are hypertensive (277).

Membranoproliferative Glomerulonephritis in Renal Allografts

The reported incidence of recurrent MPGN in renal allografts varies in different series (222,278,279). It depends on the renal transplant biopsy policy and on accurate morphologic diagnosis of the primary renal disease. Recurrence of type I MPGN occurs with a frequency, that varies 18% to 30% (222,280) and the rate of graft loss due to recurrence is higher than 50%. The true frequency of type I recurrence may be difficult to establish because of its similarity of its clinical and histologic features to those of chronic allograft glomerulopathy (281). A primary cytomegalovirus infection can induce an apparent recurrence of type I MPGN (282). If patients with type I MPGN have had a rapid deterioration in native kidney function, a similar pattern is more likely to occur in their transplant allograft. Type II MPGN recurs in the renal allograft with a frequency of 80% to 90% (48,278,279). Dense deposits are easy to recognize and are the earliest histologic marker. Other morphologic changes, such as mesangial hypercellularity and matrix interposition come later (16, 283, 284). In some patients, recurrence is limited to the presence of deposits in the mesangium without GBM abnormalities, whereas in one-quarter the presence of diffuse crescents causes loss of graft (285). Serum complement levels or presence of C3 nephritic factor are not reported to be predictors or markers of dense deposit disease recurrence (286), but some authors do not agree with this observation (287). Renal failure in transplanted patients is much more often the consequence of rejection, rather than secondary to recurrence (283).

Late in the course of successful transplantation, the appearance of heavy proteinuria, decline of renal function, hypertension, and abnormal urinary sediment can be attributed to a distinct glomerular disease, called *glomerular transplant disease or allograft glomerulopathy*, rather than to the recurrence of primary MPGN (288,289). This condition has many histologic features similar to those of idiopathic MPGN, but mesangial changes are less conspicuous and consist of rarefaction followed by sclerosis, with little cell proliferation (208).

De novo type I MPGN has been observed only rarely in transplanted patients, and type II has never been reported (290,291). Elimination of MPGN as the primary disease obviously is necessary to establish the diagnosis of *de novo* MPGN.

TREATMENT

The efficacy of therapeutic regimens in MPGN is difficult to assess because of the small number of patients in short-term, controlled clinical trials reported in the literature; the larger trials have been uncontrolled. Moreover, spontaneous fluctuations of disease activity in natural history of patients with MPGN and the morphologic heterogeneity of the disease make the analysis of therapeutic results more difficult. There is no proven successful treatment for MPGN but examination of single drugs or groups of drugs represents a simple way to assess their efficacy in therapeutic approach to MPGN.

Corticosteroids

Long-term, uncontrolled studies of corticosteroids therapy were performed in children with types I, II, and III diseases by the Cincinnati group (263), using an alternate-day regimen (2.0 to 2.5 mg/kg). The dose was slowly reduced to 1.5 mg/kg at 2 years and to 0.8 to 1.0 mg/kg at 4 years, always administered every other day. The authors' latest results (258) indicate an improvement in renal function and glomerular morphology with prolonged renal survival and reduced severity of proteinuria. In the absence of a control untreated group, survival was compared with previously reported series of untreated children (2). The beneficial effect of alternate-day steroids was more evident after 3 years of treatment and only if prednisone was started within 12 months from clinical onset. A prospective, multicenter, randomized trial was carried out by the International Study of Kidney Disease in Children (ISKDC) (292). Patients were children affected with type I MPGN, with a GFR of a least 70 mL/minute/1.73 m^2 and a persistent proteinuria over 40 mg/hour/m^2. Eighty children were randomized to receive prednisone 40 mg/m^2 every other day or placebo for a mean of 41 months, with termination of treatment for occurrence of renal failure. All three types of MPGN were included. Thirty-three percent of the treated patients had a treatment failure (30% increase in serum creatinine) and the same event occurred in 58% in the placebo group. At 130 months, 61% of patients under steroids had a stable renal function, whereas the rate of preserved renal function among those taking placebo was 12%. Nevertheless, in the treated group the interval between apparent onset of disease and study entry was only 8.9 ± 1.3 months, as opposed to 18.1 ± 3.9 months in the control group. The researchers concluded that long-term treatment with prednisone appears to improve the outcome of children with MPGN (292,293). Ford et al. (294) conducted another uncontrolled study in 19 children with type I MPGN, tailoring the dose of steroids based on renal function and proteinuria of single subjects. Treatment was usually started within 1 year of diagnosis. The highest dose was intravenous pulses methylprednisolone, 30 mg/kg for three doses, followed by oral prednisone 2 mg/kg/day. The lowest dosage was prednisone 20 mg every other day. The mean follow-up was 6.5 years, and the total duration of treatment was 38 ± 3 months. Repeat renal biopsies, performed after approximately 3 years, showed a reduced histologic activity in most patients. Forty-two percent of the treated patients had a complete remission, with protein-free urines. No patient had uremia. The mean creatinine clearance rose from 78 to 126 mL/minute during the course of treatment. This study suggests that in children with type I MPGN, aggressive and early steroid treatment, with a dosage tailored to severity of disease, may be of some benefit. Nevertheless, no control group was included and patients' outcomes had been favored by a better control of hypertension and the use of angiotensin-converting enzyme inhibitors (ACEI). A recent comparison of the long-term effects of an alternate-day prednisone regimen in types I and III MPGN in children, gave clear evidence of a significant difference with respect to changes in urinalysis, serum creatinine, and C3 levels (195). The outcome of patients with type I MPGN patients treated with prednisone was in general good, whereas similarly treated patients with type III showed reduced renal function, slower rise of serum C3 levels, and more persistent urinary abnormalities. They also experienced more disease relapses. These data confirm the clinical differences between types I and III MPGN.

In adults, steroids trials are very limited. Results have been reviewed by Donadio and Offord (295), who concluded that available information does not support a favorable effect of glucocorticoids. Nevertheless, in many studies treatment was started too late in the course of disease. The early use of methylprednisolone pulse therapy in patients with nephrotic syndrome or severe proliferative lesions, followed by oral alternate-day prednisone, can improve the prognosis and presumably exert an "antiinflammatory" effect over glomerular lesions (296).

Alkylating Agents

The use of alkylating drugs had been poorly investigated until comparatively recently in MPGN because of unfavorable results obtained by these agents in combination with others such as warfarin, heparin, or dipyridamole (252,297). More recently, uncontrolled trials were conducted using oral cyclophosphamide in combination with methylprednisolone in pulses, followed by oral prednisone. Faedda et al. (298) treated 19 patients between 9 and 65 years of age with various types of MPGN with this aggressive regimen, and obtained a complete remission in 15 of 19 patients and a partial remission in 3 of 19 patients. Four patients progressed to uremia and some of the responders had a relapse. The survival rate, after a mean follow-up of 7.4 years, was 79%. The rate of remission was higher than that reported for untreated "historical" series, but the overall survival rate did not differ greatly from that observed in children treated with steroids alone.

Anticoagulants and Antithrombotics

Available data involve patients with type I MPGN. Dipyridamole and warfarin were used in one study, in a randomized, crossover, prospective trial that enrolled 22 patients; only 13 of whom completed both a control and a treatment year (299). The treated group showed a better preserved renal function, but the rate of complications was high, with significant hemorrhagic problems in 37% of treated patients. A combination of aspirin 975 mg/day and dipyridamole 325 mg/day was studied in 40 patients who were treated for 1 year in a well-designed randomized trial. In the treated group, GFR, measured by the iothalamate method, was better preserved and platelet survival time was normalized. After an average extended follow-up period of 4 years, treated patients had a lower percentage of advanced renal failure than the placebo group. There was no change in proteinuria, hematuria, or complement profile; 15% of patients had to discontinue the trial because of bleeding complications. Dipyridamole combined with steroids proved to be useful in children with type I MPGN (300).

More recently (301), a nonblinded multicentric prospective controlled trial randomly assigned 18 adult patients either to aspirin (500 mg/day) plus dipyridamole (75 mg/day) or to placebo for a period of 36 months. Fifteen patients had type I and 3 had type II MPGN. All patients had impaired renal function and nephrotic proteinuria. Treated patients had a greater drop in proteinuria, and a partial remission was observed in 7 of 10 patients in the aspirin-dipyridamole group and in 2 of 8 in the placebo group. The treatment time and follow-up period were too short to observe the postrandomization effect on renal function. Donadio and Offord (295) stressed that these studies (aspirin plus dipyridamole) followed the course of disease from introduction of therapy and not from the diagnosis. The follow-up period was too brief to offer any conclusion on the long-term effect of this therapy on the natural history of MPGN.

Other Therapeutic Approaches

A few uncontrolled trials have been reported the use of cyclosporine in various types of primary glomerular disease (302,303). Cyclosporine affects proteinuria, whose reduction is related to a reversible lowering of GFR. It may act through its suppression of T-cell activity. This drug, used at the dosage of 4 mg/kg/day for 3 to 6 months, because of its potential nephrotoxicity and aggravation of hypertension, should be carefully employed in MPGN.

Levin presented successful treatment of a patient with MPGN and severe nephrotic syndrome using mycophenolate mofetil (304). A beneficial effect on proteinuria was reported for other anecdotal cases (305,306).

Jones et al. (307) recently treated five adult MPGN patients with mycophenolate plus oral steroids and compared outcome measures with six control untreated patients. A significant reduction in proteinuria was observed during an 18-month follow-up. No significant difference between the two groups was found for creatinine clearance, but a decrease was present in the control group, though without reaching a statistical significance.

In conclusion, preliminary data indicated that mycophenolate, a well-tolerated but expensive drug, in cases of MPGN has a favorable effect in reducing proteinuria and in stabilizing renal function.

Angiotensin-converting enzyme inhibitors could be used for their effect in reducing proteinuria and in preserving renal function (308). Experimental and clinical data indicate that angiotensin II receptor antagonists (AIIRA) added to ACEI have an additional protective effect (309,310). As in other glomerular diseases, combined therapy have an additive efficacy in reducing proteinuria and slowing the progression of renal decline (311). A low-protein diet can also play a role in lowering proteinuria and possibly slowing the rate of progression of renal disease.

Conclusions

In conclusion, from available data we can recommend three main lines of treatment in idiopathic MPGN, depending on clinical presentation:

1. Children with preserved renal function and nephrotic proteinuria should be given a long-term, alternate-day corticosteroid treatment with careful monitoring of blood pressure.

A period of 6 to 12 months of such therapy has been suggested (312), rather than the longer time of treatment recommended previously.

2. Adults with proteinuria and reduced GFR, could be treated with a combination of aspirin and dipyridamole, with attention to potential hemorrhagic complications. Patients with low proteinuria and normal renal function do not need any treatment, except diet and ACEI and/or AIIRA.

3. In patients with rapidly progressive renal failure or a recent sharp reduction in renal function, aggressive treatment with methylprednisolone pulse therapy followed by oral prednisone plus oral cyclophosphamide is an appropriate therapeutic approach, especially if crescents are present on histologic investigation, indicating more severe disease.

References

1. Cameron JS, et al. Membranoproliferative glomerulonephritis and persistent hypocomplementemia. *BMJ* 1970;4:7.
2. Habib R, et al. Idiopathic membranoproliferative glomerulonephritis in children: report of 105 cases. *Clin Nephrol* 1973;1:194.
3. Habib R, et al. Idiopathic membranoproliferative glomerulonephritis: morphology and natural history. In: Kincaid-Smith P, Mathew TH, Becker EL, eds. *Glomerulonephritis: morphology, natural history, and treatment.* New York, John Wiley & Sons, 1973:491
4. Monga G, et al. The presence and possible role of monocyte infiltration in human chronic proliferative glomerulonephritides: light microscopic, immunofluorescence, and histochemical correlations. *Am J Pathol* 1979;94:271.
5. Berger J, Galle P. Dépôts denses au sein des membranes basales du rein: étude en microscopies optique et électronique. *Presse Med* 1963;71:2351.
6. West CD, et al. Hypocomplementemic and normocomplementemic persistent (chronic) glomerulonephritis: clinical and pathologic characteristics. *J Pediatr* 1965;67:1089.
7. Mandalenakis N, et al. Lobular glomerulonephritis and membranoproliferative glomerulonephritis: a clinical and pathologic study based on renal biopsies. *Medicine (Baltimore)* 1971;50:319.
8. Bohle A, et al. The morphological and clinical features of membranoproliferative glomerulonephritis in adults. *Virchows Arch* 1974;363:213.
9. Donadio JV, et al. Idiopathic membranoproliferative (mesangiocapillary) glomerulonephritis a clinicopathologic study. *Mayo Clin Proc* 1979;54:141.
10. Cameron, JS, et al. Mesangiocapillary glomerulonephritis and persistent hypocomplementemia. In: Kincaid-Smith P, Mathew TH, Becker EL, eds: *Glomerulonephritis: morphology, natural history and treatment.* New York: John Wiley & Sons; 1973:541.
11. Pickering, RJ, et al. Chronic glomerulonephritis associated with low serum complement activity (chronic hypocomplementemic glomerulonephritis). *Medicine (Baltimore)* 1970;49:207.
12. Michael AF, et al. Chronic membranoproliferative glomerulonephritis with hypocomplementemia. *Transplant Proc* 1969;1:925.
13. Westberg NG, et al. Glomerular deposition of properdin in acute and chronic glomerulonephritis with hypocomplementemia. *J Clin Invest* 1971; 50:642.
14. Mahieu P. Biochemical structure of glomerular basement membrane in chronic glomerulonephritis: I. Lobular and membranoproliferative glomerulonephritis. *Kidney Int* 1972;1:115.
15. Burkholder PM, Marchand A, Krueger RP. Mixed membranous and proliferative glomerulonephritis: a correlative light, immunofluorescence, and electron microscopic study. *Lab Invest* 1970;23:459.
16. Habib R, et al. Dense deposit disease: a variant of membranoproliferative glomerulonephritis. *Kidney Int* 1975;7:204.
17. Lamb V, et al. Membranoproliferative glomerulonephritis with dense intramembranous alterations: a clinicopathologic study. *Lab Invest* 1977; 36:607.
18. Churg J, Duffy JL, Bernstein J. Identification of dense deposit disease: A report for the International Study of Kidney Diseases in Children. *Arch Pathol Lab Med* 1979;103:67.
19. Kim Y, et al. Immunofluorescence studies of dense deposit disease. The presence of railroad tracks and mesangial rings. *Lab Invest* 1979;40:474.
20. Mazzucco G, et al. Glomerulonephritis with dense deposits: a variant of membranoproliferative glomerulonephritis or a separate morphological entity? Light, electron microscopic and immunohistochemical study of eleven cases. *Virchows Arch (A)* 1980;387:17.
21. Holley KE, Donadio JV Jr. Membranoproliferative glomerulonephritis. In: Tisher CC, Brenner BM. eds. *Renal pathology: clinical and functional correlates,* 2nd ed. Philadelphia: JB Lippincott, 1994:294.
22. Simon P, et al. Epidemiological data in population of 250.000 on minimal change nephrotic syndrome, IgA nephropathy, idiopathic membranous, and membranoproliferative glomerulonephritis. *Kidney Int* 1984;26:512 (abstr).
23. Jungers P, et al. Is membranoproliferative glomerulonephritis disappearing in France? *Kidney Int* 1982;21:899 (abstr).
24. Jungers P, et al. Rarefaction of membranoproliferative glomerulonephritis (MPGN) in France. *Kidney Int* 1985;28:264 (abstr).
25. Barbiano di Belgiojoso G, et al. Is membranoproliferative glomerulonephritis really decreasing? A multicentre study of 1548 cases of primary glomerulonephritis. *Nephron* 1985;40:380.
26. Gonzalo A, et al. Incidence of membranoproliferative in a Spanish population. *Clin Nephrol* 1986;26:161.
27. Simon P, et al. Variations of primary glomerulonephritis incidence in a rural area of 400.000 inhabitants in the last decade. *Nephron* 1987;45:171.
28. Study Group of the Spanish Society Nephrology. Progressively decreasing incidence of membranoproliferative glomerulonephritis in Spanish adult population. *Nephron* 1989;52:370.
29. Study Group of the Spanish Society Nephrology. Decreasing incidence of membranoproliferative GN in Spanish children. *Pediatr Nephrol* 1990;4:266.
30. Simon P, et al. Epidemiology of primary glomerular diseases in a French region. Variations according to period and age. *Kidney Int* 1994;46:1192.
31. Iitaka K, et al. Decreasing hypocomplementemia and membranoproliferative glomerulonephritis in Japan. *Pediatr Nephrol* 2000;14:794.
32. Gesualdo L, et al. The Italian experience of the national registry of renal biopsies. *Kidney Int* 2004;66:890.
33. Jungers P, et al. Epidemiology of primary glomerulonephritis (GN) in a French urban area (abstr). Eliahou HE, Iaina A, Bar-Khayim (eds). *Proc XXIInd Int Congr of Nephrology,* Jerusalem 1993:77.
34. Simon P, et al. Epidemiologic data of primary glomerular diseases in western France. *Kidney Int* 2004;66:905.
35. Haas M, et al. Changing etiologies of unexplained adult nephrotic syndrome: a comparison of renal biopsy findings from 1976–1979 and 1995–1997. *Am J Kidney Dis* 1977;30:621.
36. Hurtado A, et al. Distinct patterns of glomerular disease in Lima, Peru. *Clin Nephrol* 2000;53:325.
37. Madala, ND, et al. The pathogenesis of membranoproliferative glomerulonephritis in KwaZulu-Natal, South Africa is unrelated to hepatitis C virus infection. *Clin Nephrol* 2003;60:69.
38. Johnson RJ, et al. Renal manifestations of hepatitis C virus infection. *Kidney Int* 1994;46:1255.
39. Johnson RJ, et al. Hypothesis: dysregulation of immunologic balance resulting from hygiene and socioeconomic factors may influence the epidemiology and cause of glomerulonephritis worldwide. *Am J Kidney Dis* 2003;42:575.
40. Holdsworth SR, Kitching AR, Tipping PG. Th1 and Th2 T helper subsets affect patterns of injury and outcomes in glomerulonephritis. *Kidney Int* 1999;55:1198.
41. Silva FG. Membranoproliferative glomerulonephritis. In: Heptinstall RH, ed. *Pathology of the kidney,* 3rd ed. Boston: Little, Brown; 1983:447.
42. Churg J, Habib R, White RH. Pathology of the nephrotic syndrome in children: a report for the International Study of Kidney Disease in Children. *Lancet* 1970;1:1299.
43. Ferrario F, et al Histopathological atlas of renal diseases. Membranoproliferative glomerulonephritis. *J Nephrol* 2004;17:483.
44. Davis AE, et al. Membranoproliferative glomerulonephritis (MPGN type 1) and dense deposit disease (DDD) in children. *Clin Nephrol* 1978;9:184.
45. Nagi AH. Histological, ultrastructural and immunofluorescence studies in membranoproliferative glomerulonephritis. *J Pathol* 1972;106:151.
46. Zucchelli C, et al. Membranoproliferative glomerulonephritis: correlations between immunological and histological findings. *Nephron* 1976;7:449.
47. Swainson CP, et al. Mesangiocapillary glomerulonephritis: a long-term study of 40 cases. *J Pathol* 1983;141:449.
48. Cameron JS, et al. Idiopathic mesangiocapillary glomerulonephritis: comparison of types I and II in children and adults and long-term prognosis. *Am J Med* 1983;74:175.
49. Chan MK, et al. Adult-onset mesangiocapillary glomerulonephritis: a disease with a poor prognosis. *QJM* 1989;72:599.
50. Antoine B, Faye C. The clinical course associated with dense deposits in the kidney basement membranes. *Kidney Int* 1972;1:420.
51. Kashtan CE, et al. Dense intramembranous deposit disease: a clinical comparison of histological subtypes. *Clin Nephrol* 1990;33:1.
52. Bennett WM, et al. Mesangiocapillary glomerulonephritis type II (dense-deposit disease): clinical features in progressive disease. *Am J Kidney Dis* 1989;6:469.
53. Fox A. Light microscopy of membranoproliferative glomerulonephritis type II (MPGN with homologous extraglomerular lesions). *Am J Clin Pathol* 1981;76:644.
54. Muda AO, Barsotti P, Marinozzi V. Ultrastructural histochemical investigations of "dense deposit disease": pathogenic approach to a special type of mesangiocapillary glomerulonephritis. *Virchows Arch (A)* 1988;413:529.
55. Burkholder PM, Bradford WD. Proliferative glomerulonephritis in children: a correlation of varied clinical and pathologic patterns utilizing light, immunofluorescence, and electron microscopy. *Am J Pathol* 1969;56:423.
56. Droz D, et al. Dense deposits disease. *Nephron* 1977;19:1.
57. Galle P, Mahieu P. Electron dense alteration of kidney basement membranes: a renal lesion specific of a systemic disease. *Am J Med* 1975;58:749.

58. Zollinger HV, Mihatsch MJ. Focally accentuated glomerulonephritis. In: Zollinger HV, Mihatsch MJ, eds. Renal pathology in biopsy: light, electron, immunofluorescent and clinical aspects. Berlin: Springer-Verlag; 1978:252.

59. Davis AE, Schneeberger EE, Grupe WE. Mesangial proliferative glomerulonephritis with irregular intramembranous deposits: another variant of hypocomplementemic nephritis. Am J Med 1977;63:481.

60. Burkholder PM, ed. Atlas of human glomerular pathology. New York: Harper & Row; 1974.

61. Burkholder PM, Hyman LR, Krueger RP. Characterization of mixed membranous and proliferative glomerulonephritis: recognition of three varieties. In: Kincaid-Smith P, Mathew H, Becker EL, eds. Glomerulonephritis: morphology, natural history, and treatment. New York: John Wiley & Sons; 1973:557.

62. Anders D, et al. Basement membrane changes in membranoproliferative glomerulonephritis: II. characterization of a third type by silver impregnation of ultrathin sections. Virchows Arch (A) 1977;376:1.

63. Strife CF, et al. Membranoproliferative glomerulonephritis with disruption of the glomerular basement membrane. Clin Nephrol 1977;7:65.

64. Jackson EC, et al. Differences between membranoproliferative glomerulonephritis types I and III in clinical presentation, glomerular morphology, and complement perturbation. Am J Kidney Dis 1987;9:115.

65. Abreo K, Moorthy AV. Type 3 membranoproliferative glomerulonephritis: clinicopathologic correlations and long-term follow-up in nine patients. Arch Pathol Lab Med 1932;106:413.

66. D'Amico G, Ferrario F. Mesangiocapillary glomerulonephritis. J Am Soc Nephrol 1992;2:S159.

67. Jones DB. Membranoproliferative glomerulonephritis: one of many diseases? Arch Pathol Lab Med 1977;101:457.

68. Watson AR, et al. Membranoproliferative glomerulonephritis type I in children: correlation of clinical features with pathologic subtypes. Am J Kidney Dis 1984;4:141.

69. Pound SE, McDonald MK, Thomson D. Diffuse proliferative glomerulonephritis. How many types? Histopathology 1987;11:227.

70. Herdman RC, et al. Chronic glomerulonephritis associated with low serum complement activity (chronic hypocomplementemic glomerulonephritis). Medicine (Baltimore) 1970;49:207.

71. Lévy M, Gubler MC, Habib R. New concepts on membranoproliferative glomerulonephritis. In: Kincaid-Smith P, d'Apice AJ, Atkins RC, eds. Progress in glomerulonephritis. New York: John Wiley & Sons; 1979:177.

72. van Acker KJ, van den Brande J, Vincke H. Membranous-proliferative glomerulonephritis. Helv Paediatr Acta 1970;25:204.

73. Kanwar YS, Garces JG, Molitch ME. Occurrence of intercapillary glomerulosclerosis in the absence of glucose intolerance. Am J Kidney Dis 1990;3:281.

74. Harrington AR, Hare HG, Chambers WN. Nodular glomerulosclerosis suspected during life in a patient without demonstrable diabetes mellitus. N Engl J Med 1966;2:206.

75. Nash DA, Rogers PW, Langlinais PC. Diabetic glomerulosclerosis without glucose tolerance. Am J Med 1975;59:191.

76. Alpers CE, Biava CG. Idiopathic lobular glomerulonephritis (nodular mesangial sclerosis): a distinct diagnostic entity. Clin Nephrol 1989;32:68.

77. Saito YS, et al. Mesangiolysis in diabetic glomeruli: its role in the formation of nodular lesions. Kidney Int 1988;34:389.

78. Herf S, et al. An evaluation of diabetic and pseudo-diabetic glomerulosclerosis. Am J Med 1979;66:1040.

79. Morita T, et al. Mesangiolysis. Sequential ultrastructural study of Habu venom-induced glomerular lesion. Lab Invest 1978;38:94.

80. Sinniah R, Cohen AH. Glomerular capillary aneurysms in light-chain nephropathy. Am J Pathol 1985;118:298.

81. Ganeval D, Noël LH, Preud-homme JL. Light-chain deposition disease: its relation with AL-type amyloidosis. Kidney Int 1984;26:1.

82. Bruneval P, et al. Glomerular matrix proteins in nodular glomerulosclerosis in association with light chain deposition disease and diabetes mellitus. Hum Pathol 1985;16:477.

83. Taguchi T, Bohle A. Evaluation of change with time of glomerular morphology in membranoproliferative glomerulonephritis: a serial biopsy study of 33 cases. Clin Nephrol 1989;31:297.

84. Strife CF, McAdams AJ, West CD. Membranoproliferative glomerulonephritis characterized by focal, segmental proliferative lesions. Clin Nephrol 1982;18:9.

85. Monga G, et al. Pattern of double glomerulopathies: a clinicopathologic study of superimposed glomerulonephritis on diabetic glomerulosclerosis. Mod Pathol 1989;2:407.

86. Laohapand T, Cattell V, Gabriel JR. Monocyte infiltration in human glomerulonephritis: alpha-1 antitrypsin as a marker for mononuclear phagocytes in renal biopsies. Clin Nephrol 1983;19:309.

87. Magil AB, Wadsworth LD, Loewen H. Monocytes and human renal glomerular disease. A quantitative evaluation. Lab Invest 1981;44:27.

88. Ferrario F, et al. The detection of monocytes in human glomerulonephritis. Kidney Int 1985;28:513.

89. Ferrario F, et al. Role of monocytes in human glomerulonephritis. Contrib Nephrol 1985;45:131.

90. Weening J. The classification of glomerulonephritis in systemic lupus erythematosus revisited. Kidney Int 2004;65:521.

91. Appel GB, et al. Renal involvement in SLE: a study of 56 patients emphasizing histologic classification. Medicine (Baltimore) 1978;57:371.

92. Balow JE, Austin HA. Renal disease in systemic lupus erythematosus. Rheum Dis Clin North Am 1988;14:117.

93. D'Amico G, et al. Renal involvement in essential mixed cryoglobulinemia. Kidney Int 1989;35:1004.

94. Ferrario F, et al. Histological and immunohistological features in essential mixed cryoglobulinemia glomerulonephritis. In: Ponticelli C, Minetti L, D'Amico G, eds. Antiglobulins, cryoglobulins and glomerulonephritis. Dordrecht: Martinus Nijhoff; 1986:193.

95. Ernst A, Radonic M, Belicza M. The syndrome of long-standing staphylococcus albus bacteremia, bacterial endocarditis and diffuse membranoproliferative glomerulonephritis complicating ventriculoatrial shunt infection: Case report and review of literature. Acta Med Iugosl 1980;34:137.

96. Zunin C, et al. Membranoproliferative glomerulonephritis associated with infected ventriculoatrial shunt. Report of two cases recovered after removal of the shunt. Pathologica 1977;69:297.

97. Yoshikawa N, et al. Focal and diffuse membranoproliferative glomerulonephritis in children. Am J Nephrol 1988;8:102.

98. Kincaid-Smith, P. The morphologic varieties, clinical features, course and treatment of mesangiocapillary (membranoproliferative) glomerulonephritis. In: The kidney: a clinico-pathological study. Oxford: Blackwell; 1975:179.

99. Korzets Z, Bernheim J, Bernheim J. Rapidly progressive glomerulonephritis (crescentic glomerulonephritis) in the course of type I idiopathic membranoproliferative glomerulonephritis. Am J Kidney Dis 1987;10:56.

100. McCoy RC, Clapp J, Seigler HF. Membranoproliferative glomerulonephritis: progression from the pure form to the crescentic form with recurrence after transplantation. Am J Med 1975;59:288.

101. Niaudet P, Lévy M. Glomérulonéphrite à croissant diffus. In: Royer P II, et al., eds. Néphrologie pediatrique. Paris: Flammarion; 1983:390.

102. Miller MN, et al. Incidence and prognostic importance of glomerular crescents in renal diseases of childhood. Am J Nephrol 1984;4:244.

103. Morrin PA, et al. Rapidly progressive glomerulonephritis. A clinical and pathologic study. Am J Med 1978;65:446.

104. Ferrario F, et al. Critical re-evaluation of 41 cases of "idiopathic" crescentic glomerulonephritis. Clin Nephrol 1994;41:1.

105. Bonsib SM. Glomerular basement membrane discontinuities. Scanning electron microscopy study of acellular glomeruli. Am J Pathol 1985;119:357.

106. Stejskal J, et al. Discontinuities (gaps) of the glomerular capillary wall and basement membrane in renal disease. Lab Invest 1973;28:149.

107. Mazzucco G, Monga G. Monocyte escape through a glomerular capillary basement membrane gap. Nephron 1985;39:272.

108. Strutz F, Muller GA. The role of tubulo-interstitial process in progression of primary renal diseases. Nephron Dial Transpl 1994;9:10.

109. Katafuchi R, et al. Structural functional correlations in serial biopsies from patients with glomerulonephritis. Clin Nephrol 1987;28:169.

110. Abe S, et al. Significance of tubulo-interstitial lesions in biopsy specimens of glomerulonephritis patients. Am J Nephrol 1989;9:30.

111. Mackensen-Haen S, et al. The consequences for renal function of widening of the interstitium and changes in the tubular epithelium of the renal cortex and outer medulla in various renal diseases. Clin Nephrol 1992;37:70.

112. Kuncio GS, Neilson EG, Haverty T. Mechanisms of tubulo-interstitial fibrosis. Kidney Int 1991;39:550.

113. Schmitt H, et al. Long-term prognosis of membranoproliferative glomerulonephritis type I. Nephron 1990;55:242.

114. Fischbach H, et al. Relationship between glomerular lesions, serum creatinine and interstitial volume in membranoproliferative glomerulonephritis. Klin Wochensschr 1977;55:603.

115. Mackensen-Haen S, et al. Impairment of glomerular filtration rate by glomerular and interstitial factors in membranoproliferative glomerulonephritis with normal serum creatinine concentration. Virchows Arch 1979;382:11.

116. Schmitt H, Cavalcanti de Oliveira V, Bohle A. Tubulointerstitial alterations in type I membranoproliferative glomerulonephritis: an investigation of 259 cases. Pathol Res Pract 1987;182:6.

117. D'Amico G. Influence of clinical and histological features on actuarial renal survival in adult patients with idiopathic IgA nephropathy, membranous nephropathy, and membranoproliferative glomerulonephritis: survey of the recent literature. Am J Kidney Dis 1992;20:315.

118. D'Amico G. Role of interstitial infiltration of leukocytes in glomerular disease. Nephrol Dial Transplant 1988;3:596.

119. Barbiano di Belgiojoso G, et al. Immunofluorescence patterns in chronic membranoproliferative glomerulonephritis (MPGN). Clin Nephrol 1976;6:303.

120. Berger J, Yaneva H, Hinglais N. Immunohistochemistry of glomerulonephritis. In: Hamburger J, Crosnier J, Maxwell MH, eds. Advances in nephrology. Chicago: Year Book Medical; 1971:11

121. Davis BK, Cavallo T. Membranoproliferative glomerulonephritis: localization of early components of complement in glomerular deposits. Am J Pathol 1976;84:283.

122. Gartner HV, Wehner H, Bohle A. The immunohistological findings in various forms of glomerulonephritis: a comparative investigation based on 335 renal biopsies. Part II: minimal proliferating intercapillary glomerulonephritis (with nephrotic syndrome), focal sclerosing, epi-extraperimembranous, membranoproliferative and extracapillary (rapidly progressive) glomerulonephritis. Pathol Res Pract 1978;162:198.

123. Morel-Maroger L, Leathem A, Richet G. Glomerular abnormalities in non-systemic diseases: relationship between findings by light microscopy and immunofluorescence in 433 renal biopsy specimens. *Am J Med* 1972;53:170.

124. Westberg NG, et al. Glomerular deposition of properdin in acute and chronic glomerulonephritis with hypocomplementemia. *J Clin Invest* 1971;50:642.

125. Lévy M, et al. Immunopathology of membranoproliferative glomerulonephritis with subendothelial deposits (type I MPGN). *Clin Immunol Immunopathol* 1978;10:477.

126. Nakamoto Y, et al. Hepatic glomerulonephritis: characteristic of hepatic IgA glomerulonephritis as the major part. *Virchows Arch* 1981;329:45.

127. Sinniah R. Heterogeneous IgA glomerulopathy in liver cirrhosis. *Histopathology* 1984;8:947.

128. Lehman DH, Wilson CB, Dixon FJ. Extraglomerular immunoglobulin deposits in human nephritis. *Am J Med* 1975;58:765.

129. Anders D, Thoenes W. Basement membrane changes in membranoproliferative glomerulonephritis: a light and electron microscopic study. *Virchows Arch (A)* 1975;369:87.

130. Magil AB, et al. Membranoproliferative glomerulonephritis type 1: comparison of natural history in children and adults. *Clin Nephrol* 1979;11:239.

131. Mrozowicz-Picken M, Wrzolkowa T. Mesangiocapillary glomerulonephritis in children. Electron microscopic studies. *Int J Pediatr Nephrol* 1980;1:204.

132. Monga G, et al. Ultrastructural glomerular findings in cryoglobulinemic glomerulonephritis. *Appl Pathol* 1987;5:108.

133. Perez GO, Pardo V, Fletcher M. Renal involvement in essential mixed cryoglobulinemia. *Am J Kidney Dis* 1987;10:276.

134. Galle P. Mise en évidence au microscope électronique d'une lésion singulière des membranes basales du rein et de la substance hyaline. Thesis in Medicine, University of Paris, 1962.

135. Sibley RK, and Kim Y. Dense intramembranous deposit disease. *Kidney Int* 1984;25:660.

136. Jenis EH, et al. Glomerulonephritis with basement membrane dense deposits. *Arch Pathol* 1974;97:84.

137. Vargas R, et al. Mesangiocapillary glomerulonephritis with dense "deposits" in the basement membranes of the kidney. *Clin Nephrol* 1976;5:73.

138. Davis AE, et al. Membranoproliferative glomerulonephritis (MPGN type 1) and dense-deposit disease (DDD) in children. *Clin Nephrol* 1978;9:84.

139. Klein M, et al. Characteristics of a benign subtype of dense deposit disease: comparison with the progressive form of this disease. *Clin Nephrol* 1983;20:163.

140. Southwest Pediatric Nephrology Study Group. Dense deposit disease in children: Prognostic value of clinical and pathologic indicators. *Am J Kidney Dis* 1985;6:161.

141. Thorner P, Baumal R. Extraglomerular dense deposits in dense deposit disease. *Arch Pathol Lab Med* 1982;106:628.

142. Campbell-Boswell MV, et al. Kidney tubule basement membrane alterations in type II membranoproliferative glomerulonephritis. *Virchows Arch (A)* 1979;382:49.

143. Jenis EH, Lowenthal DT. Renal basement membrane dense-deposit disease. In: Jenis EH, Lowenthal DR, eds. *Kidney biopsy interpretation*. Philadelphia. Davis, 1977:63.

144. Wyatt RJ, et al. Glomerular deposition of complement-control proteins in acute and chronic glomerulonephritis. *Kidney Int* 1979;16:505.

145. Date A, Neela P, Shastry JC. Thioflavin T fluorescence in membranoproliferative glomerulonephritis. *Nephron* 1982;32:90.

146. Nevins TE. Lectin binding in membranoproliferative glomerulonephritis: evidence for N-acetylglucosamine in dense intramembranous deposits. *Am J Pathol* 1985;118:325.

147. Duvall-Young J, MacDonald MK, McKechnie NM. Fundus changes in (type II) mesangiocapillary glomerulonephritis simulating drusen: a histopathologic report. *Br J Ophthalmol* 1989;73:297.

148. Leys A, et al. Specific eye fundus lesions in type II membranoproliferative glomerulonephritis. *Pediatr Nephrol* 1991;5:89.

149. Brouet JC, et al. Biological and clinical significance of cryoglobulins. A report of 86 cases. *Am J Med* 1974;57:775.

150. D'Amico G, et al. L'atteinte rénal dans la cryoglublinémie mixte essentielle: un type particulière de néphropathie à médiation immunologique. In: Crosnier J, Funk-Brentano JL, Bach JF, et al., eds. *Actualités néphrologique de l'Hôpital Necker*. Paris: Flammarion; 1987:201.

151. Gorevic PD, et al. Mixed cryoglobulinemia: clinical aspects and long-term follow-up of 40 patients. *Am J Med* 1980;69:287.

152. D'Amico G, et al. Glomerulonephritis in essential mixed cryoglobulinemia (EMC). In: Davison PJ, Guillon PJ, eds. *Proceedings of the XXI Congress of the European Dialysis and Transplant Association*. London: Pitman; 1985:527.

153. Cordonnier D, et al. Cryoglobulines et glomérulonéphrites. Etude particulière des cryoglobulines mixtes à composant monoclonal IgM. In: Hamburger J, Crosnier J, Funk-Brentano JL, eds. *Actualités néphrologiques de l'Hôpital Necker*. Paris: Flammarion; 1982:349.

154. Monga G, et al. Glomerular findings in mixed IgG-IgM cryoglobulinemia. Light, electron microscopy, immunofluorescence and histochemical correlations. *Virchows Arch Zell Pathol* 1986;20:185.

155. Mazzucco G, et al. Cell interposition in glomerular capillary walls in cryoglobulinemic glomerulonephritis. Ultrastructural investigation of 23 cases. *Ultrastruct Pathol* 1986;10:355.

156. Tarantino A, et al. Renal disease in essential mixed cryoglobulinemia. Long-term follow-up of 44 patients. *QJM* 1981;50:1.

157. Castiglione A, et al. The relationship of infiltrating renal leucocytes to disease activity in lupus and cryoglobulinemic glomerulonephritis. *Nephron* 1988;50:14.

158. Morel-Maroger L, Méry JP. Renal lesions in mixed IgG-IgM essential cryoglobulinemia. In: Villarreal H, ed. *Proceedings of the 5th Congress of Nephrology*. Basel: Karger; 1972:249.

159. Barbiano di Belgiojoso G, et al. Immunohistological patterns in mixed IgG-IgM essential cryoglobulinemia glomerulonephritis. In: Leaf A, Giebisch G, Bolis L, et al., eds. *Renal pathophysiology*. New York: Raven Press; 1980:245.

160. Barbiano di Belgiojoso G, et al. Clinical and histological correlations in essential mixed cryoglobulinemia (EMC) glomerulonephritis. In: Ponticelli C, Minetti L, D'Amico G, eds. *Antiglobulins, cryoglobulins and glomerulonephritis*. Dordrecht: Martinus Nijhoff; 1986:203.

161. Ben Bassat M, et al. The clinicopathological features of cryoglobulinemic nephropathy. *Am J Clin Pathol* 1983;79:147.

162. Cordonnier D, et al. Mixed IgG-IgM cryoglobulinemia with glomerulonephritis. Immunochemical fluorescent and ultrastructural study of kidney and in vitro cryoprecipitate. *Am J Med* 1975;59:867.

163. Feiner H, Gallo G. Ultrastructure in glomerulonephritis associated with cryoglobulinemia. *Am J Pathol* 1977;88:145.

164. Mihatsch MJ, Banfi G. Ultrastructural features in glomerulonephritis in essential mixed cryoglobulinemia. In: Ponticelli C, Minetti L, D'Amico G, eds. *Antiglobulins, cryoglobulins and glomerulonephritis*. Dordrecht: M. Nijhoff; 1986:211.

165. Austin H, et al. Diffuse proliferative lupus nephritis: identification of specific pathologic features affecting renal outcome. *Kidney Int* 1984;25:689.

166. Baldwin DS, et al. Lupus nephritis: clinical course as related to morphologic forms and their transitions. *Am J Med* 1977;62:12.

167. Baumal R, Farine M, Poucell S. Clinical significance of renal biopsies showing mixed mesangial and global proliferative lupus nephritis. *Am J Kidney Dis* 1987;10:236.

168. Cameron JS. The nephritis of systemic lupus erythematosus. In: Kincaid-Smith P, d'Apice AJ, Atkins RC, eds. *Progress in glomerulonephritis*. New York: John Wiley & Sons; 1979:387.

169. Alexopoulos E, et al. Lupus nephritis: correlation of interstitial cells with glomerular function. *Kidney Int* 1990;37:100.

170. Hill GS, et al. Systemic lupus erythematosus: morphologic correlations with immunologic and clinical data at the time of biopsy. *Am J Med* 1978;64:61.

171. Lewis EJ, Busch GJ, Schur PH. Gamma G globulin subgroup composition of the glomerular deposits in human renal disease. *J Clin Invest* 1970;49:1103.

172. Morel-Maroger L, Méry JP, Richet G. Lupus nephritis: immunofluorescence study of 54 cases. In: Kincaid-Smith P, Mathew TH, Becker EL, eds. *Glomerulonephritis: morphology, natural history and treatment*. New York: John Wiley & Sons; 1973:1183.

173. Cameron JS, Jones MD. The course of lupus nephritis. In: Kincaid-Smith P, Mathew TH, Becker EL, eds. *Glomerulonephritis: morphology, natural history and treatment*. New York: John Wiley & Sons; 1973:1187.

174. Comerford FR, Cohen AS. The nephropathy of systemic lupus erythematosus: an assessment by clinical, light and electron microscopic criteria. *Medicine (Baltimore)* 1967;46:425.

175. Gallo GR. Nodular glomerulopathy associated with nonamyloidotic kappa light chain deposits and excess immunoglobulin light chain synthesis. *Am J Pathol* 1980;99:621.

176. Ganeval D, et al. Systemic light chain deposition disease developing in the course of a lambda light chain myeloma. *BMJ* 1981;282:681.

177. Noël LH, et al. Renal granular monoclonal light chain deposits: morphological aspects of 11 cases. *Clin Nephrol* 1984;21:263.

178. Randall RE, et al. Manifestations of systemic light chain deposition. *Am J Med* 1976;60:293.

179. Gallo G, et al. The spectrum of monoclonal immunoglobulin deposition disease associated with immunocytic dyscrasias. *Semin Hematol* 1989;26:234.

180. Silver MM, et al. Renal and systemic kappa light chain deposits and their plasma cell origin identified by immunoelectron microscopy. *Am J Pathol* 1986;122:17.

181. Fries D, et al. Ultrastructure des lésions glomérulaires dans un cas de myélome avec syndrome néphrotique. *J Urol Néphrol* 1967;73:839.

182. Schuurmans-Stekhoven JH, van Haelst UJ. Unusual findings in the human renal glomerulus in multiple myeloma: A light and electron microscopy study. *Virchows Arch (A)* 1971;9:311.

183. Seymour AE, et al. Kappa light chain glomerulosclerosis in multiple myeloma. *Am J Pathol* 1980;101:557.

184. Montoliu J, et al. Glomerular disease in cirrhosis of the liver: low frequency of IgA deposits. *Am J Nephrol* 1986;6:199.

185. West CD. Idiopathic membranoproliferative glomerulonephritis in childhood. *Pediatr Nephrol* 1992;6:96.

186. Kim Y, Michael AF, Fish AJ. Idiopathic membranoproliferative glomerulonephritis. *Contemp Issues Nephrol* 1982;9:237.

187. Abderrahim E, et al. Glomérulonéphrite membrano-proliférative chez deux frères. *Néphrologie* 1990;11:227.

188. Power DA, Ng YC, Simpson JG. Familial incidence of C3 nephritic factor, partial lipodystrophy and membranoproliferative glomerulonephritis. *QJM* 1990;75:387.

189. Welch TR, et al. Major histocompatability-complex extended haplotypes in membranoproliferative glomerulonephritis. *N Engl J Med* 1986;314:1476.

190. Yata N, et al. Typical MPGN with few urinary abnormalities. *Am J Kidney Dis* 2004;43:918.

191. Leys A, et al. Fundus changes in membranoproliferative glomerulonephritis type II: a fluorescein angiographic study of 23 patients. *Graefes Arch Clin Exp Ophthalmol* 1991;229:406.

192. Ulbig MR, et al. Membranoproliferative glomerulonephritis type II associated with central serous retinopathy. *Am J Ophthalmol* 1993;116:410.

193. Michielsen B, et al. Fundus changes in chronic membranoproliferative glomerulonephritis type II. *Doc Ophthalmol* 1990–1991;76:219.

194. Leys A, et al. Subretinal neovascular membranes associated with chronic membranoproliferative glomerulonephritis type II. *Graefes Arch Clin Exp Ophthalmol* 1990;228:499.

195. Braun MC, West CD, Strife F. Differences between membranoproliferative glomerulonephritis types I and III in long-term response to an alternate-day prednisone regimen. *Am J Kidney Dis* 1999;34:1022.

196. Varade WS, Forristal J, West CD. Patterns of complement activation in idiopathic membranoproliferative glomerulonephritis, type I, II and III. *Am J Kidney Dis* 1990;16:196.

197. Clardy CW, et al. A properdin dependent nephritic factors slowly activating C3, C5 and C9 in membranoproliferative glomerulonephritis, types I and III. *Clin Immunopathol* 1989;50:333.

198. Clardy CW, et al. Serum terminal complement component levels in hypocomplementemic glomerulonephritis. *Clin Immunol Immunopathol* 1989;50:307.

199. Strife CF, et al. Autoantibody to complement neoantigens in membranoproliferative glomerulonephritis. *J Pediatr* 1990;116:S98.

200. Meyers KE, Finn L, Kaplan BC. Membranoproliferative glomerulonephritis type III. *Pediatr Nephrol* 1998;12:512.

201. Kobayashi Y, Hasegawa O, Honda M. Clinical significance of the terminal complement complex in children with type I membranoproliferative glomerulonephritis. *Nippon Jinzo Gakkai Shi* 2004;46:419.

202. Yasuda K. Terminal complement complex (TCC) levels in urine in patients with renal diseases. *Hokkaido Igaku Zasshi* 2001;76:71.

203. Davis CA, Marder H, West CD. Circulating immune complexes in membranoproliferative glomerulonephritis. *Kidney Int* 1981;20:728.

204. Solling J. Circulating immune complexes in glomerulonephritis: a longitudinal study. *Clin Nephrol* 1983;20:177.

205. West CD. Pathogenesis and approaches to therapy of membranoproliferative glomerulonephritis. *Kidney Int* 1976;9:1.

206. Ooi YM, Vallota EH, West CD. Classical complement pathway activation in membranoproliferative glomerulonephritis. *Kidney Int* 1976;9:46.

207. Fearon DT, et al. Pathways of complement activation in membranoproliferative glomerulonephritis and allograft rejection. *Transplant Proc* 1977;9:729.

208. Dawson KP, et al. Glomerulonephritis associated with an infected ventriculo-atrial shunt. *NZ Med J* 1980;91:342.

209. WyszynskaT, et al. Hepatitis B mediated glomerulonephritis in children. *Int J Pediatr Nephrol* 1984;5:147.

210. West CD, Mc Adams AJ. Glomerular paramesangial deposits: association with hypocomplementemia in membranoproliferative glomerulonephritis type I and III. *Am J Kidney Dis* 1998;31:427.

211. West CD, Mc Adams AJ. Membranoproliferative glomerulonephritis type III: association of glomerular deposits with circulating nephritic factor-stabilized convertase. *Am J Kidney Dis* 1998;32:56.

212. Kim Y, et al. Inherited deficiency of the second component of complement (C2) with membranoproliferative glomerulonephritis. *Am J Med* 1977;62:765.

213. Borzy MS, Houghton D. Mixed-pattern immune deposit glomerulonephritis in a child with inherited deficiency of the third component of complement. *Am J Kidney Dis* 1985;5:54.

214. Coleman TH, et al. Inherited complement component deficiencies in membranoproliferative glomerulonephritis. *Kidney Int* 1983;24:681.

215. Pussell BA, et al. Complement deficiency and nephritis: A report of a family. *Lancet* 1980;1:675.

216. Loirat C, et al. Deficiency of the second component of complement: its occurrence with membranoproliferative glomerulonephritis. *Arch Pathol Lab Med* 1980;104:467.

217. Suzuki J, et al. Membranoproliferative glomerulonephritis associated with hereditary deficiency of the 4th component of complement. *Clin Nephrol* 2003;60:279.

218. Angus KW, et al. Mesangiocapillary glomerulonephritis in lambs: the ultrastructure and immunopathology of diffuse glomerulonephritis in newly born Finnish Landrace lambs. *J Pathol* 1980;131:65.

219. Berry PL, et al. Membranoproliferative glomerulonephritis in two sibships. *Clin Nephrol* 1981;16:101.

220. Rennke HG. Secondary membranoproliferative glomerulonephritis. *Kidney Int* 1995;47:643.

221. Hunter AM, Lawson AA, Thomson D. Partial lipodystrophy with nephrotic syndrome. *Postgrad Med J* 1978;54:286.

222. Cameron JS. Glomerulonephritis in renal transplants. *Transplantation* 1982;34:237.

223. Dragon-Durey MA, et al. Heterozygous and homozygous factor H deficiencies associated with hemolytic uremic syndrome or membranoprolifer-ative glomerulonephritis: report and genetic analysis of 16 cases. *J Am Soc Nephrol* 2004;15:787.

224. West CD, McAdams AJ. Paramesangial glomerular deposits in membranoproliferative glomerulonephritis type II correlate with hypocomplementemia. *Am J Kidney Dis* 1995;25:853.

225. West CD, Witte DP, McAdams AJ. Composition of nephritic factor-generated glomerular deposits in membranoproliferative glomerulonephritis type 2. *Am J Kidney Dis* 2001;37:1120.

226. Johnson RJ, et al. Membranoproliferative glomerulonephritis associated with hepatitis C virus infection. *N Engl J Med* 1993;328:465.

227. Yamabe H, et al. Hepatitis C virus infection and membrano-proliferative glomerulonephritis in Japan. *J Am Soc Nephrol* 1995;6:2220.

228. Fabrizi F, et al. Hepatitis C virus infection and acute or chronic glomerulonephritis: an epidemiological and clinical appraisal. *Nephrol Dial Transplant* 1998;13:1991.

229. D'Amico G. Is type II mixed cryoglobulinemia an essential part of hepatitis C virus (HCV) associated glomerulonephritis?. *Nephrol Dial Transplant* 1995;10:1279.

230. Rostoker G, et al. Low prevalence of antibodies to hepatitis C virus among adult patients with idiopathic membranoproliferative type I glomerulonephritis in France (letter). *Nephron* 1995;69:97.

231. Gonzalo A, et al. Searching for hepatitis C virus antibodies in chronic primary glomerular disease (letter). *Nephron* 1995;69:96.

232. Paydas S, et al. The frequencies of hepatitis B virus markers and hepatitis C virus antibody in patients with glomerulonephritis. *Nephron* 1996;74:617.

233. Mac-Moune Lai F, et al. Low prevalence of hepatitis virus antibodies with primary membranous nephropathy and membranoproliferative glomerulonephritis in Hong Kong. *Nephron* 1995;70:367.

234. Cosio FG, et al. Prevalence of hepatitis C in patients with idiopathic glomerulopathies in native and transplant kidneys. *Am J Kidney Dis* 1996;28:752.

235. Lopes LM, et al. Prevalence of viral hepatitis markers in primary glomerulonephritis. (Abstr 27th Ann Meet ASN). In: *J Am Soc Nephrol* 1994;5:354.

236. Arima S, et al. Glomerular impairment in patients with hepatitis C virus (HCV) infection in Japan. *J Am Soc Nephrol* 1994;5:346 (abstr).

237. Wang H, Yin X, Zhang G. Is there hepatitis C virus associated glomerulonephritis? *J Am Soc Nephrol* 1994;5:363(abstr).

238. D'Amico, G. Renal involvement in hepatitis C infection: cryoglobulinemic glomerulonephritis. *Kidney Int* 1998;54:650.

239. Sabry AA, et al. A comprehensive study of the association between hepatitis C virus and glomerulopathy. *Nephrol Dial Transplant* 2002;17:239.

240. Garozzo M, et al. HCV and renal disease: not always associated with mixed cryoglobulinemia. *Clin Nephrol* 2003;60:361.

241. Dohi K, et al. Natural killer activity and antibody-dependent cell-mediated cytotoxicity in primary glomerular diseases. *Clin Nephrol* 1987;27:11.

242. Chatenoud L, Bach MA. Abnormalities of T-cell subsets in glomerulonephritis and systemic lupus erythematosus. *Kidney Int* 1981;20:267.

243. Imai H, et al. IgG subclasses in patients with membranoproliferative glomerulonephritis, membranous nephropathy, and lupus nephritis. *Kidney Int* 1997;51:270.

244. Kawasaki Y, et al. Evaluation of helper -1/-2 balance on the basis of IgG subclasses and serum cytokines in children with glomerulonephritis. *Am J Kidney Dis* 2004;44:42.

245. Cameron JS. Platelets in glomerular disease. *Annu Rev Med* 1984;35:175.

246. Cameron JS. The pathogenesis of glomerulonephritis. In: Bertani T, Remuzzi G, eds. *Glomerular injury 300 years after Morgagni.* Milano: Wichtig; 1983:18.

247. Nakashima Y, Hirose S, Hamashima Y. Proliferation of cultured rabbit renal glomerular cells stimulated by platelet factor. *Acta Pathol Jpn* 1980;30:1.

248. Deuel TF, et al. Chemotaxis of monocytes and neutrophils to platelet-derived growth factor. *J Clin Invest* 1982;69:1046.

249. George CR, et al. A kinetic evaluation of hemostatis in renal disease. *N Engl J Med* 1974;291:1111.

250. Donadio JV Jr, et al. Membranoproliferative glomerulonephritis: a prospective clinical trial of platelet-inhibitor therapy. *N Engl J Med* 1984;310:1421.

251. Droz D, et al. Évolution à long terme des glomérulonéphrites 0membranoproliferatives de l'adulte: Remission spontanée durable chez 13 malades avec étude de biopsies rénales itératives dans 5 cas. *Néphrologie* 1982;3:6.

252. Cattran DC, et al. Results of a controlled drug trial in membranoproliferative glomerulonephritis. *Kidney Int* 1985;27:436.

253. McAdams AJ, McEnery PT, West CD. Mesangiocapillary glomerulonephritis: changes in glomerular morphology with long-term alternate-day prednisone therapy. *J Pediatr* 1975;86:23.

254. McEnery PT, McAdams AJ, West CD. The effect of prednisone in a high-dose, alternate-day regimen on the natural history of idiopathic membranoproliferative glomerulonephritis. *Medicine (Baltimore)* 1985,64:401.

255. Barbiano di Belgiojoso G, et al. The prognostic value of some clinical and histological parameters in membranoproliferative glomerulonephritis (MPGN): report of 112 cases. *Nephron* 1977;19:250.

256. Cansick JC, et al. Prognosis, treatment and outcome of childhood mesangio-capillary (membranoproliferative) glomerulonephritis. *Nephrol Dial Transplant* 2004;19:2769.

257. Iitaka K, et al. Idiopathic membranoproliferative glomerulonephritis in Japanese children. *Pediatr Nephrol* 1995;9:272.

258. McEnery PT. Membranoproliferative glomerulonephritis: the Cincinnati experience cumulative renal survival from 1957 to 1989. *J Pediatr* 1990;116:S109.

259. Ferrario F. Le glomerulonefriti membranoproliferative. Studio multicentrico del Gruppo di Immunopatologia Renale. *Giorn It Nefrologia* 1990;7:67.

260. Miller MN, et al. Incidence and prognostic importance of glomerular crescents in renal diseases of childhood. *Am J Nephrol* 1984;4:244.

261. Williams DG, Bartlett A, Duffus P. Identifications of nephritic factor as an immunoglobulin. *Clin Exp Immunol* 1978;33:425.

262. Bennett WM, et al. Mesangiocapillary glomerulonephritis type II (dense-deposits disease): clinical features of progressive disease. *Am J Kidney Dis* 1989;13:469.

263. West CD. Childhood membranoproliferative glomerulonephritis: an approach to management. *Kidney Int* 1986;29:1077.

264. Vallota EH, et al. The C3 nephritic factor and membranoproliferative nephritis: correlation of serum levels of the nephritic factor with C3 levels, with therapy and with progression of the disease. *J Pediatr* 1972;80:947.

265. Schena FP, et al. Biological significance of the C3 nephritic factor in membranoproliferative glomerulonephritis. *Clin Nephrol* 1982;18:240.

266. Wehrmann M, et al. Long-term prognosis of focal sclerosing glomerulonephritis. An analysis of 250 cases with particular regard to tubulo-interstitial changes. *Clin Nephrol* 1990;33:115.

267. Alexopoulos E, Seron D, Hartley RB. Immune mechanisms in idiopathic membranous nephropathy: the role of the interstitial infiltrates. *Am J Kidney Dis* 1989;13:404.

268. Sabadini E, et al. Characterization of interstitial infiltrating cells in Berger's disease. *Am J Kidney Dis* 1988;12:307.

269. Alexopoulos E, Seron D, Hartley RB. The role of interstitial infiltrates in IgA nephropathy: a study with monoclonal antibodies. *Nephrol Dial Transplant* 1989;4:187.

270. D'Amico G. Clinical factors in progressive renal injury: the role of proteinuria. *Am J Kidney Dis* 1991;17(Suppl 1):48.

271. Alpers CE, Biava CG. Idiopathic lobular glomerulonephritis (nodular mesangial sclerosis): a distinct diagnostic entity. *Clin Nephrol* 1989;32:68.

272. Surian M, et al. Glomerular disease and pregnancy. A study of 123 pregnancies in patients with primary and secondary glomerular diseases. *Nephron* 1984;36:101.

273. Jungers P, Forget D, Houillier P. Risques foetal et maternel de la grossesse chez les femmes atteintes de glomérulonéphrite chronique primitive (II). *Néprologie* 1990;11:171.

274. Becker GJ, Fairley KF, Whitworth JA. Pregnancy exacerbates glomerular disease. *Am J Kidney Dis* 1985;6:266.

275. Fairley KF. Hypertension and renal disease in pregnancy. In: Zurukzoglu W, Papadimitriou M, Pyrpasopoulos M, et al., eds. Proceedings of the VIII International Congress Nephrology, Athens. Basel: Karger; 1981:440.

276. Cameron JS, Hicks J. Pregnancy in patients with pre-existing glomerular disease. *Contrib Nephrol* 1984;37:149.

277. Hayslett JP. Interaction of renal disease and pregnancy. *Kidney Int* 1984;25:579.

278. Cameron JS, Turner DR. Recurrent glomerulonephritis in allografted kidneys. *Clin Nephrol* 1977;7:47.

279. Curtis JJ, et al. Renal transplantation for patients with type I and type II membranoproliferative glomerulonephritis: serial complement and nephritic factor measurements and the problem of recurrence of disease. *Am J Med* 1979;66:216.

280. Hamburger J, Crosnier J, Noël LH. Recurrent glomerulonephritis after renal transplantation. *Annu Rev Med* 1978;29:67.

281. Petersen VP, et al. Late failure of human renal transplants: an analysis of transplant disease and graft failure among 125 recipients surviving for one to eight years. *Medicine (Baltimore)* 1975;54:45.

282. Andresdottir MB, et al. Type I Membranoproliferative glomerulonephritis in a renal allograft: a recurrence induced by a cytomegalovirus infection? *Am J Kidney Dis* 2000;35:E6.

283. Broyer M, et al. Kidney transplantation in children: results of 383 grafts performed at Enfants Malades Hopital from 1973 to 1984. *Adv Nephrol* 1987;16:307.

284. Turner DR, et al. Transplantation in mesangiocapillary glomerulonephritis with intramembranous dense "deposit": recurrence of disease. *Kidney Int* 1976;9:439.

285. Andresdottir MB, et al. Renal transplantation in patients with dense deposit disease: morphologic characteristics of recurrent disease and clinical outcome. *Nephrol Dial Transplant* 1999;14:1723.

286. Leibowitch J, et al. Recurrence of dense deposits of transplanted kidney: II. Serum complement and nephritic factor profiles. *Kidney Int* 1979;15:396.

287. Berthoux FC, et al. Renal transplantation in mesangioproliferative glomerulonephritis (MPGN): relationship between the high frequency of recurrent glomerulonephritis and hypocomplementemia. *Kidney Int* 1975;(Suppl 7):S-323.

288. Olsen S, Bohman SO, Petersen VP. Ultrastructure of the glomerular basement membrane in long-term renal allografts with transplant glomerular disease. *Lab Invest* 1974;30:176.

289. Busch GJ, Galvanek EG Raynolds ES Jr. Human renal allografts: Analysis of lesions in long-term survivors. *Hum Pathol* 1971;2:253.

290. Pommer W, et al. De novo membranoproliferative glomerulonephritis in a renal allograft. *Int Urol Nephrol* 1983;15:359.

291. Honkanen E, et al. Glomerulonephritis in renal allografts: results of 18 years of transplantations. *Clin Nephrol* 1984;21:210.

292. Tarshish P, et al. Treatment of mesangiocapillary glomerulonephritis with alternate-day prednisone. A report of the International Study of Kidney Disease in Children. *Pediatr Nephrol* 1992;6:123.

293. Bergstein JM, Andreoli SP. Response of type I membranoproliferative glomerulonephritis to pulse methylprednisolone and alternate-day prednisone therapy. *Pediatr Nephrol* 1995;9:268.

294. Ford DM, et al. Childhood membranoproliferative glomerulonephritis type I: limited steroid therapy. *Kidney Int* 1992;41:1606.

295. Donadio JV Jr, Offord KP. Reassessment of treatment results in membranoproliferative glomerulonephritis, with emphasis on life-table analysis. *Am J Kidney Dis* 1989;14:445.

296. Glassock RJ. Membranoproliferative glomerulonephritis. In: Ponticelli C, Glassock RJ, eds. *Treatment of primary glomerulonephritis*. Oxford: Oxford University Press; 1997:218.

297. Tiller DJ, et al. A prospective randomized trial in the use of cyclophosphamide, dipyridamole and warfarin in membranous and mesangiocapillary glomerulonephritis. In: Zurukzoglu W, et al., eds. *Proceedings of the VIIIth International Congress Nephrology, Athens*. Basel: Karger; 1981:345.

298. Faedda R, et al. Immunosuppressive treatment of membranoproliferative glomerulonephritis. *Nephron* 1994;67:59.

299. Zimmermann SW, et al. Prospective trial of warfarin and dipyridamole in patients with membranoproliferative glomerulonephritis. *Am J Med* 1983;75:920.

300. Takeda A, Niimura F, Matsutani H. Long term corticosteroid and dipyridamole treatment of membranoproliferative glomerulonephritis type I in children. *Nippon Jinzo Gakkai Shi Jpn J Nephrol* 1995;37:330.

301. Zäuner I, et al. Effect of aspirin and dipyramidole on proteinuria in idiopathic membranoproliferative glomerulonephritis: a multicentre prospective clinical trial. *Nephrol Dial Transplant* 1994;6:619.

302. Meyrier A. Treatment of glomerular disease with cyclosporin A. *Nephrol Dial Transplant* 1989;4:923.

303. Cattran DC. Current status of Cyclosporin A in the treatment of membranous, IgA and membranoproliferative glomerulonephritis. *Clin Nephrol* 1991;35(Suppl 1):S43.

304. Levin ML Mycophenolate mofetil treatment for primary glomerular diseases. *Kidney Int* 2002;61:1475.

305. Choi MJ, et al. Mycophenolate mofetil treatment for primary glomerular diseases. *Kidney Int* 2002;61:1098.

306. Valentin M, et al. Membranoproliferative glomerulonephritis associated with autoimmune thyroiditis. *Nefrologia* 2004;24:43.

307. Jones G, et al. Treatment of idiopathic membranoproliferative glomerulonephritis with mycophenolate mofetil and steroids. *Nephrol Dial Transplant* 2004;19:3160.

308. Bedogna V, et al. Effects of ACE inhibition in normotensive patients with chronic glomerular disease and normal renal function. *Kidney Int* 1990;38:101.

309. Zoja C, et al. Pharmacologic control of angiotensin II ameliorates renal disease while reducing renal TGF-(in experimental mesangioproliferative glomerulonephritis. *Am J Kidney Dis* 1998;31:453.

310. Nakao N, et al. Combination treatment of angiotensin II receptor blocker and angiotensin-converting enzyme inhibitor in non-diabetic renal disease (COOPERATE): a randomised controlled trial. *Lancet* 2003;361:117.

311. Kincaid-Smith P, Fairley KF, Packham D. Dual blockade of the renin-angiotensin system compared with a 50% increase in the dose of angiotensin-converting enzyme inhibitor: effects on proteinuria and blood pressure. *Nephrol Dial Transplant* 2004;19:2272.

312. Levin A. Management of membranoproliferative glomerulonephritis: evidence-based recommendations. *Kidney Int* 1999;55:S41.

CHAPTER 63 ■ MEMBRANOUS NEPHROPATHY

MITCHELL ROSNER AND WARREN KLINE BOLTON

Membranous nephropathy (MN), also know as membranous glomerulonephritis, represents the most common cause of the nephrotic syndrome in elderly adults, representing up to 30% of all cases in patients over age 50 (1–4). It is recognized by its characteristic pathological findings of diffuse subepithelial immune deposits without glomerular hypercellularity (5–7). It occurs most commonly in isolation (idiopathic MN, 80%), but may be a feature of an underlying disease (secondary MN, 20%), most often either autoimmune, infectious or malignant (8–10). The pathogenesis of MN is likely autoimmune in nature based upon animal models where the disease can be reproduced with antibodies that react to antigens expressed on the glomerular epithelial cell (GEC) (11–15). Interestingly, a recent case of congenital MN in humans has also been determined to be secondary to a passively transmitted maternal antibody that reacted to an endogenous antigen on the GEC (16). In animal models, immune complex deposition leads to complement activation and subsequent injury to the GEC and the glomerular basement membrane with the resulting expression of proteinuria and depressed glomerular filtration rate (17–21). Its course is variable with spontaneous remissions and relapses and leads to end-stage renal disease (ESRD) in up to 30% to 40% of patients over an extended period of time (22–24). Despite this good prognosis, the high incidence of MN makes it the second or third most common primary glomerular disease to progress to ESRD (25). Additional morbidity and mortality from the nephrotic syndrome accrues from accelerated vascular disease, hyperlipidemia, and the occurrence of thromboembolic events (26). Despite numerous clinical trials, therapeutic approaches remain controversial and the subject of much debate.

EPIDEMIOLOGY

Idiopathic (or primary) MN is the cause of nephrotic syndrome in approximately 25% of adults (1,27). It is a disease that affects patients most commonly around the fourth and fifth decade (median age approximately 40) but can present at any age (28,29). In patients older than age 60, MN can be seen in up to 35% of biopsy specimens (4). Secondary MN (either related to autoimmune disease, infections, malignancy, or drugs) is seen more commonly at the extremes of young and old age. In younger patients, especially in Asia, hepatitis B infection is a much more common etiology (30,31). In older patients, related malignancies are more commonly seen and may be responsible for up to 20% to 30% of all cases in patients older than age 60 years of age (32,33). MN is more common in men than in women (2 or 3:1) (34).

Determining the true incidence and prevalence of MN is difficult. In Victoria, Australia over a 2-year period, the incidence of MN identified by renal biopsy was 13.27 cases per million person-years (35). A larger study from the United Kingdom gave an annual incidence of 11 cases per million population per year (36). While the majority of patients (80%) present with signs and symptoms of the nephrotic syndrome, up to 20% to 25% of patients may be detected as having asymptomatic proteinuria from urinalysis as part of a medical examination (37). Since most physicians do not routinely screen for proteinuria and the onset of the disease is insidious, these numbers are likely an underestimate. Furthermore, many of these patients never develop the nephrotic syndrome and would go unbiopsied and undetected.

The United States Renal Data Service records MN as the cause of 0.6% of all of the ESRD population (25). This number has remained constant over the past decade.

Geographic variations in the prevalence of MN have been reported and may, in part, be related to differences in the rate of secondary MN due to infectious diseases such as hepatitis B and malaria (38).

SECONDARY MEMBRANOUS NEPHROPATHY

In over 75% of MN cases, no etiological agents can be determined. However, certain underlying conditions have been reported to be associated with the development of MN and account for up to 25% of cases (Table 63-1) (37). In many of these cases, the causal link is tenuous and consists only of isolated case reports making causation speculative. In other cases, the condition has been described so frequently as being associated with MN that causation is more definitive. The best evidence comes from conditions in which treatment of the underlying process (infection, malignancy, autoimmune disease) or removal of an offending agent or drug is associated with resolution of the nephropathy. Furthermore, in some cases (such as hepatitis B infection and malignancy) an associated antigen can be localized to the glomerular site of injury further substantiating causality (30,39–41).

In most cases, the lesion of secondary MN appears pathologically identical to the idiopathic form. The notable exception to this is MN associated with underlying systemic lupus erythematosus in which subendothelial and mesangial immune deposits as well as mesangial hypercellularity are seen (42,43).

Autoimmune Conditions

Various rheumatologic disorders have been described in association with MN (Table 63-1). Systemic lupus erythematosus (SLE) is the most common rheumatologic disease associated with MN (43–48). About 15% to 25% of patients with lupus nephritis are classified with a class V (membranous) World Health Organization (WHO) lesion with predominately subepithelial deposits (49,50). Clinically, the presentation is that of the nephrotic syndrome and is indistinguishable from idiopathic MN. The majority of these patients are young females and in a substantial number the onset of the nephrotic

TABLE 63-1

AUTOIMMUNE DISEASES ASSOCIATED WITH MEMBRANOUS NEPHROPATHY

Systemic lupus erythematosus (43–56)
Rheumatoid arthritis (57,58)
Mixed connective tissue disease (101)
Dermatomyositis (102)
Ankylosing spondylitis (103,104)
Systemic sclerosis (105)
Myasthenia gravis (79)
Bullous pemphigoid (106)
Autoimmune thyroid disease (75,76)
Sjögren's syndrome (107,108)
Temporal arteritis (109)
Crohn's disease (77)

(Adapted from: Short C, Mallick NP. Membranous nephropathy. In: Schrier RW, ed. *Diseases of the kidney.* 7th ed. Philadelphia: Lippincott Williams and Wilkins; 2001:1743.)

TABLE 63-2

INFECTIOUS DISEASES ASSOCIATED WITH MEMBRANOUS NEPHROPATHY

Hepatitis B (81–84)
Hepatitis C (96–98)
Human immunodeficiency virus (114)
Malaria (115)
Schistosomiasis (116)
Filariasis (117)
Syphilis (110–113)
Enterococcal endocarditis (118)
Hydatid disease (119,120)
Leprosy (121)

(Adapted from: Short C, Mallick NP. Membranous nephropathy. In: Schrier RW, ed. *Diseases of the kidney.* 7th ed. Philadelphia: Lippincott Williams and Wilkins; 2001:1743.)

syndrome predates the development of other signs of SLE (51,52). Thus, there should be a high degree of suspicion for SLE in any young female who presents with the nephrotic syndrome and MN on renal biopsy. Up to 25% to 50% of patients have negative anti-nuclear antibody levels, and often the antibody, if present, is of low avidity (51,52). Complement levels are usually normal. Morphologically, the lesion in class V lupus nephritis can look identical to that of idiopathic MN, but more often there are distinguishing features on renal biopsy (43). Light microscopy can reveal mesangial hypercellularity and expansion. Immunofluorescence reveals a more varied immunoglobulin response with the presence of immunoglobulin A (IgA), immunoglobulin G (IgG), and immunoglobulin M (IgM) as well as C1q deposition. Electron microscopy can reveal typical tuboreticular inclusions in glomerular endothelial cells. Otherwise, the clinical course of lupus MN mirrors that of the idiopathic form with an excellent long-term prognosis in excess of 85% renal survival at 10 years (53–56).

When patients with rheumatoid arthritis develop MN, it is usually in the setting of treatment with agents such as gold, penicillamine, bucillamine, or nonsteroidal antiinflammatory agents (57–68). Recently, cyclo-oxygenase-2 (COX-2) inhibitors have also been associated with a lesion of MN in conjunction with acute interstitial nephritis (69). In these cases, proteinuria develops soon after exposure to the drug and resolves slowly over a period of months after withdrawal of the offending agent. The pathologic lesion is identical to idiopathic MN.

The association of MN with other autoimmune disorders is less definitive. The immune response that leads to immune complex formation in MN has been linked to the human leukocyte antigen (HLA) class II antigen DR3 (70–71). There is a threefold or greater increase in the relative risk for MN is patients with HLA-DR3 (70–72). HLA-DR3 has also been associated with several other autoimmune conditions such as Sjögren's syndrome, dermatitis herpetiformis, and Grave's disease (36). Interestingly, many of the patients with rheumatoid arthritis who develop MN in the setting of drug therapy are also HLA-DR3 positive (60–62). Thus, the association of MN with these disorders may simply reflect this common HLA association.

Many other miscellaneous conditions that have an autoimmune basis have been associated with MN. These include diverse diseases such as Grave's disease, sarcoidosis, Crohn's disease, myasthenia gravis and multiple sclerosis (73–80).

Infectious Diseases

Numerous infectious diseases have been associated with the development of MN (Table 63-2). In all cases, these represent chronic infections with long-standing and persistent antigenemia. The etiological role of these infectious diseases is strengthened when the nephrotic syndrome resolves with treatment of the infection.

The association of MN with hepatitis B viral (HBV) chronic infection is particularly strong having been first described by Combes et al. in 1971 (81). HBV infection may account for up to 30%–40% of cases on MN in Asia (but less than 1% of MN in the United States) and is particularly prevalent in childhood cases of MN throughout the world (accounting for 80% of cases in Asia, and 20% of cases in the United States) (30,31,38,82). Patients present with the nephrotic syndrome and have a history of viral hepatitis with laboratory evidence of chronic active or persistent hepatitis. Serologically, these patients are usually positive for HB surface antigen (HBsAg) and in 60% to 80% of patients, HBeAg as well (30,83–84). In contrast to idiopathic MN, C3 and C4 levels are mildly depressed and immune deposits can be found in the mesangium and subendothelial regions of the glomeruli (30). The pathogenesis of HBV-associated MN is unknown. However, HBsAg, HBcAg and HBeAg have been localized by immunofluorescence to the glomerular capillary wall in patients with HBV-associated MN supporting a possible role for these antigens in leading to immune complex formation in the glomerulus (39–41). HBeAg seems to have a particularly strong predilection to localize to the capillary wall (41). It is also possible that autoantibodies could be induced secondary to chronic liver disease and that the findings of viral antigens in capillary walls may reflect passive trapping in damaged glomerular tissue (85). Adults with HBV associated MN generally have a good prognosis (30). However, up to 10% of untreated patients may require dialysis. Children have a better prognosis with the majority undergoing spontaneous remission within 5 years (30). Remission is often associated with clearance of HBeAg (30). Treatment of HBV infection with either alpha-interferon or lamivudine has been associated with remission of the nephrotic syndrome in a number of cases (86–91).

Hepatitis C viral (HCV) infection has been associated with mixed cryoglobulinemia and the development of membranoproliferative glomerulonephritis (MPGN) (92–95). However, HCV has also been associated with MN (96–98). These patients are anti-HCV IgG and HCV RNA positive. Core antigen, which is strongly cationic, has been localized to the glomerular capillary wall in two patients with MN associated with HCV (99). Unlike HCV-associated MPGN, cryoglobulin is undetectable and complement levels are normal. Combination alpha-interferon and ribavirin therapy has led to significant reduction in proteinuria and improved renal function in several patients (100).

Syphilis has rarely been associated with the development of MN (110–113). This association is strengthened both by the demonstration of treponemal antigens in the glomeruli of patients with MN and the resolution of the nephrotic syndrome with treatment of the infection (110–112). Human immunodeficiency viral (HIV) infection has also been rarely described in association with MN (114).

Malignancy

In patients older than age 60, up to 20% of patients with MN may have an occult or diagnosed malignancy (Table 63-3) (85). The majority of these cancers are carcinomas of the gastrointestinal tract, lung or breast. The incidence of carcinoma in patients diagnosed with MN is 10-fold higher than that expected for an age-matched normal population (32,33,122–125). In up to 70% of patients, the malignancy may be occult at the time of diagnosis of the nephrotic syndrome and thus careful follow-up of elderly patients with MN is warranted (125). Anecdotal evidence supports the view that the majority of these cancers manifest within 2 years after the diagnosis of MN (33,125). There are rare reports of resolution of the nephrotic syndrome after tumor resection or chemotherapy (126–128). Whether these represent evidence of true causation or simply spontaneous remission of MN is unknown. Supporting a direct role in the causation of MN is the finding of tumor-related antigens, including carcinoembryonic antigen, in glomerular deposits in several patients (129–132). Whether this may simply represent passive trapping of antigen to a damaged glomerulus rather than a direct role in pathogenesis is not known. A recent case of MN in association with an adrenal ganglioneuroma demonstrated the presence of an antibody from the patient's serum that reacted against the tumor as well as the glomerular basement membrane (127). Resection of the tumor was associated with disappearance of this antibody from the serum along with clinical remission of the nephrotic syndrome. The pathological

TABLE 63-3

MALIGNANCIES ASSOCIATED WITH MEMBRANOUS NEPHROPATHY

Carcinomas	Noncarcinomas
Lung (135,136)	Hodgkin's lymphoma (143)
Esophageal (137)	Non-Hodgkin's lymphoma (144)
Colon (129,130)	Leukemia (145)
Breast (138)	Mesothelioma (146)
Stomach (131,134)	Melanoma (147,148)
Renal (139)	Wilm's tumor (149)
Ovary (140)	Hepatic adenoma (150)
Prostate (141)	Angiolymphatic hyperplasia (151)
Oropharynx (142)	Schwannoma (152)
	Neuroblastoma (153)
	Adrenal ganglioneuroma (127)
	Associated with graft-versus-host disease after stem cell transplant (154)

(Adapted from: Short C, Mallick NP. Membranous nephropathy. In: Schrier RW, ed. *Diseases of the kidney,* 7th ed. Philadelphia: Lippincott Williams & Wilkins; 2001:1743.)

TABLE 63-4

DRUGS/TOXINS ASSOCIATED WITH MEMBRANOUS NEPHROPATHY

Gold (59,60,156)
Penicillamine (157–159)
Bucillamine (61)
Mercury compounds (160)
Captopril (161–163)
Probenicid (164)
Trimethadione (165)
Non-steroidal anti-inflammatory drugs (65–68)
Cyclooxygenase-2 inhibitors (69)
Clopidogrel (166)
Lithium (167)
Formaldehyde (168)
Hydrocarbons (169)

(Adapted from: Short C, Mallick NP. Membranous nephropathy. In: Schrier RW, ed. *Diseases of the kidney,* 7th ed. Philadelphia: Lippincott Williams & Wilkins; 2001:1743.)

lesion was identical to that of idiopathic MN. There are no data on the response of malignancy associated MN to steroids or immunosuppressive therapy (33). Unfortunately, malignant disease is often advanced in patients with MN with a 75% mortality 12 months after the diagnosis of MN (33,122,133).

Drugs

Drug-associated MN can develop at any age and typically develops soon after exposure to the offending agent (Table 63-4) (155). The most commonly implicated drugs are gold, penicillamine, and NSAIDs (68,156–159). Mercury compounds have also been implicated (160). In these cases, removal of the offending drug usually leads to resolution of the nephrotic syndrome over a prolonged period of months to even years. Once again, caution should be exercised in attributing causation based upon isolated case reports alone.

Miscellaneous Conditions

MN has also been associated with diabetes mellitus, with or without associated diabetic nephropathy (170,171). Other diverse diseases that have been described in association with MN are listed in Table 63-5. Whether these are merely fortuitous associations or true causation is a matter of speculation, especially given the rarity of these reports.

Renal Allograft Membranous Nephropathy

While MN can recur in the renal allograft, a more common occurrence is the appearance of *de novo* membranous nephropathy (185–191). Prevalence rates for *de novo* MN in renal transplant recipients vary from 0.4% to 9.2% (185–191). In renal transplant patients who develop the nephrotic syndrome, *de novo* MN is the diagnosis in up to 30% and is the second most common cause of the nephrotic syndrome in renal transplant recipients, behind chronic allograft nephropathy (185–191). In the majority of cases, no secondary cause has been identified, although hepatitis B, C, and HIV infection have been identified in some patients (190,192). The pathogenesis is unknown but may relate to chronic production of low-avidity

TABLE 63-5

MISCELLANEOUS CONDITIONS ASSOCIATED WITH MEMBRANOUS NEPHROPATHY

Diabetes mellitus (170,171)
Sarcoidosis (73,74)
Sickle cell disease (172)
Polycystic kidney disease (173)
Alpha1-antitrypsin deficiency (174)
Weber-Christian disease (175)
Primary biliary cirrhosis (176,177)
Systemic mastocytosis (178)
Guillain-Barré syndrome (179,180)
Urticarial vasculitis (181)
Hemolytic-uremic syndrome (182)
Dermatitis herpetiformis (183)
Myelodysplasia (184)

(Adapted from: Short C, Mallick NP. Membranous nephropathy. In: Schrier RW, ed. *Diseases of the kidney,* 7th ed. Philadelphia: Lippincott Williams & Wilkins; 2001:1743.)

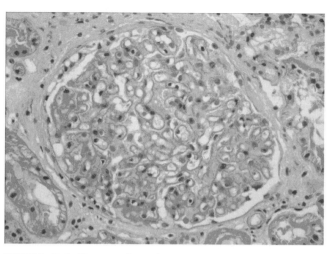

FIGURE 63-1. Hematoxylin and eosin stain (×250) of a glomerulus from a patient with idiopathic MN. There is diffuse thickening of the basement membrane without associated hypercellularity of the glomerular tuft. Inflammatory infiltrates are not seen and the capillary loops are widely patent. (Courtesy of Dr. Helen Cathro.)

antibodies to histocompatibility antigens. While recurrent MN usually develops in the allograft within the first 6–12 months post-transplant, *de novo* disease usually occurs 2 or more years after transplantation (193–195). The majority of patients develop nephrotic-range proteinuria. Graft outcome in *de novo* disease is variable, with some patients progressing to graft failure (usually in the setting of heavy proteinuria and preexisting graft dysfunction), and others maintaining stable graft function (196,197). Overall, the bulk of data reveals no increased risk in graft failure in patients with *de novo* MN. Alteration of immunosuppression or additional cytotoxic therapy has not demonstrated any benefit and treatment should focus on reduction of proteinuria, control of blood pressure, and management of complications such as hyperlipidemia and venous thrombosis (198–200).

PATHOLOGY

It is essential that all histologic techniques be utilized in examining the renal tissue of patients with the nephrotic syndrome. While MN derives its name by the characteristic global thickening of the basement membrane on light microscopy, early in the course of the disease glomeruli may appear normal and the diagnosis can only be made with electron microscopy and/or immunofluorescence (201–203). Conceptually, it is useful to think of membranous nephropathy as beginning with the deposition of immune complexes in the subepithelial region of the glomerular basement membrane followed by the response of the basement membrane and glomerular epithelial cell to this deposition. Subsequent histologic changes are due to this response.

Light Microscopy

Light microscopy, with either hematoxylin and eosin (H&E) or periodic acid-Schiff (PAS) staining, reveals diffuse and uniform thickening of the glomerular basement membrane (Fig. 63-1). The basement membrane takes on the appearance of a thick eosinophilic loop (Fig. 63-2). These stains, however, do not distinguish the etiology of the basement membrane thickening (i.e., thickening due to deposition of immune complexes or increased basement membrane matrix production). These

changes are best seen with silver methenamine, which binds to basement membrane matrix but not to immune complexes (Fig. 63-3). With this staining technique, characteristic ultrastructural changes in the basement membrane have been described by Ehrenreich and Churg (Table 63-6) (5). These stages represent a morphological but not necessarily a pathophysiological continuum (204). The initial stage is the formation of subepithelial immune complexes which is followed by the synthesis of new basement membrane that ultimately surrounds the complexes and is followed by the eventual digestion and disappearance of the immune complexes. On light microscopy with silver staining these changes can appear as a spectrum ranging from projections of the basement membrane ("spikes") (Fig. 63-3) corresponding to new basement membrane matrix synthesized by the GEC, to a chainlike appearance where the basement membrane completely incorporates the immune complexes (5). Later stages result in areas of lucency within the basement membrane that represent resolving immune complexes. These morphologic stages have not been correlated with

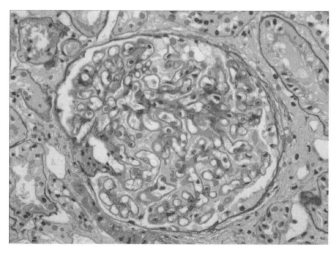

FIGURE 63-2. Periodic acid-Schiff stain of a glomerulus from a patient with idiopathic MN (×250). The basement membrane surrounding the capillary loops is diffusely thickened giving the appearance of "wire loops." (Courtesy of Dr. Helen Cathro.)

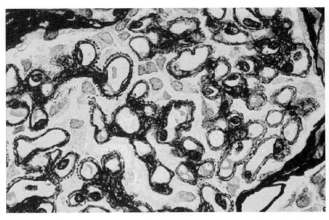

FIGURE 63-3. Jones silver stain (×250) of a glomerulus from a patient with idiopathic MN demonstrating "spikes" corresponding to newly synthesized basement membrane surrounding immune complexes. (Courtesy of Dr. Edward Klatt.)

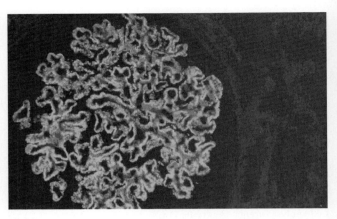

FIGURE 63-4. Immunofluorescence staining (anti-IgG) of a glomerulus from a patient with idiopathic MN (×250). Diffuse granular staining along the basement membrane is evident and corresponds to the deposition of immune complexes. Mesangial areas are free of immune deposits.

clinical findings and do not predict the degree of proteinuria, changes in renal function, responses to therapy or prognosis (204).

Other compartments of the glomerulus usually appear normal. There is usually no evidence of mesangial cell proliferation or expansion, except in the setting of SLE (205). There is also no evidence of inflammatory cell infiltrates which may relate to the fact that subepithelial immune complexes are unable to transmit chemotactic signals to effector cells in the circulation (as opposed to subendothelial deposits). In some cases, concurrent focal and segmental glomerulosclerosis can be seen and if present portends a worse prognosis (206,207).

Over time, the interstitial compartment develops fibrotic changes along with tubular atrophy. It is thought that these changes may reflect chronic, toxic effects of proteinuria on tubule cells (208–210). These tubulointerstitial changes correlate best with changes in renal function and offer important prognostic information (208–212).

Immunofluorescence Microscopy

Immunofluorescence (IF) microscopy reveals fine granular deposits of IgG and often complement components that follow

the glomerular basement membrane and spares the mesangium (Fig. 63-4) (213). The predominant immunoglobulin is always IgG (often IgG4 subclass) with minimal staining for IgA and IgM (214,215). The presence of strong staining for other immunoglobulins and C1q is suggestive of MN due to SLE or other secondary causes (216). In approximately 50% of cases, staining for C3 is seen and tends to be a marker for active and more severe disease (217,218). If performed, staining for the membrane attack complex (C5b-9) is usually positive and likely reflects the important role of this complex in mediating injury to the GEC (217–219).

Electron Microscopy

As noted above, Ehrenreich and Churg described a morphologic continuum of evolutionary stages of MN by electron microscopy (5). Four stages (I through IV) are described ranging from early changes (stage I) to advanced and late changes (stage IV) (Table 63-6). These stages serve as a useful descriptive tool but have not been correlated with clinical features of MN (211).

The hallmark of MN is the finding of electron-dense deposits corresponding to immune complexes (Fig. 63-5). These deposits are located along the glomerular basement membrane in a subepithelial location adjacent to the GEC (220). Electron-dense deposits are not found in the mesangium except in the case of SLE (221). In stage I lesions, the deposits tend to be small and finely granular and there is no response of the basement membrane. However, there is evidence of GEC injury as foot cell processes are effaced. Progressive changes to the glomerular basement membrane then ensue. The basement membrane begins to project between the immune deposits (stage II) forming the characteristic spikes seen on silver staining. Eventually these outgrowths of new basement membrane matrix material begin to coalesce and completely surround the immune deposits (stage III). Over time, the immune deposits undergo dissolution leaving electron lucent areas in the basement membrane (stage IV). At this stage, the glomerular basement membrane is thickened and considerably disrupted. While it is generally believed that these stages develop in a continuum, there are no studies of follow-up biopsies in single patients over time.

The changes to the glomerular basement membrane seen on light or electron microscopy do not relate to the degree of proteinuria or to renal function (211). While it is believed that

TABLE 63-6

PATHOLOGICAL STAGING OF MEMBRANOUS NEPHROPATHY

Stage	Electron microscopy
I	Subepithelial electron-dense deposits
II	Subepithelial electron-dense deposits with intervening basement membrane ("spikes")
III	Incorporation of subepithelial electron-dense deposits into the basement membrane
IV	Reabsorption of deposits with loss of electron-dense deposits and development of lucent area in the basement membrane
	Remodeling of basement membrane and loss of electron-dense deposits

(From: Ehreneich T, Churg J. Pathology of membranous nephropathy. *Pathol Annu* 1968;3:145.)

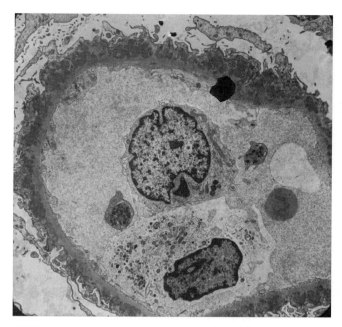

FIGURE 63-5. Electron micrograph of a glomerulus from a patient with idiopathic MN revealing characteristic electron-dense subepithelial deposits (×5000). In this micrograph, basement membrane can be seen to encircle the deposits forming the spikes seen on Jones silver staining (stages II and III). (Courtesy of Dr. Helen Cathro.)

patients with earlier stage lesions may have a better prognosis, it has been demonstrated that patients can go into clinical remission at any morphological stage (204). Renal function and prognosis is more dependent on the extent of interstitial damage.

PATHOGENESIS

Various lines of evidence support the idea that MN represents an autoimmune disorder. There is an association with other autoimmune diseases and a strong association with HLA-DR3 (70-72). There is characteristic deposition of immune complexes in the glomerular basement membrane and a strikingly similarity of the human lesion to the rat lesion of Heymann nephritis mediated by antibodies to the GEC (11–15). The recent finding of a human case of antenatal MN induced by maternally transmitted antibodies also supports an autoimmune etiology (16).

The majority of experimental work on the pathogenesis of MN has been performed in rats utilizing the Heymann nephritis model (11–15). In this model, a crude preparation of tubular brush-border extract (Fx1α) is injected into allogeneic animals. The injected animals then develop pathogenic antibody-antigen complexes that are localized to the subepithelial space and a lesion identical to MN develops (11–15). How immune complexes localize to their unique position in the subepithelial region has been the object of much speculation (222–226). First, intact circulating immune complexes could become trapped as a preformed entity in the subepithelial space. Alternatively, these immune complexes could dissociate and then reform after traversing the basement membrane. Finally, immune complexes could form in situ in the subepithelial space with circulating antibodies reacting to intrinsic glomerular antigens or to extrinsic antigens (either endogenous or exogenous) that become planted in the subepithelial space. Further work on the Heymann nephritis model supports the model that circulating antibodies react with either intrinsic glomerular epithelial

cell antigens or to planted extrinsic antigens (227). An accelerated form of this nephritis can be induced by the injection of preformed antibody into rats (passive Heymann's nephritis), suggesting that subepithelial immune deposits can be formed without the formation of circulating immune complexes (228–230). The antigen responsible for the development of the immune complex in the rat model has been determined to be a large glycoprotein (megalin or gp330) complexed to a smaller receptor associated protein (RAP) which is expressed in the clathrin-coated pits of the glomerular epithelial cell foot processes (231–235). Once antibody binds this antigen complex, the complex is patched in the clathrin-coated pits, capped and extruded from the cell membrane (227,236). The complexes then lie in the subepithelial region where they persist as the electron-dense deposits seen on electron microscopy. Although megalin has been found in human proximal tubules, it has not been detected in human glomeruli or in immune deposits in patients with MN, thus limiting the applicability of the Heymann nephritis model (237). However, a recent case of antenatal MN in humans has been described in which maternal antibodies to neutral endopeptidase (NEP) were passively transferred to the infant (16). These antibodies reacted against NEP antigen on the glomerular epithelial cell with the formation of subepithelial immune complexes and the development of the nephrotic syndrome. The mother had no apparent renal abnormalities since she was deficient in NEP and had previously been sensitized to this antigen from a prior miscarriage (238). Thus, one mechanism of subepithelial immune complex formation in MN is the reaction of circulating antibody with antigens expressed on the GEC. Whether exogenous antigens (especially small cationic proteins) can localize to the subepithelial region and also elicit immune complex formation is still unknown.

In the rat model, once immune complexes form in the subepithelial space, complement activation occurs and is necessary to produce proteinuria (239–243). Complement activation leads to the cleavage of C5 with the formation of C5a and C5b. Given the absence of inflammatory cells in MN, it seems plausible that the chemotactic factor C5a is filtered in the urine and does not move backwards across the basement membrane to attract inflammatory cells. C5b then combines with other complement components to form the membrane attack complex (C5b-C9) which inserts into the membrane of the GEC (244–248). The complex is endocytosed into the GEC and then extruded into the urinary space where it can be identified in the urine (249–254). The GEC is resistant to the lytic effects of the C5b-C9 complex but instead undergoes metabolic activation with the resulting production of proteases (matrix metalloprotease 9), prostaglandin metabolites, oxidants, growth factors, and cytokines (255–258). A protein that is upregulated in response to GEC activation is cytochrome b$_{558}$, an integral component of the NAPDH oxidoreductase complex that leads to the formation of toxic reactive oxygen species that damage the basement membrane (259). Transforming growth factors are also produced by the GEC and lead to formation of new basement membrane matrix components such as type I and IV collagen (260). Finally, the podocyte slit diaphragm, an important barrier to proteinuria, is altered by the activation of complement (261). Nephrin, a major and essential component of the slit diaphragm, is linked to the actin cytoskeleton of the GEC via adapter molecules that include CD2AP and podocin (262–264). In passive Heymann nephritis, activation of complement led to alteration in the distribution of nephrin and in its association with actin, thus disrupting the slit diaphragms (261). This dissociation of nephrin from actin was not seen if complement was depleted. Thus the consequences of injury induced by C5b-9 are multifaceted and ultimately lead to the clinical expression of proteinuria and altered renal function.

Antigens on the surface of the GEC may have important enzymatic roles and antibodies to these proteins may lead to important alterations in function that may have pathogenic significance (238). For instance, NEP is a metallopeptidase that is responsible for the cleavage and inactivation of vasoactive mediators such as bradykinin and endothelin (265). Neutralizing antibodies to this antigen would result in higher local concentrations of these vasoactive mediators that could alter glomerular hemodynamics and capillary wall permeability. Whether these mechanisms are operative in the pathogenesis of MN remains speculative.

CLINICAL FEATURES

The onset of clinical disease is usually insidious with the majority of patients (70% to 80%) presenting with peripheral edema and the nephrotic syndrome (266). In 20% of cases, non-nephrotic range proteinuria is found and usually these patients are identified through an abnormal urinalysis that is performed for an unrelated reason such as an insurance examination (267). Secondary causes of MN may present with a more abrupt onset (268). The proteinuria tends to be nonselective and averages 5 to 10 g/day (although this can vary widely depending upon salt and protein intake and medications that the patient may be taking). Microscopic hematuria occurs in up to 50%, but macroscopic hematuria is rare. Hypertension may be seen in up to 30% of patients but is usually mild. Renal function at the time of presentation is usually well preserved and when impaired often reflects prerenal factors, such as over zealous diuretic use, more than intrinsic renal disease. Proteinuria is usually present for an extended period of time (months to years) before renal impairment develops (269–271).

Thromboembolic complications, such as deep vein thrombosis, pulmonary embolism, and especially renal vein thrombosis, can be the presenting feature in some patients (272, 273). These complications are more common in patients with heavy, persistent proteinuria and serum albumin concentrations below 2.5 g/dL (274,275). These patients tend to have hyperfibrinogenemia with increases in procoagulant factors (factors V and VIII), along with decreases in anticoagulant factors (such as antithrombin III) (276,277). High levels of lipoprotein (a) in MN patients may serve as an inhibitor of plasminogen and thus inhibit thrombolysis (278). Renal vein thrombosis (RVT) is especially common in MN, developing in anywhere from 5 to 50% of cases (279–281). MN is the most common associated condition seen in patients with RVT. Patients may be asymptomatic or present with flank pain, hematuria, or deterioration in renal function (279–281). Alternatively, patients may present with embolic complications such as pulmonary emboli (279–281). The diagnosis can be made with noninvasive imaging studies such as Doppler ultrasonography, spiral computerized tomography, or magnetic resonance angiography. Venous angiography is the gold standard and is reserved for diagnostic dilemmas.

Uncommonly, patients with MN may present with or develop a superimposed rapidly progressive glomerulonephritis usually in the presence of anti–glomerular basement membrane antibodies (282–286). Renal biopsy will demonstrate typical crescents as well as subepithelial immune deposits.

LABORATORY FINDINGS

Laboratory findings in patients with MN generally reflect the ongoing proteinuria and nephrotic syndrome. Thus, hypoalbuminemia, hyperlipidemia and lipiduria are common findings (287). A typical lipid profile will reveal increased levels of total cholesterol, low-density lipoproteins (LDL), and very-low-density lipoproteins (VLDL) (288). High-density lipoprotein levels are either normal or low (288). The elevation in LDL

is thought to be secondary to hepatic overproduction and is stimulated by the low serum albumin level and reduced oncotic pressure (289). Lipoprotein (a) levels are also elevated (290,291).

Studies should be performed to exclude secondary causes of MN and include: anti-nuclear antibody, C3 and C4 levels, hepatitis B and C profiles, and age-appropriate cancer screening (mammography, prostate-specific antigen, chest radiography, colonoscopy, and careful thyroid examination). In those patients over age 60, an underlying malignancy should always be suspected. Syphilis serologies may also be useful in selected patients. Since the differential diagnosis of MN includes other causes of the nephrotic syndrome such as minimal change disease, focal glomerulosclerosis, membranoproliferative glomerulonephritis, diabetic glomerulosclerosis, monoclonal immunoglobulin deposition diseases, and amyloid; other useful laboratory tests include assessment of HIV status and serum and urine protein electrophoresis. Renal biopsy is essential for the correct diagnosis and biopsy material must be analyzed by all histologic techniques. Unlike the diagnosis of other renal diseases, sample size is not a problem in making the pathologic diagnosis of MN. The diagnosis can be made on a single glomerulus with typical subepithelial immune deposits.

Given the importance of the membrane attack complex (C5b-C9) in the pathogenesis of MN, there has been much interest in measuring the levels of this complex in the urine of patients with MN (250–254,292,293). In experimental animals, the appearance of C5b-9 in the urine closely parallels the level of disease activity and the formation of new immune deposits (250). In one human study, C5b-9 levels in the urine were elevated in 12 of 17 patients with progressive disease and in only 2 of 18 patients with stable disease (254). This assay is not widely available and further studies are still needed before this assay can be routinely used in the diagnosis and treatment of MN.

NATURAL HISTORY AND PROGNOSIS

The clinical course of MN is quite varied and complex (37). Various natural history studies have been performed and describe several possible outcomes (9,10,23,24,124,125,294–297). These include: (a) complete and lasting remission of the nephrotic syndrome with stable renal function; (b) complete remission of the nephrotic syndrome punctuated by one or more relapses but with stable renal function; (c) a partial remission of the nephrotic syndrome (generally defined as greater than a 50% reduction in proteinuria and proteinuria ≤3.5 g/day) with either stable or slowly deteriorating renal function; (d) persistence of nonnephrotic range proteinuria with or without progressive deterioration in renal function; (e) persistence of nephrotic range proteinuria with slowly progressive deterioration of renal function; or (f) persistence of nephrotic range proteinuria with development of superimposed acute or rapidly progressive renal failure (37). The approximate prevalence of these outcomes in untreated patients has been determined from several natural history studies and from placebo arms of intervention studies (9,10,23,24,124,125,294–297). Spontaneous complete remissions are seen in approximately 25% to 30% of patients within 3 to 5 years after presentation. Another 20% to 25% of patients will have partial remissions with persistent proteinuria ≤3.5 grams per day and stable renal function. However, of these patients who undergo remissions, nephrotic-range proteinuria may recur in 15% to 30% of patients. Thus, nearly 50% of patients will have persistent nephrotic syndrome. These latter patients are at much higher risk of developing progressive renal dysfunction (298).

In fact, 25% to 40% of these patients will develop end-stage renal disease (ESRD) or death within 5 years. This number rises to 50% or more after 10 years of persistent proteinuria. Progression to ESRD is uncommon (<1%) in patients who experience at least one complete remission and in those with persistent non-nephrotic-range proteinuria (299). One caveat to these natural history studies is that many of these patients did not receive aggressive anti-proteinuric therapies such as angiotensin-converting enzyme inhibitors (ACE-inhibitors) or angiotensin receptor blockers (ARBs). Furthermore, lipid abnormalities were not aggressively treated with statin drugs. Whether the natural history would be altered by these therapies is not known.

Several prognostic factors have been identified that when present are associated with an unfavorable course (9,10,23,24,124,125,294–303). These include: advanced age, male sex, reduced renal function at presentation or within 5 years of presentation, nephrotic range proteinuria (especially if persistent), excretion of increased quantities of low-molecular-weight proteins (signifying tubular abnormalities), hypertension, persistent hyperlipidemia, persistently elevated urinary C5b-C9 excretion, chronic tubulointerstitial fibrosis or focal sclerosis on renal biopsy, and the presence of HLA-B18 DRw3, or BfF1 DR5. The factors that seem to be most important in predicting both a spontaneous remission and its durability are persistent, low-grade (subnephrotic) proteinuria and female gender (9,10,23,24,124,125,294–302).

The natural history of MN makes treatment decisions difficult. Since only a subset of patients will progress to renal failure and this progression occurs over an extended period of time, therapy (especially with potentially toxic immunosuppressants) must be tailored to those patients at greatest risk for a poor outcome. Thus, efforts to identify these patients are critically important. In this regard, several of the prognostic features listed above have greater predictive ability than others. The most important prognostic variables have proven to be: age, male sex, level of renal function, and degree of proteinuria (9,10,23,24,124,125,294–303). The likelihood of progression to renal failure in those patients with an elevated serum creatinine level may be as high as 70% as compared to less than 20% in patients with normal renal function (298,304). Proteinuria is excess of 3.5 grams per day is associated with a two- to threefold increased risk of progressive disease and has often been used as criteria to initiate therapy. If the proteinuria is massive (>8 g/day) and persistent (lasting >6 months) the risk for progression is especially high (84%) (298,304). Cattran et al. have developed a predictive model using data from 184 patients with MN from the Metro Toronto Glomerulonephritis Registry (305,306). This model had 85% accuracy in predicting which patients will subsequently develop renal insufficiency. The model has also been validated in a total of 179 patients from Italy and Finland (306). The model calculates a probability of progression from knowledge of the highest level of persistent (≥6 months) proteinuria, the creatinine clearance at the beginning of this period and the slope of the creatinine clearance during the observation period. Based upon calculations from this model, if immunosuppressive agents were restricted to only those patients at high risk for progressive disease, then of the 363 patients analyzed, only 100 patients would receive potentially toxic therapy (305). This model has not been applied prospectively and thus cannot be widely recommended at this time.

THERAPY

The goal of therapy for patients with MN is the prevention of renal failure as well as the reduction of proteinuria and minimization of the complications associated with MN. These aims must be weighed against the risk of therapy, especially given the variable natural history of the disease. Multiple controlled trials have investigated numerous therapeutic approaches to patients with MN. Despite the wealth of trials, therapy for MN remains controversial with proponents advocating a spectrum of therapy ranging from aggressive immunosuppressive therapy to no disease-specific therapy. In part, these divergent opinions are due to difficulty in interpreting the trial data. Many trials enroll small numbers of patients with limited periods of follow-up. Given a slowly progressive disease with spontaneous remissions and relapses, long-term studies with comparable control groups are needed to adequately evaluate interventions. In many studies, many of the variables that determine prognosis are not controlled. Thus, the risk of progression in the control and intervention groups may be quite different. Finally, in many older studies, non-disease-specific therapies such as antihypertensive therapy with ACE-inhibitors or ARBs, lipid-lowering therapy, and dietary manipulations are not incorporated into the treatment regimen. Despite these limitations, several options for the treatment of MN exist.

Non-Disease-Specific Therapy

These nonimmunosuppressive therapies should be implemented in all patients with MN and include strategies to lower proteinuria, decrease the rate of disease progression, and prevent complications of the nephrotic syndrome, especially hyperlipidemia (307). Numerous studies have documented the role of ACE-inhibitors and ARBs in reducing proteinuria and the rate of renal disease progression in both diabetic and nondiabetic nephropathy (308–312). These drugs reduce intraglomerular pressure, improve glomerular barrier size selectivity, and have antiinflammatory properties (309,310,313). The benefit of ACE-inhibitors seems to be greatest in those patients with the greatest degree of proteinuria (308–312). Few studies specifically comment on the use of ACE-inhibitors in patients with MN. In one small study of 14 patients with MN, enalapril decreased proteinuria from 7.1 to 5.0 g/day (314). This was accompanied by an improvement in glomerular membrane size-selectivity as determined by dextran sieving coefficients. Given that the goal of therapy is to reduce proteinuria to non-nephrotic ranges or ideally to less than 500 mg per day, it is unlikely that ACE-inhibitors alone will be able to achieve this goal in nephrotic patients. Furthermore, the goal blood pressure in proteinuric patients should be 125/75 mm Hg, a difficult goal on a single antihypertensive medication. Recent evidence supports that combination therapy with both ACE-inhibitors and ARBs may affect more complete blockade of the renin–angiotensin–aldosterone system (315). Several trials have shown a synergistic reduction of proteinuria using this combination. In one trial, including 28 patients with MN, this translated into slower progression of nephropathy (316). One small study also investigated the addition of the aldosterone antagonist spironolactone to ACE-inhibitor therapy in 11 patients with MN. In this trial, blood pressure fell with the addition of spironolactone but urine protein excretion remained unchanged (317). In all cases, a low-sodium diet (100 mEq/day) should be instituted to maximize the antiproteinuric effects of these medications.

Nonsteroidal antiinflammatory agents also have been shown to have antiproteinuric effects (318–320). Their role in the treatment of MN is controversial. In one study where indomethacin was added to ramipril therapy, there was no additional reduction in proteinuria (321). However, there was a higher risk of side effects including hyperkalemia and a reversible rise in serum creatinine. These agents are not routinely recommended.

Patients with MN and the nephrotic syndrome typically have elevated cholesterol levels, with 66% of patients having total cholesterol levels greater than 300 mg/dL, and 70% of patients with low-density lipoprotein (LDL) levels greater than 160 mg/dL (288,322). This translates into an increased risk for cardiovascular events (288,322). In a prospective cohort study of 142 nephrotic patients the relative risk for myocardial infarction versus controls was 5.5 and for cardiac death it was 2.8 (323). Furthermore, in patients reaching ESRD, the leading cause of mortality is cardiovascular disease (25). Finally, hyperlipidemia has also been associated with an increased risk for declining GFR, and a meta-analysis has concluded that lipid reduction may have a role in reducing the rate of progression of renal disease (324–328). Treatment of hyperlipidemia rests on treatment of the underlying nephrotic syndrome, dietary modification, and antihyperlipidemic medications (329–332). 3-hydroxy-3-methylglutaryl coenzyme A (HMG-CoA) reductase inhibitors can lower LDL and total cholesterol levels by up to 50% in nephrotic patients and are the cornerstone of antihyperlipidemic therapy (329–332). Other agents include: ezetimibe, fibric acid derivatives, and bile acid sequestrants (329–334). While target goals for LDL have not been set for patients with the nephrotic syndrome, it seems reasonable to place these patients in the group at high risk for cardiovascular events with a goal LDL of less than 100 mg/dL (335).

Patients with MN are clearly at higher risk for venous thromboembolism (279–281). Whether to initiate prophylactic anticoagulation with warfarin at time of diagnosis of MN or to postpone treatment until a thrombotic event occurs remains controversial. Some clinicians recommend prophylactic anticoagulation in patients with serum albumin levels less than 2 g/dL and nephrotic range proteinuria, believing that the risk of thromboembolism in this group is greater than any risk of bleeding events (336). However, no prospective trial has examined this question. In those patients who do develop a thrombotic event, anticoagulation with warfarin to a goal international normalized ratio (INR) of 2 to 3 should be initiated (279–281). There are no data on the use of antiplatelet agents in this setting.

Corticosteroids

Two early controlled trials in the United Kingdom reported a small but statistically insignificant benefit in patients with MN treated with corticosteroids (336,337). However, these study were small (15 patients in one study and 19 in the other), used low doses of corticosteroid (20 to 30 mg/day) and had short-term follow-up. In 1979, the Collaborative Study of the Adult Idiopathic Nephrotic Syndrome was performed (338). In this prospective, randomized, placebo-controlled trial, 72 patients with the nephrotic syndrome due to MN were randomized to either an 8- week course of high-dose alternate-day prednisone (125 mg) followed by a tapering dose or a placebo. In the prednisone-treated group there were an increased number of remissions of the nephrotic syndrome. Over time, there were also an increased number of relapses in this group, so that at the end of 2 years, the prevalence of both complete and partial remissions were identical in the two groups. The major difference between the groups was in the level of renal function. After 6 months of therapy, the serum creatinine had doubled in only 2 of 34 steroid-treated patients, as compared to 11 of the 38 patients who received placebo. This study has been widely criticized since the risk and rate of progression of the control group was much higher than previous studies had reported for an untreated cohort of MN patients. Thus, the risk for disease progression was likely different in the two groups.

Subsequently, two other trials have examined the role of corticosteroids in the treatment of MN. In 1990, the MRC study evaluated 103 patients with MN using a similar protocol to the U.S. Collaborative Study (339). Patients were followed for a mean of 4 years and during this time there were no significant differences in either urinary protein excretion or rate of renal loss between the treatment and control groups. The Toronto Glomerulonephritis Study Group examined 158 patients with MN (340). Patients received either a 6-month course of prednisone (45 mg /m^2 of body-surface area) or placebo and were followed for a mean of 48 months. The proportion of patients with complete remission of proteinuria was similar in the two groups, as was the annual change in creatinine clearance. Progression to ESRD was identical in the two groups. A multivariate analysis adjusting for factors that may be related to the risk of disease progression failed to show any effect of prednisone on the outcome. One important difference between the U.S. Collaborative Study and the Toronto Study was that patients in the Toronto study had a longer median duration of disease prior to treatment (15 to 17 months vs. 6 months in the U.S. Collaborative Study) and more advanced glomerular changes (stage III to stage IV) on biopsy. Whether corticosteroid therapy is beneficial in patients with early lesions and a short duration of disease is not known. A meta-analysis of trials using corticosteroids for MN could find no evidence of benefit (341–342). Overall, the balance of evidence does not support the utility of corticosteroid therapy alone in either leading to remission of the nephrotic syndrome or in improving renal survival.

Cytotoxic Therapy

Initial trials of cytotoxic agents with or without corticosteroids generally involved small numbers of patients with short follow-up. In 1971, the MRC investigated the role of prednisone plus azathioprine in 14 patients with MN with no statistically significant effect of therapy on the rate of disease progression, although there was a trend toward lower serum creatinine in the treated group (337). A study from the Canadian Medical Association also found no benefit from azathioprine therapy (343). A more promising approach has been the use of either cyclophosphamide or chlorambucil. In 1975, Lagrue et al. studied the effects of a 1-year course of azathioprine (11 patients), chlorambucil (16 patients), or no treatment (14 patients) (344). There was no effect of azathioprine with 25% of patients in both the azathioprine-treated and control groups achieving a remission. However, 81% of patients treated with chlorambucil achieved either a partial or complete remission. Several subsequent studies utilized cyclophosphamide (often in addition to warfarin and dipyridamole) and found that active treatment tended to diminish proteinuria while having no effect on renal function (346–349). The interpretation of these studies is hampered by the small numbers of patients studied, the short duration of follow-up and lack of appropriate control groups.

The most effective regimen utilizing cytotoxic agents has been reported by Ponticelli et al. (350). This complex protocol involves three doses of intravenous methylprednisolone (1.0 gram daily), followed by oral prednisone (0.4 to 0.5 mg/kg/day) for a month. This regimen is then alternated monthly with oral chlorambucil (0.2 mg/kg/day) for a month. The entire treatment protocol lasts 6 months. The first report of this protocol was published in 1984 (349). Sixty-seven patients were randomized to either treatment with methylprednisolone plus chlorambucil or to placebo. After a mean follow-up of 31.4 months, 23 of 32 treated patients were in complete (12 patients) or partial remission as compared with 9 of 30 control patients. Renal function remained stable in the treated patients whereas there was progressive deterioration in the control group. Five years later, a larger cohort of patients that had received this protocol for an average of 5 years was reported (350). Plasma creatinine increased by 50% or more in 19 (49%) control patients but in only 4 (10%) treated patients. In the control group, only 9 patients (23%) achieved remission of the nephrotic syndrome versus 67% of the treated patients. Follow-up of this protocol has now been extended out to 10 years with 40% of the control patients reaching an endpoint of either death or dialysis as compared with 8% of the treated patients (351). When patients with MN were treated with either methylprednisolone versus methylprednisolone plus chlorambucil it was clear that the beneficial effects of this regimen were related to the alkylating agent (352).

There have been concerns over the use of chlorambucil given its potential toxicity (leukopenia and risk of infectious complications). Furthermore, most clinicians in the United States have had little experience with this drug. Ponticelli et al compared oral chlorambucil and cyclophosphamide in a head–to-head trial utilizing the same 6-month protocol as prior studies (353). Cyclophosphamide was dosed orally at a daily dose of 2.5 mg/kg. In this study, 36 of 44 (82%) patients on chlorambucil achieved a complete or partial remission versus 40 of 43 (93%) patients assigned to cyclophosphamide. Relapses occurred in 30.5% of the chlorambucil-treated patients and in 25% of cyclophosphamide-treated patients over 6 to 30 months of follow-up. Renal function remained stable in both groups. Importantly, herpes zoster infections were more common (9%) in patients treated with chlorambucil. A similar study from Williams et al. also compared chlorambucil and cyclophosphamide as given by the Ponticelli protocol (354). After a mean follow-up of 32 months, the cyclophosphamide group had better renal function, with ESRD occurring in only 1 of 17 patients as compared to 5 of 15 patients treated with chlorambucil. Infectious complications were less common in the cyclophosphamide group (354). Several other studies have confirmed the benefit of oral cyclophosphamide in protocols similar to that of Ponticelli et al. (355,356). Interestingly, two controlled studies have not shown a benefit of monthly intravenous pulse cyclophosphamide therapy (357,358).

A regimen of corticosteroids and cytotoxic agents has been studied in patients with progressive renal insufficiency. Bruns et al. studied in 11 patients with MN and rising serum creatinines and showed a decline in serum creatinine as well as proteinuria with a regimen of one year of cyclophosphamide 100 mg orally a day along with daily prednisone (359). Branten et al. treated 39 patients with a 1-year course of oral cyclophosphamide with corticosteroids and demonstrated a 38% median reduction of proteinuria (360). Jindal et al. treated 9 patients with MN with a mean baseline creatinine of 2.6 mg/dL with oral cyclophosphamide and corticosteroids (355). At the end of the treatment period there was a fall in mean creatinine to 2.2 mg/dL and proteinuria fell from 11.1 to 2.2 g/day. However, after treatment there was a progressive rise in creatinine levels to 2.9 mg/dL after 83 months.

In those patients who do suffer a relapse after a course of cytotoxic therapy, a second course of cytotoxic agents has been shown to be beneficial in reduction of proteinuria and in extending dialysis-free survival (361–363). However, these studies are small, uncontrolled, and subject patients to the risks of cumulative cytotoxic therapy.

Two meta-analyses of cytotoxic therapy for MN have shown that cytotoxic therapy leads to a more frequent remission of the nephrotic syndrome (342,364). However, a conclusion regarding the effects of therapy on renal function could not be drawn given the lack of large, prospective trials with long-term follow-up.

Mycophenolate Mofetil

Mycophenolate mofetil (MMF), an inhibitor of purine biosynthesis in activated lymphocytes, has also been studied in the treatment of resistant MN. Many of the published reports describing the efficacy of this agent are uncontrolled case reports subject to reporting bias. Choi et al. studied 17 patients with MN that were either resistant or intolerant to therapy with corticosteroids or cytotoxic agents. There was a significant reduction in proteinuria with two patients achieving a complete remission and 8 achieving a partial remission (365). Renal function remained stable in the treated patients. Miller et al. studied 16 patients with MN at high risk of progression with baseline proteinuria over 9 g/day (366). All patients had failed corticosteroid therapy, six patients had failed cytotoxic therapy, and five patients had failed cyclosporine. Patients were treated for a mean of 8 months with MMF with a target dose of 2 g/day. There was no change in mean proteinuria during the study and only six patients had a partial response. There was no change in serum creatinine during the study. At this time, the experience with MMF is too limited to draw any firm conclusions.

Cyclosporine

Cyclosporine has been studied in several randomized prospective clinical trials in patients with MN (367–373). Generally, the patients who have been studied are those that have moderate or high degrees of risk for progressive disease and had often failed other therapies such as cytotoxic agents.

Patients that had failed an 8-week course of corticosteroid therapy and had persistent nephrotic-range proteinuria were randomized to either cyclosporine (CSA) (28 patients) or placebo (23 patients) (371). Cyclosporine trough levels were maintained between 125 and 225 ng/mL (average dose 3.7 mg/kg/day) for a total of 6 months of therapy. Patients also received prednisone therapy, up to a maximum of 15 mg/day. Therapy was well tolerated with no patients discontinuing therapy. At the end of 6 months of therapy, 75% of the CSA-treated patients versus 22% of the control group had a remission in proteinuria. After 1 year, remission rates fell to 48% in the CSA-treated group and 13% of the placebo group. The overall rate of the change in renal function between the two groups was identical. Another trial from China randomized 30 patients to either CSA (initial dose of 5 mg/kg/day which was tapered after 3 months to 2 mg/kg/day and continued for a total of 15 months) or captopril (373). At the end of 15 months, 11 of 15 patients in the CSA-treated group were in either complete or partial remission as compared to 2 of 15 patients treated with captopril alone. In both trials there was a high rate of relapse (up to 50%) with longer follow-up after CSA withdrawal. Despite this, there remained a larger fraction of patients in remission after CSA treatment than with placebo.

Rostoker et al. performed an open-label study in patients with MN at high risk for progression (369). These patients had shown a progressive rise in serum creatinine before the initiation of therapy. Fifteen patients were treated with CSA to maintain a 12-hour trough level between 100 and 250 ng/mL. Four of the 15 patients showed no response to therapy and the drug was discontinued after 4 months. In the remaining 11 patients, CSA was continued for 6 months, followed by tapering over 6 months. In this group, four patients had a complete remission and seven had a partial remission. Nine patients discontinued CSA, and 33% had a relapse of their proteinuria that responded to reintroduction of the drug.

Another open-label study in patients at high-risk for progressive disease studied 41 patients with a mean urine protein excretion of 10.9 g/day (375). Patients received a mean CSA dose of 3.3 mg/kg/day for 1 year. At the end of therapy, 14 patients had entered a complete remission with a mean decrease in proteinuria of 6 g/day. In those patients who entered a complete remission, the mean treatment time before a response was seen was 225 days. There was only a small rise in serum creatinine (0.3 mg/dL) during the trial.

Only one randomized controlled trial has been performed in patients at high risk for progressive renal disease (372). Entry criteria for this trial included an absolute fall in creatinine clearance of 8 mL/minute or greater over a 4- to 12-month observation period. Furthermore, patients had persistent nephrotic-range proteinuria. Seventeen patients were selected for randomization to either CSA alone (trough level of 110 to 170 ng/mL) or placebo. Proteinuria fell in the treatment group by an average of 4.5 g/day as compared to a rise in proteinuria of 0.7 g/day in the placebo group. Most importantly, CSA therapy improved the average change in the slope of creatinine clearance versus time (from −2.4 mL/min/month prior to therapy to −0.7 mL/min/month with therapy). There was no change in the rate of decline in renal function in the placebo group. Importantly, the effects of CSA on improved renal function were maintained for up to 2 years after the medication was stopped.

In these trials, CSA therapy has been associated with transient increases in serum creatinine, hypertension, and gingival hyperplasia (368-375). Infectious complications were not seen and overall the medication has been well tolerated. The major drawback has been a relapse rate as high as 50% within 2 years of drug withdrawal (368–376). This may be minimized by extended therapy but further trials are needed. The mechanism by which CSA may decrease proteinuria and preserve renal function is unclear. The drug may act to decrease T cell–derived cytokine production as well as directly altering glomerular permeability to proteins through an unknown mechanism (376).

Alternative Therapies

Several alternative therapies have been studied in patients with MN. These are generally small, uncontrolled trials with short follow-up but have provided interesting results and point the direction for future therapies.

Intravenous immunoglobulin has been given in repeated doses to patients with severe MN (377,378). In these cases, both proteinuria and renal function has shown improvement. There are no reports of the long-term outcome of these patients.

Pentoxifylline, a phosphodiesterase inhibitor, was given to 10 patients with MN for 6 months and significantly reduced proteinuria from 11 to 1.8 g/day (379). Renal function remained stable in these patients. Pentoxifylline is an inhibitor of tumor necrosis factor-alpha (TNF-α) and plasma and urinary levels of TNF-α significantly fell in the treated patients (380). Whether pentoxifylline may serve as a useful adjunct to cytotoxic or CSA therapy has not been studied.

Based upon the experimental data demonstrating the importance of B cell activation and immunoglobulin production in the pathogenesis of MN, a monoclonal antibody that targets the B cell surface antigen CD20 has been employed in the treatment of patients with MN (381–383). Eight patients with MN and persistent nephrotic-range proteinuria were treated with four weekly infusions of the anti-CD20 monoclonal antibody rituximab. Two patients entered complete remission and three patients had a partial remission. In all patients, there was a substantial fall in urinary protein excretion with the mean protein excretion falling from 8.6 to 3.0 g/day at 1 year of follow-up. Renal function remained stable in all patients. The drug was well tolerated with no major adverse events during the trial. This therapy, which may specifically target autoreactive B cell clones, holds great promise for a disease-specific therapy that may have minimal long-term side effects. Obviously, larger randomized controlled trials with extended periods of follow-up are needed.

Future therapies are being developed that target the immune system. Eculizumab is a humanized C5 complement inhibitor that prevents the cleavage of C5 into its proinflammatory components (385). It has undergone phase II testing in patients with membranous nephropathy and 12 months of therapy with the agent resulted in an increased remission rate (386). Future clinical trials with this agent are anticipated.

Other targets for therapy include the induction of immune tolerance, modulation of inflammatory mediators (such as anti-TNF-α therapy with infliximab), blockade of co-stimulation (with anti-CD40L or CTLA4-Ig) or blockade of mechanism that lead to progressive glomerular scarring and tubulointerstitial injury (384).

Treatment Recommendations

In recent years the treatment of autoimmune diseases has undergone a revolution and new therapies that specifically target the molecular pathways involved in inflammation and immunologic regulation have become available (385). In MN, where immune complex localization to the subepithelial region of the glomerulus leads to complement activation and subsequent damage to the glomerular basement membrane and epithelial cell, therapies that intervene in the various steps in the process could be envisioned. Such therapies are being developed but have not been subject to human trials. Thus, current treatment of MN relies on nonspecific antiproteinuric strategies as well as global immunosuppression. Most clinicians reserve treatment with cytotoxic agents to those patients at greatest risk for progressive renal disease. Thus, patients with persistent high-grade proteinuria and/or worsening renal function should receive steroids and cytotoxic therapy. In those patients who do not respond to therapy or who are intolerant these drugs, cyclosporine and MMF are additional options. In the future, therapies that directly target the pathogenic mechanisms involved in glomerular injury will hopefully be available.

References

1. Braden Gl, et al. Changing incidence of glomerular diseases in adults. *Am J Kidney Dis* 2000;35:878.
2. Yamagata K. A long-term follow-up study of asymptomatic hematuria and/or proteinuria in adults. *Clin Nephrol* 1996;45:281.
3. Haas M. Changing etiologies of unexplained adult nephrotic syndrome: a comparison of renal biopsy findings from 1976–1979 and 1995–1997. *Am J Kidney Dis* 1997;30:621.
4. Preston RA, et al. Renal biopsy in patients 65 years of age or older: an analysis of the results of 334 biopsies. *J Am Geriatr Soc* 1990;38:669.
5. Ehrenreich T, Churg J. Pathology of membranous nephropathy. *Pathol Annu* 1968;3:145.
6. Movat H, McGregor D. The fine structure of the glomerulus in membranous glomerulonephritis (lipoid nephritis) in adults. *Am J Clin Pathol* 1959;32:109.
7. Heptinstall RH. *Pathology of the kidney*, 2nd ed. Boston: Little, Brown; 1974.
8. Abrass C, Couser W. Pathogenesis of membranous nephropathy. *Annu Rev Med* 1998;39:517.
9. Row P, et al. Membranous nephropathy: long-term follow-up and association with neoplasia. *Q J Med* 1975;44:215.
10. Murphy B, Fairley K, Kincaid-Smith P. Idiopathic membranous glomerulonephritis: Long-term follow-up in 139 cases. *Clin Nephrol* 1988;30:175.
11. Heymann W, et al. Production of the nephrotic syndrome in rats by Freund's adjuvants and rat kidney suspensions. *Proc Soc Exp Biol Med* 1959;100:660.
12. Couser W, Stilmant M, Darby C. Autologous immune complex nephropathy I: Sequential study of immune complex deposition, ultrastructural changes, proteinuria and alterations in glomerular sialoprotein. *Lab Invest* 1976;34:23.
13. Van Damme B, et al. Experimental glomerulonephritis in the rat induced by antibodies directed against tubular antigens IV: Fixed glomerular antigens in the pathogenesis of heterologous immune complex glomerulonephritis. *Lab Invest* 1978;38:502.
14. Couser W, et al. Experimental glomerulonephritis in the isolated perfused rat kidney. *J Clin Invest* 1978;62:1275.
15. Cavallo T. Membranous nephropathy: Insights for Heymann nephritis. *Am J Pathol* 1994;144:651.
16. Debiec H, et al. Antenatal membranous glomerulonephritis from maternal anti-neutral endopeptidase antibodies. *N Engl J Med* 2002;346:2053.
17. Couser W, Salant D. In situ immune complex formation and glomerular injury. *Kidney Int* 1980;17:1.
18. Couser W. In situ formation of immune complexes and the role of complement activation in glomerulonephritis. *Clin Immunol Allergy* 1986;6:267.
19. Couser W, Baker P, Adler S. Complement and the direct mediation of immune glomerular injury. *Kidney Int* 1985;28:879.

20. Adler S, et al. Mediation of proteinuria in membranous nephropathy due to a planted glomerular antigen. *Kidney Int* 1983;23:807.
21. Perkinson DT, et al. Membrane attack complex deposition in experimental glomerular injury. *Am J Pathol* 1985;120:1221.
22. Wehrmann M, et al. Long-term prognosis of idiopathic membranous glomerulonephritis: an analysis of 334 cases with regard to tubulo-interstitial changes. *Clin Nephol* 1989;31:67.
23. Donadio J, et al. Idiopathic membranous nephropathy: The natural history of untreated patients. *Kidney Int* 1988;33:708.
24. Schieppati A, et al. Prognosis of untreated patients with idiopathic membranous nephropathy. *N Engl J Med* 1993;329:85.
25. United States Renal Data System. Annual data report 2003. http://www.usrds.org.
26. Orth SR, Ritz E. The nephrotic syndrome. *N Engl J Med* 1998;338:1202.
27. Couser WG, Alpers CE. Membranous nephropathy. In: Neilson EG, Couser WG, eds. *Immunologic renal diseases,* 2nd ed. Philadelphia, PA: Lippincott Williams and Wilkins; 2001:1029.
28. Gluck MC, et al. Membranous glomerulonephritis: evolution of clinical and pathologic features. *Ann Intern Med* 1973;78:1.
29. Cattran DC. Idiopathic membranous glomerulonephritis. *Kidney Int* 2001;59:1983.
30. Johnson RJ, Couser WG. Hepatitis B infection and renal disease: Clinical, immunopathogenetic, and therapeutic considerations. *Kidney Int* 1990;37:663.
31. Southwest Pediatric Nephrology Study Group: Hepatitis B surface antigenemia in North American children with membranous glomerulonephropathy. *J Pediatr* 1985;106:571.
32. Lee J, Yamauchi H, Hopper JJ. The association of cancer and nephrotic syndrome. *Ann Intern Med* 1966;64:41.
33. Burstein DM, Korbet SM, Schwartz MM. Membranous glomerulonephritis and malignancy. *Am J Kidney Dis* 1993;22:5.
34. Coggins C, Frommer J, Glassock R. Membranous nephropathy. *Semin Nephrol* 1982;2:264.
35. Briganti EM, et al. The incidence of biopsy proven glomerulonephritis in Australia. *Nephrol Dial Transplant* 2001;16:1364.
36. Short C, Mallick NP. Membranous nephropathy. In: Schrier RW, ed. *Diseases of the kidney,* 7th ed. Philadelphia: Lippincott Williams and Wilkins; 2001:1743.
37. Glassock RJ. Diagnosis and natural course of membranous nephropathy. *Semin Nephrol* 2003;23:324.
38. Abe S. Idiopathic membranous glomerulonephritis: aspects of geographical differences. *J Clin Pathol* 1986;39:1193.
39. Hattori S, Furuse A, Matsuda I. Presence of HB e antibody in glomerular deposits in membranous glomerulonephritis is associated with hepatitis B infection. *Am J Nephrol* 1988;8:384.
40. Hirose H, et al. Deposition of HB e antigen in membranous glomerulonephritis: identification by F (abl)2 fragments of monoclonal antibody. *Kidney Int* 1984;26:338.
41. Ito H, et al. Hepatitis B e antigen-mediated membranous glomerulonephritis: correlation of ultrastructural changes with HBeAg in the serum and glomeruli. *Lab Invest* 1981;44:214.
42. Schwartz MM. Nephrotic syndrome and proteinuria. In: Silva FG, D'Agati VD, Nadasdy T, eds. *Renal biopsy interpretation.* New York: Churchill Livingstone; 1996:115.
43. Jennette JC, Iskandar SS, Dalldorf FG. Pathologic differentiation between lupus and non-lupus membranous glomerulopathy. *Kidney Int* 1983;24:377.
44. Austin HC, et al. Prognostic factors in lupus nephritis: contribution of renal histologic data. *Am J Med* 1983;75:382.
45. Baldwin DS, et al. Lupus nephritis: clinical course as related to morphologic forms and their transitions. *Am J Med* 1977;62:12.
46. Balow JE, Austin HA. Therapy of membranous nephropathy in systemic lupus erythematosus. *Semin Nephrol* 2003;23:386.
47. Adler SG, et al. Lupus membranous glomerulonephritis: different prognostic subgroups obscured by imprecise histologic classifications. *Mod Pathol* 1990;3:186.
48. Pasquali S, et al. Lupus membranous nephropathy: long-term outcome. *Clin Nephrol* 1993;39:175.
49. Korbet SM. Membranous lupus glomerulonephritis. In: Lewis EJ, Schwartz MM, Korbet SM, eds. *Lupus nephritis.* Oxford: Oxford University Press; 1999:219.
50. Huong DL, et al. Renal involvement in systemic lupus erythematosus: A study of 180 patients from a single center. *Medicine (Baltimore)* 1999;78:148.
51. Shearn MA, Hopper J Jr, Biava GG. Membranous lupus nephropathy initially seen as idiopathic membranous nephropathy. *Arch Intern Med* 1980;140:1521.
52. Adu D, et al. Late onset systemic lupus erythematosus and lupus-like disease in patients with apparent idiopathic glomerulonephritis. *QJM* 1983;52:471.
53. Bakir AA, Levy PS, Dunea G. The prognosis of lupus nephritis in African-Americans: A retrospective analysis. *Am J Kidney Dis* 1994;24:159.
54. Sloan RP, et al. Long-term outcome in systemic lupus erythematosus membranous glomerulonephritis. *J Am Soc Nephrol* 1996;7:299.
55. Bono LS, Cameron JS, Hicks JA. The very long-term prognosis and complications of lupus nephritis and its treatment. *QJM* 1999;92:211.
56. Appel GB, et al. Long-term follow-up of patients with lupus nephritis: A study based on the classification of the World Health Organization. *Am J Med* 1987;83:877.
57. Figueroa JE, Waxman J. Membranous nephropathy in rheumatoid arthritis. *South Med J* 1982;75:480.
58. Sellars L, et al. Renal biopsy appearances in rheumatoid disease. *Clin Nephrol* 1983;20:114.
59. Samuels B, et al. Membranous nephropathy in patients with rheumatoid arthritis: relationship to gold therapy. *Medicine (Baltimore)* 1978;57:319.
60. Lee JC, et al. Renal lesions associated with gold therapy: light and electron microscopic studies. *Arthritis Rheum* 1965;8:1.
61. Yoshida A, et al. Clinicopathological findings of bucillamine-induced nephrotic syndrome in patients with rheumatoid factor. *Am J Nephrol* 1991;11:284.
62. Ross JH, McGinty F, Brewer DG. Penicillamine nephropathy. *Nephron* 1980;26:184.
63. Hall CL, et al. Natural course of penicillamine nephropathy: a long-term study of 33 patients. *BMJ* 1988;296:1083.
64. Higuchi A, Suzuki Y, Okada T. Membranous glomerulonephritis in rheumatoid arthritis unassociated with gold or penicillamine treatment. *Ann Rheum Dis* 1987;46:488.
65. Ducret F, Pointet P, Pichot C. Membranous glomerulonephritis during rheumatoid arthritis: probably toxicity of diclofenac. *Nephrologie* 1984;5:135.
66. Campistol JM, et al. Reversible membranous nephritis associated with diclofenac. *Nephrol Dial Transplant* 1989;4:393.
67. Cahen R, et al. Fenoprofen induced membranous glomerulonephritis. *Nephrol Dial Transplant* 1988;3:705.
68. Radford MG Jr, et al. Reversible membranous nephropathy associated with the use of non-steroidal anti-inflammatory drugs. *JAMA* 1996;276:466.
69. Markowitz GS, et al. Membranous glomerulopathy and acute interstitial nephritis following treatment with celecoxib. *Clin Nephrol* 2003;59:137.
70. Freedman B, et al. HLA associations in end-stage renal disease due to membranous glomerulonephritis: HLA-DR3 associations with progressive renal injury. *Am J Kidney Dis* 1994;23:797.
71. Klouda P, et al. Strong association between idiopathic membranous nephropathy and HLA-DRW3. *Lancet* 1979;2:770.
72. Berthoux F, et al. Immunogenetics and immunopathology of human primary membranous glomerulonephritis: HLA-A, B, DR antigens: functional activity of splenic macrophage Fc-receptor and peripheral blood T-lymphocyte subpopulations. *Clin Nephrol* 1984;22:15.
73. Taylor RG, Fisher C, Hoffbrand BI. Sarcoidosis and membranous glomerulonephritis: a significant association. *BMJ* 1982;284:1297.
74. Khan IH, et al. Membranous nephropathy and granulomatous interstitial nephritis in sarcoidosis. *Nephron* 1994;66:459.
75. Jordan SC, Johnston WH, Bergstein JM. Immune complex glomerulonephritis mediated by thyroid antigens. *Arch Pathol Lab Med* 1978;102:530.
76. Becker BA, Fenves AZ, Breslau NA. Membranous glomerulonephritis associated with Graves' disease. *Am J Kidney Dis* 1999;33:369.
77. O'Loughlin EV, et al. Membranous glomerulonephritis in a patient with Crohn's disease of the small bowel. *J Pediatr Gastroenterol Nutr* 1985;4:135.
78. Witte AS, Burke JF. Membranous glomerulonephritis associated with chronic progressive demyelinating neuropathy. *Neurology* 1987;37:342.
79. Chen WY, et al. Membranous glomerulonephritis and myasthenia gravis. *Taiwan I Hseuh Hui Tsa Chih* 1980;79:667.
80. Campos A. et al. Membranous nephropathy associated with multiple sclerosis. *Pediatr Neurol* 1993;9:64.
81. Combes B, et al. Glomerulonephritis with deposition of Australian antigen-antibody complexes in glomerular basement membrane. *Lancet* 1971;2:234.
82. Hsu HC, et al. Membranous nephropathy in 52 hepatitis B surface antigen (HBsAg) carrier children in Taiwan. *Kidney Int* 1989;36:1103.
83. Bhimma R, et al. Characterization of proteinuria in asymptomatic family members and household contacts of children with hepatitis B virus-associated membranous nephropathy. *Am J Kidney Dis* 2001;37:125.
84. Lai Kn, et al. Membranous nephropathy related to hepatitis B virus in adults. *N Engl J Med* 1991;324:1457.
85. Jefferson JA, Couser WG. Therapy of membranous nephropathy associated with malignancy and secondary causes. *Semin Nephrol* 2003;23:400.
86. Lin CY. Treatment of hepatitis B virus-associated membranous nephropathy with recombinant alpha-interferon. *Kidney Int* 1995;47:225.
87. de Man RA, et al. Improvement of hepatitis B-associated glomerulonephritis after antiviral combination therapy. *J Hepatol* 1989;8:367.
88. Conjeevaram HS, et al. Long-term outcome of hepatitis B virus-related glomerulonephritis after therapy with interferon alpha. *Gastroenterology* 1995;109:540.
89. Lisker-Melman M, et al. Glomerulonephritis caused by chronic hepatitis B virus infection: Treatment with recombinant human alpha-interferon. *Ann Intern Med* 1989;111:479.
90. Ben-Ari Z, et al. An open-label study of lamivudine for chronic hepatitis B in six patients with chronic renal failure before and after kidney transplantation. *Am J Gastroenterol* 2000;95:3579.

91. Gumber SC, Chopra S. Hepatitis C: a multifaceted disease. Review of extrahepatic manifestations. *Ann Intern Med* 1995;123:615.

92. D'Amico G, Fornasieri A. Cryoglobulinemic glomerulonephritis: a membranoproliferative glomerulonephritis induced by hepatitis C virus. *Am J Kidney Dis* 1995;25:361.

93. Johnson R, et al. Renal manifestations of hepatitis C virus infection. *Kidney Int* 1994;46:1255.

94. Johnson RJ, et al. Membranoproliferative glomerulonephritis associated with hepatitis C virus infection (see comments). *N Engl J Med* 1993;328:465.

95. Rollino C, et al. Hepatitis C virus infection and membranous glomerulonephritis. *Nephron* 1991;59:319.

96. Davda R, et al. Membranous glomerulonephritis in association with hepatitis C virus infection. *Am J Kidney Dis* 1993;17:452.

97. Stehmann-Breen C, et al. Hepatitis C virus associated membranous glomerulonephritis. *Clin Nephrol* 1995;44:141.

98. Okada K, et al. Detection of hepatitis C virus core protein in the glomeruli of patients with membranous glomerulonephritis. *Clin Nephrol* 1996;45:71.

99. Jefferson JA, Johnson RJ. Treatment of hepatitis C-associated glomerular disease. *Semin Nephrol* 2000;20:286.

100. Kobayashi S, et al. Renal involvement in mixed connective tissue disease: report of 5 cases. *Am J Nephrol* 1985;5:282.

101. Rose JD. Membranous glomerulonephritis, dermatomyositis and bronchial carcinoma. *BMJ* 1979;2:641.

102. Botey A, Torras A, Reverl L. Membranous nephropathy in ankylosing spondylitis. *Nephron* 1981;29:203.

103. Lemmer JP, Irby WR. Coexistence of HLA-B27 ankylosing spondylitis and DR4 seropositive nodular rheumatoid arthritis in a patient with membranous nephropathy. *J Rheumatol* 1981;8:661.

104. Akikusa B, et al. Hashimoto's thyroiditis and membranous nephropathy developed in progressive systemic sclerosis (PSS). *Am J Clin Pathol* 1984;81:260.

105. Singhal PC, Scharschmidt LA. Membranous nephropathy associated with primary biliary cirrhosis and bullous pemphigoid. *Ann Allergy* 1985;55:484.

106. Bonet Sol J, et al. Sjögren's syndrome and membranous glomerulonephritis. *Rev Clin Esp* 1985;177:191.

107. Bloch KJ, et al. Sjögren's syndrome: a clinical, pathological and serological study of 62 cases. *Medicine (Baltimore)* 1965;44:187.

108. Truong L, et al. Temporal arteritis and renal disease: case report and review of the literature. *Am J Med* 1985;78:171.

109. Gamble CN, Reardon JB. Immunopathogenesis of syphilitic glomerulonephritis: elution of antitreponemal antibody from glomerular immune complex deposits. *N Engl J Med* 1975;292:499.

110. Losito A, et al. Membranous glomerulonephritis in congenital syphilis. *Clin Nephrol* 1979;12:32.

111. O'Regan S, et al. Treponemal antigens in congenital and acquired syphilitic nephritis. *Ann Intern Med* 1976;85:325.

112. Sanchez-Bayle M, et al. Incidence of glomerulonephritis in congenital syphilis. *Clin Nephrol* 1983;20:27.

113. Mattana J, et al. AIDS-associated membranous nephropathy with advanced renal failure: response to prednisone. *Am J Kidney Dis* 1997;30:116.

114. Hendrickise RG, Adeniyi A. Quartan malarial nephrotic syndrome in children. *Kidney Int* 1979;16:67.

115. Andrade ZA, Rocha H. Schistosomal glomerulopathy. *Kidney Int* 1979;16:23.

116. Ngu JL, et al. Nephropathy in Cameroon: evidence for filarial derived immune complex pathogenesis in some cases. *Clin Nephrol* 1985;24:128.

117. Iida H, et al. Membranous glomerulonephritis associated with enterococcal endocarditis. *Nephron* 1985:40:88.

118. Viatel P, et al. Membranous nephropathy associated with hydatid disease. *N Engl J Med* 1981;304:610.

119. Sanchez Ibarrola A, et al. Membranous glomerulonephritis secondary to hydatid disease. *Am J Med* 1981;70:311.

120. Shwe T. Immune complexes in glomeruli of patients with leprosy. *Lepr Rev* 1972;42:282.

121. Eagen JW. Glomerulopathies of neoplasia. *Kidney Int* 1977;11:297.

122. Cahen R, et al. Aetiology of membranous glomerulonephritis: A prospective study of 82 adult patients. *Nephrol Dial Transplant* 1989;4:172.

123. Zech P, et al. The nephrotic syndrome in adults over 60: etiology, evolution, and treatment of 76 cases. *Clin Nephrol* 1982;17:232.

124. Row PG, et al. Membranous nephropathy. Long-term follow-up and association with neoplasia. *QJM* 1975;44:207.

125. Yamauchi H, et al. Cure of membranous nephropathy after resection of carcinoma. *Arch Intern Med* 1985;145:2061.

126. Wadhwa NK, et al. Membranous glomerulonephritis in a patient with an adrenal ganglioneuroma. *Am J Kidney Dis* 2004;44:363.

127. Robinson WL, et al. Remission and exacerbation of tumor-related nephrotic syndrome with treatment of the neoplasm. *Cancer* 1984;54:1082.

128. Couser WG, et al. Glomerular deposition of tumor antigen in membranous nephropathy associated with colonic carcinoma. *Am J Med* 1974;57:962.

129. Costanza ME, et al. Carcinoembryonic antigen-antibody complexes in a patient with colonic carcinoma and nephrotic syndrome. *N Engl J Med* 289;520.

130. Pascal RR, Slovin SF. Tumor directed antibody and carcinoembryonic antigen in the glomeruli of a patient with gastric carcinoma. *Hum Pathol* 1980;11:69.

131. Lewis MG, Loughridge LW, Phillips TM. Immunological studies in nephrotic syndrome associated with extrarenal malignant disease. *Lancet* 1971;2:134.

132. Sawyer N, et al. Prevalence, concentration and prognostic importance of proteinuria in patients with malignancies. *Br Med J* 1988;296:1295.

133. Wakashin M, et al. Association of gastric cancer and nephrotic syndrome. An immunologic study in three patients. *Gastroenterology* 1980;78:749.

134. Da Costa CR, et al. Nephrotic syndrome in bronchogenic carcinoma: report of two cases with immunochemical studies. *Clin Nephrol* 1974;2:245.

135. Higgins MR, Randall RE Jr, Still WJ. Nephrotic syndrome with oat cell carcinoma. *BMJ* 1974;3:450.

136. Ducret F, et al. Membranous glomerulonephritis associated with esophageal carcinoma. *Praxis* 1981;70:519.

137. Barton CH, Vaziri ND, Spear GS. Nephrotic syndrome associated with adenocarcinoma of the breast. *Am J Med* 1980;68:308.

138. Kerpen HO, et al. Membranous nephropathy associated with renal cell carcinoma: evidence against a role of renal tubular or tumor antibodies in pathogenesis. *Am J Med* 1978;64:863.

139. Beauvais P, et al. Membranous nephropathy associated with ovarian tumor in a young girl, recovery after removal. *Eur J Pediatr* 1989;148:624.

140. Stuart K, Fallon BG, Cardi MA. Development of the nephrotic syndrome in a patient with prostate carcinoma. *Am J Med* 1986;80:295.

141. Borochovitz D, et al. Adenocarcinoma of the palate associated with nephrotic syndrome and epimembranous carcinoembryonic antigen deposits. *Cancer* 1982;49:2097.

142. Hotta O, et al. Membranous nephropathy associated with nodular sclerous Hodgkin's disease. *Nephron* 1993;63:347.

143. Rosenman E, et al. Atypical membranous glomerulonephritis with fibrillar subepithelial deposits in a patient with malignant lymphoma. *Nephron* 1988;48:226.

144. White CA, Dillman RO, Royston I. Membranous nephropathy associated with an unusual phenotype of chronic lymphocyte leukemia. *Cancer* 1983;52:2253.

145. Venzano C, et al. Nephrotic syndrome associated with pleural mesothelioma: an unusual paraneoplastic event. *Recenti Prog Med* 1990;81:325.

146. Weksler ME, et al. Nephrotic syndrome in malignant melanoma: demonstration of melanoma antigen-antibody complexes in kidney. *Kidney Int* 1974;6:112A.

147. Olson JL, et al. Malignant melanoma with renal dense deposits containing tumor antigens. *Clin Nephrol* 1979;12:74.

148. Lopez JA, et al. Tumor de Wilms asociado a una glomerulonefritis membranosa. *Arch Esp Urol* 1989;42:163.

149. Coma-del-Corral MJ, et al. Liver cell adenoma associated with membranous nephropathy. *Nephron* 1991;57:117.

150. Weisenburger DD. Membranous nephropathy: its association with multicentric angiofollicular lymph node hyperplasia. *Arch Pathol Lab Med* 1979;103:591.

151. Lai KN, et al. Membranous nephropathy associated with spinal schwannoma. *Pathology* 1991: 23:250.

152. Zheng HL, et al. Neuroblastoma presenting with the nephrotic syndrome. *J Pediatr Surg* 1979;14:414.

153. Lin J, et al. Membranous glomerulopathy associated with graft-versus host disease following allogeneic stem cell transplantation. Report of 2 cases and review of the literature. *Am J Nephrol* 2001;21:351.

154. Gartner HV, et al. Drug-associated nephropathy. Part I: glomerular lesions. *Curr Top Pathol* 1980;69:143.

155. Tornroth T, Skrivfars B. Gold nephropathy prototype of membranous glomerulonephritis. *Am J Pathol* 1974;75:573.

156. Bacon PA, et al. Penicillamine nephropathy in rheumatoid arthritis: a clinical, pathological and immunopathological study. *QJM* 1976;45:661.

157. Lachmann PJ. Nephrotic syndrome from penicillamine. *Postgrad Med J* 1968;44(Suppl):235.

158. Mathieson PW, et al. Coexistent membranous nephropathy and ANCA-positive glomerulonephritis in association with penicillamine. *Nephrol Dial Transplant* 1996;11:863.

159. Tubbs RR, et al. Membranous glomerulonephritis associated with industrial mercury exposure: study of pathogenetic mechanisms. *Am J Clin Pathol* 1982;77:409.

160. Textor SC, et al. Membranous glomerulopathy associated with captopril therapy. *Am J Med* 1983;74:705.

161. Hoorntje SJ, et al. Immune complex glomerulopathy in patients treated with captopril. *Lancet* 1980;1:1212.

162. Joyce DA, Beilin LJ, Vandongen R. Captopril induced nephrotic syndrome. *Med J Aust* 1981;1:190.

163. Sokol A, Bashner MH, Okun R. Nephrotic syndrome caused by probenecid. *JAMA* 1967;199:43.

164. Bar-Khayim Y, et al. Trimethadione-induced nephrotic syndrome: a report of a case with unique ultrastructural renal pathology. *Am J Med* 1973;54:272.

165. Tholl U, Anlauf M, Helmchen U. Clopidogrel and membranous nephropathy. *Lancet* 1999;354:1443.

166. Phan L, et al. Extramembranous glomerulonephritis induced by lithium. *Nephrologie* 1991;12:185.

167. Breyesse P, et al. Membranous nephropathy and formaldehyde exposure. *Ann Intern Med* 1994;120:396.
168. Ehrenreich T. Renal disease from exposure to solvents. *Ann Clin Lab Sci* 1977;7:6.
169. Venkateswara K, Crosson JT. Idiopathic membranous glomerulonephritis in diabetic patients: report of three cases and review of the literature. *Arch Intern Med* 1980;140:624.
170. Kobayashi K, et al. Idiopathic membranous glomerulonephritis associated with diabetes mellitus: light, immunofluorescence and electron microscopic study. *Nephron* 1981;28:163.
171. Kleinknecht C, et al. Membranous glomerulonephritis with extrarenal disorders in children. *Medicine (Baltimore)* 1979;58:219.
172. Saxena S, et al. Membranous glomerulonephritis associated with autosomal dominant polycystic kidney disease. *Nephron* 1993;62:316.
173. Rodriguez-Soriano J, et al. Juvenile cirrhosis and membranous glomerulonephritis in a child with alpha-1-antitrypsin deficiency. *Acta Paediatr Scand* 1978;67:793.
174. Dupont AG, Verbeelen DL, Six RO. Weber-Christian panniculitis with membranous glomerulonephritis. *Am J Med* 1983;75:527.
175. Reitsma D, Gratama S, Vroom TM. Clinical remission of membranous glomerulonephritis in primary biliary cirrhosis with cutaneous vasculitis. *BMJ* 1984;288:27.
176. Bindi D, et al. Membranous glomerulonephritis associated with primary biliary cirrhosis: a pathogenic role of anti-M2 antibodies? *Gastroenterol Clin Biol* 1993;17:142.
177. Lal SM, et al. Systemic mastocytosis associated with membranous nephropathy and peripheral neuropathy. *Am J Kidney Dis* 1988;12:538.
178. Talamo TS, Borochovits D. Membranous glomerulonephritis associated with the Guillain-Barré syndrome. *Am J Clin Pathol* 1982;78:563.
179. Haslitt J. Membranous glomerulopathy associated with Landry-Guillain-Barre syndrome. *Am J Kidney Dis* 1987;9:445.
180. Kobayashi S, et al. Membranous nephropathy associated with hypocomplementemic urticarial vasculitis: report of two cases and a review of the literature. *Nephron* 1994;66:1.
181. Dische FE, Cuilliford EJ, Parsons V. Haemolytic uraemic syndrome and idiopathic membranous glomerulonephritis. *BMJ* 1978;1: 1112.
182. Combs RC, Hazelrigg DW. Dermatitis herpetiformis and membranous glomerulonephritis. *Cutis* 1980;25:660.
183. Paydas S, et al. A case of membranous glomerulonephritis and myelodysplastic anemia. *Nephron* 1992;62:231.
184. Hariharan S, et al. Recurrent and de novo glomerular disease after renal transplantation: a report from Renal Allograft Disease Registry (RADR). *Transplantation* 1999;68:635.
185. Briganti EM, et al. Risk of renal allograft loss from recurrent glomerulonephritis. *N Engl J Med* 2002;347:103.
186. Hariharan S, et al. Recurrent and de novo renal diseases after transplantation: a report from the renal allograft disease registry. *Am J Kidney Dis* 1998;31:928.
187. Truong L, et al. De novo membranous glomerulopathy in renal allografts: a report of ten cases and review of the literature. *Am J Kidney Dis* 1989;14:131.
188. Davison AM, Johnson PA. Allograft membranous nephropathy. *Nephrol Dial Transplant* 1992;(Suppl 1):114.
189. Poduval RD, Josephson MA, Javaid B. Treatment of de novo and recurrent membranous nephropathy in renal transplant patients. *Semin Nephrol* 2003;23:392.
190. Monga G, et al. Membranous glomerulonephritis in transplanted kidneys: morphologic investigation on 256 renal allografts. *Mod Pathol* 1993;6:249.
191. Morales JM, et al. Membranous glomerulonephritis associated with hepatitis C virus infection in renal transplant patients. *Transplantation* 1997;63:1634.
192. Marcen R, et al. Membranous nephropathy: recurrence after kidney transplantation. *Nephrol Dial Transplant* 1996;11:1129.
193. Lieberthal W, et al. Rapid recurrence of membranous nephropathy in a related renal allograft. *Clin Nephrol* 1979;12:222.
194. Cosyns JP, et al. Recurrence of membranous nephropathy after renal transplantation: probability, outcome and risk factors. *Clin Nephrol* 1998;50:144.
195. Schwartz A, et al. Impact of de novo membranous glomerulonephritis on the clinical course after kidney transplantation. *Transplantation* 1994;58:650.
196. Cheigh JS, et al. Kidney transplant nephrotic syndrome: relationship between allograft histopathology and natural course. *Kidney Int* 1980;18:358.
197. Johnston PA, et al. Membranous allograft nephropathy: remission of nephrotic syndrome with pulsed methylprednisolone and high-dose alternate day steroids. *Transplantation* 1993;55:214.
198. Montagnino G, et al. Membranous nephropathy in cyclosporine-treated renal transplant recipients. *Transplantation* 1989;4:725.
199. Freedman BI, et al. The impact of different immunosuppressant regimens on recurrent glomerulonephritis. *Transplant Proc* 1989;1:2121.
200. Tornroth T, Skrifars B. The development and resolution of glomerular basement membrane damage associated with subepithelial immune deposits. *Am J Pathol* 1975;79:219.
201. Tornroth T, et al. Nonprogressive, histologically mild membranous glomerulonephritis appearing in all evolutionary phases as histologically "early" membranous glomerulonephritis. *Kidney Int* 1978;14:511.
202. Tornroth T, Honkanen E, Pettersson E. The evolution of membranous glomerulonephritis reconsidered: new insights from a study on relapsing disease. *Clin Nephrol* 1987;28:107.
203. Zucchelli P, et al. Clinical and morphologic evolution of idiopathic membranous nephropathy. *Clin Nephrol* 1986;25:282.
204. Jennette JC, Iskandar SS, Dalldorf FG. Pathologic differentiation between lupus and non-lupus membranous glomerulopathy. *Kidney Int* 1983;24:377.
205. Van Damme B, et al. Adhesions, focal sclerosis, protein crescents and capsular lesions in membranous glomerulopathy. *J Pathol* 1990;161:47.
206. Wakai S, Magil AB. Focal glomerulosclerosis in idiopathic membranous glomerulonephritis. *Kidney Int* 1992;41:428.
207. Couser WG, Johnson RJ. Mechanism of progressive renal disease in glomerulonephritis. *Am J Kidney Dis* 1994;46:1255.
208. Pichler R, et al. The pathogenesis of tubulointerstitial disease associated with glomerulonephritis: the glomerular cytokine theory. *Miner Electrolyte-Metab* 1995;21:317.
209. Ruggenenti P, et al. Chronic proteinuric nephropathies: outcomes and response to treatment in a prospective cohort of 352 patients with different patterns of renal injury. *Am J Kidney Dis* 2000;35:1155.
210. Gartner HV, et al. Correlations between morphologic and clinical features in idiopathic perimembranous glomerulonephritis: a study on 403 renal biopsies of 367 patients. *Curr Top Pathol* 1977;1.
211. Magil A. Tubulointerstitial lesions in human membranous glomerulonephritis: relationship to proteinuria. *Am J Kidney Dis* 1995;25:375.
212. Harrison DJ, Thomson D, MacDonald MK. Membranous glomerulonephritis. *J Clin Pathol* 1986;39:167.
213. Bannister KM, et al. Glomerular IgG subclass distribution in human glomerulonephritis. *Clin Nephrol* 1983;161.
214. Noel LH, et al. Glomerular and serum immunoglobulin G subclasses in membranous nephropathy and anti-glomerular basement membrane nephritis. *Clin Immunol Immunopathol* 1988;46:186.
215. Roberts JL, et al. Differential characteristics of immune-bound antibodies in diffuse proliferative and membranous forms of lupus glomerulonephritis. *Clin Immunol Immunopathol* 1983;29:223.
216. Schulze M, et al. Glomerular C3c localization indicates ongoing immune deposit formation and complement activation in experimental glomerulonephritis. *Am J Pathol* 1993;142:179.
217. Doi T, et al. Demonstration of C3d deposits in membranous nephropathy. *Nephron* 1984;37:323.
218. Couser W, Baker P, Adler S. Complement and the direct mediation of immune glomerular injury. *Kidney Int* 1985;28:879.
219. Bonsib SM. Segmental subepithelial deposits in primary glomerulonephritis: scanning electron microscopic examination of acellular glomeruli. *Hum Pathol* 1985;16:1115.
220. Honig C, et al. Mesangial electron-dense deposits in membranous nephropathy. *Lab Invest* 1980;42:427.
221. Cairns S, London A, Mallick N. Circulating immune complexes in idiopathic glomerular disease. *Kidney Int* 1982;21:507.
222. Vogt A. New aspects of the pathogenesis of immune complex glomerulonephritis. Formation of subepithelial deposits. *Clin Nephrol* 1984;21:15.
223. Oite T, et al. Quantitative studies of in-situ immune complex glomerulonephritis in the rat induced by planted cationized antigen. *J Exp Med* 1982;155:460.
224. Caulin-Glaser T, Gallo G, Lamm M. Non-dissociating cationic immune complexes can deposit in glomerular basement membrane. *J Exp Med* 1983;158:1561.
225. Couser WG. In situ formation of immune complexes and the role of complement activation in glomerulonephritis. *Clin Immunol Allergy* 1986;6:267.
226. Kerjaschki D, Miettinen A, Farquhar MG. Initial events in the formation of immune deposits in passive Heymann nephritis: gp-330-anti-gp-330 immune complexes form in epithelial coated pits and rapidly become attached to the glomerular basement membrane. *J Exp Med* 1987;166:109.
227. Sugisaki T, et al. Passive transfer of Heymann nephritis with serum. *Kidney Int* 1973;3:66.
228. Barabas AZ, Lannigan R. Induction of an autologous immune complex glomerulonephritis in the rat by intravenous injection of heterologous anti-rat tubular antibody. *Br J Exp Pathol* 1974;55:4y.
229. Makker SP, Moorthy B. In situ immune complex formation in isolated perfused kidney using homologous antibody. *Lab Invest* 1981;44:1.
230. Farquhar M, et al. The Heymann nephritis antigenic complex: Megalin (gp330) and RAP. *J Am Soc Nephrol* 1995;6:35.
231. Kerjaschki D, Farquhar M. The pathogenic antigen of Heymann nephritis is a membrane glycoprotein of the renal proximal tubule brush border. *Proc Natl Acad Sci* 1982;79:5557.
232. Kerjaschki D, Farquhar M. Immunocytochemical localization of the Heymann nephritis antigen (gp330) in glomerular epithelial cells of normal Lewis rats. *J Exp Med* 1983;157:667.
233. Farquhar ML. The unfolding story of megalin (gp330): now recognized as a drug receptor. *J Clin Invest* 1995;96:1404.
234. Orlando R, Kerjaschki D, Farquhar M. Megalin (gp330) possess antigenic epitopes capable of inducing passive Heymann nephritis independent of the nephritogenic epitope in RAP. *J Am Soc Nephrol* 1995;6:61.
235. Camussi G, et al. Antibody-induced redistribution of Heymann antigen on the surface of cultured visceral epithelial cells: possible role in the pathogenesis of Heymann glomerulonephritis. *J Immunol* 1985;135:2409.

236. Kerjaschki D, et al. Identification of a 400-kD protein in the brush borders of human kidney tubules that is similar to gp330, the nephritogenic antigen of rat Heymann nephritis. Am J Pathol 1987;129:183.
237. Debiec H, et al. Antenatal membranous glomerulonephritis with vascular injury induced by anti-neutral endopeptidase antibodies: toward new concepts in the pathogenesis of glomerular diseases. J Am Soc Nephrol 2003;14:S27.
238. Salant D, et al. A new role for complement in experimental membranous nephropathy in rats. J Clin Invest 1980;66:1339.
239. Susani M, et al. Antibodies to glycolipids activate complement and promote proteinuria in passive Heymann nephritis. Am J Pathol 1994;144:807.
240. Adler S, et al. Mediation of proteinuria in membranous nephropathy due to a planted glomerular antigen. Kidney Int 1983;23:807.
241. Baker P, et al. Depletion of C6 prevents development of proteinuria in experimental membranous nephropathy in rats. Am J Pathol 1989;135:185.
242. Couser WG, et al. Depletion of C6 reduces proteinuria in a model of membranous nephropathy induced with a non-glomerular antigen. J Am Soc Nephrol 1991;2:894.
243. Savin V, Johnson R, Couser W. C5b-9 increases albumin permeability of isolated glomeruli in vitro. Kidney Int 1994;46:382.
244. Schiller B, et al. Inhibition of complement regulation is key to the pathogenesis of active Heymann nephritis. J Exp Med 1998;188:1353.
245. Perkinson DT, et al. Membrane attack complex deposition in experimental glomerular injury. Am J Pathol 1985;120:121.
246. Falk R, et al. Localization of S protein and its relationship to the membrane attack complex of complement in renal tissue. Am J Pathol 1987;127:182.
247. Adler S, et al. Presence of terminal complement components in complement-dependent experimental glomerulonephritis. Kidney Int 1984;26:830.
248. Kerjaschki D, et al. Transcellular transport and membrane insertion of the C5b-9 membrane attack complex of complement by glomerular epithelial cells in experimental membranous nephropathy. J Immunol 1989;143:546.
249. Schulze M, et al. Increased urinary excretion of C5b-9 distinguished passive Heymann nephritis in the rat. Kidney Int 1989;35:60.
250. Schulze M, et al. Elevated urinary excretion of the C5b-9 complex in membranous nephropathy. Kidney Int 1991;40:533.
251. Brenchley P, et al. Urinary C3dg and C5b-9 indicate active immune disease in human membranous nephropathy. Kidney Int 1992;41:933.
252. Kon S, et al. Urinary C5b-9 excretion and clinical course in idiopathic human membranous nephropathy. Kidney Int 1995;48:1953.
253. Morita YM, et al. Complement activation products in the urine from proteinuric patients. J Am Soc Nephrol 2000;11:700.
254. McMillan JI, et al. Characterization of a glomerular epithelial cell metalloproteinase as matrix metalloproteinase-9 with enhanced expression in a model of membranous nephropathy. J Clin Invest 1996;1094.
255. Shankland S, et al. Differential expression of transforming growth factor-beta isoforms and receptors in experimental membranous nephropathy. Kidney Int 1996;50:116.
256. Cybulsky AV, et al. Complement C5b-9 activates phospholipase in glomerular epithelial cells. Am J Physiol (Renal Fluid Electrolyte Physiol) 1989;257:F826.
257. Peng H, et al. Complement activates the c-Jun N-terminal kinase/stress-activated protein kinase in glomerular epithelial cells. J Immunol 2002;169:2594.
258. Neale TJ, et al. Reaction oxygen species and neutrophil respiratory burst cytochrome b558 are produced by kidney glomerular cells in passive Heymann nephritis. Proc Natl Acad Sci USA 1993;90:3645.
259. Kim TS, et al. mRNA expression of glomerular basement membrane proteins and TGF-beta1 in human membranous nephropathy. J Pathol 1999;189:425.
260. Saran AM, et al. Complement mediates nephrin redistribution and actin dissociation in experimental membranous nephropathy. Kidney Int 2003;64:2072.
261. Ruotsalainen V, et al. Nephrin is specifically located at the slit diaphragm of glomerular podocytes. Proc Natl Acad Sci USA 1999;96:7962.
262. Schwartz K, et al. Podocin, a raft-associated component of the glomerular slit diaphragm, interacts with CD2AP and nephrin. J Clin Invest 2001;108:1621.
263. Yuan H, Takeuchi E, Salant DJ. The podocyte slit-diaphragm protein nephrin is linked to the actin cytoskeleton. Am J Physiol Renal Physiol 2002;282:F585.
264. Erdos EG, Skidgel RA. Neutral endopeptidase 24.11 (enkephalinase) and related regulators of peptide hormones. FASEB J 1989;3:145.
265. Gartner H, et al. Comparison of clinical and morphological features of peri-(epi-extra) membranous glomerulonephritis. Nephron 1974;13:288.
266. Glassock RJ. Diagnosis and natural course of membranous nephropathy. Semin Nephrol 2003;23:324.
267. Glassock RJ. Secondary membranous glomerulonephritis. Nephol Dial Transplant 1992;7:64.
268. Noel LH, et al. Long-term prognosis of idiopathic membranous glomerulonephritis. Am J Med 1979;66:82.
269. Ramzy MH, et al. The long-term prognosis of idiopathic membranous nephropathy. Clin Nephrol 1981;16:13.
270. Kida H, et al. Long-term prognosis of membranous nephropathy. Clin Nephrol 1986;25:64.
271. Velasquez FF, et al. Idiopathic nephrotic syndrome of the adult with asymptomatic thrombosis of the renal vein. Am J Nephrol 1988;8:457.
272. Llach F. Hypercoagulability, renal vein thrombosis, and other complications of the nephrotic syndrome. Kidney Int 1985;28:429.
273. Wagoner RD, et al. Renal vein thrombosis in idiopathic membranous glomerulopathy and nephrotic syndrome: Incidence and significance. Kidney Int 1983;23:368.
274. Llach F, Papper S, Massry SG. The clinical spectrum of renal vein thrombosis: Acute and chronic. Am J Med 1980;69:819.
275. Kafner A. Coagulation factors in nephrotic syndrome. Am J Nephrol 1990;10(Suppl):S63.
276. Kaufman RH, et al. Acquired antithrombin III deficiency and thrombosis in the nephrotic syndrome. Am J Med 1978;65:607.
277. McLean JW, et al. cDNA sequence of human apolipoprotein (a) is homologous to plasminogen. Nature 1987;300:132.
278. Llach F, ed. Renal vein thrombosis. Mount Kisco, NY: Futura Publishing; 1983.
279. Trew P, et al. Renal vein thrombosis in membranous glomerulonephropathy: incidence and association. Medicine 1978;57:69.
280. Llach F, Arieff A, Massry S. Renal vein thrombosis and nephrotic syndrome: a prospective study of 36 adult patients. Ann Intern Med 1975;83:8.
281. Pettersson E, Tornroth T, Miettinen A. Simultaneous anti-glomerular basement membrane and membranous glomerulonephritis: case report and literature review. Clin Immunol Immunopathol 1984;31:171.
282. Klassen J, et al. Evolution of membranous nephropathy into anti-glomerular basement membrane glomerulonephritis. N Engl J Med 1974;1340.
283. Moorthy AV, et al. Association of crescentic glomerulonephritis with membranous glomerulonephropathy: A report of three cases. Clin Nephrol 1976;6:319.
284. Koethe JD, et al. Progression of membranous nephropathy to acute crescentic rapidly progressive glomerulonephritis and response to pulse methylprednisolone. Am J Nephrol 1986;6:224.
285. Pasternack A, Tornroth T, Linder E. Evidence of both anti-GBM and immune complex mediated pathogenesis in the initial phase of Goodpasture's syndrome. Clin Nephrol 1978;9:77.
286. Bernard D. Extrarenal complications of the nephrotic syndrome. Kidney Int 1988;33:1184.
287. Radhakrishnan J, et al. The nephrotic syndrome, lipids and risk factors for cardiovascular disease. Am J Kidney Dis 1993;22:135.
288. Appel GB, et al. The hyperlipidemia of the nephrotic syndrome. Relation to plasma albumin, oncotic pressure and viscosity. N Engl J Med 1985;312:1544.
289. Wanner C, et al. Elevated plasma lipoprotein (a) in patients with the nephrotic syndrome. Ann Intern Med 1993;119:263.
290. De Sain-van der Velden MG, et al. Evidence for increased synthesis of lipoprotein (a) in the nephrotic syndrome. J Am Soc Nephrol 1998;9:1474.
291. Coupes B, et al. Temporal relationship between urinary C5b-9 and C3dg and clinical parameters in human membranous nephropathy. Nephrol Dial Transplant 1993;8:397.
292. Montinaro V, et al. Renal C3 synthesis in idiopathic membranous nephropathy: correlation to urinary C5b-9 excretion. Kidney Int 2000;57:137.
293. Mallick N, Short C, Manos J. Clinical membranous nephropathy. Nephron 1983;34:209.
294. Hopper JJ, Trew P, Biava C. Membranous nephropathy: its relative benignity in women. Nephron 1981;29:18.
295. Honkanen E. Survival in idiopathic membranous glomerulonephritis. Clin Nephrol 1986;25:122.
296. Erwin D, Donadio JJ, Holley KE. The clinical course of idiopathic membranous nephropathy. Mayo Clin Proc 1973;48:697.
297. Cattran DC. Idiopathic membranous glomerulonephritis. Kidney Int 2001;59:1983.
298. Troyanov SW, Cattran DC. Natural history of patients with idiopathic membranous nephropathy who never become nephrotic. J Am Soc Nephrol 2003;14:287A.
299. Cattran DC. Outcomes research in glomerulonephritis. Semin Nephrol 2003;23:340.
300. Marx BE, Marx M. Prediction in idiopathic membranous nephropathy. Kidney Int 1999;56:666.
301. Tu WH, et al. Membranous nephropathy: predictors of terminal renal failure. Nephron 1984;36:118.
302. MacTier R, et al. The natural history of membranous nephropathy in the West of Scotland. Q J Med 1986;60:793.
303. Geddes CC, Cattran DC. The treatment of idiopathic membranous nephropathy. Semin Nephrol 2000;20:299.
304. Pei Y, Cattran C, Greenwood C. Predicting chronic renal insufficiency in idiopathic membranous glomerulonephritis. Kidney Int 1992;42:960.
305. Cattran DC, et al. Validation of a predictive model of idiopathic membranous nephropathy: its clinical and research implications. Kidney Int 1997;51:901.
306. Schieppati A, et al. Nonimmunosuppressive therapy of membranous nephropathy. Semin Nephrol 2003;23:333.
307. Remuzzi G, Bertani T. Pathophysiology of progressive nephropathies. N Engl J Med 1998;339:1448.

308. Taal MW, Brenner BM. Renoprotective benefits of RAS inhibition: from ACEI to angiotensin II antagonists. *Kidney Int* 2000;57:1803.
309. DeZeeuw D, et al. Mechanism of the antiproteinuric effect of angiotensin-converting enzyme inhibition. *Contrib Nephrol* 1990;83:160.
310. Gansevoort RT, deZeeuw D, de Jong PE. Long-term benefits of the antiproteinuric effect of angiotensin-converting enzyme inhibition in nondiabetic renal disease. *Am J Kidney Dis* 1993;22:202.
311. Lewis EJ, et al. The effect of angiotensin-converting enzyme inhibition on diabetic nephropathy. *N Engl J Med* 1993;329:1456.
312. Ruggenenti P, et al. ACE inhibition improves glomerular size selectivity in patients with idiopathic membranous nephropathy and persistent nephrotic syndrome. *Am J Kidney Dis* 2000;35:381.
313. Thomas D, et al. Enalapril treats the proteinuria of membranous glomerulonephritis without detriment to systemic or renal hemodynamics. *Am J Kidney Dis* 1991;18:38.
314. Campbell R, et al. Effects of combined ACE inhibitor and angiotensin II antagonist treatment in human chronic nephropathies. *Kidney Int* 2003;63:1094.
315. Nakao N, et al. Combination treatment of angiotensin-II receptor blocker and angiotensin-converting-enzyme inhibitor in non-diabetic renal disease (COOPERATE): a randomized controlled trial. *Lancet* 2003;361:117.
316. Chrysostomou A, Becker G. Spironolactone in addition to ACE inhibitors to reduce proteinuria in patients with chronic renal disease. *N Engl J Med* 2001;345:925.
317. Neugarten J, Kozin A, Cook K. Effect of indomethacin on glomerular permselectivity and hemodynamics in nephrotoxic serum nephritis. *Kidney Int* 1989;36:51.
318. Golbetz H, et al. Mechanism of the antiproteinuric effect of indomethacin in nephrotic humans. *Am J Physiol* 1989;256:F44.
319. Remuzzi A, Remuzzi G. The effects of nonsteroidal anti-inflammatory drugs on glomerular filtration of proteins and their therapeutic utility. *Semin Nephrol* 1995;15:236.
320. Pisoni R, et al. Effect of high dose ramipril with or without indomethacin on glomerular selectivity. *Kidney Int* 2002;62:1010.
321. Nickolas TL, Radhakrishnan J, Appel GB. Hyperlipidemia and thrombotic complications in patients with membranous nephropathy. *Semin Nephrol* 2003;23:406.
322. Ordonez JD, et al. The increased risk of coronary heart disease associated with nephrotic syndrome. *Kidney Int* 1993;44:638.
323. Mantarri M, et al. Effects of hypertension and dyslipidemia on the decline in renal function. *Hypertension* 1995;26:670.
324. Kamanna VS, Roh DD, Kirschenbaum MA. Atherogenic lipoproteins: mediators of glomerular injury. *Am J Nephol* 1993;13:1.
325. Samuelsson O, et al. Lipoprotein abnormalities are associated with increased rate of progression of human chronic renal insufficiency. *Nephrol Dial Transplant* 1997;12:1908.
326. Muntner P, et al. Plasma lipids and risk of developing renal dysfunction: The Atherosclerosis Risk in Communities Study. *Kidney Int* 2000;58:293.
327. Fried LF, Orchard TJ, Kasiske BL. Effect of lipid reduction on the progression of renal disease: a meta-analysis. *Kidney Int* 2001;59:260.
328. Massy ZA, et al. Lipid-lowering therapy in patients with renal disease. *Kidney Int* 1995;48:188.
329. Thomas ME, et al. Simvastatin therapy for hypercholesterolemic patients with nephrotic syndrome or significant proteinuria. *Kidney Int* 1993;44:1124.
330. Spitalewitz S, et al. Treatment of hyperlipidemia in the nephrotic syndrome: The effects of pravastatin therapy. *Am J Kidney Dis* 1993;22:143.
331. Valeri A, et al. Treatment of hyperlipidemia of the nephrotic syndrome: a controlled trial. *Am J Kidney Dis* 1986;8:388.
332. Knopp RH. Ezetimibe. *N Engl J Med* 1995;341:498.
333. Gagne C, et al. Efficacy and safety of ezetimibe added to ongoing statin therapy for treatment of patients with primary hypercholesterolemia. *Am J Cardiol* 2002;90:1084.
334. Third Report of the Expert Panel on Detection, Evaluation, and Treatment of High Blood Cholesterol in Adults (Adult Treatment Panel III) Full Report, www.nhlbi.nih.gov/guidelines/cholesterol/atp3_rpt.htm, 2004.
335. Sarasin FR, Schifferli JA. Prophylactic oral anticoagulation in nephrotic patients with idiopathic membranous nephropathy. *Kidney Int* 1994;45:578.
336. Black DA, Rose G, Brewer DB. Controlled trial of prednisone in adult patients with the nephrotic syndrome. *Br Med J* 1970;3:421.
337. Medical Research Council Working Party. Controlled trial of azathioprine and prednisone in chronic renal disease. *Br Med J* 1971;2:239.
338. Collaborative Study of the Adult Idiopathic Nephrotic Syndrome. A controlled study of short-term prednisone treatment in adults with membranous nephropathy. *N Engl J Med* 1979;301:1031.
339. Cameron JS, Healy MJR, Adu D. The Medical Research Council trial of short-term high-dose alternate-day prednisolone in idiopathic membranous nephropathy with nephrotic syndrome in adults. *QJM* 1990;74:133.
340. Cattran DC, et al. A randomized controlled trial of prednisone in patients with idiopathic membranous nephropathy. *N Engl J Med* 1989;320:210.
341. Bolton WK, et al. Therapy of the idiopathic nephrotic syndrome with alternate day steroids. *Am J Med* 1977;62:60.
342. Hogan SL, et al. A review of therapeutic studies of idiopathic membranous nephropathy. *Am J Kidney Dis* 1995;25:862.
343. Canadian Medical Association. Controlled trial of azathioprine in the nephrotic syndrome secondary to idiopathic membranous glomerulonephritis. *CMAJ* 1976;115:1209.
344. Lagrue G, et al. Traitement par le chlorambucil et l'azathioprine dans les glomerulonephrites primitives. *J Urol Nephrol* 1975;9:655.
345. Tiller DJ, et al. A prospective randomized trial in the use of cyclophosphamide, dipyridamole, and warfarin in membranous and mesangiocapillary glomerulonephritis. *Proc 8th Int Congr Nephrol* 1981;S7:345.
346. Donadio JV, et al. Controlled trial of cyclophosphamide in idiopathic membranous nephropathy. *Kidney Int* 1987;32:579.
347. Murphy BF, et al. Randomized controlled trial of cyclophosphamide, warfarin and dipyridamole in idiopathic membranous glomerulonephritis. *Clin Nephrol* 1992;37:229.
348. Shearman JD, et al. The effect of treatment with prednisolone or cyclophosphamide-warfarin-dipyridamole combination on the outcome of patients with membranous nephropathy. *Clin Nephrol* 1988;30:320.
349. Ponticelli C, et al. Controlled trial of methylprednisolone and chlorambucil in idiopathic membranous nephropathy. *N Engl J Med* 1984;310:946.
350. Ponticelli C, et al. A randomized trial of methylprednisolone and chlorambucil in idiopathic membranous nephropathy. *N Engl J Med* 1989l320:8.
351. Ponticelli C, et al. A 10-year follow-up of a randomized study with methylprednisolone and chlorambucil in membranous nephropathy. *Kidney Int* 1995;48:1600.
352. Ponticelli C, et al. Methylprednisolone plus chlorambucil as compared with methylprednisolone alone for the treatment of idiopathic membranous nephropathy. *N Engl J Med* 1992;327:599.
353. Ponticelli C, et al. A randomized study comparing methylprednisolone plus chlorambucil versus methylprednisolone plus cyclophosphamide in idiopathic membranous nephropathy. *J Am Soc Nephrol* 1998;9:444.
354. Williams PS, Bone JM. Immunosuppression can arrest progressive renal failure due to idiopathic membranous glomerulonephritis. *Nephrol Dial Transplant* 1989;43:181.
355. Jindal K, et al. Long-term benefits of therapy with cyclophosphamide and prednisone in patients membranous glomerulonephritis and impaired renal function. *Am J Kidney Dis* 1992;19:61.
356. West ML, et al. A controlled trial of cyclophosphamide in patients with membranous glomerulonephritis. *Kidney Int* 1987;32:579.
357. Falk RJ, et al. Treatment of progressive membranous glomerulopathy: A randomized trial comparing cyclophosphamide and corticosteroids with corticosteroids alone. *Ann Intern Med* 1992;116:438.
358. Reichert LJ, et al. Preserving renal function in patients with membranous nephropathy: daily oral chlorambucil compared with intermittent monthly pulses of cyclophosphamide. *Ann Intern Med* 1994;121:328.
359. Bruns FJ, et al. Sustained remission of membranous glomerulonephritis after cyclophosphamide and prednisone. *Ann Intern Med* 1991;114:725.
360. Branten AJ, et al. Oral cyclophosphamide versus chlorambucil in the treatment of patients with membranous nephropathy and renal insufficiency. *Q J Med* 1998;91:359.
361. du Buf-Vereijken PW, Wetzels JF. Efficacy of a second course of immunosuppressive therapy in patients with membranous nephropathy and persistent or relapsing disease activity. *Nephrol Dial Transplant* 2004;19:2036.
362. Suki WN, Trimarchi H, Frommer JP. Relapsing membranous nephropathy. Response to therapy of relapses compared to that of the original disease. *Am J Nephrol* 1999;19:474.
363. Faedda R, et al. Immunosuppressive treatment of membranous glomerulonephritis. *J Nephrol* 1995;8:107.
364. Imperiale TF, Goldfarb S, Berns J. Are cytotoxic agents beneficial in idiopathic membranous nephropathy? A meta-analysis of the controlled trials. *J Am Soc Nephrol* 1995;5:1553.
365. Choi MJ, et al. Mycophenolate mofetil treatment for primary glomerular diseases. *Kidney Int* 2002;61:1098.
366. Miller G, et al. Use of mycophenolate mofetil in resistant membranous nephropathy. *Am J Kidney Dis* 2000: 36:250.
367. DeSanto NG, Capodicasa G, Giordano C. Treatment of idiopathic membranous nephropathy unresponsive to methylprednisolone and chlorambucil with cyclosporine. *Am J Nephrol* 1987;7:74.
368. Guasch A, et al. Short-term responsiveness of membranous nephropathy to cyclosporine. *Am J Kidney Dis* 1992;20:472.
369. Rostoker G, et al. Long-term cyclosporin A therapy for severe idiopathic membranous nephropathy. *Nephron* 1993;63:335.
370. Cattran DC, et al. A controlled trial of cyclosporine in patients with progressive membranous nephropathy. *Kidney Int* 1995;47:1130.
371. Cattran DC, et al. Cyclosporine in patients with steroid-resistant membranous nephropathy: a randomized trial. *Kidney Int* 2001;59:1484.
372. Radhakrishnan J, et al. Cyclosporine treatment of lupus membranous nephropathy. *Clin Nephrol* 1994;42:147.
373. Yao X, et al. Cyclosporin A treatment for idiopathic membranous nephropathy. *Chin Med J (Engl)* 2001;114:1305.
374. Fritsche L, et al. Treatment of membranous nephropathy with cyclosporine A: How much patience is required? *Nephrol Dial Transplant* 1999;14:1036.
375. Cattran DC. Mycophenolate mofetil and cyclosporine therapy in membranous nephropathy. *Semin Nephrol* 2003;23:272.
376. Ambalavanan S, et al. Mechanism of the antiproteinuric effect of cyclosporine in membranous nephropathy. *J Am Soc Nephrol* 1996;7:290.
377. Palla R, et al. Intravenous immunoglobulin therapy of membranous nephropathy: efficacy and safety. *Clin Nephrol* 1991: 35:98.
378. Yokoyama H, et al. The short- and long-term outcomes of membranous

nephropathy treated with intravenous immunoglobulin therapy. Kanazawa Study Group for Renal Diseases and Hypertension. *Nephrol Dial Transplant* 1999;14:2379.

379. Ducloux D, Bresson-Vautrin C, Chalopin JM. Use of pentoxifylline in membranous nephropathy. *Lancet* 2001;357:1672.

380. Waage A, Sorensen M, Stordal B. Differential effect of pentoxifylline on tumor necrosis factor and interleukin-6 production. *Lancet* 1990;335:543.

381. Johnson PW, Glennie MJ. Rituximab: mechanisms and applications *Br J Cancer* 2001;85:1619.

382. Remuzzi G, et al. Rituximab for idiopathic membranous nephropathy. *Lancet* 2002;360:923.

383. Ruggenenti P, et al. Rituximab in idiopathic membranous nephropathy: a one-year prospective study. *J Am Soc Nephrol* 2003;14:1851.

384. Kshirsagar AV, Nachman PH, Falk RJ. Alternative therapies and future intervention for treatment of membranous nephropathy. *Semin Nephrol* 2003;23:362.

385. Kaplan M. Eculizumab (Alexion). *Curr Opin Investig Drugs* 2002;3:1017.

386. http://www.alexionpharmaceuticals.com/products/index.cfm?pagename=nephritis

CHAPTER 64 ■ NEPHROTIC SYNDROME: MINIMAL CHANGE NEPHROPATHY, FOCAL SEGMENTAL GLOMERULOSCLEROSIS, AND COLLAPSING GLOMERULOPATHY

H. WILLIAM SCHNAPER, ALAN M. ROBSON, AND JEFFREY B. KOPP

The term *nephrotic syndrome* refers to a classic tetrad of proteinuria, hypoproteinemia, edema, and hyperlipidemia. Although a relationship among these findings was recognized as early as the 15th century, the term *nephrosis* first achieved widespread acceptance in the early part of the 20th century, when Volhard and Fahr employed it as one of the major divisions of bilateral kidney disease (1). Later developments, notably the advent of percutaneous renal biopsy, facilitated further delineation of the many forms of kidney disease that result in the nephrotic syndrome (2,3). We have divided these diseases into three general categories, as shown in Table 64-1: (a) primary nephrotic syndrome, in which the process that initiates proteinuria is not immediately apparent from histopathologic evaluation; (b) inflammatory glomerular lesions; and (c) glomerulopathy secondary to other diseases that affect the kidney. Regardless of the underlying cause, all of these diseases share a common denominator in that each involves proteinuria of sufficient severity to produce hypoproteinemia. Typically, when the serum albumin concentration falls below a critical level of approximately 2 g/dL, the other clinical features of the nephrotic syndrome appear.

An analysis of the diseases underlying nephrosis is complicated because studies have used varied definitions; different methods of acquiring patient populations; and groupings that reflect clinical, functional, or histologic criteria. Clearly, the relative frequency of different causes of nephrosis varies with age and has changed over time. The data in Table 64-1 were developed more than 25 years ago and indicated that approximately 80% of children with renal disease had primary nephrotic syndrome, as opposed to only 25% of adults. Chronic glomerulonephritis was responsible for about half of the cases of nephrotic syndrome in adults but only 10% to 15% of childhood cases. These glomerulonephritides may result from a systemic disease, such as systemic lupus erythematosus, or they may be idiopathic, such as in membranous nephropathy. The remaining cases of nephrotic syndrome were associated with diseases such as diabetes mellitus and amyloidosis. They accounted for up to 20% of adult cases but a very small percentage of childhood cases. This general pattern of causes for nephrotic syndrome is still observed in most industrial countries; additional causes are more likely to be seen in developing nations (4–8).

This chapter focuses on the group of diseases subsumed under the category of *primary nephrotic syndrome*. We employ this term to describe the clinical picture of nephrotic syndrome that occurs in the absence of evidence for glomerulonephritis or systemic disease that would be sufficient to account for massive proteinuria. Primary nephrotic syndrome includes patients who have been described as having *minimal change nephropathy* (MCN), also called lipoid nephrosis, "nil"

disease, idiopathic nephrotic syndrome of childhood, minimal change nephrotic syndrome (MCNS), or steroid-sensitive or steroid-responsive nephrotic syndrome. We have chosen to use MCN as the preferred term for this entity. We will reserve the alternate term, MCNS, for the clinical presentation in which MCN has caused the nephrotic syndrome. Nephrosis is not always present, particularly in adult patients (9,10). Although most pathologists require at least the presence of nephrotic-range proteinuria prior to treatment to make the diagnosis of MCN, occasional patients may lack edema, hypoalbuminemia, or hypercholesterolemia but have renal histology and ultrastructure that are otherwise typical. Furthermore, describing the lesion as a nephropathy offers a descriptor that is in parallel with the other forms of primary nephrotic syndrome, in that it is based upon the defined histopathology rather than a potentially variable clinical picture. Some patients with primary nephrotic syndrome have only a small amount of immunoglobulin M (IgM) deposited in the glomeruli, which usually is believed to be insignificant; some biopsy specimens reveal mild mesangial hypercellularity. These patients are considered to represent variants of MCN. A larger group of patients have significant extracellular matrix accumulation or glomerular capillary collapse. These patients are defined as having *focal segmental glomerulosclerosis* (FSGS), also called focal sclerosis and hyalinosis; and *collapsing glomerulopathy*, respectively. A spectrum of pathologic findings may be observed. Moreover, some patients, regardless of the underlying pathology, respond to treatment with corticosteroids; others with an apparently identical histologic lesion are resistant to steroid therapy.

Examination of the incidence of these diseases illustrates both the age-dependence of diagnoses and the changing nature of the underlying lesion. A large series of adults in Chicago is depicted in Table 64-2, in which was evaluated the renal biopsies of 1,000 consecutive patients who presented with the nephrotic syndrome. At this referral center, the relative incidence of different causes of nephrosis is changing, with significantly more FSGS and less MCN (10). Although this study could reflect some degree of referral bias, it is likely that these numbers approximate the general distribution of histologic diagnoses in nephrotic patients. The data for children shown in this table describe all children 0.5 to 19 years of age in the province of Ontario who were diagnosed as having nephrotic syndrome. In this group, the incidence of FSGS also is increasing. Consistent with the data shown in Table 64-1, the overall proportion of patients with primary nephrotic syndrome in children is greater than 90% (11) compared with 50% in the adult study. The increasing incidence of FSGS (more than doubled in both children and adults) is considered further in the section on Focal Segmental Glomerulosclerosis and Collapsing Glomerulopathy, later in this chapter.

TABLE 64-1

TYPES OF KIDNEY DISEASE CAUSING THE NEPHROTIC SYNDROME IN PEDIATRIC AND ADULT PATIENTS

	Relative incidence	
	Children	Adults
Primary nephrotic syndrome	79	24
Nephrotic syndrome associated with a glomerulopathy		
Chronic glomerulonephritis and systemic inflammatory disease	13	52
Secondary glomerulopathy	8	24

(Data derived from: International Study of Kidney Disease in Children. A controlled therapeutic trial of cyclophosphamide plus prednisone vs. prednisone alone in children with focal segmental glomerulonephritis. *Pediatr Res* 1980;14:1006; and Glassock RJ. The nephrotic syndrome. *Hosp Pract* 1979;14:105.)

In addition to the clinical observation that inflammation does not underlie the proteinuria of primary nephrotic syndrome, advances in our understanding of these disorders suggest that the origin of all these diseases resides in the specialized visceral epithelial cell of the glomerular filter—the podocyte. This cell contributes to the final barrier that determines the nature of the glomerular filtrate, and podocyte lesions appear to play a critical role in progressive forms of primary nephrotic syndrome. In Table 64-3 is shown a taxonomy of the primary podocyte diseases, grouped according to histologic characteristics. An analysis of the pathology, physiology, and genetics of these diseases, and insight derived from examining acquired causes of each lesion, was utilized in this categorization. Patients who show few or no glomerular abnormalities by use of light microscopy include those with classical MCN and its histologic variants, and patients with Finnish-type congenital nephrotic syndrome. A second group has diffuse mesangial sclerosis and represents mostly young children with congenital forms of nephrosis, frequently resulting from a single gene mutation. The third category, FSGS, represents an entity the incidence of which is rising rapidly throughout the world. We have chosen to define a fourth group: patients with collapsing glomerulopathy. Although this diagnosis previously has been thought to be a part of FSGS, the histo-

logic appearance and clinical course strongly suggest that it represents a distinct lesion. Further details regarding the definition of the categories in this table will be provided in this chapter.

It is important to note that the nephrotic syndrome has many physiologic consequences that are not limited to the classic tetrad of proteinuria, hypoalbuminemia, edema, and hyperlipidemia. These include abnormalities of electrolyte balance, coagulation, hormonal function, and immunity. This chapter reviews the mechanisms underlying these manifestations of nephrosis, our understanding of the pathogenesis of different forms of primary nephrotic syndrome, and the clinical features and management of patients with this entity.

PATHOPHYSIOLOGY OF THE NEPHROTIC SYNDROME

Virtually every abnormality observed in primary nephrotic syndrome can be traced directly or indirectly to the urinary loss of protein. Thus, the mechanisms responsible for this proteinuria have systemic consequences that are manifested in the clinical signs and symptoms of nephrosis.

TABLE 64-2

CHANGING ETIOLOGIES OF NEPHROTIC SYNDROME

	Percentage of total sample			
	Children[a]		Adults[b]	
Diagnosis	1985–1993	1993–2002	1976–1979	1995–1997
Minimal change nephropathy	81[c]	65[c]	23	15
Diffuse mesangial hypercellularity	3	7	—	—
Focal segmental glomerulosclerosis	11	25	15	35
Membranous nephropathy	1	2	36	33
Membranoproliferative glomerulonephritis	1	0	6	2
Chronic glomerulonephritis	—	—	5	<1
IgA Nephropathy	—	—	3	9
Amyloid Nephropathy	0	0	7	4
Other	3	1	7	2

[a]Data from: Ontario (Filler G, Young E, Geier P, et al. Is there really an increase in nonminimal change nephrotic syndrome in children? *Am J Kidney Dis* 2003;42:1107).
[b]Data from: Chicago (Haas M, Meehan SM, Karrison TG, et al. Changing etiologies of unexplained adult nephrotic syndrome: a comparison of renal biopsy findings from 1976–1979 and 1995–1997. *Am J Kidney Dis* 1997;30:621).
[c]Includes children with steroid-sensitive nephrotic syndrome and presumed minimal change nephropathy.

TABLE 64-3

CLASSIFICATION OF PRIMARY PODOCYTE DISEASES

Pathology	Genetic (Mendelian inheritance)	Acquired	Medication-induced

Minimal change histology	• Congenital NS, Finnish type
	 NPHS1
	 NPHS1 + NPHS2
		• MCN
		 • MCN variants
		    Mesangial hypercellularity
		    IgM nephropathy
		    Glomerular tip lesion
		    C1q nephropathy
		 • MCN, association
		    Hodgkin disease
		    Infection (see Table 64-5)
			• Nonsteroidal anti-inflammatory agents
			 • Gold
			 • Penicillamine
			 • Lithium
			 • Interferon-α and -β

Diffuse mesangial sclerosis (DMS) histology	• Congenital presentation *LAMB2* (Pierson syndrome) • Childhood presentation *WT1* (Denys-Drash syndrome, isolated DMS)	• Isolated DMS	

Focal segmental glomerulosclerosis (FSGS)	• Congenital presentation
	 ITGB4
	 • Infancy/childhood presentation
	 NPHS2
	 NPHS1 + NPHS2
	 WT1 (Denys-Drash syndrome, Frasier syndrome)
	 PAX2 (renal-coloboma syndrome with oligomeganephronia)
	 mtDNA (MELAS syndrome)
	 COQ2
	 • Adult presentation
	 ACTN4
	 CD2AP
	 TRPC6
	 mtDNA (MELAS syndrome)
		• Idiopathic FSGS
		   Columbia classification
		    1. Not otherwise specified
		    2. Perihilar variant
		    3. Cellular variant
		    4. Tip lesion variant
		    5. Collapsing FSGS
		
		 • C1q nephropathy
		 • Postadaptive FSGS
		   Follows an adaptive response consisting of glomerular hyperperfusion and hypertrophy
		
		 (a) Reduced nephron mass: renal dysplasia, oligomeganephronia, surgical renal mass reduction, reflux nephropathy, chronic interstitial nephritis
		 (b) Initially normal nephron mass: obesity, increased muscle mass, sickle cell anemia, cyanotic congenital heart disease, hypertension*
			• Cyclosporine, tacrolimus
			 • Interferon-α
			 • Lithium
			 • Pamidronate

Collapsing glomerulopathy	• Action myoclonus-renal failure syndrome	• Idiopathic collapsing glomerulopathy
		 • C1q nephropathy
		 • Collapsing glomerulopathy associated with infection
		    HIV-1
		    parvovirus B19*
		    Loa loa filariasis
		    Visceral leishmaniasis
		 • Collapsing glomerulopathy, other associations
		    Adult Still disease*
		    Allograft vascular diseases*
		    Multiple myeloma*
			• Interferon-α
			 • Pamidronate

ACTN4, α-actinin-4; *CD2AP*, CD2 associated protein; *COQ2*, coenzyme Q synthetase 2; *FSGS*, focal segmental glomerulosclerosis; *ITGB4*, integrin β4; *LAMB2*, laminin β2; *NPHS1*, nephrin; *NPHS2*, podocin; *MCN*, minimal change nephropathy; *mtDNA*, mitochondrial DNA; *TRPC6*, transient receptor patontial cation channel 6; *WT1*, Wilms tumor 1.

A classification scheme for the MCN/FSGS/collapsing glomerulopathy spectrum is presented. The forms of FSGS that are assigned to the acquired and medication-induced categories may have genetic risk components that have not been well-defined at present. The Columbia classification divides idiopathic FSGS into five variants; in the present classification system the fifth variant, collapsing FSGS, has been termed idiopathic collapsing glomerulopathy. In recognition that there may be distinct forms of glomerular tip lesion with divergent prognoses, this entity has been divided into two forms, glomerular tip lesion MCN variant and glomerular tip lesion FSGS variant (these forms may have distinct clinical outcomes but similar pathologic appearance). The diagnosis of postadaptive FSGS requires the exclusion of specific glomerular disease, for example, immune-mediated glomerulonephritis and diabetic nephropathy (which may manifest focal and segmental scarring but are not considered FSGS). Possible associations of idiopathic FSGS and collapsing glomerulopathy with other disease states have been treated somewhat conservatively, so that associations based on isolated case reports and controversial associations are excluded or designated with an asterisk. C1q nephropathy can present as MCN, FSGS, and collapsing glomerulopathy, as well as other forms of glomerulopathy.

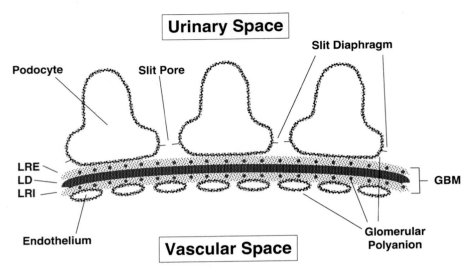

FIGURE 64-1. The glomerular filtration barrier. The distribution of glomerular polyanion in the glomerular basement membrane and on the endothelial and epithelial cell layers is shown. *LRE*, lamina rara externa; *LD*, lamina densa; *LRI*, lamina rara interna; *GBM*, glomerular basement membrane.

Mechanisms for Proteinuria

The renal factors contributing to albumin homeostasis include both glomerular filtration and tubular reabsorption. In its simplest form, the glomerulus functions as a means to promote fluid and solute flux from the blood vessel to the urinary space, from where most constituents of the filtrate are then reabsorbed. This model acquires significant complexity as solute particles approach the size limits that are characteristic of the glomerular filter. Further, recent progress in understanding tubular handling of protein has demonstrated that the reabsorptive component also has a significant impact on albumin homeostasis.

Renal Handling of Macromolecules

The glomerular barrier to filtration consists of three layers: fenestrated endothelial cells, the trilaminar glomerular basement membrane (GBM), and the epithelial cell layer (Fig. 64-1). The epithelium does not constitute a continuous layer; rather, the interdigitating extensions from adjacent epithelial cells or podocytes are separated by spaces readily apparent on electron microscopy. The GBM has been considered a major barrier to filtration (12). Experimental evidence supports a hypothetical construct in which the GBM is a thixotropic gel (one containing spicules that retard the passage of macromolecules through it) (13). Diffusion through this gel plays a significant role in restricting protein passage (14). Thus, the filtration of protein is restricted in the same manner that regulates protein movement during gel electrophoresis, where small molecules most easily penetrate (15). At the same time, other studies support a model in which macromolecules encounter a porous structure that limits the passage of larger molecules by steric hindrance (16). Glomerular filtration is possible because the interdigitations of the podocytes are separated by a small portion of the urinary space. These spaces are partly occluded by the epithelial slit diaphragm (Fig. 64-1), which has rectangular pores (17) that likely constitute the limiting barrier structure causing steric hindrance (18). The barrier itself is composed primarily of nephrin, a cell–cell adhesion molecule that interdigitates between adjacent cell processes (19), and is supported by accessory molecules including CD2-associated protein (CD2AP), FAT, Neph1, and P-cadherin (20). The result is a latticework of proteins with openings of approximately 4 × 14 nm (21). Therefore, both the GBM and the slit diaphragm contribute to steric influences on macromolecular filtration.

The porous component is demonstrated by permselectivity curves that plot the renal clearance of macromolecules, relative to the glomerular filtration rate (GFR), against molecular radius, describing a sigmoid shape (Fig. 64-2) between approximately 2 and 5 nm (20 and 50Å) (22). Therefore, some restriction in filtration of dextrans occurs with molecules of about

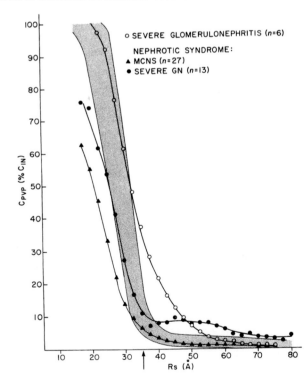

FIGURE 64-2. Permselectivity curves for patients with severe proliferative glomerulonephritis and for those with nephrotic syndrome secondary either to the minimal change nephropathy (MCN) or to glomerulonephritis. Normal values are depicted by the *shaded area*. The *arrow* indicates the molecular size of albumin. The fractional clearance of larger macromolecules is increased in severe glomerulonephritis. In minimal change nephrotic syndrome, the fractional clearance of smaller molecules is decreased. Patients with nephrotic syndrome secondary to glomerulonephritis show a hybrid curve. (Data modified from: Robson AM, Cole BR. Pathologic and functional correlations in the glomerulopathies. In: Cummings NB, Michael AF, Wilson CB, eds. *Immune Mechanisms in Renal Disease.* New York: Plenum; 1982:109, with permission.)

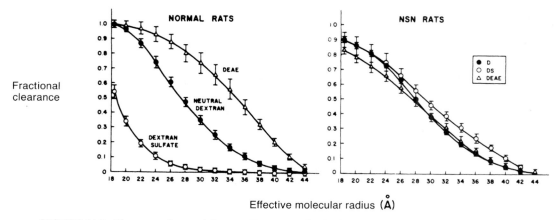

FIGURE 64-3. Clearance of neutral dextran (*D*), negatively charged dextran sulfate (*DS*), and positively charged diethylaminoethyl (*DEAE*) dextran of varying molecular size in normal rats and in those made albuminuric by treatment with nephrotoxic serum (NSN). In normal animals, clearance of negatively charged dextrans is retarded, and that of cationic dextrans is enhanced, demonstrating charge selectivity by the glomerular filter. In NSN, charge discrimination is lost. (Reprinted from: Bohrer MP, Baylis C, Humes HD, et al. Permselectivity of the glomerular capillary wall: facilitated filtration of circulating polycations. *J Clin Invest* 1978;61:72; by copyright permission of the American Society for Clinical Investigation.)

a 2-nm radius; restriction increases with increasing molecular size and approaches 100% for molecules of a radius of 5 nm (23). In addition to size, the ability of macromolecules to cross the glomerular barrier is affected by molecular configuration, shape, deformability, and flexibility (24). Permselectivity also is modified by glomerular hemodynamic factors, although the mechanism for this effect remains a subject of some controversy (15).

Initially, it was believed that macromolecule handling could be accounted for by an isoporous model for glomerular filtration, one in which steric hindrance of glomerular passage of macromolecules results from the presence of uniform pores in the barrier, each with a radius of approximately 5 nm. The size of these pores may be increased in models of increased permeability of the GBM (25). However, it has become apparent that a heteroporous model may be more appropriate (26). In this model, there are two pathways: one subject to classic steric hindrance, and a "shunt" pathway unaffected by size selectivity. As demonstrated by clearance of very large dextrans, glomerular filtration of macromolecules through this second pathway is enhanced in most forms of nephrosis and exacerbated by colloid volume expansion (27), and is ameliorated in humans by antihypertensive therapy (28), pressor doses of angiotensin II (in contrast to the effect in rats) (29), or indomethacin (30). Therefore, there appears to be a hemodynamic component to activation of this mechanism for proteinuria. The impact of this shunt is most noticeable for large molecules (greater than 6 nm); its effect on albumin clearance remains to be determined.

Steric hindrance is not sufficient to account for all aspects of permselectivity. Although proteins are handled in a manner similar to that for inert macromolecules (31), protein clearances tend to be less than those of dextrans of comparable size (24). Part of this difference is explained by the relatively rigid structure of the proteins. However, albumin, which has an effective molecular radius of 3.6 nm, is cleared by the normal kidney considerably less than are the equivalent-sized dextran molecules. Albumin carries a negative electrostatic charge, and its clearance is only slightly less than that of similarly sized dextran carrying a negative charge (32). This apparent charge selectivity has been attributed to negatively charged sialoglycoproteins in the glomerular filter (33), which are present at regularly spaced intervals in the laminae rarae of the basement membrane (34), at the endothelial fenestrae (35), and lining the epithelial podocytes (36). Collectively, these con-

stitute the glomerular polyanion (Fig. 64-1). The presence of such negative-charge sites was proposed to be responsible for both the facilitated transport of polycations (37) and the restricted transport of polyanions (38) relative to that of neutral molecules of comparable size (Fig. 64-3). These effects are most apparent in the size range that is affected by some degree of steric hindrance. Thus the determinants of glomerular permeability for a given particle are steric hindrance, glomerular hemodynamics, and electrostatic charge.

Tubular Handling of Protein. Renal protein metabolism also is affected significantly by tubular function. The glomerular filtrate normally contains a small amount of protein. A proximal tubular system has sufficient capacity that, under physiologic conditions, little intact protein from the filtrate is present in the urine. For example, filtered albumin is subject to lysosomal degradation in the proximal tubule, with fragments appearing in both the plasma and the urine (39). However, studies of rat kidneys, isolated but perfused *in situ* with radiolabeled albumin, indicate that some albumin is reabsorbed intact (40). One mechanism of tubular protein reabsorption is demonstrated by its absence in Dent disease, a defect in chloride transport resulting from a mutation in the gene for a renal-specific, voltage-gated chloride channel, CLC-5, leading to hypercalciuric nephrolithiasis (41). Proteinuria in this disease results from disruption of both receptor-mediated and fluid-phase endocytosis (42). Patients with Dent disease have characteristic urinary losses of retinol-binding protein (RBP) and albumin (43). The failure of protein reabsorption in this lesion has permitted an estimate that the glomerular filtrate contains 22 to 32 mg/L of albumin, or roughly 3 to 6 g per day in the normal human adult, virtually all of which is reabsorbed under normal conditions. This represents greater than 4% of the total plasma albumin (44).

This saturable mechanism for albumin reabsorption is mediated by two proteins that are associated with clathrin-coated pits in the proximal tubular cell (45). Megalin is a 600-kDa, transmembrane protein and a member of the low-density lipoprotein-receptor family. It co-localizes in cultured opossum kidney (OK) cells with exogenous albumin and with cubilin, a 460-kDa protein that does not have a transmembrane domain. Ligands for cubilin in the glomerular filtrate include not only albumin but also immunoglobulin light chain and apoA-I. Megalin binds to the vitamin-binding proteins, RBP and vitamin

D-binding protein, hormones, enzymes and β_2- and α_1-microglobulin, as well as albumin (46,47). As will be discussed in the section to follow on Consequences of Proteinuria, the loss of many of these proteins has clinical significance in nephrotic syndrome. Another albumin "rescue" pathway that appears to facilitate reabsorption of intact albumin has been attributed to the FcRn immunoglobulin receptor (48).

Altered Permselectivity in Nephrosis

Permselectivity patterns obtained in patients with MCNS (49,50) (Fig. 64-2) or animal models of selective albuminuria (Fig. 64-3) (38) show a relative decrease in macromolecular clearance even in the presence of marked proteinuria. In contrast, patients with glomerulonephritis show increased macromolecular clearances (Fig. 64-2), presumably due to structural damage to the GBM, which may be visible in renal biopsy material from patients in these disease states; this concept is supported by work in animals (51). Thus the mechanisms for proteinuria in both MCN and FSGS appear to be distinct from those in glomerulonephritis. In the former, proteinuria is relatively selective for albumin and occurs even though clearance of macromolecules comparable in size to albumin is decreased. In the latter, permselectivity of macromolecules that are 2.5 nm (25 Å) or larger is increased, resulting in poorly selective proteinuria. Patients with glomerulonephritis and proteinuria that is sufficiently severe to cause the nephrotic syndrome may show a pattern of permselectivity (Fig. 64-2) that is a hybrid between those found in MCNS and those found in uncomplicated glomerulonephritis (49). In these patients, as in MCNS, clearance of smaller molecules is relatively decreased. However, in contrast to the situation in MCNS, the relative clearance of larger molecules is increased. Similar hybrid curves have been described in diabetic glomerulosclerosis (52).

Therefore, nephrotic proteinuria does not result from a simple defect in glomerular filter steric hindrance. Several theories have been advanced to account for albumin loss. A prominent one is a decrease in glomerular electrostatic charge selectivity. Renal biopsy material from patients with nephrotic syndrome shows decreased staining for glomerular polyanion (53–56). Indeed, studies in MCNS patients suggested that albuminuria results from a reduction of fixed negative charge by approximately 50% (57). Rats with nephrotic syndrome induced by puromycin aminonucleoside (PAN), which causes predominant albuminuria, show decreased staining by cationic dyes (58) and decreased sialic acid content (59). Animals with puromycin nucleoside (PAN)-induced nephrotic syndrome (60) as well as those with acute heterologous nephrotoxic serum nephritis (32) show increased clearance of negatively charged dextrans, with permselectivity curves approximating those of neutral dextrans. Further, intravenous infusion of various polycations into animals results in loss of staining for glomerular polyanion, increased porosity of the glomerular filter, and heavy proteinuria (61–63). Unilateral renal artery infusion of the polycation protamine sulfate causes ipsilateral albuminuria and depletion of glomerular polyanion (63). Finally, studies in patients suggest that neutralization of vascular anionic charges may be systemic in nature (64,65) rather than confined to the kidney. This could result from effects of a protease present in the circulation such as hemopexin (66,67). However, sieving curves generated in rats by glomerular localization of neutral or negatively charged polysaccharides were unable to demonstrate charge selectivity of the glomerular filter (68), suggesting that technical factors or differences in experimental approach could significantly affect the validity of experiments demonstrating charge selectivity. In these studies, bovine serum albumin (BSA) "uptake" was extremely high relative to other markers. Another study found a role for negative charge in

modulating renal protein handling in rats infused with neutral or anionic horseradish peroxidase. These results suggested that proteins may be more affected than polysaccharides by charge, but in this model charge selectivity was lost after inhibiting tubular protein uptake with lysine or ammonium chloride, suggesting the conclusion that charge selectivity does not reside in the glomerulus (69).

In mice, the plasma elimination rate of albumin (effective molecular radius of 36 Å) was comparable to that of much larger Ficoll molecules ($\geq$65 Å). When the animals were treated with PAN, albumin clearance increased through an unknown renal mechanism (70). Although charge selectivity could explain these findings, any mechanism that is involved could have affected either the glomerulus or the tubule. A study in analbuminemic rats treated with PAN showed no effect on renal size selectivity with treatment. There also was no change in the characteristics of urinary protein excretion (71). Previously, it has been assumed that greatly increased delivery of albumin to the proximal tubule saturated transport mechanisms or that the other proteins lost in the urine were bound to albumin, in either case causing loss of the nonalbumin proteins. However, the pattern of proteinuria observed in this study was similar to the findings in the CLC-5-null mouse, where low-molecular-weight proteinuria occurs, and suggests that at least some protein losses in nephrosis result from specific tubular mechanisms. These data support a significant role for derangement of tubular protein handling in nephrotic syndrome.

Several investigators have suggested that impairment of the rescue pathway and other tubular mechanisms are a significant cause of nephrotic proteinuria (15,72). However, several lines of evidence suggest that this is not the case. Patients with Dent disease, and the CLC-5-null mouse, have "nephrotic-range" proteinuria but do not have nephrosis. The salvage of some of the 4% of the plasma albumin that is filtered per day (44) is likely to contribute positively to homeostasis, but a significant portion of albumin rescued by the tubule is degraded (39). Assuming that half of the albumin is reclaimed intact, it is unlikely that losing 2% of plasma albumin per day will have a major effect on plasma albumin concentration. Finally, Deen and Lazzara (73) modeled the sieving coefficient for albumin. They performed a mass-transfer analysis to determine whether the sieving coefficient could be similar to, rather than greatly less than, that for neutral Ficoll of the same size. The higher value, which would have been required in the models supported by adherents of a causal role for tubular proteinuria, would generate tubular albumin concentrations located 1 mm distal to the glomerulus that are 20-fold higher than has been measured by rat micropuncture studies. The authors concluded that the glomerulus was the primary restricting site for albuminuria (73). Although the possibility of charge selectivity was considered, it could not be tested by this analysis. Therefore, the mechanism of nephrotic proteinuria remains uncertain.

Even if glomerular charge neutralization does not cause proteinuria, it could account for other aspects of nephrosis. Electron micrographs of renal tissue obtained after protamine sulfate infusion sufficient to deplete glomerular polyanion show podocyte alterations identical to those seen in nephrotic syndrome (74). Perfusion of the kidney with heparin (which is negatively charged) after infusion of polycation results in reestablishment of the normal podocyte structure (74). Furthermore, chemical removal of the sialic acid coating also causes foot-process fusion/effacement (75). These findings support the notion that repelling electrostatic effects of the negatively charged cellular coating may contribute to the normal separation between adjacent podocyte foot processes. An alternative view holds that albuminuria itself may cause foot-process fusion (76).

Alteration of podocyte architecture also may account for the generally decreased fractional clearance of smaller macromolecules in nephrotic syndrome cited previously. It has been suggested that simplification of the foot process makes the glomerular pore less complex, thereby allowing for increased clearance of some long, narrow, rigid molecules. However, most plasma proteins are prolate ellipsoids (stubby cigar-shaped) and show decreased clearance (77). The effective pore radius was reported to be decreased in both MCNS and FSGS (78). In this study, the ratio of total pore area to pore length was reduced by more than 50%. Further support for decreased pore area is found in studies indicating decreased filtration slit frequency (likely secondary to foot-process fusion) (79) or decreased pore number (80). These findings would account for decreased macromolecular clearance but not enhanced albumin clearance.

An alternative to charge neutralization as an explanation of proteinuria is suggested by the data indicating that permselectivity patterns show enhanced clearance of larger neutral dextrans in FSGS (80). Studies by Yoshioka and colleagues (81) suggest that there is enhanced clearance of albumin by less-affected glomeruli, implicating hemodynamic factors related to hyperfiltration in remnant nephrons (82). This could be accounted for by the heteroporous model, in which a different class of pores greater than 60Å in radius is increasingly utilized. This shunt pathway is active in angiotensin II-stimulated proteinuria (83) and Heymann nephritis (84). Further, the hemodynamic implications of proposing a role for the shunt pathway are supported by the salient effect of angiotensin converting enzyme inhibition on glomerular size selectivity in disease (85). However, since patients with MCN do not necessarily have increased utilization of the shunt pathway (80), it is not clear that shunting represents a mechanism of proteinuria common to all causes of the nephrotic syndrome, or is the major cause of nephrotic albuminuria.

A third hypothesis regarding the stimulus for proteinuria could account for changes in both charge and steric hindrance in the glomerular filtration barrier. Small anions such as Cl^- are freely filtered by the glomerulus, whereas negatively charged molecules such as albumin that are large enough to interact with the filtration barrier (but pass through) are affected by electrostatic hindrance. Modest increases in slit diaphragm pore size, perhaps mediated by alterations in cytoskeletal function (86), may be sufficient to both decrease steric hindrance of, and reduce electrostatic interference with, albumin transit, even before considering the amplifying effects of barrier charge neutralization or increased shunt pathway utilization.

Consequences of Proteinuria

It is generally accepted that the central feature of the nephrotic syndrome, irrespective of its underlying renal cause, is hypoalbuminemia resulting from urinary loss. There is increased fractional catabolism of albumin in nephrotic syndrome (87), mostly within the renal tubule after increased filtration of plasma proteins (88). Rates of hepatic synthesis of albumin are increased (89), but this increase is inadequate to compensate for urinary losses (90). Although gastrointestinal losses are possible through transudation of albumin across the bowel wall in nephrosis, these are not likely to contribute significantly to decreased plasma albumin concentrations.

Nonetheless, urinary losses cannot be considered an isolated phenomenon. It is apparent that a special relationship exists among protein synthetic capability, urinary loss of protein, and plasma protein concentrations. For example, patients undergoing chronic peritoneal dialysis lose "nephrotic range" amounts of protein, yet they usually have close to normal serum albumin concentrations (91). In nephrosis, the rate of hepatic albumin synthesis is related to dietary protein intake. However, increasing protein intake leads to glomerular hyperfiltration (92,93) and enhanced loss of protein in the urine, resulting in lower serum albumin concentrations in patients on high-protein diets (94). The increase in dietary intake appears to stimulate selective hepatic expression of messenger ribonucleic acid (mRNA) for albumin, indicating that the stimulus is specific for albumin production and not generalized to other proteins as well (95). The dietary stimulus can be dissociated from potential effects of alterations in plasma oncotic pressure (96). Although specific plasma amino acid content is unchanged, nitrogen balance is rendered more positive by angiotensin-converting enzyme (ACE) inhibition (97), which decreases hyperfiltration and thus the amount of protein lost in the urine. Indeed, enalapril decreases $U_{Albumin}V$ (absolute albumin excretion) and fractional catabolism of albumin in normal or nephrotic rats on high-protein diets (98,99).

Edema Formation

One of the major consequences of hypoalbuminemia is edema formation. The major forces that maintain vascular volume are believed to be those described by Starling (100), namely, the algebraic sum of hydrostatic and oncotic pressures acting at the level of the peripheral capillary beds (Fig. 64-4). Hydrostatic pressure is the dominant force at the arteriolar end of the capillary, where it is generated by arterial blood pressure. Pressure

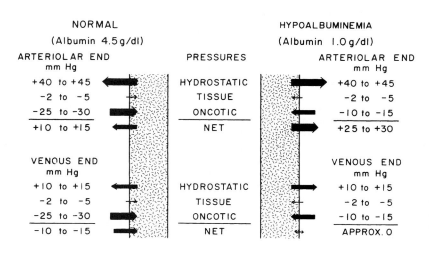

FIGURE 64-4. The forces that govern the movement of fluid across the peripheral capillary wall in healthy persons and in patients with primary nephrotic syndrome. The *shaded area* represents the lumina of the capillaries. The size and direction of the *arrows* are in proportion to the magnitude and direction of the force described by that arrow. In MCNS, hypoalbuminemia causes a marked reduction in oncotic pressure. This increases the driving force for fluid out of the arteriolar end of the capillary and decreases the forces available for return of fluid at the venous end. The result is the development of increased amounts of fluid in the interstitial space and the beginning of edema formation. See text for more details. (From: Robson AM. Edema and edema forming states. In: Klahr S, ed. *The kidney and body fluids in health and disease.* New York: Plenum; 1984:119, with permission.)

is lower in the capillaries (40 to 45 mm Hg) than in the arterial system, but it is markedly higher than tissue pressure, which ranges from 2 to 5 mm Hg. Hydrostatic pressure is opposed by plasma oncotic pressure (the osmotic pressure generated by colloidal solute), which is 25 to 30 mm Hg in healthy individuals. The resulting net force (10 to 15 mm Hg) drives an ultrafiltrate of blood from the capillaries into the interstitial fluid space. By the venous end of the capillary, hydrostatic pressure has been further dissipated (Fig. 64-4) and is exceeded by oncotic pressure, so that there is a net force for return of fluid into the capillaries. In health, the loss of fluid at the arteriolar end of the capillaries slightly exceeds the amount resorbed at the venous end. The difference is returned to the circulation through the lymphatic system (101).

Albumin, because of its abundance and its relatively small molecular size, is the plasma protein primarily responsible for the generation of oncotic pressure (102). A decrease in plasma albumin concentration thus results in a decrease in oncotic pressure, so that the net driving force for loss of fluid at the arteriolar end of the capillary bed is increased and that for return of fluid at the venous end is reduced. Consequently, fluid accumulates in the interstitial space, initiating edema formation. This accumulation occurs first where tissue pressure is lowest, for example, in the eyelids or in the scrotum; it also appears in the most dependent parts of the body because venous hydrostatic pressure is highest at these sites and is transmitted to the venous end of the capillaries.

In this traditional model of nephrotic edema formation, often referred to as "underfilling" (103), the translocation of fluid from the vascular to the interstitial fluid space as edema forms should decrease blood volume. The physiologic responses precipitated by such a reduction would then be important factors in producing the massive amounts of edema often seen in nephrotic syndrome. These changes include the release of antidiuretic hormone (ADH), the release of renin with increased production of angiotensin II, and decreases in renal blood flow and GFR (104–106). All these changes favor renal retention and positive balances of both sodium and water unless intakes are decreased. Indeed, patients may exhibit increased thirst, which is probably stimulated both by angiotensin II (107) and by the decrease in blood volume monitored through baroreceptors and volume receptors. Retained sodium and water do not remain in the vascular space. Because of the hypoalbuminemia, they add to the edema.

In practice, the pathophysiology of edema formation in nephrotic syndrome is more complex than this traditional concept. Animal studies have documented that hypoproteinemia alone does not result in edema (108). Humans with congenital analbuminemia do not develop nephrosis-like edema and have a normal plasma volume even in the virtual absence of serum albumin (109). Furthermore, if the traditional theory is correct, patients in relapse of nephrotic syndrome should have decreased blood volumes and values should return to normal during remission from the disease. Although reduced values for blood volume have been reported (110), normal or even increased levels have been documented, too (111,112). A survey of the literature (113) found that only 38% of patients with nephrosis had measurements indicating blood volumes reduced by 10% or more from normal; 48% had normal values and 14% had increased values. Furthermore, patients with carefully documented MCNS studied during relapse and again during remission did not show a consistent increase in blood volumes with remission; indeed, in most, the values did not change (113,114). Therefore, in contrast to the "underfilling" model, others have proposed an "overflow" hypothesis, in which the vascular tree is filled to excess, with increased hydrostatic pressure leading to fluid extravasation. Remarkably, nail-bed micropuncture measurements in nephrotic patients did not support the notion that capillary overfilling occurs, but capillary

leak appeared more important than underfilling in differentiating nephrotic from normal subjects (115).

There are several possible explanations for these conflicting models, each of which appears valid in some cases. One is that the reported patients had varying underlying causes of their nephrotic syndrome, in some cases involving significantly decreased renal function. Nephrotic syndrome secondary to glomerulonephritis usually is associated with a normal or expanded blood volume (116). A second potential confounding factor is that some patients were receiving treatment when studied. In addition to specific treatments, albumin infusion might enhance volume, and diuretic therapy may reduce both blood and interstitial fluid volume in nephrotic subjects (117). A third issue is that measurements of blood volume are difficult to interpret because of methodologic problems. Labeled red cells may not circulate ideally in volume-depleted states, so that peripheral hematocrit may not reflect total body hematocrit; labeled albumin may have an increased volume of distribution in nephrotic syndrome, especially if vascular integrity to albumin is decreased (118). Thus both methods could be subject to errors (116). Indeed, if the suggestion that nephrotic syndrome results from a generalized loss of negative-charge sites (65) is correct, loss of such charge sites in capillary beds could cause increased losses of albumin into edema fluid (119). This occurrence not only would alter the apparent volume of distribution for albumin, but also might increase net extravascular oncotic pressure at the level of the capillaries. Support for this hypothesis is found in the observation that large changes in extracellular fluid volume cause little change in plasma volume in nephrotic patients (120).

An attractive explanation for variations in reported blood volume is that the patients were studied in different phases of their disease process. Blood volume could be reduced during the pathogenesis of the nephrotic state, particularly in MCNS, but return to normal as anasarca develops. Therefore, the decrease in plasma volume after experimental depletion of serum proteins can be prevented by massive expansion of the extracellular fluid with saline solution (121). Nephrotic subjects progress through a sodium-retaining phase but eventually enter into a new steady state in which they no longer accumulate edema and once again demonstrate the ability to excrete a sodium load (106). With this new steady state, sodium and water retention may be so marked and edema accumulation so massive that tissue hydrostatic pressure is increased and blood volume is returned to normal. This may explain reports in which nephrotic subjects could be separated into those with high and those with low urine sodium concentrations (114). The high-volume state, whether from massive fluid intake or decreased renal function, represents the overflow pathogenesis of nephrotic edema. It is likely that both underfilling and overflow occur, perhaps at different times in the same patient.

Hormonal mechanisms. Regardless of whether underfilling or overflow is paramount, a third model suggests that hormonal mechanisms are of primary importance. Although we have emphasized a primary role for hypoalbuminemia in oliguria and sodium retention, patients with MCNS often undergo a marked, remission-induced diuresis beginning as soon as urinary albumin concentrations start to decrease and before normalization of serum albumin. Initial studies of the pathophysiology of nephrosis suggested that fluid redistribution results in aldosterone-mediated sodium retention designed to replenish vascular volume (122,123). Accordingly, aldosterone activity was thought to be more important in the genesis of fluid retention than either serum albumin or colloid osmotic pressure (114). Consistent with this notion, patients with nephrotic syndrome show an increase in distal renal tubular sodium reabsorption (106,124). Increased tubular sensitivity to aldosterone may further enhance edema formation (125).

Renin–angiotensin–aldosterone system. Inconsistencies in reported plasma renin activity (PRA) results could be due to clinical factors similar to those that confound interpretation of blood volume measurement. These include different stages of both disease process and sodium balance as well as variations in therapeutic regimen. For example, immunofluorescence staining of renin-producing cells in renal biopsy material from nephrotic patients revealed increased numbers of these cells in hypoalbuminemic states. However, the increase correlated with a number of variables, most notably the presence of vascular disease (126). In an attempt to standardize some of these variables, renin–sodium profiles were performed on patients with nephrotic syndrome. Two groups of patients were identified. In keeping with traditional concepts, the classic form was typically seen in patients with MCNS, in whom high levels of PRA and aldosterone activity were associated with vasoconstriction and hypoalbuminemia; values were further stimulated rather than suppressed by salt loading and decreased spontaneously before the occurrence of steroid-induced diuresis. In the hypervolemic, overfilling, form, seen typically with chronic glomerulonephritis and renal insufficiency, low renin activity was associated with sodium retention and increased normally with sodium depletion (116). Other studies correlated PRA with plasma volume, serum albumin concentration (127), or the state of sodium balance (113). Natriuresis in MCNS was associated with an increase in PRA and presumably a decrease in plasma volume (113), whereas that induced by water immersion, presumably mediated by an increase in blood volume, was associated with a measured decrease in PRA (128). Therefore, PRA appears to correlate better with plasma volume than with rate of urinary sodium excretion.

Difficulties in confirming a definitive role for the renin–angiotensin system in the genesis of nephrotic edema are similar to those in explaining edema formation in cirrhosis (129). A multiplicity of interacting factors may be responsible in both of these disease states. Therefore, plasma renin levels could be controlled tightly by a variety of feedback mechanisms so that subtle changes, too small to be detected by current laboratory methods, are all that occur to maintain the altered homeostasis.

Other Hormonal Regulators of Fluid and Electrolyte Balance.

In addition to renin, other factors affecting volume status may include abnormal vascular tone (130) and altered levels of catecholamines (131).

Antidiuretic hormone secretion. Nephrotic patients with MCN may show decreased solute-free water excretion, although the capacity to generate solute-free water remains intact (105). Increased ADH secretion may reflect a physiological response to decreased intravascular volume (110). In contrast, maximal urine osmolarity may be decreased in experimental rat nephrosis due to decreased renal tubular expression of aquaporin (132,133).

Prostaglandin metabolism. Elevated levels of prostaglandin E_2 (PGE_2) were found in the serum of patients with nephrotic syndrome, the majority of whom had MCN (134). The highest values were observed when the patients had clinically apparent edema. Urinary PGE_2 levels were increased in patients with idiopathic nephrotic syndrome who had a low urine sodium concentration as well as elevated plasma renin–aldosterone activity (135). The observation that the administration of indomethacin to nephrotic patients results in an increase in body weight and decrease in GFR suggests that prostaglandins may play a role in either maintenance of GFR or amelioration of edema in nephrotic syndrome. Indomethacin also decreased proteinuria and PRA (135). Response to indomethacin is dependent on concurrent sodium intake. When the agent was given to nephrotic patients on sodium-restricted diets, it resulted in a decrease in GFR; a similar drug regimen for patients with more liberal sodium intake did not affect renal hemodynamics (136).

Atrial natriuretic peptide. Because atrial natriuretic peptide (ANP) causes renal vasodilation, an increase in GFR, and increased sodium excretion (137), it has been suggested that abnormal metabolism of this hormone could mediate sodium retention in nephrosis. The acute increase of plasma volume following albumin infusion in nephrotic children is accompanied by a fivefold increase in ANP levels (138). However, this may simply reflect a change from low plasma volume status before the infusion is begun in patients who likely have MCNS. Plasma concentrations of ANP were determined to be low in nephrotic patients compared to patients who had acute glomerulonephritis, and ANP levels correlated well with the degree of edema in nephritis but not in nephrosis (139). Therefore, regulation of ANP appeared to be appropriate for presumed volume status. In rats with adriamycin-induced nephrotic syndrome, changes in GFR after infusion of ANP were similar to those in control animals, indicating that nephrosis does not alter glomerular filtration by changing ANP sensitivity (140). In a similar model, no change was detected in ANP receptor density in nephrotic kidneys (141). Nephrotic patients respond physiologically to ANP infusion (142), although the mechanism by which this occurs may be different from that in normal subjects (143). It has been proposed that ANP mediates the diuretic response to head-out immersion in nephrosis (144), but the effect of ANP infusion, unlike that of immersion, is blocked by enalapril (145).

Physical and Anatomic Factors Affecting Glomerular Filtration Rate.

Taken together, these findings suggest that, although secretion of ANF may in part mediate diuresis, physical factors are of greatest importance in the fluid retention of nephrosis, with abnormalities of ANF representing appropriate responses for the patient's physiology (146). These physical factors may include a significant intrarenal component. Children with MCNS have decreases in both GFR and filtration fraction (104,147,148). Decreased GFR could be due to a decrease in the ultrafiltration coefficient (K_f), causing a reduction in single-nephron GFR (146), and has been suggested to result from effacement of the glomerular epithelial cell foot processes (149). Alternatively, the decreased GFR could be a consequence of raised intratubular hydrostatic pressure in the proximal tubule secondary to the presence of filtered albumin, an increase in resistance to tubular flow (150), or decreased proximal reabsorption of tubular fluid as a result of a reduction in peritubular capillary oncotic pressure (146). There also may be a local role for the renin–angiotensin system, as saralasin infusion in experimental unilateral PAN-induced nephrotic syndrome resulted in an increase in single-nephron GFR in the experimental, but not the control, kidney (146). In another animal model of nephrotic syndrome, that of nephrotoxic serum nephritis, the K_f was reduced, but compensatory mechanisms maintained renal blood flow and whole-kidney and single-nephron GFR. These responses appeared to be intrarenal in origin and caused an increase in glomerular capillary pressure (151).

Another factor affecting GFR is plasma albumin concentration. Hypoalbuminemia has been postulated to decrease glomerular plasma flow, thereby decreasing GFR. However, lower albumin also decreases plasma oncotic pressure, which should increase GFR. Löwenborg and Berg report that GFR and filtration fraction vary directly with serum albumin but inversely with mean arterial blood pressure in children with MCNS (152). This finding supports a role for altered K_f in relapse, consistent with foot-process effacement. K_f is determined by the total filtration slit length, as shown by mathematical modeling of experimental data (153). Some studies suggest that there is a weak correlation between the amount of proteinuria and the extent of foot-process effacement, but these studies included patients in relapse and in remission with MCN (154) and with multiple nephrotic diseases (155). A recent study of 23 MCN patients in relapse showed no correlation between proteinuria and foot-process effacement ($r = 0.25$, $p = 0.25$) (156). The authors make the important point that assessment of the quantitative relationship between podocyte foot-process effacement and proteinuria should exclude patients in remission, as these patients have normal podocyte morphology (and therefore do not address the hypothesis that the degree of effacement correlates with proteinuria). Foot-process effacement reverses when patients undergo spontaneous remission or glucocorticoid-induced remission.

Other Physiologic Changes in Fluid and Electrolyte Metabolism

A curious phenomenon in primary nephrotic syndrome, perhaps related to decreased filtration fraction, is the occurrence of reversible or permanent renal failure unexplained by the underlying disease process. This has been reported in association with both MCN (157–159) and FSGS (130). In some patients, renal failure was associated with the use of nonsteroidal antiinflammatory drug (NSAID) therapy (160,161). These episodes occur in the absence of renal vein thrombosis (vide infra) or other systemic symptoms. Because fractional excretion of sodium is low in these patients (162), it is likely that the marked decrease in GFR occurs for hemodynamic reasons (163) rather than because of acute tubular necrosis or vasomotor nephropathy. In a study of 15 patients with MCNS and renal failure, GFR measured by inulin clearance was decreased out of proportion to clearance of *para*-aminohippurate (PAH), with filtration fraction reduced to between 3% and 9% (164). Improvement of renal function occurred in association with diuretic therapy either with or without albumin infusion. In patients who improved with pharmacologic diuresis, the serum creatinine level again rose on return to an edematous state. The authors postulate that glomerular hemodynamics was altered by the presence of intrarenal edema, which occurred when peripheral edema developed.

Other circulatory abnormalities have been observed in patients with nephrotic syndrome. The occurrence of hypovolemic shock and hypotension has been related to a variety of medical procedures (165). However, hypotension may occur spontaneously. These episodes usually are seen in patients during relapse who have an intercurrent illness causing fluid loss, such as emesis or diarrhea. The patients usually show marked responsiveness to small amounts of intravenous saline that are insufficient to replenish all fluid losses, suggesting a failure in maintenance of vascular tone. Recovery usually occurs if this complication is identified early and treated promptly. Sequelae may include acute tubular necrosis, renal vein thrombosis (RVT), or death.

Hyperlipidemia

Lipemic serum has long been recognized as a cardinal feature of the nephrotic syndrome (166). Abnormalities in postprandial lipid metabolism were described more than 40 years ago (167). Biochemical evaluation has shown that all lipid components of the plasma are increased, with cholesterol increasing more rapidly than phospholipid. Thus, as acute severity of the disease worsens, the ratio of cholesterol to phospholipid increases (168). Triglycerides are relatively normal at the initiation of relapse but increase as the disease continues (169); lactescence occurs when the plasma triglyceride content exceeds 400 mg/dL. Hyperlipidemia may persist well into remission (170), suggesting a residual effect of nephrosis on lipoprotein transport (171).

Depending on the classification employed, the most common patterns of hyperlipoproteinemia seen in nephrosis are types II and IV (172) or types IIa, IIb, and V (173). Low-density lipoproteins (LDLs) and very low-density lipoproteins (VLDLs) show the greatest increase in concentration. Values for high-density lipoprotein (HDL) cholesterol have been reported to be elevated (174,175), normal (176,177), or decreased (169,178,179). This variation may relate to the age of the patients studied, the underlying cause of the nephrotic syndrome, patient treatment, and whether renal insufficiency is present. Studies of lipoprotein cholesterol have produced conflicting results (169,174–179). The ratio of cholesterol to phospholipid or to triglyceride in various lipoproteins is altered, indicating abnormalities in quality as well as quantity of lipoproteins.

Several events may contribute to these abnormalities. Lipid metabolism is normally accomplished through a series of complex steps (Fig. 64-5). Through the action of 3-hydroxy-3-methylglutaryl coenzyme A (HMG CoA) reductase, mevalonate is produced from acetate in the liver. This in turn is used to make cholesterol, which is incorporated into lipoproteins. The greater the triglyceride content of the lipoprotein, the less dense it is. Dietary fat absorbed from the intestine is formed into chylomicrons by being surrounded with a coat of apolipoprotein that is critical for transport of the hydrophobic lipid. The triglyceride content of the chylomicron is reduced in the periphery (mainly by the action of lipoprotein lipase [LPL]), and the resulting particle containing apolipoprotein (apo) B-48

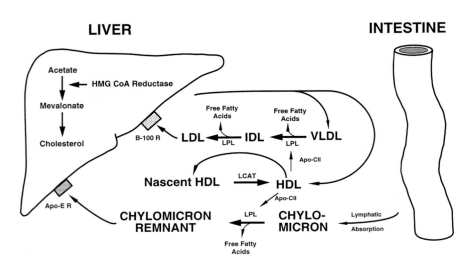

FIGURE 64-5. Normal pathways of lipid metabolism. *apo-CII*, Apolipoprotein C-II; *Apo-E R*, chylomicron remnant (apo E) receptor; *B-100 R*, apolipoprotein B-100 (LDL) receptor; *HDL*, high-density lipoprotein; *IDL*, intermediate-density lipoprotein; *HMG CoA reductase*, 3-hydroxy-3-methylglutaryl coenzyme A reductase; *LCAT*, lecithin-cholesterol acyltransferase; *LDL*, low-density lipoprotein; *LPL*, lipoprotein lipase; *VLDL*, very-low-density lipoprotein. Figure composed with the assistance of Nader Rifai.

and apo E binds to the hepatocyte via a chylomicron remnant receptor. VLDL is synthesized in the liver and metabolized in the periphery through the action of LPL to intermediate-density lipoprotein (IDL), and then to LDL. LDL is bound to apo B-100, which is then taken up by the hepatocyte LDL receptor (180,181). This brings additional cholesterol back to the liver, suppressing HMG CoA reductase activity and decreasing new cholesterol synthesis. The liver also produces HDL, which participates as a transport protein in catabolism of lower-density moieties, being regenerated by lecithin-cholesterol acyltransferase (LCAT). HDL also carries apo C-II, which activates LPL. Abnormalities at any step of metabolism from lipid uptake to the enterohepatic secretion of bile could result in the hyperlipidemia of nephrosis. Likely contributing factors include increased hepatic synthesis of lipoprotein; abnormal transport of lipid through the metabolic pathway; and abnormal catabolism secondary to decreased enzyme activity.

Lipoprotein Synthesis. It is clear that hepatic synthesis of lipoproteins is increased in nephrotic patients (168,182–185). The signal for this event appears to be related to hypoalbuminemia because daily infusion of albumin into nephrotic patients, sufficient to raise serum levels, also decreases serum lipid, triglyceride, and cholesterol levels (186). Increasing the plasma oncotic pressure in nephrotic patients or animals, by infusion of dextrans, decreases hepatic lipoprotein synthesis (167,187). Additional laboratory studies suggest that the regulatory signal could be viscosity rather than oncotic pressure (186,188,189). Cholesterol biosynthesis also has been investigated (190,191). These studies show increased incorporation of ^{14}C from labeled mevalonate into cholesterol by the liver in experimental nephrosis. Although this result is consistent with the interpretation that rates of hepatic cholesterol synthesis are increased in nephrosis, artifactual changes due to the addition of exogenous substrate (mevalonate) could not be ruled out in these experiments.

Lipid Transport. Several aspects of lipid transport may be impaired in nephrosis. The major cholesterol-transporting protein associated with the LDLs in the plasma is apo B-100 (192). This also has been implicated as a significant apolipoprotein in atherogenesis. A recent study of nephrotic patients found that elevated serum concentrations of cholesterol, triglycerides, and phospholipids resulted mostly from changes in apo B-100-containing lipoproteins. The size of the apo B-100 pool in patients was two to three times that found in healthy subjects or in patients in remission. Fractional catabolism was decreased only slightly, suggesting that the major problem was overproduction rather than decreased breakdown (193). Hepatic uptake of LDLs may be decreased (194) if the structural composition of LDLs in the circulating pool is abnormal, or if systemic neutralization of membrane negative charge leads to less efficient uptake of the largely cationic liposomes (195); this would exacerbate hypercholesterolemia by decreasing negative feedback affecting hepatic synthesis. Alternatively, decreased hepatic uptake of LDLs could result from, rather than cause, hepatic overproduction of cholesterol (192).

Metabolism of Lipids. At least one report indicates that while LDL synthesis may be increased in nephrosis, VLDL catabolism is decreased (185). Another study demonstrates that apolipoprotein E-rich IDL from nephrotic patients, but not from normal controls, inhibits sterol synthesis and cholesterol esterification (196). This finding suggests that cellular apo E metabolism may be deranged in nephrosis. Consistent with this finding, genetic variations in the expression of *apo E* alleles may influence the degree of lipid abnormality in nephrotic patients (197).

Interest regarding catabolism of lipids in nephrosis has focused on two enzymes: LPL, which facilitates the breakdown of ester bonds in glycerides, and LCAT, which catalyzes the reaction of lecithin and cholesterol to form lysolecithin and cholesterol ester (198). In nephrotic children, elevated serum lipid levels correlate with decreased postheparin LPL activity (199). In another study of nephrotic patients, most of whom had MCNS, hepatic LPL activity was normal, but serum and adipose tissue LPL activities were decreased in association with elevated plasma triglycerides (174). Decreased hepatic (200) and adipose tissue (199) LPL activity in experimental rat models of nephrosis may contribute to altered lipoprotein levels in these animals. LCAT activity also is decreased in experimental nephrosis (201), with levels appearing to correlate with serum albumin concentration (202).

Activity of these enzymes may be affected both directly and indirectly by urinary protein loss. Albumin binds to free fatty acids (FFAs); decreases in serum albumin concentration lead to FFA accumulation, thereby inhibiting LPL activity (203). LPL activity also may be inhibited by cholesterol (202). LCAT activity is inhibited by the accumulation of triglyceride and cholesterol esters (204), suggesting that abnormal LCAT activity could be a result, rather than a cause, of nephrotic hyperlipidemia. However, lysolecithin, a reaction product that binds to albumin, inhibits LCAT activity *in vitro*; this feedback mechanism is blocked by addition of physiologic levels of albumin (204,205). Therefore, urinary loss of albumin may lead to inhibition of lipolytic enzyme function.

Albumin loss does not account entirely, however, for the elevated lipid levels. Although infusion of albumin decreased serum lipid levels in an acute animal model of nephrotic syndrome, normalization occurred only after simultaneous infusion of heparin. This suggests the need for an additional factor that aids in clearing lipid from the plasma (206). In further experiments with this model, nephrectomy resulted in greater improvement of the hyperlipidemia than did albumin infusions alone (207), indicating that the factor may be lost in the urine. Further support for loss of a specific regulatory molecule in the urine is provided by the observation that alteration of dietary protein intake markedly modulates the hepatic albumin synthetic rate but does not alter the hepatic synthesis of lipoproteins (208). In this study, lipoprotein synthesis correlated directly with the urinary clearance of albumin, suggesting that albumin, or another substance lost in parallel with albumin, was needed to suppress lipoprotein synthesis. Experiments with analbuminemic rats indicate that albumin itself is not likely to be the critical molecule (209). It has been suggested that the lost factor is LCAT (168). HDL, which plays an essential role in catabolism of VLDL, also may be lost in the nephrotic urine (210,211). Conversely, other studies indicate that HDL excretion is low (187), especially in MCNS (212). Apo C-II also may be lost in the urine (192,213).

Clinical Significance. Regardless of the cause, the clinical significance of the lipid abnormalities in nephrosis must be considered. Hyperlipidemia has been associated with cardiovascular disease in otherwise healthy young adults, but studies evaluating such a correlation in nephrotic patients produced conflicting results. Premature coronary atherosclerosis (214) and a high incidence of myocardial infarction and other cardiovascular diseases (215,216) have been documented in nephrotic subjects, as well as a higher incidence of hypertension in nephrotic men than in control subjects (217). In this respect, the observation that macrophage morphology and function are altered by the hyperlipidemia of nephrosis (218) could relate to the development of atheromatous plaques. In addition, plasma levels of lipoprotein(a), a strong risk factor in cardiovascular disease, are increased (219). In contrast, other studies have not confirmed a predisposition to atherosclerosis in patients with nephrosis (220,221). These discrepant results may reflect limitations of population base or selection bias (174,212). In the studies that did not demonstrate an increased risk, it is unclear whether stratification of the patients into cohorts according to the degree of lipid abnormality would have shown an increased risk in patients with the highest consistent elevations in lipoprotein levels. Age, underlying diagnosis, disease course, and incidence of other complicating factors such as hypertension also may be important. Another significant consideration is the possible ameliorating effect of HDL on hyperlipidemia (220–223). In several studies (174,212), HDL levels were normal or increased in MCNS. This could have a protective effect and decrease the likelihood of cardiovascular complications. Further study of larger groups of nephrotic patients would allow differentiation among patients with other cardiac risk factors in addition to the potential hazard of elevated serum lipid levels.

A second risk involves the role of lipids in causing or enhancing the progression of the renal disease itself. Rats with PAN nephrosis fed high-cholesterol diets develop mesangial foam cells and mesangial proliferative changes (224). The relationship of systemic hypertension and hyperlipidemia to atherosclerosis parallels the relationship of intraglomerular hypertension and high lipid levels to focal sclerosis (224). Effective therapy of hyperlipidemia ameliorates single-nephron hyperfiltration (225) and retards progression of renal failure in obese Zucker rats (226) and in nephrotic rats with reduced renal mass (227). In obese Zucker rats, a relative decrease in polyunsaturated fatty acids (PUFAs), rather than high cholesterol levels, may be the most important lipid-related factor in progression of renal disease, since dietary supplementation with n-6 PUFA (sunflower oil) or n-3 PUFA (fish oil) slowed progression of renal disease but only fish oil decreased serum cholesterol levels (225).

In view of these considerations, and the fact that treatments for nephrosis such as steroids and diuretics may exacerbate hyperlipidemia, clinicians have invested increasing effort in controlling the lipid abnormalities of nephrosis (228). Traditional dietary therapy is of marginal value, and may actually worsen the hyperlipidemia (229). Cholestyramine may, by increasing secretion of cholesterol into the bile, predispose toward the development of cholesterol gallstones (192). Nicotinic acid has significant side effects and has not been studied extensively. Probucol may cause concomitant loss of HDLs (229). However, it has been shown experimentally to reverse lipid-mediated vasoconstriction (230), and to be effective in treating patients who were 5 to 20 years old (231). Two other classes of drugs found to be effective in treating nephrotic hyperlipidemia are fibric acids and HMG CoA reductase inhibitors. Gemfibrozil, a fibric acid, caused a 51% reduction in serum triglyceride levels but only a 15% decrease in cholesterol when given at a dose of 600 mg twice a day to adult nephrotic patients; a 26% reduction in apo B was achieved (232). Lovastatin, an inhibitor of HMG CoA reductase, caused a 27% to 29% reduction in total cholesterol, LDL cholesterol, and apo B at a dose of 20 mg twice daily in adult patients with nephrosis due to MCNS or other diseases (193). In patients with nephrotic-range proteinuria, doses up to 40 mg twice daily caused similar decreases regardless of whether the patients were on corticosteroid therapy. A slight increase was noted in serum HDL concentrations (233). Kinetic studies showed that lovastatin enhances the catabolism of VLDL triglycerides and lowers LDL cholesterol by decreasing input rates for LDLs (234), most likely through inhibition of LDL–apo B synthesis from VLDL (235). Atorvastatin also is effective in nephrotic hyperlipidemia (236). In children, HMG CoA reductase inhibitors may be effective, but some clinicians have urged caution regarding their use in the very young child, raising the possibility that inhibiting cholesterol synthesis might impair neural myelination. This concern needs to be

weighed against the more immediate issues of cardiovascular complications and renal disease progression.

Disorders of Hemostasis

The association between nephrotic syndrome and intravascular coagulation has been known for more than a century, but it was not until 1948 that the concept of a thrombotic diathesis in nephrotic patients was proposed (237). In a review of 3,377 children with nephrotic syndrome, the incidence of thromboembolic complications was 1.8% (238). The prevalence of such complications in adult nephrotic subjects is much higher and averaged 26% in eight series of patients (239). Thrombosis may occur at any stage during the course of the nephrotic syndrome, but it is most frequent in the early months.

Extent of Clinical Involvement. Deep vein thrombosis of the leg is the most common thrombotic complication in the nephrotic adult and was responsible for one third of the thromboembolic complications in the largest published series of nephrotic children (238). Other reported sites of venous thromboses include the subclavian, axillary, external jugular, portal, splenic, hepatic, and mesenteric veins as well as the superficial cerebral cortical sinus, where thrombosis has been observed in both children and adults and may be fatal (240,241). Arterial thrombosis occurs less frequently and is seen primarily in children. Thrombosis of the aorta and of the mesenteric, axillary, femoral, ophthalmic, carotid, cerebral, renal, pulmonary, and coronary arteries has been reported, as has intracardiac thrombosis (240,241). The pulmonary (242) and femoral arteries are particularly susceptible, the former potentially resulting in infarction (243) and the latter usually as a complication of attempted blood sampling from the femoral vein. Although recanalization of the artery does occur, a relatively high proportion of patients with arterial thrombi die (242).

The lesion that has attracted the most attention, however, is RVT or renal vein thrombosis. It is most often seen with membranous glomerulopathy (244), to the extent that at one time there was some controversy about whether RVT was the cause, rather than a complication, of the glomerular lesion. The reported frequency of RVT in patients with membranous disease has ranged from 4% to 51%, depending on the methods used to establish the diagnosis and to select the patient population for study (245). The mean prevalence is 12%. There is a high incidence of RVT in mesangiocapillary glomerulonephritis and the nephritis of systemic lupus erythematosus, and renal vein thrombosis can complicate numerous other renal diseases (240). It is relatively uncommon in nephrotic children except in those with congenital nephrotic syndrome of the Finnish type (246).

The thrombosis may involve only the renal venous system or it may extend into the inferior vena cava. Therefore it is not surprising that pulmonary emboli develop in about 40% of adult patients with RVT, although pulmonary emboli occur rarely in children. Death from pulmonary emboli is uncommon (238,240).

Diagnosis of acute RVT is suggested by flank pain, costovertebral angle tenderness, gross hematuria, increased proteinuria, and acute reduction in renal function; intravenous pyelography may show ureteral notching or pelvocaliceal irregularities (245). Ultrasonography may demonstrate only a large kidney or may visualize the thrombus if it extends to the renal vein or inferior vena cava. However, Doppler ultrasound analysis often shows decreased venous blood flow. A more chronic form of RVT may be asymptomatic and may be identifiable only by venography (245,247). The mode of presentation of other thromboses depends on their site. Diagnosis can be difficult and the existence of arterial thrombosis may not be realized until

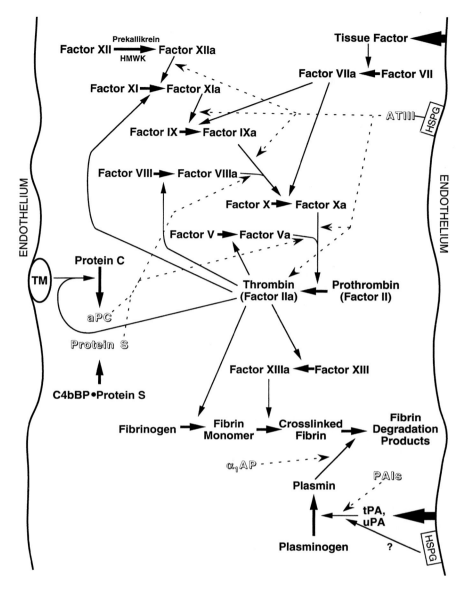

FIGURE 64-6. Interactions among circulating participants in the coagulation cascade. The intrinsic pathway begins in the upper left; the contact system of factor XII, prekallikrein, and high-molecular-weight kininogen (HMWK) that initiates the intrinsic cascade is shown in condensed form. The extrinsic pathway begins in the upper right. The action of factor VIIa on the activation of factor IX has blurred the distinction between these two limbs of the cascade. The common pathway begins with activation of factor X and results in thrombin activity and fibrin crosslinking. Coagulation is counteracted by the fibrinolytic pathway, including plasminogen activators and plasminogen/plasmin. In addition, there are several anticoagulant pathways, most notably inhibition of factors Va and VIIIa by the inhibitory cofactors protein S and activated protein C (aPC). Alpha-2-macroglobulin, which binds to and inhibits most of the enzymes in this system, is not shown here for the purpose of simplicity. The relationship between heparan sulfate proteoglycans (HSPGs) and plasminogen activator activity shown in the lower right should be regarded as hypothetical for human pathophysiology. *Thick solid lines with arrows* indicate reactions; *thin solid lines with triangular arrows* denote catalytic effects; *joining lines* show cofactors in catalysis. *Broken lines with fork-tailed arrows* represent inhibitory actions. α_1 AP, α_1-antiplasmin; ATIII, antithrombin III; C4bBP, complement factor 4b-binding protein; PAIs, plasminogen activator inhibitors; TM, thrombomodulin; tPA, tissue-type plasminogen activator; uPA, urokinase plasminogen activator. PAI-1 and PAI-3 bind to aPC; this interaction may cause mutual inhibition of the action of these proteins. (Figure composed with the assistance of G.A. Soff.)

autopsy. Ultrasonography and angiography are the preferred studies.

Regulators of Coagulation. The blood coagulation pathway represents a complex series of events that regulate the dynamic balance between the ability of the blood to remain fluid and its tendency to assume a gelled state in the presence of altered flow conditions or exposure to nonendothelial surfaces. Contributing to hemostatic balance are several opposing systems that contribute to a cascade through which a series of enzymes regulates fibrin polymerization (Fig. 64-6). Coagulation is initiated by activation of prekallikrein to kallikrein (intrinsic pathway), or by exposure to nonendothelial tissues (extrinsic pathway). These pathways meet in the activation of factor IX, initiating a common pathway in which a central role is played by thrombin (factor IIa). This enzyme stimulates activation of fibrinogen to fibrin and aggregation of platelets. It also activates factors V, VIII, and XIII. Factor XIIIa triggers crosslinking of fibrin monomer into a stable polymer. Two systems oppose clot formation and stability. Protein C is processed to activated protein C (aPC) by thrombin complexed with thrombomodulin. With free protein S as a cofactor, aPC inactivates

factors Va and VIIIa. The other system that opposes coagulation is the fibrinolytic pathway, in which plasminogen activators convert plasminogen to plasmin, which degrades fibrin polymer. Several proteins inhibit these pathways: Antithrombin III and α_2-macroglobulin inhibit thrombin; α_1-antiplasmin and α_2-macroglobulin inhibit plasmin; and the plasminogen activator inhibitors (PAIs) inhibit plasminogen activators and aPC. Activated protein C, in turn, opposes PAI effects. Many of the components of these pathways are altered in nephrosis. In addition, physical conditions of the nephrotic syndrome, such as venous stasis, hemoconcentration, increased blood viscosity, and possibly the administration of steroids, may also contribute to enhanced blood clotting. These nephrotic effects on coagulation pathways, which are listed in Table 64-4 and discussed in detail elsewhere (240,247,248), are considered here briefly.

Platelet Aggregation. Platelets may play a role in the genesis of the coagulopathy of nephrotic syndrome. Thrombocytosis is commonly found, especially early in the disease course (249), and platelets show markers of activation (250). Platelet aggregability is increased and platelet degranulation has been described (251). In addition, plasma levels of the platelet release

TABLE 64-4

COAGULATION SYSTEM ABNORMALITIES IN THE
NEPHROTIC SYNDROME

Increased platelet aggregation
Thrombocytosis
β-Thromboglobulin
Platelet factor 4
Increased procoagulant activity
Physical factors
Hemoconcentration
Hyperviscosity
Increased factor production
   Intrinsic pathway—factors VII and IX (variably)
   Extrinsic pathway—factor VII (variably)
   Common pathway
      Fibrinogen
      Factors V and VIII
      Factors X and II (variably)
Urinary loss of anticoagulants
   Antithrombin III
   Free protein S
Increased inhibitors of anticoagulation
   α_2-Macroglobulin
   C4b-binding protein
Increased plasminogen

substance β-thromboglobulin are increased (249,252). Levels of platelet factor 4 are normal (253) or increased (249). In contrast, platelet calcium ion release and ATP secretion have been found to be decreased in nephrosis (254). The authors of that report suggest that platelets may become desensitized to platelet activating factor (PAF) because of exposure to consistently high ambient concentrations.

Platelet hyperaggregability correlates with the degree of proteinuria and with plasma cholesterol levels. It can be reversed by the addition of urine protein (253). These findings suggest that the urinary loss of albumin (255) or of some factor that normally inhibits platelet aggregation is responsible for the changes seen in nephrotic syndrome. Alternatively, hyperlipidemia could result in the changes, as platelet aggregation is increased in patients with type II hyperlipoproteinemia to a degree that is comparable to that seen in nephrotic syndrome (256). Altered platelet function could be a response to hypoalbuminemia, because the conversion of arachidonic acid into metabolites that aggregate platelets is known to be regulated by albumin (257,258). Thus platelets show greater production of thromboxane B_2 and malondialdehyde in nephrotic plasma than in normal plasma when challenged with arachidonic acid. Addition of albumin to the nephrotic plasma corrects this abnormality (259). Finally, it is possible that alterations in platelet membranes could be responsible for increased platelet activity. Platelet membranes contain a sialoglycoprotein with a pK of 1.8 to 2.2 (260). This may be important in preventing spontaneous platelet aggregation or platelet interaction with the vessel wall (261). Because systemic negative-charge sites may be reduced during relapses of nephrotic syndrome (65), the same mechanism responsible for the reduction of negative-charge sites in the GBM could enhance platelet aggregation.

Coagulation Factors. Evidence that various functions of blood coagulation are activated in nephrosis is provided by increased concentration of the D-dimer of fibrinogen (262). Elevated levels of this breakdown product of crosslinked fibrin indicate that both the coagulation and fibrinolytic pathways are concur-

rently activated. Plasma fibrinogen is consistently elevated in nephrotic syndrome due to increased hepatic synthesis. Chromatography demonstrates both increased polymerization and increased proteolytic derivatives of fibrinogen or fibrin. These changes reverse as patients with nephrotic syndrome enter remission (263). This evidence for increased intravascular fibrin formation is supported by the finding of increased plasma levels of fibrinopeptide A, at least in FSGS (263).

The concentration in nephrotic patients of coagulation factors that initiate fibrin formation likely reflects the balance between the increased hepatic synthesis of these proteins, triggered as part of a nonspecific response to hypoproteinemia as described previously for lipoproteins, and urinary losses. Therefore, lower molecular-size proteins (approximately less than 70 kDa) may be lost in the urine, whereas higher molecular-size proteins (greater than 300 kDa) are likely to be increased in the plasma. For example, most studies agree that levels of factors V and VIII are increased in the plasma, whereas those of factors IX, XI, and XII are decreased (264) despite the possibility that production may still be increased. The magnitude of the increase in concentration of factors V and VIII, for example, correlates with the degree of reduction in serum albumin and the likely resulting increased hepatic synthesis of these factors, stimulated by hypoalbuminemia (265). Plasma levels of factors II, VII, X, and XIII are often found to be increased (266–268). There is no direct evidence that any of these changes are responsible for the hypercoagulable state. Indeed, the alterations in blood levels of these factors are often inconsistent and of minor degree. Therefore, these abnormalities may be of more biochemical than clinical interest. Most of the changes in concentration of these zymogen factors reverse with clinical remission of the nephrotic syndrome.

Inhibitors of Coagulation. The most well-studied biologic antagonist of coagulation, antithrombin III, is decreased in the plasma of nephrotic patients (269–273). This is presumed to be due to urinary loss of antithrombin III, which has a relatively low molecular weight. Indeed, plasma antithrombin III levels in nephrotic syndrome correlate well with those of serum albumin and inversely with the renal clearance of antithrombin III. Because hereditary antithrombin III deficiency is associated with frequent thrombosis, it was hypothesized that the low plasma antithrombin III levels were insufficient to inactivate procoagulant factors and were the major cause for the hypercoagulable state and the development of thrombosis in nephrotic syndrome (271). However, only patients with plasma albumin levels below 2 g/dL show significant reductions in plasma antithrombin III levels (274), whereas hypercoagulability may be present in patients with albumin levels exceeding this value. Further, normal plasma levels of antithrombin III were found in nephrotic subjects who had loss of antithrombin III in the urine and who had thromboembolic complications (275). Indeed, decreases in antithrombin III levels may be compensated for by increased plasma levels of α_2-macroglobulin (268), leading to increased total antithrombin activity (263).

A complex effect of nephrosis has been noted on the anticoagulation pathway by which protein C is activated by thrombin and thrombomodulin to aPC. Activated protein C and protein S combine to inhibit factor VIIIa (decreasing activation of factor X) and factor Va (decreasing activation of factor XI). Protein S exists in circulation in two forms: free and bound to C4b binding protein. Only the free protein S can serve as a cofactor with protein C to inactivate factors Va and VIIIa (276). In nephrotic syndrome, although small amounts of protein C are lost in the urine, serum concentrations are normal (277,278), indicating that hepatic synthesis is able to compensate. In contrast, although plasma levels of C4b binding protein–protein S complex are usually normal to elevated, free levels are markedly decreased (279). This finding is consistent with the molecular sizes of the complex (640 kDa) and the free protein S (69 kDa). Acquired dysfunction of this system is a common cause of thrombotic diathesis (276,280). Indeed, intractable deep vein thrombosis in an unusual nephrotic child with decreases in both protein S and C4b-binding protein concentrations (281) supports the notion that abnormalities of this system are clinically significant.

Fibrinolysis. Alterations in the concentrations of several of the components of the fibrinolytic system have been documented (282). Decreased fibrinolytic activity has been associated with hypertriglyceridemia (283). Of the individual components of the fibrinolytic system, decreased concentrations of plasminogen have been found (270,284); levels of tissue-type plasminogen activator (262) and PAI-1 (285) are elevated. Varying levels of α_2-antiplasmin have been reported (262,263), possibly depending on whether thrombosis has occurred. Of the serine protease inhibitors that modulate both the fibrinolytic and thrombin systems, levels of α_2-macroglobulin are increased and those of α_1-antitrypsin are decreased (268). Again, this probably reflects the effect of urinary loss on plasma concentrations. It also is possible that local vascular conditions affect fibrinolysis. Infusion of a variety of polyanions causes an immediate local increase in release of plasminogen activator and PAI activity in the sow ear. The PAI activity immediately returns to normal but the increase in plasminogen activator activity is sustained (286), suggesting that negative charges in the vascular tree are important for inducing the plasminogen activator pathway. If nephrosis is associated with a generalized reduction of fixed negative charge sites in the vascular space (65), it is likely that decreased negative charges could have an impact on induction of fibrinolysis. Coupled with increased α_2-antiplasmin concentrations, decreased tissue-type plasminogen activator activity would significantly impair fibrin degradation. However, the increase in circulating D-dimer cited previously indicates that at least some fibrinolysis occurs in nephrosis. It also is possible that fibrin polymerization is impaired in nephrotic patients. In one study of a broad spectrum of adults with nephrosis, most had prolonged thrombin times. Half of the patients showed decreased ability to polymerize fibrin monomer. There was no correlation of this finding with prothrombin time, partial thromboplastin time, fibrin degradation products, antithrombin III concentration, or platelet count (287).

Environmental Factors Affecting Coagulation. Physical factors such as increased blood viscosity also may contribute to the generation of thromboembolic complications (288). Both children and adults with MCNS and well-preserved renal function may have marked hemoconcentration with elevated hematocrit and hemoglobin concentrations. Such changes are associated with disproportionate increases in viscosity and could be aggravated by the therapeutic use of diuretics, especially if these cause further hemoconcentration. In addition, when plasma fibrinogen levels increase, especially to values as high as 1 g/dL as can be seen in nephrotic syndrome, they cause increased erythrocyte aggregation and marked increases in plasma viscosity (289). A role for physical factors is supported by the high incidence of renal vein thrombosis, as hemoconcentration of the blood and the effect of urinary inhibitor loss will be most pronounced in the radicles of the renal vein (290).

Steroid administration increases the concentrations of several clotting factors and modifies coagulation mechanisms (240). Moreover, a high incidence of thromboses was recorded after these drugs were first used to treat nephrotic syndrome (291). Both arterial and venous thromboses, however, have been found in nephrotic subjects not receiving steroids. Furthermore, a hypercoagulable state is present in untreated MCNS patients, and levels of the coagulation factors do not change after steroid treatment is implemented (263).

Except for the protein S data, the potential relationship between various biochemical findings and the clinical importance of thrombus formation remains largely theoretical. For example, the biochemical abnormalities in children may be more severe than those in adults with the nephrotic syndrome, whereas the incidence of thromboembolic phenomena is worse in adults (292). This may reflect the fact that MCN is more common in children, whereas membranous nephropathy (see Chapter 63) is more common in adults. Therefore, the underlying nature of the disease may be important in determining the occurrence of intravascular coagulation. Finally, it is important to consider the physiologic conditions within the circulatory tree. For example, one study suggested that although platelet aggregation is increased in nephrosis, fibrin conversion inhibits platelet interaction with the vessel wall extracellular matrix, actually decreasing the likelihood of platelet participation in thrombus formation. In this system, the data suggest that increased fibrin formation, but not increased platelet aggregation, contributes to the hypercoagulability of the nephrotic syndrome (293). In support of a primary role for the coagulation cascade, nephrotic patients show biochemical evidence for endothelial injury (294). The effects of negative-charge sites must also be considered. Like plasminogen activator activity, antithrombin III is active in association with vascular wall heparan sulfate proteoglycans. If MCNS involves a generalized decrease in negative-charge sites, antithrombin III activity may be impaired.

Infections

It has long been known that patients with MCNS have increased susceptibility to infection. This increase may be related to the prolonged presence of gross edema or ascites, which is composed of fluids that represent ideal culture media for bacterial growth. Infection risk may be potentiated by therapy with steroids or immunosuppressive drugs, although the high incidence of infections was noted in the era before these drugs were available. Humoral responses to bacteria may be defective. Plasma concentrations of IgG are markedly reduced during relapse (295), and the ability of MCN patients to generate specific antibodies is impaired (296) between as well as during relapses. Although the role of these abnormalities in predisposing nephrotic subjects to infections remains to be elucidated, it may be significant that boys with MCN respond poorly to hepatitis B vaccine (297). This same population has a higher incidence of chronic hepatitis B surface antigenemia than that found in a control population (298). Another factor that could contribute to a high rate of infections in patients with nephrosis is a decreased serum level of alternative complement pathway factor B. Absence of this factor has been linked to defective opsonization of *Escherichia coli* in nephrotic patients (299) and to defective neutrophil function (300). Serum levels of hemolytic factor D also are decreased in patients during relapse and return to normal with remission (301). Levels of both of these factors correlate strongly with serum albumin concentration, suggesting that decreased serum levels result from urinary loss. These concerns have led to recommendations that both pediatric and adult patients with nephrosis should receive pneumococcal vaccine (302,303). In addition, the use of penicillin prophylaxis may be required in children younger than 2 years of age, or in older patients who have low antibody titers or recurrent pneumococcal infection (304). Immune system abnormalities more specifically associated with MCN are unlikely to result entirely from albuminuria, since they are specific for that disease; these will be considered in the section on MCN later in this chapter.

Consequences of Loss of Other Proteins

Numerous proteins in addition to albumin are lost in the urine. In most instances, these proteins are of a similar or smaller size than albumin. Such losses could alter function in the endocrine system or in metabolic pathways. Therefore, loss of insulin-like growth factors could contribute to poor growth in some nephrotic children (305). The urinary loss of thyroxin-binding globulin (TBG) correlates well with total urinary protein excretion (306). In addition to TBG, losses of thyroxine (T_4) and triiodothyronine (T_3) in nephrotic urine are associated with decreased serum levels of T_3 and TBG. Most of the patients studied were clinically euthyroid and their serum levels of free T_4 and thyroid-stimulating hormone (TSH) did not differ from those in normal control subjects (307). In addition, their values for T_3 uptake were normal. Another study documented urinary losses, but normal serum concentrations of TBG (308). The patients had low or low-normal T_4 levels. Such differences in findings could relate to the underlying cause for nephrotic syndrome, whether it is associated with selective or nonselective proteinuria and whether it is accompanied by uremia. Children with MCNS have serum T_4 or free T_4 levels that are marginally low (309). They have been interpreted as having mild thyroid failure based on increased baseline TSH levels and their response to thyrotropin-releasing hormone (310). In patients who have congenital nephrotic syndrome, nephrectomy to eliminate proteinuria is associated with normalization of thyroid status, indicating that these abnormalities result from massive proteinuria rather than an intrinsic glandular defect (311).

Total serum calcium is markedly reduced, primarily because of hypoalbuminemia and the consequent decrease in protein-bound calcium. Serum ionized calcium levels may be reduced as well (312,313), even in nephrotic subjects with normal renal function; this may result in symptomatic hypocalcemia. At least some of the reduction in ionized calcium is the consequence of loss of 25-hydroxyvitamin D (25-[OH]-D) in nephrotic urine (314,315); other metabolites of vitamin D may be lost, as well (316). Low plasma levels of 25-(OH)-D, $1,25(OH)_2$-D, and $24,25$-$(OH)_2$-D have been reported in patients with nephrotic syndrome (314), and intestinal absorption of calcium is reduced (312); serum parathyroid hormone levels are increased (313). From these observations, it has been postulated (317) that urinary loss of vitamin D complex results in decreased absorption of intestinal calcium, skeletal resistance to parathyroid hormone, and reduced serum calcium levels. In turn, these changes cause increased parathyroid hormone (PTH) production and could result in defective bone mineralization. Although it has not been proved that the changes described cause significant bone disease (318), ongoing steroid therapy may increase the likelihood of clinically significant problems (319,320). In 60 children and adolescents with relapsing nephrotic syndrome, bone mineral density (BMD) was decreased but whole-body bone mineral content was higher because of an increase in the body-metabolic index (321). In patients with unremitting proteinuria and low 25-OH-D levels, supplementation with oral calcium and 25-OH-D should be considered (322).

Carbohydrate metabolism also may be deranged. Of 38 adult nephrotic patients who had not received any drugs, including glucocorticoids, for at least 2 months, 14 had oral glucose tolerance test results that were similar to those found in diabetic patients (323). Affected patients had increased insulin secretion that was thought to be secondary to increased growth hormone levels. The initiating event for these changes was not determined. There was no correlation of these findings with either serum albumin levels or renal histopathology. This observation raises the question of whether nephrotic hyperlipidemia could contribute to the development of noninsulin-dependent (type 2) diabetes mellitus.

Alterations in trace metal metabolism may be due to urinary losses of either the metals or their carrier proteins. Decreased serum levels of both iron and copper, associated with a low serum iron-binding capacity and low erythrocyte copper content, have been documented in nephrotic syndrome (324). Serum levels of copper, but not iron, were improved by oral administration of the metal. Urinary iron and copper concentrations correlated with protein excretion. The intravenous infusion of albumin led to increased albuminuria and increased metal excretion. In each case, the abnormalities appeared to be related to urinary protein loss. Nephrotic children may develop anemia secondary to urinary loss of transferrin and iron (325,326). Serum zinc levels are low in nephrotic syndrome, but urinary excretion of zinc is not elevated. Zinc binds to albumin so that serum zinc levels change with alterations in albumin levels, regardless of the etiology of the nephrotic syndrome. However, decreased zinc content in the hair of these patients suggests that other aspects of zinc metabolism also may be deranged (327).

Many drugs are protein-bound in the plasma. Hypoalbuminemia decreases the number of drug-binding sites and could result in increased toxicity of drugs that normally are bound to protein. For example, digoxin is 25% bound to proteins in the plasma, digitoxin is 90% bound, hydrochlorothiazide is 60% bound, and furosemide is 96% bound; hydralazine, prazosin, and diazoxide are all approximately 90% bound, whereas the binding of barbiturates varies from 5% to 80% depending on molecular structure (328).

General Approach to the Treatment of Nephrotic Syndrome

Based on the consequences of proteinuria described in the preceding text, symptomatic treatment regimens have been developed for the care of all nephrotic patients, even beyond those classified as having a form of primary nephrotic syndrome. These treatments, which are aimed at the physiology of nephrosis rather than the etiology of the disease, have implications beyond the reduction of nephrotic proteinuria and edema.

Diuretics and Fluid Management

Many patients with nephrotic syndrome respond to the acute use of diuretics with increased urinary losses of sodium and water. Although diuretics may be effective, there are limited indications for their use in the acute treatment of nephrotic subjects, especially children. The degree of diuresis and natriuresis they induce is small compared to that observed when the patient responds to treatment directed at the underlying cause. Furthermore, it is possible that diuretic use, by depleting intravascular as well as interstitial fluid volume, may contribute to the development of shock seen in some patients with MCNS (165).

Nonetheless, oral or parenteral diuretics are effective and often are indicated in the management of persistent edema. Parenteral furosemide is more effective than orally administered drug. Treatment may be initiated at 1 mg/kg (up to 40 mg) with judicious increases up to three to four times the usual dose (329) in an effort to elicit a response. Diuretic therapy may be less effective in patients with primary nephrotic syndrome than in most other patients, in part because of a combination of factors resulting in a physiologically decreased ability to excrete sodium. This is especially true of the loop diuretics such as furosemide, which also may be inhibited by its binding to albumin present in the tubular lumen (330). Although spironolactone interferes with distal nephron sodium reabsorption and thus is a theoretically useful diuretic, in practice its delayed onset of action and relatively weak potency limit its usefulness to being a potentiating agent with loop diuretics. Metolazone, a thiazide-like drug that impedes both proximal and late distal nephron sodium absorption (331), is a singularly effective oral diuretic in patients with sodium retention secondary to nephrotic syndrome. There is a possibility that diuretic therapy will deplete the intravascular volume without significantly reducing the tissue edema. Therefore, diuretics should be administered with care and withheld in patients for whom a rapid response to steroids is anticipated.

If the patient has anasarca, if respiratory embarrassment results from ascites or pleural effusion, if scrotal or vulval edema is sufficiently severe to threaten tissue breakdown (332), or if peritonitis is present, then more aggressive therapy is warranted to decrease the amount of edema. A useful regimen consists of oral spironolactone, 1 mg/kg per day, and daily intravenous infusions of albumin, 0.5 g/kg initially and increasing, if well tolerated, to 1 g/kg per day. The albumin infusion should be preceded by the intravenous infusion of furosemide, 0.5 mg/kg. A repeated dose of diuretic is given toward the end of the albumin infusion. Blood pressure should be monitored throughout the albumin infusion to help avoid complications from rapid mobilization of edema fluid into the circulation, although the regimen usually is free from significant side effects when used in children and young adults. Recent observations suggest that the administration of albumin may result in more severe glomerular epithelial changes, raise the oncotic pressure of the tissue space, delay the response to corticosteroid therapy, and induce more frequent relapses after remission (333). In view of the potential for complications of albumin infusion (334), this treatment should be reserved for the specific indications of respiratory embarrassment, tissue breakdown, or the need to elicit urine output to confirm the diagnosis of nephrosis.

Management of the acute phase of nephrotic syndrome should include dietary sodium restriction. During relapse, dietary sodium intake optimally should be reduced to about 0.5 g per/day, which is approximately equivalent to a 1-g salt diet or about 20 mEq of sodium per day. Such severe dietary restriction is difficult to accomplish even in a carefully controlled hospital setting. It is important to emphasize that severe restriction of sodium intake will not result in weight loss when nephrotic patients are in the sodium-retaining phase of their disease. In such patients, the normal extrarenal losses of sodium may amount to less than 10 mEq per/day. Therefore, severe dietary sodium restriction is intended to prevent further accumulation of edema. Use of a salt substitute may facilitate compliance with the sodium-restricted diet, but in patients with renal insufficiency it must be limited because these preparations consist of potassium and ammonium salts.

At home, most patients can rarely manage dietary restriction below that of a no-added-salt diet. This provides a sodium intake of 40 to 60 mEq per/day depending on the patient's size. Even in remission, it should be employed not only to lessen the risk of edema formation if the patient has a relapse, but also to reduce side effects from steroid administration.

Although there is some debate regarding fluid management, we believe that fluid intake also should be restricted, at least initially. If intake equals insensible fluid losses plus urine output, the patient's weight will remain stable without further accumulation of edema. To accomplish loss of weight, fluid intake must be reduced below this level. Some nephrotic patients experience intense thirst. If sodium intake is limited and fluid intake is great, the patient can become hyponatremic and will remain edematous.

Anecdotal experience suggests that bed rest may potentiate a diuresis, perhaps by redistributing fluid from the peripheral tissues to the vascular space, thereby increasing renal blood flow. Bed rest also may accelerate a response to steroids and, when practical, should be advised for patients with anasarca. Other therapies that may facilitate a diuresis in some patients by mobilizing tissue fluid include local pressure using surgical elastic stockings or immersion up to the neck in warm water (128). After remission is induced, a high-protein diet may increase the rate at which plasma protein concentration returns to normal (335).

Dietary Treatment

As already indicated, dietary sodium and water restriction is important in the management of the acute phase of nephrotic syndrome. Long-term reduction of dietary sodium intake in combination with diuretics can be most effective in controlling edema in patients resistant to steroids and other pharmacologic agents.

Other dietary manipulations have received attention. High-protein diets can be beneficial in special groups of patients such as those with congenital nephrotic syndrome (336). The concept of increasing dietary protein in all nephrotic subjects has not proved to be beneficial. Although albumin synthesis increases with such diets, urinary protein excretion increases too, possibly due to an angiotensin II-induced increase in glomerular permeability. Therefore, it has been proposed that inhibitors of ACE should be used in conjunction with the high protein intake (94).

Conversely, low-protein diets will decrease albuminuria and increase albumin mass (337). This reflects conservation of essential amino acids in response to proteinuria (338). The use of soy-based, low-protein, low-fat diets rich in polyunsaturated fats and supplemented with essential amino acids or keto analogs results in decreases in urinary protein excretion and in serum total and LDL cholesterol levels (339–341). Supplementing diets with fish oils containing omega ω-3 fatty acids has not proved beneficial (342). Concerns about such dietary manipulations include their cost, the lack of patient acceptance, and whether strict adherence might result in specific nutritional deficiencies (337,343). Reducing dietary fat intake in hyperlipidemic but otherwise healthy children to the levels recommended by the National Cholesterol Education Program is safe and does not affect the children's growth or development (344). The safety of more stringent restrictions in children with renal disease remains to be determined.

Lowering dietary fat intake has a limited effect on reducing serum lipids in the nephrotic patient. Therefore, attention has focused on whether there is a role for lipid-lowering drugs in managing hyperlipidemia in these patients (see following paragraph). The efficacy of oligoantigenic diets or those that eliminate specific antigens has been tested in nephrotic subjects (see section on Atopy and Minimal Change Nephropathy). This approach is based on the possibility that some cases of nephrotic syndrome may be the consequence of food allergies, especially to milk and dairy products.

Lipid-Lowering Drugs

Long-term administration of HMG CoA reductase inhibitors in nephrotic patients will induce reductions of serum triglycerides as well as serum total and LDL cholesterol levels; HDL cholesterol values are maintained (192,236,345,346). Long-term benefits from this therapy have yet to be proved, although anecdotal experience suggests that it may help to reduce proteinuria and maintain GFR (347), as observed in experimental animals (see section on Hyperlipidemia).

Other Medical Therapy

Anticoagulation has been employed as indicated in patients with intravascular thromboses. Some clinicians utilize small doses of aspirin in an effort to prevent repeated thromboembolic episodes (348), but there are no studies confirming the efficacy of this approach.

Although hypocalcemia is common in relapses of nephrotic syndrome, it is likely that most patients in relapse of brief duration do not require routine treatment with calcium or with vitamin D or one of its metabolites (349). Supplementation with oral calcium (1 g per day) and 25-OH-vitamin D (25 μg per day) maintains normal bone status in steroid-dependent nephrotic patients (322). Vitamin D treatment may be more routinely necessary in patients who are steroid-resistant (350) (see section on Consequences of Loss of Other Proteins previously in this chapter). Similarly, patients who develop other deficiencies secondary to renal losses, such as iron-deficiency anemia, will require appropriate treatment.

Medical Treatment to Reduce Proteinuria. In patients who prove to be unresponsive to therapy directed at the underlying cause of proteinuria, efforts have been employed to decrease protein loss by employing drugs that appear to be directed against the physiology of glomerular proteinuria. The intent behind this treatment is to facilitate general medical management by decreasing proteinuria, increasing serum albumin, and thereby lessening edema formation. Thus, indomethacin is effective in ameliorating intractable nephrosis (351). Because of the association of nonsteroidal agents with renal failure in some nephrotic patients as described in the section on Complications, more recently clinicians have emphasized the use of ACE inhibition (97,352). Each of these treatments appears to reduce glomerular capillary hydraulic pressure, by different mechanisms. ACE inhibitors act by decreasing post-glomerular arteriolar resistance, whereas nonsteroidal drugs enhance preglomerular capillary resistance (353). Consistent with these mechanisms, Garini and colleagues (354) compared the effects of indomethacin, captopril and the calcium-channel blocker, nifedipine, on the changes in renal hemodynamics and proteinuria induced by a high-protein mean. The increases in GFR and renal blood flow were not blocked by captopril or nifedipine, but were blocked by indomethacin. The increase in protein excretion was blocked by indomethacin and captopril but not by nifedipine (354). Indeed, dihydropyridine calcium channel blockers do not decrease proteinuria (355) and may even increase it. Therefore, the effects on hemodynamics were different and the effect on proteinuria could be distinguished from both systemic effects on blood pressure and effects on GFR and RBF. In patients with membranous nephropathy, ACE inhibition may have a size-selective effect (356), decreasing the fractional clearance of larger (>60 Å) molecules, suggesting an effect on the shunt pathway of macromolecular clearance. Such studies have supported efforts by clinicians to utilize ACE inhibitors to decrease proteinuria not only for symptomatic management but also in an effort to delay or prevent the progression of chronic kidney disease. The efficacy of this treatment will be considered further in the section on FSGS.

It is possible that at least a part of the antiproteinuric effect of ACE inhibition is not mediated by the glomerulus. Angiotensin blockade enhances megalin expression and albumin reabsorption (357).

Nephrectomy. Unilateral nephrectomy has proved beneficial in some infants presenting with nephrotic syndrome in the first year of life (358), and bilateral nephrectomy may be a useful part of the aggressive approach required in patients with congenital nephrotic syndrome if they are to survive to an age when transplantation is feasible (359,360) (see section on Nephrotic Syndrome in the First Year of Life in the Clinical Variants of FSGS, later in this chapter). Bilateral embolization of renal arteries can be an important therapeutic option in carefully selected patients with nephrotic syndrome who appear destined to progress to end-stage renal failure (361).

MINIMAL CHANGE NEPHROPATHY

Although MCN is often thought of as a pediatric disease, it is one of the most common causes of nephrotic syndrome in adults as well. It is now the third most common cause of nephrosis in adults (10) and remains the most common cause of nephrotic syndrome in children younger than 16 years of age. Indeed, it is the second most common primary renal parenchymal disease in that age group. Two to seven new cases occur annually per 100,000 children (362), and the prevalence is about 15 cases per 100,000 children. Although most children with MCN achieve permanent remission of symptoms by the time they reach puberty, some cases persist into adulthood (363). Furthermore, new cases have been reported in the eighth decade of life (364). However, the relative incidence of MCN as the etiology of nephrotic syndrome decreases with age in both children and adults (10,364–366). Although it is not clear that adult-onset disease represents the same entity as that found in childhood, or that all patients with the clinical picture of MCNS have an identical disease, the clinical course and outcome of pediatric and adult cases appear to be sufficiently similar (364) to consider all cases together.

Minimal change disease can appear in the first year of life, but it is more common later, with a peak incidence at 2 years of age. Most pediatric surveys report that it occurs twice as often in boys as in girls, whereas it has an equal sex incidence in adults (367). Although no precipitating cause may be apparent in many children, it is not unusual for the development of edema and proteinuria to be preceded by an upper respiratory tract infection, an allergic reaction to an insect sting or other immunogenic stimuli, or the use of certain drugs (367–394) (Table 64-5). In both adult and pediatric patients, malignancies, especially Hodgkin disease, have been associated with the development of MCNS (see section on Nephrotic Syndrome and Malignancies).

Clinical Findings

Edema formation may begin within a few days of the inciting event. Facial edema usually is noted first, with few other indications of an ongoing disease process. This can be confused with allergic symptoms, especially if associated with an upper respiratory tract infection. Edema usually increases gradually. It becomes detectable in the adult only when several liters of fluid have accumulated; by the time medical advice is sought, the patient typically has pitting edema involving the sacrum and the lower extremities. When anasarca is present, periorbital edema can be so severe that the eyelids are swollen shut, scrotal or vulval edema may be marked, and there may be significant abdominal distension. Respiratory embarrassment may occur from accumulation of either pleural or ascitic fluid, although the infrequency of dyspnea or orthopnea in the setting of massive fluid retention is striking. This reflects the absence of increased pulmonary capillary wedge pressure needed to generate pulmonary edema. Headaches and irritability are common accompanying complaints of edema. The patient may note vague symptoms such as malaise, easy fatigability, irritability, and depression. Rarely,

TABLE 64-5

DRUGS AND OTHER FACTORS REPORTED TO HAVE PRECIPITATED MINIMAL CHANGE NEPHROPATHY (MCN)

Drugs
  Gold (368)
  Penicillamine (369)
  Ampicillin (370)
  Mercury-containing compounds (371)
  Nonsteroidal antiinflammatory agents (372–375)
  Trimethadione, paramethadione (376)

Atopy
  Pollen (377)
  Food allergy (378,379)
  House dust (380)
  Contact dermatitis (poison ivy and oak) (381)
  Bee (382) or wasp (395) stings

Tumors
  Lymphoma (384,385)
  Others (383)

Infections
  Various viral infections (386)
  Schistosomiasis (387)
  Ehrlichiosis (388)

Stimuli-associated with immune activation or inflammation
  Guillain-Barré syndrome (389)
  Still disease (390)
  Immunizations (391,396)
  Dermatitis herpetiformis (393)
  Epidermolysis bullosa (394)
  Thyroiditis (397,398)
  Sclerosing cholangitis (399)

the development of cellulitis, peritonitis, or pneumonia may be the first indication of an underlying nephrotic syndrome. The pallor resulting from edema can be misinterpreted as indicating anemia.

On physical examination, dependent edema is the most prominent finding. The retina has a characteristic "wet" appearance. Subungual edema may reverse the usual color pattern on the fingernails—the normally white lunulae may be pink and the rest of the nail bed white. Horizontal white lines that may be seen on both the fingernails and the toenails are referred to as *Muehrcke bands*. Inguinal and umbilical hernias may be present, especially if the patient has had severe ascites for a prolonged period. The elasticity of the cartilage in the ear appears to be decreased.

Blood pressure in patients with MCN usually is normal, but elevated systolic pressure has been recorded in 21% and elevated diastolic pressure in 14% of the children evaluated by the International Study of Kidney Disease in Children (ISKDC) (400). Hypertension is seen more commonly in adult patients with MCN (401).

Growth failure occasionally may be found in children, most often in those who have had multiple relapses of MCNS requiring frequent courses of steroids (321). Evidence for infection, especially peritonitis, cellulitis, or pneumonia, should be sought as part of the physical examination. These infections may be associated with septicemia and shock.

In MCNS, the chest radiograph usually shows a small or normal-sized heart; pleural effusions may be present, as may pneumonic infiltrates. The presence of an increased heart size

and congestive changes in the hilar regions suggests that the nephrotic syndrome is secondary to glomerulonephritis.

Laboratory Findings

Urinalysis. Clinicians who first characterized the nephrotic syndrome noted that the urine often foams excessively when voided and that it coagulates when heated. These findings result from marked proteinuria, now indicated by a dipstick reading of 3+. Other edema-forming, hypoalbuminemic states, such as malnutrition, milk protein sensitivity, and protein-losing enteropathy, can mimic nephrotic syndrome but do not manifest significant proteinuria. The amount of protein in the urine of nephrotic patients can range from less than 1 to more than 25 g per/day. The value for adult patients usually is between 3.5 and 16 g per/day; that for children typically is lower than this amount, even when allowances are made for body size (402), and averages about 50 mg/kg of body weight per/day (403). Because urine protein is a function of plasma, and thus of filtrate, protein concentration (404), children with MCNS, who may have serum albumin levels of 1 g/dL or less, may occasionally have amounts of urinary protein as low as 100 to 200 mg per/day. This finding in patients with low plasma albumin concentrations also reflects removal of much of the protein from the glomerular filtrate as it traverses the proximal convoluted tubule (405) (see previous section on Tubular Handling of Protein in Mechanisms for Proteinuria). As a consequence of proteinuria, the urine specific gravity in nephrosis usually is high, often exceeding 1.035. Exceptions include patients who are not in an edema-accumulating state (see section on Consequences of Proteinuria, earlier in this chapter) and the patient with nephrotic syndrome and renal failure or tubular dysfunction, in whom lower (but not isosthenuric) values of urine specific gravity are found. Physiologic responses of the kidney to the nephrotic state may cause further urine concentration.

The spectrum of excreted proteins depends on the renal disease responsible for the nephrotic syndrome. In primary nephrotic syndrome, most of the urine protein is albumin; in other diseases, such as glomerulonephritis, both albumin and globulins are lost in increased amounts. This occurrence has led to determination of "protein selectivity" being proposed as a noninvasive method to separate MCNS from other causes of nephrotic syndrome (406). By comparing clearance of albumin to that of larger molecules such as IgG or transferrin, a curve can be generated, indicating whether the protein loss is *selective* and restricted to small molecules, or *nonselective*, consisting of both large and small molecules. Patients with MCNS tend to show more selective proteinuria, whereas those with nephrotic syndrome from other causes have nonselective proteinuria. Unfortunately, this generalization is limited by considerable overlap in results from patients in different diagnostic categories, so that clinical determination of protein selectivity has limited value for individual patients. This limitation may reflect factors other than molecular size that also affect entry of proteins into the glomerular filtrate, and differences in tubular function, which modify reabsorption of filtered protein (407). A refined electrophoretic technique has been used to indicate protein selectivity and to predict outcome. Patients with primarily albumin and transferrin in urine as determined by sodium dodecyl sulfate-polyacrylamide gel electrophoresis (SDS-PAGE) proved to be steroid-sensitive, whereas patients who were steroid-resistant also excreted considerable amounts of IgG, lysozyme, and other larger molecules (408). Some of these larger molecules could be derived from tubular cells, reflecting tubulointerstitial injury rather than glomerular filtration, or from activation of the shunt pathway for filtration of macromolecules discussed earlier in this chapter. In analbuminemic rats with PAN nephrosis, fractional clearances of various macromolecules are similar to those in normoalbuminemic rats. The absence of competition for albumin implied by this finding suggests that urinary loss of these proteins in nephrotic patients does not result from "overload" of tubular reabsorption by filtered albumin (71).

The urine sediment from nephrotic subjects often contains oval fat bodies. Lipiduria is better diagnosed, however, using a microscope equipped with polarized light to demonstrate doubly refractile fat bodies ("Maltese crosses") in degenerative fatty vacuoles in the cytoplasm of desquamated renal epithelial cells or free in the urine as neutral fat droplets. Frequently, urine with large amounts of protein also contains hyaline casts.

Other urinary findings vary with the cause of the disease. Up to one third of patients with MCN may have microscopic hematuria. Gross hematuria may be seen in patients with uncomplicated MCN but is extremely rare (409). By contrast, it is more common in patients with prominent mesangial proliferation. Hematuria is more likely to be seen with FSGS than MCN (410). In patients with nephrotic syndrome secondary to glomerulonephritis, the urine shows more abnormalities, with cellular elements and granular, cellular, and mixed hyaline casts being present. However, patients with MCN cannot always be differentiated from those with glomerulonephritis on the basis of urine sediment abnormalities alone.

Blood Studies. Hypoproteinemia is common to all nephrotic patients and is caused, primarily, by hypoalbuminemia. Total serum protein is characteristically reduced to between 4.5 and 5.5 g/dL; serum albumin concentrations usually fall to below 2 g/dL, and, in children, may be less than 1 g/dL (363). Although serum albumin concentrations are usually decreased, those of total globulins are remarkably well preserved in MCN despite massive proteinuria. Typically, serum α_1-globulin concentrations are normal or slightly decreased, whereas levels of serum α_2- and β-globulins are increased. Although the concentration of γ-globulin determined by electrophoresis is normal or reduced, the levels of individual components vary. In MCN (295,386), serum IgG levels average approximately 20% of normal, whereas IgA levels are less severely reduced; IgM and possibly IgE levels are increased. The changes in serum IgG and IgA concentrations are less pronounced in patients with nephrotic syndrome of other causes; IgM and IgE are typically normal in these subjects (295,386).

Hyperlipidemia is one of the findings that define the nephrotic syndrome. Serum total cholesterol level is usually elevated, especially when the serum albumin level has fallen to 2 g/dL or less (167,295,386). Values average 400 mg/dL, but levels in excess of 1,000 mg/dL have been recorded. Other changes in plasma lipids are summarized in the section on Consequences of Proteinuria.

Most often, serum electrolyte concentrations are within the normal range even when anasarca is present, indicating proportionate retention of sodium and water. Factitiously low serum sodium concentrations (~130 mEq/L) may be measured with marked hyperlipidemia. This pseudohyponatremia results from the nonaqueous, nonsodium-containing component of the serum or plasma (lipid) being increased. It does not require treatment, because the sodium concentration in the aqueous phase of blood is normal, as is plasma osmolality. This artifact is not observed when sodium levels are determined by techniques that measure sodium activity with ion-specific electrodes or after sample ultracentrifugation. Low serum sodium may be an accurate finding in the case of excess free water ingestion relative to dietary sodium intake (411), compounded by potential effects of elevated plasma vasopressin (412). This problem may be exacerbated by diuretic therapy. A decreased anion gap is associated with decreased total serum protein or albumin levels. This finding is common to all hypoalbuminemic states and does not directly reflect either renal dysfunction or altered serum lipid levels (413). Serum calcium may be low, mainly as a result of the hypoalbuminemia. Normally, 40% of total serum calcium is bound to protein. A decrease in serum albumin concentration of 1 g/dL results in a decrease in total serum calcium of 0.8 mg/dL. In contrast, 1 g of globulin binds only 0.16 mg of calcium. In some cases, the hypocalcemia may be out of proportion to the hypoalbuminemia and is caused by a reduction of ionized calcium levels (414) by as much as 5% to 20%, possibly because of urinary loss of 25-OH-D (see section on Consequences of Proteinuria). Acute symptoms of hypocalcemia rarely occur. Total and ionized calcium levels return to normal with remission. Serum phosphorus is normal unless the nephrotic syndrome is associated with renal insufficiency.

Blood urea nitrogen (BUN) and serum creatinine values are usually close to normal in MCN, but may be mildly elevated if decreased intravascular volume from nephrosis causes prerenal azotemia. The BUN may be elevated because of either increased intrarenal urea circulation or increased protein catabolism if the patient has received steroids. Glomerular filtration rate measured by inulin clearance is reduced to an average of 80% of normal (147); occasionally values are reduced to 20% to 30% of normal. This may represent decreased renal perfusion secondary to hypovolemia. Reduced GFR at the onset of MCN is reversible and does not imply an unfavorable outcome (104). The presence or absence of azotemia therefore cannot be used as a reliable indicator in the differential diagnosis of the nephrotic syndrome.

Hemoglobin levels and hematocrit values may be normal or even increased if there is hemoconcentration secondary to loss of fluid into the peripheral tissues. This factor may help to differentiate azotemic patients with MCN from those who have severe renal insufficiency from parenchymal disease, in whom anemia is more typical. However, as noted previously, iron deficiency may cause nephrotic patients with normal renal function to become anemic.

Measured concentrations of serum complement and its components are generally considered to be normal in MCN. Although urinary losses cause decreases in low-molecular-weight complement components, serum concentrations of the components measured to detect activation of the complement cascade are unchanged (415). Thus, reduced levels of the third component of complement (β-1-C globulin; C3) or C4 indicate that a glomerulonephritis underlies the nephrotic syndrome; conversely, such changes do not occur invariably with glomerulonephritis. Circulating immune complexes may be elevated in MCN or in FSGS (416,417). Plasma renin activity may be increased in some patients who manifest physiologic changes consistent with decreased intravascular volume.

Histopathology

Minimal Change Nephropathy

The morphologic classification of nephrotic syndrome in childhood derives from classic papers by Churg and colleagues (418) and White and colleagues (419). The term *minimal change nephrotic syndrome* was used to describe the pathologic appearance on light microscopy of biopsies from nephrotic patients in which there are no definitive changes from normal in glomeruli (Fig. 64-7). Here, we have chosen to use the term *minimal change nephropathy* because some adult patients have been reported with proteinuria but no nephrosis (9,10) and in order to describe a histologic and functional entity in parallel to FSGS. The degree of change from normal histology that is considered significant remains the subject of some controversy. The spectrum of these changes is classified in Table 64-3 at the beginning of this chapter. Other terms that have

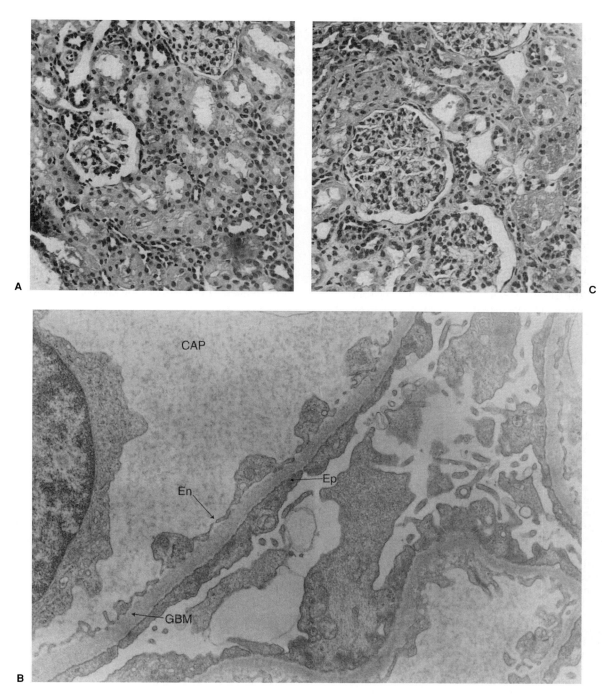

FIGURE 64-7. Findings on renal biopsies from three children with the clinical features of minimal change nephropathy. **A:** Light microscopy of a patient with MCN. Portions of two glomeruli are shown. Cellularity is normal and the capillary loops are patent. Tubular and interstitial structures are normal in appearance. (Magnification for all light microscopy ×350.) **B:** Electron microscopy from the same patient. The endothelial cells (En) lining the capillary loop show a normal fenestrated structure; the glomerular basement membrane (GBM) is uniform in thickness and structure. The epithelial cell (Ep) layer shows characteristic fusion of the epithelial foot processes, with the podocytes being in continuous contact with the GBM. Proteinaceous material and a nucleated cell are present in the capillary lumen (CAP). **C:** Light microscopy in a patient with mesangial hypercellularity. The tubular and glomerular capillary structures are normal, but an increased number of nuclei are present in the mesangial areas of the glomeruli. Immunofluorescent microscopy was negative for immunoglobulins and C3. The patient behaved clinically as one with MCNS. (Histology courtesy of Dr. John M. Kissane.)

been used to describe this general entity include *nil disease* and *steroid-sensitive nephrotic syndrome*. Changes in the proximal tubule cells reflect increased reabsorption of protein. Tubular cells may contain apparent vacuoles that are doubly refractile and are similar to the fine lipid droplets seen in oval fat bodies in the urine. This pathologic abnormality generated the term *lipoid nephrosis*, in which there is no tubular atrophy and the renal interstitium is normal. Older patients may show some globally fibrosed glomeruli with associated nephron loss. This finding is rare in children and should not involve more than 5% to 10% of glomeruli, even in elderly patients (3). Staining for glomerular polyanion with Alcian blue, colloidal iron, or ruthenium red may be reduced in the glomerular tufts. No immunoglobulin or complement deposition is observed by immunofluorescence. Electron microscopy (Fig. 64-7) reveals only glomerular epithelial cell foot-process effacement (see next paragraph) (420). Recent advances may permit this finding to be visualized by high-resolution light microscopy (421). The diffuse effacement of the podocytes that often contain protein-reabsorptive droplets typically results in the appearance of an almost continuous layer of cytoplasm on the urinary side of the GBM. Epithelial cells may appear detached in segments, producing denuded areas of the GBM. The GBM itself, however, appears normal. There are no electron-dense deposits adjacent to the GBM (422). Historically, 65% to 85% of children with primary nephrotic syndrome have this lesion (423), compared to a prevalence of about 30% of primary nephrotic syndrome and 15% of all nephrosis in adults (10).

Podocyte Foot Process Effacement

Podocyte foot process effacement is due to retraction, widening, and shortening of foot processes and is not due to fusion, as reviewed recently (424). With complete effacement, the GBM is covered by thin, sheetlike processes of podocyte cytoplasm, with gaps between the processes of adjacent cells (where protein filtration presumably occurs). Foot-process effacement is associated with a reduction in GFR, which is caused mainly by a reduction in the ultrafiltration coefficient K_f (see section on Physiologic and Anatomic Factors Affecting GFR in Consequences of Proteinuria, earlier in this chapter).

Podocyte effacement is accompanied by striking morphologic changes in the cellular cytoskeleton. The continuous layer of podocyte cytoplasm that overlies the GBM shows an increase in microfilaments and the appearance of a dense cytoskeletal band located within the basal portion of the podocyte, adjacent to the GBM. The cytoskeletal band has regions of high density at regular intervals. *En face* views demonstrate that the filaments are distributed radially from these central densities, suggesting that they may function to distribute mechanical strain and thereby prevent glomerular capillary expansion (425). Endlich et al. exposed cultured podocytes to biaxial cyclic stress, in order to model stress that might be experienced by podocytes in glomerulomegaly (426). Transverse stress fibers disappeared and were replaced by radial stress fibers connected to a single actin-rich center. The stress fibers were composed of myosin II, α-actinin, and synaptopodin. These findings differ in important ways from podocytes *in vivo*, where the actin-rich center is absent and actin is confined to the foot processes. Nevertheless, the results do suggest that podocyte response to stress consistently involves formation of radial cytoskeletal structures.

It appears likely that podocyte foot process effacement arises by different mechanisms in different settings. Certain podocyte injury models (protamine infusion, reactive oxygen species infusion, PAN administration) are associated with redistribution of α-dystroglycan from the basal surface of the podocyte, a process that occurs within as little as 15 minutes (427). MCN but not FSGS is associated with loss of podocyte dystroglycan

expression (428). Kojima and Kerjaschki (429) have suggested that polycations compete with GBM laminin for binding to its receptor, dystroglycan; free dystroglycan is then internalized into podocyte endosomes. This process is dependent upon cellular ATP and participation of the actin cytoskeleton.

Related but distinct mechanisms may explain foot process effacement in FSGS, particularly postadaptive FSGS. Shirato (424) and Kriz et al. (430) have proposed that the podocyte supports the essential but contradictory functions of structural stability and leakiness (hydraulic conductivity). Cytoskeletal hypertrophy represents cellular adaptation to increased stress. The source of stress might be glomerular enlargement, increased glomerular P_{GC} (associated with the overload state) or increased GBM distensibility (due to GBM damage). Johnson has pointed out that the transmembrane oncotic pressure gradient influences the net filtration pressure (P_{UF}) and thereby might also contribute to net hydraulic stress (431). P_{UF} is the difference between transmembrane hydraulic pressure and the transmembrane oncotic pressure gradient. In the setting of nephrotic-range proteinuria, plasma albumin is reduced, which reduces the transmembrane oncotic pressure gradient across the capillary wall and thereby increases P_{UF}. In the face of mechanical or hydraulic stress, the capillary wall has three defenses: the mesangial cell, the podocyte, and the GBM. The mesangial cell may undergo proliferation and hypertrophy. Little is known about how the GBM responds to stress. The podocyte cannot proliferate and adapts by elaborating a more complex cytoskeleton to defend the structural integrity of the capillary wall. This occurs, however, at the cost of a reduction in total slit diaphragm width, podocyte effacement, and reduced K_f.

Variations in Histopathology

Immunoglobulin Deposition. Some patients with all the clinical features of MCN may have minor morphologic differences from those already described. A common variation is the presence of IgM in the glomerular mesangium. An early report (432) suggested that this variant represents a separate entity, which was termed mesangial IgM nephropathy. All of the patients, whose ages ranged from 1.5 to 59 years, showed a slight increase in mesangial matrix, and in addition to the IgM deposits, some had C3 and rare IgA deposition. Dense mesangial deposits were noted by electron microscopy in 9 of the 12 subjects. Subsequent observations did not support this as being a separate entity. In one study, 40% of 149 consecutive patients with the clinical picture of primary nephrotic syndrome were found on biopsy to have mesangial IgM deposits. Of these, 20 had mostly or entirely IgM without complement. They could not be differentiated clinically from other MCN patients (433). Because the presence of mesangial IgM deposit in patients with clinical MCN does not appear to affect either the patient's response to treatment or the disease outcome (434), it is now believed that this finding has little significance.

Mesangial IgM deposits in apparent MCN may, in some cases, be associated with immune complexes (435). Because deposits are often found in patients who undergo biopsy after receiving a trial of corticosteroid therapy, it is of interest that experimental models of immune complex metabolism suggest that steroid administration may prolong the systemic half-life of larger complexes and increase and sustain their appearance in the mesangium (436). The presence in the glomeruli of immunoglobulins in addition to IgM usually indicates a diagnosis of a disease other than MCN (437). One group of patients with a clinical diagnosis of MCN showed some glomerular proliferation associated with immunoglobulin deposits, primarily IgG, in the glomeruli. This lesion was more often observed in African American children (119), whereas a racial predilection may not be present in adults (438). Although the patients described in this report responded to treatment with steroids initially, their subsequent course was one of frequent relapses or the development of resistance to treatment.

Mesangial Proliferation. Some patients with otherwise typical MCN have increased numbers of mesangial cells in the glomeruli. One study that correlated glomerular morphometry with the patient's clinical course found increased numbers of mesangial nuclei and smaller nuclear size in patients who had frequent relapses. The authors proposed that this indicated mesangial cell activation. They cautioned, however, that disease duration could play a role in the development of this finding, because the frequently relapsing patients had a 4-year course compared to 1.4 years in the population with infrequent relapses (439). Mesangial hypercellularity may be associated with a decreased response to steroid therapy (134,440,441), frequent relapse (441), steroid dependency (442), or a poorer prognosis (442–444). The ISKDC found that approximately 2.5% of children with nephrotic syndrome had mesangial hypercellularity (445).

Mechanisms of mesangial proliferation. Based on the finding of identical immunohistochemistry in patients with or without mesangial proliferation, it has been argued that mesangial IgM deposition does not appear to play a role in the induction of the mesangial cell response (440). Intrinsic kidney cells and cells migrating into the kidney as part of the inflammatory response, release factors that regulate mesangial cell proliferation. Mesangial cells produce platelet-derived growth factor (PDGF), a stimulant of mesangial and endothelial cell growth and wound healing (446); prostacyclin and thromboxane, produced by a variety of cells, are stimulatory cofactors for mesangial cell proliferation (447). In addition, two autocrine growth mechanisms have been defined. The first involves interleukin (IL)-1. Mesangial cells in culture secrete a mesangial cell growth factor with characteristics identical to those of IL-1 (448). Indeed, these cells express messenger RNA (mRNA) for IL-1 *in vivo* (449). The second autocrine system involves IL-6. Mesangial cell-derived IL-6 stimulates mesangial cell growth *in vitro* (450). Moreover, mice transgenic for the human IL-6 gene show marked mesangial proliferation (451). In human disease, urinary excretion of IL-6 and mesangial staining of biopsy material for IL-6 were associated with mesangial proliferation by some (452), but not all (453) authors. Because mesangial proliferative changes are associated with steroid resistance, it is noteworthy that IL-6-induced cell activation is not inhibited by steroids (454). Finally, negative regulation of mesangial cell growth may be provided by the GBM itself, as proliferation of mesangial cells is decreased by heparan sulfate (455).

Tip Lesion. A group of patients has been described as having steroid-responsive nephrotic syndrome with intercapillary foam cells adherent to Bowman's capsule in a tuft near the tubular origin (the glomerular tip lesion). Although this adhesion is irreversible, the patients appear to have a good prognosis closer to that of MCN than that of steroid-resistant nephrotic syndrome (9,456). Tip lesion is considered more extensively in the section on Selected Clinical Variants of FSGS.

C1q Nephropathy. Biopsies from some nephrotic patients show mesangial deposits of the complement component, C1q, despite the presence of normal serum complement levels and the absence of complement-activating diseases such as systemic lupus erythematosus. Accompanying pathologic findings can be protean (457), including FSGS (458), crescentic glomerulopathy (459), or minimal changes (460). Patients may present with congenital nephrotic syndrome (461), steroid-sensitive disease (460), or steroid resistance (462). It is not certain whether C1q deposits represent a distinct entity or an incidental finding.

Disease Processes and Other Findings Associated with MCN

Several clinical findings have been associated with MCN, including specific malignancies, atopy, various HLA haplotypes, and abnormalities in immune function. These associations, which could elucidate issues of both causality and treatment, will be considered here.

Malignancy. Several glomerulopathies, notably membranous glomerulopathy, have been associated with neoplasia. A significant number of patients with cancer-related nephrotic syndrome, however, have MCN (Table 64-6). The relationship between MCN and lymphomatous disorders, particularly Hodgkin disease, is especially striking (383). In a survey of the literature, 33 of 134 patients with cancer-related nephrotic syndrome had MCN, as determined by biopsy (385). Of the patients with MCN, 26 had Hodgkin disease and an additional two had non-Hodgkin lymphoma. In another review (384), 36 of 44 patients who had Hodgkin disease and the nephrotic syndrome had MCN and only two had membranous glomerulonephritis. There was a much higher incidence of nephritic diseases in patients with other types of neoplasia. Nonlymphomatous tumors that have been associated rarely with MCN include renal oncocytoma (463), embryonal cell tumors (385), pancreatic carcinoma (464), nephroblastoma (465), Waldenström's macroglobulinemia (466), bronchogenic carcinoma (467), and cecal adenocarcinoma (468).

TABLE 64-6

NEPHROTIC SYNDROME IN PATIENTS WITH MALIGNANCY

Type of malignancy	Renal histology[a]		
	Minimal change disease	Membranous nephropathy	Membranoproliferative glomerulonephritis
Hodgkin lymphoma	26	4	0
Non-Hodgkin lymphoma	2	2	1
Leukemia	1	4	1
Multiple myeloma	0	0	1
Carcinoma	3	33	4
Benign or embryonal tumors	1	1	0

[a]Only cases with defined renal pathology and without amyloidosis are shown.
(Data from: Eagen JW, Lewis EJ. Glomerulopathies of neoplasia. *Kidney Int* 1977;11:297.)

Evidence suggests that in these cases the tumor may be directly involved in the pathogenesis of the MCN. MCN can be the initial presenting sign of a lymphomatous disorder (469) and may precede clinical evidence of lymphoma by several years (470). With appropriate and successful antineoplastic therapy, either medical or surgical, the proteinuria in tumor-related MCN resolves, renal function remains normal, and the nephrotic syndrome remits (385,463,467,470). The relationship between relapse of the tumor and of the nephrotic syndrome (471,472) also strongly suggests an etiologic role for the tumor in the pathogenesis of MCN in these patients. These observations indicate the importance of considering a malignancy as an underlying cause in any adult (471–474) and, rarely, in pediatric (475) patients who present with apparent primary nephrotic syndrome. If Hodgkin lymphoma is the cause, it is essential to treat the neoplasm rather than the renal disease.

Atopy and MCN. A relationship between allergy and MCN has long been suspected. Anecdotal reports suggest that exposure to allergens may precipitate the nephrotic syndrome (377,379,475,476); rhinorrhea and allergic skin reactivity frequently precede relapses (477), and a high prevalence of allergic symptoms has been observed in nephrotic patients. Highly allergic patients who had a pathologic diagnosis of MCN based on renal biopsy experienced a decrease in urinary protein excretion when placed on an elemental diet and did not require treatment with corticosteroids. Challenge with milk led to a decrease in serum C3 and increased protein excretion, strongly suggesting that hypersensitivity was causally linked to proteinuria (378). A human basophil degranulation test was positive in 16 of 28 adults with MCN and 14 of 18 with FSGS; in contrast, only 5 of 29 patients with glomerulonephritis and 1 of 11 healthy donors showed a positive response (478). In addition, atopy and MCN were associated with increased frequency of expression of human leukocyte antigen (HLA)-B12 and -DRw7 (478–480).

Although values ranged widely, mean serum IgE levels were significantly elevated in patients with MCN compared to those with other renal problems (481); elevated levels also are associated with frequent relapse in children (482). In one study, the majority of adult MCN patients had serum IgE levels more than two standard deviations above the normal mean; of these, more than 70% had associated allergic symptoms (483). Other investigators have made similar observations, but sought to draw a distinction between primary allergic disease and the elevated IgE levels found in nephrotic syndrome. They suggest that because IgE deposition in the glomerulus is rare (484), elevated serum IgE levels could represent not the causal factor in MCN but rather evidence of more generalized derangement in the immune system (485). This concept is supported by a finding that increased serum IgE may persist even with remission. If this view is correct, it could explain why attempts to treat MCN in atopic patients with inhaled disodium cromoglycate (486) or an orally administered analog (477) were unsuccessful.

These apparently conflicting observations may be resolved by study of specific antigens. Therefore, a majority of adult nephrotic patients studied by Meadow et al., and Lagrue, Laurent, et al. had detectable elevations of specific IgE titers, with the most common sensitizing agent being house dust or dust mites. After remission induced by institution of specific desensitization and sodium cromolyn, several of these patients had a relapse on re-exposure to the allergen (477,487,488).

Immunogenetics. There may be a familial incidence of MCN. A survey from Europe, which excluded patients with the congenital nephrotic syndrome (489), found that 63 of 1,877 nephrotic children had affected family members. This prevalence of 3.35% was higher than that predicted from the frequency with which MCN occurs in the general population. Siblings were most often affected. The similarity of pathologic findings and clinical course for affected members within a family was striking (490), although in at least one report siblings showed differences in these features (491). Familial nephrotic syndrome in children has been divided into two broad categories: (a) patients with an infantile onset and a poor prognosis regardless of renal morphology and (b) patients with a juvenile onset and a generally good response to conventional therapy, provided MCN is found by renal biopsy.

An indication of a possible genetic predisposition for development of MCN is the reported association of MCN, and in some cases atopy (480,508), with certain histocompatibility-complex antigens. The most commonly cited are HLA-B8 (480 493,495,508), and -DRw7 (494,496). Not all studies have confirmed these associations. Indeed, a variety of HLA antigens have been associated with MCN (479,480,492–500,505,507) (Table 64-7) and negative associations have been reported, too. HLA-B8 was found frequently in families with more than one member having childhood nephrosis (509). In one study the combined occurrence of B8 with DR3 and DR7 produced a relative risk of 21.5 (500). In another study DR7 was linked to steroid-sensitive disease and DR3 to steroid-resistant disease (498). In French and German patients, specific DQB1 alleles have been associated with MCNS, most strongly in steroid-dependent or frequently relapsing patients (501). German studies also suggested that patients with HLA-DR7/-DR3 together are less steroid-sensitive (504) and those with HLA-DR7 are less likely to respond permanently to alkylating agent treatment of frequent relapse (506).

MCN was associated with HLA-DQB1*0601, -DRB1*01 and -DRB1*07011 in Egyptian children (507,510,511) and -DQA*0201 in German children (505,507,510). Studies from Japan linked steroid-sensitive MCN in adult patients to HLA-DRw8 and -DQw3 (497) and to specific DQB1 alleles (502,503). Different results obtained in Singaporean (512) or Bengali (513) children are likely due in part to racial or geographic differences. The observation that two extended HLA haplotypes (HLA-A1, -B8, -DR3, -DRw52, SCO1; and HLA-B44, -DR7, -DRw53, FC31) occurred with higher than expected frequency in children with steroid-sensitive, frequently relapsing MCN provides the strongest evidence to date for an immunogenetic predisposition to the disease (499).

The association between HLA type and MCN has been made primarily in children, with some studies being unable to make similar correlations in adult patients. This finding suggests that MCN in adult and pediatric patients could represent different diseases that share common pathologic and clinical features. For example, HLA-DR7, which has been linked to MCN (Table 64-7), was observed in only 18% of adult European MCN patients, a frequency not different from that of control subjects. If the data were analyzed according to age at onset of the nephrotic syndrome, 45% of patients in whom onset was before the age of 15 years were HLA-DR7, whereas the equivalent incidence in adult-onset patients was only 7% (514). It remains unclear whether these associations represent linkage disequilibrium with another gene or reflect potential underlying immune influences on the development and response of MCN.

Disordered Immunity in MCN. It has long been recognized that immunogenic stimuli may precipitate presentation or relapse of MCN. In addition to the frequent association with atopy discussed previously, episodes may follow upper respiratory tract infections, bee stings, or diseases linked with abnormal immune responses. The relationship of immunogenic events to onset of disease and the finding of disordered immune responses in these patients led Shalhoub (515) to propose a unifying hypothesis relating MCN to the immune

TABLE 64-7

RELATIONSHIP BETWEEN MINIMAL CHANGE NEPHROPATHY AND HUMAN LEUKOCYTE ANTIGEN (HLA) TYPE

Author (ref.)	Year	Country of origin	No. of patients	HLA association	Relative risk	Children	Comments
Thomson, et al. (480)	1976	England	71	B12	6.3	Yes	Relative risk with B12 and atopy—13
Trompeter, et al. (492)	1980	England	116	B12	3.1	Yes	Could not confirm atopy data
O'Regan, et al. (493)	1980	Ireland	54	B8	3.5	Yes	—
Alfiler, et al. (494)	1980	Australia	42	B18	3.16	Yes	MCN confirmed by biopsy; decreased DR2
				DRw7	5.9		
Noss, et al. (495)	1981	Germany	45	B8	2.81	Yes	
deMouzon-Cambon, et al. (479)	1981	France	54	DRw7	4.4	Yes	Related to atopy; decreased DR2
Nunez-Roldan, et al. (496)	1982	Spain	50	DRw7	4.5	Yes	Decreased DR2
Kobayashi, et al. (497)	1985	Japan	40	DRw8	3.74	No	Studied adult subjects
Cambon-Thomsen, et al. (498)	1986	France	72	DQw3	1.11	Yes	Steroid-sensitive
				DR7	6.9		
Lagueruela, et al. (499)	1990	United States	27	DR3	3.0	Yes	Steroid-resistant
			32	A1, B8, DR3, DRw52, SCO1, and/or B44, DR7, DRw53, FC31	—	Yes	Steroid-sensitive, frequently relapsing
Ruder, et al. (500)	1990	Germany	91	B8, DR3, DR7	21.5	Yes	Steroid-sensitive
Konrad (501)	1994	France, Germany	161	DQR1*07	6.2	Yes	RR = 16.5 with both DRB1*0301 and DRB1*07
				DQB1*0201	7.8		
				DQA*0201, *0301, *0302	4.1		
Abe (502)	1995	Japan	24	DQB1*0302	6.2	Yes	DQA1*0103 decreased
Kobayashi (503)	1995	Japan	30	DQB1*0301, *0601	8.6	Yes	—
Bouissou (504)	1995	Germany	152	DR3/DR7	5.6	Yes	Less steroid-sensitive; Decreased association with DR2. DR6, DQ1
		France	199		7.7		
Haeffner, et al. (505)	1997	Germany	167	DQB1*0601	38.9	Yes	DQA1*0102 and DQB1*0602 decreased
				DQA1*0201	3.8		
				DQB1*0201	8.5		
Konrad (506)	1997	Germany	54	DR7	—	—	Poor response to alkylating agents
Bakr and El-Chenawy (507)	1998	Egypt	121	DRB1*01	23.4	Yes	—

MCN, minimal change nephropathy.

system. He cited four points: (a) evidence for abnormal humoral immune responsiveness; (b) marked sensitivity of the disease process to treatment with corticosteroids or immunosuppressive agents; (c) remission of MCN upon infection with measles, an inhibitor of cell-mediated immunity; and (d) the association of MCN with Hodgkin disease. In view of the lack of significant morphologic evidence of renal damage, Shalhoub suggested that MCN represents the renal manifestation of a systemic immunologic abnormality, perhaps a T-lymphocyte disorder, rather than a primary renal parenchymal disorder. Although subsequent investigation has not yet demonstrated a causal immunologic event, numerous abnormalities in both humoral and cellular immune responses (516) have been noted in nephrotic patients (295,296,299–301,416,417,517–520) (Table 64-8). These may, in time, provide a pathogenetic mechanism.

TABLE 64-8

IMMUNOLOGIC ABNORMALITIES IN MINIMAL CHANGE NEPHROPATHY

Defective opsonization
  Decreased factor B (299,300)
  Decreased factor D (301)
Decreased neutrophil chemiluminescence (300)
Abnormal reticuloendothelial function (518)
Circulating immune complexes (416,417,519,520)
Abnormal immunoglobulin production
  Altered serum immunoglobulin concentrations
    (295,521–524)
  Decreased specific antibody reactivity (296,525,526)
  Decreased synthesis stimulated *in vitro* (527,528)
  Increased spontaneous *in vitro* synthesis (521,528)
  Alterations in cell-surface markers (527,529–532)
Altered cellular immunity
  Cytotoxicity to renal tubular epithelium (533)
  Proliferation in response to glomerular basement membrane
    (534)
  Decreased delayed-type hypersensitivity (535–537)
  Decreased experimental local graft-versus-host disease (538)
  Decreased induced lymphocyte blast transformation
    (517,539)
  Increased inducible suppressor cell activity (540)
Humoral immune abnormalities
  Serum toxicity to lymphocytes (541)
  Inhibition of rosette formation by serum (518,542,543)
  Altered antibody-dependent cellular cytotoxicity (544)
  Increased interleukin (IL) production (545)
  Decreased IL production (546,547)
Suppressor lymphokines (548–550)
  Monocyte migration inhibitory factor (534,551)
  Vascular permeability factor (552,553)
  Soluble immune-response suppressor (554,555)
  Tumor necrosis factor (556)
Lymphocyte activation
  Increased secretion of β_2-microglobulin (557)
  Soluble IL-2 receptor production (558–561)
  Increased production of IL-2, IL-4, and IFN-γ (562) IL-13
    (563)

IFN, interferon; *IL,* interleukin.

Immunoglobulin synthesis. Clinical and *in vitro* assays show impaired immunoglobulin synthesis in MCN. Serum IgG levels are decreased significantly in children with MCNS, whereas IgM levels are markedly increased (295,522–524). These values return toward normal with remission, although the IgM levels may remain elevated. Not all studies have found an equal tendency toward normalization with remission, nor is this abnormality confined to MCN in all cases (564,565). Although nephrotic proteinuria may be associated with urinary loss of IgG (566), such losses are insufficient to explain the very low serum IgG levels often found in MCN (521). This pattern of increased IgM and decreased IgG levels in the serum also is associated with some other immune-deficient states, most notably X-linked immunodeficiency disease (521).

Depression of specific antibody titers, such as those to the common streptococcal antigens endostreptosin, streptolysin O, and streptozyme, was observed in children and adults with idiopathic nephrotic syndrome (526). Levels were low during active disease, remained low for up to 20 years afterward, and were not changed by steroid therapy. Patients who were nephrotic from chronic glomerulonephritis, systemic lupus erythematosus, membranous nephropathy, diabetes mellitus, or amyloido-

sis did not have depressed titers. These data suggest a chronic, specific impairment of response in patients with MCN. Inability to generate (296) or to maintain (525) specific titers against pneumococcal polysaccharide has been described in MCN, but not all studies confirmed this observation (567). Thus depression of specific antibody titers may be restricted to certain patients or certain antigens.

Several groups evaluated the *in vitro* secretion of immunoglobulins by lymphocytes activated with lectins. Consistent with the decrease in serum IgG levels, pokeweed mitogen-stimulated synthesis of IgG by patient lymphocytes was decreased in MCN patients during the active stage of disease, returning toward normal with remission (521,523,527). Unstimulated secretion of immunoglobulin may be increased (521,528), suggesting spontaneous activation of lymphocytes in MCN. Studies of IgA and IgM synthesis by lymphocytes obtained from patients with nephrotic syndrome of other causes produced more variable results (568). Decreased immunoglobulin production *in vitro* or *in vivo* could result from either abnormalities of lymphocytes or the presence of inhibitory agents systemically or on the cell surface. Evidence suggests that both mechanisms may be present in MCN.

Studies of lymphocyte surface marker expression. These studies were employed to determine whether the immunoglobulin abnormalities in MCN reflect some form of immune cell dysfunction. Cells infiltrating the renal interstitium are predominantly T lymphocytes (569). The ratio of helper cells to suppressor cells in the glomerulus can be similar to that found in lymphocytes in the peripheral circulation (569) but may vary from one patient to another (570). Circulating lymphocyte subsets in MCN were initially reported to show no significant alterations in helper–suppressor cell ratios (571). Studies of B-cell and T-cell subpopulations also produced conflicting data, regardless of whether patients with MCN or FSGS were studied (527,529,532,535,572). A potential increase in the number of cells co-expressing B-cell and T-cell surface markers has been reported, comparable to findings in X-linked immunodeficiency (531). However, in most studies of lymphocyte subpopulations in primary nephrotic syndrome, there are few significant changes. The meaning of the differences that were found remains to be determined. In general, studies showing alterations in lymphocyte subpopulations may be useful in suggesting the possible presence of immune derangement, but inferences of a potential role for these changes in disease pathogenesis should be made with caution unless corroborated by accompanying functional analysis. Some progress in this direction is provided by reports of two-color flow cytometry indicating that the counts for circulating activated total T cells and suppressor or suppressor/inducer T cells are increased, whereas those for activated helper T cells are decreased, during relapse (530,573). Another study found that populations of activated suppressor-inducer cells and suppressor-effector cells are increased in patients whose nephrosis was sensitive to steroid treatment, accompanied by decreased memory T cells and decreased lymphocyte proliferation in response to tetanus toxoid. Lymphocytes of steroid-resistant patients also had increased suppressor-inducer cells, but decreased suppressor-effector cells and increased memory T cells, with increased responses to tetanus toxoid (574).

Cellular immunity. In studies of delayed-type hypersensitivity to common antigens, MCN patients in relapse had decreased skin reactivity to purified protein derivative of tuberculin (PPD), *Candida,* live varicella vaccine, streptokinase-streptodornase, and topical dinitrochlorobenzene (535–537). Reactivity returns when the patient enters remission (537). In addition, the lymphocytes of patients with MCN manifest decreased local graft-versus-host activity when injected into rats, a finding that can be normalized by preincubation of the cells with thymic humoral factor (575). These observations may not be restricted to MCN (576).

In vitro studies also showed abnormal cellular responses in nephrotic patients. Lymphocytes from MCN patients, but not from normal control subjects or patients who were nephrotic secondary to proliferative glomerulonephritis, were toxic to cultured renal tubular epithelial cells (533). Lymphocytes from some patients also proliferated on exposure to GBM (534). It is not clear from these reports whether the findings represent a primary process or the result of immunologic sensitization after renal damage. Blast transformation of patient lymphocytes was decreased in the presence of control or nephrotic serum (539), returning to normal after entry of the patient into remission (535). Other results showed that MCN is associated with increased concanavalin A-activated suppressor cell activity. This finding demonstrates at least the potential for exaggerated suppressor lymphocyte responses and is not consistently found in other renal diseases (540,577).

Evidence for abnormal lymphokine activity. Serum from adult nephrotic patients inhibits leukocyte migration in the presence of renal antigens (551), and serum monocyte migration inhibitory factor activity present during relapse of MCN disappears with remission of the disease (534). Furthermore, serum from most patients with MCN as well as some with diffuse proliferative glomerulonephritis is lymphocytotoxic, whereas serum from patients with acute tubular necrosis or urologic disease is not (541). These findings suggest that an immune inhibitory agent, or a series of such agents, is present in the circulation of patients with primary nephrotic syndrome. Sera from nephrotic patients may inhibit the ability of cells to form rosettes (542,543), although this is not specific for MCN, and patient sera do not support *in vitro* antibody-dependent cell-mediated cytotoxicity (ADCC) assays (544). Decreased splenic uptake of radiolabeled complexes was correlated with deficient Fc receptor function in nephrotic patients and could be due to the presence of an inhibitory protein that attaches to cell surfaces (518). Finally, multiple studies demonstrate a suppressive effect of patient sera on blastogenesis by normal lymphocytes (548,578–580). The specificity of this phenomenon for MCN varies from one study to another. Efforts to attribute suppressive activity in nephrotic sera to a lymphokine should attempt to exclude the possibility that the observed effects are caused by nonspecific toxicity to immune responses, resulting from the biochemical abnormalities that occur in nephrotic syndrome. For example, the suppressive activity in plasma from nephrotic children segregates in the lipid-rich fraction (581). It could thus be derived from constituents of LDLs and VLDLs that are present in increased concentrations in nephrotic plasma and suppress *in vitro* cellular immune responses (582,583). However, this finding also is consistent with migration of an immunosuppressive agent with the lipid-rich fraction. Alternatively, oxidized LDL could itself affect lymphocyte function. In either case, it is noteworthy that a patient with refractory nephrotic syndrome entered remission after LDL apheresis (584).

Several studies that partially characterized the suppressive activity suggested the production of a suppressor lymphokine. A heat-stable substance, present in the serum of nephrotic patients, inhibits lymphocyte proliferation. It binds to lymphocytes in the assay system and is not removed by washing (549). One study found a heat-stable inhibitory substance in the plasma of 51 (76%) of 67 children with MCN and six of nine children with FSGS (550). Only one sample from seven patients with membranous glomerulonephritis or 31 healthy adults and children showed similar activity. The factor was toxic to normal lymphocytes and was between 100 and 300 kDa. The presence of tumor necrosis factor (556), IL-4 (563,585), and IL-13 (565)

in the serum of some patients may be related to suppressive activity.

Urine and serum samples from children and adults with steroid-sensitive nephrotic syndrome, but not other causes for proteinuria, contain the lymphokine soluble immune response suppressor (SIRS) (554). This factor, which inhibits antibody production (586) and delayed-type hypersensitivity responses (587), is secreted by patient lymphocytes without a requirement for exogenous stimulating agents. SIRS production thus could account for the suppression of immune responses seen in nephrotic patients. Suppressive activity disappears from the urine after initiation of corticosteroid therapy but before urinary protein loss decreases significantly. Patient serum activates normal lymphocytes to produce SIRS by a steroid-sensitive process (555), and a regulatory mechanism has been proposed by which CD4+ T lymphocytes from patients in relapse secrete a protein that activates CD8+ T cells to produce SIRS (588). Although the parallel between the sensitivity of SIRS production to steroids and steroid responsiveness of nephrotic proteinuria in patients who produce SIRS is striking, there is no evidence to indicate that SIRS itself causes nephrotic proteinuria. It is, however, a clear marker for steroid-sensitive mechanisms of proteinuria. The means by which SIRS acts on immune responses is not known. Although this issue remains intriguing, little recent progress has been made in this area.

Circulating immune complexes. A variety of glomerular diseases have been associated with soluble circulating immune complexes. The circulating complexes reflect immunoglobulins found in the kidney; patients with MCN had little or no IgG or IgA complexes but did have marked variation with regard to circulating IgM complexes (589). Although circulating immune complexes have been documented in some patients with MCN or FSGS (520), not all studies have confirmed this observation (519) and the relationship of this finding to mesangial immune complexes remains uncertain. A possible reason for varied results is the use of different assay systems (416). In screening studies that employed liquid-phase and solid-phase C1q binding and Raji cell assays, at least one assay was positive in serum from 11 of 14 adults with MCN, 13 of 27 patients with FSGS, and 26 of 55 patients with membranous nephropathy. Prednisone treatment did not affect the prevalence of circulating immune complexes in this study (590). In another report, 17 of 18 MCN patients had IgG immune complexes that did not bind to C1q; in seven of nine patients assessed longitudinally, immune complexes disappeared within 6 weeks of entry into remission (417). This temporal relationship and the absence of glomerular IgG in patients with MCN suggest that circulating immune complexes could be a result rather than a cause of the disease. Although they may not cause the disease, some circulating immune complexes could account for the apparently nonspecific presence of IgM in the mesangium of some patients. In support of this is the finding that large, neutral, or anionic complexes show focal to diffuse mesangial localization (591,592). Complexes containing IgM tend to be large. In contrast, low-avidity, polycationic, and small immune complexes tend to deposit in capillary or mesangiocapillary distribution.

Other findings related to immunity. Further evidence of a potential role for the immune system in MCN is the possible relationship between this disease and allergic phenomena, already discussed, as well as the unique association between MCN and tumors of immune cell origin. Impaired lymphocyte blast transformation was found in the presence of plasma from patients with MCN and Hodgkin's disease (473,593); *in vitro* responses improved significantly after antitumor therapy (594). The strong association of lymphoid tumor, abnormal cellular immune responses, and MCN supports a role for deranged immunity. The nature of this derangement is unclear. Despite the clinical evidence of suppressed immune responses, the underlying abnormality paradoxically may be general immune system activation. In support of such an event, production of a number of specific cytokines and their regulators may be elevated. Increased IL-2 mRNA expression in patient lymphocytes (595), increased IL-8 production in steroid-resistant patients (596), and increased occurrence of one polymorphism of IL-1 receptor antagonist (597) have been reported. Circulating soluble IL-2 receptor concentrations are increased in MCN (558–561). Production of gamma interferon (IFN-γ) may also be increased in nephrotic children. Further, although various responses of stimulated patient lymphocytes are decreased, unstimulated cells from patients show, for example, increased immunoglobulin production relative to that of unstimulated control cells. Taken together, these findings suggest that in MCN, the immune system is generally activated, whereas the induction of responses to specific stimuli is impaired (516).

Relationship of the immunologic abnormalities to disease pathogenesis. Despite all of these studies, Shalhoub's hypothesis has not yet been proved. There is strong support, however, for the concept that cellular immunity may be a mediator of proteinuria. Monocytes or macrophages are important in the pathogenesis of some forms of glomerulonephritis (598) and in the genesis of proteinuria (599,600). These studies imply a role for mononuclear cells but do not explain how they may act. One possibility is through release of the lymphokine, vascular permeability factor (VPF), which is produced by activated lymphocytes from some nephrotic patients and which, when injected intradermally, causes increased permeability of vessels to macromolecules (601). This protein, usually referred to by its function as an endothelial cell stimulant called vascular endothelial cell growth factor (VEGF) (553), was detected in supernatants of unstimulated cultures of patients' cells but not those of normal controls (602). A VEGF-like serine protease in patient serum decreased staining for polyanion when used to treat histologic sections of normal glomerular tissue (603). However, the effect of VEGF does not appear to be specific for permeability of albumin, making it an unlikely cause of selective proteinuria. VEGF activates endothelial cells in numerous ways; by causing the cells to "round up" it disrupts tight cell–cell adhesions, promoting permeability of an endothelial monolayer (604). It also promotes the formation of endothelial fenestrae (605). However, since the glomerular capillary endothelium is not the final barrier to glomerular permeability, it is not clear how increased fenestration would cause albuminuria in primary nephrotic syndrome. Furthermore, a similar substance was described in IgA nephropathy, even in the absence of nephrotic syndrome (606), indicating that VEGF activity could be secondary to renal disease rather than a cause of proteinuria. VEGF production could be enhanced by IL-12 (607) or IL-15 (608). Substances produced by T-cell hybridomas derived from the lymphocytes of nephrotic patients (609) or found in culture media conditioned by mononuclear cells from nephrotic children (610), may prove to represent one or more selective permeability factors. One such factor could be IL-8, which is produced by lymphocytes from patients with steroid-responsive nephrosis (611) and increases renal clearance of protein in an *ex vivo* model (612). However, varied circulating levels have been reported in disease (596,613). IL-2 (562) and TNFα (614) production by patient lymphocytes normalized after the patients entered remission. A single case report describes remission of steroid-resistant disease after infliximab anti-TNFα therapy (615).

Despite the absence of proof for Shalhoub's hypothesis, the indirect evidence of an immunogenic basis for many cases of MCN remains compelling. Onset is often preceded by an immunogenic stimulus. Measles, which induces remission, inhibits lymphokine production but not proliferation by lymphocytes (616). Studies of MCN induced by nonsteroidal anti-inflammatory drugs (617) or cimetidine (618) indicated that these cases of disease may be associated with abnormal T-cell function. The relationship of disease to altered immunity is particularly striking with regard to suppressor cell activity. A good therapeutic response to cyclophosphamide was associated with decreased suppressor cell activity after treatment (619), although others were unable to confirm this finding (620). Furthermore, as described previously, cellular and humoral immune responses are suppressed in MCN. Thus it is intriguing that recombinant leukocyte interferon A, an agent that induces production of SIRS, caused nephrotic syndrome with minimal glomerular changes in a patient with T-lymphocyte malignancy (621) and that the antihelminthic agent levamisole, which inhibits SIRS activity (586), has been used successfully to treat MCN (622,623). Despite evidence suggesting that cytokines may be involved in promoting vascular permeability (624), the data regarding lymphokines do not address their role as a pathogenic agent in nephrosis and are equally consistent with the interpretation that production of these substances is an epiphenomenon of the derangement that causes albuminuria. In addition, the existence of differences between studies or even within a patient group in a given study suggest that multiple etiologies may exist for MCN, only one (or several) of which may be immunologic. Furthermore, the pathogenesis of proteinuria remains unclear. Given the importance of the epithelial slit diaphragm in the integrity of the glomerular filter, the podocyte is likely the target cell. However, the way in which the podocyte is affected is unknown. Considerable work remains to be done in this area.

Treatment of Minimal Change Nephropathy

Indications for Renal Biopsy

Although most older children and adults will undergo renal biopsy prior to starting treatment, the indications for and benefits of this procedure in patients with primary nephrotic syndrome remain somewhat controversial (625). Children 1 to 9 years old with all the features of MCNS and no atypical features Table 64-9 may be given a therapeutic trial of steroids without prior histologic confirmation of the diagnosis. Induction of a complete remission by steroids in such patients is considered to be adequate confirmation of the diagnosis of MCN (423), although other benign conditions may occasionally appear to respond to steroid therapy (626). A histologic diagnosis by renal biopsy is recommended in all patients who present with nephrotic syndrome in the first year of life or after the age of 9 years. Risk–benefit analysis at one point suggested that biopsy may not be diagnostically superior to a therapeutic trial of steroids, even in adults (627), but the increasing incidence of FSGS in nephrotic adults has led most clinicians to perform a biopsy at the time of presentation. All patients who are steroid-resistant (see Table 64-10 for some commonly used descriptors of nephrotic patients and their responses) should undergo biopsy, although the timing of this decision remains uncertain. Although steroid resistance in children usually is defined by 8 weeks of nonresponse, many clinicians recognize that most children who respond do so by 4 weeks. Therefore, it may be appropriate to perform a biopsy after 4 weeks or less, since those who have not responded by then are more likely to have a different disease that might require an alternative treatment. Other pediatric patients who may require a biopsy include those who have frequent relapses, or who are candidates for therapy with immunosuppressive drugs. Some experts have suggested that any steroid-dependent pediatric patients who continue to be steroid-sensitive are, statistically, so likely to have MCN (400,445) that biopsy is not indicated.

TABLE 64-9

FEATURES SUGGESTING THAT NEPHROTIC SYNDROME IS CAUSED BY A DISEASE OTHER THAN MINIMAL CHANGE NEPHROPATHY (MCN)

History
  Onset: before 1 year or after 9 years of age[a]
  History: skin rashes, joint pains, "nephritis," or hematuria[a]
  Family history: family member with Alport's syndrome or development of end-stage renal disease[a]

Physical examination
  General: clinical features of collagen vascular disease
  Blood pressure: marked elevation or evidence of vascular changes in fundi[a]
  Skin: purpura[a]
  Subcutaneous tissue: lipodystrophy

Laboratory findings
  Urine: dilute urine sediment containing more than 10 red blood cells per high-power field; cylindruria[a]; nonselective proteinuria[a]
  Renal function: markedly decreased[a]

Chest X-ray: enlarged heart, vascular engorgement, pulmonary edema
Serology: decreased C3 or C4, antinuclear antibody or anti-DNA positive
Serum cholesterol: only mild increase[a]
Plasma protein: only mild decrease in albumin[a] markedly decreased or increased globulin

[a]Although these features are unusual for MCN, their presence does not exclude the lesion.

TABLE 64-10

SOME DEFINITIONS USED TO DESCRIBE PATIENTS WITH PRIMARY NEPHROTIC SYNDROME

Nephrotic-range proteinuria
  Pediatric: Urine protein: creatinine ratio >2
  Adult: 24-hour protein excretion >3.5 g

Relapse
  Proteinuria (>1+ on dipstick or >4 mg/hr/m^2 surface area) for at least 1 week

Complete remission (CR)
  Pediatric: Protein-free urine (<1$^+$ on dipstick or <4 mg/hr/m^2 surface area) for at least 3 days
  Or, Urine protein: creatinine ratio <0.2
  Adult: 24-hour protein excretion <0.3 g

Partial remission (PR)
  Pediatric: ≥50% fall from baseline and/or <2.0 (or <0.3) and/or loss of edema and/or serum albumin >2.5 mg/dL
  Adult: PR 50%: 50% fall from baseline and <3.5 g/day
  Or, PR2: ≤2.0 g/1.73m^2

Limited response (LR)
  Pediatric and Adult: Fall to ≤50% baseline but not PR

Steroid-sensitive nephrotic syndrome (SSNS)
  Response to prednisone (60 mg/m^2 surface area/day) within 8 weeks of starting treatment[a]

Steroid-resistant nephrotic syndrome (SRNS)
  Pediatric: No response to prednisone (60 mg/m^2 surface area/day) within 8 weeks of starting treatment (ISKDC)[a]
  Adult: No change or increased proteinuria compared to baseline

Frequent relapsing nephrotic syndrome
  Initially responsive to prednisone: At least two relapses in a subsequent 6-month period or five relapses in 18 months

Steroid-dependent nephrotic syndrome
  Initially responsive to prednisone
  Either two consecutive relapses during period of steroid taper, or two consecutive relapses, each occurring within 2 weeks of ending a course of corticosteroid therapy

ISKDC, International Study of Kidney Disease in Children.
[a]Some studies define steroid-sensitive patients as those responding within 4 weeks of starting treatment. Those responding between 5 and 8 weeks are referred to as late responders.

Alternatively, response to steroids may itself be a more important determinant of disease process and outcome than is histopathology (628).

A renal biopsy may be technically difficult to perform in the patient with anasarca; surrounding fluid allows the kidney to be balloted by the biopsy needle. In such subjects, it is preferable to delay the attempted biopsy until after a spontaneous or drug-induced diuresis has occurred and most of the ascites has resolved.

Treatment of Minimal Change Disease

The optimal treatment for MCN is based on corticosteroids but continues to evolve. It is noteworthy that in the era before current drugs were available, 25% of children with idiopathic nephrotic syndrome underwent a spontaneous remission (629). Even today, a careful history will often suggest that prior to the presenting episode, the nephrotic patient has had one or more periods of edema that resolved without treatment. The association between MCN and both allergy and malignancy was reviewed earlier in this chapter. An occasional patient with frequently relapsing MCN may enter long-term remission only when a dietary allergen is withdrawn (379) or an underlying malignancy is identified and treated (472,475). Therefore, the possibility that either of these conditions is responsible for the patient's symptoms should be considered before any drug therapy is instituted.

Prior to 1940, the mortality rate for nephrotic syndrome was 40%; the major cause of death was infection (630). After the introduction of antibiotics, mortality was reduced by more than 50%. The development of corticosteroids has further reduced mortality to between 3% and 7% (409,419,630). The major benefits of steroids, however, may well be the faster in-

duction of a remission and reduction of morbidity, although this has never been subjected to a controlled trial. In the older adult nephrotic patient, the risk of undesirable steroid side effects could outweigh the benefits of these drugs (631). Despite these caveats, adrenocorticosteroids remain the therapeutic agent of choice for MCN in patients of all ages.

Corticosteroid Therapy. As stated in the preceding text, cessation of urinary protein excretion in response to the oral administration of prednisone is virtually diagnostic of this entity in children (632). The standard dosage regimen for inducing a remission is 2 mg/kg of body weight per day or 60 mg/m^2 of body surface area per day (maximum of 80 mg per day) (633). Although the initial ISKDC studies used the same daily dose but divided it into three equal parts, we prefer the alternative approach of giving the entire daily amount in a single dose. The Cochrane group has reported that the single daily dose is as effective as a more complex dosing schedule (634). Furthermore, short-term side effects such as hunger and hypomania are more manageable with use of the single daily dose. In addition, a single dose is more convenient to administer, with a greater likelihood of compliance. The daily dose is rounded up to the nearest multiple of 20 mg. Because nephrotic patients may be anergic, a chest radiograph should be obtained to rule out the possibility of subclinical pulmonary tuberculosis before prednisone therapy is begun. Typically, patients respond with a diuresis (114) followed by resolution of proteinuria. In most instances, response can be considered to have occurred if the patient has had protein-free urine for at least 3 days (Table 64-10). There are as yet no universally agreed-upon definitions for complete remission (CR) or partial remission (PR). Nevertheless, those presented in Table 64-10 represent a starting point for discussion. Among children, CR is commonly defined as the absence of proteinuria on dipstick or alternatively of random (or first-void) urine protein/creatinine ratio of <0.2. Among adults, where 24-hour urine collections remain the standard for definition, CR is commonly defined as <0.3 g per/day (although the upper limits of normal protein excretion at various clinical laboratories may be 150–250 mg per/day). The definitions of PR are much more problematic. Cattran et al. have argued for a 50% decrease in proteinuria from baseline and becoming subnephrotic (634a).

This definition has the merit of capturing the benefit of a substantial reduction in proteinuria, for example from 10 to 3 g per/day, and has been recently shown to correlate with long-term preservation of kidney function. Others have used a more restrictive definition of PR, for example, proteinuria <2g per/day. There may be some utility to capturing lesser degrees of benefit (e.g., limited response (LR),defined as a 50% fall in proteinuria that does not reach subnephrotic levels) but such a benefit has not been tested in longitudinal studies. In children, CR may occur within 1 week of starting treatment, and is seen within 2 weeks of treatment in 75% of responders and by 4 weeks in more than 90% (Fig. 64-8).

According to the definitions derived by the ISKDC and others (Table 64-10), patients who do not respond after 4 weeks of glucocorticoid therapy considered to be steroid-resistant. However, response may be delayed for up to 8 weeks or more in a small percentage of patients, so that approximately 95% of patients with MCNS eventually will prove to be steroid-sensitive. Serum albumin levels may not return to normal for up to 3 months (114), and serum lipid abnormalities may persist for protracted periods (170).

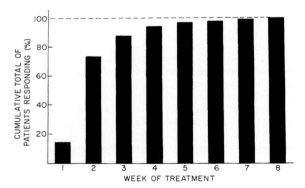

FIGURE 64-8. The cumulative rate of response to treatment with prednisone of children with primary nephrotic syndrome. Only steroid-sensitive patients are included in this analysis. The majority of patients respond in the second or third week of treatment. A small percentage, however, may take 7 or 8 weeks to respond. (Data derived from: International Study of Kidney Disease in Children. The primary nephrotic syndrome in children: identification of patients with minimal change nephrotic syndrome from initial response to prednisone. *J Pediatr* 1981;98:561, with permission.)

The persistence of some proteinuria does not necessarily indicate steroid resistance. Postural proteinuria may persist in a minority of patients and, in others, contraction of blood volume consequent to a brisk diuresis may result in renin-mediated proteinuria (635). In either case, the degree of proteinuria is modest, typically registering 1+ to 2+ on dipstick and being <1 g per/day. This should not be misinterpreted as partial responsiveness and should not be used to justify continuing steroid therapy in high doses. Alternatively, failure to respond to steroids may indicate the presence of an occult infection (633).

Studies in children have demonstrated that, *for the initial episode only*, a prolonged period of treatment with a full dose of daily corticosteroids decreases the incidence or frequency of subsequent relapses. After 6 weeks of daily treatment (rather than the standard 4 weeks of daily treatment) with prednisone, 60 mg/m^2, the patient is switched to 40 mg/m^2 on alternate days (636). Although some controlled studies may disagree (637), meta-analysis by the Cochrane Group has determined that initial treatment with high-dose daily and then prolonged alternate-day oral prednisone decreases the likelihood of relapse over the first 12 to 24 months, and suggests that long-term continuation of alternate-day steroids has increasing benefit for up to 7 months (634). Most groups continue prednisone (total of daily and alternate day) for about 3 months and then discontinue the drug. For subsequent relapses, the steroids are tapered beginning with a switch to alternate-day therapy only a few days after the response to treatment. The dose is then reduced in stepwise fashion during the next 4 to 8 weeks. Longer tapering periods may decrease the likelihood of subsequent relapses (636,638,639). For example, in a relapsed patient treated initially with prednisone, 60 mg per day, the dose is reduced to 40 mg daily after response (3 days of protein-free urine) for 2 weeks, then to 40 mg on alternate days. At 2-week intervals the doses are reduced by 50%, with the final dose of 5 mg on alternate days being given for 3 weeks. It should be noted that this regimen is a matter of preference. The only regimen that has been established by a controlled trial as efficacious is the prolonged course for children of daily and then alternate-day steroids in the initial episode. It is of interest that although prolonged treatment of the first episode seems to consolidate remission in children, those children who respond most rapidly to the initial course of corticosteroids tend to have longer remissions (640). This relationship was not observed in adults (641).

The presence of IgM deposits does not have an effect on response to steroids (642). Although initial observations suggested that patients with mesangial hypercellularity respond to treatment in a manner similar to that seen with MCN (643), subsequent studies indicated that a considerable proportion of these patients may be steroid-resistant (441,644). Conversely, evaluation of large groups of children indicated that persistence of proteinuria is only weakly predictive of mesangial hypercellularity on biopsy (168,445).

Because bacterial peritonitis is a relatively common occurrence in patients with MCN (see Complications of MCN later in this chapter), many clinicians support immunization with pneumococcal polysaccharide vaccines. Concern regarding possible poor response to immunogens in nephrotic patients, and the potential for an immunogenic stimulus to trigger a relapse, has made the issue of childhood immunization in nephrotic patients somewhat controversial. A survey of North American pediatric nephrologists indicated that most modified their approach to immunization but that there was little evidence upon which to base a standard approach (645). However, a recent British study suggests that administration of meningococcal C conjugate vaccine may increase the likelihood of relapse (396). Current recommendations on vaccination in children and adults and use of immunoglobulins (646) support the use of polyvalent pneumococcal vaccine (302,303) and (in the case of children) *Haemophilus influenzae* type B vaccine. Live virus vaccines should not be given to immunocompromised patients.

Frequent Relapse. Although earlier reports suggested that as high as 50% of steroid-sensitive children do not have a relapse after the initial episode of nephrotic syndrome, subsequent observations indicate that this figure approximates only 25% (362). The difference could be due to an altering pattern of disease but also may reflect the types of patients being referred to reporting centers. Another 25% to 30% of children have infrequent relapses and usually respond well to further courses of steroids, as already described. The remaining patients have either frequently relapsing or steroid-dependent nephrotic syndrome (Table 64-10). Several attempts have been made to correlate pathology with response to steroids or with the pattern of relapses (647). Frequency of relapse showed no correlation with histopathology in a study by the ISKDC (648), but early relapse after the initial episode was predictive of more frequent relapses subsequently.

Attempts to control frequent relapses with steroids may result in their protracted use and possible steroid toxicity. In an effort to minimize these side effects, alternative regimens have been proposed using smaller doses of steroids to treat relapses. Unfortunately the lower response and higher relapse rates associated with most of these approaches usually result in higher cumulative doses of steroids and may not be justified (638). One study suggested that for some frequently relapsing patients, maintenance on daily rather than alternate-day steroids during the tapering regimen can result in a less frequent relapse rate and an equal or lesser cumulative steroid dose (649).

Corticotropin (adrenocorticotropic hormone, ACTH) stimulation tests suggest that prolonged postprednisone adrenocortical suppression may predispose to frequent relapses. A normal response to ACTH predicted a remission for 6 months or longer; a subnormal response was associated with remissions of less than 6 months (650). Early relapse in children with poor adrenal function can be prevented with low-dose maintenance hydrocortisone administration (651).

Nitrogen mustard was found to prolong the duration of remission in patients with MCN (652), but less toxic alternatives such as cyclophosphamide and related drugs are now used in frequently relapsing and steroid-dependent nephrotic patients, especially in those with marked steroid side effects (653). Ideally, cyclophosphamide should not be used until a patient has been followed for 2 to 3 years to document a frequently relapsing course. Although some centers prefer histologic confirmation of MCN before the drug is used, steroid responsiveness may eliminate the need to obtain a biopsy specimen in children, since the disease remains overwhelmingly likely to be MCN (654).

The original cyclophosphamide regimen used doses of 5 mg/kg per day, but it was associated with a high incidence of leukopenia, hair loss, and cystitis (655). Most centers obtain satisfactory results with a dosage of 2 mg per kg per day for children (1.5 mg/kg/d for adults) given for no more than 90 consecutive days; others reported equally good results with 2.5 mg per kg per day for 8 weeks (655–658). At 2 mg/kg per day, a course of cyclophosphamide limited to 8 weeks is followed by a higher relapse rate (659). Most centers utilize cyclophosphamide in conjunction with steroids (657). The induction of a remission with steroids before therapy with cyclophosphamide is instituted, permits a liberal fluid intake to induce a high urine flow rate during treatment with the immunosuppressive agent, thereby reducing the risk of cystitis. The steroid taper is accomplished more rapidly, over a 6-week period.

Approximately 65% of frequently relapsing patients remain in remission for at least 5 years after a course of cyclophos-

phamide (657,660,661). Response to cyclophosphamide may be predictable from the patterns of relapse after steroids. Of patients who have a relapse immediately after tapering of steroids, two-thirds also have a relapse quickly after cyclophosphamide treatment. Conversely, frequently relapsing patients who can maintain remission for more than 14 days after steroid therapy is discontinued have longer remissions and fewer relapses after cyclophosphamide treatment (659).

It is rare to see acute side effects with the current cyclophosphamide regimens, although white blood cell counts should be monitored at least weekly, especially early in the course of therapy. The frequency of cystitis, alopecia, and leukopenia has been reduced markedly by institution of smaller daily and cumulative doses of the drug, and is further minimized by encouraging fluid intake and frequent voiding for 4 hours after administration. The gonadal toxicity of cyclophosphamide also appears to be cumulative-dose related; testicular and ovarian toxicity is uncommon if the total dose is less than 200 mg/kg (639,662,663). However, such doses do decrease sperm counts (664), and some men experience gonadal toxicity even at low doses (665). Higher doses lead to more significant testicular dysfunction (666). In children, the drug is usually given well before puberty to minimize the risk of gonadal toxicity, although it has been suggested that prepubertal males are more sensitive than pubertal males (667). Injection of slowly absorbed testosterone may protect against iatrogenic azoospermia (668). Female patients treated with a mean total dose of 439 mg/kg at an average age of 8.7 years were followed for a mean of 12.3 years. All had normal pubertal development and regular menstrual patterns. Hormonal studies did not show obvious ovarian or pituitary–gonadal dysfunction, and two patients gave birth to normal children (666). There are no data available to convincingly demonstrate a protective effect of ovarian suppression with oral contraceptives during alkylating agent therapy (669). Concern has been expressed about the potential for cyclophosphamide to induce malignancies. It remains uncertain whether this is a major risk of therapeutic regimens currently used in nephrotic syndrome, although leukemia occurred in at least one child treated for nephrotic syndrome with prednisone and cyclophosphamide (670). Furthermore, the use of cyclophosphamide may be associated with findings of increased sister chromatid exchange (671) and long-lasting immunosuppressive effects (517).

Anecdotal experience in patients who are refractory to conventional therapies suggests that adding six monthly intravenous injections of cyclophosphamide, 0.5 g/m² of body surface area per injection, to the oral steroid regimen may result in prolonged remission of the nephrotic syndrome even after discontinuation of the steroids (672). This bolus therapy has potential advantages related to facilitated compliance and the availability of newer agents to counter drug toxicity.

An alternative alkylating agent, chlorambucil, shares many of the side effects seen with cyclophosphamide but does not induce cystitis. Unlike cyclophosphamide, however, it may produce seizures in some patients (673) and induces electroencephalographic changes in the absence of seizures in others (674). Malignancies have developed in at least three nephrotic children treated with this drug (650,675,676). However, the overall incidence of serious complications with chlorambucil is low, especially when it is used in a dosage of 0.1 to 0.2 mg/kg per day for an 8-week course. It may produce a more stable remission than cyclophosphamide does (677,678) and be effective in some steroid-dependent and cyclophosphamide-resistant children with nephrotic syndrome (679). A meta-analysis found that both cyclophosphamide and chlorambucil are effective in frequently relapsing patients and was unable to discern a difference between the two treatments (680).

Cyclosporine and other calcineurin inhibitors can be beneficial in the management of patients with frequent relapses, especially those who do not achieve a long-term remission with an alkylating agent. The usual dose of cyclosporine, 150 mg/m^2 per day (7 mg/kg per day), is effective in inducing and sustaining remissions in these patients. An analysis of 129 children from nine studies showed complete remission in 84.5% (681). With cessation of the cyclosporine, however, there is a high rate of relapse, the subsequent relapses possibly being more difficult to control than those prior to cyclosporine treatment. Although some reports have indicated that cyclosporine is a safe, steroid-sparing agent for treating steroid-dependent nephrotic syndrome (682), others suggest that prolonged use can be associated with nephrotoxicity (683,684). An alternative and successful approach to management is the long-term use of low-dose cyclosporine combined with low-dose, alternate-day prednisone. Because of the potential for toxicity, serum creatinine should be monitored periodically in patients receiving cyclosporine.

Levamisole, an antihelminthic drug and immunopotentiating agent, can be used to treat children with MCN, especially those who have frequent relapses (623,685). The usual dose is 2.5 mg/kg of body weight given by mouth on alternate days. The drug may be valuable as a steroid-sparing agent. In a controlled trial, 14 of 31 patients taking levamisole were able to discontinue steroids and remain in remission for the 112 days of the trial, compared to only four of the 30 control subjects taking placebo (622). When the drug was added to the regimen of patients after a steroid-induced remission, the relapse rate fell from 5.2 episodes to less than 0.7 episodes per year during a 2-year period of treatment. The beneficial effect appeared to last beyond completion of the course of levamisole (686). Side effects of levamisole include a decreased neutrophil count or transient granulocytopenia in two-thirds of patients. More severe complications such as skin rash, a flu-like illness, vomiting, thrombopenia, and neurologic symptoms (insomnia, hyperactivity, and seizures) have been reported (687).

Mycophenolate mofetil has been reported to successfully treat frequently relapsing minimal change disease in adults (688,689) and children (690,691). No results of extensive controlled trials are yet available.

The use of intravenous immunoglobulin as an adjunct to steroids has not resulted in any clinically important extension of the period of remission in patients with frequent relapses (692).

Steroid-Dependent Patients. The management of these patients is similar in many respects to that of frequently relapsing patients. A minority of these individuals can be controlled with long-term, low-dose oral prednisone. Unfortunately the dose of prednisone required to maintain a remission is usually sufficiently high to result in unacceptable side effects. Therefore, alternative approaches to management are required.

Methylprednisolone pulses have not been shown to be beneficial in this population of patients (693). Some patients respond to cyclophosphamide and, as is the case with frequent relapses, the likelihood of a prolonged remission is increased if the course of drug is extended to 12 weeks (694).

The results of using cyclosporine in steroid-dependent patients are similar to those in the frequently relapsing group. Some clinicians advocate a course of alkylating agents before resorting to cyclosporine (695). Remissions can be maintained for 2 years or longer, especially if the cyclosporine is given continuously. However, 40% of these patients also require low-dose, alternate-day steroids to stay in remission. Unfortunately, long-term remission after discontinuing the cyclosporine is relatively rare (696). Treated patients show an average 20% decline in GFR after 3 months of therapy, but GFR stabilizes during subsequent therapy and has the potential to return toward normal with discontinuation of the drug (697). Nonethe-

less, toxicity may be chronic (698). A controlled multicenter study evaluating both pediatric and adult patients with either frequently relapsing or steroid-dependent nephrotic syndrome documented that cyclosporine and cyclophosphamide have a similar degree of efficacy but that more patients given cyclophosphamide have stable remissions (699). One study has suggested that cyclosporine given concomitantly with cytotoxic agents may diminish the efficacy of the latter treatment (700).

For most clinicians, when a steroid-dependent or frequently relapsing patient shows signs of steroid toxicity, the next drug to be used is cyclophosphamide, given for 12 weeks. If frequent relapses recur, cyclosporine in the lowest possible dose would be the next therapy utilized (701). Levamisole is reserved for patients who continue to have relapses. Mycophenolate also has been effective in steroid-dependent disease (690,691).

A significant number of patients who are steroid-dependent are resistant to all alternative forms of treatment and must be controlled symptomatically on a chronic basis with dietary sodium restriction and diuretics. Oral furosemide or metolazone, used alone or in combination, or in conjunction with spironolactone, is usually effective. Most patients learn to individualize their dosage. Unless there is evidence for progressive loss of renal function, this regimen probably is preferable to attempting control of the nephrotic syndrome with longer-term steroid therapy because of the significant complication rate of this latter approach. However, progressive interstitial nephritis has occurred in nephrotic patients chronically treated with diuretics, especially furosemide (702).

Treatment of Adult Patients with MCN. Most of the recommendations made for pediatric patients are equally applicable to their adult counterparts because there are remarkable similarities of MCN in the different age groups. In general, the response rates to steroids in adult and pediatric patients with MCN are comparable (657,703). However, the prevalence of relapses has not been documented systematically in adults. Differences between pediatric and adult patients with MCN may include a less rapid response to corticosteroids in adults (704) and a more effective response in adults to cyclophosphamide used alone (705,706); however, these differences may reflect technical or experimental design issues. For example, adults generally receive a lower dose of steroids on a per-weight basis.

Adult patients may be somewhat more prone to steroid complications (707), particularly in the skeleton. This has resulted in a philosophical debate about how aggressive one should be in the use of these drugs as well as immunosuppressants when treating nephrotic syndrome. However, given (a) the possibility of irreversible glomerular lesions from prolonged heavy proteinuria, (b) undesirable and potentially harmful effects of hyperlipidemia and protein deficiencies, and (c) the potential reduction of side effects from glucocorticoids and cytotoxic alkylating agents if the course of drugs is brief and the dosage not excessive (708), most internists employ aggressive therapy in treating patients with MCN.

Treatment of Steroid-Resistant MCN

Approximately 5% of children with MCN are unresponsive to a standard steroid regimen. Before considering a patient to be steroid-resistant, infection or occult malignancy must be ruled out. A small but significant percentage of those who initially are steroid-responsive will become steroid-resistant after one or more subsequent relapses. This development is an indication for renal biopsy and often denotes the presence of FSGS.

Alternative steroid regimens have been attempted to improve response to therapy. High-dose boluses of intravenous methylprednisolone induced remission in five of eight corticosteroid-resistant children (693). In another experience, methylprednisolone pulses reduced proteinuria but did not result in remission (709). One major problem in this group of patients is the development of severe side effects from protracted use of steroids. Therefore, regimens combining drugs in an attempt to reduce the amount of steroid administered, or alternative drugs to steroids, have been tried.

Occasionally a patient with biopsy-confirmed MCN who does not respond to oral steroid therapy will respond to an equivalent dose of the drug given as methylprednisolone by intramuscular injection. In several patients we have found that a tapered course of parenteral, sustained-release, methylprednisolone in combination with prolonged chlorambucil (3 months at a dose sufficient to decrease the peripheral white blood count to $<5,000/mm^3$) either induced remission or decreased proteinuria sufficiently that the patient was edema-free with little or no additional diuretic therapy. The effects appear to be long-lasting. This treatment must be employed cautiously after full consideration of its potential long-term side effects such as risk of neoplasm. It is not clear whether this improved response to injected steroids relates to the patient's compliance, to poor absorption of oral drugs, or to the metabolism of steroids by the liver. The routine measurement of prednisolone kinetics (710), however, does not appear to help in the management of children with MCN.

Cyclosporine therapy in steroid-resistant MCN has had disappointing results. In a summary of nine studies, only 12 of 60 (20%) children had complete remission and many had a relapse with cessation of therapy. Cyclosporine in association with prednisone is more effective in inducing remission than is cyclosporine alone (653), and some steroid-resistant patients became steroid-sensitive after a course of cyclosporine. Potential nephrotoxicity is of concern in any patient receiving cyclosporine for protracted periods. Tacrolimus has been reported anecdotally to be effective (711).

Therapy with nonsteroidal antiinflammatory drugs also has produced variable results in patients with MCN (712). Some patients with frequently relapsing or steroid-resistant MCNS who were treated with one of these drugs demonstrated a reduction in proteinuria, but all remained nephrotic and a high percentage had no response (713). Thus, drugs such as indomethacin and meclofenamate may at best represent a useful adjunct in selected patients who are receiving symptomatic treatment only. One potential explanation for the disappointing results is that patients selected for this therapy typically are unresponsive to all standard forms of treatment and may represent a recalcitrant population (713). NSAID should be used cautiously because of association with renal failure in nephrotic patients (see section on Consequences of Proteinuria).

Steroid-resistant patients who do not respond to alternative therapies often have to be maintained on a regimen of sodium and fluid restriction combined with judicious use of diuretics. Balancing the desire to minimize tissue edema against the importance of avoiding intravascular volume depletion is a rigorous challenge for the clinician (see section on Symptomatic Treatment of Nephrotic Syndrome).

Outcomes

Although late relapses of MCN have been reported (714,715), the majority of children with MCN enter permanent remission either before or at puberty. Their long-term prognosis is good, with at least 70% entering adult life without renal or urinary abnormalities. This finding contrasts with the much less favorable outcome if the nephrotic syndrome is associated with glomerulonephritis (716). A minority of pediatric patients who are initially steroid-responsive eventually progress to re-

nal failure. Most are found to have FSGS (443,717), although this lesion is not always present (718).

There have been many attempts to predict the long-term course either from renal histology or from patterns of response to treatment with steroids. For example, in one study of children, the presence of mesangial hypercellularity and immune complexes in the glomeruli was associated with an increased relapse rate (441). In contrast, the ISKDC (648) was unable to correlate frequency of relapse with (a) the histopathologic subgroups of MCN, (b) clinical or laboratory characteristics present at the time of diagnosis, (c) the timing of initial response, or (d) the interval between the initial response and the first relapse. Frequent relapses in the first 6 months, however, were highly predictive of frequent relapses subsequently. In contrast, children who present with minimal edema and are steroid-sensitive follow an extremely favorable clinical course (719).

Adult patients with MCN also have a good prognosis; in one series, more than 90% survived for 10 years or more without development of end-stage renal disease (ESRD) (720,721).

Complications

The most common complications observed in patients with nephrotic syndrome are secondary to therapy. Steroid-induced side effects are well known and include the typical changes in facies, obesity, hirsutism, striae, and pseudotumor cerebri. Acutely, patients receiving large doses of corticosteroids may complain of difficulty sleeping or abdominal distress from high gastric acidity. Hypertension can occur but is seen less often in patients adhering to a sodium-restricted diet. Although growth retardation may be seen in children, especially if they receive high doses of steroids for protracted periods (722), the incidence of significantly decreased height in prepubertal children is relatively low, even with repeated courses of corticosteroid therapy (723), particularly when the prednisone is given on alternate days (724). Catch-up growth often occurs when steroid therapy is discontinued (725). Patients with steroid-responsive nephrotic syndrome who had received repeated courses of high-dose steroids during childhood and who had completed growth had a mean height equivalent to the 40th percentile (726); total corticosteroid dose, however, correlated only weakly with the height scores. In another study, patients were slightly but significantly shorter than their peers. More importantly, they had a higher BMI than controls (321). Corticosteroid-induced cataracts were found in a high percentage of children (727), although visual acuity was not impaired. The complications of cytotoxic drugs were discussed previously.

Peritonitis is a particularly important complication of nephrotic syndrome in children (728). Patients who have one such episode are at increased risk for subsequent episodes. Peritonitis typically occurs during relapses of the disease associated with gross edema and ascites. Clinical evidence of peritoneal irritation usually is present even in patients receiving steroids. The most common infecting agent remains *Streptococcus pneumoniae*, which is found in approximately half of the affected patients (728); *Escherichia coli* is cultured in an additional 25%; a variety of other organisms, including *Haemophilus influenzae*, may be found in a small percentage of patients, and the peritoneal fluid may be culture-negative in some patients. Interestingly, this complication is far less common in adults; the basis for this disparity is not known.

Infections were responsible for the majority of deaths in nephrotic patients in the preantibiotic era. Although infections occur with much less frequency now, they continue to have serious implications. For example, in a report on long-term outcomes of treatment from the ISKDC in which 389 children with MCNS were followed for 5 to 15 years, 6 of the 10 deaths were due to infections. Other causes of death included one episode of dural sinus thrombosis and one incident of cardiorespiratory failure following infusion of salt-poor albumin. One child died in chronic renal failure after development of FSGS not seen in initial biopsy specimens, and one death was from uncertain causes. Five initially nonresponsive patients and four patients manifesting early relapse died. The number of fatalities among nonresponders was particularly striking; 20% of all initial nonresponders in the study died (729). Nonrenal causes of death not mentioned in this study but that may be encountered include other thromboembolic phenomena, hemorrhagic pancreatitis (403), and hypovolemic shock.

Nonfatal complications of MCNS include azotemia, hypovolemic shock, thrombosis, anemia, and effects of decreased vitamin D levels. These were discussed in the section on Consequences of Proteinuria.

FSGS AND COLLAPSING GLOMERULOPATHY

Focal segmental glomerulosclerosis (FSGS) is a common cause of nephrotic syndrome in children and adults. Synonyms for this lesion include *focal and segmental glomerulosclerosis with hyalinosis*, *focal sclerosing glomerulonephritis*, and *focal sclerosing glomerulopathy*. Some patients, particularly adults, may present with subnephrotic proteinuria or may lack other features of nephrotic syndrome. This is particularly true of postadaptive FSGS, as compared with idiopathic FSGS.

FSGS should be distinguished from the finding of occasional globally sclerosed (obsolescent) glomeruli, a benign pattern that is seen in the United States in up to 1% to 3% of glomeruli until age 40 to 55 years and then rises steadily, reaching 30% in individuals 80 years of age (730,731). Howie makes the point that FSGS "cannot be defined in a sensible, useful, unambiguous way" (456). The problem is that there are at least three meanings to the term and that definitions must include both pathologic description and clinical information: (a) idiopathic nephrotic syndrome with segmental glomerulosclerosis (which in this chapter will be termed *idiopathic FSGS*), (b) FSGS arising as a consequence of structural and function adaptation to various conditions, all of which are characterized by glomerular hypertrophy and hyperfiltration (which in this chapter will be termed *postadaptive FSGS*), and (c) segmental glomerulosclerosis arising in the setting of other glomerular diseases, such as proliferative glomerulonephritis, membranous nephropathy, and diabetic nephropathy (which are not dealt with in this chapter, out of the belief that they should not be considered part of the spectrum of primary podocyte diseases).

A related histologic entity has been termed *collapsing focal segmental glomerulosclerosis* or *collapsing glomerulopathy* (as suggested by Detwiler et al (732). We have chosen the latter term because we believe that the histology, biology, and etiology of collapsing glomerulopathy are sufficiently distinct to merit a separate classification. Moreover, the glomerular lesions may be global rather than segmental and the defining lesions are podocyte hyperplasia and capillary collapse rather than sclerosis, all of which make the use of the term FSGS inappropriate. Nonetheless, the nephrology and pathology literature continues to most commonly include collapsing glomerulopathy within FSGS, and, therefore, in this chapter will follow that convention when necessary.

Another disorder is *diffuse mesangial sclerosis* (DMS), an uncommon syndrome generally restricted to the pediatric population. Many cases of DMS are associated with genetic mutations in podocyte genes, placing this syndrome within the spectrum of podocyte diseases.

Presentation and Epidemiology

The clinical presentation of FSGS is highly variable. Nephrotic range proteinuria is seen in approximately 90% of children and 70% of adults (733), although this fraction of non-nephrotic patients in a particular practice will clearly depend upon the inclination of the nephrologist to perform a renal biopsy in the setting of subnephrotic proteinuria. Common associated features include microscopic hematuria (55% children, 45% adults) and renal insufficiency (20% children, 30% adults) (733).

FSGS is now the leading cause of primary nephrotic syndrome among adults, as shown by review of renal biopsy archives from Chicago (10), Springfield, Massachusetts (734), and New York (365). Therefore, it has replaced membranous nephropathy as the leading cause of adult nephrotic syndrome in the United States, with a relative incidence of 30% to 40% among patients undergoing renal biopsy.

A similar pattern has been seen among children. In Houston, FSGS was present in 35% of renal biopsies in children with primary nephrotic syndrome prior to 1990, rising to 47% (and the leading diagnosis) among biopsies performed after 1990 (735). In India, the prevalence of FSGS on kidney biopsy rose from 20% to 47% during the 1990s (736). In South Africa, over the period from 1970 to 1995, FSGS as a cause of nephrotic syndrome rose from 2% to 20% among Indian children and from 5% to 28% among black children (737). Among children in Ontario (with a largely Caucasian population), who represent a closed population evaluated by single pathology center, FSGS now represents 18% of the renal biopsies performed for nephrotic syndrome. This is a 2.5-fold increase in incidence, from 0.37 cases/100,000 during 1985 to 1993 to 0.94 from 1993 to 2002 (11). Furthermore, FSGS remains a leading cause of ESRD in children ages 0 to 19 (738). Over the period from 1999 to 2002, 4,859 children progressed to ESRD; in 1,262 children the cause was glomerulonephritis, of which 592 cases were FSGS (representing 47% of glomerulonephritis ESRD and 12% of all ESRD in children). By comparison, other major ESRD categories included "other cause" (including chiefly congenital renal and urologic abnormalities), 1,262 children and "missing or unknown cause," 670 children.

To date, there has not been a population-based study of FSGS incidence in the United States and there is no national registry for glomerular disease. Therefore, the increased relative incidence of FSGS could represent a decline in other diagnostic entities or an absolute increase in FSGS incidence (other possibilities, such as a change in biopsy practice or diagnostic classification, seem unlikely to account for more than a small fraction of the changes). However, as a proxy for incident FSGS trends, Kitiyakara and colleagues examined the incidence of FSGS ESRD (excluding AIDS nephropathy) and found a steady increase over the last two decades (739,740). This was not unique to FSGS (e.g., there was a similar increase in the category, "other glomerular disease") but it contrasts with a more modest increase in membranous nephropathy ESRD and a drop in ESRD due to glomerular disease, "histologically not examined." Thus, it appears to be likely that there has been a true increase in incident FSGS cases in recent years. The reasons behind these trends are not understood.

Worldwide, there is considerable heterogeneity in the relative incidence of FSGS compared to other causes of adult nephrotic syndrome, ranging from 10% to 45% (Fig. 64-9). Factors contributing to this variability likely include population genetic differences, renal biopsy practices, and environmental factors including HIV-1 infection. There are also

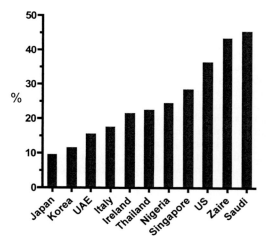

FIGURE 64-9. Relative incidence of FSGS as a cause of adult nephrotic syndrome. The fraction of adult nephrotic syndrome attributed to FSGS (which probably includes collapsing glomerulopathy in most or all series) is presented in select countries.

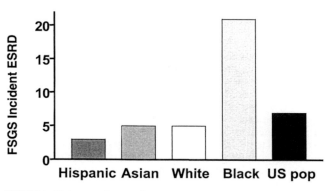

FIGURE 64-11. Incidence of FSGS ESRD by age and race in the United States. The incidence of ESRD (cases/million population/year) attributed to FSGS is presented by age and race; data from the USRDS. (Reprinted from: Kitiyakara C, Kopp JB, Eggers P, et al. Trends in the epidemiology of focal segmental glomerulosclerosis. *Semin Nephrol* 2003;23:172, with permission.)

striking racial differences in the incidence of FSGS ESRD. In the United States, blacks are at approximately fourfold increased risk for FSGS ESRD compared to whites, Hispanics (who may be of any race), and Native Americans (Fig. 64-10). Presumably genetic factors contribute to this risk. Progress is being made in identifying loci that contribute to the increased risk for ESRD among African Americans (741) and in FSGS in particular (discussed in subsequent text). Differences in FSGS ESRD can be resolved, at least in theory, into differences in FSGS incidence and differences in the progression of FSGS to ESRD. The FSGS incidence data, relative to other nephrotic diseases, that were cited previously from various U.S. cities suggest that blacks are at a higher risk for FSGS than are other racial groups. With regard to progression to ESRD, studies of adults (742) and children (743,744) have suggested that blacks are more likely to progress to ESRD than are those of other races, by a factor of approximately two- to fourfold. The reasons for these ethnic disparities remain to be elucidated; genetic differences likely contribute but environmental factors such as access to medical care, differences in the types of FSGS, and the presence of comorbid conditions could play a role. Interestingly, there also is a racial difference in the age of onset of FSGS ESRD (Fig. 64-11). In blacks, the incidence peaks in the early 50s, whereas in whites incidence peaks two decades later (when there is a second peak among blacks).

Histopathology

Fahr, writing in 1925, first noted that patients with lipoid nephrosis who progress to renal failure showed focal glomerular damage (745). In 1957, Rich examined autopsy tissues from 20 children with nephrotic syndrome and otherwise typical lipoid nephrosis and described progressive sclerosis of glomeruli, affecting first the juxtamedullary glomeruli. Heptinstall, in the 1966 edition of his renal pathology textbook, confirmed that some patients with lipoid nephrosis had hyalinization of the glomerular tuft, particularly affecting the juxtamedullary glomeruli (746). McGovern (747) and Hayslett et al. (748) showed that in some patients whose initial renal biopsy was consistent with MCN, a later renal biopsy showed FSGS. In 1970, two reports demonstrated that FSGS was the second most common cause of nephrotic syndrome in children (418,419). Thus, by 1970, it was clear that FSGS was a distinct and common glomerular disease.

Classically, the pathologic abnormalities affect only some glomeruli (focal), with only part of the glomerular tuft involved (segmental). There may be accumulation of acellular hyaline subendothelial deposits within glomerular capillaries; these represent the insudation of plasma protein below an injured endothelium. Tubular atrophy and interstitial inflammatory infiltrates are common (418). The first glomeruli affected are those located near the medulla. As a consequence, an early or superficial renal biopsy may miss the lesion. Furthermore, evaluation of sclerosis on the basis of one section or a few

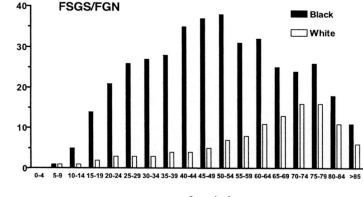

FIGURE 64-10. Racial differences (cases/million population/year) in FSGS ESRD in the United States. The annual incidence of ESRD attributed to FSGS for the years 1995 to 2000 are shown.

sections, as is typical of routine pathologic analysis, will significantly underestimate the fraction of glomeruli that are affected (749,750).

Immunofluorescent microscopy may demonstrate IgM and C3 deposits in a granular pattern, particularly within affected sclerotic segments (751). Unaffected glomerular areas also may reveal IgM and C3 in a mesangial distribution. Electron microscopy shows epithelial cell foot-process effacement that in patients with heavy proteinuria is diffuse and involves areas of the glomeruli that do not demonstrate sclerosis. Mesangial hypercellularity is present variably. In a patient with otherwise normal glomeruli, the presence of glomerular hypertrophy, focal interstitial fibrosis or tubular atrophy may reflect FSGS that is not present in the glomeruli that are sampled in the renal biopsy (752).

The incidence of FSGS in a subsequent biopsy when the original biopsy shows MCN has varied from less than 10% to more than 40% in individual studies (702), which may reflect whether each report presents a primary or referral population.

Histopathologic Variants: FSGS and Collapsing Glomerulopathy

It is now clear that the spectrum of primary podocyte diseases (MCN, DMS, FSGS, and collapsing glomerulopathy) represent several histopathologic patterns, each including multiple disease entities. The relationships among these entities remain enigmatic; we present one schema (Table 64-3). We have excluded other disorders that might otherwise be placed in the MCN/FSGS spectrum, such as idiopathic nodular sclerosis, which has been proposed to have a vascular etiology (753). Others have presented parallel but distinct approaches (754–756).

The existing classification schemes for the primary podocyte diseases, including the one presented here, rely upon a mixture of morphologic, immunologic, genetic, and historical criteria in ways that are not ideally integrated. Importantly, the presence of a risk factor for a diagnostic entity in a particular case under investigation will not always mean that that particular factor has been responsible. Therefore, although obese patients are at increased risk to develop postadaptive FSGS, they remain at some risk for other FSGS variants. Likewise many patients with FSGS have hypertension, and distinguishing hypertension-associated FSGS from other variants can be problematic. As a practical matter, information about genetic history and the presence of relevant comorbid conditions may not be available to the pathologist at the time of diagnosis. All of these comments point out the limitations of relying upon clinical factors in determining pathologic diagnosis or, conversely, determining disease based solely on histopathology. This issue may be successfully addressed by new molecular diagnostic techniques, which may improve the accuracy of clinical diagnosis and may generate more useful classification schemes in the future. Immunostaining to evaluate protein expression is one approach. For example, dystroglycan, a podocyte membrane protein contributing to cellular adhesion to the GBM, is reduced in MCN but not in FSGS (428). Another approach is quantitative analysis of RNA extracted from microdissected glomeruli. Kretzler and colleagues showed that the ratio of podocin/synaptopodin mRNA distinguished MCN from FSGS and predicted steroid-responsiveness in cases where the distinction of MCN from FSGS was uncertain (757).

Columbia Classification

D'Agati and colleagues have proposed a working classification (the Columbia classification) for idiopathic FSGS, which comprises five categories: collapsing variant, tip lesion, cellular lesion, perihilar variant, plus a final category for those cases

that do not have the diagnostic criteria for the other categories, not otherwise specified (NOS), corresponding to classic FSGS. (Table 64-11, Fig. 64-12) (754).

Evaluation of the renal biopsy requires immunologic and ultrastructural studies to exclude other disease entities. The Columbia classification of FSGS variants is based solely on semiquantitative analysis of morphology by light microscopy. There is no minimum glomerular number required to make a diagnosis, but obviously diagnostic accuracy will increase with larger sample size. A single glomerulus with the defining characteristic findings is sufficient, as long as the other criteria are met. This classification scheme was not specifically designed to serve clinical or research purposes, but rather to address both needs.

The collapsing variant of idiopathic FSGS is defined by the presence of at least one glomerulus with segmental or global collapse *and* with podocyte hypertrophy or hyperplasia. Thus podocyte changes alone are insufficient to make the diagnosis (such findings would indicate cellular FSGS). This entity is termed idiopathic collapsing glomerulopathy in Table 64-3. HIV-associated collapsing glomerulopathy has an identical histologic appearance, so that the appearance of classic or other forms of FSGS in a patient with HIV-1 infection is sufficiently unusual to raise the issue of coincidental idiopathic FSGS. Both idiopathic collapsing FSGS and HIV-associated FSGS are frequently associated with tubulointerstitial injury and fibrosis that is out of proportion to the extent of glomerular involvement.

The glomerular tip variant of idiopathic FSGS is defined by the presence of at least one glomerulus with segmental scar involving the glomerular tuft adjacent to the proximal tubule. The collapsing variant must be excluded (it would take precedence over the diagnosis of the tip variant). Most tip variants have increased cellularity as well as the required sclerosis. Mesangial hypercellularity may be present. Perihilar sclerosis cannot be present but other peripheral (non-tip, non-hilar) lesions containing IgM and C3 may be present within the tip lesion. Heavy proteinuria and extensive foot-process effacement is typically present.

The cellular variant of idiopathic FSGS has had a complicated history. Grishman and Churg described the ultrastructure of 16 patients with FSGS and found that 5 patients had podocyte abnormalities, including cellular degeneration and detachment, together with glomerular capillary collapse; 3 of these patients exhibited rapid clinical deterioration (758). Schwartz and Lewis coined the term *cellular lesion of FSGS*. The original cellular definition included segmental or global hypercellularity (representing proliferation and/or infiltration, or hypercellularity within Bowman's space overlying segmental scar, or capillary collapse) (759). Thus, many of these cases meet the Columbia criteria for collapsing variant. In the Columbia framework, diagnosis of cellular variant requires the presence of endocapillary proliferation (segmental or global) in at least one glomerulus; these cells include endothelial cells, macrophages, and foam cells. Podocyte hypertrophy and hyperplasia may be present. Mesangial hypercellularity may also be present but is uncommon. Consequently, the focus of the Columbia definition of cellular variant has shifted away from podocytes to endocapillary cells, although abnormalities of both cellular compartments may be present. A tubulopathy is present that may be disproportionate to the extent of glomerular involvement. This may include a focal microcystic dilation and tubular epithelial cells manifesting acute injury (including focal acute tubular necrosis), regeneration, and chronic injury (cellular atrophy and thickening of the tubular basement membrane). Tip variant and collapsing variant must be excluded (these diagnoses would take precedence over cellular variant).

The Columbia classification makes the perihilar variant a formal diagnostic entity. This variant is diagnosed when

TABLE 64-11

COLUMBIA CLASSIFICATION OF THE MORPHOLOGIC VARIANTS OF FSGS

Variant	Positive criteria	Negative criteria
FSGS, Not otherwise specified	• At least one glomerulus with segmental increase in matrix obliterating the capillary lumina • There may be segmental GBM collapse without podocyte hyperplasia	Exclude other defined variants below
Perihilar variant	• At least one glomerulus with perihilar hyalinosis, with or without hyalinosis • Perihilar sclerosis and hyalinosis involving >50% of segmentally sclerotic glomeruli	Exclude cellular, tip, and collapsing variants
Cellular variant	• At least one glomerulus with segmental endocapillary hypercellularity occluding lumina, with or without foam cells and karyorrhexis	Exclude tip and collapsing variants
Tip variant	• At least one segmental lesion involving the tip domain (outer 25% of the tuft next to the origin of the proximal tubule) • The tubular pole must be identified in the defining lesion • The lesion must have either an adhesion or confluence of podocytes with parietal or tubular cells at the tubular lumen or neck • The tip lesion may be sclerosing or cellular	Exclude collapsing variant Exclude if any glomeruli show perihilar sclerosis
Collapsing variant	• At least one glomerulus with segmental or global collapse and podocyte hypertrophy or hyperplasia	No exclusions

FSGS, focal segmental glomerulosclerosis; *GBM*, glomerular basement membrane.
(Adapted from: D'Agati V. Pathologic classification of focal segmental glomerulosclerosis. *Semin Nephrol* 2003;23:117; and D'Agati V, et al. Pathologic classification of focal segmental glomerulosclerosis: a working proposal. *Am J Kidney Dis* 2004;43:368.) The flow of diagnostic decision-making begins at the bottom, as the pathologist diagnoses or excludes collapsing variant, then tip variant, then cellular variant, then perihilar variant, and, finally, FSGS, not otherwise specified (NOS).

perihilar hyalinosis is present in one or more glomeruli and perihilar sclerosis and/or hyalinosis is present in at least 50% of segmentally sclerotic glomeruli. Hyalinosis represents the accumulation of glassy, homogeneous, eosinophilic material within the capillary wall and is believed to consist of plasma proteins. In the remnant rat model, hyalinosis appears first as the accumulation of PAS-positive and electron-dense material beneath damaged glomerular capillary endothelial cells, with later expansion and encroachment on the capillary lumen (760). Glomerulomegaly is common. The perihilar variant is commonly associated with what we describe as *postadaptive* FSGS (defined in subsequent text). Cellular variant, tip variant, and collapsing variants must be excluded (these diagnoses would take precedence over perihilar variant).

The most common variant of FSGS (NOS) may include features of any of the prior variants, but lacks sufficient criteria to make a more specific diagnosis. The term *classic FSGS* would include FSGS NOS.

The Columbia classification represents a very important step forward in the process of developing a robust, consistent, and clinically useful diagnostic classification system for FSGS. By laying out consensus diagnostic criteria for FSGS for the first time, D'Agati and colleagues have framed the issues that the field will address in the coming years. As the authors recognize, this is a working proposal that will almost certainly undergo revision. The next iteration might usefully address some of the following issues, and may well make use of use molecular markers to refine the classification system.

First, the relationship between the cellular variant and collapsing FSGS (collapsing glomerulopathy) remains controversial. Schwartz and colleagues note that in their terminology, the cellular lesion includes collapsing FSGS, whereas the Columbia classification includes cellular lesion and collapsing FSGS as distinct entities. (761). No patient series has yet been published that describes the clinical characteristics and outcome of patients with the cellular lesion, as defined by the Columbia classification, and so this syndrome is not yet well-characterized.

Second, and related to the previous issue, the importance of different forms of podocyte injury has become apparent as we have developed new understanding of the biologic processes underlying FSGS (podocyte depletion) and collapsing glomerulopathy (podocyte proliferation). Morphologically, podocyte proliferation is characteristic of the collapsing variant, but must be coupled with capillary loop collapse for the diagnosis to be made. When capillary loop collapse is absent and podocyte changes are coupled with endothelial cell proliferation, the diagnosis of cellular lesion is made. Thus, when podocyte hyperplasia is present, the diagnosis depends upon whether capillary collapse or endocapillary proliferation is present (762). The biologic rationale for this distinction is not immediately clear, as we do not understand the mechanisms responsible for glomerular collapse. If further studies indicate that the podocyte phenotype is similar in collapsing FSGS and those cases of cellular variant FSGS with podocyte hyperplasia, and that response to therapy and prognosis are also similar, it is probably more logical to combine these categories.

Third, the stability of classification when serial biopsies are performed needs to be defined. The few studies available suggest that patients may change diagnostic categories on

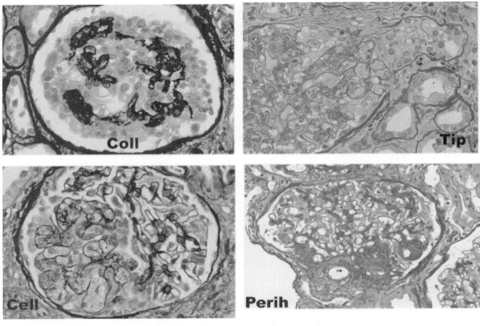

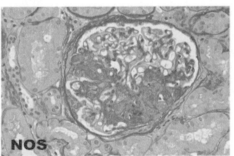

FIGURE 64-12. Variants of FSGS: the Columbia classification. This classification was developed for diagnostic purposes and involves the stepwise consideration of collapsing variant (coll), tip lesion (tip), cellular variant (cell), perihilar variant (perih) and FSGS not otherwise specified (NOS). (Figure reproduced from: D'Agati V, Fogo AB, Bruijn JA, et al. Pathologic classification of focal segmental glomerulosclerosis: a working proposal, *Am J Kidney Dis* 2004;368:43, with permission.)

subsequent biopsies (discussed in subsequent text). Future studies involving serial renal biopsies of FSGS patients would be an essential starting point. Careful consideration must be given as to whether these events represent disease evolution (category change) or disease progression (progressive scarring), and what the implication for the classification system might be.

Fourth, inter-rater reliability needs to be rigorously evaluated by practicing pathologists to ensure that the existing diagnostic framework yields reproducible results. Finally, the ability of diagnostic categories to make predictions as to etiology and prognosis, based solely on morphology and independent of clinical history, must be tested both retrospectively and prospectively on patient cohorts drawn from diverse ethnic and racial populations. Despite these considerations, the Columbia classification remains an excellent starting point, providing a common set of diagnostic criteria with which the field can advance.

Postadaptive FSGS

We propose the term *postadaptive FSGS* to include those forms of FSGS that are believed to arise as a consequence of structural adaptation (glomerular hypertrophy) and functional adaptation (glomerular hyperperfusion and hyperfiltration) to either reduced nephron mass or particular disease states (obesity, sickle cell anemia, cyanotic congenital heart disease, and others). The term *secondary FSGS* has also been used to describe this form of FSGS, although the term sometimes

has been extended to HIV-associated nephropathy, to drug-associated FSGS, and to segmental scarring arising in proliferative glomerulonephritis; these varied uses have diminished the utility of the term.

The diagnosis of postadaptive FSGS remains a challenge. Ideally, the diagnosis would be made on pathologic grounds alone. The problem with relying upon clinical factors in reaching a diagnosis is that patients with obesity, hypertension, and other disorders might present with either idiopathic FSGS or postadaptive FSGS. As these entities may have different responses to therapy, particularly immunosuppressive therapy, the distinction becomes important. Three approaches are available at present.

First, postadaptive FSGS may manifest less foot-process effacement than idiopathic FSGS. Chiang et al. studied renal biopsies obtained from 30 children and found that the extent of foot process effacement was similar in MCN (63% ± 21%), FSGS (70% ± 25%), and MCN that subsequently evolved into FSGS (56% ± 23%) (763). The large standard deviation suggests that many patients in all three disease categories had <50% effacement. Furthermore, the extent of foot-process effacement did not correlate with proteinuria, although only 15 patients were included in the analysis. D'Agati and colleagues defined obesity-associated glomerulopathy as glomerulomegaly in the setting of BMI >30 kg/m², with or without FSGS (764). They found that obesity-associated glomerulomegaly cases had a mean foot-process effacement 40% (range 10% to 100%), whereas idiopathic FSGS patients had mean foot-process effacement 75%, range 30% to 100%). Importantly, although there were significant differences in the group means for the extent of podocyte foot-process effacement in idiopathic FSGS versus postadaptive FSGS, there was much overlap, so the utility of particular diagnostic criteria (such as podocyte foot process effacement >50% in the former and <50% in the latter) is limited (765).

Second, the initial lesion in postadaptive FSGS is preferentially localized to the hilum. Rat models of FSGS that are characterized by increased transcapillary hydraulic pressure are associated with predominant or exclusive perihilar sclerosis. This is probably explained by the observation that the first capillary branches of the afferent arteriole are the largest, and thus by Laplace's law these branches would have the highest wall tension and be the most susceptible to podocyte injury (766,767). The problems in clinical use are that correctly identifying the location of the sclerosis, even with multiple sections, and the number of glomeruli available for study is limited. (It remains to be determined whether the perihilar variant of idiopathic FSGS also arises as a consequence of glomerular overload from an unrecognized risk factor or biologic process. In this context, it would be interesting to see a detailed analysis of the clinical and physiological characteristics of these patients.)

Third, glomerulomegaly can be demonstrated by direct measurement of glomerular size. D'Agati has proposed defining glomerulomegaly as 1.5-fold increase in glomerular diameter over control (comparable to a 2.5-fold increase in glomerular area and 3.4-fold increase in glomerular volume, assuming that the glomerulus is a sphere) (765). D'Agati and colleagues have also defined glomerulomegaly as average glomerular diameter >180 μm, based on study of four biopsy levels and the measurement limited to glomeruli in which hilus was identified (764). In normal controls, glomerular diameter averaged 168 μm (range 138 to 186 um), and in obese subjects with glomerulomegaly, glomerular diameter averaged 226 μm (range 172 to 300 μm).

Therefore, presently available methods to identify postadaptive FSGS include determining the fraction of glomeruli with perihilar sclerosis and measuring glomerular size. Needed are prospective studies evaluating each of these approaches, and defining the receiver-operating characteristic (ROC) curves for the diagnostic thresholds. Even with these data, a major limitation remains the requirement for sufficient numbers of intact glomeruli. An important research goal will be to identify molecular markers that reflect the glomerular adaptation; these might include proteins that are upregulated by podocytes or mesangial cells in response to mechanical stress.

Diffuse Mesangial Sclerosis and Related Disorders

Diffuse mesangial sclerosis represents a small fraction of pediatric renal biopsies (0.9% in India [768]) and all-age renal biopsies (0.45% in the United States [753]). In the pediatric population, many cases are associated with *WT1* and *LAMB2* mutations, as discussed elsewhere in this chapter. Some cases seen in children and adults are idiopathic. Unidentified genetic mutations may contribute. Two adult cases have been reported in association with multiple myeloma (769). One note of diagnostic caution is that it may be difficult to exclude advanced FSGS in renal biopsies lacking glomeruli with segmental sclerosis.

Disease Mechanisms of FSGS and Collapsing Glomerulopathy

Animal Models

A number of animal models have been used to delineate the mechanisms of FSGS and collapsing glomerulopathy, as has been reviewed recently (770). These models have been crucial for elucidating mechanisms, particularly for postadaptive FSGS, HIV-associated collapsing glomerulopathy and, most recently, for genetic causes of FSGS. In particular, they have led the field to highlight the central role of podocytes in FSGS and collapsing glomerulopathy. A significant gap is the absence of generally accepted animal models for MCN, idiopathic classic FSGS, or recurrent FSGS after renal transplantation.

Available animal models include experimentally induced disease (Table 64-12) (771–783), spontaneous genetic models

TABLE 64-12

ANIMAL MODELS OF FOCAL SEGMENTAL GLOMERULOSCLEROSIS (FSGS): INDUCED

Model	Species	Comment	Reference
Remnant nephron, excision	Rat	Hyperfiltration	(771)
Remnant nephron, infarction	Rat	Hyperfiltration	(773)
Remnant nephron, ligation and cautery	Mouse	Hyperfiltration	(774)
Aging plus uninephrectomy	Rat		(775)
Aging plus uninephrectomy	Mouse		(776)
Doxorubicin (Adriamycin)	Rat		(777)
Doxorubicin (Adriamycin)	Mouse	Less consistent than rat	(778)
Bromethylamine-induced papillary necrosis	Rat	Probable hyperfiltration associated with nephron loss	(779)
Cyclosporine (chronic)	Rat	Probable hyperfiltration associated with nephron loss	(780)
FGF-2 (chronic)	Rat		(781)
Puromycin aminonucleoside, single dose	Rat		(782)
Puromycin aminonucleoside, multiple dose	Rat	Glomerular hypertrophy	(783)

TABLE 64-13

ANIMAL MODELS OF FOCAL SEGMENTED GLOMERULOSCLEROSIS (FSGS): SPONTANEOUS GENETIC MODELS

Model	Comment	Reference
Spontaneously hypertensive rat (SHR)	Hypertensive	(824)
Dahl salt-sensitive rat	Hypertensive	(784)
Fawn-hooded hypertensive rat	Hypertensive, perihilar scar	(766)
Sabra hypertensive rat	Hypertensive	(785)
Munich-Wistar-Frömter rat	Normotensive	(786)
Spontaneously hypercholesterolemic rat (SHC)	Hyperlipidemic	(787)
Imai rat	Hyperlipidemic	(788)
Obese, fa/fa Zucker rat	Hyperlipidemic, nonhypertensive	(789)
Buffalo MNA rat	Normotensive, recurs after renal transplant	(790,791)
FSGS/Kist mouse or Nga mouse		(792)
APA strain, Syrian hamsters		(793)

(Table 64-13) (766,784–793), null mutation animals (Table 64-14) (794–804), and transgenic animals (Table 64-15) (798,805–823). Each model has particular strengths and limitations and reflects a certain portion of the spectrum of human podocyte disease. The interested reader is referred to the provided references; here we will consider the pathogenesis of FSGS and collapsing glomerulopathy by considering the structural and functional processes involved, rather than a detailed review of particular molecular pathways.

A critical aspect of these models is disordered podocyte function. Direct injury to the podocyte underlies many of the animal models of glomerulosclerosis, including toxic injury (adriamycin, PAN), proliferation (FGF-2 administration), viral gene expression (HIV-1 accessory genes, SV40 T antigen) and gene (*NPHS2, CD2AP, ACTN4*) deletion or modification. Podocyte stress likely contributes in models of postadaptive FSGS associated with nephron loss (remnant nephron, aging plus uninephrectomy, bromo-ethylamine-induced papillary necrosis). The genetic rat models demonstrate the importance of systemic and glomerular hypertension and hyperlipidemia, although the restriction of these traits to particular strains suggests that particular genetic loci are required for the full interaction of the hypertension and lipids with renal injury.

Glomerular Adaptation: Glomerular Overload and Glomerulomegaly

Reduction in nephron mass is a well-established model of postadaptive FSGS in experimental animal models (Table 64-12). In 1952, Platt and colleagues noted in rats subjected to 5/6 nephrectomy, creatinine clearance fell to a lesser degree than the reduction in renal mass would predict (825). Subsequently, Morrison and Howard reported similar findings using inulin clearance and went on to suggest that hyperfiltration might play a role in glomerulomegaly, podocyte hypertrophy, and the subsequent appearance of glomerulosclerosis (771,826). In 1981, in a highly influential study, Hostetter

TABLE 64-14

ANIMAL MODELS OF FOCAL SEGMENTAL GLOMERULOSCLEROSIS (FSGS): NULL MUTATIONS AND KNOCK-IN MUTATIONS

Gene class	Gene	Histology	Reference
Podocyte slit diaphragm and cytoskeletal genes	*CD2AP*	Diffuse global glomerulosclerosis (homozygotes) FGGS (heterozygotes)	(794,795)
	NPHS2	Mesangial sclerosis	(796)
	ACTN4	Podocyte injury, foot process effacement	(797,798)
	WT1 mutant knock-in	Mesangial sclerosis	(799)
	WT1 mutant knock-in (R394W)	Mesangial sclerosis	(800)
Other	MPV17	Mesangiolysis, focal global glomerulosclerosis	(801)
	BCL2	Oligomeganephronia	(802)
	LCAT	Mesangial proliferation and sclerosis	(803)
	Rrm2b	Collapsing glomerulopathy	(804)

TABLE 64-15

ANIMAL MODELS OF FOCAL SEGMENTAL GLOMERULOSCLEROSIS (FSGS): TRANSGENIC MICE AND RATS

Protein class	Species	Promoter	Transgene	Histology	Reference
Podocyte protein	Mouse	Nephrin	Mutant *ACTN4*	FSGS; proteinuria	(798,805)
Ligands and receptors	Rat	Renin-2	Murine renin-2		(806,807)
	Rat	Renin and angiotensin	Human renin and angiotensin	Nephrosclerosis	(808)
	Mouse	Albumin	*TGFB1*	Diffuse global glomerulosclerosis	(809)
	Mouse	PEPCK	*TGFB1*	GS	(810)
	Mouse	Metallothionein-1	Hepatocyte growth factor	FSGS	(811)
	Mouse	Endothelin-1	Endothelin-1	GS	(812)
	Mouse	Metallothionein-1	Growth hormone	GS	(813)
	Mouse	Metallothionein-1	Growth hormone releasing factor	GS	(813)
	Mouse	CMV/actin/globin	Macrophage migration inhibition factor	Mesangial expansion	(814)
	Rat	Nephrin	Angiotensin receptor type 1	FSGS	(815)
Other proteins	Mouse	MMTV	p53	FSGS	(816)
	Mouse	CMV	Cux-1	Mesangial expansion	(817)
	Mouse	Hemoglobin	Hemoglobin SAD (triple mutant)	FSGS	(818)
	Mouse	Thy1.1	Thy1.1	FSGS	(819)
Viral proteins	Mouse	SV40 early region	SV40 T Ag	FSGS	(820)
	Mouse	HIV-1 LTR	HIV-1 *env* + 6 regulatory genes	Collapsing glomerulopathy	(821)
	Rat	HIV-1 LTR	HIV-1 *env* + 6 regulatory genes	Collapsing glomerulopathy	(822)
	Mouse	HIV-1 LTR	HIV-1 *tat/vpr*	Collapsing glomerulopathy	(823)

FSGS, focal segmental glomerulosclerosis; *DMS*, diffuse mesangial sclerosis; *GS*, glomerulosclerosis is not otherwise described; *CMV*, cytomegalovirus; *LTR*, long terminal repeat; *MMTV*, mouse mammary tumor virus; *PEPCK*, phosphoenolpyruvate carboxylase.
Histology is as described in the original or subsequent publications. Models of diabetic glomerulosclerosis have been excluded.

et al. demonstrated that the remnant nephron model is characterized by increased single nephron SNGFR, due to increased transcapillary hydraulic pressure (772). The glomerular overload (or glomerular hyperfiltration) hypothesis states that some feature of adaptation to reduced renal mass, including possibly hyperperfusion, hyperfiltration, glomerulomegaly, and/or podocyte mechanical stretch, underlies some forms of FSGS and accounts for the progressive nature of chronic kidney disease in general.

In human subjects, removal of one kidney (e.g., with donor nephrectomy) is not associated with increased risk of renal disease after long-term follow-up. There is a poorly defined boundary of minimal renal mass, below which patients are at risk for progressive renal disease. It is quite possible that the boundary differs among patients, based on various factors including nephron endowment. Novick et al. studied 14 patients who had a solitary kidney and then underwent partial nephrectomy for cancer, with 25% to 75% of the solitary kidney having been removed (827). Five patients subsequently developed proteinuria, including three with biopsy-proven FSGS (828).

The Barker hypothesis proposes that prenatal programming influences fetal development in ways that influence adult susceptibility to diseases, including hypertension, coronary heart disease, and type 2 diabetes (829). The Brenner corollary of this hypothesis proposes that a reduced number of nephrons at birth predisposes to hypertension and progressive renal disease during adult life (830). Low birth weight may be a predictor of low nephron number, although studies in various human populations have come to discrepant findings (831,832). Studies support a relationship between low birth weight and essential hypertension (833), and between low birth weight and end-stage renal disease (odds ratio 1.4 for birth weight <2.5 kg compared to birth weight 3 to 3.5 kg) (834), but no data have been published that relate to birth weight to FSGS risk.

Glomerulomegaly. Human glomeruli increase in size during childhood, with mean diameters increasing from 112 μm at birth to 167 μm at age 15, as assessed in an autopsy study where maximal glomerular diameter was measured (835). In normal kidney donors ages 24 to 53, mean glomerular area was not correlated with age or sex (836). When assessed by microdissection, mean glomerular diameter remains stable until about age 40 to 50, after which there is a modest decline (837). The mechanism of age-associated decline in glomerular diameter is unknown, but could be due to an increasing fraction of obsolescent glomeruli. By contrast, children with FSGS have increased glomerular size and there is no correlation with age (838).

Glomerulomegaly is a hallmark of adaptation to reduced nephron mass. Glomerular enlargement may arise as a consequence of widening of the glomerular capillaries, increasing glomerular capillary length, or some combination of both. Experimental rat models suggest that both mechanisms occur with adaptation to reduced renal mass, at different ages. In *young rats* there are large increases in capillary length and only small increases in capillary diameter (839,840). In *older rats*, the major change is increased capillary diameter (841,842). In *children* undergoing uninephrectomy for postadaptive FSGS in the setting of reflux nephropathy, the nephrectomized kidney shows glomerulomegaly without increased capillary diameter (843). In *adults* with FSGS, glomerulomegaly is associated primarily with an increase in capillary diameter (844). Kidneys showing greater numbers of sclerotic glomeruli (more advanced disease), however, showed greater capillary lengthening, whereas there was no relationship between extent of sclerosis and capillary diameter. In conclusion, (a) the results in rats and humans show similar age-dependent patterns, with capillary lengthening predominantly in the young individual and capillary lumen increase predominating in the mature individual and (b) the results in adults with FSGS suggests that the increase in capillary lumen diameter may occur early (as a consequence of unknown mechanisms) and capillary lengthening may later occur in response to reduced functional nephron mass.

Glomerulomegaly is also present in experimental and clinical settings characterized by glomerular overload (defined as an increase in glomerular blood flow or glomerular filtration or both). These settings include obesity, sickle cell anemia, and cyanotic congenital heart disease. Thus in obese patients with glomerular disease and proteinuria, mean glomerular diameter has been reported as 226 μm (range 172 to 300 μm), compared to a mean of 168 μm (range 138 to 186 μm) in age-matched normal subjects (764), and 256 μm (range 192 to 280 μm) (845).

Glomerular Overload: Hyperperfusion and Hyperfiltration. Glomerular hyperperfusion and hyperfiltration are present at the *single nephron level* in animal models of reduced nephron mass. Under normal circumstances in the rat, the pressure gradient across the glomerular capillary wall (P_{GC}) is approximately 50 mm Hg and SNGFR is approximately 30 nl/min; in the remnant nephron model P_{GC} exceeds 60 mm Hg and SNGFR exceeds 60 nl/min (772). Furthermore, glomerular hyperfiltration is present at the *whole kidney level* early in the disease course in experimental models of postadaptive FSGS and most, if not all, human forms of postadaptive FSGS.

Conversely, there are several experimental settings where glomerular hyperperfusion, glomerular hyperfiltration, glomerulomegaly, and FSGS are less closely correlated. Yoshida et al. compared two rat models, both with 1/3 left nephrectomy: in one group the right kidney was removed and in the other group the right ureter was diverted into the peritoneum (846). SNGFR and P_{GC} increased to an equivalent degree in both models, but glomerulomegaly and glomerulosclerosis were blunted (although present) in the urinary diversion group. Thus, remnant nephrons in the left kidney acted differently in the presence of a filtering but nonexcreting right kidney. It remains unclear by what mechanism the remnant nephrons apparently sense total body functioning nephron mass; perhaps a circulating molecular product of glomerular cells contributes. In any case, although this experiment suggests caution in assuming that hyperfiltration will necessarily lead to glomerulomegaly and FSGS, the urinary diversion model has uncertain relevance to clinical situations involving glomerular adaptation.

Furthermore, glomerular hyperperfusion and hyperfiltration are clearly not essential for the development of all forms of FSGS. In rats with PAN nephrosis and rats with adriamycin nephrosis, average P_{GC} values remain normal despite the subsequent appearance of sclerosis (847). In the former model, increased single nephron GFR was uniformly absent and in the latter model, although some glomeruli exhibit increased GFR, these glomeruli did not have elevated P_{GC} and did not subsequently develop sclerosis, at least within the time-frame of the study. Consequently, hyperperfusion and hyperfiltration appear to characterize most if not all postadaptive FSGS models, but are absent from FSGS models that involve direct podocyte injury (presumably models of idiopathic FSGS).

In obese human subjects, absolute GFR (without correction for body size) has been reported to be increased by 25% to 60% (848–850), and this is partially returned to normal values by weight loss (850). Obese subjects have both increased GFR and increased filtration fraction, whereas even in nonobese subjects there is a positive correlation between BMI and filtration fraction (but not GFR) (851). Others have not found an increase in absolute GFR, despite similar levels of BMI, although the reasons for the discrepant findings are not apparent (852). The increased GFR is more striking in central compared to peripheral obesity (853). The mechanisms of obesity-related glomerular hyperfiltration are unknown but may include protein intake, various features of the metabolic syndrome (discussed in subsequent text) and possibly particular adipokines.

Most but not all studies suggest that early in the course of children with sickle cell anemia, GFR and renal plasma flow are increased (854–856). Limited data available in children with cyanotic congenital heart disease suggest that glomerular filtration may be slightly impaired (857) or normal (858). In the latter study, GFR was normal and renal plasma flow was decreased, indicating an increased filtration fraction. The authors proposed that increased blood viscosity associated with polycythemia increases renal vascular resistance and intraglomerular blood pressure.

There is at least one clinical situation in which the link between glomerulomegaly and glomerular overload is absent. Fogo et al. studied 42 pediatric MCN patients, of whom 10 subsequently experienced renal functional decline and a repeat renal biopsy showed FSGS (859). In those patients who later developed FSGS, glomerular area was on average 76% larger (which would correspond to a 1.3-fold increased diameter, assuming the glomerulus was spherical). Although the data on creatinine clearances were not provided, there is no reason to suspect hyperfiltration, and these patients had no obvious clinical features that would suggest reduced renal mass. It remains uncertain what processes might account for glomerulomegaly in this setting.

Podocyte Depletion Hypothesis

The podocyte depletion hypothesis proposes that an absolute or relative reduction in podocyte number is a critical process in FSGS of all types. Furthermore, as podocytes undergo dedifferentiation and loss of matrix adhesiveness in collapsing glomerulopathy, a loss of functional podocytes may contribute. Finally, it now appears that podocyte depletion also is present in other glomerular diseases, including diabetic nephropathy (860) and primary glomerulonephritis (861), and may promote sclerosis in these settings.

Podocytes are postmitotic cells in normal human kidney. In a study of 164 kidneys, podocyte mitoses were found in one kidney (the diagnosis was given as FSGS) and binucleate cells were found in four kidneys (FSGS, lupus nephritis, and IgA nephropathy) (862). In a seminal study, Fries et al. noted that in rats subjected to 3/4 nephrectomy plus adriamycin, the remnant nephrons undergo compensatory hypertrophy, more than doubling tuft volume (863). As part of this process, endothelial cells and mesangial cells proliferate but podocytes do not. As podocyte volume density declines, each podocyte must cover a larger capillary surface area. Areas of podocyte detachment were present, particularly in areas of segmental sclerosis. Extending these studies to human renal biopsies, Bhathena found that the unit distance of GBM covered by podocytes increased in oligomeganephronia, unilateral renal agenesis with FSGS (but not unilateral renal agenesis without FSGS), uninephrectomy with FSGS (but not uninephrectomy without FSGS), and renal transplantation with late (nonrecurrent) FSGS (but not without FSGS) (864). Thus, podocyte hypertrophy characterizes human forms of postadaptive FSGS. Podocyte depletion is also characteristic of idiopathic FSGS. Reduced podocyte numbers are present in children with FSGS compared to those with MCN (838).

Evolution of Segmental Sclerosis: The Misdirected Filtration Hypothesis

Kriz and Lemley, and Kriz et al. have proposed an intriguing model of misdirected glomerular filtration to explain the propensity for segmental sclerotic scars of FSGS to expand, to progress to global sclerosis, and to be associated with tubular damage and interstitial inflammation (767,865–867). This model was developed from intensive study of rat models of FSGS, including the hypertensive Fawn hooded rat and the normotensive Milan rat, with more limited studies of human FSGS.

The process begins when one or more podocytes undergo apoptosis or necrosis, or loses adhesion and is released into Bowman's space. Naked GBM tends to lie in apposition to the parietal cells lining Bowman's capsule, perhaps due to the ballooning of the glomerular capillary in response to the loss of mechanical restraint consequent to podocyte loss or perhaps due to a response on the part of the parietal cells to contact the GBM. This manifests as tuft adhesion (synechia). Tuft adhesion involves a loosening of contacts between parietal cells, allowing glomerular ultrafiltrate to penetrate between parietal cells. A loop of glomerular capillary also penetrates between parietal cells, leading to an expanding paraglomerular space located beneath the parietal cells or extending between layers of Bowman's capsule. These capillary loops remain perfused, at least for a time, and this allows continued delivery of glomerular filtrate into the paraglomerular space. This filtrate, having passed through an abnormal capillary wall lacking podocytes, is likely enriched in growth factors, chemokines, and other inflammatory mediators. These mediators promote the recruitment and activation of fibroblasts and leukocytes, both within the paraglomerular space and in the surrounding interstitium.

Once the paraglomerular space has formed, there are several possible outcomes. First, the process may stabilize and a segmental scar may remain. Second, the enlarging paraglomerular space may engulf additional capillary loops, thereby compromising podocyte integrity in those loops and eventually leading to global sclerosis. Third, and overlapping with the preceding outcomes, the paraglomerular space may expand and encircle the proximal tubule. This has the potential of separating the tubule from peritubular capillary, leading to tubular atrophy and the development of an atubular glomerulus. This model has considerable power to explain the pathology of FSGS. It remains to be determined which forms of human idiopathic FSGS, postadaptive FSGS, genetic FSGS, and medication-associated FSGS follow this model.

Cellular Injury and Response

A consensus has emerged that podocyte injury plays a central role in the pathogenesis of FSGS. This notion is supported by animal models and genetic mutations in human FSGS (all mutations identified to date are in genes that are exclusively expressed in the podocyte or that play critical roles in the podocyte). Pavenstadt et al. (868) provide a superb comprehensive review of podocyte cell biology.

In vivo, podocyte abnormalities are most prominent in cellular FSGS and collapsing glomerulopathy, where podocyte dedifferentiation and proliferation are characteristic, but podocyte abnormalities are seen in FSGS as well (428,869–883) (Table 64-16).

Podocyte proliferation and associated dedifferentiation are likely the critical biologic process in the pathogenesis of collapsing glomerulopathy. This striking distinction between podocyte depletion without proliferation in FSGS and podocyte hyperplasia in collapsing glomerulopathy provides the rationale for separating these diagnostic categories.

Contribution of Other Glomerular and Nonresident Cells. Mesangial cell injury and response is an important component of progressive glomerular injury in FSGS. There is extensive literature on the role of mesangial cells in elaborating extracellular matrix. It remains unclear by what pathways

TABLE 64-16

EXPRESSION OF PODOCYTE DIFFERENTIATION, INJURY, AND PROLIFERATION MARKERS IN HUMAN DISEASE

	Normal	MCN	Idiopathic FSGS	Collapsing glomerulopathy and/or cellular FSGS	Reference
Nephrin	Present	Unchanged or irregular (LM) ↓ per μm (EM)[a]	Unchanged; lost in sclerotic areas	ND	(869,870)
Podocin	Present	Unchanged or ↓	↓ In all glomeruli, absent from sclerotic areas	ND	(871,872)
Synaptopodin	Present	↓	↓ Or absent from all glomeruli	Absent in abnormal podocytes; ↓ in some podocytes in unaffected glomeruli	(872–877)
Podocalyxin	Present	ND	Absent	Absent in abnormal podocytes	(873)
GLEPP 1	Present	ND		Absent in abnormal podocytes	(873)
αβ Dystroglycan	Present	Reduced	Normal	ND	(428)
α5 Integrin	Present	ND	↓, Lost with progressive sclerosis	ND	(878)
WT-1	Present	Unchanged	Absent in sclerotic areas	Absent in abnormal podocytes, ↓ in some podocytes in unaffected glomeruli	(873,877)
Pax-2	Absent	Absent	Absent	Present in abnormal podocytes	(877)
Vimentin	Present	Present	Variably ↓ in sclerotic areas	↓	(877)
Cytokeratin	Absent	ND	ND	Present in abnormal podocytes	(874,879)
Ki67	Absent	Absent	ND	Present in abnormal podocytes	(873)
Cyclin D1	Present	ND	ND	↓ in abnormal podocytes, ↓ in some unaffected glomeruli	(875,880)
Cyclin E	Present	ND	ND	↑ in abnormal podocytes	(880)
p21	Absent	Unchanged	ND	↑ In abnormal podocytes	(882)
p27kip1, p57kip1	Present	Unchanged	ND	↓ In normal and abnormal glomeruli, absent in proliferating podocytes	(875,879,882)
p57kip2	Present	Unchanged	ND	↓ in normal podocytes, absent in proliferating podocytes, ↓ in occasional podocytes, normal glomeruli	(879,882,883)

Podocyte proteins were localized by immunostaining or by ultrastructural labeling in human tissue. Diagnoses are shown as identified in the references; in some references the type of FSGS was not specified. For simplicity, details of altered subcellular distribution of proteins have been omitted. In some cases, discrepant findings were reported. ND, not determined; LM, light microscopy; EM, electron microscopy.
[a] Absent in congenital nephrotic syndrome due to nephrin mutations.

podocyte injury stimulates mesangial cell activation. One possibility, relevant to postadaptive FSGS, is that glomerulomegaly may lead to mechanical stretch being imposed on mesangial cells (reviewed in [884]). Cultured mesangial cells respond to stretch with an increase in expression of collagens, fibronectin, laminin, transforming growth factor (TGF)-β1, connective tissue growth factor (CTGF), macrophage chemotactic protein (MCP)-1, and intercellular adhesion molecule (ICAM)-1, the latter two capable of promoting leukocyte immigration and attachment (885–890). The role of mesangial cell proliferation in progressive scarring is less certain; it could simply be an index of mesangial cell activation. The mechanisms stimulating mesangial proliferation are discussed in the section on the histopathology of MCN.

Endothelial cell injury and response are also important components of progressive glomerular injury. In the remnant nephron model, the glomerular capillary endothelial cell manifests the first structural changes (760) and the first upregulation in mRNAs for extracellular matrix genes (fibronectin, laminin-β1) and TGF-β1, occurring 24 days after ablation (891). In this model, there is an early and rapid increase in endothelial cell number and total capillary surface per glomerulus in parallel with glomerular hypertrophy; enalapril therapy partially reverses these established changes (892).

Lymphocytes, particularly CD8+ T cells, and monocyte/macrophages may be present in human glomeruli affected by FSGS (893,894). The latter may be recognized within capillary loops as lipid-laden foam cells. In the rat remnant nephron model, bone marrow suppression via X-irradiation is associated with a transient reduction in glomerular macrophage numbers and mesangial matrix scores, suggesting that macrophages might contribute to glomerular matrix expansion (895). Conversely, blockade of chemokine (C-C motif) receptor (CCR)-1 (the major receptor for macrophage inflammatory protein [MIP]-1 alpha and Regulated on Activation, Normal T cell Expressed and Secreted [RANTES]) in murine adriamycin nephropathy reduced interstitial fibrosis but had no effect on proteinuria or glomerulosclerosis (896). Therefore, the pathophysiologic role of infiltrating glomerular leukocytes in FSGS remains to be established. The potential role of infiltrating tubulointerstitial leukocytes in the progression of chronic renal disease is considered elsewhere in this text.

Cytokines and Other Mediators

Although many mediators have been implicated in glomerulosclerosis and progressive kidney disease, there is a paucity of data directly defining a role for these mediators on FSGS. Experimental data indicate that these mediators could play a role in regulating the balance between *extracellular matrix (ECM) synthesis and degradation* in the glomerulus. The most prominent of these mediators is TGF-β (897), which both directly (898) and indirectly, through induction of the cytokine CTGF (899) and generation of reactive oxygen species (900), stimulates mesangial and additional cell types to produce collagens, laminin and other ECM proteins. There are two parallel systems regulating ECM degradation (901). The balance between the matrix metalloproteinases and the tissue inhibitors of matalloproteinases (TIMPs), has been implicated in animal models of progressive kidney disease (902,903). The plasmin system enhances glomerular ECM turnover (904), and is inhibited by the plasminogen activator inhibitor, PAI-1 (905). Biologic roles for these molecules in regulating cellular functions beyond matrix turnover also have been proposed.

Cytokine mediators play a role in *proliferative changes* in the glomerulus, although the data have been limited to effects on mesangial cells. Interestingly, despite the significance of podocyte proliferation in collapsing glomerulopathy, no data are available to convincingly link a particular mediator with this proliferation. Basic fibroblast growth factor (bFGF, FGF-2) has been linked with multiple podocyte abnormalities, including proliferation, in experimental membranous nephropathy (906). Another important aspect of glomerulosclerosis is the possible loss of a continuous podocyte support structure for the glomerular capillaries. Cytokines have equally important and complex roles in podocyte *apoptosis and phenotypic changes*, as shown for TGF-β1 (907) and endothelin-1 (ET-1) (908).

Other systems play a significant part in glomerulosclerosis. An important one is the multiple potential roles of the renin-angiotensin-aldosterone system (RAAS). Spironolactone decreases fibrosis in some animal models. Aldosterone stimulates expression of TGF-β and PAI-1, and fibrotic changes mediated through the generation of reactive oxygen species (909). A role for the RAAS is supported by the strong data demonstrating that angiotensin converting enzyme inhibition and angiotensin receptor blockade ameliorate progressive glomerulosclerosis and renal fibrosis in multiple diseases. These data support a role for the RAAS in altering glomerular cell phenotypes (e.g., angiotensin II stimulates mesangial cell TGF-β production [910]), as well as in hemodynamic mechanisms that relate to glomerular perfusion and filtration. Further, it is not clear whether the RAAS stimulates glomerular hypertrophy through its effects on hemodynamics or via direct, growth factorlike effects on resident cells. Other systems regulating hemodynamics that also may have direct effects upon cellular fibrogenic activity include those representing the balance between nitric oxide and ET-1 (911), or those involving arachidonic acid metabolites (912). Leptin also has multiple effects relevant to glomerulosclerosis (913).

Recent studies demonstrated an interaction between putatively hemodynamic and sclerogenic mediators (Fig. 64-13).

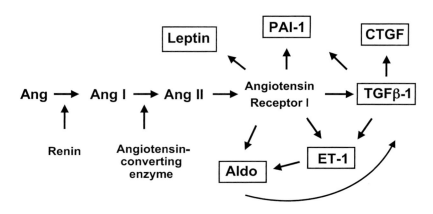

FIGURE 64-13. The renin-angiotensin system and interaction with profibrotic cytokines. In addition to the role of renin-angiotensin-aldosterone system in regulating extracellular fluid volume and potassium homeostasis, it has been become clear that this system also influences vascular remodeling and tissue fibrosis. These vascular and profibrotic effects are mediated by at least five effector molecules (*shown within boxes*), which are present in the plasma and also produced locally in tissues. *Aldo*, aldosterone; *Ang*, angiotensinogen; *ET-1*, endothelin-1; *TGF-β1*, transforming growth factor-β1; *CTGF*, connective tissue growth factor; *PAI-1*, plasminogen activator inhibitor-1.

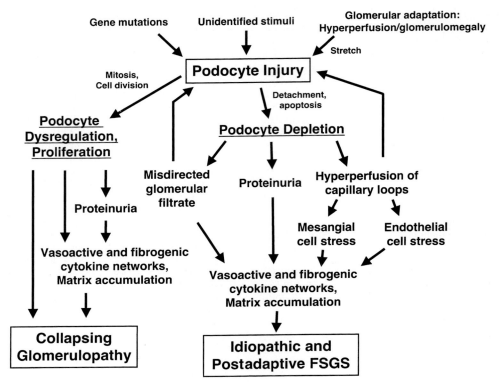

FIGURE 64-14. Proposed pathogenetic schema for FSGS and collapsing glomerulopathy. Both lesions begin with podocyte injury, resulting from a mutated gene, glomerular hyperperfusion (postadaptive) or an unidentified stimulus. Depending upon the nature of the injury, this may lead to podocyte dysregulation and proliferation, causing collapsing glomerulopathy; or relative podocyte depletion in the case of FSGS (note that podocyte depletion can be absolute, resulting from either decreased numbers of podocytes, or relative, when there are a fixed number of podocytes but a larger glomerular capillary surface area). In either FSGS or collapsing glomerulopathy, the result is a decrease in the integrity of the glomerular filtration barrier and proteinuria. Misdirected glomerular filtrate, exposure of the podocyte to excess protein, and cellular stretch/stress lead to glomerular cellular activation, changes in glomerular perfusion, and extracellular matrix accumulation. Thus, podocyte injury evolves into distinct glomerular diseases by various mechanisms, some of which are pathway-specific and others are common.

Angiotensin activation leads to the activation of the type I angiotensin receptor, which leads directly or indirectly to the production of aldosterone, ET-1, PAI-1, and TGF-β, with subsequent production of CTGF and reactive oxygen species, and extracellular matrix accumulation. This one system can thus contribute to glomerular hypertension/hyperfiltration, sodium retention, glomerular hypertrophy, podocyte dysfunction/apoptosis, and fibrosis—all of the manifestations of FSGS.

Based on the data presented in this section, a pathogenetic schema for FSGS and collapsing glomerulopathy can be proposed (Fig. 64-14). Both lesions begin with podocyte injury, resulting from a mutated gene, adaptive glomerular hyperperfusion, or an unidentified stimulus. Depending upon the nature of the injury, this may lead to podocyte dysregulation and proliferation, causing collapsing glomerulopathy, or podocyte depletion in the case of FSGS. Podocyte depletion may be absolute or relative, in the latter case when glomerulomegaly increases capillary surface area. It is noteworthy that, despite significant differences in disease etiology and course for FSGS and collapsing glomerulopathy, both manifest decreased integrity of the glomerular filtration barrier and proteinuria. Misdirected glomerular filtrate, exposure of the podocyte to excess protein, and cellular stretch/stress lead to glomerular cellular activation, changes in perfusion, and extracellular matrix accumulation. Therefore, distinct pathways may utilize similar mechanisms

that result in distinct diseases, with the critical difference being the presence or absence of podocyte proliferation.

Selected Clinical Variants of FSGS and Collapsing Glomerulopathy

Glomerular Tip Lesion: A Diagnostic Cluster

The glomerular tip lesion has been a controversial subject since its description by Howie in 1986 (914). In the intervening years, as Howie has recently pointed out, the term *glomerular tip lesion* has been used in three senses, which are given distinct names here (915,916). Estimates of the incidence of glomerular tip lesion vary enormously by definition and population: 13% of FSGS patients in Chicago (761) and 66% of patients with segmental lesions (cellular or sclerosis) in Britain (915).

First, the *glomerular tip lesion MCN variant* (term introduced here but with a definition that follows Howie's original description) is situated at the portion of the glomerular tuft located adjacent to the origin of the proximal convoluted tubule and consists of a localized collection of vacuolated podocytes and intracapillary foam cells. In some cases the podocytes rest in apposition to tubular epithelial cells. The lesion may consist partly or predominantly of sclerosis. Importantly, other glomerular lesions must be absent, including mesangial hypercellularity and sclerosis located elsewhere in the glomerulus. IgM and C3 may be present within the tip lesion. Both affected and unaffected glomeruli typically show diffuse foot-process effacement.

Second, a *glomerular tip lesion FSGS variant* has been recognized and made part of the Columbia classification. There are several differences from the preceding entity: mesangial hypercellularity may be present and peripheral scars (non-tip, non-hilar) can be present in other glomeruli. D'Agati and colleagues identified 49 cases (0.46% of their biopsy archive). There were 45 adults and 2 children. Cellular lesions (81% average per biopsy) were more typical than scarring lesions (19%). Twelve cases had glomerular tip lesion only, 18 had peripheral lesions, and 17 had associated indeterminate lesions (i.e., in some glomeruli the tip and the hilum could not be identified.) Focal mild mesangial hypercellularity was present in 45%; no cases exhibited diffuse mesangial hyperplasia. At presentation, the clinical features of glomerular tip lesion were more like those of MCN than other idiopathic FSGS: Caucasian race 77% and 59% versus 52% ($p =$ NS), mean age 48 and 48 versus 33 ($p < 0.001$ overall) and nephrotic syndrome in 89% and 97% versus 54% ($p < 0.001$ overall). Among those with the glomerular tip lesion, 59% of patients entered CR with steroids, in some cases supplemented with other therapies, and 14% of patients entered PR. Therefore, the response to therapy is much better than classic FSGS and worse than MCN. Patients with glomerular tip lesion alone versus those with peripheral and/or indeterminate lesions had similar likelihood of CR versus PR versus nonresponse ($p = 0.88$), but this may be due to small numbers in this two-by-three group analysis. Importantly, those with other glomerular lesions had higher initial serum creatinine and higher likelihood of nonresponse ($p < 0.02$). The authors conclude that the glomerular tip lesion occupies an intermediate location along the MCN/FSGS spectrum and that the presence of sclerosis in a non-tip location confers a worse prognosis. These data can be interpreted to argue for distinguishing between a glomerular tip lesion MCN variant (lacking non-tip sclerosis) and a glomerular tip lesion FSGS variant (allowing peripheral and indeterminant scars but not perihilar scars), as these forms appear to have distinct outcomes.

Another study of the outcome of glomerular tip lesion published by Howie and colleagues came to generally similar conclusions (915). Two biopsy series of adult nephrotic syndrome comprised 108 patients, with biopsies showing segmental lesions and lacking a non-FSGS diagnosis (e.g., classic MCN, collapsing glomerulopathy, or other glomerular disease). Segmental cellular or scarring lesions at first or only biopsy were divided into two categories: tip lesions (confined to the tubular pole) and multiple lesions (at least one non-tip lesion, a lesion extending from the tubular pole to the hilum, and lesions at various sites). After 10 years, renal survival was 84% in those with tip lesions and 45% in those with multiple lesions ($p < 0.001$ by Cox proportional hazards analysis). The statistical significance of the beneficial effect of tip lesion was lost in multivariable analysis, when other variables (number of segmental lesions, extent of global sclerosis, and chronic tubular damage) were included in the model. No other factor showed an independent association with outcome; instead, all these variables showed correlation with each other. Therefore, the presence of a tip lesion conferred a favorable diagnosis when it was narrowly defined (no other segmental lesions). Forty patients underwent repeat biopsies, generally for declining renal function, but also in some cases when proteinuria recurred in an allograft. Tip lesions were frequently (perhaps always, given the uncertainty of localizing all lesions) the initial segmental lesions. With progressive loss of renal function, lesions at other glomerular locations appeared. These data are important, as

they suggest that in some cases tip lesion can evolve into classic FSGS. Like the preceding paper, these data can be read as supporting a glomerular tip lesion MCN variant and glomerular tip FSGS variant, although it is unclear whether the two can be reliably distinguished at initial biopsy.

These findings support a third category, various nondiagnostic *glomerular tip changes* (Howie's suggested term), which have been described in other proteinuric conditions, including membranous nephropathy (present in 64% of cases) (917), IgM variant of MCN (918), postinfectious glomerulonephritis (919), and diabetic nephropathy (920). Experimentally, glomerular tip lesions develop in rats with crescentic glomerulonephritis; Howie showed that the initial change involves prolapse of injured podocytes into the tubule, followed by localization of macrophages to the adjacent capillary tuft and adhesion of the tuft to Bowman's capsule (921). The predisposition to injury of the podocytes at the glomerular tip remains unexplained. Haas has argued that the tip lesion is a response to prolonged heavy proteinuria and does represent a specific disease entity. In autopsy cases of severe, untreated MCN from patients who died before 1950, Haas and colleagues identified tip lesions in 5 of 8 cases (922). Among those with tip lesion, the average number of affected glomeruli was 1.8% (range 0.3% to 4.4%); there was no predilection for juxtamedullary glomeruli (unlike FSGS lesions). Thus there is a consensus that proteinuric states are commonly associated with tip changes.

In conclusion, a consensus probably exists that there is a glomerular tip lesion MCN variant and a glomerular tip lesion FSGS variant, with the former having a distinctly better prognosis but both exhibiting some degree of steroid-sensitivity. Some glomerular tip MCN variants progress over time to glomerular tip FSGS variants or classic FSGS. Important questions, however, remain to be resolved. Is it clinically useful to identify a glomerular tip lesion MCN variant rather than identify this morphology as a consequence of heavy proteinuria; in other words, is the prognosis affected, independent of the degree of proteinuria? This question remains open, as there is no published case series that compares the outcome of typical MCN patients with the glomerular tip lesion to MCN patients lacking this feature. Can we distinguish glomerular tip FSGS variants that will progress to classic FSGS? Finally, what molecular diagnostic markers might help us to differentiate between forms of tip lesion, to improve our understanding, classification, and prognostication of these disorders?

FSGS, Cellular Variant

As noted in the preceding text, the cellular variant of FSGS was first described by Schwartz and colleagues to include segmental or global endocapillary proliferation, hypercellularity in Bowman's space, or podocytes manifesting a reactive phenotype. Clinically, these patients were more likely than were those with only segmental scars (90% versus 49%) to have nephrotic range proteinuria. Compared to patients with classic FSGS, patients with cellular lesion FSGS were more likely to be black (70% versus 49%), to have a higher likelihood of proteinuria >10 g per/day (44% versus 11%), and to have a higher likelihood of progression to ESRD (40% versus 18%) (761,923). Steroid sensitivity (remission defined as CR or PR) was similar in cellular FSGS and classic FSGS (53% versus 52%). The fraction of glomeruli involved was an important predictor: >20% glomerular involvement involved defined a group that was almost exclusively black (94%), had heavier proteinuria (67% with >10 g per/day), and were less responsive to treatment (23% remission), compared to those with a lesser degree of glomerular involvement.

It appears that most or all of these patients would be classified as collapsing glomerulopathy (collapsing FSGS in the

Columbia classification). There are as yet no published data on the clinical characteristics or outcomes of patients with the cellular lesion as defined in the Columbia classification.

Postadaptive FSGS

As detailed earlier in this chapter, data as disparate as the remnant kidney model of glomerulosclerosis and epidemiologic evidence for a relationship among low nephron number, hypertension, and progressive renal scarring support the notion that increased workload per nephron can lead to glomerulosclerosis. Some clinical criteria have been developed for identifying postadaptive FSGS (Table 64-17). Here, we consider two clinical circumstances in which this can occur: reduction of nephron number or increased workload with a fixed number of nephrons.

Postadaptive FSGS with Reduced Nephron Mass. There are characteristic features of FSGS associated with reduced nephron mass. First, glomerular enlargement is common in this setting. Bhathena studied patients with FSGS appearing more than 2 years after renal transplantation, in association with chronic allograft nephropathy and interstitial nephritis (925). These patients had larger glomeruli compared to those without FSGS or those with recurrent FSGS, diagnosed within 2 years of transplantation. Subsequently Bhathena showed that glomeruli are larger in unilateral renal agenesis and following uninephrectomy when FSGS is present compared to patients with the same disorders when FSGS is lacking (926). Second, the segmental scars are preferentially located adjacent to the vascular hilum. In the rat nephrectomy model, the sclerosis preferentially affects the vascular pole (927). When colloidal carbon is injected immediately after nephrectomy, it is found preferentially within perihilar sclerotic lesions 4 months later (928). These findings suggest that some feature of this glomerular zone, possibly related to hemodynamic stress, leads to increased uptake (presumably by mesangial cells) long before the appearance of sclerotic lesions. Third, podocyte effacement is modest, typically involving <50% of the interface between podocyte and GBM, as discussed previously. There is considerable variability, however, so that this characteristic may be of limited value in clinical diagnosis. Fourth, hypoalbuminemia and edema are uncommon despite nephrotic range proteinuria (924).

Postadaptive FSGS Associated with Obesity. Obesity is associated with increased renal blood flow, glomerular filtration rate, and microalbuminuria, features that it shares with diabetes mellitus. The mechanisms for these renal abnormalities are not well understood (recently reviewed [929]). Contributing factors may include increased renal venous pressure, hyperlipidemia, and increased production of vasoactive and fibrogenic substances by adipocytes, including angiotensin II, insulin, leptin, and TGF-β1. Dogs fed a high-fat diet to produce a 60% increase in body weight manifested an increased blood pressure, plasma renin activity, and GFR, together with increased mesangial matrix and TGF-β expression (glomerular size was unchanged) (930). Obese, pre-diabetic monkeys manifest hyperinsulinemia and glomerulomegaly, suggesting that some feature of the insulin-resistant state may contribute to glomerular hypertrophy (931). Leptin is of particular interest, as it acts on cultured glomerular endothelial cells to stimulate proliferation and production of TGF-β1 and collagen I, and it stimulates expression of TGF-β type II receptor and collagen I by mesangial cells (913). Furthermore, leptin also stimulates production of angiotensin II. Therefore, leptin may initiate a pro-fibrogenic circuit within the glomerulus.

D'Agati and colleagues reviewed their experience with obesity-related glomerular disease, including 14 patients with glomerulomegaly alone and 57 patients with glomerulomegaly plus FSGS (764). The combined prevalence of these disorders

---

TABLE 64-17

CLINICAL RECOGNITION OF POSTADAPTIVE FOCAL SEGMENTAL GLOMERULOSCLEROSIS (FSGS)

Feature	Utility	Limitations
High-risk clinical setting: (a) Reduced nephron mass: renal dysplasia, ureteral reflux (b) Initially normal renal mass: sickle cell anemia, cyanotic congenital heart disease	++	The life-time incidence of postadaptive FSGS in these uncommon or rare conditions is probably relatively high, although precise incidence values are not available
Moderate-or low-risk clinical setting: obesity, hypertension	+	These are common clinical conditions, where the lifetime incidence of postadaptive FSGS is probably low; idiopathic FSGS may also occur in these individuals
Nephrotic proteinuria without edema or hypoalbuminemia	+	This pattern is more common in postadaptive FSGS but also occurs in idiopathic FSGS (924)
Perihilar FSGS variant: At least one glomerular showing perihilar hyalinosis and perihilar hyalinosis and/or sclerosis involving >50% glomeruli	++	Sensitivity and specificity remain to be determined
Glomerulomegaly (average glomerular diameter >185 μm)	+++	Requires a sufficient number of glomeruli (probably 5–10), multiple levels (possibly 4), and measurement of glomeruli cut at or near hilus (764)
Podocyte foot-process effacement	+	There are significant group differences between idiopathic FSGS and postadaptive FSGS, but there is considerable overlap between the groups, so this has limited utility in a particular case (764)

When confronted with a renal biopsy that shows FSGS, no history suggesting a genetic cause of FSGS (onset in childhood, family history of FSGS, extrarenal manifestations) and no use of FSGS-associated medication, the pathologist and clinician must weigh the likelihood of idiopathic FSGS versus postadaptive FSGS. Multiple features must be considered in making this distinction.

rose from 0.2% of all renal biopsies during the period from 1986 to 1990 to 2% during the period from 1996 to 2000; 53% had BMI >40 kg/m² (morbid obesity) and 47% had BMI 30 to 40 kg/m². Therefore morbid obesity is not required for the diagnosis. Compared to patients with idiopathic FSGS, patients with obesity-associated glomerulopathy had lower levels of proteinuria (nephrotic-range proteinuria in 48% compared to 66%), less foot-process effacement, and a more indolent course (progression to ESRD 4% versus 42%). By contrast, Praga et al. found that the outcome in obesity-related disease was almost as poor as that of idiopathic FSGS (845). Over an 82-month observation period, 8 of 15 patients maintained stable renal function and 7 of 15 patients demonstrated progressive loss of GFR, with five reaching ESRD. Proteinuria was in the nephrotic range at presentation or on follow-up in 80% of patients. The level of proteinuria correlated with BMI (R = 0.45, p <0.05). Despite heavy proteinuria, >10 g per day in three patients, edema and hypoalbuminemia were uniformly absent. With the epidemic of obesity spreading to adolescents in the United States, particularly in minority populations, obesity-associated FSGS is appearing in that age range also (932).

Recently, glomerular hypertrophy and FSGS also have been reported in patients with increased BMI associated with increased muscle mass but without increased body fat, suggesting that adiposity is not required (933). Important questions remain. We do not know whether glomerulomegaly is a precursor lesion to FSGS, although that appears likely; we do not know whether there is a threshold BMI for the appearance of glomerulomegaly and FSGS; and we do not understand the molecular signals by which increased fat mass or BMI lead to glomerular hyperfiltration.

Hypertension and FSGS

Hypertension is the attributed cause of approximately 15% of incident ESRD cases in Europe and approximately 30% of incident ESRD cases in the United States (discussed in depth in Chapter 51). Few of these patients, however, undergo renal biopsy and there remains doubt about the nature of the role of hypertension in initiating renal injury. It is undisputed that malignant hypertension can lead to ESRD; it is more controversial whether benign nephrosclerosis leads to ESRD. This controversy has been the subject of several thoughtful reviews in recent years (934–936). Hypertensive nephrosclerosis (benign nephrosclerosis) is defined by the presence of arteriolar changes consisting of hyaline arteriosclerosis and myointimal hypertrophy that particularly affect the afferent arteriole and small arterioles lacking an internal elastic lamina. The initial glomerular morphologic changes include thickening and wrinkling of the GBM, following by contraction of the capillary tuft toward the vascular pole. As the tuft contracts, fibrotic material accumulates within Bowman's space. The glomerulus ultimately shrinks to a hyalinized mass at the vascular pole. In contrast to FSGS, glomerular tufts showing global glomerulosclerosis in hypertensive nephrosclerosis are not enlarged, but rather are shrunken (937).

In recent biopsy series a substantial fraction of patients with a diagnosis of hypertensive nephrosclerosis manifested segmentally sclerosed glomeruli. In a study from Brazil of 90 hypertensive patients with renal insufficiency and subnephrotic proteinuria, 19% were found to have segmental sclerosis, most of whom also had vascular features of hypertensive injury (938). In a study from Japan, 33% of patients with hypertensive nephrosclerosis had segmental sclerotic lesions; these patients had significantly higher serum creatinine values (939). Patients who experienced progressive loss of renal function during follow-up had larger glomeruli, but the authors did not state whether those with segmental sclerosis had larger glomeruli. In a study from Tennessee, Fogo and colleagues found segmental

sclerosis in 34% of patients with hypertensive nephrosclerosis (940). The authors excluded idiopathic FSGS on the following grounds: lack of nephrotic range proteinuria, lack of extensive foot-process effacement, and glomerulosclerosis in proportion to vascular lesions. Segmental sclerosis was associated with global sclerosis and was more common in blacks than in whites. Importantly, the authors found that the extent of vascular injury did not correlate with the extent of global and segmental glomerulosclerosis, and statistical modeling failed to identify a link between blood pressure and the severity of the glomerular lesions. The authors concluded that a simple causal pathway, whereby hypertension causes vascular sclerosis which in turn causes glomerulosclerosis, is not supported by their data.

Kincaid-Smith noted that the original description of hypertensive nephrosclerosis, made 50 years ago, did not include segmental sclerosis. She makes the provocative proposal that many cases that are clinically diagnosed as hypertensive nephrosclerosis without renal biopsy, or pathologically diagnosed as hypertension-associated FSGS, may in fact be postadaptive FSGS due to obesity and associated conditions, including insulin resistance associated with the metabolic syndrome and hyperuricemia (936). This hypothesis is testable, with closer attention to clinical factors (obesity, proteinuria, uric acid levels, and levels of insulin and other endocrine factors) and pathologic variables (glomerular size, podocyte number, and extent of foot-process effacement) in patients with FSGS arising in the setting of hypertension. In conclusion, it remains uncertain whether hypertension causes a form of postadaptive FSGS, or whether hypertensive vascular changes coexist with segmental sclerosis lesions, which arise as a consequence of obesity and other clinical factors associated with hypertension.

C1q Nephropathy

C1q nephropathy was first described by Jennette and Hipp at Chapel Hill as the presence of mesangial C1q staining, either dominant or co-dominant with IgG, IgM, and/or C3 and the lack of serologic or clinical findings of lupus (462). The immune deposits were predominantly mesangial, although occasionally the deposits extended into glomerular capillary loops. In this series of 15 patients (2% of renal biopsies, age range 14–27 years), the glomerular histology ranged from normal to mesangial proliferation to focal or diffuse proliferative glomerulonephritis.

Two subsequent series have suggested that the disease probably fits best in the MCN/FSGS/collapsing glomerulopathy spectrum. Iskandar et al. at Winston-Salem reported on 15 children with prominent mesangial C1q staining and histology consistent with MCN (8 cases) and FSGS (7 cases) (941). Markowitz et al. in New York described 19 patients (9 children, 10 adults), representing 0.2% of all renal biopsies (458). Histologies ran the gamut of podocyte diseases, including MCN (2 patients), FSGS (2 patients with the cellular variant, 9 patients with the NOS variant), and collapsing glomerulopathy (6 patients). Mesangial hypercellularity was seen in one MCN case and 10 of the other cases.

In the series from Chapel Hill, North Carolina; Winston-Salem, North Carolina; and New York, blacks were generally over-represented (60%, 27%, and 74%, respectively) compared to their presence in the local populations. Nephrotic-range proteinuria was common (71%, 80%, and 79%, respectively), although many patients (particularly adults) did not have nephrotic syndrome. Response to therapy is variable but has improved in the most recent series, with CR or PR seen in 0% (0/9 patients treated) at Chapel Hill, 44% (4/9 patients treated) at Winston-Salem, and 57% in New York (7/13 with available data; 2 additional patients progressed to ESRD during follow-up), respectively. In the New York series, CR or PR occurred in 2/2 patients with MCN, 4/11 with FSGS, and

1/6 with collapsing glomerulopathy, mirroring the steroid responses typical of other forms of these diseases. Other reports have also suggested that some patients with C1q nephropathy remit spontaneously or with therapy, but some of these patients had atypical features, such as prominent subendothelial or subepithelial deposits (457,942).

C1q and other members of the newly recognized C1q/TNF superfamily share a structurally similar globular domain (943). C1q, a portion of the tripartite C1 molecule, functions as major link between innate and acquired immunity, as it binds a range of ligands via the globular domain and promotes apoptosis and phagocytosis of cells and cellular debris (944–946). Human genetic C1q deficiency is associated with lupus, presumably by impairing apoptotic cell clearance and thereby exposing the immune system to nuclear and cytoplasmic antigens. Interestingly, the classical swine fever virus may provide an animal model of C1q nephropathy. Pigs experimentally infected with classical swine fever virus develop immune complex glomerulonephritis characterized by viral infection of glomerular endothelial cells and podocytes, macrophage infiltration, and deposition of IgG, IgM, and C1q in mesangial, subendothelial, and subepithelial locations (947).

Therefore, by histology and clinical course, C1q nephropathy would appear to fit into the spectrum of MCN/FSGS/collapsing glomerulopathy, as D'Agati and colleagues have proposed (458). The pathogenesis remains poorly understood, and specifically it is unclear how to link C1q mesangial deposits with podocyte injury.

Idiopathic Collapsing Glomerulopathy

HIV-associated nephropathy was the first recognized form of collapsing glomerulopathy, and this topic is covered in Chapter 59. Idiopathic collapsing glomerulopathy was first described in Ohio (948), with subsequent reports from elsewhere within the United States and Europe (732,949–952). A retrospective review of the renal biopsy archive at Columbia University found the first case to have been seen in 1979, with a rapid increase to causing approximately 25% of idiopathic FSGS by the early 1990s (949). This epidemiologic pattern strongly suggests a new environmental agent, possibly a virus or toxin, although little progress has been reported in identifying what that agent might be. De novo collapsing glomerulopathy also has been described following renal transplantation (953,954). Recent reviews are available (955,956).

Idiopathic collapsing glomerulopathy presents clinically as the sudden onset of heavy proteinuria, although some patients have subnephrotic proteinuria. Progression to ESRD may be rapid but this in not invariably the case. Some patients report a viral-like prodrome occurring prior to presentation, with symptoms that may include fever, cough, and diarrhea.

Collapsing glomerulopathy occurs in several distinct clinical settings. It has been associated with systemic diseases, particularly adult Still's disease (957,958). Parvovirus B19 infection has the been linked with collapsing glomerulopathy (959), although controversy remains about the strength and specificity of the association (960). Most recently SV40 infection has been linked to both collapsing glomerulopathy and other forms of FSGS; these data await replication (961).

The mechanism of podocyte proliferation remains largely unexplained. Hattori et al. studied patients with cellular lesion, although it is likely that many or all of these had collapsing glomerulopathy (962). They noted that glomerular expression of smooth muscle α-actin (a marker for activated mesangial cells, exhibiting a myofibroblastic phenotype) was much greater in cellular FSGS compared to those with classic FSGS. Expression of collagen III was similar. Therefore, intense mesangial activation is part of the process and may account for the propensity to rapid progression.

Medication-associated FSGS and Collapsing Glomerulopathy

A number of medications have been associated with FSGS and collapsing glomerulopathy, as shown in Table 64-3. Cyclosporine is associated with FSGS in renal transplant patients and nonrenal organ transplant patients. In renal transplant recipients, cyclosporine contributes to the pathogenesis of chronic allograft nephropathy, but the role of other factors makes the specific role of these agents difficult to determine. The appearance of FSGS in nonrenal organ transplant recipients and its link to cyclosporine (963–965) makes the relationship more compelling. Tacrolimus likely has a very similar risk but fewer data are available. Cyclosporine induces FSGS following chronic administration to rats (966). The mechanism of glomerular toxicity may include increased matrix synthesis by glomerular cells (966) and glomerular ischemia. The 5-year risk for chronic renal failure in nonrenal organ transplantation ranges from 7% to 21% (967). The use of a calcineurin inhibitor was significantly associated with increased risk, but the degree of relative risk was modest (1.25), probably due to the study design (only use on initial hospitalization was available) and the fact that 98% of patients used these agents.

Lithium has been associated with FSGS (968–970). Chronic exposure to lithium causes tubulointerstitial injury in rats (971), which would be evidence in favor of a postadaptive mechanism. Conversely, some patients have extensive foot-process effacement (969), and nephrotic syndrome may resolve with cessation of therapy (972). These findings suggest the alternate possibility of a direct toxicity to glomerular cells.

Interferon-α has been associated with both FSGS (973–978) and collapsing glomerulopathy (979). Pamidronate has been associated with collapsing glomerulopathy (956,980). Very little is known about mechanism of renal injury with these medications.

Medications associated with idiopathic collapsing glomerulopathy include pamidronate (981) and interferon-α (979). The mechanism is unknown.

Nephrotic Syndrome in the First Year of Life

Nephrotic syndrome may occur in the first year of life and can result from MCN. Much more often, however, it is due to congenital nephrotic syndrome, especially that associated with infantile microcystic disease (982–984). This lesion is most commonly found in Finland and in people of Finnish ancestry, but it has been documented as well in many other ethnic groups throughout Europe and North America. The disease is inherited as an autosomal-recessive trait. Affected infants typically have a large placenta (983), with the placental–fetal weight ratio ranging from 0.25 to 0.43, compared to a normal ratio of 0.14. They often are born prematurely, may show signs of perinatal asphyxia, and have a high perinatal mortality rate. Indeed, the incidence of early death from congenital nephrotic syndrome may be higher than that reported, as edema and failure to thrive may not become apparent for several weeks or months, even though proteinuria is present from birth. The natural course in infancy is usually one of progressive deterioration, with hypoalbuminemia, edema, and wasting dominating the clinical picture and being more significant than decreasing renal function. In the past, half of the patients died before the age of 6 months and few survived past 2 years. However, aggressive management has dramatically improved the outlook (336).

The majority of patients with this disease have abnormal expression of the gene for nephrin, a putative cell–cell adhesion molecule that is expressed only by the glomerular podocytes (985). The gene is located on chromosome 19q13.1 (986). Histologic changes of congenital nephrotic syndrome can be subtle in the newborn. They may include dilated cortical tubules (the origin of the term *microcystic*), mesangial hypercellularity, and glomerulosclerosis, none of which are pathognomonic for congenital nephrotic syndrome of the Finnish type. A significant reduction in the number of negative-charge sites in the GBM has been reported (56). Prenatal diagnosis has been obtained by finding increased α-fetoprotein levels in the amniotic fluid. However, levels may be high in amniotic fluid from pregnancies with heterozygous (carrier) phenotype (987). Studies of patients and their families suggest that direct analysis of the fetal nephrin gene can be used for prenatal diagnosis in many patients (988).

Other idiopathic types of congenital nephrotic syndrome have been described. These are less well defined and probably represent a heterogeneous group of diseases, most of which do not appear to be inherited (985). They are distinguished from the Finnish type by the combination of clinical characteristics and histologic picture. Most have a poor prognosis, but the clinical course is often more protracted. Attempts have been made to classify these lesions according to the dominant pathologic findings. According to this approach, the presence of microcystic disease has been used to diagnose the Finnish type of congenital nephrotic syndrome. In the absence of microcystic tubules, the disease has been classified on the basis of the most prominent glomerular lesion, for example, mesangial proliferation, DMS, FSGS, or global glomerular sclerosis. Without such changes, the patient is diagnosed as having MCNS. A study that summarized the problems of this classification system emphasized that microcystic tubules are neither specific nor diagnostic for the Finnish lesion and may be acquired as a consequence of severe proteinuria in the immature kidney (989).

In many cases DMS is the dominant pathologic picture. Prognosis is poor, irrespective of whether the onset of disease is congenital or infantile. Congenital glomerulosclerosis characterized by hyalinized glomeruli in otherwise normal kidneys also has been found in infants developing nephrotic syndrome and renal failure early in life. Although such lesions could be the consequence of intrauterine infections (990), the development of DMS more frequently reflects a genetically determined metabolic or structural abnormality. It is found in a variety of syndromes associated with the gene for the WT-1 transcription factor (see discussion of *WT1* and Denys-Drash and Frasier syndromes in the next section). Other entities that have been associated with the nephrotic syndrome in the first year of life (246,465,989,991–999) are summarized in Table 64-18.

Age at presentation is an important factor in outcome. In one study, 97% of 177 patients died or subsequently required care for ESRD if they presented with nephrotic syndrome in the first 3 months of life (1000). In contrast, death or end-stage disease occurred in only 31% of patients with onset of nephrotic syndrome between the ages of 3 and 12 months. In an effort to identify children with the most severe, progressive disease, the ratio of urinary heparan sulfate to chondroitin sulfate was measured in 37 patients and 17 healthy controls. Patients with Finnish-type disease, DMS, and focal sclerosis had elevated ratios, whereas children with MCNS had results similar to those of normal subjects (1001).

However, it is advisable to determine the nature of the lesion by tissue diagnosis as early as possible after the initial presentation, since early intervention is optimal. Congenital nephrotic syndrome is associated with profound malnutrition, dehydration, hypercoagulability, and hypothyroidism. All of these problems are amenable to medical therapy. Patients may be stabilized with daily or even more frequent albumin infusions, enteral hyperalimentation, anticoagulants, and thyroid replacement. In some cases, uninephrectomy or even bilateral nephrectomy is required to overcome the effects of severe protein loss. It is our practice to begin with albumin infusions and

TABLE 64-18

CAUSES OF THE NEPHROTIC SYNDROME IN THE FIRST YEAR OF LIFE

Relatively common
  Congenital nephrotic syndrome of the Finnish (inherited) type
  Other congenital nephrotic syndromes
Less common
  Diffuse mesangial sclerosis
  Focal segmental glomerulosclerosis, congenital glomerulosclerosis, and hyalinosis
  Minimal change nephrotic syndrome (MCNS)
  Acquired immunodeficiency syndrome
Rare
  Cytomegalic inclusion disease (277)
  Hemolytic–uremic syndrome (278)
  Mercury intoxication (279)
  Nail–patella syndrome (280)
  Pseudohermaphroditism (281,282)
  Renal vein thrombosis (283)
  Syphilis (284,285)
  Toxoplasmosis (286)
  Wilms tumor (50,287)
  XY Gonadal dysgenesis (287)

progress to uninephrectomy in the hope that the child will be permitted to grow for as much as a year before entering into ESRD care.

Kidney transplantation for children with congenital nephrotic syndrome usually is effective with the nephrotic syndrome rarely recurring in the recipient. The major exception is the child with Finnish-type congenital nephrotic syndrome. Because such children are born without full-length nephrin, they may recognize intact nephrin in the transplanted kidney as foreign, developing anti-nephrin antibodies. This problem is treated most effectively with a combination of plasmapheresis and alkylating agents (987).

Genetics of FSGS and Collapsing Glomerulopathy

A major advance in the last decade has been the recognition of loci responsible for FSGS with Mendelian inheritance (Table 64-19). Molecular diagnosis of mutations, particularly podocin (*NPHS2*) and *WT1*, has now become an important part of the evaluation of pediatric FSGS. Genotyping for *NPHS1* and *NPHS2* is commercially available and is rapidly becoming a routine part of clinical practice.

As shown in Tables 64-3 and 64-19, the age at presentation and renal histology help identify the most likely genetic causes:

- Congenital nephrotic syndrome: *NPHS1* homozygous mutations or *NPHS1* + *NPHS2* compound heterozygous mutations
- DMS, congenital presentation: *LAMB2*
- DMS, congenital presentation: *WT1*
- FSGS, congenital presentation: *ITGB4*
- FSGS, infancy/childhood presentation: *NPHS2*, *NPHS1* + *NPHS2*, *WT1*, *PAX2*, mtDNA, COQ2
- FSGS, adult presentation: *ACTN4*, *CD2AP*, *TRPC6*, mtDNA

Collapsing glomerulopathy rarely presents with familial inheritance (1002–1004). A single genetic syndrome has been reported, action-myoclonus-renal failure syndrome, in which

TABLE 64-19

GENETIC CAUSES OF HUMAN PODOCYTE DISEASES

Gene	Gene product	Function	Inheritance (chromosome)	Renal syndrome	Prevalence	Extrarenal findings
NPHS1	Nephrin	Slit diaphragm complex	AR 19q13.1	Congenital nephrotic syndrome; infantile onset FSGS	Insufficient data	None
NPHS2	Podocin	Slit diaphragm complex	AR 1q25-31	FSGS onset <20 year	Up to 20% of familial or sporadic pediatric FSGS	None
CD2AP	CD2 associated protein	Slit diaphragm complex	AD 6	FSGS onset >20 year	Two reported cases, one with family history	None
ACTN4	α-Actinin-4	Cytoskeleton	AD 19q13	FSGS onset >20 year	Five reported families	None
TRPC6	Transient receptor, cationic, 6	Channel	AD 11q21-q22		Six reported families	None
WT1	Wilms tumor–1	Transcription factor	AD 11p13	DMS or less commonly FSGS (Denys-Drash syndrome); FSGS (Frasier syndrome)	Uncommon	Wilms tumor, gonadal abnormalities
ITGB4	β-1 integrin	Matrix protein receptor	AR 17q11-qter	Congenital FSGS	Uncommon	Epidermolysis bullosa, pyloric atresia
LAMB2	Laminin β2	Basement membrane component	AR 3p21	Congenital mesangial sclerosis	Five reported cases	Ophthalmic defects (Pierson syndrome)
PAX2	Pax2 homeobox protein	Transcription factor	AR 10q24.3-25.1	Renal dysplasia, oligomeganephronia		Ophthalmic defects (coloboma)
mtDNA	Mitochondrial tRNA	Protein synthesis	Maternal	FSGS	>40 Reported cases	MELAS syndrome, diabetes mellitus, cardiomyopathy
COQ2	COQ2 Synthetase	Enzyme	AR 11	FSGS, infantile or early childhood		Myopathy, central nervous system disorders
Galloway-Mowat syndrome	Unknown	Unknown	AR	DMS or FSGS, congenital, infancy, or early childhood		Microcephaly, hypotonia
Action myoclonus–renal failure syndrome	Unknown	Unknown	AR	Collapsing glomerulopathy, onset 9–30 years	Nine families	Myoclonus, seizures

AD, autosomal dominant; *AR*, autosomal recessive; *DMS*, diffuse mesangial sclerosis; *MELAS* syndrome, myopathy, encephalopathy, lactic acidosis, stroke.

renal failure occurred in 12 patients from 8 families of diverse European ethnic background; the gene responsible has not been identified (1005).

NPHS2

In 2000, Antignac and colleagues identified *NPHS2*, encoding podocin, by positional cloning in the evaluation of 14 of 16 families with autosomal recessive steroid-resistant nephrotic syndrome (1006). Subsequently, NPHS2 mutations have been identified in steroid-resistant nephrotic syndrome and FSGS from patients from a wide variety of racial and ethnic backgrounds (1007–1021). Homozygous or compound heterozygous mutations have been found in 35% of familial autosomal recessive FSGS and 8% of sporadic FSGS (1022,1023). To date, all patients have presented by age 25 and most patients present before age 10.

NPHS2 is a highly polymorphic gene. In Figure 64-15 is shown the location of 58 *NPHS2* sequence variants within the exon structure, including mutations (defined as variants associated with renal disease either in homozygosity or in compound heterozygosity, which involves two distinct *NPHS2* mutations on different alleles) and sequence variants (nucleotide variants, which are present in healthy individuals and do not meet the criteria for mutations). Podocin is a transmembrane protein, restricted to the podocyte that contributes to the maintenance of a normal slit diaphragm. Podocin is located within lipid rafts and interacts with other molecules that constitute the slit diaphragm complex, including nephrin and CD2AP (1024,1025). Further, podocin facilitates the signaling of nephrin and CD2AP via phosphatidylinositol and AKT (1026,1027). *NPHS2* mutants are either retained within the endoplasmic reticulum or delivered to the plasma membrane but fail to associate with lipid rafts (1028). *NPHS2* mutants that are retained within the endoplasmic reticulum are associated with earlier onset of FSGS compared to those that are targeted to the plasma membrane (1029).

In patients with *NPHS2* mutations, FSGS can recur following renal transplantation, but the risk appears to be lower than in patients with idiopathic FSGS. Hildebrandt reported recurrence in 7 of 20 (35%) patients without *NPHS2* mutations and 2 of 24 (8%) patients with *NPHS2* mutations (1021). In an update of an earlier publication that reported a surprisingly high rate of recurrence (1030), Ghiggeri and colleagues reported that 5 of 65 (8%) of subjects with homozygous or compound heterozygous mutations had recurrence (1022).

The *NPHS2 R229Q* variant is a common polymorphism, occurring in approximately 7% of European-derived populations and approximately 3% of African-derived populations (1014,1031). The pathologic significance of this variant remains unclear. FSGS has been associated with homozygous *R229Q* mutation in only one individual (1021); if this common polymorphism were sufficient to induce FSGS, one would expect more cases to have been identified. Tsukaguchi et al. (1014) found that 11 of 91 African Americans with idiopathic FSGS were R229Q heterozygotes, of whom two were compound heterozygotes with A248V. The prevalence of simple R229Q heterozygous was not statistically different from the control population. Conversely, two infants with congenital FSGS were found to have tri-allelic mutations (compound *NPHS1* heterozygotes with the *NPHS2* R229Q mutation), suggesting that the R229Q variant may modify the typical *NPHS1* presentation (1013). This finding of gene interaction between *NPHS1* and *NPHS2* has recently been challenged (1032). Finally, the R229Q variant may be associated with microalbuminuria in the Brazilian population (relative risk 2.8-fold, *p* <0.01) (1031). Therefore, it may be that the R229Q variant acts in concert with other genetic and environmental factors to compromise glomerular function but the hypothesis will require further testing.

WT1

Mutations in *WT1*, the gene encoding the Wilms tumor suppressor gene 1, cause four syndromes: WAGR (Wilms tumor, aniridia, genitourinary malformations, retardation), Beckwith-Wiedemann syndrome, Denys-Drash syndrome, and Frasier syndrome (1033). The rates of Wilms tumor among these syndromes are widely divergent, ranging from <5% in Beckwith-Wiedemann syndrome to >90% in Denys-Drash syndrome. Patients have a single mutant *WT1* allele; in XX female patients with heterozygous *WT1* mutations, Wilms tumors frequently have mutations in both alleles, suggesting that loss of heterozygosity has occurred. The WT1 protein is a transcriptional regulator of genes important in renal development, including amphiregulin (1034) and *PAX2*, and genes important

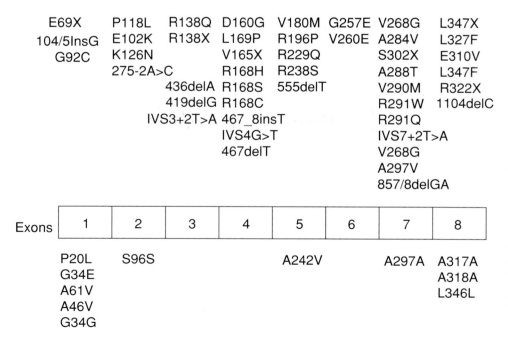

FIGURE 64-15. *NPHS2* (podocin) gene structure and variants. The eight exons of podocin are shown schematically, without portraying relative size. Mutations within the coding region (defined as variants which are associated with FSGS, when present in homozygosity or compound heterozygosity) are shown above the structure. Variants not associated with FSGS are shown below. Missense mutations are shown by the change in amino acid at the given position, with X denoting a premature stop codon. Insertions, deletions and splice site variants are also shown.

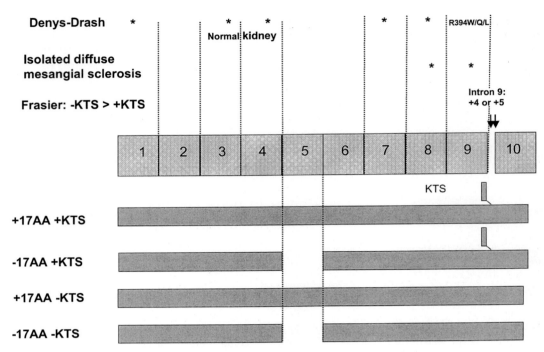

FIGURE 64-16. *WT1* gene structure, mRNA structure, and mutations associated with kidney disease. The *WT1* gene contains 10 exons (*shaded boxes*). At least 24 distinct mRNAs are generated, of which 4 predominate (*bottom*): these either do or do not contain the 17 amino acids encoded by exon 5, based on alternate splicing, and do or do not contain the three amino acids lysine-threonine-serine (KTS), based on the use of alternate splice acceptor sites located within intron 9. mRNAs lacking KTS generate more potent transcriptional activators. The Denys-Drash syndrome is associated with mutations in exons 3 and 4 (associated with normal kidneys) and in exons 7, 8, and 9 (especially the hotspot *R394W/Q/L* mutation; all are associated with DMS). Isolated diffuse mesangial sclerosis is also associated with mutations in exons 8 and 9. Frasier syndrome is associated with mutations in intron 9 at position +4 or +5, which disrupt the second splice acceptor site and lead to an excess of mRNAs that do not encode KTS (KTS-).

in maintaining the differentiated podocyte phenotype, including p21^{Cip1}, nephrin (*NPHS1*), and podocalyxin (1035). As shown in Figure 64-16, the *WT1* gene is composed of 10 exons, with the last 5 exons encoding the 4 C_2H_2 fingers comprising the zinc finger domain responsible for transcriptional regulation.

As depicted in Figure 64-16, the *WT1* gene undergoes a complex pattern of alternate splicing, producing at least 24 distinct mRNAs. Four mRNAs predominate: these do or do not contain the 17 amino acids encoded by exon 5, based on alternate splicing, and do or do not contain the three amino acids lysine-threonine-serine (KTS) located between zinc fingers 3 and 4, based on the use of alternate splice acceptor sites located within intron 9. mRNAs that do not encode KTS (KTS-) generate more potent transcriptional activators (1036). In cells from normal individuals, the +KTS/-KTS ratio ranges from 1.5 to 2; in cells from Frasier syndrome patients with intron 9 splice-site mutations, the ratio falls below 1, which would increase transcriptional activity (1037). By contrast, Denys-Drash syndrome is associated with point mutations and premature stop codon mutations, particularly involving zinc fingers 2 and 3. Many of the involved mutations disrupt the zinc finger structures, suggesting that the mutant protein might act in a dominant negative fashion to suppress or alter activation of target genes (although this has not been formally demonstrated) (1038).

The Denys-Drash syndrome is a triad composed of nephropathy (DMS or FSGS), male pseudohermaphroditism, and Wilms tumor, although many patients lack the full triad and some may have isolated DMS. Most patients have a 46, XY karyotype but a 46, XX karyotype can occur. Patients present commonly with ambiguous genitalia at birth, although

up to 40% are phenotypically female and may present with primary amenorrhea. Rare patients are phenotypically male. Nephropathy typically presents in infancy or early childhood, occasionally at birth. The renal biopsy shows focal or DMS, or less commonly, FSGS. Patients typically progress rapidly to ESRD, often within months and almost always by age 10. Mutations in *WT1* are found in 90% of patients with Denys-Drash syndrome (1039–1043). The locations of the mutations are either in the N-terminal domain (exons 1-3, often in patients lacking nephropathy) or the exons 7-9, disrupting the zinc finger domains (especially at R394). Podocyte proliferation has also been reported, with the development of pseudocrescents and shrunken glomeruli (881). The authors did not specifically describe capillary collapse, but these findings suggest that the Denys-Drash phenotype may occasionally extend to collapsing glomerulopathy. Slowly progressive FSGS has been reported with a *F392L* mutation (1044).

The Frasier syndrome is a triad composed of nephropathy, male pseudohermaphroditism, and gonadoblastoma, although many patients lack the full triad. Patients are most often phenotypically female. Wilms tumors are not seen. Mutations in the intron 9 splice donor site are uniformly present (1037,1039,1045,1046). The mutations are usually *de novo*, but in one case, maternal inheritance has been described (1047). Onset of proteinuria is typically between 2 and 18 years of age, with ESRD reached between 8 and 20 years. FSGS is most common and occasionally DMS is present. In one case, a patient with Wilms tumor was shown to have MCN with mild segmental hypercellularity (1048). FSGS was not demonstrated in a sample that included more than 100 glomeruli; nevertheless the patient progressed to ESRD.

WT1 mutations have not been identified in sporadic FSGS or collapsing glomerulopathy, but this genomic region may harbor susceptibility loci. Denamur et al. found only 1 of 37 children with steroid-resistant nephrotic syndrome (SRNS) or FSGS to have a *WT1* intron 9 mutation, and this child had other manifestations including genitourinary abnormalities (1049). Orloff et al. studied 218 African American FSGS patients, mostly with adult-onset kidney disease, and found no pathogenic mutations (1050). They studied two candidate genes *WT1* and *WIT1*, which lie in close proximity on chromosome 11, by genotyping subjects for seven SNPs in *WT1* and one SNP in *WIT1*. Three SNPs were associated with idiopathic FSGS or collapsing glomerulopathy (but not HIV-associated collapsing glomerulopathy): two SNPs in the *WT1* gene (OR 1.7) and OR 1.9) and one SNP in *WT1* (OR 1.8). One SNP within a *WT1* intron was associated with HIV-associated collapsing glomerulopathy (OR 4.3). Extending these analyses to haplotypes (particular allelic combinations at multiple loci along a chromosomal segment), they observed that a haplotype comprising one *WIT1* SNP and four *WT1* SNPs was associated with HIV-associated collapsing glomerulopathy, but not idiopathic FSGS or collapsing glomerulopathy. These data suggest that genetic variation within *WT1*, *WIT1*, or nearby genes, may contribute to susceptibility to both idiopathic and HIV-associated glomerular diseases in African Americans, but that the contributions of particular genetic variants are complex.

ACTN4

Pollak and colleagues identified *ACTN4* mutations in three families with FSGS showing autosomal dominant inheritance (1051). The mutations (K228E, T232I, R235P, recently renumbered as K256E, T260E, S263P) were in exon 8 (out of 21 exons). Affected individuals showed a range of phenotypes, from microalbuminuria and subnephrotic proteinuria (including elderly individuals) to ESRD. Penetrance was incomplete, as some patients with mutations lack proteinuria. Importantly, in the cases identified to date, proteinuria does not develop until adulthood. The α-actinins are actin-binding and cross-linking proteins; α-actinin-4 is expressed in many tissues. Podocytes express α-actinin-4 in abundant amounts and the mutant α-actinin-4 variants were initially shown to bind actin more tightly than does the wild-type protein. Mutant proteins also have an increased propensity to form aggregates, which Pollak and colleagues suggest could explain the apparent increase in actin binding, and the mutant molecules have a greatly decreased half-life (798). Two models are proposed: the mutant protein is unavailable for cytoskeletal interactions or alternatively aggregates are cytotoxic.

ACTN4 null mice develop glomerular disease, consisting of foot-process effacement and GBM duplication, but in contrast to humans, two abnormal genes are required (797). Interestingly, heterozygous transgenic mice expressing the mouse homolog of the human K256E *ACTN4* mutation develop proteinuria and FSGS (805). Nephrin mRNA and protein expression, but not synaptopodin protein expression, were reduced in mouse podocytes *in vivo*, suggesting that cytoskeletal alterations affect the podocyte transcriptional program. By contrast, homozygous knock-in mice bearing ACTN4 K228E manifested proteinuria and podocyte abnormalities but did not develop FSGS (798). These discrepancies between the two mouse models may indicate the limitations of this model system, perhaps due to the short life of the rodents, to model a disease that takes decades to develop in humans.

CD2AP

CD2-associated protein (CD2AP) was first identified as an adaptor protein that interacts with the cytoplasmic tail of CD2. Surprisingly, homozygous *CD2AP* null mutation mice develop diffuse global glomerulosclerosis (794) and heterozygotes develop FSGS (795). Subsequently it was demonstrated that CD2AP is expressed in podocytes, co-localized with F-actin in lamellipodia of cultured podocytes (1052) and to the slit diaphragm *in vivo* (1053). CD2AP interacts with F-actin (1054) and nephrin (1027,1055). CD2AP interacts with phosphatidylinositol 3-kinase, stimulating the AKT signaling pathway and suppressing apoptosis (1056). In a study of 45 African Americans with FSGS and collapsing glomerulopathy, 6 *CD2AP* variants were identified. One variant, affecting the splice effector site in exon 7, changes amino acid coding (P243S) and generates a truncated protein (795). Two unrelated FSGS patients had the *P234S* variant; one patient lacked a family history of kidney disease and the other patient had two family member with kidney disease of uncertain cause. Family studies of these individuals have not been performed, and so it remains unclear whether the variant is truly pathogenic.

TRPC6

Winn et al. recently reported that a missense mutation (*P112G*) in *TRCP6* (a member of the transient receptor potential channel protein family) was responsible for autosomal dominant FSGS in a New Zealand family of British origin (1057). Affected individuals presented in the third or fourth decades of life with heavy proteinuria and 60% progressed to ESRD. TRPC proteins are nonselective cation channels, which increase calcium flux in response to diacylglycerol. TRCP6 is expressed in the glomerular cells, probably including the podocyte, and the P112G mutant protein exhibits increased activity (1057). TRCP6 participates in VEGF receptor signaling (1058). Thus, it is possible that increased signaling via the VEGF or other receptors induces podocyte injury.

Mitochondrial Proteins: Mutations in Mitochondrial and Nuclear Genomes

The mitochondrial genome consists of a circular DNA molecule, approximately 16 kb in length. Mitochondrial DNA (mtDNA) encodes 13 essential subunits of the respiratory chain, 22 transfer RNA (tRNA) molecules, and 2 ribosomal RNA molecules. Cellular DNA replication is accompanied by mtDNA replication. mtDNA has a high rate of mutation when compared to nuclear DNA. Somatic cells possess 10 to 1,000 copies of mtDNA, whereas the oocyte has ~100,000 copies. When an mtDNA mutant arises or is inherited from a precursor cell, it exists in pool of mtDNA that includes wild type and mutant; this variety is termed *heteroplasmy*, and at least theoretically can range from near 0% to near 100%.

The MELAS syndrome involves children who present with mitochondrial encephalopathy, lactic acidosis, and strokelike episodes. In 1990, Goto et al. identified an mtDNA mutation in 26 of 31 MELAS patients; this mutation is located at position 3243 of mtDNA (A3243G) and involves mitochondrial $tRNA^{Leu}$ (1059). MELAS has been associated with FSGS in both children and adults, with at least 14 reports describing patients with FSGS (1060–1074). Of a total of 30 patients with FSGS described in these reports, 17 children had typical MELAS syndrome and FSGS and 13 pediatric and adult patients presented in an atypical fashion, either with isolated FSGS or with deafness or type 2 diabetes or both. Importantly, the extrarenal manifestations may become apparent only after renal disease has appeared, with a lag time in some cases of many years. The diagnosis requires evaluation of mtDNA by re-sequencing or by other molecular techniques. Due to heteroplasmy, leukocyte DNA may or may not show the mutation, and it may be important to test urinary cells or kidney tissue. Of the 30 patients with FSGS, all but 2 patients have had the *A3243G* mutation; single patients have been described with other tRNA mutations: tRNA[Ile] A269G (1063) and tRNA[Tyr] A5843G (1064).

The mechanism of glomerular injury is not well understood, but giant (and presumably abnormal) mitochondria are present in podocytes and tubular epithelial cells (1072). Some patients have isolated tubulointerstitial nephritis, raising the possibility that in some cases FSGS could arise as a postadaptive response to nephron loss.

Recently, a mutation in the nuclear gene encoding the enzyme coenzyme Q synethase 2 (COQ2) has been indentified as cause of at least some cases of autosomal recessive infantile encephalopathy and nephropathy syndrome, where the renal histology typically shows FSGS (1074a). COQ2 is an essential enzyme in the synthesis of COQ10, also known as ubiquinone. COQ10 plays an important role in electron transport within the mitochondrion, and also serves as an antioxidant. Children with the syndrome present as infants or in some cases as young children; they may also manifest with cerebellar ataxia, sensorineural deafness, and myopathy involving skeletal muscle and heart. Other mutations in COQ10 synthetic enzymes may well exist and will likely present as phenocopies, with similar syndromic features.

Oligomeganephronia

Oligomeganephronia is characterized by bilateral renal hypoplasia without dysplasia or urinary tract abnormalities. Pathologic findings include diminished nephron number and glomerulomegaly, leading ultimately to postadaptive FSGS. Renal function is typically impaired from birth, rises as an absolute value during development, reaches a plateau in early childhood, and begins to decrease in middle or late childhood. By contrast, children and adults who present with a single kidney most commonly have renal aplasia rather than renal agenesis; the distinction lies in the fact that a small kidney is present at birth and subsequently undergoes regression (1075). This is a common finding, affecting 1:1,300 newborns, and does not appear to be associated with oligomeganephronia or FSGS.

Oligomeganephronia occurs in the setting of several congenital syndromes. The *renal-coloboma syndrome* is due to mutations in *PAX2*, one of a family of homeobox genes, encoding paired-box-containing transcription factors (1076). These children may present with syndromic oligomeganephronia, accompanied by ocular defects, or isolated oligomeganephro-

nia (1077,1078). The *acro-renal ocular syndrome* may include various urinary tract abnormalities including renal hypoplasia (1079); some cases overlap with syndromes associated with *SALL4* mutations (1080). Patients with *branchio-oto-renal syndrome* present with mixed hearing loss, bilateral branchial cleft fistulas, and bilateral renal dysplasia; the gene responsible is unknown. The *bilateral renal agenesis or dysplasia syndrome* may be familial, with dominant inheritance (1081). The locus has not been identified.

FSGS Susceptibility Genes

The mutations listed in Table 64-19 have been associated with FSGS that is inherited in typical Mendelian fashion, and additional genes are likely to be identified in the years ahead. As noted in the preceding text, there are striking racial discrepancies in the incidence of FSGS that may be due to genetic variation, but the loci responsible are not well understood. It is likely that there is a subtle interplay between genetic susceptibility factors (genes, nephron number), environmental factors (viruses, toxins), and risk factors (obesity, hypertension, dietary protein) that determines risk for both idiopathic FSGS and postadaptive FSGS. Therefore, FSGS likely fits the pattern of a complex genetic disease, like hypertension, type 2 diabetes, and asthma, in which multiple genes are believed to interact with each other and with environmental factors. The search for susceptibility genes is challenging and requires convincing evidence of association. The probability of false positive identification is high, given the many genes and the many polymorphisms that can be tested. A convincing case that a polymorphism (or better, a haplotype covering most or all of a gene) is relevant, requires significant associations that are reproduced in multiple studies, ideally in geographically (and possibly racially) diverse populations.

The *ACE* gene is highly polymorphic, but most published renal disease association studies have focused on a single polymorphism: the intron 16 *Alu* element insertion/deletion polymorphism. This variant has not been shown to alter gene expression, but could conceivably be in linkage disequilibrium with pathogenic mutations. In Table 64-20 are presented the results of eight studies including a total of 324 patients (1082,1083) and other references. Although the results are not consistent in all populations, some evidence suggests that the D allele is weakly associated with FSGS in Asian populations and stronger evidence indicates that the D allele (or perhaps the DD genotype) may increase the risk for progressive loss of renal function.

TABLE 64-20

ASSOCIATION STUDIES OF *ACE* INSERTION/DELETION GENOTYPES AND FOCAL SEGMENTAL GLOMERULOSCLEROSIS (FSGS) AND FSGS PROGRESSION RISK

Country, year	FSGS cases (N)	Disease association	Progression association	Reference
Germany, 1997	17	No association	No association	(1084)
Korea, 1997	30	DD	DD	(1083)
Israel, 1998	47	No association	ID, DD	(1085)
Croatia, 2000	39	No association	DD	(1086)
USA, 2002	47	No association	DD	(744)
Japan, 2001	43	DD, ID	No association	(1082)
Germany, 2003	71	No association	ID, DD	(1087)
Turkey, 2004	30	No association	DD	(1088)

Eight published studies were identified that correlated the prevalence of the insertion/deletion *ACE* genotypes (II, DD, or ID) in FSGS cases and controls or progression risk (variously assessed as glomerular filtration rate [GFR] decline slope or end stage renal disease [ESRD] incidence).

Treatment of FSGS and Collapsing Glomerulopathy

The goal of treatment of all podocyte diseases is to reduce proteinuria to normal (ideally) or alternatively to the lowest level possible. There is increasing evidence that the level of proteinuria predicts long term outcome. The definitions of response are presented in Table 64-10.

Treatment of Children

Approaches to pediatric FSGS show considerable heterogeneity. In 1997, Vehaskari surveyed 181 members of the American Society of Pediatric Nephrology to learn their therapeutic practices (1089). Daily glucocorticoid therapy lasting more than 3 months was used often or sometimes by 50% of respondents (which the author found surprising, as there are no trials of this approach in children). Intravenous glucocorticoids were used often or sometimes by 52% of respondents. Oral cytotoxic therapy (cyclophosphamide or chlorambucil) were used often or sometimes by 85% of respondents. The combination of intravenous glucocorticoids plus oral cytotoxic therapy (the Tune-Mendoza protocol and variants) was used often or sometimes by 44% of respondents. Cyclosporine was used often or sometimes by 74% of respondents. ACE inhibitors were used often or sometimes by 92% of respondents.

Glucocorticoids. Because younger children undergo a therapeutic trial of corticosteroid prior to biopsy, they may be considered by the standard ISKDC nomenclature to be steroid resistant by the time they are diagnosed as having FSGS. How-

ever, most pediatricians do not wait for 8 to 12 weeks of nonresponse before performing a biopsy, and the ISKDC standard is sufficiently narrow that it does not preclude the possibility that patients will respond to some form of glucocorticoid therapy. Of those patients who are found to have FSGS, about 15% will respond to conventional oral steroid therapy and have a high likelihood of retaining kidney function long term. The remaining 85% of patients are steroid-resistant and are at substantial risk to progress to ESRD (1090).

More commonly, however, a more aggressive regimen is necessary for steroids to be effective. In the Tune-Mendoza treatment regimen (Table 64-21), patients receive high-dose, intravenous boluses of methylprednisolone (1093) with or without an accompanying alkylating agent (1091). On this regimen, more than half of patients developed stable remission and the majority had normal renal function several years later (1094,1095). However, treatment is accompanied by significant steroid toxicity, including neoplasm (1095) and serious infection (1096). The frequent administration of high-dose, intravenous medications also is labor-intensive. Nonetheless, this protocol continues to be used by a significant number of pediatric nephrologists (1097).

Calcineurin Inhibitors. As an alternative to prolonged glucocorticoid therapy, cyclosporine has been the subject of several randomized trials in pediatric SRNS. The New York–New Jersey Pediatric Nephrology study group randomized 25 patients to cyclosporine (3 mg/kg, to achieve a trough level of 300 to 500 ng/mL) or placebo treatment for 6 months (1098). Proteinuria decreased by 71% in the cyclosporine group and was unchanged in the placebo group, although the CR and

TABLE 64-21

COMPARISON OF STEROID DOSES FOR STEROID-RESISTANT NEPHROTIC SYNDROME OR FSGS

Protocol	Ref.	Age group	Duration	Child, (28 kg, 128 cm = 1 m²) Total prednisone equivalent (g)	Adult (80 kg, 180 cm = 2 m²) Total prednisone equivalent (g)
Tune-Mendoza MP 30 mg/kg IV three times weekly W1–2 MP 30 mg/kg IV weekly W3–10 MP 30 mg/kg IV every 2W W11–18 MP 30 mg/kg IV every 4W W19–50 MP 30 mg/kg IV every 8W W51–82	(1091)	Children	82 weeks	43.9	NA
Waldo MP 20 mg/kg IV three times weekly W1–2 MP 20 mg/kg IV weekly W3–10 MP 20 mg/kg IV every 2W W11–26 MP 20 mg/kg IV every 4W W27–78	(1092)	Children	78 weeks	24.0	NA
Commonly-used adult regimen Prednisone 1 mg/kg orally, W1–16 Prednisone 0.5 mg/kg orally, W17–24 Prednisone taper off, W26–32	(1148)	Adults	32 weeks	NA	12.6
NIH FSGS Dexamethasone 25 mg/m2, 4 pulses orally every 4 W	Unpub.	Adults	32 weeks	(5.0) No pediatric patients treated	10.0

MP, methylprednisolone; *W*, weeks. In the Tune-Mendoza and Waldo protocols, MP doses are capped at 1 g/dose. The conversion to prednisone-equivalent doses assumes 100% bioavailability and that the equipotent antiinflammatory doses are as follows: hydrocortisone 1, prednisone 4, methylprednisolone 5, and dexamethasone 25. Importantly, the Tune-Mendoza protocol also involves intermittent cyclophosphamide therapy.

PR responses are not provided. In one uncontrolled pediatric study, very high-dose cyclosporine was used to counteract the hyperlipidemia of unresponsive nephrotic patients (1099). In a smaller, double-blind controlled study, significant reduction in urinary protein was accomplished in patients receiving cyclosporine treatment (1100). Large, prospective studies have shown that cyclosporine may be at least as effective as high-dose methylprednisolone in treating FSGS (1101,1102). Tacrolimus has been used in a small number of steroid-resistant nephrotic patients including some with FSGS. The drug helped to control the level of urinary protein loss in some of these patients (1103). Given the positive results with cyclosporine and the potential benefits of tacrolimus data, calcineurin inhibitors are used frequently by the clinician treating steroid-resistant FSGS in children.

Cytotoxic Therapy. The response of children with FSGS to treatment with cytotoxic drugs has been extensively studied. A review of nine series involving children (702) revealed that 23% of 247 children with FSGS were steroid-responsive; 70 of the patients were treated with cytotoxic drugs, and 21 (30%) of the 70 responded; at the time of their last examination, 19.5% of the 247 children were in remission. It was not possible to determine how many of these children had FSGS documented when they presented with nephrotic syndrome and how many were found to have this lesion only when they became steroid-resistant after having previous episodes of steroid-responsive nephrotic syndrome. Although chlorambucil (1104) and intravenous boluses of cyclophosphamide (12) have been reported to be effective, these agents have not been evaluated in a larger, prospective controlled trial.

Treatment of Adults

There is a wide range of therapeutic approaches to adults with FSGS and collapsing glomerulopathy. (For simplicity, the following discussion will use the term FSGS for both conditions, as most references have not distinguished between the two disorders.)

Glucorticoids. Glucocorticoids are widely accepted as initial therapy for adult FSGS and collapsing glomerulopathy, although there is considerable controversy as to dose and duration of therapy and no randomized controlled trials have been carried out. The mechanism of action is unclear. Possible mechanisms include immunosuppression, activation of podocyte anti-oxidant enzymes (1105), and stabilization of the podocyte cytoskeleton (1106).

In Table 64-22 are summarized nine studies of glucocorticoid therapy for adult FSGS that have been reported in the last 20 years. Two studies included patients who received additional immunosuppressive therapy: 10% of patients in the Chicago study and 41% of patients in the Toronto study received such therapy; studies with more than 50% of patients treated with nonglucocorticoid therapy were excluded from this summary. Eight reports provide attained CR and PR rates, with relapse rates provided in four studies; the North Carolina study provided only sustained CR rates at follow-up. Two studies were prospective, uncontrolled trials and seven studies were retrospective analyses. Entry criteria included nephrotic-range proteinuria in five studies. Exclusion criteria included collapsing glomerulopathy in the North Carolina study, postadaptive FSGS, variously defined, in all but the Toronto study, and impaired GFR in the Italian study (patients with serum creatinine levels of >3 mg/dL). Although most patients in these studies likely had idiopathic FSGS, diagnostic standards for postadaptive FSGS have differed, so it is quite possible that some patients had postadaptive FSGS. The mean or median duration of high-dose daily glucocorticoid therapy (generally prednisolone

or prednisone 1 mg/kg/day) was 2 to 4 months, and the duration of total therapy was a mean or median 3 to 9 months. Two studies used pulse therapy, either as initiation or as sole treatment.

Does glucocorticoid therapy increase the likelihood of remission? Spontaneous remission is rare, occurring with conservative treatment in 4% (two patient with CR) (1090) and 6% (two patients with PR) (1108). As shown in Table 64-22, with treatment, CR rates ranged from 0% to 44% and combined remission rates (CR plus PR) ranged from 33% to 59% (with data on PR lacking from two studies). None of the studies were randomized, but three studies described the outcome in a comparison group that did not receive immunosuppressive treatment. Rydel et al. reported that remission rates were higher with treatment (CR 33%, PR 17%) than with conservative treatment (CR 0%, PR 7%) (1108). Conversely, Stiles et al. noted that remission rates were similar in patients receiving either prednisone (0% CR, 42% PR) or conservative therapy including ACE inhibitors (0%, 60% PR) (1111). Franceschini et al. found that CR rates at 18 months of observation were similar with prednisone (11%) and conservative therapy (11%), but did not provide PR rates; it appears that CR is uncommon with ACE inhibitor and angiotensin receptor blocker (ARB) therapy (1110). One consideration is that aggressive use of ACE inhibitors for proteinuric patients is a relatively recent phenomenon, becoming more common after the publication of the landmark captopril trial in diabetic nephropathy in 1993 (1112). This might explain the lower response rate in the conservative treatment group observed by Rydel and colleagues (patients diagnosed 1975 to 1993), compared to Stiles and colleagues (patients diagnosed from 1992 to 1999).

Does a longer total duration of glucocorticoid therapy improve the chance of remission (combined CR plus PR) or CR? Two intrastudy comparisons argue for this hypothesis and two argue against this hypothesis. In the Italian study, patients treated longer than 16 weeks were also more likely to reach CR than those treated less than 16 weeks (61% versus 15%, relative risk 4.0, p <0.01). Multivariate analysis indicated that only duration of glucocorticoid therapy (and not other clinical or histologic variables) predicted CR. These authors found that most responders entered remission after 6 months of therapy, although this observation derives from all treated patients (adults and children, glucocorticoids and other immunosuppressive therapy). In the Lucknow study, patients treated for more than 16 weeks were more likely to remit than those treated for less than 16 weeks (p <0.01); the relative risk of remission was similar in nephrotic and non-nephrotic patients (1.6 and 1.5, respectively), although treatment duration was not significantly different between remitters and nonremitters in either group studied alone. Conversely, in the Chicago study, duration of daily prednisone therapy was similar in remitting patients and in nonremitting patients (5.7 versus 5.5 months). In the Toronto study, the median duration of daily prednisone was similar for those patients in CR at follow-up and those not in CR (5 months compared to 6 months). Furthermore, the median time to CR was 4 months, with a range of 0.5 to 6 months, which the authors interpreted to mean that therapy beyond 6 months is unlikely to add to the response rate.

Does a longer duration of high-dose daily therapy improve the chance of remission? Only one (retrospective) study addresses this hypothesis. In the Chicago study, duration of daily prednisone at a dose of ≥60 mg per day was greater in remitting patients than in nonremitting patients (mean 2.7 months versus mean 1.5 months, p <0.01, and median 3 months versus median 1 month).

How do the high-response rate studies differ from the low-response rate studies? The studies can be arbitrarily dichotomized into four high-response studies (CR ≥25%) and

TABLE 64-22

CLINICAL TRIALS OF GLUCOCORTICOID THERAPY FOR ADULTS WITH FOCAL SEGMENTAL GLOMERULOSCLEROSIS (FSGS): REGIMEN, REMISSION, RELAPSE, AND LONG-TERM OUTCOME

First author, location, year	Design	N	Black subjects	Nephrotic proteinuria	Glucocorticoid therapy	Total prednisone dose equivalent	Other immuno-supressive therapy	CR definition	CR	PR definition	PR	CR+PR	Relapse	Final status (duration observation)	Reference
Agarwal, New Dehli, 1993	Prospective	65 (23 lost)	0%	100%	High dose 8–12 w Taper to 6 m	ND	None	<0.3 g/d	18%	2 g/d	15%	33%	NS	ESRD 5% (34 m)	(1107)
Rydel, Chicago, 1995	Retrospective	30	63%	100%	High dose ≥8 w in 67%, total therapy mean 5 m	ND	Cytotoxic therapy (10%)	<0.25 g/d	33%	<2.5 g/d	17%	50%	From CR or PR: 67%	CR 30%, PR 16% ESRD 20% (79 m) (additional therapy used)	(1108)
Cattran, Toronto, 1998	Retrospective	17	0%	100%	Total therapy median 5 m range 2–50 m	6.4 g	Cyclophosphamide (41%)	<0.2 g/d	47%	ND	ND	ND	From CR: 38%	CR: 47% ESRD 29% (155 m)	(1090)
Ponticelli, Italy, 1999	Retrospective	53	0%	100%	A) High dose for 8 w, total therapy mean of 6 m B) High dose for 8 w, total therapy mean of 5 m	A) 6.4 g B) ND	None	<0.2 g/d	40%	<2 g/d	19%	58%	From CR or PR: 55%	ND	(1109)
Chitalia, New Zealand, 1999	Retrospective	28	0%	ND	High dose 6–8 w, maximum duration 12 w	ND	None	<0.3 g/d	21%	ND	ND	ND	ND	ND	(1166)
Stiles Washington DC, 2001	Retrospective	12	83%	100%	High dose prednisone mean 4 m (alternate day in 17%)	8.4 g	None	<0.2 g/d	0%	<3 g/d	42%	42%	ND	ND	(1111)
Pokhariyal, Lucknow, India, 2003	Retrospective	83 (12 lost)	0%	59%	High dose prednisolone mean 3 m	5.6 g	None	<0.3 g/d	25%	<2 g/d or 50% decrease if sub-nephrotic	25%	50%	ND	ND	(1114)
Franceschini, North Carolina, 2003	Retrospective	36	31%	ND	High dose daily or alternate day for mean of 9 m	10.6 g	Cyclophos-phamide 3, cyclosporine 3 (17%)	<0.6 g/d	ND	ND	ND	ND	ND	CR 11% ESRD 18% (27 m)	(1110)
Smith, Bethesda, 2003	Prospective	14	50%	100%	Pulse oral dexmaethsone for 8 m	8.6 g	None	<0.3 g/d	7%	<2 g/d	29%	36%	From CR or PR: 60%	CR 7%, PR: 14% ESRD 0% (20 m)	(1117)

The results of nine studies, describing 338 adult FSGS patients with nephrotic range proteinuria who were treated primarily with glucocorticoids, are presented in chronological order. The number (N) of patients with nephrotic range proteinuria who were treated with glucocorticoids is shown. Nephrotic range proteinuria was variously defined as >3 g/d, >3.5 g/d or >3 g/d/1.73 m^2. High dose prednisone is defined as prednisone or prednisolone at a dose of ~1 mg/kg/d. In the Italian study, patients received either regimen A) prednisone 1 mg/kg/d for 8 weeks, followed by a taper to a mean of 24 weeks, or regimen B) 3 doses of intravenous methylprednisolone, followed by prednisolone 0.5 mg/kg for 8 weeks, and then a taper to a mean of 19 weeks. In the Bethesda study, patients received oral dexamethasone at a dose of 100 mg/m^2 monthly. For total mean prednisone dose, the value was provided by the reference or was calculated from the mean duration and assumes a mean weight of 70 kg if the reference described the total dose in mg/kg, or a mean body size of 1.73 m^2 if the dosing was by body surface area. The definitions of complete remission (CR) and partial remission (PR) are shown. The two studies from India lacked complete follow-up for end-point determination; for the present analysis, calculation of outcome made here on the conservative intention to treat basis with the assumption that patients lost to follow-up were non-responders. The mean duration of follow-up is shown and percent of patients who achieved remission are shown. CKD, chronic kidney disease; ESRD, end-stage renal disease; ND, no data provided.

four low-response studies (CR <25%). The North Carolina study is excluded because it did not provide attained response rates and provided sustained response rates at follow-up. The high-response studies (Chicago, Toronto, Italy, and Lucknow) showed CR rates of 25% to 44% and combined response rates of 50% to 59% (PR data were not provided in the Toronto study). The low-response studies (New Delhi, New Zealand, Washington DC, and Bethesda) showed attained CR rates of 0% to 21% and combined response rates of 33% to 42%. (The Lucknow study would have been classified as a high-response study (31% CR) if the analysis excluded lost patients, as the authors proposed). A qualitative interstudy comparison of the high-response studies with the low-response studies follows:

- Similar prevalence of African Americans in high-response studies (0, 0, 0, 63%) and low response studies (0, 0, 50, 83%)
- Similar *mean duration of high dose* daily glucocorticoid therapy (approximately 1 mg/kg) in high-response studies (8, 8, 12, 12 weeks) compared to low-response studies (7, 10, 16 weeks; not applicable in the Bethesda study)
- Similar *minimum duration of high dose* daily glucocorticoid therapy (approximately 1 mg/kg), specified in only three studies: high-response studies (8 weeks in the Chicago study) versus low-response studies (6 weeks in the New Zealand study, 8 weeks in the New Delhi study)
- Similar use of *daily* glucocorticoid therapy (as opposed to alternate day or intermittent pulse therapy) in high response studies (3 of 3 studies, excluding the Italian study which used both) and low response studies (3 of 4 studies; the Washington DC study used alternate day therapy in 17% and the Bethesda study using pulse therapy in 100%)
- Similar *mean/median total duration* of glucocorticoid therapy in high-response studies (3, 5, 5.5, 5 months) compared to low-response studies (4, 6 months; not applicable in the Bethesda study and no data from the New Zealand study)
- Similar total prednisone equivalent doses in high-response studies, when data were provided (5.6, 6.4, 6.4 g) compared to low-response studies (8.4, 8.6 g)
- More use of other immunosuppressive therapy in high response studies (2 of 4 studies) than in the low-response studies (0 of 4 studies)

Although these interstudy comparisons are qualitative in nature, because of the limitations of varying study design and study reporting, they do not suggest any compelling hypotheses to explain the difference between high-response and low-response studies.

Relapses were common, occurring in 38% to 67% of remitting patients. Often, patients who experienced relapse were brought back into remission with additional glucocorticoid therapy or other treatment. Surprisingly, remission status at last follow-up was generally higher with greater length of observation (duration from presentation or from initiation of therapy), ranging from 11% (CR only, mean 18 months observation) through 21% (CR plus PR, mean 20 months observation) to 46% (CR plus PR, mean 79 months observation) and 44% (CR only, 155 months).

Do children respond better than adults to therapy, including with glucocorticoids? In the only study that compared children and adults, Cattran et al. suggested that CR rates were similar in children (47%) and adults (44%) (1090).

Can clinicians identify patients who are most likely to respond to glucocorticoid therapy? Shiiki et al. studied the likelihood of response to any immunosuppressive therapy in 35 adults with idiopathic FSGS, of whom 66% experienced a CR or PR, and found the following were significant predictors of nonresponse on multivariate logistic regression analysis: larger mean glomerular diameter (OR 2.93, CI 1.07–7.92, $p = 0.04$)

and more severe tubulointerstitial changes (OR 8.86, CI 1.06–43.9, $p = 0.04$) (1113). By contrast, other investigators studying 30 adult FSGS patients (1108) and 81 adult FSGS patients (1114) could not identify any clinical or histologic features that predicted response to therapy on multivariate analysis.

What is the toxicity of a prolonged course of glucocorticoid therapy in adults? There are few published data on the toxicity of daily prednisone when used for FSGS. The Toronto study, with mean observation time of 155 months, reported four deaths (two patients who received only glucocorticoids, one patient who had received glucocorticoids and cyclophosphamide, and one patient who received neither). The Washington, DC study, with a mean observation time of 18 months, reported that 41% of patients experienced severe adverse events (diabetes mellitus, hypertension exacerbation, cellulitis, and severe myopathy). In the Lucknow study, 16% of patients experienced significant adverse events (diabetes mellitus, infections, Cushingoid facies, and dyspepsia).

Is alternative day glucocorticoid therapy an effective option, with the prospect of less toxicity? This regimen is widely used, particularly for patients who are at increased risk of adverse events, but the published data supporting this regimen are sparse. In 1977, Bolton et al. reported on the treatment of 81 adult patients with nephrotic syndrome, including 10 patients with FSGS, using prednisone 60 to 120 mg on alternate days for up to 10 years (1115). In the FSGS group, CR or PR (defined as a >50% decrease and <3 g/day) occurred in 3 (30%). In the entire patient group, the regimen was well tolerated, being associated with one adverse event per 12 patient-years of therapy. These adverse events included Cushingoid facies (10%), cataracts (6%), bone disease (5%), psychosis (1%), cytopenia (7%), infection (2%), and stroke (2%). Nagai et al. reported a case series of 17 patients older than age 60 with FSGS; 82% were nephrotic. Nine patients received 100 mg prednisone on alternate days, with two patients also receiving oral cyclophosphamide (1116). Five patients entered remission (4 CR, 1 PR), all of whom received prednisone only. A control group of 8 patients did not receive treatment and experienced only 1 PR. Two patients died during follow-up (of pancreatic cancer and stroke); other adverse events were not described. These limited data do support further studies of alternate-day therapy. Some patients in the North Carolina study received alternate-day prednisone, but there no data were presented comparing daily and alternate day therapy (1110).

If the high response-rate studies suggest that total therapy duration in excess of 4 months is desirable, does intermittent pulse therapy for an extended duration offer similar efficacy with an acceptable safety profile? The Bethesda study was a small open-label study of oral pulse dexamethasone (25 mg/m², given on each of the first 4 days of each 4 week cycle), administered over 32 weeks to 14 patients (1117). A distinguishing feature of the inclusion criteria was nephrotic proteinuria despite aggressive ACE inhibitor or ARB therapy, which might be expected to reduce the PR rate compared to studies that added these agents as part of the regimen. The efficacy outcomes would place this study in the low-response category: CR response rate (7%) and combined CR and PR response rates (36%). A low rate of adverse events was observed, limited to bone loss exceeding 3% in one patient (7%) and no hypertension, diabetes mellitus, avascular necrosis, glaucoma, cataract, or adrenal suppression.

Calcineurin Inhibitors and Cytotoxic Therapy. The literature on glucocorticoids is extensive due to the number of studies available and the controversies involved. By contrast, calcineurin inhibitors, and cyclosporine in particular, are generally accepted as standard therapy, although these agents do have significant limitations. Cyclosporine has been used to treat FSGS for approximately 20 years, as reviewed recently (1118).

Six studies have suggested combined CR and PR rates of 30% to 80%, CR rates of 0% to 25%, and relapse rates of 43% to 100% (699,1119–1123). Two of these trials were prospective trials. Ponticelli et al. studied 28 adult patients and 19 pediatric patients with FSGS; of those receiving cyclosporine 57% experienced CR or PR and 40% of these remained in remission after 2 years (1124). In the highest quality study, Cattran et al. studied 49 adult FSGS patients with steroid resistance, defined as nephrotic proteinuria despite ≥8 weeks of glucocorticoid therapy (1123). Patients were randomized to cyclosporine or placebo, together with low-dose prednisone (0.15 mg/kg/day). At the end of the study, CR occurred in 12% of the treatment arm and 0% of the control arm, whereas PR (defined as a 50% decrease in proteinuria, becoming subnephrotic, and a preserved GFR) occurred in 57% of the treatment arm and 4% of the control arm. At 78 weeks and again at 104 weeks of follow-up, 50% of those with CR and PR had experienced relapse. Cyclosporine also significantly reduced the chance of doubling serum creatinine over a 2-year period. Taken together, these six studies show a consistent effect of cyclosporine to reduce proteinuria in patients with FSGS (and possibly collapsing glomerulopathy, although this diagnosis was not standard when these trials were carried out).

Current recommendations are typically to initiate cyclosporine therapy at a dose of 3.5 mg/kg per day in a divided dose, with dose adjustment to achieve trough levels of 125 to 225 ng/mL (some nephrologists might aim for the slightly lower level, perhaps 100 to 150 ng/mL) (1125). Prednisone is not generally added, unless a patient is already receiving it. Given the high relapse rate, many nephrologists opt to extend therapy to 1 or 2 years, or in some cases for a longer duration. A note of caution about pursuing prolonged cyclosporine therapy was raised by Meyrier and colleagues, who noted that histologic injury progressed in some patients, including some patients who remained in CR (1126). Risk factors for histologic progression included cyclosporine dose >5.5 mg per day, renal insufficiency prior to initiating cyclosporine therapy, and a high percentage of glomeruli with FSGS on initial renal biopsy. It seems prudent to taper cyclosporine over several months when a patient has been in CR or PR, rather than abrupt cessation of therapy, but there are no published data that support this recommendation.

There are limited data addressing the use of tacrolimus in FSGS. Three studies involving a total 29 patients have been published: one study in children (711) and two studies in adults (1103,1127). There is no reason to predict that tacrolimus would be superior to cyclosporine in terms of nephrotoxicity, and the response rates appear to be similar to those seen with cyclosporine. The toxicity profile differs between cyclosporine and tacrolimus and this may influence the selection medication for a particular patient.

The mechanisms by which cyclosporine and tacrolimus reduce proteinuria, in primary podocyte diseases and in other glomerular diseases, are unknown. The immunosuppressive action of these agents may contribute, but there is no evidence that this is the case. Sharma et al. demonstrated that cyclosporine antagonizes the permeability enhancing properties of FSGS permeability factor on isolated rat glomeruli, suggesting that cyclosporine may have direct effects on glomerular cells (1128,1129).

Cytotoxic therapy, including cyclophosphamide and chlorambucil, plays a very limited role in adults with steroid-resistant FSGS and collapsing glomerulopathy. Korbet et al. reviewed the literature and found that among 105 steroid-resistant patients, cytotoxic therapy was associated with CR in 11% and PR in 11% (1130). By contrast, the responses were better among 33 steroid-responsive patients (CR 52%, PR 24%), suggesting that in the patient with steroid-dependent or frequently relapsing FSGS, these agents may be a reasonable choice.

Mycophenolate Mofetil. Cyclosporine has demonstrated but limited efficacy in treatment of FSGS, and has the drawbacks of exacerbating hypertension and potential nephrotoxicity with prolonged therapy. Mycophenolate mofetil (MMF) is an appealing alternative therapy. Choi et al. in Baltimore reported results with MMF used in clinical practice in 18 adults with FSGS (at least one of these patients had collapsing glomerulopathy) (1131). CR was defined as a urine protein/creatinine ratio of <0.3; PR was defined as a ≥50% fall in the urine protein/creatinine ratio. MMF was administered for a mean of 8 months (range 4 to 22 months) to 9 nephrotic patients, 7 of whom also received glucocorticoids. At the end of treatment, 1 patient was in CR, 3 in PR, and 5 did not respond (response rate 44%). At follow-up, 2 patients were in CR (MMF continued and 8 months after MMF withdrawal, respectively) and 1 patient was in PR (12 months after MMF withdrawal), for a sustained response rate of 33%.

Cattran et al. reported the results of a prospective, multicenter uncontrolled study of patients with glucocorticoid-resistant FSGS in Toronto, Baltimore, and New York (1132); 18 patients participated, of whom only 22% were African American. Therapy consisted of 6 months of MMF (dosage 1.5 g/day, actual duration 3 to 18 months, as two patients were noncompliant) combined with prednisone (0.25 mg/kg/day, tapered to a maximum of 10 mg/day over 6 weeks). Inclusion criteria included nephrotic range proteinuria and creatinine clearance ≥30 mL/minute/1.73 m². Outcomes included 0 CR; 6 PR (defined as 50% fall, becoming subnephrotic, and stable GFR), 33%; 2 patients with proteinuria response (defined as 50% fall in proteinuria), 11%; and 10 patients with no response, 56%. Among the 6 PR, further follow-up included 1 CR on MMF plus cyclosporine, 1 continued PR on MMF, 2 sustained PR off MMF (duration of observation off therapy approximately 10 months) and 2 relapses off MMF. Therefore, the sustained PR off-therapy was 12% (2/16 patients, with 2 patients continuing therapy). These results are less favorable than those from the initial single-center report. Further studies are needed to examine efficacy, in particular, sustained remission rates, in additional populations.

Effect of Immunosuppressive Therapy on Renal Survival. Does immunosuppressive therapy (glucocorticoids alone or glucocorticoids combined with other therapy) increase the likelihood of renal survival? There are no randomized controlled studies that address this question, and, therefore, the possibility of treatment selection bias limits the utility of the four nonrandomized studies that are available. Alexopoulos et al., in a study from Greece, found improved survival in treated nephrotic patients compared with untreated nephrotic patients, with 5-year renal survival of 86% versus 65% (p <0.03 by Kaplan Meier survival analysis (1133). Four retrospective studies were identified that provided outcome analysis for immunosuppressive treatment and control groups, with separate identification of nephrotic and non-nephrotic patients (Table 64-23). A pooled analysis of these studies shows that immunosuppressive therapy is associated with relative risk of ESRD of 0.52 (CI 0.32–0.84, $p = 0.02$) in nephrotic patients and 0.45 (CI 0.11–1.84, p = NS) in non-nephrotic patients. Therefore, the treatment-effect size is similar in nephrotic and non-nephrotic patients, but only in nephrotic patients is the treatment effect statistically significant. The Greek study is an outlier in two respects: use of other immunosuppressive therapy (70% of patients, compared with 10% in the other three studies combined) and the effect size (no ESRD observed with treatment of nephrotic patients). If the Greek study is omitted from analysis, the relative risk of ESRD with treatment in the remaining three studies is 0.59 (CI 0.36–0.97), which remains statistically significant ($p = 0.02$) and clinically significant.

TABLE 64-23

EFFECT OF IMMUNOSUPPRESSIVE TREATMENT ON LONG-TERM RENAL SURVIVAL IN FSGS

Location, year	Population	Immunosuppressive treatment	Duration of observation	Nephrotic, treated	Nephrotic, untreated	Relative risk of ESRD in treatment group (CI)	Nonnephrotic, treated	Nonnephrotic, untreated	Relative risk of ESRD in treatment group (CI)	Reference
Washington, DC, 2001	Adults	Prednisone	~20 F/U	ESRD 2 No ESRD 10	ESRD 3 No ESRD 7	0.55 (0.11–2.70)	ND	ND		(1111)
Greece, 2000	Adults	Prednisolone; CSA, CTX in some patients	57 mo	ESRD 0 No ESRD 11	ESRD 3 No ESRD 3	0.43 (0.12–1.5)	ESRD 2 No ESRD 5	ESRD 6 No ESRD 3	0.43 (0.12–1.51)	(1133)
Chicago, 1995	Adults	Prednisone cytotoxic therapy in some patients	79 mo	ESRD 6 No ESRD 24	ESRD 10 No ESRD 20	0.80 (0.33–2.0)	ND	ND		(1108)
Ontario, 1998	Children, adults	Prednisone; cyclophosphamide in some patients	155 mo	ESRD 16 No ESRD 33	ESRD 15 No ESRD 15	0.65 (0.38–1.11)	ESRD 1 No ESRD 2	ESRD 4 No ESRD 7	0.92 (0.15–5.4)	(1090)
Total				ESRD 24 No ESRD 78	ESRD 31 No ESRD 45	0.58 (0.37–0.90) p = 0.02	ESRD 3 No ESRD 7	ESRD 10 No ESRD 10	0.60 (0.27–1.70) p = 0.44	

Four retrospective studies are presented in order of increasing mean duration of observation (months). All treatment regimens included glucocorticoids; other immunosuppressive agents were used in selected patients as shown. The relative risk of end-stage renal disease (ESRD) and the 95% confidence interval (CI) for the outcome data from each study are shown; none of the individual studies showed a significant treatment effect when analyzed by Fisher exact test (not shown). Although each study individually is underpowered, there is a consistent pattern favoring treatment in both nephrotic and non-nephrotic patients. Pooled analyses suggest a clinically and statistically significant treatment effect in nephrotic patients, with relative risk for ESRD of 0.58. The treatment effect was of the same magnitude in non-nephrotic patients, although the group size is smaller and the results were not statistically significant.

Without randomized trials, the problem of treatment selection bias is a major concern and greatly limits the impact of these findings. In this regard, the authors of the North Carolina study carried out proportional hazards analysis and found that when other controlling for relevant clinical factors (age, sex, race, smoking status, use of ACE inhibitors or ARB, entry serum creatinine level, and entry proteinuria), immunosuppressive therapy had no effect on renal survival (1110).

Other Therapies. Several other therapeutic approaches have been tried for therapy-resistant FSGS patients. In an uncontrolled pilot study, the nonsteroidal anti-inflammatory agent meclofenamate reduced urinary protein loss by 40% without decreasing GFR in more than half of the 30 steroid-resistant nephrotic adults studied, 16 of whom had FSGS (1134). The antioxidant vitamin E, 200 IU twice daily, was studied in an open-label study involving 11 therapy-resistant pediatric FSGS patients and was associated with a fall in the mean protein/creatinine ratio from 9.7 to 4.1 (p <0.005) (1135). The antifibrotic agent pirfenidone was also studied in an open-label trial involving 20 adult FSGS patients and was found to slow progressive loss of GFR by 35% (p <0.03) without affecting proteinuria (1136).

Although plasmapheresis has been used to treat recurrent FSGS in patients undergoing transplantation (see Transplantation section, later in this chapter), there is no evidence to support routine use of this treatment in FSGS occurring in native kidneys (1137).

Conservative Therapy. All patients, whether they are receiving immunosuppressive therapy or not, should adhere to a conservative regimen if they have proteinuria (best evidence for this recommendation if proteinuria >1 g/day) or impaired GFR. Blood pressure should be controlled to <130/80 mm Hg as recommended by the Joint National Committee VII (1138). ACE inhibitors and ARB reduce proteinuria and slow progression in both diabetic and nondiabetic nephropathies, and the COOPERATE study demonstrated that the combination was superior to either agent alone in slowing progression a combined endpoint of creatinine doubling or ESRD (1139).

Although certain ACE inhibitor trials have included FSGS among multiple diagnoses (1140), few studies have provided data on substantial numbers of idiopathic FSGS patients (reviewed in [1141]). Stiles et al. retrospectively compared the results in 22 nephrotic adults with idiopathic FSGS, of whom 10 received prednisone at a dose of approximately 1 mg/kg per day for a mean of 4 months (range 1 to 6 months) plus ACE inhibitors and 10 received ACE inhibitors alone (1111). Outcomes were similar, with no CR, and PR occurring in 5 patients and 6 patients, respectively. Proteinuria fell by 33% with glucocorticoids and 65% with ACE inhibitors. The patient population at the Walter Reed Army Medical Center was predominantly young and male and disproportionately (86%) African American. The authors concluded that while the study was too small for definitive conclusions, conservative therapy was not inferior to glucocorticoids in this population. In a small controlled trial, losartan reduced proteinuria from 3.6 to 1.9 g per day in 13 FSGS patients, whereas a control group experienced an increase in proteinuria (1142). Conversely, a retrospective study of 42 African American patients treated with ACE inhibitors, glucocorticoids, both, or neither, was unable to demonstrate a protective effect of ACE inhibitors in delaying progression to ESRD compared to 6 untreated patients (1143).

ACE inhibitors and ARB have a major role to play in postadaptive FSGS. Praga et al. showed that captopril therapy over 12 months reduced proteinuria to greater extent in postadaptive FSGS (associated with reduced nephron mass and reflux nephropathy) compared to idiopathic FSGS (1144). Next Praga and colleagues studied 17 patients with obesity-associated proteinuria (>1 g/day); renal histology obtained from 5 patients documented FSGS in only 2 patients (1145). Captopril therapy in 8 patients lowered proteinuria by 79% (mean 3.4 g/day falling to 0.7 g/day); interestingly, weight loss in 9 patients (mean BMI falling from 37 kg/m^2 to 33 kg/m^2) was associated with a similar fall in proteinuria, by 86% (mean 2.9 g/day falling to 0.4 g/day). Unfortunately, Praga and colleagues subsequently reported that the proteinuria reduction induced by ACE inhibitors is lost after 12 months (845). Still, early treatment with ACE inhibitors appeared to preserve renal function in obesity-associated FSGS, although appropriate controls are lacking.

Current Therapeutic Recommendations. Some experts propose that nephrotic adults with idiopathic FSGS who have preserved renal function and lack prominent contraindications, receive 4 to 6 months of daily therapy with glucocorticoids beginning with prednisone at a dose of 1 mg/kg per day (maximum 80 mg) (1141,1146,1147). Many experts would recommend a dose reduction after 3 to 4 months, particularly for those who have not shown a significant reduction in urine protein. Those who fail 4 to 6 months of daily glucocorticoid therapy are then labeled steroid-resistant and progress to other therapies.

The Nephrology and Hypertension Medical Knowledge Self-Assessment Program expresses reluctance to endorse this aggressive approach in the absence of a controlled trial demonstrating efficacy and safety (1148). Instead, this text recommends, for adults with FSGS and serum creatinine <2.5 mg/dL and <20% interstitial fibrosis area on renal biopsy, a trial of daily prednisone at a dose of 1 mg/kg of ideal body weight (to a maximum dose of 80 mg/day), until CR or *8 weeks* have been reached. In the case of a CR, the recommendation is to prescribe an ~20-week tapering schedule of prednisone on alternate days, tapering at a rate of 20 mg every month. If there is no CR, the recommendation is to reduce the dose to 0.5 mg/kg until a CR or PR or *another 8 weeks* have been reached. If there is a CR or PR, the recommendation is to prescribe an ~20-week tapering schedule of alternate day prednisone, which would require tapering at a rate of 10 mg every other month. If there is no response, the recommendation, is a slow taper involving ~40 *weeks* of alternative-day prednisone while adjunctive therapy (ACE inhibitors or ARB are initiated). Therefore, patients with steroid-resistance would receive 16 weeks of daily prednisone and up to 40 weeks of alternate daily prednisone, for a total dose in an 80-kg person of 7.7 g. Further options during prolonged taper would include cyclosporine for 1 year or oral cyclophosphamide or chlorambucil for 8 to 12 weeks. A newer option that was not included would be mycophenolate mofetil.

Hildebrandt and colleagues noted that that pediatric patients with homozygous or compound heterozygous *NPHS2* mutations appear refractory to glucocorticoids (defined as 6 weeks of therapy) and have only limited responsiveness to cyclosporine (1021). By contrast, *NPHS2* homozygous and compound heterozygous mutations were absent from 124 children with steroid-sensitive nephrotic syndrome. Although these data are not representative of all racial and ethnic groups, it would appear at the present time that immunosuppressive treatment is of limited benefit in children with *NPHS2* homozygous and compound heterozygous mutations.

We have few data about the adult patients with *ACTN4*, *CD2AP*, *TRPC6*, and mtDNA mutations, but it would seem prudent to withhold or limit the duration of immunosuppressive therapy, particularly glucocorticoids. Similarly, FSGS or collapsing glomerulopathy associated with medication is probably best managed by withdrawing the implicated medication and instituting conservative therapy.

It should be noted that there are significant parallels but some differences between the approach to pediatric and adult patients. In particular, the majority of nephrotic children (those age 1 to 9 years) will have received an empirical trial of corticosteroids for 4 to 8 weeks before biopsy, and already been defined as being steroid resistant, albeit by ISKDC criteria rather than by response to the longer course used in adults. This may be appropriate given the relatively aggressive course of classical FSGS often observed in young children. There are many areas of uncertainty where there are no published data to determine the balance between the risks and benefits of immunosuppressive therapy, including the following patient populations:

■ Patients with subnephrotic proteinuria at presentation, especially those with proteinuria <2 g per/day; most experts would not use immunosuppressive therapy
■ Patients who become subnephrotic with therapy with ACE inhibitors, ARB, or the combination, coupled with sodium restriction and blood pressure control to <130/80 mm Hg, particularly those proteinuria falls to <2 g per/day
■ Patients with postadaptive FSGS, with the diagnosis established by compatible history and glomerulomegaly on renal biopsy
■ Patients with idiopathic FSGS who are at significantly increased risk of toxicity associated with glucocorticoid therapy, including with those with obesity (particularly BMI >35 kg/m²), diabetes mellitus or a pre-diabetic state, severe osteoporosis, prominent peptic ulcer diathesis, or advanced age

Novel Therapies. New approaches to therapy may supplement existing medication in one of several ways: (a) agents that induce a durable CR with less toxicity than glucocorticoids and cyclosporine, (b) agents that reduce proteinuria to a greater extent than ACE inhibitors and ARBs, and (c) agents that slow progressive renal scarring in patients who have proven refractory to remittive therapy. In Table 64-24 is provided a nonexhaustive list of 21 agents, including small molecules, peptides, and other biologics, which have shown promise in animal models of glomerulosclerosis, including but not exclusively FSGS, either reducing proteinuria or retarding progression of fibrosis or both (1149–1167). For some agents, further animal testing is required to define efficacy. For other agents, human trials in one or more forms of podocyte disease are probably warranted.

Clinical Course and Outcome

FSGS and collapsing glomerulopathy have the worst prognosis of the common primary nephrotic diseases. Ten-year event rates for reaching a combined endpoint of ESRD or death are as follows: for children, USA study, 21% (410) and Toronto study, 32% (1090), and for adults, Toronto study, ~28% (1090), New Zealand study, 38% (1166), Hong Kong study, 40% (1167), and Chicago study, 43% (ESRD only) for nephrotic patients (compared with 8% for nonnephrotic patients) (1108) (Table 64-25).

It has been known for some time that FSGS patients who enter a CR, even if they experience a relapse, have an excellent chance of renal survival. Recently, Cattran et al. showed that patients who experience a PR (defined as a 50% fall in proteinuria and a fall to <3.5 g/day) have a significantly improved renal survival (Fig. 64-17). These data provide justification for considering the combined response rate (CR plus PR) as well as CR alone in weighing the relative costs and benefits of particular therapeutic approaches.

What clinical factors predict long-term prognosis for renal survival? The conflicting data on the impact of treatment on outcome have been reviewed in the preceding text. In

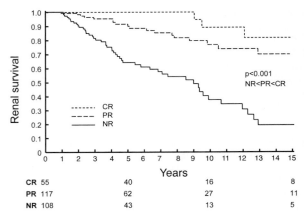

FIGURE 64-17. Long-term renal survival in FSGS by remission status. The fraction of patients with renal function is shown in nephrotic FSGS patients who enter CR (defined as <0.3 g/day) or PR50% (defined as a 50% fall in proteinuria and falling to <3.5 g/day), and those who never reach either remission (NR). (Adapted from: Troyanov S, Wall CA, Miller JA, et al. Focal and segmental glomerulosclerosis: definition and relevance of a partial remission. *J Am Soc Nephrol* 2005;16:1061, with permission.)

Table 64-26 are summarized the findings of 10 studies that have sought clinical and histologic variables that predict long-term renal function. The variables that consistently appear as significant predictors include baseline serum creatinine, baseline proteinuria, and tubulointerstitial damage/fibrosis score. The role of black race has been controversial. Ingulli and Tejani found that among children, progression to ESRD occurred in 78% of blacks and 33% of whites, despite similar baseline serum creatinine and proteinuria values (743). Conversely, Korbet and colleagues have found that in adults the progression rates are similar among blacks (64%) and whites (55%) (1108). They did find that blacks were more likely to be nephrotic at presentation (88% versus 55%). Earlier in the chapter, data were reviewed from nonrandomized controlled studies that treatment may improve renal survival. Thus, patients who enter CR have an excellent outcome, with few developing ESRD on follow-up (1090,1102).

Recurrent FSGS After Renal Transplantation

FSGS recurs following renal transplantation with a frequency that ranges from 15% to 50% depending upon the population, with the average figure cited typically being approximately 25%. When a prior allograft has manifested recurrent FSGS, the risk of recurrence rises to 70% to 80%. Recurrence is heralded by the sudden appearance of heavy proteinuria, often within the first week after transplantation. Renal biopsy obtained within the first few weeks of recurrence uniformly shows extensive foot process effacement without other changes. Subsequent biopsies commonly demonstrate FSGS. Most recurrent FSGS appears within the first 6 months following renal transplantation, as shown in the graphic depiction of data abstracted from 13 reports (1173–1186), and unpublished data kindly provided by Dr. Alok Kalia (Fig. 64-18). FSGS that appears more than 12 months after renal transplantation is typically not considered recurrent FSGS; alternative diagnoses include *de novo* FSGS and FSGS appearing as a manifestation of progressive chronic allograft nephropathy.

In patients with low-level proteinuria originating from their native kidneys, screening for recurrent FSGS may be done via urine dipstick testing performed by the patient (or parents). For those with significant proteinuria from their native kidneys, it is advisable to obtain monthly urine protein/creatinine

TABLE 64-24

NOVEL THERAPIES FOR PROGRESSIVE GLOMERULOSCLEROSIS

Class	Agent	Molecular target or pathway	Animal model	Ref.	Proteinuria	Matrix	Human use
Small molecules	Bosentan	ET_A, ET_B receptor antagonist	Ren-2 transgenic rats	(1149)	Reduced	Reduced	Approved
	Darusentan	ET_A receptor antagonist	Puromycin (rat)	(908)	Reduced	Reduced	IND
	Thiazolidine-diones	PPAR-gamma agonist	Remnant nephron (rat)	(1150)			Approved
	Eplerenone	Mineralocorticoid receptor	Uninephrectomy plus NaCl (rat)	(1151)	Reduced	ND	Approved
	Isotretinoin	Retinoid acid receptor	Thy-1 nephritis (rat)	(1152)	Reduced	Reduced	Approved
	Gefitinib	EGF-receptor tyrosine kinase inhibitor	L-NAME induced hypertension (rat)	(1153)		Reduced	Approved
	Pirfenidone	TGF-β expression? TNF signaling?	Remnant nephron, KIST mouse	(1154)	Reduced	Reduced	IND
	Tranilast	TGF-β antagonist	Remnant nephron	(1155)	Reduced	Reduced	IND
	AVE 7688	ACE and NEP inhibitor	Remnant nephron	(1156)	Reduced	Reduced	Pre-clinical
	CDK inhibitors	Cell cycle	HIV-transgenic mouse	(1157)			Pre-clinical
	Fasudil	Rho-kinase inhibitor	Dahl rat	(1158)	Reduced	Reduced	Pre-clinical
	Prolyl hydroxylase inhibitors	Collagen cross-linking	Chronic allograft nephropathy (mouse)	(1159)	ND	Reduced	Pre-clinical
	BX471	CCR1 antagonist	Adriamycin	(896)	No effect	Reduced	Pre-clinical
Peptides	IFN-γ	Fibroblasts	Remnant nephron	(1160)	Reduced	Reduced	Approved
	Bone morphogenetic protein 7	Possible TGF-β antagonist	COL4A3 null mutation mouse	(1161)	Reduced	Reduced	IND
	Hepatocyte growth factor	Possible TGF-β antagonist	ICGN mouse	(1162)	ND	Reduced	Pre-clinical
	Relaxin	Not defined	Remnant nephron (rat)	(1163)	ND	Reduced	Pre-clinical
	Decorin (proteoglycan)	Binds TGF-β	Thy-1 nephritis	(1164)	ND	ND	Pre-clinical
Monoclonal Ab and others	Etanercept, Infliximab	Binds TNF-α	ND	ND	ND	ND	Approved
	Anti-TGF-β	Binds TGF-β	Puromycin	(1165)	ND	Reduced	IND
	Sulodexide (GAG)	Unknown	ND	ND	ND	ND	IND

Approved denotes approved by the FDA for a nonrenal indication. *IND* denotes under study for any indication under the Investigational New Drug process of the FDA. *CCR1*, chemokine receptor; *CDK*, cyclin-dependent kinase; *ET*, endothelin; *GAG*, glycosaminoglycan; L-*NAME*, NG-nitro-L-arginine methyl-ester; *ND*, no data.

ratios during the first 12 months, and particularly for the first 6 months following renal transplantation. In either case, a significant worsening of proteinuria is an indication for immediate renal biopsy to establish the diagnosis. Response to therapy appears substantially greater if initiated within 2 to 4 weeks of clinical recurrence.

Pretransplantation risk factors for recurrent FSGS include the following: rapid progression of initial disease, typically defined as <3 years from diagnosis to ESRD; age of onset of FSGS between 6 and 15 years; mesangial hyperplasia; white race and recurrent FSGS in a prior renal transplant (1187). The risk of recurrence for individuals with FSGS associated with podocin mutations is controversial. Although an initial report suggested

a higher rate of recurrence (1188), there is now a consensus that the risk of recurrent FSGS in individuals with *NPHS2* mutations is lower than in other patients with FSGS, ranging from 0% (1006) to 8% (1015,1021).

Older studies suggested that living donor transplants may be associated with a higher rate of FSGS recurrence, but recent data suggest that living donor transplants still retain an overall advantage in outcomes for the FSGS patient with ESRD. A review of data from the U.S. Renal Data System (USRDS) found a higher rate of allograft loss due to FSGS recurrence with living donor allografts (19% of graft loss due to recurrence) compared to cadaveric allografts (8% of graft loss due to recurrence), but overall allograft survival remained higher

TABLE 64-25

LONG-TERM OUTCOMES IN FOCAL SEGMENTAL GLOMERULOSCLEROSIS (FSGS)

Location, year	Population	Average observation (yr)	Complete remission	Persistent renal abnormalities	CKD	ESRD	Non-renal death	Lost to follow-up	Reference
North Carolina, 1976	16 children	7 (children)	56%	24%	19%	0%	(6%)	0%	(1168)
	17 adults	3.8 (adults)	0%	0%	76%	24%	0%		
London, 1978	12 children 28 adults	9.5	10%	18%	20%	50%	2%	0%	(720)
Montreal 1981	25 children	7.4	24%	40%	4%	20%	12%	0%	(1169)
USA, 1985	75 children	4.8	11%	37%	23%	21%	0%	8%	(410)
Hong Kong, 1991	2 children 30 adults	6.8	9%	ND	ND	16%	ND	ND	(1167)
Chicago, 1995	81 adults	5.1	ND	ND	ND	17%	ND	ND	(1108)
Toronto, 1998	38 children	11	42%	13%	11%	34%	0%	0%	(1090)
	55 adults		22%	24%	13%	42%	(4%)		
Christchurch, New Zealand, 2000	165 adults	6.9	29%	8%	16%	44%			(1166)

All reports that included at least 30 patients and provided group outcomes after average duration of >4 years are presented in chronologic order. Most patients appear to have had idiopathic FSGS but some reports included a limited number of post-adaptive FSGS or focal global glomerulosclerosis. Children are variously defined as individuals <15–18 yr at the time of initial presentation, depending upon reference. When data are presented for children and adults separately, the data for children are presented first. Chronic kidney disease (CKD) is defined as impaired GFR. The percentage of patients experiencing non-renal deaths is shown in parentheses when these patients are also included in another category. Empty cells indicate that no data were provided from the report.

for living donor allografts (1189). Recipient factors that contribute to increased FSGS recurrence risk include prior recurrence, younger age and white race (1189). Also, there was an increased FSGS recurrence risk with black donor kidney and white recipient.

Posttransplantation risk factors for recurrent FSGS remain controversial; the studies are difficult to interpret in that none are controlled and many rely upon historical controls. Some observers have suggested that recurrence has increased in the recent years and this has been linked to particular lymphocyte depletional therapies. Raafat et al. found that recurrence was greater in patients who receive antilymphocyte serum (53% compared to those who did not (11%) (1178). The Miami group suggests that recurrence rose from 38% to 83% after the introduction of daclizumab (1190).

FSGS Permeability Factor

The rapid recurrence of FSGS following renal transplantation appears to be due to a circulating molecule. Molecular identification has been elusive and the activity has been referred to by various names; we will use the term FSGS permeability factor (FPF). A critical advance was the development by Savin and colleagues of an *in vitro* assay, which relies on the albumin permeability of isolated rat glomeruli as reflected by volume changes induced by an oncotic gradient (1191). There is a correlation between the level of FPF and the likelihood of recurrent FSGS following renal transplantation (1184,1192). FPF is unique to FSGS, being absent from patients with membranous nephropathy and with ESRD due to other causes. Dantal and colleagues developed a variation on Savin's assay. In contrast to the findings of Savin and colleagues, they reported that although FPF levels were higher in FSGS patients with ESRD compared to patients with other causes of ESRD, FPF levels did not predict recurrence of FSGS (1193). The reasons for the discrepant findings might include subtle differences in assay conditions and differences in patient populations. Resolving these discrepancies may not be possible until the molecular

identity of FPF is established. In summary the FPF assay has important limitations: it is laborious; it lacks high specificity, sensitivity, and precision; and it has not been validated by all centers that work with it. Therefore, the assay must be viewed as a research tool, with limited clinical utility to supplement clinical indicators of risk for recurrence FSGS.

FPF is a protein, as shown by sensitivity to proteolytic enzymes and heat (1194). Immunoadsorption of patient plasma using a protein A column reduces proteinuria in recurrent FSGS, which is a characteristic of immunoglobulin, but plasma fractionation to remove immunoglobulin does not remove FPF

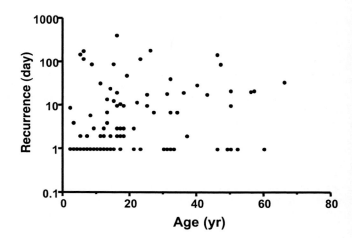

FIGURE 64-18. Timing of FSGS recurrence following renal transplant, correlated with age. Data on the timing of recurrent FSGS and patient age at renal transplantation were available for 101 patients, including 55 children <18 years of age and 46 adults. There was no relationship between age and time to FSGS recurrence (R = 0.01). In 63 cases (62%) recurrent FSGS was diagnosed within one week of renal transplantation.

TABLE 64-26

CLINICAL AND HISTOLOGIC PREDICTORS OF RENAL SURVIVAL IN FOCAL SEGMENTAL GLOMERULOSCLEROSIS (FSGS)

Location, year	N	Population	Analytic approach	Baseline clinical variables	Histologic variables	Reference
London, 1978	40	Children, adults	Univariate analysis	• Proteinuria	None tested	(720)
Rochester, Minnesota, 1983	64	Children, adults	Univariate analysis	• Proteinuria • Serum creatinine	• Tubulointerstitial damage (only severe)	(1170)
Tübingen, Germany, 1990	250	Adults	Multivariate analysis	• Proteinuria	• Tubulointerstitial damage (fibrosis, atrophy)	(1171)
New York, 1991	57	Children	Multivariate analysis	• Serum creatinine • Serum cholesterol	None tested	(743)
Hong Kong, 1991	32	Children, adults	Multivariate analysis	• Serum creatinine	None tested	(1167)
Chicago, 1995	81	Adults	Multivariate analysis	• Serum creatinine • Proteinuria (only when those entering remission were excluded)	None predictive	(1108)
Columbus, Ohio, 1996	49	Adults	Multivariate analysis	• Serum C3 (high normal levels are protective)	• Combined glomerular, tubular, interstitial, and vascular score	(1172)
Christchurch, New Zealand, 1999	111	Children, adults	Multivariate analysis	• Serum creatinine	• Interstitial fibrosis	(1166)
Thessaloniki, Greece, 2000	33	Adult	Multivariate analysis	• Serum creatinine (only nephrotic patients) • Age	• Mesangial sclerosis (only non-nephrotic patients) • Interstitial infiltrates (only non-nephrotic patients)	(1133)
Jackson, Mississippi, 2000	42	Adults	Multivariate analysis	• Serum creatinine	• Interstitial fibrosis • Global glomerulosclerosis	(1143)

Each study shown tested either clinical variables alone or both clinical and histologic variables, using either univariate analysis or multivariate analysis (in the latter case only variables that contributed to the model are shown).

activity (1195). Savin and colleagues have used sequential column chromatography to generate plasma fractions that have increased activity (10,000-fold purification) but these fractions remain complex, with multiple proteins and glycoproteins of <30 kDa (1196,1197). Some of these glycoproteins are absent from normal plasma and from sera following therapeutic plasma exchange. Ghiggheri and colleagues have taken a similar approach and identified a number of proteins (albumin isoforms, vitronectin, fibrinogen gamma chain, fibulin, and mannan-binding lectin-associated serine protease), but have not demonstrated activity *in vivo* (1198). Partially purified fractions are able to induce proteinuria in rats (1199,1200).

There also may be plasma factors that antagonize FPF activity, and it remains possible that recurrent FSGS is due to a deficiency of such a molecular inhibitor. Thus normal serum blocks the activity in the rat glomerulus assay (1201). Ghiggerhi and colleagues confirmed these findings, and reported that inhibitory proteins include the apo allelic variants E2 and E4 and apo J (1202). Nephrotic urine but not normal urine contains inhibitory activity (1203). Pharmacologic inhibitors of FPF activity *in vitro* include cyclosporine, indomethacin, cAMP

analogs, 12-HETE, and serine protease inhibitors (1129,1204–1206).

Therapy of Recurrent FSGS

The recurrence of nephrotic syndrome after renal transplantation is particularly refractory to treatment, and none of the available therapies can be recommend without serious qualifications. Plasma exchange (using either plasma or albumin as replacement solution) or immunoabsorption (using columns bearing ligands such as protein A, which bind immunoglobulins) have been used with limited success. A single course of plasma exchange or immunoabsorption is associated with response rates (CR and PR) of approximately 58% (Table 64-27) (1173,1175–1177,1186,1207,1208). The number of plasma exchange treatments has varied greatly among different centers, and has not been subjected to careful studies. Davenport reviewed the literature and identified 44 recurrent FSGS cases, using a (liberal) definition of response as a 50% fall in proteinuria in 32 patients (73%) (1209). He concluded that optimal apheresis dose was nine treatments, which he proposed

TABLE 64-27

PLASMA EXCHANGE AND IMMUNOADSORPTION THERAPY FOR RECURRENT FOCAL SEGMENTAL GLOMERULOSCLEROSIS (FSGS)

Report	Location	Modality	N	Age (y)	Complete response	Partial response	Prolonged response
Dantal, 1991 (1173)	France	PE	9	A	4	1	1 PR
Artero, 1994 (1186)	Italy	PE	9	P, A	3	3	3CR/2PR
Dantal, 1994 (1195)	France	Adsorption	8	A	2	4	1 CR
Dantal, 1998 (1174)	France	Adsorption	4	A	2	2	0
Andresdottir, 1999 (1175)	The Netherlands	PE	7	A	5	0	3 CR
Greenstein, 2000 (1176)	New York	PE	6	P	5	0	ND
Matalon, 2001 (1177)	New York	PE	13	A	1	1	ND
Shariatmadar, 2002 (1207)	Miami	PE	11	A	5	2	ND
Total			67		27 (40%)	13 (19%)	10 CR (27%) 3 PR (8%)

This table summarizes the studies that used plasma exchange or plasma absorption to treat recurrent FSGS, in studies that treated more than three patients. CR is defined as proteinuria <0.5 g/day and PR is defined as a fall in proteinuria to <2 g/day. *PE*, plasma exchange. Long-term outcome was at ≥1 year following recurrence. Chronic therapy includes that for patients who had subsequent repeat course of PE or who required intermittent, maintenance PE.

be delivered as three daily treatments followed by six treatments delivered on alternate days. Unfortunately, most patients relapse. In some patients, particularly children, a maintenance schedule of plasma modulating therapy may sustain a remission.

The limitations of this approach have led to the empiric use of cyclophosphamide, with or without plasma exchange, in four trials of pediatric patients (Table 64-28) (1181,1183, 1184,1210). The long-term outcome appears to be markedly better than those studies using only plasma exchange or immunoadsorption. This approach has not been reported in adults. Clearly randomized trials are needed before firm conclusions can be reached about either approach.

High-dose cyclosporine has been used in two pediatric trials. Salomon et al. administered intravenous cyclosporine, dose adjusted to achieve trough levels of 250 to 350 ng/mL, and achieved CR in 14 of 17 (82%) of consecutive patients with recurrent FSGS (1211). Plasma exchange was also used in 4 patients. Sustained remission was noted in 11 of 17 (65%) of patients. Raafat et al. administered oral cyclosporine, with the dose increased until proteinuria resolved or nephrotoxicity (rising serum creatinine) was noted (1212). They found that 13 of 16 (81%) of patients entered remission, either CR (11 patients) or PR (2 patients). Cyclosporine doses ranged from 6 to 25 mg/kg per day and cyclosporine trough levels

ranged from 200 to 1000 ng/mL. Remission was sustained in all patients with CR, with conversion to tacrolimus in some patients. Toxicity included hirsutism and gingival hypertrophy in all patients. Although these are intriguing data, more experience is needed, especially in view of the potential toxicity of such high cyclosporine doses; whether adults would tolerate this approach without unacceptable adverse events is unclear.

Prophylactic Therapy to Prevent Recurrent FSGS

Toma and colleagues assigned FSGS ESRD patients to undergo plasma exchange prior to or immediately after renal transplantation (1213). Recurrent FSGS was seen in 4 of 19 treated patients and 9 of 19 in untreated patients. Ohta et al. reported data from 21 patients and compared patients undergoing prophylactic plasma exchange (transplantations from 1991 to publication) with historical controls (transplantation prior to 1991) (1214). Recurrence was seen in 5 of 15 versus 4 of 6 patients. Neither study had sufficient power for a definitive result, and a prospective, adequately powered trial remains to be done. If prophylactic plasma exchange is effective, the mechanism of benefit remains somewhat puzzling. Evidence suggests that the permeability factor returns following plasma exchange; therefore, any benefit from transient reduction would

TABLE 64-28

CYCLOPHOSPHAMIDE, WITH OR WITHOUT PLASMA EXCHANGE, FOR RECURRENT FOCAL SEGMENTAL GLOMERULOSCLEROSIS (FSGS)

Report	Population	Treatment	N	Complete response	Partial response	No response	Long term response	Graft preservation
Cochat, 1993 (1181)	Children	PE + CTX 3 mo	3	3	0	0	3 CR (1 retreatment)	3
Kershaw, 1994 (1183)	Children	CTX 2–3 mo	3	3	0	0	3 CR (1 relapse)	3
Dall'Amico, 1999 (1184)	Children	PE + CTX 2 mo	11	9	0	2	7 CR	7
Cheong, 2000 (1210)	Children	PE + CTX 3 mo	6	3	3	0	2 CR	5
Total			23	18 (78%)	3 (13%)	2 (9%)	15 CR (60%)	18 (78%)

suggest that the factor is particularly injurious in the immediate peritransplantation period.

CONCLUSIONS

From the discussion in this chapter, several conclusions can be drawn regarding the group of diseases under consideration. First, the nephrotic syndrome represents a complex of symptoms resulting from urinary protein loss rather than a disease entity characterized by specific pathology. The abnormalities found include not only the hypoalbuminemia, edema, and hyperlipidemia classically associated with nephrotic syndrome, but also derangements of hemostasis, metabolism, and endocrine function. All of these findings can be attributed to the characteristics and effects of nephrotic proteinuria. Second, we have defined a group of diseases in which the common attribute is that the lesion appears to initiate with the podocyte. In MCN, the restrictive component of the glomerular filtration barrier fails, yet podocyte effacement decreases the area of the GBM that is open to the urinary space, decreasing effective filtration surface area. In FSGS genetic, morphologic and functional data all suggest that podocyte abnormality initiates the disease. Like MCN, there is massive proteinuria, but in contrast to the more benign condition, there is disruption of podocyte architecture. FSGS is accompanied by podocyte injury and depletion, whereas collapsing glomerulopathy manifests podocyte proliferation and capillary collapse. In both cases, these changes are accompanied by the extracellular matrix accumulation that is a hallmark of this disease. Multiple cell types may serve as effector cells for fibrosis, but the common denominator of podocyte involvement suggests that a more appropriate appellation for these diseases might be *podocytopathies* (1215).

A third conclusion relates to the observation that these conditions are characterized by heterogeneity of therapeutic response and prognosis. Although certain subgroups may be associated more often with specific patterns of response to treatment and outcome, such categorizations are not absolute. Most of the patients with MCN and some of those with FSGS are steroid-sensitive. The remaining patients with MCN and a larger proportion of those with FSGS are steroid-resistant. Of particular distinction is the group of patients who have collapsing glomerulopathy. Few of these patients respond to treatment, and the nature of their lesion is so distinctive that we have chosen to consider them as belonging to an entirely separate subgroup of primary nephrotic syndrome. It should be clear that all of the patients having a poor prognosis with regard to long-term renal function are steroid resistant. Moreover, a few patients with MCN, and more with FSGS, particularly those with postadaptive FSGS, may not have nephrotic syndrome. These findings suggest heterogeneity of pathogenetic mechanisms, even within a given histopathologic subgroup.

In view of the differences among MCN, FSGS, and collapsing glomerulopathy, the assumption previously held by many clinicians that patients may move from one disorder to another should be revisited. Collapsing glomerulopathy, the rapidly progressing lesion, appears quite distinct. There are many features that also differentiate MCN from FSGS. These include (a) differences in permselectivity curves, where patients with FSGS demonstrate greater utilization of the shunt pathway (78); (b) association of FSGS with podocyte gene mutations, whereas mutations have not yet been defined for classical MCN (as opposed to congenital nephrotic syndrome); and (c) more clearly defined and more likely irreversible podocyte abnormalities in FSGS. In particular, as technical capability for detecting subtle mutations or polymorphisms in podocyte-specific genes improves, it is likely that mutations will be associated with FSGS with increasing frequency (1019). Therefore, although both MCN and FSGS initiate with a podocyte lesion, the ab-

normalities in FSGS appear more profound, either leading to or reflecting the pathogenetic mechanism(s) of FSGS. Given these differences, it is likely that many, perhaps a great majority, of observations of progression from MCN to FSGS have represented sampling error or early lesion on biopsy.

An unanswered question is the basis for the presently surging incidence of FSGS. Clearly, there is a still-unknown risk factor for progressive renal disease. Hypertension, increasing obesity and perhaps environmental factors may contribute. This interpretation suggests a model in which FSGS is, finally, an idiopathic form of progressive renal disease.

ACKNOWLEDGMENTS

The authors wish to thank Dr. Laura Barisoni's essential insights into the classification scheme for podocyte diseases, Dr. Nader Rifai for suggestions about hyperlipidemia, Dr. Gerard Soff for suggestions about coagulation abnormalities, and Dr. Alok Kalia for sharing unpublished data.

References

1. Arneil GC. The nephrotic syndrome. *Pediatr Clin North Am* 1971;18: 547.
2. International Study of Kidney Disease in Children. A controlled therapeutic trial of cyclophosphamide plus prednisone vs. prednisone alone in children with focal segmental glomerulonephritis (abstract). *Pediatr Res* 1980;14:1006.
3. Glassock RJ. The nephrotic syndrome. *Hosp Pract* 1979;14:105.
4. Seggie J, Davies PG, Ninin D, et al. Patterns of glomerulonephritis in Zimbabwe: survey of disease characterized by nephrotic syndrome. *Q J Med* 1984;53:109.
5. Prathap K, Looi LM. Morphological patterns of glomerular disease in renal biopsies from 1,000 Malaysian patients. *Ann Acad Med Singapore* 1982;11:52.
6. Morgan AG, Shah DJ, Williams W, et al. Proteinuria and glomerular disease in Jamaica. *Clin Nephrol* 1984;21:205.
7. Hendrickse RG, Adenyi A, Edington GM, et al. Quartan malarial nephrotic syndrome. A collaborative clinicopathologic study in Nigerian children. *Lancet* 1972;1:1143.
8. Adu D, Anin-Addo Y, Foli AK, et al. The nephrotic syndrome in Ghana: clinical and pathological aspects. *Q J Med* 1981;50:297.
9. Stokes MB, Markowitz GS, Lin J, et al. Glomerular tip lesion: a distinct entity within the minimal change disease/focal segmental glomerulosclerosis spectrum. *Kidney Int* 2004;65:1690.
10. Haas M, Meehan SM, Karrison TG, et al. Changing etiologies of unexplained adult nephrotic syndrome: a comparison of renal biopsy findings from 1976–1979 and 1995–1997. *Am J Kidney Dis* 1997;30:621.
11. Filler G, Young E, Geier P, et al. Is there really an increase in non-minimal change nephrotic syndrome in children? *Am J Kidney Dis* 2003;42:1107.
12. Rennert WP, Kala UK, Jacobs D, et al. Pulse cyclophosphamide for steroid-resistant focal segmental glomerulosclerosis. *Pediatr Nephrol* 1999;13:113.
13. Simpson LO. Glomerular permeability: an alternate to the pore theory. *Lancet* 1981;ii:251.
14. Edwards A, Deen WM, Daniels BS. Hindered transport of macromolecules in isolated glomeruli. I. Diffusion across intact and cell-free capillaries. *Biophys J* 1997;72:204.
15. Smithies O. Why the kidney glomerulus does not clog: a gel permeation/diffusion hypothesis of renal function. *Proc Natl Acad Sci U S A* 2003;100:4108.
16. Brenner BM, Hostetter TH, Humes HD. Glomerular permselectivity: barrier function based on discrimination of molecular size and charge. *Am J Physiol* 1978;234:F455.
17. Schneeberger EE, Levey RH, McCluskey RT, et al. The isoporous substructures of the human glomerular slit diaphragm. *Kidney Int* 1975;8:48.
18. Schneeberger EE. Glomerular permeability to protein molecules—Its possible structural basis. *Nephron* 1974;13:7.
19. Reiser J, Kriz W, Kretzler M, et al. The glomerular slit diaphragm is a modified adherens junction. *J Am Soc Nephrol* 2000;11:1.
20. Khoshnoodi J, Sigmundsson K, Ofverstedt LG, et al. Nephrin promotes cell-cell adhesion through homophilic interactions. *Am J Pathol* 2003;163:2337.
21. Rodewald R, Karnovsky M. Porous substructure of the glomerular slit diaphragm in the rat and mouse. *J Cell Biol* 1974;60:423.
22. Deen WM, Myers BD, Brenner BM. The glomerular barrier to macromolecules: theoretical and experimental considerations. In: Brenner BM,

Stein JH, eds. *Contemporary issues in nephrology. IX. Nephrotic syndrome*. New York: Churchill Livingstone; 1982:1.

23. Wallenius G. Renal clearance of dextran as a measure of glomerular permeability. *Acta Soc Med Ups* 1954;4(Suppl):1–91.

24. Rennke HG, Venkatachalam MA. Glomerular permeability of macromolecules. Effect of molecular configuration on the fractional clearance of uncharged dextran and neutral horseradish peroxidase in the rat. *J Clin Invest* 1979;63:713.

25. Bridges CR, Rennke HG, Deen WM, et al. Reversible hexadimethrine-induced alterations in glomerular structure and permeability. *J Am Soc Nephrol* 1991;1:1095.

26. Deen WM, Bridges CR, Brenner BM, et al. Heteroporous model of glomerular size selectivity: application to normal and nephrotic humans. *Am J Physiol* 1985;249:F374.

27. Shemesh O, Deen WM, Brenner BM, et al. Effect of colloid volume expansion on glomerular barrier size selectivity in humans. *Kidney Int* 1986;29:916.

28. Alfino PA, Neugarten J, Schacht RG, et al. Glomerular size-selective barrier dysfunction in nephrotoxic serum nephritis. *Kidney Int* 1988;34:151.

29. Loon N, Shemesh O, Morelli E, et al. Effect of angiotensin II infusion on the human glomerular filtration barrier. *Am J Physiol* 1989;257: F608.

30. Golbetz H, Black V, Shemesh O, et al. Mechanism of the antiproteinuric effect of indomethacin in nephrotic humans. *Am J Physiol* 1989;256: F44.

31. Rennke HG, Venkatachalam MA. Glomerular permeability: in vivo tracer studies with polyanionic and polycationic ferritins. *Kidney Int* 1977;11:44.

32. Brenner BM, Hostetter TH, Humes HD. Molecular basis of proteinuria of glomerular origin. *N Engl J Med* 1978;298:826.

33. Mohos SC, Skoza L. Glomerular sialoprotein. *Science* 1969;164:1519.

34. Kanwar YS, Farquhar MG. Anionic sites in the glomerular basement membrane. In vivo and in vitro localization to the laminae rarae by cationic probes. *J Cell Biol* 1979;81:137.

35. Latta H, Johnston WH. The glycoprotein inner layer of glomerular capillary basement membrane as a filtration barrier. *J Ultrastruct Res* 1976;57:65.

36. Latta H, Johnston WH, Stanley TM. Sialoglycoproteins and filtration barriers in the glomerular capillary wall. *J Ultrastruct Res* 1975;51:354.

37. Bohrer MP, Baylis C, Humes HD, et al. Permselectivity of the glomerular capillary wall. Facilitated filtration of circulating polycations. *J Clin Invest* 1978;61:72.

38. Chang RL, Deen WM, Robertson CR, et al. Permselectivity of the glomerular capillary wall: III. Restricted transport of polyanion. *Kidney Int* 1975;8:212.

39. Gudehithlu KP, Pegoraro AA, Dunea G, et al. Degradation of albumin by the renal proximal tubule cells and the subsequent fate of its fragments. *Kidney Int* 2004;65:2113.

40. Eppel GA, Osicka TM, Pratt LM, et al. The return of glomerular-filtered albumin to the rat renal vein. *Kidney Int* 1999;55:1861.

41. Wang SS, Devuyst O, Courtoy PJ, et al. Mice lacking renal chloride channel, CLC-5, are a model for Dent's disease, a nephrolithiasis disorder associated with defective receptor-mediated endocytosis. *Hum Mol Genet* 2000;9:2937.

42. Piwon N, Gunther W, Schwake M, et al. ClC-5 Cl- channel disruption impairs endocytosis in a mouse model for Dent's disease. *Nature* 2000;408:369.

43. Norden AG, Scheinman SJ, Deschodt-Lanckman MM, et al. Tubular proteinuria defined by a study of Dent's (CLCN5 mutation) and other tubular diseases. *Kidney Int* 2000;57:240.

44. Gekle M. Renal tubule albumin transport. *Annu Rev Physiol* 2005;67: 573.

45. Zhai XY, Nielsen R, Birn H, et al. Cubilin- and megalin-mediated uptake of albumin in cultured proximal tubule cells of opossum kidney. *Kidney Int* 2000;58:1523.

46. Christensen EI, Birn H. Megalin and cubilin: Synergistic endocytic receptors in renal proximal tubule. *Am J Physiol Renal Physiol* 2001; 280:F562.

47. Birn H, Fyfe JC, Jacobsen C, et al. Cubilin is an albumin binding protein important for renal tubular albumin reabsorption. *J Clin Invest* 2000;105:1353.

48. Chaudhury C, Mehnaz S, Robinson JM, et al. The major histocompatibility complex-related Fc receptor for IgG (FcRn) binds albumin and prolongs its lifespan. *J Exp Med* 2003;197:315.

49. Robson AM, Cole BR. Pathologic and functional correlations in the glomerulopathies. In: Cummings NB, Michael AF, Wilson CB, eds. *Immune mechanisms in renal disease*. New York: Plenum; 1982:109.

50. Robson AM, Vehaskari VM. The role of charge sites in vascular permeability. In: Brodehl J, Ehrich JH, eds. *Pediatric nephrology*. New York: Springer-Verlag; 1983.

51. Kelley VE, Cavallo T. Glomerular permeability. Ultrastructural studies in New Zealand black/white mice using polyanionic ferritin as a molecular probe. *Lab Invest* 1977;37:265.

52. Scandling JD, Myers BD. Glomerular size-selectivity and microalbuminuria in early diabetic glomerular disease. *Kidney Int* 1992;41:840.

53. Blau EB, Haas JE. Glomerular sialic acid and proteinuria in human renal disease. *Lab Invest* 1973;38:477.

54. Carrie BJ, Salyer WR, Myers BD. Minimal change nephropathy: an electrochemical disorder of the glomerular membranes. *Am J Med* 1981;70:262.

55. Mahan JD, Sisson SP, Vernier RL. Altered glomerular basement membrane (GBM) anionic sites in the minimal change nephrotic syndrome (MCNS) in man (abstract). *Kidney Int* 1985;27:217.

56. Vernier RL, Klein DJ, Sisson SP, et al. Heparan sulfate-rich anionic sites in the human glomerular basement membrane. Decreased concentrations in congenital nephrotic syndrome. *N Engl J Med* 1983;309:1001.

57. Bridges CR, Myers BD, Brenner BM, et al. Glomerular charge alterations in human minimal change nephropathy. *Kidney Int* 1982;22:677.

58. Michael AF, Blau E, Vernier RL. Glomerular polyanion: alteration in aminonucleoside nephrosis. *Lab Invest* 1970;23:649.

59. Blau EB, Michael AF. Rat glomerular glycoprotein composition and metabolism in aminonucleoside nephrosis. *Proc Soc Exp Biol Med* 1972; 141:164.

60. Bohrer MP, Baylis C, Robertson CR, et al. Mechanism of the puromycin-induced defects in the transglomerular passage of water and macromolecules. *J Clin Invest* 1977;60:152.

61. Barnes JL, Radnik RA, Gilchrist EP, et al. Size and charge selective permeability defects induced in glomerular basement membrane by a polycation. *Kidney Int* 1984;25:11.

62. Hunsicker LG, Shearer TP, Shaffer SJ. Acute reversible proteinuria induced by infusion of the polycation hexadimethrine. *Kidney Int* 1981;20:7.

63. Vehaskari VM, Chang CT, Stevens JK, et al. The effect of polycation on vascular permeability in the rat: a proposed role for charge sites. *J Clin Invest* 1984;73:1053.

64. Levin M, Gascoine P, Turner MW, et al. A highly cationic protein in plasma and urine of children with steroid-responsive nephrotic syndrome. *Kidney Int* 1989;36:867.

65. Levin M, Smith C, Walters MD, et al. Steroid-responsive nephrotic syndrome: a generalised disorder of membrane negative charge. *Lancet* 1985;ii:239.

66. Cheung PK, Stulp B, Immenschuh S, et al. Is 100KF an isoform of hemopexin? Immunochemical characterization of the vasoactive plasma factor 100KF. *J Am Soc Nephrol* 1999;10:1700.

67. Cheung PK, Klok PA, Baller JF, et al. Induction of experimental proteinuria in vivo following infusion of human plasma hemopexin. *Kidney Int* 2000;57:1512.

68. Schaeffer RC, Jr, Gratrix ML, Mucha DR, et al. The rat glomerular filtration barrier does not show negative charge selectivity. *Microcirculation* 2002;9:329.

69. Osicka TM, Comper WD. Tubular inhibition destroys charge selectivity for anionic and neutral horseradish peroxidase. *Biochim Biophys Acta* 1998;1381:170.

70. Koltun M, Nikolovski J, Strong KJ, et al. Mechanism of hypoalbuminemia in rodents. *Am J Physiol Heart Circ Physiol* 2005;288:H1604.

71. Osicka TM, Strong KJ, Nikolic-Paterson DJ, et al. Renal processing of serum proteins in an albumin-deficient environment: an in vivo study of glomerulonephritis in the Nagase analbuminaemic rat. *Nephrol Dial Transplant* 2004;19:320.

72. Russo LM, Bakris GL, Comper WD. Renal handling of albumin: a critical review of basic concepts and perspective. *Am J Kidney Dis* 2002;39:899.

73. Deen WM, Lazzara MJ. Glomerular filtration of albumin: how small is the sieving coefficient? *Kidney Int Suppl* 2004;92:S63.

74. Seiler MW, Rennke HG, Venkatachalam MA, et al. Pathogenesis of polycation-induced alterations ("fusion") of glomerular epithelium. *Lab Invest* 1977;36:48.

75. Andrews PM. Glomerular epithelial alterations resulting from sialic acid surface coat removal. *Kidney Int* 1979;15:376.

76. Roy LP, Vernier RL, Michael AF. Effect of protein-load proteinuria on glomerular polyanion. *Proc Soc Exp Biol Med* 1972;141:870.

77. Luke RL. Permselectivity: relation between foot process simplification and macromolecular configuration. *Renal Physiol* 1984;7:129.

78. Winetz JA, Robertson CR, Golbetz HV, et al. The nature of the glomerular injury in minimal change and focal sclerosing glomerulopathies. *Am J Kidney Dis* 1981;1:91.

79. Drummond MC, Kristal B, Myers BD, et al. Structural basis for reduced glomerular filtration capacity in nephrotic humans. *J Clin Invest* 1994;94:1187.

80. Guasch A, Hashimoto H, Sibley RK, et al. Glomerular dysfunction in nephrotic humans with minimal changes or focal glomerulosclerosis. *Am J Physiol* 1991;260:F728.

81. Yoshioka T, Shiraga H, Yoshida Y, et al. "Intact nephrons" as the primary origin of proteinuria in chronic renal disease. Study in the rat model of subtotal nephrectomy. *J Clin Invest* 1988;82:1614.

82. Robson AM, Mor J, Root ER, et al. Mechanism of proteinuria in nonglomerular renal disease. *Kidney Int* 1979;16:416.

83. Yoshioka T, Mitarai T, Kon V, et al. Role for angiotensin II in an overt functional proteinuria. *Kidney Int* 1986;30:538.

84. Yoshioka T, Rennke HG, Salant DJ, et al. Role of abnormally high transmural pressure in the permselectivity defect of glomerular capillary wall: a study in early passive Heymann nephritis. *Circ Res* 1987;61:531.

85. Remuzzi A, Puntorieri S, Battaglia C, et al. Angiotensin converting enzyme inhibition ameliorates glomerular filtration of macromolecules and

water and lessens glomerular injury in the rat. *J Clin Invest* 1990;85: 541.

86. Smoyer WE, Mundel PE, Gupta A, et al. Podocyte alpha-actinin induction precedes foot process effacement in experimental nephrotic syndrome. *Am J Physiol* 1997;273:F150.
87. Gitlin D, Janeway CA, Farr LE. Studies on the metabolism of plasma proteins in the nephrotic syndrome. I. Albumin, g-globulin and iron-binding globulin. *J Clin Invest* 1956;35:44.
88. Galaske RG, Baldamus CA, Stolte H. Plasma protein handling in the rat kidney: micropuncture experiments in the acute heterologous phase of anti-GBM nephritis. *Pfluegers Arch* 1978;375:269.
89. Jensen H, Rossing N, Andersen SB, et al. Albumin metabolism in the nephrotic syndrome in adults. *Clin Sci* 1967;33:445.
90. Walker WA, Lowman JT, Hong RA. Measuring albumin turnover rates in patients with hypoproteinemia. *Am J Dis Child* 1973;125:51.
91. Dulaney JT, Hatch FE, Jr. Peritoneal dialysis and loss of protein: a review. *Kidney Int* 1984;26:253.
92. Jaffa AA, Harvey JN, Sutherland SE, et al. Renal kallikrein responses to dietary protein: a possible mediator of hyperfiltration. *Kidney Int* 1989;36:1003.
93. Mizuiri S, Hayashi I, Ozawa T, et al. Effects of an oral protein load on glomerular filtration rate in healthy controls and nephrotic patients. *Nephron* 1988;48:101.
94. Kaysen GA, Gambertoglio J, Jimenez I, et al. Effect of dietary protein intake on albumin homeostasis in nephrotic patients. *Kidney Int* 1986;29:572.
95. Kaysen GA, Jones HJ, Hutchison FN. High protein diets stimulate albumin synthesis at the site of albumin mRNA transcription. *Kidney Int* 1989;36:S168.
96. Kaysen GA, Jones HJ, Martin V, et al. A low-protein diet restricts albumin synthesis in nephrotic rats. *J Clin Invest* 1990;83:1623.
97. Don BR, Wada L, Kaysen GA, et al. Effect of dietary protein restriction and angiotensin converting enzyme inhibition on protein metabolism in the nephrotic syndrome. *Kidney Int* 1989;36(Suppl 27):S163.
98. Hutchison FN, Schambelan M, Kaysen GA. Modulation of albuminuria by dietary protein and converting enzyme inhibition. *Am J Physiol* 1987;253:F719.
99. Hutchison FN, Martin VI, Jones HJ, et al. Differing actions of dietary protein and enalapril on renal function and proteinuria. *Am J Physiol* 1990;258:F126.
100. Starling EH. On the absorption of fluids from the connective tissue space. *J Physiol (Lond.)* 1986;19:312.
101. Robson AM. Edema and edema-forming states. In: Klahr S, ed. *The kidney and body fluids in health and disease.* New York: Plenum; 1983: 119.
102. Landis EM, Pappenheimer JR. Exchange of substances through the capillary walls. In: Hamilton WF, Dow P, eds. *Handbook of Physiology, Section Z, Circulation* Washington, DC: American Physiological Society; 1963:961.
103. Schrier RW, Fassett RG. A critique of the overfill hypothesis of sodium and water retention in the nephrotic syndrome. *Kidney Int* 1998;53:1111.
104. Bohlin AB. Clinical course and renal function in minimal change nephrotic syndrome. *Acta Paediatr Scand* 1984;73:631.
105. Bohlin AB, Berg U. Renal water handling in minimal change nephrotic syndrome. *Int J Pediatr Nephrol* 1984;2:93.
106. Bohlin AB, Berg U. Renal sodium handling in minimal change nephrotic syndrome. *Arch Dis Child* 1984;59:825.
107. Johnson AK, Mann JFE, Rascher W, et al. Plasma angiotensin II concentrations and experimentally induced thirst. *Am J Physiol* 1981;240:R229.
108. Kaysen GA, Paukert TT, Menke DJ, et al. Plasma volume expansion is necessary for edema formation in the rat with Heymann nephritis. *Am J Physiol* 1985;248:F247.
109. Keller H, Morell A, Noseda G, et al. Analbuminamie Pathophysiologische Untersuchungen an einem Fall. *Schweiz Med Wochenschr* 1972;102:71.
110. Usberti M, Federico S, Meccariello S, et al. Role of plasma vasopressin in the impairment of water excretion in nephrotic syndrome. *Kidney Int* 1984;25:422.
111. Geers AB, Koomans HA, Roos JC, et al. Functional relationships in the nephrotic syndrome. *Kidney Int* 1984;26:324.
112. Eisenberg S. Blood volume in persons with the nephrotic syndrome. *Am J Med Sci* 1968;255:320.
113. Dorhout Mees EJ, Roos JC, Boer P, et al. Observations on edema formation in the nephrotic syndromes in adults with minimal lesion. *Am J Med* 1979;67:378.
114. Oliver WJ. Physiologic responses associated with steroid-induced diuresis in the nephrotic syndrome. *J Lab Clin Med* 1963;62:449.
115. Lewis DM, Tooke JE, Beaman M, et al. Peripheral microvascular parameters in the nephrotic syndrome. *Kidney Int* 1998;54:1261.
116. Meltzer JI, Keim HJ, Laragh JH, et al. Nephrotic syndrome: vasoconstriction and hypervolemia types indicated by renin-sodium profiling. *Ann Intern Med* 1979;91:688.
117. Garnett ES, Webber CE. Changes in blood-volume produced by treatment of the nephrotic syndrome. *Lancet* 1967;ii:798.
118. Fleck A, Raines G, Hawker F. Increased vascular permeability: a major cause of hypoalbuminemia in disease and injury. *Lancet* 1985;ii:781.
119. Vehaskari VM, Robson AM. The nephrotic syndrome in children. *Ann Pediatr* 1981;10:42.
120. Koomans HA, Braam B, Geers AB, et al. The importance of plasma protein for blood volume and blood pressure homeostasis. *Kidney Int* 1986;30:730.
121. Warren JV, Merrill AJ, Stead EA, Jr. Role of extracellular fluid in maintenance of normal plasma volume. *J Clin Invest* 1943;22:635.
122. Metcoff J, Janeway CA. Studies on the pathogenesis of nephrotic edema. *J Pediatr* 1961;58:640.
123. Luetscher JA, Jr. Johnson BB. Chromatographic separation of the sodium-retaining corticoid from the urine of children with nephrotic syndrome, compared with observations in normal children. *J Clin Invest* 1954;33:276.
124. Paller MS, Schrier RW. Pathogenesis of sodium and water retention in edematous disorders. *Am J Kidney Dis* 1982;2:241.
125. Shapiro M, Hasbargen J, Cosby R, et al. Role of aldosterone in the Na retention of patients with nephrotic syndrome. *Am J Nephrol* 1990;10: 44.
126. Nochy D, Barres D, Camilleri JP, et al. Abnormalities of renin-containing cells in human glomerular and vascular renal diseases. *Kidney Int* 1983;23:375.
127. Brown EA, Markandu ND, Roulston JE. Is the renin-angiotensin system involved in the sodium retention in the nephrotic syndrome? *Nephron* 1982;32:102.
128. Krishna GG, Danovitch GM. Effects of water immersion and renal function in the nephrotic syndrome. *Kidney Int* 1982;21:395.
129. Epstein EH. Underfilling vs. overflow in hepatic ascites. *N Engl J Med* 1982;307:1577.
130. Raij L, Keane WF, Leonard A, et al. Irreversible acute renal failure in idiopathic nephrotic syndrome. *Am J Med* 1976;61:207.
131. Oliver WJ, Kelsch RC, Chandler JP. Demonstration of increased catecholamine excretion in the nephrotic syndrome. *Proc Soc Exp Biol Med* 1967;125:1176.
132. Fernandez-Llama P, Andrews P, Nielsen S, et al. Impaired aquaporin and urea transporter expression in rats with adriamycin-induced nephrotic syndrome. *Kidney Int* 1998;53:1244.
133. Apostol E, Ecelbarger CA, Terris J, et al. Reduced renal medullary water channel expression in puromycin aminonucleoside—induced nephrotic syndrome. *J Am Soc Nephrol* 1997;8:15.
134. Garin EH, Donnelly WH, Geary D, et al. Nephrotic syndrome and diffuse mesangial proliferative glomerulonephritis in children. *Am J Dis Child* 1983;137:109.
135. Arisz I, Donker AJ, Brentjens JR, et al. The effect of indomethacin on proteinuria and kidney function in the nephrotic syndrome. *Acta Med Scand* 1976;199:121.
136. Gutierrez Millet V, Ruilope LM, Alcazar JM, et al. Effect of indomethacin administration upon renal function, proteinuria, renin-angiotensin-aldosterone axis, and urinary prostaglandin E2 in nephrotic syndrome. *Kidney Int* 1982;22:213.
137. Needleman P, Adams SP, Cole BR, et al. Atriopeptins as cardiac hormones. *Hypertension* 1985;7:469.
138. Tulassay T, Rascher W, Lang RE, et al. Atrial natriuretic peptide and other vasoactive hormones in nephrotic syndrome. *Kidney Int* 1987;31:1391.
139. Rodriguez-Iturbe B, Colic D, Parra G, et al. Atrial natriuretic factor in the acute nephritic and nephrotic syndromes. *Kidney Int* 1990;38: 512.
140. Perico N, Delaini F, Lupini C, et al. Blunted excretory response to atrial natriuretic peptide in experimental nephrosis. *Kidney Int* 1989;36: 5764.
141. Perico N, Delaini F, Lupini C, et al. Renal response to atrial peptides is reduced in experimental nephrosis. *Am J Physiol* 1987;252: F654.
142. Zietse R, Schalekamp MA. Effect of synthetic human atrial natriuretic peptide (102–126) in nephrotic humans. *Kidney Int* 1988;34:717.
143. Peterson C, Madsen B, Perlman A, et al. Atrial natriuretic peptide and the renal response to hypervolemia in nephrotic humans. *Kidney Int* 1988;34:825.
144. Epstein M, Loutzenhiser R, Friedland E, et al. Relationship of increased plasma atrial natriuretic factor and renal sodium handling during immersion-induced central hypervolemia in normal humans. *J Clin Invest* 1987;79:738.
145. Rabelink TJ, Koomans HA, Boer P, et al. Role of ANP in natriuresis of head-out immersion in humans. *Am J Physiol* 1989;257:375.
146. Ichikawa I, Rennke HG, Hoyer JR, et al. Role for intrarenal mechanisms in the impaired salt excretion of experimental nephrotic syndrome. *J Clin Invest* 1983;71:91.
147. Robson AM, Giangiacomo J, Kienstra RA, et al. Normal glomerular permeability and its modification by minimal change nephrotic syndrome. *J Clin Invest* 1974;54:1190.
148. Berg U, Bohlin AB. Renal hemodynamics in minimal change nephrotic syndrome in childhood. *Int J Pediatr Nephrol* 1982;3:187.
149. Bohman SO, Jeremko G, Bohlin AB, et al. Foot process fusion and glomerular filtration rate in minimal change nephrotic syndrome. *Kidney Int* 1984;25:696.

150. Kuroda S, Aynedjian HS, Bank N. A micropuncture study of renal sodium retention nephrotic syndrome in rats: evidence for increases resistance to tubular fluid flow. *Kidney Int* 1979;16:561.

151. Sakai T, Harris FH, Jr, Marsh DJ, et al. Extracellular fluid expansion and autoregulation in nephrotoxic serum nephritis in rats. *Kidney Int* 1984; 25:619.

152. Löwenborg EK, Berg UB. Influence of serum albumin on renal function in nephrotic syndrome. *Pediatr Nephrol* 1999;13:19.

153. Drumond MC, Kristal B, Myers BD, et al. Structural basis for reduced glomerular filtration capacity in nephrotic humans. *J Clin Invest* 1994;94:1187.

154. Powell HR. Relationship between proteinuria and epithelial cell changes in minimal lesion glomerulopathy. *Nephron* 1976;16:310.

155. Koop K, Eikmans M, Baelde HJ, et al. Expression of podocyte-associated molecules in acquired human kidney diseases. *J Am Soc Nephrol* 2003;14:2063.

156. van den Berg JG, van den Bergh Weerman MA, Assmann KJ, et al. Podocyte foot process effacement is not correlated with the level of proteinuria in human glomerulopathies. *Kidney Int* 2004;66:1901.

157. Dash SC, Molhotra KK, Sharma RK, et al. Reversible acute renal failure in idiopathic nephrotic syndrome with minimal change nephropathy. *J Assoc Physicians India* 1982;30:399.

158. Sjoberg RJ, McMillan VM, Bartram LS, et al. Renal failure with minimal change nephrotic syndrome: reversal with hemodialysis. *Clin Nephrol* 1983;20:98.

159. Steele BT, Bacheyie GS, Baumal R, et al. Acute renal failure of short duration in minimal lesion nephrotic syndrome of childhood. *Int J Pediatr Nephrol* 1982;3:59.

160. Vande Walle J, Mauel R, Raes A, et al. ARF in children with minimal change nephrotic syndrome may be related to functional changes of the glomerular basal membrane. *Am J Kidney Dis* 2004;43:399.

161. Whelton A. Renal and related cardiovascular effects of conventional and COX-2-specific NSAIDs and non-NSAID analgesics. *Am J Ther* 2000;7:63.

162. Hulter HN, Bonner EL, Jr. Lipoid nephrosis appearing as acute oliguric renal failure. *Arch Intern Med* 1980;140:403.

163. Editorial. More about minimal change. *Lancet* 1981;1:1298.

164. Lowenstein J, Schacht RG, Baldwin DS. Renal failure in minimal change nephrotic syndrome. *Am J Med* 1981;70:227.

165. Yamauchi H, Hopper J, Jr. Hypovolemic shock and hypotension as a complication in the nephrotic syndrome: Report of ten cases. *Ann Intern Med* 1964;60:242.

166. Epstein AA. The nature and treatment of chronic parenchymatous nephritis (nephrosis). *JAMA* 1917;69:444.

167. Baxter JH, Goodman HC, Havel RJ. Serum lipid and lipoprotein alterations in nephrosis. *J Clin Invest* 1960;39:455.

168. Bernard DB. Metabolic abnormalities in nephrotic syndrome: pathophysiology and complications. In: Brenner BM, Stein JH, eds. *Contemporary Issues in Nephrology. IX. Nephrotic syndrome*. New York: Churchill Livingstone; 1982:85.

169. Baxter JH. Hyperlipoproteinemia in nephrosis. *Arch Intern Med* 1962; 109:742.

170. Zilleruelo G, Hsia SL, Freundlich M, et al. Persistence of serum lipid abnormalities in children with ideopathic nephrotic syndrome. *J Pediatr* 1984;104:61.

171. Joven J, Vilella E. Hyperlipidaemia of the nephrotic syndrome—the search for a nephrotic factor. *Nephrol Dial Transplant* 1995;10:314.

172. Chopra JS, Mallick NP. Hyperlipoproteinemias in the nephrotic syndrome. *Lancet* 1971;1:317.

173. Newmark SR, Anderson CF, Donadio JV, et al. Lipoprotein profiles in adult nephrotics. *Mayo Clin Proc* 1975;50:359.

174. Oetliker OH, Mordasini R, Lutschg J, et al. Lipoprotein metabolism in nephrotic syndrome in childhood. *Pediatr Res* 1980;14:64.

175. Michaeli J, Bar-On H, Shafrir EL. Lipoprotein profiles in a heterogeneous group of patients with nephrotic syndrome. *Isr J Med Sci* 1981;17: 1001.

176. Cameron JS, Wass V, Jarrett RJ, et al. Nephrotic syndrome and cardiovascular disease. *Lancet* 1979;2:1017.

177. Ohta T, Matsuda I. Lipid and apolipoprotein levels in patients with nephrotic syndrome. *Clin Chim Acta* 1981;117:133.

178. Chan MK, Persuad JW, Ramdial L, et al. Hyperlipidemia in untreated nephrotic syndrome, increased production or decreased removal? *Clin Chim Acta* 1981;117:317.

179. Gherardi E, Rota E, Calandra S, et al. Relationship among the concentrations of serum lipoproteins and changes in their chemical composition in patients with untreated nephrotic syndrome. *Eur J Clin Invest* 1977;7:563.

180. Rifai N. Lipoproteins and apolipoproteins: Composition, metabolism, and association with coronary heart disease. *Arch Pathol Lab Med* 1986;110:694.

181. Kaysen GA. Hyperlipidemia in the nephrotic syndrome. *Am J Kidney Dis* 1988;12:548.

182. Marsh JB, Sparks CE. Hepatic secretion of lipoproteins in the rat and the effect of experimental nephrosis. *J Clin Invest* 1979;64:1229.

183. Marsh JB, Sparks CE. Lipoproteins in experimental nephrosis: plasma levels and composition. *Metabolism* 1979;28:1040.

184. Kekki M, Nikkila EA. Plasma triglyceride metabolism in the adult nephrotic syndrome. *Eur J Clin Invest* 1971;1:345.

185. Velden MG, Kaysen GA, Barrett HA, et al. Increased VLDL in nephrotic patients results from decreased catabolism while increased LDL results from increased synthesis. *Kidney Int* 1998;53:994.

186. Appel GB, Blum CB, Chien S, et al. The hyperlipidemia of the nephrotic syndrome. Relation to plasm albumin concentration, oncotic pressure and viscosity. *N Engl J Med* 1985;312:1544.

187. deMendoza SG, Kashyap ML, Chen CY, et al. High density lipoproteinuria in nephrotic syndrome. *Metabolism* 1976;25:1143.

188. Davis RA, Engelhorn SC, Weinstein DB, et al. Very low density lipoprotein secretion by cultured rat hepatocytes. Inhibition by albumin and other macromolecules. *J Biol Chem* 1980;255:2039.

189. Yedgar S, Weinstein DB, Patsch W, et al. Vicosity of culture medium as a regulation of synthesis and secretion of very low density lipoproteins by cultured hepatocytes. *J Biol Chem* 1982;257:2188.

190. Golper TA, Swartz SH. Impaired renal mevalonate metabolism in nephrotic syndrome: A stimulus for increased hepatic cholesterogenesis independent of GFR and hypoalbuminemia. *Metabolism* 1982;31:471.

191. Golper TA, Feingold KR, Fulford MH, et al. The role of circulating mevalonate in nephrotic hypercholesterolemia. *J Lipid Res* 1986;27: 1044.

192. Grundy SM. Management of hyperlipidemia of kidney disease. *Kidney Int* 1990;37:847.

193. Joven J, Villabona C, Vilella E, et al. Abnormalities of lipoprotein metabolism in patients with the nephrotic syndrome. *N Engl J Med* 1990;323:579.

194. Warwick GL, Caslake MJ, Boulton-Jones JM, et al. Low-density lipoprotein metabolism in the nephrotic syndrome. *Metabolism* 1990;39:187.

195. Moorehead JF, Wheeler DC, Varghese Z. Glomerular structures and lipids in progressive renal disease. *Am J Med* 1989;87:12N.

196. Wanner C, Kramer-Guth A, Nauck M, et al. Cholesterol metabolism in glomerular cells: effect of lipoproteins from nephrotic patients. *Miner Elect Metab* 1996;22:39.

197. Joven J, Vilella E. The influence of apoprotein epsilon 2 homozygosity on nephrotic hyperlipidemia. *Clin Nephrol* 1997;48:141.

198. Cohen L, Cramp DG, Lewis AD, et al. The mechanism of hyperlipidemia in nephrotic syndrome—Role of low albumin and the LCAT reaction. *Clin Chim Acta* 1980;104:393.

199. Yamada M, Matsuda I. Lipoprotein lipase in clinical and experimental nephrosis. *Clin Chim Acta* 1970;30:787.

200. Garber DW, Gottleib BA, Marsh JB, et al. Catabolism of very low density lipoproteins in experimental nephrosis. *J Clin Invest* 1984;74:1375.

201. Sestak TL, Alavi N, Subbaiah PV. Plasma lipids and acyltransferase activities in experimental nephrotic syndrome. *Kidney Int* 1989;36:240.

202. Fielding CJ. Human lipoprotein lipase inhibition of activity by cholesterol. *Biochim Biophys Acta* 1970;218:221.

203. Gitlin D, Cornwell DG, Nakasato D, et al. Studies on the metabolism of plasma proteins in the nephrotic syndrome. II. The lipoproteins. *J Clin Invest* 1958;37:172.

204. Fielding CJ, Shore VG, Fielding PE. Lecithin: cholesterol acyltransferase: Effects of substrate upon enzyme activity. *Biochim Biophys Acta* 1972;270:513.

205. Dixit VM, Hettiaratchi ES. The mechanism of hyperlipidemia in the nephrotic syndrome. *Med Hypotheses* 1979;5:1327.

206. Rosenman RH, Byers SO, Friedman M. Plasma lipid interrelationships in experimental nephrosis. *J Clin Invest* 1957;36:1558.

207. Rosenman RH, Friedman M. In vivo studies of the roles of albumin in endogenous heparin-activated lipaemia clearing in nephrotic rats. *J Clin Invest* 1957;36:700.

208. Kaysen GA, Gambertoglio J, Felts J, et al. Albumin synthesis, albuminuria and hyperlipemia in nephrotic patients. *Kidney Int* 1987;31: 1368.

209. Davies RW, Staprans I, Hutchison FN, et al. Proteinuria, not altered albumin metabolism, affects hyperlipidemia in the nephrotic rat. *J Clin Invest* 1990;86:600.

210. Felts JM, Mayerle JA. Urinary loss of plasma high density lipoprotein—A possible cause of hyperlipidemia in the nephrotic syndrome. *Circulation* 1974;49/50(Suppl III):263.

211. Gherardi E, Vecchia L, Calandra S. Experimental nephrotic syndrome in the rat induced by puromycin aminonucleoside. Plasma and urinary lipoproteins. *Exp Mol Pathol* 1980;32:128.

212. Lopes-Virella M, Virella G, Debeukelaer M, et al. Urinary high density lipoprotein in minimal change glomerular disease and chronic glomerulopathies. *Clin Chim Acta* 1979;94:73.

213. Kashyap ML, Srivastava LS, Hynd BA. Apolipoprotein C-II and lipoprotein lipase in human nephrotic syndrome. *Atherosclerosis* 1980;35:29.

214. Kallen RJ, Brynes RK, Aronson AJ, et al. Premature coronary atherosclerosis in a 5-year-old with corticosteroid-refractory nephrotic syndrome. *Am J Dis Child* 1977;131:976.

215. Alexander JH, Schapel GJ, Edwards DG. Increased incidence of coronary heart disease associated with combined elevation of serum triglyceride and cholesterol concentrations in the nephrotic syndrome in man. *Med J Aust* 1974;2:119.

216. Berlyne GM, Mallick NP. Ischaemic heart disease as a complication of nephrotic syndrome. *Lancet* 1969;ii:399.

217. Wass VJ, Jarrett RJ, Chilvers C, et al. Does the nephrotic syndrome increase the risk of cardiovascular disease? *Lancet* 1979;ii:664.

218. Bass JE, Fisher EA, Prack MM, et al. Macrophages from nephrotic rats regulate apolipoprotein E biosynthesis and cholesterol content independently. *J Clin Invest* 1991;87:470.

219. Nakahara C, Kobayashi K, Hamaguchi H, et al. Plasma lipoprotein (a) levels in children with minimal lesion nephrotic syndrome. *Pediatr Nephrol* 1999;13:657.

220. Gilboa N. Incidence of coronary heart disease associated with the nephrotic syndrome. *Med J Aust* 1976;1:207.

221. Vosnides G, Cameron JS. Hyperlipidemia in renal disease (letter). *Med J Aust* 1974;2:855.

222. Mallick NP, Short CD. The nephrotic syndrome and ischaemic heart disease. *Nephron* 1981;27:54.

223. Wass VJ, Cameron JS. Cardiovascular disease and the nephrotic syndrome: The other side of the coin. *Nephron* 1981;27:58.

224. Diamond JR, Karnovsky MJ. Focal and segmental glomerulosclerosis: Analogies to atherosclerosis. *Kidney Int* 1988;33:917.

225. Kasiske BL, O'Donnell MP, Garvis WJ, et al. Pharmacologic treatment of hyperlipidemia reduces glomerular injury in rat 5/6 nephrectomy model of chronic renal failure. *Circulation Res* 1988;62:367.

226. Kasiske BL, O'Donnell MP, Lee H, et al. Impact of dietary fatty acid supplementation in obese Zucker rats. *Kidney Int* 1991;39:1125.

227. Harris KP, Purkerson ML, Yates J, et al. Lovastatin ameliorates the development of glomerulosclerosis and uremia in experimental nephrotic syndrome. *Am J Kidney Dis* 1990;15:16.

228. Querfeld U. Should hyperlipidemia in children with the nephrotic syndrome be treated? *Pediatr Nephrol* 1999;13:77.

229. Grundy SM, Vega GL. Rationale and management of hyperlipidemia of the nephrotic syndrome. *Am J Med* 1989;87:3N.

230. Kaplan R, Aynedjian HS, Schlondorff D, et al. Renal vasoconstriction caused by short-term cholesterol feeding is corrected by thromboxane antagonist or probucol. *J Clin Invest* 1990;86:1707.

231. Querfeld U, Kohl B, Fiehn W, et al. Probucol for treatment of hyperlipidemia in persistent childhood nephrotic syndrome. Report of a prospective uncontrolled multicenter study. *Pediatr Nephrol* 1999;13:7.

232. Groggel GC, Cheung AK, Ellis-Benigni K, et al. Treatment of nephrotic hyperlipoproteinemia with gemfibrozil. *Kidney Int* 1989;36:266.

233. Golper TA, Illingworth R, Morris CD, et al. Lovastatin in the treatment of multifactorial hyperlipidemia. *Am J Kidney Dis* 1989;13:312.

234. Vega GL, Grundy SM. Lovastatin therapy in nephrotic hyperlipidemia: Effects on lipoprotein metabolism. *Kidney Int* 1988;33:1160.

235. Aguilar-Salinas CA, Barrett PH, Kelber J, et al. Physiologic mechanisms of action of lovastatin in nephrotic syndrome. *J Lipid Res* 1995;36:188.

236. Valdivielso P, Moliz M, Valera A, et al. Atorvastatin in dyslipidaemia of the nephrotic syndrome. *Nephrology (Carlton)* 2003;8:61.

237. Addis T. *Glomerular Nephritis, Diagnosis and Treatment.* New York: MacMillan; 1948:216.

238. Egli F, Eiminger P, Stalder G. Thromboembolism in the nephrotic syndrome. *Pediatr Res* 1974;8:903.

239. Llach FH. Hypercoagulability, renal vein thrombosis, and thrombotic complications of nephrotic syndrome. *Kidney Int* 1985;28:429.

240. Cameron JS. Coagulation and thromboembolic complications in the nephrotic syndrome. *Adv Nephrol* 1984;13:75.

241. Sung SF, Jeng JS, Yip PK, et al. Cerebral venous thrombosis in patients with nephrotic syndrome—case reports. *Angiology* 1999;40:427.

242. Jones CL, Hebert D. Pulmonary thrombo-embolism in the nephrotic syndrome. *Pediatr Nephrol* 1991;5:56.

243. Apostol EL, Kher KK. Cavitating pulmonary infarction in nephrotic syndrome. *Pediatr Nephrol* 1994;8:347.

244. Wagoner RD, Stanson AW, Holley KE. Renal vein thrombosis in idiopathic membranous glomerulopathy and nephrotic syndrome. Incidence and significance. *Kidney Int* 1983;23:368.

245. Cade R, Spooner G, Juncos L, et al. Chronic renal vein thrombosis. *Am J Med* 1977;63:387.

246. Lewy PR, Jao W. Nephrotic syndrome in association with renal vein thrombosis in infancy. *J Pediatr* 1974;85:359.

247. Llach F, Arieff AI, Massry SG. Renal vein thrombosis and nephrotic syndrome: a prospective study of 36 adult patients. *Ann Intern Med* 1975;83:8.

248. Kanfer A. Coagulation factors in nephrotic syndrome. *Am J Nephrol* 1990;10(Suppl 1):63.

249. De Mattia D, Penza R, Giordano P, et al. Thromboembolic risk in children with nephrotic syndrome. *Hemostasis* 1991;21:300.

250. Tracy M, Baja Z. Surface markers of platelet function in idiopathic nephrotic syndrome in children. *Pediatr Nephrol* 2002;17:673.

251. Richman AV, Kasnic G, Jr. Endothelial and platelet reactions in the idiopathic nephrotic syndrome: an ultrastructural study. *Hum Pathol* 1982;13:548.

252. Adler AJ, Lundin AP, Feinroth MV, et al. β–Thromboglobulin levels in the nephrotic syndrome. *Am J Med* 1980;69:551.

253. Andrassy K, Depperman D, Ritz E, et al. Different effects of renal failure on beta-thromboglobulin and high affinity platelet factor 4 (HA-PF4) concentrations. *Thromb Res* 1980;18:469.

254. Svetlov SI, Moskaleva ES, Pinelas VG, et al. Decreased intraplatelet Ca^{2+} release and ATP secretion in pediatric nephrotic syndrome. *Pediatr Nephrol* 1999;13:205.

255. Kuhlmann U, Steurer J, Rhyner K, et al. Platelet aggregation and beta thromboglobulin levels in nephrotic patients with and without thrombosis. *Clin Nephrol* 1981;15:229.

256. Carvalho A, Colman R, Lees R. Platelet function in hyperlipoproteinemia. *N Engl J Med* 1974;290:434.

257. Yoshida A, Aoki N. Release of arachidonic acid from human platelets. A key role for the potentiation of platelet aggregating ability in normal subjects as well as in those with nephrotic syndrome. *Blood* 1978;52:969.

258. Jorgensen KA, Stofferson E. On the inhibitory effect of albumin on platelet aggregation. *Thromb Res* 1980;17:13.

259. Schieppati A, Dodesini P, Benigni A, et al. The metabolism of arachidonic acid by platelets in nephrotic syndrome. *Kidney Int* 1984;25:671.

260. Pepper DS, Jamieson GA. Studies on glycoproteins. III. Isolation of sialoglycopeptides from human platelet membranes. *Biochemistry* 1969;8:3362.

261. George JN, Nurden AT, Phillips DR. Molecular defects in interactions of platelets with the vessel wall. *N Engl J Med* 1984;311:1084.

262. Vaziri ND, Gonzales EC, Shayestehfar B, et al. Plasma levels and urinary excretion of fibrinolytic and protease inhibitory proteins in nephrotic syndrome. *J Lab Clin Med* 1994;124:118.

263. Alkjaersig N, Fletcher AP, Narayanan M, et al. Course and resolution of the coagulopathy in nephrotic children. *Kidney Int* 1987;31:772.

264. Vaziri ND, Ngo JC, Ibsen KH, et al. Deficiency and urinary loss of factor XII in nephrotic syndrome. *Nephron* 1982;32:342.

265. Kanfer A, Kleinknecht D, Broyer M, et al. Coagulation studies in 45 cases of nephrotic syndrome without uremia. *Thromb Diathes Haemorrh* 1970;24:562.

266. Kendall AG. Nephrotic syndrome: a hypercoagulable state. *Arch Intern Med* 1971;127:1021.

267. Coppola R, Guerra L, Ruggeri ZM, et al. Factor VIII/von Willebrand factor in glomerular nephropathies. *Clin Nephrol* 1981;16:217.

268. Thomson C, Forbes CD, Prentice CR, et al. Changes in blood coagulation and fibrinolysis in the nephrotic syndrome. *Q J Med* 1974;43:399.

269. Thaler E, Balzar E, Kopsa H, et al. Acquired antithrombin III deficiency in patients with glomerular proteinuria. *Haemostasis* 1978;7:257.

270. Lau SO, Tkachuck MT, Hasegawa DK, et al. Plasminogen and antithrombin III deficiencies in the childhood nephrotic syndrome associated with plasminogenuria and antithrombinuria. *J Pediatr* 1980;96:390.

271. Kauffman RH, Veltkamp JJ, Van Tilburg N. Acquired antithrombin III deficiency and thrombosis in the nephrotic syndrome. *Am J Med* 1978;65:607.

272. Jorgensen KA, Stofferson E. Antithrombin III and the nephrotic syndrome. *Scand J Haematol* 1979;22:442.

273. Boneu B, Boissou F, Abbal M, et al. Comparison of progressive antithrombin activity and the concentration of three thrombin inhibitors in nephrotic syndrome. *Thromb Haemost* 1981;46:623.

274. Andrassy K, Ritz E, Bommer J. Hypercoagulability in the nephrotic syndrome. *Klin Wochenchr* 1980;58:1029.

275. Panicucci F, Sagripanti A, Vispi M, et al. Comprehensive study of haemostasis in nephrotic syndrome. *Nephron* 1983;33:9.

276. Dahlbeck B. Physiological anticoagulation. Resistance to protein C and venous thromboembolism. *J Clin Invest* 1994;94:923.

277. Cosio FG, Harker C, Batard MA, et al. Plasma concentrations of the natural anticoagulants protein C and protein S in patients with proteinuria. *J Lab Clin Med* 1985;106:218.

278. Soff GA, Jackman RW, Rosenberg RD. Expression of thrombomodulin by smooth muscle cells in culture. *Blood* 1991;77:515.

279. Vigano-D'Angelo S, D'Angelo A, Kaufman CE, et al. Protein S deficiency occurs in the nephrotic syndrome. *Ann Intern Med* 1987;107:42.

280. Kemkes-Matthes B. Acquired protein S deficiency. *Clin Invest* 1992;70:529.

281. Garbrecht F, Gardner S, Johnson V, et al. Deep venous thrombosis in a child with nephrotic syndrome associated with a circulating anticoagulant and acquired protein S deficiency. *Am J Pediatr Hematol Oncol* 1991;13:330.

282. Scheinman KI, Stiehm ER. Fibrinolytic studies in the nephrotic syndrome. *Pediatr Res* 1971;5:206.

283. Simpson HC, Mann JI, Meade IW, et al. Hypertriglyceridaemia and hypercoagulability. *Lancet* 1983;i:786.

284. Shimamatsu K, Onoyama K, Maeda T, et al. Massive pulmonary embolism occurring with corticosteroid and diuretics therapy in a minimal-change nephrotic syndrome. *Nephron* 1982;32:78.

285. Yoshida Y, Shiiki H, Iwano M, et al. Enhanced expression of plasminogen activator inhibitor 1 in patients with nephrotic syndrome. *Nephron* 2001;88:24.

286. Klocking HP, Hoffmann A, Fareed J. Influence of hypersulfated lactobionic acid amides on tissue plasminogen activator release. *Semin Thrombosis Hemostasis* 1991;17:379.

287. Mysliwiec M, Ralston A, Ackrill P, et al. A study of impaired fibrin polymerization in patients with the nephrotic syndrome. *Blut* 1990;117:S73.

288. Llach F, Papper S, Massry SG. The clinical spectrum of renal vein thrombosis. Acute and chronic. *Am J Med* 1980;69:819.

289. Ozanne P, Francis RB, Meiselman HJ. Red blood cell aggregation in nephrotic syndrome. *Kidney Int* 1983;23:519.

290. Elliott GB, Grant-Tyrell J, Ringer G. Congenital lipoid nephrosis with left renal vein thrombosis and Chiari's syndrome. *J Can Assoc Radiol* 1979;30:175.

291. Cosgriff SW. Thromboembolic complications associated with ACTH and cortisone therapy. *JAMA* 1951;147:924.

292. Eldrissy AT, Abdurrahman MB, Bahakim HM, et al. Haemostatic measurements in childhood nephrotic syndrome. *Eur J Pediatr* 1991;150:374.

293. Zwaginga JJ, Koomans HA, Sixma JJ, et al. Thrombus formation and platelet-vessel wall interaction in the nephrotic syndrome under flow conditions. *J Clin Invest* 1994;93:204.

294. Malyszko J, Malyszko JS, Mysliwiec M. Markers of endothelial cell injury and thrombin activatable fibrinolysis inhibitor in nephrotic syndrome. *Blood Coagul Fibrinolysis* 2002;13:615.

295. Giangiacomo J, Cleary TG, Cole BR, et al. Serum immunoglobulins in the nephrotic syndrome. A possible cause of minimal change nephrotic syndrome. *N Engl J Med* 1975;293:8.

296. Spika JS, Halsy NA, Fish AJ, et al. Serum antibody response to pneumococcal vaccine in children with nephrotic syndrome. *Pediatrics* 1982;69:219.

297. La Manna A, Polito C, Foglia AC, et al. Reduced response to HBV vaccination in boys with steroid-sensitive nephrotic syndrome. *Pediatr Nephrol* 1992;6:251.

298. La Manna A, Polito C, Del Gado R, et al. Hepatitis B surface antigenaemia and glomerulopathies in children. *Acta Paediatr Scand* 1985;74:122.

299. McLean RH, Forsgren A, Bjorksten B, et al. Decreased serum factor B concentration associated with decreased opsonization of *Escherichia coli* in the idiopathic nephrotic syndrome. *Pediatr Res* 1977;11:910.

300. Anderson DC, York TL, Rose G, et al. Assessment of serum factor B, serum opsonins, granulocyte chemotaxis and infection in nephrotic syndrome of children. *J Infect Dis* 1979;140:1.

301. Ballow M, Kennedy TL, Gaudio KM, et al. Serum hemolytic factor D values in children with steroid-responsive idiopathic nephrotic syndrome. *J Pediatr* 1982;100:192.

302. Pediatrics AAO. Active and passive immunization. In: Peter G, ed. Red Book: report of the Committee on Infectious Diseases. Elk Grove Village, IL: American Academy of Pediatrics, 1997:50.

303. Prevention CfDCa. Prevention of pneumococcal disease: recommendations of the Advisory Committee on Immunization Practices (ACIP). *MMWR Morb Mortal Wkly Rep* 1997;46 (RR-8):1.

304. McIntyre P, Craig JC. Prevention of serious bacterial infection in children with nephrotic syndrome. *J Paediatr Child Health* 1998;34:314.

305. Garin EH, Grant MB, Silverstein JH. Insulinlike growth factors in patients with active nephrotic syndrome. *Am J Dis Child* 1989;143:865.

306. Gavin LA, McMahon FA, Castle JN, et al. Alterations in serum hormones and serum thyroxine-binding globulin in patients with nephrosis. *J Clin Endocrinol Metab* 1978;46:125.

307. Afrasiabi MA, Vaziri ND, Gwinup G, et al. Thyroid function studies in the nephrotic syndrome. *Ann Intern Med* 1979;90:335.

308. Musa BU, Seal US, Doe RP. Excretion of corticosteroid-binding globulin, thyroxine-binding globulin and total protein in adult males with nephrosis: Effect of sex hormones. *J Clin Endocrinol* 1967;27:768.

309. Ito S, Kano K, Ando T, et al. Thyroid function in children with nephrotic syndrome. *Pediatr Nephrol* 1994;8:412.

310. DeLuca F, Gemelli M, Pandullo E, et al. Changes in thyroid function tests in infantile nephrotic syndrome. *Horm Metab Res* 1983;15:258.

311. Chadha V, Alon US. Bilateral nephrectomy reverses hypothyroidism in congenital nephrotic syndrome. *Pediatr Nephrol* 1999;13:209.

312. Lim P, Jacob E, Tock EP, et al. Calcium and phosphorus metabolism in nephrotic syndrome. *Q J Med* 1977;46:327.

313. Malluche HH, Goldstein DA, Massry SG. Osteomalacia and hyperparathyroid bone disease in patients with nephrotic syndrome. *J Clin Invest* 1979;63:494.

314. Goldstein DA, Oda Y, Kurokawa K, et al. Blood levels of 25-hydroxyvitamin D in nephrotic syndrome. *Ann Intern Med* 1977;86:664–667.

315. Barragry JM, France MW, Carter ND, et al. Vitamin D metabolism in nephrotic syndrome. *Lancet* 1977;2:629.

316. Chan YL, Mason RS, Parmentier M, et al. Vitamin D metabolism in nephrotic rats. *Kidney Int* 1983;24:336.

317. Goldstein DA, Haldimann B, Sherman D, et al. Vitamin D metabolites and calcium metabolism in patients with nephrotic syndrome and normal renal function. *J Clin Endocrinol Metab* 1981;52:116.

318. Korkor A, Schwartz J, Bergfeld M, et al. Absence of metabolic bone disease in adult patients with nephrotic syndrome and normal renal function. *J Clin Endocrinol Metab* 1983;56:496.

319. Freundlich M, Bourgoignie JJ, Zilleruelo G, et al. Bone histopathology in children with nephrotic syndrome and normal glomerular filtration rate. Calcium and vitamin D metabolism in children with nephrotic syndrome. *J Pediatr* 1996;108:383.

320. Lettgen B, Jeken C, Reiners C. Influence of steroid medication on bone mineral density in children with nephrotic syndrome. *Pediatr Nephrol* 1994;8:667.

321. Leonard MB, Feldman HI, Shults J, et al. Long-term, high-dose glucocorticoids and bone mineral content in childhood glucocorticoid-sensitive nephrotic syndrome. *N Engl J Med* 2004;351:868.

322. Polito C, LaManna A, Todisco N, et al. Bone mineral content in nephrotic children on long-term, alternate-day prednisone therapy. *Clin Pediatr* 1995;34:234.

323. Loschiavo C, Lupo A, Valvo E, et al. Carbohydrate metabolism in patients with nephrotic syndrome and normal renal function. *Nephron* 1983;33:257.

324. Cartwright GE, Gubler CJ, Wintrobe MM. Studies on copper metabolism XI. Copper and iron metabolism in the nephrotic syndrome. *J Clin Invest* 1954;33:685.

325. Ellis D. Anemia in the course of nephrotic syndrome secondary to transferrin depletion. *J Pediatr* 1977;90:953.

326. Rifkind D, Kravetz HM, Knight V, et al. Urinary excretion of iron-binding protein in nephrotic syndrome. *N Engl J Med* 1961;265:115.

327. Reimold EW. Changes in zinc metabolism during the course of nephrotic syndrome. *Am J Dis Child* 1980;134:46.

328. Gilman AG, Goodman LS, Rall TW, et al. *Goodman and Gilman's, The Pharmacological Basis of Therapeutics,* 7th Edition. New York: MacMillan; 1985:1668.

329. Ellison DH. Diuretic drugs and the treatment of edema: from clinic to bench and back again. *Am J Kidney Dis* 1994;23:623.

330. Kirchner KA, Voelker JR, Brater DC. Binding inhibitors restore furosemide potency in tubule fluid containing albumin. *Kidney Int* 1991;40:418.

331. Bennett WM, Porter GA. Efficacy and safety of metolazone in renal failure and the nephrotic syndrome. *J Clin Pharmacol* 1973;13:357.

332. Welch TR, Gianis J, Sheldon CA. Perforation of the scrotum complicating nephrotic syndrome. *J Pediatr* 1988;113:336.

333. Yoshimura A, Ideura T, Iwasaki S. Aggravation of minimal change nephrotic syndrome by administration of human albumin. *Clin Nephrol* 1992;37:109.

334. Haws RM, Baum M. Efficacy of albumin and diuretic therapy in children with nephrotic syndrome. *Pediatrics* 1993;91:1142.

335. Blainey JD, Brewer DB, Hardwicke J, et al. The nephrotic syndrome: Diagnosis by renal biopsy and biochemical and immunologic analyses related to the response to steroid therapy. *Am J Med* 1960;29:235.

336. Mahan JD, Mauer SM, Sibley RK, et al. Congenital nephrotic syndrome: evaluation of medical management and results of renal transplantation. *J Pediatr* 1984;105:549.

337. Mansy H, Goodship TH, Tapson JS, et al. Effect of a high protein diet in patients with nephrotic syndrome. *Clin Sci* 1989;77:445.

338. Maroni BJ, Staffeld C, Young VR, et al. Mechanisms permitting nephrotic patients to achieve nitrogen equilibration with a protein-restricted diet. *J Clin Invest* 1997;99:2479.

339. Barsotti G, Morelli E, Cupisti A, et al. A special, supplemented 'vegan' diet for nephrotic patients. *Am J Nephrol* 1991;11:380.

340. D'Amico G, Gentile MG. Effect of dietary manipulation on the lipid abnormalities and urinary protein loss in nephrotic patients. *Miner Elect Metab* 1992;18:203.

341. Dwyer J. Vegetarian diets for treating nephrotic syndrome. *Nutrition Rev* 1993;51:44.

342. Hall AV, Parbtani A, Clark WF, et al. Omega-3 fatty acid supplementation in primary nephrotic syndrome: effects on plasma lipids and coagulopathy. *J Am Soc Nephrol* 1992;3:1321.

343. Feehally J, Baker F, Walls J. Dietary manipulation in experimental nephrotic syndrome. *Nephron* 1988;50:247.

344. Group DW. Efficacy and safety of lowering dietary intake of fat and cholesterol in children with elevated low-density lipoprotein cholesterol: the dietary intervention study in children. *JAMA* 1995;273:1429.

345. Wanner C, Bohler J, Eckardt HG, et al. Effects of simvastatin on lipoprotein (a) and lipoprotein composition in patients with nephrotic syndrome. *Clin Nephrol* 1994;41:138.

346. Prata MM, Nogueira AE, Pinto JR, et al. Long-term effect of lovastatin on lipoprotein profile in patients with primary nephrotic syndrome. *Clin Nephrol* 1994;41:277.

347. Rabelink AJ, Hene RJ, Erkelens DW, et al. Partial remission of nephrotic syndrome in patients on long-term simvastatin. *Lancet* 1990;1:1045.

348. Hodson E. The management of idiopathic nephrotic syndrome in children. *Paediatr Drugs* 2003;5:335.

349. Grymonprez A, Proesmans W, Van Dyck M, et al. Vitamin D metabolites in childhood nephrotic syndrome. *Pediatr Nephrol* 1995;9:278.

350. Mehls O. Is it correct to supplement patients with nephrotic syndrome with vitamin D and calcium? *Pediatr Nephrol* 1990;4:519.

351. Torres VE, Velosa JA, Holley KE, et al. Meclofenamate treatment of recurrent idiopathic nephrotic syndrome with focal segmental glomerulosclerosis after renal transplant. *Mayo Clin Proc* 1984;59:146.

352. Trachtman H, Gauthier B. Effect of angiotensin converting enzyme inhibitor therapy on proteinuria in children with renal disease. *J Pediatr* 1988;112:295.

353. deJong PE, Anderson S, deZeeuw D. Glomerular preload and afterload reduction as a tool to lower urinary protein leakage: Will such treatments also help to improve renal function outcome? *J Am Soc Nephrol* 1993;3:1333.

354. Garini G, Mazzi A, Buzio C, et al. Renal effects of captopril, indomethacin and nifedipine in nephrotic patients after an oral protein load. *Nephrol Dial Transplant* 1996;11:628.

355. Bakris GL, Weir MR, Secic M, et al. Differential effects of calcium antagonist subclasses on markers of nephropathy progression. *Kidney Int* 2004;65:1991.

356. Ruggenenti P, Mosconi L, Vendramin G, et al. ACE inhibition improves glomerular size selectivity in patients with idiopathic membranous nephropathy and persistent nephrotic syndrome. *Am J Kidney Dis* 2000;35:381.

357. Tikkanen MJ. The menopause and hormone replacement therapy: lipids, lipoproteins, coagulation and fibrinolytic factors. *Maturitas* 1996;23:209.

358. Mattoo TK, al-Sowallem AM, al-Harbi MS, et al. Nephrotic syndrome in first year of life and the role of bilateral nephrectomy. *Pediatr Nephrol* 1992;6:16.

359. Kim MS, Primack W, Harmon WE. Congenital nephrotic syndrome: Preemptive bilateral nephrectomy and dialysis before renal transplantation. *J Am Soc Nephrol* 1992;3:260.

360. Holmberg C, Laine J, Ronnholm K, et al. Long-term results of active treatment of congenital nephrotic syndrome of the Finnish type (abstract). *J Am Soc Nephrol* 1994;5:646.

361. Olivero JJ, Frommer JP, Gonzalez JM. Medical nephrectomy: the last resort for intractable complications of the nephrotic syndrome. *Am J Kidney Dis* 1993;21:260.

362. Hoyer JR. Idiopathic nephrotic syndrome with minimal glomerular changes. In: Brenner BM, Stein JH, eds. *Contemporary Issues in Nephrology. Nephrotic Syndrome.* New York: Churchill Livingstone; 1982: 145.

363. Barnett HL, Schoeneman M, Bernstein J, et al. Minimal change nephrotic syndrome. In: Edelmann CM, ed. *Pediatric Kidney Disease.* Boston: Little, Brown, and Co.; 1978:695.

364. Cameron JS. Nephrotic syndrome in the elderly. *Semin Nephrol* 1996;16:319.

365. Dragovic D, Rosenstock JL, Wahl SJ, et al. Increasing incidence of focal segmental glomerulosclerosis and an examination of demographic patterns. *Clin Nephrol* 2005;63:1.

366. Kari JA. Changing trends of histopathology in childhood nephrotic syndrome in western Saudi Arabia. *Saudi Med J* 2002;23:317.

367. Cameron JS, Turner DR, Ogg CS, et al. The nephrotic syndrome in adults with "minimal change glomerular lesion". *Q J Med* 1974;43:461.

368. Francis KL, Jenis EH, Jensen GE. Gold-associated nephropathy. *Arch Pathol Lab Med* 1984;108:234.

369. Falck HM, Tornroth T, Kock B, et al. Fatal renal vasculitis and minimal change glomerulonephritis complicating treatment with penicillamine. Report on two cases. *Acta Med Scand* 1979;205:133.

370. Rennke HG, Roos PC, Wall SG. Drug-induced interstitial nephritis with heavy glomerular proteinuria. *N Engl J Med* 1980;302:691.

371. Barr RD, Rees PH, Cordy PE, et al. Nephrotic syndrome in adult Africans in Nairobi. *Br Med J* 1972;2:131.

372. Lomvardias S, Pinn VW, Wadhwa ML, et al. Nephrotic syndrome associated with sulindac. *N Engl J Med* 1981;304:424.

373. Feinfeld DA, Olesnicky L, Pirani CL, et al. Nephrotic syndrome associated with use of the nonsteroidal anti-inflammatory drugs. Case report and reviews of the literature. *Nephron* 1984;37:174.

374. Curt GA, Kaldany A, Whitley LG, et al. Reversible rapidly progressive renal failure with nephrotic syndrome due to fenoprofen calcium. *Ann Intern Med* 1980;92:72.

375. Morgenstern SJ, Bruns FJ, Fraley DS, et al. Ibuprofen-associated lipoid nephrosis without interstitial nephritis. *Am J Kidney Dis* 1989;14:50.

376. Heymann W. Nephrotic syndrome after use of trimethadione and paramethadione in petit mal. *JAMA* 1967;202:893.

377. Reeves WG, Cameron JS, Johansson SG, et al. Seasonal nephrotic syndrome. Description and immunological findings. *Clin Allergy* 1975;5:121.

378. Sandberg DH, McIntosh RM, Bernstein CW, et al. Severe steroid-responsive nephrosis associated with hypersensitivity. *Lancet* 1977;i:388.

379. Howanietz H, Lubec G. Idiopathic nephrotic syndrome, treated with steroids for five years, found to be allergic reaction to pork. *Lancet* 1985;ii:450.

380. Laurent J, Lagrue G, Belghiti D, et al. Is house dust allergen a possible causal factor for relapses in lipoid nephrosis? *Allergy* 1984;39:231.

381. Rytand DA. Fatal anuria, the nephrotic syndrome and glomerular nephritis as sequels of the dermatitis of poison oak. *Am J Med* 1948;5:548.

382. Rytand DA. Onset of the nephrotic syndrome during a reaction to bee sting. *Stanford Med Bull* 1955;13:224.

383. Gagliano RG, Costanzi JJ, Beathard GA, et al. The nephrotic syndrome associated with neoplasia: an unusual paraneoplastic syndrome. *Am J Med* 1976;60:1026.

384. Cale WF, Ullrich IH, Jenkings JJ. Nodular sclerosing Hodgkin's disease presenting as nephrotic syndrome. *South Med J* 1982;75:604.

385. Eagen JW, Lewis EJ. Glomerulopathies of neoplasia. *Kidney Int* 1977;11:297.

386. Grupe WE. Childhood nephrotic syndrome: clinical associations and response to therapy. *Postgrad Med* 1979;65:229.

387. Magalhaes-Filho AG, Barbosa AB, Ferreira TC. Glomerulonephritis in schistosomiasis with mesangial IgM deposits. *Mem Inst Oswaldo Cruz* 1981;76:181.

388. Scaglia F, Vogler LB, Hymes LC, et al. Minimal change nephrotic syndrome: a possible complication of ehrlichiosis. *Pediatr Nephrol* 1999;13:600.

389. Froelich CJ, Searles RP, Davis LE, et al. A case of Guillain-Barre syndrome with immunologic abnormality. *Ann Intern Med* 1980;93:563.

390. Jassim A, Kumar N, Kelly C. Adult Still's disease with nephrotic syndrome at presentation. *Rheumatology (Oxford)* 1999;38:283.

391. Habib R, Bois E. Heterogeneite des syndromes nephrotiques a debut precoce du nourisson (syndrome nephrotique "infantile"). *Helv Paediatr Acta* 1973;28:91.

392. Jennette JC, Charles L, Grubb W. Glomerulomegaly and focal segmental glomerulosclerosis associated with sleep-apnea syndrome. *Am J Kidney Dis* 1987;10:470.

393. Gaboardi F, Perletti L, Cambie M, et al. Dermatitis herpetiformis and nephrotic syndrome. *Clin Nephrol* 1983;20:49.

394. Khambam N, Tanji N, Seigle RL, et al. Congenital focal segmental glomerulosclerosis associated with b4 integrin mutation and epidermolysis bullosa. *Am J Kidney Dis* 2000;36:190.

395. Zaman F, Saccaro S, Latif S, et al. Minimal change glomerulonephritis following a wasp sting. *Am J Nephrol* 2001;21:486.

396. Abeyagunawardena AS, Goldblatt D, Andrews N, et al. Risk of relapse after meningococcal C conjugate vaccine in nephrotic syndrome. *Lancet* 2003;362:449.

397. Kuzmanovska DB, Shahpazova EM, Kocova MJ, et al. Autoimmune thyroiditis and vitiligo in a child with minimal change nephrotic syndrome. *Pediatr Nephrol* 2001;16:1137.

398. Tanwani LK, Lohano V, Broadstone VL, et al. Minimal change nephropathy and graves' disease: report of a case and review of the literature. *Endocr Pract* 2002;8:40.

399. Fracchia M, Manganaro M, Poccardi G, et al. Minimal change nephropathy presenting in a patient with primary sclerosing cholangitis. *Ital J Gastroenterol Hepatol* 1997;29:267.

400. ISKDC. Nephrotic syndrome in children: prediction of histopathology from clinical and laboratory characteristics at time of diagnosis. *Kidney Int* 1978;13:159.

401. Danielsen H, Kornerup HJ, Olsen S, et al. Arterial hypertension in chronic glomerulonephritis. An analysis of 310 cases. *Clin Nephrol* 1983;19:284.

402. Dennis VW, Robinson RR. Proteinuria. In: Edelmann CM, ed. *Pediatric Kidney Disease.* Boston: Little, Brown; 1978:306.

403. Habib R, Kleinknecht C. The primary nephrotic syndrome in childhood. classification and clinicopathologic study of 406 cases. In: Somers SC, ed. Pathology Annual. New York: Appleton-Century Crofts, 1971: 417.

404. Chinard FP, Lauson HD, Eder HA, et al. A study of the mechanism of proteinuria in patients with the nephrotic syndrome. *J Clin Invest* 1954;33:621.

405. Cortney MA, Sawin LL, Weiss DD. Renal tubular protein absorption in the rat. *J Clin Invest* 1970;49:1.

406. Cameron JS, Blandford G. The simple assessment of selectivity in heavy proteinuria. *Lancet* 1966;ii:242.

407. Pesce AJ, Gaizutis M, Pollak VE. Selectivity of proteinuria: an evaluation of the immunochemical gel filtration techniques. *J Lab Clin Med* 1970;75:586.

408. Ramjee G, Coovadia HM, Adhikari M. Sodium dodecyl sulfate polyacrylamide gel electrophoresis of urine proteins in steroid-responsive and steroid-resistant nephrotic syndrome in children. *Pediatr Nephrol* 1994;8:653.

409. Habib R. Focal glomerulosclerosis. *Kidney Int* 1973;4:355.

410. Southwest Pediatric Nephrology Study Group. Focal segmental glomerulosclerosis in children with idiopathic nephrotic syndrome. A report of the southwest pediatric nephrology study group. *Kidney Int* 1985;27:442.

411. Pedersen EB, Danielsen H, Sorenson SS, et al. Renal water excretion before and after remission of nephrotic syndrome: relationship between free water clearance and kidney function, arginine vasopressin, angiotensin II and aldosterone in plasma before and after water loading. *Clin Sci* 1986;71:97.

412. Trachtman H, Gauthier B. Platelet vasopressin levels in childhood idiopathic nephrotic syndrome. *Am J Dis Child* 1988;142:1313.

413. Sheth KJ, Kher KK. Anion gap in nephrotic syndrome. *Int. J. Pediatr Nephrol* 1984;2:89.

414. Alon U, Chan JC. Calcium and vitamin D metabolism in nephrotic syndrome. *Int. J. Pediatr Nephrol* 1983;4:115.

415. Strife CF, Jackson EC, Forristal J, et al. Effect of the nephrotic syndrome on the concentration of serum complement components. *Am J Kidney Dis* 1986;8:37.

416. Cairns SA, London RA, Mallick NP. Circulating immune complexes in idiopathic glomerular disease. *Kidney Int* 1982;21:507.

417. Levinsky RJ, Malleson PN, Barratt TM, et al. Circulating immune complexes in steroid-responsive nephrotic syndrome. *N Engl J Med* 1978;298:126.

418. Churg J, Habib R, White RH. Pathology of the nephrotic syndrome

in children. A report for the International Study of Kidney Disease in Children. *Lancet* 1970;1:1299.

419. White RH, Glasgow EF, Mills RJ. Clinicopathologic study of nephrotic syndrome in children. *Lancet* 1970;i:1353.

420. Farquhar MG, Vernier RL, Good RA. An electron microscope study of the glomerulus in nephrosis, glomerulonephritis, and lupus erythematosus. *J Exp Med* 1957;106:649.

421. Hoffmann EO. The detection of effaced podocytes by high resolution light microscopy. *Am J Clin Pathol* 1982;78:508.

422. Churg J, Grishman E, Goldstein MH, et al. Idiopathic nephrotic syndrome in adults. *N Engl J Med* 1965;272:165.

423. International Study of Kidney Disease in Children. The primary nephrotic syndrome in children. Identification of patients with minimal change nephrotic syndrome from initial response to prednisone. *J Pediatr* 1981;98:561.

424. Shirato I. Podocyte process effacement in vivo. *Microsc Res Tech* 2002;57:241.

425. Shirato I, Hosser H, Kimura K, et al. The development of focal segmental glomerulosclerosis in Masugi nephritis is based on progressive podocyte damage. *Virchows Arch* 1996;429:255.

426. Endlich N, Kress KR, Reiser J, et al. Podocytes respond to mechanical stress in vitro. *J Am Soc Nephrol* 2001;12:413.

427. Kojima K, Davidovits A, Poczewski H, et al. Podocyte flattening and disorder of glomerular basement membrane are associated with splitting of dystroglycan-matrix interaction. *J Am Soc Nephrol* 2004;15:2079.

428. Regele HM, Fillipovic E, Langer B, et al. Glomerular expression of dystroglycans is reduced in minimal change nephrosis but not in focal segmental glomerulosclerosis. *J Am Soc Nephrol* 2000;11:403.

429. Kojima K, Kerjaschki D. Is podocyte shape controlled by the dystroglycan complex? *Nephrol Dial Transplant* 2002;17(Suppl 9):23.

430. Kriz W, Kretzler M, Provoost AP, et al. Stability and leakiness: opposing challenges to the glomerulus. *Kidney Int* 1996;49:1570.

431. Johnson RJ. Have we ignored the role of oncotic pressure in the pathogenesis of glomerulosclerosis? *Am J Kidney Dis* 1997;29:147.

432. Cohen AH, Border WA, Glassock RJ. Nephrotic syndrome with glomerular mesangial IgM deposits. *Lab Invest* 1978;38:610.

433. Murphy MJ, Bailey RR, McGiven AR. Is there an IgM nephropathy? *Aust NZ J Med* 1983;13:35.

434. Pardo V, Reisgo I, Zilleruello G, et al. The clinical significance of mesangial IgM deposits and mesangial hypercellularity in minimal change nephrotic syndrome. *Am J Kidney Dis* 1984;3:264.

435. Cavallo T, Johnson MP. Immunopathologic study of minimal change of glomerular disease with mesangial IgM deposits. *Nephron* 1981;27:281.

436. Haakenstad AO, Case JB, Mannik M. Effect of cortisone on the disappearance kinetics and tissue localization of soluble immune complexes. *J Immunol* 1975;114:1153.

437. Larsen S. Immunofluorescent microscopy findings in minimal or no change disease and slight generalized mesangioproliferative glomerulonephritis. Fluorescent microscopy results correlated to symptoms and clinical cause. *Acta Pathol Microbiol Scand* 1978;86A:531.

438. Korbet SM, Genchi RM, Borok RZ, et al. The racial prevalence of glomerular lesions in nephrotic adults. *Am J Kidney Dis* 1996;27:647.

439. Fydryk J, Waldherr R, Mall G, et al. Mesangial alterations in steroid-responsive minimal change nephrotic syndrome. *Virchow's Arch* (Pathol Anat) 1982;397:193.

440. Ji-Yun Y, Melvin T, Sibley R, et al. No evidence for a specific role of IgM in mesangial proliferation of idiopathic nephrotic syndrome. *Kidney Int* 1984;25:100.

441. Allen WR, Travis LB, Cavallo T, et al. Immune deposits and mesangial hypercellularity in minimal change nephrotic syndrome: Clinical relevance. *J Pediatr* 1982;100:188.

442. Vangelista A, Frasca G, Biagini G, et al. Long-term study of mesangial proliferative glomerulonephritis with IgM deposits. *Proc Eur Dial Transplant Assoc* 1981;18:503.

443. Waldherr R, Gubler MC, Levy M, et al. The significance of pure diffuse mesangial proliferation in idiopathic nephrotic syndrome. *Clin Nephrol* 1978;10:171.

444. Hirszel P, Yamase HT, Carney WR, et al. Mesangial proliferative glomerulonephritis with IgM deposits. Clinicopathologic analysis and evidence for morphologic transitions. *Nephron* 1984;38:100.

445. International Study of Kidney Disease in Children. Primary nephrotic syndrome in children: clinical significance of histopathologic variants of minimal change and of diffuse mesangial hypercellularity. *Kidney Int* 1981;20:765.

446. Abboud HE, Poptic E, DiCorleto P. Production of platelet-derived growth factorlike protein by rat mesangial cells in culture. *J Clin Invest* 1987; 80:675.

447. Mene P, Abboud HE, Dunn MJ. Regulation of human mesangial cell growth in culture by thromboxane A$_2$ and prostacyclin. *Kidney Int* 1990;38:232.

448. Lovett DH, Szamel M, Ryan JL, et al. Interleukin 1 and the glomerular mesangium: I. Purification and characterization of a mesangial cell-derived autogrowth factor. *J Immunol* 1986;136:3700.

449. Werber HI, Emancipator SN, Tykocinski ML, et al. The interleukin 1 gene is expressed by rat glomerular mesangial cells and is augmented in immune complex glomerulonephritis. *J Immunol* 1987;138:3207.

450. Ruef C, Budde K, Lacy J, et al. Interleukin 6 is an autocrine growth factor for mesangial cells. *Kidney Int* 1990;38:249.

451. Suematsu S, Matsuda T, Aozasa K, et al. IgG1 plasmacytosis in interleukin 6 transgenic mice. *Proc Natl Acad Sci U S A* 1989;86:7547.

452. Horii Y, Muraguchi A, Iwano M, et al. Involvement of IL-6 in mesangial proliferative glomerulonephritis. *J Immunol* 1989;143:3949.

453. Gordon C, Richards N, Howie AT, et al. Urinary IL-6: a marker for mesangial proliferative glomerulonephritis. *Clin Exp Immunol* 1991;86:145.

454. Jevnikar AM, Singer GG, Brennan DC, et al. Dexamethasone prevents autoimmune nephritis and reduces renal expression of Ia but not costimulatory signals. *Am J Pathol* 1992;141:743.

455. Groggel GC, Marinides GN, Hovingh P, et al. Inhibition of rat mesangial cell growth by heparan sulfate. *Am J Physiol* 1990;259:F259.

456. Howie AJ. Pathology of minimal change nephropathy and segmental sclerosing glomerular disorders. *Nephrol Dial Transplant* 2003;18 (Suppl 6):vi,33.

457. Davenport A, Maciver AG, Mackenzie JC. C1q nephropathy: do C1q deposits have any prognostic significance in the nephrotic syndrome? *Nephrol Dial Transplant* 1992;7:391.

458. Markowitz GS, Schwimmer JA, Stokes MB, et al. C1q nephropathy: a variant of focal segmental glomerulosclerosis. *Kidney Int* 2003;64:1232.

459. Srivastava T, Chadha V, Taboada EM, et al. C1q nephropathy presenting as rapidly progressive crescentic glomerulonephritis. *Pediatr Nephrol* 2000;14:976.

460. Hashimoto S, Ogawa Y, Ishida T, et al. Steroid-sensitive nephrotic syndrome associated with positive C1q immunofluorescence. *Clin Exp Nephrol* 2004;8:266.

461. Kuwano M, Ito Y, Amamoto Y, et al. A case of congenital nephrotic syndrome associated with positive C1q immunofluorescence. *Pediatr Nephrol* 1993;7:452.

462. Jennette JC, Hipp CG. C1q nephropathy: A distinct pathologic entity usually causing nephrotic syndrome. *Am J Kidney Dis* 1985;6:103.

463. Forland M, Bannayan GA. Minimal-change lesion nephrotic syndrome with renal oncocytoma. *Am J Med* 1983;75:715.

464. Whelan TV, Hirszel P. Minimal-change nephropathy associated with pancreatic carcinoma. *Arch Intern Med* 1988;148:975.

465. Lines DR. Nephrotic syndrome and nephroblastoma. Report of a case. *J Pediatr* 1968;72:264.

466. Hory B, Saunier F, Wolff R, et al. Waldenstrom macroglobulinemia and nephrotic syndrome with minimal change lesion. *Nephron* 1987;45:68.

467. Moorthy AV. Minimal change glomerular disease: a paraneoplastic syndrome in two patients with bronchogenic carcinoma. *Am J Kidney Dis* 1983;3:58.

468. Gandini E, Allaria P, Castilioni A, et al. Minimal change nephrotic syndrome with cecum adenocarcinoma. *Clin Nephrol* 1996;45:268.

469. Ghosh L, Muehrcke RC. The nephrotic syndrome: a prodrome to lymphoma. *Ann Intern Med* 1970;72:379.

470. Huisman RM, deJong PE, de Zeeuw D, et al. Nephrotic syndrome preceding Hodgkin's disease by 42 months. *Clin Nephrol* 1986;26:311.

471. Hyman LR, Burkholder PM, Joo PA, et al. Malignant lymphoma and nephrotic syndrome. A clinicopathologic analysis with light, immunofluorescence and electron microscopy of the renal lesion. *J Pediatr* 1973;82:207.

472. Delmez JA, Safdar SH, Kissane JM. The successful treatment of recurrent nephrotic syndrome with the MOPP regimen in a patient with remote history of Hodgkin's disease. *Am J Kidney Dis* 1994;23:743.

473. Moorthy AV, Zimmerman SW, Burkholder PM. Nephrotic syndrome in Hodgkin's disease: evidence for pathogenesis alternative to immune complex deposition. *Am J Med* 1976;61:471.

474. Kiely JM, Wagoner RD, Holley KE. Renal complications of lymphoma. *Ann Intern Med* 1969;71:1159.

475. Mori T, Yabuhara A, Nakayama J, et al. Frequently relapsing minimal change nephrotic syndrome with natural killer cell deficiency prior to the overt relapse of Hodgkin's disease. *Pediatr Nephrol* 1995;9:619.

476. Richards W, Olson D, Church JA. Improvement of idiopathic nephrotic syndrome following allergy therapy. *Ann Allergy* 1977;39:332.

477. Meadow SR, Brocklebank JT, Wainscott G. Anti-allergic drugs in idiopathic nephrotic syndrome of childhood. *Lancet* 1978;i:1200.

478. Pirotzky E, Hieblot C, Benveniste J, et al. Basophil sensitization in idiopathic nephrotic syndrome. *Lancet* 1982;1:358.

479. deMouzon-Cambon A, Bouissou F, Dutau G, et al. HLA-DR7 in children with idiopathic nephrotic syndrome. Correlation with atopy. *Tissue Antigens* 1981;17:518.

480. Thomson PD, Barratt TM, Stokes CR, et al. HLA antigens and atopic features in steroid-responsive nephrotic syndrome of childhood. *Lancet* 1976;ii:765.

481. Groshong T, Mendelson L, Mendoza S, et al. Serum IgE in patients with minimal-change nephrotic syndrome. *J Pediatr* 1973;83:767.

482. Meadow SR, Sarsfield JK. Steroid-responsive nephrotic syndrome and allergy: Clinical studies. *Arch Dis Child* 1981;56:509.

483. Lagrue G, Laurent G, Hirbec G, et al. Serum IgE in primary glomerular disease. *Nephron* 1984;36:5.

484. Gerber MA, Paronetto F. IgE in glomeruli of patients with nephrotic syndrome. *Lancet* 1971;i:1097.

485. Schulte-Wisserman H, Gortz W, Straub E. IgE in patients with glomerulonephritis and minimal-change nephrotic syndrome. *Eur. J Pediatr* 1979;131:105.

486. Trompeter RS, Thomson PD, Barratt TM, et al. Controlled trial of disodium cromoglycate in prevention of relapse of steroid-responsive nephrotic syndrome of childhood. *Arch Dis Child* 1978;53:430.

487. Lagrue G, Laurent J. Allergy and lipoid nephrosis. *Adv Nephrol* 1983;12:151.

488. Laurent J, Rostoker G, Robeva R, et al. Is adult idiopathic nephrotic syndrome food allergy? Value of oligoantigenic diets. *Nephron* 1987;47:7.

489. White RH. The familial nephrotic syndrome. I. A European survey. *Clin Nephrol* 1973;1:215.

490. Moncrieff MW, White RH, Glasgow EF, et al. The familial nephrotic syndrome: II. A clinicopathologic study. *Clin Nephrol* 1973;1:220.

491. Kleinknecht C, Gonzales G, Gubler MC. Familial nephrosis (abstract). *Pediatr Res* 1980;14:1003.

492. Trompeter RS, Barratt TM, Kay R, et al. HLA, atopy and cyclophosphamide in steroid-responsive childhood nephrotic syndrome. *Kidney Int* 1980;17:113.

493. O'Regan D, O'Callaghan U, Dundon S, et al. HLA antigens and steroid responsive nephrotic syndrome of childhood. *Tissue Antigens* 1980;16:147.

494. Alfiler CA, Roy LP, Doran T, et al. HLA-DRw7 and steroid-responsive nephrotic syndrome of childhood. *Clin Nephrol* 1980;14:71.

495. Noss G, Bachmann HJ, Olbing H. Association of minimal change nephrotic syndrome (MCNS) with HLA-B8 and B-13. *Clin Nephrol* 1981;15:172.

496. Nunez-Roldan A, Villechenous E, Fernandez-Andrade C, et al. Increased HLA-DR7 and decreased DR2 in steroid-responsive nephrotic syndrome. *N Engl J Med* 1982;306:366.

497. Kobayashi Y, Chen XM, Hiki Y, et al. Association of HLA-DRw8 and DQw3 with minimal change nephrotic syndrome in Japanese adults. *Kidney Int* 1985;28:193.

498. Cambon-Thomsen A, Boissou F, Abbal M, et al. HLA et Bf dans le syndrome nephrotique idiopathique de l'enfant: differences entre les formes corticosensibles et corticoresistantes. *Path Biol* 1986;34:725.

499. Lagueruela CC, Buettner TL, Cole BR, et al. HLA extended haplotypes in steroid-sensitive nephrotic syndrome of childhood. *Kidney Int* 1990;38:145.

500. Ruder H, Scharer K, Opelz G, et al. Human leukocyte antigens in idiopathic nephrotic syndrome in children. *Pediatr Nephrol* 1990;4:478.

501. Konrad M, Mytilineos J, Bouissou F, et al. HLA class II associations with idiopathic nephrotic syndrome in children. *Tissue Antigens* 1994;43:275.

502. Abe KK, Michinaga I, Hiratsuka T, et al. Association of DQB1*0302 alloantigens in Japanese pediatric patients with steroid-sensitive nephrotic syndrome. *Nephron* 1995;70:28.

503. Kobayashi T, Ogawa A, Takahashi K, et al. HLA-DQB1 allele associates with idiopathic nephrotic syndrome in Japanese children. *Acta Paediatr Jpn* 1995;37:293.

504. Bouissou F, Meissner I, Konrad M, et al. Clinical implications from studies of HLA antigens in idiopathic nephrotic syndrome in children. *Clin Nephrol* 1995;44:279.

505. Haeffner A, Abbal M, Mytilineos J, et al. Oligotyping for HLA-DQA, -DQB, and -DPB in idiopathic nephrotic syndrome. *Pediatr Nephrol* 1997;11:291.

506. Konrad M, Mytilineos J, Ruder H, et al. HLA-DR7 predicts the response to alkylating agents in steroid-sensitive nephrotic syndrome. *Pediatr Nephrol* 1997;11:16.

507. Bakr AM, El-Chenawy F. HLA-DQB1 and DRB1 alleles in Egyptian children with steroid-sensitive nephrotic syndrome. *Pediatr Nephrol* 1998;12:234.

508. Chandra M, Mouradian J, Hoyer FR. Familial nephrotic syndrome and focal segmental glomerulosclerosis. *J Pediatr* 1981;98:556.

509. McEnery PT, Welch TE. Major histocompatibility complex antigens in steroid-responsive nephrotic syndrome. *Pediatr Nephrol* 1989;3:33.

510. Cameron JS, Hicks J. Pregnancy in patients with pre-existing glomerular disease. *Contrib Nephrol* 1984;37:149.

511. Bakr AM, El-Chenawi F, Al-Husseni F. HLA alleles in frequently relapsing steroid-dependent and -resistant nephrotic syndrome in Egyptian children. *Pediatr Nephrol* 2005;20:159.

512. Cheung W, Ren EC, Chan SH, et al. Increased HLA- A*11 in Chinese children with steroid-responsive nephrotic syndrome. *Pediatr Nephrol* 2002;17:212.

513. Kari JA, Sinnott P, Khan H, et al. Familial steroid-responsive nephrotic syndrome and HLA antigens in Bengali children. *Pediatr Nephrol* 2001;16:346.

514. Laurent J, Ansquer JC, deMouzon-Cambon A, et al. Adult onset lipoid nephrosis is not DR7 associated. *Tissue Antigens* 1983;22:229.

515. Shalhoub RJ. Pathogenesis of lipoid nephrosis: a disorder of T-cells function. *Lancet* 1976;ii:556.

516. Schnaper HW. The immune system in minimal change nephrotic syndrome. *Pediatric Nephrol* 1989;3:101.

517. Chapman S, Taube D, Brown Z, et al. Impaired lymphocyte transformation in minimal change nephropathy in remission. *Clin Nephrol* 1982;18:34.

518. Davin JC, Foidart JB, Mahieu PR. Fc receptor function in minimal change nephrotic syndrome of childhood. *Clin Nephrol* 1983;20:280.

519. Madalinski K, Wyszynska T, Mikulska B, et al. Immune complexes in children with different forms of glomerulonephritis. *Arch Immunol Ther Exp (Warsz)* 1983;31:191.

520. Slling J. Molecular weight of immune complexes in patients with glomerulonephritis. *Nephron* 1982;30:137.

521. Brouhard BH, Goldblum RM, Bunce H, III, et al. Immunoglobulin synthesis and urinary IgG excretion in the idiopathic nephrotic syndrome of children. *Int. J. Pediatr Nephrol* 1981;2:163.

522. Ganguly NK, Singhal PC, Tewari SC, et al. Serum immunoglobulins in glomerulonephritis with special reference to minmal lesion glomerulonephritis. *J Assoc Physicians India* 1979;27:1003.

523. Heslan JM, Lautie JP, Intrator L, et al. Impaired IgG synthesis in patients with the nephrotic syndrome. *Clin Nephrol* 1982;18:144.

524. Rashid H, Skillen AW, Morley AR, et al. Serum immunoglobulins in minimal change nephrotic syndrome—A possible defect in T-cell function. *Bangladesh Med Res Council Bull* 1982;8:15.

525. Moore DH, Shackelford PG, Robson AM, et al. Recurrent pneumococcal sepsis and defective opsonization after pneumococcal capsular polysaccharide vaccine in a child with nephrotic syndrome. *J Pediatr* 1980;96:882.

526. Lange K, Ahmed U, Seligson G, et al. Depression of endostreptosin, streptolysin O and streptozyme antibodies in patients with idiopathic nephrosis with and without nephrotic syndrome. *Clin Nephrol* 1981;15:279.

527. Dall'Aglio P, Chizzolini C, Brigati C et al. Minimal change glomerulonephritis and focal glomerulosclerosis markers and 'in vitro' activity of peripheral blood mononuclear cells. *Proc Eur Dial Transplant Assoc* 1983;19:673.

528. Beale MG, Nash GS, Bertovich MJ, et al. Immunoglobulin synthesis by peripheral blood mononuclear cells in minimal change nephrotic syndrome. *Kidney Int* 1983;23:380.

529. Herrod HG, Stapleton FB, Trouy RL, et al. Evaluation of T lymphocyte subpopulations in children with nephrotic syndrome. *Clin Exp Immunol* 1983;52:581.

530. Fiser RT, Arnold WC, Charlton RW, et al. T-lymphocyte subsets in nephrotic syndrome. *Kidney Int* 1991;40:913.

531. Kerpen HO, Bhat JG, Kantor R, et al. Lymphocyte subpopulations in minimal change nephrotic syndrome. *Clin Immunol Immunopathol* 1979;14:130.

532. Tani Y, Kida H, Abe T, et al. B-lymphocyte subset patterns and their significance in idiopathic glomerulonephritis. *Clin Exp Immunol* 1982;48:201.

533. Eyres K, Mallick NP, Taylor G. Evidence for cell-mediated immunity to renal antigens in minimal-change nephrotic syndrome. *Lancet* 1976;1:1158.

534. Eyres K, Mallick NP, Taylor G. Studies of cellular immune responses in patients with minimal change nephropathy. *Dial Transplant Nephrol* 1976;13:533.

535. Matsumoto K, Osakabe K, Harada M, et al. Impaired cell-mediated immunity in lipoid nephrosis. *Nephron* 1981;29:190.

536. Lin TY, Wang YM, Lin ST. Application of a live varicella vaccine in children with acute leukemia or nephrotic syndrome. *J Formosan Med Assoc* 1981;70:683.

537. Fodor P, Saitua MT, Rodriguez E, et al. T-cell dysfunction in minimal-change nephrotic syndrome of childhood. *Am J Dis Child* 1982;136:713.

538. Matsumoto K, Katayama H, Hatano M. Effect of thymic humoral factor on a local graft-versus-host reaction of lymphocytes in patients with lipoid nephrosis (Letter). *Nephron* 1982;32:279.

539. Minchin MA, Turner KJ, Bower GD. Lymphocyte blastogenesis in nephrotic syndrome. *Clin Exp Immunol* 1980;42:241.

540. Osakabe K, Matsumoto K. Concanavalin A-induced suppressor cell activity in lipoid nephrosis. *Scand J Immunol* 1981;14:161.

541. Ooi BS, Orlina AR, Masaitis L. Lymphocytotoxins in primary renal disease. *Lancet* 1974;ii:1348.

542. Smith MD, Barratt TM, Hayward AR, et al. The inhibitions of complement-dependent lymphocyte rosette formation by the sera of children with steroid-sensitive nephrotic syndrome and other renal diseases. *Clin Exp Immunol* 1975;21:236.

543. Tomizawa S, Suzuki S, Oguri M, et al. Studies of T lymphocyte function and inhibitory factors in minimal change nephrotic syndrome. *Nephron* 1979;24:179.

544. Lin CY. Decreased antibody-dependent cellular cytotoxicity in minimal change nephrotic syndrome. *Pediatric Nephrol* 1988;2:224.

545. Saxena S, Mittal A, Andal A. Pattern of interleukins in minimal-change nephrotic syndrome of childhood. *Nephron* 1993;65:56.

546. Matsumoto K. Decreased production of interleukin-1 by monocytes from patients with lipoid nephrosis. *Clin Nephrol* 1989:292.

547. Hinoshita F, Noma T, Tomura S, et al. Decreased production and responsiveness of interleukin 2 in lymphocytes of patients with nephrotic syndrome. *Nephron* 1990;54:122.

548. Martini A, Vitiello MA, Siena S, et al. Multiple serum inhibitors of lectin-induced lymphocyte proliferation in nephrotic syndrome. *Clin Exp Immunol* 1981;45:178.

549. Iitaka K, West CD. A serum inhibitor of blastogenesis in idiopathic nephrotic syndrome transferred by lymphocytes. *Clin Immunol Immunopathol* 1979;12:62.

550. Barna BP, Makker S, Kallen R, et al. A lymphocytotoxic factor(s) in plasma of patients with minimal change nephrotic syndrome: partial characterization. *Clin Immunol Immunopathol* 1983;27:272.

551. Mallick NP, Williams RJ, McFarlane H, et al. Cell-mediated immunity in nephrotic syndrome. *Lancet* 1972;i:507.

552. Lagrue G, Xheneumont S, Branellec A, et al. A vascular permeability factor elaborated from lymphocytes. I. Demonstration in patients with nephrotic syndrome. *Biomedicine* 1975;23:37.

553. Monacci WT, Merrill MJ, Oldfield EH. Expression of vascular permeability factor/vascular endothelial growth factor in normal rat tissues. *Am J Physiol* 1993;264:C995.

554. Schnaper HW, Aune TM. Identification of the lymphokine soluble immune response suppressor in urine of nephrotic children. *J Clin Invest* 1985;76:341.

555. Schnaper HW, Aune TM. Steroid-sensitive mechanism of soluble immune response suppressor production in patients with steroid-responsive nephrotic syndrome. *J Clin Invest* 1987;79:256.

556. Suranyi MG, Gausch A, Hall BM, et al. Elevated levels of tumor necrosis factor-alpha in the nephrotic syndrome in humans. *Am J Kidney Dis* 1993;21:251.

557. Robeva R, Heslan JM, Branellec A, et al. Enhanced β2-microglobulin levels in lymphocyte culture supernatants from patients with idiopathic nephrotic syndrome; inhibition of lymphocyte activation by cyclosporine. *Clin Nephrol* 1988;30:211.

558. Bock GH, Ongkingco JR, Patterson LT, et al. Serum and urine soluble interleukin-2 receptor in idiopathic nephrotic syndrome. *Pediatr Nephrol* 1993;7:523.

559. Hulton SA, Shah V, Byrne MR, et al. Lymphocyte subpopulations, interleukin-2 and interleukin-2 receptor expression in childhood nephrotic syndrome. *Pediatr Nephrol* 1994;8:135.

560. Mandreoli M, Beltrandi E, Casadei-Maldini M, et al. Lymphocyte release of soluble IL-2 receptors in patients with minimal change nephropathy. *Clin Nephrol* 1992;37:177.

561. Ohno I, Gomi H, Matsuda H, et al. Soluble IL-2 receptor in patients with primary nephrotic syndrome. *Nippon Jinzo Gakkai Shi* 1991;33:483.

562. Neuhaus JT, Wadhwa M, Callard R, et al. Increased IL-2, IL-4 and interferon gamma (IFN-g) in steroid-sensitive nephrotic syndrome. *Clin Exp Immunol* 1995;100:475.

563. Yap KK, Cheung W, Murugasu B, et al. Th1 and Th2 cytokine mRNA profiles in childhood nephrotic syndrome: evidence for increased IL-13 mRNA expression in relapse. *J Am Soc Nephrol* 1999;10:529.

564. Chan MK, Chan KW, Jones B. Immunoglobulins (IgG, IgA, IgM, IgE) and complement components (C3, C4) in nephrotic syndrome due to minimal change and other forms of glomerulonephritis, a clue for steroid therapy? *Nephron* 1987;47:125.

565. Harris HW, Umetsu D, Geha R, et al. Altered immunoglobulin status in congenital nephrotic syndrome. *Clin Nephrol* 1986;25:308.

566. Al-Bander HA, Martin VI, Kaysen GA. Plasma IgG pool is not defended from urinary loss in nephrotic syndrome. *Am J Physiol* 1992;262:F333.

567. Tejani A, Fikrig S, Schiffman G, et al. Persistence of protective pneumococcal antibody following vaccination in patients with nephrotic syndrome. *Am J Nephrol* 1984;4:32.

568. Lin CY, Chen CH, Lee PP. In vitro B-lymphocyte switch disturbance from IgM into IgG in IgM mesangial nephropathy. *Pediatr Nephrol* 1989;3:254.

569. Stachura I, Si L, Madan E, et al. Mononuclear cell subsets in human renal disease. Enumeration in tissue sections with monoclonal antibody. *Clin Immunol Immunopathol* 1984;30:362.

570. Nagata K, Platt JL, Michael AF. Interstitial and glomerular immune cell populations in idiopathic nephrotic syndrome. *Kidney Int* 1984;25:88.

571. Cagnoli L, Tabacchi P, Pasquali S, et al. T cell subset alterations in idiopathic glomerulonephritis. *Clin Exp Immunol* 1982;50:70.

572. Kemper MJ, Meyer-Jark T, Lilova M, et al. Combined T- and B-cell activation in childhood steroid-sensitive nephrotic syndrome. *Clin Nephrol* 2003;60:242.

573. Kobayashi K, Yoshikawa N, Nakamura H. T-cell subpopulations in childhood nephrotic syndrome. *Clin Nephrol* 1994;41:253.

574. Stachowski J, Barth C, Michalkiewicz J, et al. Th1/Th2 balance and CD45-positive T cell subsets in primary nephrotic syndrome. *Pediatr Nephrol* 2000;14:779.

575. Matsumoto K. Impaired local graft-versus host reaction in lipoid nephrosis. (Letter) *Nephron* 1982;31:281.

576. Matsumoto K, Osakabe K, Hatano M. Impaired cell-mediated immunity in idiopathic membranous nephropathy mediated by suppressor cells. *Clin Nephrol* 1983;19:213.

577. Wu MJ, Moorthy AV. Suppressor cell function in patients with primary glomerular disease. *Clin Immunol Immunopathol* 1982;22:442.

578. Beale MG, Hoffsten PE, Robson AM, et al. Inhibitory factors of lymphocyte transformation in sera from patients with minimal change nephrotic syndrome. *Clin Nephrol* 1980;13:271.

579. Moorthy AV, Zimmerman SW, Burkholder PM. Inhibition of lymphocyte blastogenesis by plasma of patients with minimal-change nephrotic syndrome. *Lancet* 1976;i:1160.

580. Taube D, Chapman S, Brown Z, et al. Depression of normal lymphocyte transformation by sera of patients with minimal change nephropathy and other forms of nephrotic syndrome. *Clin Nephrol* 1981;15:286.

581. Lenarsky C, Jordan SC, Ladisch S. Plasma inhibition of lymphocyte proliferation in nephrotic syndrome: correlation with hyperlipidemia. *J Clin Immunol* 1982;2:276.

582. Chisari FV. Immunoregulatory properties of human plasma in very low density lipoproteins. *J Immunol* 1977;119:2129.

583. Curtiss LK, Edgington TS. Regulatory serum lipoproteins: regulation of lymphocyte stimulation by a species of low density lipoprotein. *J Immunol* 1976;118:1452.

584. Faucher C, Albert C, Beaufils H, et al. Remission of a refractory nephrotic syndrome after low-density lipoprotein apheresis based on dextran sulphate adsorption. *Nephrol Dial Transpl* 1997;12:1037.

585. Cho BS, Yoon SR, Jang JY, et al. Up-regulation of interleukin-4 and CD23/FcεRII in minimal change nephrotic syndrome. *Pediatr Nephrol* 1999;13:199.

586. Schnaper HW, Pierce CW, Aune TM. Identification and initial characterization of concanavalin A- and interferon-induced human suppressor factors: evidence for a human equivalent of murine soluble immune response suppressor (SIRS). *J Immunol* 1984;132:2429.

587. Schnaper HW, Aune TM. Suppression of immune responses to sheep erythrocytes by the lymphokine soluble immune response suppressor (SIRS) in vivo. *J Immunol* 1986;137:863.

588. Schnaper HW. A regulatory system for soluble immune response suppressor production in steroid-responsive nephrotic syndrome. *Kidney Int* 1990;38:151.

589. Doi T, Kanatsu K, et al. Circulating immune complexes of IgG, IgA and IgM classes in various glomerular diseases. *Nephron* 1982;32:335.

590. Abrass CK, Hall CL, Border WA, et al. Circulating immune complexes in adults with idiopathic nephrotic syndrome. *Kidney Int* 1980;17:545.

591. Isaacs KL, Miller F. Antigen size and charge in immune complex glomerulonephritis. *Am J Pathol* 1983;111:298.

592. Iskander SS, Jenette JC. Influence of antibody avidity on glomerular immune complex formation. *Am J Pathol* 1983;112:155.

593. Sherman RL, Susin M, Wexler ME. Lipoid nephrosis in Hodgkin's disease. *Am J Med* 1972;52:699.

594. Crowley JP, Ree HJ, Esparza A. Monocyte-dependent serum suppression of lymphocyte blastogenesis in Hodgkin's disease: An association with nephrotic syndrome. *J Clin Immunol* 1982;2:270.

595. Shimoyama H, Nakajima M, Naka H, et al. Up-regulation of interleukin-2 mRNA in children with idiopathic nephrotic syndrome. *Pediatr Nephrol* 2004;19:1115.

596. Sakurai M, Muso E, Matushima H, et al. Rapid normalization of interleukin-8 production after low-density lipoprotein apheresis in steroid-resistant nephrotic syndrome. *Kidney Int* (Suppl) 1999;71:S210.

597. Kim SD, Park JM, Kim IS, et al. Association of IL-1beta, IL-1ra, and TNF-alpha gene polymorphisms in childhood nephrotic syndrome. *Pediatr Nephrol* 2004;19:295.

598. Kawasaki K, Yaoita E, Yamamoto T, et al. Antibodies against intercellular adhesion molecule-1 and lymphocyte function-associated antigen-1 prevent glomerular injury in rat experimental crescentic glomerulonephritis. *J Immunol* 1993;150:1074.

599. Holdsworth SR, Neale TJ, Wilson CB. Abrogation of macrophage-dependent injury in experimental glomerulonephritis in the rabbit. *J Clin Invest* 1981;68:686.

600. Kreisberg JE, Wayne DB, Karnovsky MJ. Rapid and focal loss of negative charge associated with mononuclear cell infiltration early in nephrotoxic serum nephritis. *Kidney Int* 1979;16:290.

601. Lagrue G, Branellec A, Blanc C, et al. A vascular permeability factor in lymphocyte culture supernatants from patients with nephrotic syndrome. II. Pharmacological and physicochemical properties. *Biomedicine* 1975;23:73.

602. Tomizawa S, Maruyama K, Nagasawa N, et al. Studies of vascular permeability factor derived from T lymphocytes and inhibitory effect of plasma on its production in minimal change nephrotic syndrome. *Nephron* 1985;41:157.

603. Bakker WW, Baller JF, vanLuijk WH, et al. A kallikrein-like molecule and vasoactivity in minimal change disease. Increased turnover in relapse vs. remission. *Contrib Nephrol* 1988;67:31.

604. Dejana E, Lampugnani MG, Martinez-Estrada O, et al. The molecular organization of endothelial junctions and their functional role in vascular morphogenesis and permeability. *Int J Dev Biol* 2000;44:743.

605. Risau W. Development and differentiation of endothelium. *Kidney Int* (Suppl), 1998;67:S3.

606. Bakker WW, Beukhof JR, VanLuijh WH, et al. Vascular permeability increasing factor (VPF) in IgA nephropathy. *Clin Nephrol* 1982;18:165.

607. Matsumoto K, Ohi H, Kanmatsuse K. Interleukin 12 upregulates the release of vascular permeability factor by peripheral blood mononuclear cells from patients with lipoid nephrosis. *Nephron* 1998;78:403.

608. Matsumoto K, Kanmatsuse K. Interleukin-15 and interleukin 12 have an additive effect on the release of vascular permeability factor by peripheral blood mononuclear cells in normals and in patients with nephrotic syndrome. *Clin Nephrol* 1999;52:10.

609. Koyama A, Fujisak M, Kobayashi M, et al. A glomerular permeability factor produced by human T-cell hybridomas. *Kidney Int* 1991;40:453.

610. Tanaka R, Yoshikawa N, Nakamura H, et al. Infusion of peripheral blood mononuclear cell products from nephrotic children increases albuminuria in rats. *Nephron* 1992;60:35.

611. Garin EH, Laflam P, Chandler L. Anti-interleukin 8 antibody abolishes effects of lipoid nephrosis cytokine. *Pediatr Nephrol* 1998;12:381.

612. Garin EH, West L, Sheng W. Effect of interleukin-8 on glomerular sulfated compounds and albuminuria. *Pediatr Nephrol* 1997;11:274.

613. Daniel V, Trautmann Y, Konrad M, et al. T-lymphocyte populations, cytokines and other growth factors in serum and urine of children with idiopathic nephrotic syndrome. *Clin Nephrol* 1997;47:289.

614. Bakr A, Shokeir M, El-Chenawi F, et al. Tumor necrosis factor-alpha production from mononuclear cells in nephrotic syndrome. *Pediatr Nephrol* 2003;18:516.

615. Raveh D, Shemesh O, Ashkenazi YJ, et al. Tumor necrosis factor-alpha blocking agent as a treatment for nephrotic syndrome. *Pediatr Nephrol* 2004;19:1281.

616. Joffe MI, Rabson AR. Dissociation of lymphokine production and blastogenesis in children with measles infection. *Clin Immunol Immunopathol* 1978;10:335.

617. Finkelstein A, Fraley DS, Stachura I. Fenprofen nephropathy: lipoid nephrosis and interstitial nephritis. A possible T-lymphocyte disorder. *Am J Med* 1982;72:81.

618. Watson AJ, Dalbow MH, Stachura I, et al. Immunologic studies in cimetidine-induced nephropathy and polymyositis. *N Engl J Med* 1983;308:142.

619. Taube D, Brown Z, Williams DG. Longterm impairment of suppressor-cell function by cyclophosphamide in minimal-change nephropathy and its association with therapeutic response. *Lancet* 1981;1:235.

620. Feehally J, Beattie TJ, Brenchley PE, et al. Modulation of cellular immune function by cyclophosphamide in children with minimal change nephropathy. *N Engl J Med* 1984;310:415.

621. Averbuch SD, Austin HA, III, Sherwin SA, et al. Acute interstitial nephritis with the nephrotic syndrome following recombinant leukocyte A interferon therapy for mycosis fungoides. *N Engl J Med* 1984;310:32.

622. British Association for Pediatric Nephrology. Levamisole for corticosteroid dependent nephrotic syndrome in childhood. *Lancet* 1991;337:1555.

623. Niaudet P, Drachman R, Gagnadoox MF, et al. Treatment of idiopathic nephrotic syndrome with levamisole. *Acta Paediatr Scand* 1984;76:637.

624. Abe Y, Sekiya S, Yamasita T, et al. Vascular hyperpermeability induced by tumor necrosis factor and its augmentation by IL-1 and IFN-g is inhibited by selective depletion of neutrophils with a monoclonal antibody. *J Immunol* 1990;145:2902.

625. Gault MH, Muehrcke RC. Renal biopsy: Current views and controversies (editorial). *Nephron* 1983;34:1.

626. Thompson AL, Durrett RR, Robinson RR. Fixed and reproducible orthostatic proteinuria. VI. Results of a 10-year follow-up evaluation. *Ann Intern Med* 1970;73:235.

627. Lau J, Levey AS, Kassirer JP, et al. Idiopathic nephrotic syndrome in a 53 year old woman. Is a kidney biopsy necessary? *Med Decision Making* 1982;2:497.

628. Webb NJ, Lewis MA, Iqbal J, et al. Childhood steroid-sensitive nephrotic syndrome: does histology matter? *Am J Kidney Dis* 1996;27:484.

629. Cornfeld D, Schwartz MW. Nephrosis: a long-term study of children treated with corticosteroids. *J Pediatr* 1966;68:507.

630. Barness LA, Moll GH, Janeway CA. Nephrotic syndrome. I. Natural history of the disease. *Pediatrics* 1949;5:486.

631. Coggins CH. Minimal change nephrosis in adults. In: Zurukzoglu W, Papadimitriou M, Pyrpasopoulis M, et al., eds. *Proceedings of the Eighth International Congress of Nephrology: advances in Basic and Clinical Nephrology.* Basel: S. Karger; 1981:336.

632. Moxey-Mims MM, Stapelton FB, Feld LD. Applying decision analysis to management of adolescent idiopathic nephrotic syndrome. *Pediatr Nephrol* 1994;8:660.

633. McEnery PT, Strife CF. Nephrotic syndrome in childhood. Management and treatment in patients with minimal change disease, mesangial proliferation, or focal glomerulosclerosis. *Pediatr Clin North Am* 1982;29:875.

634. Hodson EM, Knight JF, Willis NS, et al. Corticosteroid therapy for nephrotic syndrome in children. *Cochrane Database Syst Rev* 2004;CD001533.

634a. Troyanov S, et al. Focal and segmental glomerulosclerosis: definition and relevance of a partial remission. *J Am Soc Nephrol* 2005;16:1061.

635. Bohrer MP, Deen WM, Robertson C, et al. Mechanism of angiotensin II-induced proteinuria in the rat. *Am J Physiol* 1977;233:F13.

636. Ehrich JH, Brodehl J. Long versus standard prednisone therapy for initial treatment of idiopathic nephrotic syndrome. Arbeitsgemeinschaft for Padiatrische Nephrologie. *Eur J Pediatr* 1993;152:357.

637. Lande MB, Gullion C, Hogg RJ, et al. Long versus standard initial steroid therapy for children with the nephrotic syndrome: a report from the Southwest Pediatric Nephrology Study Group. *Pediatr Nephrol* 2003;18:342.

638. Arbeitsgemeinschaft fur Padiatrische Nephrologie. Short versus standard prednisone therapy for initial treatment of idiopathic nephrotic syndrome in children. *Lancet* 1988;i:380.

639. International Study of Kidney Disease in Children. Nephrotic syndrome in children: a randomized trial comparing two prednisone regimens in steroid-responsive patients who relapse early. *J Pediatr* 1979;95:239.

640. Constantinescu AR, Shah HB, Foote EF, et al. Predicting first-year relapses in children with nephrotic syndrome. *Pediatrics* 2000;105:492.

641. Nakayama M, Katafuchi R, Yanase T, et al. Steroid responsiveness and frequency of relapse in adult-onset minimal change nephrotic syndrome. *Am J Kidney Dis* 2002;39:503.

642. Kim PK, Kim NA, Kim KS, et al. Steroid effects on minimal lesion nephrotic syndrome with and without immune deposits. *Int J Pediatr Nephrol* 1983;3:257.

643. Brown EA, Upadhyaya K, Hayslett JP, et al. The clinical course of mesangial proliferative glomerulonephritis. *Medicine (Baltimore)* 1979;58:295.

644. Hopper J Jr, Ryan P, Lee JC. Lipoid nephrosis in 31 adult patients: renal biopsy study by light, electron and fluorescence microscopy with experience in treatment. *Medicine* 1970;49:321.

645. Schnaper HW. Immunization practices in childhood nephrotic syndrome: a survey of North American pediatric nephrologists. *Pediatr Nephrol* 1994;8:4.

646. Steele RW. Current status of vaccines and immune globulins in children with renal disease. *Pediatr Nephrol* 1994;8:7.

647. Koskimies O, Vilska J, Rapola J, et al. Long-term outcome of primary nephrotic syndrome. *Arch Dis Child* 1982;57:544.

648. International Study of Kidney Disease in Children. Early identification of frequent relapsers among children with minimal change nephrotic syndrome. *J Pediatr* 1982;101:514.

649. Wingen AM, Muller-Wiefel DE, Scharer K. Comparison of different regimens of prednisone therapy in frequently relapsing nephrotic syndrome. *Acta Paediatr Scand* 1990;79:305.

650. Leisti S, Vilska J, Hallman N. Adrenocortical insufficiency and relapsing in the idiopathic nephrotic syndrome of childhood. *Pediatrics* 1977;60:334.

651. Schoeneman MJ. Minimal change nephrotic syndrome: Treatment with low doses of hydrocortisone. *J Pediatr* 1983;102:791.

652. West CD. Use of combined hormone and mechlorethamine (nitrogen mustard) therapy in lipoid nephrosis. *Am J Dis Child* 1958;95:498.

653. Lewis EJ. Chlorambucil for childhood nephrotic syndrome. A word of caution. *N Engl J Med* 1980;302:963.

654. Schulman SL, Kaiser BA, Polinsky MS, et al. Predicting the response to cytotoxic therapy for childhood nephrotic syndrome: superiority of response to corticosteroid therapy over histopathologic patterns. *J Pediatr* 1988;113:996.

655. McCrory WW, Shibuya M, Lu WH, et al. Therapeutic and toxic effects observed with different dosage programs of cyclophosphamide in treatment of steroid-responsive but frequently relapsing nephrotic syndrome. *J Pediatr* 1973;82:614.

656. International Study of Kidney Disease in Children. Prospective, controlled trial of cyclophosphamide therapy in children with the nephrotic syndrome. *Lancet* 1974;ii:423.

657. Cameron JS, Chantler C, Ogg CS, et al. Long-term remission in nephrotic syndrome after treatment with cyclophosphamide. *Br Med J* 1974;4:7.

658. Barratt TM, Soothill JF. Controlled trial of cyclophosphamide in steroid-sensitive relapsing nephrotic syndrome of childhood. *Lancet* 1970;2:479.

659. Arbeitsgemeinschaft fur Paediatrische Nephrologie. Effect of cytoxic drugs in frequently relapsing nephrotic syndrome with and without steroid dependence. *N Engl J Med* 1982;306:451.

660. McDonald J, Murphy AV, Arneil GC. Long-term assessment of cyclophosphamide therapy for nephrosis in children. *Lancet* 1974;ii:980.

661. Dundon S, O'Callaghan U, Raftery J. Stability of remission in minimal lesion nephrotic syndrome after treatment with prednisone and cyclophosphamide. *Int J Pediatr Nephrol* 1980;1:22.

662. Etteldorf JN, West CD, Pitcock JA, et al. Gonadal function, testicular histology and meiosis following cyclophosphamide. *J Pediatr* 1976;88:206.

663. Lentz RD, Bergstein J, Steffes MW, et al. Postpubertal evaluation of gonadal function following cyclophosphamide therapy before and during puberty. *J Pediatr* 1977;91:385.

664. Trompeter RS, Evans PR, Barratt TM. Gonadal function in boys with steroid-responsive nephrotic syndrome treated with cyclophosphamide for short periods. *Lancet* 1981;i:1177.

665. Rivkees SA, Crawford JD. The relationship of gonadal activity and chemotherapy-induced gonadal damage. *JAMA* 1988;259:2123.

666. Bogdanovic R, Banicevic M, Cvoric A. Pituitary-gonadal function in women following cyclophosphamide treatment for childhood nephrotic syndrome: Long-term follow-up study. *Pediatr Nephrol* 1990;4:455.

667. Parra A, Santos D, Cervantes C, et al. Plasma gonadotropins and gonadal steroids in children treated with cyclophosphamide. *J Pediatr* 1978;92:117.

668. Masala A, Faedda R, Alagna S, et al. Use of testosterone to prevent cyclophosphamide-induced azoospermia. *Ann Intern Med* 1997;126:292.

669. Blumenfeld Z, Haim N. Prevention of gonadal damage during cytotoxic therapy. *Ann Med* 1997;29:199.

670. Kuis W, DeKraker J, Kuijten RH, et al. Acute lymphoblastic leukemia after treatment of nephrotic syndrome with immunosuppressive drugs. *Helv Paediatr Acta* 1976;31:91.

671. Elzouki AY, Al-Nassar K, Al-Ali M, et al. Sister chromatid exchange

analysis in monitoring chlorambucil therapy in primary nephrotic syndrome of childhood. *Pediatr Nephrol* 1991;5:59.

672. Jones BF. Cyclophosphamide pulse therapy in frequently relapsing nephrotic syndrome. *Nephron* 1993;63:472.

673. Williams SA, Makker SP, Grupe WE. Seizures: a significant side effect of chlorambucil therapy in children. *J Pediatr* 1978;93:516.

674. Matsui A, Takezawa N, Suzuki K, et al. Neurotoxicity of chlorambucil and cyclophosphamide therapy in steroid-dependent and/or frequently relapsing nephrotic syndrome. *Pediatr Nephrol* 1989;3:C167.

675. Muller W, Brandis MX. Acute leukemia after cytotoxic treatment for nonmalignant disease in childhood. A case report and review of the literature. *Eur J Pediatr* 1981;136:105.

676. Kleinknecht C, Guesry P, Lenoir G, et al. High-cost benefit of chlorambucil in frequently relapsing nephrotic syndrome. *N Engl J Med* 1977;296:48.

677. Grupe WE, Makker SP, Ingelfinger IR. Chlorambucil treatment of frequently relapsing nephrotic syndrome. *N Engl J Med* 1976;295:746.

678. Williams SA, Makker SP, Inglefinger JR, et al. Long-term evaluation of chlorambucil plus prednisone in the idiopathic nephrotic syndrome of childhood. *N Engl J Med* 1980;302:929.

679. Elzouki AT, Jaiswal OP. Evaluation of chlorambucil therapy in steroid-dependent and cyclophosphamide-resistant children with nephrosis. *Pediatr Nephrol* 1990;4:459.

680. Durkan AM, Hodson EM, Willis NS, et al. Immunosuppressive agents in childhood nephrotic syndrome: a meta-analysis of randomized controlled trials. *Kidney Int* 2001;59:1919.

681. Niaudet P, Habib R, Tete MJ, et al. Cyclosporin in the treatment of idiopathic nephrotic syndrome in children. *Pediatr Nephrol* 1987;1:566.

682. Rinaldi S, Sesto A, Barsotti P, et al. Cyclosporine therapy monitored with abbreviated area under curve in nephrotic syndrome. *Pediatr Nephrol* 2005;20:25.

683. Hymes LC. Steroid-resistant, cyclosporine-responsive, relapsing nephrotic syndrome. *Pediatr Nephrol* 1995;9:137.

684. Gregory MJ, Smoyer WE, Sedman A, et al. Long-term cyclosporine therapy for pediatric nephrotic syndrome: a clinical and histologic analysis. *J Am Soc Nephrol* 1996;7:543.

685. Filler G. Treatment of nephrotic syndrome in children and controlled trials. *Nephrol Dial Transplant* 2003;18(Suppl 6):vi75.

686. Ginevri F, Trivelli A, Ciardi MR, et al. Protracted levamisole in children with frequently relapsing nephrotic syndrome. *Pediatr Nephrol* 1996;10:550.

687. Palcoux JB, Niaudet P, Goumy P. Side effects of levamisole in children with nephrosis. *Pediatr Nephrol* 1994;8:263.

688. Day CJ, Cockwell P, Lipkin GW, et al. Mycophenolate mofetil in the treatment of resistant idiopathic nephrotic syndrome. *Nephrol Dial Transplant* 2002;17:2011.

689. Pesavento TE, Bay WH, Agarwal G, et al. Mycophenolate therapy in frequently relapsing minimal change disease that has failed cyclophosphamide therapy. *Am J Kidney Dis* 2004;43:e3.

690. Barletta GM, Smoyer WE, Bunchman TE, et al. Use of mycophenolate mofetil in steroid-dependent and -resistant nephrotic syndrome. *Pediatr Nephrol* 2003;18:833.

691. Bagga A, Hari P, Moudgil A, et al. Mycophenolate mofetil and prednisolone therapy in children with steroid-dependent nephrotic syndrome. *Am J Kidney Dis* 2003;42:1114.

692. Rowe PC, McLean RH, Ruley EJ, et al. Intravenous immunoglobulin in minimal change nephrotic syndrome: a crossover trial. *Pediatr Nephrol* 1990;4:32.

693. Murnaghan K, Vasmant D, Bensman A. Pulse methylprednisolone therapy in severe idiopathic childhood nephrotic syndrome. *Acta Paediatr Scand* 1984;73:733.

694. Arbeitsgemeinschaft fur Paediatrische Nephrologie. Cyclophosphamide treatment of steroid dependent nephrotic syndrome: comparison of eight week with 12 week course. *Arch Dis Child* 1987;62:1102.

695. Niaudet P. Comparison of cyclosporine and chlorambucil in the treatment of steroid dependent idiopathic nephrotic syndrome: a multicenter randomized controlled trial. The French Society of Paediatric Nephrology. *Pediatr Nephrol* 1992;6:1.

696. Hulton SA. Long-term cyclosporin A treatment of minimal-change nephrotic syndrome of childhood. *Pediatr Nephrol* 1994;8:401.

697. Hulton SA. Effect of cyclosporin A on glomerular filtration rate in children with minimal change nephrotic syndrome. *Pediatr Nephrol* 1994;8:404.

698. Inoue Y, Iijima K, Nakamura H, et al. Two-year cyclosporin treatment in children with steroid-dependent nephrotic syndrome. *Pediatr Nephrol* 1999;13:33.

699. Ponticelli C, Rissoni G, Edefonti A, et al. A randomized trial of cyclosporin in steroid-resistant nephrotic syndrome. *Kidney Int* 1993;43:1377.

700. Takeda A, Ohgushi H, Niimura F, et al. Long-term effects of immunosuppressants in steroid-dependent nephrotic syndrome. *Pediatr Nephrol* 1998;12:746.

701. Brodehl J. In what order should one introduce cyclophosphamide, or chlorambucil, cyclosporine or levamisole in a child with steroid-dependent, frequently relapsing nephrotic syndrome? *Pediatr Nephrol* 1993;7:514.

702. Melvin T, Sibley R, Michael AF. Nephrotic syndrome. In: Tune BM, Mendoza SA, eds. *Contemporary Issues in Nephrology. Pediatric Nephrology.* New York: Churchill Livingstone; 1984:191.

703. Zech P, Colon S, Pointet P, et al. The nephrotic syndrome in adults aged over 60: etiology, evolution, and treatment of 76 cases. *Clin Nephrol* 1982;17:232.

704. Yeung CK, Wong KL, Ng WL. Intravenous methylprednisolone pulse therapy in minimal change nephrotic syndrome. *Aust NZ J Med* 1983;13:349.

705. Al-Khader AA, Lien JW, Aber GM. Cyclophosphamide alone in the treatment of adult patients with minimal change glomerulonephritis. *Clin Nephrol* 1979;11:26.

706. Nolasco F, Cameron JS, Heywood EF, et al. Adult-onset minimal change nephrotic syndrome: a long-term follow-up. *Kidney Int* 1986;29:1215.

707. Black DA. Controlled trial of prednisone in adult patients with the nephrotic syndrome. *Br Med J* 1970;3:421.

708. Glassock RJ. Therapy of idiopathic nephrotic syndrome in adults: a conservative or aggressive therapeutic approach. *Am J Nephrol* 1993;13:422.

709. Rose GM, Cole BR, Robson AJ. The treatment of renal glomerulopathies in children using high dose intravenous methylprednisolone pulses. *Am J Kidney Dis* 1981;1:148.

710. Rostin M, Barthe P, Houin G, et al. Pharmacokinetics of prednisolone in children with the nephrotic syndrome. *Pediatr Nephrol* 1990;4:470.

711. Loeffler K, Gowrishankar M, Yiu V. Tacrolimus therapy in pediatric patients with treatment-resistant nephrotic syndrome. *Pediatr Nephrol* 2004;19:281.

712. Bergstein JM. Prostaglandin inhibitors in the treatment of nephrotic syndrome. *Pediatr Nephrol* 1991;5:335.

713. Garin EH, Williams RL, Rennell RS, III, et al. Indomethacin in the treatment of idiopathic minimal lesion nephrotic syndrome. *J Pediatr* 1978;93:138.

714. Cuoghi D, Evangelista A, Baraldi A, et al. Relapse of nephrotic syndrome following remission for 20 years. *Int J Pediatr Nephrol* 1983;4:211.

715. Pru C, Kjellstrand CM, Cohn RA, et al. Late recurrence of minimal lesion nephrotic syndrome. *Ann Intern Med* 1984;100:69.

716. Scharer K, Minges U. Long-term prognosis of the nephrotic syndrome in childhood. *Clin Nephrol* 1973;1:182.

717. Trainin EB, Gomez-Leon G. Development of renal insufficiency after long-standing steroid-responsive nephrotic syndrome. *Int J Pediatr Nephrol* 1982;3:55.

718. Mauer SM, Hellerstein S, Cohen RA, et al. Recurrence of steroid-responsive nephrotic syndrome after renal transplantation. *J Pediatr* 1979;95:261.

719. Hiraoka M, Takeda N, Tsukahara H, et al. Favorable course of steroid-responsive nephrotic children with mild attack. *Kidney Int* 1995;47:1392.

720. Cameron JS, Turner DR, Ogg CS, et al. The long-term prognosis of patients with focal segmental glomerulosclerosis. *Clin Nephrol* 1978;10:213.

721. Idelson BA, Smithline N, Smith GW. Prognosis in steroid-treated idiopathic nephrotic syndrome in adults. *Arch Intern Med* 1977;137:891.

722. Hyams JS, Carey DE. Corticosteroids and growth. *J Pediatr* 1988;113:249.

723. Saha MT, Laippala P, Lenko HL. Normal growth of prepubertal nephrotic children during long-term treatment with repeated courses of prednisone. *Acta Paediatr* 1998;87:545.

724. Polito C, Oporto MR, Totino SF, et al. Normal growth of nephrotic children during long-term alternate-day prednisone therapy. *Acta Pediatr Scand* 1986;75:245.

725. Fleisher DS, McCrory WW, Rapoport M. The effects of intermittent doses of adrenocortical steroids on the statural growth of nephrotic children. *J Pediatr* 1960;57:192.

726. Foote KD, Brocklebank JT, Meadow SR. Height attainment in children with steroid-responsive nephrotic syndrome. *Lancet* 1985;ii:917.

727. Brocklebank JT, Harcourt RB, Meadow SR. Corticosteroid-induced cataracts in idiopathic nephrotic syndrome. *Arch Dis Child* 1982;53:30.

728. Krensky AM, Inglefinger JR, Grupe WE. Peritonitis in childhood nephrotic syndrome. *Am J Dis Child* 1982;136:732.

729. International Study of Kidney Disease in Children. Minimal change nephrotic syndrome in children: deaths during the first 5 to 15 years' observation. *Pediatrics* 1984;73:497.

730. Kappel B, Olsen S. Cortical interstitial tissue and sclerosed glomeruli in the normal human kidney, related to age and sex. A quantitative study. *Virchows Arch A Pathol Anat Histol* 1980;387:271.

731. Smith SM, Hoy WE, Cobb L. Low incidence of glomerulosclerosis in normal kidneys. *Arch Pathol Lab Med* 1989;113:1253.

732. Detwiler RK, Falk RJ, Hogan SL, et al. Collapsing glomerulopathy: a clinically and pathologically distinct variant of focal segmental glomerulosclerosis. *Kidney Int* 1994;45:1416.

733. Korbet SM. Clinical picture and outcome of primary focal segmental glomerulosclerosis. *Nephrol Dial Transplant* 1999;14(Suppl 3):68.

734. Braden GL, Mulhern JG, O'Shea MH, et al. Changing incidence of glomerular diseases in adults. *Am J Kidney Dis* 2000;35:878.

735. Bonilla-Felix M, Parra C, Dajani T, et al. Changing patterns in the

histopathology of idiopathic nephrotic syndrome in children. *Kidney Int* 1999;55:1885.

736. Gulati S, Sharma AP, Sharma RK, et al. Changing trends of histopathology in childhood nephrotic syndrome. *Am J Kidney Dis* 1999;34:646.

737. Adhikari M, Bhimma R, Coovadia HM. Focal segmental glomerulosclerosis in children from KwaZulu/Natal, South Africa. *Clin Nephrol* 2001;55:16.

738. US Renal Data System. USRDS 2004 Annual Data Report: Atlas of End-Stage Renal Disease in the United States. National Institutes of Health, National Institute of Diabetes and Digestive and Kidney Diseases. 2004.

739. Kitiyakara C, Kopp JB, Eggers P. Trends in the epidemiology of focal segmental glomerulosclerosis. *Semin Nephrol* 2003;23:172.

740. Kitiyakara C, Eggers P, Kopp JB. Twenty-one-year trend in ESRD due to focal segmental glomerulosclerosis in the United States. *Am J Kidney Dis* 2004;44:815.

741. Freedman BI, Bowden DW, Rich SS, et al. A genome scan for all-cause end-stage renal disease in African Americans. *Nephrol Dial Transplant* 2005; 20:712.

742. Korbet SM. Primary focal segmental glomerulosclerosis. *J Am Soc Nephrol* 1998;9:1333.

743. Ingulli E, Tejani A. Racial differences in the incidence and renal outcome of idiopathic focal segmental glomerulosclerosis in children. *Pediatr Nephrol* 1991;5:393.

744. Dixit M, Mansur A, Dixit N, et al. The role of ACE gene polymorphism in rapidity of progression of focal segmental glomerulosclerosis. *J Postgrad Med* 2002;48:266; discussion 269.

745. Fahr T. Pathologische anatomie des morbus brightii. In: Henke F LO, ed. *Handbuch*. Berlin, 1925.

746. Heptinstall RH. *Nephrotic Syndrome. Pathology of the Kidney*. Boston: Little Brown; 1966:355.

747. McGovern VJ. Persistent nephrotic syndrome: a renal biopsy study. *Australas Int Med* 1964;13:306.

748. Hayslett JP, Krassner LS, Bensch KG, et al. Progression of "lipoid nephrosis" to renal insufficiency. *N Engl J Med* 1969;281:181.

749. Fogo A, Glick AD, Horn SL, et al. Is focal segmental glomerulosclerosis really focal? Distribution of lesions in adults and children. *Kidney Int* 1995;47:1690.

750. Remuzzi A, Mazerska M, Gephardt GN, et al. Three-dimensional analysis of glomerular morphology in patients with subtotal nephrectomy. *Kidney Int* 1995;48:155.

751. Morel-Maroger L, Leathem A, Richet G. Glomerular abnormalities in non-systemic diseases. Relationship between findings by light microscopy and immunofluorescence in 433 renal biopsy specimens. *Am J Med* 1972;53:170.

752. Fogo A, Hawkins EP, Berry PL, et al. Glomerular hypertrophy in minimal change disease predicts subsequent progression to focal glomerular sclerosis. *Kidney Int* 1990;38:115.

753. Markowitz GS, Lin J, Valeri AM, et al. Idiopathic nodular glomerulosclerosis is a distinct clinicopathologic entity linked to hypertension and smoking. *Hum Pathol* 2002;33:826.

754. D'Agati VD, Fogo AB, Bruijn JA, et al. Pathologic classification of focal segmental glomerulosclerosis: a working proposal. *Am J Kidney Dis* 2004;43:368.

755. Jennette JC, Mandal AK. The nephrotic syndrome. In: Mandal AK, Jennette JC, eds. *Diagnosis and Management of Renal Disease and Hypertension*. Durham, NC: Carolina Academic Press; 1994:235.

756. Barisoni L, Kopp JB. Modulation of podocyte phenotype in collapsing glomerulopathies. *Microsc Res Tech* 2002;57:254.

757. Schmid H, Henger A, Cohen CD, et al. Gene expression profiles of podocyte-associated molecules as diagnostic markers in acquired proteinuric diseases. *J Am Soc Nephrol* 2003;14:2958.

758. Grishman E, Churg J. Focal glomerular sclerosis in nephrotic patients: an electron microscopic study of glomerular podocytes. *Kidney Int* 1975;7:111.

759. Schwartz MM, Lewis EJ. Focal segmental glomerular sclerosis: the cellular lesion. *Kidney Int* 1985;28:968.

760. Olson JL, de Urdaneta AG, Heptinstall RH. Glomerular hyalinosis and its relation to hyperfiltration. *Lab Invest* 1985;52:387.

761. Chun MJ, Korbet SM, Schwartz MM, et al. Focal segmental glomerulosclerosis in nephrotic adults: Presentation, prognosis, and response to therapy of the histologic variants. *J Am Soc Nephrol* 2004;15:2169.

762. Meyrier A. E pluribus unum: The riddle of focal segmental glomerulosclerosis. *Semin Nephrol* 2003;23:135.

763. Chiang ML, Hawkins EP, Berry PL, et al. Diagnostic and prognostic significance of glomerular epithelial cell vacuolization and podocyte effacement in children with minimal lesion nephrotic syndrome and focal segmental glomerulosclerosis: An ultrastructural study. *Clin Nephrol* 1988;30:8.

764. Kambham N, Markowitz GS, Valeri AM, et al. Obesity-related glomerulopathy: an emerging epidemic. *Kidney Int* 2001;59:1498.

765. D'Agati V. Pathologic classification of focal segmental glomerulosclerosis. *Semin Nephrol* 2003;23:117.

766. Kriz W, Hosser H, Hahnel B, et al. Development of vascular pole-associated glomerulosclerosis in the Fawn-hooded rat. *J Am Soc Nephrol* 1998;9:381.

767. Kriz W, Lemley KV. The role of the podocyte in glomerulosclerosis. *Curr Opin Nephrol Hypertens* 1999;8:489.

768. Gulati S, Sharma AP, Sharma RK, et al. Do current recommendations for kidney biopsy in nephrotic syndrome need modifications? *Pediatr Nephrol* 2002;17:404.

769. Au WY, Chan KW, Lui SL, et al. Focal segmental glomerulosclerosis and mesangial sclerosis associated with myeloproliferative disorders. *Am J Kidney Dis* 1999;34:889.

770. Fogo AB. Animal models of FSGS: Lessons for pathogenesis and treatment. *Semin Nephrol* 2003;23:161.

771. Shimamura T, Morrison AB. A progressive glomerulosclerosis occurring in partial five-sixths nephrectomized rats. *Am J Pathol* 1975;79:95.

772. Hostetter TH, Olson JL, Rennke HG, et al. Hyperfiltration in remnant nephrons: a potentially adverse response to renal ablation. *Am J Physiol* 1981;241:F85.

773. Meyer TW, Rennke HG. Progressive glomerular injury after limited renal infarction in the rat. *Am J Physiol* 1988;254:F856.

774. Ma LJ, Fogo AB. Model of robust induction of glomerulosclerosis in mice: importance of genetic background. *Kidney Int* 2003;64:350.

775. Okuda S, Motomura K, Sanai T, et al. Influence of age on deterioration of the remnant kidney in uninephrectomized rats. *Clin Sci (Lond)* 1987;72:571.

776. Zheng F, Plati AR, Potier M, et al. Resistance to glomerulosclerosis in B6 mice disappears after menopause. *Am J Pathol* 2003;162:1339.

777. O'Donnell MP, Michels L, Kasiske B, et al. Adriamycin-induced chronic proteinuria: a structural and functional study. *J Lab Clin Med* 1985;106:62.

778. Chen A, Sheu LF, Ho YS, et al. Experimental focal segmental glomerulosclerosis in mice. *Nephron* 1998;78:440.

779. Garber SL, Mirochnik Y, Arruda JA, et al. Evolution of experimentally induced papillary necrosis to focal segmental glomerulosclerosis and nephrotic proteinuria. *Am J Kidney Dis* 1999;33:1033.

780. Backman L, Sundelin B, Bohman SO. Focal glomerulosclerosis and nephron atrophy in rats on long-term cyclosporine treatment. *APMIS Suppl* 1988;4:27.

781. Kriz W, Hahnel B, Rosener S, et al. Long-term treatment of rats with FGF-2 results in focal segmental glomerulosclerosis. *Kidney Int* 1995;48:1435.

782. Diamond JR, Karnovsky MJ. Focal and segmental glomerulosclerosis following a single intravenous dose of puromycin aminonucleoside. *Am J Pathol* 1986;122:481.

783. Cahill MM, Ryan GB, Bertram JF. Biphasic glomerular hypertrophy in rats administered puromycin aminonucleoside. *Kidney Int* 1996;50:768.

784. O'Donnell MP, Kasiske BL, Keane WF. Risk factors for glomerular injury in rats with genetic hypertension. *Am J Hypertens* 1989;2:9.

785. Yagil C, Sapojnikov M, Katni G, et al. Proteinuria and glomerulosclerosis in the Sabra genetic rat model of salt susceptibility. *Physiol Genomics* 2002;9:167.

786. Remuzzi A, Puntorieri S, Alfano M, et al. Pathophysiologic implications of proteinuria in a rat model of progressive glomerular injury. *Lab Invest* 1992;67:572.

787. Kondo S, Yoshizawa N, Wakabayashi K. Natural history of renal lesions in spontaneously hypercholesterolemic (SHC) male rats. *Nippon Jinzo Gakkai Shi* 1995;37:91.

788. Yoshikawa Y, Yamasaki K. Renal lesions of hyperlipidemic Imai rats: a spontaneous animal model of focal glomerulosclerosis. *Nephron* 1991;59:471.

789. Shimamura T. Focal glomerulosclerosis in obese Zucker rats and prevention of its development. *Kidney Int Suppl* 1983;16:S259.

790. Nakamura Y, Oite T, Shimizu F, et al. Sclerotic lesions in the glomeruli of Buffalo/Mna rats. *Nephron* 1986;43:50.

791. Le Berre L, Godfrin Y, Perretto S, et al. The Buffalo/Mna rat, an animal model of FSGS recurrence after renal transplantation. *Transplant Proc* 2001;33:3338.

792. Yoshida F, Matsuo S, Fujishima H, et al. Renal lesions of the FGS strain of mice: a spontaneous animal model of progressive glomerulosclerosis. *Nephron* 1994;66:317.

793. Nishida E, Yamanouchi J, Ogata S, et al. Age-related histochemical and ultrastructural changes in renal glomerular mesangium of APA hamsters. *Exp Anim* 1996;45:339.

794. Shih NY, Li J, Karpitskii V, et al. Congenital nephrotic syndrome in mice lacking CD2-associated protein. *Science* 1999;286:312.

795. Kim JM, Wu H, Green G, et al. CD2-associated protein haploinsufficiency is linked to glomerular disease susceptibility. *Science* 2003;300:1298.

796. Roselli S, Heidet L, Sich M, et al. Early glomerular filtration defect and severe renal disease in podocin-deficient mice. *Mol Cell Biol* 2004;24:550.

797. Kos CH, Le TC, Sinha S, et al. Mice deficient in alpha-actinin-4 have severe glomerular disease. *J Clin Invest* 2003;111:1683.

798. Yao J, Le TC, Kos CH, et al. Alpha-actinin-4-mediated FSGS: an inherited kidney disease caused by an aggregated and rapidly degraded cytoskeletal protein. *PLoS Biol* 2004;2:e167.

799. Patek CE, Little MH, Fleming S, et al. A zinc finger truncation of murine WT1 results in the characteristic urogenital abnormalities of Denys-Drash syndrome. *Proc Natl Acad Sci U S A* 1999;96:2931.

800. Gao F, Maiti S, Sun G, et al. The Wt1+/R394W mouse displays glomerulosclerosis and early-onset renal failure characteristic of human Denys-Drash syndrome. *Mol Cell Biol* 2004;24:9899.

801. O'Bryan T, Weiher H, Rennke HG, et al. Course of renal injury in the Mpv17-deficient transgenic mouse. *J Am Soc Nephrol* 2000;11:1067.

802. Gassler N, Elger M, Inoue D, et al. Oligonephronia, not exuberant apoptosis, accounts for the development of glomerulosclerosis in the bcl-2 knockout mouse. *Nephrol Dial Transplant* 1998;13:2509.

803. Lambert G, Sakai N, Vaisman BL, et al. Analysis of glomerulosclerosis and atherosclerosis in lecithin cholesterol acyltransferase-deficient mice. *J Biol Chem* 2001;276:15090.

804. Powell DR, Desai U, Sparks MJ, et al. Rapid development of glomerular injury and renal failure in mice lacking p53R2. *Pediatr Nephrol* 2005;20:432.

805. Michaud JL, Lemieux LI, Dube M, et al. Focal and segmental glomerulosclerosis in mice with podocyte-specific expression of mutant alpha-actinin-4. *J Am Soc Nephrol* 2003;14:1200.

806. Mullins JJ, Peters J, Ganten D. Fulminant hypertension in transgenic rats harbouring the mouse Ren-2 gene. *Nature* 1990;344:541.

807. Wagner J, Klotz S, Haufe CC, et al. Progression of renal failure after subtotal nephrectomy in transgenic rats carrying an additional renin gene (TGR[mREN2]27). *J Hypertens* 1997;15:441.

808. Mervaala E, Muller DN, Park JK, et al. Cyclosporin A protects against angiotensin II-induced end-organ damage in double transgenic rats harboring human renin and angiotensinogen genes. *Hypertension* 2000;35:360.

809. Kopp JB, Factor VM, Mozes M, et al. Transgenic mice with increased plasma levels of TGF-beta 1 develop progressive renal disease. *Lab Invest* 1996;74:991.

810. Clouthier DE, Comerford SA, Hammer RE. Hepatic fibrosis, glomerulosclerosis, and a lipodystrophy-like syndrome in PEPCK-TGF-beta1 transgenic mice. *J Clin Invest* 1997;100:2697.

811. Takayama H, LaRochelle WJ, Sabnis SG, et al. Renal tubular hyperplasia, polycystic disease, and glomerulosclerosis in transgenic mice overexpressing hepatocyte growth factor/scatter factor. *Lab Invest* 1997;77:131.

812. Hocher B, Thone-Reineke C, Rohmeiss P, et al. Endothelin-1 transgenic mice develop glomerulosclerosis, interstitial fibrosis, and renal cysts but not hypertension. *J Clin Invest* 1997;99:1380.

813. Doi T, Striker LJ, Quaife C, et al. Progressive glomerulosclerosis develops in transgenic mice chronically expressing growth hormone and growth hormone releasing factor but not in those expressing insulinlike growth factor-1. *Am J Pathol* 1988;131:398.

814. Sasaki S, Nishihira J, Ishibashi T, et al. Transgene of MIF induces podocyte injury and progressive mesangial sclerosis in the mouse kidney. *Kidney Int* 2004;65:469.

815. Hoffmann S, Podlich D, Hahnel B, et al. Angiotensin II type 1 receptor overexpression in podocytes induces glomerulosclerosis in transgenic rats. *J Am Soc Nephrol* 2004;15:1475.

816. Godley LA, Kopp JB, Eckhaus M, et al. Wild-type p53 transgenic mice exhibit altered differentiation of the ureteric bud and possess small kidneys. *Genes Dev* 1996;10:836.

817. Brantley JG, Sharma M, Alcalay NI, et al. Cux-1 transgenic mice develop glomerulosclerosis and interstitial fibrosis. *Kidney Int* 2003;63:1240.

818. Trudel M, De Paepe ME, Chretien N, et al. Sickle cell disease of transgenic SAD mice. *Blood* 1994;84:3189.

819. Smeets B, Te Loeke NA, Dijkman HB, et al. The parietal epithelial cell: a key player in the pathogenesis of focal segmental glomerulosclerosis in Thy-1.1 transgenic mice. *J Am Soc Nephrol* 2004;15:928.

820. MacKay K, Striker LJ, Pinkert CA, et al. Glomerulosclerosis and renal cysts in mice transgenic for the early region of SV40. *Kidney Int* 1987;32:827.

821. Kopp JB, Klotman ME, Adler SH, et al. Progressive glomerulosclerosis and enhanced renal accumulation of basement membrane components in mice transgenic for human immunodeficiency virus type 1 genes. *Proc Natl Acad Sci U S A* 1992;89:1577.

822. Reid W, Sadowska M, Denaro F, et al. An HIV-1 transgenic rat that develops HIV-related pathology and immunologic dysfunction. *Proc Natl Acad Sci U S A* 2001;98:9271.

823. Dickie P, Roberts A, Uwiera R, et al. Focal glomerulosclerosis in proviral and c-fms transgenic mice links Vpr expression to HIV-associated nephropathy. *Virology* 2004;322:69.

824. Komatsu K, Frohlich ED, Ono H, et al. Glomerular dynamics and morphology of aged spontaneously hypertensive rats. Effects of angiotensin-converting enzyme inhibition. *Hypertension* 1995;25:207.

825. Platt R, Roscoe MH, Smith FW. Experimental renal failure. *Clin Sci (Lond)* 1952;11:217.

826. Morrison AB, Howard RM. The functional capacity of hypertrophied nephrons. Effect of partial nephrectomy on the clearance of inulin and PAH in the rat. *J Exp Med* 1966;123:829.

827. Novick AC, Gephardt G, Guz B, et al. Long-term follow-up after partial removal of a solitary kidney. *N Engl J Med* 1991;325:1058.

828. Howie AJ, Kizaki T, Beaman M, et al. Different types of segmental sclerosing glomerular lesions in six experimental models of proteinuria. *J Pathol* 1989;157:141.

829. Barker DJ, Osmond C, Golding J, et al. Growth in utero, blood pressure in childhood and adult life, and mortality from cardiovascular disease. *BMJ* 1989;298:564.

830. Brenner BM, Mackenzie HS. Nephron mass as a risk factor for progression of renal disease. *Kidney Int Suppl* 1997;63:S124.

831. Manalich R, Reyes L, Herrera M, et al. Relationship between weight at birth and the number and size of renal glomeruli in humans: a histomorphometric study. *Kidney Int* 2000;58:770.

832. Jones SE, Nyengaard JR, Flyvbjerg A, et al. Birth weight has no influence on glomerular number and volume. *Pediatr Nephrol* 2001;16:340.

833. Keller G, Zimmer G, Mall G, et al. Nephron number in patients with primary hypertension. *N Engl J Med* 2003;348:101.

834. Lackland DT, Bendall HE, Osmond C, et al. Low birth weights contribute to high rates of early-onset chronic renal failure in the Southeastern United States. *Arch Intern Med* 2000;160:1472.

835. Moore L, Williams R, Staples A. Glomerular dimensions in children under 16 years of age. *J Pathol* 1993;171:145.

836. Ellis EN, Mauer SM, Sutherland DE, et al. Glomerular capillary morphology in normal humans. *Lab Invest* 1989;60:231.

837. Cortes P, Zhao X, Dumler F, et al. Age-related changes in glomerular volume and hydroxyproline content in rat and human. *J Am Soc Nephrol* 1992;2:1716.

838. Yoshikawa N, Cameron AH, White RH. Glomerular morphometry I: Nephrotic syndrome in childhood. *Histopathology* 1981;5:239.

839. Olivetti G, Anversa P, Melissari M, et al. Morphometry of the renal corpuscle during postnatal growth and compensatory hypertrophy. *Kidney Int* 1980;17:438.

840. Nyengaard JR. Number and dimensions of rat glomerular capillaries in normal development and after nephrectomy. *Kidney Int* 1993;43:1049.

841. Bidani AK, Mitchell KD, Schwartz MM, et al. Absence of glomerular injury or nephron loss in a normotensive rat remnant kidney model. *Kidney Int* 1990;38:28.

842. Daniels BS, Hostetter TH. Adverse effects of growth in the glomerular microcirculation. *Am J Physiol* 1990;258:F1409.

843. Akaoka K, White RH, Raafat F. Glomerular morphometry in childhood reflux nephropathy, emphasizing the capillary changes. *Kidney Int* 1995;47:1108.

844. Matsumae T, Fukuzaki M, Takebayashi S, et al. Two different pathways of glomerular enlargement in adults with focal and segmental glomerulosclerosis: A morphometric study. *Am J Nephrol* 1998;18:21.

845. Praga M, Hernandez E, Morales E, et al. Clinical features and long-term outcome of obesity-associated focal segmental glomerulosclerosis. *Nephrol Dial Transplant* 2001;16:1790.

846. Yoshida Y, Fogo A, Ichikawa I. Glomerular hemodynamic changes vs. hypertrophy in experimental glomerular sclerosis. *Kidney Int* 1989;35:654.

847. Fogo A, Yoshida Y, Glick AD, et al. Serial micropuncture analysis of glomerular function in two rat models of glomerular sclerosis. *J Clin Invest* 1988;82:322.

848. Stokholm KH, Brochner-Mortensen J, Hoilund-Carlsen PF. Increased glomerular filtration rate and adrenocortical function in obese women. *Int J Obes* 1980;4:57.

849. Chagnac A, Weinstein T, Korzets A, et al. Glomerular hemodynamics in severe obesity. *Am J Physiol Renal Physiol* 2000;278:F817.

850. Chagnac A, Weinstein T, Herman M, et al. The effects of weight loss on renal function in patients with severe obesity. *J Am Soc Nephrol* 2003;14:1480.

851. Bosma RJ, van der Heide JJ, Oosterop EJ, et al. Body mass index is associated with altered renal hemodynamics in non-obese healthy subjects. *Kidney Int* 2004;65:259.

852. Anastasio P, Spitali L, Frangiosa A, et al. Glomerular filtration rate in severely overweight normotensive humans. *Am J Kidney Dis* 2000;35:1144.

853. Scaglione R, Ganguzza A, Corrao S, et al. Central obesity and hypertension: Pathophysiologic role of renal haemodynamics and function. *Int J Obes Relat Metab Disord* 1995;19:403.

854. Morgan AG, Serjeant GR. Renal function in patients over 40 with homozygous sickle-cell disease. *Br Med J (Clin Res Ed)* 1981;282:1181.

855. Guasch A, Cua M, Mitch WE. Early detection and the course of glomerular injury in patients with sickle cell anemia. *Kidney Int* 1996;49:786.

856. Herrera J, Avila E, Marin C, et al. Impaired creatinine secretion after an intravenous creatinine load is an early characteristic of the nephropathy of sickle cell anaemia. *Nephrol Dial Transplant* 2002;17:602.

857. Passwell J, Orda S, Modan M, et al. Abnormal renal functions in cyanotic congenital heart disease. *Arch Dis Child* 1976;51:803.

858. Burlet A, Drukker A, Guignard JP. Renal function in cyanotic congenital heart disease. *Nephron* 1999;81:296.

859. Fogo A, Hawkins EP, Berry PL, et al. Glomerular hypertrophy in minimal change disease predicts subsequent progression to focal glomerular sclerosis. *Kidney Int* 1990;38:115.

860. Pagtalunan ME, Miller PL, Jumping-Eagle S, et al. Podocyte loss and progressive glomerular injury in type II diabetes. *J Clin Invest* 1997;99:342.

861. Lemley KV, Lafayette RA, Safai M, et al. Podocytopenia and disease severity in IgA nephropathy. *Kidney Int* 2002;61:1475.

862. Nagata M, Yamaguchi Y, Komatsu Y, et al. Mitosis and the presence of

binucleate cells among glomerular podocytes in diseased human kidneys. *Nephron* 1995;70:68.

863. Fries JW, Sandstrom DJ, Meyer TW, et al. Glomerular hypertrophy and epithelial cell injury modulate progressive glomerulosclerosis in the rat. *Lab Invest* 1989;60:205.

864. Bhathena DB. Glomerular basement membrane length to podocyte ratio in human nephronopenia: Implications for focal segmental glomerulosclerosis. *Am J Kidney Dis* 2003;41:1179.

865. Kriz W, Kretzler M, Nagata M, et al. A frequent pathway to glomerulosclerosis: deterioration of tuft architecture-podocyte damage-segmental sclerosis. *Kidney Blood Press Res* 1996;19:245.

866. Kriz W, Hosser H, Hahnel B, et al. From segmental glomerulosclerosis to total nephron degeneration and interstitial fibrosis: a histopathological study in rat models and human glomerulopathies. *Nephrol Dial Transplant* 1998;13:2781.

867. Kriz W. The pathogenesis of 'classic' focal segmental glomerulosclerosis-lessons from rat models. *Nephrol Dial Transplant* 2003;18(Suppl 6):vi,39.

868. Pavenstadt H, Kriz W, Kretzler M. Cell biology of the glomerular podocyte. *Physiol Rev* 2003;83:253.

869. Hingorani SR, Finn LS, Kowalewska J, et al. Expression of nephrin in acquired forms of nephrotic syndrome in childhood. *Pediatr Nephrol* 2004;19:300.

870. Huh W, Kim DJ, Kim MK, et al. Expression of nephrin in acquired human glomerular disease. *Nephrol Dial Transplant* 2002;17:478.

871. Guan N, Ding J, Zhang J, et al. Expression of nephrin, podocin, alpha-actinin, and WT1 in children with nephrotic syndrome. *Pediatr Nephrol* 2003;18:1122.

872. Horinouchi I, Nakazato H, Kawano T, et al. In situ evaluation of podocin in normal and glomerular diseases. *Kidney Int* 2003;64:2092.

873. Barisoni L, Kriz W, Mundel P, et al. The dysregulated podocyte phenotype: a novel concept in the pathogenesis of collapsing idiopathic focal segmental glomerulosclerosis and HIV-associated nephropathy. *J Am Soc Nephrol* 1999;10:51.

874. Kihara I, Yaoita E, Kawasaki K, et al. Origin of hyperplastic epithelial cells in idiopathic collapsing glomerulopathy. *Histopathology* 1999;34:537.

875. Barisoni L, Mokrzycki M, Sablay L, et al. Podocyte cell cycle regulation and proliferation in collapsing glomerulopathies. *Kidney Int* 2000;58:137.

876. Srivastava T, Garola RE, Whiting JM, et al. Synaptopodin expression in idiopathic nephrotic syndrome of childhood. *Kidney Int* 2001;59:118.

877. Yang Y, Gubler MC, Beaufils H. Dysregulation of podocyte phenotype in idiopathic collapsing glomerulopathy and HIV-associated nephropathy. *Nephron* 2002;91:416.

878. Kemeny E, Mihatsch MJ, Durmuller U, et al. Podocytes loose their adhesive phenotype in focal segmental glomerulosclerosis. *Clin Nephrol* 1995;43:71.

879. Nagata M, Horita S, Shu Y, et al. Phenotypic characteristics and cyclin-dependent kinase inhibitors repression in hyperplastic epithelial pathology in idiopathic focal segmental glomerulosclerosis. *Lab Invest* 2000;80:869.

880. Wang S, Kim JH, Moon KC, et al. Cell-cycle mechanisms involved in podocyte proliferation in cellular lesion of focal segmental glomerulosclerosis. *Am J Kidney Dis* 2004;43:19.

881. Yang AH, Chen JY, Chen BF. The dysregulated glomerular cell growth in Denys-Drash syndrome. *Virchows Arch* 2004;445:305.

882. Shankland SJ, Eitner F, Hudkins KL, et al. Differential expression of cyclin-dependent kinase inhibitors in human glomerular disease: role in podocyte proliferation and maturation. *Kidney Int* 2000;58:674.

883. Hiromura K, Haseley LA, Zhang P, et al. Podocyte expression of the CDK-inhibitor p57 during development and disease. *Kidney Int* 2001;60:2235.

884. Riser BL, Cortes P, Yee J. Modelling the effects of vascular stress in mesangial cells. *Curr Opin Nephrol Hypertens* 2000;9:43.

885. Riser BL, Varani J, Cortes P, et al. Cyclic stretching of mesangial cells up-regulates intercellular adhesion molecule-1 and leukocyte adherence: a possible new mechanism for glomerulosclerosis. *Am J Pathol* 2001;158:11.

886. Yasuda T, Kondo S, Homma T, et al. Regulation of extracellular matrix by mechanical stress in rat glomerular mesangial cells. *J Clin Invest* 1996;98:1991.

887. Suda T, Osajima A, Tamura M, et al. Pressure-induced expression of monocyte chemoattractant protein-1 through activation of MAP kinase. *Kidney Int* 2001;60:1705.

888. Hishikawa K, Oemar BS, Nakaki T. Static pressure regulates connective tissue growth factor expression in human mesangial cells. *J Biol Chem* 2001;276:16797.

889. Riser BL, Cortes P, Zhao X, et al. Intraglomerular pressure and mesangial stretching stimulate extracellular matrix formation in the rat. *J Clin Invest* 1992;90:1932.

890. Riser BL, Cortes P, Heilig C, et al. Cyclic stretching force selectively up-regulates transforming growth factor-beta isoforms in cultured rat mesangial cells. *Am J Pathol* 1996;148:1915.

891. Lee LK, Meyer TW, Pollock AS, et al. Endothelial cell injury initiates glomerular sclerosis in the rat remnant kidney. *J Clin Invest* 1995;96:953.

892. Adamczak M, Gross ML, Amann K, et al. Reversal of glomerular lesions involves coordinated restructuring of glomerular microvasculature. *J Am Soc Nephrol* 2004;15:3063.

893. Magil AB, Cohen AH. Monocytes and focal glomerulosclerosis. *Lab Invest* 1989;61:404.

894. Markovic-Lipkovski J, Muller CA, Risler T, et al. Mononuclear leukocytes, expression of HLA class II antigens and intercellular adhesion molecule 1 in focal segmental glomerulosclerosis. *Nephron* 1991;59:286.

895. van Goor H, van der Horst ML, Fidler V, et al. Glomerular macrophage modulation affects mesangial expansion in the rat after renal ablation. *Lab Invest* 1992;66:564.

896. Vielhauer V, Berning E, Eis V, et al. CCR1 blockade reduces interstitial inflammation and fibrosis in mice with glomerulosclerosis and nephrotic syndrome. *Kidney Int* 2004;66:2264.

897. Branton MH, Kopp JB. TGF-beta and fibrosis. *Microbes Infect* 1999;1:1349.

898. Poncelet AC, Schnaper HW. Regulation of mesangial cell collagen turnover by transforming growth factor-b1. *Am J Physiol* 1998;275(44):F458.

899. Leask A, Abraham DJ. The role of connective tissue growth factor, a multifunctional matricellular protein, in fibroblast biology. *Biochem Cell Biol* 2003;81:355.

900. Diamond JR. The role of reactive oxygen species in animal models of glomerular disease. *Am J Kidney Dis* 1992;19:292.

901. Schnaper HW. Balance between matrix synthesis and degradation: a determinant of glomerulosclerosis. *Pediatr Nephrol* 1995;9:104.

902. Eddy AA. Molecular basis of renal fibrosis. *Pediatr Nephrol* 2000;15:290.

903. Lovett DH, Johnson RJ, Marti HP, et al. Structural characterization of the mesangial cell type IV collagenase and enhanced expression in a model of immune complex-mediated glomerulonephritis. *Am J Pathol* 1992;141:85.

904. Baricos WH, Cortez SL, El-Dahr SS, et al. ECM degradation by cultured human mesangial cells is mediated by a plasminogen activator/plasmin/matrix metalloproteinase 2 cascade. *Kidney Int* 1995;47:1039.

905. Ma LJ, Fogo AB. Angiotensin as inducer of plasminogen activator inhibitor-1 and fibrosis. *Contrib Nephrol* 2001;161.

906. Floege J, Kriz W, Schulze M, et al. Basic fibroblast growth factor augments podocyte injury and induces glomerulosclerosis in rats with experimental membranous nephropathy. *J Clin Invest* 1995;96:2809.

907. Schiffer M, Bitzer M, Roberts IS, et al. Apoptosis in podocytes induced by TGF-beta and Smad7. *J Clin Invest* 2001;108:807.

908. Ortmann J, Amann K, Brandes RP, et al. Role of podocytes for reversal of glomerulosclerosis and proteinuria in the aging kidney after endothelin inhibition. *Hypertension* 2004;44:974.

909. Hollenberg NK. Aldosterone in the development and progression of renal injury. *Kidney Int* 2004;66:1.

910. Weigert C, Brodbeck K, Klopfer K, et al. Angiotensin II induces human TGF-beta 1 promoter activation: similarity to hyperglycaemia. *Diabetologia* 2002;45:890.

911. Sorokin A, Kohan DE. Physiology and pathology of endothelin-1 in renal mesangium. *Am J Physiol Renal Physiol* 2003;285:F579.

912. Sraer JD, Kanfer A, Rondeau E, et al. Mechanisms of glomerular injury: Overview and relation with hemostasis. *Ren Fail* 1993;15:343.

913. Wolf G, Chen S, Han DC, et al. Leptin and renal disease. *Am J Kidney Dis* 2002;39:1.

914. Howie AJ, Brewer DB. The glomerular tip lesion: a previously undescribed type of segmental glomerular abnormality. *J Pathol* 1984;142:205.

915. Howie AJ, Pankhurst T, Sarioglu S, et al. Evolution of nephrotic-associated focal segmental glomerulosclerosis and relation to the glomerular tip lesion. *Kidney Int* 2005;67:987.

916. Haas M. The glomerular tip lesion: what does it really mean? *Kidney Int* 2005;67:1188.

917. Howie AJ. Changes at the glomerular tip: a feature of membranous nephropathy and other disorders associated with proteinuria. *J Pathol* 1986;150:13.

918. Thomsen OF, Ladefoged J. Glomerular tip lesions in renal biopsies with focal segmental IgM. *APMIS* 1991;99:836.

919. Howie AJ, Ferreira MA, Majumdar A, et al. Glomerular prolapse as precursor of one type of segmental sclerosing lesions. *J Pathol* 2000;190:478.

920. Najafian B, Kim Y, Crosson JT, et al. Atubular glomeruli and glomerulotubular junction abnormalities in diabetic nephropathy. *J Am Soc Nephrol* 2003;14:908.

921. Howie AJ, Lee SJ, Sparke J. Pathogenesis of segmental glomerular changes at the tubular origin, as in the glomerular tip lesion. *J Pathol* 1995;177:191.

922. Haas M, Yousefzadeh N. Glomerular tip lesion in minimal change nephropathy: a study of autopsies before 1950. *Am J Kidney Dis* 2002;39:1168.

923. Schwartz MM, Evans J, Bain R, et al. Focal segmental glomerulosclerosis: prognostic implications of the cellular lesion. *J Am Soc Nephrol* 1999;10:1900.

924. Praga M, Morales E, Herrero JC, et al. Absence of hypoalbuminemia

despite massive proteinuria in focal segmental glomerulosclerosis secondary to hyperfiltration. *Am J Kidney Dis* 1999;33:52.

925. Bhathena DB. Glomerular size and the association of focal glomerulosclerosis in long-surviving human renal allografts. *J Am Soc Nephrol* 1993;4:1316.

926. Bhathena DB. Focal glomerulosclerosis and maximal glomerular hypertrophy in human nephronopenia. *J Am Soc Nephrol* 1996;7:2600.

927. Elema JD, Arends A. Focal and segmental glomerular hyalinosis and sclerosis in the rat. *Lab Invest* 1975;33:554.

928. Grond J, Schilthuis MS, Koudstaal J, et al. Mesangial function and glomerular sclerosis in rats after unilateral nephrectomy. *Kidney Int* 1982;22:338.

929. Bagby SP. Obesity-initiated metabolic syndrome and the kidney: a recipe for chronic kidney disease? *J Am Soc Nephrol* 2004;15:2775.

930. Henegar JR, Bigler SA, Henegar LK, et al. Functional and structural changes in the kidney in the early stages of obesity. *J Am Soc Nephrol* 2001;12:1211.

931. Cusumano AM, Bodkin NL, Hansen BC, et al. Glomerular hypertrophy is associated with hyperinsulinemia and precedes overt diabetes in aging rhesus monkeys. *Am J Kidney Dis* 2002;40:1075.

932. Adelman RD, Restaino IG, Alon US, et al. Proteinuria and focal segmental glomerulosclerosis in severely obese adolescents. *J Pediatr* 2001;138:481.

933. Schwimmer JA, Markowitz GS, Valeri AM, et al. Secondary focal segmental glomerulosclerosis in non-obese patients with increased muscle mass. *Clin Nephrol* 2003;60:233.

934. Freedman BI, Iskandar SS, Appel RG. The link between hypertension and nephrosclerosis. *Am J Kidney Dis* 1995;25:207.

935. Hsu CY. Does non-malignant hypertension cause renal insufficiency? Evidence based perspective. *Curr Opin Nephrol Hypertens* 2002;11:267.

936. Kincaid-Smith P. Hypothesis: obesity and the insulin resistance syndrome play a major role in end-stage renal failure attributed to hypertension and labelled "hypertensive nephrosclerosis." *J Hypertens* 2004;22:1051.

937. Hughson MD, Johnson K, Young RJ, et al. Glomerular size and glomerulosclerosis: relationships to disease categories, glomerular solidification, and ischemic obsolescence. *Am J Kidney Dis* 2002;39:679.

938. Caetano ER, Zatz R, Saldanha LB, et al. Hypertensive nephrosclerosis as a relevant cause of chronic renal failure. *Hypertension* 2001;38:171.

939. Takebayashi S, Kiyoshi Y, Hisano S, et al. Benign nephrosclerosis: incidence, morphology and prognosis. *Clin Nephrol* 2001;55:349.

940. Marcantoni C, Ma LJ, Federspiel C, et al. Hypertensive nephrosclerosis in African Americans versus Caucasians. *Kidney Int* 2002;62:172.

941. Iskandar SS, Browning MC, Lorentz WB. C1q nephropathy: a pediatric clinicopathologic study. *Am J Kidney Dis* 1991;18:459.

942. Nishida M, Kawakatsu H, Komatsu H, et al. Spontaneous improvement in a case of C1q nephropathy. *Am J Kidney Dis* 2000;35:E22.

943. Kishore U, Gaboriaud C, Waters P, et al. C1q and tumor necrosis factor superfamily: modularity and versatility. *Trends Immunol* 2004;25:551.

944. Navratil JS, Watkins SC, Wisnieski JJ, et al. The globular heads of C1q specifically recognize surface blebs of apoptotic vascular endothelial cells. *J Immunol* 2001;166:3231.

945. Sato T, van Dixhoorn MG, Heemskerk E, et al. C1q, a subunit of the first component of complement, enhances antibody-mediated apoptosis of cultured rat glomerular mesangial cells. *Clin Exp Immunol* 1997;109:510.

946. Cortes-Hernandez J, Fossati-Jimack L, Carugati A, et al. Murine glomerular mesangial cell uptake of apoptotic cells is inefficient and involves serum-mediated but complement-independent mechanisms. *Clin Exp Immunol* 2002;130:459.

947. Ruiz-Villamor E, Quezada M, Bautista MJ, et al. Classical swine fever: pathogenesis of glomerular damage and immunocharacterization of immunocomplex deposits. *J Comp Pathol* 2001;124:246.

948. Weiss MA, Daquioag E, Margolin EG, et al. Nephrotic syndrome, progressive irreversible renal failure, and glomerular "collapse:" a new clinicopathologic entity? *Am J Kidney Dis* 1986;7:20.

949. Valeri A, Barisoni L, Appel GB, et al. Idiopathic collapsing focal segmental glomerulosclerosis: a clinicopathologic study. *Kidney Int* 1996;50:1734.

950. Grcevska L, Polenakovik M. Collapsing glomerulopathy: clinical characteristics and follow-up (see comments). *Am J Kidney Dis* 1999;33:652.

951. Laurinavicius A, Hurwitz S, Rennke HG. Collapsing glomerulopathy in HIV and non-HIV patients: a clinicopathological and follow-up study. *Kidney Int* 1999;56:2203.

952. Singh HK, Baldree LA, McKenney DW, et al. Idiopathic collapsing glomerulopathy in children. *Pediatr Nephrol* 2000;14:132.

953. Meehan SM, Pascual M, Williams WW, et al. De novo collapsing glomerulopathy in renal allografts. *Transplantation* 1998;65:1192.

954. Stokes MB, Davis CL, Alpers CE. Collapsing glomerulopathy in renal allografts: a morphological pattern with diverse clinicopathologic associations. *Am J Kidney Dis* 1999;33:658.

955. Laurinavicius A, Rennke HG. Collapsing glomerulopathy–a new pattern of renal injury. *Semin Diagn Pathol* 2002;19:106.

956. Schwimmer JA, Markowitz GS, Valeri A, et al. Collapsing glomerulopathy. *Semin Nephrol* 2003;23:209.

957. Kumar S, Sheaff M, Yaqoob M. Collapsing glomerulopathy in adult still's disease. *Am J Kidney Dis* 2004;43:e4.

958. Bennett AN, Peterson P, Sangle S, et al. Adult onset Still's disease and collapsing glomerulopathy: successful treatment with intravenous immunoglobulins and mycophenolate mofetil. *Rheumatology (Oxford)* 2004;43:795.

959. Moudgil A, Nast CC, Bagga A, et al. Association of parvovirus B19 infection with idiopathic collapsing glomerulopathy. *Kidney Int* 2001;59:2126.

960. Tanawattanacharoen S, Falk RJ, Jennette JC, et al. Parvovirus B19 DNA in kidney tissue of patients with focal segmental glomerulosclerosis. *Am J Kidney Dis* 2000;35:1166.

961. Li RM, Branton MH, Tanawattanacharoen S, et al. Molecular identification of SV40 Infection in human subjects and possible association with kidney disease. *J Am Soc Nephrol* 2002;13:2320.

962. Hattori M, Horita S, Yoshioka T, et al. Mesangial phenotypic changes associated with cellular lesions in primary focal segmental glomerulosclerosis. *Am J Kidney Dis* 1997;30:632.

963. Griffiths MH, Crowe AV, Papadaki L, et al. Cyclosporin nephrotoxicity in heart and lung transplant patients. *Q J Med* 1996;89:751.

964. Falkenhain ME, Cosio FG, Sedmak DD. Progressive histologic injury in kidneys from heart and liver transplant recipients receiving cyclosporine. *Transplantation* 1996;62:364.

965. Paller MS, Cahill B, Harmon KR, et al. Glomerular disease and lung transplantation. *Am J Kidney Dis* 1995;26:527.

966. Ghiggeri GM, Altieri P, Oleggini R, et al. Cyclosporine enhances the synthesis of selected extracellular matrix proteins by renal cells "in culture." Different cell responses and phenotype characterization. *Transplantation* 1994;57:1382.

967. Ojo AO, Held PJ, Port FK, et al. Chronic renal failure after transplantation of a nonrenal organ. *N Engl J Med* 2003;349:931.

968. Santella RN, Rimmer JM, MacPherson BR. Focal segmental glomerulosclerosis in patients receiving lithium carbonate. *Am J Med* 1988;84:951.

969. Markowitz GS, Radhakrishnan J, Kambham N, et al. Lithium nephrotoxicity: a progressive combined glomerular and tubulointerstitial nephropathy. *J Am Soc Nephrol* 2000;11:1439.

970. Schreiner A, Waldherr R, Rohmeiss P, et al. Focal segmental glomerulosclerosis and lithium treatment. *Am J Psychiatry* 2000;157:834.

971. Christensen S, Marcussen N, Petersen JS, et al. Effects of uninephrectomy and high protein feeding on lithium-induced chronic renal failure in rats. *Ren Physiol Biochem* 1992;15:141.

972. Sakarcan A, Thomas DB, O'Reilly KP, et al. Lithium-induced nephrotic syndrome in a young pediatric patient. *Pediatr Nephrol* 2002;17:290.

973. Willson RA. Nephrotoxicity of interferon alfa-ribavirin therapy for chronic hepatitis C. *J Clin Gastroenterol* 2002;35:89.

974. Shah M, Jenis EH, Mookerjee BK, et al. Interferon-alpha-associated focal segmental glomerulosclerosis with massive proteinuria in patients with chronic myeloid leukemia following high dose chemotherapy. *Cancer* 1998;83:1938.

975. Coroneos E, Petrusevska G, Varghese F, et al. Focal segmental glomerulosclerosis with acute renal failure associated with alpha-interferon therapy. *Am J Kidney Dis* 1996;28:888.

976. Haas M, Jager U, Mayer G. Interferon alfa-2c and proteinuria in a patient with focal and segmental glomerulosclerosis. *Lancet* 1997;349:1147.

977. Jadoul M. Interferon-alpha-associated focal segmental glomerulosclerosis with massive proteinuria in patients with chronic myeloid leukemia following high dose chemotherapy. *Cancer* 1999;85:2669.

978. Bremer CT, Lastrapes A, Alper AB, Jr., et al. Interferon-alpha-induced focal segmental glomerulosclerosis in chronic myelogenous leukemia: a case report and review of the literature. *Am J Clin Oncol* 2003;26:262.

979. Stein DF, Ahmed A, Sunkhara V, et al. Collapsing focal segmental glomerulosclerosis with recovery of renal function: an uncommon complication of interferon therapy for hepatitis C. *Dig Dis Sci* 2001;46:530.

980. Kunin M, Kopolovic J, Avigdor A, et al. Collapsing glomerulopathy induced by long-term treatment with standard-dose pamidronate in a myeloma patient. *Nephrol Dial Transplant* 2004;19:723.

981. Markowitz GS, Appel GB, Fine PL, et al. Collapsing focal segmental glomerulosclerosis following treatment with high-dose pamidronate. *J Am Soc Nephrol* 2001;12:1164.

982. Zwacka RM, Reuter A, Pfaff E, et al. The glomerulosclerosis gene *Mpv17* encodes a peroxisomal protein producing reactive oxygen species. *EMBO J* 1994;13:5129.

983. Huttunen NP. Congenital nephrotic syndrome of the Finnish type: study of 75 patients. *Arch Dis Child* 1976;51:344.

984. Habib R. Nephrotic syndrome in the first year of life. *Pediatr Nephrol* 1993;7:347.

985. Kestila M, Lenkkeri U, Mannikko M, et al. Positionally cloned gene for a novel glomerular protein–nephrin–is mutated in congenital nephrotic syndrome. *Mol Cell* 1998;1:575.

986. Lenkkeri U, Mannikko M, McCready P, et al. Structure of the gene for congenital nephrotic syndrome of the Finnish type (NPHS1) and characterization of mutations. *Am J Hum Genet* 1999;64:51.

987. Patrakka J, Martin P, Salonen R, et al. Proteinuria and prenatal diagnosis of congenital nephrosis in fetal carriers of nephrin gene mutations. *Lancet* 2002;359:1575.

988. Kestila M, Jarvela I. Prenatal diagnosis of congenital nephrotic syndrome (CNF, NPHS1). *Prenat Diagn* 2003;23:323.
989. DeLuca G, Delinid N, D'Andrea S. Un raro caso di nefrosi congenita e malattia de inclusioni citomegalicho. *Minerva Pediatr* 1964;16:1164.
990. Beale MG, Strayer DS, Kissane JM, et al. Congenital glomerulosclerosis and nephrotic syndrome in two infants. *Am J Dis Child* 1979;133:842.
991. Gianantonio C, Vitacco M, Mendilaharzu F, et al. The hemolytic uremic syndrome. *J Pediatr* 1964;64:478.
992. Wilson VK, Thomson ML, Hohlzel A. Mercury nephrosis in young children. *Br Med J* 1952;1:358.
993. Simila S, Vesa L, Wasz-Hockert O. Hereditary onycho-osteodysplasia (nail-patella syndrome) with nephrosis-like renal disease in a newborn boy. *Pediatrics* 1970;46:61.
994. Spear GS, Hyde TP, Gruppo RA, et al. Pseudohermaphroditism, glomerulonephritis with the nephrotic syndrome, and Wilms' tumor in infancy. *J Pediatr* 1971;79:677.
995. Gotloib L, London R, Rosenmann E. Infantile nephrotic syndrome due to glomerulonephritis in a male pseudohermaphrodite. *Isr J Med Sci* 1976;12:52.
996. Taitz LS, Isaacson C, Stein H. Acute nephritis associated with congenital syphilis. *Br Med J* 1961;2:152.
997. Kaplan BS, Wiglesworth FW, Marks MI, et al. The glomerulopathy of congenital syphilis: an immune deposit disease. *J Pediatr* 1972;81:1154.
998. Shahin B, Papadopulous ZL, Jenis EH. Congenital nephrotic syndrome associated with congenial toxoplasmosis. *J Pediatr* 1974;85:366.
999. Gentner JM, Kauschowsky A, Gresher DW, et al. XY gonadal dysgenesis associated with the congenital nephrotic syndrome. *Obstet Gynecol* 1980;35:65S.
1000. Sibley RK, Mahan J, Mauer SM, et al. A clinicopathologic study of forty-eight infants with nephrotic syndrome. *Kidney Int* 1985;27:544.
1001. Jadresic LP, Filler G, Barratt TM. Urine glycosaminoglycans in congenital and acquired nephrotic syndrome. *Kidney Int* 1991;40:280.
1002. Ekim M, Ozcakar ZB, Acar B, et al. Three siblings with steroid-resistant nephrotic syndrome: new NPHS2 mutations in a Turkish family. *Am J Kidney Dis* 2004;44:e22.
1003. Weber S, Gribouval O, Esquivel EL, et al. NPHS2 mutation analysis shows genetic heterogeneity of steroid-resistant nephrotic syndrome and low post-transplant recurrence. *Kidney Int* 2004;66:571.
1004. Aucella F, De Bonis P, Gatta G, et al. Molecular analysis of NPHS2 and ACTN4 genes in a series of 33 Italian patients affected by adult-onset nonfamilial focal segmental glomerulosclerosis. *Nephron Clin Pract* 2005;99:c31.
1005. Badhwar A, Berkovic SF, Dowling JP, et al. Action myoclonus-renal failure syndrome: characterization of a unique cerebro-renal disorder. *Brain* 2004;127:2173.
1006. Boute N, Gribouval O, Roselli S, et al. NPHS2, encoding the glomerular protein podocin, is mutated in autosomal recessive steroid-resistant nephrotic syndrome (published erratum appears in *Nat Genet* 2000;1:125). *Nat Genet* 2000;4:349.
1007. Caridi G, Bertelli R, Carrea A, et al. Prevalence, genetics, and clinical features of patients carrying podocin mutations in steroid-resistant nonfamilial focal segmental glomerulosclerosis. *J Am Soc Nephrol* 2001;12:2742.
1008. Fuchshuber A, Gribouval O, Ronner V, et al. Clinical and genetic evaluation of familial steroid-responsive nephrotic syndrome in childhood. *J Am Soc Nephrol* 2001;12:374.
1009. Wu MC, Wu JY, Lee CC, et al. Two novel polymorphisms (c954T>C and c1038A>G) in exon 8 of NPHS2 gene identified in Taiwan Chinese. *Hum Mutat* 2001;17:237.
1010. Wu MC, Wu JY, Lee CC, et al. A novel polymorphism (c288C>T) of the NPHS2 gene identified in a Taiwan Chinese family. *Hum Mutat* 2001;17:81.
1011. Frishberg Y, Rinat C, Megged O, et al. Mutations in NPHS2 encoding podocin are a prevalent cause of steroid-resistant nephrotic syndrome among Israeli-Arab children. *J Am Soc Nephrol* 2002;13:400.
1012. Karle SM, Uetz B, Ronner V, et al. Novel mutations in NPHS2 detected in both familial and sporadic steroid-resistant nephrotic syndrome. *J Am Soc Nephrol* 2002;13:388.
1013. Koziell A, Grech V, Hussain S, et al. Genotype/phenotype correlations of NPHS1 and NPHS2 mutations in nephrotic syndrome advocate a functional inter-relationship in glomerular filtration. *Hum Mol Genet* 2002;11:379.
1014. Tsukaguchi H, Sudhakar A, Le TC, et al. NPHS2 mutations in late-onset focal segmental glomerulosclerosis: R229Q is a common disease-associated allele. *J Clin Invest* 2002;110:1659.
1015. Caridi G, Perfumo F, Ghiggeri GM. NPHS2 (Podocin) Mutations in Nephrotic Syndrome. Clinical Spectrum and Fine Mechanisms. *Pediatr Res* 2005;54R.
1016. Caridi G, Bertelli R, Perfumo F, et al. Heterozygous NPHS1 or NPHS2 mutations in responsive nephrotic syndrome and the multifactorial origin of proteinuria. *Kidney Int* 2004;66:1715.
1017. Caridi G, Berdeli A, Dagnino M, et al. Infantile steroid-resistant nephrotic syndrome associated with double homozygous mutations of podocin. *Am J Kidney Dis* 2004;43:727.
1018. Caridi G, Bertelli R, Scolari F, et al. Podocin mutations in sporadic focal-segmental glomerulosclerosis occurring in adulthood. *Kidney Int* 2003;64:365.
1019. Caridi G, Bertelli R, Di Duca M, et al. Broadening the spectrum of diseases related to podocin mutations. *J Am Soc Nephrol* 2003;14:1278.
1020. Lowik MM, Levtchenko EN, Monnens LA, et al. WT-1 and NPHS2 mutation analysis in patients with non-familial steroid-resistant focal-segmental glomerulosclerosis. *Clin Nephrol* 2003;59:143.
1021. Ruf RG, Lichtenberger A, Karle SM, et al. Patients with mutations in NPHS2 (podocin) do not respond to standard steroid treatment of nephrotic syndrome. *J Am Soc Nephrol* 2004;15:722.
1022. Caridi G, Perfumo F, Ghiggeri GM. NPHS2 (Podocin) mutations in nephrotic syndrome. Clinical spectrum and fine mechanisms. *Pediatr Res* 2005;57:54R.
1023. Ruf RG, Schultheiss M, Lichtenberger A, et al. Prevalence of WT1 mutations in a large cohort of patients with steroid-resistant and steroid-sensitive nephrotic syndrome. *Kidney Int* 2004;66:564.
1024. Schwarz K, Simons M, Reiser J, et al. Podocin, a raft-associated component of the glomerular slit diaphragm, interacts with CD2AP and nephrin. *J Clin Invest* 2001;108:1621.
1025. Roselli S, Gribouval O, Boute N, et al. Podocin localizes in the kidney to the slit diaphragm area. *Am J Pathol* 2002;160:131.
1026. Huber TB, Kottgen M, Schilling B, et al. Interaction with podocin facilitates nephrin signaling. *J Biol Chem.* 2001;276:41543.
1027. Huber TB, Hartleben B, Kim J, et al. Nephrin and CD2AP associate with phosphoinositide 3-OH kinase and stimulate AKT-dependent signaling. *Mol Cell Biol* 2003;23:4917.
1028. Huber TB, Simons M, Hartleben B, et al. Molecular basis of the functional podocin-nephrin complex: mutations in the NPHS2 gene disrupt nephrin targeting to lipid raft microdomains. *Hum Mol Genet* 2003;12:3397.
1029. Roselli S, Moutkine I, Gribouval O, et al. Plasma membrane targeting of podocin through the classical exocytic pathway: effect of NPHS2 mutations. *Traffic* 2004;5:37.
1030. Carraro M, Caridi G, Bruschi M, et al. Serum glomerular permeability activity in patients with podocin mutations (NPHS2) and steroid-resistant nephrotic syndrome. *J Am Soc Nephrol* 2002;13:1946.
1031. Pereira AC, Pereira AB, Mota GF, et al. NPHS2 R229Q functional variant is associated with microalbuminuria in the general population. *Kidney Int* 2004;65:1026.
1032. Schultheiss M, Ruf RG, Mucha BE, et al. No evidence for genotype/phenotype correlation in NPHS1 and NPHS2 mutations. *Pediatr Nephrol* 2004;19:1340.
1033. Wagner KD, Wagner N, Schedl A. The complex life of WT1. *J Cell Sci* 2003;116:1653.
1034. Lee SB, Huang K, Palmer R, et al. The Wilms tumor suppressor WT1 encodes a transcriptional activator of amphiregulin. *Cell* 1999;98:663.
1035. Palmer RE, Kotsianti A, Cadman B, et al. WT1 regulates the expression of the major glomerular podocyte membrane protein Podocalyxin. *Curr Biol* 2001;11:1805.
1036. Hammes A, Guo JK, Lutsch G, et al. Two splice variants of the Wilms' tumor 1 gene have distinct functions during sex determination and nephron formation. *Cell* 2001;106:319.
1037. Barbaux S, Niaudet P, Gubler MC, et al. Donor splice-site mutations in WT1 are responsible for Frasier syndrome. *Nat Genet* 1997;17:467.
1038. Little MH, Williamson KA, Mannens M, et al. Evidence that WT1 mutations in Denys-Drash syndrome patients may act in a dominant-negative fashion. *Hum Mol Genet* 1993;2:259.
1039. McTaggart SJ, Algar E, Chow CW, et al. Clinical spectrum of Denys-Drash and Frasier syndrome. *Pediatr Nephrol* 2001;16:335.
1040. Pelletier J, Bruening W, Kashtan CE, et al. Germline mutations in the Wilms' tumor suppressor gene are associated with abnormal urogenital development in Denys-Drash syndrome. *Cell* 1991;67:437.
1041. Jeanpierre C, Denamur E, Henry I, et al. Identification of constitutional WT1 mutations, in patients with isolated diffuse mesangial sclerosis, and analysis of genotype/phenotype correlations by use of a computerized mutation database. *Am J Hum Genet* 1998;62:824.
1042. Schumacher V, Scharer K, Wuhl E, et al. Spectrum of early onset congenital nephrotic syndrome associated with WT1 missense mutations. *Kidney Int* 1998;53:1594.
1043. Jadresic L, Leake J, Gordon I, et al. Clinicopathologic review of twelve children with nephropathy, Wilms tumor, and genital abnormalities (Drash syndrome). *J Pediatr* 1990;117:717.
1044. Kaltenis P, Schumacher V, Jankauskiene A, et al. Slow progressive FSGS associated with an F392L WT1 mutation. *Pediatr Nephrol* 2004;19:353.
1045. Klamt B, Koziell A, Poulat F, et al. Frasier syndrome is caused by defective alternative splicing of WT1 leading to an altered ratio of WT1 +/−KTS splice isoforms. *Hum Mol Genet* 1998;7:709.
1046. Kikuchi H, Takata A, Akasaka Y, et al. Do intronic mutations affecting splicing of WT1 exon 9 cause Frasier syndrome? *J Med Genet* 1998;35:45.
1047. Denamur E, Bocquet N, Mougenot B, et al. Mother-to-child transmitted WT1 splice-site mutation is responsible for distinct glomerular diseases. *J Am Soc Nephrol* 1999;10:2219.
1048. Loirat C, Andre JL, Champigneulle J, et al. WT1 splice site mutation in a 46, XX female with minimal-change nephrotic syndrome and Wilms' tumour. *Nephrol Dial Transplant* 2003;18:823.

1049. Denamur E, Bocquet N, Baudouin V, et al. WT1 splice-site mutations are rarely associated with primary steroid-resistant focal and segmental glomerulosclerosis. *Kidney Int* 2000;57:1868.

1050. Orloff MS, Iyengar SK, Winkler CA, et al. Variants in the Wilms tumor gene are associated with focal segmental glomerulosclerosis in the African American population. *Physiol Genomics* 2005;21:212.

1051. Kaplan JM, Kim SH, North KN, et al. Mutations in ACTN4, encoding alpha-actinin-4, cause familial focal segmental glomerulosclerosis. *Nat Genet* 2000;24:251.

1052. Welsch T, Endlich N, Kriz W, et al. CD2AP and p130Cas localize to different F-actin structures in podocytes. *Am J Physiol Renal Physiol* 2001;281:F769.

1053. Shih NY, Li J, Cotran R, et al. CD2AP localizes to the slit diaphragm and binds to nephrin via a novel C-terminal domain. *Am J Pathol* 2001;159:2303.

1054. Lehtonen S, Zhao F, Lehtonen E. CD2-associated protein directly interacts with the actin cytoskeleton. *Am J Physiol Renal Physiol* 2002;283:F734.

1055. Palmen T, Lehtonen S, Ora A, et al. Interaction of endogenous nephrin and CD2-associated protein in mouse epithelial M-1 cell line. *J Am Soc Nephrol* 2002;13:1766.

1056. Schiffer M, Mundel P, Shaw AS, et al. A novel role for the adaptor molecule CD2-associated protein in transforming growth factor-beta-induced apoptosis. *J Biol Chem* 2004;279:37004.

1057. Winn MP, Conlon PJ, Lynn KL, et al. A mutation in the TRPC6 cation channel causes familial focal segmental glomerulosclerosis. *Science* 2005;308;801.

1058. Pocock TM, Foster RR, Bates DO. Evidence of a role for TRPC channels in VEGF-mediated increased vascular permeability in vivo. *Am J Physiol Heart Circ Physiol* 2004;286:H10156.

1059. Goto Y, Nonaka I, Horai S. A mutation in the tRNA(Leu)[UUR] gene associated with the MELAS subgroup of mitochondrial encephalomyopathies. *Nature* 1990;348:651.

1060. Inui K, Fukushima H, Tsukamoto H, et al. Mitochondrial encephalomyopathies with the mutation of the mitochondrial tRNA(Leu[UUR]) gene. *J Pediatr* 1992;120:62.

1061. Kobayashi Y, Momoi MY, Tominaga K, et al. A point mutation in the mitochondrial tRNA(Leu)(UUR) gene in MELAS (mitochondrial myopathy, encephalopathy, lactic acidosis and stroke-like episodes). *Biochem Biophys Res Commun* 1990;173:816.

1062. Ban S, Mori N, Saito K, et al. An autopsy case of mitochondrial encephalomyopathy (MELAS) with special reference to extra-neuromuscular abnormalities. *Acta Pathol Jpn* 1992;42:818.

1063. Taniike MF, Yanagihara I, Tsukamoto H, et al. Mitochondrial rRNA Ile mutations in fatal cardiomyopathy. *Biochem Biophys Res Commun* 1992;186:47.

1064. Scaglia F, Vogel H, Hawkins EP, et al. Novel homoplasmic mutation in the mitochondrial tRNATyr gene associated with atypical mitochondrial cytopathy presenting with focal segmental glomerulosclerosis. *Am J Med Genet A* 2003;123:172.

1065. Mochizuki H, Joh K, Kawame H, et al. Mitochondrial encephalomyopathies preceded by de-Toni-Debre-Fanconi syndrome or focal segmental glomerulosclerosis. *Clin Nephrol* 1996;46:347.

1066. Kurogouchi F, Oguchi T, Mawatari E, et al. A case of mitochondrial cytopathy with a typical point mutation for MELAS, presenting with severe focal-segmental glomerulosclerosis as main clinical manifestation. *Am J Nephrol* 1998;18:551.

1067. Hotta O, Inoue CN, Miyabayashi S, et al. Clinical and pathologic features of focal segmental glomerulosclerosis with mitochondrial tRNALeu(UUR) gene mutation. *Kidney Int* 2001;59:1236.

1068. Doleris LM, Hill GS, Chedin P, et al. Focal segmental glomerulosclerosis associated with mitochondrial cytopathy. *Kidney Int* 2000;58:1851.

1069. Yamagata K, Muro K, Usui J, et al. Mitochondrial DNA mutations in focal segmental glomerulosclerosis lesions. *J Am Soc Nephrol* 2002;13:1816.

1070. Dinour D, Mini S, Polak-Charcon S, et al. Progressive nephropathy associated with mitochondrial tRNA gene mutation. *Clin Nephrol* 2004;62:149.

1071. Ueda Y, Ando A, Nagata T, et al. A boy with mitochondrial disease: asymptomatic proteinuria without neuromyopathy. *Pediatr Nephrol* 2004;19:107.

1072. Guery B, Choukroun G, Noel LH, et al. The spectrum of systemic involvement in adults presenting with renal lesion and mitochondrial tRNA(Leu) gene mutation. *J Am Soc Nephrol* 2003;14:2099.

1073. Cheong HI, Chae JH, Kim JS, et al. Hereditary glomerulopathy associated with a mitochondrial tRNA(Leu) gene mutation. *Pediatr Nephrol* 1999;13:477.

1074. Jansen JJ, Maassen JA, van der Woude FJ, et al. Mutation in mitochondrial tRNA(Leu[UUR]) gene associated with progressive kidney disease. *J Am Soc Nephrol* 1997;8:1118.

1074a. Quinzii C, Naini A, Salviati L, et al. A mutation in para-hydroxybenzoate-polyprenyl transferase (COQ2) causes primary coenzyme Q10- deficiency. *Am J Human Genetics* 2005;78:345.

1075. Hiraoka M, Tsukahara H, Ohshima Y, et al. Renal aplasia is the predominant cause of congenital solitary kidneys. *Kidney Int* 2002;61:1840.

1076. Favor J, Sandulache R, Neuhauser-Klaus A, et al. The mouse Pax2(1Neu) mutation is identical to a human PAX2 mutation in a family with renal-coloboma syndrome and results in developmental defects of the brain, ear, eye, and kidney. *Proc Natl Acad Sci U S A* 1996;93:13870.

1077. Salomon R, Tellier AL, Attie-Bitach T, et al. PAX2 mutations in oligomeganephronia. *Kidney Int* 2001;59:457

1078. Nishimoto K, Iijima K, Shirakawa T, et al. PAX2 gene mutation in a family with isolated renal hypoplasia. *J Am Soc Nephrol* 2001;12:1769.

1079. Miltenyi M, Balogh L, Schmidt K, et al. A new variant of the acrorenal syndrome associated with bilateral oligomeganephronic hypoplasia. *Eur J Pediatr* 1984;142:40.

1080. Kohlhase J, Schubert L, Liebers M, et al. Mutations at the SALL4 locus on chromosome 20 result in a range of clinically overlapping phenotypes, including Okihiro syndrome, Holt-Oram syndrome, acro-renal-ocular syndrome, and patients previously reported to represent thalidomide embryopathy. *J Med Genet* 2003;40:473.

1081. McPherson E, Carey J, Kramer A, et al. Dominantly inherited renal adysplasia. *Am J Med Genet* 1987;26:863.

1082. Hori C, Hiraoka M, Yoshikawa N, et al. Significance of ACE genotypes and medical treatments in childhood focal glomerulosclerosis. *Nephron* 2001;88:313.

1083. Lee DY, Kim W, Kang SK, et al. Angiotensin-converting enzyme gene polymorphism in patients with minimal-change nephrotic syndrome and focal segmental glomerulosclerosis. *Nephron* 1997;77:471.

1084. Burg M, Menne J, Ostendorf T, et al. Gene-polymorphisms of angiotensin converting enzyme and endothelial nitric oxide synthase in patients with primary glomerulonephritis. *Clin Nephrol* 1997;48:205.

1085. Frishberg Y, Becker-Cohen R, Halle D, et al. Genetic polymorphisms of the renin-angiotensin system and the outcome of focal segmental glomerulosclerosis in children. *Kidney Int* 1998;54:1843.

1086. Kuzmanic D, Jelakovic B, Borzo G, et al. ACE gene polymorphisms in focal segmental glomerulosclerosis and membranous glomerulonephritis—is the observed difference of clinical significance? *Periodicum Biologorium* 2000;102:67.

1087. Luther Y, Bantis C, Ivens K, et al. Effects of the genetic polymorphisms of the renin-angiotensin system on focal segmental glomerulosclerosis. *Kidney Blood Press Res* 2003;26:333.

1088. Oktem F, Sirin A, Bilge I, et al. ACE I/D gene polymorphism in primary FSGS and steroid-sensitive nephrotic syndrome. *Pediatr Nephrol* 2004;19:384.

1089. Vehaskari VM. Treatment practices of FSGS among North American pediatric nephrologists. *Pediatr Nephrol* 1999;13:301.

1090. Cattran DC, Rao P. Long-term outcome in children and adults with classic focal segmental glomerulosclerosis. *Am J Kidney Dis* 1998;32:72.

1091. Tune BM, Lieberman E, Mendoza SA. Steroid-resistant nephrotic focal segmental glomerulosclerosis: a treatable disease. *Pediatr Nephrol* 1996;10:772.

1092. Waldo FB, Benfield MR, Kohaut EC. Methylprednisolone treatment of patients with steroid-resistant nephrotic syndrome. *Pediatr Nephrol* 1992;6:503.

1093. Griswold WR, Tune BM, Reznik VM, et al. Treatment of childhood prednisone-resistant nephrotic syndrome and focal segmental glomerulosclerosis with intravenous methylprednisolone and oral alkylating agents. *Nephron* 1987;46:73.

1094. Mendoza SA, Reznik VM, Griswold WR, et al. Treatment of steroid-resistant focal segmental glomerulosclerosis with pulse methylprednisolone and alkylating agents. *Pediatr Nephrol* 1990;4:303.

1095. Waldo FB, Benfield MR, Kohaut EC. Therapy of focal and segmental glomerulosclerosis with methylprednisolone, cyclosporine A and prednisone. *Pediatr Nephrol* 1998;12:397.

1096. Murphy JL, Kano HL, Chenaille PJ, et al. Fatal *Pneumocystis* pneumonia in a child treated for focal segmental glomerulosclerosis. *Pediatr Nephrol* 1993;7:444.

1097. Vehaskari VM. Treatment practices of FSGS among North American pediatric nephrologists. *Pediatr Nephrol* 1999;13:301.

1098. Lieberman KV, Tejani A. A randomized double-blind placebo-controlled trial of cyclosporine in steroid-resistant idiopathic focal segmental glomerulosclerosis in children. *J Am Soc Nephrol* 1996;7:56.

1099. Ingulli E, Baqi N, Ahmad H, et al. Aggressive, long-term cyclosporine therapy for steroid-resistant focal segmental glomerulosclerosis. *J Am Soc Nephrol* 1995;5:1820.

1100. Lieberman KV, Tejani A. A randomized double-blind placebo-controlled trial of cyclosporine in steroid-resistant idiopathic focal segmental glomerulosclerosis in children. *J Am Soc Nephrol* 1995;7:56.

1101. Singh A, Tejani C, Tejani A. One-center experience with cyclosporine in refractory nephrotic syndrome in children. *Pediatr Nephrol* 1999;13:26.

1102. Cattran DC, Appel GB, Hebert LA, et al. A randomized trial of cyclosporine in patients with steroid-resistant focal segmental glomerulosclerosis. *Kidney Int* 1999;56:2220.

1103. McCauley J, Shapiro R, Ellis D. Pilot trial of FK 506 in the management of steroid-resistant nephrotic syndrome. *Nephrol Dial Transplant* 1993;8:1286.

1104. Baluarte HJ, Gruskin AB, Polinsky MS, et al. Chlorambucil therapy in the nephrotic syndrome. In: Gruskin AB, Norman M, eds. *Pediatric Nephrology*. Boston: Martinus Nyhoff; 1981:429.

1105. Kawamura T, Yoshioka T, Bills T, et al. Glucocorticoid activates glomerular antioxidant enzymes and protects glomeruli from oxidant injuries. *Kidney Int* 1991;40:291.

1106. Ransom RF, Vega-Warner V, Klein J, et al. Increased hsp27 expression mimics the protection from injury and actin filament disruption conferred by dexamethasone. *J Am Soc Nephrol*. In press.

1107. Agarwal SK, Dash SC, Tiwari SC, et al. Idiopathic adult focal segmental glomerulosclerosis: a clinicopathological study and response to steroid. *Nephron* 1993;63:168.

1108. Rydel JJ, Korbet SM, Borok RZ, et al. Focal segmental glomerulosclerosis in adults: presentation, course and response to treatment. *Am J Kidney Dis* 1995;25:534.

1109. Ponticelli C, Villa M, Banfi G, et al. Can prolonged treatment improve the prognosis in adults with focal segmental glomerulosclerosis? *Am J Kidney Dis* 1999;34:618.

1110. Franceschini N, Hogan SL, Falk RJ. Primum non nocere: Should adults with idiopathic FSGS receive steroids? *Semin Nephrol* 2003;23:229.

1111. Stiles KP, Abbott KC, Welch PG, et al. Effects of angiotensin-converting enzyme inhibitor and steroid therapy on proteinuria in FSGS: a retrospective study in a single clinic. *Clin Nephrol* 2001;56:89.

1112. Lewis EJ, Hunsicker LG, Bain RP, et al. The effect of angiotensin-converting-enzyme inhibition on diabetic nephropathy. The Collaborative Study Group. *N Engl J Med* 1993;329:1456.

1113. Shiiki H, Nishino T, Uyama H, et al. Clinical and morphological predictors of renal outcome in adult patients with focal and segmental glomerulosclerosis (FSGS). *Clin Nephrol* 1996;46:362.

1114. Pokhariyal S, Gulati S, Prasad N, et al. Duration of optimal therapy for idiopathic focal segmental glomerulosclerosis. *J Nephrol* 2003;16:691.

1115. Bolton WK, Atuk NO, Sturgill BC, et al. Therapy of the idiopathic nephrotic syndrome with alternate day steroids. *Am J Med* 1977;62:60.

1116. Nagai R, Cattran DC, Pei Y. Steroid therapy and prognosis of focal segmental glomerulosclerosis in the elderly. *Clin Nephrol* 1994;42:18.

1117. Smith D, Branton M, Fervenza F, et al. Pulse dexamethasone for focal segmental glomerulosclerosis. *J Am Soc Nephrol* 2003;14.

1118. Cattran DC. Cyclosporine in the treatment of idiopathic focal segmental glomerulosclerosis. *Semin Nephrol* 2003;23:234.

1119. Lee HY, Kim HS, Kang CM, et al. The efficacy of cyclosporine A in adult nephrotic syndrome with minimal change disease and focal-segmental glomerulosclerosis: a multicenter study in Korea. *Clin Nephrol* 1995;43:375.

1120. Walker RG, Kincaid-Smith P. The effect of treatment of corticosteroid-resistant idiopathic (primary) focal and segmental hyalinosis and sclerosis (focal glomerulosclerosis) with cyclosporin. *Nephron* 1990;54:117.

1121. Meyrier A, Noel LH, Auriche P, et al. Long-term renal tolerance of cyclosporin A treatment in the adult idiopathic nephrotic syndrome. *Kidney Int* 1994;45:1446.

1122. Ittel TH, Clasen W, Fuhs M, et al. Long-term cyclosporine A treatment in adults with minimal change nephrotic syndrome or focal segmental glomerulosclerosis. *Clin Nephrol* 1995;44:156.

1123. Cattran DC, Appel GB, Hebert LA, et al. A randomized trial of cyclosporin in patients with steroid-resistant focal segmental glomerulosclerosis. North America Nephrotic Syndrome Study Group. *Kidney Int* 1999;56:2220.

1124. Ponticelli C, Rizzoni G, Edefonti A, et al. A randomized trial of cyclosporin in steroid-resistant idiopathic nephrotic syndrome. *Kidney Int* 1993;43:1377.

1125. Matalon A, Valeri A, Appel GB. Treatment of focal segmental glomerulosclerosis. *Semin Nephrol* 2000;20:309.

1126. Meyrier A, Noel LH, Auriche P, et al. Long-term renal tolerance of cyclosporin A treatment in adult idiopathic nephrotic syndrome. Collaborative Group of the Societe de Nephrologie. *Kidney Int* 1994;45:1446.

1127. Duncan N, Dhaygude A, Owen J, et al. Treatment of focal and segmental glomerulosclerosis in adults with tacrolimus monotherapy. *Nephrol Dial Transplant* 2004;19:3062.

1128. Sharma R, Savin VJ. Cyclosporine prevents the increase in glomerular albumin permeability caused by serum from patients with focal segmental glomerular sclerosis. *Transplantation* 1996;61:381.

1129. Sharma R, Sharma M, Ge X, et al. Cyclosporine protects glomeruli from FSGS factor via an increase in glomerular cAMP. *Transplantation* 1996;62:1916.

1130. Korbet SM, Schwartz MM, Lewis EJ. Primary focal segmental glomerulosclerosis: clinical course and response to therapy. *Am J Kidney Dis* 1994;23:773.

1131. Choi MJ, Eustace JA, Gimenez LF, et al. Mycophenolate mofetil treatment for primary glomerular diseases. *Kidney Int* 2002;61:1098.

1132. Cattran DC, Wang MM, Appel G, et al. Mycophenolate mofetil in the treatment of focal segmental glomerulosclerosis. *Clin Nephrol* 2004;62:405.

1133. Alexopoulos E, Stangou M, Papagianni A, et al. Factors influencing the course and the response to treatment in primary focal segmental glomerulosclerosis. *Nephrol Dial Transplant* 2000;15:1348.

1134. Velosa JA, Torres VE, Donadio JV, et al. Treatment of severe nephrotic syndrome with meclofenamate: an uncontrolled pilot study. *Mayo Clin Proc* 1985;60:586.

1135. Tahzib M, Frank R, Gauthier B, et al. Vitamin E treatment of focal segmental glomerulosclerosis: results of an open-label study. *Pediatr Nephrol* 1999;13:649.

1136. Cho M, Smith D, Branton M, et al. Pirfenidone slows progressive loss of renal function in focal segmental glomerulosclerosis. *J Am Soc Nephrol* 2004;15.

1137. Feld SM, Figueroa P, Savin V, et al. Plasmapheresis in the treatment of steroid-resistant focal segmental glomerulosclerosis in native kidneys. *Am J Kidney Dis* 1998;32:230.

1138. Chobanian AV, Bakris GL, Black HR, et al. Seventh report of the Joint National Committee on Prevention, Detection, Evaluation, and Treatment of High Blood Pressure. *Hypertension*. 2003;42:1206.

1139. Nakao N, Yoshimura A, Morita H, et al. Combination treatment of angiotensin-II receptor blocker and angiotensin-converting-enzyme inhibitor in non-diabetic renal disease (COOPERATE): a randomised controlled trial. *Lancet* 2003;361:117.

1140. GISEN. Randomised placebo-controlled trial of effect of ramipril on decline in glomerular filtration rate and risk of terminal renal failure in proteinuric, non-diabetic nephropathy. *Lancet* 1997;349:1857.

1141. Korbet SM. Angiotensin antagonists and steroids in the treatment of focal segmental glomerulosclerosis. *Semin Nephrol* 2003;23:219.

1142. Usta M, Ersoy A, Dilek K, et al. Efficacy of losartan in patients with primary focal segmental glomerulosclerosis resistant to immunosuppressive treatment. *J Intern Med* 2003;253:329.

1143. Crenshaw G, Bigler S, Salem M, et al. Focal segmental glomerulosclerosis in African Americans: effects of steroids and angiotensin converting enzyme inhibitors. *Am J Med Sci* 2000;319:320.

1144. Praga M, Hernandez E, Montoyo C, et al. Long-term beneficial effects of angiotensin-converting enzyme inhibition in patients with nephrotic proteinuria. *Am J Kidney Dis* 1992;20:240.

1145. Praga M, Hernandez E, Andres A, et al. Effects of body-weight loss and captopril treatment on proteinuria associated with obesity. *Nephron* 1995;70:35.

1146. Ponticelli C, Passerini P. Alternative treatments for focal and segmental glomerular sclerosis. *Clin Nephrol* 2001;55:345.

1147. Burgess E. Management of focal segmental glomerulosclerosis: evidence-based recommendations. *Kidney Int Suppl* 1999;70:S26.

1148. Kunau RT, ed. *Nephrology and Hypertension Medical Knowledge Self-Assessment Program.* 1998, American College of Physicians: Philadelphia. 6.

1149. Dvorak P, Kramer HJ, Backer A, et al. Blockade of endothelin receptors attenuates end-organ damage in homozygous hypertensive ren-2 transgenic rats. *Kidney Blood Press Res* 2004;27:248.

1150. Ma LJ, Marcantoni C, Linton MF, et al. Peroxisome proliferator-activated receptor-gamma agonist troglitazone protects against nondiabetic glomerulosclerosis in rats. *Kidney Int* 2001;59:1899.

1151. Blasi ER, Rocha R, Rudolph AE, et al. Aldosterone/salt induces renal inflammation and fibrosis in hypertensive rats. *Kidney Int* 2003;63:1791.

1152. Schaier M, Lehrke I, Schade K, et al. Isotretinoin alleviates renal damage in rat chronic glomerulonephritis. *Kidney Int* 2001;60:2222.

1153. Francois H, Placier S, Flamant M, et al. Prevention of renal vascular and glomerular fibrosis by epidermal growth factor receptor inhibition. *FASEB J* 2004;18:926.

1154. Park HS, Bao L, Kim YJ, et al. Pirfenidone suppressed the development of glomerulosclerosis in the FGS/Kist mouse. *J Korean Med Sci* 2003;18:527.

1155. Kelly DJ, Zhang Y, Gow R, et al. Tranilast attenuates structural and functional aspects of renal injury in the remnant kidney model. *J Am Soc Nephrol* 2004;15:2619.

1156. Benigni A, Zoja C, Zatelli C, et al. Vasopeptidase inhibitor restores the balance of vasoactive hormones in progressive nephropathy. *Kidney Int* 2004;66:1959.

1157. Gherardi D, D'Agati V, Chu TH, et al. Reversal of collapsing glomerulopathy in mice with the cyclin-dependent kinase inhibitor CYC202. *J Am Soc Nephrol* 2004;15:1212.

1158. Nishikimi T, Akimoto K, Wang X, et al. Fasudil, a Rho-kinase inhibitor, attenuates glomerulosclerosis in Dahl salt-sensitive rats. *J Hypertens* 2004;22:1787.

1159. Franceschini N, Cheng O, Zhang X, et al. Inhibition of prolyl-4-hydroxylase ameliorates chronic rejection of mouse kidney allografts. *Am J Transplant* 2003;3:396.

1160. Oldroyd SD, Thomas GL, Gabbiani G, et al. Interferon-gamma inhibits experimental renal fibrosis. *Kidney Int* 1999;56:2116.

1161. Zeisberg M, Bottiglio C, Kumar N, et al. Bone morphogenic protein-7 inhibits progression of chronic renal fibrosis associated with two genetic mouse models. *Am J Physiol Renal Physiol* 2003;285:F1060.

1162. Mizuno S, Kurosawa T, Matsumoto K, et al. Hepatocyte growth factor prevents renal fibrosis and dysfunction in a mouse model of chronic renal disease. *J Clin Invest* 1998;101:1827.

1163. Garber SL, Mirochnik Y, Brecklin CS, et al. Relaxin decreases renal interstitial fibrosis and slows progression of renal disease. *Kidney Int* 2001;59:876.

1164. Border WA, Noble NA, Yamamoto T, et al. Natural inhibitor of transforming growth factor-beta protects against scarring in experimental kidney disease. *Nature* 1992;360:361.

1165. Ma LJ, Jha S, Ling H, et al. Divergent effects of low versus high dose anti-TGF-beta antibody in puromycin aminonucleoside nephropathy in rats. *Kidney Int* 2004;65:106.

1166. Chitalia VC, Wells JE, Robson RA, et al. Predicting renal survival in primary focal glomerulosclerosis from the time of presentation. *Kidney Int* 1999;56:2236.

1167. Chan PC, Chan KW, Cheng IK, et al. Focal sclerosing glomerulopathy. Risk factors of progression and optimal mode of treatment. *Int Urol Nephrol* 1991;23:619.

1168. Newman WJ, Tisher CC, McCoy RC, et al. Focal glomerular sclerosis: Contrasting clinical patterns in children and adults. *Medicine (Baltimore)* 1976;55:67.

1169. Mongeau JG, Corneille L, Robitaille P, et al. Primary nephrosis in childhood associated with focal glomerular sclerosis: Is long-term prognosis that severe? *Kidney Int* 1981;20:743.

1170. Velosa JA, Holley KE, Torres VE, et al. Significance of proteinuria on the outcome of renal function in patients with focal segmental glomerulosclerosis. *Mayo Clin Proc* 1983;58:568.

1171. Wehrmann M, Bohle A, Held H, et al. Long-term prognosis of focal sclerosing glomerulonephritis. An analysis of 250 cases with particular regard to tubulointerstitial changes. *Clin Nephrol* 1990;33:115.

1172. Cosio FG, Hernandez RA. Favorable prognostic significance of raised serum C3 concentration in patients with idiopathic focal glomerulosclerosis. *Clin Nephrol* 1996;45:146.

1173. Dantal J, Baatard R, Hourmant M, et al. Recurrent nephrotic syndrome following renal transplantation in patients with focal glomerulosclerosis. A one-center study of plasma exchange effects. *Transplantation* 1991;52:827.

1174. Dantal J, Godfrin Y, Koll R, et al. Antihuman immunoglobulin affinity immunoadsorption strongly decreases proteinuria in patients with relapsing nephrotic syndrome. *J Am Soc Nephrol* 1998;9:1709.

1175. Andresdottir MB, Ajubi N, Croockewit S, et al. Recurrent focal glomerulosclerosis: natural course and treatment with plasma exchange. *Nephrol Dial Transplant* 1999;14:2650.

1176. Greenstein SM, Delrio M, Ong E, et al. Plasmapheresis treatment for recurrent focal sclerosis in pediatric renal allografts. *Pediatr Nephrol* 2000;14:1061.

1177. Matalon A, Markowitz GS, Joseph RE, et al. Plasmapheresis treatment of recurrent FSGS in adult renal transplant recipients. *Clin Nephrol* 2001;56:271.

1178. Raafat R, Travis LB, Kalia A, et al. Role of transplant induction therapy on recurrence rate of focal segmental glomerulosclerosis. *Pediatr Nephrol* 2000;14:189.

1179. Pradhan M, Petro J, Palmer J, et al. Early use of plasmapheresis for recurrent post-transplant FSGS. *Pediatr Nephrol* 2003;18:934.

1180. Kooijmans-Coutinho MF, Tegzess AM, Bruijn JA, et al. Indomethacin treatment of recurrent nephrotic syndrome and focal segmental glomerulosclerosis after renal transplantation. *Nephrol Dial Transplant* 1993;8:469.

1181. Cochat P, Kassir A, Colon S, et al. Recurrent nephrotic syndrome after transplantation: early treatment with plasmaphaeresis and cyclophosphamide. *Pediatr Nephrol* 1993;7:50.

1182. Marcen R, Navarro JF, Mampaso F, et al. Recurrence of focal-segmental glomerulosclerosis in kidney transplant patients on ciclosporin. *Nephron* 1994;68:497.

1183. Kershaw DB, Sedman AB, Kelsch RC, et al. Recurrent focal segmental glomerulosclerosis in pediatric renal transplant recipients: successful treatment with oral cyclophosphamide. *Clin Transplant* 1994;8:546.

1184. Dall'Amico R, Ghiggeri G, Carraro M, et al. Prediction and treatment of recurrent focal segmental glomerulosclerosis after renal transplantation in children. *Am J Kidney Dis* 1999;34:1048.

1185. Saleem MA, Ramanan AV, Rees L. Recurrent focal segmental glomerulosclerosis in grafts treated with plasma exchange and increased immunosuppression. *Pediatr Nephrol* 2000;14:361.

1186. Artero ML, Sharma R, Savin VJ, et al. Plasmapheresis reduces proteinuria and serum capacity to injure glomeruli in patients with recurrent focal glomerulosclerosis. *Am J Kidney Dis* 1994;23:574.

1187. Seikaly MG. Recurrence of primary disease in children after renal transplantation: an evidence-based update. *Pediatr Transplant* 2004;8:113.

1188. Bertelli R, Ginevri F, Caridi G, et al. Recurrence of focal segmental glomerulosclerosis after renal transplantation in patients with mutations of podocin. *Am J Kidney Dis* 2003;41:1314.

1189. Abbott KC, Sawyers ES, Oliver JD, 3rd, et al. Graft loss due to recurrent focal segmental glomerulosclerosis in renal transplant recipients in the United States. *Am J Kidney Dis* 2001;37:366.

1190. Hubsch H, Montane B, Abitbol C, et al. Recurrent focal glomerulosclerosis in pediatric renal allografts: the Miami experience. *Pediatr Nephrol* 2005;20:210.

1191. Savin VJ, Sharma R, Lovell HB, et al. Measurement of albumin reflection coefficient with isolated rat glomeruli. *J Am Soc Nephrol* 1992;3:1260.

1192. Savin VJ, Sharma R, Sharma M, et al. Circulating factor associated with increased glomerular permeability to albumin in recurrent focal segmental glomerulosclerosis. *N Engl J Med* 1996;334:878.

1193. Godfrin Y, Dantal J, Perretto S, et al. Study of the in vitro effect on glomerular albumin permselectivity of serum before and after renal transplantation in focal segmental glomerulosclerosis. *Transplantation* 1997;64:1711.

1194. Sharma M, Sharma R, McCarthy ET, et al. "The FSGS factor:" enrichment and in vivo effect of activity from focal segmental glomerulosclerosis plasma. *J Am Soc Nephrol* 1999;10:552.

1195. Dantal J, Bigot E, Bogers W, et al. Effect of plasma protein adsorption on protein excretion in kidney-transplant recipients with recurrent nephrotic syndrome. *N Engl J Med* 1994;330:7.

1196. Savin VJ, McCarthy ET, Sharma M. Permeability factors in focal segmental glomerulosclerosis. *Semin Nephrol* 2003;23:147.

1197. Sharma M, Sharma R, McCarthy ET, et al. The focal segmental glomerulosclerosis permeability factor: biochemical characteristics and biological effects. *Exp Biol Med (Maywood)* 2004;229:85.

1198. Musante L, Candiano G, Bruschi M, et al. Characterization of plasma factors that alter the permeability to albumin within isolated glomeruli. *Proteomics* 2002;2:197.

1199. Le Berre L, Godfrin Y, Lafond-Puyet L, et al. Effect of plasma fractions from patients with focal and segmental glomerulosclerosis on rat proteinuria. *Kidney Int* 2000;58:2502.

1200. Sharma M, Sharma R, Reddy SR, et al. Proteinuria after injection of human focal segmental glomerulosclerosis factor. *Transplantation* 2002;73:366.

1201. Sharma R, Sharma M, McCarthy ET, et al. Components of normal serum block the focal segmental glomerulosclerosis factor activity in vitro. *Kidney Int* 2000;58:1973.

1202. Candiano G, Musante L, Carraro M, et al. Apolipoproteins prevent glomerular albumin permeability induced in vitro by serum from patients with focal segmental glomerulosclerosis. *J Am Soc Nephrol* 2001;12:143.

1203. Carraro M, Zennaro C, Candiano G, et al. Nephrotic urine prevents increased rat glomerular albumin permeability induced by serum from the same patient with idiopathic nephrotic syndrome. *Nephrol Dial Transplant* 2003;18:689.

1204. Sharma BR. Ethical and practical principles underlying the end of life decisions. *Am J Forensic Med Pathol* 2004;25:216.

1205. Carraro M, Zennaro C, Artero M, et al. The effect of proteinase inhibitors on glomerular albumin permeability induced in vitro by serum from patients with idiopathic focal segmental glomerulosclerosis. *Nephrol Dial Transplant* 2004;19:1969.

1206. McCarthy ET, Sharma M. Indomethacin protects permeability barrier from focal segmental glomerulosclerosis serum. *Kidney Int* 2002;61:534.

1207. Shariatmadar S, Noto TA. Therapeutic plasma exchange in recurrent focal segmental glomerulosclerosis following *Transplantation J Clin Apheresis*. 2002;17:78.

1208. Dantal J, Bigot E, Bogers W, et al. Effect of plasma protein adsorption on protein excretion in kidney-transplant recipients with recurrent nephrotic syndrome (see comments). *N Engl J Med* 1994;330:7.

1209. Davenport RD. Apheresis treatment of recurrent focal segmental glomerulosclerosis after kidney transplantation: re-analysis of published case-reports and case-series. *J Clin Apheresis* 2001;16:175.

1210. Cheong HI, Han HW, Park HW, et al. Early recurrent nephrotic syndrome after renal transplantation in children with focal segmental glomerulosclerosis. *Nephrol Dial Transplant* 2000;15:78.

1211. Salomon R, Gagnadoux MF, Niaudet P. Intravenous cyclosporine therapy in recurrent nephrotic syndrome after renal transplantation in children. *Transplantation* 2003;75:810.

1212. Raafat RH, Kalia A, Travis LB, et al. High-dose oral cyclosporin therapy for recurrent focal segmental glomerulosclerosis in children. *Am J Kidney Dis* 2004;44:50.

1213. Otsubo S, Tanabe K, Tokumoto T, et al. Long-term outcome in renal transplant recipients with focal and segmental glomerulosclerosis. *Transplant Proc* 1999;31:2860.

1214. Ohta T, Kawaguchi H, Hattori M, et al. Effect of pre-and postoperative plasmapheresis on posttransplant recurrence of focal segmental glomerulosclerosis in children. *Transplantation* 2001;71:628.

1215. Pollak MR. Inherited podocytopathies: FSGS and nephrotic syndrome from a genetic viewpoint. *J Am Soc Nephrol* 2002;13:3016.

CHAPTER 65 ■ RENAL INVOLVEMENT IN SYSTEMIC LUPUS ERYTHEMATOSUS

STERLING G. WEST, GREGORY A. ACHENBACH, AND CHARLES L. EDELSTEIN

Systemic lupus erythematosus (SLE) is an autoimmune disease of unknown etiology, characterized by the involvement of multiple organ systems. Glomerulonephritis is a frequent and important complication of SLE, and the presence and extent of kidney involvement greatly influence the long-term outcome of this disease. Systemic lupus erythematosus is caused by the production of autoantibodies, and a hallmark of the disease is the presence of serum antibodies directed to nuclear constituents (i.e., antinuclear antibodies, ANAs). The clinical presentation and course of SLE are extremely variable. For example, some patients have spontaneous remissions, others may have mild skin and joint involvement that respond favorably to conservative measures, and a few die from progressive multisystem disease unresponsive to high-dose corticosteroids and cytotoxic drugs. Variability is also a feature of renal involvement in SLE, and the evaluation, treatment, and prognosis for each patient need to be individualized. In this chapter, we review current ideas regarding the immunopathogenesis and pathology of glomerulonephritis in SLE. We also describe lupus nephritis in terms of clinical and laboratory findings and current approaches to therapy.

Criteria for the classification of SLE (Table 65-1) have been established by the American College of Rheumatology (ACR) to facilitate the uniform reporting of SLE cases (1). A patient is said to have SLE if four of the 11 criteria shown in Table 65-1 are satisfied. Although not designed for diagnosis, these criteria have helped physicians recognize and diagnose this disease. It is emphasized, however, that these criteria occasionally lack sensitivity for diagnosing early or mild cases of SLE, and occasional patients may fulfill four criteria and still not have SLE.

The preceding criteria emphasize that patients with lupus nephritis usually demonstrate nonrenal manifestations of SLE. The physician must be aware of these other nonrenal problems because they can be serious and can greatly complicate the evaluation and management of the disease. The reader is referred to several general reviews of the clinical manifestations of SLE (2–4).

Women of childbearing age are primarily affected, although SLE can occur at nearly any age. In cases that begin between ages 15 and 40 years, more than 90% of the patients are female (5). The female-to-male ratio is closer to 2:1 for disease that develops during childhood and after the age of 65. Epidemiologic studies have shown that the incidence of disease increases in women of childbearing age and then decreases after menopause, whereas the incidence for men is more evenly distributed and may continue to rise through the seventh decade. Together, these data strongly suggest that sex hormones influence the probability of developing or expressing SLE, and studies in animal models of lupus have supported a potential role for estrogens enhancing and androgens protecting against expression of disease (6). It should be emphasized that although men develop SLE less frequently than do women, their illness, including extent of renal involvement, may be severe (7).

The overall prevalence rate of SLE in the continental United States has been reported to range between 15 and 50 cases per 100,000 persons, and overall incidence has been estimated to be 1.8 to 7.6 cases per 100,000 persons per year (5). These rates can vary greatly depending on the risk of the population being studied. The chance that a white woman in the United States will develop SLE in her lifetime is approximately one in 700. The incidence is three to four times greater for black women, who are also more likely to demonstrate severe renal involvement and have higher disease-related mortality rates (5). Certain Asian populations, North American Indian tribes, and Hispanic individuals also may have a greater predisposition toward SLE compared to individuals of mixed-European descent. These racial differences are consistent with the known importance of genetic factors in disease development (discussed in the following section), but also partly may result from environmental influences.

PATHOGENESIS

Overview

Similar to other autoimmune diseases, the development of SLE is a complicated and multistep process (8). Major events believed to be important in the immunopathogenesis of SLE are shown in Figure 65-1. Considerable evidence indicates that the development and progression of SLE have a strong genetic basis and that these genetic contributions may operate at several different levels. The T-cell driving force in SLE involves CD4$^+$ T cells, which interact with autoreactive B cells to cause immunoglobulin G (IgG) autoantibody production and various disease manifestations. IgG autoantibody production is the central immunologic problem in SLE. These autoantibodies may mediate pathology, for example, by binding directly to their cell-surface target or by forming immune complexes, although the mechanism by which many autoantibodies are associated with particular disease manifestations in SLE is unknown. The heterogeneity in clinical manifestations among SLE patients is likely related to differences in the types and amounts of autoantibodies produced.

Studies using several murine models have contributed greatly to the elucidation of SLE pathogenesis (6,9–11). The most well-characterized lupus-prone models are New Zealand hybrid, MRL, and BXSB mice. The New Zealand murine model was first described more than 40 years ago, and usually involves crosses or recombinant strains of New Zealand black (NZB) and New Zealand white (NZW) mice. MRL-*lpr/lpr* (currently referred to as MRL-Fas^{lpr}) mice, which are homozygous for the *lymphoproliferation (lpr)* mutation in the gene encoding Fas, demonstrate an accelerated form of disease compared to non-*lpr* litter mates (10). BXSB mice most frequently studied carry the *Yaa* accelerating gene encoded on the Y chromosome

TABLE 65-1

THE 1982 REVISED CRITERIA FOR CLASSIFICATION OF SYSTEMIC LUPUS ERYTHEMATOSUS (SLE)[a]

Criterion	Definition
Malar rash	Fixed erythema, flat or raised over the malar eminences, tending to spare the nasolabial folds
Discoid rash	Erythematous raised patches with adherent keratotic scaling and follicular plugging; atrophic scarring may occur in older lesions
Photosensitivity	Skin rash a result of unusual reaction to sunlight, by patient history or physician observation
Oral ulcers	Oral or nasopharyngeal ulceration, usually painless, observed at physical examination
Arthritis	Nonerosive arthritis, involving two or more peripheral joints, characterized by tenderness, swelling, or effusion
Serositis	Pleuritis: convincing history of pleuritic pain or rub heard by a physician or evidence of pleural effusion
	Pericarditis documented by electrocardiography or rub or evidence of pericardial effusion
Renal disorder	Persistent proteinuria greater than 0.5 g/day or >3+ if quantitation not performed OR
	Cellular casts (red blood cell, hemoglobin, granular, tubular or mixed)
Neurologic disorder	Seizures in the absence of offending drugs or known metabolic derangements (e.g., uremia, ketoacidosis, or electrolyte imbalance) OR
	Psychosis in the absence of offending drugs or known metabolic derangements (e.g., uremia, ketoacidosis, or electrolyte imbalance)
Hematologic disorder	Hemolytic anemia with reticulocytosis OR
	Leukopenia: WBCs, <4,000/μL total on two or more occasions OR
	Lymphopenia: <1,500/μL on two or more occasions OR
	Thrombocytopenia: <100,000/μL in the absence of offending drugs
Immunologic disorder	Positive LE cell preparation[b] Anti-DNA: antibody to DNA in abnormal titer OR
	Anti-Sm: presence of antibody to Sm nuclear antigen OR
	False-positive serologic test for syphilis known to be positive for at least 6 months and confirmed by TPI or FTA-ABS
Antinuclear antibody	An abnormal titer of ANA by immunofluorescence or an equivalent assay at any point in time and in the absence of drugs known to be associated with "drug-induced lupus" syndrome

LE, lupus erythematosis; *TPI, Treponema pallidum* immobilization test; *FTA-ABS*, fluorescent treponemal antibody absorption test; *ANA*, antinuclear antibody.

[a]For the purpose of identifying patients in clinical studies, a person shall be said to have SLE if any four or more of the 11 criteria are present, serially or simultaneously, during any interval of observation. Taken from Tan et al. (1).

[b] The Diagnostic and Therapeutic Criteria Committee of the American College of Rheumatology (ACR) has suggested that this criterion be replaced with a positive test for antiphospholipid antibodies (elevated serum level of anticardiolipin antibodies or positive test for lupus anticoagulant using a standard method).

(From: Tan EM, et al. The 1982 revised criteria for the classification of systemic lupus erythematosus. *Arthritis Rheum* 1982;25:1271, with permission; and Rus V, Hochberg MC. The epidemiology of systemic lupus erythematosus. In: Wallace DJ, Hahn BH, eds. *Dubois' Lupus Erythematosus*, 6th ed. Philadelphia: Lippincott Williams & Wilkins; 2002.)

(11). All of these murine lupus models develop a lupus-like immune-complex-mediated glomerulonephritis associated with high levels of IgG autoantibodies to nuclear antigens, including double stranded DNA (dsDNA).

The animal models of lupus have provided systems for dissecting genetic contributions to disease, understanding the immunopathogenesis of autoimmunity, and characterizing the pathogenic events in lupus nephritis. The ability to study many related offspring with similar disease manifestations after directed breeding of autoimmune and nonautoimmune strains is a great advantage compared to genetic studies of the human disease, in which many multiplex families with heterogeneous disease manifestations must be studied (12). Studies of these animal models, in contrast to patients, also offer the opportunity to control environmental exposures. In addition, spontaneous animal models permit the characterization of immunologic changes before, during, and after disease development. Therefore, one can attempt to distinguish the early immunologic abnormalities that are central to disease development from later defects that are secondary to disease. Studies involving these animal models that emphasize certain principles are discussed in the following sections.

Genetic Contributions

Evidence for a strong genetic predisposition in SLE has come from genetic epidemiology studies that determine: (a) disease prevalence within families in which there is an affected individual, when compared with the prevalence in the general population; and (b) disease prevalence in identical versus nonidentical twins (12,13). The increased risk for a sibling of an SLE patient

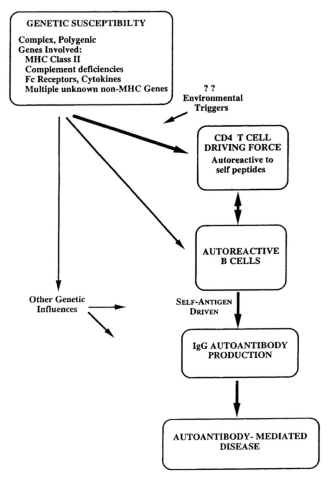

FIGURE 65-1. Genetic and immunologic events in the pathogenesis of systemic lupus erythematosus. *shape MHC*, major histocompatibility complex. (From: Kotzin BL. Systemic lupus erythematosus. *Cell* 1996;85:303, with permission).

to develop the same disease is estimated to be 15- to 20-fold greater than for the general population (12–14). Recent studies also have suggested concordance rates for identical twins of ~24% compared with ~2% for dizygotic twins (15). These results strongly support the importance of genetic contributions to disease development, but the twin data also suggest a role for other factors and/or stochastic processes in disease expression. Serologic studies indicate that identical twins discordant for disease expression may still demonstrate similar autoantibody profiles, supporting the hypothesis that certain genetic contributions operate at the level of autoantibody production.

Systemic lupus erythematosus, like other autoimmune diseases, is a complex genetic trait, which by definition is not inherited in a simple Mendelian way (12–14). Multiple genes, including major histocompatibility complex (MHC) and non-MHC genes, determine susceptibility to SLE, and no particular gene is necessary or sufficient for disease expression. The low penetrance of each contributing gene, that is, the small increase in probability of disease expression given a particular disease allele, is the main reason why diseases such as SLE are so complex genetically. Furthermore, as exemplified by the concordance rates in identical twins, overt autoimmune disease frequently does not occur even in the presence of a full complement of susceptibility alleles. Genetic complexity in SLE is also determined by genetic heterogeneity, in which the same phenotype (e.g., anti-dsDNA autoantibody production or lupus nephritis) is the result of a different set of genes in different individuals.

Many genetic studies in human SLE have focused on genes that affect immune responses, particularly those encoded within the MHC. Associations of disease with particular MHC class II alleles have been demonstrated in studies of total populations of SLE patients (i.e., inclusion of patients is based solely by meeting classification criteria) (14,16,17). However, these associations generally have been weak and consistent only within a given ethnic group. For example, in some populations, associations with HLA-DR2 and/or HLA-DR3 have been observed, but increased relative risks for disease development generally have been less than five (16,17). Furthermore, it has been suggested that the association with DR3 may be related to a null allele of complement C4A (C4A*QO), which is inherited on some extended MHC haplotypes in linkage disequilibrium with HLA-DR3 (14) or a particular allele of the gene encoding tumor necrosis factor-α (TNF-α) frequently linked with DR2 (14,18). In contrast to these weak associations with disease susceptibility in general, MHC class II genes exert a decisive influence on the production of specific types of autoantibodies in SLE (16,17). The antibody response to several autoantigens, including dsDNA, in SLE has been associated with particular MHC class II (HLA-DQ) alleles or combinations of these alleles. Overall, the data suggest that the contribution of MHC class II molecules in SLE is predominantly at the level of specific autoantibody production, perhaps reflecting the presentation of specific autoantigens.

Inherited deficiencies of classic pathway complement components, some of which are encoded within the MHC, have a significant effect on susceptibility to SLE and lupuslike disease (14,19). For example, most individuals with genetically determined complete deficiencies of complement C1q, C1r/C1s, or C4 (both C4A and C4B) develop a syndrome resembling SLE. C2 deficiency has been associated with a more than 40-fold increased risk of developing SLE. These complete deficiencies of complement components are, however, rare and account for only a very small percentage of SLE patients. In contrast, C4A deficiency may be present in as many as 13% to 15% of SLE patients (versus 1% of the general population) and studies have suggested a 15- to 20-fold increased risk of developing SLE. Furthermore, heterozygous C4A deficiency (one C4A*QO allele) is present in 35% to 60% of SLE patients compared to 13% to 20% of controls (relative risk for developing SLE is approximately two to three), although the interpretation of these data is more difficult because of the linkage disequilibrium of C4A with other possible predisposing MHC genes.

The association of complement deficiency states and SLE is likely to be etiologic, but the mechanism for this influence is unknown. Some investigators have postulated defects in the clearance of infectious particles, immune complexes, or apoptotic cells as leading to enhanced autoantibody production (20). Complement deficiencies also could affect B-cell function and the tolerance process. Alternatively, complement gene defects may exemplify genetic defects that operate distal to autoantibody production by allowing enhanced formation or deposition of immune complexes in various organs. It is emphasized that, although complement deficiencies can predispose to the development of SLE, complement activation is important for the pathogenic effects of autoantibodies and immune complexes in this disease. In SLE patients with certain types of complement deficiencies, clinical manifestations may be altered. In addition, inhibition of complement activation has been shown to suppress lupus nephritis in animal models (21), and therapeutic trials with blocking monoclonal antibodies to C5 are in progress in human SLE.

Patients with lupus nephritis have autoantibodies to the complement classical pathway protein C1q. It is not known whether these anti-C1q antibodies can cause lupus nephritis. Trouw et al. (22) developed a murine mAb, JL-1, that recognizes the tail domain of C1q. JL-1 administered alone in normal control mice resulted in glomerular deposition of C1q and anti-C1q antibodies without inducing glomerular damage. Combination of JL-1 with a subnephritogenic dose of C1q-fixing anti-glomerular basement membrane (anti-GBM) antibodies caused renal damage manifested by decreased renal function and increased albuminuria. The glomerular injury was not seen when a non-C1q-fixing anti-GBM preparation was used. Therefore, anti-C1q autoantibodies deposit in glomeruli together with C1q but induce overt renal disease only in the context of glomerular immune complex disease. This study demonstrates, for the first time, a causal link between anti-C1q antibodies and lupus nephritis (22).

Associations also have been demonstrated between SLE and alleles of the genes encoding cell-surface receptors for IgG (i.e., Fcγ receptors) (23,24). For example, investigators have demonstrated an association between SLE and alleles of the gene encoding Fcγ RIIA (CD32), expressed on monocytes–macrophages and neutrophils (23). Alleles of this gene differ substantially in the ability to bind human IgG2, and studies found a decrease in the prevalence of the high affinity binding allele in SLE, particularly in patients with lupus nephritis. Thus, possibly similar to complement deficiencies, the genetic contribution of this Fcγ receptor deficiency may reflect a relatively late event in the pathophysiologic scheme of SLE-related immune-complex damage in lupus nephritis. Consistent with this hypothesis, other studies have noted the under representation of a high-binding Fcγ RIIIA allele (expressed on NK cells and monocytes) in patients with SLE, especially with lupus nephritis (24). The Fcγ receptor molecules and related pathways appear to be extremely important in immune-complex-mediated glomerulonephritis and the generation of lupuslike disease. In studies of the (NZB × NZW)F$_1$ murine model, knockout of Fcγ RIII function had no apparent effect on the deposition of immune complexes in glomeruli but nearly completely prevented the development of severe glomerular damage (25). In contrast, knockout of the gene encoding Fcγ RIIb, which negatively regulates B-cell activation, results in lupuslike renal disease in normal mice (26).

Association studies have also focused on other immunologically relevant genes in the pathogenesis of SLE. In addition to classical complement component deficiencies, alleles of mannan binding protein have been associated with susceptibility to SLE and infection in the setting of SLE (27). Studies of genetic polymorphisms that affect expression of certain cytokines such as TNF-α, IL-10, and IL-6 have also been suggested to be associated with disease (28–30), although further confirmation of these effects are needed. In contrast, most mouse and human studies have not found a major role for polymorphisms in either the T-cell receptor (TCR) gene complex or immunoglobulin (Ig) gene complex. This is consistent with a large amount of evidence that abnormalities in these lymphocyte receptors are not required for expression of disease (8). A number of different Ig genes can be utilized to encode pathogenic autoantibodies in lupus, and multiple different TCR variable regions appear to be sufficient for disease development.

The development of techniques to map the position of disease susceptibility loci in genome-wide screens without regard to candidate genes has been a significant advance in genetic analysis in the last few years (12,13). Genetic mapping studies, including genome-wide scans, have been reported in SLE as well as murine models of these diseases (14,31–33). Unfortunately, the susceptibility genes underlying most mapped loci have not been identified to date. Except for the lpr mutation of the gene encoding Fas and gld mutation in the Fas ligand gene, none of the approximately 15 to 20 non-MHC susceptibility loci mapped in murine models of lupus have been identified with any certainty to date. In addition, although multiple loci have been suggested in mapping studies in human SLE, no non-MHC genes have yet been identified. In a recent follow-up study of a directed linkage study in SLE (34), transmission disequilibrium testing was used to implicate the gene encoding poly-ADP-ribose polymerase (PARP or ADPRT) on distal human chromosome 1 (35), but other investigator groups have not been able to confirm this observation (36).

A possible step forward in understanding genetic contributions in lupus relates to the identification of lpr and gld in murine studies as mutations in the genes encoding Fas and Fas ligand, respectively. These genes are involved in programmed cell death (apoptosis); the traits resulting from these mutations have been described extensively (10). Homozygosity for these mutations results in the acceleration of lupuslike autoimmunity as well as a massive accumulation of CD4– CD8– (double-negative) T cells. Although the mechanism by which mutations in Fas lead to accelerated autoimmunity is unknown, the strongest hypothesis is that self-reactive T and B cells arise when they fail to undergo apoptosis normally (8). Studies have shown that both T and B cells must carry the lpr mutation for maximal autoantibody production to occur (37,38). The evidence indicates that Fas is not critically important in central (intrathymic) tolerance during T-cell development (8,39,40). Instead, studies support the contention that peripheral T-cell tolerance mechanisms are primarily affected by the lpr mutation (40). In a similar manner, studies also suggest that central B-cell tolerance may be relatively independent of Fas (41,42), and surface expression of Fas on B cells may be most important in preventing inappropriate CD4$^+$ T-cell-dependent expansion of autoreactive B cells in the periphery (43). Fas mutations have been identified in a few children with lymphoproliferative syndromes and evidence of autoimmunity (44). However, it is important to emphasize that there is really no counterpart to the lpr or gld phenotype in human SLE, and recent studies have not found defects of these genes in SLE patients. Still, there is a belief that other genes involved in apoptosis or related cell-signaling pathways may be involved in the genetic susceptibility and pathogenesis of the human disease.

In animal models, many single gene knockout and transgenic manipulations have resulted in systemic autoimmune syndromes with lupuslike autoantibody production and immune-complex renal disease (14,20,26,31). Targeted perturbations of genes involved in apoptosis, T- or B-cell signaling, B-cell activation, cell cycle processes, as well as genes encoding complement components, Fc receptors, and cytokine or cytokine receptor expression have been reported to cause the development of lupuslike disease. In many studies, the background of the strain in which the knockout is placed can greatly alter the expression of disease (20,26). Although single gene models of lupus have pointed to particular genes and mechanistic pathways for study in human disease, as discussed, genetic contributions to human SLE are generally complex and determined by the combination of multiple susceptibility genes (14,31,32).

Overall, there is great optimism that a number of non-MHC alleles that contribute to SLE will be defined in the next few years. Multiple abnormalities of both B- and T-cell phenotype and function have been described in SLE and murine models of lupus. However, many of these defects probably reflect secondary events in the disease process, and it is unclear which of these lymphocyte abnormalities are primary checkpoints in the pathogenesis of disease. The genes that predispose to autoimmunity are likely related to primary events in pathogenesis; therefore, their identification will almost certainly provide important insight into the development of autoimmunity and the cause of autoimmune disease.

Environmental Triggers and Influences

In the proposed model of pathogenesis (Fig. 65-1), environmental factors interact with susceptibility genes to result in autoimmune disease; however, the existence and importance of any particular environmental trigger in SLE has yet to be defined. Geographic clustering has not been documented in SLE, and a number of postulated chemical exposures or dietary effects have not been confirmed to be associated with SLE when careful epidemiologic studies were performed. The possible viral etiology of SLE has been vigorously investigated. One recent study has shown that children with SLE have a higher prevalence of Epstein-Barr virus (EBV) infection compared to control groups (45). Although the studies are harder to perform in adults (because of the higher frequency of EBV in the general adult population), preliminary studies suggest a similar conclusion. The basis for these interesting findings in terms of which condition is predisposing to the other has yet to be clarified.

Environmental influences on the expression of disease manifestations are clearly seen in SLE. These include the exacerbation of skin rash (or even systemic symptoms) after sun exposure, exacerbations of disease after viral or bacterial infections, and changes in disease activity after administration of exogenous hormones. Several important pieces of evidence also support the contention that estrogens increase the risk of developing SLE and/or exacerbate disease. Epidemiologic studies have documented an increased frequency of disease in postmenopausal women taking estrogen supplementation (46) and in women taking birth control pills (47,48). These studies are consistent with the known increased expression of disease in women of childbearing age (5) and studies in certain animal models showing that estrogens enhance disease expression (6). There is also evidence from animal models that androgens may have a suppressive effect on disease course. Perhaps related, treatment of patients with dehydroepiandrosterone (DHEA), an abundant adrenal steroid with slight androgenic activity, has been shown in at least one controlled study to be mildly effective in patients with mild to moderate disease activity (49).

A large number of drugs have been associated with the production of ANA and development of a lupuslike syndrome (50) (see discussion later in this chapter). Drug-induced lupus, however, is not the induction of lupus in individuals predisposed to develop SLE. Compared to SLE, drug-induced lupus occurs in older patients (related to the age of patients using the offending medication) and the sex ratio is close to unity. Drug-induced lupus in general also differs from idiopathic SLE in that it tends to cause predominantly joint and pleural–pericardial involvement, and the development of lupus nephritis is very unusual. The disease remits with time when the offending drug is discontinued. The mechanism for how drugs, such as procainamide and hydralazine, induce lupuslike disease remains poorly understood.

T Cells and T-Cell Cytokines

Studies showing the association of autoantibody production with particular class II MHC genes, the requirement for class II MHC molecules in murine models of lupus, as well as the characteristics of IgG autoantibodies in SLE strongly suggest that CD4$^+$ T cells are critically involved in the pathogenesis of this SLE (8). Moreover, treatment of murine models with monoclonal anti-CD4 antibodies can ameliorate the disease, documenting an important role for CD4$^+$ T cells in the disease process (8,51–53). The specificities of the CD4$^+$ T cells involved in SLE induction have not been fully defined. The nature of T-cell help in lupus may differ from conventional responses to foreign antigens because of the unusual structure of the target autoantigens, and the T-cell specificities may not necessarily match the antigens that are stimulating and driving B cells. There is no evidence, for example, that T cells specific for DNA are involved in the anti-DNA antibody re-

sponse in spontaneous murine lupus. Most lupus antigens exist as a component of large complexes (such as nucleosomes or spliceosomes), containing multiple protein as well as nucleic acid molecules. These complexes may be more capable of cross-linking Ig receptors on B cells, making the specific B cells more susceptible to T-cell help. Proteins within these complexes may also be internalized, processed, and presented for T-cell recognition. In recent studies, pathogenic T cells recognizing peptides derived from histones (the major protein component of chromatin) have been identified in both murine and human lupus (54,55), and these T cells were capable of helping B cells produce anti-DNA antibodies.

Current theories to explain the development of autoreactive T cells in SLE are based on the mechanisms of T-cell tolerance that operate in normal individuals. For example, it is conceivable that there is a generalized failure of negative selection in the thymus. However, studies in lupus mice have repeatedly shown that high-affinity responses to self-antigens are tolerized normally in the thymus (8,39,40,56,57). Similar to other autoimmune diseases, lupus more likely involves a failure of peripheral tolerance mechanisms, including a failure to maintain T-cell ignorance, a failure to induce anergy after exposure to self-antigens in the periphery, or a failure of normal regulatory (suppressor T-cell) mechanisms. To date, there is little information to pinpoint a particular defect, and research on these questions remains an extremely active area of investigation.

Any self-antigen needs to be processed and presented with MHC molecules to allow for negative selection in the thymus. Cryptic determinants are not presented adequately, and cells capable of recognizing these peptides escape central tolerance and are part of the normal peripheral T-cell repertoire (58). Immunization of normal mice with cryptic peptides of nuclear antigens has been shown to result in lupuslike autoantibody production that can spread to other determinants on the same molecule and spread to other nuclear antigens (intramolecular and intermolecular determinant spreading) (59–62). The ability to stimulate T cells that are reactive with cryptic epitopes through molecular mimicry has been suggested as a possible initiating event in the pathogenesis of SLE.

Numerous quantitative, phenotypic, and functional abnormalities of T cells in SLE and murine models of lupus have been documented (63). Studies have suggested that T-cell signaling through the TCR and CD3 is defective, associated with deficient TCR ζ-chain expression, protein kinase A activity, and downstream activation steps (64,65). Other work has documented abnormally increased expression and release of costimulatory molecules, such as CD40 ligand (CD40L; CD156), in SLE patients versus controls, which could allow for increased T-cell activation and T-cell dependent activation of B cells (66–68). Additional T-cell–related abnormalities reported in SLE include T-cell lymphopenia, alterations in CD4$^+$ T-cell numbers and certain CD4$^+$ T-cell subsets, increased numbers of activated CD4$^+$ T cells, increased numbers of CD4– CD8– (double-negative T cells) and aberrant T-cell help from this subset, defective T helper cell activity, aberrant helper activity from CD8$^+$ T cells, defective T-cell suppressor activity, deficient *in vitro* IL-2 production and response to IL-2, and abnormal *in vitro* production of other cytokines (63). It remains unclear which of these defects are important events in disease pathogenesis and which are just secondary abnormalities induced by the markedly abnormal immune state of lupus.

Although more sharply defined in mice compared to humans, it is clear that T cells after activation may evolve into two major subsets of T helper cells, distinguished by the cytokines that they produce. Type 1 helper T (Th1) cells mainly synthesize interleukin-2 (IL-2) and interferon-γ (IFN-γ), as well as other proinflammatory cytokines such as lymphotoxin and tumor necrosis factor (TNF). Type 2 helper T (Th2) cells are distinguished primarily by their secretion of IL-4, IL-5, IL-10, and

IL-13. Th1 cells appear to be critically important in autoimmune diseases such as multiple sclerosis and type 1 diabetes (69). Th2-type responses may be relatively more important in SLE compared to these organ-specific diseases. However, in spontaneous murine models of lupus, the IgG isotypes involved in pathogenicity suggest the additional influence of Th1-type cytokines and especially the importance of interferon-γ (IFN-γ) (70,71). It is important to note the critical involvement of IFN-γ in the pathogenesis of disease in murine models of lupus (71), and evidence supports a role for this cytokine in human SLE (72) as well as its potential as a therapeutic target (71). The mechanism for the influence of IFN-γ in SLE has not been defined.

T-Cell Co-stimulation and T-Cell–B-Cell Interactions

Autoreactive T cells, like T cells specific for foreign antigens, must receive several signals to be activated. One signal is antigen-specific and provided by engagement of the T-cell receptor for antigen (TCR). Costimulatory molecules and their interactions provide additional signals. Two of the most important costimulatory interactions involve CD28 and CD40 ligand on the T cell, which bind to B7 (B7-1 CD80 and B7-2 CD86) and CD40, respectively, on antigen-presenting cells and B cells. The interaction of CD40 ligand with CD40 is clearly bidirectional in that it provides signals important for both T- and B-cell activation (73). Studies in human SLE have suggested that cell-surface CD40 ligand expression may be aberrantly increased (66,67) and that soluble CD40 ligand levels may be increased with resultant excessive B-cell activation (68). In murine models of lupus, blocking of the CD40 ligand–CD40 interaction or the CD28–B7 interaction suppresses disease activity (73,74), and currently these therapies are being developed to treat human SLE patients. Blocking both these costimulatory interactions in combination is one of the most potent treatment strategies in murine lupus at present (75).

B Cells

Generalized polyclonal B-cell hyperactivity and activation are frequently present in SLE (76), and some patients demonstrate markedly increased serum immunoglobulin levels, probably reflecting this process. However, the majority of available data also indicate that pathogenic autoantibody production in SLE is selective for only certain self-antigens and driven by self-antigen at the B-cell level. In SLE and lupus mice, for example, a subset of B cells producing IgG anti-DNA antibodies are clonally expanded and their Ig genes are modified by somatic mutation (77–79). This IgG autoantibody production appears to mimic a normal T-cell–dependent response to foreign antigen and involves similar mechanisms of somatic mutation, affinity maturation, and IgM to IgG class switching. Studies by several groups have indicated that anti-DNA autoantibodies in lupus preferentially utilize a subset of immunoglobulin heavy- and light-chain variable region gene segments (77–79). In addition, the generation of high affinity anti-DNA antibodies through immunoglobulin gene rearrangement and somatic mutation involves the accumulation of basic arginine residues in the immunoglobulin regions that bind antigen (complementarity determining regions), suggesting selection by anionic antigens, perhaps DNA itself.

B cells capable of secreting pathogenic autoantibodies characteristic of SLE are present and can develop from the normal B-cell repertoire (8). The transfer of alloreactive CD4$^+$ T cells and generation of chronic graft-versus-host disease causes pathogenic lupuslike autoantibody production in normal recipient animals (80,81). Other studies have shown that immunization of normal animals to certain peptides derived from nuclear antigens can result in spreading autoantibody responses to other determinants on the same molecule and to other molecules in the same nuclear complex (e.g., anti-Sm to anti-U1RNP and anti-Ro/SS-A to anti-La/SS-B) and can lead to lupuslike disease (59–62). This epitope spreading shows the presence of self-reactive B cells in these normal mice. Therefore, defects in central B-cell tolerance do not appear to be necessary to allow for pathogenic autoantibody production (8). Similar to regulation of autoreactive T cells, studies suggest that regulation of B cells in peripheral lymphoid tissues may be most important for the prevention of B-cell autoimmunity. Evidence also suggests that one of the genetically determined immune defects in SLE may cause generalized B-cell dysfunction and disrupt the peripheral B-cell tolerance process (26,38,76).

B cells are more important in the development of SLE than just as a source of autoantibodies (82). Studies in murine lupus have indicated that disease-related CD4$^+$ T-cell activation is dependent on the presence of B cells (82). Studies also have demonstrated an important role for B cells in epitope spreading (59), probably related to the effectiveness of antigen-specific B cells to present additional determinants after binding and internalizing antigenic complexes.

Autoantibodies

Among autoantibodies produced in SLE, those directed against components of the cell nucleus are the most characteristic and are found in more than 95% of patients (2,83–85). These antinuclear antibodies can be directed to DNA, RNA, as well as multiple different proteins contained in protein–nucleic acid complexes (Table 65-2). Cytoplasmic proteins associated with RNA also can be targets of autoantibodies in SLE (86). In general, these nuclear and cytoplasmic molecules are involved in critically important cell functions, including storage of genetic material, cell division, regulation of gene expression, RNA transcription, and RNA processing. The third major group of autoantigens in SLE is cell surface molecules (e.g., those on the surface of red blood cells, platelets, or lymphocytes). In general, the only well-studied autoantibody specificities relevant to renal involvement are antibodies to double-stranded DNA (dsDNA). In a subset of SLE patients with renal involvement, antiphospholipid antibodies may contribute to renal pathology by causing thrombosis and a thrombotic microangiopathy (discussed in more detail later in this chapter).

Antibodies to Double-Stranded DNA and Their Role in the Pathogenesis of Lupus Glomerulonephritis

Anti-dsDNA antibodies (87–89), especially when present in high levels in serum, are found essentially only in SLE patients. The titer of these antibodies fluctuate with disease activity, including systemic disease activity, but appear to correlate best with expression of glomerulonephritis in SLE. In some patients, serial measurements are useful in predicting disease flares, and quantitation of anti-dsDNA antibody activity in serum may be useful in the management of individual patients with SLE. It is clear, however, that some patients with active nephritis lack detectable serum anti-dsDNA activity, whereas other patients demonstrate persistently high levels without clinical evidence of nephritis. Some of these discrepancies may reflect problems with the assays used to measure anti-dsDNA activity, and studies have demonstrated that anti-dsDNA antibodies vary greatly in their pathogenic potential. In contrast to anti-dsDNA antibodies, antibodies to single-stranded DNA (ssDNA) have little

TABLE 65-2

EXAMPLES OF AUTOANTIBODIES IN SYSTEMIC LYPUS ERYTHEMATOSUS (SLE) AND THEIR CLINICAL ASSOCIATIONS

Target	Clinical associations
sDNA	High diagnostic specificity for SLE Correlation with disease activity (especially nephritis)
sDNA	Low diagnostic specificity
Histones	SLE and drug-induced lupus
Sm (snRNP proteins B, B′, D, E)	High diagnostic specificity for SLE No correlation with disease activity
U1 RNP Sm (snRNP proteins A, C, 70 kDa)	MCTD or other overlap syndrome (when not accompanied by anti-Sm)
SS-A/Ro (60-kDa and 50-kDa proteins)	Neonatal lupus (with anti-SS-B/La) Photosensitivity and subacute cutaneous LE
SS-B/La (48-kDa protein)	Associated with Sjögren's syndrome Neonatal lupus (with anti-SS-A/Ro)
Ku	High diagnostic specificity for SLE
PCNA/cyclin	High diagnostic specificity for SLE
Ribosomal P	High diagnostic specificity for SLE Cytoplasmic staining Psychiatric disease
Phospholipids (β2-glycoprotein 1)	Lupus anticoagulant Thrombosis Recurrent abortions/fetal wasting Focal neurologic deficits Thrombocytopenia Livido reticularis
Cell surface antigens	
Platelets	Thrombocytopenia
Red blood cells	Hemolytic anemia
Lymphocytes	Lymphopenia
Neuronal cells	Diffuse neurologic deficits

SnRNP, small nuclear ribonucleoprotein; *MCTD*, mixed connective tissue disease.
(From: Kotzin BL, O'Dell JR. Systemic lupus erythematosus. In: Frank MM, et al., eds. *Samter's Immunologic Diseases*, 5th ed. Boston: Little, Brown; 1994, with permission.)

diagnostic specificity and correlate poorly with renal disease activity.

IgG antibodies directed to dsDNA appear to play a prominent role in lupus nephritis (2,87–89). The evidence for this includes: (a) detection of anti-dsDNA antibodies in the glomeruli of patients and animals with active disease; (b) studies showing enrichment of IgG anti-dsDNA antibodies in glomerular tissues relative to serum and other organs; (c) longitudinal studies in a subset of SLE patients demonstrating that high levels of circulating anti-dsDNA antibodies frequently precede, or coincide with, active glomerulonephritis; and (d) demonstration in animals that injection of certain monoclonal IgG anti-dsDNA antibodies or expression of genes that encode pathogenic IgG anti-dsDNA activity, can lead to glomerular pathology.

Anti-DNA antibodies do not appear to mediate renal damage in SLE through the deposition of circulating immune complexes. Even in patients with active glomerulonephritis or animal models with actively increasing amounts of anti-DNA antibodies in the glomerulus, DNA–anti-DNA complexes have been difficult to demonstrate in the circulation (87,90). Two alternative theories have been proposed to explain the pathogenic

mechanisms of these antibodies. In the first, anti-DNA–DNA complexes are proposed to form in the glomerulus (*in situ* complex formation) rather than being deposited from the blood (91). Evidence supports a model in which DNA first binds to the glomerulus and is then recognized and bound by anti-DNA antibodies (92–94). Recent studies suggest that the negatively charged DNA may be binding to the glomerular basement membrane through positively charged histones, and that the target of autoantibodies is a DNA–histone–Type IV collagen complex within the glomerular basement membrane (94–97). It is of interest that increased amounts of circulating DNA have been detected in the blood of patients with SLE, which appears to be in the form of nucleosomes and therefore mostly composed of DNA and histones (98,99). The circulating nuclear material thus could become the planted renal target for a subset of pathogenic anti-DNA antibodies. This model also opens the possibility that selected antihistone, antichromatin, or other antinuclear specificities also could be pathogenic with mechanisms of damage similar to anti-DNA antibodies. There is evidence also that qualitative differences in anti-dsDNA antibodies are critically important in determining potential pathogenicity, and these differences may operate at the level of *in situ* complex formation. Other properties that have been proposed to affect pathogenicity include charge (cationic antibodies appear to be more pathogenic), avidity for DNA, idiotypes carried by the autoantibody, and the epitopes on DNA being recognized (87,88). Finally, in the planted antigen model, the release of antigen (i.e., DNA or nucleosomes) may be an additional variable in determining pathogenicity in lupus nephritis. This variable may explain studies in mice showing that "pathogenic" anti-dsDNA antibodies (either administered or induced) are not sufficient for the induction of severe renal disease (100,101). Analogous situations in human lupus nephritis also seem likely.

In an alternative model, the subset of pathogenic anti-DNA antibodies has been hypothesized to cross-react with glomerular antigens that are not DNA in origin. Thus, the potential to cross-react would be the determinant of pathogenicity. This model is supported by data showing that anti-DNA antibodies do contain other specificities and can bind to different glomerular structures (87,88,102–104). The model is also supported by data from other disease systems in which antibodies to intracellular antigens have been associated with glomerulonephritis, through cross-reactivity with glomerular antigens.

It should be emphasized that the correlation of anti-dsDNA autoantibody levels with activity of lupus nephritis is a general one. For example, numerous studies have shown that glomerulonephritis in SLE can occur in the absence of detectable anti-DNA antibodies (87,88). Although these cases may represent a failure of the sensitivity of currently available techniques to measure anti-DNA antibodies, it also suggests that autoantibodies directed to non-DNA antigens may participate in lupus renal damage in some cases. In most spontaneous murine models of lupus nephritis, antibodies to a self-retroviral envelope glycoprotein (gp70), and gp70-anti-gp70 immune complexes, are important in the development of severe nephritis (105). As discussed in the preceding paragraphs, there is reason to believe that a subset of antibodies directed to non-DNA antigens of chromatin also may be pathogenic. The relative contribution of autoantibody systems in addition to anti-DNA antibodies in lupus nephritis needs to be clarified.

Complement Activation and Fcγ Receptors in Renal Damage

The activation of complement components through the classical pathway appears to be critically involved in the pathogenesis of immune complex-mediated glomerular damage in lupus. Direct damage as well as recruitment of inflammatory cells are likely to be involved. Thus, IgG anti-DNA antibodies that are complement-fixing are most likely to be pathogenic (88). Studies in murine lupus nephritis have shown dramatic suppression of renal disease after injection of blocking monoclonal antibodies specific for complement factor C5 (21). Inhibition of complement activation in a similar fashion has been proposed as a possible therapy for patients with lupus nephritis, and studies are in progress to test this idea. In addition to the role of complement, murine studies have shown that effector cells bearing Fcγ receptors for IgG (Fcγ receptors), particularly FcγRIII, are necessary for immune complexes to mediate the full extent of damage in lupus nephritis (25).

CLINICAL–PATHOLOGIC CORRELATION IN LUPUS NEPHRITIS

Almost all patients with SLE demonstrate abnormalities on renal biopsy, especially if immunofluorescence and electron microscopy analyses are performed. Approximately half of all patients have clinically significant renal involvement at time of diagnosis. Importantly, lupus nephritis demonstrates remarkable variability in its pathologic appearance, clinical presentation, and course. Morphologic differences can be apparent among biopsies from different patients as well as among glomeruli in the same biopsy.

In order to confidently classify lupus glomerulonephritis, the renal biopsy should contain a minimum of 10 glomeruli for light microscopic analysis (106). Immunofluorescence is necessary for complete analysis and should include staining for IgG, IgA, and IgM isotypes, kappa and lambda light chains, and complement components C3 and C1q. Glomerular immune deposits in lupus nephritis should always contain dominant polyclonal IgG as well as C3 and usually C1q with lesser amounts of IgM and IgA (i.e., full house pattern). Immunofluorescence patterns not containing IgG should suggest an alternative diagnosis.

Each of the histologic types of lupus nephritis represents a nonspecific response to immune complex deposition. The one pathologic finding that is relatively specific for lupus is the presence of tubuloreticular structures in the glomerular endothelial cells seen on electron microscopy. These structures are composed of ribonucleoprotein and membrane and their synthesis is stimulated by alpha interferon (107).

World Health Organization Pathologic Classification

The World Health Organization (WHO) pathologic classification system for lupus nephritis was formulated in 1974 and modified in 1982 and 1995 (Table 65–3) (108,109). This histologic scheme addresses only glomerular lesions and in general correlates with clinical severity and prognosis in patients with lupus nephritis (110–115). However, it has been emphasized that knowledge of the WHO histologic type of renal disease may add little clinically useful information over and above that already known from clinical laboratory studies (urinalysis, protein excretion, and especially renal function studies) (113–117). When interpreting histologic findings, one must keep in mind that the renal biopsy is only a reflection of what is going on in the kidney at the time it is done and that changes from one pathologic stage to another over time are well documented in patients with lupus nephritis (110–112,118–121). In patients

TABLE 65-3

MODIFIED WORLD HEALTH ORGANIZATION (WHO) MORPHOLOGIC CLASSIFICATION OF LUPUS NEPHRITIS[a]

CLASS I	Normal glomeruli a. Nil (by all techniques) b. Normal by light microscopy, but deposits by electron or immunofluorescence microscopy
CLASS II (12%–25%)	Pure mesangial alterations (mesangiopathy) a. Mesangial widening and/or mild hypercellularity (+) b. Moderate hypercellularity (++)
CLASS III (16%–22%)	Focal segmental glomerulonephritis (associated with mild or moderate mesangial alterations) a. With "active" necrotizing lesions b. With "active" and sclerosing lesions c. With sclerosing lesions
CLASS IV (37%–46%)	Diffuse glomerulonephritis (severe mesangial, endocapillary or mesangiocapillary proliferation and/or extensive subendothelial deposits) a. Without segmental lesions b. With "active" necrotizing lesions c. With "active" and sclerosing lesions d. With sclerosing lesions
CLASS V (11%–21%)	Diffuse membranous glomerulonephritis a. Pure membranous glomerulonephritis b. Associated with lesions of class II c. Associated with lesions of class III d. Associated with lesions of class IV
CLASS VI (3%–4%)	Advanced sclerosing glomerulonephritis

[a]Percentages under each WHO class represent frequency of biopsy results in various genes of systemic lupus erythematosus (SLE) patients in which biopsies were systematically performed (105–111,114–117).

who undergo biopsy a second time, up to 40% may have undergone a change to another histologic class. This consideration is particularly true if patients are biopsied early in the course of their lupus and before therapy.

Renal biopsies showing normal glomeruli by light microscopy are designated WHO Class I. These are subdivided into completely normal by all techniques and those that have deposits demonstrated by immunofluorescence and/or electron microscopy. Mesangial nephritis (WHO Class II) (Figs. 65-2 and 65-3) is characterized by immune deposits in the mesangium that are best seen by immunofluorescence and electron microscopy. Light microscopy reveals mesangial hypercellularity and/or increased/expanded matrix. Deposits in the capillary loops are not apparent or minimal in this class of disease. Patients with mesangial nephritis usually demonstrate little clinical evidence of renal involvement, with normal or near normal urinalysis and renal function, and rarely require any treatment for their renal disease. It should be emphasized that mesangial changes represent a common denominator in lupus nephritis, and other lesions described subsequently are superimposed on these abnormalities.

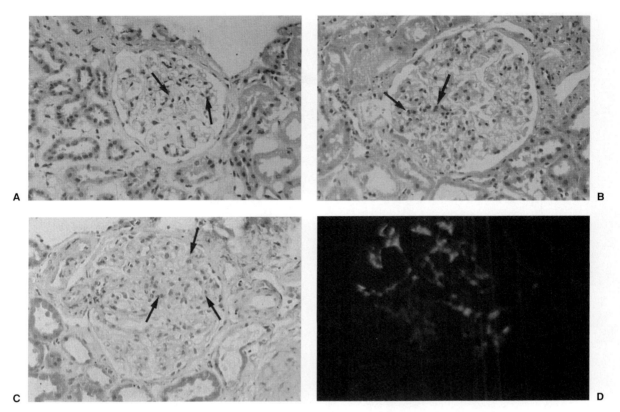

FIGURE 65-2. Histologic characteristics of mesangial glomerulonephropathy (World Health Organization Class II) in a patient with systemic lupus erythematosus. **A:** A normal glomerulus for comparison. Note the number and distribution of mesangial cells (*arrows*). (Hematoxylin and eosin, magnification ×200.) **B:** An early mesangial nephropathy displaying a subtle increase of mesangial cells (*arrows*). Compare with the normal glomerulus in **A**. (Hematoxylin and eosin, magnification ×200.) **C:** Another glomerulus from the same patient as in **B** but with a segmental accentuation of mesangial cells (*arrows*). This would be classified as a World Health Organization Class IIb lesion. (Hematoxylin and eosin, magnification ×200.) **D:** The mesangial matrix is accentuated by immunofluorescent deposits of IgG. This is an immunofluorescence analysis of the biopsy material shown in **B**. (Anti-IgG, magnification ×200.) (See Color Plate.)

Focal segmental (proliferative) glomerulonephritis (WHO Class III) (Fig. 65-4) is characterized histologically by hypercellularity owing to increases in mesangial, endocapillary, and/or infiltrating cells. These changes result in encroachment of the glomerular capillary space. Active inflammatory lesions are present. Lesions involve less than 50% of the glomeruli and are usually apparent in a segmental pattern (i.e., involve less than 50% of the glomerular tuft). Some investigators consider segmental glomerular necrosis to be the defining feature of WHO Class II lesions. Consequently, this class of lupus nephritis is further subdivided into those with active necrotizing lesions, combined active and sclerosing lesions, and primarily sclerosing lesions. Patients with this pattern frequently demonstrate proteinuria and hematuria, but severe (nephrotic range) proteinuria or progressive loss of renal function is less common. However, focal proliferative nephritis should be viewed as on a continuum with diffuse proliferative glomerulonephritis because the lesions are qualitatively similar (Figs. 65-5 and 65-6) and may progress to the more severe category with time.

Diffuse proliferative glomerulonephritis (DPGN) (WHO Class IV) is seen in about 35% to 45% of lupus patients with clinical renal disease and in most SLE patients who progress to renal failure (108–113,119–121). Diffuse proliferative glomerulonephritis is characterized by involvement of more than 50% of the glomeruli, with generalized hypercellularity of mesangial and endothelial cells. Inflammation with in-

flammatory cellular infiltrates, cellular destruction with nuclear fragmentation, and areas of fibrinoid necrosis are common in severe disease (Fig. 65-5). These changes ultimately may lead to obliteration of the capillary loops and sclerosis. Subendothelial deposits within the capillary loops and the resultant thickening of the membrane contour can result in "wire loop" lesions (Figs. 65-5 and 65-6A). Hyaline thrombi from massive aggregates of intraluminal immune complex deposits also may be present. Regions of basement membrane thickening are usually present. Crescents also may be seen in a subset of patients with progressive glomerulonephritis (Chapter 60). A subset of patients may demonstrate histologic abnormalities characteristic of true membranoproliferative (mesangiocapillary) glomerulonephritis (Chapter 62). Similar to Class III, WHO Class IV is further subdivided based on the presence of active, sclerosing, or mixed types of glomerular injury. Immunofluorescence microscopy demonstrates extensive deposition of immunoglobulin and complement in the mesangium and capillary loops, and electron microscopy frequently shows immune complex deposits in both subendothelial and subepithelial distributions (Figs. 65-5 and 65-6). Clinically, patients almost always have proteinuria and hematuria and not infrequently have decreases in renal function. Hypertension is common. Rarely, patients with no clinical evidence of renal disease have been biopsied and found to have focal or even diffuse proliferative glomerulonephritis (122), but progression does not occur without the development of urinalysis abnormalities.

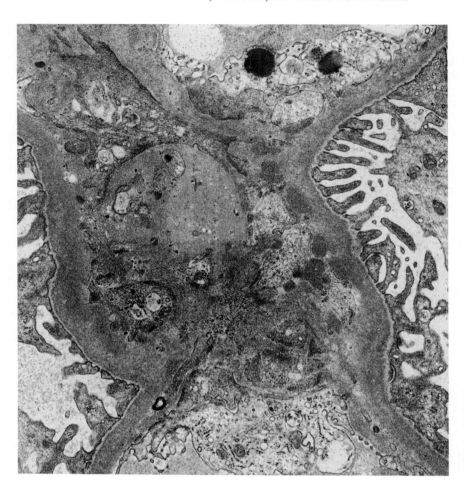

FIGURE 65-3. Electron microscopic analysis of mesangial glomerulonephropathy in a patient with systemic lupus erythematosus. Multiple electron-dense deposits are evident in the mesangium of a WHO Class IIb lesion. (Magnification ×9,000.) Light microscopic and immunofluorescence analyses of mesangial glomerulonephropathy are shown in Figure 65-2.

Membranous nephropathy (WHO Class V) (Figs. 65-7 and 65-8) is characterized histologically by diffuse thickening of the basement membrane (108–112,123–125) (Chapter 63). Glomeruli usually have normal cellularity. Lesions are further subdivided based on the presence of mesangial hypercellularity (Class II) and overlaps with focal proliferative (Class III) and diffuse proliferative (Class IV) lupus nephritis. Subepithelial deposits containing immunoglobulin and complement are apparent along the basement membrane on electron microscopy and immunofluorescence microscopy (Figs. 65-7 and 65-8). Immune deposits are also seen in the mesangium helping to separate it from idiopathic membranous nephropathy.

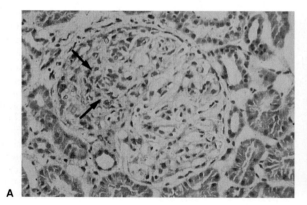
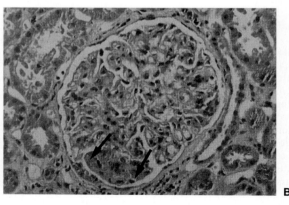

FIGURE 65-4. Histologic characteristics of focal proliferative glomerulonephritis (World Health Organization Class III) in a patient with systemic lupus erythematosus. **A:** Approximately one-half of this glomerular tuft is involved by mesangial proliferation (*arrows*), which at medium power is discernible as a segmental lesion. (Hematoxylin and eosin, magnification ×200.) **B:** Another glomerulus from the same patient. Here there is a mild global increase of mesangial cells and a segmental lesion with a suggestion of early tuft necrosis (*arrows*). (Hematoxylin and eosin, magnification ×200.) Less than half of the glomeruli in this biopsy demonstrated segmental lesions. (See Color Plate.)

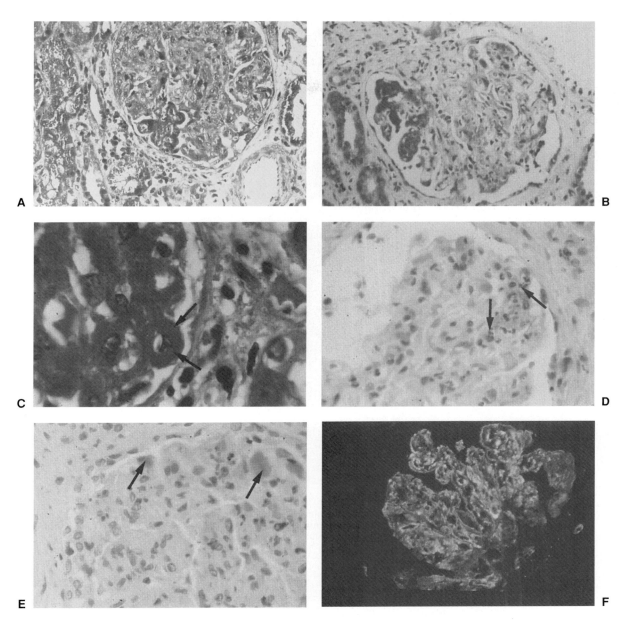

FIGURE 65-5. Histologic characteristics of diffuse proliferative glomerulonephritis (World Health Organization Class IV) in a patient with systemic lupus erythematosus. This plate also shows examples of the abnormalities used in the scoring of the activity index (Table 65-4). A: The majority of glomeruli in this case were involved by a global proliferation of mesangial cells and varying indicators of acute activity. (Trichrome, magnification ×200.) B: This trichrome stain accentuates the intracapillary thrombi present in the same biopsy as A. C: Subendothelial deposits are seen within the capillary loop (*arrows*). The resultant thickening of the membrane contour is the source of the descriptive term "wire loop." (Trichrome, magnification ×800.) D: Multiple neutrophils are apparent within the mesangium and capillary lumens (*arrows*). (Hematoxylin and eosin, magnification ×400.) E: Hematoxylin bodies (*arrows*) are not often seen in biopsy material. They are the result of altered nuclear DNA and are considered pathognomonic of lupus nephritis. Notice also the neutrophilic infiltrates and cellular proliferation, both features of an active lesion. (Hematoxylin and eosin, magnification ×400.) F: Extensive glomerular deposition of immunoglobulin demonstrated by immunofluorescent staining for IgG. Compare the distribution and intensity of staining with the immunofluorescence analysis of mesangial nephropathy shown in Figure 65-2D. (From: Kotzin BL, O'Dell JR. Systemic lupus erythematosus. In: Frank MM, et al, eds. *Samter's Immunologic Diseases*, 5th ed. Boston: Little, Brown; 1994, with permission.) (See Color Plate.)

Clinically, patients who have pure membranous disease frequently have extensive proteinuria but only minimal hematuria or functional renal abnormalities. Complement levels and titers of anti-dsDNA antibodies are frequently normal and do not correlate with the activity of this type of nephropathy. A subset of patients, estimated at 10% to 30%, slowly progresses to chronic renal failure within a 10-year period. The natural history of this form of membranous disease is somewhat unclear because nearly all patients with severe clinical manifestations are treated. Membranous disease also can be observed as a transition stage after treatment for proliferative glomerulonephritis (121,126).

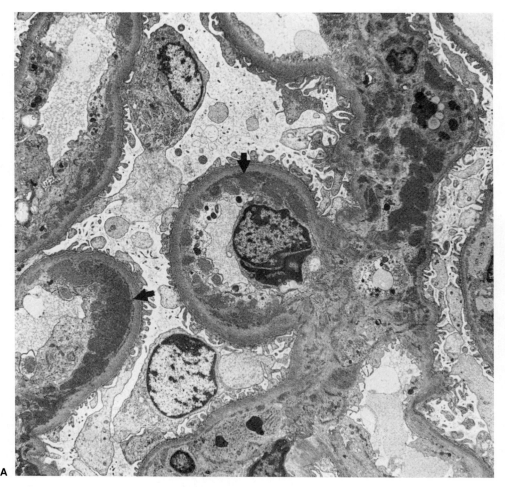

FIGURE 65-6. Electron microscopic analysis of diffuse proliferative glomerulonephritis (World Health Organization Class IV) in a patient with systemic lupus erythematosus. **A:** In this electron microscopic view of a wire-loop lesion, prominent electron-dense deposits (*arrows*) partially fill the subendothelial space. Dense deposits are also seen throughout the mesangium, which is characteristic of lupus nephritis. (Magnification ×9,000.) (*continued*)

Advanced sclerosing glomerulonephritis (WHO Class VI) was introduced when the WHO classification was first modified. This lesion is the result of progressive Class III, IV, or V glomerulonephritis. The use of numerous subdivisions has made the modified WHO classification system cumbersome and not widely accepted by all pathologists.

In 2003, an international group of renal pathologists, nephrologists, and rheumatologists developed an expanded classification system shown in Table 65-4 (127). This revised classification preserves the six WHO classes of lupus nephritis but introduces and defines important differences between Class III and IV lesions that are clinically relevant. In addition, activity and chronicity lesions are further described. This classification builds on the widely accepted WHO classification, attempts to eliminate the ambiguity about the definitions of classes III and IV lupus nephritis and includes segmental glomerulonephritis with 50% or greater glomerular involvement. A new subdivision of class IV as segmental or global has been included based on evidence that global involvement may have a different prognosis compared to segmental. This classification system is based on glomerular pathology, but the group strongly recommended separate documentation on the extent and severity of tubulointerstitial

and vascular lesions, which can clearly affect renal prognosis. Whether this system is accepted by pathologists, improves uniformity of reporting between centers, and reflects clinical outcomes better than the previous classifications is under investigation.

Lupus can also involve the renal tubules, kidney interstitium, and blood vessels (108–112,128–130). Areas of lymphocytic interstitial infiltration may be apparent, and immunofluorescence may demonstrate antibodies bound to renal tubular cells (128,129). However, this almost always occurs in conjunction with glomerular involvement, and, in general, renal outcome is determined by the severity of the glomerular lesion. Interstitial features of the chronicity index (described subsequently) appear to be closely related to glomerular damage and glomerular dropout rather than secondary to chronic interstitial inflammation; these features of irreversible damage predict a poor outcome. The role of mononuclear cell infiltrates in the pathogenesis of lupus nephritis remains poorly understood. Vascular involvement in renal biopsies from patients with SLE can vary considerably, being related to hypertension, hyperlipidemia, a small-vessel vasculopathy or small-vessel thrombosis associated with antiphospholipid antibodies, or rarely vasculitis (130,131).

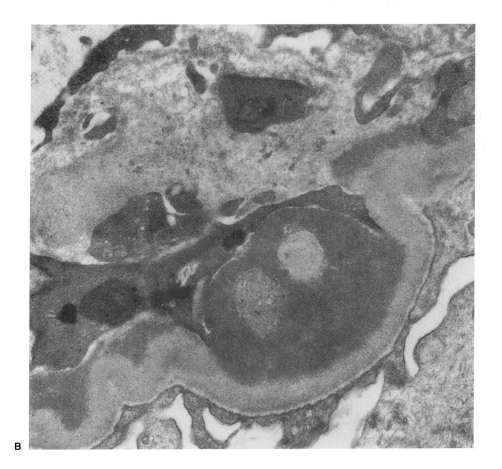

B

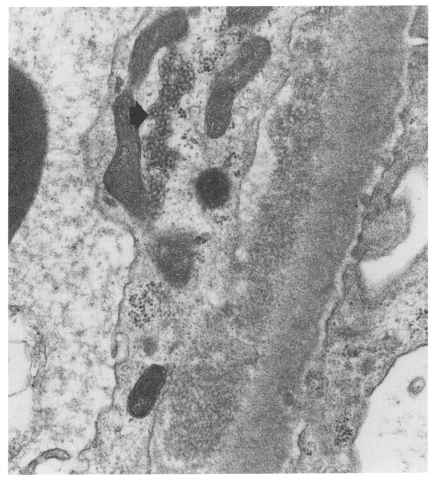

FIGURE 65-6. (*Continued*) **B:** Subendothelial deposits in a moderately active Class IV lesion, which show the concentric and swirling laminations dubbed "fingerprinting." Although not pathognomonic, they are commonly associated with lupus. (Magnification ×39,000.) **C:** Tubuloreticular structures within subendothelial cells (*arrows*). (Magnification ×62,000.) (Courtesy of Dr. William Hammond, Denver, CO.) Light microscopic and immunofluorescence analyses of diffuse proliferative glomerulonephritis are shown in Figure 65-5.

C

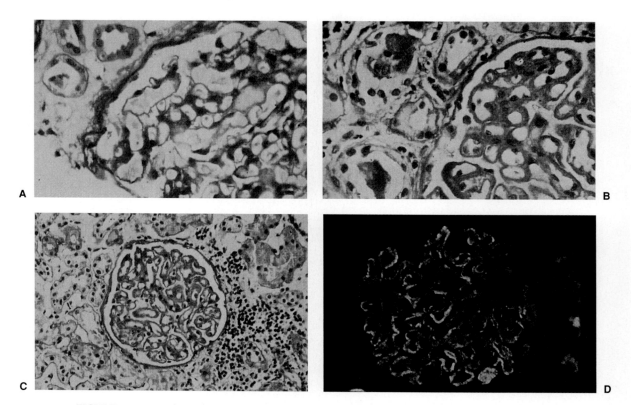

FIGURE 65-7. Histologic characteristics of membranous nephropathy (World Health Organization Class V) in a patient with systemic lupus erythematosus. **A:** Normal glomerulus for comparison. Notice the thin, delicate profile of the basement membranes. (Periodic acid–Schiff, magnification ×400.) **B:** Membranous nephropathy with thickened basement membranes. (Periodic acid–Schiff, magnification ×400.) Compare with the normal glomerulus in **A. C:** The thickened, rigid-appearing basement membranes of advanced membranous nephropathy are obvious even at medium power. (Periodic acid–Schiff, magnification ×200.) Lymphocytes are seen in the interstitium, and there is a hint of tubular dropout, an indicator that this is a chronic lesion. **D:** Immunofluorescence study of the same patient illustrated in **C.** The membranes are highlighted by fluorescent deposits of IgG. (Anti-IgG, magnification ×200.) (See Color Plate.)

Pathologic Indices of Activity and Chronicity

A semiquantitative histologic scoring system for lupus nephritis has been developed in an effort to more accurately predict renal outcome and to help determine which patients are most likely to benefit from aggressive therapy (7,119,132,133). In this system, a *chronicity index* measures four histologic components of chronic irreversible renal damage, and an *activity index* measures six histologic components of activity of lupus nephritis (Table 65-5, Figs. 65-5,65-6,65-9). In the last several years, these systems have come into major use, and a number of studies have reported on their predictive associations and usefulness. Most, but not all, studies have found that a higher chronicity index is associated with greater risk for progression to renal failure (7,113,114,117,132–144). For example, Austin and coworkers (133) showed that none of 29 patients with lupus nephritis and a low chronicity index (defined as scores of 0 to 1) progressed to renal failure over a 5-year period. In contrast, 40% of the patients with scores greater than 3 progressed to renal failure. Based on its apparent validity as a prognostic indicator as well as the fact that the presence of chronic damage identifies disease with destructive potential, several investigators have recommended the use of the chronicity index as a guide to the aggressiveness of therapy. In particular, treatment with agents such as cyclophosphamide was predicted to be most beneficial for pa-

tients with intermediate chronicity index scores (7,133). In contrast to the chronicity index, the validity of the activity index as a predictor of renal outcome is less clear; approximately half of these studies have shown that a higher score correlates with increased risk of renal failure (7,117,132–144). This may relate to the caveat that active lesions are amenable to therapy, whereas chronic lesions represent irreversible destruction. It seems likely that increased activity index scores identify patients most likely to respond to aggressive treatment.

Some studies have not been able to confirm the usefulness of the chronicity index for prognosis and management of patients with lupus nephritis (140–143). Most of the preceding studies validating this scoring system were performed in specialized academic centers with pathologists educated and skilled in the use of this histologic grading system. There is limited information on treatment and prognosis of lupus nephritis in primary care facilities. At least one study of renal pathologists from a nonreferral setting has suggested that problems with interreader reliability could explain some of the conflicting reports regarding the usefulness of the chronicity index scoring system (145). Importantly, small differences in chronicity index scoring could result in major differences in risk group assignment, and such differences in scoring could prevent the chronicity index from being a guide to therapy.

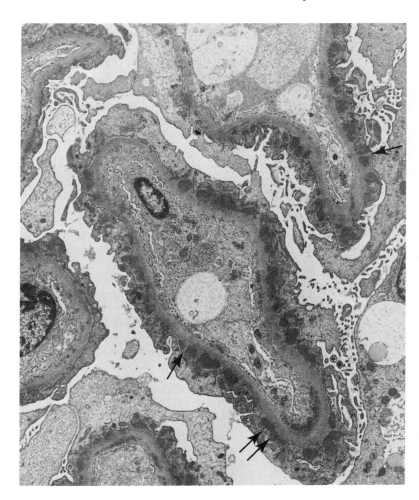

FIGURE 65-8. Ultrastructure of membranous nephropathy (World Health Organization Class V) in a patient with systemic lupus erythematosus, displaying numerous dark deposits along the outer aspect of the glomerular basement membrane. Basement membrane material has been formed and is insinuating itself between the deposits, forming so-called spikes (*single arrows*). The spikes will coalesce and envelop the deposits (*double arrows*), eventually incorporating the deposits into the membrane itself, where it will then be absorbed. (Magnification ×9,000.) Light microscopic and immunofluorescence analyses of membranous nephropathy are shown in Figure 65-7.

CLINICAL AND LABORATORY ABNORMALITIES IN LUPUS NEPHRITIS

Clinical Features

The development of lupus nephritis greatly influences long-term outcome in patients with SLE and is the most frequent reason for patients to be treated with high-dose corticosteroids and cytotoxic medications. At time of diagnosis, 50% of patients have an abnormal urinalysis with or without an elevated serum creatinine. Over the course of the disease, nearly 75% of all SLE patients demonstrate evidence of renal involvement, with urinalysis abnormalities (proteinuria (80%), hematuria (40%), or casts) or functional impairment with decreased glomerular filtration rate (GFR), as measured by creatinine clearance. Although clinically significant nephritis can occur at any time in the course of SLE, it usually occurs in the first few years (<3 years) of disease, rarely develops after 5 years, and can be the presenting feature of disease in 5% of patients (110,146–150). However, urinalysis screening at regular intervals is mandatory, since the onset of nephritis is frequently asymptomatic. Examination of an early morning, second voided urine is recommended to ensure a concentrated acidic urine specimen, which is the best condition to find urinary casts. Patients can also present with foamy urine (proteinuria), nocturia (tubular dysfunction), nephrotic syndrome, or nephritic syndrome with hypertension, depending on the extent of immune deposits and inflammation within the glomerulus. Rarely patients can present with macroscopic hematuria, rapidly progressive glomerulonephritis (doubling of creatinine within 3 months), or acute renal failure. Renal tubular acidosis is unusual and usually does not require therapy.

Individual studies have indicated that renal disease is more frequent and severe in childhood onset than adult onset SLE patients (149). In adults, young age at onset (<33 years old), male sex and nonwhite race or socioeconomic status are risk factors for developing early and more severe nephritis (5,7,144,147,150). Alternatively, patients with onset after age 50 usually have milder disease, including nephritis, although some patients can develop renal damage (151). Except for hypertension, no nonrenal clinical manifestation of SLE is reasonably reliable in predicting the likelihood of developing lupus nephritis or predicting the severity of renal involvement and renal outcome (152). As discussed in the preceding section, variability and unpredictability are major features of the course of SLE.

Hypertension is common in patients with lupus nephritis and may be important in the progression of renal damage in patients with severe disease (153). Several studies have suggested that it predicts a poor renal outcome (143,154,155). Hypertension also plays a significant role in the increased incidence of coronary artery disease seen in the SLE population. Control of hypertension is critically important for a successful outcome in lupus nephritis.

TABLE 65-4

INTERNATIONAL SOCIETY OF NEPHROLOGY/RENAL PATHOLOGY CLASSIFICATION OF LUPUS NEPHRITIS (2003)

CLASS I	**MINIMAL MESANGIAL LUPUS NEPHRITIS** Normal glomeruli by light microscopy, but mesangial immune deposits by immunofluorescence
CLASS II	**MESANGIAL PROLIFERATIVE LUPUS NEPHRITIS** Purely mesangial hypercellularity of any degree or mesangial matrix expansion by light microscopy, with mesangial immune deposits A few isolated subepithelial or subendothelial deposits may be visible by immunofluorescence or electron microscopy, but not by light microscopy
CLASS III	**FOCAL LUPUS NEPHRITIS**[a] Active or inactive focal, segmental or global endo- or extracapillary glomerulonephritis involving <50% of all glomeruli, typically with focal subendothelial immune deposits, with or without mesangial alterations
Class III (A)	Active lesions: focal proliferative lupus nephritis
Class III (A/C)	Active and chronic lesions: focal proliferative and sclerosing lupus nephritis
Class III (C)	Chronic inactive lesions with glomerular scars: focal sclerosing lupus nephritis
CLASS IV	**DIFFUSE LUPUS NEPHRITIS**[b] Active or inactive diffuse, segmental or global endo- or extracapillary glomerulonephritis involving ≥50% of all glomeruli, typically with diffuse subendothelial immune deposits, with or without mesangial alterations. This class is divided into diffuse segmental (IV-S) lupus nephritis when ≥50% of the involved glomeruli have segmental lesions, and diffuse global (IV-G) lupus nephritis when ≥50% of the involved glomeruli have global lesions. Segmental is defined as a glomerular lesion that involves less than half of the glomerular tuft. This class includes cases with diffuse wire loop deposits but with little or no glomerular proliferation.
Class IV-S (A)	Active lesions: diffuse segmental proliferative lupus nephritis
Class IV-G (A)	Active lesions: diffuse global proliferative lupus nephritis
Class IV-S (A/C)	Active and chronic lesions: diffuse segmental proliferative and sclerosing lupus nephritis
Class IV-G (A/C)	Active and chronic lesions: diffuse global proliferative and sclerosing lupus nephritis
Class IV-S (C)	Chronic inactive lesions with scars: diffuse segmental sclerosing lupus nephritis
Class IV-G (C)	Chronic inactive lesions with scars: diffuse global sclerosing lupus nephritis
CLASS V	**MEMBRANOUS LUPUS NEPHRITIS** Global or segmental subepithelial immune deposits or their morphologic sequelae by light microscopy and by immunofluorescence or electron microscopy, with or without mesangial alterations Lupus nephritis may occur in combination with class III or IV in which case both will be diagnosed Class V lupus nephritis may show advanced sclerosis
CLASS VI	**ADVANCED SCLEROTIC LUPUS NEPHRITIS** ≥ 90% of glomeruli globally sclerosed without residual activity

Indicate and grade (mild, moderate, severe) tubular atrophy, interstitial inflammation and fibrosis, severity of arteriosclerosis or other vascular lesions.
[a]Indicate the proportion of glomeruli that are active and with sclerotic lesions.
[b]Indicate the proportion of glomeruli with fibrinoid necrosis and/or cellular crescents.

Pregnancy is not an infrequent occurrence in SLE patients and can be a difficult management problem (156,157). Pregnancy in the setting of active disease, especially active or progressive renal disease, can result in severe problems and a bad outcome for both the mother and baby. Among women with lupus nephritis, the incidence of preeclampsia can be as high as 66%. It may be difficult to distinguish preeclampsia from an exacerbation of lupus nephritis, although the presence of an active urinary sediment, elevated anti-dsDNA antibody levels, and hypocomplementemia favor lupus nephritis (158). Patients with active lupus nephritis have up to a 52% risk of fetal loss during pregnancy (159). Furthermore, disease flares and exacerbations of glomerulonephritis may occur, particularly in the third trimester and immediate postpartum period, even in patients who have been clinically quiescent (160). Notably, these flares can also occur following elective termination of pregnancy. Therefore, women with lupus nephritis should be encouraged to delay pregnancy until their disease is treated and inactive for at least 6 months (156).

Autoantibodies

As reviewed in the preceding text, antinuclear antibodies (ANAs) are the hallmark of autoantibody production in SLE, and more than 98% of SLE patients with nephritis demonstrate a positive ANA test (83–85). Antinuclear antibodies are detected in most laboratories by an indirect immunofluorescence assay with human tumor cells (usually HEP-2 cells) as the substrate fixed to the slide. These cells allow the greatest sensitivity and best definition of binding patterns. A variety of immunofluorescent staining patterns (e.g., peripheral or rim, diffuse, speckled, or nucleolar) can be observed on ANA testing. However, because of the development of tests that measure

PATHOLOGIC INDICES OF ACTIVITY AND CHRONICITY IN LUPUS NEPHRITIS

Chronicity index[a]	Activity index[b]
Glomerular sclerosis	Cellular proliferation
Fibrous crescents	Fibrinoid necrosis, karyorrhexis
Tubular atrophy	Cellular crescents
Interstitial fibrosis	Hyaline thrombi, wire loop lesions
	Leukocyte infiltration in glomerulus
	Mononuclear-cell infiltration in interstitium

[a]To obtain a chronicity score, each parameter is graded 0 to 3 depending on severity of involvement, and the grades are added. Glomerular sclerosis and fibrous crescents are graded as follows: 0, absent; 1+, <25% of glomeruli involved; 2+, 25% to 50% of glomeruli involved; 3+, >75% of glomeruli involved. Tubular atrophy and interstitial fibrosis are graded as follows: 0, absent; 1+, mild; 2+, moderate; 3+, severe. The maximum chronicity score is 12.
[b]To obtain an activity score, each parameter is graded 0 to 3 depending on severity of involvement, and the individual grades are added. Fibrinoid necrosis and cellular crescents have been given a "weighting" factor of 2. The maximum activity score is 24.

specific ANA specificities, these patterns have less clinical significance today. Although elevated serum levels of ANA are very sensitive for the diagnosis of SLE, it is emphasized that this test is not at all specific for SLE or other connective tissue diseases. In a study of 15 international laboratories, nearly one-third of healthy individuals were found to have a positive ANA test at a serum dilution of 1:40 (161). The frequency of a positive ANA in healthy individuals was 5% at a serum dilution of 1:160 and 3% at 1:320. The sensitivity for the diagnosis of SLE at a 1:40 serum dilution was 97% compared to 87% at 1:320 (161). The specificity for SLE was only 68% at a titer of 1:40 but was 95% at 1:320. These results indicate that a low dilution (1:40) is most valuable for excluding the diagnosis of SLE, whereas titers higher than 1:160 have the best positive-likelihood ratio for the diagnosis of SLE.

If the screening ANA test is determined to be positive, many clinical laboratories will offer a panel to detect various specific ANAs, including antibodies to dsDNA, Sm, U1 RNP, SS-A/Ro, and SS-B/La (Table 65-2). A number of different techniques are used to detect and quantitate anti-DNA antibodies, including immunoprecipitation, radioimmunoassay (RIA), enzyme-linked immunoabsorbent assay (ELISA), and immunofluorescence staining. Using the hemoflagellate *Crithidia luciliae*, which has a kinetoplast containing only dsDNA, an indirect immunofluorescence assay has also been developed to specifically detect antibodies to dsDNA. Although ELISA and *Crithidia* techniques can be made specific and sensitive for antibodies that bind dsDNA, these assays may not best measure the subset of potentially pathogenic anti-dsDNA antibodies that correlate with lupus nephritis (88); for example, these assays may be capable of detecting lower avidity anti-dsDNA antibodies compared to other detection techniques (e.g., a modified Farr assay) that rely on precipitation of antibodies bound to DNA. Some studies have suggested that anti-DNA antibodies with high avidity have greater pathogenic potential (88).

Antiribosomal P is a highly specific lupus autoantibody that reacts with the 60S ribosomal subunit located in the cell's cytoplasm. Antiribosomal P antibodies are detected in about 15% of lupus patients and correlate with disease activity, particularly lupus cerebritis, and, more recently, nephritis. Reichlin

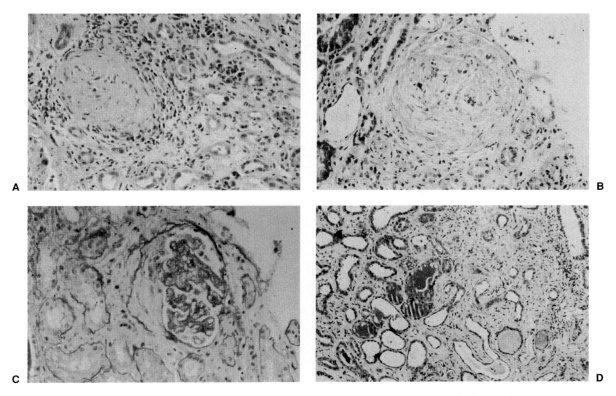

FIGURE 65-9. Examples of histologic features utilized in the chronicity index. **A:** An obsolescent glomerulus is surrounded by small strophic tubules. (Hematoxylin and eosin, magnification ×200.) **B:** The residuum of a glomerulus is barely visible in this example of a fibrous crescent. (Trichrome, magnification ×200.) **C:** A shrunken glomerular tuft is displaced by a fibrous crescent. **D:** Simplified, dilated tubules in a fibrotic stroma. (Hematoxylin and eosin, magnification ×200.) (See Color Plate.)

and Wolfson-Reichlin reported that the occurrence of both antiribosomal P and anti-ds DNA antibodies together were more associated with lupus nephritis than was the presence of either one alone (162). Interestingly, antiribosomal P antibodies can cross-react with DNA and are capable of penetrating live cells resulting in suppression of protein synthesis (163).

Serial monitoring of specific ANA in SLE should probably be limited to anti-dsDNA as there is no evidence that changes in the levels of other ANAs correlate with renal disease activity. Monitoring of anti-DNA antibody levels appears to be of most value in a subset of patients with lupus nephritis. They occur more frequently and in higher titers in patients with Class III or IV proliferative nephritis than with Class V (membranous) glomerulonephritis. Changes, particularly an increase in titer of anti-dsDNA antibodies, are more valuable than the absolute height of the antibody level (164.) Importantly, some patients with high titers of anti-dsDNA antibodies never develop nephritis, whereas severe nephritis can occasionally occur in patients with low titers of these antibodies. However, in general, patients with rising titers should be followed more closely for disease exacerbation.

The value of antichromatin/nucleosome and anti-C1q antibodies for assessing lupus nephritis activity and predicting flares is being actively investigated. Chromatin is the native histone-DNA complex organized into a repeating series of nucleosome in the nucleus of eukaryotic cells. Nucleosomes (chromatin) from apoptotic cells are autoantigens in SLE patients. Immune complexes composed of antichromatin antibodies and chromatin can bind to the glomerular basement membrane. Antichromatin antibodies have been reported to be associated with lupus nephritis with a sensitivity of up to 81% (165). Patients with antichromatin antibodies have a twofold higher prevalence of lupus nephritis and higher disease activity scores than patients without these antibodies. Similarly, anti-C1q antibodies are present in 30% to 45% of patients with SLE. These antibodies are strongly associated with lupus nephritis, and rising titers appear to predict renal flares (166). In addition, these antibodies appear to predispose patients to more severe forms of proliferative lupus nephritis. The binding of anti-C1q to C1q on immune complexes may facilitate immune complex deposition and/or amplify pathogenic complement activation once the immune complex has deposited or formed in the glomerulus (167).

Complement

Complement is consumed primarily via the classical pathway during active immune complex deposition disease; therefore, patients with active SLE characteristically have decreased levels of C3, C4, and total hemolytic complement. Low complement levels are associated with active disease, especially when active lupus nephritis is present. However, hypocomplementemia may be present in SLE patients with active cutaneous disease and other types of clinical activity and occasional patients who do not have clinical activity. Therefore, the presence of hypocomplementemia should alert the clinician to the possibility of active organ involvement but should not by itself dictate therapy. As discussed, a subset of SLE patients demonstrates hereditary deficiencies of complement components. The presence of normal levels of C3 and undetectable hemolytic complement activity (e.g., CH50) levels should alert the clinician to the possibility of a hereditary complete complement component deficiency. In these situations, assays for the individual complement components should be performed. Studies have suggested distinguishing clinical and laboratory characteristics, including less renal disease, in SLE patients with complete complement deficiencies. Serial monitoring of complement levels is discussed in the section on management.

SLE is a disease characterized by complement activation when active. Consequently, measurement of complement split products, complement receptors (CR1 on erythrocytes), and the complement membrane attack complex (C5b-9) is presently being studied for monitoring disease activity. Of these, measurement of C4d on erythrocytes (E-C4d) holds the most promise. The complement split product, C4d, has the capacity to attach covalently to cell surface components and persist longer than soluble split products in plasma. Recent studies have demonstrated that abnormally high E-C4d levels have a diagnostic sensitivity and specificity of 70% to 80% (168). In addition, the levels fluctuate over time and correlate with disease activity. Due to the short half-life of reticulocytes (2 days) compared to erythrocytes (120 days), measurement of reticulocyte-bound C4d may be an even better measure of current and ongoing disease activity. The value of measuring membrane-bound C4d levels to monitor lupus nephritis is currently being evaluated.

Tests Monitoring Renal Involvement

Routine laboratory tests used to diagnose and monitor the extent of glomerulonephritis in patients with SLE are similar to those used for other renal diseases (Chapters 10 and 11). Frequent urinalyses with microscopic examination, serum creatinines, and 24-hour creatinine clearance and urinary protein excretion studies usually are necessary in SLE patients with renal involvement. Scrupulous monitoring for changes in kidney function is critical in the management of patients with lupus nephritis. Similar to other types of glomerular disease, advanced lupus nephritis may also be associated with excessive tubular creatinine secretion, owing to tubular dysfunction (169,170); therefore, both the creatinine clearance and serum level of creatinine may overestimate true GFR in these patients. The insidious and persistent loss of GFR in lupus patients is an important marker of poor outcome and is closely related to the presence of chronic destructive lesions seen histologically (7,114,117,134,135,143,144,154). In contrast, acute decreases in kidney function often indicate the presence of newly active and potentially treatable disease.

As discussed, severe glomerulonephritis in SLE is unusual in the absence of proteinuria, and nephrotic-range proteinuria may occur in up to 25% of patients (147,148). Reduction in proteinuria is an important measure of favorable response to treatment in lupus nephritis. Studies have shown that initially severe proteinuria and persistent proteinuria (>1 g/24 hours) after treatment place patients at high risk for the development of progressive disease (143,171). Decreases in kidney function in the absence of proteinuria should alert the clinician to drug-related effects, especially when nonsteroidal antiinflammatory drugs (NSAIDs) or ACE inhibitors are being taken. Patients with SLE are at higher risk for developing decreasing renal function with these medications (Chapter 44).

RENAL INVOLVEMENT IN CLINICAL SYNDROMES CLOSELY RELATED TO SYSTEMIC LUPUS ERYTHEMATOSUS

Overlap Syndromes and Mixed Connective Tissue Disease

Patients with features of SLE or even those classified as SLE by the ACR criteria may demonstrate manifestations of other rheumatic diseases, including systemic sclerosis, polymyositis–dermatomyositis, rheumatoid arthritis, and Sjögren's syndrome. One type of overlap syndrome, referred to as mixed connective tissue disease (MCTD), has distinguishing clinical and serologic characteristics (172). This disease is partially defined by the presence of specific autoantibodies to U1 RNP in the absence of antibodies to Sm and the relative absence of other types of ANA. Features of SLE, systemic sclerosis, polymyositis/dermatomyositis, and, less commonly, a destructive arthropathy resembling rheumatoid arthritis characterize these patients clinically. Especially early in the disease process, patients tend to resemble each other with common features that include Raynaud's phenomena, puffy or edematous hands, arthritis involving the small joints of the hands, and serositis. Sclerodactyly and esophageal dysfunction also may be present. As the syndrome evolves, one type of disease process may predominate. In up to one-third of cases, patients develop a disease in which features of systemic sclerosis predominate. Severe lupuslike glomerulonephritis is much less common in MCTD as compared with SLE.

Drug-Induced Lupus

A large number of drugs have been associated with the production of ANA and development of a lupuslike syndrome (50). Most of the cases have been associated with hydralazine or procainamide. Drug-induced lupus in general differs from idiopathic lupus in that it tends to cause predominantly joint and pleural–pericardial involvement. Lupus nephritis and central nervous system manifestations are very unusual in drug-induced lupus. The disease remits when the offending drug is discontinued, but the time to remission may be prolonged (months), and manifestations may require a period of treatment with NSAIDs or steroids. Drug-induced disease is associated with positive ANA tests, and antihistone antibodies are present in almost all patients (50). Other autoantibodies frequently seen in SLE (e.g., anti-dsDNA and anti-Sm) usually are absent. Recently, minocycline has been added to the list of drugs causing a lupuslike syndrome. In addition to arthritis and a positive ANA, minocycline-induced lupus is frequently associated with hepatitis, a positive pANCA without myeloperoxidase specificity, and negative antihistone antibodies.

Antiphospholipid Antibodies and the Antiphospholipid Antibody Syndrome

Antiphospholipid antibodies are associated with an increase in thrombotic events resulting in a variety of clinical problems, including recurrent venous and arterial thrombosis, repeated spontaneous miscarriages, and focal neurologic findings secondary to cerebrovascular occlusion (173,174). Less common features associated with these autoantibodies are livedo reticularis, thrombocytopenia, verrucous thickening of cardiac valves, and Coombs-positive hemolysis. Antiphospholipid autoantibodies are present in more than 30% of patients with SLE, and complications are seen in a significant subset of these patients. Kidney involvement related to the presence of these antibodies may contribute to progressive renal damage in patients with lupus nephritis (130,131,174). The antiphospholipid antibody syndrome (APS) with complications can occur in patients without SLE or a related autoimmune disease (e.g. primary APS), and these autoantibodies are an important health problem in the general population. Prospective studies have found lupus anticoagulants in 8.5% to 14% of patients who presented with venous thromboembolism for the first time (up to 35,000 of the 250,000 cases per year) (175).

Kidney involvement related to the presence of antiphospholipid antibodies can occur in 25% of patients with primary APS (176,177). This renal involvement is characterized by noninflammatory occlusion of renal blood vessels that can range from the main renal artery and vein to a thrombotic microangiopathy affecting the glomerular capillaries (178). Histopathologic evaluation shows the vessels to have a reactive intimal mucoid thickening, medial hyperplasia, and thrombosis. The clinical presentation depends on the size of blood vessel involved.

Patients with SLE and antiphospholipid antibodies can develop any of the renal complications seen in primary APS (179). An isolated thrombotic microangiopathy causing significant renal dysfunction occurs in up to 10% of SLE patients with these antibodies. In addition, up to one-third of biopsies in lupus patients with renal abnormalities due to lupus nephritis have glomerular capillary thrombi. Lupus nephritis patients with these microthrombi were significantly more likely to have antiphospholipid antibodies (particularly lupus anticoagulant) and to have a history of previous thrombotic episodes. It is important to note that patients with lupus nephritis, glomerular vessel thrombi, and antiphosholipid antibodies were more likely to have an elevated serum creatinine, hypertension, interstitial fibrosis on renal biopsy, and the eventual development of chronic renal failure (180).

Antiphospholipid antibodies are usually detected as antibodies to cardiolipin in ELISA or as the "lupus anticoagulant" (173,174,181). Lupus anticoagulants interfere with phospholipid-dependent coagulation tests without inhibiting the activity of specific coagulation factors. The name is misleading in that it is not at all specific for SLE, and, paradoxically, it is clinically associated with venous and arterial thrombosis rather than bleeding problems. These antibodies are usually detected initially by finding an elevated partial thromboplastin test (PTT), and the abnormal PTT is not corrected by mixing the patient's plasma with normal plasma, implicating a circulating inhibitor. Antiphospholipid antibodies inhibit *in vitro* coagulation tests at the level of activation of prothrombin to thrombin (i.e., inhibit the prothrombin activator complex), dependent on the amount of phospholipid in the assay. Dilution of the phospholipid (which increases the inhibiting activity of these antibodies) or adding excess phospholipid (which saturates the antibodies) are methods used to specifically screen for this type of lupus anticoagulant. One example is the Russel viper venom test. It is emphasized that inhibition of coagulation by these antibodies is an *in vitro* phenomenon, because thrombosis and not bleeding represent their clinical consequences.

The mechanism for the recurrent thrombotic events observed in these patients is not well understood but likely involves autoantibody-mediated alterations in anticoagulant activity (181). Studies have shown that the antiphospholipid antibodies detected in the various assays are mostly directed to β 2-glycoprotein I (usually with bound phospholipid), and newer assays that specifically detect autoantibodies to β 2-glycoprotein I may increase the accuracy of predicting which patients will suffer complications from these antibodies (i.e., thrombosis) (181). Several studies have suggested that these antibodies may promote thrombosis by inhibiting activation of the protein C/protein S system, which is involved in inactivation of clotting factors Va and VIIIa. Alternatively, it has been suggested that antiphospholipid antibodies promote thrombosis by interacting with platelet phospholipid and inducing platelet aggregation. Finally, complement activation by these antibodies may contribute to the propensity to clot.

Prophylaxis in patients who demonstrate antiphospholipid antibodies but no prior clotting episodes may include antiplatelet agents. Treatment and prevention of recurrent thrombosis usually requires full anticoagulation with heparin (and subsequent warfarin), antiplatelet agents, or both, depending on the severity of the episode. Although high-dose corticosteroids can be shown to decrease antiphospholipid antibodies, the effect is frequently lost as the drug is tapered. Therefore, corticosteroid treatment is usually not a reasonable long-term therapeutic approach to prevent or treat thrombotic complications in these patients. In patients with lupus nephritis and glomerular capillary microthrombi due to these antibodies, anticoagulation may be an important addition to standard immunosuppressive therapy.

MANAGEMENT

Overview

The management of lupus nephritis is complicated by extreme variability in clinical presentation, course of disease, and response to therapy. Treatment must be tailored to the individual patient. The goal of therapy is to suppress disease while minimizing the cumulative toxicity of treatment, especially that resulting from high-dose corticosteroids. In addition, appropriate treatment of complicating problems, such as hypertension, hyperlipidemia, osteopenia, as well as pneumococcal prophylaxis, is crucial for a successful outcome in the treatment of SLE and lupus nephritis.

Outcome in SLE has been steadily improving over the last 30 years. In patients with lupus nephritis, 5- and 10-year renal survival rates have been reported as high as ~90% and ~80%, respectively (154). Substantially worse renal outcomes have been reported in centers with a high proportion of black patients (150). Some studies have emphasized the bimodal pattern of mortality in SLE and lupus nephritis, with those dying early in their disease from active lupus, whereas coronary artery disease is the major cause of death after years of disease and treatment (5,182,183). A large fraction of the deaths now occur secondary to large-vessel atherosclerotic disease or infection. Factors playing roles in the coronary disease include corticosteroid therapy, hypertension, hyperlipidemia, coagulation abnormalities, obesity, and possible vasculopathy from inflammation and immune injury (5,184). Aggressive treatment, especially with corticosteroids, has clearly contributed to the increased number of infectious deaths. Physicians also have become aware that infection can mimic manifestations of the disease as well as result in disease flares. The possibility of infection should always be considered in the management of SLE, and infection must be excluded prior to institution of corticosteroids or cytotoxic drugs.

Many aspects of the management of lupus nephritis are controversial, including the clinical value of renal biopsy, the use of certain serologic correlates of renal disease activity, and choice of therapeutic agents.

Use of the Renal Biopsy to Guide Management

Studies have suggested that the WHO histologic classification of lupus nephritis (Table 65-3) generally correlates with the clinical severity of renal disease and prognosis (108–114). However, knowledge of the histologic subtype appears to add little to the treatment plan beyond the information already known from the urinalysis, 24-hour protein excretion values, and studies of renal function (113–117). Furthermore, use of the histologic classification alone cannot reliably predict progression to renal failure and thus identify patients who should be treated more aggressively. In contrast, as discussed, the extent of chronic damage on renal biopsy (Table 65-5) may provide important prognostic information and help in treatment

considerations (7,113,114,117,132–139,144). This incremental information from a biopsy may be most valuable for patients who do not demonstrate a persistent decrease in renal function (7,114). It has been suggested that patients with no evidence of chronic damage may do well with corticosteroid therapy alone. In contrast, those who demonstrate a limited degree of sclerosis and fibrosis may benefit most from cytotoxic drugs in addition to corticosteroids to reduce the risk of renal failure. Additional studies are required to verify these predictions.

We believe that initial treatment can be started without the need of a renal biopsy in many patients with renal disease. Immediate histologic information may be helpful for those patients with factors associated with an adverse prognosis, such as decreased renal function, hypertension, or black race. Histologic information may be most useful in those patients with evidence of continuing renal disease activity despite treatment with high doses of corticosteroids. At such a time of therapeutic decision making, a renal biopsy may be particularly valuable in identifying patients with nephritis of destructive potential (increased chronicity index), who have an increased chance of progression to renal failure and may most benefit from the addition of cytotoxic drugs. The renal biopsy also is useful to determine the extent of irreversible versus active disease, particularly in those patients who have lost renal function slowly (over months to years) or for whom the duration of loss is unknown. Renal biopsy may be useful for patients with SLE who have another possible cause of renal disease and for patients with glomerulonephritis of unknown etiology in whom the diagnosis of SLE is being considered.

Monitoring Serum Levels of Anti-dsDNA Antibodies and Complement

As discussed, most patients with active proliferative glomerulonephritis have elevated serum levels of antibodies to dsDNA and decreased serum complement levels. At the time therapy is initiated, however, the levels of these markers do not have prognostic significance (114,117). These tests may aid in predicting disease flares in some patients in clinical remission (185,186). Clearly, the chance of exacerbation is less in patients who normalize anti-dsDNA and complement levels with therapy, and progression of renal disease is more likely to occur in patients with persistent serologic abnormalities, especially decreased complement levels (144,187,188). The clinical usefulness of this information is, however, limited because: (a) these serologic results are frequently redundant to what is known clinically, and (b) a significant percentage of patients with abnormal tests do not have an exacerbation of lupus nephritis during extended follow-up periods. There is no evidence, at present, to suggest that therapy for lupus nephritis should be directed at normalizing the anti-dsDNA or complement levels. If there is a lack of correlation between serum anti-dsDNA or complement levels and clinical or routine laboratory evidence of nephritis, we recommend that parameters of glomerular filtration and permeability (i.e., serum creatinine, creatinine clearance, urinary sediment, and 24-hour levels of proteinuria) be used as the most important indicators of response. Increasing anti-dsDNA antibody titers or decreasing complement levels in an otherwise stable patient, however, should prompt closer follow-up.

Drug Therapy

Not all patients with lupus nephritis need to be treated aggressively with corticosteroids and/or cytotoxic drugs. Initial therapy should be tailored to the clinical severity of glomerular involvement. For example, patients with low levels of protein-uria (<1 g/24 hours), minimal urinary sediment abnormalities, and normal stable renal function may not need aggressive therapy directed at the kidney involvement. Close monitoring is critical, especially early in the disease course. Not infrequently, treatment in these patients may need to be directed at extrarenal manifestations. At the other end of the spectrum are patients with late-stage lupus nephropathy who have gradually progressed to chronic renal insufficiency (serum creatinine >3 to 4 mg/dL) with renal biopsy showing extensive irreversible chronic damage and little activity. These patients should not be candidates for immunosuppressive therapy, as these drugs have little effect on the progression to end-stage renal failure but do increase the likelihood of infection. Systemic lupus erythematosus patients who have slowly progressed to end-stage renal failure frequently demonstrate a marked decrease in serologic abnormalities, and clinical evidence of extrarenal disease is usually minimal. Dialysis and renal transplantation for these patients are discussed elsewhere in this chapter.

The first line of therapy for previously untreated patients with active lupus nephritis and severe clinical manifestations (i.e., decreasing renal function and/or high-grade proteinuria) is high doses of corticosteroids. An attempt should be made to control disease activity quickly. The initial dosage of the most commonly used drug, prednisone, should be approximately 1 mg/kg per day (~60 to 80 mg/day) in three divided doses. It may take several weeks to achieve control of active nephritis. The rate at which the steroid dose can be decreased is dependent on the response to therapy. An initial taper should include changing a divided dose to a one-dose-per-day (AM) schedule. After the serum creatinine has returned to normal and proteinuria has decreased to low levels, initial reductions can be relatively large (e.g., ~10 mg every 2 weeks) to a dosage of 40 mg per/day. As the daily dose decreases, reductions should be at progressively smaller increments. The goal is to achieve the lowest daily dose that maintains adequate control of renal disease activity. Occasional patients can be tapered to an alternate-day schedule as a maintenance regimen. In those instances in which a 6- to 8-week course of high-dose prednisone has not restored serum creatinine levels to normal or the proteinuria continues at greater than 1 g per/day, a renal biopsy can be performed to determine whether glomerular sclerosis, fibrous crescents, and irreversible tubulointerstitial changes are present. If these poor prognostic indicators are observed, especially with evidence of continued activity, the addition of cytotoxic drugs or other immunosuppressive modalities should be considered.

The toxicity of continuous high-dose corticosteroid therapy is cumulative and severe (189). Perhaps most serious in SLE patients is the associated immune suppression and increased susceptibility to severe infections. Endocrine and metabolic problems are numerous, and include truncal obesity, moon facies, acne, hirsutism, menstrual irregularities, and impotence. Patients may also demonstrate a catabolic state with negative nitrogen balance, hyperglycemia, and hyperlipidemia, which may contribute to the increased mortality from coronary artery disease in long-term treated SLE patients. Steroid-induced osteopenia can result in an increased incidence of bone fractures, and high-risk patients should be evaluated for the need for early prophylaxis. Fluid and electrolyte abnormalities secondary to corticosteroids include sodium and water retention and rarely hypokalemia. These alterations can result in or exacerbate hypertension. Corticosteroid therapy, especially high doses, has been associated with psychological problems ranging from anxiety and insomnia to frank psychosis. Patients are also at risk for the development of a proximal myopathy, avascular necrosis, and ophthalmologic complications such as glaucoma and cataracts. Less common complications

include pancreatitis, peptic ulcer disease, and pseudotumor cerebri.

Although shown to be associated with less toxicity than daily administration, alternate-day steroid therapy is usually not successful in suppressing severe disease activity. Some patients, however, can be tapered to alternate-day therapy as a maintenance regimen. It was originally believed that pulse intravenous corticosteroid therapy (e.g., 1 g of methylprednisolone per day for 3 days) might obviate the need for continuous high-dose daily treatment. This does not appear to be true in the majority of cases. Furthermore, the addition of pulse steroids may add significantly to certain steroid toxicities such as increased susceptibility to infection and avascular bone necrosis. Complications such as sudden death rarely have been associated with these large boluses of drug. Although pulse corticosteroid therapy may improve efficacy when added to maintenance oral prednisone in a small subgroup of patients, its long-term benefit in most patients appears to be minimal. At this time, despite its relatively widespread use, alternate-day steroid therapy cannot be recommended as a routine therapy in patients with lupus nephritis. Controlled trials have demonstrated that monthly pulse methylprednisolone is not as effective as intermittent cyclophosphamide in preserving renal function (190,191).

The use of cytotoxic drugs in the treatment of lupus nephritis should be reserved for the subgroup of patients with severe, refractory disease. These include: (a) patients with evidence of active and severe glomerulonephritis (see preceding discussion) despite treatment with high-dose prednisone, (b) patients who have responded to corticosteroids but who require an unacceptably high dose to maintain a response, and (c) patients with unacceptable side effects from corticosteroids. In addition, as discussed, evidence of chronic damage on the renal biopsy or other indicators of a poor prognosis may suggest the need for early introduction of cytotoxic drug therapy. The most commonly studied cytotoxic drugs have been oral azathioprine, oral cyclophosphamide, and intermittent intravenous cyclophosphamide. These drugs are given in association with a dose of prednisone (usually 0.5 mg/kg/day) required to control extrarenal manifestations. Cytotoxic drugs, especially cyclophosphamide in combination with prednisone, have been shown to prevent progression to renal failure more effectively than prednisone alone (7,190–199). However, because of potentially severe toxicity, proportional improvements in mortality have been more difficult to demonstrate (196). It is recommended that intravenous cyclophosphamide be given under the supervision of a physician experienced in its use.

Azathioprine is rapidly converted to 6-mercaptopurine after absorption. It should be initiated at 1.0 to 1.25 mg/kg/day. Maximal clinical benefit may not be observed for weeks to months. If the clinical response is unsatisfactory, the dosage can be slowly increased to a maximal level of 3.0 mg/kg/day. The most serious toxicity during therapy is bone marrow suppression, primarily leukopenia; therefore, complete blood counts must be followed regularly during treatment. Gastrointestinal intolerance is common, but giving the dose at bedtime can decrease this. Some patients develop elevated liver enzymes early in therapy, which usually resolves during continued treatment. The major long-term risk of azathioprine use is the potential for developing a malignancy, especially lymphoma. This risk appears to be extremely low, and lower than that with cyclophosphamide. The risk also appears to be less in patients with SLE than in patients who have undergone renal transplantation. Azathioprine appears to be less toxic than cyclophosphamide. It has not been associated with hemorrhagic cystitis and has a much lower incidence of premature ovarian failure compared with cyclophosphamide. At this time, azathioprine might be recommended for a patient who wishes to preserve ovarian function; however, available data also suggest that cyclophosphamide is more potent in suppressing lupus renal disease activity compared with azathioprine (195). Cyclophosphamide, therefore, should be preferentially considered for patients with continued deterioration of renal function and those at high risk for progression to renal failure.

Recent studies have indicated that when given correctly, intermittent intravenous cyclophosphamide has a lower incidence of hemorrhagic cystitis compared with daily oral cyclophosphamide (195,196). Furthermore, recent experience indicates that improvement may be more rapid after intravenous boluses compared with daily oral administration. There is little evidence for additional toxicities with intravenous cyclophosphamide not encountered during oral administration. Therefore, the intravenous regimen is recommended in patients for whom cyclophosphamide is being considered. In current protocols, the initial dosage of cyclophosphamide is 0.5 to 0.75 g/m^2 of body surface area given intravenously over approximately 60 minutes. The lower dose should be employed in patients whose creatinine clearance is less than 33 mL/minute. The dose can be gradually increased to 1.0 g/m^2, but the leukocyte nadir should be no lower than 2,000 cells/mm^3 (>1,500 neutrophils/mm^3). Following the initial pulse, five additional doses are given at monthly intervals, and additional infusions usually are given at 3-month intervals (190,191). Each cyclophosphamide infusion must be accompanied by vigorous hydration (3 L/m^2 with half normal saline in 5% dextrose) over the subsequent 24-hour period to prevent hemorrhagic cystitis. The cyclophosphamide metabolite acrolein appears to be the major irritant responsible for damage to the bladder wall. Studies have suggested that the concomitant use of mesna (2-mercaptoethane sulfonate) likely reduces the risk of bladder complications of cyclophosphamide therapy, and in many centers, this drug is given during the cyclophosphamide infusion and early postinfusion period. Prophylaxis for nausea and vomiting frequently include dexamethasone and serotonin receptor antagonists, such as granisetron or ondansetron.

The most serious toxicity related to cyclophosphamide therapy is leukopenia, which can further predispose patients to serious infections. Even in the absence of leukopenia, an increased incidence of bacterial infections and especially herpes zoster has been reported (191,195,196). Ovarian or testicular damage is also a relatively common problem with long-term therapy; this problem correlates with age and cumulative dose (200). A long-term risk of cyclophosphamide may relate to the induction of malignancy, including acute leukemia and non-Hodgkin lymphoma, but the risk in SLE patients appears to be low.

It is currently unclear how long to continue any regimen of cytotoxic drugs in the treatment of lupus nephritis. Short courses of cyclophosphamide (<6 months) have been associated with frequent relapses and the need for repeat induction therapy (190,191). Some protocols have recommended continuing treatment for 1 year of remission and no longer than 4 years of total treatment duration (190). The cytotoxic drugs then should be slowly tapered. Replacement of maintenance therapy with less toxic regimens such as azathioprine or mycophenolate mofetil has been considered because of the potential toxicity of prolonged cyclophosphamide therapy. It remains unclear whether these approaches to reduce toxicity will be successful at maintaining remission and preventing long-term progression.

Limitations of the intravenous high-dose cyclophosphamide regimens include (192): (a) no effect on survival rates; (b) no differences in outcome compared to oral cytotoxics; (c) risk of severe infections; (d) no high relapse rate. Thus the Euro-Lupus Nephritis Trial has studied low-dose cyclophosphamide followed by azathioprine. Specifically, intravenous pulses of 500 mg cyclophosphamide weekly or fortnightly for a few months followed by oral azathioprine maintenance therapy was compared to high-dose intravenous cyclophosphamide. In the Euro-Lupus Nephritis Trial, after a median follow-up of 73 months, there was no significant greater cumulative probability of end-stage renal disease (ESRD) or doubling of serum creatinine in the low-dose versus high-dose regimens (193).

High-dose corticosteroids are the mainstay of drug therapy in a pregnant patient who demonstrates severe exacerbations of lupus nephritis. Azathioprine also appears to be an acceptable adjunct, if necessary, based on the experience in female patients receiving renal transplants. Cyclophosphamide and other cytotoxic drugs should not be used in pregnant patients.

Newer Therapies

A variety of experimental therapies have been utilized in SLE, especially in patients with severe lupus nephritis. Studies have shown that plasmapheresis does not have long-term benefit in the treatment of lupus nephritis (201), and it cannot be recommended as a routine adjunct to drug treatment. Therapies utilized in the setting of transplantation, such as cyclosporin A, tacrolimus (FK506), and total lymphoid irradiation, have been reported in the treatment of lupus nephritis as alternatives to cyclophosphamide therapy with at least anecdotal efficacy (202–209); however, none has been shown to be an acceptable alternative to the therapies described. Animal studies and anecdotal case series initially suggested that mycophenolate mofetil might be efficacious in lupus nephritis (205,210). A follow-up controlled study in patients with relatively mild DPGN showed that initial remission rates with this drug and prednisolone were comparable to responses with oral cyclophosphamide and prednisolone (followed by azathioprine and prednisolone) (206). The 1-year follow-up reported, which is early in the course of treated lupus nephritis, and study design does not allow conclusions regarding whether mycophenolate mofetil will be able to prevent progression to renal failure similar to cyclophosphamide, especially in patients with more severe disease.

Mycophenolate mofetil has recently been studied as maintenance therapy. Fifty-nine patients with lupus nephritis (12 in World Health Organization class III, 46 in class IV, and 1 in class Vb) received induction therapy consisting of four-to-seven monthly boluses of high-dose intravenous cyclophosphamide (0.5 to 1.0 g/m^2 body surface area) plus corticosteroids. The patients were then randomly assigned to one of three maintenance therapies: quarterly intravenous injections of cyclophosphamide, oral azathioprine (1 to 3 mg/kg body weight/day) or oral mycophenolate mofetil (500 to 3,000 mg/day) for 1 to 3 years. Five patients died (four in the cyclophosphamide group and one in the mycophenolate mofetil group) and chronic renal failure developed in five (three in the cyclophosphamide group and one each in the azathioprine and mycophenolate mofetil groups). The 72-month event-free survival rate for the composite end point of death or chronic renal failure was higher in the mycophenolate mofetil and azathioprine groups than in the cyclophosphamide group ($p = 0.05$ and $p = 0.009$, respectively). The rate of relapse-free survival was higher in the mycophenolate mofetil group than in the cyclophosphamide group ($p = 0.02$). The incidence of hospitalization, amenorrhea, infections, nausea, and vomiting was significantly lower in the mycophenolate mofetil and azathioprine groups than in the cyclophosphamide group. No statistically significant differences were found between the mycophenolate mofetil and azathioprine groups (207). A study comparing mycophenolate mofetil and azathioprine for maintenance therapy is underway (192).

Mycophenolate mofetil has recently been studied as induction and maintenance therapy (208). Sixty-four Chinese patients with biopsy proven diffuse proliferative lupus nephritis were studied with a median follow-up of 63 months. Thirty-three patients were randomized to receive mycophenolate mofetil and 31 were randomized to receive high-dose oral Cytoxan (2.5 mg/kg/day) followed by azathioprine. Both regimens were equally effective in induction-maintenance therapy. The mycophenolate mofetil group had fewer infections.

A 24-week randomized, open-label, noninferiority trial comparing oral mycophenolate mofetil (initial dose, 1000 mg/day, increased to 3000 mg/day) with monthly intravenous cyclophosphamide (0.5 g per square meter of body-surface area, increased to 1.0 g per square meter) as induction therapy for active lupus nephritis, has recently been completed (211). The primary end point was complete remission at 24 weeks (normalization of abnormal renal measurements and maintenance of baseline normal measurements). A secondary end point was partial remission at 24 weeks. Of 140 patients recruited, 71 were randomly assigned to receive mycophenolate mofetil and 69 were randomly assigned to receive cyclophosphamide. In this 24-week trial, mycophenolate mofetil was more effective than intravenous cyclophosphamide in inducing remission of lupus nephritis and had a more favorable safety profile.

Recent work has suggested that very-high-dose (immunoablative) cyclophosphamide, with or without bone marrow transplantation, may provide long-term benefit for patients with very severe disease, and trials are in progress to test this idea (212). Trayner et al. reported 15 patients with persistently active SLE after intravenous cyclophosphamide (CYC) therapy who underwent immunoablation and autologous hematopoietic stem cell transplantation (HSCT) (213). Seven of the patients were critically ill. There were no deaths. After a median follow-up of 36 months, all patients had a gradual, but marked, improvement. The SLE Disease Activity Index decreased to less than 6 in 12 patients. Serology normalized and marked improvements in end-organ function occurred in all subjects. Ten patients were able to discontinue immunosuppressive medications after 1 year.

Immunoablative doses of cyclophosphamide without HSCT have been studied in lupus nephritis (214). Fourteen patients with refractory SLE were treated. There were no deaths or fungal infections. In nine patients with lupus nephritis there was marked improvement in proteinuria.

There is also great excitement about several new biologic inhibitors being developed for therapy of patients with SLE. For example, inhibitors of the CD40-CD40 ligand interaction with monoclonal antibodies to CD40 ligand (73) and the CD28-B7 interaction with CTLA4-Ig (74), especially in combination (75), have demonstrated potent suppression of lupus nephritis in murine models (see previous discussion of pathogenesis). In a clinical study, a short course of BG9588 (anti-CD40 ligand antibody) improved serology in patients with proliferative lupus nephritis. However, the study was discontinued prematurely because of thromboembolic events (215). Based on studies in murine lupus, clinical trials are also being started with biologic agents that inhibit the production or signaling of interferon-γ (71) and the activation of complement C5 (21).

PROGNOSIS

Clinical Remission and Renal Flares

Clinical remission is defined by some investigators as an inactive urine sediment, a creatinine level of less than or equal to $\leq$ 1.4 mg/dL, and protein excretion of less than 330 mg per/day.

Patients who achieved a remission had a greater than 90% renal survival at 5 and 10 years compared to 46% and 31% of patients who did not achieve remission (216). In addition, overall patient survival was much improved at 10 years in those in renal remission (95% versus 60%).

Relapse of lupus nephritis after initial immunosuppression occurs in 27% to 66% of patients (217–219). In patients receiving maintenance immunosuppression the rate of relapse is decreased to 20% to 25%. Renal flares have been classified as nephritic or proteinuric (nephrotic). Nephritic flares are subgrouped into mild, moderate, or severe. A mild/moderate nephritic flare is characterized by active urinary sediment (>10 RBCs/HPF or cellular casts), an increase in proteinuria (<2 g/day for mild, >2 g/day for moderate, and stable serum creatinine level). Severe nephritic flares are accompanied by active urine sediment, increased proteinuria, and a creatinine level of greater than 30% over baseline. Most nephritic flares are associated with low C3 and elevated anti-dsDNA antibodies. Nephrotic (or proteinuric) flares are characterized by only an increase in proteinuria (>2g/day) (220).

Risk factors for patients likely to have flares of lupus nephritis have been identified (217–219). Demographically, young age, male sex, and nonwhite race are significant risk factors for relapse. Disease activity factors include severe SLE, a high activity score, rising anti-dsDNA antibodies, and arterial hypertension. A delay (>5 months) in initiating treatment and difficulty or failure to achieve a complete remission of lupus nephritis are also significant risk factors for future renal relapses.

Patients who develop a flare of their lupus nephritis need to be treated aggressively to preserve renal function (221). Patients who relapse frequently take up to three times longer to remit compared to their initial episode of nephritis. Up to 35% fail to remit or progress to end-stage renal disease in spite of reinstitution of immunosuppressive therapy. Nephritic flares with a rapid increase in creatinine (doubling or >2 mg/dL) associated with a high activity score and/or chronicity index at baseline biopsy are especially likely to progress to ESRD (218).

Rituximab is an anti-CD20 monoclonal antibody that depletes B cells. It is used to treat Hodgkin lymphoma. In a prospective observational study of 8 patients with idiopathic membranous nephropathy, rituximab treatment resulted in a significant decrease in proteinuria. (222). In an open-label trial, 10 patients with active proliferative lupus nephritis were treated with rituximab (223). Rituximab was well tolerated and resulted in B-cell depletion for 1 to 7 months. Five patients had a complete remission (normal serum creatinine level, inactive urine sediment, 24-hour urine protein <500 mg). Three patients had a partial remission (50% improvement in renal parameters). Therefore, there is preliminary evidence supporting the safety and efficacy of rituximab as monotherapy in proliferative lupus nephritis. Randomized controlled studies are needed comparing rituximab with cyclophosphamide and mycophenolate mofetil for induction and maintenance therapy.

LJP 394 selectively eliminates pathogenic autoantibody-producing B cells, sparing the non-autoimmune B-cell compartment. LJP 394 selectively decreases anti-dsDNA antibodies. In a randomized, double-blind placebo-controlled study, 230 patients were studied (224). In the intent-to-treat population, the time to institution of high-dose steroid and/or cyclophosphamide therapy was significantly prolonged and the number of treatments was significantly lower than placebo. In 189 patients with high-affinity antibodies to LJP 394, the time to renal flare was significantly longer compared to placebo, and the number of renal flares and treatments with high-dose steroid and/or cyclophosphamide therapy was significantly lower compared to placebo. A multinational, prospective, randomized study is ongoing in SLE patients with a history of renal disease and high-affinity antibodies at baseline.

End-Stage Renal Disease and Transplantation in Lupus Nephritis

Approximately 20% to 30% of patients with severe lupus nephritis progress to ESRD over a 10-year follow-up period (7,113,114,117,132–144,146,150,154,155,190,194–196,198,225). Lupus nephritis accounts for up to 3% of cases of end-stage renal failure requiring dialysis or transplantation. In a subset of patients, active lupus early in the dialysis period may require treatment with corticosteroids and/or other immunosuppressive medications. The use of these medications is associated with increased morbidity, especially infectious complications. For unclear reasons, SLE patients with progressive renal failure and those on dialysis frequently demonstrate a decrease in nonrenal clinical manifestations of active SLE as well as a decrease in serologic markers of active disease (226–231), although some patients fail to improve (232). In SLE patients with absent or minimal disease activity, clinical course and survival on dialysis (hemodialysis or continuous ambulatory peritoneal dialysis [CAPD]) compare favorably to other patient groups (230). However, SLE patients with antiphospholipid antibodies have an increased incidence of recurrent thrombosis in arteriovenous grafts, which may be lessened with warfarin therapy, and patients receiving CAPD have increased infectious complications if on immunosuppressive medications (233,234).

Although controversial, it has been recommended that patients with SLE should wait 6 to 12 months while on dialysis prior to transplantation. With time, SLE patients appear to be excellent candidates for transplantation. Recurrence of active lupus nephritis in the transplant occurs in 10% to 30% of patients (226–236). It is important to note that recurrence contributed to graft loss in less than half of these patients. However, in contrast to earlier studies (226–232), more recent follow-up studies have suggested that renal allograft survival in SLE patients is lower compared to most other patient groups (237,238). This is particularly true in patients with antiphospholipid antibodies who may lose their allograft due to renal thrombosis if not adequately anticoagulated (239–241).

ACKNOWLEDGMENT

The authors acknowledge Brian Kotzin, MD, for his contribution to the previous editions of this chapter.

References

1. Tan EM, et al. The 1982 revised criteria for the classification of systemic lupus erythematosus. *Arthritis Rheum* 1982;25:1271.
2. Kotzin BL, West SG. Systemic lupus erythematosus. In: Rich RR, Fleisher TA, Shearer WT, et al., eds. *Clinical Immunology: Principles and Practice,* 2nd ed. London: Mosby; 2001:60.
3. Gladman DD, Urowitz MB. Systemic lupus erythematosus. Hochberg MC, Silman AJ, Smolen JS, Weinblatt ME, Weisman MH, eds. *Rheumatology,* 3rd ed. London: Mosby; 2003:1359.
4. Wallace DJ, Hahn BH, eds. *Dubois' Lupus Erythematosus,* 6th ed. Philadelphia: Lippincott Williams & Wilkins; 2002.
5. Rus V, Hochberg MC. The epidemiology of systemic lupus erythematosus. In: Wallace DJ, Hahn BH, eds. *Dubois' Lupus Erythematosus,* 6th ed. Philadelphia: Lippincott Williams & Wilkins; 2002:65.
6. Hahn BH. Animal models of systemic Lupus Erythematosus. In: Wallace DJ, Hahn BH, eds. *Dubois' Lupus Erythematosus,* 6th ed. Philadelphia: Lippincott Williams & Wilkins; 2002:339.
7. Austin HA III, et al. Prognostic factors in lupus nephritis: contribution of renal histologic data. *Am J Med* 1983;75:382.
8. Kotzin BL. Systemic lupus erythematosus. *Cell* 1996;85:303.
9. Theofilopoulos AN, Dixon FJ. Murine models of systemic lupus erythematosus. *Adv Immunol* 1985;37:269.
10. Cohen PL, Eisenberg RA. Lpr and gld: single gene models of systemic autoimmunity and lymphoproliferative disease. *Annu Rev Immunol* 1991;9:243.
11. Izui S, et al. The Yaa model of systemic lupus erythematosus. *Immunol Rev* 1995;144:137.
12. Vyse TJ, Todd JA, Kotzin BL. Non-MHC genetic contributions to autoimmune disease. In: Rose NR, Mackay IR, eds. *The Autoimmune Diseases,* 3rd ed. San Diego: Academic Press; 1998:85.
13. Vyse TJ, Todd JA. Genetic analysis of autoimmune disease. *Cell* 1996;85:311.
14. Vyse TJ, Kotzin BL. Genetic susceptibility to systemic lupus erythematosus. *Annu Rev Immunol* 1998;16:261.
15. Deapen D, et al. A revised estimate of twin concordance in systemic lupus erythematosus. *Arthritis Rheum* 1992;35:311.
16. Tsao BP. Update on human systemic lupus erythematosus genetics. *Curr Opin Rheumatol* 2004;16:513.
17. Tsao BP. The genetics of human lupus. In: Wallace DJ, Hahn BH, eds. *Dubois' Lupus Erythematosus,* 6th ed. Philadelphia: Lippincott Williams & Wilkins; 2002:97.
18. Jacob CO, et al. Heritable major histocompatibility complex class II–associated differences in production of tumor necrosis factor α: relevance to genetic predisposition to systemic lupus erythematosus. *Proc Natl Acad Sci USA* 1990;87:1233.
19. Pickering MC, Walport MJ. Links between complement abnormalities and systemic lupus erythematosus. *Rheumatology* 2000;39:133.
20. Botto M, et al. Homozygous C1q deficiency causes glomerulonephritis associated with multiple apoptotic bodies. *Nat Genet* 1998;19:56.
21. Wang Y, et al. Amelioration of lupuslike autoimmune disease in NZB/W F1 mice after treatment with a blocking monoclonal antibody specific for complement C5. *Proc Natl Acad Sci U S A* 1996;93:8563.
22. Trouw LA, et al. Anti-C1q autoantibodies deposit in glomeruli but are only pathogenic in combination with glomerular C1q-containing immune complexes. *J Clin Invest.* 2004;114(5):679.
23. Karassa FB, et al. Role of the Fc gamma receptor IIa polymorphism in susceptibility to systemic lupus erythematosus and lupus nephritis. A meta-analysis. *Arthritis Rheum* 2002;46:1563.
24. Karassa FB, et al. The FcgammaRIIIA-F158 allele is a risk factor for the development of lupus nephritis: A meta-analysis. *Kidney Int* 2003;63:1475.
25. Clynes R, Dumitru C, Ravetch JV. Uncoupling of immune complex formation and kidney damage in autoimmune glomerulonephritis. *Science* 1998;279:1052.
26. Bolland S, Ravetch JV. Spontaneous autoimmune disease in FcγRIIB-deficient mice results from strain-specific epistasis. *Immunity* 2000;13:277.
27. Holers VM. Complement deficiency states, disease susceptibility, and infection risk in systemic lupus erythematosus. *Arthritis Rheum* 1999;42:2023.
28. Rood MJ, et al. TNF-308A and HLA-DR3 alleles contribute independently to susceptibility to systemic lupus erythematosus. *Arthritis Rheum* 2000;43:129.
29. D'Alfonso S, et al. Systemic lupus erythematosus candidate genes in the Italian population. *Arthritis Rheum* 2000;43:120.
30. Bidwell J, et al. Cytokine gene polymorphism in human disease: on-line databases. *Genes Immunol* 1999;1:3.
31. Theofilopoulos AN, Kono DH. The genes of systemic autoimmunity. *Proc Assoc Am Phys* 1999;111:228.
32. Wakeland EK, et al. Genetic dissection of systemic lupus erythematosus. *Curr Opin Immunol* 1999;10:718.
33. Harley JB, et al. The genetics of human systemic lupus erythematosus. *Curr Opin Immunol* 1998;10:690.
34. Tsao BP, et al. Evidence for linkage of a candidate chromosomal region to human systemic lupus erythematosus. *J Clin Invest* 1997;99:725.
35. Tsao BP, et al. PARP alleles within the linked chromosomal region are associated with systemic lupus erythematosus. *J Clin Invest* 1999;103:1135.
36. Criswell LA, et al. PARP alleles and SLE: failure to confirm association with disease susceptibility. *J Clin Invest* 2000;105:1501.
37. Sobel ES, Cohen PL, Eisenberg RA. Lpr T cells are necessary for autoantibody production in lpr mice. *J Immunol* 1993;150:4160.
38. Sobel ES, et al. An intrinsic B cell defect is required for the production of autoantibodies in the lpr model of murine systemic autoimmunity. *J Exp Med* 1991;173:1441.
39. Herron LR, et al. Selection of the T cell receptor repertoire in lpr mice. *J Immunol* 1994;151:3450.
40. Singer GG, Abbas AK. The *Fas* antigen is involved in peripheral but not thymic deletion of T lymphocytes in T cell receptor transgenic mice. *Immunity* 1994;1:365.
41. Goodnow CC, et al. Self-tolerance checkpoints in B lymphocyte development. *Adv Immunol* 1995;59:279.
42. Rubio CF, et al. Analysis of central B cell tolerance in autoimmune-prone MRL/lpr mice bearing autoantibody transgenes. *J Immunol* 1996;157:65.
43. Rathmell JC, Goodnow CC. The in vivo balance between B cell clonal expansions and elimination is regulated by CD95 both on B cells and their micro-environment. *Immunol Cell Biol* 1998;76:387.
44. Straus SE, et al. An inherited disorder of lymphocyte apoptosis: the autoimmune lymphoproliferative syndrome. *Ann Intern Med* 1999;130:591.

45. James JA, et al. An increased prevalence of Epstein-Barr virus infection in young patients suggests a possible etiology for systemic lupus erythematosus. *J Clin Invest* 1997;100:3019.
46. Sanchez-Guerrero J, et al. Postmenopausal estrogen therapy and the risk for developing systemic lupus erythematosus. *Ann Intern Med* 1995;122:430.
47. Sanchez-Guerrero J, et al. Past use of oral contraceptives and the risk of developing systemic lupus erythematosus. *Arthritis Rheum* 1997;40:804.
48. Petri M, Robinson C. Oral contraceptives and systemic lupus erythematosus. *Arthritis Rheum* 1997;40:797.
49. Vollenhoven RF, Engleman EG, McGuire JL. Dehydroepiandrosterone in systemic lupus erythematosus. *Arthritis Rheum* 1995;38:1826.
50. Rubin RR. Drug-induced lupus. In: Wallace DJ, Hahn BH, eds. *Dubois' Lupus Erythematosus*, 6th ed. Philadelphia: Lippincott Williams & Wilkins; 2002:885.
51. Wofsy D, Seaman WE. Successful treatment of autoimmunity in NZB/NZW F1 mice with monoclonal antibody to L3T4. *J Exp Med* 1985;161:378.
52. Wofsy D. Administration of monoclonal anti-T cell antibodies retards murine lupus in BXSB mice. *J Immunol* 1986;136:4554.
53. Santoro TJ, Portanova JP, Kotzin BL. The contribution of L3T4+ T cells to lymphoproliferation and autoantibody production in MRL- *lpr/lpr* mice. *J Exp Med* 1988;167:1713.
54. Kaliyaperumal A, et al. Nucleosomal peptide epitopes for nephritis-inducing T helper cells of murine lupus. *J Exp Med* 1996;183:2459.
55. Lu L, et al. Major peptide autoepitopes for nucleosome-specific T cells of human lupus. *J Clin Invest* 1999;104:345.
56. Kotzin BL, et al. T cell tolerance to self antigens in New Zealand hybrid mice with lupuslike disease. *J Immunol* 1989;143:89.
57. Fatenejad S, et al. Central T cell tolerance in lupus-prone mice: Influence of autoimmune background and the lpr mutation. *J Immunol* 1998;161:6427.
58. Sercarz EE, et al. Dominance and crypticity of T cell antigenic determinants. *Annu Rev Immunol* 1993;11:729.
59. Mamula MJ. Epitope spreading: the role of self peptides and autoantigen processing by B lymphocytes. *Immunol Rev* 1998;164:231.
60. James JA, Harley JB. B-cell epitope spreading in autoimmunity. *Immunol Rev* 1998;164:185.
61. Craft J, Fatenejed S. Self antigens and epitope spreading in systemic autoimmunity. *Arthritis Rheum* 1997;40:1374.
62. Topfer F, Gordon T, McCluskey J. Intra- and intermolecular spreading of autoimmunity involving the nuclear self-antigens La (SS-B) and Ro (SS-A). *Proc Natl Acad Sci U S A* 1995;92:875.
63. Horwitz DA, Stohl W, Gray JD. T lymphocytes, natural killer cells, and immune regulation. In: Wallace DJ, Hahn BH, eds. *Dubois' Lupus Erythematosus*, 6th ed. Philadelphia: Lippincott Williams & Wilkins; 2002:157.
64. Dayal AK, Kammer GM. The T cell enigma in lupus. *Arthritis Rheum* 1996;39:23.
65. Tsokos GC, Liossis SN. Immune cell signaling defects in lupus: activation, anergy, and death. *Immunol Today* 1999;20:119.
66. Desai-Mehta A, et al. Hyperexpression of CD40 ligand by B and T cells in human lupus and its role in pathogenic autoantibody production. *J Clin Invest* 1996;97:2063.
67. Koshy M, Berger D, Crow MK. Increased expression of CD40 ligand on systemic lupus erythematosus lymphocytes. *J Clin Invest* 1996;98:826.
68. Kato K, et al. The soluble CD40 ligand sCD154 in systemic lupus erythematosus. *J Clin Invest* 1999;104:947.
69. O'Garra A, Steinman L, Gijbels K. CD4+ T-cell subsets in autoimmunity. *Curr Opin Immunol* 1997;9:872.
70. Theofilopoulos AN, Lawson BR. Tumor necrosis factor and other cytokines in murine lupus. *Ann Rheum Dis* 1999;58:149.
71. Lawson BR, et al. Treatment of murine lupus with cDNA encoding IFN-γR/Fc. *J Clin Invest* 2000;106:207.
72. Kelley VR, Wuthrich RP. Cytokines in the pathogenesis of systemic lupus erythematosus. *Semin Nephrol* 1999;19:57.
73. Datta SK, Kalled SL. CD40-CD40 ligand interaction in autoimmune disease. *Arthritis Rheum* 1997;40:1735.
74. Finck BK, Linsley PS, Wofsy D. Treatment of murine lupus with CTLA4Ig. *Science* 1994;265:1225.
75. Daikh DI, et al. Long-term inhibition of murine lupus by brief simultaneous blockade of the B7/CD28 and CD40/gp39 costimulation pathways. *J Immunol* 1997;159:3104.
76. Liossis SN, Tsokos GC. B-cell abnormalities in systemic lupus erythematosus. In: Wallace DJ, Hahn BH, eds. *Dubois' Lupus Erythematosus*, 6th ed. Philadelphia: Lippincott Williams & Wilkins; 2002:205.
77. Diamond B, et al. The role of somatic mutation in the pathogenic anti-DNA response. *Ann Rev Immunol* 1992;10:731.
78. Shlomchik M, et al. Anti-DNA antibodies from autoimmune mice arise by clonal expansion and somatic mutation. *J Exp Med* 1990;171:265.
79. Radic MZ, Weigert M. Genetic and structural evidence for antigen selection of anti-DNA antibodies. *Annu Rev Immunol* 1994;12:5487.
80. Portanova J, Kotzin BL. Lupuslike autoimmunity in murine graft-versus-host disease. *Concepts Immunopathol* 1988;6:119.
81. Shustov A, et al. Role of perforin in controlling B-cell hyperactivity and humoral autoimmunity. *J Clin Invest* 2000;106:R39.
82. Chan OT, Madaio MP, Shlomchik MJ. The central and multiple roles of B cells in lupus pathogenesis. *Immunol Rev* 1999;169:107.
83. Tan EM. Antinuclear antibodies: diagnostic markers for autoimmune diseases and probes for cell biology. *Adv Immunol* 1989;44:93.
84. Pisetsky DS, ed. Antinuclear antibodies. *Rheum Dis Clin North Am* 1992;18:1.
85. Giles I, Isenberg D. Antinuclear antibodies: An overview. In: Wallace DJ, Hahn BH, eds. *Dubois' Lupus Erythematosus*, 6th ed. Philadelphia: Lippincott Williams & Wilkins; 2002:415.
86. Elkon KB, Bonfa E, Brot N. Antiribosomal antibodies in systemic Lupus Erythematosus. *Rheum Dis Clin North Am* 1992;18:377.
87. Emlen W, Pisetsky DS, Taylor RP. Antibodies to DNA. A perspective. *Arthritis Rheum* 1986;29:1417.
88. Hahn BH, Tsao BP. Antibodies to DNA. Wallace DJ, Hahn BH, eds. *Dubois' Lupus Erythematosus*, 6th ed. Philadelphia: Lippincott Williams & Wilkins; 2002:425.
89. Pisetsky DS. Anti-DNA and autoantibodies. *Curr Opin Rheumatol* 2000;12:364.
90. Izui S, Lambert PH, Miescher PA. Failure to detect circulating DNA-anti-DNA complexes by four radioimmunological methods in patients with lupus erythematosus. *Clin Exp Immunol* 1977;30:384.
91. Salmon JE. Abnormalities in immune complex clearance and Fcgamma receptor function. In: Wallace DJ, Hahn BH, eds. *Dubois' Lupus Erythematosus*, 6th ed. Philadelphia: Lippincott Williams & Wilkins; 2002:219.
92. Izui S, Lambert PH, Miescher PA. *In vitro* demonstration of a particular affinity of glomerular basement membrane and collagen for DNA. A possible basis for a local formation of DNA-anti-DNA complexes in systemic lupus erythematosus. *J Exp Med* 1976;144:428.
93. Termaat RM, et al. Anti-DNA antibodies can bind to the glomerulus via two distinct mechanisms. *Kidney Int* 1992;42:1363.
94. Bernstein KA, Valerio RD, Lefkowith JB. Glomerular binding activity in MRL lpr serum consists of antibodies that bind to a DNA/histone/type IV collagen complex. *J Immunol* 1995;154:2424.
95. Schmiedeke TM, et al. Histones have high affinity for the glomerular basement membrane. Relevance for immune complex formation in lupus nephritis. *J Exp Med* 1989;169:1879.
96. Termaat RM, et al. Cross-reactivity of monoclonal anti-DNA antibodies with heparan sulfate is mediated via bound DNA/histone complexes. *J Autoimmun* 1990;3:531.
97. Kramers C, et al. Anti-nucleosome antibodies complexed to nucleosomal antigens show anti-DNA reactivity and bind to rat glomerular basement membrane in vivo. *J Clin Invest* 1994;94:568.
98. Rumore PM, Steinman CR. Endogenous circulating DNA in systemic lupus erythematosus. Occurrence as multimeric complexes bound to histone. *J Clin Invest* 1990;86:69.
99. Fournie, GJ. Circulating DNA and lupus nephritis. *Kidney Int* 1988;33:487.
100. Tsao BP, et al. Structural characteristics of the variable regions of immunoglobulin genes encoding a pathogenic autoantibody in murine lupus. *J Clin Invest* 1990;85:530.
101. Portanova JP, et al. Allogeneic MHC antigen requirements for lupuslike autoantibody production and nephritis in murine graft-vs-host disease. *J Immunol* 1988;141:3370.
102. Eilat D. Cross-reactions of anti-DNA antibodies and the central dogma of lupus nephritis. *Immunol Today* 1985;6:123.
103. Pankewycz OG, Migliorini P, Madaio MP. Polyreactive autoantibodies are nephritogenic in murine lupus nephritis. *J Immunol* 1987;139:3287.
104. Madaio MP, et al. Murine monoclonal anti-DNA antibodies bind directly to glomerular antigens and form immune deposits. *J Immunol* 1987;38:2883.
105. Vyse TJ, et al. Control of separate pathogenic autoantibody responses marks MHC gene contributions to murine lupus. *Proc Natl Acad Sci U S A* 1999;96:8098.
106. Corwin HL, Schwartz MM, Lewis E. The importance of sample size in the interpretation of the renal biopsy. *Am J Nephrology* 1988;8:85.
107. Rich SA. De novo synthesis and secretion of a 36kD protein by cells that form lupus inclusions in response to alpha-interferon. *J Clin Invest* 1995;95:219.
108. Pirani CL, Pollak VE. Systemic lupus erythematosus (SLE) glomerulonephritis (lupus nephritis). In: McCluskey RT, Ardes GA, eds. *Immunologically Mediated Renal Diseases*. New York: Marcel Dekker; 1975:117.
109. Churg J, Bernstein J, Glassock RJ. *Renal Disease: Classification and Atlas of Glomerular Diseases*, 2nd ed. New York: Igaku-Shoin; 1995.
110. Baldwin DS, et al. Lupus nephritis. Clinical course as related to morphologic forms and their transition. *Am J Med* 1977;62:12.
111. Appel GB, et al. Renal involvement in systemic lupus erythematosus (SLE): a study of 56 patients emphasizing histologic classification. *Medicine (Baltimore)* 1978;57:371.
112. Appel GB, et al. Long-term follow-up of patients with lupus nephritis. A study based on the classification of the World Health Organization. *Am J Med* 1987;83:877.
113. McLaughlin J, et al. Kidney biopsy in systemic lupus erythematosus. II. Survival analysis according to biopsy results. *Arthritis Rheum* 1991;34:1268.
114. McLaughlin JR, et al. Kidney biopsy in systemic lupus erythematosus. III. Survival analysis controlling for clinical and laboratory variables. *Arthritis Rheum* 1994;37:559.
115. Najafi CC, et al. Significance of histologic patterns of glomerular injury upon long-term prognosis in severe lupus glomerulonephritis. *Kidney Int* 2001;59:2156.

116. Fries JF, Porta J, Liang MH. Marginal benefit of renal biopsy in systemic lupus erythematosus. *Arch Intern Med* 1978;138:1386.
117. Whiting-O'Keefe Q, et al. The information content from renal biopsy in systemic lupus erythematosus. *Ann Intern Med* 1982;96:718.
118. Ginzler EM, et al. Progression of mesangial and focal to diffuse nephritis. *N Engl J Med* 1974;291:696.
119. Morel-Maroger L, et al. The course of lupus nephritis: contribution of serial renal biopsies. *Adv Nephrol* 1976;6:79.
120. Lee HS, et al. Course of renal pathology in patients with systemic lupus erythematosus. *Am J Med* 1984;77:612.
121. Esdaile JM, et al. The pathogenesis and prognosis of lupus nephritis: information from repeat renal biopsy. *Semin Arthritis Rheum* 1993;23:135.
122. Mahajan SK, et al. Lupus nephropathy without clinical renal involvement. *Medicine* 1977;56:493.
123. Glassock RJ. Treatment of immunologically mediated glomerular disease. *Kidney Int* 1992;38:S121.
124. Austin HA, et al. NIH conference. Membranous nephropathy. *Ann Intern Med* 1992;116:672.
125. Schwartz MM, et al. Clinical and pathological features of membranous glomerulonephritis of systemic lupus erythematosus. *Am J Nephrol* 1984;4:301.
126. Hecht B, et al. Prognostic indices in lupus nephritis. *Medicine (Baltimore)* 1976;55:163.
127. Weening JJ, et al. The classification of glomerulonephritis in systemic lupus erythematosus revisited. *J Am Soc Nephrol* 2004;15:241.
128. Park MH, et al. Tubulointerstitial disease in lupus nephritis: relationship to immune deposits, interstitial inflammation, glomerular changes, renal function, and prognosis. *Nephron* 1986;44:309.
129. Brentjens JR, et al. Interstitial immune complex nephritis in patients with systemic lupus erythematosus. *Kidney Int* 1975;7:342.
130. Appel GB, Pirani CL, D'Agati V. Renal vascular complications of systemic lupus erythematosus. *J Am Soc Nephrol* 1994;4:1499.
131. Descombes E, et al. Renal vascular lesions in lupus nephritis. *Medicine* 1997;76:355.
132. Pirani CL, Pollak VE, Schwartz FD. The reproducibility of semiquantitative analyses of renal histology. *Nephron* 1964;1:230.
133. Austin HA, et al. Diffuse proliferative lupus nephritis: identification of specific pathologic features affecting renal outcome. *Kidney Int* 1984;25:689.
134. Nossent HC, et al. Contribution of renal biopsy data in predicting outcome in lupus nephritis. *Arthritis Rheum* 1990;33:970.
135. Nossent JC, et al. Relation between serological data at the time of biopsy and renal histology in lupus nephritis. *Rheumatol Int* 1991;11:77.
136. Rush PJ, et al. Correlation of renal histology with outcome in children with lupus nephritis. *Kidney Int* 1986;29:1066.
137. Carette S, et al. Controlled studies of oral immunosuppressive drugs in lupus nephritis. A long-term follow-up. *Ann Intern Med* 1983;99:1
138. Banfi G, et al. Morphological parameters in lupus nephritis: their relevance for classification and relationship with clinical and histological findings and outcome. *Q J Med* 1985;55:153.
139. Alexopoulos E, et al. Lupus nephritis: correlation of interstitial cells with glomerular function. *Kidney Int* 1990;37:100.
140. Levey AS, et al. Progression and remission of renal disease in the Lupus Nephritis Collaborative Study. Results of treatment with prednisone and short-term oral cyclophosphamide. *Ann Intern Med* 1992;116:114.
141. Schwartz MM, et al. Predictive value of renal pathology in diffuse proliferative lupus glomerulonephritis. Lupus Nephritis Collaborative Study Group. *Kidney Int* 1989;36:891.
142. Schwartz MM, et al. Irreproducibility of the activity and chronicity indices limits their utility in the management of lupus nephritis. Lupus Nephritis Collaborative Study Group. *Am J Kidney Dis* 1993;21:374.
143. Esdaile JM, et al. The clinical and renal biopsy predictors of long-term outcome in lupus nephritis: a study of 87 patients and review of the literature. *Q J Med* 1989;72:779.
144. Austin HA, et al. Predicting renal outcomes in severe lupus nephritis: contributions of clinical and histologic data. *Kidney Int* 1994;45:544.
145. Wernick RM, et al. Reliability of histologic scoring for lupus nephritis: a community-based evaluation. *Ann Intern Med* 1993;119:805.
146. Nossent JC, Bronsveld W, Swaak AJ. Systemic lupus erythematosus. III. Observations on clinical renal involvement and follow up of renal function: Dutch experience with 110 patients studied prospectively. *Ann Rheum Dis* 1989;48:810.
147. Wallace DJ, et al. Lupus nephritis. Experience with 230 patients in a private practice from 1950 to 1980. *Am J Med* 1982;72:209.
148. Wallace DJ. The clinical presentation of systemic lupus erythematosus. In: Wallace DJ, Hahn BH, eds. *Dubois' Lupus Erythematosus,* 6th ed. Philadelphia: Lippincott Williams & Wilkins; 2002:621.
149. Perfumo F Martini A. Lupus nephritis in children. *Lupus* 2005;14:83.
150. Dooley MA, et al. Cyclophosphamide therapy for lupus nephritis: poor renal survival in black Americans. *Kidney Int* 1997;51:1188.
151. Boddaert J, et al. Late-onset systemic lupus erythematosus: a personal series of 47 patients and pooled analysis of 714 cases in the literature. *Medicine (Baltimore)* 2004;83:348.
152. Mok CC. Prognostic factors in lupus nephritis. *Lupus* 2005;14:39.
153. Budman DR, Steinberg AD. Hypertension and renal disease in systemic lupus erythematosus. *Arch Intern Med* 1976;136:1003.
154. Gruppo Italiano per lo Studio Della Nefrite Lupica. Lupus nephritis: prognostic factors and probability of maintaining life-supporting renal function 10 years after the diagnosis. *Am J Kidney Dis* 1992;19:473.
155. Ward MM, Studenski S. Clinical prognostic factors in lupus nephritis. The importance of hypertension and smoking. *Arch Intern Med* 1992;152:2082.
156. Kitridou RC. The mother in systemic lupus erythematosus. In: Wallace DJ, Hahn BH, eds. *Dubois' Lupus Erythematosus,* 6th ed. Philadelphia: Lippincott Williams & Wilkins; 2002:985.
157. Packham DK, et al. Lupus nephritis and pregnancy. *Q J Med* 1992;83:315.
158. Repke JT. Hypertensive disorders in pregnancy. Differentiating preeclampsia from active systemic lupus erythematosus. *J Reprod Med* 1998;43:350.
159. Moroni G, Ponticelli C. The risk of pregnancy in patients with lupus nephritis. *J Nephrol* 2003;16:161.
160. Moroni G, et al. Pregnancy in lupus nephritis. *Am J Kidney Dis* 2002;40:713.
161. Tan EM, Feltkamp TE, Smolen JS. Range of antinuclear antibodies in healthy individuals. *Arthritis Rheum* 1997;40:1601.
162. Reichlin M, Wolfson-Reichlin M. Correlations of anti-dsDNA and anti-ribosomal P autoantibodies with lupus nephritis. *Clin Immunol* 2003;108:69.
163. Reichlin M. Cellular dysfunction induced by penetration of autoantibodies into living cells: cellular damage and dysfunction mediated by antibodies to ds DNA and ribosomal P proteins. *J Autoimmun* 1998;11:557.
164. Hahn B. Antibodies to DNA. *N Engl J Med* 1998;338:1359.
165. Cervera R, et al. Antichromatin antibodies in systemic lupus erythematosus: a useful marker for lupus nephropathy. *Ann Rheum Dis* 2003;62:431.
166. Coremans IE, et al. Changes in antibodies to C1q predict renal relapses in systemic lupus erythematosus. *Am J Kidney Dis* 1995;26:595.
167. Holers VM. Anti C1q autoantibodies amplify pathogenic complement activation in systemic lupus erythematosus. *J Clin Invest* 2004;114:616.
168. Manzi S, et al. Measurement of erythrocyte C4d and complement receptor 1 in systemic lupus erythematosus. *Arthritis Rheum* 2004;50:3596.
169. Shemesh O, et al. Limitations of creatinine as a filtration marker in glomerulopathic patients. *Kidney Int* 1985;28:830.
170. Myers BD, et al. Extent of glomerular injury in active and resolving lupus nephritis: a theoretical analysis. *Am J Physiol* 1991;260:F717.
171. Fraenkel L, et al. Response to treatment as a predictor of long-term outcome in patients with lupus nephritis. *J Rheumatol* 1994;21:2052.
172. Hoffman RW, Greidinger EL. Mixed connective tissue disease. *Curr Opin Rheumatol* 2000;12:396.
173. Love PE, Santoro SA. Antiphospholipid antibodies: anticardiolipin and the lupus anticoagulant in systemic lupus erythematosus (SLE) and in non-SLE disorders. *Ann Intern Med* 1990;112:682.
174. Amigo MC, Khamashta MA. Antiphospholipid (Hughes) syndrome in systemic lupus erythematosus. *Rheum Dis Clin North Am* 2000;26:331.
175. Moll S, Ortel TL. Monitoring warfarin therapy in patients with lupus anticoagulants. *Ann Intern Med* 1997;127:177.
176. Amigo MC, et al. Renal involvement in primary antiphospholipid syndrome. *J Rheumatol* 1992;19:1181.
177. Nicholls K, Kincaid-Smith P. Antiphospholipid syndrome and renal thrombotic microangiopathy. *J Nephrol* 1995;8:123.
178. Nzerue CM, et al. Black swan in the kidney: renal involvement in the antiphospholipid antibody syndrome. *Kidney Int* 2002;62:733.
179. Tektonidou MG, et al. Antiphospholipid syndrome nephropathy in patients with systemic lupus erythematosus and antiphospholipid antibodies: prevalence, clinical associations, and long-term outcome. *Arthritis Rheum* 2004;50:2569.
180. Daugas E, et al. Antiphospholipid syndrome nephropathy in systemic lupus erythematosus. *J Am Soc Nephrol* 2002;13:42.
181. Mackworth-Young CG. Antiphospholipid syndrome: multiple mechanisms. *Clin Exp Immunol* 2004;136:393.
182. Ginzler EM, Schorn K. Outcome and prognosis in systemic lupus erythematosus. *Rheum Dis Clin North Am* 1988;14:67.
183. Rubin LA, Urowitz MB, Gladman DD. Mortality in systemic lupus erythematosus: the bimodal pattern revisited. *Q J Med* 1985;55:87.
184. Petri M, et al. Risk factors for coronary artery disease in patients with systemic lupus erythematosus. *Am J Med* 1992;93:513.
185. Lightfoot RW, Hughes GV. Significance of persisting serologic abnormalities in SLE. *Arthritis Rheum* 1976;19:837.
186. ter Borg EJ, et al. Measurement of increases in anti-double-stranded DNA antibody levels as a predictor of disease exacerbation in systemic lupus erythematosus. A long-term, prospective study. *Arthritis Rheum* 1990;33:634.
187. Pillemer SR, et al. Lupus nephritis: Association between serology and renal biopsy measures. *J Rheumatol* 1988;15:284.
188. Laitman RS, et al. Effect of long-term normalization of serum complement levels on the course of lupus nephritis. *Am J Med* 1989;87:132.
189. Kirou KA, Boumpas DT. Systemic glucocorticoid therapy in systemic lupus erythematosus. In Wallace DJ, Hahn BH, eds. *Dubois' Lupus Erythematosus,* 6th ed. Philadelphia: Lippincott Williams & Wilkins; 2002:1173.
190. Boumpas DT, et al. Controlled trial of pulse methylprednisolone versus two regimens of pulse cyclophosphamide in severe lupus nephritis. *Lancet* 1992;340:741.
191. Gourley MF, et al. Methylprednisolone and cyclophosphamide, alone or in combination, in patients with lupus nephritis: a randomized, controlled trial. *Ann Intern Med* 1996;125:549.

192. Houssiau FA. Management of lupus nephritis: an update. *J Am Soc Nephrol* 2004;15:2694.
193. Houssiau FA, et al. Early response to immunosuppressive therapy predicts good renal outcome in lupus nephritis: lessons from long-term followup of patients in the Euro-Lupus Nephritis Trial. *Arthritis Rheum* 2004;50:3934.
194. Felson DT, Anderson J. Evidence for the superiority of immunosuppressive drugs and prednisone over prednisone alone in lupus nephritis: results of pooled analysis. *N Engl J Med* 1984;311:1528.
195. Austin HA, et al. Therapy of lupus nephritis. Controlled trial of prednisone and cytotoxic drugs. *N Engl J Med* 1986;314:614.
196. Balow JE, et al. NIH conference. Lupus nephritis. *Ann Intern Med* 1987;106:79.
197. McCune WJ, et al. Clinical and immunologic effects of monthly administration of intravenous cyclophosphamide in severe systemic lupus erythematosus. *N Engl J Med* 1988;318:1423.
198. Steinberg AD, Steinberg SC. Long-term preservation of renal function in patients with lupus nephritis receiving treatment that includes cyclophosphamide versus those treated with prednisone only. *Arthritis Rheum* 1991;34:945.
199. Brooks EB, Liang MH. Evaluation of recent clinical trials in lupus. *Curr Opin Rheum* 1999;11:341.
200. Mok CC, Lau CS, Wong RW. Risk factors for ovarian failure in patients with systemic lupus erythematosus receiving cyclophosphamide therapy. *Arthritis Rheum* 1998;41:831.
201. Lewis EJ, et al. A controlled trial of plasmapheresis therapy in severe lupus nephritis. *N Engl J Med* 1992;326:1373.
202. Caccavo D, et al. Long-term treatment of systemic lupus erythematosus with cyclosporin A. *Arthritis Rheum* 1997;40:27.
203. Tam LS, et al. Long-term treatment of lupus nephritis with cyclosporin A. *Q J Med* 1998;91:573.
204. Fu LW, et al. Clinical efficacy of cyclosporine A in the treatment of paediatric lupus nephritis with heavy proteinuria. *Br J Rheumatol* 1998;37:217.
205. Dooley MA, et al. Mycophenolate mofetil therapy in lupus nephritis: clinical observations. *J Am Soc Nephrol* 1999;10:833.
206. Chan TM, et al. Efficacy of mycophenolate mofetil in patients with diffuse proliferative lupus nephritis. *N Engl J Med* 2000;343:1156.
207. Contreras G, et al. Sequential therapies for proliferative lupus nephritis. *N Engl J Med* 2004;350:971.
208. Chan TM, et al. Long-term study of mycophenolate mofetil as continuous induction and maintenance treatment for diffuse proliferative lupus nephritis. *J Am Soc Nephrol* 2005;16:1076.
209. Strober S, et al. Treatment of lupus nephritis with total lymphoid irradiation. *Arthritis Rheum* 1988;31:850.
210. Coma D, et al. Mycophenolate mofetil limits renal damage and prolongs life in murine lupus autoimmune disease. *Kidney Int* 1997;51:1583.
211. Ginzler EM, et al. Mycophenolate mofetil or intravenous cyclophosphamide for lupus nephritis. *N Engl J Med* 2005;353:2219.
212. McSweeney PA, Furst DE, West SG. High-dose immunosuppressive therapy for rheumatoid arthritis: some answers, more questions. *Arthritis Rheum* 1999;42:2269.
213. Traynor AE, et al. Hematopoietic stem cell transplantation for severe and refractory lupus. Analysis after five years and fifteen patients. *Arthritis Rheum* 2002;46:2917.
214. Petri M, Jones RJ, Brodsky RA. High-dose cyclophosphamide without stem cell transplantation in systemic lupus erythematosus. *Arthritis Rheum* 2003;48:166.
215. Boumpas DT, et al. A short course of BG9588 (anti-CD40 ligand antibody) improves serologic activity and decreases hematuria in patients with proliferative lupus glomerulonephritis. *Arthritis Rheum* 2003;48:719.
216. Korbet SM, et al. Factors predictive of outcome in severe lupus nephritis. Lupus Nephritis Collaborative Study Group. *Am J Kidney Dis* 2000;35:904.
217. Sidiropoulos PI, Kritikos HD, Boumpas DT. Lupus nephritis flares. *Lupus* 2005;14:49.
218. Illei GG, et al. Renal flares are common in patients with severe proliferative nephritis treated with pulse immunosuppressive therapy: long-term followup of a cohort of 145 patients participating in randomized controlled studies. *Arthritis Rheum* 2002;46:995.
219. Ciruelo E, et al. Cumulative rate of relapse of lupus nephritis after successful treatment with cyclophosphamide. *Arthritis Rheum* 1996;39:2028.
220. Boumpas DT, Illei GG, Balow JE. Treatment-renal involvement. In Hochberg MC, et al., eds. *Rheumatology*, 3rd ed. London: Mosby; 2003:1405.
221. Ioannidis JP, et al. Remission, relapse, and re-remission of proliferative lupus nephritis treated with cyclophosphamide. *Kidney Int* 2000;57:258.
222. Ruggenenti P, et al. Rituximab in idiopathic membranous nephropathy: a one-year prospective study. *J Am Soc Nephrol* 2003;14:1851.
223. Sfikakis PP, et al. Remission of proliferative lupus nephritis following B cell depletion therapy is preceded by down-regulation of the T cell costimulatory molecule CD40 ligand: an open-label trial. *Arthritis Rheum* 2005;52:501.
224. Alarcon-Segovia D, et al. LJP 394 for the prevention of renal flare in patients with systemic lupus erythematosus: results from a randomized, double-blind, placebo-controlled study. *Arthritis Rheum* 2003;48:442.
225. Neumann K, et al. Lupus in the 1980s. III. Influence of clinical variables, biopsy, and treatment on the outcome of 150 patients with lupus nephritis seen at a single center. *Semin Arthritis Rheum* 1995;25:47.
226. Coplon NS, et al. The long-term clinical course of systemic lupus erythematosus in end-stage renal disease. *N Engl J Med* 1983;308:186.
227. Jarrett MP, Santhanam S, Del Greco F. The clinical course of end-stage renal disease in systemic lupus erythematosus. *Arch Intern Med* 1983;143:1353.
228. Nossent HC, Swaak TJ, Berden JH. Systemic lupus erythematosus: analysis of disease activity in 55 patients with end-stage renal failure treated with hemodialysis or continuous ambulatory peritoneal dialysis. Dutch Working Party on SLE. *Am J Med* 1990;89:169.
229. Nossent HC, Swaak TJ, Berden JH. Systemic lupus erythematosus after renal transplantation: patient and graft survival and disease activity. The Dutch Working Party on Systemic Lupus Erythematosus. *Ann Intern Med* 1991;114:183.
230. Cheigh JS, Stenzel KH. End-stage renal disease in systemic lupus erythematosus. *Am J Kidney Dis* 1993;21:2.
231. Mocjik CF, Klippel JH. End-stage-renal disease and systemic lupus erythematosus. *Am J Med* 1996;101:100.
232. Krane NK, et al. Persistent lupus activity in end-stage renal disease. *Am J Kidney Dis* 1999;33:872.
233. Prakash R, Miller CC, Suki WN. Anticardiolipin antibody in patients on maintenance hemodialysis and its association with recurrent arteriovenous graft thrombosis. *Am J Kidney Dis* 1995;26:347.
234. Huang JW, et al. Systemic lupus erythematosus and peritoneal dialysis: outcomes and infectious complications. *Perit Dial Int* 2001;21:143.
235. Stone JH, et al. Frequency of recurrent lupus nephritis among ninety-seven renal transplant patients during the cyclosporine era. *Arthritis Rheum* 1998;41:678.
236. Goral S, et al. Recurrent lupus nephritis in renal transplant recipients revisited: it is not rare. *Transplantation* 2003;75:651.
237. Lockhead KM, et al. Risk factors for allograft loss in patients with systemic lupus erythematosus. *Kidney Int* 1996;45:512.
238. Stone JH, Amend WC, Criswell LA. Outcome of renal transplantation in ninety-seven cyclosporine-era patients with systemic lupus erythematosus and matched controls. *Arthritis Rheum* 1998;41:1438.
239. Vella J. Significance of anticardiolipin antibodies on short- and long-term allograft survival and function following kidney transplantation. *Am J Transplant* 2004;4:1731.
240. Vaidya S, Gugliuzza K, Daller JA. Efficacy of anticoagulation in end-stage renal disease patients with antiphospholipid antibody syndrome. *Transplantation* 2004;77:1046.
241. Friedman GS, et al. Hypercoagulable states in renal transplant candidates: impact of anticoagulation upon incidence of renal allograft thrombosis. *Transplantation* 2001;72:1073.

CHAPTER 66 ■ RENAL DISORDERS ASSOCIATED WITH SYSTEMIC SCLEROSIS, RHEUMATOID ARTHRITIS, SJÖGREN'S SYNDROME, AND POLYMYOSITIS-DERMATOMYOSITIS

ROBERT W. JANSON AND WILLIAM P. AREND

SYSTEMIC SCLEROSIS

Systemic sclerosis (SSc) is a relatively rare disorder of connective tissue, the clinical hallmark of which is fibrotic skin induration (scleroderma). This manifestation in some patients is no less dramatic than that described by Osler (1), who wrote that "to be 'beaten down and marred and wasted' until one is literally a mummy, encased in an ever-shrinking, slowly contracting skin of steel, is a fate not pictured in any tragedy, ancient or modern." Although such skin involvement is a cruel form of morbidity, visceral involvement of this systemic disease equally influences morbidity and frequently determines mortality. Organ systems other than the skin—including the gastrointestinal tract, kidneys, lung, and heart—may be affected by characteristic and widespread fibrotic, inflammatory, and vascular changes. The etiology of this pathologic process remains elusive (2).

Renal involvement remains one of the most feared complications in SSc. Scleroderma renal crisis (SRC), once a uniformly fatal process and the leading cause of death in SSc, is now a form of renal failure that can be treated successfully in a substantial proportion of patients in whom it develops. However, prevention of permanent renal failure rests on early recognition of SRC and prompt, aggressive treatment with angiotensin-converting enzyme (ACE) inhibitors. It is beyond the scope of this chapter to give a detailed account of all the manifestations of SSc or an in-depth examination of its pathogenesis; therefore, the following is an overview with focus on renal involvement. Readers are encouraged to refer to recent texts and reviews for a broader discourse on this disorder (2–4).

Classification

Scleroderma occurs in localized and systemic forms. In the former, involvement is isolated to the skin and subcutaneous tissue and can be classified as *morphea* or *linear scleroderma*. In the systemic form *(systemic sclerosis)*, visceral involvement occurs in addition to skin induration. Further classification of systemic sclerosis divides this entity into two relatively distinct clinical variants: systemic sclerosis with *limited* scleroderma (lSSc) and systemic sclerosis with *diffuse* scleroderma (dSSc), based on extent of skin involvement (5). Although significant overlap exists, type and frequency of various clinical manifestations differ between these variants to the extent that they behave as two distinct clinical entities. Therefore, the pattern of ex-

tradermal involvement, in addition to characteristic serologic findings, can be of diagnostic utility to help distinguish lSSc from dSSc. An overview of these characteristics is outlined in Table 66-1.

Limited systemic sclerosis has replaced the acronymic term CREST syndrome, which remains a useful reminder of this variant's typical features of subcutaneous *c*alcinosis, *R*aynaud's phenomenon, *e*sophageal hypomotility, *s*clerodactyly (skin induration limited to the digits), and *t*elangiectasias. Raynaud's phenomenon and telangiectasias often precede by years the skin involvement, which is limited to the distal extremities and face. Visceral involvement occurs late in the course of lSSc and differs from dSSc by the rarity of renal and myocardial involvement. A leading cause of late mortality in lSSc is pulmonary hypertension occurring in the relative absence of interstitial lung disease. Such isolated pulmonary hypertension, which develops rarely in dSSc, affects 8% to 16% of patients with lSSc (6,7). The immunologic marker for lSSc is the anticentromere antibody, which is detected in 20% to 40% of affected individuals (8).

In *diffuse systemic sclerosis,* more widespread skin induration develops within months to a few years of disease onset, by definition involving the trunk and/or extremities proximal to the elbows and knees (5). Typically, Raynaud's phenomenon develops concomitantly with distal skin signs of edema and early induration. A more notable contrast to lSSc is early visceral involvement of the gastrointestinal tract, kidneys, heart, and lungs in dSSc. Anti-Scl-70 antibodies are relatively specific for dSSc and are detectable in 20% to 40% of those with this variant (8,9). The antigen to which this antibody is directed has been identified as topoisomerase I, a DNA gyrase (10). More recently, anti-RNA polymerase antibodies, particularly anti-RNA polymerase III, have been found to be relatively specific and somewhat more sensitive serologic markers for dSSc, and are detectable in approximately 20% of individuals with dSSc (11). Regarding prognosis, it has been generally accepted that dSSc is associated with a higher mortality rate than limited disease, with 10-year survival rates on the order of 55% and 70% in dSSc and lSSc, respectively (12,13). The major causes of death in dSSc are pulmonary, cardiac, and renal involvement, whereas pulmonary hypertension is the leading cause of death in lSSc. Recent studies have suggested that the two variants may now have nearly equal survival rates, which likely reflects decreasing mortality of SRC in dSSc as a result of earlier and more effective treatments (14–16). Poor prognosis is often associated with diffuse skin involvement, late age of onset of disease, African American descent, lung vital capacity of less than

TABLE 66-1

SYSTEMIC SCLEROSIS (SSC) SUBSETS

Organ system/manifestation	dSSc	lSSc
Skin	Trunk and/or proximal extremity induration	Distal extremity induration (may include face) Calcinosis Telangiectasias
Raynaud's phenomenon	Onset within 1 year of skin involvement	Frequently precedes skin involvement by years
Pulmonary	Early development of pulmonary fibrosis (>50%)	Late development of isolated pulmonary hypertension (10% to 20%); pulmonary fibrosis (<40%)
Renal	Scleroderma renal crisis (10% to 20%)	Rare involvement
Gastrointestinal	Involvement of esophagus, small intestine, colon	Involvement usually limited to the esophagus
Cardiac	Primary involvement of the myocardium/microvasculature	Secondary involvement owing to pulmonary hypertension
Musculoskeletal	Joint contractures; arthralgias/arthritis; tendon friction rubs; myositis	Acral joint contractures; arthralgias/arthritis less common; myositis
Nail-fold capillaries	Dilation and dropout	Dilation without dropout
Serologic studies		
Antinuclear antibody	>90%	>90%
Anti-topoisomerase	20% to 40%	<15%
Anticentromere	<5%	20% to 40%
Anti-RNA polymerase III	20%	6%
10-Year survival	55%	70%

55% predicted, and significant renal, cardiac, gastrointestinal, or pulmonary disease (8).

Discussion of classification must not exclude those patients with normal skin who have typical internal organ changes, and vascular, and serologic features of SSc. *Sine scleroderma* is the term used to refer to this uncommon presentation (3). It should also be noted that systemic sclerosis may occasionally occur in *overlap* with features of other autoimmune rheumatic disorders such as rheumatoid arthritis, systemic lupus erythematosus, polymyositis-dermatomyositis, and Sjögren's syndrome.

Epidemiology

Systemic sclerosis is a rare disorder that has a worldwide distribution affecting all racial groups. Epidemiologic studies of SSc have likely underestimated its true incidence and prevalence because many such studies have been based on referral center data. The published incidences range from 1 to 19 cases per million, with an estimated prevalence of about 250 cases per million (16). Peak age of onset occurs in the fourth and fifth decades, with women being affected more commonly than men at a ratio of approximately 4:1. Although SSc affects all races, certain racial groups, such as African Americans, appear to have a higher incidence compared to whites (16). Disease occurs without identifiable environmental exposures in the majority of patients. However, certain environmental and occupational factors are associated with development of SSc and SSc-like disorders. These include exposure to silica dust and various organic compounds such as vinyl chloride, epoxy resins, and organic solvents (8). It should be noted that there has yet to be shown a convincing link between SSc and silicone breast implants (17–19).

Genetic predispositions and familial clustering have been well described in other rheumatic diseases such as rheumatoid arthritis and systemic lupus erythematosus; however, genetic associations have been weak and familial clustering rare in SSc.

Relatively weak human leukocyte antigen (HLA) associations have been demonstrated in SSc, and findings have varied among ethnic groups, geographic regions, and investigating centers. Reported associations have included certain HLA-DR2, HLA-DR3, and HLA-DR5 haplotypes in addition to the C4 null alleles C4AQ0 and C4BQ0 (20,21). These HLA associations may be more related to the presence of particular autoantigens than to the disease (20). Environmental factors may play a more prominent role in the pathogenesis of this disease because there are only scarce reports of SSc occurring in familial clusters (22) and concordance in monozygotic twins is an infrequent observation (16).

Pathogenesis

One of the striking observations in SSc is the similarity of pathologic lesions in the various affected organs, that is the ubiquitous presence of vasculopathy and fibrosis. Although the inciting event triggering such systemic injury is unknown, a working hypothesis has been proposed that attempts to integrate the pathogenic abnormalities affecting the immune system, microvasculature, and connective tissue (2,23).

Immune System

Because of the observation that 95% of patients with SSc have detectable antinuclear antibodies (ANAs) using the widely used Hep-2 cell line as the detection substrate (24), SSc has long been viewed as an autoimmune disorder. Supporting this view is the observation that SSc occurs in overlap with other ANA-associated autoimmune disorders such as polymyositis, systemic lupus erythematosus, and Sjögren's syndrome. As discussed, relatively specific autoantibodies (anticentromere, anti-Scl-70, and anti-RNA polymerase III) are present in SSc, more strongly suggesting a role for the immune system in pathogenesis. However, these autoantibodies have not been shown to be pathogenic per se, at least not in the usual sense of immune complex-mediated tissue injury (25). Although circulating immune complexes have been detected in SSc (26), and immunofluorescence studies have demonstrated vascular deposition of immunoglobulins and complement components, the characteristic inflammatory sequelae expected as the result of immune-complex deposition are absent by histologic examination. Thus, convincing evidence is lacking for immune complex-mediated vascular injury in SSc.

The potential role of cellular immunity in the pathogenesis of SSc was first suggested by the observation of perivascular dermal mononuclear cell infiltrates in the early edematous phase of skin involvement (27). The extent of these dermal infiltrates has been shown to correlate with the severity of subsequent skin induration. Phenotypic examinations have shown activated CD4-positive T cells to be the predominant cell type (23,28). Elevated levels of interleukin-2 (IL-2) and its soluble receptor (sIL-2R) have been demonstrated in SSc sera and correlate with disease severity and patient survival, supporting the concept of a T-cell contribution to tissue injury in SSc (29). Perhaps the strongest evidence that cell-mediated immune injury is of pathogenic importance in SSc comes from reports of SSc-like manifestations occurring in chronic graft-versus-host disease (GVHD). Features of this disease include Raynaud's phenomenon, dermal sclerosis (particularly in the digits), positive ANA test, and vascular changes similar to those seen in SSc (30,31). A similar syndrome in mice with chronic GVHD is dependent on the presence of immunocompetent donor T cells reactive to incompatible recipient H-2 locus antigens (32). The finding that a T-cell response to cellular antigens can induce a syndrome similar to SSc, combined with the knowledge that major histocompatability complex (MHC) antigens can be expressed on activated endothelial cells, has obvious implications regarding the potential role for cell-mediated immunity in the pathogenesis of SSc. Furthermore, recent research suggests that microchimerism, the persistence of circulating fetal immune cells in previously pregnant women, could possibly, when activated by a second event, induce a GVHD-like response contributing to the development of SSc (2,23,33).

Endothelial Cell and Vasculature

The nearly universal manifestation of Raynaud's phenomenon in SSc and the finding of abnormal nail-fold capillaries in greater than 85% of patients, both usually developing early in the course of disease and often before the onset of dermal sclerosis, emphasize the importance of vasculopathy in SSc (34). The three most apparent manifestations of widespread vascular abnormalities in SSc are: (a) vasomotor instability leading to transient ischemia not only of the digits but also of the viscera, (b) structural abnormalities of small vessels characterized by endothelial cell damage and obliterative intimal proliferation, and (c) intravascular abnormalities such as enhanced coagulability and platelet activation. Development of this systemic vasculopathy, with its resultant tissue ischemia, may be the most important pathogenic mechanism of visceral organ damage in SSc, with scleroderma renal crisis being one of its more dramatic consequences.

Vasoreactivity is enhanced in SSc. Easily provoked by cold exposure, vasospasm of structurally abnormal vessels results in transient tissue hypoperfusion, with Raynaud's phenomenon being the most familiar clinical consequence. The enhanced vasoreactivity is likely multifactorial in nature, as suggested by the variety of vasopressors that have been proposed as mediators of this phenomenon, including serotonin (35), catecholamines (36), prostaglandins (37), thromboxane A_2 (38), and angiotensin (39). In addition, serum levels of endothelin, an endothelium-derived peptide and the most potent vasoconstrictor yet discovered, have been shown to be elevated in individuals with primary Raynaud's phenomenon and SSc (40,41). Kahaleh (41) demonstrated that endothelin is mitogenic for fibroblasts and stimulates collagen synthesis, thereby invoking a potential link between vascular and connective tissue abnormalities in SSc.

Morphologic studies in SSc have revealed evidence of endothelial cell (EC) injury and altered EC function. Additional observations include EC swelling and retraction with loss of intercellular junctions, ECs in various stages of cell death or apoptosis, and basement membrane abnormalities (34). The first in vivo evidence to support EC injury in SSc was the finding of elevated plasma levels of EC-specific von Willebrand's factor (42), a phenomenon seen in other disorders associated with underlying EC damage such as vasculitis (43). Interest in EC "activation" has led to the finding of increased expression of intercellular adhesion molecule-1 (ICAM-1), among other integrins, in the skin of individuals with recent onset SSc (44), suggesting a homing mechanism for pathogenic lymphocytes. Other investigators have demonstrated that serum levels of soluble ICAM-1 (s-ICAM-1), E-selectin, and P-selectin are increased in patients with SSc compared to controls and correlate both with their in situ activity and with clinical disease activity (45,46). Therefore, s-ICAM-1 and other selectins may be useful markers of EC activation.

Damaged and activated endothelial cells are potentially capable of stimulating intimal proliferation directly by elaboration of EC-derived growth factors and indirectly by triggering platelet activation and degranulation (34). This process results in the characteristic obliterative intimal lesion of SSc. Compounding the effect of the vascular structural changes is that of intravascular coagulation abnormalities. Histologically, this is indicated by the formation of luminal thrombi in affected vessels. Clinically, this is manifested by the development of microangiopathic hemolytic anemia and supported by the findings of increased fibrinogen turnover (47), increased circulating platelet aggregates, and elevated levels of ß-thromboglobulin (48).

Although EC injury and activation appear to be of primary importance in the development of vascular abnormalities in SSc, the mechanisms by which such injury occurs are not clear. As discussed previously, immune complex injury seems unlikely. Antibodies directed against EC have been detected by several investigators but have not been shown to be directly cytotoxic (49). However, a potential role for antibody-mediated damage has been implied by the observation that SSc sera are capable of mediating antibody-dependent cellular cytotoxicity against EC, although sera from only about 20% of patients exhibit this property (49,50). Cytokine-mediated EC injury may be a contributing factor based on the findings that transforming growth factor-β (TGF-β) and tumor necrosis factor-α (TNF-α) can inhibit endothelial cell growth in vitro (2). Nonimmune mechanisms of EC damage have also been described. Over the last decade, contradictory reports have appeared regarding evidence for a nonimmunoglobulin serum factor in SSc that is cytotoxic to EC (49). One group of investigators partially purified a low-molecular-weight ($\leq$5 kDa) cytotoxic factor from SSc sera, which led to elevated plasma levels of von Willebrand's factor, capillary dilation, and arterial/arteriolar intimal hyperplasia when serially injected into rabbits (51).

Fibroblast

Perhaps the most characteristic feature of SSc is that of widespread fibrosis, the result of faulty regulation of collagen synthesis leading to excessive accumulation of types I and III collagen and other extracellular matrix components in the skin and visceral organs (52). LeRoy was the first of several investigators to show that cultured dermal fibroblasts from SSc patients synthesized two to fourfold more collagen than control fibroblasts, and that this ability persisted for several cell passages before declining toward control levels (53). Evidence has accumulated to indicate that this increased collagen production by SSc fibroblasts occurs as a result of enhanced messenger RNA (mRNA) transcription (54), the probable result of cytokine stimulation. The potential ability for mast cell–elaborated products, such as heparin, to stimulate fibroblast collagen production in SSc has been reviewed (55). Of potential fibroblast stimulatory cytokines, TGF-β has been found to be the most potent inducer of collagen synthesis, likely because of its ability to upregulate the transcription of collagen mRNA (56). Recently, it has been shown that cultured scleroderma fibroblasts possess increased levels of membrane TGF-β receptors (57). Unfortunately, the finding of elevated TGF-β receptor levels in patients with SSc has not been universally reproduced (58). Transforming growth factor-β can also induce endothelial cell production of endothelin, the most potent vasoconstrictor known (59). Other soluble mediators—including the interleukins 1, 2, 4 (a profibrotic cytokine), 6, 8, and 17 (enhances the proliferation of fibroblasts), TNF-α, platelet-derived growth factor (PDGF), and fibronectin—may play a role in the pathogenesis of SSc (2,34).

A working hypothesis has been proposed in an attempt to unify the pathogenic abnormalities in SSc discussed in the preceding paragraphs (2,23). An unidentified inciting event may trigger both EC injury and immune system activation, with the latter potentiating and/or perpetuating EC damage. A cytokine cascade, the result of immune cell activation and platelet degranulation triggered by EC damage, then provokes systemic fibroblast activation and proliferation, the end result being fibrosis. Whether the associated autoantibodies are pathogenic or merely an epiphenomenon remains unclear.

Renal Involvement

Historical Perspective

Descriptions of cutaneous manifestations compatible with those of systemic sclerosis were noted in writings as early as those of Hippocrates (460–370 BC) and Galen (131–201 AD) (60). The earliest convincing description of a patient with SSc appeared in a 1753 monograph written by Carlo Curzio (61). In 1847, Gintrac (62) coined the descriptive term *sclérodermie,* which soon thereafter became the widely accepted term of reference. The earliest description of renal involvement in SSc is attributed to Auspitz (63), who in 1863 described a 29-year-old locksmith with tightness and hyperpigmentation of the skin who succumbed to "Bright's disease." Later in that century, in the first edition of his renowned medical text, Osler (64) mentioned that patients with scleroderma "are apt to succumb to pulmonary complaints or to nephritis." Although other authors subsequently acknowledged the visceral manifestations of SSc, it was not until well into this century that more detailed attention was given to renal disease in SSc. Moore and Sheehan (65) provided the first detailed clinical and pathologic description of renal involvement in three patients with SSc who developed acute hypertension and died 6 to 8 weeks later of renal failure. The concept that a direct relationship exists between SSc and renal disease became widely accepted subsequent to this convincing report.

Frequency and Type of Renal Involvement

Review of the literature makes it clear that clinically significant renal disease develops much less commonly in SSc than do the renal pathologic abnormalities. Multiple autopsy studies in SSc

have demonstrated the frequency of typical renal histopathologic lesions to be in the range of 50% to 80%; these studies have been previously reviewed (66,67). In an attempt to better estimate this frequency and understand the natural history of scleroderma renal disease, Kovalchik and colleagues (68) performed renal biopsies in nine normotensive SSc patients in whom there was no evidence for renal disease. Six of the nine biopsies demonstrated presence of vascular changes, and mild nonspecific glomerular lesions were seen in all nine. Despite the frequency of these findings, only one of these patients eventually developed SRC.

In SSc, clinical renal disease ranges from less severe renal abnormalities including hypertension, proteinuria, and azotemia (serum creatinine >1.2 mg/dL) unrelated to SRC, to overt life-threatening SRC. Cannon et al. (69) found that 45% to 60% of 210 patients with SSc had hypertension, proteinuria, or azotemia unrelated to SRC. Common causes of these abnormalities in patients with SSc include prerenal effects from congestive heart failure, diarrhea or dehydration from scleroderma gastrointestinal involvement, volume depletion from infection, and drug reactions resulting from the use of diuretics, D-penicillamine, cyclosporine, or nonsteroidal antiinflammatory drugs (NSAIDs) (70). Despite classic renal pathologic changes occurring in a large number of patients, chronic progressive renal insufficiency is rare outside of the setting of SRC. Because hypertension, proteinuria, and azotemia can all result from causes other than SSc, their use as specific indicators likely overestimates true SSc-related renal disease. However, the diagnosis of SRC always should be considered in the setting of these renal abnormalities, particularly if they are abrupt in onset.

The frequency of SRC in a University of Pittsburgh cohort of 1,118 SSc patients followed between 1972 and 1990 was 10%; the frequency in dSSc was 10-fold higher than in lSSc (19% and 2%, respectively) (71). There is much less risk of SRC in lSSc, particularly if the patient is anticentromere antibody positive. Langevitz et al. (72) reported SRC developing in only 7 (3%) of 243 SSc patients (5% frequency in dSSc) followed prospectively between 1979 and 1989, leading to the suggestion that the incidence of SRC may be declining. This observation may be due to earlier diagnosis and treatment with ACE inhibitors.

Several cases of pauci-immune crescentic glomerulonephritis associated with myeloperoxidase-specific anti-neutrophil cytoplasmic antibodies (MPO-ANCA) have also been reported in patients with SSc (73–76). Although this entity was originally thought to be a complication of treatment with D-penicillamine, occurrence in the absence of D-penicillamine has been reported (75,76). In contrast to SRC, patients with this disorder are typically normotensive with nephrotic range proteinuria and renal insufficiency, and do not have microangiopathic hemolytic anemia or thrombocytopenia. Treatment regimens for microscopic polyangiitis with corticosteroids and immunosuppressive agents may be beneficial.

Scleroderma Renal Crisis

Clinical Features. Renal crisis in SSc is a distinct clinical syndrome of abrupt onset representing a medical emergency, which inexorably results in renal failure and death if left untreated. The best predictor of the development of SRC is rapid progression of cutaneous involvement in patients with dSSc (77). The highest risk occurs early in the course of disease, with greater than 70% of cases developing within 4 years of disease onset (70,77). Investigation of multiple other clinical parameters has identified as other apparent risk factors diffuse skin involvement, anemia, pericardial effusions, congestive heart failure, the presence of anti-RNA polymerase III antibodies, and use of high-dose corticosteroids (prednisone, ≥30 mg/day) especially

TABLE 66-2

CLINICAL FACTORS AND SCLERODERMA RENAL CRISIS (SRC)

Factors predictive of SRC	Factors not predictive of SRC
Diffuse cutaneous Involvement	Baseline renal function
Early disease: within 4 years of disease onset	Urinalysis abnormalities
Rapidly progressive skin induration	Baseline blood pressure
Cardiac involvement Congestive heart failure Pericardial effusion	Plasma renin activity
New anemia	Renal pathologic abnormalities
Possibly high-dose corticosteroids (normotensive SRC)	Anti-topoisomerase antibodies (in diffuse systemic sclerosis)
Anti-RNA polymerase III antibodies	

in normotensive patients (70,77–79) (Table 66-2). Case reports of rapidly progressive SSc with SRC associated with a malignancy (breast, ovarian, lung, and renal cell carcinoma) suggest that screening for occult malignancy should be considered in this population and that SSc patients with malignancies should be monitored closely for renal, cardiac, and pulmonary complications (80).

The syndrome of SRC is classically characterized by the precipitous onset of severe hypertension, rapidly progressive renal failure, microangiopathic hemolytic anemia, consumptive thrombocytopenia (rarely <50,000 platelets/mm^3), and hyperreninemia. Although symptoms may be absent at the onset of SRC, most patients experience fatigue, headache, visual disturbances, encephalopathy, or seizures, all of which may be secondary to marked hypertension. Hypertensive funduscopic changes are frequently noted and may include hemorrhages, exudates, and papilledema. Signs and symptoms of left ventricular failure are not infrequent at presentation or shortly after onset of SRC. Pulmonary hemorrhage, which is not usually seen in SSc, can be a rare life-threatening complication (78,81).

The diagnosis of SRC is easily made when typical manifestations develop in a patient with known or obvious SSc. Diagnosis of normotensive SRC, which accounts for approximately 10% of presentations (78), depends on identification of other clinical features of SRC such as new-onset azotemia and microangiopathic hemolytic anemia. Renal crisis may occasionally develop in the setting of minimal signs of SSc or in the absence of skin involvement, termed sine scleroderma. In such cases, making an early and correct diagnosis hinges on recognition of noncutaneous manifestations of SSc such as the presence of Raynaud's phenomenon, tendon friction rubs, carpal tunnel syndrome, nail-fold capillary abnormalities, and supporting serologic findings such as antitopoisomerase (anti-Scl-70) and anti-RNA polymerase III antibodies (70,82).

Hypertension in the absence of SRC has a frequency in SSc similar to the prevalence of essential hypertension in the general adult population, in the range of 15% to 20% (69,77). Hypertension may or may not be present before SRC onset, and its presence does not appear to predict development of SRC or overall survival (77,83). A number of cases of SRC occurring in the absence of concomitant hypertension have been reported, beginning with two of the original three patients described by Moore and Sheehan (65). Helfrich et al. (78) at the University of Pittsburgh reported that of 131 pa-

tients with SRC, 15 (11%) had normal blood pressure during the complication. Compared with hypertensive SRC patients, these patients demonstrated a higher frequency of microangiopathic hemolytic anemia, thrombocytopenia, and previous corticosteroid exposure along with a poorer 12-month survival rate.

Laboratory Features. Azotemia and the hematologic manifestations of SRC have been mentioned previously. The serum creatinine concentration tends to rise rapidly and may continue to rise for several days, even after effective control of the hypertension. Proteinuria occurs frequently in SRC, but is not usually greater than 2.5 g per/24 hours. The finding of proteinuria on urinalysis is definitely not specific for SRC; mild degrees of proteinuria may be present in 20% to 36% of SSc patients in whom SRC is absent (69,71). Proteinuria has not been found to be a helpful predictor of SRC development, although its presence has been suggested to be a marker for higher mortality (77). Urinalysis may also reveal the presence of microscopic hematuria or granular casts; RBC casts are an unusual finding and would suggest a scleroderma-overlap syndrome. Abnormalities of the renin–angiotensin system are described in the following.

Course and Prognosis. As mentioned, untreated SRC is a uniformly fatal disorder. Uremia, hypertensive complications, and congestive heart failure can lead to death within 7 to 10 days. Prior to the last decade and antecedent to use of ACE inhibitors, the average survival after SRC onset was 1 to 3 months (84), despite availability of antihypertensive agents and hemodialysis. The first indication that disrupting the renin–angiotensin system was of therapeutic importance in SRC came when it was shown that bilateral nephrectomy improved mortality (84,85). LeRoy and Fleischman (85) showed that survival beyond 6 months was only 10% in those without nephrectomy, compared to 43% in those who had undergone the procedure.

A revolution in treatment of SRC began with the first report of captopril therapy reversing SRC (86). Subsequently, it was confirmed that ACE inhibition was the most effective therapy for SRC. Steen and colleagues (87) reviewed outcomes in 108 patients with SSc before and after availability of ACE inhibitors. The cumulative 1-year survival rate in 55 patients receiving ACE inhibition therapy was 76% compared to 15% in 53 patients not treated. Moreover, of 20 ACE inhibitor-treated patients requiring dialysis and surviving for 3 or more months, 11 (55%) were eventually able to discontinue dialysis; none of 15 patients who were not treated with an ACE inhibitor were able to do so. Subsequently, Steen and Medsger (88) reported the outcomes of 145 patients with SRC treated with ACE inhibitors: 61% of patients with SRC had good outcomes (55 patients received no dialysis, and 34 patients received temporary dialysis) and 39% of patients had bad outcomes (permanent dialysis or early death). The 34 patients who received temporary dialysis continued taking ACE inhibitors, and dialysis was discontinued after 2 to 18 months. The 5-year cumulative survival rate was 90% in the no dialysis and temporary dialysis groups, similar to their cohort of patients with SSc without renal crisis. Patients who had SRC requiring permanent dialysis had a 5-year cumulative survival rate of only 40%.

It seems clear that treatment with ACE inhibitors has rendered SRC a much less ominous manifestation of SSc. The use of ACE inhibitors, combined with the observation that SRC may be declining in frequency, appears to account for the recent observation that renal disease has been superseded by cardiopulmonary complications as the leading cause of death in SSc (14,72,89).

Pathophysiology of Renal Involvement

Renal Circulation

Both functional and structural vascular abnormalities contribute to impaired renal cortical perfusion in SSc, setting the stage for the development of clinical renal disease. Urai et al. (90) were the first to demonstrate reduced renal plasma flow in SSc. Their study of 25 SSc patients without evidence of renal disease revealed reduced *p*-aminohippurate clearances in 23 (92%). In a supporting study, Cannon et al. (69) demonstrated normal to slightly diminished renal cortical perfusion using a xenon-133 washout technique in patients with markers of renal involvement in the absence of renal failure. In contrast, extreme to absent renal cortical perfusion was noted in those patients with SRC. This dramatic observation was corroborated by Woolfson et al. (91), who showed almost complete loss of renal perfusion and parenchymal uptake in three SRC patients studied by dynamic renal scintigraphy. Unfortunately, these techniques have not been successful in predicting the development of SRC.

The angiographic appearance of the scleroderma kidney demonstrates well the underlying structural abnormalities of the renal vasculature. Lester and Koehler (92) first reported the striking angiographic findings of irregular narrowing of the interlobular and arcuate arteries with prolonged contrast transit time. Winograd et al. (93) described abnormal cortical lucencies of the nephrogram in two SSc patients having undergone arteriography. This "spotted nephrogram" is suggestive of focal cortical necrosis and appears to be relatively specific for SSc, particularly when seen in the absence of large vessel abnormalities (69,94).

Vasospasm may contribute to renal hypoperfusion in SSc. In a study of renal perfusion, Cannon et al. (69) found that induction of Raynaud's phenomenon by cold exposure resulted in an acute reduction in cortical perfusion. In addition, they showed that intrarenal infusion of a vasodilator resulted in increased blood flow. Vasospasm leading to decreased renal perfusion could result in the release of renin. These and other investigators have observed a higher frequency of SRC during the cold months of the year, suggesting that vasospasm may play an initiating role in SRC (84); others have not found as strong an association (77).

Renin–Angiotensin System

Plasma renin activity (PRA) acutely and rapidly rises to values 2 to 100 times that of normal during SRC (84). However, in the absence of renal involvement, PRA is frequently normal, and levels do not appear to predict development of SRC. Traub et al. (84) reported that baseline PRA determinations were normal in all 13 SRC patients who happened to have had PRA measured from 1 week to 1 year prior to SRC onset. Other investigators have confirmed this observation (95). Supporting the concept of a Raynaud's-like renal vasoconstriction, Kovalchik et al. (68) observed significant PRA elevations with cold pressor testing in four of their patients with SSc, with evidence of vasculopathy on renal biopsy, but not in those without such histologic changes. As discussed, all of the subjects in this study lacked clinical evidence of renal disease.

Considering the preceding observations, it is reasonable to conclude that in the setting of SRC, both structural and functional renal vascular abnormalities lead to hypoperfusion of the juxtaglomerular apparatus, stimulating renin secretion. With marked elevation of PRA, excessive angiotensin II is formed, exacerbating systemic and renal vasoconstriction. A self-perpetuating cycle is initiated with the resultant systemic hypertension and worsened renal cortical ischemia. The bene-

ficial therapeutic effects of ACE inhibition support the importance of this mechanism in the pathophysiology of SRC.

Histopathology

Gross Appearance

The gross appearance of the scleroderma kidney varies depending on the relative chronicity and severity of disease. In patients with acute SRC, the kidneys are generally normal in size with a smooth to finely granular surface. In florid cases of SRC with associated renal failure, the renal cortex may display areas of hemorrhagic or yellow-gray infarction. The kidneys become shrunken in size and may exhibit coarsely granular surfaces in patients who have survived SRC but have been left with chronic renal disease. These gross changes are not specific for the scleroderma kidney because they also are seen in other forms of chronic renal failure, such as malignant nephrosclerosis (66).

Microscopic Appearance

Arteries. The small interlobular and arcuate arteries, measuring 150 to 500 μm in outer diameter, exhibit the characteristic lesions of scleroderma renal involvement (69). Intimal edema is the earliest abnormality seen. This is followed by cellular intimal proliferation with associated deposition of mucoid ground substance composed primarily of mucopolysaccharide and, to a lesser extent, glycoprotein. The cellular component of this process arises from proliferation of myointimal cells, which ultrastructurally can resemble either smooth muscle cells or fibroblasts (66). The myointimal cells often arrange themselves in a concentrically whorled or "onionskin" configuration (Fig. 66-1). As a consequence, the vascular lumen becomes markedly narrowed. Endothelial cells lining the lumen are typically swollen, and in some areas may have sloughed. The internal elastic lamina is intact. The media becomes thinned, often to one or two cell layers. Typically, no significant inflammatory cell infiltrates (lymphocytes or other mononuclear cells) are present. Mild adventitial and periadventitial fibrosis may be seen, a finding reported to be relatively specific for SSc and rarely noted in malignant hypertension not associated with SSc. The nonfibrotic arterial abnormalities described are much less specific because they are difficult to distinguish from those seen

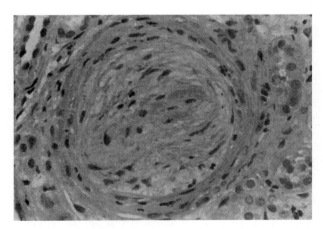

FIGURE 66-1. Photomicrograph of the kidney from a patient with systemic sclerosis with diffuse scleroderma and scleroderma renal crisis. The small muscular artery demonstrates intimal edema and concentric proliferation of myointimal cells with complete occlusion of the lumen (hematoxylin and eosin, magnification ×300). (Courtesy of William S. Hammond.)

in association with essential hypertension. In contrast to essential hypertension, where development of these renal vascular changes appears to be dependent on the level of blood pressure elevation, the lesions in SSc appear to precede or occur in the complete absence of hypertension (68,96).

With more chronic renal involvement, mucoid edematous intimal proliferation of the arteries is replaced by a dense, concentric, intimal fibroelastosis that continues to narrow the lumen. Moderate concentric reduplication of the internal elastic lamina usually can be demonstrated. In contrast to acute lesions, the media in chronic SSc renal disease lacks a stretched appearance and may appear mildly sclerotic. The adventitia is unremarkable and no inflammatory infiltration is present in the vessel wall (66).

Arterioles. Arterioles (external diameter of 50 to 150 μm) rarely display mucoid intimal proliferation. Rather, subintimal and, to a lesser degree, intramural fibrinoid necrosis affects vessels of this size, but vasculitis is rarely seen. This process, frequently extending to the hilus of the glomerulus, severely narrows the arteriolar lumen, which also may be occluded by intraluminal fibrin thrombi. These changes are indistinguishable from those found in malignant hypertension (66) (Fig. 66-2).

Glomeruli and Interstitium. Acutely the histologic characteristics of glomeruli in SSc renal disease range from normal to showing areas of infarction and necrosis. Juxtaglomerular apparatus hyperplasia is seen, nonspecific to SSc, and consistent with the hyperreninemia found in SRC. Chronically the glomeruli exhibit progressive glomerulosclerosis, a finding in common with malignant hypertension and hemolytic–uremic syndrome. Basement membrane wrinkling and thickening are noted, which in the past have improperly been referred to as "wire looping," a term now reserved for the glomerular capillary wall thickening caused by subendothelial deposits in active lupus nephritis (66). The renal tubular epithelial cells may be flattened and may exhibit hyaline droplet degeneration. The latter finding preferentially affects certain nephrons and not others, suggesting a greater degree of protein leakage from the more severely affected glomeruli. The interstitium may show varying degrees of fibrosis and mild chronic inflammatory infiltrates consisting primarily of lymphocytes and plasma cells.

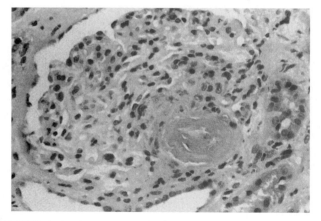

FIGURE 66-2. Photomicrograph of the kidney from the same patient as in Figure 66-1. The glomerular afferent arteriole demonstrates fibrinoid necrosis (hematoxylin and eosin, magnification ×300). (Courtesy of William S. Hammond.)

Immunofluorescence and Elution Studies. Studies utilizing immunofluorescence microscopy in SSc have described nonspecific focal deposits of immunoglobulins (primarily IgM), complement components (C1q, C3, and C4), and fibrinogen in the intima and lumina of small renal arteries and arterioles (66). Glomerular staining is more inconsistent and less intense for these components compared to vascular staining. Elution of immunoglobulin (primarily IgG) and antinuclear antibodies from kidneys of SSc patients has been reported (97–99). Although these findings have been interpreted as providing evidence for immune complex injury in the pathogenesis of SSc renal vasculopathy, this interpretation is now viewed with less certainty. Electron-dense deposits suggesting immune-complex deposition have not been demonstrated on electron microscopic examination of vessels and glomeruli in SSc (66). In addition, immunofluorescence staining in the early stages of malignant nephrosclerosis is quite similar to that seen in SSc, suggesting that this finding is nonspecific and the likely result of disruption of vascular integrity with increased vascular permeability (66,96).

Management of Renal Crisis

For reasons previously discussed, ACE inhibition is the most important intervention in the management of SRC treatment. Short-acting ACE inhibitors that can be easily titrated, such as captopril, should be started immediately on SRC diagnosis. Later, longer-acting agents may be substituted without loss of efficacy. The dose of the ACE inhibitor should be increased every 6 to 12 hours as needed to reduce the systolic blood pressure by about 10 to 20 mm Hg per day to achieve a normal blood pressure (about 120/70 mm Hg) within 48 to 72 hours (70). Although this control may be achieved with maximum ACE inhibition alone, other antihypertensives (calcium channel blockers, hydralazine, minoxidil) may be necessary while continuing the ACE inhibitor if this treatment does not normalize the blood pressure within 48 hours. Nitroprusside and lobetolol are not usually required as they may lead to arterial vasodilation with arterial underfilling resulting in further renal hypoperfusion (100). Excessive falls in blood pressure should be avoided and volume status should be monitored to maximize renal perfusion. For this reason, diuretic therapy is contraindicated. In the case of normotensive SRC, it is advised that the highest possible dose of ACE inhibitor be used that avoids hypotension. Other treatments such as corticosteroids, immunosuppressives, anticoagulation, and plasmapheresis have no role in the therapy of SRC. The use of angiotensin II receptor blockers (ARBs), such as losartan, or the combination of an ACE inhibitor with an ARB has not been extensively studied in SRC. Caskey et al. (101) reported the failure of losartan to control blood pressure in one patient with SRC. Although both ACE inhibitors and ARBs diminish the effects of angiotensin II, only ACE inhibitors increase levels of the potent renal vasodilator, bradykinin (102). Despite normalization of the blood pressure with ACE inhibition, the serum creatinine concentration may continue to rise for 7 to 10 days prior to returning toward normal. This rise in creatinine level usually is not attributable to ACE inhibitor therapy, which should be continued (70,72).

Factors associated with early death or dialysis in patients with SRC treated with ACE inhibitors include male sex, older age, congestive heart failure, inability to control blood pressure within 72 hours, and a pretreatment serum creatinine level of greater than 3 mg/dL (70). Renal replacement therapy, when needed, may take the form of either hemodialysis or continuous ambulatory peritoneal dialysis (CAPD). Although these interventions are successful in many patients with SSc, complications may occur more frequently than in end-stage renal failure patients without SSc. With hemodialysis, there may be difficulty fashioning and maintaining adequate vascular access and problems with hemodynamic instability. With CAPD, altered peritoneal permeability, caused by sclerosis, and diminished peritoneal blood flow, caused by underlying vasculopathy and vasospasm, may decrease effectiveness of this intervention (103). It should be reiterated that continuing ACE inhibition to avoid any hyperreninemia during renal replacement therapy appears to be of therapeutic importance. Steen and coworkers (87) described that by continuing ACE inhibitor therapy, patients surviving more than 3 months have a 55% chance of becoming independent of dialysis.

Renal transplantation should be considered in those patients with SRC who remain dependent on dialysis for greater than 18 to 24 months and in whom there are no disease-related contraindications such as significant pulmonary, cardiac, or intestinal involvement. Richardson (104) reported the first successful case of renal transplantation for SRC-induced renal failure in 1973. Subsequently, small numbers of other cases have been reported (105–107). Tsakiris et al. (106) reported graft survival greater than 50% at 1 year and 44% at 3 years in 28 patients with SSc who underwent renal transplantation between 1977 and 1993. Recently, Chang and Spiera (107) reported on 86 SSc renal transplant recipients who were monitored by the United Network for Organ Sharing (UNOS) Scientific Registry from 1987 through 1997. This study showed graft survival rates of 62%, 57%, and 47% at 1, 3, and 5 years, respectively. Unfortunately, data regarding characteristics of the patient population, length of time to graft failure, the cause of graft failure, and the immunosuppressive therapy regimen were lacking from this registry. In comparison, graft survival rates in patients with systemic lupus erythematosus (SLE) from the UNOS registry were 82%, 73%, and 62% at 1, 3, and 5 years, respectively (107). Similarly, Bleyer et al. (108), using the UNOS registry from 1987 through 1996, showed decreased patient and graft survival (84% and 72%, respectively) at 3 years in scleroderma patients in comparison to a reference condition, immunoglobulin A (IgA) nephropathy. The survival rate of patients with SSc on hemodialysis is approximately 35% to 40% at 3 to 5 years (88,106).

There have been several reports of a possible recurrence of SSc in renal allografts; however, the histologic changes suggesting recurrence are not easily differentiated from those found with chronic graft rejection or malignant hypertension in renal disease (103,105,107). In addition, the glomerular and vascular histologic abnormalities seen in cyclosporine-induced nephrotoxicity can appear similar to those seen in the scleroderma kidney (109). This observation and the known cyclosporine-related adverse effects of vasoconstriction and endothelial injury notwithstanding, it remains unclear whether cyclosporine increases the risk of recurrence of SSc in the allograft and whether SSc renal transplant recipients are more vulnerable to cyclosporine toxicity (110).

Conclusion

Systemic sclerosis is a disorder of unclear etiology that can vary widely in its severity. To date, no therapy, when tested in a prospective controlled fashion, has been shown to halt or reverse the vasculopathy or fibrotic process. The long-term hope is that further understanding of the pathophysiology of SSc will lead to a therapy that will arrest these processes. Current treatment is limited to those agents that may alleviate specific clinical manifestations (e.g., calcium channel blockers for Raynaud's phenomenon and potent antacids or proton-pump inhibitors for gastroesophageal reflux symptoms). Of such interventions, only the use of ACE inhibition for SRC has made a significant difference in the long-term outcome of this disorder. Although no study has been performed to address whether

"prophylactic" use of ACE inhibitors prevents SRC, it is recommended that even mild hypertension in a patient with SSc be treated with an ACE inhibitor, particularly if SRC risk factors are present. Diuretics should be avoided in the routine management of hypertension in patients with SSc because hypovolemia could potentially precipitate the onset of SRC.

RHEUMATOID ARTHRITIS

Rheumatoid arthritis (RA) is a chronic inflammatory disease of unknown etiology, characterized primarily by symmetric polyarthritis. Rheumatoid arthritis is also a systemic disease with extraarticular manifestations in up to 40% of patients, including constitutional symptoms, serositis, vasculitis, ocular involvement, rheumatoid nodules, pulmonary lesions, and cardiac disease (111). Rheumatoid arthritis is the most common of the inflammatory rheumatic diseases, with a prevalence of 1% and more than 3 million cases in the United States alone. This disease is more common in women by a ratio of 2.5:1 and can occur at any age, although the peak onset is in the fourth and fifth decades (112).

Renal involvement is generally considered to be quite rare, although RA is often characterized by the presence of rheumatoid factors and circulating immune complexes (113). Clinically, renal disease attributable to RA itself usually is mild and not a major problem in clinical management. However, studies showed that measurement of serum creatinine concentrations might underestimate renal impairment in patients with RA, possibly because of the decreased muscle mass of these patients (114,115). Furthermore, population-based studies have shown that patients with RA have an increased mortality relative to age-matched controls and that a significant proportion of this increased mortality can be attributed to renal disease (116,117). These studies suggest that a combination of insults to the kidneys over time in rheumatoid patients may contribute to renal compromise and make the kidneys more susceptible to subsequent diseases such as infection, hypertension, or atherosclerosis (116–119).

Two broad categories of renal disorders can be distinguished in RA: lesions caused by the disease itself and lesions occurring as a result of side effects of therapeutic agents. In Table 66-3 are listed the types of renal lesions that have been described in RA. It is often difficult to distinguish between disease-associated and drug-associated renal lesions because patients with RA are frequently treated with multiple drugs for many years. Many studies in the literature suffer from a failure to make this distinction. In addition, many studies from the 1940s and 1950s included a significant number of patients with other connective tissue diseases such as SLE in their series of patients with RA, thereby further confusing the definition of RA-associated renal

TABLE 66-3

RENAL INVOLVEMENT IN RHEUMATOID ARTHRITIS (RA)

Renal disorders related to RA
Amyloidosis
Glomerular lesions
Vascular lesions
Tubulointerstitial lesions
Renal disorders related to drug therapy
Nonsteroidal antiinflammatory drugs
Analgesics
Gold/penicillamine
Cyclosporine

disease. Nevertheless, substantial literature exists describing renal lesions in RA.

Renal Disorders Related to Rheumatoid Arthritis

Amyloidosis

Amyloidosis is a syndrome characterized by deposition of an insoluble proteinaceous material in the extracellular matrix of multiple organs. These deposits have a unique fibrillar ultrastructure characterized by a rigid, nonbranching filament of about 100 Å in diameter. Amyloidosis is generally classified according to the type of fibril deposited in tissue, being either secondary amyloidosis (AA amyloidosis) or primary amyloidosis associated with plasma cell dyscrasias (AL amyloidosis). Rheumatoid arthritis is one of a number of chronic inflammatory or neoplastic diseases that may eventually lead to secondary amyloidosis (AA amyloidosis). The initial manifestation of renal involvement in amyloidosis is proteinuria; it progresses at a variable rate and most patients eventually develop the nephrotic syndrome and/or uremia (Chapter 75).

The frequency with which amyloidosis is found at postmortem examination of patients with RA varies widely from 10% to 60%, although most authors report a prevalence of 10% to 20% (117,120–124). The reported frequency of amyloidosis is considerably lower in living patients. Using a Congo red stain on liver biopsies, Unger et al. (124) found amyloidosis in six of 56 patients with RA, all of whom had proteinuria. Fearnley and Lackner (122) surveyed 183 patients with RA, of whom 24 had persistent proteinuria. Eight of these patients were found to have amyloidosis, giving an overall prevalence of eight of 183, or 4%. Arapakis and Tribe (120) performed rectal biopsies on 115 patients with RA in search of amyloidosis; six patients were positive, only three of these patients had proteinuria. A recent study from Finland reported the prevalence of amyloidosis to be 5.8% in 1,666 patients with RA who died during 1989 (125). In this study, more than 90% of the cases of amyloidosis were diagnosed during life. Thus, although more frequent at autopsy, clinically significant amyloid renal disease may occur in only 3% to 6% of living patients with RA.

Amyloidosis is seen with increasing frequency in patients with long-standing RA (>10 years' duration) and is also more common in patients who are positive for rheumatoid factor (RF) and who have significant joint destruction (126). This observation implies that if arthritis is kept under good control, the frequency of secondary amyloidosis can be reduced. Parkins and Bywaters (127) described two patients in whom proteinuria and clinical renal disease improved when their arthritis went into remission, but renal disease recurred when the RA relapsed. Recently, Elkayam et al. (128) reported resolution of proteinuria and stabilization of amyloid deposits by serial ^{123}I-labeled serum amyloid P scintigraphy in a woman with rheumatoid arthritis of 10 years' duration and proteinuria (900 mg per 24 hours) treated with infliximab. Wright and Calkins (129), in a series of patients (1967 to 1979) in which management of RA was presumably more aggressive and more successful, reported a lower frequency of amyloidosis at autopsy (3.6%) than in earlier studies. These data are consistent with the hypothesis that aggressive management of active joint inflammation may decrease the frequency and severity of AA amyloidosis in patients with RA.

The clinical course of AA amyloidosis in patients with RA is usually one of progressive renal failure, as there are no satisfactory treatments aside from aggressive treatment of the underlying disorder. Cardiac involvement and serum creatinine level greater than 2.0 mg/dL at presentation appear to be poor prognostic factors (130). Patients with amyloidosis generally do poorly on dialysis, and recurrence of amyloid deposits has been reported in transplanted kidneys (131). However, because there are other causes of proteinuria in RA, the diagnosis of amyloidosis as a cause of clinical renal disease should be made only with biopsy confirmation and after other conditions have been excluded.

Glomerular Lesions

The existence of a glomerular lesion specific for RA has been debated for a number of years. Early studies reported nonspecific glomerulitis on kidney biopsy or autopsy and decreased renal function in 20% to 60% of patients with rheumatoid arthritis (132–139). However, a number of these patients may have had SLE, casting doubt on the conclusions of these studies. Subsequent studies have demonstrated either membranous or mesangial nephritis in some patients with RA (140–150). Membranous glomerulonephritis is almost always secondary to drug therapy with gold or penicillamine. A few cases of membranous glomerulonephritis occurring independent of drugs have been reported that present with mild proteinuria (140–143). Mesangial glomerulonephritis is common on renal biopsies from patients with RA (142–150). This lesion is characterized by increased mesangial matrix and/or hypercellularity and mesangial deposits of IgM, IgA, and C3 (146–150). Korpela et al. (147,150) have shown that 5% to 8% of patients with RA have histologic features of IgA nephropathy. However, whether this prevalence of IgA nephropathy is greater than that in the normal population is not clear.

Despite the findings of glomerulitis on renal biopsy, the clinical consequences of these lesions are minor. The most frequent manifestations of glomerulitis in RA are microscopic hematuria and low-grade proteinuria. Follow-up of these patients has shown a benign course, with progression to renal insufficiency and/or increasing of proteinuria occurring only rarely (145,146,148,149).

Proliferative glomerulonephritis is a rare cause of renal disease in RA. Davis et al. (151) reviewed the records of 5,232 patients with the diagnosis of RA who were hospitalized over a 22-year period. Proliferative glomerulonephritis was diagnosed in only four patients, most of whom met the criteria for SLE or mixed connective tissue disease. However, a well-documented case of proliferative glomerulonephritis in RA in the absence of any other disorder was reported (151). Although this patient was on gold therapy at the time of the renal biopsy, proteinuria and hematuria both preceded initiation of gold therapy. The renal biopsy showed mesangial hypercellularity along with proliferative changes in the glomeruli, and electron microscopy revealed subendothelial deposits. The authors raised the question as to why a proliferative glomerulonephritis is not seen more often in RA, because circulating immune complexes frequently are present in this disease. Weisman and Zvaifler (152) speculated that reduced complement-fixing ability of the immune complexes in RA might explain the paucity of renal lesions. However, the reason why immune complex nephritis is not seen more often in RA remains unclear (153).

Necrotizing glomerulonephritis complicating RA appears to be an uncommon entity. There are several reported cases of necrotizing glomerulonephritis occurring in RA associated with concurrent systemic vasculitis (154–156) and additional cases occurring in the absence of systemic vasculitis (156–159). Of interest, the majority of the renal biopsies from these cases revealed a pauci-immune necrotizing glomerulonephritis. Furthermore, the patients in the more recent case reports were perinuclear-ANCA (p-ANCA) positive (156,159). Although rare, p-ANCA positive pauci-immune necrotizing glomerulonephritis should be considered in all patients with RA and acute renal insufficiency with proteinuria and/or microscopic hematuria.

In summary, early studies describing a rheumatoid glomerulopathy are clouded by the inclusion of patients with diseases other than RA and by the inclusion of patients taking a variety of potentially nephrotoxic drugs. It appears that proliferative and necrotizing glomerulonephritis are extremely rare in RA, occurring only in isolated cases. A mild form of mesangial or membranous glomerulopathy does appear to occur in RA independent of drug therapy. Functionally, this disease is usually mild, presents with microscopic hematuria and low-grade proteinuria, and follows a benign course.

Vascular Lesions

Systemic vasculitis is the most feared of all the complications of RA and is associated with an appreciable morbidity and mortality. Schmid et al. (160) described 34 patients with RA and arteritis in whom extraarticular disease was present. The most common clinical symptoms were peripheral neuritis in 16 patients, episcleritis and pericarditis in five patients, and hypertension in four patients. Eight patients in their series were found to have proteinuria (24%), and this occurred in 43% of patients with extraarticular manifestations of RA summarized from the literature. No mention was made, however, of impaired renal function in any patient. Scott et al. (161) reviewed 50 cases of systemic rheumatoid vasculitis; 12 (24%) of their cases had clinical features of renal disease. Four patients had amyloidosis, two had chronic renal failure of undetermined cause, and six developed proteinuria or hematuria when typical lesions of cutaneous vasculitis appeared. Renal function was not impaired in these six patients.

There are, however, a few reports in which patients with RA developed a polyarteritis-like clinical syndrome with renal vessel involvement. A case report described a patient with rheumatoid vasculitis who presented with abdominal pain and had intrarenal aneurysms on arteriography (162). Ball (163) reported five cases of rheumatoid arthritis with diffuse vasculitis. Only one of the five patients had clinical renal involvement during life, but all had microscopic evidence of renal artery vasculitis.

Tubulointerstitial Lesions

Tubulointerstitial disease of the kidneys is common in RA. However, the primary cause of these changes is Sjögren's syndrome, which is seen as a secondary manifestation in up to 35% of RA patients. The renal lesions of Sjögren's syndrome are discussed elsewhere in this chapter. Another major cause of tubulointerstitial disease in RA is the use of NSAIDs. Although interstitial nephritis may occur with any of these agents, it appears to be most frequently associated with fenoprofen. Investigators examining renal changes in biopsy or autopsy specimens described some degree of interstitial fibrosis in 20% to 46% of rheumatoid patients (164,165). However, none of these studies excluded patients taking NSAIDs or patients with Sjögren's syndrome. It is, therefore, unclear as to whether RA itself causes a tubulointerstitial lesion distinct from that associated with medications or Sjögren's syndrome.

Renal Disorders Related to Drug Therapy

Nonsteroidal Antiinflammatory Drugs and Salicylates

Nonsteroidal antiinflammatory drugs (NSAIDs) are widely used in the treatment of RA. The antiinflammatory properties of these drugs result, in part, from their ability to inhibit cyclooxygenase, one of the major enzymes involved in the synthesis of prostaglandins. Inhibition of renal prostaglandin synthesis by NSAIDs may result in reduced glomerular blood flow and elevation of serum creatinine levels (166,167) (discussed in more detail in Chapter 44). In addition to this reversible rise in serum creatinine, NSAIDs also can cause an interstitial nephritis. Interstitial nephritis has also been shown to be reversible when the drugs are discontinued (Chapter 44). Although all NSAIDs and salicylates (168) can induce a rise in serum creatinine and/or an interstitial nephritis, there is some evidence that sulindac may result in a less severe decrease in renal blood flow than may occur with other NSAIDs (169–171). However, this point is controversial and may depend on the duration of therapy and severity of any underlying renal or liver disease (172). All NSAIDs should be regarded as potential inducers of renal dysfunction. The selective cyclooxygenase-2 inhibitors have the same risk for adverse effects on renal function, as do other NSAIDs (167). As mentioned, the use of NSAIDs has made analysis of renal lesions in RA more difficult to interpret. Practically, when a patient with RA presents with evidence of decreased renal function or interstitial changes, discontinuation of NSAIDs should be one of the first steps before further diagnostic or therapeutic maneuvers are undertaken.

Analgesic Nephropathy

Analgesic nephropathy is characterized by a combination of papillary necrosis and interstitial nephritis (Chapter 44). This type of injury is most widely attributed to phenacetin but may also be seen with NSAIDs (173,174). Rare cases of papillary necrosis have been reported in association with ibuprofen, phenylbutazone, fenoprofen, naproxen, and mefenamic acid, as well as with several combinations of NSAIDs. The risk of rheumatoid patients developing analgesic nephropathy appears to be lower than would be expected on the basis of their regular consumption of NSAIDs (116). This observation may be due to less frequent use of analgesic combinations or to closer physician monitoring. However, the frequency of subclinical renal disorders in patients with RA should raise the possibility that chronic NSAID therapy may cause some additional degree of renal damage.

Renal Lesions Associated with Gold Therapy

Gold salts have been advocated for the treatment of many diseases including pulmonary tuberculosis. In the belief that tuberculosis and RA had a common infectious etiology, Forestier in 1935 first described the use of gold salts in the treatment of RA (175). He noted improvement in 70% to 80% of more than 500 cases, a finding that has been confirmed in multiple studies since that time. With the availability of newer effective therapies, gold treatment is used less often in selected patients with RA, psoriatic arthritis, or juvenile chronic arthritis. It is referred to as a "disease-modifying antirheumatic drug," or DMARD, because some studies have shown healing of bone erosions after its use (176). The clinical effects of weekly gold injections do not develop until after 3 to 6 months of therapy, and the patient must receive maintenance monthly injections for years. Recent studies have shown that relatively few patients are able to remain on gold therapy for the long term, however, owing to the cumulative incidence of side effects, including nephropathy, bone marrow suppression, rash, and stomatitis. An oral form of gold (auranofin) introduced in the early 1980s has a lower incidence of serious toxicity than parenteral gold but is less effective (177,178).

Clinically, the hallmark of renal toxicity from gold is proteinuria, occurring in 3% to 10% of RA patients receiving gold injections (177,179–183). Although microscopic hematuria can accompany proteinuria, isolated hematuria or the appearance of cellular casts is rare and should prompt an investigation into other causes of renal disease. Nephrotic syndrome develops in up to one-third of patients with gold-induced proteinuria (116). The onset of proteinuria is most common 4 to 6 months after the initiation of gold therapy (total dose 1,000 to 1,500 mg at 50 mg/week), although it may occur at any time during therapy. Furthermore, the severity of proteinuria is not proportional to the dose of gold received. The frequency of proteinuria in patients receiving oral gold (auranofin) appears to be very similar to the frequency in those patients receiving injectable gold (177).

Hall et al. have extensively studied the natural history of gold nephropathy (184–187); the proteinuria resolves gradually with discontinuation of gold. Proteinuria resolved completely by 21 months in all 21 patients studied, with the mean time to resolution of proteinuria being 11 months (185). In those patients who developed the nephrotic syndrome, treatment with a high-protein diet and diuretics was sufficient to control symptoms; steroids were not required. No changes in creatinine clearance were observed in any patient during or after the resolution of proteinuria. Despite these reports, high-dose glucocorticoid therapy (prednisone 60 mg daily) may be beneficial in gold-induced nephrotic syndrome. Hall and Tighe (187) examined the outcome of nephropathy when gold was continued after the onset of proteinuria. Follow-up of these patients indicated an identical pattern of resolution of renal disease even when discontinuation of gold was delayed for up to 11 months after the onset of proteinuria. Indeed, a number of reports suggest that the continuation of gold after proteinuria develops does not necessarily lead to progressive proteinuria and renal deterioration. Klinkhoff and Teufel (188) successfully reinstituted parenteral gold therapy at a lower dose in five of eight patients with gold-induced proteinuria once their proteinuria had resolved (4 to 12 months). However, because nephrotic syndrome and renal failure can occur, it is recommended that gold therapy be discontinued if progressive proteinuria develops because a number of alternative DMARDs that are not nephrotoxic are now available for the treatment of RA.

The renal histology associated with gold-induced proteinuria and the nephrotic syndrome is membranous glomerulopathy. Light microscopy shows basement membrane thickening, and electron microscopy shows subepithelial deposits (189–191). When proteinuria is of short duration, the only changes noted are subepithelial deposits on electron microscopy. Basement membrane thickening can be detected on light microscopy with long-standing disease. Light and electron microscopy revealed no correlation between the site or degree of deposition of gold particles in the kidney and the presence of proteinuria. These observations suggest that gold nephropathy is an immune complex disease, although the inciting antigen remains unknown.

Wooley et al. (192) have offered a potential explanation for the finding of proteinuria in only some patients with RA receiving gold. They found that 14 of 15 episodes of gold-induced proteinuria occurred in patients who possessed the HLA antigens B8 and DR3. The relative risk of proteinuria during gold therapy was increased 32 times in patients with the DR3 antigen. An increased frequency of an extended haplotype containing a specific *DQA1* allele (as well as DR3 and DR5) has been found in patients with gold nephropathy (193).

In summary, it appears that gold-induced glomerulopathy is mediated by immune complexes and is more prevalent in those patients with a specific genetic background that predisposes them to the development of autoantibodies. The association of gold-induced nephropathy with the B8/DR3 haplotype may also help to explain the predilection of patients with gold nephropathy to develop renal disease when treated subsequently with penicillamine because penicillamine nephrotoxicity is associated with the same haplotype (see the following section). However, the risk of developing gold nephropathy in patients with the B8/DR3 or DQA extended haplotype does

not merit HLA typing in rheumatoid patients before instituting gold therapy.

Renal Lesions Associated with Methotrexate and Other DMARD Therapy

Methotrexate is a folic acid antagonist that has become the major DMARD used in the treatment of RA over the last two decades. Although high-dose methotrexate used in the treatment of neoplasia has been associated with renal failure, renal failure associated with the low doses of methotrexate (5 to 25 mg/week) used to treat RA is extremely rare. It was shown, however, in 13 patients with RA that doses of 15 mg/week of methotrexate reduced glomerular filtration rate (GFR) by an average of 10% (194). Renal impairment can increase the risk of side effects of low-dose weekly methotrexate therapy, particularly respiratory and hematologic toxicities (195). Bressolle et al. (196,197) have shown in patients with RA that methotrexate clearance decreases with decreasing GFR. These authors suggest a 50% dose reduction of methotrexate in patients with a GFR of less than 45 mL/minute (197). Methotrexate therapy should be avoided in patients with severe renal dysfunction. Renal function should be monitored periodically in patients taking the drug, particularly in those patients with preexisting renal insufficiency, because methotrexate is primarily excreted unchanged in the urine. Other commonly used DMARDs such as antimalarials, azathioprine, leflunomide, sulfasalazine, and the newer biologic agents etanercept and infliximab appear to have little or no renal toxicity (198).

Renal Lesions Associated with Penicillamine Therapy

Penicillamine was introduced into clinical medicine in the 1950s for the treatment of Wilson's disease (199). Within a few years it had been tried in RA, and it became accepted as a disease-modifying drug in the 1970s. However, the use of penicillamine has declined because of the recent addition of a number of other less toxic DMARDs to treat RA. It is a slow-acting drug with responses generally not observed until after 3 to 6 months of therapy (200–202).

Clinically and histologically, penicillamine-induced nephropathy is similar to gold nephropathy. The initial clinical manifestation is hematuria or proteinuria, occurring in 5% to 30% of patients receiving penicillamine. Nephrotic syndrome occurs in one-third to two-thirds of patients who develop proteinuria (186,200–204). The onset of proteinuria is usually within the first 12 months of therapy (average, 8 months), but it may occur at any time. Initial studies using high doses of penicillamine (>1,000 mg/day) indicated a rapid onset of proteinuria with a higher frequency of this complication (200,201,203). With newer treatment regimens starting therapy at lower doses, toxicity has decreased but proteinuria has been reported at doses as low as 125 mg per day. Penicillamine-induced proteinuria resolves spontaneously after the discontinuation of penicillamine, with a mean time to resolution being 8 months (range, 1 to 21 months) (184,186). No patients demonstrated changes in creatinine clearance owing to penicillamine, and no patients required steroid therapy. Continuation of penicillamine after the onset of proteinuria has been shown to have a benign outcome, similar to gold (187). Several investigators have advocated that penicillamine can be continued in patients with proteinuria if renal function is closely monitored. However, as with gold therapy, this usage rarely seems justified in light of other agents presently available for the treatment of RA.

Histologically, penicillamine-induced renal lesions appear similar to those of gold-induced nephropathy. In the studies by Hall et al. (184,185), 29 of 33 patients with proteinuria secondary to penicillamine had membranous glomerulonephritis,

2 of 33 had minimal change nephropathy, and 2 of 33 patients had only mesangial changes. Studies by Dische et al. (205) showed glomerular capillary wall thickening and increased mesangial matrix, with electron microscopy revealing subepithelial deposits, similar to gold-induced nephropathy or idiopathic membranous glomerulonephritis. The possible genetic predisposition to membranous glomerulopathy seen with gold therapy is also present with penicillamine (192). Penicillamine-induced rapidly progressive MPO-ANCA-positive crescentic glomerulonephritis that requires aggressive immunosuppressive therapy is a rare occurrence (74,206).

Cyclosporine

Cyclosporine is an immunosuppressive agent that primarily affects T cells and has been used for a number of years in transplantation medicine to prevent allograft rejection (207). A number of studies have shown that cyclosporine may be beneficial in refractory RA (208–211). It has also been used to treat other rheumatic diseases such as refractory psoriatic arthritis and polymyositis-dermatomyositis. However, cyclosporine should be reserved for those patients who have not responded to more conventional therapy owing to its potential renal and hypertensive toxicities. The major factor preventing more widespread trials of cyclosporine in RA has been nephrotoxicity, which has been reported to occur in 30% to 70% of patients receiving this drug (207,212–214). The mechanism of cyclosporine nephrotoxicity is not clear but appears to be primarily vascular, resulting in decreased GFR, decreased creatinine clearance, increased serum creatinine, hypertension, and hyperkalemia (207,215). The severity and frequency with which nephrotoxicity occurs are directly related to the dose of cyclosporine administered. Gordon et al. (216) reported that in renal transplantation patients, nephrotoxicity correlated best with trough serum levels of cyclosporine. Patients displaying cyclosporine nephrotoxicity showed trough serum levels of greater than 200 ng/mL; 96% of patients who developed impaired renal function owing to cyclosporine had trough serum levels greater than or equal to 250 ng/mL.

Treatment regimens employing cyclosporine at 2.5 to 10.0 mg/kg per day have been investigated in RA. Berg et al. (212) showed that patients receiving 5 mg/kg per day had a mean increase in serum creatinine of 19.7% and a decrease in creatinine clearance of 22%. Patients receiving 10 mg/kg per day had a mean increase in serum creatinine of 59.5%. Of note is that patients taking NSAIDs with cyclosporine demonstrated increased serum creatinine levels of only 16.6%. Renal dysfunction usually occurred within 2 to 3 weeks after the initiation of cyclosporine therapy and remained stable during the full course of treatment. After discontinuation of therapy, serum creatinine levels improved but remained slightly higher than baseline for up to 12 weeks. Boers et al. (217) demonstrated that renal function remained stable for up to 2 years after discontinuation of the drug; no improvement was noted in those patients who had developed renal impairment, but no further deterioration occurred. In a study by the International Kidney Biopsy Registry, cyclosporine nephropathy was rare in patients who did not take a daily dose in excess of 5 mg/kg per day (218,219). Renal biopsies of RA patients on cyclosporine have shown only minimal changes (tubular atrophy and interstitial fibrosis) (219,220).

In summary, cyclosporine is still an experimental drug in refractory RA. If prescribed, it should be used at a low initial dosage (2.5 to 3.5 mg/kg), and the maximum dose should not exceed 5 mg/kg per day (218,221–223). The maximum dose of the oral cyclosporine preparation Neoral should not exceed 4 mg/kg per day (223). Plasma creatinine levels should be closely monitored throughout the course of therapy. Cyclosporine dosage should be decreased if serum creatinine levels increase by greater than 30% above baseline. Concurrent use of NSAIDs should be discouraged because this may exacerbate nephrotoxicity. Cyclosporine should be used with extreme caution in older patients with RA or in patients with preexisting hypertension or renal disease. Adjustment of cyclosporine dosage based on serum creatinine levels is mandatory to minimize renal toxicity. The need to monitor trough plasma cyclosporine levels at these doses is controversial.

Renal Disease in Juvenile Chronic Arthritis

Juvenile chronic arthritis (JCA), also called juvenile rheumatoid arthritis (JRA), is defined as an inflammatory arthropathy occurring in individuals less than 16 years old. JCA can be divided into three types: (a) polyarticular (five or more joints), which resembles adult RA; (b) oligoarticular (four or fewer joints), which primarily affects young females and is associated with antinuclear antibodies and chronic iritis; and (c) systemic onset disease (Still's disease), characterized by arthritis, fever, rheumatoid rash, leukocytosis, splenomegaly, and serositis. Clinically significant renal disease in children with any of the forms of JCA is rare, although as in adults, proteinuria, hematuria, and amyloidosis have been reported. Studies in children have the same problems as studies in adults with RA; frequently the effects of drug therapy cannot be separated from the spontaneous variations of the disease itself.

Anttila (224) studied 165 children with JCA treated in Finland between 1967 and 1970. Proteinuria was observed in 42.5% of the children on at least one occasion during the 3-year period. Persistent proteinuria, however, occurred in only 2.4% of the total patient population. None of the children developed the nephrotic syndrome, although on renal biopsy two patients were found to have amyloidosis as a cause of proteinuria. Hematuria was found in 38 patients with JCA (23%). Seven of these children had two or more episodes of hematuria, whereas 31 had only one episode. Of the seven patients with JCA with more than one episode of hematuria, amyloidosis was present in two patients and coagulopathy in one, with four patients receiving treatment with gold. Repeated episodes of pyuria occurred in 10 children, or 6% of the patients with JCA. Creatinine clearance was diminished in 5.6% of the group who exhibited only joint symptoms and in 18.5% of the group who demonstrated extraarticular manifestations of JCA. Creatinine clearance was more often depressed in patients receiving salicylate therapy.

Renal biopsies were performed on 57 of the 165 patients with JCA, and autopsy specimens were obtained from three patients (224). Amyloidosis was observed in one biopsy and one autopsy specimen. Except for proteinuria, hematuria, and pyuria, amyloidosis had not caused major impairment of renal function. Glomerular changes were observed in 28% of the cases. In 13 cases it was described as a "local glomerulitis," which would now be described as mesangial changes. Twelve of these 13 patients with JCA had proteinuria and/or hematuria. Other renal biopsy changes included mild basement membrane thickening in 4 patients and interstitial changes in 8 patients. No vascular abnormalities were noted in any biopsy. Overall, approximately 40% of JCA patients in this study had an abnormal kidney biopsy, although renal function was not significantly compromised in any patient.

Amyloidosis in JCA is the subject of many reports (225–231). Of 1,272 patients with JCA, Schnitzer and Ansell (226) observed 51 who had developed amyloidosis, a cumulative incidence of 4%. A large amount of geographic variation in the incidence of amyloidosis in JCA has been reported. In North America, the frequency is estimated to be as low as 0.1%, compared to 0.25% in France, 3% in Germany, and up to 10% in Poland (225,227). Because of the poor prognosis of amyloidosis associated with JCA, Schnitzer and Ansell initiated therapy with chlorambucil in selected patients in 1967. An 8-year survival rate of 80% was reported for those patients given chlorambucil, as compared to 55% to 60% for those patients receiving intermittent or no chlorambucil therapy. Several studies since that time have indicated that chlorambucil can improve survival and decrease renal disease in a significant percentage of these patients (225,229–231). In a study by Deschénes et al. (225), 8 patients with JCA and systemic amyloidosis were treated with chlorambucil. After a mean 10-year follow-up period, one patient had died from renal disease, two had persistent nephrotic syndrome, and five were free of proteinuria or renal disease. It is of interest that the three patients who did poorly all had persistent activity of their arthritis, suggesting, as has been the experience in adult RA, that control of joint inflammation in JCA can improve renal amyloidosis. A retrospective study of 79 JCA patients with amyloidosis revealed a 10-year survival rate of 80% in those patients treated with chlorambucil compared to 23.5% in patients not treated with chlorambucil (229). In this study, the cause of death was renal failure in 82% and infection in 12% of patients. Serious side effects of chlorambucil therapy include leukopenia, thrombocytopenia, acute leukemia, and infections.

In 1985, Stapleton et al. (232) described 2 patients with JCA who had hematuria, hypercalciuria, and urolithiasis. They subsequently studied 38 children with JCA and found increased urinary calcium-creatinine ratios in 12 (32%). Six of the 12 patients with hypercalciuria had hematuria, compared to three of the 26-normocalciuric patients. Detailed studies of calcium metabolism in four of the hypercalciuric patients showed normal serum calcium levels, normal parathyroid function, and no evidence of acidosis or vitamin D abnormalities. The authors speculated that the hypercalciuria in JCA might result from immobilization and bone demineralization rather than renal calcium wasting. In an earlier paper, Lorenz and Schneider (233) reported kidney stone formation in six of 89 German children with JCA. Taken together, these reports suggest that hypercalciuria should be considered in the evaluation of children with JCA and that such children may be at risk for developing urolithiasis.

In conclusion, clinically significant renal disease in JCA is uncommon. Reports of frequent proteinuria, hematuria, and mesangial nephropathy are clouded by the inclusion of patients taking a variety of potentially nephrotoxic drugs. Although a few cases of crescentic glomerulonephritis in patients with JCA have been reported, a direct association has not been established (234,235). Renal amyloidosis can occur in JCA in frequencies ranging from as low as 0.1% in North America to 3% to 10% in Europe. There is some evidence that aggressive control of the inflammatory arthritis in patients with amyloidosis can improve outcome. Finally, children with JCA may become hypercalciuric and be at risk for the development of renal stones.

SJÖGREN'S SYNDROME

Sjögren's syndrome is a chronic systemic autoimmune disease characterized by the infiltration of lymphocytes into multiple organs, primarily the exocrine glands (236,237). The salivary and lacrimal glands are most frequently involved, resulting in the clinical symptoms of dry eyes (keratoconjunctivitis sicca) and dry mouth (xerostomia). The presence of these two symptoms together is known as the sicca complex. Although dry eyes and dry mouth are the major features of Sjögren's syndrome, in up to one-fourth of patients other organs also may be affected by the systemic autoimmune process including the lungs, gastrointestinal tract, pancreas, liver, central nervous system, and kidneys. Histologically, the salivary glands are infiltrated with

CD4+ T cells and B cells with the salivary epithelial cells expressing high levels of HLA-DR. This and other findings have led to the hypothesis that Sjögren's syndrome may be triggered by an immune response to foreign antigens or altered self-antigens in the exocrine glands (237). Rarely, the lymphoid infiltrates may distort the normal architecture of the organ or of lymph nodes, resulting in a syndrome known as pseudolymphoma (238). When this occurs, the distinction between benign and malignant tissue lesions can be difficult. Patients with Sjögren's syndrome have a 44-fold higher risk for the development of non-Hodgkin B-cell lymphomas in comparison to age- and sex-matched control subjects.

In addition to the local cellular immune response, Sjögren's syndrome is characterized by the presence of autoantibodies to tissue-specific antigens (salivary duct antibodies) and to non–tissue-specific antigens, represented by ANA and RF. Antibodies to two nuclear antigens, SS-A and SS-B, are particularly characteristic of this disease, although they also may be found in other autoimmune diseases, including SLE. Patients with Sjögren's syndrome frequently develop hypergammaglobulinemia and mild anemia indicative of a generalized inflammatory state (237).

Sjögren's syndrome can be broadly divided into two categories. Primary Sjögren's syndrome is diagnosed when the symptom complex exists in the absence of another autoimmune disease. Secondary Sjögren's syndrome can occur in primary biliary cirrhosis or in conjunction with another autoimmune disease such as RA, SLE, or scleroderma. Sjögren's syndrome has been reported to occur in up to 35% of patients with RA and is frequently seen in patients with SLE, mixed connective tissue disease, or SSc. In these diseases, the presence of Sjögren's syndrome is considered to be an additional feature of the underlying autoimmune disease process.

Renal Abnormalities in Sjögren's Syndrome

The renal abnormalities in Sjögren's syndrome arise as a result of either lymphocytic infiltration into the renal parenchyma or immune-complex deposition in the glomeruli (Table 66-4). The renal abnormalities owing to secondary Sjögren's syndrome are often minor in comparison to the renal abnormalities caused by the primary rheumatic disease such as SLE or SSc. For this reason, the following discussion will focus on the renal abnormalities seen in primary Sjögren's syndrome. There is no evidence, however, that the renal abnormalities caused by primary Sjögren's syndrome differ in any way from those of secondary Sjögren's syndrome. It must also be noted that many patients with Sjögren's syndrome are taking medications such as NSAIDs that may further contribute to renal pathology.

Tubular Dysfunction

Histologic studies of the kidneys in patients with Sjögren's syndrome have demonstrated mild to moderate interstitial infiltration of lymphocytes, with varying degrees of tubular

TABLE 66-4

RENAL ABNORMALITIES IN SJÖGREN'S SYNDROME

Tubulointerstitial disease
Hyposthenuria
Renal tubular acidosis
Fanconi's syndrome
Interstitial nephritis
Glomerulonephritis

atrophy and interstitial fibrosis (239). Immunofluorescence studies of the infiltrating cells have indicated that they are CD4+ T and B cells, a pattern identical to that seen in the exocrine glands (240,241). This type of cellular infiltration is different from that seen in many other forms of interstitial nephritis in which cytotoxic T cells are the predominant cell type (240). This finding has led several authors to postulate that the pathogenesis of renal disease in Sjögren's syndrome is similar to that seen in the salivary glands and arises as a direct result of lymphocytic infiltration into the renal interstitium. The frequency with which lymphocytic infiltrates occur in the kidney in Sjögren's syndrome has not been extensively examined. Tu et al. (239) studied nine patients with Sjögren's syndrome and found interstitial changes in six patients. There are numerous other small series of patients with Sjögren's syndrome and abnormal findings on renal biopsy. Although the presence of interstitial infiltrates appears to be common, the exact frequency cannot be determined from the present literature.

Clinically, renal dysfunction in Sjögren's syndrome is usually mild and subclinical. The most frequently reported functional abnormalities are hyposthenuria, renal tubular acidosis (RTA), Fanconi's syndrome, and interstitial nephritis.

Hyposthenuria. In 1962, a patient with Sjögren's syndrome who had nephrogenic diabetes insipidus was reported. Detailed studies on eight additional patients demonstrated that four demonstrated a persistently impaired ability to concentrate urine with water deprivation (242). This defect was not associated with proteinuria or other clinically apparent renal abnormalities. In 1965, Shearn and Tu (243) reported a case of a young woman whose presenting manifestation of Sjögren's syndrome was vasopressin-resistant nephrogenic diabetes insipidus. Her polydipsia and polyuria antedated the symptoms of dryness of the eyes and mouth by 10 years. Although hyposthenuria may exist as an isolated abnormality in Sjögren's syndrome, in many of the reported cases it has been associated with other tubular abnormalities including RTA and aminoaciduria.

Renal Tubular Acidosis. Distal RTA (type I) has been reported to occur in up to 20% to 25% of patients with Sjögren's syndrome (244), and proximal RTA (type II) can also occur (although less frequently). Shearn and Tu (245) used an acid-loading test to detect latent RTA in 10 patients with Sjögren's syndrome who lacked overt abnormalities of acid–base balance. They found impairment of acid excretion in three of the 10 patients studied. Many of these patients also demonstrated a defect in renal concentrating ability. Urinary acidification was impaired in six of 12 patients with Sjögren's syndrome studied by Talal et al. (246). The RTA was clinically evident in three patients, subclinical in two, and associated with glomerulonephritis in one patient. Creatinine clearance was not altered in those patients with RTA. Distal tubular acidosis can be associated with hypocitraturia, renal stones, nephrocalcinosis, and rare cases of osteomalacia. Hypokalemic paralysis and respiratory arrest owing to distal RTA in patients with Sjögren's syndrome have been reported (247–249).

Two studies have examined Sjögren's syndrome patients for the presence of renal tubular acidification defects by ammonium chloride loading (250,251). Shiozawa et al. (250) showed that six of 17 patients with Sjögren's syndrome had abnormal urine acidification, and a higher incidence of abnormal concentrating ability, although this defect was not clinically evident. In this study, the presence of RTA and abnormal concentrating ability did not necessarily correlate with one another, suggesting that Sjögren's syndrome may affect tubular function at multiple functional and anatomic sites.

Hypergammaglobulinemia, which is common in Sjögren's syndrome, has also been associated with RTA (252–255). It is unlikely, however, that the development of RTA in Sjögren's syndrome is simply due to the associated hypergammaglobulinemia. Tubular dysfunction can occur in the absence of hypergammaglobulinemia, and tubular dysfunction is frequently not present despite significant degrees of hypergammaglobulinemia (254,256).

Other Tubular Defects. Fanconi's syndrome (aminoaciduria, glycosuria, and phosphaturia) has been reported in several patients with Sjögren's syndrome (257), although it appears to be uncommon. In Shiozawa's study (250), six of 17 patients with Sjögren's syndrome showed decreased tubular reabsorption of phosphate.

Interstitial Nephritis. Although infiltration of the interstitium with lymphocytes is common in Sjögren's syndrome, severe interstitial nephritis resulting in impaired creatinine clearance is relatively rare. Gentric et al. (258) reported five patients with primary Sjögren's syndrome who developed severe interstitial nephritis with decreased creatinine clearance, proteinuria, and hematuria. Two patients eventually required chronic hemodialysis, but three patients improved after taking corticosteroids. Other cases of this unusual complication of Sjögren's syndrome have recently been summarized (259,260).

Glomerulonephritis

Glomerulonephritis is rare in patients with primary Sjögren's syndrome, with only scattered cases reported in the literature (261–264). The histologic types of glomerulonephritis are usually membranoproliferative, mesangial, or membranous. These patients may present with heavy proteinuria, active urinary sediment, or renal insufficiency. Renal biopsy specimens in patients with Sjögren's-associated glomerulonephritis have shown glomerular deposits of immunoglobulins and C3 on immunofluorescence studies (262,263). It is hypothesized that the pathogenesis is most likely due to deposition of immune complexes formed by cryoprecipitable monoclonal IgM RF along with polyclonal IgG and IgA (263). Cryoglobulinemia, associated with hypocomplementemia, is often found in these patients. There may be a correlation between glomerulonephritis and the development of lymphoma (263). Treatment of the glomerulonephritis with corticosteroids and cytotoxic drugs has been reported to be successful in some patients (261,263). Rare cases of ANCA-positive crescentic glomerulonephritis in patients with primary Sjögren's syndrome have been reported (265).

In summary, some form of renal involvement can occur in 30% to 50% of patients with Sjögren's syndrome. Inability to concentrate the urine, RTA, and other tubular dysfunctions can be demonstrated frequently with stress testing. However, clinically significant tubular dysfunction appears to be unusual in Sjögren's syndrome and severe interstitial nephritis resulting in renal insufficiency is rare. Glomerulonephritis is distinctly unusual. Drug-induced renal abnormalities always should be considered in these patients (see section on Rheumatoid Arthritis), because many patients with Sjögren's syndrome are treated with NSAIDs and other drugs.

POLYMYOSITIS-DERMATOMYOSITIS

The inflammatory myopathies are a heterogeneous group of diseases in which the muscles are diffusely damaged by an endomysial and occasional perivascular infiltration of inflammatory cells, which are predominantly lymphocytes (266). The clinical syndrome associated with these pathologic changes is termed *polymyositis*. Although this syndrome is frequently pleomorphic in presentation, the cardinal feature in essentially all patients (98%) is muscle weakness. When the syndrome occurs in association with characteristic skin lesions it is termed *dermatomyositis*.

Five clinical or laboratory abnormalities are present in most patients with polymyositis and dermatomyositis and thus are used to define or diagnose the disease (267). The first criterion is symmetric proximal muscle weakness, which is the initial manifestation in up to 69% of patients and is present overall in 98% at some time during the course of the disease. The second criterion is abnormal myopathic electromyographic findings, present in 90% of patients. The third criterion is elevated serum muscle enzymes (creatine kinase, aldolase), found in 95% of patients with myositis. The fourth criterion is the muscle biopsy, which should show evidence of necrosis of type 1 and 2 muscle fibers, areas of degeneration and regeneration of fibers, phagocytosis, and an interstitial or perivascular inflammatory process. The fifth criterion consists of the characteristic skin changes seen in dermatomyositis. These skin lesions include: an erythematous, scaly rash over the face, neck, and shawl area, as well as the extensor surfaces of the knees, elbows, and medial malleoli; a heliotrope rash (a periorbital violaceous discoloration, often with associated edema); and Gottron's papules (scaly erythematous flat plaques over the dorsum of the metacarpophalangeal and proximal interphalangeal joints).

Although a number of different classification schemes of polymyositis-dermatomyositis have been suggested, the scheme proposed by Bohan and Peter and Bohan et al. (267,268) is the most widely used (Table 66-5).

Organ systems other than skin and muscle may be involved in patients with polymyositis or dermatomyositis (266). This is true even when those patients with overlap syndrome (Group V) are excluded. The more common organ systems involved include the joints, with up to 35% of patients experiencing arthralgias. Synovitis can occur but is uncommon. Gastrointestinal manifestations are also common, with involvement of both the proximal and distal esophagus in adults and abdominal crisis secondary to vasculitis sometimes seen in children (266–268). Pulmonary involvement may be found in up to 50% of patients with polymyositis or dermatomyositis, with interstitial lung disease being the most common abnormality (269). Rare cardiac manifestations include electrocardiographic abnormalities and cardiomyopathy.

Renal Disease

Involvement of the kidneys in polymyositis-dermatomyositis is distinctly uncommon and in fact is not mentioned in some reviews or chapters on polymyositis-dermatomyositis in standard textbooks. Early references to renal disease with dermato-

myositis have included patients who would now be classified as having mixed connective tissue disease, including SLE or scleroderma in association with myositis (270,271). Dyck et al. (272) identified five patients with primary idiopathic polymyositis who developed proteinuria associated with urinary sediment abnormalities. Renal biopsies from these patients showed a focal mesangial proliferative glomerulonephritis with deposits of both immunoglobulin and complement. After treatment of the polymyositis with corticosteroids, the proteinuria and urinary sediment changes disappeared as the muscle disease improved. These authors speculated that immune complexes might be implicated in the etiology of this renal disease, although results of serum complement studies and serum cryoglobulins were normal in all patients except one. Other rare cases of mesangial and membranous glomerulonephritis have been reported in patients with polymyositis and dermatomyositis (273–276).

Membranous glomerulopathy is reported in up to 10% of all malignancies (277). A case report by Rose (278) describes a 58-year-old woman who presented with the nephrotic syndrome with renal biopsy features of membranous glomerulopathy who subsequently developed dermatomyositis and shortly thereafter an oat cell tumor in her lung. The relationship between these three conditions is unclear, although some interesting speculations are possible. Membranous nephropathy is thought to be an immune complex disease, which in this case may have resulted from the deposition of immune complexes induced by the tumor. Similarly, dermatomyositis is known to exhibit both humoral and cell-mediated abnormalities. Therefore, membranous glomerulonephritis may be seen in conjunction with polymyositis-dermatomyositis because both disorders may be associated with an underlying neoplasm (Group III).

Myoglobinemia and myoglobinuria may be present in up to 50% of patients with dermatomyositis and polymyositis (279). The degree of myoglobinuria is usually mild except in acute, severe disease. Myoglobinuric acute renal failure has been reported in a few cases of polymyositis (280–283).

Childhood dermatomyositis (Group IV) is frequently associated with vasculitis involving the muscles and gastrointestinal tract. Bitnum et al. (284) studied 13 children with dermatomyositis and performed percutaneous renal biopsy in six of these children because of proteinuria. All six of the biopsies were abnormal, showing mild to moderate cellular proliferation of the glomerular tuft. The glomerular basement membrane also was thickened in two patients. The authors were unsure of the implications of their findings but did note that none of the patients developed signs of clinical renal failure. Others investigators have also described diffuse glomerular changes in patients with juvenile dermatomyositis (285). As in the study by Bitnum et al. (284), these authors also found that renal function was maintained, although proteinuria was present in the children.

In summary, renal involvement in polymyositis-dermatomyositis is distinctly uncommon. It may occur in the setting of another connective tissue disease (Group V) in which the renal lesion is found to be that of either SSc or SLE. Membranous glomerulonephritis may occur in association with malignancy (Group III). In acute fulminant myositis, tubular dysfunction or acute renal failure may be associated with myoglobinemia and myoglobinuria. This usually responds to treatment of the myositis and progression to chronic renal failure is rare.

TABLE 66-5

CLASSIFICATION OF POLYMYOSITIS/DERMATOMYOSITIS

Group I	Primary idiopathic polymyositis
Group II	Primary idiopathic dermatomyositis
Group III	Dermatomyositis or polymyositis associated with malignancy
Group IV	Childhood dermatomyositis or polymyositis often associated with vasculitis
Group V	Dermatomyositis or polymyositis associated with another connective tissue disease

References

1. Osler W. On diffuse scleroderma: with special reference to diagnosis and use of thyroid-gland extract. *J Cut Genitourinary Dis* 1898;16:49.
2. Smith EA. Systemic sclerosis: etiology and pathogenesis. In: Hochberg MC, Silman AJ, Smolen JS, et al., eds. *Rheumatology*. 3rd ed. London: Mosby; 2003:1481.

3. Wigley FM, Hummers LK. Clinical features of systemic sclerosis. In: Hochberg MC, Silman AJ, Smolen JS, et al., eds. *Rheumatology.* 3rd ed. London: Mosby; 2003:1463.

4. Denton CP, Black CM. Scleroderma-clinical and pathological advances. *Best Pract Res Clin Rheumatol* 2004;18:271.

5. LeRoy EC, Black C, Fleischmajer R, et al. Scleroderma (systemic sclerosis): classification, subsets and pathogenesis. *J Rheumatol* 1988;15:202.

6. MacGregor AJ, Canovan R, Knight C, et al. Pulmonary hypertension in systemic sclerosis: risk factors for progression and consequences for survival. *Rheumatology (Oxford)* 2001;40:453.

7. Mukerjee D, St. George D, Colerio B, et al. Prevalence and outcome in systemic sclerosis associated pulmonary arterial hypertension: application of a registry approach. *Ann Rheum Dis* 2003;62:1088.

8. Steen VD. Epidemiology of systemic sclerosis. In: Hochberg MC, Silman AJ, Smolen JS, et al., eds. *Rheumatology.* 3rd ed. London: Mosby; 2003: 1455.

9. Seibold JR. Scleroderma. In: Harris ED Jr, Budd RC, Firestein GS, et al., eds. *Kelley's Textbook of Rheumatology.* 7th ed. Philadelphia: Elsevier Saunders, 2005;1279.

10. Maul GG, French BT, van Venrooij WJ, et al. Topoisomerase I identified by scleroderma 70 antisera: enrichment of topoisomerase I at the centromere in mouse mitotic cells before anaphase. *Proc Natl Acad Sci U S A* 1986;83:5145.

11. Okano Y. Antinuclear antibody in systemic sclerosis (scleroderma). *Rheum Dis Clin N Am* 1996;22:709.

12. Silman AJ. Scleroderma and survival. *Ann Rheum Dis* 1991;50:267.

13. Barrett AJ, Miller MH, Littlejohn GO. A survival study of patients with scleroderma diagnosed over 30 years (1953–1983). The value of single cutaneous classification in the early stages of the disease. *J Rheumatol* 1988;15:276.

14. Lee P, Langevitz P, Alderdice CA, et al. Mortality in systemic sclerosis (scleroderma). *Q J Med* 1992;82:139.

15. Bulpitt KJ, Clements PJ, Lachenbruch PA, et al. Early undifferentiated connective-tissue disease. III. Outcome and prognostic indicators in early scleroderma (systemic sclerosis). *Ann Intern Med* 1993;118:602.

16. Mayes MD. Scleroderma epidemiology. *Rheum Dis Clin N Am* 2003;29: 239.

17. Gabriel SE, O'Fallon WM, Kurland LT, et al. Risk of connective-tissue disease and other disorders after breast implantation. *N Engl J Med* 1994;330:1697.

18. Hochberg MC, Perlmutter DL, Medsger TA Jr, et al. Lack of associations between augmentation mammoplasty and systemic sclerosis (scleroderma). *Arthritis Rheum* 1996;39:1125.

19. Janowsky EC, Kupper LL, Hulka BS, et al. Meta-analyses of the relation between silicone breast implants and the risk of connective-tissue diseases. *N Engl J Med* 2000;342:781.

20. Johnson RW, Tew MB, Arnett FC, et al. The genetics of systemic sclerosis. *Curr Rheumatol Rep* 2002;4:99.

21. Silman AJ, Newman J. Epidemiology of systemic sclerosis. *Curr Opin Rheumatol* 1996;8:585.

22. Arnett FC, Cho M, Chatterjee S, et al. Familial occurrence frequencies and relative risks for systemic sclerosis (scleroderma) in three United States cohorts. *Arthritis Rheum* 2001;44:1359.

23. Jimenez SA, Derk CT. Following the molecular pathways toward an understanding of the pathogenesis of systemic sclerosis. *Ann Intern Med* 2004;140:37.

24. Tan EM, Rodnan GP, Garcia I, et al. Diversity of antinuclear antibodies in progressive systemic sclerosis: anticentromere antibody and its relationship to CREST syndrome. *Arthritis Rheum* 1980;23:617.

25. Cepeda EJ, Reveille JD. Autoantibodies in systemic sclerosis and fibrosing syndromes: clinical implications and relevance. *Curr Opin Rheumatol* 2004;16:723.

26. Seibold JR, Medsger TA Jr, Winkelstein A, et al. Immune complexes in progressive systemic sclerosis (scleroderma). *Arthritis Rheum* 1982;25:1167.

27. Fleishmajor R, Perlish JS, Reeves JR. Cellular infiltrates in scleroderma skin. *Arthritis Rheum* 1977;20:975.

28. Sakkas LI, Platsoucas CD. Is systemic sclerosis an antigen-driven T cell disease? *Arthritis Rheum* 2004;50:1721.

29. Kahaleh MB, LeRoy EC. Presence of interleukin-2 in scleroderma: correlation of serum level with extent of skin involvement and disease duration. *Ann Intern Med* 1989;110:446.

30. Furst DE, Clements PJ, Graze P, et al. A syndrome resembling progressive systemic sclerosis after bone marrow transplantation: a model for scleroderma? *Arthritis Rheum* 1979;22:904.

31. Jaffee BD, Claman HN. Chronic graft-versus-host disease (GVHD) as a model for scleroderma. I. Description of model systems. *Cell Immunol* 1983;77:1.

32. Gleichmann E. Capacity of genetically different T lymphocytes to induce lethal graft-versus-host disease correlates with their capacity to generate suppression but not with their capacity to generate anti-F₁ killer cells: a non-H-2 locus determines the inability to induce lethal graft-versus-host disease. *J Exp Med* 1981;153:1474.

33. Sawaya HH, Jimenez SA, Artlett CM. Quantification of fetal microchimeric cells in clinically affected and unaffected skin of patients with systemic sclerosis. *Rheumatology (Oxford)* 2004;43:965.

34. LeRoy EC. Systemic sclerosis: a vascular perspective. *Rheum Dis Clin N Am* 1996;22:675.

35. Fries JF, Lindgren JA, Bull JM. Scleroderma-like lesions and the carcinoid syndrome. *Arch Intern Med* 1973;131:550.

36. Winkelmann RK, Goldyne M, Linscheid RL. Influence of cold on catecholamine response of vascular smooth muscle strips from resistance vessels of scleroderma skin. *Angiology* 1977;29:330.

37. Jayson MI. The microcirculation in systemic sclerosis. *Clin Exp Rheumatol* 1984;2:85.

38. Reilly IA, Roy L, Fitzgerald GA. Biosynthesis of thromboxane in patients with systemic sclerosis and Raynaud's phenomenon. *Br Med J* 1986;292:1037.

39. Stone RA, Tisher CC, Hawkins HK, et al. Juxtaglomerular hyperplasia and hyperreninemia in progressive systemic sclerosis complicated by acute renal failure. *Am J Med* 1974;56:119.

40. Zamora MR, O'Brien RF, Rutherford RB, et al. Serum endothelin-1 concentrations and cold provocation in primary Raynaud's phenomenon. *Lancet* 1990;336:1144.

41. Kahaleh MB. Endothelin, an endothelial-dependent vasoconstrictor in scleroderma: enhanced production and profibrotic action. *Arthritis Rheum* 1991;34:978.

42. Kahaleh MB, Osborn I, LeRoy EC. Increased factor VIII/von Willebrand factor antigen and von Willebrand factor activity in scleroderma and Raynaud's phenomenon. *Ann Intern Med* 1981;94:482.

43. Gordon JL, Pottinger BE, Woo P, et al. Plasma von Willebrand factor in connective tissue disease. *Ann Rheum Dis* 1987;46:491.

44. Sollberg S, Peltonen J, Uitto J, et al. Elevated expression of β1 and β2 integrins, intercellular adhesion molecule 1, and endothelial leukocyte adhesion molecule 1 in the skin of patients with systemic sclerosis of recent onset. *Arthritis Rheum* 1992;35:290.

45. Sfikakis PP, Tesar J, Baraf H, et al. Circulating intercellular adhesion molecule-1 in patients with systemic sclerosis. *Clin Immunol Immunopathol* 1993;68:88.

46. Gruschwitz MS, Hornstein OP, van Den Diesch P. Correlation of soluble adhesion molecules in the peripheral blood of scleroderma patients with their in situ expression and with disease activity. *Arthritis Rheum* 1995;38:184.

47. Gratwick GM, Klein R, Sergent JS, et al. Fibrinogen turnover in progressive systemic sclerosis. *Arthritis Rheum* 1978;21:343.

48. Kahaleh BM, Osborn I, LeRoy EC. Elevated levels of circulating platelet aggregates and beta thromboglobulin in scleroderma. *Ann Intern Med* 1982;96:610.

49. Pearson JD. The endothelium: its role in scleroderma. *Ann Rheum Dis* 1991;50:866.

50. Holt CM, Lindsey N, Moult J, et al. Antibody dependent cellular cytotoxicity of vascular-endothelium. Characterization and pathogenic associations in systemic sclerosis. *Clin Exp Immunol* 1989;78:359.

51. Drenk F, Deicher HR. Pathophysiological effects of endothelial cytotoxic activity derived from sera of patients with progressive systemic sclerosis. *J Rheumatol* 1988;15:468.

52. Strehlow D, Korn JH. Biology of the scleroderma fibroblast. *Curr Opin Rheumatol* 1998;10:572.

53. LeRoy EC. Connective tissue synthesis by scleroderma skin fibroblasts in cell culture. *J Exp Med* 1972;135:1351.

54. de Crombrugghe B, Vuorio T, Karsenty G. Control of type I collagen genes in scleroderma and normal fibroblasts. *Rheum Dis Clin N Am* 1990;16: 109.

55. Claman HN. Mast cells and fibrosis: the relevance to scleroderma. *Rheum Dis Clin N Am* 1990;16:141.

56. Ignotz RA, Massague J. Transforming growth factor beta stimulates the expression of fibronectin and collagen and their incorporation into the extracellular matrix. *J Biol Chem* 1986;261:4337.

57. Kawakami T, Ihn H, Xu W, et al. Increased expression of TGF-beta receptors by scleroderma fibroblasts: evidence for contribution of autocrine TGF-beta signaling to scleroderma phenotype. *J Invest Dermatol* 1998;110:47.

58. Pannu J, Trojanowska M. Recent advances in fibroblast signaling and biology in scleroderma. *Curr Opin Rheumatol* 2004;16:739.

59. Kurihara H, Yoshizumi M, Sugiyama T, et al. Transforming growth factor β stimulates the expression of endothelin mRNA by vascular endothelial cells. *Biochem Biophys Res Commun* 1989;159:1435.

60. Rodnan GP, Benedek TG. An historical account of the study of progressive systemic sclerosis (diffuse scleroderma). *Ann Intern Med* 1962;57:305.

61. Curzio C. *Discussion: anatomico-pratiche di un raro, e stravagante morbo cutaneo in una giovane donna filicemente curato in questo grande ospedale degl' incurabili.* Napoli: Giovanne di Simone, 1753.

62. Gintrac E. Note sur la sclérodermie. *Rev Med Chir* 1847;2:263.

63. Auspitz H. Ein beitrag zur lehre von haut-sklerem der erwachsenen. *Wien Med Wschr* 1863;13:739.

64. Osler W. *The Principles and Practice of Medicine.* New York: Appleton; 1892:993.

65. Moore HC, Sheehan HL. The kidney of scleroderma. *Lancet* 1952;1:68.

66. D'Agati VD, Cannon PJ. Scleroderma (systemic sclerosis). In: Tisher CC, Brenner BM, eds. *Renal Pathology with Clinical and Functional Correlations.* Philadelphia: Lippincott; 1994.

67. Steigerwald JC. Renal involvement in systemic sclerosis (scleroderma). In: Jayson MIV, Black CM, eds. *Systemic sclerosis: scleroderma.* Chichester, New York: John Wiley & Sons, 1988.

68. Kovalchik MT, Guggenheim SJ, Silverman MH, et al. The kidney in progressive systemic sclerosis. A prospective study. *Ann Intern Med* 1978;89:881.

69. Cannon PJ, Hassar M, Case DB, et al. The relationship of hypertension and renal failure in scleroderma (progressive systemic sclerosis) to structural and functional abnormalities of the renal cortical circulation. *Medicine* 1974;53:1.

70. Steen VD. Scleroderma renal crisis. *Rheum Dis Clin N Am* 2003;29:315.

71. Shapiro AP, Medsger TA, Steen VD. Renal involvement in systemic sclerosis. In: Schrier R, Gottschalk C, eds. *Diseases of the Kidney.* 5th ed. Boston: Little, Brown; 1993.

72. Langevitz P, Buskila D, Lee P, et al. Scleroderma hypertensive renal crisis and the changing pattern of mortality in systemic sclerosis (scleroderma). *Nephron* 1991;57:111.

73. Hillis GS, Khan IH, Simpson JG, et al. Scleroderma, D-penicillamine treatment, and progressive renal failure associated with positive antimyeloperoxidase antineutrophil cytoplasmic antibodies. *Am J Kidney Dis* 1997;30:279.

74. Karpinski J, Jothy S, Radoux V, et al. D-penicillamine-induced crescentic glomerulonephritis and antimyeloperoxidase antibodies in a patient with scleroderma. Case report and review of the literature. *Am J Nephrol* 1997;17:528.

75. Maes B, Van Mieghem A, Messiaen T, et al. Limited cutaneous systemic sclerosis associated with MPO-ANCA positive renal small vessel vasculitis of the microscopic polyangiitis type. *Am J Kidney Dis* 2000;36:E16.

76. Tomioka M, Hinoshita F, Miyauchi N, et al. ANCA-related crescentic glomerulonephritis in a patient with scleroderma without marked dermatologic change and malignant hypertension. *Intern Med* 2004;43:496.

77. Steen VD, Medsger TA Jr, Osiah TA Jr, et al. Factors predicting development of renal involvement in progressive systemic sclerosis. *Am J Med* 1984;76:779.

78. Helfrich DJ, Banner B, Steen VD, et al. Normotensive renal failure in systemic sclerosis. *Arthritis Rheum* 1989;32:1128.

79. Steen VD, Medsger TA Jr. Case-controlled study of corticosteroids and other drugs that either precipitate or protect from the development of scleroderma renal crisis. *Arthritis Rheum* 1998;41:1613.

80. Booton R, Jeffrey R, Prabhu PN. Systemic sclerosis and scleroderma renal crisis associated with carcinoma of the breast. *Am J Kidney Dis* 1999;34:937.

81. Bar J, Ehrenfeld M, Rozman J, et al. Pulmonary renal syndrome in systemic sclerosis. *Semin Arthritis Rheum* 2001;30:403.

82. Phan TG, Cass A, Gillin A, et al. Anti-RNA polymerase III antibodies in the diagnosis of scleroderma renal crisis sine scleroderma. *J Rheumatol* 1999;26:2489.

83. Altman RD, Medsger TA, Bloch DA. Predictors of survival in systemic sclerosis (scleroderma). *Arthritis Rheum* 1991;34:403.

84. Traub YH, Shapiro AP, Rodnan GP, et al. Hypertension and renal failure (scleroderma renal crisis) in progressive systemic sclerosis. Review of a 25-year experience with 68 cases. *Medicine* 1983;62:335.

85. LeRoy EC, Fleischman RM. The management of renal scleroderma: experience with dialysis, nephrectomy and transplantation. *Am J Med* 1978;64:974.

86. Lopez-Ovejero JA, Saal SD, D'Angelo WA, et al. Reversal of vascular and renal crises of scleroderma by oral angiotensin-converting-enzyme blockade. *N Engl J Med* 1979;300:1417.

87. Steen VD, Costantino JP, Shapiro AP, et al. Outcome of renal crisis in systemic sclerosis: relation to availability of angiotensin converting enzyme (ACE) inhibitors. *Ann Intern Med* 1990;113:552.

88. Steen VD, Medsger TA Jr. Long-term outcomes of scleroderma renal crisis. *Ann Intern Med* 2000;133:600.

89. Steen VD, Conte C, Owens GR. Severe restrictive lung disease in systemic sclerosis. *Arthritis Rheum* 1994;37:1283.

90. Urai L, Munkasci I, Szinay G. New data on the pathology of "true scleroderma kidney." *Br Med J* 1961;1:713.

91. Woolfson RG, Cairns HS, Williams DJ. Renal scintigraphy in acute scleroderma: report of three cases. *J Nucl Med* 1993;34:1163.

92. Lester PD, Koehler PR. The renal angiographic changes in scleroderma. *Radiology* 1971;99:517.

93. Winograd J, Sckimmel DH, Polubinskas AJ. The spotted nephrogram of renal scleroderma. *Am J Roentgenol* 1976;126:734.

94. Warren BH, Rösch J. Angiography in the diagnosis of renal scleroderma. *Radiol Clin* 1977;46:194.

95. Clements PJ, Lachenbruch PA, Furst DE, et al. Abnormalities of renal physiology in systemic sclerosis: a prospective study with 10-year follow-up. *Arthritis Rheum* 1994;37:67.

96. Helmchen U, Wenzel UO. Benign and malignant nephrosclerosis and renovascular disease. In: Tisher CC, Brenner BM, eds. *Renal Pathology with Clinical and Functional Correlations.* Philadelphia: Lippincott; 1994.

97. Lapenas D, Rodnan GP, Cavello T. Immunopathology of the renal vascular lesion of progressive systemic sclerosis (scleroderma). *Am J Pathol* 1978;91:243.

98. McCoy RC, Tisher CC, Pepe PF, et al. The kidney in progressive systemic sclerosis: immunohistochemical and antibody elution studies. *Lab Invest* 1976;35:124.

99. McGiven AR, deBoer WG, Barnett AJ. Renal immune deposits in scleroderma. *Pathology* 1971;3:145.

100. Denton CP, Black CM. Management of systemic sclerosis. In: Hochberg MC, Silman AJ, Smolen JS, et al., eds. *Rheumatology.* 3rd ed. London: Mosby; 2003:1493.

101. Caskey FJ, Thacker EJ, Johnston PA, et al. Failure of losartan to control blood pressure in scleroderma renal crisis. *Lancet* 1997;349:620.

102. Siragy HM, de Gasparo M, El-Kersh M, et al. Angiotensin-converting enzyme inhibition potentiates angiotensin II Type 1 receptor effects on renal bradykinin and cGMP. *Hypertension* 2001;38:183.

103. Donohoe JF. Scleroderma and the kidney. *Kidney Int* 1992;41:462.

104. Richardson JA. Hemodialysis and kidney transplantation for renal failure from scleroderma. *Arthritis Rheum* 1973;15:265.

105. Paul M, Bear RA, Sugar L. Renal transplantation in scleroderma. *J Rheumatol* 1984;11:406.

106. Tsakiris D, Simpson KL, Jones EH, et al. Rare diseases in renal replacement therapy in ERA-EDTA registry. *Nephrol Dial Transplant* 1996;11:4.

107. Chang YJ, Spiera H. Renal transplantation in scleroderma. *Medicine* 1999;78:382.

108. Bleyer AJ, et al. Relationship between underlying renal disease and renal transplantation outcome. *Am J Kidney Dis* 2001;37:1152.

109. Kopp JB, Klotman PE. Cellular and molecular mechanisms of cyclosporin nephrotoxicity. *J Am Soc Nephrol* 1990;1:162.

110. Ruiz JC, de Francisco AL, de Bonies E, et al. Progressive systemic sclerosis and renal transplantation: a contraindication to cyclosporin. *Nephron* 1991;59:330.

111. Mattteson EL. Extra-articular features of rheumatoid arthritis and systemic involvement. In: Hochberg MC, Silman AJ, Smolen JS, et al., eds. *Rheumatology.* 3rd ed. London: Mosby; 2003:781.

112. Gordon DA, Hastings DE. Clinical features of rheumatoid arthritis. In: Hochberg MC, Silman AJ, Smolen JS, et al., eds. *Rheumatology.* 3rd ed. London: Mosby; 2003:765.

113. Steiner G. Autoantibodies in rheumatoid arthritis. In: Hochberg MC, Silman AJ, Smolen JS, et al., eds. *Rheumatology.* 3rd ed. London: Mosby; 2003:833.

114. Boers M, Dijkmans BA, Breedveld FC, et al. Errors in the prediction of creatinine clearance in patients with rheumatoid arthritis. *Br J Rheumatol* 1988;27:233.

115. Nived O, Sturfelt G, Westling H, et al. Is serum creatinine concentration a reliable index of renal function in rheumatic diseases? *Br Med J* 1983;286:684.

116. Boers M. Renal disorders in rheumatoid arthritis. *Semin Arthritis Rheum* 1990;20:57.

117. Laakso M, Mutru O, Isomäki H, et al. Mortality from amyloidosis and renal diseases in patients with rheumatoid arthritis. *Ann Rheum Dis* 1986;45:663.

118. Boers M, Croonen AM, Dijkmans BA, et al. Renal findings in rheumatoid arthritis: clinical aspects of 132 necropsies. *Ann Rheum Dis* 1987;46:658.

119. Boers M, Dijkmans BA, Breedveld FC, et al. Subclinical renal dysfunction in rheumatoid arthritis. *Arthritis Rheum* 1990;33:95.

120. Arapakis G, Tribe CR. Amyloidosis in rheumatoid arthritis investigated by means of rectal biopsy. *Ann Rheum Dis* 1963;22:256.

121. Ennevarra K, Oka M. Rheumatoid arthritis with amyloidosis. *Ann Rheum Dis* 1964;23:131.

122. Fearnley GR, Lackner R. Amyloidosis in rheumatoid arthritis, and significance of "unexplained" albuminuria. *Br Med J* 1955;1:1129.

123. Teilum G, Lindahl A. Frequency and significance of amyloid changes in rheumatoid arthritis. *Acta Med Scand* 1954;149:449.

124. Unger PN, et al. Amyloidosis in rheumatoid arthritis. *Am J Med Sci* 1948;216:51.

125. Myllykangas-Luosujarvi R, Aho K, Kantiainen H, et al. Amyloidosis in a nationwide series of 1666 subjects with rheumatoid arthritis who died during 1989 in Finland. *Rheumatology (Oxford)* 1999;38:499.

126. Bourke BE, Woodrow DF, Scott JT. Proteinuria in rheumatoid arthritis: drug-induced or amyloid? *Ann Rheum Dis* 1981;40:240.

127. Parkins RA, Bywaters EG. Progression of amyloidosis secondary to rheumatoid arthritis. *Br Med J* 1959;1:536.

128. Elkayam O, Hawkins PN, Lachmann H, et al. Rapid and complete resolution of proteinuria due to renal amyloidosis in a patient with rheumatoid arthritis treated with infliximab. *Arthritis Rheum* 2002;46:2571.

129. Wright JR, Calkins E. Clinical-pathologic differentiation of common amyloid syndrome. *Medicine* 1981;60:429.

130. Tanaka F, Migeta K, Honda S, et al. Clinical outcome and survival of secondary (AA) amyloidosis. *Clin Exp Rheumatol* 2003;21:343.

131. Light PD, Hall-Craggs M. Amyloid deposition in a renal allograft in a case of amyloidosis secondary to rheumatoid arthritis. *Am J Med* 1979;66:532.

132. Baggenstoss AH, Rosenberg EF. Visceral lesions associated with chronic infectious (rheumatoid) arthritis. *Arch Pathol* 1943;35:503.

133. Sorensen AW. The Waaler-Rose test in patients suffering from rheumatoid arthritis in relationship to 24-hour endogenous creatinine clearance (III). *Acta Rheum Scand* 1961;7:304.

134. Sorensen AW. Investigation of the kidney function in rheumatoid arthritis (II). *Acta Rheum Scand* 1961;7:138.

135. Sorensen AW. Investigation of the kidney function in rheumatoid arthritis. *Acta Rheum Scand* 1960;6:115.

136. Salomon MI, Gallo G, Poon TP, et al. The kidney in rheumatoid arthritis: a study based on renal biopsies. *Nephron* 1974;12:297.

137. Ting HC, Wang F. Mesangiocapillary (membranoproliferative) glomerulonephritis and rheumatoid arthritis. *Br Med J* 1977;1:270.

138. Whaley K, Webb J. Liver and kidney disease in rheumatoid arthritis. *Clin Rheum Dis* 1977;3:527.

139. Sellars L, Siamopoulos K, Wilkinson R, et al. Renal biopsy appearances in rheumatoid disease. *Clin Nephrol* 1983;20:114.
140. Heaney DJ, Kupor LR, Gyorkey F, et al. Membranous nephropathy associated with rheumatoid arthritis. *South Med J* 1978;71:467.
141. Pollak VE, Pirani CL, Steck IE, et al. The kidney in rheumatoid arthritis: studies by renal biopsy. *Arthritis Rheum* 1962;5:1.
142. Helin H, Korpela M, Mustonen J, et al. Mild mesangial glomerulopathy—a frequent finding in rheumatoid arthritis patients with hematuria or proteinuria. *Nephron* 1986;42:224.
143. Hordon LD, Sellars L, Morley AR, et al. Haematuria in rheumatoid arthritis: an association with mesangial glomerulonephritis. *Ann Rheum Dis* 1984;43:440.
144. Pollet S, Depuer T, Moore P, et al. Mesangial glomerulopathy and IgM rheumatoid factor in rheumatoid arthritis. *Nephron* 1989;51:107.
145. Kelly CA, Mooney P, Hordon LD, et al. Haematuria in rheumatoid arthritis: a follow up study. *Ann Rheum Dis* 1988;47:993.
146. Helin HJ, Korpela MM, Mustonen JT, et al. Renal biopsy findings and clinicopathologic correlations in rheumatoid arthritis. *Arthritis Rheum* 1995;38:242.
147. Korpela M, Mustonen JT, Helin H, et al. Immunological comparison of patients with rheumatoid arthritis with and without nephropathy. *Ann Rheum Dis* 1990;49:214.
148. Korpela M, Mustonen L, Pasternack A, et al. Mesangial glomerulopathy in rheumatoid arthritis patients. Clinical follow-up and relations to antirheumatic therapy. *Nephron* 1991;59:46.
149. Jorgensen C, Anaya JM, Cognot C, et al. Rheumatoid arthritis associated with high levels of immunoglobulin A: clinical and biological characteristics. *Clin Exp Rheum* 1992;10:571.
150. Korpela M, Mustonen J, Teppo AM, et al. Mesangial glomerulonephritis as an extraarticular manifestation of rheumatoid arthritis. *Br J Rheumatol* 1997;36:1189.
151. Davis JA, Cohen AH, Weisbart R, et al. Glomerulonephritis in rheumatoid arthritis. *Arthritis Rheum* 1979;22:1018.
152. Weisman M, Zvaifler N. Cryoimmunoglobulins in rheumatoid arthritis. *J Clin Invest* 1975;56:725.
153. Miyazaki M, Endoh M, Suga T, et al. Rheumatoid factors and glomerulonephritis. *Clin Exp Immunol* 1990;81:250.
154. Breedveld FC, Valentijn RM, Westedt ML, et al. Rapidly progressive glomerulonephritis with glomerular crescent formation in rheumatoid arthritis. *Clin Rheumatol* 1985;4:353.
155. Adu D, Berisa F, Howie AJ, et al. Glomerulonephritis in rheumatoid arthritis. *Br J Rheumatol* 1993;32:1008.
156. Harper L, Cockwell P, Howie AJ, et al. Focal segmental necrotizing glomerulonephritis in rheumatoid arthritis. *GJM* 1997;90:125.
157. Kuznetsky KA, Schwartz MM, Lohmann LA, et al. Necrotizing glomerulonephritis in rheumatoid arthritis. *Clin Nephrol* 1986;26:257.
158. Tebib JG, Trolliet, Bouvier M, et al. Necrotizing glomerulonephritis as a complication of rheumatoid arthritis vasculitis. *Br J Rheumatol* 1993;32:765.
159. Qarni MU, Kahan PE. Pauci-immune necrotizing glomerulonephritis complicating rheumatoid arthritis. *Clin Nephrol* 2000;54:54.
160. Schmid FR, Cooper NS, Ziff M, et al. Arteritis in rheumatoid arthritis. *Am J Med* 1961;30:56.
161. Scott DG, Bacon PA, Tribe CR. Systemic rheumatoid vasculitis: a clinical and laboratory study of 50 cases. *Medicine* 1981;60:288.
162. Moreland L, DiBartolomeo A, Brick J. Rheumatoid vasculitis with intrarenal aneurysm formation. *J Rheumatol* 1988;15:845.
163. Ball J. Rheumatoid arthritis and polyarteritis nodosa. *Ann Rheum Dis* 1954;13:277.
164. Brun C, Olsen TS, Raaschou F, et al. Renal biopsy in rheumatoid arthritis. *Nephron* 1965;2:65.
165. Ramirez G, Lambert R, Bloomer HA. Renal pathology in patients with rheumatoid arthritis. *Nephron* 1981;29:124.
166. Clive DM, Stoff JS. Renal syndromes associated with nonsteroidal anti-inflammatory drugs. *N Engl J Med* 1984;310:563.
167. Brater DC. Anti-inflammatory agents and renal function. *Semin Arthritis Rheum* 2002;32(3 suppl 1):33.
168. Csuka ME, McCarty DJ. Aspirin and the treatment of rheumatoid arthritis. *Rheum Dis Clin N Am* 1989;15:439.
169. Bunning RD, Barth WF. Sulindac: a potentially renal-sparing nonsteroidal anti-inflammatory drug. *JAMA* 1982;248:2864.
170. Ciabattoni G, Cinotti GA, Pierucci A, et al. Effects of sulindac and ibuprofen in patients with chronic glomerular disease. *N Engl J Med* 1984;310:279.
171. Whelton A, Stout RL, Spilman PS, et al. Renal effects of ibuprofen, piroxicam, and sulindac in patients with asymptomatic renal failure. *Ann Intern Med* 1990;112:568.
172. Roberts DG, Gerber JG, Barnes JS, et al. Sulindac is not renal sparing in man. *Clin Pharmacol Ther* 1985;38:258.
173. Nanra RS. Pathology, aetiology and pathogenesis of analgesic nephropathy. *Aust NZ Med* 1976;6:33.
174. Sandler DP, Smith JC, Weinberg CR, et al. Analgesic use and chronic renal disease. *N Engl J Med* 1989;320:1238.
175. Forestier J. Rheumatoid arthritis and its treatment by gold salts. *J Lab Clin Med* 1935;20:827.
176. Empire Rheumatism Council. Gold therapy in rheumatoid arthritis. *Ann Rheum Dis* 1960;19:95.
177. Heuer MA, Pietrusko RG, Morris RW, et al. An analysis of worldwide safety experience with auranofin. *J Rheumatol* 1985;12:695.
178. Suarez-Almazor ME, Spooner CH, Belseck E, et al. Auranofin versus placebo in rheumatoid arthritis. *Cochrane Database Syst Rev* 2000;2:CD002048.
179. The Cooperative Clinics Committee of the ARA. A controlled trial of gold salt therapy in rheumatoid arthritis. *Arthritis Rheum* 1973;16:353.
180. Furst D, Levine S, Srinivasan R, et al. A double-blind trial of high versus conventional dosages of gold salts for rheumatoid arthritis. *Arthritis Rheum* 1977;20:1473.
181. Ganley CJ, Paget SA, Reidenberg MM. Increased renal tubular cell excretion by patients receiving chronic therapy with gold and with nonsteroidal anti-inflammatory drugs. *Clin Pharmacol Ther* 1989;46:51.
182. Sharp JT, Lidsky MD, Duffy J, et al. Comparison of two dosage schedules of gold salts in the treatment of rheumatoid arthritis. *Arthritis Rheum* 1977;20:1179.
183. Silverberg DS, Kidd EG, Shnitka TK, et al. Gold nephropathy—a clinical and pathologic study. *Arthritis Rheum* 1970;13:812.
184. Hall CL. The natural course of gold and penicillamine nephropathy: a long term study of 54 patients. *Adv Exp Med Biol* 1989;252:247.
185. Hall CL, Fotahergill NJ, Blackwell MM, et al. The natural course of gold nephropathy: long term study of 21 patients. *Br Med J* 1987;295:745.
186. Hall CL, Jawad S, Harrison PR, et al. Natural course of penicillamine nephropathy: a long term study of 33 patients. *Br Med J* 1988;296:1083.
187. Hall CL, Tighe R. The effect of continuing penicillamine and gold treatment on the course of penicillamine and gold nephropathy. *Br J Rheumatol* 1989;28:53.
188. Klinkhoff AV, Teufel A. Reinstitution of gold after gold induced proteinuria. *J Rheumatol* 1997;24:1277.
189. Vaamonde CA, Hunt FR. The nephrotic syndrome as a complication of gold therapy. *Arthritis Rheum* 1970;13:826.
190. Tornroth T, Skrifvars B. Gold nephropathy prototype of membranous glomerulonephritis. *Am J Pathol* 1974;75:573.
191. Lee JC, Dushkin M, Eyring EJ, et al. Renal lesions associated with gold therapy—light and electron microscopic studies. *Arthritis Rheum* 1965;8:1.
192. Wooley PH, Griffin J, Panayi GS, et al. HLA-DR antigens and toxic reaction to sodium aurothiomalate and D-penicillamine in patients with rheumatoid arthritis. *N Engl J Med* 1980;303:300.
193. Sakkas LI, Chikanza IC, Vaughan RW, et al. Gold induced nephropathy in rheumatoid arthritis and HLA class II genes. *Ann Rheum Dis* 1993;52:300.
194. Seidman P. Renal effects of low dose methotrexate in rheumatoid arthritis. *J Rheumatol* 1993;20:1126.
195. Rheumatoid Arthritis Clinical Trial Archive Group. The effect of age and renal function on the efficacy and toxicity of methotrexate in rheumatoid arthritis. *J Rheumatol* 1995;22:218.
196. Bressolle F, Bologna C, Kinowski JM, et al. Total and free methotrexate pharmacokinetics in elderly patients with rheumatoid arthritis. A comparison with young patients. *J Rheumatol* 1997;24:1903.
197. Bressolle F, Bologna C, Kinowski JM, et al. Effects of moderate renal insufficiency on pharmacokinetics of methotrexate in rheumatoid arthritis patients. *Ann Rheum Dis* 1998;57:110.
198. Schiff MH, Whelton A. Renal toxicity associated with disease-modifying antirheumatic drugs used for the treatment of rheumatoid arthritis. *Semin Arthritis Rheum* 2000;30:196.
199. Walshe JM. Wilson's disease—new oral therapy. *Lancet* 1956;1:25.
200. Golding JR, Wilson JV, Day AT. Observations on the treatment of rheumatoid disease with penicillamine. *Postgrad Med J* 1970;46:599.
201. Hill HF. Treatment of rheumatoid arthritis with penicillamine. *Semin Arth Rheum* 1977;6:361.
202. Stein HB, Patterson AC, Offer RC, et al. Adverse effects of D-penicillamine in rheumatoid arthritis. *Ann Intern Med* 1980;92:24.
203. Bacon PA, Tribe CR, Mackenzie JC, et al. Penicillamine nephropathy in rheumatoid arthritis. *QJM* 1976;45:661.
204. Barraclough D, Cunningham TJ, Muirden KD. Microscopic hematuria in patients with rheumatoid arthritis on D-penicillamine. *Aust NZ J Med* 1981;11:706.
205. Dische FE, Swinson DR, Hamilton EB, et al. Immunopathology of penicillamine-induced glomerular disease. *J Rheumatol* 1976;3:145.
206. Nanke Y, Akama H, Terai C, et al. Rapidly progressive glomerulonephritis with D-penicillamine. *Am J Med Sci* 2000;320:398.
207. Myers BD. Cyclosporine nephrotoxicity. *Kidney Int* 1986;30:964.
208. Dougados M, Duchesne L, Awada H, et al. Assessment of efficacy and acceptability of low dose cyclosporin in patients with rheumatoid arthritis. *Ann Rheum Dis* 1989;48:550.
209. Weinblatt ME, Coblyn JS, Fraser PA, et al. Cyclosporin A treatment of refractory rheumatoid arthritis. *Arthritis Rheum* 1987;30:11.
210. van Rijthoven AW, Dijkmans BA, Goei The HS, et al. Cyclosporin treatment for rheumatoid arthritis: a placebo controlled, double blind, multicentre study. *Ann Rheum Dis* 1986;45:726.
211. Yocum DE, Klippel JH, Wilder RL, et al. Cyclosporin A in severe, treatment-refractory rheumatoid arthritis. *Ann Intern Med* 1988;109:863.
212. Berg KJ, Forre O, Djoseland O, et al. Renal side effects of high and low cyclosporin A doses in patients with rheumatoid arthritis. *Clin Nephrol* 1989;31:232.
213. Ludwin D, Bennett KJ, Grace EM, et al. Nephrotoxicity in patients with rheumatoid arthritis treated with cyclosporine. *Transplant Proc* 1988;20:367.

214. Ludwin D, Alexopoulou I. Cyclosporin-A nephropathy in patients with rheumatoid arthritis. *Br J Rheumatol* 1993;32:60.
215. Kahan BD. Cyclosporine nephrotoxicity: pathogenesis, prophylaxis, therapy, and prognosis. *Am J Kidney Dis* 1986;8:323.
216. Gordon RD, Iwatsuki S, Shaw BW Jr, et al. Cyclosporine-steroid combination therapy in 84 cadaveric renal transplants. *Am J Kidney Dis* 1985;5:307.
217. Boers M, van Rijthonen AW, Goei The HS, et al. Serum creatinine levels two years later: follow-up of a placebo-controlled trial of cyclosporine in rheumatoid patients. *Transplant Proc* 1988;20:371.
218. International Kidney Biopsy Registry of Cyclosporin (Sandimmun®) in Autoimmune Diseases. Renal morphology after cyclosporin A therapy in rheumatoid arthritis patients. *Br J Rheumatol* 1993;32(suppl 1):65.
219. Rodriguez F, Krayenbuhl JC, Harrison WB, et al. Renal biopsy findings and followup of renal function in rheumatoid arthritis patients treated with cyclosporin A. An update from the International Kidney Biopsy Registry. *Arthritis Rheum* 1996;39:1491.
220. Ludwin D, Alexpoulou I, Esdaile JM, et al. Renal biopsy specimens from patients with rheumatoid arthritis and apparently normal renal function after therapy with cyclosporine. *Am J Kidney Dis* 1994;23:260.
221. Panayi GS, Tugwell P. An International Consensus Report: the use of cyclosporin A in rheumatoid arthritis. *Br J Rheumatol* 1993;32:65.
222. van den Borne BE, Landewe RB, Goei The HS, et al. Cyclosporin A therapy in rheumatoid arthritis: only strict application of the guidelines for safe use can prevent irreversible renal function loss. *Rheumatology (Oxford)* 1999;38:254.
223. Cush JJ, Tugwell P, Weinblatt M, et al. US consensus guidelines for the use of cyclosporin A in rheumatoid arthritis. *J Rheumatol* 1999;26:1176.
224. Anttila R. Renal involvement in juvenile rheumatoid arthritis—a clinical and histopathological study. *Acta Paediatr Scand* 1972;227:3.
225. Deschênes G, Prieur AM, Hayem F, et al. Renal amyloidosis in juvenile chronic arthritis: evolution after chlorambucil treatment. *Pediatr Nephrol* 1990;4:463.
226. Schnitzer TJ, Ansell BM. Amyloidosis in juvenile chronic polyarthritis. *Arthritis Rheum* 1977;20:245.
227. Trainin EB, Spitzer A, Greifer I. Amyloidosis in juvenile rheumatoid arthritis. *NY State J Med* 1978;78:72.
228. David J. Amyloidosis in juvenile chronic arthritis. *Clin Exp Rheumatol* 1991;9:73.
229. David J, Vouyiouka O, Ansell BM, et al. Amyloidosis in juvenile chronic arthritis: a morbidity and mortality study. *Clin Exp Rheumatol* 1993;11:85.
230. Savolainen HA. Chlorambucil in severe juvenile chronic arthritis: long term followup with special reference to amyloidosis. *J Rheumatol* 1999;26:898.
231. Packham JC, Hall MA, Pimm TJ, et al. Long-term follow-up of 246 adults with juvenile idiopathic arthritis: functional outcome. *Rheumatology (Oxford)* 2002;41:1428.
232. Stapleton FB, Hanissian AS, Miller LA. Hypercalciuria in children with juvenile rheumatoid arthritis: association with hematuria. *J Pediatr* 1985;107:235.
233. Lorenz VK, Schneider F. Nephrolithiasis bei juveniler rheumatoid-arthritis. *Kinderartzl Prax* 1975;43:450.
234. Mertens JC, Huizinga TW, Hagen EC, et al. Extracapillary glomerulonephritis in a patient with juvenile chronic arthritis. *J Rheumatol* 1996;23:1633.
235. Dhib M, Prieur AM, Courville S, et al. Crescentic glomerulonephritis in juvenile chronic arthritis. *J Rheumatol* 1996;23:1636.
236. Sjögren H. Zur kenntis de keratoconjunctivitis sicca (keratitio filemormis bei hypunfunktion der tranendrusen). *Acta Ophthalmol* 1933;11:1.
237. Tzioufas AG, Moutsopoulos HM. Sjögren's syndrome. In: Hochberg MC, Silman AJ, Smolen JS, et al., eds. *Rheumatology.* 3rd ed. London: Mosby; 2003:1431.
238. Talal N, Sokoloff L, Barth WF. Extra-salivary lymphoid abnormalities in Sjögren's syndrome (reticulum cell sarcoma, "pseudolymphoma," macroglobulinemia). *Am J Med* 1966;43:50.
239. Tu WH, Shearn MA, Lee JC, et al. Interstitial nephritis in Sjögren's syndrome. *Ann Intern Med* 1968;69:1163.
240. Matsumura R, Kondo Y, Sugiyama T, et al. Immunohistochemical identification of infiltrating mononuclear cells in tubulointerstitial nephritis associated with Sjögren's syndrome. *Clin Nephrol* 1988;6:335.
241. Rosenberg ME, Schendel PB, McCurdy FA, et al. Characterization of immune cells in kidneys from patients with Sjögren's syndrome. *Am J Kidney Dis* 1988;11:20.
242. Kahn J, Merritt AD, Wohl MJ, et al. Renal concentrating defects in Sjögren's syndrome. *Ann Intern Med* 1962;56:883.
243. Shearn MA, Tu WH. Nephrogenic diabetes insipidus and other defects of renal tubular function in Sjögren's syndrome. *Am J Med* 1965;39:312.
244. Talal N. Sjögren's syndrome, lymphoproliferation, and renal tubular acidosis. *Ann Intern Med* 1971;74:663.
245. Shearn MA, Tu WH. Latent renal tubular acidosis in Sjögren's syndrome. *Ann Rheum Dis* 1968;27:27.
246. Talal N, Zisman E, Schur PH. Renal tubular acidosis, glomerulonephritis, and immunologic factors in Sjögren's syndrome. *Arthritis Rheum* 1968;11:774.
247. Al-Jubouri MA, Jones S, Macmillan R, et al. Hypokalaemic paralysis revealing Sjögren syndrome in an elderly man. *J Clin Pathol* 1999;52:157.
248. Zimhony O, Sthoeger Z, Ben David D, et al. Sjögren's syndrome presenting as hypokalemic paralysis due to distal renal tubular acidosis. *J Rheumatol* 1995;22:2366.
249. Ohtani H, Imai H, Kodama T, et al. Severe hypokalaemia and respiratory arrest due to renal tubular acidosis in a patient with Sjögren syndrome. *Nephrol Dial Transplant* 1999;14:2201.
250. Shiozawa S, Shiozawa K, Shimizu S, et al. Clinical studies of renal disease in Sjögren's syndrome. *Ann Rheum Dis* 1987;46:768.
251. Siamopoulos KC, Mavridis AK, Elisaf M, et al. Kidney involvement in primary Sjögren's syndrome. *Scand J Rheumatol Suppl* 1986;61:156.
252. Golding PL, Mason AM. Hyperglobulinemic renal tubular acidosis: a report of nine cases. *Br Med J* 1970;3:143.
253. McCurdy DK, Cornwell GG III, DePratti VJ. Hyperglobulinemic renal tubular acidosis. *Ann Intern Med* 1967;67:110.
254. Morris RC Jr, Fudenberg HH. Impaired renal acidification in patients with hypergammaglobulinemia. *Medicine* 1967;46:57.
255. Pasternack A, Linder E. Renal tubular acidosis: an immunopathological study on four patients. *Clin Exp Immunol* 1970;7:115.
256. Sjioji R, Furuyama T, Onodera S, et al. Sjögren's syndrome and renal tubular acidosis. *Am J Med* 1970;48:456.
257. Walker BR, Alexander F, Tannebaum PJ. Fanconi syndrome with renal tubular acidosis and light chain proteinuria. *Nephron* 1971;8:103.
258. Gentric A, Herve JP, Pannec YL, et al. Severe renal involvement in primary Sjögren's syndrome. *Adv Exp Med Biol* 1989;252:73.
259. Rayadurg J, Koch AE. Renal insufficiency from interstitial nephritis in primary Sjögren's syndrome. *J Rheumatol* 1990;17:1714.
260. Cacoub P, Ginsburg C, Tazi Z, et al. Sjögren's syndrome with acute renal failure caused by renal pseudolymphoma. *Am J Kidney Dis* 1996;28:762.
261. Khan MA, Akhtar M, Taher SM. Membranoproliferative glomerulonephritis in a patient with primary Sjögren's syndrome. *Am J Nephrol* 1988;8:235.
262. Moutsopoulos HM, Balow JE, Lawley TJ, et al. Immune complex glomerulonephritis in sicca syndrome. *Am J Med* 1978;64:955.
263. Goules A, Masouride S, Tzioufar AG, et al. Clinically significant and biopsy-documented renal involvement in primary Sjögren's syndrome. *Medicine* 2000;79:241.
264. Schwartzberg M, Burnstein SL, Calabro JJ, et al. The development of membranous glomerulonephritis in a patient with rheumatoid arthritis and Sjögren's syndrome. *J Rheumatol* 1979;6:65.
265. Tatsumi H, Taneno S, Hiki Y, et al. Crescentic glomerulonephritis and primary Sjögren's syndrome. *Nephron* 2000;86:505.
266. Oddis CV, Medsger TA Jr. Inflammatory muscle disease: clinical features. In: Hochberg MC, Silman AJ, Smolen JS, et al., eds. *Rheumatology.* 3rd ed. London: Mosby; 2003:1532.
267. Bohan A, Peter JB. Polymyositis and dermatomyositis. *N Engl J Med* 1975;292:344.
268. Bohan A, Peter JB, Bowman RL, et al. A computer-assisted analysis of 153 patients with polymyositis and dermatomyositis. *Medicine* 1977;56:255.
269. Dickey BF, Myers AR. Pulmonary disease in polymyositis/dermatomyositis. *Semin Arthritis Rheum* 1984;14:60.
270. O'Dell JR, Hays RC, Guggenheim SJ, et al. Tubulo-interstitial disease in systemic lupus erythematosus. *Arch Intern Med* 1985;145:1995.
271. Talbott JH, et al. Dermatomyositis with scleroderma, calcinosis and renal endarteritis associated with cortical necrosis. *Arch Intern Med* 1939;63:476.
272. Dyck RF, Katz A, Gordon DA, et al. Glomerulonephritis associated with polymyositis. *J Rheumatol* 1979;6:336.
273. Pasquali JL, Meyer P, Christmann D, et al. Renal manifestations in dermatomyositis and polymyositis. *Ann Med Interne (Paris)* 1987;138:109.
274. Valenzuela OF, Reiser IW, Porush JG. Idiopathic polymyositis and glomerulonephritis. *J Nephrol* 2001;14:120.
275. Makino H, Hirata K, Matsuda M, et al. Membranous nephropathy developing during the course of dermatomyositis. *J Rheumatol* 1994;21:1377.
276. Akashi Y, Inoh M, Gamo N, et al. Dermatomyositis associated with membranous nephropathy in a 43-year-old female. *Am J Nephrol* 2002;22:385.
277. Row PG, Cameron JS, Turner DR, et al. Membranous nephropathy. Long-term follow-up and association with neoplasias. *QJM* 1971;44:207.
278. Rose JD. Membranous glomerulonephritis, dermatomyositis and bronchial carcinoma. *Br Med J* 1979;2:641.
279. Kagen LJ. Myoglobinemia and myoglobulinemia in patients with myositis. *Arthritis Rheum* 1971;14:457.
280. Kessler E, Weinberger I, Rosenfeld JB. Myoglobinuric acute renal failure in a case of dermatomyositis. *Isr J Med Sci* 1972;8:978.
281. Sloan MF, Franks AJ, Exley KA, et al. Acute renal failure due to polymyositis. *Br Med J* 1978;1:1457.
282. Thakur V, DeSalvo J, McGrath H, et al. Case report: polymyositis-induced myoglobinuric acute renal failure. *Am J Med Sci* 1996;312:85.
283. Lewington AJ, D'Souza R, Carr S, et al. Polymyositis: a cause of acute renal failure. *Nephrol Dial Transplant* 1996;11:699.
284. Bitnum S, Daeschner CW Jr, Travis LB, et al. Dermatomyositis. *J Pediatr* 1964;64:101.
285. Dodge WF, Daeschner CW Jr, Brennan JI, et al. Percutaneous renal biopsy in children—the collagen diseases, juvenile diabetes mellitus, and idiopathic hematuria and proteinuria. *Pediatrics* 1962;30:477.

CHAPTER 67 ■ THROMBOTIC THROMBOCYTOPENIC PURPURA, HEMOLYTIC-UREMIC SYNDROME, AND ACUTE CORTICAL NECROSIS

PIERO RUGGENENTI, MICHELE CERUTI, AND GIUSEPPE REMUZZI

HISTORICAL PERSPECTIVE AND DEFINITIONS

Thrombotic thrombocytopenia purpura (TTP) and hemolytic-uremic syndrome (HUS) have been considered to be indistinguishable or separate entities. No pathologic feature is specific to one of the two entities, but they actually have different clinical manifestations. Several research studies have been performed in attempt to discover new parameters or methodological approaches for the distinction of the two entities. Hemolytic-uremic syndrome has been defined as the consequence of some infections due to an *Escherichia coli* strain. Conditions in which cerebral symptoms predominated were thought to be more specific for TTP, but HUS has been described with the same pathologic features. Familial forms of both entities have been discovered and studied. Thrombotic thrombocytopenia purpura or HUS has been found in nonhereditary subjects as adverse effects of some drugs. Posttransplantation forms have been found in subjects with different underlying pathologies.

Recently, a new paradigm of distinction has been proposed according to the plasma activity of a von Willebrand factor protease. The decrease of this parameter may be associated with the diagnosis of TTP, but a significant number of patients with clinical features of HUS has been found with the same laboratory finding.

Thus, there are forms that, regardless of the underlying etiology, cannot be definitively assigned to TTP or to HUS. Consequently, it may be better to use the broader term of thrombotic microangiopathy (TMA). This form defines lesions, common to both TTP and HUS, characterized by vessel wall thickening (mainly arterioles or capillaries), with endothelial cell swelling and/or detachment from the basement membrane with accumulation of fluffy material in subendothelial space, intraluminal platelet thrombosis, and partial or complete obstruction of the vessel lumina. Thrombotic microangiopathy was introduced in 1952 by Summers to replace thrombotic thrombopenic purpura and revived in 1979 by E. Rossi. It provides a natural link between the two syndromes and is still the best term to encompass all of the lesions just described.

A classification into subgroups may be performed according to laboratory and genetic findings with no aim to overlap old classifications that distinguished TTP and HUS according to clinical features. The new classification attempts to distinguish TMA subgroups according to genomics and molecular biologic findings.

The term thrombotic thrombocytopenic purpura (TTP) was first introduced in 1925 by Moschcowitz (1), who described a 16-year-old female patient with a fulminant febrile attack, hemolytic anemia, bleeding, renal failure, and neurologic involvement. Pathologic changes were characterized by widespread hyaline thrombosis of small vessels. In Moschcowitz's view, thrombi were constituted by agglutinated hyalinized erythrocytes. The disease was believed to be caused by a powerful "toxin that has both agglutinative and hemolytic properties" (1). Since then and up to 1980 almost 500 cases of TTP have been reported in the literature, and several criteria have been proposed for the diagnosis (2–4). The term TTP should be used when two of the three major criteria (thrombocytopenia, microangiopathic anemia, and neurologic involvement) are associated with two minor criteria (fever, renal changes, and presence of thrombi in the circulation) (5). The term hemolytic-uremic syndrome (HUS) is most commonly used when renal changes result in severe renal insufficiency. Hemolytic-uremic syndrome is more frequent in children and TTP in adults, but this is not a general rule (1,3,6–8). The same patients may be classified as having TTP or HUS during different episodes of disease exacerbation (9–11). There are also cases with severe renal failure that have been classified as TTP, and cases of HUS often have neurologic symptoms (12,13).

Idiopathic TTP has been separated from secondary TTP (5). TTP may occur in pregnancy or may complicate the postpartum period (14,15). Cases of TTP have been discovered in association with neoplastic disorders such as lymphoma (16), Sjögren's syndrome (17), rheumatoid arthritis (18), polyarteritis (19), and systemic lupus erythematosus (SLE) (20,21). Thrombotic thrombocytopenic purpura has been recognized in patients with endocarditis (22) or after treatment with sulfonamide (23,24), iodine (25), oral contraceptives (26), and some poisons (27).

The disease is more common in women, with a female to male ratio of 3:2 (3). Although the peak incidence occurs in the third decade of life, cases of TTP have been described in patients ranging from 1 to 90 years (2,28). Recurrent episodes of TTP are not exceptions, but relapses cannot be predicted by any clinical or hematologic feature (29–31). Based on cases of TTP occurring in siblings, a genetic predisposition has been suggested, and some reports indicate that there is a possibility that an autosomal recessive trait underlies TTP (32–34).

However, there are forms that, regardless of the underlying etiology, cannot be surely assigned to TTP or to HUS. In such cases, it may be better to use the broader term of TMA. As already noted, TMA defines histopathologic lesions common to both TTP and HUS. These histopathologic changes are almost invariably accompanied by thrombocytopenia and hemolytic anemia. Thrombocytopenia derives from platelet consumption in the microcirculation. The reason of hemolytic anemia is not as clear, but it may be a consequence of the mechanical fragmentation of erythrocytes during flow through partially

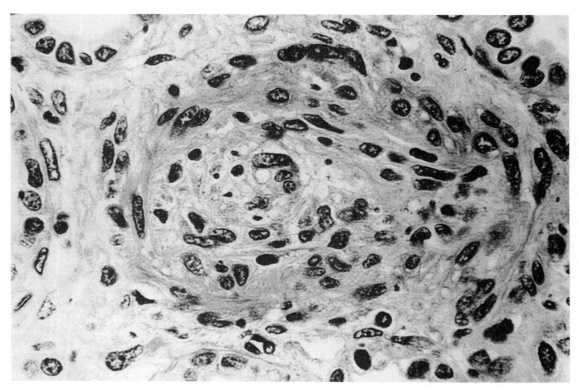

FIGURE 67-1. Marked endothelial and myointimal cell proliferation with occlusion of the lumen of an interlobular artery in a case of thrombotic thrombocytopenic purpura (trichrome, ×375).

occluded microvessels. Peripheral smear shows fragmented red blood cells with the typical aspect of burr or helmet cells. Elevations in lactate dehydrogenase (LDH) and low or undetectable haptoglobin levels are markers of hemolysis (2). Reticulocyte count is almost invariably elevated. Coomb's test is negative. Prothrombin time, partial thromboplastin time (PTT), factor V, factor VIII, and fibrinogen are normal in most cases. In some patients, high levels of fibrin degradation products and prolonged thrombin time have been observed

PATHOLOGY

Thrombotic Thrombocytopenic Purpura

The typical pathologic changes of TTP are the thrombi that occlude capillaries and arterioles in many organs and tissues (35,36). These thrombi are constituted by fibrin and platelets, and their distribution is widespread. They are most commonly detected in kidneys, pancreas, heart, adrenals, and brain (35,37,38). Compared to HUS, pathologic changes of TTP are more extensively distributed, probably reflecting the more systemic nature of the disease.

Other types of lesions have been described in TTP; the subendothelial accumulation of hyaline material has led to the term prethrombotic lesions (35), and frequently microaneurysms (36) or glomeruloid structures (10) are found. Altogether thrombi, prethrombotic changes, aneurysmal dilation of vessels, and glomeruloid structures have been considered typical of TTP, but recent studies cast doubt on the specificity of these lesions (38,39). Recently, it has been observed that gingival biopsies and bone marrow clot sections have the highest percentage of positivity for microthrombi (39,40).

Fibrin has been detected in the thrombi by immunofluorescence (41–43). Although the presence of platelets in the thrombi has been shown by electron microscopy (41), staining with antiplatelet sera is often negative (41,42,44). C3, C1q, and immunoglobulin deposits have been occasionally detected (42,45). In the kidney, fibrin–platelet thrombi are more frequent in arterioles than in glomerular capillaries (46). Reflecting the more chronic and relapsing character of the disease, proliferation of endothelial and myointimal cells (Fig. 67-1) is more pronounced in TTP than in HUS (47).

Hemolytic Uremic Syndrome

The kidneys are the main target organs involved in HUS. Pathologic changes originally described by Gasser et al. (48) in children with HUS were consistent with a picture of cortical necrosis. Since then, lesions of HUS have been described in more detail (49–53), and a term that successfully defines the characteristic pathologic changes of HUS is thrombotic microangiopathy (54). The classic lesion is characterized by thickening of the capillary walls secondary to the presence of a fluffy material in the subendothelial space (53,55,56). These changes, plus occasional thrombi, lead to occlusion of the glomerular capillary lumen. In the vessels from the tissue section, fragmented red blood cells or cells at different degrees of hemolysis may be detected (Fig.67-2). In the acute phase, arteriolar and capillary thrombi are more common, whereas the subendothelial fluff is the dominant lesion seen days or weeks after the acute attack. A widening and fibrillar appearance of the mesangium coexists with the glomerular capillary wall alterations (54,57). The vascular lesions may be differently distributed (55,58,59), and the percentage of affected glomeruli may influence the prognosis (59).

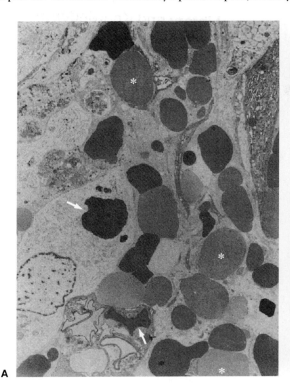
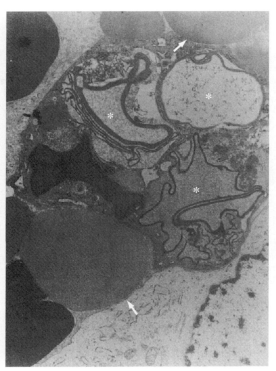

FIGURE 67-2. A: Electron micrograph showing fragmented red blood cells (*arrows*) and red cells at different stages of hemolysis (*asterisks*) in a small renal vein from a patient with hemolytic uremic syndrome (×5,000). **B:** High magnification of inset of Figure 67-2A showing red blood cells at different stages of hemolysis (*arrow*) and the presence of "ghosts" of red blood cells (*asterisks*) in a small renal vein from a patient with hemolytic-uremic syndrome (×12,000). (Both micrographs courtesy of Dr. C. L. Pirani and Dr. V. D'Agati.)

The finding of pure thrombotic microangiopathic lesions derives mainly from studies in children, especially children younger than the age of 2 years. However, in older children and adults, the histologic pattern is usually more complex and is characterized by a prevalence of arterial involvement with necrosis and thrombosis of interlobular arteries associated with ischemic changes in glomeruli.

Three patterns of renal lesions can be found in HUS—one with prevalent glomerular lesions of the microangiopathic type, one with predominant arterial involvement, and a third with simultaneous glomerular and arterial involvement. Other tentative classifications for HUS have been proposed (59). Recently, Thoenes and John (60) proposed the term endotheliotropic hemolytic nephroangiopathy. In the opinion of the authors, this term, in addition to including the main clinical features of the disease, also emphasizes the decisive pathogenetic role of endothelial damage. To emphasize the pathogenetic role of vascular changes in HUS, Bohle et al. (61) used the definition primary malignant nephrosclerosis.

A detailed analysis of renal changes in younger children includes swelling of glomerular endothelial cells leading to narrowing or complete occlusion of glomerular capillary lumens (Fig.67-3). Glomerular capillary walls are thickened, and often the endothelial cells are separated from the glomerular basement membrane (GBM). A fluffy material accumulates in the subendothelial space, giving a double-contoured appearance to the glomerular capillary walls (Fig.67-4). Together with the swelling of the endothelial cells, the widening of the subendothelial space contributes to the occlusion of the glomerular lumen. Thrombi having the characteristic staining for fibrin are occasionally seen. Mesangial matrix has a fibrillar appearance without any sign of mesangial hypercellularity.

Occasionally red blood cells and platelets are seen in the glomerular capillary lumens. Not all glomeruli are equally affected. In some cases damage is more severe, whereas in others less-pronounced changes (see Fig 67-4) are found. Arterial involvement is extremely variable, but some widening of the subendothelial space containing fluffy material is observed.

In older children and in adults, the major changes are restricted to the arteries (59,62). Interlobular arteries are often occluded by thrombosis, necrosis, or intimal edema or proliferation (62) (Figs. 67-5 and 67-6). In the more chronic phases, fibroplasia of small arteries and arteriosclerotic changes are seen. In some cases glomeruloid structures of the small arteries are observed, probably as a result of endothelial and myointimal proliferation of small arteries adjacent to the glomeruli (47). Glomerular lesions are ischemic, as shown by the thickening and wrinkling of the glomerular capillary walls, by atrophy of the glomerular tufts, and by thickening of Bowman's capsule (Fig.67-7). In a small number of patients a histologic pattern of cortical or tubular necrosis is detected (59). Not infrequently, however, the pattern of glomerular involvement coexists in the same patient with significant arterial damage (58,59).

Immunofluorescence shows fibrinogen almost invariably present in the glomeruli, along the glomerular capillary walls, and in the thrombi and vessel lumina (63). Granular deposits of C3 and immunoglobulin M (IgM) are also found in glomeruli and vessels (64,65). Ultrastructural injury to glomerular endothelial cells is pronounced. Endothelial cells are swollen and are often detached from the underlying GBM (Fig. 67-8). Beneath, the endothelium is an electron-lucent fluffy material that may be associated with a thin, newly formed GBM (Fig. 67-9). The composition of this fluffy material is not known, but it has been suggested that it might consist of fibrinogen–fibrin

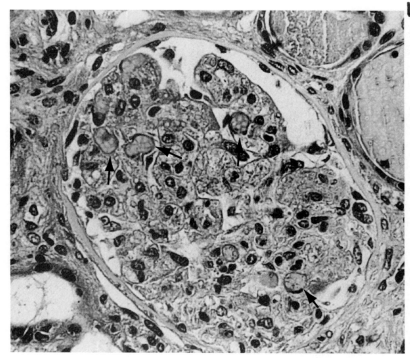

FIGURE 67-3. Swelling of glomerular endothelial cells and occlusion of almost all capillary lumens packed with red blood cells (*arrows*) in a case of hemolytic-uremic syndrome. (Trichrome, ×250.)

breakdown products as well as fibronectin (47). Glomerular capillary lumens are markedly narrowed by the combination of endothelial and subendothelial changes. Foam cells can be detected within the glomeruli, generally in the late stages of the disease, and contain lipid droplets and myelin figures. Glomerular mesangium may be the site of fibrin deposits, but

the most common lesion is edema of the mesangial matrix, leading to marked reticulation and even complete dissolution, called "mesangiolysis" (66). Endothelial damage predominates in arteries and arterioles, which demonstrate detachment of endothelium, swelling of endothelial cells, and subendothelial fluffy deposits.

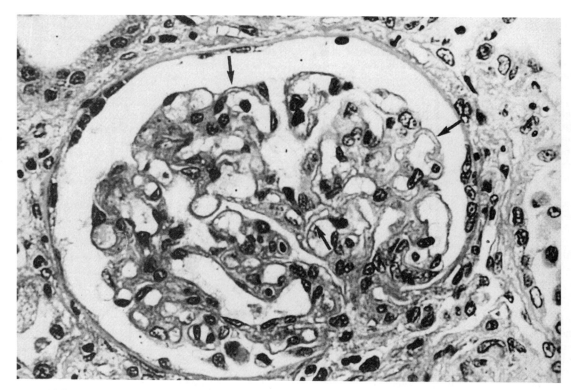

FIGURE 67-4. Double tracks (*arrows*) in some areas of glomerular capillary walls of a patient with hemolytic-uremic syndrome. (Trichrome, ×375.)

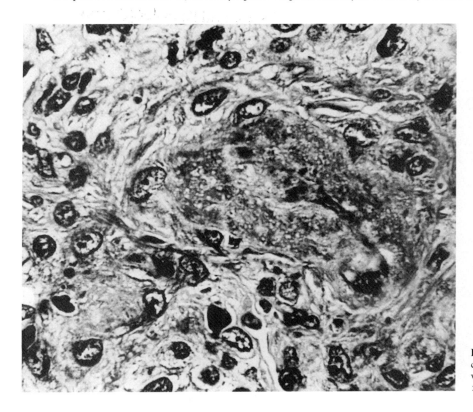

FIGURE 67-5. Thrombotic and necrotic changes in a small artery from an adult patient with hemolytic-uremic syndrome. (Trichrome, ×375.)

PATHOGENETIC MECHANISMS

The Central Role of Endothelial Damage

Toxins, immune reactants, and drugs may cause endothelial damage, which, in turn, may result in decreased prostacyclin bioavailability, increased shear stress, and oxidative stress that contribute to amplify the damage in a vicious circle resulting in microvascular thrombosis.

Toxins

Shigatoxin. In 1978, Koster et al. (67) found an association between Shigella dysenteriae type 1, severe colitis, and children with HUS, which is now reported quite frequently in India (68,69) where HUS is epidemic). Further studies (70) found that *E. coli* can produce exotoxins related to the 70-kDa protein encoded in *S. dysenteriae* DNA. In 1983, Riley et al. (71) reported the association of *E. coli* (serotype O157:H7) infection and two outbreaks of hemorrhagic colitis, and a paper in *The Lancet* described verotoxin-producing *E. coli* (VTEC)

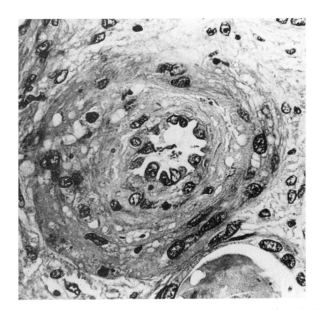

FIGURE 67-6. Occlusion of an interlobular artery with intimal swelling and myointimal proliferation in a case of adult hemolytic-uremic syndrome. (Trichrome, ×375.)

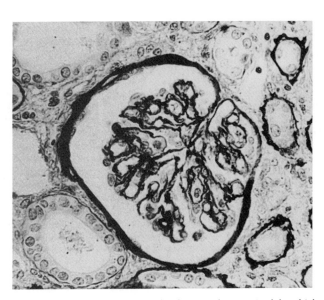

FIGURE 67-7. Ischemic glomerular lesions characterized by thickening and wrinkling of glomerular capillary walls and atrophy of glomerular tuft in a case of adult hemolytic-uremic syndrome. (Silver, ×250.)

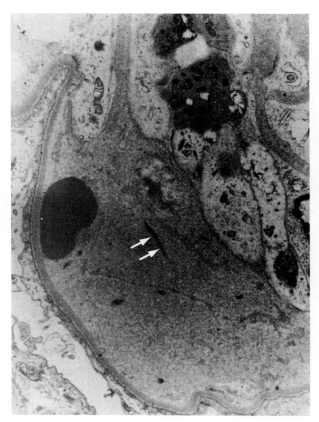

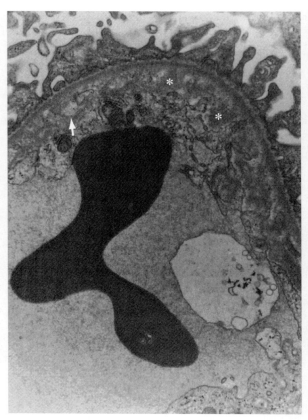

FIGURE 67-8. Detachment of endothelial cell from the underlying glomerular basement membrane in a case of hemolytic-uremic syndrome. A red blood cell is in close contact with the glomerular basement membrane. Electron-lucent "fluffy" material and a few strands of ⌐brin (*arrows*) are present in subendothelial space (×7,000). (Courtesy of Dr. C. L. Pirani and Dr. V. D'Agati.)

FIGURE 67-9. Electron-lucent "fluffy" material (*arrow*) with some electron-dense deposits (*asterisks*) is located between the cytoplasm of an endothelial cell and the glomerular basement membrane in a segment of glomerular capillary from a patient with hemolytic-uremic syndrome (×12,000). (Courtesy of Dr. C. L. Pirani and Dr. V. D'Agati.)

infection (72) in 11 of 15 cases of sporadic HUS. From now on, only the term Shigatoxin (or Stx) should be used to name exotoxins produced both *S. dysenteriae* and by *E. coli*, and the other terms such as Shiga-like toxin, verotoxin, or VTEC should be abandoned (73).

Humans may be infected from contaminated milk, meat, and fecally contaminated water, or from contact with infected animals, humans, or the excreta of either (74–76). Rowe et al. (77) found that undercooked meat and foods are not necessarily implicated in the transmission of the disease, which is more likely to occur in patients who have been exposed to a family member with diarrhea in the 7 days before the onset of symptoms than in healthy controls. This suggested a person-to-person transmission of Stx-producing *E. coli* that is also a plausible explanation for most cases of sporadic HUS (78–81). It can be estimated that in North America and western Europe about 90% of children with HUS have some evidence of Stx infection, with the serotype O157:H7 in 70% of cases (82–85). O157:H7 serotype is not common in Argentinian cases of Stx-induced diarrhea (but without hemorrhagic colitis) complicated or not by HUS (86). This would suggest that Stx of serotypes other than O157:H7 is mostly associated with nonbloody diarrhea.

Following ingestion, *E. coli* and *S. dysenteriae* localize on the colonic mucosa, invade epithelial cells, multiply, and cause cell death. (The action of such organisms normally gives diarrhea), but only strains that produce Stx's damage the vasculature of the mucosa so as to cause hemorrhagic colitis (87). Shigatoxins are picked up by polarized gastroin-

testinal cells via transcellular pathways and translocate into the circulation, probably facilitated by the transmigration of polymorphonuclear cells (PMNs), which increase paracellular permeability (88,89).

Although it has been shown *in vitro* that Stx can bind to human erythrocytes, platelets, and activated monocytes, recent studies have underpinned a role for PMN in Stx carriage in blood, since Stx rapidly and completely binds to PMN when incubated with human blood (90). Consistently, circulating PMN-bound Stx has been detected in blood of Stx-HUS patients (91). Moreover, PMN Stx receptor has a 100-fold lower affinity to the ligand than the high-affinity receptor expressed on glomerular endothelial cells, thereby facilitating the intercellular transition. Actually, *in vitro* and in co-cultures, PMN loaded with Stx transfer the ligand to glomerular endothelial cells so that at the end of the incubation Stx molecules were found on glomerular endothelial cells but no longer on PMN (90).

The human disease is caused by two distinct exotoxins— Stx-1 and Stx-2—almost identical to the toxin produced by *S. dysenteriae* type 1 (92). Stx DNA is incorporated into the genoma of a restricted number of some *E. coli* O:H serotypes, which can produce Stx-1 alone or Stx-2, or both. Both Stx-1 and Stx-2 are 70-kDa AB5 holotoxins comprising a single A subunit of 32 kDa and a five 7.7-kDa A subunit. Interestingly, a new AB5 toxin comprising a single 35-kDa A subunit and a pentamer of 13-kDa B subunits have been recently isolated from a highly virulent *E. coli* strain (O113:H21) responsible for an outbreak of HUS, which may represent the prototype of a new class of toxins, accounting for HUS associated with strains of *E. coli* that do not produce Stx's (93). Despite their similar sequences, Stx-1 and Stx-2 cause different degrees and types of tissue damage as documented by the higher pathogenicity of strains of *E. coli* that produce only Stx-2 than of those that produce Stx-2 alone (94–96). In a recent study in children who became infected by Stx-*E. coli*, *E. coli* strains producing Stx-2 were most commonly associated with HUS, whereas most strains isolated from children with diarrhea alone or remaining asymptomatic only produced Stx-1 (97). This is also true in mice and baboons (98).

Stx-1 and Stx-2 bind to different epitopes on the Gb3 molecules and they also differ in binding affinity and kinetics (99). Surface plasmon resonance analysis showed that Stx-1 easily binds to and detaches from Gb3, in contrast to Stx-2, which binds slowly but also dissociates very slowly, thus leaving time enough for the cell's incorporation (99).

After binding to endothelial cell receptors, the toxin is internalized in the cytosol by endocytosis (100) within 2 hours (101) and inhibits protein synthesis within 30 minutes (Fig. 67-10). The number of high-affinity receptors is a major determinant of susceptibility of cells to Stx (102). Therefore, cell viability and protein synthesis of endothelial cells of the kidney were reduced by 50% upon exposure to 1 pM Stx, unlike endothelial cells of umbilical vein that were viable up to greater than 1 nM exposure to the toxin. These findings are consistent with basal levels of Stx receptors 50 times higher in renal endothelium than in the umbilical cord endothelium (103). During internalization, the alpha subunit of the toxin dissociates from the beta subunits. Approximately 10% of the alpha subunit protein is removed in a trypsinlike process, resulting in a maximally ac-

tive 27-kDa subunit enzyme. It is well established that this fragment is a direct inhibitor of protein synthesis and is responsible for the cytotoxic action of the toxin. Stx selectively inactivates 60S ribosomal subunits by removing one nucleotide in the 28S ribosomal RNA in a nucleotide-specific manner (104).

For many years it was assumed that the only relevant biologic activity of Stx was the block of protein synthesis and destruction of endothelial cells. Recently, however, it has been shown that treatment of endothelial cells with sublethal doses of Stx, exerting minimal influence on protein synthesis, leads to increased mRNA levels and protein expression of chemokines, such as interleukin (IL)-8 and monocyte chemoattractant protein-1 (MCP-1) and cell adhesion molecules, a process preceded by NF-kB activation (105). Analysis of genome wide expression pattern of human endothelial cells stimulated with sublethal doses of Stx evidenced 25 and 24 genes upregulated by Stx-1 and Stx-2, respectively, mostly encoding for chemokines and cytokines, cell adhesion molecules, including P-selectin and intercellular adhesion molecule 1 (ICAM-1), and transcription factors (EGR-1, NFkB2, and NFkBIA) (106).

Adhesion molecules seem to play a critical role in mediating binding of inflammatory cells to endothelium. This is supported by adhesion experiments under flow showing that Stx-2 treatment enhanced the number of leukocytes adhering and migrating across a monolayer of human endothelial cells (107). Moreover, preventing IL-8 and MCP-1 overexpression by adenovirus-mediated NF-kB blocking, inhibited adhesion and transmigration of leukocytes (105).

Therefore, it can be inferred that Stx, by altering endothelial cell adhesion properties and metabolism, favor leukocyte-dependent inflammation and induce loss of thromboresistance

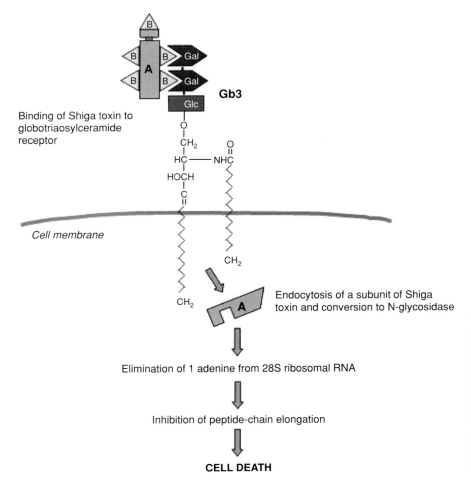

Binding of Shiga toxin to globotriaosylceramide receptor

Gb3

Cell membrane

Endocytosis of a subunit of Shiga toxin and conversion to N-glycosidase

Elimination of 1 adenine from 28S ribosomal RNA

Inhibition of peptide-chain elongation

CELL DEATH

FIGURE 67-10. Binding and mechanism of action of Shiga-like toxin. The B subunits of Shiga toxin molecules attach to galactose (gal) disaccharides of globotriaosylceramide (Gb3) receptors on the membrane of monocytes, polymorphonuclear cells, platelets, glomerular endothelial cells, and tubular epithelial cells. The toxin is internalized via retrograde transport through the Golgi complex. Then the A and B subunits dissociate, and the A subunit is translocated to the cytosol. The A subunit blocks peptide chain elongation by eliminating one adenine from the 28S ribosomal RNA.

in endothelial cells, leading to microvascular thrombosis. Evidence for such sequence of events has been obtained in experiments of whole blood flowing on human microvascular endothelial cells, pre-exposed to Stx-1, at high shear stress (108). In these circumstances early platelet activation and adhesion occurs, followed by formation of organized endothelial P-selectin and platelet-endothelial cell adhesion molecule (PECAM)-1-dependent thrombi. This offers a likely pathophysiologic pathway for microvascular thrombosis in HUS. This report may also be taken as a demonstration of a link between bacteria and their products and arterial thrombosis, as suggested by the evidence of *in vivo* coagulation disturbances, that is, increase of prothrombin fragment 1+2, found in children who developed HUS upon infection with *E. coli* O157:H7 (109–111). Although early studies suggested that fibrinolysis is augmented in Stx-HUS, more recent work revealed the presence of higher than normal levels of plasminogen-activator inhibitor type 1, indicating that fibrinolysis is substantially inhibited (111).

Endotoxins. Endotoxemia is often associated with HUS (112), which would suggest that endothelial cell damage is the result of the toxic effect of Stx, added to that of endotoxin (113). Lipopolysaccharide (LPS, endotoxin) may combine with Stx to amplify its cytotoxic potential. Such a synergism was dose-dependent on umbilical vein and renal endothelial cells in culture and was maximal after preincubation of cells with endotoxin (114). A similar synergism has also been demonstrated between Stx and tumor necrosis factor-α (TNF-α) (113). This increase occurs mainly via TNF receptor 55 upon protein kinase C activation (115). Of interest to understanding the pathogenesis of renal lesions in HUS are findings that Stx induces TNF-α biosynthesis in the kidney, but not in other organs or tissues (116).

TNF-α, IL-1 and IL-6 have been demonstrated to upregulate the expression of globotriaosylceramide on renal endothelial cells and increase the binding of Stx-1 (108,117). According to recent studies, Stx-1 may induce the endothelial cells to secrete unusually large multimers of von Willebrand factor and enhance the expression of vitronectin (αvβ3 integrin) receptors, P-selectin, and PECAM-1 on cell surfaces (108). Moreover, in another study (118) Stx-1 was shown to bind to and activate platelets through globotriaosylceramide or globotriaosylceramide-like receptors.

Yamada et al. (119) documented that endotoxin requires the presence of granulocytes to damage endothelial cells in culture. Because the damage could be reduced by suppressing granulocyte adhesiveness or by oxygen free-radical scavengers, the authors concluded that cytotoxic activity of endotoxin could be due in part to its capability of promoting granulocyte adhesion to endothelium and stimulating granulocyte production of toxic oxygen radicals. Moreover, neutrophils from children with diarrhea-associated HUS have an enhanced capacity to adhere to endothelial cells and cause injury (120).

Meyrick (121), using both *in vitro* and *in vivo* models, showed that endotoxin can cause a direct injury to pulmonary endothelium and that this damage is enhanced by activated complement and granulocytes by their interaction with the altered endothelium. In more recent years data became available indicating that similar to cytokines such as TNF and IL-1, endotoxin induces a dramatic increase in endothelial cell adhesiveness for leukocytes by stimulating the expression of endothelial cell adhesion molecules. Specifically, endotoxin acts directly upon endothelium *in vitro* to induce the expression of E-selectin, ICAM-1, and P-selectin (122–124). Munro et al. (125) showed that endotoxin injection into baboon skin resulted in the *de novo* endothelial expression of E-selectin, which was associated with concurrent extensive adhesion and extravasation of neutrophils. In another model in which en-

dotoxin was administered by intravenous injection to rats, Coughlan et al. (124) documented a rapid onset of neutropenia in association with induction of P-selectin expression on microvascular endothelial cells in kidney, liver, and lung. Treatment with an antibody to P-selectin blocked neutropenia and neutrophil accumulation in tissues.

Neuraminidase

Neuraminidase, produced by some bacteria and viruses, also can damage vascular endothelium. Klein et al. found that neuraminidase, by removing sialic acids from the cell membranes exposes the Thomsen-Friedenreich receptor present on glomeruli, red cells, and platelets (127). The formation of an anti-Thomsen-Friedenreich IgM antibody would promote agglutination of red cells and platelets.

Immune Reactants

Antibodies (128–132) and immune complexes (133–135) can induce endothelial injury and trigger massive sequestration of platelets and polymorphonuclear leukocytes in the microvasculature (131), as in acute allograft rejection in humans (132). It is likely that circulating antibodies or immune complexes or both play a pathogenetic role in the development of thrombotic microangiopathies in the course of connective tissue disorders, such as SLE (20,21), Sjögren's syndrome (17), rheumatoid arthritis (18), polyarteritis (19), the most frequent association being with SLE, although the percentage incidence varies in the different reports (136,137).

Occasional patients with TTP have cytotoxic antibody to cultured endothelial cells *in vitro* (138,139). This cytotoxicity is complement dependent and related to the IgG fraction of immunoglobulins. That autoimmune-mediated endothelial damage may be the cause of microvascular injury is supported by the findings of Leung et al. (140), who described the consistent presence of cytotoxic anti-endothelial cell antibodies in the serum of patients in the acute phase of TMA. The same authors found that sera from 13 of 14 children with acute HUS contained complement-fixing IgG and IgM antibodies that specifically injured cultured human umbilical vein endothelial cells. The endothelial cell antigen was lost after treatment of the cells with gamma interferon. In contrast, only 3 of 5 adult patients with acute, nonrelapsing TTP had lytic anti-endothelial antibodies, and only one of these recognized an antigen lost upon treatment with gamma interferon. None of 32 control sera contained lytic anti-endothelial cells antibodies. These data suggest that, at least in some children, HUS may involve a disorder of immunoregulation so that a unique class of anti-endothelial cell antibodies is detectable in such patients. The possibility of an antibody mediated injury to endothelial cells is supported by the findings of Platt et al. (141) who recently showed that exposing cultured porcine endothelium to human serum as a source of natural antibodies and complement caused cleavage and release of endothelial cell proteoglycans that preceded irreversible cell injury. These *in vitro* findings might be interpreted to indicate that the loss of endothelial cell proteoglycan is critical to the pathogenesis of vascular damage and that stimuli other than endotoxins can also induce endothelial injury.

Experimental endothelial damage can also be induced by immune complexes. A model of endothelial damage probably due to immune-complex deposition has been described in rabbits treated with BSA, which classically induces acute serum sickness (133,134). In this model, endothelial damage is probably mediated by basophil and platelet activation. These cells release vasoactive amines responsible for increasing vascular permeability and facilitating the further localization of immune complexes at the level of endothelial injury. In these animals there is extensive endothelial destruction and exfoliation with fibrin deposits in the glomerular capillaries and mesangium (133).

Hyperacute renal allograft rejection and acute serum sickness are examples of immunologically mediated endothelial damage. Hyperacute rejection of the kidney is mediated by secondary injury following antigen–cytotoxic antibody reaction at the interface of the recipient's blood and the donor's endothelium (129,130). The earliest event after fixation of antibodies and complement to the endothelium is believed to be massive sequestration of platelets and, to a lesser extent, of polymorphonuclear leukocytes in the microvasculature of the graft (131,132). Widespread microthrombosis with concomitant vasoconstriction is a crucial event leading to vascular occlusion and ischemia (142). The endothelial injury has been observed in several experimental models, such as hyperacute cardiac allograft rejection and skin allograft rejection; information obtained from rejection of these organs has greatly helped in our understanding of the mechanisms and targets of renal rejection. Dvorak et al. (143), in a model of skin allograft rejection, found diffuse microvascular damage preceding infarction of skin allograft. Vascular damage associated with hypertrophy, necrosis, and sloughing of endothelial cells was the major cause of skin graft rejection. Forbes et al. (144), studying cardiac allograft rejection in the rat, observed extensive endothelial injury that was complement dependent and associated with platelet aggregation.

Drugs

About 200 cases of TMA have been described in the course of neoplastic diseases and appear to depend on the use of some anticancer drugs, such as mitomycin, vinblastine, cisplatin, bleomycin, cytosine arabinoside, and daunorubicin (145–151). Cancer-associated TMA has been reported in 4% to 15% of patients given mitomycin. Most patients develop TMA after cumulative doses that exceed 60 mg (151). Mytomycin added to cultured endothelial cells of human umbilical cord vein inhibits prostacyclin production and cell proliferation in a dose-dependent manner (152). Perfusion of the renal artery *in vivo* also induces structural abnormalities reminiscent of HUS, which include endothelial injury followed by platelet deposition, subendothelial expansion, and obliteration of arterioles and capillaries (153). Immunotherapeutic drugs, namely cyclosporine, tacrolimus, OKT3, interferon, and quinidine, have been frequently reported to induce non–Stx-HUS (126).

Thrombotic microangiopathy has been described in women using an estrogen-containing birth control pill (154,155,156,157), but the incidence, prevalence, and strength of this association are not known. Possible predisposing factors other than birth control pills, such as "flu-like illness" (154,158), pregnancy (157), or severe hypertension (159–161), were recognized in most reports. Hence, some cases defined as "birth control pill–associated HUS" were actually forms of familial (162–164) or recurrent (165) HUS. In turn, evidence that the prevalence of women who use the birth control pill and developed HUS or TTP is comparable with the prevalence of age-matched women who use the birth control pill in the general population (166) strongly argues against a direct cause and effect relationship between birth control pill and TMA.

The platelet anti-aggregating agent ticlopidine has been associated to the development of TTP with an estimated incidence of 1 case per 1,600 to 5,000 (167–170). The first occurrence of TTP in association with ticlopidine was clearly recognized only 7 years after the approval of the drug (167–170). Thrombocytopenic purpura developed within 2 weeks after the initiation of treatment in 15% of reported cases and within one month in 80% of cases. The overall mortality rate for ticlopidine-associated cases of TTP has been estimated as 33%. Fifty-seven percent of the reported cases were treated with plasma ex-

change (167,170). Although a comparison is faulted by the use of a retrospective analysis, it should be noted that among the patients who received plasmapheresis the mortality rate was 18%, whereas it was 58% among those who did not.

A new antiplatelet agent, clopidogrel, whose mechanism of action and indications are similar to those of ticlopidine, was very recently associated with 11 cases of TTP (171); 10 of them developed TTP within 2 weeks of the beginning of treatment with the drug. All were treated with plasma exchange; one died and all the other recovered, although for two cases 20 exchanges or more were required before recovery.

Quinine was recently described to induce TMA characterized by predominant renal impairment. Despite the dramatic presenting symptoms and severe renal failure, the outcome is usually good if cessation of quinidine and institution of plasma exchange are provided early enough (73).

Recently, the use of antimotility agents has been described to be associated with an increased risk of HUS following E. coli infection (74,172). A very recent report described a case of TTP associated with treatment with zoledronic acid in which an immune-mediated reaction was suspected (173). The clinical course of a patient who presented a TTP pattern after being started on simvastatin, a HMG-CoA inhibitor, is described (174).

The Role of Platelet Activation

Damaged endothelial cells may favor platelet activation and aggregation at the site of endothelial injury. Therefore, "exhausted platelets" from patients with acute HUS contain less βbeta-thromboglobulin and serotonin and poorly aggregate in vitro (175–177). Elevated plasma levels of platelet derived proteins, beta-thromboglobulin, and platelet factor 4, and low platelet–plasma serotonin ratios in children with acute HUS (176,178), further indicate that intravascular platelet activation is a prominent pathophysiologic feature that may contribute to the genesis of the thrombocytopenia.

Platelet activating factor (PAF), a lipid mediator of inflammation released from injured endothelial cells, platelets, and leukocytes that *in vitro* induces platelet and neutrophil adhesion on the endothelial cell surface (179), is excreted in increased amounts in the urine of children during the acute phase of HUS (180). However, although PAF promotes platelet activation and impairs renal function, whether PAF release from renal vascular endothelial cells has a role in the pathogenesis of the disease or is rather a specific marker of endothelial injury has not been established to date.

Specific platelet activators have also been identified in TTP. Lian et al. (181) found that plasmas from 3 patients with acute TTP induce *in vitro* clumping of platelets from both normal subjects or from the same patients during remission. The platelet clumping substance was not adenosine diphosphate (ADP) or collagen and its activity was not inhibited by antiplatelet agents. The same authors identified a 37-kDa protein (p37) with platelet agglutinating activity that was independent from ADP release, energy metabolism, and the cyclooxygenase pathway. In turn, p37 was completely inhibited by IgG from healthy human adults or from TTP patients after recovery, likely through the formation of a p37-IgG complex (182). p37 activity is likely mediated by a specific and concentration-dependent binding to a 97-kDa platelet membrane protein. Because this protein was identified by anti-glycoprotein IV (GPIV) antibodies on either platelet or endothelial cell membranes, Lian hypothesized that p37-GPIV binding on endothelial cells may cause endothelial injury and mediate platelet–endothelial cell interaction. Also a of 59-kDa protein purified from plasma of some patients with acute TTP was found to cause the aggregation of platelets from healthy subjects. Its activity was calcium dependent, required energy metabolism and fibrinogen, and was inhibited by prostacyclin, normal plasma, and monoclonal antibodies against the GPIIb/IIa complex, but not by heparin and aspirin. Further studies are needed to better characterize these proteins and their role in the pathogenesis of TTP.

The Role of Deficient ADAMTS13 Activity

The relationship between unusually large (UL) von Willebrand factor (vWF) multimers and thrombotic microangiopathies remained elusive until the recent demonstration of the presence in human plasma of a vWF-cleaving protease (183,184), which was first partially characterized in 1996, and then identified in 2001 and shown to be a member of the so-called ADAMTS (a disintegrin and metalloprotease with thrombospondin type 1 domains family of protease) (184). This metalloprotease was shown to cleave vWF physiologically at the peptide bond between amino acid residues 842Thr and 843Met in the A2 domain of the subunit (183). ADAMTS13 is expressed by the homonymous gene restricted on chromosome 9q34. Mutations in this gene lead to an inactive enzyme as it was demonstrated in available data (185).

Two primary mechanisms for deficiency of the ADAMTS13 activity have been identified, namely a constitutive deficiency and the presence of a circulating acquired inhibitory antibody. Whereas patients affected by Upshaw-Schulman syndrome (186), which is synonymous with hereditary TTP (117), and by recurrent and familial HUS (183) have a severe deficiency of ADAMTS13 caused by heterozygous or homozygous ADAMTS13 gene defect, the role of antibody-mediated ADAMTS13 deficiency in the pathogenesis of sporadic TTP continues to be a disputed topic of discussion (184). IgG antibodies inhibiting the metalloprotease has been found in 48% to 80% of patients with acquired idiopathic TTP (117,187); these data are controversial. Moreover, a decrease in ADAMTS13 antibody titers has not been demonstrated consistently during plasma exchange procedures, which are the most effective therapeutic techniques (117,183,184).

The discovery of deficient ADAMTS13 activity in TTP has been rapidly integrated into the prevailing model of the pathophysiology of vWF-mediated thrombotic microangiopathies. According to this model, congenital or autoimmune dysfunction of ADAMTS13 prevents the normal proteolysis of large vWF multimers as they are secreted from injured endothelial cells. This ultimately causes the development of circulating UlvWFs multimers. Such material does not normally circulate but is stored in endothelial Weibel-Palade bodies, and its presence in the peripheral blood reflects endothelial cell injury. In conditions of high shear stress, ULvWF multimers are capable of supporting platelet aggregation more efficiently than normal multimers, by means of glycoprotein Ib receptors on platelet membrane (117). This condition would predispose patients to microvascular thrombosis at sites of endothelial cell injury. However, direct proof of this has never been provided.

Results of analysis of the relationship between vWF multimeric pattern and ADAMTS13 activity in TTP and HUS patients may offer alternative opportunities. On one hand, UL multimers in 2 patients with recurrent TTP have been found with normal ADAMTS13 activity. On the other hand, many patients with either TTP or HUS, with complete or severe deficiency of the ADAMTS13 activity, did not have UL multimers in their circulation. In addition, patients with deficiency of ADAMTS13 activity showed increased vWF fragmentation during the acute phase, as indirectly documented by a lower high molecular weight–low molecular weight (HMW–LMW) multimer ratio, rather than in remission. The same results were reported by Veyradier et al., who found no correlation between ADAMTS13 activity levels and ULvWF multimers in their large series. It was also found that the normal 189-, 176-, and 140-kDa (187) fragments were present in the blood of all patients with deficient ADAMTS13 activity, and the percentage of the native intact vWF subunit was even lower than in healthy subjects, at least in the acute phase. These results indicate that besides ADAMTS13, other proteases are present in the blood of patients with TMA that cleave vWF to the normal fragments and support the possibility that deficiency of the ADAMTS13 activity is not the only determinant of vWF abnormalities in these diseases. Consistent with the present findings, many studies have documented that in sporadic (190), recurrent (189–191), and familial (189) TMA, and in the acute phase of HUS resistant to plasma therapy (192), rather than the presence of ULvWF multimers, there is a loss of such multimers and an increase of LMW forms that indicate enhanced proteolytic fragmentation of the molecule.

In two large clinical studies (189,193), deficiency of ADAMTS13 activity was found in patients with diagnosis of TTP but not in those with HUS. These data seemed to indicate that the presence or absence of this activity could be used to classify patients as having TTP or HUS (183). Nevertheless, severe deficiency of ADAMTS13 activity was found in patients with disorders of thrombocytopenia other than TTP and HUS, including idiopathic thrombocytopenia (one case), SLE (two cases), and disseminated intravascular coagulation (three cases) (188,194). It is important however to recall that microvascular platelet thrombi in disseminated intravascular coagulation are vWF negative and fibrinogen positive, the opposite of thrombi in TTP patients (195). In addition, deficient ADAMTS13 activity is not the only determinant of the presence of ultralarge ULvWF multimers in some phases of the clinical disease of these patients (183).

It may be concluded that low values of ADAMTS13 activity may not be specific for TTP, at least in recurrent and familial forms. However, there is evidence of a link between ADAMTS13 and vWF, and this may be studied using the broader term of TMA (thrombotic microangiopathies), classifying patients in ADAMTS13-associated TMA, as well as in Stx-TMA or HF-dependent TMA (see the following text).

No ADAMTS13 inhibitor was found in patients with familial TTP, despite a complete deficiency of activity of the protease. However, the method used in this study would not detect the presence of antibodies that do not inhibit ADAMTS13 activity but do enhance the clearance of the protease *in vivo*, so that the prevalence of antibodies might have been underestimated in this study. However, in the available asymptomatic parents of the patients described in the preceding text, levels of ADAMTS13 activity were consistent with carriership (approximately 50% activity), indicating that the ADAMTS13 defect was inherited. These results support the view that the deficiency of ADAMTS13 activity in thrombotic microangiopathies may be acquired as a result of an autoimmune mechanism or may be inherited (183).

The Role of Uncontrolled Complement Activation

Genetically determined defects in some components of the complement system such as the factor H 1 (HF1) and the membrane cofactor protein (MCP) may result in uncontrolled complement activation, secondary endothelial damage, and eventual microvascular thrombosis.

Defective Factor H Bioavailability

HF1 consists of 20 homologous units, named short consensus repeats (SCRs). Human glomerular endothelial cells and

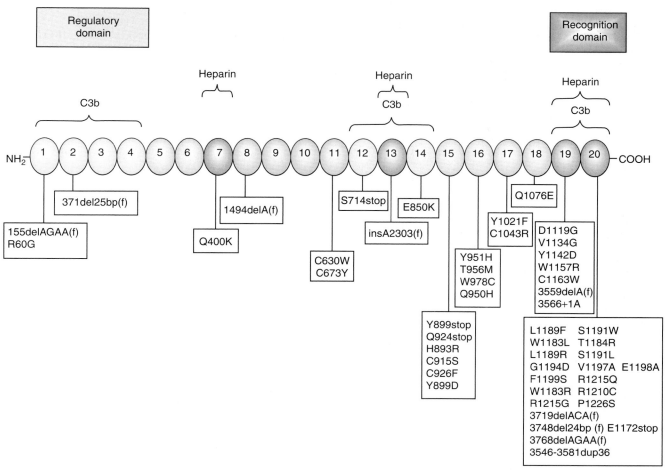

FIGURE 67-11. Factor H mutations associated with HUS. The figure shows the structure of human factor H with the 20 short consensus repeats. The locations of the N-terminal regulatory domain responsible for cofactor activity and the binding sites for C3b and polyanions (heparin) are indicated. The majority of the mutations found in patients with HUS clusters in the C-terminus of factor H that is important for binding to polyanions and to surface bound C3b and for the control of C3b deposition on cell membranes and extracellular matrix.

kidney glomerular basement membrane are rich in polyanionic molecules so that HF1 deposited on their surface would provide an efficient shield against complement attack (196,197). Fifty different HF1 mutations have been found to date in 80 patients who had familial (36 patients) and sporadic (44 patients) forms of non-Stx-HUS (198–201) (Fig. 67-11). Alterations in other genes encoding for complement regulatory proteins could theoretically be involved in determining predisposition to sporadic non-Stx-HUS. Alternatively, these forms could be caused by an acquired autoimmune HF1 defect similar to what has been observed in some patients with TTP in whom the acute episode is triggered by antibodies against ADAMTS13 (202). HF1 mutations are heterozygous in most HUS patients, who are commonly presenting normal HF1 plasma levels, in opposition to patients with type II membranoproliferative glomerulonephritis who carry homozygous HF1 mutations causing severely reduced HF1 levels (200). In a recent study (203), it has been proposed that HF1-related complement regulatory defects could be detected in serum with an *ex vivo* hemolytic assay, which may point out a more severe lysis of sheep erythrocytes with serum of patients with HF1 mutation than with serum from patients with normal HF1 activity. This, if confirmed, could represent a useful tool to select HUS patients who deserve studies of HF1 and other complement regulatory proteins.

Membrane Cofactor Protein Abnormalities

A heterozygous mutation has been recently found in MCP, a widely expressed transmembrane glycoprotein that regulates complement activation, in two patients with familial history of HUS. The mutation determines a 3-amino acid change at position 233–235 followed by a premature stop-codon that causes loss of MCP transmembrane domain and results in severely reduced MCP cell-surface expression (204). Membrane cofactor protein could be the second putative candidate gene for TMA associated with genetic defects; it is highly expressed in the kidney and plays a main role in regulating glomerular C3 activation. Reduced expression of MCP upon complement-activating stimuli may fail to restrict complement deposition on glomerular endothelial cells, leading to microvascular cell damage and tissue injury (204).

Pathophysiology of the Damaged Endothelium

Decreased Prostacyclin Bioavailability

In both TTP and HUS, damaged vessels form less than normal prostacyclin (PGI2) and serum binding capacity for

PGI2 is reduced (205–209). Although the former are indirect measurements, data of reduced urinary excretion of the renal metabolite of PGI2, 6-Keto PGF1-alpha (that normalizes in remission) (210) strongly support that, in vivo, children with acute HUS form less PGI2 than normal. PGI2, an inhibitor of platelet aggregation (211), is the major product of arachidonic acid formed by vascular endothelium in physiologic states, which inhibits platelet–platelet interaction, thereby limiting thrombus formation at the site of endothelial injury.

Shear Stress

A major factor to explain perpetuation of endothelial cell dysfunction in HUS is fluid shear stress. Shear stress changes, the force produced by flowing blood upon endothelial cell surface, have a profound influence on the pathophysiology of vascular endothelium and act as a determinant of vWF handling by enhancing the susceptibility of vWF to proteolytic cleavage (212). Specifically, a recent study found a shear-rate dependent loss of the largest multimers when normal plasma was perfused through long capillary tubings achieving shear rates normally encountered in the circulation. As the large multimers decreased, an increase in the smaller multimers was detected, including 200 and 350-kDa bands. These bands are the dimers of the 140-kDa and of the 176-kDa fragments (212). One can speculate that increased shear forces in damaged microvessels account for abnormal vWF fragmentation observed during the acute phase of TMA and serve to amplify and propagate microvascular lesions.

Oxidative Stress

There are recent data that increased flow rate *in vitro* caused a consistent release of nitric oxide (NO), a potent vasoactive derivative of L-arginine, from vascular endothelial cells (213) and upregulated NO synthase mRNA (214). Since, as documented by animal experiments, NO is a potent mediator of vascular damage (215), it derives that shear-stress mediated overproduction of endothelial NO can act as a major toxic factor for microvascular endothelium. Furthermore, convincing evidence is available that most of the toxic effects of neutrophil-derived oxygen radicals on vascular endothelium are mediated by the interaction of NO with O_2^- to form peroxynitrite, which is further transformed into HO•, the most potent and toxic oxygen-derived product radical so far known (216). It is conceivable that in HUS, NO released by endothelial cells upon the initial insult, serves to amplify endothelial damage via its direct cytotoxic potential as well as by interacting with leukocyte-derived oxygen radicals.

THE KEY SYNDROMES

TMA may be considered an idiopathic genetic or disimmune disease, or a secondary microangiopathic complication of systemic infectious or neoplastic diseases, according to the pathogenic mechanisms that have been discussed in the preceding text. In an attempt to sort out these topics, TMA may be divided according to key syndromes: TMA associated with infectious diseases or exogen infection-related toxins; TMA associated with or secondary to genetic defects; TMA associated with autoantibodies, suggesting an autoimmune disorder; TMA associated with pregnancy; TMA associated with transplant; and forms of TMA secondary to systemic diseases, such as cancer, malignant hypertension, HIV and dysimmune systemic diseases, such as scleroderma, SLE, and antiphospho-

---

TABLE 67-1

A SUGGESTED CLASSIFICATION OF THROMBOTIC MICROANGIOPATHIES (TMA) BASED ON THE UNDERLYING PATHOGENETIC MECHANISMS

TMA associated with infectious diseases
  Stx-associated HUS
  Neuraminidase-associated HUS
  HIV infection-associated TMA

TMA associated with ADAMTS 13 abnormalities
  TMA associated with genetically determined ADAMTS 13 abnormalities
  TMA associated with immune-mediated ADAMTS 13 abnormalities

TMA associated with abnormalities of the complement system
  HUS associated with genetically determined factor H deficiency
  HUS associated with immune-mediated factor H deficiency
  HUS associated with membrane cofactor protein (MCP) abnormalities

TMA associated with pregnancy
  Pregnancy associated TTP
  The Hemolysis, Elevated Liver enzymes and Low Platelet count (HELLP) syndrome
  Postpartum HUS

TMA associated with transplanation
  De novo HUS
  Recurrent HUS

TMA associated with metastatic cancer, chemotherapy, or radiotherapy

TMA associated with systemic diseases (scleroderma, systemic lupus erythematosus, vasculitis, malignant hypertension)
Idiopathic TMA
Post-TMA chronic nephropathy

---

lipid syndrome; lastly, if no clear triggering condition could be found, then idiopathic TMA. Post-HUS chronic nephropathy is the common sequela of any form of TMA resulting in chronic kidney damage after resolution of the acute microangiopathic episode (Table 67-1).

TMA Associated with Infectious Diseases

Associations between TMA and Coxsackie A (217), Coxsackie B (218), other unspecified viruses (219), microtatobiotes (9), *Mycoplasma pneumoniae* (220), *Legionella pneumophila* (221), and with recent vaccinations (222,223) have been described, and fatal simultaneous occurrence of TTP in a husband and wife (224) and in siblings (225) argue further for an infectious etiology in some cases. Neame hypothesized that viruses may cause the syndrome by producing platelet aggregation, endothelial cell damage, or the production of immune complexes (14). Circulating immune complexes are probably involved in the pathogenesis of TTP associated with bacterial endocarditis (226). TMA may complicate human immunodeficiency virus (HIV) type 1 infection as well as acquired immunodeficiency syndrome (AIDS) related complex (227–229). Elevated platelet-associated levels of IgG and IgM and of the third and fourth complements component suggest an immune-mediated pathogenesis of the syndrome (229). Among the different forms associated with infectious diseases, Stx-associated

HUS and neuraminidase-associated HUS deserve particular attention.

Stx-associated HUS

Epidemiology and Clinical Features. Typical (epidemic) HUS is also referred as D+HUS, since it is associated with prodromal diarrhea. D+HUS is mainly a disease of childhood (but no age group is exempt), with a slight prevalence in females among older children. Caucasians are more commonly affected with peak incidence in Britain, America, and India. It is now clear that Stx is associated with illnesses that include asymptomatic infection, diarrhea, hemorrhagic colitis, and HUS. Stx infection from O26, O111, O113, O121, O145, and O157 serotypes was recognized in 30 of 40 patients from Ontario and Quebec with classical HUS (230).

Gastrointestinal symptoms usually precede full manifestation of the disease and may be followed by a symptom-free period. Hemorrhagic colitis presents with abdominal cramps and watery diarrhea followed by a discharge resembling lower gastrointestinal bleeding. Barium enema reveals filling defects (pseudotumors) that are also features of HUS with bloody diarrhea. In some instances Stx-associated colitis may mimic surgical emergencies including appendicitis (231), acute ulcerative colitis with megacolon (232), and intestinal intussusception (233), which may occasionally call for unnecessary laparotomy that increases mortality. However, some individuals may well require a hemicolectomy for bowel infarction or perforation (234). These cases carry the worst prognosis. Shigellosis-associated HUS also has a high mortality rate (about 30%) and may be associated with systemic intravascular coagulation, acute cortical necrosis, and renal death (235,236). Gastrointestinal losses may cause hypovolemia, and, in combination with hemoglobinemia, hyperbilirubinemia, and hyperuricemia, may favor acute renal failure. Renal symptoms include macro- or micronematuria, proteinuria (occasionally nephrotic), oligoanuria, or polyuria. Oligoanuria, fluid retention, and hypertension may precipitate congestive heart failure. Prolonged oligoanuria and/or persistent hypertension are markers of more severe disease that often lead to residual renal impairment. Some patients with D+HUS have leukocyte counts of greater than 20,000 units and this is considered a predictor of poor outcome, especially in male patients (237). The yearly incidence of the disease (according to an epidemiologic survey in the United Kingdom) was of about 1/100,000, with a peak in children of 1 to 2 years of age (3.3/100.000/year) and between April and October (238). Diarrhea was bloody in 71.6% of cases. Stx infection was demonstrated in 62% of cases; 62% of children needed dialysis and 5% died during the acute phase of the disease. Hyponatremia was associated with an increased risk of seizures. At 1 year no patient was on chronic dialysis. All the available data indicate that patients with D+HUS tends to recover within 2 or 3 weeks without sequelae. Mortality today approaches about 6% of cases (239). However, at 10-year follow-up only 60% of patients have a normal glomerular filtration rate (GFR), whereas the rest have a GFR less than 80 mL/minute per 1.73 sqm (240). In a French series, 15 to 25 years after an episode of classical childhood HUS, only 10 of 25 patients had no renal abnormalities. Of the remaining 15 patients, four had reached end-stage renal failure, four had chronic renal failure, and eight had residual proteinuria or hypertension. All of these patients with residual renal disease had either patched cortical necrosis (11) or TMA involving at least 50% of the glomeruli at the time of disease presentation (241). Somnolence, confusion, and occasionally seizures and coma may be the consequence of uremia or hyponatremia and, in some cases, of TMA of the brain, occasionally with infarctions or hemorrhages (242). The neurologic symptoms usually subside with the remission of the disease, but sequelae including developmental retardation, learning and behavioral problems, focal motor deficits, and convulsions may persist for years (243).

Prognosis and Treatment. A recent meta-analysis of 49 published studies (3,476 patients, mean follow-up of 4.4 years) describing long-term prognosis of patients who survived an episode of Stx-HUS, reported death or permanent end-stage renal disease (ESRD) in 12% of patients and GFR of less than 80mL/minute per 1.73 m² in 25% (244). Correction of fluid and electrolyte abnormalities and dialysis played a major role in better short-term outcomes of children with HUS.

There is no clear consensus on whether antibiotics should be administered to treat Stx-E. coli infection. There are data indicating that exposure of E. coli O157:H7 to sulfamethoxazole/trimethoprim *in vitro* increases toxin production, whereas ciprofloxacin may reduce it (245). In a prospective cohort study of 71 children who had E. coli O157:H7 associated diarrhea, Wong et al. showed that antibiotic treatment was significantly associated with an increased incidence of HUS (246). The cohort comprised children infected with E. coli O157:H7, 9 of whom were treated with antibiotics. HUS developed in 10, 5 of 9 (56%) of those were treated with antibiotics and 5 of 62 (8%) of those were not treated. It was postulated that antibiotic-induced injury to the bacterial membrane might favor the acute release of large amounts of toxins. Conversely, a recent meta-analysis on 26 reports failed to show a higher risk of HUS associated with antibiotic treatment (247). Of note, in the study by Wong et al., no patient had bacteremia. Although bacteremia is very common in Stx-HUS precipitated by Shigella dysenteriae type 1, in which patients eventually progress to death if antibiotics are not started early enough, it is only rarely found in Stx-HUS caused by E. coli O157:H7 infection. A recent report of an adult patient with E. coli O157:H7-induced HUS with bacteremia and urinary tract infection showed that early antibiotic therapy rapidly resolved hematologic and renal abnormalities (248). Consequently, it may be suggested that in patients with Stx-E. coli gastrointestinal infection antibiotics should be avoided unless the patient presents with severe systemic bacteremia.

In occasional cases, enterohemorrhagic colitis progresses to severe ischemic bowel disease and perforation, which may require colectomy. Specific therapies, including corticosteroids, heparin, streptokinase, antiplatelet agents, and prostacyclin, were found of no benefit in cases of typical HUS of childhood (249,250). Only three prospective studies are available on the use of heparin. In one study (251) heparin was used in 10 of 30 severe cases of childhood HUS and appeared to worsen the outcome of the disease. Loirat et al. (252) failed to find differences in duration of hemolysis, thrombocytopenia, and oliguria, as well as differences in renal pathology and long-term renal function in 15 children with HUS given heparin and urokinase as compared to 18 controls who only had symptomatic treatment. Of note, in four patients antithrombotic therapy was associated with severe hemorrhages and was discontinued. Similarly, Van Damme-Lombaerts (253) did not find differences in duration of disease, outcome, and renal pathology in 58 children with HUS randomly given heparin plus dipyridamole or supportive therapy alone. Streptokinase and urokinase have definitely been associated with more hemorrhages and should no longer be used. Infusion of vitamin E (alpha-tocopherol, which prevents lipid peroxidation) was encouraging in uncontrolled studies. In 16 children with HUS, 14 of whom were oliguric and 11 required dialysis, oral vitamin E at the dose of 1g/m² per day for at least 1 week was associated with a good clinical course (254). All patients survived, with normal renal function in all but one 3 months later. These results appear better than those of a comparable group of children given heparin, streptokinase, or antiplatelet agents, but, in the absence of larger controlled studies, the role of vitamin E remains elusive. A double-blind controlled study by Sheth et al. (255) found that intravenous infusion of gamma-globulins had no long-term benefits in 20 children with HUS. Therefore, the risk of anaphylaxis and infection (256) provides support against their use as first choice therapy for HUS. A study with SYNSORB-Pk, a synthetic material composed of particles of silicon linked to globotriaosyl-ceramide, given orally failed to find any effect of SYNSORB over placebo (257).

Since 1980 some patients were given plasma infusion or plasma exchange with fresh frozen plasma (258,259). Published literature on pediatric cases with classic HUS given plasma manipulation is sparse. Sheth et al. (260) found that duration of anemia and thrombocytopenia and incidence of residual renal or neurologic abnormalities were comparable in 12 children given fresh-frozen plasma and in 31 historical controls. Ogborn et al. (261) compared retrospectively the outcomes of 18 children with typical HUS treated with hemodialysis and plasma infusion to that of 18 children treated with hemodialysis alone. Severity of the disease, length of hospital stay, duration of renal dysfunction, and disease-related complications were comparable. At discharge the prevalence of hypertension was higher in the plasma group than in the control. In a controlled study of plasma infusion in 32 children with severe HUS (262) the study group was given 30 mL/kg of plasma at admission and then 10 mL/kg per day until the platelet count exceeded 150,000. The average number of infusion days was 9.7. The control group had supportive therapy alone. No significant benefit of plasma could be demonstrated in the acute phase at 24 months follow-up. Renal biopsies taken one month after the onset of the disease showed comparable lesions at light microscopy. Ultrastructural studies of renal tissue, however, revealed arteriolar damage in 5 of 7 control patients, whereas none of the plasma-treated patients had such lesions. The French study by Loirat et al. (263) showed comparable blood pressure, serum creatinine, and proteinuria at 1 year follow-up in 39 children treated with plasma infusion (10 mL/kg/day for 7 days) and in 40 controls. However, renal biopsy studies revealed extensive cortical necrosis in 7 of 27 control patients, whereas no cases of cortical necrosis were found in the 27 patients who were given plasma. Therefore, despite plasma infusion in these preliminary studies appearing to ameliorate renal sequelae in children with HUS, none of the studies performed so far could demonstrate significant differences in major clinical end points, and none had the appropriate sample size to demonstrate differences, if one existed. Side effects of plasma treatment in children can be relevant and include risk of infection and fluid overload. The latter can be avoided by plasma exchange. Due to the benign course of typical HUS, risks and costs of specific treatments outweigh the potential benefits. Until new strategies become available for clinical practice, it appears that for the moment careful supportive management is still the most appropriate form of treatment.

Neuraminidase-Associated HUS

This is a rare but potentially fatal complication of pneumonia or, less frequently, meningitis caused by *Streptococcus pneumoniae*. The clinical picture is usually severe with respiratory distress, anuria, neurologic involvement, and coma (264). The outcome is strongly dependent on the effectiveness of antibiotic therapy. In theory, plasma infusion or exchange is contraindicated, since adult plasma contains antibodies against the Thomsen-Friedenreich antigen that may accelerate agglutination and hemolysis (265). Therefore, patients should be treated only with antibiotics and washed red cells. In some cases, however, plasma therapy, occasionally in combination with steroids, has been associated with recovery.

TMA Associated with Genetic or Immune-Mediated ADAMTS 13 Abnormalities

Differential diagnosis between TMA associated with genetic or immune-mediated ADAMTS 13 abnormalities is important to predict disease outcome and to guide specific treatments. Disease related to genetic defects may affect different members of the same family and tend to recur more times in the same individual (familial and recurrent TMA). Immune-mediated disease does not cluster in families, may unmask an underlying autoimmune disease or follow the exposure to certain drugs and may have a chronic, relentless course that parallels the continuous production of the anti-ADAMTS 13 autoantibody. The rationale of treatment is also different, replacement of the defective activity being the key component of treatment of genetic disease and inhibition of the autoantibody production being the main target of treatment in immune-mediated disease. Monitoring the severity of ADAMTS 13 deficiency and the levels of the autoantibodies is also important in following the patient response to treatment.

TMA Associated with Genetically Determined ADAMTS 13 Abnormalities

A recent large series of patients showed a 91% specificity of the ADAMTS13 defect in distinguishing between TTP and HUS (187), leading Veyradier et al. to conclude that "vWF-cleaving protease deficiency specifically concerns a subgroup of TMA corresponding to the TTP entity" and to formulate the paradigm that "a single laboratory test may enable physicians to distinguish TTP from HUS," according to ADAMTS13 activity. However, a few recent studies have challenged this paradigm, showing that patients with a diagnosis of HUS may have complete ADAMTS13 deficiency (183), albeit less frequently (187). Actually, in a recent study, most patients with a clinical diagnosis of recurrent or familial TTP had complete or severe deficiency of the ADAMTS13 activity during the acute phase of the disease, and in a subgroup the defect persisted at remission. Complete deficiency of ADAMTS13 activity was also found in plasma samples from 5 of 9 patients with recurrent and familial HUS during the acute phase and in 5 patients during remission. These results have been confirmed by evaluating the cleavage of recombinant vWF A1-A2-A3 domains, which overcomes possible artefacts of the collagen-binding assay due to the presence of endogenous undegraded vWF in test samples (202,274,275). In the series of the same authors each of two studied families had one patient with TTP and one with HUS who completely lacked ADAMTS13 activity (183). Because the patients within each family inherited the same genetic defect, these data can be taken to indicate that deficiency of ADAMTS13 may lead to either the TTP or the HUS phenotype. At variance with the series of Veyradier et al. showing 91% specificity of the ADAMTS13 defect in distinguishing between TTP and HUS, in the study previously described, a 44% specificity was found, thus challenging the quoted paradigm put forward by Veyradier and indicating that the protease defect cannot be narrowed to specific subtypes of TMAs. Differences in patient population, including only familial and recurrent TTP and HUS in one series (183), and mostly sporadic cases in the other one (187), may account for discrepancies in results.

TMA Associated with Immune-Mediated ADAMTS13 Abnormalities

IgG autoantibodies have been shown to react with different antigenic regions of the ADAMTS13 molecule in patients with acute TTP, suggesting an autoimmune pathogenesis for acute TTP (184,187,193,202). Further evidence of the pathogenetic role of this autoantibody is that it usually disappears from the circulation when remission is achieved by effective treatment and this occurs in parallel with the normalization of plasma vWF-cleaving protease activity. Of note, autoantibodies against ADAMTS13 have also been observed in patients developing TTP during treatment with antiplatelet drugs such as ticlopidine and clopidogrel (276).

Clinical Features

The syndrome manifests in most cases with the features of TTP. The clinical presentation is dominated in most patients by hemorrhages and neurologic symptoms (2,3). In more than 90% of cases purpura is the initial manifestation, which may or may not be associated with retinal hemorrhage, epistaxis, gingival bleeding, hematuria, gastrointestinal hemorrhage, menorrhagia, and hemoptysis (2,3,45,277). More rare symptoms are malaise, fatigue, pallor, abdominal pain, arthralgia, myalgia, and jaundice (2,3,278). Although fever is not frequently seen at onset, it is almost always present during the illness (2,3,40,45,277). Anemia is severe, with average values between 7 and 9 g/dL of hemoglobin (2,4,279). Transient and fluctuating neurologic manifestations are present in almost all patients (8). These include confusion, headache, paresis, aphasia, dysarthria, visual problems, and coma. Angiographic and electroencephalographic studies have not been performed extensively but do not appear to offer major diagnostic contributions. Ocular involvement is frequent, retinal and choroid hemorrhages being the most common manifestations (280).

Laboratory findings show microangiopathic hemolytic anemia in almost all patients (Table 67-1). A detailed analysis (5) of all the reported series of patients with TTP revealed that hemoglobin levels are less than 10 g/dL in 99% of patients and less than 6.5 g/dL in 38%. Reticulocyte counts are elevated and in 35% of patients are greater than 20% of circulating red blood cells. Serum levels of lactate dehydrogenase (LDH) are frequently correlated with the course of the disease (2,281). Leukocytosis is relatively frequent, but the white blood cell counts rarely exceed 20,000/mm^3 (3). The platelet count is generally low (2,4,40,45,277) and only rarely exceeds 60,000/mm^3. Platelet survival studies have shown reduced platelet survival, suggesting peripheral destruction or consumption (218,283). The complement system has not been studied extensively, but in most instances appears to be normal (14,284,285). Positive lupus erythematosus (LE) cell preparations and antinuclear antibody factors have been reported in a few cases (2,3,286).

Renal involvement is common, with proteinuria and microhematuria the most constant findings (2,40,198,279). Renal function is depressed in 40% to 80% of patients, although severe renal insufficiency is rare (2,4,40,277). Heart involvement is infrequent, although congestive heart failure and conduction disturbances have occasionally been reported (287,288). In rare instances, lungs may contain some alveolar and interstitial infiltrates (289). Abdominal pain has been reported in 10% to 30% of cases (2,3,286) and has been interpreted as secondary to the involvement of small vessels of the gastrointestinal tract (290,291). Pancreatitis has also been described (292).

Prognosis and Treatment

Historical Perspective. Amorosi and Ultmann (3) reported only 10% survival in 1964, but Ridolfi and Bell (277) documented a 46% survival between 1964 and 1980, that increased up to 90% in two large series published in 1991 (293,294). Factors that have improved survival in TTP include intensive care units and recent technical advances in the care of critically ill patients, but it seems unlikely that an eightfold increase in survival is merely the result of improved supportive care or statistical artefact.

Some authorities believe that antiplatelet agents have improved the prognosis of TTP. Dextran 70 was apparently used successfully (295), and subsequent reports described remissions following aspirin—alone or in combination with dipyridamole, sulfinpyrazone, and ticlopidine (296). However, cases in which the disease progressed while the patients were on antiplatelet agents as well as the increasing number of patients experiencing HUS onset with ticlopidine and clopidogrel (126) clearly challenge the significance of the previously described observations (296). Moreover, the 108 patients reported by Bell et al. (294) who never received antiplatelet agents had the same survival rate (90%) as the 102 patients of Rock et al. (293), all of whom had aspirin (325 mg per day) and dipyridamole (400 mg per day) plus steroids and plasma manipulation. All these observations seriously question the value of antiplatelet agents in the treatment of TTP.

Findings of reduced PGI2 activity have stimulated research on the possible use of PGI2 infusion as a substitutive therapy (297). PGI2 (usually as epoprostenol) was given to several patients with TTP with conflicting results (298–302). Because only a limited number of patients have been treated, there is not enough information to draw conclusions about the possible effectiveness of PGI2.

The Role of Plasma Therapy. The most effective form of treatment is plasma exchange or infusion. Exchange transfusion was first attempted in 1956 by Wile and Sturgeon in a 10-month-old infant but attracted greater attention only in 1976 when Bukowski et al. reported a 50% survival in 16 patients treated with this procedure (286). Thereafter many reports described favorable results with exchange transfusion and plasma exchange. The overall response rate to plasma exchange procedures that was 76% in 1981 (303), is 90% in the most recent series with fresh-frozen plasma as replacement therapy (293). A recent randomized trial of plasma exchange versus plasma infusion documented an apparent superiority of exchange over infusion (293). However, the total volume of plasma infused was three times more during exchange than during infusion alone (21.5 ± 7.8 L versus 6.7 ± 3.3 L), which suggested that exchange appeared more effective because more plasma was infused. Alternatively, plasma exchange may be more effective because toxic substances are removed from the circulation. The case of a patient with chronic relapsing TTP (304) who received many courses of plasma exchange or infusion during different relapsing episodes documented that infusion rather than removal of plasma is the effective maneuver (305).

Patients who properly respond to plasma therapy usually have a good prognosis if the patient survives the acute episode. Recent data have indicated that infusion of cryosupernatant of plasma (i.e., plasma devoid of vWF multimers, fibrinogen, and fibronectin, which remain in the cryoprecipitate) induced prompt remission in a small series of patients who either did not respond or did not respond adequately to repeated plasma exchanges with fresh-frozen plasma (306). Patients who do not respond to plasma therapy usually have a very poor prognosis, but occasional responses to splenectomy (4,220,295,307) or vincristine (308) have been reported. A 79% response has been reported in 19 patients who had a relapse after withdrawal of plasma therapy (309). However, the results of delayed splenectomy are possibly biased by patient selection and normally evade the early mortality of TTP. Bell et al. (294) reported a pronounced deterioration in clinical status

TABLE 67-2

A SUGGESTED ALGORITHM TO GUIDE TREATMENT OF TMA ASSOCIATED WITH DEFECTIVE ADAMTS 13 ACTIVITY

Form	Treatment[a]	Comment
Genetically determined	Plasma exchange or infusion	To replace defective activity, the exchange procedure allowing more plasma supply without risk of fluid overload
Immune mediated	Plasma exchange	To remove the autoantibody and replace the inactivated protease
	Steroids/immunosuppressive agents (?)	To aspecifically inhibit the production of the autoantibody
	Rituximab (?)	To specifically inhibit CD20 lymphocyte clones possibly involved in the production of the autoantibody
	Splenectomy (?)	Rescue therapy of unproven benefit for refractory and life-threatening forms

[a]Regardless of the underlying etiology, plasma exchange is first therapy in any severe case with neurologic signs or acute renal failure
(?) Unproven efficacy.

accompanied by a decrease in hematocrit and platelet count and an increase in serum LDH levels in six patients undergoing splenectomy because of refractoriness to corticosteroids and plasma exchange; four patients became comatose and one died suddenly. The five patients who survived progressively recovered after the reinstitution of plasma exchange. Splenectomy was not further considered by these authors to treat TTP refractory to plasma therapy. A recent study showed a higher mortality rate and longer disease duration in 13 patients undergoing splenectomy to treat their first episode of TTP as compared to 39 patients continuing on plasma therapy (310). Despite that this study is far from conclusive due to its retrospective design, the role of splenectomy remains most debated until new data becomes available.

A New Rationale for Established Treatments. Better understanding of the pathogenetic mechanisms may help explain the heterogeneous responses to treatment of apparently similar diseases. Patients with genetically determined ADAMTS 13 deficiency, such as the case with chronic relapsing TTP described in the preceding text (304), may benefit from both plasma infusion or exchange, since both procedures may replace the defective activity, the exchange procedure offering the possibility of supplying larger amounts of plasma without the risk of fluid overload (Table 67-2). Those with immune-mediated deficiency definitely benefit the most from the exchange procedure that, in addition to supplying an extra amount of protease that may saturate the autoantibody activity, may also remove the autoantibody from the circulation. Therefore, future trials of plasma therapy should consider separately genetic from immune-mediated forms. The same considerations apply to the use of steroids (3,294), vincristine (311–313), immunoglobulins (314–317), immunosuppressants, and splenectomy (4,220,294,295,307,310). In particular steroids have been extensively used in the past to cure patients with the so called idiopathic TTP, with inconsistent results. Indeed, in immune forms these treatments may aim at inhibiting the production of the autoantibody and, combined with plasma exchange, may result in an effective clearance of the autoantibody from the circulation. However, they are not effective for treatment for genetic forms. Trials considering the two forms together invariably diluted the potential benefits of steroids or immunosuppressive therapy in subjects with immune-mediated disease. This may explain the inconclusive results of previous studies in

TTP. Novel studies should likely focus on the role of steroids as first-line therapy, and on vincristine, high-dose immunoglobulins, or other immunosuppressants as second-line therapy, with splenectomy considered as rescue therapy for those patients with refractory disease and life-threatening thrombocytopenia or neurologic involvement (Table 67-2).

TMA Associated with Genetic or Immune-Mediated Abnormalities of the Complement System

TMA associated with abnormalities of the complement system usually manifests with the clinical features of HUS.

HUS Associated with Genetically Determined Factor H Deficiency

In 35 cases of familial TMA belonging to 10 families, identified through the Italian Registry of Recurrent and Familial TMA, decreased serum level of the third component of complement (C3) was associated with an increased risk of the disease (266). This was initially attributed to an inherited defect in C3 synthesis (267), but much more convincing data are now available that low C3 in HUS derives from either lack (268–270) or altered function (271) of factor H, a regulatory component of the alternative pathway of the complement system (272,273), which protects host tissues (126). Compelling molecular evidence is available that genetic alterations in factor H are involved in both autosomal dominant and recessive HUS.

Familial forms have been reported to occur in children and adults (33,163,318,319–325). Both are uncommon and share a poor prognosis. A hereditary autosomal recessive form, which may present as the relapsing variant, is most common in children (163,319). In adults the inheritance of HUS appears of autosomal dominant model (321) and male predominance has been found in a few kindreds (320). Malignant hypertension is a frequent complication of the syndrome, and the prognosis is extremely poor. Irreversible renal failure has been reported in five members of two families with autosomal dominant HUS (324). The syndrome was triggered by a virus-like disease and was complicated, despite good control of arterial blood pressure, by severe retinopathy with exudates and hemorrhages. In two cases, severe lung involvement with hemoptysis, respiratory failure, and x-ray findings of diffuse shadows were reported and improved following bilateral nephrectomy (324).

Plasma infusion or exchange has been used in patients with HUS and factor H_1 (HF_1) mutations, with the rationale to provide normal plasma HF1 activity to correct the genetic deficiency (126). In one study patients died or developed ESRD (326). In very recent studies, patients remained chronically ill or required infusion of plasma at weekly intervals in order to raise protein HF1 plasma levels enough to maintain remission (327). Only one case of total sustained remission in a patient with acute HUS and HF_1 mutation after plasma exchange has been described by Stratton and Warwicker (328). After 3 months of weekly plasma exchange in conjunction with intravenous immunoglobulins, the patient had normal renal function and hemodialysis was not needed. At one year after stopping plasma therapy, the patient did not have any relapse and remained dialysis independent.

Graft failure occurs in 30% to 100% of kidney transplants, according to different surveys (126). Given the fact that HF1 is a plasma protein mainly of liver origin, indirect evidence is available that a kidney transplantation does not correct the HF1 genetic defect (204). Simultaneous kidney and liver transplantation has been recently performed in two young children with non-Stx HUS and HF_1 mutations, with the objective of correcting the genetic defect and preventing disease recurrences. However, for reasons that possibly involve an increased liver susceptibility to immune or ischemic injury related to uncontrolled complement activation, both cases (329,330) treated with this procedure were complicated by premature irreversible liver failure. In the first case (329), the child developed hepatic encephalopathy and coma that recovered with a second, uneventful, liver transplantation. The second case (330) was complicated by a fatal, primary nonfunction of the liver graft. Graft hypoperfusion, due to a sudden drop of arterial blood pressure soon after reperfusion, triggered severe ischemia/reperfusion damage and complement deposition in the liver, conceivably as the result of defective HF1 complement regulatory potential. Thus, combined kidney and liver transplantation should not be performed unless the patient with HF1-dependent HUS is at imminent risk of life-threatening complications (126).

HUS Associated with Immune-Mediated Factor H Deficiency

An autoimmune mechanism involving regulatory proteins of the complement alternative pathway, that is, factor H (HF) and membrane co-factor protein (CD46), was first studied in familial and recurrent HUS (see subsequent text), and then it was surveyed in sporadic forms in which it was demonstrated in several studies (126,331). In a recent French study, Dragon-Durey et al. investigated the presence of HF autoantibodies by enzyme-linked immunosorbent assay (ELISA) using coated purified human HF in a series of 48 children who presented with atypical HUS (331). IgG antibodies reacting with HF were detected in the plasma of three children who presented with recurrent HUS. The HF plasma activity was found to be decreased, whereas plasma HF antigenic levels and HF gene analysis were normal (332). This report supports the possible occurrence of sporadic HUS as an autoimmune disease through the development of anti-HF antibodies.

HUS Associated with Membrane Cofactor Protein (MCP) Abnormalities

HUS may also occur in patients with a genetic abnormality of the membrane cofactor protein (MCP). The disease manifests with fever, hemolytic anemia, and thrombocytopenia (333), and the outcome is usually poor (126). Plasma infusion or ex-

change still remains a valid therapy that may have some effect. Unlike cases associated with congenital abnormalities of HF1 in which the microangiopathic process invariably recurs after kidney transplantation, it is tempting to speculate that forms associated with MCP abnormalities can be corrected by transplanting a normal kidney. Four successful kidney transplantations have been performed to date in such patients with no disease recurrence (334). Because MCP is a membrane-bound protein highly expressed in the kidney, a kidney graft would reasonably correct local MCP dysfunction. The graft, which is physiologically bearing wild-type MCP, highly expressed in the kidney, should conceivably be protected from the recurrence of a microangiopathic process (204,333).

TMA Associated with Pregnancy

Pregnancy-associated TTP may be distinguished from preeclampsia, the hemolysis elevated liver enzymes and low platelet (HELLP) syndrome (usually near term), and postpartum HUS (usually within 3 months after delivery).

Pregnancy-associated TTP

TTP develops during the antepartum period in 89% of cases, usually within 24 weeks. Measurement of plasma antithrombin III (AT III) activity has been suggested as a useful tool to differentiate TTP and preeclampsia. Before gestational week 28 and when AT III plasma activity is normal, TTP is most likely (73). After week 34 of gestation, preeclampsia is most likely. In pregnant patients with TTP, despite limited experience, available series show that the maternal mortality rate has fallen from 68% to almost zero with the institution of plasma therapy (335). Plasma therapy could be continued until term and/or complete remission of the disease. Delivery can be considered as "rescue" after failure of plasma therapy (73).

The HELLP Syndrome

The HELLP syndrome (an acronym for hemolysis, elevate liver enzymes and low platelet count) is simply a form of severe preeclampsia in which in addition to hypertension and renal dysfunction, there is evidence of microangiopathic hemolysis and liver involvement. It arises in the antepartum period in 70% of cases. Symptoms can arise within 24 to 48 hours postpartum, occasionally after an uncomplicated pregnancy (335). Diagnosis is based on: (a) hemolysis (defined as fragmented erythrocytes in the circulation and lactic dehydrogenase ≥ 600 U/L), (b) elevated liver enzymes (serum glutamicoxaloacetic transaminase >70 U/L), and (c) low platelets (platelet count $<10^3/mm^3$) (191). Overt disseminated intravascular coagulation (DIC) is reported in 25% of cases. Intrahepatic hemorrhage, subcapsular liver hematoma, and liver rupture are rare, life-threatening complications. The maternal and perinatal mortality rates range from 0% to 24% and from 7.7% to 60%, respectively (73). In the HELLP syndrome, termination of pregnancy is the only definitive therapy, but by no means the treatment of choice. Hydralazine or dihydralazine are the first choice drugs to control pregnancy-induced hypertension, and magnesium sulfate is the first choice to prevent and treat convulsions. Both peritoneal dialysis and hemodialysis have been used to treat acute renal failure. Platelet transfusions are needed for clinical bleeding or severe thrombocytopenia (platelet count $<20.000/\mu L$). In approximately 5% of patients with HELLP syndrome, symptoms and laboratory abnormalities do not improve after delivery. There are cases with central nervous system abnormalities, associated with renal and cardiopulmonary dysfunction and activation of coagulation. Uncontrolled studies suggest that plasma exchange may help recovery in patients with persistent evidence of disease 72 hours or more after delivery. However, plasma therapy is ineffective during pregnancy and may increase fetal and maternal risk when used to delay delivery. Preliminary evidence suggests that, postpartum, corticosteroids may speed up disease recovery, and, antepartum, may postpone delivery of pre-viable fetuses and reduce the mother's need for blood products (73).

Between 28 and 34 weeks of gestation, because the differential diagnosis between the HELLP syndrome and TTP is ambiguous, the optimal treatment is controversial. If there is no evidence of fetal distress and plasma AT III activity is normal, a course of plasma therapy can be reasonably attempted before inducing delivery (336).

Postpartum HUS

Postpartum HUS is a rare event that manifests within 3 months after delivery. When it ensues early postpartum it can be considered a late manifestation of severe preeclampsia or the HELLP syndrome and may recover spontaneously or with plasma therapy. On the contrary, the relationship with pregnancy is uncertain for cases that ensue in the later postpartum period. In most of these cases renal failure and neurologic symptoms are severe and are associated with severe hypertension (318). The mortality rate has ranged from 50% to 60% in the various reports (337,338). Patients who survive the acute phase of the disease have residual renal dysfunction and hypertension (337,339,340). The best management of patients with postpartum HUS is a supportive treatment (i.e., dialysis if necessary and careful fluid management). A 53% survival in heparin-treated patients versus 17% survival in untreated patients was found in a retrospective analysis of uncontrolled studies in post-partum HUS (341). However, because of severe hypertension and thrombocytopenia, heparin and antiplatelet agents enhance the risk of intracranial hemorrhage in these patients. Isolated reports of successful therapy of postpartum HUS with plasma infusion or exchange are available, but data are not as convincing as for TTP.

TMA Associated with Transplantation

Transplantation-associated HUS usually ensues with the clinical features of HUS. The disease may occur *de novo* or may recur in the transplanted kidney in subjects who progressed to ESRD because of HUS. The underlying etiology and the outcome may differ substantially. *De novo* HUS may complicate a toxic or immune-mediated damage to the kidney (such as in subjects on immunosuppressive therapy with cyclosporin A or tacrolimus, or with vascular rejection of the kidney graft) and may recover with the resolution of the underlying disease. Recurrent HUS almost invariably affects subjects with a genetic predisposition and results in irreversible graft failure regardless of treatment.

De novo HUS

De novo HUS may occur in patients receiving renal transplants and other organs, as a consequence of the use of calcineurin inhibitors (CsA and tacrolimus) or due to humoral (C4b positive) rejection (126,342). Since the first description of thrombocytopenia, hemolytic anemia, and renal failure in a patient treated with CsA for preventing graft-versus-host disease after allogenic bone marrow transplantation (343), several cases of HUS have been reported in patients given CsA to prevent bone marrow (343,344), liver, heart, and kidney graft rejection (345). It is known that cyclosporine at pharmacologic doses induces a potent vasoconstrictory effect that may result in kidney hypoperfusion and ischemia. Enhanced release of endothelin

and other mediators might then amplify endothelial damage and sustain the microangiopathic process (346). In addition, HUS has been described to occur in approximately 1% of renal transplantation patients receiving tacrolimus (342). Recently, Hochstetler et al. (347) reported the onset of thrombotic microangiopathy in 4.1% of 512 patients receiving a cadaveric renal transplant, usually in the first posttransplantation month. There were 5 deaths (24%) and 7 transplant nephrectomies (33%), resulting in an overall graft loss of 57%. These values exceeded the 6-month posttransplantation mortality rate (4%) and graft loss (12%) experienced by renal allograft recipients without TMA. Evidence of cytomegalovirus (CMV) infection during their acute TMA was found in 42% of the patients and, in combination with CsA therapy, might have favored the onset of the disease.

Removal or treatment of the underlying cause of renal damage is the key component of treatment. In most cases associated with calcineurin inhibitor therapy, early withdrawal of cyclosporine or tacrolimus may result in full recovery. Plasma therapy is usually recommended, in particular in those cases in which there is not prompt recovery with treatment withdrawal. Replacing calcineurin inhibitors with other inhibitors of IL-2 activity that are free of direct nephrotoxicity such as rapamycin and specific monoclonal antibodies against IL-2 receptors (346), may help disease recovery without increasing the risk of graft rejection. Noteworthy, two cases successfully treated with intravenous IgG infusion and without CsA discontinuation, have been recently reported (347). The outcome of *de novo* HUS associated with vascular rejection is most often severe and closely reflects the outcome of the underlying disease. Lymphocytolytic therapy and plasma exchange may help limiting the disease, but graft failure is the most common outcome.

Recurrent HUS

HUS may recur in 0% to 25% of renal grafts (348). However, the risk of recurrence, which is minimal in cadaveric kidney grafts (349,350), may approximate 50% in living related kidney transplants (351). Comparable rates of recurrence are reported among patients with or without CsA therapy (351). Miller et al. (348) found HUS to recur in 12 of 18 patients with non-Stx-HUS and only in 1 of 6 with Stx-HUS, usually within the first 2 months posttransplantation. Ten of the grafts had severe vascular lesions and 9 were irreversibly lost. Life-time analysis showed significantly poorer graft survival for HUS patients compared to overall renal transplantation population, but surprisingly this was not associated with an increased risk of graft loss due to disease recurrence. These data were confirmed by Gagnadoux et al. (350) who found that 1- and 5-year graft survival was 66% and 37% in 25 HUS children versus 80% and 69%, respectively, in all other pediatric recipients. These authors concluded that although recurrence of disease is a relatively uncommon cause of graft loss in HUS patients, actually only the minority with atypical non-Stx HUS would be at risk (348), as compared to chronic vascular rejection. For unknown reasons, it is remarkably more frequent in HUS patients as compared to the general transplantation population. One should also consider that some of the graft losses attributed to HUS in the literature are likely the consequence of allograft rejection. Actually, difficulties in differentiating recurrent HUS from antibody-mediated acute vascular rejection may account for the different rates of HUS recurrences reported in the various series.

A genetic predisposition to develop HUS after exposure to Stx has been proven in a small proportion of patients with Stx-HUS. There is concern whether this predisposition may favor recurrence of disease in such patients after kidney transplantation. However, because patients who received a kidney transplant because of ESRD secondary to Stx-associated HUS are relatively few, numbers of series are too small to definitely establish the role of genetic predisposition in posttransplantation recurrence (346). Neurologic and other extrarenal manifestations are relatively uncommon in posttransplantation HUS. However, central nervous system involvement has been described in both adults and children and has presented with spontaneous cerebral hemorrhage (352,353).

Some of the therapies effective in other forms of HUS have been empirically tried in recurrent posttransplantation HUS, but only a minority of patients recovered renal function, whereas most of them lost their graft suddenly.

Plasma infusion or exchange is the first used treatment approach in this setting but there is still no definite evidence of effectiveness. Adding plasma infusion/exchange might limit the microangiopathic process in cases sustained by plasma abnormalities (such as defective factor H activity) that can be corrected by normal plasma (346). Whether this may apply to other familial/recurrent forms is reasonable, but not proven.

Other treatments, such as immunoperfusion, that is, perfusion of autologous plasma over filters containing staphylococcal protein A, have been attempted, but there is no reason to believe that this procedure may offer any advantage as compared to plasma exchange. Finally, high-dose intravenous immunoglobulin infusion has been reported to be effective in some cases associated with CMV infection. It is possible, but not proven, that this treatment was effective by limiting viral replication (346). Combined liver and kidney transplantations have been performed in children with factor H associated HUS with the rationale to replace the defective activity with the factor H produced by the transplanted liver (354,355).

However, this procedure is not recommended due to the unacceptably high risk of premature and irreversible failure of the liver graft (see TMA associated with genetic or immune-mediated defects of the complement system).

TMA Associated with Cancer

Cancer-associated HUS complicates almost 6% of cases of metastatic carcinoma (356). Gastric cancer alone accounts for about half such cases. These patients have an extremely poor prognosis and most of them die within weeks. A form of TMA resembling HUS has also been described in cancer patients given the anticancer drug mitomycin. Platinum- and bleomycin-containing chemotherapeutic combinations may also trigger HUS. The risk of developing HUS following mitomycin-C therapy is 2% to 10% (357). Manifestations of the disease are dose related, so that cumulative doses higher than 60 mg are almost invariably associated with the disease. The case fatality rate of mitomycin HUS is 60% to 70%, and the median time to death is about 4 weeks. Deaths occurring within the first few months is usually related to complications of the syndrome, including renal failure and pulmonary edema, or sepsis. Patients surviving the acute phase of the syndrome, may have remission of the microangiopathic process but remain on chronic dialysis.

Specific therapy is minimally effective. Blood transfusions often exacerbate the disease and may trigger pulmonary edema (358). Perfusion of autologous plasma over filters containing staphylococcal protein A, which binds the Fc portion of immunoglobulin G, has been attempted to remove circulating immune complexes with encouraging results (359). HUS may also be a complication of radiation nephritis. It usually occurs late after radiotherapy and is invariably associated with irreversible kidney failure.

TMA Associated with Systemic Diseases, Including HIV Infection

TMA may complicate SLE, scleroderma (sclerodermic crisis), malignant hypertension or vasculitis. Clinical features and outcomes strongly depend on the underlying disease. Seventy percent of patients may require dialysis during the acute phase of the disease (360). The mortality rate from neurologic complications is high during the acute phase of the disease, and residual kidney dysfunction is frequent, with death or ESRD an almost invariably outcome of scleroderma or malignant hypertension. Older age is also associated with an increased mortality.

HIV infection-associated HUS was firstly reported in 1984 in a homosexual man (227). Since then, TMA diagnosed as either TTP or HUS is part of the complications of AIDS and accounts for up to 30% of hospitalized cases of TMA at least in some institutions (229). Stx infection (361) and cocaine abuse (362) are possible triggers. The clinical course is poor and depends heavily on the severity of the underlying disease. Management is the same as recommended for non-AIDS cases. However, steroids, vincristine, and immunoglobulins may increase the risk of opportunistic infection in already immunosuppressed patients and should be given with caution. Plasma exchange or infusion is likely the only feasible therapy for AIDS-associated TMA. In one series of seven patients with HIV-associated TMA the short-term response rate to plasma exchange (86%) was comparable to the response rate (80%) reported in the pooled literature of non-HIV cases (363). However, none of these patients survived more than 2 years after remission was achieved. Due to sporadic reports of remission of the syndrome after treatment with the antiretroviral agent zidovudine (364) and of recurrence of the disease after its withdrawal (365), it has been suggested that zidovudine may play a role in the management of HIV-related TMA. However, cases of TMA ensuing during zidovudine therapy make this possibility very unlikely (366).

Idiopathic TMA

Idiopathic forms of TMA encompass all thrombotic microangiopathies with an unclear etiologic pattern. It mainly consists of "non-Stx-HUS" forms in which no clear link was found with any genetic or immune-based mechanism. In opposition to genetic and familial forms, sporadic TMA appears in patients with no history of TMA in their family. Sporadic TMA manifests at all ages, but is more frequent in adults. According to a recent U.S. study, the incidence of sporadic TMA in children is approximately two cases/year/1,000,000 total population (204).

The disease manifests without prodromal diarrhea in children of all ages and in adults, and accounts for approximately 5% to 10% of all cases (238). Typically there is no evidence of Stx infection and the mortality rate may be high (260). Plasma therapy is the treatment of choice, but whether it effectively helps renal function recovery is unknown.

Post-HUS Chronic Nephropathy

Chronic sequelae may complicate any form of TMA, including Stx-associated HUS. Hypertension, proteinuria, and worsening renal function are the typical features and relentless progression to ESRD may occur over years or decades. Careful blood pressure control and renin–angiotensin system blockade may be particularly beneficial in the long term for those patients with chronic renal disease after an acute episode of HUS. A recent study (367) in 45 children with renal sequelae of HUS followed for 9 to 11 years documented that early restriction of proteins and use of ACE inhibitors may have a beneficial effect on long-term renal outcome, as documented by a positive slope of 1/Serum Cr values over time in treated patients. In another study, 8- 15-year treatment with ACE-inhibitors after severe Stx-HUS normalized blood pressure, reduced proteinuria and improved GFR (368). Finally, kidney transplantation should be considered as an effective and safe treatment for those children with Stx-HUS who progress to ESRD. The recurrence rates actually range from 0% to 10% and graft survival at 10 years is even better than in control transplanted children with other disease (369–371).

In occasional patients, severe vascular changes in the kidney may sustain refractory hypertension and microangiopathic hemolysis even after recovery from the acute phase of the disease. In those patients with extensive microvascular thrombosis at renal biopsy, refractory hypertension, and signs of hypertensive encephalopathy when conventional therapies including plasma manipulation are not enough to control the disease (i.e., persistent severe thrombocytopenia and hemolytic anemia), bilateral nephrectomy has been performed with excellent follow-up in some patients (192). When the genetic studies exclude a congenital predisposition to the disease, these patients may eventually benefit with a kidney transplant.

ACUTE CORTICAL NECROSIS

Acute cortical necrosis represents a rare cause of acute renal failure (ARF), occurring in about 2% of patients (372). The term acute cortical necrosis defines a condition of destruction of the renal cortex except for a thin tissue rim under the capsule and usually a thicker layer under the corticomedullary junction. This phenomenon reflects a disturbed blood flow to interlobular and afferent arterioles, whereas the arcuate arteries, which supply blood to the juxtamedullary nephrons, are usually spared. The lack of necrosis in subcapsular nephrons is due to the presence of anastomoses with extrarenal vessels that allow minimal perfusion to superficial nephrons, just enough to prevent necrotic changes. In 50% to 70% of the series considered, acute cortical necrosis is a complication of pregnancy (especially in multiparous women older than 30 years of age). Abruptio placentae is the most common prior complication of the ARF (372,373). Preexisting toxemia seems to be an important predisposing factor (66,374,375), but there is no general agreement on this issue (372). Intrauterine death, hemorrhage from placenta previa, septic abortion, postpartum hemorrhage, and, occasionally hyperemesis, are other conditions that may be complicated by acute cortical necrosis (372, 376–379).

Recently, Donohoe (380) followed pregnant women throughout the two decades from 1961 to 1980. Comparing the incidence of acute cortical necrosis during these periods, he found that in the second group (1971–1980) abruptio placentae occurred almost three times less often than in the first group. Acute renal failure and acute cortical necrosis also decreased further in these 10 years (1971–1980), proving that not only a better management of pregnancy but also a prompter and more appropriate approach may prevent the occurrence of necrotic changes in the cortex. In contrast, a recent experience (337) has indicated that cases of cortical necrosis associated with pregnancy are increasing despite an overall reduction in the number of patients suffering from ARF after pregnancy.

Bacterial and postoperative shock, pancreatitis, dissecting aneurysms, gastrointestinal hemorrhage, trauma, burns, phosphorus and diethylene glycol poisoning, snake venom bites, and sometimes TTP and HUS are other conditions that can be complicated by acute cortical necrosis (373,381–392). In children, cases of cortical necrosis have been reported, most frequently after protracted vomiting and diarrhea with marked dehydration. Moreover, as in adults, the disease has been seen concomitantly with infections such as peritonitis, septicemia, pharyngitis, transfusion reactions, and phosphorus poisoning (391,393–397).

The generalized Shwartzman reaction (GSR) is an experimental model of bilateral cortical necrosis of the kidneys induced in rabbits by two intravenous doses, spaced 18 to 24 hours apart, of endotoxin from gram-negative bacteria (398).

The earliest histologic lesion in the GSR is the deposition of a homogeneous, eosinophilic material with the staining properties of fibrinoid within the lumen of the glomerular capillaries of the kidneys (399). Similar material is deposited in the vessels in other visceral organs in association with necrotizing and hemorrhagic lesions (398,399).

There is experimental evidence that in pregnant animals (rabbits and rats) (400,401) or in animals pretreated with corticosteroids (398), sympathomimetics (alpha-agonists) (402), or synthetic acid polymers (403), the GSR can be triggered by a single dose of endotoxin, whereas two spaced endotoxin injections are required in nonpregnant or untreated animals. Although recent studies have emphasized the role of endothelial injury that follows the exposure of endothelium to endotoxin, direct and definitive evidence of this mechanism is still lacking. Raij et al. (404), in a model of unilateral cortical necrosis in rabbits, showed that after an *in situ* perfusion of one kidney with endotoxin followed by a systemic injection of endotoxin 24 hours later, the GSR was confined to that kidney. Therefore, it appears that endotoxin might have a specific local effect on the vascular endothelium that is sufficient as an initial event that predisposes to cortical necrosis. In agreement with this view is the finding of Arhelger et al. (405) that in rats after an injection of nephrotoxic serum, which is known to induce immediate endothelial injury, a single dose of endotoxin was sufficient to elicit the GSR. Hoyer et al. (406) extended this experiment by infusing nephrotoxic serum into the left renal artery of pregnant rats and obtained a Shwartzman reaction restricted to the left kidney. More recently, Campos et al. (407) demonstrated that vascular prostacyclin (PGI_2) infusion prior to endotoxin significantly inhibited the GSR in pregnant rats. Although the lesions of the GSR were not completely abolished, the extent and severity of the histologic changes were significantly less than in PGI_2-untreated animals.

PGI_2 might exert its protective effect against the GSR by inhibiting platelet aggregation, regulating polymorphonuclear leukocyte adherence to endothelial cells, and influencing the participation of leukocytes in the GSR. The relevance of PGI_2 in antagonizing the occurrence of the GSR is strengthened by the observation that bradykinin, which increases the synthesis of renal prostaglandins (408), prevents the GSR elicited by a single injection of endotoxin in pregnant rats and cortisone-sensitized rabbits (409). The protective effect of bradykinin on the GSR seems to be mediated by prostaglandins, since it is abolished after administration of aspirin.

Pathogenesis

The pathogenesis of cortical necrosis still remains a mystery. The two major theories proposed to date only partially explain the disease. According to Sheehan and Moore (373), who studied specimens from patients who died after abruptio placentae, vasospasm is the primary event causing cortical necrosis.

Alternatively, it has been suggested that acute vascular injury followed by activation of coagulation and thrombosis plays a key role in the development of cortical necrosis (403,410). Both these theories do not convincingly account for the fact that after the initial "trigger" a cascade of events takes place leading to a necrotic process localized at the renal cortex.

Sheehan and Davis (411) observed that prolonged experimental clamping of the renal pedicle can produce cortical necrosis. The same lesion was obtained in experimental animals by the infusion of a large amount of vasoactive substances such as epinephrine and oxytocin (412–414). However, no convincing evidence is available so far to support the idea that vasospasm is the key event in acute cortical necrosis in humans (380).

Experimental Shwartzman reaction produced in pregnant rabbits after a single injection of bacterial toxin supports the theory that vascular injury is the major etiologic event in cortical necrosis (415). The Shwartzman reaction produces DIC. The crucial role of the latter in the development of cortical necrosis is documented by the fact that heparin reduces the incidence of cortical necrosis in the model of GSR of nonpregnant rabbits (416). However, the main difference between experimental Shwartzman reaction and cortical necrosis in humans is that in animals the necrotic process involves also the renal medulla and organs other than the kidney. Probably in humans selective damage of the cortical vasculature predisposes to the subsequent development of localized damage as soon as a "trigger event," for example, abruptio placentae, occurs. In this context, recent experimental data are particularly relevant. Unilateral Shwartzman phenomenon confined to a single kidney has been produced by local perfusion of low-dose endotoxin before systemic injection of endotoxin (404). Cortical necrosis in experimental animals has also been obtained using liquid or diethylene glycol (383,417). The mechanisms by which these toxic agents lead to cortical necrosis are far from being understood, but these agents are known to cause endothelial damage.

Another intriguing issue is the significance of glomerular fibrin thrombi. Early reports have focused on the possible crucial role of glomerular thrombosis in the pathogenesis of the disease (376,418). However, a detailed analysis of the most representative series reported in the literature revealed that glomerular fibrin thrombi are relatively rare in cortical necrosis. Only occasionally have extensive intraglomerular thrombi been documented (372,378). Altogether, the available data do not support the idea that cortical necrosis is the consequence of a mechanical blockage of glomeruli by fibrin thrombi. Moreover, in the two largest series (378,419) reported so far of patients affected by DIC with glomerular fibrin thrombi, the majority of which had bacterial sepsis, cortical necrosis was found in only four of the 63 cases studied.

Finally, it has been suggested that cortical necrosis might be a consequence of immunologic mechanisms. Most evidence in support of this hypothesis comes from the observation that pathologic findings similar to cortical necrosis have been found in hyperacute rejection of renal allografts (420). Cortical necrosis in these cases presumably results from direct immunologic injury to transplanted cortical vessels by preformed antibodies. This event occurs in completely denervated allografts, and, therefore, vascular endothelial damage rather than vasospasm may be the primary event in the overall pathogenesis of at least some forms of this dramatic disease.

Clinical Features

The most typical clinical sign of acute cortical necrosis is sudden oliguria, the amount of urine ranging from 0 to 100 mL per day (421). Sometimes this is preceded by gross hematuria. Lumbar pain, if present, constitutes a rather nonspecific symptom and may be associated with fever and leukocytosis. Urine contains protein, red blood cells, white blood cells, epithelial cells, and various types of casts. Hypertension may occur, but generally the blood pressure is only slightly elevated. A picture of acute renal failure with hyperazotemia, metabolic acidosis, and hyperkalemia emerges from laboratory data. LDH and glutamic oxaloacetic transaminases in serum are elevated during the first days of the disease (417). DIC is frequent, especially in obstetric patients. Fibrinogen and platelet counts fall very low, prothrombin time is prolonged, and fibrinogen degradation products (FDPs) in serum are often elevated (380).

Acute cortical necrosis must be suspected when oliguria or anuria tends to persist for a long period. Renal biopsy provides the definitive diagnosis. However, the patient's clinical condition may not always permit the performance of a biopsy, and in some cases the diagnosis may be missed because, especially in the incomplete form of disease, the specimen does not allow for detection of the typical changes. Radiologic techniques are very useful in the evaluation of the diagnosis of acute cortical necrosis (372,422,423). Renal echography may exclude obstruction. Selective arteriography may provide information about the extent of lesions, permitting a distinction between the complete and incomplete forms. The most typical radiologic sign of acute cortical necrosis is the renal cortical calcification, which, however, is uncommon and does not occur in the early phases of the disease (417).

Hemodynamic studies with krypton or xenon washout techniques indicate reduced renal blood flow; however, these techniques, except in cases of complete acute cortical necrosis, may not differentiate between patients with incomplete acute cortical necrosis and those with acute tubular necrosis (372).

Pathology

In 1953 Sheehan and Moore (373) described in detail the pathologic changes characteristic of cortical necrosis. In massive or complete cortical necrosis, almost the whole cortex is affected by necrosis except the corticomedullary junction and a thin rim of cortical tissue under the capsule. On gross examination, the kidneys are enlarged and weigh 200 to 300 g. The cortex has a yellowish-white appearance, but congested areas are detected in the periphery. Moreover, the columns of Bertin are necrosed. The main renal arteries—the lobar and the arciform—are generally spared. Microscopic examination shows pathologic changes appearing 48 to 72 hours after the initial injury. Glomeruli and tubules show extensive necrotic changes, whereas the afferent arterioles are occluded by thrombi extending to the interlobular arteries. At the periphery of the necrosis, large-scale infiltration of polymorphonuclear leukocytes fully develops after 3 to 4 days.

In addition to the pattern of complete cortical necrosis, Sheehan and Moore (373) described other forms of acute cortical necrosis characterized by more limited necrotic changes, the so-called incomplete acute cortical necrosis. The latter includes the focal form, in which the necrotic lesion can reach a diameter ranging from 3.0 to 0.5 mm, and the patchy form, with much larger necrotic areas. The authors described an additional variant of acute cortical necrosis called confluent focal cortical necrosis, which differs from the forms previously described in the following aspects: (a) The focal lesions are so numerous that they merge with one another, (b) the typical changes are present in tubules and glomeruli but not in the arterioles and arteries and appear at different stages in the course of the disease, and (c) the pattern is not associated with abruptio placentae.

Histologically, the lesions of incomplete cortical necrosis are essentially the same as those in the complete form. The edge of the necrotic area forms a sharp border with normal renal tissue. In the late phases of the disease, kidneys are reduced in size, interstitial fibrosis occurs in the injured areas, and sclerotic substitutions occur in glomeruli and in vessels. Calcium deposits detected by Kossa stain can be found in glomeruli or in arteries.

Obviously the organ most often affected by acute cortical necrosis is the kidney; however, though to a lesser extent and more mildly, other organs are sometimes injured too, such as the adrenals, spleen, liver, large intestine, and particularly the pituitary gland sinusoids (372,424–426).

Prognosis and Treatment

The course of acute cortical necrosis is characterized by death during the first days of the disease unless dialysis treatment is undertaken. Death was almost unavoidable in the past before dialysis and better management of acute renal failure (372,386). In one of the largest series, reported by Kleinknecht et al. (372), 21 of 38 patients died. However, almost all these patients were seen before dialysis was available for the treatment of acute renal failure. The most typical clinical course, especially in the obstetric forms, is characterized by prolonged oliguria requiring dialysis. After a period of 1 to 3 months, renal function may partially recover, so that patients become dialysis independent. Urine output progressively increases, and renal function may improve over a period of 1 to 2 years, to a final plateau of 20 to 25 mL/minute (380,417). Hypertrophy of the juxtamedullary nephrons has been suggested as a factor contributing to the partial restoration of renal function (380).

A large percentage of patients require chronic dialysis, and these patients are probably those with the most severe and diffuse form of acute cortical necrosis. In this context two opposite possibilities must be mentioned: (a) the late return to dialysis a number of years after the occurrence of cortical necrosis; and (b) the late resumption of a degree of renal function sufficient to maintain patients off dialysis (380). Many patients have received renal transplants, and the prognosis of such patients has greatly improved during the last few years (417).

No specific therapeutic approaches are available for acute cortical necrosis. All the supportive maneuvers commonly employed in ARF are performed. Substitutive treatment must be started as early as possible, and daily dialytic therapy may be necessary considering the high catabolic rate often present in these patients. In experimental models of cortical necrosis, many measures favorably affect pathologic changes. These include employment of anticoagulants, general anesthesia, β-blocker agents, mannitol-induced diuresis, and the use of nitrogen mustards to induce leukopenia (416,427–430). However, none of these measures has been employed with unequivocal beneficial effects in humans.

References

1. Moschcowitz E. Acute febrile pleiochromic anemia with hyaline thrombosis of a terminal arterioles and capillaries: An underscribed disease. *Arch Intern Med* 1925;36:89.
2. Kennedy SS, Zacharski LR, Beck JR. Thrombotic thrombocytopenic purpura: Analysis of 48 unselected cases. *Semin Thromb Hemost* 1980;6:341.
3. Amorosi EL, Ultmann JE. Thrombotic thrombocytopenic purpura: report of 16 cases and review of the literature. *Medicine* 1966;45:139.
4. Cuttner J. Thrombotic thrombocytopenic purpura: a ten-year experience. *Blood* 1980;56:302.
5. Bukowski RM. Thrombotic thrombocytopenic purpura: a review. In: Spaet TH, ed. *Progress in Hemostasis and Thrombosis*, New York: Grune & Stratton; 1982:287.
6. Remuzzi G. HUS and TTP: variable expression of a single entity. *Kidney Int* 1987;32:292.
7. Fong JS, de Chadarevian JP, Kaplan BS. Hemolytic-uremic syndrome. Current concepts and management. *Pediatr Clin North Am* 1982;29:835.
8. Silverstein A. Thrombotic thrombocytopenic purpura: the initial neurologic manifestations. *Arch Neurol* 1968;18:358.
9. Mettler NE. Isolation of a microtatobiotie from patients with hemolytic-uremic syndrome and thrombotic thrombocytopenic purpura and from mites in the United States. *N Engl J Med* 1969;281:1023.
10. MacWhinney JB, Packer JT, Miller G. Thrombotic thrombocytopenic purpura in childhood. *Blood* 1962;19:181.
11. Shumway CN Jr, Miller G. An unusual syndrome of hemolytic anemia, thrombocytopenic purpura and renal disease. *Blood* 1957;12:1045.
12. Dunea G, Muerke RC, Nakamoto S, et al. Thrombotic thrombocytopenic purpura with acute anuric renal failure. *Am J Med* 1966;41:1000.
13. Sheth KJ, Swick HM, Haworth N. Neurological involvement in hemolytic-uremic syndrome. *Ann Neurol* 1986;19:90.
14. Neame PD. Immunologic and other factors in thrombotic thrombocytopenic purpura (TTP). *Semin Thromb Hemost* 1980;6:416.
15. Schwartz ML, Brenner WE. The obfuscation of eclampsia by thrombotic thrombocytopenic purpura. *Am J Obstet Gynecol* 1978;131:18.
16. Crain SM, Choudnury AM. Thrombotic thrombocytopenic purpura in a splenectomized patient with Hodgkin's disease. *Am J Med Sci* 1980;280:35.
17. Steinberg AD, Green WT, Talal N. Thrombotic thrombocytopenic purpura complicating Sjogren's syndrome. *JAMA* 1971;215:757.
18. Morey DA, Withe JB, Daily WM. Thrombotic thrombocytopenic purpura diagnosed by random lymph node biopsy. *Arch Intern Med* 1956;98:821.
19. Benitez L, Mathews M, Mallory GK. Platelet thrombosis with polyarteritis nodosa: report of a case. *Arch Pathol* 1964;77:116.
20. Dekker A, O'Brien ME, Cammarata RJ. The association of thrombotic thrombocytopenic purpura with systemic lupus erythematosus. *Am J Med Sci* 1974;267:243.
21. Laszlo MH, Alvarez A, Feldman F. The association of thrombotic thrombocytopenic purpura and disseminated lupus erythematosus: report of a case. *Ann Intern Med* 1955;42:1308.
22. Moore MR, Poon MC. Syndrome resembling thrombotic thrombocytopenic purpura associated with bacterial endocarditis. *South Med J* 1980;73:541.
23. Burke HA, Hartmann RC. Thrombotic thrombocytopenic purpura. Two patients with remission associated with the use of large amounts of steroids. *Arch Intern Med* 1959;103:105.
24. Lorber J, Emery JL. Thrombotic thrombocytopenic purpura. *Proc R Soc Med* 1959;52:301.
25. Ehrich WE, Seifter J. Thrombotic thrombocytopenic purpura caused by iodine. *Arch Pathol* 1949;47:446.
26. Caggiano V, Chosney B, Way LW. Thrombotic thrombocytopenic purpura, cholangiocarcinoma, and oral contraceptives. *Lancet* 1980;2:365.
27. Stonesifer LD, Bone RC, Hiller FC. Thrombotic thrombocytopenic purpura in carbon monoxide poisoning. *Arch Intern Med* 1980;140:104.
28. Monnens LA, Retera RJ. Thrombotic thrombocytopenic purpura in a neonatal infant. *J Pediatr* 1967;71:118.
29. Chen YC, McLeod B, Hall ER, et al. Accelerated prostacyclin degradation in thrombotic thrombocytopenic purpura. *Lancet* 1981;2:267.
30. Cuttner J. Chronic thrombotic thrombocytopenic purpura: report of a case with five relapses and review of the literature. *Mt Sinai J Med* 1978;45:418.
31. Meacham GC, Orbison JL, Heinle RW, et al. Thrombotic thrombocytopenic purpura: a disseminated disease of arterioles. *Blood* 1952;6:706.
32. Fuchs WE, George JN, Dotin LN, et al. Thrombotic thrombocytopenic purpura—occurrence two years apart during late pregnancy in two sisters. *JAMA* 1976;235:2126.
33. Hellman RM, Jackson DV, Buss DH. Thrombotic thrombocytopenic purpura and hemolytic uremic syndrome in HLA-identical siblings. *Ann Intern Med* 1980;93:283.
34. Wallace DC, Lovric A, Clubb JS, et al. Thrombotic thrombocytopenic purpura in four siblings. *Am J Med* 1975;58:724.
35. Gore I. Disseminated arteriolar and capillary platelet thrombosis: a morphological study of its histogenesis. *Am J Pathol* 1950;26:155.
36. Orbison JL. Morphology of thrombotic thrombocytopenic purpura with demonstration of aneurysms. *Am J Pathol* 1952;28:129.
37. Berkowitz LR, Dalldorf FG, Blatt PM. Thrombotic thrombocytopenic purpura: a pathology review. *JAMA* 1979;241:1709.
38. Umlas J, Kaiser J. Thrombohemolytic thrombocytopenic purpura (TTP): a disease or a syndrome? *Am J Med* 1970;49:723.
39. Goodman A, Ramos R, Petrelli M, et al. Gingival biopsy in thrombotic thrombocytopenic purpura. *Ann Intern Med* 1978;89:501.
40. Petitt RM. Thrombotic thrombocytopenic purpura: a thirty-year review. *Semin Thromb Hemost* 1980;6:350.
41. Gadek JE, Klein HG, Holland PV, et al. Replacement therapy of alpha 1-antitrypsin deficiency: reversal of protease-antiprotease imbalance within the alveolar structures of PiZ subjects. *J Clin Invest* 1981;68:1158.

42. Mant MJ, Couchi MN, Medley G. Thrombotic thrombocytopenic purpura: report of a case with possible immune etiology. *Blood* 1972;40:416.
43. Weisenburger DD, O'Conner ML, Hart MH. Thrombotic thrombocytopenic purpura with C3 vascular deposits: report of a case. *Am J Clin Pathol* 1977;67:61.
44. Craig JM, Gitlin D. The nature of the hyaline thrombi in thrombotic thrombocytopenic purpura. *Am J Pathol* 1957;33:251.
45. Kwaan HC. Role of fibrinolysis in thrombotic thrombocytopenic purpura. *Semin Thromb Hemost* 1979;6:395.
46. Alfrey AC. The renal response to vascular injury. In: Brenner BM, Rector FC, eds. *The Kidney.* 2nd ed. Philadelphia: Saunders; 1981:1668.
47. Pirani CL. Coagulation and renal disease. In: Bertani T, Remuzzi G, eds. *Glomerular Injury 300 Years After.* Morgagni, Milano: Wichtig; 1983; 119.
48. Gasser C, Gautier E, Steck A, et al. Hamolytisch-uramische syndromes bilaterale Nierenrindennekrosen bei akuten erworbenchen hamolytischen Anamien. *Schweiz Med Wschr* 1955;85:905.
49. Gervais M, Richardson JB, Chiu J, et al. Immunofluorescent and histologic findings in the hemolytic uremic syndrome. *Pediatrics* 1971;47:352.
50. Habib R, Cortecuisse V, Leclerc F, et al. Etude anatomopathologique de 35 observations de syndrome hémolytique et urémique de l'enfant. *Arch Franc Pediatr* 1969;26:391.
51. Hadley WK, Rosenan W. Study of human renal disease by immunofluorescent methods. *Arch Pathol* 1967;83:342.
52. Robson JS, Martin AM, Ruckley VA. Irreversible post partum renal failure. A new syndrome. *Q J Med* 1968;137:423.
53. Vitsky BH, Suzuki Y, Strauss L, et al. The hemolytic-uremic syndrome: a study of renal pathologic alterations. *Am J Pathol* 1969;57:627.
54. Waxman L. Calcium-activated proteases in mammalian tissues. *Methods Enzymol* 1981;80:664.
55. Goldstein MH, Churg J, Strauss L, et al. Hemolytic-uremic syndrome. *Nephron* 1979;23:263.
56. Habib R, Mathieu H, Royer P. Le syndrome hémolytique et urémique de l'enfant: aspects cliniques et anatomiques dans 27 observations. *Nephron* 1967;4:139.
57. Shigematsu H, Dikman SH, Churg J, et al. Mesangial involvement in hemolytic-uremic syndrome. *Am J Pathol* 1976;85:349.
58. Baldwin TJ, Ward W, Aitken A, et al. Elevation of intracellular free calcium levels in HEp-2 cells infected with enteropathogenic *Escherichia coli. Infect Immun* 1991;59:1599.
59. Levy M, Gagnadoux MF, Habib R. Pathology of hemolytic-uremic syndrome in children. In: Remuzzi G, Mecca G, de Gaetano G, ed. *Hemostasis, Prostaglandins and Renal Disease,* New York: Raven Press; 1980: 383.
60. Thoenes W, John HD. Endotheliotropic (hemolytic) nephroangiopathy and its various manifestation forms (Thrombotic microangiopathy, primary malignant nephrosclerosis, hemolytic uremic syndrome). *Klin Wochenschr* 1980;58:173.
61. Bohle A, Helmchen U, Grund KE. Malignant nephrosclerosis in patients with hemolytic-uremic syndrome (primary malignant nephrosclerosis). *Curr Top Pathol* 1977;65:81.
62. Kanfer A, Morel-Maroger L, Solez K, et al. The value of renal biopsy in hemolytic-uremic syndrome in adults. In: Remuzzi G, Mecca G, de Gaetano G, eds. *Hemostasis, Prostaglandins and Renal Disease,* New York: Raven Press; 1980:399.
63. Koffler D, Paronetto F. Fibrinogen deposition in acute renal failure. *Am J Pathol* 1966;49:383.
64. Gonzalo A, Mampaso F, Gallego N, et al. . Hemolytic uremic syndrome with hypocomplementemia and deposits of IgM and C3 in the involved renal tissue. *Clin Nephrol* 1981;16:193.
65. Rosenmann E, Kanter A, Bacani RA, et al. Fatal late postpartum intravascular coagulation with acute renal failure. *Am J Med Sci* 1969;257: 259.
66. Chugh KS, Singhal PC, Sharma BK, et al. Acute renal failure of obstetric origin. *Obstet Gynecol* 1976;48:642.
67. Koster F, Levin J, Walker L, et al. Hemolytic uremic syndrome after shigellosis: relation to endotoxemia and circulating immune complexes. *N Engl J Med* 1978;298:927.
68. Raghupathy P, Date A, Shastry JC, et al. Haemolytic-uraemic syndrome complicating shigella dysentery in south Indian children. *Br Med J* 1978;1:1518.
69. Rahaman MM, Jamiulalam AK, Islam MR, et al. Shiga bacillus dysentery associated with marked leukocytosis and erythrocyte fragmentation. *Johns Hopkins Med J* 1975;136:65.
70. Konowalchuk J, Speirs JI, Stavric S. Vero response to a cytotoxin of *Escherichia coli. Infect Immun* 1977;18:775.
71. Riley LW, Remis RS, Helgerson SD, et al. Hemorrhagic colitis associated with a rare *Escherichia coli* O157:H7 serotype. *N Engl J Med* 1983;308: 681.
72. Karmali MA, Steele BT, Petric M, et al. Sporadic cases of hemolytic-uraemic syndrome associated with faecal verotoxin and cytotoxin producing *Escherichia coli* in stools. *Lancet* 1983;1:619.
73. Ruggenenti P, Noris M, Remuzzi G. Thrombotic microangiopathies. In: *Therapy in Nephrology and Hypertension.* 2nd ed. Bredy HR and Wilcox CS. London; Saunders; 2003:283.
74. Mead PS, Griffin PM. *Escherichia coli* O157:H7. *Lancet* 1998;352:1207.
75. Locking ME, O'Brien SJ, Reilly WJ, et al. Risk factors for sporadic cases of *Escherichia coli* O157 infection: the importance of contact with animal excreta. *Epidemiol Rev* 2001;127:215,
76. Mead PS, Finelli L, Lambert-Fair MA, et al. Risk factors for sporadic infection with *Escherichia coli* O157:H7. *Arch Intern Med* 1997;157:204.
77. Rowe PC, Orrbine E, Ogborn M, et al. Epidemic *Escherichia coli* O157:H7 gastroenteritis and hemolytic-uremic syndrome in a Canadian Inuit community: intestinal illness in family members as a risk factor. *J Pediatr* 1994;124:21.
78. Pavia AT, Nichols CR, Green DP, et al. Hemolytic-uremic syndrome during an outbreak of *Escherichia coli* 0157:H7 infections in institutions for mentally retarded persons: clinical and epidemiologic observations. *J Pediatr* 1990;116:544.
79. Belongia EA, Osterholm MT, Soler JT, et al. Transmission of *Escherichia coli* 0157:H7 in Minnesota child day-care facilities. *JAMA* 1993;269:883.
80. Rowe PC, Orrbine E, Lior H, et al. Diarrhoea in close contacts as a risk factor for childhood haemolytic uraemic syndrome. *Epidemiol Infect* 1993;110:9.
81. Pai CH, Gordon R, Sims HV, et al. Sporadic cases of hemorrhagic colitis associated with *Escherichia coli* 0157:H7: clinical, epidemiologic, and bacteriologic features. *Ann Intern Med* 1984;101:738.
82. Remuzzi G, Ruggenenti P. The hemolytic uremic syndrome. *Kidney Int* 1995;48:2.
83. Lior H, Rowe PC, Orrbine E, et al. Microbiology of hemolytic uremic syndrome (HUS) in Canada (abstract). VTEC 94, 2nd International Symposium and Workshop on "Verocytotoxin (Shiga-like toxin)-producing Escherichia coli infections" June 27–30, Seminario Vescovile "Giovanni XXIII" Bergamo, Italy, 1994;45.
84. Shapiro AP, Medsger TA Jr, Steen VD. Renal involvement in systemic sclerosis. In: Schrier RW, Gottschalk CW, eds. *Diseases of the Kidney.* 5th ed. Boston: Little, Brown & Company; 1993:2039.
85. van de Kar NC, Roelofs H, Muytjens HL, et al. Verocytotoxin producing *E. coli* infection in patients with hemolytic uremic syndrome in western Europe: a four year prospective study (abstract). VTEC 94, 2nd International Symposium and Workshop on "Verocytotoxin (Shiga-like toxin)-producing Escherichia coli infections" June 27–30, Seminario Vescovile "Giovanni XXIII" Bergamo, Italy, 1994;45.
86. Lopez EL, Diaz M, Grinstein S, et al. Hemolytic uremic syndrome and diarrhea in argentine children: the role of Shiga-like. *J Infect Dis* 1989;160: 469.
87. Sherman P, Soni R, Karmali MA. Attaching and effacing adherence of verocytotoxin-producing *Escherichia coli* to rabbit intestine in-vivo. *Infect Immun* 1988;56:756.
88. Acheson DW, Moore R, De Brueker S, et al. Translocation of Shiga toxin across polarized cells in tissue culture. *Infect Immun* 1996;64:3294.
89. Hurley BP, Thorpe CM, Acheson DW. Shiga toxin translocation across intestinal epithelial cells is enhanced by neutrophil transmigration. *Infect Immun* 2001;69:6148.
90. te Loo DM, Monnens LA, van Der Velden TJ, et al. Binding and transfer of verocytotoxin by polymorphonuclear leukocytes in hemolytic uremic syndrome. *Blood* 2000;95:3396.
91. te Loo DM, van Hinsberg VW, van den Heuvel LP, et al. Detection of verocytotoxin bound to circulating polymorphonuclear leukocytes of patients with hemolytic uremic syndrome. *J Am Soc Nephrol* 2001;12:800.
92. O'Brien AD, Lively TA, Chen ME, et al. *Escherichia coli* 0157:H7 strains associated with haemorrhagic colitis in the United States produce a *Shigella dysenteriae* I (Shiga) like cytotoxin. *Lancet* 1983;1:702.
93. Paton AW, Srimanote P, Talbot UM, et al. A new family of potent AB5 cytotoxins produced by Shiga toxigenic Escherichia coli. *J Exp Med* 2004;200:35.
94. Scotland SM, Willshaw GA, Smith HR, et al. Properties of strains of Escherichia coli belonging to serogroup 0157 with special reference to production of Vero cytotoxins VT1 and VT2. *Epidemiol Infect* 1987;99:613.
95. Ostroff SM, Kobayashi JM, Lewis JH. Infections with Escherichia coli 0157:H7 in Washington State. The first year of statewide disease surveillance. *JAMA* 1989;262:355.
96. Cimolai N, Carter JE, Morrison BJ, et al. Risk factors for the progression of Escherichia coli 0157:H7 enteritis to hemolytic-uremic syndrome. *J Pediatr* 1990;116:589.
97. Jenkis C, Willshaw GA, Evans J, et al. Subtyping of virulences genes in verocytotoxin-producing Escherichia coli (VTEC) other than serogroup 0157 associated with disease in the United Kingdom. *J Med Microbiol* 2003;52:941.
98. Siegler RL, Obrig TG, Pysher TJ, et al. Response to Shiga toxin 1 and 2 in a baboon model of hemolytic uremic syndrome. *Pediatr Nephrol* 2003;18: 92.
99. Nakajima H, Kiyokawa N, Katagiri YU, et al. Kinetic analysis of binding between Shiga toxin and receptor glycolipid G3bCer by surface plasmon resonance. *J Biol Chem* 2001;276:42915.
100. Sandvig K, Olsnes S, Brown JE, et al. Endocytosis from coated pits of Shiga Toxin: a glycolipid-binding protein from Shigella dysenteriae 1. *J Cell Biol* 1989;108:1331.
101. Obrig TG, Del Vecchio PJ, Brown JE, et al. Direct cytotoxic action of Shiga toxin on human vascular endothelial cells. *Infect Immun* 1988;56:2373.
102. Lingwood CA. Verotoxin-binding in human renal sections. *Nephron* 1994; 66:21.

103. Mahan JD, van Setten PA, McAllister C, et al. Effect of verotoxin-1 on viability and protein synthesis of human glomerular capillary endothelial cells (abstract). VTEC 94, 2nd International Symposium and Workshop on "Verocytotoxin (Shiga-like toxin)-producing Escherichia coli infections" June 27-30, Seminario Vescovile "Giovanni XXIII" Bergamo, Italy, 1994:31.

104. Eason RJ, Tan PL, Gow PJ. Progressive systemic sclerosis in Auckland: a ten-year review with emphasis on prognostic features. *Aust New Zealand J Med* 1981;11:657.

105. Zoja C, Angioletti S, Donadelli R, et al. Shiga toxin-2 triggers endothelial leukocyte adhesion and transmigration via NF-kappaB dependent up-regulation of IL-8 and MCP-1. *Kidney Int* 2002;62:846.

106. Matussek A, Lauber J, Bergau A, et al. Molecular and functional analysis of Shiga toxin-induced response patterns in human vascular endothelial cells. *Blood* 2003;102:13232.

107. Morigi M, Micheletti G, Figliuzzi M, et al. Verotoxin-1 promotes leukocyte adhesion to cultured endothelial cells under physiologic flow conditions. *Blood* 1998;86:4553.

108. Morigi M, Galbusera M, Binda E, et al. Verotoxin-1-induced up-regulation of adhesive molecules renders microvascular endothelial cells thrombogenic at high shear stress. *Blood* 2001;98:1828.

109. Ruggeri Z. Endothelial cells: they only look all alike. *Blood* 2001;98:1644.

110. Bergstein JM, Riley M, Bang NU. Role of plasminogen-activator inhibitor type-1 in the pathogenesis and outcome of the hemolytic uremic syndrome. *N Engl J Med* 1992;327:755.

111. Chandler WL, Jelacic S, Boster DR, et al. Prothrombotic coagulation abnormalities preceding the hemolytic-uremic syndrome. *N Engl J Med* 2002;346:23.

112. Koster F, Boonpucknavig V, Suiaho S, et al. Renal histopathology in the hemolytic uremic syndrome following shigellosis. *Clin Nephrol* 1984;21:126.

113. Louise CB, Obrig TG. Shiga toxin-associated hemolytic uremic syndrome: combined cytotoxic effects of Shiga toxin, interleukin-1b, and tumor necrosis factor alpha on human vascular endothelial cells in vitro. *Infect Immun* 1991;59:4173.

114. Louise CB, Obrig TG. Shiga toxin-associated hemolytic uremic syndrome: combined cytotoxic effects of Shiga toxin and lipopolysaccharide (endotoxin) on human vascular endothelial cells in vitro. *Infect Immun* 1992;60:1536.

115. van de Kar NC, Kooistra T, Monnens LA, et al. Role of TNF receptors and protein kinase C in the induction of the verocytotoxin receptor, GB3, in human endothelial cells (abstract). VTEC 94, 2nd International Symposium and Workshop on "Verocytotoxin (Shiga-like toxin)-producing Escherichia coli infections" June 27–30, 1994 Seminario Vescovile "Giovanni XXIII" Bergamo, Italy, 1994:23.

116. Harel Y, Silva M, Giroir B, et al. A reporter transgene indicates renal-specific induction of tumor necrosis factor (TNF) by Shiga-like toxin. *J Clin Invest* 1993;92:2110.

117. Moake, et al. Thrombotic microangiopathies. *N Engl J Med* 2002;347(8):589.

118. Karpman D, Padapopulou D, Nilsson K, et al. Platelet activation by Shiga toxin and circulatory factors as a pathogenetic mechanism in the hemolytic-uremic syndrome. *Blood* 2001;97:3100.

119. Yamada O, Moldow CF, Sacks T, et al. Deleterious effects of endotoxin on cultured endothelial cells: an in vitro model of vascular injury. *Inflammation* 1981;5:115.

120. Forsyth KD, Simpson AC, Fitzpatrick MM, et al. Neutrophil-mediated endothelial injury in haemolytic uraemic syndrome. *The Lancet* 1989;II:411.

121. Meyrick BO. Endotoxin-mediated pulmonary endothelial cell injury. *Fed Proc* 1986;45:19.

122. Schleimer RP, Rutledge BK. Cultured human vascular endothelial cells acquire adhesiveness for neutrophils after stimulation with interleukin 1, endotoxin, and tumor-promoting phorbol diesters. *J Immunol* 1986;136:649.

123. Brady HR. Leukocyte adhesion molecules: potential targets for therapeutic intervention in kidney diseases. *Curr Opin Nephrol and Hypertens* 1993;2:171.

124. Coughlan AF, Hau H, Dunlop LC, et al. P-selectin and platelet-activating factor mediate initial endotoxin-induced neutropenia. *J Exp Med* 1994;179:329.

125. Munro JM, Pober JS, Cotran RS. Recruitment of neutrophils in the local endotoxin response: association with de novo endothelial expression of endothelial leukocyte adhesion molecule-1. *Lab Invest* 1991;64:295.

126. Hemolytic Uremic Syndrome: review, Noris M, Remuzzi G. *J Am Soc Nephrol* 2005;16:1035.

127. Klein PJ, Bulla M, Newman RA, et al. Thomsen-Friedenreich antigen in haemolytic uraemic syndrome. *Lancet* 1977;2:1024.

128. Neild GH. Mechanisms and models of endothelial injury. In: Bertani T, Remuzzi G, eds. *Glomerular Injury 300 Years After Morgagni*. Milano: Wichtig; 1983;139.

129. Kissmeyer-Nielsen F, Olsen S, et al. Hyperacute rejection of kidney allografts, associated with pre-existing humoral antibodies against donor cells. *Lancet* 1966;2:662.

130. Milgrom F, Kano K, Klassen J. Role of humoral antibodies in rejection of renal allografts. *Transplant Proc* 1969;1:1013.

131. Lowenhaupt R, Nathan P. The participation of platelets in the rejection of dog kidney allotransplants: hematologic and electron microscopic studies. *Transplant Proc* 1969;1:305.

132. Sharma HM, Moore S, Merrick HW, et al. Platelet in early hyperacute allograft rejection in kidneys and their modification by sulfinpyrazone (Anturan) therapy: an experimental study. *Am J Pathol* 1972;66:445.

133. Kniker WT, Cochrane CG. Pathogenetic factors in vascular lesions of experimental serum sickness. *J Exp Med* 1965;122:83.

134. Neild GH, Ivory K, Hiramatsu M, et al. Cyclosporin A inhibits acute serum sickness nephritis in rabbits. *Clin Exp Immunol* 1983;52:586.

135. Kniker WT, Cochrane CG. The localization of circulating immune complexes in experimental serum sickness. The role of vasoactive amines and hydrodynamic forces. *J Exp Med* 1968;127:119.

136. Levine S, Shearn MA. Thrombotic thrombocytopenic purpura and systemic lupus erythematosus. *Arch Intern Med* 1964;113:826.

137. Rothfield NF. Systemic lupus erythematosus. In: McCarey DJ, ed. *Arthritis and Allied Conditions*. Philadelphia: Lea and Febiger; 1979;706.

138. Wall RT, Harker LA. The endothelium and thrombosis. *Annu Rev Med* 1980;31:361.

139. Foster PA, Anderson JC. Effects of plasma from patients with thrombotic thrombocytopenic purpura (TTP) on cultured human endothelial cells (abstract). *Blood* 1979;54:240a.

140. Leung YD, Moake JL, Havens PL, et al. Lytic anti-endothelial cell antibodies in haemolytic-uraemic syndrome. *Lancet* 1988;2:183.

141. Platt JL, Vercellotti GM, Lindman BJ, et al. Release of heparan sulfate from endothelial cells. Implications for pathogenesis for hyperacute rejection. *J Exp Med* 1990;171:1363.

142. Busch GJ, Martins AC, Hollenberg NK, et al. A primate model of hyperacute renal allograft rejection. *Am J Pathol* 1975;79:31.

143. Dvorak HF, Mihn MC, Dvorak AM, et al. Rejection of first-set skin allografts in man. The microvasculature is the critical target of the immune response. *J Exp Med* 1979;150:322.

144. Forbes RD, Kuramochi T, Guttmann RD, et al. A controlled sequential morphologic study of hyperacute cardiac allograft rejection in the rat. *Lab Invest* 1975;33:280.

145. Byrnes JJ, Baquerizo H, Gonzales M, et al. Thrombotic thrombocytopenic purpura subsequent to acute myelogenous leukemia chemotherapy. *Am J Hematol* 1986;21:299.

146. Harrell N, Sibley R, Vogelzang NJ. Renal vascular lesions after chemotherapy with vinblastine, bleomycin and cisplatin. *Am J Med* 1982;73:429.

147. Cantrell JE Jr, Phillips TM, Schein PS. Carcinoma associated hemolytic-uremic syndrome: a complication of mitomycin-C chemotherapy. *J Clin Oncol* 1985;3:723.

148. Hamner RW, Verani R, Weinman EJ. Mitomycin-associated renal failure: case report and review. *Arch Intern Med* 1983;143:803.

149. Rabadi SJ, Khandekar JD, Miller HJ. Mitomycin-induced hemolytic-uremic syndrome: case presentation and review of literature. *Cancer Treat Rep* 1982;66:1244.

150. Jackson AM, Rose BD, Graff LG, et al. Thrombotic microangiopathy and renal failure associated with antineoplastic chemotherapy. *Ann Intern Med* 1984;101:41.

151. Lesesne JB, Rothschild N, Erickson B, et al. Cancer-associated hemolytic-uremic syndrome: analysis of 85 cases from a national registry. *J Clin Oncol* 1989;7:781.

152. Duperray A, Tranqui L, Alix JL, et al. Effect of mitomycin C on the biosynthesis of prostacyclin by primary cultures of human umbilical cord vein endothelial cell (abstract). *Kidney Int* 1984;25:730.

153. Cattell V. Mitomycin-induced hemolytic uremic kidney. An experimental model in the rat. *Am J Pathol* 1985;121:88.

154. Brown CB, Clarkson AR, Robson JS, et al. Haemolytic uraemic syndrome in women taking oral contraceptives. *Lancet* 1973;1:1479.

155. Morel-Maroger L. Adult hemolytic-uremic syndrome. *Kidney Int* 1980;18:125.

156. Ponticelli C, Rivolta E, Imbasciati E, et al. Hemolytic uremic syndrome in adults. *Arch Intern Med* 1980;140:353.

157. Boyd WN, Burden RP, Aber GM. Intrarenal vascular changes in patients receiving oestrogen—containing compounds—a clinical, histological and angiographic study. *Q J Med* 1975;44:415.

158. Giromini M, Hapenouza C. Prolonged survival after bilateral nephrectomy in an adult with haemolytic uraemic syndrome. *Lancet* 1969;2:169.

159. Schoolwerth AC, Sandler RS, Klahr S, et al. Nephrosclerosis postpartum and in women taking oral contraceptives. *Arch Intern Med* 1976;136:178.

160. Hauglustaine D, Van Damme B, Vanrenterghem Y, et al. Recurrent hemolytic uremic syndrome during oral contraception. *Clin Nephrol* 1981;15:148.

161. Sevitt LH, Evans DJ, Wrong OM. Acute oliguric renal failure due to accelerated (malignant) hypertension. *Q J Med* 1971;40:127.

162. Farr MJ, Roberts S, Morley AR. The haemolytic-uraemic syndrome—a family study. *Q J Med* 1975;44:161.

163. Edelsten AD, Tuck S. Familial haemolytic uraemic syndrome. *Arch Dis Child* 1978;53:255.

164. Carreras L, Romero R, Requesens C. Familial hypocomplementemic hemolytic uremic syndrome with HLA-A3, B7 haplotype. *JAMA* 1981;245:602.

165. Rifle G, Chalopin JM, Genin R, et al. Hemolytic uremic syndrome and recurrent uremia. Irreversible cortical necrosis due to estro-progestational hormones (abstract). *J Urol Nephrol* 1979;85:331.

166. Kaplan BS. An analysis of the association of the hemolytic uremic syndrome and the birth control pill. In: Kaplan BS, Trompeter RS, Moake JL, eds.

Hemolytic Uremic Syndrome and Thrombotic Thrombocytopenic Purpura. New York: Marcel Dekker Inc.; 1992:227.

167. Bennett CL, Weinberg PD, Rozenberg-Ben-Dror K, et al. Thrombotic thrombocytopenic purpura associated with ticlopidine: a review of 60 cases. *Ann Intern Med* 1998;128:541.

168. Steinhubl SR, Tan WA, Foody JM, et al. Incidence and clinical course of thrombotic thrombocytopenic purpura due to ticlopidine following coronary stenting. *JAMA* 1999;281:806.

169. Bennett CL, Kiss JE, Weinberg PD, et al. Thrombotic thrombocytopenic purpura after stenting and ticlopidine. *Lancet* 1998;352:1036.

170. Bennett CL, Davidson CJ, Raisch DW, et al. Thrombotic thrombocytopenic purpura associated with ticlopidine in the setting of coronary artery stents and stroke prevention. *Arch Intern Med* 1999;159:2524.

171. Bennett CL, Connors JM, Carwile JM, et al. Thrombotic thrombocytopenic purpura associated with clopidogrel. *N Engl J Med* 2000;342(24):1773.

172. Beatty ME, Griffin PM, Tulu AN, et al. Culturing practises and antibiotic use in children with diarrhea. *Pediatrics* 2004;113:628.

173. Ferretti G, Petti MC, Carlini P, et al. Zoledronic acid-associated thrombotic thrombocytopenic purpura. *Ann Oncol* 2004;15:1847.

174. Sundram F, Roberts P, Kennedy B, et al. Thrombotic thrombocytopenic purpura associated with statin treatment. *Postgrad Med J* 2004;80:551.

175. Kaplan BS, Fong JS. Reduced platelet aggregation in hemolytic uremic syndrome. *Thromb Haemostas* 1980;43:154.

176. Edefonti A, Tentori F, Bettinelli A, et al. Pattern of platelet serotonin (5TH), plasma beta-thromboglobulin (betaTG) and platelet factor (PG4) in hemolytic-uremic syndrome (HUS) in children. *Int J Pediatr Nephrol* 1981;2:149.

177. Fong JS, Kaplan BS. Impairment of platelet aggregation in hemolytic uremic syndrome. Evidence for platelet 'exhaustion'. *Blood* 1982;60:564.

178. Beattie TJ, Murphy AV, Willoughby ML, et al. Prostacyclin infusion in haemolytic-uraemic syndrome of children. *Br Med J* 1981;283:470.

179. Zimmermann GA, McIntyre TM, Mehra M, et al. Endothelial cell-associated platelet-activating factor: a novel mechanism for signaling intercellular adhesion. *J Cell Biol* 1990;110:529.

180. Benigni A, Boccardo P, Noris M, et al. Urinary excretion of platelet-activating factor in haemolytic uraemic syndrome. *Lancet* 1992;339:835.

181. Lian EC, Harkness DR, Byrnes JJ, et al. Presence of a platelet aggregating factor in the plasma of patients with thrombotic thrombocytopenic purpura (TTP) and its inhibition by normal plasma. *Blood* 1979;53:333.

182. Lian EC, Siddiqui FA, Chen SH, et al. Platelet-agglutinating/aggregating proteins from the plasma of patients with thrombotic thrombocytopenic purpura. In: Kaplan BS, Trompeter RS, Moake JL, eds. *HUS and TTP.* New York: Marcel Dekker, Inc.; 1992:473.

183. Remuzzi G, Galbusera M, Noris M, et al. Von Willebrand factor cleaving protease (ADAMTS13) is deficient in recurrent and familial thrombotic thrombocytopenic purpura and hemolytic uremic syndrome. *Blood* 2002;100(3):778.

184. Lämmle B, Kremer Hoviga J, Studt JD, et al. Thrombotic thrombocytopenic purpura. *Hematol J* 2004;5:S6.

185. Levy GG, Nichols WC, Lian EC, et al. Mutations in a member of the ADAMTS gene family cause thrombotic thrombocytopenic purpura. *Nature* 2001;413:488.

186. Upshaw JD. Congenital deficiency of a factor in normal plasma that reverses microangiopathic hemolysis and thrombocytopenia. *N Engl J Med* 1978;298:1350.

187. Veyradier A, Obert B, Houiller A, et al. Specific von Willebrand factor-cleaving protease in thrombotic microangiopathies: a study of 111 cases. *Blood* 2001;98:1765.

188. Remuzzi G. Is severe deficiency of ADAMTS-13 specific for thrombotic thrombocytopenic purpura? *J Thromb Haemost* 2003;1:632.

189. Galbusera M, Noris M, Rossi C, et al. Increased fragmentation of von Willebrand factor, due to abnormal cleavage of the subunit, parallels disease activity in recurrent hemolytic uremic syndrome and thrombotic thrombocytopenic purpura and discloses predisposition in families. The Italian Registry of Familial and Recurrent HUS/TTP. *Blood* 1999;94:610.

190. Galbusera M, Benigni A, Paris S, et al. Unrecognized pattern of von Willebrand factor abnormalities in hemolytic uremic syndrome and thrombotic thrombocytopenic purpura. *J Am Soc Nephrol* 1999;10:1234.

191. Furlan M, Robles R, Solenthaler M, et al. Acquired deficiency of von Willebrand factor-cleaving protease in a patient with thrombotic thrombocytopenic purpura. *Blood* 1998;91:2839.

192. Remuzzi G, Galbusera M, Salvadori M, et al. Bilateral nephrectomy stopped disease progression in plasma-resistant hemolytic uremic syndrome with neurological signs and coma. *Kidney Int* 1996;49:282.

193. Furlan M, Robles R, Galbusera M, et al. von Willebrand factor-cleaving protease in thrombotic thrombocytopenic purpura and the hemolytic-uremic syndrome. *N Engl J Med* 1998;339:1578.

194. Moore JC, Hayward CP, Warketin TE, et al. Decreased von Willebrand factor protease activity associated with thrombocytopenic disorders. *Blood* 2001;98:1842.

195. Moake JL. Thrombotic thrombocytopenic purpura and the hemolytic uremic syndrome. *Arch Pathol Lab Med* 2002;126:1430.

196. Joszi M, Manuelian T, Heinen S, et al. Attachment of the soluble complement regulator factor H to cell and tissue surfaces: relevance for pathology. *Histol Histopathol* 2004;19:251.

197. Manuelian T, Hellwage J, Meri S, et al. Mutations in factor H reduce binding affinity to C3b and heparin and surface attachment to endothelial cells in hemolytic uremic syndrome. *J Clin Invest* 2003;111:1181.

198. Caprioli J, Castelletti F, Bucchioni S, et al. Complement factor H mutations and gene polymorphisms in hemolytic uremic syndrome: the C-257T, the A2089G and the G2881T polymorphisms are strongly associated with the disease. *Hum Mol Genet* 2003;12:3385.

199. Neumann HP, Salzmann M, Bohnert-Iwan B, et al. Haemolytic uraemic syndrome and mutations of the factor H gene: a registry-based study of German speaking countries. *J Med Genet* 2003;40:676.

200. Dragon-Durley MA, Fremeaux-Bacchi V, Loirat C, et al. Heterozygous and homozygous factor H deficiencies associated with hemolytic uremic syndrome or membranoproliferative glomerulonephritis: report and genetic analysis of 16 cases. *J Am Soc Nephrol* 2004;15:787.

201. Perez-Caballero D, Gonzalez-Rubio C, Gallardo ME, et al. Clustering of missense mutations in the C-terminal region of factor H in atypical hemolytic-uremic syndrome. *Am J Hum Genet* 2001;68:478.

202. Tsai Hm, Lian EC. Antibodies to von Willebrand factor-cleaving protease in acute thrombotic thrombocytopenic purpura. *N Engl J Med* 1998;339:1585.

203. Sanchez-Corral P, Gonzales-Rubio C, Rodriguez de Cordoba S, et al. Functional analysis in serum from atypical hemolytic uremic syndrome patients reveals impaired protection of host cells associated with mutations in factor H. *Mol Immunol* 2004;41:81.

204. Contantinescu AR, Bitzan M, Weiss LS, et al. Non-enteropathic hemolytic uremic syndrome: causes and short-term courses. *Am J Kidney Dis* 2004;43:976.

205. Remuzzi G, Misiani R, Marchesi D, et al. Haemolytic-uraemic syndrome: deficiency of plasma factor(s) regulating prostacyclin activity? *Lancet* 1978;2:871.

206. Defreyn G, Proesmans W, Machin SJ, et al. Abnormal prostacyclin metabolism in the hemolytic uremic syndrome: equivocal effect of prostacyclin infusion. *Clin Nephrol* 1982;18:43.

207. Levin M, Elkon KB, Nokes TJ, et al. Inhibitor of prostacyclin production in sporadic haemolytic uraemic syndrome. *Arch Dis Child* 1983;58:703.

208. Chen YC, McLeod B, Hall ER, et al. Accelerated prostacyclin degradation in thrombotic thrombocytopenic purpura. *Lancet* 1981;2:267.

209. Wu KK, Hall ER, Rossi EC, et al. Serum prostacyclin binding defects in thrombotic thrombocytopenic purpura. *J Clin Invest* 1985;75:168.

210. Noris M, Benigni A, Siegler R, et al. Renal prostacyclin biosynthesis is reduced in children with hemolytic-uremic syndrome in the context of systemic platelet activation. *Am J Kidney Dis* 1992;20:144.

211. Moncada S. Prostacyclin and thromboxane A2 in the regulation of platelet-vascular interactions. In: Remuzzi G, Mecca G, de Gaetano G, eds. *Hemostasis, Prostaglandins and Renal Disease.* New York: Raven Press; 1980;175.

212. Tsai HM, Sussman II, Nagel RL. Shear stress enhances the proteolysis of von Willebrand factor in normal plasma. *Blood* 1994;83:2171.

213. Rubanyi GM, Romero JC, Vanhoutte PM. Flow-induced release of endothelium relaxing factor. *Am J Physiol* 1986;250:H1145.

214. Noris M, Morigi M, Zoja C, et al. Modulation of nitric oxide (NO) synthesis by endothelial cells in vitro is a function of flow conditions (abstract). *J Am Soc Nephrol* 1993;4:562.

215. Mulligan MS, Hevel JM, Marletta MA, et al. Tissue injury caused by deposition of immune complexes is L-arginine dependent. *Proc Natl Acad Sci USA* 1991;88:6338.

216. Beckman JS, Beckman TW, Chen J, et al. Apparent hydroxyl radical production by peroxynitrite: implications for endothelial injury from nitric oxide and superoxide. *Proc Natl Acad Sci USA* 1990;87:1620.

217. Glasgow LA, Balduzzi P. Isolation of Coxsackie virus group A, type 4 from a patient with hemolytic-uremic syndrome. *N Engl J Med* 1965;273:754.

218. Berberich FR, Cuene SA, Chard RL. Thrombotic thrombocytopenic purpura. Three cases with platelet and fibrinogen survival studies. *J Pediatr* 1974;84:503.

219. Wasserstein A, Hill G, Goldfarb S, et al. Recurrent thrombotic thrombocytopenic purpura after viral infection. Clinical and histologic simulation of chronic glomerulonephritis. *Arch Intern Med* 1981;141:685.

220. Reynolds PM, Jackson JM, Brine JA, et al. Thrombotic thrombocytopenic purpura-remission following splenectomy. *Am J Med* 1976;61:439.

221. Riggs SA, Wray NP, Waddell CC, et al. Thrombotic thrombocytopenic purpura complicating Legionnaires' disease. *Arch Intern Med* 1982;142:2275.

222. Antes EH. Thrombotic thrombocytopenic purpura: a review of the literature with report of a case. *Ann Intern Med* 1958;48:512.

223. Brown RC, Blecher TE, French EA, et al. Thrombotic thrombocytopenic purpura after influenza vaccination. *Br Med J* 1973;2:303.

224. Watson CG, Cooper WW. Thrombotic thrombocytopenic purpura: concomitant occurrence in husband and wife. *JAMA* 1971;215:1821.

225. Paz RA, Elijovic F, Barcat JA, et al. Fatal simultaneous thrombocytopenic purpura in siblings. *Br Med J* 1969;4:727.

226. Bayer AS, Theofilopoulous AN, Eisenberg R. Thrombotic thrombocytopenic purpura-like syndrome associated with infective endocarditis: a possible immune complex disorder. *JAMA* 1977;238:408.

227. Boccia RV, Gelmann EP, Baker CC, et al. A hemolytic uremic syndrome with the acquired immunodeficiency syndrome. *Ann Intern Med* 1984;101:716.

228. Jokela J, Flynn T, Henry K. Thrombotic thrombocytopenic purpura in a human immunodeficiency virus (HIV)-seropositive homosexual man. *Am J Hematol* 1987;25:341.

229. Leaf AN, Laubenstein LJ, Raphael B, et al. Thrombotic thrombocytopenic purpura associated with human immunodeficiency virus type 1 (HIV-1) infection. *Ann Intern Med* 1988;109:194.

230. Karmali MA, Petric M, Lim C, et al. The association between idiopathic hemolytic uremic syndrome and infection by verotoxin-producing *Escherichia coli*. *J Infect Dis* 1985;151:775.

231. Edmonson MB, Chesney RW. Hemolytic-uremic syndrome confused with acute appendicitis. *Arch Surg* 1978;113:754.

232. Helfrich DJ, Banner B, Steen VD, et al. Normotensive renal failure in systemic sclerosis. *Arthritis Rheum* 1989;32:1128.

233. Gianantonio CA, Vitacco M, Mendilaharzu F, et al. The hemolytic-uremic syndrome. In: Proceedings of the Third International Congress of Nephrology, Washington D.C.; 1966;24.

234. Medsger TA Jr, Masi AT, Rodnan GP, et al. Survival with systemic sclerosis (scleroderma). *Ann Intern Med* 1971;75:369.

235. Date A, Raghupathy P, Jadhan M, et al. Outcome of the hemolytic uremic syndrome complicating bacillary dysentery. *Ann Trop Paediatr* 1982;2:1.

236. Badami G, Srivastava RN, Kumar R, et al. Disseminated intravascular coagulation in post-dysenteric hemolytic uremic syndrome. *Acta Pediatr Scand* 1987;76:919.

237. Coad NA, Marshall T, Rowe B, et al. Changes in the postenteropathic form of the hemolytic uremic syndrome in children. *Clin Nephrol* 1991;35:10.

238. Hall S, Glickman M. The British Paediatric Surveillance Unit. *Arch Dis Child* 1988;63:344.

239. Kaplan BS, Thomson PD, de Chadarevian JP. The hemolytic uremic syndrome. *Pediatr Clin North Am* 1976;23:761.

240. O'Regan S, Blais N, Russo P, et al. Hemolytic uremic syndrome: glomerular filtration rate, 6 to 11 years later measured by 99mTcDTPA plasma slope clearance. *Clin Nephrol* 1989;32:217.

241. Gagnadoux MF, Habib R, Gubler MC, et al. Long-term (15–25 years) prognosis of childhood hemolytic-uremic syndrome (HUS) (abstract). *J Am Soc Nephrol* 1993;4:275.

242. Rasoulpour M, Leichtner A, San Jorge M, et al. Cerebral vascular accident during the recovery phase of the hemolytic uremic syndrome. *Int J Pediatr Nephrol* 1985;6:287.

243. Kahn SI, Tolkan SR, Kothari Q, et al. Spontaneous recovery of the hemolytic-uremic syndrome with prolonged renal and neurological manifestations. *Nephron* 1982;32:188.

244. Garg AX, Suri RS, Barrowman N, et al. Long-term renal prognosis of diarrhea-associated hemolytic uremic syndrome: a systemic review, meta-analysis, and meta-regression. *JAMA* 2003;290:1360.

245. Karch H, Goroncy-Bermes P, Operkuch W, et al. Subinhibitory concentrations of antibiotics modulate amount of Shiga-like toxin produced by Escherichia coli. In: Adam Y, Halin H, Opterkudi W, eds. *The Influence of Antibiotics on the Host-Parasite Relationship II*. Berlin: Springer Verlag; 1985;239.

246. Wong CS, Jelacic S, Habeeb RL, et al. The risk of the hemolytic-uremic syndrome after antibiotic treatment of *Escherichia coli* O157:H7 infections. *N Engl J Med* 2000:342(26):1930.

247. Safdar N, Said A, Gangnon RE, et al. Risk of hemolytic uremic syndrome after antibiotic treatment of *Escherichia coli* O157:H7 enteritis: a meta-analysis. *JAMA* 2002;288:996.

248. Chiurchiu C, Firrincieli A, Santostefano M, et al. Adult nondiarrhea hemolytic uremic syndrome associated with Shiga toxin *Escherichia coli* O157:H7 bacteremia and urinary tract infection. *Am J Kidney Dis* 2003;41:E4.

249. Gomperts ED, Lieberman E. Hemolytic uremic syndrome and thrombotic thrombocytopenic purpura. In: Suki WN, Massry SG, eds. *Therapy of Renal Diseases and Related Disorders*. Boston: Nijhoff; 1984:297.

250. Miller K, Kim Y. Hemolytic uremic syndrome. In: Holliday MA, Barratt TM, Vernier RL, eds. *Pediatric Nephrology*. 2nd ed. Baltimore: Williams & Wilkins; 1987:482.

251. Vitacco M, Sanchez-Avalos J, Gianantonio CA. Heparin therapy in the hemolytic uremic syndrome. *J Pediatr* 1973;83:271.

252. Loirat C, Beaufils F, Sonsino E, et al. Traitement du syndrome hémolytique et urémique de l'enfant par l'urokinase. Essai contrôlé coopératif. *Arch Fr Pédiatr* 1984;41:15.

253. Van Damme-Lombaerts R, Proesmans W, Van Damme B, et al. Heparin plus dipyridamole in childhood hemolytic uremic syndrome: a prospective, randomized study. *J Pediatr* 1988;113:913.

254. Powell HR, McCredie DA, Taylor CM, et al. Vitamin E treatment of haemolytic uraemic syndrome. *Arch Dis Child* 1984;59:401.

255. Sheth KJ, Gill JC, Leichte HE. Randomized double blind controlled study of intravenous gamma globulin (IVGG) infusions in hemolytic uremic syndrome (HUS) (abstract). *J Am Soc Nephrol* 1990;1:342.

256. Berkman SA, Lee ML, Gale RP. Clinical uses of intravenous immunoglobulins. *Ann Intern Med* 1990;112:278.

257. Trachtman H, Cnaan A, Christen E, et al. Effect of an oral Shiga toxin-binding agent on diarrhea-associated hemolytic-uremic syndrome in children: a randomized controlled trial. *JAMA* 2003;290:1337.

258. Beattie TJ, Murphy AV, Willoughby MC, et al. Plasmapheresis in the haemolytic uremic syndrome in children. *Br Med J* 1981;282:1667.

259. Gillor A, Bulla M, Roth B, et al. Plasmapheresis as a therapeutic measure in hemolytic uremic syndrome in children. *Klin Wochenschr* 1983;61:363.

260. Sheth KJ, Gill JC, Hanna J, et al. Failure of fresh frozen plasma infusions to alter the course of hemolytic uremic syndrome. *Child Nephrol Urol* 1988;9:38.

261. Ogborn MR, Crocker JF, Barnard DR. Plasma therapy for severe hemolytic-uremic syndrome in children in Atlantic Canada. *Can Med Assoc J* 1990;143:1323.

262. Rizzoni G, Claris-Appiani A, Edefonti A, et al. Plasma infusion for hemolytic-uremic syndrome in children: results of a multicenter controlled trial. *J Pediatr* 1988;112:284.

263. Loirat C, Sonsino E, Hinglais N, et al. Treatment of the childhood haemolytic uraemic syndrome with plasma. A multicenter randomized controlled trial. *Pediatr Nephrol* 1988;2:279.

264. Erickson LC, Smith WS, Biwas A, et al. Streptococcus pneumoniae-induced hemolytic-uremic syndrome: a case for early diagnosis. *Pediatr Nephrol* 1994;8:211.

265. McGraw ME, Lendon M, Stevens RF, et al. Hemolytic uremic syndrome and the Thomas Friedenreich antigen. *Pediatr Nephrol* 1989;3:135.

266. Noris M, Ruggenenti P, Perna A, et al. Hypocomplementemia discloses genetic predisposition to hemolytic uremic syndrome and thrombotic thrombocytopenic purpura: role of factor H abnormalities. Italian Registry of Familial and Recurrent Hemolytic Uremic Syndrome/Thrombotic Thrombocytopenic Purpura. *J Am Soc Nephrol* 1999;10:281.

267. Roodhooft AM, McLean RH, Elst E, et al. Recurrent hemolytic uremic syndrome and acquired hypomorphic variant of the third component of complement. *Pediatr Nephrol* 1990;4:597.

268. Pichette V, Quérin S, Schürch W, et al. Familial hemolytic-uremic syndrome and homozygous factor H deficiency. *Am J Kidney Dis* 1994;26:936.

269. Thompson RA, Winterborn MH. Hypocomplementaemia due to a genetic deficiency of b1H globulin. *Clin Exp Immunol* 1981;46:110.

270. Rougier N, Kazatchkine MD, Rougier JP, et al. Human complement factor H deficiency associated with hemolytic uremic syndrome. *J Am Soc Nephrol* 1998;9:2318.

271. Warwicker P, Goodship TH, Donne RL, et al. Genetic studies into inherited and sporadic hemolytic uremic syndrome. *Kidney Int* 1998;53:836.

272. Zipfel PF, Jokiranta TS, Hellwage J, et al. The factor H-protein family. *Immunopharmacology* 1999;42:53.

273. Vik DP, Munor-Canoves P, Chaplin DD, et al. *Curr Top Microbiol* 1989;153:147.

274. Gerritsen HE, Turecek PL, Schwarz HP. Assay of von Willebrand factor (vWF)-cleaving protease based on decreased collagen binding affinity of degraded vWF. *Thromb Haemost* 1999;82:1386.

275. Obert B, Tout H, Veyradier A, et al. Estimation of the von Willebrand factor-cleaving protease in plasma using monoclonal antibodies to vWF. *Thromb Haemost* 1999;82:1382.

276. Tsai HM, Rice L, Sarode R, et al. Antibody inhibitors to von Willebrand factor metalloproteinase and increased binding of von Willebrand Factor to platelets in ticlopidine-associated thrombotic thrombocytopenic purpura. *Ann Intern Med* 2000;132:794.

277. Ridolfi RL, Bell WR. Thrombotic thrombocytopenic purpura. Report of 25 cases and review of the literature. *Medicine* 1981;60:413.

278. Nalbandian RM, Henry RL, Bick RL. Thrombotic thrombocytopenic purpura: an extended editorial. *Semin Thromb Hemost* 1979;5:216.

279. Peterson J, Amare M, Henry J, et al. Splenectomy and antiplatelet agents in thrombotic thrombocytopenic purpura. *Am J Med Sci* 1979;277:75.

280. Percival SP. Ocular findings in thrombotic thrombocytopenic purpura (Moschowitz's disease). *Br J Ophthalmol* 1970;54:73.

281. Taft EG. Thrombotic thrombocytopenic purpura and dose of plasma exchange. *Blood* 1979;54:842.

282. Keene ER, Willis R, Aster RH. Platelet kinetics (51Cr) in thrombocytopenic purpura. *Lahey Clin Found Bull* 1968;17:51.

283. Neame PB, Hirsh J, Browman G, et al. Thrombotic thrombocytopenic purpura: a syndrome of intravascular platelet consumption. *Canada Med Assoc J* 1976;114:1108.

284. Ansell J, Beaser RS, Pechet L. Thrombotic thrombocytopenic purpura fails to respond to fresh frozen plasma infusion. *Ann Intern Med* 1978;89:647.

285. Celada A, Perrin LH. Circulating immune complexes in thrombotic thrombocytopenic purpura (TTP). *Blood* 1978;52:855.

286. Bukowski RM, Hewlett JS, Harris JW. Exchange transfusions in the treatment of thrombotic thrombocytopenic purpura. *Semin Hematol* 1976;13:219.

287. Gendel BR, Young JM, Kraus AP. Thrombotic thrombocytopenic purpura. *Am J Med* 1952;13:3.

288. Ridolfi RL, Hutchins GM, Bell WR. The heart and cardiac conduction system in thrombotic thrombocytopenic purpura. A clinicopathologic study of 17 autopsied patients. *Ann Intern Med* 1979;91:357.

289. Bone RC, Henry JE, Petterson J, et al. Respiratory dysfunction in thrombotic thrombocytopenic purpura. *Am J Med* 1978;65:262.

290. Civin H, Gotshalk HC. "Platelet thromboses" involving the gastrointestinal tract: report of a case. *Hawaii Med J* 1953;13:119.

291. Whitington PF, Friedman AL, Chesney RW. Gastrointestinal disease in the hemolytic uremic syndrome. *Gastroenterology* 1979;76:728.

292. Harrison HN. Thrombotic thrombocytopenic purpura occurring in the puerperium associated with pancreatic islet-cell necrosis. *Arch Intern Med* 1958;102:124.
293. Rock GA, Shumak KH, Buskard NA, et al. Comparison of plasma exchange with plasma infusion in the treatment of thrombotic thrombocytopenic purpura. *N Engl J Med* 1991;325:393.
294. Bell WR, Braine HG, Ness PM, et al. Improved survival in thrombotic thrombocytopenic purpura-hemolytic uremic syndrome. Clinical experience in 108 patients. *N Engl J Med* 1991;325:398.
295. Cuttner J. Splenectomy, steroids, and dextran 70 in thrombotic thrombocytopenic purpura. *JAMA* 1974;227:397.
296. Phillips MD. Antiplatelet agents in thrombotic thrombocytopenic purpura. In: Kaplan BS, Trompeter RS, Moake JL, eds. *Hemolytic Uremic Syndrome and Thrombotic Thrombocytopenic Purpura* New York: Marcel Dekker, Inc.; 1992:531.
297. Wu KK. Role of prostacyclin in the pathogenesis and therapy of thrombotic thrombocytopenic purpura. In: Kaplan BS, Trompeter RS, Moake JL, eds. *Hemolytic Uremic Syndrome and Thrombotic Thrombocytopenic Purpura,* New York: Marcel Dekker, Inc.; 1992:483.
298. Budd GT, Bukowsky RM, Lucas FV, et al. Prostacyclin therapy of thrombotic thrombocytopenic purpura. *Lancet* 1980;2:915.
299. Cocchetto DM, Cook L, Cato AE, et al. Rationale and proposal for use of prostacyclin in thrombotic thrombocytopenic purpura therapy. *Semin Thromb Hemost* 1981;7:43.
300. Fitzgerald GA, Maas RL, Stein R, et al. Intravenous prostacyclin in thrombotic thrombocytopenic purpura. *Ann Intern Med* 1981;95:319.
301. Hensby CN, Lewis PJ, Hilgard P, et al. Prostacyclin deficiency in thrombotic thrombocytopenic purpura. *Lancet* 1979;2:748.
302. Johnson JE, Mills GM, Batson AG, et al. Ineffective epoprostenol therapy for thrombotic thrombocytopenic purpura. *JAMA* 1983;250:3089.
303. Bukowski RM, Hewlett JS, Reimer RR. Therapy of thrombotic thrombocytopenic purpura: an overview. *Semin Thromb Hemost* 1981;7:1.
304. Ruggenenti P, Remuzzi G, Rossi EC. Epidemiology of the hemolytic-uremic syndrome. *N Engl J Med* 1991;324:1065.
305. Ruggenenti P, Galbusera M, Plata Cornejo R, et al. Thrombotic thrombocytopenic puerpura: evidence that infusion rather than removal of plasma induces remission of the disease. *Am J Kidney Dis* 1993;21:314.
306. Byrnes JJ, Moake JL, Klug P, et al. Effectiveness of the cryosupernatant fraction of plasma in the treatment of refractory thrombotic thrombocytopenic purpura. *Am J Hematol* 1990;34:169.
307. Rutkow IM. Thrombotic thrombocytopenic purpura (TTP) and splenectomy. A current appraisal. *Ann Surg* 1978;188:701.
308. Gutterman LA, Stevenson TD. Treatment of thrombotic thrombocytopenic purpura with vincristine. *JAMA* 1982;247:1433.
309. Raniele DP, Opsahl JA, Kjellstrand CM. Should intravenous immunoglobulin be first-line treatment for acute thrombotic thrombocytopenic purpura? Case report and review of the literature. *Am J Kidney Dis* 1991;18:264.
310. Hayward CP, Sutton DM, Carter WH, et al. Treatment outcomes in patients with adult thrombotic thrombocytopenic purpura-hemolytic uremic syndrome. *Arch Intern Med* 1994;154:982.
311. Gutterman LA, Stevenson TD. Vincristine in the treatment of thrombotic thrombocytopenic purpura (abstract). *Blood* 1979;54:242A.
312. Perneger TV, Klag MJ, Whelton PK. Race and socioeconomic status in hypertension and renal disease. *Curr Opin Nephrol Hypertens* 1995;4:235.
313. Berns JS, Tomaszewski JE. Hemolytic uremic syndrome and thrombotic thrombocytopenic purpura associated with human immunodeficiency virus infection and acquired immunodeficiency syndrome. In: Kaplan BS, Trompeter RS, Moake JL, eds. *Hemolytic Uremic Syndrome and Thrombotic Thrombocytopenic Purpura.* New York: Marcel Dekker, Inc.; 1992:299.
314. Nosari A, Muti G, Busnach G et al. Intravenous gamma globulin in refractory thrombotic thrombocytopenic purpura. *Acta Haematol* 1996;96:255.
315. Messmore HL, Yeshwant C, Remlinger K, et al. Intravenous gamma globulin in refractory thrombotic thrombocytopenic purpura (TTP) (abstract). *Thromb Haemost* 1985;54:127.
316. Finn NG, Wang JC, Hong KJ. High-dose intravenous gamma-immunoglobulin infusion in the treatment of thrombotic thrombocytopenic purpura. *Arch Intern Med* 1987;147:2165.
317. Chin D, Chyczij H, Etches W, et al. Treatment of thrombotic thrombocytopenic purpura with intravenous gamma globulin. *Transfusion* 1987;27:115.
318. Belobradkova J. The hemolytic uremic syndrome in sibs. Sb Ved Pr Lek Fak Karlovy Univerzity Hradci Kralove 1977;20(Suppl):445.
319. Kaplan BS, Chesney RW, Drummond KN. Hemolytic uremic syndrome in families. *N Engl J Med* 1975;292:1090.
320. Karlsberg RP, Lacher JW, Bartecchi CE. Adult Hemolytic-uremic syndrome familial variant. *Arch Intern Med* 1977;137:1155.
321. Hogewind BL, de la Riviere GB, Van Es LA, et al. Familial occurrence of the haemolytic uraemic syndrome. *Acta Med Scand* 1980;207:73.
322. Hagge WW, Holley KE, Burke EC, et al. . Hemolytic uremic syndrome in two siblings. *N Engl J Med* 1967;277:138.
323. Tune BM, Groshong T, Plumer L, et al. The hemolytic uremic syndrome in siblings: a prospective survey. *J Pediatr* 1974;85:682.
324. Feest TG, Hamilton W, Imong S. Severe ocular and pulmonary manifestations of familial haemolytic uraemic syndrome: possible benefit of bi-lateral nephrectomy. Proceedings of the XXIIIrd Congress of EDTA-ERA-Budapest, June 29-July 3, 1986;26.
325. Wyatt RJ, Jones D, Stapleton FB, et al. Recurrent hemolytic-uremic syndrome with the hypomorphic fast allele of the third component of complement. *J Pediatr* 1985;107:564.
326. Landau D, Shalev H, Levy-Finer G, et al. Familial hemolytic uremic syndrome associated with complement factor H deficiency. *J Pediatr* 2001;138:412.
327. Nathanson S, Fremeaux-Bacchi V, Deschenes G. Successful plasma therapy in hemolytic uremic syndrome with factor H deficiency. *Pediatr Nephrol* 2001;16:554.
328. Stratton JD, Warwicker P. Successful treatment of factor H-related hemolytic uraemic syndrome. *Nephrol Dial Transplant* 2002;17:684.
329. Remuzzi G, Ruggenenti P, Codazzi D, et al. Combined kidney and liver transplantation for familial haemolytic uraemic syndrome. *Lancet* 2002;359:1671.
330. Remuzzi G, Ruggenenti P, Gridelli B, et al. Hemolytic uremic syndrome: a fatal outcome after kidney and liver transplantation performed to correct factor H gene mutation. *Am J Transplant* 2005;5(5):1146.
331. Dragon-Durey MA, Loirat C, Cloarec S, et al. Anti-factor H autoantibodies associated with atypical hemolytic uremic syndrome. *J Am Soc Nephrol* 2004;16:555.
332. Brioschi S, Porrati F, Bresin E, et al. Mutations in membrane cofactor protein in atypical hemolytic uremic syndrome (abstract). Presented at the 7th Congress of the Italian Society of Human Genomics, October 13–15, 2004.
333. Noris M, Brioschi S, Caprioli J, et al. Mutation in membrane cofactor protein of the complement system in familial haemolytic uraemic syndrome. Identification of a second-disease-associated gene; Mechanisms of disease. *Lancet* 2003;362:1542.
334. Richards A, Kemp EJ, Liszewski MK, et al. Mutations in human complement regulator, membrane cofactor protein (CD46), predispose to development of familial hemolytic uremic syndrome. *Proc Natl Acad Sci U S A* 2003;100:12966.
335. Weiner CP. Thrombotic microangiopathy in pregnancy and the postpartum period. *Semin Hematol* 1987;24:119.
336. Ruggenenti P, Remuzzi G. The pathophysiology and management of thrombotic thrombocytopenic purpura. *Eur J Haematol* 1996;56:191.
337. Grunfeld JP, Ganeval D, Bournerias F. Acute renal failure in pregnancy. *Kidney Int* 1980;18:179.
338. Segonds A, Louradour N, Suc JM, et al. Post-partum Hemolytic uremic syndrome: a study of three cases with a review of the literature. *Clin Nephrol* 1979;12:229.
339. Clarkson AR, Meadows R, Lawrence JR. Post partum renal failure. The generalized Shwartzman reaction. *Aust Ann Med* 1969;18:209.
340. Morel-Maroger L, Kanfer A, Solez K, et al. Prognostic importance of vascular lesions in acute renal failure with microangiopathic hemolytic anemia (hemolytic uremic syndrome): clinicopathologic study in 20 adults. *Kidney Int* 1979;15:548.
341. Ponticelli C, Imbasciati E, Rivolta E. Long-term follow-up of postpartum hemolytic uremic syndrome treated with heparin and antiplatelet agents. In: Remuzzi G, Mecca G, de Gaetano G, eds. *Hemostasis, Prostaglandins and Renal Disease.* New York: Raven Press; 1980:433.
342. Ruggenenti P. Post-transplant hemolytic-uremic syndrome. *Kidney Int* 2002;62:1093.
343. Obrador GT, Zeigler ZR, Shadduck RK, et al. Effectiveness of cryosupernatant therapy in refractory and chronic relapsing thrombotic thrombocytopenic purpura. *Am J Hematol* 1993;42:217.
344. Moody H, Matz L, Hurst P. Vascular lesions as manifestations of cyclosporin nephrotoxicity. *Lancet* 1986;1:1221.
345. Bonser RS, Adu D, Franklin L, et al. Cyclosporin-induced haemolytic uraemic syndrome in liver allograft recipient. *Lancet* 1984;2:1337.
346. Ruggenenti P. Post-Transplant Hemolytic Uremic Syndrome. *Kidney Intern* 2002,62:1093.
347. Hochstetler LA, Flanigan MJ, Lager DJ. Transplant-associated thrombotic microangiopathy: the role of IgG administration as initial therapy. *Am J Kidney Dis* 1994;23:444.
348. Miller R, Burke B, Schmidt NJ, et al. Recurrence (R) of hemolytic uremic syndrome (HUS) in renal transplants: a single centre report. *Nephrol Dial Transplant* 1997;12:1425.
349. Pirson Y, Leckercq B, Squifflet JP, et al. Good prognosis of the hemolytic uremic syndrome after renal transplantation (abstract). Proceedings of the XXIIIrd Congress of EDTA-ERA, Budapest, June 29-July 3, 1986: 197.
350. Gagnadoux MF, Broyer M, Habib R. Renal transplantation in hemolytic-uremic syndrome. Report of 31 cases (abstract). Proceedings of the VIII Congress of the International Pediatric Nephrology Association. Toronto; 1989:August 27–September 1.
351. Hebert D, Sibley RK, Mauer SM. Recurrence of hemolytic uremic syndrome in renal transplant recipients. *Kidney Int* 1986;30:S51.
352. Grino JM, Caralps A, Carreras L, et al. Apparent recurrence of hemolytic uremic syndrome in azathioprine treated allograft recipients. *Nephron* 1998;49:301.
353. Mochon M, Kaiser B, Dunn S, et al. Cerebral infarct with recurrence of hemolytic uremic syndrome in a child following renal allograft (abstract). *J Am Soc Nephrol* 1990;1:765.

354. Remuzzi G, Ruggenenti P, Codazzi D, et al. Related articles, links combined kidney and liver transplantation for familial haemolytic uraemic syndrome. *Lancet* 2002;359(9318):1671.
355. Remuzzi G, Ruggenenti P, Colledan M, et al. Hemolytic uremic syndrome: a fatal outcome after kidney and liver transplantation performed to correct factor H gene mutation. *Am J Transplant* 2005;5(5):1146.
356. Lohrmann HP, Adam W, Heymer B, et al. Microangiopathic hemolytic anemia in metastatic carcinoma: report of eight cases. *Ann Intern Med* 1973;79:368.
357. Murgo AJ. Cancer- and chemotherapy-associated thrombotic microangiopathy. In: Kaplan BS, Trompeter RS, Moake JL, eds. *Hemolytic Uremic Syndrome and Thrombotic Thrombocytopenic Purpura*. New York: Marcel Dekker Inc.; 1992:271.
358. Bruntsch U, Groos G, Tigges FJ, et al. Microangiopathic hemolytic anemia, a frequent complication of mitomycin therapy in cancer patients. *Eur J Cancer Clin Oncol* 1984;20:905.
359. Korec S, Schein PS, Smith FP. Treatment of cancer-associated hemolytic-uremic syndrome with staphylococcal protein A immunoperfusion. *J Clin Oncol* 1986;4:210.
360. Schieppati A, Ruggenenti P, Plata Cornejo R, et al. For the Italian Registry of Haemolytic Uremic Syndrome: renal function at hospital admission as a prognostic factor in adult hemolytic uremic syndrome. *J Am Soc Nephrol* 1992;2:1640.
361. Farina C, Gavazzeni G, Caprioli A, et al. Hemolytic uremic syndrome associated with verocytotoxin-producing Escherichia coli infection in acquired immunodeficiency syndrome. *Blood* 1990;75:2465.
362. Tumlin JA, Sands JM, Someren A. A hemolytic-uremic syndrome following "crack" cocaine inhalation. *Am J Med Sci* 1990;299:366.
363. Thompson CE, Damon LE, Ries CA, et al. Thrombotic microangiopathies in the 1980s: clinical features, response to treatment, and the impact of the human immunodeficiency virus epidemic. *Blood* 1992;80:1890.
364. Salem G, Terebelo H, Raman S. Human immunodeficiency virus associated with thrombotic thrombocytopenic purpura: successful treatment with zidovudine. *South Med J* 1991;84:493.
365. Segal GH, Tubbs RR, Ratliff NB, et al. Thrombotic thrombocytopenic purpura in a patient with AIDS. *Cleve Clin J Med* 1990;57:360.
366. Charasse C, Michelet C, LeTulzo Y, et al. Thrombotic thrombocytopenic purpura with the acquired immunodeficiency syndrome: a pathologically documented case report. *Am J Kidney Dis* 1991;17:80.
367. Caletti MG, Lejarraga H, Kelmansky D, et al. Two different therapeutic regimes in patients with sequelae of hemolytic-uremic syndrome. *Pediatr Nephrol* 2004;19:1148.
368. Van Dyck M, Proesmans W. Renoprotection by ACE inhibitors after severe hemolytic uremic syndrome. *Pediatr Nephrol* 2004;19:688.
369. Loirat C, Niaudet P. The risk of recurrence of hemolytic uremic syndrome after renal transplantation in children. *Pediatr Nephrol* 2003;18:1095.
370. Artz MA, Steenbergen EJ, Hoitsma AJ, et al. Renal transplantation in patients with hemolytic uremic syndrome: high rate of recurrence and increased incidence of acute rejections. *Transplantation* 2003;76:821.
371. Ferraris JR, Ramirez JA, Ruiz S, et al. Shiga toxin-associated hemolytic uremic syndrome: absence of recurrence after renal transplantation. *Pediatr Nephrol* 2002;17:809.
372. Kleinknecht D, Grunfeld JP, Gomez PC, et al. Diagnostic procedures and long-term prognosis in bilateral renal cortical necrosis. *Kidney Int* 1973;4:390.
373. Sheehan HL, Moore HC. Renal Cortical Necrosis and the Kidney of Concealed Hemorrhage. Springfield: Charles C. Thomas; 1953.
374. Ferris TF. The kidney and pregnancy. In: Earley LE, Gottschalk CW, eds. *Strauss and Welt's Diseases of the Kidney*. Boston: Little, Brown; 1979; 1321.
375. Ober WE, Reid DE, Romney SL, et al. Renal lesions and acute renal failure in pregnancy. *Am J Med* 1956;21:781.
376. McKay DG. Disseminated Intravascular Coagulation: an Intermediary Mechanism of Disease. New York: Harper and Row; 1965:431.
377. Mookerjee BK, Bilefsky R, Kendall AG. Generalized Shwartzman reaction due to gram-negative septicemia after abortion: recovery after bilateral cortical necrosis. *Can Med Assoc J* 1968;98:578.
378. Solez K. Acute renal failure ("Acute tubular necrosis" infarction and cortical necrosis). In: Heptinstall RH, ed. *Pathology of the Kidney*. 3rd ed. Boston: Little Brown; 1983;1069.
379. Yoshikawa T, Tanaka KR, Guze LB. Infection and disseminated intravascular coagulation. *Medicine* 1971;50:237.
380. Donohoe JF. Acute bilateral cortical necrosis. In: Brenner BM, Lazarus JM, eds. *Acute Renal Failure*. Philadelphia: Saunders; 1983:252.
381. Brown CE, Crane GL. Bilateral cortical necrosis following severe burns. *JAMA* 1943;122:871.
382. Da Silva OA, Lopez M, Godoy P. Bilateral cortical necrosis and calcification of the kidney following snakebite: a case report. *Clin Nephrol* 1979;11:136.
383. Geiling EM, Cannon PR. Pathologic effects of elixir of sulfanilamide (diethylene glycol) poisoning. A clinical and experimental correlation. Final report. *JAMA* 1938;111:919.
384. Godwin B, McCall AJ. Cortical necrosis complicating perforated gastric ulcer. *Lancet* 1941;2:512.
385. Lauler DP, Schreiner GE. Bilateral renal cortical necrosis. *Am J Med* 1958;24:519.
386. Matlin RA, Gary NE. Acute cortical necrosis. Case report and review of the literature. *Am J Med* 1974;56:110.
387. Moss SW, Gary NE, Eisinger RP. Renal cortical necrosis following streptococcal infection. *Arch Intern Med* 1977;137:1196.
388. Oram S, Ross G, Pell L, et al. Renal cortical calcification after snake bite. *Br Med J* 1963;1:1647.
389. Rosello SG, Piulats EL, Gomez I, et al. Renal cortical necrosis and right nephrectomy with survival, in a man. *Am J Med* 1969;45:309.
390. Sporn IN. Renal cortical necrosis. *Arch Intern Med* 1978;138:1866.
391. Walls J, Schorr WJ, Kerr DN. Prolonged oliguria with survival in acute bilateral cortical necrosis. *Br Med J* 1968;4:220.
392. Woods JW, Williams TF. Hypertension due to renal vascular diseases, renal infarction and renal cortical necrosis. In: Strauss MB, Welt LG, eds. *Diseases of the Kidney*. 2nd ed. Boston: Little Brown; 1971:769.
393. Campbell AC, Henderson JL. Symmetrical cortical necrosis of the kidneys in infancy and childhood. *Arch Dis Child* 1941;24:269.
394. Groshong TD, Taylor AA, Nolph KD, et al. Renal function following cortical necrosis in childhood. *J Pediatr* 1971;79:267.
395. Perry JW. Phosphorus poisoning with cortical necrosis of the kidney: a report of two fatal cases. *Aust Ann Med* 1953;2:94.
396. Wahle GH, Muirhead EE. Bilateral renal cortical necrosis in a child associated with an incompatible blood transfusion. *Texas J Med* 1953;49:770.
397. Zuelzer WW, Charles S, Kurnetz R, et al. Circulatory diseases of the kidneys in infancy and childhood. *Am J Dis Child* 1951;81:1.
398. Thomas L, Good RA. Studies on the generalized Shwartzman reaction. I. General observations concerning the phenomenon. *J Exp Med* 1952;96:605.
399. Brunson JG, Thomas L, Gamble CN. Morphological changes in rabbits following the intravenous administration of meningococcal toxin. II. Two appropriately spaced injections; the role of fibrinoid in the generalized Shwartzman reaction. *Am J Pathol* 1955;31:655.
400. Galton M, Wong TC, McKay DG. Vasomotor changes in the pregnant rabbit induced by bacterial endotoxin. *Fed Proc* 1960;19:246.
401. Fontaine A, Arondel J, Sansonetti PJ. Role of Shiga toxin in the pathogenesis of bacillary dysentery, studied by using a tox mutant of Shigella dysenteriae 1. *Infect Immun* 1988;56:3099.
402. Whitaker AN. Acute renal failure in disseminated intravascular coagulation: experimental studies of the induction and prevention of renal fibrin deposition. *Progr Biochem Pharmacol* 1974;9:45.
403. Thomas L, Brunson J, Smith RT. Studies on the generalized Shwartzman reaction. VI Production of the reaction by synergistic action of endotoxin with three synthetic acid polymers (sodium polyanethol sulfonate, dextran sulfate, and sodium polyvinyl alcohol sulfonate). *J Exp Med* 1952;96:249.
404. Raij L, Keane WF, Michael AF. Unilateral Shwartzman reaction: cortical necrosis in one kidney following in vivo perfusion with endotoxin. *Kidney Int* 1977;12:91.
405. Arhelger RB, Brunson JG, Good RA. Influence of gram-negative endotoxin on pathogenesis of nephrotoxic serum nephritis in rats. *Lab Invest* 1961;10:669.
406. Hoyer JR, Bergstein JM, Michael AF, et al. Immunofluorescent localization of factor VIII-related antigen and fibrinogen in hyperacute xenograft rejection and in the Shwartzman reaction in the rat. *Clin Immunol Immunopathol* 1978;9:454.
407. Campos A, Kim Y, Azar SH, et al. Prevention of the generalized Shwartzman reaction in pregnant rats by prostacyclin infusion. *Lab Invest* 1983;48:705.
408. McGiff JC, Itskovitz HD, Terragno A, et al. Modulation and mediation of the action of the renal kallikrein-kinin system by prostaglandins. *Fed Proc* 1976;35:175.
409. Latour JG, Leger-Gauthier C. Prostaglandins in the pathogenesis of the generalized Shwartzman reaction. *Am J Obstet Gynecol* 1979;135:577.
410. Rohrer H. Kidney necrosis in acute hog cholera. *Virchows Arch A Pathol Anat Histol.* 1983;284:203.
411. Sheehan HL, Davis JC. Renal ischaemia with failed reflow. *J Pathol Bacteriol* 1959;78:105.
412. Byrom FB. Morbid effects of vasopressin in the organs and vessels of rats. *J Pathol Bacteriol* 1937;45:1.
413. Byrom FB, Pratt OE. Oxytocin and renal cortical necrosis. *Lancet* 1959;1:753.
414. Penner A, Bernheim AI. Acute ischaemic necrosis of the kidney: a clinico-pathologic and experimental study. *Arch Pathol* 1940;30:465.
415. Shwartzman G. Phenomenon of Local Tissue Reactivity, and its Immunological, Pathological and Clinical Significance. New York: Paul B Hoebner; 1937.
416. Corrigan JJ Jr. Effect of anticoagulating and non-anticoagulating concentrations of heparin on the generalized Shwartzman reaction. *Thromb Diath Haemorrh* 1970;24:136.
417. Schreiner GE. La Necrose Corticale Bilaterale des Reins. In: Hamburger J, Crosnier J, eds. *Nephrologie*, Paris: Editions Medicale Flammarion; 1979;422.
418. Marcussen H, Asnaes S. Renal cortical necrosis: an evaluation of the possible relation to the Shwartzman reaction. *Acta Pathol Microbiol Scand* 1972;80:351.
419. Robboy SJ, Major MC, Colman RW, et al. Pathology of disseminated intravascular coagulation (DIC): analysis of 26 cases. *Hum Pathol* 1972;3:327.

420. Gelfand MD, Friedman EA, Knepshield JH, et al. Detection of antiplatelet antibody activity in patients with renal cortical necrosis. *Kidney Int* 1974; 6:426.
421. Levinsky NG, Alexander EA. Acute renal failure. In: Brenner BM, Rector FC, eds. *The Kidney*. Philadelphia: Saunders; 1981;1181.
422. Moell H. Gross bilateral renal cortical necrosis during long period of oliguria-anuria. Roentgenologic observations in two cases. *Acta Radiol* 1957;48:355.
423. Whelan JG, Ling JT, Davis LA. Antemortem roentgen manifestation of bilateral renal cortical necrosis. *Radiology* 1967;89:682.
424. Duff GL, Murray EG. Bilateral cortical necrosis of the kidneys. *Am J Med Sci* 1941;201:428.
425. MacGillivray I. Combined renal and anterior pituitary necrosis. *J Obstet Gynaecol Br Commonw* 1950;57:924.
426. Sheldon WH, Hertig AT. Bilateral cortical necrosis of the kidney: a report of 2 cases. *Arch Pathol* 1942;34:866.
427. Hatcher CR Jr, Gagnon JA, Clarke RW. The effects of hydration in epinephrine-induced renal shutdown in dogs. *Surg Forum* 1958;9:106.
428. Palmerio C, Ming SC, Frank E. The role of sympathetic nervous system in the generalized Shwartzman reaction. *J Exp Med* 1962;115:609.
429. Sheehan HL, Davis JC. The protective effect of anesthesia in experimental renal ischaemia. *J Pathol Bacteriol* 1960;79:337.
430. Stetson CA, Good RA. Studies on the mechanism of the Shwartzman phenomenon. *J Exp Med* 1951;93:49.

CHAPTER 68 ■ VASCULITIC DISEASES OF THE KIDNEY

PATRICK H. NACHMAN, J. CHARLES JENNETTE, AND RONALD J. FALK

The last decade has witnessed an explosion of knowledge in the field of vasculitis. The advent of antineutrophil cytoplasmic antibodies (ANCA) has led to new approaches in the clinical diagnosis of the vasculitides. There has been a reclassification of vasculitis, and modern tools of molecular immunology are shedding light on the pathogenesis of these disorders. Treatment strategies are slowly changing, no longer aimed only at improving patient and renal survival, but also at decreasing the short- and long-term toxicity of current therapies. This chapter focuses on the many facts of small-, medium-, and large-vessel vasculitis.

DIAGNOSTIC CLASSIFICATION AND PATHOLOGY OF VASCULITIDES

Vasculitis can affect any vessels in the body and thus can cause various clinical signs and symptoms. Most of these manifestations are indicative of vessel involvement in a particular organ rather than a specific pathologic category of disease. Therefore, vasculitis cannot be accurately diagnosed on the basis of clinical features alone. Serologic and other laboratory data can be very helpful in narrowing the differential diagnosis or providing additional support to a presumptive diagnosis, but data are rarely definitive. As with all tissues, vessels have a limited number of nonspecific patterns of response to injury. For example, many different inflammatory stimuli cause histologically indistinguishable acute and chronic inflammation with and without necrotizing or granulomatous features. To further complicate pathologic evaluation, vasculitic lesions evolve through various stages of active (Fig. 68-1) and sclerosing injury (Fig. 68-2). Specific categories of vasculitis have a particular predilection for involvement of certain types of vessels, although there is so much overlap that type of vessel involvement alone does not provide adequate categorization (Table 68-1, Fig. 68-3). Therefore, vasculitis cannot be diagnosed accurately on the basis of pathologic features alone, especially if these are evaluated only by routine light microscopy. The best current approach to a specific diagnosis is to combine clinical, laboratory, and histologic data to identify distinctive clinicopathologic categories of vasculitis. Vasculitis categorization schemes will certainly be improved in the future; however, current systems provide valuable guidance for prognostication and for determining the most effective management strategy.

There are a number of approaches to the diagnostic categorization of vasculitis. The system that we use in this chapter is the so-called Chapel Hill Nomenclature System, which was agreed on by an international group of clinicians and pathologists with a special interest in vasculitis (Table 68-2) (1).

Knowledge of the historical evolution of vasculitis categorization is helpful to understand the current diagnostic criteria for the classification of vasculitides. The following discussion of diagnostic classification includes a brief review of the his-

torical events in the recognition of each category. The discussion is divided into sections dealing with large-vessel vasculitis, medium-sized vessel vasculitis, and small-vessel vasculitis (Tables 68-1, 68-2, Fig. 68-3). Large-vessel vasculitides were first recognized because of the reduced pulses and ischemic manifestations caused by chronic narrowing of major arteries. Medium-sized vessel vasculitides were first recognized because of the pseudoaneurysms caused by necrotizing lesions of medium-sized arteries, and small-vessel vasculitides were first recognized because of the glomerulonephritis and purpura caused by involvement of glomerular capillaries and dermal venules, respectively. Most of the discussion focuses on small-vessel vasculitides because these cause a higher frequency of renal disease.

Large-Vessel Vasculitis: Takayasu's Arteritis and Giant Cell Arteritis

Large-vessel vasculitis affects the aorta and its major branches, such as the arteries to the extremities and to the head and neck (1,2). During the acute phase of disease, large-vessel vasculitis is characterized pathologically by chronic granulomatous inflammation that often contains giant cells in the inflammatory infiltrates during the active phase of disease. The chronic phase is characterized by extensive vascular sclerosis with little or no active inflammation. Inflammatory and sclerotic thickening of the aorta and the arteries causes narrowing of lumina, which in turn causes ischemia and the resultant clinical manifestations. Involvement of the renal artery may cause renovascular hypertension. The two major categories of large-vessel vasculitis are Takayasu's arteritis and giant cell arteritis.

In 1856, William Savory described patients with diminished peripheral pulses who probably had Takayasu's arteritis involving the major arteries to the extremities (3). However, this category of vasculitis is named for Mikito Takayasu, a Japanese ophthalmologist who reported the ocular ischemic effects of this chronic granulomatous arteritis in 1908 (4). Takayasu's arteritis, which also includes "aortic arch syndrome" and "pulseless disease," most often involves the aorta and its major branches, although the pulmonary arteries may be affected (2,5–7). Takayasu's arteritis is most common in Asia, although it occurs worldwide. It rarely occurs in patients older than 40 years and is usually diagnosed during the second decade of life. Clinically, it often presents with reduced pulses, vascular bruits, claudication, and renovascular hypertension.

Giant cell arteritis rarely occurs in patients younger than 50 years and is most common in patients of northern European ethnicity (8,9). Like Takayasu's arteritis, giant cell arteritis affects the aorta and its major branches; however, it has a much greater predilection for the extracranial branches of the carotid artery. Frequent clinical manifestations include headache, jaw claudication, blindness, deafness, tongue dysfunction, extremity claudication, and reduced peripheral pulses. Pathologic

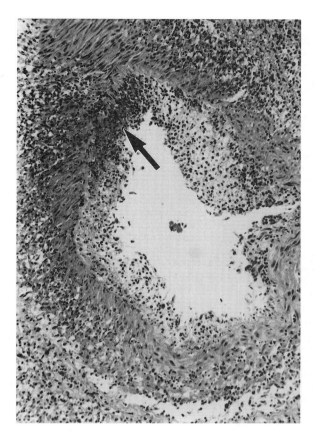

FIGURE 68-1. Acute necrotizing arteritis affecting a renal interlobar artery in a patient with Kawasaki's disease. There is (*arrow*) transmural inflammation and necrosis. (Hematoxylin and eosin stain, magnification ×125.)

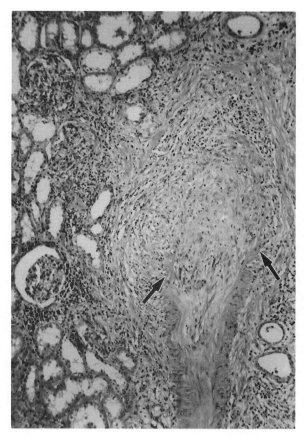

FIGURE 68-2. Chronic scarring in an arcuate artery from a patient with polyarteritis nodosa. The muscularis is completely destroyed (*arrows*), indicating that the sclerosis is secondary to a necrotizing arteritis rather than severe arteriosclerosis. (Hematoxylin and eosin stain, magnification ×75.)

involvement of the renal artery is common in giant cell arteritis, but symptomatic renovascular hypertension is rare. This is in contradistinction to Takayasu's arteritis, which often causes renovascular hypertension.

Giant cell arteritis has also been called "temporal arteritis," partly because one of the earliest descriptions of this type of vasculitis in 1890 by Hutchinson emphasized temporal artery involvement (10). However, the term "giant cell arteritis" is more appropriate than "temporal arteritis" because a) not all patients with giant cell arteritis have temporal artery involvement and b) vasculitides other than giant cell arteritis can cause temporal artery inflammation, such as polyarteritis nodosa, Wegener's granulomatosis, and microscopic polyangiitis (MPA) (1). If a patient with clinical manifestations of temporal artery inflammation is found by temporal artery biopsy to have a necrotizing rather than a granulomatous arteritis, the differential diagnosis should include polyarteritis nodosa, MPA, Wegener's granulomatosis, and other forms of necrotizing vasculitis. The frequent association of polymyalgia rheumatica with giant cell arteritis is a useful diagnostic aid, although not all patients with giant cell arteritis have polymyalgia rheumatica and not all patients with polymyalgia rheumatica have giant cell arteritis.

Takayasu's arteritis and giant cell arteritis cannot be accurately distinguished on the basis of pathologic evaluation of involved arteries. Polymyalgia rheumatica and involvement of branches of the carotid artery are more in favor of giant cell arteritis, and preferential involvement of the aorta and arteries to the extremities is slightly in favor of Takayasu's arteritis. However, the best diagnostic discriminator is age. If a patient

with clinical or pathologic features of chronic granulomatous arteritis is older than 50 years, a diagnosis of giant cell arteritis is warranted, whereas a diagnosis of Takayasu's arteritis is warranted if the patient is younger than 50 years (1). The presence of renovascular hypertension in a child or a young adult is suggestive of Takayasu's arteritis. In a patient older than 50 years, renal artery involvement by a chronic sclerosing process is more likely secondary to atherosclerosis than to giant cell arteritis, and Takayasu's arteritis is essentially ruled out by the age of the patient.

Medium-Sized Vessel Vasculitis: Polyarteritis Nodosa and Kawasaki's Disease

The medium-sized vessel vasculitides are necrotizing arteritides that have a predilection for arteries that lead to major viscera and their initial branches. In the kidneys, the major targets are the interlobar and arcuate arteries, with less frequent involvement of the main renal artery and interlobular arteries (Fig. 68-3). The two major categories of medium-sized vessel vasculitis are polyarteritis nodosa and Kawasaki's disease. Pathologically, both are characterized in the acute phase by necrotizing arteritis with transmural inflammation that initially includes neutrophils and foci of fibrinoid necrosis (Fig. 68-1). The acute necrotizing inflammation often erodes completely through the artery wall and into the adjacent perivascular tissue, thereby forming a pseudoaneurysm (Fig. 68-4). Secondary

TABLE 68-1

MAJOR DIAGNOSTIC CATEGORIES OF VASCULITIS

Large-vessel vasculitis (chronic granulomatous arteritis)
Giant cell arteritis
Takayasu's arteritis
Medium-sized vessel vasculitis (necrotizing arteritis)
Polyarteritis nodosa
Kawasaki disease
Small-vessel vasculitis (necrotizing polyangiitis)
Pauciimmune small-vessel vasculitis (usually antineutrophil
    cytoplasmic antibody (ANCA) positive)
Microscopic polyangiitis
Wegener's granulomatosis
Churg-Strauss syndrome
Drug-induced ANCA vasculitis
Immune complex small-vessel vasculitis
Henoch-Schönlein purpura
Cryoglobulinemic vasculitis
Lupus vasculitis
Rheumatoid vasculitis
Goodpasture's syndrome
Serum sickness vasculitis
Hypocomplementemic urticarial vasculitis
Drug-induced immune complex vasculitis
Infection-induced immune complex vasculitis
Behçet's disease
Paraneoplastic small-vessel vasculitis
Lymphoproliferative neoplasm-induced vasculitis
Carcinoma-induced vasculitis
Myeloproliferative neoplasm-induced vasculitis
Inflammatory bowel disease vasculitis

complications of the arteritis include thrombosis, infarction, and hemorrhage. In only a few days, the lesions evolve from an acute neutrophil-rich inflammation to a "chronic" inflammation with predominantly mononuclear leukocytes. Sites of thrombosis and necrosis develop progressive scarring (Fig. 68-2). By definition, medium-sized vessel vasculitides do not cause glomerulonephritis, although they can cause hematuria, proteinuria (usually less than 2 g per 24 hours), and renal insufficiency as a result of renal infarction. Pseudoaneurysms near the renal surface may rupture and cause severe, even fatal, retroperitoneal and intraperitoneal hemorrhage.

The meaning of the diagnostic term "polyarteritis nodosa" has evolved over the past century, and substantial confusion continues over how best to use it (11). The problem and the solution that we propose is best understood in historical context. Systemic necrotizing arteritis was first clearly described by Kussmaul and Maier in the mid-1800s (12). They reported a patient with widespread visceral nodules caused by acute inflammation of arteries and called the process "periarteritis nodosa." Ferrari introduced the term "polyarteritis nodosa" (13), which is more appropriate because the inflammation is transmural rather than perivascular. For approximately 50 years, essentially all patients with any pattern of necrotizing arteritis were included in the polyarteritis nodosa category. During the early to mid-1900's, astute investigators recognized that many patients with necrotizing arteritis had distinctive distributions of vascular inflammation or characteristic pathologic processes that warranted their separation from patients with arteritis alone. For example, Kawasaki's disease, Wegener's granulomatosis, Churg-Strauss syndrome, and MPA were initially included in the category of polyarteritis nodosa but now are recognized as distinct entities (1). The removal of these vasculitides from the polyarteritis nodosa category is justified not only on the basis of different patterns and distributions of ves-

sel involvement, but also because they have different natural histories, prognoses, and treatment requirements.

The reduction of polyarteritis nodosa to a more homogeneous and clinically useful category of vasculitis began when Arnaout, among others, recognized that some patients with necrotizing arteritis had lesions that could be seen only by microscopic examination (14). In about 1950, Zeek et al. (15,16) and Godman and Churg (17) carried out careful evaluations of patients with arteritis and concluded that polyarteritis nodosa should be separated from the "microscopic" form of vasculitis that was characterized by involvement of not only small arteries but also venules and capillaries. As discussed later in the section on small-vessel vasculitis, Godman and Churg also concluded that polyarteritis nodosa was distinct not only from MPA but also from Wegener's granulomatosis and Churg-Strauss syndrome, and that MPA, Wegener's granulomatosis, and Churg-Strauss syndrome were related to one another.

The diagnostic approach that we advocate defines polyarteritis nodosa as necrotizing inflammation of medium-sized or small arteries without glomerulonephritis or vasculitis in arterioles, capillaries, or venules (Table 68-2.) (1). This allows the separation of polyarteritis nodosa from other types of vasculitis, such as Wegener's granulomatosis, MPA, and Churg-Strauss syndrome, which have necrotizing arteritis as a component of a systemic polyangiitis that affects capillaries, venules, and arteries. By using this approach, the presence of glomerulonephritis rules out a diagnosis of polyarteritis nodosa and indicates the presence of some type of small-vessel vasculitis. In Table 68-3 are compared some of the features of polyarteritis nodosa and MPA. Note that glomerular capillaritis (glomerulonephritis) or pulmonary alveolar capillaritis with pulmonary hemorrhage rule out a diagnosis of polyarteritis nodosa and raise the possibility of MPA. Peripheral neuropathy is not a discriminator, because involvement of small epineural arteries in peripheral nerves may occur with polyarteritis nodosa or MPA. As we discuss in more detail later, testing for ANCA is useful for distinguishing between polyarteritis nodosa and the ANCA-associated small-vessel vasculitides (11,18–21). In a patient with necrotizing arteritis, a positive ANCA result decreases the likelihood of polyarteritis nodosa and increases the likelihood of MPA, Wegener's granulomatosis, or Churg-Strauss syndrome, i.e.; increases the likelihood that the patient has or will develop necrotizing inflammation of vessels other than arteries, such as pulmonary alveolar capillaritis or glomerular capillaritis (glomerulonephritis).

Necrotizing arteritis that is pathologically indistinguishable from the necrotizing arteritis of polyarteritis nodosa can occur in patients with Kawasaki's disease (Figs. 68-1, 68-3). Kawasaki's disease is an acute febrile illness of childhood that is characterized by the mucocutaneous lymph node syndrome, which includes nonsuppurative lymphadenopathy, polymorphous erythematous rash, erythema of the oropharyngeal mucosa, erythema of the palms and soles, conjunctivitis, and indurative edema and desquamation of the extremities (22–25). A major cause for morbidity and mortality in patients with Kawasaki's disease is the development of a necrotizing arteritis (24–27). This arteritis has a predilection for coronary arteries but can occur anywhere, including the kidney (Figs. 68-1, 68-3). Symptomatic renal involvement is rare in Kawasaki's disease.

The treatment of Kawasaki's disease is different from the treatment of polyarteritis nodosa. Kawasaki's disease usually is treated with aspirin and intravenous γ-globulin therapy (28–31), whereas polyarteritis nodosa usually is treated with high-dose corticosteroids and cyclophosphamide. Therefore, differentiation between the arteritis of Kawasaki's disease and that of polyarteritis nodosa is very important. The presence or absence of the mucocutaneous lymph node syndrome is an effective diagnostic discriminator between Kawasaki's disease and polyarteritis nodosa.

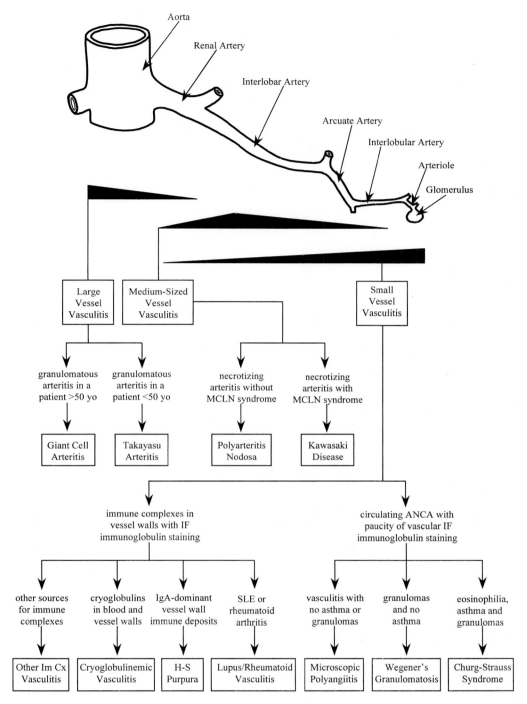

FIGURE 68-3. Predominant vascular involvement by large-vessel vasculitides, medium-sized vessel vasculitides, and small-vessel vasculitides as indicated by the positions and heights of the solid triangles. The algorithm suggests clinical and pathologic features that discriminate among different diagnostic categories of vasculitis. *yo*, years old; *MCLN*, mucocutaneous lymph node syndrome; *IF*, immunofluorescence microscopy; *ANCA*, antineutrophil cytoplasmic autoantibodies; *Im Cx*, immune complex; *SLE*, systemic lupus erythematosus; *H-S*, Henoch-Schönlein. (From: Jennette JC, Falk RJ. Renal involvement in systemic vasculitis. In: Greenberg A, Cheung AK, Coffman TM, et al, eds. *National Kidney Foundation Nephrology Primer.* 2nd ed. San Diego, CA: Academic Press; 1998:200, with permission.)

Small-Vessel Vasculitis: Microscopic Polyangiitis, Wegener's Granulomatosis, and Churg-Strauss Syndrome

Small-vessel vasculitides are characterized by necrotizing inflammation of multiple types of vessels. Arteries, veins, ar-terioles, venules, and capillaries may be affected; however, venules and capillaries are the most frequent targets (11). An understanding of the small-vessel vasculitides is important for nephrologists because these diseases often involve the kidneys and frequently cause glomerulonephritis (11,32). All of the small-vessel vasculitides listed in Table 68-1 can involve the kidneys. As mentioned earlier in the discussion about the

TABLE 68-2

NAMES AND DEFINITIONS OF VASCULITIS ADOPTED BY THE CHAPEL HILL CONSENSUS CONFERENCE ON THE NOMENCLATURE OF SYSTEMIC VASCULITIS

Large-vessel vasculitis[a] Giant cell arteritis	Granulomatous arteritis of the aorta and its major branches, with a predilection for the extracranial branches of the carotid artery. Often involves the *temporal artery*. *Usually occurs in patients older than 50 years and often is associated with polymyalgia rheumatica.*
Takayasu's arteritis	Granulomatous inflammation of the aorta and its major branches. Usually occurs in patients younger than 50 years.
Medium-sized vessel vasculitis[a] Polyarteritis nodosa	Necrotizing inflammation of medium-sized or small arteries without glomerulonephritis or vasculitis in arterioles, capillaries, or venules.
Kawasaki's disease	Arteritis involving large, medium-sized, and small arteries, and associated with mucocutaneous lymph node syndrome. *Coronary arteries are often involved*. Aorta and veins may be involved. Usually occurs in children.
Small-vessel vasculitis[a] Wegener's granulomatosis[b]	Granulomatous inflammation involving the respiratory tract, and necrotizing vasculitis affecting small-to medium-sized vessels, for example, capillaries, venules, arterioles, and arteries. Necrotizing glomerulonephritis is common.
Churg-Strauss syndrome[b]	Eosinophil-rich and granulomatous inflammation involving respiratory tract and necrotizing vasculitis affecting small-to medium-sized vessels, and associated with asthma and blood eosinophilia.
Microscopic polyangiitis[b]	Necrotizing vasculitis with few or no immune deposits affecting small vessels, for example, capillaries, venules, or arterioles. Necrotizing arteritis involving small- and medium-sized arteries may be present. Necrotizing glomerulonephritis is very common. Pulmonary capillarities often occurs.
Henoch-Schönlein purpura	Vasculitis with IgA-dominant immune deposits affecting small vessels, for example, capillaries, venules, or arterioles. Typically involves skin, gut, and glomeruli and is associated *with arthralgias or arthritis*.
Cryoglobulinemic vasculitis	Vasculitis with cryoglobulin immune deposits affecting small vessels, for example, capillaries, venules, or arterioles, and associated with cryoglobulins in serum. *Skin and glomeruli are often involved.*
Cutaneous leukocytoclastic angiitis	Isolated cutaneous leukocytoclastic angiitis without systemic vasculitis or glomerulonephritis.

[a] "Large artery" refers to the aorta and the largest branches directed toward major body regions (e.g., to the extremities and the head and neck); "medium-sized artery" refers to the main visceral arteries (e.g., renal, hepatic, coronary, and mesenteric arteries); and "small artery" refers to the distal arterial radicals that connect with arterioles. Note large and medium-sized vessel vasculitides do not involve vessels other than arteries.
[b] Strongly associated with ANCA.
(From: Jennette JC, Falk RJ, Andrassy K, et al. Nomenclature of systemic vasculitides. Proposal of an international consensus conference. *Arthritis Rheum* 1994;37:187, with permission.)

evolution of the definition of polyarteritis nodosa, small-vessel vasculitides with arterial involvement once were subsumed in the polyarteritis nodosa category. Zeek et al. (15,16) and Godman and Churg (17) were among the first to recognize that vasculitides that involve capillaries and venules in addition to arteries have clinical and pathologic features that are clearly distinct from those of polyarteritis nodosa.

The two major categories of small-vessel vasculitis include the "pauciimmune small vessel vasculitides" and the "immune complex–mediated small vessel vasculitides" (Table 68-1) (11). Immune complex–mediated vasculitides, such as Henoch-Schönlein purpura (HSP), cryoglobulinemic vasculitis, lupus vasculitis, and antiglomerular basement membrane (anti-GBM) vasculitis, have extensive localization of immunoglobulin and complement in vessel walls as a consequence of deposition of circulating immune complexes or *in situ* immune-complex formation between circulating antibodies and planted or constitutive antigens. The pauciimmune small-vessel vasculitides have little or no vascular wall localization of immunoglobulins (11,33–35). The pauciimmune small-vessel vasculitides often have necrotizing and crescentic glomerulonephritis as a component of the systemic necrotizing vasculitis. A pathologically identical pauciimmune necrotizing and crescentic

glomerulonephritis also occurs as a renal limited process, which has sometimes been referred to as "idiopathic crescentic glomerulonephritis" or "renal vasculitis" (11,34–38). Pauciimmune crescentic glomerulonephritis, which usually is a component of systemic pauciimmune small-vessel vasculitis, is the most common type of crescentic glomerulonephritis (Table 68-4).

The three major categories of systemic pauciimmune small-vessel vasculitis are MPA, Wegener's granulomatosis, and Churg-Strauss syndrome (CSS) (17,34,39). Table 68-2 and Figure 68-3 provide an approach for differentiating these three vasculitides and for distinguishing them from other types of vasculitis (11). MPA, Wegener's granulomatosis, and Churg-Strauss syndrome share a histologically identical necrotizing vasculitis that can affect arteries (Fig. 68-5), arterioles (Fig. 68-6), venules (Fig. 68-7), and capillaries, especially glomerular capillaries (Fig. 68-8). At all of these sites, the acute lesion is characterized by segmental necrosis with mural and perivascular fibrinoid material, sometimes accompanied by thrombosis in the vascular lumen. The initial inflammatory infiltrate has conspicuous neutrophils, often undergoing leukocytoclasia (Fig. 68-7), but this usually transforms into a predominantly mononuclear leukocyte infiltrate within a few days. The

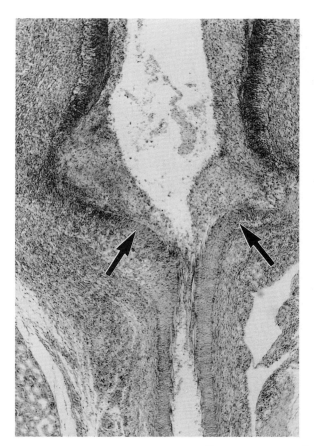

FIGURE 68-4. Acute necrotizing arteritis affecting a renal interlobar artery in a patient with Kawasaki's disease. The necrotizing inflammation (*arrows*) has eroded into the perivascular tissue to produce a pseudoaneurysm. (Hematoxylin and eosin stain, magnification ×350.)

TABLE 68-3

CLINICAL DIFFERENCES BETWEEN POLYARTERITIS NODOSA AND MICROSCOPIC POLYANGIITIS

Clinical feature	Polyarteritis nodosa	Microscopic polyangiitis
Rapidly progressive nephritis	No	Very common
Pulmonary hemorrhage	No	Yes
Peripheral neuropathy	Yes	Yes
Microaneurysms by angiography	Yes	Rare
Renovascular hypertension	Occasional	No
Positive hepatitis B serology	Uncommon	No
Positive antineutrophil cytoplasmic antibodies serology results	Rare	Frequent
Relapses	Rare	Frequent

(From: Guillevin L, Lhote F, Amouroux J, et al. Antineutrophil cytoplasmic antibodies, abnormal angiograms and pathological findings in polyarteritis nodosa and Churg-Strauss syndrome: Indications for the classification of vasculitides of the polyarteritis nodosa group. *Br J Rheumatol* 1996;35:958, with permission.)

glomerular lesion of pauciimmune ANCA-associated glomerulonephritis begins with segmental fibrinoid necrosis (Fig. 68-8) that quickly leads to crescent formation (Fig. 68-9). At the time of renal biopsy, approximately 90% of patients with pauciimmune crescentic glomerulonephritis have some degree of glomerular necrosis and crescent formation, although this may involve fewer than 50% of glomeruli (34,40). Arteritis, arteriolitis, and medullary angiitis are seen in less than 20% of renal biopsy specimens. Medullary angiitis can be severe enough to cause focal papillary necrosis.

In addition to the renal vasculitic lesions illustrated in Figures 68-5–68-9, patients with all three systemic pauciimmune small-vessel vasculitides share histologically identical inflammatory vascular lesions in other tissues, such as pulmonary

TABLE 68-4

FREQUENCY OF IMMUNOPATHOLOGIC CATEGORIES OF CRESCENTIC GLOMERULONEPHRITIS IN MORE THAN 3,000 CONSECUTIVE NONTRANSPLANT RENAL BIOPSIES EVALUATED BY IMMUNOFLUORESCENCE MICROSCOPY IN THE UNIVERSITY OF NORTH CAROLINA NEPHROPATHOLOGY LABORATORY

	Any crescents (N = 540)	>50% crescents (N = 195)	Arteritis in biopsy (N = 37)
Immunohistology			
Pauciimune (<2 positive immunoglobulin)	51% (277/540)	61% (118/195)[a]	84% (31/37)
Immune complex (≤2 positive immunoglobulin)	44% (238/540)	29% (56/195)	14% (5/37)[c]
Antiglomerular basement membrane	5% (25/540)[b]	11% (21/195)	3% (1/37)[d]

[a]70 of 77 patients tested for antineutrophilic cytoplasmic antibodies (ANCA. were positive (91%) (44 p-ANCA and 26 c-ANCA).
[b]3 of 19 patients tested for ANCA were positive (16%) (2 p-ANCA and 1 c-ANCA).
[c]4 patients had lupus and 1 poststreptococcal glomerulonephritis.
[d]This patient also had a p-ANCA (myeloperoxidase-ANCA).
(From: Jennette JC, Falk RJ. The pathology of vasculitis involving the kidney. *Am J Kidney Dis* 1991;24:130, with permission.)

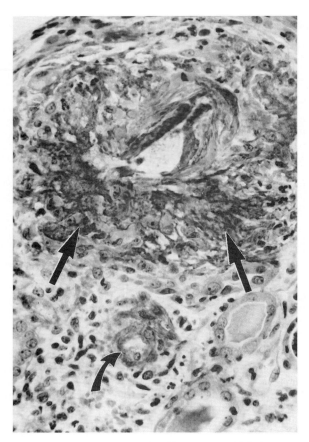

FIGURE 68-5. Necrotizing arteritis affecting an interlobular artery in a patient with microscopic polyangiitis. Note the extension of fibrinoid material into perivascular interstitium (*straight arrows*). Also note the necrotizing arteriolitis (*curved arrow*). (Masson trichrome, magnification ×350.)

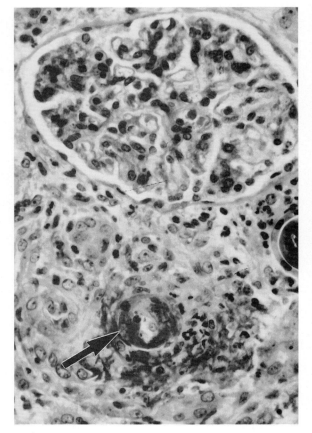

FIGURE 68-6. Necrotizing arteriolitis (*arrow*) affecting an arteriole in the renal cortex of a patient with microscopic polyangiitis. Note the fibrinoid material in the vessel wall and adjacent interstitium, and the focal perivascular leukocytoclasia. (Masson trichrome stain, magnification ×350.)

hemorrhagic alveolar capillaritis, dermal leukocytoclastic venulitis, and necrotizing inflammation of arteries in many tissues, including but not limited to peripheral nerves, skeletal muscle, gut, liver, pancreas, and skin. The diagnostic distinctions among the three diseases are not based on the pathologic or clinical features of vasculitis *per se*, but on the presence or absence of accompanying features, specifically granulomatous inflammation, asthma, and blood eosinophilia (1;11). As detailed in Table 68-2 and diagrammed in Figure 68-3, a diagnosis of MPA is warranted if a patient has systemic pauciimmune small-vessel vasculitis with no evidence for necrotizing granulomatous inflammation or asthma. A diagnosis of Wegener's granulomatosis is warranted if a patient has systemic pauciimmune small-vessel vasculitis with necrotizing granulomatous inflammation, usually in the upper or lower respiratory tract, and no asthma. A diagnosis of CSS is warranted if a patient has systemic pauciimmune small-vessel vasculitis with asthma and blood eosinophilia. Reaching these diagnostic conclusions does not necessarily require pathologic documentation of the lesions if reasonable clinical surrogates are identified. For example, in a patient with a renal biopsy that demonstrates pauciimmune necrotizing and crescentic glomerulonephritis, radiographic demonstration of cavitary lung nodules (in the absence of infection) or lytic bone lesions in the nasal septum are reasonable evidence for necrotizing granulomatous inflammation and thus warrant a diagnosis of Wegener's granulomatosis.

Serologic testing for ANCA is useful for making the diagnosis of pauciimmune small-vessel vasculitis or renal-limited pauciimmune crescentic glomerulonephritis. As discussed in more detail elsewhere in this chapter, the major types of ANCA are those that have specificity for proteinase 3 (PR3-ANCA) and for myeloperoxidase (MPO-ANCA) (18–21,41). In an indirect immunofluorescence microscopy assay, PR3-ANCA usually causes cytoplasmic staining of neutrophils (c-ANCA. and MPO-ANCA usually causes perinuclear staining (p-ANCA).

The clinical differential diagnosis of ANCA-associated pauciimmune small-vessel vasculitis also includes immune-complex small-vessel vasculitis. In Table 68-5 is demonstrated a great deal of overlap in organ system involvement among different types of pauciimmune small-vessel vasculitis and immune-complex small-vessel vasculitis. Upper or lower respiratory tract involvement has the greatest discriminatory value because respiratory tract involvement is common with pauciimmune small-vessel vasculitis and rare with immune-complex small-vessel vasculitis. In Table 68-6 and Figure 68-3 are detailed a number of observations that can be used to conclusively differentiate among MPA, Wegener's granulomatosis, CSS, cryoglobulinemic vasculitis, and HSP (11). Direct immunofluorescence microscopy of vessels in biopsy specimens, such as glomerular capillaries or dermal venules, is useful because this demonstrates immunoglobulin A (IgA)-dominant vascular immunoglobulin deposits in HSP, IgG and IgM deposits in cryoglobulinemic vasculitis, and little or no

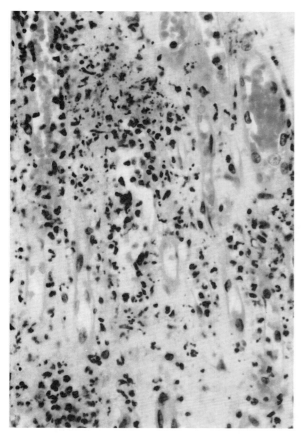

FIGURE 68-7. Leukocytoclastic medullary angiitis affecting the peritubular vasa recta in a patient with Wegener's granulomatosis. (Hematoxylin and eosin stain, magnification ×350.)

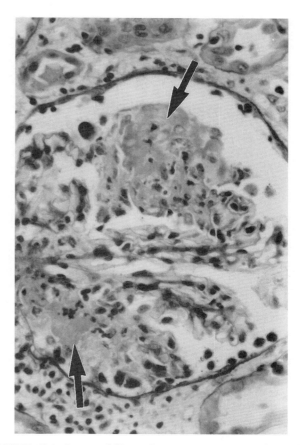

FIGURE 68-8. Segmental fibrinoid necrosis (*arrows*) in a glomerulus from a patient with microscopic polyangiitis. (Hematoxylin and eosin stain, magnification ×350.)

immunoglobulin in pauciimmune small-vessel vasculitis. Serologic testing also helps to focus the differential diagnosis, for example, testing for ANCA, anti-GBM, cryoglobulins, hepatitis C or B, antinuclear antibodies (ANA), and complement component levels.

In summary, the precise and accurate diagnosis of different categories of vasculitis, including small-vessel vasculitis, requires the knowledgeable integration of clinical, laboratory, and pathologic data.

EPIDEMIOLOGY OF SYSTEMIC VASCULITIS

In the past, the incidence of systemic vasculitis was difficult to determine, largely because of an inconsistent classification strategy. The advent of the Chapel Hill Nomenclature System allowed for a more precise estimation of incidence and prevalence. The incidence of giant cell arteritis varies from 15 to 30 per 100,000 in individuals older than 50 years. There is an increased incidence with age and a female-to-male ratio of 2:1 (42). Giant cell arteritis is more common in Caucasians and is uncommon in African Americans. Takayasu's arteritis has been described worldwide, but the disease is much more prevalent in Japan, where there are approximately 150 new cases per year. In Olmstead County, Minnesota, the incidence is 2.6 cases per million per year.

The incidence of the small-vessel vasculitides associated with ANCA (Wegener's granulomatosis, MPA, and CSS) appears to be on the order of 20 cases per million (42,43). In contrast, polyarteritis nodosa has become a rare disease. It is possible that the perceived increase in the incidence of MPA is a consequence of the development and widespread use of ANCA testing. Nonetheless, the incidence of MPA appeared to be more common in the 1990's than in the 1980's (19.8 versus 7 cases per million). Two interesting studies reported a much higher incidence of ANCA-associated vasculitis. One study reported a much higher incidence in Alaskan Indians, in which all cases were associated with hepatitis B (43). The other report from Kuwait after the Gulf War found an increased incidence of 16 cases per million of polyarteritis nodosa and 24 cases per million of MPA (44). The incidence of Wegener's granulomatosis was 0.7 per million per year from 1980 to 1986, increasing to 2.8 million per year from 1987 to 1989. In the 1990s, the prevalence of Wegener's granulomatosis was closer to 10.6 cases per million in the United Kingdom. The annual incidence of (CSS) is on the order of 4 cases per million (45). A recent study estimated the prevalence of polyarteritis nodosa (PAN), MPA, Wegener's granulomatosis and CSS in a large multiethnic suburb of Paris based on a three-source capture-recapture method. During the calendar year 2000, the prevalences per 1,000,000 adults were estimated to be 30 for PAN, 25 for MPA, 24 for Wegener's granulomatosis, and 11 for CSS. The overall prevalence was 2.0 times higher for subjects of European ancestry than for non-Europeans (P = 0.01) (46).

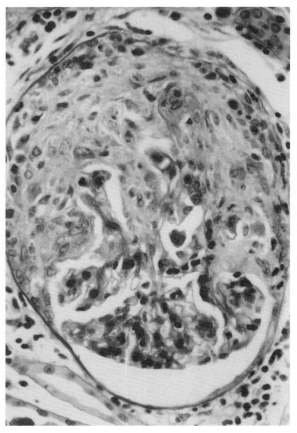

FIGURE 68-9. Cellular crescent in a glomerulus from a patient with microscopic polyangiitis. (Hematoxylin and eosin stain, magnification ×350.)

SMALL-VESSEL VASCULITIDES ASSOCIATED WITH ANCA

Demographics

ANCA-associated small-vessel vasculitis affects men and women equally. All ages are susceptible to disease, although the mean age of our population is 55 years. Almost 90% of our population is Caucasian, and 10% is African American. There appears to be a seasonal variation of the onset of disease, most commonly occurring in the late fall and early spring (47). It is possible but not proven that in northern latitudes, Wegener's granulomatosis predominates, whereas MPA is more common in southern climes.

Clinical Features

Renal Disease

The renal manifestations of small-vessel vasculitis are several. Many, if not most, patients present with rapidly progressive glomerulonephritis with hematuria, proteinuria, and a rising serum creatinine over the course of days to weeks. This clinical presentation is associated with the pathologic findings of glomerular necrosis and crescent formation. Invariably, interstitial inflammation results in interstitial fibrosis. At the other end of the spectrum are patients who present with much milder disease marked by isolated hematuria and low-grade proteinuria. On biopsy, these patients have focal areas of necrosis that result in areas of focal glomerulosclerosis.

Persistent microscopic hematuria can be the harbinger of different renal outcomes. In some patients, persistent hematuria correlates with focal inflammation in the kidney that with additional inflammatory stimuli (e.g., infection and environmental exposure. transforms into an aggressive acute nephritis. The acute nephritic presentation is usually associated with renal insufficiency, hypertension, and, on biopsy, with diffuse glomerular necrosis and crescent formation. In contrast, some patients with persistent microscopic hematuria without proteinuria have a clinically indolent disease that in the absence of a renal biopsy is ascribed to IgA nephropathy or thin basement membrane disease. Frequently, a renal biopsy is delayed until azotemia or significant proteinuria develops. By then, the biopsy reveals a picture of chronic glomerulonephritis with widespread glomerular sclerosis and only focal necrosis. Unfortunately, in such cases, the persistent microscopic hematuria was a reflection of unrecognized, unchecked glomerular inflammation. The treatment of such patients must be evaluated on a case-by-case basis depending on the degree of scarring and renal insufficiency, as the risks of aggressive antiinflammatory and immunosuppressive treatment may outweigh the potential benefits.

Proteinuria in ANCA glomerulonephritis is usually due to glomerular sclerosis or severe necrotizing and crescentic glomerulonephritis. In most cases of acute nephritis or rapidly progressive glomerulonephritis, the amount of proteinuria is on

TABLE 68-5

COMPARISON OF APPROXIMATE FREQUENCY OF MANIFESTATIONS OF MICROSCOPIC POLYANGIITIS WITH SEVERAL OTHER FORMS OF SMALL VESSEL VASCULITIS

	Microscopic polyangiitis	Wegener's granulomatosis	Churg-Strauss syndrome	Henoch-Schönlein	Cryoglobulin vasculitis
Cutaneous	40%	40%	60%	90%	90%
Renal	90%	80%	45%	50%	55%
Pulmonary	50%	90%	70%	<5%	<5%
Ear, nose, and throat	35%	90%	50%	<5%	<5%
Musculoskeletal	60%	60%	50%	75%	70%
Neurologic	30%	50%	70%	10%	40%
Gastrointestinal	50%	50%	50%	60%	30%

(From: Jennette JC, Falk RJ. Small vessel vasculitis. *N Engl J Med* 1997;337:1512, with permission.)

TABLE 68-6

FEATURES THAT ALLOW DIFFERENTIATION OF MICROSCOPIC POLYANGIITIS FROM SEVERAL OTHER FORMS OF SMALL-VESSEL VASCULITIS

	Henoch-Schönlein purpura	Cryoglobuline vasculitis	Microscopic polyangiitis	Wegener's granulomatosis	Churg-Strauss syndrome
Small-vessel vasculitis signs and symptoms[a]	+	+	+	+	+
IgA-dominant immune deposits	+	0	0	0	0
Cryoglobulins in blood and vessels	0	+	0	0	0
ANCA in blood	0	0	+	+	+
Necrotizing granulomas	0	0	0	+	+
Asthma and eosinophilia	0	0	0	0	+

[a] All of these small-vessel vasculitides can manifest any or all of the shared features of small-vessel vasculitides, such as purpura, nephritis, abdominal pain, peripheral neuropathy, myalgias and arthralgias. Each is distinguished by the presence and just as importantly the absence of certain specific features.
(From: Jennette JC, Falk R. Small vessel vasculitis. *N Engl J Med* 1997;337:1512, with permission.)

the order of 500 to 3,000 mg per 24 hours. The mean 24-hour urine protein excretion of our entire population at presentation is only 800 mg per 24 hours. Certainly there are cases of nephrotic-range proteinuria typically associated with diffuse glomerulosclerosis.

Acute interstitial nephritis is an unusual expression of small-vessel vasculitis. These patients generally present with pyuria and white blood cell casts without evidence of hematuria or proteinuria. In these cases, the glomeruli are completely spared, and inflamed vasa rectae are accountable for the clinical findings.

There are many examples of patients in whom ANCA-associated small-vessel vasculitis coexists with other forms of glomerular injury, the most common of these being anti-GBM disease. Typically these patients with both ANCA and anti-GBM have vasculitis affecting vascular beds other than the kidney and the lung. Their clinical course is more consistent with an ANCA glomerulonephritis than with anti-GBM disease. However, a recent retrospective analysis of patients with both ANCA and anti-GBM suggests that these patients have more severe renal disease and a poorer prognosis than patients with ANCA alone (48). It is unclear whether patients with both antibodies and severe renal failure share the poor renal prognosis of dialysis-dependent patients with anti-GBM disease alone. Indeed, some patients may respond to treatment with a dialysis-free interval of months to years.

Similarly, there are patients with ANCA-associated small-vessel vasculitis and immune complex forms of glomerulonephritis (e.g., membranous glomerulopathy or IgA nephropathy). Typically, the renal biopsy reveals areas of crescent transformation or glomerular necrosis. The clinical finding of a sudden decrease in renal function and worsening of the hematuria herald this pathologic event. ANCA glomerulonephritis may occur in patients with scleroderma, in whom the renal dysfunction is not attributable to a thrombotic microangiopathy, but to ANCA-induced necrosis and crescent formation.

As noted previously in this chapter, vessels larger than capillaries and venules are targets of inflammation. Small arteries, including the renal artery, can be injured. The most common clinical consequence of this process is renal infarction resulting in flank pain and renal insufficiency. Persistent disease of the renal artery causes stenosis and poststenotic dilation, with the clinical presentation of renovascular hypertension. Renal arteriography is necessary to delineate the degree of renal artery disease. Angioplasty or surgical correction of the stenotic vessel is frequently curative.

Skin Disease

Because the most commonly affected vessels of ANCA-associated small-vessel vasculitis are capillaries and postcapillary venules, the typical skin lesion is palpable purpura. Lesions tend to occur in "crops," primarily on the lower extremities. With time, the lesions flatten and either disappear or leave small hyperpigmented areas. In addition to this classic dermal presentation, there are several other cutaneous lesions, including petechiae, ecchymosis, ulceration, nodules, and plaquelike lesions, livido reticularis, and urticaria. Several cases of urticarial vasculitis have been observed in the absence of hypocomplementemia and immune-complex deposition. In unusual circumstances, vasculitic lesions give rise to erythema nodosum or pyoderma gangrenosum–like lesions. Biopsy of the affected area reveals a leukocytoclastic angiitis. However, in the case of nodular lesions, a simple punch biopsy may not provide sufficiently deep material to sample an involved vessel of larger caliber. A deep "excisional" biopsy is necessary.

The differential diagnosis of renal dermal vasculitic syndromes is important. In addition to the ANCA-associated small-vessel vasculitides, SLE, cryoglobulinemia, and HSP cause cutaneous vasculitides and renal disease. Each of these conditions is associated with a different natural history and treatment approach. For instance, many patients with HSP require only supportive care. If the renal dermal vasculitic syndrome is a consequence of ANCA-associated small-vessel vasculitis or lupus, immunosuppressive therapy is warranted. In addition, cutaneous vasculitis is frequently the consequence of a drug reaction. There are numerous classes of drugs that cause leukocytoclastic lesions, the most common being propylthiouracil, minocycline, phenytoin, and penicillamine.

Pulmonary Disease

The pulmonary consequences of ANCA-associated small vessel vasculitis are numerous and involve not only the lung parenchyma, but also the respiratory tract from the subglottis to the alveolar sacs. Several clinical presentations are common. Patients with MPA typically present with pulmonary infiltrates that are frequently initially ascribed to an infectious process. Generally, these patients describe hemoptysis, although many patients have no overt evidence of pulmonary bleeding. In some cases, the infiltrates wax and wane spontaneously. Infiltrates may coalesce, resulting in dyspnea and hypoxemia. The most alarming consequence of pulmonary capillaritis is the development of massive pulmonary hemorrhage. In our series, the occurrence of pulmonary hemorrhage was the most powerful predictor of death (49). As is discussed later, the prompt institution of plasmapheresis substantially decreased the mortality rate when compared with conventional immunosuppressive treatments.

Necrotizing granulomatous inflammation is a hallmark of Wegener's granulomatosis. Focal necrotizing lesions progress to confluent areas of necrosis that when surrounded by palisading histocytes, are called "geographic necrosis" (50). Nodular lesions are of varying size, from those that can only be seen by spiral computed tomography (CT) to those that occupy a complete lobe of the lung. In general, the larger lesions tend to cavitate. The differential diagnosis must include aspergillus or tuberculous infection, as well as other opportunistic infections. Determining whether the nodular and cavitary lesions are due to granulomatous infection or are a consequence of an opportunistic infection can present a difficult diagnostic dilemma. These two processes may coexist at times.

Similarly, recurrent alveolar hemorrhage in immunosuppressed patients may be attributable to infection. Alveolar lavage is useful in determining an infectious cause of alveolar hemorrhage rather than as a consequence of small-vessel vasculitis alone. Bronchioalveolar lavage should be performed, carefully considering the possible deterioration in oxygenation immediately after the procedure. Careful attention to the protection of airway patency for modern ventilatory support is mandatory. Transbronchial biopsy of the lung in patients with these diseases often results in non-diagnostic results. Open lung biopsy or procedures play a role in the diagnosis of these diseases.

In addition to the characteristic pulmonary nodules of Wegener's granulomatosis, endobronchial lesions, similar to those found in the subglottic region and trachea, can cause airway obstruction and may result in areas of collapsed lung. The lesions are usually quite sensitive to systemic glucocorticosteroid treatment (51).

CSS is characterized by the presence of asthma and eosinophilia in the circulation and within tissues. The pulmonary infiltrates tend to result in diffuse alveolar involvement but nodules and cavitations also occur. Eosinophilic pneumonia of other causes can be indistinguishable from the pulmonary presentation of CSS. Therefore, it is important to verify that a small-vessel vasculitis exists before determining that the patient has CSS (52).

Patients with subglottic masses or stenosis present with stridor or a sense of breathlessness. Results of flow–volume loop study results are abnormal. These lesions necessitate emergent attention to avoid life-threatening critical airway narrowing. Direct laryngoscopy with fiberoptic instrumentation allows visualization of the lesion. Glucocorticoid treatment is usually effective, but surgical intervention may be necessary. Areas of tracheal and bronchial granulomatous lesions can occur throughout the respiratory tree and result in bronchial obstruction.

The long-term consequences of intermittent pulmonary capillaritis result in pulmonary fibrosis. In some individuals, the diagnosis of idiopathic pulmonary fibrosis prompts consideration of ANCA-associated small-vessel vasculitis. Similarly, some patients with bronchiolitis obliterans with organizing pneumonia have had an underlying small-vessel vasculitis.

Upper Respiratory Tract Disease

Vasculitis frequently affects the areas of the ear, nose, and throat. By far the most common localization occurs in the nose, especially in patients with Wegener's granulomatosis. Other areas of involvement include the nasopharynx, the paranasal sinuses, and within the larynx. With respect to the nose, persistent or repetitive episodes of rhinosinusitis are one of the first symptoms. Small ulcerations lead to a nasal discharge that becomes hemorrhagic. Once these lesions become inflamed, a thick purulent material oozes from bloody crusts covering much larger areas of ulceration and granulation tissue. Histologic evaluation of these tissues most commonly reveals nonspecific acute and chronic inflammation. With a good sample, one may find areas of fibrinoid necrosis or granulomatous inflammation. Focal areas of ischemia and infarction occur. Repetitive bouts of inflammation eventually lead to septal perforations, the loss of turbinates, and may result in a loss of support of the nasal bridge (saddle nose deformity of Wegener's granulomatosis). Even with treatment, the nasal mucosa becomes atrophic and crusty. The crusts cause epistaxis when patients sneeze or blow their nose. *Staphylococcus aureus* superinfections may be the root cause of these ulcerations and an important factor in their development. Topical treatment with antibacterial ointments or systemic treatment with antibiotics decreases nasal symptoms and limits the number of relapses (53).

Sinusitis typically occurs with bloody nasal or postnasal discharge. Computed tomography may reveal bony erosions caused by granulomatous lesions typical of Wegener's granulomatosis. Necrotizing capillaritis associated with MPA or CSS frequently causes necrotizing lesions in the sinuses as well but do not lead to bony erosions. Granulomatous inflammation that blocks the eustachian tubes leads to serous otitis media. Bacterial superinfections lead to infectious otitis media. Ventilating tubes placed in the tympanic membrane may lessen the problem. Facial nerve paralysis may occur as a result of entrapment of the nerve by granulomatous inflammation anywhere along the course of the nerve. Large granulomatous pseudotumors invade the orbit and may lead to loss of an eye.

Gastrointestinal Tract Disease

The gastrointestinal tract represents one of the least well-studied areas of involvement of small-vessel vasculitis. In our experience, at least one-third of patients with active necrotizing glomerulonephritis have abdominal complaints, either on presentation or at some point during the course of disease. One of the more common areas of vasculitic involvement is the gastric mucosa, causing non-healing gastric or peptic ulcers. It is sometimes difficult to determine whether these ulcers are the consequence of vascular inflammation or glucocorticoid treatment. Endoscopic biopsy can provide a diagnosis, yet a presumptive diagnosis is made by a favorable response to glucocorticoid therapy. Similarly, pancreatitis, small bowel infarction, and ulcers throughout the gastrointestinal tract lead to abdominal pain. The most catastrophic of all abdominal vasculitic disease is transmural infarction of the bowel, leading to viscus perforation and polymicrobial sepsis. Prompt diagnosis and treatment is mandatory.

Autoimmune hepatitis and sclerosing cholangitis occur with p-ANCA that is not specific for MPO. The liver is usually not involved with necrotizing vasculitis.

Patients with small-vessel vasculitis may have medium-sized artery involvement as well. Aneurysmal dilation and fibrinoid necrosis of mesenteric or renal arteries results in infarction of the affected organ. If a mesenteric artery is involved, infarctions cause substantial abdominal pain or an ischemic colitis. These patients require mesenteric arteriography to identify the areas of arteritic involvement.

Neurologic Disease

Mononeuritis multiplex, or a pattern of multiple mononeuropathies, is caused by nerve impairment in anatomically separate regions. Most commonly, these areas of peripheral nerve ischemia are found in areas in the midthigh or mid upper arm, in watershed zones of poor vascular perfusion. Lesions of peripheral neuropathy occur abruptly and are very painful. The pain is described as a deep ache that is difficult to localize. Symptoms of the cutaneous distribution of the nerve occur several days after the onset of weakness and are described as a burning pain. Nerve biopsy should be performed in individuals with neuropathy as the major manifestation of vasculitis. A negative sural nerve biopsy result does not rule out the diagnosis. Repetitive biopsy of the nerve is almost useless. In a series of 200 patients with vasculitis and a neuropathy, only 27% had a vasculitis demonstrated in a muscular specimen only, 35% in a nerve only, and 27% in the nerve and the muscle (54). Many patients develop distal peripheral sensory neuropathies. Whether these symptoms are a consequence of vasculitis, pharmaceutical treatment, or malnutrition is not clear.

The central nervous system is an uncommon locus for vasculitis disease. Vasculitis involving the central nervous system usually results in a headache (55), without which the diagnosis is unlikely. Rarely, seizures are the presenting manifestation of central nervous system vasculitis. In Wegener's granulomatosis, meningeal disease can occur. Magnetic resonance imaging (MRI. with gadolinium infusion may reveal enhancing lesions in many separate foci. Most commonly, however, small-vessel vasculitis affects vessels that are too small to produce a positive magnetic resonance imaging (MRI) scan. Cerebral angiography may reveal abnormalities in less than half of patients. If the patient has systemic hypertension, cerebrovascular disease from atherosclerosis, or renal insufficiency resulting in uremia, it may not be possible to ascertain the precise cause of central nervous system symptoms. Treatment with antihypertensive agents and dialysis can exclude or decrease the possibility that hypertension and uremia are the cause of the symptoms. Many patients with ANCA-associated small-vessel vasculitis are older adults, and vasculitis may be impossible to differentiate from atherosclerosis in that population.

Other Organ System Diseases

Any organ system or capillary bed may be inflamed by small vessel vasculitis, resulting in numerous other clinical manifestations. Ocular manifestations of disease include iritis, uveitis, and peripheral keratitis. These lesions result in a red eye and are observed using a slit lamp by a qualified ophthalmologist.

Cardiac vasculitic disease results in subendocardial ischemia. The lesions can be difficult to see by using coronary arteriogram. Whether patients have coronary vascular disease as a consequence of atherosclerotic disease or of vasculitis is difficult to determine. In our population, 5% of patients had myocardial infarction at the time of their generalized disease process. Pericarditis is much less common in patients with ANCA-associated small-vessel vasculitis than in those with lupus vasculitis. A pericardial friction rub should raise the specter of a separate disease process.

In more than 90% of our patients, constitutional features are hallmarks of disease. Fatigue represents a ubiquitous finding that persists even after all of the other specific manifestations of vasculitis appear to be in remission. In addition, fever, myalgias, and arthralgias are common. Arthralgias are frequently migratory in which joint pain occurs in one joint,

only to resolve and appear in another joint at another time. Frank arthritis with synovial thickening occurs in at least 10% of patients.

LABORATORY FINDINGS

Abnormal laboratory findings in patients with small vessel vasculitis include normochromic and normocytic anemia, mild to marked leukocytosis, and mild thrombocytosis. Eosinophilia is uncommon in patients with Wegener's granulomatosis and MPA but is required for the diagnosis of CSS. Several markers of inflammation such as the C-reactive protein and the erythrocyte sedimentation rate are elevated, especially at times of disease exacerbation. Rheumatoid factor levels are positive in some individuals.

In the differential diagnosis of ANCA-associated small-vessel vasculitis, a number of other vasculitic syndromes can be excluded by serologic tests. These include tests for lupus, including ANA, anti–double-stranded DNA (dsDNA. antibodies, serum complement levels, and cryoglobulins. Rarely, a patient may have an overlap syndrome of SLE and ANCA-associated small-vessel vasculitis, with positive ANA, anti-dsDNA, and usually anti-MPO antibodies. Unlike with polyarteritis nodosa, screening for infectious diseases usually yields negative results, including assays for hepatitis B and hepatitis C. Anti-GBM antibodies should be measured at least once in the differential diagnosis of crescentic glomerulonephritis. Tests for circulating immune complexes are not reliable.

The laboratory findings in patients with CSS include eosinophilia in all patients. The degree of eosinophilia may reach 50% of the total leukocyte count. Elevated serum IgE levels and IgA containing immune complexes are found in some patients (56).

ANCA Serologic Studies

Since Richard Davies reported eight patients with antibodies to neutrophils associated with necrotizing glomerulonephritis (57), substantial advances have been made in the serologic analysis of ANCA. ANCA reacts not only to neutrophils, but also to monocytes. Effective ANCA testing must use both indirect immunofluorescent microscopy in conjunction with antigen-specific tests using highly purified MPO and PR3 antigens (18–21,41,58). Indirect immunofluorescent microscopy has elucidated two different ANCA patterns. On ethanol-fixed human neutrophils, cytoplasmic ANCA (c-ANCA) result in diffuse immunofluorescent staining of the cytoplasm. In contrast, perinuclear ANCA (p-ANCA) stain the periphery of the nucleus using ethanol-fixed cells but have a cytoplasmic pattern when using formalin-fixed leukocytes. Most c-ANCA react with PR3, a serine proteinase found within the primary granule of neutrophils and monocytes. This serine proteinase has substantial homology with elastase and cathepsin G. Some c-ANCA (less than 10%) react with bacterial/permeability increasing protein. This pattern of reactivity is found mainly in patients with cystic fibrosis and inflammatory bowel disease (59).

p-ANCA react with MPO in more than 90% of cases. The MPO is a member of a multichain peroxidase family that also includes thyroperoxidase, eosinophil peroxidase, and lactoperoxidase. Many if not most of the p-ANCA found in diseases other than pauciimmune necrotizing glomerulonephritis and vasculitis do not react with MPO, such as in ulcerative colitis, primary sclerosing cholangitis, and Felty's syndrome. The most confusing situation occurs in patients with lupus erythematosus. In these patients, p-ANCA are usually attributable to ANA, although in some rare cases, antilactoferrin and antielastase

TABLE 68-7

APPROXIMATE FREQUENCY OF ANTINEUTROPHIL CYTOPLASMIC ANTIBODIES (ANCAS) WITH SPECIFICITY FOR PROTEINASE 3 (PR3-ANCA, c-ANCA) OR MYELOPEROXIDASE (MPO-ANCA, p-ANCA) IN PATIENTS WITH ACTIVE UNTREATED MICROSCOPIC POLYANGIITIS, WEGENER'S GRANULOMATOSIS, AND CHURG-STRAUSS SYNDROME

	Microscopic polyangiitis	Wegener's granulomatosis	Churg-Strauss syndrome	Renal-limited vasculitis[a]
PR3-ANCA c-ANCA	40%	75%	10%	20%
MPO-ANCA p-ANCA	50%	20%	60%	70%
Negative ANCA	10%	5%	30%	10%

[a] Renal-limited vasculitis refers to pauciimmune necrotizing and crescentic glomerulonephritis with no apparent extrarenal vasculitis.

antibodies are found. Patients with lupus may have a false-positive anti-MPO test result by enzyme-linked immunosorbent assay (ELISA) (60).

The antigen specificity of circulating ANCA is not diagnostic for a particular clinicopathologic variant of ANCA-associated small vessel vasculitis, although there are differences in the relative frequency of PR3-ANCA and MPO-ANCA in different types of pauciimmune small-vessel vasculitis (Table 68-7). For example, most patients with Wegener's granulomatosis have PR3-ANCA (c-ANCA), whereas most patients with renal-limited pauciimmune crescentic glomerulonephritis have MPO-ANCA (p-ANCA).

A positive ANCA result in a patient with strong clinical evidence for crescentic glomerulonephritis or another manifestation of small-vessel vasculitis, such as purpura or pulmonary hemorrhage, has a high positive predictive value. A positive ANCA result in a patient with weak evidence for crescentic glomerulonephritis or small-vessel vasculitis, such as isolated hematuria and proteinuria with normal renal function, has a much lower positive predictive value (Table 68-8). However, in a patient with weak clinical evidence for crescentic glomerulonephritis or small-vessel vasculitis, a positive result increases the likelihood to a level that requires expeditious additional diagnostic evaluation, possibly including a renal biopsy, to confirm or refute the presence of a pauciimmune small-vessel vasculitis or crescentic glomerulonephritis. A negative ANCA result is more effective at ruling out pauciimmune crescentic glomerulonephritis in a patient with weak clinical evidence of

small-vessel vasculitis than in a patient with strong clinical evidence for small-vessel vasculitis (Table 68-8).

The ANCA result is typically negative in patients with polyarteritis nodosa, Takayasu's arteritis, or giant cell arteritis. There are individuals who have an overlapping disease with vasculitic involvement not only of large vessels, but also of small arteries. These patients have either PR3- or MPO-ANCA.

PATHOGENESIS

There has been an explosion of knowledge pertaining to the pathogenesis of ANCA small-vessel vasculitis and pauciimmune necrotizing glomerulonephritis, but much still remains to be discovered. While Wegener's granulomatosis, microscopic polyangiitis, and CSS share the hallmark of pauciimmune necrotizing small-vessel vasculitis, each presents phenotypic differences. It is still unclear what causes the granulomatous lesions of Wegener's granulomatosis or stimulates the eosinophilia and asthma in CSS. Furthermore, the severity of disease varies from one patient to another. To date, the host factors that produce minimal disease in some patients and severe disease in others remain unknown. More intriguing is the observation that while vasculitis affects many capillary beds (e.g., kidney, skin, or lung) in some patients, it is limited to one organ in others. In many instances, the disease processes are focal. For example, only a segment of a capillary bed is affected,

TABLE 68-8

PREDICTIVE VALUE OF COMBINED INDIRECT FLUORESCENT ANTIBODY (IFA) AND ENZYME IMMUNOASSAY (EFA) ANTINEUTROPHIL CYTOPLASMIC ANTIBODY TESTING FOR PAUCIIMMUNE CRESCENTIC GLOMERULONEPHRITIS

Adult with	Prevalence pretest likelihood	Positive predictive value post-test likelihood	Negative predictive value post-test unlikelihood
RPGN	47%	95%	85%
Hematuria, Proteinuria, (creatinine >3 mg/dL)	21%	84%	95%
Hematuria, Proteinuria, (creatinine 1.5–3 mg/dL)	7%	60%	99%
Hematuria, Proteinuria, (creatinine <1.5 mg/dL)	2%	29%	100%

Data derived from an analysis of 2,315 patients, with ANCA assay sensitivity 81% and specificity 96%.
(From: Lim LC, Taylor JG III, Schmitz JL, et al. Diagnostic usefulness of antineutrophil cytoplasmic autoantibody serology. Comparative evaluation of commercial indirect fluorescent antibody (IFA) kits and enzyme immunoassay (EIA) kits. *Am J Clin Pathol* 1999;111(3):363, with permission.)

leaving an adjacent segment spared. This is exemplified by the observation that a segmental necrotizing lesion in a glomerulus may sit adjacent to an ostensibly normal glomerular segment.

A number of clinical and basic science observations suggest that ANCA play a pivotal role in the pathogenesis of pauciimmune vasculitis and glomerulonephritis (11,61–63). ANCA are found in 85% to 90% of patients with pauciimmune glomerulonephritis and small-vessel vasculitis. There is an absence of evidence for more clearly delineated pathogenetic mechanisms, such as immune-complex disease or direct antibody attack–mediated disease. ANCA titers tend to correlate with disease activity in most but not all patients, yet the most convincing human data come from patients who develop a drug-induced ANCA-vasculitis. In some cases, cessation of the offending agent is associated with remission of small-vessel vasculitis and diminution of ANCA titers. Finally, there is a clear description of trans-placental transfer of MPO-ANCA from a mother with active MPA during pregnancy resulting in a pulmonary-renal vasculitic syndrome in the newborn infant (64,65).

ANCA more than likely participate in the pathogenesis of vasculitis by activation of primed leukocytes and monocytes in the circulation and increasing their adherence or leukocytes adherent to the vascular endothelium. A number of laboratories have confirmed that ANCA induce neutrophil and monocyte activation using various methods. These include analysis of respiratory burst and degranulation and measurement of several chemokines and cytokines (66–69). How these antibodies bind to cognate antigens is likely a consequence of a number of factors. It is possible that there is a genetic increase in the expression of PR3 on the surface of neutrophils and monocytes (70,71). Another possibility stems from the observations that in patients with ANCA vasculitis, neutrophils and monocytes have substantially increased expression of genes for MPO and PR3. In fact, the expression of RNA from these cells was correlated with disease activity. Interestingly, while the MPO and PR3 genes are on different chromosomes, message from both of these genes was coordinately increased, suggesting a similar, but unrecognized, transcription factor that may be regulating the production of many granular constituents (72).

Once antigen is available for antibody binding, neutrophils and monocytes are then activated by two coordinated and separate signal transduction pathways. In the past, controversy abounded as to whether ANCA activation of neutrophils and monocytes occurred by the Fc receptor alone or whether there was F(ab')2 stimulation (73). Human neutrophils constitutively express receptors for IgG, including FcRIIa and FcRIIIb. The former is a widely expressed receptor, whereas the latter is a low-affinity receptor with expression that is restricted to neutrophils and eosinophils (74). Engagement of the Fc receptor results in a number of neutrophil-activation events, including respiratory burst, degranulation, phagocytosis, cytokine production, and upregulation of adhesion molecules. Fc receptors are thus likewise engaged in the activation of neutrophils and monocytes by ANCA (75,76). Polymorphisms of the Fc receptors could play an important role in the development of ANCA vasculitis. Whereas the FcRIIa single nucleotide polymorphisms do not appear to be important (77,78), some evidence suggests that the FcRIIIb polymorphism may influence disease severity (79,80). In addition to Fc receptor–induced activation, there are substantial data that the F(ab')$_2$ portion of the antibody molecule also plays a role in leukocyte activation. ANCA F(ab')$_2$ not only induce oxygen radical production (73), but also induce the transcription of cytokine genes in normal human neutrophils and monocytes. Whereas some genes are upregulated by both whole ANCA immunoglobulin and ANCA F(ab')$_2$, other genes are upregulated by only one or the other (81). It is most likely that F(ab')$_2$ portions of ANCA are capable of low-level neutrophil and monocyte activation (73). The Fc portion of the molecule almost certainly causes leukocyte activation once the F(ab')$_2$ portion of the immunoglobulin

has interacted with the antigen, either on the cell surface or in the microenvironment (75). Recently, the signal transduction pathways of F(ab')2 and Fc receptor activation have been nicely elucidated. Both of these possible activation pathways appear to activate a specific p21ras (Kristen-ras) through separate but coordinated pathways (82). This is an important observation in that it may provide a focus for a therapeutic target.

As described in several studies, once neutrophils and monocytes are activated by ANCA, they interact with endothelial cells causing damage to the endothelium (83–86). It has been thought that it is possible that endothelial cells expressed ANCA antigens, especially PR3, but this observation has been excluded by a number of investigators. What has emerged, however, is the possibility that, in addition to direct damage of the endothelium by the respiratory burst properties of leukocytes, ANCA antigens released from neutrophils and monocytes enter endothelial cells and cause endothelial cell damage. For example, PR3 released into the microenvironment enters endothelium, resulting in IL-8 production (87) and chemoattractant protein-1. PR3 is also capable of inducing apoptotic events from both proteolytic and non-proteolytic mechanisms (88,89). The internalization of PR3 into endothelial cells is receptor mediated (90–92).

Similarly, MPO has been shown to be internalized into endothelial cells by an energy-dependent process (93), and to transcytose intact endothelium to localize within the extracellular matrix. There, in the presence of the substrates H_2O_2 and NO_2-, MPO catalyzes nitration of tyrosine residues on extracellular matrix proteins (94), resulting in the fragmentation of extracellular matrix protein (95).

There have been a number of in vitro models of ANCA neutrophil and endothelial cell interaction using flow models and intravital microscopy. With treatment using tumor necrosis factor (TNF), endothelial cells capture neutrophils from the circulation. With the addition of ANCA over these rolling neutrophils, a more substantial adhesion of leukocytes to endothelial cells and transmigration of leukocytes occur. This occurs through a conformational change on CD11b that reveals an activation epitope (86).

The Role of T Cells

It has long been known that there are circulating T cells in patients with ANCA small-vessel vasculitis that have a Th1-type cytokine profile (96–101). Within tissues, Th-1 cytokine profiles have also been reported, especially in T cells from granulomatous tissue of patients with Wegener's granulomatosis (102). Very little is known, however, about T cells and ANCA vasculitis since it has been difficult to demonstrate that circulating T cells derived from affected patients are activated by the ANCA target antigens. There is mounting evidence implicating T cells in the pathogenesis of ANCA glomerulonephritis. T cells and monocytes are the predominant cell types in inflammatory vascular and perivascular lymphoid infiltrates in ANCA glomerulonephritis (103). The predominance of IgG1 and IgG4 subclasses of ANCA denotes the effects of T-cell help and IL-4 on isotype switching (104). Furthermore, in patients with ANCA glomerulonephritis, the concentrations of soluble IL-2 receptor, which is a marker of T-cell activation, correlate well with disease activity (105).

In vitro analyses of peripheral blood T-cell proliferation in response to MPO and PR3 yielded conflicting results. Recent studies have shown little or no difference in T-cell reactivity to PR3 between patients with ANCA-disease and controls (106,107). In the largest study looking at T-cell proliferative responses in 45 patients at various stages of disease (with and without treatment), PR3 responses were seen at all stages of disease activity, and to a lesser degree in healthy controls (108).

Interestingly, T cells from only two patients with PR3-ANCA, and none of the controls, proliferated in response to MPO.

Analysis of the profile of cytokine secretion by T cells derived from tissue with granulomatous inflammation (nasal mucosa or bronchiolar lavage fluid. as well as from peripheral blood T cells revealed a T-helper 1 (T_H1) pattern of cytokines (99,101). This is corroborated by the finding that T cells from patients with Wegener's granulomatosis have a decreased expression of CD28 as compared to healthy controls (102). CD28 costimulation promotes the production of T_H2 cytokines (109). Conversely, a recent study looking at the cytokine profile of T cells from patients with ANCA disease in complete remission and receiving *no* immunosuppressants revealed a T_H2 cytokine profile with elevated production of IL-6 and IL-10 and low production of interferon gamma (IFN-γ) (110). These differences in the detected cytokine profiles could be due to the state of disease activity.

Antiendothelial Cell Antibodies

Antiendothelial cell antibodies (AECA) have been recognized for some time in several autoimmune diseases. AECA are more common in vasculitides associated with SLE, rheumatoid arthritis, systemic sclerosis, and antiphospholipid-induced vasculopathy (111,112). These antibodies recognize endothelial cell antigens expressed on large arterial vessel endothelial cells (Takayasu's arteritis) and on microvascular cells from both the arterial and the venous system. The precise nature of the target antigen has still not been elucidated. However, it is reasonable to presume that planted antigens complex with AECA resulting in *in situ* immune complex formation. Such antigens include DNA or DNA-histone complexes in SLE (113). Once AECA react with the surface of the endothelium, they likely induce a pathogenetic event by fixing complement.

When endothelial cells are cultured from a variety of tissues, including those from the human kidney, liver, lung, and nasal carriage, there is increased binding of AECA to unstimulated cells and cytokine-treated lung endothelial cells when compared to human umbilical vein endothelial cells or liver sinusoidal cells (114). These observations provide a newer concept: that AECA are specific for certain endothelial cells in target organ and may recruit leukocytes to their site of engagement.

Role of *Staphylococcus aureus* and Superantigens

Clinical studies reveal that 60% to 70% of patients with Wegener's granulomatosis have a chronic nasal carriage of *S. aureus* (53) that is associated with an eightfold increased rate of relapse (115). Importantly, in a placebo-controlled randomized trial, patients with nasal carriage of *S. aureus* treated with trimethoprim-sulfamethoxazole had a significantly lower rate of relapse of the nasal or upper respiratory tract disease. *S. aureus* superantigens are most likely implicated in disease activity. For instance, patients with superantigen-positive *S. aureus* strains are more likely to have a relapse of disease than carriers of superantigen-negative strains (116). The staphylococcal acid phosphatase appears to bind to the endothelium as a consequence of its cationic nature and is recognized by the sera of patients with Wegener's granulomatosis (116). In addition, Brown-Norway rats immunized with staphylococcal acid phosphatase and then perfused with this same protein developed severe crescentic glomerulonephritis (117).

Environmental Factors (Including Infections)

The first report of ANCA was an association in eight patients with necrotizing glomerulonephritis and arbovirus infection with the Ross River virus (55). Several animal models suggest an association of arteritis and infection. For instance, parvovirus B19 is associated with a vasculopathy not only in humans, but also in the Aleutian mink (118). These animals develop a chronic parvovirus illness that results in immune complex–mediated vasculitis. There are several animal models of infection-mediated vasculitis in which there may be direct invasion of the vascular wall.

Environmental factors, particularly exposure to silica dust and other silica-containing compounds, may increase the risk of developing a number of different autoimmune diseases including scleroderma, rheumatoid arthritis, systemic sclerosis, SLE, and vasculitis (119). The early data were derived from studies that primarily evaluated cohorts of workers in occupations with high exposure to silica dust. This type of study is not ideal for assessing rare outcomes, such as autoimmune diseases. Case-control studies of specific autoimmune disorders have offered more insight into diseases potentially associated with silica dust exposure. Previous case-control studies have shown an association between ANCA-associated diseases and exposure to silica dust or other silica-containing compounds (120–122) with odds ratios ranging from 4.4 to 14.0. More recently, a case-control study reported an association between primary systemic vasculitis and farming activities and exposure to occupational solvents (the association with exposure to silica could not be ascertained (123). In a study involving 129 patients with ANCA-vasculitis with glomerulonephritis and 109 matched controls, only prolonged silica exposure (>23 years) was statistically significantly more common among patients than controls. There was no difference between the two groups in exposure to silica of shorter duration (124). In contrast, exposure to silica dust was not associated with the development of lupus nephritis, which is in contrast to reports from occupational cohorts (122,125,126).

Many drugs can induce vasculitis. In fact, 10% to 20% of cutaneous reactions to drug exposure are vasculitic in nature. A list of the most frequently implicated drugs includes anticonvulsants, antibiotics, penicillamine, hydralazine, nonsteroidal antiinflammatory drugs, and propylthiouracil (127). One of the drugs most commonly related to the development of anti-MPO–induced disease is propylthiouracil (127).

Animal Models

There are now excellent animal models of ANCA-induced small-vessel vasculitis. The most direct evidence of the pathogenic role of anti-MPO antibodies stems from a model of transfer of either splenocytes or anti-MPO antibodies into Rag 2−/− mice (128). In this model, MPO knockout mice (MPO−/−) were immunized with purified mouse MPO, and developed mouse anti-mouse -MPO antibodies. When splenocytes from these mice were transferred into Rag2−/− mice, which lack functioning T and B cells, these animals developed a systemic necrotizing vasculitis and severe necrotizing and crescentic glomerulonephritis. When anti-MPO antibodies derived from immunized MPO knockout mice were transferred into Rag 2-/- mice, a pauciimmune necrotizing and crescentic glomerulonephritis was induced. This disease process occurred without antigen-driven T cells. Several follow-up studies have now been performed using this mouse model. In particular, the disease process was aggravated by the administration of lipopolysaccharide (LPS) into recipient mice by increasing the percentage of glomeruli involved with necrotizing and

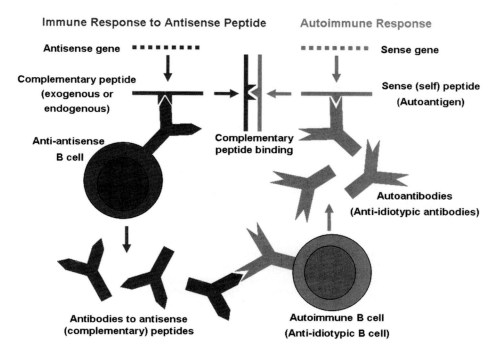

Immune Response to Antisense Peptide   Autoimmune Response

FIGURE 68-10. Schematic of a mechanism for the development of autoimmunity (theory of autoantigen complementarity) as a consequence of an immune response to a protein whose amino acid sequence is complementary to a self protein.

crescentic glomerulonephritis when anti-MPO antibodies were transferred into these mice (129). The role of neutrophils in this response was highlighted by the abrogation of disease when the neutrophils of anti-MPO recipient mice were depleted by a selective anti-neutrophil monoclonal antibody (NIMP-R14) (130).

The pathogenic role of anti-MPO antibodies is also documented in a second animal model (131). In this model, rats immunized with human MPO developed anti-rat-MPO antibodies. These animals then developed a necrotizing and crescentic glomerulonephritis, as well as pulmonary capillaritis. Microscopy of superior mesenteric vessels demonstrated that when a chemokine was applied to the vessel, the anti-MPO antibodies induced adherence and margination of leukocytes to the vessel wall. These two animal models document that anti-MPO antibodies are capable of causing a necrotizing and crescentic glomerulonephritis and a widespread systemic vasculitis, and also demonstrate that cytokines and chemokines exacerbate the injury in a manner that mimics the *in vitro* studies of ANCA-induced leukocyte activation. A model of anti-PR3-induced vascular injury was developed in which a perivascular infiltrate was observed around cutaneous vessels in the setting of anti-PR3 antibodies and cytokine exposure (62,132). In summary, these animal studies document that both anti-MPO and proteinase-3 antibodies are capable of causing disease.

Theory of Autoantigen Complementarity

For all autoimmune diseases, the critical question is, is the most proximate cause of the formation of the autoantibody or the abnormal T cell clone. There have been a number of theories that may provide a basis for the alteration of self antigens, the most plausible of which is known as the theory of molecular mimicry (133–135). This theory suggests that there is an immune response directed against a microbial antigen that mimics the amino acid sequence or structure of a self protein. To date, it has been difficult to demonstrate this theory in human autoimmune disease. A serendipitous finding in ANCA vasculitis has spawned a theory of autoantigen complementarity. While

the details of this theory and the proof that it may pertain to ANCA vasculitis is beyond the scope of this chapter, a brief description of this observation is germane for the understanding of ANCA vasculitis (136,137) (Fig. 68-10).

It has been known for decades that proteins transcribed and translated from the sense strand of DNA bind to proteins that are transcribed and translated from the anti-sense strand of DNA. Some patients with PR3 ANCA harbored antibodies to an antigen complementary to the middle portion of PR3. These anti-complementary PR3 antibodies formed an anti-idiotypic pair with PR3-ANCA. Moreover, cloned complementary PR3 proteins bind to PR3 and function as a serine proteinase inhibitor. What is the source of the complementary PR3 antigen? Preliminary data suggest that these proteins are found on a variety of microbes, some of which have been associated with ANCA vasculitis and also found in the genome of some patients with both PR3- and MPO-ANCA (137). These studies need to be confirmed and expanded to understand what the source of the complementary PR3 antigen is in any given person, and just as importantly, whether these complementary proteins are capable of inducing disease. If these observations remain true, they may provide a promising avenue for the detection of the proximate cause of the autoimmune response in any given person.

TREATMENT

The treatment of ANCA-associated small-vessel vasculitis and glomerulonephritis rests primarily on the use of induction methylprednisolone, high-dose corticosteroids, and cyclophosphamide. Considering the importance of the serum creatinine concentration at the time treatment is initiated as a determinant of long-term renal outcome (49), pulse methylprednisolone (7 mg/kg per day for 3 days) is used to curb the active inflammation as soon as possible. This is followed by instituting prednisone at a daily dosage of 1 mg/kg per day (not to exceed 80 mg per day for the first month of therapy) Corticosteroids are then tapered over the second month to an alternate-day dosing schedule and subsequently decreased every week by

10 to 20 mg per day until they are eventually discontinued by the end of the fourth to fifth month. The rate of decrease in corticosteroid dosing should be tailored based on an assessment of each patient's disease activity.

The beneficial role of cyclophosphamide in the treatment of acute ANCA-associated small-vessel vasculitis is evidenced by the substantial improvement in the rate of remission (56% to 85%) and a threefold decrease in the risk of relapse is associated with the use of this drug (138). Cyclophosphamide may be administered as a daily oral regimen or as monthly intravenous pulses. When the intravenous route is used, it is usually started at a dose of 0.5 g/m^2 of body surface area, which is subsequently increased to a maximal dosage of 1 g/m^2. This dose is adjusted to maintain the 2-week leukocyte nadir at more than 3,000/mm^3. When the daily oral regimen is used, cyclophosphamide is given at a daily dosage of 1.5 to 2 mg/kg (139). To prevent severe leukopenia, careful attention to the leukocyte count must be maintained throughout this therapy. Cyclophosphamide is usually continued for a total of 6 to 12 months, depending on the patient's response to treatment. Whether one form of cyclophosphamide therapy is superior to the other is a subject of continued investigation. In general, the intravenous regimen allows for a 2 to 3 times smaller total dose of cyclophosphamide than the oral regimen. In prospective and retrospective analyses, intravenous therapy was associated with a significant decrease in the rate of clinically significant neutropenia and other complications. A regimen of daily oral cyclophosphamide may be associated with a decreased risk of relapse (140). However, in a meta-analysis of three randomized controlled trials comparing pulse versus oral continuous cyclophosphamide, pulse cyclophosphamide attained a statistically higher rate of remission, and lower rates of leucopenia and infections. Pulse cyclophosphamide was associated with a higher rate of relapse which was not statistically significant (141). The final outcomes of patients (death or end stage renal disease [ESRD]) were no different in the two groups despite the lower rate of relapse in the oral cyclophosphamide group (141).

Patients presenting with pulmonary hemorrhage also benefit from the institution of plasmapheresis in a regimen similar to that used for patients with Goodpasture's disease. Although no controlled data are available, early and aggressive institution of plasmapheresis has in our experience substantially diminished the mortality rate associated with massive pulmonary hemorrhage (142). Plasmapheresis is typically performed daily until the pulmonary hemorrhage ceases and then every other day for a total of seven to ten treatments. Plasma is replaced with a solution of 5% albumin, but two units of fresh-frozen plasma are administered at the end of the treatment to replace clotting factors and minimize the risk of persistent or renewed bleeding. On the basis of several relatively small studies, plasmapheresis does not seem to be of added benefit over the use of corticosteroids and cyclophosphamide in patients without pulmonary hemorrhage (143–145) or severe renal involvement. In a randomized trial of plasma exchange versus methylprednisolone as additional therapy in patients with severe ANCA glomerulonephritis (creatinine >500 μmol/L or dialysis), the of use plasma exchange was associated with a significant improvement in the recovery of renal function and dialysis-free survival (146).

Once remission is attained, an alternative maintenance regimen consists of switching cyclophosphamide to oral azathioprine at the end of 3 months. Azathioprine is then continued for 12 to 24 months. This regimen offers the advantage of a limited use of cyclophosphamide and results in similar rates of remission and relapse as the cyclophosphamide-only–based therapies (147).

Patients suffering primarily from mild ANCA-associated small-vessel vasculitis without renal involvement may benefit from the use of methotrexate in lieu of cyclophosphamide. In an uncontrolled study, methotrexate afforded rates of remission comparable to those published for cyclophosphamide (148). An open-label study suggests that methotrexate could be used for maintenance therapy after the induction of remission with cyclophosphamide and corticosteroids (149), but may be associated with a relatively high rate of relapse. In a randomized controlled trial of induction therapy among patients with "early" ANCA-associated vasculitis comparing weekly methotrexate (15 mg/week escalating to a maximum of 20 to 25 mg/week by 12 weeks) to daily oral cyclophosphamide (2 mg/kg/day to a maximum of 150 mg/day), the rate of remission at 6 months was comparable among the two treatment groups (89.8% for methotrexate vs. 93.5% for cyclophosphamide, p = 0.041). However, the onset of remission in methotrexate-treated patients with relatively extensive disease or pulmonary involvement was delayed. Methotrexate was associated with a significantly higher rate of relapse than cyclophosphamide (69.5% vs. 46.5%), and 45% of relapses occurred while patients were receiving methotrexate (150). Importantly, patients enrolled in this trial did not have organ- or life-threatening manifestations, or significant renal involvement. The dose of methotrexate must be reduced in patients whose creatinine clearance is less than 80 ml/min, and its use is contraindicated when creatinine clearances are less than 10 ml/min. Most experience of methotrexate in Wegener's granulomatosis has involved patients with no renal involvement or with glomerulonephritis and near-normal renal function.

With the use of an alkylating agent, the rate of remission is on the order of 70% to 85%. Patients who require dialysis at the time of diagnosis have a decreased probability of recovering sufficient renal function to discontinue dialysis (about 50%). Patients that do recover sufficient renal function, do so within the first 3 months of treatment. For that reason, and in the absence of active extrarenal vasculitis, immunosuppression may be stopped after 3 months if no signs of renal recovery have occurred.

Relapse of ANCA-associated small-vessel vasculitis occurs in about 30% of patients (138). In our experience, 80% of relapses occur in the first 18 months after immunosuppressive therapy is discontinued. Other authors did not detect such a clustering of relapses in the early months after discontinuing therapy (151). Recurrent disease may resemble clinically the initial presentation but is sometimes associated with new organ involvement.

The risk of relapse is not uniform among patients with ANCA-associated vasculitis. Multivariate analysis of 258 patients with the disease who were treated and attained remission showed that presence of PR3-ANCA antibody and involvement of the lungs and upper respiratory tract were independent risk factors for relapse. Of the patients who presented none of these risk factors, 26% relapsed in a median of 62 months (median among those who relapsed was 20 months). In contrast, 47% of the patients who presented with a single risk factor experienced a risk for relapse (95% CI 1.1-3.9, p = 0.038). Of patients presenting with all three risk factors, 73% relapsed in a median of 17 months (median among those who relapsed was 15 months), corresponding to a 3.7-times increased risk of relapse (95% CI 1.4-9.7, p = 0.007) compared to those with no risk factors (152).

Whether ANCA titers are predictive of a relapse is a matter of controversy. To determine the occurrence of a relapse, serial measurements of ANCA titers should be interpreted only in the context of the clinical history and physical and laboratory examination of the patient. Recurrent glomerulonephritis is usually indicated by the recurrence or worsening of hematuria with an increase in serum creatinine. An increase in proteinuria alone or the gradual increase in serum creatinine without hematuria may be the result of progressive chronic scarring, rather than recurrent active inflammation. Repeated renal biopsy is sometimes indicated to best differentiate between recurrent disease and progressive scarring and to avoid unnecessary immunosuppression in the latter case.

Whether ANCA titers are clinically useful in ascertaining the occurrence of relapse or of predicting its occurrence in the future remains a subject of investigation. Although ANCA titers correlate with disease activity when a group of patients are considered, the ANCA titer may not correlate in an individual patient. Some patients maintain a high titer level despite clinical remission, whereas others exhibit clinical evidence of active vasculitis in the absence of a rise in titer. ANCA titers are best used in serial measurements and interpreted in consideration with each patient's pattern.

Several studies have addressed whether ANCA could reliably predict the future occurrence of a relapse (153). Although a rise in ANCA titer tends to predict recurrent disease, the relapse may not occur for several months. In a study by Cohen Tervaert et al., one-third of patients with a rise in titer did not experience clinical signs of relapse even after 18 months (154). In this context, and considering the toxicities of immunosuppression, the prophylactic use of high-dose corticosteroids or cyclophosphamide to prevent relapse would needlessly expose many patients to their toxic side effects. If alternative, less-toxic therapies are shown to be effective in the treatment of ANCA vasculitis, the risk–benefit ratio may make such a preemptive or prophylactic approach more appealing. To date, the evidence does not support the use of preemptive immunosuppressive therapy to prevent a relapse in patients with an increase in ANCA titer.

Relapsing ANCA-associated vasculitis responds to immunosuppression with corticosteroids and cytotoxic agents with a similar response rate as the initial disease. The decision regarding the repeated use of pulse methylprednisolone can be based on the total amount of corticosteroid that has been administered to the patient over the course of the disease, as well as the severity of the relapse. Patients with a history of relapsing disease pose a particular challenge because they are particularly subject to the cumulative toxic effects of cytotoxic agents and corticosteroids. Some may require the use of long-term "maintenance" immunosuppressive therapy with either low-dose prednisone or azathioprine. Although the use of trimethoprim-sulfamethoxazole or cotrimoxazole is beneficial in the prevention of relapses involving the nose and upper respiratory tract, no benefit is seen in disease affecting the kidneys or other organ systems (52). The concomitant use of trimethoprim-sulfamethoxazole and methotrexate is contraindicated because it may result in severe bone marrow toxicity.

In an effort to limit the exposure to cytotoxic agents, a number of immunomodulatory drugs and antibodies are being evaluated for the treatment of patients with recurrent vasculitis. The various studies can conceptually be divided into two categories: studies aimed at treating patients who are resistant to conventional treatment with cyclophosphamide and corticosteroids, and studies aimed at the prevention of relapse. Table 68-9 summarizes various "novel" therapies that have been or are being evaluated. The efficacy of any such agents is currently

TABLE 68-9

A SUMMARY OF VARIOUS "NOVEL" THERAPIES THAT HAVE BEEN OR ARE BEING EVALUATED IN THE TREATMENT OF ANCA-ASSOCIATED SMALL-VESSEL VASCULITIS AND GLOMERULONEPHRITIS

Therapy	Possible role	References
Plasmapheresis	Adjunctive therapy in patients with pulmonary hemorrhage or advanced renal disease	Gaskin 2001(266); Frasca 1992, 1993(267,268); Pusey 1991(145); Zauner 2002(269); Klemmer 2003(142); Cole 1992(144)
Intravenous Immunoglobulin	Adjunctive therapy in patients with persistent disease on standard therapy	Jayne et al. (155)
Methotrexate	Alternative to cyclophosphamide in patients with 'early disease' and without significant renal or pulmonary disease.	Sneller 1995(148); Langford 2000(270); DeGroot 2005(150)
	Prevention of relapse?	Isaacs 1996(161), Booth 2002(167), Stegeman 1997(271)
Azathioprine	Prevention of relapse?	Jayne 2003(147)
Mycophenolate mofetil	Prevention of relapse?	Nowack 1999(170); Langford 2004(272)
Leflunomide	Prevention of relapse?	Metzler 2004(273).
Rituximab	Adjunctive therapy for cyclophosphamide-resistant or relapsing patients?	Specks 2001(274), Keogh 2005(156); Eriksson 2005(157)
Infliximab	Adjunctive therapy for cyclophosphamide-resistant or relapsing patients?	Lamprecht 2002(164); Bartolucci 2002(165); Booth 2004(166); D'Haens 1999(275)
Alemtuzumab	Adjunctive therapy for cyclophosphamide-resistant or relapsing patients?	Kirk 2003(160)
Etanercept	Shown NOT to be efficacious in the prevention of relapse	WGET(276)
Trimethoprim-sulfamethoxazole	Prevention of relapses that affect the upper respiratory tract.	DeRemee 1985(277), Reinhold-Keller 1996(278); Stegeman 1996(53)

not established, and they should not be considered as first-line therapies.

Potential Adjunctive Treatment for Patients with Resistant Disease or Contraindications to Conventional Therapy

Several agents have been evaluated as adjunctive therapy for patients with resistant forms of ANCA vasculitis. Adjunctive therapy with intravenous immunoglobulin (IVIg) (single course of a total of 2 gm/kg) was evaluated in a randomized controlled trial in patients with persistently active ANCA vasculitis despite conventional therapy. Patients treated with IVIg experienced a more rapid decline in disease activity (as measured by a 50% reduction in Birmingham Vasculitis Activity Score [BVAS]) and C-reactive protein at 1 and 3 months, but there was no significant difference between the two groups after 3 months with respect to disease activity or frequency of relapse (155).

Rituximab, a chimeric monoclonal antibody directed against the CD20 antigen, effectively depletes B lymphocytes, but not plasma cells. Preliminary evidence indicates that rituximab may have a role in the management of ANCA-associated vasculitis that is resistant to or relapsing after standard therapy based on small, uncontrolled case series (156–158). In these studies, the use of rituximab (375mg/m^2 IV weekly × 4 or 500 mg IV weekly × 4 fixed doses) in conjunction with corticosteroids, resulted in remission in the majority of patients and was generally well tolerated. In contrast, in a fourth open label study of 8 patients with severe, refractory Wegener's granulomatosis, the addition of rituximab (375mg/m2 every four weeks × 4 doses) to cyclophosphamide, mycophenolate mofetil or methotrexate was associated with limited benefit (159). The use of rituximab as induction therapy is currently compared to cyclophosphamide in an ongoing multicenter, randomized controlled trial.

Alemtuzumab (Campath-1H) is a humanized monoclonal IgG1 antibody directed against the CD52 antigen expressed on the surface of peripheral blood lymphocytes, monocytes and macrophages (160). Treatment with alemtuzumab results in complement-mediated lysis, antibody-dependent cellular cytotoxicity and induction of apoptosis of target cells and results in depletion of T cells and B cells (161). Alemtuzumab has been used to treat a select group of patients with refractory or relapsing autoimmune diseases, including 70 patients with ANCA-associated vasculitis (162). These patients received at least one course of 135 mg intravenous alemtuzumab over 5 days. Remission was achieved by 83% of surviving patients. Unfortunately, this treatment regimen was associated with high rates of serious infections and death (18% at 1 year) and a 43% rate of relapse.

Similarly, the chimeric monoclonal antibody directed against TNF-α (163) Infliximab was been evaluated in four open-label uncontrolled trials of small numbers of patients (164–167). In these studies, the treatment regimen included infliximab plus corticosteroids, and either cyclophosphamide or other immunosuppressive agents. In the largest of these trials, which included 32 patients with acute or resistant disease, infliximab was associated with a remission rate of 88% and a relapse rate of 20% (166). These promising results are mitigated, however, by an elevated rate of serious infectious complications.

The immunosuppressant, 15-Deoxyspergualin, used in Japan for the treatment of steroid-resistant renal transplant rejection, was also evaluated for the treatment of refractory Wegener's granulomatosis in a small uncontrolled trial (168).

Potential Agents for the Prevention of Relapse

Preliminary small-scale pilot studies suggest that mycophenolate mofetil may have a role in the treatment of mild or moderate ANCA-associated small-vessel vasculitis (169) or as "maintenance" therapy to prevent relapse (170). Currently there are not sufficient data to support its use in the treatment of life- or organ-threatening disease or as a first-line drug. The efficacy and safety of the TNF receptor–Fc fusion protein etanercept (171) in the treatment of patients with ANCA-associated vasculitis was compared in a controlled trial to that of the traditional regimen of daily oral cyclophosphamide or methotrexate and corticosteroids. Although the rate of remission was comparable in the two treatment groups, patients treated with etanercept had a higher rate of solid tumors (172).

RENAL TRANSPLANTATION

Renal transplantation has been recognized as an option of renal replacement therapy in patients with ANCA-associated Wegener's granulomatosis, MPA, or necrotizing crescentic glomerulonephritis. Successful renal transplantation in patients with ANCA-associated small-vessel vasculitis has been reported in patients who were in full remission and with negative ANCA test results, in patients with positive ANCA test results (173–175), and even in patients with evidence of active vasculitis at the time of transplantation (176). Recurrent disease after transplantation has also been described as occurring as early as a few days posttransplantation (177) and as late as several years posttransplantation (178). Just as with the initial ANCA-associated small-vessel vasculitis, reported recurrences after transplantation involve a spectrum of various organs and are not limited to the transplanted kidney (179).

Based on a pooled analysis (180), ANCA-associated small-vessel vasculitis recurs in about 19% of all patients, with an average time from transplantation to relapse of 31 months. The presence of ANCA at transplantation does not appear to increase the rate of relapse posttransplantation. Therapy with cyclosporine does not appear to have a significant protective effect on recurrent ANCA-associated small-vessel vasculitis over that afforded by other immunosuppressant regimens (corticosteroids and azathioprine). The evaluation of the role of mycophenolate mofetil in the treatment of ANCA-associated vasculitis is in its infancy, and it remains to be seen whether this drug will reduce the incidence of recurrent disease posttransplantation. Patients with Wegener's granulomatosis had a relative risk of relapse of 2.75 when compared with patients with MPA or necrotizing crescentic glomerulonephritis alone. Conversely, ANCA pattern (c-ANCA or p-ANCA) or antigen specificity (PR3 or MPO) was not associated with differences in relapse rate posttransplantation.

A review of the reports of recurrent ANCA-associated small-vessel vasculitis posttransplantation reveal a good response to cyclophosphamide in the treatment of relapsing disease, although recurrent disease can lead to graft loss and even patient death (181).

In summary, renal transplantation is a beneficial option in the management of patients with ANCA-associated small-vessel vasculitis and end-stage renal disease. Although the presence of circulating ANCA is not a sufficient contraindication to transplantation, it is current practice not to perform transplantation in patients with active vasculitis, but to delay surgery until the disease is in remission. No data are currently available about the need to wait a certain period of time after remission is attained and before proceeding to transplantation.

POLYARTERITIS NODOSA

Clinical Features

Patients with polyarteritis nodosa typically have constitutional symptoms, including fever and weight loss. The presence of mononeuritis multiplex, myalgias, and arthralgias, as well as nodular skin lesions in half of patients, characterize the disease. Vasculitis of the coronary arteries may lead to cardiac symptoms. The renal disease seen in polyarteritis nodosa is primarily related to vasculitis of the renal arteries resulting in renovascular hypertension and/or renal parenchymal infarction. Patients with polyarteritis nodosa do not have evidence of small-vessel vasculitis, glomerulonephritis, or pulmonary capillaritis. In fact, the lung is rarely injured in polyarteritis nodosa, in contrast to the frequency of pulmonary disease in patients with Wegener's syndrome, MPA, or CSS (182). Although not distinguishing features, gastrointestinal complaints and peripheral neuropathy are more common among patients with polyarteritis nodosa than patients with MPA (182). The prognosis of polyarteritis is really a reflection of the involvement of kidneys, heart, central nervous system, or gastrointestinal tract (183,184).

Pathogenesis

The etiology of polyarteritis nodosa remains unclear, and most cases of polyarteritis nodosa are probably idiopathic. An association between polyarteritis nodosa and hepatitis B infection is evident by the fact that patients with hepatitis B antigenemia are at greater risk of developing polyarteritis nodosa. However, the incidence of polyarteritis nodosa among these patients varies in different populations worldwide (185–187). A role for hepatitis B antigenemia in the pathogenesis of polyarteritis nodosa is further suggested by reports of vasculitis after hepatitis B vaccination (188). Furthermore, treatment with antiviral agents and plasma exchange has led to resolution of the vasculitis in patients whose serology converts from being positive for the HBe or HBs antigens to the corresponding antibodies (189,190).

Polyarteritis nodosa has been associated with a number of cancers, especially hairy cell leukemia (191–194). Treatment of hairy cell leukemia with interferon-alpha (INF-α) may be associated with resolution of polyarteritis nodosa (195). As opposed to patients with small-vessel vasculitis, patients with polyarteritis nodosa are ANCA-negative (182).

Renal Manifestations

Both polyarteritis nodosa and Kawasaki's disease are medium-sized vessel vasculitides that affect the kidney. These arteritides result in necrotizing lesions in the major renal arteries and aneurysm formation with thrombosis and renal infarction. The aneurysms are not true aneurysms but pseudoaneurysms. The arteritis of Kawasaki's disease most commonly involves the coronary arteries, but in at least 25% of patients the lesions also involve the kidney. Kawasaki's disease is distinguished from polyarteritis nodosa by the pathognomonic *sine qua non* feature of mucocutaneous lymph node syndrome. Renal arterial involvement by polyarteritis nodosa, including interlobar and arcuate arteries, results in renal ischemia, infarction, and hemorrhage. One of the most painful and catastrophic consequence of this disease is rupture of an arterial pseudoaneurysm that causes retroperitoneal and sometimes intraperitoneal hemorrhage.

Treatment

The treatment of classic polyarteritis nodosa has been based on the use of high-dose corticosteroids with the addition, in moderate to severe or organ-threatening cases, of cyclophosphamide. Unfortunately, most studies pertinent to the treatment of polyarteritis nodosa antedate the 1994 Chapel Hill consensus conference, which classified MPA among the small-vessel vasculitides separate from classic polyarteritis nodosa. Consequently, most of the older studies and reports include a substantial number of patients who would now be diagnosed with MPA and not classic polyarteritis nodosa. As a result of the consensus conference, the incidence of classic polyarteritis nodosa involving medium-sized vessels alone and without evidence for glomerulonephritis is very low and is not readily amenable to large-scale evaluation of various therapies. The problem is compounded by the relatively recent recognition of the association of polyarteritis nodosa with hepatitis B virus (HBV) infection in a subset of patients with polyarteritis nodosa that varies from 10% to 50%, depending on the population studied.

In the absence of HBV infection, the mainstay of treatment of classic polyarteritis nodosa continues to rest on the use of high doses of corticosteroids. Typically, prednisone is initiated at a dosage of 1 mg/kg per day for the first month. Over the course of the second month, the dosage is tapered to an alternate-day regimen so that the patient is receiving 1 mg/kg every other day by the end of the second month. It is subsequently tapered slowly by 5 mg per day weekly as tolerated. The addition of an alkylating agent such as cyclophosphamide in the treatment of polyarteritis nodosa is not as well established as in the treatment of MPA or Wegener's granulomatosis, although some studies report improved patient survival when immunosuppressive drugs were added (196). In another study, the addition of cyclophosphamide to corticosteroids and plasma exchange led to decreased relapse in the cyclophosphamide-treated group, but no improvement in the 10-year survival rate (197). The beneficial effects of cyclophosphamide were also demonstrated when this drug was added to the corticosteroid regimen of patients who failed to respond to corticosteroids alone (198). No randomized study exists to critically assess the value of a daily oral regimen of cyclophosphamide compared with pulse cyclophosphamide in the outcome of patients with classic polyarteritis nodosa. Plasma exchange does not seem to improve the outcome, decrease relapse, or improve long-term survival of patients with polyarteritis nodosa not associated with HBV (199).

In current practice, cyclophosphamide should be reserved for patients with severe or organ-threatening disease, patients with disease that fails to respond to treatment with corticosteroids alone, patients who require unacceptably high doses of corticosteroids, or patients who are intolerant to corticosteroid side effects (200). Although azathioprine has been used in the treatment of classic polyarteritis nodosa, this agent is better reserved for maintenance therapy or as a steroid-sparing agent. The successful use of infliximab in PAN resistant to "conventional therapy" has been reported in a small number of cases (201,202).

In the setting of HBV-associated polyarteritis nodosa, treatment with immunosuppression consisting of corticosteroids with or without cyclophosphamide is thought to be deleterious because it facilitates viral replication, delays the development of protective anti–hepatitis B antibodies, and may lead to an aggravation of hepatic involvement (203). For this reason, it has been advocated that only a short course of corticosteroids (1 mg/kg per day) be used for 1 week, followed by a rapid taper over the following week. The prompt institution of antiviral therapy may ameliorate the vascular inflammation.

Treatment with plasma exchange has been advocated to clear circulating immune complexes thought to be important in the pathogenesis of this disease (204), although no controlled trial has critically assessed the need for plasmapheresis. The antiviral agents used have included vidarabine, INF-α-2b, or more recently combination therapy of INF-α-2b in addition to lamivudine (205) or famciclovir (190). No large-scale trials of antiviral therapy are available to critically assess the efficacy of these combinations in patients with HBV-related polyarteritis nodosa. Current work in the treatment of chronic HBV is focusing on the use of INF-α-2b, modified purine analogs such as famciclovir or L-stereoisomers of pyrimidine derivatives such as lamivudine (206). In an uncontrolled study, the combination of a short course of corticosteroids followed by a 6-month course of lamivudine and scheduled plasma exchange (until hepatitis B antigen or anti-HBe antibody seroconversion) resulted in a clinical remission of the vasculitis (207). In a recent retrospective analysis of 115 patients with HBV-associated polyarteritis nodosa (according to the Chapel Hill nomenclature) followed by the French Vasculitis Study Group between 1972 and 2002, the overall remission rate was 80.9% with a subsequent overall 9.7% relapse rate (208). The rates of relapse or death were not significantly different among patients treated with antiviral agents (vidarabine, INF-α, or lamivudine) (n = 80) when compared to patients treated with corticosteroids alone, or with cyclophosphamide, or plasma exchanges (n = 35) (5% vs. 14.3% relapse; and 30% vs. 48.6% death, respectively). However, the use of antiviral agents has led to a significantly higher rate of seroconversions from HBeAg to anti-HBeAb (49.4% vs. 14.7%; p <0.001). Such seroconversion was associated with a clinical remission and absence of relapse.

Outcome

Most studies examining patient outcome and predictors of patient survival in polyarteritis nodosa antedate the Chapel Hill consensus conference of 1994. These studies are based on cohorts of patients that include those with MPA, CSS, and hepatitis B–associated classic polyarteritis nodosa. Earlier studies report a 5-year survival rate of approximately 55% in patients primarily treated with corticosteroids alone (209). The addition of cyclophosphamide or immunosuppressive therapy to glucocorticoids seems to have improved the 5-year survival rate to about 80%. Patients with bowel infarction, serious gastrointestinal bleeding, or renal insufficiency had particularly poor prognosis. In a more recent prospective study including 342 patients, of whom 119 had classic polyarteritis nodosa without HBV (89 patients with HBV, 52 patients with MPA, 82 patients with CSS) (183), proteinuria of 10 g per day, renal insufficiency, and gastrointestinal tract involvement were the major prognostic markers for a worse outcome.

BEHÇET'S DISEASE

Behçet's disease is a systemic vasculitic syndrome classically characterized by a triad of recurrent oral ulcerations, genital ulcerations, and ocular lesions usually consisting of uveitis, iritis, or retinal vasculitis. Behçet's disease can present with protean manifestations with multiple organ involvement, either concomitantly or consecutively. Other organ system involvement includes the skin, musculoskeletal system with arthralgias and myalgias, central nervous system, and lungs, and gastrointestinal, cardiac, and genitourinary systems. Vascular involvement may affect large blood vessels, capillaries, venules, and veins. The diagnosis of Behçet's disease is based on an established set of criteria (210). The criteria include the presence of oral ulcerations, and two or more of the following: recurrent genital ulcerations, eye lesions, skin lesions, and positive pathergy test results. The latter test represents a nonspecific skin hyperreactivity induced by intradermal needle prick (211).

Epidemiology

Although Behçet's disease has been reported worldwide, the highest incidence of disease appears to be in Japan, the Middle East, and around the Mediterranean basin. The incidence ranges from 1 to 2 per 10,000 in Japan and Saudi Arabia to as low as 0.3 per 100,000 in Northern Europe. The peak age of onset is within the third decade, and there is a male preponderance in most published case series. Men are also reported to have more severe disease than women.

Pathogenesis

The etiology of Behçet's disease remains unknown. Associations with infectious agents such as herpes simplex virus I, *Streptococcus sanguis*, parvovirus B19, and *Mycobacterium tuberculosis* have been hypothesized and evaluated to various degrees. However, no direct link has been convincingly established. Human leukocyte antigen (HLA) typing reveals a close association between Behçet's disease and HLA-B51 (especially the allelic variants HLA-B*5101) (212) and HLA-B*5108 and HLA-B*57 among Caucasians (213). Other studies point to an association with a microsatellite located between the HLA-B locus and the TNF gene rather than an association with the HLA-B*51 gene itself (214). Therefore, the TNF promoter allele TNF-1031 was found to be independently associated with susceptibility to Behçet's disease among Caucasians (213). The presence of antibodies to a number of autoantigens such as alpha-tropomyosin (215) has been described. The role of such autoantibodies in the pathogenesis of the disease is unclear. Similarly, T cells are likely involved in the pathogenesis of Behçet's disease as evidenced by an increase in γδT cells (216), a predominance of Th1 cell phenotype (217) and autoreactive T cells (218).

Renal Involvement

Renal involvement in Behçet's disease appears to be more frequent than previously recognized. The spectrum of involvement ranges from subtle urinary abnormalities to end-stage renal disease and can conceptually be divided into five categories: (i) glomerulonephritis, (ii) amyloidosis, (iii) renal vascular involvement, (iv) interstitial nephritis, and (v) other problems, such as complications of drug therapy or genitourinary system abnormalities (219). The nephrotic syndrome and renal failure occurring in the setting of Behçet's disease can be associated with the presence of AA amyloidosis more typically found in patients with long-standing disease (220). Based on an extensive review of the published case reports (totaling 159 patients), amyloidosis was the most commonly reported lesion (43% of cases), whereas glomerulonephritis accounted for 32% of cases (219). Although an early study reported the presence of hematuria, proteinuria, or both in about one-third of patients (221), a recent extensive retrospective review of more than 4200 cases identified such urinary abnormalities in about 11% of patients tested and documented glomerulonephritis in only 7 (0.16%) patients (222). The pathologic lesions associated with Behçet's disease include focal and diffuse proliferative glomerulonephritis, membranoproliferative glomerulonephritis, focal segmental necrotizing glomerulonephritis with crescents, and minimal change disease. In Benekli's review, predominant IgA deposits are reported in 11 of 40 cases of glomerulonephritis associated with Behçet's disease. The report of several cases of focal segmental necrotizing and crescentic glomerulonephritis (223,224) in the absence of immune complex deposition raises the question of an association with ANCA. The presence of such autoantibodies has been reported in rare cases (225), but not in systematic screening of patients with Behçet's disease (226).

Treatment

A number of immunomodulatory and immunosuppressant agents are used in the treatment of Behçet's disease. These include corticosteroids, calcineurin inhibitor, azathioprine, and interferon-alpha (227,228). More recently the use of agents that block the TNF pathway has also been reported (229). Because of the rarity of glomerular involvement in Behçet's disease, no definitive data for treatment are available. The use of corticosteroids has been reported with variable outcomes. In cases of Behçet's disease with severe vasculitic disease or glomerulonephritis, the use of corticosteroids and immunosuppressive therapy with azathioprine or cyclophosphamide may be justified.

TAKAYASU'S ARTERITIS AND TEMPORAL (GIANT CELL) ARTERITIS

Aortitis is a common feature of Takayasu's and giant cell arteritis but is also associated with other vasculitides such as syphilis, tuberculosis, mycosis, Behçet's disease, and Kawasaki's disease. The most commonly involved vessels are the subclavian arteries in more than 90% of patients. Diagnostic differentiation between Takayasu's and giant cell arteritis is largely based on age, with patients younger than 40 years having Takayasu's arteritis and those older than 50 having giant cell arteritis. Aortic aneurysm rupture represents a morbid complication of giant cell arteritis. Aortitis may result in ischemic symptoms or infarction of the area supplied by the involved vessel. Asymptomatic aortitis may be a more common phenomenon than previously thought (230).

Laboratory Findings

Laboratory findings in large-vessel vasculitis include a mild anemia, elevated levels of C-reactive protein, elevated erythrocyte sedimentation rate, and a generalized elevation in γ-globulin levels. Other serologic study results, including those from tests for lupus and infections, are typically negative. Patients typically present with only mild proteinuria and hematuria. The most common presentation is associated with hypertension and renal insufficiency, whereas renal failure is uncommon.

Pathogenesis

The pathogenesis of giant cell and Takayasu's arteritis is not known. However, there are several tantalizing clues that infectious agents may play a role in these diseases. In animals, there is evidence that gamma herpes virus 68 causes arteritis in mice lacking the interferon-γ receptor. In humans, an association exists between giant cell arteritis and parvovirus B19 infection (231). However a recent study using polymerase chain reaction

(PCR) and immunohistochemistry techniques on 147 temporal artery biopsies found no evidence of parvovirus B19 DNA in the arteries of patients with giant cell arteritis (232). A cyclic occurrence of disease, with a peak incidence occurring every 5 to 7 years, suggests an infectious cycle. Certain genetic factors are associated with the development of giant cell arteritis. This form of vasculitis is more common in individuals of Northern European descent living in Europe or the United States (233), and there is clustering of cases among families (234). The development of giant cell arteritis also correlates with the expression of HLA-DR4, which is also found in high frequency among patients with polymyalgia rheumatica (235).

Giant cell arteritis may be a consequence of either or both the humoral and cellular immune responses. The clinical and experimental findings suggest that a cell-mediated process is most likely (236). Most inflammatory cells that invade the vessel walls are CD4-positive T cells. Elevated levels of IL-6 correlate with the severity of the disease and decrease quite rapidly when glucocorticoids are administered (237). Levels of several other cytokines and chemokines are similarly elevated. It is hypothesized that activated monocytes infiltrate the adventitia of large vessel walls via the vasa vasorum and become macrophages that then produce interferon-γ and recruit additional leukocytes, including macrophages. Unfortunately, the antigen responsible for these interactions has yet to be elucidated.

Renal Involvement

Renal involvement in Takayasu's arteritis and giant cell arteritis is usually a consequence of inflammation and scarring of the aorta adjacent to the orifice of the renal artery, leading to stenosis of the renal artery and ischemic renal failure. One of the most common clinical presentations of this phenomenon is renovascular hypertension affecting more than 50% of patients with Takayasu's arteritis (238). In Japan, Takayasu's arteritis is an important cause of hypertension in adolescents.

Glomerular lesions and necrosis occurs in patients with large-vessel vasculitis, but this may be an overlap of a small-vessel vasculitis. Several cases of glomerulonephritis in the setting of Takayasu's arteritis have been reported in the literature. The renal pathology in these cases varies from case to case, including focal segmental sclerosis (239), mesangial proliferation (240), membranoproliferative lesions (241), and crescentic lesions (242).

Treatment

The cornerstone of treatment of giant cell arteritis is based on the use of high-dose corticosteroids. Several guidelines or recommendations have been published. Typically, prednisone is started at 1 to 1.5 mg/kg per day, until the erythrocyte sedimentation rate is normal and the patient is asymptomatic. Initial treatment on an alternate-day basis is ineffective in the treatment of giant cell arteritis. When compared with patients receiving daily corticosteroids, only 30% (versus 85%) of patients treated with an alternate-day dosing enter an early remission, and 75% (versus 15%) experience a flare of disease activity (243). Intravenous pulses of methylprednisolone (1 g per day for 3 to 5 days) is recommended for patients with severe visual loss, because this treatment seems to prevent additional visual loss or fellow-eye involvement after initiation of corticosteroids (244). The initiation of corticosteroids within 2 weeks before a temporal artery biopsy does not change the characteristic pathologic findings (245,246). A delay in treatment to obtain a temporal artery biopsy is therefore not warranted.

Once a clinical remission is attained, a subsequent slow taper of corticosteroids is undertaken by decreasing the dose by 10% every 2 weeks to a dose of 10 mg per day, then by 1 mg per day. Other similar tapering protocols have been suggested, but no critical assessment of these recommendations is available. A switch to an alternate-day regimen may be similarly efficacious and perhaps less toxic (247). Symptoms usually resolve within 2 to 3 days and the erythrocyte sedimentation rate usually normalizes within 4 to 6 weeks. Most patients with giant cell arteritis require 2 years of corticosteroids, and a few remain on a low-dose regimen indefinitely. Patients who continue to require "maintenance" dosages of more than 15 mg per day may be considered "steroid resistant."

The high rate of complications attributable to the prolonged duration of corticosteroid therapy and the age distribution of patients with giant cell arteritis has led to an interest in identifying steroid-sparing alternative drugs. Dapsone, azathioprine, cyclosporine, antimalarials, cyclophosphamide, or gold have not been found to reduce corticosteroid toxicity and still maintain therapeutic effectiveness (248). The reported beneficial effect on the rate of relapse of adding methotrexate to corticosteroids (249), was not confirmed by a multicenter, placebo-controlled trial (250). A retrospective study suggests that the concomitant use of low-dose aspirin decreases the rate of visual loss and cerebrovascular events in patients with giant cell arteritis (251). Information on the use of TNF-alpha-blocking agents in the treatment of giant cell arteritis is currently limited to very small case series (252–254).

The treatment of Takayasu's arteritis is similarly based on high-dose corticosteroids. In a National Institutes of Health study, treatment was initiated at 1 mg/kg (up to 60 mg per day) for 1 to 3 months, followed by a slow taper to an alternate-day regimen over the following 4 to 8 weeks, and a subsequent slow taper over the following 6 to 12 months. This regimen is associated with a remission rate of 60% and an estimated median time to remission of 22 months (238).

Unfortunately, relapses occur in as much as 45% of patients, leading to multiple or prolonged courses of corticosteroids. Up to 40% of patients require the addition of cytotoxic drugs such as cyclophosphamide or methotrexate. In an open-label study of 18 patients with persistent or refractory Takayasu's arteritis despite treatment with corticosteroids alone, the use of methotrexate was associated with an 81% remission rate (255). Fifty percent of patients achieved a corticosteroid-free remission on methotrexate, and half of these patients remained in remission after methotrexate was withdrawn. About 20% of patients did not attain remission despite corticosteroids and methotrexate. The successful use of infliximab has been reported in several case reports of patients with active Takayasu arteritis despite conventional therapy with corticosteroids and cyclophosphamide (256) or methotrexate (257). The use of anti-TNF therapy was assessed in a pilot, open-label trial involving a total of 15 patients with active, relapsing Takayasu's arteritis. Seven patients were initially treated with etanercept and eight with infliximab. The use of anti-TNF agents led to remission in 10 of the 15 patients that was sustained for 1 to 3.3 years without glucocorticoid therapy. Four patients achieved partial remission, with a >50% reduction in the glucocorticoid requirement. Two relapses occurred during periods when etanercept was interrupted, but remission was reestablished upon reinstitution of therapy (258).

The optimal treatment of patients with Takayasu's arteritis is further complicated by the results of biopsies of affected vessels obtained at the time of bypass surgery. These data revealed evidence of persistent vascular inflammation even in the absence of clinical signs or symptoms of active disease and in the setting of a normal erythrocyte sedimentation rate (238,259,260).

The diagnosis and treatment of hypertension represents a very important aspect of the care of patients with Takayasu's arteritis because congestive heart failure, ischemic or hemorrhagic stroke, and renal failure account for most of the deaths from this disease (261). The diagnosis of hypertension may be missed if it is based on measurement of blood pressure in the upper extremities alone, because of the high incidence of subclavian artery stenoses, which may be bilateral. In some cases, lesions in the thoracic or abdominal aorta or the iliac or femoral arteries may give misleading normal blood pressures in the lower extremities as well. It is thus recommended that arteriographic studies be performed with pressure transducers so that aortic pressures can be compared with extremity pressures, and to identify the extremity where blood pressure monitoring is most reliable and reflective of true blood pressure (261).

THERAPEUTIC CONSIDERATIONS COMMON TO ALL VASCULITIC SYNDROMES

As the mainstay of therapy of severe vasculitis remains based on corticosteroids and alkylating agents, it is associated with short- and long-term complications. The most prominent side effects of this form of therapy are infection, ovarian failure (especially with a prolonged course of cyclophosphamide), bone disease, and cataract formation. In addition, the prolonged use of cyclophosphamide is associated with a 15% risk of developing a transitional cell carcinoma of the bladder over the course of 5 to 10 years (214). Whether the use of monthly pulse intravenous cyclophosphamide (which is associated with a smaller incidence cumulative dose and a lower incidence of hemorrhagic cystitis) can reduce the rate of bladder cancer is not yet ascertained.

The institution of attentive supportive care is crucial in minimizing the short- and long-term complications. Compulsive attention must be paid to the early detection and aggressive treatment of infections, because they remain an important cause of morbidity and death (262). Whenever possible, the use of trimethoprim-sulfamethoxazole for the prevention of *Pneumocystis carinii* pneumonia should be considered.

Whenever corticosteroids are used, measures must be taken to minimize the development of osteoporosis (263). Specific recommendations include calcium (1.2 g per day) and vitamin D supplementation, and, in selected patients with established osteoporosis, calcitonin nasal spray or alendronate for patients in whom the drug is not contraindicated (e.g., azotemia or esophagitis). Rigorous control of blood pressure with sodium restriction and antihypertensive therapy is essential to minimize the additive effect of hypertension in loss of renal function after active nephritis. Current research directions include the preservation of gonadal function by hormonal manipulation during cytotoxic therapy. In a small study, the use of testosterone during cyclophosphamide treatment appeared to prevent azoospermia (264). The gonadotropin-releasing hormone agonist leuprolide appears to be effective in the prevention of cyclophosphamide-induced ovarian failure based on a small prospective uncontrolled trial of patients with lupus nephritis (265).

References

1. Jennette JC, Falk RJ, Andrassy K, et al. Nomenclature of systemic vasculitides: proposal of an international consensus conference. *Arthritis Rheum* 1994;37(2):187.
2. Churg J. Large vessel vasculitis. *Clin Exp Immunol* 1993;93(Suppl 1):11.

3. Savory WS. Case of a young woman in whom the main arteries of both upper extremities and of the left side of the neck were throughout completely obliterated. *Med Chir Trans Lond* 1856;39:205.

4. Takayasu M. Case with unusual changes of the central vessels in the retina. *Acta Soc Opthamology* 1908;12:554.

5. Arend WP, Michel BA, Bloch DA, et al. The American College of Rheumatology 1990 criteria for the classification of Takayasu arteritis. *Arthritis Rheum* 1990;33(8):1129.

6. Lie JT. Takayasu arteritis. In: Churg A, Churg J, eds, *Systemic Vasculitides*. New York: Igaku-Shoin, 1991:159.

7. Lupi-Herrera E, Sanchez-Torres G, Marcushamer J, et al. Takayasu's arteritis: clinical study of 107 cases. *Am Heart J* 1977;93(1):94.

8. Hamilton CR, Jr, Shelley WM, Tumulty PA. Giant cell arteritis: including temporal arteritis and polymyalgia rheumatica. *Medicine (Baltimore)* 197150(1):1.

9. Hunder GG, Bloch DA, Michel BA, et al. The American College of Rheumatology 1990 criteria for the classification of giant cell arteritis. *Arthritis Rheum* 1990;33(8):1122.

10. Hutchinson J. Diseases of the arteries: on a peculiar form of thrombotic arteries of the aged which is sometimes productive of gangrene. *Arch Surg* 1890;1:323.

11. Jennette JC, Falk RJ. Small-vessel vasculitis (see comments). *N Engl J Med* 1997; 337(21):1512.

12. Kussmaul A, Maier R. Uber eine bisher nicht beschreibene eigenthumliche Arterienerkrankung (Periarteritis nodosa), die mit Morbus Brightii und rapid fortschreitender allgemeiner Muskellahmung einhergeht. *Dtsch Arch Klin Med* 1866;1:484.

13. Ferrari E. Ueber Polyarteritis actua nodosa (sogenannte Periarteriitis nodosa), und ihre Beziehungen zur Polymyositis and Polyneuritis acuta. 1903;34:350.

14. Arnaout MA. A clinical and pathological study of periarteritis nodosa: a report of five cases, one histologically healed. *Am J Pathol* 1930;6:426.

15. Zeek PM, Smithh CC, Weeter JC. Studies on periarteritis nodosa. III: the differentiation between the vascular lesions of periarteritis nodosa and of hypersensitivity. *Am J Pathol* 1948;24:889.

16. Zeek PM. Periarteritis nodosa: a critical review. *Am J Clin Pathol* 1952; 22:777.

17. Godman GC, Churg J. Wegener's granulomatosis: pathology and review of the literature. *Arch Pathol Lab Med* 1954;58:533.

18. Guillevin L, Lhote F, Amouroux J, et al. Antineutrophil cytoplasmic antibodies, abnormal angiograms and pathological findings in polyarteritis nodosa and Churg-Strauss syndrome: indications for the classification of vasculitides of the polyarteritis Nodosa Group. *Br J Rheumatol* 1996;35(10):958.

19. Kirkland GS, Savige J, Wilson D, et al. Classical polyarteritis nodosa and microscopic polyarteritis with medium vessel involvement: a comparison of the clinical and laboratory features. *Clin Nephrol* 1997;47(3):176.

20. Jennette JC, Falk RJ. Anti-neutrophil cytoplasmic autoantibodies: discovery, specificity, disease associations and pathogenic potential. *Adv Pathol Lab Med* 1995;8:363.

21. Kallenberg CG, Brouwer E, Weening JJ, et al. Anti-neutrophil cytoplasmic antibodies: current diagnostic and pathophysiological potential. *Kidney Int* 1994;46(1):1.

22. Bell DM, Brink EW, Nitzkin JL, et al. Kawasaki syndrome: description of two outbreaks in the United States. *N Engl J Med* 1981;304(26):1568.

23. Gribetz D, Landing B, Larson E. Kawasaki disease: mucocutaneous lymph node syndrome (MCLNS). In: Churg A, Churg J, eds. *Systemic Vasculitides*. New York: Igaku-Shoin; 1991:257.

24. Naoe S, Takahashi K, Masuda H, et al. Kawasaki disease: with particular emphasis on arterial lesions. *Acta Pathol Jpn* 1991;41(11):785.

25. Rauch AM, Hurwitz ES. Centers for Disease Control (CDC) case definition for Kawasaki syndrome (letter). *Pediatr Infect Dis* 1985;4(6):702.

26. Tanaka N, Naoe S, Kawasaki T. Pathological study on autopsy cases of mucocutaneous lymph node syndrome. *J Jap Red Cross Cent Hosp* 1971;2:85.

27. Nagashima M, Matsushima M, Matsuoka H, et al. High-dose gammaglobulin therapy for Kawasaki disease. *J Pediatr* 1987;110(5):710.

28. Tanemoto M, Miyakawa H, Hanai J, et al. Myeloperoxidase-antineutrophil cytoplasmic antibody-positive crescentic glomerulonephritis complicating the course of Graves' disease: report of three adult cases. *Am J Kidney Dis* 1995;26(5):774.

29. Newburger JW, Takahashi M, Burns JC, et al. The treatment of Kawasaki syndrome with intravenous gamma globulin. *N Engl J Med* 1986;315(6):341.

30. Rowley AH, Duffy CE, Shulman ST. Prevention of giant coronary artery aneurisms in Kawasaki disease by intravenous gamma globulin therapy (see comments). *J Pediatr* 1988;113(2):290.

31. Fujiwara H, Hamashima Y. Pathology of the heart in Kawasaki disease. *Pediatrics* 1978;61(1):100.

32. Jennette JC, Falk RJ. The pathology of vasculitis involving the kidney. *Am J Kidney Dis* 1994;24(1):130.

33. Ronco P, Mougenot B, Bindi P, et al. "Idiopathic" extracapillary glomerulonephratides without immune deposits are vascularities: clinical and serologic analysis. *Bull Acad Natl Med* 1993;177:481.

34. Savage CO, Winearls CG, Evans DJ, et al. Microscopic polyarteritis: presentation, pathology and prognosis. *Q J Med* 1985;56(220):467.

35. Croker BP, Lee T, Gunnells JC. Clinical and pathologic features of polyarteritis nodosa and its renal-limited variant: primary crescentic and necrotizing glomerulonephritis. *Hum Pathol* 1987;18(1):38.

36. Stilmant MM, Bolton WK, Sturgill BC, et al. Crescentic glomerulonephritis without immune deposits: clinicopathologic features. *Kidney Int* 1979; 15(2):184.

37. Cameron JS. Renal vasculitis: microscopic polyarteritis and Wegener's granuloma. *Contrib Nephrol* 1991;94:38.

38. D'Amico G, Sinico RA, Ferrario F. Renal vasculitis. *Nephrol Dial Transplant* 1996;11(Suppl 9):69.

39. Churg J, Strauss L. Allergic granulomatosis, allergic angiitis and periarteritis nodosa. *Am J Pathol* 1951;27:277.

40. Jennette JC, Wilkman AS, Falk RJ. Anti-neutrophil cytoplasmic autoantibody-associated glomerulonephritis and vasculitis. *Am J Pathol* 1989; 135(5):921.

41. Hagen EC, Daha MR, Hermans J, et al. Diagnostic value of standardized assays for anti-neutrophil cytoplasmic antibodies in idiopathic systemic vasculitis. EC/BCR Project for ANCA Assay Standardization (see comments). *Kidney Int* 1998;53(3):743.

42. Scott DG, Watts RA. Systemic vasculitis: epidemiology, classification and environmental factors. *Ann Rheum Dis* 2000;59(3):161.

43. Scott DG. Epidemiology of systemic vasculitis: increasing evidence? *Clin Exp Immunol* 2000;120(Suppl 1):19.

44. el Reshaid K, Kapoor MM, el Reshaid W, et al. The spectrum of renal disease associated with microscopic polyangiitis and classic polyarteritis nodosa in Kuwait. *Nephrol Dial Transplant* 1997;12(9):1874.

45. Satterly KK, Hogan SL, Nachman PH, et al. ANCA-associated diseases with renal involvement but not lupus nephritis are associated with silica exposure. *Clin Exp Immunol* 1998;112:25.

46. Mahr A, Guillevin L, Poissonnet M, et al. Prevalences of polyarteritis nodosa, microscopic polyangiitis, Wegener's granulomatosis, and Churg-Strauss syndrome in a French urban multiethnic population in 2000: a capture-recapture estimate. *Arthritis Rheum* 2004;51(1):92.

47. Izzedine H, Rosenheim M, Launay-Vacher V, et al. Epidemiology of microscopic polyangiitis: a 16-year study. *Kidney Int* 2004;65(2):741.

48. Levy JB, Hammad T, Coulthart A, et al. Clinical features and outcome of patients with both ANCA and anti-GBM antibodies. *Kidney Int* 2004;66(4):1535.

49. Hogan SL, Nachman PH, Wilkman AS, et al. Prognostic markers in patients with antineutrophil cytoplasmic autoantibody-associated microscopic polyangiitis and glomerulonephritis. *J Am Soc Nephrol* 1996;7(1):23.

50. Colby TV, Specks U. Wegener's granulomatosis in the 1990s: a pulmonary pathologist's perspective. *Monogr Pathol* 1993;(36):195.

51. Daum TE, Specks U, Colby TV, et al. Tracheobronchial involvement in Wegener's granulomatosis. *Am J Respir Crit Care Med* 1995;151(2, Pt 1):522.

52. Guillevin L, Cohen P, Gayraud M, et al. Churg-Strauss syndrome: clinical study and long-term follow-up of 96 patients. *Medicine (Baltimore)* 1999;78(1):26.

53. Stegeman CA, Tervaert JW, De Jong PE, et al. Trimethoprim-sulfamethoxazole (co-trimoxazole) for the prevention of relapses of Wegener's granulomatosis. Dutch Co-Trimoxazole Wegener Study Group. *N Engl J Med* 1996;335(1):16.

54. Said G. Vasculitis neuropathies. In: Latov N, Wokke JH, Kelly JJ, eds. *Immunologic and Infectious Diseases of the Peripheral Nerves*. Cambridge: Cambridge University Press; 1998:158.

55. Calabrese LH, Duna GF, Lie JT. Vasculitis in the central nervous system (see comments). *Arthritis Rheum* 1997;40(7):1189.

56. Chumbley LC, Harrison EG, Jr, DeRemee RA. Allergic granulomatosis and angiitis (Churg-Strauss syndrome): report and analysis of 30 cases. *Mayo Clin Proc* 1977;52(8):477.

57. Davies DJ, Moran JE, Niall JF, et al. Segmental necrotising glomerulonephritis with antineutrophil antibody: possible arbovirus aetiology? *Br Med J (Clin Res Ed)* 1982;285(6342):606.

58. Falk RJ, Jennette JC. Anti-neutrophil cytoplasmic autoantibodies with specificity for myeloperoxidase in patients with systemic vasculitis and idiopathic necrotizing and crescentic glomerulonephritis. *N Engl J Med* 1988;318(25):1651.

59. Cooper T, Savige J, Nassis L, et al. Clinical associations and characterisation of antineutrophil cytoplasmic antibodies directed against bactericidal/permeability- increasing protein and azurocidin. *Rheumatol Int* 2000; 19(4):129.

60. Jethwa HS, Nachman PH, Falk RJ, et al. False-positive myeloperoxidase binding activity due to DNA/anti-DNA antibody complexes: a source for analytical error in serologic evaluation of anti-neutrophil cytoplasmic autoantibodies. *Clin Exp Immunol* 2000;121(3):544.

61. Morgan MD, Harper L, Williams J, et al. Anti-neutrophil cytoplasm-associated glomerulonephritis. *J Am Soc Nephrol* 2006;17(5):1224.

62. Jennette JC, Xiao H, Falk RJ. Pathogenesis of vascular inflammation by anti-neutrophil cytoplasmic antibodies. *J Am Soc Nephrol* 2006; 17(5):1235.

63. Feldmann M, Pusey CD. Is there a role for TNF-α in anti-neutrophil cytoplasmic antibody-associated vasculitis?: lessons from other chronic inflammatory diseases. *J Am Soc Nephrol* 2006;17(5):1243.

64. Bansal PJ, Tobin MC. Neonatal microscopic polyangiitis secondary to transfer of maternal myeloperoxidase-antineutrophil cytoplasmic antibody resulting in neonatal pulmonary hemorrhage and renal involvement. *Ann Allergy Asthma Immunol* 2004;93(4):398.

65. Schlieben DJ, Korbet SM, Kimura RE, et al. Pulmonary-renal syndrome in a newborn with placental transmission of ANCAs. *Am J Kidney Dis* 2005;45(4):758.

66. Falk RJ, Terrell RS, Charles LA, et al. Anti-neutrophil cytoplasmic autoantibodies induce neutrophils to degranulate and produce oxygen radicals in vitro. *Proc Natl Acad Sci U S A* 1990;87(11):4115.

67. Ewert BH, Jennette JC, Falk RJ. Anti-myeloperoxidase antibodies stimulate neutrophils to damage human endothelial cells. *Kidney Int* 1992;41(2):375.

68. Savage CO, Pottinger BE, Gaskin G, et al. Autoantibodies developing to myeloperoxidase and proteinase 3 in systemic vasculitis stimulate neutrophil cytotoxicity toward cultured endothelial cells. *Am J Pathol* 1992;141(2):335.

69. Cockwell P, Brooks CJ, Adu D, et al. Interleukin-8: a pathogenetic role in antineutrophil cytoplasmic autoantibody-associated glomerulonephritis (see comments). *Kidney Int* 1999;55(3):852.

70. Schreiber A, Otto B, Ju X, et al. Membrane proteinase 3 expression in patients with Wegener's granulomatosis and in human hematopoietic stem cell-derived neutrophils. *J Am Soc Nephrol* 2005;16(7):2216.

71. Witko-Sarsat V, Lesavre P, Lopez S, et al. A large subset of neutrophils expressing membrane proteinase 3 is a risk factor for vasculitis and rheumatoid arthritis. *J Am Soc Nephrol* 1999;10(6):1224.

72. Yang JJ, Pendergraft WF, Alcorta DA, et al. Circumvention of normal constraints on granule protein gene expression in peripheral blood neutrophils and monocytes of patients with antineutrophil cytoplasmic antibody-associated glomerulonephritis. *J Am Soc Nephrol* 2004;15(8):2103.

73. Kettritz R, Jennette JC, Falk RJ. Crosslinking of ANCA-antigens stimulates superoxide release by human neutrophils. *J Am Soc Nephrol* 1997;8(3):386.

74. Kimberly RP. Fcgamma receptors and neutrophil activation. *Clin Exp Immunol* 2000;120(Suppl 1):18.

75. Porges AJ, Redecha PB, Kimberly WT, et al. Anti-neutrophil cytoplasmic antibodies engage and activate human neutrophils via Fc gamma RIIa. *J Immunol* 1994;153(3):1271.

76. Kocher M, Edberg JC, Fleit HB, et al. Antineutrophil cytoplasmic antibodies preferentially engage Fc gammaRIIIb on human neutrophils. *J Immunol* 1998;161(12):6909.

77. Edberg JC, Wainstein E, Wu J, et al. Analysis of FcgammaRII gene polymorphisms in Wegener's granulomatosis. *Exp Clin Immunogenet* 1997;14(3):183.

78. Tse WY, Abadeh S, McTiernan A, et al. No association between neutrophil FcgammaRIIa allelic polymorphism and anti-neutrophil cytoplasmic antibody (ANCA)-positive systemic vasculitis. *Clin Exp Immunol* 1999;117(1):198.

79. Wainstein E, Edberg J, Csernok E, et al. FcgammaRIIIb alleles predict renal dysfunction in Wegener's granulomatosis (WG). *Arthritis Rheum* 1995;39:210.

80. Dijstelbloem HM, Scheepers RH, Oost WW, et al. Fcgamma receptor polymorphisms in Wegener's granulomatosis: risk factors for disease relapse. *Arthritis Rheum* 1999;42(9):1823.

81. Yang JJ, Alcorta DA, Preston GA, et al. Genes activated by ANCA IgG amd ANCA F(ab')2 fragments (abstract). *J Am Soc Nephrol* 2000;11:485A.

82. Williams JM, Savage CO. Characterization of the regulation and functional consequences of p21ras activation in neutrophils by antineutrophil cytoplasm antibodies. *J Am Soc Nephrol* 2005;16(1):90.

83. Mayet WJ, Schwarting A, Meyer zum Buschenfelde KH. Cytotoxic effects of antibodies to proteinase 3 (C-ANCA) on human endothelial cells. *Clin Exp Immunol* 1994;97(3):458.

84. King WJ, Adu D, Daha MR, et al. Endothelial cells and renal epithelial cells do not express the Wegener's autoantigen, proteinase 3. *Clin Exp Immunol* 1995;102(1):98.

85. Pendergraft WF, Alcorta DA, Segelmark M, et al. ANCA antigens, proteinase 3 and myeloperoxidase, are not expressed in endothelial cells (see comments). *Kidney Int* 2000;57(5):1981.

86. Calderwood JW, Williams JM, Morgan MD, et al. ANCA induces beta2 integrin and CXC chemokine-dependent neutrophil-endothelial cell interactions that mimic those of highly cytokine-activated endothelium. *J Leukoc Biol* 2005;77(1):33.

87. Ballieux BE, Hiemstra PS, Klar-Mohamad N, et al. Detachment and cytolysis of human endothelial cells by proteinase 3. *Eur J Immunol* 1994;24(12):3211.

88. Yang JJ, Kettritz R, Falk RJ, et al. Apoptosis of endothelial cells induced by the neutrophil serine proteases proteinase 3 and elastase. *Am J Pathol* 1996;149(5):1617.

89. Taekema-Roelvink ME, van Kooten C, Janssens MC, et al. Effect of antineutrophil cytoplasmic antibodies on proteinase 3-induced apoptosis of human endothelial cells. *Scand J Immunol* 1998;48(1):37.

90. Taekema-Roelvink ME, van KC, Heemskerk E, et al. Proteinase 3 interacts with a 111-kD membrane molecule of human umbilical vein endothelial cells. *J Am Soc Nephrol* 2000;11(4):640.

91. Kurosawa S, Esmon CT, Stearns-Kurosawa DJ. The soluble endothelial protein C receptor binds to activated neutrophils: involvement of proteinase-3 and CD11b/CD18. *J Immunol* 2000;165(8):4697.

92. Esmon CT. Structure and functions of the endothelial cell protein C receptor. *Crit Care Med* 2004;32(Suppl 5):S298.

93. Baldus S, Eiserich JP, Mani A, et al. Endothelial transcytosis of myeloperoxidase confers specificity to vascular ECM proteins as targets of tyrosine nitration. *J Clin Invest* 2001;108(12):1759.

94. Brennan ML, Wu W, Fu X, et al. A tale of two controversies: defining both the role of peroxidases in nitrotyrosine formation in vivo using eosinophil peroxidase and myeloperoxidase-deficient mice, and the nature of peroxidase-generated reactive nitrogen species. *J Biol Chem* 2002;277(20):17415.

95. Woods AA, Linton SM, Davies MJ. Detection of HOCl-mediated protein oxidation products in the extracellular matrix of human atherosclerotic plaques. *Biochem J* 2003;370(Pt 2):729.

96. Gutfleisch J, Baumert E, Wolff-Vorbeck G, et al. Increased expression of CD25 and adhesion molecules on peripheral blood lymphocytes of patients with Wegener's granulomatosis (WG) and ANCA positive vasculitides. *Adv Exp Med Biol* 1993;336:397.

97. Schlesier M, Kaspar T, Gutfleisch J, et al. Activated CD4+ and CD8+ T-cell subsets in Wegener's granulomatosis. *Rheumatol Int* 1995;14(5):213.

98. Ikeda M, Watanabe Y, Kitahara S, et al. Distinctive increases in HLA-DR+ and CD8+57+ lymphocyte subsets in Wegener's granulomatosis. *Int Arch Allergy Immunol* 1993;102(2):205.

99. Ludviksson BR, Sneller MC, Chua KS, et al. Active Wegener's granulomatosis is associated with HLA-DR+ CD4+ T cells exhibiting an unbalanced Th1-type T cell cytokine pattern: reversal with IL-10. *J Immunol* 1998;160(7):3602.

100. Popa ER, Stegeman CA, Bos NA, et al. Differential B- and T-cell activation in Wegener's granulomatosis. *J Allergy Clin Immunol* 1999;103(5 Pt 1):885.

101. Csernok E, Trabandt A, Muller A, et al. Cytokine profiles in Wegener's granulomatosis: predominance of type 1 (Th1) in the granulomatous inflammation. *Arthritis Rheum* 1999;42(4):742.

102. Moosig F, Csernok E, Wang G, et al. Costimulatory molecules in Wegener's granulomatosis (WG): lack of expression of CD28 and preferential up-regulation of its ligands B7-1 (CD80) and B7-2 (CD86) on T cells. *Clin Exp Immunol* 1998;114(1):113.

103. Gephardt GN, Ahmad M, Tubbs RR. Pulmonary vasculitis (Wegener's granulomatosis): immunohistochemical study of T and B cell markers. *Am J Med* 1983;74(4):700.

104. Brouwer E, Tervaert JW, Horst G, et al. Predominance of IgG1 and IgG4 subclasses of anti-neutrophil cytoplasmic autoantibodies (ANCA) in patients with Wegener's granulomatosis and clinically related disorders. *Clin Exp Immunol* 1991;83(3):379.

105. Schmitt WH, Heesen C, Csernok E, et al. Elevated serum levels of soluble interleukin-2 receptor in patients with Wegener's granulomatosis. Association with disease activity. *Arthritis Rheum* 1992;35(9):1088.

106. Brouwer E, Stegeman CA, Huitema MG, et al. T cell reactivity to proteinase 3 and myeloperoxidase in patients with Wegener's granulomatosis (WG). *Clin Exp Immunol* 1994;98(3):448.

107. Mathieson PW, Oliveira DB. The role of cellular immunity in systemic vasculitis. *Clin Exp Immunol* 1995;100(2):183.

108. King WJ, Brooks CJ, Holder R, et al. T lymphocyte responses to antineutrophil cytoplasmic autoantibody (ANCA) antigens are present in patients with ANCA-associated systemic vasculitis and persist during disease remission. *Clin Exp Immunol* 1998;112(3):539.

109. Rulifson IC, Sperling AI, Fields PE, et al. CD28 costimulation promotes the production of Th2 cytokines. *J Immunol* 1997;158(2):658.

110. Popa ER, Franssen CF, Limburg PC, et al. In vitro cytokine production and proliferation of T cells from patients with anti-proteinase 3- and antimyeloperoxidase-associated vasculitis, in response to proteinase 3 and myeloperoxidase. *Arthritis Rheum* 2002;46(7):1894.

111. Meroni PL. Antiendothelial cell antibodies (AECA): from a laboratory curiosity to another useful autoantibody. In: Shoenfeld Y, ed. *The Decade of Autoimmunity.* Amsterdam: Elsevier Science; 1998:227.

112. Constans J, Dupuy R, Blann AD, et al. Anti-endothelial cell autoantibodies and soluble markers of endothelial cell dysfunction in systemic lupus erythematosus. *J Rheumatol* 2003;30(9):1963.

113. Del Papa N. Antiendothelial cell IgG fractions from systemic lupus erythematosus patients bind to human endothelial cells and induce a pro-adhesive and a pro-inflammatory phenotype in vitro (abstract). *Lupus* 1999;8:1.

114. Holmen C, Christensson M, Pettersson E, et al. Wegener's granulomatosis is associated with organ-specific antiendothelial cell antibodies. *Kidney Int* 2004;66(3):1049.

115. Stegeman CA, Cohen Tervaert JW, Manson WL, et al. Chronic nasal carriage of *Staphylococcal aureus* in Wegener's granulomatosis identifies a subgroup of patients more prone to relapse. *Ann Intern Med* 1994;120:12.

116. Popa ER, Stegeman CA, Bos NA. Staphylococcal superantigens: a risk factor for disease reactivation in Wegener's granulomatosis (abstract). *Clin Exp Immunol* 2000;120:44.

117. Brons RH, Klok PA, vanDijk NW, et al. Staphylococcal acid phosphatase induces a severe crescentic glomerulonephritis in immunized Brown-Norway rats: relevance for Wegener's granulomatosis (abstract)? *Clin Exp Immunol* 2000;120(Suppl 1):44.

118. Dal Canto AJ, Virgin HW. Animal models of infection-mediated vasculitis. *Curr Opin Rheumatol* 1999;11(1):17.

119. Parks CG, Cooper GS, Nylander-French LA, et al. Occupational exposure

to crystalline silica and risk of systemic lupus erythematosus: a population-based, case-control study in the southeastern United States. *Arthritis Rheum* 2002;46(7):1840.

120. Gregorini G, Ferioli A, Donato F, et al. Association between silica exposure and necrotizing crescentic glomerulonephritis with p-ANCA and anti-MPO antibodies: a hospital-based case-control study. *Adv Exp Med Biol* 1993;336:435.

121. Nuyts GD, Van Vlem E, De Vos A, et al. Wegener granulomatosis is associated to exposure to silicon compounds: a case-control study (see comments) (published erratum appears in *Nephrol Dial Transplant* 1995 Nov;10(11):2168). *Nephrol Dial Transplant* 1995;10(7):1162.

122. Hogan SL, Satterly KK, Dooley MA, et al. Silica exposure in anti-neutrophil cytoplasmic autoantibody-associated glomerulonephritis and lupus nephritis. *J Am Soc Nephrol* 2001;12(1):134.

123. Lane SE, Watts RA, Bentham G, et al. Are environmental factors important in primary systemic vasculitis?: a case-control study. *Arthritis Rheum* 2003;48(3):814.

124. Hogan SL, Cooper GS, Nylander-French LA, et al. Duration of silican exposure and development of ANCA-associated small vessel vasculitis with glomerular involvement: a case-control study (abstract). *J Am Soc Nephrol* 2004;15:16.

125. Sanchez-Roman J, Wichmann I, Salaberri J, et al. Multiple clinical and biological autoimmune manifestations in 50 workers after occupational exposure to silica (see comments). *Ann Rheum Dis* 1993;52(7):534.

126. Conrad K, Mehlhorn J, Luthke K, et al. Systemic lupus erythematosus after heavy exposure to quartz dust in uranium mines: clinical and serological characteristics. *Lupus* 1996;5(1):62.

127. ten Holder S, Joy MS, Falk RJ. Drug-induced vasculitis: a review of cutaneous and systemic manifestations (abstract). *Clin Exp Immunol* 2000;120(Suppl 1):60.

128. Xiao H, Heeringa P, Hu P, et al. Antineutrophil cytoplasmic autoantibodies specific for myeloperoxidase cause glomerulonephritis and vasculitis in mice. *J Clin Invest* 2002;110(7):955.

129. Huugen D, Xiao H, van EA, et al. Aggravation of anti-myeloperoxidase antibody-induced glomerulonephritis by bacterial lipopolysaccharide: role of tumor necrosis factor-alpha. *Am J Pathol* 2005;167(1):47.

130. Xiao H, Heeringa P, Liu Z, et al. The role of neutrophils in the induction of glomerulonephritis by anti-myeloperoxidase antibodies. *Am J Pathol* 2005;167(1):39.

131. Little MA, Smyth CL, Yadav R, et al. Antineutrophil cytoplasm antibodies directed against myeloperoxidase augment leukocyte-microvascular interactions in vivo. *Blood* 2005;106(6):2050.

132. Pfister H, Ollert M, Froehlich LF, et al. Anti-neutrophil cytoplasmic autoantibodies (ANCA) against the murine homolog of proteinase 3 (Wegener's autoantigen) are pathogenic in vivo. *Blood* 2004;104(5):1411.

133. Oldstone MB. Molecular mimicry and autoimmune disease. *Cell* 1987; 50(6):819.

134. Oldstone MB. Molecular mimicry, microbial infection, and autoimmune disease: evolution of the concept. *Curr Top Microbiol Immunol* 2005;296:1.

135. Prinz JC. Disease mimicry: a pathogenetic concept for T cell-mediated autoimmune disorders triggered by molecular mimicry? *Autoimmun Rev* 2004;3(1):10.

136. Pendergraft WF, Pressler BM, Jennette JC, et al. Autoantigen complementarity: a new theory implicating complementary proteins as initiators of autoimmune disease. *J Mol Med* 2005;83(1):12.

137. Pendergraft WF, Preston GA, Shah RR, et al. Autoimmunity is triggered by cPR-3(105-201), a protein complementary to human autoantigen proteinase-3. *Nat Med* 2004;10(1):72.

138. Nachman PH, Hogan SL, Jennette JC, et al. Treatment response and relapse in antineutrophil cytoplasmic autoantibody-associated microscopic polyangiitis and glomerulonephritis. *J Am Soc Nephrol* 1996;7(1):33.

139. Hoffman GS, Kerr GS, Leavitt RY, et al. Wegener granulomatosis: an analysis of 158 patients (see comments). *Ann Intern Med* 1992;116(6):488.

140. Guillevin L, Cordier JF, Lhote F, et al. A prospective, multicenter, randomized trial comparing steroids and pulse cyclophosphamide versus steroids and oral cyclophosphamide in the treatment of generalized Wegener's granulomatosis (see comments). *Arthritis Rheum* 1997;40(12):2187.

141. de Groot K, Adu D, Savage CO. The value of pulse cyclophosphamide in ANCA-associated vasculitis: meta-analysis and critical review. *Nephrol Dial Transplant* 2001;16(10):2018.

142. Klemmer PJ, Chalermskulrat W, Reif MS, et al. Plasmapheresis therapy for diffuse alveolar hemorrhage in patients with small-vessel vasculitis. *Am J Kidney Dis* 2003;42(6):1149.

143. Glockner WM, Sieberth HG, Wichmann HE, et al. Plasma exchange and immunosuppression in rapidly progressive glomerulonephritis: a controlled, multi-center study. *Clin Nephrol* 1988;29(1):1.

144. Cole E, Cattran D, Magil A, et al. A prospective randomized trial of plasma exchange as additive therapy in idiopathic crescentic glomerulonephritis. *Am J Kidney Dis* 1992; 20(3):261.

145. Pusey CD, Rees AJ, Evans DJ, et al. Plasma exchange in focal necrotizing glomerulonephritis without anti-GBM antibodies. *Kidney Int* 1991;40(4):757.

146. Gaskin G, Jayne DR. European Vasculitis Study Group: Adjunctive plasma exchange is superior to methylprednisolone in acute renal failure due to ANCA-associated glomerulonephritis. *J Am Soc Nephrol* 2002;13:2A.

147. Jayne D, Rasmussen N, Andrassy K, et al. A randomized trial of maintenance therapy for vasculitis associated with antineutrophil cytoplasmic autoantibodies. *N Engl J Med* 2003;349(1):36.

148. Sneller MC, Hoffman GS, Talar-Williams C, et al. An analysis of forty-two Wegener's granulomatosis patients treated with methotrexate and prednisone. *Arthritis Rheum* 1995;38(5):608.

149. Langford CA, Talar-Williams C, Barron KS, et al. Use of a cyclophosphamide-induction methotrexate-maintenance regimen for the treatment of Wegener's granulomatosis: extended follow-up and rate of relapse. *Am J Med* 2003;114(6):463.

150. de GK, Rasmussen N, Bacon PA, et al. Randomized trial of cyclophosphamide versus methotrexate for induction of remission in early systemic antineutrophil cytoplasmic antibody-associated vasculitis. *Arthritis Rheum* 2005;52(8):2461.

151. Gordon M, Luqmani RA, Adu D, et al. Relapses in patients with a systemic vasculitis. *Q J Med* 1993;86(12):779.

152. Hogan SL, Falk RJ, Chin H, et al. Predictors of relapse and treatment resistance in antineutrophil cytoplasmic antibody-associated small-vessel vasculitis. *Ann Intern Med* 2005;143(9):621.

153. Boomsma MM, Stegeman CA, van der Leij MJ, et al. Prediction of relapses in Wegener's granulomatosis by measurement of antineutrophil cytoplasmic antibody levels: a prospective study. *Arthritis Rheum* 2000;43(9):2025.

154. Tervaert JW, Huitema MG, Hene RJ, et al. Prevention of relapses in Wegener's granulomatosis by treatment based on antineutrophil cytoplasmic antibody titre. *Lancet* 1990;336(8717):709.

155. Jayne DR, Chapel H, Adu D, et al. Intravenous immunoglobulin for ANCA-associated systemic vasculitis with persistent disease activity. *QJM* 2000;93(7):433.

156. Keogh KA, Wylam ME, Stone JH, et al. Induction of remission by B lymphocyte depletion in eleven patients with refractory antineutrophil cytoplasmic antibody-associated vasculitis. *Arthritis Rheum* 2005;52(1):262.

157. Eriksson P. Nine patients with anti-neutrophil cytoplasmic antibody-positive vasculitis successfully treated with rituximab. *J Intern Med* 2005;257(6):540.

158. Stasi R, Stipa E, Poeta GD, et al. Long-term observation of patients with anti-neutrophil cytoplasmic antibody-associated vasculitis treated with rituximab. *Rheumatol (Oxford)* 2006.

159. Aries PM, Hellmich B, Both M, et al. Lack of efficacy of Rituximab in Wegener's Granulomatosis with refractory granulomatous manifestations. *Ann Rheum Dis* 2006;65(7):853.

160. Kirk AD, Hale DA, Mannon RB, et al. Results from a human renal allograft tolerance trial evaluating the humanized CD52-specific monoclonal antibody alemtuzumab (CAMPATH-1H). *Transplantation* 2003;76(1):120.

161. Isaacs JD, Manna VK, Rapson N, et al. CAMPATH-1H in rheumatoid arthritis—an intravenous dose-ranging study. *Br J Rheumatol* 1996;35(3):231.

162. Jayne DR: Campath-1H (anti-CD52) for refractory vasculitis: retrospective Cambridge experience 1989-1999. *Cleve Clin J Med* 2002;69(Suppl II):SII.

163. Scallon BJ, Moore MA, Trinh H, et al. Chimeric anti-TNF-alpha monoclonal antibody cA2 binds recombinant transmembrane TNF-alpha and activates immune effector functions. *Cytokine* 1995;7(3):251.

164. Lamprecht P, Voswinkel J, Lilienthal T, et al. Effectiveness of TNF-alpha blockade with infliximab in refractory Wegener's granulomatosis. *Rheumatol (Oxford)* 2002;41(11):1303.

165. Bartolucci P, Ramanoelina J, Cohen P, et al. Efficacy of the anti-TNF-alpha antibody infliximab against refractory systemic vasculitides: an open pilot study on 10 patients. *Rheumatol (Oxford)* 2002;41(10):1126.

166. Booth A, Harper L, Hammad T, et al. Prospective study of TNF alpha blockade with infliximab in anti-neutrophil cytoplasmic antibody-associated systemic vasculitis. *J Am Soc Nephrol* 2004;15(3):717.

167. Booth AD, Jefferson HJ, Ayliffe W, et al. Safety and efficacy of TNF alpha blockade in relapsing vasculitis. *Ann Rheum Dis* 2002;61(6):559.

168. Birck R, Warnatz K, Lorenz HM, et al. 15-Deoxyspergualin in patients with refractory ANCA-associated systemic vasculitis: a six-month open-label trial to evaluate safety and efficacy. *J Am Soc Nephrol* 2003;14(2):440.

169. Nachman PH, Joy MS, Hogan SL, et al. Preliminary results of a pilot study on the use of mycophenolate mofetil (MMF) in relapsing ANCA small vessel vasculitis (ANCA-SVV) (abstract). *J Am Soc Nephrol* 2000;11:158.

170. Nowack R, Gobel U, Klooker P, et al. Mycophenolate mofetil for maintenance therapy of Wegener's granulomatosis and microscopic polyangiitis: a pilot study in 11 patients with renal involvement. *J Am Soc Nephrol* 1999;10(9):1965.

171. Etanercept. Soluble tumour necrosis factor receptor, TNF receptor fusion protein, TNFR-Fc, TNR 001, Enbrel: *Drugs R D* 1999;3(3):258.

172. Stone JH. Limited versus severe Wegener's granulomatosis: baseline data on patients in the Wegener's granulomatosis etanercept trial. *Arthritis Rheum* 2003;48(8):2299.

173. Frasca GM, Neri L, Martello M, et al. Renal transplantation in patients with microscopic polyarteritis and antimyeloperoxidase antibodies: report of three cases. *Nephron* 1996;72(1):82.

174. Rostaing L, Modesto A, Oksman F, et al. Outcome of patients with antineutrophil cytoplasmic autoantibody- associated vasculitis following cadaveric kidney transplantation. *Am J Kidney Dis* 1997;29(1):96.

175. Morin MP, Thervet E, Legendre C, et al. Successful kidney transplantation in a patient with microscopic polyarteritis and positive ANCA (letter). *Nephrol Dial Transplant* 1993;8(3):287.

176. Schmitt WH, Haubitz M, Mistry N, et al. Renal transplantation in Wegener's granulomatosis (letter). *Lancet* 1993;342(8875):860.

177. Reaich D, Cooper N, Main J. Rapid catastrophic onset of Wegener's granulomatosis in a renal transplant. *Nephron* 1994;67(3):354.

178. Fogazzi GB, Banfi G, Allegri L, et al. Late recurrence of systemic vasculitis after kidney transplantation involving the kidney allograft. *Adv Exp Med Biol* 1993;336:503.

179. Rich LM, Piering WF. Ureteral stenosis due to recurrent Wegener's granulomatosis after kidney transplantation. *J Am Soc Nephrol* 1994;4(8):1516.

180. Nachman PH, Segelmark M, Westman K, et al. Recurrent ANCA-associated small vessel vasculitis after transplantation: a pooled analysis. *Kidney Int* 1999;56(4):1544.

181. Steinman TI, Jaffe BF, Monaco AP, et al. Recurrence of Wegener's granulomatosis after kidney transplant. Successful re-induction of remission with cyclophosphamide. *Am J Med* 1980;68(3):458.

182. Agard C, Mouthon L, Mahr A, et al. Microscopic polyangiitis and polyarteritis nodosa: how and when do they start? *Arthritis Rheum* 2003;49(5):709.

183. Guillevin L, Lhote F, Gayraud M, et al. Prognostic factors in polyarteritis nodosa and Churg-Strauss syndrome: a prospective study in 342 patients. *Medicine (Baltimore)* 1996;75(1):17.

184. Guillevin L, Lhote F, Cohen P, et al. Polyarteritis nodosa related to hepatitis B virus: a prospective study with long-term observation of 41 patients. *Medicine (Baltimore)* 1995;74(5):238.

185. Duffy J, Lidsky MD, Sharp JT, et al. Polyarthritis, polyarteritis and hepatitis B. *Medicine (Baltimore)* 1976;55(1):19.

186. McMahon BJ, Bender TR, Templin DW, et al. Vasculitis in Eskimos living in an area hyperendemic for hepatitis B. *JAMA* 1980;244(19):2180.

187. Johnson RJ, Couser WG. Hepatitis B infection and renal disease: clinical, immunopathogenetic and therapeutic considerations. *Kidney Int* 1990;37(2):663.

188. De Keyser F, Naeyaert JM, Hindryckx P, et al. Immune-mediated pathology following hepatitis B vaccination: two cases of polyarteritis nodosa and one case of pityriasis rosea-like drug eruption. *Clin Exp Rheumatol* 2000;18(1):81.

189. Guillevin L, Lhote F, Sauvaget F, et al. Treatment of polyarteritis nodosa related to hepatitis B virus with interferon-alpha and plasma exchanges. *Ann Rheum Dis* 1994;53(5):334.

190. Kruger M, Boker KH, Zeidler H, et al. Treatment of hepatitis B-related polyarteritis nodosa with famciclovir and interferon alfa-2b. *J Hepatol* 1997;26(4):935.

191. Hasler P, Kistler H, Gerber H. Vasculitides in hairy cell leukemia. *Semin Arthritis Rheum* 1995;25(2):134.

192. Thorwarth WT, Jr, Jaques PF, Orringer EP. Polyarteritis nodosa in hairy cell leukemia. *J Can Assoc Radiol* 1983;34(2):151.

193. Le Pogamp P, Ghandour C, Le Prise PY. Hairy cell leukemia and polyarteritis nodosa. *J Rheumatol* 1982;9(3):441.

194. Wooten MD, Jasin HE. Vasculitis and lymphoproliferative diseases. *Semin Arthritis Rheum* 1996;26(2):564.

195. Carpenter MT, West SG. Polyarteritis nodosa in hairy cell leukemia: treatment with interferon-alpha. *J Rheumatol* 1994;21(6):1150.

196. Leib ES, Restivo C, Paulus HE. Immunosuppressive and corticosteroid therapy of polyarteritis nodosa. *Am J Med* 1979;67(6):941.

197. Guillevin L, Jarrousse B, Lok C, et al. Longterm followup after treatment of polyarteritis nodosa and Churg-Strauss angiitis with comparison of steroids, plasma exchange and cyclophosphamide to steroids and plasma exchange: a prospective randomized trial of 71 patients. The Cooperative Study Group for Polyarteritis Nodosa (see comments). *J Rheumatol* 1991;18(4):567.

198. Guillevin L, Fain O, Lhote F, et al. Lack of superiority of steroids plus plasma exchange to steroids alone in the treatment of polyarteritis nodosa and Churg-Strauss syndrome: a prospective, randomized trial in 78 patients. *Arthritis Rheum* 1992;35(2):208.

199. Guillevin L, Lhote F, Cohen P, et al. Corticosteroids plus pulse cyclophosphamide and plasma exchanges versus corticosteroids plus pulse cyclophosphamide alone in the treatment of polyarteritis nodosa and Churg-Strauss syndrome patients with factors predicting poor prognosis: a prospective, randomized trial in sixty-two patients. *Arthritis Rheum* 1995;38(11):1638.

200. Balow JE, Fouci A. Vasculitic diseases of the kidney. In: Schrier RW, Gottscholk CW, eds. *Diseases of the Kidney*. New York: Little, Brown and Company; 1997:1851.

201. Al-Bishri J, le RN, Pope JE. Refractory polyarteritis nodosa successfully treated with infliximab. *J Rheumatol* 2005;32(7):1371.

202. Keystone EC. The utility of tumour necrosis factor blockade in orphan diseases. *Ann Rheum Dis* 2004;63(Suppl 2):ii79.

203. Lam KC, Lai CL, Trepo C, et al. Deleterious effect of prednisolone in HBsAg-positive chronic active hepatitis. *N Engl J Med* 1981;304(7):380.

204. Guillevin L, Lhote F, Jarrousse B, et al. Polyarteritis nodosa related to hepatitis B virus: a retrospective study of 66 patients. *Ann Med Interne (Paris)* 1992;143(Suppl 1):63.

205. Wicki J, Olivieri J, Pizzolato G, et al. Successful treatment of polyarteritis nodosa related to hepatitis B virus with a combination of lamivudine and interferon alpha (letter). *Rheumatol (Oxford)* 1999;38(2):183.

206. Torresi J, Locarnini S. Antiviral chemotherapy for the treatment of hepatitis B virus infections. *Gastroenterology* 2000;118(2 Suppl 1):83.

207. Guillevin L, Mahr A, Cohen P, et al. Short-term corticosteroids then lamivudine and plasma exchanges to treat hepatitis B virus-related polyarteritis nodosa. *Arthritis Rheum* 2004;51(3):482.

208. Guillevin L, Mahr A, Callard P, et al. Hepatitis B virus-associated polyarteritis nodosa: clinical characteristics, outcome, and impact of treatment in 115 patients. *Medicine (Baltimore)* 2005;84(5):313.

209. Cohen RD, Conn DL, Ilstrup DM. Clinical features, prognosis, and response to treatment in polyarteritis. *Mayo Clin Proc* 1980;55(3):146.

210. Criteria for diagnosis of Behcet's disease. International Study Group for Behcet's Disease: *Lancet* 1990;335(8697):1078.

211. Kaklamani VG, Vaiopoulos G, Kaklamanis PG. Behcet's Disease. *Semin Arthritis Rheum* 1998;27(4):197.

212. Koumantaki Y, Stavropoulos C, Spyropoulou M, et al. HLA-B*5101 in Greek patients with Behcet's disease. *Hum Immunol* 1998;59:250.

213. Ahmad T, Wallace GR, James T, et al. Mapping the HLA association in Behcet's disease: a role for tumor necrosis factor polymorphisms? *Arthritis Rheum* 2003;48(3):807.

214. Mizuki N, Ota M, Yabuki K, et al. Localization of the pathogenic gene of Behcet's disease by microsatellite analysis of three different populations. *Invest Ophthalmol Vis Sci* 2000;41(12):3702.

215. Mor F, Weinberger A, Cohen IR. Identification of alpha-tropomyosin as a target self-antigen in Behcet's syndrome. *Eur J Immunol* 2002;32(2):356.

216. Freysdottir J, Lau S, Fortune F. Gammadelta T cells in Behcet's disease (BD) and recurrent aphthous stomatitis (RAS). *Clin Exp Immunol* 1999;118(3):451.

217. Frassanito MA, Dammacco R, Cafforio P, et al. Th1 polarization of the immune response in Behcet's disease: a putative pathogenetic role of interleukin-12. *Arthritis Rheum* 1999;42(9):1967.

218. de Smet MD, Dayan M. Prospective determination of T-cell responses to S-antigen in Behcet's disease patients and controls. *Invest Ophthalmol Vis Sci* 2000;41(11):3480.

219. Akpolat T, Akkoyunlu M, Akpolat I, et al. Renal Behcet's disease: a cumulative analysis. *Semin Arthritis Rheum* 2002;31(5):317.

220. Akpolat I, Akpolat T, Danaci M, et al. Behcet's disease and amyloidosis. *Review of the literature. Scand J Rheumatol* 1997;26(6):477.

221. Rosenthal T, Weiss P, Gafni J. Renal involvement in Behcet's syndrome. *Arch Intern Med* 1978;138(7):1122.

222. Altiparmak MR, Tanverdi M, Pamuk ON, et al. Glomerulonephritis in Behcet's disease: report of seven cases and review of the literature. *Clin Rheumatol* 2002;21(1):14.

223. Kansu E, Deglin S, Cantor RI, et al. The expanding spectrum of Behcet syndrome: a case with renal involvement. *JAMA* 1977;237(17):1855.

224. Herreman G, Beaufils H, Godeau P, et al. Behcet's syndrome and renal involvement: a histological and immunofluorescent study of eleven renal biopsies. *Am J Med Sci* 1982;284(1):10.

225. Burrows NP, Zhao MH, Norris PG, et al. ANCA associated with Behcet's disease. *J R Soc Med* 1996;89(1):47P.

226. Ben Hmida M, Hachicha J, Kaddour N, et al. ANCA in Behcet's disease (letter). *Nephrol Dial Transplant* 1997;12(11):2465.

227. Barnes CG. Treatment of Behcet's syndrome. *Rheumatol (Oxford)* 2006;45(3):245.

228. Pipitone N, Olivieri I, Cantini F, et al. New approaches in the treatment of Adamantiades-Behcet's disease. *Curr Opin Rheumatol* 2006;18(1):3.

229. Melikoglu M, Fresko I, Mat C, et al. Short-term trial of etanercept in Behcet's disease: a double blind, placebo controlled study. *J Rheumatol* 2005;32(1):98.

230. Rojo-Leyva F, Ratliff NB, Cosgrove DM, et al. Study of 52 patients with idiopathic aortitis from a cohort of 1,204 surgical cases. *Arthritis Rheum* 2000;43(4):901.

231. Gabriel SE, Espy M, Erdman DD, et al. The role of parvovirus B19 in the pathogenesis of giant cell arteritis: a preliminary evaluation. *Arthritis Rheum* 1999;42(6):1255.

232. Rodriguez-Pla A, Bosch-Gil JA, Echevarria-Mayo JE, et al. No detection of parvovirus B19 or herpesvirus DNA in giant cell arteritis. *J Clin Virol* 2004;31(1):11.

233. Salvarani C, Gabriel SE, O'Fallon WM, et al. The incidence of giant cell arteritis in Olmsted County, Minnesota: apparent fluctuations in a cyclic pattern (see comments). *Ann Intern Med* 1995;123(3):192.

234. Mathewson JA, Hunder GG. Giant cell arteritis in two brothers. *J Rheumatol* 1986;13(1):190.

235. Weyand CM, Hunder NN, Hicok KC, et al. HLA-DRB1 alleles in polymyalgia rheumatica, giant cell arteritis, and rheumatoid arthritis. *Arthritis Rheum* 1994;37(4):514.

236. Weyand CM, Goronzy JJ. Giant cell arteritis as an antigen-driven disease. *Rheum Dis Clin North Am* 1995;21(4):1027.

237. Roche NE, Fulbright JW, Wagner AD, et al. Correlation of interleukin-6 production and disease activity in polymyalgia rheumatica and giant cell arteritis (see comments). *Arthritis Rheum* 1993;36(9):1286.

238. Kerr GS, Hallahan CW, Giordano J, et al. Takayasu arteritis. *Ann Intern Med* 1994;120(11):919.

239. Zilleruelo GE, Ferrer P, Garcia OL, et al. Takayasu's arteritis associated with glomerulonephritis. *A case report. Am J Dis Child* 1978;132(10):1009.

240. Lai KN, Chan KW, Ho CP. Glomerulonephritis associated with Takayasu's arteritis: report of three cases and review of literature. *Am J Kidney Dis* 1986;7(3):197.

241. Kerr GS. Takayasu's arteritis. *Rheum Dis Clin North Am* 1995;21(4):1041.
242. Hellmann DB, Hardy K, Lindenfeld S, et al. Takayasu arteritis associated with crescentic glomerulonephritis. *Arthritis Rheum* 1987;30(4):451.
243. Hunder GG, Sheps SG, Allen GL, et al. Daily and alternate-day corticosteroid regimens in treatment of giant cell arteritis: comparison in a prospective study. *Ann Intern Med* 1975;82(5):613.
244. Liu GT, Glaser JS, Schatz NJ, et al. Visual morbidity in giant cell arteritis: clinical characteristics and prognosis for vision. *Ophthalmolo* 1994;101(11):1779.
245. Achkar AA, Lie JT, Hunder GG, et al. How does previous corticosteroid treatment affect the biopsy findings in giant cell (temporal) arteritis? *Ann Intern Med* 1994;120(12):987.
246. Ray-Chaudhuri N, Kine DA, Tijani SO, et al. Effect of prior steroid treatment on temporal artery biopsy findings in giant cell arteritis. *Br J Ophthalmol* 2002;86(5):530.
247. Wilke WS, Hoffman GS. Treatment of corticosteroid-resistant giant cell arteritis. *Rheum Dis Clin North Am* 1995;21(1):59.
248. Nesher G, Sonnenblick M. Steroid-sparing medications in temporal arteritis–report of three cases and review of 174 reported patients. *Clin Rheumatol* 1994;13(2):289.
249. Jover JA, Hernandez-Garcia C, Morado IC, et al. Combined treatment of giant cell arteritis with methotrexate and prednisone: a randomized, double-blind, and placebo-controlled study (abstract). *Arthritis Rheum* 2000;43:S365.
250. Hoffman GS, Cid M, Hellmann DB, et al. A multicenter, placebo-controlled study of methotrexate (Mtx) in giant cell arteritis (GCA) (abstract). *Arthritis Rheum* 2000;43:S115.
251. Nesher G, Berkun Y, Mates M, et al. Low-dose aspirin and prevention of cranial ischemic complications in giant cell arteritis. *Arthritis Rheum* 2004;50(4):1332.
252. Tan AL, Holdsworth J, Pease C, et al. Successful treatment of resistant giant cell arteritis with etanercept. *Ann Rheum Dis* 2003;62(4):373.
253. Cantini F, Niccoli L, Salvarani C, et al. Treatment of longstanding active giant cell arteritis with infliximab: report of four cases. *Arthritis Rheum* 2001;44(12):2933.
254. Andonopoulos AP, Meimaris N, Daoussis D, et al. Experience with infliximab (anti-TNF alpha monoclonal antibody) as monotherapy for giant cell arteritis. *Ann Rheum Dis* 2003;62(5):1116.
255. Hoffman GS, Leavitt RY, Kerr GS, et al. Treatment of glucocorticoid-resistant or relapsing Takayasu arteritis with methotrexate. *Arthritis Rheum* 1994;37(4):578.
256. Della RA, Tavoni A, Merlini G, et al. Two Takayasu arteritis patients successfully treated with infliximab: a potential disease-modifying agent? *Rheumatol (Oxford)* 2005;44(8):1074.
257. Tanaka F, Kawakami A, Iwanaga N, et al. Infliximab is effective for Takayasu arteritis refractory to glucocorticoid and methotrexate. *Intern Med* 2006;45(5):313.
258. Hoffman GS, Merkel PA, Brasington RD, et al. Anti-tumor necrosis factor therapy in patients with difficult to treat Takayasu arteritis. *Arthritis Rheum* 2004;50(7):2296.
259. Lagneau P, Michel JB, Vuong PN. Surgical treatment of Takayasu's disease. *Ann Surg* 1987;205(2):157.
260. Kieffer E, Piquois A, Bertal A, et al. Reconstructive surgery of the renal arteries in Takayasu's disease. *Ann Vasc Surg* 1990;4(2):156.
261. Hoffman GS. Treatment of resistant Takayasu's arteritis. *Rheum Dis Clin North Am* 1995;21(1):73.
262. Ward MM, Pyun E, Studenski S. Causes of death in systemic lupus erythematosus: long-term followup of an inception cohort. *Arthritis Rheum* 1995;38(10):1492.
263. Recommendations for the prevention and treatment of glucocorticoid-induced osteoporosis. American College of Rheumatology Task Force on Osteoporosis Guidelines. *Arthritis Rheum* 1996;39(11):1791.
264. Masala A, Faedda R, Alagna S, et al. Use of testosterone to prevent cyclophosphamide-induced azoospermia. *Ann Intern Med* 1997;126(4):292.
265. Dooley MA, Patterson CC, Hogan SL, et al. Preservation of ovarian function using depot leuprolide acetate during cyclophosphamide therapy for severe lupus nephritis (abstract). *Arthritis Rheum* 2000;43.
266. Gaskin G, Pusey CD. Plasmapheresis in antineutrophil cytoplasmic antibody-associated systemic vasculitis. *Ther Apher* 2001;5(3):176.
267. Frasca GM, Zoumparidis NG, Borgnino LC, et al. Plasma exchange treatment in rapidly progressive glomerulonephritis associated with anti-neutrophil cytoplasmic autoantibodies. *Int J Artif Organs* 1992;15(3):181.
268. Frasca GM, Zoumparidis NG, Borgnino LC, et al. Combined treatment in Wegener's granulomatosis with crescentic glomerulonephritis: clinical course and long-term outcome. *Int J Artif Organs* 1993;16(1):11.
269. Zauner I, Bach D, Braun N, et al. Predictive value of initial histology and effect of plasmapheresis on long-term prognosis of rapidly progressive glomerulonephritis. *Am J Kidney Dis* 2002;39(1):28.
270. Langford CA, Talar W, Sneller MC. Use of methotrexate and glucocorticoids in the treatment of Wegener's granulomatosis: long-term renal outcome in patients with glomerulonephritis. *Arthritis Rheum* 2000;43(8):1836.
271. Stegeman CA, Tervaert JW, Kallenberg CG. Co-trimoxazole and Wegener's granulomatosis: more than a coincidence? *Nephrol Dial Transplant* 1997;12(4):652.
272. Langford CA, Talar-Williams C, Sneller MC. Mycophenolate mofetil for remission maintenance in the treatment of Wegener's granulomatosis. *Arthritis Rheum* 2004;51(2):278.
273. Metzler C, Fink C, Lamprecht P, et al. Maintenance of remission with leflunomide in Wegener's granulomatosis. *Rheumatol (Oxford)* 2004;43(3):315.
274. Specks U, Fervenza FC, McDonald TJ, et al. Response of Wegener's granulomatosis to anti-CD20 chimeric monoclonal antibody therapy. *Arthritis Rheum* 2001;44(12):2836.
275. D'Haens G, Van DS, Van HR, et al. Endoscopic and histological healing with infliximab anti-tumor necrosis factor antibodies in Crohn's disease: a European multicenter trial. *Gastroenterology* 1999;116(5):1029.
276. Wegener's granulomatosus Etanercept Trial (WGET). Etanercept plus standard therapy for Wegener's granulomatosis: *N Engl J Med* 2005;352(4):351.
277. DeRemee RA, McDonald TJ, Weiland LH. Wegener's granulomatosis: observations on treatment with antimicrobial agents. *Mayo Clin Proc* 1985;60(1):27.
278. Reinhold-Keller E, DeGroot K, Rudert H, et al. Response to trimethoprim/sulfamethoxazole in Wegener's granulomatosis depends on the phase of disease. *QJM* 1996;89(1):15.

CHAPTER 69 ■ MIXED CRYOGLOBULINEMIA

GIUSEPPE D'AMICO

The term "cryoglobulinemia" describes a group of proteins with the common property of precipitating from cooled serum (1–5). On the basis of immunochemical studies, Brouet et al. (6) identified three types of cryoglobulins.

In type I, the cryoprecipitated immunoglobulin is a single monoclonal immunoglobulin. Types II and III cryoglobulinemias are both mixed types with at least two immunoglobulins; in both types, polyclonal immunoglobulin G (IgG) is bound to another immunoglobulin, which is an antiglobulin, acting as an anti-IgG rheumatoid factor (RF). The important difference between these two types of mixed cryoglobulins (MCs) is that in type II the antiglobulin component, which usually is of the IgM class, is monoclonal, whereas in type III it is polyclonal. Both components of MCs, IgG and IgM RF, are necessary for precipitation in the cold, whereas the individual components do not have this property.

The majority of MCs, defined as "secondary mixed cryoglobulins," have been detected in patients with connective tissue disorders, lymphoproliferative disorders, noninfectious hepatobiliary diseases, or immunologically mediated glomerular diseases.

Until the end of the 1980s, the cause of approximately 30% of both type II and type III mixed cryoglobulinemias was not clear; this subset of cryoglobulinemias was called "essential" (7). Over the past 10 years, anti-hepatitis C virus (HCV) antibodies and HCV RNA (a marker of active viremia) have been detected in the great majority (up to 90%) of patients with "essential" mixed cryoglobulinemia of both types (8–17). Positivity for HCV RNA was even greater in the cryoprecipitate (11,13,16).

The clinical syndrome of mixed cryoglobulinemia (MC) was first described by Meltzer et al. in 1966 (7). It was characterized by purpura, weakness, arthralgias, and, in several patients, proliferative glomerulonephritis (GN). Many subsequent reports further defined this syndrome, confirming that renal involvement is particularly frequent in MC (18–37). Kidney involvement ranges from 8% to 58% in large series of patients and is more frequent in women and in type II MC. The incidence of MC nephritis varies in different geographic areas, probably reflecting a different distribution of hepatitis C. The disease seems to be more frequent in some Mediterranean countries such as France, Spain, and, particularly, Italy, whereas it is very rare in northern Europe and in North America. Although the glomerular lesions are variable and nonspecific in the few cases of type III MC with renal involvement, in type II MC in which IgMk is the monoclonal component, a particularly well-characterized pattern of glomerular disease has been described (24,26,27,31,38,39), that Mazzucco et al. (39) termed "cryoglobulinemic glomerulonephritis."

RENAL HISTOLOGY

Light Microscopy Findings

Glomeruli

Cryoglobulinemic glomerulonephritis is a membranoproliferative, exudative GN. It is different from the idiopathic type of membranoproliferative GN as well as from the diffuse proliferative GN of systemic lupus by having the following features:

1. Endocapillary hypercellularity mainly due to a frequently massive infiltration of monocytes and sometimes T lymphocytes (38–44) (Fig 69-1). Some of the infiltrating monocytes express anti-tissue factor procoagulant activity and are therefore activated cells (44).
2. Large, amorphous, eosinophilic, periodic acid-Schiff (PAS)–positive, Congo red-negative deposits lying against the inner side of glomerular capillary wall and filling the capillary lumen, the so-called *intraluminal thrombi*, seen in about one-third of all patients and especially in those with more acute renal disease and more massive proliferation and exudation (26,27,31,43,45,46) (Fig. 69-2).
3. Thickening of the glomerular basement membrane, with a "double contour" appearance, which is more diffuse and evident than in lupus nephritis and idiopathic membranoproliferative GN (Fig. 69-3). As seen by electron microscopy, the double contour is mainly due to the peripheral interposition of monocytes, whereas mesangial matrix and cell interposition are less evident than in lupus nephritis and in idiopathic membranoproliferative GN (37,39,43,47,48).

Not all patients with type II MC have these characteristic glomerular lesions. In about 10% of patients only a mild segmental mesangial proliferation, without significant monocytes infiltration, is found. In another 10% of patients the glomerular pattern is that of a lobular GN, with mesangial expansion and centrolobular sclerosis. With the exception of this small group of patients, glomerular segmental and global sclerosis is rather mild and inconstant even many years after the onset of renal disease (26,31,43).

Interstitium and Vessels

Monocytes and T lymphocytes accumulate in the interstitium in the acute stages (44). Interstitial fibrosis, however, is not a prominent finding, even in late biopsy specimens.

An acute vasculitis of small and medium-sized arteries is present in at least one-third of patients who are biopsied

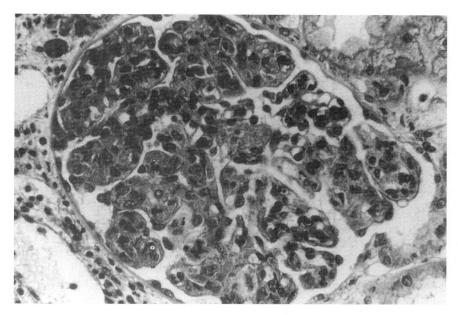

FIGURE 69-1. Cryoglobulinemic glomeru-lonephritis. Note the marked infiltration of the glomerular tuft with mononuclear cells. Light microscopy. (Masson trichrome, magnification ×320.)

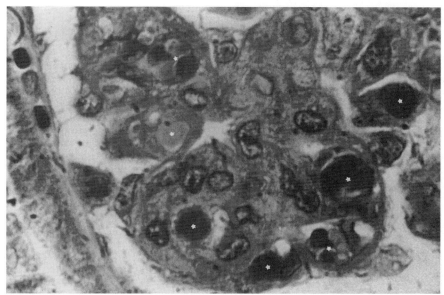

FIGURE 69-2. Numerous hyaline thrombi (∗) occluding many capillary lumina. Note their different tinctorial affinity. Light microscopy. (Masson trichrome, magnification ×750.)

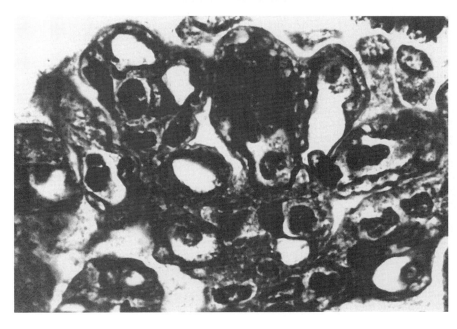

FIGURE 69-3. Glomerular capillary walls with "double-contour" appearance. Light microscopy. (Jones silver methenamine, magnification ×750.)

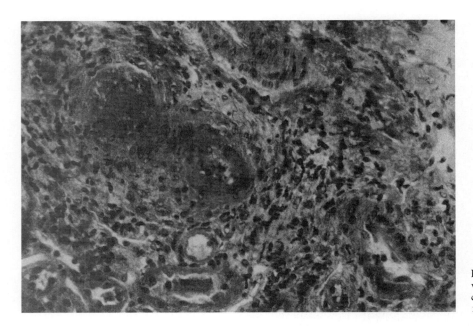

FIGURE 69-4. Severe necrotizing arteritis involving an interlobular artery. Light microscopy. (Masson trichrome, magnification ×320.)

during the acute stage of the renal disease, and in a larger percentage of postmortem specimens (31,47). It can be found even in the absence of obvious glomerular damage. The acute vasculitis is characterized by fibrinoid necrosis of the arteriolar wall, with infiltration of monocytes around the wall (Fig. 69-4). Even when the fibrinoid necrosis of the arterial wall is severe, the lesions of segmental necrosis of the capillary loops, with crescentic extracapillary proliferation (now considered the equivalent of vasculitic damage of the glomerular capillaries), is absent, suggesting that the vasculitic damage is limited to arterial vessels of larger size.

Electron Microscopic Findings

Electron-dense deposits can be found in the capillary lumen, usually in a subendothelial position but sometimes also filling the capillary lumen. They are sometimes amorphous immune complex-like deposits, but often they have a peculiar fibrillar or crystalloid structure (24,26,27,31,49,50), which is identical to that seen in the *in vitro* cryoprecipitate in the same patients, consisting of cylinders that are 100 or 1000 nm long and having a hollow axis (Fig. 69-5). In cross-sections they look like annular bodies with a light center, a dense ring, and lighter peripheral protein coat. The crystalloid deposits, when present, are often surrounded by areas of amorphous, weakly osmiophilic and translucent material, attributed to degradation of the deposits. Both types of deposits are infrequently seen in mesangial area, and subepithelial deposits are quite unusual. Circulating aggregates or structured material can sometimes be found in peritubular capillaries and arterioles. Ultrastructural examination confirms that monocytes in the capillary lumina are responsible mainly for the intracapillary proliferation, and increase in mesangial matrix can also be found. Monocytes very often appear to be in close contact with subendothelial and intraluminal amorphous or crystalloid deposits. In fact, these cells appear to be filled with large amorphous protein droplets with different osmiophilia, which are probably products of phagocytosis (phagolysosomes) (38,40,50). These intracellular protein droplets do not have a crystalloid structure, suggesting that the cryoglobulins lose their structure during phagocytosis. When a large number of these monocytes with giant protein droplets accumulate in the capillary lumen with the amorphous or crystalloid deposits, they contribute to the complete occlusion of the lumen. Monocytes can frequently be found interspersed with the subendothelial deposits, between the glomerular basement membrane and the endothelial cells or the newly formed basement membrane-like material in those areas in which capillary walls are double-contoured.

Immunohistologic Features

Three patterns of glomerular deposition can be seen by immunofluorescence (30,31,45,51,52).

1. Intensive, massive staining of huge deposits that fill the capillary lumen (intraluminal thrombi), usually associated with faint, irregular, segmental parietal staining of some peripheral loops, in a subendothelial position (Fig. 69-6).
2. The same pattern of faint, irregular, segmental parietal staining of some peripheral loops, in a subendothelial position, but without any intraluminal staining.
3. Intense granular diffuse staining of peripheral loops, with a subendothelial pattern (Fig. 69-7).

IgM and IgG are the prevailing immunoreactants in type II MC, suggesting that they are locally trapped or precipitated cryoglobulins. This identity was confirmed by the demonstration (53) that the immune deposits have antiglobulin activity similar to that of the serum cryo-IgM. More recently, using monoclonal antibodies against cross-reactive idiotypes present on rheumatoid factors, we identified the same idiotype of the circulating monoclonal rheumatoid factors in renal biopsy specimens from patients with MC-GN (54). C3 is present very frequently in the parietal deposits, with a distribution similar to that of immunoglobulins, although with a lower intensity. Intraluminal thrombi only occasionally show positive fluorescence for complement components. Deposits of earlier complement components (C1 and C4) and fibrinogen are also found in the parietal deposits in about 30% of cases. Vascular deposits of IgM, IgG, C3, and fibrinogen are detected in about one-third of cases.

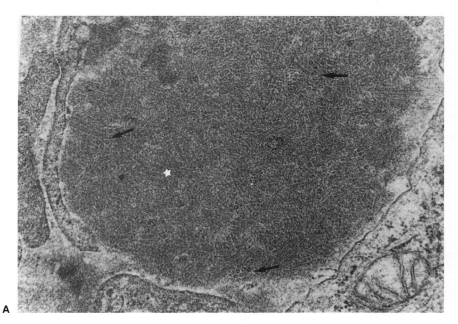

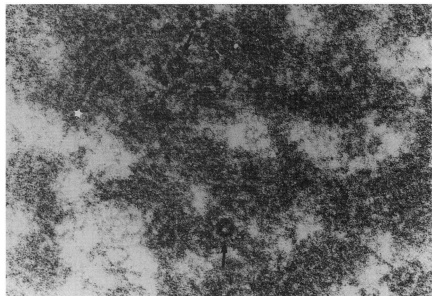

FIGURE 69-5. A: Crystalloid structure of deposits in the glomerulus. **B:** Identical structure in the *in vitro* cryoprecipitate of the same patient. The deposits consist of straight or slightly curved paired cylinders (✷) and annular structures (→).

CLINICAL MANIFESTATION

Clinical Features at Presentation

In most patients, type II MC is diagnosed between the fifth and the sixth decades of life, but in many patients some symptoms of the disease may first appear some 10 to 20 years before a correct diagnosis is made. Renal involvement usually manifests many years after the first symptoms develop. In some cases, however, renal and extrarenal manifestations appear concomitantly. More rarely, renal disease may be the first presenting manifestation.

The most frequent presenting renal syndrome is isolated proteinuria with microscopic hematuria, sometimes associated with signs of moderate chronic renal insufficiency. An acute nephritic syndrome characterized by severe proteinuria, micro-

scopic or macroscopic hematuria, arterial hypertension, and a sudden rise in serum creatinine is the first renal manifestation in about 20% to 30% of patients and may be complicated by oliguria in some 5% of cases. In another 20% of patients, renal involvement presents with a nephrotic syndrome (26,27,30,34,37).

Arterial hypertension is observed in more than 80% of patients at the time of onset of renal disease (31,34,37). Extrarenal symptoms and signs are usually observed at presentation (Table 69-1).

Natural History and Prognosis

The severity of the disease may be remarkably variable. Extrarenal symptoms may show a fluctuating course with alternations of quiescence and exacerbation. Most patients have

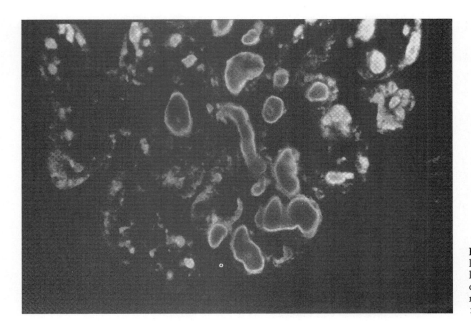

FIGURE 69-6. Large thrombi in many capillary lumina and scanty deposits along glomerular basement membranes. The antiserum stains only the periphery of the thrombi. Immunofluorescence study. (Anti-IgM serum, magnification ×450.)

recurrent, nonpruritic, palpable purpura or petechiae, usually affecting the lower extremities. Joints involved in MC include the hands, knees, ankles, and elbows, often in a migratory fashion. Fever is a relatively frequent manifestation of MC. About one-fourth of patients in whom infection can be excluded may present with prolonged episodes of fever. Liver involvement is frequent and can have serious consequences, but very often, despite the concomitant HCV infection, liver function abnormalities are mild and rarely symptomatic. Abnormal liver function tests were detected in about 25% of cases in two large series (27,34) of patients with renal involvement, in higher percentages of patients in other series of nonselected patients (25,35,36). Eighty to 100% of patients tested with antibodies or polymerase chain reaction have been found to be positive for HCV (8,9,11–15). An association with hepatitis B surface antigen has been reported in the past by some investigators (55,56), but this association was not confirmed. It is possible

that some HBV-positive patients were also HCV positive. Histology shows a chronic hepatitis with a striking mononuclear cell infiltrate (56). In rare cases patients with MC may develop severe intestinal vasculitis with consequent ischemia, which can pose problems of differential diagnosis. Lung involvement is frequent in MC, probably as a consequence of immune complex deposition. Tests that are considered to be indicative of small airways disease frequently demonstrate abnormalities in MC (35). Several patients can show attack of spasmodic asthma, pleurisy, and hemoptysis with roentgenographic or histologic abnormalities (35,57). An acute respiratory distress syndrome requiring mechanical ventilation may rarely occur (58). Peripheral neuropathy was considered to be a rare complication of MC in the past, but when electromyography was routinely made, an abnormal peripheral nerve conductivity was found in 68% to 82% of patients (59,60). Lymphadenopathy, thrombocytopenia, Sjögren syndrome, Raynaud phenomenon, retinal vasculitis, and central nervous system involvement are rarely observed (32,34,61,62).

Kidney involvement in MC often heralds an ominous prognosis, although renal disease may have a variable course. Some 10% to 15% of patients may attain complete or partial remission of renal symptoms even though some of them presented with an acute nephritic syndrome (23,29). In another 30% of patients the renal disease follows an indolent course and does not progress to end-stage renal failure despite the persistence of urinary abnormalities and even some degree of renal dysfunction. In about 20% of patients, several episodes of an acute nephritic syndrome can occur, sometimes associated with flare-ups of the systemic signs of the disease. These episodes may be treated with high-dose corticosteroids and/or plasmapheresis but sometimes may spontaneously reverse and reappear; a moderate degree of renal insufficiency is rather frequent, usually long after the onset of the disease. However, the development of terminal renal failure is relatively rare. In the large series of patients with MC nephritis studied in Milan, Tarantino et al (29) reported that after a mean follow-up of 131 months only 15 of 105 patients required regular dialysis. However, in the meantime, 42 patients died because of extrarenal complications. Cardiovascular complications, infections, liver failure, and neoplasia were the most important causes of death (Table 69-2). Cardiovascular and cerebrovascular accidents were particularly frequent in patients with

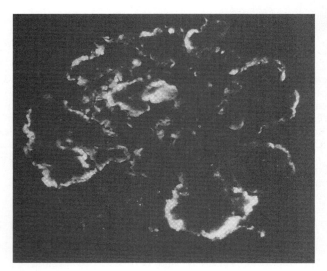

FIGURE 69-7. Diffuse granular deposits irregularly distributed on peripheral capillary loops. Immunofluorescence study. (Anti-IgM serum, magnification ×320.)

TABLE 69-1

EXTRARENAL SIGNS AND SYMPTOMS IN 116 PATIENTS WITH ESSENTIAL MIXED CRYOGLOBULINEMIA NEPHRITIS

Purpura	88%	Raynaud's phenomenon	35%
Hepatomegaly	88%	Nervous system involvement	31%
Arthralgias	78%	Abdominal pain	27%
Weakness	67%	Thrombocytopenia	26%
Fever	56%	Increase in liver enzymes	25%
Anemia	53%	Weight loss	23%
Splenomegaly	50%	Pleurisy	23%

(From: Tarantino A, et al. Prognostic factors in essential mixed cryoglobulinemia nephropathy. In Ponticelli C, Minetti L, D'Amico G, eds. *Antiglobulins, Cryoglobulins and Glomerulonephritis.* Dordrecht: M. Nijhoff; 1986:219.)

arterial hypertension, which occurs early in MC and is often severe and difficult to control. In that study, the 10-year probability of being alive without dialysis was 49%. Older patients, those with purpura, splenomegaly, high serum cryocrit, low serum C3 levels, and high serum creatinine were more likely to die or to reach end-stage renal failure. An even higher mortality rate in patients with MC nephritis has been reported by others. Death was reported in 18 of 22 patients by Gorevic et al. (20) in 12 of 15 patients by Cordonnier et al. (22), and in 8 of 12 patients by Frankel et al. (27).

In summary, two groups of patients with MC nephritis can be identified: (a) those with multisystemic involvement including renal disease who have a tumultuous course and may die before end-stage renal failure develops, and (b) those with fewer signs of systemic vasculitis who generally have a benign course

TABLE 69-2

CAUSES OF DEATH IN 42 PATIENTS WITH MIXED CRYOGLOBULINEMIA NEPHRITIS

Cause of death	No. of patients
Cardiovascular accidents	12
Cerebral hemorrhage	4
Heart failure	3
Intestinal infarction	2
Myocardial infarction	2
Pulmonary embolism	1
Infections	9
Sepsis	5
Tuberculosis	1
Meningitis	1
Pneumonia	1
Peritonitis	1
Liver failure	8
Neoplasia	4
Chronic lymphatic	1
Leukemia	1
Non-Hodgkin's lymphoma	1
Laryngeal cancer	1
Acute respiratory distress	1
Unknown	8

(Data from: Tarantino A, et al. Long-term predictors of survival in essential mixed cryoglobulinemic nephritis. *Kidney Int* 1995;47:618.)

without developing renal failure. Whether these differences are correlated to the nature of immunoglobulins involved in the phenomenon of cryoprecipitation or to the physicochemical characteristics and other properties of cryoglobulins remains to be ascertained.

Laboratory Data

As already discussed, cryoglobulins in type II MC are composed of two immunoglobulins, one of which is monoclonal and acts as an antiglobulin against polyclonal IgG. The monoclonal immunoglobulin is usually an IgM but can also be an IgG or IgA (18,63–66). Characterization of the cryoglobulins in patients with renal disease shows the exclusive monoclonal nature of antiglobulin IgM, which is nearly always an IgM-k (26,27,31). On the contrary, in rheumatologic surveys, patients with polyclonal IgM (type III cryoglobulinemia) outnumber those with monoclonal IgM. Serum titers of IgM rheumatoid factor (RF) activity are usually elevated and there are high serum levels of immune complex material as assessed by the C1q-binding assay (69–71).

The cryocrit value may vary considerably from 2% to 80% in different patients and can fluctuate over time in single patients. Also characteristic, although not invariable, is the pattern of complement activation in serum, with selective depletion of early components of the classic pathway and normal factor B levels (70). The serum pattern of complement is rather specific for MC. C1q, C4, and CH50 are usually low; C3 may be slightly low or normal; and the late components (C5-C9) C3PA and C1NH tend to be higher than in normal controls. The C3 breakdown product C3d is sometimes increased (26,70–72). These complement component abnormalities have been attributed to complement hyposynthesis (70,73), but it is also possible that the consumption of the early serum complement components with the characteristic sparing of C3 might be attributed to the C4-binding protein that controls the mechanism of the classic pathway C3 convertase (71,74). A retarded clearance of IgG coated autologous erythrocytes, indicative of abnormal Fc receptor function, is specific for patients with MC and renal involvement or motor neuropathy (75).

A peculiar hematologic finding of all types of cryoglobulinemias is represented by pseudoleukocytosis and/or pseudothrombocytosis, with an abnormal histogram as determined by a Coulter Counter (76,77). These abnormalities, which disappear if the blood sample is warmed at 37°C, can alert the clinician to the possible diagnosis of MC. Therefore, particular attention should be paid to the leukocytes and platelet counts in patients with MC (78).

No correlation has been found between the degree of activity of MC and the values for cryocrit, IgM rheumatoid factor, or early complement components (21,25,29,70). However, patients who have died had significantly higher cryocrit values and lower levels of IgG than did those who have survived, thereby suggesting a possible prognostic value of these parameters (79).

PATHOGENESIS

The Role of Hepatitis C Virus (HCV) Infection in Inducing Mixed Cryoglobulinemia

The polyclonal anti-IgG immunoglobulins involved in type III MC are derived from perturbation and magnification of the physiologic mechanism of production of antigloblulins concerned with immunoregulation and are antigen-driven, whereas the monoclonal anti-IgG immunoglobulins of type II MC may be derived from abnormal proliferation of a special clone of B lymphocytes, probably as a consequence of lymphoproliferative disorder (even though only a small number of patients with type II MC develop lymphoid malignancy) (37,80). Obviously, the same chronic antigen stimulation that induces the production of polyclonal RFs by B lymphocytes might in some cases favor the growth and amplification of a specific clone of B cells that produces a monoclonal RF. With a panel of mouse monoclonal anti-RF idiotypes, an increased percentage of idiotype-positive ($\mu +$) B cells has been found in patients with type II MC (81). Peripheral B lymphocytes from MC patients produce larger quantities of IgM-RF than normal B lymphocytes, both spontaneously and after *in vitro* stimulation with pokeweed mitogen (82). Moreover, Agnello's group in the United States found the same cross-idiotype (WA) in the monoclonal IgM of type II essential MC and of type II MC secondary to malignancies of the immune system (83). It has been suspected that some antigen, possibly the same antigen that triggers the production of RFs, is bound to the polyclonal IgG of the MC of type II or III, so that the IgM RFs acts as anti-immune complex antibody. The recent demonstration of a very high rate of positivity of anti-hepatitis C virus (HCV) antibodies and of HCV RNA in the sera of patients with all type of mixed cryoglobulinemia suggests a direct role of such chronic infection in their pathogenesis.

Because it has been found recently that peripheral blood mononuclear leukocytes, and, especially B lymphocytes, can be the site for extrahepatic viral replication of HCV (84–86), particularly when there is chronic infection (84), we have postulated (32,80,87) that in a subgroup of patients with chronic infection direct active viral replication in B lymphocytes induces type III MC by triggering the activation of clones of B cells to hyperproduce polyclonal IgM RF. We have further postulated,that some additional, as yet uncharacterized, events might induce, in a small subgroup of this population of patients with polyclonal B cell activation due to viral infection, the shift to the abnormal proliferation of a clone of B cells producing a monoclonal IgM rheumatoid factor (type II MC).

The Role of HCV Infection for the Pathogenesis of Cryoglobulinemic Glomerulonephritis (and Other Types of Membranoproliferative Glomerulonephritis?)

It is now accepted that the large majority of patients with type II mixed cryoglobulinemia and membranoproliferative glomerulonephritis (MPGN) have an active HCV infection; however, in almost 10% of our large group of patients with cryoglobulinemic GN, we found constant and protracted negativity of all signs of HCV infection (80).

The role of the virus in inducing renal lesions is still a matter of controversy. It is still debated whether HCV antigens are directly involved in mediating the immune complex glomerular lesions, independent of the concomitant existence of a cryoglobulinemia (as HBV antigens do in chronic hepatitis B infection), or whether the renal lesion is mediated by the virus through induction of the lymphoproliferative disorder, which activates the B-cell clones that produce monoclonal IgM, and is present only when a type II mixed cryoglobulinemia is also present. Data from the United States (88,89) and from Japan (90) show that, although type II MC and MPGN usually coexist in patients with HCV infection, the same type of glomerulonephritis can be found even in the absence of cryoglobulins. On the contrary, no cases of idiopathic MPGN concomitant with HCV infection, in the absence of type II MC, were found in another report from the United States (91), in Italy (32), in France (92), in Spain (93), in Turkey (94), and in Hong Kong (95).

In an experimental mouse model recently developed by Fornasieri et al. (96), an MPGN very similar to human cryoglobulinemic GN could be induced by intravenous injection of 37°C solubilized cryoglobulins from patients with this renal disease and HCV infection; IgMk isolated from such cryoglobulins, and certainly not containing any viral antigenic component, when injected separately could deposit in the glomerulus, suggesting a specific affinity of IgMk RF components of the cryoglobulins for some glomerular structure, as has been demonstrated for light chain disease (97). These investigators demonstrated also that the same purified IgMk binds to cellular fibronectin, a known constituent of mesangial matrix (98).

On the basis of this preliminary evidence, we hypothesize that cryoglobulinemic GN might be initiated by the binding, either *in situ* or in circulation, of IgG antibodies-HCV complexes to IgMk RF, the nephrotoxicity being due to the particular affinity of the IgMk RF for the glomerular matrix.

Treatment

Antiviral Therapy of Hepatitis C Viral Infection with Associated Mixed Cryoglobulinemia. It is probable that eradication of the viral infection can affect production of new cryoglobulins, and thus also systemic and renal damage.

In 1987, before the viral cause of essential MC had been proved, Bonomo et al. (99) had already reported a remarkable improvement of clinical signs in seven cryoglobulinemic patients treated with interferon alfa (IFNα), used for its potential antiproliferative and immunoregulatory effects.

After the viral etiopathogenesis of MC was demonstrated, the same antiviral drug, interferon-α, was used extensively. However, only three controlled trials in patients with HCV infection and associated MC have been reported in the literature (100–102). All of them showed a significant improvement of systemic signs, mainly purpura, with a reduction of cryoglobulins and transaminases. However, although eradication of viremia was obtained in only a fraction of patients, a recurrence of viremia and a rebound of the clinical signs, and of cryocrit, was reported by all these investigators. With the exception of the study of Misiani et al. (101), no clear renal involvement was present in the treated patients.

More extensive information (103–124) has been accumulated in these last years on the effect of interferon-α, administered alone or in association with another antiviral agent, ribavirin, in reducing the viremia and the liver damage in patients with HCV infection, and in controlling the systemic symptoms of MC in the subgroup of patients with associated cryoglobulinemia.

The most effective standard treatment is the combination of pegylated IFNα and ribavirin (125). In the pegylated form of interferon, the interferon-a molecule is linked to a polyethylene glycol molecule to ensure sustained interferon concentrations after single weekly injection (126–133).

Pegylated interferon-α potently inhibits the replication of HCV and has immunomodulatory properties that probably accelerate the clearance of infected cells. Ribavirin exerts a weak and transient early antiviral effect and acts primarily by preventing relapses during and after therapy in patients who have had an initial response. Ribavirin's mechanisms of action are unknown.

The main end-point of therapy is a "sustained virologic response," defined by an undetectable HCV RNA level in the patient's blood 24 weeks after the end of treatment. In most patients in whom a sustained virologic response is achieved, HCV infection appears to be definitively cured. Sustained virologic response, that did not exceed 40% to 45% of patients when the association nonpegylated IF-α-ribavirin was used, has been increased to 55% to 60% of them. In patients with no sustained virologic response with standard therapy, the lack of efficaciousness can be predicted already after 3 months of treatment. It has been found that in patients who do not have a reduction in HCV RNA of at least 2 $\log_{10}$ international units or an undetectable HCV RNA level by 12th week of treatment, there is virtually no chance of achieving a sustained virologic response. These patients can stop therapy at week 12. However, not all patients who have a reduction or disappearance of the virus at week 12 will subsequently have a sustained virologic response (125). Two pegylated interferon molecules have been commercialized. The recommended dose of peginterferon-α 2a is of 180 μg/week, that of peginterferon-α 2b is 1.5 μg/kg/week. The recommended dose of ribavirin is 1,000 to 1,200 mg/daily, based on body weight.

It has been found that both race and viral genotype influence the response to antiviral therapy. Blacks have been reported to have significantly lower response rates than the white and Asian populations. Treatment failure is more frequent among patients infected with HCV genotype 1.

As for the control of the extrarenal clinical manifestations of cryoglobulinemia, one study (133) suggested that improvement in cryoglobulinemia-related symptoms can be achieved, even without complete biochemical or virologic response.

Treatment of the Renal Complications of Mixed Cryoglobulinemia Associated with Hepatitis C Virus Infection

Although a sustained virologic response to the standard viral therapy described in the preceding text can interrupt the progression of the hepatic damage, and frequently improves the extrarenal signs of cryoglobulinemia, the results on the control of the clinical signs of the renal complication and on its progression are still controversial. Improvement, sometimes even protracted, of the renal disease has been reported in some anecdotal cases (134–137). In a more recent study in 25 consecutive patients with mixed cryoglobulinemia and proteinuria in the nephrotic range due to MPGN bioptically documented (138), a significant reduction of proteinuria and cryocrit after the standard combined antiviral therapy, without modifications of the serum creatinine, was found in the subgroup with sustained virologic response. The reduction in cryoglobulin level was sometimes persistent. Other clinical manifestations of cryoglobulinemia, such as arthralgia and polyneuropathy, were not clearly influenced by antiviral treatment.

There is now clear evidence that, when acute exacerbations of the glomerular disease occur, especially if they are associated with signs of acute systemic vasculitis, the antiviral therapy is not sufficient to control the disease (17,133,138–140), and may even exacerbate it (141–143).

According to our experience, steroids, and, in most severe cases, also plasmapheresis and cyclophosphamide, extensively used by us and by many others to treat "essential" MC in the 1980s, are still necessary to control flare-ups of cryoglobulinemic GN, despite the potential detrimental effect of the immunosuppressive drugs in increasing viral titers and aggravating hepatic damage.

Let us consider each of them separately.

Steroids. After the initial report by De Vecchi et al. (144), the subsequent experience of treatment of acute flare-ups of cryoglobulinemic GN and vasculitis has demonstrated that intravenous high-dose methylprednisolone (usually 1g per/day given every 24 hours for 3 consecutive days), followed by oral prednisone (0.5 mg/kg/day, rapidly tapered to 0.1 to 0.2 mg/kg/day) for at least 6 months, allows rapid improvement of the renal damage (serum creatinine and proteinuria) together with dramatic amelioration of the extrarenal symptoms.

Cyclophosphamide. This cytotoxic drug is usually in addition to steroid treatment, at the dose of 2 to 3 mg/kg per/day, for a minimum of 4 months, in the most severe cases of renal involvement, and in particular when renal and/or systemic vasculitis coexist. It has been accepted as a valid remedy despite the lack of controlled trials.

Plasmapheresis. The removal of significant amounts of cryoproteins from the blood, thereby preventing local cryoprecipitation in small renal vessels and restoring reticuloendothelial system functions that have been saturated by the chronic overload of circulating cryoglobulins, has been accepted as a useful therapy for the last 20 years. Many uncontrolled studies have reported good results, with improvements in serum creatinine, proteinuria, and cryocrit (7,30,145–151), and a very transient reduction of HCV viremia (152). Although in the majority of cases intensive plasma exchange (exchanges of 3 L of plasma per week for 2 to 3 weeks) has been performed in association with steroids and cyclophosphamide to block the production of new cryoglobulins

---

TABLE 69-3

THERAPY OF THE ACUTE FLARE-UPS OF CRYOGLOBULINEMIC GLOMERULONEPHRITIS AND VASCULITIS ASSOCIATED WITH HEPATITIS C VIRUS (HCV) INFECTION

INTERFERON-α
3 million units 3 times a week or peginterferon-α 2a 180 μg/week for 1 year (drug can be discontinued after 6 months if HCV-RNA does not disappear from the blood), and can be associated from the beginning to *ribavirin* (0.8–1.0 g/day)

STEROIDS
0.75–1.0 g/day of *methylprednisolone*, intravenously, for 3 consecutive days, followed by oral *prednisone* for 6 months (0.5 mg/kg of body weight daily, tapered over a few weeks until small maintenance doses are achieved)

CYCLOPHOSPHAMIDE
2 mg/kg of body weight, for 3 to 4 months (especially when signs of severe renal and systemic vasculitis are present)

PLASMAPHERESIS
Exchanges of 3 L of plasma 3 times/week, for 2 to 3 weeks (only most severe cases of acute renal involvement)

by the immunocomponent cells and the possible rebound, one group of investigators from Pisa, ltaly (147,153) has used plasmapheresis alone, repeated every few weeks for 2 to 24 months, to prevent clinical relapses.

Our current policy, derived from an extensive experience accumulated also with the treatment of "essential" MC in the 1980s, is to use antiviral agents (possibly a combination of IFNα and ribavirin), associated with small doses of oral steroids when necessary to control the systemic signs of MC. When an acute flare-up of the renal disease is present, with rapid deterioration of renal function and/or proteinuria in the nephrotic range, the schema indicated in Table 69-3 is used.

There was no evidence of any worsening of the liver involvement, as indicated by the level of hepatic enzymes in more than 50 patients treated with such a therapy, even though the potential increase of HCV replication in peripheral blood mononuclear cells, both *in vitro* and *in vivo*, after corticosteroid boluses has been recently reported (154).

References

1. Zinneman HH, Levi D, Seal U. On the nature of cryoglobulins. *J Immunol* 1968;100:594.
2. Abraham, GN, et al. Immunological structural properties of human monoclonal IgG cryoglobulins. *Clin Exp Immunol* 1979;36:63.
3. Saulk PA, Clem W. Studies on the cryoprecipitation of human IgG cryoglobulins: the effects of temperature-induced conformational changes of primary interaction. *Immunochemistry* 1975;12:29.
4. Litman GW, et al. Molecular basis for the temperature-dependent insolubility of cryoglobulins. XII. *Immunol Commun* 1981;10:707.
5. Grey HH, Kohler PE. Cryoimmunoglobulins. *Semin Hematol* 1973;10:87.
6. Brouet JC, et al. Biological and clinical significance of cryoglobulins. A report of 86 cases. *Am J Med* 1974;57:775.
7. Meltzer M, et al. Cryoglobulinemia—a clinical and laboratory study. II. Cryoglobulins with rheumatoid factor activity. *Am J Med* 1966;40:837.
8. Ferri C, et al. Antibodies against hepatitis C virus in mixed cryoglobulinemia patients. *Infection* 1991;19:417.
9. Misiani R, et al. Hepatitis C virus infection in patients with essential mixed cryoglobulinemia. *Ann Intern Med* 1992;117:573.
10. Dammacco F, Sansonno D. Antibodies to hepatitis C virus in essential mixed cryoglobulinemia. *Clin Exp Immunol* 1992;87:352.
11. Marcellin P, et al. Cryoglobulinemia with vasculitis associated with hepatitis C virus infection. *Gastroenterology* 1993;104:272.
12. Pechére-Bertschi A, et al. Hepatitis C: a possible etiology for cryoglobulinemia type II. *Clin Exp Immunol* 1992;89:419.
13. Agnello V, Chung RT, Kaplan ML. A role for hepatitis C virus infection in type II cryoglobulinemia. *N Engl J Med* 1992;327:1490.
14. Cacoub P, et al. Mixed cryoglobulinemia and hepatitis C virus. *Am J Med* 1996;96:124.
15. D'Amico G. Hepatitis C virus and essential mixed cryoglobulinemia. *Nephrol Dial Transplant* 1993;8:579.
16. Bichard P, et al. High prevalence of hepatitis C virus RNA in the supernatant and the cryoprecipitate of patients with essential and secondary type II mixed cryoglobulinemia. *J Hepatol* 1994;21:58.
17. Meyers CM, et al. Hepatitis C and renal disease: an update. *Am J Kidney Dis* 2003;42:631.
18. Bengtsson U, et al. Monoclonal IgG cryoglobulinemia with secondary development of glomerulonephritis and nephrotic syndrome. *Q J Med* 1975;175:491.
19. Cordonnier D, et al. Mixed IgG-IgM cryoglobulinemia with glomerulonephritis. Immunochemical fluorescent and ultrastructural study of kidney and in vitro cryoprecipitate. *Am J Med* 1975;59:867.
20. Gorevic PD, et al. Mixed cryoglobulinemia: Clinical aspects and long-term follow-up of 40 patients. *Am J Med* 1980;69:287.
21. Tarantino A, et al. Renal disease in essential mixed cryoglobulinemia. Long-term follow-up of 44 patients. *Q J Med* 1981;50:1.
22. Cordonnier S, et al. Lésions rénales chez 18 malades porteurs de cryoglobulines mixtes (IgM-IgG) de Type II. In: Hamburger J, Crosnier J, Funck-Brentano JL, eds. *Actualités Néphrologique de Hôpital Necker*. Paris: Flammarion; 1982.
23. Tarantino A, Ponticelli C. Kidney involvement in essential cryoglobulinemia. In: Bacon PA, Hadler NM, eds. *The Kidney and Rheumatic Disease*. London: Butterworth Scientific; 1982.
24. Ben Bassat M, et al. The clinicopathologic features of cryoglobulinemic nephropathy, *Am J Clin Pathol* 1983;79:147.
25. D'Amico G, et al. Glomerulonephritis in essential mixed cryoglobulinemia (EMC). In: Davison AM, Guillon PJ, eds. *Proceedings of European Dialysis and Transplant Association. European Renal Association*. London: Pitman; 1984.
26. D'Amico G, et al. Renal involvement in essential mixed cryoglobulinemia. *Kidney Int* 1989;35:1004.
27. Frankel AH, et al. Type II essential mixed cryoglobulinemia: presentation, treatment and outcome in 13 patients. *Q J Med* 1992;298:101.
28. Levey JM, et al. Mixed cryoglobulinemia in chronic hepatitis C infection. *Medicine* 1994;73:53.
29. Tarantino A, et al. Long-term predictors of survival in essential mixed cryoglobulinemic nephritis. *Kidney Int* 1995;47:618.
30. Bombardieri S, et al. Lung involvement in essential mixed cryoglobulinemia. *Am J Med* 1979;66:748.
31. Invernizzi F, et al. A long term follow-up study in essential mixed cryoglobulinaemia. *Acta Haematol* 1979;61:93.
32. D'Amico G, Fornasieri A. Cryoglobulinemic glomerulonephritis: a membrano-proliferative glomerulonephritis induced by hepatitis C virus. *Am J Kidney Dis* 1995;25:361.
33. Rieu V, et al. Characteristics and outcome of 49 patients with symptomatic cryoglobulinemia. *Rheumatology* 2002;41:290.
34. Dispenzieri A, Gorevic PD. Cryoglobulinemia. *Hematol Oncol Clin North Am* 1999;13(6):1315.
35. Morales JM, et al. Glomerulonephritis associated with hepatitis C virus infection. *Nephrol Hypertens* 1999;8:205.
36. Lamprecht P, et al. Immunological and clinical follow up of hepatitis C virus associated cryoglobulinaemic vasculitis. *Ann Rheum Dis* 2001;60:385.
37. Ferri C, Zignego AL, Pileri SA. Cryoglobulins. *J Clin Pathol* 2002;55:4.
38. Monga G, et al. Glomerular findings in mixed IgG-IgM cryoglobulinemia. Light, electron microscopy, immunofluorescence and histochemical correlations. *Virchows Arch Zell Pathol* 1976;20:185.
39. Mazzucco G, et al. Cell interposition in glomerular capillary walls in cryoglobulinemic glomerulonephritis. Ultrastructural investigation of 23 cases. *Ultrastruct Pathol* 1986;10:355.
40. Monga G, et al. The presence and possible role of monocyte infiltration in human chronic proliferative glomerulonephritis. *Am J Pathol* 1979;94:271.
41. Magil AB. Monocytes and glomerulonephritis associated with remote visceral infection. *Clin Nephrol* 1984;22:169.
42. Ferrario F, et al. The detection of monocytes in human glomerulonephritis. *Kidney Int* 1985;28:513.
43. Ferrario F, et al. Histological and immunohistological features in essential mixed cryoglobulinemia glomerulonephritis. In: Ponticelli C, Minetti L, D'Amico G, eds. *Antiglobulins, Cryoglobulins and Glomerulonephritis*. Dordrecht: M Nijhoff; 1986.
44. Castiglione A, et al The relationship of infiltrating renal leukocytes to disease activity in lupus and cryoglobulinemic glomerulonephritis. *Nephron* 1988;50:14.
45. Morel-Maroger L, Méry JP. Renal lesions in mixed IgG-IgM essential cryoglobulinemia. In *Proceedings of the Fifth Congress of Nephrology, Mexico, 1972*. Basel: Karger; 1972.
46. Morel-Maroger L, Verroust P. Glomerular lesions in dysproteinemias. *Kidney Int* 1974;5:249.
47. Zollinger HU, Mihatsch MJ. Immunohistopathologic parameters. In: Zollinger HU, Mihatsch MJ, eds. *Renal Pathology in Biopsy*. Berlin: Springer; 1978.
48. Faraggiana T, et al. Light and electron microscopic findings in five cases of cryoglobulinemic glomerulonephritis. *Virchows Arch Pathol Anat* 1979;384:29.
49. Feiner H, Gallo, G. Ultrastructure in glomerulonephritis associated with cryoglobulinemia. *Am J Pathol* 1977;88:145.
50. Mihatsch MJ, Banfi, G. Ultrastructural features in glomerulonephritis in essential mixed cryoglobulinemia. In: Ponticelli C, Minetti L, D'Amico G, eds. *Antiglobulins, Cryoglobulins and Glomerulonephritis*. Dordrecht: M. Nijhoff; 1986.
51. Barbiano di Belgiojoso G, et al. Immunohistological patterns in mixed IgG-IgM essential cryoglobulinemia glomerulonephritis. In: Leaf A, Giebisch G, Bolis L, Gorini S, eds. *Renal Pathophysiology*. New York: Raven; 1980.
52. Barbiano di Belgiojoso G, et al. Clinical and histological correlations in essential mixed cryoglobulinemia (EMC) glomerulonephritis. In: Ponticelli C, Minetti L, D'Amico G eds. *Antiglobulins, Cryoglobulins and Glomerulonephritis*. Dordrecht: M. Nijhoff; 1986.
53. Maggiore Q, et al. HbsAG glomerular deposits in glomerulonephritis: Fact or artifact? *Kidney Int* 1981;19:579.
54. Sinico AR, et al. Identification of glomerular immune deposits in cryoglobulinemia glomerulonephritis. *Kidney Int* 1988;34:109.
55. Levo Y, et al. Association between hepatitis B virus and essential mixed cryoglobulinemia. *N Engl J Med* 1977;296:1501.
56. Gorevic P. Mixed cryoglobulinemia: an update of recent clinical experience. In Ponticelli C, Minetti L, D'Amico G, eds. *Antiglobulins, Cryoglobulins and Glomerulonephritis*. Dordrecht: M. Nijhoff; 1986.
57. Martinez JS, Kohler PF. Variant "Goodpasture's syndrome?" The need for immunologic criteria in rapidly progressive glomerulonephritis and hemorrhagic pneumonitis. *Ann Intern Med* 1971;75:67.
58. Stagg MP, Lauber J, Michaliski JP. Mixed essential cryoglobulinemia and adult respiratory distress syndrome: a case report. *Am J Med* 1988;87:445.
59. Valli G, et al. Peripheral nervous system involvement in essential cryoglobulinemia and nephropathy. *Clin Exp Rheumatol* 1989;7:479.
60. Ferri C, et al. Peripheral neuropathy in mixed cryoglobulinemia: clinical and electrophysiologic investigations. *Rheumatol* 1992;19:889.

61. Reik L Jr, Korn JH. Cryoglobulinemia with encephalopathy: successful treatment by plasma exchange. *Ann Neurol* 1981;10:488.
62. Invernizzi F, et al. Secondary and essential cryoglobulinemias. *Acta Haematol* 1983;70:73.
63. Cream JJ, Howard A, Virella G. IgG heavy chain subclasses in mixed cryoglobulins. *Immunology* 1972;23:405.
64. Franklin EC, Frangione B. Common structural and antigenic properties of human M anti-γ-globulins. *J Immunol* 1971;107:1527.
65. Klein F, et al. IgM-IgG cryoglobulinemia with paraprotein component. *Clin Exp Immunol* 1968;3:703.
66. Trieshmann HW Jr, Abraham GN, Santucci EA. The characterization of human anti IgG autoantibodies by liquid isoelectric focusing. *J Immunol* 1975;114:176.
67. Aho K, Simons K. Studies of the nature of the rheumatoid factor. Reaction of the rheumatic factor with human specific precipitates and with native human gamma globulin. *Arthritis Rheum* 1963;6:676.
68. Lawley TJ, et al. Multiple types of immune complexes in patients with mixed cryoglobulinemia. *J Invest Dermatol* 1980;75:297.
69. McDuffie FC, Hunder GG, Clark JR. Complement fixing material in the sera of patients with rheumatoid arthritis. *Clin Exp Immunol* 1978;32:218.
70. Tarantino A, et al. Serum complement pattern in essential mixed cryoglobulinemia. *Clin Exp Immunol* 2978;32:77.
71. Gigli I. Complement activation in patients with mixed cryoglobulinemia (cryoglobulins and complement). In: Ponticelli C, Minetti L, D'Amico G, eds. *Antiglobulins, Cryoglobulins and Glomerulonephritis*. Dordrecht: M. Nijoff; 1986.
72. Linscott WD, Kane JP. The complement system in cryoglobulinemia: interaction with immunoglobulins and lipoproteins. *Clin Exp Immunol* 1975;21:510.
73. Ruddy S, et al. Human complement metabolism: an analysis of 144 studies. *Medicine* 1975;54:165.
74. Haydey RP, Patarroyo de Royas M, Gigli IA. A newly described control mechanism of complement activation in patients with mixed cryoglobulinemia (cryoglobulins and complement). *J Invest Dermatol* 1980;74:328.
75. Hamburger MI, et al. Mixed cryoglobulinemia. Association of glomerulonephritis with defective reticuloendothelial system Fc-receptor function. *Trans Assoc Am Physicians* 1979;62:104.
76. Banfi G, Bonini PA. Detection of cryoglobulins by Coulter Counter model S-Plus IV/D. *Clin Lab Haematol* 1988;10:453.
77. Montecucco C, Cherie-Ligniere EL, Ascari E. Pseudo-leucocytosis in essential mixed cryoglobulinemia may simulate chronic lymphocytic leukemia. *Clin Exp Rheumat* 1985;3:278.
78. Zandechi M, et al. Numération leucocytaire et plaquettaire artificiellement augmentées, rélévatrices d'une cryoglobulinemie de type II. *Nouv Presse Med* 1989;35:1756.
79. Tarantino A, et al. Prognostic factors in essential mixed cryoglobulinemia nephropathy. In: Ponticelli C, Minetti L, D'Amico G, eds. *Antiglobulins, Cryoglobulins and Glomerulonephritis*. Dordrecht: M Nijhoff; 1986.
80. D'Amico, G. Renal involvement in hepatitis C infection: cryoglobulinemic glomerulonephritis. *Kidney Int* 1998;54:650.
81. Winearls CG, et al. Numeration of circulating MRF-producing cells in essential mixed cryoglobulinemia. *Nephrol Dial Transplant* 1986;1:78.
82. Meroni PL, et al. In vitro synthesis of IgM rheumatoid factor by lymphocytes from patients with essential mixed cryoglobulinemia. *Clin Exp Immunol* 1986;65:303.
83. Abel G, Zhang Q, Agnello V. Hepatitis C virus infection in type II mixed cryoglobulinemia. *Arthritis Rheum* 1993;36:1341.
84. Müller HM, et al. Peripheral blood leukocytes serve as possible extrahepatic site for hepatitis C virus replication. *J Gen Virol* 1993;74:669.
85. Zignego AL, et al. Infection of peripheral mononuclear blood cells by hepatitis C virus. *J Hepatol* 1992;15:382.
86. Shimizu YK, et al. Evidence for *in vitro* replication of hepatitis C virus genome in human T-cell line. *Proc Natl Acad Sci U S A* 1992;89:5477.
87. D'Amico G. Is type II mixed cryoglobulinemia an essential part of hepatitis C virus (HCV) associated glomerulonephritis? *Nephrol Dial Transplant* 1995;10:1279.
88. Johnson RJ, et al. Membranoproliferative glomerulonephritis associated with hepatitis C virus infection. *N Engl J Med* 1993;328:465.
89. Johnson RJ, et al. Renal manifestation of hepatitis C virus infection. *Kidney Int* 1994;46:1255.
90. Yamabe H, et al. Hepatitis C virus (HCV) infection may be an important cause of membrano-proliferative glomerulonephritis (MPGN) in Japan (abstract). *J Am Soc Nephrol* 1993;4:2911.
91. Cosio FG, et al. Prevalence of hepatitis C in patients with idiopathic glomerulopathies in native and transplant kidneys. *Am J Kidney Dis* 1996;28:752.
92. Rostoker G, et al. Low prevalence of hepatitis C virus antibodies among adult patients with primary glomerulonephritis in France. *Nephron* 1993;63:367.
93. Gonzalo A, et al. Searching for hepatitis C virus antibodies in chronic primary glomerular diseases (letter). *Nephron* 1995;69:96.
94. Paydas S, et al. The frequencies of hepatitis B virus markers and hepatitis C virus antibody in patients with glomerulonephritis. *Nephron* 1996;74:617.
95. Mac-Moune Lai F, et al. Low prevalence of hepatitis virus antibodies with primary membranous nephropathy and membranoproliferative glomerulonephritis in Hong Kong. *Nephron* 1995;70:367.
96. Fornasieri A, et al. Glomerulonephritis induced by human IgMk-IgG cryoglobulins in mice. *Lab Invest* 1993;69:531.
97. Solomon A, Weiss DT, Kattine AA. Nephrotoxic potential of Bence Jones proteins. *N Engl J Med* 1991;324:1845.
98. Fornasieri A, et al. High binding of immunoglobulin Mκ rheumatoid factor from type II cryoglobulins to cellular fibronectin: a mechanism for induction of in situ immune complex glomerulonephritis? *Am J Kidney Dis* 1996;27:476.
99. Bonomo L, et al. Treatment of idiopathic mixed cryoglobulinemia with alpha interferon. *Am J Med* 1987;83:726.
100. Ferri C, Marzo E, Longobardo G. Interferon-alpha in mixed cryoglobulinemia patients: a randomized, crossover-controlled trial. *Blood* 1993;81:1132.
101. Misiani R, et al. Interferon alfa-2a therapy in cryoglobulinemia associated with hepatitis C virus. *N Engl J Med* 1994;330:751.
102. Dammacco F, et al. Natural interferon-alpha versus its combination with 6-methyl-prednisolone in the therapy of type II mixed cryoglobulinemia: a long-term, randomized, controlled study. *Blood* 1994;84:3336.
103. McHutchison JG, et al. Interferon alfa-2b alone or in combination with ribavirin as initial treatment for chronic hepatitis C. *N Engl J Med* 1998;21:1485.
104. Jake Liang T. Combination therapy for hepatitis C infection. *N Engl J Med* 1998;339:1549.
105. Mazzella G, et al. Long term results with interferon therapy in chronic type B hepatitis: a prospective randomized trial. *Am J Gastroenterol* 1999;8:2246.
106. Shiffman ML, et al. A randomized, controlled trial of maintenance interferon therapy for patients with chronic hepatitis C virus and persistent viremia. *Gastroenterology* 1999;5:1164.
107. Morisco F, et al. Clinical outcome of chronic hepatitis C in patients treated with interferon: Comparison between responders and non-responders. *Ital J Gastroenterol Hepatol* 1999;6:454.
108. Barnes E, et al. Long-term efficacy of treatment of chronic hepatitis C with alpha interferon or alpha interferon and ribavirin. *J Hepatol* 1999;1:244.
109. Jensen DM, et al. Biochemical and viral response to consensus interferon (CIFN) therapy in chronic hepatitis C patients: effect of baseline viral concentration. Consensus Interferon Study Group. *Am J Gastroenterol* 1999;12:3583.
110. Pol S, et al. A randomized trial of ribavirin and interferon-alpha vs. interferon-alpha alone in patients with chronic hepatitis C who were nonresponders to a previous treatment. Multicenter Study Group under the coordination of the Necker Hospital, Paris, France. *J Hepatol* 1999;1:1.
111. Camma C, et al. Chronic hepatitis C: interferon retreatment of relapsers. A meta-analysis of individual patient data. European Concerted Action on Viral Hepatitis (Eurohelp). *Hepatology* 1999;3:801.
112. Spadaro A, et al. Interferon retreatment of patients with chronic hepatitis C. A long-term follow-up. *Hepatogastroenterology* 1999;30:3229.
113. Daniel C, Cattran, MD. Interferon therapy: a double-edged sword? *Am J Kidney Dis* 1999;33:1174.
114. Bacon B, R. Available options for treatment of interferon nonresponders. *Am J Med* 1999;(6B):67S.
115. Jacobson I. Management of interferon relapsers. *Am J Med* 1999;6B:62S.
116. Lawrence SP. Advances in the treatment of hepatitis C. *Adv. Intern. Med.* 2000;45:65.
117. Pagliaro L, et al. Interferon-α for chronic hepatitis C: an analysis of pretreatment clinical predictors of response. *Hepatology* 1994;19:820.
118. Mc Hutchison J. Hepatitis C therapy in treatment-naïve patients. *Am J Med* 1999;6B:56S.
119. Polzien F, et al. Interferon-alpha treatment of hepatitis C virus-associated mixed cryoglobulinemia. *J Hepatol* 1997;27:63.
120. Casato M, et al. Predictors of long-term response to high-dose interferon therapy in type II cryoglobulinemia associated with hepatitis C virus infection. *Blood* 1997;10:3865.
121. Durand JM, et al. Ribavirin in hepatitis C-related cryoglobulinemia. *J Rheumat* 1998;6:1115.
122. Calleja JL, et al. Sustained response to interferon-alpha or to interferon-alpha plus ribavirin in hepatitis C virus-associated symptomatic mixed cryoglobulinemia. *Aliment Pharmacol Ther* 1999;9:1179.
123. Sabry AA, et al. Effect of combination therapy (ribavirin and interferon) in HCV-related glomerulopathy. *Nephrol Dial Transplant* 2002;17:1924.
124. D'Amico G, Fornasieri A. Cryoglobulinemia. In: Brady HR, Wilcox CS. *Therapy in Nephrology and Hypertension*. 2nd ed. Philadelphia: Saunders Co.; 2003:147.
125. Pawlotsky JM. Hepatitis C in "difficult to treat" patients. *N Engl J Med* 2004;351:421.
126. Glue P, et al. Pegylated interferon-alpha2b: pharmacokinetics, pharmacodynamics, safety, and preliminary efficacy data. Hepatitis C Intervention Therapy Group. *Clin Pharmacol Ther* 2000;68:556.
127. Zeuzem S, et al. Peginterferon alfa-2a in patients with chronic hepatitis C. *N Engl J Med* 2000;343:1666.
128. Heathcote EJ, et al. Peginterferon alfa-2ᵈ in patients with chronic hepatitis C and cirrhosis. *N Engl J Med* 2000;343:1673.
129. Lindsay KL, et al. A randomized, double-blind trial comparing pegylated interferon alfa-2b to interferon alfa-2b as initial treatment for chronic hepatitis C. *Hepatology* 2001;34:395.

130. Manns MP, et al. Peginterferon alfa-2b plus ribavirin for initial treatment of chronic hepatitis C: a randomized trial. *Lancet* 2001;358:395.
131. Fried MW, et al. Peginterferon alfa-2^a plus ribavirin for chronic hepatitis C virus infection. *N Engl J Med* 2002;347:975.
132. Hadziyannis SJ, et al. Peginterferon alfa-2^a (40 kD) (PEGASYS) in combination with ribavirin (RBV): efficacy and safety results from phase III, randomized, double-blind, multicenter study examining effect of duration of treatment and RBV dose (abstract). *J Hepatol* 2002;36(suppl):S3A.
133. Zuckerman E, et al. Treatment of refractory, symptomatic, hepatitis C virus related mixed cryoglobulinemia with ribavirin and interferon-alpha. *J Rheumatol* 2000;27:2172.
134. Johnson RJ, et al. Hepatitis C virus-associated glomerulonephritis. Effect of α-interferon therapy. *Kidney Int* 1994;46:1700.
135. Sarac E, Bastacky S, Johnson JP. Response to high-dose interferon-alpha after failure of standard therapy in MPGN associated with hepatitis C virus infection. *Am J Kidney Dis* 1997;1:113.
136. Misiani R, et al. Successful treatment of HCV-associated cryoglobulinaemic glomerulonephritis with a combination of interferon-α and ribavirin. *Nephrol Dial Transplant* 1999;14:1558.
137. Rossi P, et al. Hepatitis C-related cryoglobulinemic glomerulonephritis. Long-term remission after antiviral therapy. *Kidney Int* 2003;63:2236.
138. Alric L, et al. Influence of antiviral therapy in hepatitis C virus-associated cryoglobulinemic MPGN. *Am J Kidney Dis* 2004;43:617.
139. Beddhu S, et al. Clinical and morphological spectrum of renal cryoglobulinemia. *Medicine* 2002;81:398.
140. Roithinger FX, et al. A lethal course of chronic hepatitis C, glomerulonephritis, and pulmonary vasculitis unresponsive to interferon treatment. *Am J Gastroenterol* 1995;90:1006.
141. Ohta S, et al. Exacerbation of glomerulonephritis in subjects with chronic hepatitis C virus infection after interferon therapy. *Am J Kidney Dis* 1999;33:1040.
142. Suzuki T, et al. Progressive renal failure and blindness due to retinal hemorrhage after interferon therapy for hepatitis C virus-associated membranoproliferative glomerulonephritis. *Intern Med* 2001;40:708.
143. Gordon AC, et al. Acute exacerbation of vasculitis during interferon-alpha therapy for hepatitis C-associated cryoglobulinaemia. *J Infect* 1998;36:229.
144. De Vecchi A, et al. Intravenous methylprednisolone pulse therapy in essential mixed cryoglobulinemia nephropathy. *Clin Nephrol* 1983;19:221.
145. Houwert DA, et al. Effect of plasmapheresis (PP), corticosteroids and cyclophosphamide in essential mixed polyclonal cryoglobulinemia associated with glomerulonephritis. In: Robinson BHB, Hawkins JB, eds. *Proceedings of European Dialysis and Transplant Association*. London: Pitman; 1980.
146. Berkman EM, Orlin JB. Use of plasmapheresis and partial plasma exchange in the management of patients with cryoglobulinemia. *Transfusion* 1980;20:171.
147. Bombardieri S, et al. Prolonged plasma exchange in the treatment of renal involvement in essential mixed cryoglobulinemia. *Intern J Artif Organs* 1983;6:47.
148. McLeod BC, Sassetti RJ. Plasmapheresis with return of cryoglobulins-depleted autologous plasma (cryoglobulin-pheresis) in cryoglobulinaemia. *Blood* 1980;55:866.
149. Pusey CD, et al. Use of plasma exchange in the management of mixed essential cryoglobulinaemia. *Artif Organs* 1981;(suppl):183.
150. Maggiore Q, et al. Effects of cryoapheresis on plasma cryoglobulins and renal function in patients with EMC glomerulonephritis. In: Ponticelli C, Minetti L, D' Amico G, eds. *Antiglobulins, Cryoglobulins and Glomerulonephritis*. Dordrecht: M Nijhoff; 1986.
151. Sinico RA, et al. Plasma exchange in the treatment of essential mixed cryoglobulinemia nephropathy. Long-term follow up. *Intern J Artif Organs* 1985;2:15.
152. Manzin A, et al. Dynamics of hepatitis C viremia after plasma exchange. *J Hepatol* 1999;3:389.
153. Ferri C, et al. Treatment of the renal involvement in mixed cryoglobulinemia with prolonged plasma exchange. *Nephron* 1986;43:246.
154. Magy N, et al. Effects of corticosteroids on HCV infection. *Int J Immunopharmacol* 1999;4:253.

CHAPTER 70 ■ RENAL ARTERY THROMBOSIS, THROMBOEMBOLISM, ANEURYSMS, ATHEROEMBOLI, AND RENAL VEIN THROMBOSIS

FRANCISCO LLACH AND MICHAEL YUDD

This chapter focuses on vascular complications of the main renal arteries and veins. The complex variety of vascular complications include (a) acute thrombosis of the renal artery, most often arising from trauma; (b) thromboembolism to the renal arterial vasculature; (c) acute dissection of the renal artery; (d) atheroembolic disease of the kidneys; (e) rupture of renal arterial aneurysms; and (f) acute and chronic renal vein thrombosis. The latter condition occurs primarily in patients with the nephrotic syndrome. Therefore, special attention is paid to the hypercoagulability of the nephrotic syndrome. In addition, other thromboembolic problems associated with this condition are examined. Furthermore, certain conditions, such as fibromuscular dysplasia and atherosclerotic disease of the renal vessels, which generally cause "renovascular" hypertension, are not considered in this chapter except as they relate to the differential diagnosis of the occlusive disorders just noted.

ACUTE THROMBOSIS OF THE RENAL ARTERY FROM TRAUMA

Acute thrombosis of the renal artery can be classified as traumatic and nontraumatic in origin. Blunt abdominal trauma of the acceleration or deceleration type is the most common cause of renal artery thrombosis (1). This occurs more often in young people, in the setting of motor vehicle accidents and falls. Thrombosis, lacerations with hemorrhage, and contusions may involve the main renal artery, branch vessels, and renal veins (2). Thrombosis is more commonly unilateral than bilateral, and is more likely to be left-sided (3), presumably because the left renal artery is shorter and more acutely angled to the aorta than the right renal artery. Thrombosis of the renal artery often occurs in conjunction with injury to other intraabdominal organs, which often obscures the diagnosis. Thrombosis may occur in 1% to 3% of severe blunt abdominal trauma (4–6). In a review of 250 patients who underwent surgery for traumatic renal artery injury, thrombosis (52%) was the most common finding, followed by avulsion (12%), and branch injury and lacerations (3%) (7). Renal lesions were bilateral in 22%, and injuries to other organs were present in 45% (7).

The rapid development of renal infarction with irreversible loss of renal function is the major concern of acute thrombosis. The maximal warm ischemic time tolerated by the human kidney before the development of infarction is uncertain, but it may be as short as 1 to 2 hours in complete occlusions (8). Incomplete occlusions or occlusions to kidneys with previous stenosis that have developed collateral circulation are viable for longer periods. Early experimental animal studies of temporary arterial occlusion shed light on this issue. Dogs that had a unilateral renal artery clamped to induce complete occlusion for variable hours had split renal function evaluated 4 days after the occlusion (9,10). When the ischemic clamp time was 1 hour, 60% of those kidneys had good function (more than two-thirds the glomerular filtration rate (GFR) of the contralateral kidney) 4 days later; in the group with 2 hours of clamping, this dropped to 38% of the kidneys, and after 3 hours of ischemia, none were functioning. Some of the acute renal failure may have been ischemic acute tubular necrosis and not infarction. Other dogs underwent partial occlusion of the suprarenal aorta, which allowed a low mean arterial pressure downstream, 17 to 30 mm Hg, to perfuse the kidneys. The kidneys tolerated 1 and 2 hours of this partial occlusion very well. Four days after the occlusion, GFR was similar to pre-ischemia control values in all the dogs. This suggests that in the dog, very low perfusion pressures that are inadequate to maintain glomerular filtration, can maintain renal viability for at least 2 hours.

There are no specific clinical or laboratory findings specific for renal artery thrombosis. Anuria or oliguria following abdominal trauma suggests the presence of bilateral thrombosis, but these can be seen in unilateral occlusion. Abdominal and flank pain are usually present. Hematuria may be noted, either gross or microscopic, but may be absent in 25% of patients (1). Elevations of creatine kinase (CK), lactate dehydrogenase (LDH), aspartate aminotransferase (AST), and alkaline phosphatase may be present.

An early diagnosis is of paramount importance if surgical revascularization is contemplated. Computed tomography with contrast is the preferred study in severe abdominal trauma (11). The main computed tomographic (CT) findings in renal artery thrombosis are the lack of renal parenchymal enhancement and the absence of contrast excretion (Fig. 70-1). Occasionally, enhancement of the peripheral renal cortex, the "cortical rim sign," may be noted, which is attributed to capsular or collateral perfusion of the cortex (12). Other renal findings can be subcapsular, perinephric and intrarenal hematomas, renal lacerations, and extravasation of contrast media (Fig. 70-2). Depending on the severity of the lesion, it may be advisable to proceed to early angiography, which can provide the definitive diagnosis. Angiography, the gold standard for occlusive renal artery disease, can identify the severity of the lesion and the presence or absence of collateral circulation (13). With digital subtraction technology, angiography can be performed using very little iodinated contrast or none at all, if carbon dioxide and/or gadolinium or one of its derivatives is used instead (14). With these methods, concerns of contrast-induced renal failure are no longer a major concern, even in patients considered to be high risk for this complication. In the critical patient

1787

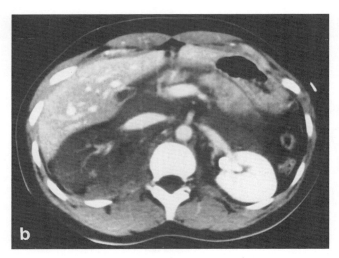

FIGURE 70-1. Arterial phase of computed tomographic (CT) image with contrast. Note the absence of enhancement of the right kidney because of renal artery thrombosis, and avulsion because of trauma. There is reflux of blood to the right kidney from the inferior vena cava because of decreased pressure in the right renal veins. (From: Lang, EK. *Radiology of the Upper Urinary Tract.* Heidelberg: Springer; 1991, with permission.)

who is too unstable to undergo these preoperative diagnostic studies, a bolus injection of contrast material followed by a "one-shot" excretory urogram may be extremely valuable to the surgeon preoperatively. A normal urogram of the kidney in question would exclude the presence of major trauma to that kidney. Alternatively, if the surgeon has to perform an emergent nephrectomy to control hemorrhage, a normal urogram of the contralateral kidney would suggest that it has good function (15).

Early surgical revascularization has been attempted to avoid renal infarction and irreversible loss of renal function, but the results for renal salvage have been mixed and often disappointing (15–18). The warm ischemic time and the size of the thrombosed artery (e.g., main renal artery or a branch), and the extent of occlusion (complete or partial) are major factors (15,17–23). Most successful revascularizations were performed within 12 hours of the onset of thrombosis. Maggio and Brosman re-

ported 80% success of renal salvage when revascularization was performed within 12 hours of trauma, 57% success for repairs performed between 12 and 18 hours, and 0% for later attempts (23). Clark et al. described a dismal 17% success rate for renal salvage even though revascularization attempts were performed early, between 3 and 18 hours after the injury (7). Hass et al. reported surgical outcomes in 20 cases of bilateral occlusion and 34 cases of unilateral renal arterial occlusion (24,25). These cases were a mixture of their own cases and data from reports in the literature. Surgical revascularization was successful in 56% of the bilateral cases and in only 26% of the unilateral cases.

Early revascularization is indicated in cases of bilateral renal artery thromboses and of thrombosis to solitary functioning kidneys in order to avoid severe irreversible renal failure. However, in patients with unilateral thrombosis and a functioning contralateral kidney, surgical outcomes may not be better than medical management alone, so the indication for surgery in this setting is not clear. Despite the concerns regarding ischemic time, there are scattered reports of restored renal function when revascularization for traumatic renal artery thrombosis was performed long after the period of injury (21,22,23,27). In these cases renal function may have been preserved by collateral circulation if preexisting stenosis was present or the occlusion was incomplete.

Surgical revascularization should not consist of a thrombectomy alone (25,26). The occluded segment of the renal artery should be resected, with reinsertion in the aorta, or, alternatively, with interposition of an aorto-renal graft, with either PTFE or great saphenous vein (28). Nephrectomy may be required in emergent situations to control hemorrhage.

NONTRAUMATIC ACUTE OCCLUSIVE DISEASES OF THE RENAL ARTERIES

Acute occlusion of the renal artery or its branches may be due to thrombosis from trauma or other causes, from acute embolic events usually arising from the heart, or from dissecting aneurysms. The major consequence of acute arterial occlusion is the rapid development of renal infarction and irreversible loss of renal function.

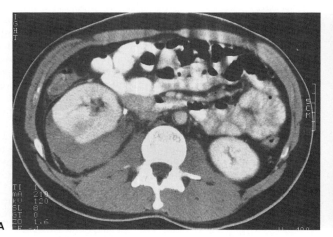
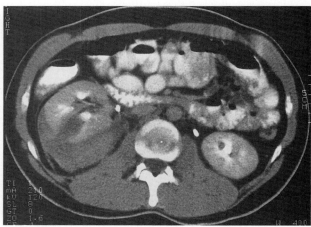

FIGURE 70-2. Computed tomography with contrast. Arterial phase (A) and late phase (B) demonstrate a wedge-shaped traumatic infarct localized to the posterolateral midpole of the right kidney. A large right perirenal hematoma is present as well. (From: Lang, EK, *Radiology of the Upper Urinary Tract.* Heidelberg: Springer; 1991, with permission.)

Nontraumatic Renal Artery Thrombosis—Causes

In Table 70-1 are listed the nontraumatic causes of renal artery thrombosis. Damage or disruption of the arterial endothelial surface initiates platelet adhesion and aggregation, and leads to thrombus formation. The most common setting for this is atherosclerotic renovascular disease. Other settings include fibromuscular dysplasia (28,29), inflammation, infection, renal artery aneurysms, and dissecting aneurysms. Thrombosis of the main renal arteries or branches has been described in the various vasculitides, including polyarteritis nodosum (30,31), Takayasu arteritis (32,33) Kawasaki's disease, and thromboangiitis obliterans. Other causes include Behçet's disease (34–37), syphilis (38), inflammatory diseases such as phycomycosis (39,40), cocaine use (41–43), neurofibromatosis (44), and infiltrating urothelial carcinoma of the renal pelvis (45). Thrombosis has been attributed to strenuous aerobic exercise (46) and to trauma from car seat belts (47). Renal infarction has been observed with sickle cell anemia (48).

Hypercoagulable states usually lead to venous thrombosis, not to arterial thrombosis. Exceptions to this include the antiphospholipid syndrome (APS) and heparin-induced thrombocytopenia. Severe cases of catastrophic diffuse arterial and venous thromboses can occur in both diseases. Thrombosis in the APS may occur in any location within the renal vasculature, that is, from the renal artery trunk to the renal veins. Renal artery thrombosis has been noted in both primary and secondary (lupus-related) APS (49–59). In a recent report of abdominal CT scan findings of abdominal thrombosis and ischemic events in patients with APS, renal infarctions of varying sizes were found in 22 of the 42 patients (60). Factor V Leiden mutation, which is associated with a short partial thrombo-

plastin time, has been implicated as the cause of renal artery thrombosis in native kidneys and in renal allografts (61). Arterial thrombosis has also been observed rarely in patients with the nephrotic syndrome (62–64).

Thromboembolism of the Renal Arteries—Causes

Emboli to the renal vasculature most commonly originate in the heart. These emboli, depending on their size, will travel downstream and obstruct arteries depending on their size. Cardiac disease and dysrhythmias, in particular atrial fibrillation, are the most common settings as an embolic source (65–67). Mural atrial and ventricular thrombi may develop in the settings of myocardial infarction or in congestive cardiomyopathy. Thrombi or vegetations may form on prosthetic or diseased heart valves and be the source of renal emboli. Before the use of antibiotics, renal emboli often occurred as a consequence of subacute bacterial endocarditis. Rarely, paradoxical renal emboli may result from venous clots passing through patent interatrial or interventricular septal defects (68). In addition to a cardiac source, peripheral emboli may originate from clots that develop along diseased endothelium or in aneurysms of the suprarenal aorta or renal artery.

Iatrogenic causes of renal artery thrombosis and thromboemboli have increased in recent years following endovascular aortic and renovascular procedures, and with stent placements by interventional radiologists and vascular surgeons. The risk of major complications associated with renal artery procedures is 7% to 10% according to a recent review. These include thrombosis, dissection, rupture, and atheroembolic showering (69,70). Morris et al. reported renal artery rupture or occlusion from acute thrombosis in 4.2% of 308 procedures of percutaneous transluminal angioplasty or stent dilatation of the renal artery (71) Two German centers reported renal complications following endovascular repair of thoracic and abdominal aortic aneurysms using a variety of endografts in 775 patients (72,73). New renal infarctions were noted in 10% of the cases when pre-procedure CT images were compared to postprocedure studies. New infarcts were considered to be the consequence of thromboembolic complications of the endovascular repair. Most of these infarctions were asymptomatic, and were small wedge-shaped findings on CT; however, one of the studies reported a 2.6% incidence of total unilateral renal artery occlusion following the procedure (72,73).

The downstream complications from renal angioplasty and stenting may be diminished with the use of distal filter protection devices. Holden and Hill reported their early experience with distal devices in 46 procedures of renal artery stent revascularization for atherosclerotic renal artery stenosis (74). Sixty-five percent of the distal protection baskets contained embolic material, including fresh and chronic thrombi and atheroemboli. More experience with distal filters is needed to determine their merit.

Pathology of Renal Infarction

Renal infarction is a fairly common autopsy finding, but an infrequent clinical diagnosis. In a review of 14,411 autopsies, renal infarctions of varying sizes were found in 1.4% of the cases, and most of them were postmortem diagnoses (75). Renal infarctions may occur in venous thrombosis, but they are much more common with arterial occlusions. Depending on the size of the occluded artery, the infarction could be a small wedge-like lesion or encompass the entire kidney. The gross appearance of the infarct depends on the size of the occluded

---

TABLE 70-1

NONTRAUMATIC CAUSES OF ACUTE OCCLUSIVE RENOVASCULAR DISEASE

1. Renal artery thrombosis
   (A) following damage/disruption of endothelial surface
   - atherosclerotic disease
   - fibromuscular dysplasia
   - renal artery aneurysms and dissecting aneurysms
   - polyarteritis nodosum
   - Takayasu's arteritis
   - Kawasaki's disease
   - thromboangiitis obliterans
   - Behçet's disease
   - syphilis
   - cocaine
   (B) specific hypercoaguable states
   - antiphospholipid antibody syndrome
   - heparin-induced thrombocytopenia
   - factor V Leiden mutation
   - nephrotic syndrome (rare)
2. Renal artery thromboembolism
   (A) cardiac origin
   - atrial fibrillation
   - endocarditis
   - myocardial infarction
   - congestive cardiomyopathy
   - paradoxical emboli through patent septal defect
   (B) aortic or renal artery source
   - severe atherosclerosis/thrombosis

artery, the age of the infarct, and whether infection is present. Early on the infarct is red and pyramidal, and within hours it becomes gray with a narrow red rim of congested parenchyma. The necrotic area is eventually replaced by collagenous tissue. The area shrinks, leaving behind a V-shaped scar. Infarctions involve only the renal cortex; the medulla is usually spared (76).

On microscopic examination, sterile infarcts have the classic picture of coagulative necrosis (76). The initial findings of marked congestion are followed by cytoplasmic and nuclear degenerative changes, with gradual loss of viable cytologic structure. The cytoplasm becomes homogeneous and eosinophilic, and the nuclei undergo condensation and karyorrhexis. Surrounding this necrotic area is a transitional zone of sublethal injury with findings similar to acute tubular necrosis. This peripheral area becomes infiltrated with polymorphonuclear leukocytes. Eventually the central necrotic area becomes smaller, with eventual collapse, and is replaced by a collagenous scar (76).

Clinical Features and Diagnosis of Acute Occlusive Renal Arterial Disease

There are no specific signs or symptoms specific for arterial occlusion (Table 70-2). Most patients with acute thrombosis or thromboembolism to the kidney seeking medical care present with flank and/or abdominal pain. The pain is not specific, and may vary in intensity from a mild dull ache to excruciating pain. Nausea and vomiting, and fever and chills, may also be present, but fever may not develop until the second or third day after the onset of pain. The patient may have noted anuria or oliguria, and gross hematuria. Anuria or severe oliguria raises the suspicion of bilateral renal artery occlusion. However, oliguria may be seen in unilateral occlusion with a normal contralateral kidney, and it may last for several days. The decreased renal function and oliguria have been attributed to arteriolar spasm of the contralateral kidney. On physical examination, blood pressure may be mildly to markedly elevated. The abdomen and/or flank are usually tender. Bowel sounds may be absent, and guarding and peritoneal signs may be elicited. Conversely, small infarcts may be painless and asymptomatic in many cases. Gorich et al. found 12 new small renal infarcts on CT imaging following endovascular procedures that were considered iatrogenic thromboemboli; all 12 patients were asymptomatic (73). Obviously, the size of the occluding artery and the extent of renal ischemia play a critical role in the patients' symptoms. Early diagnosis of acute arterial occlusion is usually missed because the initial diagnostic considerations are typically directed toward other more common diseases such as gastroenteritis, pancreatitis, cholecystitis, nephrolithiasis, and pyelonephritis.

Laboratory abnormalities include an elevated LDH level, which may rise to 2,000 IU/L in cases of large infarctions. Serum AST and alanine aminotransferase (ALT) levels may be increased, but usually not to the same extent as LDH. Moderate elevations of alkaline phosphatase occur in 30% to 50% of patients, and may persist for up to 10 days. The course of changes of various serum enzymes in a patient with thromboembolic disease is shown in Figure 70-3. Most patients have microscopic hematuria (77), and mild proteinuria and leukocytosis are frequent. A low urinary sodium concentration, suggestive of renal hypoperfusion, is occasionally noted (Fig. 70-4) (78).

Imaging with CT with contrast, magnetic resonance angiography (MRA), or angiography, are the best means of diagnosis (Figs. 70-5 and 70-6). Angiography has the added advantage in that thrombolytic agents can be infused directly to

TABLE 70-2

CLINICAL AND LABORATORY FEATURES OF THROMBOEMBOLIC DISEASES OF THE KIDNEY

Feature	Approximate incidence[a]
History and physical findings	
Pain and tenderness (flank, abdominal, chest, or back)	75%
Nausea and vomiting	50%
Gross hematuria	20%
Cardiac disease (myocardial infarction, atrial fibrillation, rheumatic valvular disease)	90%
Laboratory features	
Leukocytosis (11,000–32,000/μL)	95%
Microscopic hematuria (>15 erythrocytes per high-power field)	90%
Pyuria (>10 leukocytes per high-power field)	80%
Proteinuria (1+ to 4+)	95%
Increased enzymes (LDH, SGOT, SGPT, alkaline phosphatase)	95%–100%

Special diagnostic procedures	Finding
Intravenous urogram	Decr. or absent function; delayed appearance
Renal ultrasonography	No obstruction; rarely, wedge-shaped mass
Isotope renal flow scan	Decreased flow to all or part of kidney
Computed tomography (with contrast material)	Area of decreased accentuation; cortical rim of accentuation

[a]Refer to text.
LDH, lactic dehydrogenase; SGOT, glutamic-oxaloacetic transaminase; SGPT, glutamic-pyruvic transaminase; Decr., decreased.

treat an occluded artery if it is found. Noncontrast studies will miss the underperfused areas of the kidney. Isotopic renal flow scans can show absent or markedly reduced perfusion defects (Fig. 70-7). Their accuracy may be limited if acute renal failure is present. Ultrasonographic evaluation of the renal arteries using color and power-Doppler techniques is of limited value because the imaging of the entire renal artery is technically difficult, the procedure takes a long time, and the quality of the studies is operator-dependent.

Therapy for Nontraumatic Acute Occlusive Renal Arterial Disease

The overwhelming concerns of renal arterial occlusion are renal ischemia and imminent infarction with irreversible loss of renal function. A rapid diagnosis and initiation of therapy, usually intraarterial thrombolysis, are critical to avert infarction and preserve renal function. The duration of warm ischemia, the size and extent of the vascular occlusion (e.g., bilateral versus unilateral; main, branch, or peripheral artery; complete versus partial occlusions) and the presence or absence of collateral

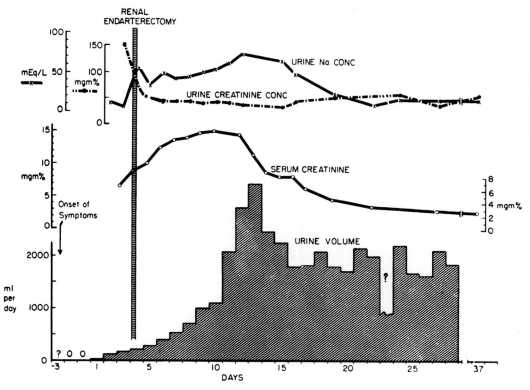

FIGURE 70-3. Course of a 56-year-old woman with abrupt onset of anuria and right lower quadrant and low back pain; she had atrial fibrillation and mitral stenosis owing to rheumatic heart disease. One year earlier she had undergone a left nephrectomy for malignant hypertension. (Earlier, she had had a stroke and blindness of the left eye owing to an embolism.) A diagnosis of thromboembolism to the renal artery was confirmed by aortography (Fig. 70-6), and surgery was perfumed with removal of the embolus and endarterectomy. The fractional excretion of sodium was 0.36% before surgery and increased to 7.3% after removal of the thrombus. There was ultimate recovery from acute tubular necrosis, as indicated. (From: Lessman, RK, et al. Renal artery embolism: clinical features and long-term follow-up in 17 cases. *Ann Intern Med* 1978;89:477, with permission.)

circulation are important factors in determining whether renal function can be preserved. The general rule is the shorter the duration of renal ischemia, the greater the chance of preserving renal function.

Blum et al. described 14 patients with acute embolic renal artery occlusion who were treated with thrombolytic therapy: intraarterial streptokinase, urokinase, or tissue-type plasminogen activator (79). The estimated ischemic time from onset of symptoms to therapy varied from 12 hours to 8 days. Recanal-

ization and adequate renal perfusion were achieved in 13 of the 14 patients. Despite these results, renal function did not improve in any patient with complete occlusion, but did stabilize in those patients with partial occlusions. In their review of the literature, the duration and degree of renal artery occlusion were crucial; in 50 patients with complete occlusion of the main renal artery and ischemic time greater than 3 hours who underwent a successful reperfusion procedure by either thrombolysis or surgery, evidence of irreversible renal damage as shown by

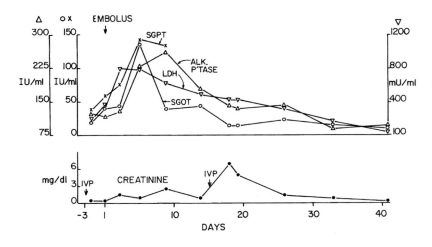

FIGURE 70-4. Serial serum levels of glutamic-oxaloacetic transaminase (SGOT, ○) glutamic-pyruvic transaminase (SGPT, X), lactic dehydrogenase (LDH, ▽), alkaline phosphatase (ALK P TASE, △) and creatinine (●) in a 62-year-old man with thromboembolism to a single kidney 10 days after a myocardial infarction. Right flank and chest pain and lower abdominal tenderness appeared on day 1. The patient also exhibited an increase in serum creatinine level following the second intravenous pyelogram (IVP). (From Lessman, RK, et al. Renal artery embolism: clinical features and long-term follow-up in 17 cases. *Ann Intern Med* 1978;89:477, with permission.)

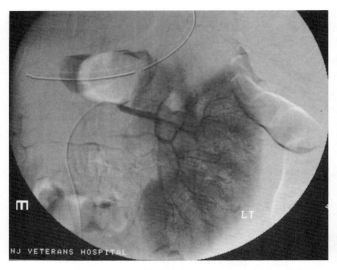

FIGURE 70-5. Left renal angiogram shows a wedge-shaped perfusion defect involving the upper pole of the kidney due to a thromboembolism.

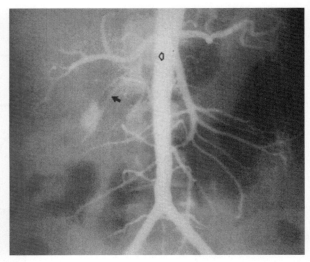

FIGURE 70-7. Aortogram of a patient with an embolism to a solitary right kidney. There is a faint lucency projecting into the lumen of the aorta (*open arrow*) at the site of an embolus to the right renal artery. The distal renal artery filled faintly (*solid arrow*), presumably via collaterals. (From: Lessman, RK, et. al. Renal artery embolism: clinical features and long-term follow-up in 17 cases. *Ann Intern Med* 1978;89:477, with permission.)

repeat scintigraphic perfusion defects was noted in all. In the small number of patients with complete occlusion of the main artery and short ischemic time, less than 3 hours, renal function was preserved. Patients with either incomplete occlusion of the main renal artery or with branch artery occlusions fared better.

Recent convincing case reports refute this "critical ischemic period" (80–83). A patient with bilateral occlusion and another with occlusion of a solitary functioning kidney with relatively

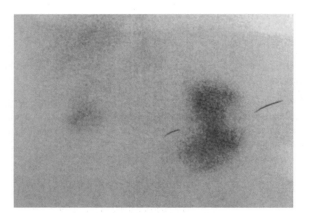

FIGURE 70-6. Renal scan with technetium 99m-labeled dimercaptosuccinic acid (DMSA) showing evidence of segmental renal infarcts of the left kidney of a 74-year-old man who was hospitalized with abrupt appearance of a supraventricular tachycardia. There was a progressive rise in serum creatinine from a baseline value of 2.2 to 4.4 mg/dL over 5 successive days. He was never oliguric; urinalysis showed 2+ proteinuria. His white blood cell count rose from 10,200/μL on admission to 15,400/μL after 4 days; there was no eosinophilia. The serum alanine aminotransferase level rose from 33 to 42 U/L and lactate dehydrogenase, from 49 to 173 U/L. A technetium-labeled "flow" scan disclosed markedly reduced flow bilaterally that was more marked on the left than the right. There was a history of emboli to his feet, with the serum creatinine level increasing from 1.2 to 2.2 mg/dL in association with an acute myocardial infarction several years earlier. On the basis of DMSA scan, a diagnosis of thromboembolism to the kidney was made; the patient received anticoagulants and his serum creatinine level gradually fell to 2.4 mg/dL.

prolonged ischemia (20 and 36 hours, respectively), underwent successful thrombolytic therapy and correction of severe renal failure to normal function. Another report describes an elderly patient with new-onset flank pain, anuria, severe acute renal failure requiring dialysis, and bilateral occlusion by angiography with a complete lack of the left nephrogram noted 4 days after the onset of pain. Following angioplasty, renal function returned to near-normal values over time, and repeated imaging studies showed normal perfusion to the whole left kidney.

Surgical outcomes for preserving renal function in acute nontraumatic obstructions are mixed. Lacombe showed very good surgical results (84). Twenty patients with acute obstruction of the main renal arteries (25 kidneys at risk), 5 from acute embolism, and 15 from acute thrombosis underwent revascularization 18 hours to 68 days after the onset of occlusion. The kidney salvage rate was 64%, but the postoperative mortality rate was 15%. It is unclear whether some of these cases may have been caused by thrombosis associated with atherosclerosis with collateral circulation, which may have a better prognosis for renal salvage than an acute occlusion without collateral circulation. Other studies do not show such optimistic outcomes. In another study, renal artery embolectomy failed to restore renal function in 13 patients with acute renal artery embolism (85).

In summary, an aggressive approach at revascularization should be attempted in bilateral occlusions or occlusions to solitary functioning kidneys, since the threat to major renal function is great. For unilateral occlusions with normal contralateral kidneys, clinical judgment is required to determine whether to intervene with one of these. Either therapy is probably futile if prolonged complete occlusion of the renal artery without collateral circulation persists for more than a day or two. Conversely, intervention may be successful for shorter ischemic durations, and the shorter the period the better. If the obstruction is incomplete or if collaterals are present, the kidney may remain viable much longer. For unilateral occlusions, thrombolysis may be preferable because of the lower risks compared to surgery. If a unilateral segmental embolus is detected, anticoagulation may be all that is necessary.

Many reports describe the rapid relief of pain, which may be very severe, during thrombolytic intervention. Severe pain, which suggests ongoing ischemia, is probably a good indication for thrombolytic intervention. In patients with embolic disease, particular attention should be paid to the source of embolization. Some patients, for example, those with atrial fibrillation, will require long-term anticoagulation to avoid future recurrences of embolization to the kidneys or other vital organs.

RENAL ARTERY ANEURYSMS

Renal artery aneurysms (RAAs) are uncommon in the general population, and are usually diagnosed serendipitously on imaging studies. From large autopsy studies, the incidence of RAAs in the general population is about 0.01% (86). In patients who have undergone renal arteriography for any reason, not uncommonly to evaluate renovascular hypertension, RAAs were found in 0.3% to 1% (87,88). In one study, RAAs were diagnosed in 83 of 8,525 patients (0.97%) who underwent renal arteriography (87). Sixty-one percent of the aneurysms were right-sided, and 7% were bilateral.

Renal artery aneurysms are classified as saccular, fusiform, dissecting, and intrarenal (88,89). Saccular aneurysms, the most common type, comprise about 80% of RAAs. They may be located anywhere along the vascular tree. About 90% are extrarenal, and most are located at the first-order bifurcation of the main renal artery. Less than 10% are within the renal parenchyma.

Fusiform aneurysms, less common, (90–94), usually follow areas of stenosis, and give the image of poststenotic dilation. In fibromuscular dysplasia there may be several series of stenoses followed by dilations, giving a "string of beads" appearance on arteriography. Fusiform aneurysms are most commonly found in young women who undergo renal angiography for the evaluation of renovascular hypertension.

Intrarenal aneurysms comprise 10% to 15% of RAAs, and are frequently multiple. They may be congenital, posttraumatic (e.g., following renal biopsies), or associated with polyarteritis nodosa (91,95) (Fig. 70-8).

The histologic findings of the RAA resemble medial fibromuscular dysplasia. In the arterial wall, degeneration of the internal elastic lamina with fragmentation, increased collagen,

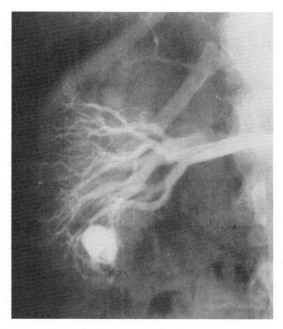

FIGURE 70-8. Renal arteriogram shows a traumatic intrarenal aneurysm located in the lower pole of the right kidney. (From: Lang, EK. *Radiology of the Upper Urinary Tract.* Heidelberg: Springer; 1991, with permission.)

and a lack of elastic tissue are observed. Atherosclerotic lesions may be the cause of the aneurysm, or more likely, may be a secondary factor (96). Calcification of the arterial walls may occur.

Table 70-3 shows demographic and clinical data of 277 patients who underwent surgical correction of renal aneurysms in three recently published studies (96–98). The mean age of the patients was around 50 years, and ranged from 13 to 78 years in one study. Women outnumbered men by 65% to 35%. Hypertension was common, present in 73% to 89%. In other series, hypertension was found in 35% to 100% of the patients (100). Medial fibromuscular dysplasia, present in 34% to 54%, was considered the major cause, and was the

TABLE 70-3

DATA FROM THREE LARGE STUDIES REPORTING THEIR SURGICAL OUTCOMES OF RENAL ARTERY ANEURYSMS IN 277 PATIENTS

Studies-Authors (ref.)	English (96)	Pfeiffer (98)	Henke (97)
No. patients	62	94	121
No. RAAs repaired	72	107	168
Time-period of surgery (yr)	1987–2003	1980–2002	1965–2000
Mean patient age (yr)	46	51	51
Male/female (%)	70/30	61/39	60/40
Hypertension (%)	89	80	73
Pathogenesis			
Fibromuscular dysplasia (%)	54	51	34
Atherosclerosis (%)	35	30	25
Outcomes			
Perioperative mortality	1 (1.6%)	0	0
Perioperative morbidity (%)	12	17	?
Hypertension improved (%)	54	22	?
Hypertension cured (%)	21	25	?
Long-term artery patency (%)	91	81	98

probable reason for the female gender preference. Atherosclerosis was present in 25% to 35%. A small number of cases were due to arteritis, including polyarteritis nodosum and giant cell arteritis, Marfan's syndrome, dissection, mycotic aneurysms, and trauma (96–100).

Most patients with RAAs are asymptomatic. Approximately 20% may complain of nonspecific flank or abdominal pain, and there may be hematuria and an abdominal bruit. Complications include rupture, renovascular hypertension, thrombosis with acute arterial occlusion and infarction, distal embolization, and erosion into adjacent veins with the formation of arteriovenous fistulae. The latter may lead to the development of high-output heart failure (89,90).

Rupture of a renal artery aneurysm, a potentially catastrophic event, is the most serious complication. This can present or quickly lead to hemorrhagic shock, irreversible loss of that kidney's function, and death. In cases of rupture, severe flank pain is usually present and flank ecchymoses may develop later.

It is generally accepted, though not proven in prospective studies, that the larger the RAA, the greater the risk of rupture. The risk of rupture of small RAAs, less than 1.5 to 2.0 cm in diameter, appears to be low based on data from several studies that followed the natural history of RAAs. However, RAAs of any size in the setting of pregnancy, and large aneurysms, especially those greater than 4.0 cm in diameter, have a greater tendency to rupture. The older literature suggested that aneurysms without calcified walls may also have a greater tendency to rupture, but this is questionable. Six studies described the natural history of small aneurysms in more than 200 patients with small aneurysms, who were followed conservatively without surgery for up to 17 years (86,97,101–104). Most of these aneurysms were less than 2.0 cm. During follow-up, none of the aneurysms ruptured, and very few of them caused symptoms or had a considerable increase in size. Henriksson et al. described 34 patients with RAAs who underwent repeat angiographic studies (102). Twenty-eight of the 34 patients exhibited no change in size of the RAA on follow-up, and 5 had slight enlargement, thrombosis, or calcification. One patient had a worrisome dilation of the RAA and underwent surgical repair. These studies suggest that small aneurysms, less than 2.0 cm in diameter, are unlikely to rupture, enlarge, or cause symptoms. It appears safe to follow them conservatively with periodic imaging studies.

Pregnant women make up a disproportionate number of cases of RAA rupture. In a review of 43 cases of rupture, 18 (42%) occurred in pregnant women (103). Most occurred during the last trimester of pregnancy, but case reports describe rupture and hemorrhage occurring earlier in pregnancy and during the postpartum period (105–108). Renal artery rupture during pregnancy has also been described in a renal transplant recipient (109). Many of the pregnant women who had RAA rupture did not have hypertension before or during their pregnancy (106,110,111). The reason for increased rupture in pregnancy is not certain. Pathogenic considerations include increased renal blood flow, particularly during the third trimester, steroid hormone effects on the vasculature, and increased intraabdominal pressure (110). The role of pressure on the pelvic vasculature caused by the enlarged uterus, particularly in certain positions, may be a factor (106, 111,112). Emergent nephrectomy is usually required in this setting to control the hemorrhage. In recent years, maternal mortality has decreased to 6% and fetal mortality to 25% if the pregnancy reached the third trimester (113,114). If rupture occurred before the third trimester, fetal mortality approaches 100%.

Renal angiography and MRA will diagnose renal artery aneurysms. Computed tomography and radionuclide scanning may be useful screening techniques.

Three surgical centers specializing in renovascular surgery recently published very good surgical outcomes in a combined number of 277 patients who underwent surgical RAA repair (96–98). The mean size of the aneurysms was reported from 1.5 cm to 2.6 cm. Primary surgical success was around 97%, and long-term arterial patency free of stenosis was 81% to 91%. In one center, unplanned nephrectomy had to be performed in 8 of 121 surgeries (6.6%), a risk for this surgery. Perioperative death rate was 0% to 1.6%, and morbidity was 12% to 17%. Hypertension was considered cured in 21% to 25%, and improved in another 22% to 54%. The specific surgical procedures are detailed in the studies (96–98,115–120). An experienced surgical team is essential for successful outcomes.

The following points should be considered in deciding whether or not to surgically correct RAA: the increased risk of rupture of large aneurysms, and the low risk of small ones, less than 1.5 cm; the increased risk of rupture in pregnancy; the benefits of curing or improving renovascular hypertension, especially in a young person; the risk of major surgery; the risk of a failed procedure, which frequently results in renal infarction and irreversible loss of renal function. There are no set criteria for surgery, but recent recommendations for surgery are the following (91,96–98):

1. RAA diameter greater than 1.5 to 2.0 cm in a healthy, normotensive person;
2. RAA greater than 1.0 cm in women of child-bearing age, since rupture during pregnancy is increased;
3. RAAs with associated renal artery stenosis or evidence of distal embolization.
4. RAA showing significant expansion during follow-up imaging studies.

If medical management is chosen, blood pressure should be well controlled, and periodic CT monitoring of the aneurysm should be undertaken.

Endovascular approaches have been used to treat RAAs as an alternative to surgery. Radiologic transcatheter placement of stent grafts, and exclusion of the aneurysm through the placement of microcoils and with Onyx, a radiopaque nonadhesive liquid embolic agent, have been described in limited cases (121–124). The long-term outcome of these procedures is not known. Superselective end-branch embolic therapy may be used to occlude intraparenchymal RAAs.

DISSECTING ANEURYSMS OF THE RENAL ARTERY

Tears of the arterial intima and medial necrosis lead to dissection of the arterial wall. Atherosclerosis and fibromuscular dysplasia are common predisposing factors that lead to intimal tears. Iatrogenic dissection due to angiographic procedures may be induced by trauma from guide wires, catheters, or angioplasty balloons (125). Rarely, dissections occur after blunt trauma of the abdomen or flank (126,127). Occasionally, renal artery dissections are found as incidental findings at autopsy, without any apparent clinical manifestations during life.

Dissecting aneurysms can cause acute or chronic occlusions of the renal artery, with consequent renal ischemia and infarction and renovascular hypertension (128). They occasionally can rupture and cause a retroperitoneal hemorrhage. The discussions in the preceding text regarding acute renal artery occlusion and renal infarction apply also to dissecting aneurysms. Chronic renal artery dissection most commonly manifests itself as renovascular hypertension (129).

In acute dissections, new-onset hypertension or worsening hypertension and flank pain are common. Occasionally, patients may experience malignant hypertension. Headache may occur, probably as a result of hypertension. Some patients, especially those who develop the lesion iatrogenically from an angiographic procedure, may show no symptoms or signs other than hypertension.

Dissections are about three times more common in males than females (128,129). They occur most commonly between 40 and 60 years of age, but young adults can be affected, particularly if fibromuscular dysplasia and hypertension are present. Dissecting aneurysms are more commonly right-sided, and are bilateral in 20% to 30% of cases (128,129).

Proteinuria may be detected, and hematuria is present in 20% to 35% of patients. Impaired renal function with serum creatinine level greater than 1.5 mg/dL was present in 9% and 33% of patients in two series (127,128).

Renal angiography or MRA may diagnose dissection. Selective arteriography typically reveals an abrupt narrowing of the arterial lumen (Fig. 70-9). Less often, both the true and false lumina fill with contrast, giving the appearance of a double lumen separated by the intimal flap. The dissection may extend from the main renal artery, distally to the first bifurcation and into the branch arteries. Follow-up arteriography may show persistent dissection, but others have described some degree of reversibility, with gradual improvement of renal function and improvement of hypertension (127,130). Renal function generally is relatively well maintained. Approximately 50% of patients in one study had lateralization of renal vein renin levels, and the isotope renogram showed unilateral abnormalities in a similar fraction (128).

The appropriate therapy depends on the severity of the hypertension and its response to medical management. Some patients have persistent severe renovascular hypertension re-sistant to antihypertensive therapy. They may benefit from surgical revascularization, or nephrectomy if renal infarction is present, with improvement or complete resolution of hypertension following these procedures (131,132). In other patients, hypertension can be controlled with medications, and these patients may become normotensive again with time. Edwards and colleagues noted an adequate response of the hypertension to medical therapy in the majority of patients (129).

ATHEROEMBOLIC RENAL DISEASE

The clinical presentation of atheroembolic disease (AED), also known as cholesterol embolic disease, differs from acute renal ischemia and infarction produced by the larger thromboemboli to the renal artery and medium-sized arteries. In atheroembolic disease, tiny cholesterol-containing plaques with fibrin slough off the aorta and large arteries and travel downstream, eventually occluding many small arteries and arterioles with diameters of 150 to 200 μm (133). Local ischemia and inflammatory reactions follow. This leads to the acute or insidious onset of renal impairment if the renal vasculature is showered, as well as a wide range of clinical manifestations depending on which other organs are showered. The presentation lacks the clinical features of a large renal infarct due to thromboemboli or acute thrombosis described in the previous sections.

Atheroembolic disease is a disease of the elderly, who typically have evidence of diffuse atherosclerosis, and especially smokers. Precipitating factors are invasive procedures with aortic or arterial catheters, vascular surgery, and therapy with thrombolytic agents or anticoagulants; less commonly, AED occurs spontaneously without a precipitating event. Clinical manifestations can be mild or severe depending on the degree of atheroemboli. Almost any organ can be involved, but the most common clinical manifestations involve the skin, kidneys, gastrointestinal tract, and central nervous system. No specific therapy is known to limit or halt the cholesterol showering and the clinical sequelae.

Pathology

Autopsy studies show that cholesterol-containing microemboli in the renal vasculature are fairly common. Large autopsy studies describe renal cholesterol emboli in 5% of men and 3% of women older than 50 years of age. (134). This is far higher than the clinically apparent disease, and it suggests that only the more severe cases of AED have clinical manifestations, whereas mild cases are asymptomatic. The incidence of symptomatic cholesterol emboli involving the skin or kidneys following cardiac catheterization was found to be 1.4% in a large prospective Japanese study (135). In autopsy studies of patients with AED, the kidney is the most commonly involved internal organ. Renal involvement was found in 75% of 173 autopsy cases of AED (136). Cholesterol emboli were widespread, and each autopsy averaged 3.4 organs with microemboli. In addition to renal involvement, other common organ sites for atheroemboli were the spleen, pancreas, and gastrointestinal tract (137).

Fragments of atheromatous plaques become embedded in small arteries, arterioles, and sometimes in the glomerular capillaries. The arcuate, interlobular, and terminal arterioles are involved (138). Pathologic examination of the occluded vessels reveals characteristic biconvex, needle-shaped clefts that remain after the lipid is dissolved during histologic processing (Fig. 70-10). Complete obstruction of the small arteries or arterioles leads to distal areas of small infarction and necrosis;

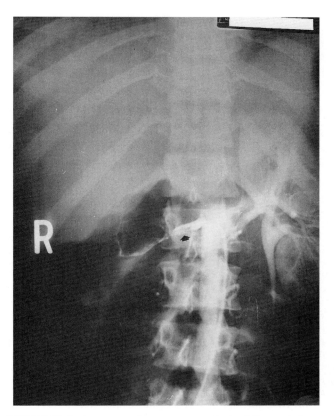

FIGURE 70-9. Aortogram demonstrates an intimal flap and dissection with thrombosis of the right renal kidney. Note the absence of enhancement of the right kidney. (From: Lang, EK. *Radiology of the Upper Urinary Tract*. Heidelberg: Springer; 1991, with permission.)

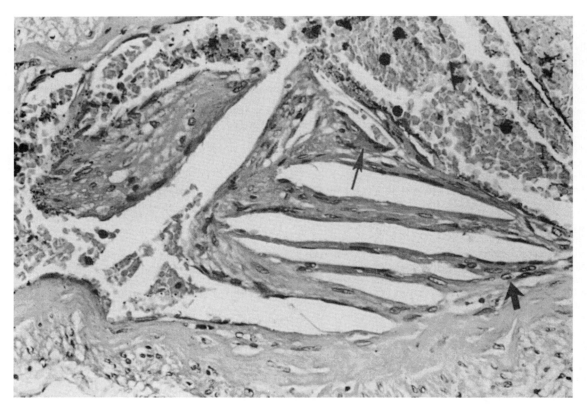

FIGURE 70-10. Light microscopy illustrates the needle-shaped clefts of atheroemboli in a renal arteriole. Foreign-body giant cells (*arrows*) surround the cholesterol clefts.

in incomplete obstruction, distal areas exhibit ischemic atrophy.

During the early period after atheroembolization, cholesterol crystals may be surrounded by eosinophilic material, with little inflammatory reaction in the surrounding interstitium. Subsequently, there is intimal thickening, and the appearance of macrophages, lymphocytes, and multinucleated giant cells of the foreign body type (138). Later there may be marked intimal thickening with concentric fibrosis. Necrosis of the arterial wall is not present. The ischemic glomeruli may become hyalinized, and the tubules become atrophic (139). Grossly, the kidney may shrink and have a rough granular surface with wedge-shaped scars. The lesions produced in experimental animals closely parallel the pathologic features observed in humans (140,141).

Renal impairment arises from recurrent and multiple episodes of cholesterol microembolization. The debris and cholesterol crystals found at the site of occlusion are identical to the material found in the severe atheromatous lesions observed in the aorta of these patients (142,143). Indeed, the incidence of AED and the severity of aortic atherosclerosis have been correlated (143,144). The irregular and ulcerating internal surface of the aorta is commonly covered with fibrin and platelet thrombi. These pliable and soft thrombi can be dislodged easily. The intima may be completely eroded, revealing direct communications between an atheroma and the lumen of the aorta.

A secondary form of focal glomerulosclerosis (FGS) has been described in cases of AED. In a report of 24 patients with renal biopsy evidence of AED, FGS was found in the majority of patients (145). In the patients with nephrotic-range proteinuria, the collapsing variant of FGS was common. The authors speculated that glomerulosclerosis and collapse were the consequences of chronic ischemia and progressive damage of the remaining glomeruli to hyperfiltration. In addition, there are

several reports of necrotizing glomerulonephritis including antineutrophil cytoplasmic antibody positive pauci-immune extracapillary glomerulonephritis associated with atheroembolic disease (146–148).

Clinical Features

Atheroembolic renal disease is a disease of the elderly, and is rare in patients younger than 50 years of age. The disorder is more common in males than females, and in a U.S. series, it is described predominantly in caucasians (137,138,149,150). Several Japanese series have been published recently (151,148). Evidence of aortic atherosclerosis is almost invariably present, and symptomatic peripheral or cerebral vascular disease, coronary artery disease, hypertension, and mild renal insufficiency are common. Most patients are smokers. In three clinical studies and one large review of AED, which jointly included 350 patients with AED, the mean age was 66 years age, more than three-fourths were male, and more than 90% were caucasian (137,138,149,152,153). Cigarette smoking was present in 79% to 92% of the patients. Hypertension was present in 61% to 100%, coronary artery disease in 44% to 73%, peripheral vascular disease in 59% to 75%, and cerebrovascular disease in 32% to 62%. Abdominal aortic aneurysms were noted in 25% to 67%, and baseline renal insufficiency was common, noted by a baseline serum creatinine of 1.8 mg/dL (137,149,153). The clinical characteristics of AED are summarized in Table 70-4.

Invasive angiographic procedures, vascular surgery, and therapy with anticoagulants or thrombolytic agents have been implicated as precipitating factors for cholesterol atheroemboli. Coronary, carotid, and aortic angiograms as well as cardiovascular, aortic, and renal artery surgery have been

TABLE 70-4

CLINICAL CHARACTERISTICS OF ATHEROEMBOLIC DISEASE AND THEIR APPROXIMATE INCIDENCE[a]

Age (yr)	60 and higher (rare lower than 50)
Male (%)	75%
Caucasian race	90%
Cigarette smoking history	70%–90%
Medical and vascular disease	
Hypertension	60%–90%
Peripheral vascular disease	60%–75%
Coronary artery disease	40%–75%
Abdominal aortic aneurysm	20%–45%
Diabetes mellitus	10%–35%
Hypercholesterolemia	20%–50%

[a] Refer to text.

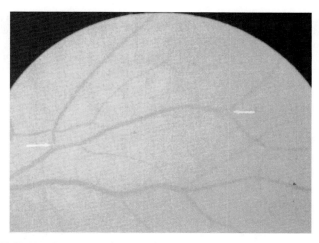

FIGURE 70-11. Retinal image shows two bright yellow cholesterol plaques (Hollenhorst plaques) at two bifurcations of retinal arterioles (*arrows*). This was noted in a 68-year-old man with progressive renal insufficiency owing to atheroembolic disease following cardiac catherization. (From: Goehagen M. Ophthalmology Service, Department of Veterans Affairs Medical Center, West Los Angeles, Wadsworth Division, with permission.)

complicated by AED (154–157). Thrombolysis and anticoagulation with heparin and Coumadin were considered sole or contributing factors in 14% to 37% of cases (158–165). Less commonly, blunt abdominal trauma, intraaortic balloon placement, cardiopulmonary resuscitation, and percutaneous renal angioplasty have been implicated as causing AED. Occasionally, AED occurs spontaneously without precipitating events. Only 13% of 95 cases were spontaneous in an Italian study (152,165).

The time from the precipitating event to clinically apparent AED is variable, with a range of 1 day to a month or two. In a study of 52 patients with AED and renal failure, clinical manifestations, most often skin manifestations, were seen within 1 day of the precipitating event in 50% of the patients (149). Skin lesions are the most common clinical finding in AED, and are described in 35% to 50% of patients (149,167). Skin findings include purpura, petechiae, violaceous mottling of the toes and feet, the so-called "purple toe syndrome," livedo reticularis, gangrene, and ulcers. The lower extremities are most commonly involved and they are frequently bilateral, although other parts of the body may be involved. Severe scrotal and penile necrosis due to AED has been described (166–168).

Renal involvement is frequently severe and often is the most critical problem. The presentation of renal failure may be acute and fulminant, or it may follow a more insidious, sometimes stepwise course. The onset of renal failure may follow the precipitating event closely, within 1 or 2 days, or it may develop weeks or months later. From three reports of 91 patients who developed acute renal failure from AED, 17% to 44% had severe failure that required dialysis (137,138,149). About 20% of these patients recovered sufficient function to no longer require dialysis, after 42 to 122 days (149). Predictors of end-stage renal disease (ESRD) among 95 patients with AED were preexisting chronic kidney disease and longstanding hypertension; use of statins was independently associated with a decreased risk of ESRD (152). Atheroemboli to transplanted renal allografts have been described (169,170).

The gastrointestinal (GI) tract is showered with microemboli in 18% and 48% of cases. (171–173). Abdominal pain and hemorrhage develop from mucosal ulcerations and small infarcts. Diarrhea and postprandial pain may also be present. Pancreatitis (174), and, less commonly, small bowel perforation, bowel obstruction, cholecystitis, and splenic infarcts have been described (172).

The central nervous system may be involved, with findings of confusion, obtundation, and focal neurologic deficits. Visual deficits and the funduscopic finding of Hollenhorst plaques,

bright copper-yellow plaques usually lodged at the bifurcations of the retinal arterioles, may be noted (175,176) (Fig. 70-11). Several cases of pulmonary involvement with hemoptysis and a pulmonary-renal presentation have been described (177–179). Patients may have nonspecific findings of weight loss, fever, and muscle aches.

Laboratory results are often abnormal but not specific. Occasionally, mild leukocytosis and eosinophilia may be present. Reports on the incidence of eosinophilia in AED have been varied. Eosinophilia was seen in only 14% of 37 patients in one report, but was found transiently in 71% of 80 patients and in 77% in another study (180–182). The erythrocyte sedimentation rate is commonly elevated, and hypocomplementemia has been observed (183). Mild proteinuria is generally present, but nephrotic-range proteinuria has also been described (145,184,185).

Microscopic hematuria occasionally occurs, and hyaline and granular casts may be found on urinalysis. Rarely, dysmorphic red blood cells and red blood cell casts, findings of a nephritic sediment, may be seen. Eosinophiluria detected by the Hansel stain was found in 8 of 9 patients with AED, but noted in only 2 of 37 patients in a report that used the Wright stain (149,186). Depending upon the site of the atheroembolic showering, increases of amylase, lipase, creatine kinase, and liver enzymes may be present.

A high index of suspicion for AED should be present when elderly patients, especially those with diffuse atherosclerotic disease, develop renal failure following a vascular procedure. On the other hand, the diagnosis of spontaneously occurring AED may be perplexing. In these latter cases, a tissue diagnosis is often necessary. The safest and easiest tissue to biopsy is the skin, which is diagnostic for AED in 90% of biopsies (137,167,187). Renal biopsies are often diagnostic, but they may miss the typical lesions because of the patchy distribution of atheroemboli. Other organs that showed cholesterol emboli were the muscle, bone marrow, prostate, stomach, and lung (177,178,188).

At present, there is no satisfactory therapy for patients with atheroembolic renal disease. General medical supportive measures and the avoidance of anticoagulants may be the best current approach, since there is the concern that these agents could worsen the atheroembolic showering (189–195).

Corticosteroids, antiplatelet agents, and vasodilators have unproven effects. If patients require dialysis, it may be safest to perform heparin-free dialysis.(152,191,195,196).

The vascular surgical literature describes improvement of renal function with revascularization of the kidney when AED is the consequence of severe atherosclerosis of the renal artery and when renal artery stenosis is present (137,197,198). In these cases, renal function was allowed to stabilize for a few months following the initial episode of atheroemboli before intervention, either surgical bypass or intra-arterial stent placement, was performed. Surgical benefit has also been described in AED, mainly for limb salvage (197–199). In a study of 100 patients with AED, surgery was attempted to remove the source of the atheroemboli. Surgical outcome and long-term prognosis, especially limb salvage, were good in the patients in whom the infrarenal aorta or iliac artery were the source of the atheroemboli. However, clinical outcomes were poor and mortality rates were high in patients who underwent suprarenal aortic surgery (197). In another study, 42 patients with AED underwent bypass surgery or endarterectomy, most of them at the level of the infrarenal aorta or more distally. They reported good limb salvage, low operative mortality, and excellent long-term relief of embolization (198). Surgical candidates among this elderly population, many with comorbid conditions, must be chosen carefully.

RENAL VEIN THROMBOSIS

Thrombosis of the renal vein was originally thought to be a relatively uncommon vascular complication of the kidney. Although the first description of thrombosis of the renal vein was made by J. Hunter (200), Rayer in 1840 was the first to make an association between renal vein thrombosis (RVT) and the nephrotic syndrome (201). Much later, Abeshouse extensively reviewed the medical literature in regard to thrombotic disease of the renal vein (202). Among the most important causes cited were infectious suppuration, malignancy, and trauma. It is important to note that in all of these patients reported to have RVT, the diagnosis was made postmortem. Later, with the development of more advanced radiographic techniques and selective catheterization, antemortem diagnosis of RVT was made possible, and the number of patients in the adult population diagnosed with RVT increased. Although RVT may be caused by trauma or tumor, it occurs most commonly in the nephrotic patient.

Because of the early descriptions, emphasis was placed on the presence of lumbar pain with flank tenderness, edema, and the appearance of a lumbar mass. As a consequence, the early reports following this description focused attention on these symptoms, and it was generally assumed that RVT always presented suddenly with florid symptomatology. However, Harrison et al. in 1956 described two groups of patients with RVT (203). The first, with complete acute thrombosis of the renal vein, was characterized by severe lumbar or abdominal pain, enlargement of the affected kidney, proteinuria, edema, and deterioration of renal function. A second group had only the nephrotic syndrome and absence of acute symptomatology.

Etiology

The incidence of RVT in the adult population is difficult to establish. A review of 29,280 necropsy studies performed in the Mayo Clinic from 1920 to 1961 revealed 17 adults with bilateral RVT, an incidence of approximately 0.6% per 1,000 necropsies (204). Among the 17 patients, only 2 had the nephrotic syndrome; however, during the last decade, prospective studies evaluated the incidence of RVT in the nephrotic patient and found it to be significant, although variable. In Table 70-5 are displayed data from various prospective studies evaluating the incidence of RVT in patients with the nephrotic syndrome and membranous nephropathy (210–216). These prospective studies evaluated patients undergoing routine renal venograms regardless of the presence or absence of symptoms suggestive of RVT. It can be appreciated that the overall incidence of RVT in both the nephrotic syndrome and membranous nephropathy is significant; however, there are marked differences, ranging from 5% to 62%. The reason for such differences is not clear. One possibility, in light of current immunologic advances, is that membranous nephropathy may include different immunologic entities and some patients may be more prone to develop RVT than others. Another possibility is that the duration of the nephrotic syndrome and the persistence and magnitude of the hypoalbuminemia may have varied in these studies. It is generally agreed that the most common underlying nephropathy associated with RVT is membranous nephropathy. A review of all our patients with

TABLE 70-5

PROSPECTIVE STUDIES EVALUATING THE INCIDENCE OF RENAL VEIN THROMBOSIS (RVT) IN PATIENTS WITH NEPHROTIC SYNDROME (NS) AND MEMBRANOUS GLOMERULOPATHY (MGN)

	Patients with RVT in NS	Incidence (%)	Patients with RVT in MGN	Incidence (%)
Bennett (4)	—	—	5/10	50
Noel et al. (154)	—	—	5/16	31
Wagoner et al. (158)	—	—	14/27	52
Cameron et al. (76)	—	—	2/15	13
Pohl et al. (155)	1/54	2	1/20	5
Llach et al. (152)	33/151	22	20/69	29
Monteon et al. (153)	15/53	28	15/24	62
Vosnides et al. (157)	7/44	16	5/30	17
Velasquez-Forero and Garcia-Prugue (156)	8/19	42	3/5	60

(From: Llach, F. The hypercoagulability and thrombotic complications of nephrotic syndrome. *Kidney Int* 1985;28:4259. Editorial review, with permission.)

TABLE 70-6

ETIOLOGY OF THE NEPHROTIC SYNDROME IN 151 PATIENTS

Renal diagnosis	Patients with renal vein thrombosis (no.)	Patients without renal vein thrombosis (no.)	Total
Membranous nephropathy	20	49	69
Membranoproliferative glomerulonephritis	6	21	27
Lipoid nephrosis	2	8	10
Rapidly progressive glomerulonephritis	1	1	2
Amyloidosis	1	5	6
Focal sclerosis	1	3	4
Renal sarcoidosis	1	0	1
Lupus nephritis	1	10	11
Diabetic nephropathy	0	15	15
Focal glomerulonephritis	0	3	3
Acute poststreptococcal glomerulonephritis	0	2	2
End-stage renal disease	0	1	1
Total	33	118	151

(From: Llach F, Koffler A, Massry SG. Renal vein thrombosis and the nephrotic syndrome. *Nephron* 1977;19:65, with permission.)

nephrotic syndrome is shown in Table 70-6. Of 151 patients with the nephrotic syndrome, 33 had RVT, and of these, 20 had membranous nephropathy (205). However, other causes such as membranoproliferative glomerulonephritis, minimal change nephrosis, and amyloidosis may be associated with RVT. Of our 33 patients with RVT, only 4 had an acute mode of presentation.

The concept of the relationship between RVT and the nephrotic syndrome has changed in the last two decades. For many years, it was thought that RVT was the cause of the nephrotic syndrome, a belief that is no longer held. Several lines of evidence seriously questioned this hypothesis. First, experimentally induced RVT causes only mild proteinuria, and renal histology by immunofluorescent findings in these cases does not resemble that of membranous nephropathy (206,207). Second, according to the surgical literature, RVT can occur in the absence of the nephrotic syndrome (208,209). Moreover, in autopsy studies of patients with RVT, nephrotic syndrome was present antemortem in only a few patients. Third, most patients with RVT and nephrotic syndrome who have been subjected to renal morphologic study exhibit an identifiable glomerulopathy, most of the time membranous nephropathy, which is responsible for the nephrotic syndrome (210–216). Finally, as shown recently, RVT occurs after the onset of the nephrotic syndrome (216). Therefore, the general view today is that the nephrotic syndrome provides a favorable milieu for the development of RVT.

Pathophysiology

An important factor in the causation of RVT in patients with the nephrotic syndrome is the presence of a hypercoagulable state. Various investigators (217–231) observed profound clotting factor abnormalities in patients with the nephrotic syndrome. There are five major functional classes of coagulation components: (a) zymogens (factors II, V, IX, XI, and XII), which are activated by enzymes and cofactors (factors V and VIII) the major role of which is to accelerate the role of enzymes; (b) fibrinogen and products from the conversion of fibrinogen

to fibrin; (c) the fibrinolytic system; (d) clotting inhibitors; and (e) components of the platelet reaction and thrombogenesis. Alterations in all of these coagulation components have been observed in the nephrotic patient.

Alterations in zymogens and cofactors include a decrease in the levels of factors IX, XI, and XII. The low levels of these proteins are due most likely to urinary loss secondary to their small molecular size rather than to impaired protein synthesis. An increase in the levels of factor II and combined factors VII and X has also been described (222–227). In general, most of these zymogen abnormalities tend to normalize with clinical remission of the nephrotic syndrome. Most consistently, increased levels of cofactors (factors V and VIII) have been noted in the nephrotic syndrome (231–233). A number of studies showed a correlation between increases in factors V and VIII and a fall in serum albumin level (232,233). These alterations in cofactors result from increased synthesis of these proteins by the liver; the mitochondria of the liver cells are the final sites of production of most of these proteins, and a decrease in plasma oncotic pressure or a decrease in serum albumin concentration or both may be sensed by these liver cells, which in turn respond with an increased production of different proteins (234).

During the earlier description of the hypercoagulable state of the nephrotic syndrome, the hypothesis was advanced that an increase in cofactors may lead to hypercoagulability and may explain the high incidence of thrombosis in these patients. However, two important points must be made regarding this hypothesis. First, all of these factors are normally present in great excess in the circulation, with only a small amount of any given factor being activated during thrombus formation. Therefore, it seems unlikely that high levels of any of these zymogens would lead to thrombosis or that reduced levels of some coagulation factors would be a sensitive marker of the presence of thrombosis. Second, there is no evidence suggesting that the increased level of cofactors may lead to thromboembolic phenomena. High levels of these factors are usually present during acute inflammatory responses because they are acute-phase reactant proteins. There is no current evidence that these conditions are associated with an increased risk of thrombosis.

An elevation of plasma ^{131}I-labeled fibrinogen levels is a consistent and significant abnormality observed in nephrotic patients (235–238). As demonstrated by the use of ^{131}I-labeled fibrinogen, the rate of fibrinogen catabolism is normal in these patients, and the observed increase in plasma fibrinogen is due to an increased liver synthesis that is proportional to the urinary protein loss (237). In addition, there is a significant correlation between fibrinogen and cholesterol levels, and both are related inversely to the levels of serum albumin. The level of fibrinogen in nephrotic patients may be as high as 1 g/dL and can alter plasma viscosity considerably (232). Therefore, increased plasma fibrinogen concentration reflects its increased hepatic synthesis; contracted intravascular distribution may be present, and there is a normal degradation rate of fibrinogen in the nephrotic patient. It is possible that the high fibrinogen levels, by significantly increasing blood viscosity, are important in the hypercoagulable state of nephrotic syndrome.

Various tests for the determination of the products of fibrinogen to fibrin conversion have been developed for diagnosis of a prethrombotic state. An increase in the plasma concentration of fibrinogen degradation products (FDPs) is not commonly observed in nephrotic patients but has been observed in the urine of patients with glomerulonephritis (238–241). Some nephrotic patients have increased urinary levels of FDPs (238). However, these findings should not be taken as definite evidence for increased fibrinolysis in the systemic or renal vasculature, because in patients with nonselective proteinuria, fibrinogen is filtered at the glomerulus and may undergo proteolytic degradation by protease. In this regard, gel chromatography shows clearly that material that in the past was interpreted as FDP is actually filtered fibrinogen that has been degraded in the tubules (238).

Alterations in the fibrinolytic system have also been observed in nephrotic patients (233). The basic reaction of the fibrinolytic system is the conversion by plasminogen activators of β-globulin, plasminogen, to an active serum protease, plasmin. This system is modulated by inhibitors of both plasminogen and plasmin. A number of clinical studies reported an association between defective fibrinolysis and thrombosis; the association included oral contraceptive ingestion (242), pregnancy (243), postoperative states (244), malignant disease (245), obesity (246), and the nephrotic syndrome (247). The data in regard to the fibrinolytic abnormalities in nephrotic patients have shown in general a decrease in plasma plasminogen concentration (248–251) that is correlated with a low serum albumin concentration and the magnitude of the proteinuria (251). The clinical significance of this abnormality is not known, and a cause–effect relationship of these abnormalities and RVT has not been made. However, Du et al. (252) identified a plasmin inhibitor that is identical to α_2-antiplasmin. They evaluated 14 nephrotic patients with RVT together with 30 nephrotic patients without RVT. In both groups the level of total fibrinolytic activity was normal and that of the plasma inhibitor (α_2-antiplasmin) of plasminogen activation was elevated. However, the plasmin inhibitor was elevated in 13 of 14 patients with RVT and in only 12 of 30 patients without RVT. The authors suggested that the increased level of α_2-antiplasmin may be a factor in determining susceptibility to the development and persistence of RVT in nephrotic patients. Further studies are needed to confirm the importance of these observations.

Alterations in coagulation inhibitors have been observed in nephrotic patients. The components of the coagulation system exist in the circulation as zymogens, and they are cleaved to form proteolytic enzymes. Activated clotting factors are inhibited by naturally occurring coagulation inhibitors (253–255). The most important physiologically of these inhibitors is antithrombin III (AT III), an α_2-globulin that is the main inhibitor of thrombin and also inhibits activated factors XII, IX, X, and

XI and plasmin (256–258). The rate of inhibition of these enzymes by AT III is markedly increased in the presence of heparin. In patients from families with an inherited deficiency of AT III, an increased incidence of thromboembolic complications is generally observed when AT III levels are less than 75% of normal (256).

Kauffman et al. studied AT III levels in 48 patients with proteinuria and their relationship with the occurrence of thromboembolic phenomena (259,260). Nine patients had evidence of thrombosis, including 4 with RVT. In 8 of these 9 patients, the serum AT III levels were less than 70% of normal. There was a significant correlation between AT III concentration and urinary protein excretion. Only 6 of the 32 patients who excreted less than 10 g per 24 hours showed depressed AT III levels of less than 85%, whereas 13 of 16 patients with a urinary protein loss higher than 10 g per 24 hours showed depressed AT III levels. Because the molecular weight of AT III is relatively low, excretion in the urine would be expected in patients with proteinuria. Because of similar molecular weights, the renal clearance of AT III and albumin was compared. A significant correlation was noted between the plasma concentrations of these two proteins. In addition, there was a significant correlation between the renal clearance of AT III and the degree of AT III deficiency. It was concluded that thrombosis in nephrotic patients may be associated with deficiency of AT III due to increased urinary loss and that low levels of AT III may be insufficient to inactivate procoagulant factors, thus resulting in the development of thrombosis. These results are in apparent conflict with those of studies showing normal or increased antithrombin activity in nephrotic children (261,262). This finding may have been due to the nonspecific in vitro inhibition of thrombin by α_2-globulin and α_2-antitrypsin (two other clotting inhibitors), and, therefore, the apparent increment in AT III activity may not have reflected a true increase in AT III levels. In addition, AT III deficiency was generally associated with a serum albumin concentration of less than 2 g/dL by other investigators (259–260), whereas in the earlier studies only a few patients had severe hypoalbuminemia. Panicucci et al. reported normal levels of AT III despite high urinary AT III levels (263). They suggested that increased AT III synthesis compensated for its renal loss. Later, Vaziri et al. observed a significant decrease in AT III plasma concentration and activity in 20 nephrotic patients compared with normal subjects (264). In addition, substantial urinary losses of AT III were demonstrated in the nephrotic patients. Therefore, although the rate of synthesis and degradation of AT III and its distribution have not been determined, it is likely that renal losses of AT III in nephrotic patients contribute to AT III deficiency. It is possible that the danger of thromboembolic phenomena may arise with sudden changes in the activity of the renal disease, resulting in abrupt renal losses of AT III while hepatic synthesis of AT III has not yet increased. An interesting observation is the increase in AT III levels in nephrotic children after steroid therapy (263). Furthermore, of interest is the recent observation in a healthy non-nephrotic 13-year-old girl presenting with acute flank pain and anuria due to RVT (265). She was noted to have a marked familial deficiency of AT III levels. Urgent surgical thrombectomy and anticoagulation resulted in recovery of renal function. Consequently, an early diagnosis of this familial condition may lead to the use of preventive measures or acute specific therapeutic intervention at the onset of the acute thrombosis.

Important data about the role of coagulation inhibitors in the development of thrombosis have been reported. Protein C and protein S have been identified as potent anticoagulants. Protein C is a vitamin K–dependent serum protease zymogen that is homologous with other known vitamin K–dependent serum proteases (266–269). This protein is an anticoagulant because it prolongs the clotting time of plasma in various clotting assays (270). The clinical role of protein C as an important antithrombotic regulatory molecule was demonstrated by identifying a familial thrombotic disease that is associated with an inherited partial deficiency of protein C (271). Consequently, families with a deficiency in plasma protein C have recurrent thrombosis. It appears that protein C levels less than 50% result in thrombosis. Although AT III appears to be a major regulatory protein in limiting the activity of procoagulant plasma enzymes, activated protein C may represent a major regulatory protein limiting the activity of activated procoagulant factors (factors V and VIII). In this respect, the anticoagulant properties of activated protein C and AT III are complementary.

The rate of inactivation of factor V by activated protein C is stimulated by another vitamin K–dependent protein, protein S (272). Protein S has no effect on factor V activity in the absence of activated protein C, indicating that it is not a protease. In protein S–deficient plasma, the anticoagulant activity of protein C is restored. It appears that the complex between protein S and activated protein C is formed only in the presence of phospholipids (266,267). Because protein S is required for the expression of the anticoagulant activity of activated protein C, it is not surprising that a deficiency of protein S predisposes to recurrent thrombosis (272). Comp and Esmon (271) identified six unrelated persons with severe, recurrent venous thrombosis who were deficient in protein S, with levels between 15% and 37%. Early high protein C and S levels were observed in the nephrotic patients (273).

Other investigators noted normal protein C levels in nephrotic patients (271). However, it was observed that the functional levels of protein S did not correlate with the immunologic levels. Further, protein S was noted in two forms in plasma, as free and functionally active protein S and complexed to C4b-binding protein. When compared with control subjects, nephrotic patients had reduced functional levels of protein S, despite having elevated levels of total protein S antigen (274). Decreased total protein S activity was caused by significant reductions in free (active) protein S levels due to selective urinary loss of free protein S and elevation of C4b-binding protein levels that favors complex formation. These authors also observed that the specific activity of protein C (activity-antigen ratio) was lower in nephrotic patients than in controls. The authors concluded that acquired protein S deficiency occurs in nephrotic syndrome and may be a risk factor for the development of the thromboembolic complications.

Platelet abnormalities have also been observed in nephrotic patients. Therefore, thrombocytosis is often present (274–276), and an increased platelet aggregation with adenosine diphosphate (ADP) and collagen but not with epinephrine has been observed (277,278). Remuzzi et al. observed that the degree of platelet function abnormalities correlates with the degree of hypoalbuminemia and the severity of the proteinuria (276). The levels of β-thromboglobulin, a specific protein released by platelets on aggregation, are significantly elevated in nephrotic patients and return to normal with clinical remission (277). This suggests that nephrotic patients have an increase in platelet aggregation. However, normal β-thromboglobulin levels have also been reported in nephrotic patients (278). One study of nephrotic patients demonstrated that thrombotic complications occur only in patients with increased platelet aggregation and elevated β-thromboglobulin levels (279). In addition, these complications occurred primarily in patients with a serum albumin level of less than 2 g/dL.

In summary, the hypercoagulable state of the nephrotic syndrome is characterized by low zymogen factors, a marked increase in cofactors, an increase in plasma fibrinogen levels, a decrease in the levels of AT III and antiplasmin activity, thrombocytosis, increased plasma aggregation, and increased levels of β-thromboglobulin. The high levels of fibrinogen leading to increased plasma viscosity may be an important factor in the hypercoagulable state. A convincing relationship has been found between low AT III and thrombosis, and it is likely that increased platelet aggregation may also be an important factor in hypercoagulability; the increased levels of β-thromboglobulin may be a reliable marker of platelet aggregation. The severity of the hypoalbuminemia, by increasing hepatic synthesis of fibrinogen and platelet aggregation, may play a pivotal role in the generation and maintenance of these abnormalities.

In regard to the role of a protein S deficiency in the hypercoagulable state, additional studies in nephrotic patients with thrombosis are necessary to reach any conclusion. However, because protein S deficiency is an acquired problem, it should be determined in patients with thromboembolic complications.

In addition to hypercoagulability, other factors may be important in the pathogenesis of RVT. Therefore, a persistent reduction in plasma volume, an important feature in some patients with the nephrotic syndrome, especially those with membranous nephropathy and normal renal function, may provide a milieu favorable to RVT. Theoretically, a sustained reduction in blood volume could lead to decreased renal venous flow, thereby favoring the development of RVT. In this regard, we have been impressed by the marked decrease in washout time in renal venograms in patients with membranous nephropathy who do not have RVT (235). Diuretics may enhance volume depletion and thereby contribute to the thromboembolic phenomena of the nephrotic syndrome. Recent preliminary data presented by Cheng et al. (280) in evaluating 97 nephrotic patients, strongly suggest that intensive diuretic therapy is associated with a high incidence of RVT. Third, the nature of the immunologic injury may also be important. One study investigating the relationship between membranous nephropathy and RVT separated a subpopulation of patients with membranous nephropathy and RVT (281). It is attractive to speculate that such complexes may be the triggering factor in the coagulation process. In one study, the presence of factor XII and prekallikrein in subepithelial deposits was observed in 29 patients with membranous nephropathy (282). It is tempting to relate the high incidence of RVT in membranous nephropathy to activation of factor XII, a factor that is at the crossroads of important proteolytic pathways. Clinically, patients with nephrotic syndrome and membranous nephropathy have a high incidence of other thromboembolic phenomena in addition to RVT (235,236). Furthermore, greater disturbances of hypercoagulability were noted in patients with membranous nephropathy than in those nephrotic patients with minimal change disease (235). An underestimated factor predisposing to acute peripheral vascular thrombosis and even RVT may be arterial diagnostic puncture as well as placement of central catheters (283). Finally, the role of steroids in the pathogenesis of RVT has not yet been defined. Steroids can aggravate the hypercoagulable state (284), and historically the advent of steroid therapy coincided with an increase in thromboembolic complications (285,286). The previously mentioned study by Cheng et al. (280) indicated that steroid therapy was associated with a high incidence of RVT. Therefore, these agents should be used cautiously in the treatment of nephrotic syndrome.

In summary, the pathogenesis of RVT in patients with nephrotic syndrome may be multifactorial. A general integrated scheme of the pathogenetic factors leading to RVT and other thromboembolic complications is displayed in Figure 70-12.

Clinical Manifestations: Acute Versus Chronic

The pattern and mode of clinical presentation of the nephrotic syndrome and RVT may differ from those mentioned in the early literature. Rayer's description of RVT included lumbar pain with tenderness, swelling, and the appearance of a lumbar

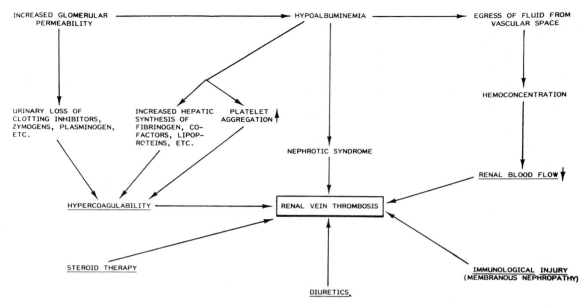

FIGURE 70-12. Schematic representation of pathogenetic factors leading to renal vein thrombosis in nephrotic syndrome.

mass (201). Subsequent reports stressed the presence of flank pain and macroscopic hematuria in the clinical presentation of RVT (287). However, descriptions of more cases revealed that many patients with RVT did not have any local symptoms and signs. The clinical spectrum of RVT varies from patient to patient. (216) The rapidity of venous occlusion and the development of venous collateral circulation determine the clinical presentation and subsequent renal function; however, in general, patients with RVT usually have two modes of clinical presentation: acute and chronic. The chronic presentation of RVT is observed most frequently and in general is asymptomatic. Acute RVT is characterized by sudden onset and usually occurs in younger patients complaining of persistent acute flank pain, which may be colicky at times; marked costovertebral angle tenderness and macroscopic hematuria are usually present. The following case is a representative example of acute RVT:

A 25-year-old white man came to the hospital with a year-long history of proteinuria and ankle swelling. Physical examination revealed no acute distress with normal blood pressure. The only physical finding was ankle edema. Urinary sediment demonstrated 3+ proteinuria. Biochemical data were consistent with the presence of nephrotic syndrome and normal renal function. Renal biopsy revealed early membranous nephropathy. Lung scan and intravenous pyelogram (IVP) were within normal limits. An inferior vena cavogram as well as a left renal venogram were within normal limits. At the time the left renal venogram was performed, the patient experienced acute left flank pain that lasted 4 to 5 hours and was accompanied by macroscopic hematuria and marked tenderness in the left costovertebral angle. The procedure was terminated and the patient was returned to the ward. A second IVP showed marked enlargement of the left kidney with poor visualization of pelvocaliceal system. A selective left renal venogram obtained 1 week later revealed complete obstruction of the main renal vein. The creatinine clearance rate was reduced, and the patient was given anticoagulant therapy. In 2 days, the flank pain resolved completely, and the creatinine clearance rate, after 6 months of anticoagulant therapy, increased from 40 to 90 mL/minute.

On occasion, acute RVT may be bilateral, resulting in marked oliguric acute renal failure and flank pain. The sever-

ity of the symptomatology and oliguria and the magnitude of renal function deterioration depend on various factors. Therefore, previously compromised renal function, absence of collateral circulation, and a large thrombus involving both renal veins may result in a florid clinical presentation as well as rapid deterioration in renal function.

Other causes of acute RVT with or without the nephrotic syndrome are trauma, ingestion of oral contraceptive agents, dehydration (mostly in infants), and steroid administration.

RVT secondary to trauma is usually accompanied by renal artery thrombosis. The history of the trauma, the severe acute flank pain, and a palpable mass are usually suggestive of this condition.

The use of oral contraceptives is implicated occasionally as a cause of RVT. In a young female on oral contraceptives without the nephrotic syndrome or any traumatic event, acute RVT developed with florid clinical manifestations (288). Whether there was a cause–effect relationship between the contraceptive agents and the RVT was not clear.

Dehydration is clearly associated with RVT in infants (289). In this condition thrombosis develops in the small renal veins, predominantly the arcuate or intralobular vein. The majority of these infants do not have nephrotic syndrome or even significant proteinuria. This syndrome develops initially in the clinical setting of diarrhea, vomiting, and often shock. Oliguria and hematuria rapidly ensue. Contributing factors are a history of maternal diabetes, congenital heart disease, and performance of angiocardiography. An enlarged palpable kidney may be found in 60% of affected infants. The common clinical presentation is a hyperosmolar hypovolemic syndrome. The mortality of RVT in infants is high. Fortunately, the frequency of this syndrome has diminished due to earlier therapy and control of volume-depleting events.

Steroid administration is clearly associated with acute and chronic RVT as well as other thrombotic complications (284,285); however, the causative role of these agents in RVT remains to be established. The role of steroids cannot be appraised until other factors influencing thrombus formation are understood. As mentioned earlier, Cheng et al. (280) presented preliminary data from 97 nephrotic patients who were prospectively evaluated. Of these, 44 patients had RVT as shown by routine renal venography. Multivariate regression analysis revealed that steroid therapy was associated with a high tendency to develop RVT ($p < 0.01$).

Recently, acute RVT was noted with increasing frequency in the transplanted kidney (290–292), which, unlike the native kidney, has a single drainage system. In this setting RVT usually leads to permanent damage of the graft within hours. Predisposing factors are the use of OKT3 and cyclosporine therapy (293). The available evidence suggests that cyclosporine may predispose to vascular thrombosis by exacerbating the hypercoagulability (294). In fact, rupture of renal allografts, an uncommon complication, usually is an early manifestation of acute RVT that often is attributable to cyclosporine therapy (293).

Finally, abdominal tumors, especially hypernephromas, are a common cause of RVT; however, in the majority of these patients chronic rather than acute RVT is the common clinical presentation.

The radiologic manifestations of acute RVT are well defined and characteristic in contrast to those of chronic RVT, which often are minimal. Experimentally, with complete occlusion of the renal vein, the kidney increases rapidly in size within the first 24 hours, reaching a peak within 1 week of renal vein occlusion (295). Thereafter, there is a progressive decrease in renal size over the next 2 months, resulting in a small, atrophic kidney. A progressive decrease in the caliber and length of the renal artery follows the occlusion.

Clinically, in a patient with acute RVT, the plain film of the abdomen and IVP initially reveal an enlarged kidney (see Fig. 70-13). In the IVP, if the obstruction is sudden and complete, there may not be any visualization of the collecting system. However, in most patients, because of the presence of some collateral circulation, there is renal enlargement and opacification of varying degree with some visualization of the kidney. Often the renal pelvis can be visualized and is usually stretched, distorted, and blurred (see Fig. 70-13). This may be the result of severe interstitial edema and swelling of the pelvocaliceal system. At this stage the radiographic appearance has been compared to that observed in polycystic kidney disease, and on occasion it has led to this mistaken diagnosis. The acute symptomatology of RVT in association with this radiologic appearance establishes the diagnosis. Ureteral edema may progress to the point at which the collecting system is completely obliterated; there have been cases of complete ureteral obstruction in which during retrograde pyelography the catheter could not be advanced into the pelvis. A characteristic radiographic finding of RVT is notching of the ureter, which usually occurs when collateral veins in close relation to the ureters become tortuous as they dilate to form an alternative drainage route. Originally the notching of the ureters was interpreted as representative of mucosal edema; however, more detailed radiographic studies have shown indentation of the ureters by the collateral venous circulation (296,297). Notching of the ureter is a very infrequent finding in nephrotic patients with RVT and usually occurs only in a minority of patients with chronic rather than acute RVT (296).

Retrograde pyelography may be useful in the patient with complete RVT who does not excrete the contrast material. In such instances, retrograde pyelography may demonstrate a rectangular, linear mucosal pattern with irregular renal pelvic outlines similar to those described with the IVP.

Inferior vena cavography with selective catheterization of the renal vein establishes the diagnosis of RVT. If the inferior vena cava is patent and free of filling defects, and if a good stream of unopacified renal blood is demonstrated to wash out contrast material from the vena cava, a diagnosis of RVT is unlikely. The Valsalva maneuver is useful during vena cavography; by increasing the intraabdominal pressure the transit of contrast agent and blood from the inferior vena cava is slowed, the proximal part of the main renal vein may be opacified, and the patency of the lumen or even the outline of the thrombus may be demonstrated. On occasion, a lack of washout in the area of the renal vein may be suggestive of RVT; sometimes partial defects in the area of the renal vein may be demonstrated, characteristic of renal venous thrombus extending into the inferior vena cava. In the presence of complete inferior vena cava obstruction below the renal vein it is desirable to demonstrate the proximal extent of the thrombus, and this can be accomplished readily by transbrachial catheterization with passage of the catheter into the inferior vena cava via the subclavian vein.

Often the inferior vena cavogram is not diagnostic and selective catheterization of the renal vein must be performed. A normal renal venogram demonstrates the entire intralobular venous system to the level of the arcuate vein. In general, use of epinephrine for better visualization of the smaller vessels is not necessary. However, in the presence of normal renal blood flow all contrast material is washed out of the renal vein within 3 seconds or less, and occasionally only the main renal vein and major branches are visualized. Therefore, in this situation there may be uncertainty about thrombi in major or smaller branches. The use of intrarenal arterial epinephrine by decreasing blood flow enhances retrograde venous filling and allows later visualization of the smaller intrarenal veins. An abnormal

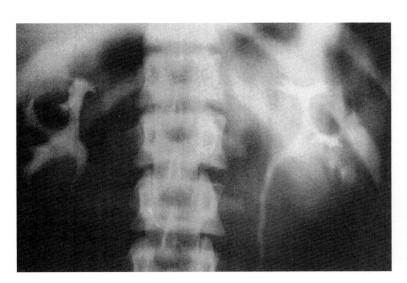

FIGURE 70-13. Intravenous pyelogram of a patient with acute renal vein thrombosis. Note blurring and irregularities of the left pelvocaliceal system as well as marked enlargement of the left kidney. (From: Llach, F. Renal vein thrombosis and the nephrotic syndrome. In: Llach, F. *Renal Vein Thrombosis.* Mount Kisco, NY: Futura; 1993: 155, with permission.)

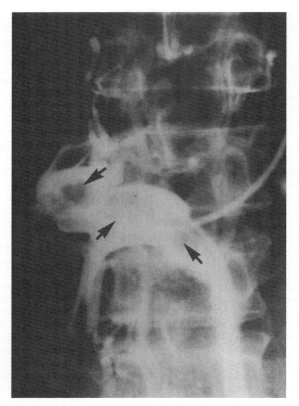

FIGURE 70-14. Left renal venography from a patient with renal vein thrombosis. Note the arrows indicating filling defects, which reflect accumulation of thrombotic material, surrounded by contrast material. There is complete obstruction of the main renal vein as well as of collateral circulation. (From: Llach, F, Papper, S, Massry, SG. The clinical spectrum of renal vein thrombosis: acute and chronic. *Am J Med* 1980;69:819, with permission.)

renal venogram usually demonstrates a thrombus within the lumen as a filling defect surrounded by contrast material (Fig. 70-14). In the presence of partial thrombosis, extensive collateral circulation can be demonstrated. Thus, the presence of such collaterals usually reflects the chronicity of the RVT and may explain the lack of renal functional deterioration.

Many investigators originally considered renal arteriography preferable to renal venography for the diagnosis of RVT. With renal arteriography important information is obtained about the status of the renal parenchyma. In addition, the theoretical danger of dislodging the clot material from the renal vein during renal venography and precipitating a pulmonary embolism is avoided. However, this complication did not occur following renal venography in several extensive radiographic series of patients with RVT (297,298). Renal arteriography may be useful in patients being evaluated for RVT associated with renal trauma or tumor because of the common involvement of the renal artery phase. Deviation and stretching of the interlobular arteries are usually observed in these conditions. In the nephrographic phase, the medullary pyramids are more densely opacified than the cortex, and instead of presenting the usual triangular appearance, they appear to bulge and sometimes are even ovoid in appearance.

Renal ultrasonography may be a useful potential diagnostic procedure for the diagnosis of RVT (297). The sonographic diagnosis of RVT is based on direct visualization of thrombi within the renal vein and inferior vena cava, demonstration of renal vein dilation proximal to the point of occlusion, loss of normal renal structure, and an increase in renal size during the

acute phase. These ultrasonography findings, however, usually have to be confirmed with other diagnostic procedures.

Preliminary information on the use of combined ultrasonic scanning and Doppler ultrasonography for the diagnosis of RVT has been advanced. This is a noninvasive technique that essentially measures the renal venous flow velocity. Although the results of this approach are not definite in RVT, some studies suggest that Doppler ultrasonography may be helpful in the diagnosis of RVT in the transplanted kidney (297).

Computed tomography is the procedure of choice for the noninvasive evaluation of acute RVT. Lower attenuation density shows a thrombus and may be identified within the renal vein and inferior vena cava, or the venous diameter may be enlarged owing to obstruction. In general, intravenous infusion of contrast material, together with computed tomography, may help to visualize the thrombus. In the near future it is likely that noninvasive diagnosis of RVT may be possible using either ultrasonography or computed tomography, or both, together with clinical findings. The radiographic findings include enlargement and distention of the affected renal vein, with visualization of the clots within the vein and sometimes extension into the inferior vena cava (297). Persistent parenchymal opacification with kidney enlargement is usually observed. Capsular venous collaterals, thickening of Gerota's fascia, and pericapsular "whiskering" are often observed.

Preliminary observations of isolated cases suggest that magnetic resonance imaging (MRI) may be, in the future, the diagnostic procedure of choice in the noninvasive diagnosis of RVT. Because MRI produces high-contrast images between flowing blood, vascular walls, and surrounding tissues, vascular patency may be best determined by this technique. A major potential advantage in using this method is the avoidance of contrast material.

Clinical Course and Treatment

The experience to date on the course, prognosis, and treatment of RVT in nephrotic patients is limited. In 1963 Kowal et al. reviewed 65 patients with RVT (296). Only 14 of these patients were alive after 2 years of follow-up. Unfortunately, clinical data and literature references were given only for the 14 surviving patients. Ten of these patients had acute RVT. Recurrent thromboembolic phenomena were cited as the most common cause of death. Later, Rosenmann et al. followed 11 of 15 nephrotic patients with RVT over a period of 24 to 115 months (287). Only 4 of these patients had symptoms suggestive of acute RVT. The incidence of thromboembolic phenomena was high and the phenomena were fatal in 7 patients. One or more episodes of pulmonary embolism occurred in 7 patients, and 4 had evidence of repeated episodes of thrombosis involving the renal venous system. Three patients received anticoagulant therapy and had no new episodes of pulmonary emboli. These data suggest that the prognosis for nephrotic patients with RVT may be poor and is determined by the presence or absence of recurrent thrombotic complications.

In 1970 Richet and Meyrier reviewed 112 cases of RVT reported in the literature. Of the 112 patients, 72 had died, constituting a 64% mortality rate (299). Earlier, McCarthy et al. estimated the average survival period after the onset of RVT to be 9 months (204). These data, however, may not be representative of the present prognosis of this entity. First, most of the earlier data about the course and prognosis of RVT were obtained from autopsy studies. Therefore, the mortality may have been overestimated. Second, renal insufficiency secondary to RVT was a common cause of death in these patients. Dialysis therapy has, of course, reduced the rate of uremic death considerably. Third, the new diagnostic techniques and better understanding of this entity together with better use of

TABLE 70-7

FOLLOW-UP DATE ON NEPHROTIC PATIENTS WITH ACUTE AND CHRONIC RENAL VEIN THROMBOSIS (RVT)

Patients	Urine protein (g/24 hr)	Creatinine clearance (mL/min)	Serum albumin (g/dL)	Serum cholesterol (g/dL)	No. of patients undergoing dialysis
29 with chronic RVT	5.9 ± 3.9[a]	71 ± 25[a]	2.4 ± 0.7[a]	370 ± 110[a]	4
	(4.8 ± 2.3)	(65 ± 29)	(2.9 ± 0.7)	(360 ± 88)	
4 with acute RVT	5.2 ± 1.2[a]	76 ± 19[a]	2.1 ± 0.2[a]	347 ± 19[a]	0
	(5.0 ± 1.2)	(98 ± 8)[b]	(2.3 ± 0.2)	(332 ± 26)	

[a] Initial laboratory data (mean ± SD). Data obtained after anticoagulant therapy are shown in parentheses.
[b] $p < 0.05$.

anticoagulant therapy have contributed to better management of these patients. Nevertheless, a serious complication in patients with RVT is still thromboembolic phenomena, most often pulmonary embolism.

Lavelle et al. recently reevaluated 27 nephrotic patients with RVT, 10 of whom had acute lumbar pain and acute renal failure (300). Eleven patients died within the first 6 months. Survivors were followed for 6 months to 19 years. Nephrotic syndrome improved or even disappeared in 12 patients, and renal function did not worsen throughout the follow-up period. The main prognostic factors were initial renal function and type of nephropathy; that is, patients with membranous nephropathy had significantly better renal function and lower mortality than did patients with other nephropathies. Initial renal insufficiency was significantly associated with a poor prognosis. In fact, 6 of the 8 patients with acute renal failure died; hemorrhagic complications were the major cause of death in these patients.

Renal function may dramatically improve in patients with acute RVT treated with anticoagulant therapy. In Table 70-7 are shown the follow-up data on patients with acute RVT who had significant improvement in renal function with anticoagulant therapy during the follow-up period, and it is recommended that these patients be maintained on long-term anticoagulant therapy (205,210,216,217,220,221,239,251). Convincing evidence has been gathered suggesting that anticoagulant therapy reduces the incidence of new thromboembolic episodes and often reverses the deterioration of renal function that occurs with acute RVT (220,301). Patients treated with anticoagulant therapy may have recanalization of the renal vein, and in some instances a total dissolution of the clot may occur (301). Heparin is the initial therapy of choice. In patients with a large RVT and pulmonary embolism, the clearance rate of heparin is increased, and these patients may need higher doses of heparin in the early stages of therapy. Although the dosage of heparin varies from patient to patient, the aim is to maintain the clotting time of two to two and one-half times normal. In general, because of fewer complications, continued infusion of heparin is preferable to intermittent intravenous administration. Warfarin therapy is instituted once the patient has been treated with heparin for 5 to 7 days and the partial thromboplastin time is within the desired range. Warfarin is started orally with small loading doses. Common clinical problems with warfarin therapy are the drug interactions related to the kinetics of warfarin such as drug absorption, protein binding, metabolism, and excretion. These drug interactions are very common and may play an important role in the enhancement of or decrease in the anticoagulant effect of heparin. It should also be remembered that drugs such as aspirin and indomethacin can increase the risk of bleeding in these patients owing to the effect on the gastrointestinal mucosa and platelet aggregation. From all these observations it is obvious that individualization

of warfarin therapy is essential, and the clinical status, patient sensitivity, metabolism, and possible drug interactions must all be taken into consideration. Once oral anticoagulant therapy is established, the prothrombin time should be kept at about one and one-half to two times normal. The recommended duration of anticoagulant therapy in these patients is difficult to establish. The severity of the hypoalbuminuria is a good indicator of the magnitude of the hypercoagulability. Thus, the nephrotic patient should probably be treated with anticoagulants as long as the serum albumin level is below 2.5 g/L. Relapses with new episodes of acute RVT have been observed after cessation of anticoagulant therapy (251). It is our belief that in general these patients should be on anticoagulation therapy as long as they have the nephrotic syndrome with significant hypoalbuminemia.

Early resolution of the acute RVT has been reported using either streptokinase or urokinase, both systemically or with selective infusion (302–304). However, it appears that selective infusion of these agents is also successful in RVT of the transplanted kidney (305,306).

Surgical treatment for RVT is rarely used today because the role of thrombectomy in the treatment of RVT has not been established as beneficial. Although marked improvement in renal function is occasionally observed after thrombectomy, the majority of these patients do not improve with surgery. This modality of therapy may be theoretically useful in patients with acute bilateral RVT who are not otherwise expected to survive the acute episode, especially when recurrent pulmonary emboli occur despite anticoagulation therapy.

Thromboembolic Complications Other than Renal Vein Thrombosis

The high cumulative risks of thromboembolic complications in the nephrotic patient have been recognized in the last three decades (217,220,251,305). These complications have been observed previously in the pulmonary arteries (307); axillary and subclavian veins (308); and femoral, coronary, and mesenteric arteries (309–310). However, the most common observation may be deep vein thrombosis of the extremities. A summary of thromboembolic complications studies is shown in Table 70-8. Therefore, Andrassy et al. studied 84 nephrotic patients and observed 37 episodes of thromboembolic complications in 30 patients during a period of 3 years (310). There were 23 episodes of deep vein thrombosis, an incidence of 44%, among the highest number encountered in medical patients. Kanfer et al. observed arterial and venous thrombosis in 5 of 8 children and in 10 of 29 adult nephrotic patients during a period of 7 years (231). Although lower (27%), this is still a significant incidence. Four other investigators observed a 17%

TABLE 70-8

SUMMARY OF PUBLISHED STUDIES EVALUATION THROMBOEMBOLIC COMPLICATIONS IN THE NEPHROTIC SYNDROME

	No. of patients	No. with thrombosis[a]	Venous			Arterial			Total no of other episodes[a]
			Renal	Pulmonary	DVT	Heart	Brain	Peripheral	
Andrassy et al. (256)	84	30 (38)	6	7	23	3	1	3	37 (44)
Kauffman et al. (206)	48	9 (19)	4	4	3	—	—	1	8 (17)
Kanfer et al. (178)	45	13 (29)	3	3	6	—	2	1	12 (27)
Pohl et al. (155)	59	5(10)	1	2	3	—	—	—	5 (8.5)
Kuhlmann (226)	17	4 (23)	1	2	1	—	—	—	3 (17)
Velasquez-Forero et al. (156)	19	8 (42)	8	1	2	—	—	—	3 (16)
Llach et al. (159)	151	41 (26)	33	18	3	2	2	1	26 (17)
Kendall et al. (179)	35	4 (23)	1	3	—	1	1	1	6 (17)

[a]Numbers in parentheses represent percentages.
DVT, deep vein thrombosis.

incidence of mostly deep venous thrombosis (210,213,214). In our prospective studies (216), 26 episodes of thromboembolic complications other than RVT were noted in 151 nephrotic patients (17%). Noteworthy is the finding that Pohl et al. reported only 1 patient with RVT of 54, but they observed 5 episodes of thrombosis, an 8.5% incidence, which is still high (212); as shown in Table 70-6 the incidence of thromboembolic complications ranges from 8.5% to 44%. Peripheral venous thrombosis and pulmonary embolism were the most frequent complications, but arterial thrombosis also occurred.

In our prospective study, ventilation-perfusion lung scanning was performed in 94 nephrotic patients, 24 with and 70 without RVT (220). Asymptomatic perfusion defects in the presence of normal-appearing chest X-ray films were observed in 12 patients, 5 with and 7 without RVT. Because pulmonary angiography was not done in these patients, a definitive interpretation of this defect is not possible. However, these data suggest a significant incidence of pulmonary embolism in the nephrotic patients. Similar observations noted (19%) of 37 nephrotic patients with abnormal ventilation-perfusion lung scans and only 1 with RVT (304).

Clearly, there is a significant incidence of thromboembolic phenomena other than RVT in nephrotic patients, but the morbidity and mortality of these complications are not well defined and prospective longitudinal studies must be done to elucidate both the magnitude of this problem and the use of appropriate prophylaxis and therapy in the patient with a high risk of thrombosis.

References

1. Stables DP, Fouche RF, de Villiers JP, et al. Traumatic renal artery occlusion: 21 cases. *Urology* 1976;115:229.
2. Dinchman KH, Spirnak JP. Traumatic renal artery thrombosis. *Semin Urol* 1995;13:90.
3. Barlow B, Gandhi R. Renal artery thrombosis following blunt trauma. *J Trauma* 1980;20:614.
4. Peterson NE, Moore EE. Bilateral renal artery thrombosis secondary to blunt trauma. *J Trauma* 1997;45:713.
5. Peters PC, Bright TC. Blunt renal injuries. *Urol Clin North Am* 1977;4:17.
6. Bretan PN, McAnineh JW, Federle MP, et al. Computerized tomographic staging of renal trauma: 85 consecutive cases. *J Urol* 1986;136:561.
7. Clark DE, Georgitis JW, Ray FS. Renal artery injuries caused by blunt trauma. *Surgery* 1981;90:87.
8. Moyer JH, Heider C, Morris GC, et al. Renal failure: I. The effect of complete renal artery occlusion for variable periods of time as compared to exposure to sub-filtration arterial pressures below 30 mm Hg for similar periods. *Ann Surg* 1957;145:41.
9. Vollmar J, Helmstadter D, Hallwacks O. Complete occlusion of the renal artery. *J Cardiovasc Surg* 1971;12:441.
10. Lang EK, Sullivan J, Frentz G. Renal trauma: radiological studies. Comparison of urographic, computed tomography, angiography, and radionuclide studies. *Radiology* 1985;154:1.
11. Kamel IR, Berkowitz JF. Assessment of the cortical rim sign in post-traumatic renal infarction. *J Comput Assist Tomogr* 1996;20:803.
12. Lang EK. Arteriography in the assessment of renal trauma. *J Trauma* 1975;15:553.
13. Spinosa DJ, Matsumoto AH, Angle JF, et al. Renal insufficiency: Usefulness of gadodiamide-enhanced renal angiography to supplement CO_2-enhanced renal angiography for diagnosis and percutaneous treatment. *Radiology* 1999;210:663.
14. Dean RH. Acute occlusive events involving the renal vessels. In: Rutherford RB, ed. *Vascular Surgery*. 4th ed. Philadelphia: Saunders; 1995:1452.
15. Spirnak JP, Resnick MI. Revascularization of traumatic thrombosis of the renal artery. *Surg Gynecol Obstet* 1987;164:22.
16. Brunetti DR, Sasaki TM, Friedlander G, et al. Successful renal autotransplantation in a patient with bilateral renal artery thrombosis. *Urology* 1994;43:235.
17. Cass AS. Renovascular injuries from external trauma: diagnosis, treatment and outcome. *Urol Clin North Am* 1989;16:213.
18. Munoz D, Gutierrez C, Hidalgo F, et al. Traumatic renal artery thrombosis. *Scand J Urol Nephrol* 1998;32:296.
19. Peterson NE. Review article: traumatic bilateral infarction. *Trauma* 1989;29:158.
20. Weimann S, Flora G, Dittrich P, et al. Traumatic renal artery occlusion: is late reconstruction advisable? *J Urol* 1987;137:727.
21. Fort J, Camps J, Ruiz P, et al. Renal artery embolism successfully revascularized by surgery after 5 days anuria. Is it never too late? *Nephrol Dial Transplant* 1996;11:1843.
22. Letsou GV, Gusberg R. Isolated bilateral renal artery thrombosis: an unusual consequence of blunt abdominal trauma—case report. *J Trauma* 1990;30:509.
23. Maggio AJ, Brosman S. Renal artery trauma. *Urology* 1978;11:125.
24. Haas CA, SPirnak JP. Traumatic renal artery occlusion: a review of the literature. *Tech Urol* 1998;4:1.
25. Haas CA, Dinchman KF, Nasrallah PF, et al. Traumatic renal artery occlusion: a 15-year review. *J Trauma* 1998;45:557.
26. Adovaso R, Pancrazio F. Acute thrombosis of renal artery: restoration of renal function after late revascularization. *Vasa* 1989;18:239.
27. van der Wal MA, Wisselink W, Rauwerda JA. Traumatic bilateral renal artery thrombosis: case report and review of the literature. *Cardiovasc Surg* 2003;11:527.
28. Vuong PN, Desoutter P, Mickley V, et al. Fibromuscular dysplasia of the renal artery responsible for renovascular hypertension: a histological presentation based on a series of 102 patients. *Vasa* 2004;33:13.
29. Stinchcome SJ, Manhire AR, Bishop MC, et al. Renal arterial fibromuscular dysplasia: acute renal infarction in three patients with angiographic evidence of medial fibroplasia. *Br J Radiol* 1992;65:81.
30. Hoover LA, Hall-Craggs M, Dagher FJ. Polyarteritis involving only the main renal arteries. *Am J Kidney Dis* 1988;11:66.
31. Templeton PA, Pats SO. Renal artery occlusion in polyarteritis nodosum. *Radiology* 1985;156:308.
32. Teoh MK. Takayasu's arteries with renovascular hypertension: results of surgical treatment. *Cardiovasc Surg* 1999;7:626.

33. Dardik A, Ballermann BJ, Williams GM. Successful delayed bilateral renal artery revascularization during active phase of Takayasu's arteritis. *J Vasc Surg* 1998;27:552.
34. El Ramahi KM, Al Dalaan A, Al Shaikh A, et al. Renal involvement in Behcet's disease: review of 9 cases. *J Rheumatol* 1998;25:2254.
35. Sherif A, Stewart P, Mendes DM. The repetitive vascular catastrophes of Behcet's disease: a case report with review of the literature. *Ann Vasc Surg* 1992;6:85.
36. Sueyoshi E, Sakamoto I, Hayashi N, et al. Rupturable renal artery aneurysm due to Behcet's disease. *Abdom Imag* 1996;21:166.
37. Akpolat T, Akkoyunlu M, Akpolat I, et al. Renal Behcet's disease: a cumulative analysis. *Semin Arthritis Rheum* 2002;31:317.
38. Price RK, Skelton R. Hypertension due to syphilitic occlusion of the main renal arteries. *Br Heart J* 1948;10:29.
39. Sane SY, Deshmukh SS. Total renal infarct and peri-renal abscess caused by phycomycosis (a case report). *J Postgrad Med* 1998;34:448.
40. Vesa J, Bielsa O, Arango O, et al. Massive renal infarction due to mucormycosis in an AIDS patient. *Infection* 1992;20:234.
41. Heng MC, Haberfeld G. Thrombotic phenomena associated with intravenous cocaine. *J Am Acad Dermatol* 1987;16:462.
42. Goodman PE, Rennie WP. Renal infarction secondary to nasal insufflation of cocaine. *Am J Emerg Med* 1995;13:421.
43. Kramer RK, Turner RC. Renal infarction associated with cocaine use and latest protein C deficiency. *South Med J* 1993;86:1436.
44. Lam J, Henriquez R, Cruzat C. Pheochromocytoma and von Recklinghausen neurofibromatosis: postpartum crisis and renal artery thrombosis. *Rev Med Child* 1998;126:1367.
45. Hitti IF, Celmer EJ, Rapuano J. Hemorrhagic infarction of the kidney: an uncommon presentation of infiltrating urothelial carcinoma of the renal pelvis. *Urol Int* 1986;41:212.
46. Montgomery JH, Moinuddin M, Buchignani JS, et al. Renal infarction after aerobics. *Clin Nucl Med* 1984;9:664.
47. Coulshed SJ, Caterson RJ, Mahony JF. Traumatic infarct at the lower pole of a renal transplant secondary to seat belt compression. *Nephrol Dial Transplant* 1995;10:1464.
48. Granfortuna J, Zamkoff K, Urrutia E. Acute renal infarction in sickle cell disease. *Am J Hematol* 1986;23:59.
49. Sa H, Freitas L, Mota A, et al. Primary antiphospholipid syndrome presented by total infarction of right kidney with nephrotic syndrome. *Clin Nephrol* 1999;52:56.
50. Klein O, Bernheim J, Strahilevitz J, et al. Renal colic in a patient with anti-phospholipid antibodies and factor V Leiden mutation. *Nephrol Dial Transplant* 1999;14:2502.
51. Karassa FB, Avdikou K, Pappas P, et al. Late renal transplant arterial thrombosis in a patient with systemic lupus erythematosus and antiphospholipid syndrome. *Nephrol Dial Transplant* 1999;14:472.
52. Remondino GI, Mysler E, Pissano MN, et al. A reversible bilateral renal artery stenosis in association with antiphospholipid syndrome (case report). *Lupus* 2000;9:65.
53. Ostuni PA, Lazzarin P, Pengo V, et al. Renal artery thrombosis and hypertension in a 13 year old girl with antiphospholipid syndrome. *Ann Rheum Dis* 1990;49:184.
54. Pous JM, Boudet R, Lacrois P, et al. Renal infarction and thrombosis of the infrarenal aorta in a 35 year old man with primary antiphospholipid syndrome. *Am J Kidney Dis* 1996;27:712.
55. Sonpal GM, Sharma A, Miller A. Primary antiphospholipid antibody syndrome, renal infarction and hypertension. *J Rheumatol* 1993;7:1221.
56. Hernandez D, Dominguez ML, Diaz F, et al. Renal infarction in a severely hypertensive patient with lupus erythematosus and antiphospholipid antibodies. *Nephron* 1996;72:298.
57. Kleinknecht D, Bobric G, Meyer O, et al. Recurrent thrombosis and renal vascular disease in patients with a lupus anticoagulant. *Nephrol Dial Transplant* 1989;4:854.
58. Arnold MH, Schreiber L. Splenic and renal infarction in systemic lupus erythematosus: association with anti-cardiolipin antibodies. *Clin Rheumatol* 1988;7:406.
59. Dasgupta B, Almond MK, Tanqeray A. Polyarteritis nodosa and the antiphospholipid syndrome. *Br J Rheumatol* 1997;36:121.
60. Kaushik SM, Federle MP, Schur PH, et al. Abdominal thrombotic and ischemic manifestations of the antiphospholipid antibody syndrome: CT findings in 42 patients. *Radiology* 2001;218(3):768.
61. Guirguis N, Budisavljevic MN, Self S, et al. Acute renal artery and vein thrombosis after renal transplant, associated with a short partial thromboplastin time and factor V Leiden mutation. *Ann Clin Lab Sci* 2000;30:75.
62. Nakamura M, Ohnishi T, Okamoto S, et al. Abdominal aortic thrombosis in a patient with nephrotic syndrome. *Clin Nephrol* 1993;39:257.
63. Temes Montes XL, Almaraz Jimenez MA, Lorenzo Aguiar MD, et al. Renal artery thrombosis occurring in an adult with the idiopathic nephrotic syndrome: results of local treatment with streptokinase. *Clin Nephrol* 1979;12:90.
64. Pochet JM, Bobrie G, Basile C, et al. Renal arterial thrombosis complicating nephrotic syndrome. *Presse Med* 1988;17:2139.
65. Morris D, Kisly A, Stoyka CG, et al. Spontaneous bilateral renal artery occlusion associated with chronic atrial fibrillation. *Clin Nephrol* 1993;39:257.
66. Argiris A. Splenic and renal infarctions complicating atrial fibrillation. *Mt Sinai J Med* 1992;64:342.
67. Cheng KL, Tseng SS, Tarng DC. Acute renal failure caused by unilateral renal artery thromboembolism. *Nephrol Dial Transplant* 2003;8:833.
68. Gill TJ, Dammin GJ. Paradoxical embolism with renal failure caused by occlusion of the renal arteries. *Am J Med* 1958;25:780.
69. Isles CG, Robertson S, Hill D. Management of renovascular disease: a review of renal artery stenting in 10 studies. *Q J Med* 1999;92:159.
70. Textor, SC. Managing renal arterial disease and hypertension. *Curr Opin Cardiol* 2003;18:260.
71. Morris CS, Bonnevie GJ, Najarian KE. Nonsurgical treatment of acute iatrogenic renal artery injuries occurring after renal artery angioplasty and stenting. *AJR Am J Roentgenol* 2001;177(6):1353.
72. Bockler D, Krauss M, Mannsmann U, et al. Incidence of renal infarctions after endovascular AAA repair. *J Endovasc Ther* 2003;10:1054.
73. Gorich J, Kramer S, Tomczak R, et al. Thromboembolic complications after endovascular aortic aneurysm repair. *J Endovasc Ther* 2002;9:180.
74. Holden A, Hill A. Renal angioplasty and stenting with distal protection of the main renal artery in ischemic nephropathy: early experience. *J Vasc Surg* 2003;38:962.
75. Hoxie HJ, Coggin CB. Renal infarction: statistical study of 255 cases and detailed report of an unusual case. *Arch Intern Med* 1940;65:587.
76. Jennette JC, Olson JL, Schwartz MM, et al. eds. *Heptinstall's Pathology of the Kidney.* 5th ed. New York: Lippincott Williams & Wilkins; 1998.
77. Abuelo JG. Diagnosing vascular causes of renal failure. *Ann Intern Med* 1995;123:601.
78. Blakely P, Cosby RL, McDonald BR. Nephritic urinary sediment in embolic renal infarction. *Clin Nephrol* 1994;42:401.
79. Blum U, Billmann P, Krause T, et al. Effect of local low-dose thrombolysis on clinical outcome in acute embolic renal artery occlusion. *Radiology* 1993;189:549.
80. Mesnard L, Delahousse M, Raynaud A, Delayed angioplasty after renal thrombosis. *Am J Kidney Dis* 2003;41:E9.
81. Pilmore HL, Walker RJ, Solomon C, et al. Acute bilateral renal artery occlusion: successful revascularization with streptokinase. *Am J Nephrol* 1995;15:90.
82. Skinner RE, Hefty T, Long TD, et al. Recovery of function in a solitary kidney after intra-arterial thrombolytic therapy. *J Urol* 1989;141:108.
83. Marron B, Ubeda I, Gallego J, et al. Functional renal recovery after spontaneous renal embolization in a sole kidney. *Nephrol Dial Transplant* 1997;12:2417.
84. Lacombe M. Acute nontraumatic obstructions of the renal artery. *J Cardiovasc Surg* 1992;33:163.
85. Ouriel K, Andrus CH, Ricotta JJ, et al. Acute renal artery occlusion: when is revascularization justified? *J Vasc Surg* 1987;5:348.
86. Tham G, Ekelund L, Herrlin K, et al. Renal artery aneurysms: natural history and prognosis. *Ann Surg* 1983;197:348.
87. Silver PR, Budin JA. Unusual manifestations of renal artery aneurysms. *Urol Radiol* 1990;12:80.
88. Cummings KB, Lecky JW, Kaufman JJ. Renal artery aneurysms and hypertension. *J Urol* 1973;109:144.
89. Erdsman G. Angionephrography and suprarenal angiography. *Acta Radiol (Stockholm)* 1957;155:104.
90. Poutasse EF. Renal artery aneurysms. *J Urol* 1975;113:443.
91. Cinat M, Yoon P, Wilson SE. Management of renal artery aneurysms. *Semin Vasc Surg* 1996;9:236.
92. Kincaid OW, Davis GD, Hallermann FJ, et al. Fibromuscular dysplasia of the renal arteries: Arteriographic features, classification and observations on natural history of the disease. *AJR Am J Roentgenol* 1968: 104:271.
93. Barth RA. Fibromuscular dysplasia with clotted renal artery aneurysm. *Pediatr Radiol* 1993;23:296.
94. Stinchcombe SJ, Manhire AR, Bishop MC, et al. Renal arterial fibromuscular dysplasia: acute renal failure in 3 patients with angiographic evidence of medial fibroplasia. *Br J Radiol* 1992;65:81.
95. Smith JN, Hinman F Jr. Intrarenal arterial aneurysms. *J Urol* 1967;97:990.
96. English W, Pearce J, Craven T, et al. Surgical management of renal artery aneurysms. *J Vasc Surg* 2004;40:53.
97. Henke P, Cardneau J, Welling T, et al. Renal artery aneurysms: a 35-year clinical experience with 252 aneurysms in 168 patients. *Ann Surg* 2001;234:454.
98. Pfeiffer T, Lutz R, Grabitz K, et al. Reconstruction for renal artery aneurysm: operative techniques and long-term results. *J Vasc Surg* 2003;37(2):293.
99. Sicard GA, Reilly JM, Picus DD, et al. Alternatives in renal revascularization. *Curr Probl Surg* 1995;32:571.
100. Henke P, Stanley J. Renal artery aneurysms: diagnosis, management and outcomes. *Minerva Chir* 2003;58:305.
101. Hubert JP Jr, Pairolera PC, Kazmier FJ. Solitary renal artery aneurysm. *Surgery* 1980;88:557.
102. Henriksson C, Lukes P, Nilson A. Angiographically discovered nonoperated renal artery aneurysms. *Scand J Urol Nephrol* 1984;18:59.
103. Martin RS, Meacitam PW, Ditesheim JA. Renal artery aneurysm: selective treatment for hypertension and prevention of rupture. *J Vasc Surg* 1989;9:26.
104. Hageman JH, Smith RF, Szilagyi E, et al. Aneurysms of the renal artery: problems of prognosis and surgical management. *Surgery* 1978;84:563.

105. Hidai H, Kindshita Y, Murayama T. Rupture of renal artery aneurysm. *Eur Urol* 1985;11:249.
106. Cohen JR, Shamash FS. Ruptured renal artery aneurysms during pregnancy. *J Vasc Surg* 1978;16:51.
107. Schoon I, Seeman T, Niemand D, et al. Rupture of renal arterial aneurysm in pregnancy: case report. *Acta Chir Scand* 1988;154:593.
108. Smith JA, Cacleish DG. Postpartum rupture of a renal artery aneurysm to a solitary kidney. *Aust N Z J Surg* 1985;55:299.
109. Richardson AJ, Liddington M, Jaskowski A, et al. Pregnancy in a renal transplant recipient complicated by rupture of a transplant renal artery aneurysm. *Br J Surg* 1990;77:228.
110. Rijbroek A, Dikh AV, Roex JM. Rupture of renal artery aneurysm during pregnancy. *Eur J Vasc Surg* 1994;8:375.
111. Love WK, Robinette MA, Vernon CP. Renal artery aneurysm rupture in pregnancy. *J Urol* 1981;126:809.
112. Milsom I, Forssman L. Factors influencing aortocaval compression in late pregnancy. *Am J Obstet Gynecol* 1984;148:764.
113. Yang JC, Hye RJ. Ruptured renal artery aneurysm during pregnancy. *Ann Vasc Surg* 1996;10:370.
114. Ortenberg J, Novick AC, Straffon RA, et al. Surgical treatment of renal artery aneurysms. *Br J Urol* 1983: 55:341.
115. Soussou ID, Starr DS, Lawrie GM, et al. Renal artery aneurysm: long term relief of renovascular hypertension by in situ operative correction. *Arch Surg* 1979;114:1410.
116. Youkey JR, Collins GJ, Orecchia PM, et al. Saccular renal artery aneurysm as a cause of hypertension. *Surgery* 1985;97:498.
117. Bulbul MA, Farrow GA. Renal artery aneurysms. *Urology* 1992;40:124.
118. Hupp T, Allenberg JR, Post K, et al. Renal artery aneurysms: surgical indications and results. *Eur J Vasc Surg* 1992;6:477.
119. Lumsden AB, Salam RA, Walton KG. Renal artery aneurysm: a report of 28 cases. *Cardiovasc Surg* 1996;4:185.
120. Dzsinich C, Gloviczki P, McKusick MA, et al. Surgical management of renal artery aneurysm. *Cardiovasc Surg* 1993;1(3):243.
121. Klein GE, Brien LE, Raith J, et al. Endovascular treatment of renal aneurysms with conventional nondetachable microcoils and Guglielmi detachable coils. *Br J Urol* 1997;79:852.
122. Lupattelli T, Abubacker Z, Morgan R, et al. Embolization of a renal artery aneurysm using ethylene vinyl alcohol copolymer (Onyx). *J Endovasc Ther* 2003;10:366.
123. Bui BT, Oliva VL, Leclerc G. Renal artery aneurysm: treatment with percutaneous placement of a stent-graft. *Radiology* 1995;195:181.
124. Vinuela F, Murayama Y, Tateshima S. Embolization of arteriovenous malformations with Onyx: clinicopathological experience in 23 patients. *Neurosurgery* 2001;48:984.
125. Smith B, Holcomb GW, Richie R. Renal artery dissection. *Ann Surg* 1984;200:134.
126. Gewertz BL, Stanley FC, Fry WJ. Renal artery dissection. *Arch Surg* 1977;122:409
127. Alamir A, Middendorf DF, Baker P, et al. Renal artery dissection causing renal infarction in otherwise healthy men. *Am J Kidney Dis* 1997;30:851.
128. Sicard GA, Reilly JM, Picus DD. Alterations in renal revascularization. *Curr Probl Surg* 1995;32:569.
129. Edwards BS, Stanson AW, Holley KE. Isolated renal artery dissection: presentation, evaluation, management and pathology. *Mayo Clin Proc* 1982;57:564.
130. Slavis S, Hodge EE, Novic AC, et al. Surgical treatment for isolated dissection of the renal artery. *J Urol* 1990;144:233.
131. Esayag-Tendler B, Yamase H, Ramsey G, et al. Accelerated hypertension with encephalopathy due to an isolated dissection of a renal artery branch vessel. *Am J Kidney Dis* 1994;23:869.
132. Reilly LM, Cummingham CG, Maggisano R, et al. The role of arterial reconstruction in spontaneous renal artery dissection. *J Vasc Surg* 1991;14:468.
133. Eliot RS, Kanjuh VI, Edwards JE. Atheromatous embolism. *Circulation* 1964;30:611.
134. Handler FP. Clinical and pathologic significance of atheromatous embolization with emphasis on the aetiology of renal hypertension. *Am J Med* 1956;20:366.
135. Fukimoto Y, Tsutsui H, Tsduchihashi M, et al. The incidence of risk factors of cholesterol embolization syndrome, a complication of cardiac catheterization: a prospective study. *J Am Coll Cardiol* 2003;42:211.
136. Chomette G, Auriol M, Trambaloc P, et al. Cholesterol emboli: anatomical locations and clinical manifestations. *Ann Med Interne (Paris)* 1980;131:17.
137. Vidt DG. Cholesterol emboli: a common cause of renal failure. *Ann Rev Med* 1997;48:375.
138. Fine MJ, Kapoor W, Falanga V. Cholesterol crystal embolization: a review of 221 cases in the English literature. *Angiology* 1987;38:769.
139. Kashgarian M. Acute tubular necrosis and ischemic renal injury. In: Jennette JC, Olson JL, Schwartz MM, et al., eds. *Heptinstall's Pathology of the Kidney*. 5th ed. New York: Lippincott Williams & Wilkins; 1998:884.
140. Gore I, Collins DP. Spontaneous atheromatous embolization: review of the literature and report of 16 additional cases. *Am J Clin Pathol* 1960;33:416.
141. Otken LB Jr. Experimental production of atheromatous embolization. *Arth Pathol* 1959;68:685.

142. Snyder HE, Shapiro JL. Correlative study of atheromatous embolism in human beings and experimental animals. *Surgery* 1961;49:195.
143. Flory CM. Arterial occlusions produced by emboli from eroded aortic atheromatous plaques. *Am J Pathol* 1945;21:549.
144. Sayre GP, Campbell DC. Multiple peripheral emboli in atherosclerosis of the aorta. *Arch Intern Med* 1959;103:799.
145. Greenberg A, Bastacky SI, Iqbal A. Focal segmental glomerulosclerosis associated with nephrotic syndrome in cholesterol atheroembolism: clinicopathological correlations. *Am J Kidney Dis* 1997;29:334.
146. Aviles B, Ubeda I, Blanco J, et al. Pauci-immune extracapillary glomerulonephritis and atheromatous embolization. *Am J Kidney Dis* 2002;40:847.
147. Kaplan-Pavlovcic S, Vizjak A, Vene N, et al. Antineutrophil cytoplasmic autoantibodies in atheroembolic disease. *Nephrol Dial Transplant* 1998;13:985.
148. Maeshima E, Yamada Y, Mune M, et al. A case of cholesterol embolism with ANCA treated with corticosteroid and cyclophosphamide. *Ann Rheum Dis* 2001;60:726.
149. Thadhani RI, Camargo CA, Xavier RJ, et al. Atheroembolic renal failure after invasive procedures. *Medicine* 1995;74:350.
150. Saklayen MG. Atheroembolic renal disease: preferential occurrence in whites only. *Am J Nephrol* 1989;9:87.
151. Hara S, Asada Y, Fujimoto S, et al. Atheroembolic renal disease: clinical findings of 11 cases. *J Atheroscler Thromb* 2002;9:288.
152. Scolari F, Ravani P, Pola A, et al. Predictors of renal and patient outcomes in atheroembolic renal disease: a prospective study. *J Am Soc Nephrol* 2003;14:1584.
153. Belenfant X, Meyrier A, Jacjuot C. Supportive treatment improves survival in multivisceral cholesterol crystal embolism. *Am J Kidney Dis* 1999;33:840.
154. Mashiah A, Pasik S, Hurwitz N. Massive atheromatous emboli to both kidneys: a fatal complication following aortic surgery. *J Cardiovasc Surg* 1988;29:60.
155. Dahlberg PJ, Frecentese DR, Cogbill TH. Cholesterol embolism: experience with 22 histologically proven cases. *Surgery* 1989;105:737.
156. Hertzer NR. Peripheral atheromatous embolization following blunt trauma. *Surgery* 1977;82:244.
157. Gupta BK, Spinowitz BS, Charytan C, et al. Cholesterol crystal embolization: associated renal failure after therapy with recombinant tissue-type plasminogen activator. *Am J Kidney Dis* 1993;21:659.
158. Rudnigk MR, Berns JS, Cohen RM, et al. Nephrotoxic risks of renal angiography: contrast media-associated nephrotoxicity and atheroembolism—a critical review. *Am J Kidney Dis* 1994;24:713.
159. Wong FK, Chan SK, Ing TS, et al. Acute renal failure after streptokinase therapy in a patient with acute myocardial infarction. *Am J Kidney Dis* 1995;26:508.
160. Larry JA, Falkenhain ME, Mazzafer EL. Acute renal failure in an elderly man taking warfarin. *Hosp Pract* 1996;52:119.
161. Schwartz MW, McDonald G. Cholesterol embolization syndrome. Occurrence after intravenous streptokinase therapy for myocardial infarction. *JAMA* 1987;258:1934.
162. Queen M, Blem HJ, Moe GW. Development of cholesterol embolization after intravenous streptokinase for acute myocardial infarction. *Am J Cardiol* 1990;65:1042.
163. Hyman B, Landas S, Ashman R, et al. Warfarin-related purple toes syndrome and cholesterol micro-embolization. *Am J Med* 1987;82:1233.
164. Tilley WS, Harston WE, Siami G. Renal failure due to cholesterol emboli following PTCA. *Am Heart J* 1985;110:1301.
165. Scolari F, Bracchi M, Valzorio B, et al. Cholesterol atheromatous embolism: an increasingly recognized cause of acute renal failure. *Nephrol Dial Transplant* 1996;11:1607.
166. Frock J, Bierman M, Hammeke M, et al. Atheroembolic renal disease: experience with 22 patients. *Neb Med J* 1994;79:317.
167. Falanga V, Fine MJ, Kapoor WN. The cutaneous manifestations of cholesterol crystal embolization. *Arch Dermatol* 1986;122:1194.
168. Quintart C, Treille S, Lefebvre P, et al. Penile necrosis following cholesterol embolism. *Br J Urol* 1997;80:347.
169. Aujla ND, Greenberg A, Banner BF, et al. Atheroembolic involvement of renal allografts. *Am J Kidney Dis* 1989;13:329.
170. Singh I, Killen PD, Leichtman AB. Cholesterol emboli presenting as acute allograft dysfunction after renal transplantation. *J Am Soc Nephrol* 1995;6:165.
171. Jiminez-Heffernan JA, Martinez-Garcia M, Burgos E. Small bowel perforation due to cholesterol atheromatous embolism. *Dig Dis Sci* 1995;40:481.
172. Mollenaar W, Lamers CB. Cholesterol crystal embolization and the digestive system. *Scand J Gastroenterol* 1991;188:69.
173. Socindki MA, Frankel JP, Morow PL, et al. Painless diarrhea secondary to intestinal ischemia. Diagnosis of atheromatous emboli by jejunal biopsy. *Dig Dis Sci* 1984;51:674.
174. Probstein JG, Joshi RA, Blumenthan HT. Atheromatous embolism: an etiology of acute pancreatitis. *Arch Surg* 1957;75:566.
175. David MJ, Klintworth GK, Friedbert SG, et al. Fatal atheromatous cerebral embolism associated with bright plaques in retinal arterioles: report of a case. *Neurology* 1963;13:708.
176. Hollenhorst RW. Significance of bright plaques in the retinal arterioles. *Trans Am Ophthalmol Soc* 1961;59:252.

177. Sabatine MS, Oelberg DA, Mark EJ, et al. Pulmonary cholesterol crystal embolization. *Chest* 1997;112:1687.
178. Vacher CH, Pache X, Dussol B, et al. Pulmonary renal syndrome responding to corticosteroids: consider cholesterol embolization. *Nephrol Dial Transplant* 1997;12:1977.
179. Stanton RC. Case records of the Massachusetts General Hospital. *N Engl J Med* 1996;334:973.
180. Kasinath BS, Lewis EJ. Eosinophils as a clue to the diagnosis of atheroembolic renal disease. *Arch Intern Med* 1987;147:1384.
181. Kasinath BS, Corwin HL, Bidani AK, et al. Eosinophilia in the diagnosis of atheroembolic renal disease. *Am J Med* 1987;7:173.
182. Levine J, Rennke HG, Idelson BA. Profound persistent eosinophilia in a patient with spontaneous renal atheroembolic disease. *Am J Nephrol* 1992;12:377.
183. Cosio F, Zager R, Sharma H. Atheroembolic renal disease causes hypocomplementemia. *Lancet* 1985;2:118.
184. Williams HH, Wall BM, Cooke CR. Reversible nephrotic range proteinuria and renal failure in atheroembolic renal disease. *Am J Med Sci* 1990;299:58.
185. Haqqie SS, Urizar RE, Singh J. Nephrotic-range proteinuria in renal atheroembolic disease: Report of four cases. *Am J Kidney Dis* 1996;28:493.
186. Wilson DM, Salazer TL, Farkooh ME. Eosinophiluria in atheroembolic renal disease. *Am J Med* 1991;91:186.
187. McGowan JA, Greenberg A. Cholesterol atheroembolic renal disease. *Am J Nephrol* 1986;6:135.
188. Knechtges TC, Defever VA. Cholesterol emboli in transurethral curettings: report of 4 cases. *J Urol* 1975;114:102.
189. Scoble JE, O'Donnell PJ. Renal atheroembolic disease: the Cinderella of nephrology? *Nephrol Dial Transplant* 1996;11:1516.
190. Scoble JE. Is Nihilism in the treatment of atheroembolic disease at an end? *Am J Kidney Dis* 1999;33:975.
191. Belenfant X, Meyrier A, Jacquot C. Supportive treatment improves survival in multivisceral cholesterol embolism. *Am J Kidney Dis* 1999;33:840.
192. Bruns FJ, Segel DP, Adler S. Control of cholesterol embolization by discontinuation of anticoagulant therapy. *Am J Med* 1978;275:105.
193. Rosansky SJ. Multiple cholesterol emboli syndrome. *South Med J* 1982;75:677.
194. Drost H, Buis B, Haan D. Cholesterol embolism as a complication of left heart catheterization: report of seven cases. *Br Heart J* 1984;52:339.
195. Smyth JS, Scoble JE. Atheroembolism. Current treatment options. *Cardiovasc Med* 2002;4:255.
196. Siemons L, Van Den Heuvel P, Parizel G, et al. Peritoneal dialysis in acute renal failure due to cholesterol embolization: two cases of recovery of renal function and extended survival. *Clin Nephrol* 1987;28:205.
197. Keen RR, McCarthy WJ, Shireman PK, et al. Surgical management of atheroembolization. *J Vasc Surg* 1995;21:773.
198. Baumann DS, McGraw D, Rubin BG, et al. An institutional experience with arterial atheroembolism. *Ann Vasc Surg* 1994;8:258.
199. Ballesteros AL, Bromsoms J, Valles M, et al. Vasculitis look-alikes: variants of renal atheroembolic disease. *Nephrol Dial Transplant* 1999;14:430.
200. Hunter J. Guide to the Hunterian Collection, Part 1: pathological Series in the Hunterian Museum. Specimen p. 389. A Case of Renal Vein Thrombosis (Lady Beauchamp). Edinburgh: Livingstone, 1966:267.
201. Rayer PR. O Traite des Maladies des Reins et des Alterations de la Secretion urinaire, Vol 2. Paris: JB Bailiere, 1840:590.
202. Abeshouse BS. Thrombosis and thrombophlebitis of the renal veins. *Urol Cutaneous Rev* 1945;49:661.
203. Harrison CV, Milne MD, Steiner RE. Clinical aspects of renal vein thrombosis. *Q J Med* 1956;25:285.
204. McCarthy LJ, Titus JL, Daugherty GW. Bilateral renal vein thrombosis and the nephrotic syndrome in adults. *Ann Intern Med* 1963;58:837.
205. Llach F, Koffler A, Massry SG. Renal vein thrombosis and the nephrotic syndrome. *Nephron* 1977;19:65.
206. Cornog JL, et al. Immunofluorescent and ultrastructural study of the renal lesions observed in human renal view thrombosis and the nephrotic syndrome. *Lab Invest* 1968;18:689.
207. Fisher ER, Sharkey D, Pardo V, et al. Experimental renal constriction. Its relation to renal lesions observed in human renal vein thrombosis and the nephrotic syndrome. *Lab Invest* 1968;18:689.
208. Deodhar KP, Bhalerao RA, Kelkar MD, et al. Inferior vena cava obstruction. *J Postgrad Med* 1969;25:64.
209. Jackson BT, Thomas ML. Post-thrombotic inferior vena cava obstruction: A review of 24 patients. *Br Med J* 1970;1:18.
210. Monteon F, et al. Nephrotic syndrome with renal vein thrombosis treated with thrombectomy and anticoagulants (abstract). 8th International Congress Nephrology, Athens; 1981:82.
211. Noel LH, Zanetti M, Droz D, et al. Long-term prognosis of idiopathic membranous glomerulonephritis: study of 116 untreated patients. *Am J Med* 1979;66:82.
212. Pohl MA, MacLaurin JP, Alfidi RJ. Renal vein thrombosis and the nephrotic syndrome (abstract). 10th Annual Meeting of the American Society of Nephrologists, Washington, DC; 1977:20A.
213. Velazquez-Forero F, Garcia Prugue N, Ruiz-Morales N. Idiopathic nephrotic syndrome of the adult with asymptomatic thrombosis of the renal vein. *Am J Nephrol* 1988;8:457.
214. Vosnides GR, et al. Renal vein thrombosis in patients with nephrotic syndrome (abstract). IX International Congress of Nephrol. Los Angeles: June, 1984:138A.
215. Wagoner RD, et al. Renal vein thrombosis in idiopathic membranes, glomerulopathy, and the nephrotic syndrome: Incidence and significance. *Kidney Int* 1983;23:368.
216. Llach F, Papper S, Massry SG. The clinical spectrum of renal vein thrombosis: acute and chronic. *Am J Med* 1980;69:819.
217. Llach R. Nephrotic syndrome: hypercoagulability, renal vein thrombosis, and other thromboembolic complications. In: Brenner B, Stein J, eds. *Contemporary Issues in Nephrology*. vol. 9. New York: Churchill-Livingston; 1982:121.
218. Gatewood OM, et al. Renal vein thrombosis in patients with nephrotic syndrome: CT diagnosis. *Radiology* 1986;159:117.
219. Hruby MA, Honig GR, Shapiro E. Immunoquantitation of Hageman factor in the urine and plasma of children with nephrotic syndrome. *J Lab Clin Med* 1980;96:501.
220. Llach F, Koffler A, Finck E, et al. On the incidence of renal vein thrombosis in the nephrotic syndrome. *Arch Intern Med* 1977;137:33.
221. Llach F, Arieff AI, Massry SG. Renal vein thrombosis and nephrotic syndrome: a prospective study of 36 adult patients. *Ann Intern Med* 1975;83:8.
222. Trew P, Biava CG, Jacobs RP, et al. Renal vein thrombosis in membranous glomerulopathy: incidence and association. *Medicine* 1978;57:69.
223. Green D, Arruda J, Honig G, et al. Urinary loss of clotting factor due to hereditary membranous nephropathy. *Am J Clin Pathol* 1976;65:376.
224. Berger J, Yneva H. Hageman factor deposition in membranous nephropathy. *Transplant Proc* 1982;3:472.
225. Handley DA, Lawrence JR. Factor IX deficiency in the nephrotic syndrome. *Lancet* 1967;1:1079.
226. Honig GR, Lindley A. Deficiency of Hageman factor (factor XII) in patients with nephrotic syndrome. *J Pediatr* 1971;78:633.
227. Lange LG III, Carvalho A, Baqdasarian A, et al. Activation of Hageman factor in the nephrotic syndrome. *Am J Med* 1974;56:565.
228. Natelson EA, Lynch EC, Hettig RA, et al. Acquired factor IX deficiency in the nephrotic syndrome. *Ann Intern Med* 1970;73:373.
229. Saito K, et al. Urinary excretion of Hageman factor (factor XII) and presence of non-functional Hageman factor in the nephrotic syndrome. *Am J Med* 1981;70:53.
230. van Royen EA, de Boer JE, Wilmink JM, et al. Acquired factor XII deficiency in a patient with nephrotic syndrome. *Acta Med Scand* 1979;205:535.
231. Kanfer A, Kleinknecht D, Broyer M, et al. Coagulation studies in 45 cases of nephrotic syndrome without uremia. *Thromb Diathes Haemorrh* 1970;24:562.
232. Kendall AG, Lohmann RE, Dossetor JB. Nephrotic syndrome: a hypercoagulable state. *Arch Intern Med* 1971;127:1021.
233. Thompson C, et al. Changes in blood coagulation and fibrinolysis in the nephrotic syndrome. *Q J Med* 1974;43:399.
234. Earley LE, et al. Nephrotic syndrome. *Calif Med* 1971;115:12.
235. Llach F. Renal vein thrombosis and the nephrotic syndrome. In: Llach, F, ed. *Renal Vein Thrombosis*. Mount Kisco, NY: Futura; 1983:155.
236. Andrassy K, Ritz E, Bommer J. Hypercoagulability in the nephrotic syndrome. *Klin Wochenschr* 1980;58:1029.
237. Takeda Y, Chen A. Fibrinogen metabolism and distribution in patients with the nephrotic syndrome. *J Lab Clin Med* 1967;70:678.
238. Clarkson A, McDonald MK, Petrie JJ, et al. Serum and urinary fibrinogen/fibrin degradation products in glomerulonephritis. *Br Med J* 1971;3:447.
239. Cade R, Spooner G, Juncos L, et al. Chronic renal vein thrombosis. *Am J Med* 1977;63:387.
240. Hall C, Pejhan N, Terry JM, et al. Urinary fibrin/fibrinogen degradation products in nephrotic syndrome. *Br Med J* 1975;1:419.
241. Wu KK, Hoak JC. Urinary plasminogen and chronic glomerulonephritis. *Am J Clin Pathol* 1973;60:915.
242. Astedt B, Issacson S, Milsson IM. Thrombosis and oral contraceptives: possible predisposition. *Br Med J* 1973;4:631.
243. Bonnar J, McNichol GP, Douglas AS. Fibrinolytic enzyme system and pregnancy. *Br Med J* 1969;3:387.
244. Ygge J. Changes in blood coagulation and fibrinolysis during the postoperative period. *Am J Surg* 1970;119:225.
245. Rennie J, Ogston D. Fibrinolytic activity in malignant disease. *J Clin Pathol* 1975;28:872.
246. Almer LO, Janzon L. Low vascular fibrinolytic activity in obesity. *Thromb Res* 1975;6:171.
247. Edward N, Young DP, Macleod M. Fibrinolytic activity in plasma and urine in chronic renal disease. *J Clin Pathol* 1961;17:365.
248. Hedner U, Nilsson IM. Antithrombin III in a clinical material. *Thromb Res* 1973;3:631.
249. Scheinman JI, Stiehm ER. Fibrinolytic studies on the nephrotic syndrome. *Pediatr Res* 1971;5:206.
250. Lau SO, Tkachuck JY, Haseqawa DK, et al. Plasminogen and antithrombin III deficiencies in the childhood nephrotic syndrome associated with plasminogenuria and antithrombinuria. *J Pediatr* 1980;96:390.
251. Llach F. The hypercoagulability and thrombotic complications of nephrotic syndrome. *Kidney Int* 1985;28:429.
252. Du XH, et al. Nephrotic syndrome with renal vein thrombosis: pathogenetic

importance of a plasmin inhibitor (abstract). IXth International Congress on Nephrology. Los Angeles: June, 1984:84A.

253. Egebert O. Inherited antithrombin deficiency causing thrombophilia. *Thromb Haemostas* 1974;13:516.

254. Godal HC, Rygh M, Laake K. Progressive inactivation of purified factor VIII by heparin and antithrombin III. *Thromb Res* 1974;5:773.

255. Marciniak E, Farley CH, Desimone PA. Familial thrombosis due to antithrombin III deficiency. *Blood* 1974;43:219.

256. Rosenberg JS, McKeena P, Rosenberg RD. The inhibition of human factor IXa by human antithrombin heparin cofactor. *J Biol Chem* 1975;250:8883.

257. Rosenberg RD. Actions and interactions of antithrombin and heparin. *N Engl J Med* 1975;292:146.

258. Yin ET, Wessler S, Stroll PJ. Identity of plasma-activated factor X inhibitor with antithrombin III and heparin cofactor. *J Biol Chem* 1971;246:3712.

259. Kauffman RH, Veltkamp JJ, Van Tilrurgh NH, et al. Acquired antithrombin III deficiency and thrombosis in the nephrotic syndrome. *Am J Med* 1978;65:607.

260. Kauffman RH, De Graeff J, Brutel G, et al. Unilateral renal vein thrombosis and nephrotic syndrome. *Am J Med* 1976;60:1048.

261. Thaler E, Blazar E, Kopsa H, et al. Acquired antithrombin III deficiency in patients with glomerular proteinuria. *Hemostasis* 1978;7:257.

262. Ellis D. Recurrent renal vein thrombosis and renal failure associated with antithrombin-III deficiency. *Pediatr Nephrol* 1992;6:131.

263. Panicucci R, Sagripanti P, Vispi M, et al. Comprehensive study of haemostasis in nephrotic syndrome. *Nephron* 1983;33:9.

264. Vaziri ND, Paule P, Toohey J, et al. Acquired deficiency and urinary excretion of antithrombin III in nephrotic syndrome. *Arch Intern Med* 1984;144:1802.

265. Stenflo J. A new vitamin K-dependent protein: purification from bovine plasma and preliminary characterization. *J Biol Chem* 1976;251:355.

266. Kisiel W, Canfield W, Ericsson L, et al. Anticoagulation properties of bovine plasma protein C following activation by thrombin. *Biochemistry* 1977;16:5824.

267. Griffin JH, et al. Deficiency of protein C in congenital thrombotic disease. *J Clin Invest* 1981;68:1370.

268. Walker FJ, Fay PJ. Regulation of blood coagulation by the protein C system. *FASEB J* 1992;6(8):2561.

269. Walker FJ. Regulation of activated protein C by a new protein. *J Biol Chem* 1980;255:5521.

270. Wardle EN, Memom IS, Ratogi SP. Study of proteins and fibrinolysis in patients with glomerulonephritis. *Br Med J* 1970;2:260.

271. Comp P, Esmon CT. Recurrent venous thromboembolism in patients with a partial deficiency of protein S. *N Engl J Med* 1984;311:1525.

272. Cosio FG. Plasma concentrations of the natural anticoagulants protein C and protein S in patients with proteinuria. *J Lab Clin Med* 1985;106:218.

273. Sorenson PJ, Knudsen F, Nielsen AH, et al. Protein C activity in renal disease. *Thromb Res* 1985;38:243.

274. Vigano-D'Angelo S, Kaufman C, et al. Protein S deficiency occurs in the nephrotic syndrome. *Am Int Med* 1987;107:42.

275. Bang N. Enhanced platelet function in glomerular renal disease. *J Lab Clin Med* 1973;81:651.

276. Remuzzi G, Mecca G, Marchest D, et al. Platelet hyperaggregability and the nephrotic syndrome. *Thromb Res* 1979;16:345.

277. Alder AJ, Lundin AP, Feinroth AP, et al. B-thromboglobulin levels in the nephrotic syndrome. *Am J Med* 1980;69:551.

278. Andrassy K, Depperman D, Walter E, et al. Is beta thromboglobulin a useful indicator of thrombosis in nephrotic syndrome? *Thromb Haemost* 1979;42:486.

279. Kuhlmann U, Stevens J, Rhyner K, et al. Platelet aggregation and B-thromboglobulin levels in nephrotic patients with and without thrombosis. *Clin Nephrol* 1981;15:229.

280. Cheng HF, Liu YG, Pan JS, et al. A prospective study of renal vein thrombosis (abstract). XIth International Congress on Nephrology. Tokyo, Japan: 1990:6A.

281. Ooi BS, Ooi YM, Pollak VE. Circulating immune complexes in renal vein thrombosis. 11th Annual Meeting of the American Society of Nephrology. New Orleans: 1978:24A.

282. Lohman RC, Kendall AG, Dosettor JB, et al. The fibrinolytic system in the nephrotic syndrome. *Clin Res* 1969;17:333.

283. Harms K, Speer CP. Thrombosis: an underestimated complication of central catheters. Suldarain vein and renal vein thrombosis after Silastic catheters. *Monatsschr Kinderheilkd* 1993;141:21.

284. Mukherjee AP, Tog BH, Chan GL. Vascular complications in nephrotic syndrome: relationship to steroid therapy and accelerated thromboplastin generation. *Br Med J* 1970;4:273.

285. Luetscher JA, Deming QB. Treatment of nephrotics with cortisone. *J Clin Invest* 1950;29:1576.

286. Cosgriff SW, Diefenbach AF, Vogt W Jr. Hypercoagulability of the blood associated with ACTH and cortisone therapy. *Am J Med* 1950;9:752.

287. Rosenmann E, Pollak VE, Pirani CL. Renal vein thrombosis in the adult: a clinical and pathological study based on renal biopsies. *Medicine* 1968;47:269.

288. Slick GL, Schnetzler DE, Koloyanides GJ. Hypertension, renal vein thrombosis and renal failure occurring in a patient on an oral contraceptive agent. *Clin Nephrol* 1975;3:70.

289. Arneil GC. Renal venous thrombosis. *Clin Nephrol* 1973;1:119.

290. Hay CR, McEvoy P. Main graft vessels thromboses due to conventional dose OKT3 in renal transplantation. *Lancet* 1992;339:1612.

291. Hollenbeck M. Doppler sonography and renal graft vessel thromboses after OKT3 treatment. *Lancet* 1992;340:619.

292. Richardson AJ, Martin J. Spontaneous rupture of renal allografts: the importance of renal vein thrombosis in the cyclosporin era. *Br J Surg* 1990;77:558.

293. Brown Z. Increased factor VIII as an index of vascular injury in cyclosporin nephrotoxicity. *Transplantation* 1986;42:150.

294. Brown Z, Neild GH. Cyclosporin inhibits prostaglandin production by cultured human endothelial cells. *Transplant Proc* 1987;19:1170.

295. Koehler PR, Bowles WT, McAlister WH. Renal arteriography in experimental renal vein occlusion. *Radiology* 1966;86:851.

296. Kowal J, Figur A, Hitzig WM. Renal vein thrombosis and the nephrotic syndrome with complete remission. *J Mt Sinai Hosp* 1963;30:47.

297. Scanlon GT. Radiographic changes in renal vein thrombosis. *Radiology* 1963;80:208.

298. MacLennan AC, Baxter BM, Harden P, et al. Renal transplant vein occlusions: an early diagnostic sign? *Clin Radiol* 1995;50:251.

299. Richet G, Meyrier A, eds. *Liposclerose retroperitoneal. Thrombose des veines renales. Deux syndromes retroperitoneaux.* Paris: Masson; 1970.

300. Lavelle M. The prognosis of renal vein thrombosis: a reevaluation of 27 cases. *Nephrol Dial Transplant* 1988;3:247.

301. Briefel GR, Manis T, Gordon DH, et al. Recurrent renal vein thrombosis consequent to membranous nephropathy. *Clin Nephrol* 1978;10:32.

302. Vogelsanc RL, Brown M. Acute renal vein thrombosis: successful treatment with intraarterial urokinase. *Radiology* 1988;169:681.

303. Kennedy JS. Simultaneous renal arterial and venous thrombosis associated with idiopathic nephrotic syndrome: treatment with intra-arterial urokinase. *Am J Med* 1991;90:124.

304. Monte XL, Groo J. Renal arterial thrombosis occurring in an adult with idiopathic nephrotic syndrome: Results of local treatment with streptokinase. *Clin Nephrol* 1979;12:90.

305. Chiu AS, Ladsberg DN. Successful treatment of acute renal vein thrombosis with selective streptokinase infusion. *Transplant Proc* 1991;23:2297.

306. Schwieger J, Reiss R, Cohen JL, et al. Acute renal allograft dysfunction in the setting of deep venous thrombosis: a case of successful urokinase thrombolysis and a review of the literature. *Am J Kidney Dis* 1993;22:345.

307. Gootman M, Groo J, Mensch A. Pulmonary artery thrombosis. *Pediatrics* 1964;34:861.

308. Coon WW, Willis PW. Thrombosis of axillary and subclavian vein. *Arch Surg* 1967;94:622.

309. Berlyne GM, Mallick NP. Ischemic heart as a complication of nephrotic syndrome. *Lancet* 1969;2:392.

310. Andrassy K, Ritz R. Biochemie und klinische bedeutung von urokinase. *Dtsch Med Wochenschr* 1978;24:1015.

CHAPTER 71 ■ THE LONG-TERM OUTCOME OF GLOMERULAR DISEASES

CHIRAG R. PARIKH, ERIC GIBNEY, AND JOSHUA M. THURMAN

At first sight, the task of describing the outcome of a particular disease seems to be a simple one; in fact, nothing could be further from the truth. First, we have the problem of definition, that is, what the "disease" under consideration may be. Without getting into a deep philosophical discussion of what the word *disease* signifies, at a practical level, a number of difficulties arise. Next, the very idea of a disease in its own right is an abstraction: As many clinicians emphasize, there are no "diseases"—only diseased patients—so in essence, we are describing the behavior and fate of groups of patients. But how are they to be defined for inclusion in a study?

Immediately new problems arise because there are no hard boundaries for the disease we are dealing with in the glomerulus. Various clinical presentations can be defined but in real life they have fluid boundaries; there are histologic appearances both on optical and immunofluorescence microscopy, between which there is no one-to-one correspondence; and finally, there are proved or (more usually) probable precipitating events, organisms, or multisystem diseases that affect other organs.

To cite an example, when we consider the outcome of acute glomerulonephritis, we meet accounts in the literature of patients with the clinical presentation of acute glomerulonephritis, many or all of whom did not have a renal biopsy; we have other accounts of patients with a similar presentation, but in whom a streptococcal etiology was established by cultures or antibody titers, with or without biopsies; and we have accounts of patients with streptococcal glomerulonephritis, some of whom had mesangioproliferative glomerulonephritis (MPGN) as shown by biopsy, or severe crescents.

Inevitably, there will be discrepancies in the conclusions drawn about the outcomes from these similar, but not identical, groups. A further difficulty arises because almost certainly some of the histologic appearances of the diseased glomerulus—for example, membranous nephropathy—are no more single diseases than the broad clinical features they present. We must think of these as appearances—patterns of glomerular injury—rather than diseases.

There may be several different pathogenic routes into a single histologic appearance, and each of these may have a different outcome. If we cannot distinguish or are ignorant of these subgroups, then a different mix of the subgroups inevitably leads to different descriptions of outcome. The second major problem is more obvious but equally neglected when we look at follow-up data from diverse sources: This is the question of patient selection (Fig. 71-1). The only unassailable data are those that derive from a population survey in which techniques that will select all the patients with a particular condition are applied, and all those patients are followed without fallout for a given period. Such studies do not exist in the study of glomerular diseases. Many of the conditions we discuss in this chapter such as IgA-associated glomerulopathy, minimal change disease, and membranous nephropathy exist in the population without ever being detected. The more diligently the population is examined, and the more frequently the urine is tested,

the more such "patients" (who are, in fact, symptomless individuals) will be detected. The second stage of selection is when these patients are discovered; just how much are they studied or referred for investigation? Many patients with proteinuria or hematuria discovered on routine examination for insurance purposes may not be followed.

Specialist centers also will attract (because of their skills in management) patients who present with considerable problems, and it is often from such centers that descriptions of outcomes are published. It is usual for these first studies to present an overly pessimistic outlook for the prognosis of disease, and subsequent recognition of milder, more indolent, forms may restore the balance, with an apparent decrease in gravity in the view of the condition. Thus, the best outlook probably approximates more closely the true description of outcome for the general worldwide population.

Even if a patient is referred, a crucial question is whether to perform a renal biopsy. Because the criteria for many of the conditions discussed in this chapter depend on the availability of renal biopsy data, this point is crucial. It is often impossible to know exactly what the criteria for renal biopsy in a health care facility at a particular time may have been, because the authors do not tell us. Usually most adult patients with a nephrotic syndrome, or profuse proteinuria, undergo renal biopsy. The policy for biopsy in patients having isolated minor (0.5 to 1.5 g per 24 hours) proteinuria, isolated hematuria, or hematuria with minor proteinuria is particularly variable, among health care facilities and in different countries, sometimes depending on non-medical factors such as the local availability of skills and funding structures for medical investigations. The presence or absence of routine screening of populations, for example, military inductees, will depend on other factors, such as whether military service is obligatory.

Even when a population of patients, however gathered, is available for study, fallout begins as patients are lost to follow-up. Diligent work will often lead, even 10 to 40 years later, to more than 90% of "lost" patients being recovered, but very often the data available may be limited to those who are entirely healthy or who are dead. Built into any system of follow-up, however, is the inevitable fact that some patients enter the study early and some later, so the length of follow-up may vary from 1 to 2 years or to several decades. How do we best handle these incomplete data in order to extract the best information?

First, it is clear that in the end all diseases result in one of two states: Either the patient is dead or cured (Fig. 71-2). The proportion of patients who follow each of these two courses can vary from 1:99 to 99:1. Equally, the time required for the progression of this disease may vary; in practice, most glomerular diseases have run their course within 15 to 20 years of apparent onset, with the possible exception of IgA-associated nephropathies, which appear to have a slower evolution. This statement brings up yet another difficulty: When did the disease really start? What we have on record is the earliest point at which it reached clinical attention or, in retrospect, when the

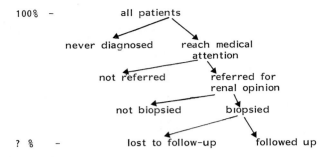

FIGURE 71-1. The various levels of patient selection that confuse descriptions of diseases and their outcome.

patient had symptoms (e.g., frothy urine or edema). In the case of symptomless hematuria and proteinuria, this point may be years or even decades from the true onset.

The next question is to describe outcome. A technique that is much used in this area and that appears throughout this chapter is that of the *actuarial life table,* usually presented in graphic form as a survival curve. It is worth discussing here the strengths and limitations of this technique, which is described in detail by Peto et al. (1). The table was developed by actuaries to provide estimates of survival of populations, for example, at different ages, mainly for insurance purposes. It was first applied in medicine to studies of cancer data and was used in renal disease in the mid-1960s to analyze transplant survival of kidney graft. Finally, in the early 1970s it was introduced to the study of glomerular and other chronic diseases, and it has become popular as its advantages have been recognized.

Life tables were originally designed to be applied to large populations—thousands or tens of thousands—whereas in medical practice, they are rarely used for the analysis of more than a few hundred persons, especially for relatively rare diseases, such as those affecting the glomeruli; many series involve less than 100 individuals. The importance of this is that as with any statistical estimate, the potential error of the estimate achieved will increase sharply when small numbers are under

consideration. In general terms, all data on glomerular diseases deal only with small (or very small) numbers of patients.

The life table technique produces an estimate often referred to as the Kaplan-Meier (2) estimate of what the behavior of the population at risk might be if all patients had been followed for the full period under analysis. As already noted, this is almost never the case, except for very short follow-up periods. The lines in a figure may be drawn in a bold fashion, but it is the possible error—usually expressed as the standard error for each point on the life table—that is crucial. For example, an estimated population survival of 60% at 10 years may have 95% confidence limits of 20% to 90%, so the estimate is almost useless for purposes of comparison; in fact, the only valid method of comparison between two life tables is to compare the whole curve with the contrasted one—that is, assuming that the two populations are comparable (1), which is almost never the case except in carefully randomized prospective controlled studies.

With all these reservations in mind, we can examine how a life table is constructed. There are several ways to do this in detail, and a number of computer programs are available. For any period under study, first the number of patients "at risk" of having the event in question is calculated. The event can be any event of interest—loss of proteinuria, absence of hypertension, entry into end-stage renal disease (ESRD), or death, for example. The number of patients at risk throughout the interval in question clearly is related to the number being followed at the start of the follow-up period but will be less than this latter number because some patients will be lost to follow-up during the interval.

The calculation of a standard error of any point on the curve is possible using the following formula:

$$\text{Cumulative survival rate} \sqrt{\frac{1 - \text{Cumulative survival rate}}{\text{Number at risk}}}$$

And two life table curves can be compared for the statistical difference between them by statistics discussed originally by Kaplan and Meier (2) and more recently by Peto et al. (1) and Breslow (3). In essence, this procedure is a χ^2 test, weighted by the distribution of the data in the life table.

Obviously it is possible, by drawing up a life table for terminal renal failure and another for loss of proteinuria, to generate a diagram of the type shown in Figure 71-2 for any given glomerular condition or group of patients. Programs are available to construct life tables on microprocessors from raw data of dates of entry and the date of event or most recent follow-up—whatever the reason for exiting from the follow-up may be. If one wishes purely to examine the rate of entry into uremia, rather than true survival, then death from unrelated causes can be treated as "lost to follow-up" for the purposes of analysis. This may seem bizarre, but a similar problem arises in the analysis of transplantation data when immunologic graft loss is being examined and a patient dies of another cause with a functioning graft.

This raises the difficult problem of deaths attributed to causes other than renal failure in any study. Clearly in the end, all the patients in the study will be dead, including those who are in remission. In addition, the numbers of those dying within a decade or two of causes other than uremia will increase sharply if the mean age of the population under study is older than 60 years. Ideally, any life table analysis should include the expected life table for the population at risk, assuming no renal diseases were present. In Western countries, at the age of 35 years, at least 95% of patients will survive 15 years; therefore, in the case of most glomerular diseases that affect predominantly a young population, the effect of neglecting expected mortality is trivial. However, only 85% of 60-year-olds will survive a decade, the average survival time being 18 years for women and 20 years for men; at 65 years old,

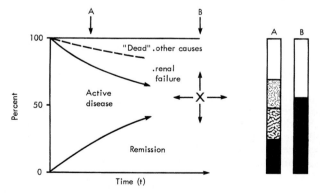

FIGURE 71-2. A generalized diagram to describe the outcome of a glomerular disease. Vertically, the proportion of patients in a given state is shown: dead (either incidentally or as a result of the glomerular disease), with continued proteinuria, or in remission. The time *(t)* at which the final state of all patients being in remission or dead will be reached will depend on the aggression of the disease; and the proportion dead or in remission, on its severity. If a cross-section of patients is studied at time A or B, a proportion of patients will still have active disease, with or without impairment of renal function, as represented in the bar graphs (**right**). Diagrams such as these can be used to summarize the outcome of glomerular diseases, the curves being calculated by the best estimate obtained from life table analysis of the necessarily incomplete data (see text).

the corresponding values are 12 and 16 years. Consequently, for some diseases, such as membranous nephropathy and vasculitis, some account of age of presentation must be taken.

It is not always clear what should be considered "other" causes of death and what role secondary hypertension may play, both as a direct cause of death and as a cause of accelerated fall-off in renal function. Similarly, vascular disease would be considered by some as a possible complication of a persisting nephrotic syndrome. How should deaths from complications of therapy be treated for statistical purposes? Clearly, they are the result of the disease, but this statistical treatment may not be appropriate to some observers.

Therefore, the technique of life tables allows us to make a description of the general average outcome of a glomerular disease or its appearances, but of course this is not what the patient wants to know. He or she wishes to know what his or her individual outcome will be, and from the data on population, the physician can make only the most general statements of risk. The possible evolution of the disease in individual patients can be made more precise by attempting to assess the predictive value of various individual characteristics. At a clinical level, such observations as the presence or absence of hematuria in a patient with proteinuria, the degree and persistence of proteinuria, and the presence or absence of hypertension or reduced renal function can be examined; and on histology, various glomerular and tubulointerstitial or vascular features can be assessed for their effect on prognosis. The crude way to do this is simply to examine the outcomes of patients with a certain feature and compare that with outcomes of patients without the same feature (univariate analysis), but this process ignores possible interactions, either purely statistical or causative, which may relate to certain features. This evaluation requires simultaneous multivariate analysis, for which a number of methods are available.

Perhaps the best technique for this type of analysis is the Cox method of proportional hazards (4). This technique has been applied surprisingly little to the study of glomerular disease (5–9), perhaps because the number of patients under study is so small that the technique may not be appropriate, but perhaps also because of ignorance of the technique. Analysis by the Cox method can be calculated only by the use of a computer program and is included in the widely available statistical software packages on the internet. A discussion on the use of the Cox model and related statistics in renal data can be found in the article by Beukhof et al. (5). It is often forgotten that when applying this type of technique, predictive variables are analyzed sequentially, so events that may be useful or convenient in the clinical sphere become nonsignificant statistically after the analysis shows they are secondarily dependent on some stronger variable. Therefore, in many analyses, only proteinuria and interstitial fibrosis emerge as independent determinants of outcome.

Obviously, the monitoring of proteinuria and indices of renal function, such as plasma creatinine and the glomerular filtration rate (GFR), followed sequentially, is among some of the most powerful tools available that allow prediction of disease course in individual patients. For example, it has become apparent that functional progression rarely, if ever, occurs in proteinuric renal disease if the excretion of protein falls to within normal limits even for a short while (10), although hypertensive damage is possible subsequently. Furthermore, the persistence of profuse proteinuria within or near the nephrotic range in patients with structurally disordered glomeruli (e.g., other than minimal change) is a clear indicator of a poorer prognosis in most patients with this phenomenon (Fig. 71-3), and in membranous nephropathy is a continuous variable—the greater the protein loss, the poorer the prognosis (see later discussion).

The behavior of the plasma creatinine concentration (P_{creat}) also has been the subject of much study. Mitch et al. reminded us 15 years ago (11) that GFR varies as $1/P_{creat}$ and several articles (11,12) have emphasized that the plot of $1/P_{creat}$ against time may be relatively linear, the slope being characteristic for each patient. The linearity of such plots has been greatly exaggerated, and the r value for correlation plots, even with the best fit, rarely if ever exceeds 0.70 (13).

Study of glomerular diseases confirms this point, and although membranous nephropathy shows relatively linear plots (14), study of data from the Medical Research Council (MRC) trial in the United Kingdom (15) showed that only 18 of 41 nephrotic membranous patients with a decline in renal function showed substantially linear fall-off in reciprocal creatinine plots. Similarly, Fellin et al. (16) found few patients with IgA nephropathy, whose decline in renal function could be described in a single slope of $1/P_{creat}$. MPGN often shows a markedly nonlinear pattern (17) with sudden falloffs in renal function that are not associated with hypertension, even after periods of relatively stable function lasting several years. In addition, the predictive value of the P_{creat} for the GFR has been overemphasized; changes occur with changes in diet and muscle mass, and, conversely, a constant plasma creatinine may conceal a fall-off in GFR. The use and misuse of reciprocal and other functions of P_{creat} have been reviewed by Walser (18), Hunsicker (19), and Levey (20).

One interesting observation (14,15) is that for the main groups of progressive, proteinuric glomerular diseases (membranous nephropathy, focal segmental glomerular sclerosis [FSGS], and MPGN), progressive disease usually reveals itself by a detectable fall-off in GFR and a rise in plasma creatinine concentration within only 3 or so years of onset. Together with the observations on the presence and persistence of proteinuria mentioned previously, this information allows a better individual prognosis to be given quite early in the course of the disease. However, this is not the case for IgA nephropathy, which generally evolves much more slowly.

In this chapter, for reasons of brevity, we deal mainly with recently published observations on the outcomes of glomerular disease, published in 1980 or later. For a more detailed consideration of the literature before 1980, the reader is referred to an earlier treatment of the subject (21). Given that an etiologic classification is still beyond our grasp, this chapter is organized in a conventional fashion around the usual histologic classification of glomerular disease (22), with the many limitations of this approach acknowledged herein.

THE OVERALL PROGNOSIS OF THE NEPHROTIC SYNDROME

Unlike symptomless patients with hematuria or proteinuria, patients who have the nephrotic syndrome are likely to be referred for medical attention and very likely to have a renal biopsy as part of the investigation of their condition. It is still common to perform a biopsy on all adult patients with onset of a nephrotic syndrome, and older data exist for unselected series of children with nephrotic syndrome who had a biopsy; however, it is now no longer common practice to perform a biopsy on all nephrotic children, especially those between the ages of 1 and 5 years.

The outcome of nephrotic syndrome generally depends on four sets of circumstances: complications of the nephrotic syndrome, the effects of proteinuria itself, the influence of underlying histopathology, and the response to treatment (23). Furthermore, there is expanding interest in identifying urinary biomarkers, which may predict progression of nephrotic syndrome. Some, including fractional excretion of immunoglobulin G (IgG), urinary N-acetyl-beta-glucosaminidase, urinary

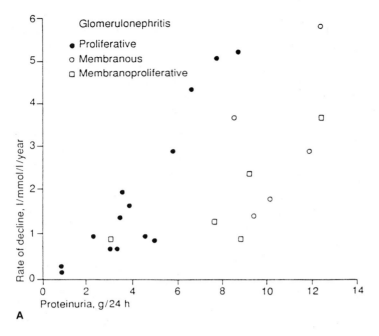

A

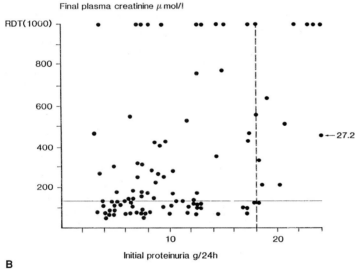

B

FIGURE 71-3. The important relationship between the outcome and the quantity of proteinuria is further examined by correlating plasma creatinine concentration during follow-up with the quantity of proteinuria at presentation. In various forms of glomerular diseases, the relationship between initial proteinuria and rate of change in the $1/P_{creat}$ holds. (From: Williams PS, Fass G, Bone JM. Renal pathology and proteinuria determine progression in untreated mild/moderate chronic renal failure. *Q J Med* 1988;67:343, with permission.)

beta-2 microglobulin, and urinary retinol-binding protein are promising as prognostic indicators (24–27).

Complications of the Nephrotic State

Now only few nephrotic children or adults die as a result of complications of the nephrotic state (28,29). In the study of Wass et al. (30), only one-third of adults with nephrotic syndrome remained nephrotic 4 years later. The remainder had either progressed to renal failure with diminution of proteinuria and disappearance of edema or had gone into remission either spontaneously or as a result of treatment. Today an even smaller proportion of children with nephrotic syndrome have a persistent course. Most children have minimal change lesions, and these children will either have a remission within 3 years spontaneously (two-thirds) or have earlier remissions secondary to treatment with corticosteroids or cytotoxic agents (95%) (see later discussion). According to the data reviewed by

Trompeter et al. (31), after 15 to 20 years, only 3% of an unselected cohort of children with biopsy-proven minimal change nephrotic syndrome still had active disease.

Similarly, in a study of 89 adults with onset of minimal change nephrotic syndrome after the age of 15 years (32), at follow-up after 2 to 24 years, 59 (80%) of 74 surviving patients were in complete remission, and only 5 had persisting nephrotic syndrome. Therefore, in contrast to past experience, neither of these groups is exposed to possible risks of complications for prolonged periods. However, the few adults and children who have severe and persistent proteinuria are at high risk for complications. Many of these individuals, especially nephrotic children and young adults, have lesions of FSGS that are resistant to treatment with corticosteroids and cytotoxic drugs; others have membranous nephropathy or MPGN. In these unfortunate individuals, a full nephrotic syndrome may progress to chronic kidney disease (CKD) or renal replacement therapy. Even nephrectomy or renal infarction has been occasionally required (33).

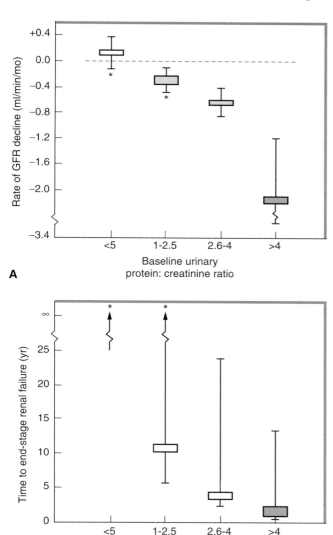

FIGURE 71-4. In chronic nondiabetic, proteinuric nephropathies, decline of glomerular filtration rate (GFR) and predicted time to end-stage renal disease (ESRD) are highly dependent on baseline urine protein/creatinine ratio. Data are from 98 patients with various glomerular diseases. Mean (±SE) Rate of Decline in the Glomerular Filtration per Patient per Month (**Panel A**) and Mean Predicted Time to End-Stage Renal Disease (Panel B). Asterisks indicate a significant difference (*p* <0.05) from a baseline urinary protein/creatinine ratio above 4. The I bars in **Panel B** are ranges. (From: Remuzzi G, Bertani T. Pathophysiology of progressive nephropathies. *N Engl J Med* 1998;339:1448–1456, with permission.)

Infections

Although their importance is still evident, in the past, infections (34) played an even more important role in determining the outcome for the nephrotic patient. For example, the data of Arneil (35) from the Sick Children's Hospital in Glasgow, Scotland, suggest that during the preantibiotic era, more than half of nephrotic children were dead by 5 years after onset, most infections occurring within the first 2 years. There are no data from this period from a single source dealing with adult-onset nephrotic patients, but perusal of accounts in the literature of the 1920s and 1930s (36) suggests that the clinical picture was similar, although (as today) primary pneumococcal

peritonitis is mostly confined to children and adolescents. This is because they have yet to develop specific antibody against pneumococcal polysaccharides and are dependent on nonspecific immunity resting on the activity of the alternative pathway of complement, which is much reduced in nephrotic patients because of protein losses into the urine (29).

Hyperlipidemia

The ubiquitous hyperlipidemia of the nephrotic syndrome (34,37,38) is usually manifest with elevated triglycerides, low-density lipoproteins (LDLs), and total cholesterol, often with low high-density lipoprotein (HDL) values (39). Any attempt to understand the clinical consequences of hyperlipidemia in relation to accelerated vascular disease must take into account the various other cardiovascular risk factors present in nephrotic patients. For example, most patients with persistent nephrotic syndrome also have hypertension, which may be a stronger risk factor for myocardial and other vascular diseases than hyperlipidemia (40). Analysis of 100 nephrotic adults demonstrated that most had one or more risks for cardiovascular disease, including hypertension, left ventricular hypertrophy (LVH), smoking, and others (41). Furthermore, nephrotic diseases with circulating immune complexes may carry their own specific risks, as shown experimentally (42,43) and in humans with systemic lupus who demonstrate premature atherosclerosis (44–46). Although studies have varied in their conclusions (30), a commonly cited study by Ordonez et al. found an elevated risk for myocardial infarction and cardiovascular death in nephrotic adults (47).

Given the information on the deleterious effects of hyperlipidemia in the general population, an exhaustive multivariate analysis implicating the hyperlipidemia of nephrotic syndrome as an *independent* risk factor for cardiovascular events is unlikely to be performed. On balance, it seems reasonable to assume that the hyperlipidemia of persistent nephrotic syndromes probably leads to an increased risk of atherosclerosis.

Thrombosis

Thrombosis is the third major risk besides infection and vascular disease (30,34,48,49). This prothrombotic state probably arises from platelet hyperaggregability, itself the result of platelet–von Willebrand factor interactions and possibly increased availability of arachidonic acid to form aggregant prostaglandins. High fibrinogen levels are also important (49). Major alterations in fluid-phase coagulation proteins are almost confined to severe nephrotic syndromes, with a serum albumin concentration of less than 2 g/dL. Unlike the risk of vascular disease, thrombosis may strike within only a few days or weeks of onset and although rare may attack most tragically those with the most reversible of nephrotic syndromes, because their urinary protein loss is great and their hypoalbuminemia and alterations in other proteins such as von Willebrand factor profound.

Prevention of Complications of the Nephrotic State

To what extent any of these risks can be minimized is controversial. Prophylactic treatment of children with a severe active nephrotic syndrome using penicillin seems sensible, and prompt treatment of cellulitis or septicemia is almost always successful. With the introduction of HMG-CoA reductase inhibitors (statins), which are effective in reversing nephrotic hyperlipidemia (50,51), therapy seems reasonable in those with persistent nephrotic syndromes or in those who are clinically likely to remain nephrotic despite treatment (i.e., MPGN). The question of prophylaxis against thrombosis with anticoagulants in patients with active severe nephrotic syndromes remains contentious (48). Especially for idiopathic membranous nephropathy, expert opinion and decision analyses have supported the use of prophylactic warfarin in high-risk patients with serum albumin level less than 2 g/dL (52). However, controlled studies are not available for warfarin, or for antiplatelet agents, which may have less toxicity but similarly unestablished efficacy.

Proteinuria as a Factor in Progression

The second major area of risk in the nephrotic syndrome is the proteinuria itself (53–55). It is well known that progression into renal failure in the absence of proteinuria almost never occurs in glomerular disease (56), although exceptions occur (57–59). One such exception is when secondary hypertension appears after apparent "healing" of the original disease. Conversely, progression is almost always accompanied by urinary protein more than 2 g per 24 hours or elevated urine protein/creatinine ratio, and usually within the nephrotic range (Figs. 71-3, 71-4). The prognosis for patients with varying glomerular lesions is worse when a nephrotic syndrome is present, as demonstrated in Figure 71-3 and confirmed by Williams et al. (60) and Hunt et al. (61). In FSGS (62,63), membranous nephropathy (64–66), and MPGN (67), the prognosis is markedly worse for nephrotic patients compared with patients who were never nephrotic. Furthermore, if one plots proteinuria against rate of progression of renal disease (60,66), one finds that the greater the proteinuria, the more rapid the decline in renal function.

Two interpretations of these data are possible (53,68): Either profuse continuing proteinuria is a marker for more severe and eventually more serious disease, or profuse persisting proteinuria is damaging and leads to acceleration of the original disease process or to secondary renal damage (69). It has been established that proteinuria leads directly to the production of chemotactic factors (70) and a damaging interstitial infiltrate (68). Transit of protein across the glomerulus may be damaging as well. The accumulating experimental evidence for a

direct role of proteinuria in initiating tubulointerstitial injury and progressive nephropathy is reviewed elsewhere (71).

There is much current interest in these hypotheses, given that it has proved possible to reduce the protein loss in patients with glomerular diseases using various agents—angiotensin-converting enzyme (ACE) inhibitors or angiotensin II receptor blockers (ARBs), nonsteroidal antiinflammatory drugs (NSAIDs), cyclosporine, and dipyridamole—and following low-protein diets (53,72). For ACE inhibitors and ARBs, evidence in treatment of type 1 and type 2 diabetes with nephropathy suggests that reduction in proteinuria slows the decline in glomerular filtration rate (GFR) independent of blood-pressure lowering effects (73–76). This is perhaps the strongest evidence that proteinuria in and of itself may be injurious. An exception to the general rule that proteinuria dominates prognosis may be lupus nephritis (77–79), in which the outcome of this disease is more affected by treatment than are all the previously mentioned progressive glomerular diseases.

Renal Histopathology

The third factor that determines prognosis for the nephrotic patient is the histologic appearance of renal biopsy specimens, which despite many reservations remains the best guide to the nature and prognosis of the syndrome, although this has been challenged (68,80,81). The general prognosis association with the various aspects of the histopathologic appearances was reviewed in detail elsewhere (82). However, a number of general points can be made.

The first point is to examine the differing underlying histologic appearances, especially because they are different at various ages and in different parts of the world. In Figure 71-5 data are shown from a series of more than 600 adult-onset nephrotic patients seen at Guy's Hospital in London between 1965 and 1984. The data for the childhood-onset cases are in Figures 71-5 and 71-6 and are from the International Study of Kidney Disease in Childhood (ISKDC) on more than 500 unselected nephrotic children and 200 childhood-onset patients seen at Guy's Hospital before 1970, during which time all

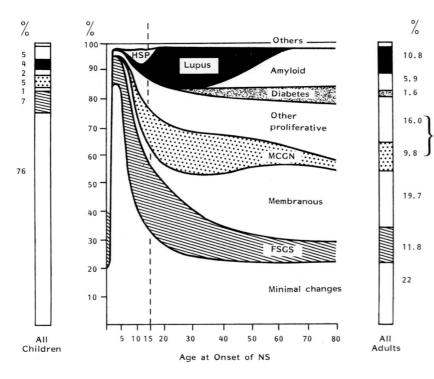

FIGURE 71-5. The underlying histopathologic appearances from a series of 607 nephrotic patients with onset after the age of 15 years, studied at Guy's Hospital from 1963 to 1984. The childhood data are derived from 521 patients studied by the International Study of Kidney Disease in Childhood and 200 patients studied at Guy's Hospital before 1970, during which time all childhood nephrotic patients underwent biopsy. The curves have been smoothed to simplify the diagram, but the adult data are shown in Table 71-2, and the childhood data are shown in more detail in Figure 71-6. (From: Cameron JS, Glassock RJ. The natural history and outcome of the nephrotic syndrome. In: Cameron JS, Glassock RJ, eds. *The Nephrotic Syndrome.* New York: Marcel Dekker; 1987, with permission.)

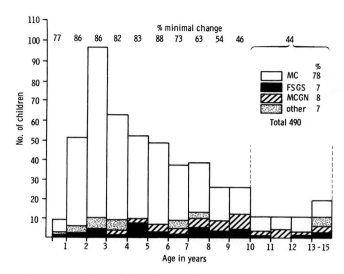

FIGURE 71-6. The underlying histopathology in more than 500 unselected nephrotic children studied by the International Study of Kidney Disease in Childhood, 1965–1976. *MC*, minimal changes; *FSGS*, focal segmental glomerulosclerosis; *MPGN*, mesangioproliferative glomerulonephritis. (From: Barnett HL, et al. Minimal change nephrotic syndrome. In: Edelmann CM, ed. *Pediatric Kidney Disease.* Boston: Little, Brown and Company; 1978:195, with permission.)

children who presented with a nephrotic syndrome underwent biopsy. The main categories shown account for almost 99% of all nephrotic patients, and a few others are discussed in subsequent text. The increase in the proportion of patients with membranous nephropathy with increasing age at onset is obvious. Although amyloidosis is rare before the age of 40, primary amyloid is a relatively common cause of a nephrotic syndrome in older adults. Lupus has the usual age distribution (ages 15 to 50 years) with or without a nephrotic syndrome. Focal segmental sclerosis is present at all ages, from neonates until old age, although the proportion of patients with minimal change lesions declines steadily from the age of 3 to the age of 20 years, but thereafter remains rather constant.

These classic descriptions on the occurrence of various histopathologic syndromes have been challenged in recent years by a growing literature suggesting that FSGS is more prevalent clinically and in large biopsy series. Although initially confined to reports in U.S. adults (83,84), similar data have emerged for nephrotic children in Canada, the United States, and India, and for adults in Peru, Korea, and other regions (85–90). Thus, the current literature strongly suggests a worldwide increase in the frequency of FSGS in both adults and children.

A number of factors distort the incidence of various diseases. First, there is a tendency not to refer older patients for biopsy. Second, the proportion of diabetic patients seen with a nephrotic syndrome depends on the referral and biopsy policy in diabetic patients with proteinuria, with or without edema. In general, many centers have avoided biopsy in diabetic nephrotic patients with retinopathy and have performed a biopsy only when there is some indication that the condition is unlikely to be diabetic nephropathy. For example, the presence of significant hematuria, or the absence of retinopathy, may be an indication for a biopsy. However, the proportion of all nephrotic patients with diabetic nephropathy, even where all nephrotic patients have undergone biopsy, does not exceed 10% in any published series. The coincidence or association of diabetes and membranous nephropathy (91) or other forms of glomerular pathology needs emphasis, and many centers are performing biopsies more often in diabetic nephrotic patients.

Although these data apply to developed Western communities, there are many variations within the much higher incidence of nephrotic syndrome found in the Tropics (92). Although poorly documented for developing countries, the admission data analyzed by Kibukamusoke (93) suggest that nephrotic syndrome may represent a much more common admission diagnosis than in Western nations. In the absence of firm data on incidence, it is difficult to judge whether minimal change disease is actually rare in the Tropics or merely submerged in a much larger number of other forms of histopathology. For example, in Malaysia (94), there may be a higher incidence of minimal change disease or very minor proliferative histology in adults. These patients are sensitive to corticosteroids in terms of decreasing urinary protein excretion and represent 40% to 50% of all nephrotic adults. Minor variations in incidence almost certainly occur throughout the Western world. For example, higher proportions of nephrotic adult patients from the United States have membranous nephropathy compared with counterparts from Europe. In the Interhospitals Study (95) of the nephrotic syndrome, 72 of 154 nephrotic patients had membranous nephropathy, whereas in U.K. data (Fig. 71-5), the proportion of adult-onset cases with this appearance remained constant at about 20% to 25%. Membranous nephropathy, unrelated to carriage of hepatitis B virus, also seems to be common in Greece (96) and the Balkans. MPGN is relatively uncommon in Japan, but in Iran, it accounts for 64% of nephrotic patients (97). Thus, it is difficult to make general assumptions regarding incidence of various diseases, given regional variations and changing frequencies of primary diseases such as FSGS.

When one is considering the histopathology of diseases that underlie a nephrotic syndrome, the general prognosis of the group of patients with any given histopathologic pattern may be estimated, but it remains the individual prognosis that is of primary concern to physician and patient. Within general statements, such as that 90% of adult type I MPGN patients with a nephrotic syndrome will be in renal failure before 10 years, or that up to 60% of adult-onset nephrotic patients with membranous nephropathy will have renal failure eventually, the prognosis and rate of progression of the individual are submerged.

Effects of Treatment

The fourth and final influence on prognosis is again an obvious one: the effect of specific treatment in resolving the nephrotic syndrome or at least diminishing the proteinuria to the point at which edema no longer forms. The treatment of nephrotic children and adults has been discussed extensively elsewhere in these volumes, but a few additional points are worth making here. Clearly, the response of the various histologic types of glomerulonephritis underlying the clinical presentations of glomerular disease differs. For example, 90% of nephrotic patients with minimal change lesions, and 45% to 65% of those with FSGS (98,99) will respond to treatment with corticosteroids, cytotoxic agents, or cyclosporine by complete or partial remission of proteinuria. As noted previously, progression into renal insufficiency is almost unknown for any patient whose proteinuria remits completely (56), and thus these patients have almost universally a good prognosis for long-term renal function. Therefore, response to early treatment is a powerful indicator of good prognosis. For example, it has been known for many years that the outlook for adult nephrotic patients who respond to corticosteroids is much superior to those who do not respond to corticosteroids (100), irrespective of renal biopsy appearances (Fig. 71-7). By the 1970s, this distinction was so clear to pediatric nephrologists that since then, it has been almost universal practice to treat all but a few

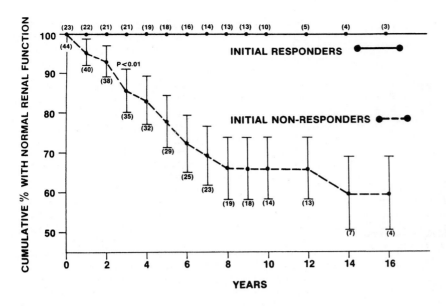

FIGURE 71-7. The long-term outcome of adult patients with a nephrotic syndrome who never underwent a biopsy and who were treated with prednisone. Those who responded to this treatment with loss of proteinuria during the initial treatment fared much better than those who did not, with respect to the outlook for renal function. (From: Idelson BA, et al. Prognosis in steroid-treated idiopathic nephrotic syndrome in adults. *Arch Intern Med* 1977;137:891, with permission.)

childhood-onset nephrotic syndrome patients with corticosteroids and to perform a biopsy at about 4 weeks in those whose proteinuria fails to remit by this time.

It has been argued (79–81) that such a policy has merit also for patients with adult-onset nephrotic syndrome, even though the proportion of adult nephrotic patients who respond to a brief course of steroids is much lower in adults than in children. Such a suggestion involves balancing the relative risks of a continuing nephrotic syndrome against the risks of renal biopsy itself and of the corticosteroid treatment to be given. Given such data as the lack of effectiveness of steroids in membranous nephropathy (101), the often protracted duration of steroid therapy required for many patients with FSGS (102), and the general safety of real-time renal biopsies using automated needles (103), it seems increasingly difficult to rationalize an empiric course of steroids in nephrotic adults. Furthermore, Nolasco (32) and Korbet et al. (104) analyzed the rates of response to corticosteroids in patients with adult-onset minimal change nephrotic syndrome treated with corticosteroids (Fig. 71-10). The response rate for adults in these series was slower and less frequently complete than that for children in the ISKDC study. Therefore, a policy of performing a renal biopsy in all adult-onset nephrotic syndrome patients without obvious diabetic nephropathy is preferred.

PROGNOSIS OF INDIVIDUAL HISTOLOGIC GROUPS

Minimal Change Lesions

Most patients who undergo biopsy and show minimal change lesions have a full nephrotic syndrome, but there are many symptomless patients with isolated proteinuria—especially adolescents and young adults (105,106), who may show appearances consistent with a diagnosis of minimal change lesions in their renal biopsy specimens (Chapter 64). However, these patients may not undergo biopsy unless the urinary protein loss is more than 2 g per 24 hours or edema appears, because of the excellent prognosis for this group (105,106) and because the changes in their renal biopsy specimens are usually benign. Therefore, this discussion is confined to patients with a minimal change lesion in the setting of a nephrotic syndrome. The

outcome of minimal change disease as observed today is very much modified from its "natural" history, both by control of infections (discussed already) and by the successful use of immunosuppressive agents to eliminate proteinuria.

Childhood-Onset Minimal Change Nephrotic Syndrome

History Without Treatment: Causes of Death. As Figure 71-6 demonstrates, the minimal change lesion is most commonly found in childhood-onset nephrotic syndrome patients but also accounts for 20% to 25% of adult nephrotic patients of all ages. As discussed already (34,82), until the era of diuretics and antibiotics, death from sepsis and occasionally from thrombosis was common in patients with nephrotic syndrome. Now death from complications is rare, although Trompeter (31) and the ISKDC (107) demonstrated that a low rate of mortality from complications persists. In Trompeter's study of 183 unselected children with a nephrotic syndrome and biopsy-proven minimal change lesions, there were 11 deaths during the subsequent 15 to 22 years, 7 of which were related to the nephrotic syndrome or its treatment (e.g., infections, septicemia, and hypovolemia). The only death from 1982 to 1990 in this group was of one boy, who had brain infarction from sagittal sinus thrombosis during a relapse. Of 10 children who died of the 389 children studied by the ISKDC (107) for 7 to 15 years, 6 died of infection, 1 died of dural sinus thrombosis, 1 died of circulatory overload precipitated by intravenous albumin infusion, and 1 died in chronic renal failure; the cause of death in the final child was undetermined. Notably, all the deaths occurred in the early part of the study (i.e., before 1972). Krensky et al. (108) and Gorensek et al. (109) confirmed the continued importance of peritonitis as a complication of childhood nephrotic syndrome. In these two series, three children died of their sepsis.

Much attention has been directed to the relapsing pattern of patients with minimal change nephrotic syndrome. It has sometimes been said that this pattern is the result of "forcing" patients into remission with corticosteroids, whose disease would otherwise have persisted. This pattern of behavior was recorded, however, well before the introduction of corticosteroids; indeed, one of the first accounts of a patient with childhood nephrotic syndrome, in Paris (1833 to 1834), described two children whose urine became completely free of albumin between relapses (110). The relapses themselves

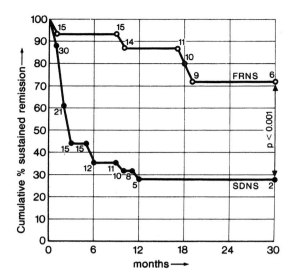

FIGURE 71-8. The stability of response of nephrotic children who have multiple relapses (Frequent Relapsing Nephrotic Syndrome [FRNS]) or have become steroid-dependent (Steroid Dependent Nephrotic Syndrome [SDNS]) (see text for definitions) treated with mustardlike agents (cyclophosphamide or chlorambucil). Those who have multiple relapses have a much superior response in the long term, compared with those who were steroid-dependent before treatment with cytotoxics. (From: Arbeitsgemeinschaft für pödiatrische nephrologie. Effect of cytotoxic drugs in frequently relapsing nephrotic syndrome with and without steroid dependence. *N Engl J Med* 1982;306:451, with permission.)

also may remit spontaneously (111). There is little doubt from the data of Arneil (35) and Schwartz (112) that the natural evolution of childhood nephrotic syndrome progresses slowly toward remission; from Arneil's data, one can calculate a spontaneous remission rate of about 65% at 3 years from onset (35).

History with Treatment. Today, this long-term natural evolution is modified by early treatment with corticosteroids. From the data of the ISKDC (113), 93% of nephrotic children will go into remission within 6 to 8 weeks on a dosage of prednisone of 60 mg/m² per 24 hours (Fig. 71-8). Thirty-six percent will never experience a relapse, 18% will have infrequent relapses, but 39% will experience multiple relapses, either with a period without treatment and free of proteinuria between relapses ("frequent relapser") or relapsing immediately when prednisone is withdrawn or even during modest doses of the drug (corticosteroid-dependent).

What the exact influence of the initial treatment on subsequent outcome may be has been debated. Early claims were made that more prolonged initial treatment resulted in fewer subsequent relapses (114). The German Arbeitsgemeinschaft für Pödiatrische Nephrologie (APN) (115) examined the ISKDC regimen of treatment for 8 weeks contrasted with treatment for a shorter period, the period of treatment being determined by how rapidly complete remission appeared. Sustained remission was significantly less frequent (19%), with the shorter course over the following 14 months of follow-up, compared with 39% for the standard protocol; when an even longer course (12 weeks of treatment) was given (116), the results were even more impressive: 64% had sustained remission. Choonara et al. (117) compared stability of remission in a group of relapsing children treated for similar lengths of time but with lower dosages (30 mg per 24 hours) with those given the "standard" ISKDC dosage of 60 mg/m²; duration of remission was similar in the two groups. The French Club for

Pediatric Nephrology reexamined the suggestion of Lange et al. (114) but found that stability of remission was no more after 1 year of alternate-day treatment than after 16 weeks (118).

Multiple Relapsing Nephrotic Syndrome. Much attention has been paid to the optimum management of frequently relapsing or corticosteroid-dependent patients (Chapter 64). Although cytotoxic agents such as *cyclophosphamide* and *chlorambucil* may induce a remission in such children (119–121), recent reports in small numbers of patients cast some doubt on the uniform effectiveness of cyclophosphamide in steroid-dependent nephrotic syndrome (122,123). Other corticosteroid-based therapy includes carefully titrated alternate-day prednisone (124) or lower dose prednisone (125) on an intermittent or continuous basis for a longer duration. This tendency has been strengthened by the observations of Garin et al. (126) and the German APN (127); the patients who need the relief from steroid dosage the most, that is, the steroid-dependent patients, achieve the least benefit from cytotoxics in terms of duration of remission (Fig. 71-8). The optimum duration of the course of cyclophosphamide has not been determined precisely. Initial data suggested that a course of only 2 weeks was without effect, and that 6 or 8 weeks at 3 mg/kg per 24 hours would achieve as much as longer courses (119). This view was challenged by the APN (115), who showed more stable remission when 12 weeks of treatment was used, but yet again a Japanese study found no difference (128). Schulman et al. (129) noted no difference in the proportion of prolonged remissions in those with or without IgM deposits or global sclerosis. Of note, a recent report found that children with a history of intrauterine growth retardation (IUGR) and minimal change disease were far more likely to become steroid-dependent or frequent relapsers, perhaps indicating a subgroup eligible for heightened monitoring and a low threshold for conversion to cytotoxic agents (130).

In the last two decades, *cyclosporine* has been used extensively in children with minimal change nephrotic syndrome (131), on the reasonable assumption that the inhibition of activated T cells achieved by this drug could be useful. Accumulated data (121,131–134) have produced a consensus that the drug has a useful place in the management of relapsing patients but makes only a small difference in the longer term evolution of the condition. Remission can usually be induced in steroid-dependent or frequently relapsing patients, but relapse is the norm when the dosage of the drug is stopped or tapered during the first year of treatment. However, cyclosporine may be useful in permitting a reduction in dosage or cessation of corticosteroids, although its use may substitute the side effects of cyclosporine and cyclosporine dependency for corticosteroid dependency and side effects. This is particularly important in permitting normal stature. There is, however, some evidence that longer courses of cyclosporine therapy may induce prolonged remission (135), as cytotoxic drugs may achieve, but at a much lower level of frequency; in most series, even after long-term (more than 1 year) treatment, withdrawal leads to relapse (136). Chronic cyclosporine therapy confers a significant risk of nephrotoxicity. As seen from one study, progressive nephrotoxicity in children on long-term cyclosporine can be minimized if patients are kept volume expanded and low doses are used with close monitoring of levels (137).

As in adults, the antiproliferative agent *mycophenolate mofetil* (MMF) has garnered interest as a treatment for children with steroid-dependent minimal change disease. Although numbers of patients are small, this agent has shown the ability to substantially reduce relapses (138). Another agent, the antihelminthic agent levamisole, is known to have immunomodulatory effects. Very few randomized or controlled studies are available in which levamisole has been used alone or in combination treatment in minimal change disease in children (139–141). It has been used mainly to prevent relapses

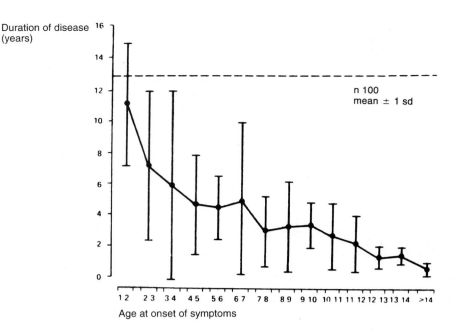

Duration of disease (years)

n 100
mean ± 1 sd

Age at onset of symptoms

FIGURE 71-9. The duration of relapsing course in relation to age at onset in minimal change nephrotic children initially treated with corticosteroids. (From: Trompeter RS, et al. Long-term outcome for children with minimal change nephrotic syndrome: a long term follow-up. *Kidney Int* 1978;29:1215, with permission.)

after remission has been obtained with the use of prednisone. But the main problem once again is occurrence of relapse once the drug has been stopped. In a recent study from India (140), alternate-day levamisole therapy in steroid-dependent nephrotic syndrome reduced the relapse rate from a mean of 3 per year to 0.9 per year. Because of unavailability controlled or new large-scale studies, the exact place of levamisole and MMF in therapy of minimal change disease is unclear.

Relapses in the Longer Term. Although the tendency to relapse is prolonged, in most patients with minimal change nephrotic syndromes, it is not indefinite, and it is striking how few childhood patients are referred to adult clinics because they are still relapsing. Siegel et al. (142,143) studied 60 nephrotic children responsive to corticosteroids for a mean of 14.5 years, with particular emphasis on the subset of 20 relapsers who received cyclophosphamide treatment. Those so treated had all gone into remission, whereas just more than half (52%) of those treated with corticosteroids alone were still having relapses.

In Trompeter's long-term study of 183 children (31), only 10 children with a duration of disease from 15.0 to 20.5 years were still having relapses. By this time, they were 17 to 27 years old. Lewis et al. (144), from Manchester, England, followed 63 children with steroid-sensitive nephrotic syndromes for 10 to 21 years and again noted a tendency for relapses to become less frequent 4 years after diagnosis, and the percentage of patients relapsing fell steadily with time (Fig. 71-9). Only two children died: one from sagittal sinus thrombosis and one from septicemia. Niali (145) reported a patient who had relapses repeatedly between the ages of 4 and 53 years, at which point he died of tuberculosis.

Another observation of practical value is how long remission must elapse before a further relapse becomes unlikely. These data are influenced by the use of cytotoxic agents, but from other published data (145), it appears that it is rare for a relapse to occur after more than 2 years in remission and almost unknown after 7 years of remission. Nevertheless, reports of relapses occurring 10 to 25 years later have been published (146–149). These very late relapses are almost always responsive to treatment with corticosteroids, but an acquired resistance to treatment has been described (149).

It would be useful to be able to predict at the outset which children will have relapses frequently, but no features of the initial nephrotic syndrome appear to distinguish frequent relapsers with any certainty from those who will have no relapses or infrequent relapses. However, in the study of Trompeter et al. (31), there was a striking relation between persistent relapsing disease and the patient's age (Fig. 71-9). All children with persisting disease had onset before the age of 6 years, and the younger the child at onset, the more likely he or she was to have a prolonged relapsing course. Data from the ISKDC show that the pattern of frequent relapses is usually established soon after an attack, with two relapses within 6 months or three within 1 year being the pattern in most patients; these data are useful in deciding which therapy to use before long-term corticosteroids are used. In a recent retrospective study of nearly 400 children, long-term outlook was excellent if there was response in the first 8 weeks and remission was maintained for the next 6 months. These patients had very few relapses. A relapse in the first 6 months predicted further relapses in the next 3 years. Of the children who failed to achieve remission, 21% progressed to renal failure. Therefore, aggressive therapy may be required in slow responders (150).

Stature and Bone Characteristics in Children with Minimal Change Nephrotic Syndrome. The terminal height attained by children with prolonged periods of relapse and consequent prolonged treatment with corticosteroids is of particular interest. Trompeter's data (31) show that the height of 10 children who had relapses for 20 to 25 years was within 2 standard deviations (SDs) of expected, although most values were on the lower side of the mean. Similarly, Manchester data (151) showed a mean height in the 40th percentile in 80 patients, most of whom were relapsers, after 5 to 24 years; the height in only six patients was more than 2 SDs below the mean. In both studies, hypertension was absent and all patients had normal renal function. The results of the study of Berns et al. (143), from Yale, were not so encouraging; the mean height of those treated with corticosteroids alone was −0.93 ± 0.3 SD, and those who had received cyclophosphamide, −0.84 ± 0.4 SD, after a mean follow-up of 14.5 years. Padilla and Brem (152) studied growth velocity before and after treatment with cyclophosphamide. They found a doubling of growth velocity from 4.3 ± 1.3 to 8.7 ± 2.5 cm per year. The negative effects of corticosteroids on stature and growth velocity have been partially ameliorated in a one-year pilot study using growth hormone in steroid-dependent children (153).

Focus has shifted in recent years to bone densitometry and markers of bone turnover. Mixed reports on bone-mineral density exist (154,155), but a recent, carefully controlled (and somewhat surprising) study suggests that bone mineral density is not affected by long-term glucocorticoids when controlling for factors such as age, sex, Tanner stage, and body mass index (BMI) (156). To date, there is no clear evidence that markers of bone turnover, such as urinary deoxypyridinoline and N-telopeptide, are clearly affected by corticosteroids in childhood nephrotic syndrome (155,157).

Evolution to Chronic Renal Failure in Corticosteroid-Sensitive Minimal Change Nephrotic Syndrome

It is very rare for a nephrotic patient with a minimal change lesion in biopsy tissue and demonstrated responsiveness to prednisone, with complete loss of proteinuria, to go into renal failure subsequently. Only a handful of such patients has been recorded in the literature (158–163). These exceptional patients are of great interest in influencing our ideas on the relationship between minimal change disease and focal segmental sclerosis (see the following discussion).

However, the experience of Tejani (161) is at variance with this general conclusion. Thirty-three of 48 children who had multiple relapses showed segmental sclerosis (164), IgM (165), or both in specimens taken at a second biopsy; in the remaining 9 children, minimal changes were still present, and third biopsies showed similar changes in 6. The reasons for this markedly poorer prognosis for frequently relapsing children, so much at variance with all other reports, is not clear, although the ethnic origins of this group of patients is different from the origins reported in most other published series (predominantly American Hispanic and black), and black adults frequently show progressive focal segmental lesions (166) (see later discussion).

Still rare but slightly more frequent is the patient who appears to have minimal changes on an initial biopsy sample but fails to respond to corticosteroids or cyclophosphamide (121). Often, these patients have a rather prominent mesangium in their biopsy specimens and sometimes mesangial deposits of IgM (see the following discussion). Material obtained at subsequent biopsies may show obvious lesions of focal and segmental glomerulosclerosis, and the question arises as to whether these lesions may have already been present in the kidney but not in the plane of the biopsy section or the entire biopsy specimen on the first occasion. Either way, the initial resistance to treatment with both agents is an important indicator of an adverse prognosis for renal function, and it exceeds in value the details of the histologic appearances in renal biopsy material.

Minimal Change Nephrotic Syndrome in Adults

Natural History Unmodified by Treatment. As with the childhood data, the bulk of information available represents the modified history of the condition after treatment including corticosteroids, cytotoxic agents, and cyclosporine. Data from untreated adult patients with minimal change syndrome are available from the preantibiotic era but are dominated by deaths from infections (34); data are also from the control cases from two controlled trials, that of the MRC in Great Britain (167) and that of the Interhospitals Study (168). Both series suggest that after 3 years, about two-thirds of patients with adult-onset disease will have gone into spontaneous remission, whereas one-third will still have proteinuria; there were no deaths among 28 untreated patients in the two trials.

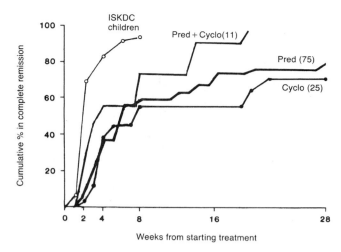

FIGURE 71-10. Rate of response (judged by loss of proteinuria) of patients with adult-onset minimal change nephrotic syndrome treated with corticosteroids, cyclophosphamide, or both, compared with data in children taken from the International Study of Kidney Disease in Childhood. Data from 89 adults in the Guy's Hospital series (32) are shown.

History Modified by Treatment. It is often forgotten that at all ages, minimal change disease accounts for one-fourth of adult nephrotic syndromes, but far fewer data are available from adults than from children with minimal change disease (32,104,121,168–170). The literature up to 1980 was reviewed by Coggins (168) and Broyer et al. (121), and Nolasco reviewed long-term follow-up of 89 adults with minimal change nephrotic syndrome (32). These cases, together with those summarized by Coggins (168), 40 cases of Korbet (104), 33 from Fujimoto et al. (169), 51 from Mak et al. (170), and 46 from Huang (171) form the bulk of the data.

Patients with adult-onset minimal change nephrotic syndrome responded more slowly and more incompletely than children to corticosteroids in all series (32,104,169,171) (Fig. 71-10). Therapy as long as 15 weeks may be required to achieve remission. This might reflect the lower dosage of prednisone normally in use on a body weight or surface area basis, when compared with pediatric use. However, the same effect was seen with cyclophosphamide, and here the dosage was identical (3 mg/kg per 24 hours for 8 weeks). In addition, a lower percentage of adult patients achieved a complete response after corticosteroid treatment. Fourteen (24%) of Nolasco's 58 patients whose proteinuria resolved completely never had a relapse, 32 (56%) had relapse on a single occasion or infrequently, and only 12 (21%) were frequent relapsers or steroid-dependent—a much lower proportion than that in children. The same gradient of a less frequent relapsing course with age was seen in patients with adult-onset minimal change syndrome, so after the age of 60, relapses were rare. Some authors also have seen this (32), in contrast to Zech et al. (172), who observed no relapses in this age group. As in children, a first relapse was uncommon after 2 years of remission and never occurred more than 8 years later.

In Nolasco's study, stability of remission after treatment with cyclophosphamide (36 patients) was superior to that found in children, with 60% of patients still in remission at 10 to 15 years. Only patients older than 55 years died, and only 5 of 15 deaths noted were related to the nephrotic syndrome, most in the period before 1975. At last follow-up, which was 1 to 24 years after onset, only 13 of 89 patients still had active disease and only 6 were still manifesting nephrotic syndrome, as were only 3 of 51 of Mak's series (170). As in children, cyclosporine has been used in frequently relapsing and steroid-dependent adults (132,135,173), and has also been used successfully in combination with steroids as primary therapy (174).

Primary Resistance to Treatment, Histologic Changes, and Acquired Resistance to Treatment in Minimal Change Nephrotic Syndrome

As mentioned already, resistance to treatment with prednisone and cyclophosphamide is usually an ominous sign in patients with minimal change disease demonstrated by biopsy. It is easy to forget that the diagnosis of minimal change disease is a diagnosis of exclusion made with varying certainty according to whether the juxtamedullary glomeruli (most frequently and earliest affected by FSGS) are included in the biopsy material, and whether immunofluorescence or electron microscopy is available to distinguish a very early membranous pattern. Therefore, some of these patients have histologic changes, other than minimal changes, which have not been detected as such. However, within the scope of what is usually regarded as minimal changes are focal global sclerosis of glomeruli, sometimes accompanied by tubular atrophy and varying mild degrees of mesangial matrix expansion and hypercellularity. The former appears to have no effect on prognosis when present in children with a nephrotic syndrome (175). In adults, with increasing age, more and more global obsolescence of glomeruli is seen (176), together with tubulointerstitial damage and vessel changes that are probably the origin of these appearances. The interpretation of "minimal changes" in adults must take into account these alterations that occur with age.

Some initially resistant patients, however, fail to respond to corticosteroids in conventional doses or have only a diminution of continuing proteinuria but then respond promptly to cyclophosphamide. They probably represent a rather resistant group of patients who require more treatment, but are at one end of the responsive spectrum and have a good prognosis according to the ISKDC data (175); 23 of 31 initial nonresponders to prednisone (no loss of abnormal proteinuria by 8 weeks) lost their abnormal proteinuria eventually. In data from the Hopital des Enfants Malades (121,177), 46 (56%) of 83 children with nonresponsive nephrotic syndrome eventually lost their abnormal proteinuria.

The presence of mesangial expansion, proliferation, or both is a more controversial topic. In childhood nephrotic syndrome, there seems to be little doubt that as the mesangial volume increases (as judged by its area in fixed material in histologic preparations), a higher proportion of patients with hematuria, hypertension, initial resistance to corticosteroid treatment, and ultimate entry into renal insufficiency is seen (159,175,178–182). The presence or absence of IgM or minor mesangial deposits on electron microscopy does not, however, seem to alter the prognosis (178–181). Because fixation techniques affect the mesangial area, and there are no absolute criteria for normality, different observers may classify the same biopsy sample in different ways. However, a remarkable unanimity on the significance of mesangial expansion for prognosis has emerged, as outlined already. What is much less clear is what pathogenic significance the mesangial expansion, proliferation, or deposits may have. Some patients with only mesangial expansion in initial biopsy specimens, and no segmental lesions, will show segmental sclerosis on subsequent specimens. This type of observation leads many observers (113,121,159,182) to treat this group of patients as a variant of the minimal change–FSGS group, and the whole as a spectrum of presentations of a single disease. The older German American name, "lipoid nephrosis," is perhaps preferable for this group, because the name used by the Parisians (113,121,145) (idiopathic nephrotic syndrome)

could equally apply to other forms of primary glomerular disease.

Late unresponsiveness to corticosteroid treatment in relapsing patients is another less common pattern of behavior in patients with minimal changes. In the ISKDC data (175), 43 of 311 initial responders acquired some degree of resistance to corticosteroid treatment during follow-up. Because only these troublesome patients usually have late biopsies, and, in many, focal segmental sclerosing lesions were found (180), it was supposed at first that this evolution was confined to resistant patients. Since then, it has become apparent that the biopsy material may remain normal in appearance in resistant patients (179) and show sclerosing lesions in responding relapsers.

The value of the presence of IgM in predicting outcome is controversial, mainly because different authors have asked different questions. There seems little doubt that within the group of patients with minimal changes on optical microscopy, the presence of IgM makes no difference to short- or long-term outlook (121,183,184). Mesangial proliferative glomerulonephritis with mesangial IgM deposition is dealt with in the following discussion.

Focal Segmental Glomerulosclerosis (FSGS)

The appearances of focal and segmental sclerosis are nonspecific (185–188), just as global glomerular sclerosis is nonspecific. Particularly in adults, this type of lesion can be found in a number of clinical and pathologic settings, such as in the presence of a reduced number of nephrons, hypertension and aging, human immunodeficiency virus (HIV) positivity, and/or intravenous drug abuse, as well as superimposed on almost any form of progressive glomerular disease. It has been suggested that the study of the details of the lesion may allow a consistent distinction between these different types of FSGS (189). Here, we exclusively discuss "primary" FSGS found as an isolated phenomenon in patients with proteinuria, usually of considerable dimensions and frequently accompanied by a nephrotic syndrome.

The relationship of this lesion to minimal changes has been much debated, and the controversy is reviewed elsewhere in detail (82,185) (Chapter 64). In short, it is not likely that we will be able to decide whether FSGS and minimal changes represent different aspects of what is pathogenically the same lesion or two distinct diseases unless and until we understand the pathogenesis of either; at the moment, despite much speculation and experimentation, this remains unknown, although a humoral factor that is possibly identical in the two appearances seems to be involved in the induction of proteinuria in both. However, data from patients with recurrent disease who underwent transplantation (190), the occasional entry of patients with a completely responsive minimal change lesion into renal failure already mentioned, the more frequent appearance of focal segmental lesions in patients with mesangial expansion, and the occasional response of even the most severe forms of FSGS to intense immunosuppression all support the thesis that FSGS and minimal changes represent aspects of the same or similar disease (121,159,185,187).

It has became obvious that the FSGS lesion is much more common in black nephrotic patients than in white patients in the United States, accounting for up to one-half of black adult nephrotic patients (166) and one-third of children (191), compared with 25% of adult whites and 10% of white children. In many of these patients, the FSGS is of what has been called the "collapsing" variety (186,187,192,193). Although it has become usual to include collapsing glomerulopathy as a variety of FSGS, it is in fact a diffuse disease in almost all instances and perhaps deserves its own category.

TABLE 71-1

INITIAL RESPONSIVENESS OF NEPHROTIC CHILDREN WITH FOCAL SEGMENTAL GLOMERULOSCLEROSIS TO CORTICOSTEROID TREATMENT

Author	Year	Reference no.	Number treated	No. responded with loss of proteinuria	Percentage
Siegel et al.	1974	(180)	22	16	73
Newman et al.	1976	(596)	15	9	60
Gubler et al.	1978	(236)	85	21	25
Tarshish et al.	1983	(150)	16	5	31
Mongeau et al.	1981	(218)	31	6	19
Arbus et al.	1982	(195)	51	19	37
Schärer et al.	1982	(627)	51	10	20
South West Pediatric Nephrology Study Group	1985	(203)	56	16	16
Trompeter (Guy's)	1987	(194)	62	10	16
Total			389	112	29

Clinical Picture

Short-Term Behavior with Treatment. Complicating the understanding of corticosteroid responsiveness in children is the reality that steroid-sensitive patients with FSGS may never receive a biopsy. Therefore, case series of FSGS in children may represent a relatively steroid-resistant group. A proportion of children with FSGS with a full nephrotic syndrome respond to treatment with the conventional 6 to 8 weeks of prednisolone, similar to those with minimal change (Table 71-1). In the published literature on 332 children, 96 (29%) responded with complete loss of proteinuria (194); many of these patients subsequently had a relapsing course, just as in the minimal change nephrotic syndrome, but some became corticosteroid-resistant later (195). In more recent series, which tend to include either higher doses or longer courses of steroids, the rate of complete remission has been higher (196), with reported completer remission rates as high as 65% (197). However, a substantial price of toxicity (growth retardation, cataracts) may be paid (197).

Whether adults can achieve high rates of sustained remission is debated in the literature (198). For example, of 39 nephrotic patients reported by Beaufils (62), 6 went into remission, but 2.5 to 10.0 years later, and only 3 of 26 treated with corticosteroids alone and 1 each treated with indomethacin and chlorambucil went into remission. In the series of Cameron (63), only 2 patients responded with loss of abnormal proteinuria, of 18 adults treated with corticosteroids alone. In an analysis of the literature (199), 17% of adult nephrotic patients with FSGS were found to have lost abnormal proteinuria completely. However, with evolution in steroid dose and duration of therapy, these pessimistic outcomes may need to be revised. Even in groups with high proportions of African Americans and nephrotic-range proteinuria, complete response rates exceeded 30%, and between 50% and 70% of patients achieved complete or partial response (196,200,201).

Almost all studies on nephrotic patients with FSGS support the idea that the prognosis of patients with complete resolution of proteinuria in response to corticosteroids is much better than the prognosis for those who do not show this initial response (Table 71-2). In contrast, however, Tejani et al. (202) and the South West Pediatric Nephrology Study Group (203) reported that the outcome in terms of renal failure was no different in those who responded initially and those who did not, so the prognosis even for those who respond must remain guarded. Both of these latter series contained, in contrast to the rest of the literature, a high proportion of black and Hispanic children. Ingulli and Tejani (191) demonstrated that as in black adults (166), FSGS is more common in black or Hispanic children with a nephrotic syndrome (57 of 177), and that 78% of this group evolved to renal failure compared with only 33% (4 of 12) of white children. However, only 30% of white children respond to initial treatment with corticosteroids, so the difference may not be as large as these authors suggest.

Therefore, the response to an initial treatment with *corticosteroids* may be a valuable indicator of likely prognosis. It also follows that the overall survival of a group of nephrotic patients with FSGS may depend on the proportion of steroid-responsive patients within the population under study. Finally, the data support the advisability of giving *all* nephrotic patients with FSGS a trial of prednisone for a minimum of 3 months; patients should not be considered steroid-resistant until a 6-month trial has been completed (200). Ponticelli et al. (201) pointed out that it may take much longer for proteinuria to resolve than with patients with minimal change disease, which highlights the difficulty of defining "corticosteroid resistance."

It is less clear whether it is worth giving *cyclophosphamide* thereafter to those who do not respond. The ISKDC, performed

TABLE 71-2

LONG-TERM OUTCOME IN NEPHROTIC PATIENTS WITH FSGS IN RELATION TO INITIAL RESPONSIVENESS TO CORTICOSTEROIDS[a]

	Responders[b]	Nonresponders	Total
All	49 (20%)	196 (80%)	245
In CRF	3 (10%)	49 (53%)	52 (45%)
"Death"[c]	2	55	57

FSGS, focal segmental glomerulosclerosis; CRF, chronic renal failure.
[a]Summary of literature on adults and children 1969–1978 and personal cases.
[b]Response equals complete loss of proteinuria, usually within 8 weeks.
[c]Death equals dead, dialyzed, or transplanted; mean follow-up, 6.4 years.
(Reprinted from: Cameron JS. The problem of focal segmental glomerulosclerosis. In: Kincaid-Smith P, D'Apice AJF, Atkins RC, eds. *Progress in Glomerulonephritis.* New York: Wiley; 1979:209 with permission.)

% Survival

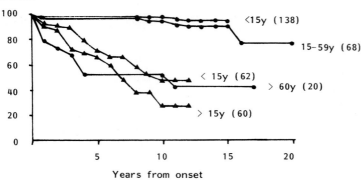

FIGURE 71-11. Survival of nephrotic children or adults with either minimal change (●) or focal segmental glomerular sclerosis (▲). (From: Cameron JS, Glassock RJ. The natural history and outcome of the nephrotic syndrome. In: Cameron JS, Glassock RJ, eds. *The Nephrotic Syndrome.* New York: Marcel Dekker Inc; 1987; unpublished data are from the Guy's Hospital series [32], with permission.)

in the 1970s, reported in 1996 that addition of cyclophosphamide to alternate-day prednisone in children resistant to 8 weeks corticosteroid therapy provided no additional benefit (204). Tune et al. used alkylating agents in 78% of children with FSGS and achieved a remission rate of 70% (197). Others have described high remission rate followed by a disappointingly high relapse rate (205), as well as low initial response rate (206). Conclusions from these scattered series are difficult to draw in children. For adult-onset patients, there is a lack of any randomized trials or even long-term prospective studies using cytotoxic agents (207). Ponticelli et al. provide some information (201). In 65 patients receiving cytotoxic agents as first-line therapy, 40% achieved a response (the majority partial remissions), and 6 of 11 patients with steroid-resistance achieved partial or complete remission. As for chlorambucil, Mendoza et al. (208) reported favorable results in white children treated with an intensive regimen of *methylprednisolone* and *chlorambucil,* but this was not confirmed in a mainly black population (205). Therefore, for both children and adults with FSGS, there is marginal evidence for benefit of cytotoxic agents after a 12- to 16-week course of steroids (207).

Cyclosporine has been used extensively in children (121,209,210) and adults (132,209) with FSGS, usually in association with corticosteroids. A higher response rate than with either corticosteroids alone or cyclophosphamide has been reported, although a reduction in urinary protein loss (see previous discussion) has often been used as a criterion for success, and this may be a purely hemodynamic event. In an analysis of the literature, 29 (27%) of 109 corticosteroid-resistant adults and 11 (25%) of 44 corticosteroid-resistant children showed complete remission (132). This benefit was confirmed by Ponticelli et al. (209): 13 of 22 treated patients attained remission of the nephrotic syndrome after 1 year of cyclosporine treatments, compared with 3 of 19 control subjects. A recent randomized controlled trial in adults supports these conclusions (211). Despite high relapse rates, a substantial lowering of the risk of active disease remained at 4 years. The French Society of Pediatric Nephrology noted remission in 42% of 65 steroid-resistant children treated with cyclosporine (210), whereas Lieberman and Tejani noted a remission rate of 66% (212). The addition of chlorambucil to a cyclosporine-containing regimen has not appeared helpful (213). In summary, there is a case for cyclosporine rather than cyclophosphamide as second-line therapy in corticosteroid-resistant patients with FSGS.

The possibility that mycophenolate mofetil (MMF) may have a future in the treatment of FSGS deserves mention. In a study of 46 patients with primary glomerular disease treated with MMF, 18 patients with FSGS experienced a decline in urinary protein excretion without a change in renal function (214). Smaller studies have also demonstrated activity against the disease (215).

Long-Term Outcome with Treatment. In adults, as with other histologic appearances, the prognosis is better for patients with FSGS if urinary protein excretion remains below the nephrotic range (62,216). Few if any patients with subnephrotic proteinuria progress to renal failure within a decade. There are only scant data on children with FSGS who are not nephrotic, perhaps because this is a rather rare finding. In the series of Yoshikawa (217), there was no difference in outcome with degree of proteinuria.

The actuarially calculated 10-year survival rates for renal function in all patients with FSGS have been reported as 38% ± 12% for adults (62) and as 45% ± 21% by Trompeter (*unpublished data, 1978*) for children. In Figure 71-11 is shown the survival curves for nephrotic adults and children with either minimal change disease or FSGS in Guy Hospital. The two curves of 60 adults and 62 children with FSGS are not statistically different. Mongeau et al. (218,219) also emphasized the better prognosis of the children in their series with FSGS, with an overall renal survival rate of 56% at 20 years, suggesting that the difference resides with the type of patient referred to some centers. Much higher rates of ultimate remission have been reported in intensively treated adults by Ponticelli et al. (201), but it must be remembered that in this series, only patients with normal or near-normal renal function were included. Recently, Chun et al. reported a 10-year renal survival of 67% in a cohort of patients mostly treated with corticosteroids; ESRD was uncommon in those who achieved either a compete or partial remission (98).

"Malignant" Focal Segmental Glomerulosclerosis. Brown et al. (220) and Saint-Hillier et al. (216) drew attention to a group of patients whose condition has been called *malignant FSGS.* These patients demonstrated complete resistance to corticosteroids and conventional cytotoxic therapy. Furthermore, they usually had torrential urinary protein loss, with frequent hypovolemic episodes, and were almost always younger than 25 years. These patients had a relentless course to renal failure within only 1 to 4 years from onset of the nephrotic syndrome, maintaining the proteinuria into terminal renal failure and even on to dialysis, so bilateral nephrectomy or renal infarction may be needed (33). Recurrence of equally torrential urinary protein loss in patients with transplanted kidneys may be immediate, with later appearance of typical lesions of FSGS in the allograft and graft failure (163,190). The term *malignant FSGS* has been used also to describe the severe form of FSGS associated in black patients with glomerular "collapse" and very rapid entry into renal failure (186,192,193). When compared with age-matched controls with classic FSGS, patients with the collapsing variant exhibited more rapid progression with a time-course of only 13 months to end-stage renal failure compared with 62.5 months (221).

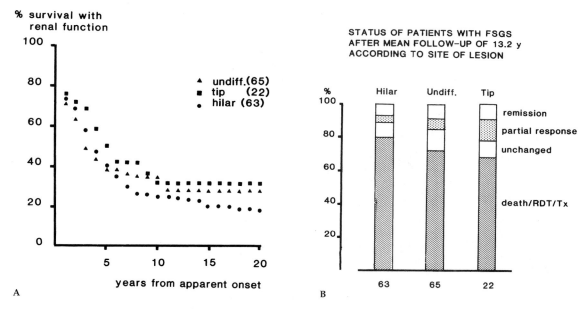

FIGURE 71-12. Data on nephrotic children and adults showing focal segmental glomerular sclerosis in their renal biopsy specimen, seen at Guy's Hospital during a 20-year period. Survival curves (**A**) and status at most recent follow-up (**B**) are shown for 22 patients in whom the site of the lesion could be localized to the glomerular "tip," 63 patients in whom the lesion was perihilar, and 65 patients in whom on the sections available no statement as to localization could be made. Patients with both tip and perihilar lesions were counted as perihilar. There is no difference in outcome between the groups. (From: Chaudhury N, Cameron JS, *unpublished data,* with permission.)

There is also a problem of recurrent FSGS in patients who have received a renal allograft (222–224). This has been attributed to the presence of a circulating factor that was identified using an *in vitro* assay measuring the permeability of rat glomeruli. It has been suggested that prophylactic use of plasmapheresis prior to transplantation may reduce early recurrence by 50% (225). Treatment of established recurrent FSGS with plasmapheresis may also be beneficial; predictors of success may include early therapy (226).

Histologic Pattern and Pathologic Markers in Relation to Outcome

Almost all biopsy tissue from patients with FSGS shows some degree of tubular atrophy, so there is not much use in determining prognosis within the group. Severe tubular atrophy is usually not a good prognostic sign. However, as in almost all other forms of progressive glomerulopathy, interstitial fibrosis emerges from multistep analysis as the major histologic determinant of outcome (227). The clinical correlate of this severe tubular disease is the finding of glycosuria, aminoaciduria (228), and excessive losses of β_2-microglobulin in the urine (229), which may be a clinical indicator of the presence of FSGS. Another important new marker of poor prognosis and poor response to therapy is an elevated fractional excretion of IgG, which is thought to represent a more severe alteration in permselectivity of the glomerular filtration barrier (230).

The lesions of FSGS have a characteristic distribution, often affecting either the perihilar area, known as *classic FSGS,* or the pole of the glomerulus opposite the hilus—named the *glomerular tip lesion* (231–235). Ito et al. (232) found that almost all those children with perihilar lesions progressed to renal failure, whereas those with "tip" lesions adjacent to the exit of the tubule from Bowman's capsule did well. These interesting observations were not confirmed by others (233). Guy's Hospital data show no difference in the rather gloomy long-term outcome of pediatric and adult patients, whatever the site of the lesion (Fig. 71-12). This area of study remains controversial, as described by Chun et al. (98), who presented a series of 87 adults with nephrotic syndrome and biopsy-proven FSGS. Patients with classic, cellular/collapsing, and tip lesions had similar prognosis and response to steroid therapy regardless of the lesion. Even those with collapsing lesions responded to steroids in 64% of cases; 80% of the collapsing patients who responded were free of ESRD at 10 years. It has also been suggested, with more general agreement, that mesangial prominence is an adverse finding (182,236,237), but again, there are data that do not agree with this conclusion (220). Finally, precocious and prominent afferent arteriolar hyalinosis has been noted in patients with a poor outcome for renal function (220), an observation that has been confirmed (238).

Membranous Nephropathy

Membranous nephropathy is a well-documented histologic appearance, presenting in general with proteinuria and affecting principally middle-aged and older adult men (Chapter 63). The short-term (less than 5-year) outcome of membranous nephropathy was extensively documented in adults during the late 1960s and 1970s; the data are reviewed elsewhere (185). In its idiopathic form, membranous nephropathy is a relatively indolent disease in most patients, with few patients entering remission or progressing to renal failure within 5 years of apparent onset; although in contrast to this statement, several observers reported 40% to 50% of patients dead or in renal failure within 5 to 6 years. Others noted a relatively benign outcome within the first 5 years, with the results in other series falling somewhere between the two extremes.

All of these older data have several handicaps. First, patients with idiopathic membranous nephropathy often were not separated from those with identifiable precipitating factors, some of which (e.g., drugs) might improve the overall prognosis and some (e.g., malignancies) might make it worse. Second, a variable proportion had been treated for varying times with a number of agents believed to affect the outcome of the condition. Third, patients with only mild proteinuria were often mixed with those showing a full nephrotic syndrome. Fourth, the numbers in most of these series were small. Finally, the effects of late referral of patients with progressive disease were not considered.

Outlook in Untreated Patients

Over the past two decades, data that avoid some of these criticisms have become available on groups of patients. Noel et al. (239) described the outcome of a group of patients with idiopathic membranous nephropathy, none of whom had received treatment that was believed to be specific. The actuarial survival rate at 10 years was estimated at 75%. Forty-eight percent of the patients were women (now known to do better, as discussed later) and only 78% had a nephrotic syndrome, which again is an indicator of poor prognosis. Donadio et al. (240) followed 140 patients (47 women, 83% nephrotic) for up to 15 years, 89 of whom had received no treatment. They made the valuable comparison between the expected survival of this middle-aged and older adult population of patients with that expected for the population as a whole: There was no difference for the whole population of patients (75% at 10 years) and no difference whether treatment was given or not. The Bergamo group (241) reviewed another large untreated group of 100 patients, of whom 63 were nephrotic, 32 were women, and none had been treated. The 8-year survival rate for renal function was 73% ± 7%, and 42% were in remission and only 30% were still nephrotic. The relatively good outlook reported in these articles contrasted with the control, untreated group in the Interhospitals Study of the nephrotic syndrome reported from the United States in 1979 (95), in which 11 (29%) of 38 untreated patients reached a renal failure endpoint (plasma creatinine concentration of more than 4 mg/dL) within 48 months of entry.

Davison et al. performed a three-center retrospective analysis of 62 untreated patients with idiopathic adult-onset membranous nephropathy, all of whom were nephrotic (242). Of 62 untreated idiopathic nephrotic patients followed for a mean of 4.5 years, only 32 (50%) showed a deterioration in renal function. The rate of change of plasma creatinine concentration was only approximately linear for each patient, but the slopes of the data vary greatly from patient to patient. Three patients went into renal failure within 2 years of onset of a nephrotic syndrome, as previously described by Coggins (168) in untreated patients, and by the end of 5 years, only 9 (14%) had started dialysis. Data on untreated patients are available from four further prospective controlled trials in nephrotic patients, from Italy (243,244), Canada (245), and the United Kingdom (164). A total of 190 control patients were entered into these trials using roughly the same criteria (data from the Canadian trial are included here only for those patients with a nephrotic syndrome). After a follow-up averaging just less than 5 years, 18 patients (11%) had actually started dialysis, and at least 9 more patients (6%) had plasma creatinine concentrations of more than 400 μmol/L (data not available in the report by Ponticelli et al. (243).

Other series of untreated patients have also been studied and reported from individual units: Donadio (240), 89 patients; Honkanen et al. (246), 19 patients; Kida et al. (247), 45 patients; Murphy et al. (248), 79 patients; and a large collected series (249). Although not all the patients in these studies had a nephrotic syndrome, these series in general confirmed the apparently better prognosis—at least during the first decade—found in recent studies of untreated membranous nephropathy.

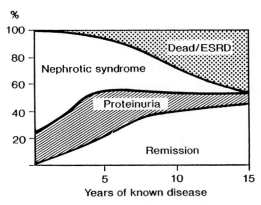

FIGURE 71-13. The course of membranous nephropathy, summarized from J.S. Cameron's data and the literature up to 1978. The evolution is relatively slow, and remissions and entry to uremia may occur more than 15 years after onset, although some patients evolve much more rapidly. *ESRD*, end-stage renal disease.

Estimated 10-year renal survival rates were 77% (249), 81% (248), 64% (240), 82% (246), and 92% (247). Figure 71-13 has thus been modified from that in previous editions of this book, in light of these more recent data, to show that more than 40% of patients with adult-onset membranous nephropathy will go into remission and only about 10% enter into renal failure or die within 10 years. Although some 10- to 15-year data are available (250–252) from long-term studies of patients studied earlier, which suggest a 50% renal failure/mortality rate at this time, little 20-year outcome is available. An exception is a recent national report on Japanese patients with idiopathic membranous nephropathy (253); the 20-year survival was 60.5%, despite excellent renal survival at 10 years (90%) and 15 years (81%). It is thus likely that only 40% of all patients with membranous nephropathy eventually experience renal failure, even if a nephrotic syndrome is present to begin with.

Relapses

Another change in the evaluation of the outcome in membranous nephropathy has been the realization that relapses and a relapsing course are not that rare. For example, of the 141 patients who went into remission in the controlled trials just cited (95,164,243,245)—either spontaneously or in apparent response to treatment—46 subsequently had relapse; of these, only 8 were among 39 untreated patients, perhaps suggesting a higher relapse rate in patients with corticosteroid-induced remissions. Passerini et al. (56) examined the prognostic implications of complete remission of proteinuria after treatment, even if it returns. In 33 patients followed for a median of 8 years, none showed an abnormal plasma creatinine concentration, although half had a relapse, 9 with a full nephrotic syndrome. Using Kaplan-Meier statistics, they estimated that two-thirds of those who go into remission will have a further relapse of proteinuria before 10 years have gone by.

Problems for Trials of Treatment of Membranous Nephropathy

The realization that the prognosis for membranous nephropathy with regard to renal function is better than formerly supposed presents formidable problems in the design and conduct of therapeutic trials. First, the rather good survival and spontaneous tendency toward remission make it difficult to show improvement in terms of renal or patient survival, at least within the usual length of trials in practice. Therefore, trial endpoints

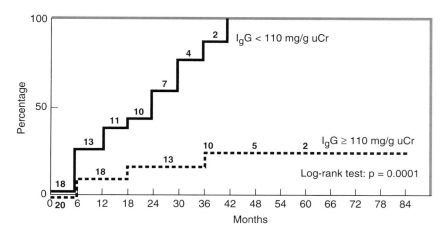

FIGURE 71-14. In a study of 38 patients with membranous nephropathy, nephrotic syndrome, and normal renal function (sCr, 0.99 ± 0.20 mg/dL), probability of complete or partial remission was highly dependent on urinary IgG excretion values less than 110 mg/g uCr versus 110 mg/g uCr or greater. (From: Bazzi C et al. Urinary excretion of IgG and alpha(1)-microglobulin predicts clinical course better than extent of proteinuria in membranous nephropathy. *Am J Kidney Dis* 2001;38:240, with permission.)

must depend on levels of renal function and urinary protein excretion. Second, any trial that randomizes patients at apparent onset will result in the control group including three or four of every 10 patients who will have a remission spontaneously within 5 years and thus can only have side effects without benefit from the treatment. Thus, it may be preferable to treat patients with nonspecific therapy (ACE-inhibition, hyperlipidemic therapies, blood pressure control) for 6 months prior to cytotoxic therapy or enrollment in a clinical trial.

Predictors of Poor Prognosis

Possible interventions and trials in membranous nephropathy are discussed in detail in Chapter 63. In this discussion, we consider which criteria might allow us to predict entry to renal failure at or near onset in idiopathic membranous nephropathy (252).

Clinically, several features seem to carry a poorer prognosis in univariate analysis: male sex (242,254–256), increasing age (242), urinary protein loss in excess of the nephrotic range (66,239,242,255), reduced renal function (239,242,249, 256,257), and raised blood pressure (240,249,255). Of these, persistent proteinuria is probably the strongest predictor of renal failure in multivariate analysis; initial creatinine clearance and decline in creatinine clearance have also been demonstrated as independent predictors (66). Kobayashi et al. (257) considered in detail the prognosis of non-nephrotic patients with membranous nephropathy. Of 123 patients with membranous nephropathy and subnephrotic proteinuria, including 18 of their own patients, only 13 (10%) had gone into renal failure over a mean follow-up of 4 years, even though 40 had later developed a full nephrotic syndrome. Twenty-five (22%) were in complete remission. In a recent update comparing Canadian data to those of other populations in Italy and Finland, a predictive model has been outlined and validated (258). The most important factor determining long-term outcome in patients with membranous nephropathy was found to be the highest level of proteinuria sustained over 6 months. The model was able to predict patients at high risk of progression with an accuracy of more than 85%, despite differences at baseline.

Genetically, in white populations a strong association between membranous nephropathy and the whole major histocompatibility complex haplotype HLA-A1, B8, DR3, and each of its component genes has been described, whereas in Japanese populations, the association is with HLA-DR2 (Chapter 63). Despite some earlier data that suggested correlations between outcome and major histocompatibility complex type among white populations (259), the largest study to date, that of the

British MRC trial (164), failed to reveal any associations between either HLA or Bf allotypes and outcome in more than 100 patients with nephrotic syndrome and idiopathic membranous nephropathy.

Urinary markers have also been explored as predictors of eventual renal failure in idiopathic membranous nephropathy. In a prospective study, urinary excretion of beta-2 microglobulin and IgG were found to have sensitivities of 88% and specificities of 88% and 91%, respectively, for the development of eventual renal failure in a group of patients with nephrotic syndrome and serum creatinine (SCr) less than 1.5 mg/dL. When the two tests were combined, specificity reached 97% (260). Similarly, excretion of N-acetyl-beta-glucosaminidase was also found to be superior to total protein excretion in predicting prognosis and response to treatment, as was IgG and beta-2 microglobulin (24, 25, 261). These studies bring optimism to the idea that prognostic information as well as selection of patients for treatment may be possible with noninvasive urinary studies (Fig. 71-14).

Patients with milder (class I and II) glomerular disease (239,249,251) as determined by histopathologic evaluation have been suggested to do better than those with class III and IV lesions, but several other groups failed to find any correlation (242,250,256). Bohle et al. (262) and others (250) noted that interstitial lesions best predicted a poor outcome, and more recently Wehrmann et al. (249) performed a multivariate analysis confirming that tubulointerstitial lesions predict a poor outcome better than any other criterion; Ponticelli et al. (244) came to the same conclusion. In addition, if phenotype of the interstitial infiltrate is determined, the numbers of both monocytes and helper T cells in the interstitium predict the GFR after 5 years of follow-up (263).

Some patients show focal sclerosing lesions (264), which may have some value in predicting outcome. Vascular lesions have also predicted outcome in a univariate analysis with long-term follow-up (250). Finally a few patients with membranous nephropathy develop crescentic nephritis (265–267), with or without circulating antiglomerular basement membrane (anti-GBM) antibody. A poorer prognosis is experienced by these unfortunate patients, but luckily they are rare.

As in most glomerular diseases, in membranous nephropathy, once renal function begins to fall, it usually continues to decline at a varying rate over the following years until ESRD is reached (242). However, one or two circumstances may lead to acute reversible declines in renal function; these include renal venous thrombosis, the appearance of a spontaneous or drug-induced acute interstitial nephritis, and the formation of new crescents, as just discussed. In the course of the tri-hospital study (242), it became apparent that some patients with membranous nephropathy might show a reversible decline in function without any of these circumstances being present; in the MRC trial (164), six patients showed remarkable slowing in renal function loss and one showed reversal of decline without any identifiable event or intervention such as control of hypertension, treatment with immunosuppressive agents, or use of low-protein diets. This obviously needs to be considered when evaluating the data of serial renal function studies in relation to late treatment interventions.

Treatment History

The treatment of membranous nephropathy is discussed in detail in Chapter 63; therefore, only salient aspects are discussed here. Whether major differences in the outcome of adult nephrotic patients with idiopathic membranous nephropathy emerge from treatment with cytotoxic agents and corticosteroids remains contentious (101,268–272).

Membranous Nephropathy in Children. In white children, membranous nephropathy is rare, accounting for only 1% of nephrotic syndromes in childhood in the unselected data of the ISKDC. However, in some areas of the world, particularly in Asia and Poland, membranous nephropathy in association with hepatitis B virus carriage accounts for 5% to 15% of nephrotic syndromes in childhood (92,271,273).

Therefore, 40% of children have some associated disease, principally infections (273), contrasting with only about 20% to 25% of adults (274,275). Because patients with such forms of membranous nephropathy usually do well, it is not surprising that the overall prognosis for children with membranous nephropathy is good; however, even in children with the apparently idiopathic form, the outlook is much better than it is in adults, with less than 10% going into renal failure. Such an evolution is almost unknown with onset before the age of 10 and rare with onset before the age of 20 (274). One interesting observation is that children with membranous nephropathy never, and adolescents very rarely, develop renal venous thrombosis.

Membranous Nephropathy in Adults. About one-third of adult patients with membranous nephropathy reach end-stage renal failure. What can be done to alter this outcome? Based on a critical review of the literature, high-dose oral steroids should not be used as sole therapy because they are ineffective in either producing a sustained remission of the nephrotic syndrome or preserving renal function (101,272). The use of azathioprine is not associated with any significant benefits and is therefore not justified. The alkylating agents cyclophosphamide and chlorambucil are efficacious in the management of membranous nephropathy (272,276,277). Because of their long-term toxicities, use of these drugs should be reserved for patients with a moderate-to-high likelihood of progression to ESRD (severe proteinuria and renal insufficiency). Alkylating agents should always be used with steroids. Cyclosporine has a growing role in the treatment of membranous nephropathy; some have suggested that it may be more effective than cytotoxic agents in patients at highest risk of progression, that is, those with renal failure and/or greater than 8 g of protein per/day (207,278). Other agents, such as MMF and rituximab, will be discussed in Chapter 63; long-term results for these agents are not yet available (279–282). Based on the decision model by Sarasin and Schifferli (52), prophylactic anticoagulation is suggested to be beneficial in membranous nephropathy patients with persistent nephrotic syndrome and albumin levels of less than 2g/dL. However, no randomized controlled trial has been done to study the effect of anticoagulation in these patients.

PROGNOSIS OF DISEASES ASSOCIATED WITH GLOMERULONEPHRITIS

IgA-Associated Nephropathy (Berger's Disease)

Despite almost 40 years of research, we still do not know whether the IgA present in the mesangium plays any role in glomerular injury or what the significance of the raised serum IgA concentrations, the IgA-containing immune complexes, or IgA autoantibodies in the serum may be (283). In addition, it must be noted that classifying patients with glomerular disease by the presence or absence of predominant IgA on immunohistology cuts across both clinical presentation and conventional histologic classifications, as outlined already here and elsewhere in this book. There is great variability in disease progression for patients who are given the diagnosis of IgA nephropathy. On the one hand, this variability of outcomes raises doubts regarding the current definition and diagnosis of IgA nephropathy. On the other hand, such diverse outcomes also emphasize the need to identify those patients with a worse prognosis whenever possible.

Because IgA-associated nephropathy commonly presents without symptoms through abnormal findings on urine tests, there is considerable possibility for variation in any population of patients under study, for example, depending on whether systematic urine testing of schoolchildren has been performed, as in some Japanese reports, or testing of the urine in all army recruits, as in Singapore. Furthermore, the local criteria for performing a renal biopsy becomes critical; if it is policy simply to watch patients with isolated hematuria, then a group with a generally favorable prognosis will be excluded. If in contrast all such patients undergo a biopsy, then the group of patients with isolated symptomless hematuria and isolated mesangial IgA will be included and "improve" the prognosis of that particular series.

The prognosis of IgA nephropathy has been examined in considerable detail, perhaps because of the large number of cases available worldwide (72). A series of conferences (held in Milan in 1983) was devoted to the subject of IgA nephropathy (284), and other useful reviews have been published (72,285–289) including two meta-analyses (287,289). The reader is also referred to Chapter 61 of this book.

IgA Nephropathy in Adults

All reports describing IgA-associated disease suggest a condition of indolent evolution toward healing or renal damage, although an aggressive course associated with extensive crescents may be seen in a few patients (290,291). In general, the entry into renal dysfunction and finally failure is slower in IgA nephropathy than in any of the other diseases discussed in this chapter (289,292), occurring over a time scale of 30 years or more (Table 71-3), in contrast to the 5 to 15 years that is more usual in other glomerulopathies. This may reflect earlier diagnosis in patients with macroscopic hematuria, but many patients with the slowest evolution into renal failure present with symptomless urinary abnormalities on casual urine testing.

The long-term outcome of several large series of adult patients with IgA nephropathy has been described (286,293–297) and the literature summarized (287,289). Schena (289) highlighted the differing proportions of patients with hypertension, already elevated plasma creatinine concentrations, macroscopic hematuria, and profuse proteinuria noted in differing

TABLE 71-3

ACTUARIAL RENAL SURVIVAL AT 10 YEARS AND CLINICAL FEATURES AT PRESENTATION IN LARGE POPULATIONS OF ADULT PATIENTS WITH IgA NEPHROPATHY ACCORDING TO THE MOST ACCURATE STUDIES IN THE LITERATURE

Reference	Country	No. of patients	Mean age at presentation (y)	High serum creatinine (%)	High blood pressure (%)	Proteinuria >3 g/24 hr (%)	History of macroscopic hematuria (%)	Mean duration of follow-up (mo)	Actuarial renal survival at 10 years (%)
Europe									
D'amico et al. (1986) (298)	Italy	365	29	24	36	7	55	79	85[a]
Beukof et al. (1986) (303)	The Netherlands	75	24	—	37	—	46	92	84[a]
Droz et al. (1984) (297), Noël et al. (1987) (628)	France	280	—	—	6	10	37	>60	85[a]
Velo et al. (1987) (629)	Spain	153	22	—	—	1	78	>60	81[a]
Bogenschütz et al. (1990) (630)	Germany	239	—	34	19	—	26	59	81[b]
Rekola et al. (1989,1990) (631,632)	Finland	209	25	16	11	1	64	76	83[c]
Alamartine et al. (1991) (304)	France	282	28	2	9	3	27	96	94[a]
Johnston et al. (1992) (296)	UK	220	30	28	26	32	—	65	83[a]
Australia									
Nicholls et al. (1984) (305)		244	32	36	43	6	39	60	87[c]
Ibels et al. (1994) (633)		121	39	36	31	16	40	107	93[a]
Asia									
Woo et al. (1986) (294)	Singapore	151	27	6	33	4	24	65	82[a]
Kusumoto et al. (1987) (320)	Japan	87	27	—	31	15	—	114	80[a]
Katafuchi et al. (1994) (308)	Japan	225	32	36	22	16	20	48	74[c]
Yagame et al. (1996) (287)	Japan	206	30	—	—	—	—	110	87[c]
Koyama et al. (1997) (634)	Japan	448	>10 in 95%	19	29	3	24	142	85[a]
United States									
Wyatt et al. (1984) (635)		58	27	—	47	—	—	>60	78[a]
Radford et al. (1997) (636)		148	39	59	49	30	—	45	67[c]
Haas et al. (1997) (637)		109	~40	Mean = 2.2 ± 1.9 mg/dL		33	35	>18	57[a]

Clinical features at presentation

[a] After the first manifestation.
[b] Not specified.
[c] After the biopsy.
(Reprinted from: D'Amico G. Natural history of idiopathic IgA nephropathy: role of clinical and histological prognostic factors. *Am J Kid Dis* 2000;36(2):227, with permission.)

parts of the world such as Europe, North America, East Asia, and Australia, which are bound to influence final data on follow-up (see later discussion). He also drew attention to the fact that in the reports from North America, follow-up was notably shorter than that elsewhere in the world, which again will affect reported outcomes. Various studies have reported renal survival rates between 57% to 94% after 10 years (287). Studies from the United States have reported worse renal outcomes than those in Europe and Asia, perhaps due to the inclusion of a more severely ill patient population (287). At least 25%—and maybe 50%—of adult patients with IgA nephropathy will end up in renal failure; the proportion of the remainder that may develop renal insufficiency as well in their third, fourth, or fifth decades is unknown.

IgA nephropathy has been examined in great detail for factors that may predict prognosis for groups of patients (294,298–302) and for individuals (303) using univariate and multivariate (72,303,304) techniques. Clinically, proteinuria (especially if profuse), hypertension, and a raised plasma creatinine concentration were determinants of a poorer prognosis in most studies. Male sex is a risk factor for a poor prognosis in several studies in which it has been examined (287). Macroscopic hematuria has given discordant results: Bennett and Kincaid-Smith (292) pointed to a poorer prognosis in patients with macroscopic hematuria, a conclusion reinforced in a later paper from this group (305), whereas all other studies, including those of D'Amico (286) and Beukhof (303), showed that macroscopic hematuria is a favorable sign. In multivariate analyses (298,303), proteinuria was the single most powerful clinical predictor of a poor outcome and the only independent clinical variable.

Pathologically, interstitial scarring is the most powerful predictor (298,303), along with number of crescents (306), vascular hyaline lesions (307), the number of obsolescent glomeruli and the degree of glomerular segmental sclerosis (308), and proliferation. Several groups (309–312) counted and determined the phenotype of the cells infiltrating the interstitium in IgA nephropathy and related these findings to prognosis. It has also been observed that only the rather small numbers of interstitial B cells correlated with rapid entry to renal failure (309), an interesting finding in view of the general B-cell overactivity in this condition. This area deserves further study.

Studies suggest that a polymorphism in the ACE gene may have an impact on the progression of IgA nephropathy. The polymorphism consists of insertion (I) or deletion (D) of a 287-bp DNA fragment, which may be the silencer portion of the ACE gene (313). The DD genotype of the ACE gene is found more frequently in patients with progressive IgA nephropathy than is the ID or II genotype. This was supported by a study done by Pei et al., in which polymorphisms in the ACE gene

were important markers for predicting progression to chronic renal failure in 168 white patients with IgA nephropathy (314). In another study and meta-analysis by Schena et al. (315), however, the ACE gene polymorphisms did not correlate with disease progression. No relationship of the disease has been found with the angiotensin II receptor gene (313,316,317).

There are surprisingly few data on entry into complete remission for adults with IgA nephropathy. Nicholls et al. (305) noted that only 6% of their patients had entered remission after 5 years of follow-up, and Kitajima et al. (318), in a collaborative study of 1,394 adults, found only 6.5% after an average of 36 months; Schena (289) did not address the question in his otherwise admirable review, perhaps because so few authors comment on this aspect. Consequently, we simply do not know what proportion of adult patients will be in complete remission with normal urine after, say, 20 years. One is left with the impression that even in those with persisting normal renal function, at least for a decade or two, urinary abnormalities persist in the great majority.

IgA nephropathy is notably uncommon in blacks, although it is frequent in whites and Asians. One study of long-term outcome in black patients with IgA nephropathy found no difference from that of white patients (319).

IgA Nephropathy in Children

Although IgA nephropathy is a common form of glomerulopathy in children, documentation of the longer term outlook has not been extensive until recently. A relatively benign outlook for children presenting with hematuria, macroscopic or microscopic, was noted in the past (290,292) but did not include histologic data or information on the presence or absence of IgA. Levy et al. (290) described one of the larger follow-up studies on 91 children with IgA nephropathy, and their data are summarized in Table 71-4. Only eight children developed renal failure (six terminal, two more modest) within the follow-up period (mean, 13.5 years); the 10-year survival rate was estimated to be 92% ± 2%. Most patients in this series had macroscopic hematuria at some point in their course, 66 at presentation, and only 7 had microscopic hematuria associated with proteinuria. Levy et al. (290) noted 800 children previously described in the literature, with only 8 patients entering renal failure 5 to 44 years after onset and another 11 showing some degree of renal insufficiency 3 to 17 years after onset.

Data are available also from Japanese children, in whom IgA-associated nephropathy is particularly common. The study of Kitajima et al. (318), included in Levy's analysis of the literature, summarized data collected from 491 Japanese children;

TABLE 71-4

PROGNOSIS OF IgA-ASSOCIATED GLOMERULONEPHRITIS IN CHILDREN

Appearance on optical microscopy	N	Subsequent behavior 1–16 (mean, 5.6) years			
		No. with recurrent macroscopic hematuria	Remission	Nephrotic syndrome	Renal failure
Minimal changes	26	25	16	0	0
Mesangial proliferation only	3	3	1	0	0
Focal segmental proliferative glomerulonephritis + mesangial proliferation	41	28	14	0	0
Proliferative glomerulonephritis + crescents	21	13	2	0	8
	91	69	33	0	8

(Reprinted from: Levy M, et al. Berger's disease in children: natural history and outcome. *Medicine (Baltimore)* 1985;64:151, with permission.)

only 9 developed chronic renal failure or died. Kusumoto et al. (320) reported on 98 children with IgA nephropathy, with renal failure occurring in only 9 and an estimated 10-year survival rate of 94%. Most of these children presented with proteinuria and hematuria, and only two with isolated hematuria. Yoshikawa et al. (321,322) reported on follow-up of 200 Japanese children with IgA-associated nephropathy. Only 2 of 83 children younger than 8 years at apparent onset went into renal failure, but follow-up was relatively short (5.5 ± 2.8 years). A much higher proportion than in an adult series (93 of 200) had normal urine by this time. Of 117 children aged 9 to 15 years at onset, 8 went into renal failure after a similar brief period. In Kusumoto's study (320), the outlook for renal function was significantly poorer in 86 patients with adult-onset disease studied in parallel, so a gradient of poorer prognosis with age at onset seems to be present.

Therefore, the overall prognosis in the medium term seems to be generally good for children with IgA-associated nephropathy. However, the very slow evolution of the disease must not be forgotten. After 10 years in Levy's study, only one-third of patients were in complete remission with normal urine, and the longer term fate (20 or 30 years) of such patients has not been established. Other authors have emphasized the poorer prognosis of their pediatric patients with IgA nephropathy (323,324), probably because of referral and biopsy policies determining that only patients with more severe disease reach tertiary referral centers. In children, the same prognostic indicators as those in adults, although less extensively studied (323), have emerged as indicators of a poorer early prognosis; on histology, extensive crescent formation, interstitial fibrosis, and sclerosing glomerular lesions carry a poorer outlook. Clinically, proteinuria, hypertension, and older age at onset seem the most important variables.

Unusual Patterns of Evolution in IgA Nephropathy

A particular feature of IgA-associated nephropathy is that although generally proteinuria has been an adverse factor in determining prognosis, a small but widespread number of patients have been described in whom a full nephrotic syndrome, normal renal function, and prompt response—and often a relapsing course—followed corticosteroid therapy (325). These patients, more often children than adults, almost always show only minimal changes on optical microscopy, although some show mesangial expansion or even FSGS. However, in the few patients examined by electron microscopy, characteristic electron-dense aggregates have been absent. Whether these patients represent a subset of IgA-associated nephropathy or the coincidence of minimal change nephropathy with symptomless IgA deposition within the mesangium, as may occur in the healthy population (e.g., organ donors), is not known. Many of the patients described in the literature, even from non-Asian countries, are ethnic Chinese.

Another unusual pattern in IgA nephropathy is recurrent attacks of acute renal failure (326), first described by Talwalkar et al. (327) in 1978. It has been proposed that the acute hematuria is toxic to renal tubules (292,301), and red blood cells ingested by the tubules have been demonstrated, which is supported by a report of a hematuric patient who did not have IgA nephropathy (328). These patients must be distinguished from those going into acute renal insufficiency because of crescentic glomerulonephritis (290,292), and thus a repeated renal biopsy is usually necessary.

Treatment of IgA Nephropathy

The reader is referred to Chapter 61 for the details of treatment. The effect of treatment on the outcomes reported in various series is difficult to determine, but recent evidence suggests that treatment does affect the long-term outcome. Although D'Amico noted that there have been similar results in those studies reported before and after the widespread use of ACE inhibitors (287), several studies have now shown a benefit for patients treated with ACE inhibitors (329–332), and all proteinuric patients should probably be treated with these agents. Previously it was felt that patients with proteinuria of more than 3 g per day and preserved renal function should be treated with steroids to reduce proteinuria and stabilize renal function (333,334). Pozzi et al. also recently reported the 10-year follow-up data for a cohort of patients with mild initial renal disease (plasma creatinine ≤1.5 mg/dL and urinary protein excretion of 1 to 3.5 g per day) who were randomized to treatment with steroids for 6 months or supportive treatment. In this study, treatment with steroids significantly improved renal survival and led to a statistically significant reduction in the percentage of patients who doubled their plasma creatinine (335). In patients with progressive disease, fish oil may be tried because there is some benefit seen in some studies (336,337). In a 6-year follow-up study of the earlier trial (338), Donadio et al. concluded that early and prolonged treatment with fish oil slows renal progression for high-risk patients with IgA nephropathy. Cyclosporine has not been shown to be of benefit.

Membranoproliferative Glomerulonephritis

Since the early 1970s it has been the practice to divide the light microscopic appearances of membranoproliferative glomerulonephritis (MPGN, also mesangiocapillary glomerulonephritis) (Chapter 62) into two categories: the more common variety with subendothelial immune aggregates (type I), and a variety with extensive replacement of the lamina densa of the capillary basement membranes and those of the tubules and Bowman's capsule, with a birefringent, rather continuous material that takes stains avidly (type II). On light microscopy, not all type I patients with MPGN show a true mesangiocapillary pattern—that is, expansion of the mesangium with a complex thickening of the glomerular capillary walls by mesangial cell cytoplasm and new material. Some authors (339–342) distinguish a "type III" MPGN in which the immune aggregates are found by electron microscopy not only at a subendothelial site, but also throughout the basement membrane with subepithelial aggregates, so that in isolation the appearances resemble those of an advanced membranous nephropathy. Some authors regard this as a later stage of type I MPGN and it is so treated in this chapter.

One striking feature of data from Europe has been the decline in the number of new patients presenting with either type of MPGN (343,344), suggesting that some precipitating environmental agent or agents, most probably infectious, has declined in frequency. MPGN has always been unusual in adults and children in Japan, although it is very common in other parts of the world: In Iran, MPGN is the underlying histologic appearance in two-thirds of adult-onset nephrotic syndromes (345). MPGN may be seen complicating various infections and as part of systemic disorders. Infection-related MPGN needs to be separated from the apparently idiopathic disorder, because the outlook for infection-related MPGN, whether from endocarditis (346), infected juguloatrial shunts (347), or deep sepsis (347), is generally good, provided that the infection can be controlled. The prognosis of MPGN in a setting of lupus or Henoch-Schönlein purpura (HSP) is considered in later sections of this chapter.

Long-Term Outcome

The survival of patients with idiopathic type I or type II MPGN was documented in a number of series during the 1970s and a

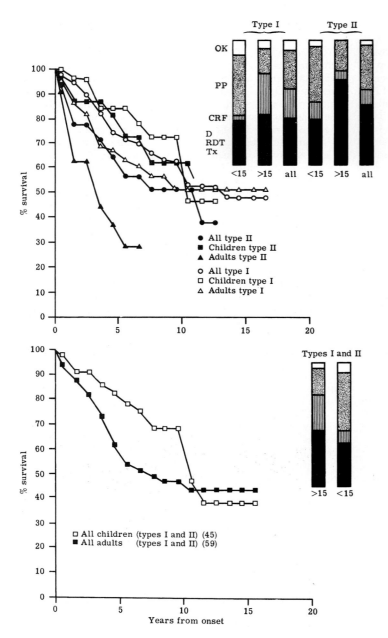

FIGURE 71-15. (Top) Survival and status at last follow-up evaluation in patients with mesangioproliferative glomerulonephritis (MPGN). The survival curves were calculated by the actuarial method. None of the curves differ from each other when tested by the log-rank method (Peto et al. [1]), although the adult patients with type II MPGN approach significance when compared with similar children ($p = 0.08$). The most recent status is shown at top right: OK, well, normal urine, normal renal function; PP, persistent proteinuria with or without a nephrotic syndrome but with normal renal function; CRF, glomerular filtration rate of less than 80 mL per minute/1.73 m² and persistent proteinuria with or without a nephrotic syndrome; D, RDT, Tx, dead, regular dialysis treatment, or transplantation. Data are presented for each of type I and II MPGN for patients older and younger than 15 years at apparent onset. In type I MPGN, children have a significantly better prognosis than adults ($p <0.01$) compared in this fashion. Similarly, data for types I and II together show a significant difference ($p = 0.003$). In the case of patients with type II alone, the differences between children ($N = 22$) and adults ($N = 13$) were not significant ($p = 0.12$). (Bottom) Survival in children and adults with MPGN. There is no significant difference between the two curves, although there is an excess of early deaths among the adult patients. When the data for most recent status are examined, there is a significantly worse prognosis for adults than children ($\kappa^2 = 7.74$; $p = 0.003$). (From: Cameron JS, et al. Idiopathic mesangiocapillary glomerulonephritis: comparison of types I and II in children and adults and long-term prognosis. *Am J Med* 1983;74:175, with permission.)

few more recent sets of data. These show that in general MPGN of either type is usually a progressive disorder in white and Chinese (67) populations, with the estimated survival rate for renal function at 10 years being about 60% and the 15-year survival rate being no more than 50%. In agreement with this, a large study from Italy (348) found an estimated 10-year survival rate of 60% to 65%. Because the patients in general are children or young adults (67,129), the impact of nonrenal deaths is minor compared with that of membranous nephropathy, for example, and near 100% survival for at least 10 years can be expected for the control population. Data from MPGN type I are rather concordant, whereas those for type II show much more varied outcomes, perhaps because of the small number of patients studied in individual series. In general, no form of treatment appears to affect the outcome of either form of MPGN, with the exception of a single series discussed later in this chapter, so untreated and treated patients are not separated in the data presented here.

Follow-up data have been reported for 104 patients (349), both children and adults (69 type I and 35 type II) who had idiopathic disease. These data (Fig. 71-15) are in general agreement with other published data, with only 7 patients showing complete remission. The group of the Hospital des Enfants Malades in Paris presented its data from children in the same year (350). Complete remission was equally rare; this occurred in only 1 patient with type II and 4 patients with type I MPGN of 44 and 84 patients with idiopathic MPGN, respectively. Of the 44 patients with type II MPGN, 18 were either dead or in ESRD, 1 was uremic, 11 had a persisting nephrotic syndrome, and 11 had persisting proteinuria and normal renal function. Of the 84 patients with type I MPGN, 21 were dead or in ESRD treatment, 9 had chronic renal failure, 18 had a persisting nephrotic syndrome, and 32 had persisting proteinuria with normal renal function.

In type II MPGN, only two groups noted a better prognosis. In children Klein et al. (351) found that 5 of 18 patients were in remission after 11 ± 1 year of follow-up. Similarly, Strife et al. (342) reported 17 children with type II MPGN, with only 4 showing progressive disease and 3 being nephrotic, whereas no child presenting with subnephrotic proteinuria showed progression.

Finally, controlled trials in the United States (352,353) gave some data on serial GFRs in adult patients with type I MPGN. In the former trial (352), over 18 months, the control group lost 9 mL/minute and the treatment group did marginally worse, at 14 mL/minute. In the Mayo Clinic trial (353), the control group lost a mean of 19 mL/minute over 1 year, whereas those treated with aspirin and dipyridamole lost only 5 mL/minute. However, long-term follow-up results were identical in the two groups despite continued treatment (353). The rate of fall-off in renal function was varied, as in membranous nephropathy; Chan et al. (67) analyzed rates of change in $1/P_{creat}$ and noted similarly wide variations in rates of decline in renal function.

Indicators of Prognosis

Several groups studying type I MPGN (67,349,354) were able to identify *clinical* indicators of a poor prognosis using univariate analysis (Table 71-5). As in most forms of progressive glomerular disease, and in most other MPGN series, a nephrotic syndrome—particularly if persistent—was a major clinical indicator of a poor outcome, but Schmitt et al. (354) did not confirm this observation. Hypertension was modestly predictive of a poor outcome in both sets of data (67,349), but there was (in sharp contrast to membranous nephropathy) no difference in outcomes between adults and children. In one series, the presence, absence, or degree of hypocomplementemia had no relation to outcomes in either type of MPGN, suggesting that the prominent *in vivo* complement breakdown is an epiphenomenon of the disease, although Swainson et al. (355) and Klein et al. (351) reported the opposite in smaller series. Magil et al. (57) found that men did worse than women, as in other forms of glomerular disease, but this trend did not reach significance.

Hardly surprising, reduced GFR or elevated plasma creatinine concentration (354) at presentation had an adverse effect on outcome. Donadio et al. (352) found that onset with an acute nephritic syndrome and macroscopic hematuria (common in children) was an adverse feature, and Bennett et al. (356) noted a higher incidence of macroscopic hematuria in patients with type II MPGN who did poorly. The presence of hypertension is controversial; Schmitt et al. found it to be a strong predictor of adverse outcome and a major direct cause of death (354), whereas others (67) found no effect on outlook.

On *histologic* evaluation, crescents have been shown to indicate a worse prognosis (67,344,350). Schmitt et al. (354) performed a more elaborate analysis of the glomerular histology, with five grades, the last of which included crescent formation; patients with this last grade did worst of all. Although Barbiano di Belgiojoso et al. (344) noted a poorer prognosis for those patients with more lobular forms of glomerulonephritis, Schmitt's data did not support this suggestion. Schmitt et al. (354) also assessed interstitial changes carefully and found, as in other glomerular diseases, that the degree of tubulointerstitial changes was strongly predictive of outcome (Fig. 71-16).

Possible Effects of Treatment

Treatment in adults and children with idiopathic MPGN is reserved for patients with nephrotic-range proteinuria, interstitial disease on biopsy, or impaired renal function—all markers for poor prognosis.

Children. One group (357–359) has consistently stated that their treatment results—using alternate-day, high-dose oral prednisolone—have been significantly better than those in children with type I MPGN managed in other centers, with a 10-year survival rate for renal function of 82% but falling to 56% after 20 years. Another group supported the idea that this may represent an improvement in prognosis induced by the high-dose, alternate-day corticosteroid regimen used (360). Likewise, the ISKDC (361), which was a prospective randomized controlled trial using steroids, showed that 61% of the treatment group and 12% of the placebo group had stable renal function at the end of the study.

Adults. A study using aspirin and dipyridamole demonstrated a clinically significant effect of reduction in proteinuria in the treatment group but no change in GFR (362). The general

---

TABLE 71-5

EFFECT OF FEATURES AT ONSET ON PROGNOSIS FOR RENAL FUNCTION IN TYPE I AND TYPE II MESANGIOCAPILLARY GLOMERULONEPHRITIS

	Type I		Type II		All	
	"Dead"[a] vs. alive	"Uremia"[b] vs. persistent proteinuria and remission	"Dead" vs. alive	"Uremia" vs. persistent proteinuria and remission	"Dead" vs. alive	"Uremia" vs. persistent proteinuria and remission
Child or adult (< or >15 yr)	NS[c]	<0.001	(0.07)	NS	NS	0.003
Hematuria at onset	NS	NS	NS	NS	0.003	NS
Nephrotic syndrome at onset	0.01	NS	NS	NS	0.02	NS
Nephrotic syndrome at any time	0.001	0.06	0.04	NS	0.0001	0.003
Blood pressure elevated at onset	0.03	NS	NS	NS	NS	NS
Glomerular filtration rate decreased at onset	(0.07)	0.002	NS	NS	NS	NS

[a] "Dead," dead, dialysis, or transplantation.
[b] "Uremia," "dead" or persistent disease with glomerular filtration rate <80 mL/minute/1.73 m^2.
[c] NS = p >0.05 (χ^2 test).
(Reprinted from: Cameron JS, et al. Idiopathic mesangiocapillary glomerulonephritis: comparison of types I and II in children and adults and long-term prognosis. *Am J Med* 1983;74:175, with permission.)

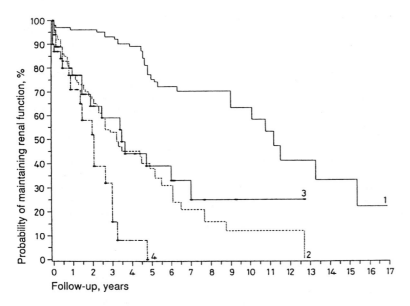

FIGURE 71-16. Probability of entering renal failure in patients with membranoproliferative glomerulonephritis type I, according to the degree of interstitial changes. Curve 1 is derived from 92 patients with a normal interstitium in the initial biopsy; curve 2, from 77 patients with interstitial fibrosis only; curve 3, from 32 patients with tubular damage only; and curve 4, from 19 patients with both tubular damage and interstitial fibrosis present. (From: Schmitt H, et al. Long-term prognosis of membranoproliferative glomerulonephritis type I. Significance of clinical and morphological parameters: an investigation of 220 cases. *Nephron* 1990;55:242, with permission.)

opinion is that no treatment reliably affects the long-term outlook of MPGN in adults.

Postinfectious Glomerulonephritis

In patients with postinfectious glomerulonephritis, there are particular problems with definition, as mentioned in the first section in this chapter (see also Chapter 58). Different observers may be writing about different types of patients, and it is essential to be absolutely clear about which are and perhaps even more important which are not the subject of study. Three main sets of observations help to define this group of patients: the clinical presentation (an acute nephritic syndrome), a precipitating event (e.g., documented antecedent streptococcal infection), and the histopathology involving exclusively, or at least predominantly, the endocapillary wall, and with infiltrates of leukocytes in the early stages.

Apart from "core" patients who satisfy all three criteria there will be other patients who variably do not. In temperate climates, most patients with an acute nephritic syndrome do not seem to have a renal disorder that has arisen from streptococcal infections, which are now rare given better hygiene and the absence of insect vectors. Patients with an acute nephritic syndrome and streptococcal infection may also present with mesangiocapillary patterns of nephritis or extensive crescent formation. Obviously, different mixes of patients within these groups will lead to different impressions of outcomes. Because this chapter is organized predominantly according to appearances viewed by light microscopy, this discussion is limited only to those patients with an exudative endocapillary pattern, because the prognosis of those patients with streptococcal infection with acute nephritis who show either MPGN or extensive crescents on biopsy specimens resembles closely that of patients without streptococcal infection with a similar histology. Even within the "core" group, there are two separate clusters to consider: those patients associated with epidemics of disease and those in whom disease appears to be sporadic. The prognosis of the latter may well be not as good as it is for those observed in an epidemic setting.

There has been some controversy regarding the frequency of occult or evident streptococcal glomerulonephritis as a cause of chronic renal failure, and, conversely, the frequency with

which persistent renal disease may be expected in patients with postinfectious glomerulonephritis (363,364). Part of the problem arises from the fact that the mix of patients observed in epidemics, mostly not in a Western urban environment, and the sporadic disease patients seen in city center referral specialist units are not the same.

Few cases of acute postinfectious nephritis are reported in industrialized countries, and most of those are not the sequel of streptococcal infection (365,366). Conversely, an unknown number of patients may have subclinical attacks of poststreptococcal nephritis; these numbers at least equal the number of obvious cases in the epidemic situation and may exceed them severalfold (367–370). The urine may show little or no abnormality (371) and hypertension may be the principal feature. Unless these atypical patients are investigated very thoroughly with serology, serial complement estimations, and renal biopsy with electron microscopy, it may be difficult to exclude other forms of glomerulonephritis. Occasional patients with a typical insidious nephrotic syndrome may show typical active diffuse endothelial nephritis in renal biopsy specimens. Some otherwise typical acute nephritic patients may have rather profuse proteinuria and show, rather briefly, a full nephrotic syndrome; this certainly can occur with the biopsy appearances discussed here, but it raises the suspicion of MPGN. An occasional patient with only acute endothelial proliferative glomerulonephritis presents with anuria and acute renal failure (372).

Childhood

Many early statements of the prognosis of acute nephritis in children are difficult to evaluate, because in almost all cases, histology was not available and the assumption was made (often without good evidence) that acute glomerulonephritis must necessarily be poststreptococcal. These early reports are summarized by Perlman et al. (373). One report is worthy of summary here, however, because it represents an early attempt to assess the very long-term prognosis of acute nephritic children (374). Twenty-seven patients who had acute nephritis in childhood severe enough to result in hospital admission were studied 19 to 32 years later. These patients represented only 25% of the 130 patients the author set out to trace. None of the 27 showed evidence of disease, and all urine test results and blood pressures were normal. Only one patient had died, and that was from tuberculosis.

Epidemic Cases. The prognosis of epidemic-proven acute streptococcal glomerulonephritis appears to be equally benign. Perlman et al. (373) studied the children who had acute glomerulonephritis 10 years previously in the streptococcal epidemic in the Red Lake Indian reservation. All children were studied initially and were shown to have streptococcal infection. After 10 years, renal function was normal in all, and the degree of proteinuria and hematuria did not differ from that in control subjects. Renal biopsies were performed in 16 of the 61 children; 12 specimens were entirely normal and 4 showed minor mesangial changes. Sanjad et al. (375) reported on 153 cases of acute glomerulonephritis from Florida. In this study, 103 patients were followed and none showed any clinical evidence of progressive disease up to 10 years later. However, ten children showed minor urinary abnormalities and all six who underwent biopsy had some glomerular abnormality.

Potter et al. (376–378), in an important study, described the 2- to 6-, 7- to 12-, and 12- to 17-year follow-up of a group of patients, mostly children, with sporadic or epidemic poststreptococcal nephritis, collected in Trinidad in 1965 and the following years. This study involved more than 700 persons, almost all of whom were still available in 1977 (378). Only 2 patients had died in renal failure, 19 had proteinuria, 3 had hematuria, and 3 had both. The incidence of hypertension (16 patients) was no higher than what is expected for the Trinidad population as a whole. The 1981 survey (377) was less complete. Only 534 patients with urinary abnormalities were identified, and all had normal plasma creatinine concentrations. It is worth noting that in the histories of the three patients who died, it was not clear whether they died of renal failure or if so, whether this was attributable to their nephritis.

An interesting observation of Nissenson et al. (378) was of 13 persons who had abnormal urine samples, but no symptoms during the attack (i.e., subclinical nephritis); none showed abnormalities 7 to 12 years later. The other study of this type of patient is that of Smith et al. (379), who performed biopsies and followed symptomless patients with acute poststreptococcal nephritis and minor urinary abnormalities. After 1 to 4 years, 8 of 28 patients showed persisting urinary abnormalities, and 2 had hypertension. Rodriguez-Iturbe et al. (369,380,381) summarized their experience of epidemic poststreptococcal glomerulonephritis in Maracaibo; only 1 of 71 patients followed for 11 to 12 years went into renal failure, but 15 (21%) still showed urinary abnormalities.

Sporadic Cases. Evidence is also available from patients with sporadic poststreptococcal glomerulonephritis in childhood. In an extensive study from Galveston (367,382), 60 patients were followed for at least 3 years, an important aspect in a condition with a relatively benign prognosis. Only 1 of 60 patients died after 2 years, and his initial biopsy specimen showed an unstated number of epithelial crescents; another child died of causes unrelated to renal disease at 18 months. At 3 years, only 8 of 45 children had urinary abnormalities (367), and at 5 years, only 2 of 32 still under observation showed proteinuria. Similarly, in the study from Lewy et al. (383) of 46 children with sporadic poststreptococcal glomerulonephritis, only 4 patients died, all showing extensive crescent formation in their biopsy samples. Two children still showed proteinuria after 5 years of follow-up. One of these two children had crescents in the initial biopsy specimen. Only three patients were lost to follow-up. Hinglais et al. (384) presented evidence from 29 children with acute nephritic syndromes; 16 of their 65 patients had raised antistreptolysin levels, but it is impossible to deduce which of these 16 patients were children. Of the 29 children, 25 had various forms of endocapillary glomerulonephritis, including exudative patterns with "humps" in 16. No patient with only endocapillary glomerulonephritis did poorly, and at the assessment point 2 years later, all those patients with en-

docapillary glomerulonephritis with humps had normal urine samples. Popovic-Rolovic et al. (385) followed 88 patients with sporadic disease in Serbia for 10 to 17 years. Only hypertension (3.4%) and proteinuria (2.3%) and microscopic hematuria were observed. The creatinine clearance was normal in all patients.

Evidence of persistent disease or progression was confined to those patients showing lesions other than endocapillary lesions, as in the series of Mota-Hernandez et al. (386). Baldwin et al. (387) included 37 children in their mainly adult study. One child required dialysis after 9 weeks, and her biopsy specimen showed extensive epithelial crescents. In six children, GFRs were measured 3 to 10 years from onset; all were more than 80 mL/minute except in one patient with a GFR of 77 mL/minute (uncorrected). In another series (388), 38 children with acute poststreptococcal glomerulonephritis were first studied between 1962 and 1970. Two patients died during the acute illness with crescentic nephritis and 33 of the remaining 36 were studied a mean of 9.4 years later (range, 6 to 13 years) (389). Two of the other three patients were known to be alive and in good health and only one was lost to follow-up. One patient showed persistent hypocomplementemia, and a second biopsy in this child revealed MPGN (390). All others showed normal blood urea and plasma creatinine concentrations, and in 21, creatinine clearance rates were normal (mean, 113 mL/minute; range, 80 to 70 mL/minute per 1.73 m^2). However, nine patients showed persisting urinary abnormalities: hematuria plus proteinuria in three, and isolated urinary protein loss in six, ranging from 0.2 to 0.5 g per 24 hours. Blood pressure was within the normal range in all patients. All of these patients were recalled for restudy a mean of 19.4 years (range, 14.6 to 22 years) later (349). Only one was hypertensive, three patients had microscopic hematuria, and the patient with MPGN had proteinuria. All showed normal plasma creatinine concentrations.

Although GFR appears to be conserved, renal reserve may be impaired. Cleper et al. (391) reported on 36 patients who had recovered from an episode of poststreptococcal glomerulonephritis 1 to 16 years earlier without apparent sequelae. Basal creatinine clearance was no different from that in control patients. However, the renal reserve in response to protein loading was significantly decreased. The magnitude of the impairment in renal reserve appeared to increase with more time since the initial episode of poststreptococcal glomerulonephritis. A similar note of caution regarding the degree of recovery was sounded by Herthelius and Berg who reported that although the GFR is normal, the filtration fraction remains high, suggesting possible glomerular hyperperfusion (392).

In summary, the accumulated evidence suggests that in epidemic and sporadic poststreptococcal glomerulonephritis and other acute nephritic syndromes in childhood, a similar pattern emerges. If the biopsy reveals endocapillary changes only, whether or not "humps" are present, then healing within 5 years is the rule. The few patients who do badly almost always show some other histologic pattern and are usually associated with other adverse features such as the appearance of a full nephrotic syndrome.

Adults

The evidence that progression can occur in acute poststreptococcal glomerulonephritis is somewhat stronger in adults, even in those with only an endocapillary glomerulonephritis demonstrated by renal biopsy. In addition, other patterns of histology such as the presence of extracapillary crescents are more common. In Jennings and Earle's classic paper of 1961 (393), the only patient of their 36 who died, still anuric, had extensive crescent formation in his biopsy specimen. Thirteen other patients had clinical evidence of continuing disease at follow-up

5 months to 4 years after onset. McCluskey and Baldwin (394) reported on a mixed group of adults showing an acute nephritic onset; 5 patients died and 14 showed evidence of progressive disease. Some of their patients showed either diffuse crescentic glomerulonephritis or MPGN. More recently, Baldwin et al. and Baldwin and Schacht (364,387,395) reported their findings in 89 adults with proven poststreptococcal nephritis, drawing the widely quoted conclusion that "up to one-half" of patients with this condition show evidence of progressive disease. This conclusion deserves careful examination.

The ten patients older than 15 years at onset who died or required dialysis had extensive crescent formation, and four of these patients had a rapidly progressive course over 3 months into renal failure. The other patient with crescentic glomerulonephritis became uremic 6 months after a second attack of glomerulonephritis. Of the other five who died, only two died later, at 2 and 6 years of follow-up. Six of these ten fatal patients showed a full nephrotic syndrome at presentation. These patients, therefore, although part of the spectrum of poststreptococcal nephritis, are not typical of this condition and were seen in a tertiary referral center.

In the remainder of the patients in this study, the evidence for persisting disease must be considered against the large fallout of patients. Unlike the childhood series discussed previously, only 56 of 126 patients completed even 1 year of follow-up, only 29 were still in contact after 5 years, and only 5 at 10 years or later. The fact that 50% of patients showed a raised blood pressure after 8 to 10 years is made less impressive if one remembers that the 10 patients studied at this point represent only 7% of the whole group; the assumption cannot be made, as discussed at the beginning of this chapter, that those patients lost to follow-up had the same characteristics as those retained. In most studies of relatively benign disease, as noted already, patients with the more severe disease progressively concentrate in the follow-up group.

However, 8 of 16 adults whose GFR was measured 3 to 15 years after their attack of glomerulonephritis showed values of less than 80 mL/minute. An inulin clearance rate of 100 mL/minute was used as the lower limit of normality. These data are not corrected for sex, surface area, or age, and other published figures suggest that this would not represent the mean minus 2 SDs, and the blood pressures were not compared with normal data for sex and age. Twenty patients still had proteinuria at 5 years, and four at 10 years, although the description of proteinuria as evidence of irreversible disease is not justified. Hypertension, judged as a diastolic blood pressure of more than 90 mm Hg, was equally common. Baldwin and Schacht (395) presented further data on this group of patients; 125 of 176 patients in the study had a renal biopsy, and 105 were followed for 2 years or longer. By 1975, nine patients entered terminal renal failure within a maximum of 6 months from onset, whereas six others progressed to uremia from 1 to 12 years after onset; all the patients in the latter group showed typical acute endocapillary glomerulonephritis in their initial biopsy specimen.

What have other authors reported? Hinglais et al. (384), in their study of 36 adults with sporadic acute nephritis, found 25 patients with only endocapillary lesions in the renal biopsy specimen. Seven of these showed persistent proteinuria when restudied at 2 years. In contrast, 10 of the other 11 patients with changes other than endocapillary glomerulonephritis (mesangiocapillary, extracapillary) had continuing disease. However, GFRs were not measured in this study. Lien et al. (396) also studied 57 patients, 52 of which were adults who had sporadic poststreptococcal glomerulonephritis, for a mean range of 7 ± 4 years. All had an initial biopsy and 33 had second biopsies. Two patients died with abnormal renal function, and 11 showed evidence of some renal damage and four additional patients had only hypertension. Vogl et al. (397) de-

scribed 2- to 13-year follow-up for 72 of 101 patients with adult-onset, sporadic acute poststreptococcal nephritis in Germany, Luxemburg, and Austria. Only three patients entered ESRD, one in only 5 months after transformation into a diffuse crescentic nephritis as shown by a second biopsy, as others have described (389,398). Only two other patients had raised plasma creatinine concentrations and continued proteinuria. Four other patients died, however: one from accelerated hypertension after only 2 months, another of sepsis, and two others of unknown causes. Vogl et al. (397) confirmed the suggestion of Hinglais et al. (384) and others that onset with a nephrotic syndrome indicates a poorer prognosis. Similarly, Rodriguez-Iturbe reported that of adult patients presenting with nephrotic-range proteinuria, as many as 77% will develop ESRD (399).

In a more recent study (400), the long-term outcomes were reported for patients diagnosed with infection-associated glomerulonephritis between 1979 and 1999. In this study, the prognosis was significantly worse for patients who also had a severe underlying disease. After a mean follow-up of more than 7 years, 64% of those without underlying disease were in complete remission, whereas only 14% of those with severe underlying disease (such as cirrhosis or malignancy) achieved complete remission.

Baldwin's group has also emphasized that widespread vascular sclerosis of arterioles may be a marker of progression (401). On the clinical side, profuse proteinuria, anuria, the persistence of low complement levels, and hypertension beyond about 4 weeks after onset are valuable indicators of a poor outlook, and many such patients show MPGN in their biopsy specimens. Patients may begin with a biopsy specimen that shows a pure endocapillary disease, which then develops into MPGN (389) or into severe crescentic nephritis (389,397,402). However, it must be emphasized again that pure endocapillary glomerulonephritis can occur with anuria and that anuria does not always indicate crescentic nephritis (403).

One practical problem in uncomplicated cases is to know just how long one has to wait before the urine can be expected to become free of blood, trace protein, or both, and whether late renal biopsy should be performed. There are surprisingly few data on this important point, but it has been known for many years that it could take up to several years for complete clinical "healing" to occur. Joseph and Polani (404) provided evidence from a trial of bedrest (which showed no effect) that more than 90% of children with sporadic poststreptococcal nephritis will be free of hematuria by 6 months.

In summary, the prognosis of acute glomerulonephritis, both epidemic and sporadic, postinfectious or poststreptococcal, probably becomes worse with age. Recovery is almost invariable in the preschool child, there is some suggestion of chronicity in older children, and the disease becomes chronic in a significant minority of adults. With increasing age, an increasing proportion of patients show diffuse extracapillary proliferation or MPGN, which accounts for an increased incidence of precocious renal failure. It is difficult to generalize from these controversial figures, but of 100 acute nephritic children, 1% or less will show crescentic glomerulonephritis and go on to early uremia; 75% will be free of proteinuria in 2 to 3 years, and a further 20% by 5 years. Only 1% or 2%, usually older children, will develop uremia later. Some of these will have shown MPGN or crescentic glomerulonephritis at onset. In adults, perhaps 5% will show persisting proteinuria, and some of these patients will have reduced renal function and hypertension. Their fate is not known, but some may progress to uremia within a decade or two. Thus, most of the difficulties and apparent inconsistencies in the various reports of the outcome of acute nephritic patients resolve themselves if the differences in age, etiology, epidemiology, and type of histology seen in renal biopsy specimens are taken into account.

TABLE 71-6

VARIOUS GLOMERULAR CONDITIONS THAT MAY BE ASSOCIATED WITH EXTENSIVE CRESCENT FORMATION

Primary crescentic glomerulonephritis
  Common
    Idiopathic[a] crescentic glomerulitis, usually necrotizing segmental
    ANCA-associated vasculitis
    Antiglomerular basement membrane nephritis
    Membranoproliferative glomerulonephritis (I or II)
  Uncommon
    IgA nephropathy
    Membranous nephropathy
    Secondary crescentic glomerulonephritis
  Common
    Henoch-Schönlein purpura
    Microscopic polyarteritis
  Uncommon
    Systemic lupus erythematosus
    Behçet's syndrome
    Mixed cryoglobulinemia
    Shunt nephritis
    Subacute bacterial endocarditis
    Neoplasia

[a]Considered by some always to represent microscopic polyarteritis (see text).

Crescentic Glomerulonephritis

The group of patients with crescentic glomerulonephritis is neither pathologically nor clinically homogeneous (Table 71-6). Only the thesis that extensive crescent formation is a dominant determinant of progression, overriding that of the underlying glomerulopathy, justifies considering them together (405–407) (Chapter 60). In practice, the outlook for patients with extensive crescent formation, whatever the underlying disease, is so much poorer than that noted for other forms of glomerulopathy (17), that this approach seems worthwhile, at least for purposes of clinical management.

Types

Three main groups of patients may be included under the heading of "crescentic glomerulonephritis." The proportion of each varies with the ages of the patients and geography. For example, crescents complicating proliferative glomerulonephritis form a greater proportion of cases in children (408–411) and in the developing world (411–414). Some degree of extracapillary proliferation is relatively common in patients with primary proliferative glomerulonephritis. This is true of postinfectious endocapillary nephritis, MPGN, and less commonly, IgA nephropathy. The changes are usually minor and often segmental. In some patients, however, a significant number of glomeruli show multilayered crescents affecting a large proportion of the glomerular circumference. In the minority of patients who are of concern, most or all glomeruli show such circumferential extracapillary proliferation.

Interpretation of the distorted and compressed glomerular tuft engulfed by a crescent is always difficult and may be impossible, but on immunohistologic examination, granular IgG and C3 are seen in various distributions in other patients with endocapillary or mesangiocapillary nephritis, or lupus, and IgA

is seen in patients with crescentic IgA nephropathy (415–417) or HSP (405,408–411).

Anti-GBM disease and *vasculitis* of various types are the other two main varieties of crescentic nephritis and form most cases in adults in developed countries (405–407). Extracapillary crescent formation is present in most patients, together with necrotizing lesions within the glomerulus. On immunohistology, fibrin is seen within the crescents; this is particularly common in crescentic nephritis associated with vasculitis (see later discussion). Linear deposits of IgG and complement, and occasionally IgA, are seen in anti-GBM disease along the capillary walls, whereas in vasculitic patients (with the exception of those with HSP), no glomerular immune aggregates are visible.

Apart from these three main groups, the so-called "idiopathic crescentic glomerulonephritis" remains. In patients with this form, there is usually a segmental necrotizing glomerulitis and collapsed but otherwise normal glomerular tufts (418–420). Many of these patients have antineutrophil cytoplasmic antibodies (ANCA) in their plasma, directed against myeloperoxidase (MPO) (see later discussion). However, very few patients do not fit this description, do not have circulating ANCA, and if untreated, do not develop vasculitis. Some authors have never seen such cases (421,422), and certainly they are very uncommon (423,424).

How Many Crescents Make Crescentic Nephritis?

It is impossible to draw a firm line at any point to distinguish what should be called "crescentic glomerulonephritis." For purposes of discussion, criteria of 50%, 60%, 70%, and 80% of glomeruli affected by crescents have been used by different authors to define crescentic glomerulonephritis. Because the prognosis, at least of the untreated disease, may depend on the proportion of affected glomeruli, this is not an academic point. Expressing the percentage involvement from a total number of glomeruli of less than, say, 10 may not seem to be a useful exercise, and reservations about the sampling error are certainly present. However, because the extent of the involvement in an individual glomerulus varies with the proportion affected (412,425), the conclusions may be more secure than at first appears. The important point made earlier is that although the presence of extensive crescent formation may dominate the histologic and clinical picture, justifying the separation of the group, the glomeruli themselves may show various changes and the patients various clinical pictures.

Clinical Presentation

Despite this heterogeneity, most patients with extensive crescent formation have a characteristic presentation and clinical course. The most common presentation is with sudden onset of rapidly progressive renal failure, sometimes with anuria. Other patients have a course over several months, which is still quick enough to justify the description of "rapidly progressive glomerulonephritis" (RPGN). Of course, the apparent onset of the disease may not be anywhere near its true beginnings. RPGN may also supervene in a patient with an indolent course of nephritis, for example, with membranous nephropathy, as discussed previously. Overall, the prognosis for patients with crescentic nephritis is poorer than that for any other form of nephropathy and relates in broad fashion in the untreated patient to the extent and severity of the crescent formation. Successful treatment of the two major groups (vasculitis and anti-GBM disease) has removed this correlation. Despite this generally poor outlook in the absence of treatment, occasionally patients make remarkable recoveries, sometimes without any specific intervention; however, few patients with crescentic nephritis escape treatment. A search of the literature from 1964 to 1980 shows 115 patients with crescentic nephritis who

TABLE 71-7

PROGNOSIS OF UNTREATED AND TREATED PATIENTS WITH
CRESCENTIC-GLOMERULONEPHRITIS

Total no. of patients	No. not treated	No. judged to have "improved"	Total no. treated	No. judged to have improved
328	115	13 (11.3%)	213	90 (42%)

Summary of treated and untreated patients with crescentic glomerulonephritis (>50% of glomeruli with crescents).
World literature 1964–1980, excluding patients with (i) anti-glomerular basement membrane disease, (ii) known or suspected vasculitis, (iii) systemic lupus erythematosus, and (iv) Henoch-Schönlein purpura.

received no specific treatment, of which thirteen (11.3%) made a spontaneous recovery (Table 71-7).

Prognostic Features

Most authors (422,426–429) reached the conclusion that within this severely affected group, the following clinical and histologic features indicate a (relatively) favorable prognosis: (a) history of prior infection, (b) presence of a urine output, (c) lesser extent of crescent formation, (d) absent or mild tubular atrophy and interstitial fibrosis, (e) presence of glomerular immune aggregates shown by immunohistology or electron microscopy, (f) presence of endocapillary proliferation, (g) intact Bowman's capsule, and (h) ANCA titers.

On *histology*, the correlation with the proportion of glomeruli affected by extensive crescents has been mentioned previously (Table 71-8). In view of the difficulty in defining "crescents," the change in number and extent of crescents with time, and the small sample available, it is not surprising that the correlation is only approximate: Even when 100% of glomeruli are so affected, a proportion of patients may yet recover function. As usual, the extent and severity of tubulointerstitial disease correlates well with outcome, as reported for almost all other forms of glomerulonephritis. In one series (418) using a scoring system for severity of tubular atrophy and interstitial fibrosis, of 26 patients with scores of less than 3 (of 8), 14 patients showed improvement in renal function, which was sustained in 12. In contrast, of 13 patients with scores of 3 or higher, only 5 showed improvement and this was sustained in only a single patient. Therefore, tubulointerstitial changes together with the extent of crescent formation can give a very good idea of which patients may respond to treatment and point to those whose disease has evolved to a point at which recovery is likely.

TABLE 71-8

FREQUENCY OF AN OLIGOANURIC PRESENTATION
IN CRESCENTIC GLOMERULONEPHRITIS

Crescents (%)	Patients with oligoanuria (%)
60–70	0
70–80	40
80–90	44
90–100	72
100	92

Excluding anti-glomerular basement membrane, polyarteritis, systemic lupus erythematosus, and Henoch-Schönlein purpura.
(Data from: Rees AJ, Cameron JS. Crescentic nephritis. In: Cameron JS, et al., eds. *Oxford Textbook of Clinical Nephrology*. London: Oxford; 1992:418, with permission.)

Persistently high or rising titers of ANCA are often associated with disease relapses (430,431). However, this association may not occur in 10% to 30% or more of those with such ANCA profiles during one or more years of follow-up, but the use of an elevation in ANCA titer as the sole parameter to justify immunosuppressive therapy cannot be endorsed. In a prospective study of 100 ANCA-positive patients observed over a 2-year period, relapse did not occur in 43% and 29% of those with a rise in ANCA titers by immunofluorescence and in PR3-ANCA titers by enzyme-linked immunosorbent assay (ELISA), respectively (430,431). Thus, treating all patients who have increases in ANCA titers would have resulted in unnecessary risks of toxicity in a substantial percentage of patients. Therapy should be instituted only on the basis of unequivocal evidence of clinical relapse, but patients with rising titers should be followed closely for signs of clinical activity. Conversely, if a patient was ANCA-positive during a period of active disease, a persistently ANCA-negative status is consistent with, but not absolutely proof of, remission. This was illustrated in a report in which 37 of 100 patients with ANCA-associated vasculitis suffered flares during the period of observation (430,431). Of these, 13 were ANCA negative at the time of relapse.

Clinical Course

Postinfectious nephritis, even when crescents are present, has a reputation of being more benign than comparable idiopathic disease; the apparently good prognosis in poststreptococcal nephritis is, however, the result—at least in part—of the inclusion in published data of patients with relatively minor degrees of crescent formation. In the analysis of Heaf et al. (432), only 51% of patients in the infection-related group had more than 80% of the glomeruli affected by crescents, compared with 69% of the anti-GBM group and 65% of the "idiopathic" group. The prognosis for recovery diminishes only when the number of glomeruli affected by occluding crescents reaches or exceeds 60%; the literature on poststreptococcal crescentic nephritis is particularly poor in its definitions of "extensive" crescent formation, as we have discussed elsewhere (17). Consequently, the prognosis for postinfectious nephritis with extensive crescent formation may not be as benign as supposed in the past.

Second, oligoanuria is a factor indicating a poor prognosis. In Table 71-8, the frequency of oligoanuria in relation to the extent of crescent formation is shown in data taken from five articles in the literature (406). Of 100 patients presenting with oliguria of less than 500 mL per 24 hours, a GFR of less than 3 mL/minute, only 20 showed any recovery of renal function, with or without treatment, which varied from series to series. Bolton and Couser (433) reached an even more pessimistic conclusion from their analysis of the literature: Only 7% of oligoanuric patients recovered function. Age, surprisingly, does not play a major part in determining recovery (432).

TABLE 71-9

PROGNOSIS OF CRESCENTIC GLOMERULONEPHRITIS IN RELATION TO ASSOCIATED GLOMERULAR DISEASE

Histologic diagnosis	No. of patients	"Improved"	Death or dialysis
Postinfectious	47	23 (49%)	24 (51%)
No immune deposits/immune deposits	70	13 (19%)	57 (81%)
Antiglomerular basement membrane disease	81	9 (11%)	72 (89%)
Vasculitis	69	4 (6%)	65 (94%)
All patients	521	124 (24%)	297 (76%)

(Reprinted from: Glassock RJ. A clinical and immunopathologic dissection of rapidly progressive glomerulonephritis. *Nephron* 1978;22:253, with permission.)

The outlook for different groups of crescentic nephritis varies, as might be expected. In Glassock's analysis (427) (Table 71-9) dating from the early and mid-1970s, the prognosis for patients with vasculitis and those with "idiopathic" immune deposit–negative crescentic glomerulonephritis—many of whom had vasculitis—was particularly poor. As shown in the next section, this "natural" history of vasculitic crescentic nephritis has been much modified for the better. Crescentic nephritis complicating proliferative glomerulonephritis, other than poststreptococcal nephritis, is rare in adults in developed countries, and few cases of crescentic MPGN (90) or IgA nephropathy (417) have been described. In general, the prognosis is worse than it is in patients not affected by crescents (see previous discussion in section on MPGN and IgA nephropathy) but the data are not extensive.

Apart from HSP, crescentic nephritis is rare in children. At least four extensive series have been published (408–411), for a total of 164 cases including 82 children with primary glomerulonephritis (postinfectious, MPGN). Only nine (5%) had anti-GBM nephritis, emphasizing the rarity of this form of nephritis in childhood. Fourteen children had crescentic nephritis without deposits, many (17%) had occult vasculitis, and the remainder had various forms of glomerulonephritis, including seven (4%) with crescentic IgA nephropathy; thus, this type of crescentic nephritis, secondary to identifiable glomerulopathy, appears relatively more common in children than in adults. Twenty-two children (13%) had postinfectious nephritis and 17 had MPGN (six had type II MPGN). One child had a juguloatrial shunt, and in 15, the crescentic nephritis could not be further characterized. Twenty-five, the largest single group, had HSP.

Clinicopathologic correlations were similar to those found in adults. A total of 84 of 158 children with follow-up entered end-stage renal failure, more than half within 1 month of onset and the remainder, from several months to 5 years later. No patient in the South West Pediatric Group series (409) entered into complete remission, but seven in the series from Paris (408) and three in London (410) did. The remainder retained proteinuria and hematuria with varying degrees of renal dysfunction. Therefore, the outlook for children with crescentic nephritis does not differ greatly from that for adults, and even patients with postinfectious glomerulonephritis may go into renal failure.

At several points in this section, the effects of *treatment* on the "natural" history of crescentic nephritis are mentioned (432–434). Of course, dialysis alone without specific treatment may allow time for spontaneous healing, when otherwise an early death from uremia could be expected. Treatment of both ANCA-related vasculitis and anti-GBM nephritis (discussed later) has had dramatic effects. What evidence is there

that treatment affects the outcome of other forms of crescentic nephritis? The earliest data comes from Heaf et al. (432) who undertook an extensive analysis of the effects of treatment in all forms of crescentic nephritis, but their analysis included patients with both anti-GBM and vasculitic nephritis (Table 71-10). The "best" results are obtained with the use of intravenous methylprednisolone, which is relatively inexpensive, safe, and simple to administer, or with plasma exchange, which is none of these things. Bolton and Sturgill (435) and Couser (436) reviewed the use and results of intravenous methylprednisolone and concluded that about three-fourths of treated patients with idiopathic crescentic nephritis maintain or recover renal function (44 of 59 in Couser's (436) analysis). Because these results are as good as or better than those of more complicated regimens including prolonged anticoagulation or plasma exchange, this form of treatment seems preferable for all forms of crescentic nephritis, with the exception of anti-GBM nephritis, in which intravenous methylprednisolone appears to have little or no effect (435) (see later discussion).

The longer term outcome of patients with crescentic nephritis has been less studied (437–439), perhaps because until recently, survival of patients with severe disease was unusual. Long-term follow-up of responders has revealed that more than one-half have a sustained improvement in renal function, whereas some patients slowly progress to ESRD. The series of Bruns et al. (437) included eight patients with crescentic nephritis without immune deposits (i.e., probable vasculitis) and two patients with anti-GBM disease. However, in the remaining 13 patients, the disease was immune complex–related and its evolution is of interest here. Seven patients entered chronic renal failure after temporary recovery, two within a few months, but five from 1 to 2 years later, and four remained in various degrees of renal failure (P_{creat} of 2 to 4 mg/dL) for 2 to 11 years. Despite the initial clinical improvement, repeated renal biopsy usually shows a marked increase in glomerulosclerosis, presumably reflecting healing of injury induced during the active stage of the disease (440). Therefore, early therapy is essential in this disorder to minimize the inflammatory damage that leads to late glomerular scarring.

Anti-GBM Nephritis

The prognosis of anti-GBM nephritis, with or without pulmonary hemorrhage (Goodpasture's syndrome), is now very different from that described two or three decades ago (441) (Chapter 60). First, many of the older descriptions were unknowingly contaminated by patients who had pulmonary hemorrhage as part of vasculitic syndromes (442). Second, as anti-GBM antibody assays have become widely available, a group of less severely affected patients have been described with more

TABLE 71-10

APPARENT INFLUENCE OF TREATMENT ON PROGNOSIS IN CRESCENTIC GLOMERULONEPHRITIS (ALL TYPES)

Treatment	No. of patients	Results Alive, normal renal function (%)	Alive, abnormal renal function (%)	In uremia (%)	In dialysis (%)	Death (%)		Uremia + dialysis + death
Symptomatic	82	3	7	3	42	45	=	90
Immunosuppression	144	11	15	4	22	47	=	71
Anticoagulation[a]	94	13	9	4	27	47	=	78
Plasma exchange	117	3	30	25	29	13	=	65
Methylprednisolone	39	20	36	7	24	12	=	43
Plasma exchange and methylprednisolone	7	0	42	0	42	14	=	56

[a] Regarding these data, it must be remembered that comparable patients were not allocated to all the treatment groups and that some data are predominantly recent (e.g., plasma exchange) and others less recent (e.g., immunosuppression alone).
Often combined with immunosuppression.
(Reprinted from: Heaf JG, Jorgensen F, Nielsen NP. Treatment and prognosis of extracapillary glomerulonephritis. *Nephrons* 1983;35:217, with permission.)

indolent disease arising from anti-GBM antibody who do not have extensive crescent formation (443). Finally, treatment has modified the "natural" history of the condition in the last 15 years.

We realize now that anti-GBM disease may present first with overt or occult pulmonary hemorrhage and with anemia, and only later will renal manifestations supervene. Some patients who show linear deposits of anti-GBM antibody along the GBM do not have clinical manifestations of renal disease. Some patients have no lung hemorrhage, some have occult lung hemorrhage detectable by the presence of severe anemia or a raised K_{co} (pulmonary carbon monoxide transfer), whereas in others the pulmonary hemorrhage is the dominant feature of the disease and may be life-threatening.

At first, the prognosis for anti-GBM nephritis was worse than that for almost any other form of nephritis, at least with regard to renal function (Table 71-9). Some additional patients died from pulmonary hemorrhage with relatively good renal function. Therefore, only 18 of 136 patients reported in the 1960s and early 1970s survived. Even as recently as 1977, Beirne et al. (426) found only 3 of 17 patients who retained independent renal function and survived. Although occasional dramatic recoveries have been described, even in those requiring dialysis (444), they usually are related to patients without very extensive crescent formation (3 of 13 glomeruli in the case just cited) (444).

Plasma exchange to remove the circulating antibody, together with cyclophosphamide to prevent its resynthesis, has changed the outlook for anti-GBM disease dramatically (Chapter 60), although no controlled studies are available. It has become evident that plasma exchange is normally effective in protecting renal function only if the patient is treated early enough, before oligoanuria and a requirement for dialysis has become established (Table 71-11). Among patients already requiring dialysis (445,446) very few recover renal function. Walker et al. (447), however, reported more encouraging results: 5 (45%) of 11 oligoanuric patients in their series of 22 patients recovered renal function. Savage et al. (448), as well as reviewing their extensive personal data from the Hammersmith Hospital (Table 71-11), reviewed collected data from other units on 59 patients presenting between 1980 and 1984. Of a total of 58 patients of 108 local and collected patients who were oligoanuric and who received treatment with plasma exchange and cyclophosphamide, 18 died and 51 continued

on dialysis; only 7 patients (13%) requiring dialysis recovered function with aggressive treatment. In the series from Herody et al. (449) in Paris, only 16 of 29 patients required dialysis, illustrating the changed presentation of anti-GBM disease. The more uremic patients did worse. Twenty-five of the 35 patients of Merkel et al. (450) developed ESRD. In both series, the combination of extensive crescents and oligoanuria predicted a poor outcome. More severe disease and a poorer outlook are associated also with the HLA type; those with HLA-DR2 along with HLA-B7 doing poorly (451).

There are few longer term data on the survival of patients with anti-GBM disease; renal survival is obviously much poorer than patient survival, even though patients are at risk from pulmonary hemorrhage and the effects of intensive immunosuppression. Turner and Rees (441) noted eight deaths (28%) during the first year among 29 patients seen at the Hammersmith Hospital between 1976 and 1988. All occurred in patients with extensive crescents, an initial plasma creatinine concentration of more than 600 μmol/L, and pulmonary hemorrhage. Similarly, 8 (36%) of 22 patients in Walker's series (447) died within 12 months. Savage et al. (448) noted 15 deaths (25%) within 8 weeks in their collected series of 59 British patients seen during 1980–1984, half of which were the result of lung hemorrhage and 14 in patients requiring dialysis. In the patients seen at the Hammersmith Hospital, 8 (16%) of 49 patients died, all but 1 among those requiring dialysis, and most dying from lung hemorrhage. The later mortality is not given for either group, so 1-year figures are not available. However, Merkel et al. (450) and Herody et al. (449) noted only four deaths in the 64 patients in their two series, with 37 remaining alive on dialysis and 23 with recovery or retention of some renal function. Only eight patients had a GFR within the normal range, including one patient without clinical renal involvement.

Therefore, an important determinant of the response to therapy is early diagnosis. There is a direct correlation between the initial plasma creatinine concentration and the percentage of glomeruli with crescents; in particular, crescents are present in more than 75% of glomeruli when the plasma creatinine concentration is greater than 5 mg/dL (442 μmol/L). Avoidance of maintenance dialysis is rare in patients who require dialysis within 72 hours of presentation, particularly in those who have crescents involving all glomeruli. In comparison, prevention of ESRD can usually be achieved in less severe

TABLE 71-11

IMMEDIATE OUTCOME IN PATIENTS WITH ANTIGLOMERULAR BASEMENT MEMBRANE NEPHRITIS

Presentation P_{creat} (μmol/L)	N	Received full treatment[a]	Outcome after 8 wk		
			Improved	Requiring dialysis	Death
Patients from British Renal units 1980–1984 (N = 59)					
Normal	3	2	3	—	—
<600	5	5	2	2	1
>600	7	7	—	4	3
Dialysis-dependent	44	33	—	33	11
Patients seen at the Royal Postgraduate Medical School 1974–1984 (N = 49)					
Normal	4	4	3	—	—
<600	15	15	13	2	—
>600	5	5	1	4	—
Dialysis-dependent	25	25	—	18	7

Treatment	5-yr survival (%)	Author	Year
Supportive only	13	Rose and Spencer	1957
	13	Frohnert and Sheps	1964
	12	Leib et al.	1979
Corticosteroids	62	MRC (U.K.)	1960
	48	Frohnert and Sheps	1967
	57	Sack et al.	1975
	61	Cohen et al.	1980
Corticosteroids plus cytotoxics	80	Leib et al.	1979
	55	Cohen et al.	1980
Corticosteroids plus cytotoxics methylprednisolone IV and plasma exchange in severe cases			
N			
53	38 Both	Serra et al.	1984
34	65 Micropolyarteritis	Savage et al.	1985
36	64 Both	Coward et al.	1986
43	62 Micropolyarteritis	Adu et al.	1987
26	80 Both	Fuiano et al.	1988
54	56 Wegener's	Gaskin and Pusey	1992
49	64 Micropolyarteritis	Gaskin and Pusey	1992
17	74 Wegener's	Cameron	1991
35	56 Micropolyarteritis	Cameron	1991

[a]Full treatment, at least 8 weeks of cyclophosphamide + plasma exchange for 2 weeks.
(Reprinted from: Savage COS, et al. Antiglomerular basement membrane antibody–mediated disease in the British Isles 1980–4. *Br Med J* 1986;292:301, with permission.)
In the earlier series (pre-1980, e.g., Leib et al.), many patients had either no renal disease or only minor renal disease. In addition, most of these early series included some patients with large-vessel vasculitis (polyarteritis nodosa). Thus, the data are not strictly comparable with those of more recent series consisting almost exclusively of patients with either Wegener's granuloma or microscopic polyarteritis, with severe (usually crescentic) glomerulonephritis.

cases, although some do progress. From all the presented data in the preceding text one can predict that about one-fourth of patients with anti-GBM nephritis can be expected to recover or maintain renal function, but only 10% of this 25% will have a normal GFR. The other 15% of the total will remain dialysis-dependent, and of these about 10% will die within 12 months, most within the first 3 months, often from pulmonary hemorrhage. Among those who recover or maintain renal function, a proportion subsequently develop uremia (447,452) and require dialysis or transplantation later. This "late" deterioration presumably arises through whatever mechanisms operate in remnant kidneys, rather than through specific immunologic attack. Return of active disease during follow-up is exceptionally rare, although it has been described (453), which agrees with the hypothesis that anti-GBM disease results from a single time-limited episode of autoimmunity, the duration and severity of which can be inhibited by removal and prevention of resynthesis of the causative autoantibody.

ANCA-mediated Vasculitis

Wegener's Granuloma, Microscopic Polyarteritis, and the Churg-Strauss Syndrome. Wegener's granulomatosis is a systemic vasculitis of the medium and small arteries, as well as the venules, arterioles, and occasionally large arteries. "Classic" Wegener's granulomatosis primarily involves the upper and lower respiratory tracts and the kidneys. A "limited" form, with clinical findings isolated to the upper respiratory tract or the lungs, occurs in approximately one-fourth of cases. Microscopic polyangiitis is a vasculitis that primarily affects capillaries, venules, or arterioles. Involvement of small and medium-sized arteries may also be present. This disorder is thought by some investigators to represent part of a clinical spectrum that includes Wegener's granulomatosis, since both are associated with the presence of ANCA, with similar histologic changes outside the respiratory tract (e.g., a focal necrotizing, pauci-immune glomerulonephritis), and have similar outcomes. Although the similarities between these diseases are generally accepted, histopathology in microscopic polyangiitis does not include granuloma formation, and the ear, nose, and throat are generally spared.

Until recently, there were few data on the long-term survival of such patients because untreated survival was so miserable (454–460). The 2-year survival rate of untreated vasculitic patients with severe nephritis was essentially zero, and there is overwhelming evidence—albeit uncontrolled—that aggressive treatment has modified the outlook dramatically over the last two decades. Although Fauci et al. (457,458) were the first to report the transformation of a 20% 2-year survival rate to a 93% survival rate at the same point in patients with vasculitis, scrutiny of their reports shows that most of their patients had no or only trivial renal disease.

Modern aggressive treatment of vasculitic nephritis is centered on the use of cytotoxic agents (usually cyclophosphamide) and corticosteroids (454,461–466). There is evidence that this more aggressive regime improves results, decreasing the number of patients who die of the vasculitis in the acute phase (463). For patients with advancing or severe renal failure, *many* units employ intravenous methylprednisolone, plasma exchange, or both (461–466). Taken together, the results of several small controlled trials (467–470) indicate that although the addition of plasmapheresis is of no benefit in the predialysis period, it may improve long-term survival in dialysis-dependent patients. In contrast, there is no evidence to suggest that intravenous administration of cyclophosphamide during the acute phase has any advantage (471), although intermittent intravenous cyclophosphamide may have benefits over long-term azathioprine in the longer term. No trial comparing the two has been performed, however.

Nachman et al. have recently published their experience with treatment of 97 patients with ANCA-associated microscopic vasculitis or ANCA-associated necrotizing crescentic nephritis (472). Patients received prednisone alone or prednisone with cyclophosphamide for about a year after the pulse therapy with methylprednisone. Because this was not a randomized controlled trial, multivariate analysis was performed to assess treatment response and relapses. Overall, 75 of the 97 patients (77%) went into remission. Of the 75 responders, 32 patients (43%) remained in long-term remission. Twenty-nine percent of the initial responders suffered a relapse that generally occurred within 18 months from the end of therapy. There was a significant difference in the remission rate between corticosteroid-treated patients and cyclophosphamide-treated patients (56% versus 89%; $p = 0.003$). The cyclophosphamide-treated patients had three times less risk of experiencing a relapse than did corticosteroid-treated patients.

Prognostic markers for patient and renal survival were analyzed in the same cohort of patients (473). The important clinical markers that predicted patient death were presentation with pulmonary hemorrhage, presence of c-ANCA (compared with p-ANCA), and treatment with steroids alone. Conversely, serum creatinine on presentation, race (African Americans worse than whites) and presence of arteriosclerosis on renal biopsy predicted renal survival.

Unlike in patients with anti-GBM nephritis, recovery of renal function in patients with vasculitis and crescentic nephritis who are already dialysis-dependent and oligoanuric is common, almost the rule (462–466,474). Death still occurs from other complications of the vasculitis, but now the main cause

of early death is sepsis from the intense immunosuppression in patients who are frequently older adults and often frail. In earlier cases, reversal of mounting uremia is also usual. About three-fourths or more of patients can be expected to survive the early phases of the disease (462,464,474–476).

The rate for longer term patient survival using these forms of treatment is between 50% and 80% at 5 years (463–466,475,476), with similar figures reported for the few patients studied for as long as 10 years. The redefinition of this group of patients using ANCA has not altered prognosis (477,478). Unlike patients with anti-GBM disease, rather few patients survive requiring dialysis after the acute attack. For example, of 60 patients with Wegener's granuloma, Gaskin and Pusey (479) noted severe renal disease in 54. Eleven patients (20%) died during the first 2 weeks, seven among the 24 requiring dialysis, mostly the result of pulmonary complications (hemorrhage and infection); only 3 of the 24 continued on dialysis. There were three additional later deaths in those who recovered function, all the result of infection. The actuarial survival rate was estimated to be 70% at 1 year and 56% at 5 years. Similarly, of their 49 patients with microscopic polyarteritis (479), 14 initially required dialysis, 4 died without recovering function, 8 recovered function, 2 died shortly thereafter, and only 2 continued on dialysis. The patient survival rate was 78% (38 of 49) at 8 week, and renal survival was 73% (36 of 49). When Wegener's granuloma and microscopic polyarteritis are compared, even when allowing for the extent of renal damage, usually the patients with Wegener's granuloma appear to do a little better (465,479), but the difference is not striking. The patients who die later (460,479) usually still have active but suppressed so-called smoldering disease (479), but the mortality rate has recently been reduced. An additional problem with Wegener's granuloma is that many patients with this condition have little or no renal involvement (480,481), and not surprisingly, the presence of renal disease is an indicator of poorer prognosis (480,481). In some patients renal vasculitis reactivates after prolonged remission (480), even after the patient has received a transplant (482,483). After the dramatic improvement in prognosis during the 1970s and 1980s for vasculitic patients, it appears that prognosis has now stabilized and further improvement was not seen during the last decade (484).

Factors that predict outcome are now obscured by the relative success of treatment. Clinically, as already mentioned, oligoanuria does not predict failure of treatment, although as a group, oligoanuric patients do rather worse. Histologically, the extent of crescent formation also has ceased to be a predictor of longer term outcome in this data (465), although it correlates with renal function at presentation (Fig. 71-17).

Patients with vasculitis who survive the initial illness may have a relapsing course, in which the frequency depends very much on the intensity of the immunosuppression. Therefore, in the series of 52 vasculitic patients seen during the 1980s, almost all of whom were maintained on prednisolone and azathioprine for 5 years or more, relapses were rare (465). ANCA titers may be of help in diagnosing the possibility of relapse early (485,486) and in modulating immunosuppression, because relapse is unlikely when the ANCA titer is normal. Persistently high or rising titers of ANCA are often associated with disease relapses (430,431). However, this association may not occur in 10% to 30% or more of those with such ANCA profiles during one or more years of follow-up. In a prospective study of 100 ANCA-positive patients observed over a 2-year period, relapse did not occur in 43% and 29% of those with a rise in ANCA titers by immunofluorescence and in PR3-ANCA titers by ELISA, respectively (430,431). Patients with rising titers should be followed closely for signs of clinical activity. Conversely, if a patient was ANCA-positive during a period of

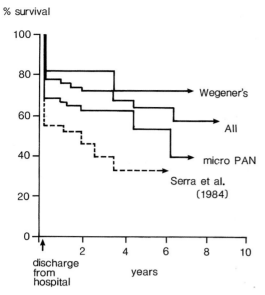

% survival

FIGURE 71-17. Probability of survival of patients presenting with renal vasculitis, 1981–1990. Guy's Hospital data are from 1980 to 1989 (429). Wegener's, 17 patients; microscopic polyarteritis (micro PAN), 34 patients; total, 51; mean age, 65 years; 19 requiring dialysis. Also shown are the data of Serra et al. (419) published in 1984 on the outcome of 53 patients presenting during the decade preceding the Guy's Hospital study. Overall survival has improved ($p<0.05$) in association with more aggressive treatment (see text), and the major cause of death is no longer the vasculitis itself but side effects of the more intense immunosuppression. Early mortality during the acute illness, although reduced, remains the main problem.

active disease, a persistently ANCA-negative status is consistent with, but not absolutely proof of, remission.

Vasculitis is rare in childhood (487), with the sole exceptions of the infantile Kawasaki disease, which usually spares the kidney, and HSP, which is addressed in the next section. Habib (488) reviewed a relatively large experience of 16 children with Wegener's granuloma or polyarteritis, whose clinical picture did not differ from that in similar adults.

There are few data on the outcome of renal disease in the Churg-Strauss syndrome, although it is now recognized that renal involvement is more common and more severe than what was thought in the past. Clutterbuck et al. (489) described the outcome of 19 patients whose renal disease resembled histologically that of Wegener's granuloma or microscopic polyarteritis. However, the prognosis was better, with only one patient requiring transplantation, five having varying degrees of chronic renal failure, and the remainder maintaining renal function for up to a decade. Only one patient died, of a restrictive cardiomyopathy.

Henoch-Schönlein Purpura Nephritis

HSP occurs more often in children than in adults, and many cases follow an upper respiratory tract infection, suggesting that the precipitating antigen may be infectious. In a review from the United Kingdom, the annual incidence was about 20 per 100,000 children (peak 70 per 100,000 between the ages of 4 and 6 years) and was little influenced by skin color or ethnicity (490). The prognosis of HSP without clinical nephritis is excellent (491,492) (Chapter 61), and nephritis forms the major cause of mortality and morbidity, apart from occasional problems with intussusception and other gastrointestinal tract complications (Chapter 61). Nephritis may appear with the initial attack but is particularly associated with recurrent attacks

of purpura (493) that may continue in exceptional patients for months or even years. Even so, compared with that for most other forms of glomerulonephritis in children or adults, the prognosis even with nephritis remains good (494). Overall, after 2 years, half the children with HSP nephritis will be in complete remission, whereas one-third show persisting urinary abnormalities with normal renal function.

Few children (perhaps 3%) progress to renal failure immediately, and their renal biopsy specimens usually show extensive crescent formation (409,410). No more than 19% show continued urinary abnormalities with reduced renal function. By the time 10 years has passed (495), most of the children who had urinary abnormalities but normal renal function at 2 years will have gone into remission, but a proportion of those with decreased renal function will have progressed to renal failure.

It is difficult to judge how many will eventually do so, but Habib and Cameron (494) reported that 32 (17%) of 188 patients went into renal failure, and the total would probably be about 20%. These data come from two highly specialized referral centers, and the proportion of children with more severe disease is inevitably exaggerated in these figures (see the first section of this chapter). The prognosis for unselected children with HSP nephritis is undoubtedly better than this, but by how much is impossible to say exactly. In the series from Kobayashi et al. (496), only 3 (2.7%) of 123 children with nephritis died, and 106 (86%) were in complete remission. In the study by Koskimies et al. (491), only 1 child of 39 still showed signs of evident nephritis and another 2 had chronic disease. Kobayashi et al. (496) calculated a final remission rate of 91%, with a 9% renal failure–death rate. However, although the benign nature of the disease is usually emphasized, HSP nephritis accounts for about 3% of children going into end-stage renal failure (497).

It would be useful to know at the outset which children would be most likely to have a severe course, so treatment could be concentrated on the minority who might require it. There is some correlation between clinical and outcome (Table 71-12). In general, patients with only symptomless urinary abnormalities do well, whereas those with a nephrotic syndrome, especially when combined with renal insufficiency, do poorly (494,495,498–500). However, there are exceptions in both directions. Another adverse feature is age at onset (Table 71-13); there was, however, no relation with serum IgA concentrations (497,499).

The best guide to outcome is a combination of clinical data (Table 71-12) and biopsy data (494,501) (Table 71-14). Almost all of those patients without diffuse glomerular proliferation and with less than 50% of glomeruli affected by segmental lesions or crescents did well. However, those with more extensive crescent formation tended to do poorly. Of children with diffuse proliferative glomerulonephritis, only half of those who had less than 50% of glomeruli affected by segmental lesions healed clinically; the remainder showed persisting disease. In those with more than 50% of glomeruli affected by segmental lesions, the evolution was favorable much less often, and in those with more than 80% of glomeruli affected by crescents, evolution was usually into renal failure (12 of 19 patients). It is in this group that aggressive treatment with intravenous methylprednisolone and plasma exchange is usually concentrated (492). Two children in this group, however, recovered completely without aggressive intervention. Overall, the greater the number of glomeruli affected by crescents, the poorer the prognosis (409,410).

There are few data on the very-long-term outcome of children with HSP nephritis, but recently 20-year data about (502) patients studied in the past (493,501) was published. One important finding was that seven children who had apparently recovered completely according to the last analysis in 1976 had deteriorated. Schaerer et al. (503) have published data on 64 children followed for two decades. Renal survival at

TABLE 71-12

OUTCOME IN RELATION TO CLINICAL ONSET (10 YEARS FROM ONSET) IN HENOCH-SCHÖNLEIN NEPHRITIS

	Outcome (no. of patients)				
	Recovery	Minor urinary abnormalities	Moderate nephropathy	Renal failure	Total
Hematuria only	4	0	1	0	5
Proteinuria + hematuria	31	3	3	3	40
Proteinuria + hypertension	7	0	0	1	8
NS + hematuria	8	0	0	1	9
"Nephritic-nephrotic" syndrome	11	3	5	7	26
Total	61	6	9	12	88

NS, nephrotic syndrome.
(Reprinted from: Counahan R, et al. Prognosis of Henoch-Schönlein nephritis in children. *Br Med J* 1977;2:11, with permission.)

10 years was 73%, with initial renal insufficiency being the most powerful predictor of an adverse outcome.

Discussion of HSP nephritis in adults is made difficult by several circumstances. First, a number of older articles that purported to deal with the topic do not distinguish between HSP, other forms of vasculitis, and essential cryoglobulinemia, even with the technology available when the data were collected (504). Second, some articles dealt with adults and children and it is impossible to separate the data. Third, in some reports, patients without renal involvement cannot be separated from those with nephritis. And finally, because of the relative rarity of HSP nephritis in adult life, no single series is large enough to form conclusions or do statistical analyses.

However, based on the published literature (505–518) and data from a national survey of 47 patients with HSP nephritis in the United Kingdom seen from 1976 to 1986 (519), the clinical manifestations do not differ much from those in children, although a history of prior drug ingestion and severe arthralgia (80%) are more common, and abdominal signs and symptoms less common (35%). The purpura more frequently ulcerates in adults with HSP, particularly older adults, than in children. The condition may be seen even in the ninth decade of life; there is some suggestion that in younger adults, older individuals with the childhood disease are present in decreasing numbers with increasing age; then there is a "bulge" of cases in the 50- to 70-year-old age-group, corresponding to that for other forms of adult vasculitis. Coppo et al. (520) examined prognosis in a collaborative study of adults and children with Henoch-Schönlein purpura, all of whom had nephritis. In

general, outcomes were similar, although slightly more adults (15.8% of 97) than children (7% of 57) entered end-stage renal failure. Two further series compared unselected adults and children with Henoch-Schönlein purpura, both with and without renal disease (521,522), noting a higher incidence of renal disease in older patients and an association of renal disease with upper body purpura. Again, most adults (89%) and children (94%) recovered completely.

However, the long-term prognosis may not be benign in all patients who appear to recover from the acute nephritic episode (523–525). A long-term retrospective study of a cohort of 250 adults with HSP and renal involvement of sufficient severity to require biopsy also reported that the renal outcome of some patients is relatively poor (523). At a median follow-up of nearly 15 years, 11% and 13% had become dialysis-dependent or had severe renal failure (creatinine clearance of less than 30 mL/minute), respectively. Sclerosis and fibrosis on initial renal biopsy correlated closely with poor outcomes.

The renal histology in adults is similar to the findings in children, and most interest has centered on whether the prognosis in the adult differs from that in children (Table 71-15). There is a suggestion that adults do a little worse than the selected children seen in referral centers, but again the adults are even more highly selected. Overall, 35 (12%) of 282 selected patients had gone into ESRD or died of renal failure, although the duration of follow-up differed greatly in the various studies included in Table 71-15. Death, as might be expected in this older population, sometimes resulted from unrelated causes (21 of 282, 7.4%). In the United Kingdom study of 43 patients (519), after 1 to 7 years of follow-up, 15 were in complete remission, 17 had urinary abnormalities (12 with normal renal function), 4 were receiving treatment for ESRD, and 7 had died (2 with normal renal function). Some patients with HSP nephritis may apparently heal but present with severe hypertension 10 to 20 years later (526), so blood pressure should be checked at least once a year, indefinitely.

TABLE 71-13

OUTCOME IN RELATION TO AGE AT ONSET IN HENOCH-SCHÖNLEIN PURPURA NEPHRITIS

	Age at onset (yr)		
	<6	6–11	<12
Recovery	19	38	3
Minor urinary abnormalities	2	4	0
Moderate nephropathy	2 (12.5%)	6 (26%)	1 (50%)
Renal failure	1	9	2
Total	24	57	6

(Reprinted from: Counahan R, Cameron JS. Henoch-Schönlein nephritis. *Contrib Nephrol* 1977;7:143, with permission.)

Systemic Lupus Erythematosus

The outlook for patients with clinically evident nephritis in a setting of systemic lupus erythematosus is difficult to summarize for several reasons (Chapter 65): First, being a multisystem disease, extrarenal organ involvement may have a major effect on the mortality and morbidity of patients with lupus, even those in whom the main involvement is in the kidney (527–530). Second, even in its "natural" untreated state, the disease may manifest over a very wide range of activity, from a limited indolent condition to a fulminant aggressive disorder affecting

TABLE 71-14

OUTCOME IN RELATION TO INITIAL BIOPSY APPEARANCE IN PATIENTS WITH HENOCH-SCHÖNLEIN NEPHRITIS FOLLOWED FOR MORE THAN 1 YEAR

	Recovery	Minimal urinary abnormalities	Persisting disease	Renal failure
Nonproliferative glomerulonephritis				
No crescents	1	0	0	0
Crescents <50%	17	9	1	2
Crescents >50%	0	0	1	3
Proliferative glomerulonephritis				
No crescents	1	1	1	0
Crescents <50%	4	4	6	1
Crescents 50–80%	3	2	3	2
Crescents >80%	2	4	1	12
Total	28	20	13	20

(Reprinted from: Levy M, et al. Anaphylactoid purpura nephritis in childhood: natural history and immunopathology. *Adv Nephrol* 1976;6:182, with permission; and from: Habib R, Broyer M, Levy M. Schönlein-Henoch purpura glomerulonephritis in children. In: Strauss J, ed. *Pediatric Nephrology 4*. New York: Garland; 1977:155, with permission.)

almost all major organ systems. Third, almost any pattern of glomerulopathy may be seen in renal biopsy specimens (Chapter 65). Fourth, the appearances may transform in sequential biopsy specimens, both spontaneously and in response to treatment (531–534).

The overall 10-year survival for patients with lupus is greater than 90% (535). Patients with nephritis still have worse survival rates than those without nephritis (88% versus 94%, p <0.05) (535). During the last 20 to 30 years, however, the major differences in outlook for those with different WHO classes of nephritis (which had been evident in earlier studies [536,537]) have disappeared (Table 71-16). This is likely be-

cause treatment has been more aggressive in those with clinically or histologically more severe forms of nephritis (538,539). Those with severe proliferative lupus nephritis (WHO class IV) appear to have benefited from improved therapies (540,541), and renal failure is no longer the principal cause of mortality in this population (538,542,543). Awareness of lupus as a diagnosis is greater now than it was 30 years ago and relatively specific tests for the condition are now widely available. Thus, it is possible that some of the "improvement" in the survival of all patients with lupus results from the inclusion of milder forms in recent series, or due to earlier diagnosis of the disease (544).

TABLE 71-15

FOLLOW-UP IN PATIENTS WITH ADULT-ONSET HENOCH-SCHÖNLEIN PURPURA NEPHRITIS

Ref.	Author	Country	Period	N	Age (yr)	Male: female ratio	f/u (yr)	Outcome in those with f/u[a]		
								Remitted	Persisting disease (reduced function)	ESRD/dead[b]
Series in which all patients had renal involvement										
(507)	Ballard	U.S.A	1954–58	14	>20	14:0	Not stated	8	1 (1)	5/0
(512)	Fillastre	France	1964–71	28	>20	22:6	?–13	8	7 (3)	2/1
(514)	Kalowski	Australia	1959–71	18	>16	13:5	Mean 3.7	5	9 (2)	1/3
(517)	Roth	U.S.A.	1968–83	9	>16	9:0	Not stated	7	2 (1)	0
(515)	Lee	Korea	1979–82	17	>16	9:8	Mean 3.2	10	7 (0)	0
(510)	Esteve	Spain	Not stated	11	>16	5:6	Not stated	3	5 (0)	3
(511)	Faull	Australia	1975–85	27[c]	>12	16:11	0.16–9.0	6	16 (6)	2/3
(519)	Knight	U.K.	1976–86	47	>20	34:13	1–7	15	17 (5)	4/7
(513)	Fogazzi	Italy	1967–88	16	>15	11:5	1–20	2	11 (9)	3/0
				187	—	133:54	—	64	75 (27)	20/14
Series in which only some patients had renal involvement										
(509)	Debray	France	?–1971	22 (10)	>15	12:10	4	5	2 (0)	0
(508)	Bar-On	Israel	1959–69	21 (12)	>15	12:9	0.5–6.0	4	2	2/0
			Totals	209	—	—	—	73	79 (27)	22/14

f/u, follow-up; *ESRD*, end-stage renal disease.
[a] Normal urine plus hypertension counted as continuing disease in f/u.
[b] Dead, dead from causes other than renal failure.
[c] 24 Patients older than 20 years.

TABLE 71-16

FIVE-YEAR ACTUARIAL SURVIVAL RATES FOR LUPUS, LUPUS NEPHRITIS, AND WORLD HEALTH ORGANIZATION CLASS IV NEPHRITIS OVER THE LAST 40 YEARS

Period	% 5-year survival (weighted mean of published series)		
	All lupus (no. of papers)	Lupus nephritis (no. of papers)	Class IV nephritis (no. of papers)
1953–1969	49% (4)	44% (3)	17% (2)
1970–1979	82% (6)	67% (13)	55% (9)
1980–1989	86% (5)	82% (6)	80% (3)
1990–1995	92% (3)	82% (5)	82% (4)

A number of new treatment regimens offer the prospect of improved outcomes, decreased toxicity, and possibly both (545). Because of the small number of patients now dying or going into ESRD, however, many of the recent studies are too short or too small to adequately compare these newer regimens. Clinicians now face the difficult decision of treating patients with less well-established therapy in order to minimize the side effects of therapy. Risk stratification and close clinical follow-up are, therefore, as important as ever.

Causes of Death

Because it is a multisystem disease, the causes of death in lupus are much more varied than those in other forms of primary glomerulonephritis that are seen in young adults and that are confined to the kidney. Sepsis, not surprisingly, emerges as one of the major causes of death (527,530,546–548) promoted or potentiated by immunosuppressive treatment. However, other manifestations of extrarenal lupus may prove fatal as well (527,530,546–548). Rather surprisingly, however, recent survival curves for renal function and for the patient are almost identical in most series (538,548,549). A number of observers have commented that in lupus patients, entry into chronic renal failure may be preceded by long periods of clinical quiescence (550,551), suggesting that the mechanisms other than continued activity of the nephritis determine the fate of the kidneys. A further cause of late death, even in young women with lupus, is severe atheromatous myocardial and other vascular diseases (44,46,527,547,548). The pathogenesis of these late vascular lesions is not clear, but corticosteroid treatment, hyperlipidemia, and immune complexes may all play a part. Interactions between immune complexes and hyperlipidemia have been shown in experimental animals to accelerate atheroma formation (42,43,552).

Predictors of Prognosis

The response to therapy and maintenance of remission are of prognostic importance, highlighting the necessity of adequate treatment. Korbet et al. (553) reported on the long-term experience of the Lupus Nephritis Collaborative Study Group. Defining remission as the combination of serum creatinine level of less than or equal to 1.4 mg/dL and proteinuria of less than or equal to 330 mg per day, these authors found a 10-year renal survival of 94% in patients achieving remission in contrast to only 31% in those failing to achieve remission. The importance of remaining in remission has been underscored by the study of Moroni et al. (554), who described the effect of renal disease "flares" (significant increase in proteinuria or serum creatinine level) on long-term renal function. In a group of 70 patients followed for a median of more than 10 years, the likelihood of

adverse renal outcome (defined as doubling of serum creatinine level) was increased nearly sevenfold in patients with a flare of renal disease compared with those with no renal disease flares. In patients with flares characterized by a rapid rise in serum creatinine level, the risk of poor renal outcome increased 27-fold. In a study of Chinese patients with WHO class IV disease who were treated with cyclophosphamide, 38% of the patients had renal flares with a mean follow-up of 8 years after the last dose of cyclophosphamide (555). Significant independent risk factors for renal flares were chronicity score, persistently positive anti-dsDNA, and the absence of maintenance therapy (azathioprine in this study). Furthermore, nephritic flares were an independent risk factor for doubling of the serum creatinine in this study. It appears clear, therefore, that the goal of therapy must be the achievement and maintenance of remission with stable renal function and minimal proteinuria.

Race is an obvious target for analysis, because the incidence and prevalence of lupus are so much higher in blacks and Asians than in whites (556–559). Although some studies comparing black and white subjects have found no difference in outcome (528,560–564), several large studies have shown a poorer outcome for black subjects (556,565). Tejani et al. (566) suggested that black children with an onset before puberty form a particularly high-risk group. Gordon et al. (567), examining national mortality from lupus in the United States, again suggested a higher mortality among black women. Similar results have been obtained from the Glomerular Disease Collaborative Network at the University of North Carolina as reported by Dooley et al. (568). In contrast to whites, in whom 95% retained renal function 5 years after the diagnosis of lupus nephritis, African Americans had a significantly worse course, with only 58% retaining renal function at 5 years. The difference was not attributable to age, duration of lupus, hypertension, or biopsy indices of disease activity or chronicity. The difference in outcomes in black Americans compared to white Americans may, in part, be confounded by socioeconomic status (561,565). Reveille et al. (569) reported black race as a risk factor for renal disease and poorer survival and systemic lupus erythematosus. This risk was independent of socioeconomic status. Barr et al. (570), however, found that race was no longer a significant predictor of progression when adjusted for socioeconomic factors. This study also concluded that socioeconomic status, itself, is an important risk factor for disease progression. The potential role of biologic or genetic factors in the observed racial heterogeneity of outcomes remains to be defined, although some genetic polymorphisms have been suggested (571).

Clinical severity of nephritis may be a predictor of outcome. Although many patients with initially severe disease may have a favorable outcome, several studies have found that a raised plasma creatinine concentration at the onset of disease is strongly associated with a poorer outcome (548,553, 556,564,572–574). The magnitude of proteinuria or the presence of nephrotic syndrome is more controversial. Several reports (78,549,562) have not noted a difference in outcome in those with nephrotic range proteinuria compared to those with lesser degrees of proteinuria in univariate analysis. However, Esdaile et al. (564) and Appel et al. (575) found poorer survival in their nephrotic patients. In the data by Appel et al. (575) this was particularly true in those whose nephrotic syndrome persisted. In multivariate analysis, the degree of proteinuria has also been shown to be a predictor of remission (553).

Indices of clinical activity of the lupus itself have been examined in a number of studies (563,564), many of which either did not deal with lupus nephritis or did not specify how many of the group studied had nephritis. However, there are clear correlations between immunologic findings such as complement concentrations and levels of circulating anti-dsDNA antibody, and the severity of the clinical picture, judged in various ways (576–579). In the analysis of Esdaile et al. (564) of a group exclusively consisting of patients with nephritis, thrombocytopenia, hypocomplementemia, and an elevated DNA binding at onset, all predicted poor outcome. Najafi et al. reported that the presence of anti-Ro antibodies was a predictor of the development of ESRD (574). Austin et al. (556) also found hypocomplementemia to be predictive of a poor renal prognosis, together with anemia, which was also a risk factor in the analysis by Donadio et al. (548) and in the report by Moroni et al. (554). Using the National Institutes of Health (le Riche) index, Goulet et al. (580) found good correlation between overall disease activity and renal outcomes. This was particularly important in patients without severe renal disease at presentation in whom higher disease activity index nevertheless portended an increased risk for subsequent renal insufficiency.

Age may also be a prognostic factor for patients with lupus. The outcome of lupus in childhood has been the subject of some controversy (581), with some series reporting poorer survival rates in children than adults. Wallace et al. (78) reported the outcome in 50 patients with onset before the age of 16 years. The survival was 73% at 5 years and 58% at 10 years. Only one-third of these patients had nephritis, however, and unlike in most North American series the children were predominantly White. Other series have shown better survival rates for childhood lupus. In a series of 80 patients who had the onset of lupus nephritis before the age of 20 years, the 5- and 10-year estimates of survival were 85% and 82%, respectively (581). In data from Minneapolis (533) on 70 childhood-onset cases, the 10- and 15-year survival rates were 85% and 77%. Esdaile et al. (564) performed a Cox analysis and noted no difference in renal failure or renal death in those older and those younger than 24 years at onset in a series of 87 patients. Austin et al. (582), however, found that age less than 24 years was a predictor of the development of renal failure. There seems to be little difference in the survival of adults and children or adolescents with lupus nephritis when other factors are also considered (78,563–565,582), although some authors (583) have interpreted the existing data as demonstrating that young age confers a poorer prognosis. Overall it seems that the difference in survival between children and adults, if there is one, is not a major one.

Hypertension, at least severe hypertension, is not as commonly present in lupus nephritis at apparent onset as in some other forms of glomerulopathy (e.g., 10 of 87 in Esdaile's study]). Hypertension was not examined as a prognostic factor in either of two of the largest studies cited previously (78, 565), and it was not mentioned in most follow-up studies. Esdaile et al. (564) did not find any association between outcome and high blood pressure itself, only with comorbid conditions. Similarly, the Glomerular Disease Collaborative Network (568) did not find hypertension to be an independent marker for poor renal outcome. In contrast, the Gruppo Italiano (549), Ward and Studenski (584), and Ginzler et al. (585) showed a markedly poorer survival in their hypertensive subgroups. In almost all

patients, if hypertension is present at the outset or appears later, it is usually treated vigorously. Nevertheless, unlike in IgA nephropathy, for example, high blood pressure does not seem to be a powerful predictor of outcome in lupus nephritis.

The number of *disease criteria* a patient demonstrates may predict a worse outcome. Esdaile et al. (564) and Ginzler et al. (565) have found that the total number of American College of Rheumatology (ACR) criteria for the diagnosis of lupus present at onset was a useful index of a poorer outcome. Swaak et al. (586) noted a poorer prognosis in those with an increasing number of clinical relapses, although this was in a population predominantly not under heavy immunosuppression. The antiphospholipid antibody syndrome (APS) has been associated with renal artery stenosis, thrombotic microangiopathy, and APS nephropathy, and the presence antiphospholipid antibodies was associated with worse renal outcomes during long-term follow-up (587).

Several authors have studied *gender* as a prognostic factor. Male patients, of course, form only a small minority of patients with lupus, which makes comparison difficult except in the largest series. In the series of Wallace et al. (78), in which only 39% of patients had evident nephritis, there was a significantly worse outcome for the 63 men compared with the 546 women, and the data of Austin et al. (582) are in agreement with this conclusion. In the study by Swaak et al. (586), 5 of 16 men and only 9 of 94 women died. The Cox analysis by Esdaile et al. (564) suggested a higher rate of renal failure in men, but no difference in nonrenal deaths. However, Ginzler et al. (565), using a stepwise linear regression model, found no difference in their large collected series. Tejani et al. (566) and other pediatricians (588) suggested a poorer outcome for male children, especially those with a prepubertal onset. In contrast, Levy et al. (589) reported a higher frequency of death or end-stage renal failure in girls. It must be recognized, however, that the numbers are small and other confusing factors such as race (see earlier discussion) are difficult to correct for.

Renal Biopsy Data

Pattern of Glomerular Disease

At a histologic level, a considerable body of data is available. The WHO classification, which includes a category of sclerosing glomerulopathy (537,590), has been studied the most. Although the overall prognosis of lupus nephritis has improved, it is clear that the outcome varies for different classes of disease (Fig. 71-18). Appel et al. (575) noted a better survival in those with class II (mesangial) nephritis compared with the other histologic classes. Similar results have been reported in a review by Berden (591). In contrast, despite recent improvement, Austin et al. (592) reported a poorer survival rate in those with class IV nephritis, as did Nossent et al. (573) and Berden (591).

A particular problem exists with regard to patients classified as having the WHO class III appearance—focal proliferative glomerulonephritis. A diverse outcome has been reported for such individuals (58,593,594), which illustrates the great variation in severity within this group. The survival of patients with class IIIa disease (by the original WHO classification system) resembles that for milder forms of lupus nephritis (595–597), whereas survival of patients with more severe focal disease is more akin to that of patients with class IV disease. In fact, in the 10-year follow-up data from the Lupus Collaborative Study (574), patients with class III disease were significantly less likely to enter remission and had significantly worse renal survival rates than patients with class IV disease. In the revised WHO classification, the activity and chronicity of class III lesions is also described (598).

Patients showing the WHO class V pattern (i.e., membranous nephropathy) almost always have a more favorable course

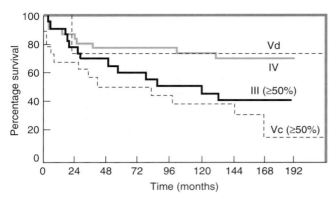

FIGURE 71-18. Renal survival based on histologic categorization and subcategorization (censoring for nonrenal death). Renal survival is shown for patients with World Health Organization (WHO) class III (≥50%; or active and/or necrotizing lesions in 50% or more of glomeruli), IV (in which there was inflammation in ≥80% of non-hyalinized glomeruli), Vc (membranous glomerulonephritis superimposed upon class III), or Vd (membranous glomerulonephritis superimposed upon class IV). Survival for class III (N = 24) was significantly worse than for class IV (N = 35) disease (P = 0.05, IV vs. III (≥50%). Class Vc (N = 20) disease had a significantly worse renal survival than class IV (p = 0.002). (From: Najafi CC, et al. Significance of histologic patterns of glomerular injury upon long-term prognosis in severe lupus glomerulonephritis. *Kidney Int* 2001;59:2156, with permission.)

(175,537,599–601), although renal failure occurs in a minority (601,602). Persistent nephrotic syndrome has been reported to be associated with a worse prognosis (564,572,575). It has recently become clear that the long-term prognosis of lupus membranous nephropathy varies depending on whether the patient exhibits pure membranous (Va) or just mild mesangial proliferation (Vb) versus those with coexisting proliferative disease, either focal (Vc) or diffuse (Vd) (601,603). The 10-year survival rate fell from 72% in patients with Va or Vb disease to 48% in those with Vc lesions and only 20% in patients with class Vd disease (603). As a consequence, in a recent revision of the WHO classification system, the grades Vc and Vd have been dropped (598). In this revised system, both pathologic grades should be reported for patients with a combination of class V disease with either class III or class IV so as to more clearly communicate the lesion.

Individual Elements of Histology

Analyses have been performed also to assess the predictive value of individual elements of the histologic picture. Two observations appear to show some reliability in predicting a poor outcome. The first of these is extensive subendothelial deposits, especially if they persist in repeated biopsy specimens (604–607). The value of this observation may now be reduced in most patients by aggressive treatment of such a histologic appearance. Still of value, however, are tubulointerstitial changes, which were noted by Muehrcke et al. (608) as long ago as 1957. These changes pointed to a poor prognosis in a number of studies (564,592,609). Magil et al. (572) found that the number of nonspecific esterase-positive cells (macrophages) correlated with outcome, and another study (610) showed, using monoclonal antibodies to determine the phenotype of the interstitial cells, correlations between both the numbers of infiltrating monocytes and T cells and subsequent GFRs. The presence of crescents has also been related to a poorer prognosis (611), as in other forms of nephritis, but very extensive crescentic disease is relatively uncommon in lupus. Vascular le-

sions within the biopsy material (612,613) and intraglomerular capillary thrombi (614) have been associated with unfavorable outcomes also, although the latter observation has been contested (595,615). In another study, the presence of intraglomerular leukocyte infiltration was found to be the strongest correlate with progression to renal insufficiency (616).

Activity/Chronicity Indices. Because of dissatisfaction with the data obtained by considering the morphologic aspects of nephritis (which is in any case variable between and within glomeruli in lupus nephritis, and also varies in sequential biopsy samples (531–534)), an alternative approach has gained support: that of assessing the histologic activity of the nephritis on the one hand, and its apparent chronicity on the other, as judged by the extent of sclerosis. This approach was pioneered by Pirani and Salinas-Madrigal (617), Morel-Maroger (590), and others in the 1960s and 1970s, but became popular after Austin et al. (592) described the calculation of activity and chronicity indices using data from glomeruli and interstitium (Table 71-17). This approach allowed these workers (592) to identify clear groups at high and low risk for a poor outcome and permitted therapeutic stratification, specifically, when and when not to use aggressive treatment.

These data were supported by Magil et al. (572), Esdaile et al. (564), and Nossent et al. (573), who all found a high chronicity index to be the best predictor of subsequent renal failure. However, several other authors found a poor or absent association of outcome with either index, or combinations of them (575,595,618), although the follow-up period in Schwartz's study (618) was only 2 years. Nevertheless, it is clear that chronic scarring is associated with poor prognosis.

Additional Value of Renal Biopsy Data. Several authors (564,572,582,606,607) using different multivariate models and different sets of data examined the additional value for predicting outcome of the information from renal biopsy specimens over that available from clinical studies. Whiting-O'Keefe et al. (606,607) concluded that only the degree of sclerosis and the presence or absence of subendothelial deposits seemed of any great value. Austin et al. (592) and Magil et al. (572) suggested that the WHO classification of biopsy data adds useful information, and that the chronicity index is an even better predictor of outcome. Esdaile et al. (564), however, found no biopsy information that added to the clinical predictions. The

TABLE 71-17

RENAL PATHOLOGY SCORING SYSTEM IN LUPUS NEPHRITIS

Activity index	Chronicity index
Glomerular abnormalities	
Cellular proliferation	Glomerular sclerosis
Fibrinoid necrosis[a]	Fibrous crescents
Karyorrhexis	
Cellular crescents[a]	
Hyaline thrombi wire loops	
Leukocyte infiltration	
Tubulointerstitial abnormalities	
Mononuclear cell infiltration	Interstitial fibrosis
	Tubular atrophy

[a]Fibrinoid necrosis and cellular crescents are weighted by a factor of 2. Maximum score of activity index is 24 and chronicity index is 12. (Reprinted from: Austin KA III, et al. Prognostic factors in lupus nephritis: contribution of renal histologic data. *Am J Med* 1983;75:382, with permission.)

TABLE 71-18

RISK FACTORS FOR PROGRESSION OF LUPUS NEPHRITIS

Strong evidence
  Response to treatment (553)
  Maintenance of remission (553–555)
  Race (556,565,566,568)
  Plasma creatinine at onset of disease (548,553,556,564, 572–574)
  Disease activity (overall disease activity [580], anemia [548,554,556], hypocomplementemia [556,564], anti-Ro antibodies [574])
  WHO histologic classification (573,574,591,592)
  Chronicity index (564,572,573,592)

Some evidence
  Socioeconomic status (570)

Conflicting evidence
  Proteinuria (549,553,562,564,575)
  Hypertension (549,564,568,584,585)
  Age (78,563–565,582,583)

value of the biopsy in directing more aggressive—and possibly more successful—therapeutic strategies is almost impossible to evaluate, but as most analysis of prognosis and response to therapy in lupus nephritis is based upon the underlying histology, evaluation of the biopsy is an essential part of risk stratification and therapeutic decision making

Inapparent Renal Disease in Lupus. A number of authors noted that patients without clinical manifestations of nephritis have changes in their glomeruli amounting to glomerular disease. There have been few follow-up studies on such patients, but the study of Leehey et al. (619) showed that most remain without clinical nephritis for some years, although even severe diffuse proliferative patterns may be observed in some patients. Similar findings have been reported by Gonzalez-Crespo et al. (620). However, it is equally obvious that all patients with clinically evident nephritis must go through a period of absent or occult disease before the disease becomes evident; it is not known how many of these patients run a subclinical course for a prolonged period.

Long-Term Outlook for Lupus Nephritis

There are some data relating to 10-year survival or longer for patients with lupus nephritis (543,548,549,621–623). The differences between the various forms of nephritis have decreased and the survival is now better than 80% at 10 years (562,595). However, recent data (543,562,595) show no further improvement in outlook during the 1990s, with a persisting minority of patients who either die or go into end-stage renal failure within a decade. There is little information on 20-year survival, although a cohort of 60 patients treated between 1976 and 1986 (543) demonstrated about 75% survival, similar to data found in the paper of Moroni et al. (623).

There are surprisingly few data also on the longer term status of patients with lupus nephritis in relation to treatment: How common is stable long-term remission after discontinuing all therapy? Is there a difference between patients treated with cyclophosphamide or azathioprine in this respect? Given the recent evidence that mycophenolate is effective for induction or maintenance therapy (624,625), the long-term outcome for patients treated with this agent are also important to know. As noted previously, in an analysis of patients treated before

1986 (543) who all had a potential follow-up of more than 15 years (actual median follow-up, 15.5 years; range, 2 to 31 years) prognosis improved in the cohort studied from 1976 compared with those who entered in 1975 or earlier, but the subsequent decade saw no further improvement (10-year survival of 57%, 81%, and 84%, respectively). After 20 years, more than three-quarters of patients can expect to be alive with renal function. Of living patients with renal function, 38% had no proteinuria, but only 11% were receiving no specific treatment. The report by Moroni and colleagues (623) on a smaller group of patients is more encouraging. Of 34 patients who had actually completed 10 years of follow-up, only 6 (17.5%) had died, 3 were receiving end-stage treatment, 6 had elevated plasma creatinine levels (3 with proteinuria), 6 had minor proteinuria with normal function, and 15 were in complete remission; 11 patients (32%) had been off all treatment for a mean of 7.5 years. None of the patients in these two series had received intravenous cyclophosphamide, and the medium-term (2 to 10 years) results are similar to those treated with this type of regimen in other hands. In a more recent report that included patients with proliferative disease who had been treated with cyclophosphamide (574), the overall 15 year renal survival was 50% and the 15-year patient survival was 70%. Unfortunately, greater detail regarding the long-term outlook for patients after receiving cyclophosphamide has not been reported. In particular, data regarding the number of patients free of treatment long term is unknown.

CONCLUSIONS

This chapter presents data suggesting that most patients with progressive forms of glomerulonephritis reach renal failure within 5 to 15 years after apparent clinical onset, and similarly, those who enter remission will usually have done so by the end of this time. Few patients show much more rapid evolution or remission, and only a few will have persisting urinary abnormalities with normal renal function.

These patients show "grumbling" nephritis, with proteinuria, hematuria, or both, persisting at various levels of apparently stable renal function for 20 years or more. This is particularly common in membranous nephropathy and in IgA-associated disease. It can also be seen in treated patients with lupus nephritis.

One major task, along with the introduction of effective treatments to slow or eliminate the deterioration in renal function, is to identify as early as possible those patients who have a progressive course so treatments can be focused on this high-risk group. Several features consistently emerge from multivariate analyses as predictors of a poor outcome in a broad range of glomerular diseases: (a) the magnitude and duration of proteinuria—although this must be interpreted in light of the renal biopsy findings, because patients with minimal change nephrotic syndrome may show the highest figures; (b) a raised plasma creatinine concentration that does not return to normal on control of the nephrotic syndrome, because reversible changes in K_f may depress the GFR temporarily; (c) tubulointerstitial damage in the renal biopsy specimen—in general the severity of glomerular changes is a much poorer indicator of outlook, with the sole exception of extensive crescent formation; and (d) a persistently raised blood pressure—again, the transient hypertension of some patients with minimal change nephrotic syndrome or reversible acute nephritis makes a period of observation necessary, and the first figures obtained on admission to hospital relatively useless.

A number of other features (e.g., male sex and increasing age) are less consistently predictive of a poor outcome. Some authors have suggested that the amount of urinary blood excreted by patients with hematuric illnesses predicts poor outcome, but others found just the opposite. Therefore, the archetypal patient with glomerulopathy and a poor outlook is a middle-aged or older adult man with sustained hypertension, an elevated plasma creatinine concentration, persistent nephrotic-range proteinuria, tubulointerstitial damage in renal biopsy specimens, and crescents if a proliferative glomerulonephritis is present. On the contrary, a young normotensive woman whose proteinuria remits or diminishes, who has normal renal function, and whose biopsy reveals only intraglomerular changes is almost certain to do well.

Glomerulonephritis, although no longer the most common single cause of end-stage renal failure, remains the most common cause in young adults. Now we need 15-, 20-, and 30-year follow-up data on patients with glomerular diseases to answer the many questions raised in this chapter about the fate of individual groups. Collecting such data is tedious, without glamor, and difficult to fund; changes in staff over the years result in many studies never being completed. Without such data, however, we will never be able to present even a 20-year picture of what happens to patients with glomerular disease.

ACKNOWLEDGMENTS

The authors are indebted to Dr. JS Cameron for his immense contribution to these chapters in previous editions.

References

1. Peto R, Pike MC, Armitage P, et al. Design and analysis of randomized clinical trials requiring prolonged observation of each patient. II. analysis and examples. Br J Cancer 1977;35:1.
2. Kaplan E, Meier P. Non-parametric estimation from incomplete observations. J Am Stat Assoc 1958;53:457.
3. Breslow N. A generalized Kruskal-Wallis test for comparing K samples subject to unequal patterns of censorship. Biometrika 1970;57(3):579.
4. Cox D. Regression models and life table (with discussion). J R Stat Soc 1972;34:187.
5. Beukhof JR, Kardaun O, Schaafsma W, et al. Toward individual prognosis of IgA nephropathy. Kidney Int 1986;29:549.
6. D'Amico G, Minetti L, Ponticelli C, et al. Prognostic indicators in idiopathic IgA mesangial nephropathy. Q J Med 1986;59:363.
7. Esdaile JM, Levinton C, Federgreen W, et al. The clinical and renal biopsy predictors of long-term outcome in lupus nephritis: a study of 87 patients and review of the literature. Q J Med 1989;72:779.
8. Magil AB, Puterman ML, Ballon HS, et al. Prognostic factors in diffuse proliferative lupus glomerulonephritis. Kidney Int 1988;34:511.
9. Wehrmann M, Bohle A, Held H, et al. Long-term prognosis of focal sclerosing glomerulonephritis. An analysis of 250 cases with particular regard to tubulointerstitial changes. Clin Nephrol 1990;33:115.
10. Passerini P, Pasquali S, Cesana B, et al. Long-term outcome of patients with membranous nephropathy after complete remission of proteinuria. Nephrol Dial Transplant 1989;4:525.
11. Mitch WE, Walser M, Buffington GA, et al. A simple method of estimating progression of chronic renal failure. Lancet 1976;2:1326.
12. Rutherford WE, Blondin J, Miller JP, et al. Chronic progressive renal disease: rate of change of serum creatinine concentration. Kidney Int 1977; 11:62.
13. Gretz N, Manz F, Strauch M. Predictability of the progression of chronic renal failure. Kidney Int 1983;15(Suppl):S2.
14. Davison AM, Cameron JS, Kerr DN, et al. The natural history of renal function in untreated idiopathic membranous glomerulonephritis in adults. Clin Nephrol 1984;22:61.
15. Cameron JS, Healy MJ, Adu D. The Medical Research Council trial of short-term high-dose alternate day prednisolone in idiopathic membranous nephropathy with nephrotic syndrome in adults. The MRC Glomerulonephritis Working Party. Q J Med 1990;74:133.
16. Fellin G, Gentile MG, Duca G, et al. Renal function in IgA nephropathy with established renal failure. Nephrol Dial Transplant 1988;3:17.
17. Cameron J. The natural history of glomerulonephritis. Contrib Nephrol 1989;75:68.
18. Walser M. Progression of chronic renal failure in man. Kidney Int 1990;37:1195.
19. Hunsicker LG. Studies of therapy of progressive renal failure in humans. Semin Nephrol 1989;9:380.
20. Levey AS. Use of glomerular filtration rate measurements to assess the progression of renal disease. Semin Nephrol 1989;9:370.
21. Cameron J. Clinicopathological correlations—problems and limitations. Clin Nephrol 1977;4:1.
22. Churg J, Sobin L. Renal disease: classification and atlas of glomerular disease. Tokyo: Igaku-Shoin Medical Publishers, 1982.
23. Cameron JS. The nephrotic syndrome: management, complications and pathophysiology. In: Davison AM, Cameron JS, Grunfeld JP, et al, eds. Oxford Textbook of Clinical Nephrology. 2nd ed. London: Oxford University Press; 1998:461.
24. Bazzi C, D'Amico G. The urinary excretion of IgG and alpha1-microglobulin predicts renal outcome and identifies patients deserving treatment in membranous nephropathy. Kidney Int 2002;61:2276.
25. Bazzi C, Petrini C, Rizza V, et al. Urinary N-acetyl-beta-glucosaminidase excretion is a marker of tubular cell dysfunction and a predictor of outcome in primary glomerulonephritis. Nephrol Dial Transplant 2002;17:1890.
26. Fede C, Conti G, Chimenz R, et al. N-acetyl-beta-D-glucosaminidase and beta2-microglobulin: prognostic markers in idiopathic nephrotic syndrome. J Nephrol 1999;12:51.
27. Mastroianni Kirsztajn G, Nishida SK, et al. Urinary retinol-binding protein as a prognostic marker in the treatment of nephrotic syndrome. Nephron 2000;86:109.
28. Harris RC, Ismail N. Extrarenal complications of the nephrotic syndrome. Am J Kidney Dis 1994;23:477.
29. Cameron JS. Clinical consequences of the nephrotic syndrome. In: Cameron JS, ed. Oxford Textbook of Clinical Nephrology. London: Oxford University Press; 1992:276.
30. Wass VJ, Jarrett RJ, Chilvers C, et al. Does the nephrotic syndrome increase the risk of cardiovascular disease? Lancet 1979;2:664.
31. Trompeter RS, Lloyd BW, Hicks J, et al. Long-term outcome for children with minimal-change nephrotic syndrome. Lancet 1985;1:368.
32. Nolasco F, Cameron JS, Heywood EF, et al. Adult-onset minimal change nephrotic syndrome: a long-term follow-up. Kidney Int 1986;29:1215.
33. McCarron DA, Rubin RJ, Barnes BA, et al. Therapeutic bilateral renal infarction in end-stage renal disease. N Engl J Med 1976;294:652.
34. Cameron JS, Ogg CS, Wass VJ. Complications of the nephrotic syndrome. In: Cameron JS, ed. The Nephrotic Syndrome. New York: Marcel Dekker Inc.; 1988:849.
35. Arneil GC. 164 children with nephrosis. Lancet 1961;2:1103.
36. Christian H. Nephrosis—a critique. JAMA 1929;93:23.
37. Wass V, Cameron JS. Cardiovascular disease and the nephrotic syndrome: the other side of the coin. Nephron 1981;27:58.
38. Keane WF. Lipids and the kidney. Kidney Int 1994;46:910.
39. Wheeler DC. Lipid abnormalities in the nephrotic syndrome: the therapeutic role of statins. J Nephrol 2001;14(Suppl 4):S70.
40. Shurtleff D. (Department of Health, Education and Welfare). Some characteristics related to the incidence of cardiovascular disease and death: framingham Study, 18 year follow-up. In: The Framingham Study: An Epidemiological Investigation of Cardiovascular Disease. 1974. Report No.: NIH publication no. 74–599.
41. Radhakrishnan J, Appel AS, Valeri A, et al. The nephrotic syndrome, lipids, and risk factors for cardiovascular disease. Am J Kidney Dis 1993;22:135.
42. Stills HF, Jr., Bullock BC, Clarkson TB. Increased atherosclerosis and glomerulonephritis in cynomolgus monkeys (Macaca fascicularis) given injections of BSA over an extended period of time. Am J Pathol 1983;113:222.
43. Fernandes G, Alonso DR, Tanaka T, et al. Influence of diet on vascular lesions in autoimmune-prone B/W mice. Proc Natl Acad Sci U S A 1983;80: 874.
44. Bonfiglio TA, Botti RE, Hagstrom JW. Coronary arteritis, occlusion, and myocardial infarction due to lupus erythematosus. Am Heart J 1972;83: 153.
45. Haider YS, Roberts WC. Coronary arterial disease in systemic lupus erythematosus: quantification of degrees of narrowing in 22 necropsy patients (21 women) aged 16 to 37 years. Am J Med 1981;70:775.
46. Meller J, Conde CA, Deppisch LM, et al. Myocardial infarction due to coronary atherosclerosis in three young adults with systemic lupus erythematosus. Am J Cardiol 1975;35:309.
47. Ordonez JD, Hiatt RA, Killebrew EJ, et al. The increased risk of coronary heart disease associated with nephrotic syndrome. Kidney Int 1993;44:638.
48. Cameron JS. Coagulation and thromboembolic complications in the nephrotic syndrome. Adv Nephrol Necker Hosp 1984;13:75.
49. Rabelink TJ, Zwaginga JJ, Koomans HA, et al. Thrombosis and hemostasis in renal disease. Kidney Int 1994;46:287.
50. Kasiske BL, Velosa JA, Halstenson CE, et al. The effects of lovastatin in hyperlipidemic patients with the nephrotic syndrome. Am J Kidney Dis 1990;15:8.
51. Chan PC, Robinson JD, Yeung WC, et al. Lovastatin in glomerulonephritis patients with hyperlipidaemia and heavy proteinuria. Nephrol Dial Transplant 1992;7:93.
52. Sarasin FP, Schifferli JA. Prophylactic oral anticoagulation in nephrotic patients with idiopathic membranous nephropathy. Kidney Int 1994;45:578.
53. Cameron JS. Proteinuria and progression in human glomerular diseases. Am J Nephrol 1990;10(Suppl 1):81.
54. De Jong PE, de Zeeuw D, Mogensen CE, eds. Proteinuria and progressive renal disease. Nephrol Dial Transplant 1996;1(Suppl 2):1.
55. Abbate M, Benigni A, Bertani T, et al. Nephrotoxicity of increased glomerular protein traffic. Nephrol Dial Transplant 1999;14:304.
56. Passerini P, Pasquali S, Cesana B, et al. Long-term outcome of patients

with membranous nephropathy after complete remission of proteinuria. *Nephrol Dial Transplant* 1989;4:525.

57. Magil AB, Price JD, Bower G, et al. Membranoproliferative glomerulonephritis type 1: Comparison of natural history in children and adults. *Clin Nephrol* 1979;11:239.

58. Magil AB, Ballon HS, Rae A. Focal proliferative lupus nephritis. A clinicopathologic study using the WHO classification. *Am J Med* 1982;72:620.

59. Treser G, Ehrenreich T, Ores R, et al. Natural history of "apparently healed" acute poststreptococcal glomerulonephritis in children. *Pediatrics* 1969;43:1005.

60. Williams PS, Fass G, Bone JM. Renal pathology and proteinuria determine progression in untreated mild/moderate chronic renal failure. *Q J Med* 1988;67:343.

61. Hunt LP, Short CD, Mallick NP. Prognostic indicators in patients presenting with the nephrotic syndrome. *Kidney Int* 1988;34:382.

62. Beaufils H, Alphonse JC, Guedon J, et al. Focal glomerulosclerosis: natural history and treatment. A report of 70 cases. *Nephron* 1978;21:75.

63. Cameron JS, Turner DR, Ogg CS, et al. The long-term prognosis of patients with focal segmental glomerulosclerosis. *Clin Nephrol* 1978;10:213.

64. Cameron JS. Pathogenesis and treatment of membranous nephropathy. *Kidney Int* 1979;15:88.

65. Erwin DT, Donadio JV, Jr., Holley KE. The clinical course of idiopathic membranous nephropathy. *Mayo Clin Proc* 1973;48:697.

66. Pei Y, Cattran D, Greenwood C. Predicting chronic renal insufficiency in idiopathic membranous glomerulonephritis. *Kidney Int* 1992;42:960.

67. Chan MK, Chan KW, Chan PC, et al. Adult-onset mesangiocapillary glomerulonephritis: a disease with a poor prognosis. *Q J Med* 1989;72:599.

68. Eddy AA, McCulloch L, Liu E, et al. A relationship between proteinuria and acute tubulointerstitial disease in rats with experimental nephrotic syndrome. *Am J Pathol* 1991;138:1111.

69. Burton CJ, Walls J. Proximal tubular cell, proteinuria and tubulo-interstitial scarring. *Nephron* 1994;68:287.

70. Kees-Folts D, Sadow JL, Schreiner GF. Tubular catabolism of albumin is associated with the release of an inflammatory lipid. *Kidney Int* 1994;45:1697.

71. Remuzzi G, Bertani T. Pathophysiology of progressive nephropathies. *N Engl J Med* 1998;339:1448.

72. de Jong PE, Anderson S, de Zeeuw D. Glomerular preload and afterload reduction as a tool to lower urinary protein leakage: will such treatments also help to improve renal function outcome? *J Am Soc Nephrol* 1993;3:1333.

73. Lewis JB, Berl T, Bain RP, et al. Effect of intensive blood pressure control on the course of type 1 diabetic nephropathy. Collaborative Study Group. *Am J Kidney Dis* 1999;34:809.

74. Lewis EJ, Hunsicker LG, Bain RP, et al. The effect of angiotensin-converting-enzyme inhibition on diabetic nephropathy. The Collaborative Study Group. *N Engl J Med* 1993;329:1456.

75. Lewis EJ, Hunsicker LG, Clarke WR, et al. Renoprotective effect of the angiotensin-receptor antagonist irbesartan in patients with nephropathy due to type 2 diabetes. *N Engl J Med* 2001;345:851.

76. Brenner BM, Cooper ME, de Zeeuw D, et al. Effects of losartan on renal and cardiovascular outcomes in patients with type 2 diabetes and nephropathy. *N Engl J Med* 2001;345:861.

77. Cameron JS, Turner DR, Ogg CS, et al. Systemic lupus with nephritis: a long-term study. *Q J Med* 1979;48:1.

78. Wallace DJ, Podell T, Weiner J, et al. Systemic lupus erythematosus—survival patterns. Experience with 609 patients. *JAMA* 1981;245:934.

79. Hlatky MA. Is renal biopsy necessary in adults with nephrotic syndrome? *Lancet* 1982;2:1264.

80. Kassirer JP. Is renal biopsy necessary for optimal management of the idiopathic nephrotic syndrome? *Kidney Int* 1983;24:561.

81. Levey AS, Lau J, Pauker SG, et al. Idiopathic nephrotic syndrome. Puncturing the biopsy myth. *Ann Intern Med* 1987;107:697.

82. Cameron J. The natural history of glomerulonephritis. In: Kincaid-Smith P DAA, Atkins RC, eds. *Progress in Glomerulonephritis*. New York: Wiley; 1979:1.

83. Haas M, Meehan SM, Karrison TG, et al. Changing etiologies of unexplained adult nephrotic syndrome: a comparison of renal biopsy findings from 1976–1979 and 1995–1997. *Am J Kidney Dis* 1997;30:621.

84. Kitiyakara C, Kopp JB, Eggers P. Trends in the epidemiology of focal segmental glomerulosclerosis. *Semin Nephrol* 2003;23:172.

85. Filler G, Young E, Geier P, et al. Is there really an increase in non-minimal change nephrotic syndrome in children? *Am J Kidney Dis* 2003;42:1107.

86. Bonilla-Felix M, Parra C, Dajani T, et al. Changing patterns in the histopathology of idiopathic nephrotic syndrome in children. *Kidney Int* 1999;55:1885.

87. Srivastava T, Simon SD, Alon US. High incidence of focal segmental glomerulosclerosis in nephrotic syndrome of childhood. *Pediatr Nephrol* 1999;13:13.

88. Gulati S, Sharma AP, Sharma RK, et al. Changing trends of histopathology in childhood nephrotic syndrome. *Am J Kidney Dis* 1999;34:646.

89. Choi IJ, Jeong HJ, Han DS, et al. An analysis of 4,514 cases of renal biopsy in Korea. *Yonsei Med J* 2001;42:247.

90. Hurtado A, Escudero E, Stromquist CS, et al. Distinct patterns of glomerular disease in Lima, Peru. *Clin Nephrol* 2000;53:325.

91. Kasinath BS, Mujais SK, Spargo BH, et al. Nondiabetic renal disease in patients with diabetes mellitus. *Am J Med* 1983;75:613.

92. Seggie J. Nephrotic syndrome in the tropics. In: Cameron JS, ed. *The Nephrotic Syndrome*. New York: Marcel Dekker Inc.; 1988:653.

93. Kibukamusoke J. Nephrotic syndrome of quartan malaria in Bristol: Edward Arnold, 1973.

94. Wang F, Looi LM, Chua CT. Minimal change glomerular disease in Malaysian adults and use of alternate day steroid therapy. *Q J Med* 1982;51:312.

95. A controlled study of short-term prednisone treatment in adults with membranous nephropathy. Collaborative Study of the Adult Idiopathic Nephrotic Syndrome. *N Engl J Med* 1979;301:1301.

96. Vosnides G. Frequency of various forms of primary glomerulonephritis (GN) in Greek adults (abstract). IX Congress of the International Society of Nephrology, 1984.

97. Broumand B. High incidence of membranoproliferative glomerulonephritis in Iran (abstract). IX Congress of the International Society of Nephrology, 1984.

98. Chun MJ, Korbet SM, Schwartz MM, et al. Focal segmental glomerulosclerosis in nephrotic adults: presentation, prognosis, and response to therapy of the histologic variants. *J Am Soc Nephrol* 2004;15:2169.

99. Pei Y, Cattran D, Delmore T, et al. Evidence suggesting under-treatment in adults with idiopathic focal segmental glomerulosclerosis. Regional Glomerulonephritis Registry Study. *Am J Med* 1987;82:938.

100. Idelson BA, Smithline N, Smith GW, et al. Prognosis in steroid-treated idiopathic nephrotic syndrome in adults. Analysis of major predictive factors after ten-year follow-up. *Arch Intern Med* 1977;137:891.

101. Perna A, Schieppati A, Zamora J, et al. Immunosuppressive treatment for idiopathic membranous nephropathy: a systematic review. *Am J Kidney Dis* 2004;44:385.

102. Burgess E. Management of focal segmental glomerulosclerosis: Evidence-based recommendations. *Kidney Int* 1999;70(Suppl):S26.

103. Whittier WL, Korbet SM. Timing of complications in percutaneous renal biopsy. *J Am Soc Nephrol* 2004;15:142.

104. Korbet SM, Schwartz MM, Lewis EJ. Minimal-change glomerulopathy of adulthood. *Am J Nephrol* 1988;8:291.

105. Antoine B, Symvoulidis A, Dardenne M. The stable evolution of asymptomatic persistent proteinuria. *Nephron* 1969;6(4):526.

106. Levitt JI. The prognostic significance of proteinuria in young college students. *Ann Intern Med* 1967;66:685.

107. Minimal change nephrotic syndrome in children: deaths during the first 5 to 15 years' observation. Report of the International Study of Kidney Disease in Children. *Pediatrics* 1984;73:497.

108. Krensky AM, Ingelfinger JR, Grupe WE. Peritonitis in childhood nephrotic syndrome: 1970–1980. *Am J Dis Child* 1982;136:732.

109. Gorensek MJ, Lebel MH, Nelson JD. Peritonitis in children with nephrotic syndrome. *Pediatrics* 1988;81:849.

110. Cameron JS. The natural history and outcome of the nephrotic syndrome. In: Cameron JS, ed. *The Nephrotic Syndrome*. New York: Marcel Dekker Inc.; 1987.

111. Wingen AM, Muller-Wiefel DE, Scharer K. Spontaneous remissions in frequently relapsing and steroid dependent idiopathic nephrotic syndrome. *Clin Nephrol* 1985;23:35.

112. Schwartz H, Kohn JL. Lipoid nephrosis. A clinical and pathological study based on fifteen years' observation with special reference to prognosis. *Am J Dis Child* 1939;49:579.

113. Nash MA, Edelman CM Jr, Bernstein J, et al. Minimal change nephrotic syndrome, diffuse mesangial hypercellularity, and focal glomerular sclerosis. In: Edelmann CM Jr, ed. *Pediatric Nephrology*. Boston: Little, Brown and Company; 1993:1267.

114. Lange K, Wasserman E, Slobody LB. Prolonged intermittent steroid therapy for nephrosis in children and adults. *JAMA* 1958;168:377.

115. Short versus standard prednisone therapy for initial treatment of idiopathic nephrotic syndrome in children. Arbeitsgemeinschaft fur Padiatrische Nephrologie. *Lancet* 1988;1:380.

116. Brodehl J. The treatment of minimal change nephrotic syndrome: lessons learned from multicentre co-operative studies. *Eur J Pediatr* 1991;150:380.

117. Choonara IA, Heney D, Meadow SR. Low dose prednisolone in nephrotic syndrome. *Arch Dis Child* 1989;64:610.

118. Kleinknecht A. Comparison of short and long treatment at onset on steroid-sensitive nephrosis (SSN). Preliminary results of a multicenter controlled trial from the French Society of Pediatric Nephrology. *Int J Pediatr Nephrol* 1982;3:45.

119. Trompeter RS. Immunosuppressive therapy in the nephrotic syndrome in children. *Pediatr Nephrol* 1989;3:194.

120. Mendoza SA, Tune BM. Treatment of childhood nephrotic syndrome. *J Am Soc Nephrol* 1992;3:889.

121. Broyer M, Naiudet P, et al. Minimal changes and focal segmental glomerular sclerosis. In: Cameron JS, ed. *Oxford Textbook of Clinical Nephrology*. London: Oxford University Press; 1992:298.

122. Bajpai A, Bagga A, Hari P, et al. Intravenous cyclophosphamide in steroid-resistant nephrotic syndrome. *Pediatr Nephrol* 2003;18:351.

123. Alshaya HO, Al-Maghrabi JA, Kari JA. Intravenous pulse cyclophosphamide—is it effective in children with steroid-resistant nephrotic syndrome? *Pediatr Nephrol* 2003;18:1143.

124. Polito C, Oporto MR, Totino SF, et al. Normal growth of nephrotic children during long-term alternate-day prednisone therapy. *Acta Paediatr Scand* 1986;75:245.

125. Warshaw BL, Hymes LC. Daily single-dose and daily reduced-dose prednisone therapy for children with the nephrotic syndrome. *Pediatrics* 1989;83:694.

126. Garin EH, Pryor ND, Fennell RS, et al. Pattern of response to prednisone in idiopathic, minimal lesion nephrotic syndrome as a criterion in selecting patients for cyclophosphamide therapy. *J Pediatr* 1978;92:304.

127. Effect of cytotoxic drugs in frequently relapsing nephrotic syndrome with and without steroid dependence. *N Engl J Med* 1982;306:451.

128. Ueda N, Kuno K, Ito S. Eight and 12 week courses of cyclophosphamide in nephrotic syndrome. *Arch Dis Child* 1990;65(10):1147.

129. Schulman SL, Kaiser BA, Polinsky MS, et al. Predicting the response to cytotoxic therapy for childhood nephrotic syndrome: superiority of response to corticosteroid therapy over histopathologic patterns. *J Pediatr* 1988;113:996.

130. Zidar N, Avgustin Cavic M, Kenda RB, et al. Unfavorable course of minimal change nephrotic syndrome in children with intrauterine growth retardation. *Kidney Int* 1998;54:1320.

131. Niaudet P, Habib R. Cyclosporine in the treatment of idiopathic nephrosis. *J Am Soc Nephrol* 1994;5:1049.

132. Meyrier A. Treatment of glomerular disease with cyclosporin A. *Nephrol Dial Transplant* 1989;4:923.

133. Hino S, Takemura T, Okada M, et al. Follow-up study of children with nephrotic syndrome treated with a long-term moderate dose of cyclosporine. *Am J Kidney Dis* 1998;31:932.

134. Aksu N, Turker M, Erdogan H, et al. Cyclosporin A plus prednisone treatment of steroid-sensitive frequently relapsing nephrotic syndrome in children. *Turk J Pediatr* 1999;41:225.

135. Ponticelli C, Edefonti A, Ghio L, et al. Cyclosporin versus cyclophosphamide for patients with steroid-dependent and frequently relapsing idiopathic nephrotic syndrome: A multicentre randomized controlled trial. *Nephrol Dial Transplant* 1993;8:1326.

136. Hulton SA, Neuhaus TJ, Dillon MJ, et al. Long-term cyclosporin A treatment of minimal-change nephrotic syndrome of childhood. *Pediatr Nephrol* 1994;8:401.

137. Gregory MJ, Smoyer WE, Sedman A, et al. Long-term cyclosporine therapy for pediatric nephrotic syndrome: a clinical and histologic analysis. *J Am Soc Nephrol* 1996;7:543.

138. Bagga A, Hari P, Moudgil A, et al. Mycophenolate mofetil and prednisolone therapy in children with steroid-dependent nephrotic syndrome. *Am J Kidney Dis* 2003;42:1114.

139. Niaudet P, Drachman R, Gagnadoux MF, et al. Treatment of idiopathic nephrotic syndrome with levamisole. *Acta Paediatr Scand* 1984;73:637.

140. Bagga A, Sharma A, Srivastava RN. Levamisole therapy in corticosteroid-dependent nephrotic syndrome. *Pediatr Nephrol* 1997;11:415.

141. Levamisole for corticosteroid-dependent nephrotic syndrome in childhood. British Association for Paediatric Nephrology. *Lancet* 1991;337:1555.

142. Siegel NJ, Goldberg B, Krassner LS, et al. Long-term follow-up of children with steroid-responsive nephrotic syndrome. *J Pediatr* 1972;81:251.

143. Berns JS, Gaudio KM, Krassner LS, et al. Steroid-responsive nephrotic syndrome of childhood: a long-term study of clinical course, histopathology, efficacy of cyclophosphamide therapy, and effects on growth. *Am J Kidney Dis* 1987;9:108.

144. Lewis MA, Baildom EM, Davis N, et al. Nephrotic syndrome: from toddlers to twenties. *Lancet* 1989;1:255.

145. Niali JF. Prolonged survival in the nephrotic syndrome. *Med J Aust* 1965;310:843.

146. Habib R, Kleinknecht C. The primary nephrotic syndrome of childhood. Classification and clinicopathologic study of 406 cases. *Pathol Annu* 1971;6:417.

147. Cuochi D. Relapsing nephrotic syndrome following remission for 20 years. *Int J Pediatr Nephrol* 1983;4:211.

148. Pru C, Kjellstrand CM, Cohn RA, et al. Late recurrence of minimal lesion nephrotic syndrome. *Ann Intern Med* 1984;100:69.

149. Shearn MA, Tu WH, Piel CF. Recurrent Nephrotic Syndrome. *Arch Intern Med* 1964;114:525.

150. Tarshish P, Tobin JN, Bernstein J, et al. Prognostic significance of the early course of minimal change nephrotic syndrome: report of the International Study of Kidney Disease in Children. *J Am Soc Nephrol* 1997;8:769.

151. Foote KD, Brocklebank JT, Meadow SR. Height attainment in children with steroid-responsive nephrotic syndrome. *Lancet* 1985;2:917.

152. Padilla R, Brem AS. Linear growth of children with nephrotic syndrome: effect of alkylating agents. *Pediatrics* 1989;84:495.

153. Loke KY, Yap HK, Zhou X, et al. Efficacy and safety of one year of growth hormone therapy in steroid-dependent nephrotic syndrome. *J Pediatr* 1997;130:793.

154. Gulati S, Godbole M, Singh U, et al. Are children with idiopathic nephrotic syndrome at risk for metabolic bone disease? *Am J Kidney Dis* 2003;46:1163.

155. Esbjorner E, Arvidsson B, Jones IL, et al. Bone mineral content and collagen metabolites in children receiving steroid treatment for nephrotic syndrome. *Acta Paediatr* 2001;90:1127.

156. Leonard MB, Feldman HI, Shults J, et al. Long-term, high-dose glucocorticoids and bone mineral content in childhood glucocorticoid-sensitive nephrotic syndrome. *N Engl J Med* 2004;351:868.

157. Fujita T, Satomura A, Hidaka M, et al. Acute alteration in bone mineral density and biochemical markers for bone metabolism in nephrotic patients

158. receiving high-dose glucocorticoid and one-cycle etidronate therapy. *Calcif Tissue Int* 2000;66:195.

159. Hayslett JP, Krassner LS, Bensch KG, et al. Progression of "lipoid nephrosis" to renal insufficiency. *N Engl J Med* 1969;281:181.

159. Kleinknecht C. La Néphrose. In: Royer P, Mathieu H, et al. eds. *Néphrologie Pédiatrique*. 3rd ed. Paris: Flammarion; 1983:274.

160. Nash MA, Bakare MA, D'Agati V, et al. Late development of chronic renal failure in steroid-responsive nephrotic syndrome. *J Pediatr* 1982;101:411.

161. Tejani A. Morphological transition in minimal change nephrotic syndrome. *Nephron* 1985;39:157.

162. Trainin EB, Gomez-Leon G. Development of renal insufficiency after long-standing steroid-responsive nephrotic syndrome. *Int J Pediatr Nephrol* 1982;3:55.

163. Cameron JS, Senguttuvan P, Hartley B, et al. Focal segmental glomerulosclerosis in fifty-nine renal allografts from a single centre; analysis of risk factors for recurrence. *Transplant Proc* 1989;21(1 Pt 2):2117.

164. Cameron JS, Healy MJ, Adu D. The Medical Research Council trial of short-term high-dose alternate day prednisolone in idiopathic membranous nephropathy with nephrotic syndrome in adults. The MRC Glomerulonephritis Working Party. *Q J Med* 1990;74:133.

165. Wehrmann M, Bohle A, Held H, et al. Long-term prognosis of focal sclerosing glomerulonephritis. An analysis of 250 cases with particular regard to tubulointerstitial changes. *Clin Nephrol* 1990;33:115.

166. Bakir AA, Bazilinski NG, Rhee HL, et al. Focal segmental glomerulosclerosis. A common entity in nephrotic black adults. *Arch Intern Med* 1989;149:1802.

167. Black DA, Rose G, Brewer DB. Controlled trial of prednisone in adult patients with the nephrotic syndrome. *Br Med J* 1970;3:421.

168. Coggins CH. Minimal change nephrosis in adults. In: Zurukzoglu W, ed. *Proceedings of the 8th International Congress of Nephrology*. Basel: Karger; 1981:336.

169. Fujimoto S, Yamamoto Y, Hisanaga S, et al. Minimal change nephrotic syndrome in adults: response to corticosteroid therapy and frequency of relapse. *Am J Kidney Dis* 1991;17:687.

170. Mak SK, Short CD, Mallick NP. Long-term outcome of adult-onset minimal-change nephropathy. *Nephrol Dial Transplant* 1996;11:2192.

171. Huang JJ, Hsu SC, Chen FF, et al. Adult-onset minimal change disease among Taiwanese: clinical features, therapeutic response, and prognosis. *Am J Nephrol* 2001;21:28.

172. Zech P, Colon S, Pointet P, et al. The nephrotic syndrome in adults aged over 60: etiology, evolution and treatment of 76 cases. *Clin Nephrol* 1982; 17:232.

173. Lee HY, Kim HS, Kang CM, et al. The efficacy of cyclosporine A in adult nephrotic syndrome with minimal change disease and focal-segmental glomerulosclerosis: a multicenter study in Korea. *Clin Nephrol* 1995;43:375.

174. Matsumoto H, Nakao T, Okada T, et al. Favorable outcome of low-dose cyclosporine after pulse methylprednisolone in Japanese adult minimal-change nephrotic syndrome. *Intern Med* 2004;43:668.

175. Lentz RD, Michael AF, Friend PS. Membranous transformation of lupus nephritis. *Clin Immunol Immunopathol* 1981;19:131.

176. Kaplan C, Pasternack B, Shah H, et al. Age-related incidence of sclerotic glomeruli in human kidneys. *Am J Pathol* 1975;80:227.

177. Gagnadoux MF. Long-term prognosis in children (abstract). 1984.

178. Hui A, Poucell S, Thorner P, et al. Clinical features and glomerular immunofluorescence of renal biopsies from children with nephrotic syndrome due to minimal change disease and two variants of mesangial proliferative glomerulonephritis. *Int J Pediatr Nephrol* 1984;5:5.

179. Trainin EB, Boichis H, Spitzer A, et al. Late nonresponsiveness to steroids in children with the nephrotic syndrome. *J Pediatr* 1975;87:519.

180. Siegel NJ, Kashgarian M, Spargo BH, et al. Minimal change and focal sclerotic lesions in lipoid nephrosis. *Nephron* 1974;13:125.

181. Childhood nephrotic syndrome associated with diffuse mesangial hypercellularity. A report of the Southwest Pediatric Nephrology Study Group. *Kidney Int* 1983;24:87.

182. Waldherr R, Gubler MC, Levy M, et al. The significance of pure diffuse mesangial proliferation in idiopathic nephrotic syndrome. *Clin Nephrol* 1978;10:171.

183. Vilches AR, Turner DR, Cameron JS, et al. Significance of mesangial IgM deposition in "minimal change" nephrotic syndrome. *Lab Invest* 1982;46:10.

184. Ji-Yun Y, Melvin T, Sibley R, et al. No evidence for a specific role of IgM in mesangial proliferation of idiopathic nephrotic syndrome. *Kidney Int* 1984;25:100.

185. Cameron J. The problem of focal segmental glomerulosclerosis. In: Kincaid-Smith P, d'Apice AJ, Atkins RC, ed. *Progress in Glomerulonephritis*. New York: Wiley; 1979:209.

186. D'Agati V. The many masks of focal segmental glomerulosclerosis. *Kidney Int* 1994;46:1223.

187. Schwartz MM, Korbet SM. Primary focal segmental glomerulosclerosis: pathology, histological variants, and pathogenesis. *Am J Kidney Dis* 1993;22:874.

188. Cameron JS. The enigma of focal segmental glomerulosclerosis. *Kidney Int* 1996;57(Suppl):S119.

189. Howie AJ, Lee SJ, Green NJ, et al. Different clinicopathological types of segmental sclerosing glomerular lesions in adults. *Nephrol Dial Transplant* 1993;8:590.

190. Cameron JS. Recurrent primary disease and de novo nephritis following renal transplantation. *Pediatr Nephrol* 1991;5:412.
191. Ingulli E, Tejani A. Racial differences in the incidence and renal outcome of idiopathic focal segmental glomerulosclerosis in children. *Pediatr Nephrol* 1991;5:393.
192. Weiss MA, Daquioag E, Margolin EG, et al. Nephrotic syndrome, progressive irreversible renal failure, and glomerular "collapse:" a new clinicopathologic entity? *Am J Kidney Dis* 1986;7:20.
193. Detwiler RK, Falk RJ, Hogan SL, et al. Collapsing glomerulopathy: a clinically and pathologically distinct variant of focal segmental glomerulosclerosis. *Kidney Int* 1994;45:1416.
194. Trompeter R. Steroid resistant nephrotic syndrome: a review of the treatment of focal segmental glomerulosclerosis (FSGS) in children. In: Murakami K, ed. *Pediatric Nephrology.* Amsterdam: Elsevier Science; 1987:363.
195. Arbus GS, Poucell S, Bacheyie GS, et al. Focal segmental glomerulosclerosis with idiopathic nephrotic syndrome: three types of clinical response. *J Pediatr* 1982;101:40.
196. Cattran DC, Rao P. Long-term outcome in children and adults with classic focal segmental glomerulosclerosis. *Am J Kidney Dis* 1998;32:72.
197. Tune BM, Kirpekar R, Sibley RK, et al. Intravenous methylprednisolone and oral alkylating agent therapy of prednisone-resistant pediatric focal segmental glomerulosclerosis: a long-term follow-up. *Clin Nephrol* 1995;43:84.
198. Korbet SM, Schwartz MM, Lewis EJ. Primary focal segmental glomerulosclerosis: clinical course and response to therapy. *Am J Kidney Dis* 1994;23:773.
199. Schena FP, Cameron JS. Treatment of proteinuric idiopathic glomerulonephritides in adults: a retrospective survey. *Am J Med* 1988;85:315.
200. Rydel JJ, Korbet SM, Borok RZ, et al. Focal segmental glomerular sclerosis in adults: presentation, course, and response to treatment. *Am J Kidney Dis* 1995;25:534.
201. Ponticelli C, Villa M, Banfi G, et al. Can prolonged treatment improve the prognosis in adults with focal segmental glomerulosclerosis? *Am J Kidney Dis* 1999;34(4):618.
202. Tejani A, Nicastri AD, Sen D, et al. Long-term evaluation of children with nephrotic syndrome and focal segmental glomerular sclerosis. *Nephron* 1983;35:225.
203. Focal segmental glomerulosclerosis in children with idiopathic nephrotic syndrome. A report of the Southwest Pediatric Nephrology Study Group. *Kidney Int* 1985;27:442.
204. Tarshish P, Tobin JN, Bernstein J, et al. Cyclophosphamide does not benefit patients with focal segmental glomerulosclerosis. a report of the International Study of Kidney Disease in Children. *Pediatr Nephrol* 1996;10:590.
205. Waldo FB, Benfield MR, Kohaut EC. Methylprednisolone treatment of patients with steroid-resistant nephrotic syndrome. *Pediatr Nephrol* 1992;6:503.
206. Martinelli R, Okumura AS, Pereira LJ, et al. Primary focal segmental glomerulosclerosis in children: prognostic factors. *Pediatr Nephrol* 2001;16:658.
207. Cattran DC. Outcomes research in glomerulonephritis. *Semin Nephrol* 2003;23:340.
208. Mendoza SA, Reznik VM, Griswold WR, et al. Treatment of steroid-resistant focal segmental glomerulosclerosis with pulse methylprednisolone and alkylating agents. *Pediatr Nephrol* 1990;4:303.
209. Ponticelli C, Rizzoni G, Edefonti A, et al. A randomized trial of cyclosporine in steroid-resistant idiopathic nephrotic syndrome. *Kidney Int* 1993;43:1377.
210. Niaudet P. Treatment of childhood steroid-resistant idiopathic nephrosis with a combination of cyclosporine and prednisone. French Society of Pediatric Nephrology. *J Pediatr* 1994;125(6, Pt 1):981.
211. Cattran DC, Appel GB, Hebert LA, et al. A randomized trial of cyclosporine in patients with steroid-resistant focal segmental glomerulosclerosis. North America Nephrotic Syndrome Study Group. *Kidney Int* 1999;56:2220.
212. Lieberman KV, Tejani A. A randomized double-blind placebo-controlled trial of cyclosporine in steroid-resistant idiopathic focal segmental glomerulosclerosis in children. *J Am Soc Nephrol* 1996;7:56.
213. Heering P, Braun N, Mullejans R, et al. Cyclosporine A and chlorambucil in the treatment of idiopathic focal segmental glomerulosclerosis. *Am J Kidney Dis* 2004;43:10.
214. Choi MJ, Eustace JA, Gimenez LF, et al. Mycophenolate mofetil treatment for primary glomerular diseases. *Kidney Int* 2002;61:1098.
215. Day CJ, Cockwell P, Lipkin GW, et al. Mycophenolate mofetil in the treatment of resistant idiopathic nephrotic syndrome. *Nephrol Dial Transplant* 2002;17:2011.
216. Saint-Hillier Y, Morel-Maroger L, Woodrow D, et al. Focal and segmental hyalinosis. *Adv Nephrol Necker Hosp* 1975;5:67.
217. Yoshikawa N, Ito H, Akamatsu R, et al. Focal segmental glomerulosclerosis with and without nephrotic syndrome in children. *J Pediatr* 1986;109:65.
218. Mongeau JG, Corneille L, Robitaille P, et al. Primary nephrosis in childhood associated with focal glomerular sclerosis: is long-term prognosis that severe? *Kidney Int* 1981;20:743.
219. Mongeau JG, Robitaille PO, Clermont MJ, et al. Focal segmental glomerulosclerosis (FSG) 20 years later. From toddler to grown up. *Clin Nephrol* 1993;40:1.
220. Brown CB, Cameron JS, Turner DR, et al. Focal segmental glomerulosclerosis with rapid decline in renal function ("malignant FSGS"). *Clin Nephrol* 1978;10:51.
221. Valeri A, Barisoni L, Appel GB, et al. Idiopathic collapsing focal segmental glomerulosclerosis: A clinicopathologic study. *Kidney Int* 1996;50:1734.
222. Savin VJ, Sharma R, Sharma M, et al. Circulating factor associated with increased glomerular permeability to albumin in recurrent focal segmental glomerulosclerosis. *N Engl J Med* 1996;334:878.
223. Lesavre P, Grunfeld JP. Idiopathic focal segmental glomerulosclerosis—new lessons from kidney transplantation. *N Engl J Med* 1996;334:914.
224. Abbott KC, Sawyers ES, Oliver JD, 3rd, et al. Graft loss due to recurrent focal segmental glomerulosclerosis in renal transplant recipients in the United States. *Am J Kidney Dis* 2001;37:366.
225. Kawaguchi H, Hattori M, Ito K, et al. Recurrence of focal glomerulosclerosis of allografts in children: the efficacy of intensive plasma exchange therapy before and after renal transplantation. *Transplant Proc* 1994;26:7.
226. Matalon A, Markowitz GS, Joseph RE, et al. Plasmapheresis treatment of recurrent FSGS in adult renal transplant recipients. *Clin Nephrol* 2001;56:271.
227. Chitalia VC, Wells JE, Robson RA, et al. Predicting renal survival in primary focal glomerulosclerosis from the time of presentation. *Kidney Int* 1999;56:2236.
228. McVicar M, Exeni R, Susin M. Nephrotic syndrome and multiple tubular defects in children: an early sign of focal segmental glomerulosclerosis. *J Pediatr* 1980;97:918.
229. Haycock GB. β2-microglobulin excretion in children with renal disease (abstract). *Int J Pediatr Nephrol* 1984;3:132.
230. Bazzi C, Petrini C, Rizza V, et al. Fractional excretion of IgG predicts renal outcome and response to therapy in primary focal segmental glomerulosclerosis: a pilot study. *Am J Kidney Dis* 2003;41:328.
231. Beaman M, Howie AJ, Hardwicke J, et al. The glomerular tip lesion: a steroid responsive nephrotic syndrome. *Clin Nephrol* 1987;27:217.
232. Ito H, Yoshikawa N, Aozai F, et al. Twenty-seven children with focal segmental glomerulosclerosis: correlation between the segmental location of the glomerular lesions and prognosis. *Clin Nephrol* 1984;22(1):9.
233. Morita M, White RH, Coad NA, et al. The clinical significance of the glomerular location of segmental lesions in focal segmental glomerulosclerosis. *Clin Nephrol* 1990;33:211.
234. Howie AJ, Brewer DB. Further studies on the glomerular tip lesion: early and late stages and life table analysis. *J Pathol* 1985;147:245.
235. Howie AJ, Brewer DB. The glomerular tip lesion: a previously undescribed type of segmental glomerular abnormality. *J Pathol* 1984;142:205.
236. Gubler MC, Habib R. Signification des lesions de sclérose/hyalinose segmentaire et focale (SHSF) dans la néphrose. Proceedings of the 6th International Congress of Nephrology. Montreal: Karger; 1978:437.
237. Schoeneman MJ, Bennett B, Greifer I. The natural history of focal segmental glomerulosclerosis with and without mesangial hypercellularity in children. *Clin Nephrol* 1978;9:45.
238. Lee HS, Spargo BH. Significance of renal hyaline arteriolosclerosis in focal segmental glomerulosclerosis. *Nephron* 1985;41:86.
239. Noel LH, Zanetti M, Droz D, et al. Long-term prognosis of idiopathic membranous glomerulonephritis. Study of 116 untreated patients. *Am J Med* 1979;66:82.
240. Donadio JV Jr, Torres VE, Velosa JA, et al. Idiopathic membranous nephropathy: the natural history of untreated patients. *Kidney Int* 1988;33:708.
241. Schieppati A, Mosconi L, Perna A, et al. Prognosis of untreated patients with idiopathic membranous nephropathy. *N Engl J Med* 1993;329:85.
242. Davison AM, Cameron JS, Kerr DN, et al. The natural history of renal function in untreated idiopathic membranous glomerulonephritis in adults. *Clin Nephrol* 1984;22:61.
243. Ponticelli C, Zucchelli P, Passerini P, et al. Methylprednisolone plus chlorambucil as compared with methylprednisolone alone for the treatment of idiopathic membranous nephropathy. The Italian Idiopathic Membranous Nephropathy Treatment Study Group. *N Engl J Med* 1992;327:599.
244. Ponticelli C, Zucchelli P, Passerini P, et al. A randomized trial of methylprednisolone and chlorambucil in idiopathic membranous nephropathy. *N Engl J Med* 1989;320:8.
245. Cattran DC, Delmore T, Roscoe J, et al. A randomized controlled trial of prednisone in patients with idiopathic membranous nephropathy. *N Engl J Med* 1989;320:210.
246. Honkanen E, Tornroth T, Gronhagen-Riska C. Natural history, clinical course and morphological evolution of membranous nephropathy. *Nephrol Dial Transplant* 1992;7(Suppl 1):35.
247. Kida H, Asamoto T, Yokoyama H, et al. Long-term prognosis of membranous nephropathy. *Clin Nephrol* 1986;25:64.
248. Murphy BF, Fairley KF, Kincaid-Smith PS. Idiopathic membranous glomerulonephritis: long-term follow-up in 139 cases. *Clin Nephrol* 1988;30:175.
249. Wehrmann M, Bohle A, Bogenschutz O, et al. Long-term prognosis of chronic idiopathic membranous glomerulonephritis. An analysis of 334 cases with particular regard to tubulo-interstitial changes. *Clin Nephrol* 1989;31:67.
250. Ramzy MH, Cameron JS, Turner DR, et al. The long-term outcome of idiopathic membranous nephropathy. *Clin Nephrol* 1981;16:13.
251. Zucchelli P, Ponticelli C, Cagnoli L, et al. Long-term outcome of idiopathic

251. membranous nephropathy with nephrotic syndrome. *Nephrol Dial Transplant* 1987;2:73.
252. Zucchelli P. Membranous nephropathy. In: Cameron JS, ed. *Oxford textbook of clinical nephrology.* London: Oxford University Press; 1992:370.
253. Shiiki H, Saito T, Nishitani Y, et al. Prognosis and risk factors for idiopathic membranous nephropathy with nephrotic syndrome in Japan. *Kidney Int* 2004;65:1400.
254. Hopper J, Jr, Trew PA, Biava CG. Membranous nephropathy: its relative benignity in women. *Nephron* 1981;29:18.
255. Toth T, Takebayashi S. Factors contributing to the outcome in 100 adult patients with idiopathic membranous glomerulonephritis. *Int Urol Nephrol* 1994;26:93.
256. Tu WH, Petitti DB, Biava CG, et al. Membranous nephropathy: predictors of terminal renal failure. *Nephron* 1984;36:118.
257. Kobayashi Y, Tateno S, Shigematsu H, et al. Prednisone treatment of non-nephrotic patients with idiopathic membranous nephropathy. a prospective study. *Nephron* 1982;30:210.
258. Cattran DC, Pei Y, Greenwood CM, et al. Validation of a predictive model of idiopathic membranous nephropathy: its clinical and research implications. *Kidney Int* 1997;51:901.
259. Papiha SS, Pareek SK, Rodger RS, et al. HLA-A, B, DR and Bf allotypes in patients with idiopathic membranous nephropathy (IMN). *Kidney Int* 1987;31:130.
260. Branten AJ, du Buf-Vereijken PW, Klasen IS, et al. Urinary excretion of beta2-microglobulin and IgG predict prognosis in idiopathic membranous nephropathy: a validation study. *J Am Soc Nephrol* 2005;16(1):169.
261. Bazzi C, Petrini C, Rizza V, et al. Urinary excretion of IgG and alpha(1)-microglobulin predicts clinical course better than extent of proteinuria in membranous nephropathy. *Am J Kidney Dis* 2001;38:240.
262. Bohle A, Grund KE, Mackensen S, et al. Correlations between renal interstitium and level of serum creatinine. Morphometric investigations of biopsies in perimembranous glomerulonephritis. *Virchows Arch A Pathol Anat Histol* 1977;373:15.
263. Alexopoulos E, Seron D, Hartley RB, et al. Immune mechanisms in idiopathic membranous nephropathy: the role of the interstitial infiltrates. *Am J Kidney Dis* 1989;13:404.
264. Gaffney EF, Panner BJ. Membranous glomerulonephritis: clinical significance of glomerular hypercellularity and parietal epithelial abnormalities. *Nephron* 1981;29:209.
265. Klassen J, Elwood C, Grossberg AL, et al. Evolution of membranous nephropathy into anti-glomerular-basement-membrane glomerulonephritis. *N Engl J Med* 1974;290:1340.
266. Moorthy AV, Zimmerman SW, Burkholder PM, et al. Association of crescentic glomerulonephritis with membranous glomerulonephropathy: a report of three cases. *Clin Nephrol* 1976;6:319.
267. Kwan JT, Moore RH, Dodd SM, et al. Crescentic transformation in primary membranous glomerulonephritis. *Postgrad Med J* 1991;67:574.
268. Ponticelli C, Passerini P. The natural history and therapy of idiopathic membranous nephropathy. *Nephrol Dial Transplant* 1990;5(Suppl 1):37.
269. Cameron JS. Membranous nephropathy—still a treatment dilemma. *N Engl J Med* 1992;327:638.
270. Lewis EJ. Idiopathic membranous nephropathy—to treat or not to treat? *N Engl J Med* 1993;329:127.
271. Cameron JS. Membranous nephropathy in childhood and its treatment. *Pediatr Nephrol* 1990;4:193.
272. Hogan SL, Muller KE, Jennette JC, et al. A review of therapeutic studies of idiopathic membranous glomerulopathy. *Am J Kidney Dis* 1995;25:862.
273. Levy M. Membranous glomerulonephritis. In: Edelmann CM, Jr, ed. *Pediatric Nephrology.* 2nd ed. Boston: Little, Brown and Company; 1993:1325.
274. Cahen R, Francois B, Trolliet P, et al. Aetiology of membranous glomerulonephritis: a prospective study of 82 adult patients. *Nephrol Dial Transplant* 1989;4:172.
275. Adu D, Cameron JS. Aetiology of membranous nephropathy. *Nephrol Dial Transplant* 1989;4:757.
276. Ponticelli C, Zucchelli P, Passerini P, et al. A 10-year follow-up of a randomized study with methylprednisolone and chlorambucil in membranous nephropathy. *Kidney Int* 1995;48:1600.
277. Imperiale TF, Goldfarb S, Berns JS. Are cytotoxic agents beneficial in idiopathic membranous nephropathy? A meta-analysis of the controlled trials. *J Am Soc Nephrol* 1995;5:1553.
278. Cattran DC, Greenwood C, Ritchie S, et al. A controlled trial of cyclosporine in patients with progressive membranous nephropathy. Canadian Glomerulonephritis Study Group. *Kidney Int* 1995;47:1130.
279. Cattran DC. Mycophenolate mofetil and cyclosporine therapy in membranous nephropathy. *Semin Nephrol* 2003;23:272.
280. Polenakovic M, Grcevska L, Dzikova S. Mycophenolate mofetil in treatment of idiopathic stages III-IV membranous nephropathy. *Nephrol Dial Transplant* 2003;18:1233.
281. Miller G, Zimmerman R, 3rd, Radhakrishnan J, et al. Use of mycophenolate mofetil in resistant membranous nephropathy. *Am J Kidney Dis* 2000;36:250.
282. Ruggenenti P, Chiurchiu C, Brusegan V, et al. Rituximab in idiopathic membranous nephropathy: a one-year prospective study. *J Am Soc Nephrol* 2003;14:1851.
283. Emancipator SN. Immunoregulatory factors in the pathogenesis of IgA nephropathy. *Kidney Int* 1990;38:1216.
284. D'Amico G, di Belgiojoso GB, Imbasciati E, et al. Idiopathic IgA mesangial nephropathy: natural history. *Contrib Nephrol* 1984;40:208.
285. D'Amico G. Idiopathic IgA mesangial nephropathy. *Nephron* 1985;41:1.
286. D'Amico G, Imbasciati E, Barbiano Di Belgioioso G, et al. Idiopathic IgA mesangial nephropathy. Clinical and histological study of 374 patients. *Medicine (Baltimore)* 1985;64:49.
287. D'Amico G. Natural history of idiopathic IgA nephropathy: role of clinical and histological prognostic factors. *Am J Kidney Dis* 2000;36:227.
288. Kincaid-Smith PS. Mesangial IgA nephropathy. *Br Med J (Clin Res Ed)* 1985;290:96.
289. Schena FP. A retrospective analysis of the natural history of primary IgA nephropathy worldwide. *Am J Med* 1990;89:209.
290. Levy M, Gonzalez-Burchard G, Broyer M, et al. Berger's disease in children. Natural history and outcome. *Medicine (Baltimore)* 1985;64:157.
291. D'Amico G, Ferrario F, Colasanti G, et al. IgA-mesangial nephropathy (Berger's disease) with rapid decline in renal function. *Clin Nephrol* 1981;16:251.
292. Bennett WM, Kincaid-Smith P. Macroscopic hematuria in mesangial IgA nephropathy: Correlation with glomerular crescents and renal dysfunction. *Kidney Int* 1983;23(2):393.
293. Rekola S, Bergstrand A, Bucht H. Deterioration of GFR in IgA nephropathy as measured by 51Cr-EDTA clearance. *Kidney Int* 1991;40:1050.
294. Woo KT, Edmondson RP, Wu AY, et al. The natural history of IgA nephritis in Singapore. *Clin Nephrol* 1986;25:15.
295. Mustonen J, Pasternack A, Rantala I. The nephrotic syndrome in IgA glomerulonephritis: response to corticosteroid therapy. *Clin Nephrol* 1983;20:172.
296. Johnston PA, Brown JS, Braumholtz DA, et al. Clinico-pathological correlations and long-term follow-up of 253 United Kingdom patients with IgA nephropathy. A report from the MRC Glomerulonephritis Registry. *Q J Med* 1992;84:619.
297. Droz D, Kramar A, Nawar T, et al. Primary IgA nephropathy: prognostic factors. *Contrib Nephrol* 1984;40:202.
298. D'Amico G, Minetti L, Ponticelli C, et al. Prognostic indicators in idiopathic IgA mesangial nephropathy. *Q J Med* 1986;59:363.
299. Alamartine E, Sabatier JC, Berthoux FC. Comparison of pathological lesions on repeated renal biopsies in 73 patients with primary IgA glomerulonephritis: value of quantitative scoring and approach to final prognosis. *Clin Nephrol* 1990;34:45.
300. Kobayashi Y, Tateno S, Hiki Y, et al. IgA nephropathy: prognostic significance of proteinuria and histological alterations. *Nephron* 1983;34:146.
301. Neelakantappa K, Gallo GR, Baldwin DS. Proteinuria in IgA nephropathy. *Kidney Int* 1988;33:716.
302. Payton CD, McLay A, Jones JM. Progressive IgA nephropathy: the role of hypertension. *Nephrol Dial Transplant* 1988;3:138.
303. Beukhof JR, Kardaun O, Schaafsma W, et al. Toward individual prognosis of IgA nephropathy. *Kidney Int* 1986;29:549.
304. Alamartine E, Sabatier JC, Guerin C, et al. Prognostic factors in mesangial IgA glomerulonephritis: an extensive study with univariate and multivariate analyses. *Am J Kidney Dis* 1991;18:12.
305. Nicholls KM, Fairley KF, Dowling JP, et al. The clinical course of mesangial IgA associated nephropathy in adults. *Q J Med* 1984;53:227.
306. Abe T, Kida H, Yoshimura M, et al. Participation of extracapillary lesions (ECL) in progression of IgA nephropathy. *Clin Nephrol* 1986;25:37.
307. Hotta O, Yoshizawa N, Oshima S, et al. Significance of renal hyaline arteriolosclerosis and tubulo-interstitial change in IgA glomerulonephropathy and focal glomerular sclerosis. *Nephron* 1987;47:262.
308. Katafuchi R, Oh Y, Hori K, et al. An important role of glomerular segmental lesions on progression of IgA nephropathy: a multivariate analysis. *Clin Nephrol* 1994;41:191.
309. Alexopoulos E, Seron D, Hartley RB, et al. The role of interstitial infiltrates in IgA nephropathy: a study with monoclonal antibodies. *Nephrol Dial Transplant* 1989;4:187.
310. Li HL, Hancock WW, Hooke DH, et al. Mononuclear cell activation and decreased renal function in IgA nephropathy with crescents. *Kidney Int* 1990;37:1552.
311. Sabadini E, Castiglione A, Colasanti G, et al. Characterization of interstitial infiltrating cells in Berger's disease. *Am J Kidney Dis* 1988;12:307.
312. Arima S, Nakayama M, Naito M, et al. Significance of mononuclear phagocytes in IgA nephropathy. *Kidney Int* 1991;39:684.
313. Yoshida H, Mitarai T, Kawamura T, et al. Role of the deletion of polymorphism of the angiotensin converting enzyme gene in the progression and therapeutic responsiveness of IgA nephropathy. *J Clin Invest* 1995;96:2162.
314. Pei Y, Scholey J, Thai K, et al. Association of angiotensinogen gene T235 variant with progression of immunoglobin A nephropathy in Caucasian patients. *J Clin Invest* 1997;100:814.
315. Schena FP, D'Altri C, Cerullo G, et al. ACE gene polymorphism and IgA nephropathy: an ethnically homogeneous study and a meta-analysis. *Kidney Int* 2001;60:732.
316. Harden PN, Geddes C, Rowe PA, et al. Polymorphisms in angiotensin-converting-enzyme gene and progression of IgA nephropathy. *Lancet* 1995;345:1540.
317. Hunley TE, Julian BA, Phillips JA, 3rd, et al. Angiotensin converting enzyme gene polymorphism: potential silencer motif and impact on progression in IgA nephropathy. *Kidney Int* 1996;49:571.

318. Kitajima T, Murakami M, Sakai O. Clinicopathological features in the Japanese patients with IgA nephropathy. *Jpn J Med* 1983;22:219.

319. Crowley-Nowick PA, Julian BA, Wyatt RJ, et al. IgA nephropathy in blacks: studies of IgA2 allotypes and clinical course. *Kidney Int* 1991;39:1218.

320. Kusumoto Y, Takebayashi S, Taguchi T, et al. Long-term prognosis and prognostic indices of IgA nephropathy in juvenile and in adult Japanese. *Clin Nephrol* 1987;28:118.

321. Yoshikawa N, Ito H, Yoshiara S, et al. Clinical course of immunoglobulin A nephropathy in children. *J Pediatr* 1987;110:555.

322. Yoshikawa N, Ito H, Nakamura H. Prognostic indicators in childhood IgA nephropathy. *Nephron* 1992;60:60.

323. Hogg RJ, Silva FG, Wyatt RJ, et al. Prognostic indicators in children with IgA nephropathy—report of the Southwest Pediatric Nephrology Study Group. *Pediatr Nephrol* 1994;8:15.

324. Linne T, Berg U, Bohman SO, et al. Course and long-term outcome of idiopathic IgA nephropathy in children. *Pediatr Nephrol* 1991;5:383.

325. Clive DM, Galvanek EG, Silva FG. Mesangial immunoglobulin A deposits in minimal change nephrotic syndrome: a report of an older patient and review of the literature. *Am J Nephrol* 1990;10:31.

326. Delclaux C, Jacquot C, Callard P, et al. Acute reversible renal failure with macroscopic haematuria in IgA nephropathy. *Nephrol Dial Transplant* 1993;8:195.

327. Talwalkar YB, Price WH, Musgrave JE. Recurrent resolving renal failure in IgA nephropathy. A case report. *J Pediatr* 1978;92:596.

328. Fogazzi GB, Imbasciati E, Moroni G, et al. Reversible acute renal failure from gross haematuria due to glomerulonephritis: not only in IgA nephropathy and not associated with intratubular obstruction. *Nephrol Dial Transplant* 1995;10:624.

329. Bannister KM, Weaver A, Clarkson AR, et al. Effect of angiotensin-converting enzyme and calcium channel inhibition on progression of IgA nephropathy. *Contrib Nephrol* 1995;111:184, Discussion192.

330. Cattran DC, Greenwood C, Ritchie S. Long-term benefits of angiotensin-converting enzyme inhibitor therapy in patients with severe immunoglobulin a nephropathy: a comparison to patients receiving treatment with other antihypertensive agents and to patients receiving no therapy. *Am J Kidney Dis* 1994;23:247.

331. Laville M, Alamartine E. Treatment options for IgA nephropathy in adults: a proposal for evidence-based strategy. *Nephrol Dial Transplant* 2004;19:1947.

332. Praga M, Gutierrez E, Gonzalez E, et al. Treatment of IgA nephropathy with ACE inhibitors: a randomized and controlled trial. *J Am Soc Nephrol* 2003;14:1578.

333. Kobayashi Y, Hiki Y, Kokubo T, et al. Steroid therapy during the early stage of progressive IgA nephropathy. A 10-year follow-up study. *Nephron* 1996;72:237.

334. Pozzi C, Bolasco PG, Fogazzi GB, et al. Corticosteroids in IgA nephropathy: a randomised controlled trial. *Lancet* 1999;353:883.

335. Pozzi C, Andrulli S, Del Vecchio L, et al. Corticosteroid effectiveness in IgA nephropathy: long-term results of a randomized, controlled trial. *J Am Soc Nephrol* 2004;15:157.

336. Hogg RJ. A randomized, placebo-controlled, multicenter trial evaluating alternate-day prednisone and fish oil supplements in young patients with immunoglobulin A nephropathy. Scientific Planning Committee of the IgA Nephropathy Study. *Am J Kidney Dis* 1995;26:792.

337. Donadio JV, Jr, Bergstralh EJ, Offord KP, et al. A controlled trial of fish oil in IgA nephropathy. Mayo Nephrology Collaborative Group. *N Engl J Med* 1994;331:1194.

338. Donadio JV, Jr, Grande JP, Bergstralh EJ, et al. The long-term outcome of patients with IgA nephropathy treated with fish oil in a controlled trial. Mayo Nephrology Collaborative Group. *J Am Soc Nephrol* 1999;10:1772.

339. Anders D, Agricola B, Sippel M, et al. Basement membrane changes in membranoproliferative glomerulonephritis. II. Characterization of a third type by silver impregnation of ultra thin sections. *Virchows Arch A Pathol Anat Histol* 1977;376:1.

340. Anders D, Thoenes W. Basement membrane-changes in membranoproliferative glomerulonephritis: a light and electron microscopic study. *Virchows Arch A Pathol Anat Histol* 1975;369:87.

341. Jackson EC, McAdams AJ, Strife CF, et al. Differences between membranoproliferative glomerulonephritis types I and III in clinical presentation, glomerular morphology, and complement perturbation. *Am J Kidney Dis* 1987;9:115.

342. Strife CF, Jackson EC, McAdams AJ. Type III membranoproliferative glomerulonephritis: long-term clinical and morphologic evaluation. *Clin Nephrol* 1984;21:323.

343. Simon P, Ramee MP, Ang KS, et al. Variations of primary glomerulonephritis incidence in a rural area of 400,000 inhabitants in the last decade. *Nephron* 1987;45:171.

344. Barbiano di Belgiojoso G, Baroni M, Pagliari B, et al. Is membranoproliferative glomerulonephritis really decreasing? A multicentre study of 1,548 cases of primary glomerulonephritis. *Nephron* 1985;40:380.

345. Broumand B, Antonovych T. High incidence of membranoproliferative glomerulonephritis in Iran (abstract). IX Congress of the International Society of Nephrology, Los Angeles, 1984.

346. Neugarten J, Gallo GR, Baldwin DS. Glomerulonephritis in bacterial endocarditis. *Am J Kidney Dis* 1984;3:371.

347. Kim Y, Michael A, Trashish P. Infection and nephritis. In: Jr CE, ed. *Pediatric Nephrology*. Boston: Little, Brown and Company; 1993:1569.

348. D'Amico G, Ferrario F. Mesangiocapillary glomerulonephritis. *J Am Soc Nephrol* 1992;2(Suppl 10):S159.

349. Cameron JS, Turner DR, Heaton J, et al. Idiopathic mesangiocapillary glomerulonephritis. Comparison of types I and II in children and adults and long-term prognosis. *Am J Med* 1983;74:175.

350. Habib R. Glomerulonephrite membranoproliferative. In: Matheiu H, ed. *Nephrologie Pediatrique*. Paris: Flammarion;1983:316.

351. Klein M, Poucell S, Arbus GS, et al. Characteristics of a benign subtype of dense deposit disease: comparison with the progressive form of this disease. *Clin Nephrol* 1983;20:163.

352. Donadio JV, Jr, Anderson CF, Mitchell JC, 3rd, et al. Membranoproliferative glomerulonephritis. A prospective clinical trial of platelet-inhibitor therapy. *N Engl J Med* 1984;310:1421.

353. Donadio JV, Jr, Offord KP. Reassessment of treatment results in membranoproliferative glomerulonephritis, with emphasis on life-table analysis. *Am J Kidney Dis* 1989;14:445.

354. Schmitt H, Bohle A, Reineke T, et al. Long-term prognosis of membranoproliferative glomerulonephritis type I. Significance of clinical and morphological parameters: an investigation of 220 cases. *Nephron* 1990;55:242.

355. Swainson CP, Robson JS, Thomson D, et al. Mesangiocapillary glomerulonephritis: a long-term study of 40 cases. *J Pathol* 1983;141:449.

356. Bennett WM, Fassett RG, Walker RG, et al. Mesangiocapillary glomerulonephritis type II (dense-deposit disease): clinical features of progressive disease. *Am J Kidney Dis* 1989;13(6):469.

357. McEnery PT, McAdams AJ, West CD. The effect of prednisone in a high-dose, alternate-day regimen on the natural history of idiopathic membranoproliferative glomerulonephritis. *Medicine (Baltimore)* 1985;64:401.

358. McEnery PT. Membranoproliferative glomerulonephritis: the Cincinnati experience—cumulative renal survival from 1957 to 1989. *J Pediatr* 1990;116(5):S109.

359. West CD. Idiopathic membranoproliferative glomerulonephritis in childhood. *Pediatr Nephrol* 1992;6:96.

360. Ford DM, Briscoe DM, Shanley PF, et al. Childhood membranoproliferative glomerulonephritis type I: limited steroid therapy. *Kidney Int* 1992;41:1606.

361. Tarshish P, Bernstein J, Tobin JN, et al. Treatment of mesangiocapillary glomerulonephritis with alternate-day prednisone—a report of the International Study of Kidney Disease in Children. *Pediatr Nephrol* 1992;6:123.

362. Zauner I, Bohler J, Braun N, et al. Effect of aspirin and dipyridamole on proteinuria in idiopathic membranoproliferative glomerulonephritis: a multicentre prospective clinical trial. Collaborative Glomerulonephritis Therapy Study Group (CGTS). *Nephrol Dial Transplant* 1994;9:619.

363. Kurtsman NA. Does acute poststreptococcal glomerulonephritis lead to chronic renal disease? *N Engl J Med* 1978;298:795.

364. Baldwin DS. Poststreptococcal glomerulonephritis. A progressive disease? *Am J Med* 1977;62:1.

365. Meadow SR. Poststreptococcal nephritis—a rare disease? *Arch Dis Child* 1975;50:379.

366. Montseny JJ, Meyrier A, Kleinknecht D, et al. The current spectrum of infectious glomerulonephritis. Experience with 76 patients and review of the literature. *Medicine (Baltimore)* 1995;74:63.

367. Dodge WF, Spargo BH, Travis LB, et al. Poststreptococcal glomerulonephritis. A prospective study in children. *N Engl J Med* 1972;286:273.

368. Kaplan EL, Anthony BF, Chapman SS, et al. Epidemic acute glomerulonephritis associated with type 49 streptococcal pyoderma. I. Clinical and laboratory findings. *Am J Med* 1970;48:9.

369. Rodriguez-Iturbe B, Rubio L, Garcia R. Attack rate of poststreptococcal nephritis in families. A prospective study. *Lancet* 1981;1:401.

370. Sagel I, Treser G, Ty A, et al. Occurrence and nature of glomerular lesions after group A streptococci infections in children. *Ann Intern Med* 1973;79:492.

371. Kandall S, Edelmann CM, Jr, Bernstein J. Acute poststreptococcal glomerulonephritis. A case with minimal urinary abnormalities. *Am J Dis Child* 1969;118:426.

372. Cameron J. Acute renal failure in glomerular disease. In: Andreucci V, ed. *Acute Renal Failure-Pathophysiology, Prevention, and Treatment*. The Hague: Martinus Nyhoff; 1984:271.

373. Perlman LV, Herdman RC, Kleinman H, et al. Poststreptococcal glomerulonephritis. A ten-year follow-up of an epidemic. *JAMA* 1965;194:63.

374. Hebert HJ. Acute glomerulonephritis in childhood: a study of the late prognosis of twenty-seven cases. *J Pediatr* 1952;40:549.

375. Sanjad S, Tolaymat A, Whitworth J, et al. Acute glomerulonephritis in children: a review of 153 cases. *South Med J* 1977;70:1202.

376. Potter EV, Abidh S, Sharrett AR, et al. Clinical healing two to six years after poststreptococcal glomerulonephritis in Trinidad. *N Engl J Med* 1978;298:767.

377. Potter EV, Lipschultz SA, Abidh S, et al. Twelve to seventeen-year follow-up of patients with poststreptococcal acute glomerulonephritis in Trinidad. *N Engl J Med* 1982;307:725.

378. Nissenson AR, Mayon-White R, Potter EV, et al. Continued absence of clinical renal disease seven to 12 years after poststreptococcal acute glomerulonephritis in Trinidad. *Am J Med* 1979;67:255.

379. Smith EC, Co BS, Freedman P. The evolution of the focal post-streptococcal glomerular lesion. *J Chron Dis* 1974;27:405.
380. Rodriguez-Iturbe B. Epidemic poststreptococcal glomerulonephritis. *Kidney Int* 1984;25:129.
381. Garcia R, Rubio L, Rodriguez-Iturbe B. Long-term prognosis of epidemic poststreptococcal glomerulonephritis in Maracaibo: follow-up studies 11–12 years after the acute episode. *Clin Nephrol* 1981;15:291.
382. Travis LB, Dodge WF, Beathard GA, et al. Acute glomerulonephritis in children. A review of the natural history with emphasis on prognosis. *Clin Nephrol* 1973;1:169.
383. Lewy JE, Salinas-Madrigal L, Herdson PB, et al. Clinico-pathologic correlations in acute poststreptococcal glomerulonephritis. A correlation between renal functions, morphologic damage and clinical course of 46 children with acute poststreptococcal glomerulonephritis. *Medicine (Baltimore)* 1971;50:453.
384. Hinglais N, Garcia-Torres R, Kleinknecht D. Long-term prognosis in acute glomerulonephritis. The predictive value of early clinical and pathological features observed in 65 patients. *Am J Med* 1974;56:52.
385. Popovic-Rolovic M, Kostic M, Antic-Peco A, et al. Medium- and long-term prognosis of patients with acute poststreptococcal glomerulonephritis. *Nephron* 1991;58:393.
386. Mota-Hernandez F, Briseno-Mondragon E, Gordillo-Paniagua G. Glomerular lesions and final outcome in children with glomerulonephritis of acute onset. *Nephron* 1976;16:272.
387. Baldwin DS, Gluck MC, Schacht RG, et al. The long-term course of poststreptococcal glomerulonephritis. *Ann Intern Med* 1974;80:342.
388. Clark G, White RH, Glasgow EF, et al. Poststreptococcal glomerulonephritis in children: clinicopathological correlations and long-term prognosis. *Pediatr Nephrol* 1988;2:381.
389. Gill DG, Turner DR, Chantler C, et al. The progression of acute proliferative post streptococcal glomerulonephritis to severe epithelial crescent formation. *Clin Nephrol* 1977;8:449.
390. Glasgow E, White R. Acute post-streptococcal glomerulonephritis with failure to resolve. In: Becker E, ed. *Glomerulonephritis.* vol. 1 New York: Wiley; 1973:345.
391. Cleper R, Davidovitz M, Halevi R, et al. Renal functional reserve after acute poststreptococcal glomerulonephritis. *Pediatr Nephrol* 1997;11:473.
392. Herthelius M, Berg U. Renal function during and after childhood acute poststreptococcal glomerulonephritis. *Pediatr Nephrol* 1999;13:907.
393. Jennings RB, Earle DP. Post-streptococcal glomerulo-nephritis: histopathologic and clinical studies of the acute, subsiding acute and early chronic latent phases. *J Clin Invest* 1961;40:1525.
394. McCluskey RT, Baldwin DS. Natural history of acute glomerulonephritis. *Am J Med* 1963;35:213.
395. Baldwin DS, Schacht RG. Late sequelae of poststreptococcal glomerulonephritis. *Annu Rev Med* 1976;27:49.
396. Lien JW, Mathew TH, Meadows R. Acute post-streptococcal glomerulonephritis in adults: a long-term study. *Q J Med* 1979;48:99.
397. Vogl W, Renke M, Mayer-Eichberger D, et al. Long-term prognosis for endocapillary glomerulonephritis of poststreptococcal type in children and adults. *Nephron* 1986;44:58.
398. Modai D, Pik A, Behar M, et al. Biopsy proven evolution of post streptococcal glomerulonephritis to rapidly progressive glomerulonephritis of a post infectious type. *Clin Nephrol* 1985;23:198.
399. Rodriguez-Iturbe B. Infection-related glomerulonephritis. In: Glassock R, ed. *Current Therapy in Nephrology and Hypertension.* 4th ed. St. Louis: Mosby; 1998:141.
400. Moroni G, Pozzi C, Quaglini S, et al. Long-term prognosis of diffuse proliferative glomerulonephritis associated with infection in adults. *Nephrol Dial Transplant* 2002;17:1204.
401. Gallo GR, Feiner HD, Steele JM, Jr, et al. Role of intrarenal vascular sclerosis in progression of poststreptococcal glomerulonephritis. *Clin Nephrol* 1980;13:49.
402. Old CW, Herrera GA, Reimann BE, et al. Acute poststreptococcal glomerulonephritis progressing to rapidly progressive glomerulonephritis. *South Med J* 1984;77:1470.
403. Ferrario F, Kourilsky O, Morel-Maroger L. Acute endocapillary glomerulonephritis in adults: a histologic and clinical comparison between patients with and without initial acute renal failure. *Clin Nephrol* 1983;19:17.
404. Joseph MC, Polani PE. The effect of bed rest on acute haemorrhagic nephritis in children. *Guys Hosp Rep* 1958;107:500.
405. Cameron JS. The nosology of crescentic nephritis. *Nephrologic* 1992;13(6):243.
406. Rees A, Cameron J. Crescentic nephritis. In: Cameron J, et al. eds. *Oxford Textbook of Clinical Nephrology.* London: Oxford University Press; 1992:418.
407. Suc JM, Ronco P. Rapidly progressive glomerulonephritis (RPGN): from crescents to polynuclear activation. *Nephrologie* 1992;13(6):241.
408. Niaudet P, Levy M. Glomerulonephrites a croissants diffus. *Nephrologie pediatrique* 1983:381.
409. Southwest Pediatric Nephrology Study Group. A clinico-pathologic study of crescentic glomerulonephritis in 50 children. A report of the Southwest Pediatric Nephrology Study Group. *Kidney Int* 1985;27:450.
410. Jardim HM. Crescentic glomerulonephritis in children. *Pediatr Nephrol* 1992:231.
411. Srivastava RN, Moudgil A, Bagga A, et al., eds. Crescentic glomerulonephritis in children: a review of 43 cases. *Am J Nephrology* 1992;12(3):155.
412. Dash SC, Malhotra KK, Sharma RK, et al. Spectrum of rapidly progressive (crescentic) glomerulonephritis in northern India. 1982.
413. Parag KB, Naran AD, Seedat YK, et al. Profile of crescentic glomerulonephritis in Natal—a clinicopathological assessment. *Q J Med* 1988;68:629.
414. Zent R, Van Zyl Smit R, Duffield M, et al. Crescentic nephritis at Groote Schuur Hospital, South Africa—not a benign disease. *Renal Unit Groote Schuur Hospital, Capetown, South Africa.*
415. Bennett WM, Kincaid-Smith P. Macroscopic hematuria in mesangial IgA nephropathy: correlation with glomerular crescents and renal dysfunction. *Kidney Int* 1983;23:393.
416. D'Amico G, Ferrario F, Colasanti G, et al. IgA-mesangial nephropathy (Berger's disease) with rapid decline in renal function. *Clin Nephrol* 1981;16:251.
417. Welch TR, McAdams AJ, Berry A. Rapidly progressive IgA nephropathy. *Am J Dis Child* 1988;142:789.
418. Neild GH, Cameron JS, Ogg CS, et al. Rapidly progressive glomerulonephritis with extensive glomerular crescent formation. *Q J Med* 1983;52:395.
419. Stilmant MM, Bolton WK, Sturgill BC, et al. Crescentic glomerulonephritis without immune deposits: clinicopathologic features. *Kidney Int* 1979;15:184.
420. Pollak VE, Mendoza N. Rapidly progressive glomerulonephritis. *Med Clin North Am* 1971;55:1397.
421. Cuochi D, et al. Relapsing nephrotic syndrome following remission for 20 years. *Int J Pediatr Nephrol* 1983;4:211.
422. Cohen AH, Border WA, Shankel E, et al. Crescentic glomerulonephritis: immune vs. nonimmune mechanisms. *Am J Nephrol* 1981;1:78.
423. Whitworth JA, Morel-Maroger L, Mignon F, et al. The significance of extracapillary proliferation. Clinicopathological review of 60 patients. *Nephron* 1976;16:1.
424. Angangco R, Thiru S, Esnault VL, et al. Does truly 'idiopathic' crescentic glomerulonephritis exist? *Nephrol Dial Transplant* 1994;9:630.
425. Ferrario F, Tadros MT, Napodano P, et al. Critical re-evaluation of 41 cases of "idiopathic" crescentic glomerulonephritis. *Clin Nephrol* 1994;41:1.
426. Beirne GJ, Wagnild JP, Zimmerman SW, et al. Idiopathic crescentic glomerulonephritis. *Medicine (Baltimore)* 1977;56:349.
427. Glassock RJ. A clinical and immunopathologic dissection of rapidly progressive glomerulonephritis. *Nephron* 1978;22:253.
428. Morrin PA, Hinglais N, Nabarra B, et al. Rapidly progressive glomerulonephritis. A clinical and pathologic study. *Am J Med* 1978;65:446.
429. Sonsino E, Nabarra B, Kazatchkine M, et al. Extracapillary proliferative glomerulonephritis so-called malignant glomerulonephritis. *Adv Nephrol Necker Hosp* 1972;2:121.
430. Han WK, Choi HK, Roth RM, et al. Serial ANCA titers: useful tool for prevention of relapses in ANCA-associated vasculitis. *Kidney Int* 2003;63:1079.
431. Boomsma MM, Stegeman CA, van der Leij MJ, et al. Prediction of relapses in Wegener's granulomatosis by measurement of antineutrophil cytoplasmic antibody levels: a prospective study. *Arthritis Rheum* 2000;43:2025.
432. Heaf JG, Jorgensen F, Nielsen LP. Treatment and prognosis of extracapillary glomerulonephritis. *Nephron* 1983;35:217.
433. Bolton WK, Couser WG. Intravenous pulse methylprednisolone therapy of acute crescentic rapidly progressive glomerulonephritis. *Am J Med* 1979;66:495.
434. Levy JB, Winearls CG. Rapidly progressive glomerulonephritis: what should be first-line therapy? *Nephron* 1994;67:402.
435. Bolton WK, Sturgill BC. Methylprednisolone therapy for acute crescentic rapidly progressive glomerulonephritis. *Am J Nephrol* 1989;9:368.
436. Couser WG. Rapidly progressive glomerulonephritis: classification, pathogenetic mechanisms, and therapy. *Am J Kidney Dis* 1988;11:449.
437. Bruns FJ, Adler S, Fraley DS, et al. Long-term follow-up of aggressively treated idiopathic rapidly progressive glomerulonephritis. *Am J Med* 1989;86:400.
438. Baldwin DS, Neugarten J, Feiner HD, et al. The existence of a protracted course in crescentic glomerulonephritis. *Kidney Int* 1987;31:790.
439. Nakamato Y, et al. Combined anticoagulant and immunosuppressive glomerulonephritis (RPGN). A long-term follow-up study. *Jpn J Med* 1979;18:210.
440. Kunis CL, Kiss B, Williams G, et al. Intravenous "pulse" cyclophosphamide therapy of crescentic glomerulonephritis. *Clin Nephrol* 1992;37:1.
441. Turner N, Rees A. Anti-glomerular basement membrane disease. In: Cameron JS, et al., eds. *Oxford Textbook of Clinical Nephrology.* London: Oxford University Press; 1992:438.
442. Holdsworth S, Boyce N, Thomson NM, et al. The clinical spectrum of acute glomerulonephritis and lung haemorrhage (Goodpasture's syndrome). *Q J Med* 1985;55:75.
443. McPhaul JJ, Jr, Mullins JD. Glomerulonephritis mediated by antibody to glomerular basement membrane. Immunological, clinical, and histopathological characteristics. *J Clin Invest* 1976;57:351.
444. Cohen LH, Wilson CB, Freeman RM. Goodpasture syndrome: recovery after severe renal insufficiency. *Arch Intern Med* 1976;136:835.
445. Levin M, Rigden SP, Pincott JR, et al. Goodpasture's syndrome: treatment

with plasmapheresis, immunosuppression, and anticoagulation. *Arch Dis Child* 1983;58:697.

446. Hind CR, Bowman C, Winearls CG, et al. Recurrence of circulating anti-glomerular basement membrane antibody three years after immunosuppressive treatment and plasma exchange. *Clin Nephrol* 1984;21:244.

447. Walker RG, Scheinkestel C, Becker GJ, et al. Clinical and morphological aspects of the management of crescentic anti-glomerular basement membrane antibody (anti-GBM) nephritis/Goodpasture's syndrome. *Q J Med* 1985;54:75.

448. Savage CO, Pusey CD, Bowman C, et al. Antiglomerular basement membrane antibody mediated disease in the British Isles 1980–84. *Br Med J (Clin Res Ed)* 1986;292:301.

449. Herody M, Bobrie G, Gouarin C, et al. Anti-GBM disease: predictive value of clinical, histological and serological data. *Clin Nephrol* 1993;40:249.

450. Merkel F, Pullig O, Marx M, et al. Course and prognosis of anti-basement membrane antibody (anti-BM-Ab)-mediated disease: report of 35 cases. *Nephrol Dial Transplant* 1994;9:372.

451. Rees AJ, Peters DK, Amos N, et al. The influence of HLA-linked genes on the severity of anti-GBM antibody-mediated nephritis. *Kidney Int* 1984;26:445.

452. Johnson JP, Moore J, Jr, Austin HA, 3rd, et al. Therapy of anti-glomerular basement membrane antibody disease: analysis of prognostic significance of clinical, pathologic and treatment factors. *Medicine (Baltimore)* 1985;64:219.

453. Dahlberg PJ, Kurtz SB, Donadio JV, et al. Recurrent Goodpasture's syndrome. *Mayo Clin Proc* 1978;53:533.

454. Balow JE. Renal vasculitis. *Kidney Int* 1985;27:954.

455. Droz D, Noel LH, Leibowitch M, et al. Glomerulonephritis and necrotizing angiitis. *Adv Nephrol Necker Hosp* 1979;8:343.

456. Fauci AS. Vasculitis. *J Allergy Clin Immunol* 1983;72:211.

457. Fauci AS, Haynes B, Katz P. The spectrum of vasculitis: clinical, pathologic, immunologic and therapeutic considerations. *Ann Intern Med* 1978;89:660.

458. Fauci AS, Haynes BF, Katz P, et al. Wegener's granulomatosis: prospective clinical and therapeutic experience with 85 patients for 21 years. *Ann Intern Med* 1983;98:76.

459. Serra A, Cameron JS. Clinical and pathologic aspects of renal vasculitis. *Semin Nephrol* 1985;5:15.

460. Serra A, Cameron JS, Turner DR, et al. Vasculitis affecting the kidney: presentation, histopathology and long-term outcome. *Q J Med* 1984;53:181.

461. Grotz W, Wanner C, Keller E, et al. Crescentic glomerulonephritis in Wegener's granulomatosis: morphology, therapy, outcome. *Clin Nephrol* 1991;35:243.

462. Hind CR, Paraskevakou H, Lockwood CM, et al. Prognosis after immunosuppression of patients with crescentic nephritis requiring dialysis. *Lancet* 1983;1:263.

463. Pinching AJ, Lockwood CM, Pussell BA, et al. Wegener's granulomatosis: observations on 18 patients with severe renal disease. *Q J Med* 1983;52:435.

464. Savage CO. Microscopic polyarteritis: presentation, pathology and prognosis. *Q J Med* 1983;56:467.

465. Fuiano G, Cameron JS, Raftery M, et al. Improved prognosis of renal microscopic polyarteritis in recent years. *Nephrol Dial Transplant* 1988;3:383.

466. Cameron JS. New horizons in renal vasculitis. *Klin Wochenschr* 1991; 69:536.

467. Pusey CD, Rees AJ, Evans DJ, et al. Plasma exchange in focal necrotizing glomerulonephritis without anti-GBM antibodies. *Kidney Int* 1991;40:757.

468. Glockner WM, Sieberth HG, Wichmann HE, et al. Plasma exchange and immunosuppression in rapidly progressive glomerulonephritis: a controlled, multi-center study. *Clin Nephrol* 1988;29:1.

469. Cole E, Cattran D, Magil A, et al. A prospective randomized trial of plasma exchange as additive therapy in idiopathic crescentic glomerulonephritis. The Canadian Apheresis Study Group. *Am J Kidney Dis* 1992;20:261.

470. Glassock RJ. Intensive plasma exchange in crescentic glomerulonephritis: help or no help? *Am J Kidney Dis* 1992;20:270.

471. Hoffman GS, Leavitt RY, Fleisher TA, et al. Treatment of Wegener's granulomatosis with intermittent high-dose intravenous cyclophosphamide. *Am J Med* 1990;89:403.

472. Nachman PH, Hogan SL, Jennette JC, et al. Treatment response and relapse in antineutrophil cytoplasmic autoantibody-associated microscopic polyangiitis and glomerulonephritis. *J Am Soc Nephrol* 1996;7:33.

473. Hogan SL, Nachman PH, Wilkman AS, et al. Prognostic markers in patients with antineutrophil cytoplasmic autoantibody-associated microscopic polyangiitis and glomerulonephritis. *J Am Soc Nephrol* 1996;7:23.

474. Coward RA, Hamdy NA, Shortland JS, et al. Renal micropolyarteritis: a treatable condition. *Nephrol Dial Transplant* 1986;1:31.

475. Adu D, Howie AJ, Scott DG, et al. Polyarteritis and the kidney. *Q J Med* 1987;62:221.

476. Bindi P, Mougenot B, Mentre F, et al. Necrotizing crescentic glomerulonephritis without significant immune deposits: a clinical and serological study. *Q J Med* 1993;86:55.

477. Falk RJ. ANCA-associated renal disease. *Kidney Int* 1990;38:998.

478. Gans RO, Kuizinga MC, Goldschmeding R, et al. Clinical features and outcome in patients with glomerulonephritis and antineutrophil cytoplasmic autoantibodies. *Nephron* 1993;64:182.

479. Gaskin G, Pusey C. Systemic vasculitis. In: Cameron J, et al., eds. *Oxford Textbook of Clinical Nephrology*. London: Oxford University Press; 1992:612.

480. Luqmani RA, Bacon PA, Beaman M, et al. Classical versus non-renal Wegener's granulomatosis. *Q J Med* 1994;87:161.

481. Anderson G, Coles ET, Crane M, et al. Wegener's granuloma. A series of 265 British cases seen between 1975 and 1985. A report by a sub-committee of the British Thoracic Society Research Committee. *Q J Med* 1992;83:427.

482. Innes A, Cotton RE, Rowe PA, et al. Very late recurrence of renal vasculitis. *Clin Nephrol* 1991;35:252.

483. Fogazzi GB, Banfi G, Allegri L, et al. Late recurrence of systemic vasculitis after kidney transplantation involving the kidney allograft. *Adv Exp Med Biol Vol*. 336; 1993;336:503.

484. McLaughlin K, Jerimiah P, Fox JG, et al. Has the prognosis for patients with pauci-immune necrotizing glomerulonephritis improved? *Nephrol Dial Transplant* . Vol 13; 1998;13:1696.

485. Cohen Tervaert JW, Huitema MG, Hene RJ, et al. Prevention of relapses in Wegener's granulomatosis by treatment based on antineutrophil cytoplasmic antibody titre. *Lancet* 1990;336:709.

486. Gaskin G, Savage CO, Ryan JJ, et al. Anti-neutrophil cytoplasmic antibodies and disease activity during long-term follow-up of 70 patients with systemic vasculitis. *Nephrol Dial Transplant* 1991;6:689.

487. Cameron JS. Renal disease and vasculitis. *Pediatr Nephrol* 1988;2:490.

488. Habib R. Periarterite noueuse et angeites necrosantes. In: Mathieu H, et al., eds. *Nephrologie Pediatrique*. 3rd ed. Paris: Flammarion; 1983:368.

489. Clutterbuck EJ, Evans DJ, Pusey CD. Renal involvement in Churg-Strauss syndrome. *Nephrol Dial Transplant* 1990;5:161.

490. Gardner-Medwin JM, Dolezalova P, Cummins C, et al. Incidence of Henoch-Schonlein purpura, Kawasaki disease, and rare vasculitides in children of different ethnic origins. *Lancet* 2002;360:1197.

491. Koskimies O, Mir S, Rapola J, et al. Henoch-Schonlein nephritis: long-term prognosis of unselected patients. *Arch Dis Child* 1981;56:482.

492. Meadow S. Schonlein-Henoch syndrome. In: Edelmann CM, Jr., eds. *Pediatric Nephrology*. 2nd ed. Boston: Little, Brown and Company; 1993:1525.

493. Meadow SR, Glasgow EF, White RH, et al. Schonlein-Henoch nephritis. *Q J Med* 1972;41:241.

494. Habib R, Cameron J. Schonlein-Henoch purpura. In: Hadler N, ed. *The Kidney in Rheumatic Disease*. London: Butterworth-Heineman; 1982:178.

495. Counahan R, Cameron JS. Henoch-Schonlein nephritis. *Contrib Nephrol* 1977;7:143.

496. Kobayashi O. Schonlein-Henoch's syndrome in children. *Contrib Nephrol* 1977;4:48.

497. Alexander SR, Arbus GS, Butt KM, et al. The 1989 report of the North American Pediatric Renal Transplant Cooperative Study. *Pediatr Nephrol* 1990;4:542.

498. Habib R, Broyer M, Levy M. Schonlein-Henoch purpura glomerulonephritis in children. In: Strauss J, ed. *Pediatric Nephrology*. 4th ed. New York: Garland; 1977:155.

499. Levy M, Broyer M, Arsan A, et al. Anaphylactoid purpura nephritis in childhood: Natural history and immunopathology. *Adv Nephrol Necker Hosp* 1976;6:183.

500. Mota-Hernandez F, Valbuena-Paz R, Gordillo-Paniagua G. Long-term prognosis of anaphylactoid purpura nephropathy. *Paediatrician* 1975;4:52.

501. Goldstein AR, White RH, Akuse R, et al. Long-term follow-up of childhood Henoch-Schonlein nephritis. *Lancet* 1992;339:280.

502. Counahan R, Winterborn MH, White RH, et al. Prognosis of Henoch-Schonlein nephritis in children. *Br Med J* 1977;2:11.

503. Scharer K, Krmar R, Querfeld U, et al. Clinical outcome of Schonlein-Henoch purpura nephritis in children. *Pediatr Nephrol* 1999;13:816–.

504. Cream JJ, Gumpel JM, Peachey RD. Schonlein-Henoch purpura in the adult. A study of 77 adults with anaphylactoid or Schonlein-Henoch purpura. *Q J Med* 1970;39:461.

505. Cameron JS. Henoch-Schonlein purpura: clinical presentation. *Contrib Nephrol* 1984;40:246.

506. Brun C, Bryld C, Fenger L, et al. Glomerular lesions in adults with the Schonlein-Henoch syndrome. A light and electron microscopy study. *Acta Pathol Microbiol Scand (A)* 1971;79:569.

507. Ballard HS, Eisinger RP, Gallo G. Renal manifestations of the Henoch-Schoenlein syndrome in adults. *Am J Med* 1970;49:328.

508. Bar-On H, Rosenmann E. Schoenlein-Henoch syndrome in adults. A clinical and histological study of renal involvement. *Isr J Med Sci* 1972;8:1702.

509. Debray J, Krulik M, Giorgi H. Rheumatoid purpura (Schonlein-Henoch syndrome) in the adult. Apropos of 22 cases. *Semin Hop* 1971;47:1805.

510. Esteve A, et al. Henoch-Schonlein nephritis in adults. *Clin Nephrol* 1986;26:313.

511. Faull RJ, Aarons I, Woodroffe AJ, et al. Adult Henoch-Schonlein nephritis. *Aust N Z J Med* 1987;17:396.

512. Fillastre JP. Atteinte renal du purpura rhumatoide chez l'adulte. Etude de 20 biopsies renales. Interet de l'examen glomerulaire en immunofluorescence. *Presse Med* 1971;78:2375.

513. Fogazzi GB, Pasquali S, Moriggi M, et al. Long-term outcome of Schonlein-Henoch nephritis in the adult. *Clin Nephrol* 1989;31:60.

514. Kalowski S, Kincaid-Smith P. Glomerulonephritis in Henoch-Schonlein syndrome. In: Becker E, ed. *Glomerulonephritis*. New York: Wiley; 1973:1123.

515. Lee HS, Koh HI, Kim MJ, et al. Henoch-Schoenlein nephritis in adults: a clinical and morphological study. *Clin Nephrol Vol*. 26; 1986;26:125.

516. Laisseur C, et al. Purpura rheumatoide chez l'adulte: a propos d'une etude de 38 malades. *Rev Med Interne* 1993;14:1019.

517. Roth DA, Wilz DR, Theil GB. Schonlein-Henoch syndrome in adults. *Q J Med* 1985;55:145.

518. Kuster S, Andrassy K, Waldherr R, et al. Contrasting clinical course of Henoch-Schonlein purpura in younger and elderly patients. *Contrib Nephrol* 1993;105:93.

519. Knight J, Cameron JS. UK Medical Research Council Glomerulonephritis Registry 1987 (unpublished data), 1987.

520. Coppo R, Mazzucco G, Cagnoli L, et al. Long-term prognosis of Henoch-Schonlein nephritis in adults and children. Italian Group of Renal Immunopathology Collaborative Study on Henoch-Schonlein purpura. *Nephrol Dial Transplant* 1997;12:2277.

521. Blanco R, Martinez-Taboada VM, Rodriguez-Valverde V, et al. Henoch-Schonlein purpura in adulthood and childhood: two different expressions of the same syndrome. *Arthritis Rheum* 1997;40:859.

522. Tancrede-Bohin E, Ochonisky S, Vignon-Pennamen MD, et al. Schonlein-Henoch purpura in adult patients. Predictive factors for IgA glomerulonephritis in a retrospective study of 57 cases. *Arch Dermatol* 1997;133:438.

523. Pillebout E, Thervet E, Hill G, et al. Henoch-Schonlein Purpura in adults: outcome and prognostic factors. *J Am Soc Nephrol* 2002;13:1271.

524. Ronkainen J, Nuutinen M, Koskimies O. The adult kidney 24 years after childhood Henoch-Schonlein purpura: a retrospective cohort study. *Lancet* 2002;360:666.

525. Ronkainen J, Ala-Houhala M, Huttunen NP, et al. Outcome of Henoch-Schoenlein nephritis with nephrotic-range proteinuria. *Clin Nephrol* 2003;60:80.

526. Trainin EB, Gomez-Leon G. Development of renal insufficiency after long-standing steroid-responsive nephrotic syndrome. *Int J Pediatr Nephrol* 1982;3:55.

527. Correia P, Cameron JS, Lian JD, et al. Why do patients with lupus nephritis die? *Br Med J (Clin Res Ed)* 1985;290:126.

528. Estes D, Christian CL. The natural history of systemic lupus erythematosus by prospective analysis. *Medicine (Baltimore)* 1971;50:85.

529. Karsh J, Klippel JH, Balow JE, et al. Mortality in lupus nephritis. *Arthritis Rheum* 1979;22:764.

530. Rosner S, Ginzler EM, Diamond HS, et al. A multicenter study of outcome in systemic lupus erythematosus. II. Causes of death. *Arthritis Rheum* 1982;25:612.

531. Baldwin DS. Clinical usefulness of the morphological classification of lupus nephritis. *Am J Kidney Dis* 1982;2(Suppl 1):142.

532. Ginzler EM, Nicastri AD, Chen CK, et. Progression of mesangial and focal to diffuse lupus nephritis. *N Engl J Med* 1974;291:693.

533. Platt JL, Burke BA, Fish AJ, et al. Systemic lupus erythematosus in the first two decades of life. *Am J Kidney Dis* 1982;2(Suppl 1):212.

534. Zimmerman SW, Jenkins PG, Shelf WD, et al. Progression from minimal or focal to diffuse proliferative lupus nephritis. *Lab Invest* 1975;32:665.

535. Cervera R, Khamashta MA, Font J, et al. Morbidity and mortality in systemic lupus erythematosus during a 10-year period: a comparison of early and late manifestations in a cohort of 1,000 patients. *Medicine (Baltimore)* 2003;82:299.

536. Pollak VE, Pirani CL. Renal histologic findings in systemic lupus erythematosus. *Mayo Clin Proc* 1969;44:630.

537. Baldwin DS, Gluck MC, Lowenstein J, et al. Lupus nephritis. Clinical course as related to morphologic forms and their transitions. *Am J Med* 1977;62:12.

538. McLigeyo SO, Cameron SJ, Williams GD, et al. Improved survival in lupus nephritis in the modern era (1979–1989). *Afr J Health Sci* 1995;2:211.

539. Martins L, Rocha G, Rodrigues A, et al. Lupus nephritis: a retrospective review of 78 cases from a single center. *Clin Nephrol* 2002;57:114.

540. Gourley MF, Austin HA, 3rd, Scott D, et al. Methylprednisolone and cyclophosphamide, alone or in combination, in patients with lupus nephritis: a randomized, controlled trial. *Ann Intern Med* 1996;125:549.

541. Boumpas DT, Austin HA, 3rd, Vaughn EM, et al. Controlled trial of pulse methylprednisolone versus two regimens of pulse cyclophosphamide in severe lupus nephritis. *Lancet* 1992;340:741–745.

542. Ponticelli C, Zucchelli P, Moroni G, et al. Long-term prognosis of diffuse lupus nephritis. *Clin Nephrol* 1987;28:263.

543. Bono L, Cameron JS, Hicks JA. The very long-term prognosis and complications of lupus nephritis and its treatment. *Q J Med* 1999;92:211.

544. Fiehn C, Hajjar Y, Mueller K, et al. Improved clinical outcome of lupus nephritis during the past decade: importance of early diagnosis and treatment. *Ann Rheum Dis* 2003;62:435.

545. Houssiau FA. Management of lupus nephritis: an update. *J Am Soc Nephrol* 2004;15:2694.

546. Rubin LA, Urowitz MB, Gladman DD. Mortality in systemic lupus erythematosus: the bimodal pattern revisited. *Q J Med* 1985;55:87.

547. Urowitz MB, Bookman AA, Koehler BE, et al. The bimodal mortality pattern of systemic lupus erythematosus. *Am J Med* 1976;60:221.

548. Donadio JV, Jr, Hart GM, Bergstralh EJ, et al. Prognostic determinants in lupus nephritis: a long-term clinicopathologic study. *Lupus* 1995;4:109.

549. Lupus nephritis: prognostic factors and probability of maintaining life-supporting renal function 10 years after the diagnosis. Gruppo Italiano per lo Studio della Nefrite Lupica (GISNEL). *Am J Kidney Dis* 1992;19:473.

550. Cheigh JS, Kim H, Stenzel KH, et al. Systemic lupus erythematosus in patients with end-stage renal disease: long-term follow-up on the prognosis of patients and the evolution of lupus activity. *Am J Kidney Dis* 1990;16:189.

551. Coplon NS, Diskin CJ, Petersen J, et al. The long-term clinical course of systemic lupus erythematosus in end-stage renal disease. *N Engl J Med* 1983;308:186.

552. Roman MJ, Shanker BA, Davis A, et al. Prevalence and correlates of accelerated atherosclerosis in systemic lupus erythematosus. *N Engl J Med* 2003;349:2399.

553. Korbet SM, Lewis EJ, Schwartz MM, et al. Factors predictive of outcome in severe lupus nephritis. Lupus Nephritis Collaborative Study Group. *Am J Kidney Dis* 2000;35:904.

554. Moroni G, Quaglini S, Maccario M, et al. "Nephritic flares" are predictors of bad long-term renal outcome in lupus nephritis. *Kidney Int* 1996;50:2047.

555. Mok CC, Ying KY, Tang S, et al. Predictors and outcome of renal flares after successful cyclophosphamide treatment for diffuse proliferative lupus glomerulonephritis. *Arthritis Rheum* 2004;50:2559.

556. Austin HA, 3rd, Boumpas DT, Vaughan EM, et al. Predicting renal outcomes in severe lupus nephritis: contributions of clinical and histologic data. *Kidney Int* 1994;45:544.

557. Fessel WJ. Systemic lupus erythematosus in the community. Incidence, prevalence, outcome, and first symptoms: the high prevalence in black women. *Arch Intern Med* 1974;134:1027.

558. Serdula MK, Rhoads GG. Frequency of systemic lupus erythematosus in different ethnic groups in Hawaii. *Arthritis Rheum* 1979;22(4):328.

559. Siegel M, Lee SL. The epidemiology of systemic lupus erythematosus. *Semin Arthritis Rheum.* 1973;3:1.

560. Urman JD, Rothfield NF. Corticosteroid treatment in systemic lupus erythematosus. Survival studies. *JAMA* 1977;238:2272.

561. Petri M, Perez-Gutthann S, Longenecker JC, et al. Morbidity of systemic lupus erythematosus: role of race and socioeconomic status. *Am J Med* 1991;91:345.

562. Adu D, Cameron JS. Lupus Nephritis. *Clin Rheum Dis* 1982;8:153.

563. Fries JF, Weyl S, Holman HR. Estimating prognosis in systemic lupus erythematosus. *Am J Med* 1974;57:561.

564. Esdaile JM, Levinton C, Federgreen W, et al. The clinical and renal biopsy predictors of long-term outcome in lupus nephritis: a study of 87 patients and review of the literature. *Q J Med* 1989;72:779.

565. Ginzler EM, Diamond HS, Weiner M, et al. A multicenter study of outcome in systemic lupus erythematosus. I. Entry variables as predictors of prognosis. *Arthritis Rheum* 1982;25:601.

566. Tejani A, Nicastri AD, Chen CK, et al. Lupus nephritis in black and hispanic children. *Am J Dis Child* 1983;137:481.

567. Gordon MF, Stolley PD, Schinnar R. Trends in recent systemic lupus erythematosus mortality rates. *Arthritis Rheum* 1981;24:762.

568. Dooley MA, Hogan S, Jennette C, et al. Cyclophosphamide therapy for lupus nephritis: poor renal survival in black Americans. Glomerular Disease Collaborative Network. *Kidney Int* 1997;51:1188.

569. Reveille JD, Bartolucci A, Alarcon GS. Prognosis in systemic lupus erythematosus. Negative impact of increasing age at onset, black race, and thrombocytopenia, as well as causes of death. *Arthritis Rheum* 1990;33:37.

570. Barr RG, Seliger S, Appel GB, et al. Prognosis in proliferative lupus nephritis: the role of socio-economic status and race/ethnicity. *Nephrol Dial Transplant* 2003;18:2039.

571. Wu J, Edberg JC, Redecha PB, et al. A novel polymorphism of FcgammaRIIIa (CD16) alters receptor function and predisposes to autoimmune disease. *J Clin Invest* 1997;100:1059.

572. Magil AB, Puterman ML, Ballon HS, et al. Prognostic factors in diffuse proliferative lupus glomerulonephritis. *Kidney Int* 1988;34:511.

573. Nossent HC, Henzen-Logmans SC, Vroom TM, et al. Contribution of renal biopsy data in predicting outcome in lupus nephritis. Analysis of 116 patients. *Arthritis Rheum* 1990;33:970.

574. Najafi CC, Korbet SM, Lewis EJ, et al. Significance of histologic patterns of glomerular injury upon long-term prognosis in severe lupus glomerulonephritis. *Kidney Int* 2001;59:2156.

575. Appel GB, Cohen DJ, Pirani CL, et al. Long-term follow-up of patients with lupus nephritis. A study based on the classification of the World Health Organization. *Am J Med* 1987;83:877.

576. Hecht B, Siegel N, Adler M, et al. Prognostic indices in lupus nephritis. *Medicine (Baltimore)* 1976;55:163.

577. Levinsky RJ, Cameron JS, Soothill JF. Serum immune complexes and disease activity in lupus nephritis. *Lancet* 1977;1:564.

578. Lloyd W, Schur PH. Immune complexes, complement, and anti-DNA in exacerbations of systemic lupus erythematosus (SLE). *Medicine (Baltimore)* 1981;60:208.

579. Swaak AJ, Aarden LA, Statius van Eps LW, et al. Anti-dsDNA and complement profiles as prognostic guides in systemic lupus erythematosus. *Arthritis Rheum* 1979;22:226.

580. Goulet JR, MacKenzie T, Levinton C, et al. The longterm prognosis of lupus nephritis: the impact of disease activity. *J Rheumatol* 1993;20:59.

581. Cameron JS. Lupus nephritis in childhood and adolescence. *Pediatr Nephrol* 1994;8:230.

582. Austin HA, 3rd, Muenz LR, Joyce KM, et al. Prognostic factors in lupus nephritis. Contribution of renal histologic data. *Am J Med* 1983;75:382.

583. Ginzler EM, Schorn K. Outcome and prognosis in systemic lupus erythematosus. *Rheum Dis Clin North Am* 1988;14(1):67.

584. Ward MM, Studenski S. Clinical prognostic factors in lupus nephritis. The importance of hypertension and smoking. *Arch Intern Med* 1992;152:2082.

585. Ginzler EM, Felson DT, Anthony JM, et al. Hypertension increases the risk of renal deterioration in systemic lupus erythematosus. *J Rheumatol* 1993;20:1694.

586. Swaak AJ, Nossent JC, Bronsveld W, et al. Systemic lupus erythematosus. I. Outcome and survival: Dutch experience with 110 patients studied prospectively. *Ann Rheum Dis* 1989;48:447.

587. Moroni G, Ventura D, Riva P, et al. Antiphospholipid antibodies are associated with an increased risk for chronic renal insufficiency in patients with lupus nephritis. *Am J Kidney Dis* 2004;43:28.

588. Celermajer DS, Thorner PS, Baumal R, et al. Sex differences in childhood lupus nephritis. *Am J Dis Child* 1984;138:586.

589. Levy M. Unfavorable outcomes (end-stage renal failure/death) in childhood onset systemic lupus erythematosus. A multicenter study in Paris and its environs. *Clin Exp Rheum* 1994;12(Suppl 10):S63.

590. Morel-Maroger L, Mery JP, Droz D, et al. The course of lupus nephritis: contribution of serial renal biopsies. *Adv Nephrol Necker Hosp* 1976;6:79.

591. Berden JH. Lupus nephritis. *Kidney Int* 1997;52:538.

592. Austin HA, 3rd, Muenz LR, Joyce KM, et al. Diffuse proliferative lupus nephritis: identification of specific pathologic features affecting renal outcome. *Kidney Int* 1984;25:689.

593. Grishman E, Churg J. Focal segmental lupus nephritis. *Clin Nephrol* 1982;17:5.

594. Appel GB, Silva FG, Pirani CL, et al. Renal involvement in systemic lupus erythematosus (SLE): a study of 56 patients emphasizing histologic classification. *Medicine (Baltimore)* 1978;57:371.

595. Leaker B, Fairley KF, Dowling J, et al. Lupus nephritis: clinical and pathological correlation. *Q J Med* 1987;62:163.

596. Balow JE, Boumpas DT, Fessler BJ, et al. Management of lupus nephritis. *Kidney Int* 1996;53(Suppl):S88.

597. Appel GB. Cyclophosphamide therapy of severe lupus nephritis. *Am J Kidney Dis* 1997;30:872, Discussion 876.

598. Weening JJ, D'Agati VD, Schwartz MM, et al. The classification of glomerulonephritis in systemic lupus erythematosus revisited. *J Am Soc Nephrol* 2004;15:241.

599. Baldwin DS, Lowenstein J, Rothfield NF, et al. The clinical course of the proliferative and membranous forms of lupus nephritis. *Ann Intern Med* 1970;73:929.

600. Donadio JV, Jr, Burgess JH, Holley KE. Membranous lupus nephropathy: a clinicopathologic study. *Medicine (Baltimore)* 1977;56:527.

601. Pasquali S, Banfi G, Zucchelli A, et al. Lupus membranous nephropathy: long-term outcome. *Clin Nephrol* 1993;39:175.

602. Wang F, Looi LM. Systemic lupus erythematosus with membranous lupus nephropathy in Malaysian patients. *Q J Med* 1984;53:209.

603. Sloan RP, Schwartz MM, Korbet SM, et al. Long-term outcome in systemic lupus erythematosus membranous glomerulonephritis. Lupus Nephritis Collaborative Study Group. *J Am Soc Nephrol* 1996;7:299.

604. Dujovne I, Pollak VE, Pirani CL, et al. The distribution and character of glomerular deposits in systemic lupus erythematosus. *Kidney Int* 1972;2:33.

605. Tateno S, Kobayashi Y, Shigematsu H, et al. Study of lupus nephritis: its classification and the significance of subendothelial deposits. *Q J Med* 1983;52:311.

606. Whiting-O'Keefe Q, Henke JE, Shearn MA, et al. The information content from renal biopsy in systemic lupus erythematosus. *Ann Intern Med* 1982;96(6, Pt 1):718.

607. Whiting-O'Keefe Q, Riccardi PJ, Henke JE, et al. Recognition of information in renal biopsies of patients with lupus nephritis. *Ann Intern Med* 1982;96(6, Pt 1):723.

608. Muehrcke RC, Kark RM, Pirani CL, et al. Lupus nephritis: a clinical and pathologic study based on renal biopsies. *Medicine (Baltimore)* 1957;36:1.

609. Park MH, D'Agati V, Appel GB, et al. Tubulointerstitial disease in lupus nephritis: relationship to immune deposits, interstitial inflammation, glomerular changes, renal function, and prognosis. *Nephron* 1986;44:309.

610. Alexopoulos E, Seron D, Hartley RB, et al. Lupus nephritis: correlation of interstitial cells with glomerular function. *Kidney Int* 1990;37:100.

611. Yeung CK, Wong KL, Wong WS, et al. Crescentic lupus glomerulonephritis. *Clin Nephrol* 1984;21:251.

612. Banfi G, Bertani T, Boeri V, et al. Renal vascular lesions as a marker of poor prognosis in patients with lupus nephritis. Gruppo Italiano per lo Studio della Nefrite Lupica (GISNEL). *Am J Kidney Dis* 1991;18:240.

613. Bhuyan UN, Malaviya AN, Dash SC, et al. Prognostic significance of renal angiitis in systemic lupus erythematosus (SLE). *Clin Nephrol* 1983;20:109.

614. Kant KS, Pollak VE, Weiss MA, et al. Glomerular thrombosis in systemic lupus erythematosus: prevalence and significance. *Medicine (Baltimore)* 1981;60:71.

615. Miranda JM, Garcia-Torres R, Jara LJ, et al. Renal biopsy in systemic lupus erythematosus: significance of glomerular thrombosis. Analysis of 108 cases. *Lupus* 1994;3:25.

616. Jacobsen S, Starklint H, Petersen J, et al. Prognostic value of renal biopsy and clinical variables in patients with lupus nephritis and normal serum creatinine. *Scand J Rheumatol* 1999;28:288.

617. Pirani C, Salinas-Madrigal L. Evaluation of percutaneous renal biopsy. *Pathol Annu* 1968;3:249.

618. Schwartz MM, Bernstein J, Hill GS, et al. Predictive value of renal pathology in diffuse proliferative lupus glomerulonephritis. Lupus Nephritis Collaborative Study Group. *Kidney Int* 1989;36:891.

619. Leehey DJ, Katz AI, Azaran AH, et al. Silent diffuse lupus nephritis: long-term follow-up. *Am J Kidney Dis* 1982;2(Suppl 1):188.

620. Gonzalez-Crespo MR, Lopez-Fernandez JI, Usera G, et al. Outcome of silent lupus nephritis. *Semin Arthritis Rheum*. 1996;26:468.

621. Kimberly RP, Lockshin MD, Sherman RL, et al. Reversible "end-stage" lupus nephritis. Analysis of patients able to discontinue dialysis. *Am J Med* 1983;74:361.

622. Correia P, Cameron JS, Ogg CS, et al. End-stage renal failure in systemic lupus erythematosus with nephritis. *Clin Nephrol* 1984;22:293.

623. Moroni G, Banfi G, Ponticelli C. Clinical status of patients after 10 years of lupus nephritis. *Q J Med* 1992;84:681.

624. Chan TM, Li FK, Tang CS, et al. Efficacy of mycophenolate mofetil in patients with diffuse proliferative lupus nephritis. Hong Kong-Guangzhou Nephrology Study Group. *N Engl J Med* 2000;343:1156.

625. Contreras G, Pardo V, Leclercq B, et al. Sequential therapies for proliferative lupus nephritis. *N Engl J Med* 2004;350:971.

626. Rutherford WE, Blondin J, Miller JP, et al. Chronic progressive renal disease: rate of change of serum creatinine concentration. *Kidney Int* 1977;11:62.

627. Schärer K. Idiopathic nephrotic syndrome associated with focal segmental glomerulosclerosis. In: Bulla M, ed. *Renal Insufficiency in Children*. Berlin: Springer; 1982:23.

628. Noel LH, Droz D, Gascon M, et al. Primary IgA nephropathy: from the first-described cases to the present. *Semin Nephrol* 1987;7:351.

629. Velo M, Lozano L, Egido J, et al. Natural history of IgA nephropathy in patients followed-up for more than ten years in Spain. *Semin Nephrol* 1987;7:346.

630. Bogenschutz O, Bohle A, Batz C, et al. IgA nephritis: on the importance of morphological and clinical parameters in the long-term prognosis of 239 patients. *Am J Nephrol* 1990;10:137.

631. Rekola S, Bergstrand A, Bucht H. Development of hypertension in IgA nephropathy as a marker of a poor prognosis. *Am J Nephrol* 1990;10:290.

632. Rekola S, Bergstrand A, Bucht H. IGA nephropathy: a retrospective evaluation of prognostic indices in 176 patients. *Scand J Urol Nephrol* 1989;23:37.

633. Ibels LS, Gyory AZ. IgA nephropathy: Analysis of the natural history, important factors in the progression of renal disease, and a review of the literature. *Medicine (Baltimore)* 1994;73:79.

634. Koyama A, Igarashi M, Kobayashi M. Natural history and risk factors for immunoglobulin A nephropathy in Japan. Research Group on Progressive Renal Diseases. *Am J Kidney Dis* 1997;29:526.

635. Wyatt RJ, Julian BA, Bhathena DB, et al. Iga nephropathy: presentation, clinical course, and prognosis in children and adults. *Am J Kidney Dis* 1984;4:192.

636. Radford MG, Jr, Donadio JV, Jr, Bergstralh EJ, et al. Predicting renal outcome in IgA nephropathy. *J Am Soc Nephrol* 1997;8:199.

637. Haas M. Histologic subclassification of IgA nephropathy: a clinicopathologic study of 244 cases. *Am J Kidney Dis* 1997;29:829.

CHAPTER 72 ■ CHRONIC TUBULOINTERSTITIAL NEPHROPATHIES

GARABED EKNOYAN AND UDAY KHOSLA

Diseases of the kidney primarily affect the glomeruli, the vasculature, or the remainder of the renal parenchyma, that is, the tubules and interstitium. The chronic forms of the latter category of diseases of the kidney are considered in this chapter. Initially referred to as *interstitial nephritis* (1,2), the more descriptive terms *tubulointerstitial diseases* (3), *nephritis,* or *nephropathies* (4) are now used to classify this heterogeneous group of disorders that in its primary form affects the renal tubules and interstitium and only secondarily involves the other structural components of the kidney.

The preferential use of the qualifier tubulointerstitial was first proposed because structurally it is the tubules, not the interstitium, that comprise the bulk of the normal kidney parenchyma and sustain the brunt of the injury; and clinically, disorders of tubular function constitute the most notable component of the disordered pathophysiology of these diseases and thereby differentiate them from other forms of kidney disease resulting from glomerular or vascular lesions (3–5). In addition, increasing evidence now indicates that the tubular epithelial cells are an integral component of the pathogenesis of these diseases, in both the processing and the presentation of foreign antigens and in the progressive interstitial changes that ensue (6–9). This is not to imply that glomerular lesions do not occur or contribute to the loss of kidney function in these diseases. Although the primary lesions originate in the tubules and interstitium, many of them eventually will develop structural and functional abnormalities of the glomeruli (3,5), whose structural alterations are characterized by glomerulosclerosis, whereas the functional changes are evidenced by a progressive reduction in the glomerular filtration rate (GFR), the development of glomerular proteinuria, and ultimately, the onset of volume-dependent hypertension (4,10,11). Early in the course of tubulointerstitial diseases of the kidney, with their characteristic insidious onset and indolent course, tubular dysfunction is almost always out of proportion to any coexistent glomerular dysfunction (3,4,11). In the later phases of tubulointerstitial diseases of the kidney in which the glomerular lesions are quite advanced, it may be difficult to differentiate them from the end-stage kidney disease of any etiology. Although diseases of the glomeruli and vasculature are excluded, by definition, from primary chronic tubulointerstitial nephropathies, the secondary forms of tubulointerstitial nephritis are an important component of diseases of the glomeruli and vasculature, and the extent and severity of concurrent tubulointerstitial changes contribute significantly to their clinical course (12). It is the development of the secondary form of tubulointerstitial nephritis that attends almost all instances of progressive glomerular and vascular diseases that determines, in large part, their outcome (12–18).

The frequency with which primary tubulointerstitial diseases affect the kidney is difficult to determine. Their importance, however, can be appreciated because an estimated 20% to 40% of all patients who develop kidney failure and become dialysis-dependent have primary tubulointerstitial disease as the cause of their kidney failure (19–21). Taken together with the demonstrated role of secondary tubulointerstitial lesions in the deterioration of kidney function in those with primary glomerular or vascular disease (8,21,22), it becomes evident why it is important to evaluate and appreciate lesions of the interstitium and tubules in chronic kidney disease of any etiology.

The preferential use of the term *tubulointerstitial* should in no way minimize the role of the interstitium, because this is where the pathogenesis and evolution of the disease is perpetuated (7,8,18), and the interstitial lesions may well account for many of the disorders of tubular function that are characteristic of these diseases. The renal interstitium as an important component of kidney function has long been appreciated. The interstitial solute concentration in the cortex and in the medulla is an integral component of the regulatory mechanisms for proximal reabsorption and for concentration and dilution of urine, respectively (23,24). Furthermore, the endocrine functions of the interstitial cells, in the release of renin and erythropoietin in the cortex and of prostaglandins in the medulla, are essential modulators in the role of the kidney in maintaining homeostasis (14,23–25). Conceptually then, interstitial events could account for the pathogenesis, progression, and clinical manifestations of chronic kidney diseases in general and of the tubulointerstitial nephropathies in particular (Fig. 72-1). Still, the tubular changes bear the brunt of the insult and, because they are functionally more important, account for the clinical and functional manifestations of any interstitial nephritis. Evaluation of tubular function is extremely important because of its predictive value of the extent of tubulointerstitial nephritis, and as such would provide a readily available, noninvasive, clinical assessment of the severity and prognosis of chronic kidney diseases (26).

STRUCTURAL FEATURES OF THE INTERSTITIUM

The interstitium of the kidney consists of peritubular and perivascular spaces. The relative contribution of each of these spaces to interstitial volume varies, reflecting in part the arbitrary boundaries used in assessing them. The portion of renal tissue occupied by interstitium increases from the cortex to the papilla. In the cortex, there is little interstitium, because the peritubular capillaries fill most of the space between the tubules and the cortical interstitial cells, which are scattered between the capillaries and tubules of the cortical labyrinth and are relatively inconspicuous. In the medulla, however, there is a noticeable increase in interstitial space, and the interstitial cells have characteristic structural features and an organized arrangement. The ground substance of the interstitium contains different types of fibrils and a basementlike material embedded in a glycosaminoglycan-rich substance (27–30).

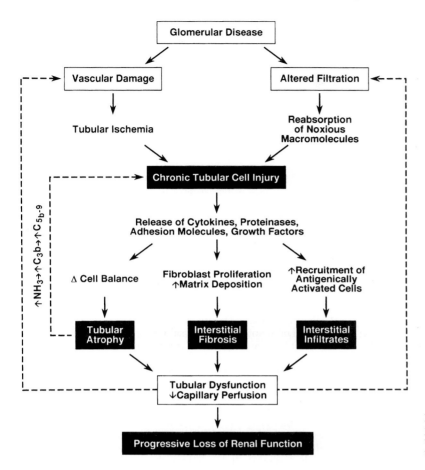

FIGURE 72-1. Schematic overview of the potential pathways in the pathogenesis of chronic tubulointerstitial nephritis due to primary tubular injury or secondary to glomerular disease.

The relative volume of the interstitium of the cortex is approximately 7%, consisting of about 3% interstitial cells and 4% extracellular space (23,31,32). The vasculature occupies another 6%; the remainder (i.e., 85% or more) is occupied by the tubules. The cortical interstitial space is distributed unevenly and has been divided into "narrow" and "wide" structural components (30,31). The tubules and peritubular capillaries are closely apposed at several points, sometimes to the point of sharing a common basement membrane, or are separated by a very narrow space, the so-called *narrow interstitium,* which occupies an estimated 0.6% of cortical volume in the rat. The narrow interstitium occupies about one-half to two-thirds of the cortical peritubular capillary surface area. The remainder of the cortical interstitium consists of irregularly shaped, clearly discernible larger areas, the so-called *wide interstitium,* which occupies an estimated 3.4% of cortical volume in the rat (30,31). Most of the cortical interstitial cells are located in the wide interstitium. The capillary wall facing the narrow interstitium is significantly more fenestrated than that facing the wide interstitium (23,30). Evidence for a possible functional heterogeneity of these interstitial spaces has been advanced on the basis of studies of the interstitial albumin pool (28). The actual significance of these findings, however, remains to be clarified.

In the medulla, the size of the interstitium increases gradually from the outer medullary stripe to the tip of the papilla (23,30), because of the increase in the relative volume contribution of both the interstitial cells and the extracellular space. Actually, in the outer stripe of the outer medulla, the relative volume of the interstitium is slightly less than that in the cortex and has been estimated to be approximately 5% in the rat. It is in the inner stripe of the outer medulla that the interstitium

begins to increase significantly in volume in increments that gradually becomes greater toward the papillary tip (23,30–34). The inner stripe of the outer medulla consists of the vascular bundles and the interbundle regions, which are occupied principally by tubules. Within the vascular bundles, the interstitial spaces are meager, whereas in the interbundle region, the interstitial spaces occupy 10% to 20% of the volume. In the inner medulla, the differentiation into vascular bundles and interbundle regions becomes gradually less obvious until the two regions merge. This is coupled by a gradual increase in the relative volume of the interstitial space from the base of the inner medulla to the tip of the papilla. In the rat, the increment in interstitial space is from 10% to 15% at the base to about 30% at the tip, and, in the rabbit, from 20% to 25% at the base to more than 40% at the tip (35).

The cortex contains two types of interstitial cells. The more abundant variety of interstitial cells are the type I or the fibroblastic cells. These have a prominent rough endoplasmic reticulum and elongated mitochondria. They appear to produce the extracellular interstitial matrix and contribute to fibrosis in response to chronic irritation as they evolve into myofibroblasts. The less common type II interstitial cells are mononuclear cells or macrophages, which have an abundant chromatin and no endoplasmic reticulum with demonstrable phagocytic ability, and through their autocrine function contribute to the fibrogenesis of tubulointerstitial nephropathy (23,30). An interstitial infiltrate of recruited mononuclear cells is a prominent feature of chronic interstitial nephritis, but some of the infiltrating cells are derived from these local precursors (6,7,19).

In the outer zone of the outer medulla, the interstitial cells are similar to those in the cortex. In the inner zone of the outer medulla and the inner medulla, the cellular content is significantly altered. A unique type of cell that is present in increasing numbers toward the tip of the papilla is the lipid-laden interstitial cell. The number of cytoplasmic lipid droplets of these cells varies from one cell to the other, and there are differences in the number of droplets among species and among individuals of the same species. A change in the number of droplets has been suggested, but not conclusively demonstrated, to occur in relation to the intake of salt and water and the level of blood pressure (36). These cells are also the source of the interstitial glycosaminoglycans in the inner medulla (30). Another characteristic feature of these medullary cells is their connection to each other in a characteristic arrangement, similar to the rungs of a ladder, with a distinct close and regular transverse apposition to their surrounding structures, specifically the limbs of the loop of Henle and capillaries, but not to the collecting duct cells (23,27). The other types of medullary cells are the mononuclear cells or macrophages and the pericytes. The latter are prominent in the descending vasa recta in the outer medulla but become rare as the vascular bundles break up in the inner medulla. The number of mononuclear cells and macrophages increases in the inner stripe of the outer medulla and is highest in the inner medulla (29). Proliferation and upregulation of resident macrophages and pericytes, in response to injury, are an essential determinant of the extent of fibrosis that characterizes tubulointerstitial nephritis.

The extracellular loose matrix is a hydrated gelatinous substance that consists of glycoproteins and glycosaminoglycans (hyaluronic acid, heparan sulfate, dermatan sulfate, and chondroitin sulfate) that are embedded within a fibrillar reticulum, which consists of collagen fibers (types I, III, and VI) and unbanded microfilaments. Collagen types IV and V are the principal components of the basement membrane lining the vessels and tubules. Glycoprotein (fibronectin, laminin) components of the basement membrane connect it to the interstitial cell membranes and to the fibrillar structures of the interstitial matrix (37). The relative increase in interstitial matrix of the medulla may be important for providing support to the delicate tubular and vascular structures in this region, and its inflammation-mediated compositional alterations might well account for the susceptibility of the structures in this region to toxic reactive metabolites (38).

FUNCTIONAL SIGNIFICANCE OF THE INTERSTITIUM

Exchange processes between the different segments of the renal tubular and vascular components are at the core of the homeostatic functions of the kidney. In most physiologic discussions, the transport of ions, water, and proteins is described as though it occurred directly from the tubule to the capillary, and the emphasis is on the permeability of the membranes concerned. In fact, the reabsorbed or secreted tubular fluid has to traverse a true interstitial space between the tubules and peritubular capillaries. The structure, composition, and permeability characteristic of the interstitial space must, of necessity, exert an effect on any such exchange. Several studies suggest that pressure and volume conditions of the interstitial space modulate renal tubule function in response to fluid-balance disturbances. The normal interstitial hydrostatic pressure of about 3 mm Hg and protein concentration of about 2 g% changes with extracellular fluid volume expansion to 5 to 10 mm Hg and 0.5 g%, respectively (39). Similarly, rapid transient changes in the hydrostatic pressure of the interstitial spaces occur after the intraaortic injection of albumin or saline solutions (39). There are also measurable changes in the volume of the medullary interstitial space during water diuresis and vasopressin-induced antidiuresis (40). Homeostasis is also controlled by paracrine

mediators according to the cytoarchitectural features between the tubules and arterioles. The site where such a structure–function mechanism has been best elucidated is the conglomerate of cells at the connection between the macula densa and the glomerular vasculature that has been considered to form an "apparatus," as reflected in its accepted name: the juxtaglomerular apparatus (41).

Although the normal structural and functional correlates of the interstitial space are poorly defined, changes in the interstitial composition and structure are bound to reflect themselves in changes of tubular function. Structural changes of the interstitium, by altering equilibration or exchange, and the release of vasoactive cytokines by the infiltrating cells, could well result in a significant alteration in the normal functions of the renal tubule. Correlation of the structural changes of the interstitium to those of kidney function may be better envisioned when the rich but delicate capillary network of the renal microcirculation is taken into consideration. The periarterial loose connective tissue that envelops the intrarenal microvasculature in the cortex is continuous with that of the sparse peritubular interstitium (23,30,31). It is possible that changes in the supporting interstitium could affect the blood flow to the adjacent tubule and thereby cause tubular dysfunction (Fig. 72-1). Angiographic studies of the renal microcirculation reveal that the number and volume of peritubular capillaries are markedly compromised in the areas of interstitial inflammation and fibrosis (42–44). Interstitial alterations also may be reflected in changes in glomerular capillary pressure and filtration rate through a tubuloglomerular feedback mechanism; specifically, as the function of the affected tubular segments becomes compromised secondary to interstitial disease, solute delivery to the macula densa may be altered (24,39,45,46). On the basis of experimental models and studies correlating morphometric analysis of human kidney biopsy specimens to kidney function, it has been suggested that obliteration of postglomerular capillaries secondary to interstitial injury and fibrosis may account for changes in kidney function (44,47), and by extension to the pathogenesis of progression of kidney disease to kidney failure (48,49).

It is of special relevance, in this regard, that attempts to correlate kidney function with histologic abnormalities of the glomeruli have been conflicting. Whereas some studies found a relationship (50,51), others were unable to document any correlation (46). Conversely, several studies of abnormalities of the tubulointerstitial tissue show a close correlation with abnormalities of kidney function in an assortment of chronic kidney diseases (13,22,52–56). A careful study of 70 patients with various renal diseases, most of which were glomerular in origin, evaluated by semiquantitative morphometric analysis of the biopsy material the changes in glomerular, tubular, vascular, and interstitial components (57). Studies of kidney function, performed within 2 days of the biopsy, included measurements of GFR, effective renal plasma flow, acidifying ability, and maximal concentrating ability. The GFR showed a higher correlation with interstitial and tubular damage, regardless of the disease process (Fig. 72-2). Interstitial fibrosis and cellular infiltration were also well correlated with GFR, whereas edema was not. In contrast to these findings, there was only a modest correlation between GFR and the glomerular injury score. As might be expected, effective renal plasma flow showed a high correlation with the degree of vascular disease (Fig. 72-3); it was also highly correlated with tubular and interstitial damage but not to glomerular lesions. The urinary concentrating ability was found to be a very sensitive indicator of the presence or absence of tubular and interstitial abnormalities (Fig. 72-4). It was the severity of tubulointerstitial damage and not the primary kidney disease that seemed to be the determinant of impairment in concentrating ability. All patients whose maximal urinary osmolality was less

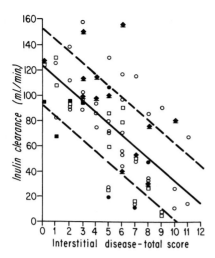

FIGURE 72-2. Relationship of inulin clearance to the severity of tubulointerstitial lesions. The regression line is $y = 122 - 8.8x$. Symbols represent categories of kidney diseases studied: ♦, acute glomerulonephritis; ○, chronic glomerulonephritis; ●, tubulointerstitial nephropathy; ■, nephrosclerosis; □, miscellaneous. (From: Schainuck LL, et al. Structural-functional correlations in renal disease. Part II: the correlations. *Hum Pathol* 1970;1:631, with permission.)

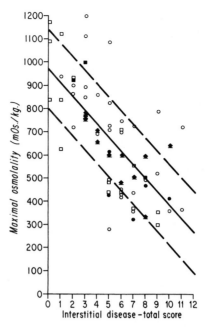

FIGURE 72-4. Relationship of the maximum ability to concentrate the urine (maximal osmolality) to the severity of tubulointerstitial lesions. The regression line is $y = 975 - 59x$. Symbols represent categories of kidney diseases studied: ♦, acute glomerulonephritis; ○, chronic glomerulonephritis; ●, tubulointerstitial nephropathy; ■, nephrosclerosis; □, miscellaneous. (From: Schainuck LL, et al. Structural-functional correlations in renal disease. Part II: the correlations. *Hum Pathol* 1970;1:631, with permission.)

than 600 mOsmol/kg of water had moderate-to-severe tubulointerstitial lesions, whereas those able to concentrate their urine to more than 800 mOsmol/kg of water had only minimal tubulointerstitial lesions. There was only a modest, albeit significant, relationship between urinary concentrating ability and the severity of the glomerular score. Finally, the impairment in the ability to excrete titratable acid and ammonium

in response to an acid load was highly correlated with the degree of interstitial and tubular lesions and to a much lesser degree with glomerular changes (Fig. 72-5). With increased awareness of the role of the interstitial lesion, these studies were expanded (12,14,58–60), and the presence of interstitial fibrosis has been documented to show a significant correlation with the progression of kidney diseases of glomerular origin (Fig. 72-6). Therefore, the presence of secondary tubulointerstitial lesions in primary glomerular diseases not only correlates with the severity of altered kidney function at the time of biopsy but also provides a prognostic index of the rate of progression to end-stage kidney failure (14,15,61–64).

Glomerular Influence on Tubulointerstitial Disease

Altered glomerular permeability with consequent proteinuria has emerged as an important contributory factor to the development of tubulointerstitial lesions in primary glomerular diseases (62,64,65) (Fig. 72-1). Glomerular diseases associated with proteinuria elicit tubulointerstitial inflammation, which when persistent will progress to interstitial fibrosis (18,66). Different potential pathways can account for this association, but an abnormal glomerular filtrate appears to mediate tubular epithelial cell injury, and their consequent antigenic activation is an important step in initiating the sequence of events that leads to fibrosis and scarring of the interstitium. Activated epithelial cells release chemokines, such as monocyte chemotactic peptide-1 (MCP-1) and osteopontin, which are capable of attracting leukocytes (67,68) and vasoactive peptides, such as endothelin-1, that alter vascular permeability (67–69). The activated epithelial cells also express major histocompatibility complex (MHC)-II molecules and act as antigen-presenting

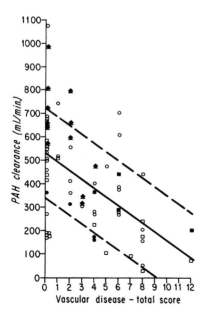

FIGURE 72-3. Relationship of effective renal plasma flow as measured by the clearance of p-aminohippurate *(PAH)* to the severity of vascular disease. The regression line is $y = 553 - 38x$. Symbols represent categories of kidney diseases studied: ♦, acute glomerulonephritis; ○, chronic glomerulonephritis; ●, tubulointerstitial nephropathy; ■, nephrosclerosis; □, miscellaneous. (From: Schainuck LL, et al. Structural-functional correlations in renal disease. Part II: the correlations. *Hum Pathol* 1970;1:631, with permission.)

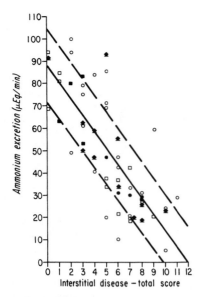

FIGURE 72-5. Relationship between ammonium excretion in response to an acute acid load and the severity of tubulointerstitial lesions. The regression line is $y = 90 - 7.6x$. Symbols represent categories of kidney diseases studied: ♦, acute glomerulonephritis; ○, chronic glomerulonephritis; ●, tubulointerstitial nephropathy; ■, nephrosclerosis; □, miscellaneous. (From: Schainuck LL, et al. Structural-functional correlations in renal disease. Part II: the correlations. *Hum Pathol* 1970;1:631, with permission.)

cells to the infiltrating interstitial T cells (70). Interstitial nephritis has been induced by protein overload in uni-nephrectomized rats (71). Significant cellular infiltration develops in the interstitium of experimental animals within 1 week of exposure to a protein overload consisting of 1 g of bovine serum albumin (BSA) injected in the peritoneum daily. The initial infiltrates consisting predominantly of macrophages are soon replaced by T lymphocytes, and by the fourth week, tubular atrophy and interstitial fibrosis is present. This has been attributed to the proximal tubular epithelial cell catabolism of the filtered

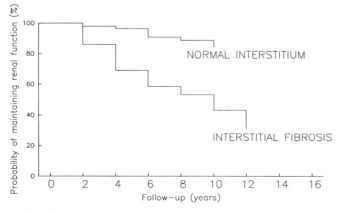

FIGURE 72-6. Effect of the presence of cortical interstitial fibrosis noted at the time of the initial diagnostic kidney biopsy on the long-term prognosis of patients with mesangioproliferative glomerulonephritis ($N = 455$), membranous nephropathy ($N = 334$), and membranoproliferative glomerulonephritis ($N = 220$). (From: Bohle A, et al. The consequences of tubulointerstitial changes for renal function in glomerulopathies: a morphometric and cytological analysis. *Pathol Res Pract* 1990;186:135, with permission.)

albumin, which results in the generation of a nonpolar lipid that is chemotactic for macrophages (72). Apart from its effect on tubular epithelial cells, the "inflammatory filtrate" of the injured glomerulus also can diffuse into the interstitial space and elicit an inflammatory response in the periglomerular interstitium (18,66).

In addition to the effect of altered glomerular permeability on interstitial fibrosis, glomerular inflammation and scarring can compromise postglomerular blood flow and initiate ischemic tubular injury. Injury to the peritubular capillaries and rarefaction of the peritubular vasculature are components of several models of experimental tubulointerstitial nephritis (73). An early angiogenic response followed by progressive endothelial cell apoptosis and regression of peritubular capillaries has been implicated as a potential contributory factor to tubulointerstitial fibrosis (73,74). In experimental models, hypoxic tubular epithelial cells increase expression of several proinflammatory molecules that promote fibrosis, such as interleukin-6 (IL-6) and tumor growth factor-β (TGF-β) (75–77). Hypoxia also leads to the increased local production of angiotensin and the transdifferentiation of tubular epithelial cells into migrating fibroblastlike cells (78). As such, tubular ischemia triggers a localized inflammation and leukocyte recruitment and promotes the deposition of extracellular matrix (67–70). The resultant tubulointerstitial nephritis correlates with reduced renal blood flow, fall in glomerular filtration rate, and altered nitric oxide (NO) activity (79).

Iron loss in the tubular fluid also has been implicated in the pathogenesis of the tubulointerstitial injury associated with primary glomerular disease. In an experimental model of glomerulonephritis in rats, the induction of iron deficiency reduced the urinary protein excretion rate and attenuated the development of tubulointerstitial lesions and attendant deterioration of kidney function (80,81). Conceivably, iron, dissociated from filtered transferrin at the more acid pH of the tubule fluid or during its absorption in the proximal tubule, contributes to the formation of free hydroxyl radicals, which account for tubular epithelial cell injury and consequent tubulointerstitial lesions. In type II diabetic patients, transferrinuria correlates with interstitial injury, perhaps through a similar free-radical mediated mechanism (82) or possibly by stimulating platelet-derived growth factor (PDGF) (83).

These experimental studies notwithstanding, severe tubulointerstitial lesions do not invariably accompany proteinuric glomerular diseases, and the search for additional factors contributory to the development of interstitial lesions deserves continuous scrutiny.

In summary, the available evidence would indicate that the normal interstitium plays an important role in kidney function and that changes in the integrity of interstitial components show a significant correlation to the severity and extent of loss of function in various diseases of the kidney. As such, tubulointerstitial nephritis can be considered the final common pathway of all forms of chronic kidney diseases associated with progressive loss of kidney function independent of the original site of injury—glomeruli, vasculature, or tubules. The importance of the interstitium in the normal and diseased kidney is now well established. The mechanisms involved in the initiation and progression of interstitial fibrosis remain to be fully elucidated.

PATHOLOGIC FEATURES OF TUBULOINTERSTITIAL NEPHROPATHIES

Independent of its initiating process, the principal morphologic feature of chronic tubulointerstitial nephropathy is an increase in the interstitial volume, mainly because of interstitial fibrosis and of varying degrees of infiltration with chronic inflammatory cells (Fig. 72-1). Tubular atrophy and degeneration are also common, if not invariable, findings, particularly in the late phases of the disease (84). As interstitial widening by fibrosis progresses, the tubular basement membrane (TBM) thickness increases as a result of deposition of type IV collagen and laminin (85). Depending on the duration, cause, and severity of the initiating disease process, the distribution of the lesions will vary from focal to diffuse but is generally patchy. This interstitial inflammatory reaction is a secondary feature of several progressive kidney diseases, including those of glomerular or vascular origin (62,86–90). There are, however, other diseases of the kidney in which primary tubulointerstitial lesions are the principal, and early in the course of the disease, usually the only detectable lesion on morphologic examination of kidney tissue (91). Changes of glomerular sclerosis, periglomerular fibrosis, and atrophy, if not present at the onset, will ultimately occur in primary tubulointerstitial diseases of the kidney (92). The final picture that emerges in the end-stage form of the disease may be indistinguishable from that of end-stage kidney disease of any etiology. As such, progressive tubulointerstitial lesions are a major contributory cause of progressive loss of kidney function and of all end-stage renal diseases, whether of primary or secondary etiology.

Immunohistologic examination, using monoclonal antibodies, coupled with conventional and electron microscopy indicates that most of the mononuclear cells making up renal interstitial infiltrates are T lymphocytes (93–97). Chronic inflammatory cell loci may be characterized by Ia antigen-positive T cells, considered to be markers of activated lymphocytes (86,98). The interstitial infiltrates contain varying numbers of activated lymphocytes in the absence of tubulointerstitial immune deposits (62), even in classic examples of immune complex–mediated diseases such as systemic lupus erythematosus (59). The extent of interstitial infiltrates shows a direct correlation between the severity of tubular atrophy and interstitial fibrosis determined semiquantitatively (86). The profile of immunocompetent cells suggests a major role for cell-mediated immunity in the tubulointerstitial lesions that are mediated by autoimmune mechanisms (99,100). Experimental studies have shown the sequential accumulation of T cells and monocytes after the initial immune insult, which would implicate an important role for T cells, both as inflammatory cells and in the progression of subsequent injury (7,94,96,97). The infiltrating lymphocytes may be of the CD4+ helper/inducer subset (78) or the CD8+ cytotoxic/suppressor subset (76), although there generally seems to be a selective prevalence of the former variety (94). A more limited number of natural killer cells are a component of the infiltrates. Lymphocytes that are peritubular and are seen invading the tubular epithelial cells, so-called *tubulitis*, are generally of the cytotoxic (CD8+) variety (100), with a contributory role of the natural killer cells. Nephritogenic CD8+ T-cell lines of distinct functional phenotypes, which are specifically cytotoxic to tubular epithelial cells, have been isolated and identified (101). The further characterization of T-cell clones from these lesions can better define the role of the infiltrating cells in the pathogenesis of tubulointerstitial diseases (Fig. 72-1). Fine-needle aspiration of the kidney can be useful in the characterization of the cellular infiltrates (102) and their sequential evolution (103). The interstitial accumulation of monocytes involves a host of chemo-attractant cytokines such as osteopontin (uropontin), a secreted cell-attachment glycoprotein whose messenger RNA expression is upregulated and levels are increased at sites of tubular injury in proportion to the severity of tubular damage (104,105). The expression of other cell adhesion molecules (intercellular adhesion molecule 1 [ICAM-1], vascular cell adhesion molecule 1 [VCAM-1], E selectin) also is increased at sites of tubular injury and may

contribute to the recruitment of mononuclear cells and increase the susceptibility of renal cells to cell-mediated injury (66–70,106,107).

In addition to the infiltrating nephritogenic lymphocytes, macrophages and mast cells are recruited and participate in the proteolytic and fibrotic injury of the normal parenchyma (97,108). The resident fibroblastic (or type I) interstitial cells, which normally produce and maintain the extracellular matrix, proliferate and increase their well-developed rough endoplasmic reticulum in response to injury (20,109) (Fig. 72-1). The number of fibroblasts derived in cell culture from kidney biopsy material obtained from patients with interstitial fibrosis is increased by a factor of five to ten, compared with that from cultures derived from normal kidney biopsy samples (19). Growth kinetic studies of these cells show a significant increase in proliferating capacity and generation time, indicating hyperproliferative growth (110).

The type of infiltrate can be characteristic and occasionally diagnostic of the kidney disease. The presence of eosinophils can be diagnostic of drug-induced acute allergic interstitial nephritis (Chapter 48). Another cell type, the presence of which may be of diagnostic importance, is the foam cell, with its characteristic vacuolated appearance. Studies using monoclonal antibodies showed these cells to be derived from macrophages (111), which have phagocytosed lipids. Macrophage-derived foam cells can perpetuate an inflammatory reaction by release of cytokines that promote vascular smooth muscle cell proliferation and matrix deposition (112). Isolated foam cells are frequently encountered in patients with heavy proteinuria of any etiology (113). Their presence in large numbers in the glomeruli and interstitium is indicative of Alport's nephritis (114). Masses of interstitial foam cells, interspersed with inflammatory cells, occur in chronic forms of pyelonephritis and, when prominent, form the characteristic lesion of xanthogranulomatous interstitial nephritis (115). A closely related condition is the appearance of large mononuclear cells with abundant cytoplasm, containing large and laminated phagolysosomes that show progressive mineralization and form the characteristic Michaelis-Gutmann bodies seen in malakoplakia (115,116). Although malakoplakia is commonly a lesion of the urinary bladder, it occasionally involves the renal interstitium and usually occurs in the context of chronic urinary tract infection (116,117). These peculiar cells have also been observed in hemolytic-uremic syndrome (118) and in transplanted kidneys (119).

The interstitial lesions of one group of tubulointerstitial diseases can be distinguished by the presence of a characteristic noncaseating granulomatous pattern, which, when present, is highly suggestive of sarcoidosis (120,121). Usually coexistent with extrarenal granulomata there are rare reports of sarcoid granulomatous lesions localized to the kidney only, in the absence of extrarenal lesions (122,123). Interstitial granulomatous reactions also occur in response to oxalate deposition (124) and to infection of the kidney by mycobacteria (125), fungus (126), or bacteria (127). Granulomatous reactions to drugs, such as methicillin (121), sulfonamides (128), and narcotics (129), have been observed in patients with acute forms of tubulointerstitial disease. In experimental models of anti–basement membrane nephritis, granulomatous inflammation develops around the immunologically altered TBM. In the course of the granulomatous reaction, tissue monocytes evolve from recruited circulating monocytes and pursue one of two independent pathways of differentiation: (a) macrophages that evolve distant from the tubules or (b) epithelioid cells that are formed adjacent to the tubules. The latter form through cell fusion and can develop into the multinucleated giant cells of Langhans (130–133). Multinucleated giant cells also are a feature of renal involvement in multiple myeloma (134,135).

Intracellular crystals can be diagnostic of some forms of tubulointerstitial diseases. Rhomboid-shaped crystals within the cell lysosomes are characteristic of cystinosis (136). Tophaceous deposits and birefringent deposits of sodium biurate are seen in hyperuricemia and gout (137). Birefringence on dark-field microscopy is observed in oxalosis (106,119,120). Gold therapy for rheumatoid arthritis can result in characteristic lysosomal crystalloid aggregates that can be seen by electron microscopy (140).

The interstitial spaces may be invaded by proliferative malignant cells in leukemias and lymphomas (141), typically causing an increase in kidney size. Interstitial infiltration by malignant cells can lead to increased interstitial pressure with resultant tubular obstruction and disruption of peritubular vasculature. Commonly found at postmortem in patients with clinically evident malignant disease, massive infiltration of the kidney with renal failure may be an initial presenting feature in some patients (141,142).

PATHOGENESIS AND MECHANISMS OF INJURY IN TUBULOINTERSTITIAL NEPHRITIS

Tubulointerstitial nephropathy is an inflammatory reaction that is perpetuated by continuous exposure to injury or a failure to respond to the usual controlling mechanisms in the feedback loop of the normal defensive response to injury. The demonstration that the infiltrating cells are antigenetically active implicates a principal role of cell-mediated immune reaction in this inappropriate response, which evolves into one progressive parenchymal injury (96,97). The gradual increase in interstitial spaces by infiltrating cells and fibrous tissue implicates a relentless fibrogenesis in replacing the regressive tubular atrophy and degeneration caused by the parenchymal injury (143).

The immune response to the initiating injury includes recognition of the insult, an integration of the response, and an effector phase, which in the kidney entails a complex integrated operation between the tubular epithelial cells, resident interstitial cells, and the recruited inflammatory cells (Fig. 72-7). This interactive process is mediated by a host of cytokines and autocoids released by the involved cells at various stages of the response and of the upregulated expression of specific receptors to them by the targeted cells. More of these stimulatory or responsive signals have been identified, with different, often overlapping, functions that modulate and amplify the inflammatory reaction that accounts for the tubulointerstitial lesions. Some of these are cell surface markers that have antigenic (MHC; human leukocyte antigen class II; osteonectin; and secreted protein acidic and rich in cysteine) or adhesive (ICAM-1, VCAM-1; integrins; osteopontin; thrombospondin; selectins) properties. Others are cytokines that are chemoattractant (monocyte chemoattractant protein-1; regulated on activation, normal T-cell expressed and secreted; osteopontin; eotaxin; fibronectin; macrophage inflammatory protein-1), *proinflammatory* (IL-6, IL-8, platelet-derived growth factor β [PDGFβ]; granulocyte monocyte colony-stimulating factor; tumor necrosis factor α [TNFα]; Tamm-Horsfall glycoprotein [TH]; transforming growth factor-α [TGF-α]), *vasoactive* (nitrous oxide [NO]; endothelin 1; angiotensin II [AII]; thromboxanes; prostaglandins; adenosine), *cytotoxic* (matrix metalloproteinases-1 and -2 [MMP-1 and MMP-2]; tissue inhibitor of metalloproteinase-1; TNFα; reactive oxygen species [ROS]; ferric ion), fibrogenetic (fibroblast growth factor-2; AII; aldosterone; TGF-β; PDGF; IL-1; IL-6; TNF; and plasminogen activator inhibitor [PAI]), *growth promoting* (AII, PDGF; TGF-β; endothelin 1), or *apoptotic* (clusterin; Fas; bax; osteopontin) (8,9,144–150).

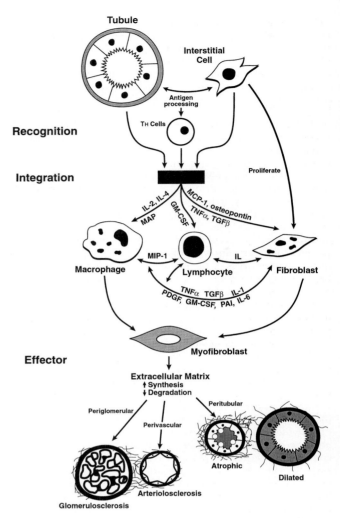

FIGURE 72-7. Pathogenesis and mechanisms of injury in tubulointerstitial nephritis. T_H, T helper cells.

The initiating insult may be a drug, an infection, a filtered noxious protein, mechanical obstruction, ischemia, or a specific antigen (41,66–70). The reactive process begins by antigenic recognition, uptake, processing, and presentation by antigen-presenting cells followed by the recruitment of T helper cells (T_H cells), which are activated and initiate the subsequent recruitment of the effector mononuclear B and T lymphocytes. In rare conditions in which the injury is induced by a specific antigen, the B cells differentiate into antibody-producing plasma cells, which result in the deposition of immunoglobulins and immune complexes along the TBM. In more common conditions, the effector mechanism is nonspecific and consists principally of inflammatory CD4+ and cytotoxic CD8+ lymphocytes, and depending on the injury, fewer and variable numbers of B cells, natural killer cells, and macrophages (96,97,145). In acute tubulointerstitial nephritis, feedback mechanisms restore this initial coordinated response to injury to its baseline steady state. In chronic tubulointerstitial nephritis, either persistent injury or perpetuation of the effector phase results in variable rates of progressive and permanent tubulointerstitial damage.

The deposition of fibrous tissue is the first indicator of progression. An integral component of this progressive stage is activation of interstitial fibroblasts, which undergo upregulation and increased expression of new or constitutive receptors for the fibrogenetic cytokines (TGF-β1, PDGF, TNF-α, IL-6,

PAI), released by the tubular epithelial cells and infiltrating cells (8,9,145–148). Infiltrating macrophages produce direct injury (proteases, ROS) and account for triggering of several fibrogenetic cytokines, among which TGF-β and PDGF appear to play a dominant role (151–153).

The subsequent evolution of the fibroblasts (derived from resident fibroblasts or the transdifferentiation into fibroblasts of epithelial cells, vascular pericytes, and recruited macrophages) into myofibroblasts, as they undergo phenotypic changes including acquisition of smooth muscle (actin), and mesenchymal cell markers (vimentin, desmin), parallels the increased deposition of extracellular matrix (66–70, 154–157). Fibronectin has been proposed as the first extracellular matrical protein to appear, and that its chemoattractant and adhesive properties then provide for the recruitment of fibroblasts and deposition of the other extracellular proteins (158). Experimental maneuvers that diminish early mediators of fibrosis (macrophages, fibronectin, myofibroblast phenotype) have been shown to attenuate interstitial fibrosis in different models of kidney disease (153,154). The deposited extracellular matrix consists principally of proteoglycans (decorin, biglycan) and collagen types I, III, and IV (143,145,155,156). In addition to the stimulated fibrogenesis, atrophy and collapse of injured tubules and contraction of the myofibroblasts have been proposed for the apparent disproportionate amount of fibrous tissue seen in the affected kidney (143).

Experimental evidence indicates that tubular epithelial cells can differentiate into interstitial fibroblasts, which contribute to the interstitial fibrosis (70,160). Hypoxia and TGF-β initiate their transdifferentiation (78,161). Inhibition of TGF-β pathways interrupts progressive fibrosis in experimental models of obstructive nephropathy (161) and glomerulonephritis (162) induced tubulointerstitial nephritis. Consequently, TGF-β has emerged as a potential target in limiting the progression of fibrosis and scarring. From a therapeutic standpoint, targeting epithelial to fibroblast differentiation and profibrotic pathways is a promising avenue of investigation. Bone morphogenic protein-7 (BMP-7), a factor expressed in tubular epithelial cells, has been shown in experimental models to inhibit this pathogenic transdifferentiation (163–165) and TGF-β synthesis (166).

In the affected kidney, myofibroblasts aggregate around the injured tubules and the arterioles. Microvascular obliteration (fibrosis) and constriction (myofibroblasts, vasoactive agents) induce ischemia, alter glomerular hemodynamics, and increase production of AII, which magnifies the fibrogenesis (144) and perpetuates (48) the injury. Although circulating levels of AII are not elevated, the concentration of AII within the kidney is several-fold higher than in plasma (147) and contributes to the proliferation of fibroblasts and their conversion into myofibroblasts (144,167,168), and to fibrosis by the activation of PDGF and TGF-β1 (169,170). In a rat experimental model, AII infusion has been shown to shift T-helper cell balance to a T_h1 subtype, an effect that could be blocked with angiotensin receptor blockers (144). Thus, the renoprotective effects of angiotensin-converting enzyme (ACE) inhibitors or angiotensin receptor blockers is not limited to their hemodynamic effect on glomerular intracapillary pressure, but perhaps more importantly to their demonstrated ability to favorably alter the lesions of tubulointerstitial nephritis through an immunomodulatory as well as vascular effect. Part of the effect of AII may be related to its action in stimulating aldosterone, which is an independent autacoid promulgator of the injury process (170,171). Aldosterone has been shown to increase TGF-β expression in the kidney, an effect that could be blocked with spironolactone (167,172). Whether the cardioprotective effect of low-dose spironolactone also can protect the kidney in humans, as suggested from experimental evidence (149,151,168), remains to be established.

Increased ammonia generation, due to proteinuria or the remaining intact tubules, has also been implicated as a cause of progressive injury (173,174). Ammonia possesses the capability to form amidated C3, which acts on C3/C5 convertase and activates through the alternate complement pathway the membrane attack complex C5b-9 (173–176). Administration of bicarbonate to correct the acidosis reduces tubular ammonia generation and has been shown to ameliorate the tubulointerstitial lesions in the remnant model of kidney disease.

The evidence for all of these pathogenetic mechanisms has been marshaled from experimental laboratory models of tubulointerstitial disease. Several of them have been confirmed to be operative in humans from *in situ* hybridization and histochemical studies of kidney biopsies. The implicated pathogenetic mechanisms provide a basis for the therapy of tubulointerstitial nephritis. The initial inflammatory cell infiltration is amenable to steroid therapy. Evidence also supports the role of other forms of cell-directed therapy with cyclosporine or cyclophosphamide. The renoprotective effects of ACE inhibitors and AII blockers make them a logical agent of choice in management, even in the absence of hypertension. Correction of acidosis to limit activation of the alternate complement pathway initiated injury by the membrane attack complex deserves attention. Finally, accrued evidence for determinants of extracellular matrix biosynthesis and degradation provides a basis for the identification of potentially effective agents in controlling interstitial fibrosis.

FUNCTIONAL MANIFESTATIONS OF TUBULOINTERSTITIAL NEPHROPATHIES

The principal manifestations of interstitial lesions are those of tubular dysfunction, which is one reason why the term *tubulointerstitial disease* is preferred to *tubulointerstitial nephritis*. Convincing evidence has been presented that there is a correlation between the structural changes in the tubulointerstitium and tubular function, and that the magnitude of tubular dysfunction tends to relate to the extent of tubulointerstitial involvement (12,13,26,57). Because of the focal nature of the lesions that occur and the segmental nature of normal tubular function, the pattern of tubular dysfunction that results will vary, depending on the major site of injury, whereas the extent of damage will determine the severity of tubular dysfunction. The hallmarks of glomerular disease, such as salt retention, edema, hypertension, proteinuria, and hematuria, are characteristically absent in the early phases of primary chronic tubulointerstitial nephropathies (4,10,11,177). However, in keeping with the intact nephron hypothesis, glomerular damage ultimately will appear. As a rule, the magnitude of glomerular function reduction seems to correlate with the magnitude of interstitial fibrosis, whereas the enlargement of the interstitium by cellular infiltrate appears to have less of a bearing on the GFR in the early stages of the disease (57,178–180).

Basically, the tubulointerstitial lesions are localized either to the cortex or to the medulla. Cortical lesions will affect, in the main, the proximal tubule or the distal tubule. Medullary lesions will affect the loop of Henle and the collecting duct. The change in the normal function of each of these affected segments then determines the manifestations of tubular dysfunction (Table 72-1). Essentially, the proximal nephron segment reabsorbs the bulk of bicarbonate, glucose, amino acids, phosphate, and uric acid. Changes in proximal tubular function, therefore, result in bicarbonaturia (proximal renal tubular acidosis), β_2-microglobinuria, glucosuria (renal glucosuria), aminoaciduria, magnesemia, phosphaturia, and uricosuria (48,181,182). The latter two can be valuable in suspecting

TABLE 72-1

PRINCIPAL SITES OF INJURY AND PATTERNS OF TUBULAR DYSFUNCTION IN CHRONIC TUBULOINTERSTITIAL NEPHROPATHIES

Site of injury	Cause	Tubular dysfunction
Cortex Proximal tubule	Heavy metals Multiple myeloma Immunologic diseases Cystinosis	↓ Reabsorption of: Bicarbonate Glucose Uric acid Phosphate Amino acids
Distal tubule	Immunologic diseases Granulomatous diseases Hereditary diseases Hypercalcemia Urinary tract obstruction Sickle cell hemoglobinopathy Amyloidosis	↓ Secretion of: Hydrogen ion Potassium ↓ Reabsorption of: Sodium
Medulla	Analgesic nephropathy Sickle hemoglobinopathy Uric acid disorders Hypercalcemia Infection Hereditary disorders Granulomatous diseases	Impaired ability to concentrate urine ↓ Reabsorption of: Sodium
Papilla	Analgesic nephropathy Diabetes mellitus Infection Urinary tract obstruction Sickle hemoglobinopathy Transplanted kidney	Impaired ability to concentrate urine ↓ Reabsorption of: Sodium

tubulointerstitial disease when the serum phosphate and urate concentrations are noted to be lower than expected, particularly in individuals with reduced GFR and azotemia (178). Measurements of the fractional clearance of uric acid from a spot urine sample can also be helpful. The normal fractional clearance of urate is about 10%; values significantly higher than normal would suggest a defect in urate handling by the proximal tubule. In addition, there is a linear correlation between the fractional excretion of magnesium and the extent of tubulointerstitial fibrosis, and an increase in the fractional excretion of magnesium has been proposed as the most sensitive index to detect an early abnormality of tubular structure and function (26). The clinical conditions in which this has best been characterized are patients receiving cisplatin or gentamicin (183,184). The distal nephron segment secretes hydrogen and potassium and regulates the final amount of sodium chloride excreted. Lesions affecting primarily this segment, therefore, result in the distal form of renal tubular acidosis, hyperkalemia, and salt wasting (185–188). Lesions that primarily involve the medulla and papilla disproportionately affect the loops of Henle, the collecting ducts, and the other medullary structures essential to attaining and maintaining medullary hypertonicity. Disruption of these structures, therefore, results in different degrees of nephrogenic diabetes insipidus and clinically manifests as polyuria and nocturia (189,190).

Although this general framework is useful in localizing the site of injury, considerable overlap may be encountered clinically, with different degrees of proximal, distal, and medullary dysfunction present. In addition, the ultimate development of kidney failure complicates the issue further because of the added effect of urea-induced osmotic diuresis on tubular function in the remaining nephrons. In this later stage of tubu-

lointerstitial diseases, the absence of glomerular proteinuria and the more common occurrence of hypertension in glomerular diseases can be helpful in the differential diagnosis of primary from secondary forms of tubulointerstitial nephritis (4,13,178). Under any circumstance though, the diagnosis and severity of tubulointerstitial disease can be established only by morphologic examination of kidney tissue.

The type of insult determines the segmental location of injury (Table 72-1). For example, agents secreted by the organic pathway in the pars recta (cephalosporins) or reabsorbed in the proximal tubule (aminoglycoside and light-chain proteins) cause predominantly proximal tubular lesions. Conditions or agents that cause hypersensitivity reactions (methicillin) or depositional disorders (amyloid and hypergammaglobulinemic states) cause predominantly distal tubular lesions. Finally, insulting agents that are affected by the urine concentrating mechanism (analgesics and uric acid) or medullary tonicity (sickle cell) cause medullary injury (11).

The clinical course of tubulointerstitial diseases depends to a great extent on the primary cause and the magnitude and persistence of the insult. In general, acute exposure to a massive insult results in the rapid deterioration of kidney function (191), whereas sporadic exposure to small amounts of the same insult results in a more indolent course, with a gradual but progressive loss of kidney function (192). Tubulointerstitial diseases are divided into acute or chronic forms on the basis of the clinical course and accompanying pathologic lesions (Table 72-2). The *acute* form is characterized by prominent interstitial edema and focal areas of varied cellular infiltrates. If the injury is severe, tubular damage and dilation are also present, and azotemia and renal insufficiency are early presenting features (Chapter 48). In the chronic form, interstitial fibrosis and tubular atrophy are

TABLE 72-2

TABLE 72-2

MORPHOLOGIC FEATURES OF TUBULOINTERSTITIAL NEPHRITIS

Feature	Acute	Chronic
Interstitium[a]		
Cellular infiltrate	$+ \to + + + +$	$+ \to + +$
Edema	$+ \to + + + +$	$\pm \to + +$
Fibrosis	$\pm$	$+ + \to + + + +$
Tubules		
Epithelium	Injury $\to$ necrosis	Atrophy
Basement membrane	Injury $\to$ disruption	Thickened
Shape	Preserved	Atrophy Dilation
Glomerulus		
Structure	None $\to$ MCD Sclerosis	Periglomerular fibrosis
Vascular		
Structure	Minimal Reversible	Variable Sclerosis

MCD, minimal change disease.
[a]The severity of the changes is given as an estimate with + for minimal to + + + + as severe.

TABLE 72-3

CONDITIONS ASSOCIATED WITH CHRONIC TUBULOINTERSTITIAL NEPHROPATHY

Immunologic diseases
  Systemic lupus erythematosus
  Sjögren's syndrome
  Transplanted kidney
  Cryoglobulinemia
  Goodpasture's syndrome
  IgA nephropathy
  Amyloidosis
  Pyelonephritis
Infection
  Systemic
  Renal
    Bacterial
    Viral
    Fungal
    Mycobacterial
Urinary tract obstructions
  Vesicoureteral reflux
  Mechanical
Drugs
  Analgesics
  Cyclosporine
  Nitrosourea
  Cisplatinum
  Lithium
  Miscellaneous
Hematopoietic diseases
  Sickle hemoglobinopathies
  Multiple myeloma
  Lymphoproliferative disorders
  Aplastic anemia
Heavy metals
  Lead
  Cadmium
  Miscellaneous
Vascular diseases
  Nephrosclerosis
  Atheroembolic disease
  Radiation nephritis
  Diabetes mellitus
  Sickle hemoglobinopathies
  Vasculitis
Metabolic disorders
  Hyperuricemia/hyperuricosuria
  Hypercalcemia/hypercalcuria
  Hyperoxaluria
  Potassium depletion
  Cystinosis
Hereditary diseases
  Medullary cystic disease
  Hereditary nephritis
  Medullary sponge kidney
  Polycystic kidney disease
  Familial juvenile nephronophthisis
Granulomatous diseases
  Sarcoidosis
  Tuberculosis
  Wegener's granulomatosis
Endemic diseases
  Balkan nephropathy
  Nephropathia epidemica
Idiopathic diseases

present, and the cellular infiltrate is uniformly mononuclear. In this more indolent form, loss of glomerular filtration is slow to develop and the early manifestations of the disease are those of tubular dysfunction that may go undetected unless specifically elicited in the history, noted in the laboratory results, or documented by specific testing (177). Ultimately, though, kidney failure will occur. The onset of heavy proteinuria is an ominous sign and is indicative of the development of glomerulosclerosis (91,193). In contrast to glomerular disease, hypertension is a late development and occurs after significant decrements in filtration rate have occurred (10). In a study of 48 patients with biopsy-proven tubulointerstitial nephritis, hypertension was present in only half the cases (178). In the other half, the blood pressure was normal even in the presence of kidney failure. Of the 15 patients with a creatinine clearance rate of less than 15 mL per minute, 7 had normal blood pressure.

ETIOLOGIC FACTORS

Arbitrarily grouped together because the predominant morphologic involvement is in the tubules and interstitium, primary tubulointerstitial nephropathies are caused by a motley group of diseases of varied and diverse etiologies (Table 72-3). The different initiating mechanisms that have been implicated include immunologic diseases, infection, toxic and metabolic perturbations, mechanical obstruction to urine flow, neoplasia, and hereditary factors.

Immunologic Diseases

Evidence exists for three immunologic mechanisms of tubulointerstitial injury: immune complex deposition, antibodies directed against the TBM, and altered cell-mediated immunity (194–196). Although the preponderance of the evidence in human tubulointerstitial nephropathy implicates a cell-mediated immune process, the best-studied experimental model is that of anti-TBM nephritis (197,198). However, anti-TBM antibodies are a rare cause of tubulointerstitial nephritis in humans, except in association with antiglomerular basement membrane (anti-GBM) disease (195), as is that of immune complex deposits (197,199).

Immune Complex Deposition

The repeated injection of homologous kidney tissue in Freund's adjuvant into rabbits (200) and rats (201) results in tubulointerstitial immune complex disease characterized by tubule cell injury, interstitial fibrosis, and mononuclear cell infiltration, with only minimal changes noted in the glomeruli. Immunofluorescent staining reveals granular deposits of immunoglobulins and complement along the TBM. Electron microscopy confirms the presence of focal electron-dense deposits along the tubule. The postulated mechanism for this model of tubulointerstitial disease is that the circulating antibodies, which are formed in response to the injection of homologous kidney tissue, diffuse across the peritubular capillaries and combine in the interstitium with a tubular cell antigen that diffuses out of the epithelial cells, thereby forming the peritubular interstitial immune complexes seen on microscopy. A similar lesion can be produced in rats immunized with Tamm-Horsfall protein (THP), a surface membrane glycoprotein of the epithelial cells of the ascending thick limb of the loop of Henle and distal tubules. These animals develop antibodies to THP and a tubulointerstitial nephritis that selectively involves the thick ascending limb (201–203). In this model, the earliest electron-dense deposits are detected in the extracellular space between the basal infoldings of the cell membranes and the TBM. Later, they are noted within the TBM. Selective mononuclear cell infiltrates occur around the tubules at the site of the deposits. Tubulointerstitial immune complex nephritis also has been produced by passive immunization of rats with antisera to rat THP (204). In these studies, the antibodies were noted to combine with THP at the base of the cells lining the thick ascending limb of the loop of Henle and to form granular immune complexes *in situ* in the spaces between the basal cell surface membrane and the TBMs. The deposits were maximal in the juxtamedullary region and least prominent in the first portion of the ascending limb in the inner zone of the outer medulla. Immune complexes also were selectively formed, at the same sites, during perfusion of the isolated kidneys with antisera to THP. The deposits of immune complexes were maximal during the first week after injection, at a time when the circulating antibody titers were highest. As the antibody titers subsequently fell to undetectable levels, tubular immune complexes cleared rapidly and were virtually absent by about 4 weeks after the injection of the anti-THP antibodies. This is in contrast to the prolonged persistence of glomerular immune complex deposits that occurs after the experimental injection of appropriate antiglomerular antisera and may account for the rapid reversibility of immune injury in tubulointerstitial nephritis when exposure to the antibody is limited (204). In addition, although immunoglobulin deposition in the glomeruli correlates with glomerular damage, a similar association is not found between the extent of tubulointerstitial deposits and interstitial inflammation and tubular injury (194,195,205,206).

A role for THP-mediated immune complex disease has been implicated in certain forms of human chronic kidney diseases. Antibodies to THP are found in sera of patients with vesicoureteral reflux (207) and pyelonephritis (208) and are demonstrated in the interstitium of patients with medullary cystic disease (209), hydronephrosis (210), diabetes (211), and hereditary nephritis (212), as well as in the glomeruli of patients with obstructive uropathy (213). However, immunoglobulins are not regularly associated with THP deposits noted in the interstitium of human kidneys (213). In addition, the frequent occurrence of mononuclear cell infiltrates surrounding the immune complex deposits may reflect a cell-mediated immune response that accounts for the progressive nature of the kidney injury in some of these clinical conditions (Fig. 72-1). In experimental tubulointerstitial nephritis induced in guinea pigs by immunization with homologous THP, the transfer of lymphocytes and spleen cells to unimmunized animals does induce a tubulointerstitial nephritis in the recipients (214), indicating a causative role of cell-mediated immunity. Finally, it is not possible to attribute a primary role to antibodies, to THP, or to that of any other cellular antigenic component, because the immune deposits could have followed primary tubular injury by another mechanism, with the subsequent release of THP or other cellular antigenic components into the interstitium and the secondary formation of autologous antibodies. Evidence has been advanced that the rise of intrarenal ammonia concentration, engendered by the adaptation to chronic kidney disease, could determine attendant immune complex deposits (215). Because ammonia attacks the reactive thioester bond of C3 (173), the direct reaction of ammonia with C3 forms amidated C3, which is sufficient to trigger the alternative complement pathway that activates the membrane attack complex of complement and thereby propagates the injury and peritubular deposition of C3 and C5b-9 (174–176), as well as the generation of other mediators of tubulointerstitial injury (216) (Fig. 72-1). As noted previously, in a study of rats with surgically reduced kidney mass, dietary supplementation with sodium bicarbonate resulted in lower tissue levels of ammonia, less deposition of complement components, and a diminution of tubulointerstitial damage (217). It is possible, therefore, that it is the local activation of the complement system, rather than THP protein, which contributes to immune complex deposition and the propagation of interstitial injury by an immune-mediated mechanism independent of the initial etiology of the kidney disease (218).

Primary tubulointerstitial nephritis mediated by immune complex deposition is rare in humans (195). The condition in which tubulointerstitial deposits are most commonly found clinically is lupus nephritis, in which interstitial infiltrates are detected by light microscopy in more than half of biopsy specimens (219–222). The deposits may be focal or diffuse. They are located either along or within the TBM, around the peritubular capillaries, or in the interstitium. They consist principally of immunoglobulin G (IgG) and C3 and often of IgM or IgA. Evidence for immune complex–mediated injury is adduced from the demonstration of DNA in the deposits. In general, the tubular and interstitial changes correlate with the magnitude of the deposits, although interstitial mononuclear cell infiltrates can be present in the kidneys of patients who have few, if any, tubulointerstitial immune complex deposits (220–222). Moreover, even in the presence of tubulointerstitial deposits, there is no correlation between the prevalence of immune complex deposits and the severity of interstitial reaction, indicating a more important role of a cell-mediated injury (59). Nevertheless, the severity of the interstitial changes, independent of the pathogenesis, correlates quite well with the degree of reduced kidney function in lupus nephritis (59,180,223), and appraisal of the disease activity may be possible by renal imaging with gallium-67 (224). Prominent tubulointerstitial nephritis also can occur in patients with systemic lupus erythematosus with only mild glomerular involvement, and generally pursues a rapid fulminant course (225).

Tubulointerstitial immune complex deposits have been also described in kidney allografts (226), Sjögren's syndrome (100, 227–229), mixed cryoglobulinemia (221), crescentic glomerulonephritis (220), IgA nephropathy (52), Wegener's granulomatosis (230), and idiopathic tubulointerstitial nephropathy (231). In addition, the sera from some patients with idiopathic tubular dysfunction contain antibodies that react with distal tubular epithelium (232–234). However, aside from systemic lupus erythematosus, in which antigen (DNA) has been demonstrated in the deposits, and mixed cryoglobulinemia, in which anti-IgG antibodies and IgG have been identified, there is no evidence to support a specific antigen responsible for the immune complex deposits. Therefore, direct proof of immune complex–mediated injury is lacking in most of the rare clinical instances in which immune complex deposits are noted on examination of the kidney tissue.

Antibodies Against Tubular Basement Membrane

Evidence for anti-TBM antibody disease was first obtained when guinea pigs were noted to develop a progressive, fatal tubulointerstitial kidney disease after they were injected with crude rabbit cortical tissue in Freund's adjuvant (235). Morphologic examination of the kidneys from these animals revealed tubular cell injury, peritubular multinucleated giant cells, interstitial fibrosis, and mononuclear cell infiltration. The infiltrating cells consisted of monocytes, macrophages, and T lymphocytes. Linear deposits of IgG were noted along the TBM on immunofluorescent study (235,236). Similar lesions were produced in guinea pigs immunized with bovine TBM (237) and in the Brown Norway strain of rats, but not Sprague-Dawley or Lewis rats immunized with homologous or heterologous TBM (197,238). In both species, the lesion could be reproduced in normal recipients by injecting them with serum from the immunized animals (168,170). Independent of the initiating role of anti-TBM antibodies, cell infiltrates are a prominent feature in all models studied, implicating a role for cell-mediated immunity in the pathogenesis and modulation of the interstitial lesions (197–199). Although the disease cannot be transmitted by cells in all species, it can be transferred by intravenous injection of lymph node and splenic cells from sensitized animals in other species (197,198), suggesting again the central role of cell-mediated immunity.

Evidence for anti-TBM antibodies causing tubulointerstitial disease in humans has been advanced from patients with Goodpasture's syndrome associated with anti-GBM antibodies (220) and patients with rapidly progressive glomerulonephritis who have associated anti-TBM antibodies (20,230). In both forms, absorption of eluates with solubilized GBM removed the anti-TBM activity (196). A target antigen in human anti-TBM disease has been identified as a 58-kDa glycoprotein (239–241), which in experimental models synthesizes as a high-molecular-weight glycoprotein that is processed to smaller forms that are secreted by proximal tubular cells into the extracellular matrix, where it attaches to the TBM (199,242). This noncollagenous glycoprotein constitutes about 9% of the TBM and accounts for 90% of the tubulointerstitial antigen to which anti-TBM antibodies are directed. Its overall composition is similar to that of laminin and nidogen (243,244). Target antigens or tubulointerstitial nephritis antigens (TIN-Ag) identified in human anti-TBM disease have been termed TIN1 and TIN2 and shown to promote cell adhesion and to interact with type IV collagen (245). Anti-TBM antibodies also have been demonstrated in some cases of glomerulonephritis without associated anti-GBM antibodies (246–249), such as kidney allografts (215,226,250), and lupus nephritis (251,252), and detected in the serum of patients with biopsy proven tubulointerstitial nephritis (253). The role of these implicated antigens in the pathophysiology of chronic tubulointerstitial nephritis remains to be elucidated.

Cell-Mediated Immunity

Although the presence of anti-TBM antibodies or immune complex deposits is a variable feature of tubulointerstitial disease, interstitial cell infiltration is an almost invariable essential component of the lesion. Most of the mononuclear cells making up the renal interstitium are T cells and are generally characterized by markers of activated lymphocytes (62,86,98). Hence, the role of cell-mediated immunologic mechanisms involved in tubulointerstitial diseases can be considered on a reasonably sound basis (199,254). Because both immune complex–mediated and anti-TBM nephritis can be transferred by lymph node and spleen cells, a cell-mediated response appears to be an essential component of the immunopathology of all tubulointerstitial nephropathies (197,199). It is evident then that even in antibody-dependent forms of the disease, recruited interstitial cells play a major role in anti-TBM and immune complex–mediated interstitial lesions. Some rats injected with homologous kidney tissue develop interstitial mononuclear cell infiltrates before there is evidence of autoantibody production (194,195). This was also noted in the early studies of nonimmunosuppressed canine experimental kidney transplants (3). In a study of guinea pigs sensitized to bovine γ-globulin, the direct injection of the heterologous globulin into the renal cortex resulted in a mononuclear interstitial infiltrate with focal tubular destruction (255). This reactivity could then be transferred to unsensitized animals with lymph node cells, but not with serum, providing direct evidence for cell-mediated tubulointerstitial injury in this experimental model.

The tubular epithelial cells appear to contribute to the recruitment of the mononuclear cells (65,110,256). Cytokines and TNFs released by the activated infiltrating cells and injured tubular epithelial cells have been implicated in the pathogenesis and progression of tubulointerstitial lesions (7,8,16,257–259). Moreover, the epithelial cells of the proximal tubule are one of the few epithelial cells in the body shown to constitutively express the class II MHC molecules required to present antigens to CD4+ T cells (6) and likely are central to the initiation and perpetuation of the sequence of events that results in chronic tubulointerstitial nephropathies (Figs. 72-1, 72-7).

Infection

Many organisms have been associated with acute tubulointerstitial nephritis, either due to their direct invasion of the kidney or due to a reactive response of the kidney to a systemic infection (Chapters 34 and 48). By contrast, the bulk of the available evidence implicates direct bacterial infection of the kidney, rather than a reactive response to systemic infections, as a cause of chronic tubulointerstitial disease.

Cellular reactivity to bacterial antigens has been implicated in the pathogenesis of interstitial lesions of pyelonephritis (260). By using an indirect fluorescent method for the detection of a common enterobacterial antigen in infected tissues, it was shown that bacterial antigen persisted in renal scars after the healing of experimental pyelonephritis (261,262). In one clinical study, bacterial antigen was found in six of seven kidneys of patients with "abacterial" pyelonephritis who had not had clinical or bacteriologic evidence of infection for as long as 19 years before the study (263). This finding, however, could not be substantiated in other studies in which the antigen could be demonstrated in kidneys from patients with acute pyelonephritis caused by enteric organisms, but not from those with chronic interstitial nephritis or nonspecific renal scars or patients with pyelonephritis who were bacteriologically free of infecting organisms (260). Experimental studies have revealed that rats with acute enteric streptococcal pyelonephritis develop cellular reactivity to bacteria, as indicated by lymphocyte stimulation *in vitro*. In these animals, bacterial antigens can be shown by immunofluorescent studies within both the infiltrating leukocytes and the interstitium. However, after eradication of the infection, bacterial antigens were not demonstrable in the interstitium, and, when present, were found only within macrophages (260–262). It would seem unlikely, therefore, that delayed reactivity against bacterial antigens could provide a mechanism for the perpetuation of the tubulointerstitial lesions of pyelonephritis beyond the period when viable organisms are present in the kidney (260–264).

Whereas the role of bacterial infection as the major determinant for the development of acute pyelonephritis is unequivocal, the role of recurrent infection as a cause of kidney damage remains doubtful. Progression from acute infection to chronic "atrophic" pyelonephritis does not appear to be a result of persistent or recurrent infection itself but may be due to chronic tubular cell injury (Figs. 72-1, 72-7), with consequent altered cellular immune mechanisms (151), and usually will develop in those with a coexistent mechanical outflow obstruction (207,264–266), thereby implicating an added role for obstruction. Several studies of many women and men with significant bacteriuria, who were followed over a decade, showed that urinary tract infection does not lead to kidney damage, provided the condition is not associated with obstruction and there are no coexistent diseases, such as diabetes and hypertension (267,268). In children, however, bacteriuria does not necessarily pursue the same relatively benign course as that seen in adults (269,270). Chronic atrophic pyelonephritis, with classic tubulointerstitial lesions, is a disease of childhood that manifests itself clinically in adult life (269). Children younger than 5 to 6 years in whom urinary tract infection coexists with vesicoureteral reflux and in whom pyelotubular backflow develops appear to be the individuals who are at increased risk of developing interstitial scarring, and, ultimately, tubular atrophy. Reflux or obstruction without complicating infection can initiate the injury to the tubules and interstitium (207,264). However, it is mainly children in whom infection and vesicoureteral reflux coexist and persist despite treatment who develop renal scars and tubulointerstitial disease (270). One study (271) with a 2-year follow-up revealed the formation of new scars in 3 of 34 children whose infection was untreated, as compared with only 1 of 26 children whose bacteriuria was treated. Therefore, the role of infection is not to be discounted. Whether urinary tract infection uncomplicated by obstruction causes sufficient interstitial injury to result in irreversible changes and progressive kidney disease is questionable (269,272–278). However, obstruction or vesicoureteral reflux can produce renal injury by causing either recurrent infection, by backpressure damage in the absence of infection, or both (207). Moreover, pyelonephritogenic strains of *Escherichia coli* that are more cytotoxic to the renal tubular epithelium because of stronger bacterial attachment and hemolysin delivery have been identified and characterized (90,279,280), as has a dysfunctional neutrophil response in pyelonephritis-prone cases (281).

Experimentally, the unmanipulated urinary tract is remarkably resistant to retrograde challenge with an infectious inoculum, whereas direct intrarenal injection of organisms causes bacterial proliferation and elicits a local cellular reaction (273). The initial inflammatory response to infection of the renal parenchyma is that of a classic acute tubulointerstitial nephritis characterized by edema, cellular infiltration, and tubular damage. To determine whether this initial response results in progressive immune-mediated injury after sterilization of the urinary tract, efforts were made to characterize the local response and the immunologic activity to the lymphoid cells isolated from the experimentally infected kidney (274–276). Within the first few days after infection, polymorphonuclear leukocytes predominate in the interstitium and tubular lumen, and the renal epithelial cells express class II MHC antigens (277) and the TNF-α gene (278), indicating their ability to act as antigen-presenting cells and to initiate the inflammatory sequence of events implicated in the pathogenesis of tubulointerstitial nephritis, such as increased excretion of TGF-β1 (282) and IL-6 and IL-8 (283). The local release of chemoattractants to recruit polymorphonuclear cells has been demonstrated to

contribute to the tubular damage that results (284), as has that of free radical mediated tissue injury by the recruited leukocytes (285). Within the subsequent days, the neutrophilic infiltrate dissipates while a dense mononuclear lymphocytic infiltrate develops, indicating an active cellular response evident by the presence of B-lymphocytes and a depression of helper T-lymphocyte activity, whereas suppressor T-cell activity is increased (275). There is also evidence for the local activation and deposition of the complement system (286) and for an increased local production of IgG, IgM, and IgA by the infected kidney (287,288). During an acute infection, an increase in the level of circulating antibodies to THP has been reported (208,289). The level of antibodies decreases once the active infection is eradicated, and clearance studies showed the rapid clearance of antibodies from local deposits (204). Whether these antibodies or the local cellular infiltrates play a role in the perpetuation of chronic kidney injury and scarring is a possibility that has been proposed by some (263) but questioned by others (260). The potential for ammonia production by urease-producing organisms has been implicated in the propensity of these organisms to produce renal injury (173,218).

Preexisting kidney disease or an immunocompromised host seems to predispose to the detrimental effect of infection (290,291). The latter is best exemplified by the unusual infections causing interstitial injury encountered in kidney allografts (291,292), the kidneys of patients with acquired immunodeficiency syndrome (AIDS) (293), and following bone marrow transplantation (294). Of the various infections that have been implicated to cause tubulointerstitial lesions in the transplanted kidney the incidence of that due to polyomavirus infection appears to have increased after the introduction of mycophenolate mofetil–based antirejection therapy (295–298), and to subside after a decrease in the dose of mycophenalate based immunosuppression or after switching to cyclosporine-based antirejection therapy (295,297). Actually, recipients of kidney allograft and patients with AIDS are prone to tubulointerstitial nephritis even in the absence of superimposed infection (299–302).

Obstruction and Reflux

Interstitial changes are a prominent feature of the kidneys in urinary tract obstruction of any etiology. The initial structural changes that follow are those of tubular dilation and cortical infiltration with lymphocytes. Later, a network of fibrosis develops, extending from the capsule through the medulla of the affected pyramids. Fibrosis gradually increases and causes contraction and scarring (264). Proliferation of interstitial cells also occurs after ureteral obstruction (109,146,303). Many quantifiable pathophysiologic events occur during the first week of unilateral ureteral obstruction, which make this an important model for the study of the mechanisms of tubulointerstitial nephritis (304,305). The whole process can occur in the absence of infection. If infection is deliberately induced, or develops spontaneously, a polymorphonuclear reaction occurs and tubular casts are noted. More importantly, in the coexistence of infection, the fibrosis is more extensive.

In vesicoureteral reflux, kidney damage depends on the degree of incompetence of the ureterovesical valve, the magnitude of pressure that develops, and the length of time that the vesicoureteral reflux persists before correction. In persons with neurogenic bladder disorders, in which a high-pressure condition develops, vesicoureteral reflux occurs as a secondary event. In one study, more than 90% of children and 50% of adults with pyelonephritic scars had vesicoureteral reflux demonstrated on voiding cystourethrograms. In 89% of adults with scars, cystoscopic examination revealed abnormal ureteral orifices, suggesting ureteral reflux (306).

The importance of reflux of infected urine in the causation of tubulointerstitial lesions and atrophic kidney is now well established (264,309). Reflux, present in about 1% of newborns, is due to a number of congenital abnormalities such as defects at the vesicoureteral junction or impaired peristalsis of the urinary outflow tract (307,308). The role of sterile urine reflux, in doing so, although supported by experimental studies in pigs, remains to be documented in humans. A role for extravasation of a potentially powerful autoantigen, THP, in causing immune-mediated injury in the absence of infection has been postulated to occur in patients with vesicoureteral reflux, urine outflow obstruction, or inadequately draining transplanted kidneys (264). However, a number of studies have failed to confirm an immediate relationship between THP deposition and subsequent inflammatory response (309).

A proinflammatory potential of THP has been proposed on the basis of its demonstrated ability to bind neutrophils *in vitro* (310). Experimental support has been advanced for the notion that THP contributes to the pathogenesis of tubulointerstitial nephritis when it is increased in the interstitium after cell injury, where it initiates an autoantibody reaction and contributes to the infiltration of polymorphonuclear leukocytes (311). The oxidative burst of the now-activated adherent leukocytes then releases proteases and ROS, which contribute to the further loss of epithelial cell integrity. The tubular rupture responsible for extravasation of THP is related to the increased pressure in the tubules when the intrapelvic pressure rises in the presence of urine flow obstruction (312). Studies in 23 human neonatal kidneys obtained at autopsy showed that the range of pressure needed to cause pyelotubular backflow, with extravasation into the interstitial tissue, was 22 to 87 mm Hg, with a mean of 47 mm Hg (313). Pyelovenous reflux occurs in about 50% of cases when intrapelvic pressures of 50 to 70 mm Hg are induced experimentally and in 100% when pressures of more than 70 mm Hg are attained (313). In humans, intrapelvic pressures of more than 70 mm Hg are attained in patients with hydronephrosis in whom focal pyelotubular backflow can be demonstrated radiologically (314). Vesicoureteral reflux of a minor degree probably causes no kidney injury, but vesicoureteral reflux in a high-pressure situation or in the presence of infection does appear to be associated with tubulointerstitial injury. Thus, whereas renal scarring as a result of intrarenal reflux does occur, secondary to urinary outflow obstruction of any cause, no comprehensive uniform explanation has been advanced for the renal scarring and atrophy that develop in some but not in others.

Most of the experimental work attempting to explore the pathogenesis of scarring due to reflux has been done on rats, in which the unilobular pelvic anatomy is different from that of human kidney, which is multilobular and has 8 to 12 calices (313,315). The pig kidney used in some studies is multilobular and therefore is considered more analogous to human anatomy (207). About 75% of human kidneys have compound papillae, which fuse to drain several papillae generally in a polar location. The ducts of Bellini in some of the composite renal papillae have wide-open orifices, as opposed to the narrow slit-like orifices of the simple single papilla (316). Consequently, if the pressure of the refluxing urine is sufficient to overcome the pressure within the nephrons of the composite renal papillae, intrarenal reflux can occur (317,318). This accounts for the experimental and clinical observations that reflux can be demonstrated in only some segments of the kidney and that these are usually at a polar location. However, if the tubular flow is high and there is a large diuresis, injury from intrarenal reflux may be prevented (319).

Inflammatory pathways also play a role in the tubulointerstitial injury of urinary tract obstruction. Of interest are the changes of parenchymal cell infiltration that accompany increased intrapelvic pressure. Mononuclear cell infiltration is one of the earliest responses of the kidney to ureteral obstruction. Fairly early following acute urinary tract obstruction, cortical tubule epithelial cells express MCP-1 and RANTES, providing an impetus for the recruitment and accumulation of inflammatory cells (304,320). The infiltrating cells are macrophages and suppressor and cytotoxic lymphocytes (321,322). In experimental models of urinary tract obstruction, an increased expression of MCP-1 and RANTES is observed simultaneously with leukocyte and macrophage infiltration, with the subsequent onset of fibrosis (305). The release of various proinflammatory and vasoactive cytokines, by the infiltrating cells of the hydronephrotic kidney, appears to exert a significant modulating role in the tubulointerstitial injury and hemodynamic changes seen early in the course of obstruction (321–328). With persistent obstruction, changes of chronic tubulointerstitial nephritis occur within weeks (329), and gradually fibrosis becomes prominent (304,330,331). Cultures of the fibroblastic type of cortical interstitial cells from explants of unilateral hydronephrotic rabbit kidneys, compared with those from the contralateral normal kidney, grow significantly faster and have increased prostaglandin E_2 production in response to bradykinin (332).

Also of note in reflux nephropathy are the glomerular changes that develop in the later phases of the disease in some patients. As a rule, the glomerular changes commonly encountered are ischemic in nature, consisting of sclerosis, periglomerular fibrosis, and obsolescence, and are associated with modest proteinuria. In a few, focal and segmental glomerulosclerosis and hyalinosis develop and are manifested clinically by massive proteinuria and rapidly progressive kidney failure. The affected glomeruli commonly contain IgM and C3 as shown by immunofluorescent microscopy, suggesting an immunologic mechanism (193,333–335). The nature of the immune reaction remains unclear. Autologous (THP, brush-border antigen) or bacterial antigen derivatives have been implicated, as have hemodynamic changes that develop in the glomeruli of remaining intact nephrons of the hydronephrotic kidney, adapting to a reduction in renal mass by hyperfiltration (333).

Drugs

Drugs that are the major cause of acute tubulointerstitial disease also produce the chronic forms of tubulointerstitial nephropathy. Patients who develop the acute form of drug-induced tubulointerstitial nephritis generally recover fully. A few, however, do not recover and progress to chronic tubulointerstitial disease, as best exemplified by cisplatin (336,337). Based on a retrospective review of kidney biopsies, it has been estimated that about a third of patients with acute tubulointerstitial nephritis develop either only partially reversible or irreversible loss of kidney function (338). Most patients who develop drug-induced chronic tubulointerstitial nephritis do so insidiously, during or after the chronic use of one or more drugs. The latter (in which exposure to a mixture of more than one agent accounts for the kidney lesions) is best exemplified by analgesic abuse nephropathy (339,340), whereas cases of chronic tubulointerstitial nephritis due to chronic use of a single drug are exemplified by prolonged exposure to cyclosporine (340,341), cisplatin (342), nitrosourea (343), herbal medications (344–347), lithium (348,349), methotrexate (350), mesalazine (351,352), 5-aminosalicylic acid (353), and nonsteroidal antiinflammatory drugs (354–356). The risk of chronic tubulointerstitial nephropathy with these therapeutic agents is quite small and often preventable, and the risk–benefit ratio associated with these agents is much too small to limit their beneficial clinical use (356). Conversely, cases occurring due to herbal medicines, which are of questionable therapeutic merit, deserve closer scrutiny (357). First reported in 1993 from Belgium, as a unique rapidly progressive, hypocellular, fibrosing interstitial nephritis in young women using a slimming regimen of Chinese herbs (356), the entity is now recognized with increasing frequency worldwide and in association with various herbal medicines (356–362). The lesions have been attributed to the content of phytotoxins—specifically aristolochic acid—which are not only nephrotoxic but also carcinogenic, in that nearly half of the patients with nephropathy have been subsequently diagnosed with transitional cell carcinomas of the urinary tract (346,358,361,362). However, aristolochic acid was not present in all herbal preparations associated with tubulointerstitial nephritis (344,346). Especially alarming is the rapid progression to end-stage kidney failure despite the discontinuation of herbal medications (363,364). The exact mechanism of aristolochic acid nephropathy is unknown. However, specific DNA adducts have been detected in the kidney of patients with aristolochic acid nephropathy that are not seen in other forms of chronic tubulointerstitial nephropathy (346). Aristolochic acid has been shown to inhibit filtered albumin reuptake by proximal tubule epithelial cells, even after cessation of its ingestion (359). Considered together with the fact that the nephropathy progresses even after cessation of aristolochic acid exposure and that uroepithelial tumors are common in these patients, it is reasonable to assume that DNA injury and mutagenesis may be an important cause of aristolochic acid nephropathy. Interestingly, the interstitial fibrosis due to aristolochic acid is not inhibited by ACE inhibition or angiotensin blockade, suggesting an injury pathway independent of the renin–angiotensin system (360).

Progressive loss of kidney function associated with a characteristic tubulointerstitial nephritis with cystic tubular dilatation and global glomerulosclerosis has been described in patients receiving chronic lithium therapy for bipolar disorders (349,365,366) and demonstrated experimentally (367). Initially, this was considered controversial because the kidney biopsies were performed in individuals whose kidney function was reduced, and similar lesions were described in psychiatric patients with reduced kidney function who had not been treated with lithium (368,369). However, confirmatory reports of loss of kidney function (365) that progresses to kidney failure and is dialysis-dependent (366,370–372) leave little doubt that lithium is nephrotoxic, particularly in those with recurrent lithium intoxication (365). The prevalence of the interstitial lesions, however, remains to be determined. Of special interest in these cases are the characteristic cystic dilations, which have been shown to be localized to the distal and collecting tubules (370). This is particularly relevant because of the commonly encountered nephrogenic diabetes insipidus that affects as many as 20% to 70% of lithium-treated patients (369), and the experimentally demonstrated lithium-induced downregulation of the vasopressin-regulated water aquaporin-2 water-channel expression in the apical plasma cells of the collecting tubules (373,374). Whereas the progression of kidney disease is dependent on the duration of therapy and cumulative dose exposure (372), the prevalence of interstitial lesions during lithium therapy remains to be determined.

The lesions of analgesic abuse deserve special consideration. To a great extent, it is the appreciation of their role in the causation of chronic interstitial nephritis that had the greatest impact in questioning the wisdom of attributing all chronic tubulointerstitial lesions to pyelonephritis. In the initial reports from Switzerland, the lesion was described as chronic interstitial nephritis (chronische interstitielle nephritis), with a high incidence of papillary necrosis (375,376). Subsequent reports established papillary necrosis as a prominent lesion of analgesic-associated nephropathy (AAN) and documented the significance and occurrence of this problem worldwide (377–

382). From the outset, it was evident that there was considerable variation in the incidence of AAN in different parts of the world (from Australia to New Zealand to Scandinavia to England to Canada to the United States), with wide regional differences within each country (18,339,383–389).

Because of the over use of analgesic compounds, a common ingredient of which was phenacetin, the lesions of AAN were initially attributed to phenacetin (379–390). Subsequent clinical studies, however, questioned the role of any single agent as the cause of kidney disease (391), and despite the withdrawal of phenacetin, AAN remained one of the main causes of end-stage renal disease in Australia, Switzerland, Belgium, and Germany (384–386). The preponderance of experimental studies indicates that phenacetin, paracetamol, and aspirin given alone are only moderately nephrotoxic, even in massive doses. Renal lesions can be much more readily induced when a mixture of aspirin and paracetamol or phenacetin is used, particularly when they are combined with water deprivation (339,392). In all experimental studies, the extent of renal injury was dose-dependent, and when examined, water diuresis protected from analgesic-induced renal injury (339,393). Actually, phenacetin itself is not toxic; it is rapidly metabolized by the liver to paracetamol (N-acetyl-p-aminophenol), which is then excreted by the kidneys either as the free compound or as its conjugate. The bulk of the latter consists of the glucuronide and a smaller portion of the sulfate. Both paracetamol and its conjugates attain significant (fourfold to fivefold) concentrations in the medulla and papilla, depending on the state of hydration of the experiment animals studied. The toxic effect of these substances is apparently related to their intrarenal oxidation to reactive intermediates, which in the absence of reducing substances such as glutathione become cytotoxic by virtue of their capacity to induce oxidation (38,393,394) and induce tubular cell apoptosis (395). Salicylates are also significantly (6-fold to 13-fold) concentrated in the medulla and papilla, where they attain a sufficient level to uncouple oxidative phosphorylation and reduce the ability of cells to generate reducing substances (393–395). Thus, both agents attain sufficient medullary concentration in the kidney to individually exert a detrimental and injurious effect on cell function. Their simultaneous presence results in an additive effect because of the salicylate-induced decrease in reducing capability at a time when the concentrations of the reactive oxidative byproducts of phenacetin are increased locally. Considered in this context, it is evident why water diuresis, by reducing the medullary tonicity and therefore the medullary concentration of drug attained, protects from analgesic-induced cell injury (339,393,396). A direct role of analgesic-induced injury can be adduced from the arrest of the progressive loss and generally improvement of kidney function that are noted after cessation of analgesic abuse (397,398). That it is the use of analgesics in combination that accounts for kidney injury is evidenced from the decrease in AAN as a cause of end-stage kidney failure in Australia and European countries since legal restrictions were imposed on the sale of over-the-counter analgesic mixtures (356,399), and the epidemiologic demonstration of a direct relationship of the prevalence of AAN to the proportion of analgesic mixtures available for sale over the counter (400).

The intrarenal distribution of analgesics provides an explanation for the medullary location of the pathologic lesions of analgesic abuse (Fig. 72-8). The initial lesions are patchy and consist of necrosis of the interstitial cells, thin limbs of the loops of Henle, and vasa rectae of the papilla. The collecting ducts are spared. The quantities of tubular and vascular basement membrane and interstitial ground substance are increased. At this stage, the kidneys are normal in size and there are no abnormalities in the renal cortex. With persistent drug exposure, the changes extend to the outer medulla. Again, the lesions are initially patchy, involving the interstitial cells, the loops of

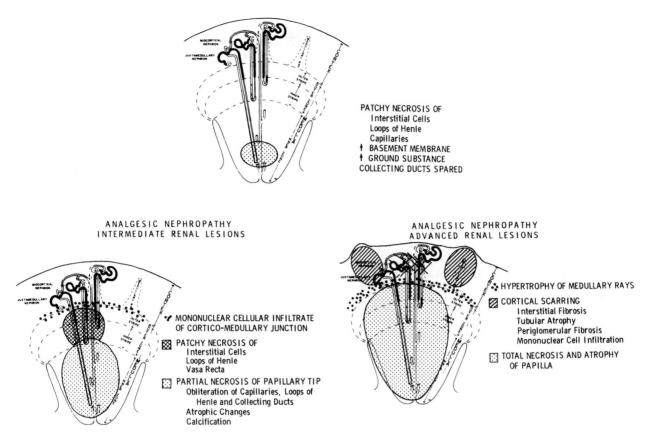

FIGURE 72-8. The course and stages of analgesic nephropathy. (From: Eknoyan G. Analgesic nephrotoxicity and renal papillary necrosis. *Semin Nephrol* 1984;4:65, with permission.)

Henle, and vascular bundles. With continued drug abuse, the severity of the inner medullary lesions increases with sclerosis and obliteration of the capillaries, atrophy and degeneration of the loops of Henle and collecting ducts, and the beginning of calcification of the necrotic foci. Ultimately, the papillae become entirely necrotic, with sequestration and demarcation of the necrotic tissue. The necrotic papillae may then slough and are excreted into the urine or remain *in situ,* where they atrophy further and become calcified. Cortical scarring, characterized by interstitial fibrosis, tubular atrophy, and periglomerular fibrosis, develops over the necrotic medullary segments. The medullary rays traversing the cortex are usually spared and become hypertrophic, thereby imparting a characteristic cortical nodularity to the now shrunken kidneys. The visualization of these configurational changes can be extremely useful in the diagnosis of AAN. A comparison of 60 analgesic abusers with 188 control subjects, using renal ultrasound and computed tomography, showed that a decrease in kidney size combined with bumpy contours of both kidneys provided a diagnostic sensitivity of 90% and a specificity of 95%. The additional finding of evidence of renal papillary necrosis resulted in an overall sensitivity of 72% and specificity of 97%, giving a positive predictive value of 92% (400). Examination of kidney tissue at this late stage of AAN reveals the classic features of cortical tubulointerstitial nephropathy (377,391,401–403).

As might be expected from the slow progressive nature of the lesion, the deterioration of kidney function is insidious. Kidney injury can be detected by appropriate testing for sterile pyuria, reduced concentrating ability, and a distal acidifying

defect. These may be evident at levels of mild functional insufficiency and become more pronounced and prevalent as kidney function deteriorates. Proximal tubular function is preserved in those with mild loss of function but can be abnormal with more advanced kidney disease (356). In all cases, there is a relationship between kidney function and the duration, intensity, and quantity of analgesic consumed (404,405). The magnitude of injury is related to the quantity of analgesic ingested chronically over the years. In persons with significant impairment of kidney function, the average dose ingested has been estimated at about 10 kg over a mean period of 13 years (406). The minimum amount of drug consumption that results in significant kidney damage is unknown. It has been estimated that a cumulative dose of 3 kg of the index compound, or a daily ingestion of 1 g per day over 3 years or more, is a minimum that can result in detectable renal impairment (18). Only a minority of persons who regularly take analgesic mixtures develop kidney injury (405). There is also considerable variation in the severity of the renal lesions in those who do develop kidney injury. One reason for this variable response may be adduced from the experimental evidence for the medullary concentration of analgesics and the prevention of renal injury by hydration (393).

It is possible that those who develop analgesic nephropathy ingest lower quantities of fluid or are subjected to dehydration due to environmental conditions. This issue has not been investigated clinically, although a role for dehydration due to the climatic conditions has been proposed as one reason for the geographic variability in the incidence of analgesic nephropathy (339). Other factors that might contribute to dehydration, such as laxative and diuretic use, have also been implicated (407,408). Differences in the content of the mixtures also could account for the geographic variation in the incidence of AAN (407,409). Finally, coexistent diseases, such as diabetes, sickle cell disease, and infection, which themselves cause tubulointerstitial nephritis, may predispose analgesic abusers to more severe kidney injury (339). An association between the ingestion of analgesic drugs and end-stage renal disease has been proposed on the basis of population-based case-control studies (385,386,410). The noted risk was greatest in heavy users of acetaminophen and nonsteroidal antiinflammatory drugs. An associated risk has also been reported with use of aspirin and salicylates (411,412). The validity of these epidemiologic observations remains to be established from prospective studies.

Consumption of phenacetin-containing analgesics has been associated with a significant increase (10% of abusers) of urothelial tumors of the renal pelvis, ureters, and bladder (37,413). The tumors occur after a latent period of decades, are typically multiple, are poorly differentiated, and spread rapidly. Epidemiologic and retrospective case-control studies of the role of paracetamol association with urothelial tumors have yielded negative results (414,415). However, paracetamol may not be free of all such side effects (413). A recent population-based case-control study showed that the risk of renal pelvic cancer was increased by phenacetin-aspirin mixtures to a greater extent than by paracetamol alone (relative risk, 12.2 versus 1.3), but the risk of renal cell carcinoma appeared to be increased to a similar degree by phenacetin-aspirin mixtures (relative risk, 1.4) and paracetamol (relative risk, 1.5) taken in any form (416). The presence of renal papillary necrosis in phenacetin abusers significantly increased the relative risk for urothelial cancer (417).

Tubulointerstitial nephritis has emerged as the most serious side effect of *cyclosporine* (418). Cyclosporine-mediated vasoconstriction of the cortical microvasculature has been implicated in the development of an occlusive arteriolopathy and tubular epithelial cell injury (419–422). Although these early lesions tend to be reversible with cessation of therapy, an irreversible interstitial fibrosis and cellular infiltrate develop with prolonged use of the drug, especially with higher doses (340,341,421–425). Cyclosporine increases the expression of renal TGF-β, which likely promotes interstitial fibrosis (426–428). The fibrosis has been shown to be inhibited by ACE inhibition (428) and by blocking the TGF-β pathway (427). The irreversible nature of this tubulointerstitial nephritis and its attendant loss of kidney function have raised serious concerns regarding the long-term use of this otherwise-efficient immunosuppressive agent (429,430), the use of which has been proposed in the treatment of tubulointerstitial nephritis (199). Chronic tubulointerstitial nephritis also occurs with tacrolimus, although kidney function is reported to be better preserved than with cyclosporine (431–433). Both agents exert a stimulatory effect on endothelin-1 (ET-1) synthesis and secretion in the kidney (434). The vasoconstrictor effect of ET-1 may account for the ischemic effect of these agents in initiating kidney injury.

Hematopoietic Disorders

The renal lesion that develops in disorders of the hematopoietic system is generally that of a tubulointerstitial nephropathy. This is by far most common in persons with a sickle cell hemoglobinopathy. Although more frequent in those with sickle cell disease, tubulointerstitial lesions also are common in those with sickle cell trait, sickle cell hemoglobin C disease, or sickle cell thalassemia (435,436). The predisposing factors that lead to the propensity of kidney involvement are the physicochemical properties of hemoglobin S that predispose its poly-

merization in an environment of low oxygen tension, hypertonicity, and low pH level (437). These conditions are characteristic to the renal medulla and therefore are conducive to the intraerythrocytic polymerization of hemoglobin S and consequent erythrocyte sickling that accounts for the development of typical vascular occlusive lesions (438–442). Although some of these lesions occur in the cortex, the lesions start and are predominantly located in the inner medulla, where they are at the core of the focal scarring and interstitial fibrosis (436,443,444), and account for the common occurrence of papillary necrosis in these persons (339). The incidence of radiographically demonstrable papillary necrosis is from 33% to 65% (436), and of increased renal echogenecity on ultrasonography is 17.6% (437). Tubular function abnormalities such as impaired concentrating ability, depressed distal potassium and hydrogen secretion, tubular proteinuria, and decreased proximal reabsorption of phosphate and increased secretion of creatinine are common and detectable early in the course of the disease (445,446).

Disorders of plasma cell function also produce tubulointerstitial disease. Actually, the pathogenesis of kidney involvement is of varied etiologies (186), and the renal complications of multiple myeloma are a major contributing factor in the morbidity and mortality of this neoplastic disorder (447–449). As might be expected, it has been shown that in those who present with kidney failure, ultimate survival depends to a great extent on the hematologic response to chemotherapy and much less on the coexistent kidney failure that is amenable to dialytic therapy (450,451). Kidney involvement depends on the tumor burden. Less than 5% of myeloma cases with a low tumorous mass have kidney involvement, whereas more than 40% of those with a high tumor mass will have reduced kidney function (452). The lesions that are directly the result of excessive production of light chains are those caused by the precipitation of the light-chain dimers in the distal tubules and result in what has been termed *myeloma cast nephropathy*. The affected tubules are surrounded by chronic inflammatory cells, interstitial fibrosis, and multinucleated giant cells (134,135,447). Adjoining tubules show varying degrees of atrophy. The propensity of light chains to lead to myeloma cast nephropathy appears to be related to their concentration in the tubular fluid, the tubular fluid pH level, and their structural configuration, rather than their intrinsic physicochemical properties, as was initially postulated (452–456). This accounts for the observation that increasing the flow rate of urine or its alkalinization will prevent or reverse the casts in their early stages of formation. Direct tubular toxicity of light chains also may contribute to the tubular injury (134). λ Light chains appear to be slightly more injurious than κ light chains (453,457), whereas the larger and heavier IgG myeloma protein is least likely to to be injurious (458). In fact, light-chain proteinuria is a highly significant risk factor for the kidney dysfunction, especially when it is more than 2 g per day (457,459). Binding of human κ and λ light chains to human and rat proximal tubule epithelial cell brush-border membrane has been demonstrated (460). Analysis of the binding data reveals a single class of low-affinity, high-capacity binding sites that are specific to light chains. Epithelial cell injury associated with their absorption has been implicated in the pathogenesis of tubulointerstitial nephritis (Fig. 72-1). Another mechanism whereby plasma cell dyscrasias cause tubulointerstitial lesions is related to the interstitial and perivascular deposition of paraproteins, either as amyloid fibrils that are derived from λ chains or as fragments of light chains that are derived from κ chains, and produce the so-called light-chain deposition disease (134,461). Of these various lesions, myeloma cast nephropathy appears to be the most common, being observed in one-third of the autopsied cases, followed by amyloid deposition, present in 10% of cases, whereas intramembranous light-chain deposition is relatively rare and present in less than 5% of cases (449,462,463).

The kidney is one of the most common extranodal sites of metastatic lymphomas (464), and it is not uncommon to diagnose occult lymphomas by kidney biopsy that clinically mimic chronic kidney disease (465). Infiltration of the kidney is frequent in patients with acute lymphoblastic leukemia and non-Hodgkin's lymphomas but less common in those with Hodgkin's disease (134). Renal infiltrates are generally clinically silent and only result in kidney failure either from vascular or ureteral compression or from extensive parenchymal infiltration (142).

Tubulointerstitial lesions are common in the acute stage of the hemolytic syndrome and are an integral feature of those who develop persistent kidney damage necessitating renal replacement therapy (398,466).

Heavy Metals

Environmental exposure to *cadmium* results in its accumulation in the body, where it is preferentially concentrated in the kidney, principally in the proximal tubule, in the form of a cadmium-metallothionein complex that has a biologic half-life of approximately 10 years (462). Because of its chronic local toxic effect, an insidious form of chronic tubulointerstitial nephropathy results, the principal manifestation of which is proximal tubule dysfunction (468–470), a distinctive form of low-molecular-weight proteinuria (471) and osteomalacia due to calciuria, which causes nephrolithiasis in 40% of such cases (472).

Exposure to *lead,* as an occupational hazard, environmental exposure, or its ingestion in homemade brew, results in its insidious accumulation in the body (139,473,474). This subclinical accumulation of lead has been implicated in the causation of hyperuricemia, hypertension, and kidney failure (5,475,476). Episodes of acute gouty attacks precede the onset of reduced kidney function, and hypertension develops early in the course of kidney disease at a time when the serum creatinine level is only slightly above the normal range. Focal tubulointerstitial lesions are present in as many as half of such patients. Actually, tubulointerstitial lesions of such cases once attributed to gouty nephropathy are now considered the consequence of lead overload (476). The infusion of calcium disodium ethylenediaminetetraacetic acid (EDTA) to mobilize body stores of lead is a useful diagnostic tool for the detection and treatment of this disorder (139,476–478). Environmental exposure appears to be associated with worsening of preexisting chronic kidney disease. In a randomized study of nondiabetic Taiwanese patients with chronic kidney disease and an elevated body lead burden, repeated EDTA chelation resulted in improved kidney function and a slower rate of progression over 24 months compared to a placebo-treated group (479).

Rare cases of tubulointerstitial nephropathy have been caused by exposure to *silicon, copper, bismuth, barium, uranium,* and *arsenic* (480,481), and possibly *organic solvents* (482). Early detection is important in all cases of heavy metal exposure because of the potential of reversibility. Unfortunately, the onset of kidney disease is insidious and often goes undetected. Urinary enzymatic markers of tubular injury and selective proteinuria (THP, retinal binding protein, alkaline phosphatase) can be useful in early detection but are not readily available (483,484).

Vascular Diseases

Tubular degeneration, interstitial fibrosis, and mononuclear cell infiltration are part of the degenerative process that affects the kidneys in vascular diseases that involve the intrarenal vasculature with any degree of severity as to result in ischemia (67,485–488) (Figs. 72-1, 72-7). Rarely, if the insult is sudden and massive, the lesions are those of infarction and acute deterioration of kidney function. More commonly, the vascular lesions develop gradually and go undetected until renal insufficiency supervenes (49). It is this chronic form that accounts for the tubulointerstitial lesions of arteriolar nephrosclerosis and hypertension (10,49,89,489) that accounts for the relatively high prevalence of end-stage renal disease in selected ethnic populations and contributes to the tubulointerstitial lesions of patients with diabetes (486), sickle cell hemoglobinopathy (436), vasculitis (487,488), and cyclosporine nephrotoxicity (421,422).

The kidney injury caused by radiation, which is characteristically one of tubulointerstitial nephropathy, is also ischemic in origin because of the radiation-induced injury of the renal vasculature (490,491). The rash of cases that were reported from the 1940s through the 1960s resulted from the failure to recognize the sensitivity of renal vessels to irradiation (492) and the then-prevailing misconception that the kidney was resistant to radiation injury (493). Recognition that the total dose and frequency of the administered radiation are important determinants of nephrotoxicity, and institution of shielding of the kidneys during radiation exposure has resulted in a dramatic decrease in the frequency with which radiation-induced tubulointerstitial lesions are currently encountered.

Metabolic Disorders

Hyperuricemia/Hyperuricosuria

The kidneys are the major organs for the excretion of uric acid and a primary target organ affected in disorders of urate metabolism. The renal lesions result from crystallization of uric acid, either in the urine outflow tract or in the kidney parenchyma (494–496). The determinants of uric acid solubility are its concentration and the pH of the medium in which it is dissolved (497). Consequently, the supersaturation of the tubular fluid, as the excreted uric acid becomes concentrated in the medulla, and the acidification of the urine in the distal tubule will be conducive to the precipitation of uric acid. Not unexpectedly then, the major sites of urate deposition are the renal medulla, the collecting tubules, and the urinary tract. The pH of uric acid is 5.4, and at the acid pH of the distal tubule fluid, the bulk of the filtered urate will be present in its unionized form as uric acid, whereas at the more alkaline pH of the blood and interstitium, it is in its ionized form as urate salts. If deposition occurs in an acid medium, as in the tubular fluid, birefringent uric acid crystals are formed, whereas in an alkaline medium, as in the interstitium, amorphous urate salts are deposited (498,499). Depending on the load of uric acid presented to the kidneys, one of three disorders results: acute uric acid nephropathy, uric acid nephrolithiasis, or chronic urate nephropathy. Whereas either one of the former two forms can produce tubulointerstitial lesions, only the latter is considered here, because uric acid nephropathy is an acute lesion and uric acid nephrolithiasis produces its effect by obstruction.

The principal lesion of chronic hyperuricemia is the deposition of microtophi of amorphous urate crystals in the interstitium, with a surrounding giant-cell reaction (133,500,501). The earlier change, however, is probably due to the precipitation of birefringent uric acid crystals in the collecting tubules, with consequent tubular obstruction, dilation, atrophy, and interstitial fibrosis (498,502). Experimental evidence in support of a role of tubular precipitation of uric acid has been advanced from studies on pigs fed a high purine diet (503). Additional support derives from the reported high incidence of uric acid crystals in the kidneys of patients with gout and those with Lesch-Nyhan syndrome (495,504). The proposal has, therefore, been made that most patients whose hyperuricemia and gout are due to decreased uric acid excretion, rather than overproduction, would be spared from renal injury. However, this is not the case because kidney lesions are encountered in these "underexcretors." The kidney injury of these individuals has been attributed to hyperacidity of the urine because of an inherent abnormality in their ability to produce ammonia (505,506). The acidity of urine is important because uric acid is 17 times less soluble than urate, and, therefore, it facilitates precipitation in the distal nephron of those who are not overproducers but have an acid urine.

The earlier notion that chronic kidney disease was common in patients with hyperuricemia (504) has been questioned in light of prolonged follow-up studies of kidney function in persons with hyperuricemia (505–507). Reduced kidney function could be documented only when the serum urate concentration was more than 10 mg/dL in women and more than 13 mg/dL in men for prolonged periods. The deterioration of kidney function in those with hyperuricemia of a lower magnitude has been attributed to the higher-than-expected occurrence of concurrent hypertension, diabetes mellitus, abnormal lipid metabolism, and nephrosclerosis (508,509). Recent experimental evidence indicates that milder hyperuricemia is associated with endothelial dysfunction, hypertension, and chronic tubulointerstitial nephritis (510–514). The development of tubulointerstitial nephritis in mild hyperuricemia is crystal-dependent and is likely secondary to activation of the renin–angiotensin system and altered production of nitric oxide (NO), since the hypertension and kidney lesions were attenuated with administration of allopurinol, ACE inhibition and the NO-substrate, l-arginine (511,512). Clinically, hyperuricemia is independently associated with hypertension and cardiovascular disease, whether its treatment affects kidney function remains to be determined (511,513). An association of kidney disease and hyperuricemia exists in persons with a history of exposure to lead and consequent subclinical lead toxicity (475,476). A series of studies from New Jersey showed that patients with coexistent hyperuricemia and reduced kidney function had lead overload, whereas those with hyperuricemia and normal kidney function had normal body lead stores. The mechanism whereby lead aggravates hyperuricemia is not clear (515).

Hyperoxaluria

The increased production or intestinal absorption of oxalate, with its consequent increased renal excretion, almost invariably results in its precipitation as calcium oxalate in the urine outflow tract (138,516). Microcrystallization first occurs in the proximal tubules where oxalate secretion occurs (516–518), but the lesions that develop are more severe in the renal medulla, where the increasing concentration of the tubular fluid and its acidification promote calcium oxalate precipitation (138,139,519), and adhesion to distal nephron epithelial cells (520), particularly in the presence of Tamm-Horsfall protein deficiency (521). The exposure of tubule epithelial cells to calcium oxalate crystals results in the increased synthesis of osteopontin, MCP-1, prostaglandin E_2, and AII receptors, which are known to activate the interstitial inflammatory process and matrix deposition (522,523). This results in atrophy of the epithelial cells lining the affected tubules, interstitial edema, and inflammatory cell infiltration (138,139,523).

Hyperoxaluria may be primary or acquired (138). The primary form is a rare inherited disorder due to an enzymatic abnormality in the metabolism of glyoxylic acid. The acquired forms of hyperoxaluria are more common and result either from the ingestion of oxalate precursors, such as ethylene glycol (524) and ascorbic acid (138), and exposure to methoxyflurane anesthesia (525) or from its increased absorption from the

intestinal tract of persons with inflammatory bowel disease or who have undergone small bowel resection (526–528). When the hyperoxaluria is sudden and massive, such as after ethylene glycol ingestion, acute renal failure develops. Otherwise, as with most cases of hyperoxaluria, the overload is insidious and chronic; as a result, interstitial fibrosis, tubular atrophy, and dilation result in a chronic tubulointerstitial nephritis, with progressive renal failure. The propensity to recurrent calcium oxalate nephrolithiasis and consequent obstructive uropathy contributes to the tubulointerstitial lesions.

Hypercalcemia/Hypercalciuria

Given the many and vital roles of calcium in normal cell function, it is evident why changes in calcium concentration, either in the blood or in the urine, produce immediate reversible changes in kidney function, which are followed by irreversible structural changes if calcium derangement goes undetected or remains untreated (529). In most instances, the severity and potential reversibility of the changes that occur are related to the degree and duration of the hypercalcemia (529,530). Several experimental studies noted the development of acute changes in tubular function and renal hemodynamics (531–533). A defect in the urinary concentration is the most notable tubular dysfunction (529,530,533). It is multifactorial in origin but results mainly from a direct inhibitory effect of calcium on the reabsorption of sodium in the tubule in general, but in the loop of Henle in particular (529,530,533), and from an altered responsiveness of the collecting duct to antidiuretic hormone due to downregulation of aquaporin-2 water channels (534–538). The hemodynamic changes result from an effect of calcium on the systemic and the renal vasculature, either directly or indirectly through its effect on cardiac function (530,532,539) and renal prostaglandin and renin–angiotensin production (540).

Focal degeneration and necrosis of the tubular epithelium, primarily in the medulla where calcium is concentrated, occur shortly after persistent hypercalcemia and have been attributed to increased intracellular and mitochondrial calcium content (539–542). The subsequent calcification and destruction of the TBM result in proliferative and infiltrative changes of the adjacent interstitium, whereas the sloughing of necrotic cells results in tubular atrophy and obstruction with consequent dilation and pressure injury to the proximal segments of the tubule (539,540). Early changes in the proximal tubule also have been noted (451,453). Deposition of calcium in the necrotic and injured areas results in the characteristic nephrocalcinosis seen on radiography or noted at autopsy (529,530,542,543). The deposition of calcium in the glomerular capillaries and vasculature probably contributes to the further progression of the injury. The final lesion of focal scarified areas of tubular atrophy, increased interstitial fibrosis, and mononuclear cell infiltration is a classic example of chronic tubulointerstitial disease. The propensity to kidney stone formation and therefore to obstructive nephropathy also can contribute to the tubulointerstitial lesions.

Potassium Depletion

Various well-documented abnormalities of kidney function accompany the development of potassium depletion (544,545), the hallmark of which is a vasopressin-resistant impairment of the ability to concentrate the urine (546–548), increased ammonia genesis (549), and a modest reduction of the GFR (544,546). The characteristic structural change that accompanies potassium depletion in humans is that of vacuolation and hypertrophy of the tubule epithelial cells due to the dilated cisternae of the endoplasmic reticulum and the basilar foldings of the cells (550). The lesions are generally limited to the proximal tubule segments, with only focal changes in the distal segment. With potassium repletion, the functional and structural changes appear to be reversible (544,545). Whether they can progress to a chronic tubulointerstitial nephropathy and result in persistent kidney dysfunction is uncertain but seems likely depending on the duration and extent of potassium depletion (544,545,551). A familial form of hypokalemic tubulointerstitial nephritis with progressive kidney disease has been described (552,553). Experimental potassium depletion in rats resulted in persistent interstitial fibrosis and scarring several months after potassium repletion (554). In rats, the lesions of acute potassium depletion are more extensive than those in humans, with vacuolation and tubular hyperplasia affecting both the proximal and the distal tubule segments (555,556). These changes have been attributed to the susceptibility of potassium-depleted rats to chronic pyelonephritis (551,556), although the evidence that potassium depletion predisposes to pyelonephritis is not well established and is controversial at best (557). A principal cause of kidney injury may well be the augmented ammonia genesis associated with hypokalemia (Fig. 72-1). Ammonia directly activates the alternative complement pathway and thereby sets off an immune-mediated process of progressive tubulointerstitial injury (218). In hypokalemic rats, suppression of ammoniagenesis with bicarbonate supplementation ameliorated the tubulointerstitial lesions (558).

Potassium depletion has also been shown to induce the production in the vasculature of the kidney of cytokines implicated in interstitial fibrosis such as TGF-β, insulin-like growth factor 1, and renin (559–561). Another contributory role to fibrosis may be that of aldosterone in cases in which potassium losses are due to either primary or secondary hyperaldosteronism. Increasing evidence for aldosterone-induced fibrogenesis and its prevention by low-dose spironolactone has been presented recently (562,563) in various experimental models of kidney disease including streptozotocin-induced diabetes (564) and obstructive nephropathy (565).

Cystinosis

Cystinosis is a rare autosomal inherited disorder of amino acid metabolism that is characterized by the deposition of cystine crystals throughout the body (136). The early lesions of the kidney in these persons is a "swan neck" deformity or atrophy of the proximal tubule segments that are adjacent to cystine-containing interstitial cells. The structural changes coincide with the development of proximal tubular dysfunction characteristic of Fanconi's syndrome (566), which is one of the eponyms used in describing this entity (136). Progressive interstitial fibrosis, tubular atrophy, and interstitial inflammatory reaction result in progression to end-stage renal failure (567,568). The characteristic rhomboid-shaped crystals of cystine that are generally seen in the interstitium also have been noted in the glomerular and tubular cells (569).

Hereditary Diseases of the Kidney

Tubulointerstitial lesions are a prominent component of the structural changes of various hereditary diseases of the kidney, such as the medullary cystic disease, familial juvenile nephronophthisis, medullary sponge kidney, and polycystic kidney disease (570–574). The primary disorder of these conditions is a tubular defect that in some patients results in the cystic dilation of the affected segment. Several of the identified genes disrupted in polycystic kidney disease and nephronophthisis encode proteins expressed in the primary cilia of epithelial cells that project into the lumen, and cilium-generated signaling has been implicated in the pathogenesis of cyst formation (572,573). Altered epithelial cell proliferation and associated TBM changes account for cyst formation (574–578). It is the continuous growth of cysts and their progressive dilation

that cause pressure-induced ischemic injury of the adjacent renal parenchyma (578–580). A defect in urinary concentrating capacity is an early functional manifestation of experimental and clinical cystic diseases of the kidney (581–583). Hypertension is common in these diseases, and the vascular lesions of nephrosclerosis may contribute further to the course of renal deterioration and development of tubulointerstitial lesions (584–589).

Tubulointerstitial lesions are also a salient feature of inherited diseases of the glomerular basement membrane (590). Notable among them are those of hereditary nephritis or Alport's syndrome, in which a mutation in the encoding gene localized to the X chromosome results in a defect in the α_5 chain of type IV collagen (591–593). Of interest are the lesions that occur in the transplanted kidney of these patients who develop antitubular and antiglomerular antibodies resulting in progressive loss of kidney function (594).

Granulomatous Diseases

Interstitial granulomatous reactions are a rare but characteristic hallmark of certain forms of tubulointerstitial disease (121). The two best-known forms are sarcoidosis and tuberculosis. Granulomatous infiltration of the renal interstitium may be present in as many as 40% of the patients with sarcoidosis, but it is rarely sufficiently extensive to cause detectable kidney dysfunction (5,120,122,595,596). The granulomatous reactions may develop after subsidence of pulmonary lesions (597). The lesions are usually responsive to steroid therapy (598,599). However, the regression of the active granulomatous reaction can result in interstitial fibrosis and progressive loss of kidney function (596,600). Interstitial nephritis also has been noted in the absence of granulomatous lesions in some patients with sarcoidosis (596); it may be due to the hypercalcemia, glomerular disease, and arteritis that occur in sarcoidosis (601–604).

A similar pathogenetic sequence of events occurs in tuberculosis of the kidney. The granulomatous reaction to the mycobacterial infection responds to antituberculous treatment, but the residual fibrosis can result in tubulointerstitial disease (125,605,606). A potential role for steroid treatment in conjunction with antituberculous therapy for attenuation of the interstitial lesions has been suggested (607). A contributory factor to the interstitial lesions of renal tuberculosis is the obstructive nephropathy that follows ureteral and caliceal scarring caused by tuberculous involvement of the genitourinary tract (270).

Interstitial granulomatous reactions also have been noted in xanthogranulomatous pyelonephritis (127), renal malakoplakia (116), Wegener's granulomatosis (608), renal candidiasis (126), heroin abuse (609), and hyperoxaluria after jejunoileal bypass surgery (610), and in association with anterior uveitis (611).

Endemic Diseases

Two endemic diseases in which tubulointerstitial lesions are a predominant component are Balkan nephropathy and nephropathia epidemica.

Endemic Balkan nephropathy is a progressive chronic tubulointerstitial nephritis, the occurrence of which is limited to a geographic area bordering the Danube River as it traverses Romania, Bulgaria, and the former Yugoslavia (612–614). The etiology of the disease remains unknown but has been attributed to genetic factors, heavy metals, trace elements, and infectious agents (612,615,616). Environmental industrial contaminants and aromatic hydrocarbons have also been implicated, and the frequent association of the nephropathy with urothelial tumors attributed to them (617). The regions where the disease occurs have a high ambient humidity and heavy rainfall, and, hence, a propensity to fungal infection of food (612,618,619). Ochratoxin A, a mycotoxin found in food, is known to be nephrotoxic and cancerogenic (620). Foods with a high content of ochratoxin A are shown to cluster in the same areas where Balkan nephropathy is prominent and this mycotoxin has been implicated as its causative agent (621). Ochratoxin A has been shown to induce tubule epithelial cell injury (622,623), to modulate a number of epithelial cellular proinflammatory signals, to enhance collagen deposition (624) and to cause vasoconstriction through an AII-dependent mechanism (623). Ochratoxin A has also been implicated in chronic tubulointerstitial nephritis of unknown etiology (620,625). The disease evolves in emigrants from endemic regions, suggesting a role for inheritance or the perpetuation of injury sustained before emigration (626). It is now evident that the disease is clustered but may not be confined to the Balkans (615).

Nephropathia epidemica, initially thought to be restricted to the Scandinavian countries and termed *Scandinavian acute hemorrhagic interstitial nephritis,* has a more universal occurrence (627,628) and has therefore been more appropriately termed by the World Health Organization (WHO) as hemorrhagic fever with renal syndrome (629,630). As a rule, the disease presents as a reversible acute tubulointerstitial nephritis after an initial febrile episode but can progress to a chronic form (631,632). It is caused by a rodent-transmitted virus of the *Hantavirus* genus of the Bunyaviridae family (633). Humans appear to be infected by respiratory aerosols contaminated by rodent excreta. Antibodies to the virus are detected in the serum of affected individuals (628), and in that of patients with varied forms of chronic kidney disease and IgA nephropathy (634). Tubulointerstitial nephropathy due to other viral infections has also been reported with polyomavirus (298,635), cytomegalovirus (636,637), herpes simplex virus (291), human immunodeficiency virus (HIV) infection, and infectious mononucleosis (638).

IDIOPATHIC

Despite extensive evaluation, in several cases of primary chronic tubulointerstitial nephritis it is not possible to determine the cause of the lesions. A potential role of Epstein-Barr virus (EBV) infection of proximal tubule cells has been implicated as a contributory factor to the irritation and/or progression of the tubulointerstitial lesion of such cases. Using *in situ* hybridization and the polymerase chain reaction, the EBV genome could be detected exclusively in kidney tissue of patients with idiopathic chronic tubulointerstitial nephropathy but not in that of cases due to glomerular disease, infection, or drug-induced tubulointerstitial nephritis (639).

Mild proteinuria and microhematuria occur in 16% of patients with clinical and serologic evidence of infectious mononucleosis (640). Except in rare cases of acute renal failure (641), kidney function is well preserved in these cases. In the rare cases that have been biopsied, a monocytic interstitial cellular infiltrate is common and can result in tubulointerstitial lesions (638), but glomerular changes have been reported also (642). Whether active EBV infection or activation of latently infected proximal tubule cells may evoke the cellular immune response that results in the tubulointerstitial lesions of some of these cases remains to be established.

PAPILLARY NECROSIS

Renal papillary necrosis develops in various diseases that cause chronic tubulointerstitial nephropathy in which the lesion is more severe in the inner medulla (189). The basic lesion is one of impairment of the vasculature and consequent focal or diffuse ischemic necrosis of the distal segments of one or more of the renal pyramids (402,643–645). In the affected papilla, the sharp demarcation of the lesion and the coagulative necrosis seen in the early stages of the disease closely resemble those of infarction (646). The cellular infiltrates that characterize tubulointerstitial lesions of the cortex are sparse in the medullary lesions (84). The fact that the necrosis is anatomically limited to the papillary tips can be attributed to various features that are unique to this site, especially those of the vasculature. The renal papilla receives its blood supply from two sources: the vasa recta and branches of the arteries in the adventitia of the minor calices. The importance of the latter is evidenced by the finding that the terminal portions of the papilla may be viable at a time when the remainder of it is necrotic, presumably because the blood supply from the minor caliceal arteries remains intact when the vascular involvement is limited to the vasa recta (647,648), and by the report of a case of renal papillary necrosis due to caliceal arteritis (649). The vascular bundles formed by the vasa recta in the outer medulla and the interbundle region form distinct compartments; in the inner medulla, a subdivision into compartments is not obvious. In addition, the vascular bundles, which are widest in the outer medulla, gradually decrease in size, and at the papillary tip only single or a few communicating vessels remain (648,650). The tapering away of the bundles is due to the gradual reduction of the vessels entering and leaving at different levels of the medullary capillary plexus. Measurements of medullary blood flow notwithstanding, it should be noted that much of the blood flow in the vasa recta serves the countercurrent exchange mechanism. Nutrient blood supply is provided by small capillary vessels that originate in each given region. The net effect is that the nutrient blood supply to the papillary tip is less than that to the rest of the medulla, and hence its predisposition to ischemic necrosis caused by diseases of the vasculature or induced by hemodynamic changes such as shock and nonsteroidal anti-inflammatory drugs (651–653).

Infection is usually, but not invariably, a concomitant finding of most cases of renal papillary necrosis (189,654–658). With few exceptions, most patients with renal papillary necrosis ultimately develop a urinary tract infection. Some authors considered the infection to be the cause of the renal papillary necrosis and the suggestion has been made that renal papillary necrosis is a form of acute pyelonephritis that is more devastating than usual because its natural course is altered by associated disease states, specifically diabetes mellitus and obstruction of the urinary tract (655,659,660). However, angiographic studies revealed that vascular deficiency contributes even to the renal papillary necrosis associated with chronic pyelonephritis (661), and the necrosis of acute pyelonephritis has been attributed to compression of the thin-walled medullary vasculature by the inflammatory reaction of the interstitium (655). In addition, in considering infection as a cause of renal papillary necrosis, one must consider that infection itself represents a complication of papillary necrosis (189); that is, the infection develops after the primary underlying disease has initiated local injury to the renal medulla, with foci of impaired blood flow and poor tubular drainage. In any case, infection, if not the cause, is a frequent and important finding in most patients with renal papillary necrosis (189). It contributes significantly to the symptomatology of renal papillary necrosis because fever and chills are the presenting symptoms in two-thirds of patients and a positive urine culture is obtained in 70% (189). However, to consider renal papillary necrosis as an extension of severe pyelonephritis is inaccurate and simplistic. In most patients with florid acute pyelonephritis, renal papillary necrosis does not occur. To classify renal papillary necrosis as a form of necrotizing pyelonephritis is archaic and

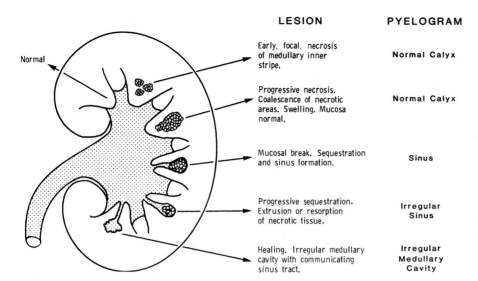

LESION	PYELOGRAM
Early, focal, necrosis of medullary inner stripe.	Normal Calyx
Progressive necrosis. Coalescence of necrotic areas. Swelling. Mucosa normal.	Normal Calyx
Mucosal break. Sequestration and sinus formation.	Sinus
Progressive sequestration. Extrusion or resorption of necrotic tissue.	Irregular Sinus
Healing. Irregular medullary cavity with communicating sinus tract.	Irregular Medullary Cavity

FIGURE 72-9. Pathogenesis and radiologic changes in the medullary form of renal papillary necrosis. (From: Eknoyan G, et al. Renal papillary necrosis: an update. *Medicine* 1982;61:55, with permission.)

has detracted from the recognition of renal papillary necrosis as a distinct clinicopathologic entity that can develop in the absence of pyelonephritis and urinary tract infection (189).

The necrotic lesion occurs in one of two forms. In the medullary form (Fig. 72-9), also termed *partial papillary necrosis*, the inner medulla is affected but the papillary tip and fornices remain intact; in the papillary form, also termed *total papillary necrosis*, the caliceal fornices and entire papillary tip are necrotic (662–664) (Fig. 72-10). In the latter form, renal papillary necrosis is characterized by necrosis, demarcation, and sequestration of the papilla, which ultimately sloughs into the pelvis and may be recovered in the urine. In most of these cases, however, the necrotic papilla is not sloughed but is either resorbed or remains *in situ*, where it becomes calcified or forms the nidus of a calculus (654,665). In these patients, excretory radiologic examination and computed tomography are diagnostic. Unfortunately, these changes may not be evident until the late stages of renal papillary necrosis, when the papillae are shrunken and sequestered (Fig. 72-8). Actually, even when the papillae are sloughed out, excretory radiography results can be negative (666,667). The passage of sloughed papillae is

associated with lumbar pain, which is indistinguishable from ureteral colic of any cause and is present in about half of the patients (189). Oliguria occurs in less than 10% of patients. Because a definitive diagnosis of renal papillary necrosis can be made by finding portions of necrotic papillae in the urine, a deliberate search should be made for papillary fragments in urine collected during or after attacks of colicky pain of all suspected cases, by straining the urine through filter paper or a piece of gauze (668,669). The separation and passage of papillary tissue may be associated with hematuria, which is microscopic in about 40% to 45% of the patients and gross in 20% (161). The hematuria can be massive, and occasional instances of exsanguinating hemorrhage requiring nephrectomy have been reported (670,671).

The necrotic lesions of renal papillary necrosis may be limited to only a few of the papillae or involve several of them in either one or both of the kidneys. In most patients, the lesions are bilateral (189,654,655,659,665,672). In patients in whom one kidney is involved at the time of initial presentation, renal papillary necrosis develops in the other kidney within the ensuing 4 years (663). This is not unexpected, considering

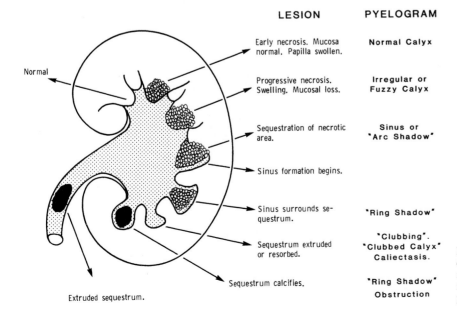

LESION	PYELOGRAM
Early necrosis. Mucosa normal. Papilla swollen.	Normal Calyx
Progressive necrosis. Swelling. Mucosal loss.	Irregular or Fuzzy Calyx
Sequestration of necrotic area.	Sinus or "Arc Shadow"
Sinus formation begins.	
Sinus surrounds sequestrum.	"Ring Shadow"
Sequestrum extruded or resorbed.	"Clubbing". "Clubbed Calyx" Caliectasis.
Sequestrum calcifies.	"Ring Shadow" Obstruction

Extruded sequestrum.

FIGURE 72-10. Pathogenesis and radiologic changes in the papillary form of renal papillary necrosis. (From: Eknoyan G, et al. Renal papillary necrosis: an update. *Medicine* 1982;61:55, with permission.)

the systemic nature of the diseases that are associated with renal papillary necrosis. Renal papillary necrosis may be unilateral in patients in whom predisposing factors, such as the infection and obstruction, are limited to one kidney. Azotemia may be absent even in bilateral papillary necrosis, because it is the total number of papillae involved that ultimately determines the level of renal insufficiency that develops (189). Each human kidney has an average of eight pyramids, such that even with bilateral renal papillary necrosis affecting one or two papillae in each kidney, sufficient unaffected renal lobules remain to maintain an adequate level of renal function. Moreover, in instances in which several papillae in each kidney are necrotic, the localization of the lesion to the inner medulla results in the loss of the juxtamedullary nephrons only, whereas the cortical nephrons, which terminate in the outer medulla, are spared, such that even in the affected pyramids, there remain several intact nephrons that are capable of contributing to the maintenance of normal homeostasis (645,665,673). Inability to concentrate the urine maximally is a more common development than kidney failure, as might be expected from the involvement of the inner medulla (665,673). Hence, a long-standing history of polyuria and nocturia can be elicited from many of these patients. With the loss of several papillae and involvement of the cortex, however, kidney failure will ultimately supervene.

The clinical course of renal papillary necrosis is variable. In its rare acute form it may occur as a rapidly progressive devastating illness that results in the death of the patient because of septicemia and kidney failure (659,660). In its more common chronic form, it will pursue a protracted course of months or years. These patients may remain totally asymptomatic, with the diagnosis made incidentally, either at autopsy or by excretory urography. Alternatively, it may be symptomatic, manifesting itself principally as episodes of nephrolithiasis or pyelonephritis (189,654,655,663,674,675). In these conditions, fever and chills or renal colic are the presenting symptoms. Of those diagnosed while living, survival is lowest and the risk of progression to end-stage kidney failure is greatest among diabetic patients (676).

Diabetes mellitus is the most common condition associated with renal papillary necrosis, accounting for some 50% to 60% of the cases reported in the major series. The occurrence of renal papillary necrosis in patients with diabetes may be more common than is generally appreciated. In an intravenous urographic study of 76 patients with longstanding insulin-dependent diabetes mellitus, renal papillary necrosis was observed in almost 25% of the patients (677). *Obstructive uropathy* has been reported as the cause of renal papillary necrosis in 15% to 40% of the major reviews. *Pyelonephritis* can result in papillary necrosis, and infection is present in most patients with renal papillary necrosis, but its exact prevalence as the cause of renal papillary necrosis is difficult to determine because infection may develop secondary to obstruction or diabetes, which remain the primary cause of renal papillary necrosis in the United States (189). Analgesic abuse accounts for about 15% to 20% of the cases of renal papillary necrosis in the United States but for as many as 70% in countries in which analgesic abuse is common (189,384,678,679), including in children exposed to analgesics and nonsteroidal anti-inflammatory drugs (680,681). Radiologic evidence for renal papillary necrosis has been reported in more than half of patients with *sickle cell hemoglobinopathy* (436,682). The transplanted kidney appears to be vulnerable to developing renal papillary necrosis, either because of allograft rejection or secondary to the usual causes of renal papillary necrosis, which may have caused the end-stage kidney disease in the first place (250,683–685). In addition, the vasculitis of allograft rejection may lead to obliteration of the vessels supplying the papilla and may result in ischemic necrosis of the papilla. Alternatively, the renal papillary necrosis may be due to the primary disease that caused end-stage kidney disease, such as analgesic abuse, sickle cell disease, or diabetes mellitus.

As a rule, renal papillary necrosis is a disease of the older age-group, with the average age of patients being 53 years. Nearly half the cases occur in persons older than 60 years, and more than 90% of cases in those older than 40 years (189). Renal papillary necrosis is rare in persons younger than 40 years, except for those cases due to sickle hemoglobinopathy (436). Renal papillary necrosis is much less common in children, in whom the chronic conditions associated with renal papillary necrosis are rare, but it has been reported in association with hypoxia and hypotension associated with dehydration and septicemia (680,686–692), particularly in children but also in adults (693,694) and in recurrent dialysis-associated hypotensive episodes (695).

Other conditions in which renal papillary necrosis has been reported are renal vein thrombosis (674,675), cryoglobulinemia (676,696), renal candidiasis (684), idiopathic acute granulomatous interstitial nephritis (697), contrast dye–induced nephropathy (698,699), Wegener's granulomatosis (608), necrotizing angiitis (700), hypotensive shock (701), pancreatitis (657), chronic alcoholism (702,703), and aplastic anemia (189). Most of these have been observed in individual patients, and at least in some of them, their association with renal papillary necrosis may have been coincidental. Actually, even in conditions commonly associated with renal papillary necrosis, more than one of the causative factors of renal papillary necrosis has been noted to be present in more than half of the patients with renal papillary necrosis (189). Therefore, in most cases of renal papillary necrosis, the lesion is multifactorial in origin and the pathogenesis of renal papillary necrosis may be considered the result of an overlap phenomenon, in which a combination of detrimental factors are operating in concert to cause renal papillary necrosis (Fig. 72-11). As such, although each of the conditions alone can cause renal papillary necrosis, the coexistence of more than one predisposing factor in any one person significantly increases the risk for renal papillary necrosis. The contribution of any one of these factors to renal papillary necrosis would be expected to differ among individuals

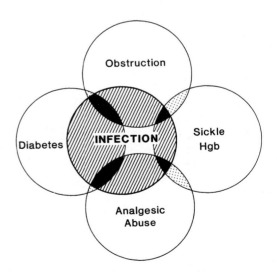

FIGURE 72-11. Spectrum of diseases that are the major causes of renal papillary necrosis, illustrating the multifactorial pathogenesis of renal papillary necrosis. Whereas each condition can, by itself, cause renal papillary necrosis, the coexistence of two (*striped areas*) or three (*black areas*) predisposing conditions increases the risk for renal papillary necrosis. (From: Eknoyan G, et al. Renal papillary necrosis: an update. *Medicine* 1982;61:55, with permission.)

and at various periods during the course of the disease. To the extent that the natural course of renal papillary necrosis itself predisposes to the development of infection of necrotic foci and obstruction by sloughed papillae, it may be difficult to assign a primary role for any of these processes in an individual patient (189). Furthermore, the occurrence of any of these factors— necrosis, obstruction, or infection—may itself initiate a vicious cycle that can lead to the other and culminate in renal papillary necrosis. Evidence that this may well be the case can be adduced not only from clinical studies (189) but also from experimental models of renal papillary necrosis. For example, in the Gunn rat with congenital hyperbilirubinemia, renal papillary necrosis occurs spontaneously secondary to the deposition of unconjugated bilirubin in the renal papillae (590). The administration of analgesics to these animals results in an acceleration of the papillary necrotic process and can be induced at doses of analgesics considerably less than those necessary to induce papillary lesions in other strains of rats (704).

References

1. Councilman WT. Acute interstitial nephritis. *J Exp Med* 1898;3:393.
2. Heptinstall RH. Interstitial nephritis. A brief review. *Am J Pathol* 1976;83:214.
3. Suki WN, Eknoyan G. Tubulo-interstitial disease. In: Brenner B, Rector F, eds. *The Kidney.* Philadelphia: WB Saunders; 1976:1113.
4. Cogan MG. Tubulo-interstitial nephropathies: a pathophysiologic approach. *West J Med* 1980;132:134.
5. Rastegar A, Kashgarian M. The clinical spectrum of tubulointerstitial nephritis. *Kidney Int* 1998;54:313.
6. Haggerty DT, Allen DM. Processing and presentation of self and foreign antigens by the renal proximal tubule. *J Immunol* 1992;148:2324.
7. Strutz F, Neilson EG. The role of lymphocytes in the progression of interstitial disease. *Kidney Int* 1994;45(Suppl):S106.
8. Palmer BF. The renal tubule in the progression of chronic renal failure. *J Invest Med* 1997;45:346.
9. Johnson DW, et al. Paracrine stimulation of renal fibroblasts by proximal tubule cells. *Kidney Int* 1998;54:747.
10. Blythe WB. Natural history of hypertension in renal parenchymal disease. *Am J Kidney Dis* 1985;5:A50.
11. Cogan MG. Classification and patterns of renal dysfunction. *Contemp Issues Nephrol* 1983;10:35.
12. Abe S, et al. Significance of tubulointerstitial lesions in biopsy specimens of glomerulonephritic patients. *Am J Nephrol* 1989;9:30.
13. Bohle A, et al. The role of the interstitium of the renal cortex in renal disease. *Contrib Nephrol* 1979;16:109.
14. Bohle A, et al. The consequences of tubulo-interstitial changes for renal function in glomerulopathies: a morphometric and cytological analysis. *Pathol Res Pract* 1990;186:135.
15. Vangelista A, et al. Clinical factors in progressive renal damage: the role of interstitial fibrosis. *Am J Kidney Dis* 1991;17(Suppl 1):62.
16. Eddy AA. Experimental insights into the tubulointerstitial disease accompanying primary glomerular lesions. *J Am Soc Nephrol* 1994;5:1273.
17. Jungthirapanich J, et al. Significance of tubulointerstitial fibrosis in paediatric IgM nephropathy. *Nephrology* 1997;3:509.
18. Kriz W, Lehir M. Pathways to nephron loss starting from glomerular diseases. *Kidney Int* 2005;67:404.
19. Murray T, Goldberg M. Chronic interstitial nephritis. Etiologic factors. *Ann Intern Med* 1975;82:453.
20. Rodeman HP, Müller GH. Abnormal growth and clonal proliferation of fibroblasts derived from kidneys with interstitial fibrosis. *Proc Soc Exp Biol Med* 1990;195:57.
21. Rostand S, et al. Racial differences in the incidence of treatment for end-stage renal disease. *N Engl J Med* 1982;306:1276.
22. Nath KA. Tubulointerstitial changes as a major determinant in the progression of renal damage. *Am J Kidney Dis* 1992;20:1.
23. Bohman S. The ultrastructure of the renal interstitium. *Contemp Issues Nephrol* 1983;10:1.
24. Persson AE. Functional aspects of the renal interstitium. In: Maunsback AB, Olsen TS, Christenson AL, eds. *Functional Ultrastructure of the Kidney.* London: Academic Press; 1980:399.
25. Koury ST, et al. Quantitation of erythropoietin-producing cells in kidneys of mice by in situ hybridization: correlation with hematocrit, renal erythropoietin mRNA, and serum erythropoietin concentration. *Blood* 1989;74:645.
26. Futrakul P, et al. Tubular function and tubulointerstitial disease. *Am J Kidney Dis* 1999;33:886.
27. Bulger RE, Nagle RB. Ultrastructure of the interstitium in the rabbit kidney. *Am J Anat* 1973;136:183.
28. Kriz W, Napiwotzky P. Structural and functional aspects of the renal interstitium. *Contrib Nephrol* 1979;16:104.
29. Lemley KV, Kriz W. Anatomy of the renal interstitium. *Kidney Int* 1991;39:370.
30. Lemley KV, Kriz W. Cycles and separations: the histotopography of the urinary concentrating process. *Kidney Int* 1987;31:538.
31. Pedersen JC, Persson AE, Maunsback AB. Ultrastructure and quantitative characterization of the cortical interstitium in the rat kidney. In: Maunsback AB, Olsen TS, Christensen AL, eds. *Functional Ultrastructure of the Kidney.* London: Academic Press; 1980:143.
32. Pfaller W, Rittinger M. Quantitative morphology of the rat kidney. *Int J Biochem* 1980;12:17.
33. Pinter GG, et al. Interstitial albumin pool in the renal cortex: its turnover and permeability of peritubular capillaries. In: Maunsback AB, Olsen TS, Christensen AL, eds. *Functional Ultrastructure of the Kidney.* London: Academic Press; 1980:411.
34. Bulger RE, et al. Human renal ultrastructure. II. The thin limb of Henle's loop and the interstitium of healthy individuals. *Lab Invest* 1967;16:124.
35. Knepper MA, et al. Quantitative analysis of renal medullary anatomy in rats and rabbits. *Kidney Int* 1977;12:313.
36. Pitcock JA, et al. The morphology and antihypertensive effect of renomedullary interstitial cells derived from salt sensitive and resistant rats. *Exp Mol Pathol* 1985;42:29.
37. Leblond CP, Inoui S. Structure, composition and assembly of basement membranes. *Am J Anat* 1989;185:367.
38. Bach PH, Bridges JW. Chemically induced renal papillary necrosis and upper urothelial carcinoma: parts 1 and 2. *Crit Rev Toxicol* 1985;15:217.
39. Persson AE, Muller-Swur R, Selen G. Capillary oncotic pressure as a modifier for tubuloglomerular feedback. *Am J Physiol* 1979;236:F97.
40. Tisher CC, Bulger RE, Valtin H. Morphology of renal medulla in water diuresis and vasopressin-induced antidiuresis. *Am J Physiol* 1971;220:87.
41. Kriz W. Adenosine and ATP: traffic regulators in the kidney. *J Clin Invest* 2004;114:611.
42. Ljungqvist A. The intrarenal arterial pattern in the normal and diseased human kidney. *Acta Med Scand* 1963;174(Suppl 401):5.
43. Mellmann J, et al. Angiographic results in interstitial, vascular and glomerular kidney disease. *Contrib Nephrol* 1979;16:115.
44. Ivanyi B. Hypoxic damage to tubules due to blockage of perfusion in acute hematogenous *E. coli* pyelonephritis of rats. *Acta Morphol Hung* 1991;39:239.
45. Bohle A, Mackensen-Haen S, von Gise H. Significance of tubulointerstitial changes in renal cortex for the excretory function and concentration ability of the kidney: a morphometric contribution. *Am J Nephrol* 1987;7:421.
46. Sahai T, et al. Extracellular fluid expansion and autoregulation in nephrotoxic nephritis in rats. *Kidney Int* 1984;25:619.
47. Bohle A, et al. The obliteration of the postglomerular capillaries and its influence upon the function of both glomeruli and tubuli: functional interpretation of morphologic findings. *Klin Wochenschr* 1981;59:1043.
48. Bohle A, Mackensen-Haen S, Wehrmann M. Significance of postglomerular capillaries in the pathogenesis of chronic renal failure. *Kidney Blood Press Res* 1996;19:191.
49. Bohle A. Change of paradigms in nephrology—a view back and a look forward. *Nephrol Dial Transplant* 1998;13:556.
50. Brod J, Benesova D. A comparative study of functional and morphologic renal changes in glomerulonephritis. *Acta Med Scand* 1957;157:23.
51. Partman RJ, Kissane JM, Robson AM. Use of β_2-microglobulin to diagnose tubulointerstitial lesions in children. *Kidney Int* 1986;30:91.
52. Frasca GM, et al. Immunological tubulo-interstitial deposits in IgA nephropathy. *Kidney Int* 1982;22:184.
53. Hutt MS, Pinniger JL, de Wardener HE. The relationship between the clinical and histological features of acute glomerular nephritis. *Q J Med* 1958;27:265.
54. Muehrcke RC, et al. Lupus nephritis: a clinical and pathologic study based on renal biopsies. *Medicine* 1957;36:1.
55. Benabe JE, Martinez-Maldonado M. Tubulointerstitial nephritis associated with systemic disease and electrolyte abnormalities. *Semin Nephrol* 1988;8:29.
56. Risdon RA, Slopper JC, de Wardener HE. Relationship between renal function and histological changes found in renal biopsy specimens from patients with persistent glomerular nephritis. *Lancet* 1968;2:363.
57. Schainuck LL, et al. Structural-functional correlations in renal disease. Part II. The correlations. *Hum Pathol* 1970;1:631.
58. Hotta O, et al. Significance of renal hyaline atherosclerosis and tubulointerstitial change in IgA glomerulonephropathy and focal glomerular sclerosis. *Nephron* 1987;47:262.
59. Park MH, et al. Tubulointerstitial disease in lupus nephritis: relationship to immune deposits, interstitial inflammation, glomerular changes, renal function and progression. *Nephron* 1986;44:309.
60. Wehrmann M, et al. Long-term prognosis of chronic idiopathic membranous glomerulonephritis: an analysis of 334 cases with particular regard to tubulo-interstitial changes. *Clin Nephrol* 1989;31:67.
61. Cameron JS. Immunologically mediated interstitial nephritis: primary and secondary. *Adv Nephrol* 1989;18:207.
62. D'Amico G. Role of interstitial filtration of leukocytes in glomerular diseases. *Nephrol Dial Transplant* 1988;3:596.

63. D'Amico G, et al. Prognostic indicators in idiopathic IgA mesangial nephropathy. *Q J Med* 1986;59:363.
64. Mera J, Uchida S, Nagase M. Clinicopathologic study on prognostic markers of IgA nephropathy. *Nephron* 2000;84:148.
65. Burton CJ, Walls J. Proximal tubular cells, proteinuria and tubulointerstitial scarring. *Nephron* 1994;68:287.
66. Kriz W, et al. From segmental glomerulosclerosis to nephron degeneration and interstitial fibrosis: a histopathological study in rat models and human glomerulonephropathies. *Nephrol Dial Transplant* 1998;13:2781.
67. Nakagawa T. Tubulointerstitial disease: role of ischemia and nonvascular disease. *Curr Opin Nephrol Hypertens* 2003;12:233.
68. Eddy AE. Proteinuria and interstitial nephritis. *Nephrol Dial Transplant* 2004;19:277.
69. Meyers CM. New insights into the pathogenesis of interstitial nephritis. *Curr Opin Nephrol Hypertens* 1999;8:287.
70. Healy E, Brady HR. Role of tubule epithelial cells in the pathogenesis of tubulointerstitial nephritis induced by glomerular diseases. *Curr Opin Nephrol Transplant* 1998;7:525.
71. Eddy AE, et al. Interstitial nephritis induced by protein-overload proteinuria. *Am J Pathol* 1989;135:719.
72. Kees-Folts D, Sadow JL, Schreiner GF. Tubular catabolism of albumin is associated with the release of an inflammatory lipid. *Kidney Int* 1994;45:1697.
73. Ohashi R, et al. Peritubular capillary regression during progression of experimental obstructive nephropathy. *J Am Soc Nephrol* 2002;13:1795.
74. Choi C, et al. Peritubular capillary loss is associated with chronic tubulointerstitial injury in human kidney: altered expression of vascular endothelial growth factor. *Human Pathol* 2000;31:1491.
75. Basile DP, et al. Renal ischemic injury results in permanent damage to tubular capillaries and influences long-term function. *Am J Physiol Renal Physiol* 2001;281:F887.
76. Barne-Taney MJ, et al. Acute renal failure after whole body ischemia is characterized by inflammation and T cell mediated injury. *Am J Physiol Renal Physiol* 2003;285:F87.
77. Orphanides C, Fine LG, Narman JT. Hypoxial stimulates proximal cell matrix production via TGF-beta 1-independent mechanism. *Kidney Int* 1997;52:637.
78. Manotham K, et al. Transdifferentiation of cultured tubular epithelial cells induced by hypoxia. *Kidney Int* 2004;65:871.
79. Gabbai FB, et al. Effect of acute iNOS inhibition on glomerular function in tubulointerstitial nephritis. *Kidney Int* 2002;61:851.
80. Alfrey AC, Froment DH, Stammond WS. Role of iron in the tubulointerstitial injury of nephrotoxic serum nephritis. *Kidney Int* 1989;36:753.
81. Baliga R, Ueda N, Shah SV. Kidney iron status in passive Heymann nephritis and the effect of iron deficient diet. *J Am Soc Nephrol* 1996;7:1183.
82. Kanauchi M, Akai Y, Hashimoto T. Transferrinuria in type 2 diabetic patients with early nephropathy and tubular injury. *Eur J Intern Med* 2002;13:190.
83. Tang S, et al. Transferrin up-regulates chemokine synthesis by human proximal tubular epithelial cells: implication on mechanism of tubuloglomerular communication in glomerular proteinuria. *Kidney Int* 2002;61:1655.
84. Eknoyan G, Truong LD. Renal interstitium and major features of chronic tubulointerstitial nephritis. In: Schrier RW, ed. *Atlas of Diseases of the Kidney*, vol 2. Philadelphia: Current Medicine; 1999.
85. Sinniah R, Khan TN. Renal tubular basement membrane changes in tubulointerstitial damage in patients with glomerular diseases. *Ultrastruct Pathol* 1999;23:359.
86. Cheng HF, et al. HLA-DR display by renal tubular epithelium and phenotype of filtrate in interstitial nephritis. *Nephrol Dial Transplant* 1989;4:205.
87. Hooke DH, Gee DC, Atkins RC. Leukocyte analysis using monoclonal antibodies in human glomerulonephritis. *Kidney Int* 1987;31:964.
88. Markovic-Lipkovski J, et al. Association of glomerular and interstitial mononuclear leukocytes with different forms of glomerulonephritis. *Nephrol Dial Transplant* 1990;5:10.
89. Mai M, et al. Early interstitial changes in hypertension-induced renal injury. *Hypertension* 1993;22:754.
90. Svanborg C, De Man P, Sandberg T. Renal involvement in urinary tract infection. *Kidney Int* 1991;39:541.
91. Sugisaki T, et al. Immunopathologic study of an autoimmune tubular and interstitial renal disease in Brown Norway rats. *Lab Invest* 1973;28:658.
92. Pfaltz M, Briner J. Glomerular changes in interstitial kidney diseases. *Schweiz Med Wochenschr* 1984;114:204.
93. Bender WL, et al. Interstitial nephritis, proteinuria and renal failure caused by nonsteroidal anti-inflammatory drugs. Immunologic characterization of the inflammatory infiltrate. *Am J Med* 1984;76:1006.
94. Mampaso FM, Wilson CB. Characterization of inflammatory cells in autoimmune tubulointerstitial nephritis in rats. *Kidney Int* 1983;23:448.
95. Pamukou R, et al. Idiopathic acute interstitial nephritis: characterization of the infiltrating cells in the renal interstitium as T helper lymphocytes. *Am J Kidney Dis* 1984;4:24.
96. Neilson EG. The nephritogenic T lymphocyte response in interstitial nephritis. *Semin Nephrol* 1992;13:496.
97. Kelly CJ. Cellular immunity and the tubulointerstitium. *Semin Nephrol* 1999;19:182.
98. Husby G, Tung KS, Williams RC. Characterization of renal tissue lymphocytes in patients with interstitial nephritis. *Am J Med* 1981;70:31.
99. Macdonegal IC, et al. Interstitial nephritis and primary biliary cirrhosis: a new association. *Clin Nephrol* 1987;27:36.
100. Matsuma R, et al. Immunohistochemical identification of infiltrating mononuclear cells in tubulointerstitial nephritis Sjögren's syndrome. *Clin Nephrol* 1988;30:335.
101. Myers CM, Kelly C. Effector mechanisms in organ-specific autoimmunity. Characterization of CD8+ T cell line that mediates murine interstitial nephritis. *J Clin Invest* 1991;88:408.
102. Grönhagen-Riska C, et al. Interstitial cellular infiltration detected by fine-needle aspiration biopsy in nephritis. *Clin Nephrol* 1990;34:189.
103. Capodicasa G, et al. Sequential fine needle aspiration biopsy in glomerulonephritis. *Int J Pediatr Nephrol* 1986;7:3.
104. Pichler R, et al. Tubulointerstitial disease in glomerulonephritis. Potential role of osteopontin (uropontin). *Am J Pathol* 1994;144:915.
105. Giachelli CM, et al. Osteopontin expression in angiotensin II-induced tubulointerstitial nephritis. *Kidney Int* 1994;45:515.
106. Gibbs P, et al. Adhesion molecule expression (ICAM-1, VCAM-1, E-selection, and PECAM) in human allografts. *Transplant Immunol* 1993;1:109.
107. Tang WW, et al. Cytokine expression, upregulation of interstitial adhesion molecule 1, and leukocyte infiltration in experimental tubulointerstitial nephritis. *Lab Invest* 1994;70:631.
108. Hiromura K, et al. Tubulointerstitial mast cell infiltration in glomerulonephritis. *Am J Kidney Dis* 1998;32:593.
109. Nagle RB, Johnson ME, Jervis HR. Proliferation of renal interstitial cells following injury induced by ureteral obstruction. *Lab Invest* 1976;35:18.
110. Müller GA, Rodeman HP. Characterization of human renal fibroblasts in health and disease. I. Immunophenotyping of cultured tubular epithelial cells and fibroblasts derived from kidneys with histologically proven interstitial fibrosis. *Am J Kidney Dis* 1991;17:680.
111. Nolasco F, et al. Interstitial foam cells in the nephrotic syndrome belong to the monocyte/macrophage lineage. *Proc Eur Dial Transplant Assoc* 1984;21:666.
112. Abrass CK. Cellular lipid metabolism and the role of lipids in progressive renal disease. *Am J Nephrol* 2004;24:46
113. Rosen S, Pirani CL, Muehrcke RC. Renal interstitial foam cells: a light and electron microscopic study. *Am J Clin Pathol* 1966;45:32.
114. Grace SG, et al. Hereditary nephritis in the Negro. Report of a kindred. *Arch Intern Med* 1970;125:451.
115. Kelly DR, Murad TM. Megalocytic interstitial nephritis, xanthogranulomatous pyelonephritis and malakoplakia. An ultrastructural comparison. *Am J Clin Pathol* 1981;75:333.
116. Dobyan DC, Truong LD, Eknoyan G. Renal malakoplakia reappraised. *Am J Kidney Dis* 1993;22:243.
117. Esparza AR, et al. Renal parenchymal malakoplakia: histologic spectrum and its relationship to megalocystic interstitial nephritis and xanthogranulomatous pyelonephritis. *Am J Surg Pathol* 1989;13:225.
118. Hill JW, Seedat YK. The diagnosis of malakoplakia of the kidney by percutaneous renal biopsy. *S Afr Med J* 1972;46:953.
119. Osborn DE, Castro JE, Ansell ID. Malakoplakia in a cadaver renal allograft: a case study. *Hum Pathol* 1977;8:341.
120. Longcope WT, Friedman DG. A study of sarcoidosis: based on a combined investigation of 160 cases including 30 autopsies from the Johns Hopkins Hospital and Massachusetts General Hospital. *Medicine* 1952;31:1.
121. Mignon F, et al. Granulomatous interstitial nephritis. *Adv Nephrol* 1984;13:219.
122. King BP, et al. Sarcoid granulomatous nephritis occurring as isolated renal failure. *Arch Intern Med* 1976;136:241.
123. Singere DR, Evans DJ. Renal impairment in sarcoidosis: granulomatous nephritis as an isolated cause (two case reports and a review of the literature). *Clin Nephrol* 1986;26:250.
124. Verani R, Nasir M, Foley R. Granulomatous interstitial nephritis after a jejunoileal bypass: an ultrastructural and histochemical study. *Am J Nephrol* 1989;9:51.
125. Latimer JK. Renal tuberculosis. *N Engl J Med* 1975;273:208.
126. Guziel LP, et al. Primary renal candidiasis with renal granulomata and salt-losing nephropathy. *Am J Med Sci* 1975;269:123.
127. Gammill S, et al. New thoughts concerning xanthogranulomatous pyelonephritis (XP). *Am J Roentgenol Radiat Ther Nucl Med* 1975;125:154.
128. More RH, McMillan GL, Duff GL. The pathology of sulfonamide allergy in man. *Am J Pathol* 1946;22:702.
129. Steinmuller DR, et al. Chronic interstitial nephritis and mixed cryoglobulinemia associated with drug abuse. *Arch Pathol Lab Med* 1979;103:63.
130. Schwaderer AL, Arend L, Lande MB. Granulomatous interstitial nephritis associated with bone marrow transplantation. *Pediatr Nephrol* 2005;20:539.
131. Baum HP, Thoenes W. Differentiation of granuloma cells (epithelioid cells and multinucleated giant cells): a morphometric analysis. Investigations using the model of experimental (anti-TMB) tubulo-interstitial nephritis. *Vichows Arch (B)* 1985;50:181.
132. Langer KH, Thoenes W. Characterization of cells involved in the formation of granuloma. *Virchows Arch (Cell Pathol)* 1981;36:179.
133. Thoenes W, et al. Cell fusion as a mechanism for the formation of giant cells (Langhan's type): autoradiographic findings in autoimmune tubulointerstitial nephritis. *Virchows Arch (Cell Pathol)* 1982;41:45.

134. Pirani CL, Silva FG, Appel GB. Tubulo-interstitial disease in multiple myeloma and other non-renal neoplasias. *Contemp Issues Nephrol* 1983; 10:287.
135. Levi DF, Williams RC, Linstrom FD. Immunofluorescence studies of the myeloma kidney with special reference to light chain disease. *Am J Med* 1968;44:922.
136. Schulman JD, Schneider JA. Cystinosis and the Fanconi syndrome. *Pediatr Clin North Am* 1976;23:779.
137. Klinenberg JR, Kippen I, Bluestone R. Hyperuricemic nephropathy: pathologic features and factors influencing urate deposition. *Nephron* 1975;14:88.
138. Hodgkinson A. *Oxalic Acid in Biology and Medicine.* New York: Academic Press; 1977.
139. Wedeen RP, Batuman V. Tubulointerstitial nephritis induced by heavy metals and metabolic disturbances. *Contemp Issues Nephrol* 1983;10:211.
140. Viol GW, Minielly JA, Bistricki T. Gold nephropathy. *Arch Pathol Lab Med* 1977;101:635.
141. Gilboa N, Lum GN, Urizar RE. Early renal involvement in acute lymphoblastic leukemia and non-Hodgkin's lymphoma in children. *J Urol* 1983;129:364.
142. Kanfer A, et al. Acute renal insufficiency due to lymphomatous infiltration of the kidneys. *Cancer* 1976;38:2588.
143. Hewitson TD, et al. Evolution of tubulointerstitial fibrosis in experimental renal infection and scarring. *J Am Soc Nephrol* 1998;9:632.
144. Shao J, et al. Imbalance of T-cell subsets in angiotensin II infused hypertensive rats with kidney injury. *Hypertension* 2003;42:31.
145. Eddy AA. Molecular insights into renal interstitial fibrosis. *J Am Soc Nephrol* 1996;7:2495.
146. Klahr S, Morrissey JJ. The role of growth factors, cytokines, and vasoactive compounds in obstructive nephropathy. *Semin Nephrol* 1998;18:622.
147. Wardle EN. Modulatory proteins and processes in alliance with immune cells, mediators, extracellular proteins in renal interstitial fibrosis. *Ren Fail* 1999;21:121.
148. Segerer S, Nelson PJ, Schlondorff D. Chemokines, chemokine receptors, and renal disease: from basic science to pathophysiologic and therapeutic studies. *J Am Soc Nephrol* 2000;11:152.
149. Mené P. Molecular cell biology of renal diseases. *J Nephrol* 1999;12:140.
150. Ortiz A, Corina L, Egido J. New kids in the block: the role of Fas L and Fas in kidney damage. *J Nephrol* 1999;12:150.
151. El-Nahas AM, et al. Phenotypic modulation of renal cells during experimental and clinical renal scarring. *Kidney Int* 1996;49(Suppl 54):S23.
152. Border WA, Noble NA. TGF-beta in kidney fibrosis: a target for gene therapy. *Kidney Int* 1997;51:1388.
153. Ludewig D, et al. PDGF receptor kinase blocker AG1295 attenuates interstitial fibrosis in rat kidney after unilateral obstruction. *Cell Tissue Res* 2000;299:97.
154. Rodeman HP, et al. Fibroblasts of rabbit kidney in cultures. I. Characteristics and identification of cell specific markers. *Am J Physiol* 1991;261:F283.
155. Hewiston TD, Becker GJ. Interstitial myofibroblasts in IgA glomerulonephritis. *Am J Nephrol* 1995;15:111.
156. Alpers CE, et al. Human renal cortical interstitial cells and some features of smooth muscle cells participate in tubulointerstitial and crescentic glomerular injury. *J Am Soc Nephrol* 1994;5:201.
157. Boukhalfa G, et al. Relationship between alpha-smooth muscle actin expression and fibrotic changes in human kidney. *Exp Nephrol* 1996;4:241.
158. Gharall-Kermoni M, et al. Fibronectin is the major fibroblast chemoattractant in rabbit anti-glomerular basement membrane disease. *Am J Pathol* 1996;148:961.
159. Stokes MB, et al. Expression of decorin, biglycan, and collagen type I in human renal fibrosing disease. *Kidney Int* 2000;57:487.
160. Harris DC. Tubulointerstitial renal diseases. *Curr Opin Nephrol Hypertens* 2001;10:303
161. Sato M, et al. Targeted disruption of TGF-β1/Smad3 signaling protects against renal tubulointerstitial fibrosis induced by unilateral ureteral obstruction. *J Clin Invest* 2003;112:486.
162. Fukusawa H, et al. Treatment with anti-TGF-beta antibody ameliorates chromic progressive nephritis by inhibiting Smad/TGF-β signaling. *Kidney Int* 2004;65:63.
163. Zeisberg M, Shah AA, Kalluri R. Bone morphogenic protein-7 induces mesenchymal to epithelial transition in adult renal fibroblasts and facilitates regeneration of injured kidney. *J Biol Chem* 2005; 280:294
164. Hruska KA. Treatment of chromic tubulointerstitial disease: a new concept. *Kidney Int* 2002;61:911.
165. Klahr S, Morrissey J. Obstructive nephropathy and renal fibrosis: the role of bone morphogenic protein-7 and hepatic growth factor. *Kidney Int* 2003;(Suppl 87):S105
166. Zhang XL, et al. Bone morphogenic protein-7 inhibits monocyte-stimulated TGF-β1 generation of renal tubular epithelial cells. *J Am Soc Nephrol* 2005;16:79.
167. Jukneius I, et al. Effect of aldosterone on renal transforming growth factor-beta. *Am J Physiol Renal Physio* 2004;286:F1059.
168. Trachtman H, et al. Prevention of renal fibrosis by spironolactone in mice with complete unilateral ureteral occlusion. *J Urol* 2004;172:1590.
169. Junaid A, Hostetter TH, Rosenberg ME. Interaction of angiotensin II and TGF-β1 in the rat remnant kidney. *J Am Soc Nephrol* 1997;8:1732.
170. Maric C, et al. Effects of angiotensin II on cultured rat renomedullary interstitial cells are mediated by ATIA receptors. *Am J Physiol* 1996;271:F1020.
171. Greene EL, Kren SM, Hostetter TH. Role of aldosterone in the remnant kidney model in the rat. *J Clin Invest* 1996;98:1063.
172. Juknevicius I, et al. Aldosterone causes TGFβ-1 expression (abstract). *J Am Soc Nephrol* 2000;11:621A.
173. Hostetter MK, et al. Binding of C3b proceeds by a transesterification reaction at the thioester site. *Nature (London)* 1982;298:72.
174. Nangaku M, Pippin J, Couser WG. Complement membrane attack complex (C5-9) mediates interstitial disease in experimental nephrotic syndrome. *J Am Soc Nephrol* 1999;10:2323.
175. Hinglais N, et al. Immunohistochemical study of the C5b-9 complex of complement in human kidneys. *Kidney Int* 1986;30:399.
176. Falk RJ, et al. Ultrastructural localization of the membrane attack complex of complement in human renal tissue. *Am J Kidney Dis* 1987;9:121.
177. Piscator M. Early detection of tubular dysfunction. *Kidney Int* 1991; 34(Suppl):S15.
178. Eknoyan G, et al. Chronic tubulointerstitial nephritis: correlation between structural and functional findings. *Kidney Int* 1990;38:736.
179. Mackensen S, et al. Influence of the renal cortical interstitium on the serum creatinine concentration and creatinine clearance in different chronic sclerosing interstitial nephritis. *Nephron* 1979;24:30.
180. Mahieu P, Darderme M, Bach JF. Detection of humoral and cell-mediated immunity of kidney basement membranes in human renal diseases. *Am J Med* 1972;53:185.
181. Parrish AE, et al. Relationship between glomerular function and histology in acute glomerulonephritis. *J Lab Clin Med* 1961;58:197.
182. Battle DC, Arruda JA, Kurtzman NA. Hyperkalemic distal renal tubular acidosis associated uropathy. *N Engl J Med* 1981;304:373.
183. Schilsky RL, Anderson T. Hypomagnesemia and renal magnesium wasting in patients receiving cisplatin. *Ann Intern Med* 1979;90:929.
184. Barr RS, Wilson HE, Mazzaferri EI. Hypomagnesemic hypocalcemia secondary to renal magnesium wasting. A possible consequence to high-dose gentamicin therapy. *Ann Intern Med* 1975;82:645.
185. Kozeny GA, et al. Occurrence of renal tubular dysfunction in lupus nephritis. *Arch Intern Med* 1987;147:891.
186. Martinez-Maldonado M, et al. Renal complications in multiple myeloma. Pathophysiology and some aspects of clinical management. *J Chronic Dis* 1971;24:221.
187. Mujais S, Battle DC. Functional correlates of tubulointerstitial damage. *Semin Nephrol* 1988;8:94.
188. Rodriguez-Soriano J, et al. Normokalemic pseudohypoaldosteronism is present in children with acute pyelonephritis. *Acta Paediatr* 1992;81: 402.
189. Eknoyan G, et al. Renal papillary necrosis: an update. *Medicine* 1982;61: 55.
190. Wang LC, et al. Downregulation of AQP 1,-2 and -3 after ureteral obstruction is associated with long term urine concentration defect. *Am J Physiol Renal Physiol* 2001;281:F163
191. Grunfeld JP, et al. Acute renal failure in McArdle's disease. Report of two cases. *N Engl J Med* 1972;286:1237.
192. McCarron DA, et al. Chronic tubulo-interstitial nephritis caused by recurrent myoglobinuria. *Arch Intern Med* 1980;140:1106.
193. Senekjian HO, et al. Irreversible renal failure following vesicoureteral reflux. *JAMA* 1979;241:160.
194. McCluskey RT. Immunologically mediated tubulo-interstitial nephritis. *Contemp Issues Nephrol* 1983;10:121.
195. McCluskey RT, Colvin RB. Immunological aspects of renal tubular and interstitial diseases. *Annu Rev Med* 1978;29:191.
196. McPhaul JJ, Dixon FJ. Characterization of human antiglomerular basement membrane antibodies eluted from glomerulonephritic kidneys. *J Clin Invest* 1970;49:308.
197. Wilson CB. Study of the immunopathogenesis of tubulointerstitial nephritis using model systems. *Kidney Int* 1989;35:938.
198. Bannister KM, Ullich TR, Wilson CB. Induction, characterization and cell transfer of autoimmune tubulointerstitial nephritis. *Kidney Int* 1987;32: 642.
199. Neilson EG. Pathogenesis and therapy of interstitial nephritis. *Kidney Int* 1989;35:1257.
200. Klassen J, McCluskey RT, Milgrom F. Nonglomerular renal disease produced in rabbits by immunization with homologous kidney. *Am J Pathol* 1971;63:333.
201. Hoyer JR. Tubulo-interstitial immune complex nephritis in rats immunized with Tamm-Horsfall protein. *Kidney Int* 1980;17:284.
202. Mayrer AR, et al. Tubulo-interstitial nephritis and immunologic response to Tamm-Horsfall protein. *J Immunol* 1982;128:2634.
203. Seiler MW, Hoyer JR. Ultrastructural studies of tubulointerstitial immune complex nephritis in rats immunized with Tamm-Horsfall protein. *Lab Invest* 1981;45:321.
204. Friedman J, Hoyer JR, Seiler MW. Formation and clearance of tubulointerstitial immune complexes in kidneys of rats immunized with heterologous antisera to Tamm-Horsfall protein. *Kidney Int* 1982;21:575.
205. Makker SP. Tubular basement membrane antibody-induced interstitial nephritis in systemic lupus erythematosus. *Am J Med* 1980;69:949.
206. Hall CL, et al. Passive transfer of autoimmune disease with isologous IgG, and IgG2 and antibodies to the tubular basement membrane in strain XIII

guinea pigs. Loss of self-tolerance induced by autoantibodies. *J Exp Med* 1977;146:1246.

207. Hodson J, et al. Reflux nephropathy. *Kidney Int* 1975;8:S50.

208. Hanson LA, Fasth A, Jodal U. Autoantibodies to Tamm-Horsfall protein, a tool of diagnosing the level of urinary tract infection. *Lancet* 1976;1:226.

209. Vernier RL, Resnick J. Medullary cystic disease: the possible role of Tamm-Horsfall protein. *Kidney Int* 1976;9:450.

210. Barne HJ. Herniations into the renal veins with special reference to hydronephrosis. *J Pathol Bacteriol* 1961;82:177.

211. Chakraborty J, Below AA, Solaiman D. Tamm-Hordfall protein in patients with kidney damage and diabetes. *Urol Res* 2004;32:79.

212. Zager RA, Cotran RS, Hoyer JR. Pathologic localization of Tamm-Horsfall protein in interstitial deposits in renal disease. *Lab Invest* 1978;38:52.

213. Resnick JS, Sisson S, Vernier RL. Tamm-Horsfall protein. Abnormal localization in renal disease. *Lab Invest* 1978;38:550.

214. Sato K, et al. Tubulointerstitial nephritis induced by Tamm-Horsfall protein sensitization in guinea pigs. *Virchows Arch (B)* 1990;58:357.

215. Klassen J, et al. Tubular lesions produced by autoantibodies to tubular basement membrane in human renal allografts. *Int Arch Allergy App Immunol* 1973;45:675.

216. Gordon DL, et al. Amidation of C_3 at the thiolester site: stimulation of phagocytosis and chemiluminescence by a new inflammatory mediator. *J Immunol* 1985;134:3339.

217. Nath KA, Hostetter MK, Hostetter TH. Pathophysiology of chronic tubulointerstitial disease in rats. Interaction of dietary acid load, ammonia and complement C_3. *J Invest* 1985;76:667.

218. Clark EC, et al. Role of ammonia in progressive interstitial nephritis. *Am J Kidney Dis* 1991;17(Suppl 1):15.

219. Bittar EE, Misanik L. Renal necrotizing papillitis. *Am J Med* 1963;34:82.

220. Lehman DH, Wilson CB, Dixon FJ. Extraglomerular immunoglobulin deposits in human nephritis. *Am J Med* 1975;58:765.

221. Klassen J, et al. An immunologic renal tubular lesion in man. *Clin Immunol Immunopathol* 1972;1:69.

222. Yeung CK, et al. Tubular dysfunction in systemic lupus erythematosus. *Nephron* 1984;36:84.

223. O'Dell JR, et al. Tubulointerstitial renal disease in systemic lupus erythematosus. *Arch Intern Med* 1985;145:1996.

224. Bakir AA, et al. Appraisal of lupus nephritis by renal imaging with gallium-67. *Am J Med* 1985;79:175.

225. Case records of the Massachusetts General Hospital, Case 2-1976. *N Engl J Med* 1976;294:100.

226. Andres GA, et al. Human renal transplants. I. Immunopathologic studies. *Lab Invest* 1970;22:588.

227. Miller TE, Stewart E, North JDK. Immunobacteriological aspects of pyelonephritis. *Contrib Nephrol* 1979;16:11.

228. Rosenberg ME, et al. Characterization of immune cells in kidneys from patients with Sjögren's syndrome. *Am J Kidney Dis* 1988;11:20.

229. Winer RL, et al. Sjögren's syndrome with immune complex tubulointerstitial renal disease. *Clin Immunol Immunopathol* 1977;8:494.

230. Andres G, et al. Histology of human tubulo-interstitial nephritis associated with antibodies to renal basement membranes. *Kidney Int* 1978;13:480, 1978.

231. Kambham N, et al. Idiopathic hypocomplmentemic interstitial nephritis with extensive tubulointerstitial deposits. *Am J Kidney Dis* 2001;37:388.

232. Chanarin I, et al. Defect of renal tubular acidification with antibody to loop of Henle. *Lancet* 1974;2:317.

233. Ford PM. A naturally occurring human antibody to loops of Henle. *Clin Exp Immunol* 1973;14:569.

234. Pasternack A, Linder E. Renal tubular acidosis: an immunologal study on four patients. *Clin Exp Immunol* 1970;7:115.

235. Steblay RW, Rudofsky U. Renal tubular disease and autoantibodies against tubular basement membrane induced in guinea pigs. *J Immunol* 1971;107:589.

236. Steblay RW, Rudofsky U. Transfer of experimental autoimmune renal cortical tubular and interstitial disease in guinea pigs by serum. *Science* 1973;180:966.

237. Lehman DH, et al. Specificity of autoantibodies to tubular and glomerular basement membranes induced in guinea pigs. *J Immunol* 1974;112:241.

238. Lehman DH, Wilson CB, Dixon FJ. Interstitial nephritis in rats immunized with heterologous tubular basement membrane. *Kidney Int* 1974;5:187.

239. Clayman MD, et al. Isolation of the target antigen of human anti-tubular basement membrane antibody-associated interstitial nephritis. *J Clin Invest* 1986;077:1143.

240. Fliger FD, et al. Identification of a target antigen in human anti-tubular basement membrane nephritis. *Kidney Int* 1987;31:800.

241. Neilson EG, et al. Molecular characterization of a major nephritogenic domain in the autoantigen of anti-tubular basement membrane disease. *Proc Natl Acad Sci U S A* 1991;88:2006.

242. Butkowski RJ, et al. Distribution of tubulointerstitial nephritis antigens and evidence for multiple forms. *Kidney Int* 1991;40:838.

243. Butkowski RJ, et al. Characterization of a tubular basement membrane component reactive with acute antibodies associated with tubulointerstitial nephritis. *J Biol Chem* 1990;265:21091.

244. Crary GS, et al. Role of a basement membrane glycoprotein in anti-tubular basement membrane nephritis. *Kidney Int* 1993;43:140.

245. Zhou B, et al. Identification of two alternatively spliced forms of tubulonterstitial antigens (TIN-Ag). *J Am Soc Nephrol* 2000;11:658

246. Bergstein JM, Litman N. Interstitial nephritis with antitubular basement membrane antibody. *N Engl J Med* 1975;292:875.

247. Morel-Maroger L, et al. Antitubular basement membrane antibodies in rapidly progressive post-streptococcal glomerulonephritis. Report of a case. *Clin Immunol Immunopathol* 1974;2:185.

248. Spital A, Panner BJ, Sterns RH. Primary acute idiopathic tubulointerstitial nephritis: report of two cases and review of the literature. *Am J Kidney Dis* 1987;9:710.

249. Lindqvist B, Lundberg L, Wieslander J. The prevalence of circulating antitubular basement membrane–antibody in renal diseases and clinical observations. *Clin Nephrol* 1994;41:199.

250. Whitworth JA, et al. Papillary necrosis in renal allografts. Reports of two cases. *Aust N Z J Med* 1975;5:69.

251. Gur H, Kopolovic Y, Gross DJ. Chronic predominant interstitial nephritis in a patient with systemic lupus erythematosus: a follow-up of three years and review of the literature. *Ann Rheum Dis* 1987;46:617.

252. Madias NE, Harrington JT. Platinum nephrotoxicity. *Am J Med* 1978;65:307.

253. Su ZM, et al. Detection of anti-tubular basement membrane antibodies in sera of patients with tubulointerstitial nephritis. *Beijing Da Xue Bao* 2004;36:177.

254. McCluskey RT, Bahn AK. Cell mediated immunity in renal disease. *Hum Pathol* 1986;17:146.

255. Van Zveiten ML, et al. Experimental cell mediated interstitial nephritis induced with exogenous antigens. *J Immunol* 1977;118:589.

256. Neilson EG. Is immunologic tolerance self-modulated through antigen presentation by parenchymal epithelium. *Kidney Int* 1993;44:927.

257. Meyers CM, Kelly CJ. Immunoregulation of TGF-β1: suppression of a nephritogenic murine T cell clone. *Kidney Int* 1994;46:1295.

258. Frank J, et al. Human renal tubular cells as a cytokine source: PDGF-B, GM-CSF, and IL-6 mRNA expression in vitro. *Exp Nephrol* 1993;1:26.

259. Chow J, et al. ICAM-1 expression in renal disease. *J Clin Pathol* 1992;45:880.

260. Schwartz MM, Cotran RZ. Common enterobacterial antigen in human chronic pyelonephritis and interstitial nephritis. An immunofluorescent study. *N Engl J Med* 1973;289:830.

261. Sanford JP, Hunter BW, Donaldson P. Localization and fate of *Escherichia coli* in hematogenous pyelonephritis. *J Exp Med* 1962;116:285.

262. Cotran RS. Retrograde proteus pyelonephritis in rats: localization of antigen and antibody in treated sterile pyelonephrotic kidneys. *J Exp Med* 1963;117:813.

263. Aoki S, et al. "Abacterial" and bacterial pyelonephritis: immunofluorescent localization of bacterial antigen. *N Engl J Med* 1969;281:1375.

264. Hodson CJ. Formation of renal scars with special reference to reflux nephropathy. *Contrib Nephrol* 1979;16:83.

265. Angell ME, Relman AS, Robbins SL. Active chronic pyelonephritis without evidence of bacterial infection. *N Engl J Med* 1968;278:1303.

266. Hodson CJ. Vesico-ureteric reflux and renal scarring with and without infection. *Kidney Int* 1974;5:308.

267. Freedman LR. Natural history of urinary infection in adults. *Kidney Int* 1975;4(Suppl):96.

268. Asscher AW. Renal damage due to urinary tract infection. *Contrib Nephrol* 1979;16:5.

269. Roberts JA. Etiology and pathophysiology of pyelonephritis. *Am J Kidney Dis* 1991;17:1.

270. Simon HB, et al. Genitourinary tuberculosis. Clinical features in a general hospital population. *Am J Med* 1977;63:410.

271. Savage DCL, et al. Controlled trial of therapy in covert bacteriuria in childhood. *Lancet* 1975;1:358.

272. Hucans H, Busch R. Chronic pyelonephritis as a cause of end-stage disease. *J Urol* 1982;127:642.

273. Miller TE, Robinson KB. Experimental pyelonephritis: a new method for inducing pyelonephritis in the rat. *J Infect Dis* 1973;127:307.

274. Miller TE, et al. Modification by suppressor cells and serum factors of cell-mediated immune response in experimental pyelonephritis. *J Clin Invest* 1978;61:964.

275. Korhonen TK, Virkola R, Holthofer H. Localization of binding sites for purified E. coli fimbriae in the human kidney. *Infect Immunol* 1986;54:328.

276. Lehman JD, et al. Local immune response in experimental pyelonephritis. *J Clin Invest* 1968;47:2541.

277. Kurnick JT, et al. *Escherichia coli* specific T lymphocytes in experimental pyelonephritis. *J Immunol* 1988;141:3220.

278. Wuthrich R, et al. MHC class II, antigen presentation and tumor necrosis factor in renal tubular epithelial cells. *Kidney Int* 1990;37:783.

279. Mobley HL, et al. Pyelonephritogenic *Eshericha coli* and killing of cultured human renal proximal tubular epithelial cells: role of hemolysin in some strains. *Infect Immun* 1990;58:1281.

280. Triffilis AL, et al. Binding to and killing of human renal epithelial cells by hemolytic P-fimbriated *E. coli*. *Kidney Int* 1994;46:1083.

281. Svenson M, et al. Natural history of renal scarring in susceptible mIL-8Rh-1 mic. *Kidney Int* 2005; 67:103.

282. Farnaki E, et al. Transforming growth factor beta 1 in the urine of young children with urinary tract infection. *Pediatr Nephrol* 2005;20:180.

283. Krzemien G, et al. Urinary levels if interleukin-8 in children with urinary tract infection to age 2. *Med Sci Monit* 2004;10:CR593.
284. Tardif M, et al. L-651, 392, a potent leukotriene inhibitor, controls inflammatory process in *Escherichia coli* pyelonephritis. *Antimicrob Agents Chemother* 1994;38:1555.
285. Gupta R, et al. Prevention of tissue injury in ascending mouse chronic pyelonephritis—role of free radical scavengers. *Comp Immunol Microbiol Infect Dis* 2004;27:225.
286. Roberts JA, et al. Immunology of pyelonephritis in primates: model IV. Effect of complement depletion. *J Urol* 1983;129:193.
287. Smellie JM. Medical aspects of urinary infection in children. *J R Coll Physicians Lond* 1967;1:189.
288. Smith J, et al. Local antibody production in experimental pyelonephritis: amount, acidity and immunoglobulin class. *Infect Immun* 1974;10:411.
289. Hanson LA, et al. Antigens to *Escherichia coli* human immune response and the pathogenesis of urinary tract infections. *J Infect Dis* 1977;136:S144.
290. Eknoyan G. The natural history of primary pyelonephritis. *Contrib Nephrol* 1989;75:82.
291. Silbert PL, et al. Herpes simplex virus interstitial nephritis in a renal allograft. *Clin Nephrol* 1990;33:264.
292. Platt JL, Sibley RK, Michael AF. Interstitial nephritis associated with cytomegalovirus infection. *Kidney Int* 1985;28:550.
293. Bourgoignie JJ. Renal complications of human immunodeficiency virus type I. *Kidney Int* 1990;37:1571.
294. Strade S, et al. Polyoma virus-associated interstitial nephritis in a patient with acute myeloid leukemia and peripheral blood stem cell transplantation. *Nephrol Dial Transplant* 2003;18:2431.
295. Mathur VS, et al. Polyomavirus-induced interstitial nephritis in two renal transplant recipients: case reports and review of the literature. *Am J Kidney Dis* 1997;29:754.
296. Drachenberg CB, et al. Human polyomavirus in renal allograft biopsies: morphological findings and correlation with urine cytology. *Hum Pathol* 1999;30:970.
297. Randhawa PS, et al. Human polyomavirus-associated interstitial nephritis in the allograft kidney. *Transplantation* 1999;67:103.
298. Howell DN, et al. Diagnosis and management of BK polyomavirus interstitial nephritis in renal transplant recipients. *Transplantation* 1999;68:1279.
299. Cohen AH, Nast CC. HIV-associated nephropathy: a unique combined glomerular, tubular and interstitial lesion. *Modern Pathol* 1988;1:87.
300. Fourman P, McCance RA, Parker RA. Chronic renal disease in rats following a temporary deficiency of potassium. *Br J Exp Pathol* 1955;37:40.
301. Ray PE, et al. bFGF and its low affinity receptors in the pathogenesis of HIV associated nephropathy in transgenic mice. *Kidney Int* 1994;46:759.
302. deCastro MC, et al. Post-traumatic neutrophilic interstitial nephritis—an important cause of graft dysfunction. *Transplant Int* 1998;11:S144.
303. Nagle RB, et al. Unilateral obstructive nephropathy in the rabbit. I. Early morphologic, physiologic, and histochemical changes. *Lab Invest* 1973;28:456.
304. Klahr S, Morrissey J. Obstructive nephropathy and renal fibrosis. *Am J Physiol Renal Physiol* 2002;283:F875.
305. Vielhauser V, et al. Obstructive nephropathy in the mouse: progressive fibrosis correlates with tubulointerstitial chemokine expression and accumulation of CC chemokine receptor 2- and 5-positive leukocytes. *J Am Soc Nephrol* 2001;12:1173.
306. Arant BS. Vesicoureteric reflux and renal injury. *Am J Kidney Dis* 1991;17:491.
307. Mendelsohn C. Functional obstruction: the renal pelvis rules. *J Clin Invest* 2004;113:957.
308. Obha K, et al. Clinicopathological study of vesicoureteral reflux (VUR)-associated pyelonephritis in renal transplantation. *Clin Transplant* 2004;18(Suppl 11):34.
309. Searafini-Cassi F, Malagolini N, Cavallone D. Tamm-Horsfalll glycoprotein: biology and clinical relevance. *Am J Kidney Dis* 2003;42:658.
310. Thomas BD, et al. Tamm-Horsfall protein binds to a single class of carbohydrate specific receptors on human neutrophils. *Kidney Int* 1993;44:423.
311. Cavallone D, Malagolini N, Serafini-Cessi F. Binding of human neutrophils to cell-surface anchored Tamm-Horsfall glycoprotein in tubulointerstitial nephritis. *Kidney Int* 1999;55:1787.
312. Gottschalk CW, Mylle M. Micropuncture study of pressures in proximal tubules and peritubular capillaries of the rat kidney and their reaction to ureteral and renal venous pressures. *Am J Physiol* 1956;185:430.
313. Moffat DB, Lawrence KM. The pathomorphology of intrarenal reflux. *Contrib Nephrol* 1979;16:78.
314. Risholm L. Studies in renal colic and its treatment by posterior splanchnic block. *Acta Chir Scand* 1954;184(Suppl):5.
315. Moffat DB, Lawrence KM. The structure of the pelvis in the immature human kidney. *Nephron* 1976;16:205.
316. Tamminen TE, Kapiro EA. The relationship of the shape of the renal papillae and of collecting duct openings to intrarenal reflux. *Br J Radiol* 1977;49:345.
317. Ransley PG, Risdon RA. Renal papillary morphology and intrarenal reflux in the young pig. *Urol Res* 1975;3:105.
318. Ransley PG, Risdon RA. Renal papillary morphology in infants and young children. *Urol Res* 1975;3:110.
319. Fairley KF, Roysmith J. The forgotten factor in the evaluation of vesicoureteral reflux. *Med J Aust* 1977;2:10.
320. Crisman JM, et al. Chemokine expression in the obstructed kidney. *Exp Nephrol* 2001;9:241.
321. Schreiner GF Jr, et al. Immunological aspects of acute ureteral obstruction: immune cell infiltrate in the kidney. *Kidney Int* 1988;34:487.
322. Rice EK, et al. Macrophage accumulation and renal fibrosis are independent of macrophage migration inhibitory factor in mouse obstructive nephropathy. *Nephrology* 2004;9:278.
323. Schreiner GF Jr, Kohan DE. Regulation of renal transport processes and hemodynamics by macrophages and lymphocytes. *Am J Physiol* 1990;258:F761.
324. Solari S, et al. Cyclooxygenase-2 up-regulation in reflux nephropathy. *J Urol* 2003;170:1624.
325. Eis V, et al. Chemokine receptor CCR1 but not CCR5 mediates leukocyte recruitment and subsequent renal fibrosis after unilateral obstruction. *J Am Soc Nephrol* 2004;15:337.
326. Seiko T, et al. Obstructive nephropathy in mice and humans: potential role of PDGF-D in the progression of tubulointerstitial injury. *J Am Soc Nephrol* 2003;14:3544.
327. Fukuda K, et al. Quantification of TGF-β1 mRNA along rat nephron in obstructive nephropathy. *Am J Physiol Renal Physiol* 2001;281:F513.
328. Guo G, et al. Contributions of angiotensin II and tumor necrosis factor alpha to the development of renal fibrosis. *Am J Physiol Renal Physiol* 2001;280:F777.
329. Klahr S. New insight into the consequences and mechanisms of renal impairment in obstructive nephropathy. *Am J Kidney Dis* 1991;18:689.
330. Klahr S. Interstitial macrophages. *Semin Nephrol* 1993;13:488.
331. Gonzalez-Avila G, Vadillo-Ortega F, Perez-Tamayo R. Experimental diffuse interstitial renal fibrosis: a biochemical approach. *Lab Invest* 1988;59:245.
332. Davis BB, Thomasson D, Zenser TV. Renal disease profoundly alters cortical interstitial cell function. *Kidney Int* 1983;23:458.
333. Cotran RS. Glomerulosclerosis in reflux nephropathy. *Kidney Int* 1982;21:528.
334. Kincaid-Smith P. Glomerular lesions in atrophic pyelonephritis and reflux nephropathy. *Kidney Int* 1975;8:S81.
335. Torres VE, et al. The progression of vesicoureteral reflux nephropathy. *Ann Intern Med* 1980;92:776.
336. Magil AB, Tyler M. Tubulo-interstitial disease in lupus nephritis. A morphometric study. *Histopathology* 1984;8:81.
337. Dentino M, et al. Long-term effect of cis-diaminedichloride platinum (CDDP) on renal function and structure in man. *Cancer* 1978;41:1274.
338. Schwarz A, et al. The outcome of acute interstitial nephritis: risk factors for the transition from acute to chronic interstitial nephritis. *Clin Nephrol* 2000;54:179.
339. Eknoyan G. Analgesic nephrotoxicity and renal papillary necrosis. *Semin Nephrol* 1984;4:65.
340. Svenson K, Bohman S, Hallgren R. Renal interstitial fibrosis and vascular changes: occurrence in patients with autoimmune disease treated with cyclosporine. *Arch Intern Med* 1986;146:2007.
341. Fellstrom B. Cyclosporine nephrotoxicity. *Transplant Proc* 2004;36(Suppl 2):220S.
342. Blachley JD, Hill JB. Renal and electrolyte disturbances associated with cisplatin. *Ann Intern Med* 1981;95:628.
343. Harmon W, et al. Chronic renal failure in children treated with methyl CCNU. *N Engl J Med* 1979;300:1200.
344. Vanherweghem JL, et al. Rapidly progressive interstitial renal fibrosis in young women: association with slimming regimen including Chinese herbs. *Lancet* 1993;341:387.
345. Depierreux M, et al. Pathologic aspects of a newly described nephropathy related to the prolonged use of Chinese herbs. *Am J Kidney Dis* 1994;24:172.
346. Bagnis IC, et al. Herbs and the kidney. *Am J Kidney Dis* 2004;44:1.
347. Colson CR, Debroe ME. Kidney injury from alternative medicines. *Adv Chronic Kidney Dis* 2005;12:261
348. Case Records of the Massachusetts General Hospital, Case 17-1981. *N Engl J Med* 1981;304:1025.
349. Hansen HE, et al. Chronic interstitial nephropathy in patients on long-term lithium treatment. *Q J Med* 1979;48:577.
350. Pitman SW, Parker LM, Tattersall MH. Clinical trial of high dose methotrexate with citrovorum factor: toxicologic and therapeutic observations. *Cancer Chemother Rep* 1975;6:43.
351. World MJ, et al. Mesalazine-associated interstitial nephritis. *Nephrol Dial Transplant* 1996;11:614.
352. Corrigan G, Stevens PE. Interstitial nephritis associated with the use of mesalazine in inflammatory bowel disease. *Aliment Pharmacol Ther* 2000;14:1.
353. DeBroe ME, et al. 5-Aminosalicylic acid (5ASA) and chronic tubulointerstitial nephritis in patients with chronic inflammatory bowel disease: is there a link? *Nephrol Dial Transplant* 1997;12:1839.
354. Clive DM, Stoff JS. Renal syndromes associated with nonsteroidal anti-inflammatory drugs. *N Engl J Med* 1984;310:563.
355. Henrich WL. Nephrotoxicity of nonsteroidal anti-inflammatory agents. *Am J Kidney Dis* 1983;2:478.
356. Eknoyan G. Current status of chronic analgesic and nonsteroidal anti-inflammatory drug nephropathy. *Curr Opin Nephrol Hypertens* 1994;3:182.

357. Eknoyan G. Alternative medicine: the renaissance of an unbroken tradition. *Adv Chronic Kidney Dis* 2005;12:247

358. Cosyns JP. Aristolochic acid and 'chinese herb nephropathy'; a review of the evidence to date. *Drug Saf* 2003;26:33.

359. Lebeau C, et al. Aristolochic acid impedes endocytosis and induces DNA adducts in the proximal tubule cells. *Kidney Int* 2001;60:1332.

360. Debelle FD, et al. The rennin-angiotensin system blockade does not prevent renal interstitial fibrosis induce by aristolochic acid. *Kidney Int* 2004;66:1815.

361. Vanherweghem J. Nephropathy and herbal medicine. *Am J Kidney Dis* 2000;35:330.

362. Arlt VM, Shirborova M, Schmeiser HH. Aristolochic acid as a probable cause of human cancer hazard in herbal remedies: a review. *Mutagenesis* 2002;17:265.

363. Yang C, et al. Rapidly progressive fibrosing interstitial nephritis associated with Chinese herbal drugs. *Am J Kidney Dis* 2000;35:313.

364. Vanherweghem JL. Nephropathy and herbal medicine. *Am J Kidney Dis* 2000;35:330.

365. DePaulo JR, Correa EI, Sapir DG. Renal toxicity of lithium and its implications. *John Hopkins Med J* 1981;149:15.

366. Boton R, Gaviria M, Battle D. Prevalence, pathogenesis and treatment of renal dysfunction associated with chronic lithium therapy. *Am J Kidney Dis* 1987;10:329.

367. Walker RG, et al. Chronic progressive renal lesions induced by lithium. *Kidney Int* 1986;29:875.

368. Walker RG, et al. A clinico-pathological study of lithium nephrotoxicity. *J Chronic Dis* 1982;35:685.

369. Timmer RT, Sands JM. Lithium intoxication. *J Am Soc Nephrol* 1999;10:666.

370. Markowitz G, et al. Lithium nephrotoxicity: a progressive combined glomerular and tubulointerstitial nephropathy. *J Am Soc Nephrol* 2000;11:1439.

371. Gitlin M. Lithium and the kidney. An updated review. *Drug Saf* 1999;20:231.

372. Presne C, et al. Lithium-induced nephropathy: rate of progression and prognostic factors. *Kidney Int* 2003;64:585.

373. Johnson GF, et al. Renal function and lithium treatment initial and follow-up tests in manic-depressive patients. *J Affective Disord* 1984;6:249.

374. Marples D, et al. Lithium-induced downregulation of aquaporin-2 water channel expression in rat kidney medulla. *J Clin Invest* 1995;95:1838.

375. Spuhler O, Zollinger HU. Die chronische interstitielle nephritis. *Z Klin Med* 1953;151:1.

376. Zollinger HU. Chronische interstitielle nephritis bei abusus von phenacetin hatingen analgetua. *Schweiz Med Woschenschr* 1955;85:746.

377. Gault MH, Blennerhasset J, Muehrcke RC. Analgesic nephropathy: a clinicopathologic study using electron microscopy. *Am J Med* 1971;51:740.

378. Gault MH, et al. Syndrome associated with the abuse of analgesics. *Ann Intern Med* 1968;68:906.

379. Jacobs LA, Morris JG. Renal papillary necrosis and abuse of phenacetin. *Med J Aust* 1962;2:531.

380. Larsen K, Moller CE. Renal lesions caused by abuse of phenacetin. *Acta Med Scand* 1959;165:321.

381. Sanerkin NG. Chronic phenacetin nephropathy with particular reference to the relationship between renal papillary necrosis and "chronic interstitial nephritis." *Br J Urol* 1966;38:361.

382. Schreiner GE. The nephrotoxicity of analgesic abuse. *Ann Intern Med* 1962;57:1047.

383. Gonwa TA, Hamilton RW, Buckalew VA. Chronic renal failure and end-stage renal disease in northwest North Carolina. *Arch Intern Med* 1981;141:462.

384. Gregg NJ, et al. Epidemiology and mechanistic basis of analgesic-associated nephropathy. *Toxicol Lett* 1989;46:141.

385. Michielsen P, Schepper P. Trends of analgesic nephropathy in two endemic regions with different legislation. *J Am Soc Nephrol* 2001;12:550.

386. Stewart JH, et al. Interpreting incidence trends for treated end-stage renal disease: implications for evaluating disease control in Australia. *Nephrology* 2004;9:238.

387. McAnally JF, Winchester JF, Schreiner GE. Analgesic nephropathy: an uncommon cause of end-stage renal disease. *Arch Intern Med* 1983;143:1897.

388. Murray TG, et al. Epidemiologic study of regular analgesic use and end-stage renal disease. *Arch Intern Med* 1983;143:1687.

389. Plotz A. Analgesic nephropathy: for this time and this place. *Arch Intern Med* 1983;143:1676.

390. Ramsay AG, Whick DF. Phenacetin nephropathy. *Can Med Assoc J* 1965;92:55.

391. Kincaid-Smith P. Pathogenesis of the renal lesions associated with the abuse of analgesics. *Lancet* 1967;1:859.

392. Bach PH, Hardy TL. Relevance of animal models to analgesic-associated renal papillary necrosis in humans. *Kidney Int* 1985;28:605.

393. Duggin GG. Mechanisms in the development of analgesic nephropathy. *Kidney Int* 1980;18:553.

394. Ford SM, Hook PB. Biochemical mechanisms of toxic nephropathies. *Semin Nephrol* 1984;4:88.

395. Lorx C, et al. Paracetamol-induced renal tubular injury: a role for ER stress. *J Am Soc Nephrol* 2004;15:380.

396. Davis BB, Mattammal MB, Zenser TV. Renal metabolism of drugs and xenobiotics. *Nephron* 1981;27:187.

397. Bell D, et al. Analgesic nephropathy: clinical course after withdrawal of phenacetin. *Br Med J* 1969;3:38.

398. Tebloeva LT, Latysheva NM. Tubulo-interstitial syndrome in children with hemolytic-uremic syndrome. *Pediatria* 1991;7:55.

399. Brummer FP, Selwood NH, for the EDTA-ERA Registree Committee. End-stage renal failure due to analgesic nephropathy, its changing pattern and cardiovascular mortality. *Nephrol Dial Transplant* 1994;9:1371.

400. Elseviers MM, et al. Diagnostic criteria of analgesic nephropathy in patients with end-stage renal failure: results of the Belgian Study. *Nephrol Dial Transplant* 1992;7:479.

401. Gloor FJ. Changing concepts in the pathogenesis and morphology of analgesic nephropathy as seen in Europe. *Kidney Int* 1978;13:27.

402. Kincaid-Smith P, Saker BM, McKenzie IF. Lesions in the vasa recta in experimental analgesic nephropathy. *Lancet* 1968;1:24.

403. Molland EA. Experimental renal papillary necrosis. *Kidney Int* 1978;13:5.

404. Dubach UC, Rosner B, Pfister E. Epidemiologic study of analgesic containing phenacetin: renal morbidity and mortality (1968–1979). *N Engl J Med* 1983;308:357.

405. Duffy WB, et al. Management of asymptomatic hyperuricemia. *JAMA* 1981;246:2215.

406. Burry AF. The evolution of analgesic nephropathy. *Nephron* 1967;5:185.

407. Murray RM. Patterns of analgesic use and abuse of medical patients. *Practitioner* 1973;211:639.

408. Wainscoat IS, Finn R. Possible role of laxatives in analgesic nephropathy. *Br Med J* 1974;4:697.

409. Nordenfelt O. Deaths from renal failure in abusers of phenacetin containing drugs. *Acta Med Scand* 1972;191:11.

410. Perneger TV, Whelton PK, Klag MJ. Risk of kidney failure associated with the use of acetaminophen, aspirin, and nonsteroidal antiinflammatory drugs. *N Engl J Med* 1994;331:1675.

411. Pommer W, Bronder E, Greiser E. Regular analgesic intake and the risk of end-stage renal failure. *Am J Nephrol* 1989;9:403.

412. Morlans M, et al. End-stage renal disease and non-narcotic analgesics: a case-control study. *Br J Clin Pharmacol* 1990;30:717.

413. Mellemgaard A, et al. Risk of kidney cancer in analgesic users. *J Clin Epidemiol* 1992;45:1021.

414. McCredie M, Stewart JH. Does paracetamol cause urothelial cancer or renal papillary necrosis? *Nephron* 1988;49:296.

415. Piper J, Tonascia J, Matanoshi G. Heavy phenacetin use and bladder cancer in women aged 20 to 49 years. *N Engl J Med* 1985;313:292.

416. McCredie M, Stewart JH, Day NE. Different roles for phenacetin and paracetamol in cancer of the kidney and renal pelvis. *Int J Cancer* 1993;53:245.

417. McCredie M, et al. Phenacetin and papillary necrosis: independent risk factors for renal pelvic cancer. *Kidney Int* 1986;30:81.

418. Mihatsch M, Thiel G, Ryffel B. Cyclosporin A: action and side effects. *Toxicol Lett* 1989;46:125.

419. Mihatsch M, et al. Morphological finding in kidney transplants after treatment with cyclosporine. *Transplant Proc* 1983;15:2821.

420. Neild GH, et al. Glomerular thrombi in renal allografts associated with cyclosporine treatment. *J Clin Pathol* 1985;38:253.

421. Shulman H, et al. Nephrotoxicity of cyclosporin A after allogenic marrow transplantation. *N Engl J Med* 1981;305:1392.

422. Wolfe JA, McCann RL, Sanfilipo F. Cyclosporine-associated microangiopathy in renal transplantation: a severe but potentially reversible form of early graft injury. *Transplantation* 1986;41:541.

423. Gillum DM, Truong L, Tasby J. Characterization of the interstitial cellular infiltrate in experimental chronic cyclosporine nephropathy. *Transplantation* 1990;49:793.

424. Klintmalm G, et al. Interstitial fibrosis in renal allografts after 12 to 46 months of cyclosporine treatment: beneficial effects of low doses in early post-transplantation period. *Lancet* 1984;2:950.

425. Ruiz P, et al. Associations between cyclosporine therapy and interstitial fibrosis in renal allograft biopsies. *Transplantation* 1988;45:91.

426. Sun BK, et al. Expression of transferring growth factor-beta inducible gene-h3 in normal and cyclosporine-treated rat kidney. *J Lab Clin Med* 2004;143:175.

427. Xin J, et al. Suppression of cyclosporine A nephrotoxicity in vivo by transforming growth factor β receptor-immunoglobulin G chimeric protein. *Transplant* 2004;77:1433.

428. Johnson DW, et al. Enalaprilat directly ameliorates in vitro cyclosporine nephrotoxicity in human tubulo-interstitial cells. *Nephron* 2000;86:473.

429. Myers BD, et al. The long-term course of cyclosporine-associated chronic nephropathy. *Kidney Int* 1988;33:590.

430. Remuzzi G, Bertani T. Renal vascular and thrombotic effects of cyclosporine. *Am J Kidney Dis* 1989;13:261.

431. Nankiwell BJ, et al. Delta analysis of posttransplantation tubulointerstitial damage. *Transplant* 2004;78:434.

432. Kim HC, et al. Primary immunosuppression with tacrolimus in kidney transplantation: three year follow up in a single center. *Transplant Proc* 2004;36:2082.

433. Martins L, et al. Cyclosporine versus tacrolimus in kidney transplantation: are there differences in nephrotoxicity? *Transpl Proc* 2004;36:877.

434. Moutabarrik A, et al. FK506 mechanism of nephrotoxicity: stimulatory effect on endothelin secretion by cultured kidney cells. *Transplant Int* 1992;5(Suppl 1):393.

435. Sergeant GR. *The Clinical Features of Sickle Cell Disease*. New York: American Elsevier; 1974:1.

436. Vaamonde CA. Renal papillary necrosis in sickle cell hemoglobinopathies. *Semin Nephrol* 1984;4:48.

437. Papadaki MG, et al. Abdominal ultrasonographic findings with sickle cell and thalassemia. *Pediatr Radiol* 2003;33:515.

438. Khademi M, Marquis JR. Renal angiography in sickle cell disease: a preliminary report correlating the angiographic and urographic changes in sickle cell nephropathy. *Radiology* 1973;107:41.

439. Statius van Eps LW, et al. Nature of concentrating defect in sickle cell nephropathy: microradioangiographic studies. *Lancet* 1970;1:450.

440. Scheinman JL. Sickle cell disease and the kidney. *Semin Nephrol* 2003;23:66.

441. Wesson D. The initiation and progression of sickle cell nephropathy. *Kidney Int* 2002;61:2277.

442. Pham PT, et al. Renal abnormalities in sickle cell disease. *Kidney Int* 2000;57:1.

443. Buckalew VM Jr, Someren A. Renal manifestations of sickle cell disease. *Arch Intern Med* 1974;133:660.

444. Kimmelstiel P. Vascular occlusion and ischemic infarction in sickle cell disease. *Am J Med Sci* 1948;216:11.

445. Allon M. Renal abnormalities in sickle cell disease. *Arch Intern Med* 1990;150:501.

446. Herrera J, et al. Impaired creatinine secretion after intravenous creatinine load is an early characteristic of the nephropathy of sickle cell anemia. *Nephrol Dial Transplant* 2002;17:602.

447. Kyle RA. Multiple myeloma: review of 869 cases. *Mayo Clin Proc* 1975;50:29.

448. Le Goas F, et al. Tubulointerstitial renal complications of myeloma. *Rev Prat* 1993;43:307.

449. Herrera G, et al. Renal pathologic spectrum in an autopsy series of patients with plasma cell dyscrasias. *Arch Pathol Lab Med* 2004;128:875.

450. Iggo N, et al. Chronic dialysis patients with multiple myeloma and renal failure: a worthwhile treatment. *Q J Med* 1989;73:903.

451. Korzets A, et al. The role of continuous ambulatory peritoneal dialysis in end-stage renal failure due to myeloma. *Am J Kidney Dis* 1990;16:216.

452. Alexanian R, Barlogie B, Dixon D. Renal failure in multiple myeloma: pathogenesis and prognostic implications. *Arch Intern Med* 1990; 150:1693.

453. Clyne DH, et al. Nephrotoxicity of Bence-Jones protein in the rat: importance of protein isoelectric point. *Kidney Int* 1979;16:345.

454. Kyle RA. Monoclonal gammopathies and the kidney. *Ann Rev Med* 1989;40:53.

455. Norden AG, et al. Renal impairment of myeloma: negative association with isoelectric point of excreted Bence-Jones protein. *J Clin Pathol* 1989;42:59.

456. Preud'Homme J, et al. Monoclonal immunoglobulin deposition disease (Randall type): relationship with structural abnormalities of immunoglobulin chains. *Kidney Int* 1994;46:965.

457. Rota S, et al. Multiple myeloma and severe renal failure: a clinicopathologic study of outcome and prognosis in 34 patients. *Medicine* 1987;66:127.

458. Sakhuja V, et al. Renal involvement in multiple myeloma: a 10 year study. *Ren Fail* 2000;22:465.

459. Pasquali S, et al. Long-term survival of patients with acute and severe renal failure due to multiple myeloma. *Clin Nephrol* 1990;34:247.

460. Batuman V, Dreishbach AW, Cryan J. Light-chain binding sites on renal brush-border membranes. *Am J Physiol* 1990;258:F1259.

461. Korbet SM, Schwartz M, Lewis EJ. The fibrillary glomerulopathies. *Am J Kidney Dis* 1994;23:751.

462. Ivanyi B. Frequency of light chain deposition nephropathy relative to renal amyloidosis and Bence-Jones cast nephropathy in a necropsy study of patients with myeloma. *Arch Pathol Lab Med* 1990;114:986.

463. Sanders PW, et al. Spectrum of glomerular and tubulointerstitial renal lesions associated with monotypical immunoglobulin light chain deposition. *Lab Invest* 1991;64:527.

464. Martinez-Maldonado M, Ramirez-Arillano GA. Renal involvement in malignant lymphoma: a survey of 49 cases. *J Urol* 1966;95:485.

465. Tomroth T, et al. Lymphoma diagnosed by percutaneous kidney biopsy. *Am J Kidney Dis* 2003;42:960.

466. Morel-Maroger L, et al. Prognostic importance of vascular lesions in acute renal failure with microangiopathic hemolytic anemia. Chemolytic-uremic syndrome: clinicopathologic study in 20 adults. *Kidney Int* 1979;15:548.

467. Bremner I. Mammalian absorption, transport and excretion of cadmium. *Top Environ Health* 1979;2:175.

468. Adams RG, Harrison F, Scott P. The development of cadmium-induced proteinuria, impaired renal function, and osteomalacia in alkaline battery workers. *Q J Med* 1969;38:425.

469. Lindquist B, et al. Cadmium concentration in human biopsies. *Scand J Urol Nephrol* 1989;23:213.

470. Kazantzis G. Cadmium nephropathy. *Contrib Nephrol* 1979;16:161.

471. Jung L, et al. Urinary proteins and enzymes as early indicators of renal dysfunction in chronic exposure to cadmium. *Clin Chem* 1993;39:757.

472. Jarup L, Elinder CG. Incidence of renal stones among cadmium exposed battery workers. *Br J Ind Med* 1993;50:598.

473. Morgan JM, Hartley MN. Etiologic factors in lead nephropathy. *South Med J* 1976;69:1445.

474. Wedeen RP, et al. Occupational lead nephropathy. *Am J Med* 1975;59:630.

475. Batuman V, et al. Contribution of lead to hypertension with renal impairment. *N Engl J Med* 1983;309:17.

476. Batuman V, et al. The role of lead in gouty nephropathy. *N Engl J Med* 1981;304:520.

477. Wedeen RP, Mallik DK, Batuman V. Detection and treatment of occupational lead nephropathy. *Arch Intern Med* 1979;139:53.

478. Sanchez-Fructuoso AI, et al. Experimental lead nephropathy: treatment with calcium disodium ethylenediaminetetraacetate. *Am J Kidney Dis* 2002;40:59.

479. Lin J, et al. Environmental lead exposure and progression of chronic renal diseases in patients without diabetes. *New Engl J Med* 2003;348:277.

480. Roxe DM, Krumlovsky FA. Toxic interstitial nephropathy from metals, metabolites and radiation. *Semin Nephrol* 1988;8:72.

481. Porter GA, ed. *Nephrotoxic Mechanisms of Drugs and Environmental Toxins*. New York: Plenum Press; 1982.

482. Navarte J, Saba SR, Ramirez G. Occupational exposure to organic solvents causing chronic tubulointerstitial nephritis. *Arch Intern Med* 1989;149:154.

483. Goyer R, et al. Urinary biomarkers to detect significant effect of environmental and occupational exposure to nephrotoxins. II. Nephrotoxins of significant frequency and economic impact. *Ren Fail* 1997;19:523.

484. Roels H, et al. Markers of early renal changes induced by industrial pollutants. *Br J Ind Med* 1993;50:37.

485. Truong LD, et al. Experimental chronic renal ischemia: morphologic and immunologic studies. *Kidney Int* 1992;41:1676.

486. Gellman DD, et al. Diabetic nephropathy. *Medicine* 1959;38:321.

487. Akikusa B, et al. Tubulointerstitial changes in systemic vasculitis disorders: a quantitative study of 18 biopsy cases. *Am J Kidney Dis* 1990;16:481.

488. Nojima Y, et al. Tubulointerstitial immune complex nephritis in a patient with cutaneous vasculitis. *Clin Nephrol* 1986;25:48.

489. Johnson RJ, et al. Hypertension: a microvascular and tubulointerstitial disease. *J Hypertens* 2002;20(Suppl 3):S1.

490. Keane WF, et al. Radiation-induced renal disease: a clinicopathologic study. *Am J Med* 1976;60:127.

491. Luxton RW. Radiation nephritis. *Q J Med* 1953;22:215.

492. Asseher AW, Wilson C, Anson SG. Sensitization of blood vessels to hypertensive damage by X-irradiation. *Lancet* 1961;1:580.

493. Arruda JA. Radiation nephritis. *Contemp Issues Nephrol* 1983;10:275.

494. Cameron JS, Simmonds HA. Gout and crystal-related nephropathy. *Contrib Nephrol* 1979;16:147.

495. Foley R, Weinman EJ. Urate nephropathy. *Am J Med Sci* 1984;288:208.

496. Yu TF, Guttman AB. Uric acid nephrolithiasis in gout: predisposing factors. *Ann Intern Med* 1967;67:1133.

497. Kippen I, et al. Factors affecting urate solubility in vitro. *Ann Rheum Dis* 1974;33:313.

498. Emmerson BT, Row PG. An evaluation of the pathogenesis of the gouty kidney. *Kidney Int* 1975;8:65.

499. Epstein FH, Pigeon G. Experimental urate nephropathy: studies of the distribution of urate in renal disease. *Nephron* 1964;1:144.

500. Barlow KA, Beilin KI. Renal disease of primary gout. *Q J Med (New Series)* 1968;37:79.

501. Gonick HC, et al. The renal lesion in gout. *Ann Intern Med* 1965;62:667.

502. Seegmiller JA, Frazier PP. Biological considerations of the renal damage of gout. *Ann Rheum Dis* 1966;25(Suppl 6):668.

503. Farebrother DA, et al. Experimental crystal nephropathy: one year study in the pig. *Clin Nephrol* 1975;4:243.

504. Talbott JH, Terplan KL. The kidney in gout. *Medicine* 1960;39:405.

505. Yu TF, Berger L. Impaired renal function in gout. *Am J Med* 1982;72:95.

506. Yu TF, et al. Renal function in gout. *Am J Med* 1979;67:766.

507. Tessel WJ. Renal outcomes of gout and hyperuricemia. *Am J Med* 1979;67:74.

508. Duffy WB, Senekjian HO, Knight TF. Management of asymptomatic hyperuricemia. *JAMA* 1981;246:2215.

509. Messerli FH, et al. Serum uric acid in essential hypertension: an indicator of renal vascular involvement. *Ann Intern Med* 1980;93:817.

510. Khosla UM, et al. Hyperuricemia induces endothelial dysfunction. *Kidney Int* 2005;67:1739.

511. Mazzali M, et al. Elevated uric acid increase blood pressure in the rat by a novel crystal-intendant mechanism. *Hypertension* 2001;38:1101.

512. Johnson RJ, et al. Reappraisal of the pathogenesis and consequences of hyperuricemia in hypertension, cardiovascular disease and renal disease. *Am J Kidney Dis* 1999;33:225.

513. Kang D, Nakagawa T. Uric acid and renal disease: possible implications of hyperuricemial on progression of renal disease. *Sem Nephrol* 2005;25:43.

514. Sanchez-Lozada LG. Mild hyperuricemia induces vasoconstriction and maintains glomerular hypertension in normal and remnant kidney. *Kidney Int* 2005;67:237.

515. Farkas WR, Stanawitz T, Schneider M. Saturnine gout: lead-induced formation of guanine crystals. *Science* 1978;199:786.

516. Fanger H, Esparza A. Crystals of calcium oxalate in the kidney in uremia. *Am J Clin Pathol* 1964;41:597.

517. Khan SR, Finlayson B, Hackett RL. Scanning electron microscopy of calcium oxalate crystal formation in experimental nephrolithiasis. *Lab Invest* 1979;41:504.

518. Thompson CS, Weinman EJ. The significance of oxalate in renal failure. *Am J Kidney Dis* 1984;4:97.

519. Hodgkinson A, Wilkinson R. Plasma oxalate concentration and renal excretion of oxalate in man. *Clin Sci Mol Med* 1974;46:61.

520. Farrel G, et al. Modulation of proliferating renal epithelial cell affinity for calcium oxalate monohydrate crystals. *J Am Soc Nephrol* 2004;15:3052.

521. Mo L, et al. Tamm-Horsfall protein is a critical renal defense factor protecting against calcium oxalate crystal formation. *Kidney Int* 2004;66:1159.

522. Khan SR. Crystal-induced inflammation of the kidneys: results from human studies, animal models and tissue culture studies. *Clin Exp Nephrol* 2004;8:75.

523. Tobilli N, et al. Effects of angiotensin II subtype 1 receptor blockade by losartan on tubulointerstitial lesions caused by hyperoxaluria. *J Urol* 2002;168:1550.

524. Wacker WE, Haynes H, Druyan R. Treatment of ethylene glycol poisoning with ethyl alcohol. *JAMA* 1965;194:1231.

525. Mazzer T, Shue GL, Jackson SH. Renal dysfunction associated with methoxyflurane anesthesia. *JAMA* 1971;216:278.

526. Cryer PE, et al. Renal failure after small intestinal bypass for obesity. *Arch Intern Med* 1975;135:1610.

527. Chadwick VS, Modha K, Dowling RH. Mechanisms for hyperoxaluria in patients with ileal dysfunction. *N Engl J Med* 1973;289:172.

528. Worcester EM. Stones from bowel disease. *Endocrinol Metab Clin North Am* 2002;31:979.

529. Benabe J, Martinez-Maldonado M. Hypercalcemic nephropathy. *Arch Intern Med* 1978;138:777.

530. Epstein FH. Calcium and the kidney. *Am J Med* 1968;45:700.

531. Levitt MF, et al. The effect of abrupt changes in plasma calcium concentrations on renal function and electrolyte excretion in man and monkey. *J Clin Invest* 1958;37:294.

532. Marone C, Beretta-Piccoli C, Weidman P. Acute hypercalcemic hypertension in man: role of hemodynamics, catecholamines and renin. *Kidney Int* 1980;20:92.

533. Suki WN, et al. The renal diluting and concentrating mechanism in hypercalcemia. *Nephron* 1969;6:50.

534. Beck N, et al. Pathogenic role of cyclic AMP in the impairment of urinary concentrating ability in acute hypercalcemia. *J Clin Invest* 1974;54:1049.

535. Berl T. Cellular calcium uptake in the action of prostaglandins on renal water excretion. *Kidney Int* 1981;19:15.

536. Dousa TP, Valtin H. Cellular action of vasopressin in the mammalian kidney. *Kidney Int* 1976;10:46.

537. Peterson MJ, Edelman IS. Calcium inhibition of the action of vasopressin on the urinary bladder of the toad. *J Clin Invest* 1964;43:583.

538. Earm JH, et al. Decreased aquaporin-2 expression and apical plasma membrane delivery in kidney collecting ducts of polyuric hypercalcemic rats. *J Am Soc Nephrol* 1998;9:2181.

539. Ganote CE, et al. Acute calcium nephrotoxicity: an electron microscopic and semiquantitative light microscopic study. *Arch Pathol Lab Med* 1975;99:650.

540. Levi M, Ellis MA, Berl T. Control of renal hemodynamics and glomerular filtration rate in chronic hypercalcemia. Role of prostaglandins, renin-angiotensin, and calcium. *J Clin Invest* 1983;71:1624.

541. Caulfield JB, Shrag PE. Electron microscopic study of renal calcification. *Am J Pathol* 1964;44:365.

542. Scarpelli DG. Experimental nephrocalcinosis: a biochemical and morphological study. *Lab Invest* 1965;14:123.

543. Giacomelli F, Spiro D, Wiener J. A study of metastatic calcification at the cellular level. *J Cell Biol* 1964;22:189.

544. Relman AS, Schwartz WB. The kidney in potassium depletion. *Am J Med* 1958;24:764.

545. Schwartz WB, Relman AS. Effect of electrolyte disorders on renal structure and function. *N Engl J Med* 1967;276:383.

546. Rubini M. Water excretion in potassium deficient man. *J Clin Invest* 1961;40:2215.

547. Raymond KH, Davidson KK, McKinney TD. *In vivo* and *in vitro* studies of urinary concentrating ability in potassium depleted rabbits. *J Clin Invest* 1985;76:561.

548. Eknoyan G, et al. Renal diluting capacity in the hypokalemic rat. *Am J Physiol* 1970;219:933.

549. Tannen RL. The effect of uncomplicated potassium depletion on urine acidification. *J Clin Invest* 1970;49:813.

550. Biava GG, et al. Kaliopenic nephropathy: a correlated light and electron microscopy study. *Lab Invest* 1963;12:443.

551. Cremer W, Bock KD. Symptoms and causes of chronic hypokalemia nephropathy in man. *Clin Nephrol* 1977;7:112.

552. Gullner HG, et al. A sibship with hypokalemic alkalosis and renal proximal tubulopathy. *Arch Intern Med* 1983;143:1534.

553. Wallace MR, et al. End-stage renal failure due to familial hypokalemic interstitial nephritis with identical HLA tissue types. *N Z Med J* 1985;98:5.

554. Fourman P, McCance RA, Parker RA. Chronic renal disease in rats following a temporary deficiency of potassium. *Br J Exp Pathol* 1955;37:40.

555. Toback FG, et al. Zonal changes in renal structure and phospholipid metabolism in potassium deficient rats. *Lab Invest* 1976;34:115.

556. Woods JW, et al. Susceptibility of rats to experimental pyelonephritis following recovery from potassium depletion. *J Clin Invest* 1960;39:28.

557. Carone FA, Kashgarian M, Epstein FH. Effect of acute potassium deficiency on susceptibility to infection with particular reference to the kidney. *Yale J Biol Med* 1959;32:100.

558. Tolins JP, Hostetter MK, Hostetter TH. Hypokalemic nephropathy in the rat: role of ammonia in chronic tubular injury. *J Clin Invest* 1987;79:1147.

559. Ray PE, et al. Renal vascular induction of TGF-beta2 and renin by potassium depletion. *Kidney Int* 1993;44:1006.

560. Tsao E, et al. Expression of insulin-like growth factor-1 and transferring growth factor beta in hypokalemic nephropathy in the rat. *Kidney Int* 2001;39:96.

561. Suga S, et al. Angiotensin II type 1 receptor blockade ameliorates tubulointerstitial injured induce by potassium deficiency. *Kidney Int* 2002;61:951.

562. Pitt B, et al. The effect of spironolactone on morbidity and mortality in patients with severe heart failure. *N Engl J Med* 1999;341:709.

563. Hollenberg N. Aldosterone in the development and progression of renal injury. *Kidney Int* 2004;66:1.

564. Fujisawa G. Spironolactone prevents early renal injury in streptozocin-induced diabetic rats. *Kidney Int* 2004;66:1493.

565. Trachtman H, et al. Prevention of renal fibrosis by spironolactone in mice with complete unilateral ureteral obstruction. *J Urol* 2004;172:1590.

566. Spear GS. Pathology of the kidney in cystinosis. *Pathol Annu* 1974;9:81.

567. Teree TM, et al. Cystinosis and proximal tubular nephropathy in siblings: progressive development of the physiological and anatomical lesions. *Am J Dis Child* 1970;119:481.

568. van't Hoff WG, et al. Early onset of chronic renal failure as presentation of infantile nephropathic cystinosis. *Pediatric Nephrol* 1995;9:483.

569. Haugulstaine D, et al. Glomerulonephritis in late-onset cystinosis: report of two cases and review of the literature. *Clin Nephrol* 1976;6:529.

570. Coles GA, Robinson K, Branch RA. Familial interstitial nephritis. *Clin Nephrol* 1976;6:513.

571. Bernstein J, Gardner KD. Hereditary tubulo-interstitial nephropathies. *Contemp Issues Nephrol* 1983;9:335.

572. Pan J, Wang Q, Snell WJ. Cilium-generated signaling and cilia-related disorders. *Lab Invest* 2005;21:452.

573. Praetorius HA, Spring KR. A physiological view of the primary cilium. *Ann Rev Physiol* 2005;67:515.

574. Carone FA. Functional changes in polycystic kidney disease are tubulo-interstitial in origin. *Semin Nephrol* 1988;8:89.

575. Carone FA, Makino H, Kanwar YS. Basement membrane antigens in renal polycystic kidney disease. *Am J Pathol* 1988;130:466.

576. Grantham JJ, Geiser JL, Evan AP. Cyst formation and growth in autosomal dominant polycystic kidney disease. *Kidney Int* 1987;31:1145.

577. Kelly CJ, Neilson EG. Medullary cystic disease: an inherited form of autoimmune interstitial nephritis? *Am J Kidney Dis* 1987;10:389.

578. Wilson PD. Polycystic kidney disease. *New Engl J Med* 2004;350:161.

579. Grantham JJ. Understanding polycystic kidney disease: a system biology approach. *Kidney Int* 2003;64:1157.

580. Igarashi P, Somlo S. Genetics and pathogenesis of polycystic kidney disease. *J Am Soc Nephrol* 2002;13:2384.

581. Eknoyan G, et al. Renal function in experimental cystic disease of the rat. *J Lab Clin Med* 1976;88:402.

582. Gabow PA, et al. The clinical utility of renal concentrating capacity of polycystic kidney disease. *Kidney Int* 1989;35:675.

583. Martinez-Maldonado M, et al. Adult polycystic disease: demonstration of a defect in urine concentration in patients without renal insufficiency and studies of its mechanism. *Kidney Int* 1972;2:107.

584. Bell PE, et al. Hypertension in autosomal dominant polycystic kidney disease. *Kidney Int* 1988;34:683.

585. Grantham JJ. Polycystic kidney disease: a predominance of giant nephrons. *Am J Physiol* 1983;244:F3.

586. Grantham JJ. Polycystic kidney disease: hereditary and acquired. *Kidney* 1984;17:19.

587. Hansson L, et al. Hypertension in polycystic kidney disease. *Scand J Urol Nephrol* 1974;8:203.

588. Seegal AJ, Spataro RF, Barbanic ZL. Adult polycystic disease: a review of 100 eases. *J Urol* 1977;118:711.

589. Suki WN. Polycystic kidney disease. *Kidney Int* 1982;22:571.

590. Bodziak KA, Hammond WS, Molitoris BA. Inherited diseases of glomerular basement membrane. *Am J Kidney Dis* 1994;23:605.

591. Chugh KS, et al. Hereditary nephritis (Alport's syndrome): clinical profile and inheritance in 28 kindreds. *Nephrol Dial Transplant* 1993;8:690.

592. Ding J, et al. A monoclonal antibody marker for Alport syndrome identifies antigen as the alpha 5 chain of type IV collagen. *Kidney Int* 1994;45:1504.

593. Gregory MC. Alport's syndrome and thin basement nephropathy: unraveling the tangled strands of type IV collagen. *Kidney Int* 2004;65:1109.

594. Diaz JI, et al. Antiglomerular and antitubular basement membrane nephritis in a renal allograft recipient with Alport's syndrome. *Arch Pathol Lab Med* 1994;118:728.

595. Coburn PW, et al. Granulomatous sarcoid nephritis. *Am J Med* 1976;42:273.

596. Muther RS, McCarron DA, Bennet WB. Renal manifestations of sarcoidosis. *Arch Intern Med* 1981;141:643.

597. Verani R, Nasir M, Foley R. Granulomatous interstitial nephritis after a je-junoileal bypass: an ultrastructural and histochemical study. *Am J Nephrol* 1989;9:51.
598. Berger KW, Relman AS. Renal impairment due to sarcoid infiltration of the kidney. *N Engl J Med* 1955;252:44.
599. Guenel J, Chevet D. Interstitial nephropathies in sarcoidosis: effect of corti-costeroid therapy and long-term evolution: retrospective study of 22 cases. *Nephrologie* 1988;9:253.
600. Muther RS, McCarron DA, Bennet WM. Granulomatous sarcoid nephritis: a cause of multiple renal tubular abnormalities. *Clin Nephrol* 1980;14:190.
601. Lebacq E, Verhaegen H, Desmet V. Renal involvement in sarcoidosis. *Post-grad Med J* 1970;46:526.
602. Lofgren S, Snellman B, Lindgren AG. Renal complications in sarcoidosis: functional and biopsy studies. *Acta Med Scand* 1957;159:295.
603. MacSearraigh ET, et al. Sarcoidosis with renal involvement. *Postgrad Med J* 1978;54:528.
604. Gobel U, et al. The protean face of renal sarcoidosis. *J Am Soc Nephrol* 2001;12:616.
605. Christensen WI. Genitourinary tuberculosis: review of 102 cases. *Medicine* 1974;53:377.
606. Eastwood JB, Corbishley CM, Grange JM. Tuberculosis and the kidney. *J Am Soc Nephrol* 2001;12:1307.
607. Mallinson WJ, et al. Diffuse interstitial renal tuberculosis: an unusual cause of renal failure. *Q J Med* 1981;198:137.
608. Watanabe T, et al. Renal papillary necrosis associated with Wegener's gran-ulomatosis. *Hum Pathol* 1983;14:551.
609. McAllister CJ, et al. Granulomatous interstitial nephritis: a complication of heroin abuse. *South Med J* 1979;72:162.
610. Sweet RM, et al. Jejunoileal bypass surgery and granulomatous disease of the kidney and liver. *Arch Intern Med* 1978;138:626.
611. Dobrin RS, Vernier RL, Fish AJ. Acute eosinophilic interstitial nephritis and renal failure with bone marrow-lymph node granulomatous and anterior uveitis: a new syndrome. *Am J Med* 1975;59:325.
612. Austwick PK, et al. Balkan (endemic) nephropathy. *Contrib Nephrol* 1979;16:154.
613. Wolstenholme GE, Knight J, eds. *The Balkan Nephropathy* (Ciba Founda-tion Study Group No. 33). Boston: Little, Brown and Company; 1967.
614. Ferluga D, et al. Renal function, protein excretion, and pathology of Balkan endemic nephropathy. III. Light and electron microscopic studies. *Kidney Int* 1991;34(Suppl):S57.
615. Stefanovic V, Polenakovic MH. Kidney disease beyond the Balkans. *Am J Nephrol* 1991;11:1.
616. Uzelac-Keserovic B, et al. Isolation of a coronavirus from kidney biopsies of endemic Balkan nephropathy patients. *Nephron* 1999;81:141.
617. Stefanovic V. Balkan endemic nephropathy: a need for novel aetiological approaches. *Q J Med* 1998;91:457.
618. Krogh P, et al. Balkan (endemic) nephropathy and food-borne ochratoxin: A. Preliminary results of a survey of foodstuffs. *Acta Pathol Microbiol Scand (Section B)* 1977;85:238.
619. Adatia R, et al. Acute histopathological changes produced by *Penicillium aurantiogriseum* nephrotoxin in the rat. *Int J Exp Pathol* 1991;72:47.
620. Hassan W, et al. Ochratoxin A and β2 microalbuminuria in healthy and in chronic interstitial nephropathy patients in the Centre of Tunisia: a hot spot of ochratoxin exposure. *Toxicology* 2004;199:185.
621. Vrabcheva T, et al. Analysis of ochratoxin A in foods consumed by in-habitants from an area with Balkan nephropathy: a 1 month followup. *J Agricult Food Chem* 2004;52:2404.
622. Domijan AM, et al. Ochratoxin A-induced apoptosis in rat kidney tissue. *Ark Hig Rada Toksikol* 2004;55:243.
623. Gekle M, Sauvant G, Schmidt G. Ochratoxin A at nanomolar concen-trations: a signal modulator in renal cells. *Mol Nutr Food Res* 2005;49:118.
624. Sauvant G, et al. Exposure to nephrotoxic ochratoxin A enhances colla-gen secretion in human renal proximal tubular cells. *Mol Nutr Food Res* 2005;49:31.
625. Adib S, et al. Ochratoxin A and human chronic nephropathy in Tunisia: is the situation endemic? *Human Exper Toxicol* 2003;22:77.
626. Adranova IE, et al. Balkan nephropathy and genetic variants of glutathione S-transferase. *J Nephrol* 2004;17:390.
627. Desmyter J, et al. Laboratory rat associated with outbreak of hemorrhagic fever with renal syndrome due to Hantaan-like virus in Belgium. *Lancet* 1983;2:1445.
628. Lahdevirta J, et al. Clinical and serological diagnosis of nephropathia epi-demica, the mild type of haemorrhagic fever with renal syndrome. *J Infect* 1984;9:230.
629. Cosgriff TM. Hemorrhagic fever with renal syndrome: four decades of research. *Ann Intern Med* 1989;110:313.
630. World Health Organization. Report of the working group on hemorrhagic fever with renal syndrome. Tokyo: World Health Organization, 1982.
631. van Ypersele de Strihou C, Mery JP. Hantavirus-related acute interstitial nephritis in Europe: expansion of a world-wide zoonosis. *Q J Med* 1989;73:941.
632. Makela S, et al. Renal function and blood pressure five years after Puumala virus induced nephropathy. *Kidney Int* 2000;58:1711.
633. Lee HW, et al. Aetiological relation between Korean hemorrhagic fever and nephropathia epidemica. *Lancet* 1979;1:186.
634. Patmaik M, Velsosa JA, Peter JB. Hantavirus-specific IgG, IgM, and IgA in acute and chronic renal disease versus congenital renal disease in the United States. *Am J Kidney Dis* 1999;33:734.
635. Rosen S, et al. Tubulo-interstitial nephritis associated with polyoma-virus (BK type) infection. *N Engl J Med* 1983;308:1192.
636. Cameron J, et al. Severe tubulo-interstitial disease in a renal allograft due to cytomegalovirus infection. *Clin Nephrol* 1982;18:321.
637. Warrell MJ, et al. The effects of viral infections of renal transplants and their recipients. *Q J Med* 1980;49:219.
638. Bennett WM, Barry JM, Joughton DC. Chronic tubulointerstitial nephritis from infectious mononucleosis. *West J Med* 1981;33:2480.
639. Becker JL, et al. Epstein-Barr virus infection of renal proximal tubule cells: possible role in chronic interstitial nephritis. *J Clin Invest* 1999;104:1673.
640. Lee S, Kjellstram CM. Renal disease in infectious mononucleosis. *Clin Nephrol* 1978;9:236.
641. Mayer HB, et al. Epstein-Barr virus-induced infectious mononucleosis com-plicated by acute renal failure: case report and review. *Clin Infect Dis* 1996;22:1009.
642. Nadasy T, et al. Epstein-Barr infection-associated renal disease: diagnostic use of molecular hybridization technology in patients with negative serol-ogy. *J Am Soc Nephrol* 1994;2:1734.
643. Lagergren C, Ljungqvist A. The intrarenal arterial pattern in renal papillary necrosis. *Am J Pathol* 1962;41:633.
644. Nanra RS, Chirawong P, Kincaid-Smith P. Medullary ischemia in experi-mental analgesic nephropathy: the pathogenesis of renal papillary necrosis. *Aust N Z J Med* 1973;3:580.
645. Waylie RG, et al. Experimental papillary necrosis of the kidney: III. Effects of reserpine and other pharmacologic agents on the lesion. *Am J Pathol* 1972;68:235.
646. Heptinstall RH. *Pathology of the Kidney*. 3rd ed. Boston: Little, Brown and Company; 1983:1149.
647. Baker SB. The blood supply of the renal papilla. *Br J Urol* 1959;31:53.
648. Fourman J, Moffat DB. *The Blood Vessels of the Kidney*. Oxford: Blackwell Science; 1971:1.
649. Heaton J, Bourke E. Papillary necrosis associated with calyceal arteritis. *Nephron* 1976;16:57.
650. Beeuwkes R III, Bonventre JV. Tubular organization and vascular-tubular relations in the dog kidney. *Am J Physiol* 1975;229:695.
651. Dobyan DC, Jamison RL. Structure and function of the renal papilla. *Semin Nephrol* 1984;4:5.
652. Kovacevic L, et al. Renal papillary necrosis induced by naproxen. *Pediatric Nephrol* 2003;18:826.
653. Brix BE. Renal papillary necrosis. *Toxicol Pathol* 2002;30:672.
654. Hultengren N. Renal papillary necrosis: a clinical study of 103 cases. *Acta Chir Scand* 1961;277(Suppl):1.
655. Lauler DP, Schreiner GE, David A. Renal medullary necrosis. *Am J Med* 1960;29:132.
656. Schourup K. Necrosis of the renal papillae: post-mortem series. *Acta Pathol Microbiol Scand* 1957;41:462.
657. Seegmiller JA, Frazier PO. Biological considerations of the renal damage of gout. *Ann Rheum Dis* 1966;25(Suppl 6):668.
658. Simon HB, Bennett WA, Emmett JL. Renal papillary necrosis: a clinico-pathologic study of 42 cases. *J Urol* 1957;77:557.
659. Harrison JH, Bailey OT. The significance of necrotizing pyelonephritis in diabetes mellitus. *JAMA* 1942;118:15.
660. Robbins SL, Mallory GK, Kinney DT. Necrotizing renal papillitis: form of acute pyelonephritis. *N Engl J Med* 1946;235:885.
661. Moffat DB. The fine structure of the blood vessels in the renal medulla. *J Ultrastruct Res* 1967;16:532.
662. Gunther GW. Die papillennekrosen der niere bei diabetes. *Munchen Med Wochnschr* 1937;84:1695.
663. Lindvall N. Renal papillary necrosis: a roentgenographic study of 155 cases. *Acta Radiol* 1960;192(Suppl 1):1.
664. Lindvall N. Radiological changes in renal papillary necrosis. *Kidney Int* 1978;13:93.
665. Rutner AB, Smith DR. Renal papillary necrosis. *J Urol* 1961;84:462.
666. Fairley KF, Kincaid-Smith P. Renal papillary necrosis with a normal pyelo-gram. *Br Med J* 1968;1:156.
667. Lalli AF. Renal papillary necrosis. *Am J Roentgenol Radiat Ther Nucl Med* 1972;114:741.
668. Bergnes MA. Recovery of papillae in renal papillary necrosis: report of two cases. *Arch Pathol* 1963;75:501.
669. Lindholm T. On renal papillary necrosis with special reference to the diag-nostic importance of papillary fragments in the urine, therapy and prognosis. *Acta Med Scand* 1960;167:319.
670. Flasters S, Lowe L. Urological complications of renal papillary necrosis. *J Urol* 1975;5:331.
671. Greenlaw WA. Renal papillary necrosis. *J Maine Med Assoc* 1979;70:72.
672. Sargent JC, Sargent JW. Unilateral renal papillary necrosis. *J Urol* 1955;73:757.
673. Martinez-Maldonado M, Stitzer O. Urine concentration and dilution in the rat: contributions of papillary structures during high rates of urine flow. *Kidney Int* 1978;13:194.
674. Bittar EE, Misanik L. Renal necrotizing papillitis. *Am J Med* 1963; 34:82.
675. Mandel EE. Renal medullary necrosis. *Am J Med* 1952;13:322.

676. Griffin MD, Bergstralh EJ, Larson TS. Renal papillary necrosis: a sixteen year clinical experience. *J Am Soc Nephrol* 1995;6:248.
677. Groop L, Laasonen L, Egren J. Renal papillary necrosis in patients with IDDM. *Diabetes Care* 1989;12:189.
678. Henry MA, Tange JD. Lesions of the renal papilla induced by paracetamol. *J Pathol* 1987;151:11.
679. Segasothy M, et al. Chronic renal disease and papillary necrosis associated with the long-term use of nonsteroidal anti-inflammatory drugs as the sole or predominant analgesic. *Am J Kidney Dis* 1994;24:17.
680. Allen RC, et al. Renal papillary necrosis in children with chronic arthritis. *Am J Dis Child* 1986;140:20.
681. Szer IS, Goldstein C, Kurtin PS. Paucity of renal complications associated with nonsteroidal anti-inflammatory drugs in children with chronic arthritis. *J Pediatr* 1991;119:815.
682. Zadeii G, Lohr JW. Renal papillary necrosis in a patient with sickle cell trait. *J Am Soc Nephrol* 1997;8:1034.
683. Kaude JV, et al. Papillary necrosis in kidney transplant patients. *Radiology* 1976;120:69.
684. Knepshield JH, Feller HA, Leb DE. Papillary necrosis due to *Candida albicans* in a renal allograft. *Arch Intern Med* 1968;122:441.
685. Tuma S, et al. Fatal papillary necrosis in a kidney graft. *JAMA* 1976;235:754.
686. Chrispin AR, et al. Renal tubular necrosis and papillary necrosis after gastroenteritis in infants. *Br Med J* 1970;1:410.
687. Davies DJ, Kennedy A, Roberts C. Renal medullary necrosis in infancy and childhood. *J Pathol* 1969;99:125.
688. Funston MR, Cremin BJ, Tidbury LJ. Renal cortical necrosis and papillary necrosis in an infant. *Br J Radiol* 1976;19:94.
689. Harris VJ, Gooneratne NS, White H. Papillary necrosis in a child with homozygous sickle cell anemia. *Radiology* 1976;121:156.
690. Kozlowski K, Brown RW. Renal medullary necrosis in infants and children. *Pediatr Radiol* 1978;7:85.
691. Marks IM. Renal medullary necrosis following exsanguination in infancy. *Lancet* 1960;2:680.
692. Mauer SM, Nogredy MB. Renal papillary and cortical necrosis in a newborn infant: report of a survivor with roentgenologic documentation. *J Pediatr* 1969;74:750.
693. Brenke B, Nahm AM, Ritz EA. Papillary necrosis in a ballet dancer with no history of analgesic abuse. *Nephrol Dial Transplant* 1996;11:2501.
694. Duclonox D, Lemouel A, Chalopin J. Renal papillary necrosis in a marathon runner. *Nephrol Dial Transplant* 1999;14:247.
695. Ifediora O, Benz RL. Renal papillary necrosis in a hemodialysis patient. *Clin Nephrol* 1993;39:279.
696. Koelz AM, Bourke E. Cryoglobinaemic nephropathy with papillary necrosis. *Nephron* 1977;19:42.
697. Fong P, Sepandj F, Trillo A. Idiopathic acute granulomatous interstitial nephritis leading to renal papillary necrosis. *Nephrol Dial Transplant* 1997;12:1043.
698. Allwall N, Erlanson P, Tomberg A. The clinical course of renal failure occurring after intravenous urography and/or retrograde pyelography. *Acta Med Scand* 1955;152:163.
699. Eskelund V. Necrosis of renal papillae following retrograde pyelography. *Acta Radiol* 1945;26:548.
700. Heppleston AG. Renal papillary necrosis associated with necrotizing angiitis and tubular necrosis. *J Pathol Bacteriol* 1955;70:401.
701. Koutsaimanis KG, De Wardener HE. Phenacetin nephropathy, with particular reference to the effect of surgery. *Br Med J* 1970;4:131.
702. Edmondson HA, Reynolds TB, Jacobson A. Renal papillary necrosis with special reference to chronic alcoholism: a report of 20 cases. *Arch Intern Med* 1966;118:255.
703. Pablo NC, et al. Renal papillary necrosis: relapsing form associated with alcoholism. *Am J Kidney Dis* 1986;7:88.
704. Axelsen RA, Burry AF. Papillary necrosis in the Gunn rat: rapid induction by analgesics. *Pathology* 1972;4:225.

■ SUBJECT INDEX

Page numbers followed by *f* indicate figures; page numbers followed by *t* indicate tables.